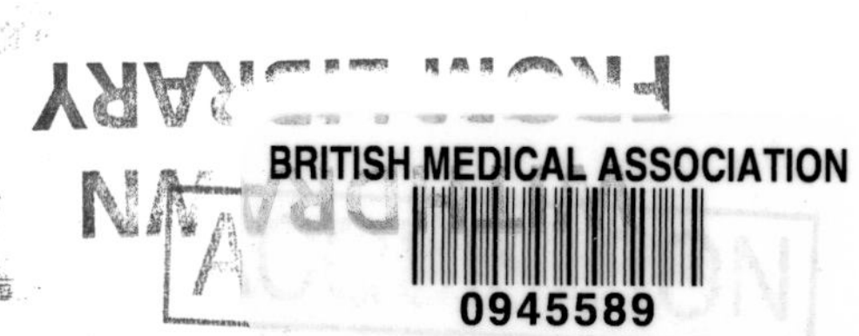

Chestnut's Obstetric Anesthesia: Principles and Practice

Chestnut's Obstetric Anesthesia: Principles and Practice

Fourth Edition

David H. Chestnut, MD
Director of Medical Education
Gundersen Lutheran Health System
Professor of Anesthesiology
Associate Dean for the Western Academic Campus
University of Wisconsin School of Medicine and Public Health
La Crosse, Wisconsin

Lawrence C. Tsen, MD
Associate Professor of Anaesthesia
Harvard Medical School
Director of Anesthesia, Center for Reproductive Medicine
Department of Anesthesiology, Perioperative and Pain Medicine
Brigham and Women's Hospital
Boston, Massachusetts

Linda S. Polley, MD
Associate Professor of Anesthesiology
University of Michigan Medical School
Director, Obstetric Anesthesiology
University of Michigan Health System
Ann Arbor, Michigan

Cynthia A. Wong, MD
Associate Professor of Anesthesiology
Northwestern University Feinberg School of Medicine
Medical Director, Obstetric Anesthesia
Northwestern Memorial Hospital
Chicago, Illinois

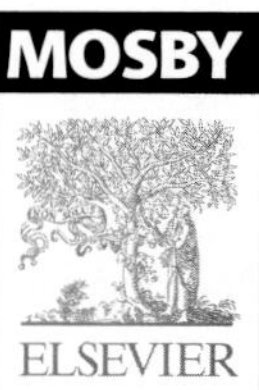

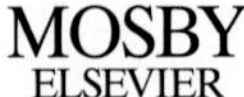

1600 John F. Kennedy Blvd.
Ste 1800
Philadelphia, PA 19103-2899

CHESTNUT'S OBSTETRIC ANESTHESIA: PRINCIPLES AND PRACTICE

ISBN: 978-0-323-05541-3

Library of Congress Cataloging-in-Publication Data

Chestnut's obstetric anesthesia : principles and practice / [edited by] David H. Chestnut ... [et al.].
– 4th ed.
p. ; cm.
Rev. ed. of: Obstetric anesthesia. 3rd ed. 2004.
Includes bibliographical references and index
ISBN 978-0-323-05541-3
1. Anesthesia in obstetrics. I. Chestnut, David H. II. Title: Obstetric anesthesia.
[DNLM: 1. Anesthesia, Obstetrical–methods. 2. Anesthetics. 3. Obstetric Labor Complications. WO 450 C525 2009].
RG732.C44 2009
617.9'682–dc22 2008050031

Acquisitions Editor: Natasha Andjelkovic
Developmental Editor: Anne Snyder
Publishing Services Manager: Tina Rebane
Project Manager: Norm Stellander
Design Direction: Louis Forgione

Printed in the United States of America

Last digit is the print number: 9 8 7 6 5 4 3 2 1

To my wife, **Janet**, and our children, **Stephen**, **Annie**, **Mary Beth**, **Michael**, and **John Mark** and **Catherine**

DHC

To my sons, **Tad** and **John**

LSP

To my wife, **Paulita**, our children, **London** and **Hamilton**, and my parents-in-law, **Deirdre** and **Oscar**

LCT

To my husband, **Lawrence**, and our children, **Anna**, **Molly**, **Leah**, and **Sofie**

CAW

Contributors

Susan W. Aucott, M.D.
Assistant Professor of Pediatrics
Johns Hopkins University School of Medicine
Director, Neonatal Intensive Care Unit
Johns Hopkins Hospital
Baltimore, Maryland

Angela M. Bader, M.D., M.P.H.
Associate Professor of Anaesthesia
Harvard Medical School
Vice Chair for Perioperative Medicine
Director, Weiner Center for Perioperative Evaluation
Department of Anesthesiology, Perioperative and Pain Medicine
Brigham and Women's Hospital
Boston, Massachusetts

Yaakov Beilin, M.D.
Professor of Anesthesiology and Obstetrics, Gynecology, and Reproductive Sciences
Vice Chair for Quality
Co-Director of Obstetric Anesthesia
Mount Sinai School of Medicine
New York, New York

David J. Birnbach, M.D., M.P.H.
Professor and Executive Vice Chair of Anesthesiology
Director, UM-JMH Center for Patient Safety
University of Miami Miller School of Medicine
Miami, Florida

David L. Brown, M.D.
Chair, Institute of Anesthesiology
Cleveland Clinic
Cleveland, Ohio

Brenda A. Bucklin, M.D.
Professor of Anesthesiology
University of Colorado School of Medicine
Denver, Colorado

Alexander Butwick, M.B.B.S., FRCA
Instructor in Anesthesia
Stanford University School of Medicine
Stanford, California

William Camann, M.D.
Associate Professor of Anaesthesia
Harvard Medical School
Director, Obstetric Anesthesia
Brigham and Women's Hospital
Boston, Massachusetts

Katherine Campbell, M.D.
Department of Obstetrics, Gynecology, and Reproductive Sciences
Yale University School of Medicine
New Haven, Connecticut

Brendan Carvalho, M.B., B.Ch., FRCA, MDCH
Assistant Professor of Anesthesia
Stanford University School of Medicine
Stanford, California

Donald Caton, M.D.
Professor Emeritus of Anesthesiology
University of Florida College of Medicine
Gainesville, Florida

Paula D. M. Chantigian, M.D., FACOG
Obstetrician and Gynecologist
Byron, Minnesota

Robert C. Chantigian, M.D.
Associate Professor of Anesthesiology
Mayo Clinic
Rochester, Minnesota

David H. Chestnut, M.D.
Director of Medical Education
Gundersen Lutheran Health System
Professor of Anesthesiology
Associate Dean for the Western Academic Campus
University of Wisconsin School of Medicine and Public Health
La Crosse, Wisconsin

Edward T. Crosby, B.Sc., M.D., FRCPC
Professor of Anesthesiology
Faculty of Medicine
University of Ottawa
Ottawa Hospital
Ottawa, Ontario, Canada

Robert D'Angelo, M.D.
Professor and Vice Chair of Anesthesiology
Section Head, Obstetric Anesthesia
Wake Forest University School of Medicine
Winston-Salem, North Carolina

Joanna M. Davies, M.B.B.S., FRCA
Assistant Professor of Anesthesiology
University of Washington School of Medicine
Seattle, Washington

Kathleen M. Davis, M.D.
Assistant Professor of Anesthesiology
University of Maryland School of Medicine
Baltimore, Maryland

David D. Dewan, M.D.
Professor of Anesthesiology (retirement status)
Wake Forest University School of Medicine
Winston-Salem, North Carolina

M. Joanne Douglas, M.D., FRCPC
Clinical Professor of Anesthesiology, Pharmacology and Therapeutics
Faculty of Medicine
University of British Columbia
British Columbia Women's Hospital and Health Centre
Vancouver, British Columbia, Canada

Sunil Eappen, M.D.
Assistant Professor of Anaesthesia
Harvard Medical School
Vice-Chair for Clinical Affairs
Department of Anesthesiology, Perioperative and Pain Medicine
Brigham and Women's Hospital
Boston, Massachusetts

James C. Eisenach, M.D.
Professor and Vice Chair for Research
Section of Obstetric Anesthesia
Wake Forest University School of Medicine
Winston-Salem, North Carolina

Roshan Fernando, M.D., FRCA
Consultant Anaesthetist and Honorary Senior Lecturer
Department of Anaesthesia
University College Hospitals
London, United Kingdom

Michael Froelich, M.D., M.S.
Associate Professor of Anesthesiology
University of Alabama at Birmingham School of Medicine
Birmingham, Alabama

Robert Gaiser, M.D.
Professor of Anesthesiology and Critical Care
University of Pennsylvania School of Medicine
Philadelphia, Pennsylvania

Carin A. Hagberg, M.D.
Professor and Chair of Anesthesiology
University of Texas Medical School at Houston
Houston, Texas

M. Shankar Hari, M.D., FRCA
Consultant in Intensive Care Medicine
Guy's and St. Thomas' NHS Trust
London, United Kingdom

Miriam Harnett, M.B., FFARCSI
Consultant Anaesthetist
Cork University Maternal Hospital
Cork, Ireland

Andrew P. Harris, M.D., M.H.S.
Professor of Anesthesiology and Critical Care Medicine
Johns Hopkins University School of Medicine
Baltimore, Maryland

Joy L. Hawkins, M.D.
Professor of Anesthesiology
Associate Chair for Academic Affairs
University of Colorado School of Medicine
Director of Obstetric Anesthesia
University of Colorado Hospital
Aurora, Colorado

David Hepner, M.D.
Assistant Professor of Anaesthesia
Harvard Medical School
Associate Director, Weiner Center for Perioperative Evaluation
Department of Anesthesiology, Perioperative and Pain Medicine
Brigham and Women's Hospital
Boston, Massachusetts

Norman L. Herman, M.D., Ph.D.
Assistant Professor of Anesthesiology (retirement status)
Cornell University Medical College
New York, New York

Paul Howell, B.Sc., M.B., Ch.B., FRCA
Consultant Anaesthetist
St. Bartholomew's Hospitals
West Smithfield
London, United Kingdom

Tanya Jones, M.B., Ch.B., MRCP, FRCA
Smiths Medical Research Fellow in Obstetric Anaesthesia
Department of Anaesthesia
Royal Free Hospital
London, United Kingdom

BettyLou Koffel, M.D.
Chief of Staff
Interstate Ambulatory Surgicenter
Portland, Oregon

Lisa R. Leffert, M.D.
Assistant Professor of Anaesthesia
Harvard Medical School
Co-Chief, Obstetric Anesthesia
Department of Anesthesia and Critical Care
Massachusetts General Hospital
Boston, Massachusetts

Karen S. Lindeman, M.D.
Associate Professor of Anesthesiology and Critical Care Medicine
Johns Hopkins University School of Medicine
Baltimore, Maryland

Elizabeth G. Livingston, M.D.
Associate Professor of Obstetrics and Gynecology
Duke University School of Medicine
Durham, North Carolina

Alison Macarthur, B.M.Sc., M.D., M.Sc., FRCPC
Associate Professor, Faculty of Medicine
University of Toronto
Department of Anesthesia
Mount Sinai Hospital
Toronto, Ontario, Canada

Andrew M. Malinow, M.D.
Professor of Anesthesiology
University of Maryland School of Medicine
Director, Obstetric Anesthesiology
University of Maryland Medical System
Baltimore, Maryland

David C. Mayer, M.D.
Professor of Anesthesiology and Obstetrics and Gynecology
University of North Carolina School of Medicine
Co-Director of Obstetric Anesthesiology
University of North Carolina Hospitals
Chapel Hill, North Carolina

Jill M. Mhyre, M.D.
Assistant Professor of Anesthesiology
University of Michigan Medical School
Women's Hospital
University of Michigan Health System
Ann Arbor, Michigan

Marie E. Minnich, M.D., M.M.M., M.B.A., C.P.E.
Division of Anesthesiology
Geisinger Health System
Danville, Pennsylvania

Holly A. Muir, M.D., FRCPC
Chief, Division of Women's Anesthesia
Vice Chair for Clinical Operations
Department of Anesthesiology
Duke University Medical Center
Durham, North Carolina

Naveen Nathan, M.D.
Instructor of Anesthesiology
Northwestern University Feinberg School of Medicine
Chicago, Illinois

Kenneth E. Nelson, M.D.
Associate Professor of Anesthesiology
Section of Obstetric Anesthesia
Wake Forest University School of Medicine
Winston-Salem, North Carolina

Warwick D. Ngan Kee, B.H.B., M.B., Ch.B., M.D., FANZCA, FHKCA, FHKAM
Department of Anaesthesia and Intensive Care
The Chinese University of Hong Kong
Prince of Wales Hospital
Shatin, Hong Kong, China

Errol R. Norwitz, M.D., Ph.D.
Associate Professor of Obstetrics, Gynecology and Reproductive Sciences
Yale University School of Medicine
New Haven, Connecticut

Geraldine O'Sullivan, M.D., FRCA
Consultant Anaesthetist
Obstetric Anaesthesia
Guy's and St. Thomas' NHS Trust
London, United Kingdom

Peter H. Pan, M.D.
Professor of Anesthesiology
Director of Clinical Research
Section of Obstetric Anesthesia
Wake Forest University School of Medicine
Winston-Salem, North Carolina

Joong Shin Park, M.D., Ph.D.
Department of Obstetrics and Gynecology
Seoul National University Hospital
Seoul, Korea

Donald H. Penning, M.D., M.Sc., FRCP
Professor of Clinical Anesthesiology
University of Miami Miller School of Medicine
Miami, Florida

Linda S. Polley, M.D.
Associate Professor of Anesthesiology
University of Michigan Medical School
Director, Obstetric Anesthesiology
University of Michigan Health System
Ann Arbor, Michigan

Roanne Preston, M.D., FRCPC
Clinical Associate Professor of Anesthesiology
Faculty of Medicine
University of British Columbia
British Columbia Women's Hospital and Health Centre
Vancouver, British Columbia, Canada

Robert W. Reid, M.D.
Consultant in Critical Care Medicine
Saint Luke's Health System
Kansas City, Missouri

Felicity Reynolds, M.B., B.S., M.D., FRCA, FRCOG ad eundem
Emeritus Professor of Obstetric Anaesthesia
St. Thomas' Hospital
London, United Kingdom

Mark A. Rosen, M.D.
Professor and Vice Chair of Anesthesia and Perioperative Care
Professor of Obstetrics, Gynecology, and Reproductive Sciences
Director of Obstetric Anesthesia
University of California San Francisco
San Francisco, California

Brian K. Ross, M.D., Ph.D.
Professor of Anesthesiology
University of Washington School of Medicine
Seattle, Washington

Dwight J. Rouse, M.D., M.S.P.H.
Professor of Obstetrics and Gynecology
University of Alabama at Birmingham School of Medicine
Birmingham, Alabama

Eduardo Salas, Ph.D.
Professor of Psychology
Program Director, Human Systems Integration Research Department
Institute for Simulation and Training
University of Central Florida
Orlando, Florida

Alan C. Santos, M.D., M.P.H.
Professor and Chair of Anesthesiology
Ochsner Clinic Foundation
New Orleans, Louisiana

Scott Segal, M.D.
Associate Professor of Anaesthesia
Harvard Medical School
Vice Chair for Education
Department of Anesthesiology, Perioperative and Pain Medicine
Brigham and Women's Hospital
Boston, Massachusetts

Shiv K. Sharma, M.D., FRCA
Professor of Anesthesiology and Pain Management
University of Texas Southwestern Medical School
Dallas, Texas

Kathleen A. Smith, M.D.
Assistant Professor of Anesthesiology and Obstetrics and Gynecology
University of North Carolina School of Medicine
Co-Director of Obstetric Anesthesiology
University of North Carolina Hospitals
Chapel Hill, North Carolina

John A. Thomas, M.D.
Assistant Professor of Anesthesiology
Section of Obstetric Anesthesia
Wake Forest University School of Medicine
Winston Salem, North Carolina

Alan T. N. Tita, M.D., M.P.H., Ph.D.
Department of Obstetrics and Gynecology
University of Alabama at Birmingham School of Medicine
Birmingham, Alabama

Lawrence C. Tsen, M.D.
Associate Professor of Anaesthesia
Harvard Medical School
Director of Anesthesia, Center for Reproductive Medicine
Department of Anesthesiology, Perioperative and Pain Medicine
Brigham and Women's Hospital
Boston, Massachusetts

Marc Van de Velde, M.D., Ph.D.
Professor of Anesthesia
Director, Obstetric Anesthesia
Catholic University Leuven
Leuven, Belgium

Robert D. Vincent, Jr., M.D.
Staff Anesthesiologist
University of South Alabama Medical Center
Mobile, Alabama

Mark S. Williams, M.D., M.B.A., J.D.
Clinical Associate Professor of Anesthesiology
University of Alabama at Birmingham School of Medicine
Senior Vice-President and Chief Medical Officer
St. Vincent's Health System
Birmingham, Alabama

Richard N. Wissler, M.D., Ph.D.
Associate Professor of Anesthesiology and Obstetrics and Gynecology
Director of Obstetric Anesthesiology
University of Rochester School of Medicine and Dentistry
Rochester, New York

David J. Wlody, M.D.
Professor of Clinical Anesthesiology
State University of New York – Downstate Medical Center
Chair of Anesthesiology
Long Island College Hospital
Brooklyn, New York

Cynthia A. Wong, M.D.
Associate Professor of Anesthesiology
Northwestern University Feinberg School of Medicine
Medical Director, Obstetric Anesthesia
Northwestern Memorial Hospital
Chicago, Illinois

Jerome Yankowitz, M.D.
Professor of Obstetrics and Gynecology
University of Iowa Roy L. and Lucille A. Carver College of Medicine
Iowa City, Iowa

Mark I. Zakowski, M.D.
Obstetric Anesthesiology
Cedars-Sinai Medical Center
Los Angeles, Callifornia

Rhonda L. Zuckerman, M.D.
Assistant Professor of Anesthesiology and Critical Care
Assistant Professor of Gynecology and Obstetrics
Johns Hopkins University School of Medicine
Baltimore, Maryland

Preface

Three decades ago, I could not decide whether I wanted to pursue a career in anesthesiology or obstetrics. So ... I decided to do both. I obtained training in both specialties largely because of my love of perinatal medicine. This text is the result of my desire to prepare a comprehensive resource for all anesthesia providers (and obstetricians) who provide care for pregnant women.

In the preface to the first edition, I identified two goals: (1) to collate the most important information that anesthesia providers should know about obstetrics, and (2) to prepare a thorough and user-friendly review of anesthesia care for obstetric patients. I asked each contributor to prepare a comprehensive, scholarly discussion of the subject and also to provide clear, practical recommendations for clinical practice. As we unveil the fourth edition, those goals remain intact. Further, the fourth edition has undergone a more extensive revision than either the second or the third edition.

First, consider the **cover**. The maternal-fetal image draws attention to the fact that the anesthesia provider and the obstetrician provide simultaneous care for two (or more) patients – both the mother and her unborn child. As I look at that image, I am awestruck by the miraculous beauty of conception, pregnancy, and childbirth.

Second, consider the **content**. At least 10 chapters – including the chapters on neuraxial labor analgesia, cesarean delivery, the difficult airway, and hypertensive disorders – have been rewritten from start to finish. The three previously published chapters on neuraxial labor analgesia have been consolidated into a single chapter, as have the two previously published chapters on anesthesia for cesarean delivery. All chapters have been updated, and most chapters have undergone extensive revision. Two new chapters address the important subjects of patient safety and maternal mortality. And the fourth edition – for the first time – features a dedicated website that includes the whole content of the book and is fully searchable. The book's interior has been enhanced by the addition of a second color, which allows a better and more attractive visual presentation.

Third, consider the **contributors**. The fourth edition includes an astounding number of 32 new contributors! Of special significance is the addition of three outstanding new editors. I hand-picked these new editors as a result of my personal interaction with them in the preparation of previous editions of this textbook, as well as my familiarity with – and respect for – the depth and breadth of their knowledge and judgment, and the quality of their scholarship. The title page lists their academic affiliations and hospital leadership positions. In addition, **Linda S. Polley, M.D.,** is the current President of the Society for Obstetric Anesthesiology and Perinatology (SOAP). **Lawrence C. Tsen, M.D.,** is the President-elect of SOAP, and he also serves as Editor-in-Chief of *International Journal of Obstetric Anesthesia*. And **Cynthia A. Wong, M.D.,** is the obstetric anesthesia section editor for *Anesthesia and Analgesia*. The addition of these extraordinary obstetric anesthesiologists to the editorial team has resulted not only in the preparation of a better product, but it also reflects the publisher's (and my own) long-term commitment to this text.

My fellow editors and I should like to acknowledge the important roles of four groups of special people. First, we should like to thank the 72 other talented and distinguished contributors to the fourth edition, as well as the contributors to previous editions of this text. Without their commitment to this project, the fourth edition would not have seen the light of day. Second, we should like to gratefully acknowledge the invaluable contributions made by our competent, loyal, and at times long-suffering assistants: Jennifer Lee and Donna Stortz (DHC); Mary Lou Greenfield (LSP); Judy Johnson (LCT); and Allison Ernt and Sean Jones (CAW). Third, we should like to acknowledge the encouragement, expertise, and attention to detail provided by the professional production team at Elsevier Mosby. And finally, we should like to thank *you*, the readers, not only for your support of this text through the years, but also for your ongoing commitment to the provision of safe and compassionate care for pregnant women and their unborn children.

David H. Chestnut, M.D.

Micah 6:8

Contents

Part I

Introduction

Chapter 1

The History of Obstetric Anesthesia

Donald Caton, M.D.

For I heard a cry as of a woman in travail, anguish as of one bringing forth her first child, the cry of the daughter of Zion gasping for breath, stretching out her hands, "Woe is me!"

—Jeremiah 4:31

"The position of woman in any civilization is an index of the advancement of that civilization; the position of woman is gauged best by the care given her at the birth of her child." So wrote Haggard[1] in 1929. If his thesis is true, Western civilization made a giant leap on January 19, 1847, when James Young Simpson used diethyl ether to anesthetize a woman with a deformed pelvis for delivery. This first use of a modern anesthetic for childbirth occurred a scant 3 months after Morton's historic demonstration of the anesthetic properties of ether at the Massachusetts General Hospital in Boston. Strangely enough, Simpson's innovation evoked strong criticism from contemporary obstetricians, who questioned its safety, and from many segments of the lay public, who questioned its wisdom. The debate over these issues lasted more than 5 years and influenced the future of obstetric anesthesia.[2]

JAMES YOUNG SIMPSON

Few people were better equipped than Simpson to deal with controversy. Just 36 years old, Simpson already had 7 years' tenure as Professor of Midwifery at the University of Edinburgh, one of the most prestigious medical schools of its day (Figure 1-1). By that time, he had established a reputation as one of the foremost obstetricians in Great Britain, if not the world. On the day he first used ether for childbirth, he also received a letter of appointment as Queen's Physician in Scotland. Etherization for childbirth was only one of Simpson's contributions. He also designed obstetric forceps (which still bear his name), discovered the anesthetic properties of chloroform, made important innovations in hospital architecture, and wrote a textbook on the practice of witchcraft in Scotland that was used by several generations of anthropologists.[3]

An imposing man, Simpson had a large head, a massive mane of hair, and the pudgy body of an adolescent. Contemporaries described his voice as "commanding," with a wide range of volume and intonation. Clearly Simpson had "presence" and "charisma." These attributes were indispensable to someone in his profession, because in the mid-nineteenth century, the role of science in the development of medical theory and practice was minimal; rhetoric resolved more issues than facts. The medical climate in Edinburgh was particularly contentious and vituperative. In this milieu, Simpson had trained, competed for advancement and recognition, and succeeded. The rigor of this preparation served him well. Initially, virtually every prominent obstetrician, including Montgomery of Dublin, Ramsbotham of London, Dubois of Paris, and Meigs of Philadelphia, opposed etherization for childbirth. Simpson called on all of his professional and personal finesse to sway opinion in the ensuing controversy.

MEDICAL OBJECTIONS TO THE USE OF ETHER FOR CHILDBIRTH

Shortly after Simpson administered the first obstetric anesthetic, he wrote, "It will be necessary to ascertain anesthesia's precise effect, both upon the action of the uterus and on the assistant abdominal muscles; its influence, if any, upon the child; whether it has a tendency to hemorrhage or other complications."[4] With this statement he identified the issues that would most concern obstetricians who succeeded him and thus shaped the subsequent development of the specialty.

Simpson's most articulate, persistent, and persuasive critic was Charles D. Meigs, Professor of Midwifery at Jefferson Medical College in Philadelphia (Figure 1-2).

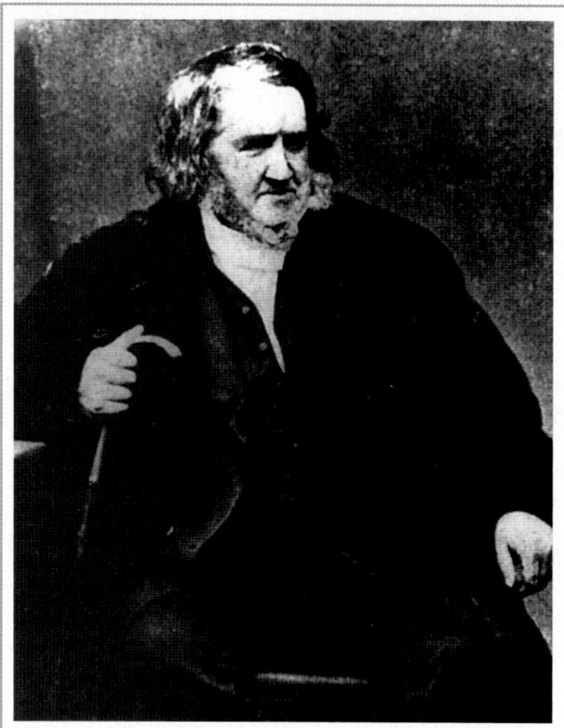

FIGURE 1-1 James Young Simpson, the obstetrician who first administered a modern anesthetic for childbirth. He also discovered the anesthetic properties of chloroform. Many believe that he was the most prominent and influential physician of his day. (Courtesy Yale Medical History Library.)

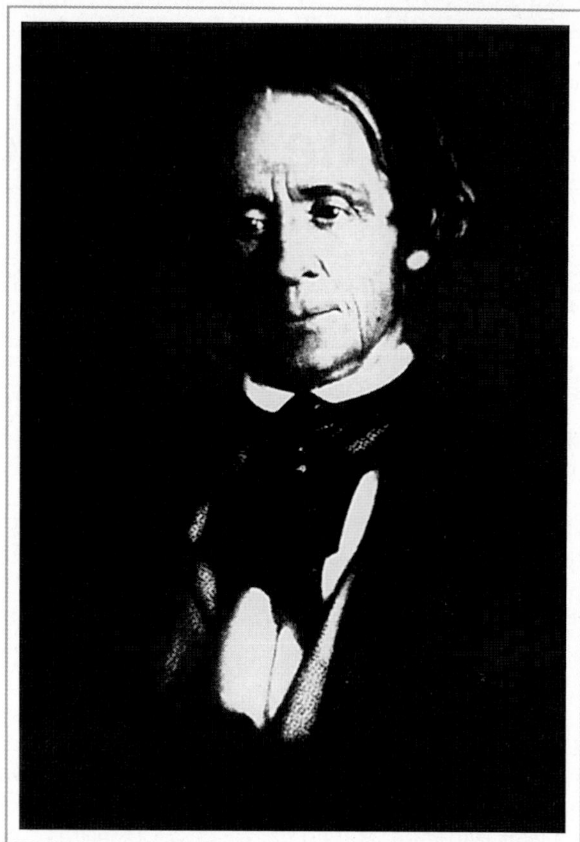

FIGURE 1-2 Charles D. Meigs, the American obstetrician who opposed the use of anesthesia for obstetrics. He questioned the safety of anesthesia and said that there was no demonstrated need for it during a normal delivery. (Courtesy Wood Library Museum.)

In character and stature, Meigs equaled Simpson. Born to a prominent New England family, Meigs' forebears included heroes of the American revolutionary war, the first governor of the state of Ohio, and the founder of the University of Georgia. His descendants included a prominent pediatrician, an obstetrician, and one son who served the Union Army as Quartermaster General during the Civil War.[5]

At the heart of the dispute between Meigs and Simpson was a difference in their interpretation of the nature of labor and the significance of labor pain. Simpson maintained that all pain, labor pain included, is without physiologic value. He said that pain only degrades and destroys those who experience it. In contrast, Meigs argued that labor pain has purpose, that uterine pain is inseparable from contractions, and that any drug that abolishes pain will alter contractions. Meigs also believed that pregnancy and labor are normal processes that usually end quite well. He said that physicians should therefore not intervene with powerful, potentially disruptive drugs (Figure 1-3). We must accept the statements of both men as expressions of natural philosophy, because neither had facts to buttress his position. Indeed, in 1847, physicians had little information of any sort about uterine function, pain, or the relationship between them. Studies of the anatomy and physiology of pain had just begun. It was only during the preceding 20 years that investigators had recognized that specific nerves and areas of the brain have different functions and that specialized peripheral receptors for painful stimuli exist.[2]

In 1850, more physicians expressed support for Meigs's views than for Simpson's. For example, Baron Paul Dubois[6] of the Faculty of Paris wondered whether ether, "after having exerted a stupefying action over the cerebro-spinal nerves, could not induce paralysis of the muscular element of the uterus?" Similarly, Ramsbotham[7] of London Hospital said that he believed the "treatment of rendering a patient in labor completely insensible through the agency of anesthetic remedies ... is fraught with extreme danger." These physicians' fears gained credence from the report by a special committee of the Royal Medical and Chirurgical Society documenting 123 deaths that "could be positively assigned to the inhalation of chloroform."[8] Although none involved obstetric patients, safety was on the minds of obstetricians.

The reaction to the delivery of Queen Victoria's eighth child in 1853 illustrated the aversion of the medical community to obstetric anesthesia. According to private records, John Snow anesthetized the Queen for the delivery of Prince Leopold at the request of her personal physicians. Although no one made a formal announcement of this fact, rumors surfaced and provoked strong public criticism. Thomas Wakley, the irascible founding editor of *The Lancet*, was particularly incensed. He "could not imagine that anyone had incurred the awful responsibility of advising the administration of chloroform to her Majesty during a perfectly natural labour with a seventh child."[9] (It was her

OBSTETRICS:

THE

SCIENCE AND THE ART.

BY

CHARLES D. MEIGS, M.D.,

PROFESSOR OF MIDWIFERY AND THE DISEASES OF WOMEN AND CHILDREN IN JEFFERSON MEDICAL COLLEGE AT PHILADELPHIA; LATELY ONE OF THE PHYSICIANS TO THE LYING-IN DEPARTMENT OF THE PENNSYLVANIA HOSPITAL; MEMBER OF THE SOCIETY OF SWEDISH PHYSICIANS AT STOCKHOLM; CORRESPONDING MEMBER OF THE HUNTERIAN SOCIETY OF LONDON; MEMBER OF THE AMERICAN PHILOSOPHICAL SOCIETY; OF THE ACADEMY OF NATURAL SCIENCES OF PHILADELPHIA; OF THE AMERICAN MEDICAL ASSOCIATION, ETC. ETC.

THIRD EDITION. REVISED.

WITH ONE HUNDRED AND TWENTY-NINE ILLUSTRATIONS.

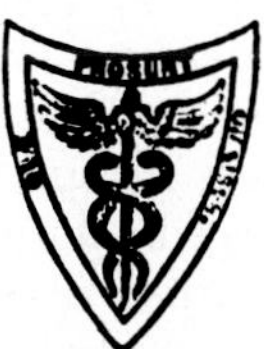

PHILADELPHIA:
BLANCHARD AND LEA.
1856.

FIGURE 1-3 Frontispiece from Meigs's textbook of obstetrics.

eighth child, but Wakley had apparently lost count—a forgivable error considering the propensity of the Queen to bear children.) Court physicians did not defend their decision to use ether. Perhaps not wanting a public confrontation, they simply denied that the Queen had received an anesthetic. In fact, they first acknowledged a royal anesthetic 4 years later when the Queen delivered her ninth and last child, Princess Beatrice. By that time, however, the issue was no longer controversial.[9]

PUBLIC REACTION TO ETHERIZATION FOR CHILDBIRTH

The controversy surrounding obstetric anesthesia was not resolved by the medical community. Physicians remained skeptical, but public opinion changed. Women lost their reservations, decided they wanted anesthesia, and virtually forced physicians to offer it to them. The change in the public's attitude in favor of obstetric anesthesia marked the culmination of a more general change in social attitudes that had been developing over several centuries.

Before the nineteenth century, pain meant something quite different from what it does today. Since antiquity, people had believed that all manner of calamities—disease, drought, poverty, and pain—signified divine retribution inflicted as punishment for sin. According to Scripture, childbirth pain originated when God punished Eve and her descendants for Eve's disobedience in the Garden of Eden. Many believed that it was wrong to avoid the pain of divine punishment. This belief was sufficiently prevalent and strong to retard acceptance of even the idea of anesthesia, especially for obstetric patients. Only when this tradition weakened did people seek ways to free themselves from disease and pain. In most Western countries, the transition occurred during the nineteenth century. Disease and pain lost their theologic connotations for many people and became biologic processes subject to study and control by new methods of science and technology. This evolution of thought facilitated the development of modern medicine and stimulated public acceptance of obstetric anesthesia.[10]

The reluctance that physicians felt about the administration of anesthesia for childbirth pain stands in stark contrast to the enthusiasm expressed by early obstetric patients. In 1847, Fanny Longfellow, wife of the American poet Henry Wadsworth Longfellow and the first woman in the United States anesthetized for childbirth, wrote:

> *I am very sorry you all thought me so rash and naughty in trying the ether. Henry's faith gave me courage, and I had heard such a thing had succeeded abroad, where the surgeons extend this great blessing more boldly and universally than our timid doctors.... This is certainly the greatest blessing of this age.*[11]

Queen Victoria, responding to news of the birth of her first grandchild in 1860 and perhaps remembering her own recent confinement, wrote, "What a blessing she [Victoria, her oldest daughter] had chloroform. Perhaps without it her strength would have suffered very much."[9] The new understanding of pain as a controllable biologic process left no room for Meigs's idea that pain might have physiologic value. The eminent nineteenth-century social philosopher John Stuart Mill stated that the "hurtful agencies of nature" promote good only by "inciting rational creatures to rise up and struggle against them."[12]

Simpson prophesied the role of public opinion in the acceptance of obstetric anesthesia, a fact not lost on his adversaries. Early in the controversy he predicted, "Medical men may oppose for a time the superinduction of anaesthesia in parturition but they will oppose it in vain; for certainly our patients themselves will force use of it upon the profession. The whole question is, even now, one merely of time."[13] By 1860, Simpson's prophecy came true; anesthesia for childbirth became part of medical practice by public acclaim, in large part in response to the demands of women.

OPIOIDS AND OBSTETRICS

The next major innovation in obstetric anesthesia came approximately 50 years later. *Dämmerschlaff,* which means "twilight sleep," was a technique developed by von Steinbüchel[14] of Graz and popularized by Gauss[15] of Freiberg. It combined opioids with scopolamine to make women amnestic and somewhat comfortable during labor (Figure 1-4). Until that time, opioids had been used sparingly for obstetrics. Although opium had been part of the medical armamentarium since the Roman Empire, it was

Vorläufige Mittheilung über die Anwendung von Skopolamin-Morphium-Injektionen in der Geburtshilfe.
Von
Dr. v. Steinbüchel,
Docent fur Geburtshilfe und Gynäkologie an der Universität Graz.

(Aus der Frauenklinik in Basel.)
II. Über Medullarnarkose bei Gebärenden.
Von
Oskar Kreis,
Assistenzarzt der geburtshilflichen Abtheilung.

FIGURE 1-4 Title pages from two important papers published in the first years of the twentieth century. The paper by von Steinbüchel introduced twilight sleep. The paper by Kreis described the first use of spinal anesthesia for obstetrics.

not used extensively, in part because of the difficulty of obtaining consistent results with the crude extracts available at that time. Therapeutics made a substantial advance in 1809 when Sertürner, a German pharmacologist, isolated codeine and morphine from a crude extract of the poppy seed. Methods for administering the drugs remained unsophisticated. Physicians gave morphine orally or by a method resembling vaccination, in which they placed a drop of solution on the skin and then made multiple small puncture holes with a sharp instrument to facilitate absorption. In 1853, the year Queen Victoria delivered her eighth child, the syringe and hollow metal needle were developed. This technical advance simplified the administration of opioids and facilitated the development of twilight sleep approximately 50 years later.[16]

Although reports of labor pain relief with hypodermic morphine appeared as early as 1868, few physicians favored its use. For example, in an article published in *Transactions of the Obstetrical Society of London*, Sansom[17] listed the following four agents for relief of labor pain: (1) carbon tetrachloride, the use of which he favored; (2) bichloride of methylene, which was under evaluation; (3) nitrous oxide, which had been introduced recently by Klikgowich of Russia; and (4) chloroform. He did not mention opioids, but neither did he mention diethyl ether, which many physicians still favored. Similarly, Gusserow,[18] a prominent German obstetrician, described using salicylic acid but not morphine for labor pain. (Von Baeyer did not introduce acetylsalicylic acid to medical practice until 1899.) In retrospect, von Steinbüchel's and Gauss's descriptions of twilight sleep in the first decade of the century may have been important more for popularizing morphine than for suggesting that scopolamine be given with morphine.

Physicians reacted to twilight sleep as they had reacted to diethyl ether several years earlier. They resisted it, questioning whether the benefits justified the risks. Patients also reacted as they had before. Not aware of, or perhaps not concerned with, the technical considerations that confronted physicians, patients harbored few doubts and persuaded physicians to use it, sometimes against the physicians' better judgment. The confrontation between physicians and patients was particularly strident in the United States. Champions of twilight sleep lectured throughout the country and published articles in popular magazines. Public enthusiasm for the therapy subsided slightly after 1920, when a prominent advocate of the method died during childbirth. She was given twilight sleep, but her physicians said that her death was unrelated to any complication from its use. Whatever anxiety this incident may have created in the minds of patients, it did not seriously diminish their resolve. Confronted by such firm insistence, physicians acquiesced and used twilight sleep with increasing frequency.[19,20]

Although the reaction of physicians to twilight sleep resembled their reaction to etherization, the medical milieu in which the debate over twilight sleep developed was quite different from that in which etherization was deliberated. Between 1850 and 1900, medicine had changed, particularly in Europe. Physiology, chemistry, anatomy, and bacteriology became part of medical theory and practice. Bright students from America traveled to leading clinics in Germany, England, and France. They returned with new facts and methods that they used to examine problems and critique ideas. These developments became the basis for the revolution in American medical education and practice launched by the Flexner report published in 1914.[21]

Obstetrics also changed. During the years preceding World War I, it had earned a reputation as one of the most exciting and scientifically advanced specialties. Obstetricians experimented with new drugs and techniques. They recognized that change entails risk, and they examined each innovation more critically. In addition, they turned to science for information and methods to help them solve problems of medical management. Developments in obstetric anesthesia reflected this change in strategy. New methods introduced during this time stimulated physicians to reexamine two important but unresolved issues, the effects of drugs on the child, and the relationship between pain and labor.

THE EFFECTS OF ANESTHESIA ON THE NEWBORN

Many physicians, Simpson included, worried that anesthetic drugs might cross the placenta and harm the newborn. Available information justified their concern. The idea that gases cross the placenta appeared long before the discovery of oxygen and carbon dioxide. In the sixteenth century, English physiologist John Mayow[22] suggested that "nitro aerial" particles from the mother nourish the fetus. By 1847, physiologists had corroborative evidence. Clinical experience gave more support. John Snow[23] observed depressed neonatal breathing and motor activity and smelled ether on the breath of neonates delivered from mothers who had been given ether. In an early paper, he surmised that anesthetic gases cross the placenta. Regardless, some advocates of obstetric anesthesia discounted the possibility. For example, Harvard professor Walter Channing denied that ether crossed the placenta because he could not detect its odor in the cut ends of the umbilical cord. Oddly enough, he did not attempt to smell ether on the child's exhalations as John Snow had done.[24]

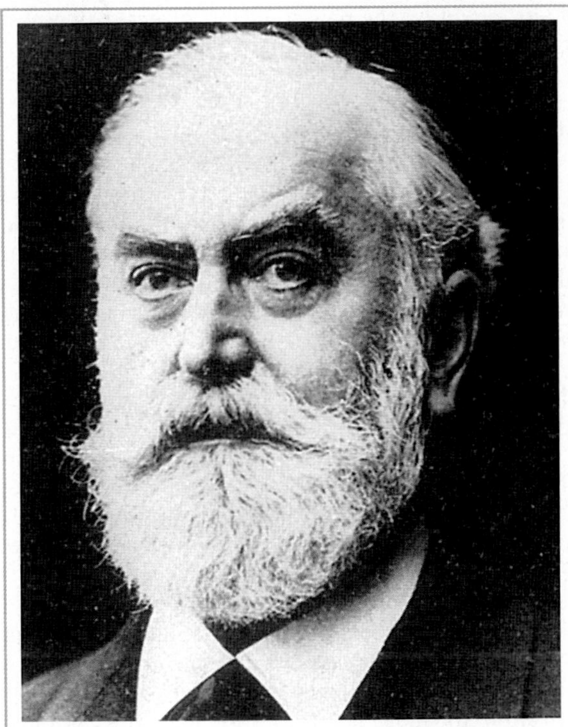

FIGURE 1-5 Paul Zweifel, the Swiss-born obstetrician who performed the first experiments that chemically demonstrated the presence of chloroform in the umbilical blood and urine of infants delivered by women who had been anesthetized during labor. (Courtesy J.F. Bergmann-Verlag, München, Germany.)

In 1874, Swiss obstetrician Paul Zweifel[25] published an account of work that finally resolved the debate about the placental transfer of drugs (Figure 1-5). He used a chemical reaction to demonstrate the presence of chloroform in the umbilical blood of neonates. In a separate paper, Zweifel[26] used a light-absorption technique to demonstrate a difference in oxygen content between umbilical arterial and venous blood, thereby establishing the placental transfer of oxygen. Although clinicians recognized the importance of these data, they accepted the implications slowly. Some clinicians pointed to several decades of clinical use "without problems." For example, Otto Spiegelberg,[27] Professor of Obstetrics at the University of Breslau, wrote in 1887, "As far as the fetus is concerned, no unimpeachable clinical observation has yet been published in which a fetus was injured by chloroform administered to its mother." Experience lulled them into complacency, which may explain their failure to appreciate the threat posed by twilight sleep.

Dangers from twilight sleep probably developed insidiously. The originators of the method, von Steinbüchel and Gauss, recommended conservative doses of drugs. They suggested that 0.3 mg of scopolamine be given every 2 to 3 hours to induce amnesia and that no more than 10 mg of morphine be administered subcutaneously for the whole labor. Gauss, who was especially meticulous, even advised physicians to administer a "memory test" to women in labor to evaluate the need for additional scopolamine. However, as other physicians used the technique, they changed it. Some gave larger doses of opioid—as much as 40 or 50 mg of morphine during labor. Others gave additional drugs (e.g., as much as 600 mg of pentobarbital during labor as well as inhalation agents for delivery). Despite administering these large doses to their patients, some physicians said they had seen no adverse effects on the infants.[28] They probably spoke the truth, but this probability says more about their powers of observation than the safety of the method.

Two situations eventually made physicians confront problems associated with placental transmission of anesthetic drugs. The first was the changing use of morphine.[29] In the latter part of the nineteenth century (before the enactment of laws governing the use of addictive drugs), morphine was a popular ingredient of patent medicines and a drug frequently prescribed by physicians. As addiction became more common, obstetricians saw many pregnant women who were taking large amounts of morphine daily. When they tried to decrease their patients' opioid use, several obstetricians noted unexpected problems (e.g., violent fetal movements, sudden fetal death), which they correctly identified as signs of withdrawal. Second, physiologists and anatomists began extensive studies of placental structure and function. By the turn of the century, they had identified many of the physical and chemical factors that affect rates of drug transfer. Thus, even before twilight sleep became popular, physicians had clinical and laboratory evidence to justify caution. As early as 1877, Gillette[30] described 15 instances of neonatal depression that he attributed to morphine given during labor. Similarly, in a review article published in 1914, Knipe[31] identified stillbirths and neonatal oligopnea and asphyxia as complications of twilight sleep and gave the incidence of each problem as reported by other writers.

When the studies of obstetric anesthesia published between 1880 and 1950 are considered, four characteristics stand out. First, few of them described effects of anesthesia on the newborn. Second, those that did report newborn apnea, oligopnea, or asphyxia seldom defined these words. Third, few used controls or compared one mode of treatment with another. Finally, few writers used their data to evaluate the safety of the practice that they described. In other words, by today's standards, even the best of these papers lacked substance. They did, however, demonstrate a growing concern among physicians about the effects of anesthetic drugs on neonates. Perhaps even more important, their work prepared clinicians for the work of Virginia Apgar (Figure 1-6).

Apgar became an anesthesiologist when the chairman of the Department of Surgery at the Columbia University College of Physicians and Surgeons dissuaded her from becoming a surgeon. After training in anesthesia with Ralph Waters at the University of Wisconsin and with E. A. Rovenstine at Bellevue Hospital, she returned to Columbia Presbyterian Hospital as Director of the Division of Anesthesia. In 1949, she was appointed professor, the first woman to attain that rank at Columbia University.[32]

In 1953, Apgar[33] described a simple, reliable system for evaluating newborns and showed that it was sufficiently sensitive to detect differences among neonates whose mothers had been anesthetized for cesarean delivery by different techniques (Figure 1-7). Infants delivered of women with spinal anesthesia had higher scores than

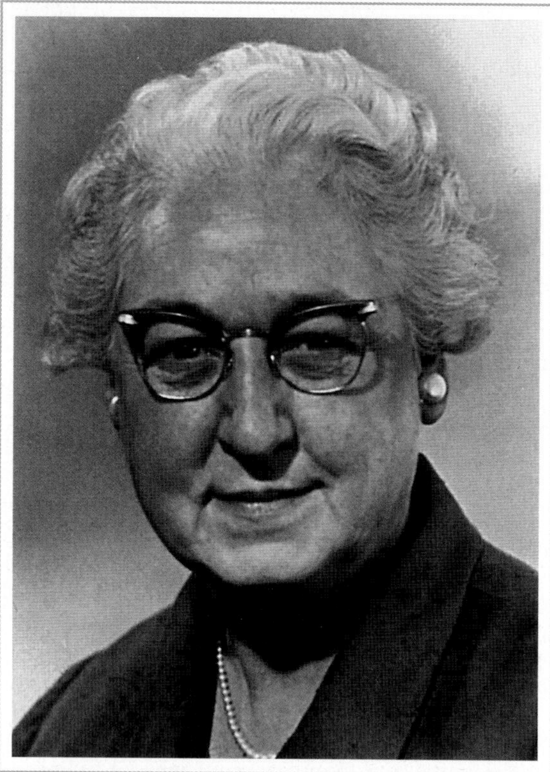

FIGURE 1-6 Virginia Apgar, whose scoring system revolutionized the practice of obstetrics and anesthesia. Her work made the well-being of the infant the major criterion for the evaluation of medical management of pregnant women. (Courtesy Wood Library Museum.)

those delivered with general anesthesia. The Apgar score had three important effects. First, it replaced simple observation of neonates with a reproducible measurement—that is, it substituted a numerical score for the ambiguities of words such as oligopnea and asphyxia. Thus it established the possibility of the systematic comparison of different treatments. Second, it provided objective criteria for the initiation of neonatal resuscitation. Third, and most important, it helped change the focus of obstetric care. Until that time the primary criterion for success or failure had been the survival and well-being of the mother, a natural goal considering the maternal risks of childbirth until that time. After 1900, as maternal risks diminished, the well-being of the mother no longer served as a sensitive measure of outcome. The Apgar score called attention to the child and made its condition the new standard for evaluating obstetric management.

Current Researches in Anesthesia and Analgesia—July-August, 1953

A Proposal for a New Method of Evaluation of the Newborn Infant.*

Virginia Apgar, M.D., New York, N. Y.

Department of Anesthesiology, Columbia University, College of Physicians and Surgeons and the Anesthesia Service, The Presbyterian Hospital

FIGURE 1-7 Title page from the paper in which Virginia Apgar described her new scoring system for evaluating the well-being of a newborn.

THE EFFECTS OF ANESTHESIA ON LABOR

The effects of anesthesia on labor also worried physicians. Again, their fears were well-founded. Diethyl ether and chloroform depress uterine contractions. If given in sufficient amounts, they also abolish reflex pushing with the abdominal muscles during the second stage of labor. These effects are not difficult to detect, even with moderate doses of either inhalation agent.

Simpson's method of obstetric anesthesia used significant amounts of drugs. He started the anesthetic early, and sometimes he rendered patients unconscious during the first stage of labor. In addition, he increased the depth of anesthesia for the delivery.[34] As many people copied his technique, they presumably had ample opportunity to observe uterine atony and postpartum hemorrhage.

Some physicians noticed the effects of anesthetics on uterine function. For example, Meigs[35] said unequivocally that etherization suppressed uterine function, and he described occasions in which he had had to suspend etherization to allow labor to resume. Other physicians waffled, however. For example, Walter Channing,[36] Professor of Midwifery and Medical Jurisprudence at Harvard (seemingly a strange combination of disciplines, but at that time neither of the two was thought sufficiently important to warrant a separate chair), published a book about the use of ether for obstetrics (Figure 1-8). He endorsed etherization and influenced many others to use it. However, his book contained blatant contradictions. On different pages Channing contended that ether had no effect, that it increased uterine contractility, and that it suspended contractions entirely. Then, in a pronouncement smacking more of panache than reason, Channing swept aside his inconsistencies and said that whatever effect ether may have on the uterus he "welcomes it." Noting similar contradictions among other writers, W. F. H. Montgomery,[37] Professor of Midwifery at the King and Queen's College of Physicians in Ireland, wrote, "By one writer we are told that, if uterine action is excessive, chloroform will abate it; by another that if feeble, it will strengthen it and add new vigor to each parturient effort."

John Snow[23] gave a more balanced review of the effects of anesthesia on labor. Originally a surgeon, Snow became the first physician to restrict his practice to anesthesia. He experimented with ether and chloroform and wrote many insightful papers and books describing his work (Figure 1-9). Snow's technique differed from Simpson's. Snow withheld anesthesia until the second stage of labor, limited administration to brief periods during contractions, and attempted to keep his patients comfortable but responsive. To achieve better control of the depth of anesthesia, he recommended using the vaporizing apparatus that he had developed for surgical cases. Snow[23] spoke disparagingly of Simpson's technique and the tendency of people to use it simply because of Simpson's reputation:

The high position of Dr. Simpson and his previous services in this department, more particularly in being the first to administer ether in labour, gave his recommendations very great influence; the consequence of which is

A TREATISE

ON

ETHERIZATION IN CHILDBIRTH.

ILLUSTRATED BY

FIVE HUNDRED AND EIGHTY-ONE CASES.

BY WALTER CHANNING, M.D.

PROFESSOR OF MIDWIFERY AND MEDICAL JURISPRUDENCE IN THE UNIVERSITY AT CAMBRIDGE.

"Give me the facts, said my Lord Judge: your reasonings are the mere guess-work of the imagination." — OLD PLAY.

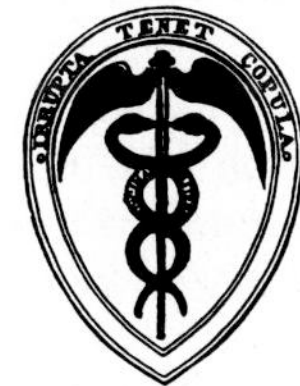

BOSTON:

WILLIAM D. TICKNOR AND COMPANY,

CORNER OF WASHINGTON AND SCHOOL STREETS.

M.DCCC.XLVIII.

FIGURE 1-8 Frontispiece from Walter Channing's book on the use of etherization for childbirth. Channing favored the use of etherization, and he persuaded others to use it, although evidence ensuring its safety was scant.

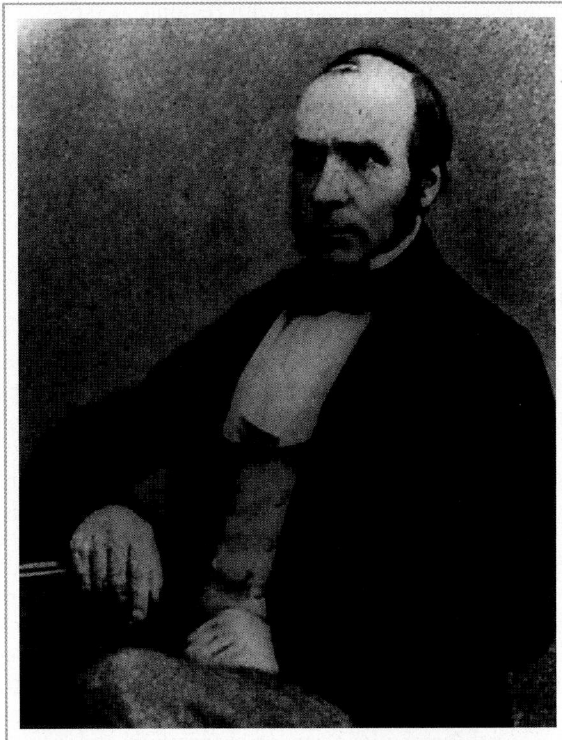

FIGURE 1-9 John Snow, a London surgeon who gave up his surgical practice to become the first physician to devote all his time to anesthesia. He wrote many monographs and papers, some of which accurately describe the effects of anesthesia on infant and mother. (Courtesy Wood Library Museum.)

> *that the practice of anesthesia is presently probably in a much less satisfactory state than it would have been if chloroform had never been introduced.*

Snow's method, which was the same one he had used to anesthetize Queen Victoria, eventually prevailed over Simpson's. Physicians became more cautious with anesthesia, reserving it for special problems such as cephalic version, the application of forceps, abnormal presentation, and eclampsia. They also became more conservative with dosage, often giving anesthesia only during the second stage of labor. Snow's methods were applied to each new inhalation agent—including nitrous oxide, ethylene, cyclopropane, trichloroethylene, and methoxyflurane—as it was introduced to obstetric anesthesia.

Early physicians modified their use of anesthesia from experience, not from study of normal labor or from learning more about the pharmacology of the drugs. Moreover, they had not yet defined the relationship between uterine pain and contractions. As physicians turned more to science during the latter part of the century, however, their strategies began to change. For example, in 1893 the English physiologist Henry Head[38] published his classic studies of the innervation of abdominal viscera. His work stimulated others to investigate the role of the nervous system in the control of labor. Subsequently, clinical and laboratory studies of pregnancy after spinal cord transection established the independence of labor from nervous control.[39] When regional anesthesia appeared during the first decades of the twentieth century, physicians therefore had a conceptual basis from which to explore its effects on labor.

Carl Koller[40] introduced regional anesthesia when he used cocaine for eye surgery in 1884. Recognizing the potential of Koller's innovation, surgeons developed techniques for other procedures. Obstetricians quickly adopted many of these techniques for their own use. The first papers describing obstetric applications of spinal, lumbar epidural, caudal, paravertebral, parasacral, and pudendal nerve blocks appeared between 1900 and 1930 (see Figure 1-4).[41-43] Recognition of the potential effects of regional anesthesia on labor developed more slowly, primarily because obstetricians seldom used it. They continued to rely on inhalation agents and opioids, partly because few drugs and materials were available for regional anesthesia at that time, but also because obstetricians did not appreciate the chief advantage of regional over general anesthesia—the relative absence of drug effects on the infant. Moreover, they rarely used regional anesthesia except for delivery, and then they often used elective forceps anyway. This set of circumstances limited their opportunity and motivation to study the effects of regional anesthesia on labor.

Among early papers dealing with regional anesthesia, one written by Cleland[44] stands out. He described his experience with paravertebral anesthesia, but he also wrote a thoughtful analysis of the nerve pathways mediating labor pain, an analysis he based on information he had gleaned from clinical and laboratory studies. Few investigators were as meticulous or insightful as Cleland. Most of those who studied the effects of anesthesia simply timed the length of the first and second stages of labor. Some timed the duration of individual contractions or estimated changes in the strength of contractions by palpation. None of the investigators measured the intrauterine pressures, even though a German physician had described such a method in 1898 and had used it to evaluate the effects of morphine and ether on the contractions of laboring women.[45]

More detailed and accurate studies of the effects of anesthesia started to appear after 1944. Part of the stimulus was a method for continuous caudal anesthesia introduced by Hingson and Edwards,[46] in which a malleable needle remained in the sacral canal throughout labor. Small, flexible plastic catheters eventually replaced malleable needles and made continuous epidural anesthesia even more popular. With the help of these innovations, obstetricians began using anesthesia earlier in labor. Ensuing problems, real and imagined, stimulated more studies. Although good studies were scarce, the strong interest in the problem represented a marked change from the early days of obstetric anesthesia.

Ironically, "natural childbirth" appeared just as regional anesthesia started to become popular and as clinicians began to understand how to use it without disrupting labor. Dick-Read,[47] the originator of the natural method, recognized "no physiological function in the body which gives rise to pain in the normal course of health." He attributed pain in an otherwise uncomplicated labor to an "activation of the sympathetic nervous system by the emotion of fear." He argued that fear made the uterus contract and become ischemic and therefore painful. He said that women could avoid the pain if they simply learned to abolish their fear of labor. Dick-Read never explained why uterine ischemia that results from fear causes pain, whereas ischemia that results from a normal contraction does not. In other words, Dick-Read, like Simpson a century earlier, claimed no necessary or physiologic relationship between labor pain and contractions. Dick-Read's book, written more for the public than for the medical profession, represented a regression of almost a century in medical thought and practice. It is important to note that contemporary methods of childbirth preparation do not maintain that fear alone causes labor pain. However, they do attempt to reduce fear by education and to help patients manage pain by teaching techniques of self-control. This represents a significant difference from and an important advance over Dick-Read's original theory.

SOME LESSONS

History is important in proportion to the lessons it teaches. With respect to obstetric anesthesia, four lessons stand out. First, every new drug and method entails risks. Physicians who first used obstetric anesthesia seemed reluctant to accept this fact, perhaps because of their inexperience with potent drugs (pharmacology was in its infancy) or because they acceded too quickly to patients, who wanted relief from pain and had little understanding of the technical issues confronting physicians. Whatever the reason, this period of denial lasted almost half a century, until 1900. Almost another half-century passed before obstetricians learned to modify their practice to limit the effects of anesthetics on the child and the labor process.

Second, new drugs or therapies often cause problems in completely unexpected ways. For example, in 1900, physicians noted a rising rate of puerperal fever.[48] The timing was odd. Several decades had passed since Robert Koch had suggested the germ theory of disease and since Semmelweis had recognized that physicians often transmit infection from one woman to the next with their unclean hands. With the adoption of aseptic methods, deaths from puerperal fever had diminished dramatically. During the waning years of the nineteenth century, however, they increased again. Some physicians attributed this resurgence of puerperal fever to anesthesia. In a presidential address to the Obstetrical Society of Edinburgh in 1900, Murray[49] stated the following:

> *I feel sure that an explanation of much of the increase of maternal mortality from 1847 onwards will be found in, first the misuse of anaesthesia and second in the ridiculous parody which, in many hands, stands for the use of antiseptics.... Before the days of anaesthesia, interference was limited and obstetric operations were at a minimum because interference of all kinds increased the conscious suffering of the patient.... When anaesthesia became possible, and interference became more frequent because it involved no additional suffering, operations were undertaken when really unnecessary ... and so complications arose and the dangers of the labor increased.*

Although it was not a direct complication of the use of anesthesia in obstetric practice, puerperal fever appeared to be an indirect consequence of it.

Changes in obstetric practice also had unexpected effects on anesthetic complications. During the first decades of the twentieth century, when cesarean deliveries were rare and obstetricians used only inhalation analgesia for delivery, few women were exposed to the risk of aspiration during deep anesthesia. As obstetric practice changed and cesarean deliveries became more common, this risk rose. The syndrome of aspiration was not identified and labeled until 1946, when obstetrician Curtis Mendelson[50] described and named it. The pathophysiology of the syndrome had already been described by Winternitz et al.,[51] who instilled hydrochloric acid into the lungs of dogs to simulate the lesions found in veterans poisoned by gas during the trench warfare of World War I. Unfortunately, the reports of these studies, although excellent, did not initiate any change in practice. Change occurred only after several deaths of obstetric patients were highly publicized in lay, legal, and medical publications. Of course, rapid-sequence induction, currently recommended to reduce the risk of aspiration, creates another set of risks—those associated with a failed intubation.

The third lesson offered by the history of obstetric anesthesia concerns the role of basic science. Modern medicine developed during the nineteenth century after physicians learned to apply principles of anatomy, physiology, and chemistry to the study and treatment of disease. Obstetric anesthesia underwent a similar pattern of development. Studies of placental structure and function called physicians' attention to the transmission of drugs and the potential effects of drugs on the infant. Similarly, studies of the physiology and anatomy of the uterus helped elucidate potential effects of anesthesia on labor. In each instance, lessons from basic science helped improve patient care.

The fourth and perhaps the most important lesson is the role that patients have played in the use of anesthesia for obstetrics. During the nineteenth century it was women who pressured cautious physicians to incorporate routine use of anesthesia into their obstetric practice. A century later, it was women again who altered patterns of practice, this time questioning the overuse of anesthesia for routine deliveries. In both instances the pressure on physicians emanated from prevailing social values regarding pain. In 1900 the public believed that pain, and in particular obstetric pain, was destructive and something that should be avoided. Half a century later, with the advent of the natural childbirth movement, many people began to suggest that the experience of pain during childbirth, perhaps even in other situations, might have some physiologic if not social value. Physicians must recognize and acknowledge the extent to which social values may shape medical "science" and practice.[52,53]

During the past 60 years, scientists have accumulated a wealth of information about many processes integral to normal labor: the processes that initiate and control lactation; neuroendocrine events that initiate and maintain labor; the biochemical maturation of the fetal lung and liver; the metabolic requirements of the normal fetus and the protective mechanisms that it may invoke in times of stress; and the normal mechanisms that regulate the amount and distribution of blood flow to the uterus and placenta. At this point, we have only the most rudimentary understanding of the interaction of anesthesia with any of these processes. Only a fraction of the information available from basic science has been used to improve obstetric anesthesia care. Realizing the rewards from the clinical use of such information may be the most important lesson from the past and the greatest challenge for the future of obstetric anesthesia.

KEY POINTS

- Physicians have debated the safety of obstetric anesthesia since 1847, when James Young Simpson first administered anesthesia for delivery. Two issues have dominated the debate: the effects of anesthesia on labor and the effects of anesthesia on the newborn.
- Despite controversy, physicians quickly incorporated anesthesia into clinical practice, largely because of their patients' desire to avoid childbirth pain.
- Only after obstetric anesthesia was in use for many years did problems become apparent.
- Important milestones in obstetric anesthesia are the introduction of inhalation agents in 1847, the expanded use of opioids in the early decades of the twentieth century, and the refinement of regional anesthesia starting in the mid-twentieth century.
- Outstanding conceptual developments are (1) Zweifel's idea that drugs given to the mother cross the placenta and affect the fetus and (2) Apgar's idea that the condition of the newborn is the most sensitive assay of the quality of anesthetic care of the mother.
- The history of obstetric anesthesia suggests that the major improvements in patient care have followed the application of principles of basic science.

REFERENCES

1. Haggard HW. Devils, Drugs, and Doctors: The Story of the Science of Healing from Medicine-Man to Doctor. New York, Harper & Brothers, 1929.
2. Caton D. What a Blessing. She Had Chloroform: The Medical and Social Response to the Pain of Childbirth from 1800 to the Present. New Haven, Yale University Press, 1999.
3. Shepherd JA. Simpson and Syme of Edinburgh. Edinburgh, London, E & S Livingstone, 1969.
4. Simpson WG, editor. The Works of Sir JY Simpson, Vol II: Anaesthesia. Edinburgh, Adam and Charles Black, 1871:199-200.
5. Levinson A. The three Meigs and their contribution to pediatrics. Ann Med Hist 1928; 10:138-48.
6. Dubois P. On the inhalation of ether applied to cases of midwifery. Lancet 1847; 49:246-9.
7. Ramsbotham FH. The Principles and Practice of Obstetric Medicine and Surgery in Reference to the Process of Parturition with Sixty-four Plates and Numerous Wood-cuts. Philadelphia, Blanchard and Lea, 1855.
8. Report of the Committee Appointed by the Royal Medical and Chirurgical Society to Inquire into the Uses and the Physiological, Therapeutical, and Toxical Effects of Chloroform, as Well as into the Best Mode of Administering it, and of Obviating Any Ill Consequences Resulting from its Administration. Med Chir Trans 1864; 47:323-442.
9. Sykes WS. Essays on the First Hundred Years of Anaesthesia, Vol I. Park Ridge, IL, Wood Library Museum of Anesthesiology, 1982.
10. Caton D. The secularization of pain. Anesthesiology 1985; 62:493-501.
11. Wagenknecht E, editor. Mrs. Longfellow: Selected Letters and Journals of Fanny Appleton Longfellow (1817-1861). New York, Longmans, Green, 1956.
12. Cohen M, editor. Nature: The Philosophy of John Stuart Mill. New York, Modern Library, 1961:463-7.
13. Simpson WG, editor. The Works of Sir JY Simpson, Vol II: Anaesthesia. Edinburgh, Adam and Charles Black, 1871:177.
14. von Steinbüchel R. Vorläufige Mittheilung über die Anwendung von Skopolamin-Morphium-Injektionen in der Geburtshilfe. Centralblatt Gyn 1902; 30:1304-6.
15. Gauss CJ. Die Anwendung des Skopolamin-Morphium-Dämmerschlafes in der Geburtshilfe. Medizinische Klinik 1906; 2:136-8.
16. Macht DI. The history of opium and some of its preparations and alkaloids. JAMA 1915; 64:477-81.
17. Sansom AE. On the pain of parturition, and anaesthetics in obstetric practice. Trans Obstet Soc Lond 1868; 10:121-40.
18. Gusserow A. Zur Lehre vom Stoffwechsel des Foetus. Arch Gyn 1871; III:241.
19. Wertz RW, Wertz DC. Lying-In: A History of Childbirth in America. New York, Schocken Books, 1979.
20. Leavitt JW. Brought to Bed: Childbearing in America, 1750-1950. New York, Oxford University Press, 1986.
21. Kaufman M. American Medical Education: The Formative Years, 1765-1910. Westport, CT, Greenwood Press, 1976.
22. Mayow J. Tractatus quinque medico-physici. Quoted in: Needham J. Chemical Embryology. New York, Hafner Publishing, 1963.
23. Snow J. On the administration of chloroform during parturition. Assoc Med J 1853; 1:500-2.

24. Caton D. Obstetric anesthesia and concepts of placental transport: A historical review of the nineteenth century. Anesthesiology 1977; 46:132-7.
25. Zweifel P. Einfluss der Chloroformnarcose Kreissender auf den Fötus. Klinische Wochenschrift 1874; 21:1-2.
26. Zweifel P. Die Respiration des Fötus. Arch Gyn 1876; 9:291-305.
27. Spiegelberg O. A Textbook of Midwifery. Translated by JB Hurry. London, The New Sydenham Society, 1887.
28. Gwathmey JT. A further study, based on more than twenty thousand cases. Surg Gynecol Obstet 1930; 51:190-5.
29. Terry CE, Pellens M. The Opium Problem. Camden, NJ, Bureau of Social Hygiene, 1928.
30. Gillette WR. The narcotic effect of morphia on the new-born child, when administered to the mother in labor. Am J Obstet, Dis Women Child, 1877; 10:612-23.
31. Knipe WHW. The Freiburg method of Däammerschlaf or twilight sleep. Am J Obstet Gynecol 1914; 70:884.
32. Calmes SH. Virginia Apgar: A woman physician's career in a developing specialty. J Am Med Wom Assoc 1984; 39:184-8.
33. Apgar V. A proposal for a new method of evaluation of the newborn infant. Curr Res Anesth Analg 1953; 32:260-7.
34. Thoms H. Anesthesia á la Reine—a chapter in the history of anesthesia. Am J Obstet Gynecol 1940; 40:340-6.
35. Meigs CD. Obstetrics, the Science and the Art. Philadelphia, Blanchard and Lea, 1865:364-76.
36. Channing W. A Treatise on Etherization in Childbirth. Boston, William D. Ticknor and Company, 1848.
37. Montgomery WFH. Objections to the Indiscriminate Administration of Anaesthetic Agents in Midwifery. Dublin, Hodges and Smith, 1849.
38. Head H. On disturbances of sensation with especial reference to the pain of visceral disease. Brain 1893; 16:1-132.
39. Gertsman NM. Über Uterusinnervation an Hand des Falles einer Geburt bei Quersnittslähmung. Monatsschrift Gebürtshüfle Gyn 1926; 73:253-7.
40. Koller C. On the use of cocaine for producing anaesthesia on the eye. Lancet 1884; 124:990-2.
41. Kreis O. Über Medullarnarkose bei Gebärenden. Centralblatt Gynäkologie 1900; 28:724-7.
42. Bonar BE, Meeker WR. The value of sacral nerve block anesthesia in obstetrics. JAMA 1923; 81:1079-83.
43. Schlimpert H. Concerning sacral anaesthesia. Surg Gynecol Obstet 1913; 16:488-92.
44. Cleland JGP. Paravertebral anaesthesia in obstetrics. Surg Gynecol Obstet 1933; 57:51-62.
45. Hensen H. Ueber den Einfluss des Morphiums und des Aethers auf die Wehenthätigkeit des Uterus. Archiv für Gynakologie 1898; 55:129-77.
46. Hingson RA, Edwards WB. Continuous caudal analgesia: An analysis of the first ten thousand confinements thus managed with the report of the authors' first thousand cases. JAMA 1943; 123:538-46.
47. Dick-Read G. Childbirth Without Fear: The Principles and Practice of Natural Childbirth. New York, Harper & Row, 1970.
48. Lea AWW. Puerperal Infection. London, Oxford University Press, 1910.
49. Murray M. Presidential address to the Obstetrical Society of Edinburgh, 1900. Quoted in: Cullingworth CJ. Oliver Wendell Holmes and the Contagiousness of Puerperal Fever. J Obstet Gyaecol Br Emp 1905; 8:387-8.
50. Mendelson CL. The aspiration of stomach contents into the lungs during obstetric anesthesia. Am J Obstet Gynecol 1946; 52:191-205.
51. Winternitz MC, Smith GH, McNamara FP. Effect of intrabronchial insufflation of acid. J Exp Med 1920; 32:199-204.
52. Caton D. "The poem in the pain": the social significance of pain in Western civilization. Anesthesiology 1994; 81:1044-52.
53. Caton D. Medical science and social values. Int J Obstet Anesth 2004; 13:167-73.

Part II

Maternal and Fetal Physiology

Metabolism was among the first areas of physiology to influence clinical practice. By the beginning of the twentieth century, physiologists had established many of the principles that we recognize today, including normal rates of oxygen consumption and carbon dioxide production, the relationship between oxygen consumption and heat production, and the relationship between metabolic rate and body weight and surface area among individuals and species. Almost simultaneously, clinicians began to apply these principles to their studies of patients in different states of health and disease.

In one early study, physiologist Magnus-Levy[1] found an exception to the rule that basal metabolic rate varied in proportion to body surface area. As he measured a woman's oxygen consumption during pregnancy, he observed that her metabolic rate increased out of proportion to increments in her body weight and surface area. Subsequent studies by other investigators established the basis of this phenomenon. Per unit of weight, the fetus, placenta, and uterus together consumed oxygen (and released carbon dioxide and heat) at a higher rate than the mother. In effect, the metabolism of a pregnant woman represented the sum of two independent organisms, each metabolizing at its own rate in proportion to its own surface area. Thus, each kilogram of maternal tissue consumed oxygen at a rate of approximately 4 mL/min, whereas the average rate for the fetus, placenta, and uterus was approximately 12 mL/min, although it could rise as high as 20 mL/min. Therefore, during pregnancy, the mother's metabolism was the sum of her metabolic rate plus that of the fetus, placenta, and uterus.[1-4] Subsequent studies established that the highest rates of fetal metabolism occurred during the periods of most rapid growth, thereby reaffirming another physiologic principle—the high metabolic cost of synthesizing new tissue.[5]

The aforementioned studies gave clinicians estimates of the stress imposed by pregnancy. To maintain homeostasis during pregnancy, a pregnant woman had to make an appropriate adjustment in each of the physiologic mechanisms involved in the delivery of substrates to the fetal placental unit and in the excretion of metabolic wastes. Thus, for every increment in fetal weight, clinicians could expect to find a proportional change in all the mechanisms involved in the delivery of substrate to the fetus and in the excretion of all byproducts. In fact, subsequent clinical studies established predictable changes in uterine blood flow, cardiac output, blood volume, minute ventilation, the dissipation of body heat, and the renal excretion of nitrogenous waste and other materials.

Donald Caton, M.D.

REFERENCES

1. Magnus-Levy A. Stoffwechsel und Nahrungsbedarf in der Schwangerschaft. A. Geburtsh. u. Gynaek lii:116-84.
2. Carpenter TM, Murlin JR. The energy metabolism of mother and child just before and just after birth. AMA Arch Intern Med 1911; 7:184-222.
3. Root H, Root HK. The basal metabolism during pregnancy and the puerperium. Arch Intern Med 1923; 32:411-24.
4. Sandiford I, Wheeler T. The basal metabolism before, during, and after pregnancy. J Biol Chem 1924; 62:329-52.
5. Caton D, Henderson DJ, Wilcox CJ, Barron DH. Oxygen consumption of the uterus and its contents and weight at birth of lambs. In Longo LD, Reneau DD, editors. Fetal and Newborn Cardiovascular Physiology, vol 2. New York, Garland STPM Press, 1978:123-34.

Chapter 2

Physiologic Changes of Pregnancy

Robert Gaiser, M.D.

Marked anatomic and physiologic changes occur in women during pregnancy. The pregnant woman must adapt to the developing fetus and provide for its increased metabolic demands. The enlarging uterus places mechanical strain on the woman's body. The greater production of various hormones by the ovaries and the placenta further alters maternal physiology. The hallmark of successful anesthetic management of the pregnant woman is recognition of these anatomic and physiologic changes and appropriate adaptation of anesthetic techniques to these changes. This chapter reviews the physiologic alterations of normal pregnancy and their anesthetic implications.

BODY WEIGHT AND COMPOSITION

The mean maternal weight increase during pregnancy is 17% of the prepregnancy weight, or approximately 12 kg.[1] Weight gain results from an increase in the size of the uterus and its contents (uterus, 1 kg; amniotic fluid, 1 kg; fetus and placenta, 4 kg); increases in blood volume and interstitial fluid (approximately 2 kg each); and deposition of new fat and protein (approximately 4 kg). Normal weight gain during the first trimester is 1 to 2 kg, and there is a 5- to 6-kg gain in each of the last two trimesters.

Obesity is a major problem in the United States and also represents a potential problem for the parturient. Obesity increases the risk of adverse pregnancy outcome, including the rate of cesarean delivery. The odds ratios for cesarean delivery are 1.46, 2.05, and 2.89 for overweight, obese, and severely obese women, respectively, compared with pregnant women of normal weight.[2] Excessive weight gain during pregnancy constitutes a major risk factor for long-term increase in body mass index (BMI).[3]

THE HEART AND CIRCULATION

Physical Examination of the Heart

Pregnancy causes cardiac hypertrophy. The hypertrophy is a result of greater blood volume as well as increased stretch and force of contraction.[4] These changes, coupled with the elevation of the diaphragm, lead to several alterations in cardiac findings.

Changes in heart sounds include accentuation of the first heart sound with exaggerated splitting of the mitral and tricuspid components (Box 2-1).[5] The second heart sound changes little, although the aortic-pulmonic interval tends to vary less with respiration during the third trimester. The third heart sound may be heard during the third trimester and does not possess any clinical significance. A fourth heart sound may be heard in 16% of pregnant women, although it typically disappears by term. A grade II systolic ejection murmur is commonly heard at the left sternal border.[6] The murmur is considered a benign flow murmur that is attributed to cardiac enlargement from increased intravascular volume, which causes dilation of the tricuspid annulus and regurgitation.

Elevation of the diaphragm shifts the heart anteriorly and to the left during pregnancy. On physical examination the point of maximal cardiac impulse is displaced cephalad to the fourth intercostal space and leftward to at least the midclavicular line.

The electrocardiogram (ECG) typically changes during pregnancy, especially during the third trimester. There is an increase in heart rate and a shortening of both the PR interval and the uncorrected QT interval. This shortening has implications for the clinical course of women with long QT syndrome.[7] During pregnancy in these women, the risk of cardiac events is reduced (risk ratio [RR] = 0.38) compared with that in periods between pregnancy. However, the initial 9 months after delivery are associated with a markedly higher risk of adverse cardiac events (RR = 2.7), suggesting that the QT interval may be prolonged in the postpartum period. Other ECG changes include an axis shift; the QRS axis shifts to the right during the first trimester but may shift to the left during the third trimester as a result of displacement by the expanding uterus.[8] Depressed ST segments and isoelectric low-voltage T waves in the left-sided precordial and limb leads are commonly observed during pregnancy.[9]

Echocardiography demonstrates left ventricular hypertrophy by 12 weeks' gestation, with a 50% increase in mass at term.[10] This hypertrophy occurs as a result of an increase in the size of the preexisting cardiomyocytes rather than in the number of cells. The hypertrophy is eccentric, resembling that developed during exercise.[1] A significant increase in the annular diameters of the mitral, tricuspid, and pulmonic valves occurs; 94% of term pregnant women exhibit tricuspid and pulmonic regurgitation, and 27% exhibit mitral regurgitation.[11] The aortic annulus is not dilated.

BOX 2-1 Changes in the Cardiac Examination in the Pregnant Patient

- Accentuation of S1 (first heart sound); exaggerated splitting of the mitral and tricuspid components
- Typical systolic ejection murmur
- Possible presence of S3 (third heart sound) and S4 (fourth heart sound) (no clinical significance)
- Leftward displacement of point of maximal cardiac impulse

Central Hemodynamics

Prerequisites for the accurate determination of hemodynamic changes during pregnancy require that measurements be made with subjects in a resting position, which minimizes compression of the aorta and inferior vena cava by the gravid uterus. Further, comparisons must be made with an appropriate control, such as the same group of women before pregnancy or a matched group of nonpregnant women. If control measurements are made during the postpartum period, a sufficient interval must have elapsed so that hemodynamic parameters return to prepregnancy values. For some measurements, this return may take 24 weeks or more.[12]

Cardiac output increases during pregnancy (Table 2-1). This change occurs by 5 weeks' gestation, with a resultant increase of 35% to 40% by the end of the first trimester of pregnancy.[10,13] Cardiac output continues to rise throughout the second trimester until it reaches a level approximately 50% greater than that of nonpregnant women (Figure 2-1).[10,12,14-16] This parameter does not change from this level during the third trimester. In the past it had been postulated that cardiac output declined during

TABLE 2-1 Central Hemodynamics at Term Gestation

Parameter	Change*
Cardiac output	+50%
Stroke volume	+25%
Heart rate	+25%
Left ventricular end-diastolic volume	Increased
Left ventricular end-systolic volume	No change
Ejection fraction	Increased
Left ventricular stroke work index	No change
Pulmonary capillary wedge pressure	No change
Pulmonary artery diastolic pressure	No change
Central venous pressure	No change
Systemic vascular resistance	−20%

*Relative to nonpregnant state.

Adapted from Conklin KA. Maternal physiological adaptations during gestation, labor, and the puerperium. Semin Anesth 1991; 10:221-34.

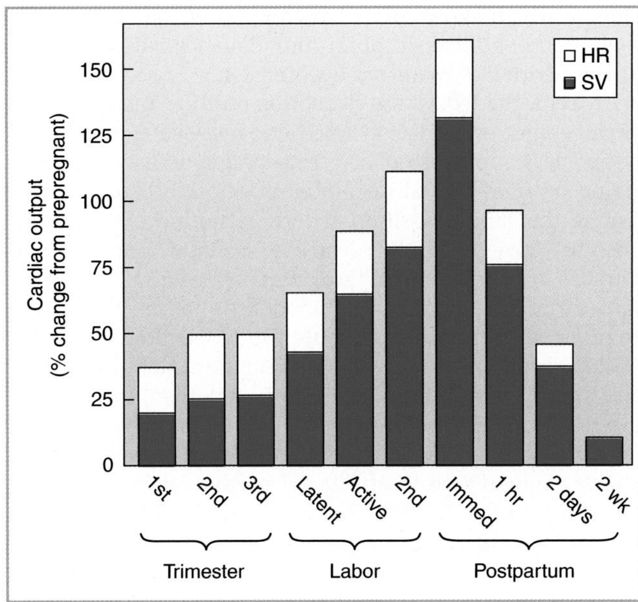

FIGURE 2-1 Cardiac output during pregnancy, labor, and the puerperium. Values during pregnancy are measured at the end of the first, second, and third trimesters. Values during labor are measured between contractions. For each measurement, the relative contributions of heart rate (HR) and stroke volume (SV) to the change in cardiac output are illustrated.

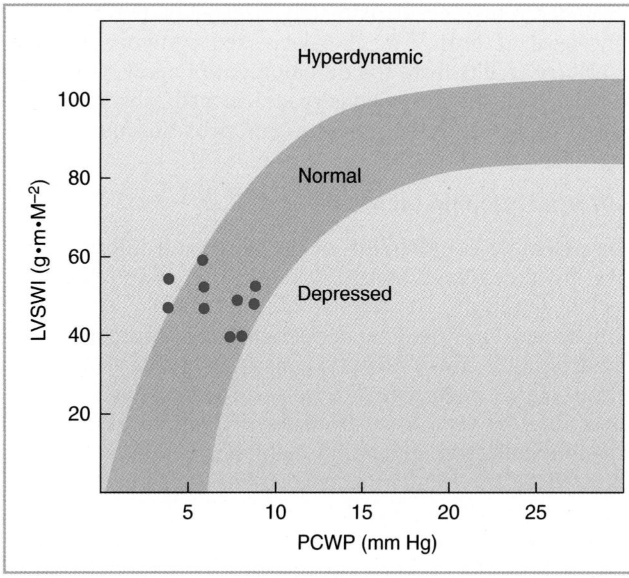

FIGURE 2-2 Left ventricular function in late phase of third-trimester normotensive pregnant patients. LVSWI, left ventricular stroke work index; PCWP, pulmonary capillary wedge pressure. (Modified from Clark SL, Cotton DB, Lee W, et al. Central hemodynamic assessment of cardiac function. Am J Obstet Gynecol 1989; 161:439-42.)

the third trimester. The problem with this supposition was that measurements were obtained with pregnant women in the supine position; thus, the observed decrease in cardiac output was a reflection of aortocaval compression rather than a true physiologic change.

Cardiac output is a reflection of heart rate and stroke volume. The earliest change in cardiac output is attributed to an increase in heart rate, which occurs by the fourth to fifth week of pregnancy.[10] The heart rate increases approximately 15% to 25% over baseline by the end of the first trimester and does not change during the third trimester.[10,12-17] Stroke volume rises by approximately 20% between the fifth and eighth weeks of gestation, and by 25% to 30% by the end of the second trimester, and then remains at this level until term.[10,12,13,17] Left ventricular mass increases by 23% from the first to the third trimester.[18] The increase in stroke volume correlates with rising estrogen levels.[1]

Left ventricular end-diastolic volume increases during gestation, whereas end-systolic volume remains unchanged, resulting in a larger ejection fraction.[10,12-15,17] Central venous, pulmonary artery diastolic, and pulmonary capillary wedge pressures during pregnancy are within the normal range for nonpregnant individuals.[16] The apparent discrepancy between left ventricular filling pressure and end-diastolic volume is explained by hypertrophy and dilation, with the dilated ventricle accommodating a greater volume without an increase in pressure.

Myocardial contractility is also increased, as demonstrated by the higher velocity of left ventricular circumferential fiber shortening (Figure 2-2).[10,14,17] Tissue Doppler imaging has been used to assess diastolic function, as this technique is relatively independent of preload.[19] Investigators found that left ventricular diastolic function was not impaired during pregnancy, whereas systolic function was increased during the second trimester.

The rise in cardiac output during pregnancy results in greater perfusion to the uterus, kidneys, and extremities. Blood flow to the brain and liver do not change. Uterine blood flow increases from a baseline of approximately 50 mL/min to 700 to 900 mL/min at term.[20-24] Approximately 90% of this flow perfuses the intervillous space, with the balance perfusing the myometrium.[22] At term, skin blood flow is approximately three to four times the nonpregnant level, resulting in higher skin temperature.[25] Renal plasma flow is increased by 80% at 16 to 26 weeks' gestation but declines to 50% above the nonpregnant baseline at term.[26]

Blood Pressure

Positioning, gestational age, and parity affect blood pressure measurements. Brachial sphygmomanometry yields the highest measurements in the supine position and the lowest measurements in the lateral position.[15,27] Blood pressure increases with maternal age, and for a given age, nulliparous women have a higher mean pressure than parous women.[28] Systolic, diastolic, and mean arterial pressures decrease during mid-pregnancy and return toward baseline as the pregnancy approaches term.[29] Diastolic blood pressure falls to a greater degree than does systolic blood pressure, with early to mid-gestational decreases of approximately 20%.[30] The changes in blood pressure are consistent with changes in systemic vascular resistance, which falls during early gestation, reaches its nadir (35% decline) at 20 weeks' gestation, and rises during late gestation. Unlike blood pressure, systemic vascular resistance remains approximately 20% below the nonpregnant level at term.[12,16] The decreased systemic vascular resistance results from the development of a low-resistance vascular bed (the intervillous space) as well as vasodilation caused by prostacyclin, estrogen, and progesterone.

Aortocaval Compression

The extent of compression of the aorta and inferior vena cava by the gravid uterus depends on positioning and weeks' gestation. At term there is partial vena caval compression in the lateral position, as documented by angiography.[31] This finding is consistent with the 75% elevation—above nonpregnant levels—of femoral venous and lower inferior vena caval pressures.[32] Despite caval compression, collateral circulation maintains venous return, as reflected by the right ventricular filling pressure, which is unaltered in the lateral position.[16]

In the supine position, there is nearly complete obstruction of the inferior vena cava at term gestation.[33] Blood return from the lower extremities occurs through the intraosseous vertebral veins, paravertebral veins, and the epidural veins.[34] However, venous return via these collaterals is less than would occur through the inferior vena cava, resulting in a decrease in right atrial pressure.[35] Compression of the inferior vena cava occurs as early as 13 to 16 weeks' gestation and is evident from the 50% increase in femoral venous pressure that occurs when a woman assumes the supine position at this stage of pregnancy (Figure 2-3).[36] By term, femoral venous and lower inferior vena cava pressures are approximately 2.5 times the nonpregnant measurements in the supine position.[32,36]

In the supine position, the aorta may be compressed by the term gravid uterus. This compression accounts for the lower femoral artery pressure compared with brachial artery pressure in the supine position.[37,38] These findings are consistent with angiographic studies in supine pregnant women, which show partial obstruction of the aorta at the level of the lumbar lordosis and enhanced compression during periods of maternal hypotension.[39]

At term, the left lateral decubitus position results in less enhancement of cardiac sympathetic nervous system activity and less suppression of cardiac vagal activity than the supine or right lateral decubitus position.[40] Women who assume the supine position at term gestation experience a 10% to 20% decline in stroke volume and cardiac output.[41,42] These effects are consistent with the fall in right atrial filling pressure. Blood flow in the upper extremities is normal, whereas uterine blood flow decreases by 20%, and lower extremity blood flow falls by 50%.[43] Perfusion of the uterus is less affected than that of the lower extremities because vena caval compression does not obstruct venous outflow via the ovarian veins.[34] The adverse hemodynamic effects of aortocaval compression are reduced once the fetal head is engaged.[37,38]

Many term pregnant women exhibit an increase in brachial artery pressure when they assume the supine position. This finding is caused by a higher systemic vascular resistance, which is attributed to compression of the aorta. Up to 15% of women at term experience bradycardia and a substantial drop in blood pressure when supine, the so-called **supine hypotension syndrome**.[44,45] It may take several minutes for the bradycardia and hypotension to develop, and the bradycardia is usually preceded by a period of tachycardia. The syndrome results from a profound drop in venous return for which the cardiovascular system cannot compensate.

Hemodynamic Changes during Labor and the Puerperium

Cardiac output during labor (but between uterine contractions) increases from prelabor measurements by approximately 10% in the early first stage, by 25% in the late first

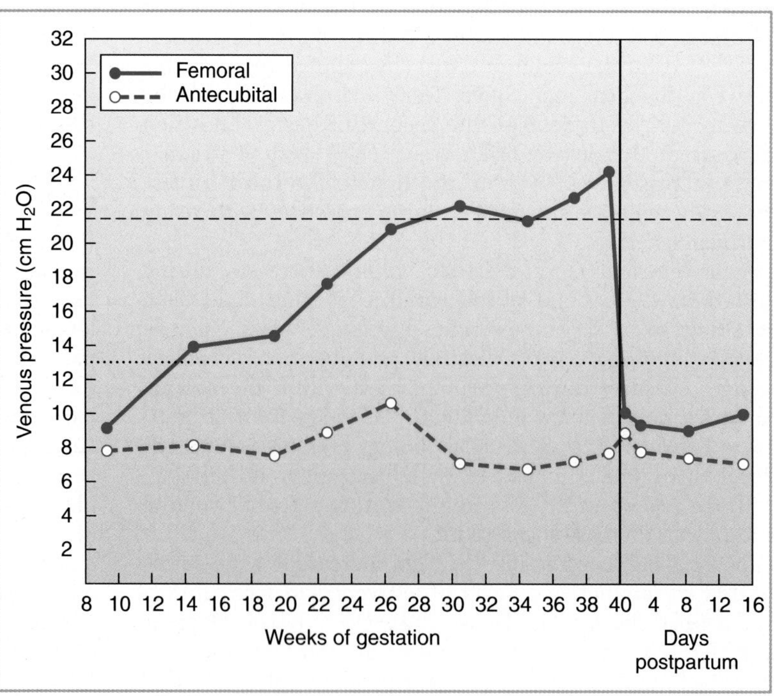

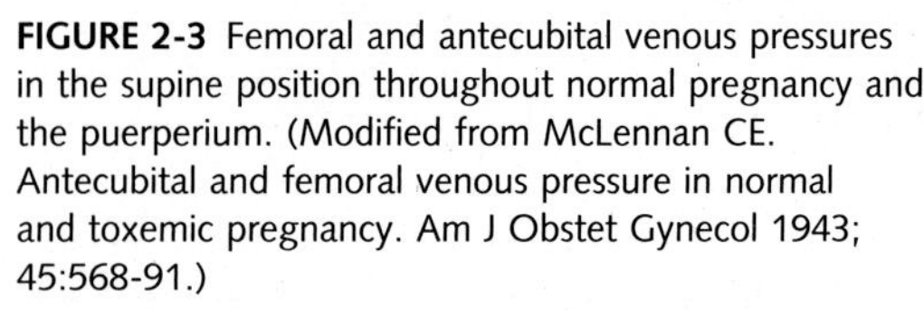
FIGURE 2-3 Femoral and antecubital venous pressures in the supine position throughout normal pregnancy and the puerperium. (Modified from McLennan CE. Antecubital and femoral venous pressure in normal and toxemic pregnancy. Am J Obstet Gynecol 1943; 45:568-91.)

stage, and by 40% in the second stage.[46-48] In the immediate postpartum period, cardiac output may be as much as 75% above predelivery measurements.[47] These changes result from an increase in stroke volume due to greater venous return and alterations in sympathetic nervous system activity. During uterine contractions, 300 to 500 mL of blood is displaced from the intervillous space into the central circulation (i.e., autotransfusion).[49-51] Increased intrauterine pressure forces blood from the intervillous space through the relatively unimpeded ovarian venous outflow system.[34] The postpartum rise in cardiac output results from relief of vena caval compression, diminished lower extremity venous pressure, and a reduction of maternal vascular capacitance.[48] Cardiac output falls to just below prelabor measurements at 24 hours postpartum.[49] It returns to prepregnancy levels between 12 and 24 weeks postpartum.[12] Heart rate falls rapidly after delivery, reaches the prepregnancy rate by 2 weeks postpartum, and is slightly below the prepregnancy rate for the next several months.[12,52] Other anatomic and functional changes of the heart are also fully reversible.[19,53]

TABLE 2-2 Effects of Pregnancy on Respiratory Mechanics

Parameter	Change*
Diaphragm excursion	Increased
Chest wall excursion	Decreased
Pulmonary resistance	Decreased 50%
FEV_1	No change
FEV_1/FVC	No change
Flow-volume loop	No change
Closing capacity	No change

FEV_1, Forced expiratory volume in 1 second; FVC, forced vital capacity.

*Relative to nonpregnant state.

Adapted from Conklin KA. Maternal physiological adaptations during gestation, labor, and the puerperium. Semin Anesth 1991; 10:221-34.

THE RESPIRATORY SYSTEM

Despite the multiple anatomic and physiologic changes that occur during pregnancy, it is remarkable that pregnancy has a relatively minor impact on lung function.

Anatomy

The thoracic cage enlarges in circumference by 5 to 7 cm during pregnancy because of increases in both anteroposterior and transverse diameters.[54,55] An increase in the hormone relaxin causes the rib cage to undergo structural changes, including relaxation of the ligamentous attachments of the ribs.[55,56] The vertical measurement of the chest decreases by as much as 4 cm as a result of the elevated position of the diaphragm.

Capillary engorgement of the larynx and the nasal and oropharyngeal mucosa begins early in the first trimester and increases progressively throughout pregnancy.[54] Voice changes frequently result from involvement of the false vocal cords and the arytenoid region of the larynx. Nasal breathing commonly becomes difficult, and epistaxis may occur. The nasal congestion may contribute to the perceived shortness of breath of pregnancy.[57]

Airflow Mechanics

Inspiration in the term pregnant woman is almost totally attributable to diaphragmatic excursion.[58] This is caused by a greater descent of the diaphragm from its elevated resting position and limitation of thoracic cage expansion because of its expanded resting position (Table 2-2). Both large- and small-airway function are minimally altered during pregnancy. The shape of flow-volume loops, the absolute flow rates at normal lung volumes,[59] forced expiratory volume in 1 second (FEV_1), and the ratio of FEV_1 to forced vital capacity (FVC) are unchanged during pregnancy, as is closing capacity.[60]

The peak expiratory flow rate achieved with a maximal effort following a maximal inspiration is often considered a surrogate for the FEV_1. The test is often used to monitor asthma therapy. Studies are conflicting as to whether peak expiratory flow rates decrease during pregnancy.[61,62] Harirah et al.[61] found that peak expiratory flow rate declined significantly throughout gestation in all positions (Figure 2-4) and that flow rates in the supine position were lower than those during standing and sitting. The mean rate of decline was 0.65 L/min per week, and peak expiratory flow remained below normal at 6 weeks postpartum.

Lung Volumes and Capacities

Tidal volume increases by 45% during pregnancy, with approximately half of the change occurring during the first trimester (Table 2-3; Figure 2-5). The early change in tidal volume is associated with a reduction in inspiratory reserve volume. Total lung capacity usually is preserved or

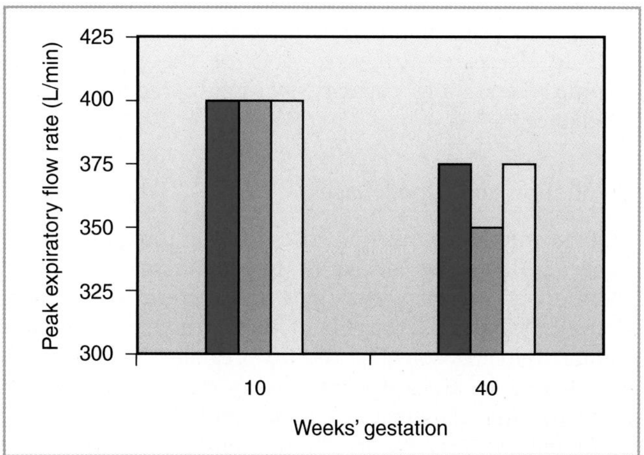

FIGURE 2-4 Peak expiratory flow rates during standing (*dark blue bars*), lying supine (*medium blue bars*), and during sitting (*gray bars*) in pregnant women. Peak expiratory flow rates declined significantly throughout gestation. The rate of decline was greater for the supine position than for the standing position. (Based on data from Harirah HM, Donia SE, Nasrallah FK, et al. Effect of gestational age and position on peak expiratory flow rate: A longitudinal study. Obstet Gynecol 2005; 10:372-6.)

TABLE 2-3 Changes in Respiratory Physiology at Term Gestation

Parameter	Change*
Lung volumes:	
Inspiratory reserve volume	+5%
Tidal volume	+45%
Expiratory reserve volume	−25%
Residual volume	−15%
Lung capacities:	
Inspiratory capacity	+15%
Functional residual capacity	−20%
Vital capacity	No change
Total lung capacity	−5%
Dead space	+45%
Respiratory rate	No change
Ventilation:	
Minute ventilation	+45%
Alveolar ventilation	+45%

*Relative to nonpregnant state.

From Conklin KA. Maternal physiological adaptations during gestation, labor, and the puerperium. Semin Anesth 1991; 10:221-34.

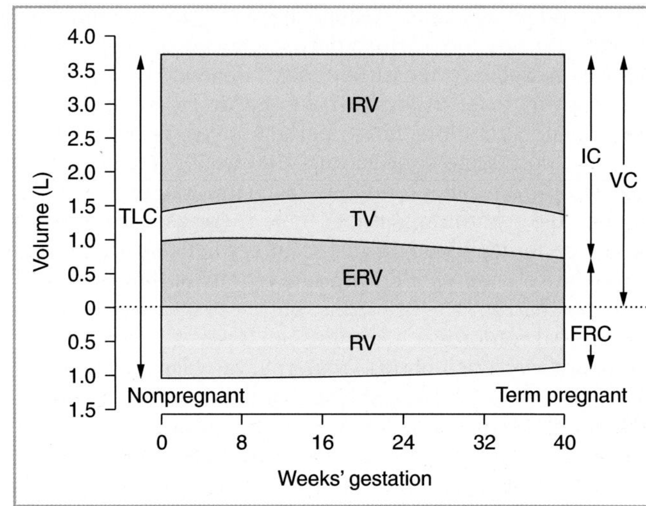

FIGURE 2-5 Lung volumes and capacities during pregnancy. ERV, expiratory reserve volume; FRC, functional residual capacity; IC, inspiratory capacity; IRV, inspiratory reserve volume; RV, residual volume; TLC, total lung capacity; TV, tidal volume; VC, vital capacity.

is decreased minimally. The residual volume tends to drop slightly, a change that maintains vital capacity. Inspiratory capacity increases by 15% during the third trimester because of increases in tidal volume and inspiratory reserve volume.[63,64] There is a corresponding decrease in expiratory reserve volume.[63,64]

Functional residual capacity (FRC) begins to fall by the fifth month of pregnancy and is decreased to 80% of the prepregnancy capacity by term.[60,63,64] This change is caused by elevation of the diaphragm, which occurs as the enlarging uterus enters the abdominal cavity. A 25% reduction in expiratory reserve volume and a 15% reduction in residual volume account for the change. It is important to remember that assumption of the supine position causes FRC to decrease further to 70% of the prepregnancy volume. Total lung capacity is slightly reduced during pregnancy.[63,65]

Ventilation and Blood Gases

Resting minute ventilation rises during pregnancy (see Table 2-3), owing primarily to an increase in tidal volume.[63,66] The inspiratory rate and pattern remain relatively unchanged. The ratio of total dead space to tidal volume remains constant during pregnancy, resulting in an increase in alveolar ventilation of approximately 30% above baseline. The rise in minute ventilation results from hormonal changes and greater carbon dioxide production. Carbon dioxide production at rest rises by about 30% to 300 mL/min[59] and is closely related to the blood level of progesterone.[67] Progesterone acts as a direct respiratory stimulant,[68] and the progesterone-induced increase in chemosensitivity results in a steeper slope and a leftward shift of the CO_2 ventilatory response curve. The greater chemosensitivity occurs early in pregnancy and remains constant until delivery.[59]

The hypoxic ventilatory response is increased during pregnancy to twice the normal level secondary to rises in estrogen and progesterone levels.[69] This increase occurs despite blood and cerebrospinal fluid (CSF) alkalosis.

The arterial pressure of oxygen increases to 100 to 105 mm Hg as a result of greater alveolar ventilation (Table 2-4).[66] The higher $Pa{O_2}$ results from the decline in $Pa{CO_2}$ and a lower arteriovenous oxygen difference, which reduces the impact of venous admixture on the $Pa{O_2}$.[70,71] As pregnancy progresses, oxygen consumption continues to increase, and cardiac output increases to a lesser extent, resulting in a reduced mixed venous oxygen content and increased arteriovenous oxygen difference. After midgestation, pregnant women in the supine position frequently exhibit a $Pa{O_2}$ less than 100 mm Hg. This occurs because the FRC may be less than closing capacity, resulting in closure of small airways during normal tidal volume ventilation.[66] Moving a pregnant woman from the supine to the erect or lateral decubitus position improves arterial oxygenation and reduces the alveolar-to-arterial oxygen gradient.

The $Pa{CO_2}$ declines to approximately 30 mm Hg by 12 weeks' gestation but does not change further during the remainder of pregnancy. Although in nonpregnant individuals a gradient exists between the end-tidal carbon dioxide tension and $Pa{CO_2}$, the two measurements are equivalent during early pregnancy,[72] at term gestation,[73]

TABLE 2-4 Blood Gas Measurements during Pregnancy

Parameter	Nonpregnant	Trimester		
		First	Second	Third
$Pa{CO_2}$ (mm Hg)	40	30	30	30
$Pa{O_2}$ (mm Hg)	100	107	105	103
pH	7.40	7.44	7.44	7.44
$[HCO_3^-]$ (mEq/L)	24	21	20	20

and in the postpartum period.[74] This finding is attributed to a reduction in alveolar dead space, which results from an increase in cardiac output during pregnancy. The mixed venous P_{CO_2} is 6 to 8 mm Hg below the nonpregnant level from the late first trimester until term.[1]

Metabolic compensation for the respiratory alkalosis of pregnancy reduces the serum bicarbonate concentration to approximately 20 mEq/L, the base excess by 2 to 3 mEq/L, and the total buffer base by approximately 5 mEq/L.[75] This compensation is incomplete, as demonstrated by the elevation of venous,[76] capillary,[77] and arterial[66] blood pH by 0.02 to 0.06 unit.

The rise in minute ventilation that accompanies pregnancy may be interpreted as shortness of breath. By 30 weeks' gestation, 75% of pregnant women have exertional dyspnea.[78] The proposed etiology is the greater drive to breathe and the increased respiratory load. Factors that contribute to the sensation of dyspnea include larger pulmonary blood volume, anemia, and nasal congestion. Exercise has no effect on pregnancy-induced changes in ventilation or alveolar gas exchange.[79]

Sleep

Sleep disturbances are a common occurrence during pregnancy owing to mechanical and hormonal factors. Pregnant women have more complaints of insomnia and daytime sleepiness. The American Academy of Sleep Medicine has established a disease entity, **pregnancy-associated sleep disorder,** defined as the occurrence of insomnia or excessive sleepiness that develops in the course of pregnancy.[80] Progesterone has a strong sedating effect, and cortisol, levels of which are higher in pregnancy, is associated with an increase in rapid eye movement (REM) sleep.[81]

Sleep quality is worsened in the first and third trimesters. Polysomnography reveals reduced slow-wave and REM phases of sleep, decreased total sleep time, and increased rate of wakening after sleep onset.[82] Sleep may be poor for up to 3 months postpartum.[82,83] Snoring is common during pregnancy, occurring in up to 20% of women by the third trimester. Pregnancy is associated with transient restless leg syndrome, a disorder in which the patient experiences the need to move her legs.[84] The incidence ranges from 15% in the first trimester to 23% in the third trimester.[84]

Metabolism and Respiration during Labor and the Puerperium

Minute ventilation of the unmedicated parturient increases by 70% to 140% in the first stage of labor and by 120% to 200% in the second stage of labor compared with prepregnancy measurements.[85] The Pa_{CO_2} may fall to as low as 10 to 15 mm Hg. Oxygen consumption increases above the prelabor value by 40% in the first stage and by 75% in the second stage.[85] The changes in oxygen consumption result from the increased metabolic demands of hyperventilation, uterine activity, and maternal expulsive efforts during the second stage. The maternal aerobic requirement for oxygen exceeds oxygen consumption during labor, as is evident from the progressive rise of blood lactate concentration, an index of anaerobic metabolism.[86-88] Initiation of neuraxial analgesia prevents these changes during the first stage of labor and mitigates the changes during the second stage of labor.[86-89]

FRC increases after delivery but remains below the prepregnancy volume for 1 to 2 weeks. Oxygen consumption, tidal volume, and minute ventilation remain elevated until at least 6 to 8 weeks after delivery. The alveolar and mixed venous P_{CO_2} rise slowly after delivery and are still slightly below prepregnancy levels at 6 to 8 weeks postpartum.[1]

HEMATOLOGY

Blood Volume

Maternal plasma volume expansion begins as early as 6 weeks' gestation and continues until it reaches a net increase of approximately 50% by 34 weeks' gestation (Table 2-5; Figure 2-6).[90-93] After 34 weeks' gestation, the plasma volume stabilizes or falls slightly. Red blood cell volume falls during the first 8 weeks of pregnancy, increases to the prepregnancy level by 16 weeks, and undergoes a further rise to 30% above the prepregnancy volume at term.[91,93,94] The plasma volume expansion increase exceeds that of the red blood cell volume increase, resulting in the **physiologic anemia of pregnancy**. With volumes expressed in milliliters per kilogram (mL/kg), pregnancy results in an increase in plasma volume from 49 to 67 mL/kg, an increase in total blood volume from 76 to 94 mL/kg, and no change in red cell volume (27 mL/kg).[91] Greater increases in blood volume occur with twin than with singleton pregnancies, and blood volume is positively correlated with the size of the fetus in singleton pregnancies.[92] The physiologic hypervolemia facilitates delivery of nutrients to the fetus, protects the mother from hypotension, and reduces the risks associated with hemorrhage at delivery. The decrease in blood viscosity from the lower hematocrit creates lower resistance to blood flow, which may be an essential component of maintaining the patency of the uteroplacental vascular bed.

The rise in plasma volume results from fetal and maternal hormone production, and several hormonal systems may play a role. Additionally, the expansion of plasma volume may be an adaptive physiologic response that helps maintain blood pressure in the presence of decreased vascular tone.[95,96] The maternal concentrations of estrogen and progesterone increase nearly 100-fold during pregnancy.[1] Estrogens increase plasma renin activity, enhancing renal sodium absorption and water retention via the renin-angiotensin-aldosterone system. Fetal adrenal production of the estrogen precursor dehydroepiandrosterone may be the

TABLE 2-5 Hematologic Parameters at Term Gestation

Parameter	Change* or Actual Measurement
Blood volume	+45%*
Plasma volume	+55%*
Red blood cell volume	+30%*
Hemoglobin	11.6 g/dL
Hematocrit	35.5%

*Relative to nonpregnant state.

From Conklin KA. Maternal physiological adaptations during gestation, labor, and the puerperium. Semin Anesth 1991; 10:221-34.

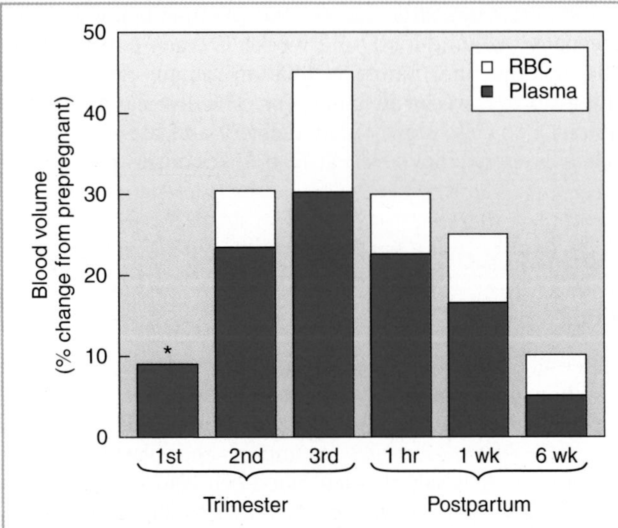

FIGURE 2-6 Blood volume during pregnancy and the puerperium. Values during pregnancy are measured at the end of the first, second, and third trimesters. Postpartum values are measured after a vaginal delivery. The values for red blood cell volume (RBC) and plasma volume (Plasma) do not represent the actual percentage of change in these parameters but instead reflect the relative contribution of each to the change in blood volume. The *asterisk* indicates that RBC volume is below the prepregnancy volume at the end of the first trimester.

underlying control mechanism. Progesterone also enhances aldosterone production. These changes result in marked increases in plasma renin activity and the aldosterone level as well as in retention of approximately 900 mEq of sodium and 7000 mL of total body water. The concentration of plasma adrenomedullin, a potent vasodilating peptide, increases during pregnancy, and correlates significantly with blood volume.[97]

Red blood cell volume increases in response to elevated erythropoietin concentration[98] and the erythropoietin effects of progesterone, prolactin, and placental lactogen. Both hemoglobin concentration and hematocrit drop after conception until they are approximately 11.2 g/dL and 34%, respectively, by mid-gestation.[1,93,94] This change represents a 15% decrease from prepregnancy levels. During late gestation the hemoglobin concentration and hematocrit increases to approximately 11.6 g/dL and 35.5%, respectively, because of a greater increase in red blood cell volume than in plasma volume after mid-gestation. Women who do not receive iron supplementation during pregnancy experience greater decreases in hemoglobin concentration and hematocrit.[93]

Plasma Proteins

Plasma albumin concentration decreases from 4.5 to 3.9 g/dL during the first trimester and to 3.3 g/dL by term (Table 2-6).[99,100] Globulins decline by 10% in the first trimester and then rise throughout the remainder of pregnancy to 10% above the prepregnancy level at term.[99] The albumin-to-globulin ratio falls during pregnancy from 1.4 to 0.9, and the total plasma protein concentration drops from approximately 7.8 to 7.0 g/dL.[99] Maternal colloid osmotic pressure decreases by approximately 5 mm Hg during pregnancy.[16,101,102] The plasma cholinesterase concentration

TABLE 2-6 Plasma Protein Values during Pregnancy

		Trimester		
Protein	**Nonpregnant**	**First**	**Second**	**Third**
Total protein (g/dL)	7.8	6.9	6.9	7.0
Albumin (g/dL)	4.5	3.9	3.6	3.3
Globulin (g/dL)	3.3	3.0	3.3	3.7
Albumin/globulin ratio	1.4	1.3	1.1	0.9
Plasma cholinesterase	—	−25%	−25%	−25%
Colloid osmotic pressure (mm Hg)	27	25	23	22

falls by approximately 25% during the first trimester and remains at that level until the end of pregnancy.[103,104]

Coagulation

Pregnancy is associated with enhanced platelet turnover, clotting, and fibrinolysis (Box 2-2). Thus, pregnancy represents a state of accelerated but compensated intravascular coagulation.

Increases in platelet factor 4 and beta-thromboglobulin signal elevated platelet activation, and the progressive increase in platelet distribution width and platelet volume are consistent with greater platelet consumption during pregnancy.[105-107] Platelet aggregation in response to collagen, epinephrine, adenosine diphosphate, and arachidonic

BOX 2-2 Changes in Coagulation and Fibrinolytic Parameters at Term Gestation*

Increased Factor Concentrations
- Factor I (fibrinogen)
- Factor VII (proconvertin)
- Factor VIII (antihemophilic factor)
- Factor IX (Christmas factor)
- Factor X (Stuart-Prower factor)
- Factor XII (Hageman factor)

Unchanged Factor Concentrations
- Factor II (prothrombin)
- Factor V (proaccelerin)

Decreased Factor Concentrations
- Factor XI (thromboplastin antecedent)
- Factor XIII (fibrin-stabilizing factor)

Other Parameters
- Prothrombin time: shortened 20%
- Partial thromboplastin time: shortened 20%
- Thromboelastography: hypercoagulable
- Fibrinopeptide A: increased
- Antithrombin III: decreased
- Platelet count: no change or decreased
- Bleeding time: no change
- Fibrin degradation products: increased
- Plasminogen: increased

*Relative to nonpregnant state.

acid is increased.[108] Despite changes in platelet count and/or function, the bleeding time measurement is not altered during normal gestation.[109] Some investigators have noted a decrease in platelet count,[107,110] whereas others have noted no change,[105,106] suggesting that increased platelet production compensates for greater activation. However, 7.6% of otherwise normal women have a platelet count less than 150,000/mm^3, and 0.9% have a platelet count less than 100,000/mm^3.[106] This so-called **gestational thrombocytopenia** appears to be an exaggerated normal response.

The concentrations of most coagulation factors, including fibrinogen (factor I), proconvertin (factor VII), antihemophilic factor (factor VIII), Christmas factor (factor IX), Stuart-Prower factor (factor X), and Hageman factor (factor XII), rise during pregnancy. The concentrations of some factors increase by more than 100%.[105,106,111-113] Prothrombin (factor II) and proaccelerin (factor V) concentrations do not change, whereas the concentrations of thromboplastin antecedent (factor XI) and fibrin-stabilizing factor (factor XIII) diminish.[112-114] An increase in most factor concentrations, shortening of the prothrombin and partial thromboplastin times,[111] an increase in fibrinopeptide A concentration, and a decrease in antithrombin III concentration suggest an activation of the clotting system.[105] Changes in thromboelastography also suggest that pregnancy is a hypercoagulable state.[115]

The greater concentration of fibrin degradation products signals increased fibrinolytic activity during gestation.[105,114] The marked rise in the plasminogen concentration also is consistent with enhanced fibrinolysis.[116]

Hematology and Coagulation during the Puerperium

Blood loss during normal vaginal delivery and the early puerperium is approximately 600 mL.[117] The normal physiologic changes of pregnancy allow the healthy parturient to compensate for this normal blood loss. However, blood loss after either vaginal or cesarean delivery is often underestimated, and the larger the blood loss, the greater the discrepancy between actual and estimated blood loss.[118]

Blood volume drops to 125% of the prepregnancy level during the first postpartum week,[91,117] followed by a more gradual decline to 110% of the prepregnancy level at 6 to 9 weeks postpartum. The hemoglobin concentration and hematocrit fall during the first 3 postpartum days, rise gradually during the next 3 days (because of a reduction in plasma volume), and continue to rise to prepregnancy measurements by 6 weeks postpartum.[119]

Cesarean delivery results in a blood loss of approximately 1000 mL within the first few hours of delivery.[117] The hematocrit in the immediate postpartum period is lower after cesarean delivery than after vaginal delivery because of the greater blood loss during cesarean delivery.[117]

Albumin and total protein concentrations and colloid osmotic pressure decline after delivery and gradually rise to prepregnancy levels by 6 weeks postpartum.[99,101] Plasma cholinesterase falls below the predelivery level by the first postpartum day and remains at that decreased level during the next week.[103,104] Globulin concentrations are elevated throughout the first postpartum week.[99]

Beginning with delivery and during the first postpartum day, there is a rapid fall in the platelet count and in the concentrations of fibrinogen, factor VIII, and plasminogen as well as an increase in antifibrinolytic activity.[120] Clotting times remain shortened during the first postpartum day,[121] and thromboelastography remains consistent with a hypercoagulable state.[115] During the first 3 to 5 postpartum days the fibrinogen concentration and platelet count rise, changes that may account for the higher incidence of thrombotic complications during the puerperium.[121] The coagulation profile returns to that of the nonpregnant state by 2 weeks postpartum.[120]

THE IMMUNE SYSTEM

The blood leukocyte count rises progressively during pregnancy from the prepregnancy level of approximately 6,000/mm^3 to 9,000 to 11,000/mm^3.[110] This increase reflects a rise in the number of polymorphonuclear cells, with the appearance of immature granulocytic forms (i.e., myelocytes and metamyelocytes) in most pregnant women. The proportion of immature forms falls during the last 2 months of pregnancy. The lymphocyte, eosinophil, and basophil counts fall, whereas the monocyte count does not change during pregnancy. The leukocyte count rises to approximately 13,000/mm^3 during labor and increases further to an average of 15,000/mm^3 on the first postpartum day.[119] By the sixth postpartum day the leukocyte count decreases to an average of 9250/mm^3, although the count is still above normal at 6 weeks postpartum.

Polymorphonuclear leukocyte function is impaired during pregnancy, as shown by depressed neutrophil chemotaxis and adherence.[122] This finding may account for the higher incidence of infection during pregnancy and the lower incidence of symptoms in some pregnant women with autoimmune diseases (e.g., rheumatoid arthritis). Although the serum concentrations of immunoglobulins A, G, and M are unchanged during gestation,[100] humoral antibody titers to certain viruses (e.g., herpes simplex, measles, influenza A) are decreased.[123]

During pregnancy, the uterine mucosa is characterized by a large number of maternal immune cells found in close contact with the trophoblast. These cells are responsible for both fetal survival and miscarriage.[124] Human CD4$^+$ T cells can be classified into Th1 and Th2 cells on the basis of their cytokine production. Successful pregnancy is associated with a predominant Th2 cytokine profile; Th1 cytokines are detrimental to pregnancy. These cells also produce natural antimicrobials within the uterus, which is important for prevention of uterine infection during pregnancy.[125]

THE GASTROINTESTINAL SYSTEM

Anatomy, Barrier Pressure, and Pyrosis

The stomach is displaced upward toward the left side of the diaphragm during pregnancy, and its axis is rotated approximately 45 degrees to the right from its normal vertical position. The altered position of the stomach displaces the intra-abdominal segment of the esophagus into the thorax in most pregnant women. This causes a reduction in tone of the *l*ower *e*sophageal *h*igh-*p*ressure *z*one (LEHPZ), which normally prevents the reflux of gastric contents. Progestins also may contribute to a relaxation of the LEHPZ.[126]

Approximately 30% to 50% of women experience gastroesophageal reflux during pregnancy.[127] In the first trimester of pregnancy, basal LEHPZ pressure may not change, but the sphincter is less responsive to physiologic stimuli that usually increase pressure.[128] In the second and third trimesters, LEHPZ pressure gradually falls to approximately 50% of basal levels, reaching a nadir at 36 weeks' gestation and returning to prepregnancy levels at 1 to 4 weeks postpartum (Table 2-7). Risk factors for gastroesophageal reflux in pregnancy include gestational age, heartburn antecedent to the pregnancy, and multiparity. Prepregnancy body mass index, weight gain during pregnancy, and rate of weight gain do not correlate with the occurrence of reflux, whereas maternal age has an inverse correlation with the incidence of reflux.[129]

Gastrointestinal Motility

The gastric emptying of liquid and solid materials is not altered at any time during pregnancy. This fact has been demonstrated in studies that measured the absorption of orally administered acetaminophen[130-132] and in studies that assessed the emptying of a test meal by radiographic,[133] ultrasonographic,[132,134] and dye dilution[135] techniques; epigastric impedance[136]; and applied potential tomography.[137] In one study of morbidly obese women at term, gastric emptying of 300 mL of water took no longer than gastric emptying of 50 mL of water.[138]

Esophageal peristalsis and intestinal transit are slowed during pregnancy.[134,139] These effects on motility have been attributed to the inhibition of gastrointestinal contractile activity by progesterone. However, this inhibition may be an indirect action that results from a negative effect of progesterone on the plasma concentration of motilin, which declines during pregnancy.[134] Up to 40% of women suffer from constipation at some time during their pregnancy.[140] The prevalence of constipation is highest in the first two trimesters of gestation and declines in the third trimester.

Gastric Acid Secretion

Early work suggested that both basal and maximal gastric acid secretion declined in mid-gestation, reaching a nadir at 20 to 30 weeks' gestation.[141] Van Thiel et al.[142] demonstrated no difference in basal or peak gastric acid secretion in four pregnant women studied in each trimester and at 1 to 4 weeks postpartum, although a plasma gastrin level significantly lower than postpartum levels was observed during the first trimester. Gastric pH and serum gastrin concentration were compared in 100 nonlaboring women scheduled for elective cesarean delivery and in 100 nonpregnant women undergoing gynecologic surgery.[143] The pH was lower in the pregnant group (2.4 versus 3.0), but serum gastrin levels were not different despite the fact that gastrin is secreted by the placenta beginning at 15 weeks' gestation.[144] Other studies that have examined stomach contents have shown that approximately 80% of both pregnant and nonpregnant women have a gastric pH of 2.5 or less, approximately 50% have gastric volumes of 25 mL or greater, and 40% to 50% exhibit both low pH and gastric volume greater than 25 mL. These results are similar to those obtained from studies of women at a mean gestational age of 15 weeks.[145]

Gastric Function during Labor and the Puerperium

Gastric emptying is slowed during labor, as shown by ultrasonographic imaging, emptying of a test meal, and the rate of absorption of oral paracetamol.[146,147] Direct measurements show that the mean gastric volume increases.[148] However, one study found that postpartum gastric volume was not different in parturients who consumed water in labor compared with those who consumed an isotonic sports drink composed of mixed carbohydrates and electrolytes.[149] Gastric acid secretion may decrease during labor, because only 25% of laboring parturients have a gastric pH of 2.5 or less.[150] Gastric emptying is delayed during the early postpartum period but returns to prepregnancy measurements by 18 hours postpartum.[151] Similarly, gastric volume and pH are similar in fasting women more than 18 hours after delivery and in nonpregnant individuals who have been without oral intake before elective surgery.[152-154]

TABLE 2-7 Changes in Gastrointestinal Physiology during Pregnancy*

	Trimester				
Parameter	**First**	**Second**	**Third**	**Labor**	**Postpartum (18 hr)**
Barrier pressure†	Decreased	Decreased	Decreased	Decreased	?
Gastric emptying	No change	No change	No change	Delayed	No change
Gastric acid secretion	No change or decreased	No change or decreased	No change	?	?
Proportion of women with gastric volume > 25 mL	No change	No change	No change	Increased	No change
Proportion of women with gastric pH < 2.5	No change	No change	No change	Decreased	No change

*Relative to nonpregnant state.

†Difference between intragastric pressure and tone of the lower esophageal high-pressure zone.

EFFECTS OF ANALGESIA ON GASTRIC FUNCTION DURING LABOR

Compared with parturients who do not receive analgesia, those who receive intramuscular opioids during labor exhibit delayed gastric emptying.[147] Epidural analgesia using local anesthetics does not delay gastric emptying; however, epidural fentanyl administered as a 100-μg bolus does delay gastric emptying,[155,156] as does intrathecal fentanyl 25 μg.[157] In one study an epidural infusion of low-dose bupivacaine and fentanyl 2.5 μg/mL, which was not preceded by a fentanyl bolus, did not slow gastric emptying during labor.[158]

THE LIVER AND GALLBLADDER

Liver size, morphology, and blood flow do not change during pregnancy, although the liver is displaced upward, posterior, and to the right during late pregnancy.

Serum levels of bilirubin, alanine aminotransferase (ALT, SGPT), aspartate aminotransferase (AST, SGOT), and lactic dehydrogenase increase to the upper limits of the normal range during pregnancy.[159] The total alkaline phosphatase activity increases twofold to fourfold, mostly from production by the placenta. Excretion of sulfobromophthalein into bile decreases, whereas hepatic extraction and retention of this compound increases.[160]

Biliary stasis and the higher secretion of bile with cholesterol raise the risk of gallbladder disease during pregnancy.[161] The incidence of gallstones is 5% to 12% of all pregnant women.[162] One in 1600 to 1 in 10,000 women undergo cholecystectomy during pregnancy. Progesterone inhibits the contractility of the gastrointestinal smooth muscle, leading to gallbladder hypomotility.[163] The size of the total bile acid pool increases by about 50% during pregnancy, and the relative proportions of the various bile acids change.[164] These changes in the composition of gallbladder bile revert rapidly after delivery, even in patients with gallstones.

THE KIDNEYS

Owing to an increase in total vascular volume, both renal vascular volume and interstitial volume increase during pregnancy. These increases are reflected in an enlarged kidney; the renal volume increases by as much as 30%.[165] The collecting system dilates, including the renal calyces, pelvis, and ureters. Hydronephrosis may occur in 80% of women by mid-pregnancy.[166]

Both glomerular filtration rate (GFR) and renal plasma flow increase markedly during pregnancy. Reduced renal vascular resistance is responsible for the increased renal blood flow and for the rise in GFR.[26] Renal plasma flow rises to 75% over nonpregnant measurements by 16 weeks' gestation and is maintained until 34 weeks, when a slight decline occurs. By the end of the first trimester, GFR is 50% higher than baseline, and this rate is maintained until the end of pregnancy. GFR does not return to prepregnancy levels until 3 months postpartum. Because GFR does not increase as rapidly or as significantly as renal plasma flow, the filtration fraction decreases from nonpregnancy levels until the third trimester.[167]

Creatinine clearance is increased to 150 to 200 mL/min from the normal baseline measurements of 120 mL/min.[168] The increase occurs early in pregnancy, reaches a maximum by the end of the first trimester, falls slightly near term, and returns to the prepregnancy level by 8 to 12 weeks postpartum.[167] These renal hemodynamic alterations are among the earliest and most dramatic maternal adaptations to pregnancy. The increased GFR results in reduced blood concentrations of nitrogenous metabolites. The blood urea nitrogen concentration falls to 8 to 9 mg/dL by the end of the first trimester and remains at that level until term.[168] Serum creatinine concentration is a reflection of skeletal muscle production and urinary excretion. In pregnancy, skeletal muscle production of creatinine remains relatively constant, but GFR is increased, resulting in a reduced serum creatinine. The serum creatinine concentration falls progressively to 0.5 to 0.6 mg/dL by the end of pregnancy. The serum uric acid level declines in early pregnancy because of the rise in GFR, and it declines to 2.0 to 3.0 mg/dL by 24 weeks' gestation.[169] After this point, the uric acid level begins to rise, reaching the prepregnancy level by the end of pregnancy. Tubular reabsorption of urate accounts for the rise during the third trimester.

Total protein excretion and urinary albumin excretion are higher than nonpregnant levels. The average 24-hour total protein and albumin excretion amounts are 200 mg and 12 mg, respectively (upper limits are 300 mg and 20 mg, respectively).[170,171] Glucose is filtered and almost completely absorbed in the proximal tubule. In the nonpregnant state, a small amount of glucose is excreted. Pregnancy imposes a change in the glucose resorptive capacity of the proximal tubules, so all pregnant women exhibit an elevation of glucose excretion. Of pregnant women who have normal glucose tolerance to an oral load and normal glucose excretion when not pregnant, approximately half will exhibit a doubling of glucose excretion. Most of the remainder have increases of 3 to 10 times the nonpregnant amount, and a small proportion (less than 10%) excrete as much as 20 times the nonpregnant amount.[172] Overall, the amount of excreted glucose in the third trimester is increased several fold over that in the nonpregnant state. The normal nonpregnant pattern of glucose excretion is reestablished within a week of delivery.

The kidney is also involved in maintenance of acid-base status during pregnancy. An increase in alveolar ventilation results in a respiratory alkalosis. A compensatory response occurs in the kidney, with greater bicarbonate excretion and a decline in serum bicarbonate levels. The decrease in serum bicarbonate affects the pregnant woman's ability to buffer an acid load.

NONPLACENTAL ENDOCRINOLOGY

Thyroid Function

The thyroid gland enlarges 50% to 70% during pregnancy because of follicular hyperplasia and greater vascularity. The estrogen-induced increase in thyroid-binding globulin results in a 50% increase in total triiodothyronine (T_3) and thyroxine (T_4) concentrations during the first trimester, and these concentrations are maintained until term.[173]

The concentrations of free T_3 and T_4 do not change. The concentration of thyroid-stimulating hormone falls during the first trimester but returns to the nonpregnant level shortly thereafter and undergoes no further change during the remainder of pregnancy.

Glucose Metabolism

Mean blood glucose concentration remains within the normal range during pregnancy, although the glucose concentration may be lower in some women during the third trimester than in nonpregnant individuals.[174] This finding is easily explained by the greater glucose demand of the fetus and the placenta. The relative hypoglycemic state results in fasting hypoinsulinemia. Pregnant women also exhibit an exaggerated starvation ketosis.

Pregnant women are insulin resistant owing to hormones secreted by the placenta, primarily placental lactogen.[175] The blood glucose levels after a carbohydrate load are greater in pregnant women than in nonpregnant women, despite a hyperinsulinemic response. These changes resolve within 24 hours of delivery.

Adrenal Cortical Function

The concentration of corticosteroid-binding globulin (CBG) doubles during gestation as a result of an estrogen-induced enhancement of hepatic synthesis.[176] The elevated CBG results in a 100% increase in the plasma cortisol concentration at the end of the first trimester and a 200% increase at term. The concentration of unbound, metabolically active cortisol at the end of the third trimester is 2.5 times the nonpregnant level. The increase in free cortisol results from greater production and reduced clearance. Protein binding of corticosteroids is affected by an increase in CBG and a decrease in serum albumin. CBG binding capacity usually saturates at low concentrations of glucocorticoids. Clearance of betamethasone is higher during pregnancy, possibly because the drug is metabolized by placental enzymes.[177]

THE MUSCULOSKELETAL SYSTEM

Back pain during pregnancy is a common problem. A cohort of 200 consecutive women without back pain at the start of pregnancy were followed throughout their pregnancy.[178] At 12 weeks' gestation, 19% of the study population complained of backache. The incidence increased to 47% at 24 weeks' gestation and peaked at 49% at 36 weeks' gestation. After delivery, the prevalence of back pain declined to 9.4%. Despite a relatively high prevalence, only 32% of women with low back pain during pregnancy reported this problem to their physicians, and only 25% of providers recommended specific therapy.[179]

The etiology of the back pain is multifactorial. One theory is that the enlarging uterus results in exaggerated lumbar lordosis, placing significant mechanical strain on the lower back. The hormonal changes of pregnancy may also play a role. Relaxin, a polypeptide hormone of the insulin-like growth factor family, is associated with remodeling of collagen fibers and pelvic connective tissue. The primary source of circulating relaxin is the corpus luteum; the placenta is a secondary major source of relaxin. Serum relaxin levels in early pregnancy are positively correlated with the presence of back pain.[180]

Women in whom low back pain develops during pregnancy may avoid subsequent pregnancy to prevent recurrence of the back pain. These women also have a very high risk for experiencing a new episode during a subsequent pregnancy.[181] In the majority of patients, low back pain during pregnancy responds to activity and postural modification. Exercise to increase the strength of the abdominal and back muscles is helpful. Scheduled rest periods with elevation of the feet to flex the hips and decrease the lumbar lordosis help relieve muscle spasm and pain.[182]

The enhancement of the lumbar lordosis during pregnancy alters the center of gravity over the lower extremities (Figure 2-7) and may lead to other mechanical problems. Exaggerated lumbar lordosis tends to stretch the lateral femoral cutaneous nerve, possibly resulting in meralgia paresthetica, with paresthesia and/or sensory loss over the anterolateral thigh. Anterior flexion of the neck and slumping of the shoulders usually accompany the enhanced lordosis, sometimes leading to a brachial plexus neuropathy.

Mobility of the sacroiliac, sacrococcygeal, and pubic joints increases during pregnancy in preparation for passage of the fetus. A widening of the pubic symphysis is evident

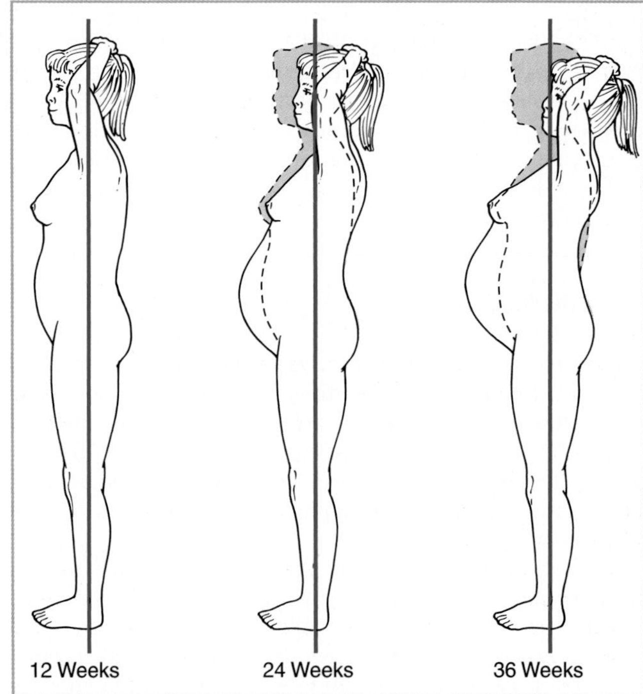

FIGURE 2-7 Changes in posture during pregnancy. The first figure and the subsequent dotted-line figures represent a woman's posture before growth of the uterus and its contents have affected the center of gravity. The second and third solid figures show that as the uterus enlarges and the abdomen protrudes, the lumbar lordosis is enhanced and the shoulders slump and move posteriorly. (Redrawn from Beck AC, Rosenthal AH. Obstetrical Practice. Baltimore, Williams & Wilkins, 1955:146.)

by 30 weeks' gestation. These changes are attributable to the hormone relaxin and the biomechanical strain of pregnancy on the ligaments.[183] Relaxin may also contribute to the higher incidence of carpal tunnel syndrome during pregnancy by changing the nature of the connective tissue so that more fluid is absorbed.[184]

THE NERVOUS SYSTEM

Pregnancy-Induced Analgesia

The minimum alveolar concentration (MAC) for inhaled anesthetics is up to 40% lower in pregnancy.[185-187] Women experience an elevation in the threshold to pain and discomfort near the end of pregnancy and during labor.[188] The mechanism is unclear, although it may be related to progesterone (which has sedative activity) and endorphins. Elevated concentrations of endorphins and enkephalins are found in the plasma and CSF of parturients.[189] Administration of opioid antagonists to experimental animals abolishes the pregnancy-induced analgesia to visceral stimulation.[190]

Pregnant women require less local anesthetic to produce the same level of epidural or neuraxial blockade.[191,192] Although anatomic and mechanical changes in the vertebral column likely play a role in this phenomenon (see later), this decreased dose requirement for local anesthetic is seen in the first trimester, well before significant mechanical changes have occurred.[193] Pregnancy-induced alterations in nerve tissue sensitivity, either directly or indirectly related to changes in hormone concentrations, likely explain this phenomenon.[191] Acid-base changes in CSF and a decrease in CSF specific gravity[194] may also influence the action of local anesthetics in the subarachnoid space.

Vertebral Column

Mechanical changes in the vertebral column also contribute to altered response to anesthetic solutions injected into the epidural or subarachnoid space. The epidural space can be regarded as a rigid tube that contains two fluid-filled distensible tubes, the dural sac and the epidural veins, in addition to epidural fat. The volume of epidural fat and the epidural veins enlarge during pregnancy, so spinal CSF volume is reduced.[195]

In the lateral position, lumbar epidural pressure is positive in term pregnant women but negative in more than 90% of nonpregnant women.[196] Turning a parturient from the lateral to the supine position increases the epidural pressure. Epidural pressure also increases during labor. The greater pressure results from increased diversion of venous blood through the vertebral plexus, specifically from either enhanced compression of the inferior vena cava in the supine position or greater intra-abdominal pressure during pain and pushing. The epidural pressure returns to the nonpregnant level by 6 to 12 hours postpartum.

Despite compression of the dural sac by the epidural veins, the CSF pressure in pregnant women is the same as in nonpregnant women.[197] Uterine contractions and pushing result in an increase in CSF pressure that is secondary to acute increases in epidural vein distention.

Sympathetic Nervous System

Dependence on the sympathetic nervous system for maintenance of hemodynamic stability increases progressively throughout pregnancy and reaches a peak at term.[198-200] The effect is primarily on the venous capacitance system of the lower extremities, which counteracts the adverse effects of uterine compression of the inferior vena cava on venous return. Thus pharmacologic sympathectomy in term pregnant women results in a marked decrease in blood pressure, whereas nonpregnant women experience a minimal decline.[198] The dependence on the sympathetic nervous system activity returns to that of the nonpregnant state by 36 to 48 hours postpartum.

ANESTHETIC IMPLICATIONS

Positioning

Aortocaval compression and impairment of uteroplacental blood flow occur when pregnant women assume the supine position. Compression of the vena cava reduces return of blood to the heart and therefore reduces cardiac output. Further decreases in uterine blood flow occur if the uterus compresses the aorta, given that the uterine artery—a branch of the hypogastric artery—emerges distal to the level of aortic compression. Objective parameters of fetal well-being,[201,202] as well as neonatal outcome,[203] are compromised when parturients are positioned supine instead of tilted during labor or cesarean delivery. Anesthetic drugs or techniques that cause venodilation further reduce venous return with caval obstruction. A drop in maternal blood pressure results in a decrease in uteroplacental perfusion. Studies performed with pregnant women in the lateral position have not noted major decreases in cardiac output.[204,205] Therefore, a pregnant woman should not lie supine after 20 weeks' gestation; the uterus should be tilted to the left, through placement of a wedge underneath the right hip (Figure 2-8), or the woman should assume the full left or right lateral position.

Blood Replacement

At delivery, maternal vascular capacitance is reduced by the volume of the intervillous space (at least 500 mL).[49,50]

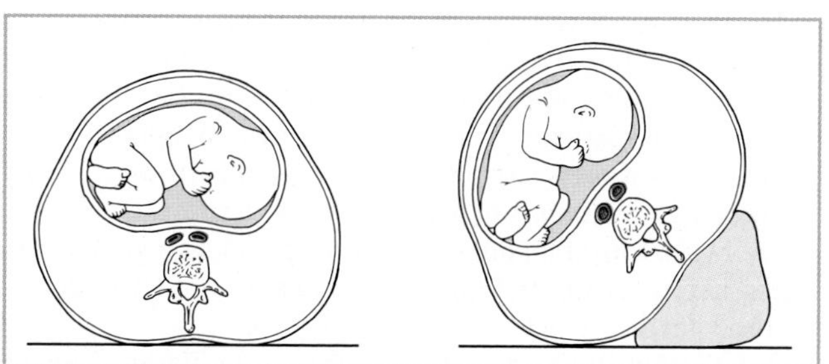

FIGURE 2-8 Compression of the aorta and inferior vena cava in the supine (*left*) and lateral tilt (*right*) positions. (Redrawn from Camann WR, Ostheimer GW. Physiologic adaptations during pregnancy. Int Anesthesiol Clin 1990; 28:2-10.)

Therefore, during vaginal or cesarean delivery, this volume of blood does not need to be replaced for hemodynamic stability, nor should it be considered in the estimation of blood loss for the purpose of replacing red blood cells. Hemoconcentration occurs as maternal blood volume declines from 94 mL/kg at term gestation to 76 mL/kg during the postpartum period; this fact should be considered in the decision whether a parturient should receive crystalloid, colloid, or blood for volume replacement.[91]

General Anesthesia

Changes in the maternal airway and respiratory physiology (Box 2-3) mandate changes in airway management during pregnancy.

ENDOTRACHEAL INTUBATION

The proportion of pregnant women with a Mallampati classification of IV increases by 34% between 12 and 38 weeks' gestation.[206] Vascular engorgement of the airway results in edema of the oral and nasal pharynx, larynx, and trachea.[207] This airway edema can lead to difficult tracheal intubation, and the mucous membranes may be quite friable. In one study, the incidence of failed intubation in obstetric patients was 1:280, compared with 1:2230 in nonpregnant patients.[208] Of the general anesthesia-related maternal deaths in the United States, approximately half occur because of failed intubation.[209,210] Airway edema may be exacerbated in patients with upper respiratory tract infection or preeclampsia and in those who have been pushing during the second stage of labor for a long time.

Capillary engorgement of airway mucosa, including the false cords, mandates the use of a smaller endotracheal tube in pregnant women. A 6.5- or 7.0-mm cuffed endotracheal tube is a good choice for most pregnant women, although a 6.0-mm tube should be readily available. Airway manipulation and instrumentation, such as nasal intubation or the insertion of a nasogastric tube, may result in excessive bleeding.

MATERNAL OXYGENATION

Pregnant women become hypoxemic more rapidly than nonpregnant women during episodes of apnea (see Box 2-3). This is caused by the reduced FRC and the higher oxygen consumption of pregnant women. Moreover, FRC is less than closing capacity in as many as 50% of supine pregnant women.[60] During periods of apnea associated with rapid-sequence induction of general anesthesia, the Pa_{O_2} falls at more than twice the rate in pregnant than in nonpregnant women (139 mm Hg/min versus 58 mm Hg/min).[211] After complete denitrogenation via inhalation of 100% oxygen, nonpregnant patients tolerate 9 minutes of apnea before oxygen saturation is less than 90%, whereas parturients tolerate only 2 to 3 minutes of apnea. Denitrogenation is achieved more rapidly in pregnant than in nonpregnant women; this difference is attributed to the elevated minute ventilation and the decreased FRC seen in pregnancy.

Ventilation during general anesthesia should be adjusted so that the Pa_{CO_2} of the pregnant woman is maintained at approximately 30 mm Hg. Allowing the Pa_{CO_2} to rise to the normal level for nonpregnant women results in respiratory acidosis. Because of the reduced serum bicarbonate concentration, the pregnant woman is less able to adapt to acidosis. A Pa_{CO_2} of 30 mm Hg during cesarean delivery can be achieved by maintaining minute ventilation at 121 mL/kg/min, whereas 77 mL/kg/min is required to maintain a comparable Pa_{CO_2} in nonpregnant women.[212]

BOX 2-3 Changes in General Anesthesia during Pregnancy

Medications
- Thiopental:
  - Induction dose decreased
  - Elimination half-life prolonged
- Propofol:
  - Induction dose unaltered
  - Elimination half-life unaltered
- Volatile anesthetic agents:
  - Minimum alveolar concentration decreased
  - Rate of uptake increased
- Succinylcholine:
  - Duration of blockade unaltered or decreased
- Rocuronium:
  - Increased sensitivity

Intubation
- Increased rate of decline of Pa_{O_2} during apnea
- Smaller endotracheal tube required (6.5 or 7.0 mm)
- Increased risk of failed intubation
- Increased risk of bleeding with nasal instrumentation

Vasopressors
- Response diminished

INHALATION AND INTRAVENOUS ANESTHETICS

The minimum alveolar concentration for volatile anesthetics is decreased up to 40% in pregnancy (see Box 2-3).[185] The rate of rise of the alveolar anesthetic concentration compared with that of inspired gas (i.e., the rate of anesthetic induction) increases during pregnancy as a result of the greater minute ventilation and the reduced FRC. This occurs despite the higher cardiac output, which slows the rate of induction.

The average induction dose of thiopental in parturients is 35% lower in term pregnant women[213] and 18% lower in pregnant women in the first trimester[214] than in nonpregnant women. This change in sensitivity to thiopental is similar to that for inhalation anesthetic agents. The elimination half-life of thiopental in pregnant women is 26.1 hours, compared with 11.5 hours in nonpregnant women.[215] The longer half-life is explained by a marked increase in the volume of distribution of thiopental despite a rise in thiopental clearance. Plasma protein binding of thiopental is similar in term pregnant and nonpregnant women.[215] In contrast, the dose of propofol required for loss of consciousness is not reduced early in pregnancy.[216] The elimination half-life of propofol is unaffected by pregnancy, although clearance of the drug may be higher.[217]

MUSCLE RELAXANTS

Pseudocholinesterase activity is decreased by 24% before delivery and by 33% on the third postpartum day.[104,218] It returns to normal 2 to 6 weeks postpartum. The reduced cholinesterase activity is usually not sufficient to result in clinically relevant prolongation of paralysis after a single dose of succinylcholine (see Box 2-3). Twitch height recovery after administration of succinylcholine does not differ significantly between normal pregnant and nonpregnant women. Recovery may even be faster in pregnant women because the larger volume of distribution results in a lower initial drug concentration and a shorter time before the threshold for recovery is attained. Pregnant women may be less sensitive than nonpregnant women to comparable plasma concentrations of succinylcholine, a feature that also would contribute to more rapid recovery during pregnancy.

Pregnant and postpartum women exhibit enhanced sensitivity to the aminosteroid muscle relaxants vecuronium and rocuronium.[219-221] The greater sensitivity to vecuronium is not explained by altered pharmacokinetics, because the drug exhibits increased clearance and a shortened elimination half-life in pregnant women.[222] In contrast, the pharmacodynamics and pharmacokinetics of the bisquaternary ammonium benzylisoquinoline compound atracurium are unaltered during pregnancy.[221] However, the mean onset time and clinical duration of cis-atracurium are significantly shorter in women immediately after delivery than in nonpregnant women.[223]

CHRONOTROPIC AGENTS AND PRESSORS

Pregnancy reduces the chronotropic response to isoproterenol and epinephrine owing to the down-regulation of beta-adrenergic receptors (see Box 2-3).[224] These agents are less sensitive markers of intravascular injection during administration of neuraxial anesthesia in pregnant patients than in nonpregnant patients.

Neuraxial Analgesia and Anesthesia

TECHNICAL CONSIDERATIONS AND POSITIONING

The enhancement of lumbar lordosis during pregnancy may reduce the vertebral interspinous gap, thus creating technical difficulty in the administration of neuraxial anesthesia (Box 2-4; Figure 2-9). Widening of the pelvis results in a head-down tilt when a pregnant woman is in the lateral position (Figure 2-10). This tilt may increase the rostral subarachnoid spread of local anesthetic solution—especially hyperbaric solution—when an injection is made with the patient in this position. The flow of CSF from a spinal needle is unchanged throughout gestation because pregnancy does not alter CSF pressure.[197] The rate of flow may rise during a uterine contraction because the CSF pressure is increased at this time.

ANESTHETIC DOSE REQUIREMENTS

Pregnant women exhibit a more rapid onset and a longer duration of spinal anesthesia than nonpregnant women who receive the same dose of local anesthetic. This finding is consistent with enhanced neural sensitivity to local anesthetics,[225,226] although the pregnancy-associated elevation in CSF pH may contribute to these effects.[227]

The dose of hyperbaric local anesthetic required in term pregnant women is 25% lower than that in nonpregnant women.[228-230] The lower segmental dose requirement can be attributed to the following factors: (1) reduction of the spinal CSF volume, which accompanies distention of the vertebral venous plexus[31-33]; (2) enhanced neural susceptibility to local anesthetics; (3) increased rostral spread, caused by the widening of the pelvis, when injections are made with the patient in the lateral position; (4) inward displacement of intervertebral foraminal soft tissue, resulting from increased abdominal pressure[195]; and (5) a higher level of the apex of the thoracic kyphosis (the lowest point of the thoracic spinal canal in the supine position) during

BOX 2-4 Neuraxial Anesthesia: Anesthetic Implications of Maternal Physiologic Changes

Technical Considerations
- Lumbar lordosis increased
- Apex of thoracic kyphosis at higher level
- Head-down tilt when in lateral position

Treatment of Hypotension
- Decreased sensitivity to vasopressors*

Local Anesthetic Dose Requirements†
- Subarachnoid dose reduced 25%
- Epidural dose:
  - Large dose unaltered
  - Small dose reduced

*Relative to that required by nonpregnant women.

†Change in the segmental dose requirement relative to that in nonpregnant women.

Adapted from Conklin KA. Maternal physiologic adaptations during gestation, labor, and the puerperium. Semin Anesth 1991; 10:221-34.

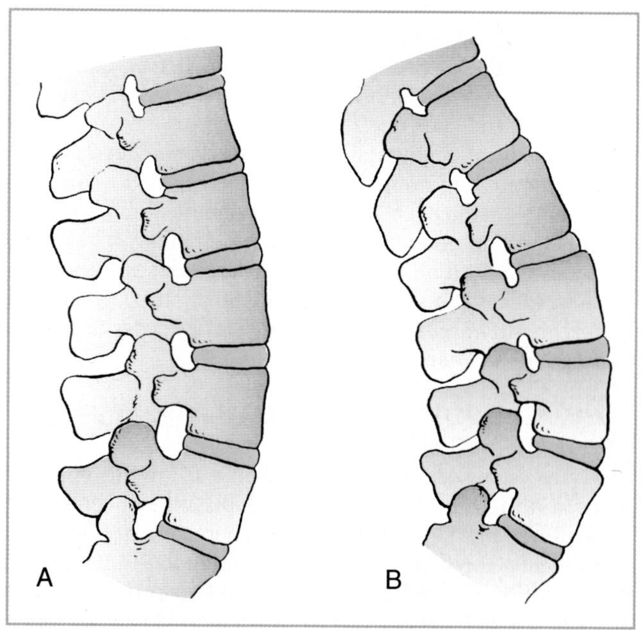

FIGURE 2-9 Effects of pregnancy on the lumbar spine. **A,** Nonpregnant. **B,** Pregnant. There is a marked increase in lumbar lordosis and a narrowing of the interspinous spaces during pregnancy. (Modified from Bonica JJ. Principles and Practice of Obstetric Analgesia and Anesthesia, Volume 1. Philadelphia, FA Davis Company, 1967:35.)

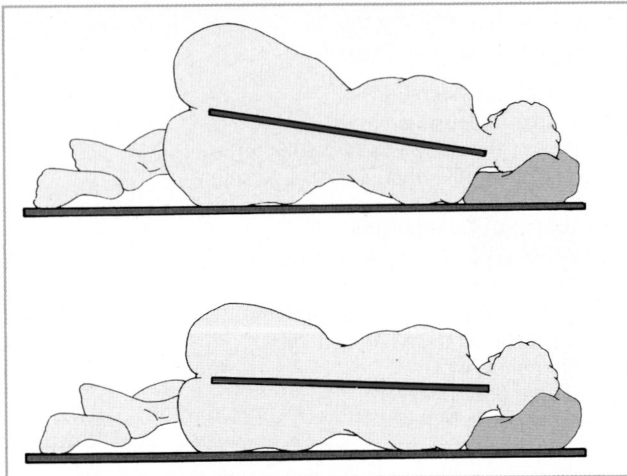

FIGURE 2-10 Pelvic widening and resultant head-down tilt in the lateral position during pregnancy. *Upper panel,* pregnant; *lower panel,* nonpregnant. (Modified from Camann WR, Ostheimer GW. Physiological adaptations during pregnancy. Int Anesthesiol Clin 1990; 28:2-10.)

late pregnancy.[231] Spinal dose requirements change rapidly in the postpartum period, with segmental dose requirements returning to those of nonpregnant women within 24 to 48 hours.[229] The postpartum change can be explained by an expansion of the spinal CSF volume that accompanies the relief of vena caval compression.

Despite enhanced neural susceptibility during pregnancy, the administration of *large doses* of local anesthetic results in the same spread of epidural anesthesia in term pregnant women as in nonpregnant women.[232] These results are consistent with the observation that it is often difficult to achieve a higher sensory level by administering additional increments of local anesthetic epidurally to any patient, whether pregnant or not.

The epidural segmental dose requirement decreases in both pregnant and nonpregnant women as the dose of local anesthetic is reduced, but pregnant women exhibit a greater decrease in segmental dose requirements. Therefore, although epidural administration of large doses of bupivacaine produces the same anesthetic spread in pregnant and nonpregnant women, the spread of *smaller* doses is greater in pregnant women.[233]

PHARMACOKINETICS AND PHARMACODYNAMICS OF LOCAL ANESTHETICS

The rate of absorption of bupivacaine from the epidural space and the time required for peak plasma concentration is unaltered during pregnancy.[234] There is no change in bupivacaine protein binding at therapeutic doses.[235] Bupivacaine is bound by the following two proteins, levels of both of which decline during pregnancy: (1) alpha-1-acid glycoprotein, a high-affinity, low-capacity site, and (2) albumin, a low-affinity, high-capacity site. The lack of reduction in the bound fraction of bupivacaine at low bupivacaine concentrations in pregnancy has been attributed to the fact that the alpha-1-acid glycoprotein is not fully saturated at this concentration.[235] Although the primary metabolites of bupivacaine are different in pregnant and nonpregnant women, the elimination half-life does not differ.[234]

Protein binding of lidocaine progressively decreases throughout gestation.[236] Ropivacaine pharmacokinetics are little affected by pregnancy.[237]

SYSTEMIC TOXICITY OF LOCAL ANESTHETICS

Pregnancy does not enhance the susceptibility of ewes to the neurotoxicity of lidocaine or to the cardiac toxicity of bupivacaine. The incidence of lethal ventricular arrhythmias is no higher in pregnant than in nonpregnant ewes treated with bupivacaine, ropivacaine, or levobupivacaine.[238,239]

HYPOTENSION DURING NEURAXIAL ANALGESIA AND ANESTHESIA

Pregnancy increases dependence on the sympathetic nervous system for the maintenance of venous return.[198-200] Thus, pregnant women require more medical intervention than nonpregnant patients to maintain hemodynamic stability during neuraxial anesthesia–induced sympathetic blockade. By 48 hours postpartum, the blood pressure response to neuraxial anesthesia returns to that of the nonpregnant state.[198]

The ideal method for augmenting central blood volume to prevent hypotension—and the ideal pharmacologic regimen to prevent and/or treat hypotension—during administration of neuraxial anesthesia in pregnant women is currently a matter of study and debate. A 2001 meta-analysis concluded that colloid infusion is more consistently effective than crystalloid in reducing the incidence of hypotension; leg wrapping or use of thromboembolic stockings was also found to be effective in reducing the occurrence of hypotension.[240] Crystalloid administered at the time of induction of spinal anesthesia (co-load) is more effective than preload (crystalloid administered before the induction of anesthesia) in preventing hypotension.[241]

Investigators have challenged the long-standing dogma that ephedrine is the vasopressor of choice for treatment of hypotension in pregnant women receiving neuraxial anesthesia. Studies now suggest that phenylephrine and ephedrine have similar efficacy in the treatment of hypotension and that use of phenylephrine is associated with a slightly higher umbilical arterial blood pH, although the incidence of frank fetal acidemia (pH < 7.2) is not lower with phenylephrine than with ephedrine.[242] Because of down-regulation of adrenergic receptors during pregnancy, treatment of hypotension requires higher doses of vasopressors in pregnant women than in nonpregnant women.

EFFECTS OF NEURAXIAL ANESTHESIA ON RESPIRATORY FUNCTION

FRC diminishes during neuraxial anesthesia,[243] resulting in an increase in respiratory dead space and a ventilation-perfusion mismatch. Abdominal muscles are important for forced expiration and coughing, and paralysis of these muscles during neuraxial anesthesia decreases the peak expiratory flow rate, the maximum expiratory pressure, and the ability to increase intra-abdominal and intrathoracic pressures during coughing.[244-246]

KEY POINTS

- Pregnancy results in various anatomic and physiologic changes that allow the mother to adapt to the growing fetus and that allow the fetus to develop.
- Cardiac output rises during pregnancy as a result of an increase in stroke volume and heart rate. A pregnant woman with cardiovascular disease may not be able to meet this greater demand.
- Beginning at mid-pregnancy, assumption of the supine position may result in compression of the inferior vena cava and aorta by the gravid uterus, which may result in decreases in both cardiac output and uteroplacental perfusion. Severe hypotension and bradycardia in the supine position is called the supine hypotension syndrome.
- Pregnant women should not lie supine after 20 weeks' gestation. Rather, the uterus should be tilted to the left by placement of a wedge underneath the right hip or the pregnant woman should assume either the full left or right lateral position.
- The greater blood volume of pregnancy allows the parturient to tolerate the blood loss of delivery with minimal hemodynamic perturbation. Maternal vascular capacitance is reduced at the time of delivery.
- Oxygen demand and delivery are higher during pregnancy.
- Minute ventilation rises while functional residual capacity diminishes during pregnancy. It is not uncommon for the pregnant woman to experience dyspnea.
- Pregnancy is a state of partially compensated respiratory alkalosis.
- Gastric volume, emptying, and pH are unaltered during pregnancy, but lower esophageal sphincter tone is reduced, thus increasing the incidence of gastroesophageal reflux.
- Mechanical changes in the vertebral column influence neuraxial analgesia and anesthesia.
- Pregnant women have higher sympathetic tone than nonpregnant women.
- Pregnant women are more sensitive to inhalation anesthetics and local anesthetics. Pregnancy results in higher levels of endorphins.
- Pregnant women have a rapid fall in Pa_{O_2} during periods of apnea.
- Pregnant women are at increased risk for failed intubation.
- Pregnant women are less responsive to vasopressors than nonpregnant women.

REFERENCES

1. Spätling L, Fallenstein F, Huch A, et al. The variability of cardiopulmonary adaptation to pregnancy at rest and during exercise. Br J Obstet Gynaecol 1992; 99(Suppl 8):1-40.
2. Chu SY, Kim SY, Schmid CH, et al. Maternal obesity and risk of cesarean delivery: A meta-analysis. Obes Rev 2007; 8:385-94.
3. Amorim AR, Rossner S, Neovius M, et al. Does excess pregnancy weight gain constitute a major risk for increasing long-term BMI? Obesity (Silver Spring) 2007; 15:1278-86.
4. Eghbali M, Wang Y, Toro L, Stefani E. Heart hypertrophy during pregnancy: A better functioning heart? Trends Cardiovasc Med 2006; 16:285-91.
5. Cutforth R, MacDonald CB. Heart sounds and murmurs in pregnancy. Am Heart J 1966; 71:741-7.
6. Northcote RJ, Knight PV, Ballantyne D. Systolic murmurs in pregnancy: Value of echocardiographic assessment. Clin Cardiol 1985; 8:327-8.
7. Seth R, Moss AJ, McNitt S, et al. Long QT syndrome and pregnancy. J Am Coll Cardiol 2007; 49:1092-8.
8. Carruth JE, Mivis SB, Brogan DR, Wenger NK. The electrocardiogram in normal pregnancy. Am Heart J 1981; 102:1075-8.
9. Oram S, Holt M. Innocent depression of the S-T segment and flattening of the T-wave during pregnancy. J Obstet Gynaecol Br Emp 1961; 68:765-70.
10. Robson SC, Hunter S, Boys RJ, Dunlop W. Serial study of factors influencing changes in cardiac output during human pregnancy. Am J Physiol 1989; 256:H1060-5.
11. Campos O, Andrade JL, Bocanegra J, et al. Physiologic multivalvular regurgitation during pregnancy: A longitudinal Doppler echocardiographic study. Int J Cardiol 1993; 40:265-72.
12. Robson SC, Hunter S, Moore M, Dunlop W. Haemodynamic changes during the puerperium: A Doppler and M-mode echocardiographic study. Br J Obstet Gynaecol 1987; 94:1028-39.
13. Capeless EL, Clapp JF. Cardiovascular changes in early phase of pregnancy. Am J Obstet Gynecol 1989; 161:1449-53.
14. Laird-Meeter K, van de Ley G, Bom TH, et al. Cardiocirculatory adjustments during pregnancy—an echocardiographic study. Clin Cardiol 1979; 2:328-32.
15. Katz R, Karliner JS, Resnik R. Effects of a natural volume overload state (pregnancy) on left ventricular performance in normal human subjects. Circulation 1978; 58:434-41.
16. Clark SL, Cotton DB, Lee W, et al. Central hemodynamic assessment of normal term pregnancy. Am J Obstet Gynecol 1989; 161:1439-42.
17. Rubler S, Damani PM, Pinto ER. Cardiac size and performance during pregnancy estimated with echocardiography. Am J Cardiol 1977; 40:534-40.
18. Shannwell CM, Schneppenhein M, Zimmerman T, et al. Left ventricular hypertrophy and diastolic dysfunction in healthy pregnant women. Cardiology 2002; 97:73-8.
19. Fok WY, Chan LY, Wong JT, et al. Left ventricular diastolic function during normal pregnancy: Assessment by spectral tissue Doppler imaging. Ultrasound Obstet Gynecol 2006; 28:789-93.
20. Assali NS, Rauramo L, Peltonen T. Measurement of uterine blood flow and uterine metabolism. VIII. Uterine and fetal blood flow and oxygen consumption in early human pregnancy. Am J Obstet Gynecol 1960; 79:86-98.
21. Thaler I, Manor D, Itskovitz J, et al. Changes in uterine blood flow during human pregnancy. Am J Obstet Gynecol 1990; 162:121-5.
22. Rekonen A, Luotola H, Pitkanen M, et al. Measurement of intervillous and myometrial blood flow by an intravenous ^{133}Xe method. Br J Obstet Gynaecol 1976; 83:723-8.
23. Kauppila A, Koskinen M, Puolakka J, et al. Decreased intervillous and unchanged myometrial blood flow in supine recumbency. Obstet Gynecol 1980; 55:203-5.
24. Palmer SK, Zamudio S, Coffin C, et al. Quantitative estimation of human uterine artery blood flow and pelvic blood flow redistribution in pregnancy. Obstet Gynecol 1992; 80:1000-6.
25. Katz M, Sokal MM. Skin perfusion in pregnancy. Am J Obstet Gynecol 1980; 137:30-3.
26. Dunlop W. Serial changes in renal haemodynamics during normal human pregnancy. Br J Obstet Gynaecol 1981; 88:1-9.
27. Wilson M, Morganti AA, Zervoudakis I, et al. Blood pressure, the renin-aldosterone system and sex steroids throughout normal pregnancy. Am J Med 1980; 68:97-104.

28. Christianson RE. Studies on blood pressure during pregnancy. I. Influence of parity and age. Am J Obstet Gynecol 1976; 125:509-13.
29. Iwasaki R, Ohkuchi A, Furuta I, et al. Relationship between blood pressure level in early pregnancy and subsequent changes in blood pressure during pregnancy. Acta Obstet Gynecol Scand 2002; 81:918-25.
30. Pyorala T. Cardiovascular response to the upright position during pregnancy. Acta Obstet Gynecol Scand 1966; 45(Suppl 5):1-116.
31. Kerr MG, Scott DB, Samuel E. Studies of the inferior vena cava in late pregnancy. Br Med J 1964; 1:532-3.
32. Kerr MG. The mechanical effects of the gravid uterus in late pregnancy. J Obstet Gynaecol Br Commonw 1965; 72:513-29.
33. Hirabayashi Y, Shimizu R, Fukada H, et al. Soft tissue anatomy within the vertebral canal in pregnant women. Br J Anaesth 1996; 77:153-6.
34. Bieniarz J, Yoshida T, Romero-Salinas G, et al. Aortocaval compression by the uterus in late human pregnancy. IV. Circulatory homeostasis by preferential perfusion of the placenta. Am J Obstet Gynecol 1969; 103:19-31.
35. Lees MM, Scott DB, Kerr MG, Taylor SH. The circulatory effects of recumbent postural change in late pregnancy. Clin Sci 1967; 32: 453-65.
36. McLennan CE. Antecubital and femoral venous pressure in normal and toxemic pregnancy. Am J Obstet Gynecol 1943; 45:568-91.
37. Eckstein KL, Marx GF. Aortocaval compression and uterine displacement. Anesthesiology 1974; 40:92-6.
38. Kinsella SM, Whitwam JG, Spencer JA. Aortic compression by the uterus: Identification with the Finapres digital arterial pressure instrument. Br J Obstet Gynaecol 1990; 97:700-5.
39. Abitbol MM. Aortic compression by pregnant uterus. NY State J Med 1976; 76:1470-5.
40. Kuo CD, Chen GY, Yang MJ, Tsai YS. The effect of position on autonomic nervous activity in late pregnancy. Anaesthesia 1997; 52:1161-5.
41. Milsom I, Forssman L. Factors influencing aortocaval compression in late pregnancy. Am J Obstet Gynecol 1984; 148:764-71.
42. Clark SL, Cotton DB, Pivarnik JM, et al. Position change and central hemodynamic profile during normal third-trimester pregnancy and post partum. Am J Obstet Gynecol 1991; 164:883-7.
43. Drummond GB, Scott SE, Lees MM, Scott DB. Effects of posture on limb blood flow in late pregnancy. Br Med J 1974; 2:587-8.
44. Kinsella SM, Lohmann G. Supine hypotensive syndrome. Obstet Gynecol 1994; 83:774-88.
45. Howard BK, Goodson JH, Mengert WF. Supine hypotensive syndrome in late pregnancy. Obstet Gynecol 1953; 1:371-7.
46. Robson SC, Dunlop W, Boys RJ, Hunter S. Cardiac output during labor. Br Med J 1987; 295:1169-72.
47. Ueland K, Hansen JM. Maternal cardiovascular dynamics. III. Labor and delivery under local and caudal analgesia. Am J Obstet Gynecol 1969; 103:8-18.
48. Kjeldsen J. Hemodynamic investigations during labour and delivery. Acta Obstet Gynecol Scand Suppl 1979; 89:1-252.
49. Adams JQ, Alexander AM Jr. Alterations in cardiovascular physiology during labor. Obstet Gynecol 1958; 12:542-9.
50. Hendricks CH. The hemodynamics of a uterine contraction. Am J Obstet Gynecol 1958; 76:969-82.
51. Lee W, Rokey R, Miller J, Cotton DB. Maternal hemodynamic effects of uterine contractions by M-mode and pulsed-Doppler echocardiography. Am J Obstet Gynecol 1989; 161:974-7.
52. Robson SC, Dunlop W, Hunter S. Haemodynamic changes during the early puerperium. Br Med J 1987; 294:1065.
53. Sadaniantz A, Saint Laurent L, Parisi AF. Long-term effects of multiple pregnancies on cardiac dimensions and systolic and diastolic function. Am J Obstet Gynecol 1996; 174:1061-4.
54. Leontic EA. Respiratory disease in pregnancy. Med Clin North Am 1977; 61:111-28.
55. Thomson K, Cohen M. Studies on the circulation in pregnancy. II. Vital capacity observations in normal pregnant women. Surg Gynaecol Obstet 1938; 66:591-603.
56. Goldsmith LT, Weiss G, Steinetz BG. Relaxin and its role in pregnancy. Endocrinol Metab Clin North Am 1995; 24:171-86.
57. Wise RA, Polito AJ, Krishnan V. Respiratory physiologic changes in pregnancy. Immunol Allergy Clin North Am 2006; 26:1-12.
58. Grenville-Mathers R, Trenchard HJ. The diaphragm in the puerperium. J Obstet Gynaecol Br Emp 1953; 60:825-33.
59. Norregaard O, Schultz P, Ostergaard A, Dahl R. Lung function and postural changes during pregnancy. Respir Med 1989; 83:467-70.
60. Russell IF, Chambers WA. Closing volume in normal pregnancy. Br J Anaesth 1981; 53:1043-7.
61. Harirah HM, Donia SE, Nasrallah FK, et al. Effect of gestational age and position on peak expiratory flow rate: A longitudinal study. Obstet Gynecol 2005; 105:372-6.
62. Brancazio LR, Laifer SA, Schwartz T. Peak expiratory flow rate in normal pregnancy. Obstet Gynecol 1997; 89:383-6.
63. Alaily AB, Carrol KB. Pulmonary ventilation in pregnancy. Br J Obstet Gynaecol 1978; 85:518-24.
64. Gee JB, Packer BS, Millen JE, Robin ED. Pulmonary mechanics during pregnancy. J Clin Invest 1967; 46:945-52.
65. Baldwin GR, Moorthi DS, Whelton JA, MacDonnell KF. New lung functions and pregnancy. Am J Obstet Gynecol 1977; 127:235-9.
66. Templeton A, Kelman GR. Maternal blood-gases (PAO_2-PaO_2), physiological shunt and VD/VT in normal pregnancy. Br J Anaesth 1976; 48:1001-4.
67. Machida H. Influence of progesterone on arterial blood and CSF acid-base balance in women. J Appl Physiol 1981; 51:1433-6.
68. Zwillich CW, Natalino MR, Sutton FD, Weil JV. Effects of progesterone on chemosensitivity in normal men. J Lab Clin Med 1978; 92:262-9.
69. Moore LG, McCullough RE, Weil JV. Increased HVR in pregnancy: Relationship to hormonal and metabolic changes. J Appl Physiol 1987; 62:158-63.
70. Bader RA, Bader ME, Rose DF, Braunwald E. Hemodynamics at rest and during exercise in normal pregnancy as studied by cardiac catheterization. J Clin Invest 1955; 34:1524-36.
71. Sady MA, Haydon BB, Sady SP, et al. Cardiovascular response to maximal cycle exercise during pregnancy and at two and seven months post partum. Am J Obstet Gynecol 1990; 162:1181-5.
72. Shankar KB, Moseley H, Vemula V, et al. Arterial to end-tidal carbon dioxide tension difference during anaesthesia in early pregnancy. Can J Anaesth 1989; 36:124-7.
73. Shankar KB, Moseley H, Kumar Y, Vemula V. Arterial to end-tidal carbon dioxide tension difference during caesarean section anaesthesia. Anaesthesia 1986; 41:698-702.
74. Shankar KB, Moseley H, Kumar Y, et al. Arterial to end-tidal carbon dioxide tension difference during anaesthesia for tubal ligation. Anaesthesia 1987; 42:482-6.
75. Dayal P, Murata Y, Takamura H. Antepartum and postpartum acid-base changes in maternal blood in normal and complicated pregnancies. J Obstet Gynaecol Br Commonw 1972; 79:612-24.
76. Seeds AE, Battaglia FC, Hellegers AE. Effects of pregnancy on the pH, pCO_2, and bicarbonate concentrations of peripheral venous blood. Am J Obstet Gynecol 1964; 88:1086-9.
77. Lim VS, Katz AI, Lindheimer MD. Acid-base regulation in pregnancy. Am J Physiol 1976; 231:1764-9.
78. Tenholder MF, South-Paul JE. Dyspnea in pregnancy. Chest 1989; 96:381-8.
79. McAuley SE, Jensen D, McGrath MJ, Wolfe LA. Effects of human pregnancy and aerobic conditioning on alveolar gas exchange during exercise. Can J Physiol Pharmacol 2005; 83:625-33.
80. Amercian Academy of Sleep Medicine: International Classification of Sleep Disorders Revised: Diagnostic and Coding Manual. Westchester, IL, American Academy of Sleep Medicine, 2000.
81. Pien GW, Schwab RJ. Sleep disorders during pregnancy. Sleep 2004; 27:1405-17.
82. Santiago JR, Nolledo MS, Kinzler W, Santiago TV. Sleep and sleep disorders in pregnancy. Ann Intern Med 2001; 134:396-408.
83. Schweiger MS. Sleep disturbance in pregnancy: A subjective survey. Am J Obstet Gynecol 1972; 114:879-82.
84. Manconi M, Govoni V, De Vito A, et al. Pregnancy as a risk factor for restless legs syndrome. Sleep Med 2004; 5:305-8.

85. Hägerdal M, Morgan CW, Sumner AE, Gutsche BB. Minute ventilation and oxygen consumption during labor with epidural analgesia. Anesthesiology 1983; 59:425-7.
86. Pearson JF, Davies P. The effect of continuous lumbar epidural analgesia on the acid-base status of maternal arterial blood during the first stage of labour. J Obstet Gynaecol Br Commonw 1973; 80:218-24.
87. Jouppila R, Hollmen A. The effect of segmental epidural analgesia on maternal and foetal acid-base balance, lactate, serum potassium and creatine phosphokinase during labour. Acta Anaesth Scand 1976; 20:259-68.
88. Thalme B, Raabe N, Belfrage P. Lumbar epidural analgesia in labour. II. Effects on glucose, lactate, sodium chloride, total protein, haematocrit and haemoglobin in maternal, fetal and neonatal blood. Acta Obstet Gynecol Scand 1974; 53:113-9.
89. Pearson JF, Davies P. The effect of continuous lumbar epidural analgesia on maternal acid base balance and arterial lactate concentrations during the second stage of labour. J Obstet Gynaecol Br Commonw 1973; 80:225-9.
90. Bernstein IM, Ziegler W, Badger GJ. Plasma volume expansion in early pregnancy. Obstet Gynecol 2001; 97:669-72.
91. Lund CJ, Donovan JC. Blood volume during pregnancy: Significance of plasma and red cell volumes. Am J Obstet Gynecol 1967; 98: 394-403.
92. Hytten FE, Paintin DB. Increase in plasma volume during normal pregnancy. J Obstet Gynaecol Br Emp 1963; 70:402-7.
93. Taylor DJ, Lind T. Red cell mass during and after normal pregnancy. Br J Obstet Gynaecol 1979; 86:364-70.
94. Pritchard JA. Changes in the blood volume during pregnancy and delivery. Anesthesiology 1965; 26:393-9.
95. Schrier RW, Berl T, Anderson RJ. Osmotic and nonosmotic control of vasopressin release. Am J Physiol 1979; 236:F321-32.
96. Duvekot JJ, Cheriex EC, Pieters FA, et al. Early pregnancy changes in hemodynamics and volume homeostasis are consecutive adjustments triggered by a primary fall in systemic vascular tone. Am J Obstet Gynecol 1993; 169:1382-92.
97. Hayashi Y, Ueyama H, Mashimo T, et al. Circulating mature adrenomedullin is related to blood volume in full-term pregnancy. Anesth 2005; 101:1816-20.
98. Cotes PM, Canning CE, Lind T. Changes in serum immunoreactive erythropoietin during the menstrual cycle and normal pregnancy. Br J Obstet Gynaecol 1983; 90:304-11.
99. Coryell M, Beach E, Robinson A, et al. Metabolism of women during the reproductive cycle. XVII. Changes in electrophoretic patterns of plasma proteins throughout the cycle and following delivery. J Clin Invest 1950; 29:1559-67.
100. Mendenhall HW. Serum protein concentrations in pregnancy. I. Concentrations in maternal serum. Am J Obstet Gynecol 1970; 106:388-99.
101. Robertson EG, Cheyne GA. Plasma biochemistry in relation to oedema of pregnancy. J Obstet Gynaecol Br Commonw 1972; 79:769-76.
102. Wu PY, Udani V, Chan L, et al. Colloid osmotic pressure: Variations in normal pregnancy. J Perinat Med 1983; 11:193-9.
103. Evans RT, Wroe JM. Plasma cholinesterase changes during pregnancy: Their interpretation as a cause of suxamethonium-induced apnoea. Anaesthesia 1980; 35:651-4.
104. Leighton BL, Cheek TG, Gross JB, et al. Succinylcholine pharmacodynamics in peripartum patients. Anesthesiology 1986; 64:202-5.
105. Gerbasi FR, Buttoms S, Farag A, Mammen E. Increased intravascular coagulation associated with pregnancy. Obstet Gynecol 1990; 75:385-9.
106. Tygart SG, McRoyan DK, Spinnato JA, et al. Longitudinal study of platelet indices during normal pregnancy. Am J Obstet Gynecol 1986; 154:883-7.
107. Fay RA, Hughes AO, Farron NT. Platelets in pregnancy: Hyperdestruction in pregnancy. Obstet Gynecol 1983; 61:238-40.
108. Norris LA, Sheppard BL, Bonnar J. Increased whole blood platelet aggregation in normal pregnancy can be prevented in vitro by aspirin and dazmegrel (UK38485). Br J Obstet Gynaecol 1992; 99:253-7.
109. Berge LN, Lyngmo V, Svensson B, Nordoy A. The bleeding time in women: An influence of the sex hormones? Acta Obstet Gynecol Scand 1993; 72:423-7.
110. Pitkin RM, Witte DL. Platelet and leukocyte counts in pregnancy. JAMA 1979; 242:2696-8.
111. Talbert LM, Langdell RD. Normal values of certain factors in the blood clotting mechanism in pregnancy. Am J Obstet Gynecol 1964; 90:44-50.
112. Kasper CK, Hoag MS, Aggeler PM, Stone S. Blood clotting factors in pregnancy: Factor VIII concentrations in normal and AHF-deficient women. Obstet Gynecol 1964; 24:242-7.
113. Stirling Y, Woolf L, North WR, et al. Haemostasis in normal pregnancy. Thromb Haemost 1984; 52:176-82.
114. Coopland A, Alkjaersig N, Fletcher AP. Reduction in plasma factor XIII (fibrin stabilizing factor) concentration during pregnancy. J Lab Clin Med 1969; 73:144-53.
115. Sharma SK, Philip J, Wiley J. Thromboelastographic changes in healthy parturients and postpartum women. Anesth Analg 1997; 85:94-8.
116. Hellgren M. Hemostasis during normal pregnancy and puerperium. Semin Thromb Hemost 2003; 29:125-30.
117. Ueland K. Maternal cardiovascular dynamics. VII. Intrapartum blood volume changes. Am J Obstet Gynecol 1976; 126:671-7.
118. Toledo P, McCarthy RJ, Hewlett BJ, et al. The accuracy of blood loss estimation after simulated vaginal delivery. Anesth Analg 2007; 105:1736-40.
119. Taylor DJ, Phillips P, Lind T. Puerperal haematological indices. Br J Obstet Gynaecol 1981; 88:601-6.
120. Ygge J. Changes in blood coagulation and fibrinolysis during the puerperium. Am J Obstet Gynecol 1969; 104:2-12.
121. Bonnar J, McNicol GP, Douglas AS. Coagulation and fibrinolytic mechanisms during and after normal childbirth. Br Med J 1970; 2:200-3.
122. Krause PJ, Ingardia CJ, Pontius LT, et al. Host defense during pregnancy: Neutrophil chemotaxis and adherence. Am J Obstet Gynecol 1987; 157:274-80.
123. Baboonian C, Griffiths P. Is pregnancy immunosuppressive? Humoral immunity against viruses. Br J Obstet Gynaecol 1983; 90:1168-75.
124. Piccinni MP. Role of T-cell cytokines in decidua and in cumulus oophorus during pregnancy. Gynecol Obstet Invest 2007; 64:144-8.
125. King AE, Kelly RW, Sallenave JM, et al. Innate immune defences in the human uterus during pregnancy. Placenta 2007; 28:1099-1106.
126. VanThiel DH, Gavaler JS, Stremple J. Lower esophageal sphincter pressure in women using sequential oral contraception. Gastroenterology 1976; 71:232-4.
127. Richter JE. Review article: The management of heartburn in pregnancy. Aliment Pharmacol Ther 2005; 22:749-57.
128. Fisher RS, Roberts GS, Grabowski CJ, Cohen S. Altered lower esophageal sphincter function during early pregnancy. Gastroenterology 1978; 74:1233-7.
129. Marrero JM, Goggin PM, de Caestecker JS, et al. Determinants of pregnancy heartburn. Br J Obstet Gynaecol 1992; 99:731-4.
130. Macfie AG, Magides AD, Richmond MN, Reilly CS. Gastric emptying in pregnancy. Br J Anaesth 1991; 67:54-7.
131. Whitehead EM, Smith M, Dean Y, O'Sullivan G. An evaluation of gastric emptying times in pregnancy and the puerperium. Anaesthesia 1993; 48:53-7.
132. Wong CA, Loffredi M, Ganchiff JN, et al. Gastric emptying of water in term pregnancy. Anesthesiology 2002; 96:1395-1400.
133. La Salvia LA, Steffen EA. Delayed gastric emptying time in labor. Am J Obstet Gynecol 1950; 59:1075-81.
134. Chiloiro M, Darconza G, Piccioli E, et al. Gastric emptying and orocecal transit time in pregnancy. J Gastroenterol 2001; 36:538-43.
135. Davison JS, Davison MC, Hay DM. Gastric emptying time in late pregnancy and labour. J Obstet Gynaecol Br Commonw 1970; 77:37-41.
136. O'Sullivan GM, Sutton AJ, Thompson SA, et al. Noninvasive measurement of gastric emptying in obstetric patients. Anesth Analg 1987; 66:505-11.

137. Sandhar BK, Elliott RH, Windram I, Rowbotham DJ. Peripartum changes in gastric emptying. Anaesthesia 1992; 47:196-8.
138. Wong CA, McCarthy RJ, Fitzgerald PC, et al. Gastric emptying of water in obese pregnant women at term. Anesth Analg 2007; 105:751-5.
139. Derbyshire EJ, Davies J, Detmar P. Changes in bowel function: Pregnancy and the puerperium. Dig Dis Sci 2007; 52:324-8.
140. Parry E, Shields R, Turnbull AC. Transit time in the small intestine in pregnancy. J Obstet Gynaecol Br Commonw 1970; 77:900-1.
141. Murray FA, Erskine JP, Fielding J. Gastric secretion in pregnancy. J Obstet Gynaecol Br Emp 1957; 64:373-81.
142. Van Thiel DH, Gavaler JS, Joshi SN, et al. Heartburn of pregnancy. Gastroenterology 1977; 72:666-8.
143. Hong JY, Park JW, Oh JI. Comparison of preoperative gastric contents and serum gastrin concentrations in pregnant and nonpregnant women. J Clin Anesth 2005; 17:451-5.
144. Attia RR, Ebeid AM, Fischer JE, Goudsouzian NG. Maternal fetal and placental gastrin concentrations. Anaesthesia 1982; 37:18-21.
145. Wyner J, Cohen SE. Gastric volume in early pregnancy: Effect of metoclopramide. Anesthesiology 1982; 57:209-12.
146. Carp H, Jayaram A, Stoll M. Ultrasound examination of the stomach contents of parturients. Anesth Analg 1992; 74:683-7.
147. Murphy DF, Nally B, Gardiner J, Unwin A. Effect of metoclopramide on gastric emptying before elective and emergency caesarean section. Br J Anaesth 1984; 56:1113-6.
148. Roberts RB, Shirley MA. Reducing the risk of acid aspiration during cesarean section. Anesth Analg 1974; 53:859-68.
149. Kubli M, Scrutton MJ, Seed PT, O'Sullivan G. An evaluation of isotonic "sport drinks" during labor. Anesth Analg 2002; 94:404-8.
150. Lahiri SK, Thomas TA, Hodgson RM. Single-dose antacid therapy for the prevention of Mendelson's syndrome. Br J Anaesth 1973; 45:1143-6.
151. Gin T, Cho AM, Lew JK, et al. Gastric emptying in the postpartum period. Anaesth Intensive Care 1991; 19:521-4.
152. James CF, Gibbs CP, Banner T. Postpartum perioperative risk of aspiration pneumonia. Anesthesiology 1984; 61:756-9.
153. Blouw R, Scatliff J, Craig DB, Palahniuk RJ. Gastric volume and pH in postpartum patients. Anesthesiology 1976; 45:456-7.
154. Lam KK, So HY, Gin T. Gastric pH and volume after oral fluids in the postpartum patient. Can J Anaesth 1993; 40:218-21.
155. Ewah B, Yau K, King M, et al. Effect of epidural opioids on gastric emptying in labour. Int J Obstet Anesth 1993; 2:125-8.
156. Wright PMC, Allen RW, Moore J, Donnelly JP. Gastric emptying during lumbar extradural analgesia in labor: Effect of fentanyl supplementation. Br J Anaesth 1992; 68:248-51.
157. Kelly MC, Carabine UA, Hill DA, Mirakhur RK. A comparison of the effect of intrathecal and extradural fentanyl on gastric emptying in laboring women. Anesth Analg 1997; 85:834-8.
158. Porter JS, Bonello E, Reynolds F. The influence of epidural administration of fentanyl infusion on gastric emptying in labour. Anaesthesia 1997; 52:1151-6.
159. Romalis G, Claman AD. Serum enzymes in pregnancy. Am J Obstet Gynecol 1962; 84:1104-10.
160. Combes B, Shibata H, Adams R, et al. Alterations in sulfobromophthalein sodium-removal mechanisms from blood during normal pregnancy. J Clin Invest 1963; 42:1431-42.
161. Blum A, Tatour I, Monir M, et al. Gallstones in pregnancy and their complications: postpartum acute pancreatitis and acute peritonitis. Eur J Intern Med 2005; 16:473-6.
162. Mendez-Sanchez N, Chavez-Tapia NC, Uribe M. Pregnancy and gallbladder disease. Ann Hepatol 2006; 5:227-30.
163. Ryan JP, Pellecchia D. Effect of progesterone pretreatment on guinea pig gallbladder motility in vitro. Gastroenterology 1982; 83:81-3.
164. Kern F Jr, Everson GT, DeMark B, et al. Biliary lipids, bile acids, and gallbladder function in the human female: Effects of contraceptive steroids. J Lab Clin Med 1982; 99:798-805.
165. Jeyabalan A, Lain KY. Anatomic and functional changes of the upper urinary tract during pregnancy. Urol Clin North Am 2007; 34:1-6.
166. Rasmussen PE, Nielsen FR. Hydronephrosis during pregnancy: A literature survey. Eur J Obstet Gynecol Reprod Biol 1988; 27:249-59.
167. Davison JM, Hytten FE. Glomerular filtration during and after pregnancy. J Obstet Gynaecol Br Commonw 1974; 81:588-95.
168. Sims EA, Krantz KE. Serial studies of renal function during pregnancy and the puerperium in normal women. J Clin Invest 1958; 37:1764-74.
169. Lind T, Godfrey KA, Otun H, Philips PR. Changes in serum uric acid concentrations during normal pregnancy. Br J Obstet Gynaecol 1984; 91:128-32.
170. Airoldi J, Weinstein L. Clinical significance of proteinuria in pregnancy. Obstet Gynecol Surv 2007; 62:117-24.
171. Higby K, Suiter CR, Phelps JY, et al. Normal values of urinary albumin and total protein excretion during pregnancy. Am J Obstet Gynecol 1994; 171:984-9.
172. Davison JM, Hytten FE. The effect of pregnancy on the renal handling of glucose. Br J Obstet Gynaecol 1975; 82:374-81.
173. Harada A, Hershman JM, Reed AW, et al. Comparison of thyroid stimulators and thyroid hormone concentrations in the sera of pregnant women. J Clin Endocrinol Metab 1979; 48:793-7.
174. Felig P, Lynch V. Starvation in human pregnancy: Hypoglycemia, hypoinsulinemia, and hyperketonemia. Science 1970; 170:990-2.
175. Fisher PM, Sutherland HW, Bewsher PD. The insulin response to glucose infusion in normal human pregnancy. Diabetologia 1980; 19:15-20.
176. Rosenthal HE, Slaunwhite WR Jr, Sandberg AA. Transcortin: A corticosteroid-binding protein of plasma. X: Cortisol and progesterone interplay and unbound levels of these steroids in pregnancy. J Clin Endocrinol Metab 1969; 29:352-67.
177. Pacheco LD, Ghulmiyyah LM, Snodgrass WR, Hankins GD. Pharmacokinetics of corticosteroids during pregnancy. Am J Perinatol 2007; 24:79-82.
178. Kristiansson P, Svardsudd K, von Schoultz B. Back pain during pregnancy: A prospective study. Spine 1996; 21:702-9.
179. Wang SM, Dezinno P, Maranets I, et al. Low back pain during pregnancy: Prevalence, risk factors, and outcomes. Obstet Gynecol 2004; 104:65-70.
180. Kristiansson P, Nilsson-Wikmar L, von Schoultz B, et al. Back pain in in-vitro fertilized and spontaneous pregnancies. Hum Reprod 1998; 13:3233-8.
181. Brynhildsen J, Hansson A, Persson A, Hammar M. Follow-up of patients with low back pain during pregnancy. Obstet Gynecol 1998; 91:182-6.
182. Borg-Stein J, Dugan SA, Gruber J. Musculoskeletal aspects of pregnancy. Am J Phys Med Rehabil 2005; 84:180-92.
183. Berg G, Hammar M, Moller-Nielsen J, et al. Low back pain during pregnancy. Obstet Gynecol 1988; 71:71-5.
184. Wilkinson M. The carpal-tunnel syndrome in pregnancy. Lancet 1960; 1:453-4.
185. Palahniuk RJ, Shnider SM, Eger EI 2nd. Pregnancy decreases the requirement for inhaled anesthetic agents. Anesthesiology 1974; 41:82-3.
186. Abboud TK, Zhu J, Richardson M, et al. Desflurane: A new volatile anesthetic for cesarean section. Maternal and neonatal effects. Acta Anaesthesiol Scand 1995; 39:723-6.
187. Preckel B, Bolten J. Pharmacology of modern volatile anaesthetics. Best Pract Res Clin Anaesthesiol 2005; 19:331-48.
188. Cogan R, Spinnato JA. Pain and discomfort thresholds in late pregnancy. Pain 1986; 27:63-8.
189. Abboud TK, Sarkis F, Hung TT, et al. Effects of epidural anesthesia during labor on maternal plasma beta-endorphin levels. Anesthesiology 1983; 59:1-5.
190. Iwasaki H, Collins JG, Saito Y, Kerman-Hinds A. Naloxone-sensitive, pregnancy-induced changes in behavioral responses to colorectal distention: Pregnancy-induced analgesia to visceral stimulation. Anesthesiology 1991; 74:927-33.
191. Datta S, Lambert DH, Gregus J, et al. Differential sensitivities of mammalian nerve fibers during pregnancy. Anesth Analg 1983; 62:1070-2.

192. Bromage PR. Spread of analgesic solutions in the epidural space and their site of action: A statistical study. Br J Anaesth 1962; 34:161-78.
193. Fagraeus L, Urban BJ, Bromage PR. Spread of epidural analgesia in early pregnancy. Anesthesiology 1983; 58:184-7.
194. Richardson MG, Wissler RN. Density of lumbar cerebrospinal fluid in pregnant and nonpregnant humans. Anesthesiology 1996; 85:326-30.
195. Hogan QH, Prost R, Kulier A, et al. Magnetic resonance imaging of cerebrospinal fluid volume and the influence of body habitus and abdominal pressure. Anesthesiology 1996; 84:1341-9.
196. Messih MN. Epidural space pressures during pregnancy. Anaesthesia 1981; 36:775-82.
197. Marx GF, Zemaitis MT, Orkin LR. Cerebrospinal fluid pressures during labor and obstetrical anesthesia. Anesthesiology 1961; 22:348-54.
198. Assali NS, Prystowsky H. Studies on autonomic blockade. I. Comparison between the effects of tetraethylammonium chloride (TEAC) and high selective spinal anesthesia on blood pressure of normal and toxemic pregnancy. J Clin Invest 1950; 29:1354-66.
199. Tabsh K, Rudelstorfer R, Nuwayhid B, Assali NS. Circulatory responses to hypovolemia in the pregnant and nonpregnant sheep after pharmacologic sympathectomy. Am J Obstet Gynecol 1986; 154:411-9.
200. Goodlin RC. Venous reactivity and pregnancy abnormalities. Acta Obstet Gynecol Scand 1986; 65:345-8.
201. Abitbol MM. Supine position in labor and associated fetal heart rate changes. Obstet Gynecol 1985; 65:481-6.
202. Huch A, Huch R, Schneider H, Rooth G. Continuous transcutaneous monitoring of fetal oxygen tension during labour. Br J Obstet Gynaecol 1977; 84(Suppl 1):1-39.
203. Crawford JS, Burton M, Davies P. Time and lateral tilt at Caesarean section. Br J Anaesth 1972; 44:477-84.
204. Lees MM, Taylor SH, Scott DB, Kerr MG. A study of cardiac output at rest throughout pregnancy. J Obstet Gynaecol Br Commonw 1967; 74:319-28.
205. Ueland K, Novy MJ, Peterson EN, Metcalfe J. Maternal cardiovascular dynamics. IV. The influence of gestational age on the maternal cardiovascular response to posture and exercise. Am J Obstet Gynecol 1969; 104:856-64.
206. Pilkington S, Carli F, Dakin MJ, et al. Increase in Mallampati score during pregnancy. Br J Anaesth 1995; 74:638-42.
207. Dobb G. Laryngeal oedema complicating obstetric anaesthesia. Anaesthesia 1978; 33:839-40.
208. Samsoon GLT, Young JRB. Difficult tracheal intubation: A retrospective study. Anaesthesia 1987; 42:487-90.
209. Ezri T, Szmuk P, Evron S, et al. Difficult airway in obstetric anesthesia: A review. Obstet Gynecol Surv 2001; 56:631-41.
210. Hawkins JL, Koonin LM, Palmer SK, Gibbs CP. Anesthesia-related deaths during obstetric delivery in the United States, 1979-1990. Anesthesiology 1997; 86:277-84.
211. Archer GW Jr, Marx GF. Arterial oxygen tension during apnoea in parturient women. Br J Anaesth 1974; 46:358-60.
212. Rampton AJ, Mallaiah S, Garrett CP. Increased ventilation requirements during obstetric general anaesthesia. Br J Anaesth 1988; 61:730-7.
213. Christensen JH, Andreasen F, Jansen JA. Pharmacokinetics of thiopental in caesarian section. Acta Anaesthesiol Scand 1981; 25:174-9.
214. Gin T, Mainland P, Chan MT, Short TG. Decreased thiopental requirements in early pregnancy. Anesthesiology 1997; 86:73-8.
215. Morgan DJ, Blackman GL, Paull JD, Wolf LJ. Pharmacokinetics and plasma binding of thiopental. II. Studies at cesarean section. Anesthesiology 1981; 54:474-80.
216. Higuchi H, Adachi Y, Arimura S, et al. Early pregnancy does not reduce the C(50) of propofol for loss of consciousness. Anesth Analg 2001; 93:1565-9.
217. Gin T, Gregory MA, Chan K, et al. Pharmacokinetics of propofol in women undergoing elective caesarean section. Br J Anaesth 1990; 64:148-53.
218. Shnider SM. Serum cholinesterase activity during pregnancy, labor and the puerperium. Anesthesiology 1965; 26:335-59.
219. Baraka A, Jabbour S, Tabboush Z, et al. Onset of vecuronium neuromuscular block is more rapid in patients undergoing caesarean section. Can J Anaesth 1992; 39:135-8.
220. Puhringer FK, Sparr HJ, Mitterschiffthaler G, et al. Extended duration of action of rocuronium in postpartum patients. Anesth Analg 1997; 84:352-4.
221. Khuenl-Brady KS, Koller J, Mair P, et al. Comparison of vecuronium- and atracurium-induced neuromuscular blockade in postpartum and nonpregnant patients. Anesth Analg 1991; 72:110-3.
222. Dailey PA, Fisher DM, Shnider SM, et al. Pharmacokinetics, placental transfer, and neonatal effects of vecuronium and pancuronium administered during cesarean section. Anesthesiology 1984; 60: 569-74.
223. Pan PH, Moore C. Comparison of cisatracurium-induced neuromuscular blockade between immediate postpartum and nonpregnant patients. J Clin Anesth 2001; 13:112-17.
224. DeSimone CA, Leighton BL, Norris MC, et al. Chronotropic effect of isoproterenol is reduced in term pregnant women. Anesthesiology 1988; 69:626-8.
225. Popitz-Bergez FA, Leeson S, Thalhammer JG, Strichartz GR. Intraneural lidocaine uptake compared with analgesic differences between pregnant and nonpregnant rats. Reg Anesth 1997; 22: 363-71.
226. Flanagan HL, Datta S, Lambert DH, et al. Effect of pregnancy on bupivacaine-induced conduction blockade in the isolated rabbit vagus nerve. Anesth Analg 1987; 66:123-6.
227. Hirabayashi Y, Shimizu R, Saitoh K, et al. Acid-base state of cerebrospinal fluid during pregnancy and its effect on spread of spinal anaesthesia. Br J Anaesth 1996; 77:352-5.
228. Barclay DL, Renegar OJ, Nelson EW Jr. The influence of inferior vena cava compression on the level of spinal anesthesia. Am J Obstet Gynecol 1968; 101:792-800.
229. Abouleish EI. Postpartum tubal ligation requires more bupivacaine for spinal anesthesia than does cesarean section. Anesth Analg 1986; 65:897-900.
230. Hirabayashi Y, Shimizu R, Saitoh K, Fukuda H. Spread of subarachnoid hyperbaric amethocaine in pregnant women. Br J Anaesth 1995; 74:384-6.
231. Hirabayashi Y, Shimizu R, Fukuda H, et al. Anatomical configuration of the spinal column in the supine position. II. Comparison of pregnant and non-pregnant women. Br J Anaesth 1995; 75:6-8.
232. Grundy EM, Zamora AM, Winnie AP. Comparison of spread of epidural anesthesia in pregnant and nonpregnant women. Anesth Analg 1978; 57:544-6.
233. Kalas DB, Senfield RM, Hehre FW. Continuous lumbar peridural anesthesia in obstetrics. IV. Comparison of the number of segments blocked in pregnant and nonpregnant subjects. Anesth Analg 1966; 45:848-51.
234. Pihlajamaki K, Kanto J, Lindberg R, et al. Extradural administration of bupivacaine: Pharmacokinetics and metabolism in pregnant and nonpregnant women. Br J Anaesth 1990; 64:556-62.
235. Tsen LC, Tarshis J, Denson DD, et al. Measurements of maternal protein binding of bupivacaine throughout pregnancy. Anesth Analg 1999; 89:965-8.
236. Fragneto RY, Bader AM, Rosinia F, et al. Measurements of protein binding of lidocaine throughout pregnancy. Anesth Analg 1994; 79:295-7.
237. Santos AC, Karpel B, Noble G. The placental transfer and fetal effects of levobupivacaine, racemic bupivacaine, and ropivacaine. Anesthesiology 1999; 90:1698-1703.
238. Santos AC, DeArmas PI. Systemic toxicity of levobupivacaine, bupivacaine, and ropivacaine during continuous intravenous infusion to nonpregnant and pregnant ewes. Anesthesiology 2001; 95:1256-64.
239. Santos AC, Arthur GR, Wlody D, et al. Comparative systemic toxicity of ropivacaine and bupivacaine in nonpregnant and pregnant ewes. Anesthesiology 1995; 82:734-40.

240. Morgan PJ, Halpern SH, Tarshis J. The effects of an increase of central blood volume before spinal anesthesia for cesarean delivery: A qualitative systematic review. Anesth 2001; 92:997-1005.
241. Dyer RA, Farina Z, Joubert IA, et al. Crystalloid preload versus rapid crystalloid administration after induction of spinal anaesthesia (coload) for elective caesarean section. Anaesth Intensive Care 2004; 32:351-7.
242. Lee A, Ngan Kee WD, Gin T. A quantitative, systematic review of randomized controlled trials of ephedrine versus phenylephrine for the management of hypotension during spinal anesthesia for cesarean delivery. Anesth Analg 2002; 94:920-6.
243. Askrog VF, Smith TC, Eckenhoff JE. Changes in pulmonary ventilation during spinal anesthesia. Surg Gynecol Obstet 1964; 119:563-7.
244. Moir D. Ventilatory function during epidural analgesia. Br J Anaesth 1963; 35:3-7.
245. Egbert LD, Tamersoy K, Deas TC. Pulmonary function during spinal anesthesia: The mechanism of cough depression. Anesthesiology 1961; 22:882-5.
246. von Ungern-Sternberg BS, Regli A, Bucher E, et al. The effect of epidural analgesia in labour on maternal respiratory function. Anaesthesia 2004; 59:350-3.

Chapter 3

Uteroplacental Blood Flow

Warwick D. Ngan Kee, B.H.B., M.B.Ch.B., M.D., FANZCA, FHKCA, FHKAM

Uteroplacental blood flow is the major determinant of oxygen and nutrient delivery to the fetus. A normal uteroplacental circulation is essential to the growth and development of a healthy fetus. Acute reductions in uteroplacental blood flow may immediately threaten fetal viability. Chronic placental insufficiency related to inadequate development or maintenance of uteroplacental blood flow is associated with disorders such as preeclampsia and intrauterine growth restriction (IUGR) and may even predispose to cardiovascular disease during subsequent adulthood.[1]

The uteroplacental circulation undergoes circadian changes[2] and may be affected by parturition, disease, and anesthetic techniques and drugs. An understanding of the regulation of uteroplacental circulation is an important foundation for the safe provision of obstetric anesthesia. In addition, knowledge of the underlying mechanisms associated with the regulation of uteroplacental blood flow assists in the treatment of many pregnancy-related diseases. Although research in this area is highly active, difficulties and ethical considerations associated with human studies have prompted many investigators to rely on studies in laboratory animals, particularly pregnant sheep and, to a lesser degree, nonhuman primates and other species. Such studies have provided invaluable insight into uteroplacental circulation. However, it is important to appreciate the possibility of interspecies differences. Further, clinicians should always examine the methodologies and contexts of animal research carefully when extrapolating findings into recommendations for clinical anesthesia care.

ANATOMY

The blood supply to the uterus is derived mainly from the uterine arteries (Figure 3-1). The ovarian arteries make a smaller, variable contribution, which increases in late pregnancy in rhesus monkeys.[3] Although the pelvic vasculature shows anatomic variation,[4] the uterine artery arises bilaterally from the anterior division of the internal iliac (hypogastric) artery, whereas the ovarian artery arises from the

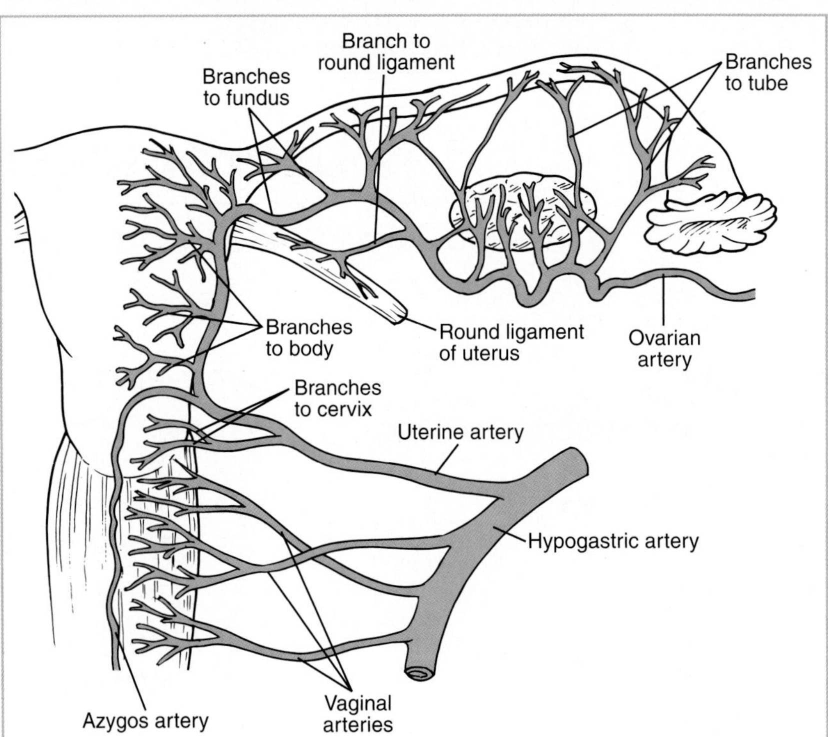

FIGURE 3-1 Arterial supply to the female reproductive tract.

anterolateral abdominal aorta below the renal arteries. The uterine artery passes medially to the side of the uterus, where it supplies branches to the cervix and vagina and ascends between the two layers of the broad ligament, yielding arcuate arteries that supply the body of the uterus to the junction with the fallopian tubes. During pregnancy, flow may differ between the right and left uterine arteries; Konje et al.[5] estimated that vessel diameter was approximately 11% greater and blood flow was approximately 18% greater in the uterine artery on the same side as the placenta than the artery on the contralateral side. Anastomoses are formed with the contralateral uterine artery, the vaginal arteries, and the ovarian arteries. The arcuate arteries give rise to small branches that supply the myometrium and large radial arteries that branch deeply and enter the endometrium to form the convoluted spiral arteries. During gestation, trophoblastic invasion of the spiral arteries results in loss of smooth muscle and the inability of these vessels to constrict; this process underlies the low-resistance nature of the uteroplacental circulation. Abnormal or inadequate trophoblastic invasion is integral to the pathophysiology of preeclampsia.[6]

From the spiral arteries, oxygenated maternal blood enters the intervillous space in fountain-like jets. Blood traveling toward the chorionic plate bathes the villi, permitting the exchange of oxygen, nutrients, and wastes between maternal and fetal blood. Maternal blood then returns to the basal plate and drains into multiple collecting veins. Venous drainage of the uterus occurs via the uterine veins to the internal iliac veins and also via the ovarian veins (utero-ovarian plexus) to the inferior vena cava on the right and the renal vein on the left.[7] In primates, the venous drainage occurs predominantly via the ovarian venous system.[8] The uterine artery and other branches of the anterior division of the internal iliac artery, as well as the ovarian artery, may be targeted during angiographic embolization procedures for treatment of obstetric and gynecologic hemorrhage.[4,9]

CHANGES AND FUNCTION DURING PREGNANCY

Uterine blood flow increases dramatically during pregnancy, rising from 50 to 100 mL/min before pregnancy to approximately 700 to 900 mL/min at term (Figure 3-2). Reported estimates of uterine blood flow vary according to the measurement method, with rates as great as 970 mL/min being observed at term.[5] Studies in sheep have shown that increases in uterine blood flow can be divided into three stages.[10] An initial phase, most likely controlled by the ovarian hormones estrogen and progesterone, occurs before and during implantation and early placentation. A second stage results from the growth and remodeling of the uteroplacental vasculature to support further placental development. A third and final stage results from progressive uterine artery vasodilation to meet the markedly increased nutrient requirements of the rapidly growing fetus. When expressed in terms of uterine weight, however, uterine flow per gram of tissue is particularly high in early gestation, and this ratio decreases as pregnancy progresses.[11] In comparison, umbilical blood flow, expressed as a function of fetal weight, is relatively constant throughout most of pregnancy and is estimated to be 110 to 120 mL/min/kg.[12] Uterine blood flow is increased in twin pregnancy, but the flow per unit of estimated fetal weight is similar to that in a singleton pregnancy.[13]

Primate studies have shown that approximately 80% to 90% of total uterine blood flow perfuses the placenta at

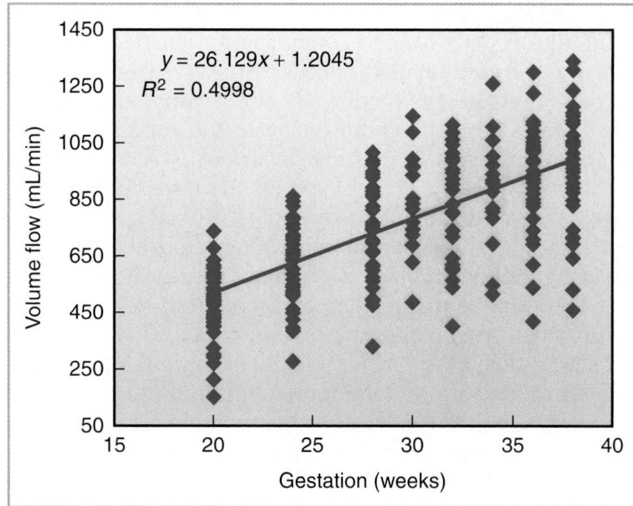

FIGURE 3-2 Changes in uterine artery blood flow with gestation. (From Konje JC, Kaufmann P, Bell SC, Taylor DJ. A longitudinal study of quantitative uterine blood flow with the use of color power angiography in appropriate for gestational age pregnancies. Am J Obstet Gynecol 2001; 185:608-13.)

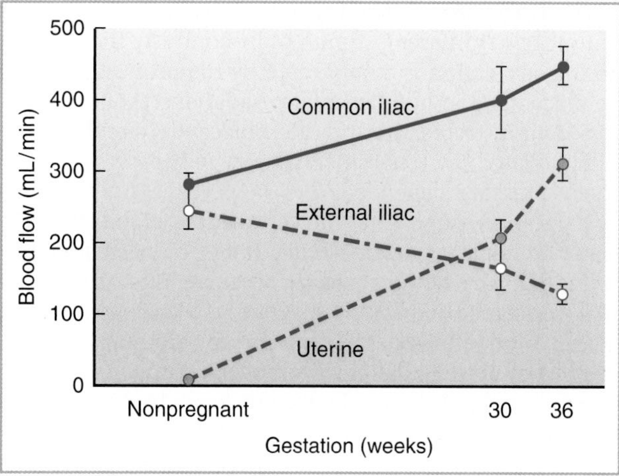

FIGURE 3-4 Redistribution of blood flow in pelvic blood vessels during pregnancy determined unilaterally by Doppler ultrasonography. Blood flow increased in the common iliac and uterine arteries but decreased in the external iliac artery, indicating that redistribution of flow favors uterine perfusion. Data are mean ± SEM. (Adapted from Palmer SK, Zamudio S, Coffin C, et al. Quantitative estimation of human uterine artery blood flow and pelvic blood flow redistribution in pregnancy. Obstet Gynecol 1992; 80:1000-6.)

term, with the remainder supplying the myometrium and nonplacental endometrium.[14] The placental and nonplacental vasculatures are anatomically and functionally distinct, and regulation of perfusion through these vascular beds differs.[14] Therefore, it is important to differentiate studies that measure total uteroplacental blood flow versus placental blood flow. Because mean arterial pressure diminishes slightly during pregnancy, increases in uterine blood flow are achieved by substantial decreases in uterine vascular resistance (Figure 3-3). This change in resistance is created by progressive increases in uterine artery diameter and the development of the widely dilated placental circulation; the hemodynamic characteristics of this placental circulation have been likened to those of an arteriovenous shunt.[15]

Distribution of Blood Flow

Important alterations in the volume and distribution of blood flow occur concomitantly. Uterine blood flow at term represents a greater proportion of cardiac output (approximately 12%) than in early pregnancy (approximately 3.5%).[16] Regional distribution of blood flow within the pelvis also changes during gestation. Palmer et al.[17] observed that increases in common iliac artery blood flow during pregnancy were associated with corresponding increases in uterine artery blood flow but also with decreases in external iliac artery blood flow. This pattern effectively constitutes a "steal" phenomenon, in which blood flow in the pelvis is preferentially redistributed toward the uterus (Figure 3-4).

Functional Classification

Placental vascular function varies among different species. The human multivillous model is commonly thought to function as a "venous equilibrator," in which oxygen tension in the umbilical vein approximates that in the uterine veins. In contrast, the placenta in some species (e.g., rodents) functions as a countercurrent exchanger. The more efficient function of the latter is reflected by the higher fetal-placental weight ratio in rodents (20:1) than in humans (6:1).[18]

Autoregulation

Studies of pressure-flow relationships suggest that the nonpregnant uterine circulation exhibits autoregulation,

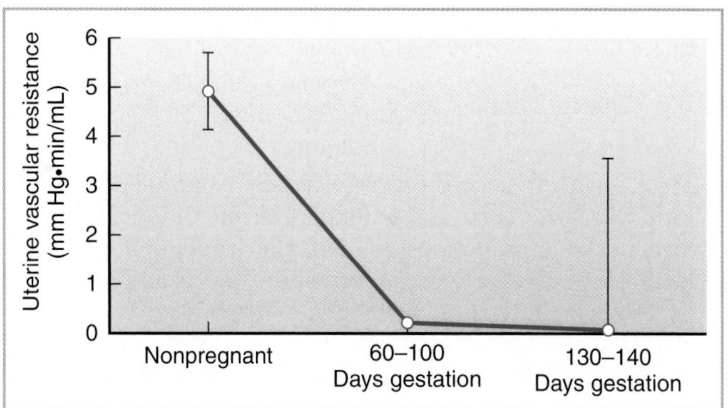

FIGURE 3-3 Changes in uterine vascular resistance with gestation. Data are mean ± SE. (Adapted from Rosenfeld CR. Distribution of cardiac output in ovine pregnancy. Am J Physiol 1977; 232:H231-5.)

alternatively vasoconstricting or vasodilating in response to a number of different stimuli.[19] In contrast, the pregnant uterine circulation is complicated by the properties of both the placental and nonplacental circulations. Animal studies have demonstrated that the uteroplacental circulation is a widely dilated low-resistance system with perfusion that is largely pressure dependent[20-22]; however, a study in pregnant rabbits found that uteroplacental blood flow was relatively constant over a wide range of perfusion pressures.[23] During hemorrhage in pregnant rats, uterine vascular resistance *increased* as systemic blood pressure and uterine blood flow decreased, thereby demonstrating an absence of autoregulation. Moreover, although the uteroplacental circulation is often considered to be maximally vasodilated with little or no ability for autoregulation,[20] further vasodilation has been observed in response to systemically administered estrogen, prostacyclin, bradykinin, and acetylcholine.[24-26] These discrepancies may be explained by changes in the nonplacental uterine vasculature, which accounts for a small fraction of total uteroplacental blood flow but appears to have similar autoregulatory responses during pregnant and nonpregnant states; this feature contrasts with the limited autoregulatory ability of the placental circulation.[27] Laird et al.[22] found that reducing arterial pressure by 22% with an inflatable aortic occluder in pregnant rabbits produced a drop in total uteroplacental and placental blood flow but no significant change in myoendometrial blood flow. Clinically, limited autoregulation results in placental blood flow that most likely decreases with reductions in maternal blood pressure (e.g., after induction of general or neuraxial anesthesia).

Margin of Safety

Studies in animals have demonstrated that, in normal physiologic conditions, uterine blood flow exceeds the minimum required to satisfy fetal oxygen demand.[28] Although this feature confers a margin of safety that protects the fetus from fluctuations in uterine blood flow,[29] decreases in fetal Po_2 and progressive metabolic acidosis can occur with reductions in uteroplacental blood flow, depending on the magnitude and duration.[30] However, the relationship between uterine blood flow and oxygen transfer appears nonlinear and suggests that uteroplacental blood flow can decrease by as much as 50% for limited periods before fetal oxygen uptake decreases and metabolic acidosis occurs.[28]

Studies in sheep have shown that although uterine blood flow varies over a wide range, fetal oxygen uptake remains relatively constant, suggesting that the efficiency of oxygen extraction is greater when perfusion decreases.[31] Using an inflatable balloon occluder around the terminal aorta to reduce uterine blood flow in sheep, Wilkening and Meschia[28] found that at high levels of oxygen delivery, fetal oxygen uptake was not significantly affected by variations in uterine blood flow; moreover, fetal oxygen uptake became flow-dependent only when uterine oxygen delivery was reduced to less than half the baseline value. Boyle et al.,[32] investigating the effects of acute uterine arterial embolization with microspheres in sheep, found a linear decrease in fetal aortic oxygen tension as uterine blood flow decreased. However, uterine oxygen consumption did not decrease and fetal hydrogen ion concentration did not increase until uterine blood flow had dropped to approximately 50% of the baseline value. As uterine blood flow diminished, a reduction in uterine venous oxygen content and a greater arteriovenous oxygen content difference were observed, indicating an increase in oxygen extraction. Gu et al.[33] reported comparable findings with the compression of the common uterine artery by an inflatable occluder in sheep.

Although the preceding experiments were conducted in sheep, the same principles may apply to humans. The human placenta, like the sheep placenta, is a relatively inefficient oxygen exchanger. Thus, in humans and sheep, the transfer rate of oxygen is affected less by decreases in placental perfusion than the transfer rate in animals with more efficient placentas, such as the rabbit and guinea pig. Of interest, this difference may afford some protection in humans, because alterations in placental perfusion in animals with more efficient placentas frequently result in spontaneous abortion.[34] Animal data would also suggest the presence of a significant physiologic buffer that protects the fetus during transient fluctuations in uteroplacental perfusion (e.g., changes in endogenous vasoconstrictor levels, uterine contractions, and parturition).[35] This may partially explain why clinical studies have failed to demonstrate fetal acidosis when alpha-adrenergic agonists are used to maintain maternal blood pressure during neuraxial anesthesia,[36] despite experimental data showing that these agents reduce uteroplacental perfusion in laboratory animals.[37] These observations are based on an assumption of normal physiology; the presence of pathology likely diminishes any margin of safety.

Changes during Parturition

With the onset of the uterine contractions of labor, uteroplacental perfusion undergoes cyclical changes. During uterine contractions, a decrease in perfusion occurs that is inversely related to the strength of the contraction and the rise in intrauterine pressure.[35] Conversely, during uterine relaxation, there is a period of hyperemia when perfusion is increased. Placental perfusion is thought to be more sensitive to these contraction-induced changes than myometrial or endometrial blood flow.[38] Within the first few hours of parturition, uterine blood flow in sheep decreases on average by 50% or more, although there is notable inter-individual variation.[39]

DETERMINANTS OF UTERINE BLOOD FLOW

In the acute setting, uterine blood flow is related to perfusion pressure (the difference between uterine arterial pressure and uterine venous pressure) and vascular resistance, as represented in the following equation:

$$\text{Uterine blood flow} = \frac{\text{Uterine perfusion pressure}}{\text{Uterine vascular resistance}} \quad (1)$$

As a result, there are several ways that uterine blood flow can decrease (Box 3-1). First, uterine blood flow may decline with reductions in perfusion pressure because of decreased uterine arterial pressure—for example, during systemic hypotension from hemorrhage, aortocaval compression, or the sympathetic blockade of neuraxial anesthesia. Second, uterine blood flow may decline with reductions in perfusion pressure caused by increased

BOX 3-1 Causes of Decreased Uterine Blood Flow

Decreased Perfusion Pressure

Decreased uterine arterial pressure:

- Supine position (aortocaval compression)
- Hemorrhage/hypovolemia
- Drug-induced hypotension
- Hypotension during sympathetic blockade

Increased uterine venous pressure:

- Vena caval compression
- Uterine contractions
- Drug-induced uterine hypertonus (oxytocin, local anesthetics)
- Skeletal muscle hypertonus (seizures, Valsalva maneuver)

Increased Uterine Vascular Resistance

Endogenous vasoconstrictors:

- Catecholamines (stress)
- Vasopressin (in response to hypovolemia)

Exogenous vasoconstrictors:

- Epinephrine
- Vasopressors (phenylephrine > ephedrine)
- Local anesthetics (in high concentrations)

uterine venous pressure—for example, with vena caval compression, increased intrauterine pressure during uterine contractions, drug effects (e.g., oxytocin, cocaine), and Valsalva maneuvers that accompany maternal expulsive efforts during the second stage of labor. Third, uterine blood flow may decline because of increased uterine vascular resistance, which may be caused by a number of factors, including endogenous vasoconstrictors that are released in response to stress or hypotension, exogenous vasoconstrictors, and compression of endometrial spiral arterioles with uterine contractions.[38]

MECHANISMS OF REGULATION OF UTEROPLACENTAL BLOOD FLOW

The mechanism by which uteroplacental blood flow increases and is maintained during pregnancy depends on the interaction of a multitude of factors and is the subject of continuing research. During early pregnancy, growth of new blood vessels contributes to increased blood flow. Blood flow continues to rise after the completion of new vessel growth, indicating that vasodilation is a fundamental component. However, the mechanism by which vasodilation is achieved and maintained is not completely understood. Many factors are thought to modulate vasodilation, including vasoconstrictors, endothelium-derived vasodilators, steroid hormones, and shear stress.

Vasoconstrictors

Pregnancy is associated with a generalized reduction in response to endogenous and exogenous vasoconstrictors, including angiotension II, endothelin, thromboxane, epinephrine, norepinephrine, phenylephrine, serotonin, thromboxane, and arginine vasopressin.[40-42] However, the relative refractoriness of the systemic and uterine circulations varies for different agents, a fact that has important implications for the regulation and maintenance of uteroplacental blood flow.

ANGIOTENSIN II

During pregnancy, concentrations of angiotensin II in maternal blood are increased twofold to threefold,[43] whereas the vasopressor response to angiotensin II is attenuated.[44] This refractoriness is diminished in patients in whom preeclampsia develops.[44] Studies have shown the uterine circulation to be *less* responsive than the systemic circulation to the vasoconstrictor effects of angiotensin II.[45] Thus, during infusion of angiotensin II at low rates, uterine blood flow actually increases because the rise in uterine perfusion pressure caused by systemic vasoconstriction has a greater effect than the rise in uterine vascular resistance caused by uterine vasoconstriction.[45] The difference in sensitivity of the uterine and systemic circulations to angiotensin II is considered an important physiologic adaptation during pregnancy that contributes to the redistribution of cardiac output, the increase in uterine blood flow, and, possibly, the maintenance of uterine blood flow during normal fluctuations in blood pressure.[46]

A number of different mechanisms may contribute to the refractoriness of the uteroplacental circulation to angiotensin II. They include alterations in angiotensin II receptor expression and binding, angiotensin II metabolism, uterine vascular smooth muscle response, and local angiotension II antagonists.[47] Although down-regulation of angiotensin II receptors is not thought to occur,[48,49] differences in the expression of angiotensin II receptor subtypes may be important. In large mammals, there are at least two distinct subtypes of angiotensin II receptors, AT_1R and AT_2R. In systemic vascular smooth muscle, AT_1R receptors are predominant and mediate vasoconstriction. In contrast, AT_2R receptors, which do not mediate smooth muscle contraction, account for 75% to 90% of angiotensin II binding in uterine artery smooth muscle.[47,48] Increases in endothelium-derived vasodilators such as prostacyclin and nitric oxide have also been described to be important in modulating uteroplacental response to angiotensin II.[47]

ALPHA-ADRENERGIC AGONISTS

The sensitivity of the vasopressor response to alpha-adrenergic agonists such as epinephrine, norepinephrine, and phenylephrine is attenuated during pregnancy.[50] However, in contrast to the responses to angiotensin II, the uterine circulation is *more* responsive to the vasoconstrictor effects of alpha-adrenergic agonists than the systemic circulation.[50] Thus, during hemorrhage or other major stresses that result in large catecholamine release, it is unlikely that uteroplacental perfusion will be preferentially preserved above essential maternal perfusion.[51] This finding also suggests that uteroplacental perfusion is vulnerable to the effects of exogenous vasoconstrictors given to maintain maternal blood pressure during neuraxial anesthesia.

Vasodilators

PROSTAGLANDINS

The greater synthesis and higher circulating concentrations of vasodilatory prostaglandins during pregnancy[52] are believed to modulate systemic and uterine vascular responses to angiotensin II and other vasoconstrictors.[53] In particular, production of prostacyclin (prostaglandin I_2 [PGI_2]) is increased, as evidenced by greater circulating and urinary concentrations of its stable metabolites.[54] Prostacyclin is produced primarily by the vascular endothelium, and during pregnancy, uterine vascular production is greater than systemic vascular production; this difference most likely underlies a role in maintaining uteroplacental blood flow against the effects of circulating vasoconstrictors.[55] The presence of angiotensin II stimulates the production of prostacyclin, which in turn attenuates the former's effects. An enhanced response to angiotensin II during pregnancy has been demonstrated with the systemic and local infusion of indomethacin, an agent that blocks prostacyclin production.[54] However, inhibition of prostaglandin synthesis by an infusion of indomethacin induces only a transient decrease in uteroplacental blood flow, indicating that uteroplacental blood flow is not solely dependent on the continued production of prostacyclin.[56]

NITRIC OXIDE

Synthesized from arginine in vascular endothelial cells, nitric oxide stimulates soluble guanylate cyclase in vascular smooth muscle, resulting in vascular relaxation through increases in cyclic guanosine monophosphate (cGMP). Synthesis of nitric oxide is an important mechanistic factor underlying changes in systemic and uterine vascular resistance, attenuated responses to vasoconstrictors, and vascular effects of estrogen during pregnancy.[57,58] During pregnancy, uterine arteries have increased endothelial nitric oxide synthase (eNOS) activity, which is associated with higher levels of eNOS messenger ribonucleic acid (mRNA) and eNOS protein; biosynthesis of nitric oxide and levels of cGMP are subsequently elevated.[59,60] Removal of the vascular endothelium diminishes or eliminates the refractoriness of the uterine artery to vasoconstrictors,[41] and inhibition of nitric oxide synthesis by *N*-nitro-L-arginine methyl ester (L-NAME) decreases uterine blood flow and also reverses refractoriness to vasoconstrictors.[61] Long-term inhibition of nitric oxide synthase causes hypertension and fetal growth restriction in rats.[62]

Steroid Hormones

Estrogen and progesterone are thought to interact in the regulation of uteroplacental blood flow in pregnancy. Plasma concentrations of estrogen, initially derived from the ovaries and later predominantly from the placenta, rise concomitantly with the increase in uterine blood flow during pregnancy. Exogenously administered estrogen promotes a marked rise in uterine blood flow that is effected by vasodilation[63] and inhibited by progesterone.[64] Acute estrogen-induced increases in uterine blood flow are associated with nitric oxide–dependent increases in cGMP synthesis and activation of high-conductance vascular smooth muscle potassium channels.[10] Estrogen and pregnancy may alter receptor-mediated G-protein coupling so that a functional decrease in guanosine triphosphatase (GTPase) activity occurs; this may be an important part of the regulatory mechanism.[65]

Vasoactive Substances

Additional vasoactive substances have been investigated for possible roles in the regulation of uteroplacental blood flow. Atrial and brain natriuretic peptides attenuate the response to angiotensin II, and intravenous infusion of atrial natriuretic peptide reduces blood pressure while increasing uterine blood flow in preeclamptic women.[66] Protein kinase C activity is decreased in uterine, but not systemic, arteries of pregnant sheep and may cause vasodilation and an increase in uterine blood flow as part of the regulatory effect on local ovarian and placental estrogen production.[67] Studies in rats have shown a decrease in endogenous endothelin–dependent vasoconstrictor tone in uteroplacental vessels, which may contribute to the increase in placental blood flow observed in late gestation.[68]

Shear Stress

Shear stress, the frictional forces on the vessel wall from blood flow, is thought to be an important stimulus for uteroplacental vasodilation.[69,70] Nitric oxide is considered an important mediator of this effect because increases in eNOS expression and nitric oxide production are witnessed with shear stress, and stripping the endothelium or pretreatment with L-NAME reduces or abolishes flow-induced vasodilation.[69] Studies *in vitro* have shown that shear stress also increases endothelial production of prostacyclin.

METHODS OF MEASUREMENT OF UTEROPLACENTAL BLOOD FLOW

Many techniques have been used to measure uteroplacental blood flow in animals and humans. The approaches used in different studies have varied according to the nature of the experimental question, the existing state of technology, and the ethical considerations and limitations. All methods have an inherent potential for error.

Many past studies of uterine artery flow have measured flow in only one uterine artery, which may not be an accurate representation of total flow, depending on the location of the placenta. The parameter of greatest clinical interest is placental perfusion, but this is not always differentiated from total uterine blood flow, from which it may vary independently. However, in most circumstances, the measurement of intervillous blood flow provides a close approximation of functional placental blood flow. Ovarian arterial blood flow is generally not measured, although it may contribute as much as one sixth of placental perfusion.[3]

Early studies relied on the Fick principle, utilizing substances such as nitrous oxide and 4-amino-antipyrine. A problem with this method is that the venous effluent of the pregnant uterus is collected by several veins, introducing the potential for error.[71] Placental perfusion can also be measured in animals by the injection of radioactive microspheres. This method allows for the separate calculation of placental and myometrial blood flows, but it provides information from only a single point in time. Total uterine arterial blood flow can also be measured (or estimated) with the use of surgically implanted electromagnetic or Doppler flow probes.

Placental perfusion can be measured in humans by the injection of trace amounts of radioactive substances, typically xenon (^{133}Xe).[72] During the washout phase, the rapid decrease in measured radioactivity over the placenta is calculated as a biexponential or triexponential process. The most rapid decay constant is ascribed to intervillous perfusion. Alternatively, radioactively tagged proteins (e.g., albumin) can be injected; scintigraphy is then performed over the placenta for the analysis of blood flow.[73] Although the accuracy of these methods for determining absolute flow is limited, the measurement of relative change over time is probably adequate.

The most common method of assessing uterine blood flow clinically in humans is Doppler ultrasonography.[74] The principle of Doppler shift enables the calculation of red blood cell velocity in blood vessels (V_{RBC}). A pulsed ultrasound signal from a stationery transducer is directed toward the vessel, and reflections scattered from the red blood cells are received (Figure 3-5). Because the red blood cells are moving, the frequency of the received signal differs from the transmitted frequency (f_0) by an amount known as the Doppler shift (Δf). This is proportional to the flow velocity according to the following equation:

$$\Delta f = \frac{2 \times f_0 \times V_{REL}}{c} \quad (2)$$

where c is the speed of sound propagation in tissue and V_{REL} is the vector component of the velocity of flow relative to the direction of the transducer. The latter takes into account the difference between the direction of the ultrasound signal from the direction of flow according to the angle of insonation (θ) (see Figure 3-5). With the use of basic trigonometry, V_{RBC} is related to the relative velocity of flow in the direction of the probe (V_{REL}) according to the following equation:

$$V_{RBC} = \frac{V_{REL}}{\cos\theta} \quad (3)$$

Combining equations 2 and 3 gives the following equation:

$$V_{RBC} = \frac{\Delta f}{f_0} \times \frac{c}{2 \times \cos\theta} \quad (4)$$

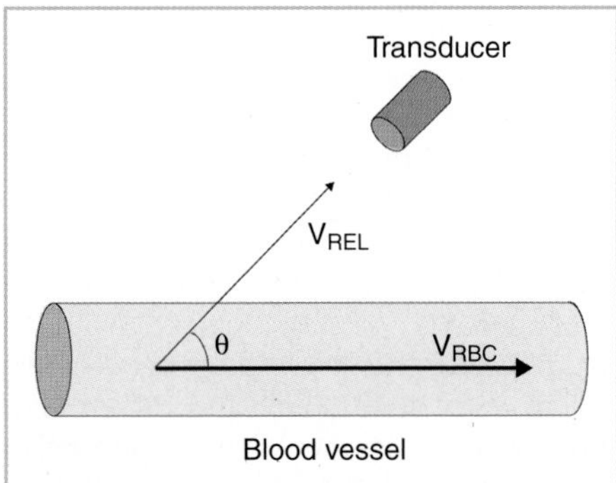

FIGURE 3-5 Principles of use of Doppler ultrasonography to estimate blood flow. Blood flow is calculated as the product of blood vessel cross-sectional area (A) and mean flow velocity in the vessel (V_{RBC}). The latter is derived from the measured flow velocity relative to the direction of the probe (V_{REL}) and requires precise determination of the angle of insonation (θ).

Thus, the flow velocity is estimated from the ratio of the Doppler shift frequency to the transmitted frequency, multiplied by the speed of sound propagation and divided by two times the cosine of the insonation angle.

Information about the velocity of flow in a blood vessel can be utilized in a number of ways. Calculating vessel cross-sectional area (A) (usually by measuring vessel diameter) with two-dimensional (B-mode) ultrasonography and multiplying this value by the mean velocity permits a noninvasive estimation of the volume of blood flow (Q), as follows:

$$Q = V_{RBC} \times A \quad (5)$$

In addition, a number of indices related to vascular impedance can be derived from the flow velocity waveform, with the advantage that the angle of insonation is not required, as follows[74]:

$$\text{Systolic-diastolic (S/D) ratio} = \frac{\text{Systolic (maximum) velocity}}{\text{Diastolic (minimum) velocity}} \quad (6)$$

$$\text{Pulsatility index (PI)} = \frac{\left(\text{Systolic (maximum) velocity} - \text{Diastolic (minimum) velocity}\right)}{\text{Mean velocity}} \quad (7)$$

$$\text{Resistance index (RI)} = \frac{\left(\text{Systolic (maximum) velocity} - \text{Diastolic (minimum) velocity}\right)}{\text{Systolic (maximum) velocity}} \quad (8)$$

There are several potential sources of error in Doppler measurements. The reproducibility of the measurement depends greatly on the examination of the same portion of the same artery each time, and accuracy requires the precise determination of mean velocity, vessel cross-sectional area, and angle of insonation. For example, small errors in the estimation of the angle of insonation can result in blood flow measurement errors as large as 30%.[17] The derived indices can be affected by both "upstream" variables (e.g., cardiac output) and "downstream" variables (e.g., changes in the number and sites of capillaries recruited and open at one time). In addition, studies that assess indices in uterine versus umbilical arteries should be carefully distinguished; the response to various stimuli may be as different as the clinical implications of their respective results. Thus, the methods used in any clinical study that employs Doppler ultrasonography to assess uterine artery blood flow should be examined critically.

NEURAXIAL ANESTHESIA

The effect of neuraxial anesthesia on uteroplacental blood flow depends on the complex interaction of many factors (Box 3-2). Pain and stress during labor may reduce

BOX 3-2 Effects of Neuraxial Anesthesia on Uterine Blood Flow

Increased uterine blood flow as a result of:
- Pain relief
- Decreased sympathetic activity
- Decreased maternal hyperventilation

Decreased uterine blood flow as a result of:
- Hypotension
- Unintentional intravenous injection of local anesthetic and/or epinephrine
- Absorbed local anesthetic (little effect)

uteroplacental blood flow through sympathetic stimulation and the release of circulating catecholamines. Shnider et al.[75] observed that acute stress increased plasma norepinephrine concentrations by 25% and uterine blood flow by 50% in gravid ewes. In laboring women, stress is associated with increased plasma epinephrine concentrations and abnormal fetal heart rate (FHR) patterns. Effective pain relief with neuraxial analgesia decreases circulating concentrations of catecholamines[76] and reduces hyperventilation, and therefore may help protect uteroplacental blood flow. In the absence of hypotension, epidural anesthesia does not change uteroplacental blood flow in pregnant sheep.[77] Human studies suffer from complex interactions of multiple clinical factors and differences in study design; however, studies in laboring women typically have shown either no change or an increase in uteroplacental blood flow following administration of epidural analgesia.[78-82] An increase in uterine vascular resistance indices, however, has been reported.[83] In women with severe preeclampsia, evidence suggests that epidural analgesia using a plain local anesthetic solution reduces indices of uterine artery resistance[79] and increases intervillous blood flow.[84]

The effect of combined spinal-epidural (CSE) anesthesia on uteroplacental blood flow is controversial. Fetal bradycardia has been reported after administration of CSE analgesia during labor,[85] which has been related to maternal hypotension and respiratory depression.[86] An additional postulated mechanism is a decrease in uteroplacental blood flow secondary to uterine hypertonus caused by a rapid decrease in circulating catecholamine concentrations associated with the rapid onset of analgesia[87]; studies are required to confirm this mechanism.

Hypotension

Hypotension occurring during neuraxial block, depending on its magnitude and duration, may decrease uteroplacental blood flow, for several reasons—the reduction in perfusion pressure,[20] reflex release of endogenous vasoconstrictors, diversion (steal) of blood to the lower limbs,[88] and response to administered vasopressors.[37] Spinal anesthesia may be expected to have more profound effects on uteroplacental blood flow than epidural anesthesia, because spinal anesthesia results in a more rapid onset of sympathetic blockade. This difference may account for the observation that umbilical arterial blood pH is lower with spinal anesthesia than with epidural or general anesthesia for cesarean delivery.[89]

Fluid Preload

Intravenous preload (prehydration) is commonly administered before neuraxial block to prevent hypotension, although the efficacy of this approach has been questioned.[90,91] Studies of the effect of fluid preload on uteroplacental blood flow have had mixed results. Most Doppler studies have shown that preload does not change vascular resistance indices,[92-95] although a decrease has been reported.[96] In their study in 14 women, Gogarten et al.[93] found that colloid preload did not affect the uterine artery pulsatility index, although uterine blood flow increased.

Vasopressors

The effects of vasopressors on uteroplacental blood flow and the resulting implications for clinical drug selection are controversial. Historically, ephedrine has been the preferred agent for the treatment of hypotension because animal and *in vitro* studies showed that ephedrine was more effective in the maintenance of uteroplacental blood flow than alpha-adrenergic agonists such as phenylephrine, metaraminol, and methoxamine.[37] Ephedrine's action is mediated predominantly by beta-adrenergic receptor stimulation and increased cardiac output, as opposed to vasoconstriction. Moreover, *in vitro* studies of the effects of ephedrine on blood vessels from pregnant sheep have demonstrated more selective vasoconstrictor activity on femoral versus uterine vessels and decreased uterine vasoconstriction as a result of the release of nitric oxide.[97,98] In contrast, pregnancy increases the uterine arteriolar vasoconstrictor response to phenylephrine.[99,100]

Despite strong experimental support for the use of ephedrine as the preferred vasopressor in obstetrics, its superiority has not been supported by clinical studies. Contrary to expectations, comparisons between ephedrine and alpha-adrenergic agonists (e.g., phenylephrine, metaraminol) have shown that umbilical arterial blood pH and base excess are significantly greater when alpha-adrenergic agonists are used to maintain maternal blood pressure during spinal anesthesia for cesarean delivery (Figure 3-6).[101-103] A comparison of different infusion regimens showed that when phenylephrine was titrated to keep maternal systolic blood pressure near baseline, fetal pH and base excess were not depressed despite the use of very large total doses of phenylephrine (up to 2500 μg) before delivery.[36] In contrast, large doses of ephedrine given at cesarean delivery depressed umbilical arterial blood pH and base excess in a dose-dependent manner.[104]

The explanation for the discrepancy between experimental and clinical data is complex and incompletely determined. Animal studies are not always appropriate models for clinical situations. Under clinical conditions, Doppler studies have shown some evidence that uterine vascular resistance is increased by alpha-adrenergic agonists,[105] but this finding has not been consistent.[103] Although data suggest that alpha-adrenergic agonists increase uterine vascular resistance more than systemic vascular resistance, the difference may be primarily due to an effect in the

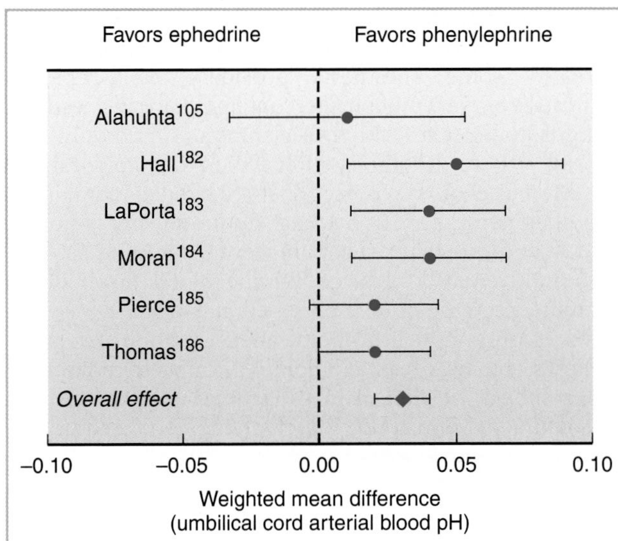

FIGURE 3-6 Results from a meta-analysis of trials comparing phenylephrine and ephedrine for the management of hypotension during spinal anaesthesia for cesarean delivery. The chart shows the effect of choice of vasopressor on umbilical cord arterial pH. Data are mean difference with 95% confidence intervals. (Modified from Lee A, Ngan Kee WD, Gin T. A quantitative systematic review of randomized controlled trials of ephedrine versus phenylephrine for the management of hypotension during spinal anesthesia for cesarean delivery. Anesth Analg 2002; 94:920-6.)

myometrium, with relative sparing of the vessels that perfuse the placenta.[106,107] In addition, the margin of safety of uteroplacental blood flow may allow modest decreases in uterine blood flow (caused by clinically appropriate doses of alpha-adrenergic agonists) without compromising oxygen transfer. Finally, the propensity of ephedrine to worsen fetal acid-base status may not be related to its effects on uteroplacental blood flow but instead may result from ephedrine's direct beta-adrenoceptor–mediated fetal metabolic effects, which follow the transfer of ephedrine across the placenta.[102,108] Ngan Kee et al.[109] found that use of ephedrine was associated with greater placental transfer and higher fetal levels of lactate, glucose, epinephrine, and norepinephrine than use of phenylephrine, a finding consistent with the hypothesis of fetal metabolic stimulation due to ephedrine. Whether the differences in human and sheep placental structures affect the placental transfer of ephedrine has yet to be determined; humans have a hemomonochorial placenta, in which a less substantial tissue layer barrier separates maternal and fetal blood, whereas sheep and other ruminants have synepitheliochorial placentas.[18]

Thus, considering the choice of vasopressor for clinical use, rather than the effect on uteroplacental blood flow in isolation, the clinician should take into account the sum effect on fetal oxygen supply and demand balance. In this respect, clinical studies do not favor the use of ephedrine. In addition, a slow onset and a long duration of action make ephedrine more difficult to titrate than phenylephrine. However, other than showing differences in acid-base measurements, studies comparing ephedrine and other vasopressors in humans have not demonstrated any clinical differences in neonatal outcome. Moreover, the vast majority of clinical data have been obtained from low-risk patients; only limited data are available on the effects of vasopressors on uteroplacental blood flow and neonatal outcome in the presence of fetal compromise or placental insufficiency.

Erkinaro et al.[110,111] developed a sheep model to compare the effects of phenylephrine and ephedrine after a period of experimental fetal hypoxia. Hypotension was induced by epidural anesthesia and then corrected with either phenylephrine or ephedrine. In an initial study, ephedrine was associated with better restoration of uterine artery blood flow, but no differences in fetal acid-base measurements or lactate concentration were observed.[110] However, in a second study, these investigators embolized the placenta with microspheres to model placental insufficiency and found that phenylephrine and ephedrine had similar effects on uterine blood flow and fetal pH and base excess as found in the initial study, with the exception that fetal lactate concentration was greater in the phenylephrine group.[111] Although Erkinaro et al.[111] speculated that this exception might reflect impaired fetal clearance of lactate, the placental embolization may have narrowed the margin of safety for uteroplacental blood flow and increased fetal lactate production in the phenylephrine group. In humans, a 2007 study compared the abilities of phenylephrine and ephedrine to maintain maternal blood pressure during spinal anesthesia for nonelective cesarean delivery.[112] Evidence of fetal compromise was present in 24% of the 204 patients. The results showed that although umbilical arterial and venous blood lactate concentrations were lower in the phenylephrine group, umbilical arterial blood pH and base excess values were similar in the two groups. However, umbilical arterial and venous blood PO_2 measurements were lower in the phenylephrine group, suggesting that although phenylephrine may potentially have caused some reduction in uteroplacental perfusion, adequate oxygen supply was likely maintained by increased oxygen extraction.

In summary, ephedrine and phenylephrine both continue to be used clinically for maintaining maternal blood pressure during administration of neuraxial anesthesia. Although most experimental data suggest that uteroplacental perfusion is likely to be better maintained with ephedrine than with alpha-adrenergic agonists, this advantage may be outweighed by other considerations, such as differences in efficacy for maintaining blood pressure and direct fetal effects that occur from placental transfer of drug.

Local Anesthetics

Studies *in vitro* have shown that local anesthetics constrict arteries directly and inhibit endothelium-mediated vasodilation.[113] High concentrations of local anesthetic can decrease uteroplacental blood flow by stimulating vasoconstriction and myometrial contractility.[114-116] A comparative study in pregnant sheep showed that bupivacaine was more potent than either lidocaine or 2-chloroprocaine in decreasing uterine blood flow (Figure 3-7).[115] However, the adverse effects of local anesthetics were seen only at concentrations in excess of those observed clinically, with two possible exceptions, (1) the unintentional intravenous injection of local anesthetic and (2) the use of paracervical block. At clinically relevant doses, no adverse effect on uteroplacental

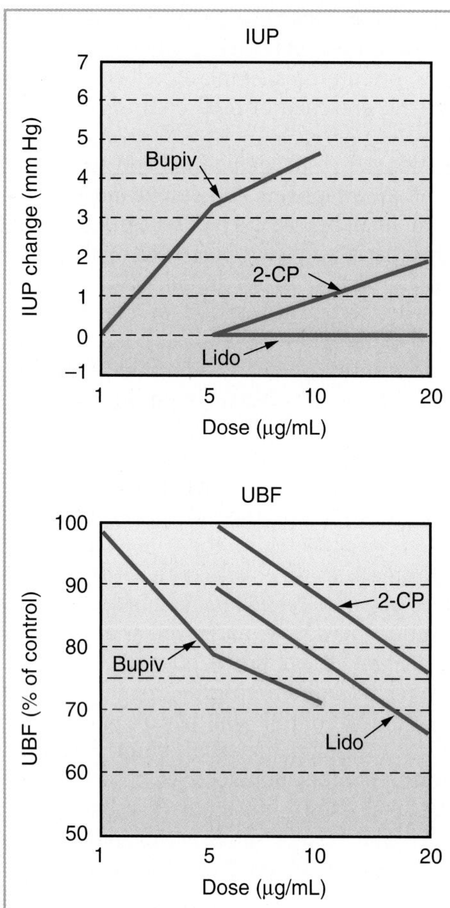

FIGURE 3-7 Effects of injection of local anesthetic agents into the common uterine artery at the aortic trifurcation in pregnant sheep. Bupivacaine (Bupiv) is more potent than lidocaine (Lido) or 2-chloroprocaine (2-CP) with regard to increasing intrauterine pressure (IUP) and decreasing uterine blood flow (UBF). (Adapted from Fishburne JI Jr, Greiss FC Jr, Hopkinson R, Rhyne AL. Responses of the gravid uterine vasculature to arterial levels of local anesthetic agents. Am J Obstet Gynecol 1979; 133:753-61.)

blood flow was reported.[117,118] Although the inherent vasoconstrictor properties of ropivacaine were initially a matter of concern, studies in animals[117] and humans[119] have not shown that administration of ropivacaine results in a reduction in uterine blood flow.

Epinephrine and Alpha$_2$-Adrenergic Agonists

Epinephrine is often combined with local anesthetic agents in obstetric anesthesia. Wallis et al.[77] found that the epidural injection of an epinephrine-containing solution of local anesthetic produced a small, brief reduction in uterine blood flow in pregnant sheep. In contrast, Alahuhta et al.[120] reported that epidural bupivacaine with epinephrine had no effect on intervillous blood flow in women undergoing cesarean delivery. Studies have not shown a reduction in uteroplacental blood flow as a result of the absorption of epinephrine from local anesthetic solutions given epidurally to healthy women during labor.[120,121] However, one study observed that the addition of epinephrine (85 to 100 µg) to epidural bupivacaine increased Doppler indices of uteroplacental vascular resistance in hypertensive parturients with chronic fetal asphyxia.[122] Therefore, some anesthesia providers avoid epidural administration of epinephrine-containing local anesthetic solutions to women with preeclampsia. Commonly, epinephrine (10 to 15 µg) is included in the epidural test dose. Marcus et al.[123] reported that repeated epidural injections of epinephrine (10 to 15 µg) did not decrease uterine blood flow in pregnant sheep; however, the same dose injected intravenously reduced uterine blood flow, with a maximum decrease of 43% observed at 1 minute.

The epidural and intrathecal administration of alpha$_2$-adrenergic agonists (e.g., clonidine, dexmedetomidine) has been a subject of clinical investigations. Intravenous, but not epidural, administration of clonidine decreased uterine blood flow in gravid ewes.[124,125]

Opioids

Opioids are often combined with local anesthetic agents for epidural and intrathecal analgesia in labor and during or after surgery. Intrathecal opioids have been implicated as contributing to a greater risk of fetal bradycardia when used for labor analgesia.[126] The mechanism for this effect has been postulated as an increase in uterine tone and a resulting decrease in uteroplacental blood flow, although further research is needed. Craft et al.[127,128] observed that neither epidural fentanyl nor morphine had a significant effect on uterine blood flow in gravid ewes. Alahuhta et al.[129] reported that epidural sufentanil 50 µg did not alter uterine artery blood flow velocity waveform indices in laboring women. Intrathecal meperidine and sufentanil, however, may be associated with hypotension that may potentially decrease uterine blood flow.[130,131]

GENERAL ANESTHESIA

Induction Agents

Available data suggest that the commonly used induction agents have minimal or no direct adverse effect on uteroplacental blood flow. Allen et al.[132] found that thiopental inhibited the response of human myometrial arteries to contractile agents *in vitro* but had no effect on relaxation induced by prostacyclin. Alon et al.[133] reported that uterine blood flow did not change significantly during induction and maintenance of propofol anesthesia in pregnant sheep. Craft et al.[134] reported that uterine tone increased but uterine blood flow remained constant after an intravenous bolus of ketamine in pregnant sheep. Similarly, Strümper et al.[135] reported that neither racemic nor S$^+$-ketamine affected uterine perfusion in pregnant sheep. Few data are available on the direct effects of etomidate on uteroplacental blood flow.

During intravenous induction of general anesthesia, uteroplacental perfusion may be affected by indirect mechanisms such as blood pressure changes and the sympathetic response to laryngoscopy and endotracheal intubation. Jouppila et al.[136] reported that intervillous blood flow decreased by 22% to 50% during induction of general anesthesia for cesarean delivery with thiopental 4 mg/kg, succinylcholine 1 mg/kg, and endotracheal intubation.

Gin et al.[137] compared thiopental 4 mg/kg and propofol 2 mg/kg in patients undergoing elective cesarean delivery. These investigators found that venous plasma concentrations of epinephrine and norepinephrine rose after endotracheal intubation in both groups, but maximum norepinephrine concentrations were lower in the propofol group; however, no differences in neonatal outcomes were observed. Levinson et al.[138] found that intravenous ketamine raised blood pressure with a concomitant rise in uterine blood flow in pregnant sheep. Addition of a rapid-acting opioid (e.g., alfentanil, remifentanil) during induction of general anesthesia may minimize the increase in circulating catecholamines that occurs after laryngoscopy and endotracheal intubation.[139,140] Although the use of such opioids might attenuate any decrease in uterine blood flow, the potential for neonatal respiratory depression should be considered.

Inhalational Agents

Studies in pregnant sheep have shown that usual clinical doses (i.e., 0.5 to 1.5 minimum alveolar concentration [MAC]) of halothane, isoflurane, enflurane, desflurane, and sevoflurane have little or no effect on uterine blood flow, although deeper planes of anesthesia are associated with reductions in cardiac output, maternal blood pressure, and uterine blood flow.[141,142] Nonetheless, high concentrations of inhalational agents (approximately 2 MAC) have been used during *ex utero* intrapartum treatment (EXIT) procedures, without evidence of impaired fetal gas exchange.[143] A dose-dependent reduction in uterine tone caused by inhalational agents would be expected to increase uterine blood flow in clinical circumstances in which tone is increased (e.g., hyperstimulation with oxytocin, cocaine overdose, placental abruption). Overall, there is little reason to choose one inhalational agent over another on the basis of an agent's effects on uterine blood flow.

Ventilation

Although moderate levels of hypoxemia and hypercapnia do not affect uteroplacental blood flow,[144,145] marked alterations may reduce blood flow indirectly by mechanisms most likely involving sympathetic activation and catecholamine release. The effect of hypocapnia on uteroplacental blood flow is controversial. Some investigators have noted that hyperventilation with hypocapnia caused fetal hypoxia and metabolic acidosis in animals,[146] whereas others have found no effect.[147,148] Levinson et al.[149] observed that positive-pressure ventilation decreased uterine blood flow in pregnant sheep; however, because the addition of carbon dioxide did not improve uterine blood flow, the reduction in blood flow was attributed to the mechanical hyperventilation rather than the hypocapnia. In general, most authorities recommend that hyperventilation be avoided in pregnancy, in part because of concerns about uterine blood flow.

EFFECTS OF OTHER DRUGS

Magnesium Sulfate

Magnesium sulfate increases uterine blood flow in normotensive and hypertensive pregnant sheep.[150,151] Although hypermagnesemia was found to exacerbate maternal hypotension during epidural anesthesia in pregnant sheep, no reduction in uterine blood flow was observed.[150] In women in preterm labor, magnesium sulfate caused a modest decrease in uterine vascular resistance, as determined by Doppler flow studies.[152] Infusion of magnesium caused an increase in uterine blood flow, which was associated with an improvement in red blood cell deformability in women with preeclampsia or IUGR.[153]

Antihypertensive Agents

The effects of hydralazine on uteroplacental blood flow have been assessed during deliberate induction of hypertension in pregnant sheep. Ring et al.[154] found that hydralazine increased uterine blood flow and lowered blood pressure to baseline measurements during an infusion of phenylephrine. Pedron et al.[155] reported an increase in total uteroplacental and myoendometrial blood flow with no change in placental blood flow when hydralazine was given to sheep during an infusion of angiotensin II. Clinical studies have demonstrated no change in uteroplacental blood flow when hydralazine was administered to women with preeclampsia.[156,157] However, Vertommen et al.[158] found that hydralazine did not restore uterine blood flow and caused a marked maternal tachycardia when given to treat cocaine-induced hypertension in pregnant sheep.

Investigations into the effects of labetalol in pregnant animals have had varying results. Labetalol decreased placental perfusion when given to hypertensive pregnant guinea pigs[159] but did not affect placental perfusion in pregnant rats.[160] In pregnant sheep made hypertensive by infusion of norepinephrine, Eisenach et al.[161] found that labetalol lowered maternal blood pressure and increased uterine blood flow. Morgan et al.[162] infused norepinephrine into pregnant baboons and found that labetalol lowered maternal blood pressure; uterine blood flow decreased when 1.0 mg/kg or more of labetalol was infused. Clinical studies in preeclamptic women have shown that labetalol reduces blood pressure without adversely affecting uteroplacental blood flow.[163,164]

Studies of methyldopa in patients with preeclampsia have found either a reduction[165,166] or no change[167] in indices of uterine and placental vascular resistance.

Calcium Entry–Blocking Agents

Murad et al.[168] observed that verapamil 0.2 mg/kg decreased maternal blood pressure and decreased uterine blood flow in pregnant sheep. Studies of nifedipine, which is commonly used as a tocolytic and antihypertensive agent, have yielded conflicting results. Some animal studies have shown that nifedipine decreases uteroplacental blood flow and worsens the fetal condition,[169,170] whereas human studies have shown either no change in uteroplacental blood flow or vascular resistance[171,172] or a decrease in vascular resistance.[173]

Vasodilators

The vasodilators nitroglycerin and sodium nitroprusside are occasionally used for acute control of severe hypertension.

Nitroglycerin has also been used to provide rapid uterine relaxation during episodes of uterine hyperstimulation. Toda et al.[174] found that nitroglycerin caused relaxation of human uterine arteries *in vitro*. Wheeler et al.[175] reported that both nitroglycerin and nitroprusside reduced systemic blood pressure but did not significantly change uterine blood flow or uterine vascular conductance (the reciprocal of resistance) in pregnant sheep; however, in the same experiment, both vasodilators antagonized the vasoconstrictor effect of norepinephrine in pregnant sheep, resulting in vasodilation and an increase in uterine blood flow.[175] Ramsay et al.[176] infused intravenous nitroglycerin in women with abnormal uterine artery blood flow at 24 to 26 weeks' gestation; decreases in the resistance index and the pulsatility index measured by Doppler ultrasonography were observed, indicating the potential for nitroglycerin to increase uterine blood flow. Cacciatore et al.[177] reported that transdermal nitroglycerin administered for 3 days to patients with preeclampsia and IUGR resulted in decreases in the mean uterine pulsatility index and resistance index; the maximal effect was observed on the last treatment day. In contrast, Grunewald et al.[178] reported that an infusion of nitroglycerin in women with severe preeclampsia did not change the pulsatility index of the uterine artery, although a reduction was observed in the umbilical artery.

When interpreting such studies, clinicians should remember that increases in total uterine blood flow do not necessarily result in enhanced placental perfusion. For example, one study noted that an intravenous infusion of adenosine in pregnant sheep also receiving angiotensin II increased total uterine blood flow without changing placental blood flow.[179] Further work is required to define the utility of systemic vasodilators for improving uteroplacental blood flow in clinical practice.

Inotropic Drugs

Positive inotropic drugs are rarely indicated in obstetric patients. On the basis of studies of normal pregnant sheep, milrinone and amrinone may increase uterine blood flow, whereas dopamine and epinephrine may diminish it.[180,181] However, any direct but negative effect of these agents on the uterine vasculature may be blunted by improvements in cardiac function and arterial oxygenation and a decrease in sympathetic outflow. The choice of an inotropic agent should be based primarily on the desired efficacy (i.e., maternal considerations) rather than the potential direct effects on uterine blood flow.

KEY POINTS

- Growth and development of the uteroplacental vasculature and progressive vasodilation allow uteroplacental blood flow to increase during pregnancy. Uteroplacental blood flow constitutes approximately 12% of maternal cardiac output at term.
- Many factors modulate the maintenance and regulation of uteroplacental blood flow, including altered responses to vasoconstrictors, increases in endothelium-derived vasodilators, and the effects of steroid hormones and shear stress.
- The uteroplacental circulation is a widely dilated, low-resistance vascular bed with limited ability for autoregulation. Flow may be reduced by a decrease in uterine arterial pressure, an increase in uterine venous pressure, or an increase in uterine vascular resistance.
- The uteroplacental circulation is comprised of placental and nonplacental circulations that are anatomically and functionally dissimilar.
- Acute or chronic reductions in uteroplacental blood flow may threaten fetal viability and predispose to disorders such as preeclampsia and intrauterine growth restriction. In situations of acute reduction in uteroplacental perfusion, there is a limited margin of safety before fetal oxygen uptake decreases and metabolic acidosis occurs.
- Animal studies are the principal source of uteroplacental blood flow data; thus, clinicians should carefully consider interspecies differences and study methodology when extrapolating experimental findings to clinical practice.
- Doppler ultrasonography is the method most commonly used to estimate uterine blood flow in humans, but the technique has several potential sources of inaccuracy.
- Neuraxial anesthesia can increase uterine blood flow by reducing pain and stress or can decrease uterine blood flow by causing hypotension.
- Although animal studies show that ephedrine protects uteroplacental blood flow better than alpha-adrenergic agonists such as phenylephrine, umbilical arterial blood pH and base excess are lower after administration of ephedrine. This effect may be related to a greater propensity of ephedrine to cross the placenta and have direct metabolic effects on the fetus. Thus, a growing number of obstetric anesthesia providers recommend phenylephrine as a first-line vasopressor for treatment of hypotension associated with neuraxial anesthesia in obstetric patients.
- The doses of general anesthetic agents used clinically have minimal direct effects on uterine blood flow. General anesthesia may reduce uterine blood flow by causing decreased cardiac output as well as hypotension. Conversely, noxious stimulation during light anesthesia may precipitate the release of catecholamines, which results in decreased uterine blood flow.
- For cardiovascular emergencies in pregnant women, the choice of inotropic drug should depend primarily on drug efficacy rather than minor differences in the drugs' direct effects on uterine blood flow.

REFERENCES

1. Couzin J. Quirks of fetal environment felt decades later. Science 2002; 296:2167-9.
2. Harbert GM Jr. Circadian changes in uteroplacental blood flow. In Rosenfeld CR. The Uterine Circulation. Ithaca, NY, Perinatology Press, 1989:157-73.
3. Wehrenberg WB, Chaichareon DP, Dierschke DJ, et al. Vascular dynamics of the reproductive tract in the female rhesus monkey: Relative contributions of ovarian and uterine arteries. Biol Reprod 1977; 17:148-53.
4. Pelage JP, Le Dref O, Soyer P, et al. Arterial anatomy of the female genital tract: Variations and relevance to transcatheter embolization of the uterus. Am J Roentgenol 1999; 172:989-94.
5. Konje JC, Kaufmann P, Bell SC, Taylor DJ. A longitudinal study of quantitative uterine blood flow with the use of color power angiography in appropriate for gestational age pregnancies. Am J Obstet Gynecol 2001; 185:608-13.
6. Brosens IA, Robertson WB, Dixon HG. The role of the spiral arteries in the pathogenesis of preeclampsia. Obstet Gynecol Annu 1972; 1: 177-91.
7. Cicinelli E, Einer-Jensen N, Galantino P, et al. The vascular cast of the human uterus: From anatomy to physiology. Ann N Y Acad Sci 2004; 1034:19-26.
8. Ramsay EM, Martin CB Jr, McGaughey HS Jr, et al. Venous drainage of the placenta in rhesus monkeys: Radiographic studies. Am J Obstet Gynecol 1966; 95:948-55.
9. Banovac F, Lin R, Shah D, et al. Angiographic and interventional options in obstetric and gynecologic emergencies. Obstet Gynecol Clin North Am 2007; 34:599-616.
10. Rosenfeld CR, Roy T, Cox BE. Mechanisms modulating estrogen-induced uterine vasodilation. Vascul Pharmacol 2002; 38:115-25.
11. Rosenfeld CR, Morriss FH Jr, Makowski EL, et al. Circulatory changes in the reproductive tissues of ewes during pregnancy. Gynecol Invest 1974; 5:252-68.
12. Gill RW, Kossoff G, Warren PS, Garrett WJ. Umbilical venous flow in normal and complicated pregnancy. Ultrasound Med Biol 1984; 10:349-63.
13. Rigano S, Boito S, Maspero E, et al. Absolute uterine artery blood flow volume is increased in twin human pregnancies compared to singletons. Ultrasound Obstet Gynecol 2007; 30:506.
14. Novy MJ, Thomas CL, Lees MH. Uterine contractility and regional blood flow responses to oxytocin and prostaglandin E_2 in pregnant rhesus monkeys. Am J Obstet Gynecol 1975; 122:419-33.
15. Longo LD. Maternal blood volume and cardiac output during pregnancy: A hypothesis of endocrinologic control. Am J Physiol 1983; 245:R720-9.
16. Thaler I, Manor D, Itskovitz J, et al. Changes in uterine blood flow during human pregnancy. Am J Obstet Gynecol 1990; 162:121-5.
17. Palmer SK, Zamudio S, Coffin C, et al. Quantitative estimation of human uterine artery blood flow and pelvic blood flow redistribution in pregnancy. Obstet Gynecol 1992; 80:1000-6.
18. Leiser R, Kaufmann P. Placental structure: In a comparative aspect. Exp Clin Endocrinol 1994; 102:122-34.
19. Greiss FC Jr, Anderson SG. Pressure-flow relationship in the nonpregnant uterine vascular bed. Am J Obstet Gynecol 1974; 118:763-72.
20. Greiss FC Jr. Pressure-flow relationship in the gravid uterine vascular bed. Am J Obstet Gynecol 1966; 96:41-7.
21. Berman W Jr, Goodlin RC, Heymann MA, Rudolph AM. Relationships between pressure and flow in the umbilical and uterine circulations of the sheep. Circ Res 1976; 38:262-6.
22. Laird MR, Faber JJ, Binder ND. Maternal placental blood flow is reduced in proportion to reduction in uterine driving pressure. Pediatr Res 1994; 36:102-10.
23. Venuto RC, Cox JW, Stein JH, Ferris TF. The effect of changes in perfusion pressure on uteroplacental blood flow in the pregnant rabbit. J Clin Invest 1976; 57:938-44.
24. Rosenfeld CR, Morriss FH Jr, Battaglia FC, et al. Effect of estradiol-17β on blood flow to reproductive and nonreproductive tissues in pregnant ewes. Am J Obstet Gynecol 1976; 124:618-29.
25. Rosenfeld CR, Worley RJ, Gant N Jr. Uteroplacental blood flow and estrogen production following dehydroisoandrosterone infusion. Obstet Gynecol 1977; 50:304-7.
26. Still JG, Greiss FC Jr. The effect of prostaglandins and other vasoactive substances on uterine blood flow and myometrial activity. Am J Obstet Gynecol 1978; 130:1-8.
27. Greiss FC Jr. Uterine blood flow: An overview since Barcroft. In Rosenfeld CR. The Uterine Circulation. Ithaca, NY, Perinatology Press, 1989:3-15.
28. Wilkening RB, Meschia G. Fetal oxygen uptake, oxygenation, and acid-base balance as a function of uterine blood flow. Am J Physiol 1983; 244:H749-55.
29. Meschia G. Safety margin of fetal oxygenation. J Reprod Med 1985; 30:308-11.
30. Skillman CA, Plessinger MA, Woods JR, Clark KE. Effect of graded reductions in uteroplacental blood flow on the fetal lamb. Am J Physiol 1985; 249:H1098-105.
31. Clapp JF III. The relationship between blood flow and oxygen uptake in the uterine and umbilical circulations. Am J Obstet Gynecol 1978; 132:410-3.
32. Boyle JW, Lotgering FK, Longo LD. Acute embolization of the uteroplacental circulation: Uterine blood flow and placental CO diffusing capacity. J Dev Physiol 1984; 6:377-86.
33. Gu W, Jones CT, Parer JT. Metabolic and cardiovascular effects on fetal sheep of sustained reduction of uterine blood flow. J Physiol 1985; 368:109-29.
34. Faber JJ. Review of flow limited transfer in the placenta. Int J Obstet Anesth 1995; 4:230-7.
35. Assali NS, Dasgupta K, Kolin A, Holms L. Measurement of uterine blood flow and uterine metabolism. V. Changes during spontaneous and induced labor in unanesthetized pregnant sheep and dogs. Am J Physiol 1958; 195:614-20.
36. Ngan Kee WD, Khaw KS, Ng FF. Comparison of phenylephrine infusion regimens for maintaining maternal blood pressure during spinal anaesthesia for Caesarean section. Br J Anaesth 2004; 92:469-74.
37. Ralston DH, Shnider SM, deLorimier AA. Effects of equipotent ephedrine, metaraminol, mephentermine, and methoxamine on uterine blood flow in the pregnant ewe. Anesthesiology 1974; 40:354-70.
38. Rosenfeld CR. Changes in uterine blood flow during pregnancy. In Rosenfeld CR. The Uterine Circulation. Ithaca, NY, Perinatology Press, 1989:135-56.
39. Caton D, Wilcox CJ, Kalra PS. Correlation of rate of uterine blood flow and plasma steroid concentrations at parturition in sheep. J Reprod Fertil 1980; 58:329-37.
40. Yang D, Clark KE. Effect of endothelin-1 on the uterine vasculature of the pregnant and estrogen-treated nonpregnant sheep. Am J Obstet Gynecol 1992; 167:1642-50.
41. Weiner CP, Thompson LP, Liu KZ, Herrig JE. Endothelium-derived relaxing factor and indomethacin-sensitive contracting factor alter arterial contractile responses to thromboxane during pregnancy. Am J Obstet Gynecol 1992; 166:1171-8.
42. Weiner CP, Martinez E, Chestnut DH, Ghodsi A. Effect of pregnancy on uterine and carotid artery response to norepinephrine, epinephrine, and phenylephrine in vessels with documented functional endothelium. Am J Obstet Gynecol 1989; 161:1605-10.
43. Wier RJ, Brown JJ, Fraser R, et al. Relationship between plasma renin, renin-substrate, angiotensin II, aldosterone and electrolytes in normal pregnancy. J Clin Endocrinol Metab 1975; 40:108-15.
44. Chesley LC, Talledo E, Bohler CS, Zuspan FP. Vascular reactivity to angiotension II and norepinephrine in pregnant women. Am J Obstet Gynecol 1965; 91:837-42.
45. Naden RP, Rosenfeld CR. Effect of angiotensin II on uterine and systemic vasculature in pregnant sheep. J Clin Invest 1981; 68:468-74.
46. Rosenfeld CR. Consideration of the uteroplacental circulation in intrauterine growth. Semin Perinatol 1984; 8:42-51.
47. Rosenfeld CR. Mechanisms regulating angiotensin II responsiveness by the uteroplacental circulation. Am J Physiol Regul Integr Comp Physiol 2001; 281:R1025-40.

48. Cox BE, Rosenfeld CR, Kalinyak JE, et al. Tissue specific expression of vascular smooth muscle angiotensin II receptor subtypes during ovine pregnancy. Am J Physiol 1996; 271:H212-21.
49. Mackanjee HR, Shaul PW, Magness RR, Rosenfeld CR. Angiotensin II vascular smooth-muscle receptors are not down-regulated in near-term pregnant sheep. Am J Obstet Gynecol 1991; 165:1641-8.
50. Magness RR, Rosenfeld CR. Systemic and uterine responses to alpha-adrenergic stimulation in pregnant and nonpregnant ewes. Am J Obstet Gynecol 1986; 155:897-904.
51. Bruce NW. Effects of acute maternal hemorrhage on uterine blood flow in the pregnant rat. J Appl Physiol 1973; 35:564-9.
52. Magness RR, Mitchell MD, Rosenfeld CR. Uteroplacental production of eicosanoids in ovine pregnancy. Prostaglandins 1990; 39:75-88.
53. Clark KE, Ryan MJ, Brody MJ. Effect of prostaglandins on vascular resistance and adrenergic vasoconstrictor responses in the canine uterus. Prostaglandins 1976; 12:71-82.
54. Magness RR, Rosenfeld CR, Faucher DJ, Mitchell MD. Uterine prostaglandin production in ovine pregnancy: Effects of angiotensin II and indomethacin. Am J Physiol 1992; 263:H188-97.
55. Magness RR, Rosenfeld CR, Hassan A, Shaul PW. Endothelial vasodilator production by uterine and systemic arteries. I. Effects of ANG II on PGI_2 and NO in pregnancy. Am J Physiol 1996; 270: H1914-23.
56. Naden RP, Iliya CA, Arant BS Jr, et al. Hemodynamic effects of indomethacin in chronically instrumented pregnant sheep. Am J Obstet Gynecol 1985; 151:484-94.
57. Weiner CP, Thompson LP. Nitric oxide and pregnancy. Semin Perinatol 1997; 21:367-80.
58. Rosenfeld CR, Cox BE, Roy T, Magness RR. Nitric oxide contributes to estrogen-induced vasodilation of the ovine uterine circulation. J Clin Invest 1996; 98:2158-66.
59. Sladek SM, Magness RR, Conrad KP. Nitric oxide and pregnancy. Am J Physiol 1997; 272:R441-63.
60. Conrad KP, Joffe GM, Kruszyna H, et al. Identification of increased nitric oxide biosynthesis during pregnancy in rats. FASEB J 1993; 7:566-71.
61. Miller SL, Jenkin G, Walker DW. Effect of nitric oxide synthase inhibition on the uterine vasculature of the late-pregnant ewe. Am J Obstet Gynecol 1999; 180:1138-45.
62. Yallampalli C, Garfield RE. Inhibition of nitric oxide synthesis in rats during pregnancy produces signs similar to those of preeclampsia. Am J Obstet Gynecol 1993; 169:1316-20.
63. Magness RR, Rosenfeld CR. Local and systemic estradiol-17 beta: Effects on uterine and systemic vasodilation. Am J Physiol 1989; 256:E536-42.
64. Resnik R, Brink GW, Plumer MH. The effect of progesterone on estrogen-induced uterine blood flow. Am J Obstet Gynecol 1977; 128: 251-4.
65. Buhimschi IA, Hall G, Thompson LP, Weiner CP. Pregnancy and estradiol decrease GTPase activity in the guinea pig uterine artery. Am J Physiol Heart Circ Physiol 2001; 281:H2168-75.
66. Grunewald C, Nisell H, Jansson T, et al. Possible improvement in uteroplacental blood flow during atrial natriuretic peptide infusion in preeclampsia. Obstet Gynecol 1994; 84:235-9.
67. Magness RR, Rosenfeld CR, Carr BR. Protein kinase C in uterine and systemic arteries during ovarian cycle and pregnancy. Am J Physiol 1991; 260:E464-70.
68. Ajne G, Nisell H, Wolff K, Jansson T. The role of endogenous endothelin in the regulation of uteroplacental and renal blood flow during pregnancy in conscious rats. Placenta 2003; 24:813-8.
69. Li Y, Zheng J, Bird IM, Magness RR. Effects of pulsatile shear stress on signaling mechanisms controlling nitric oxide production, endothelial nitric oxide synthase phosphorylation, and expression in ovine fetoplacental artery endothelial cells. Endothelium 2005; 12:21-39.
70. Joyce JM, Phernetton TM, Magness RR. Effect of uterine blood flow occlusion on shear stress-mediated nitric oxide production and endothelial nitric oxide synthase expression during ovine pregnancy. Biol Reprod 2002; 67:320-6.
71. Meschia G. Techniques for the study of the uteroplacental circulation. In Rosenfeld CR. The Uterine Circulation. Ithaca, NY, Perinatology Press, 1989:35-51.
72. Jouppila R, Jouppila P, Hollmen A, Kuikka J. Effect of segmental extradural analgesia on placental blood flow during normal labour. Br J Anaesth 1978; 50:563-7.
73. Skjoldebrand A, Eklund J, Johansson H, et al. Uteroplacental blood flow measured by placental scintigraphy during epidural anaesthesia for caesarean section. Acta Anaesthesiol Scand 1990; 34:79-84.
74. Boote EJ. AAPM/RSNA physics tutorial for residents: Topics in US: Doppler US techniques: Concepts of blood flow detection and flow dynamics. Radiographics 2003; 23:1315-27.
75. Shnider SM, Wright RG, Levinson G, et al. Uterine blood flow and plasma norepinephrine changes during maternal stress in the pregnant ewe. Anesthesiology 1979; 50:524-7.
76. Shnider SM, Abboud TK, Artal R, et al. Maternal catecholamines decrease during labor after lumbar epidural anesthesia. Am J Obstet Gynecol 1983; 147:13-5.
77. Wallis KL, Shnider SM, Hicks JS, Spivey HT. Epidural anesthesia in the normotensive pregnant ewe: Effects on uterine blood flow and fetal acid-base status. Anesthesiology 1976; 44:481-7.
78. Jouppila R, Jouppila P, Kuikka J, Hollmen A. Placental blood flow during caesarean section under lumbar extradural analgesia. Br J Anaesth 1978; 50:275-9.
79. Ramos-Santos E, Devoe LD, Wakefield ML, et al. The effects of epidural anesthesia on the Doppler velocimetry of umbilical and uterine arteries in normal and hypertensive patients during active term labor. Obstet Gynecol 1991; 77:20-6.
80. Hollmen AI, Jouppila R, Jouppila P, et al. Effect of extradural analgesia using bupivacaine and 2-chloroprocaine on intervillous blood flow during normal labour. Br J Anaesth 1982; 54:837-42.
81. Hughes AB, Devoe LD, Wakefield ML, Metheny WP. The effects of epidural anesthesia on the Doppler velocimetry of umbilical and uterine arteries in normal term labor. Obstet Gynecol 1990; 75: 809-12.
82. Patton DE, Lee W, Miller J, Jones M. Maternal, uteroplacental, and fetoplacental hemodynamic and Doppler velocimetric changes during epidural anesthesia in normal labor. Obstet Gyecol 1991; 77:17-9.
83. Chen LK, Lin CJ, Huang CH, et al. The effects of continuous epidural analgesia on Doppler velocimetry of uterine arteries during different periods of labour analgesia. Br J Anaesth 2006; 96:226-30.
84. Jouppila P, Jouppila R, Hollmen A, Koivula A. Lumbar epidural analgesia to improve intervillous blood flow during labor in severe preeclampsia. Obstet Gynecol 1982; 59:158-61.
85. Clarke VT, Smiley RM, Finster M. Uterine hyperactivity after intrathecal injection of fentanyl for analgesia during labor: A cause of fetal bradycardia? Anesthesiology 1994; 81:1083.
86. Lu JK, Manullang TR, Staples MH, et al. Maternal respiratory arrests, severe hypotension, and fetal distress after administration of intrathecal sufentanil, and bupivacaine after intravenous fentanyl. Anesthesiology 1997; 87:170-2.
87. Friedlander JD, Fox HE, Cain CF, et al. Fetal bradycardia and uterine hyperactivity following subarachnoid administration of fentanyl during labor. Reg Anesth 1997; 22:378-81.
88. Baumann H, Alon E, Atanassoff P, et al. Effect of epidural anesthesia for cesarean delivery on maternal femoral arterial and venous, uteroplacental, and umbilical blood flow velocities and waveforms. Obstet Gynecol 1990; 75:194-8.
89. Reynolds F, Seed PT. Anaesthesia for Caesarean section and neonatal acid-base status: A meta-analysis. Anaesthesia 2005; 60:636-53.
90. Jackson R, Reid JA, Thorburn J. Volume preloading is not essential to prevent spinal-induced hypotension at Caesarean section. Br J Anaesth 1995; 75:262-5.
91. Ngan Kee WD, Khaw KS, Lee BB, et al. Metaraminol infusion for maintenance of arterial pressure during spinal anesthesia for cesarean delivery: The effect of a crystalloid bolus. Anesth Analg 2001; 93:703-8.

92. Tercanli S, Schneider M, Visca E, et al. Influence of volume preloading on uteroplacental and fetal circulation during spinal anaesthesia for caesarean section in uncomplicated singleton pregnancies. Fetal Diagn Ther 2002; 17:142-6.
93. Gogarten W, Struemper D, Gramke HF, et al. Assessment of volume preload on uteroplacental blood flow during epidural anaesthesia for Caesarean section. Eur J Anaesthesiol 2005; 22:359-62.
94. Long MG, Price M, Spencer JA. Uteroplacental perfusion after epidural analgesia for elective caesarean section. Br J Obstet Gynaecol 1988; 95:1081-2.
95. Morrow RJ, Rolbin SH, Ritchie JW, Haley S. Epidural anaesthesia and blood flow velocity in mother and fetus. Can J Anaesth 1989; 36:519-22.
96. Giles WB, Lah FX, Trudinger BJ. The effect of epidural anaesthesia for caesarean section on maternal uterine and fetal umbilical artery blood flow velocity waveforms. Br J Obstet Gynaecol 1987; 94:55-9.
97. Tong C, Eisenach JC. The vascular mechanism of ephedrine's beneficial effect on uterine perfusion during pregnancy. Anesthesiology 1992; 76:792-8.
98. Li P, Tong C, Eisenach JC. Pregnancy and ephedrine increase the release of nitric oxide in ovine uterine arteries. Anesth Analg 1996; 82:288-93.
99. D'Angelo G, Osol G. Regional variation in resistance artery diameter responses to alpha-adrenergic stimulation during pregnancy. Am J Physiol 1993; 264:H78-85.
100. Wang SY, Datta S, Segal S. Pregnancy alters adrenergic mechanisms in uterine arterioles of rats. Anesth Analg 2002; 94:1304-9.
101. Lee A, Ngan Kee WD, Gin T. A quantitative systematic review of randomized controlled trials of ephedrine versus phenylephrine for the management of hypotension during spinal anesthesia for cesarean delivery. Anesth Analg 2002; 94:920-6.
102. Cooper DW, Carpenter M, Mowbray P, et al. Fetal and maternal effects of phenylephrine and ephedrine during spinal anesthesia for cesarean delivery. Anesthesiology 2002; 97:1582-90.
103. Ngan Kee WD, Lau TK, Khaw KS, Lee BB. Comparison of metaraminol and ephedrine infusions for maintaining arterial pressure during spinal anesthesia for elective cesarean section. Anesthesiology 2001; 95:307-13.
104. Ngan Kee WD, Khaw KS, Lee BB, et al. A dose-response study of prophylactic intravenous ephedrine for the prevention of hypotension during spinal anesthesia for cesarean delivery. Anesth Analg 2000; 90:1390-5.
105. Alahuhta S, Räsänen J, Jouppila P, et al. Ephedrine and phenylephrine for avoiding maternal hypotension due to spinal anaesthesia for caesarean section: Effects on uteroplacental and fetal haemodynamics. Int J Obstet Anesth 1992; 1:129-34.
106. Rosenfeld CR, West J. Circulatory response to systemic infusion of norepinephrine in the pregnant ewe. Am J Obstet Gynecol 1977; 127:376-83.
107. Greiss FC Jr. Differential reactivity of the myoendometrial and placental vasculatures: Adrenergic responses. Am J Obstet Gynecol 1972; 112:20-30.
108. Ngan Kee WD, Lee A. Multivariate analysis of factors associated with umbilical arterial pH and standard base excess after Caesarean section under spinal anaesthesia. Anaesthesia 2003; 58:125-30.
109. Ngan Kee WD, Khaw KS, Tan P, Ng FF. Vasopressor drugs in regional anaesthesia for obstetrics: Quantification of transplacental transfer and determination of metabolic effects on the fetus. Asian J Anaesthesiol 2007; 8:13.
110. Erkinaro T, Mäkikallio K, Kavasmaa T, et al. Effects of ephedrine and phenylephrine on uterine and placental circulations and fetal outcome following fetal hypoxaemia and epidural-induced hypotension in a sheep model. Br J Anaesth 2004; 93:825-32.
111. Erkinaro T, Kavasmaa T, Päkkilä M, et al. Ephedrine and phenylephrine for the treatment of maternal hypotension in a chronic sheep model of increased placental vascular resistance. Br J Anaesth 2006; 96:231-7.
112. Ngan Kee W, Khaw K, Ng K, et al. Randomized double-blinded comparison of phenylephrine versus ephedrine for treating hypotension during spinal anaesthesia for emergency Caesarean section (abstract). Eur J Anaesthesiol 2007; 24(Suppl S39):143.
113. Johns RA. Local anesthetics inhibit endothelium-dependent vasodilation. Anesthesiology 1989; 70:805-11.
114. Greiss FC Jr, Still JG, Anderson SG. Effects of local anesthetic agents on the uterine vasculatures and myometrium. Am J Obstet Gynecol 1976; 124:889-99.
115. Fishburne JI Jr, Greiss FC Jr, Hopkinson R, Rhyne AL. Responses of the gravid uterine vasculature to arterial levels of local anesthetic agents. Am J Obstet Gynecol 1979; 133:753-61.
116. Chestnut DH, Weiner CP, Herrig JE. The effect of intravenously administered 2-chloroprocaine upon uterine artery blood flow velocity in gravid guinea pigs. Anesthesiology 1989; 70:305-8.
117. Santos AC, Arthur GR, Roberts DJ, et al. Effect of ropivacaine and bupivacaine on uterine blood flow in pregnant ewes. Anesth Analg 1992; 74:62-7.
118. Biehl D, Shnider SM, Levinson G, Callender K. The direct effects of circulating lidocaine on uterine blood flow and foetal well-being in the pregnant ewe. Can Anaesth Soc J 1977; 24:445-51.
119. Alahuhta S, Räsänen J, Jouppila P, et al. The effects of epidural ropivacaine and bupivacaine for cesarean section on uteroplacental and fetal circulation. Anesthesiology 1995; 83:23-32.
120. Alahuhta S, Räsänen J, Jouppila R, et al. Effects of extradural bupivacaine with adrenaline for caesarean section on uteroplacental and fetal circulation. Br J Anaesth 1991; 67:678-82.
121. Albright GA, Jouppila R, Hollmen AI, et al. Epinephrine does not alter human intervillous blood flow during epidural anesthesia. Anesthesiology 1981; 54:131-5.
122. Alahuhta S, Räsänen J, Jouppila P, et al. Uteroplacental and fetal circulation during extradural bupivacaine-adrenaline and bupivacaine for caesarean section in hypertensive pregnancies with chronic fetal asphyxia. Br J Anaesth 1993; 71:348-53.
123. Marcus MA, Gogarten W, Vertommen JD, et al. Haemodynamic effects of repeated epidural test-doses of adrenaline in the chronic maternal-fetal sheep preparation. Eur J Anaesthesiol 1998; 15:320-3.
124. Eisenach JC, Castro MI, Dewan DM, et al. Intravenous clonidine hydrochloride toxicity in pregnant ewes. Am J Obstet Gynecol 1989; 160:471-6.
125. Eisenach JC, Castro MI, Dewan DM, Rose JC. Epidural clonidine analgesia in obstetrics: Sheep studies. Anesthesiology 1989; 70:51-6.
126. Mardirosoff C, Dumont L, Boulvain M, Tramèr MR. Fetal bradycardia due to intrathecal opioids for labour analgesia: A systematic review. Br J Obstet Gynaecol 2002; 109:274-81.
127. Craft JB Jr, Coaldrake LA, Bolan JC, et al. Placental passage and uterine effects of fentanyl. Anesth Analg 1983; 62:894-8.
128. Craft JB Jr, Bolan JC, Coaldrake LA, et al. The maternal and fetal cardiovascular effects of epidural morphine in the sheep model. Am J Obstet Gynecol 1982; 142:835-9.
129. Alahuhta S, Räsänen J, Jouppila P, et al. Epidural sufentanil and bupivacaine for labor analgesia and Doppler velocimetry of the umbilical and uterine arteries. Anesthesiology 1993; 78:231-6.
130. Ngan Kee WD. Intrathecal pethidine: A review of pharmacology and clinical applications. Anaesth Intensive Care 1998; 26:137-46.
131. D'Angelo R, Anderson MT, Philip J, Eisenach JC. Intrathecal sufentanil compared to epidural bupivacaine for labor analgesia. Anesthesiology 1994; 80:1209-15.
132. Allen J, Svane D, Petersen LK, et al. Effects of thiopentone and chlormethiazole on human myometrial arteries from term pregnant women. Br J Anaesth 1992; 68:256-60.
133. Alon E, Ball RH, Gillie MH, et al. Effects of propofol and thiopental on maternal and fetal cardiovascular and acid-base variables in the pregnant ewe. Anesthesiology 1993; 78:562-76.
134. Craft JB Jr, Coaldrake LA, Yonekura ML, et al. Ketamine, catecholamines, and uterine tone in pregnant ewes. Am J Obstet Gynecol 1983; 146:429-34.

135. Strümper D, Gogarten W, Durieux ME, et al. The effects of S+-ketamine and racemic ketamine on uterine blood flow in chronically instrumented pregnant sheep. Anesth Analg 2004; 98: 497-502.
136. Jouppila P, Kuikka J, Jouppila R, Hollmén A. Effect of induction of general anesthesia for cesarean section on intervillous blood flow. Acta Obstet Gynecol Scand 1979; 58:249-53.
137. Gin T, O'Meara ME, Kan AF, et al. Plasma catecholamines and neonatal condition after induction of anaesthesia with propofol or thiopentone at Caesarean section. Br J Anaesth 1993; 70:311-6.
138. Levinson G, Shnider SM, Gildea JE, deLorimier AA. Maternal and foetal cardiovascular and acid-base changes during ketamine anaesthesia in pregnant ewes. Br J Anaesth 1973; 45:1111-5.
139. Gin T, Ngan Kee WD, Siu YK, et al. Alfentanil given immediately before the induction of anesthesia for elective cesarean delivery. Anesth Analg 2000; 90:1167-72.
140. Ngan Kee WD, Khaw KS, Ma KC, et al. Maternal and neonatal effects of remifentanil at induction of general anesthesia for cesarean delivery: A randomized, double-blind, controlled trial. Anesthesiology 2006; 104:14-20.
141. Palahniuk RJ, Shnider SM. Maternal and fetal cardiovascular and acid-base changes during halothane and isoflurane anesthesia in the pregnant ewe. Anesthesiology 1974; 41:462-72.
142. Stein D, Masaoka T, Wlody D, et al. The effects of sevoflurane and isoflurane in pregnant sheep: Uterine blood flow and fetal well-being. Anesthesiology 2007; 75:851.
143. Dahlgren G, Tornberg DC, Pregner K, Irestedt L. Four cases of the ex utero intrapartum treatment (EXIT) procedure: Anesthetic implications. Int J Obstet Anesth 2004; 13:178-82.
144. Greiss FC Jr, Anderson SG, King LC. Uterine vascular bed: Effects of acute hypoxia. Am J Obstet Gynecol 1972; 113:1057-64.
145. Makowski EL, Hertz RH, Meschia G. Effects of acute maternal hypoxia and hyperoxia on the blood flow to the pregnant uterus. Am J Obstet Gynecol 1973; 115:624-31.
146. Motoyama EK, Rivard G, Acheson F, Cook CD. Adverse effect of maternal hyperventilation on the foetus. Lancet 1966; 1(7432): 286-8.
147. Parer JT, Eng M, Aoba H, Ueland K. Uterine blood flow and oxygen uptake during maternal hyperventilation in monkeys at cesarean section. Anesthesiology 1970; 32:130-5.
148. Lumley J, Renou P, Newman W, Wood C. Hyperventilation in obstetrics. Am J Obstet Gynecol 1969; 103:847-55.
149. Levinson G, Shnider SM, deLorimier AA, Steffenson JL. Effects of maternal hyperventilation on uterine blood flow and fetal oxygenation and acid-base status. Anesthesiology 1974; 40:340-7.
150. Vincent RD Jr, Chestnut DH, Sipes SL, et al. Magnesium sulfate decreases maternal blood pressure but not uterine blood flow during epidural anesthesia in gravid ewes. Anesthesiology 1991; 74: 77-82.
151. Dandavino A, Woods JR Jr, Murayama K, et al. Circulatory effects of magnesium sulfate in normotensive and renal hypertensive pregnant sheep. Am J Obstet Gynecol 1977; 127:769-74.
152. Keeley MM, Wade RV, Laurent SL, Hamann VD. Alterations in maternal-fetal Doppler flow velocity waveforms in preterm labor patients undergoing magnesium sulfate tocolysis. Obstet Gynecol 1993; 81:191-4.
153. Schauf B, Mannschreck B, Becker S, et al. Evaluation of red blood cell deformability and uterine blood flow in pregnant women with preeclampsia or IUGR and reduced uterine blood flow following the intravenous application of magnesium. Hypertens Pregnancy 2004; 23:331-43.
154. Ring G, Krames E, Shnider SM, et al. Comparison of nitroprusside and hydralazine in hypertensive pregnant ewes. Obstet Gynecol 1977; 50:598-602.
155. Pedron SL, Reid DL, Barnard JM, et al. Differential effects of intravenous hydralazine on myoendometrial and placental blood flow in hypertensive pregnant ewes. Am J Obstet Gynecol 1992; 167:1672-8.
156. Jouppila P, Kirkinen P, Koivula A, Ylikorkala O. Effects of dihydralazine infusion on the fetoplacental blood flow and maternal prostanoids. Obstet Gynecol 1985; 65:115-8.
157. Janbu T, Nesheim BI. The effect of dihydralazine on blood velocity in branches of the uterine artery in pregnancy induced hypertension. Acta Obstet Gynecol Scand 1989; 68:395-400.
158. Vertommen JD, Hughes SC, Rosen MA, et al. Hydralazine does not restore uterine blood flow during cocaine-induced hypertension in the pregnant ewe. Anesthesiology 1992; 76:580-7.
159. Verkeste CM, Peeters LL. The effect of labetalol on maternal haemodynamics and placental perfusion in awake near term guinea pigs. Eur J Obstet Gynecol Reprod Biol 1995; 58:177-81.
160. Ahokas RA, Mabie WC, Sibai BM, Anderson GD. Labetalol does not decrease placental perfusion in the hypertensive term-pregnant rat. Am J Obstet Gynecol 1989; 160:480-4.
161. Eisenach JC, Mandell G, Dewan DM. Maternal and fetal effects of labetalol in pregnant ewes. Anesthesiology 1991; 74:292-7.
162. Morgan MA, Silavin SL, Dormer KJ, et al. Effects of labetalol on uterine blood flow and cardiovascular hemodynamics in the hypertensive gravid baboon. Am J Obstet Gynecol 1993; 168:1574-9.
163. Jouppila P, Kirkinen P, Koivula A, Ylikorkala O. Labetalol does not alter the placental and fetal blood flow or maternal prostanoids in pre-eclampsia. Br J Obstet Gynaecol 1986; 93:543-7.
164. Lunell NO, Nylund L, Lewander R, Sarby B. Acute effect of an antihypertensive drug, labetalol, on uteroplacental blood flow. Br J Obstet Gynaecol 1982; 89:640-4.
165. Günenc O, Çiçek N, Görkemli H, et al. The effect of methyldopa treatment on uterine, umblical and fetal middle cerebral artery blood flows in preeclamptic patients. Arch Gynecol Obstet 2002; 266:141-4.
166. Rey E. Effects of methyldopa on umbilical and placental artery blood flow velocity waveforms. Obstet Gynecol 1992; 80:783-7.
167. Montan S, Anandakumar C, Arulkumaran S, et al. Effects of methyldopa on uteroplacental and fetal hemodynamics in pregnancy-induced hypertension. Am J Obstet Gynecol 1993; 168:152-6.
168. Murad SH, Tabsh KM, Shilyanski G, et al. Effects of verapamil on uterine blood flow and maternal cardiovascular function in the awake pregnant ewe. Anesth Analg 1985; 64:7-10.
169. Blea CW, Barnard JM, Magness RR, et al. Effect of nifedipine on fetal and maternal hemodynamics and blood gases in the pregnant ewe. Am J Obstet Gynecol 1997; 176:922-30.
170. Harake B, Gilbert RD, Ashwal S, Power GG. Nifedipine: Effects on fetal and maternal hemodynamics in pregnant sheep. Am J Obstet Gynecol 1987; 157:1003-8.
171. Lindow SW, Davies N, Davey DA, Smith JA. The effect of sublingual nifedipine on uteroplacental blood flow in hypertensive pregnancy. Br J Obstet Gynaecol 1988; 95:1276-81.
172. Moretti MM, Fairlie FM, Akl S, et al. The effect of nifedipine therapy on fetal and placental Doppler waveforms in preeclampsia remote from term. Am J Obstet Gynecol 1990; 163:1844-8.
173. Guclu S, Gol M, Saygili U, et al. Nifedipine therapy for preterm labor: Effects on placental, fetal cerebral and atrioventricular Doppler parameters in the first 48 hours. Ultrasound Obstet Gynecol 2006; 27:403-8.
174. Toda N, Kimura T, Yoshida K, et al. Human uterine arterial relaxation induced by nitroxidergic nerve stimulation. Am J Physiol 1994; 266:H1446-50.
175. Wheeler AS, James FM III, Meis PJ, et al. Effects of nitroglycerin and nitroprusside on the uterine vasculature of gravid ewes. Anesthesiology 1980; 52:390-4.
176. Ramsay B, De Belder A, Campbell S, et al. A nitric oxide donor improves uterine artery diastolic blood flow in normal early pregnancy and in women at high risk of pre-eclampsia. Eur J Clin Invest 1994; 24:76-8.
177. Cacciatore B, Halmesmaki E, Kaaja R, et al. Effects of transdermal nitroglycerin on impedance to flow in the uterine, umbilical, and fetal middle cerebral arteries in pregnancies complicated by preeclampsia and intrauterine growth retardation. Am J Obstet Gynecol 1998; 179:140-5.

178. Grunewald C, Kublickas M, Carlström K, et al. Effects of nitroglycerin on the uterine and umbilical circulation in severe preeclampsia. Obstet Gynecol 1995; 86:600-4.
179. Landauer M, Phernetton TM, Rankin JH. Maternal ovine placental vascular responses to adenosine. Am J Obstet Gynecol 1986; 154:1152-5.
180. Fishburne JI Jr, Dormer KJ, Payne GG, et al. Effects of amrinone and dopamine on uterine blood flow and vascular responses in the gravid baboon. Am J Obstet Gynecol 1988; 158:829-37.
181. Santos AC, Baumann AL, Wlody D, et al. The maternal and fetal effects of milrinone and dopamine in normotensive pregnant ewes. Am J Obstet Gynecol 1992; 166:257-62.
182. Hall PA, Bennett A, Wilkes MP, Lewis M. Spinal anaesthesia for caesarean section: Comparison of infusions of phenylephrine and ephedrine. Br J Anaesth 1994; 73:471-4.
183. LaPorta RF, Arthur GR, Datta S. Phenylephrine in treating maternal hypotension due to spinal anaesthesia for caesarean delivery: Effects on neonatal catecholamine concentrations, acid-base status and Apgar scores. Acta Anaesthesiol Scand 1995; 39:901-5.
184. Moran DH, Perillo M, LaPorta RF, et al. Phenylephrine in the prevention of hypotension following spinal anesthesia for cesarean delivery. J Clin Anaesth 1991; 3:301-5.
185. Pierce ET, Carr DB, Datta S. Effects of ephedrine and phenylephrine on maternal and fetal atrial natriuretic peptide levels during elective cesarean section. Acta Anaesthesiol Scand 1994; 38:48-51.
186. Thomas DG, Robson SC, Redfern N, et al. Randomized trial of bolus phenylephrine or ephedrine for maintenance of arterial pressure during spinal anaesthesia for caesarean section. Br J Anaesth 1996; 76:61-5.

Chapter 4

The Placenta: Anatomy, Physiology, and Transfer of Drugs

Mark I. Zakowski, M.D.
Norman L. Herman, M.D., Ph.D.

The placenta, which presents unceremoniously after delivery of the neonate, has been given the undignified name *afterbirth.* This often ignored structure is, in fact, a critical organ that should not be an afterthought in the study of obstetric anesthesia. Revered by ancient cultures as *the seat of the external soul* or *the bundle of life*, the placenta has been the subject of many cultural rituals.[1] However, a true understanding of the indispensable role of the placenta in the development of the fetus did not evolve until the seventeenth century. Much of the placenta's function remained a mystery until the development of microanatomic, biochemical, and molecular biologic techniques during the past 50 years. The concept of the placenta as a passive sieve (which does little more than serve as a conduit for oxygen, nutrients, and waste) has been dispelled with the realization that the placenta is a complex and dynamic organ.

The placenta brings the maternal and fetal circulations into close apposition, without substantial interchange of maternal and fetal blood, for the physiologic transfer of gases, nutrients, and wastes.[2] This important exchange is accomplished within a complex structure that is almost entirely of fetal origin.

ANATOMY

Embryology

At implantation, the developing blastocyst erodes the surrounding decidua, leaving the cellular debris on which it survives. The placenta develops in response to the embryo's outstripping its ability to gain oxygen and nutrients by simple diffusion. The syncytiotrophoblasts (invasive cells located at the margin of the growing conceptus) continue to erode the surrounding decidua and its associated capillaries and arterioles until the blastocyst is surrounded by a sea of circulating maternal blood (trophoblastic lacunae). The vitelline vein system develops in the yolk sac of the embryo to enhance the transport of nutrients, which diffuse from the maternal blood through the trophoblast layer and chorionic plate into the chorionic cavity. The embryo undergoes a dramatic acceleration in growth as its dependence on simple diffusion diminishes.[3]

At 2 weeks of development, the primitive extraembryonic mesoderm (cytotrophoblast layer) begins to proliferate as cellular columns into the syncytiotrophoblast. These columns with their syncytiotrophoblast covering extend

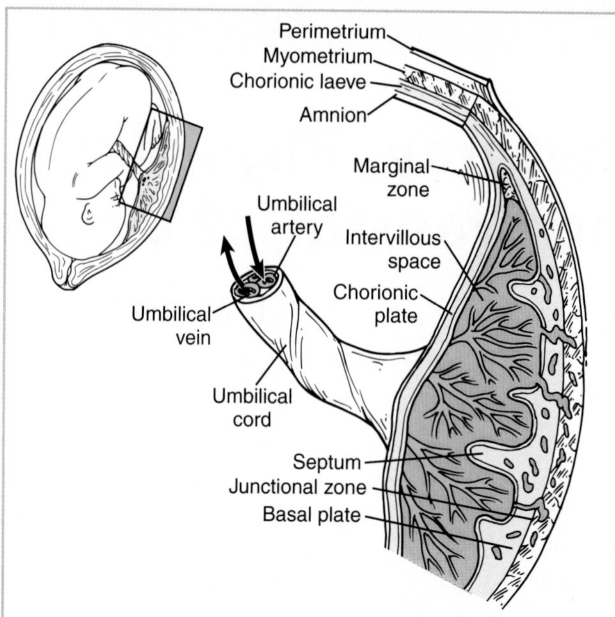

FIGURE 4-1 The placenta is a complex structure that brings the maternal and fetal circulations into close apposition for exchange of substances. (Redrawn from Kaufmann P, Scheffen I. Placental development. In Polin RA, Fox WW, editors. Fetal and Neonatal Physiology. 2nd edition. Philadelphia, WB Saunders, 1998:59-70.)

into the maternal blood lacunae and represent *primary* villi. Further mesodermal invasion into the core of these primary villi marks the metamorphosis into *secondary* villi. Cellular differentiation of the villi mesoderm results in the formation of a network of blood cells and vessels; this transition allows their classification as *tertiary* villi. The vascular components of each villus develop connections within the chorionic plate and into the stalk that connects the developing embryo and primitive placenta. Penetration of the cytotrophoblast continues through the syncytiotrophoblastic layer until many of the villi reach the decidua and form *anchoring* villi (Figure 4-1).[2,3]

Villi continue to develop and undergo extensive branching into treelike structures; the branches, which extend into the lacunar (or intervillous) spaces, enlarge the surface area available for exchange. Further villous maturation results in a marked reduction in the cytotrophoblastic component and a shortening of the distance between the fetal villi and maternal intervillous blood.[3]

The growing embryo within the blastocyst attaches to the chorion through a connecting or body stalk. Mesodermal components of this stalk coalesce to form the allantoic (or rudimentary umbilical) vessels. As the embryo continues its exponential growth phase, the connecting stalk shifts ventrally from its initial posterior attachment. The expansive open region at the ventral surface of the embryo constricts as the body wall grows and closes. By so doing, the body wall surrounds the yolk stalk, allantois, and developing vessels within the connecting stalk to form the primitive umbilicus. As the expanding amnion surrounds and applies itself over the connecting stalk and yolk sac, the cylindrical umbilical cord takes on its mature form.[3]

The placenta grows dramatically from the third month of gestation until term. A direct correlation exists between the growth of the placenta and the growth of the fetus. By term, the mature placenta is oval and flat, with an average diameter of 18.5 cm, weight of 500 g, and thickness of 23 mm.[4] Wide variations in size and shape are within the range of normal and make little difference in function.

Comparative Anatomy

The placentas of different species differ greatly, beginning with their method of uterine attachment, which can include adhesion, interdigitation, and fusion. In addition, the number of tissue layers between the maternal and fetal circulations at their point of apposition can differ. The most commonly used placental categorization system, the Grossner classification, uses the number of tissue layers in the placental barrier to determine the species (Figure 4-2).[5] Although still imperfect in modified form, this system remains a useful means of placental classification.

The functional ability of the placenta to transfer various substances differs among species. The markedly thicker epitheliochorial placenta found in sheep, which is the most common animal species used for placental transfer studies, has three maternal layers (epithelium, connective tissues, and endothelium) that separate maternal from fetal blood. By contrast, the human hemochorial placenta lacks these maternal layers, allowing maternal blood to directly bathe fetal tissues (see Figure 4-2). As a result, the substances that are able to transfer through the placenta differ; for example, fatty acids cannot cross through the placenta in sheep as they do in humans.[6] This wide diversity in placental structure and function among species makes extrapolation from animal investigations to clinical medicine tenuous.

Vascular Architecture

MATERNAL

Under the initial hormonal influences of the corpus luteum, the spiral arteries of the uterus become elongated and more extensively coiled. In the area beneath the developing conceptus, the compression and erosion of the decidua induces lateral looping of the already convoluted spiral arteries.[7] These vessels under the placenta gain access to the intervillous spaces. In late pregnancy, the growing demands of the developing fetus require the 200 spiral arteries that directly feed the placenta to handle a blood flow of approximately 600 mL/min.[7] The vasodilation required to accommodate this flow is the result of the replacement of the elastic and muscle components of the artery, initially by cytotrophoblast cells and later by fibroid cells. This replacement reduces the vasoconstrictor activity of these arteries and exposes the vessels to the dilating forces of the greater blood volume of pregnancy, especially at the terminal segments, where they form funnel-shaped sacs that enter the intervillous space.[7] The increased diameter of the vessels slows blood flow and reduces blood pressure.

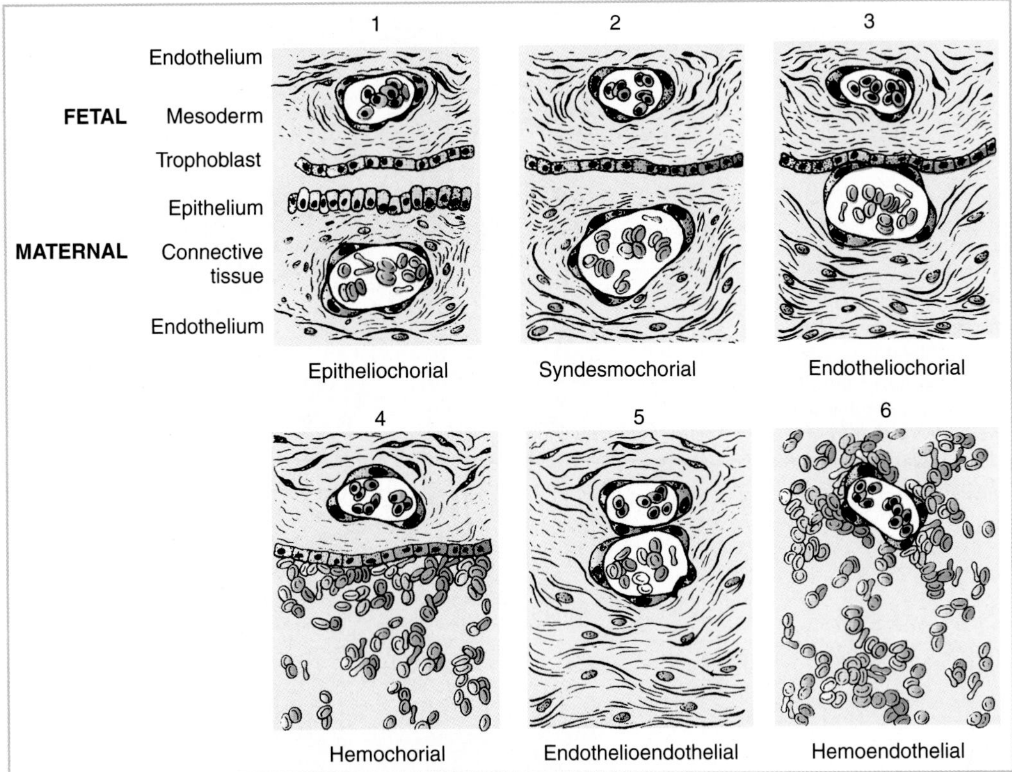

FIGURE 4-2 Modification of Grossner's original classification scheme, showing the number and types of tissue layers between the fetal and maternal circulations. Examples of each are as follows: (1) epitheliochorial, sheep; (2) syndesmochorial, no known examples; (3) endotheliochorial, dogs and cats; (4) hemochorial, human and hamster; (5) endothelioendothelial, bandicoot (Australian opossum); and (6) hemoendothelial, Rocky Mountain pika. (Modified from Ramsey EM. The Placenta: Human and Animal. New York, Praeger Publishers, 1982.)

The **intervillous space** is a large cavernous expanse that develops from the fusion of the trophoblastic lacunae and the erosion of the decidua by the expanding blastocyst. This space, which is essentially a huge blood sinus, is bounded by the chorionic plate and the decidua basalis (i.e., the maternal or basal plate). Folds in the basal plate form septa that separate the space into 13 to 30 anatomic compartments known as *lobules*. Each lobule contains numerous villous trees that are also known as *cotyledons* or *placentones*. Although tightly packed with highly branched villous trees, the intervillous space of the mature placenta can accommodate approximately 350 mL of maternal blood.[8]

Maternal arterial blood leaves the funnel-shaped spiral arteries and enters the intervillous space. The blood moves into the nearly hollow, low-resistance area, where villi are very loosely packed (the intercotyledonary space), prior to entering another region of densely packed intermittent and *terminal* villi (Figure 4-3).[9] The terminal villi represent the areas where placental exchange predominates. After passing through this dense region, maternal venous blood collects between neighboring villous trees in an area called the *perilobular zone*.[10] Collecting veins penetrate the maternal plate at the periphery of the villous trees to drain perilobular blood from the intervillous space.

Blood from the intervillous space is drained through fenestrations in the decidual veins; however, as pregnancy progresses, the total number of veins contributing to blood return is dramatically reduced by rising uterine wall pressure from intrauterine contents. Of interest, veins exhibit the same changes witnessed in the spiral arteries (i.e., atrophy of the tunica media and replacement with fibroid cells),[4,10] which reduce vasoconstrictive abilities and enhance the dilation of patent veins to accommodate venous return from the placenta.[7]

FETAL

Two coiled arteries bring fetal blood within the umbilical cord toward the placenta. On the placental surface, these arteries divide into **chorionic arteries** that ultimately supply the vessels of the 50 villous trees located in the placental lobules (Figure 4-4).[4,11] At the base of each villous tree, the chorionic arteries are considered the *main villous stem* or *truncal arteries* (first-order vessels), which in turn branch into four to eight *ramal* or *cotyledonary arteries* (second-order vessels); as they pass toward the maternal plate, they further subdivide into *ramulus chorii* (third-order vessels) and finally, *terminal arterioles*.[4] The terminal arterioles lead through a neck region into a bulbous enlargement where they form two to four narrow capillary loops. Here the large endothelial surface area and the near absence of connective tissue allow optimal maternal-fetal exchange (Figure 4-5).[10,12]

The **venous end of the capillaries** loops, narrows, and returns through the neck region to the collecting venules, which coalesce to form the larger veins in the stem of the villous trees. Each villous tree drains into a large vein,

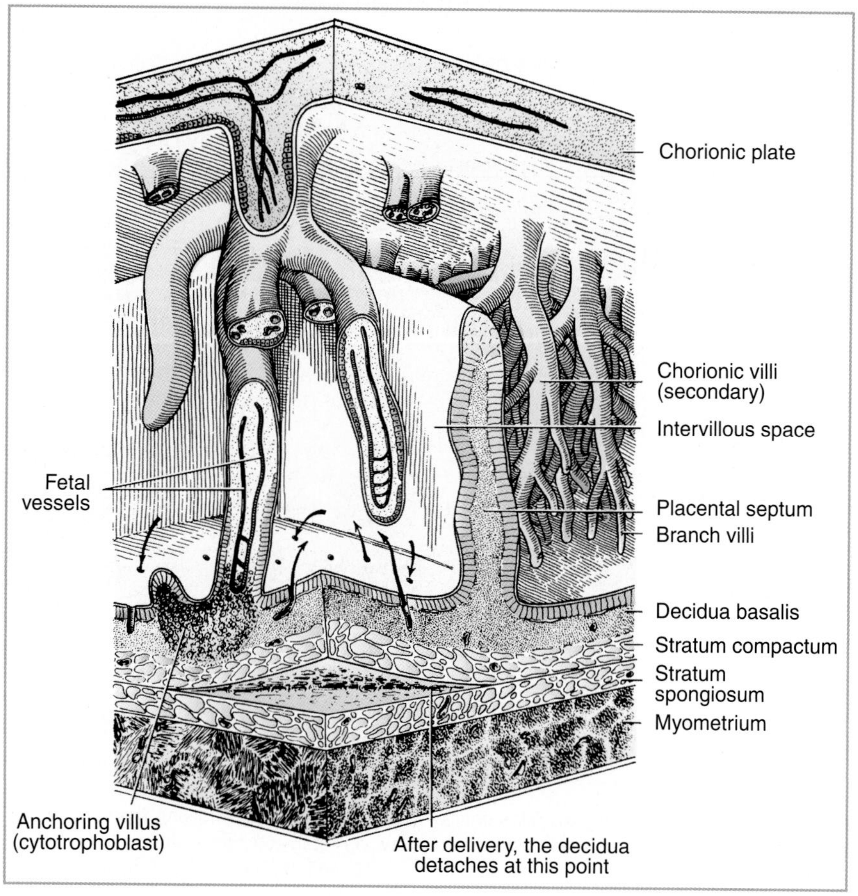

Chorionic plate
Chorionic villi (secondary)
Intervillous space
Placental septum
Branch villi
Decidua basalis
Stratum compactum
Stratum spongiosum
Myometrium
Fetal vessels
Anchoring villus (cytotrophoblast)
After delivery, the decidua detaches at this point

FIGURE 4-3 The relationship between the villous tree and maternal blood flow. *Arrows* indicate the maternal blood flow from the spiral arteries into the intervillous space and out through the spiral veins. (Modified from Tuchmann-Duplessis H, David G, Haegel P. Illustrated Human Embryology. Vol 1: Embryogenesis. New York, Springer Verlag, 1972:73.)

which, as it perforates the chorionic plate, becomes a **chorionic vein**. All of the venous tributaries course toward the umbilical cord attachment site, where they empty into one umbilical vein that delivers blood to the fetus.

PHYSIOLOGY

Barrier Function

The placenta is an imperfect barrier that allows almost all substances to cross, including an occasional red blood cell.

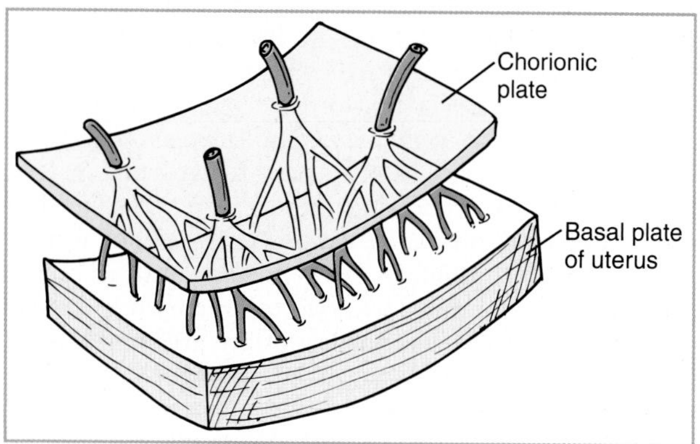

FIGURE 4-4 The dispersal of chorionic arteries through the chorionic plate and into the villous trees (or placentones or cotyledons) of the human placenta.

The rate and amount of placental transfer depend on the level of permeability and the ability of various mechanisms to restrict movement. A vast array of cytochrome P-450 isoenzymes are found within the placenta; some of these are inducible, whereas others are constitutive. The inducible enzymes are mainly of the 3-methylcholanthrene–inducible type rather than the phenobarbital-inducing variety found in the liver. These enzymes may play a role in metabolizing agents and decreasing fetal exposure, but the extent to which this involvement occurs is poorly understood.[13] In addition, a number of substances undergo specific or nonspecific binding within the placental tissues, thereby minimizing fetal exposure to and accumulation of the substances.[14] Finally, the thickness of the placental membranes, which diminishes as gestation progresses, may influence the rate of diffusion.[15] Of interest, the rate of transfer of certain substances (e.g., glucose, water) differs very little among species, even though the placental thickness varies greatly.[16]

Hormonal Function

A sophisticated transfer of precursor and intermediate compounds in the maternal-fetal-placental unit allows placental enzymes to convert steroid precursors into estrogen and progesterone. This steroidogenic function of the placenta begins very early during pregnancy; by 35 to 47 days after ovulation, the placental production of estrogen and progesterone exceeds that of the corpus luteum (i.e., the ovarian-placental shift).[17]

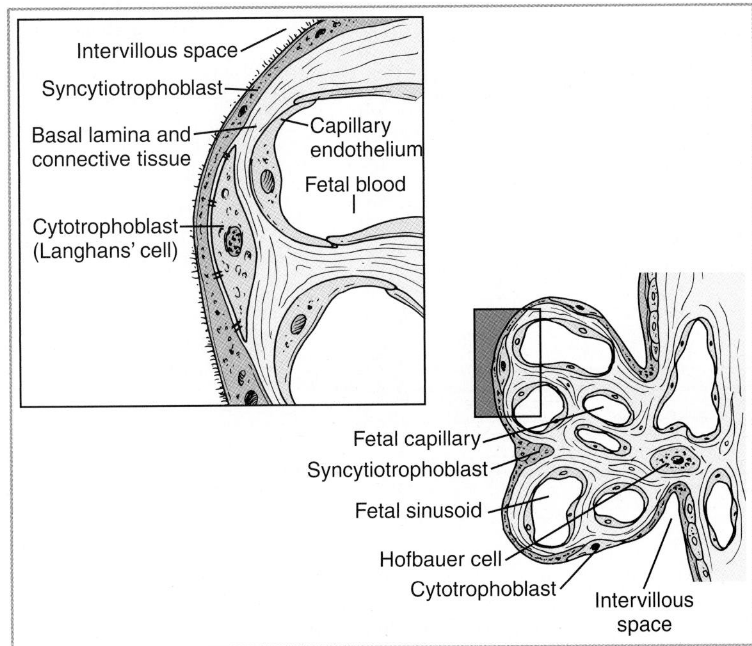

FIGURE 4-5 *Near left,* Cellular morphology of two terminal villi. *Far left,* Higher magnification of the boxed region exhibiting the placental barrier between fetal and maternal blood. (Redrawn from Kaufmann P. Basic morphology of the fetal and maternal circuits in the human placenta. Contrib Gynecol Obstet 1985; 13:5-17. Reproduced with permission of S. Karger AG, Basel, Switzerland.)

The placenta also produces a wide array of enzymes, binding proteins, and polypeptide hormones. For example, the placenta produces human chorionic gonadotropin, human placental lactogen (a growth hormone also known as human chorionic somatomammotropin), and factors that control hypothalamic function.[17] This ability to produce proteins and steroid hormones allows the placenta to influence and control the fetal environment.

Regulation of Placental Blood Flow

MATERNAL BLOOD FLOW

The trophoblastic invasion and functional denervation of the musculoelastic lining of the spiral arteries may represent adaptive mechanisms to decrease vascular reactivity and promote vasodilation.[18,19] These alterations allow the spiral arteries to vasodilate as much as 10 times their normal diameter, thereby lowering resistance for the passage of blood through the intervillous spaces.[20]

Maternal blood enters the intervillous cotyledon space at a pressure of 70 to 80 mm Hg in an area that has relatively few villi.[7] This pressure, and the subsequent velocity of blood flow, rapidly diminishes to approximately 10 mm Hg as the blood passes into an area of higher resistance created by the densely packed villi of the placentone.[15]

FETAL BLOOD FLOW

In contrast to maternoplacental blood flow, the gestational increases in fetoplacental blood flow are more the result of vascular growth, rather than vasodilation, of the villous beds.[21] Fetoplacental blood flow is autoregulated, but the process is not well defined; however, the maintenance of basal arteriolar tone is known to be independent of catecholamines or angiotensin.[22] Maternal hyperglycemia[23] and hypoxemia[24] are examples of derangements that can alter regional fetal blood flow, probably through vascular mediators. Endothelium-derived relaxing factors, especially prostacyclin[25] and nitric oxide,[26] appear to be important in the control of fetoplacental circulation. Evidence suggests that hypoxia-induced fetoplacental vasoconstriction is mediated by a reduction in the basal release of nitric oxide.[27,28] This vasoconstrictor activity is functionally similar to that found in the lung and allows optimal fetal oxygenation through redistribution of fetal blood flow to better-perfused lobules.[24]

Transport Mechanisms

Substances are transferred across the placenta by one of several mechanisms.[29-32] These processes are summarized in this section.

PASSIVE TRANSPORT

The passive transfer of molecules across a membrane depends on (1) concentration and electrochemical differences across the membrane, (2) molecular weight, (3) lipid solubility, (4) level of ionization, and (5) membrane surface area and thickness. This process requires no expenditure of cellular energy, with transfer driven principally by the concentration gradient across a membrane. Simple transmembrane diffusion can occur either through the lipid membrane (e.g., lipophilic molecules and water) or within protein channels that traverse the lipid bilayer (e.g., charged substances such as ions) (Figure 4-6).[31,33]

FACILITATED TRANSPORT

Carrier-mediated transport of relatively lipid-insoluble molecules down their concentration gradient is called *facilitated diffusion*.[33] Facilitated diffusion differs from simple diffusion in several ways. Specifically, this mode of transfer exhibits (1) saturation kinetics, (2) competitive and noncompetitive inhibition, (3) stereospecificity, and (4) temperature influences (e.g., a higher temperature results in greater transfer).[29] With *simple diffusion*, the net rate of diffusion is proportional to the difference in concentration between the two sides of the membrane. This rate

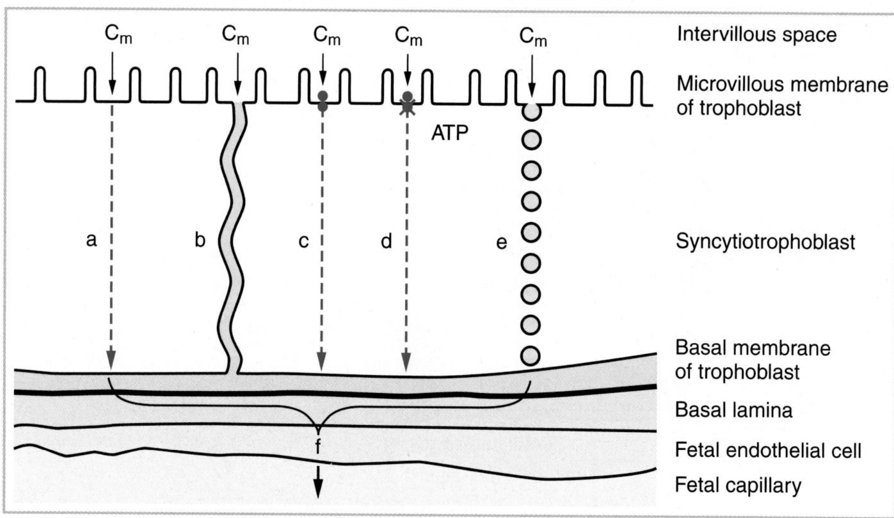

FIGURE 4-6 The transfer mechanisms used for the transfer of substances across the placental barrier: a, simple diffusion; b, simple diffusion through channels; c, facilitated diffusion; d, active transport; e, endocytosis; f, substance available for transfer into fetal circulation; C_m, intervillous concentration of substance at the trophoblastic membrane. (Modified from Morriss FH Jr, Boyd RDH, Mahendran D. Placental transport. In Knobil E, Neill JD, editors. The Physiology of Reproduction. 2nd edition. New York, Raven Press, 1994; 2:813-61.)

limitation is valid for facilitated diffusion only when transmembrane concentration differences are small. At higher concentration gradients, a maximum rate of transfer (V_{max}) is reached; thereafter, further rises in the concentration gradient do not affect the rate of transfer. The rate of transfer is determined by the number of membranous carrier protein complexes and the extent of interaction between the carrier and the substance undergoing transport.[31] An example of facilitated diffusion is the transplacental transfer of glucose.

A special type of facilitated diffusion involves the "uphill" transport of a molecule linked to another substance traveling down its concentration gradient. As such, the transfer is not directly driven by cellular energy expenditure. In most cases, sodium is the molecule that facilitates transport. For the membrane-bound carrier to transfer these molecules, both molecules must be bound to the carrier. This hybrid system is called *secondary active transport* or *co-transport*.[30,31] The transplacental transport of amino acids appears to occur principally through secondary active transport.

ACTIVE TRANSPORT

Active transport involves the movement of any substance across a cell membrane being linked with cellular metabolic activity. In general, active transport occurs against a concentration, electrical, or pressure gradient, although not necessarily in all circumstances.[30] Active transport requires cellular energy.

Like facilitated diffusion, active transport requires a protein membrane carrier that exhibits saturation kinetics and competitive inhibition (see Figure 4-6).[33] However, unlike secondary active transport, this movement of a substance against its concentration gradient is directly linked to the hydrolysis of high-energy phosphate bonds of adenosine triphosphate (ATP). The best known example of primary active transport is the translocation of sodium and potassium through the Na^+/K^+ ATPase pump.

New active transport proteins that have been identified include P-glycoprotein, breast cancer resistance protein, and the sodium/multivitamin transporter, as well as the many proteins involved in monoamine transport and multidrug resistance. These transport proteins play an important role in protecting the fetus from foreign and potentially teratogenic compounds. P-glycoprotein exists on the maternal side of the trophoblastic cell membrane of the placenta, and prevents compounds such as methadone and saquinavir (a protease inhibitor) from leaving the maternal blood, thus limiting fetal exposure.[34] Inhibition of these transporter proteins (e.g., inhibition of P-glycoprotein by verapamil) can significantly increase the fetal transfer of certain drugs, including midazolam, which is a substrate for P-glycoprotein.

PINOCYTOSIS

Large macromolecules (e.g., proteins that exhibit negligible diffusion properties) can cross cell membranes via the process of pinocytosis (a type of endocytosis). Pinocytosis is an energy-requiring process whereby the cell membrane invaginates around the macromolecule. Although the contents of pinocytotic vesicles are subject to intracellular digestion, electron microscopic studies have demonstrated that vesicles can move across the cytoplasm and fuse with the membrane at the opposite pole.[35] This appears to be the mechanism by which immunoglobulin G is transferred from the maternal to the fetal circulation.[33,36]

OTHER FACTORS THAT INFLUENCE PLACENTAL TRANSPORT

Other factors that affect maternal-fetal exchange are (1) maternal and fetal blood flow,[37] (2) placental binding,[14] (3) placental metabolism,[13,38] (4) diffusion capacity,[15] (5) maternal and fetal plasma protein binding,[29] and (6) gestational age (i.e., the placenta is more permeable in early pregnancy).[39] Lipid solubility, pH gradients between the maternal and fetal environments for certain basic drugs ("ion trapping"), and alterations in maternal or fetal plasma protein concentrations found in normal pregnancy[40] and other disease states (e.g., preeclampsia) may also alter placental transport.

Transfer of Respiratory Gases and Nutrients

OXYGEN

As the "lung" for the fetus, the placenta has only one fifth of the oxygen transfer efficiency of the adult lung,[41] yet must

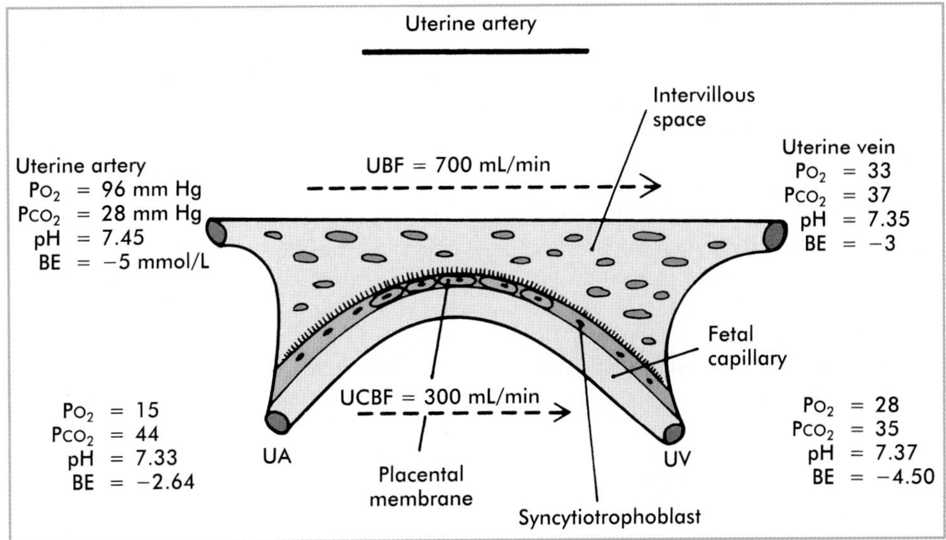

FIGURE 4-7 The concurrent relationship between the maternal and fetal circulations within the placenta and the way this arrangement affects gas transfer. These values were obtained from patients breathing room air during elective cesarean delivery. BE, Base excess; UA, umbilical artery; Po_2, partial pressure of oxygen; Pco_2, partial pressure of carbon dioxide; UBF, uterine blood flow; UCBF, umbilical cord blood flow; UV, umbilical vein. (Modified from Ramanathan S. Obstetric Anesthesia. Philadelphia, Lea & Febiger, 1988:27.)

provide approximately 8 mL O_2/min per kg fetal body weight for fetal growth and development.[42] To determine the transplacental diffusion capacity for oxygen, the oxygen tension on both sides of the diffusional surface (i.e., within the placenta itself) must be determined. Because this approach is not practical, investigators have used surrogate measurements of oxygen content taken from blood in the uterine and umbilical vessels. One study in sheep demonstrated a transplacental pressure gradient of 37 to 42 mm Hg,[43] which suggests poor oxygen diffusion capacity. This gradient is believed to be an inaccurate measure of true end-capillary O_2 tensions for at least three reasons. First, approximately 16% and 6% of uterine blood flow and umbilical blood flow, respectively, are shunted through diffusional areas of the placenta, resulting in an admixture.[15] Second, unlike the lung, the placenta consumes a significant amount (20% to 30%) of transferred oxygen.[44] Third, the uterus also consumes oxygen. Consequently, placental diffusion capacity is significantly higher than a simple measurement of uterine venous Po_2 would suggest.

By contrast, as a gas not used by any organ, carbon monoxide is not affected by shunt or consumption. When placental diffusion capacity was estimated using carbon monoxide, it was found to be four times greater than that obtained with calculations made from arterial-venous Po_2 differences.[45] Because oxygen and carbon monoxide have similar diffusion coefficients, the placental diffusion capacity for oxygen must be essentially the same as that for carbon monoxide. Therefore, as with carbon monoxide, the transfer of oxygen is limited by flow and not by diffusion.[15]

Oxygen transfer across the placenta depends on the oxygen partial pressure gradient between maternal blood and fetal blood. As physically dissolved oxygen diffuses across the villous membranes, bound oxygen is released by maternal hemoglobin in the intervillous space and also diffuses across the placenta. Several factors affect the fetal blood Po_2 once it reaches equilibration in the villi end-capillaries. First, the concurrent and countercurrent arrangements of maternal and fetal blood flow play a key role for placental oxygen transfer in various species. The almost complete equilibration of maternal and fetal Po_2 values suggests that a concurrent (or parallel) relationship between maternal blood and fetal blood exists within the human placenta (Figure 4-7) [15,46]; however, one study demonstrated that umbilical venous Po_2 was slightly higher than intervillous Po_2, suggesting a more complex, multivillous pool relationship.[47] Second, the differences between the oxyhemoglobin dissociation curves of maternal and fetal blood may influence transplacental oxygen transfer to the fetus,[48] although this proposal is a matter of some dispute.[15] The fetal oxyhemoglobin dissociation curve is positioned to the left of the maternal curve because of the lower P_{50} (partial pressure of oxygen in the blood at which the hemoglobin is 50% saturated) for fetal blood (see Figure 5-4). In theory, this difference enhances oxygen uptake by fetal red blood cells and promotes the transfer of additional oxygen across the placenta. Third, the **Bohr effect** may also augment the transfer of oxygen across the placenta. Specifically, fetal-to-maternal transfer of carbon dioxide makes maternal blood more acidic and fetal blood more alkalotic, differences that in turn cause right and left shifts in the maternal and fetal oxyhemoglobin dissociation curves, respectively. This "double" Bohr effect enhances the transfer of oxygen from mother to fetus and accounts for 2% to 8% of the transplacental transfer of oxygen.[49]

The maximum fetal arterial Po_2 (Pao_2) is never greater than 50 to 60 mm Hg, even when maternal fractional inspired oxygen concentration (Fio_2) is 1.0, for several reasons. First, the placenta tends to function as a venous rather than arterial equilibrator. Because of the shape of the maternal oxyhemoglobin dissociation curve, a rise in maternal Pao_2 above 100 mm Hg does not result in a substantial increase in maternal arterial oxygen content.

Therefore, under conditions of constant uterine and umbilical blood flow and fetal oxygen consumption, fetal Pa_{O_2} rises only slightly when maternal F_{IO_2} is increased. Although this rise in Pa_{O_2} is of limited significance at normal levels of fetal Pa_{O_2}, it is more important at decreased levels closer to the P_{50} of fetal blood (approximately 21 mm Hg in humans) because of the steep slope of the fetal oxyhemoglobin dissociation curve within that range. Second, the placenta has a relatively high rate of oxygen consumption, which lowers the amount of oxygen available for transfer (see Chapter 5). Third, fetal arterial blood represents a mixture of oxygenated umbilical venous blood and deoxygenated inferior vena caval blood (which returns centrally from the fetal lower extremities).

CARBON DIOXIDE

The transfer of carbon dioxide occurs through a number of different forms, including dissolved CO_2, carbonic acid (H_2CO_3), bicarbonate ion (HCO_3^-), carbonate ion (CO_3^{2-}), and carbaminohemoglobin. Dissolved CO_2 (8%) and HCO_3^- (62%) are the predominant forms involved in transplacental transfer because the concentrations of H_2CO_3 and CO_3^{2-} are almost negligible and carbaminohemoglobin (30%) is present only within red blood cells.[15,38] Equilibrium between CO_2 and HCO_3^- is maintained by a reaction catalyzed by carbonic anhydrase in red blood cells. A difference in P_{CO_2} normally exists between fetal and maternal blood (i.e., 40 versus 34 mm Hg, respectively); this gradient favors fetal-to-maternal transfer. Carbon dioxide is 20 times more diffusible than oxygen and readily crosses the placenta,[38] although dissolved CO_2 is the form that actually crosses. The rapid movement of CO_2 from fetal capillary to maternal blood invokes a shift in the equilibrium of the carbonic anhydrase reaction (i.e., La Chatelier's principle) that produces more CO_2 for diffusion. The transfer of CO_2 is augmented further by the production of deoxyhemoglobin in the maternal blood, which has a higher affinity for CO_2 than oxyhemoglobin (i.e., the **Haldane effect**). The resulting affinity may account for as much as 46% of the transplacental transfer of carbon dioxide.[46] Although a significant fetal-maternal concentration gradient exists for HCO_3^-, its charged nature impedes its transfer and contribution to carbon dioxide transport except as a source for CO_2 production through the carbonic anhydrase reaction.[50]

GLUCOSE

Simple diffusion alone cannot account for the amount of glucose required to meet the demands of the placenta and fetus. To assist the movement of glucose down its concentration gradient, a stereospecific facilitated diffusion system has been described, which is independent of insulin, a sodium gradient, or cellular energy.[51,52] In addition, D-glucose transport proteins have been identified within the trophoblast membrane.[53] The placenta, which must maintain its own metabolic processes, competes with the fetus for maternal glucose, and consequently only 28% of the glucose absorbed from the maternal surface is transferred through the umbilical vein to the term fetus.[33] The placenta may also produce glucose via a different mechanism from the conventional hepatic glucose-6-phosphatase reaction.[54]

AMINO ACIDS

Concentrations of amino acids are highest in the placenta, followed by umbilical venous blood and then maternal blood.[55] The maternal-fetal transplacental transfer of amino acids is an active process that occurs principally through a linked translocation with sodium. The energy required for this transfer comes from the large sodium gradient established by the Na^+/K^+ ATPase pump.[56] This results in increased intracellular concentrations of amino acids, which then "leak" down their gradients into the fetal circulation. This transport mechanism may not be viable for all amino acids and may be susceptible to inhibitors; for example, histidine does not exhibit elevated intracellular concentrations.[15]

FATTY ACIDS

Free fatty acids, such as palmitic and linoleic acids, readily cross the human, but not ovine, placenta.[6,57-59] A concentration gradient from mother to fetus exists for most fatty acids (with arachidonic acid being a notable exception[60]), and the rate of transfer appears to depend on the magnitude of the gradient.[58] These findings imply that fatty acids cross the placenta by means of simple diffusion, although the actual mechanism remains unclear.

DRUG TRANSFER

Placental permeability and pharmacokinetics help determine the fetal exposure to maternal drugs. Animal models (e.g., pregnant ewes, guinea pigs) have been used to assess the placental transport of drugs; however, interspecies differences in placental anatomy and physiology may limit the application of these data to humans.[61] Investigations of transport within the human placenta have been performed on placental slices, isolated villi, membrane vesicles, homogenates, and tissue culture cells. The direct application of these data, however, is in question because these methods do not account for the dual (i.e., maternal and fetal) perfusion of the intact placenta *in situ*.[61]

The inaccessibility of the placenta *in situ* and concerns for maternal and fetal safety have limited direct studies of the placenta in humans. Only one published study has reported the real-time transfer pharmacokinetics of an anesthetic drug across the human placenta *in vivo*.[62] Data regarding the transplacental transfer of anesthetic agents have been extrapolated primarily from single measurements of drug concentrations in maternal and umbilical cord blood samples obtained at delivery. Most studies have reported fetal-maternal (F/M) ratios of the drug concentration. In these studies, the umbilical vein blood concentration represents the fetal blood concentration of the drug.

Single-measurement studies obtain only one set of measurements for each parturient. Maternal and fetal concentrations of a drug are influenced by drug metabolism in the mother, the placenta, and the fetus, and also by changes during delivery (e.g., altered uteroplacental blood flow).[61,63] Unless a study includes a large number of patients with variable durations of exposure, it is difficult to reach conclusions about the type and time course of transplacental transfer of an individual drug from its results. In addition, single-measurement studies provide information only on the net transfer of a drug across the maternal-placental-fetal unit and do not allow for the determination of unidirectional fluxes at any point (i.e., maternal-to-fetal or fetal-to-maternal). Nonetheless, these studies have provided the best data available for most anesthetic agents.

BOX 4-1 Transplacental Transfer of Anesthetic Drugs

Drugs that Cross the Placenta

Anticholinergic agents
- Atropine
- Scopolamine

Antihypertensive agents
- Beta-adrenergic receptor antagonists
- Nitroprusside
- Nitroglycerin

Benzodiazepines
- Diazepam
- Midazolam

Induction agents
- Propofol
- Thiopental

Inhalational anesthetic agents
- Halothane
- Isoflurane
- Nitrous oxide

Local anesthetics

Opioids

Vasopressor
- Ephedrine

Drugs that Do Not Cross the Placenta

Anticholinergic agent
- Glycopyrrolate

Anticoagulants
- Heparin

Muscle relaxants
- Depolarizing—succinylcholine
- Nondepolarizing agents

A dual-perfused, *in vitro* human placental model has been developed to allow for the independent perfusion of the maternal and fetal sides of the placenta and thereby investigate maternal-to-fetal (or fetal-to-maternal) transport. The validity of this method for the study of placental transfer has been well established.[61] Equilibration studies (i.e., recirculating maternal and fetal perfusates) using this model are not directly applicable to the placenta *in vivo*.[64] However, when a nonrecirculating scheme is used, steady-state drug clearance can be determined for either direction (maternal-to-fetal or fetal-to-maternal) and may have direct clinical application. This method has been used to assess the placental transfer of anesthetic agents (e.g., thiopental,[65] methohexital,[66] propofol,[67] bupivacaine,[68] ropivacaine,[69] alfentanil,[70] sufentanil[71,72]). Transfer across the placenta may be reported as drug clearance or as a ratio referred to as the **transfer index** (i.e., drug clearance/reference compound clearance). The use of a transfer index allows for interplacental comparisons by accounting for differences between placentas (e.g., lobule sizes). Commonly used reference compounds are either flow-limited (e.g., antipyrine, tritiated water) or membrane-limited (e.g., creatinine). These studies have enhanced our understanding of the placental transfer of anesthetic drugs (Box 4-1).

Pharmacokinetic Principles

Factors affecting drug transfer across the human placenta include lipid solubility, protein binding, tissue binding, pKa, pH, and blood flow (Table 4-1). High lipid solubility may enable easy cell membrane (lipid bilayer) penetration but may also cause the drug (e.g., sufentanil) to be trapped within the placental tissue.[72] Highly protein-bound drugs are affected by the concentration of maternal and fetal plasma proteins, which varies with gestational age and disease. Some drugs (e.g., diazepam) bind to albumin, whereas others (e.g., sufentanil, cocaine) bind predominantly to alpha-1-acid glycoprotein (Table 4-2). Although the free, unbound fraction of drug equilibrates across the placenta,

TABLE 4-1 Factors Affecting Placental Transfer of Drug (Maternal to Fetal)

	Increased Transfer	Decreased Transfer
Size—molecular weight (Da)	<1000	>1000
Charge of molecule	Uncharged	Charged
Lipid solubility	Lipophilic	Hydrophilic
pH vs. drug pKa*	Higher proportion of un-ionized drug in maternal plasma	Higher proportion of ionized drug in maternal plasma
Placental efflux transporter† proteins (e.g., P-glycoprotein)	Absent	Present
Binding protein type	Albumin (lower binding affinity)‡	Alpha-1-acid glycoprotein (AAG) (higher binding affinity)
Free (unbound) drug fraction	High	Low

Da, dalton;

*The pH relative to the pKa datermines the amount of drug that is ionized and un-ionized in both maternal and fetal plasma. Fetal acidemia enhances the maternal-to-fetal transfer (i.e., "ion trapping") of basic drugs such as local anesthetics and opioids.

†The efflux transporter pumps substances in a fetal-to-maternal direction.

‡Note: albumin concentration is higher in the fetus and AAG concentration is higher in the maternal circulation.

TABLE 4-2 Concentrations of Proteins that Bind Drugs

	Maternal	Umbilical Cord
Albumin	33.1 g/L	37.1 g/L*
Alpha-1-acid glycoprotein (AGP)	0.77 g/L	0.26 g/L*

*$P < .05$.

Data from Sudhakaran S, Rayner CR, et al. Differential protein binding of indinavir and saquinavir in matched maternal and umbilical cord plasma. Br J Clin Pharmacol 2006:63:315-21.

the total drug concentration is greatly affected by both the extent of protein binding and the quantity of maternal and fetal proteins; fetal blood typically contains less than half the concentration of alpha-1-acid glycoprotein than in maternal blood.[73] One study of the placental transfer of sufentanil *in vitro* noted different results when fresh frozen plasma, rather than albumin, was used as a perfusate.

The pKa of a drug determines the fraction of drug that is nonionized at physiologic pH. Thus, fetal acidemia greatly enhances the maternal-to-fetal transfer (i.e., "ion trapping") of many basic drugs, such as local anesthetics and opioids (Figure 4-8).[74] Most anesthetic drugs are passively transferred, with the rate of blood flow (hence drug delivery) affecting the amount of drug that crosses the placenta.[75] One of the authors (M.I.Z.) has used the *in vitro* perfused human placenta model to perform a number of studies of the placental transfer of opioids (Table 4-3).

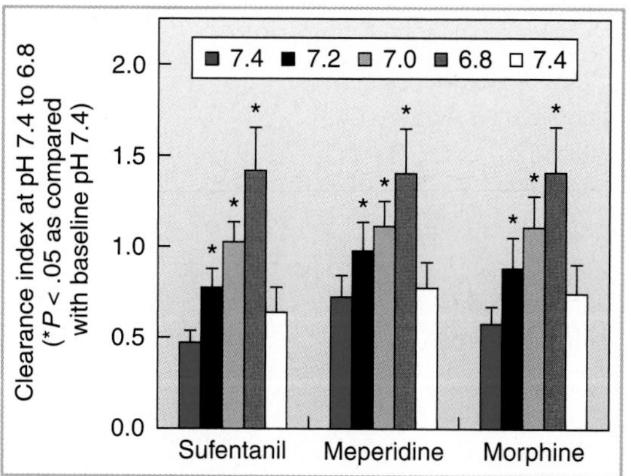

FIGURE 4-8 The effects of changes in fetal pH on the transfer of opioids during *in vitro* perfusion of the human placenta. This figure demonstrates the "ion trapping" of opioids, which is similar to that of local anesthetics. Clearance index = clearance drug/clearance creatinine (a reference compound). (Modified from Zakowski MI, Krishna R, Grant GJ, Turndorf H. Effect of pH on transfer of narcotics in human placenta during in vitro perfusion [abstract]. Anesthesiology 1995; 85:A890.)

Inhalation Anesthetic Agents

When general anesthesia is necessary in a pregnant patient, maintenance of anesthesia is often provided with inhalation agents. The lipid solubility and low molecular weight of these agents facilitate rapid transfer across the placenta. A prolonged induction-to-delivery interval results in lower Apgar scores in infants exposed to general anesthesia.[76]

When administered during cesarean delivery, **halothane** is detectable in both umbilical venous blood and arterial blood within 1 minute. Even with relatively short induction-to-delivery times, an F/M ratio of 0.71 to 0.87 is established.[77,78] **Enflurane** also exhibits unrestricted transfer across the placenta, with even brief exposures resulting in an F/M ratio of approximately 0.6.[79] **Isoflurane** distributes rapidly across the placenta during cesarean delivery, resulting in an F/M ratio of approximately 0.71.[78] To our knowledge, there are no published data regarding the placental transfer of either **desflurane** or **sevoflurane**.

Nitrous oxide also rapidly crosses the placenta, with an F/M ratio of 0.83 expected within 3 minutes.[80] Maternal administration of nitrous oxide decreases fetal central vascular resistance by 30%,[81] and a prolonged induction-to-delivery interval may cause neonatal depression.[82] Diffusion hypoxia may occur during the rapid elimination of nitrous oxide from the neonate; therefore, the administration of supplemental oxygen to any neonate exposed to nitrous oxide immediately before delivery appears prudent.[83]

TABLE 4-3 Opioid Transfer during *In Vitro* Perfusion of the Human Placenta

	Morphine	Meperidine	Alfentanil	Fentanyl	Sufentanil
Lipid solubility	1.4	39	129	816	1727
Percent nonionized at pH 7.4	23%	7.4%	89%	8.5%	20%
Percent protein binding	30%	70%	93%	84%	93%
Placenta drug ratio	0.1	0.7	0.53	3.4	7.2
F/M ratio, MTF	0.08	0.27	0.22	0.19	0.14
F/M ratio, FTM	0.08	0.13	0.11	0.08	0.18
Minutes to steady state	30	20	20	40-60	40-60
Clearance index, MTF	0.4	0.95	0.75	0.76	0.41
Clearance index, FTM	0.5	0.91	0.78	0.61	0.76

Clearance index, clearance drug/clearance antipyrine (a flow-limited reference compound); FTM, fetal-to-maternal (direction); MTF, maternal-to-fetal (direction); Placenta drug ratio, placenta drug concentration/g placental tissue/maternal drug concentration.

Data from nonrecirculated experiments, using perfusate Media 199 without protein, with maternal flow 12 mL/min and fetal flow 6 mL/min.[67,69,104,107,113]

Induction Agents

The lipophilic characteristics that make anesthetic agents ideal for the induction of anesthesia also enhance their transfer across the placenta. The understanding of the transplacental transfer of these drugs is better than for any other group of anesthetic agents.

BARBITURATES

A popular agent used for the induction of general anesthesia in parturients, **thiopental** is the most extensively studied barbiturate. An extremely short-acting agent, it quickly appears in umbilical venous blood after maternal injection,[84,85] with mean F/M ratios between 0.4 and 1.1.[86,87] High F/M ratios suggest that thiopental is freely diffusible; however, factors other than simple diffusion must play a role, because there is wide intersubject variability in umbilical cord blood concentrations at delivery. Both maternal-to-fetal and fetal-to-maternal transfer of thiopental are strongly influenced by maternal and fetal protein concentrations.[65]

The rapid transfer of the oxybarbiturate **methohexital** into the fetal circulation, with simultaneous peak concentrations in maternal blood and fetal blood, has been demonstrated by *in vivo* studies.[62] Human placental perfusion studies *in vitro* confirm that methohexital rapidly crosses the placenta in both maternal-to-fetal and fetal-to-maternal directions, with transfer indices of 0.83 and 0.61, respectively,[66] when the concentration of albumin is equal in the two perfusates. This transfer asymmetry disappears when physiologic albumin concentrations in maternal and fetal blood (8 g/100 mL and 4 g/100 mL, respectively) are used; such conditions significantly increase fetal-to-maternal transfer so that it approximates maternal-to-fetal transfer.[66]

KETAMINE

Ketamine, a phencyclidine derivative, rapidly crosses the placenta. Although less lipid soluble than thiopental, ketamine (2 mg/kg) reaches a mean F/M ratio of 1.26 in as little as 97 seconds when administered to the mother for vaginal delivery.[88]

PROPOFOL

Review of published evidence suggests that the role of propofol in obstetric anesthesia practice remains unclear.[89] Maternal administration of propofol in a bolus dose of 2 to 2.5 mg/kg results in a mean F/M ratio between 0.65 and 0.85.[90-92] When given in a bolus dose of 2 mg/kg followed by a continuous infusion of either 6 mg/kg/hr or 9 mg/kg/hr, propofol results in mean F/M ratios of 0.50 and 0.54, respectively.[93] These F/M ratios are similar to those found in early gestation (i.e., 12 to 18 weeks).[94] Propofol may have sedative effects on the neonate; the maternal administration of propofol (2.8 mg/kg) for the induction of general anesthesia for elective cesarean delivery has resulted in lower 1- and 5-minute Apgar scores than the administration of thiopental (5 mg/kg).[89] The plasma levels of propofol in the neonate depend on the maternal dose and resulting plasma level as well as on the time elapsed between drug administration and delivery of the neonate. In one study, when delivered within 10 minutes of induction, neonates whose mothers were given propofol (2 mg/kg) had an average umbilical vein propofol concentration of 0.32 μg/mL.[95]

Several factors that affect propofol transfer have been investigated with *in vitro* human placental perfusion models.[96-98] Increased maternal blood flow and reduced protein binding increase both placental tissue uptake and transplacental transfer of propofol.[93] The effect of propofol's high protein binding varies with alterations in fetal and maternal protein concentrations. Greater *fetal* albumin concentrations increase the total, but not free, concentration of propofol in umbilical venous blood,[97] whereas doubling the *maternal* albumin concentration decreases the umbilical venous blood concentration of propofol by approximately two thirds.[98]

ETOMIDATE

The use of etomidate, a carboxylated imidazole, for the induction of general anesthesia in obstetric patients was first described in 1979.[99] A dose of 0.3 to 0.4 mg/kg administered before cesarean delivery results in an F/M ratio of approximately 0.5,[100] which is similar to the ratio found in sheep.[101]

Benzodiazepines

Highly un-ionized and lipophilic, **diazepam** is associated with F/M ratios of 1.0 within minutes and 2.0 within 60 minutes of maternal administration.[102,103] Less lipophilic, **lorazepam** takes almost 3 hours after administration for the F/M ratio to reach unity.[104] **Midazolam** is more polarized, with an F/M ratio of 0.76 at 20 minutes after administration. Unlike that of other benzodiazepines, however, midazolam's F/M ratio falls quickly; by 200 minutes, it is only 0.3.[105]

Opioids

Opioids have long been used for systemic pain relief in obstetric patients. More detailed pharmacokinetic data, enhanced monitoring, and the ability to reverse adverse effects with opioid antagonists have reduced the adverse side effects associated with their use.

Administration of **meperidine** has been associated with neonatal central nervous system and respiratory depression. Intravenous administration of meperidine results in rapid transfer across the human placenta; the drug can be detected in the umbilical venous blood as soon as 90 seconds after maternal administration.[106] F/M ratios for meperidine may exceed 1.0 after 2 to 3 hours; maternal levels fall more rapidly than fetal levels because of the mother's greater capacity for metabolism of the drug.[107] Human placental perfusion studies *in vitro* have demonstrated rapid placental transfer in both maternal-to-fetal and fetal-to-maternal directions with equal clearance profiles, minimal placental tissue binding, and no placental drug metabolism.[108]

Morphine also rapidly crosses the placenta. One study demonstrated a mean F/M ratio of 0.61, a mean umbilical venous blood concentration of 25 ng/mL, and a significant reduction in the biophysical profile score (primarily as a result of decreased fetal breathing movements and fewer fetal heart rate accelerations) within 20 to 30 minutes.[109] Intrathecal administration of morphine results in a high

F/M ratio (0.92), although the absolute fetal concentrations are less than those associated with fetal and neonatal side effects.[110] Human placental perfusion studies *in vitro* have demonstrated that morphine, which is a hydrophilic compound, exhibits membrane-limited transfer with a low placental tissue content and a fast washout.[111] Concurrent naloxone administration apparently does not affect the placental transfer of morphine.[112]

Fentanyl and its analogues are administered through epidural, intrathecal, and intravenous routes. Fentanyl has a high level of lipophilicity and albumin binding (74%).[113] Maternal epidural administration of fentanyl results in an F/M ratio between 0.37 and 0.57.[114,115] During early pregnancy, fentanyl is rapidly transferred and may be detected not only in the placenta but also in the fetal brain.[116] Perfusion of the human placenta *in vitro* results in rapid transfer in both maternal-to-fetal and fetal-to-maternal directions, with the placenta acting as a moderate drug depot.[117]

Despite a relatively low F/M ratio (0.30),[118] maternal administration of **alfentanil** has been associated with a reduction of 1-minute Apgar scores.[119] Perfusion of the human placenta *in vitro* shows rapid and symmetric maternal-to-fetal and fetal-to-maternal transfers of alfentanil, with low placental drug uptake and rapid washout.[70]

Maternal administration of **sufentanil** results in a very high F/M ratio, 0.81. Compared with fentanyl, sufentanil has higher lipid solubility and more rapid uptake by the central nervous system, thereby resulting in less systemic absorption from the epidural space; less systemic absorption lowers both maternal and umbilical vein concentrations and reduces fetal exposure and the associated potential risk for neonatal respiratory depression.[114] Human placental perfusion studies *in vitro* have confirmed the rapid transplacental transfer of sufentanil, which is influenced by differences in maternal and fetal plasma protein binding and fetal pH. High placental tissue uptake suggests that the placenta serves as a drug depot.[71,72]

Remifentanil undergoes rapid placental transfer, with an average F/M ratio of 0.88 observed when it is given by intravenous infusion (0.1 μg/kg/min) before cesarean delivery.[120] Excessive maternal sedation without adverse neonatal effects has been reported with the use of remifentanil during labor.[120,121] Remifentanil has been used for patient-controlled analgesia (PCA) during labor, with patient-controlled bolus doses of 0.5 μg/kg resulting in an F/M ratio of approximately 0.5 and a 20% incidence of fetal heart rate (FHR) tracing changes.[122]

The systemic administration of an opioid agonist/antagonist for labor analgesia has been associated with few maternal, fetal, and neonatal side effects. Both **butorphanol** and **nalbuphine** rapidly cross the placenta, with mean F/M ratios of 0.84 and 0.74 to 0.97, respectively.[123-125] In one study, maternal administration of nalbuphine resulted in "flattening" of the FHR tracing in 54% of cases.[125]

Local Anesthetics

Local anesthetic agents readily cross the placenta (see Chapter 13). The enantiomers of bupivacaine cross the placenta at the same rate as racemic bupivacaine.[126]

Muscle Relaxants

As fully ionized, quaternary ammonium salts, muscle relaxants do not readily cross the placenta; however, maternal administration of single clinical doses of muscle relaxants can result in detectable fetal blood concentrations. Maternal administration of muscle relaxants for the induction of general anesthesia for cesarean delivery rarely affects neonatal muscle tone at delivery.

A single induction dose of **succinylcholine** is not detected in umbilical venous blood at delivery[127]; maternal doses larger than 300 mg are required before the drug can be detected in umbilical venous blood.[128] Neonatal neuromuscular blockade can occur when high doses are given repeatedly or when the fetus has a pseudocholinesterase deficiency.[129,130] One report described maternal masseter muscle rigidity and neonatal fasciculations after administration of succinylcholine for an emergency cesarean delivery; however, both the mother and the newborn were diagnosed with central core myopathy and malignant hyperthermia susceptibility.[131]

The administration of nondepolarizing muscle relaxants results in low F/M ratios: 0.12 for **d-tubocurare**[132]; 0.19 to 0.26 for **pancuronium**[133-135]; 0.06 to 0.11 for **vecuronium**[135,136]; and 0.07 for **atracurium**.[137] The F/M ratio may be the result of expedient fetal/neonatal blood sampling; in a study in rats, the F/M ratio of vecuronium nearly doubled as the induction-to-delivery interval increased from 180 to 420 seconds.[136] To our knowledge, no published study has investigated the placental transfer of the atracurium isomer **cisatracurium. Rapacuronium,** a short-acting analogue of vecuronium advocated as an alternative to succinylcholine for rapid-sequence induction,[138,139] has an F/M ratio of 0.09 and is associated with increased maternal heart rate.[140] Although no published reports have documented problems with rapacuronium in parturients or neonates, reports of bronchospasm resulted in the withdrawal of rapacuronium from the market.

Nondepolarizing muscle relaxants are frequently administered in bolus form; although the transfer rates are low, the fetal blood concentrations increase over time.[136] Fetal blood concentrations of nondepolarizing muscle relaxants can be minimized by giving succinylcholine to facilitate intubation, followed by the administration of small doses of either succinylcholine or a nondepolarizing muscle relaxant to maintain paralysis.[134]

Anticholinergic Agents

The placental transfer rate of anticholinergic agents directly correlates with their ability to cross the blood-brain barrier. **Atropine** is detected in the umbilical circulation within 1 to 2 minutes of maternal administration, and an F/M ratio of 0.93 is attained at 5 minutes.[141] **Scopolamine,** the other commonly used tertiary amine, also crosses the placenta easily. Intramuscular administration of scopolamine results in an F/M ratio of 1.0 within 55 minutes.[142] By contrast, **glycopyrrolate** is poorly transferred across the placenta with maternal intramuscular administration, resulting in a mean F/M ratio of only 0.22.[143] Maternal intravenous administration of glycopyrrolate does not result in a detectable fetal hemodynamic response.[144]

Anticholinesterase Agents

Neostigmine, pyridostigmine, and **edrophonium** are quaternary ammonium compounds that are ionized at physiologic pH and consequently undergo limited transplacental transfer.[145] For example, maternal administration of neostigmine does not reverse atropine-induced fetal tachycardia. However, small amounts of these agents do cross the placenta, and fetal bradycardia after maternal administration of neostigmine and glycopyrrolate has been reported.[146] Because neostigmine may cross the placenta to a greater extent than glycopyrrolate, the combination of neostigmine and atropine should be considered for the reversal of nondepolarizing muscle relaxants in pregnant patients.[146]

Antihypertensive Agents

Beta-adrenergic receptor antagonists are commonly used as antihypertensive agents in pregnancy, despite early investigations noting an association with intrauterine growth restriction and neonatal bradycardia, hypoglycemia, and respiratory depression.[147,148] Although a single dose of **propranolol** administered 3 hours before cesarean delivery has been shown to lead to an F/M ratio of 0.26,[149] long-term administration during pregnancy results in F/M ratios greater than 1.0.[147] Maternal administration of **atenolol** and **metoprolol** leads to mean F/M ratios of 0.94 and 1.0, respectively.[150,151]

The maternal administration of **labetalol** for the treatment of either chronic or acute hypertension in pregnant women has been supported by a low F/M ratio, 0.38, with long-term oral administration, despite mild neonatal bradycardia.[152,153]

The short-acting beta-adrenergic receptor antagonist **esmolol** has been used to attenuate the hypertensive response to laryngoscopy and intubation. A mean F/M ratio of 0.2 after maternal administration of esmolol was observed in gravid ewes.[154] However, a few cases of significant and prolonged fetal bradycardia requiring the performance of emergency cesarean delivery have been reported.[155]

Clonidine and **methyldopa** act through the central stimulation of alpha$_2$-adrenergic receptors; studies have reported mean F/M ratios of 0.89[156] and 1.17,[157] respectively, for these agents. In concentrations likely present in maternal blood with clinical use, magnesium and nifedipine, but not clonidine, produce fetal vasodilation in human placental perfusion studies *in vitro*.[158] **Dexmedetomidine,** an alpha$_2$-adrenergic agonist, has an F/M ratio of 0.12, with evidence of significant placental tissue binding due to high lipophilicity.[159] **Phenoxybenzamine,** an alpha-adrenergic receptor antagonist, is commonly used to treat hypertension in patients with pheochromocytoma and has an F/M ratio of 1.6 with long-term maternal administration.[160]

Direct-acting vasodilators are used for short-term management of severe hypertension in pregnant women. Administration of **hydralazine,** which is often given to lower blood pressure in preeclamptic women, results in an F/M ratio of 1.0[161] and causes fetal vasodilation in *in vitro* studies.[162] **Sodium nitroprusside** is lipid soluble, rapidly crosses the placenta, and can produce cyanide as a byproduct.[163] Sodium thiosulfate, the agent used to treat cyanide toxicity, does not cross the placenta in a maternal-to-fetal direction in gravid ewes, but it can treat fetal cyanide toxicity by lowering maternal cyanide levels, thereby enhancing fetal-to-maternal transfer of cyanide.[164]

Glyceryl trinitrate (nitroglycerin) crosses the placenta to a limited extent, with an F/M ratio of 0.18, and results in minimal changes in fetal umbilical blood flow, blood pressure, heart rate, and blood gas measurements in gravid ewes.[165] However, dinitrate metabolites found in both maternal and fetal venous blood indicate the capacity for placental biotransformation.[166] Indeed, placental tissue production of nitric oxide may be an important factor that enhances the uterine relaxation caused by nitroglycerin *in vivo*.[167] In one *in vitro* study, in which prostaglandin $F_{2\alpha}$ was used to create fetal vasoconstriction, the following order of nitrovasodilator compound potency was observed: glyceryl trinitrate $\geq$ sodium nitroprusside $\geq$ sodium nitrate ($NaNO_2$) $\geq$ S-nitroso-*N*-acetylpenicillamine (SNAP) = S-nitroso-*N*-glutathione (SNG).[162] SNG and $NaNO_2$ were significantly more potent under conditions of low oxygen tension. The antioxidants cysteine, glutathione, and superoxide dismutase significantly enhanced the vasodilatory effects of $NaNO_2$ only.[168]

Placental transfer of angiotensin-converting enzyme (ACE) inhibitors may adversely affect fetal renal function. **Enalaprilat** rapidly crosses the placenta, and its maternal administration in high doses resulted in a 20% reduction in fetal arterial pressure in rhesus monkeys.[169]

Vasopressor Agents

Vasopressor agents are often administered to prevent or treat hypotension during the administration of neuraxial anesthesia in obstetric patients; however, few studies have evaluated their transplacental transfer. **Ephedrine** easily crosses the placenta and results in an F/M ratio of approximately 0.7.[170] To our knowledge, no studies have evaluated the transfer of **phenylephrine** across the placenta.

Cocaine, a common drug of abuse during pregnancy (see Chapter 53), has potent vasoconstrictor activity. Human placenta perfusion studies *in vitro* have demonstrated the rapid transfer of cocaine without metabolism in both maternal-to-fetal and fetal-to-maternal directions; transfer is constant over a wide range of concentrations.[171] The active cocaine metabolites norcocaine and cocaethylene, but not the inactive metabolite benzoylecgonine, are also rapidly transferred across the placenta.[172,173] Chronic maternal administration of cocaine increases fetal concentrations; however, they remain lower than maternal peak levels.[174]

In a study using the *in vitro* dually perfused human placental lobule, fetal-side administration of vasoconstrictors was found to raise fetal placental perfusion pressure, thus causing a shift of fluid from the fetus to the maternal circulation.[175]

Anticoagulants

Anticoagulation therapy during pregnancy is often necessary despite its association with maternal and fetal morbidity. Maternal administration of **warfarin** results in a higher rate of fetal loss and congenital anomalies[176]; these findings indirectly confirm the transplacental transfer of warfarin, because no direct measurements of the F/M ratio have been performed. In contrast, **heparin** does not appear to cross the placenta, as measured by neonatal coagulation studies[177] and the measurement of radiolabeled heparin in fetal lambs.[178] **Low-molecular-weight heparin (LMWH)** appears to have limited placental transfer; however, maternal administration of **enoxaparin** does not alter fetal anti-IIa or anti-Xa activity.[179] Even when enoxaparin or **fondaparinux** (a new pentasaccharide that selectively inhibits factor Xa) are given at doses used for acute thromboembolic therapy, human placental perfusion studies *in vitro* have demonstrated no placental transfer of the drugs.[180]

Drug Delivery Systems

New drug delivery systems may influence drug transfer and distribution across the human placenta. Liposome encapsulation, depending on the type and ionic charge, can affect placental transfer; anionic and neutral liposomes increase placental transfer, whereas cationic liposomes decrease placental transfer and placental tissue uptake.[181] Liposome encapsulation of valproic acid significantly reduces drug transfer and placental uptake.[182]

Disease States

Disease states, such as diabetes, may affect the placental transfer of drugs. **Glyburide,** a second-generation sulfonylurea, is partially dependent on a P-glycoprotein active transport mechanism and demonstrates a lower F/M ratio of 0.3 than the first-generation agents, even in the presence of a P-glycoprotein inhibitor.[183] A high level of protein binding (99.8%) may also account for the low transplacental transfer of glyburide; when protein levels are reduced *in vitro,* higher transfer rates are observed.[184,185] Some investigators have speculated that the thickened placenta found in diabetic patients is a cause of low transfer rates; however, no difference in maternal-to-fetal transfer of **metformin** has been observed between placentas from parturients with gestational diabetes and those from healthy parturients.[186]

Gestational age may alter placental transfer, although the direction of the alteration requires further evaluation. Although existing belief holds that placentas from younger fetuses are more likely to transfer substances, one study has demonstrated that methadone transfer is 30% lower in human preterm placentas than in term placentas.[187]

PLACENTAL PATHOLOGY

There has been a growing interest in the clinical-pathologic correlation between placental abnormalities and adverse obstetric outcomes.[188,189] In some cases, a skilled and systematic examination of the umbilical cord, fetal membranes, and placenta may provide insight into antepartum pathophysiology; in most of these cases, examination of the placenta confirms the clinical diagnosis (e.g., chorioamnionitis). When adverse outcomes occur, often the "disorder that was not suspected clinically may be revealed by placental pathology" (e.g., microabscesses of listeriosis; amnion nodosum, which suggests long-standing oligohydramnios).[188] Drugs may produce placental abnormalities (e.g., cocaine causes chorionic villus hemorrhage and villous edema).[190] The significance of many findings (e.g., villous edema, hemorrhagic endovasculitis, chronic villitis), however, is unclear.

The following factors limit the assessment of placental pathology: (1) "the paucity of properly designed studies of adequate size with appropriate outcome parameters,"[188] which impairs the correlation of placental abnormalities with adverse clinical outcomes; (2) the limited number of pathologists with expertise in the recognition and interpretation of subtle abnormalities of the placenta; and (3) the cost associated with a routine assessment of placental pathology. The American College of Obstetricians and Gynecologists Committee on Obstetrics has concluded, "An examination of the umbilical cord, membranes, and placenta may assist the obstetric care provider in clinical-pathologic correlation when there is an adverse perinatal outcome. However, the scientific basis for clinical correlation with placenta pathology is still evolving, and the benefit of securing specimens on a routine basis is as yet unproven."[188]

KEY POINTS

- The placenta is a dynamic organ with a complex structure. It brings two circulations close together for the exchange of blood gases, nutrients, and other substances (e.g., drugs).
- During pregnancy, anatomic adaptations result in substantial (near maximal) vasodilation of the uterine spiral arteries; this leads to a low-resistance pathway for the delivery of blood to the placenta. Therefore, adequate uteroplacental blood flow depends on the maintenance of a normal maternal perfusion pressure.
- The marked diversity in placental structure and function among various animal species limits clinicians' ability to extrapolate the results of animal investigations to human pregnancy and clinical practice.
- Placental transfer involves all of the physiologic transport mechanisms that exist in other organ systems.
- Physical factors (e.g., molecular weight, lipid solubility, level of ionization) affect the placental transfer of drugs and other substances. In addition, other factors affect maternal-fetal exchange, including changes in maternal and fetal blood flow, placental binding, placental metabolism, diffusion capacity, and extent of maternal and fetal plasma protein binding.
- Lipophilicity, which enhances the central nervous system uptake of general anesthetic agents, also heightens the transfer of these drugs across the placenta. However, the placenta itself may take up highly lipophilic drugs, thereby creating a placental drug depot that limits the initial transfer of drug.
- Fetal acidemia can result in the "ion trapping" of both local anesthetics and opioids.
- Vasoactive drugs cross the placenta and may affect the fetal circulation.

REFERENCES

1. Haynes DM. The human placenta: Historical considerations. In Lavery JP, editor. The Human Placenta: Clinical Perspectives. Rockville, MD, Aspen Publishers, 1987:1-10.
2. Kaufmann P, Scheffen I. Placental development. In Polin RA, Fox WW, editors. Fetal and Neonatal Physiology. 2nd edition. Philadelphia, WB Saunders, 1998:59-70.
3. Sadler TW. Langman's Medical Embryology. 7th edition. Baltimore, Williams & Wilkins, 1995.
4. Boyd JD, Hamilton WJ. The Human Placenta. Cambridge, W. Heffer and Sons Ltd., 1970.
5. Flexner LB, Gellhorn A. The comparative physiology of placental transfer. Am J Obstet Gynecol 1942; 43:965-74.
6. James E, Meschia G, Battaglia FC. A-V differences of free fatty acids and glycerol in the ovine umbilical circulation. Proc Soc Exp Biol Med 1971; 138:823-6.
7. Ramsey EM, Donner MW. Placental Vasculature and Circulation: Anatomy, Physiology, Radiology, Clinical Aspects. Atlas and Textbook. Philadelphia, WB Saunders, 1980.
8. Arey LB. Developmental Anatomy: A Textbook and Laboratory Manual of Embryology. Philadelphia, WB Saunders, 1974.
9. Freese UE. The fetal-maternal circulation of the placenta. I. Histomorphological, plastoid injection, and x-ray cinematographic studies on human placentas. Am J Obstet Gynecol 1966; 94:354-60.
10. Leiser R, Kosanke G, Kaufmann P. Human placental vascularization: Structural and quantitative aspects. In Soma H, editor. Placenta: Basic Research for Clinical Application. Basel, Switzerland, Karger, 1991:32-45.
11. Gruenwald P. Lobular architecture of primate placentas. In Gruenwald P, editor. The Placenta and Its Maternal Supply Line: Effects of Insufficiency on the Fetus. Baltimore, University Park Press, 1975:35-55.
12. Kaufmann P. Basic morphology of the fetal and maternal circuits in the human placenta. Contrib Gynecol Obstet 1985; 13:5-17.
13. Juchau MR, Namkung MJ, Rettie AE. P-450 cytochromes in the human placenta: Oxidation of xenobiotics and endogenous steroids: A review. Trophoblast Res 1987; 2:235-63.
14. Wier PJ, Miller RK. The pharmacokinetics of cadmium in the dually perfused human placenta. Trophoblast Res 1987; 2:357-66.
15. Faber JJ, Thornburg KL. Placental Physiology: Structure and Function of Fetomaternal Exchange. New York, Raven Press, 1983.
16. Russo P. Maternal-fetal exchange of nutrients. In Nutrition and Metabolism in Pregnancy: Mother and Fetus. New York, Oxford University Press, 1990:133-67.
17. Siler-Khodr TM. Endocrine and paracrine function of the human placenta. In Polin RA, Fox WW, editors. Fetal and Neonatal Physiology. 2nd edition. Philadelphia, WB Saunders, 1998:89-102.
18. O'Shaughnessy RW, O'Toole R, Tuttle S, Zuspan FP. Uterine catecholamines in normal and hypertensive human pregnancy. Clin Exp Hypertens 1983; 82:447-57.
19. Thorbert G, Alm P, Björklund AB, et al. Adrenergic innervation of the human uterus: Disappearance of the transmitter and transmitter-forming enzymes during pregnancy. Am J Obstet Gynecol 1979; 135:223-6.
20. Greiss FC Jr. Uterine blood flow in pregnancy: An overview. In Moawad AH, Lindheimer MD, editors. Uterine and Placental Blood Flow. New York, Masson Publishing, 1982:19-26.
21. Rosenfeld CR. Regulation of placental circulation. In Polin RA, Fox WW, editors. Fetal and Neonatal Physiology. 2nd edition. Philadelphia, WB Saunders, 1998:70-7.
22. Rankin JHG, McLaughlin MK. The regulation of the placental blood flows. J Dev Physiol 1979; 1:3-30.
23. Roth JB, Thorp JA, Palmer SM, et al. Response of placental vasculature to high glucose levels in the isolated human placental cotyledon. Am J Obstet Gynecol 1990; 163:1828-30.
24. Howard RB, Hosokawa T, Maguire MH. Hypoxia-induced fetoplacental vasoconstriction in perfused human placental cotyledons. Am J Obstet Gynecol 1987; 157:1261-6.
25. Kuhn DC, Stuart MJ. Cyclooxygenase inhibition reduces placental transfer: Reverse by carbacyclin. Am J Obstet Gynecol 1987; 157: 194-8.
26. Myatt L, Brewer A, Brockman DE. The action of nitric oxide in the perfused human fetal-placental circulation. Am J Obstet Gynecol 1991; 164:687-92.
27. Byrne BM, Howard RB, Morrow RJ, et al. Role of the L-arginine nitric oxide pathway in hypoxic fetoplacental vasoconstriction. Placenta 1997; 18:627-34.
28. Coumans AB, Garnier Y, Supçun S, et al. The role of nitric oxide on fetal cardiovascular control during normoxia and acute hypoxia in 0.75 gestation sheep. J Soc Gynecol Investig 2003; 10:275-82.
29. Miller RK, Koszalka TR, Brent RL. The transport of molecules across the placental membranes. In Poste G, Nicolson GL, editors. The Cell Surface in Animal Embryogenesis and Development. Amsterdam, Elsevier/North-Holland Biomedical Press, 1976:145-223.
30. Schuster VL. Properties and functions of cell membranes. In West JB, editor. Best and Taylor's Physiological Basis of Medical Practice. 12th edition. Baltimore, Williams & Wilkins, 1991:14-30.
31. Guyton AC, Hall JE. Transport of ions and molecules through the cell membrane. In Textbook of Medical Physiology. 9th edition. Philadelphia, WB Saunders, 1996:43-55.
32. van Kreel BK. Basic mechanisms of placental transfer. Int J Biol Res Pregnancy 1981; 2:28-36.
33. Morriss FH Jr, Boyd RDH, Mahendran D. Placental transport. In Knobil E, Neill JD, editors. The Physiology of Reproduction. 2nd edition. New York, Raven Press, 1994:813-61.
34. Wang JS, Newport D, Stowe ZN, et al. The emerging importance of transporter proteins in the psychopharmacological treatment of the pregnant patient. Drug Metab Rev 2007; 39:723-46.
35. Casley-Smith JR, Chin JC. The passage of cytoplasmic vesicles across endothelial and mesothelial cells. J Microsc 1971; 93:167-89.
36. Griffiths GD, Kershaw D, Booth AG. Rabbit peroxidase-antiperoxidase complex (PAP) as a model for the uptake of immunoglobulin G by the human placenta. Histochem J 1985; 17:867-81.
37. Illsley NP, Hall S, Stacey TE. The modulation of glucose transfer across the human placenta by intervillous flow rates: An in vitro perfusion study. Trophoblast Res 1987; 2:535-44.
38. Battaglia FC, Meschia G. Foetal and placental metabolism: Their interrelationship and impact upon maternal metabolism. Proc Nutr Soc 1981; 40:99-113.
39. Jauniaux F, Gulbis B. In vivo investigation of placental transfer early in human pregnancy. Eur J Obstet Gynecol Reprod Biol 2000; 92:45-9.
40. Tsen LC, Tarshis J, Denson DD, et al. Measurements of maternal protein binding of bupivacaine throughout pregnancy. Anesth Analg 1999; 89:965-8.
41. Dancis J, Schneider H. Physiology: Transfer and barrier function. In Gruenwald P, editor. The Placenta and Its Maternal Supply Line: Effects of Insufficiency on the Fetus. Baltimore, University Park Press, 1975:98-124.
42. Longo LD. Respiration in the fetal-placental unit. In Cowett RM, editor. Principles of Perinatal-Neonatal Metabolism. New York, Springer-Verlag, 1991:304-15.
43. Barron DH, Alexander G. Supplementary observations on the oxygen pressure gradient between the maternal and fetal blood of sheep. Yale J Biol Med 1952; 25:61-6.
44. Campbell AGM, Dawes GS, Fishman AP, et al. The oxygen consumption of the placenta and foetal membranes in the sheep. J Physiol 1966; 182:439-64.
45. Longo LD, Power GG, Forster RE II. Respiratory function of the placenta as determined with carbon monoxide in sheep and dogs. J Clin Invest 1967; 46:812-28.
46. Wilkening RB, Meschia G. Current topic: Comparative physiology of placental oxygen transport. Placenta 1992; 13:1-15.
47. Nicolaides KH, Soothill PW, Rodeck CH, Campbell S. Ultrasound-guided sampling of umbilical cord and placental blood to assess fetal well-being. Lancet 1986; 1(8489):1065-7.
48. Longo LD, Hill EP, Power GG. Theoretical analysis of factors affecting placental O_2 transfer. Am J Physiol 1972; 222:730-9.

49. Hill EP, Power GG, Longo LD. A mathematical model of carbon dioxide transfer in the placenta and its interaction with oxygen. Am J Physiol 1973; 224:283-99.
50. Longo LD, Delivoria-Papadopoulos M, Forster RE II. Placental CO_2 transfer after fetal carbonic anhydrase inhibition. Am J Physiol 1974; 226:703-10.
51. Rice PA, Rourke JE, Nesbitt REL Jr. In vitro perfusion studies of the human placenta. VI. Evidence against active glucose transport. Am J Obstet Gynecol 1979; 133:649-55.
52. Challier JC, Nandakumaran M, Mondon F. Placental transport of hexoses: A comparative study with antipyrine and amino acids. Placenta 1985; 6:497-504.
53. Johnson LW, Smith CH. Glucose transport across the basal plasma membrane of human placental syncytiotrophoblast. Biochim Biophys Acta 1985; 815:44-50.
54. Leonce J, Brockton N, Robinson S, et al. Glucose production in the human placenta. Placenta 2006; 27(Suppl A):S103-8.
55. Reynolds ML, Young M. The transfer of free a-amino nitrogen across the placental membrane in the guinea-pig. J Physiol 1971; 214:583-97.
56. Yudilevich DL, Sweiry JH. Transport of amino acids in the placenta. Biochim Biophys Acta 1985; 822:169-201.
57. Leat WMF, Harrison FA. Transfer of long-chain fatty acids to the fetal and neonatal lamb. J Dev Physiol 1980; 2:257-74.
58. Elphick MC, Hull D, Sanders RR. Concentrations of free fatty acids in maternal and umbilical cord blood during elective caesarean section. Br J Obstet Gynaecol 1976; 83:539-44.
59. Booth C, Elphick MC, Hendrickse W, Hull D. Investigation of [14C]linoleic acid conversion into [14C]arachidonic acid and placental transfer of linoleic and palmitic acids across the perfused human placenta. J Dev Physiol 1981; 3:177-89.
60. Filshie GM, Anstey MD. The distribution of arachidonic acid in plasma and tissues of patients near term undergoing elective or emergency caesarean section. Br J Obstet Gynaecol 1978; 85:119-23.
61. Dancis J. Why perfuse the human placenta? Contrib Gynecol Obstet 1985; 13:1-4.
62. Marshall JR. Human antepartum placental passage of methohexital sodium. Obstet Gynecol 1964; 23:589-92.
63. Tropper PJ, Petrie RH. Placental exchange. In Lavery JP, editor. The Human Placenta: Clinical Perspectives. Rockville, MD, Aspen Publishers, 1987:199-206.
64. Reynolds F, Knott C. Pharmacokinetics in pregnancy and placental drug transfer. Oxf Rev Reprod Biol 1989; 11:389-449.
65. Herman NL, Li A-T, Bjoraker R, et al. The effects of maternal-fetal perfusate protein differences on the bidirectional transfer of thiopental across the human placenta (abstract). Anesthesiology 1998; 89:A1046.
66. Herman NL, Li AT, Van Decar TK, et al. Transfer of methohexital across the perfused human placenta. J Clin Anesth 2000; 12:25-30.
67. Herman N, Van Decar TK, Lanza M, et al. Distribution of propofol across the perfused human placenta (abstract). Anesthesiology 1994; 81:A1140.
68. Johnson RF, Herman N, Johnson HV, et al. Bupivacaine transfer across the human term placenta: A study using the dual human placental model. Anesthesiology 1995; 82:459-68.
69. Johnson RF, Cahana A, Olenick M, et al. A comparison of the placental transfer of ropivacaine versus bupivacaine. Anesth Analg 1999; 89:703-8.
70. Zakowski MI, Ham AA, Grant GJ. Transfer and uptake of alfentanil in the human placenta during in vitro perfusion. Anesth Analg 1994; 79:1089-93.
71. Johnson RF, Herman N, Arney TL, et al. The placental transfer of sufentanil: Effects of fetal pH, protein binding, and sufentanil concentration. Anesth Analg 1997; 84:1262-8.
72. Krishna BR, Zakowski MI, Grant GJ. Sufentanil transfer in the human placenta during in vitro perfusion. Can J Anaesth 1997; 44:996-1001.
73. Yang Y, Schenker S. Effects of binding on human transplacental transfer of cocaine (letter). Am J Obstet Gynecol 1995; 172:720-2.
74. Zakowski MI, Krishna R, Grant GJ, Turndorf H. Effect of pH on transfer of narcotics in human placenta during in vitro perfusion (abstract). Anesthesiology 1995; 85:A890.
75. Giroux M, Teixera MG, Dumas JC, et al. Influence of maternal blood flow on the placental transfer of three opioids—fentanyl, alfentanil, sufentanil. Biol Neonate 1997; 72:133-41.
76. Lumley J, Walker A, Marum J, Wood C. Time: An important variable at Caesarean section. J Obstet Gynaecol Br Commonw 1970; 77:10-23.
77. Kangas L, Erkkola R, Kanto J, Mansikka M. Halothane anaesthesia in caesarean section. Acta Anaesthesiol Scand 1976; 20:189-94.
78. Dwyer R, Fee JP, Moore J. Uptake of halothane and isoflurane by mother and baby during caesarean section. Br J Anaesth 1995; 74:379-83.
79. Dick W, Knoche E, Traub E. Clinical investigations concerning the use of Ethrane for cesarean section. J Perinat Med 1979; 7:125-33.
80. Marx GF, Joshi CW, Orkin LR. Placental transmission of nitrous oxide. Anesthesiology 1970; 32:429-32.
81. Polvi HJ, Pirhonen JP, Erkkola RU. Nitrous oxide inhalation: Effects on maternal and fetal circulations at term. Obstet Gynecol 1996; 87:1045-8.
82. Stenger VG, Blechner JN, Prystowsky H. A study of prolongation of obstetric anesthesia. Am J Obstet Gynecol 1969; 103:901-7.
83. Mankowitz E, Brock-Utne JG, Downing JW. Nitrous oxide elimination by the newborn. Anaesthesia 1981; 36:1014-6.
84. Flowers CE Jr. The placental transmission of barbiturates and thiobarbiturates and their pharmacological action on the mother and the infant. Am J Obstet Gynecol 1959; 78:730-42.
85. Finster M, Mark LC, Morishima HO, et al. Plasma thiopental concentrations in the newborn following delivery under thiopental-nitrous oxide anesthesia. Am J Obstet Gynecol 1966; 95:621-9.
86. Morgan DJ, Blackman GL, Paull JD, Wolf LJ. Pharmacokinetics and plasma protein binding of thiopental. II. Studies at cesarean section. Anesthesiology 1981; 54:474-80.
87. Levy CJ, Owen G. Thiopentone transmission through the placenta. Anaesthesia 1964; 19:511-23.
88. Ellingson A, Haram K, Sagen N, Solheim E. Transplacental passage of ketamine after intravenous administration. Acta Anaesthesiol Scand 1977; 21:41-4.
89. Celleno D, Capogna G, Tomassetti M, et al. Neurobehavioural effects of propofol on the neonate following elective caesarean section. Br J Anaesth 1989; 62:649-54.
90. Dailland P, Cockshott ID, Lirzin JD, et al. Intravenous propofol during cesarean section: Placental transfer, concentration in breast milk, and neonatal effects. A preliminary study. Anesthesiology 1989; 71:827-34.
91. Valtonen M, Kanto J, Rosenberg P. Comparison of propofol and thiopentone for induction of anaesthesia for elective caesarean section. Anaesthesia 1989; 44:758-62.
92. Gin T, Gregory MA, Chan K, Oh TE. Maternal and fetal levels of propofol at caesarean section. Anaesth Intensive Care 1990; 18:180-4.
93. Gin T, Yau G, Chan K, et al. Disposition of propofol infusions for caesarean section. Can J Anaesth 1991; 38:31-6.
94. Jauniaux E, Gulbis B, Shannon C, et al. Placental propofol transfer and fetal sedation during maternal general anaesthesia in early pregnancy. Lancet 1998; 352:290-1.
95. Sanchez-Alcaraz A, Quintana MB, Laguarda M. Placental transfer and neonatal effects of propofol in caesarean section. J Clin Pharm Ther 1998; 23:19-23.
96. He YL, Seno H, Tsujimoto S, Tashiro C. The effects of uterine and umbilical blood flows on the transfer of propofol across the human placenta during in vitro perfusion. Anesth Analg 2001; 93:151-6.
97. He YL, Tsujimoto S, Tanimoto M, et al. Effects of protein binding on the placental transfer of propofol in the human dually perfused cotyledon in vitro. Br J Anaesth 2000; 85:281-6.
98. He YL, Seno H, Sasaki K, Tashior C. The influences of maternal albumin concentrations on the placental transfer of propofol in the human dually perfused cotyledon in vitro. Anesth Analg 2002; 94:1312-4.

99. Downing JW, Buley RJR, Brock-Utne JG, Houlton PC. Etomidate for induction of anaesthesia at caesarean section: Comparison with thiopentone. Br J Anaesth 1979; 51:135-40.
100. Gregory MA, Davidson DG. Plasma etomidate levels in mother and fetus. Anaesthesia 1991; 46:716-8.
101. Fresno L, Andaluz A, Moll X, et al. Placental transfer of etomidate in pregnant ewes after an intravenous bolus dose and continuous infusion. Vet J 2008; 175:395-402.
102. Mandelli M, Morselli PL, Nordio S, et al. Placental transfer to diazepam and its disposition in the newborn. Clin Pharmacol Ther 1975; 17:564-72.
103. Erkkola R, Kangas L, Pekkarinen A. The transfer of diazepam across the placenta during labour. Acta Obstet Gynecol Scand 1973; 52:167-70.
104. McBride RJ, Dundee JW, Moore J, et al. A study of the plasma concentrations of lorazepam in mother and neonate. Br J Anaesth 1979; 51:971-8.
105. Wilson CM, Dundee JW, Moore J, et al. A comparison of the early pharmacokinetics of midazolam in pregnant and nonpregnant women. Anaesthesia 1987; 42:1057-62.
106. Shnider SM, Way EL, Lord MJ. Rate of appearance and disappearance of meperidine in fetal blood after administration of narcotics to the mother (abstract). Anesthesiology 1966; 27:227-8.
107. Caldwell J, Wakile LA, Notarianni LJ, et al. Transplacental passage and neonatal elimination of pethidine given to mothers in childbirth (abstract). Br J Clin Pharmacol 1977; 4:715P-6P.
108. Zakowski MI, Krishna BR, Wang SM, et al. Uptake and transfer of meperidine in human placenta during in vitro perfusion (abstract). Annual Meeting of the Society for Obstetric Anesthesia and Perinatology. Vancouver, 1997; 104.
109. Kopecky EA, Ryan ML, Barrett JFR, et al. Fetal response to maternally administered morphine. Am J Obstet Gynecol 2000; 183:424-30.
110. Hée P, Sørensen SS, Bock JE, et al. Intrathecal administration of morphine for the relief of pains in labour and estimation of maternal and fetal plasma concentration of morphine. Eur J Obstet Gynecol Reprod Biol 1987; 25:195-201.
111. Bui T, Zakowski MI, Grant GJ, Turndorf H. Uptake and transfer of morphine in human placenta during in vitro perfusion (abstract). Anesthesiology 1995; 83:A932.
112. Kopecky EA, Simone C, Knie B, Koren G. Transfer of morphine across the human placenta and its interaction with naloxone. Life Sci 1999; 65:2359-71.
113. Bower S. Plasma protein binding of fentanyl. J Pharm Pharmacol 1981; 33:507-14.
114. Loftus JR, Hill H, Cohen SE. Placental transfer and neonatal effects of epidural sufentanil and fentanyl administered with bupivacaine during labor. Anesthesiology 1995; 83:300-8.
115. Bang U, Helbo-Hansen HS, Lindholm P, Klitgaard NA. Placental transfer and neonatal effects of epidural fentanyl-bupivacaine for cesarean section (abstract). Anesthesiology 1991; 75:A847.
116. Cooper J, Jauniaux E, Gulbis B, et al. Placental transfer of fentanyl in early human pregnancy and its detection in fetal brain. Br J Anaesth 1999; 82:929-31.
117. Zakowski M, Schlesinger J, Dumbroff S, et al. In vitro human placental uptake and transfer of fentanyl (abstract). Anesthesiology 1993; 79:A1006.
118. Gepts E, Heytens L, Camu F. Pharmacokinetics and placental transfer of intravenous and epidural alfentanil in parturient women. Anesth Analg 1986; 65:1155-60.
119. Gin T, Ngan-Kee WD, Siu YK, et al. Alfentanil given immediately before the induction of anesthesia for elective cesarean delivery. Anesth Analg 2000; 90:1167-72.
120. Kan RE, Hughes SC, Rosen MA, et al. Intravenous remifentanil: Placental transfer, maternal and neonatal effects. Anesthesiology 1998; 88:1467-74.
121. Santos Iglesias LJ, Sanchez LJ, Reboso Morales JA, et al. General anesthesia with remifentanil in two cases of emergency cesarean section [Spanish]. Rev Esp Anestesiol Reanim 2001; 48:244-7.
122. Volikas I, Butwick A, Wilkinson C, et al. Maternal and neonatal side-effects of remifentanil patient controlled analgesia in labour. Br J Anaesth 2005; 95:504-9.
123. Pittman KA, Smyth RD, Losada M, et al. Human perinatal distribution of butorphanol. Am J Obstet Gynecol 1980; 138:797-800.
124. Wilson SJ, Errick JK, Balkon J. Pharmacokinetics of nalbuphine during parturition. Am J Obstet Gynecol 1986; 155:340-4.
125. Nicolle E, Devillier P, Delanoy B, et al. Therapeutic monitoring of nalbuphine: Transplacental transfer and estimated pharmacokinetics in the neonate. Eur J Clin Pharmacol 1996; 49:485-9.
126. de Barro Duarte L, Moises EC, Carvalho-Cavalli R, et al. Placental transfer of bupivacaine enantiomers in normal pregnant women receiving epidural anesthesia for cesarean section. Eur J Clin Pharmacol 2007; 63:523-6.
127. Moya F, Kvisselgaard N. The placental transmission of succinylcholine. Anesthesiology 1961; 22:1-6.
128. Kvisselgaard N, Moya F. Investigation of placental thresholds to succinylcholine. Anesthesiology 1961; 22:7-10.
129. Owens WD, Zeitlin GL. Hypoventilation in a newborn following administration of succinylcholine to the mother: A case report. Anesth Analg 1975; 54:38-40.
130. Baraka A, Haroun S, Dassili M, Abu-Haider G. Response of the newborn to succinylcholine injection in homozygotic atypical mothers. Anesthesiology 1975; 43:115-6.
131. Hinkle AJ, Dorsch JA. Maternal masseter muscle rigidity and neonatal fasciculations after induction for emergency cesarean section. Anesthesiology 1993; 79:175-7.
132. Kivalo I, Saarikoski S. Placental transfer of 14C-dimethyltubocurarine during Caesarean section. Br J Anaesth 1976; 48:239-42.
133. Duvaldestin P, Demetriou M, Henzel D, Desmonts JM. The placental transfer of pancuronium and its pharmacokinetics during caesarian section. Acta Anaesthesiol Scand 1978; 22:327-33.
134. Abouleish E, Wingard LB Jr, de la Vega S, Uy N. Pancuronium in caesarean section and its placental transfer. Br J Anaesth 1980; 52:531-6.
135. Dailey PA, Fisher DM, Shnider SM, et al. Pharmacokinetics, placental transfer, and neonatal effects of vecuronium and pancuronium administered during cesarean section. Anesthesiology 1984; 60:569-74.
136. Iwama H, Kaneko T, Tobishima S, et al. Time dependency of the ratio of umbilical vein/maternal artery concentration of vecuronium in caesarean section. Acta Anaesthesiol Scand 1999; 43:9-12.
137. Shearer ES, Fahy LT, O'Sullivan EP, Hunter JM. Transplacental distribution of atracurium, laudanosine and monoquaternary alcohol during elective caesarean section. Br J Anaesth 1991; 66:551-6.
138. Abouleish E, Abboud T, Lechevalier T, et al. Rocuronium (Org 9426) for caesarean section. Br J Anaesth 1994; 73:336-41.
139. Baraka AS, Sayyid SS, Assaf BA. Thiopental-rocuronium versus ketamine-rocuronium for rapid-sequence intubation in parturients undergoing cesarean section. Anesth Analg 1997; 84:1104-7.
140. Abouleish EI, Abboud TS, Bikhazi G, et al. Rapacuronium for modified rapid sequence induction in elective caesarean section: Neuromuscular blocking effects and safety compared with succinylcholine, and placental transfer. Br J Anaesth 1999; 83:862-7.
141. Kivalo I, Saarikoski S. Placental transmission of atropine at full-term pregnancy. Br J Anaesth 1977; 49:1017-21.
142. Kanto J, Kentala E, Kaila T, Pihlajamäki K. Pharmacokinetics of scopolamine during caesarean section: Relationship between serum concentration and effect. Acta Anaesthesiol Scand 1989; 33:482-6.
143. Ali-Melkkilä T, Kaila T, Kanto J, Iisalo E. Pharmacokinetics of glycopyrronium in parturients. Anaesthesia 1990; 45:634-7.
144. Abboud TK, Read J, Miller F, et al. Use of glycopyrrolate on the parturient: Effect on the maternal and fetal heart and uterine activity. Obstet Gynecol 1981; 57:224-7.
145. Briggs GG, Freeman RK, Yaffee SJ. Drugs in Pregnancy and Lactation: A Reference Guide to Fetal and Neonatal Risk. 4th edition. Baltimore, Williams & Wilkins, 1994.
146. Clark RB, Brown MA, Lattin DL. Neostigmine, atropine, and glycopyrrolate: Does neostigmine cross the placenta? Anesthesiology 1996; 84:450-2.

147. Cottrill CM, McAllister RGJ, Gettes L, Noonan JA. Propranolol therapy during pregnancy, labor, and delivery: Evidence for transplacental drug transfer and impaired neonatal drug disposition. J Pediatr 1977; 91:812-4.
148. Witter FR, King TM, Blake DA. Adverse effects of cardiovascular drug therapy on the fetus and neonate. Obstet Gynecol 1981; 58:100S-5S.
149. Erkkola R, Lammintausta R, Liukko P, Anttila M. Transfer of propranolol and sotalol across the human placenta. Their effect on maternal and fetal plasma renin activity. Acta Obstet Gynecol Scand 1982; 61:31-4.
150. Melander A, Niklasson B, Ingemarsson I, et al. Transplacental passage of atenolol in man. Eur J Clin Pharmacol 1978; 14:93-4.
151. Lindeberg S, Sandström B, Lundborg P, Regårdh C-G. Disposition of the adrenergic blocker metoprolol in the late-pregnant woman, the amniotic fluid, the cord blood and the neonate. Acta Obstet Gynecol Scand Suppl 1984; 118:61-4.
152. Macpherson M, Broughton-Pipkin F, Rutter N. The effect of maternal labetalol on the newborn infant. Br J Obstet Gynaecol 1986; 93:539-42.
153. Michael CA. Use of labetalol in the treatment of severe hypertension during pregnancy. Br J Clin Pharmacol 1979; 8:211S-5S.
154. Östman PL, Chestnut DH, Robillard JE, et al. Transplacental passage and hemodynamic effects of esmolol in the gravid ewe. Anesthesiology 1988; 69:738-41.
155. Ducey JP, Knape KG. Maternal esmolol administration resulting in fetal distress and cesarean section in a term pregnancy. Anesthesiology 1992; 77:829-32.
156. Hartikainen-Sorri A-L, Heikkinen JE, Koivisto M. Pharmacokinetics of clonidine during pregnancy and nursing. Obstet Gynecol 1987; 69:598-600.
157. Jones HMR, Cummings AJ, Setchell KD, Lawson AM. A study of the disposition of (alpha-methyldopa in newborn infants following its administration to the mother for the treatment of hypertension during pregnancy. Br J Clin Pharmacol 1979; 8:433-40.
158. David R, Leitch IM, Read MA, et al. Actions of magnesium, nifedipine and clonidine on the fetal vasculature of the human placenta. Aust N Z J Obstet Gynaecol 1996; 36:267-71.
159. Ala-Kokko TI, Pienimaki P, Lampela E, et al. Transfer of clonidine and dexmedetomidine across the isolated perfused human placenta. Acta Anaesthesiol Scand 1997; 41:313-9.
160. Santeiro ML, Stromquist C, Wyble L. Phenoxybenzamine placental transfer during the third trimester. Ann Pharmacother 1996; 30:1249-51.
161. Liedholm H, Wahlin-Boll E, Hanson A, et al. Transplacental passage and breast milk concentrations of hydralazine. Eur J Clin Pharmacol 1982; 21:417-9.
162. Magee KP, Bawdon RE. Ex vivo human placental transfer and the vasoactive properties of hydralazine. Am J Obstet Gynecol 2000; 182:167-9.
163. Naulty J, Cefalo RC, Lewis PE. Fetal toxicity of nitroprusside in the pregnant ewe. Am J Obstet Gynecol 1981; 139:708-11.
164. Gracine KA, Curry SC, Bikin DS, et al. The lack of transplacental movement of the cyanide antidote thiosulfate in gravid ewes. Anesth Analg 1999; 89:1448-52.
165. Bootstaylor BS, Roman C, Parer JT, Heymann MA. Fetal and maternal hemodynamic and metabolic effects of maternal nitroglycerin infusion in sheep. Am J Obstet Gynecol 1997; 176:644-50.
166. Bustard MA, Farley AE, Smith GN. The pharmacokinetics of glyceryl trinitrate with the use of the in vitro term human placental perfusion setup. Am J Obstet Gynecol 2002; 187:187-90.
167. Segal S, Csavoy AN, Datta S. Placental tissue enhances uterine relaxation by nitroglycerin. Anesth Analg 1998; 86:304-9.
168. Zhang XQ, Kwek K, Read MA, et al. Effects of nitrovasodilators on the human fetal-placental circulation in vitro. Placenta 2001; 22:337-46.
169. Ducsay CA, Umezaki H, Kanshal KM, et al. Pharmacokinetic and fetal cardiovascular effects of enalaprilat administration to maternal rhesus macaques. Am J Obstet Gynecol 1996; 175:50-5.
170. Hughes SC, Ward MG, Levinson G, et al. Placental transfer of ephedrine does not affect neonatal outcome. Anesthesiology 1985; 63: 217-9.
171. Krishna RB, Levitz M, Dancis J. Transfer of cocaine by the perfused human placenta: The effect of binding to serum proteins. Am J Obstet Gynecol 1995; 172:720-2.
172. Schenker S, Yang Y, Johnson RF, et al. The transfer of cocaine and its metabolites across the term human placenta. Clin Pharmacol Ther 1993; 53:329-39.
173. Simone C, Derewlany LO, Oskamp M, et al. Transfer of cocaine and benzoylecgonine across the perfused human placental cotyledon. Am J Obstet Gynecol 1994; 170:1404-10.
174. Zhou M, Song ZM, Lidow MS. Pharmacokinetics of cocaine in maternal and fetal rhesus monkeys at mid-gestation. J Pharmacol Exp Ther 2001; 297:556-62.
175. Brownbill P, Sibley CP. Regulation of transplacental water transfer: The role of fetoplacental venous tone. Placenta 2006; 27:560-7.
176. Hall JG, Pauli RM, Wilson KM. Maternal and fetal sequelae of anticoagulation during pregnancy. Am J Med 1980; 68:122-40.
177. Flessa HC, Kapstrom AB, Glueck HI, Will JJ. Placental transport of heparin. Am J Obstet Gynecol 1965; 93:570-3.
178. Andrew M, Boneu B, Cade J, et al. Placental transport of low molecular weight heparin in the pregnant sheep. Br J Haematol 1985; 59:103-8.
179. Dimitrakakis C, Papageorgiou P, Papageorgiou I, et al. Absence of transplacental passage of the low molecular weight heparin enoxaparin. Haemostasis 2000; 30:243-8.
180. Lagrange F, Vergnes C, Brun JL, et al. Absence of placental transfer of pentasaccharide (fondaparinux, Arixtra®) in the dually perfused human cotyledon in vitro. Thromb Haemost 2002; 87:831-5.
181. Bajoria R, Contractor SF. Effect of surface change on small unilamellar liposome on uptake and transfer of carboxyfluorescein across the perfused human term placenta. Pediatr Res 1997; 42:520-7.
182. Barzago MM, Bortolotti A, Stellari FF, et al. Placental transfer of valproic acid after liposome encapsulation during in vitro human placenta perfusion. J Pharmacol Exper Ther 1996; 277:79-86.
183. Kraemer J, Klein J, Lubetsky A, Koren G. Perfusion studies of glyburide transfer across the human placenta: Implications for fetal safety. Am J Obstet Gynecol 2006; 195:270-4.
184. Nanovskaya TN, Nekhayeva I, Hankins GDV, Ahmed MS. Effect of human serum albumin on transplacental transfer of glyburide. Biochem Pharmacol 2006; 72:632-9.
185. Gedeon C, Behravan J, Koren G, Piqueette-Miller M. Transport of glyburide by placental ABC transporters: Implication in fetal drug exposure. Placenta 2006; 27:1096-102.
186. Nanovskaya TN, Nekhayeva IA, Patriekeeva SL, et al. Transfer of metformin across the dually perfused human placental lobule. Am J Obstet Gynecol 2006; 195:1081-5.
187. Nanovskaya TN, Nekhayeva IA, Hankins GD, Ahmed MS. Transfer of methadone across the dually perfused preterm human placental lobule. Am J Obstet Gynecol 2008; 198:126.
188. American College of Obstetricians and Gynecologists Committee on Obstetrics: Maternal and Fetal Medicine. Placental pathology. ACOG Committee Opinion No. 125, July 1993. (Int J Gynaecol Obstet 1993; 42:318-9.)
189. The examination of the placenta: Patient care and risk management. College of American Pathologists Conference XIX: Northfield, Illinois, September 6-7, 1990. Proceedings. Arch Pathol Lab Med 1991; 115:660-721.
190. Mooney EE, Boggess KA, Herbert WN, Layfield LJ. Placental pathology in patients using cocaine: An observational study. Obstet Gynecol 1998; 91:925-9.

Chapter 5

Fetal Physiology

Kenneth E. Nelson, M.D.
Andrew P. Harris, M.D., M.H.S.

The fetus relies completely on maternal sources of metabolic substrate to maintain viability and consequently depends on special physiology patterns that differ from those in postnatal animals. The fetus must also be prepared to undergo an abrupt transition to a state of physiologic independence through the process of birth. This transition necessarily involves adaptive mechanisms that ameliorate the stress that occurs during the change from intrauterine to postnatal life.

FETAL OXIDATIVE METABOLISM

Oxygen Uptake and Substrate Use

Like postnatal animals, the fetus depends on the metabolism of oxygen to provide the energy necessary to maintain life. Unlike postnatal animals, however, the fetus has almost no oxygen reservoir and thus is totally dependent on ongoing transplacental oxygen from the mother. When this transfer is hindered significantly, the fetus attempts to preserve oxygen transport to vital organ systems for as long as possible (see later).

Oxygen is transferred from the uterine circulation to the umbilical circulation by passive diffusion (see Chapter 4). Under chronic basal conditions, fetal arterial Po_2 is much lower than that in postnatal life. However, fetal tissues are not ischemic because of an increased hemoglobin concentration (compared with that in adults) as well as the presence of hemoglobin F, which has greater oxygen affinity than adult hemoglobin. Evidence supporting a normoxemic fetal state includes the following: (1) net lactate uptake (not production) by the fetus occurs, (2) only small amounts of hydrogen ion are transferred from the fetus to the mother, (3) no increase in oxygen consumption ($\dot{V}o_2$) occurs when more oxygen is made available to the fetus, and (4) the healthy fetus has a normal basal pH.[1]

Total uterine oxygen uptake can be divided into two components: placental consumption and umbilical oxygen uptake (i.e., uptake by the fetus). At term, placental oxygen consumption accounts for approximately 40% of total uterine oxygen uptake,[2] but at midgestation, an even higher uptake is observed.[3] The placenta is metabolically active and plays an important role in carbohydrate and amino acid metabolism and substrate transport; all of these functions depend on the energy produced through oxidative metabolism.

Umbilical $\dot{V}o_2$ is fairly constant and varies little among different mammalian species when it is corrected for fetal weight.[4] Human fetal $\dot{V}o_2$ is estimated to be approximately 6.8 to 8.0 mL O_2/kg/min.[5,6] By contrast, there is a clear inverse relationship between weight and metabolic rate in adult mammals.

Factors that influence fetal $\dot{V}o_2$ include (1) fetal growth, (2) fetal activity (e.g., breathing movements, limb movements, cardiac activity), (3) substrate availability, (4) fetal organ metabolism, and (5) fetal hormonal status. Growth and activity account for a significant portion of $\dot{V}o_2$[7,8]; however, the use of oxygen for growth and activity is not necessary for survival and can be eliminated in times of stress.

Studies in sheep suggest that approximately 10% to 15% of total $\dot{V}o_2$ is used for striated muscle activity.[7] The fetal brain accounts for approximately 8% to 9% of total $\dot{V}o_2$,

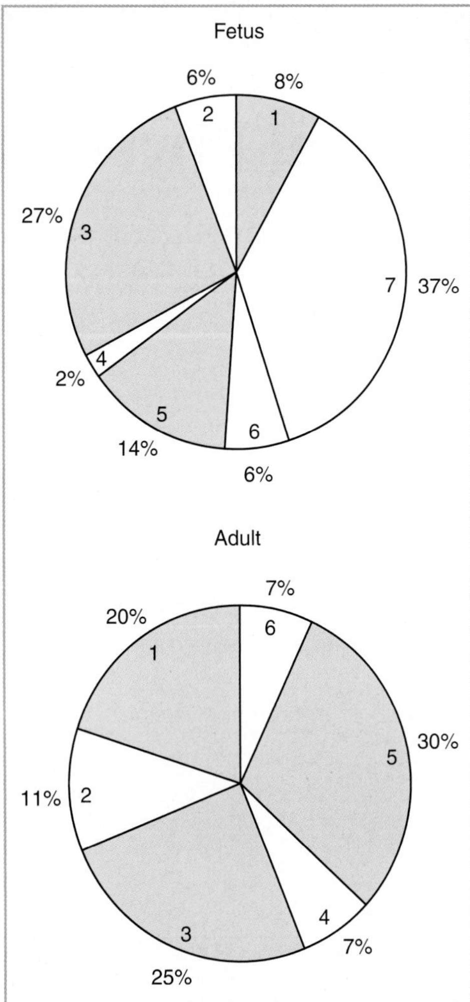

FIGURE 5-1 Tissue-specific oxygen consumption in continuously instrumented fetal lambs and resting adult humans. 1, Brain; 2, heart; 3, liver and intestines; 4, kidney; 5, muscle; 6, other; 7, growth (fetus only). (Data from Edelstone DI, Holzman IR. Fetal intestinal oxygen consumption at various levels of oxygenation. Am J Physiol 1982; 242:H50-4; and Philipps AF. Carbohydrate metabolism of the fetus. In Polin RA, Fox WW, editors. Fetal and Neonatal Physiology. Vol 1. Philadelphia, WB Saunders, 1992:373-84.)

and the liver, intestines, and kidneys together account for approximately 29% (Figure 5-1).[1,9-13]

Fetal $\dot{V}O_2$ rises above normal levels *in utero* in at least three circumstances: (1) increased fetal activity, (2) increased glucose uptake, and (3) increased secretion of various hormones. Maternal hyperglycemia results in excessive maternal-fetal glucose transfer; the subsequent hyperinsulinemia can raise fetal $\dot{V}O_2$ by as much as 30%.[14] Although such large increases in fetal $\dot{V}O_2$ can result in acidosis and even death in fetal lambs, the same does not consistently occur in humans.[15] Excessive secretion of catecholamines or thyroid hormones can also result in 20% to 30% increases in $\dot{V}O_2$ in fetal lambs; thus the higher fetal catecholamine concentrations witnessed during labor and delivery may adversely affect fetal oxygenation, especially if oxygen transport is reduced and the fetal response to the reduced oxygen transport is impaired.

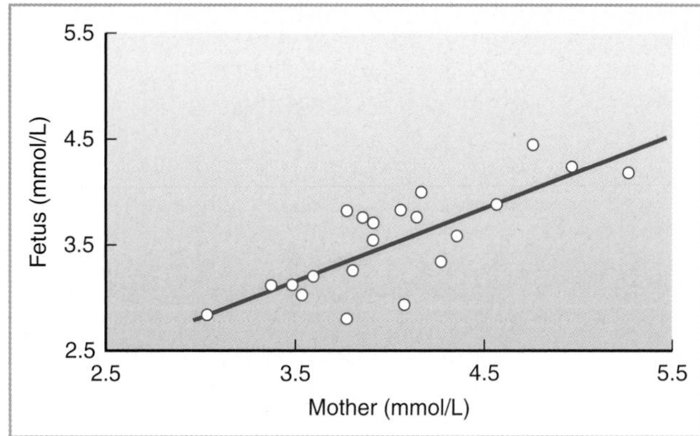

FIGURE 5-2 The linear relationship between maternal and fetal blood glucose concentrations during the third trimester. Fetal blood was obtained by percutaneous umbilical cord blood sampling. (From Kalhan SC. Metabolism of glucose and methods of investigation in the fetus and newborn. In Polin RA, Fox WW, editors. Fetal and Neonatal Physiology. Vol. I. Philadelphia, WB Saunders, 1992:477-88.)

Fetal $\dot{V}O_2$ does not change during fetal hypoglycemia, because hypoglycemia stimulates glycogenolysis and gluconeogenesis. By contrast, during severe fetal hypoxemia, $\dot{V}O_2$ may be depressed by as much as 40% in fetal lambs.[16] Such hypoxemia-related decreases in fetal $\dot{V}O_2$ are associated with lower metabolism in the fetal liver, intestine, and kidney, and reduced fetal skeletal muscle activity[11,16,17]; cerebral and myocardial oxygen uptake are unchanged. If bradycardia occurs, myocardial oxygen uptake diminishes. The ability of the cerebral and myocardial organ systems to continue functioning in the setting of hypoxia, coupled with ongoing glycogenolysis to produce energy substrates for their maintenance, give the fetus the best opportunity for survival under conditions of stress.

Glucose-Lactate Metabolism

Under normal conditions, gluconeogenesis does not occur to any significant extent in mammalian fetuses. During normal fasting conditions in a term, human gestation, the sole fetal source of glucose is whatever is transferred across the placenta.[18] Fetal glucose concentrations are linearly related to maternal concentrations over the range of 3 to 5 mmol/L (Figure 5-2), with studies in isolated placentas suggesting that this relationship continues up to a glucose concentration of 20 mmol/L.[19] Glucose is transferred across the placenta by facilitated, carrier-mediated diffusion. An analysis of total uterine glucose uptake reveals that the majority of the glucose is used by the placenta and that the remainder is transferred to the umbilical circulation. Glucose is used by the placenta for oxidation, glycogen storage, and conversion to lactate. Interestingly, when ovine uterine blood flow is reduced by 50%, there is no corresponding effect on fetal glucose uptake or fetal arterial glucose concentration.[20] However, when uterine blood flow is decreased further or when umbilical arterial flow is reduced by ligation of one of the umbilical arteries, fetal glucose uptake diminishes.[20,21]

The umbilical glucose uptake is approximately 5 mg/kg/min at normal maternal arterial plasma glucose concentrations.[22] Because the umbilical glucose-oxygen quotient varies from approximately 0.5 in sheep[23] to 0.8 in human fetuses during labor,[24] it must be assumed that substrates other than glucose (e.g., lactate, amino acids) fuel a significant amount of fetal oxidative metabolism. Lactate and amino acids may each account for approximately 25% of total fetal $\dot{V}O_2$.[25,26]

Lactate is produced even in well-oxygenated fetal lambs, with total lactate production being approximately 4 mg/kg/min.[27] Although the exact origin of fetal lactate is unclear, skeletal muscles and bones are definite sources of lactate production under resting conditions; other organs probably produce lactate as well. Lactate production increases during episodes of acute hypoxemia, although this response may be blunted in fetuses previously exposed to oxidative stress.[28] In terms of lactate use, the fetal myocardium is a net consumer of lactate, and the fetal liver also is a likely site of lactate utilization.[29] Exogenous lactate infusion in fetal lambs (sufficient to lower the pH to 7.20) results in transient fetal bradycardia and increased fetal breathing movements but no adverse effects.[30]

Amino Acid and Lipid Metabolism

Amino acids are taken up by the fetus for protein synthesis, growth, and oxidation. Most maternal-to-fetal amino acid transfer occurs against a concentration gradient and involves energy-dependent transfer mechanisms. Under conditions in which fetal aerobic metabolism is decreased, amino acid uptake by the placenta and fetus may be reduced because it involves an expenditure of energy. Hypoxia results in a large reduction in nitrogen uptake in fetal lambs.[31] During maternal fasting, fetal amino acid uptake does not change; however, enhanced fetal proteolysis may occur, which subsequently results in amino acid oxidation or gluconeogenesis.

Lipid products also are transferred from the mother to the fetus. The fetus requires free fatty acids for growth, brain development, and the deposition of body fat for postnatal life. Fatty acids are transferred across the placenta by simple diffusion. Ketones are also transferred by simple diffusion; in humans, the maternal-fetal ketone ratio is approximately 2.0.[32] The fetus can use ketones as energy or as lipogenic substrates.[33] Fetal tissues that can oxidize ketones include the brain, kidney, heart, liver, and placenta. Beta-hydroxybutyrate (fatty acid) metabolism can replace glucose metabolism deficits in the placenta, brain, and liver during episodes of fetal hypoglycemia that result from maternal fasting.[33] Cholesterol synthesis or free cholesterol diffusion does not appear to occur in the placenta.[34] However, there is a significant correlation between maternal and fetal concentrations of lipoprotein(a), implying that diffusion of lipoprotein(a) may occur.[34]

GENERAL GROWTH AND DEVELOPMENT

Normal growth and development occur when the fetus has an adequate supply of metabolic substrate and is able to use it. Conversely, growth and development are abnormal when adequate supplies are not available or when the fetus is unable to use the available substrate. Fetal measurements allow not only a dynamic assessment of fetal growth but also a static indication of fetal well-being. Normal fetal growth curves have been constructed with the use of birth weights in a large series of newborns at varying weeks of gestation; these curves indicate a normal rate of human fetal growth of approximately 1.45% per day.

Such growth curves are useful in defining static categorizations of infant size. For example, infants who are appropriate for gestational age (AGA) are those with weights between the 10th and 90th percentiles for their gestational age. Infants who are small (SGA) and large (LGA) for gestational age are those with weights less than the 10th percentile and more than the 90th percentile for their gestational age, respectively. Infants at both extremes are at increased risk of complications in postnatal life; at the lower end of the spectrum, evidence suggests that the 15th percentile would be a more useful threshold, because fetuses between the 10th and 15th percentiles have higher risk for fetal death.[35] These terms—AGA, LGA, and SGA—should not be confused with terms used to describe birth weight independent of gestational age. Specifically, low-birth-weight (LBW) infants are those who weigh less than 2500 g, regardless of gestational age. Very low-birth-weight (VLBW) infants are those who weigh less than 1500 g, and extremely low-birth-weight (ELBW) infants are those who weigh less than 1000 g, regardless of gestational age. These last terms may not indicate abnormal growth. For example, although it would be normal for a newborn at 25 weeks' gestation to be an ELBW infant, it would not be normal at term. SGA or LGA infants may not have suffered from pathophysiologic processes; rather these infants may represent a normal phenotypic expression of size.[36]

However, the diagnosis of intrauterine growth restriction (IUGR) signals an ongoing process of subnormal fetal growth over time. IUGR is more likely than birth weight to represent an underlying physiologic abnormality. Any process that results in a chronically inadequate availability of substrate or that impedes the fetus's ability to use substrate will cause the fetus to grow at a less-than-normal rate. For example, the plasma concentrations of a number of amino acids (but not glucose) are decreased in cases of IUGR, possibly as a result of reduced placental transport. In cases of IUGR, the activity of placental microvillous transport system A is reduced *in vitro*.[37] Fetuses who suffer intrauterine oxidative stress also have a reduction in oxygen consumption, even after the stress is removed.[28] Of course, if an affected fetus remains *in utero* long enough, it will probably be SGA at birth. Most cases of IUGR result in the delivery of an SGA infant.

IUGR may be **asymmetric** or **symmetric**. In cases of asymmetric IUGR, fetal brain growth is relatively preserved, but growth of the remainder of the body is diminished, resulting in an asymmetry between head growth and body growth. An asymmetric growth pattern may be the consequence of a constantly decreased supply of substrate, which may occur for a variety of reasons. In cases of symmetric IUGR, head circumference and body length are reduced proportionately to overall weight. In some instances, this may be a normal growth pattern (e.g., genetic predisposition); in other cases, it may signal an insult that began early in gestation (e.g., genetic abnormality, congenital infection, prolonged uteroplacental insufficiency). Either category of IUGR makes the fetus less tolerant of a superimposed acute substrate deprivation, which may occur in a variety of circumstances, including labor and delivery. The diagnosis of IUGR is associated with a higher risk of fetal death.[38]

The diagnosis of IUGR, although more useful than static measurements, is also more difficult to ascertain. Various diagnostic techniques are used to assess intrauterine fetal growth. Physical examination (e.g., serial measurement of fundal height) is an inexpensive but nonsensitive and nonspecific means of assessment. Serial sonographic examinations represent the most reliable method for the diagnosis of IUGR. During early gestation, a sonographic examination involves the measurement of crown-rump length, with subsequent examinations including assessment of head size, abdominal circumference, and femur length. These measurements may be used to provide an estimate of fetal weight.

Other methods may be used to study fetuses in whom abnormalities of growth are suspected. Doppler ultrasonography can be used to study both the uteroplacental and umbilical vessels. Although ultrasonography cannot measure fetal size or growth, it can identify abnormal flow patterns[39,40] or pulse waveforms,[41] which correlate with adverse fetal outcomes. In growth-restricted fetuses, there may be increased resistance in the umbilical arteries and descending aorta, with relatively normal internal carotid[42] or middle cerebral[43] (especially the subcortical segment[44]) artery flow; these findings are consistent with the brain sparing that occurs with asymmetric IUGR. In SGA infants, abnormalities of both umbilical and middle cerebral artery velocimetry predict adverse fetal outcome.[45] Abnormal Doppler flow studies of the fetal aorta are associated with poor perinatal outcome, especially when associated with abnormal umbilical artery flow.[46]

FETAL HEAT PRODUCTION AND THERMOREGULATION

At term, the human fetus consumes oxygen at the rate of approximately 6.8 to 8.0 mL/kg/min, which is approximately twice the rate of adult oxygen consumption. Fetal heat production, as a byproduct of oxygen metabolism, is consequently large relative to that of an adult. Assuming that approximately 5 cal of heat are produced for each milliliter of oxygen consumed, a 4-kg human fetus produces approximately 136 cal/min, which is approximately 10 watts. Fetal heat accumulates until a relatively constant temperature gradient of approximately 0.5° C is established, after which heat is dissipated into the mother. Because the gradient remains relatively constant, fetal heat dissipation depends on maternal temperature; this relationship is sometimes referred to as a "heat clamp," which prevents independent fetal thermoregulation *in utero*.

Heat dissipates from the fetus by means of two possible avenues: (1) the umbilical circulation (and therefore the placenta) and (2) fetal skin (by means of the amniotic fluid). Of these two, experimental evidence suggests that the umbilical circulation is the major source of fetal heat loss. In both baboons[47] and sheep,[48] fetal temperature rises shortly after umbilical cord occlusion, which may result in part from the activation of normal postnatal thermogenic mechanisms.[49] A decrease in uterine blood flow likewise would be expected to increase fetal temperature, but this issue has not been studied directly. However, the maternal-fetal temperature gradient does increase during uterine contractions in humans,[50] a finding that indirectly confirms the importance of the placenta as a heat exchanger for the fetus. Heat loss through the skin and amniotic fluid represents only a small portion (15%) of fetal-maternal heat exchange.[49] Epidural anesthesia during labor may result in increased fetal temperature,[51] possibly because epidural anesthesia "alters the [maternal] thermoregulatory response to warming by increasing the threshold for thermoregulatory sweating and in some cases, [by] preventing leg sweating"[52] (see Chapter 36).

FETAL CIRCULATION

The fetal circulation allows the fetus to match the local supply of metabolic substrate to local demand. An understanding of fetal circulation requires an understanding of the following: (1) fetal oxygen transport, (2) the regulation of fetal blood volume, (3) the unique fetal circulatory pattern, and (4) the various factors that control the distribution of blood flow. These factors become critically important when substrate demand exceeds substrate supply during periods of fetal stress.

Fetal Oxygen Transport

Oxygen delivery to a fetal organ is the product of blood flow to that organ multiplied by the oxygen content of fetal arterial blood. The oxygen content of fetal blood is largely determined by the product of the concentration of hemoglobin (the predominant vehicle of oxygen transport in blood), the percentage of hemoglobin that is bound to oxygen, and a constant of approximately 1.39 mL O_2/g Hgb (the oxygen-carrying capacity of hemoglobin). In adults, as the Po_2 is increased toward 1 atm, the oxygen content of arterial blood is augmented significantly by the presence of oxygen dissolved in plasma. Plasma oxygen content increases by approximately 0.003 mL O_2/dL blood per mm Hg increase in Pao_2. In theory, an increased Pao_2 allows adult animals to augment their total blood oxygen content by 1.5 to 1.8 mL O_2/dL (i.e., by approximately one third of adult oxygen consumption). In contrast, fetal umbilical venous Po_2 does not increase by more than 50 to 60 mm Hg, even when maternal oxygenation is optimized under isobaric oxygen conditions. The amount of oxygen dissolved in fetal plasma is insignificant relative to fetal oxygen demand or fetal hemoglobin oxygen-carrying capacity. The normal fetal hemoglobin concentration is approximately 18 g/dL. The oxygen-carrying capacity of fetal blood should be approximately 25 mL O_2/dL, greater than that of adults. However, this is only a theoretical capacity, because fetal hemoglobin never approaches complete saturation at the relatively low levels of Po_2 *in utero*.

At the low Po_2 of the intervillous space, a higher affinity of fetal blood for oxygen would augment the transfer of oxygen from the mother to the fetus. In fact, fetal blood has a higher affinity for oxygen than does maternal blood *in vivo*. The P_{50} of human fetal blood (partial pressure of oxygen in the blood at which the hemoglobin is 50% saturated) is approximately 19 to 21 mm Hg, in contrast to the 27 mm Hg found in adult blood (Figure 5-3). This observed difference in affinity for oxygen is largely a result of the relatively high concentration of hemoglobin F in fetal blood (i.e., approximately 75% to 84% of total hemoglobin

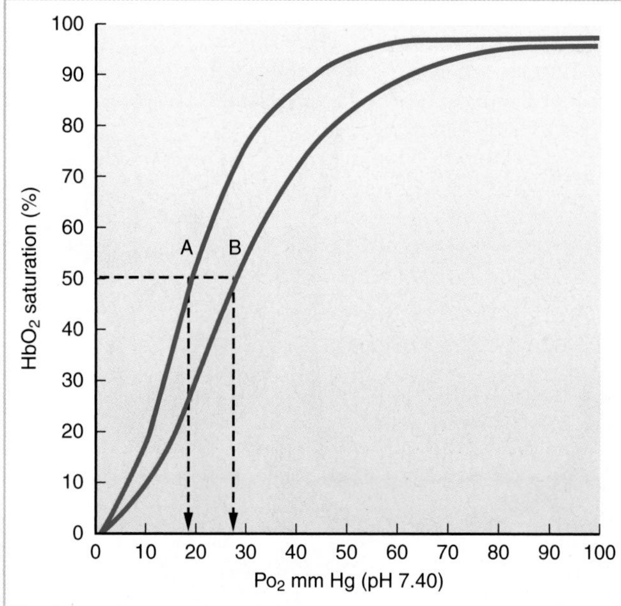

FIGURE 5-3 Oxyhemoglobin saturation curves for fetal (A) and adult (B) human blood. The P_{50} is indicated by the *dashed vertical line*. (Modified from Delivoria-Papadopoulos M, DiGiacomo JE. Oxygen transport. In Polin RA, Fox WW, editors. Fetal and Neonatal Physiology. Vol. 1. Philadelphia, WB Saunders, 1992:807.)

at term).[53] The tetramer for hemoglobin F consists of two alpha chains and two gamma chains, whereas the tetramer for adult hemoglobin A includes two alpha chains and two beta chains. This change in globin composition does not result in a change in the absorption spectra of oxygenated and reduced hemoglobin[54] or in a change in oxygen affinity outside of the erythrocyte *in vitro*.[55] Instead, the shift in fetal blood oxygen affinity *in vivo* can be explained by a decreased interaction between hemoglobin F and intra-erythrocyte 2,3-diphosphoglycerate (DPG), which normally acts to lower oxygen affinity by binding to and stabilizing the deoxygenated hemoglobin tetramer. The gamma chains of hemoglobin F do not bind as readily to 2,3-DPG. The net effect is that 2,3-DPG does not decrease the oxygen affinity of hemoglobin F as much as it reduces the oxygen affinity of hemoglobin A. Thus, although fetuses and adults have similar intraerythrocyte 2,3-DPG concentrations, fetal blood exhibits a lower P_{50} than adult blood. *In utero*, this greater affinity of fetal blood for oxygen results in a 6% to 8% higher saturation of hemoglobin on the fetal side of the intervillous membrane.

Hemoglobin A levels begin to increase and 2,3-DPG concentrations transiently increase above fetal and adult levels during the first few months of life. Therefore, the affinity of neonatal blood for oxygen is equivalent to that of the adult within 3 to 4 months of birth, despite the persistence of approximately 25% hemoglobin F.

Regulation of Extracellular Fluid Volume

Extracellular fluid volume consists of both interstitial fluid and intravascular volume. The distribution between these two compartments is determined predominantly by the colloid osmotic pressure in the intravascular compartment, the capillary hydrostatic pressure, and the capillary membrane permeability according to the Starling equation, as follows:

$$Q = K_f[(P_c - P_t) - \delta(\pi_c - \pi_t)]$$

where Q is fluid flux; K_f is the filtration coefficient (which expresses the membrane permeability to water flux); P_c and P_t are capillary and tissue hydrostatic pressures, respectively; δ is the reflection coefficient (which expresses the membrane's permeability to protein); and π_c and π_t are capillary and tissue oncotic pressures, respectively.

The intravascular volume of the term human fetus is approximately 100 to 110 mL/kg. This volume is larger than the blood volume in either the newborn or the adult, but approximately one third of fetal blood volume is contained outside the fetal body, in the umbilical cord and placenta.

Blood volume is regulated by the balance between interstitial volume and intravascular volume and is determined by plasma fluid loss across the capillaries. Given the relative stability of colloid osmotic pressure and capillary permeability, changes in hydrostatic pressure predominantly affect fetal blood volume. For example, blood volume decreases when hydrostatic pressure is transiently increased; such transient increases in hydrostatic pressure can occur during uterine contractions as blood is transferred from the placental vascular bed into the fetal body. Another cause of decreased blood volume is an increase in capillary pressure due to release of vasoconstrictive hormones, which occurs during periods of stress. Both factors may account for the observed drop in circulating blood volume during labor and delivery.[56]

Infusion of water or crystalloid in the mother also changes fetal extracellular fluid volume. Under these conditions, transient changes in colloid osmotic pressure lead to transplacental osmotic gradients, and rapid equilibration occurs across the placenta. When this fluid is transferred to the fetus, its disposition differs from that found in adults. Adults who receive an intravenous infusion of crystalloid retain approximately 25% of the infused volume in the intravascular space at 30 minutes. By contrast, in unanesthetized fetal lambs, a crystalloid infusion increases blood volume by only 6% to 7%; the remainder of the infusion rapidly enters the interstitial space.[57] This difference can be explained by the relatively high interstitial space compliance in the fetus and an apparently higher capillary filtration coefficient.[58] Thus, maternal infusion of crystalloid may ultimately result in significant increases in fetal extracellular fluid volume. Anesthesia providers should consider this potential effect when giving a large volume of crystalloid to the mother.

Circulatory Pattern *In Utero*

The most striking difference between the fetal circulation and the postnatal circulation is that systemic and pulmonary circulations are not completely separated in the fetus (Figure 5-4), whereas postnatal circulations are in series. Blood flowing through the fetal right atrium is directed either through the foramen ovale into the left atrium or through the right ventricle into the pulmonary artery.

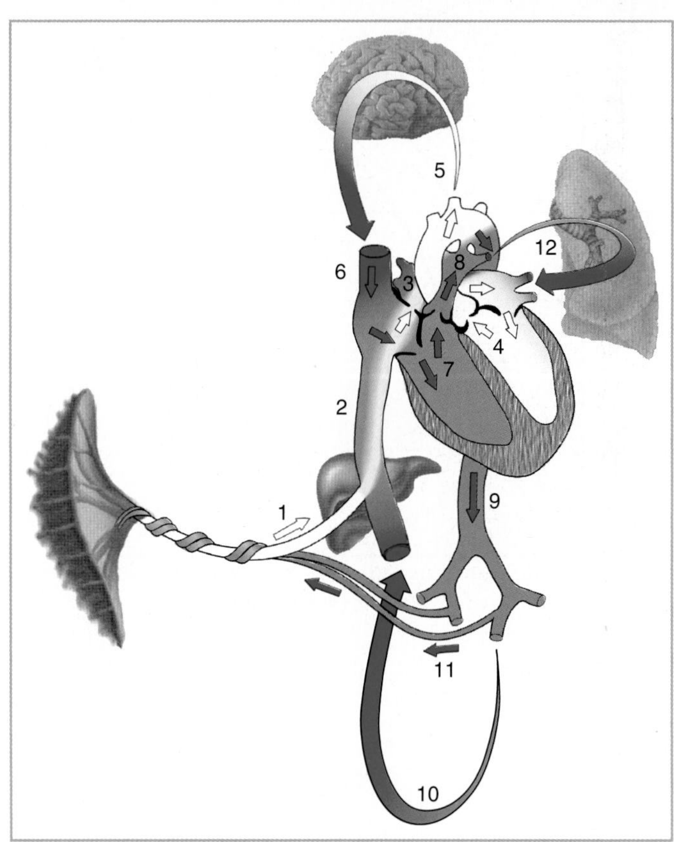

FIGURE 5-4 Oxygenated blood leaves the placenta via the fetal umbilical vein (1), enters the liver where flow divides between the portal sinus and the ductus venosus, and then empties into the inferior vena cava (2). Inside the fetal heart, blood enters the right atrium, where most of the blood is directed through the foramen ovale (3) into the left atrium and ventricle (4), and then enters the aorta. Blood is then sent to the brain (5) and myocardium, ensuring that these cells receive the highest oxygen content available. Deoxygenated blood returning from the lower extremities and the superior vena cava (6) is preferentially directed into the right ventricle (7) and pulmonary trunk. The majority of blood passes through the ductus arteriosus (8) into the descending aorta (9), which in turn supplies the lower extremities (10) and the hypogastric arteries (11). Blood returns to the placenta via the umbilical arteries for gas and nutrient exchange. A small amount of blood from the pulmonary trunk travels through the pulmonary arteries (12) to perfuse the lungs. *Arrows* in this figure depict the direction and oxygen content [*white* (oxygenated), *teal* (deoxygenated)] of the blood in circulation. (Drawing by Naveen Nathan, M.D., Northwestern University Feinberg School of Medicine, Chicago, IL.)

The majority of pulmonary artery blood flow crosses the ductus arteriosus into the descending aorta and the left side of the circulation; only a small percentage travels through the lungs into the left atrium. The fetal systemic and pulmonary circulations are not completely separated because the fetal lungs do not participate in blood oxygenation; instead, this role is met by the umbilical circulation, which is a component of the systemic circulation.

To maximize the efficiency of cardiac work and transplacental oxygen transfer, almost all deoxygenated blood from the fetal head and upper extremities enters the right atrium by means of the superior vena cava. Moving from the right atrium to the right ventricle, blood then travels through the ductus arteriosus into the distal aorta, from which a significant percentage goes to the placenta to be reoxygenated. By contrast, the oxygenated umbilical venous blood returns from the placenta, enters the right atrium by means of the inferior vena cava, and preferentially flows across the foramen ovale into the left atrium. The blood then enters the left ventricle and is distributed through the preductal circulation, which includes the two organs with the highest oxygen requirements, the brain and myocardium. This circulatory pattern facilitates the delivery of highly oxygenated blood to areas of high oxygen consumption and allows for the delivery of deoxygenated blood to the placenta, where oxygen uptake occurs. At birth, the circulatory pattern changes dramatically (see Chapter 9).

Cardiac Output

In postnatal mammals, the right and left ventricular outputs are approximately equal. Therefore, *cardiac output* is defined as the output of either the **right ventricle** (commonly measured with a thermodilution technique using a pulmonary artery catheter) or the **left ventricle** (measured with a green dye technique). By contrast, the fetus has an almost complete right-to-left shunt at the level of the ductus arteriosus. Therefore, fetal systemic flow consists of the sum of right and left ventricular outputs. Fetal cardiac output to the systemic circulation is **biventricular** and consequently called **combined ventricular output (CVO)**. The CVO is approximately 500 mL/min/kg in near-term fetal lambs.[59-61] Right ventricular output is greater than left ventricular output, and right ventricular coronary blood flow is 50% greater than left ventricular coronary blood flow.[62] In fetal lambs, approximately two thirds of CVO originates from the right ventricle.[63] The primary function of the right ventricle (both *in utero* as well as after delivery) is to deliver blood for oxygen uptake. The purpose of the left ventricle is to deliver oxygenated blood.

CVO *in utero* is approximately equal to the output of each individual ventricle after birth.[64] Although total ventricular output doubles immediately after birth, it appears that the fetus is unable to increase CVO *in utero*, even during periods of stress. To understand why cardiac output cannot be augmented *in utero*, one must consider the following four major determinants of ventricular function: **preload, afterload, contractility,** and **heart rate**. The fetal response to changes in each of these factors differs from that of postnatal mammals.

VENTRICULAR RESPONSE TO CHANGES IN PRELOAD

According to the Frank-Starling curve, ventricular distention lengthens the diastolic fibers and results in augmented contractility. Whereas decreases in preload (i.e., fetal hemorrhage) lead to an immediate drop in fetal cardiac output, increases in preload (i.e., intravenous volume infusion) in normovolemic fetuses do not consistently result in higher ventricular output, for reasons that are not clear.[65-68]

Several factors, however, may help explain this finding. First, the fetal myocardium demonstrates diminished tension development at all muscle lengths compared with that in the adult[69]; this decreased tension response may be due to a significantly greater proportion of noncontractile proteins in fetal myocytes. Further, at any given level of developed tension, myocardial shortening velocity and the extent of shortening are decreased in the fetus relative to those in the adult.[69] The velocity of force development is determined primarily by adenosine triphosphatase (ATPase) activity that is present in the myosin heavy chain. The myosin heavy chain isoform is different in fetuses from that in adults, perhaps explaining the difference in myocardial shortening.

Second, the highly compliant placental vascular bed accommodates even large increases in intravascular volume, thus limiting significant alterations in filling pressures and myocardial end-diastolic fiber length. Even when end-diastolic pressures are raised as a result of intravascular transfusion, cardiac output does not change to any significant degree, in part because of the relatively stiff fetal myocardium.[70]

Third, volume infusion in the fetus typically results in a simultaneous increase in afterload, and the fetal heart is quite sensitive to any increase in afterload.[71] Fourth, a large interatrial shunt allows right and left ventricular end-diastolic pressures to increase equally during volume infusion. This biventricular filling, particularly in the stiff fetal ventricles, may limit the overall distention of the heart and ventricles.

VENTRICULAR RESPONSE TO CHANGES IN AFTERLOAD

The second determinant of ventricular systolic function is afterload, which can be approximated by systemic vascular resistance (SVR). In normal adults, increases in afterload result in little if any decrease in cardiac output; however, decreases in afterload typically result in an increase in cardiac output. By contrast, in fetal animals, the ventricles respond to an increase in afterload with a decrease in cardiac output.[65,66] Conversely, the fetal right ventricle responds to a decrease in afterload with little change in right ventricular output; the fetal left ventricle responds similarly.[65,66]

FETAL CARDIAC CONTRACTILITY

The third determinant of ventricular function is contractility. At all muscle lengths, significantly less active tension is generated by fetal myocardium than by the myocardium of the mature heart. The sarcoplasmic reticulum is relatively immature in both structure and function. In addition, myofibrils are structurally and functionally immature in the fetus.[72,73] Finally, the beta-adrenergic receptors may be relatively unresponsive. Isoproterenol infusion does not lead to an increase in cardiac output in fetal lambs.[74]

VENTRICULAR RESPONSE TO ALTERED HEART RATES

The fourth determinant of ventricular function is heart rate. In adult mammals, significant heart rate changes do not cause proportional changes in cardiac output. A decreased heart rate results in increases in diastolic filling time, end-diastolic volume, and end-diastolic fiber length. These changes result in an increase in stroke volume, which compensates for the decreased heart rate and helps keep cardiac output constant. A higher heart rate is accompanied by an increase in intrinsic myocardial contractility, but decreased diastolic filling time results in reduced end-diastolic and stroke volumes. The net result is no change or a slight increase in cardiac output. At either extreme of heart rate, cardiac output decreases.

By contrast, fetal ventricular output appears to be more sensitive to changes in heart rate. As heart rate increases, cardiac output increases.[75-77] As heart rate decreases, stroke volume increases only slightly, most likely because of the lower compliance of the fetal myocardium and the ventricular diastolic interaction described previously. Although fetal bradycardia leads to an extended diastolic filling time, the stiff, interactive ventricles are limited in their ability to distend. Therefore, fetal bradycardia is associated with a marked drop in fetal cardiac output.

DISTRIBUTION OF CARDIAC OUTPUT

Figure 5-5 shows the distribution of CVO in near-term fetal lambs and resting adult humans. Approximately 41% of fetal CVO perfuses the placenta, and another 38% perfuses the skeletal muscle and bone. Renal, gastrointestinal, myocardial, and cerebral blood flow account for 2%, 6%, 4%, and 3% of CVO, respectively. The fetal systemic circulation is considered a low-resistance circuit, because a large fraction of CVO perfuses the relatively compliant placental circulation. In both fetal and adult animals, approximately equal volumes of blood proceed to the oxygen-uptake organs (i.e., the placenta before delivery, the lungs after delivery) and to the oxygen-consuming organs (i.e., the remainder of the body before delivery, the systemic circulation after delivery).

Control of the Systemic Circulation and the Fetal Response to Stress

Fetal cardiovascular function adapts to varying metabolic and environmental conditions through neuroregulation and endocrine regulation. The predominant form of neuroregulation occurs in response to baroreceptor and chemoreceptor afferent input to the autonomic nervous system and through modulation of myocardial adrenergic receptor activity. Thus, the autonomic nervous system functions to reversibly redirect blood flow and oxygen delivery where and when required.

Arterial baroreceptor function has been demonstrated in several different fetal animal models. The predominant baroreceptors are located in the aortic arch and at the bifurcation of the common carotid arteries. These receptors project signals to the vasomotor center in the medulla, from which autonomic responses emanate. Functioning relatively early in fetal development, the baroreceptors reset as blood pressure increases during normal gestation.[78] A sudden increase in fetal mean arterial pressure (MAP)—as occurs with partial or complete occlusion of the umbilical arteries—results in cholinergic stimulation and subsequent fetal bradycardia.

Chemoreceptor activity is also present in many animal species. Peripheral chemoreceptors are present in at least two locations, (1) between the aortic arch and the main pulmonary artery and (2) at the bifurcation of the common

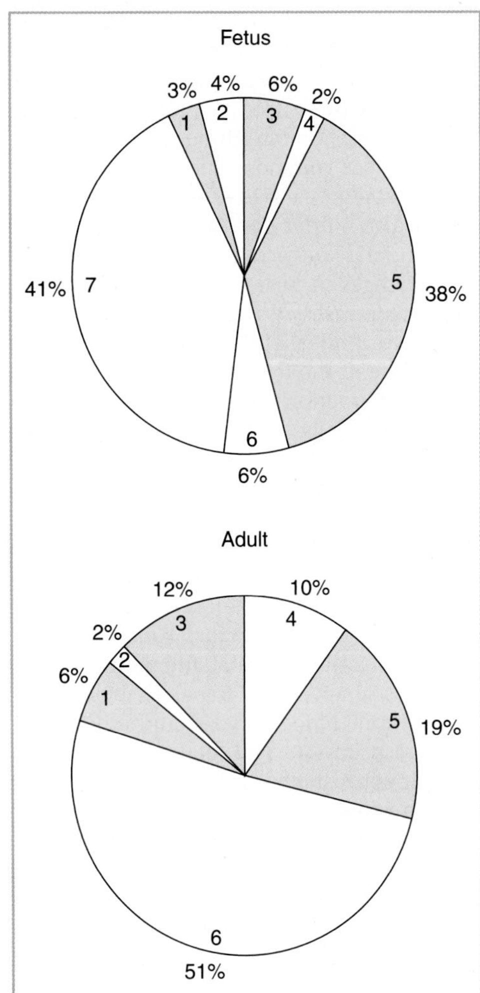

FIGURE 5-5 Regional distribution of the combined ventricular output in fetal lambs and resting adult humans. 1, Brain; 2, heart; 3, liver and intestines; 4, kidney; 5, muscles and other; 6, lungs; 7, placenta. (Data from Peltonen R. The difference between fetal and maternal temperatures during delivery (abstract). Fifth European Congress of Perinatal Medicine, Uppsala, Sweden, June 1976:188; and Philipps AF. Carbohydrate metabolism of the fetus. In Polin RA, Fox WW, editors. Fetal and Neonatal Physiology. Philadelphia, WB Saunders, 1992:373-84.)

carotid arteries. Also, in some species a peripheral chemoreceptor is present in the adrenal gland that disappears after birth.[79] The fetal aortic chemoreceptors are quite active and respond to small changes in arterial oxygenation.[80,81] Fetal carotid chemoreceptors are less active. Dawes et al.[82] concluded that carotid chemoreceptors are important for postnatal respiratory control, whereas aortic chemoreceptors are important in cardiovascular control and the regulation of oxygen delivery. Central chemoreceptors appear to play little if any role in the fetal chemoreceptor response.

Hypoxemia is the most common fetal stress occurring during labor and delivery. In continuously instrumented pregnant sheep, a number of investigators have evaluated the response to fetal hypoxemia produced by a variety of methods (e.g., administration of a hypoxic gas mixture to the mother, partial occlusion of the umbilical cord, partial occlusion of the uterine artery). Fetal hypoxemia redistributes blood flow from the kidneys, spleen, carcass, and skin toward the heart, brain, placenta, and adrenal glands. Nitric oxide and prostaglandins appear to be important mediators in the coronary[83] and cerebral[84-86] circulatory responses to hypoxia.

To a large extent, myocardial and cerebral blood flows can increase to compensate for decreased blood oxygen content, even during episodes of severe hypoxemia. At modest levels of hypoxemia, CVO is not affected, and blood pressure and heart rate are unchanged. However, extreme hypoxemia causes chemoreceptor stimulation, which results in bradycardia and a reduction in cardiac output. This decrease in CVO can be exacerbated by the presence of acidemia[87] and increased afterload resulting from umbilical cord occlusion. Combined blood flow to the heart and brain, which accounts for 7% to 8% of cardiac output under baseline conditions, increases to approximately 25% of cardiac output when oxygen content is reduced by 80% (Figure 5-6).[88] The absolute placental blood flow does not change during hypoxemia; however, when CVO decreases, the fraction of CVO distributed to the placenta increases. In part, this altered distribution is produced by changes in placental vascular resistance, which rises slightly during acute hypoxemia[87,88]; this response can be reversed by fetal alpha-adrenergic receptor blockade.[89] Chronic hypoxemia *in utero* may lead to vascular remodeling that maintains the ability of the coronary circulation to dilate in response to superimposed acute hypoxemia, even in the presence of a preexisting increase in flow that has occurred in response to the chronic hypoxemia.[83]

Sympathetic and Parasympathetic Development

Autonomic regulation of the peripheral circulation occurs predominantly through adrenergic mechanisms. The contractile response of the fetal vasculature to norepinephrine is present although it is somewhat less functional than the adult response.[90,91] Administration of alpha-adrenergic agonists results in the redistribution of fetal blood flow away from the kidneys, skin, and splanchnic organs and toward the heart, brain, placenta, and adrenal glands.[92]

Parasympathetic tone also affects the circulation, predominantly through an effect on heart rate. Parasympathetic activity first appears at approximately 16 weeks' gestation, when fetal administration of atropine leads to fetal tachycardia. Sympathetic innervation of the heart becomes significant at the end of the second trimester. At this time, the fetal administration of a beta-adrenergic receptor antagonist causes fetal bradycardia. Inotropic and chronotropic responses to adrenergic agents are present much earlier in gestation, having been measured as early as 4 to 5 weeks' gestation.[93] Likewise, the fetal myocardial pacemaker can be inhibited by the cholinergic agonists carbamylcholine and acetylcholine as early as 4 weeks' gestation.[94] Therefore, it is clear that autonomic receptor function appears much earlier than functional autonomic tone. Autonomic function is delayed even though nerve cells have been identified in the human heart as early as 5 to 6 weeks' gestation,[95] with parasympathetic cholinergic nerves present by 8 weeks' gestation[96,97] and sympathetic adrenergic nerves present by 9 to 10 weeks' gestation.[93]

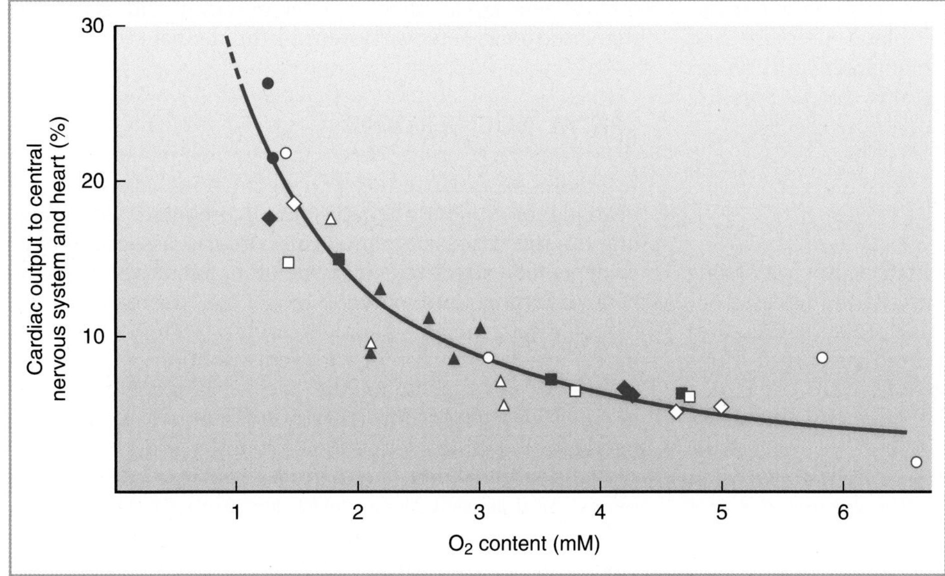

FIGURE 5-6 The redistribution of cardiac output to the heart and central nervous system during hypoxemia in fetal lambs. Each symbol represents a measurement from an individual fetal lamb. (Modified from Sheldon RE, Peeters LLH, Jones MD Jr, et al. Redistribution of cardiac output and oxygen delivery in the hypoxic fetal lamb. Am J Obstet Gynecol 1979; 135:1071-8.)

Most studies have confirmed that parasympathetic innervation occurs earlier than sympathetic innervation and is more completely functional at birth. As pregnancy progresses, fetal parasympathetic activity becomes more dominant; thus the baseline fetal heart rate (FHR) at 40 weeks' gestation is less than the baseline FHR at 26 weeks' gestation. This decrease in FHR is reversible with administration of atropine (Figure 5-7). Adrenergic innervation is relatively incomplete at birth.

Endocrine Control and the Response to Stress

Epinephrine released by the adrenal medulla is present in fetal plasma but at much lower concentrations than norepinephrine. Stress (e.g., hypoxemia, hemorrhage) may engender release of epinephrine.

Arginine vasopressin (AVP) is detectable as early as 11 weeks' gestation in the posterior pituitary of human fetuses.[98] Prior to midgestation, hemorrhage can be a potent stimulus of vasopressin release in fetal lambs.[99] Under normal conditions, however, vasopressin is not an important regulator of fetal circulation, as demonstrated by the little or no effect of vasopressin-receptor antagonists on arterial blood pressure in fetal lambs. Vasopressin is released during episodes of acute fetal hypoxia and hypotension,[100,101] resulting in fetal hypertension and decreases in splanchnic and skin blood flow. These changes are accompanied by proportionate increases in cerebral, myocardial, and placental blood flows.[102] As a result of these changes, fetal PO_2 rises significantly, implying that vasopressin may be an important mediator of the fetal response to acute hypoxemia.[87]

The renin-angiotensin system appears to be active under basal conditions in fetal animals. Renin activity is present and circulating angiotensin II concentrations can be measured in fetal lambs just after midgestation.[103] Stress results in increased renin-angiotensin system activity in fetal lambs, with the response to hypotension[101] being greater than that to hypoxemia.[100] Interestingly, angiotensin II constricts the umbilical circulation when it is infused to achieve plasma concentrations similar to those observed during hemorrhage.[104] Basal concentrations of angiotensin II

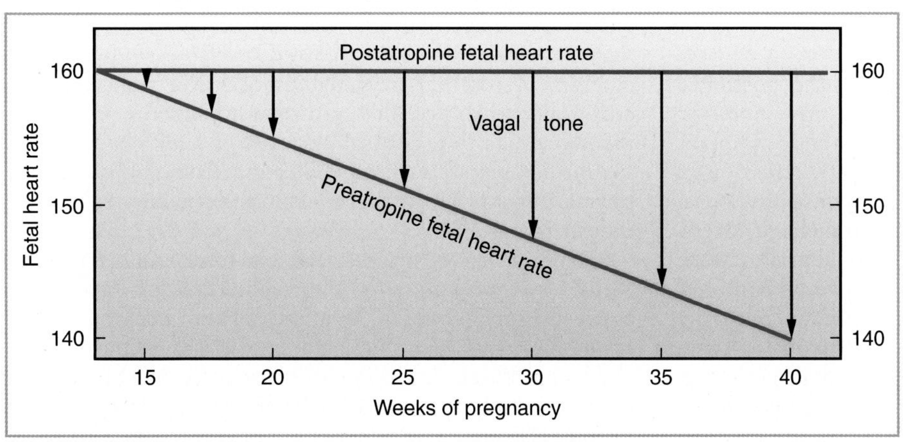

FIGURE 5-7 The growing influence of the parasympathetic nervous system on fetal heart rate as gestation progresses. This parasympathetic activity is reversible with administration of atropine. (From Schifferli P, Caldeyro-Barcia R. Effects of atropine and beta-adrenergic drugs on the heart rate of the human fetus. In Broeus L, editor. Fetal Pharmacology. New York, Raven Press, 1973:264.)

maintain chronic vasoconstriction of the peripheral circulation, which helps maintain arterial blood pressure and umbilical-placental blood flow. When angiotensin II receptors are blocked under basal conditions, blood pressure decreases and umbilical-placental blood flow falls.[105]

Circulatory Responses to Increased Intracranial Pressure

As the fetal head descends into the maternal pelvis during normal labor, fetal intracranial pressure (ICP) increases out of proportion to the rises in intrauterine pressure. Pressures measured at the equator of the fetal head far exceed intra-amniotic pressure.[106] These observations were confirmed in a study that used an intracranial catheter to measure ICP in two hydrocephalic fetuses during labor.[107] Outside the range of cerebral autoregulation, cerebral perfusion pressure (defined as the MAP minus the greater of either cerebral venous pressure or ICP) is the determining factor in cerebral perfusion. Large increases in ICP in postnatal animals cause a transient decrease in cerebral perfusion pressure; this decrease results in a Cushing response (i.e., vasoconstriction, increased MAP and cardiac output, and decreased heart rate), which acts to return cerebral perfusion pressure toward normal. During labor, the fetal response to increased ICP may be important in preserving cerebral viability.

In fetal lambs, increased ICP leads to a dramatic redistribution of the circulation. During gradual increases in ICP, MAP rises to maintain a cerebral perfusion pressure of approximately 26 mm Hg. Under these conditions, the redistribution of circulation consists of (1) decreased perfusion of the splanchnic organs, kidneys, and skin; (2) preservation of blood flow to the skeletal muscle and bone; and (3) augmented blood flow to the heart, brain, placenta, and adrenal glands.[108] Cardiac output does not change. Over time, fetal pH decreases as a result of these compensatory mechanisms. Nonetheless, cerebral oxygen delivery and uptake are maintained. In a similar model, when ICP is periodically increased to the level of MAP (in an oscillatory pattern), similar redistributions of blood flow occur over time; cardiac output does not change.[109] Experiments involving alpha-adrenergic receptor blockade indicate that the alpha-adrenergic system is primarily responsible for mediating this redistribution of the circulation,[101] which appears effective in preserving cerebral oxygen uptake despite the increased ICP.

Postnatal Effects of Intrauterine Stress

Investigators have expressed an interest in the postnatal effect of intrauterine stress on the autonomic nervous system. In one study, the postnatal sympathetic nervous system response to postural change (tilt) stress was enhanced, and the parasympathetic response to odor blunted, in infants who had chronic intrauterine stress (CIUSTR) from causes such as maternal smoking or maternal hypertension.[110] In a similar study,[111] a painful stimulus elicited a greater sympathetic response (i.e., increase in heart rate and blood pressure) in CIUSTR neonates than in a control group. In this study, an altered response to ocular compression indicated an enhanced parasympathetic response in the CIUSTR neonates. Thus, it appears that intrauterine stress affects the maturation and activity of the autonomic nervous system in the neonate.

FETAL NOCICEPTION

In studies of intrauterine fetal blood transfusion, surgical needling of the intrahepatic vein (compared with needling of the insensate umbilical cord) is associated with evidence of a stress response, including increases in plasma beta-endorphin and cortisol levels and decreases in the Doppler-determined middle cerebral artery pulsatility index, which is consistent with redistribution of blood flow to vital organs, including the brain.[112] Administration of fentanyl (10 μg/kg) blunts this stress response to intrahepatic needling.[113] Human fetuses demonstrate pituitary-adrenal, sympathoadrenal, and circulatory stress responses to noxious stimuli as early as 18 weeks' gestation.[114-117]

The withdrawal from noxious stimuli or an increased release of stress hormones does not necessarily reflect an *awareness* of pain, because local spinal reflexes and hormonal release can occur without cortical involvement.[118,119] The experience of pain is a conscious subjective experience with emotional and affective components that requires higher-level cortical processing. Nociceptive processing begins in the peripheral neurons, which relay signals through the spinothalamic tract, the thalamus, and ultimately the cerebral cortex, where conscious perception of pain occurs.[120]

Evidence suggests that thalamocortical axons reach the somatosensory cortex at 24 to 26 weeks' gestation.[121-123] Methods used to assess whether these fibers are functionally active include electroencephalography (EEG), somatosensory evoked potentials (SSEPs), behavioral responses, and near-infrared measurement of changes in cerebral oxygenation. Although the presence of pain does not correlate with a specific EEG response, the EEG pattern associated with wakefulness has been used as a surrogate indicator of the thalamocortical connections necessary for pain perception.[118,124] This pattern first appears in preterm neonates at approximately 30 weeks' postmenstrual age. Similarly, SSEPs do not specifically demonstrate the capacity to feel pain; however, they do reflect somatosensory cortex processing of a peripheral somatic stimulus. Such patterns are present at 29 weeks' postmenstrual age.[125,126] Behavioral responses, such as specific facial movements, have also been used to demonstrate pain perception in neonates.[127,128] Facial expressions during heel lancing, similar to those that occur in adults experiencing pain, are found in neonates at 28 to 30 weeks' postmenstrual age, but not at 25 to 27 weeks.[127] Recent studies using near-infrared spectroscopy to measure changes in cerebral oxygenation over the somatosensory cortex demonstrated that noxious stimulation of preterm infants results in a cortical response that differs from that to non-noxious stimulation, indicating that noxious information is transmitted to the infant cortex at 25 weeks' postmenstrual age.[129,130]

Current evidence suggests that fetal nociception at the level of the cortex occurs after the midpoint of pregnancy (i.e., between 24 and 30 weeks' gestation). Of note, maternal administration of general anesthesia does not guarantee the presence of fetal anesthesia or analgesia. For example, most infants are clearly awake and cry loudly immediately after cesarean delivery during maternal administration of general anesthesia.

KEY POINTS

- Unlike postnatal animals, the fetus has no effective oxygen reservoir.
- The basal rate of oxygen uptake in the fetus is approximately twice that in the adult but may decrease significantly during episodes of hypoxemia.
- Lactate is produced and consumed even in well-oxygenated fetuses.
- The diagnosis of intrauterine growth restriction signals a greater fetal susceptibility to physiologic stress.
- Although the level of fetal PaO_2 is low *in utero*, the fetus is neither hypoxemic nor hypoxic under basal conditions.
- The P_{50} of fetal blood is significantly lower than that of adult blood.
- Fluid moves readily between the maternal intravascular and fetal interstitial spaces.
- The fetal circulation directs oxygenated blood toward the brain and heart and directs deoxygenated blood to the umbilical circulation and placenta.
- The fetus cannot significantly increase its combined ventricular output above basal levels.
- Hypoxemia results in chemoreceptor stimulation, which leads to significant redistribution of cardiac output towards the heart, brain, placenta, and adrenal glands.
- Even at term, the fetal autonomic nervous system is relatively immature.
- As pregnancy progresses, tonic parasympathetic activity increases; thus the baseline fetal heart rate is slower at 40 weeks' gestation than at 26 weeks' gestation.
- Increased fetal intracranial pressure can significantly alter the fetal circulatory pattern.
- Intrauterine stress affects the maturation and activity of the autonomic nervous system in the neonate.

REFERENCES

1. Philipps AF. Carbohydrate metabolism of the fetus. In Polin RA, Fox WW, editors. Fetal and Neonatal Physiology. Vol 1. Philadelphia, WB Saunders, 1992:373-84.
2. Meschia G, Battaglia FC, Hay WW Jr, Sparks JW. Utilization of substrates by the ovine placenta in vivo. Fed Proc 1980; 39:245-9.
3. Molina RD, Meschia G, Wilkening RB. Uterine blood flow, oxygen and glucose uptakes at mid-gestation in the sheep. Proc Soc Exp Biol Med 1990; 195:379-85.
4. Battaglia FC, Meschia G. An Introduction to Fetal Physiology. Orlando, FL, Academic Press, 1986:65.
5. Sandiford I, Wheeler T. The basal metabolism before, during and after pregnancy. J Biol Chem 1924; 62:329-50.
6. Bonds DR, Crosby LD, Cheek TG, et al. Estimation of human fetal-placental unit metabolic rate by application of the Bohr principle. J Dev Physiol 1986; 8:49-54.
7. Brooke OG. Energy expenditure in the fetus and neonate: Sources of variability. Acta Paediatr Scand Suppl 1985; 319:128-34.
8. Rurak DW, Gruber NC. The effect of neuromuscular blockage on oxygen consumption and blood gases in the fetal lamb. Am J Obstet Gynecol 1983; 145:258-62.
9. Jones MD Jr, Traystman RJ. Cerebral oxygenation of the fetus, newborn, and adult. Semin Perinatol 1984; 8:205-16.
10. Battaglia FC, Meschia G. An Introduction to Fetal Physiology. New York, Academic Press, 1986:136-53.
11. Bristow J, Rudolph AM, Itskovitz J. A preparation for studying liver blood flow, oxygen consumption, and metabolism in the fetal lamb in utero. J Dev Physiol 1981; 3:255-66.
12. Edelstone DI, Holzman IR. Fetal intestinal oxygen consumption at various levels of oxygenation. Am J Physiol 1982; 242:H50-4.
13. Milnor WR. Normal circulatory function. In Mountcastle VB, editor. Medical Physiology. 13th edition. St. Louis, Mosby, 1974:34.
14. Philipps AF, Porte PJ, Stabinsky S, et al. Effects of chronic fetal hyperglycemia upon oxygen consumption in the ovine uterus and conceptus. J Clin Invest 1984; 74:279-86.
15. Philipson EH, Kalhan SC, Riha MM, Pimentel R. Effects of maternal glucose infusion on fetal acid-base status in human pregnancy. Am J Obstet Gynecol 1987; 157:866-73.
16. Edelstone DI. Fetal compensatory responses to reduced oxygen delivery. Semin Perinatol 1984; 8:184-91.
17. Peeters LL, Sheldon RE, Jones MD Jr, et al. Blood flow to fetal organs as a function of arterial oxygen content. Am J Obstet Gynecol 1979; 135:637-46.
18. Kalhan SC, D'Angelo LJ, Savin S, Adam PAJ. Glucose production in pregnant women at term gestation: Sources of glucose for the human fetus. J Clin Invest 1979; 63:388-94.
19. Hauguel S, Desmaizieres V, Challier JC. Glucose uptake, utilization, and transfer by the human placenta as functions of maternal glucose concentration. Pediatr Res 1986; 20:269-73.
20. Wilkening RB, Battaglia FC, Meschia G. The relationship of umbilical glucose uptake to uterine blood flow. J Dev Physiol 1985; 7:313-9.
21. Oh W, Omori K, Hobel CJ, et al. Umbilical blood flow and glucose uptake in lamb fetus following single umbilical artery ligation. Biol Neonate 1975; 26:291-9.
22. Hay WW Jr, Sparks JW, Wilkening RB, et al. Fetal glucose uptake and utilization as functions of maternal glucose concentration. Am J Physiol 1984; 246:E237-42.
23. Boyd RDH, Morriss FH Jr, Meschia G, et al. Growth of glucose and oxygen uptakes by fetuses of fed and starved ewes. Am J Physiol 1973; 225:897-907.
24. Morriss FH Jr, Makowski EL, Meschia G, Battalgia FC. The glucose/oxygen quotient of the term human fetus. Biol Neonate 1975; 25:44-52.
25. Burd LI, Jones MD Jr, Simmons MA, et al. Placental production and foetal utilization of lactate and pyruvate. Nature 1975; 254:710-1.
26. Gresham EL, James EJ, Raye JR, et al. Production and excretion of urea by the fetal lamb. Pediatrics 1972; 50:372-9.
27. Battaglia FC, Meschia G. An Introduction to Fetal Physiology. Orlando, FL, Academic Press, 1986:91.
28. Gardner DS, Giussani DA, Fowden AL. Hindlimb glucose and lactate metabolism during umbilical cord compression and acute hypoxemia in the late-gestation ovine fetus. Am J Physiol Regul Integr Comp Physiol 2003; 284:R954-64.
29. Sparks JW, Hay WW Jr, Bonds D, et al. Simultaneous measurements of lactate turnover rate and umbilical lactate uptake in the fetal lamb. J Clin Invest 1982; 70:179-92.
30. Bocking AD, Challis JR, White SE. Effect of acutely-induced lactic acidemia on fetal breathing movements, heart rate, blood pressure, ACTH and cortisol in sheep. J Dev Physiol 1991; 16:45-50.
31. Milley JR. Protein synthesis during hypoxia in fetal lambs. Am J Physiol 1987; 252:E519-24.
32. Palacin M, Lasuncion MA, Herrara E. Lactate production and absence of gluconeogenesis from placental transferred substrates in fetuses from fed and 48-h starved rats. Pediatr Res 1987; 22:6-10.
33. Shambaugh GE III, Mrozak SC, Freinkel N. Fetal fuels. I. Utilization of ketones by isolated tissues at various stages of maturation and maternal nutrition during late gestation. Metabolism 1977; 26:623-35.

34. Neary RH, Kilby MD, Kumpatula P, et al. Fetal and maternal lipoprotein metabolism in human pregnancy. Clin Sci 1995; 88:311-8.
35. Seeds JW, Peng T. Impaired growth and risk of fetal death: Is the tenth percentile the appropriate standard? Am J Obstet Gynecol 1998; 178:658-69.
36. Klebanoff MA, Schulsinger C, Mednick BR, Secher NJ. Preterm and small-for-gestational-age birth across generations. Am J Obstet Gynecol 1997; 176:521-6.
37. Jansson T, Ylven K, Wennergren M, et al. Glucose transport and system A activity in syncytiotrophoblast microvillous and basal plasma membranes in intrauterine growth restriction. Placenta 2002; 23:392-9.
38. Ferguson R, Myers SA. Population study of the risk of fetal death and its relationship to birth weight, gestational age, and race. Am J Perinatol 1994; 11:267-72.
39. Zelop CM, Richardson DK, Heffner LJ. Outcomes of severely abnormal umbilical artery Doppler velocimetry in structurally normal singleton fetuses. Obstet Gynecol 1996; 87:434-8.
40. Poulain P, Palaric JUC, Paris-Liado J, Jacquemart F, and the Doppler Study Group. Fetal umbilical Doppler in a population of 541 high-risk pregnancies: Prediction of perinatal mortality and morbidity. Doppler Study Group. Eur J Obstet Gynecol Reprod Biol 1994; 54:191-6.
41. Madazli C, Sen S, Uludag V, et al. Doppler dynamics: Their clinical significance and relationship with fetal blood gases and pH measurements. J Obstet Gynaecol 2001; 21:448-52.
42. Wladimiroff JW, Wijngaard JAGW, Degani S, et al. Cerebral and umbilical arterial blood flow velocity waveforms in normal and growth retarded pregnancies. Obstet Gynecol 1987; 69:705-9.
43. Yoshimura S, Masuzaki H, Miura K, et al. Fetal blood flow redistribution in term intrauterine growth retardation (IUGR) and post-natal growth. Int J Gynaecol Obstet 1998; 60:3-8.
44. Luzi G, Coata G, Caserta G, et al. Doppler velocimetry of different sections of the fetal middle cerebral artery in relation to perinatal outcome. J Perinat Med 1996; 24:327-34.
45. Strigini FA, De Luca G, Lencioni G, et al. Middle cerebral artery velocimetry: Different clinical relevance depending on umbilical velocimetry. Obstet Gynecol 1997; 90:953-7.
46. Madazli R, Uludag S, Ocak V. Doppler assessment of umbilical artery, thoracic aorta and middle cerebral artery in the management of pregnancies with growth restriction. Acta Obstet Gynecol Scand 2001; 80:702-7.
47. Morishima HO, Yeh M-N, Niemann WH, James LS. Temperature gradient between fetus and mother as an index for assessing intrauterine fetal condition. Am J Obstet Gynecol 1977; 129:443-8.
48. Power GG, Kawamura T, Dale PS, et al. Temperature responses following ventilation of the fetal sheep in utero. J Dev Physiol 1986; 8:477-84.
49. Schroder HJ, Power GG. Engine and radiator: Fetal and placental interactions for heat dissipation. Exp Physiol 1997; 82:403-14.
50. Peltonen R. The difference between fetal and maternal temperatures during delivery (abstract). Fifth European Congress of Perinatal Medicine, Uppsala, Sweden, June 1976:188.
51. Camann WR, Hortvet LA, Hughes N, et al. Maternal temperature regulation during extradural analgesia for labour. Br J Anaesth 1991; 67:565-8.
52. Glosten B, Savage M, Rooke GA, Brengelmann GL. Epidural anesthesia and the thermoregulatory responses to hyperthermia: Preliminary observations in the volunteer subjects. Acta Anaesthesiol Scand 1998; 42:442-6.
53. Kirschbaum TH. Fetal hemoglobin composition as a parameter of the oxyhemoglobin dissociation curve of fetal blood. Am J Obstet Gynecol 1962; 84:477-85.
54. Harris AP, Sendak MJ, Donham RT, et al. Absorption characteristics of human fetal hemoglobin at wavelengths used in pulse oximetry. J Clin Monit 1988; 4:175-7.
55. Allen DW. The oxygen equilibrium of fetal and adult human hemoglobin. J Br Chem 1953; 203:81-7.
56. Comline RS, Silver M. The composition of foetal and maternal blood during parturition in the ewe. J Physiol 1972; 222:233-56.
57. Brace RA. Fetal blood volume responses to intravenous saline solution and dextran. Am J Obstet Gynecol 1983; 147:777-81.
58. Brace RA, Gold PS. Fetal whole-body interstitial compliance, vascular compliance, and capillary filtration coefficient. Am J Physiol 1984; 247:R800-5.
59. Anderson DF, Bissonette JM, Faber JJ, Thornburg KL. Central shunt flows and pressures in the mature fetal lamb. Am J Physiol 1981; 241:H60-6.
60. Gilbert RD. Control of fetal cardiac output during changes in blood volume. Am J Physiol 1980; 238:H80-6.
61. Rudolph AM, Heymann MA. Circulatory changes during growth in the fetal lamb. Circ Res 1970; 26:289-99.
62. Thornburg KL, Reller MD. Coronary flow regulation in the fetal sheep. Am J Physiol 1999; 277:R1249-60.
63. Rasanen J, Wood DC, Weiner S, et al. Role of the pulmonary circulation in the distribution of human fetal cardiac output during the second half of pregnancy. Circulation 1996; 94:1068-73.
64. Klopfenstein HS, Rudolph AM. Postnatal changes in the circulation and the responses to volume loading in sheep. Circ Res 1978; 42:839-45.
65. Thornburg KL, Morton MJ. Filling and arterial pressures as determinants of RV stroke volume in the sheep fetus. Am J Physiol 1983; 244:H656-63.
66. Gilbert RD. Effects of afterload and baroreceptors on cardiac function in fetal sheep. J Dev Physiol 1982; 4:299-309.
67. Heymann MA, Rudolph AM. Effects of increasing preload on right ventricular output in fetal lambs in utero (abstract). Circulation 1973; 48(Suppl 4):37.
68. Kirkpatrick SE, Pitlick PT, Naliboff J, Friedmon WF. Frank-Starling relationship as an important determinant of fetal cardiac output. Am J Physiol 1976; 231:495-500.
69. Friedman WF. The intrinsic physiologic properties of the developing heart. Prog Cardiovasc Dis 1982; 15:87-111.
70. Kilby MD, Szware RS, Benson LN, Morrow RJ. Left ventricular hemodynamic effects of rapid, in utero intravascular transfusion in anemic fetal lambs. J Matern Fetal Med 1998; 7:51-8.
71. Hawkins JA, Van Hare GF, Rudolph AM. The effect of preload and afterload on left ventricular output in the fetal lamb. Pediatr Res 1988; 23:244A.
72. Friedman WF, Pool PE, Jacobowitz D, et al. Sympathetic innervation of the developing rabbit heart. Circ Res 1968; 23:25-32.
73. Nassar R, Reedy MC, Anderson PAW. Developmental changes in the ultrastructure and sarcomere shortening of the isolated rabbit ventricular myocyte. Circ Res 1987; 61:465-83.
74. Picardo S, Li C, Tyndall M, Rudolph AM. Fetal cardiovascular response to beta adrenoreceptor (BAR) stimulation. Pediatr Res 1986; 20:371A.
75. Anderson PAW, Glick KL, Killam AP, Mainwaring RD. The effect of heart rate on in utero left ventricular output in the fetal sheep. J Physiol 1986; 372:557-73.
76. Anderson PAW, Killam AP, Mainwaring RD, Oakeley AE. In utero right ventricular output in the fetal lamb: The effect of heart rate. J Physiol 1987; 387:297-316.
77. Rudolph AM, Heymann MA. Cardiac output in the fetal lamb: The effects of spontaneous and induced changes of heart rate on right and left ventricular output. Am J Obstet Gynecol 1976; 124:183-92.
78. Blanco CE, Dawes GS, Hanson MA, McCooke HB. Studies of carotid baroreceptor afferents in fetal and newborn lambs. In Jones CT, Nathaniels PW, editors. The Physiological Development of the Fetus and Newborn. Orlando, FL, Academic Press, 1985:595-8.
79. Long WA. Developmental pulmonary circulatory physiology. In Long WA, editor. Fetal and Neonatal Cardiology. Philadelphia, WB Saunders, 1990:76-96.
80. Walker AM. Physiological control of the fetal cardiovascular system. In Beard RW, Nathanielsz PW, editors. Fetal Physiology and Medicine. New York, Marcel Dekker, 1984:287-316.
81. Boekkooi PF, Baan J Jr, Teitel D, Rudolph AM. Chemoreceptor responsiveness in fetal sheep. Am J Physiol 1992; 263:H162-7.
82. Dawes GS, Duncan SLD, Lewis BV, et al. Cyanide stimulation of the systemic arterial chemoreceptors in foetal lambs. J Physiol (Lond) 1969; 201:117-28.

83. Thornburg KL, Jonker S, Reller MD. Nitric oxide and fetal coronary regulation. J Card Surg 2002; 17:307-16.
84. van Bel F, Sola A, Roman C, et al. Perinatal regulation of the cerebral circulation: Role of nitric oxide and prostaglandins. Pediatr Res 1997; 42:299-304.
85. Gardner DS, Fowden AL, Giussani DA. Adverse intrauterine conditions diminish the fetal defense against acute hypoxia by increasing nitric oxide activity. Circulation 2002; 106:2278-83.
86. van Bel F, Sola A, Roman C, et al. Role of nitric oxide in the regulation of the cerebral circulation in the lamb fetus during normoxemia and hypoxemia. Biol Neonate 1995; 68:200-10.
87. Cohn HE, Sacks EJ, Heymann MA, Rudolph AM. Cardiovascular responses to hypoxemia and acidemia in fetal lambs. Am J Obstet Gynecol 1974; 120:817-24.
88. Sheldon RE, Peeters LLH, Jones MD Jr, et al. Redistribution of cardiac output and oxygen delivery in the hypoxemic fetal lamb. Am J Obstet Gynecol 1979; 135:1071-8.
89. Reuss ML, Parer JT, Harris JL, Krueger TR. Hemodynamic effects of alpha-adrenergic blockade during hypoxia in fetal sheep. Am J Obstet Gynecol 1982; 142:410-5.
90. Assali NS, Brinkman CR III, Wood R Jr, et al. Ontogenesis of the autonomic control of cardiovascular functions in the sheep. In Longo LD, Reneau DD, editors. Fetal and newborn cardiovascular physiology: Proceedings of a symposium to honor Donald H. Barron. Held in conjunction with the fall meeting of the American Physiological Society, August 11-14, 1976, Bryn Mawr, PA. New York, Garland STPM, 1978:47-91.
91. Van Petten GR, Harris WH, Mears GJ. Development of fetal cardiovascular responses to alpha-adrenergic agonists. In Longo LD, Reneau DD, editors. Fetal and newborn cardiovascular physiology: Proceedings of a symposium to honor Donald H. Barron. Held in conjunction with the fall meeting of the American Physiological Society, August 11-14, 1976, Bryn Mawr, PA. New York, Garland STPM, 1978:158-66.
92. Lorijn RHW, Longo LD. Norepinephrine elevation in the fetal lamb: Oxygen consumption and cardiac output. Am J Physiol 1980; 239: R115-22.
93. Papp JG. Autonomic responses and neurohumoral control in the human early antenatal heart. Basic Res Cardiol 1988; 83:2-9.
94. Long WA, Henry GW. Autonomic and central neuroregulation of fetal cardiovascular function. In Polin RA, Fox WW, editors. Fetal and Neonatal Physiology. Vol 1. Philadelphia, WB Saunders, 1992: 629-45.
95. Walls EW. The development of the specialized conducting tissue of the human heart. J Anat 1947; 81:93-107.
96. Smith RB. The development of the intrinsic innervation of the human heart between the 10- and 70- mm stages. J Anat 1970; 107: 271-9.
97. Taylor IM, Smith RB. Cholinesterase activity in the human fetal heart rate between the 35- and 160- mm crown-rump length stages. J Histochem Cytochem 1971; 19:498-503.
98. Levina SE. Endocrine features in development of human hypothalamus, hypophysis, and placenta. Gen Comp Endocrinol 1968; 11:151-9.
99. Drummond WH, Rudolph AM, Keil LC, et al. Arginine vasopressin and prolactin after hemorrhage in the fetal lamb. Am J Physiol 1980; 238:214-9.
100. Raff H, Wood CE. Effect of age and blood pressure on the heart rate, vasopressin, and renin response to hypoxia in fetal sheep. Am J Physiol Regul Integr Comp Physiol 1992; 263:R880-4.
101. Wood CE, Tong H. Central nervous system regulation of reflex responses to hypotension during fetal life. Am J Physiol 1999; 277:R1541-52.
102. Iwamoto HS, Rudolph AM, Keil LC, Heymann MA. Hemodynamic responses of the sheep fetus to vasopresssin infusion. Circ Res 1979; 44:430-6.
103. Robillard JE, Gomez RA, Meernik JG, et al. Role of angiotensin II on adrenal and vascular responses to hemorrhage during development in fetal lambs. Circ Res 1982; 50:645-50.
104. Iwamoto HS, Rudolph AM. Effects of angiotensin II on the blood flow and its distribution in fetal lambs. Circ Res 1981; 48:183-9.
105. Iwamoto HS, Rudolph AM. Effects of endogenous angiotensin II on the fetal circulation. J Dev Physiol 1979; 1:283-93.
106. Schwarcz RL, Strada-Saenz G, Althabe O, et al. Pressure exerted by uterine contractions on the head of the human fetus during labor. In Perinatal Factors Affecting Human Development (PAHO Scientific Publication No. 185). Proceedings of the Special Session, 18th Meeting of the PAHO Advisory Committee on Medical Research. Washington, DC, World Health Organization, 1969:115-26.
107. Mocsary P, Gaal J, Komaromy B, et al. Relationship between fetal intracranial pressure and fetal heart rate during labor. Am J Obstet Gynecol 1970; 106:407-11.
108. Harris AP, Koehler RC, Gleason CA, et al. Cerebral and peripheral circulatory responses to intracranial hypertension in fetal sheep. Circ Res 1989; 64:991-1000.
109. Harris AP, Koehler RC, Nishijima MK, et al. Circulatory dynamics during periodic intracranial hypertension in fetal sheep. Am J Physiol 1992; 263:R95-102.
110. Van Reempts PJ, Wouters A, De Cock W, Van Acker KJ. Stress responses to tilting and odor stimulus in preterm neonates after intrauterine conditions associated with chronic stress. Physiol Behav 1997; 61:419-24.
111. Van Reempts PJ, Wouters A, De Cock W, Van Acker KJ. Stress responses in preterm neonates after normal and at-risk pregnancies. J Paediatr Child Health 1996; 32:450-6.
112. Giannakoulopoulos X, Sepulveda W, Kourtis P, et al. Fetal plasma cortisol and beta-endorphin response to intrauterine needling. Lancet 1994; 344:77-81.
113. Fisk NM, Gitau R, Teixeira JM, et al. Effect of direct fetal opioid analgesia on fetal hormonal and hemodynamic stress response to intrauterine needling. Anesthesiology 2001; 95:828-35.
114. Teixeria J, Fogliani R, Giannakoulopoulos X, et al. Fetal haemodynamic stress response to invasive procedures. Lancet 1996; 347:624.
115. Giannakoulopoulos X, Teixeira J, Fisk N, Glover V. Human fetal and maternal noradrenaline response to invasive procedures. Pediatr Res 1999; 45:494-9.
116. Teixeria JM, Glover V, Fisk NM. Acute cerebral redistribution in response to invasive procedures in the human fetus. Am J Obstet Gynecol 1999; 181:1018-25.
117. Gitau R, Fisk NM, Teixeira JM, et al. Fetal hypothalmic-pituitary-adrenal stress responses to invasive procedures are independent of maternal responses. J Clin Endocrinol Metab 2001; 86:104-9.
118. Benatar D, Benatar M. A pain in the fetus: Toward ending confusion about fetal pain. Bioethics 2001; 15:57-76.
119. Carrasco GA, Van de Kar LD. Neuroendocrine pharmacology of stress. Eur J Pharmacol 2003; 463:235-72.
120. Fitzgerald M, Howard RF. The neurobiologic basis of pediatric pain. In Schechter NL, Berde CB, Yaster M, editors. Pain in Infants, Children and Adolescents. 2nd edition. Philadelphia, Lippincott Williams & Wilkins, 2003:19-42.
121. Kostovic I, Rakic P. Development of prestriate visual projections in the monkey and human fetal cerebrum revealed by transient cholinesterase staining. J Neurosci 1984; 4:25-42.
122. Mrzljak L, Uylings HB, Kostovic I, Van Eden CG. Prenatal development of neurons in the human prefrontal cortex. I. A qualitative Golgi study. J Comp Neurol 1988; 271:355-86.
123. Lee SJ, Ralston HJP, Drey EA, et al. Fetal pain: A systemic multidisciplinary review of the evidence. JAMA 2005; 294:947-54.
124. Burgess JA, Tawia SA. When did you first begin to feel it? Locating the beginning of human consciousness. Bioethics 1996; 10:1-26.
125. Clancy RR, Bergqvist AGC, Dlugos DJ. Neonatal electroencephalography. In Ebersole JS, Pedley TA, editors. Current Practice of Clinical Electroencephalography. 3rd edition. Philadelphia, Lippincott Williams & Wilkins, 2003:160-234.
126. Hrbek A, Karlberg P, Olsson T. Development of visual and somatosensory evoked responses in preterm newborn infants. Electroenceph Clin Neurophysiol 1973; 34:225-32.

127. Craig KD, Whitfield MF, Grunau RV, et al. Pain in the preterm neonate: Behavioural and physiological indices. Pain 1993; 52:287-99.
128. Hadjistavropoulos HD, Craig KD, Grunau RE, Whitfield MF. Judging pain in infants: Behavioural, contextual, and developmental determinants. Pain 1997; 73:319-24.
129. Merker B. Consciousness without a cerebral cortex: A challenge for neuroscience and medicine. Behav Brain Sci 2007; 30:63-134.
130. Bartocci M, Bergqvist L, Lagercrantz H, Anand KJS. Pain activates cortical areas in the preterm newborn brain. Pain 2006; 122:109-17.

Part III

Fetal and Neonatal Assessment and Therapy

Ostensibly, concern for the neonate began in 1861, when London physician W. J. Little published a paper entitled "On the influence of abnormal parturition, difficult labors, premature birth, and asphyxia neonatorum, on the mental and physical condition of the child, especially in relation to deformities."[1] Hailed as "an original field of observation," Little's paper was among the first to identify antepartum asphyxia as the cause of problems in the neonate.

Almost half a century passed, however, before clinicians developed a sustained interest in fetal oxygenation. This development came through the influence of Sir Joseph Barcroft and his book *Researches on Prenatal Life.*[2] A professor of physiology at Cambridge University, Barcroft was already highly respected for his studies of respiration when this book was published.

From his laboratory studies, Barcroft discovered a progressive decrease in fetal oxygen saturation during the last half of pregnancy. He attributed this finding to the fetal demands for oxygen, which slowly increased until the capacity of the placenta was exhausted. Barcroft compared the fetus to a mountaineer climbing Mt. Everest, in that the oxygen environment of the fetus became progressively less dense. He suggested that the term fetus faced either asphyxia *in utero* or escape through the initiation of labor. Barcroft's depiction of the fetal environment disturbed clinicians who were already well aware of the additional stress imposed by labor.

Ironically, one of Barcroft's own students proved him wrong. D. H. Barron, Professor of Physiology at Yale, suggested that Barcroft's data had been skewed by the conditions of his experiments, all of which had been conducted on animals anesthetized for immediate surgery. Barron and his colleagues developed methods to sample fetal blood in awake, unstressed animals. Under these circumstances, they observed no deterioration in the fetal environment until the onset of labor. Oxygen saturation, hemoglobin concentration, and pH remained stable and normal.[3]

Barcroft's data have had the greatest impact on clinical practice. Virtually all current methods of fetal monitoring grew out of the belief that oxygen availability is the single most important factor influencing the well-being of the newborn. However, Barron's studies affected physiologists, who began to study the mechanisms that maintained the stability of the intrauterine environment in the presence of increasing fetal demands.

Donald Caton, M.D.

REFERENCES

1. Little WJ. On the influence of abnormal parturition, difficult labours, premature birth and asphyxia neonatorum, on the mental and physical condition of the child, especially in relation to deformities. Trans Obstet Soc Lond 1862; 3:293-344.
2. Barcroft J. Researches on Prenatal Life, Vol. I. Springfield, IL, Charles C Thomas, 1947.
3. Barron DH. The environment in which the fetus lives: Lessons learned since Barcroft in prenatal life. In Mack H, editor. Prenatal Life: Biological and Clinical Perspectives. Detroit, Wayne State University Press, 1970;109-28.

Chapter 6

Antepartum Fetal Assessment and Therapy

Katherine Campbell, M.D.
Joong Shin Park, M.D., Ph.D.
Errol R. Norwitz, M.D., Ph.D.

Obstetric care providers have two patients, the mother and the fetus. Although assessment of maternal health is relatively straightforward, assessment of fetal well-being is far more challenging. Several tests have been developed to assess the fetus during pregnancy, including some that are recommended for all pregnancies (e.g., ultrasonography for pregnancy dating) and others that are reserved only for women with pregnancy complications (e.g., middle cerebral artery Doppler velocimetry in pregnancies with isoimmunization). In addition, a limited number of fetal interventions are employed to improve fetal outcome, including some that are used frequently, such as maternal corticosteroid administration, and others much more rarely, such as intrauterine fetal procedures. This chapter reviews the tests available to assess fetal well-being in both low- and high-risk pregnancies and the fetal therapies used during the antepartum period.

PRENATAL CARE IN LOW-RISK PREGNANCIES

Determination of Gestational Age

The mean duration of a singleton pregnancy is 280 days (40 weeks) from the first day of the last normal menstrual period. *Term*, defined as the period from 37 weeks' (259 days') to 42 weeks' (294 days') gestation, is the optimal time for delivery. Both preterm births (defined as delivery before 37 weeks' gestation) and post-term births (delivery after 42 weeks' gestation) are associated with higher perinatal and neonatal morbidity and mortality. Evaluation of fetal growth, efficient use of screening and diagnostic tests, appropriate initiation of fetal surveillance, and optimal timing of delivery all depend on accurate dating of the pregnancy.

A number of clinical, biochemical, and radiologic tests are available to determine gestational age (Box 6-1).[1,2] Determination of gestational age is most accurate in early pregnancy, and the estimated date of delivery (EDD) should be established at the first prenatal visit. Embryo transfer dating in women undergoing *in vitro* fertilization (IVF) is the most accurate clinical dating criterion. Among women with regular menstrual cycles who conceive spontaneously, if the first day of the last menstrual period (LMP) is known and if uterine size is consistent with dates by clinical examination, then Naegele's rule (subtract 3 months and add 7 days to the LMP) can be used to determine the EDD. However, menstrual dating is known to be inaccurate in women taking oral contraceptives, in women who conceive in the immediate postpartum period, and in women who

BOX 6-1 Clinical Criteria Commonly Used to Confirm Gestational Age

- Reported date of last menstrual period (estimated due date can be calculated by subtracting 3 months and adding 7 days to the first day of the last normal menstrual period [Naegele's rule]) or date of assisted reproductive technology (intrauterine insemination or embryo transfer).
- The size of the uterus as estimated on bimanual examination in the first trimester, which should be consistent with dates.
- The perception of fetal movement ("quickening"), which usually occurs at 18 to 20 weeks in nulliparous women and at 16 to 18 weeks in parous women.
- Fetal heart activity, which can be detected with a nonelectronic fetal stethoscope by 18 to 20 weeks and with Doppler ultrasonography by 10 to 12 weeks.
- Fundal height; at 20 weeks, the fundal height in a singleton pregnancy should be approximately 20 cm above the pubic symphysis (usually corresponding to the umbilicus).
- Ultrasonography, involving crown-rump length measurement of the fetus during the first trimester, or fetal biometry (biparietal diameter, head circumference, and/or femur length) during the second trimester.

Data from American College of Obstetricians and Gynecologists. Antepartum fetal surveillance. ACOG Practice Bulletin No. 9. Washington, DC, ACOG, 1999; and American College of Obstetricians and Gynecologists. Management of postterm pregnancy. ACOG Practice Bulletin No. 55. Washington, DC, ACOG, 2004.

have irregular menstrual cycles or a history of intermenstrual bleeding. Moreover, clinical examination of uterine size can be inaccurate in women with a high body mass index (BMI), uterine fibroids, or a multifetal pregnancy. For these reasons, reliance on standard clinical criteria alone to determine the EDD will lead to an inaccurate diagnosis, with a tendency to overestimate gestational age.[3-6] For example, one study reported that reliance on LMP alone leads to a false diagnosis of preterm birth and post-term pregnancy in one quarter and one eighth of cases, respectively.[7] Use of other historic factors (such as the date of the first positive pregnancy test result or the first perceived fetal movements ["quickening"]) and physical findings (such as the date when fetal heart sounds are first audible) may help obstetric providers determine the EDD more accurately (see Box 6-1).

Most early pregnancy tests involve the identification and quantification of human chorionic gonadotropin (hCG), a hormone produced by the syncytiotrophoblast of the fetoplacental unit.[8,9] Levels in the maternal circulation increase exponentially to a peak of 80,000 to 100,000 mIU/mL at 8 to 10 weeks' gestation and then decrease to a level of 20,000 to 30,000 mIU/mL for the remainder of the pregnancy. Commercially available hCG test kits can detect concentrations as low as 25 to 50 mIU/mL in serum or urine, which are typically seen 8 to 9 days after conception.

Uncertainty in dating parameters should prompt ultrasonographic assessment of gestational age. Transabdominal ultrasonography can identify an intrauterine sac in 94% of eutopic (intrauterine) pregnancies once the serum hCG concentration is 6000 mIU/mL or higher.[10] With the use of transvaginal ultrasonography, an intrauterine pregnancy can typically be confirmed at a serum hCG level of 1500 to 2000 mIU/mL.[11] Failure to confirm an intrauterine sac at these hCG levels should raise concerns about an abnormal pregnancy (e.g., ectopic pregnancy, missed abortion) and requires further evaluation. A fetal pole and cardiac activity should be visible at a serum hCG concentration of approximately 1700 mIU/mL (5 to 6 weeks) and 5400 mIU/mL (6 to 8 weeks), respectively.

In the first trimester, the fetal crown-rump length (CRL) is the most accurate determinant of gestational age (±3 to 5 days). In the second trimester, the biparietal diameter (BPD) and length of the long bones (especially femur length) are the sonographic measurements used most often to determine gestational age. Of these, the BPD is the more accurate indicator with a variation of ±7 to 10 days.[12] Two large clinical studies of approximately 50,000 pregnancies demonstrated that a second-trimester BPD measurement, when used instead of menstrual dating to establish the EDD, resulted in a significant increase in the number of women who delivered within 7 days of their due dates and a 60% to 70% reduction in the number of pregnancies continuing post-term.[13,14] Moreover, because it is unaffected by fetal Down syndrome,[15] the BPD is particularly useful for determining the timing of serum analyte screening for fetal aneuploidy. After 26 weeks' gestation, the variation in the BPD measurement is greater (±14 to 21 days), thereby making it less valuable in estimating gestational age.[12] Both femur length and humerus length correlate strongly with the BPD and gestational age and are sometimes used for additional confirmation.[16] By contrast, because abdominal circumference (AC) reflects fetal nutritional status and growth, it is less accurate than either BPD or femur length. All fetal biometric measurements are subject to some degree of error, so a number of techniques have been used to predict gestational age more accurately. These include using an average of several measurements or a ratio of two measurements, such as femur length to BPD. Serial determinations of gestational age at weekly to biweekly intervals may be more accurate than a single determination, especially in the third trimester.

Routine Ultrasonography

Routine early ultrasonography significantly improves the accuracy of gestational age dating.[3-6,17-20] Early ultrasonography can also detect pregnancy abnormalities (e.g., molar pregnancy), major fetal structural abnormalities (e.g., anencephaly), and multiple pregnancy. Although recommended in Europe, the practice of routine ultrasonography for pregnancy dating has not been recommended as a standard of prenatal care in the United States.[21,22]

The utility of routine second-trimester ultrasonography in all pregnant women remains a subject of debate. Early studies suggested an improvement in perinatal outcome with its use.[18,23-26] For example, one prospective clinical trial in Helsinki, Finland, randomly assigned 9310 low-risk women either to a single screening ultrasonographic examination at 16 to 20 weeks' gestation or to ultrasonography for obstetric indications only; a significantly lower perinatal mortality rate was found in the screening ultrasonography group (4.6 versus 9.0 per 1000 births, respectively).[19] This difference was due in part to earlier detection of major fetal malformations (which prompted elective abortion) and multiple pregnancies (which resulted in more appropriate antenatal care) with the screening examination. As expected, routine ultrasonography also led to improved pregnancy dating and a lower rate of induction of labor for post-term pregnancy.[19]

In contrast, a subsequent large multicenter randomized clinical trial involving 15,151 low-risk women in the United States (designated as the RADIUS study) concluded that screening ultrasonography did *not* improve perinatal outcomes and had no impact on the management of the anomalous fetus.[20,27,28] Although this trial was adequately powered, it has been criticized for the highly selective entry criteria (by one estimate, less than 1% of pregnant women in the United States would have been eligible[29]) and the selection of primary outcomes (perinatal morbidity and mortality) that were inappropriate for the low-risk population studied. In addition, only 17% of major congenital anomalies were detected before 24 weeks' gestation in the routine ultrasonography group, so the rate of elective pregnancy termination for fetal anomalies was significantly lower than that in the Helsinki study. The skill and experience of the sonographer is also an important variable in these studies. The utility of routine second-trimester ultrasonography remains controversial.

Evaluation of Fetal Growth

Normal fetal growth is a critical component of a healthy pregnancy and the subsequent long-term health of the child. Maternal weight gain during pregnancy is at best an indirect measure of fetal growth, because much of the weight gain during pregnancy is the result of fluid (water) retention. Recommendations for weight gain in pregnancy are based on the Institute of Medicine guidelines published in 1990 (Table 6-1).[30] Weight gain should be accompanied by an increase in fundal height.

The size, presentation, and lie of the fetus can be assessed with abdominal palpation. A systematic method of examination of the gravid abdomen was first described by Leopold and Sporlin in 1894.[31] Although the abdominal examination has several limitations (especially in the setting of a small fetus, maternal obesity, multiple pregnancy, uterine fibroids, or polyhydramnios), it is safe, is well tolerated,

TABLE 6-1 Recommendations for Weight Gain in Pregnancy

Mother's Body Mass Index	Recommended Weight Gain
18.5 to 24.9 kg/m² (normal weight)	25 to 35 lbs (11.2 to 15.9 kg)
25 to 29.9 kg/m² (overweight)	15 to 25 lbs (6.8 to 11.2 kg)
>30 kg/m² (obesity)	15 lbs (6.8 kg)

Data from the Institute of Medicine. Nutritional status and weight gain. In: Nutrition During Pregnancy. Washington, DC, National Academies Press, 1990:27-233.

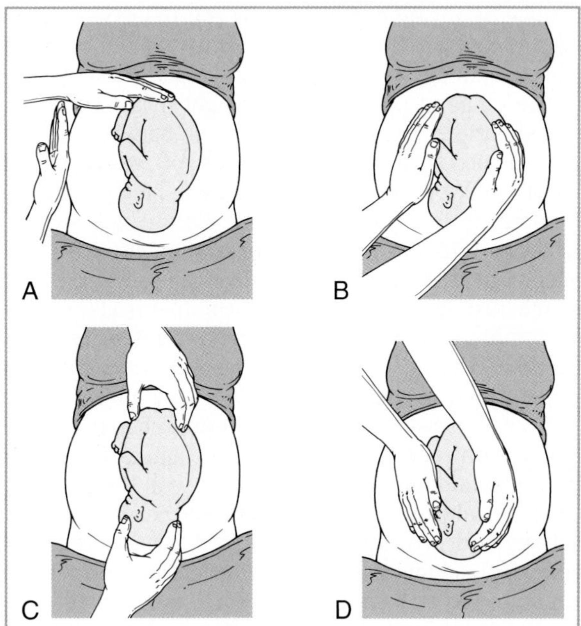

FIGURE 6-1 Leopold's maneuvers for palpation of the gravid abdomen.

and may add valuable information to assist in antepartum management. Palpation is divided into four separate Leopold's maneuvers (Figure 6-1). Each maneuver is designed to identify specific fetal landmarks or to reveal a specific relationship between the fetus and mother. The first maneuver, for example, involves measurement of the fundal height. The uterus can be palpated above the pelvic brim at approximately 12 weeks' gestation. Thereafter, fundal height should increase by approximately 1 cm per week, reaching the level of the umbilicus at 20 to 22 weeks' gestation (Figure 6-2). Between 20 and 32 weeks' gestation,

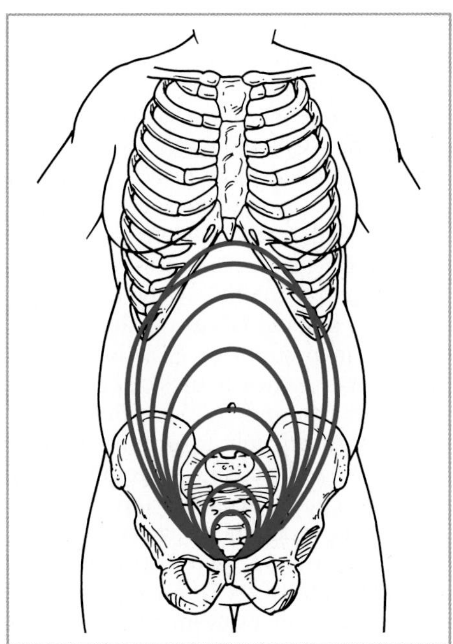

FIGURE 6-2 Fundal height measurements in a singleton pregnancy with normal fetal growth.

the fundal height (in centimeters) is approximately equal to the gestational age (in weeks) in healthy women of average weight with an appropriately growing fetus. However, there is a wide range of normal fundal height measurements. In one study, there was a 6-cm difference between the 10th and 90th percentiles at each week of gestation after 20 weeks.[32] Moreover, maximal fundal height occurs at approximately 36 weeks' gestation, after which time the fetus drops into the pelvis in preparation for labor—this development is known as "lightening." For all of these reasons, reliance on fundal height measurements alone fails to identify more than 50% of fetuses with intrauterine growth restriction (IUGR).[33] Serial fundal height measurements by an experienced obstetric care provider are more accurate than a single measurement and will lead to better diagnosis of IUGR, with reported sensitivities as high as 86%.[34]

If clinical findings are not consistent with the stated gestational age, ultrasonography is indicated to confirm gestational age and provide a more objective measure of fetal growth. Ultrasonography may also identify an alternative explanation for the discrepancy, such as multifetal pregnancy, fetal demise, and uterine fibroids. For many years, obstetric ultrasonography has used fetal biometry to define fetal size by weight estimations. This approach has a number of limitations. First, regression equations used to create weight estimation formulas are derived primarily from cross-sectional data for infants being delivered within an arbitrary period after the ultrasonographic examination. Second, these equations assume that body proportions (fat, muscle, bone) are the same for all fetuses.[34-45] Finally, growth curves for "normal" infants between 24 and 37 weeks' gestation rely on data collected from pregnancies delivered preterm, which are abnormal and probably complicated by some element of uteroplacental insufficiency, regardless of whether the delivery was spontaneous or iatrogenic. Despite these limitations, if the gestational age is well validated, the prevailing data suggest that prenatal ultrasonography can be used to verify an alteration in fetal growth in 80% of cases and to exclude abnormal growth in 90% of cases.[46]

Sonographic estimates of fetal weight are commonly derived from mathematical formulas that use a combination of fetal measurements, especially the BPD, AC, and femur length.[47] The AC is the single most important measurement and is weighted more heavily in these formulas. Unfortunately, the AC is also the most difficult measurement to acquire, and small differences in the measured value result in large changes in the estimated fetal weight (EFW). The accuracy of the EFW depends on a number of variables, including gestational age (in absolute terms, EFW is more accurate in preterm or growth-restricted fetuses than in term or macrosomic fetuses), operator experience, maternal body habitus, and amniotic fluid volume (measurements are more difficult to acquire if the amniotic fluid volume is low). Objective sonographic EFW estimations are not particularly accurate and have an error of 15% to 20%, even in experienced hands.[48] Indeed, a sonographic EFW at term is no more accurate than a clinical estimate of fetal weight made by an experienced obstetric care provider or the mother's estimate of fetal weight if she has delivered before.[49] Sonographic estimates of fetal weight must therefore be evaluated within the context of the clinical situation and balanced against the clinical estimate. Serial sonographic evaluations of fetal weight are more useful than a single measurement in diagnosing abnormal fetal growth. The ideal interval for fetal growth evaluations is every 3 to 4 weeks, because more frequent determinations may be misleading. Similarly, the use of population-specific growth curves, if available, improves the ability of the obstetric care provider to identify abnormal fetal growth. For example, growth curves derived from a population that lives at high altitude, where the fetus is exposed to lower oxygen tension, will be different from those derived from a population at sea level. Abnormal fetal growth can be classified as insufficient (IUGR) or excessive (fetal macrosomia).

INTRAUTERINE GROWTH RESTRICTION

The definition of *intrauterine growth restriction* (IUGR) has been a subject of long-standing debate. Distinguishing the healthy, constitutionally small-for-gestational-age (SGA) fetus, defined as having an EFW below the 10th percentile for a given week of gestation, from the nutritionally deprived, truly growth-restricted fetus has been particularly difficult. Fetuses with an EFW less than the 10th percentile are not necessarily pathologically growth restricted. Conversely, an EFW above the 10th percentile does not necessarily mean that an individual fetus has achieved its growth potential, and such a fetus may still be at risk for perinatal mortality and morbidity. Therefore, IUGR is best defined as either (1) an EFW less than the 5th percentile for gestational age in a well-dated pregnancy or (2) an EFW less than the 10th percentile for gestational age in a well-dated pregnancy with evidence of fetal compromise, such as oligohydramnios or abnormal umbilical artery Doppler velocimetry.

Fetal growth restriction has traditionally been classified as either asymmetric or symmetric IUGR. **Asymmetric IUGR,** characterized by normal head growth but suboptimal body growth, is seen most commonly in the third trimester. It is thought to result from a late pathologic event (such as chronic placental abruption leading to uteroplacental insufficiency) in an otherwise uncomplicated pregnancy and normal fetus. In cases of **symmetric IUGR,** both the fetal head size and body weight are reduced, indicating a global insult that likely occurred early in gestation. Symmetric IUGR may reflect an inherent fetal abnormality (e.g., fetal chromosomal anomaly, inherited metabolic disorder, early congenital infection) or long-standing severe placental insufficiency due to an underlying maternal disease (e.g., hypertension, pregestational diabetes mellitus, or collagen vascular disorder). In practice, the distinction between asymmetric and symmetric IUGR is not particularly useful.

Early and accurate diagnosis of IUGR coupled with appropriate intervention leads to an improvement in perinatal outcome. If IUGR is suspected clinically and on the basis of ultrasonography, a thorough evaluation of the mother and fetus is indicated. Referral to a maternal-fetal medicine specialist should be considered. Every effort should be made to identify the cause of the IUGR and to modify or eliminate contributing factors. Up to 20% of cases of severe IUGR are associated with fetal chromosomal abnormalities or congenital malformations, 25% to 30% are related to maternal conditions characterized by vascular disease, and a smaller proportion are the result of abnormal placentation.

However, in a substantial number of cases (greater than 50% in some studies), the etiology of the IUGR remains unclear even after a thorough investigation.[50]

FETAL MACROSOMIA

Fetal macrosomia is defined as an EFW (not birth weight) of 4500 g or greater measured either clinically or by ultrasonography, and is independent of gestational age, diabetic status, and actual birth weight.[51] Fetal macrosomia should be differentiated from the large-for-gestational age (LGA) fetus, in whom the EFW is greater than the 90th percentile for gestational age. By definition, 10% of all fetuses are LGA at any given gestational age. Fetal macrosomia is associated with an increased risk of cesarean delivery, instrumental vaginal delivery, and birth injury to both the mother (including vaginal, perineal, and rectal trauma) and the infant (orthopedic and neurologic injury).[52-56] Shoulder dystocia with resultant brachial plexus injury (Erb's palsy) is a serious consequence of fetal macrosomia; it is more likely in the setting of diabetes because of the larger diameters of the fetal upper thorax and neck.

Fetal macrosomia can be determined clinically (with abdominal palpation using Leopold's maneuvers) or with ultrasonography, and these two techniques appear to be equally accurate.[57] However, EFW measurements are less accurate in large (macrosomic) fetuses than in normally grown fetuses, and factors such as low amniotic fluid volume, advancing gestational age, maternal obesity, and the position of the fetus can compound these inaccuracies. Indeed, clinical examination has been shown to underestimate the birth weight by more than 0.5 kg in almost 80% of macrosomic fetuses.[58] For all these reasons, prediction of fetal macrosomia is not particularly accurate, with a false-positive rate of 35% and a false-negative rate of 10%.[57,58] A number of alternative sonographic measurements have therefore been proposed in an attempt to better identify the macrosomic fetus, including fetal AC alone,[59] umbilical cord circumference,[60] cheek-to-cheek diameter,[61] and upper arm circumference.[62] However, these measurements remain investigational.

Despite the inaccuracy in the prediction of fetal macrosomia, an EFW should be documented by either clinical estimation or ultrasonography in all high-risk women at approximately 38 weeks' gestation. Suspected fetal macrosomia is not an indication for induction of labor, because induction does not improve maternal or fetal outcomes.[51] However, if the EFW is excessive, an elective cesarean delivery should be considered to prevent fetal and maternal birth trauma. Although controversy remains as to the precise EFW at which an elective cesarean delivery should be recommended, a suspected birth weight in excess of 4500 g in a diabetic woman or 5000 g in a nondiabetic woman is a reasonable threshold.[51,52,63]

Assessment of Fetal Well-Being

All pregnant women should receive regular antenatal care throughout their pregnancy, and fetal well-being should be evaluated at every visit. Fetal heart activity should be assessed at each visit and the fetal heart rate (FHR) estimated. A low FHR (less than 100 bpm) is associated with an increased risk of pregnancy loss, although congenital complete heart block should be excluded. In the latter half of pregnancy, physical examination of the abdomen using the Leopold's maneuvers should be performed at each prenatal visit to document fetal lie and presentation and to estimate amniotic fluid volume and fetal size.

Fetal movements ("quickening") are typically reported at 18 to 20 weeks' gestation by nulliparous women and at 16 to 18 weeks' gestation by parous women, and the presence of fetal movements is strongly correlated with fetal health. Although the mother appreciates only 10% to 20% of total fetal movements,[64-67] such movements are almost always present when she does report them.[67] Factors associated with a diminution in perceived fetal movements include increasing gestational age, smoking, decreased amniotic fluid volume, anterior placentation, and antenatal corticosteroid therapy. However, decreased fetal movements may also be a harbinger of an adverse pregnancy event (e.g., stillbirth) that can be averted if detected early. For these reasons, a subjective decrease in perceived fetal movements in the third trimester should prompt an immediate investigation.

Published studies support the value of **fetal movement** charts ("kick counts") in the detection and prevention of fetal complications (including stillbirth) in both high- and low-risk populations.[68-73] The normal fetus exhibits an average of 20 to 50 (range of 0 to 130) gross body movements per hour, with fewer movements during the day and increased activity between 9:00 PM and 1:00 AM.[74] Several different schemes have been proposed and evaluated for routine daily assessment of fetal activity after 28 weeks' gestation. The goal of these schemes is to determine the baseline fetal activity pattern for an individual fetus and to evaluate activity patterns that may represent fetal compromise. One commonly used scheme ("count-to-10") instructs the mother to rest quietly on her left side once each day in the evening (between 7:00 PM and 11:00 PM) and to record the time interval required to feel 10 fetal movements. Most patients with a healthy fetus will feel 10 movements in approximately 20 minutes; 99.5% of women with a healthy fetus feel this amount of activity within 90 minutes.[75] Under this scheme, failure to appreciate 10 fetal movements in 2 hours should prompt an immediate office or hospital visit for further evaluation. In one large clinical trial, institution of this fetal activity monitoring scheme resulted in a significant increase in hospital visits, labor induction, and cesarean deliveries, but also in a reduction in perinatal mortality from 44.5 to 10.3 per 1000 births.[75] Taken together, these data suggest that daily or twice-daily fetal "kick counts" should be performed after 32 weeks' gestation in all high-risk pregnancies. Whether fetal "kick counts" should be recommended after 36 weeks' gestation in all low-risk pregnancies remains controversial.

PRENATAL CARE IN HIGH-RISK PREGNANCIES

Approximately 20% of all pregnancies should be regarded as high risk (Box 6-2). Because of the attendant risks to both the mother and fetus, additional efforts should be made to confirm fetal well-being throughout such pregnancies. In addition to the testing outlined previously, high-risk pregnancies should be monitored closely and regularly by a multidisciplinary team, including subspecialists in maternal-fetal medicine and neonatology, if indicated.

BOX 6-2 High-Risk Pregnancies

Maternal Factors
- Preeclampsia (gestational proteinuric hypertension)
- Chronic hypertension
- Diabetes mellitus (including gestational diabetes)
- Maternal cardiac disease
- Chronic renal disease
- Chronic pulmonary disease
- Active thromboembolic disease

Fetal Factors
- Nonreassuring fetal testing (fetal compromise)
- Intrauterine growth restriction
- Isoimmunization
- Intra-amniotic infection
- Known fetal structural anomaly
- Prior unexplained stillbirth
- Multiple pregnancy

Uteroplacental Factors
- Premature rupture of fetal membranes
- Unexplained oligohydramnios
- Prior classic (high vertical) hysterotomy
- Placenta previa
- Placental abruption
- Vasa previa

Goals of Antepartum Fetal Testing

The goal of antepartum fetal surveillance is the early identification of a fetus at risk for preventable neurologic morbidity or mortality. Numerous causes of neonatal cerebral injury exist, including congenital abnormalities, chromosomal abnormalities, intracerebral hemorrhage, hypoxia, infection, drugs, trauma, hypotension, and metabolic derangements (e.g., hypoglycemia, thyroid dysfunction). Antenatal fetal testing cannot reliably predict or detect all of these causes; however, those specifically associated with uteroplacental vascular insufficiency should be identified when possible. Antenatal fetal testing makes the following assumptions: (1) pregnancies may be complicated by progressive fetal asphyxia that can lead to fetal death or permanent neurologic handicap; (2) current antenatal tests can adequately discriminate between asphyxiated and nonasphyxiated fetuses; and (3) detection of asphyxia at an early stage can lead to an intervention that is capable of reducing the likelihood of an adverse perinatal outcome.

Of interest, it is not clear whether any of these assumptions are true, and nonreassuring fetal test results may reflect existing but not ongoing neurologic injury. At most, 15% of cases of cerebral palsy are thought to result from antepartum or intrapartum hypoxic-ischemic injury.[75-78] Despite these limitations, a number of antepartum tests have been developed in an attempt to identify fetuses at risk. These include the nonstress test (NST), biophysical profile (BPP), and contraction stress test (CST). Such tests can be used either individually or in combination. There is no consensus as to which of these modalities is preferred, and no single method has been shown to be superior.[1]

Antepartum Fetal Tests

All antepartum fetal tests should be interpreted in light of the gestational age, the presence or absence of congenital anomalies, and underlying clinical risk factors.[79] For example, a nonreassuring NST in a pregnancy complicated by severe IUGR and heavy vaginal bleeding at 32 weeks' gestation has a much higher predictive value in identifying a fetus at risk for subsequent neurologic injury than an identical tracing in a well-grown fetus at 40 weeks, because of the higher prevalence of this condition in the former situation. It should be remembered that, in many cases, the efficacy of antenatal fetal testing in preventing long-term neurologic injury has not been validated by prospective randomized clinical trials. Indeed, because of ethical and medicolegal concerns, there are no studies of pregnancies at risk that include a non-monitored control group, and it is highly unlikely that such trials will ever be performed.

NONSTRESS TEST

The fetal nonstress test, also known as fetal cardiotocography, investigates changes in the FHR pattern with time and reflects the maturity of the fetal autonomic nervous system. For this reason, it is less useful in the extremely premature fetus (< 28 weeks) before the autonomic nervous system has matured sufficiently to influence the FHR. The NST is noninvasive, simple to perform, inexpensive, and readily available in all obstetric units. However, interpretation of the NST is largely subjective. Although a number of different criteria have been used to evaluate these tracings, most obstetric care providers have used the definitions for FHR interpretation established in 1997 by the National Institute of Child Health and Human Development (NICHD) Research Planning Workshop (Table 6-2).[80,*]

By definition, an NST is performed before the onset of labor and does not involve invasive (intrauterine) monitoring. The test is performed as follows: The FHR is recorded for a period of 30 to 40 minutes and evaluated for a number of periodic changes. The FHR is determined externally with use of Doppler ultrasonography, in which sound waves emitted from the transducer are deflected by movements of the heart and heart valves. The shift in frequency of these deflected waves is detected by a sensor and converted into heart rate. The FHR is printed on a strip-chart recorder running at 3 cm/min. A single mark on the FHR tracing therefore represents the average rate in beats per minute (bpm) of 6 fetal heart beats. The presence or absence of uterine contractions is typically recorded at the same time with an external tonometer. This tonometer records myometrial tone and provides information about the timing and duration of contractions, but it does not measure intrauterine pressure or the intensity of the contractions.

Visual interpretation of the FHR tracing involves the following components: (1) baseline FHR, (2) baseline FHR variability, (3) presence of accelerations, (4) presence of periodic or episodic decelerations, and (5) changes of FHR pattern over time. The definitions of each of these variables are summarized in Table 6-2.[80] The patterns are

*A 2008 report summarized terminology and nomenclature used in contemporary clinical practice and research. This report described a three-tier system for FHR tracing interpretation: Category I (normal), Category II (indeterminate), and Category III (abnormal). (The 2008 National Institute of Child Health and Human Development Workshop on Electronic Fetal Monitoring. Obstet Gynecol 2008; 112:661-6.)

TABLE 6-2 Interpretation of Antepartum Nonstress Test (NST) Results

Criterion	Definition
• Baseline fetal heart rate (FHR)	Defined as the approximate mean FHR during a 10-minute segment and lasting at least 2 minutes in duration. The normal FHR is defined as 110 to 160 bpm.
• Baseline FHR variability	Described as fluctuations in the baseline FHR of $\geq$2 cycles/min. It is quantified visually as the amplitude of peak-to-trough in bpm. Variability is classified as follows: • Absent: amplitude range undetectable • Minimal: amplitude range detectable but $\leq$5 bpm • Moderate: amplitude range 6 to 25 bpm • Marked: amplitude range $>$25 bpm The normal baseline FHR variability is defined as moderate variability.
• Accelerations	Defined as an abrupt increase in FHR above baseline. • At and after 32 weeks' gestation, an acceleration is defined as $\geq$15 bpm above baseline for $\geq$15 seconds but $<$2 minutes. • Before 32 weeks' gestation, an acceleration is defined as $\geq$10 bpm above baseline for $\geq$10 seconds but $<$2 minutes. A **prolonged acceleration** is defined as an acceleration lasting $\geq$2 minutes but $<$10 minutes. If the duration is longer than 10 minutes, it is referred to as a "change in baseline" and not a prolonged acceleration.
• Decelerations	Decelerations are not normal. However, some decelerations are a more serious sign of fetal compromise than others. The following three types of decelerations are recognized: • **Early decelerations** are characterized by a gradual decrease and return to baseline FHR associated with a uterine contraction. The onset, nadir, and recovery of the deceleration are coincident with the beginning, peak, and ending of the uterine contraction. • **Variable decelerations** are characterized by an abrupt decrease in the FHR to $\geq$15 bpm below the baseline and lasting for $\geq$15 seconds but $<$2 minutes. Abrupt is defined as $<$30 seconds from baseline to the nadir of the deceleration. When variable decelerations are associated with uterine activity, their onset, depth, and duration commonly vary with successive contractions. • **Late decelerations** are characterized by a gradual decrease and return to baseline FHR associated with a uterine contraction. Importantly, the deceleration is delayed in timing, with the nadir of the deceleration occurring after the peak of the contraction. Onset, nadir, and recovery of the deceleration occur after the beginning, peak, and ending of the uterine contraction. A **prolonged deceleration** is defined as a deceleration lasting $\geq$2 minutes but $<$10 minutes. If the duration is longer than 10 minutes, it is referred to as a "change in baseline" and not a prolonged deceleration. **Recurrent decelerations** describe the presence of decelerations with more than 50% of uterine contractions in any 20-minute period.

Data from the National Institute of Child Health and Human Development Research Planning Workshop. Electronic fetal heart rate monitoring: Research guidelines for interpretation. Am J Obstet Gynecol 1997; 177:1385-90.

categorized as baseline, periodic (i.e., associated with uterine contractions), or episodic (i.e., not associated with uterine contractions). Periodic changes are described as *abrupt* or *gradual* (defined as onset-to-nadir time less than 30 seconds or more than 30 seconds, respectively). In contrast to earlier classifications, this classification makes no distinction between short-term and long-term variability, and certain characteristics (such as the definition of an acceleration) depend on gestational age (see Table 6-2).[80]

A normal FHR tracing is defined as having a normal baseline rate (110 to 160 bpm), normal baseline variability (i.e., moderate variability, defined as 6 to 25 bpm from peak to trough), presence of accelerations, and absence of decelerations. The FHR typically accelerates in response to fetal movement. Therefore, FHR accelerations usually indicate fetal health and adequate oxygenation.[80-82] An FHR tracing is designated *reactive* if there are two or more accelerations in a 20-minute period (Figure 6-3). *At risk* FHR patterns demonstrate recurrent late decelerations with absence of baseline variability, recurrent variable decelerations with absence of baseline variability, or substantial bradycardia with absence of baseline variability (Figure 6-4). *Intermediate* FHR patterns have characteristics between the two extremes of normal and *at risk* already described.[80]

Persistent fetal tachycardia (defined as an FHR > 160 bpm) may be associated with fetal hypoxia, maternal fever, chorioamnionitis (intrauterine infection), administration of an anticholinergic or beta-adrenergic receptor agonist, fetal anemia, or tachyarrhythmia. Persistent fetal bradycardia (FHR < 110 bpm) may be a result of congenital

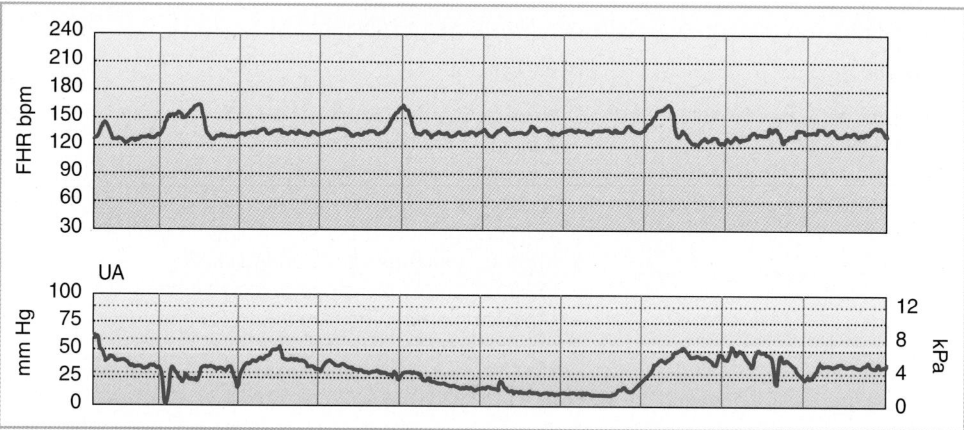

FIGURE 6-3 A normal (reactive) fetal heart rate (FHR) tracing. The baseline FHR is normal (between 110 and 160 bpm), there is moderate variability (defined as 6 to 25 bpm from peak to trough), there are no decelerations, and there are two or more accelerations (defined as an increase in FHR of ≥ 15 bpm above baseline lasting at least 15 seconds) in a 20-minute period.

heart block, administration of a beta-adrenergic receptor antagonist, hypoglycemia, or hypothermia (Table 6-3). However, it may also indicate fetal hypoxia.[81] Both tachyarrhythmias and bradyarrhythmias require immediate evaluation.

Baseline FHR variability, perhaps the most important component of the NST, is determined on a beat-to-beat basis by the competing influences of the sympathetic and parasympathetic nervous systems on the fetal sinoatrial node. A variable FHR, characterized by fluctuations that are irregular in both amplitude and frequency,[80] indicates that the autonomic nervous system is functioning and that the fetus has normal acid-base status. Variability is defined as absent, minimal, moderate, or marked (see Table 6-2) (Figure 6-5).[80] The older terms short-term variability and long-term variability are no longer used.[80] Normal (moderate) variability indicates the absence of cerebral hypoxia. With acute hypoxia, variability may be minimal or marked. Persistent or chronic hypoxia is typically associated with loss of variability. Reduced variability also may be the result of other factors, including maternal drug administration (see Table 6-3), fetal arrhythmia, and neurologic abnormality (e.g., anencephaly).[1,80,81]

An NST is performed when formal documentation of the fetal condition is necessary. Because most healthy fetuses move within a 75-minute period, the testing period for an NST should not exceed 80 minutes.[83] The NST is most useful in cases of suspected uteroplacental insufficiency. A reactive NST is regarded as evidence of fetal health,[84,85] but the interpretation of a nonreactive NST remains controversial. Determination of a nonreactive NST must consider the gestational age, the underlying clinical circumstance, and the results of previous FHR tracings. Only 65% of fetuses have a reactive NST by 28 weeks' gestation, whereas 95% do so by 32 weeks.[79,86] However, once a reactive NST has been documented in a given pregnancy, the NST should remain reactive throughout the remainder of the pregnancy. A nonreactive NST at term is associated with poor perinatal outcome in only 20% of cases. The significance of such a result at term depends on the clinical endpoint under investigation. If the clinical endpoint of interest is a 5-minute Apgar score less than 7, a nonreactive NST at term has a sensitivity of 57%, a positive predictive value of 13%, and a negative predictive value of 98% (assuming a prevalence of 4%). If the clinical endpoint is permanent neurologic injury, a nonreactive NST at term has a 99.8% false-positive rate.[87] Nonetheless, FHR monitoring remains the test most commonly used to document fetal well-being in the antepartum period.

VIBROACOUSTIC STIMULATION

Fetal vibroacoustic stimulation (VAS) refers to the response of the FHR to a vibroacoustic stimulus (82 to 95 dB for 3 seconds) applied to the maternal abdomen in the region of the fetal head. An FHR acceleration in response to VAS represents a positive result and is suggestive of fetal health. VAS is a useful adjunct to shorten the time needed to achieve a reactive NST and to decrease the proportion of

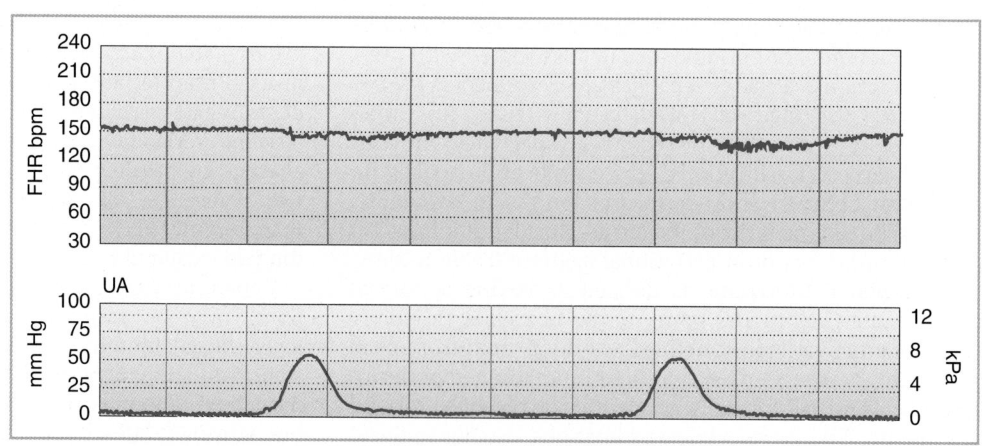

FIGURE 6-4 An "at risk" fetal heart rate (FHR) tracing. The baseline FHR is normal (between 110 and 160 bpm), but the following abnormalities can be seen: minimal baseline FHR variability (defined as 0 to 5 bpm from peak to trough), no accelerations, and decelerations that are late in character (start after the peak of the contraction) and repetitive (occur with more than half of the contractions).

TABLE 6-3 Drugs that Affect the Fetal Heart Rate Tracing

Effect on the Fetus	Drug
Fetal tachycardia	Atropine Epinephrine (adrenaline) Beta-adrenergic agonists (ritodrine, terbutaline)
Fetal bradycardia	Antithyroid medications (including propylthiouracil) Beta-adrenergic antagonists (e.g., propranolol) Intrathecal or epidural analgesia Methylergonovine (contraindicated prior to delivery) Oxytocin (if associated with excessive uterine activity)
Sinusoidal fetal heart rate pattern	Systemic opioid analgesia
Diminished variability	Atropine Anticonvulsants (but not phenytoin) Beta-adrenergic antagonists Antenatal corticosteroids (betamethasone, dexamethasone) Ethanol General anesthesia Hypnotics (including diazepam) Insulin (if associated with hypoglycemia) Magnesium sulfate Systemic opioid analgesia Promethazine

nonreactive NSTs at term, thereby precluding the need for further testing. In one study of low-risk women at term, VAS reduced the proportion of nonreactive NSTs over a 30-minute period by 50% (from 14% to 9%), and shortened the time needed to achieve a reactive NST by an average of 4.5 minutes.[88] VAS has no adverse effect on fetal hearing. The absence of an acceleration in response to VAS at term is associated with an 18-fold higher risk of nonreassuring fetal testing in labor[89] and a 6-fold higher risk of cesarean delivery.[90]

BIOPHYSICAL PROFILE

An NST alone may not be sufficient to confirm fetal well-being. In such cases, a biophysical profile (BPP) may be performed. The BPP is a sonographic scoring system performed over a 30- to 40-minute period designed to assess fetal well-being. It was initially described for testing of the post-term fetus but has since been validated for use in both term and preterm fetuses.[91-97] It is not validated for use in active labor. The five variables described in the original BPP were (1) gross fetal body movements, (2) fetal tone (i.e., flexion and extension of limbs), (3) amniotic fluid volume, (4) fetal breathing movements, and (5) the NST.[97] More recently, the BPP has been interpreted without the NST (Table 6-4).

The individual variables of the BPP become apparent in the normal fetus in a predictable sequence: Fetal tone appears at 7.5 to 8.5 weeks' gestation, fetal movement at 9 weeks, fetal breathing at 20 to 22 weeks, and FHR reactivity at 24 to 28 weeks. In the setting of antepartum hypoxia, these characteristics typically disappear in the reverse order of their appearance (i.e., FHR reactivity is lost first, followed by fetal breathing, fetal movements, and finally fetal tone).[93] The amniotic fluid volume, which is composed almost entirely of fetal urine in the second and third trimesters, is not influenced by acute fetal hypoxia or acute fetal central nervous system dysfunction. Rather, oligohydramnios (decreased amniotic fluid volume) in the latter half of pregnancy and in the absence of ruptured membranes is a reflection of chronic uteroplacental insufficiency and/or increased renal artery resistance leading to diminished urine output.[98] It predisposes to umbilical cord compression, thus leading to intermittent fetal hypoxemia, meconium passage, or meconium aspiration. Adverse pregnancy outcome (including a nonreassuring FHR tracing, low Apgar scores, and/or admission to the neonatal intensive care unit) is more common when oligohydramnios is present.[98-101] Serial (weekly) screenings of high-risk pregnancies for oligohydramnios is important because amniotic fluid can become drastically reduced within 24 to 48 hours.[102]

Although each of the five features of the BPP are scored equally (2 points if the variable is present or normal, and 0 points if absent or abnormal, for a total of 10 points), they are not equally predictive of adverse pregnancy outcome. For example, amniotic fluid volume is the variable that correlates most strongly with adverse pregnancy events. The management recommended on the basis of the BPP score is summarized in Table 6-5.[97] A score of 8 or 10 is regarded as reassuring; a score of 4 or 6 is suspicious and requires reevaluation; and a score of 0 or 2 suggests nonreassuring fetal status (previously referred to as "fetal distress").[91,92] Evidence of nonreassuring fetal status or oligohydramnios in the setting of otherwise reassuring fetal testing should prompt evaluation for immediate delivery.[93,94]

CONTRACTION STRESS TEST

Also known as the oxytocin challenge test (OCT), the contraction stress test is an older test of uteroplacental function. It assesses the response of the FHR to uterine contractions artificially induced by either intravenous oxytocin administration or nipple stimulation (which causes release of endogenous oxytocin from the maternal neurohypophysis). A minimum of three contractions of minimal-to-moderate strength in 10 minutes is required to interpret the test. A negative CST (no decelerations with contractions) is reassuring and suggestive of a healthy, well-oxygenated fetus. A positive CST (repetitive late or severe variable decelerations with contractions) is suggestive of a fetus suffering from impaired maternal-fetal oxygen exchange during uterine contractions and is associated with adverse perinatal outcome in 35% to 40% of cases (Figure 6-6). The combination of a positive CST and absence of FHR variability is especially ominous. Consideration should be given to immediate and urgent delivery of a fetus with a positive CST, with or without FHR variability. It should be noted, however, that the false-positive rate of this test exceeds 50%.[84] If the CST is uninterpretable or equivocal, the test should be repeated in 24 to 72 hours. Studies suggest that more than 80% of results of repeated tests are negative.

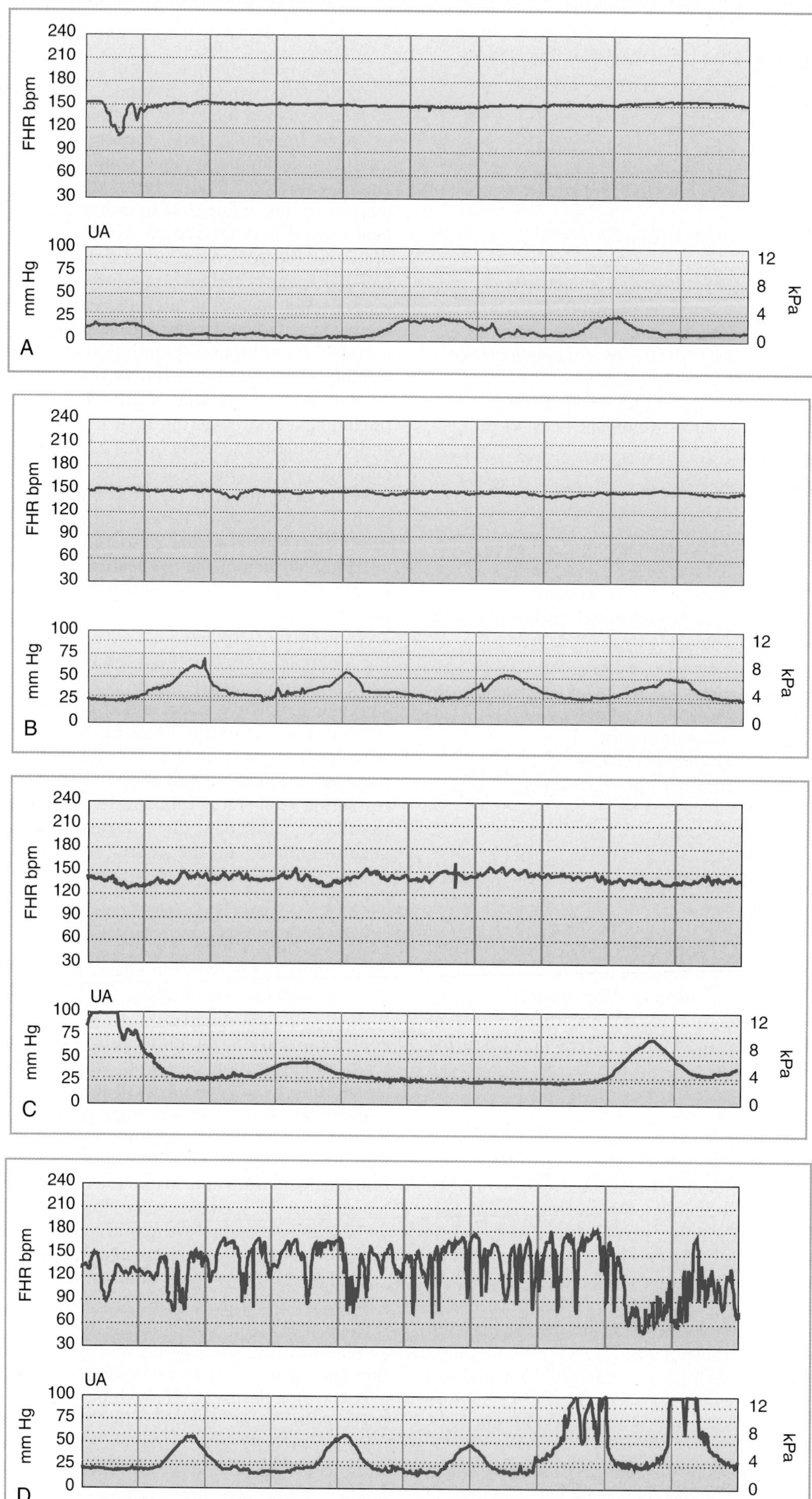

FIGURE 6-5 Components of baseline fetal heart rate (FHR) variability. **A,** Absence of variability. **B,** Minimal variability (0 to 5 bpm from peak to nadir). **C,** Moderate variability (6 to 25 bpm from peak to nadir). **D,** Marked variability (>25 bpm from peak to nadir).

TABLE 6-4 Characteristics of the Biophysical Profile (BPP)

Biophysical Variable	Normal Score (Score = 2)	Abnormal Score (Score = 0)
Fetal breathing movements (FBMs)	At least one episode of FBM lasting at least 30 seconds in duration	Absence of FBM altogether or no episode of FBM lasting ≥30 seconds
Gross body movements	At least 3 discrete body/limb movements in 30 minutes (episodes of active continuous movements should be regarded as a single movement)	Less than 3 episodes of body/limb movements over a 30-minute period
Fetal tone	At least one episode of active extension with return to flexion of fetal limbs or trunk; opening and closing of hand are considered normal tone	Slow extension with return to partial flexion, movement of limb in full extension, or absence of fetal movements
Qualitative amniotic fluid (AF) volume	At least one pocket of AF that measures ≥1 cm in two perpendicular planes	No AF pockets or an AF pocket measuring <1 cm in two perpendicular planes
Reactive nonstress test	At least two episodes of FHR acceleration of ≥15 bpm lasting ≥15 seconds associated with fetal movements over 30 minutes of observation	Less than two episodes of FHR accelerations or accelerations of <15 bpm over 30 minutes of observation

Data from Manning FA. Fetal biophysical assessment by ultrasound. In Creasy RK, Resnik R, editors. Maternal-Fetal Medicine: Principles and Practice. 2nd edition. Philadelphia, WB Saunders, 1989:359.

TABLE 6-5 Recommended Management Based on Biophysical Profile (BPP)

Score	Interpretation	Recommended Management
8 or 10	Normal	No intervention
6	Suspect asphyxia	Repeat in 4 to 6 hours Consider delivery for oligohydramnios
4	Suspect asphyxia	If ≥36 weeks' gestation or mature pulmonary indices, deliver immediately If <36 weeks' gestation, repeat BPP in 4 to 6 hours versus delivery with mature pulmonary indices If score persistently ≤4, deliver immediately
0 or 2	High suspicion of asphyxia	Evaluate for immediate delivery

Data from Manning FA. Fetal biophysical assessment by ultrasound. In Creasy RK, Resnik R, editors. Maternal-Fetal Medicine: Principles and Practice. 2nd edition. Philadelphia, WB Saunders, 1989:359.

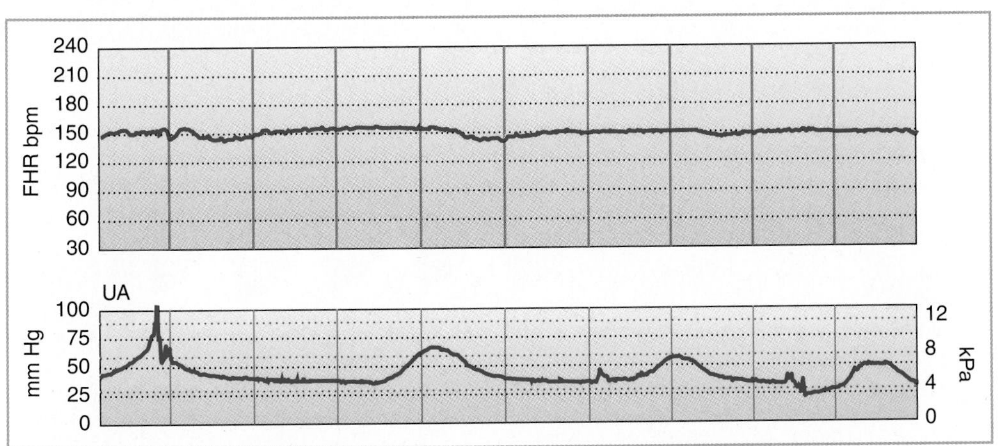

FIGURE 6-6 A positive contraction stress test (CST) result. There are at least 3 contractions in a 10-minute period. The baseline fetal heart rate is 130 bpm, there is minimal baseline FHR variability (defined as as 0 to 5 bpm from peak to trough), and there are decelerations that are late in character (start after the peak of the contraction) and repetitive (occur with more than half of the contractions).

TABLE 6-6 False-Positive and False-Negative Rates for the Nonstress Test, Biophysical Profile, and Contraction Stress Test

Test	False-Positive Rate (%)	False-Negative Result (per 1000 live births)*
Nonstress test (NST)	58	1.4 to 6.2
Biophysical profile (BPP):		0.7 to 1.2
• Score 6/10	45	
• Score 0/10	0	
Contraction stress test (CST)	30	0.4 to 0.6

*Data are presented as perinatal mortality rate within one week of a reactive NST, a BPP score of 8 or 10, or a negative CST after adjustments for congenital anomalies and known causes.

Data from references 1, 84, 95, and 103.

Because this test is time consuming, requires skilled nursing care, and necessitates an inpatient setting owing to the possibility of precipitating fetal compromise requiring emergency cesarean delivery, the CST is rarely used in clinical practice. Moreover, there are a number of contraindications to its use, including placenta previa, placental abruption, prior classic (high-vertical) cesarean delivery, and risk of preterm labor. Despite these limitations, the CST allows for indirect evaluation of fetal oxygenation during periods of uterine contractions and diminished uteroplacental perfusion and may therefore provide a better assessment of fetal well-being and fetal reserve than either the NST or the BPP (Table 6-6).[1,84,95,103]

UMBILICAL ARTERY DOPPLER VELOCIMETRY

Doppler velocimetry shows the direction and characteristics of blood flow and can be used to examine the maternal, uteroplacental, or fetal circulation. The umbilical artery is one of the few arteries that normally has diastolic flow and consequently is one of the vessels most frequently evaluated during pregnancy. Umbilical artery Doppler velocimetry measurements reflect resistance to blood flow from the fetus to the placenta. Factors that affect placental vascular resistance include gestational age, placental location, pregnancy complications (e.g., placental abruption, preeclampsia), and underlying maternal disease (chronic hypertension).

Doppler velocimetry of umbilical artery blood flow provides an indirect measure of fetal status. Decreased diastolic flow with a resultant increase in the systolic-to-diastolic (S/D) ratio suggests an increase in placental vascular resistance and fetal compromise. Severely abnormal umbilical artery Doppler velocimetry (defined as absence of or reversed diastolic flow) is an especially ominous observation and is associated with poor perinatal outcome in the setting of IUGR (Figure 6-7).[104-108] The role of ductus venosus and/or middle cerebral artery (MCA) Doppler velocimetry in the management of IUGR pregnancies is not well defined. An urgent delivery should be considered when Doppler findings are severely abnormal in the setting of IUGR, regardless of gestational age. However, in the presence of a normally grown fetus, it is unclear how to interpret such findings. For these reasons, umbilical artery

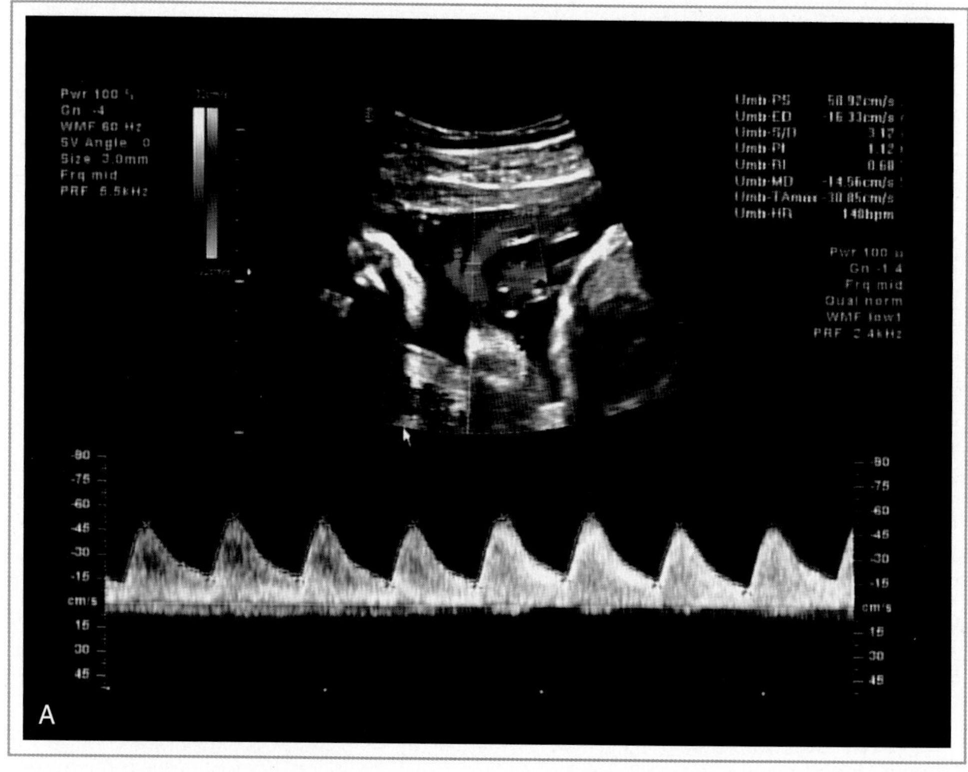

FIGURE 6-7 Umbilical artery Doppler velocimetry. **A,** Normal waveform in the umbilical artery as shown on Doppler velocimetry. Forward flow can be seen during both fetal systole (S) and diastole (D).

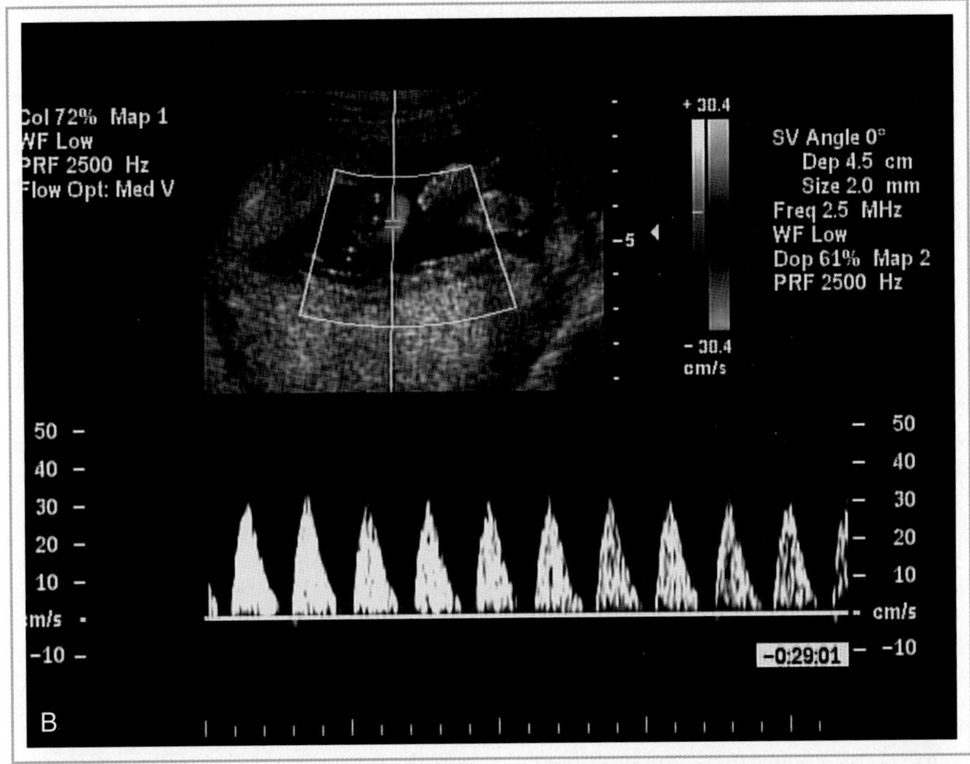

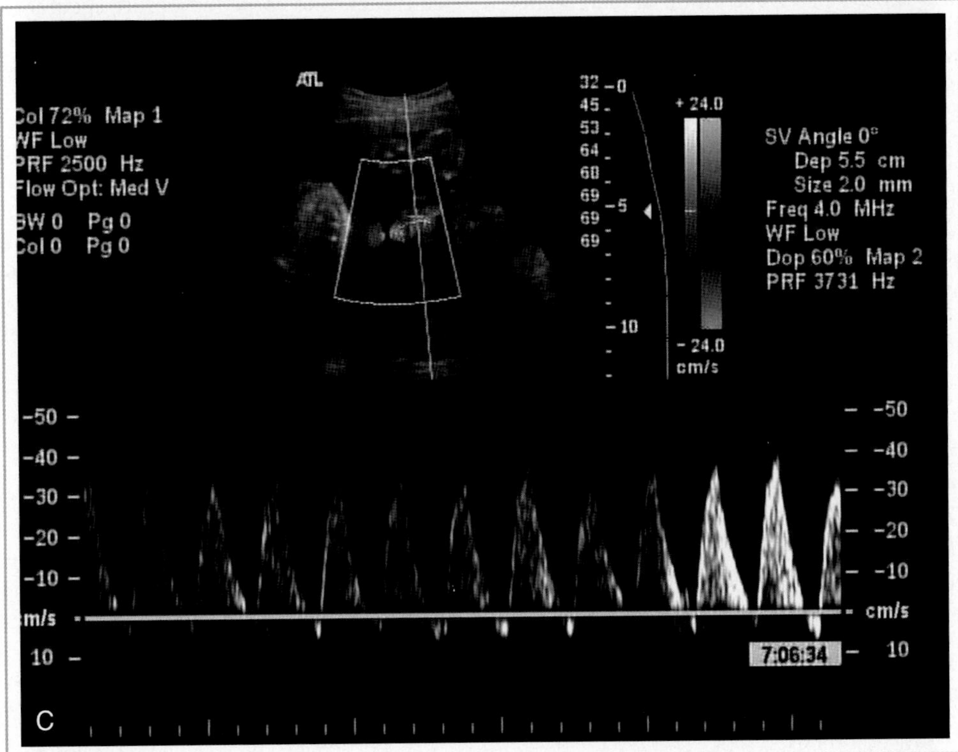

FIGURE 6-7, cont'd B, Absent end-diastolic flow. Forward flow can be seen during systole (S), but there is no flow during diastole (D). **C,** Reverse diastolic flow. Forward flow can be seen during systole (S), but there is reverse flow in the umbilical artery during diastole (D), which is suggestive of high resistance to blood flow in the placenta.

Doppler velocimetry should not be performed routinely in low-risk women. Appropriate indications include IUGR, cord malformations, unexplained oligohydramnios, suspected or established preeclampsia, and, possibly, fetal cardiac anomalies.

Umbilical artery Doppler velocimetry has not been shown to be useful in the evaluation of some high-risk pregnancies, including diabetic and post-term pregnancies, primarily owing to a high false-positive rate.[2,109-112] Thus, in the absence of IUGR, obstetric management decisions are not usually made on the basis of Doppler velocimetry findings alone. Nonetheless, new applications for Doppler technology are currently under investigation. A new application that has proved useful is the noninvasive evaluation of fetal anemia resulting from isoimmunization. When severe anemia develops in a fetus, blood is preferentially shunted to the vital organs, such as the brain, and the shunt can be demonstrated by an increase in peak MCA flow velocity.[113] This finding can help the perinatologist counsel affected patients about the need for cordocentesis and fetal blood transfusion. Doppler studies of other vessels (including the uterine artery, fetal aorta, ductus venosus, and fetal carotid arteries) have contributed to our knowledge of maternal-fetal physiology but as yet have resulted in few clinical applications.

MULTIPLE MODALITIES TO ASSESS FETAL WELL-BEING

All standard tests to assess antepartum fetal well-being (i.e., NST, BPP, CST) are evaluated according to their ability to predict the absence of fetal death during the 1-week period after the test. The false-negative rate (defined as a reassuring test result with a subsequent bad outcome) and false-positive rate (an abnormal result with a subsequent normal outcome) for each of these tests are listed in Table 6-6.[1,84,95,103] The false-negative rates for all three tests are relatively low. Because the NST has a high false-positive rate, some authorities consider it a screening test to identify fetuses requiring further assessment with either a BPP or a CST. No method of fetal assessment is perfect, and clinical judgment plays a large role in any management decision.

SPECIAL TECHNIQUES FOR ANTEPARTUM FETAL SURVEILLANCE

Perinatal Ultrasonography

Ultrasonography uses high-frequency sound waves (3.5 to 5 MHz for transabdominal transducers and 5 to 7.5 MHz for transvaginal transducers) that are directed into the body by a transducer, reflected by maternal and fetal tissue, detected by a receiver, processed, and displayed on a screen. Increasing the wave frequency results in greater display resolution at the expense of diminished tissue penetration. Interpretation of images requires operator experience. Widespread clinical application of two-dimensional ultrasonography began in the 1960s after pioneering work by researchers in the United States and Great Britain.[114] Although no deleterious biologic effects have been associated with obstetric ultrasonography, the rates of false-positive and false-negative diagnoses based on the images are a major limitation.

Perinatal ultrasonography can be classified broadly into three types of examinations: basic, targeted (comprehensive), and limited. The **basic examination** (level I) involves determination of fetal number, viability, position, gestational age, and gross malformations. Placental location, amniotic fluid volume, and the presence of abnormal maternal pelvic masses can be evaluated as well.[21] Most pregnancies can be evaluated adequately with this type of examination alone. If the patient's history, physical findings, or basic ultrasonographic results suggest the presence of a fetal malformation, a **targeted** or **comprehensive examination** (level II) should be performed by an ultrasonographer who is skilled in fetal evaluation. During a targeted ultrasonographic examination, which is best performed at 18 to 20 weeks' gestation, fetal structures are examined in detail to identify and characterize any fetal malformation. Ultrasonographic markers of fetal aneuploidy (see later) can be evaluated as well. In some situations, a **limited examination** may be appropriate to answer a specific clinical question (e.g., fetal viability, amniotic fluid volume, fetal presentation, placental location, cervical length) or to provide ultrasonographic guidance for an invasive procedure (e.g., amniocentesis).

Current debate centers on identifying those patients who would benefit from an ultrasonographic evaluation and determining what type of evaluation would be optimal. Advocates of the universal application of ultrasonography cite the advantages of more accurate dating of pregnancy (see earlier) and earlier and more accurate diagnosis of multiple gestation, structural malformations, and fetal aneuploidy (see later). Opponents of routine ultrasonographic examination view it as an expensive screening test ($100 to $250 for a basic examination) that is not justified by published research, which suggests that routine ultrasonography does not change perinatal outcome significantly.[20,27,28] Although routine ultrasonography for all low-risk pregnant women is controversial, few would disagree that the benefits far outweigh the costs for selected patients.

First-trimester ultrasonography is indicated to confirm an intrauterine pregnancy (i.e., exclude ectopic pregnancy), confirm fetal viability, document fetal number, estimate gestational age, and evaluate the maternal pelvis and ovaries (see earlier).

Second-trimester ultrasonography is indicated in patients with an uncertain LMP date, uterine size larger or smaller than expected for the estimated gestational age, a medical disorder that can affect fetal growth and development (e.g., diabetes, hypertension, collagen vascular disorders), a family history of an inherited genetic abnormality, and suspected fetal malformation or growth disturbance.[21] Most patients undergo a detailed fetal anatomy survey at 18 to 20 weeks' gestation to screen for structural defects. An understanding of normal fetal physiology is critical to the diagnosis of fetal structural anomalies. For example, extra-abdominal herniation of the midgut into the umbilical cord, which occurs normally in the fetus at 8 to 12 weeks' gestation, can be misdiagnosed as an abdominal wall defect. Placental location should be documented with the bladder empty, because overdistention of the maternal bladder or a lower uterine contraction can give a false impression of placenta previa. If placenta previa is identified at 18 to 22 weeks' gestation, serial ultrasonographic examinations should be performed to follow placental location. Only 5% of cases of placenta previa identified in the second trimester persist to term.[115] The umbilical cord should also be imaged and the number of vessels, placental insertion, and fetal insertion should be noted. A single umbilical artery may suggest fetal aneuploidy, especially if associated with other structural anomalies. In pregnancies at high risk for fetal cardiac anomalies or preterm birth, fetal echocardiography and/or cervical length measurements should be performed, respectively (see later).

The indications for **third-trimester ultrasonography** are similar to those for second-trimester ultrasonography. Fetal anatomic surveys and EFW become less accurate with higher gestational age, especially in obese women or pregnancies complicated by oligohydramnios. Fetal biometry and detailed anatomic surveys are still performed in late gestation, however, because certain fetal anomalies (e.g., achondroplasia) become evident for the first time during this period. Transvaginal ultrasonographic measurement of cervical length (performed to identify women at risk for preterm birth) is of little utility after 30 to 32 weeks' gestation.[116]

Screening for Fetal Chromosomal Abnormalities

Fetal chromosomal abnormalities are a major cause of perinatal morbidity and mortality, accounting for 50% of first-trimester spontaneous abortions, 6% to 12% of all stillbirths and neonatal deaths, 10% to 15% of structural anomalies in live-born infants, and more than 60 clinical syndromes characterized by developmental delays and anatomic malformations.[117] The most common aneuploidy encountered during pregnancy, autosomal trisomy, results primarily from nondisjunction during meiosis I, an event that occurs with growing frequency in older women. Women of advanced maternal age (defined as 35 years of age or older at delivery) are at higher risk of having a pregnancy complicated by fetal aneuploidy and are commonly offered a primary invasive diagnostic procedure, either amniocentesis or chorionic villus sampling (CVS). However, because only 8% to 12% of all births occur in women age 35 and older, at most 20% to 25% of all cases of trisomy 21 (Down syndrome) would be identified if all women of advanced maternal age agreed to amniocentesis.[118] Many older women are now opting for serum analyte screening for fetal aneuploidy, which is equally accurate in older women.[119]

SECOND-TRIMESTER FETAL ANEUPLOIDY SCREENING

Methods have been developed to help identify women at high risk for fetal aneuploidy. The major focus of attention has been the detection of Down syndrome, because it is the most common chromosomal abnormality manifesting at term and because, unlike the less common disorders trisomy 13 and 18, its diagnosis can be very difficult to make with ultrasonography. In all of these screening tests, one or more serum analytes are used to adjust the *a priori* risk for fetal aneuploidy in a given pregnancy, which depends primarily on maternal age. The maternal serum analytes used most commonly in second-trimester aneuploidy screening protocols are maternal serum alpha-fetoprotein (MS-AFP), total or free β-hCG, unconjugated estriol, and dimeric inhibin A (collectively known as the quadruple or "quad" screen). If the adjusted risk of fetal aneuploidy exceeds the rate of amniocentesis procedure–related pregnancy loss, which is currently defined as 1 or more in 400 (i.e., if the chance of finding a chromosomal abnormality on fetal karyotype is higher than the risk of the invasive procedure), then genetic amniocentesis is recommended.[120] If all screen-positive women undergo amniocentesis and if the fetal karyotype analysis is successful in all cases, this protocol can identify 60% of all Down syndrome cases with a screen-positive (amniocentesis) rate of approximately 5%. Older women are more likely to be screen positive but also have higher detection rates. In women older than 35 years, this protocol identifies 75% of aneuploid fetuses with a screen-positive rate of approximately 25%.[118,121,122]

SECOND-TRIMESTER ULTRASONOGRAPHIC SCREENING FOR FETAL ANEUPLOIDY

Second-trimester ultrasonographic findings are not generally incorporated into standard algorithms to predict risk for fetal aneuploidy. Multiple major structural abnormalities, such as those often found in fetuses with trisomy 13 or 18, can be detected easily and reliably by perinatal ultrasonography. However, approximately 50% of fetuses with Down syndrome appear structurally normal on ultrasonography[123]; when ultrasonographic findings are abnormal, they involve major anomalies suggestive of Down syndrome (such as duodenal atresia and endocardial cushion defect), or "soft markers" (Table 6-7).[123-125] The clinical significance of an isolated "soft" ultrasonographic marker for Down syndrome is unclear, and whether its identification should be followed by genetic amniocentesis is controversial. If more than one "soft" ultrasonographic marker is evident, the risk of Down syndrome rises substantially, and genetic amniocentesis is indicated.

FIRST-TRIMESTER FETAL ANEUPLOIDY SCREENING

First-trimester fetal aneuploidy screening is a more recent development. The screening protocol involves the following three steps undertaken at 11 to 14 weeks' gestation: (1) maternal serum analyte screening for pregnancy-associated placental protein-A (PAPP-A) and total or free β-hCG; (2) ultrasonographic assessment of nuchal translucency (NT); and (3) genetic counseling.[126] The measurement of free rather than total β-hCG provides a small statistical advantage without apparent clinical benefit.[127] First-trimester aneuploidy screening appears as good as, and possibly better than, second-trimester serum analyte screening in identifying fetuses with Down syndrome.[128,129] Currently, there are no studies comparing first-trimester aneuploidy screening with second-trimester screening incorporating both serum analyte measurements and second-trimester ultrasonography.

The advantage of first-trimester aneuploidy screening is that it is performed early in pregnancy, allowing for the option of CVS and early pregnancy termination if desired. The screening test most commonly used in Europe for identifying pregnancies at risk of Down syndrome is the "integrated" test, which combines first-trimester screening with second-trimester serum analyte screening into a single adjusted risk in the mid to late second trimester. The integrated test can identify approximately 85% to 90% of fetuses with Down syndrome with a false-positive rate of 2% (Table 6-8).[129-135] However, the true application of the integrated

TABLE 6-7 Accuracy Measurements of Second-Trimester Ultrasonographic "Soft Markers" for Trisomy 21 (Down Syndrome) when Identified as Isolated Anomalies

Ultrasonographic Marker	Sensitivity (95% CI)	Specificity (95% CI)	Positive LR (95% CI)	Negative LR (95% CI)
Thickened nuchal fold	0.04 (0.02-0.10)	0.99 (0.99-0.99)	17 (8.0-38.0)	0.97 (0.94-1.00)
Choroid plexus cyst	0.01 (0.00-0.03)	0.99 (0.97-1.00)	1.00 (0.12-9.40)	1.00 (0.97-1.00)
Short femur length	0.16 (0.05-0.40)	0.96 (0.94-0.98)	2.7 (1.2-6.0)	0.87 (0.75-1.00)
Short humeral length	0.09 (0.00-0.60)	0.97 (0.91-0.99)	7.5 (4.7-12.0)	0.87 (0.67-1.10)
Echogenic bowel	0.04 (0.01-0.24)	0.99 (0.97-1.00)	6.1 (3.0-12.6)	1.00 (0.98-1.00)
Echogenic intracardiac focus	0.11 (0.06-0.18)	0.96 (0.94-0.97)	2.8 (1.5-5.5)	0.95 (0.89-1.00)
Renal pyelectasis (pelviceal dilation)	0.02 (0.01-0.06)	0.99 (0.98-1.00)	1.9 (0.7-5.1)	1.00 (1.00-1.00)

CI, confidence interval; LR, likelihood ratio.

Data from Smith-Bindman P, Hosmer W, Feldstein VA, et al. Second-trimester ultrasound to detect fetuses with Down syndrome: A meta-analysis. JAMA 2001; 285:1044-55; and Vintzeleos AM, Campbell WA, Rodis JF, et al. The use of second-trimester genetic sonogram in guiding clinical management of patients at increased risk for fetal trisomy 21. Obstet Gynecol 1996; 87:948-52.

screening test requires that the first-trimester test results, *even if abnormal,* be withheld from the patient until combined with the second-trimester test results; this practice of withholding information has generated controversy, particularly in the United States. To overcome this objection, *sequential* and *contingent* integrated screening tests have been developed, whereby the second-trimester test is performed after disclosure of the first-trimester screening result or if the first test result is abnormal, respectively. It remains unclear, however, whether the detection rates for these integrated tests are any better than those of the first-trimester screening test alone (see Table 6-8).[129-132] Indeed, if the first-trimester aneuploidy screen result is negative (indicating low risk), the sensitivity of second-trimester

TABLE 6-8 Detection Rate of Down Syndrome Screening Tests

Screening Test	Detection Rate (%)*	False-Positive Rate (%)†
Maternal age >35 years	30-40	10-15
First Trimester		
NT assessment	64-70	5-10
NT assessment, PAPP-A, and total or free β-hCG measurements	82-87	5-6
Second Trimester		
Triple screen (measurements of MS-AFP, total or free β-hCG, unconjugated estriol)	69-77	9
Quadruple screen (measurements of MS-AFP, total or free β-hCG, unconjugated estriol, inhibin A)	79-83	6
Combined First and Second Trimesters		
Integrated (NT assessment, PAPP-A measurement, quadruple screen)	93-96	1-2
Serum integrated (PAPP-A measurement, quadruple screen)	84-88	2-3
Stepwise sequential: • If first-trimester test result positive, diagnostic test offered • If first-trimester test result negative, second-trimester test offered, and final risk assessment incorporates both first- and second-trimester results	84-95	1
Contingent sequential: • If first-trimester test result positive, diagnostic test offered • If first-trimester test result negative, no further testing • If first-trimester test result intermediate, second-trimester test offered, and final risk assessment incorporates both first- and second-trimester results	88-94	1

hCG, human chorionic gonadotropin; MS-AFP, maternal serum level of alpha-fetoprotein; NT, nuchal translucency; PAPP-A, pregnancy-associated placental protein-A.

*Assuming a 5% false-positive rate.

†Assuming an 85% detection rate.

Data from references 128, 130-132.

serum analyte screening is reduced fivefold.[136] For this reason, many authorities suggest that no further aneuploidy screening be done if the first-trimester screen result is negative, with the exception of the second-trimester fetal anatomy survey and possibly isolated MS-AFP serum screening for open neural tube defects at 15 to 20 weeks' gestation.

In addition to the nuchal translucency (NT) measurement, absence of the nasal bone on first-trimester ultrasonography has been correlated with Down syndrome. However, whether this ultrasonographic marker adds to the predictive value of first-trimester risk assessment in either low- or high-risk populations has been questioned.[137,138] At this time, the presence or absence of the nasal bone is not included in the first-trimester screening test.

Risk assessment for Down syndrome can be performed in multiple pregnancies using either first- or second-trimester serum analyte measurements but is less accurate than in singleton pregnancies.[132] However, such screening has not been validated for use in higher-order multiple pregnancies (triplets and up) or in multiple pregnancies with a nonviable fetus (either due to spontaneous demise or following a multifetal pregnancy reduction). In such cases, Down syndrome risk assessment can be achieved using first-trimester NT measurements only, although this is not a particularly good screening test and has a lower sensitivity even than NT alone in singleton pregnancies.[132]

Definitive Diagnosis of Fetal Chromosomal Abnormalities

Although an abnormal screening test result or the presence of ultrasonographic abnormalities may signal an increased risk of Down syndrome or other chromosomal abnormality, the majority of fetuses with such findings are chromosomally normal. To provide a definitive diagnosis, an invasive procedure is needed to obtain the fetal karyotype; generally amniocentesis or CVS is used, although in rare cases a cordocentesis is performed.

All invasive procedures are associated with risks to the pregnancy. Risks common to all invasive procedures include the chance of bleeding, isoimmunization (especially in women who are Rh-negative), and infection. All women who are Rh-negative should receive Rh_0(D) immune globulin prior to the procedure. Although the risk of vertical transmission of viral infections (e.g., hepatitis B, hepatitis C, human immunodeficiency virus) with invasive procedures is thought to be low,[139] every effort should be made to avoid invasive procedures in such patients, especially if there is a high viral load in the maternal circulation.

AMNIOCENTESIS

Amniotic fluid is composed of fetal urine, lung fluid, skin transudate, and water that is filtered across the amniotic membranes. It contains electrolytes, proteins, and desquamated fetal cells (amniocytes). Sampling of amniotic fluid **(amniocentesis)** can be used to measure various substances such as lecithin and sphingomyelin for assessing fetal lung maturity, to look for pathogenic bacteria for confirmation of an intra-amniotic infection, and to obtain fetal cells for determination of fetal karyotype or performance of specific genetic analyses.

Cell culture with karyotype analysis typically takes 10 to 14 days, although a small chance exists that the cells will fail to grow, resulting in an inconclusive result. Fluorescence *in situ* hybridization (FISH) does not require that the cells be cultured for any length of time, and its results can be obtained within a few days. This technique uses a series of chromosome-specific fluorescent probes to analyze the metaphase spread in fetal cells to determine fetal gender and detect common trisomies (X, Y, 13, 18, and 21). It can also be used to identify chromosome deletions or duplications in pregnancies at risk for a specific genetic disorder because of a family history or suspicious ultrasonographic findings, such as the 22q11 deletion in DiGeorge's syndrome.[140-142] Although FISH is highly sensitive (trisomy present on FISH testing is invariably present in the fetus), it is not particularly specific, with a false-negative rate of approximately 15%. For this reason, the American College of Medical Genetics and the American Society of Human Genetics recommend that all FISH results be confirmed by complete karyotype analysis.[142]

The most common indication for second-trimester amniocentesis is cytogenetic analysis of fetal cells, although on occasion it is performed to determine amniotic fluid AFP levels and acetylcholinesterase activity for the diagnosis of fetal neural tube defects. Amniocentesis later in pregnancy is usually performed for nongenetic indications, such as (1) to document fetal pulmonary maturity prior to elective delivery before 39 weeks' gestation, (2) for amnioreduction in pregnancies complicated by severe polyhydramnios, (3) to confirm preterm premature rupture of membranes (PROM), (4) to exclude intra-amniotic infection, or (5) to perform spectrophotometric analysis of amniotic fluid bilirubin and to determine fetal Rh type (by direct DNA analysis of fetal amniocytes) in pregnancies complicated by isoimmunization.

Genetic amniocentesis typically involves the insertion of a 20- or 22-gauge spinal needle through the maternal abdominal wall and into the uterine cavity at 15 to 20 weeks' gestation. The procedure is now commonly performed under ultrasonographic guidance, which allows the operator to choose the safest site, preferably in the fundus and away from the placenta and fetal head. The greatest risk of amniocentesis is spontaneous abortion; however, the procedure-related pregnancy loss rate for genetic amniocentesis performed before 24 to 28 weeks' gestation is low (0.25% to 1.0%).[120,143-145] Of interest, the pregnancy loss rate is not influenced by operator experience or needle placement through the placenta,[145,146] but is higher in the presence of first-trimester bleeding or recurrent miscarriage, ultrasonographic demonstration of chorioamniotic separation, discolored amniotic fluid at the time of the procedure, and an unexplained elevation in MS-AFP.[144,147] Whether this risk is higher in twin pregnancies is not clear. Transient leakage of amniotic fluid can be seen in 1% to 2% of procedures, although this leakage usually stops after 48 to 72 hours, and infection is extremely rare (< 0.1% of cases).[148-152]

Compared with late second-trimester amniocentesis, early amniocentesis (before 15 weeks' gestation) is associated with significantly higher procedure-related pregnancy loss rates, ranging from 2.2% to 4.8%.[148-151] This rate is fourfold higher than that of late amniocentesis and twice as high as that of CVS. Early amniocentesis has also been shown to be associated with higher rates of rupture of membranes, club foot, and amniocyte culture failures (2% to 5%) than late amniocentesis.[148-153] For these reasons, amniocentesis before 15 weeks' gestation is not recommended.

If early karyotyping is desired, CVS is preferred over early amniocentesis. Amniocentesis in the third trimester is technically easier and is associated with fewer complications. If a late amniocentesis is being performed for any reason (e.g., to confirm fetal pulmonary maturity), consideration should be given to obtaining the karyotype if indicated, even though the pregnancy is too far along to be ended electively.

CHORIONIC VILLUS SAMPLING

Like that of amniocentesis, the goal of CVS is to provide fetal cells for genetic analysis, although in this case the cells are trophoblasts (placental cells) rather than amniocytes. The technique entails ultrasound-guided aspiration of chorionic villi by means of a 16-gauge catheter inserted transcervically or a 20-gauge spinal needle inserted transabdominally into the placenta. The 15 to 30 mg of villous material collected can be examined in two ways: (1) by direct cytogenetic analysis after an overnight incubation, which yields results in 2 to 3 days; and (2) by longer-term culture followed by cytogenetic analysis, which yields results in 6 to 8 days.[154] To provide rapid and accurate results, many centers report the results of both methods. The main advantage of CVS over amniocentesis is that it allows for fetal karyotyping results in the first trimester, thereby allowing decisions about pregnancy termination to be made earlier if chromosomal abnormalities are detected. Moreover, although rare, certain genetic disorders (such as osteogenesis imperfecta) can be diagnosed antenatally only through analysis of placental tissue.

CVS is best performed between 10 and 12 weeks' gestation. CVS performed before 10 weeks' gestation has been associated with limb reduction defects,[155,156] whereas no such association exists if the procedure is performed after 66 days' gestation.[157] Transabdominal CVS can also be performed in the second or third trimester and is a reasonable alternative to cordocentesis for obtaining tissue for an urgent fetal karyotype.[158]

The most common complication of CVS is vaginal spotting, which occurs in 10% to 25% of patients within the first few days after the procedure. Fortunately, the bleeding is usually mild and resolves spontaneously with no long-term sequelae. The incidences of amnionitis (0.3%) and rupture of membranes (0.3%) after CVS do not differ significantly from those seen with late amniocentesis, and are significantly lower than those reported after early amniocentesis.[157] As with amniocentesis, the most serious complication of CVS is spontaneous abortion. CVS appears to be associated with a higher risk of pregnancy loss than late amniocentesis; the procedure-related loss rate in CVS performed prior to 24 to 28 weeks' gestation is reported as 1.0% to 1.5%.[157,159-164] This rate is significantly higher (0.6% to 0.8%) than that seen after late amniocentesis, with an adjusted odds ratio of 1.30 (95% confidence interval [CI], 1.17 to 1.52).[163] Factors that increase the procedure-related loss rate are operator inexperience, number of needle passes, and a history of bleeding prior to the procedure.[163] By contrast, the risk does not appear to be increased in twin gestations or with the anatomic approach used (i.e., transabdominal versus transcervical catheter placement).[162,165] Some investigators have suggested that the apparently higher pregnancy loss related to CVS (compared with late amniocentesis) is a function of the earlier gestational age at which the procedure is performed.[120]

One complication unique to CVS involves the interpretation of the genetic test results. Because the fetus and placenta both arise from the same cell, it is assumed that the genetic complements of these two tissues are identical, but this is not always the case. **Confined placental mosaicism** (CPM) refers to the situation in which the karyotype of the chorionic villus is a mosaic (i.e., it contains two or more populations of cells with different karyotypes, usually one normal and one trisomic), but the karyotype of the fetus is normal. The incidence of CPM may be as high as 1% to 2% with the direct cytogenetic analysis method, but most cases are not confirmed by the long-term tissue-culture method,[157,161] suggesting a methodologic error. For this reason, many centers report only the long-term culture results. On occasion, it may be necessary to repeat the fetal karyotype, either with a second CVS or with amniocentesis, to resolve the dilemma. The reverse situation, in which the CVS result is normal but the fetus has aneuploidy (a false-negative result), has also been reported[166] but is rare. It may occur from contamination with maternal cells or from inadvertent sampling of a twin placenta.

CORDOCENTESIS

In cases in which pregnancy complications or fetal abnormalities are discovered late in gestation, **cordocentesis** (also known as percutaneous umbilical blood sampling [PUBS]) is an option for rapid evaluation of the fetal karyotype. Cordocentesis involves the insertion of a 22-gauge spinal needle through the maternal abdominal and uterine walls and into the umbilical vein, preferably at the insertion site on the placenta, under direct ultrasonographic guidance. Considerable training and expertise are needed to perform this procedure.

The first cordocentesis was reported in 1983.[167] Although this procedure was originally considered superior to amniocentesis for a number of diagnostic indications, advances in laboratory analysis have allowed more information to be obtained through amniocentesis.[168] For example, cordocentesis was commonly used to obtain a sample of fetal blood for rapid karyotyping when a major structural anomaly or severe IUGR was identified late in pregnancy; however, this sample can be obtained as rapidly from amniocentesis or CVS samples using FISH analysis. Similarly, DNA analysis of amniocytes can rapidly and accurately determine the fetal Rh status as well as the presence of other red cell and platelet antigens,[169] which in the past was an absolute indication for cordocentesis. Now employed primarily for therapeutic indications, cordocentesis is most commonly used to transfuse fetuses with severe anemia from isoimmunization, parvovirus infection, or fetomaternal hemorrhage. This intravascular route of fetal transfusion is preferred to the older technique of intraperitoneal transfusion.[170] Other indications for cordocentesis are to measure drug concentrations in the fetal circulation, to document response to pharmacologic therapy, and to administer drugs directly to the fetus (such as adenosine to treat resistant fetal tachydysrhythmia).[171]

When cordocentesis is performed by skilled operators, complications are infrequent and similar to those encountered with amniocentesis. Specifically, there is risk of bleeding, infection, and preterm PROM. The risk of pregnancy loss as a result of the procedure is estimated to be 1.4%,[172] although fetuses with severe IUGR or major structural anomalies are at higher risk, especially in comparison with well-grown, structurally normal fetuses. Operator experience is an important determinant of success, as are logistical issues (e.g., volume of amniotic fluid, placental position, location of the cord insertion site within the placenta). A transient fetal bradycardia may occur during the procedure, often resulting from unintentional placement of the needle into one of the umbilical arteries and leading to arterial vasospasm. Although this bradycardia invariably resolves, if the fetus is at a favorable gestational age (> 24 weeks), the procedure should be performed at a facility with the capacity to perform an emergency cesarean delivery. No consistent data or recommendations exist regarding the use of prophylactic antibiotics, tocolysis, and maternal sedation during cordocentesis.

Other Tests

THREE-DIMENSIONAL ULTRASONOGRAPHY

Compared with standard two-dimensional ultrasonography, three-dimensional (3D) ultrasonography (or four-dimensional, if fetal movements are included) allows for concurrent visualization of fetal structures in all three dimensions for improved characterization of complex fetal structural anomalies. Unlike two-dimensional ultrasonographic images, 3D images are greatly influenced by fetal movements and are subject to more interference from structures such as fetal limbs, umbilical cord, and placental tissue. Because of movement interference, visualization of the fetal heart with 3D ultrasonography is suboptimal.

In addition to rapid acquisition of images that can be later reconstructed and manipulated, 3D ultrasonography has the following potential advantages:

1. The ability to provide clearer images of soft tissue structures through surface rendering. Such images may improve the diagnosis of certain fetal malformations, especially craniofacial anomalies (e.g., cleft lip and palate, micrognathia, ear anomaly, facial dysmorphism, intracranial lesions), club foot, finger and toe anomalies, spinal anomalies, ventral wall defects, and fetal tumors.
2. The ability to provide more accurate measurements of the gestational sac, yolk sac, and crown-rump length and to obtain a midsagittal view for measuring NT.
3. The ability to measure tissue volume. Preliminary data suggest that assessment of cervical volume may identify women at risk for cervical insufficiency,[173] and measurement of placental volume in the first trimester may determine fetuses at risk for IUGR.[174]

Despite these advantages, 3D ultrasonography has been used primarily as a complementary technique rather than the standard technique for ultrasonographic imaging. In the future, technical improvements should provide higher-quality images, perhaps similar to those offered by computed tomography and magnetic resonance imaging (MRI).

COMPLEMENTARY RADIOGRAPHIC IMAGING

Ultrasonography remains the first-line imaging modality during pregnancy. In certain situations, however, enhanced imaging may be required to better define a particular fetal anomaly. For example, radiographic imaging is superior to ultrasonography in evaluating the fetal skeleton and may provide valuable information in the evaluation of a fetus with a suspected bony dystrophy. At least 25 different forms of osteochondrodysplasia are identifiable at birth, 11 of which are lethal in the peripartum period.[175] Although some of these forms can be identified from their unusual appearance on ultrasonography (such as cloverleaf skull and small thorax in thanatophoric dysplasia), the majority are missed. Timely radiographic imaging may allow an experienced pediatric radiologist to more thoroughly evaluate the fetal skeleton and determine the correct diagnosis. A simple maternal abdominal radiograph may be all that is required, because ossification is sufficient by 20 weeks' gestation to allow good visualization of the fetal bones.

Although computed tomography is best avoided in pregnancy because it exposes the fetus to ionizing radiation (albeit at small doses), MRI is regarded as safe. This latter technology relies on the interaction between an applied magnetic field and the inherent nuclear magnetism of atomic nuclei within the patient's tissues to generate a high-resolution anatomic image. Because MRI is particularly good at visualizing soft tissue rather than bony structures, it is uniquely suited to the evaluation of fetal intracranial defects and the soft tissues of the maternal pelvis (Figure 6-8).[176,177] Although fetal motion artifact has previously been a major limitation in the use of MRI, new ultrafast technology allows for rapid image acquisition and has largely overcome this problem.

FETAL ECHOCARDIOGRAPHY

Cardiac anomalies are the most common major congenital defects encountered in the antepartum period. A four-chamber ultrasonographic view of the heart during the fetal anatomy survey at 18 to 20 weeks' gestation detects only 30% of congenital cardiac anomalies, although the detection rate can be increased to approximately 60% to 70% if the outflow tracts are adequately visualized.[178] Owing to the number of congenital cardiac anomalies that would be missed, however, fetal echocardiography should be performed by a skilled and experienced sonologist at 20 to 22 weeks' gestation in all pregnancies at high risk for a fetal cardiac anomaly—pregnancies complicated by pregestational diabetes mellitus, with a personal or family history of congenital cardiac disease (regardless of the nature of the lesion or whether it has been repaired), with maternal exposure to certain drugs (e.g., lithium, paroxetine),[179] and with conception by *in vitro* fertilization (but not if the pregnancy was conceived through the use of clomiphene citrate or ovarian stimulation/intrauterine insemination alone).[180]

FETAL CELLS OR DNA IN THE MATERNAL CIRCULATION

To minimize the fetal risks of invasive prenatal diagnosis (amniocentesis and CVS), noninvasive tests are being developed for definitive fetal aneuploidy genetic testing. Fetal cells are known to be present in the maternal circulation throughout pregnancy at a concentration of approximately 1 fetal cell for every 10,000 maternal cells.[181] Of interest,

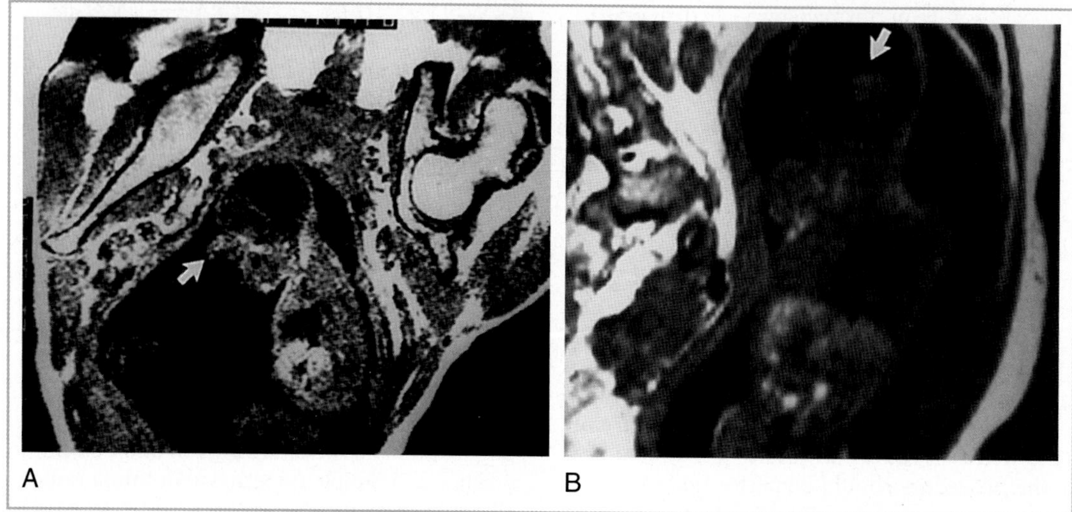

FIGURE 6-8 Magnetic resonance imaging of a fetus with holoprosencephaly. **A,** Sagittal view showing the proboscis (*arrow*). **B,** Coronal view showing the single ventricle and fused thalami (*arrow*). (From Wenstrom KD, Williamson RA, Weiner CP, et al. Magnetic resonance imaging of fetuses with intracranial defects. Reprinted with permission from the American College of Obstetricians and Gynecologists. Obstet Gynecol 1991; 77:529-32.)

fetal DNA accounts for 3% to 6% of all free DNA in maternal serum but up to 20% in the setting of preeclampsia or major fetomaternal hemorrhage. Because of its relative abundance, purity, and short half-life (precluding contamination from a prior pregnancy), fetal DNA may be superior to fetal cells for genetic analysis.[182] Attempts at identifying and isolating fetal cells and/or DNA from the maternal circulation for use in genetic testing have been largely unsuccessful, however.[183,184]

An alternative approach under investigation for definitive genetic testing is the isolation of trophoblast cells from the cervicovaginal discharge of women in early pregnancy.[185-188] Provisional studies have isolated these cells from the maternal cervix with cervical canal lavage at 7 to 10 weeks' gestation[185] or with the use of a brush-type collection device (Cytobrush, Medscand, Inc., Monroe, CT) at 5 to 12 weeks (the "genetic Pap smear").[188] With this technique, such cells have been isolated in 86% (195/227) of samples by immunocytochemistry with trophoblast-specific antibodies, and results agreed with those of placental tissue karyotyping via CVS in 95% (186/195) of cases.[188] The ability to successfully collect trophoblast cells from the cervicovaginal discharge of women in early pregnancy may provide a simple, reliable, noninvasive, yet definitive genetic test for fetal aneuploidy in a singleton pregnancy with no risk to the mother or fetus.

SPECIAL CIRCUMSTANCES REQUIRING ADDITIONAL FETAL SURVEILLANCE

Under certain circumstances, additional antenatal fetal surveillance may be required (see Box 6-2). If appropriate, early consultation with a specialist (such as a maternal-fetal medicine specialist, medical geneticist, pediatric surgeon, pediatric urologist, pediatric cardiologist, or infectious disease specialist) and delivery at a tertiary care center should be considered.

Abnormal Serum Analyte Screening Result with Normal Fetal Karyotype

Pregnancies with abnormal serum analyte screening in the first or second trimester are at increased risk for adverse outcomes, including preterm birth, preeclampsia, and stillbirth, *even if the karyotype is normal* (Tables 6-9 and 6-10).[189-191] Such pregnancies therefore require more intensive fetal monitoring (Table 6-11) and consideration for early delivery. Fetuses with an NT measurement of 3.5 mm or higher in the first trimester have a higher risk of congenital heart defects, even with a negative aneuploidy screening test result and normal fetal chromosomes.[132,192] Women with such pregnancies should be offered a fetal echocardiogram at 20 to 22 weeks' gestation in addition to a routine targeted fetal anatomy survey at 18 to 20 weeks.

Hydrops Fetalis

Hydrops fetalis (Latin for "edema of the fetus") is a rare pathologic condition that complicates approximately 0.05% of all pregnancies. It is an ultrasonographic diagnosis requiring the presence of an abnormal accumulation of fluid in more than one fetal extravascular compartment, including ascites, pericardial effusion, pleural effusion, subcutaneous edema, and/or placental edema. Polyhydramnios is seen in 50% to 75% of cases. Although classically seen in fetuses with severe anemia resulting from Rh isoimmunization, the introduction of $Rh_0(D)$ immune globulin has led to a substantial decrease in the incidence of immune hydrops. Indeed, 90% of hydrops fetalis cases are due to nonimmune causes, such as maternal infection (e.g., with parvovirus B19, cytomegalovirus, syphilis), massive fetomaternal hemorrhage, and fetal abnormalities (e.g., congenital cardiac defects, fetal thalassemia, twin-to-twin transfusion syndrome). Although the overall perinatal mortality rate in the setting of hydrops fetalis exceeds 50%, the prognosis depends on the underlying cause, the severity, and gestational age.

TABLE 6-9 Relationship between First-Trimester PAPP-A Level at or below Fifth Percentile (0.42 MoM) and Risks of Adverse Pregnancy Outcomes

Adverse Outcome	Adjusted Odds Ratio	95% Confidence Interval
Spontaneous loss < 24 weeks	2.50	1.76-3.56
Fetal death ≥ 24 weeks	2.15	1.11-4.15
Preterm birth ≤ 37 weeks	1.87	1.61-2.17
Preterm birth ≤ 32 weeks	2.10	1.59-2.76
Preeclampsia	1.54	1.16-2.03
Gestational hypertension	1.47	1.20-1.82
Placental abruption	1.80	1.15-2.84
Intrauterine growth restriction	3.22	2.38-4.36

MoM, multiple of the median; PAPP-A, pregnancy-associated placental protein-A test.

Data from Dugoff L, Hobbins JS, Malone FD, et al. First-trimester maternal serum PAPP-A and free beta-subunit human chorionic gonadotropin concentrations and nuchal translucency are associated with obstetric complications: A population-based screening study (the FASTER Trial). Am J Obstet Gynecol 2004; 191:1446-51.

Immune hydrops occurs when fetal erythrocytes express a protein that is not present on maternal erythrocytes. The maternal immune system can become sensitized and produce antibodies against these "foreign" proteins. These immunoglobulin (Ig) G antibodies can cross the placenta and destroy fetal erythrocytes, leading to fetal anemia and high-output cardiac failure. Immune hydrops is typically associated with a fetal hematocrit less than 15% (normal fetal hematocrit is 50%). The most antigenic protein on the surface of fetal erythrocytes is the D antigen of the Rhesus protein complex, also known as Rh(D). Other antigens that can cause severe immune hydrops are Kell ("Kell kills"), Rh(E), Rh(c), and Duffy ("Duffy dies"). Antigens causing less severe hydrops are ABO, Rh(e), Rh(C), Ce, k, and s. Lewis a and b (Le^a, Le^b) incompatibility can cause mild anemia but not hydrops, because this condition primarily results in production of IgM antibodies, which do not cross the placenta ("Lewis lives"). For identification of women at risk of isoimmunization, every pregnant woman should undergo blood type and antibody screening at the first prenatal visit and again in the third trimester.

Sixty percent of cases of immune hydrops result from ABO incompatibility; however, only Rh(D) isoimmunization can be prevented. The Rh(D) antigen is expressed only on primate erythrocytes and becomes evident by 38 days of intrauterine life. A mutation in the Rh(D) gene on chromosome 1 results in lack of expression of Rh(D) antigen on circulating erythrocytes (Rh[D]-negative). This mutation arose in the Basque region of Spain, and the difference in prevalence of Rh(D)-negative individuals between the races likely reflects the amount of Spanish blood in their ancestry: Caucasian, 15%; African-American, 8%; African, 4%; Native American, 1%; and Asian, less than 1%.[193] If the fetus of an Rh(D)-negative woman is Rh(D)-negative, Rh(D) sensitization will not occur. However, 60% of Rh(D)-negative women have Rh(D)-positive fetuses, and exposure of these women to as little as 0.25 mL of Rh(D)-positive blood may induce an antibody response. Because the initial immune response is production of IgM, the index pregnancy is rarely affected. However, immunization in subsequent pregnancies triggers an IgG response that crosses the placenta and causes

TABLE 6-10 Second-Trimester Serum Analyte (Marker) Screening and Adverse Pregnancy Outcome

Adverse Outcome	Marker	Odds Ratio
Spontaneous loss < 24 weeks	MS-AFP	7.8
Fetal death ≥ 24 weeks	Inhibin A	3.7
Preterm birth ≤ 32 weeks	Inhibin A	5.0
Preterm premature rupture of membranes	MS-AFP	1.9
Preeclampsia	Inhibin A	3.8
Gestational hypertension	Inhibin A	1.7
Placental abruption	MS-AFP	1.9
Placenta previa (confirmed at delivery)	MS-AFP	3.1
Intrauterine growth restriction	Inhibin A	3.0
Birth weight ≤ 5th percentile	Inhibin A	2.3
• Delivery < 37 weeks	Inhibin A	8.0
• Delivery < 32 weeks	Inhibin A	18.6

MS-AFP, maternal serum level of alpha-fetoprotein.

Data from Dugoff L, Hobbins JS, Malone FD, et al; FASTER Trial Research Consortium. Quad screen as a predictor of adverse pregnancy outcome. Obstet Gynecol 2005; 106:260-7.

TABLE 6-11 Special Circumstances Requiring Additional Fetal Surveillance during Pregnancy

Pregnancy-Related Condition	Additional Testing Recommended	Gestational Age at Which Testing Should Be Started
Maternal Conditions		
Chronic hypertension	Growth scans q3-4 weeks Weekly NST ± AFV	24 weeks 32 weeks
Diabetes mellitus:		
Pregestational diabetes	Growth scans q3-4 weeks Weekly NST ± AFV	24 weeks 32 weeks
Gestational diabetes	Growth scans q3-4 weeks Weekly NST ± AFV	From diagnosis 36 weeks
Maternal obesity (body mass index > 30 kg/m^2)	Weekly NST ± AFV	36 weeks
Advanced maternal age	Weekly NST ± AFV	38 weeks
Abnormal serum analyte screening result (maternal serum level of alpha-fetoprotein [MS-AFP] > 2.0 MoM; pregnancy-associated placental protein-A [PAPP-A] < 0.4 MoM) with normal fetal karyotype	Growth scans q3-4 weeks Weekly NST ± AFV	24 weeks 36 weeks
Prior unexplained preterm birth < 35 weeks	Weekly to biweekly cervical length measurements ± Weekly to biweekly fFN	16-18 weeks to 30-32 weeks 24 weeks to 32-34 weeks
Prior cervical cone biopsy	Weekly to biweekly cervical length measurements ± Weekly to biweekly fFN	16-18 weeks to 30-32 weeks 24 weeks to 32-34 weeks
Post-term pregnancy	Twice-weekly NST and AFV	41-42 weeks
Isoimmunization	Weekly middle cerebral artery Doppler velocimetry	18-20 weeks
Uteroplacental Conditions		
Chronic abruption	Growth scans q3-4 weeks Weekly NST ± AFV	From diagnosis 28-32 weeks
Uterus didelphys	Weekly to biweekly cervical length measurements	16-18 weeks to 30-32 weeks
Preterm premature rupture of membranes	Daily NST Growth scans q3-4 weeks Weekly AFV	From diagnosis From diagnosis From diagnosis
Unexplained oligohydramnios	Growth scans q3-4 weeks Weekly AFV Weekly NST with AFV Weekly UA Doppler velocimetry	From diagnosis From diagnosis 32 weeks From diagnosis
Fetal Conditions		
Twin pregnancy:		
Dichorionic, diamniotic twin pregnancy	Biweekly AFV Growth scans q3-4 weeks Weekly NST with AFV Weekly to biweekly cervical length measurements ± Weekly to biweekly fFN	18-20 weeks 24 weeks 32 weeks 16-18 weeks to 30-32 weeks 22-24 weeks to 30-32 weeks
Monochorionic, diamniotic twin pregnancy	Weekly AFV Growth scans q3-4 weeks Weekly NST with AFV Weekly to biweekly cervical length measurements ± Weekly to biweekly fFN	16-18 weeks 24 weeks 28-32 weeks 16-18 weeks to 30-32 weeks 22-24 weeks to 30-32 weeks
Monochorionic, monoamniotic twin pregnancy	Weekly AFV Growth scans q3-4 weeks Weekly to biweekly cervical length measurements ± Weekly to biweekly fFN ± Continuous fetal heart rate monitoring	16-18 weeks 24 weeks 16-18 weeks to 30-32 weeks 22-24 weeks to 30-32 weeks 24-26 weeks to delivery

TABLE 6-11—cont'd Special Circumstances Requiring Additional Fetal Surveillance during Pregnancy

Pregnancy-Related Condition	Additional Testing Recommended	Gestational Age at Which Testing Should Be Started
Twin pregnancy complicated by demise of one twin	Weekly NST with AFV	From diagnosis
	Growth scans q3-4 weeks	From diagnosis
Higher-order multiple pregnancy (≥ triplets)	Weekly AFV	16-18 weeks
	Growth scans q3-4 weeks	24 weeks
	Weekly NST with AFV	28-32 weeks
	Weekly to biweekly cervical length measurements	16-18 weeks to 30-32 weeks
	± Weekly to biweekly fFN	22-24 weeks to 30-32 weeks
Intrauterine growth restriction:		
< 10th percentile	Growth scans q3-4 weeks	From diagnosis
	Weekly NST with AFV	From diagnosis
< 5th percentile	Growth scans q3-4 weeks	From diagnosis
	Weekly to twice weekly NST with AFV	From diagnosis
	Weekly to twice weekly UA Doppler velocimetry	From diagnosis
Major fetal structural anomaly	Growth scans q3-4 weeks	24 weeks
	Weekly NST with AFV	32 weeks
	± Weekly UA Doppler velocimetry	32 weeks

AFV, amniotic fluid volume; biweekly, every 2 weeks; fFN, fetal fibronectin; MoM, multiple of median; NST, nonstress test; UA, umbilical artery.

hemolysis. Risk factors for Rh(D) sensitization include a mismatched blood transfusion (95% sensitization rate), ectopic pregnancy (< 1%), abortion (3% to 6%), amniocentesis (1% to 3%), and pregnancy itself (16% to 18% sensitization rate after normal pregnancy without Rh_0(D) immune globulin, 1.3% with Rh_0(D) immune globulin at delivery only, and 0.13% with anti-Rh_0(D) immune globulin at 28 weeks and again at delivery).[193,194] The risk of isoimmunization depends on the volume of fetomaternal hemorrhage (Table 6-12). Passive immunization with Rh_0(D) immune globulin can destroy fetal erythrocytes before they evoke a maternal immune response, thereby preventing sensitization. Therefore, Rh_0(D) immune globulin should be given within 72 hours of potential exposure; 300 μg given intramuscularly is adequate for exposure to as much as 30 mL of fetal whole blood or 15 mL of fetal red blood cells.

TABLE 6-12 Fetal-Maternal Transfusion Volume and Risk of Rh(D) Isoimmunization in an Rh(D)-Negative Woman

Transfusion Volume	Incidence at Delivery (%)	Risk of Isoimmunization (%)*
Unmeasurable	50	Minimal
< 0.1 mL	45-50	3
> 5.0 mL	1	20-40
> 30 mL	0.25	60-80

*Without Rh_0(D) immune globulin.

Data from American College of Obstetricians and Gynecologists. Prevention of Rh D alloimmunization. ACOG Practice Bulletin No. 4. Washington, DC, ACOG, 1999 (Int J Gynaecol Obstet 1999; 66:63-70); and Moise KJ. Red blood cell alloimmunization in pregnancy. Semin Hematol 2005; 42:169-78.

Once isoimmunization has occurred, passive immunoglobulin is not useful. Such pregnancies should be followed closely for evidence of fetal compromise. Fetal hemolysis results in release of bile pigment into the amniotic fluid, which can be quantified as a change in optical density measured at wavelength 450 nm. Traditionally, the extent of hemolysis has been measured with serial amniocenteses, with amniotic fluid optical density plotted against gestational age; increased density (upper 80% of zone 2 or zone 3 of the Liley curve) is associated with a poor prognosis,[195,196] and prompt intervention is indicated. Measurements of peak flow velocity in the fetal MCA by means of noninvasive Doppler velocimetry have now been shown to accurately identify fetuses with severe anemia requiring urgent intervention, regardless of the cause of the anemia.[113,194,197] Depending on gestational age, these interventions may include immediate delivery or intrauterine blood transfusion.

Post-Term Pregnancy

Post-term (prolonged) pregnancy is defined as any pregnancy that continues to or beyond 42 weeks (294 days) from the first day of the last normal menstrual period or 14 days beyond the best obstetric estimate of the EDD.[2,198] The prevalence of post-term pregnancy depends on the patient population (e.g., percentage of primigravidas, incidence of pregnancy complications, frequency of spontaneous preterm births) and the local practice patterns (e.g., use of ultrasonographic assessment of gestational age, cesarean delivery rates, use of labor induction). Approximately 10% (range, 3% to 14%) of all pregnancies continue beyond 42 weeks, and 4% (range, 2% to 7%) continue beyond 43 weeks in the absence of obstetric intervention.[2] Compared with delivery at 40 weeks, post-term pregnancies pose significant risks to both the mother (including higher risk of cesarean delivery, severe perineal injury, and postpartum hemorrhage) and the fetus (including stillbirth, fetal macrosomia, birth injury, and meconium aspiration syndrome).[2,198-201] The risks to the fetus can be largely prevented by routine induction of labor for all low-risk pregnancies at 40 to 41 weeks' gestation.[2,199]

Post-term pregnancy is a universally accepted indication for antenatal fetal surveillance,[2] although the efficacy of this approach has not been validated by prospective randomized trials. Options for evaluating fetal well-being include NST with or without amniotic fluid volume assessment, BPP, CST, and a combination of these modalities. There is no consensus as to which of these modalities is preferred, and no single method has been shown to be superior.[2] The American College of Obstetricians and Gynecologists (ACOG) has recommended that antepartum fetal surveillance be initiated by 42 weeks' gestation, without making a specific recommendation about the type of test or frequency.[2] Many investigators would advise twice-weekly testing with some evaluation of amniotic fluid volume at least weekly. Doppler ultrasonography has no benefit in monitoring the post-term fetus and is not recommended for this indication.[109,110] Although the data are inconsistent, there is a suggestion that antenatal testing at 40 to 42 weeks' gestation may be associated with improvements in perinatal outcome. In one retrospective study, women with routine antenatal testing beginning at 41 weeks had lower rates of cesarean delivery for nonreassuring fetal test results than women in whom testing was started at 42 weeks (2.3% versus 5.6%, respectively; $P < .01$).[202] Additionally, in this study, the group with delayed antenatal testing experienced three stillbirths and seven other neonatal major morbidity events, compared with none in the group who had antenatal testing from 41 weeks ($P < .05$).[202]

In the post-term period, evidence of fetal compromise (nonreassuring fetal test results) or **oligohydramnios** (e.g., low amniotic fluid volume) should prompt delivery.[2] Oligohydramnios may result from uteroplacental insufficiency or increased renal artery resistance and may predispose to umbilical cord compression, thus leading to intermittent fetal hypoxemia, meconium passage, and meconium aspiration. A uniform definition for oligohydramnios has not been established; however, options are as follows: (1) a depth of less than 2 cm for the largest vertical fluid pocket; (2) amniotic fluid index (AFI) less than 5 cm (i.e., < 5 cm for the sum of the depths in cm of the largest vertical pocket in each of four uterine quadrants); and (3) product of length times width times depth of the largest pocket (in cm) less than 60. Adverse pregnancy outcomes (nonreassuring FHR tracing, low Apgar score, and neonatal intensive care unit admission) are more common when oligohydramnios is present. Frequent (twice-weekly) screening of post-term patients for oligohydramnios is important, because amniotic fluid can become dramatically reduced within 24 to 48 hours. One prospective, double-blind, cohort study of 1584 women after 40 weeks' gestation found that an AFI less than 5 with no largest vertical fluid pocket depth less than 2 cm was associated with birth asphyxia and meconium aspiration, although the sensitivity for adverse outcomes was low.[203]

Intrauterine Fetal Demise

Intrauterine fetal demise (IUFD), also known as stillbirth, is defined in the United States as demise of the fetus after 20 weeks' gestation and prior to delivery.[204-206] In Europe, only fetuses more than 24 weeks' gestation are included. The stillbirth rate in the United States diminished from 15.8 per 1000 total births in 1960 to 7.5 per 1000 births in 1990.[205,206] However, it remains a vastly underappreciated clinical problem, with antepartum stillbirths accounting for more perinatal deaths than either complications of prematurity or sudden infant death syndrome (SIDS).[207] Risk factors for stillbirth include extremes of maternal age, chromosomal disorders, congenital malformations, antenatal infection, multiple pregnancy, prior unexplained IUFD, post-term pregnancy, fetal macrosomia, male fetus, umbilical cord and placental abnormalities, and underlying maternal medical conditions (e.g., chronic hypertension, pregestational or gestational diabetes mellitus, autoimmune disorders, inherited or acquired thrombophilias).[204,208,209]

Although older studies observed that approximately 50% of cases of IUFD were unexplained, an aggressive approach may identify the cause in up to 80% to 90% of cases (Table 6-13).[209-212] Pathologic examination of the fetus and the placenta/fetal membranes is the single most useful means of identifying a cause for the IUFD.[210,211] Early detection and appropriate management of underlying maternal disorders (e.g., diabetes, preeclampsia) may also reduce the risk. Fetal karyotyping should be considered in all cases of fetal death to identify chromosomal abnormalities, particularly in cases with documented fetal structural abnormalities. Approximately 6% to 10% of stillborn fetuses

TABLE 6-13 Causes of Intrauterine Fetal Demise

Maternal causes	Underlying medical conditions (diabetes mellitus, thyroid disease, antiphospholipid antibody syndrome) Preeclampsia Isoimmunization Illicit drug use (cocaine) Antepartum drug/toxin exposure
Uteroplacental causes	Placental abruption Placenta previa Vasa previa Fetomaternal hemorrhage Cord accident
Fetal causes	Fetal chromosomal/genetic anomalies Fetal structural abnormalities Intra-amniotic infection Complications of multiple pregnancies (including twin-to-twin transfusion syndrome)

have an abnormal karyotype.[212] On occasion, amniocentesis may be recommended to salvage viable amniocytes for cytogenetic analysis before delivery. Fetomaternal hemorrhage (spilling of fetal blood cells into the maternal circulation) occurs in all pregnancies, but is usually minimal (< 0.1 mL total volume). In rare instances, fetomaternal hemorrhage may be massive, leading to fetal demise. The Kleihauer-Betke (acid elution) test allows an estimate of the volume of fetal blood in the maternal circulation, and a maternal blood sample should be drawn within 6 to 8 hours of the purported bleeding episode because of rapid clearance of fetal cells from the maternal circulation.[213] Intra-amniotic infection resulting in fetal death is usually evident on clinical examination. Placental membrane culture and autopsy examination of the fetus, placenta/fetal membranes, and umbilical cord may be useful. Fetal radiographic or MRI may sometimes be valuable if autopsy is declined.[214,215]

The inability to identify fetal heart activity or the absence of uterine growth may suggest the diagnosis. Ultrasonography is the "gold standard" for confirming IUFD by documenting the absence of fetal cardiac activity. Other ultrasonographic findings in late pregnancy include Spalding's sign (overlapping of the cranial sutures), scalp edema, and soft tissue maceration, although these usually take a few days to develop. Every effort should be made to avoid cesarean delivery in the setting of IUFD. Thus, in the absence of a contraindication, expectant management is often recommended. Latency (the period from fetal demise to delivery) varies according to the underlying cause and gestational age. In general, the earlier the gestational age, the longer the latency period. Overall, more than 90% of women go into spontaneous labor within 2 weeks of fetal death. However, many women find the prospect of carrying a dead fetus distressing and want the pregnancy terminated as soon as possible. Management options include surgical dilation and evacuation or induction of labor with cervical ripening, if indicated. Disseminated intravascular coagulation (DIC) develops in approximately 20% to 25% of women who retain a dead singleton fetus for longer than 3 weeks, because of excessive consumption of clotting factors.[216,217] Therefore, delivery should be effected within this period. Induction of labor with prostaglandins or oxytocin has been shown to be safe in the setting of an IUFD.

The death of one twin poses a particular challenge. In this setting, the surviving twin is at significant risk of major morbidity, including IUFD, neurologic injury, multiorgan system failure, thromboembolic events, placental abruption, and preterm birth.[218-220] The prognosis for the surviving twin depends on the cause of death, gestational age, chorionicity, and the time between death of the first twin and delivery of the second. Dizygous twin pregnancies do not share a circulation, and death of one twin may have little impact on the surviving twin. The dead twin may be resorbed completely or may become compressed and incorporated into the membranes (*fetus papyraceus*). Disseminated intravascular coagulation in the surviving fetus and/or mother is rare.[221] On the other hand, some level of shared circulation can be demonstrated in almost all monozygous twin pregnancies, and death of one fetus in this setting raises the risk of death of its co-twin owing to profound hypotension and/or purported transfer of thromboplastic proteins from the dead fetus to the live fetus.[222] If it survives, the co-twin has a 40% risk for development of permanent neurologic injury (multicystic encephalomalacia), which may not be prevented by immediate delivery.[223,224] Therefore, management of a surviving co-twin depends on chorionicity and gestational age. Regular fetal surveillance (kick counts, NST, BPP) should be instituted (see Table 6-11), and delivery considered in the setting of nonreassuring fetal test results or at a favorable gestational age.

FETAL THERAPY

Continued assessment of the fetus throughout pregnancy is critical to optimizing pregnancy outcomes. In most cases, evidence of fetal compromise prompts delivery. However, in certain situations, treatment may be available to improve or even correct the underlying problem *in utero*. These interventions can be noninvasive (e.g., administration of digoxin to the mother to treat a fetal supraventricular tachycardia) or invasive (e.g., placement of a vesico-amniotic shunt), and are summarized in Tables 6-14 and 6-15, respectively.[225-260] Some of these interventions have been subjected to rigorous clinical trials and have been shown to be effective, whereas others remain investigational. The intervention that has perhaps had the greatest effect on perinatal outcome is antenatal maternal administration of corticosteroids.

Antenatal Corticosteroids

Respiratory distress syndrome (RDS) refers to respiratory compromise presenting at or shortly after delivery due to a deficiency of pulmonary surfactant, an endogenous detergent that serves to decrease the surface tension within alveoli, thereby preventing alveolar collapse. Overall, neonatal RDS affects approximately 1% of live births, but not all infants are at equal risk. The pulmonary system is among the last of the fetal organ systems to become functionally mature. Thus, RDS is primarily, although not exclusively, a disease of premature infants, with the incidence and severity highly dependent on gestational age. For example, RDS affects more than 80% of infants younger than 28 weeks' gestation and 10% to 15% of all infants weighing less than 2500 g.[261,262] RDS remains a major cause of perinatal morbidity and mortality in extremely premature infants. In addition to gestational age, a number of other factors influence the risk for RDS in a given fetus. For reasons that are not clear, African-American ethnicity, female gender, preeclampsia, and intrauterine exposure to cigarette smoke are protective against the development of RDS.

In 1972, Liggins and Howie[263] demonstrated that the administration of a single course of two antenatal doses of a corticosteroid (betamethasone) reduced the incidence of RDS by 50%. This original observation has since been confirmed by a number of investigators.[225,264-267] A meta-analysis of 12 randomized controlled trials with more than 3000 participants concluded that antenatal administration of corticosteroids to women in preterm labor reduced the incidence of neonatal RDS by 40% to 60% and resulted in an improvement in overall survival.[225] In one study, a single course of antenatal corticosteroids resulted in a threefold

TABLE 6-14 Noninvasive Treatment Options to Improve Perinatal Outcome

Clinical Condition	Treatment	Efficacy
Imminent risk of preterm birth < 34 weeks	Antenatal corticosteroids	Effective in decreasing respiratory distress syndrome, intraventricular hemorrhage, necrotizing enterocolitis[225]
Pregestational diabetes mellitus	Strict glycemic control	Effective in decreasing rate of stillbirths and birth defects[226]
Phenylketonuria (autosomal recessive disorder due to phenylalanine hydroxylase deficiency)	Dietary manipulation (low-phenylalanine diet)	Effective in decreasing birth defects and brain damage in affected fetuses[227]
Alloimmune thrombocytopenia	Maternal intravenous immunoglobulin ± corticosteroids	Data conflicting on effect of intravenous immunoglobulin on fetal platelets; steroids probably of no benefit[228,229]
Fetal thyrotoxicosis	Maternal propylthiouracil	Effective in decreasing intrauterine growth restriction and subsequent neurodevelopmental defects[230,231]
Congenital adrenal hyperplasia (due usually to 21-hydroxylase deficiency)	Maternal dexamethasone	Effective in preventing virilization of female fetus if given prior to 8 to 9 weeks' gestation[232]
Fetal supraventricular tachycardia (SVT)	Maternal digoxin	Data conflicting on effect of digoxin to correct fetal SVT

TABLE 6-15 Invasive Treatment Options to Improve Perinatal Outcome

Clinical Condition	Treatment	Efficacy
Severe fetal anemia with or without hydrops fetalis	Intrauterine transfusion	Effective[233,234]
Fetal supraventricular tachycardia	Digoxin given directly to fetus by intramuscular injection	Effective
Severe obstructive uropathy	Vesicoamniotic shunt	Effective in preventing renal injury and improving survival[235]
Isolated fluid collection in the fetus (severe ascites, hydrothorax)	Fetoamniotic shunting	Effective[236]
Severe valvular stenosis	Fetal surgery (*in utero* valvuloplasty)	Investigational[237]
Fetal lung masses (congenital cystic adenomatous malformation, pulmonary sequestration)	Fetal surgery (*in utero* resection of lesion)	Investigational[238,239]
Congenital hydrocephalus	Fetal surgery (*in utero* shunting)	Investigational[240]
Congenital diaphragmatic hernia	Fetal surgery (*in utero* repair; tracheal occlusion)	Investigational[241,242]
Fetal neural tube defect	Fetal surgery (*in utero* repair)	Investigational[243-245]
Higher-order multiple pregnancy (≥ triplets)	Multifetal pregnancy reduction	Effective in improving perinatal outcomes with reduction to twins[246-249]
Twin-to-twin transfusion syndrome (TTTS)	Serial amnioreduction vs. septostomy vs. fetal surgery (endoscopic laser ablation, cord ligation)	Effective Laser ablation appears to give the best chance of intact survival in severe TTTS[250-255]
Preterm premature rupture of membranes	Serial amnioinfusion vs. fetal surgery (laser coagulation, intra-amniotic amniopatch)	Investigational[256-258]
Ex utero intrapartum therapy (EXIT)	To facilitate oxygenation at delivery prior to ligation of the umbilical cord when the infant's airway is obstructed; may facilitate transition to extracorporeal membrane oxygenation (ECMO) in infants with severe pulmonary or cardiac malformations	Case reports of success[259,260]

rise in the chance of unaffected survival in neonates with a birth weight less than 1500 g.[264] Certain steroids cross the placenta and induce cellular differentiation at the expense of growth. Type II pneumocytes in the lungs differentiate and begin making pulmonary surfactant, which accounts for the decrease in risk of RDS, and endothelial cells lining the vasculature undergo cellular maturation and stabilization, which explains the concomitant drop in incidence of bleeding into the brain (intraventricular hemorrhage) or gastrointestinal tract (necrotizing enterocolitis).[265] Prednisone does not cross the placenta and therefore does not have a similar protective effect.

The National Institutes of Health and the American College of Obstetricians and Gynecologists have recommended that a single course of antenatal corticosteroids, defined as either betamethasone (12 mg intramuscularly every 24 hours × 2 doses) or dexamethasone (6 mg intramuscularly every 12 hours × 4 doses), be given after 23 to 24 weeks' gestation to any pregnant woman in whom delivery before 34 weeks' gestation is threatening.[266,267] There is as yet no proven benefit to antenatal administration of steroids after 34 weeks' gestation[266,267] or between 32 to 34 weeks in the setting of preterm PROM,[268] but this situation is largely due to the absence of data in these subgroups. Although the maximum benefit of antenatal corticosteroids is achieved 24 to 48 hours after the first injection, as little as 4 hours of treatment exerts some protective effect. This protective effect lasts for 7 days, after which further benefit is unclear. Multiple (three or more) courses of antenatal corticosteroids have been associated with growth restriction, smaller head circumference, and (in animals) abnormal myelination of the optic nerves; consequently, multiple courses are not routinely recommended. If the initial course was completed before 28 weeks' gestation and the clinical situation dictates, however, a single second course or a single "rescue" dose may provide additional protection against RDS.[269-273]

Fetal Surgery

Fetal surgery has been proposed in selected cases to prevent progressive organ damage or to restore normal anatomy and fetal development (see Chapter 7). The ideal case for fetal surgery consists of a singleton pregnancy prior to fetal viability (i.e., before 23 to 24 weeks' gestation) in which the fetus has a normal karyotype and an isolated malformation that, if untreated, will result in fetal or neonatal demise. A detailed understanding of the natural history of the malformation is essential when one is considering whether or not to recommend surgery. Fetal surgery should not be attempted if the natural history of the disorder is unknown or if the chances of survival without *in utero* treatment are equal to or greater than the risks of the procedure. Repair of lesions that are not believed to be life-threatening (e.g., cleft lip and palate) should be deferred until after delivery to minimize risks to the mother.

Before *in utero* surgery can be recommended, a thorough evaluation must be performed to (1) precisely characterize the defect, (2) exclude associated malformations, (3) perform a fetal karyotype analysis, and (4) eliminate the possibility that the condition can be treated using less aggressive technologies. Detailed counseling about the risks and benefits of the proposed procedure is required, and written informed consent is mandatory. Such a discussion must include a detailed review of the risks to both the fetus and the mother, including preterm PROM (28% to 100%), preterm labor and delivery (> 50%), maternal pulmonary edema (20% to 30%), placental abruption (5% to 10%), chorioamnionitis and sepsis (< 5%), and maternal death (rare).[242,244] Specific examples of fetal surgical procedures are summarized in Table 6-15.

KEY POINTS

- Accurate determination of gestational age is essential for the management of pregnancy complications and the effective use of antepartum fetal testing.
- Ultrasonography can be used to estimate gestational age, assess fetal growth, monitor amniotic fluid volume, and detect and characterize fetal anomalies.
- Appropriate fetal growth is strongly correlated with fetal health and can be assessed either clinically or with ultrasonography. Inappropriate fetal growth requires further evaluation.
- Fetal movement charts ("kick counts") can be used to confirm fetal well-being in both high- and low-risk populations. High-risk pregnancies may require additional fetal monitoring such as the nonstress test (NST), biophysical profile (BPP), or contraction stress test (CST).
- A fetal karyotype can be obtained by chorionic villus sampling, amniocentesis, or fetal blood sampling (cordocentesis).
- Doppler velocimetry has advanced our understanding of maternal-fetal physiology, but its role in confirming fetal well-being is unclear.
- Additional radiologic imaging (especially magnetic resonance imaging) may be used in selected cases to better define fetal malformations.
- A number of *in utero* therapies have been shown to improve perinatal outcome in selected cases, including antenatal corticosteroid administration, intrauterine transfusion, and fetal surgery (such as laser photocoagulation for twin-to-twin transfusion syndrome).
- The appropriate timing of delivery is a critical determinant of perinatal outcome. In general, delivery is indicated when the benefits of delivery to the fetus or mother outweigh the risks of continuing the pregnancy. Simply stated, delivery is indicated when the fetus is better off outside the uterus than inside. A number of variables should be considered in such a decision, the most important of which are gestational age and fetal well-being.

REFERENCES

1. American College of Obstetricians and Gynecologists. Antepartum fetal surveillance. ACOG Practice Bulletin No. 9. Washington, DC, ACOG, 1999.
2. American College of Obstetricians and Gynecologists. Management of postterm pregnancy. ACOG Practice Bulletin No. 55. Washington, DC, ACOG, 2004.
3. Neilson JP. Ultrasound for fetal assessment in early pregnancy. Cochrane Database Syst Rev 2000; (2):CD000182.
4. Hertz RH, Sokol RJ, Knoke JD, et al. Clinical estimation of gestational age: Rules for avoiding preterm delivery. Am J Obstet Gynecol 1978; 131:395-402.
5. Gardosi J, Vanner T, Francis A. Gestational age and induction of labor for prolonged pregnancy. Br J Obstet Gynaecol 1997; 104:792-7.
6. Taipale P, Hiilermaa V. Predicting delivery date by ultrasound and last menstrual period on early gestation. Obstet Gynecol 2001; 97:189-94.
7. Kramer MS, Mclean FH, Boyd ME, Usher RH. The validity of gestational age estimation by menstrual dating in term, preterm, and post-term gestations. JAMA 1988; 260:3306-8.
8. Rasor JL, Farber S, Braunstein GD. An evaluation of 10 kits for determination of human chorionic gonadotropin in serum. Clin Chem 1983; 29:1828-31.
9. American College of Obstetricians and Gynecologists. Medical management of tubal pregnancy. ACOG Practice Bulletin No. 3. Washington, DC, ACOG, 1998.
10. Kadar N, DeVore G, Romero R. Discriminating hCG zone: Its use in the sonographic evaluation for ectopic pregnancy. Obstet Gynecol 1981; 58:156-61.
11. Fossum GT, Davajan V, Kletzky OA. Early detection of pregnancy with transvaginal ultrasound. Fertil Steril 1988; 49:788-91.
12. Sabbaha RE, Hughey M. Standardization of sonar cephalometry and gestational age. Obstet Gynecol 1978; 52:402-6.
13. Mongelli M, Wilcox M, Gardosi J. Estimating the date of confinement: Ultrasonographic biometry versus certain menstrual dates. Am J Obstet Gynecol 1996; 174:278-81.
14. Tunon K, Eik-Nes SH, Grottum P. A comparison between ultrasound and a reliable last menstrual period as predictors of the day of delivery in 15,000 examinations. Ultrasound Obstet Gynecol 1996; 8:178-85.
15. Cuckle HS, Wald NJ. The effect of estimating gestational age by ultrasound cephalometry on the sensitivity of alpha fetoprotein screening for Down's syndrome. Br J Obstet Gynaecol 1987; 94:274-6.
16. Seeds JW, Cefalo RC. Relationship of fetal limb lengths to both biparietal diameter and gestational age. Obstet Gynecol 1982; 60:680-5.
17. Bennett KA, Crane JM, O'Shea P, et al. First trimester ultrasound screening is effective in reducing postterm labor induction rates: A randomized controlled trial. Am J Obstet Gynecol 2004; 190: 1077-81.
18. Waldenström U, Axelsson O, Nilsson S, et al. Effects of routine one-stage ultrasound screening in pregnancy: A randomised controlled trial. Lancet 1988; 2:585-8.
19. Saari-Kemppainen A, Karjalainen O, Ylostalo P, Heinonen OP. Ultrasound screening and perinatal mortality: Controlled trial of systematic one-stage screening in pregnancy. The Helsinki Ultrasound Trial. Lancet 1990; 336:387-91.
20. Ewigman BG, Crane JP, Frigoletto FD, et al. Effect of prenatal ultrasound screening on perinatal outcome. RADIUS Study Group. N Engl J Med 1993; 329:821-7.
21. American College of Obstetricians and Gynecologists. Ultrasonography in pregnancy. ACOG Technical Bulletin No. 187. Washington, DC, ACOG, 1993.
22. American Academy of Pediatrics and American College of Obstetricians and Gynecologists. Guidelines for Perinatal Care. 4th edition. Washington, DC, ACOG, 1997.
23. Persson PH, Kullander S. Long-term experience of general ultrasound screening in pregnancy. Am J Obstet Gynecol 1983; 146:942-7.
24. Belfrage P, Fernström I, Hallenberg G. Routine or selective ultrasound examinations in early pregnancy. Obstet Gynecol 1987; 69:747-50.
25. Thacker SB. Quality of controlled clinical trials: The case of imaging ultrasound in obstetrics: A review. Br J Obstet Gynaecol 1985; 92:432-44.
26. Kieler H, Axelsson O, Nilsson S, Waldenström U. The length of human pregnancy as calculated by ultrasonographic measurement of the fetal biparietal diameter. Ultrasound Obstet Gynecol 1995; 6:353-7.
27. Crane JP, LeFevre ML, Winborn RC, et al. A randomized trial of prenatal ultrasonographic screening: Impact on the detection, management, and outcome of anomalous fetuses. Am J Obstet Gynecol 1994; 171:392-9.
28. LeFevre ML, Bain RP, Ewigman BG. A randomized trial of prenatal ultrasonographic screening: Impact on maternal management and outcome. Am J Obstet Gynecol 1993; 169:483-9.
29. American Institute of Ultrasound in Medicine Bioeffects Committee. Review of the Radius Study. AIUM Reporter 1994; 10:2-4.
30. Institute of Medicine. Nutritional status and weight gain. In: Nutrition During Pregnancy. Washington, DC, National Academies Press, 1990:27-233.
31. Leopold, Sporlin. Conduct of normal births through external examination alone. Arch Gynaekol 1894; 45:337.
32. Belizan JM, Villar J, Nardin JC, et al. Diagnosis of intrauterine growth retardation by a simple clinical method: Measurement of fundal height. Am J Obstet Gynecol 1978; 1313:643-6.
33. Gardosi J, Francis A. Controlled trial of fundal height measurement plotted on customised antenatal growth charts. Br J Obstet Gynaecol 1999; 106:309-17.
34. Warsof SL, Gohari P, Berkowitz RL, Hobbins JC. The estimation of fetal weight by computer-assisted analysis. Am J Obstet Gynecol 1977; 128:881-92.
35. Shepard MJ, Richards VA, Berkowitz RL. An evaluation of two equations for predicting fetal weight by ultrasound. Am J Obstet Gynecol 1982; 142:47-54.
36. Jeanty P, Cousaert E, Cantraine F, et al. A longitudinal study of fetal limb growth. Am J Perinatol 1984; 1:136-44.
37. Lockwood CJ, Weiner S. Assessment of fetal growth. Clin Perinatol 1986; 13:3-35.
38. Bahado-Singh RO, Dashe J, Deren O, et al. Prenatal prediction of neonatal outcome in the extremely low-birth-weight infant. Am J Obstet Gynecol 1998; 178:462-8.
39. Ehrenkranz RA. Estimated fetal weights versus birth weights: Should the reference intrauterine growth curves based on birth weights be retired? Arch Dis Child Fetal Neonatal Ed 2007; 92:161-2.
40. Deter RL, Hadlock FP, Harrist RB, Carpenter RJ. Evaluation of three methods for obtaining fetal weight estimates using dynamic image ultrasound. J Clin Ultrasound 1981; 9:421-5.
41. Deter RL, Rossavik IK, Harrist RB, Hadlock FP. Mathematic modeling of fetal growth: Development of individual growth curve standards. Obstet Gynecol 1986; 68:156-61.
42. Rossavik IK, Deter RL. Mathematical modeling of fetal growth. I. Basic principles. J Clin Ultrasound 1984; 12:529-33.
43. Gardosi J. Customized fetal growth standards: Rationale and clinical application. Semin Perinatol 2004; 28:33-40.
44. Nyberg DA, Abuhamad A, Ville Y. Ultrasound assessment of abnormal fetal growth. Semin Perinatol 2004; 28:3-22.
45. Deter RL. Individualized growth assessment: Evaluation of growth using each fetus as its own control. Semin Perinatol 2004; 28:23-32.
46. Sabbagha RE. Intrauterine growth retardation. In Sabbagha RE, editor. Diagnostic Ultrasound Applied to Obstetrics and Gynecology. 2nd edition. Philadelphia, JB Lippincott, 1987:112.
47. Hadlock FP, Harrist RB, Carpenter RJ, et al. Sonographic estimation of fetal weight. The value of femur length in addition to head and abdomen measurements. Radiology 1984; 150:535-40.
48. Anderson NG, Jolley IJ, Wells JE. Sonographic estimation of fetal weight: Comparison of bias, precision and consistency using 12 different formulae. Ultrasound Obstet Gynecol 2007; 30:173-9.
49. Chauhan SP, Lutton PM, Bailey KJ, et al. Intrapartum clinical, sonographic, and parous patients' estimates of newborn birth weight. Obstet Gynecol 1992; 79:956-8.

50. Resnik R. Intrauterine growth restriction. Obstet Gynecol 2002; 99:490-6.
51. American College of Obstetricians and Gynecologists. Fetal macrosomia. ACOG Practice Bulletin No. 22. Washington, DC, ACOG, 2000.
52. American College of Obstetricians and Gynecologists. Gestational diabetes. ACOG Practice Bulletin No. 30. Washington, DC, ACOG, 2001.
53. Magee MS, Walden CE, Benedetti TJ, Knopp RH. Influence of diagnostic criteria on the incidence of gestational diabetes and perinatal morbidity. JAMA 1993; 269:609-15.
54. O'Sullivan JB, Mahan CM, Charles D, Dandrow RV. Screening criteria for high-risk gestational diabetic patients. Am J Obstet Gynecol 1973; 116:895-900.
55. Kjos SL, Buchanan TA. Gestational diabetes mellitus. N Engl J Med 1999; 341:1749-56.
56. Widness JA, Cowett RM, Coustan DR, et al. Neonatal morbidities in infants of mothers with glucose intolerance in pregnancy. Diabetes 1985; 34:61-5.
57. Watson WJ, Soisson AP, Harlass FE. Estimated weight of the term fetus. Accuracy of ultrasound vs clinical examination. J Reprod Med 1988; 33:369-71.
58. Niswander KR, Capraro VJ, Van Coevering RJ. Estimation of birth weight by quantified external uterine measurements. Obstet Gynecol 1970; 36:294-8.
59. Jazayeri A, Heffron JA, Phillips R, Spellacy WN. Macrosomia prediction using ultrasound fetal abdominal circumference of 35 centimeters or more. Obstet Gynecol 1999; 93:523-6.
60. Cromi A, Ghezzi F, Di Naro E, et al. Large cross-sectional area of the umbilical cord as a predictor of fetal macrosomia. Ultrasound Obstet Gynecol 2007; 30:861-6.
61. Abramowicz JS, Robischon K, Cox C. Incorporating sonographic cheek-to-cheek diameter, biparietal diameter and abdominal circumference improves weight estimation in the macrosomic fetus. Ultrasound Obstet Gynecol 1997; 9:409-13.
62. Sood AK, Yancey M, Richards D. Prediction of fetal macrosomia using humeral soft tissue thickness. Obstet Gynecol 1995; 85:937-40.
63. American College of Obstetricians and Gynecologists. Shoulder dystocia. ACOG Practice Bulletin No. 40. Washington, DC, ACOG, 2002. (Int J Gynaecol Obstet 2003; 80:87-92.)
64. Sadovsky E, Polishuk WZ, Mahler Y, Malkin A. Correlation between electromagnetic recording and maternal assessment of fetal movement. Lancet 1973; 1(7813):1141-3.
65. Hertogs K, Roberts AB, Cooper D, et al. Maternal perception of fetal motor activity. Br Med J 1979; 2:1183-5.
66. Schmidt W, Cseh I, Hara K, Kubli F. Maternal perception, tocodynamic findings and real-time ultrasound assessment of total fetal activity. Int J Gynaecol Obstet 1984; 22:85-90.
67. Rayburn WF. Clinical significance of perceptible fetal motion. Am J Obstet Gynecol 1980; 138:210-2.
68. Frøen JF. A kick from within—fetal movement counting and the cancelled progress in antenatal care. J Perinat Med 2004; 32:13-24.
69. Sadovsky E. Fetal movement in utero—A review. II. Fetal movements and fetal distress. Isr J Obstet Gynecol 1992; 3:75-8.
70. Harper RG, Greenberg M, Farahani G, et al. Fetal movement, biochemical and biophysical parameters, and the outcome of pregnancy. Am J Obstet Gynecol 1981; 141:39-42.
71. Sadovsky E, Yaffe H, Plushuk W. Fetal movements in pregnancy and urinary estriol in prediction of impending fetal death in utero. Isr J Med Sci 1974; 10:1096-9.
72. Moore T, Piacquadio K. A prospective evaluation of fetal movement screening to reduce the incidence of antepartum fetal death. Am J Obstet Gynecol 1990; 163:264-5.
73. Liston R, Cohen A, Mennuti M, Gabbe S. Antepartum fetal evaluation by maternal perception of fetal movement. Obstet Gynecol 1982; 60:424-6.
74. Patrick J, Campbell K, Carmichael L, et al. Patterns of gross fetal body movements over 24-hour observation intervals during the last 10 weeks of pregnancy. Am J Obstet Gynecol 1982; 142:363-71.
75. Moore TR, Piacquadio K. A prospective evaluation of fetal movement screening to reduce the incidence of antepartum fetal death. Am J Obstet Gynecol 1989; 160:1075-80.
76. American College of Obstetricians and Gynecologists and American Academy of Pediatrics. Neonatal encephalopathy and cerebral palsy: Defining the pathogenesis and pathophysiology. ACOG Task Force on Neonatal Encephalopathy and Cerebral Palsy. Washington, DC, ACOG, 2003.
77. Nelson KB. Can we prevent cerebral palsy? N Engl J Med 2003; 349:1765-9.
78. Hankins GDV, Speer M. Defining the pathogenesis and pathophysiology of neonatal encephalopathy and cerebral palsy. Obstet Gynecol 2003; 102:628-36.
79. Leveno KJ, Cunningham FG, Nelson S, et al. A prospective comparison of selective and universal electronic fetal monitoring in 34,995 pregnancies. N Engl J Med 1986; 315:615-9.
80. National Institute of Child Health and Human Development Research Planning Workshop. Electronic fetal heart rate monitoring: Research guidelines for interpretation. Am J Obstet Gynecol 1997; 177:1385-90.
81. Parer JT. Fetal heart rate. In Creasy RK, Resnik R, editors. Maternal Fetal Medicine: Principles and Practice. 2nd edition. Philadelphia, WB Saunders, 1989:314-43.
82. Lee CY, DiLoreto PC, Logrand B. Fetal activity acceleration determination for the evaluation of fetal reserve. Obstet Gynecol 1976; 48:19-26.
83. Brown R, Patrick J. The nonstress test: How long is enough? Am J Obstet Gynecol 1981; 141:646-51.
84. Freeman RK, Anderson G, Dorchester W. A prospective multi-institutional study of antepartum fetal heart rate monitoring. I. Risk of perinatal mortality and morbidity according to antepartum fetal heart rate test results. Am J Obstet Gynecol 1982; 143:771-7.
85. Boehm FH, Salyer S, Shah DM, Vaughn WK. Improved outcome of twice weekly nonstress testing. Obstet Gynecol 1986; 67:566-8.
86. Smith CV, Phelan JP, Paul RH. A prospective analysis of the influence of gestational age on the baseline fetal heart rate and reactivity in a low-risk population. Am J Obstet Gynecol 1985; 153:780-2.
87. Nelson KB, Dambrosia JM, Ting TY, Grether JK. Uncertain value of electronic fetal monitoring in predicting cerebral palsy. N Engl J Med 1996; 334:613-8.
88. Smith CV, Phelan JP, Platt LD, et al. Fetal acoustic stimulation testing. II. A randomized clinical comparison with the nonstress test. Am J Obstet Gynecol 1986; 155:131-4.
89. Ingemarsson I, Arulkumaran S, Paul RH, et al. Fetal acoustic stimulation in early labor in patients screened with the admission test. Am J Obstet Gynecol 1988; 158:70-4.
90. Sarno AP, Ahn MO, Phelan JP, Paul RH. Fetal acoustic stimulation in the early intrapartum period as a predictor of subsequent fetal condition. Am J Obstet Gynecol 1990; 162:762-7.
91. Manning FA, Baskett TF, Morrison I, Lange I. Fetal biophysical profile scoring: A prospective study in 1,184 high-risk patients. Am J Obstet Gynecol 1981; 140:289-94.
92. Manning FA, Morrison I, Harman CR, et al. Fetal assessment based on fetal biophysical profile scoring: Experience in 19,221 referred high-risk pregnancies. Am J Obstet Gynecol 1987; 157:880-4.
93. Vintzileos AM, Campbell WA, Nochimson DJ, Weinbaum PJ. The use and misuse of the fetal biophysical profile. Am J Obstet Gynecol 1987; 156:527-33.
94. Vintzileos AM, Gaffney SE, Salinger LM, et al. The relationships among the fetal biophysical profile, umbilical cord pH, and Apgar scores. Am J Obstet Gynecol 1987; 157:627-31.
95. Manning FA, Morrison I, Lagne IR, et al. Fetal assessment based on fetal biophysical profile scoring: Experience in 12,620 referred high-risk pregnancies. I. Perinatal mortality by frequency and etiology. Am J Obstet Gynecol 1985; 151:343-50.
96. Vintzileos AM, Campbell WA, Ingardia CJ, Nochimson DJ. The fetal biophysical profile and its predictive value. Obstet Gynecol 1983; 62:271-8.
97. Manning FA. Fetal biophysical assessment by ultrasound. In Creasy RK, Resnik R, editors. Maternal-Fetal Medicine: Principles and Practice. 2nd edition. Philadelphia, WB Saunders, 1989:359.
98. Oz AU, Holub B, Mendilcioglu I, et al. Renal artery Doppler investigation of the etiology of oligohydramnios in postterm pregnancy. Obstet Gynecol 2002; 100:715-8.

99. Tongsong T, Srisomboon J. Amniotic fluid volume as a predictor of fetal distress in postterm pregnancy. Int J Gynaecol Obstet 1993; 40:213-7.
100. Bochner CJ, Medearis AL, Davis J, et al. Antepartum predictors of fetal distress in postterm pregnancy. Am J Obstet Gynecol 1987; 157:353-8.
101. Morris JM, Thompson K, Smithey J, et al. The usefulness of ultrasound assessment of amniotic fluid in predicting adverse outcome in prolonged pregnancy: A prospective blinded observational study. Br J Obstet Gynaecol 2003; 110:989-94.
102. Clement D, Schifrin BS, Kates RB. Acute oligohydramnios in postdate pregnancy. Am J Obstet Gynecol 1987; 157:884-6.
103. Eden RD, Boehm FH, editors. Assessment and Care of the Fetus; Physiological, Clinical, and Medicolegal Principles. East Norwalk, CT, Appleton & Lange, 1990:351-96.
104. McCallum WD, Williams CS, Nagel S, Daigle RE. Fetal blood velocity waveforms and intrauterine growth retardation. Am J Obstet Gynecol 1978; 132:425-9.
105. Rochelson B, Schulman H, Fleischer A, et al. The clinical significance of Doppler umbilical artery velocimetry in the small for gestational age fetus. Am J Obstet Gynecol 1987; 156:1223-6.
106. Ducey J, Schulman H, Farmalcaides G, et al. A classification of hypertension in pregnancy based on Doppler velocimetry. Am J Obstet Gynecol 1987; 157:680-5.
107. Wenstrom KD, Weiner CP, Williamson RA. Diverse maternal and fetal pathology associated with absent diastolic flow in the umbilical artery of high risk fetuses. Obstet Gynecol 1991; 77:374-8.
108. Zelop CM, Richardson DK, Heffner LJ. Outcomes of severely abnormal umbilical artery Doppler velocimetry in structurally normal singleton fetuses. Obstet Gynecol 1996; 87:434-8.
109. Farmakides G, Schulman H, Ducey J, et al. Uterine and umbilical artery Doppler velocimetry in postterm pregnancy. J Reprod Med 1988; 33:259-61.
110. Stokes HJ, Roberts RV, Newnham JP. Doppler flow velocity waveform analysis in postdate pregnancies. Aust N Z J Obstet Gynaecol 1991; 31:27-30.
111. Baschat AA. Doppler application in the delivery timing of the preterm growth-restricted fetus: Another step in the right direction. Ultrasound Obstet Gynecol 2004; 23:111-8.
112. Landon MB, Gable SG, Bruner JP, Ludmir J. Doppler umbilical artery velocimetry in pregnancy complicated by insulin-dependent diabetes mellitus. Obstet Gynecol 1989; 73:961-5.
113. Mari G, Adrignolo A, Abuhamad AZ, et al. Diagnosis of fetal anemia with Doppler ultrasound in the pregnancy complicated by maternal blood group immunization. Ultrasound Obstet Gynecol 1995; 5:400-5.
114. Donald I. On launching a new diagnostic science. Am J Obstet Gynecol 1969; 103:609-28.
115. Zelop CC, Bromley B, Frigoletto FD Jr, Benacerraf BR. Second trimester sonographically diagnosed placenta previa: Prediction of persistent previa at birth. Int J Gynaecol Obstet 1994; 44:207-10.
116. Berghella V, Roman A, Daskalakis C, et al. Gestational age at cervical length measurement and incidence of preterm birth. Obstet Gynecol 2007; 110:311-7.
117. American College of Obstetricians and Gynecologists. Invasive prenatal testing for aneuploidy. ACOG Practice Bulletin No. 88. Washington, DC, ACOG, 2007. (Obstet Gynecol 2007; 110:1459-67.)
118. Haddow JE, Palomake GE, Knight GJ, et al. Prenatal screening for Down's syndrome with use of maternal serum markers. N Engl J Med 1992; 327:588-93.
119. Rose NC, Palomaki GE, Haddow JE, et al. Maternal serum alpha-fetoprotein screening for chromosomal abnormalities: A prospective study in women aged 35 and older. Am J Obstet Gynecol 1994; 170:1073-8.
120. Eddleman KA, Malone FD, Sullivan L, et al. Pregnancy loss rates after midtrimester amniocentesis. Obstet Gynecol 2006; 108: 1067-1072.
121. Canick JA, Palomaki GE, Osathanondh R. Prenatal screening for trisomy 18 in the second trimester. Prenat Diag 1987; 7:623-30.
122. Haddow JE, Palomaki GE, Knight GJ, et al. Reducing the need for amniocentesis in women 35 years of age or older with serum markers for screening. N Engl J Med 1994; 330:1114-8.
123. Drugan A, Johnson MP, Reichler A, et al. Second trimester minor ultrasound abnormalities: Impact on the risk of aneuploidy associated with advanced age. Obstet Gynecol 1996; 88:203-6.
124. Smith-Bindman P, Hosmer W, Feldstein VA, et al. Second-trimester ultrasound to detect fetuses with Down syndrome: A meta-analysis. JAMA 2001; 285:1044-55.
125. Vintzeleos AM, Campbell WA, Rodis JF, et al. The use of second-trimester genetic sonogram in guiding clinical management of patients at increased risk for fetal trisomy 21. Obstet Gynecol 1996; 87:948-52.
126. Wapner R, Thom E, Simpson JL, et al. First Trimester Serum Biochemistry and Fetal Nuchal Translucency Screening (BUN) Study Group: First trimester screening for trisomies 21 and 18. N Engl J Med 2003; 349:1405-13.
127. Canick JA, Lambert-Messerlian GM, Palomaki GE, et al. First- and Second-Trimester Evaluation of Risk (FASTER) Research Consortium. Comparison of serum markers in first-trimester Down syndrome screening. Obstet Gynecol 2006; 108:1192-9.
128. Malone FD, Canick JA, Ball RH, et al. First- and Second-Trimester Evaluation of Risk (FASTER) Research Consortium. First-trimester or second-trimester screening, or both, for Down's syndrome. N Engl J Med 2005; 353:2001-11.
129. American College of Obstetricians and Gynecologists. First-trimester screening for fetal aneuploidy. ACOG Committee Opinion No. 296. Washington, DC, ACOG, 2004. (Obstet Gynecol 2004;104:215-7.)
130. Evans MI, Cuckle HS. Biochemical screening for aneuploidy. Expert Rev Obstet Gynecol 2007; 2:765-72.
131. Wald NJ, Rodeck DH, Hackshaw AK, et al. SURUSS Research Group: First and second trimester antenatal screening for Down syndrome: The results of the Serum, Urine, and Ultrasound Screening Study (SURUSS). Health Technol Assess 2003; 7:1-7.
132. American College of Obstetricians and Gynecologists. Screening for fetal chromosomal abnormalities. ACOG Practice Bulletin No. 77. Washington, DC, ACOG, 2007. (Obstet Gynecol 2007; 109:217-27.)
133. Wald NJ, Hackshaw AK. Combining ultrasound and biochemistry in first-trimester screening for Down's syndrome. Prenat Diagn 1997; 17:821-9.
134. De Biasio P, Siccardi M, Volpe G, et al. First-trimester screening for Down syndrome using nuchal translucency measurement with free beta-hCG and PAPP-A between 10 and 13 weeks of pregnancy—the combined test. Prenat Diagn 1999; 19:360-6.
135. Krantz DA, Hallahan TW, Orlandi F, et al. First-trimester Down syndrome screening using dried blood biochemistry and nuchal translucency. Obstet Gynecol 2000; 96:207-13.
136. Ball RH, Caughey AB, Malone FD, et al. First- and Second-Trimester Evaluation of Risk (FASTER) Research Consortium. First- and second-trimester evaluation of risk for Down syndrome. Obstet Gynecol 2007; 110:10-7.
137. Malone FD, Ball RH, Nyberg DA, et al. FASTER Research Consortium. First-trimester nasal bone evaluation for aneuploidy in the general population. Obstet Gynecol 2004; 104:1222-8.
138. Prefumo F, Sairam S, Bhide A, Thilaganathan B. First-trimester nuchal translucency, nasal bones, and trisomy 21 in selected and unselected populations. Am J Obstet Gynecol 2006; 194:828-33.
139. Towers CV, Asrat T, Rumney P. The presence of hepatitis B surface antigen and deoxyribonucleic acid in amniotic fluid and cord blood. Am J Obstet Gynecol 2001; 184:1514-8.
140. D'Alton ME, Malone FD, Chelmow DM, et al. Defining the role of fluorescence in situ hybridization on uncultured amniocytes for prenatal diagnosis of aneuploidies. Am J Obstet Gynecol 1997; 176:769-76.
141. Oh DC, Min JY, Lee MH, et al. Prenatal diagnosis of tetralogy of Fallot associated with chromosome 22q11 deletion. J Korean Med Sci 2002; 17:125-8.
142. ACMG/ASHG Test and Technology Transfer Committee. Technical and clinical assessment of fluorescence in situ hybridization: An ACMG/ASHG position statement. I. Technical considerations. Genet Med 2000; 2:356-61.

143. Tabor A, Philip J, Madsen M, et al. Randomised controlled trial of genetic amniocentesis in 4606 low-risk women. Lancet 1986; 1(8493):1287-93.
144. Antsaklis A, Papantoniou N, Xygakis A, et al. Genetic amniocentesis in women 20-34 years old: Associated risks. Prenat Diagn 2000; 20:247-50.
145. Daegan A, Johnson MP, Evans MI. Amniocentesis. In Eden RD, Boehm FH, editors. Assessment and Care of the Fetus: Physiological, Clinical, and Medicolegal Principles. East Norwalk, CT, Appleton & Lange, 1990:283-90.
146. Giorlandino C, Mobili L, Bilancioni E, et al. Transplacental amniocentesis: Is it really a higher-risk procedure? Prenat Diagn 1994; 14:803-6.
147. Zorn EM, Hanson FW, Greve LC, et al. Analysis of the significance of discolored amniotic fluid detected at midtrimester amniocentesis. Am J Obstet Gynecol 1986; 154:1234-40.
148. Alfirevic Z. Early amniocentesis versus transabdominal chorion villus sampling for prenatal diagnosis. Cochrane Database Syst Rev 2000; (2):CD000077.
149. Sundberg K, Bang J, Smidt-Jensen S, et al. Randomised study of risk of fetal loss related to early amniocentesis versus chorionic villus sampling. Lancet 1997; 350:697-703.
150. Tharmaratnam S, Sadek S, Steele EK, et al. Early amniocentesis: Effect of removing a reduced volume of amniotic fluid on pregnancy outcome. Prenat Diagn 1998; 18:773-8.
151. Yoon G, Chernos J, Sibbald B, et al. Association between congenital foot anomalies and gestational age at amniocentesis. Prenat Diagn 2001; 21:1137-41.
152. The Canadian Early and Mid-Trimester Amniocentesis Trial (CEMAT) Group. Randomized trial to assess safety and fetal outcome of early and midtrimester amniocentesis. Lancet 1998; 351:242-7.
153. Farrell SA, Summers AM, Dallaire L, et al. Club foot, an adverse outcome of early amniocentesis: Disruption or deformation? J Med Genet 1999; 36:843-6.
154. Wapner RJ, Jackson L. Chorionic villus sampling. Clin Obstet Gynecol 1988; 31:328-44.
155. Firth HV, Boyd PA, Chamberlain P, et al. Severe limb abnormalities after chorion villus sampling at 56-66 days' gestation. Lancet 1991; 337:762-3.
156. Burton BK, Schulz CJ, Burd LI. Limb anomalies associated with chorionic villus sampling. Obstet Gynecol 1992; 79:726-30.
157. Kuliev A, Jackson L, Froster U, et al. Chorionic villus sampling safety. Report of World Health Organization/EURO meeting in association with the Seventh International Conference on Early Prenatal Diagnosis of Genetic Diseases, Tel-Aviv, Israel, May 21, 1994. Am J Obstet Gynecol 1996; 174:807-11.
158. Carroll SGM, Davies T, Kyle PM, et al. Fetal karyotyping by chorionic villus sampling after the first trimester. Br J Obstet Gynaecol 1999; 106:1035-40.
159. Multicentre randomised clinical trial of chorion villus sampling and amniocentesis. First report. Canadian Collaborative CVS-Amniocentesis Clinical Trial Group. Lancet 1989; 1(8628):1-6.
160. Rhoads GG, Jackson LG, Schlesselman SE, et al. The safety and efficacy of chorionic villus sampling for early prenatal diagnosis of cytogenetic abnormalities. N Engl J Med 1989; 320:609-17.
161. MRC Working Party on the Evaluation of Chorion Villus Sampling. Medical Research Council European trial of chorion villus sampling. Lancet 1991; 337:1491-9.
162. Jackson LG, Zachary JM, Fowler SE, et al. A randomized comparison of transcervical and transabdominal chorionic-villus sampling. The U.S. National Institute of Child Health and Human Development Chorionic-Villus Sampling and Amniocentesis Study Group. N Engl J Med 1992; 327:594-8.
163. Alfirevic Z, Sundberg K, Brigham S. Amniocentesis and chorionic villus sampling for prenatal diagnosis. Cochrane Database Syst Rev 2003; (3):CD003252.
164. American College of Obstetricians and Gynecologists. Prenatal diagnosis of fetal chromosomal abnormalities. ACOG Practice Bulletin No. 97. Washington, DC, ACOG, 2001. (Obstet Gynecol 2001; 97:1-12.)
165. Wapner RJ, Johnson A, Davis G, et al. Prenatal diagnosis in twin gestations: A comparison between second-trimester amniocentesis and first-trimester chorionic villus sampling. Obstet Gynecol 1993; 82:49-56.
166. Martin AO, Elias S, Rosinsky B, et al. False negative findings on chorion villus sampling. Lancet 1986; 2(8503):391-2.
167. Daffos F, Capella-Bilovsky M, Forestier F. A new procedure for fetal blood sampling in utero: Preliminary results of fifty three cases. Am J Obstet Gynecol 1983; 146:985-7.
168. Fisk N, Bower S. Fetal blood sampling in retreat. Br Med J 1993; 307:143-4.
169. Van den Veyver IB, Moise KJ. Fetal RhD typing by polymerase chain reaction in pregnancies complicated by rhesus alloimmunization. Obstet Gynecol 1996; 88:1061-7.
170. Harman CR, Bowman JM, Manning FA, Menticoglou SM. Intrauterine transfusion—intraperitoneal versus intravascular approach: A case-control comparison. Am J Obstet Gynecol 1990; 162:1053-9.
171. Weiner CP, Thompson MIB. Direct treatment of fetal supraventricular tachycardia after failed transplacental therapy. Am J Obstet Gynecol 1988; 158:570-3.
172. Ghidini A, Sepulveda W, Lockwood C, Romero R. Complications of fetal blood sampling. Am J Obstet Gynecol 1993; 168:1339-44.
173. Rovas L, Sladkevicius P, Strobel E, Valentin L. Intraobserver and interobserver reproducibility of three-dimensional gray-scale and power Doppler ultrasound examinations of the cervix in pregnant women. Ultrasound Obstet Gynecol 2005; 26:132-7.
174. Schuchter K, Metzenbauer M, Hafner E, Philipp K. Uterine artery Doppler and placental volume in the first trimester in the prediction of pregnancy complications. Ultrasound Obstet Gynecol 2001; 18:590-2.
175. Rimoin DL, Lachman RS. The chondrodysplasias. In Emergy AE, Rimoin DL, editors. Principles and Practice of Medical Genetics. 2nd edition. New York, Churchill Livingstone, 1990:895-932.
176. Levine D, Barnes PD, Edelman RR. Obstetric MR imaging. Radiology 1999; 211:609-17.
177. Levine D. Fetal magnetic resonance imaging. J Matern Fetal Neonatal Med 2004; 15:85-94.
178. Kirk JS, Riggs TW, Comstock CH, et al. Prenatal screening for cardiac anomalies: The value of routine addition of the aortic root to the four-chamber view. Obstet Gynecol 1994; 84:427-31.
179. Bérard A, Ramos E, Rey E, et al. First trimester exposure to paroxetine and risk of cardiac malformations in infants: The importance of dosage. Birth Defects Res B Dev Reprod Toxicol 2007; 80:18-27.
180. Olson CK, Keppler-Noreuil KM, Romitti PA, et al. In vitro fertilization is associated with an increase in major birth defects. Fertil Steril 2005; 84:1308-15.
181. Guetta E, Gutstein-Abo L, Barkai G. Trophoblasts isolated from the maternal circulation: In vitro expansion and potential application in non-invasive prenatal diagnosis. J Histochem Cytochem 2005; 53:337-9.
182. Christensen B, Kolvraa S, Lykke-Hansen L, et al. Studies on the isolation and identification of fetal nucleated red blood cells in the circulation of pregnant women before and after chorion villus sampling. Fetal Diagn Ther 2003; 18:376-84.
183. Dhallan R, Au WC, Mattagajasingh S, et al. Methods to increase the percentage of free fetal DNA recovered from the maternal circulation. JAMA 2004; 291:1114-9.
184. Siva SC, Johnson SI, McCracken SA, Morris JM. Evaluation of the clinical usefulness of isolation of fetal DNA from the maternal circulation. Aust N Z J Obstet Gynaecol 2003; 43:10-5.
185. Bahado-Singh RO, Kliman H, Feng TY, et al. First-trimester endocervical irrigation: Feasibility of obtaining trophoblast cells for prenatal diagnosis. Obstet Gynecol 1995; 85:461-4.
186. Sherlock J, Halder A, Tutschek B, et al. Detection of fetal aneuploidies using transcervical cell samples. J Med Genetics 1997; 34:302-5.
187. Holzgreve W, Hahn S. Fetal cells in cervical mucus and maternal blood. Baillieres Best Pract Res Clin Obstet Gynaecol 2000; 14:709-22.
188. Fejgin MD, Diukman R, Cotton Y, et al. Fetal cells in the uterine cervix: A source for early non-invasive prenatal diagnosis. Prenat Diagn 2001; 21:619-21.

189. Dugoff L, Hobbins JS, Malone FD, et al. First-trimester maternal serum PAPP-A and free beta-subunit human chorionic gonadotropin concentrations and nuchal translucency are associated with obstetric complications: A population-based screening study (the FASTER Trial). Am J Obstet Gynecol 2004; 191:1446-51.
190. Dugoff L, Hobbins JS, Malone FD, et al. FASTER Trial Research Consortium. Quad screen as a predictor of adverse pregnancy outcome. Obstet Gynecol 2005; 106:260-7.
191. Duric K, Skrablin S, Lesin J, et al. Second trimester total human chorionic gonadotropin, alpha-fetoprotein and unconjugated estriol in predicting pregnancy complications other than fetal aneuploidy. Eur J Obstet Gynecol Reprod Biol 2003; 110:12-5.
192. Galindo A, Comas C, Martínez JM, et al. Cardiac defects in chromosomally normal fetuses with increased nuchal translucency at 10-14 weeks of gestation. J Matern Fetal Neonatal Med 2003; 13:163-70.
193. American College of Obstetricians and Gynecologists. Prevention of Rh D alloimmunization. ACOG Practice Bulletin No. 4. Washington, DC, ACOG, 1999. (Int J Gynaecol Obstet 1999; 66:63-70.)
194. Moise KJ. Red blood cell alloimmunization in pregnancy. Semin Hematol 2005; 42:169-78.
195. Spinnato JA, Clark AL, Ralston KK, et al. Hemolytic disease of the fetus: A comparison of the Queenan and extended Liley methods. Obstet Gynecol 1998; 92:441-5.
196. American College of Obstetricians and Gynecologists. Management of alloimmunization. ACOG Practice Bulletin No. 75. Washington, DC, ACOG, 2006. (Obstet Gynecol 2006; 108:457-64.)
197. Bullock R, Martin WL, Coomarasamy A, Kilby MD. Prediction of fetal anemia in pregnancies with red-cell alloimmunization: Comparison of middle cerebral artery peak systolic velocity and amniotic fluid OD450. Ultrasound Obstet Gynecol 2005; 25:331-4.
198. Eden RD, Seifert LS, Winegar A, Spellacy WN. Perinatal characteristics of uncomplicated postdate pregnancies. Obstet Gynecol 1987; 69:296-9.
199. Rand L, Robinson JN, Economy KE, Norwitz ER. Post-term induction of labor revisited. Obstet Gynecol 2000; 96:779-83.
200. Smith GC. Life-table analysis of the risk of perinatal death at term and post term in singleton pregnancies. Am J Obstet Gynecol 2001; 184:489-96.
201. Caughey AB, Bishop JT. Maternal complications of pregnancy increase beyond 40 weeks of gestation in low-risk women. J Perinatol 2006; 26:540-5.
202. Bochner CJ, Williams J, Castro L, et al. The efficacy of starting post-term antenatal testing at 41 weeks as compared with 42 weeks of gestational age. Am J Obstet Gynecol 1988; 159:550-4.
203. Morris JM, Thompson K, Smithey J, et al. The usefulness of ultrasound assessment of amniotic fluid in predicting adverse outcome in prolonged pregnancy: A prospective blinded observational study. Br J Obstet Gynaecol 2003; 110:989-94.
204. Pitkin RM. Fetal death: Diagnosis and management. Am J Obstet Gynecol 1987; 157:583-9.
205. Spong CY, Erickson K, Willinger M, et al. Stillbirth in obstetric practice: Report of survey findings. J Matern Fetal Neonatal Med 2003; 14:39-44.
206. MacDorman MF, Hoyert DL, Martin JA, et al. Fetal and perinatal mortality, United States, 2003. Natl Vital Stat Rep 2007; 55:1-17.
207. Cotzias CS, Paterson-Brown S, Fisk NM. Prospective risk of unexplained stillbirth in singleton pregnancies at term: Population based analysis. Br Med J 1999; 319:287-8.
208. Huang DY, Usher RH, Kramer MS, et al. Determinants of unexplained antepartum fetal deaths. Obstet Gynecol 2000; 95:215-21.
209. Frøen JF, Arnestad M, Frey K, et al. Risk factors for sudden intrauterine unexplained death: Epidemiologic characteristics of singleton cases in Oslo, Norway, 1986-1995. Am J Obstet Gynecol 2001; 184:694-702.
210. Faye-Petersen OM, Guinn DA, Wenstrom KD. The value of perinatal autopsy. Obstet Gynecol 1999; 96:915-20.
211. Craven CM, Demsey S, Carey JC, Kochenour NK. Evaluation of perinatal autopsy protocol: Influence of the prenatal diagnosis conference team. Obstet Gynecol 1990; 76:684-8.
212. Wapner RJ, Lewis D. Genetics and metabolic causes of stillbirth. Semin Perinatol 2002; 26:70-4.
213. Kolialexi A, Tsangaris GT, Antsaklis A, Mavroua A. Rapid clearance of fetal cells from maternal circulation after delivery. Ann N Y Acad Sci 2004; 1022:113-8.
214. Brookes JS, Hagmann C. MRI in fetal necropsy. J Magn Reson Imaging 2006; 24:1221-8.
215. Cernach MC, Patricio FR, Galera MF, et al. Evaluation of a protocol for postmortem examination of stillbirths and neonatal deaths with congenital anomalies. Pediatr Dev Pathol 2004; 7:335-41.
216. Reid DE, Weiner AE, Roby CC, Diamond LK. Maternal afibrinogenemia associated with long-standing intrauterine fetal death. Am J Obstet Gynecol 1953; 66:500-6.
217. Pritchard JA. Fetal death in utero. Obstet Gynecol 1959; 14:573-80.
218. Carlson NJ, Towers CV. Multiple gestation complicated by the death of one fetus. Obstet Gynecol 1989; 73:685-9.
219. D'Alton ME, Newton ER, Cetrulo CL. Intrauterine fetal demise in multiple gestation. Acta Genet Med Gemellol (Roma) 1984; 33:43-9.
220. Bejar R, Vigliocco G, Gramajo H, et al. Antenatal origin of neurologic damage in newborn infants. II. Multiple gestations. Am J Obstet Gynecol 1990; 162:1230-6.
221. Romero R, Duffy TP, Berkowitz RL, et al. Prolongation of a preterm pregnancy complicated by death of a single twin in utero and disseminated intravascular coagulation. Effects of treatment with heparin. N Engl J Med 1984; 310:772-4.
222. Benirschke K. Intrauterine death of a twin: Mechanisms, implications for surviving twin, and placental pathology. Semin Diagn Pathol 1993; 10:222-31.
223. Szymonowicz W, Preston H, Yu VY. The surviving monozygotic twin. Arch Dis Child 1986; 61:454-8.
224. Ben-Shlomo I, Alcalay M, Lipitz S, et al. Twin pregnancies complicated by the death of one fetus. J Reprod Med 1995; 40:458-62.
225. Crowley PA, Chalmers I, Kierse MJNC, et al. The effects of corticosteroid administration before preterm delivery: An overview of the evidence from controlled trials. Br J Obstet Gynaecol 1990; 97:11-25.
226. Greene MF, Hare JW, Cloherty JP, et al. First-trimester hemoglobin A1 and risk for major malformation and spontaneous abortion in diabetic pregnancy. Teratology 1989; 39:225-31.
227. Leuke RR, Levy HL. Maternal phenylketonuria and hyperphenylalaninemia. N Engl J Med 1980; 303:1202-8.
228. Bussel JB, Berkowitz RL, McFarland JG, et al. Antenatal treatment of neonatal alloimmune thrombocytopenia. N Engl J Med 1988; 319:1374-8.
229. Bussel JB, Berkowitz RL, Lynch L, et al. Antenatal management of alloimmune thrombocytopenia with intravenous gammaglobulin: A randomized trial of the addition of low dose steroid to intravenous gammaglobulin. Am J Obstet Gynecol 1996; 174:1414-23.
230. Bruinse HW, Vermeulen-Meiners C, Wit JM. Fetal treatment for thyrotoxicosis in non-thyrotoxic pregnant women. Fetal Ther 1988; 3:152-7.
231. Wenstrom KD, Weiner CP, Williamson RA, Grant SS. Prenatal diagnosis of fetal hyperthyroidism using funipuncture. Obstet Gynecol 1990; 76:513-7.
232. Pang S, Pollack MS, Marshall RN, Immken L. Prenatal treatment of congenital adrenal hyperplasia due to 21-hydroxylase deficiency. N Engl J Med 1990; 322:111-5.
233. Weiner CP, Williamson RA, Wenstrom KD, et al. Management of hemolytic disease by cordocentesis. I. Prediction of fetal anemia. Am J Obstet Gynecol 1991; 165:546-53.
234. Weiner CP, Williamson RA, Wenstrom KD, et al. Management of hemolytic disease by cordocentesis. II. Outcome of treatment. Am J Obstet Gynecol 1991; 165:1303-7.
235. Johnson MP, Bukowski TP, Reitleman C, et al. In utero surgical treatment of fetal obstructive uropathy: A new comprehensive approach to identify candidates for vesicamniotic shunt therapy. Am J Obstet Gynecol 1994; 170:1770-9.
236. Rodeck CH, Fisk NM, Fraser DI, Nicolini U. Long term in utero drainage of fetal hydrothorax. N Engl J Med 1988; 319:1135-8.

237. Tworetzky W, Wilkins-Haug L, Jennings RW, et al. Balloon dilation of severe aortic stenosis in the fetus: Potential for prevention of hypoplastic left heart syndrome. Candidate selection, technique, and results of successful intervention. Circulation 2004; 110:2125-31.
238. Romero R, Pilu G, Jeanty P, et al. Congenital cystic adenomatoid malformation of the lung. Prenatal Diagnosis of Congenital Anomalies. Norwalk, CT, Appleton Lange, 1988:198-201.
239. Adzick NS, Harrison MR, Crombleholme TM, et al. Fetal lung lesions: Management and outcome. Am J Obstet Gynecol 1998; 179:884-9.
240. Manning FA, Harrison MR, Rodeck CR, et al. Catheter shunts for fetal hydronephrosis and hydrocephalus: Report of the international fetal surgery registry. N Engl J Med 1986; 315:336-40.
241. Dommergues M, Louis-Sylvestre C, Mandelbrot L, et al. Congenital diaphragmatic hernia: Can prenatal ultrasonography predict outcome? Am J Obstet Gynecol 1996; 174:1377-81.
242. Harrison MR, Keller RL, Hawgood SB, et al. A randomized trial of fetal endoscopic tracheal occlusion for severe fetal congenital diaphragmatic hernia. N Engl J Med 2003; 349:1916-24.
243. Meuli M, Meuli-Simmen C, Hutchins GM, et al. The spinal cord lesion in fetuses with meningomyelocele: Implications for fetal surgery. J Pediatr Surgery 1997; 32:448-52.
244. Bruner JP, Tulipan N, Paschall RL, et al. Fetal surgery for myelomeningocele and the incidence of shunt-dependent hydrocephalus. JAMA 1999; 282:1819-25.
245. Hirose S, Farmer DL, Albanese CT. Fetal surgery for meningomyelocele. Curr Opin Obstet Gynecol 2001; 13:215-22.
246. American College of Obstetricians and Gynecologists. Multifetal pregnancy reduction and selective fetal termination. ACOG Committee Opinion No. 94. Washington, DC, ACOG, 1991. (Int J Gynaecol Obstet 1992; 38:140-2.)
247. Boulot P, Hedon B, Pelliccia G, et al. Effects of selective reduction in triplet gestation: A comparative study of 80 cases managed with or without this procedure. Fertil Steril 1993; 60:497-503.
248. Berkowitz RL, Lynch L, Lapinski R, Bergh P. First-trimester transabdominal multifetal pregnancy reduction: A report of two hundred completed cases. Am J Obstet Gynecol 1993; 169:17-21.
249. Smith-Levitin M, Kowalik A, Birnholz J, et al. Selective reduction of multifetal pregnancies to twins improves outcome over nonreduced triplet gestations. Am J Obstet Gynecol 1996; 175:878-82.
250. Quintero RA, Dickinson JE, Morales WJ, et al. Stage-based treatment of twin-twin transfusion syndrome. Am J Obstet Gynecol 2003; 188:1333-40.
251. Moise KJ Jr, Dorman K, Lamvu G, et al. A randomized trial of amnioreduction versus septostomy in the treatment of twin-twin transfusion syndrome. Am J Obstet Gynecol 2005; 193:701-7.
252. Roberts D, Neilson JP, Weindling AM. Interventions for the treatment of twin-twin transfusion syndrome. Cochrane Database Syst Rev 2001; (1):CD002073.
253. Dickinson JE, Duncombe GJ, Evans SF, et al. The long term neurologic outcome of children from pregnancies complicated by twin-to-twin transfusion syndrome. Br J Obstet Gynaecol 2005; 112:63-8.
254. Senat MV, Deprest J, Boulvain M, et al. Endoscopic laser surgery versus serial amnioreduction for severe twin-to-twin transfusion syndrome. N Engl J Med 2004; 351:136-44.
255. Foley MR, Clewell WH, Finberg HJ, Mills MD. Use of the Foley Cordostat grasping device for selective ligation of the umbilical cord of an acardiac twin: A case report. Am J Obstet Gynecol 1995; 172:212-4.
256. Quintero RA, Morales WJ, Kalter CS, et al. Transabdominal intra-amniotic endoscopic assessment of previable premature rupture of membranes. Am J Obstet Gynecol 1998; 179:71-6.
257. Quintero RA, Morales WJ, Allen M, et al. Treatment of iatrogenic previable premature rupture of membranes with intra-amniotic injection of platelets and cryoprecipitate (amniopatch): Preliminary experience. Am J Obstet Gynecol 1999; 181:744-9.
258. Locatelli A, Vergani P, Di Pirro G, et al. Role of amnioinfusion in the management of premature rupture of the membranes at <26 weeks' gestation. Am J Obstet Gynecol 2000; 183:878-92.
259. Oepkes D, Teunissen AK, Van De Velde M, et al. Congenital high airway obstruction syndrome successfully managed with ex-utero intrapartum treatment. Ultrasound Obstet Gynecol 2003; 22:437-9.
260. Kanamori Y, Kitano Y, Hashizume K, et al. A case of laryngeal atresia (congenital high airway obstruction syndrome) with chromosome 5p deletion syndrome rescued by ex utero intrapartum treatment. J Pediatr Surg 2004; 39:25-8.
261. American College of Obstetricians and Gynecologists. Fetal maturity assessment prior to elective repeat cesarean delivery. ACOG Committee Opinion No. 98. Washington, DC, ACOG, 1991.
262. American College of Obstetricians and Gynecologists. Assessment of fetal lung maturity. Educational Bulletin No. 230. Washington, DC, ACOG, 1996.
263. Liggins GC, Howie RN. A controlled trial of antepartum glucocorticoid treatment for prevention of the respiratory distress syndrome in premature infants. Pediatrics 1972; 50:515-25.
264. Rennie JM. Perinatal management at the lower end of viability. Arch Dis Child Fetal Neonatal Ed 1996; 74:214-8.
265. Leviton A, Kuban KC, Pagano M, et al. Antenatal corticosteroids appear to reduce the risk of postnatal germinal matrix hemorrhage in intubated low birth weight newborns. Pediatrics 1993; 91:1083-8.
266. NIH Consensus Development Panel on the Effect of Corticosteroids for Fetal Maturation on Perinatal Outcomes. Effect of corticosteroids for fetal maturation on perinatal outcomes. JAMA 1995; 273:413-8.
267. American College of Obstetricians and Gynecologists. Committee on Obstetric Practice. Antenatal corticosteroid therapy for fetal maturation. ACOG Committee Opinion. (Int J Gynaecol Obstet 2002; 78:95-7.)
268. American College of Obstetricians and Gynecologists. Premature rupture of membranes. ACOG Practice Bulletin No. 1. Washington, DC, ACOG, 1998.
269. Vermillion ST, Bland ML, Soper DE. Effectiveness of a rescue dose of antenatal betamethasone after an initial single course. Am J Obstet Gynecol 2001; 185:1086-9.
270. Guinn DA, Atkinson MW, Sullivan L, et al. Single vs weekly courses of antenatal corticosteroids for women at risk of preterm delivery. JAMA 2001; 286:1581-7.
271. Wapner R, Sorokin Y, Thom EA, et al. National Institutes of Child Health and Human Development Maternal-Fetal Medicine Units Network. Single versus weekly courses of antenatal corticosteroids: Evaluation of efficacy and safety. Am J Obstet Gynecol 2006; 195:633-42.
272. Crowther CA, Haslam RR, Hiller JE, et al. Australasian Collaborative Trial of Repeat Doses of Steroids (ACT ORDS) Study Group. Neonatal respiratory distress syndrome after repeat exposure to antenatal corticosteroids: A randomised controlled trial. Lancet 2006; 367:1913-9.
273. Crowther CA, Harding JE. Repeat doses of prenatal corticosteroids for women at risk of preterm birth for preventing neonatal respiratory disease. Cochrane Database Syst Rev 2007; (3):CD003935.

Chapter 7

Anesthesia for Fetal Surgery and Other Intrauterine Procedures

Mark A. Rosen, M.D.

Fetal therapy originated in 1963 with Sir William Liley's successful intraperitoneal blood transfusion to a fetus with erythroblastosis fetalis.[1] This event was followed by (indirect) fetal administration of corticosteroids—via the mother—to increase fetal surfactant production. Fetal surgery and anesthesia for fetal surgery began in 1981 after careful experimentation and practice in sheep and rhesus monkey models.[2] The first successful human fetal surgery was a vesicostomy to treat a fetus with bilateral hydronephrosis due to a lower urinary tract obstruction.[3] Fundamentally, the anesthetic approach for fetal surgery has not changed since it was originally described.[2-4]

Advances in prenatal diagnostic technology contribute to an increasingly sophisticated capability for prenatal diagnosis of fetal disorders that are amenable to antenatal therapy. These advances have included chorionic villus sampling, biochemical and cytogenetic analyses of amniotic fluid (amniocentesis) and fetal blood (cordocentesis), and fetoscopy as well as imaging techniques such as ultrasonography, computed tomography, single-shot rapid-acquisition magnetic resonance imaging (MRI), and fetal echocardiography. With these advances, substantial improvements have been made in the ability to recognize and precisely delineate fetal anatomy and anomalies. Some identified disorders are amenable to antenatal therapy, such as intrauterine surgery for fetal structural anomalies. However, fetal therapy is largely nonsurgical (e.g., administration of medications, nutrients, blood, stem cells) (see Chapter 6), and most anatomic malformations diagnosed *in utero* remain unsuitable for antenatal intervention. Furthermore, correction of an anatomic malformation *in utero* is technically more difficult.

Prenatal diagnosis of a serious malformation (i.e., one that is neither correctable nor compatible with normal postnatal life) allows the choice of termination of pregnancy. Some fetal malformations cause dystocia and require cesarean delivery. Some defects, especially those that cause airway obstruction, can be treated with intrapartum intervention, in which the fetus undergoes repair of the defect and/or the airway is secured during birth, while the uteroplacental unit remains functional. Many correctable malformations are best managed after delivery at term gestation; their recognition and diagnosis allow time for the coordination of appropriate prenatal and postnatal care, including transportation of the fetus to a medical center while *in utero* rather than as a newly delivered, fragile neonate. When early correction or treatment of a malformation can minimize the progressive impairment associated with continued gestation, preterm delivery is considered; however, the risks of prematurity must be weighed against the risks of continued gestation. Only certain fetal anomalies are amenable to *in utero* intervention that results in improved outcome.

Fetal surgical intervention can be broadly categorized into three different kinds of procedures. **Open surgical procedures** involve both a laparotomy and a hysterotomy.

The uterine incision is made anteriorly or posteriorly, depending on the position of the fetus and placenta as located by intraoperative ultrasonography. Absorbable staples are used to open the uterus; they compress the myometrium and membranes and maintain hemostasis. After surgery on the fetus, the uterus is closed in two layers, and warm fluid is instilled to replace lost amniotic fluid. Intraoperative and postoperative tocolysis is crucial for success. These procedures are typically performed at midgestation. Open procedures entail the greatest maternal and fetal risks, including postoperative membrane separation, preterm premature rupture of the membranes (PROM), and preterm delivery.

Minimally invasive procedures involve either endoscopic or percutaneous procedures guided by ultrasonography, typically performed at midgestation. These procedures reduce the risk of preterm labor and delivery because they do not involve a hysterotomy, yet the risk of preterm PROM remains.

Midgestation fetal surgery is a reasonable alternative for selected fetal anomalies that might result in fetal death, severe disability, or irreversible harm before the adequate development of fetal lung maturity necessary for extrauterine survival. Fetal surgery is reasonable only with informed consent and only if (1) the lesion is diagnosed accurately; (2) the lesion's severity is assessed correctly; (3) associated anomalies that contraindicate intervention are excluded; (4) maternal risk is acceptably low; and (5) neonatal outcome would be better with *in utero* surgery than with surgery performed after delivery. As with all fetal surgical procedures, emphasis must be placed on maternal welfare to guard against undue maternal risk.[5,6]

The third kind of procedure is a modification of cesarean delivery to allow various interventions during birth, which we called the **EXIT procedure**, for *ex* utero *i*ntrapartum *t*herapy.[7] EXIT procedures are most often employed (1) to secure an airway by intubation, bronchoscopy, or tracheostomy or (2) to perform a procedure while gas exchange continues in the placenta (placental bypass). The EXIT procedure enables the prevention of postnatal asphyxia for lesions such as cystic hygroma, lymphangioma, cervical teratoma, and congenital syndromes in which securing an airway after birth can be problematic. The procedure is also used as a bridge to extracorporeal membrane oxygenation (ECMO) for a fetus with cardiopulmonary disease at risk for postnatal cardiac failure or failure of adequate gas exchange in the lungs. The EXIT procedure has become the most widely practiced fetal intervention for a growing list of indications.

Fetal surgery is a reasonable therapeutic intervention for certain correctable fetal anomalies with predictable, life-threatening, or serious developmental consequences. Examples of anatomic anomalies currently considered suitable for antepartum correction are obstructive hydronephrosis, diaphragmatic hernia, cystic adenomatoid malformation or other thoracic mass lesions, sacrococcygeal teratoma, myelomeningocele, twin-to-twin transfusion syndrome, and valvular cardiac stenosis. If untreated, these lesions can interfere with fetal organ development or cause high-output cardiac failure. Their correction *in utero* may prevent irreversible organ damage or fetal demise. In the future, antenatal intervention may prove beneficial for other malformations that interfere with organ development or cause fetal cardiac failure as well as for other nonlethal defects, such as craniofacial deformities. However, controlled clinical trials are needed to establish efficacy and substantiate the safety of fetal surgery for each of these lesions.

INDICATIONS AND RATIONALE FOR FETAL SURGERY

Bilateral Hydronephrosis–Obstructive Uropathy

Congenital bilateral hydronephrosis results from fetal urethral obstruction at the bladder outlet, most often by posterior urethral valves in male fetuses or urethral obstruction in females. Other causes of fetal obstructive uropathy are obstruction at the ureteropelvic or vesicoureteric junction and more complex disorders (e.g., cloacal plate anomalies) in females. These uropathies are easily detected by ultrasonography, which is often performed to investigate the associated oligohydramnios resulting from decreased fetal urine output. These lesions often have devastating developmental consequences, with high morbidity associated with progressive renal dysplasia and dysfunction and oligohydramnios causing pulmonary hypoplasia that can prevent postnatal survival (Figure 7-1).[8] Preterm delivery of the fetus allows early urinary tract decompression *ex utero*, but fetal pulmonary immaturity

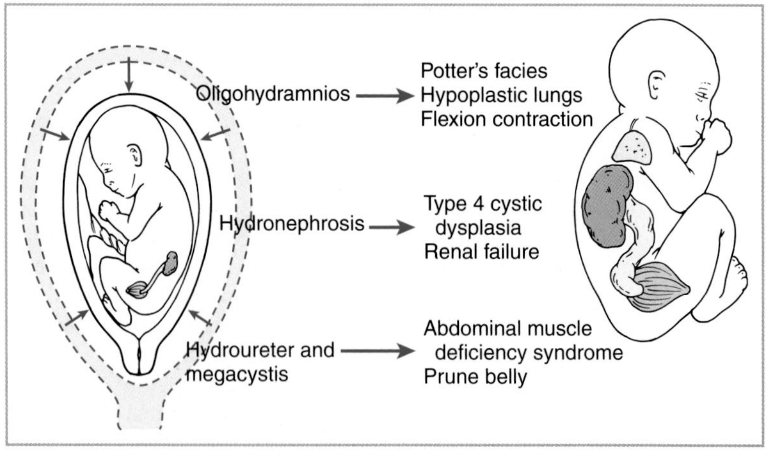

FIGURE 7-1 Developmental consequences of fetal urethral obstruction. Obstructed fetal urinary flow results in hydronephrosis, hydroureter, megacystis, oligohydramnios, and pulmonary hypoplasia. (Redrawn from Harrison MR, Filly RA, Parer JT, et al. Management of the fetus with a urinary tract malformation. JAMA 1981; 246:635-9.)

limits the efficacy of this approach. Early intrauterine intervention allows drainage of urine from the fetal bladder into the amniotic cavity, which decompresses the urinary tract and allows fetal renal development. It can also restore normal amniotic fluid volume and prevent the sequelae of oligohydramnios (e.g., pulmonary hypoplasia, umbilical cord compression). Animal models of obstructive uropathy demonstrate changes in renal histology similar to those seen in kidneys of human neonates with congenital hydronephrosis. Relief of obstruction *in utero* ameliorates but does not eliminate the dysplastic changes in these animal models.[9] Restoration of normal urine flow and amniotic fluid volume allows the lungs to grow and prevents the development of pulmonary hypoplasia. However, the applicability of these animal models to human fetal obstructive uropathy remains unclear and controversial.[10]

Methods used to assess renal function include measurement of fetal urine volume and electrolytes, and ultrasonographic and MRI assessment of the renal parenchyma. Even fetal renal biopsies are possible. However, the prognostic value of these assessments remains unclear. Earlier presentation during gestation and a greater severity of oligohydramnios and associated structural abnormalities have been correlated with poor outcomes.

Vesicoamniotic catheter shunts have been utilized for intrauterine treatment of bilateral hydronephrosis since the early 1980s.[11] These valveless, double-coiled catheters are placed percutaneously with the use of ultrasonographic guidance. One coil is lodged in the urinary bladder and the other in the amniotic space. Common problems associated with these catheters include difficult placement, occlusion, displacement, and infection. Some difficult placements have resulted in iatrogenic abdominal wall defects and maternal amnioperitoneal leaks. The open surgical procedures fetal vesicostomy and ureterostomies were performed as an alternative to catheter decompression of fetal obstructive uropathy.[12]

Despite some early problems,[13] success has been reported with careful selection and the use of techniques including fetoscopic vesicostomy, cystoscopic laser ablation of valves,[14] and placement of wire-mesh stents. However, overall survival was only about 45%, and 40% of the survivors had end-stage renal disease.[15,16]

Clinical experience suggests that fetal surgery for the correction of obstructive uropathy is feasible, safe, and perhaps effective in the restoration of amniotic fluid volume and the prevention of pulmonary hypoplasia.[17] However, the potential for reversal of long-term renal morbidity remains unclear.

Congenital Diaphragmatic Hernia

Approximately 1 or 2 of 2500 newborn infants has a congenital diaphragmatic hernia (CDH) causing varying degrees of pulmonary parenchymal and vascular hypoplasia. Without fetal intervention, this anomaly has a significant mortality from pulmonary hypoplasia and insufficiency, ranging from 40% to 60%.[18,19] High mortality rates occur despite optimal postnatal surgical management (removal of the herniated viscera from the chest and closure of the diaphragm) at a tertiary care medical center and the use of ECMO. Intrauterine correction of CDH has the potential of preventing the development of pulmonary hypoplasia, allowing the fetal lung to develop before delivery.

Through the use of a fetal lamb model, it was demonstrated that the broad range of severity of CDH is explained by the timing and extent of visceral herniation and pulmonary compression, and that fatal pulmonary hypoplasia is caused by compression of the developing lung. Further studies demonstrated that parenchymal hypoplasia and associated pulmonary vascular changes may be reversed by correction *in utero*.[20]

Primary repairs of CDH *in utero* were undertaken only for fetuses with severe disease, with limited success but many lessons learned.[21] Enlargement of the fetal abdomen using an abdominal patch was necessary to accommodate the added abdominal contents without increasing intra-abdominal pressure, which compromises ductus venosus blood flow.[21] The procedure was technically difficult and usually unsuccessful when the liver had herniated into the fetal chest. Reduction of the herniated liver compromised umbilical circulation, with devastating consequences; many fetuses died intraoperatively because of this problem. Careful evaluation of the umbilical vein by color Doppler imaging allows more accurate preoperative assessment of the extent of liver herniation. Performing both subcostal and thoracotomy incisions on the fetus improves surgical exposure, allows the reduction of viscera by pushing and pulling techniques, and facilitates the reconstruction of a diaphragm with a prosthetic patch.[22] Other lessons learned from this experience are as follows: (1) the advantages of opening the uterus with a stapling device to ensure effective hemostasis, (2) improved techniques of uterine closure, and (3) use of fibrin glue to help prevent amniotic fluid leaks. However, adequate control of postoperative uterine tone remained a substantial problem. In a prospective trial, survival after open fetal surgery did not improve over that after standard postnatal treatment for fetuses without herniation of the liver into the thorax.[23]

Given the difficulties encountered with primary repair of CDH *in utero*, another approach was developed, taking a clue from fetuses with *c*ongenital *h*igh *a*irway *o*bstruction *s*yndrome (CHAOS). Fetal tracheal occlusion impedes the normal egress of fetal lung fluid and results in expansion of the hypoplastic lung. In experimental animals, fetal tracheal occlusion induced lung growth and morphologic maturation.

This technique replaced primary repair *in utero* for the correction of the pulmonary hypoplasia associated with CDH. It is a less extensive, palliative fetal surgical procedure that enhances lung growth to improve postnatal survival, allowing postponement of the definitive repair until after birth.[24,25] Once the trachea is occluded, fetal pulmonary fluid slowly accumulates and expands the lung, pushing the viscera out of the thorax, a technique called "*p*lug the *l*ung *u*ntil it *g*rows" (i.e., PLUG).[26] In the first attempts at establishing reversible, controlled tracheal occlusion techniques, a foam plug was placed in the trachea during open fetal surgery, but it failed to completely occlude the trachea. An open procedure was used to place metallic hemoclips around the trachea after meticulous neck dissection to avoid injury to the recurrent laryngeal and vagus nerves. Subsequently, *fet*al *endo*scopic (i.e., FETENDO) surgical techniques replaced the open technique for placement of the clips.[27] Currently, a small detachable balloon is placed in the trachea via percutaneous endoscopic endotracheal intubation for endoluminal tracheal occlusion and is either left in place until delivery or deflated earlier.[28,29]

A prospective randomized trial evaluated fetal tracheal occlusion for intrauterine treatment of severe CDH. Severe CDH was defined as a (1) diagnosis before 25 weeks' gestation, (2) presence of liver herniated into the hemithorax, and (3) low ultrasonographically measured lung-to-head ratio (LHR), a ratio of the contralateral lung size compared with head circumference, which is an indicator of the severity of pulmonary hypoplasia.[30,31] Fetal tracheal occlusion resulted in modest improvements in neonatal pulmonary function,[32] but the lung probably remained abnormal with low radial alveolar counts and greater alveolar size.[33] Fetal intervention did not improve survival or reduce morbidity when compared with postnatal treatment with ECMO at a tertiary care center.[34] Further, at 1 and 2 years of age, comprehensive evaluation was conducted to assess chronic morbidity.[35] Infants who underwent tracheal occlusion *in utero* were more premature at birth than the control group (31 versus 37 weeks), but hearing impairment, chronic lung disease, and growth failure were severe in both groups, and there were no differences in neurodevelopmental outcomes.

Preliminary results from Europe using percutaneous *f*etal *e*ndoscopic *t*racheal *o*cclusion (FETO) for severe CDH with smaller-gauge endoscopes and reversal of the tracheal occlusion before birth show great promise for reduction in the risk of preterm delivery due to rupture of the fetal membranes.[36,37] A tracheal balloon is placed at 26 to 28 weeks' gestation and retrieved before birth by a second fetal tracheoscopy or by ultrasonography-guided puncture of the balloon at 34 weeks (if still *in utero*) to avoid the need for the EXIT procedure, and perhaps to improve lung growth and minimize the reduction of type II alveolar cells associated with prolonged tracheal occlusion. This "plug-unplug" sequence or temporary tracheal occlusion may be one step closer to an ideal sequence of cyclical occlusion and release for optimal pulmonary structural maturation, pulmonary artery remodeling, and pneumocyte maturation.

Ex Utero Intrapartum Treatment Procedure

First described as a method to remove the iatrogenic airway obstruction created for intrauterine treatment of CDH,[38,39] the EXIT procedure has evolved into a technique useful for a number of fetal disorders. During the EXIT procedure, a uterine incision is made with a stapling device to ensure hemostasis, and the baby is partially delivered (or sometimes fully delivered and placed on the maternal abdomen). The baby continues to exchange gases (including inhaled anesthetic agents) via the placenta rather than via the lungs, thereby providing time to secure the airway while the infant remains on "placental bypass." In the setting of a tracheal balloon placed for CDH, the surgeons perform fetal bronchoscopy to pierce the balloon and retrieve it from the trachea. The trachea is then secured with an endotracheal tube, surfactant is administered if indicated, and the lungs are ventilated with oxygen. The cord is clamped after the baby's oxygen saturation increases, and the baby is delivered.

This technique is now widely used for a variety of fetal problems (e.g., embryonic cervical tumors, laryngeal atresia) that compress the airway and/or render neonatal intubation unfeasible, and has generated numerous published case reports of success.[39-42] During the EXIT procedure for airway obstruction, either the fetal trachea is intubated directly with a laryngoscope or bronchoscope, or a tracheostomy is performed.

Since the successful use of the EXIT procedure for management of airway compromise, the procedure has become useful for a wide variety of other problems, including thoracotomy for cystic adenomatoid malformation, transitioning from placental gas exchange to ECMO for anticipated pulmonary insufficiency, as a bridge for the separation of conjoined twins, and excision of a giant cervical teratoma.[43] Several surgical procedures lasting more than 2.5 hours have been performed, while the placental circulation has been maintained without evidence of neonatal hypercarbia or acidosis at delivery.[44]

Maternal outcomes after EXIT procedures have been very good. There may be a slightly higher rate of wound complications than in women undergoing routine cesarean delivery, but transfusion requirements, postoperative hematocrit levels, and lengths of hospital stay do not differ.[45,46]

Congenital Cystic Adenomatoid Malformation

Congenital *c*ystic *a*denomatoid *m*alformation (CCAM) is a pulmonary tumor with cystic and solid components. Lesions identified *in utero* can either regress and cause minimal morbidity or progress and enlarge, often causing hydrops fetalis. Small lesions detected *in utero* or in the newborn infant are treated after birth by surgical excision of the affected pulmonary lobe. Large lesions can cause mediastinal shift, hydrops, and pulmonary hypoplasia and can interfere with fetal or neonatal survival.[47] Untreated, fetal mass lesions associated with hydrops have a survival rate less than 5%. Macrocystic lesions have been decompressed *in utero* by the placement of shunt catheters between large cysts and the amniotic cavity, resulting in sustained decompression and resolution of hydrops; these procedures are followed by postnatal surgery.[48] However, not all lesions can be decompressed successfully by thoracentesis because the cysts are not always contiguous (i.e., in communication with each other) and can refill rapidly. *In utero* pulmonary lobectomy for lesions associated with hydrops has resulted in 50% survival, allowing compensatory lung growth and resolution of hydrops.[49] Refined selection criteria, as well as the potential for radiofrequency ablation of the tumor by means of a minimally invasive technique, hold promise for improved outcomes.

Intralobar and extralobar pulmonary sequestrations (bronchopulmonary sequestrations) in the fetus are rarer congenital lung anomalies than CCAM and involve nonfunctional lung tissue (disconnected from the bronchial tree) that derives blood supply from an artery, typically directly from the aorta. As with CCAM, therapeutic options depend on fetal morbidity, hydrops fetalis, and/or pulmonary hypoplasia.

Sacrococcygeal Teratoma

Some fetuses with sacrococcygeal teratoma undergo massive tumor enlargement, experience hydrops and placentomegaly, and die *in utero*. These tumors function as large arteriovenous fistulas, and fetal demise results from high-output cardiac failure. Fetuses with large lesions are at risk for intrapartum dystocia or tumor rupture and hemorrhage; these fetuses may require cesarean delivery. Fetuses with lesions diagnosed before 30 weeks' gestation have a poor prognosis and may benefit from surgical excision *in utero*. However, fetal surgical techniques have not reached the necessary level of sophistication to allow resection of lesions that deeply invade the pelvis, where considerable fetal blood loss would be expected. In addition, the "maternal mirror syndrome," a hyperdynamic state (e.g., hypertension, peripheral and pulmonary edema) in which the maternal physiology mirrors the abnormal circulatory physiology of the hydropic fetus, does not resolve with rapid correction of the fetal pathophysiology.[50] Successful operations for large sacrococcygeal teratomas have been performed with catheterization of a fetal hand or umbilical cord vein for blood and crystalloid transfusion during tumor resection; however, there has been no significant improvement in outcome with fetal intervention in hydropic fetuses with sacrococcygeal teratoma.

Myelomeningocele

Although not lethal, a myelomeningocele is a protrusion of meninges and spinal cord through a congenital defect in the vertebrae and overlying muscles and skin. It can result in lifelong morbidity and disability, including paraplegia, incontinence, hydrocephalus, and, occasionally, impaired cognition. Relatively common, with an incidence of about 1 in 2000 births, myelomeningocele is becoming less common owing to folate supplementation of maternal diet and early detection of the lesion by alpha-fetoprotein screening of maternal blood, which allows the option of pregnancy termination. Experimental work has demonstrated that the associated neurologic damage may result from exposure of the spinal cord to amniotic fluid, suggesting that the spinal cord is not inherently defective. The purpose of *in utero* surgery for myelomeningocele is to cover the cord, preventing its further contact with amniotic fluid. Primarily open fetal surgical techniques have been employed to repair this lesion. Preliminary results from the pioneering work at Vanderbilt University suggest that *in utero* repair successfully reverses the hindbrain herniation of the Arnold-Chiari II malformation, probably through normalization of cerebrospinal fluid flow, and decreases the need for ventriculoperitoneal shunt placement before 1 year of age.[51] However, it remains unclear whether *in utero* correction reduces the likelihood of paraplegia and whether the benefits (e.g., improved neurologic function) outweigh the risks and complications.[52] A multicenter, prospective trial conducted at Vanderbilt, Children's Hospital of Philadelphia, and the University of California–San Francisco (UCSF) is currently assessing the efficacy of *in utero* myelomeningocele repair.[53]

Twin-to-Twin Transfusion Syndrome

Abnormal connection of chorionic blood vessels in the placenta between two monochorionic twins results in a substantial incidence of mortality (i.e., as high as 75% for anatomically normal twins). The *t*win-to-*t*win *t*ransfusion *s*yndrome (TTTS) usually manifests in the second trimester of monochorionic twin gestation. Intertwin transfusion, common between monochorionic twins, is usually balanced through arterioarterial and venovenous connections but unidirectional and imbalanced through arteriovenous chorionic vessels. These abnormal vascular communications between the twins result in imbalanced twin-to-twin transfusion and TTTS, with one twin (the recipient) demonstrating polycythemia, polyuria, polyhydramnios, and hypertrophic cardiomyopathy. This twin is at risk for hydrops fetalis and fetal death. The donor twin is typically hypovolemic, oliguric, growth-restricted, and stuck against the endometrium in an oligohydramniotic sac (hence the designation "stuck twin") and often has a velamentous cord insertion. This twin is at risk for neonatal renal failure or renal tubular dysgenesis and dysfunction.

For unclear reasons, the survivors are at risk for neurologic injury with white-matter lesions and long-term disability. If TTTS occurs before 25 weeks' gestation and is untreated, fetal mortality is very high. A variety of therapeutic management techniques have been developed, including (1) serial amnioreduction to control polyhydramnios and reduce the risk of preterm labor, (2) surgical septostomy of the amnions to equalize amniotic pressures, (3) selective feticide to allow the other fetus to survive, and (4) *s*elective *f*etoscopic *l*aser *p*hotocoagulation (SFLP) of the vascular anastomoses between the two twins.[54] The laser can be inserted either percutaneously or through a maternal laparotomy or minilaparotomy incision, depending on placental location. However, results of two prospective, randomized multicenter trials did not conclusively determine whether SFLP was superior to amnioreduction.[55,56] There was an increase in fetal recipient mortality with SFLP, offset by an increase in neonatal recipient mortality in the amnioreduction group. The presence or absence of hypertensive cardiomyopathy of the recipient twin was the important factor in survival. (Vasoactive hormones [renin-angiotensin system factors] from the donor compromise the recipient, causing hypertension and cardiomyopathy.[57]) SFLP has the advantage of being one procedure, whereas amnioreduction requires serial procedures.

Twin Reversed Arterial Perfusion Sequence

In monozygotic twins, one twin can perfuse the other by retrograde blood flow though arterioarterial anastomoses. *T*win *r*eversed *a*rterial *p*erfusion sequence (i.e., TRAP) affects 1% of monozygotic twins and 1 in 30 triplets. Inadequate perfusion to the perfused twin via retrograde flow results in the development of a lethal set of anomalies that include acardia and acephalus. The normal ("pump") twin, which perfuses both itself and the nonviable twin, is at risk for high-output congestive heart failure, which if untreated is associated with a risk of *in utero* death exceeding 50%. Cardiovascular failure in the normal twin is the indication for intervention. The goal of therapy is interruption of the vascular communication between the two twins. In contrast to the treatment of TTTS, treatment of TRAP results in the death of the anomalous fetus. It is most readily achieved by percutaneous endoscopic laser or radiofrequency coagulation of the umbilical cord and/or placental vascular anastomoses. Alternative therapy has included *sectio parva* (selective cesarean delivery of one of multiple fetuses), percutaneous thrombosis of the acardiac twin's umbilical cord with coils or other thrombogenic material, and alcohol-impregnated suture cord ligation. Without treatment, the normal fetus invariably dies *in utero*. Surgical endoscopy for cord ligation via laser or radiofrequency coagulation is relatively simple and very effective, with overall survival rates approaching 80% and a median gestational age at delivery of 37.4 weeks.[58]

Congenital Heart Defects

Congenital heart defects that are considered amenable to antepartum therapy include ventricular outflow tract obstruction, aortic stenosis with developing hypoplastic left heart syndrome, pulmonary atresia without ventricular septal defect, and evolving hypoplastic right heart syndrome. Other defects possibly amenable to therapy *in utero* are mitral stenosis, premature closure of the foramen ovale, and tetralogy of Fallot. However, *in utero* balloon catheter valvuloplasties have been performed for more than a decade and have had limited technical success with discouraging results.[59] The best results have been achieved with aortic stenosis by the fetal treatment group at Boston Children's Hospital, who have reported successful outcomes consisting of improved left ventricular systolic function.[60] Initially a percutaneous approach was used but had limited success. Use of a laparotomy to expose the uterus improved success by allowing better ultrasonographic guidance and better fetal positioning.[61] Techniques for extracorporeal circulation have undergone investigation in fetal lambs and have been attempted in a human fetus.[62]

Other Lesions

Placement of thoracoamniotic shunts has resulted in successful decompression of massive congenital pleural effusions caused by fetal chylothorax that otherwise would have resulted in hydrops, pulmonary compression, and fetal or neonatal death.[63] Refractory cardiac arrhythmias can be treated by transplacental administration of medication to restore sinus rhythm and improve survival. Along with a long list of many other possibilities, placement of pacemakers for complete heart block; correction of gastroschisis, cleft lip and palate, or other craniofacial anomalies; and correction of skeletal anomalies by allogenic bone grafting are potentially feasible *in utero*.

SURGICAL BENEFITS AND RISKS

Fetal surgery *in utero* has some unique advantages. The primary advantage is to improve neonatal outcome over that of surgery performed after a preterm or term delivery. The intrauterine environment supports rapid wound healing (i.e., without scarring before midgestation), and the umbilical circulation meets nutritional and respiratory needs without outside assistance. The poorly developed fetal immune surveillance system may facilitate certain invasive procedures. Intrauterine cleft palate or lip surgery may restore normal form without scarring, allow midfacial growth without restriction or scar formation, and prevent associated nasal deformities. However, continued refinement of surgical and anesthetic techniques and reduction of maternal and fetal risk must occur before fetal surgery can be performed on a more routine basis, or for less severe fetal anomalies.

The fetal risks of fetal surgery remain relatively high. Although the mother is also at risk, serious maternal complications are relatively uncommon. Maternal risks include blood loss, infection, placental abruption, and pulmonary edema secondary to tocolytic therapy.[64] Open fetal surgery involves a hysterotomy that is not a lower uterine segment incision, and therefore all deliveries after performance of open procedures must be cesarean deliveries. However, future reproductive capabilities are not compromised. It cannot be overstated that maternal welfare must always be emphasized.[5,6]

The most common postoperative complications are fetal central nervous system injuries, postoperative amniotic fluid leaks, membrane separation, preterm PROM, preterm labor, and preterm delivery. Preterm delivery accounts for significant morbidity and mortality among fetuses that might otherwise benefit from the therapeutic effects of intervention. Chorioamniotic membrane separation can cause amniotic bands, umbilical cord strangulation, and fetal demise.[65] Better techniques for sealing the membranes are being devised; to date, improvements have included better surgical techniques, fibrin glue, and intra-amniotic injection of platelets and cryoprecipitate.[66]

ANESTHETIC MANAGEMENT

Fundamental considerations for anesthetic management of fetal surgery are similar to those for nonobstetric surgery during pregnancy (see Chapter 17). Maternal safety is paramount. Women at increased risk are excluded after preoperative assessment by the anesthesiologist. Anesthesiologists must participate in determining whether maternal risk is acceptably low for potential fetal benefit. To ensure both maternal and fetal safety, the anesthesiologist must understand the physiologic changes of pregnancy and their effects on anesthetic management and must take an active role in perioperative management.

Unlike other surgical procedures (e.g., appendectomy) performed during pregnancy in which the fetus is an innocent bystander, fetal surgery involves two surgical patients, requiring the anesthesiologist to balance the needs of both and preserve their gas exchange and cardiovascular stability. Further, for fetal surgery, the anesthesiologist must consider the anesthetic requirements of the fetus, including amnesia, analgesia, and immobility. Additionally, fetal surgery necessitates control of uterine tone. For open procedures, complete uterine relaxation (i.e., atony) is necessary. This concern for uterine tone continues postoperatively.

Maternal analgesia/anesthesia can involve local infiltration, intravenous sedation, neuraxial anesthesia, general anesthesia, or a combination, depending on the procedure and the position of the placenta. Fetal analgesia/anesthesia can be achieved via direct fetal intravenous or intramuscular administration of agents, placental transfer of anesthetic agents given to the mother, and possibly, intra-amniotic administration of agents.[67]

There are a number of fetal treatment centers in the world; they include University Hospitals Leuven (Belgium),

Imperial and King's Colleges London (UK), University Medical Centre Hamburg (Germany), Vall D'Hebron Hospital Barcelona (Spain), Hôpital Necker Enfants Malades Paris (France), University of Basel (Switzerland), University of South Florida, Vanderbilt University, University of North Carolina, Children's Hospital of Philadelphia, Boston Children's Hospital, and University of California–San Francisco. This is not an exhaustive list and does not include all the medical centers that perform EXIT procedures. What follows are generic descriptions of anesthetic approaches to the various fetal procedures, without consideration of local variations.

Anesthesia for Minimally Invasive and Percutaneous Procedures

Local anesthetic infiltration of the abdominal wall is sufficient to reduce maternal discomfort for many percutaneous procedures (e.g., amniocentesis, cordocentesis, intrauterine blood transfusion, needle aspiration of cysts, shunt placement into the fetal bladder or thorax, surgery on the placental vessels for TTTS). However, it does not provide fetal analgesia or immobility. Supplemental maternal analgesia and anxiolysis can be achieved by maternal administration of an opioid, a benzodiazepine, or a low-dose propofol infusion, which may confer some fetal immobility and analgesia via placental transfer.[68] Continuous infusion of remifentanil has been shown to improve fetal immobility and provide effective maternal sedation in comparison with diazepam.[69] Direct fetal paralysis has replaced reliance on placental transfer of agents used for maternal sedation to achieve fetal immobilization for many percutaneous procedures that do not involve noxious stimulation of the fetus. Fetal immobilization is not necessary for laser surgery involving the chorionic plate, such as for TTTS.

When larger needles and/or multiple attempts are necessary for a percutaneous procedure or a minilaparotomy, maternal comfort can be difficult to achieve with local infiltration and/or sedation. In these circumstances, neuraxial anesthesia is administered. Most fetal treatment centers use spinal or epidural anesthesia for percutaneous or minilaparotomy approaches for endoscopic surgery when large or multiple access ports are required, provided the placenta is positioned so that access can be achieved without requiring uterine exteriorization.[70] General anesthesia is preferred when surgical exposure requires a laparotomy and uterine exteriorization, both for maternal comfort and to block the uterine response to the requisite greater manipulation.

Unfortunately, fetal activity may render the procedure technically difficult or impossible. Placental transfer of the opioid and/or benzodiazepine does not ensure an immobile fetus. Fetal movement may be hazardous for the fetus because displacement of the needle or catheter may lead to trauma, bleeding, or compromise of the umbilical circulation. Fetal movement can be safely controlled with the use of direct fetal intramuscular or umbilical venous administration of pancuronium or vecuronium (0.3 mg/kg intramuscularly or 0.05 to 0.25 mg/kg intravenously). The onset of fetal paralysis occurs in approximately 2 minutes, with a duration of 1 to 2 hours.[71] For procedures that can cause noxious stimulation of the fetus, such as shunt catheter placement or cardiac septoplasty, fetal intramuscular or intravascular opioid administration (fentanyl 10 to 25 μg/kg) can supplement medications given to the mother if the procedure is performed with maternal local infiltration or neuraxial anesthesia. If general anesthesia is employed, placental transfer of a volatile halogenated agent may be sufficient.

Cordocentesis occasionally results in prolonged fetal bradycardia, especially if the needle punctures the umbilical artery rather than the umbilical vein. Persistent fetal bradycardia may prompt performance of emergency cesarean delivery if the gestational age is compatible with extrauterine viability. For patients with a viable fetus, the mother is fasted overnight, intravenous access is established, medication for aspiration prophylaxis is administered, and the patient is fully monitored in case general anesthesia is required for emergency cesarean delivery. Rarely, "prophylactic" spinal or epidural anesthesia is administered before cordocentesis, especially at later gestational ages (i.e., 30 weeks' gestation or later).

Anesthesia for Open Fetal Surgery

When corrective fetal surgery or an *in utero* procedure requires surgical access through a hysterotomy, high concentrations of a volatile anesthetic agent are administered to provide both maternal and fetal anesthesia as well as the required uterine relaxation.[2] Volatile anesthetic agents produce a dose-dependent depression of uterine myometrial contractility. At equal minimum alveolar concentrations (MAC), sevoflurane and desflurane are comparable to halothane, but isoflurane is less potent.[72] Preoperatively, the mother receives medication for aspiration prophylaxis and rectal indomethacin for prophylactic tocolysis, and an epidural catheter is placed primarily for postoperative analgesia. Minimal doses of preanesthetic medication and adjuvant anesthetic agents are given to supplement the volatile halogenated agent. This approach allows administration of maximum doses of a volatile halogenated agent to achieve effective uterine relaxation. With left uterine displacement—and following denitrogenation of the lungs—rapid-sequence induction of general anesthesia and tracheal intubation are performed. Anesthesia is maintained with a low concentration of a volatile halogenated agent while further preparations for surgery are undertaken, including (1) obtaining additional vascular access, (2) prophylactic antibiotic administration, (3) urinary bladder catheterization, and (4) performance of ultrasonography to assess fetal presentation and placental location. Additional medications to provide fetal anesthesia (e.g., fentanyl 10 to 25 μg/kg), immobility (e.g., vecuronium 0.2 mg/kg), and resuscitation (atropine 0.02 mg/kg, epinephrine 1 μg/kg, and crystalloid 10 mL/kg) are delivered to the scrub nurse or surgeon in a sterile fashion for subsequent fetal administration, as per the anesthesiologist's direction. Each syringe should contain one dose. Multiple doses should be placed in multiple, single-dose syringes to avoid accidental overdosing. Occasionally, it is important to have ready access to O-negative, cytomegalovirus-negative, leukocyte-depleted blood for fetal transfusion.

In anticipation of maternal skin incision, the concentration of the volatile halogenated agent is increased to 2 to 3 MAC. Any volatile halogenated agent can be used. Maternal blood pressure is supported with ephedrine or phenylephrine as needed to maintain adequate mean arterial pressures (>65 mm Hg). Before surgery begins, it is important to achieve an increased end-tidal concentration of the volatile halogenated agent to provide both fetal anesthesia and uterine relaxation. Fetal uptake of anesthetic gases takes longer than maternal uptake, but fetal MAC is lower. Fetal well-being is assessed with pulse oximetry, fetal heart rate (FHR) monitoring using ultrasonography, fetal echocardiography to assess ventricular contractility, and/or direct fetal electrocardiography (ECG).

Prior to the uterine incision, the uterus is assessed both visually and by palpation for contractions or increased tone. The inspired concentration of the volatile halogenated agent is increased if the uterus is not soft and flaccid. If a uterine contraction band is seen or higher uterine tone is palpated after the hysterotomy incision is made, supplemental tocolysis is achieved with the administration of nitroglycerin in small boluses (50 to 200 μg intravenously) or by infusion. With the use of ultrasonographic guidance or under direct vision, fentanyl and vecuronium are administered to the fetus intramuscularly prior to uterine incision or after the uterus is open and before surgery on the fetus. The uterine incision is made (remote from the location of the placenta) with a stapling device that prevents excessive bleeding and seals the membranes to the endometrium. During surgery, the exposed fetus and uterus are bathed with warmed fluids.

When uterine closure is initiated at the conclusion of the procedure, a loading dose of magnesium sulfate is administered (4 to 6 g intravenously over 20 minutes), followed by an intravenous infusion of 1 to 2 g/hr. The volatile halogenated agent can be discontinued after the magnesium sulfate bolus is given, and maternal anesthesia can be maintained with fentanyl and nitrous oxide in oxygen as well as with activation of epidural anesthesia with a bolus dose of local anesthetic and opioid. This regimen (1) allows time for elimination of the high concentrations of volatile halogenated agent; (2) facilitates tracheal extubation shortly after surgery is completed, with a fully awake patient who is capable of protecting her airway with minimal coughing or straining that might jeopardize the integrity of the watertight uterine closure; and (3) allows the patient to awaken without pain.

Intraoperative maternal intravenous fluids are restricted to minimize the risk for the postoperative pulmonary edema associated with tocolytic agents. Other postoperative concerns are maternal and fetal pain, preterm labor, rupture of membranes, infection, and a variety of potential fetal complications, including heart failure, intracranial hemorrhage, constriction of the ductus arteriosus from indomethacin, and fetal demise. Analgesia can be maintained with a continuous epidural infusion of a dilute solution of local anesthetic and opioid for the first several days. Effective analgesia may help prevent postoperative preterm labor.[73] Early postoperative uterine contractions are expected, and tocolysis is provided with an infusion of magnesium sulfate, which may be supplemented with indomethacin and, occasionally, terbutaline or nifedipine. Uterine activity and FHR are monitored closely during the first 2 to 3 postoperative days. The fetus is evaluated postoperatively by ultrasonography and MRI; the latter is performed to look for evidence of intracranial hemorrhage.

Administration of nitroglycerin is an alternative technique for providing open fetal surgery or the EXIT procedure. With this technique, high concentrations of volatile agents that can cause ventricular dysfunction in the fetus are avoided.[74] Instead, nitrous oxide, fentanyl, and a low concentration of the volatile halogenated agent are used. Intraoperative uterine relaxation is achieved by administration of intravenous nitroglycerin in large doses (as much as 20 μg/kg/min), and blood pressure is supported with vasopressors. Fetal anesthesia is achieved primarily by intramuscular administration of an opioid such as fentanyl. This technique has been used successfully, but it does not have a clear advantage for fetal outcome and may be associated with more maternal and, perhaps, fetal morbidity. For example, postoperative administration of such high doses of nitroglycerin for tocolysis can cause maternal nonhydrostatic pulmonary edema, possibly owing to peroxynitrite, a nitroglycerin metabolite.[64] Fetal intraventricular and periventricular hemorrhage and cerebral ischemia can result from changes in fetal cerebral blood flow, and concern has been raised that tocolytic agents that affect vascular tone and cross the placenta may be harmful to the fetus.[75] This technique has been used for unusual circumstances, such as in patients at risk for malignant hyperthermia, when it is necessary to avoid use of volatile halogenated agents.[76]

Further studies are needed to determine the optimal anesthetic technique that ensures maternal and fetal cardiovascular stability, optimal uteroplacental perfusion, total uterine relaxation, adequate fetal anesthesia and immobility, minimal fetal myocardial depression, and adequate blockade of the fetal stress response. Direct fetal administration of vasoactive agents may block the fetal autonomic response to stress, but may redistribute blood flow away from the placenta.[77] Total fetal spinal anesthesia would block the fetal autonomic response to noxious stimuli, but it does not seem feasible technically at this time.

Anesthesia for the *Ex Utero* Intrapartum Treatment Procedure

Anesthesia for EXIT procedures can be achieved two ways, the conventional method and an alternative. The **conventional method** has been a modification of a general anesthetic technique for cesarean delivery. An epidural catheter is placed preoperatively for postoperative analgesia. Unlike with general anesthesia for cesarean delivery, sufficient time must be allowed after induction of anesthesia—before surgery commences—to achieve the high end-tidal concentration of volatile halogenated agent needed to ensure uterine relaxation and allow time for fetal anesthesia; surgery does not start immediately after induction and intubation of the mother's trachea. However, the techniques of pulmonary denitrogenation (preoxygenation), rapid-sequence induction, and tracheal intubation are not different from those typically used for cesarean delivery. Fetal anesthesia can be supplemented by intramuscular administration of an opioid, and immobility can be ensured with administration of a paralytic agent, administered either prior to uterine incision with ultrasonographic guidance or after incision under direct vision. After adequate uterine relaxation has been achieved, a uterine incision is made with the stapling device, and the fetal head and shoulders are delivered in preparation for tracheal intubation. For more extensive procedures, such as fetal thoracotomy, or when there is fetal bradycardia suggestive of umbilical cord compression, the fetus is completely delivered and placed on the maternal chest and abdomen. The umbilical cord is not manipulated; it is kept wet with warmed fluids, and the fetoplacental circulation is maintained. The fetus is monitored with (1) a pulse oximeter probe placed on the fetal hand, (2) periodic ultrasonography, and (3) direct visualization.

The fetal procedure can range from a few minutes, to perform bronchoscopy or secure an airway (e.g., cervical neck mass), to several hours, to resect a neck or thoracic mass or to perform a tracheostomy and/or obtain subclavian intravenous access. This anesthetic technique can provide maternal, fetal, and uteroplacental stability over several hours. Once surgery is completed, with the baby's trachea intubated, surfactant is given if indicated and the baby's lungs are ventilated. When the baby's oxygen saturation increases (typically above 90%), the umbilical cord is cut and the (already intubated) newborn infant is transferred to the neonatologist for further resuscitation.

Once the umbilical cord is clamped, the maternal anesthetic technique is changed, and the uterine relaxation is rapidly reversed to avoid postpartum hemorrhage, as follows:

1. The inspired concentration of the volatile halogenated agent is substantially reduced or discontinued.
2. Nitrous oxide 70% and an opioid are administered.
3. Ventilation is increased to facilitate elimination of the volatile agent.
4. Oxytocin is administered in the usual fashion.
5. Epidural anesthesia is activated with a bolus dose of a local anesthetic agent and an opioid administered through the epidural catheter, if one has been placed.

With this technique, postpartum uterine atony, excessive blood loss, and requirement for methylergonovine or a prostaglandin to achieve adequate uterine tone are rare.[45]

The **alternative technique** for EXIT procedures involves use of neuraxial anesthesia and nitroglycerin.[77-81] It has the advantage of avoiding the risks associated with general anesthesia administration to the mother but may require large doses of nitroglycerin to achieve adequate uterine atony. Fetal analgesia and immobility can be achieved via intramuscular drug administration as described previously. Prospective trials are necessary to delineate the advantages and disadvantages of these two anesthetic approaches to the EXIT procedure.

Fetal Response to Surgical Stimulation

The subjective phenomenon of pain has not been, and perhaps cannot be, assessed adequately in human fetuses. Pioneering studies of preterm *neonates* undergoing surgery with minimal anesthesia found circulatory, sympathoadrenal, and pituitary adrenal responses characteristic of stress (e.g., increased release of catecholamines, growth hormone, glucagon, cortisol, aldosterone, and other corticosteroids; decreased secretion of insulin).[82,83] Administration of adequate anesthesia blunts the neonatal stress response,[84] and in preterm neonates, attenuation of the stress response with opioids might improve outcome.[85]

In studies of intrauterine blood transfusion in the human fetus, surgical needling of the intrahepatic vein (compared with needling of the insensate umbilical cord) is associated with evidence of a stress response, including increases in plasma beta-endorphin and cortisol concentrations and diminution in the Doppler imaging–determined middle cerebral artery pulsatility index, consistent with redistribution of blood flow to vital organs, including the brain.[86] Administration of fentanyl (10 μg/kg) blunts this stress response to intrahepatic needling.[87] Human fetuses elaborate pituitary-adrenal, sympathoadrenal, and circulatory stress responses to noxious stimuli as early as 18 weeks' gestation.[88-91] Further, during late gestation, fetuses respond to environmental stimuli such as noises, light, music, pressure, touch, and cold.[92] However, these physiologic responses associated with stress are not necessarily equivalent to the multidimensional, subjective phenomenon called pain, and a reduction in stress hormones is not necessarily an indicator of adequate analgesia.[93] The stress response is mediated largely in the spinal cord, brainstem, and/or basal ganglia, without cortical involvement. The experience of pain is a conscious subjective experience that has emotional and affective components and requires higher-level cortical processing.

When is the fetus adequately developed to feel pain? Is cortical development necessary? Thalamocortical axons reach the somatosensory cortex at 24 to 26 weeks' gestation,[94] and the cortex subsequently undergoes further development to establish its enormously complex and highly integrated neural networking. Of course, the presence of neural networks, no matter how sophisticated, are not functional without electrical activity. Studies of fetal electroencephalograms (EEGs) at 24 weeks' gestation show electrical activity only 2% of the time, with periods of inactivity lasting up to 8 minutes and bursts of activity of only 20 seconds in duration. By 30 weeks' gestation, although not completely continuous, EEGs begin showing patterns of wakefulness and sleep, but these are not concordant with fetal behavior. By 34 weeks' gestation, electrical activity is present 80% of the time, with more distinct sleep/wake cycles similar to adult patterns.

Can the fetus experience pain before development of this final anatomic link from periphery to cortex or before the existence of significant brain electrical activity? It has been postulated that nociceptive information may be transmitted earlier than 30 weeks' gestation through a complete neurologic connection from the peripheral tissue through the brainstem and the thalamus to the cerebral cortex via transient thalamocortical fibers that disappear before birth, and that the midbrain reticular system rather than the thalamocortical system is responsible for consciousness.[95,96] However, although the midbrain systems are crucial for the waking state, instincts, orienting, goal-directed control, and purposeful behavior, consciousness is regarded as a more complex phenomenon in which experience, perception, context-sensitive brain dynamics involved in cognitive control, and recursive object-related consciousness are key elements, and for which the cerebral cortex is indispensable. Awareness and awakeness are not necessarily synonymous.

Two studies using near-infrared spectroscopy to measure changes in cerebral oxygenation over the somatosensory cortex demonstrated that noxious stimulation of preterm infants results in a cortical response that differs from that after non-noxious stimulation, indicating that noxious information is transmitted to the infant cortex at 25 weeks' gestation.[97,98] However, the subjects were preterm neonates, not fetuses. Some observers have suggested that the low level of oxygenation *in utero* might preclude awareness and the ability to experience pain. Additionally, endogenous neuroinhibitors such as adenosine and pregnenolone, produced in the placenta, might sustain fetal sleep and suppress fetal awareness.[99] In contrast to their effect in the newborn, noxious stimuli do not appear to cause fetal cortical arousal to an awake state. Thus, some observers have suggested that the intrauterine environment might keep the fetus from being awake or aware, although this issue is a matter of some dispute.

Even if noxious stimulation does not affect consciousness, can it influence development? For example, circumcision in a nonanesthetized neonate increases the infant's pain response to injections 6 months later,[100] and fetal stress has long-term adverse hormonal effects in young monkeys.[101] Clearly, many questions remain unanswered. However, it is possible that noxious stimuli can have adverse long-term neurodevelopmental consequences that could be attenuated or blocked by anesthesia.[102]

It seems doubtful that fetal exposure to general anesthesia for fetal surgery would be more harmful to the fetus than direct exposure to anesthesia in neonates or the indirect exposure in fetuses of mothers who undergo nonobstetric surgery during pregnancy (see Chapter 17).[103,104] It seems best to err on the side of administering adequate fetal anesthesia.[105] Altogether, clinical observations of fetal and neonatal behavior, information about the development of mechanisms of pain perception, and studies of fetal and neonatal responses to noxious stimuli provide a compelling physiologic and philosophic rationale for the provision of adequate fetal anesthesia, especially after 24 to 26 weeks' gestation. Although we do not know exactly when the fetus can experience pain, noxious stimulation during fetal life causes a stress response, which could have both short- and long-term adverse effects on the developing central nervous system. Although the link between the stress response and pain is not always predictable, the threshold for pain relief is typically below that for stress response ablation, and the stress response to noxious stimulation is clear evidence that the fetal nervous system is reactive.[106] Administration of fetal anesthesia has been the standard practice since the inception of fetal surgery more than 25 years ago,[2-4] and it is practiced worldwide.[107] The importance of fetal immobility, cardiovascular homeostasis, analgesia, and, perhaps, amnesia have always been emphasized in fetal surgery practice.

Effects of Anesthesia on Fetal Circulation

In fetal lambs, the concentration of halothane required to prevent movement in response to painful stimuli is lower than that for adult sheep or newborn lambs (Table 7-1).[108] Despite rapid placental transfer of volatile halogenated agents, fetal concentrations of these agents remain lower than maternal concentrations for significant periods after maternal administration (Figures 7-2 and 7-3).[109,110]

Experimental studies of the fetal effects of maternal administration of a volatile halogenated agent have not produced uniform results.[109-112] In one study, maternal administration of 0.7% halothane or 1.0% isoflurane (i.e., 1.0 MAC for sheep) caused a modest decrease in fetal blood pressure with no change in fetal heart rate, oxygen saturation, or acid-base status. However, another study demonstrated that maternal administration of 1.5% halothane or 2.0% isoflurane decreased fetal blood pressure, heart rate, oxygen saturation, and base excess, with development of progressive fetal acidosis.[111] Other studies of maternal administration of 1.5% halothane demonstrated decreased fetal arterial pressure caused by reduced peripheral vascular resistance, with no change in fetal heart rate, cardiac output, oxygenation, acid-base status, or blood flow to the fetal brain or other major fetal organs (Figures 7-4 to 7-6).[109,112] Another study noted decreased fetal cardiac output and placental blood flow and progressive fetal acidosis during maternal administration of 2% isoflurane for 90 minutes. Exposures lasting as long as 30 minutes did not significantly decrease fetal cardiac output or result in fetal acidosis.[110]

TABLE 7-1 Fetal Anesthetic Requirement (MAC) for Halothane in Sheep (Mean ± SE)·

	Blood Concentration at MAC (mg/L)*	Theoretical (Calculated) End-Tidal Concentration (%)*
Mothers	133 ± 5	0.69 ± 0.25
Fetuses	49 ± 28	0.33 ± 0.29

MAC, minimal anesthetic concentration.

*Maternal and fetal values are significantly different ($P < .001$).

Modified from Gregory GA, Wade JG, Biehl DR, et al. Fetal anesthetic requirement (MAC) for halothane. Anesth Analg 1983; 62:9-14.

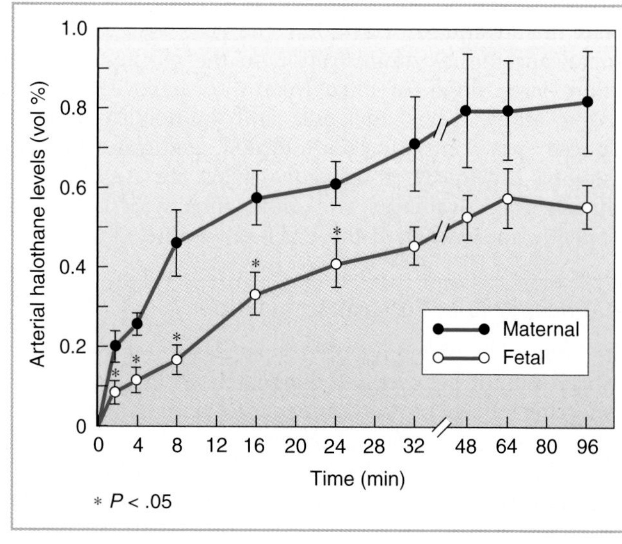

FIGURE 7-2 Maternal and fetal arterial halothane concentrations in sheep during maternal administration of 1.5% halothane (mean ± SE). (From Biehl DR, Cote J, Wade JG, et al. Uptake of halothane by the foetal lamb in utero. Can Anaesth Soc J 1983; 30:24-7.)

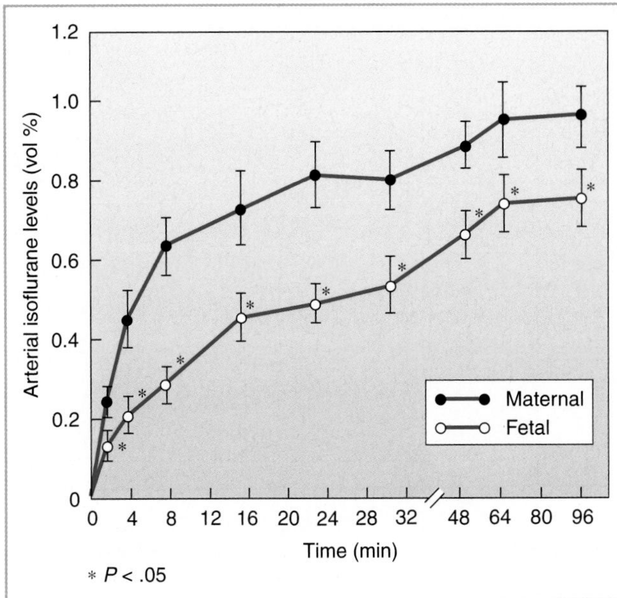

FIGURE 7-3 Maternal and fetal arterial isoflurane concentrations in sheep during maternal administration of 2.0% isoflurane (mean ± SE). (From Biehl DR, Yarnell R, Wade JG, Sitar D. The uptake of isoflurane by the foetal lamb in utero: Effect on regional blood flow. Can Anaesth Soc J 1983; 30:581-6.)

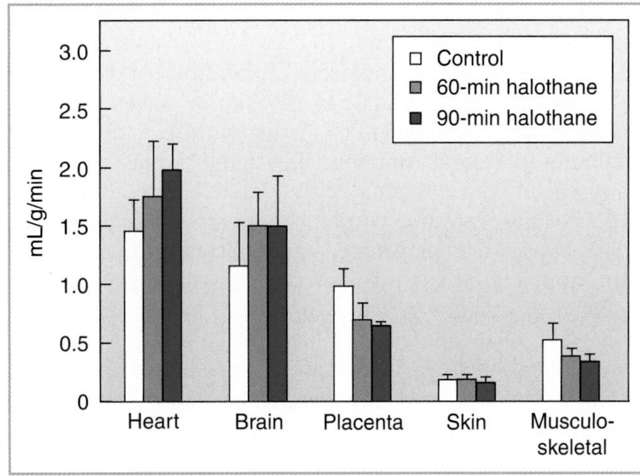

FIGURE 7-5 Fetal sheep regional blood flow during maternal administration of 1.5% halothane (mean ± SE). Measurements made at control and after 60 and 90 minutes of halothane anesthesia using the labeled microsphere injection technique. (From Biehl DR, Tweed WA, Cote J, et al. Effect of halothane cardiac output and regional flow in the fetal lamb in utero. Anesth Analg 1983; 62:489-92.)

In the chronic maternal-fetal sheep model, with no surgical stimulus to either the mother or fetus, it appears that prolonged, deep maternal inhalation anesthesia (i.e., 2.0 MAC) results in progressive fetal acidosis and is unsafe. Whether this adverse response results from direct impairment of fetal myocardial contractility, adverse redistribution of fetal blood flow, or reduced maternal uterine blood flow remains unclear. Light maternal inhalation anesthesia (i.e., 1.0 MAC) may be undesirable because it does not block the fetal response to a painful stimulus (e.g., surgery), which includes increased fetal catecholamines, vasoconstriction, and redistribution of fetal blood flow.[113] Fetal exposure to light maternal inhalation

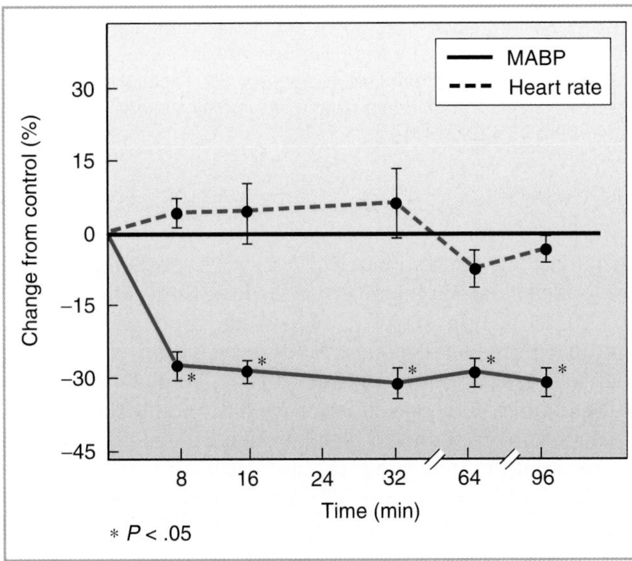

FIGURE 7-4 Changes in fetal sheep mean arterial blood pressure (MABP) and heart rate during maternal administration of 1.5% halothane, expressed as percentage change from control levels (mean ± SE). (From Biehl DR, Tweed WA, Cote J, et al. Effect of halothane on cardiac output and regional flow in the fetal lamb in utero. Anesth Analg 1983; 62:489-92.)

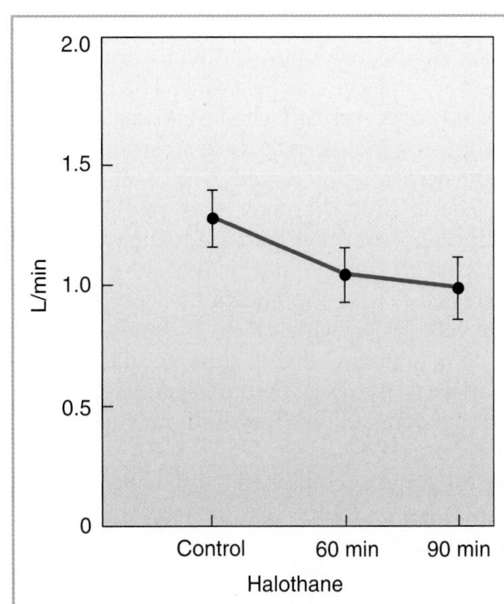

FIGURE 7-6 Fetal sheep cardiac output calculated using the labeled microsphere injection technique during maternal administration of 1.5% halothane (mean ± SE). Measurements made at control and after 60 and 90 minutes of halothane anesthesia. (From Biehl DR, Tweed WA, Cote J, et al. Effect of halothane on cardiac output and regional flow in the fetal lamb in utero. Anesth Analg 1983; 62:489-92.)

anesthesia (i.e., 1.0 MAC), without fetal stimulation, or brief fetal exposure to deep maternal inhalation anesthesia (i.e., 2.0 to 3.0 MAC) seems safe. Inhibition of the stress response via fetal spinal anesthesia in sheep achieves better fetal hemodynamic status during surgery and facilitates placental function after fetal cardiac bypass in comparison with a technique of fetal ketamine administration.[114] However, the combined effect of adequate fetal anesthesia with a halogenated agent, intrauterine manipulation, and fetal stress on fetal cardiovascular stability and regional blood flow remains unknown. In our experience, long and deep maternal inhalation anesthesia has not caused fetal hypoxia, hypercarbia, or acidosis even after exposures of 2 hours. However, others have seen acidosis after 45 minutes of fetal exposure to anesthesia.[115]

Fetal Monitoring

Maternal and fetal anesthesia, uterine incision, fetal manipulation, and surgical stress may adversely affect uteroplacental and fetoplacental circulation by several mechanisms. Maternal hypotension, increased uterine activity, and maternal hyperventilation and hypocarbia impair uteroplacental and/or umbilical blood flow. Fetal manipulation may affect fetal cardiac output, regional distribution of cardiac output, and/or umbilical blood flow. Direct compression of the umbilical cord, inferior vena cava, and/or mediastinum adversely affects fetal circulation.

Current methods of intraoperative fetal monitoring include FHR monitoring, pulse oximetry, ultrasonography (echocardiography), and blood gas and pH determinations.

In the early days of fetal surgery, monitoring of the FHR was attempted with a standard fetal corkscrew electrode processed by a standard FHR cardiotachometer, but signal failure was frequent, because the signal was of low amplitude and very sensitive to movement artifact. Using modified, atrial pacing wires, direct fetal ECG monitoring was more reliable. The distal ends of the bare wires were sutured subcutaneously onto the fetal shoulders and flank in standard lead placement locations. The proximal ends of the insulated wires were attached to coaxial shielded cables, which connected the three leads to a cardiotachometer that was modified with an increased gain to allow signal amplification. The cardiotachometer was modified further with the addition of a fixed low-pass frequency filter and a variable high-pass frequency filter, which substantially reduced motion artifact. These modifications allowed more reliable display of fetal ECG, with visible P waves and QRS complexes. Unfortunately, this technique did not eliminate motion artifact. Analysis of the fetal ECG using the ST waveform analysis (STAN) system may prove beneficial for fetal surgery.[116]

Plethysmography combined with spectrophotometric oximetry (pulse oximetry) has proved to be very useful, particularly for the EXIT procedure. In the early 1980s, before commercial availability of the pulse oximeter, this author developed a flat sensor for placement over any exposed fetal part to measure light by *reflectance* rather than *transmittance*.[117] This instrument became the foundation for fetal pulse oximetry now used in labor.[118] Later, the commercially available noninvasive neonatal digital sensor was used, wrapped around a fetal foot or the palm of the hand. With pulse oximetry, fetal oxygen saturations

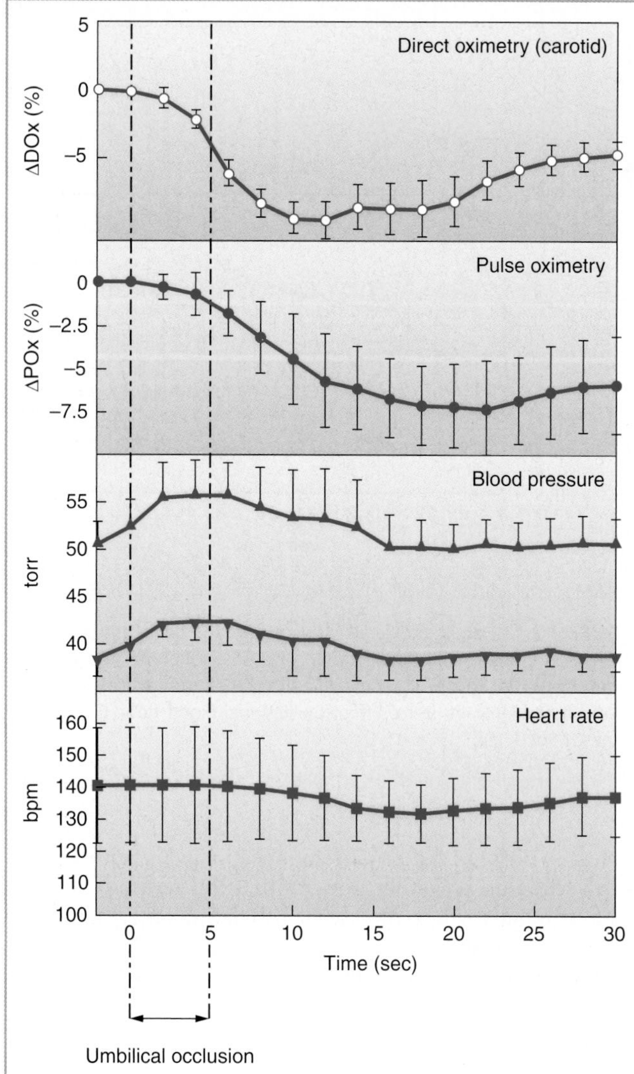

FIGURE 7-7 Response to 5 seconds of umbilical cord occlusion in the fetal lamb. Direct oximetry and pulse oximetry are expressed as delta saturation ($T_x - T_0$). (From Luks FI, Johnson BD, Papadakis K, et al. Predictive value of monitoring parameters in fetal surgery. J Pediatr Surg 1998; 33:1297-1301.)

sustained at approximately 75% were observed during prolonged fetal surgery with high-dose isoflurane (i.e., 2.0 to 3.0 MAC) in oxygen, suggesting good fetal cardiac output, perfusion pressure, and oxygenation despite the high concentration of isoflurane. The predictive value of pulse oximetry may be superior to FHR monitoring; bradycardia has been found to be a late sign of fetal compromise in fetal lambs subjected to umbilical cord compression (Figure 7-7).[119] However, bradycardia can precede desaturation during human fetal surgery (Figures 7-8 to 7-10).[120]

Ultrasonography is a crucial intraoperative fetal monitoring device. The FHR can be determined with visualization of the heart or with Doppler assessment of umbilical cord blood flow. Fetal cardiac contractility and volume also can be assessed qualitatively by echocardiography. Unfortunately, the sterile transducer cannot be positioned continuously because it often interferes with surgery.

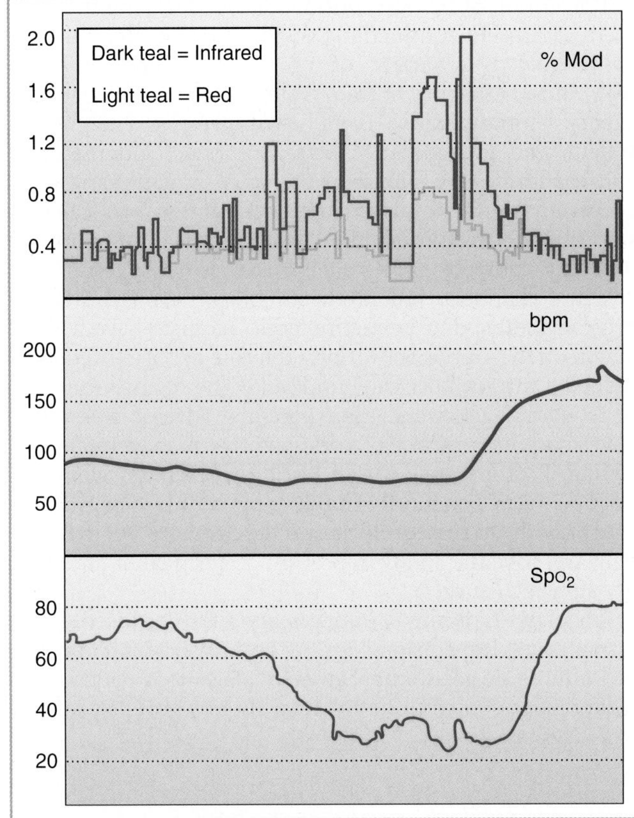

FIGURE 7-8 Two-minute tracing showing (*top*) modulation of red and infrared light signals (light = red; dark = infrared; scale 0% to 2%), (*middle*) fetal heart rate (FHR) (beats per minute [bpm]; scale 0 to 250), and (*bottom*) oxygen saturation (SpO_2; scale 0% to 100%), in a fetus of 24 weeks' gestation undergoing open diaphragmatic hernia repair. The decrease in FHR from about 90 to 70 bpm precedes the decrease in oxygen saturation from about 70% to 22%, and recovery in FHR to about 160 bpm precedes the recovery in oxygen saturation. This pattern may represent a transport delay in propagation of blood to the peripheral SpO_2 sensor. FHR may be a better monitor than SpO_2 for acute changes. (From Rosen MA. Anesthesia for fetal surgery. In Hughes SC, Levinson G, Rosen MA, editors. Shnider and Levinson's Anesthesia for Obstetrics. 4th edition. Philadelphia, Lippincott Williams & Wilkins, 2002.)

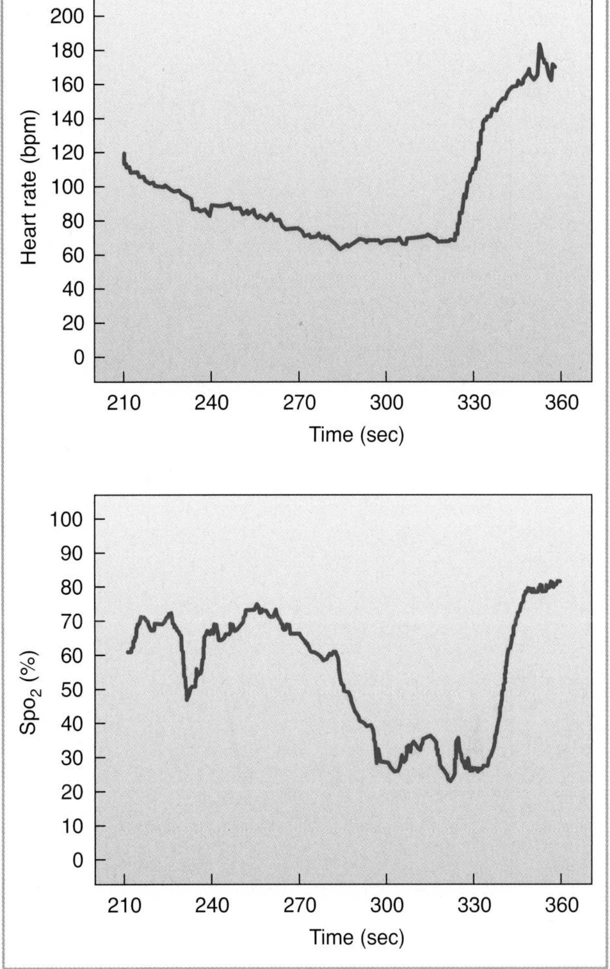

FIGURE 7-9 Graphic representation of the data in Figure 7-8 showing fetal heart rate (bpm) and oxygen saturation (SpO_2) more precisely detailed over the 120-second period. (From Rosen MA. Anesthesia for fetal surgery. In Hughes SC, Levinson G, Rosen MA, editors. Shnider and Levinson's Anesthesia for Obstetrics. 4th edition. Philadelphia, Lippincott Williams & Wilkins, 2002.)

Fetal monitoring has been limited; fetal blood pressure is a basic vital sign not currently monitored. Invasive methods used in experimental fetal animal preparations require indwelling catheters that have not been used routinely for human fetal surgery to date. Capillary or umbilical venous blood samples have been obtained for blood gas, pH, electrolyte, and glucose determinations. Vascular access has been achieved by surgical cutdown on the internal jugular vein for fluid, blood, and/or drug administration during prolonged procedures (e.g., correction of a diaphragmatic hernia). On several occasions, intravenous catheters have been placed in a fetal arm vein, and blood has been administered to replace blood lost during procedures such as sacrococcygeal teratoma resection. In the future, placental vessels may be catheterized for continuous blood pressure monitoring and blood gas determinations, and more information may be obtained from waveform analysis of the fetal ECG. Intraosseous access has been investigated in fetal sheep,[121] and long-term fetal vascular access has been achieved with use of laparoscopic techniques to cannulate chorionic vessels via an extra-amniotic approach in fetal rhesus monkeys.[122] New devices may become available for monitoring fetal blood pressure and fetal EEG; for continuous monitoring of arterial blood oxygen saturation, PO_2, and PCO_2; and for monitoring cerebral oxygenation, blood volume, and blood flow with near-infrared spectroscopy.

PRETERM LABOR

The human uterus has a thick, muscular layer that is sensitive to stimulation or manipulation. Uterine incision and stimulation may result in strong uterine contractions,

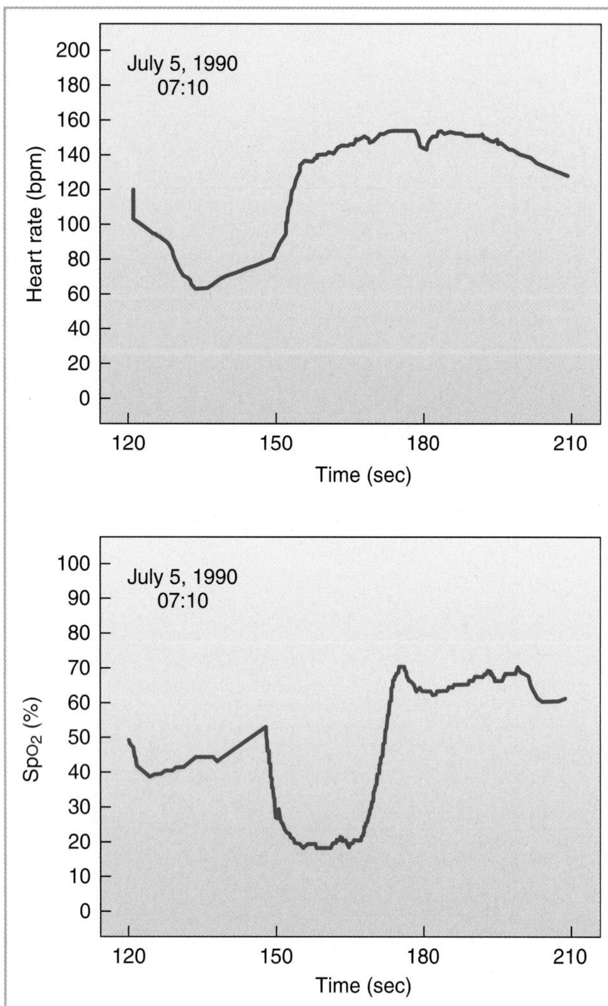

FIGURE 7-10 Data similar to those in Figure 7-9 from the same fetus a few minutes earlier, showing an acute decrease in fetal heart rate (FHR) with an associated decrease in fetal oxygen saturation (Spo_2). The onset of the desaturation detected in the fetal hand is delayed in relation to the onset of the bradycardia. Similarly, the recovery in FHR precedes the onset of the rapid increase in saturation. This pattern most likely represents a transport delay of the blood from the heart to the fetal hand. (From Rosen MA. Anesthesia for fetal surgery. In Hughes SC, Levinson G, Rosen MA, editors. Shnider and Levinson's Anesthesia for Obstetrics. 4th edition. Philadelphia, Lippincott Williams & Wilkins, 2002.)

which have resulted in a high incidence of postoperative abortion in studies of primate fetuses. Therefore, fetal surgery entails a high risk for preterm labor. Uterine contractions may also impede uterine blood flow and/or induce partial placental separation. Management of postoperative preterm labor has been the "Achilles heel" of fetal surgery.[123] The size of the uterine incision appears to directly relate to the likelihood and intensity of preterm labor. Less preterm labor (or more easily treated preterm labor) has been observed among women who have undergone minimally invasive surgery than among those who have undergone open procedures involving a large hysterotomy.

Prevention of uterine contractions is ideal, and the treatment of uterine contractions is essential. Tocolytic therapy has involved a variety of agents, including preoperative indomethacin; intraoperative volatile halogenated agents; intraoperative and postoperative magnesium sulfate; and postoperative beta-adrenergic, indomethacin, and calcium entry–blockade therapies. Volatile anesthetic agents may inhibit myometrial contractility via calcium-sensitive potassium channel modulation.[124] Magnesium probably competes with calcium at these voltage-operated calcium channels, indomethacin blocks the synthesis of prostaglandins, and beta-adrenergic agonists have a direct action on the uterus, activating adenylate cyclase and thereby reducing intracellular calcium levels. The relative inefficacy of tocolytic agents and their potential adverse side effects have made this aspect of postoperative management frustrating. Postoperative use of nitric oxide donor agents has not been very beneficial. The development of new tocolytic agents with increased efficacy and selectivity will substantially improve the ability to prevent preterm labor and delivery after fetal surgery.

Tocolysis typically is unnecessary after cordocentesis or intrauterine transfusion. For more invasive percutaneous procedures (e.g., shunt catheter placement, endoscopic techniques), some but not all fetal surgery groups use tocolytic agents.

THE FUTURE OF FETAL THERAPY

Despite more than 25 years of experience, fetal surgery and anesthesia for fetal surgery are still in the infant stages as fields of medicine. Success in these endeavors relies on a multidisciplinary team whose members communicate and work together to improve fetal outcome without incurring substantive maternal risk. A well-organized, multidisciplinary, professional, and comprehensive fetal treatment program at an academic medical center facilitates continued innovation for new techniques and helps ensure ongoing success. More potent tocolytics and greater use of the fetoscopic approach with improved techniques of visualization are the future for fetal surgery.[125,126] For example, closure of a myelomeningocele, a procedure that has been preformed only by an open technique for many years, has now been performed successfully via fetoscope.[127]

Although the rationale for fetal surgery seems straightforward, many issues remain problematic. Questions remain regarding maternal and fetal rights, safety, efficacy, cost-effectiveness, and societal resource allocation. Societal expectations and the availability of therapy must be balanced against the greater budgetary constraints in health care. In addition, there is concern about the sensitivity, specificity, and appropriate use of diagnostic testing. Fetal therapy raises complex social, ethical, and legal issues that go beyond those customary for therapeutic intervention. There is considerable controversy about fetal surgery, particularly for nonlethal lesions such as myelomeningocele.[128,129]

In some cases, distinguishing innovative therapy from experimentation is difficult. The ethical framework for the transition from innovation in fetal surgery to clinical trials to offering fetal surgery as a standard of care must be managed thoughtfully and responsibly.[130,131] Fetal therapy must be evaluated carefully in properly conducted trials and undertaken only with great caution and informed maternal consent. Publication in scientific journals and open communication with colleagues nationally and internationally facilitates the moral obligation of researchers to report all results to allow peer review of the merits and liabilities of fetal surgery.

Advances in fetal treatment continue to receive widespread attention within the scientific community as well as the popular news media. This fascination represents a transition from the former perception of the fetus as secluded from medical treatment to the recognition of the fetus as a patient—an individual for whom medical treatment has become possible. However, associated with these possibilities are new considerations that have legal, moral, and ethical effects. Fetal surgical and anesthetic techniques and tocolytic therapy continue to evolve. More therapeutic procedures are likely to become available in the future. Fetuses that may benefit from invasive therapy must be carefully distinguished from those that will not. Intervention should be undertaken only when there is a reasonable probability of fetal benefit and minimal maternal risk. Despite more than two decades of experience, there remains much to study, a great deal to learn, and, hopefully, a lot to achieve.

KEY POINTS

- Advances in antenatal diagnostic technology have led to the recognition and delineation of fetal disorders amenable to treatment *in utero*.
- Most malformations diagnosed *in utero* are not suitable for antenatal intervention. Fetal surgery is a reasonable option for anomalies that cause harm to the fetus before adequate development necessary for extrauterine survival (particularly lung maturity).
- Local or neuraxial anesthesia is often suitable for minimally invasive, endoscopic intrauterine procedures. Open intrauterine procedures typically require general anesthesia.
- Anesthetic considerations for intrauterine fetal surgery are similar to those for nonobstetric surgery in pregnant women. However, fetal surgery typically requires: (1) provision of analgesia for the fetus, (2) more intensive intraoperative fetal monitoring, and (3) intraoperative uterine relaxation. Also, the patient is at high risk for preterm labor or rupture of membranes after surgery.
- There are many medical, social, ethical, and legal questions regarding the efficacy and safety of intrauterine fetal surgery. Careful evaluation of fetal benefits and maternal risks is fundamental to the decision as to when and whether fetal intervention is appropriate.

REFERENCES

1. Liley AW. Intrauterine transfusion of foetus in haemolytic disease. Br Med J 1963; 2:1107-9.
2. Harrison MR, Anderson J, Rosen MA, et al. Fetal surgery in the primate. I. Anesthetic, surgical, and tocolytic management to maximize fetal-neonatal survival. Pediatr Surg 1982; 17:115-22.
3. Harrison MR, Golbus MS, Filly RA, et al. Fetal surgery for congenital hydronephrosis. N Engl J Med 1982; 306:591-3.
4. Rosen MA. Anesthesia and tocolysis for fetal intervention. In Harrison MR, Golbus MS, Filly RA, editors. The Unborn Patient. Orlando, FL, Grune & Stratton, 1984:417-34.
5. Longaker MT, Golbus MS, Filly RA, et al. Maternal outcome after open fetal surgery: A review of the first 17 human cases. JAMA 1991; 265:737-41.
6. Golombeck K, Ball RH, Lee H, et al. Maternal morbidity after maternal-fetal surgery. Am J Obstet Gynecol 2006; 194:834-9.
7. Mychaliska GB, Bealer JF, Graf JL, et al. Operating on placental support: The ex utero intrapartum treatment procedure. J Pediatr Surg 1997; 32:227-30.
8. Harrison MR, Filly RA, Parer JT, et al. Management of the fetus with a urinary tract malformation. JAMA 1981; 246:635-9.
9. Glick PL, Harrison MR, Adzick NS, et al. Correction of congenital hydronephrosis in utero. IV. In utero decompression prevents renal dysplasia. J Pediatr Surg 1984; 19:649-57.
10. Lissauer D, Morris RK, Kilby MD. Fetal lower urinary tract obstruction. Semin Fetal Neonatal Med 2007; 12:464-70.
11. Golbus MS, Harrison MR, Filly RA, et al. In utero treatment of urinary tract obstruction. Am J Obstet Gynecol 1982; 142:383-8.
12. Crombleholme TM, Harrison MR, Langer JC, et al. Early experience with open fetal surgery for congenital hydronephrosis. J Pediatr Surg 1988; 23:1114-21.
13. Johnson MD, Birnbach DJ, Burchman C, et al. Fetal surgery and general anesthesia: A case report and review. J Clin Anesth 1989; 1:363-7.
14. Quintero RA, Shukla AR, Homsy YL, Bukkapatnam R. Successful in utero endoscopic ablation of posterior urethral valves: A new dimension in fetal urology. Urology 2000; 55:774.
15. Manning FA, Harrison MR, Rodeck C. Catheter shunts for fetal hydronephrosis and hydrocephalus. Report of the International Fetal Surgery Registry. N Engl J Med 1986; 315:336-40.
16. Coplen DE. Prenatal intervention for hydronephrosis. J Urol 1997; 157:2270-7.
17. Agarwal SK, Fisk NM. In utero therapy for lower urinary tract obstruction. Prenat Diagn 2001; 21:970-6.
18. Harrison MR, Adzick NS, Estes JM, Howell LJ. A prospective study of the outcome for fetuses with diaphragmatic hernia. JAMA 1994; 271:382-4.
19. Stege G, Fenton A, Jaffray B. Nihilism in the 1990s: The true mortality of congenital diaphragmatic hernia. Pediatrics 2003; 112:532-5.
20. Harrison MR, Bressack MA, Churg AM, de Lorimier AA. Correction of congenital diaphragmatic hernia in utero. II. Simulated correction permits fetal lung growth with survival at birth. Surgery 1980; 88:260-8.
21. Harrison MR, Adzick NS, Flake AW, et al. Correction of congenital diaphragmatic hernia in utero. VI. Hard-earned lessons. J Pediatr Surg 1993; 28:1411-8.
22. Harrison MR, Adzick NS, Flake AW, Jennings RW. The CDH two-step: A dance of necessity. J Pediatr Surg 1993; 28:813-6.
23. Harrison MR, Adzick NS, Bullard KM, et al. Correction of congenital diaphragmatic hernia in utero. VII. A prospective trial. J Pediatr Surg 1997; 32:1637-42.
24. Wilson JM, DiFiore JW, Peters CA. Experimental fetal tracheal ligation prevents the pulmonary hypoplasia associated with fetal nephrectomy: Possible application for congenital diaphragmatic hernia. J Pediatr Surg 1993; 28:1433-40.
25. DiFiore JW, Fauza DO, Slavin R, et al. Experimental fetal tracheal ligation reverses the structural and physiological effects of pulmonary hypoplasia in congenital diaphragmatic hernia. J Pediatr Surg 1994; 29:248-57.

26. Bealer JF, Skarsgard ED, Hedrick MH, et al. The "PLUG" odyssey. Adventures in experimental fetal tracheal occlusion. J Pediatr Surg 1995; 30:361-5.
27. Harrison MR, Adzick NS, Flake AW, et al. Correction of congenital diaphragmatic hernia in utero. VIII. Response of the hypoplastic lung to tracheal occlusion. J Pediatr Surg 1996; 31:1339-48.
28. Deprest JA, Evrad VA, Van Ballaer PP, et al. Tracheoscopic endoluminal plugging using an inflatable device in the fetal lamb model. Eur J Obstet Gynaecol Reprod Biol 1998; 81:165-9.
29. Harrison MR, Albanese CT, Hawgood SB, et al. Fetoscopic temporary tracheal occlusion by means of detachable balloon for congenital diaphragmatic hernia. Am J Obstet Gynecol 2001; 185:730-3.
30. Keller RL, Glidden DV, Paek BW, et al. The lung-to-head ratio and fetoscopic temporary tracheal occlusion: Prediction of survival in severe left congenital diaphragmatic hernia. Ultrasound Obstet Gynecol 2003; 21:244-9.
31. Yang SH, Nobuhara KK, Keller RL, et al. Reliability of the lung-to-head ratio as a predictor of outcome in fetuses with isolated left congenital diaphragmatic hernia at gestation outside 24-26 weeks. Am J Obstet Gynecol 2007; 197:30. e1-7.
32. Keller RL, Hawgood S, Neuhaus JM, et al. Infant pulmonary function in a randomized trial of fetal tracheal occlusion for severe congenital diaphragmatic hernia. Pediatr Res 2004; 56:818-25.
33. Heerema AE, Rabban JT, Sydorak RM, et al. Lung pathology in patients with congenital diaphragmatic hernia treated with fetal surgical intervention, including tracheal occlusion. Pediatr Develop Pathol 2003; 6:536-46.
34. Harrison MR, Keller RL, Hawgood SB, et al. A randomized trial of fetal endoscopic tracheal occlusion for severe fetal congenital diaphragmatic hernia. N Engl J Med 2003; 349:1916-24.
35. Cortes RA, Keller RL, Townsend T, et al. Survival of severe congenital diaphragmatic hernia has morbid consequences. J Pediatr Surg 2005; 40:36-46.
36. Jani J, Gratacos E, Greenough A, et al. Percutaneous fetal endoscopic tracheal occlusion (FETO) for severe left-sided congenital diaphragmatic hernia. Clin Obstet Gynecol North Am 2005; 48:910-22.
37. Deprest J, Jani J, Cannie M, et al. Prenatal intervention for isolated congenital diaphragmatic hernia. Curr Opin Obstet Gynecol 2006; 18:355-67.
38. Norris MC, Joseph J, Leighton BL. Anesthesia for perinatal surgery. Am J Perinatol 1989; 6:39-40.
39. Schulman SR, Jones BR, Slotnick N, et al. Fetal tracheal intubation with intact uteroplacental circulation. Anesth Analg 1993; 76:197-9.
40. Gaiser RR, Cheek TG, Kurth CD. Anesthetic management of cesarean delivery complicated by ex utero intrapartum treatment of the fetus. Anesth Analg 1997; 84:1150-3.
41. Midrio P, Zadra N, Grismondi G, et al. EXIT procedure in a twin gestation and review of the literature. Am J Perinatol 2001; 18:357-62.
42. Bouchard S, Johnson MP, Flake AW, et al. The EXIT procedure: Experience and outcome in 31 cases. J Pediatr Surg 2002; 37:418-26.
43. MacKenzie TC, Crombleholme TM, Flake AW. The ex-utero intrapartum treatment. Curr Opin Pediatr 2002; 14:453-8.
44. Hirose S, Sydorak RM, Tsao K. Spectrum of intrapartum management strategies for giant fetal cervical teratoma. J Pediatr Surg 2003; 38:446-50.
45. Noah MM, Norton ME, Sandberg P, et al. Short-term maternal outcomes that are associated with the EXIT procedure, as compared with cesarean delivery. Am J Obstet Gynecol 2002; 186:773-7.
46. Hirose S, Farmer DL, Lee H, et al. The ex utero intrapartum treatment procedure: Looking back at the EXIT. J Pediatr Surg 2004; 39:375-80.
47. Harrison MR, Adzick NS, Jennings RW, et al. Antenatal intervention for congenital cystic adenomatoid malformation. Lancet 1990; 336:965-7.
48. Clark SL, Vitale DJ, Minton SD, et al. Successful fetal therapy for cystic adenomatoid malformation associated with second trimester hydrops. Am J Obstet Gynecol 1987; 157:294-5.
49. Grethel RJ, Wagner AJ, Clifton M, et al. Fetal intervention for mass lesions and hydrops improves outcome: A 15-year experience. J Pediatr Surg 2007; 42:117-23.
50. Langer JC, Harrison MR, Schmidt KG, et al. Fetal hydrops and death from sacrococcygeal teratoma: Rationale for fetal surgery. Am J Obstet Gynecol 1989; 160:1145-50.
51. Bruner JP. Intrauterine surgery in myelomeningocele. Semin Fetal Neonatal Med 2007; 12:471-6.
52. Mazzola CA, Albright AL, Sutton LN, et al. Dermoid inclusion cysts and early spinal cord tethering after fetal surgery for myelomeningocele. N Engl J Med 2002; 347:256-9.
53. Jobe AH. Perspective: Fetal surgery for myelomeningocele. N Engl J Med 2002; 347:230-1.
54. Ville Y, Hyett J, Hecher K, Nicolaides K. Preliminary experience with endoscopic laser surgery for severe twin-twin transfusion syndrome. N Engl J Med 1995; 332:224-7.
55. Moise KJ Jr, Dorman K, Lamvu G, et al. A randomized trial of amnioreduction versus septostomy in the treatment of twin-twin transfusion syndrome. Am J Obstet Gynecol 2005; 193:701-7.
56. Crombleholme TM, Shera D, Lee H, et al. A prospective, randomized, multicenter trial of amnioreduction vs selective fetoscopic laser photocoagulation for the treatment of severe twin-twin transfusion syndrome. Am J Obstet Gynecol 2007; 197:396. e1-9.
57. Mahieu-Caputo D, Meulemans A, Martinovic J, et al. Paradoxic activation of the renin-angiotensin system in twin-twin transfusion syndrome: An explanation for cardiovascular disturbances in the recipient. Pediatr Res 2005; 58:685-8.
58. Diehl W, Hecher K. Selective cord coagulation in acardiac twins. Semin Fetal Neonatal Med 2007; 12:458-63.
59. Matsui H, Gardiner H. Fetal intervention for cardiac disease: The cutting edge of perinatal care. Semin Fetal Neonatal Med 2007; 12:482-9.
60. Tworetzky W, Wilkins-Haug L, Jenkins R. Balloon dilation of severe aortic stenosis in the fetus: Potential for prevention of hypoplastic left heart syndrome. Candidate selection, technique, and results of successful intervention. Circulation 2004; 110:2125-31.
61. Wilkins-Haug LE, Tworetzky W, Benson CB, et al. Factors affecting technical success of fetal aortic valve dilation. Ultrasound Obstet Gynecol 2006; 28:47-52.
62. Fenton KN, Heinemann MK, Hickey PR, et al. Inhibition of the fetal stress response improves cardiac output and gas exchange after fetal cardiac bypass. J Thorac Cardiovasc Surg 1994; 107:1416-22.
63. Rodeck CH, Fisk NM, Fraser DI, Nicolini U. Long-term in utero drainage of fetal hydrothorax. N Engl J Med 1988; 319:1135-8.
64. DiFederico EM, Harrison M, Matthay MA. Pulmonary edema in a woman following fetal surgery. Chest 1996; 109:1114-7.
65. Sydorak RM, Hirose S, Sandberg PL, et al. Chorioamniotic membrane separation following fetal surgery. J Perinatol 2002; 22:407-10.
66. Cortes RA, Wagner AJ, Lee H, et al. Pre-emptive placement of a presealant for amniotic access. Am J Obstet Gynecol 2005; 193:1197-203.
67. Strumper D, Durieux ME, Gogarten W, et al. Fetal plasma concentrations after intraamniotic sufentanil in chronically instrumented pregnant sheep. Anesthesiology 2003; 98:1400-6.
68. Spielman FJ, Seeds JW, Corke BC. Anaesthesia for fetal surgery. Anaesthesia 1984; 39:756-9.
69. Van de Velde M, Van Schoubroeck D, Lewi LE, et al. Remifentanil for fetal immobilization and maternal sedation during fetoscopic surgery: A randomized, double-blind comparison with diazepam. Anesth Analg 2005; 101:251-8.
70. Myers LB, Watcha MF. Epidural versus general anesthesia for twin-twin transfusion syndrome requiring fetal surgery. Fetal Diagn Ther 2004; 19:286-91.
71. Leveque C, Murat I, Toubas F, et al. Fetal neuromuscular blockade with vecuronium bromide: Studies during intravascular intrauterine transfusion in isoimmunized pregnancies. Anesthesiology 1992; 76:642-4.
72. Yoo KY, Lee JC, Yoon MH, et al. The effects of volatile anesthetics on spontaneous contractility of isolated human pregnant uterine muscle: A comparison among sevoflurane, desflurane, isoflurane, and halothane. Anesth Analg 2006; 103:443-7.
73. Tame JD, Abrams LM, Ding XY, et al. Level of postoperative analgesia is a critical factor in regulation of myometrial contractility after laparotomy in the pregnant baboon: Implications for human fetal surgery. Am J Obstet Gynecol 1999; 180:1196-201.

74. Rychick J, Tian Z, Cohen MS, et al. Acute cardiovascular effects of fetal surgery in the human. Circulation 2004; 110:1549-56.
75. Bealer JF, Raisanen J, Skarsgard ED, et al. The incidence and spectrum of neurological injury after open fetal surgery. J Pediatr Surg 1995; 30:1150-4.
76. Rosen MA, Andreae M, Cameron A. Nitroglycerin for fetal surgery: Fetoscopy and ex utero intrapartum treatment procedure with malignant hyperthermia precautions. Anesth Analg 2003; 96:698-700.
77. Bradley SM, Hanley FL, Duncan BW, et al. Fetal cardiac bypass alters regional blood flows, arterial blood gases, and hemodynamics in sheep. Am J Physiol 1992; 263:H919-28.
78. Clark KD, Viscomi CM, Lowell J, Chien EK. Nitroglycerin for relaxation to establish a fetal airway (EXIT). Obstet Gynecol 2004; 103:1113-5.
79. Benonis JG, Habib AS. Ex utero intrapartum treatment procedure in a patient with arthrogryposis multiplex congenita, using spinal anesthesia and intravenous nitroglycerin for uterine relaxation. Int J Obstet Gynecol 2008; 17:53-6.
80. Okutomi T, Saito M, Kuczkowski KM. The use of potent inhalational agents for the ex-utero intrapartum treatment (EXIT) procedures: What concentrations? Acta Anaesthesiol Belg 2007; 58:97-9.
81. George RG, Melnick AH, Rose EC, Habib AS. Case series: Combined spinal epidural anesthesia for cesarean delivery and ex utero intrapartum treatment procedure. Can J Anaesth 2007; 54:218-22.
82. Anand KJ, Brown MJ, Bloom SR, Aynsley-Green A. Studies on the hormonal regulation of fuel metabolism in the human newborn infant undergoing anaesthesia and surgery. Horm Res 1985; 22:115-28.
83. Anand KJ, Brown MJ, Causon RC, et al. Can the human neonate mount an endocrine and metabolic response to surgery? J Pediatr Surg 1985; 20:41-8.
84. Anand KJ, Sippell WG, Aynsley-Green A. Randomised trial of fentanyl anaesthesia in preterm neonates undergoing surgery: Effects on the stress response. Lancet 1987; 1(8524):62-6.
85. Anand KJ, Hickey PR. Pain and its effects in the human neonate and fetus. N Engl J Med 1987; 317:1321-9.
86. Giannakoulopoulos X, Sepulveda W, Kourtis P, et al. Fetal plasma cortisol and beta-endorphin response to intrauterine needling. Lancet 1994; 344:77-81.
87. Fisk NM, Gitau R, Teixeira JM, et al. Effect of direct fetal opioid analgesia on fetal hormonal and hemodynamic stress response to intrauterine needling. Anesthesiology 2001; 95:828-35.
88. Teixeira J, Fogliani R, Giannakoulopoulos X, et al. Fetal haemodynamic stress response to invasive procedures. Lancet 1996; 347:624.
89. Giannakoulopoulos X, Teixeira J, Fisk N, Glover V. Human fetal and maternal noradrenaline responses to invasive procedures. Pediatr Res 1999; 45:494-9.
90. Teixeira JM, Glover V, Fisk NM. Acute cerebral redistribution in response to invasive procedures in the human fetus. Am J Obstet Gynecol 1999; 181:1018-25.
91. Gitau R, Fisk NM, Teixeira JM, et al. Fetal hypothalamic-pituitary-adrenal stress responses to invasive procedures are independent of maternal responses. J Clin Endocrinol Metab 2001; 86:104-9.
92. Liley AW. The foetus as a personality. Aust N Z J Psych 1972; 6:99-105.
93. Derbyshire SW. Locating the beginnings of pain. Bioethics 1999; 13:1-31.
94. Lee SJ, Ralston HJP, Drey EA, et al. Fetal pain: A systematic multidisciplinary review of the evidence. JAMA 2005; 294:947-54.
95. Kostovic I, Rakic P. Developmental history of the transient subplate zone in the visual and somatosensory cortex of the macaque monkey and human brain. J Comp Neurol 1990; 297:441-70.
96. Merker B. Consciousness without a cerebral cortex: A challenge for neuroscience and medicine. Behav Brain Sci 2007; 30:63-134.
97. Slater R, Cantarella A, Gallella S, et al. Cortical pain response in human infants. J Neurosci 2006; 26:3662-6.
98. Bartocci M, Bergqvist L, Lagercrantz H, Anand KJS. Pain activates cortical areas in the preterm newborn brain. Pain 2006; 122:109-17.
99. Mellor DJ, Diesch TJ, Gunn AJ, Bennet L. The importance of 'awareness' for understanding fetal pain. Brain Res Rev 2005; 49:455-71.
100. Taddio A, Katz J, Ilersich AL, et al. Effect of neonatal circumcision on pain response during subsequent routine vaccination. Lancet 1997; 349:599-603.
101. Clarke AS, Wittwer DJ, Abbott DH, Schneider ML. Long-term effects of prenatal stress in HPA axis activity in juvenile rhesus monkeys. Dev Psychobiol 1994; 27:257-69.
102. Lowery CL, Hardman MP, Manning N, et al. Neurodevelopmental changes of fetal pain. Semin Perinatol 2007; 31:275-82.
103. Bhutta AT, Anand KJ. Vulnerability of the developing brain: Neuronal mechanisms. Clin Perinatol 2002; 29:357-72.
104. Lidow MS. Long-term effects of neonatal pain on nociceptive systems. Pain 2002; 99:377-83.
105. Glover V, Fisk NM. Do fetuses feel pain? We don't know: Better to err on the safe side from mid-gestation. Br Med J 1996; 313:796.
106. White MC, Wolf AR. Pain and stress in the human fetus. Best Prac Res Clin Anaesthesiol 2004; 18:205-20.
107. Van de Velde M, Jani J, De Buck F, Deprest J. Fetal pain perception and pain management. Semin Fetal Neonatal Med 2006; 11:232-6.
108. Gregory GA, Wade JG, Biehl DR, et al. Fetal anesthetic requirement (MAC) for halothane. Anesth Analg 1983; 62:9-14.
109. Biehl DR, Cote J, Wade JG, et al. Uptake of halothane by the foetal lamb in utero. Can Anaesth Soc J 1983; 30:24-7.
110. Biehl DR, Yarnell R, Wade JG, Sitar D. The uptake of isoflurane by the foetal lamb in utero: Effect on regional blood flow. Can Anaesth Soc J 1983; 30:581-6.
111. Palahniuk RJ, Shnider SM. Maternal and fetal cardiovascular and acid-base changes during halothane and isoflurane anesthesia in the pregnant ewe. Anesthesiology 1974; 41:462-72.
112. Biehl DR, Tweed WA, Cote J, et al. Effect of halothane on cardiac output and regional flow in the fetal lamb in utero. Anesth Analg 1983; 62:489-92.
113. Sabik J, Assad RS, Hanley FL: Halothane as an anesthetic for fetal surgery. J Pediatr Surg 1993; 28:542-7.
114. Fenton KN, Zinn HE, Heinemann MK, et al. Long-term survivors of fetal cardiac bypass in lambs. J Thorac Cardiovasc Surg 1994; 107:1423-7.
115. Gaiser TT, Kurth CD, Cohen D, Crombleholme T. The cesarean delivery of a twin gestation under 2 minimum alveolar anesthetic concentration of isoflurane: One normal and one with a large anesthetic neck mass. Anesth Analg 1999; 88:584-6.
116. Rosen KG, Amer-Wahlin I, Luzietti R, Noren H. Fetal ECG waveform analysis. Best Pract Res Clin Obstet Gynaecol 2004; 18:485-514.
117. Rosen MA. Reflectance oximetry for fetal monitoring. First International Symposium on Intrapartum Surveillance, Nottingham, UK, October 18/19, 1990. Nottingham, Nottingham Press, 1990.
118. Johnson N, Johnson VA, Fisher J, et al. Fetal monitoring with pulse oximetry. Br J Obstet Gynaecol 1991; 98:36-41.
119. Luks FI, Johnson BD, Papadakis K, et al. Predictive value of monitoring parameters in fetal surgery. J Pediatr Surg 1998; 33:1297-301.
120. Izumi A, Minakami H, Sato I. Fetal heart rate decelerations precede a decrease in fetal oxygen content. Gynecol Obstet Invest 1997; 44:26-31.
121. Jennings RW, Adzick NS, Longaker MT, et al. New techniques in fetal therapy. J Pediatr Surg 1992; 27:1329-33.
122. Hedrick MH, Jennings RW, MacGillivray TE, et al. Chronic fetal vascular access. Lancet 1993; 342:1086-7.
123. Harrison MR. Fetal surgery. Am J Obstet Gynecol 1996; 174:1255-64.
124. Kafali H, Kaya T, Gursoy S, et al. The role of K^+ channels on the inhibitor effect of sevoflurane in pregnant rat myometrium. Anesth Analg 2002; 94:174-8.
125. Deprest J, Jani J, Lewi L, et al. Fetoscopic surgery: Encouraged by clinical experience and boosted by instrument innovation. Semin Fetal Neonatal Med 2006; 11:398-412.
126. Gratocos E, Wu J, Devlieger R, et al. Nitrous oxide amniodistention compared with fluid amniodistention reduces operation time while inducing no changes in fetal acid-base status in a sheep model for endoscopic fetal surgery. Am J Obstet Gynecol 2002; 186:538-43.

127. Kohl T, Tchatcheva K, Merz W, et al. Percutaneous fetoscopic patch closure of human spina bifida aperta: Advances in fetal surgical techniques may obviate the need for early postnatal neurosurgical intervention. Surg Endosc 2008 Sep 26 (Epub ahead of print).
128. Lyerly AD, Cefalo RC, Socol M, et al. Attitudes of maternal-fetal specialists concerning maternal-fetal surgery. Am J Obstet Gynecol 2001; 185:1052-8.
129. Chervenak FA, McCullough LB. Ethics of maternal-fetal surgery. Semin Fetal Neonatal Med 2007; 12:426-31.
130. Lyerly AD, Gates EA, Cefalo RC, et al. Toward the ethical evaluation and use of maternal-fetal surgery. Obstet Gynecol 2001; 98:689-97.
131. Chervenak FA, McCullough LB. A comprehensive ethical framework for fetal research and its application to fetal surgery for spina bifida. Am J Obstet Gynecol 2002; 187:10-4.

Chapter 8

Intrapartum Fetal Assessment and Therapy

Elizabeth G. Livingston, M.D.

The value of obstetric interventions during labor and delivery has been scrutinized in recent years. Old technologies have been reassessed, and new ones have been introduced. A rising cesarean delivery rate, persistent cases of fetal/neonatal neurologic injury, and excessive litigation have prompted an ongoing search for optimal methods of intrapartum fetal assessment and therapy.

FETAL RISK DURING LABOR

Historical epidemiologic data suggest that the fetus is at increased risk for morbidity and mortality during labor and delivery. In 1963, the British Perinatal Mortality Survey reviewed autopsy data for 1400 stillborn infants and concluded that slightly more than 30% of these losses resulted from intrapartum asphyxia.[1] Delivery outcomes in the industrialized world have improved over the past 40 years. A Canadian database covering 1981 to 2002 identified approximately 80 intrapartum stillbirths per 120,000 live births, a rate of 0.67/1000; some 11 of the infants were considered viable (i.e., not severely preterm or anomalous), so the preventable death rate was 0.09/1000.[2] In 1991, the intrapartum death rate of nonmalformed fetuses in Scandinavia ranged from 1.9 to 4.2 per 10,000.[3] A Norwegian audit suggested that the decline in stillbirths was mostly a result of a reduction in intrapartum stillbirths.[4] Intrapartum stillbirths are rare in developed countries, constituting less than 10% of all stillbirths. By contrast, in some developing countries, as many as 50% of stillbirths occur intrapartum.[5] According to a World Health Organization report, intrapartum-related neonatal deaths account for almost 10% of deaths in children less than 5 years of age.[6]

Experimental models lend support to the hypothesis that intrapartum events can have long-term neurologic sequelae. Fetal monkeys subjected to hypoxia *in utero* suffer neurologic injuries similar to those seen in children who presumably suffered asphyxia *in utero*.[7,8] Work with rodent models has shown similar patterns of damage.[9] Epidemiologic and experimental data suggest that the fetus is at significant jeopardy during labor and delivery.

Studies also suggest that some fetuses are at greater risk for adverse intrapartum events than others. Older studies report that high-risk mothers constitute 20% of the pregnant population, but their offspring represent 50% of the cases of perinatal morbidity and mortality.[10] Various schemes for identification of high-risk pregnancies have been published (Box 8-1).[11,12] High-risk pregnancies include, but are not limited to, women with (1) **medical complications** (e.g., hypertension, preeclampsia, diabetes, autoimmune disease, hemoglobinopathy); (2) **fetal complications** (e.g., intrauterine growth restriction, nonlethal anomalies, prematurity, multiple gestation, postdatism, hydrops); and (3) **intrapartum complications** (e.g., abnormal vaginal bleeding, maternal fever, meconium-stained amniotic fluid, oxytocin augmentation of labor). Owing to inadequate sensitivity, poor positive predictive values, and the inability to modify risk-factor related outcomes, high-risk scoring systems have not been shown to improve pregnancy outcomes.[13] In one study, more than half of infants with asphyxia had no clinical risk factors.[14] However, scoring systems may be of use in the management of low-risk parturients who do not want continuous monitoring during labor.[13] An additional strategy for identifying high-risk parturients in European centers is the analysis of a fetal heart rate (FHR) tracing at the time of admission; if the FHR tracing is abnormal, patients receive intensive monitoring, and if the tracing is normal, they may receive less monitoring.[15]

The magnitude of risk for intrapartum fetal neurologic injury is a matter of some dispute. In 2003, the American

BOX 8-1 Independent Risk Factors with a Significant Effect on Perinatal Outcome

Maternal Demographic Factors
- Age < 18 or > 39 years
- Unmarried
- Weight < 50 kg
- Smoking
- No education beyond primary school

Past Obstetric History
- History of perinatal loss
- History of infant < 2500 g
- History of preterm birth (< 28 weeks' gestation)
- Repeat pregnancy within 1 year

Past Medical History
- Rh negative with antibodies
- Renal disease
- Thyroid disease
- Cardiac disease
- Previous cervical cone biopsy

Risk Factors During Pregnancy
- Pyelonephritis
- Multiple gestation
- Anemia (hemoglobin < 8 g/dL)
- Hypertension (diastolic pressure > 90 mm Hg)
- Proteinuria (> 500 mg/day)
- Gestational or established diabetes
- Placental abruption
- Placenta previa
- Bleeding before 28 weeks' gestation
- Delivery before 37 or after 42 weeks' gestation

From Knox AJ, Sadler L, Pattison NS, et al. An obstetric scoring system: Its development and application in obstetric management. Reprinted with permission from the American College of Obstetricians and Gynecologists. Obstet Gynecol 1993; 81:195-9.

BOX 8-2 Criteria that Define an Acute Intrapartum Hypoxic Event as Sufficient to Cause Cerebral Palsy

Essential Criteria
1. Evidence of metabolic acidosis in umbilical cord arterial blood obtained at delivery (i.e., pH < 7.00, base deficit > 12 mmol/L)
2. Early onset of encephalopathy in an infant delivered at > 34 weeks' gestation
3. Cerebral palsy of the spastic quadriplegia or dyskinetic type
4. Exclusion of other identifiable etiologies

Criteria that Suggest Intrapartum Timing of Insult
1. Sentinel hypoxic event occurring immediately before or during labor
2. Sudden, sustained bradycardia or absence of fetal heart rate variability with persistent late or variable decelerations
3. Apgar scores of 0-3 beyond 5 minutes of life
4. Evidence of multisystem involvement within 72 hours of delivery
5. Early imaging study that shows evidence of acute, nonfocal cerebral abnormality

Adapted from American College of Obstetricians and Gynecologists Task Force on Neonatal Encephalopathy and Cerebral Palsy. Neonatal Encephalopathy and Cerebral Palsy: Defining the Pathogenesis and Pathophysiology. The American College of Obstetricians and Gynecologists and the American Academy of Pediatrics, Washington, D.C., January 2003; and MacLennan A. A template for defining a causal relation between acute intrapartum events and cerebral palsy: International consensus statement. Br Med J 1999; 319:1054-9.

College of Obstetricians and Gynecologists (ACOG) Task Force on Neonatal Encephalopathy and Cerebral Palsy concluded that 70% of these types of fetal neurologic injuries result from events that occur before the onset of labor.[16,17] Examples of antepartum events that may cause fetal neurologic injury include congenital anomalies, chemical exposure, infection, and fetal thrombosis/coagulopathy. Only 4% of cases of neonatal encephalopathy result solely from intrapartum hypoxia, an incidence of approximately 1.6/1000.[16-18] Approximately 25% of fetuses may have antepartum and intrapartum risk factors for neurologic injury. Box 8-2 lists the criteria required to define an acute intrapartum hypoxic event as sufficient to cause cerebral palsy.[16,17,19]

The ability of contemporary obstetricians to recognize and treat pregnancies at risk during labor is an evolving science. With the current understanding of pathophysiology and the contemporary technology used clinically, the extent to which obstetricians can prevent intrapartum injury is unclear. It is hoped that a clearer definition of intrapartum injury will lead to more precise identification of fetuses at risk and allow the development of strategies and interventions that can correct reversible pathophysiology.

Efforts to understand placental physiology and pathophysiology are central to the efforts to support the health of the pregnant woman and her fetus, both antepartum and intrapartum. The fetus depends on the placenta for the diffusion of nutrients and for respiratory gas exchange. Many factors affect placental transfer, including concentration gradients, villus surface area, placental permeability, and placental metabolism (see Chapter 4). Maternal hypertensive disease, congenital anomalies, and intrauterine infection are examples of conditions that may impair placental transfer.

One of the most important determinants of placental function is uterine blood flow.[20] A uterine contraction results in a transient decrease in uteroplacental blood flow. A placenta with borderline function before labor may be unable to maintain gas exchange adequate to prevent fetal asphyxia during labor. The healthy fetus may compensate for the effects of hypoxia during labor.[21,22] The compensatory response includes (1) decreased oxygen consumption, (2) vasoconstriction of nonessential vascular beds, and (3) redistribution of blood flow to the vital organs (e.g., brain, heart, adrenal glands, placenta).[23,24] Humoral responses (e.g., release of epinephrine from the adrenal medulla, release of vasopressin and endogenous opioids) may enhance fetal cardiac function during hypoxia.[20]

Prolonged or severe hypoxia overwhelms these compensatory mechanisms, resulting in fetal injury or death.

INTRAPARTUM FETAL ASSESSMENT

Electronic Fetal Heart Rate Monitoring

An optimal, yet practical method for assessing fetal health during labor and delivery has not been developed.[25] Most contemporary methods include assessment of the FHR. The FHR can be monitored intermittently with a simple DeLee stethoscope. Alternatively, either Doppler ultrasonography or a fetal electrocardiography (ECG) electrode can be used to monitor the FHR intermittently or continuously.

Experimental models have provided insight into the regulation of the FHR. Both neuronal and humoral factors affect the intrinsic FHR. Parasympathetic outflow by means of the vagus nerve decreases the FHR, whereas sympathetic activity increases FHR and cardiac output.[20] Baroreceptors respond to increased blood pressure and chemoreceptors respond to decreased $Pa{O_2}$ and increased $Pa{CO_2}$ to modulate the FHR through the autonomic nervous system. Cerebral cortical activity and hypothalamic activity affect the FHR through their effects on integrative centers in the medulla oblongata (Figure 8-1).[20] Both animal studies and clinical observations have helped establish a correlation between FHR and perinatal outcome.

An electronic monitor simultaneously records the FHR and uterine contractions. Use of an electronic monitor allows determination of the **baseline rate** and **patterns** of the FHR and their relationship to uterine contractions. External or internal techniques can assess the FHR and uterine contractions (Figure 8-2). Doppler ultrasonography detects the changes in ventricular wall motion and blood flow in major vessels during each cardiac cycle. The monitor calculates the FHR by measuring the intervals between fetal myocardial contractions. Alternatively, an ECG lead attached to the fetal scalp enables the cardiotachometer to calculate the FHR by measuring each successive R-R interval. Both external and internal methods allow continuous assessment of the FHR.

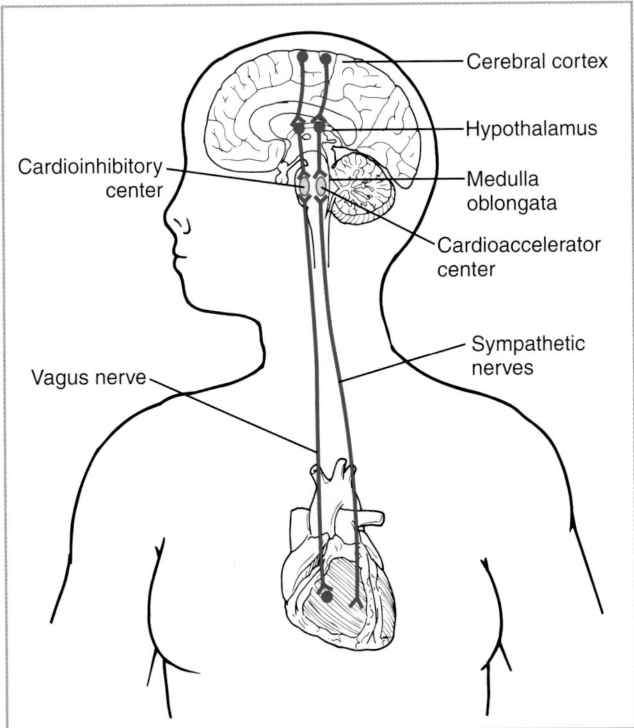

FIGURE 8-1 Regulation of fetal heart rate. (Redrawn from Parer JT. Physiological regulation of fetal heart rate. JOGN Nurs 1976; 5:26S-9S.)

The FHR is superimposed over the uterine contraction pattern. Uterine contractions can be monitored externally with a tocodynamometer or internally with an intrauterine pressure catheter. The tocodynamometer allows determination of the approximate onset, duration, and offset of each uterine contraction. An intrauterine pressure catheter must be used to determine the strength of uterine contractions. In some cases, an intrauterine pressure catheter is needed to determine the precise onset and offset of each uterine contraction. Such information may be needed to distinguish among early, variable, and late FHR decelerations.

The following features of the FHR pattern can be assessed: (1) **baseline** measurements, (2) **variability** (the extent to which the rate changes both instantaneously and over longer periods), and (3) **periodic changes** (i.e., patterns of acceleration or deceleration) and their association with uterine contractions.

BASELINE FETAL HEART RATE

A normal baseline FHR is defined as 110 to 160 beats per minute (bpm) and is determined by assessing the mean heart rate over a 10-minute period rounded to increments of 5 bpm.[26] In general, term fetuses have a lower baseline FHR than preterm fetuses because of greater parasympathetic nervous system activity. Laboratory studies suggest that bradycardia (caused by increased vagal activity) is the initial fetal response to acute hypoxemia. After prolonged hypoxemia, the fetus may experience tachycardia as a result of catecholamine secretion and sympathetic nervous system activity.[22] Changes in baseline FHR may also be caused by fetal anatomic or functional heart pathology, maternal fever and/or intrauterine infections, or maternally administered medications, such as the beta-adrenergic receptor agonist terbutaline (given to treat preterm labor) or the anticholinergic agent atropine.

FETAL HEART RATE VARIABILITY

Fetal heart rate variability is the fluctuation in the FHR of 2 cycles or greater per minute.[25,27] Previously, FHR variability was divided into *short term* (from one beat, or R wave, to the next) and *long term* (occurring over the course of 1 minute), but this distinction is no longer made because in clinical practice variability is visually assessed as a unit (Figure 8-3). The presence of normal FHR variability reflects the presence of normal, intact pathways from—and within—the fetal cerebral cortex, midbrain, vagus nerve, and cardiac conduction system (see Figure 8-1).[20] Variability is greatly influenced by the parasympathetic tone, by means of the vagus nerve; maternal administration of atropine, which readily crosses the placenta, can eliminate some variability. In humans, the sympathetic nervous system appears to have a lesser role in influencing variability.[20] Maternal administration of the beta-adrenergic receptor antagonist propranolol has little effect on FHR variability.[20]

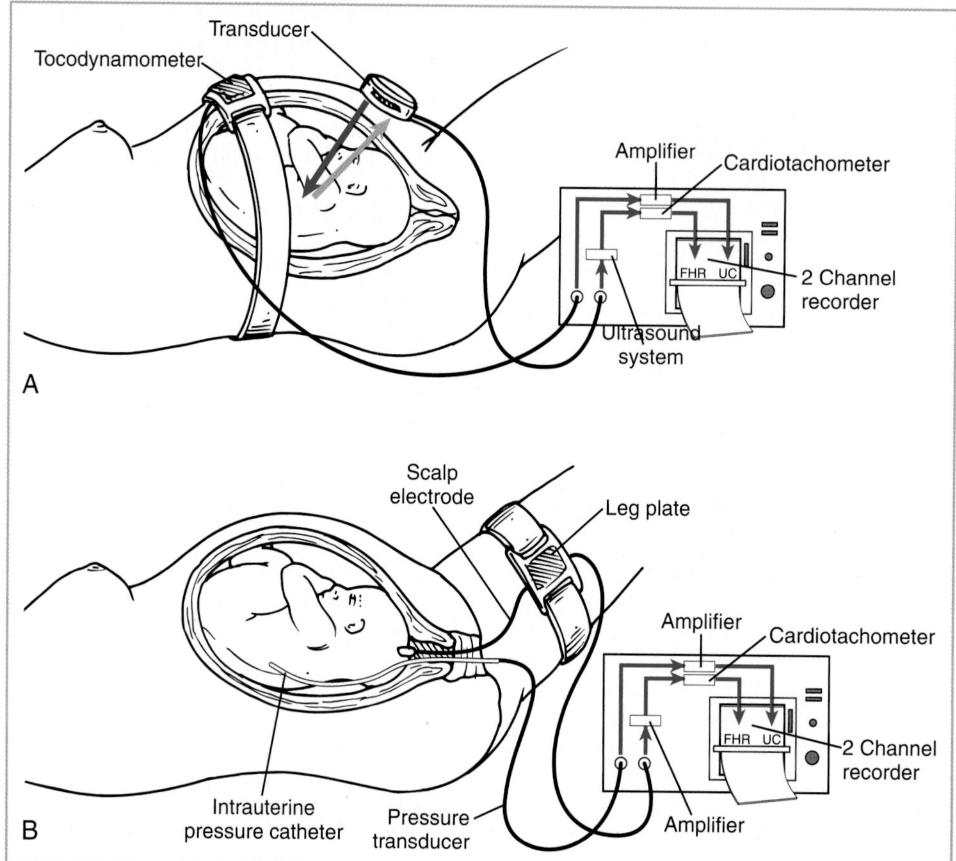

FIGURE 8-2 Electronic fetal monitoring apparatus. **A,** Instrumentation for external monitoring. Contractions are detected by the pressure-sensitive tocodynamometer, amplified, and then recorded. The fetal heart rate (FHR) is monitored with the Doppler ultrasound transducer, which emits and receives the reflected ultrasound signal that is then counted and recorded. **B,** Techniques used for direct monitoring of FHR and uterine contractions (UC). Uterine contractions are assessed with an intrauterine pressure catheter connected to a pressure transducer. This signal is then amplified and recorded. The fetal electrocardiogram (ECG) is obtained by direct application of the scalp electrode, which is then attached to a leg plate on the mother's thigh. The signal is transmitted to the monitor, where it is amplified, counted by the cardiotachometer, and recorded. (Redrawn from Reiss RE, Gabbe SG, Petrie RH. Intrapartum fetal evaluation. In Gabbe SG, Niebyl JR, Simpson JL, editors. Obstetrics: Normal and Problem Pregnancies. 3rd edition. New York, Churchill Livingstone, 1996:401-2.)

During hypoxemia, myocardial and cerebral blood flows increase to maintain oxygen delivery.[28,29] With severe hypoxemia, however, blood flow cannot increase sufficiently to maintain oxygen delivery. The decompensation of cerebral blood flow and oxygen delivery results in a loss of FHR variability.[20] The absence of variability in an anencephalic fetus also suggests that the presence of FHR variability reflects the integrity of the central nervous system (CNS). In animal models, perfusion of the CNS with calcium results in depolarization of electroencephalographic (EEG) activity, which abolishes FHR variability.

Clinically, the presence of normal FHR variability predicts early neonatal health, as defined by an Apgar score of greater than 7 at 5 minutes.[30,31] In a case series of monitored fetal deaths, no fetus had normal variability immediately before demise.[20] The differential diagnosis of decreased variability includes fetal hypoxia, fetal sleep state, fetal neurologic abnormality, and decreased CNS activity that results from exposure to drugs such as opioids.

PERIODIC CHANGES

Periodic FHR changes include accelerations and early, late, or variable decelerations. **Early decelerations** occur simultaneously with uterine contractions and usually are less than 20 bpm below baseline. The onset and offset of each deceleration coincides with the onset and offset of the uterine contraction (see Figure 8-3). In animal models, head compression can precipitate early decelerations.[22] In humans, early decelerations are believed to result from reflex vagal activity secondary to mild hypoxia. Early decelerations are not ominous.

Late decelerations begin 10 to 30 seconds after the beginning of uterine contractions, and end 10 to 30 seconds after the end of uterine contractions. Late decelerations are smooth and repetitive (i.e., they occur with each uterine contraction). Animal studies suggest that late decelerations represent a response to hypoxemia. The delayed onset of the deceleration reflects the time needed for the chemoreceptors to detect decreased oxygen tension and mediate the change in FHR by means of the vagus nerve.[22,32] Late decelerations may also result from decompensation of the myocardial circulation and myocardial failure. Unfortunately, clinical and animal studies suggest that late decelerations may be an oversensitive indication of fetal asphyxia.[22] However, the combination of late decelerations and decreased or absent FHR variability is an accurate, ominous signal of fetal compromise.[21,33,34]

Variable decelerations vary in depth, shape, and duration. They often are abrupt in onset and offset. Variable decelerations result from baroreceptor- or chemoreceptor-mediated vagal activity. Experimental models and clinical studies suggest that **umbilical cord occlusion,** either partial or complete, results in variable decelerations. During the second stage of labor, variable decelerations may result from compression of the fetal head. In this situation, dural stimulation leads to increased vagal discharge.[35] The healthy fetus can typically tolerate mild to moderate variable decelerations (not below 80 bpm) without decompensation. With prolonged, severe variable decelerations (less than 60 bpm) or persistent fetal bradycardia, it is difficult for the fetus to maintain cardiac output and umbilical blood flow.[35]

During the antepartum period, the heart rate of the healthy fetus accelerates in response to fetal movement. Antepartum FHR **accelerations** signal fetal health, and their presence indicates a reactive nonstress test. During the intrapartum period, the significance of FHR accelerations is less clear.[22,31] Whereas intrapartum accelerations may indicate a vulnerable umbilical cord in some cases, their presence most commonly precludes the existence of significant fetal metabolic acidosis.

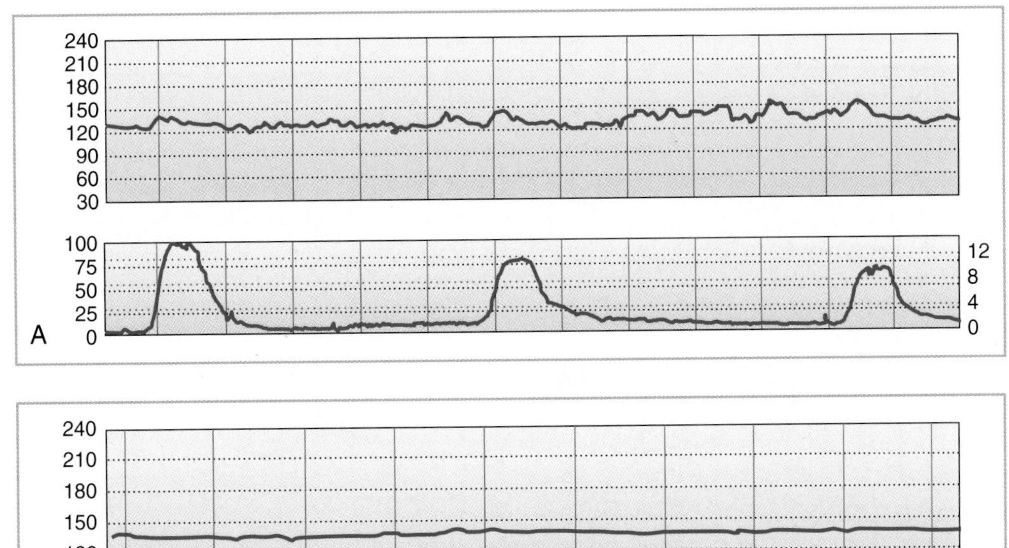

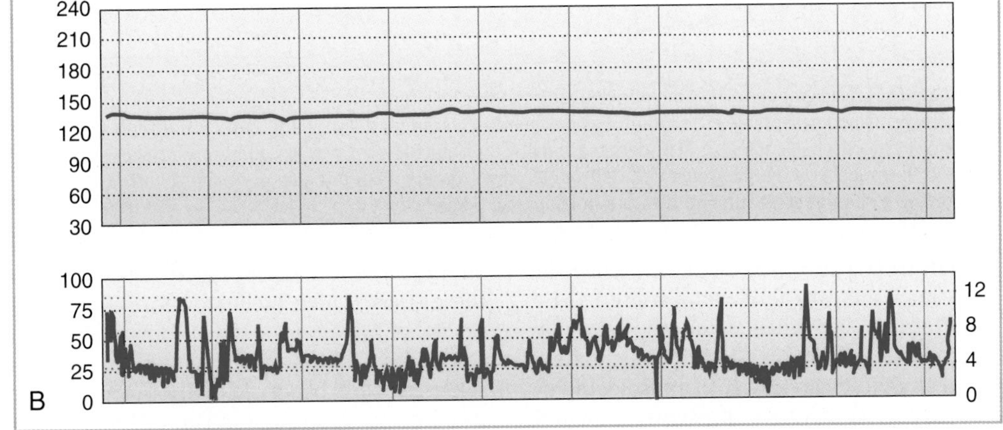

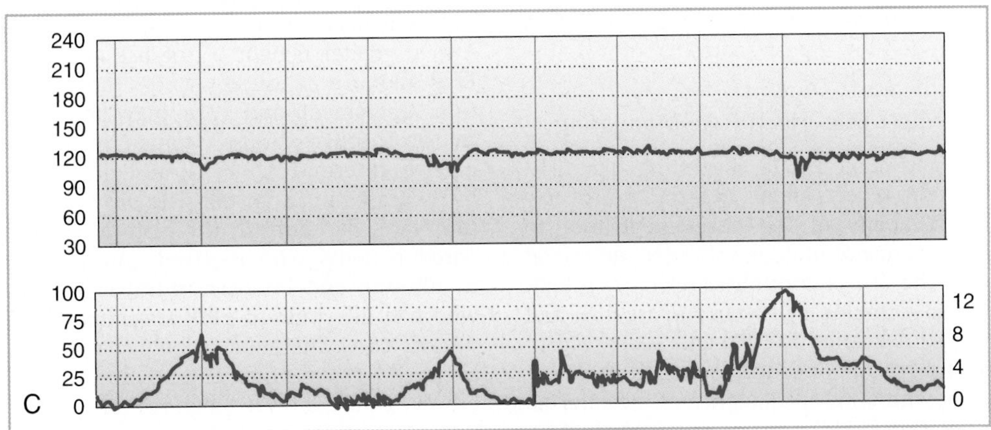

FIGURE 8-3 A, Normal intrapartum fetal heart rate (FHR) tracing. The infant had Apgar scores of 8 and 8 at 1 and 5 minutes, respectively. **B,** Absence of variability in a FHR tracing. Placental abruption was noted at cesarean delivery. The infant had an umbilical arterial blood pH of 6.75 and Apgar scores of 1 and 4, respectively. **C,** Early FHR decelerations. After a normal spontaneous vaginal delivery, the infant had Apgar scores of 8 and 8, respectively.

(Continued)

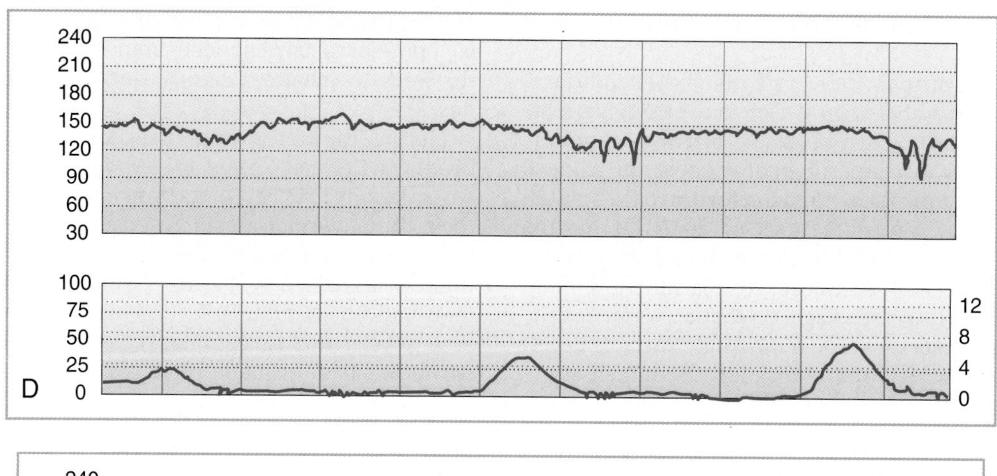

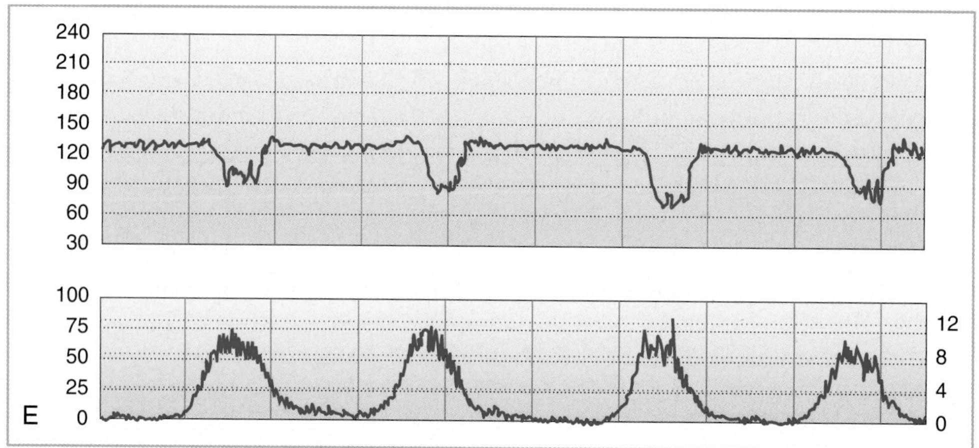

FIGURE 8-3, cont'd D, Late FHR decelerations. The amniotic fluid surrounding this fetus was meconium-stained. Despite the late FHR decelerations, the variability remained acceptable. The infant was delivered by cesarean delivery and had an umbilical venous blood pH of 7.30. Apgar scores were 9 and 9, respectively. **E,** Variable FHR decelerations. A tight nuchal cord was noted at low-forceps vaginal delivery. The infant had Apgar scores of 6 and 9, respectively. Numerical scales: *Left upper panel margin*, FHR in beats per minute; *left lower panel margin*, uterine pressure in mm Hg; *right lower panel margin*, uterine pressure in kilopascal (kPa).

Sinusoidal and **saltatory** patterns are two unusual FHR tracing results that may indicate fetal compromise. The sinusoidal FHR pattern is a regular, smooth, wavelike pattern that may signal fetal anemia.[20] Occasionally, maternal administration of an opioid can lead to a sinusoidal FHR pattern. The saltatory pattern consists of excessive swings in variability (more than 25 bpm) and may signal the occurrence of acute fetal hypoxia; there is a weak association between this pattern and low Apgar scores.[20]

Limitations of Electronic Fetal Heart Rate Monitoring

Despite laboratory and clinical data suggesting that FHR monitoring accurately reflects fetal health, controversy exists regarding the ability of this assessment tool to improve fetal and neonatal outcomes. First described some 40 years ago, the use of continuous electronic FHR monitoring increased dramatically to encompass 45% and 85% of the monitored deliveries by 1980 and 2002, respectively.[25] Retrospective reports of continuous FHR monitoring associate its use with a lower incidence of intrauterine fetal demise, neonatal seizures, and neonatal death.[36-38] By contrast, the only consistent finding from multiple case-control studies and more than a dozen prospective, randomized trials of electronic FHR monitoring (with control arms that employed intermittent FHR auscultation[39-41]) is an increased rate of operative delivery. In a meta-analysis of these trials, which included more than 50,000 women from several continents, a decreased incidence of 1-minute Apgar scores less than 4 and a decreased incidence of neonatal seizures were observed with the use of continuous FHR monitoring.[39-42] These results appear to suggest a correlation between abnormal FHR tracings and fetal acidemia.[34,43]

It remains unclear why prospective studies have not confirmed greater benefit of the use of continuous electronic FHR monitoring during labor; the intensity of intrapartum assessment and care may be partially responsible. In prospective trials, women randomly assigned to receive intermittent FHR auscultation were monitored by dedicated nursing staff who provided intensive intrapartum care. By contrast, the historical cohort studies compared patients who received continuous electronic FHR monitoring and intensive intrapartum care with patients who had intermittent FHR auscultation with *non*intensive nursing care. There are no published studies that randomly assigned a group of patients to receive no FHR monitoring; however, the continued high rate of intrapartum stillbirth in unmonitored births in the developing world suggests that FHR assessment may be beneficial.

Consistent with the results of the prospective trials, the ACOG endorses the use of either intermittent auscultation or continuous electronic FHR monitoring during labor.

In high-risk patients, the ACOG guidelines recommend that the obstetrician or nurse review the electronic FHR tracing every 15 minutes during the first stage of labor and every 5 minutes during the second stage. For low-risk patients, the intervals may be lengthened to 30 minutes for the first stage and 15 minutes for the second stage.[25] The optimal interval for intermittent FHR monitoring has not been studied, but the intervals suggested within the ACOG guidelines have some indirect support.[44] Adherence to these standards for intermittent auscultation may be difficult to achieve in the clinical setting; in one study, only 3% of parturients met this standard.[45]

Several hypotheses to account for the apparent failure of intrapartum FHR monitoring to reduce the incidence of cerebral palsy have been proposed, as follows: (1) a large proportion of the asphyxial damage begins before the onset of labor; (2) catastrophic events (e.g., cord prolapse, placental abruption, uterine rupture) may not allow sufficient time for intervention before neurologic damage occurs; (3) a larger proportion of very low-birth-weight (VLBW) infants survive and thus contribute to the numbers with cerebral palsy; (4) infection is associated with abnormal FHR patterns and the subsequent development of cerebral palsy, and it is unclear that early intervention offers any benefit in such cases; and (5) the amount of asphyxia required to cause permanent neurologic damage approximates the amount that causes fetal death, leaving a narrow window for intervention.[46] The number of patients in whom cerebral palsy develops from intrapartum asphyxia is probably quite small.[46]

Limitations of FHR monitoring include a poor positive predictive value in distinguishing between abnormal FHR tracings and abnormal outcomes. Because of this imprecision, the ACOG has recommended that abnormal FHR tracings be described with the term *nonreassuring fetal status* rather than *fetal distress* or *birth asphyxia*.[47] In one population-based study of California children with cerebral palsy, FHR tracings were retrospectively reviewed and compared with those of neurologically normal children (controls). A markedly higher incidence of tracings with late decelerations and decreased variability was found in children with cerebral palsy than in controls. However, of the estimated 10,791 monitored infants weighing 2500 g or more who had these FHR abnormalities, only 21 (0.19%) had cerebral palsy, representing a false-positive rate of 99.8%.[48] Later case-control studies have yielded similar results.[14,49] Therefore, use of electronic FHR monitoring in combination with clinical and laboratory assessments has been proposed to enhance the prediction and prevention of severe asphyxia.[14]

Further limitations of continuous FHR monitoring include: (1) the poor intraobserver and interobserver agreement despite the use of trained observers,[50] especially when FHR patterns are observed[51,52]; (2) the required continual presence of a nurse or physician to assess the FHR tracing; (3) the inconvenience to the patient (e.g., confinement to bed and the application of monitor belts or a scalp electrode); and (4) the need to maintain the FHR tracings as legal documents.

Despite little evidence for its efficacy, Parer and King[53] have noted that obstetricians continue to heavily rely on FHR monitoring for at least the following three reasons: (1) professional obstetric organizations (e.g., ACOG) advise some form of monitoring during labor, (2) electronic FHR monitoring is logistically easier and less expensive than one-on-one nursing care during labor, and (3) individual (often anecdotal) experiences cause "many obstetricians [to] believe that in their own hands FHR monitoring is . . . efficacious."[53] In an effort to improve the utility of FHR monitoring, a 1997 National Institutes of Health workshop recommended standardization of nomenclature regarding the FHR interpretation, followed by research into the validity of electronic FHR monitoring as a predictor of fetal health.[27] Such research has been directed to include quantitation of abnormal patterns, correlation with short- and long-term outcomes, and evaluation of the role of ancillary techniques of fetal health evaluation.[27,54]

In 2008 the National Institute of Child Health and Human Development sponsored a workshop that resulted in the publication of updated definitions, interpretation, and research guidelines for intrapartum electronic FHR monitoring. The published report[55] proposed a three-tier system for the categorization of FHR patterns:

- **Category I (normal):** Strongly predictive of *normal* fetal acid-base status at the time of observation
- **Category II (indeterminate):** Not predictive of *abnormal* fetal acid-base status, but without adequate evidence to classify as normal or abnormal
- **Category III (abnormal):** Predictive of *abnormal* fetal acid-base status at the time of observation, and thus requiring prompt evaluation[55]

Methods for Improving the Efficacy of Electronic Fetal Heart Rate Monitoring

Several technologies have been employed to enhance the value of electronic FHR monitoring. To facilitate continual FHR assessment, many labor-and-delivery units transmit the tracings from the bedside to the nurses' station. Presumably, this practice facilitates a rapid response to worrisome FHR tracings.

Computerized algorithms may assist in the interpretation of FHR tracings. Although some studies have suggested that computerized analysis may be more accurate than traditional methods in identifying pregnancies with a pathologic neonatal outcome, others have not confirmed this finding.[56-60] As a result, none of these computerized methods has achieved widespread use.

Continuous FHR monitoring requires the patient to wear FHR and uterine contraction monitoring devices and to remain within several feet of the monitor. An alternative is the use of telemetry, which transmits the FHR from the patient to the monitor and consequently allows ambulation. The low-risk patient who wishes to ambulate probably does not require continuous electronic FHR monitoring.

Electronic archiving allows for the electronic storage and retrieval of FHR tracings and eliminates the need for long-term storage of the paper record. The FHR tracing is a medicolegal document, and if it is lost, the plaintiff's lawyer may allege that the tracing was discarded intentionally because it was detrimental to the defendant.[61]

Supplemental Methods of Fetal Assessment

Electronic FHR monitoring is very accurate in the identification of a healthy fetus and in the prediction of the birth of a healthy infant. It is more than 99% accurate in predicting a 5-minute Apgar score higher than 7. Unfortunately, electronic FHR monitoring suffers from a lack of specificity; an abnormal FHR tracing has a false-positive rate of more than 99%.[25] Adding other fetal assessment tools may help identify the compromised fetus with greater specificity.

An older method used to confirm or exclude the presence of fetal acidosis when FHR monitoring suggests the presence of fetal compromise is the **fetal scalp blood pH determination**. Suggested indications include the presence of decreased or absent FHR variability or persistent late or variable FHR decelerations.[20] The obstetrician inserts an endoscope into the vagina, makes a small laceration in the fetal scalp (or buttock), and uses a capillary tube to collect a sample of fetal capillary blood (Figure 8-4). The obstetrician cannot perform this procedure if there is minimal cervical dilation. Relative contraindications include (1) the presence of intact membranes and an unengaged vertex presentation; (2) fetal coagulopathy (which entails the potential for fetal exsanguination); (3) infection, such as chorioamnionitis, human immunodeficiency virus, or herpes simplex virus (disruption of the fetal scalp allows a portal of entry for infection); and (4) an anticipated need for many samples, which might result in significant fetal trauma.[20] The technical challenges of obtaining the sample and having readily available instrumentation to conduct the test have led many centers to abandon this technique.

In general, a fetal scalp blood pH measurement more than 7.25 is acceptable and indicates that the patient may continue to labor. If the FHR tracing abnormalities continue, repeated sampling is recommended approximately every 30 minutes. A pH measurement less than 7.20 is considered abnormal, and delivery should be expedited if the measurement is confirmed by a second pH determination. A pH between 7.20 and 7.25 usually warrants a second scalp pH determination. Interpretation of the fetal scalp blood pH requires consideration of conditions that may give a false-positive result (e.g., abnormalities of the maternal pH, an inadequate sample, contamination with amniotic fluid, sampling from the caput succedaneum). Although early studies suggested that fetal scalp sampling may decrease the cesarean delivery rate,[62] a 1994 study from a clinically active maternity hospital reported that there was no change in the rate of cesarean delivery or perinatal asphyxia when the technique was abandoned.[63]

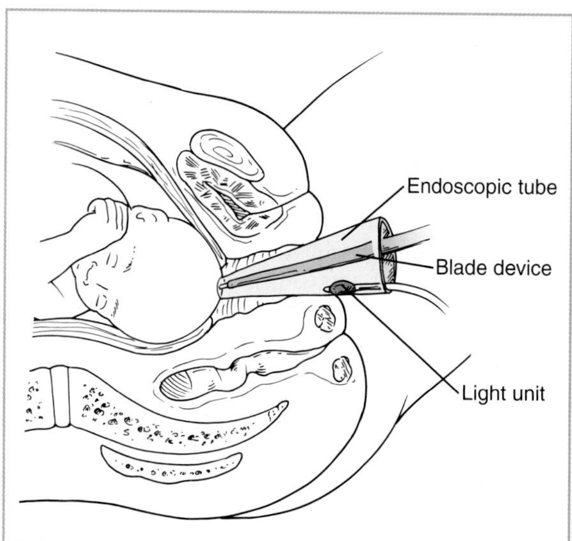

FIGURE 8-4 Technique of obtaining fetal scalp blood during labor. (Redrawn from Creasy RK, Parer JT. Perinatal care and diagnosis. In Rudolph AM, editor. Pediatrics. 16th edition. New York, Appleton-Century-Crofts, 1977:121.)

An alternative to fetal scalp blood sampling is **fetal scalp stimulation** (although fetal scalp blood sampling is a form of fetal scalp stimulation). The fetal scalp can be digitally stimulated during vaginal examination or squeezed with an Allis clamp. The heart rate of a healthy, nonacidotic fetus accelerates in response to scalp stimulation; FHR acceleration is associated with a fetal pH of at least 7.19.[64,65]

Vibroacoustic stimulation is another method for assessing a worrisome FHR tracing. Advocates of this technique contend that the application of an artificial larynx to the maternal abdomen results in an FHR acceleration in a healthy fetus and improves the specificity of FHR monitoring.[66] The use of scalp stimulation or vibroacoustic stimulation has largely replaced the use of fetal scalp blood pH determination in most centers. A meta-analysis of intrapartum stimulation tests (i.e., fetal scalp blood pH determination, Allis clamp scalp stimulation, vibroacoustic stimulation, and digital fetal scalp stimulation) found the tests to be equivalent at predicting fetal acidemia, with digital fetal scalp stimulation having the greatest ease of use.[67]

The intrapartum use of **umbilical artery velocimetry** has been used as an adjunct to FHR monitoring, with mixed results (see Chapter 6).[68,69] Just as the antenatal use of the **biophysical profile (BPP)** decreases the false-positive rate of a positive nonstress test, the BPP has been proposed as a potential tool to assist with intrapartum management.[70,71]

The presence of **meconium-stained amniotic fluid** has long been associated with an increased risk for depression at birth. Moderate to thick meconium is associated with lower Apgar scores, lower umbilical arterial blood pH, an increased incidence of neonatal seizures, and higher rates of cesarean delivery and admission to an intensive care nursery.[72-74] Although approximately 5% to 20% of all deliveries are complicated by meconium-stained amniotic fluid, few of these infants experience neonatal depression. The odds ratio for complications is increased with meconium, but the majority of infants with neonatal complications have clear fluid.[72] Meconium-stained fluid has a poor positive predictive value and poor sensitivity in predicting adverse neonatal outcomes.[72] The physiology associated with the passage of meconium is incompletely understood. Ultrasonographic imaging suggests that the fetus regularly passes rectal contents into the amniotic fluid throughout gestation.[72] However, meconium-stained amniotic fluid is more common in pregnancies complicated by postdatism or intrauterine growth restriction (IUGR). Putative triggers for the passage of meconium include umbilical cord compression and hypoxia. The presence of meconium combined with an abnormal FHR tracing or another risk factor (e.g., IUGR, postdatism) appears to be associated with an increased likelihood of neonatal depression.[73,74]

Among the 5% to 20% of pregnancies with meconium-stained amniotic fluid, the neonatal respiratory compromise termed **meconium aspiration syndrome** develops in approximately 5%.[75-77] Antenatal risk factors for this syndrome include moderate or thick meconium (suggesting recent passage and lower amniotic fluid volume) and abnormal FHR tracings.[76] The lung injury likely originates from intrapartum fetal hypoxia.[76,78,79] Oropharyngeal suctioning at delivery has not proved beneficial[80]; randomized controlled trials have suggested that vigorous neonates do not need aggressive airway cleansing with endotracheal intubation (see Chapter 9).[76] Aggressive management of postdate pregnancies has led to a decreased incidence of meconium-stained amniotic fluid over the past decade.[77]

New Technologies for Fetal Assessment

Because FHR monitoring provides only an *indirect* measure of fetal oxygenation and acid-base status, alternative technologies, such as transcutaneous PO_2, PCO_2, and pH monitors, have been developed to provide a more direct assessment.[81-83] These new monitors, however, are limited by technical difficulties in application of the probe(s), drift of the baseline, artifactual measurements, and a slow response time.

Reflectance pulse oximetry has been adapted for assessment of fetal oxygenation. The U.S. Food and Drug Administration (FDA) has approved the Nellcor N-400 fetal pulse oximeter (Nellcor, Puritan Bennett, Pleasanton, CA) for use in the setting of a term, singleton fetus at more than 36 weeks' gestation with a vertex presentation and a nonreassuring FHR pattern after rupture of membranes.[84,85] The most commonly used probes are held in place against the fetal head or cheek with pressure from the cervix. A reliable pulse oximetry signal can be obtained in 60% to 70% of cases; however, environmental factors and physiologic events (e.g., fetal scalp congestion, thick fetal hair, vernix caseosa, uterine activity, movement artifacts) may affect the accuracy.[85] The saturation measurements are averaged every 45 seconds,[84] with the human fetus typically demonstrating an oxygen saturation of 35% to 65%. Animal and human data suggest that metabolic acidosis does not occur until the oxygen saturation has fallen below 30% for at least 10 minutes as measured with this device.[86,87] Pulse oximetry does not predict acidosis accurately in fetuses with severe variable decelerations during the second stage of labor.[88] Moreover, the accuracy of fetal pulse oximetry readings lower than 30% in human fetuses has been challenged.[84,89] Fetal pulse oximetry used in conjunction with FHR monitoring appears to reduce the rate of cesarean delivery for a nonreassuring FHR tracing; however, this reduction is offset by an increased rate of cesarean delivery for dystocia.[90-92] The absence of an effect on the overall cesarean delivery rate prompted the ACOG to withhold an endorsement of fetal pulse oximetry pending further investigation of its utility.[85]

ST waveform analysis of fetal electrocardiography (ECG) is another technique proposed to enhance intrapartum fetal assessment. Fetal hypoxia induces changes in the ECG morphology of the ST segment and T wave. ST waveform analysis enhances the specificity of FHR tracings,[93,94] but not the sensitivity.[95] A meta-analysis of randomized controlled trials, accounting for almost 10,000 deliveries, of automatic ST waveform analysis (the STAN S21 system, Neoventa Medical, Göteborg, Sweden) demonstrated that a combination of FHR monitoring and ST waveform analysis reduced the risk of severe fetal acidosis and the incidence of newborn infants with encephalopathy.[96-98] No differences in the rates of cesarean delivery, 5-minute Apgar scores less than 7, or admission to the neonatal special care unit were observed.[94,96,97,99,100] Other components of the fetal ECG waveform have also been investigated.[101] Combining computer analysis of FHR tracings with pulse oximetry may improve specificity and sensitivity for the prediction of fetal acidosis.[102]

Near-infrared spectroscopy (NIRS) has the potential to measure fetal cerebral oxygenation directly.[103] NIRS can detect changes in the ratio of reduced to oxygenated cytochrome-*c* oxidase in the brain and in the ratio of oxygenated to deoxygenated hemoglobin in the blood perfusing the brain. This technique can also measure the total amount of hemoglobin in the tissue, which provides an estimate of tissue blood perfusion.[103] In theory, NIRS offers the opportunity to determine whether neurons are at risk for hypoxic damage, and currently, the technique is being correlated with other measures of fetal well-being, such as periodic FHR changes and umbilical cord blood pH measurements at delivery. Similar to fetal pulse oximetry, current NIRS technology is limited by a frequent inability to obtain interpretable measurements (approximately 20% of the time) and the need to correlate the measurements with long-term neurodevelopmental outcomes. Therefore, NIRS remains a research rather than a clinical tool at this time.[103]

Proton magnetic resonance spectroscopy (^{1}H MRS) can obtain metabolic information from the brains of humans and animals, and early investigations suggest an ability to assess fetal brain oxygenation.[104,105] ^{1}H MRS has proved useful in the evaluation of hypoxic-ischemic encephalopathy and metabolic disorders in pediatric patients. This technique can also measure levels of the metabolites *N*-acetylaspartate, creatine, choline, and inositol in fetal and neonatal neural tissue. Although these measurements can be correlated with the level of tissue oxygenation,[106] the clinical utility of this technique as a means of fetal assessment remains unclear.

INTRAPARTUM FETAL THERAPY

The identification of intrapartum fetal compromise should prompt a careful assessment of maternal, placental, and fetal factors. Clinical history, physical findings, laboratory findings, and fetal monitoring (e.g., FHR, ultrasonography) should be used to identify the etiology.

Correctable **maternal factors** that may contribute to fetal compromise include pathologic states that result in hypoxemia or decreased oxygen delivery to the placenta (Table 8-1). **Respiratory failure** due to long-standing diseases (e.g., asthma) can be determined from the history and physical findings, whereas additional laboratory measurements may be necessary to diagnose pneumonia or pulmonary edema as an underlying cause. **Decreased oxygen delivery** to the placenta may result from acute (e.g., sepsis, hypotension) or chronic conditions. **Decreased uteroplacental perfusion** can result from reduced maternal cardiac output (e.g., cardiovascular disease) or chronic vascular disease (e.g., chronic hypertension, diabetes). Dehydration from prolonged labor is a more subtle cause of diminished uteroplacental perfusion.

TABLE 8-1 Intrauterine Treatment for Abnormal Fetal Heart Rate (FHR) Patterns

Causes	Resulting FHR Patterns	Corrective Maneuver	Mechanism
Hypotension (e.g., supine hypotension, neuraxial anesthesia)	Bradycardia, late decelerations	Intravenous fluids, position change, vasopressor (phenylephrine or ephedrine)	Return of uterine blood flow toward normal
Excessive uterine activity (tachysystole)	Bradycardia, late decelerations	Decrease in oxytocin, lateral position, tocolysis (e.g., terbutaline, nitroglycerin)	Return of uterine blood flow toward normal
Transient umbilical cord compression	Variable decelerations	Change in maternal position (e.g., left or right lateral or Trendelenburg position), amnioinfusion	Return of umbilical blood flow toward normal
Head compression, usually during the second stage of labor	Variable decelerations	Pushing only with alternate contractions	Return of umbilical blood flow toward normal
Decreased uterine blood flow associated with uterine contractions, below limits of fetal basal oxygen needs	Late decelerations	Change in maternal position (e.g., left lateral position), administration of supplemental oxygen	Return of uterine blood flow toward normal, increase in maternal-fetal O_2 gradient
		Tocolysis (e.g., terbutaline, nitroglycerin)	Decrease in contractions or uterine tone, thus abolishing the associated drop in uterine blood flow
Prolonged asphyxia	Decreased FHR variability*	Change in maternal position (e.g., left lateral or Trendelenburg position), administration of supplemental oxygen	Return of uterine blood flow toward normal, increase in maternal-fetal O_2 gradient

*During labor, this development is typically preceded by a heart rate pattern that signals asphyxial stress (e.g., late decelerations or a prolonged bradycardia). Such a signal does not necessarily appear in the antepartum period, before the onset of uterine contractions.

Modified from Parer JT. Fetal heart rate. In Creasy RK, Resnik R, editors. Maternal-Fetal Medicine. Philadelphia, WB Saunders, 1989:332.

Attention to the etiology of fetal hypoxemia and institution of appropriate treatments may mitigate fetal compromise. Administration of supplemental oxygen may enhance fetal oxygenation, even in the previously normoxemic mother[107]; however, whether maternal oxygen therapy improves fetal outcome remains unclear.[107-109]

Uterine hypertonus or **frequent uterine contractions (tachysystole),** which may result in decreased uteroplacental perfusion, are known risks of oxytocin or prostaglandin compounds used for the induction of labor. Uterine contractions constrict the uterine spiral arteries, decreasing oxygen delivery to the placenta. A rare cause of fetal compromise is **uterine rupture,** which may result from uterine hyperstimulation, particularly in the setting of a uterine scar. **Placental abruption,** which may result in a partial or complete cessation of oxygen transfer to the fetus, can be associated with chronic or acute diseases. Long-standing vascular diseases produced by chronic hypertension or smoking, as well as acute factors such as cocaine abuse and abdominal trauma, can precipitate a placental abruption.

The treatment of uteroplacental causes of fetal compromise includes correction of uterine hypertonus or tachysystole by cessation of oxytocin infusion (see Table 8-1). Oxytocin has a plasma half-life of 1 to 6 minutes, and consequently, it may take several minutes for the hypertonus to be relieved. Alternatively, a tocolytic agent (e.g., terbutaline, nitroglycerin) may be administered. Normal maternal circulation should be maintained by avoiding aortocaval compression, expanding intravascular volume, and giving a vasopressor (e.g., phenylephrine, ephedrine) if indicated.[110]

Fetal factors may contribute to fetal hypoxemia and acidosis. **Umbilical cord prolapse** through the cervix causes cord compression and often results in sudden fetal bradycardia. In the vast majority of circumstances, treatment of a prolapsed cord consists of manual elevation of the fetal head until emergency cesarean delivery can be accomplished. Only rarely should the umbilical cord be returned into the uterus and expectant care be attempted.[111] Reports from the developing world indicate that, in some cases, expeditious vaginal delivery may produce acceptable neonatal outcome.[112] Alternative methods to decompress a prolapsed umbilical cord include the use of the Trendelenburg position or an infusion of 500 to 700 mL of 0.9% saline into the maternal bladder.[111,113]

Umbilical cord prolapse is not the only cause of **umbilical cord compression**. Much more commonly, such compression occurs within the uterus and manifests as variable FHR decelerations or bradycardia. **Oligohydramnios** is a risk factor for this type of cord compression, and a **change in maternal position** or the use of **saline amnioinfusion** may be therapeutic. Amnioinfusion presumably restores the natural cushion of amniotic fluid, and studies suggest that it reduces the frequency of severe variable decelerations and the incidence of cesarean delivery, and increases the umbilical cord blood pH in women with preterm premature rupture of membranes (PROM), oligohydramnios, or variable decelerations during labor.[114,115] Systematic reviews have produced different conclusions as to whether *prophylactic* intrapartum amnioinfusion in patients with oligohydramnios is superior to *therapeutic* amnioinfusion in patients with both oligohydramnios and FHR abnormalities.[116,117]

Initial studies suggested that in patients with thick, meconium-stained amniotic fluid, amnioinfusion might decrease the incidence of meconium aspiration syndrome and fetal acidosis.[118-120] Later studies, however, have suggested no benefit of amnioinfusion in the setting of meconium unless decelerations due to oligohydramnios are present.[121-125]

Saline amnioinfusion requires a dilated cervix, ruptured membranes, and the placement of an intrauterine catheter. Equipment that allows simultaneous saline amnioinfusion and measurement of intrauterine pressure is preferred. Either normal saline or Ringer's lactate may be infused as a bolus or as a continuous infusion.[26] The ideal rate of infusion has not been determined, but a commonly used regimen consists of a bolus of as much as 800 mL (infused at a rate of 10 to 15 mL/min) followed by either a continuous infusion at a rate of 3 mL/min or repeated boluses of 250 mL, as needed.[26] The necessity of either an infusion pump or a fluid warmer has not been demonstrated.[26] Alleviation of abnormal FHR patterns generally requires 20 to 30 minutes.[26]

Although most studies suggest that amnioinfusion is safe for the mother and fetus, some complications have been reported. Overdistention of the uterus, a higher rate of maternal infections, and respiratory distress, including cases of fatal amniotic fluid embolism, have occurred.[123,126-128] A causal relationship between amniotic fluid embolism and amnioinfusion has yet to be determined. Overdistention of the uterus may be controlled with proper documentation of fluid loss from the uterus during infusion, the provision of amnioinfusion by gravity instead of an infusion pump, and the use of ultrasonography to evaluate the fluid volume.[126]

Maternal fever may increase fetal oxygen consumption. Obstetricians should treat maternal fever with acetaminophen, a cooling blanket, and antibiotics as indicated to maintain maternal and fetal euthermia. **Hyperglycemia** also increases fetal oxygen consumption, so administration of a large bolus of a glucose-containing solution is contraindicated.

Fetal cardiac failure results in inadequate umbilical blood flow and fetal hypoxemia and acidosis. **Fetal anemia** due to maternal isoimmunization, fetal hemoglobinopathy, or fetal hemorrhage results in diminished fetal oxygen-carrying capacity. There are few options for the treatment of fetal cardiac failure or anemia during labor.

A scheme for categorizing and responding to various findings on the FHR tracing has been proposed, and standardization of FHR tracing interpretation and staged levels of intervention could improve research and future management.[129] If intrapartum assessment suggests the presence of fetal compromise and fetal therapy is unsuccessful, the obstetrician should affect an expeditious, atraumatic delivery.

KEY POINTS

- A normal FHR tracing accurately predicts fetal well-being. An abnormal tracing is not very specific in the prediction of fetal compromise. Exceptions include the fetus with a prolonged bradycardia or the fetus with late FHR decelerations and absence of variability; both suggest a high likelihood of fetal distress.
- Large, prospective, randomized studies have not confirmed that continuous electronic FHR monitoring confers substantial clinical benefit over intermittent FHR auscultation as performed by dedicated labor nurses.
- The specificity of FHR monitoring may be augmented by the use of fetal scalp stimulation, fetal vibroacoustic stimulation, and fetal scalp blood sampling. Pulse oximetry increases the specificity of FHR monitoring but does not reduce the rate of cesarean delivery.
- When possible, FHR resuscitation *in utero* is preferable to emergency delivery of an acidotic fetus.
- Saline amnioinfusion effectively prevents or relieves variable decelerations caused by umbilical cord compression, and it may improve perinatal outcome in patients with oligohydramnios.

REFERENCES

1. Bonham DG, Butler NR. Perinatal Mortality: The First Report of the 1958 British Perinatal Mortality Survey. Edinburgh, Livingstone, 1963.
2. Mattatall FM, O'Connell CM, Baskett TF. A review of intrapartum fetal deaths, 1982 to 2002. Am J Obstet Gynecol 2005; 192:1475-7.
3. Westergaard HB, Langhoff-Roos J, Larsen S, et al. Intrapartum death of nonmalformed fetuses in Denmark and Sweden in 1991: A perinatal audit. Acta Obstet Gynecol Scand 1997; 76:959-63.
4. Dahl LB, Berge LN, Dramsdahl H, et al. Antenatal, neonatal and post neonatal deaths evaluated by medical audit: A population-based study in northern Norway—1976 to 1997. Acta Obstet Gynecol Scand 2000; 79:1075-82.
5. McClure EM, Wright LL, Goldenberg RL, et al. The global network: A prospective study of stillbirths in developing countries. Am J Obstet Gynecol 2007; 197:247.e1-5.
6. Lawn J, Shibuya K, Stein C. No cry at birth: Global estimates of intrapartum stillbirths and intrapartum-related neonatal deaths. Bull World Health Organ 2005; 83:409-17.
7. Juul SE, Aylward E, Richards T, et al. Prenatal cord clamping in newborn *Macaca nemestrina*: A model of perinatal asphyxia. Dev Neurosci 2007; 29:311-20.
8. Brann AW Jr, Myers RE. Central nervous system findings in the newborn monkey following severe in utero partial asphyxia. Neurology 1975; 25:327-38.
9. Bernert G, Hoeger H, Mosgoeller W, et al. Neurodegeneration, neuronal loss, and neurotransmitter changes in the adult guinea pig with perinatal asphyxia. Pediatr Res 2003; 54:523-8.
10. Nesbitt RE Jr, Aubry RH. High-risk obstetrics. II. Value of semiobjective grading system in identifying the vulnerable group. Am J Obstet Gynecol 1969; 103:972-85.
11. Gomez JL, Young BK. A weighted risk index for antenatal prediction of perinatal outcome. J Perinat Med 2002; 30:137-42.

12. Knox AJ, Sadler L, Pattison NS, et al. An obstetric scoring system: Its development and application in obstetric management. Obstet Gynecol 1993; 81:195-9.
13. Koong D, Evans S, Mayes C, et al. A scoring system for the prediction of successful delivery in low-risk birthing units. Obstet Gynecol 1997; 89:654-9.
14. Low JA, Pickersgill H, Killen H, Derrick EJ. The prediction and prevention of intrapartum fetal asphyxia in term pregnancies. Am J Obstet Gynecol 2001; 184:724-30.
15. Gourounti K, Sandall J. Admission cardiotocography versus intermittent auscultation of fetal heart rate: Effects on neonatal Apgar score, on the rate of caesarean sections and on the rate of instrumental delivery—a systematic review. Int J Nurs Stud 2007; 44:1029-35.
16. American College of Obstetricians and Gynecologists. Neonatal encephalopathy and cerebral palsy: Executive summary. Obstet Gynecol 2004; 103:780-1.
17. American College of Obstetricians and Gynecologists Task Force on Neonatal Encephalopathy and Cerebral Palsy. Neonatal Encephalopathy and Cerebral Palsy: Defining the Pathogenesis and Pathophysiology. Washington, DC, American College of Obstetricians and Gynecologists, 2003.
18. Perlman JM. Intrapartum asphyxia and cerebral palsy: Is there a link? Clin Perinatol 2006; 33:335-53.
19. Strijbis EM, Oudman I, van Essen P, MacLennan AH. Cerebral palsy and the application of the international criteria for acute intrapartum hypoxia. Obstet Gynecol 2006; 107:1357-65.
20. Parer JT. Handbook of Fetal Heart Rate Monitoring. 2nd edition. Philadelphia, WB Saunders, 1997.
21. Parer JT, Livingston EG. What is fetal distress? Am J Obstet Gynecol 1990; 162:1421-7.
22. Court DJ, Parer JT. Experimental studies of fetal asphyxia and fetal heart rate interpretation. In Nathanielsz PW, Parer JT, editors. Research in Perinatal Medicine I. Ithaca, NY, Perinatology Press, 1984:113-69.
23. Peeters LL, Sheldon RE, Jones MD Jr, et al. Blood flow to fetal organs as a function of arterial oxygen content. Am J Obstet Gynecol 1979; 135:637-46.
24. Cohn HE, Sacks EJ, Heymann MA, Rudolph AM. Cardiovascular responses to hypoxemia and acidemia in fetal lambs. Am J Obstet Gynecol 1974; 120:817-24.
25. American College of Obstetricians and Gynecologists. Intrapartum fetal heart rate monitoring. ACOG Practice Bulletin No. 70. Washington, DC, ACOG, December 2005. (Replaces Practice Bulletin No. 62, May 2005). (Obstet Gynecol 2005; 106:1453-60.)
26. American College of Obstetricians and Gynecologists. Fetal heart rate patterns: Monitoring, interpretation, and management. ACOG Technical Bulletin No. 207. Washington, DC, July 1995. (Int J Gynaecol Obstet 1995; 51:65-74.)
27. National Institute of Child Health and Human Development Research Planning Workshop. Electronic fetal heart rate monitoring: Research guidelines for interpretation. Am J Obstet Gynecol 1997; 177:1385-90.
28. Jones M Jr, Sheldon RE, Peeters LL, et al. Fetal cerebral oxygen consumption at different levels of oxygenation. J Appl Physiol 1977; 43:1080-4.
29. Fisher DJ, Heymann MA, Rudolph AM. Fetal myocardial oxygen and carbohydrate consumption during acutely induced hypoxemia. Am J Physiol 1982; 242:H657-61.
30. Hammacher K, Huter KA, Bokelmann J, Werners PH. Foetal heart frequency and perinatal condition of the foetus and newborn. Gynaecologia 1968; 166:349-60.
31. Krebs HB, Petres RE, Dunn LJ, et al. Intrapartum fetal heart rate monitoring. I. Classification and prognosis of fetal heart rate patterns. Am J Obstet Gynecol 1979; 133:762-72.
32. Westgate JA, Wibbens B, Bennet L, et al. The intrapartum deceleration in center stage: A physiologic approach to the interpretation of fetal heart rate changes in labor. Am J Obstet Gynecol 2007; 197:236.e1-11.
33. Williams KP, Galerneau F. Intrapartum fetal heart rate patterns in the prediction of neonatal acidemia. Am J Obstet Gynecol 2003; 188:820-3.
34. Sameshima H, Ikenoue T. Predictive value of late decelerations for fetal acidemia in unselective low-risk pregnancies. Am J Perinatol 2005; 22:19-23.
35. Ball RH, Parer JT. The physiologic mechanisms of variable decelerations. Am J Obstet Gynecol 1992; 166:1683-9.
36. Renou P, Chang A, Anderson I, Wood C. Controlled trial of fetal intensive care. Am J Obstet Gynecol 1976; 126:470-6.
37. Paul RH, Huey JR Jr, Yaeger CF. Clinical fetal monitoring: Its effect on cesarean section rate and perinatal mortality: Five-year trends. Postgrad Med 1977; 61:160-6.
38. Yeh SY, Diaz F, Paul RH. Ten-year experience of intrapartum fetal monitoring in Los Angeles County/University of Southern California Medical Center. Am J Obstet Gynecol 1982; 143:496-500.
39. Vintzileos AM, Nochimson DJ, Guzman ER, et al. Intrapartum electronic fetal heart rate monitoring versus intermittent auscultation: A meta-analysis. Obstet Gynecol 1995; 85:149-55.
40. Thacker SB, Stroup DF, Peterson HB. Efficacy and safety of intrapartum electronic fetal monitoring: An update. Obstet Gynecol 1995; 86:613-20.
41. Graham EM, Petersen SM, Christo DK, Fox HE. Intrapartum electronic fetal heart rate monitoring and the prevention of perinatal brain injury. Obstet Gynecol 2006; 108:656-66.
42. Alfirevic Z, Devane D, Gyte GM. Continuous cardiotocography (CTG) as a form of electronic fetal monitoring (EFM) for fetal assessment during labour. Cochrane Database Syst Rev 2006; (3):CD006066.
43. Sameshima H, Ikenoue T, Ikeda T, et al. Unselected low-risk pregnancies and the effect of continuous intrapartum fetal heart rate monitoring on umbilical blood gases and cerebral palsy. Am J Obstet Gynecol 2004; 190:118-23.
44. Vintzileos AM, Nochimson DJ, Antsaklis A, et al. Comparison of intrapartum electronic fetal heart rate monitoring versus intermittent auscultation in detecting fetal acidemia at birth. Am J Obstet Gynecol 1995; 173:1021-4.
45. Morrison JC, Chez BF, Davis ID, et al. Intrapartum fetal heart rate assessment: Monitoring by auscultation or electronic means. Am J Obstet Gynecol 1993; 168:63-6.
46. Freeman RK. Problems with intrapartum fetal heart rate monitoring interpretation and patient management. Obstet Gynecol 2002; 100:813-26.
47. American College of Obstetricians and Gynecologists Committee on Obstetric Practice. Inappropriate use of the terms fetal distress and birth asphyxia. ACOG Committee Opinion No. 197. Washington, DC, ACOG, February 1998. (Replaces Committee Opinion No. 137, April 1994). (Int J Gynaecol Obstet 1998; 61:309-10.)
48. Nelson KB, Dambrosia JM, Ting TY, Grether JK. Uncertain value of electronic fetal monitoring in predicting cerebral palsy. N Engl J Med 1996; 334:613-8.
49. Larma JD, Silva AM, Holcroft CJ, et al. Intrapartum electronic fetal heart rate monitoring and the identification of metabolic acidosis and hypoxic-ischemic encephalopathy. Am J Obstet Gynecol 2007; 197:301.e1-8.
50. Palomaki O, Luukkaala T, Luoto R, Tuimala R. Intrapartum cardiotocography—the dilemma of interpretational variation. J Perinat Med 2006; 34:298-302.
51. Figueras F, Albela S, Bonino S, et al. Visual analysis of antepartum fetal heart rate tracings: Inter- and intra-observer agreement and impact of knowledge of neonatal outcome. J Perinat Med 2005; 33:241-5.
52. Blix E, Oian P. Interobserver agreements in assessing 549 labor admission tests after a standardized training program. Acta Obstet Gynecol Scand 2005; 84:1087-92.
53. Parer JT, King T. Fetal heart rate monitoring: Is it salvageable? Am J Obstet Gynecol 2000; 182:982-7.
54. Parer JT, King T, Flanders S, et al. Fetal acidemia and electronic fetal heart rate patterns: Is there evidence of an association? J Matern Fetal Neonatal Med 2006; 19:289-94.
55. Macones GA, Hankins GDV, Spong CY, Hauth J. The 2008 National Institute of Child Health and Human Development Workshop Report on Electronic Fetal Monitoring: Update on Definitions, Interpretation, and Research Guidelines. Obstet Gynecol 2008; 112:661-6.

56. Tongsong T, Iamthongin A, Wanapirak C, et al. Accuracy of fetal heart-rate variability interpretation by obstetricians using the criteria of the National Institute of Child Health and Human Development compared with computer-aided interpretation. J Obstet Gynaecol Res 2005; 31:68-71.
57. Giannubilo SR, Buscicchio G, Gentilucci L, et al. Deceleration area of fetal heart rate trace and fetal acidemia at delivery: A case-control study. J Matern Fetal Neonatal Med 2007; 20:141-4.
58. Georgoulas G, Stylios CD, Groumpos PP. Predicting the risk of metabolic acidosis for newborns based on fetal heart rate signal classification using support vector machines. IEEE Trans Biomed Eng 2006; 53:875-84.
59. Agrawal SK, Doucette F, Gratton R, et al. Intrapartum computerized fetal heart rate parameters and metabolic acidosis at birth. Obstet Gynecol 2003; 102:731-8.
60. Salamalekis E, Hintipas E, Salloum I, et al. Computerized analysis of fetal heart rate variability using the matching pursuit technique as an indicator of fetal hypoxia during labor. J Matern Fetal Neonatal Med 2006; 19:165-9.
61. Phelan JP. Confronting medical liability. Contemp Obstet Gynecol 1991; 36:70-81.
62. Young DC, Gray JH, Luther ER, Peddle LJ. Fetal scalp blood pH sampling: Its value in an active obstetric unit. Am J Obstet Gynecol 1980; 136:276-81.
63. Goodwin TM, Milner-Masterson L, Paul RH. Elimination of fetal scalp blood sampling on a large clinical service. Obstet Gynecol 1994; 83:971-4.
64. Clark SL, Gimovsky ML, Miller FC. The scalp stimulation test: A clinical alternative to fetal scalp blood sampling. Am J Obstet Gynecol 1984; 148:274-7.
65. Rice PE, Benedetti TJ. Fetal heart rate acceleration with fetal blood sampling. Obstet Gynecol 1986; 68:469-72.
66. Smith CV, Nguyen HN, Phelan JP, Paul RH. Intrapartum assessment of fetal well-being: A comparison of fetal acoustic stimulation with acid-base determinations. Am J Obstet Gynecol 1986; 155:726-8.
67. Skupski DW, Rosenberg CR, Eglinton GS. Intrapartum fetal stimulation tests: A meta-analysis. Obstet Gynecol 2002; 99:129-34.
68. Ogunyemi D, Stanley R, Lynch C, et al. Umbilical artery velocimetry in predicting perinatal outcome with intrapartum fetal distress. Obstet Gynecol 1992; 80:377-80.
69. Dawes GS, Moulden M, Redman CW. Short-term fetal heart rate variation, decelerations, and umbilical flow velocity waveforms before labor. Obstet Gynecol 1992; 80:673-8.
70. Tongprasert F, Jinpala S, Srisupandit K, Tongsong T. The rapid biophysical profile for early intrapartum fetal well-being assessment. Int J Gynaecol Obstet 2006; 95:14-7.
71. Kim SY, Khandelwal M, Gaughan JP, et al. Is the intrapartum biophysical profile useful? Obstet Gynecol 2003; 102:471-6.
72. Greenwood C, Lalchandani S, MacQuillan K, et al. Meconium passed in labor: How reassuring is clear amniotic fluid? Obstet Gynecol 2003; 102:89-93.
73. Nathan L, Leveno KJ, Carmody TJ 3rd, et al. Meconium: A 1990s perspective on an old obstetric hazard. Obstet Gynecol 1994; 83:329-32.
74. Berkus MD, Langer O, Samueloff A, et al. Meconium-stained amniotic fluid: Increased risk for adverse neonatal outcome. Obstet Gynecol 1994; 84:115-20.
75. Halliday HL. Endotracheal intubation at birth for preventing morbidity and mortality in vigorous, meconium-stained infants born at term. Cochrane Database Syst Rev 2000; (2):CD000500. (Update in Cochrane Database Syst Rev. 2001; [1]:CD000500.)
76. Wiswell TE, Gannon CM, Jacob J, et al. Delivery room management of the apparently vigorous meconium-stained neonate: Results of the multicenter, international collaborative trial. Pediatrics 2000; 105:1-7.
77. Yoder BA, Kirsch EA, Barth WH, Gordon MC. Changing obstetric practices associated with decreasing incidence of meconium aspiration syndrome. Obstet Gynecol 2002; 99:731-9.
78. Ahanya SN, Lakshmanan J, Morgan BL, Ross MG. Meconium passage in utero: Mechanisms, consequences, and management. Obstet Gynecol Surv 2005; 60:45-56.
79. Ross MG. Meconium aspiration syndrome—more than intrapartum meconium. N Engl J Med 2005; 353:946-8.
80. Vain NE, Szyld EG, Prudent LM, et al. Oropharyngeal and nasopharyngeal suctioning of meconium-stained neonates before delivery of their shoulders: Multicentre, randomised controlled trial. Lancet 2004; 364:597-602.
81. Nickelsen C, Thomsen SG, Weber T. Continuous acid-base assessment of the human fetus during labour by tissue pH and transcutaneous carbon dioxide monitoring. Br J Obstet Gynaecol 1985; 92:220-5.
82. Mueller-Heubach E, Caritis SN, Edelstone DI, et al. Comparison of continuous transcutaneous Po_2 measurement with intermittent arterial Po_2 determinations in fetal lambs. Obstet Gynecol 1981; 57:248-52.
83. Stamm O, Latscha U, Janecek P, Campana A. Development of a special electrode for continuous subcutaneous pH measurement in the infant scalp. Am J Obstet Gynecol 1976; 124:193-5.
84. Stiller R, von Mering R, Konig V, et al. How well does reflectance pulse oximetry reflect intrapartum fetal acidosis? Am J Obstet Gynecol 2002; 186:1351-7.
85. American College of Obstetricians and Gynecologists. Fetal pulse oximetry. ACOG Committee Opinion No. 258. Washington, DC, ACOG, September 2001. (Obstet Gynecol 2001; 98:523-4.)
86. Kuhnert M, Seelbach-Goebel B, Butterwegge M. Predictive agreement between the fetal arterial oxygen saturation and fetal scalp pH: Results of the German multicenter study. Am J Obstet Gynecol 1998; 178:330-5.
87. Nijland R, Jongsma HW, Nijhuis JG, et al. Arterial oxygen saturation in relation to metabolic acidosis in fetal lambs. Am J Obstet Gynecol 1995; 172:810-9.
88. Salamalekis E, Bakas P, Saloum I, et al. Severe variable decelerations and fetal pulse oximetry during the second stage of labor. Fetal Diagn Ther 2005; 20:31-4.
89. Luttkus AK, Lubke M, Buscher U, et al. Accuracy of fetal pulse oximetry. Acta Obstet Gynecol Scand 2002; 81:417-23.
90. East CE, Brennecke SP, King JF, et al. FOREMOST Study Group: The effect of intrapartum fetal pulse oximetry, in the presence of a nonreassuring fetal heart rate pattern, on operative delivery rates: A multicenter, randomized, controlled trial (the FOREMOST trial). Am J Obstet Gynecol 2006; 194:606.e1-16.
91. Kuhnert M, Schmidt S. Intrapartum management of nonreassuring fetal heart rate patterns: A randomized controlled trial of fetal pulse oximetry. Am J Obstet Gynecol 2004; 191:1989-95.
92. Garite TJ, Dildy GA, McNamara H, et al. A multicenter controlled trial of fetal pulse oximetry in the intrapartum management of nonreassuring fetal heart rate patterns. Am J Obstet Gynecol 2000; 183:1049-58.
93. Kwee A, van der Hoorn-van den Beld CW, Veerman J, et al. STAN S21 fetal heart monitor for fetal surveillance during labor: An observational study in 637 patients. J Matern Fetal Neonatal Med 2004; 15:400-7.
94. Luttkus AK, Noren H, Stupin JH, et al. Fetal scalp pH and ST analysis of the fetal ECG as an adjunct to CTG: A multi-center, observational study. J Perinatal Med 2004; 32:486-94.
95. Westerhuis ME, Kwee A, van Ginkel AA, et al. Limitations of ST analysis in clinical practice: Three cases of intrapartum metabolic acidosis. Br J Obstet Gynaecol 2007; 114:1194-201.
96. Ojala K, Vaarasmaki M, Makikallio K, et al. A comparison of intrapartum automated fetal electrocardiography and conventional cardiotocography—a randomised controlled study. Br J Obstet Gynaecol 2006; 113:419-23.
97. Neilson JP. Fetal electrocardiogram (ECG) for fetal monitoring during labour. Cochrane Database Syst Rev 2006; (3):CD000116.
98. Noren H, Amer-Wahlin I, Hagberg H, et al. Fetal electrocardiography in labor and neonatal outcome: Data from the Swedish randomized controlled trial on intrapartum fetal monitoring. Am J Obstet Gynecol 2003; 188:183-92.
99. Vayssiere C, David E, Meyer N, et al. A French randomized controlled trial of ST-segment analysis in a population with abnormal cardiotocograms during labor. Am J Obstet Gynecol 2007; 197:299.e1-6.
100. Su LL, Chong YS, Biswas A. Use of fetal electrocardiogram for intrapartum monitoring. Ann Acad Med Singapore 2007; 36:416-20.

101. Oudijk MA, Kwee A, Visser GH, et al. The effects of intrapartum hypoxia on the fetal QT interval. Br J Obstet Gynaecol 2004; 111:656-60.
102. Salamalekis E, Siristatidis C, Vasios G, et al. Fetal pulse oximetry and wavelet analysis of the fetal heart rate in the evaluation of abnormal cardiotocography tracings. J Obstet Gynaecol Res 2006; 32:135-9.
103. Wolfberg AJ, du Plessis AJ. Near-infrared spectroscopy in the fetus and neonate. Clin Perinatol 2006; 33:707-28.
104. Roelants-van Rijn AM, Groenendaal F, Stoutenbeek P, van der Grond J. Lactate in the foetal brain: Detection and implications. Acta Paediatr 2004; 93:937-40.
105. Borowska-Matwiejczuk K, Lemancewicz A, Tarasow E, et al. Assessment of fetal distress based on magnetic resonance examinations: Preliminary report. Acad Radiol 2003; 10:1274-82.
106. Wolfberg AJ, Robinson JN, Mulkern R, et al. Identification of fetal cerebral lactate using magnetic resonance spectroscopy. Am J Obstet Gynecol 2007; 196:e9-11.
107. Haydon ML, Gorenberg DM, Nageotte MP, et al. The effect of maternal oxygen administration on fetal pulse oximetry during labor in fetuses with nonreassuring fetal heart rate patterns. Am J Obstet Gynecol 2006; 195:735-8.
108. Dildy GA, Clark SL, Loucks CA. Intrapartum fetal pulse oximetry: The effects of maternal hyperoxia on fetal arterial oxygen saturation. Am J Obstet Gynecol 1994; 171:1120-4.
109. Thorp JA, Trobough T, Evans R, et al. The effect of maternal oxygen administration during the second stage of labor on umbilical cord blood gas values: A randomized controlled prospective trial. Am J Obstet Gynecol 1995; 172:465-74.
110. Thurlow JA, Kinsella SM. Intrauterine resuscitation: Active management of fetal distress. Int J Obstet Anesth 2002; 11:105-16.
111. Lin MG. Umbilical cord prolapse. Obstet Gynecol Surv 2006; 61:269-77.
112. Enakpene CA, Omigbodun AO, Arowojolu AO. Perinatal mortality following umbilical cord prolapse. Int J Gynaecol Obstet 2006; 95:44-5.
113. Katz Z, Shoham Z, Lancet M, et al. Management of labor with umbilical cord prolapse: A 5-year study. Obstet Gynecol 1988; 72:278-81.
114. Hofmeyr GJ. Amnioinfusion for umbilical cord compression in labour. Cochrane Database Syst Rev 2000 (2):CD000013.
115. Puertas A, Tirado P, Perez I, et al. Transcervical intrapartum amnioinfusion for preterm premature rupture of the membranes. Eur J Obstet Gynecol Reprod Biol 2007; 131:40-4.
116. Hofmeyr GJ. Prophylactic versus therapeutic amnioinfusion for oligohydramnios in labour. Cochrane Database Syst Rev 1996; (1):CD000176.
117. Pitt C, Sanchez-Ramos L, Kaunitz A, Gaudier F. Prophylactic amnioinfusion for intrapartum oligohydramnios: A meta-analysis of randomized controlled trials. Obstet Gynecol 2000; 96:861-6.
118. Pierce J, Gaudier FL, Sanchez-Ramos L. Intrapartum amnioinfusion for meconium-stained fluid: Meta-analysis of prospective clinical trials. Obstet Gynecol 2000; 95:1051-6.
119. Eriksen NL, Hostetter M, Parisi VM. Prophylactic amnioinfusion in pregnancies complicated by thick meconium. Am J Obstet Gynecol 1994; 171:1026-30.
120. Cialone PR, Sherer DM, Ryan RM, et al. Amnioinfusion during labor complicated by particulate meconium-stained amniotic fluid decreases neonatal morbidity. Am J Obstet Gynecol 1994; 170:842-9.
121. Hofmeyr GJ. Amnioinfusion for meconium-stained liquor in labour. Cochrane Database Syst Rev 2002; (2):CD000014. (Update in: Cochrane Database Syst Rev 2004; [1]:CD000184.)
122. Fraser WD, Hofmeyr J, Lede R, et al. Amnioinfusion for the prevention of the meconium aspiration syndrome. N Engl J Med 2005; 353:909-17.
123. Spong CY, Ogundipe OA, Ross MG. Prophylactic amnioinfusion for meconium-stained amniotic fluid. Am J Obstet Gynecol 1994; 171:931-5.
124. Usta IM, Mercer BM, Aswad NK, Sibai BM. The impact of a policy of amnioinfusion for meconium-stained amniotic fluid. Obstet Gynecol 1995; 85:237-41.
125. American College of Obstetricians and Gynecologists. Amnion infusion does not prevent meconium aspiration syndrome. ACOG Committee Opinion No. 346. Washington, DC, ACOG, October 2006. (Obstet Gynecol 2006;108:1053.)
126. Maher JE, Wenstrom KD, Hauth JC, Meis PJ. Amniotic fluid embolism after saline amnioinfusion: Two cases and review of the literature. Obstet Gynecol 1994; 83:851-4.
127. Dorairajan G, Soundararaghavan S. Maternal death after intrapartum saline amnioinfusion—report of two cases. Br J Obstet Gynecol 2005; 112:1331-3.
128. Dragich DA, Ross AF, Chestnut DH, Wenstrom K. Respiratory failure associated with amnioinfusion during labor. Anesth Analg 1991; 72:549-51.
129. Parer JT, Ikeda T. A framework for standardized management of intrapartum fetal heart rate patterns. Am J Obstet Gynaecol 2007; 197:26.e1-6.

Chapter 9

Neonatal Assessment and Resuscitation

Susan W. Aucott, M.D.
Rhonda L. Zuckerman, M.D.

The transition from intrauterine to extrauterine life represents the most important adjustment that the newborn will make in its life. It is remarkable that this transition occurs uneventfully after most deliveries. Satisfactory transition depends on (1) the anatomic and physiologic condition of the infant at delivery, (2) the ease or difficulty of the delivery itself, and (3) the extrauterine environment. When transition is unsuccessful, prompt assessment and supportive care must be initiated immediately.

At least one person skilled in neonatal resuscitation should be present at every delivery.[1] Available individuals include personnel from the pediatrics, anesthesiology, obstetrics, respiratory therapy, and nursing services. The composition of the resuscitation team varies from place to place, but some type of in-house, 24-hour coverage is essential for all hospitals that have labor and delivery services.[1] The departments of pediatrics, anesthesiology, and obstetrics should participate in the process of ensuring that appropriate personnel and equipment are available for neonatal resuscitation.[2]

All personnel working in the delivery area should receive training in neonatal resuscitation so as to be able to facilitate its prompt initiation when the appointed resuscitation team has not arrived in time for the delivery. The 2005 American Heart Association (AHA) Conference on Cardiopulmonary Resuscitation and Emergency Cardiovascular Care led to the publication of revised guidelines for neonatal resuscitation.[3] Changes in these guidelines reflect the careful review of scientific evidence by members of the American Academy of Pediatrics (AAP), the AHA, and the International Liaison Committee on Resuscitation. The new guidelines have been included in the Neonatal Resuscitation Program (NRP), which is the standardized training and certification program administered by the AAP. The NRP, which was originally sponsored by the AAP and the AHA in 1987, is designed to be appropriate for all personnel who attend deliveries. To ensure the implementation of current guidelines for neonatal resuscitation, the AAP recommends that at least one NRP-certified practitioner attend every delivery.[4]

Both the American Society of Anesthesiologists (ASA) and the American College of Obstetricians and Gynecologists (ACOG) have published specific goals and guidelines for neonatal resuscitation (Box 9-1).[5] The ASA has emphasized that a single anesthesiologist should not be expected to assume responsibility for the concurrent care of both the mother and her child. Rather, a second anesthesia provider or a qualified individual from another service should assume responsibility for the care of the newborn, except in an unforeseen emergency.

In clinical practice, anesthesiologists often are involved in resuscitation of the newborn.[6,7] In 1991, Heyman et al.[6] noted that anesthesia personnel were involved in newborn resuscitation in 99 (31%) of 320 selected Midwestern community hospitals. The individual who administered anesthesia to the mother was also responsible for the care of the newborn in 13.4% of these hospitals. In 6.8% of these institutions, a second anesthesia provider routinely assumed primary responsibility for the infant. In a survey of the obstetric anesthesia workforce in the United States, Hawkins et al.[7] found that fewer anesthesiologists were involved in neonatal resuscitation in 1992 than in 1981,

BOX 9-1 Optimal Goals for Anesthesia Care in Obstetrics: Neonatal Resuscitation

Personnel other than the surgical team should be immediately available to assume responsibility for resuscitation of the depressed newborn. The surgeon and anesthesiologist are responsible for the mother and may not be able to leave her to care for the newborn, even when a neuraxial anesthetic is functioning adequately. Individuals qualified to perform neonatal resuscitation should demonstrate:

- Proficiency in rapid and accurate evaluation of the newborn's condition, including Apgar scoring.
- Knowledge of the pathogenesis of a depressed newborn (acidosis, drugs, hypovolemia, trauma, anomalies, and infection) as well as specific indications for resuscitation.
- Proficiency in newborn airway management, laryngoscopy, endotracheal intubations, suctioning of airways, artificial ventilation, cardiac massage, and maintenance of thermal stability.

In larger maternity units and those functioning as high-risk centers, 24-hour in-house anesthesia, obstetric, and neonatal specialists are usually necessary.

Modified from a joint statement from the American College of Obstetricians and Gynecologists and the American Society of Anesthesiologists. Optimal goals for anesthesia case in obstetrics. Approved by the American Society of Anesthesiologists in October 2008. (See Appendix C for full document.)

although anesthesiologists still provided neonatal resuscitation in 10% of cesarean deliveries.

Even when the anesthesiologist is not primarily responsible for neonatal resuscitation, he or she is often asked to provide assistance in cases of difficult airway management or in emergency cases, when members of the neonatal resuscitation team have not arrived. The anesthesiologist should be prepared to offer assistance to those in charge of neonatal resuscitation, provided that such care does not compromise the care of the mother. A study of University of Pennsylvania residency graduates from 1989 to 1999 revealed that most anesthesiologists were not certified in neonatal resuscitation, although they would have liked to have been.[8] It is hoped that opportunities for anesthesiologists to become NRP-certified will increase; the NRP course is now offered at the annual meeting of the Society for Obstetric Anesthesiology and Perinatology (SOAP).[9]

In the ASA Closed-Claims Database, 13% of obstetric anesthesia malpractice claims were related to neonatal resuscitation.[10] Of the five cases listed, three involved delayed or failed tracheal intubation, and one involved an unrecognized esophageal intubation. A review of obstetric anesthesia–related lawsuits from 1985 to 1993 showed that 12 (17%) of the 69 obstetric anesthesia cases involved claims of inadequate neonatal resuscitation by anesthesia personnel[11]; 10 of these 12 cases resulted in payment to the plaintiff. Written hospital policies should identify the personnel responsible for neonatal resuscitation, and obstetric anesthesia providers should maintain a high level of skill in neonatal resuscitation.

TRANSITION FROM INTRAUTERINE TO EXTRAUTERINE LIFE

Circulation

At birth, the circulatory system changes from fetal circulation (which is in parallel), through a transitional circulation, to adult circulation (which is in series) (Figure 9-1).[12,13] In the fetus, blood from the placenta travels through the umbilical vein and the ductus venosus to the inferior vena cava and the right side of the heart. The anatomic orientation of the inferior vena caval–right atrial junction favors the shunting (i.e., streaming) of this well-oxygenated blood through the foramen ovale to the left side of the heart. This well-oxygenated blood is pumped through the ascending aorta, where branches that perfuse the upper part of the body (e.g., heart, brain) exit proximal to the entrance of the ductus arteriosus.[14] Desaturated blood returns to the heart from the upper part of the body by means of the superior vena cava. The anatomic orientation of the superior vena caval–right atrial junction favors the streaming of blood into the right ventricle. Because fetal pulmonary vascular resistance is higher than systemic vascular resistance (SVR), approximately 90% of the right ventricular output passes through the ductus arteriosus and enters the aorta distal to the branches of the ascending aorta and aortic arch; therefore, less well-oxygenated blood perfuses the lower body, which consumes less oxygen than the heart and brain.

At the time of birth and during the resulting circulatory transition, the amount of blood that shunts through the foramen ovale and ductus arteriosus diminishes, and the flow becomes bidirectional. Clamping the umbilical cord (or exposing the umbilical cord to room air) results in increased SVR. Meanwhile, expansion of the lungs and increased alveolar oxygen tension and pH result in decreased pulmonary vascular resistance.[15,16] Decreased pulmonary vascular resistance allows a greater flow of pulmonary artery blood through the lungs. Increased pulmonary artery blood flow results in improved oxygenation and higher left atrial pressure; the latter leads to a diminished shunt across the foramen ovale. Increased $Pa{O_2}$ and SVR and decreased pulmonary vascular resistance result in a constriction of the ductus arteriosus.[17,18] Together, these changes in vascular resistance result in functional closure of the foramen ovale and the ductus arteriosus. This process does not occur instantaneously, and arterial oxygen saturation ($Sa{O_2}$) remains higher in the right upper extremity (which is preductal) than in the left upper extremity and the lower extremities until blood flow through the ductus arteriosus is minimal.[19] Differences in $Sa{O_2}$ are usually minimal by 10 minutes and absent by 24 hours after birth. Provided that there is no interference with the normal drop in pulmonary vascular resistance, both the foramen ovale and the ductus arteriosus close functionally, and the infant develops an adult circulation (which is in series).

Persistent fetal circulation—more correctly called **persistent pulmonary hypertension of the newborn**—can occur when the pulmonary vascular resistance remains elevated at the time of birth. Factors that may contribute to this problem include hypoxia, acidosis, hypovolemia, and hypothermia.[15,20,21] Maternal use of nonsteroidal anti-inflammatory drugs may also be problematic, because these agents may cause premature constriction of the

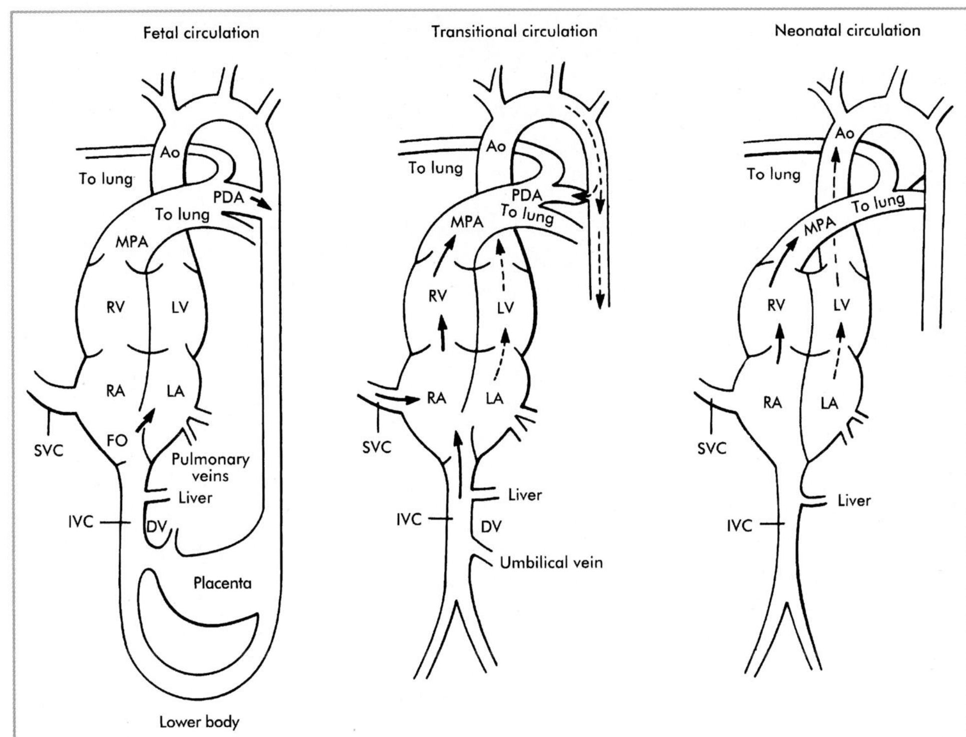

FIGURE 9-1 Transition of the circulation from the fetal to the normal postnatal flow patterns. During the normally short-lived transitional period, the patent ductus arteriosus (PDA) and foramen ovale (FO) may be significant conduits. Ao, aorta; DV, ductus venosus; IVC, inferior vena cava; LV, left ventricle; LA, left atrium; MPA, main pulmonary artery; RA, right atrium; RV, Right ventricle; SVC, superior vena cava. (Adapted from Polin RA, Burg FD. Workbook in Practical Neonatology. Philadelphia, WB Saunders, 1983:156-7.)

ductus arteriosus in the fetus and thus may predispose to persistent pulmonary hypertension of the newborn.[22]

Respiration

Fetal breathing movements have been observed *in utero* as early as 11 weeks' gestation. These movements increase with advancing gestational age, but they are markedly reduced within days of the onset of labor. They are stimulated by hypercapnia and maternal smoking and are inhibited by hypoxia and central nervous system (CNS) depressants (e.g., barbiturates). Under normal conditions, this fetal breathing activity results only in the movement of pulmonary dead space.[23] The fetal lung contains a liquid composed of an ultrafiltrate of plasma, which is secreted by the lungs *in utero*[24]; the volume of this lung liquid is approximately 30 mL/kg. Partial reabsorption of this liquid occurs during labor and delivery, and approximately two thirds is expelled from the lungs of the term newborn by the time of delivery.[25] Small preterm babies and those requiring cesarean delivery may have greater residual lung liquid after delivery. These infants experience less chest compression at delivery than larger infants and infants delivered vaginally; this difference can lead to difficulty in the initiation and maintenance of a normal breathing pattern. Retained fetal lung liquid is the presumed cause of **transient tachypnea of the newborn (TTN)**.[26]

The first breath occurs approximately 9 seconds after delivery. Air enters the lungs as soon as the intrathoracic pressure begins to fall. This air movement during the first breath is important, because it establishes the newborn's functional residual capacity (FRC) (Figure 9-2).

Lung inflation is a major physiologic stimulus for the release of lung surfactant into the alveoli.[27] Surfactant, which is necessary for normal breathing, is present within the alveolar lining cells by 20 weeks' gestation[28] and within the lumen of the airways by 28 to 32 weeks' gestation. However, significant amounts of surfactant do not appear in terminal airways until 34 to 38 weeks' gestation unless surfactant production has been stimulated by chronic stress or maternal corticosteroid administration.[29]

Stress during labor and delivery can lead to gasping efforts by the fetus, which may result in the inhalation of amniotic fluid into the lungs.[30] This event can produce problems if the stress causes the fetus to pass meconium into the amniotic fluid before gasping.

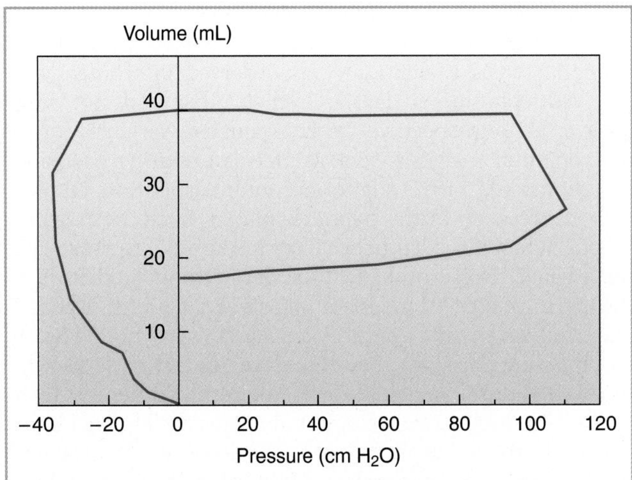

FIGURE 9-2 Typical pressure-volume loop of the first breath. The intrathoracic pressure falls to −30 to −40 cm H_2O, drawing air into the lungs. The expiratory pressure is much greater than the inspiratory pressure. (Modified from Milner AD, Vyas H. Lung expansion at birth. J Pediatr 1982; 101:881.)

Catecholamines

Transition to extrauterine life is associated with a catecholamine surge. Catecholamines may be necessary for the transition process to be successful. In chronically catheterized sheep, catecholamine levels begin to rise a few hours before delivery. At the time of delivery, the catecholamine levels may be higher than at any other time during life.[31] Catecholamines have an important role in the following areas: (1) the production and release of surfactant; (2) the mediation of preferential blood flow to vital organs during the period of stress that occurs during every delivery; and (3) thermoregulation of the newborn.

Thermal Regulation

Thermal stress challenges the newborn in the extrauterine environment. Newborns raise their metabolic rates and release norepinephrine in response to cold; this response facilitates the oxidation of brown fat, which contains numerous mitochondria. The oxidation results in **nonshivering thermogenesis,** the major mechanism for newborn heat regulation.[32] This process may lead to significant oxygen consumption, especially if the newborn has not been dried off and kept in an appropriate thermoneutral environment, such as a radiant warmer. Thermal stress is an even greater problem in infants with low fat stores, such as preterm infants or infants who are small for gestational age (SGA). It is important to maintain a neutral thermal environment (i.e., 34° to 35° C) for newborns. Studies of perinatal brain injury suggest that mild hypothermia may be neuroprotective in the setting of hypoxia-ischemia.[33,34] This therapy must be initiated in the first 6 hours of life in order to provide neuroprotection. Hyperthermia, which may worsen neurologic outcome, should be avoided.[3,35]

Administration of epidural analgesia during labor is associated with an increase in maternal and fetal temperature.[36] Concern has been expressed that the temperature elevation associated with intrapartum epidural analgesia might result in an increase in frequency of neonatal sepsis evaluations.[36,37] In one study, such an increase was observed only when the mother developed fever (body temperature > 38° C).[36] In another study, a higher frequency of neonatal sepsis evaluations was observed in women who received epidural analgesia, even if they did not have fever.[37] A retrospective study evaluated variables other than epidural analgesia, such as preeclampsia/hypertension, gestational age, birth weight, meconium aspiration, respiratory distress at birth, hypothermia at birth, and group B beta-hemolytic streptococcal colonization of the maternal birth canal. These other factors were strong predictors of the performance of neonatal sepsis evaluations, whereas maternal fever and epidural analgesia were not.[38] Many confounding variables may influence results; patients who receive epidural analgesia are inherently different from those who do not receive epidural analgesia. The incidence of actual neonatal sepsis is not higher in term infants whose mothers received epidural analgesia than in infants whose mothers did not receive epidural analgesia. At this time, there is no evidence to suggest that parturients should hesitate to receive epidural analgesia because of concerns about an epidural analgesia–associated rise in maternal temperature.

BOX 9-2 Risk Factors Suggesting a Greater Need for Neonatal Resuscitation

Antepartum Risk Factors

- Maternal diabetes
- Hypertensive disorder of pregnancy
- Chronic hypertension
- Chronic maternal illness (e.g., cardiovascular, thyroid, neurologic, pulmonary, renal)
- Anemia or isoimmunization
- Previous fetal or neonatal death
- Bleeding in second or third trimester
- Maternal infection
- Polyhydramnios
- Oligohydramnios
- Premature rupture of membranes
- Post-term gestation
- Multiple gestation
- Discrepancy between fetal size and dates (i.e., last menstrual period)
- Drug therapy (e.g., lithium carbonate, magnesium, adrenergic-blocking drugs)
- Maternal substance abuse
- Fetal malformation
- Diminished fetal activity
- No prenatal care
- Maternal age < 16 or > 35 years

Intrapartum Risk Factors

- Emergency cesarean delivery
- Forceps or vacuum-assisted delivery
- Breech or other abnormal presentation
- Preterm labor
- Precipitous labor
- Chorioamnionitis
- Prolonged rupture of membranes (> 18 hours before delivery)
- Prolonged labor (> 24 hours)
- Prolonged second stage of labor (> 2 hours)
- Fetal bradycardia
- Nonreassuring fetal heart rate pattern
- Use of general anesthesia
- Uterine tetany
- Maternal administration of opioids within 4 hours of delivery
- Meconium-stained amniotic fluid
- Prolapsed cord
- Placental abruption
- Placenta previa

Adapted from Niermeyer S, Kattwinkel J, Van Reempts P, et al. International Guidelines for Neonatal Resuscitation: An excerpt from the Guidelines 2000 for Cardiopulmonary Resuscitation and Emergency Cardiovascular Care: International Consensus on Science. Pediatrics 2000; 106:E29:1-16.

ANTENATAL ASSESSMENT

Approximately 10% of newborns require some level of resuscitation.[3] The need for resuscitation can be predicted before labor and delivery with approximately 80% accuracy on the basis of a number of antepartum factors (Box 9-2).

Preterm delivery increases the likelihood that the newborn will require resuscitation. When a mother is admitted with either preterm labor or premature rupture of membranes (PROM), plans should be made for neonatal care in the event of delivery. The antenatal assessment of gestational age is based on the presumed date of the last menstrual period, the fundal height, and ultrasonographic measurements of the fetus. Unfortunately, it may be difficult to assess gestational age accurately, because menstrual dates may be unknown or incorrect, the fundal height may be affected by abnormalities of fetal growth or amniotic fluid volume, and ultrasonographic assessment of fetal age is less precise after mid-pregnancy. The assessment of gestational age is most accurate in patients who receive prenatal care early in pregnancy. An accurate approximation of gestational age enables the health care team to plan for the needs of the newborn and to counsel the parents regarding neonatal morbidity and mortality. These plans and expectations must be formulated with caution and flexibility, because the antenatal assessment may not accurately predict the size, maturity, and/or condition of the newborn at delivery.

A variety of **intrauterine insults** can impair the fetal transition from intrauterine to extrauterine life. For example, neonatal depression at birth can result from acute or chronic uteroplacental insufficiency or acute umbilical cord compression. Chronic uteroplacental insufficiency, regardless of its etiology, may result in fetal growth restriction. Fetal hemorrhage, viral or bacterial infection, meconium aspiration, and exposure to opioids or other CNS depressants also can result in neonatal depression. Although randomized trials have not confirmed that fetal heart rate (FHR) monitoring improves neonatal outcome, a nonreassuring FHR tracing is considered a predictor of the need for neonatal resuscitation.[39]

Studies have evaluated the use of fetal pulse oximetry for the evaluation of fetal well-being during labor. This technique involves insertion of a flexible fetal oxygen sensor transcervically until it rests against the fetal cheek. A randomized trial found that use of the fetal pulse oximeter in conjunction with FHR monitoring led to a reduction in the number of cesarean deliveries performed because of a nonreassuring FHR tracing.[40] However, an increase in the number of cesarean deliveries performed for dystocia was seen in the fetal pulse oximeter group, so that the overall cesarean delivery rates were no different in the two groups. The concern was raised that the probe might predispose to dystocia. Consequently the ACOG recommended further study before fetal pulse oximetry is used in clinical practice, because of the potential for higher cost without any improvement in outcome.[41] A meta-analysis of five trials also concluded that there was some benefit to fetal pulse oximetry in the presence of a nonreassuring FHR tracing, but the use of fetal pulse oximetry did not lead to an overall reduction in the cesarean delivery rate.[42]

Infants with **congenital anomalies** (e.g., tracheoesophageal fistula, diaphragmatic hernia, CNS and cardiac malformations) may need resuscitation and cardiorespiratory support. Improved ultrasonography allows for the antenatal diagnosis of many congenital anomalies and other fetal abnormalities (e.g., nonimmune hydrops). Obstetricians should communicate knowledge or suspicions regarding these entities to those who will provide care for the newborn in the delivery room to allow the resuscitation team to make specific resuscitation plans.

In the past, infants born by either elective or emergency cesarean delivery were considered more likely to require resuscitation than infants delivered vaginally. Later evidence suggests that repeat cesarean deliveries and cesarean deliveries performed for dystocia—in patients without FHR abnormalities—result in the delivery of infants at low risk for neonatal resuscitation, especially when those cesarean deliveries are performed with neuraxial anesthesia.[43,44] However, infants born through elective repeat cesarean delivery are at higher risk for subsequent respiratory problems (e.g., transient tachypnea of the newborn) than similar infants whose mothers had a trial of labor before cesarean delivery.[45] Emergency cesarean delivery is considered a risk factor for the need for neonatal resuscitation.

ASSESSMENT OF THE NEWBORN

Apgar Score

Resuscitative efforts typically precede the performance of a thorough physical examination of the newborn. Because NRP instructions require simultaneous assessment and treatment, it is important that assessment of the newborn be both simple and sensitive. In 1953, Dr. Virginia Apgar, an anesthesiologist, described a simple method for the assessment of the newborn that could be performed while care was being delivered.[46] She developed this system to provide a standardized and relatively objective method of assessing the newborn's clinical status. Dr. Apgar suggested that this scoring system would differentiate between infants who require resuscitation and those who need only routine care.[47]

The Apgar score is based on five parameters that are assessed at 1 and 5 minutes after birth. Further scoring at 5- or 10-minute intervals may be done if initial scores are low. The parameters are heart rate, respiratory effort, muscle tone, reflex irritability, and color. A score of 0, 1, or 2 is assigned for each of these five entities (Table 9-1). A total score of 8 to 10 is normal; a score of 4 to 7 indicates moderate impairment; and a score of 0 to 3 signals the need for immediate resuscitation. Dr. Apgar emphasized that this system does not replace a complete physical examination and serial observation of the newborn for several hours after birth.[48]

The Apgar score is widely used to assess newborns, although its value has been questioned repeatedly. The scoring system may help predict mortality and neurologic morbidity in *populations* of infants, but Dr. Apgar cautioned against the use of the Apgar score to make these predictions in an *individual* infant. She noted that the risk of neonatal mortality was inversely proportional to the 1-minute score.[48] In addition, the 1-minute Apgar score was a better predictor of mortality within the first 2 days of life than within 2 to 28 days of life.

Several studies have challenged the notion that a low Apgar score signals perinatal asphyxia. In a prospective study of 1210 deliveries, Sykes et al.[49] noted a poor correlation between the Apgar score and the umbilical cord blood pH. Several studies, including those of low-birth-weight (LBW) infants, have found that a low Apgar

TABLE 9-1 Apgar Scoring System

Parameter	Score 0	1	2
Heart rate (bpm)	Absent	< 100	> 100
Respiratory effort	Absent	Irregular, slow, shallow, or gasping respirations	Robust, crying
Muscle tone	Absent, limp	Some flexion of extremities	Active movement
Reflex irritability (nasal catheter, oropharyngeal suctioning)	No response	Grimace	Active coughing and sneezing
Color	Cyanotic	Acrocyanotic (trunk pink, extremities blue)	Pink

bpm, beats per minute.

Adapted from Tabata BK. Neonatal resuscitation. In Rogers MC, editor. Current Practice in Anesthesiology. 2nd edition. St. Louis, Mosby, 1990:368.

score is a poor predictor of neonatal acidosis, although a high score is reasonably specific for the exclusion of the presence of severe acidosis.[50-56] By contrast, the fetal biophysical profile has a good correlation with the acid-base status of the fetus and the newborn (see Chapter 6).[57] The biophysical profile includes performance of a nonstress test (NST) and ultrasonographic evaluation of fetal tone, fetal movement, fetal breathing movements, and amniotic fluid volume.[57]

Other studies that have evaluated the relationship between Apgar scores and neurologic outcome suggest that Apgar scores are poor predictors of long-term neurologic impairment.[58,59] The Apgar score is more likely to predict a poor neurologic outcome when the score remains 3 or less at 10, 15, and 20 minutes. However, when a child has cerebral palsy, low Apgar scores alone are not adequate evidence that perinatal hypoxia was responsible for the neurologic injury.

The ACOG Task Force on Neonatal Encephalopathy and Cerebral Palsy published criteria for defining an intrapartum event sufficient to cause cerebral palsy.[60] An Apgar score of 0 to 3 beyond 5 minutes of age is not included in the list of "essential criteria"; rather, it is one of five criteria that "collectively suggest an intrapartum timing (within close proximity to labor and delivery . . .) but are nonspecific to asphyxial insults."[60-65]

In a retrospective analysis of 151,891 singleton infants born at 26 weeks' gestation or later between 1988 and 1998, Casey et al.[66] examined the relationship between Apgar scores and neonatal death rates during the first 28 days of life. The highest relative risk for neonatal death was observed in infants with an Apgar score of 3 or less at 5 minutes of age. The 5-minute Apgar score was a better predictor of neonatal death than the umbilical arterial blood pH. In term infants, the relative risk was eight times higher in infants with a 5-minute Apgar score of 3 or less than in those with an umbilical arterial blood pH of 7.0 or less.[66,67] In preterm infants, lower 5-minute Apgar scores were associated with younger gestational age (i.e., mean score 6.6 ± 2.1 for infants born at 26 to 27 weeks' and 8.7 ± 0.8 for infants born at 34 to 36 weeks' gestation).[66] Similarly, earlier studies found that preterm infants were more likely than term infants to have low 1- and 5-minute Apgar scores, independent of neonatal oxygenation and acid-base status. Respiratory effort, muscle tone, and reflex irritability are the components of the score that are most influenced by gestational age.[68]

The earlier the gestational age, the greater the likelihood of a low Apgar score, even in the presence of a normal umbilical cord blood pH. Preterm infants often require active resuscitation efforts immediately after delivery, and these manipulations may affect the components of the Apgar score. For example, pharyngeal and tracheal stimulation may cause a reflex bradycardia, which affects the heart rate score.[52] In addition, it is difficult to judge respiratory effort during suctioning or endotracheal intubation. Likewise, it is difficult to assess respiratory effort in infants (either preterm or term) who require laryngoscopy for the removal of meconium.

During cases of active neonatal resuscitation, the Apgar scores often are not assigned at the appropriate times; rather, these scores may be assigned retrospectively. In these situations, the individual must rely on recall of the infant's condition at earlier times, introducing inaccuracy. Even if the scores are assigned at the appropriate times, there may be disagreement among the several individuals who are providing care for the infant. To avoid bias, Dr. Apgar recommended that the score be assigned by someone not involved in the care of the mother.

Noninvasive monitoring of newborn heart rate and $Sa{O_2}$ (the latter a more objective criterion than assessment of color) can be accomplished with a pulse oximeter. These measurements, coupled with the other components of the Apgar score (i.e., muscle tone, reflex irritability, respiratory effort) may strengthen the correlations between Apgar scores and other outcome predictors, such as umbilical cord blood pH measurements.[69] Although there is some appeal to the use of objective measurements (e.g., $Sa{O_2}$, heart rate) rather than subjective observations, it should not be inferred that the subjective components of the Apgar score (e.g., muscle tone) are less important than the objective measurements. Also, there are some practical limitations to the usefulness of pulse oximetry in the delivery room (e.g., movement artifact).[19] However, newer-generation pulse oximeters provide more accurate estimations of $Sa{O_2}$ (see later).[70]

In summary, the usefulness of the Apgar score is still being debated more than 50 years after its inception.[66,67,71] The Apgar scoring system is used throughout the world, but its limitations must be kept in mind. Low Apgar scores alone do not provide sufficient evidence of perinatal asphyxia; rather, Apgar scores can be low for a variety of reasons. Preterm delivery, congenital anomalies, neuromuscular diseases, antenatal drug exposure, manipulation at delivery, and subjectivity and error may influence the Apgar score.

Umbilical Cord Blood Gas and pH Analysis

Some obstetricians routinely assess umbilical cord blood gas and pH measurements immediately after delivery. Others obtain these measurements only in cases of neonatal depression. Umbilical cord blood gas and pH measurements reflect the fetal condition immediately before delivery and may be a more objective indication of a newborn's condition than the Apgar score. However, there is a lag between the time that the samples are obtained and the time that analysis is complete; during this interval, decisions must be made on the basis of clinical assessment. In 2006, the ACOG recommended that cord blood gas measurements be obtained in circumstances of cesarean delivery for fetal compromise, low 5-minute Apgar score, severe growth restriction, abnormal FHR tracing, maternal thyroid disease, intrapartum fever, and/or multiple gestation.[72]

Acids produced by the fetus include carbonic acid (produced during oxidative metabolism) and lactic and beta-hydroxybutyric acids (which result primarily from anaerobic metabolism). Carbonic acid, which is often called **respiratory acid,** is cleared rapidly by the placenta as carbon dioxide, provided that placental blood flow is normal. However, metabolic clearance of lactic and beta-hydroxybutyric acids requires hours; thus, these acids are called **metabolic** or **fixed acids**. In the fetus, metabolic acidemia is more ominous than respiratory acidemia, because the former reflects a significant amount of anaerobic metabolism.

The measured components of umbilical cord blood gas analysis are pH, P_{CO_2}, P_{O_2}, and HCO_3^-. Bicarbonate (HCO_3^-) is a major buffer in fetal blood. The measure of change in the buffering capacity of umbilical cord blood is reflected in the delta base, which is also known as the base excess or deficit. This value can be calculated from the pH, P_{CO_2}, and HCO_3^-. Ideally, blood samples from both the umbilical artery and vein are collected. Umbilical artery blood gas measurements represent the fetal condition, whereas umbilical vein measurements reflect the maternal condition and uteroplacental gas exchange. Unfortunately, it may be difficult to obtain blood from the umbilical artery, especially when it is small, as it is in very LBW (VLBW) infants. Caution should be used in the interpretation of an isolated umbilical venous blood pH measurement, which can be normal despite the presence of arterial acidemia.

The blood samples should be drawn and handled properly for accurate measurements to be obtained. The measurements should be accurate, provided that (1) the umbilical cord is double-clamped immediately after delivery[73-75]; (2) the samples are drawn, within 15 minutes of delivery,[76] into a syringe containing the proper amount of heparin[77]; and (3) the samples are analyzed within 30 to 60 minutes.[78-80] The P_{O_2} measurement is more accurate if residual air bubbles are removed from the syringe.

Historically, the normal umbilical cord blood pH measurement was thought to be 7.2 or higher[81,82]; however, investigators have challenged the validity of this number. The assumption that 7.2 was the lower limit of normal made no distinction between umbilical arterial blood and umbilical venous blood, although there are clear differences between the normal measurements for the two.[83] One study noted that the median umbilical arterial blood pH in vigorous infants (those with 5-minute Apgar scores of 7 or higher) was 7.26, with a 2.5th percentile measurement of 7.10.[84] Published studies suggest that the lower limit of normal umbilical arterial blood pH may range from 7.02 to 7.18 (Table 9-2).[49,85-94] Other factors may also influence the umbilical arterial blood pH measurement. A fetus subjected to the stress of labor has lower pH measurements than one born by cesarean delivery without labor.[91] Offspring of nulliparous women tend to have a lower pH than offspring of parous women, a difference that is likely related to a difference in the duration of labor.[95]

Some studies have suggested that preterm infants have a higher incidence of acidemia. Later studies show that term and preterm infants have similar umbilical cord blood gas and pH measurements.[86,87,95] Preterm infants often receive low Apgar scores despite the presence of normal umbilical cord blood gas and pH measurements; therefore, assessment of umbilical cord blood is especially helpful in the evaluation of preterm neonates.

Physicians should use strict definitions when interpreting umbilical cord blood gas and pH measurements. Terms such as "birth asphyxia" should be avoided in most cases.[60] **Acidemia** refers to an increase in the hydrogen ion concentration in the blood. **Acidosis** occurs when there is an increased hydrogen ion concentration in *tissue*. *Asphyxia* is a clinical situation that involves hypoxia (i.e., a decreased level of oxygen in tissue), damaging acidemia, and metabolic acidosis.

When acidemia is present, the type—respiratory, metabolic, or mixed—must be identified (Table 9-3). Metabolic acidemia is more likely to be associated with acidosis than respiratory acidemia and is clinically more significant. Similarly, mixed acidemia with a high P_{CO_2}, an extremely low HCO_3^-, and a high base deficit is more ominous than a mixed acidemia with a high P_{CO_2} but only a slightly reduced HCO_3^- and a low base deficit. Mixed or metabolic acidemia (but not respiratory acidemia) is associated with an increased incidence of neonatal complications and death.[95] In their study of 3506 term neonates, Goldaber et al.[96] noted that an umbilical arterial blood pH measurement less than 7.00 was associated with a significantly higher incidence of neonatal death. All neonatal seizures in their study occurred in infants with an umbilical arterial blood pH less than 7.05. By contrast, a short-term outcome study failed to show a good correlation between arterial blood pH and the subsequent health of an infant.[56] In the previously discussed large study reported by Casey et al.,[66] an umbilical arterial blood pH of 7.0 or less was a poorer predictor of the relative risk of neonatal death during the first 28 days of life than a 5-minute Apgar score of 3 or less. However, 6264 infants were excluded from their study because umbilical arterial

TABLE 9-2 Studies Reporting Umbilical Cord Arterial Blood Gas Measurements*

Study	Sample Size	pH	P_{CO_2}	Bicarbonate	Base Deficit	P_{O_2}
Huisjes and Aarnoudse (1979)[88]	852	7.20 ± 0.09 (7.02-7.38)				
Sykes et al. (1982)[49]	899	7.20 ± 0.08 (7.04-7.36)			8.3 ± 4.0 (0.3-16.3)	
Eskes et al. (1983)[89]	4667	7.23 ± 0.07 7.09-7.37				
Yeomans et al. (1985)[85]	146	7.28 ± 0.05 (7.18-7.38)	49.2 ± 8.4 (32.4-66.0)	22.3 ± 2.5 (17.3-27.3)		
Low (1988)[90]	4500	7.26 ± 0.07 (7.12-7.40)	54.9 ± 9.9 (35.1-74.7)			15.1 ± 4.9 (5.3-24.9)
Ruth and Raivio (1988)[94]	106	7.29 ± 0.07 (7.15-7.43)			4.7 ± 4.0 (−3.3-12.7)	
Thorp et al. (1989)[91]	1694	7.24 ± 0.07 (7.10-7.38)	56.3 ± 8.6 (39.1-73.5)	24.1 ± 2.2 (19.7-28.5)	3.6 ± 2.7 (−1.8-9.0)	17.9 ± 6.9 (4.1-31.7)
Ramin et al. (1989)[86]	1292	7.28 ± 0.07 (7.14-7.42)	49.9 ± 14.2 (21.5-78.3)	23.1 ± 2.8 (17.5-28.7)	3.6 ± 2.8 (−2.0-9.4)	23.7 ± 10.0 (3.7-43.7)
Riley and Johnson (1993)[92]	3522	7.27 ± 0.07 (7.13-7.41)	50.3 ± 11.1 (28.1-72.5)	22.0 ± 3.6 (14.8-29.2)	2.7 ± 2.8 (−2.9-8.3)	18.4 ± 8.2 (2.0-34.8)
Nagel et al. (1995)[93]	1614	7.21 ± 0.09 (7.03-7.39)				

*Data are presented as mean ± 1 SD and (−2 to +2 SD). *Sample size* pertains to cord arterial pH and not necessarily to other parameters. Some studies report selected low-risk populations with normal vaginal deliveries only,[82,83] unselected patients with vaginal deliveries,[89] and unselected nulliparous patients,[88] and others report all deliveries at one hospital.[47,87,90,91]

Adapted from Thorp JA, Dildy BA, Yeomans ER, et al. Umbilical cord blood gas analysis at delivery. Am J Obstet Gynecol 1996; 175:517-22.

blood gas measurements could not be obtained, and these infants had a higher incidence of neonatal death than those for whom blood gas measurements were available (4.5 per 1000 versus 1.2 per 1000, respectively).

According to the ACOG Task Force, an umbilical arterial blood pH less than 7.0 and a base deficit greater than or equal to 12 mmol/L at delivery are considered one part of the definition of an acute intrapartum hypoxic event sufficient to cause cerebral palsy.[60] The base deficit and bicarbonate (the metabolic component) values are the most significant factors associated with neonatal morbidity in newborns with an umbilical arterial blood pH less than 7.0. Ten percent of infants with an umbilical arterial base deficit of 12 to 16 mmol/L have moderate to severe complications, which increases to 40% when the deficit is greater than 16 mmol/L.[72]

TABLE 9-3 Criteria Used to Define Types of Acidemia in Newborns with an Umbilical Arterial pH Measurement Less than 7.20

Classification	P_{CO_2} (mm Hg)	HCO_3^- (mEq/L)	Base Deficit (mEq/L)*
Respiratory	High (> 65)	Normal (≥ 22)	Normal (−6.4 ± 1.9)
Metabolic	Normal (< 65)	Low (≤ 17)	High (−15.9 ± 2.8)
Mixed	High (≥ 65)	Low (≤ 17)	High (−9.6 ± 2.5)

*Means ± SD given in parentheses.

From the American College of Obstetricians and Gynecologists. Assessment of fetal and newborn acid-base status. ACOG Technical Bulletin No. 127. Washington, DC, ACOG, April 1989.

There is a lack of consistent correlation between abnormal FHR patterns and umbilical cord blood gas measurements and newborn outcome.[39] Because the correlation is poor, it is important to remember that a newborn may suffer multi-organ system damage, including neurologic injury, even in the absence of a low pH and a low Apgar score.

As Dr. Apgar emphasized in 1962, the most important components of newborn assessment are a careful physical examination and continued observation for several hours.[48] Additional information can be gained from the antenatal history, Apgar scores, and umbilical cord blood gas and pH measurements, provided that clinicians are aware of the proper methods of interpretation as well as the limitations of these methods of assessment.

Respiration and Circulation

There are some similarities between the initial assessment of the newborn and the initial assessment of an adult who requires resuscitation. In both situations, the physician should give immediate attention to the ABCs of resuscitation (i.e., airway, breathing, circulation).

The normal respiratory rate of the newborn is between 30 and 60 breaths per minute. Breathing should begin by 30 seconds and be regular by 90 seconds of age. The newborn who is not breathing by 90 seconds of age has either primary or secondary apnea. These two distinct apneic states have been observed in a neonatal rhesus monkey model.[12]

During intrauterine surgery, a plastic bag was placed over the fetal head, and intravascular catheters were placed for post-delivery monitoring and blood sampling. After surgery, the fetus was delivered vaginally. Immediately after delivery, gasping motions were observed for approximately 1 minute; this was followed by a 1-minute period of apnea, then 5 minutes of gasping motions, and a final period of apnea. The two periods of apnea have been called primary and secondary (or terminal) apnea.

During **primary apnea,** tactile stimulation of the newborn monkey initiated breathing efforts. This was not the case during **secondary apnea**. The heart rate was low during both periods of apnea; however, blood pressure dropped only during secondary apnea. By the time of the onset of secondary apnea (approximately 8 minutes after birth), the pH was 6.8 and the Pa_{O_2} and Pa_{CO_2} measurements were less than 2 and 150 mm Hg, respectively. This experimental model illustrates two important points. First, distinguishing primary from secondary apnea is not possible unless blood pressure and/or blood gases and pH are measured. Second, by the time secondary apnea has begun, blood gas measurements have deteriorated significantly. Therefore, during evaluation of the apneic newborn, aggressive resuscitation must be initiated promptly if tactile stimulation does not result in the initiation of spontaneous breathing.

Assessment of the adequacy of respiratory function requires comprehensive observation for signs of newborn respiratory distress. These signs include cyanosis, grunting, flaring of the nares, retracting chest motions, and unequal breath sounds. The adequacy of respiratory function can also be assessed by the estimation of Sa_{O_2}. The reliability of pulse oximetry for the assessment of newborn Sa_{O_2} was questioned initially because of concerns about the accuracy of spectrophotometric assessments of fetal hemoglobin and the difficult signal detection caused by the rapidity of the newborn's heart rate.[97-99] Newer-generation pulse oximeters, which employ signal extraction and averaging techniques, provide more reliable measurements than conventional oximeters, especially when poor perfusion, patient movement, and ambient light artifacts are present.[70,100]

Pulse oximetry provides accurate estimates of Sa_{O_2} during periods of stability, but it may overestimate Sa_{O_2} during periods of a rapid decrease in saturation.[101] The Sa_{O_2} (Sp_{O_2}) measurements may fluctuate in the delivery room as a result of the ongoing transition from the fetal to the adult circulation, and it may take more than 10 minutes to achieve a preductal Sa_{O_2} greater than 95% in a healthy term infant. Overall, the newer-generation pulse oximeters reliably provide continuous noninvasive Sa_{O_2} measurements and are useful for monitoring the newborn.[102]

The pulse oximeter sensor should be applied to the newborn's right upper extremity. This extremity receives preductal blood flow (see earlier discussion); therefore, right upper extremity Sa_{O_2} measurements provide a more accurate assessment of CNS oxygenation, because CNS blood flow is also preductal.[19] Sensor placement can be difficult on skin that is wet and that may be covered with vernix caseosa. It may be easier to place the sensor over the right radial artery rather than on a finger, especially in preterm infants.[100]

It is technically difficult to obtain an arterial blood sample from a newborn; thus, neonatal arterial blood samples are rarely obtained in the delivery room. Cannulation of the umbilical artery is useful in infants who will require frequent blood sampling. This procedure often requires the use of microinstruments (especially in preterm and VLBW infants) and the ability to monitor an infant's condition while the infant is obscured from view by surgical drapes; therefore, this procedure is usually performed in the neonatal intensive care unit (NICU).

The normal heart rate in the newborn is 120 to 160 beats per minute (bpm). The heart rate may be greater than 160 bpm in the tiny preterm newborn, but it should be within the range of 120 to 160 bpm by 28 weeks' gestational age. The heart rate can be determined in several ways. The clinician can lightly grasp the base of the umbilical cord to feel the arterial pulsations. (This method cannot be used in situations in which the pulsations become difficult to feel, such as in an infant with a low cardiac output.) Alternatively, the clinician can listen to the apical heartbeat. When either of these two methods is used, the evaluator should tap a hand with each heartbeat so that other members of the resuscitation team are aware of the rate. A third method involves the use of a cardiotachometer, a monitor that detects the heart rate by means of electrodes taped to the chest and emits a sound for each beat. Use of this monitor—unlike the use of the first two methods—eliminates the need for an additional team member.

Measurement of arterial blood pressure is not a priority during the initial assessment and resuscitation of the newborn.[3] However, observation for signs of abnormal circulatory function is considered essential. These signs include cyanosis, pallor, mottled coloring, prolonged capillary refill time, and weakness or absence of pulses in the extremities. One of the causes of abnormal circulatory function is hypovolemia. Hypovolemia should be anticipated in cases of bleeding from the umbilical cord or the fetal side of the placenta or whenever a newborn does not respond appropriately to resuscitation. The hypovolemic newborn may exhibit not only signs of abnormal circulatory function but also tachycardia and tachypnea. (Neonatal hypovolemia usually does not accompany placental abruption, which may cause maternal bleeding or other conditions associated with fetal asphyxia.)

Neurologic Status

The initial neurologic assessment of the newborn requires only simple observation. The newborn should demonstrate evidence of vigorous activity, including crying and active flexion of the extremities. Signs of possible neurologic abnormality include apnea, seizures, hypotonia, and unresponsiveness. Newborns should be assessed for physical signs of hypoxic-ischemic encephalopathy (HIE) (Table 9-4). The different stages of HIE are associated with different outcomes: stage I, good; stage II, moderate; and stage III, poor.[103] Although detailed neurologic assessment is performed after the newborn is transferred to the NICU, assessment of tone, baseline heart rate, respirations, and reflex activity is part of both the Apgar scoring system and the HIE assessment and is made initially in the delivery room.

TABLE 9-4 Stages of Neonatal Hypoxic-Ischemic Encephalopathy

Stage I	Stage II	Stage III
Irritable	Lethargic/obtunded	Coma
Normal respirations	Depressed respirations	Apnea
Hypertonic	Hypotonic	Flaccid
Increased reflexes	Decreased reflexes	Absence of reflexes
No seizures	Occasional seizures	Status epilepticus or nearly isoelectric electroencephalogram
Good outcome	Moderate outcome	Poor outcome

Adapted from Eicher DJ, Wagner C. Update on neonatal resuscitation. J S C Med Assoc 2002; 98:115.

Gestational Age

When assessing a very small newborn whose gestational age appears to be lower than that of viability, the evaluator must consider whether it is appropriate to initiate and maintain resuscitation efforts. The neonatal gestational age is often assessed with the use of the scoring systems described by Dubowitz et al.[104] and Ballard et al.[105] The **Dubowitz system** makes use of an external score based on physical characteristics described previously by Farr et al.[106,107] and a neurologic score. The **Ballard system** uses simplified scoring criteria to assess gestational age. Ballard et al.[105] eliminated certain physical criteria such as edema and skin color because of the unreliability of these criteria in some clinical conditions. In addition, they abbreviated the neurologic criteria, on the basis of observations by Amiel-Tison.[108]

Both the Dubowitz and Ballard scores are most accurate when they are used to estimate gestational age at 30 to 42 hours after delivery rather than during the first several minutes after birth[104,105]; therefore, these scores are of limited value in determining the gestational age immediately after delivery.

These scoring systems are also less accurate in very small, preterm infants. In one study of 100 preterm babies with birth weights less than 1500 g, agreement among antenatal measures of gestational age (e.g., last menstrual period, ultrasonography determination) and postnatal measures (e.g., Dubowitz and Ballard scores) was poor.[109] Both scoring systems overestimated gestational age in this subset of VLBW babies. Ballard et al.[110] refined the Ballard score to provide a more accurate estimate of gestational age in preterm babies (Figure 9-3). The new Ballard score assesses **physical criteria,** such as eyelid fusion, breast tissue, lanugo hair, and genitalia, and **neurologic criteria,** such as wrist "square window." (The square window assessment is performed by flexing the infant's wrist on the forearm and noting the angle between the hypothenar eminence and the ventral aspect of the forearm). Although the new Ballard score may be more accurate than the older score for the assessment of preterm infants, inconsistencies occur with all of these methods. Of particular interest is the observation that fetuses of different racial origin mature at different rates (i.e., black fetuses mature faster than white fetuses), which suggests that gestational-age scoring systems should be race specific.[111]

Another commonly used criterion for the estimation of gestational age is birth weight. Normal values for birth weight are published and readily available.[112] Although birth weight may help physicians estimate the gestational age of an otherwise healthy preterm baby, physicians cannot rely on birth weight to provide an accurate estimate of gestational age in a baby who suffered from intrauterine growth restriction (IUGR) or who is large for gestational age (LGA).

Because of the potential for inaccurate gestational age estimation in the delivery room, it is best not to use these scoring systems to guide decisions regarding the initiation or continuation of neonatal resuscitation immediately after delivery. In most circumstances, the newborn's response to resuscitative efforts is the best indicator as to whether further intervention is warranted.

NEONATAL RESUSCITATION

The equipment and medications needed for neonatal resuscitation are listed in Box 9-3. Equipment, supplies, and medications should be checked regularly to ensure that all components are available and functional.

Care of the newborn ideally begins as soon as the head is delivered, before the baby takes its first breath. First the mouth and then the nose should be suctioned gently with a bulb syringe to remove residual amniotic fluid, mucus, blood, and meconium. (The management of the newborn who has expelled meconium into the amniotic fluid is discussed separately.)

After delivery is complete, the newborn is transferred to the resuscitation area. The availability of sterile blankets allows the individual performing the delivery to remain sterile while transferring the newborn; this issue is especially important during cesarean deliveries. The timing of delivery should be noted, assessment and appropriate resuscitative measures should continue, and Apgar scores should be assigned at the appropriate intervals (Figure 9-4).

The neonatal examination table should be adjustable to allow for 30-degree Trendelenburg and reverse Trendelenburg positioning. The former favors the drainage of secretions, and the latter may increase Pa_{O_2} during spontaneous ventilation.[113] The physician or nurse should promptly dry the skin of a healthy, vigorous baby delivered at term gestation and wrap the baby in a warm, dry blanket. The baby who is delivered preterm or who is depressed should also be placed beneath an overhead radiant warmer, which maintains body temperature while allowing access to the baby during resuscitation. Hypothermia can result in greater oxygen consumption and metabolic acidosis,[114,115] and leads to a significantly higher mortality among preterm infants.[116]

Studies now suggest that selective cerebral hypothermia[117] or whole-body hypothermia[33,34] may protect against brain injury in the asphyxiated infant. This treatment is not yet recommended in the neonatal resuscitation guidelines, because which infants would benefit most from these therapies is unclear. On the other hand, the current guidelines recommend avoidance of hyperthermia.[3]

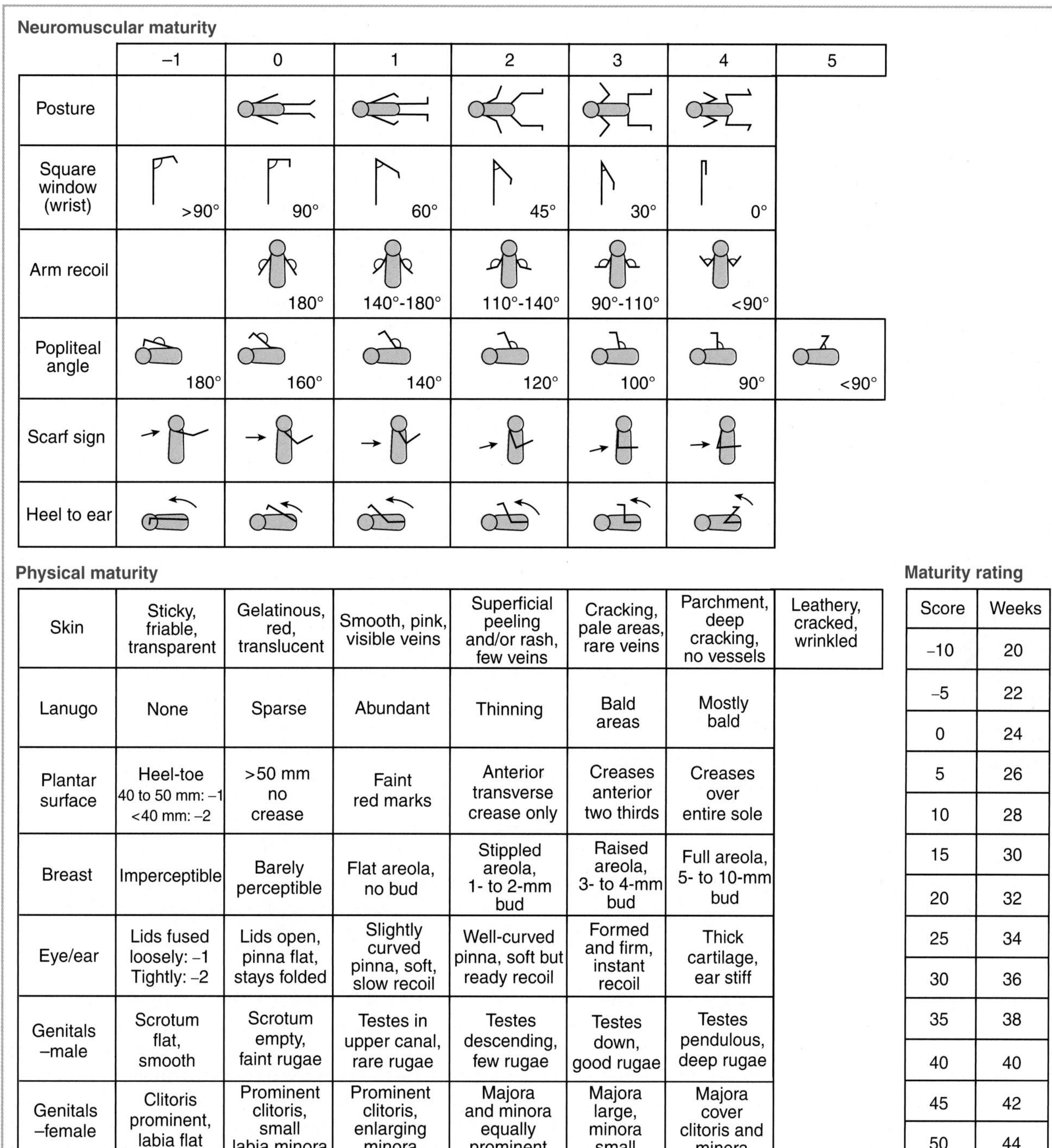

Neuromuscular maturity

	−1	0	1	2	3	4	5
Posture							
Square window (wrist)	>90°	90°	60°	45°	30°	0°	
Arm recoil		180°	140°-180°	110°-140°	90°-110°	<90°	
Popliteal angle	180°	160°	140°	120°	100°	90°	<90°
Scarf sign							
Heel to ear							

Physical maturity

Skin	Sticky, friable, transparent	Gelatinous, red, translucent	Smooth, pink, visible veins	Superficial peeling and/or rash, few veins	Cracking, pale areas, rare veins	Parchment, deep cracking, no vessels	Leathery, cracked, wrinkled
Lanugo	None	Sparse	Abundant	Thinning	Bald areas	Mostly bald	
Plantar surface	Heel-toe 40 to 50 mm: −1 <40 mm: −2	>50 mm no crease	Faint red marks	Anterior transverse crease only	Creases anterior two thirds	Creases over entire sole	
Breast	Imperceptible	Barely perceptible	Flat areola, no bud	Stippled areola, 1- to 2-mm bud	Raised areola, 3- to 4-mm bud	Full areola, 5- to 10-mm bud	
Eye/ear	Lids fused loosely: −1 Tightly: −2	Lids open, pinna flat, stays folded	Slightly curved pinna, soft, slow recoil	Well-curved pinna, soft but ready recoil	Formed and firm, instant recoil	Thick cartilage, ear stiff	
Genitals −male	Scrotum flat, smooth	Scrotum empty, faint rugae	Testes in upper canal, rare rugae	Testes descending, few rugae	Testes down, good rugae	Testes pendulous, deep rugae	
Genitals −female	Clitoris prominent, labia flat	Prominent clitoris, small labia minora	Prominent clitoris, enlarging minora	Majora and minora equally prominent	Majora large, minora small	Majora cover clitoris and minora	

Maturity rating

Score	Weeks
−10	20
−5	22
0	24
5	26
10	28
15	30
20	32
25	34
30	36
35	38
40	40
45	42
50	44

FIGURE 9-3 New Ballard scoring system for clinical assessment of maturation in newborns. This scoring system has been expanded to include extremely preterm infants, and it has been refined to improve the accuracy of assessment of more mature infants. (Adapted from Ballard JL, Khoury JC, Wedig K, et al. New Ballard score, expanded to include extremely premature infants. J Pediatr 1991; 119:418.)

The newborn should be positioned in a way that allows the airway to remain open, with the head in the "sniffing" position (the neck flexed on the chest and the head extended on the neck, thereby aligning the oropharynx, pharynx, and hypopharynx). Additional suctioning of the mouth and nose with a bulb syringe may be necessary if secretions accumulate.

The newborn with a normal respiratory pattern, heart rate, and color requires no further intervention. However, evaluation for choanal atresia can be performed at this time; it is accomplished by gentle insertion of a small suction catheter through each nostril into the nasopharynx. Vigorous nasal suctioning should be avoided, because it can cause trauma to the nasal mucosa and result in progressive edema and airway obstruction. The newborn is an obligate nasal breather; thus, choanal atresia is a potentially lethal anomaly that requires immediate attention. If this anomaly is present (as evidenced by failure of nasal passage of the

BOX 9-3 Equipment and Drugs Needed for Neonatal Resuscitation

Suction Equipment
Bulb syringe
Mechanical suction and tubing
Suction catheters, 5F or 6F, 8F, and 10F or 12F
8F feeding tube and 20-mL syringe
Meconium aspiration device

Bag-and-Mask Equipment
Neonatal resuscitation bag with a pressure-release valve or pressure manometer (the bag must be capable of delivering 90% to 100% oxygen)
Face masks, newborn and preterm sizes (masks with cushioned rim preferred)
Oxygen with flowmeter (flow rate up to 10 L/min) and tubing (including portable oxygen cylinders)

Intubation Equipment
Laryngoscope with straight blades, No. 0 (preterm) and No. 1 (term)
Extra bulbs and batteries for laryngoscope
Tracheal tubes, 2.5, 3.0, 3.5, and 4.0 mm ID
Stylet (optional)
Scissors
Tape or securing device for tracheal tube
Alcohol sponges
CO_2 detector (optional)
Laryngeal mask airway (optional)

Medications
Epinephrine 1:10,000 (0.1 mg/mL), 3- or 10-mL ampules
Isotonic crystalloid (normal saline or Ringer's lactate) for volume expansion, 100 or 250 mL
Sodium bicarbonate 4.2% (5 mEq/10 mL), 10-mL ampules
Naloxone hydrochloride 0.4 mg/mL, 1-mL ampules (or 1.0 mg/ml, 2-mL ampules)
Normal saline, 30 mL
Dextrose 10%, 250 mL
Normal saline "fish" or "bullet" (optional)
Feeding tube, 5F (optional)
Umbilical vessel catheterization supplies:
- Sterile gloves
- Scalpel or scissors
- Povidone-iodine solution
- Umbilical tape
- Umbilical catheters, 3.5F, 5F
- Three-way stopcock

Syringes, 1-, 3-, 5-, 10-, 20-, and 50-mL
Needles, 25-, 21-, and 18-gauge, or puncture device for needleless system

Miscellaneous
Gloves and appropriate personal protection
Radiant warmer or other heat source
Firm, padded resuscitation surface
Clock (timer optional)
Warmed linens
Stethoscope
Tape, ½- or ¾-inch
Cardiac monitor and electrodes and/or pulse oximeter with probe (optional for delivery room)
Oropharyngeal airways

ID, internal diameter.

Adapted from Niermeyer S, Kattwinkel J, Van Reempts P, et al. International Guidelines for Neonatal Resuscitation: An excerpt from the Guidelines 2000 for Cardiopulmonary Resuscitation and Emergency Cardiovascular Care: International Consensus on Science. Pediatrics 2000; 106:E29:1-16.

catheter), an oral airway or endotracheal tube should be inserted, and the newborn should be evaluated for repair of the obstruction. The classic clinical presentation for choanal atresia is an infant with cyanosis and respiratory distress at rest who becomes pink when crying.

Often the newborn has a normal respiratory pattern and heart rate but may not be pink. Acrocyanosis often persists for several minutes after delivery. If the newborn is breathing but not vigorous (i.e., Apgar score less than 8), the administration of supplemental oxygen may be beneficial. It is preferable to use a flow-through system, which does not require positive pressure for the delivery of oxygen. Indeed, administration of "blow-by" oxygen, without positive pressure, is adequate for most newborns.

Tactile stimulation should be used if the newborn does not breathe immediately; this consists of rubbing the back and flicking the soles of the feet. Tactile stimulation does not trigger respiratory efforts during secondary apnea in the newborn. Therefore, if the newborn does not begin to breathe spontaneously after tactile stimulation, the evaluator should begin positive-pressure mask ventilation. If the newborn has an abnormally slow heart rate (i.e., less than 100 bpm), positive-pressure ventilation should be performed until the heart rate rises to the normal range. Overzealous tactile stimulation (e.g., slapping the back) is not useful; it provides no advantage over the more moderate methods and can cause traumatic injury.

High concentrations of oxygen (as opposed to ambient air) can raise production of oxygen free radicals, which have been linked to hypoxia-reoxygenation injury. Additionally, an association between neonatal oxygen supplementation and childhood cancer has been noted when oxygen exposure occurred for 3 minutes or longer.[118,119] Because of these concerns, the use of room air rather than 100% oxygen for neonatal resuscitation has been evaluated.[120,121] In a randomized trial of 609 term infants, no major outcome difference was found between the infants who received 100% oxygen and those who received room air for resuscitation.[121] A meta-analysis of four human trials showed a lower mortality rate with no evidence of harm when resuscitation was performed with room air rather than 100% oxygen.[122] The current guidelines for neonatal resuscitation continue to recommend the use of 100% oxygen for assisted ventilation during neonatal resuscitation but allow for the option of resuscitation with room air. If room air is used, an oxygen source should be available for

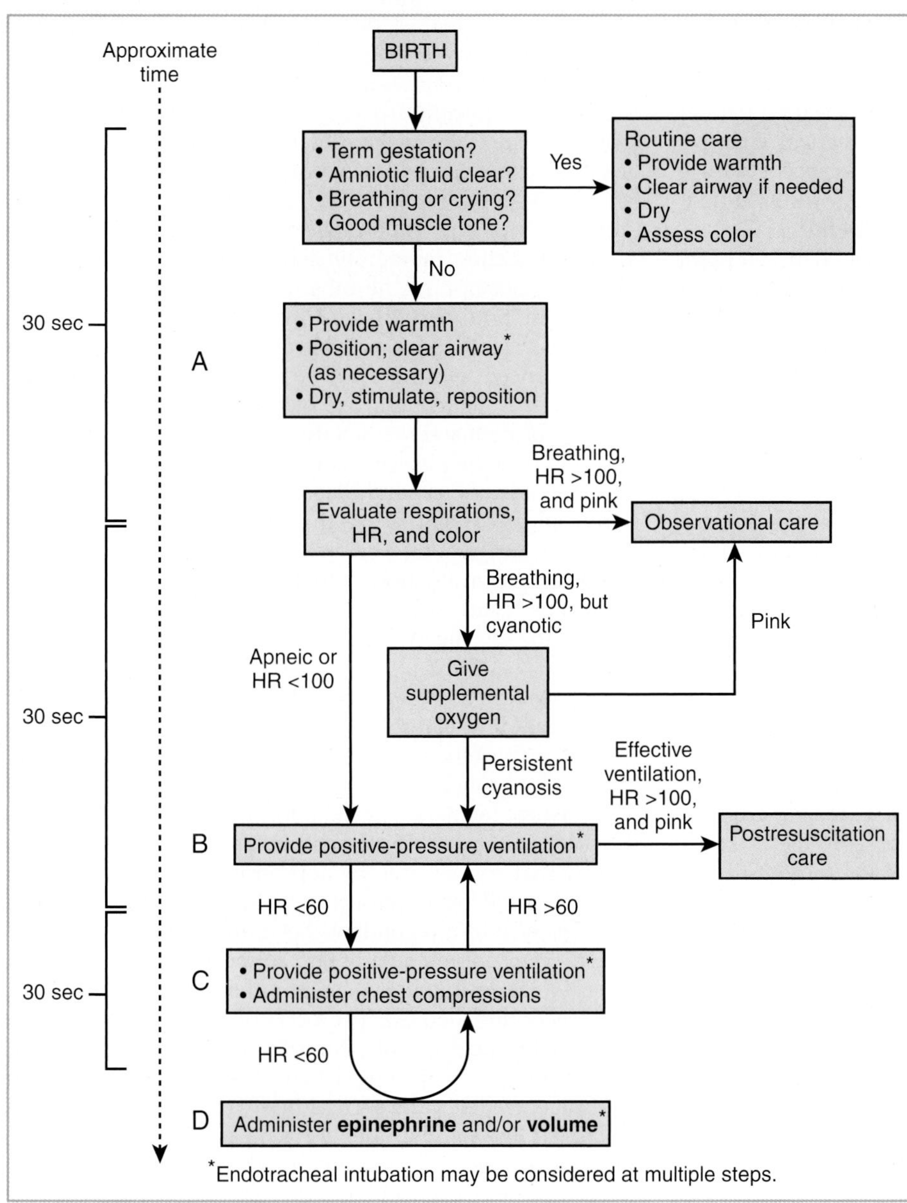

FIGURE 9-4 Algorithm for resuscitation of the newly born infant. HR, heart rate. (From American Heart Association and American Academy of Pediatrics. 2005 American Heart Association guidelines for cardiopulmonary resuscitation (CPR) and emergency cardiovascular care (ECC) of pediatric and neonatal patients: Neonatal resuscitation guidelines. Pediatrics 2006;117;e1029-38.)

use if there is no improvement after 90 seconds. The inspired oxygen concentration should be lowered as soon as possible—especially in preterm newborns—to reduce the risk of retinopathy of prematurity and pulmonary toxicity.[123] Sa_{O_2} measurements of 85% to 92% are thought to be adequate and appropriate for newborns of less than 34 weeks' gestation.[120,121,123]

Positive-pressure ventilation must be performed correctly to ensure that it is effective and does not cause barotrauma. A ventilation bag with a volume of 250 to 500 mL may be used. The circuit must contain a safety pop-off pressure valve (e.g., at 35 cm H_2O), a visible pressure gauge, or both. An oxygen flow rate of 5 to 10 L/min is adequate. Alternatively, a T-piece, which is a valved mechanical device, may be used; it allows more consistent delivery of target inflation pressures and long inspiratory times. The mask must be of appropriate size and shape to ensure a good seal around the nose and mouth. A variety of masks should be available to accommodate infants of all sizes and gestational ages. For the infant with excessive occipital scalp edema (e.g., caput succedaneum), placing a small roll under the shoulders to alleviate hyperflexion of the neck may be helpful.

During the first assisted breath, positive pressure at 30 to 40 cm H_2O should be maintained for 4 to 5 seconds at the end of inspiration to overcome the surface tension of the lungs and open the alveoli.[124] The neonatal response to a large, rapid inflation of the lungs is a sharp inspiration of its own (Head's paradoxical reflex).[2] Subsequent breaths should be delivered at a rate of 40 to 60 per minute, with intermittent inspiratory pauses to prevent the development of atelectasis. The maximum pressure generated should range between 20 and 30 cm H_2O, with an inspiration-to-expiration ratio of approximately 1:1. In preterm infants, whose lungs may be more easily injured, initial inflation pressures of 20 to 25 cm H_2O may be adequate. If mask ventilation is needed for longer than 2 to 3 minutes, the stomach should be emptied with an orogastric catheter. Distention of the stomach with oxygen or air can compromise respiratory function in the newborn. This maneuver should be performed with care, because pharyngeal stimulation can result in arrhythmias and apnea.[125]

The adequacy of respiratory resuscitation can be monitored from observation of its effect on heart rate; an increase in heart rate is the first reliable sign of effective oxygenation. By contrast, changes in color occur slowly and are a relatively poor index of successful resuscitation. Color is also difficult to assess in many newborns.

When the newborn's heart rate is higher than 100 bpm, positive-pressure ventilation can be stopped, and the newborn can be reevaluated for spontaneous respiratory effort. If the newborn does not begin to breathe and if an opioid effect is the suspected etiology, administration of **naloxone** (0.1 mg/kg) may be considered, but it is not recommended as part of the initial resuscitation. Naloxone may be given intravenously, or, if perfusion is adequate, intramuscularly.[3] Naloxone should be given only if it is indicated and with caution, because it can worsen the neurologic damage caused by asphyxia.[126,127] The duration of action of naloxone is shorter than that of many opioids. A newborn who shows response to naloxone requires observation for as long as 24 hours, especially if he or she was exposed to a relatively long-acting opioid or a large dose of opioid *in utero* or both, to avoid recurrent respiratory depression. Use of naloxone is contraindicated in cases of maternal opioid abuse, because the agent can precipitate acute neonatal opioid withdrawal, which may include seizures.

If positive-pressure mask ventilation does not improve oxygenation (as reflected by an increase in heart rate), prompt endotracheal intubation is indicated. Endotracheal intubation must be performed gently to avoid damage to the delicate newborn neck and airway. The size of the newborn's head is large relative to that of its body; therefore, the newborn is in the "sniffing" position when it lies supine. In most cases, it is not necessary to elevate or hyperextend the newborn's head during laryngoscopy. The neonatal larynx is more anterior than that of the adult, and visualization often is easier when cricoid pressure is applied. The practitioner should hold the laryngoscope and apply cricoid pressure with the same hand. The thumb and first two fingers hold the base of the laryngoscope, the third finger rests on the mandible, and the fourth finger applies cricoid pressure. This technique promotes gentleness during airway manipulation. The distance from the gums to the larynx often is surprisingly short. A common mistake is to advance the laryngoscope blade too deeply—past the larynx and into the esophagus. When this error occurs, the larynx falls into view if the laryngoscope blade is withdrawn slowly to allow a second attempt.

The diameter of the endotracheal tube should be large enough to allow adequate ventilation and insertion of a suction catheter (if needed) but small enough to avoid causing trauma and subsequent subglottic stenosis. The ratio of internal diameter to gestational age should be less than 0.1 (e.g., 3.0 mm tube/35 weeks' gestation = 0.09).[128,129]

After endotracheal intubation, positive-pressure ventilation should be resumed by means of an appropriate circuit, as described earlier for mask ventilation. Assessment of proper tube placement is accomplished by listening for breath sounds in both axillae. Exhaled CO_2 detection is the recommended method for confirming placement of the tube in the trachea.[3] False-negative results can occur in situations in which the infant is correctly intubated, with the tube in the trachea, but pulmonary blood flow is poor or absent. This may lead to unnecessary extubation in critically ill infants. As noted previously, the fractional inspired oxygen concentration (F_{IO_2}) should be reduced as soon as possible, especially in the preterm neonate. The addition of a pulse oximeter and an oxygen blender allows more targeted oxygen delivery for the preterm infant immediately after birth. If the endotracheal tube is to remain in the newborn, a chest radiograph should be obtained to confirm the exact position of the tube.

Because both endotracheal intubation and effective bag-and-mask ventilation may be difficult for those who are inexperienced with neonatal resuscitation, some investigators have evaluated the use of the laryngeal mask airway (LMA) for neonatal resuscitation.[130,131] The LMA is blindly inserted into the pharynx, and a cuff is inflated to provide a low-pressure seal around the larynx. This method allows for more effective ventilation than bag-and-mask ventilation but does not require the skill and experience needed for endotracheal intubation. When evaluated in term infants requiring resuscitation at delivery, use of the LMA was found to be highly successful and without complications.[130,131] A 2002 report described the successful use of a size 1 LMA in a preterm newborn (35 weeks' gestation).[132] Endotracheal intubation via direct laryngoscopy was unsuccessful, but intubation was accomplished successfully, with fiberoptic bronchoscopy performed through the LMA. The revised neonatal resuscitation guidelines state that the LMA is an acceptable alternative means of establishing an airway that can be used by appropriately trained providers when bag-and-mask ventilation is ineffective or attempts at endotracheal intubation have been unsuccessful.[3]

One cause of unequal breath sounds and eventual circulatory collapse is tension pneumothorax. Some physicians have recommended that providers of neonatal resuscitation be skilled in needle aspiration of a tension pneumothorax.[2] This maneuver is accomplished by placement of a 22- or 25-gauge needle in the second intercostal space in the midclavicular line (on the side where no breath or heart sounds are heard). Air will rush out of the needle hub, thereby reducing the tension pneumothorax.

In the vast majority of resuscitations, the neonates respond to ventilatory support. Chest compressions are needed in only 0.03% of deliveries.[133] Chest compressions are indicated when the heart rate is less than 60 bpm despite adequate ventilation with supplemental oxygen for 30 seconds.[3]

Chest compressions can be given either with the first two fingers of one hand or with the thumbs of both hands; the latter method generates a better cardiac output and is preferred.[3,134] Pressure is applied over the sternum just below an imaginary line drawn between the nipples; pressure applied over the lower part of the sternum or xiphoid can injure the abdomen. The sternum should be compressed to approximately one-third to one-half the anterior-posterior dimension of the chest, and the compression depth must be adequate to produce a palpable pulse.[3,135-137] The compression time should be slightly shorter than the release time; this may be the best timing for improving blood flow in the very young infant.[138] Ventilation is compromised if the chest is compressed simultaneously with the administration of positive-pressure ventilation. The recommended ratio of compressions to breaths is 3:1.[139,140] This pattern is given at a rate of 120 events per minute, with 90 chest compressions and 30 breaths administered each minute. Respirations, heart rate, and color should be rechecked every 30 seconds. Compressions should be resumed until the heart rate is 60 bpm or higher. Positive-pressure ventilation with supplemental oxygen should be continued until the heart rate is higher than 100 bpm.

Medications are rarely required during neonatal resuscitation, because most newborns who require resuscitative measures respond well to satisfactory oxygenation and ventilation alone.[141] However, a variety of pharmacologic agents should be available in the delivery room (see Box 9-3). **Epinephrine** is the drug recommended for use during neonatal resuscitation.[3] The current recommended practice is to administer epinephrine (0.01 to 0.03 mg/kg or 0.1 to 0.3 mL/kg of a 1:10,000 solution) if the heart rate remains lower than 60 bpm after 30 seconds of adequate ventilation and chest compressions. Intravenous administration is the preferred route (via an umbilical venous line). While access is being established, endotracheal administration may be considered. Administration of epinephrine is especially important if the heart rate is zero. Epinephrine both raises the heart rate (the major determinant of newborn cardiac output) and restores coronary and cerebral blood flow.[142]

Sodium bicarbonate is used infrequently during resuscitation. Because of its high osmolarity, this agent can cause hepatic injury at any gestational age, and cerebral hemorrhage in the preterm newborn[143,144]; it may also compromise myocardial and cerebral function.[145,146] It should be given only during prolonged resuscitation and only when adequate ventilation and circulation have been established. Arterial blood gas measurements and serum chemistry determinations should guide the use of sodium bicarbonate. The current recommended dose is 1 to 2 mEq/kg of a 0.5 mEq/mL solution given over at least 2 minutes by slow intravenous push.

Atropine is no longer recommended for use during the resuscitation of the newborn. Epinephrine is considered the drug of choice for the treatment of bradycardia.

Calcium administration is no longer recommended for neonatal resuscitation, unless it is given specifically to reverse the effect of magnesium (which may have crossed the placenta from the mother to the fetus). Evidence suggests that calcium administration causes cerebral calcification and decreases survival in stressed newborns.[147]

Volume expanders must be given strictly according to recommended dosage. A continuous infusion is dangerous in the newborn, because it can easily result in the administration of an excessive fluid volume. Fluid overload can cause hepatic capsular rupture, brain swelling in the asphyxiated infant, or intracranial hemorrhage in the preterm infant. Fluids and medications can be administered either intravenously (most commonly through the umbilical vein) or, if necessary, intraosseously.

There are at least two ways to cannulate the umbilical vein. The first requires that an ample length of umbilical cord be left attached to the newborn at delivery; this issue should be discussed with the obstetrician before delivery, especially if resuscitation is anticipated. A 20- or 22-gauge catheter can be inserted into the umbilical vein via the same technique that is used to cannulate a peripheral vein. The standard intravenous catheter is relatively stiff; therefore, it must be inserted into the distal cord so that the tip does not extend into the abdomen, where it could cause trauma. The second method involves insertion of a soft catheter into the cut end of the vein (Figure 9-5). The catheter is advanced until blood return is noted, but no more than 2 cm past the abdominal surface. If central venous pressure (CVP) monitoring is required during the newborn's hospital course, the soft umbilical catheter can be advanced through the ductus venosus into the inferior vena cava. Care must be taken to avoid leaving the tip in an intermediate location because of possible hepatic damage if a high-osmolarity substance (e.g., improperly diluted sodium bicarbonate) were injected. Other complications of umbilical venous catheterization are hemorrhage and sepsis.

Intraosseous access is accomplished by insertion of a 20-gauge needle into the proximal tibia approximately 1 cm below the tibial tuberosity.[148] This technique may be easier to perform than umbilical venous cannulation for practitioners who have little experience with intravenous catheterization in the newborn. Absorption from the newborn bone marrow into the general circulation occurs almost immediately.[149-152] This rapid absorption results from the preponderance of red bone marrow over yellow bone marrow, which is less vascular and is the dominant form of marrow after age 5 years. Complications related to this technique are rare and include tibial fracture

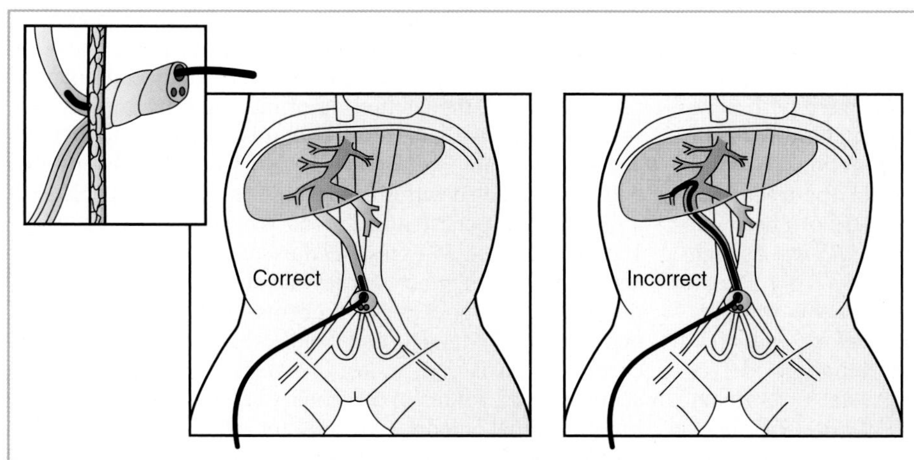

FIGURE 9-5 Cannulation of the umbilical vein. A 3.5F or 5F umbilical catheter with a single end-hole and a radiopaque marker should be used. For emergency use, the catheter should be inserted into the vein of the umbilical stump until the tip of the catheter is just below the skin level but free flow of blood is present. If the catheter is inserted farther, there is a risk of infusing solutions into the liver and possibly causing damage. (Adapted from Kattwinkel J, editor. Textbook of Neonatal Resuscitation. 4th edition. Elk Grove Village, IL, American Heart Association and American Academy of Pediatrics, 2000:6-6.)

(which occurs more often in older children)[153] and osteomyelitis. The risk of infection is proportional to the duration of intraosseous infusion[154-156]; therefore, the needle should be removed after 1 to 2 hours, and if necessary, a more conventional route of access should be established. Current guidelines state that intraosseous access should be used for medication administration or volume expansion when venous access is difficult to achieve.[3]

Volume expanders should be considered when the infant demonstrates signs of shock, such as pale skin, poor perfusion, and weak pulse, or has not shown adequate response to other resuscitative measures. **Normal saline** and **Ringer's lactate** are the preferred volume expanders, given initially at 10 mL/kg over 5 to 10 minutes, with doses repeated as necessary after reassessment for ongoing hypovolemia. Intravascular volume should be assessed through evaluation of heart rate, capillary refill time, and color. If heavy blood loss is suspected, **O-negative packed red blood cells** may be used according to the same dosage regimen.[3] Red blood cells replete the oxygen-carrying capacity as well as the intravascular volume. O-negative blood should be available at all times for emergency use during neonatal resuscitation. Placental blood has been used for newborn volume expansion,[157] but this practice is discouraged in most institutions because of the risks of infection or transfusion of clotted blood. Albumin administration is no longer recommended, because it carries a risk of infectious disease and has been associated with higher mortality.[158]

SPECIAL RESUSCITATION CIRCUMSTANCES

Meconium Aspiration

A great deal of interest has centered on the management of the newborn whose airway has been exposed to meconium-containing amniotic fluid. Meconium is present in the intestinal tract of the fetus after approximately 31 weeks' gestation. Meconium-stained amniotic fluid is present in approximately 10% to 15% of all pregnancies; the incidence is higher in post-term pregnancies. Intrapartum passage of meconium may be associated with fetal stress and hypoxia.[159,160] Among newborns exposed to meconium in the amniotic fluid, as many as 60% have meconium in the trachea.

Meconium aspiration syndrome (MAS) is defined as respiratory distress in a newborn whose airway was exposed to meconium and whose chest radiographic study exhibits characteristic findings, including pulmonary consolidation and atelectasis.[161] Treatment of MAS often involves the use of positive-pressure ventilation and is associated with a 5% to 20% incidence of pneumothorax from pulmonary air leaks.[162] Extracorporeal membrane oxygenation (ECMO) and inhaled nitric oxide have been used for the treatment of MAS.[163-165] In one study of 176,790 infants born between 1973 and 1987, the annual death rate from MAS was as high as 6 per 10,000 live infants.[166]

Prevention of MAS is preferable to treatment, and preventive measures should be taken both before and after delivery. FHR monitoring and fetal scalp blood pH determination (when indicated) help detect fetal stress that can lead to the passage of meconium.[167] Since 1974, neonatologists have attempted to determine whether peripartum suctioning of the newborn's airway reduces the risk of developing MAS. Gregory et al.[166] published the original study of 80 meconium-exposed newborns who were born either vaginally or by cesarean delivery. All infants underwent endotracheal intubation and suctioning after delivery. In 34 infants, no meconium was observed below the vocal cords; none of these infants demonstrated MAS. Meconium was noted below the cords in the remaining 46 infants, and MAS developed in a total of 16 (35%) of these infants. These investigators concluded that "all infants born through thick, particulate, or 'pea soup' meconium should have the trachea aspirated immediately after birth."[166]

Another study conducted soon thereafter reviewed the delivery room airway management of newborns who required NICU admission for the treatment of MAS.[168] The investigators observed that 37% of infants in whom MAS developed had undergone endotracheal suctioning, whereas 85% of those in whom MAS did not develop had undergone endotracheal suctioning. Almost 20% of the infants with MAS died; most of those who died had not undergone endotracheal suctioning. The investigators concluded that immediate endotracheal suctioning is indicated for infants exposed to meconium.[168]

A third study investigated the effect of pharyngeal suctioning (immediately after delivery of the fetal head) on the incidence of MAS.[169] The purpose of this early suctioning (before delivery of the thorax) was to remove the meconium from the pharynx before the newborn took the first breath; this would prevent meconium passage into the distal areas of the lung and therefore prevent MAS. In this study, 273 meconium-exposed infants underwent early pharyngeal suctioning. Afterward, all underwent laryngoscopy, but only those who had visible meconium below the cords (2 of the 273 infants) underwent endotracheal intubation and suctioning. MAS developed in only 1 of these 2 infants, and in none of the 271 who received only pharyngeal suctioning. None of the infants died.[169]

There has been controversy regarding whether severe MAS is caused by meconium aspiration or whether the pathophysiologic changes in the lung may be caused by intrauterine stress such as asphyxia or sepsis. Two schools of thought have emerged. One school holds that the development of MAS is primarily an intrauterine event caused by fetal stress. Hypoxia induces pathologic changes in the pulmonary vasculature, which results in pulmonary hypertension and respiratory distress after birth. The pulmonary damage is independent of meconium aspiration; therefore, it is not prevented by the suctioning of meconium. The other school holds that MAS is the direct result of meconium aspiration and that the suctioning of meconium is indicated in selected high-risk cases of meconium-stained amniotic fluid.

Murphy et al.[170] examined the lungs of 11 newborns who had MAS and died within 4 days of birth. Of those, 10 also had a diagnosis of persistent pulmonary hypertension, and these 10 had evidence of excessive muscularization of the intra-acinar arteries. Previous studies had shown that muscularization of these arteries is not a normal finding in the fetus or neonate.[171,172] Meyrick and Reid[173] had earlier shown that chronic hypoxia (i.e., at least 4 weeks' duration), but not acute hypoxia, results in pulmonary vascular muscularization in an animal model. Murphy et al.[170] concluded that the observed changes in the 1- to 4-day-old human lung could not be explained by the postdelivery effects of meconium aspiration but, rather, the pathologic findings in MAS must result from intrauterine maldevelopment of the pulmonary vasculature. They suggested a potential link between greater intestinal motility, passage of meconium, and precocious muscularization of the intra-acinar arteries.

Perlman et al.[174] have challenged the belief that muscularization of the intra-acinar arteries is an abnormal event in the newborn. They examined lung tissue from 62 newborns; 24 had meconium aspiration, 20 had meconium staining but no aspiration, and 18 had placental abruption without meconium aspiration or staining. The newborns with meconium aspiration or staining died within 48 hours of birth. Meconium was found in the lungs of all newborns with meconium aspiration. Lungs of newborns with either meconium aspiration or staining showed a greater inflammatory response than those of newborns with placental abruption. These researchers identified muscularized intra-acinar arteries in all newborns except for 1 infant in the group with meconium staining. They observed no difference in the degree of muscularization among these three groups. Perlman et al.[174] stated that this increased muscularization is not an abnormal finding indicative of intrauterine stress. They also noted that muscularization of intra-acinar arteries normally occurs in the fetus,[175-177] but its level is underestimated when the pulmonary vessels are injected and distended before examination.[178,179] They concluded that the etiology of pulmonary hypertension in newborns with MAS lies in the pathophysiology of meconium aspiration and its associated events, and not in pulmonary vascular structural changes.

Some investigators have not confirmed that airway suctioning at birth prevents MAS and its associated mortality. One retrospective study examined the outcome of 1420 meconium-exposed live-born infants between 1977 and 1981.[180] The airway management involved early pharyngeal suctioning followed by endotracheal intubation and suctioning if meconium was present in the pharynx. If necessary, repetitive intubations were performed until no meconium was seen during endotracheal suctioning. MAS occurred in 30 (2.1%) of the meconium-exposed newborns; approximately 40% of those newborns died. The investigators compared these results with those from studies in which combined obstetric and pediatric suctioning was not used. They concluded that vigorous airway management does not always prevent either MAS or death from MAS, but that the incidence of symptomatic MAS is reduced by early pharyngeal suctioning followed by endotracheal intubation and suctioning.

Falciglia et al.[181] compared the incidence of MAS in newborns who underwent early pharyngeal suctioning with the incidence among those who underwent delayed suctioning after delivery of the thorax and the onset of breathing. Both groups of infants received subsequent endotracheal inspection and suctioning. There was no difference in the incidence of MAS between the two groups. The investigators concluded that, because early suctioning did not reduce the incidence of MAS, it is likely that MAS is primarily the result of intrauterine events.

Linder et al.[182] performed a prospective study to assess the efficacy of routine endotracheal suctioning of meconium to prevent MAS. These investigators randomly divided 572 meconium-exposed newborns into two groups. All had been delivered vaginally, all had 1-minute Apgar scores higher than 8, and all had received early pharyngeal suctioning. Infants in one group also underwent endotracheal suctioning, whereas those in the other group did not. Among the infants in the first group, 4 experienced MAS, and 2 had laryngeal stridor. None of the infants in the second group had complications. The investigators cautioned practitioners about the hazards of endotracheal intubation and suction. They suggested that vigorous newborns who have begun breathing before transfer to the resuscitation table derive little or no benefit from endotracheal suctioning and, in fact, may suffer some harm.

Ghidini and Spong[183] reviewed studies published between 1980 and 1999 to determine whether a causal relationship exists between meconium aspiration and MAS. They found that most cases of severe MAS were not causally related to meconium aspiration but rather resulted from intrauterine stress. They concluded that severe MAS is a misnomer because, in most cases, much more than meconium aspiration has contributed to the damage to the lung. The implication is that when severe MAS occurs, inadequate suctioning at delivery or during resuscitation should not be considered the cause, and therefore, other causes of intrauterine lung damage should be investigated.

Amnioinfusion—the instillation of saline into the amniotic cavity—has been used successfully for reduction of cord compression in the presence of oligohydramnios during labor. It has also been proposed as a potential treatment to reduce the incidence of MAS in infants born to women with thick meconium staining of the amniotic fluid. Potential benefits include (1) the reduction of cord compression, thus alleviating fetal compromise and acidemia that contribute to MAS; and (2) the dilution or washing out of the meconium in the amniotic fluid. A large multicenter randomized trial found no difference in rates of MAS or other neonatal disorders with the use of amnioinfusion.[184,185] Thus, the routine practice of amnioinfusion for meconium-stained fluid alone is not recommended.[186]

The 2005 neonatal resuscitation guidelines include revision of the recommendations for the suctioning of meconium at birth. Suctioning of the infant's oropharynx after delivery of the head is no longer recommended,[3,187] given that a large multicenter randomized trial showed no benefit to this practice.[188] If the infant is not vigorous at birth (i.e., absence or depression of respirations, a heart rate less than 100 bpm, or poor muscle tone), direct tracheal suctioning should be performed to remove meconium from the airway prior to initiating positive-pressure ventilation.[3] If the infant is vigorous at birth, it is not necessary to perform endotracheal suctioning. Because of the potential harm of endotracheal intubation, this practice is no longer recommended for the vigorous infant, regardless of the presence of thick or particulate meconium. In this latter situation, meconium should be cleared from the mouth and then the nose by means of a bulb syringe or a large suction catheter (e.g., 12F to 14F).[189]

The preferred method of applying suction to the endotracheal tube has changed since the early 1970s. Originally, meconium was removed by means of oral suctioning performed by the resuscitator. A face mask and a DeLee trap were often used to prevent the transmission of newborn secretions into the resuscitator's mouth, although it was not always successful.[190] Conversely, secretions apparently can be transmitted from the resuscitator to the newborn, as noted in a case report of a newborn to whom herpes simplex virus infection was transmitted from the resuscitating physician.[191] In contemporary practice, endotracheal suctioning is performed via an endotracheal tube connected to a meconium aspirator, which has been connected to a regulated suction source.[192] Suction is then applied as the endotracheal tube is withdrawn from the newborn's mouth. Repeated endotracheal suctioning is performed until little additional meconium is recovered, or until the heart rate indicates that other resuscitative measures (e.g., oxygenation, ventilation) should be begun.[3] If a vigorous meconium-stained newborn subsequently has apnea or respiratory distress, endotracheal suctioning of meconium should be performed before the administration of positive-pressure ventilation.

Because the passage of meconium has been associated with fetal stress and hypoxia, the liberal administration of supplemental oxygen to meconium-exposed newborns is recommended (after suctioning). Once the newborn has a normal heart rate, the resuscitator should gently pass a soft nasogastric or orogastric catheter to remove gastric meconium that may have been swallowed and could later be regurgitated and aspirated.

Preterm Infant

The preterm newborn, especially the VLBW infant, is at higher risk for problems with multiple organ systems simply because of immaturity. During resuscitation, the physician should give special attention to the effect of prematurity on the lungs and the brain. Before the addition of surfactant and high-frequency ventilation to the therapeutic armamentarium of the neonatologist, pulmonary hyaline membrane disease (also known as neonatal respiratory distress syndrome) was the overwhelming obstacle to the attempted salvage of the very preterm newborn.

Between 1970 and 2005, the proportion of infants weighing less than 1500 g at delivery rose from 1.17% to 1.5%.[193] The survival rate of these 500- to 1500-g infants has increased to approximately 85%.[193] Of these, approximately 5% to 10% have what is characterized as cerebral palsy, and 25% to 50% exhibit behavioral and cognitive deficits that lead to important school problems (see Chapter 10).[194-196] These VLBW infants constitute a tiny proportion of the birth population, but they are at the highest risk for development of cerebral palsy; infants weighing less than 1500 g at birth account for 25% of cases of this disorder.[61]

Markers for brain injury affecting preterm infants are germinal matrix intraventricular hemorrhage (IVH) and periventricular leukomalacia. The brain injury may occur either as a consequence of the IVH and its sequelae or as an associated finding.[194] The incidence of germinal matrix IVH in preterm infants declined from 35% to 50% in the late 1970s and early 1980s to approximately 15% in the mid-1990s.[197] Volpe[194,197] has stated that this decrease in the incidence of IVH does not mean that the problem is becoming less important, given that the incidence is directly related to the extent of prematurity[198] and that survival rates for very preterm infants continue to rise. Periventricular leukomalacia, which is the classic neuropathology associated with hypoxic-ischemic cerebral injury in the preterm infant, commonly accompanies IVH.[199]

The fragility of the immature subependymal germinal matrix predisposes the preterm newborn to the development of IVH. The hemorrhage originates from the endothelial cell–lined vessels that course through the germinal matrix in free communication with the venous circulation (i.e., the capillary-venule junction). The mechanism of damage to these endothelial cells and to the integrity of these capillaries has been investigated in the fetal lamb[200] and beagle puppy[201] models, and in newborn humans by means of Doppler velocimetry.[202]

Volpe,[203,204] who has reviewed the theories of the pathogenesis of germinal matrix IVH, has concluded that the pathogenesis is multifactorial; different combinations of factors are relevant in different patients. The three major categories in the pathogenesis of IVH are intravascular, vascular, and extravascular. **Intravascular factors** include fluctuating cerebral blood flow (CBF), which can result from respiratory disturbances in the ventilated preterm infant with neonatal respiratory distress syndrome[202,205]; increases in CBF[201,206]; increases in cerebral venous pressure[207]; decreases in CBF followed by reperfusion; and platelet and coagulation disturbances.[208] **Vascular factors** include the tenuousness of the capillary integrity of the germinal matrix and the vulnerability of the matrix capillaries to hypoxic-ischemic injury.[209] **Extravascular factors** include deficient vascular support, excessive fibrinolytic activity, and a possible postnatal decrease in extravascular tissue pressure.[210]

Of special interest in the discussion of antepartum and intrapartum care and neonatal resuscitation are the possible interventions that may prevent or lessen the severity of IVH. The best way to prevent germinal matrix IVH is to prevent preterm birth. Infection and inflammation are the most common identified causes of preterm birth at the lowest relevant gestational age.[211] Antenatal treatment of infections has not been proved to prevent preterm labor or premature rupture of membranes.[61] Prevention of infection, if possible, may be an important way to reduce the risk of IVH. Another intervention that lowers the incidence of IVH is the transportation of the preterm mother while the fetus is still *in utero* to a center that specializes in the care of high-risk newborns.[194]

Various antenatal pharmacologic interventions have been evaluated for the prevention of IVH. Clinical trials of antenatal maternal administration of phenobarbital[212,213] and vitamin K[213-215] have yielded conflicting results, and their routine use is not currently recommended.[61]

Corticosteroids are currently the most clearly beneficial antenatal pharmacologic intervention for the prevention of IVH. This effect was first noticed when obstetricians began giving betamethasone and dexamethasone to pregnant women to help accelerate fetal lung maturity. The mechanism behind this protection is thought to be improved neonatal cardiovascular stability, which results in less hypotension and less need for blood pressure treatment in these infants.[216] Antenatal betamethasone administration leads to lower placental vascular resistance and higher placental blood flow.[217] This improvement in placental blood flow may decrease impairment of the preterm infant's cerebral autoregulation. In addition, corticosteroids may stimulate the maturation of the germinal matrix.[194] There is consensus regarding the efficacy of a single course of corticosteroids in patients at risk for preterm delivery, but the risks and benefits of multiple courses of steroids for women who remain undelivered 7 days after the initial dose are still controversial. Obstetricians must balance the possible benefits of these agents against their potentially deleterious effects on neuronal and organ growth (see Chapter 34).

Some studies have noted a lower incidence of cerebral palsy in infants of mothers given magnesium sulfate for the treatment of preeclampsia or for tocolysis.[218,219] However, most evidence does not suggest that maternal magnesium sulfate administration results in a decreased incidence of IVH, although the incidence of high-grade (grade III or IV) lesions may be reduced.[220] At least one group of investigators has suggested that antenatal exposure to magnesium sulfate results in a higher risk of adverse neonatal outcome (see Chapter 34).[221]

Volpe[194] has also noted that the avoidance of prolonged labor or vaginal breech delivery may help prevent IVH. Some investigators have suggested that early cesarean delivery—performed before the onset of the active phase of labor—may help prevent IVH in preterm infants. Data are needed to confirm this hypothesis before this practice can be recommended.[222]

Postnatal interventions that may prevent IVH include the avoidance of overly rapid infusion of volume expanders or hypertonic solutions such as sodium bicarbonate.[143,194] The establishment of adequate ventilation is the most beneficial immediate intervention that helps preserve cerebrovascular autoregulation in the preterm infant. The prevention of hypoxemia and hypercarbia is essential, because they are both linked to pressure-passive cerebral circulation, which in turn leads to the development of IVH.[194]

Among infants who exhibit fluctuating CBF velocity, Perlman et al.[223] have found that treatment with pancuronium bromide, which corrects this fluctuation, reduced both the incidence and severity of IVH.[223] Volpe[194] has emphasized that the future direction of IVH prevention should involve trials of other pharmacologic agents for correction of fluctuating hemodynamic disturbances. Studies with meperidine[224] and fentanyl[225] have shown some benefit, but the side effects and need for prolonged ventilation associated with these agents must be weighed against any potential benefits.

If the use of antepartum and intrapartum pharmacologic prophylaxis against IVH becomes part of preterm delivery management, the practice of obstetric anesthesia for preterm patients will be directly affected. For example, the conventional wisdom is that preterm infants are more sensitive than term infants to the effects of maternally administered agents such as analgesics[226] and that this effect is inherently deleterious. However, if this effect is found to protect the preterm infant brain from factors that may lead to IVH (e.g., hemodynamic instability), perhaps obstetric anesthesia providers will no longer attempt to avoid the placental transfer of pharmacologic agents but will deliberately administer these agents to the mother with the intent that they reach the fetus.

Congenital Anomalies

Occasionally, resuscitation of the newborn is complicated by congenital anomalies of the airway or diaphragm. These anomalies may manifest as respiratory distress, which resolves only when appropriate resuscitation techniques are used. For example, newborns are obligatory nose breathers. The diagnosis and management of choanal stenosis and atresia include placement of an oral airway or endotracheal intubation until a definitive surgical procedure can be performed.

Other congenital anomalies that cause upper airway obstruction include (1) micrognathia, as in Pierre Robin syndrome; (2) macroglossia, as in Beckwith-Wiedemann syndrome or glycogen storage disease type II; (3) laryngeal webs; (4) laryngeal atresia; (5) stenosis or paralysis at the level of the vocal cords; (6) subglottic stenosis; (7) subglottic webs; (8) tracheal agenesis; and (9) tracheal rings. Obstruction also can occur as a result of tumors such as subglottic hemangiomas. The presence of a cleft palate may lead to difficulty with manual ventilation. In an infant with micrognathia or macroglossia, airway patency may be maintained if the newborn is kept in the prone position, which reduces posterior movement of the tongue into the pharynx. If macroglossia is extreme, use of an oral airway or a small nasogastric or orogastric suction catheter may be necessary to prevent complete obstruction of the pharynx by the tongue.

When respiratory distress and difficulty with bag-and-mask ventilation are encountered, laryngoscopy should be performed. The cause of the obstruction may be evident if it is supraglottic. Some supraglottic entities (e.g., laryngeal webs) may be treated successfully by forcing an endotracheal tube through the obstruction and into the trachea. Subglottic lesions may require tracheostomy. The help of an otolaryngologist may be invaluable during resuscitation of a newborn with congenital airway obstruction. If there is evidence of such a condition (e.g., laryngeal stenosis[227]) antepartum, it is best to have an otolaryngologist present at the time of delivery. If obstruction is first noted after delivery, the resuscitator should not hesitate to call for surgical assistance.

Fetal neck masses such as cervical teratoma and lymphangioma can lead to extrinsic airway compression. The resulting distortion of the airway can result in airway obstruction, and it may be difficult—if not impossible—to secure an airway in a timely fashion at the time of delivery. These masses often are diagnosed before delivery because of the associated occurrence of polyhydramnios resulting from esophageal compression. In these rare cases, a multidisciplinary team should be assembled before delivery to assist in securing the airway. Leichty et al.[228] described a way of providing the time to secure an airway, known as the ***ex utero* intrapartum treatment (EXIT) procedure**. The procedure was used initially for the delivery of fetuses with diaphragmatic hernia who had undergone intrauterine tracheal clip application for the induction of fetal lung growth (see Chapter 7).

Use of the EXIT procedure by Leichty et al.[228] in the management of five infants with life-threatening neck masses can be summarized as follows: The multidisciplinary team consisted of two or three pediatric surgeons, an obstetrician, a neonatologist, and an anesthesiologist. After rapid-sequence induction of anesthesia and endotracheal intubation, maternal anesthesia was maintained with 50% nitrous oxide and isoflurane at 0.3% to 1.9% expired. Maternal muscle relaxation was maintained with vecuronium.

The isoflurane concentration was titrated to achieve and maintain uterine relaxation to preserve uteroplacental circulation and fetal gas exchange. At the time of hysterotomy, nitrous oxide administration was discontinued. The fetal head and shoulders were delivered while the umbilical cord and lower torso remained in the uterus. The fetus was given additional agents intramuscularly (fentanyl, vecuronium, and atropine) to provide fetal analgesia and to prevent movement and breathing. The FHR and Sa_{O_2} were monitored continuously via a pulse oximeter probe attached to the fetal hand. The surgeon performed direct laryngoscopy in an attempt to secure the airway with a 2.5- to 3.5-mm endotracheal tube. If the airway was not visualized adequately, a rigid bronchoscope was used. If an endotracheal tube still could not be passed, tracheostomy was performed. After establishment of the airway, the infant was completely delivered. Maternal isoflurane was decreased to 0.3% expired, and oxytocin was administered to prevent uterine atony and excessive maternal bleeding.

Since its initial description, the EXIT procedure has been considered an option for fetuses with other congenital anomalies.[229] A common indication for the EXIT procedure is intrinsic airway obstruction. High intrinsic airway obstruction from defects such as laryngeal webs, subglottic cysts, and tracheal atresias is classified as the **congenital high airway obstruction syndrome (CHAOS)**.[229] Use of the EXIT procedure resulted in the first long-term survival of a child with this syndrome.[230]

The EXIT procedure may also be useful in conditions such as severe congenital heart disease, in which the need for emergency ECMO at birth is anticipated. The EXIT procedure allows for the placement of arterial and venous cannulas before umbilical cord clamping, thereby avoiding an unstable period between the termination of placental perfusion and the institution of ECMO.[229] Other possible indications for the EXIT procedure include the resection of congenital cystic adenomatoid malformations and as a first step in separation procedures for conjoined twins with cardiovascular involvement.

Noah et al.[231] reviewed maternal outcomes associated with the EXIT procedure. In 34 patients who underwent the EXIT procedure between 1994 and 1999, short-term outcomes were compared with those in a control group who underwent nonemergency primary cesarean delivery. The EXIT procedure group had higher estimated blood loss, but there was no difference in postoperative hematocrit or duration of hospital stay. The EXIT procedure group also had a higher rate of superficial wound infection (15% versus 2%), but there was no difference between the two groups in the incidence of endometritis.

Anesthetic considerations for the mother during the EXIT procedure include those relevant to general anesthesia for the mother undergoing cesarean delivery or other surgical procedures during pregnancy (see Chapters 17 and 26). Several volatile halogenated agents have been used for the EXIT procedure, including isoflurane, desflurane, and sevoflurane.[229] Sevoflurane has the advantage of providing uterine relaxation similar to that achieved with isoflurane without the resulting tachycardia associated with isoflurane and desflurane. Sevoflurane also has the advantage of being eliminated quickly once the procedure is completed, so that the uterus can readily contract in response to oxytocin.[232]

George et al.[233] described an alternative approach for the EXIT procedure. Specifically, they reported three cases performed with combined spinal-epidural anesthesia (1.5 mL of bupivacaine 0.75%, fentanyl 15 µg, and morphine 0.15 mg, administered intrathecally, followed by placement of a multi-orifice epidural catheter). Supplemental oxygen was provided through a face mask at 6 L/min. Immediately before uterine incision, the patients were given intravenous nitroglycerin 50 to 100 µg, followed by an infusion of nitroglycerin (0.5 to 1.5 µg/kg/min), allowing adequate uterine relaxation for partial delivery of the infant's head. Maternal hypotension occurred in two of the three women and required vasopressor administration. After the infant's airway was secured and the infant was completely delivered, the nitroglycerin was discontinued at the time of umbilical cord clamping.

Esophageal atresia and **tracheoesophageal fistula** occur in 1 out of every 3000 births.[234] There are many variations of these anomalies, the most common being esophageal atresia with a distal tracheoesophageal fistula (80% to 90% of cases). Newborns with a tracheoesophageal fistula are at increased risk for the pulmonary aspiration of gastric contents through the fistula into the lung. When the presence of a tracheoesophageal fistula is not known antepartum, it should be suspected if bubbling secretions are noted during spontaneous or bag-and-mask ventilation. Once a tracheoesophageal fistula is suspected, bag-and-mask ventilation should be discontinued, because its use may contribute to overdistention of the gastrointestinal tract with air, possibly leading to difficulty in ventilation from impingement of the enlarged stomach on the diaphragm. The newborn should be kept in the reverse Trendelenburg position, and a suction catheter should be placed in the esophageal pouch to facilitate the removal of oral secretions. If mechanical ventilation is necessary, an endotracheal tube should be inserted, and the tip should be distal to the entrance of the fistula. This positioning usually can be accomplished by the performance of a right mainstem bronchial intubation followed by a slow withdrawal of the tube until breath sounds are auscultated on the left; a lack of breath sounds over the stomach should then be confirmed. Percutaneous gastrostomy placement may be necessary during resuscitation to facilitate decompression of the gastrointestinal tract.

Congenital diaphragmatic hernia (CDH) occurs in approximately 1 in 4000 live births.[235] The mortality rate from CDH is 30% to 60%. Approximately 80% to 90% of cases occur on the left side and are the result of herniation of the gut through the posterolateral defect of Bochdalek. During formation of the lung, herniation of the gut into the thoracic cavity results in hypoplasia of the lung tissue and pulmonary vasculature. This hypoplasia may be unilateral, but often it is bilateral because of the shift of mediastinal structures to the other side. CDH should be suspected when a newborn has respiratory difficulty and a scaphoid abdomen; this abnormal abdominal shape results from the presence of abdominal contents in the thorax.

During resuscitation of the newborn with CDH, bag-and-mask ventilation is contraindicated, because it allows further distention of the gut, which would further impinge on the lung. If mechanical ventilation is required, endotracheal intubation should be performed and followed by the placement of a nasogastric or orogastric tube to ensure decompression of the gastrointestinal tract. Ventilation should consist of low-positive-pressure breaths (e.g., less than 15 cm H_2O, if possible) delivered at a rapid rate (e.g., 60 to 100 per minute). This low-pressure ventilation may decrease the risk of causing a pneumothorax on the side contralateral to the CDH. If a pneumothorax does occur, it must be evacuated promptly. In the newborn, evacuation is accomplished initially by placement of a 22-gauge needle into the second intercostal space in the midclavicular line and aspiration of air with an attached stopcock and syringe. Severe pulmonary hypertension often accompanies CDH. Maintenance of euthermia, normoxia, and adequate systemic blood pressure promotes pulmonary artery blood flow.

Whenever congenital anomalies of the respiratory tract are noted, the presence of other anomalies should be suspected. It is important to evaluate the newborn promptly for cardiac malformations, especially if appropriate resuscitative efforts are not successful. Echocardiography is used to evaluate cardiac structures and function.

ETHICAL CONSIDERATIONS

The current neonatal resuscitation guidelines address the ethical considerations of non-initiation or discontinuation of resuscitation in the delivery room.[3] Extremes of prematurity (< 23 weeks' confirmed gestation) and severe congenital anomalies (e.g., anencephaly, confirmed trisomy 13 or 18) are examples of circumstances when non-initiation of resuscitation is considered appropriate. Because intrapartum confirmation of pertinent information may not be possible, it is recognized that initiation of resuscitation may occur and that its discontinuation may then be appropriate after further information has been obtained and discussion with family has occurred. In some cases, a trial of therapy may be appropriate, which does not always mandate continued support. In situations or conditions in which there is a high rate of survival and acceptable morbidity (i.e., 25 or more weeks' gestation and most congenital malformations), resuscitation is generally indicated. For those situations with a poor prognosis, including unlikely survival and potentially high morbidity (i.e., 23 to 25 weeks' gestation), the parents' desires as to initiation of resuscitation should be supported (Table 9-5).

Discontinuation of resuscitation of an infant with cardiopulmonary arrest may be appropriate if spontaneous circulation has not occurred in 15 minutes. After 10 minutes of asystole, survival itself and survival without severe disabilities are very unlikely.[236-239]

NEUROBEHAVIORAL TESTING

It is difficult to detect subtle neurobehavioral differences among newborns during the assignment of Apgar scores or the performance of the initial neurologic examination; therefore, investigators have developed and studied methods of documenting newborn neurobehavioral status (Table 9-6). In the past, the newborn was considered incapable of exhibiting higher cortical function. However, investigators have noted that the term newborn is able to sense and respond to a variety of stimuli in a well-organized fashion.[240-242]

In 1973, Brazelton[243] described the Neonatal Behavioral Assessment Scale (NBAS). Brazelton listed the following four variables as key determinants of newborn neurobehavior: (1) various prenatal influences (e.g., infection); (2) the maturity of the infant, especially its CNS; (3) the effects of analgesics and anesthetics administered to the mother before and during delivery; and (4) the effects of difficulties encountered during delivery (e.g., trauma).[244] The NBAS was developed as a tool to detect neurobehavioral abnormalities that resulted from any of these four variables.

This scale consists of 47 individual tests, 27 evaluating behavior, and the remaining 20 evaluating elicited or provoked responses. The 47 tests can be completed in approximately 45 minutes. The NBAS evaluates the ability of the newborn to perform complex motor behaviors, to alter the state of arousal, and to suppress meaningless stimuli. The goal is to provide an extensive evaluation of newborn cortical function and to detect subtle differences among groups of infants. Habituation (i.e., the ability to suppress the response to meaningless, repetitive stimuli) is considered an excellent indicator of normal early cortical function.[244]

In 1974, Scanlon et al.[245] described the Early Neonatal Behavioral Scale (ENNS). The ENNS is based on descriptions of newborn neurobehavioral activity by Prechtal and Beintema,[246] Beintema,[247] and Brazelton.[244] Scanlon et al.[245] selected tests that are easy to perform and score quantitatively during the neonatal period. The ENNS was

TABLE 9-5 Guidelines for Withholding or Discontinuing Resuscitation

Conditions with high survival, acceptable risk of morbidity	≥ 25 weeks' gestational age Most congenital malformations	Resuscitation nearly always indicated
Conditions with poor prognosis, high risk of morbidity	23 to 25 weeks' gestational age	Parental desires about initiating/continuing resuscitation should be supported
Conditions with almost certain death or unacceptably high morbidity	< 23 weeks' gestational age Birth weight < 400 g Anencephaly Chromosomal abnormalities incompatible with life (e.g., trisomy 13)	Resuscitation not indicated

Adapted from American Heart Association and American Academy of Pediatrics. 2005 AHA guidelines for cardiopulmonary resuscitation (CPR) and emergency cardiovascular care (ECC) of pediatric and neonatal patients: Neonatal resuscitation guidelines. Pediatrics 2006; 117:e1035.

TABLE 9-6 Neurobehavioral Tests for Neonates

Neurobehavioral Test	Items Tested	Focus	Uses
Brazelton (Neonatal Behavioral Assessment Scale)	45 individual tests taking 45 minutes	Early cortical function	Evaluates prenatal influences, effects of maturity, maternal medications, effects of difficult delivery
Scanlon (Early Neonatal Behavior Scale)	26 observations taking 6-10 minutes	Early cortical function	Evaluates effects of maternal medications
Amiel-Tison (Neurologic and Adaptive Capacity Score)	20 criteria taking 3-4 minutes	Motor tone	Differentiates drug-induced depression from depression related to asphyxia, trauma, or neurologic disease

developed primarily for the evaluation of the effects of maternal medications (e.g., analgesic and anesthetic agents) on newborn neurobehavior. The ENNS consists of (1) 15 observations of muscle tone and power, reflexes (e.g., rooting, sucking, Moro), and response to stimuli (e.g., light, sound, pinprick); (2) 11 observations of the infant's state of wakefulness; (3) an assessment of the ability of the newborn to habituate to repetitive stimuli; and (4) an overall general assessment of neurobehavioral status. This test can be performed in 6 to 10 minutes.

In 1982, Amiel-Tison et al.[248] described the Neurologic and Adaptive Capacity Score (NACS). It was intended to differentiate drug-induced depression from depression due to asphyxia, birth trauma, or neurologic disease. The ENNS concentrates on the infant's habituation ability, but the NACS emphasizes motor tone as a key indicator of drug-induced abnormal neurobehavior. The basis for this emphasis on newborn motor tone is explained as follows: Unilateral or upper body hypotonus may occur as a result of either birth trauma or anoxia, but global motor depression is more likely a result of anesthetic- or analgesic-induced depression. A total of 20 criteria are tested in the areas of adaptive capacity, passive tone (e.g., scarf sign), active tone (e.g., assessment of the flexor and extensor muscles of the neck), primary reflexes (e.g., Moro), and alertness. The total possible score is 40, and a score of 35 to 40 is considered normal. The NACS can be performed in 3 to 4 minutes.

Amiel-Tison et al.[248] examined interobserver reliability and assessed the correlation of results between the NACS and ENNS. A total of 61 infants underwent 183 NACS and 122 ENNS examinations; this yielded 3660 joint observations for the NACS examinations and 2074 joint observations for the ENNS examinations. The interobserver reliability was 93% for the NACS and 88% for the ENNS. Approximately 92% of infants with high scores on the ENNS scored equally well on the NACS. Reviews of studies that have relied on the NACS have questioned its reliability.[249,250] Halpern et al.[251] examined 200 healthy term infants with the NACS and found poor interobserver reliability. Amiel-Tison[252] has reported her ongoing experience with the NACS, in which she has documented good interobserver reliability.

Anesthesiologists have used neurobehavioral testing primarily to document the effects of analgesic and anesthetic agents and techniques on newborn neurobehavior (see Table 9-6); the American Academy of Pediatrics[253] and the U.S. Food and Drug Administration[254,255] have recommended that these investigations be performed. Investigators have evaluated the effects of maternally administered systemic agents (e.g., meperidine, diazepam) on newborn neurobehavior, and many of these studies have demonstrated a transient serum concentration–dependent depression of newborn neurobehavior.[256-259] However, one study that controlled for differences in patient and labor and delivery characteristics noted only decreased habituation during NBAS examination after systemic administration of meperidine to the mother.[260] Similarly, maternal systemic administration of fentanyl minimally affects performance on the NACS.[261]

As is the case with many studies of systemic agents, studies of epidural anesthesia are often confounded by variables that are difficult to control, such as different patient populations, varied durations of labor, and multiple drug administrations. Scanlon et al.[245] introduced the ENNS in a study of the effect of maternal epidural anesthesia on newborn neurobehavior. The researchers concluded that epidural anesthesia was associated with lower ENNS scores because of decreased muscle strength and tone. In this study, all patients who had received epidural anesthesia were considered part of one group, although 9 patients had received lidocaine and 19 had received mepivacaine. Further investigation showed that epidural lidocaine, even when administered in larger doses for cesarean delivery, does not affect ENNS scores.[262] The difference in ENNS scores between the epidural and nonepidural groups noted in the earlier study[245] was most likely related to the use of mepivacaine rather than lidocaine.[263] As was observed with lidocaine, epidurally administered bupivacaine, 2-chloroprocaine, and etidocaine—when given for cesarean delivery—do not affect ENNS scores.[262,264] Kuhnert et al.[265] assessed performance on the NBAS in a group of infants exposed to either epidural lidocaine or 2-chloroprocaine. Although the investigators observed subtle changes in neurobehavior in the group of infants whose mothers had received lidocaine, they concluded that other variables (e.g., mode of delivery) are more likely to affect performance on neurobehavioral testing.

Sepkoski et al.[266] compared NBAS scores between two groups of vaginally delivered infants. In one group, the mothers had received epidural bupivacaine, and in the other group, the mothers had received no anesthesia or analgesia. The infants in the epidural group showed less alertness, less orientation ability, and less motor function maturity than the infants in the control group. However, variables such as duration of labor, incidence of oxytocin administration, and incidence of instrumental delivery were not similar in the two groups. Earlier, Abboud et al.[267] performed ENNS examinations on vaginally delivered infants whose mothers had received epidural bupivacaine. In this study, epidural administration of bupivacaine did not affect the ENNS scores. The maternal doses of epidural bupivacaine and the maternal venous and umbilical cord blood bupivacaine concentrations were similar to those noted by Sepkoski et al.[266] Abboud et al.[267] also noted normal ENNS scores for infants whose mothers had received epidural lidocaine or 2-chloroprocaine.

Critics of the ENNS and the NACS claim that these examinations fail to show subtle differences in neurobehavior that would be detected by the more comprehensive NBAS.[268] However, although some investigators have observed differences in NBAS performance among groups of infants exposed or not exposed to local anesthetics, confounding variables have prevented clear conclusions as to cause and effect.

Hodgkinson et al.[269] observed that the subarachnoid administration of tetracaine for cesarean delivery did not adversely affect ENNS performance. Other studies have used the NACS to evaluate the effects of maternal epidural opioids[270-276] and epinephrine (in combination with a local anesthetic).[277-280] These drugs did not significantly affect NACS performance in these studies.

Other studies have used the ENNS and NACS to study the effects of general anesthetic agents on newborn neurobehavior. In a prospective, randomized study, Abboud et al.[281] assessed NACS performance at 15 minutes, 2 hours, and 24 hours of age in infants whose mothers received general, epidural, or spinal anesthesia for cesarean delivery. Women who underwent general anesthesia received thiopental 4 mg/kg followed by enflurane 0.5% with nitrous oxide 50% in oxygen. Although the NACS was lower at both 15 minutes and 2 hours of age in the infants in the general anesthesia group than in the infants in either neuraxial anesthesia group, no difference in NACS results was noted at 24 hours of age.

Hodgkinson et al.[269] used the ENNS to evaluate outcomes among three groups of infants, all of whom were delivered by elective cesarean delivery. One group of women received general anesthesia with thiopental 4 mg/kg followed by 50% nitrous oxide. A second group received general anesthesia with ketamine 1 mg/kg followed by 50% nitrous oxide. A third group received spinal anesthesia with tetracaine 6 to 8 mg. The ENNS evaluations were conducted at 4 to 8 hours of age and again at 24 hours. During the 4- to 8-hour examination, infants in the spinal anesthesia group scored significantly higher on multiple components of the ENNS than did infants in either of the general anesthesia groups. At 24 hours, infants in the spinal anesthesia group scored significantly higher than those in the thiopental group in alertness, total decrement score, and overall assessment. Similarly, infants in the spinal anesthesia group scored higher than those in the ketamine group in alertness and overall assessment. No significant differences existed between the scores of the thiopental group infants and the ketamine group infants.[269] Palahniuk et al.[282] observed similar results in a study that compared groups of infants whose mothers received either epidural anesthesia or general anesthesia for elective cesarean delivery. Infants whose mothers had received thiopental and nitrous oxide scored significantly lower in the alertness component of the ENNS than infants whose mothers had received epidural lidocaine with epinephrine.

Stefani et al.[283] observed that subanesthetic maternal doses of enflurane or nitrous oxide did not affect newborn neurobehavior (as assessed by ENNS and NACS) at 15 minutes, 2 hours, and 24 hours of age. Abboud et al.[284] obtained similar results from NACS examinations of infants whose mothers had received subanesthetic doses of isoflurane.

In summary, subtle changes in newborn neurobehavior may result from factors such as antepartum maternal drug exposure. Parent-infant bonding and the ability of the infant to breast-feed may be adversely affected by these neurobehavioral changes.[244] These transient effects may seem trivial to some observers but important to others. With regard to the long-term neurologic outcome of individual infants, performance during neurobehavioral assessment may aid the observer in the formulation of a prognosis. However, as demonstrated with Apgar scores, the prognostic value of an isolated test score is likely to be lower than the prognostic value of multiple factors considered together during the overall assessment of an individual infant.

KEY POINTS

- The anesthesia provider attending the mother should not be responsible for resuscitation of the newborn. However, all anesthesia providers should be prepared to provide assistance during neonatal resuscitation when it is needed.
- Adverse conditions at birth (e.g., hypoxia, acidosis, profound hypovolemia, hypothermia) may impair the transition from intrauterine to extrauterine life. Impaired transition may manifest as persistent pulmonary hypertension of the newborn.
- The Apgar scoring system gives the practitioner a standard guide for assessing the need for newborn resuscitation.
- No single factor should be considered prognostic of poor neurologic outcome. A combination of factors, including severe metabolic acidemia and Apgar scores of 3 or less beyond 5 minutes, are included among the criteria that suggest the occurrence of intrapartum hypoxia of sufficient severity to cause long-term neurologic impairment. However, not all infants who fulfill these criteria suffer permanent neurologic injury.
- Severe mixed or metabolic acidemia—but not respiratory acidemia alone—is associated with a higher incidence of neonatal complications and death.
- During evaluation of the apneic newborn, assisted ventilation should be initiated promptly if tactile stimulation does not result in the initiation of spontaneous breathing.

- During the first assisted breath, positive pressure (30 to 40 cm H_2O) should be maintained for 4 to 5 seconds at the end of inspiration to overcome the surface tension of the lungs and open the alveoli. Thereafter, the maximum pressure generated for all assisted breaths should range between 20 and 30 cm H_2O.
- Meconium-exposed newborns no longer undergo nasopharyngeal and oropharyngeal suctioning before delivery of the thorax. Suctioning by means of endotracheal intubation may be necessary, especially for those meconium-exposed newborns believed to be at highest risk for development of meconium aspiration syndrome (i.e., those who have respiratory depression, bradycardia, or poor muscle tone).
- In most circumstances, decisions about the initiation or continuation of resuscitation in the delivery room should be based on the newborn's response to resuscitative efforts rather than an estimation of gestational age. Parental desires should be considered when the prognosis for infant survival is poor.

REFERENCES

1. American Academy of Pediatrics and American College of Obstetricians and Gynecologists. Guidelines for Perinatal Care. 6th edition. Elk Grove Village, IL, American Academy of Pediatrics and American College of Obstetricians and Gynecologists, 2007:22.
2. Ostheimer GW. Resuscitation of the newborn. In Stanley TH, Schafer PG, editors. Pediatric and Obstetrical Anesthesia. Dordrecht, Netherlands, Kluwer Academic, 1995:159-86.
3. American Heart Association and American Academy of Pediatrics. 2005 American Heart Association (AHA) guidelines for cardiopulmonary resuscitation (CPR) and emergency cardiovascular care (ECC) of pediatric and neonatal patients: Neonatal resuscitation. Pediatrics 2006; 117:e1029-38.
4. Eicher DJ, Wagner CL. Update on neonatal resuscitation. J S C Med Assoc 2002; 98:114-20.
5. American College of Obstetricians and Gynecologists Committee on Obstetric Practice and American Society of Anesthesiologists Committee on Obstetric Anesthesia. Optimal goals for anesthesia care in obstetrics. ACOG Committee Opinion No. 256, May 2001. (Obstet Gynecol 2001; 97:Suppl 1-3.)
6. Heyman HJ, Joseph NJ, Salem MR, Heyman K. Anesthesia personnel, neonatal resuscitation, and the courts (abstract). Anesthesiology 1991; 75:A1074.
7. Hawkins JL, Gibbs CP, Orleans M, et al. Obstetric anesthesia work force survey, 1981 versus 1992. Anesthesiology 1997; 87:135-43.
8. Gaiser RR, Lewis SB, Cheek TG, Gutsche BB. Neonatal resuscitation and the anesthesiologist (abstract). Anesthesiology 2001; 94:A80.
9. Gaiser RR, Lewin SB, Cheek TG, Gutsche BB. Anesthesiologists' interest in neonatal resuscitation certification. J Clin Anesth 2001; 13:374-6.
10. Chadwick HS, Posner K, Caplan RA, et al. A comparison of obstetric and nonobstetric anesthesia malpractice claims. Anesthesiology 1991; 74:242-9.
11. Heyman HJ. Neonatal resuscitation and anesthesiologist liability. Anesthesiology 1994; 81:783.
12. Dawes GS. Foetal and Neonatal Physiology. Chicago, Year Book Medical Publishers, 1968:160-76.
13. Rudolph AM, Heymann MA. Fetal and neonatal circulation and respiration. Annu Rev Physiol 1974; 36:187-207.
14. Rudolph AM. The changes in the circulation after birth: Their importance in congenital heart disease. Circulation 1970; 41:343-59.
15. Rudolph AM, Yuan S. Response of the pulmonary vasculature to hypoxia and H^+ ion concentration changes. J Clin Invest 1966; 45:399-411.
16. Cassin S, Dawes GS, Mott JC, et al. The vascular resistance of the foetal and newly ventilated lung of the lamb. J Physiol 1964; 171:61-79.
17. Assali NS, Morris JA, Smith RW, Manson WA. Studies on ductus arteriosus circulation. Circ Res 1963; 13:478-89.
18. Boréus LO, Malmfors T, McMurphy DM, Olson L. Demonstration of adrenergic receptor function and innervation in the ductus arteriosus of the human fetus. Acta Physiol Scand 1969; 77:316-21.
19. Dimich I, Singh PP, Adell A, et al. Evaluation of oxygen saturation monitoring by pulse oximetry in neonates in the delivery system. Can J Anaesth 1991; 38:985-8.
20. Brady JP, Rigatto H. Pulmonary capillary flow in infants. Circulation (Suppl) 1969; 3:50.
21. Walsh-Sukys MC. Persistent pulmonary hypertension of the newborn: The black box revisited. Clin Perinatol 1993; 20:127-43.
22. Alano MA, Ngougmna E, Ostrea EM Jr, Konduri GG. Analysis of nonsteroidal anti-inflammatory drugs in meconium and its relation to persistent pulmonary hypertension of the newborn. Pediatrics 2001; 107:519-23.
23. Adams FH, Moss AJ, Fagan L. The tracheal fluid of the foetal lamb. Biol Neonate 1963; 5:151-8.
24. Ross BB. Comparison of foetal pulmonary fluid with foetal plasma and amniotic fluid. Nature 1963; 199:1100.
25. Karlberg P. The adaptive changes in the immediate postnatal period, with particular reference to respiration. J Pediatr 1960; 56:585-604.
26. Usher RH, Allen AC, McLean FH. Risk of respiratory distress syndrome related to gestational age, route of delivery, and maternal diabetes. Am J Obstet Gynecol 1971; 111:826-32.
27. Lawson EE, Birdwell RL, Huang PS, Taeusch HW Jr. Augmentation of pulmonary surfactant secretion by lung expansion at birth. Pediatr Res 1979; 13:611-4.
28. Platzker ACG, Kitterman JA, Mescher EJ, et al. Surfactant in the lung and tracheal fluid of the fetal lamb and acceleration of its appearance by dexamethasone. Pediatrics 1975; 56:554-61.
29. Platzker ACG, Kitterman JA, Clements JA, Tooley WH. Surfactant appearance and secretion in fetal lamb lung in response to dexamethasone. Pediatr Res 1972; 6:406.
30. Turbeville DF, McCaffree MA, Block MF, Krous HF. In utero distal pulmonary meconium aspiration. South Med J 1979; 72:535-6.
31. Lagercrantz H, Bistoletti P. Catecholamine release in the newborn infant at birth. Pediatr Res 1977; 11:889-93.
32. Dahm LS, James LS. Newborn temperature and calculated heat loss in the delivery room. Pediatrics 1972; 49:504-13.
33. Shankaran S, Laptook AR, Ehrenkranz RA, et al. Whole-body hypothermia for neonates with hypoxic-ischemic encephalopathy. N Engl J Med 2005; 353:1574-84.
34. Papile LA. Systemic hypothermia: A "cool" therapy for neonatal hypoxic-ischemic encephalopathy. N Engl J Med 2005; 353:1619-20.
35. Volpe JJ. Perinatal brain injury: From pathogenesis to neuroprotection. Ment Retard Dev Disabil Res Rev 2001; 7:56-64.
36. Philip J, Alexander JM, Sharma SK, et al. Epidural analgesia during labor and maternal fever. Anesthesiology 1999; 90:1271-5.
37. Lieberman E, Lang JM, Frigoletto F Jr, et al. Epidural analgesia, intrapartum fever, and neonatal sepsis evaluation. Pediatrics 1997; 99:415-9.
38. Kaul B, Vallejo M, Ramanathan S, Mandell G. Epidural labor analgesia and neonatal sepsis evaluation rate: A quality improvement study. Anesth Analg 2001; 93:986-90.
39. Huddleston JF. Intrapartum fetal assessment: A review. Clin Perinatol 1999; 26:549-68.
40. Garite TJ, Dildy GA, McNamara H, et al. A multicenter controlled trial of fetal pulse oximetry in the intrapartum management of nonreassuring fetal heart rate patterns. Am J Obstet Gynecol 2000; 183:1049-58.
41. American College of Obstetricians and Gynecologists Committee on Obstetric Practice. Fetal pulse oximetry. ACOG Committee Opinion No. 258, September 2001. (Obstet Gynecol 2001; 98:523-4.)
42. East CE, Chan FY, Colditz PB, Begg LM. Fetal pulse oximetry for assessment on labour. Cochrane Database Syst Rev 2007; (2):CD004075.

43. Jacob J, Pfenninger J. Cesarean deliveries: When is a pediatrician necessary? Obstet Gynecol 1997; 89:217-20.
44. Gordon A, McKechnie EJ, Jeffery H. Pediatric presence at cesarean section: Justified or not? Am J Obstet Gynecol 2005; 193:599-605.
45. Hook B, Kiwi R, Amini SB, et al. Neonatal morbidity after elective repeat cesarean section and trial of labor. Pediatrics 1997; 100:348-53.
46. Apgar V. A proposal for a new method of evaluation of the newborn infant. Curr Res Anesth Analg 1953; 32:260-7.
47. Apgar V. The newborn (Apgar) scoring system: Reflections and advice. Pediatr Clin North Am 1966; 13:645-50.
48. Apgar V, James LS. Further observations on the newborn scoring system. Am J Dis Child 1962; 104:419-28.
49. Sykes GS, Johnson P, Ashworth F, et al. Do Apgar scores indicate asphyxia? Lancet 1982; 1(8270):494-6.
50. Lauener PA, Calame A, Janecek P, et al. Systematic pH-measurements in the umbilical artery: Causes and predictive value of neonatal acidosis. J Perinat Med 1983; 11:278-85.
51. Suidan JS, Young BK. Outcome of fetuses with lactic acidemia. Am J Obstet Gynecol 1984; 150:33-7.
52. Fields LM, Entman SS, Boehm FH. Correlation of the one-minute Apgar score and the pH value of umbilical arterial blood. South Med J 1983; 76:1477-9.
53. Boehm FH, Fields LM, Entman SS, Vaughn WK. Correlation of the one-minute Apgar score and umbilical cord acid-base status. South Med J 1986; 79:429-31.
54. Page FO, Martin JN, Palmer SM, et al. Correlation of neonatal acid-base status with Apgar scores and fetal heart rate tracings. Am J Obstet Gynecol 1986; 154:1306-11.
55. Luthy DA, Shy KK, Strickland D, et al. Status of infants at birth and risk for adverse neonatal events and long-term sequelae: A study in low birth weight infants. Am J Obstet Gynecol 1987; 157:676-9.
56. Josten BE, Johnson TRB, Nelson JP. Umbilical cord blood pH and Apgar scores as an index of neonatal health. Am J Obstet Gynecol 1987; 157:843-8.
57. Vintzileos AM, Gaffney SE, Salinger LM, et al. The relationships among the fetal biophysical profile, umbilical cord pH, and Apgar scores. Am J Obstet Gynecol 1987; 157:627-31.
58. Drage JS, Kennedy C, Berendes H, et al. The Apgar score as an index of infant morbidity: A report from the collaborative study of cerebral palsy. Dev Med Child Neurol 1966; 8:141-8.
59. Drage JS, Kennedy C, Schwarz BK. The Apgar score as an index of neonatal mortality: A report from the collaborative study of cerebral palsy. Obstet Gynecol 1964; 24:222-30.
60. American College of Obstetricians and Gynecologists, American Academy of Pediatrics. Neonatal Encephalopathy and Cerebral Palsy: Defining the Pathogenesis and Pathophysiology. Washington, DC, American College of Obstetricians and Gynecologists, 2003.
61. Freeman JM, Nelson KB. Intrapartum asphyxia and cerebral palsy. Pediatrics 1988; 82:240-9.
62. Gilstrap LC, Leveno KJ, Burris J, et al. Diagnosis of birth asphyxia on the basis of fetal pH, Apgar score, and newborn cerebral dysfunction. Am J Obstet Gynecol 1989; 161:825-30.
63. Nelson KB, Ellenberg JH. Antecedents of cerebral palsy: Multivariate analysis of risk. N Engl J Med 1986; 315:81-6.
64. American College of Obstetricians and Gynecologists Committee on Obstetric Practice. The Apgar score. ACOG Committee Opinion No. 333, May 2006. (Obstet Gynecol 2006; 107:1209-12.)
65. Finister M, Wood M. The Apgar score has survived the test of time. Anesthesiology 2005; 102:855-7.
66. Casey BM, McIntire DD, Leveno KJ. The continuing value of the Apgar score for the assessment of newborn infants. N Engl J Med 2001; 344:467-71.
67. Papile LA. The Apgar score in the 21st century. N Engl J Med 2001; 344:519-20.
68. Catlin EA, Carpenter MW, Brann BS IV, et al. The Apgar score revisited: Influence of gestational age. J Pediatr 1986; 109:865-8.
69. Helmy SAK, Ebeid AM. Modified Apgar score using pulse oximetry (abstract). Anesth Analg 1995; 80:S179.
70. Urschitz MS, Von Einem V, Seyfang A, Poets CF. Use of pulse oximetry in automated oxygen delivery to ventilated infants. Anesth Analg 2002; 94:S37-40.
71. Macarthur A, Halpern S. Obstetrical and pediatric anesthesia: Best evidence in anesthetic practice: Prognosis: The Apgar score predicts 28-day neonatal mortality (editorial). Can J Anesth 2002; 49:46-8.
72. American College of Obstetricians and Gynecologists Committee on Obstetric Practice. Umbilical cord blood gas and acid-base analysis. ACOG Committee Opinion No. 348, November 2006. (Obstet Gynecol 2006; 108:1319-22.)
73. Lievaart M, de Jong PA. Acid-base equilibrium in umbilical cord blood and time of cord clamping. Obstet Gynecol 1984; 63:44-7.
74. Ackerman BD, Sosna MM, Ullrich JR. A technique for serial sampling of umbilical artery blood at birth. Biol Neonate 1972; 20:458-65.
75. Chou PJ, Ullrich JR, Ackerman BD. Time of onset of effective ventilation at birth. Biol Neonate 1974; 24:74-81.
76. Santos DJ. Discussion of: Page FO, Martin JN, Palmer SM, et al: Correlation of neonatal acid-base status with Apgar scores and fetal heart rate tracings. Am J Obstet Gynecol 1986; 154:1309-10.
77. Kirshon B, Moise KJ. Effect of heparin on umbilical arterial blood gases. J Reprod Med 1989; 34:267-9.
78. Strickland DM, Gilstrap LC, Hauth JC, Widmer K. Umbilical cord pH and pCO_2: Effect of interval from delivery to determination. Am J Obstet Gynecol 1984; 148:191-4.
79. Hilger JS, Holzman IR, Brown DR. Sequential changes in placental blood gases and pH during the hour following delivery. J Reprod Med 1981; 26:305-7.
80. Sato I, Saling E. Changes of pH value during storage of fetal blood samples. J Perinatal Med 1975; 3:211-4.
81. Gilstrap LC, Hauth JC, Hankins GDV, Beck AW. Second-stage fetal heart rate abnormalities and type of neonatal acidemia. Obstet Gynecol 1987; 70:191-5.
82. Wible JL, Petrie RH, Koons A, Perez A. The clinical use of umbilical cord acid-base determinations in perinatal surveillance and management. Clin Perinatol 1982; 9:387-97.
83. Miller JM, Bernard M, Brown HL, et al. Umbilical cord blood gases for term healthy newborns. Am J Perinatol 1990; 7:157-9.
84. Helwig JT, Parer JT, Kilpatrick SJ, Laros RK. Umbilical cord blood acid-base state: What is normal? Am J Obstet Gynecol 1996; 174:1807-14.
85. Yeomans ER, Hauth JC, Gilstrap LC, Strickland DM. Umbilical cord pH, pCO_2 and bicarbonate following uncomplicated term vaginal deliveries. Am J Obstet Gynecol 1985; 151:798-800.
86. Ramin SM, Gilstrap LC, Leveno KJ, et al. Umbilical artery acid-base status in the preterm infant. Obstet Gynecol 1989; 74:256-8.
87. Thorp JA, Dildy GA, Yeomans ER, et al. Umbilical cord blood gas analysis at delivery. Am J Obstet Gynecol 1996; 175:517-22.
88. Huisjes HJ, Aarnoudse JG. Arterial or venous umbilical pH as a measure of neonatal morbidity? Early Hum Dev 1979; 3:155-61.
89. Eskes TKAB, Jongsma HW, Houx PCW. Percentiles for cord gas values in human umbilical cord blood. Eur J Obstet Gynecol Reprod Biol 1983; 14:341-6.
90. Low JA. The role of blood gas and acid-base assessment in the diagnosis of intrapartum fetal asphyxia. Am J Obstet Gynecol 1988; 159:1235-40.
91. Thorp JA, Sampson JE, Parisi VM, Creasy RK. Routine umbilical cord blood gas determinations? Am J Obstet Gynecol 1989; 161:600-5.
92. Riley RJ, Johnson JWC. Collecting and analyzing cord blood gases. Clin Obstet Gynecol 1993; 36:13-23.
93. Nagel HTC, Vandenbussche FPHA, Oepkes D, et al. Follow-up of children born with an umbilical arterial blood pH <7. Am J Obstet Gynecol 1995; 173:1758-64.
94. Ruth VJ, Raivio KO. Perinatal brain damage: Predictive value of metabolic acidosis and the Apgar score. Br Med J 1988; 297:24-7.
95. Vintzileos AM, Egan JFX, Campbell WA, et al. Asphyxia at birth as determined by cord blood pH measurements in preterm and term gestations: Correlation with neonatal outcome. J Matern Fetal Med 1992; 1:7-13.
96. Goldaber KG, Gilstrap LC, Leveno KJ, et al. Pathologic fetal acidemia. Obstet Gynecol 1991; 78:1103-7.

97. Zwart A, Buursma A, Oeseburg B, Zijlstra WG. Determination of hemoglobin derivatives with the IL 282 CO-Oximeter as compared with a manual spectrophotometric five-wavelength method. Clin Chem 1981; 27:1903-7.
98. Huch R, Huch A, Tuchschmid P, et al. Carboxyhemoglobin concentration in fetal cord blood (letter). Pediatrics 1983; 71:461-2.
99. Zijlstra WG, Buursma A, Koek JN, et al. Problems in the spectrophotometric determination of HbO_2 and HbCO in fetal blood. In Maas AHJ, Kofstad J, Siggard-Andersen O, et al, editors. Proceeding of the Ninth Meeting of the IFCC Expert Panel on pH and Blood Gases. Oslo, Norway, Private Press, 1984:44-55.
100. Kopotic RJ, Lindner W. Assessing high-risk infants in the delivery room with pulse oximetry. Anesth Analg 2002; 94:S31-6.
101. Jennis MS, Peabody JL. Pulse oximetry: An alternative method for the assessment of oxygenation in newborn infants. Pediatrics 1987; 79:524-8.
102. Severinghaus JW, Naifeh KH. Accuracy of response of six pulse oximeters to profound hypoxia. Anesthesiology 1987; 67:551-8.
103. Sarnat HB, Sarnat MS. Neonatal encephalopathy following fetal distress: A clinical and electroencephalographic study. Arch Neurol 1976; 33:696-705.
104. Dubowitz LMS, Dubowitz V, Goldberg C. Clinical assessment of gestational age in the newborn infant. J Pediatr 1970; 77:1-10.
105. Ballard JL, Novak KK, Driver M. A simplified score for assessment of fetal maturation of newly born infants. J Pediatr 1979; 95:769-74.
106. Farr V, Mitchell RG, Neligan GA, Parkin JM. The definition of some external characteristics used in the assessment of gestational age in the newborn infant. Dev Med Child Neurol 1966; 8:507-11.
107. Farr V, Kerridge DF, Mitchell RG. The value of some external characteristics in the assessment of gestational age at birth. Dev Med Child Neurol 1966; 8:657-60.
108. Amiel-Tison C. Neurological evaluation of the maturity of newborn infants. Arch Dis Child 1968; 43:89-93.
109. Sanders M, Allen M, Alexander GR, et al. Gestational age assessment in preterm neonates weighing less than 1500 grams. Pediatrics 1991; 88:542-6.
110. Ballard JL, Khoury JC, Wedig K, et al. New Ballard Score, expanded to include extremely premature infants. J Pediatr 1991; 119:417-23.
111. Alexander GR, de Caunes F, Hulsey TC, et al. Ethnic variation in postnatal assessments of gestational age: A reappraisal. Paediatr Perinat Epidemiol 1992; 6:423-33.
112. Battaglia FC, Lubchenco LO. A practical classification of newborn infants by weight and gestational age. J Pediatr 1967; 71:159-163.
113. Thoresen M, Cowan F, Whitelaw A. Effect of tilting on oxygenation in newborn infants. Arch Dis Child 1988; 63:315-7.
114. Schubring C. Temperature regulation in healthy and resuscitated newborns immediately after birth. J Perinat Med 1986; 14:27-33.
115. Leuthner SR, Jansen RD, Hageman JR. Cardiopulmonary resuscitation of the newborn: An update. Pediatr Clin North Am 1994; 41:893-907.
116. Hazan J, Maag U, Chessex P. Association between hypothermia and mortality rate of premature infants: Revisited. Am J Obstet Gynecol 1991; 164:111-2.
117. Gluckman PD, Wyatt JS, Azzopardi D, et al. Selective head cooling with mild systemic hypothermia after neonatal encephalopathy: Multicentre randomised trial. Lancet 2005; 365:663-70.
118. Spector LG, Klebanoff MA, Feusner JH, et al. Childhood cancer following neonatal oxygen supplementation. J Pediatr 2005; 147:27-31.
119. Paneth N. The evidence mounts against use of pure oxygen in newborn resuscitation. J Pediatr 2005; 147:4-6.
120. Saugstaad OD, Rootwelt T, Aalen O. Resuscitation of asphyxiated newborn infants with room air or oxygen: An international controlled trial: The Resair 2 study. Pediatrics 1998; 102:e1.
121. Vento M, Asensi M, Sastre J, et al. Resuscitation with room air instead of 100% oxygen prevents oxidative stress in moderately asphyxiated term neonates. Pediatrics 2001; 107:642-7.
122. Davis PG, Tan A, O'Donnell CP, Schulze A. Resuscitation of newborn infants with 100% oxygen or air: A systematic review and meta-analysis. Lancet 2004; 364:1329-33.
123. Weinberger B, Laskin DL, Heck DE, Laskin JD. Oxygen toxicity in premature infants. Toxicol Appl Pharmacol 2002; 181:60-7.
124. Vyas H, Milner AD, Hopkin IE, Boon AW. Physiologic responses to prolonged and slow-rise inflation in the resuscitation of the asphyxiated newborn infant. J Pediatr 1981; 99:635-9.
125. Cordero L, Hon EH. Neonatal bradycardia following nasopharyngeal stimulation. J Pediatr 1971; 78:441-7.
126. Young RS, Hessert TR, Pritchard GA, Yagel SK. Naloxone exacerbates hypoxic-ischemic brain injury in the neonatal rat. Am J Obstet Gynecol 1984; 150:52-6.
127. Chernick V, Manfreda J, De Booy V, et al. Clinical trial of naloxone in birth asphyxia. J Pediatr 1988; 113:519-25.
128. Sherman JM, Lowitt S, Stephenson C, Ironson G. Factors influencing acquired subglottic stenosis in infants. J Pediatr 1986; 109:322-7.
129. Laing IA, Cowan DL, Ballantine GM, Hume R. Prevention of subglottic stenosis in neonatal ventilation. Int J Pediatr Otorhinolaryngol 1986; 11:61-6.
130. Paterson SJ, Byrne PJ, Molesky MG, et al. Neonatal resuscitation using the laryngeal mask airway. Anesthesiology 1994; 80:1248-53.
131. Brimacombe J, Berry A. The laryngeal mask airway for obstetric anaesthesia and neonatal resuscitation. Int J Obstet Anesth 1994; 3:211-8.
132. Fernández-Jurado MI, Fernández-Baena M. Use of laryngeal mask airway for prolonged ventilatory support in a preterm newborn. Paediatr Anaesth 2002; 12:369-70.
133. Jain L, Vidyasagar D. Cardiopulmonary resuscitation of newborns: Its application to transport medicine. Pediatr Clin North Am 1993; 40:287-302.
134. David R. Closed chest cardiac massage in the newborn infant. Pediatrics 1988; 81:552-4.
135. Orlowski JP. Optimum position for external cardiac compression in infants and young children. Ann Emerg Med 1986; 15:667-73.
136. Phillips GWL, Zideman DA. Relation of infant heart to sternum: Its significance in cardiopulmonary resuscitation. Lancet 1986; 1(8488):1024-5.
137. Finholt DA, Kettrick RG, Wagner R, Swedlow DB. The heart is under the lower third of the sternum: Implications for external cardiac massage. Am J Dis Child 1986; 140:646-9.
138. Dean JM, Koehler RC, Schleien CL, et al. Age-related effects of compression rate and duration in cardiopulmonary resuscitation. J Appl Physiol 1990; 68:554-60.
139. Fitzgerald KR, Babbs CF, Frissora HA, et al. Cardiac output during cardiopulmonary resuscitation at various compression rates and durations. Am J Physiol 1981; 241:H442-8.
140. Babbs CF, Tacker WA, Paris RL, et al. CPR with simultaneous compression and ventilation at high airway pressure in four animal models. Crit Care Med 1982; 10:501-4.
141. Burchfield DJ. Medication use in neonatal resuscitation. Clin Perinatol 1999; 26:683-91.
142. Schleien CL, Dean JM, Koehler RC, et al. Effect of epinephrine on cerebral and myocardial perfusion in an infant animal preparation of cardiopulmonary resuscitation. Circulation 1986; 73:809-17.
143. Simmons MA, Adcock EW, Bard H, Battaglia FC. Hypernatremia and intracranial hemorrhage in neonates. N Engl J Med 1974; 291:6-10.
144. Papile LA, Burstein J, Burstein R, et al. Relationship of intravenous sodium bicarbonate infusions and cerebral intraventricular hemorrhage. J Pediatr 1978; 93:834-6.
145. Kette F, Weil MH, von Planta M, et al. Buffer agents do not reverse intramyocardial acidosis during cardiac resuscitation. Circulation 1990; 81:1660-6.
146. Kette F, Weil MH, Gazmuri RJ. Buffer solutions may compromise cardiac resuscitation by reducing coronary perfusion pressure. JAMA 1991; 266:2121-6 (erratum in JAMA 1991; 266:3286).
147. Changaris DG, Purohit DM, Balentine JD, et al. Brain calcification in severely stressed neonates receiving parenteral calcium. J Pediatr 1984; 104:941-6.
148. Fiser DH. Intraosseous infusion. N Engl J Med 1990; 322:1579-81.
149. Tocantins LM. Rapid absorption of substances injected into the bone marrow. Proc Soc Exp Biol Med 1940; 45:292-6.

150. Papper EM. The bone marrow route for injecting fluids and drugs into the general circulation. Anesthesiology 1942; 3:307-13.
151. Hodge D III, Delgado-Paredes C, Fleisher G. Intraosseous infusion flow rates in hypovolemic "pediatric" dogs. Ann Emerg Med 1987; 16:305-7.
152. Redmond AD, Plunkett PK. Intraosseous infusion. Arch Emerg Med 1986; 3:231-3.
153. La Fleche FR, Slepin MJ, Vargas J, Milzman DP. Iatrogenic bilateral tibial fractures after intraosseous infusion attempts in a 3-month-old infant. Ann Emerg Med 1989; 18:1099-101.
154. Rosetti VA, Thompson BM, Miller J, et al. Intraosseous infusion: An alternative route of pediatric intravascular access. Ann Emerg Med 1985; 14:885-8.
155. Quilligan JJ Jr, Turkel H. Bone marrow infusion and its complications. Am J Dis Child 1946; 71:457-65.
156. Heinild S, Sndergaard T, Tudvad F. Bone marrow infusion in childhood: Experiences from a thousand infusions. J Paediatr 1947; 30:400-12.
157. Golden SM, O'Brien WF, Metz SA. Anticoagulation of autologous cord blood for neonatal resuscitation. Am J Obstet Gynecol 1982; 144:103-4.
158. Human albumin administration in critically ill patients: Systematic review of randomised controlled trials. Cochrane Injuries Group Albumin Reviewers. BMJ 1998; 317:235-40.
159. Brown CA, Desmond MM, Lindley JE, Moore J. Meconium staining of the amniotic fluid: A marker of fetal hypoxia. Obstet Gynecol 1957; 9:91-103.
160. Matthews TG, Warshaw JB. Relevance of the gestational age distribution of meconium passage in utero. Pediatrics 1979; 64:30-1.
161. Yeh TF, Harris V, Srinivasan G, et al. Roentgenographic findings in infants with meconium aspiration syndrome. JAMA 1979; 242:60-3.
162. Wiswell TE, Tuggle JM, Turner BS. Meconium aspiration syndrome: Have we made a difference? Pediatrics 1990; 85:715-21.
163. Short BL, Miller MK, Anderson KO. Extracorporeal membrane oxygenation in the management of respiratory failure in the newborn. Clin Perinatol 1987; 14:737-48.
164. Truog WE. Inhaled nitric oxide: A tenth anniversary observation. Pediatrics 1998; 101:696-7.
165. Wessel DL, Adatia I, Van Marter LJ, et al. Improved oxygenation in a randomized trial of inhaled nitric oxide for persistent pulmonary hypertension of the newborn. Pediatrics 1997; 100:E7.
166. Gregory GA, Gooding CA, Phibbs RH, Tooley WH. Meconium aspiration in infants: A prospective study. J Pediatr 1974; 85:848-52.
167. Gadzinowski J. Contemporary treatment options for meconium aspiration syndrome. Croat Med J 1998; 39:158-64.
168. Ting P, Brady JP. Tracheal suction in meconium aspiration. Am J Obstet Gynecol 1975; 122:767-71.
169. Carson BS, Losey RW, Bowes WA Jr, Simmons MA. Combined obstetric and pediatric approach to prevent meconium aspiration syndrome. Am J Obstet Gynecol 1976; 126:712-5.
170. Murphy JD, Vawter GF, Reid LM. Pulmonary vascular disease in fatal meconium aspiration. J Pediatr 1984; 104:758-62.
171. Hislop A, Reid L. Intra-pulmonary arterial development during fetal life: Branching pattern and structure. J Anat 1972; 113:35-48.
172. Hislop A, Reid L. Pulmonary arterial development during childhood: Branching pattern and structure. Thorax 1973; 28:129-35.
173. Meyrick B, Reid L. The effect of continued hypoxia on rat pulmonary arterial circulation: An ultrastructural study. Lab Invest 1978; 38:188-200.
174. Perlman EJ, Moore GW, Hutchins GM. The pulmonary vasculature in meconium aspiration. Hum Pathol 1989; 20:701-6.
175. O'Neal RM, Ahlvin RC, Bauer WC, Thomas WA. Development of fetal pulmonary arterioles. AMA Arch Pathol 1957; 63:309-15.
176. Naeye RL. Arterial changes during the perinatal period. Arch Pathol 1961; 71:121-8.
177. Davies G, Reid L. Growth of the alveoli and pulmonary arteries in childhood. Thorax 1970; 25:669-81.
178. Haworth SG, Hislop AA. Pulmonary vascular development: Normal values of peripheral vascular structure. Am J Cardiol 1983; 52:578-83.
179. Wagenvoort CA, Dingemans KP. Pulmonary vascular smooth muscle and its interaction with endothelium: Morphologic considerations. Chest 1985; 88:200S-2S.
180. Davis RO, Philips JB, Harris BA, et al. Fatal meconium aspiration syndrome occurring despite airway management considered appropriate. Am J Obstet Gynecol 1985; 151:731-6.
181. Falciglia HS, Henderschott C, Potter P, Helmchen R. Does DeLee suction at the perineum prevent meconium aspiration syndrome? Am J Obstet Gynecol 1992; 167:1243-9.
182. Linder N, Aranda JV, Tsur M, et al. Need for endotracheal intubation and suction in meconium-stained neonates. J Pediatr 1988; 112:613-5.
183. Ghidini A, Spong CY. Severe meconium aspiration syndrome is not caused by aspiration of meconium. Am J Obstet Gynecol 2001; 185:931-8.
184. Fraser WD, Hofmeyr J, Lede R, et al. Amnioinfusion for the prevention of the meconium aspiration syndrome. N Engl J Med 2005; 353:909-17.
185. Ross MG. Meconium aspiration syndrome: More than intrapartum meconium. N Engl J Med 2005; 353:946-8.
186. American College of Obstetricians and Gynecologists Committee on Obstetric Practice. Amnioinfusion does not prevent meconium aspiration syndrome. ACOG Committee Opinion No. 346, October 2006. (Obstet Gynecol 2006; 108:1053-5.)
187. American College of Obstetricians and Gynecologists Committee on Obstetric Practice. Management of delivery of a newborn with meconium-stained amniotic fluid. ACOG Committee Opinion No. 379, September 2007. (Obstet Gynecol 2007; 110:739.)
188. Vain NE, Szyld EG, Prudent LM, et al. Oropharyngeal and nasopharyngeal suctioning of meconium-stained neonates before delivery of their shoulders: Multicentre, randomised controlled trial. Lancet 2004; 364:597-602.
189. Locus P, Yeomans E, Crosby U. Efficacy of bulb versus DeLee suction at deliveries complicated by meconium stained amniotic fluid. Am J Perinatol 1990; 7:87-91.
190. Ballard JL, Musial MJ, Myers MG. Hazards of delivery room resuscitation using oral methods of endotracheal suctioning. Pediatr Infect Dis 1986; 5:198-200.
191. Van Dyke RB, Spector SA. Transmission of herpes simplex virus type 1 to a newborn infant during endotracheal suctioning for meconium aspiration. Pediatr Infect Dis 1984; 3:153-6.
192. Oriol NE. Aspiration of meconium from the trachea of neonates. Anesthesiology 1990; 73:1294.
193. Hamilton BE, Minino AM, Martin JA, et al. Annual summary of vital statistics: 2005. Pediatrics 2007; 119:345-60.
194. Volpe JJ. Neurology of the Newborn. 4th edition. Philadelphia, WB Saunders, 2001.
195. Wolke D, Meyer R. Cognitive status, language attainment, and prereading skills of 6-year-old very preterm children and their peers. The Bavarian Longitudinal Study. Dev Med Child Neurol 1999; 41:94-109.
196. Paneth N. Classifying brain damage in preterm infants. J Pediatr 1999; 134:527-9.
197. Volpe JJ. Brain injury in the premature infant: Overview of clinical aspects, neuropathology, and pathogenesis. Semin Pediatr Neurol 1998; 5:135-51.
198. Vohr BR, Wright LL, Dusick AM, et al. Neurodevelopmental and functional outcomes of extremely low birth weight infants in the National Institute of Child Health and Human Development Neonatal Research Network, 1993-1994. Pediatrics 2000; 105:1216-26.
199. Chen CH, Shen WC, Wang TM, Chi CS. Cerebral magnetic resonance imaging of preterm infants after corrected age of one year. Acta Paed Sin 1995; 36:261-5.
200. Reynolds ML, Evans CAN, Reynolds EOR, et al. Intracranial haemorrhage in the preterm sheep fetus. Early Hum Dev 1979; 3:163-86.
201. Goddard J, Lewis RM, Armstrong DL, Zeller RS. Moderate, rapidly induced hypertension as a cause of intraventricular hemorrhage in the newborn beagle model. J Pediatr 1980; 96:1057-60.
202. Perlman JM, McMenamin JB, Volpe JJ. Fluctuating cerebral bloodflow velocity in respiratory-distress syndrome: Relation to the

development of intraventricular hemorrhage. N Engl J Med 1983; 309:204-9.
203. Volpe JJ. Neurologic outcome of prematurity. Arch Neurol 1998; 55:297-300.
204. Volpe JJ. Brain injury in the premature infant: Neuropathology, clinical aspects, pathogenesis, and prevention. Clin Perinatol 1997; 24:567-87.
205. Perlman JM, Volpe JJ. Are venous circulatory abnormalities important in the pathogenesis of hemorrhagic and/or ischemic cerebral injury? Pediatrics 1987; 80:705-11.
206. Goldberg RN, Chung D, Goldman SL, Bancalari E. The association of rapid volume expansion and intraventricular hemorrhage in the preterm infant. J Pediatr 1980; 96:1060-3.
207. Nakamura Y, Okudera T, Fukuda S, Hashimoto T. Germinal matrix hemorrhage of venous origin in preterm neonates. Hum Pathol 1990; 21:1059-62.
208. van de Bor M, Briet E, Van Bel F, Ruys JH. Hemostasis and periventricular-intraventricular hemorrhage of the newborn. Am J Dis Child 1986; 140:1131-4.
209. Goldstein GW. Pathogenesis of brain edema and hemorrhage: Role of the brain capillary. Pediatrics 1979; 64:357-60.
210. Gould SJ, Howard S. An immunohistochemical study of the germinal layer in the late gestation human fetal brain. Neuropathol Appl Neurobiol 1987; 13:421-37.
211. Goldenberg RL, Hauth JC, Andrews WW. Intrauterine infection and preterm delivery. N Engl J Med 2000; 342:1500-7.
212. Shankaran S, Cepeda E, Muran G, et al. Antenatal phenobarbital therapy and neonatal outcome. I. Effect on intracranial hemorrhage. Pediatrics 1996; 97:644-8.
213. Shankaran S, Woldt E, Nelson J, et al. Antenatal phenobarbital therapy and neonatal outcome. II. Neurodevelopmental outcome at 36 months. Pediatrics 1996; 97:649-52.
214. Morales WJ, Angel JL, O'Brien WF, et al. The use of antenatal vitamin K in the prevention of early neonatal intraventricular hemorrhage. Am J Obstet Gynecol 1988; 159:774-9.
215. Thorp JA, Parriott J, Ferrette-Smith D, et al. Antepartum vitamin K and phenobarbital for preventing intraventricular hemorrhage in the premature newborn: A randomized, double-blind, placebo-controlled trial. Obstet Gynecol 1994; 83:70-6.
216. Moïse AA, Wearden ME, Kozinetz CA, et al. Antenatal steroids are associated with less need for blood pressure support in extremely premature infants. Pediatrics 1995; 95:845-50.
217. Wallace EM, Baker LS. Effect of antenatal betamethasone administration on placental vascular resistance. Lancet 1999; 353:1404-7.
218. Nelson KG, Grether JK. Can magnesium sulfate reduce the risk of cerebral palsy in very low birthweight infants? Pediatrics 1995; 95:263-9.
219. Paneth N, Jetton J, Pinto-Martin J, et al. Magnesium sulfate in labor and risk of neonatal brain lesions and cerebral palsy in low birth weight infants. Pediatrics 1997; 99:e1.
220. Hirtz DG, Nelson K. Magnesium sulfate and cerebral palsy in premature infants. Curr Opin Pediatr 1998; 10:131-7.
221. Mittendorf R, Dambrosia J, Pryde PG, et al. Association between the use of antenatal magnesium sulfate in preterm labor and adverse health outcomes in infants. Am J Obstet Gynecol 2002; 186:1111-8.
222. Anderson GD, Bada HS, Shaver DC, et al. The effect of cesarean section on intraventricular hemorrhage in the preterm infant. Am J Obstet Gynecol 1992; 166:1091-1101.
223. Perlman JM, Goodman S, Kreusser KL, Volpe JJ. Reduction in intraventricular hemorrhage by elimination of fluctuating cerebral bloodflow velocity in preterm infants with respiratory distress syndrome. N Engl J Med 1985; 312:1353-7.
224. Miall-Allen VM, Whitelaw AG. Effect of pancuronium and pethidine on heart rate and blood pressure in ventilated infants. Arch Dis Child 1987; 62:1179-80.
225. Saarenmaa E, Huttunen P, Leppäluoto J, et al. Advantages of fentanyl over morphine in analgesia for ventilated newborn infants after birth: A randomized trial. J Pediatr 1999; 134:144-50.
226. Myers RE, Myers SE. Use of sedative, analgesic, and anesthetic drugs during labor and delivery: Bane or boon? Am J Obstet Gynecol 1979; 133:83-104.
227. Richards DS, Yancey MK, Duff P, Stieg FH. The perinatal management of severe laryngeal stenosis. Obstet Gynecol 1992; 80:537-40.
228. Leichty KW, Crombleholme TM, Flake AW, Adzick NS. Intrapartum airway management for giant fetal neck masses: the EXIT (ex utero intrapartum treatment) procedure. Am J Obstet Gynecol 1997; 177:870-4.
229. MacKenzie TC, Crombleholme TM, Flake AW. The ex-utero intrapartum treatment. Curr Opin Pediatr 2002; 14:453-8.
230. Crombleholme TM, Sylvester K, Flake AW, et al. Salvage of a fetus with congenital high airway obstruction syndrome by ex utero intrapartum treatment (EXIT) procedure. Fetal Diagn Ther 2000; 15:280-2.
231. Noah MMS, Norton ME, Sandberg P, et al. Short-term maternal outcomes that are associated with the EXIT procedure, as compared with cesarean delivery. Am J Obstet Gynecol 2002; 186:773-7.
232. Sakawi Y, Boyd G, Shaw B, et al. Use of sevoflurane to provide uterine relaxation for the ex-utero intrapartum procedure. Am J Anesthesiol 2001; 28:195-8.
233. George RB, Melnick AH, Rose EC, Habib AS. Case series: Combined spinal epidural anesthesia for cesarean delivery and ex utero intrapartum treatment procedure. Can J Anaesth 2007; 54:218-22.
234. Gregory GA. Esophageal atresia and tracheoesophageal fistula. In Rogers MC, editor. Current Practice in Anesthesiology. 2nd edition. St. Louis, Mosby-Year Book, 1990:218-22.
235. Haberkern CM, Crone RK. Congenital diaphragmatic hernia. In Rogers MC, editor. Current Practice in Anesthesiology. 2nd edition. St. Louis, Mosby-Year Book, 1990:211-7.
236. Davis DJ. How aggressive should delivery room cardiopulmonary resuscitation be for extremely low birth weight neonates? Pediatrics 1993; 92:447-50.
237. Jain L, Ferre C, Vidyasagar D, Nath S, Sheftel D. Cardiopulmonary resuscitation of apparently stillborn infants: Survival and long-term outcome. J Pediatr 1991; 118:778-82.
238. Yeo CL, Tudehope DI. Outcome of resuscitated apparently stillborn infants: A ten-year review. J Paediatr Child Health 1994; 30:129-33.
239. Casalaz DM, Marlow N, Speidel BD. Outcome of resuscitation following unexpected apparent stillbirth. Arch Dis Child Fetal Neonatal Ed 1998; 78:F112-5.
240. Brazelton TB, Scholl ML, Robey JS. Visual behavior in the neonate. Pediatrics 1966; 37:284-90.
241. Ball W, Tronick E. Infant response to impending collision: Optical and real. Science 1971; 171:818-20.
242. Kearsley RB. The newborn's response to auditory stimulation: A demonstration of orienting and defensive behavior. Child Dev 1973; 44:582-90.
243. Brazelton TB. Neonatal behavioral assessment scale. (Clinics in Developmental Medicine, No. 50.) London, Spastics International Medical Publications, William Heinemann Medical Books, 1973.
244. Brazelton TB. Psychophysiologic reactions in the neonate. II. Effect of maternal medication on the neonate and his behavior. J Pediatr 1961; 58:513-8.
245. Scanlon JW, Brown WU Jr, Weiss JB, Alper MH. Neurobehavioral responses of newborn infants after maternal epidural anesthesia. Anesthesiology 1974; 40:121-8.
246. Prechtal HFR, Beintema D. The neurological examination of the full term infant. (Clinics in Developmental Medicine, No. 12.) London, Spastics International Medical Publications, William Heinemann Medical Books, 1964.
247. Beintema DJ. A neurological study of newborn infants. (Clinics in Developmental Medicine, No. 28.) London, Spastics International Medical Publications, William Heinemann Medical Books, 1968.
248. Amiel-Tison C, Barrier G, Shnider SM, et al. A new neurologic and adaptive capacity scoring system for evaluating obstetric medications in full-term newborns. Anesthesiology 1982; 56:340-50.
249. Brockhurst NJ, Littleford JA, Halpern SH. The neurologic and adaptive capacity score. Anesthesiology 2000; 92:237-46.
250. Camann W, Brazelton TB. Use and abuse of neonatal neurobehavioral testing (editorial). Anesthesiology; 2000; 92:3-5.

251. Halpern SH, Littleford JA, Brockhurst NJ, et al. The neurologic and adaptive capacity score is not a reliable method of newborn evaluation. Anesthesiology 2001; 94:958-62.
252. Amiel-Tison C. Update of the Amiel-Tison neurologic assessment for the term neonate or at 40 weeks corrected age. Pediatr Neurol 2002; 27:196-212.
253. American Academy of Pediatrics Committee on Drugs. Effects of medication during labor and delivery on infant outcome. Pediatrics 1978; 62:402-3.
254. US Department of Health and Human Services, Public Health Service, Food and Drug Administration. Guidelines for the Clinical Evaluation of Local Anesthetics. Rockville, MD, US Dept of Health and Human Services, FDA, 1977:82-3053.
255. US Department of Health and Human Services, Public Health Service, Food and Drug Administration. Guidelines for the Clinical Evaluation of General Anesthetics. Rockville, MD, US Dept of Health and Human Services, FDA, 1977:82-3052.
256. Brackbill Y, Kane J, Manniello RL, Abramson D. Obstetric meperidine usage and assessment of neonatal status. Anesthesiology 1974; 40:116-20.
257. Rolbin SH, Wright RG, Shnider SM, et al. Diazepam during cesarean section: Effects on neonatal Apgar scores, acid-base status, neurobehavioral assessment and maternal and fetal plasma norepinephrine levels. Abstracts of Scientific Papers. New Orleans, American Society of Anesthesiologists, 1977:449.
258. Dailey PA, Baysinger CL, Levinson G, Shnider SM. Neurobehavioral testing of the newborn infant: Effects of obstetric anesthesia. Clin Perinatol 1982; 9:191-214.
259. Hodgkinson R, Bhatt M, Wang CN. Double-blind comparison of the neurobehaviour of neonates following the administration of different doses of meperidine to the mother. Can Anaesth Soc J 1978; 25:405-11.
260. Lieberman BA, Rosenblatt DB, Belsey E, et al. The effects of maternally administered pethidine or epidural bupivacaine on the fetus and newborn. Br J Obstet Gynaecol 1979; 86:598-606.
261. Rayburn WF, Smith CV, Leuschen MP, et al. Comparison of patient-controlled and nurse-administered analgesia using intravenous fentanyl during labor. Anesthesiol Rev 1991; 18:31-6.
262. Kileff ME, James FM, Dewan DM, Floyd HM. Neonatal neurobehavioral responses after epidural anesthesia for cesarean section using lidocaine and bupivacaine. Anesth Analg 1984; 63:413-7.
263. Brown WU Jr, Bell GC, Lurie AO, et al. Newborn blood levels of lidocaine and mepivacaine in the first postnatal day following maternal epidural anesthesia. Anesthesiology 1975; 42:698-707.
264. Datta S, Corke BC, Alper MH, et al. Epidural anesthesia for cesarean section: A comparison of bupivacaine, chloroprocaine, and etidocaine. Anesthesiology 1980; 52:48-51.
265. Kuhnert BR, Harrison MJ, Linn PL, Kuhnert PM. Effects of maternal epidural anesthesia on neonatal behavior. Anesth Analg 1984; 63:301-8.
266. Sepkoski CM, Lester BM, Ostheimer GW, Brazelton TB. The effects of maternal epidural anesthesia on neonatal behavior during the first month. Dev Med Child Neurol 1992; 34:1072-80.
267. Abboud TK, Khoo SS, Miller F, et al. Maternal, fetal, and neonatal responses after epidural anesthesia with bupivacaine, 2-chloroprocaine, or lidocaine. Anesth Analg 1982; 61:638-44.
268. Tronick E. A critique of the neonatal Neurologic and Adaptive Capacity Score (NACS). Anesthesiology 1982; 56:338-9.
269. Hodgkinson R, Bhatt M, Kim SS, et al. Neonatal neurobehavioral tests following cesarean section under general and spinal anesthesia. Am J Obstet Gynecol 1978; 132:670-4.
270. Hughes SC, Rosen MA, Shnider SM, et al. Maternal and neonatal effects of epidural morphine for labor and delivery. Anesth Analg 1984; 63:319-24.
271. Preston PG, Rosen MA, Hughes SC, et al. Epidural anesthesia with fentanyl and lidocaine for cesarean section: Maternal effects and neonatal outcome. Anesthesiology 1988; 68:938-43.
272. Murakawa K, Abboud TK, Yanagi T, et al. Clinical experience of epidural fentanyl for labor pain. J Anesth 1987; 1:93-5.
273. Cohen SE, Tan S, Albright GA, Halpern J. Epidural fentanyl/bupivacaine mixtures for obstetric analgesia. Anesthesiology 1987; 67:403-7.
274. Abboud TK, Afrasiabi A, Zhu J, et al. Epidural morphine or butorphanol augments bupivacaine analgesia during labor. Reg Anesth 1989; 14:115-20.
275. Abboud TK, Zhu J, Afrasiabi A, et al. Epidural butorphanol augments lidocaine sensory anesthesia during labor. Reg Anesth 1991; 16:265-7.
276. Little MS, McNitt JD, Choi HJ, Tremper KK. A pilot study of low dose epidural sufentanil and bupivacaine for labor anesthesia (abstract). Anesthesiology 1987; 67:A444.
277. Abboud TK, David S, Nagappala S, et al. Maternal, fetal and neonatal effects of lidocaine with and without epinephrine for epidural analgesia in obstetrics. Anesth Analg 1984; 63:973-9.
278. Abboud TK, Sheik-ol-Eslam A, Yanagi T, et al. Safety and efficacy of epinephrine added to bupivacaine for lumbar epidural analgesia in obstetrics. Anesth Analg 1985; 64:585-91.
279. Abboud TK, DerSarkissian L, Terrasi J, et al. Comparative maternal, fetal and neonatal effects of chloroprocaine with and without epinephrine for epidural anesthesia in obstetrics. Anesth Analg 1987; 66:71-5.
280. Abboud TK, Afrasiabi A, Zhu J, et al. Bupivacaine/butorphanol/epinephrine for epidural anesthesia in obstetrics: Maternal and neonatal effects. Reg Anesth 1989; 14:219-24.
281. Abboud TK, Nagappala S, Murakawa K, et al. Comparison of the effects of general and regional anesthesia for cesarean section on neonatal neurologic and adaptive capacity scores. Anesth Analg 1985; 64:996-1000.
282. Palahniuk RJ, Scatliff J, Biehl D, et al. Maternal and neonatal effects of methoxyflurane, nitrous oxide and lumbar epidural anaesthesia for Caesarean section. Can Anaesth Soc J 1977; 24:586-96.
283. Stefani SJ, Hughes SC, Shnider SM, et al. Neonatal neurobehavioral effects of inhalation analgesia for vaginal delivery. Anesthesiology 1982; 56:351-5.
284. Abboud TK, Gangolly J, Mosaad P, Crowell D. Isoflurane in obstetrics. Anesth Analg 1989; 68:388-91.

Chapter 10

Fetal and Neonatal Neurologic Injury

Donald H. Penning, M.D., M.Sc., FRCP

The detection and diagnosis of fetal and newborn brain injury have been advanced by improvements in functional imaging and the identification of potential biochemical markers. The pathophysiology of fetal brain injury, including responsible factors and clinical associations, indicates that inflammatory mediators play an important role. Controversy exists regarding the use of hypothermia for therapy and the possible effects of magnesium sulfate and anesthetic agents on neurologic outcomes. Overall, little progress has been made to reduce the incidence of fetal brain injury and cerebral palsy.

HISTORY, DEFINITIONS, AND SIGNIFICANCE

In 1861, an orthopedic surgeon named John Little first described cerebral palsy in a report to the Obstetrical Society of London. Described as a newborn neurologic disorder associated with difficult labor or birth trauma, the disorder was known as Little's disease until William Osler coined the term *cerebral palsy* in 1888.[1] The definition and classification of cerebral palsy has proved to be elusive. In the "Report on the Definition and Classification of Cerebral Palsy," published in 2007 in *Developmental Medicine and Child Neurology*, Peter Baxter[2] wrote, "This [supplement] illustrates the difficulties inherent in trying to agree what we mean by the terms we use and that a classification that suits one purpose, such as a diagnostic approach, may not always be ideal for others, such as therapy issues. Defining and classifying cerebral palsy is far from easy. We do need a consensus that can be used in all aspects of day-to-day care and for future research on cerebral palsy."

Today, **cerebral palsy** can be defined as a nonprogressive disorder of the central nervous system (CNS) present since birth that includes some impairment of motor function or posture.[3] *Intellectual disability* (formerly known as *mental retardation*) may be present but is not an essential diagnostic criterion. Various forms of cerebral palsy exist, with differences in pathology, pathophysiology, and potential relationships with intrapartum events. Rosen and Dickinson[4] reviewed studies from Europe, Australia, and the United States that were published between 1985 and 1990 and that included data from 1959 to 1982 (Table 10-1). The rate of cerebral palsy ranged from 1.8 to 4.9 (composite rate of 2.7) cases per 1000 live births. The incidence of certain conditions was as follows: birth weight less than 2500 g, 26%; diplegia, 34%; hemiplegia, 30%; quadriplegia, 20%; and extrapyramidal forms, 16%.[5-15] The data from individual studies are difficult to compare owing to variations in the duration of follow-up evaluations, birth weight classifications, inclusion criteria for congenital abnormalities, and exclusion criteria for various causes of death.

The literature on cerebral palsy is difficult to review and understand. Terms such as *hypoxic-ischemic encephalopathy (HIE) of the newborn, newborn asphyxia, birth asphyxia*, and *asphyxia neonatorum* are difficult to distinguish. Some authorities have argued that the term *birth asphyxia* should be abandoned. The American College of Obstetricians and Gynecologists (ACOG) prefers the use of the more descriptive and less pejorative terms **hypercarbia, hypoxia, metabolic acidemia,** and **respiratory** or **lactic acidosis.**[16,17] However, the term *birth asphyxia* continues

TABLE 10-1 Cumulative Incidence of Cerebral Palsy per 1000 Live Births

Study	Birth Years	Year Published	Country	Length of Follow-Up (Years)	Rate (per 1000), Excluding Acquired
Jarvis et al.[5]	1972-1975	1985	England	5	1.8
Nelson and Ellenberg[6]*	1959-1966	1986	United States	7	4.6
Emond et al.[7]	1970	1989	England	7	2.5
Hagberg et al.[8]†	1979-1982	1989	Sweden	4	2.2
Holst et al.[9]	1978	1989	Denmark	4	4.9
Dowding and Barry[10]‡	1979-1981	1988	Ireland	4	1.9
Stanley and Watson[11]	1979-1981	1988	West Australia	5	2.3
Riikonen et al.[12]	1978-1982	1989	Finland	5	2.5
Torfs et al.[13]§	1959-1966	1990	United States	5	2.0
Pharoah et al.[14]	1984	1990	England	5	1.9
Meberg[15]	1980-1984	1990	Norway	4	2.1
Composite rate					**2.7**

*Collaborative Perinatal Project.

†Excluded deaths before age 2 years.

‡Excluded all congenital anomalies.

§Did not indicate whether deaths were included.

Modified from Rosen MG, Dickinson JC. The incidence of cerebral palsy. Am J Obstet Gynecol 1992; 167:417-23.

to be used, and in this chapter, the term *asphyxia* has been retained as a reflection of our incomplete knowledge of the factors responsible for neurologic injury.

Intrapartum misadventures continue to receive the blame for some cases of cerebral palsy. It is a logical and widely believed theory that an intrapartum reduction in fetal oxygen delivery may cause cerebral palsy, and early reports in primates demonstrated that perinatal asphyxia could cause brain injury.[18] Electronic fetal heart rate (FHR) monitoring, which has largely replaced intermittent FHR auscultation during labor (despite the fact that studies have failed to demonstrate its clear superiority), is believed to prompt the delivery of at-risk fetuses and thus prevent asphyxial events. However, despite a higher incidence of cesarean delivery prompted by nonreassuring FHR tracings, no reduction in the incidence of cerebral palsy has been observed.[19,20] Further, among patients with new-onset late FHR decelerations, an estimated 99% of tracings would be false positive "if used as an indicator for subsequent development of cerebral palsy."[21] This information is probably surprising to the lay public and trial lawyers as well as obstetricians; a survey of maternal-fetal medicine fellows showed that they, too, have greatly overestimated the diagnostic accuracy of FHR monitoring.[21]

Large randomized trials have not demonstrated better fetal and neonatal outcomes with continuous electronic FHR monitoring than with intermittent FHR auscultation.[22,23] In an editorial citing observations made by Schifrin and Dame,[24] Friedman[25] opined, "The absence of either suggestive or overtly ominous fetal heart rate patterns is reliably reassuring." Unfortunately, there is little objective evidence that reassuring FHR tracings exclude the subsequent occurrence of cerebral palsy. In a review of published FHR monitoring studies, Rosen and Dickinson[26] could not identify FHR patterns that were consistently associated with neurologic injuries. Moreover, no consistent FHR pattern was observed in a subset of 55 brain-damaged infants. These investigators concluded, "We do not advocate the abandonment of the use of electronic fetal monitoring, but we do believe that it is yet to be proved to be of value in predicting or preventing neurologic morbidity." A more focused application of FHR monitoring may ultimately be found useful. For example, fetal inflammatory changes, which can be associated with neurologic injury, may be associated with characteristic FHR findings.[27]

Electronic FHR monitoring provides incomplete data that should be evaluated in clinical context. When FHR tracings (for infants with neurologic impairment) are evaluated retrospectively, it is appropriate to ask the following questions:

1. Was the tracing normal on admission? If not, perhaps injury occurred earlier and no intervention would be effective.
2. When were abnormalities detected in relation to interventions or delivery?
3. Was the uterus hyperstimulated?
4. Was oxytocin infusion discontinued or reduced?
5. Was delivery imminent? If not, were preparations made for expedited delivery if the FHR abnormalities were not corrected?

Despite significant limitations in the use of intrapartum electronic FHR monitoring, there is no doubt that it will continue to be used for the foreseeable future. In a review of medicolegal issues in FHR monitoring, Schifrin and Cohen[28] noted that despite its limitations, "Monitoring deserves credit for reducing intrapartum death, one of the original rationales for its development. In contrast to the studies showing either no benefit of [electronic FHR monitoring] or no advantage over auscultation, there are studies that show that hospitals [that] use monitors have improved outcomes in litigation-based studies of individual cases . . . in which glaring failures of monitoring and communication among providers of obstetric care lead to presumably preventable adverse outcomes."[28] One thing seems clear: Nonreassuring changes in FHR tracings must be identified, and clear communication of those changes must occur. As these investigators concluded, "It seems that we best protect ourselves in medicolegal matters when we protect the mother and the fetus during labor."

In a separate report, Schifrin and Cohen[29] described "the 100% cesarean solution," which might reduce the risks of intrapartum asphyxia, birth trauma, and pelvic floor injury, and thus, in theory, might reduce the number of lawsuits for bad outcomes associated with vaginal delivery. Elective cesarean delivery is convenient for the patient and obstetrician and, at least for the first pregnancy, poses a relatively low risk. However, in subsequent pregnancies, patients may be at higher risk for maternal morbidity and mortality from uterine rupture, placenta accreta, catastrophic bleeding and transfusion, and other surgical complications (e.g., infection) as well as for increased neonatal morbidity from iatrogenic prematurity.

It is understandable that many cesarean deliveries are performed in an effort to avoid significant mediocolegal judgments against obstetricians for fetal/neonatal neurologic injury. These awards are not limited to the United States; in the United Kingdom, payments to plaintiffs "regularly exceed £3 million, and in some cases lawyers' fees exceed the award."[1] Many attorneys and physicians contend that most cases of cerebral palsy are a direct result of a perinatal complication or misadventure.[30] One plaintiff's attorney stated, "If the doctor does not know or is not apprised of the possibility of a depressed fetus and does not remove the fetus by cesarean [delivery] so that the baby can survive the birth process, then that doctor has committed malpractice."[31] Clearly this represents an extreme view. Intrapartum events are responsible for some cases of cerebral palsy[32]; however, these cases are few in number. After exclusion of infants with significant congenital anomalies, intrapartum events—including asphyxial insults—likely account for only 6% to 10% of cases of cerebral palsy.[33,34] Of interest, fetal neurologic abnormalities that are potentially the result of intrapartum events have been described and published as templates (see later).[35]

EPIDEMIOLOGY AND ETIOLOGY OF CEREBRAL PALSY

The causes of cerebral palsy are not known, but the varying forms suggest a multifactorial etiology. The Collaborative Perinatal Project still represents one of the largest studies of the antecedent factors associated with cerebral palsy. The investigators in this study evaluated the outcomes of 54,000 pregnancies among patients who delivered at 12 university hospitals between 1959 and 1966. They evaluated more than 400 variables in a univariate analysis,[36] which identified potential risk factors that were then subjected to a more rigorous multivariate analysis.[37] The univariate analysis did not suggest that maternal age, parity, socioeconomic status, smoking history, maternal diabetes, duration of labor, or use of anesthesia was associated with cerebral palsy. The multivariate analysis determined that the leading factors associated with cerebral palsy were (1) maternal mental retardation (now known as intellectual disability), (2) birth weight of 2000 g or less, and (3) fetal malformations. Other factors associated with cerebral palsy included (1) breech presentation (but not vaginal breech delivery), (2) severe proteinuria (more than 5 g/24 hr) during the second half of pregnancy, (3) third-trimester bleeding, and (4) a gestational age of 32 weeks or less. There was a slight association between cerebral palsy and fetal bradycardia, chorioamnionitis, and low placental weight. However, only 34% of the cases of cerebral palsy occurred among the 5% of the population deemed to be at highest risk before pregnancy; this proportion increased to 37% when the investigators included factors identified during pregnancy or postpartum. These data suggest that most cases of cerebral palsy cannot be predicted and that the identification of pregnancy-related conditions contributes minimally to the identification of patients at risk for having a child with cerebral palsy. A large epidemiologic study noted an incidence of neonatal encephalopathy of 3.8 per 1000 term births.[38] The investigators identified certain preconception and antepartum factors that were associated with neonatal encephalopathy (Box 10-1). Intrapartum factors alone are associated with neonatal encephalopathy in less than 5% of cases.[38,39]

BOX 10-1 Western Australian Risk Factors for Newborn Encephalopathy

Preconception Factors*

- Increasing maternal age
- Mother unemployed, unskilled laborer, or housewife
- No private health insurance
- Family history of seizures
- Family history of neurologic disorders
- Infertility treatment

Antepartum Factors*

- Maternal thyroid disease
- Severe preeclampsia
- Bleeding in pregnancy
- Viral illness in pregnancy
- Postdates pregnancy
- Fetal growth restriction
- Placental abnormalities

*Significantly and independently associated with newborn encephalopathy in multiple logistic regression analysis.

Information compiled from Badawi N, Kurinczuk JJ, Keogh JM, et al. Antepartum risk factors for neonatal encephalopathy: The Western Australia case-control study. BMJ 1998; 317:1549-53.

In 2000, the ACOG and the American Academy of Pediatrics convened the Neonatal Encephalopathy and Cerebral Palsy Task Force. The resulting landmark report,[39] which was released in January 2003, was reviewed and endorsed by such groups as the U.S. Department of Health, the Child Neurology Society, the March of Dimes Birth Defects Foundation, the National Institutes of Health, the Royal Australian and New Zealand College of Obstetricians and Gynaecologists, the Society for Maternal-Fetal Medicine, and the Society of Obstetricians and Gynaecologists of Canada. The Task Force extended the earlier international consensus statement regarding the requirements for establishing a causal relationship between

BOX 10-2 Criteria to Define an Acute Intrapartum Hypoxic Event as Sufficient to Cause Cerebral Palsy

Essential Criteria (All Four Must Be Met)

1. Evidence of metabolic acidosis in fetal umbilical cord arterial blood obtained at delivery (pH < 7 and base deficit ≥ 12 mmol/L)*
2. Early onset of severe or moderate neonatal encephalopathy in infants born at 34 or more weeks' gestation
3. Cerebral palsy of the spastic quadriplegic or dyskinetic type†
4. Exclusion of other identifiable etiologies, such as trauma, coagulation disorders, infectious conditions, and genetic disorders

Criteria that Collectively Suggest an Intrapartum Event—within Close Proximity to Labor and Delivery (e.g., 0 to 48 Hours)—but Are Nonspecific to Asphyxial Insults

1. A sentinel (signal) hypoxic event occurring immediately before or during labor
2. A sudden and sustained fetal bradycardia or the absence of fetal heart rate variability in the presence of persistent, late, or variable decelerations, usually after a hypoxic sentinel event when the pattern was previously normal
3. Apgar scores of 0 to 3 beyond 5 minutes
4. Onset of multisystem involvement within 72 hours of birth
5. Early imaging study showing evidence of acute nonfocal cerebral abnormality

*Buffer base is defined as the amount of buffer in blood available to combine with nonvolatile acids. A buffer base of 34 mmol/L is equivalent to a whole blood base deficit of 12 mmol/L.

†Spastic quadriplegia and, less commonly, dyskinetic cerebral palsy are the only types of cerebral palsy associated with acute hypoxic intrapartum events. Spastic quadriplegia is not specific to intrapartum hypoxia. Hemiparetic cerebral palsy, hemiplegic cerebral palsy, spastic diplegia, and ataxia are unlikely to result from acute intrapartum hypoxia. (Nelson KB, Grether JK. Potentially asphyxiating conditions and spastic cerebral palsy in infants of normal birth weight. Am J Obstet Gynecol 1998; 179:507-13.)

Modified from the American College of Obstetricians and Gynecologists Taskforce on Neonatal Encephalopathy and Cerebral Palsy. Neonatal Encephalopathy and Cerebral Palsy: Defining the Pathogenesis and Pathophysiology. Washington, DC, American College of Obstetricians and Gynecologists, 2003. Modified from MacLennan A. A template for defining a causal relation between acute intrapartum events and cerebral palsy: International consensus statement. BMJ 1999; 319:1054-9.

intrapartum events and cerebral palsy.[35] The most important results are summarized in Box 10-2. They lead to several medicolegal conclusions[35,39]:

1. The only types of cerebral palsy associated with intrapartum hypoxia are spastic quadriplegia, and less commonly, dyskinesia.
2. Intellectual disability, learning disorders, and epilepsy should not be ascribed to birth asphyxia unless accompanied by spastic quadriplegia.
3. No statements about severity should be made before an affected child is 3 to 4 years of age, because mild cases may improve and dyskinesia may not be evident until then.
4. Intrapartum hypoxia sufficient to cause cerebral palsy is always accompanied by neonatal encephalopathy and seizures.

Peripartum Asphyxia and Cerebral Palsy

In 1953, Dr. Virginia Apgar, an anesthesiologist, introduced her scoring system to identify newborn infants in need of resuscitation and to assess the adequacy of subsequent resuscitation efforts.[40] Although the Apgar score has also been used to identify infants at risk for cerebral palsy, only a weak association could be found[41,42]; in the Collaborative Perinatal Project, only 1.7% of children with a 1-minute Apgar score of 3 or less demonstrated cerebral palsy.[3] Among infants who weighed more than 2500 g at delivery, the incidence of cerebral palsy was 4.7% if the 5-minute Apgar score was 0 to 3, but 0.2% if the Apgar score was at least 7; among infants who weighed less than 2500 g with the same 5-minute Apgar scores, the incidence of cerebral palsy was 6.7% and 0.8%, respectively. Among all infants, a higher incidence of cerebral palsy was observed if the Apgar score remained 3 or less for longer than 5 minutes. Likewise, the incidence of early neonatal death increased among those infants with prolonged neonatal depression.

Most infants who subsequently manifest evidence of cerebral palsy have a normal 5-minute Apgar score. In the Collaborative Perinatal Project, only 15% of the infants in whom cerebral palsy later developed had a 5-minute Apgar score of 3 or less, approximately 12% had a score of 4 to 6, and the remaining 73% had a score of at least 7.[3]

The Apgar scoring system should be modified for the assessment of preterm newborns. Even under ideal circumstances, preterm neonates are more likely to have hypotonia and peripheral cyanosis and to be less responsive than infants delivered at term; thus, even healthy preterm infants are unlikely to have Apgar scores higher than 7.[43] Current guidelines for both term and preterm neonatal resuscitation delineate assessment on the basis of heart rate, respiration, and color.[44,45]

Although most cases of cerebral palsy are attributed to insults that predate the intrapartum period, intrapartum asphyxia does occur and can have serious consequences; however, the amount of asphyxia necessary to produce irreversible CNS injury is unclear. In some cases, an intrapartum insult that might have otherwise been innocuous might be superimposed on subclinical chronic fetal compromise and result in permanent injury.

The definition of *asphyxia* may be reduced to "insufficient exchange of respiratory gases."[46] Although accurate, this definition does not include an index of severity or have any predictive value. Unfortunately, most studies have not used a uniform definition of *birth asphyxia*.[47-49] Moreover, what constitutes *normal* umbilical cord blood gas and pH measurements remains unclear.[46] In one study of 16,060 *vigorous* neonates (arbitrarily defined as having a

5-minute Apgar score of 7 or more) conducted between 1977 and 1993, the median umbilical arterial blood measurements (with the 2.5th percentile in parentheses) of the 15,073 (94%) of neonates who met the inclusion criteria were as follows: pH 7.26 (7.10), PO_2 17 (6) mm Hg, PCO_2 52 (74) mm Hg, and base excess −4 (−11) mEq/L.[46] Only small differences in median pH and other measurements were present when infants were grouped according to gestational age. It would have been useful if the investigators had reported data for all newborns, including those with Apgar scores less than 7, even though Apgar scores are not good predictors of the development of cerebral palsy.

Although intrapartum events are most likely associated with a minority of cerebral palsy cases, clinical studies have attempted to define the associated extent and duration of perinatal asphyxia. Fee et al.[50] defined asphyxia as an umbilical arterial blood pH of less than 7.05 with a base deficit greater than 10 mEq/L, and they concluded that this threshold was a poor predictor of adverse neurologic outcomes. Goodwin et al.[51] defined asphyxia as an umbilical arterial blood pH of less than 7.00, and they found a greater frequency of morbidity with increases in the severity of acidemia. Goldaber et al.[52] also observed greater neonatal morbidity and mortality among term infants (birth weight more than 2500 g) with an umbilical arterial blood pH of less than 7.00. In summary, asphyxia, by definition, represents an insufficient exchange of respiratory gases; however, the magnitude of impairment that results in clinically significant outcomes remains unclear.

Low et al.[53,54] attempted to further evaluate the role of perinatal asphyxia in cases of neurologic injury through the use of a unique, but not universally accepted, definition of asphyxia. At their institution, a buffer base of less than 36 mmol/L is more than two standard deviations below the mean for "clinically normal" term infants at delivery.[55] Lactic acid contributes to the metabolic acidosis produced by asphyxia; however, because approximately one third of lactate may be derived from pyruvate, the buffer base threshold was reduced to less than 34 mmol/L to "serve as a measure of metabolic acidosis due to hypoxia."[56] With this definition, the incidence of asphyxia in term newborns was found to be approximately 2%; but in a much smaller cohort of preterm infants (less than 2000 g at birth), the incidence was approximately 6%.[56,57] Neurodevelopmental studies in term infants at 1 year of age observed a higher incidence of neurologic deficits among those infants in whom an umbilical artery buffer base value was less than 34 mmol/L at birth; the relationship was especially strong when the umbilical artery buffer base was less than 20 mmol/L at birth.[58] The same investigators observed a similar relationship in a study of preterm newborns.[59]

Low et al.[60,61] also studied complications of intrapartum asphyxia in term and preterm infants; they developed a complication score that expressed the magnitude of neonatal complications. Among term infants, the frequency and severity of newborn complications increased with the severity and duration of metabolic acidosis at birth. A low Apgar score at 1 minute was a better predictor of neonatal complications than a low score at 5 minutes. Of interest, respiratory acidosis at birth did not predict complications in newborns. Similar results were noted for preterm infants delivered between 32 and 36 weeks' gestation. With infants delivered before 32 weeks' gestation, complications were similar in the control and asphyxia groups. When this scoring system was used in term infants, the predicted threshold for moderate or severe newborn complications was an umbilical arterial blood base deficit of 12 mmol/L.[62]

Although Low's definition of asphyxia has not been universally accepted, few studies have followed neurodevelopment examinations for a sufficient duration to refute or accept these associations. Nagel et al.[63] performed such examinations in 30 children in whom umbilical arterial blood pH had been less than 7.00 at delivery, 28 of whom survived the neonatal period. Evaluation at 1 to 3 years of age detected 3 children who had experienced an episode of hypertonia. The majority of children exhibited no major problems, with only 1 child displaying a mild motor developmental delay. Another study examined neonatal complications in 35 newborns with an umbilical arterial blood pH of less than 7.00 at delivery,[64] 3 of whom died during the neonatal period. These investigators did not perform any follow-up neurologic examinations after the neonatal period.[64]

Because metabolic acidosis may be a predictor of complications in newborns, the severity of intrapartum acidosis could be an important variable. Gull et al.[65] studied a small cohort of 27 patients with "terminal bradycardia" who were delivered vaginally. Not surprisingly, the umbilical arterial blood base deficit was greater in infants with end-stage bradycardia than in controls. The loss of short-term FHR variability for more than 4 minutes during end-stage bradycardia correlated with the development of metabolic acidosis.

The relationship between umbilical arterial blood base excess values and the timing of hypoxic injury has been estimated in human and animal studies.[66] Unfortunately, this relationship does not consider the role of previous or repetitive hypoxic episodes before the episode in question and therefore cannot accurately time the injury. In general, the human fetus is quite robust, and episodes of intrauterine asphyxia yield a normal neonate; a much smaller number of fetuses experiencing such episodes die *in utero*. Blumenthal[1] concluded, "There is a fine threshold between normality and death from asphyxia."

The increased presence of nucleated red blood cells in the umbilical circulation at delivery has been proposed as a marker of the occurrence and timing of intrauterine asphyxia.[67-69] However, data from these investigations have demonstrated considerable variability and are influenced by birth weight and gestational age.[70] Furthermore, the timing of the injury may be difficult to express with confidence, because multiple episodes of asphyxia may have occurred. In such cases, the nucleated red blood cell count may reflect and implicate only the most recent, but possibly least important, event. Both nucleated red blood cell and lymphocyte counts appear to undergo more sustained elevations in cases of antepartum than intrapartum asphyxia.[39]

Chorioamnionitis, Fever, and Cerebral Palsy

An association between cerebral palsy and chorioamnionitis has been demonstrated in preterm infants and term infants of normal birth weight.[71,72] An elevated maternal temperature is one sign of chorioamnionitis, but alone it is insufficient for the diagnosis. Other signs include, but are not limited to, maternal and fetal tachycardia, foul-smelling amniotic fluid, uterine tenderness, and maternal leukocytosis. The diagnosis remains unproven until confirmed by placental culture or histologic examination; a Gram stain examination of the amniotic fluid may be useful. The mechanism by which chorioamnionitis is associated with cerebral palsy is unclear; however, inflammatory cytokines may play a role.[73-75]

Several studies have demonstrated a tendency for maternal temperature to rise after administration of epidural analgesia during labor.[76,77] Although the relationship and mechanism of epidural analgesia–associated maternal pyrexia remain unclear, it would be erroneous to suggest a further association with chorioamnionitis and a subsequent risk of cerebral palsy.[78] Moreover, epidural analgesia has been blamed for the common obstetric practice of administering antibiotics to mothers with fever but no other evidence of chorioamnionitis; this practice may lead to unnecessary neonatal sepsis evaluations and antibiotic exposure.[79] Mayer et al.[80] correctly stated that "rather than treating all women with temperature elevations and epidurals for presumed chorioamnionitis," physicians should make an effort to differentiate true chorioamnionitis from incidental maternal fever. These investigators found that additional signs of chorioamnionitis were present in all cases in which the diagnosis was later confirmed by culture or pathologic examination. The influence of epidural analgesia–associated maternal fever on the incidence of cerebral palsy has not been studied directly; however, the largest univariate analysis did not identify neuraxial anesthesia as a risk factor for cerebral palsy.[36]

The mode of delivery has been examined as an independent risk factor for periventricular leukomalacia, the most common form of ischemic brain injury in surviving preterm infants in whom cerebral palsy later develops. In 99 women meeting the criteria for chorioamnionitis and delivering at 25 to 32 weeks' gestation, vaginal delivery had a significant association with periventricular leukomalacia.[81] Because the cesarean delivery group likely included a substantial number of infants with nonreassuring FHR tracings, the better outcomes in these infants is striking; prospective trials are needed to confirm these retrospective observations.

Advances in the Radiologic Diagnosis of Cerebral Injury

Magnetic resonance imaging (MRI) is a useful tool in the diagnosis of neonatal brain injury.[82-84] Although most commonly used during the neonatal period, MRI can also provide an intrauterine diagnosis of fetal brain injury.[85] MRI can assist in the diagnosis of HIE in newborn infants,[86] provide three-dimensional evaluations to determine the volume of gray matter and the extent of white matter myelination (thus providing valuable insights into normal and abnormal brain development),[87] and estimate the timing of the brain injury in patients with cerebral palsy.[88] The presence of cerebral edema confirms recent-onset brain injury; edema develops 6 to 12 hours after injury and resolves within 4 days.[1] Unfortunately, the changes are subtle and the time frame of interest may extend before or after the intrapartum period. Nonetheless, the information can be quite helpful, and early imaging should be performed in cases of suspected brain injury. There is a strong correlation between anatomic brain lesions detected on MRI and specific types of cerebral palsy.[89] MRI is particularly sensitive in the detection of periventricular leukomalacia, although many children with this MRI abnormality have clinically normal neurologic development.[90]

New imaging techniques, such as diffusion tensor imaging and magnetic resonance spectroscopy, may offer advantages over conventional MRI when performed early (i.e., hours) after a hypoxic-ischemic insult. These methods, developed in rabbit[91] and sheep[92] models of intrauterine hypoxia, may accurately predict motor outcome in preterm infants.[93] Injuries detected with these methods are present for a couple of days and resolve over the next week, at which point they may become visible with conventional MRI. Injuries apparent with these newer techniques can therefore support the hypothesis that an injury occurred within days of delivery.[94] Both magnetic resonance spectroscopy and diffusion tensor imaging are powerful new tools for timing the occurrence and understanding the pathophysiology of perinatal brain injury.[95] Cerebral ultrasonography remains a useful technique in the early neurologic assessment of the newborn,[96] especially for the critically ill infant who might not be a candidate for transfer to an MRI facility.

PATHOPHYSIOLOGY OF FETAL ASPHYXIA

Much of our knowledge of the fetal response to asphyxia has been gained through the use of animal models; however, the limitations of these models must be acknowledged. Raju[97] has reviewed the various animal models of fetal brain injury. One advantage of the chronically instrumented fetal lamb is that it is similar in size to the human fetus, facilitating the placement of electrodes and vascular catheters in both the fetus and the mother. Investigators may obtain measurements while the mother (and fetus) remains anesthetized, or from awake animals that have recovered from surgery. Studies of animals with continuous instrumentation allow the assessment of fetal breathing movements, gross body movements, brain electrical activity (electroencephalogram), and blood gas and pH measurements. Blood concentrations of glucose, lactate, and various hormones can also be determined.[98-100] Newer studies have used microdialysis techniques to evaluate neurotransmitter release within the fetal brain *in vivo* in acute, exteriorized, and chronic preparations.[101-103] Other studies have measured fetal cerebral blood flow *in vivo* during episodes of hypoxemia[104] and during maternal infusion of ethanol.[105] Together, these studies have enhanced the understanding of the fetal brain response to pathophysiologic insults *in utero*. Ultimately, these new insights may lead to improved diagnoses, treatment, and prevention of fetal brain injury.

Studies have used a variety of methods to produce fetal hypoxemia and acidemia in fetal lambs. Each method may mimic one or more clinically relevant situation(s), including (1) decreased concentration of maternal inspired oxygen for several hours[98] or days[99]; (2) decreased uterine blood flow, which may be accomplished by placement of an adjustable clamp on the common iliac artery[106]; (3) decreased umbilical blood flow, either by total obstruction[107] or by means of a slow, progressive obstruction[108,109]; (4) selective uteroplacental embolization[110]; (5) maternal hemorrhage[111]; and (6) a combination of two insults, such as hypoxemia plus hypotension.[112]

Care must be exercised in the application of knowledge gained from hypoxia-ischemia studies conducted on nonfetal models (e.g., rat pups) to the problem of intrauterine asphyxia. The fetus and the fetal brain exist in a relatively hypoxemic environment. Despite preferential streaming of the most highly oxygenated blood to the brain and heart, the average Po_2 measured in the carotid artery of fetal lambs at term is approximately 22 mm Hg.[113] Furthermore, unlike adult conditions, in which global anoxia (i.e., cardiac arrest) or focal ischemia (i.e., stroke) is the clinical correlate, fetal asphyxia typically involves diminution, but not absence, of delivery of oxygen with variable degrees of respiratory or metabolic acidosis. A complete loss of cerebral blood flow rarely occurs, except as a terminal event. Of course, prolonged hypoxemia and decreased oxygen delivery can lead to acidemia and myocardial failure, followed by ischemia and rapid fetal demise. Fetal hypoxemia may result from the compromise of any or all of the steps involved in maternal-fetal oxygen transport (Box 10-3).[114] The impact of repeated hypoxic-ischemic insults should not be underestimated, and numerous clinical scenarios can be envisioned whereby this might occur (e.g., repetitive cord occlusion). Moreover, brief insults that may be harmless could cause damage if repeated, as has been demonstrated in adult rats[115] and in fetal lambs.[116]

The fetus takes advantage of several adaptive responses for survival and growth in the relatively hypoxemic intrauterine environment. These responses may be categorized as an alteration of fetal metabolism or maximization of fetal oxygen transport (Box 10-4).[114] Richardson[117] has defined the *oxygen margin of safety* as the extent to which fractional oxygen extraction can increase and fetal arterial Po_2 can decrease before tissue oxygen supplies are inadequate. Regardless of the etiology of decreased oxygen delivery to the fetus, fetal oxygen consumption is maintained by increasing oxygen extraction until oxygen delivery is approximately 50% of normal.[118] Lower levels of tissue oxygen tension result in progressive metabolic acidemia and a terminal decrease in oxygen consumption.[117]

BOX 10-3 Factors Decreasing Oxygen Transfer to the Fetus

Environmental Po_2
- High altitude

Maternal Cardiopulmonary Function
- Cyanotic heart disease

O_2 Transport by Maternal Blood
- Anemia
- Cigarette smoking

Placental Blood Flow
- Hypertension
- Diabetes
- Placental abruption
- Uterine contractions

Placental O_2 Transfer
- Placental abruption
- Placental infarcts

Umbilical Blood Flow and Fetal Circulation
- Umbilical cord occlusion
- Heart disease

O_2 Transport by Fetal Blood
- Anemia
- Hemorrhage

From Richardson B. The fetal brain: Metabolic and circulatory responses to asphyxia. Clin Invest Med 1993; 16:103-14.

BOX 10-4 Fetal Cerebral Responses to Asphyxia

Fetal Cerebral Metabolism
- Increased oxygen extraction
- Use of alternative energy sources
- Decreased growth
- Altered behavioral state

Fetal Cerebral O_2 Transport
- Redistribution of cerebral blood flow

Modified from Richardson B. The fetal brain: Metabolic and circulatory responses to asphyxia. Clin Invest Med 1993; 16:103-14.

Alterations in substrate use may affect the fetal response to asphyxia. Unlike the adult brain, the fetal brain can use ketone bodies and lactate as alternative energy sources.[39] In gravid ewes, reductions in uterine blood flow result in reduced fetal glucose consumption.[119] Current opinion holds that hyperglycemia should be avoided in adult humans at risk for ischemia.[120] Hyperglycemia may exacerbate metabolic acidosis by providing substrate for anaerobic metabolism, which increases lactic acid production. However, Vannucci and Mujsce,[121] citing experiments in neonatal rat pups, suggested that the immature brain may respond differently and that glucose administration may actually reduce hypoxic-ischemic brain injury. These investigators did not consider earlier work by Blomstrand et al.,[122] who studied the effects of hypoxia in the anesthetized, exteriorized fetal lamb. In that study, hyperglycemia accelerated the loss of somatosensory evoked potentials, the onset of metabolic acidosis, and the reduction of cerebral oxygen consumption. Until these different observations are reconciled, the maintenance of normoglycemia *in utero* appears prudent.

During chronic hypoxemia, the fetus may also restrict the use of energy derived from oxidative metabolism to maintain essential cellular processes; this may lead to decreased somatic growth and intrauterine growth restriction. Using an ovine model of asphyxia, Hooper[123] detected a decreased incorporation of tritiated [^{3}H]-thymidine (which reflects decreased DNA turnover and, presumably, decreased cell division) in fetal tissue. The decrease in incorporation of tritiated [^{3}H]-thymidine was not uniform in all tissues. The rates of DNA synthesis were maintained in most fetal tissues (including the fetal brain) but were greatly reduced in the lung, the skeletal muscle, and the thymus gland.

The fetus can conserve additional energy by decreasing breathing and gross body movements. Rurak and Gruber[124] demonstrated a 17% reduction in fetal oxygen consumption in fetal lambs that were paralyzed by a neuromuscular blocking agent. Perceptible fetal movements represent an index of fetal health. Many obstetricians instruct their patients to count episodes of fetal activity for specified periods and to consult them immediately if fetal movements are decreased or absent (see Chapter 6). Fetal hypoxemia results in decreases in both activity and rapid eye movement (REM) sleep in fetal lambs. REM sleep states are associated with an increased cerebral metabolic rate for oxygen ($CMRO_2$).[104] Thus, during periods of fetal stress, reductions in fetal body movements or REM sleep lead to a significant decline in fetal energy expenditure.

Oxygen deprivation typically results in a change in and/or redistribution of fetal cardiac output[125]; the magnitude of these changes depends on the mechanism and severity of oxygen deprivation. Sheldon et al.[126] demonstrated that experimental fetal hypoxemia (produced by the administration of a decreased maternal-inspired concentration of oxygen) resulted in greater blood flow to the brain, myocardium, and adrenal glands. In fetal lambs, a brief (4-minute) complete arrest of uterine and ovarian blood flow resulted in a decrease in blood flow to all organs except the myocardium and adrenal glands.[127]

Adaptive changes to intrauterine hypoxemia vary between immature and mature fetuses. The neuropathology of intrauterine asphyxia depends, to some extent, on gestational age. The neuropathologic response to sustained hypoxemia with developing acidemia was studied in mid-gestation and near-term fetal lambs.[128] In this study, immature fetuses demonstrated a predominantly periventricular injury, whereas mature fetuses had a primarily cortical injury, although there was some overlap (Figure 10-1).[128] This finding is consistent with injury patterns in humans. It is not surprising that the biophysical and biochemical responses to hypoxemia vary between preterm and term fetuses. Matsuda et al.[98] observed that the development of metabolic acidemia, reduced fetal breathing and body movements, and an altered sleep state were much less pronounced in mid-gestation fetal lambs subjected to hypoxemia than in fetal lambs at term.

Studies of fetal lambs are valuable and have provided data that cannot be obtained from human fetuses. The role of the fetal lamb preparation has been reviewed[129]; the ability to measure fetal blood pressure, oxygenation, and blood flow represents a distinct advantage of this model over small rodent models. However, the limitations of all animal models should be understood before one extrapolates experimental findings to the human fetus. At birth, sheep and guinea pig brains are much closer to maturity than the human brain. In this regard, rat pup and human brains are more similar to each other because they both undergo significant extrauterine development (Figure 10-2).[130] Nevertheless, the importance of this

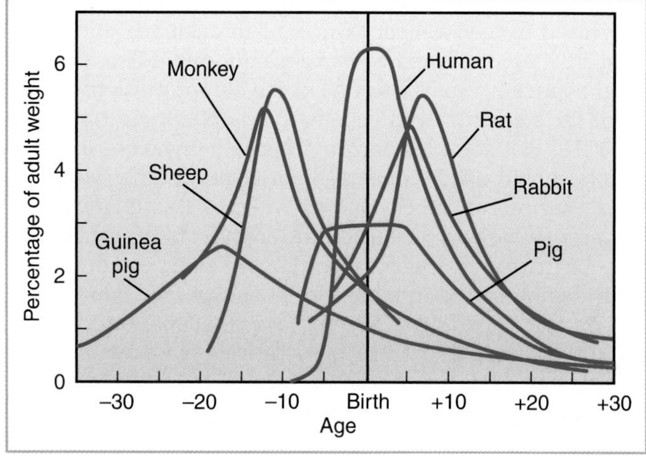

FIGURE 10-2 Brain growth spurts of seven mammalian species expressed as first-order velocity curves of the increase in weight with age. The units of time for each species are as follows: guinea pig (days); rhesus monkey (4 days); sheep (5 days); pig (weeks); human (months); rabbit (2 days); rat (days). Rates are expressed as a percentage of adult weight for each unit of time. (Modified from Dobbing J, Sands S. Comparative aspects of the brain growth spurt. Early Hum Dev 1979; 3:79-83.)

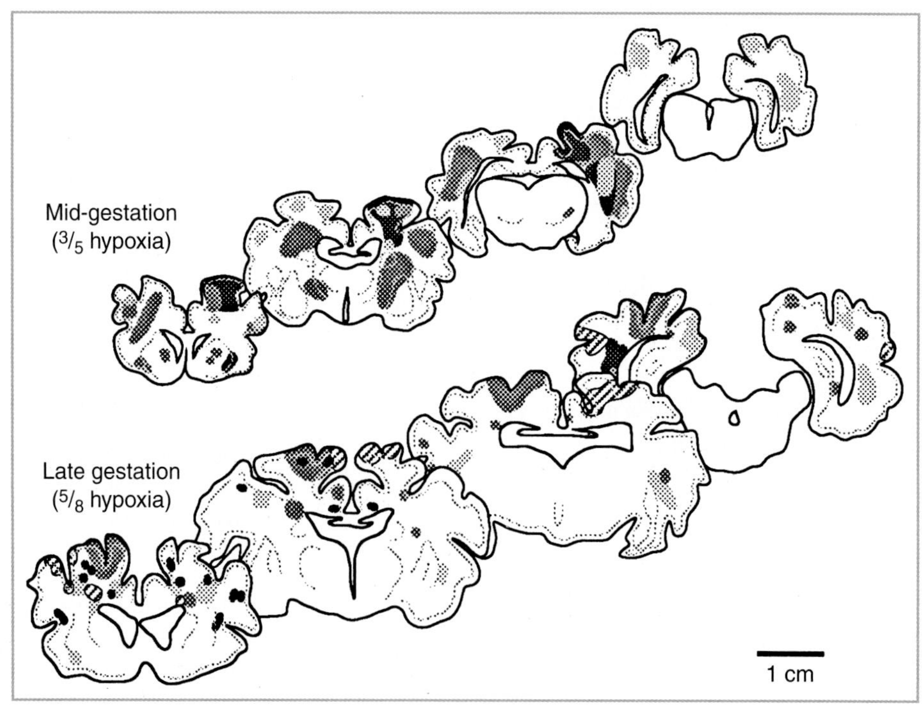

FIGURE 10-1 Composite diagram showing distribution of hypoxic injury in mid-gestation (*top*) and near-term (*bottom*) fetal lambs at 3 days following 8 hours of arterial hypoxemia. Hypoxemia was produced by placing the pregnant ewe in a chamber with reduced ambient oxygen. Each shading pattern represents an individual animal. The severity of injury is not indicated in this diagram. (From Penning DH, Grafe MR, Hammond R, et al. Neuropathology of the near-term and midgestation ovine fetal brain after sustained in utero hypoxemia. Am J Obstet Gynecol 1994; 170:1425-32.)

distinction has been challenged. Previously, investigators relied mainly on morphologic milestones (e.g., the brain growth spurt) to compare species at different stages of development. A new computerized method attempts to more accurately compare observations among 10 species (including humans) by evaluating the mathematical relationships of more than 100 developmental events and factors (e.g., evolutionary, genetic, neurochemical, and neuroanatomical).[131] Although all events have not been catalogued for any one species, the iterative process allows information to be added to improve the theoretic model and is freely available on-line (http://www.translatingtime.net/). The new method is not completely understood or accepted but may explain some of the variability seen between various models of developmental brain injury.

Exchange of nutrients, including oxygen, between the mother and fetus takes place through the placenta, and the efficiency of this process is vital. Because placentation varies among animal species, the type of placentation affects the extent of transplacental transfer of various substances (see Chapter 4). Moreover, the relationship of maternal and fetal blood flows varies among species. Among animals used for studies of fetal physiology, the morphology of the placenta may be either hemochorial or epitheliochorial (see Figure 4-2). In hemochorial forms, the fetal chorion invades the uterine stroma, thereby destroying the maternal endothelium and coming in direct contact with maternal blood. By contrast, epitheliochorial placentas have an intact maternal vascular epithelium.[132]

Maternal blood and fetal blood can flow past each other in an efficient countercurrent pattern, or the exchange can be less well coordinated and efficient, as occurs in the concurrent (or venous equilibration) pattern.[132] The importance of maternal influences on fetal growth and development is lacking in all models of extrauterine "fetal" asphyxia. Thus, in our view, a clinically relevant model of cerebral palsy should be a pregnant intrauterine model; however, identification of such a model has proved elusive. Although the pregnant ewe has been the "gold standard" for years, difficulties remain in translating intrauterine events to functional measurements in postnatal lambs. One group of investigators has described a new animal model that may identify the missing element[133-135]; in their pregnant rabbit model, inflation of an aortic balloon above the uterine arteries produces uterine ischemia *in vivo*. The balloon inflation can mimic various ischemic regimens (sustained or repetitive) and produce fetal hypoxia, bradycardia, and a reduction in cerebral cortical blood flow. Most important, the rabbit babies can be born alive and spontaneously and can be reared prior to neuroradiologic investigations. The experiments have yielded babies with motor deficits and hypertonia comparable to severe forms of cerebral palsy, with evidence of white matter injury on tensor magnetic imaging. This model shows great promise for advancing our knowledge of the pathophysiology of cerebral palsy.

Magnesium Sulfate and Cerebral Palsy

Some controversy exists about the role of magnesium sulfate in preventing or possibly exacerbating fetal brain injury. Two reports documented a decreased incidence of cerebral palsy in surviving very low-birth-weight (VLBW) infants who were exposed to magnesium sulfate *in utero*.[136,137] In a retrospective study, Nelson and Grether[137] reviewed the outcomes of a cohort of San Francisco–area VLBW children born between 1983 and 1985 who had survived to at least 3 years of age. Of the 155,636 live births during this period, 881 VLBW survivors met the study criteria, and 42 of those children had moderate to severe cerebral palsy. These children were matched with 75 randomly selected VLBW controls. Magnesium sulfate had been administered to 7% of the children in the cerebral palsy group and to 36% of the controls (odds ratio [OR], 0.14; 95% confidence interval [CI], 0.05 to 0.51), suggesting that magnesium sulfate had a protective effect. In the majority of cases, magnesium sulfate was administered for seizure prophylaxis in preeclamptic patients. The number of subjects was too small to separate the possible effect of preeclampsia from the proposed protective effect of magnesium sulfate. However, a separate analysis of patients who received magnesium sulfate only for preterm labor tocolysis found that magnesium sulfate was responsible for the protective effect. Further, when a covariate analysis was performed to assess the potential contribution of antenatal corticosteroids administered to accelerate fetal lung maturity, the protective effect of magnesium remained evident.

In a study that has received international attention,[138] Schendel et al.[136] evaluated all VLBW infants born in Atlanta, Georgia, and surrounding counties during a 2-year period to examine the relationship between prenatal exposure to magnesium sulfate and the risk for development of cerebral palsy or intellectual disability among survivors. Among the children who were alive at 3 to 5 years of age, the presence or absence of cerebral palsy, intellectual disability, and intrauterine exposure to magnesium sulfate was determined. The incidence of cerebral palsy for groups exposed and not exposed to magnesium sulfate was 0.9% and 7.7%, respectively (OR, 0.11; 95% CI, 0.02 to 0.81). The incidence of intellectual disability for groups exposed and not exposed to magnesium sulfate was 1.8% and 5.8%, respectively (OR, 0.3; 95% CI, 0.07 to 1.29). The investigators performed a multivariate analysis to assess the contribution of risk factors, including preeclampsia/eclampsia; antihypertensive therapy; maternal drug administration (i.e., antibiotics, other tocolytic agents, corticosteroids); maternal age, education, and race; and infant birth weight, gender, and gestational age at delivery. All of these factors had a negligible effect on the relative risk for either cerebral palsy or intellectual disability. Because the selective mortality of magnesium sulfate–exposed children could have created bias in favor of a protective effect of magnesium sulfate, the investigators also determined whether there was any difference in mortality between magnesium sulfate–exposed and unexposed children; they found no association between prenatal magnesium sulfate exposure and infant mortality.

In an editorial accompanying the publication of the Schendel study, Nelson[139] delineated several possible interpretations of these data, including the possibility that magnesium or preeclampsia per se protects against fetal neurologic injury. The small sample size in this study precluded a definite conclusion, but the results suggested that magnesium exerted an independent protective effect. The potential contribution of concurrent corticosteroid therapy, which is most often combined with magnesium sulfate when the latter is used for tocolysis, was also discussed, with the notation that other studies have not demonstrated a neuroprotective effect of corticosteroids.

More recently, a randomized, controlled multicenter trial[140] found that fetal exposure to magnesium sulfate before anticipated early preterm delivery did not reduce the combined risk of moderate or severe cerebral palsy or death, although the rate of cerebral palsy was reduced among surviving children. The investigators suggested that "magnesium sulfate may reduce the chance that cerebral palsy will subsequently be diagnosed in a child who was at high risk for preterm birth."[140]

Whether a potential fetal therapeutic role for magnesium sulfate exists during term pregnancy is unresolved. At term, the effect of magnesium sulfate is difficult to separate from the effects of preeclampsia per se, because this disease is essentially the only indication for magnesium sulfate use at this gestational age.

These studies[137,141] have also prompted interest in the potential of magnesium sulfate to protect the fetal brain during pathophysiologic insults such as hypoxia. A neuroprotective effect of magnesium appears to result primarily from an interaction with the glutamate neuronal system. When present in the synapse at a high concentration, glutamate can produce excitotoxic neuronal cell death by means of excessive calcium ion influx, primarily because of *N*-methyl-D-aspartate (NMDA) receptor overactivation. The developing CNS is also vulnerable to the excitotoxic actions of glutamate. In fact, areas such as the cerebral cortex are much more susceptible to glutamate/NMDA receptor–induced excitotoxic injury during the period of rapid fetal brain growth and development than in adulthood.[142]

The fetus reacts to decreased arterial oxygen content by centralizing blood flow to the vital organs, including the brain.[125] Reynolds et al.[111] performed a study of the effect of fetal hypermagnesemia on this compensatory mechanism during an episode of hypoxia in fetal lambs. The results were disturbing; the administration of magnesium sulfate increased the proportion of fetal deaths produced by maternal hemorrhage. Furthermore, among surviving fetuses, hypermagnesemia inhibited the compensatory increase in fetal cerebral blood flow that was observed in the saline-treated animals. Although caution must be used in extrapolating these data to humans, the results suggest that magnesium sulfate may not be entirely beneficial or benign.

By contrast, de Haan et al.[143] did not observe any effect (either positive or negative) of magnesium sulfate on fetal survival or compensatory cerebral blood flow in fetal lambs subjected to umbilical cord occlusion. However, these investigators used different methods of producing fetal hypoxemia and measuring changes in blood flow (i.e., Doppler measurements of carotid artery flow instead of radioactive microspheres). Moon et al.[144] also found that magnesium sulfate did not impair the redistribution of cardiac output or cause fetal death in response to maternal hemorrhage in gravid ewes. A study in rats found magnesium sulfate to be protective if given *before* a hypoxic-ischemic insult but associated with greater neuronal injury if given *after* the insult.[145] These findings indicate that magnesium may have intrinsic neuroprotective properties at the cellular and molecular level but may impair important compensatory responses at the whole-organism level.

In a controversial randomized, controlled trial, Mittendorf et al.[146] observed that women randomly assigned to receive magnesium sulfate for tocolysis experienced worse perinatal outcomes and that this effect was dose-related. It seems intuitive that women having refractory preterm labor would be expected to have higher magnesium sulfate requirements and possibly also worse outcomes. This was a small study, but its results should give practitioners pause in view of the conflicting data regarding the efficacy of magnesium sulfate for tocolysis.[147]

In summary, the preponderance of evidence supports the continued use of magnesium sulfate for seizure prophylaxis in women with preeclampsia. Some clinical evidence suggests that the antenatal use of magnesium sulfate confers some protection against neonatal demise.[148] However, in certain situations that may produce fetal hypoxemia (e.g., maternal hemorrhage), magnesium sulfate may inhibit the expected compensatory increase in fetal cerebral blood flow.

NEUROPATHOLOGY OF PERINATAL ASPHYXIA

The mechanism and timing of an asphyxial insult can affect the resulting fetal or neonatal pathology. Acute, complete asphyxia must be distinguished from incomplete, brief, or intermittent asphyxia or chronic hypoxemia. **Complete asphyxia** may occur in the setting of a total placental abruption or umbilical cord occlusion, which if unrecognized and untreated rapidly leads to fetal demise. **Incomplete asphyxia** may occur in any setting in which oxygen delivery to the fetus is inadequate to meet all of its needs (e.g., brief and/or repeated episodes of umbilical cord occlusion, placental embolization, or incomplete placental abruption). This latter category of asphyxia most likely contributes to the largest proportion of cases of cerebral palsy. In these cases, the insult is not severe enough to lead to immediate fetal death but can profoundly affect fetal brain growth and development. Ongoing studies are attempting to determine whether there is a period of time *in utero* when the fetus is especially vulnerable to neurologic injury.

Using a primate model to perform seminal research on the subject of perinatal brain injury, Myers[18] identified two patterns of injury according to whether the fetus suffered complete or partial asphyxia. The first pattern was demonstrated in fetal monkeys at term subjected to varying durations (0 to 25 minutes) of **complete asphyxia**. These fetuses were resuscitated when possible, a procedure that often required the use of cardiac massage and epinephrine, and postmortem examinations revealed extensive pathology in brainstem areas. In humans, such a severe intrauterine insult would most likely be incompatible with extrauterine survival. If survival did occur, the infant would show obvious encephalopathy and multiorgan system dysfunction at birth. The second pattern is more relevant to the discussion of cerebral palsy and was observed in fetal monkeys subjected to **partial asphyxia**; a number of these animals demonstrated cortical necrosis, subcortical white matter damage, and basal ganglia damage.[149] Although these two studies form the core of our knowledge of perinatal brain injury in primates, there were relatively few animals in each experimental group, and considerable variation in response occurred; some animals suffered no injury, whereas others could not be resuscitated.

Several investigators have attempted to summarize the neuropathology of fetal and newborn asphyxia.[149-151] Volpe[152] has emphasized that the variation in neuropathology after intrauterine asphyxia depends on the gestational age of the fetus. Volpe has also proposed a framework for these variations; the principal sites of injury in preterm fetuses are the white matter (especially periventricular white matter) and the basal ganglia, whereas older fetuses demonstrate injury primarily in the gray matter of the cortex and cerebellum.

Two pathologic entities deserve additional discussion: periventricular leukomalacia and selective neuronal injury. **Periventricular leukomalacia** is the most common pathologic finding in preterm infants with brain injury.[153] This lesion is characterized by coagulative necrosis of the white matter adjacent to the lateral ventricles and around the foramen of Monro, especially at the external angle of the lateral ventricles and the optic radiation.[154] With long-term survival, the lesion may progress to a widening of the ventricles and hydrocephalus *ex vacuo*. Clinically, periventricular leukomalacia may not be apparent at birth.[150] Developing hydrocephalus may be detected on computed tomography or ultrasonographic examination. In more subtle cases, MRI may show decreased myelination (see earlier discussion).[155]

The pathophysiology of periventricular leukomalacia is unclear. Conventional wisdom has held that periventricular leukomalacia is an ischemic lesion unique to preterm infants.[156] The insult is thought to occur in an arterial border zone perfused by end-arterial branches of the middle and posterior cerebral arteries. This border zone has been identified by DeReuck,[156] who demonstrated periventricular arborizations between vessels penetrating to the ventricles (i.e., ventriculopedal vessels) and between vessels arising from the ventriculochoroidal arteries (i.e., ventriculofugal vessels). Others have challenged DeReuck's anatomic findings and have questioned whether periventricular leukomalacia is a purely ischemic lesion.[157,158]

White matter in the immature fetal brain may be at increased risk for hypoxic-ischemic injury because of a limited ability of its vessels to vasodilate.[153] If this is true, autoregulation would be precluded in situations of hypotension. However, at least one study has shown that blood flow to white matter actually may increase (relative to gray matter) during fetal asphyxia.[160] Fetal white matter may be more metabolically active than gray matter because of large numbers of actively myelinating cells.[153] In situations of marginal oxygen supply, glia are subsequently at greater risk for injury. One study has suggested that immature astrocytes are more susceptible to ischemic death than mature astrocytes.[160] Studies in fetal lambs have successfully produced pathologic changes similar to those present in infants with periventricular leukomalacia[128]; these models may help clarify the mechanism of this common pathologic correlate of cerebral palsy in the preterm infant.

Selective neuronal injury, which may also occur during the perinatal period, refers to neuronal death without infarction (i.e., without any obvious disturbance of the associated glia or vascular elements). This entity is most often associated with glutamate-induced neuronal death (see later).[161,162] The human brain sites most vulnerable to selective neuronal injury are difficult to identify, because this injury often occurs in infants with severe HIE, multiorgan system failure, and a prolonged intensive care unit stay, which may confound the eventual findings at autopsy. Box 10-5 lists the brain sites known to exhibit selective neuronal necrosis.[152]

BOX 10-5 Major Sites for Selective Neuronal Necrosis in Neonatal Hypoxic-Ischemic Encephalopathy

Cerebral Cortex
- Hippocampus more than supralimbic cortex

Diencephalon
- Thalamus
- Hypothalamus
- Lateral geniculate body

Basal Ganglia
- Caudate
- Putamen
- Globus pallidus

Midbrain
- Inferior colliculus
- Oculomotor and trochlear nuclei
- Red nucleus
- Substantia nigra
- Reticular formation

Pons
- Motor nuclei of trigeminal and facial nerves
- Dorsal more than ventral cochlear nuclei
- Reticular formation
- Pontine nuclei

Medulla
- Dorsal motor nucleus of vagus nerve
- Nucleus ambiguus
- Inferior olivary nuclei
- Cuneate and gracilis nuclei

Cerebellum
- Purkinje cells
- Dentate nuclei
- Other roof nuclei

Modified from Volpe JJ. Hypoxic-ischemic encephalopathy: Neuropathology and pathogenesis. In Volpe JJ. Neurology of the Newborn. 2nd edition. Philadelphia, WB Saunders, 1987:209-35.

GLUTAMATE-INDUCED NEURONAL INJURY

Glutamate, the most prevalent neurotransmitter in the CNS, has excitatory (i.e., depolarizing) actions on postsynaptic neurons.[163] Hypoxia has been demonstrated to raise extracellular glutamate levels and arrest synaptic activity within *in vitro* preparations.[164] The role of glutamate in ischemic neuronal injury has been reviewed extensively.[161,162,165-168] Figures 10-3 and 10-4 depict the

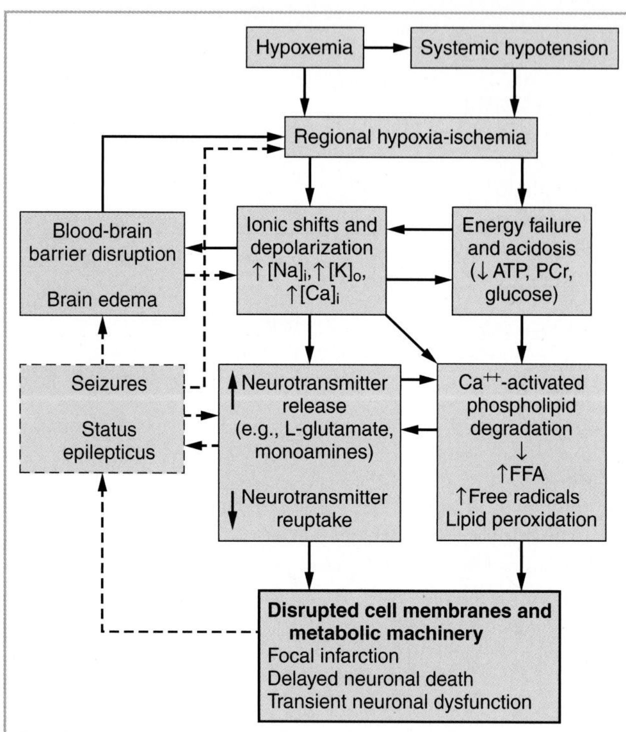

FIGURE 10-3 Pathogenesis of events that may mediate hypoxic-ischemic injury to neurons and other tissues in the brain in the hours after asphyxia. ATP, adenosine triphosphate; $[Ca]_i$, calcium concentration inside neuron; FFA, free fatty acids; $[K]_o$, potassium concentration outside neuron; $[Na]_i$, sodium concentration inside neuron; PCr, phosphocreatine. (From Nelson N, editor. Current Therapy in Neonatal-Perinatal Medicine, Vol 2. Toronto, B.C. Decker, 1990:276.)

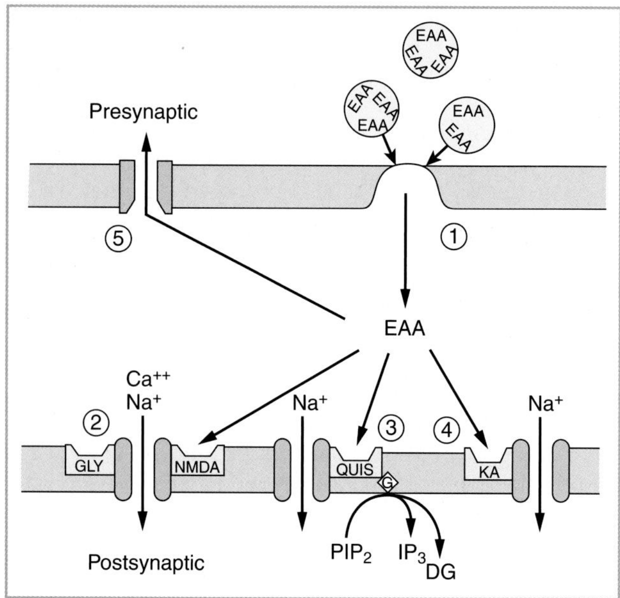

FIGURE 10-4 Excitatory amino acid (EAA) synaptic components that contribute to synaptic transmission, second messenger generation, and cessation of these responses. 1, Glutamate and related excitatory amino acids are released from presynaptic neuronal terminals in a calcium-dependent process by depolarization of the presynaptic neuron. 2 to 4, Once released into the synaptic cleft, glutamate can depolarize the postsynaptic neuronal membrane by binding to at least three subsets of excitatory amino acid receptors. Activation of the *N*-methyl-D-aspartate (NMDA) receptor channel complex (2), quisqualate (QUIS) receptors (3), or kainate (KA) receptors (4) can produce cationic fluxes through receptor-associated ionophores. Alternatively, a subset of quisqualate receptors are linked with phospholipase C, which activates phosphoinositol hydrolysis and generates the second messengers inositol triphosphate (IP_3) and diacylglycerol (DG). The distribution of these subtypes of excitatory amino acid receptors in brain can be examined with radiolabeled ligands specific to each receptor subtype. 5, The excitatory action of glutamate on postsynaptic membranes is inactivated by a presynaptic, high-affinity, energy-dependent transport process. GLY, glycine; PIP_2, phosphatidylinositol biphosphate. (From McDonald JW, Johnston MV. Physiological and pathophysiologic roles of excitatory amino acids during central nervous system development. Brain Res Rev 1990; 15:41-70.)

pathogenesis of hypoxic-ischemic injury and the function of excitatory amino acid (EAA) receptors.[169,170] Figure 10-5 gives an overview of the cascade of events that result from the pathologic activation of EAA receptors.[170]

More than 60 years ago, investigators observed that immature animals are more likely to withstand asphyxia than adult animals.[171-173] The evidence for the role of EAAs in the pathophysiology of hypoxic-ischemic brain injury in adults has stimulated research on the development (ontogeny) of these neurotransmitter systems in the fetus. Results of experiments in rat pups indicate that asphyxia causes a disruption in EAA receptors, suggesting a susceptibility to hypoxic-ischemic injury.[174] Hypoxia-ischemia is known to reduce glutamate reuptake, thus inhibiting the normal process that terminates glutamate's action at the synapse.[175]

The ontogeny of EAA systems has been studied in many species, including fetal lambs.[176] Anatomically distinct binding patterns exist for each of the major glutamate receptor subtypes (Box 10-6).[169,177] These receptors are commonly referred to as **NMDA** or **non-NMDA** types. Non-NMDA types include kainate, alpha-amino-3-hydroxy-5-methyl-4-isoxazole-propionic acid (AMPA), and metabotropic subtypes. The metabotropic subtype is unique; whereas activation of other receptors is linked to ion flow across the postsynaptic membrane, activation of metabotropic receptors is linked to turnover of phosphoinositol (an intracellular second messenger) in the postsynaptic cell. The metabotropic subclass of glutamate receptor shows developmental alterations.[178] The changing pattern of the glutamate receptor profile may explain, in part, why some neuronal populations are more sensitive to injury at different stages of brain development. Cells with EAA receptors may have an enhanced susceptibility to ischemic injury during specific periods of development[179]; this possibility underlines the importance of determining the developmental profile of these neurotransmitter systems in the fetus.

The chronic intrauterine microdialysis technique has been used to document the accumulation of glutamate in the fetal brain after a pathophysiologic insult. Increases in cortical glutamate concentrations occur after acute fetal hypoxemia caused by severe maternal hemorrhage[102] and during chronic hypoxemia produced by restriction of uterine artery blood flow for 24 hours.[106] Presumably, the released glutamate is free to participate in processes that ultimately lead to fetal brain injury.

Lee and Choi[180] have identified the density and distribution of EAA receptors in the developing human brain.

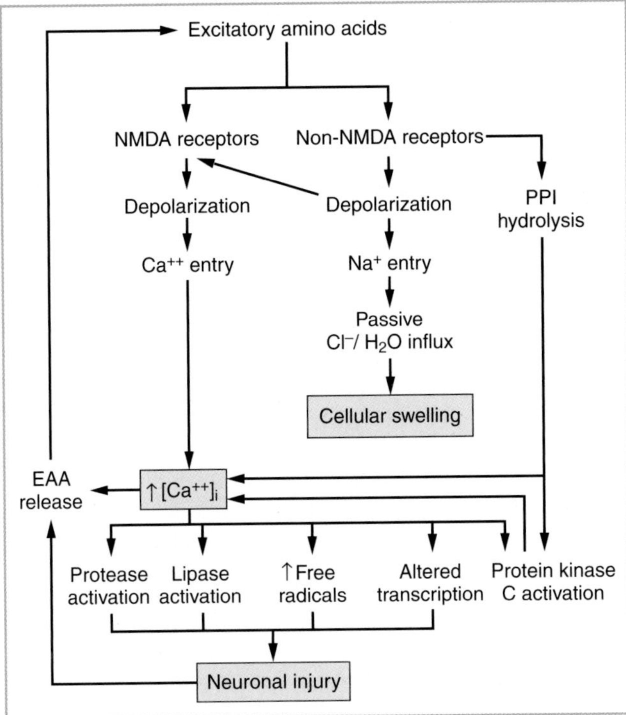

FIGURE 10-5 Some of the mechanisms that may contribute to excitatory amino acid (EAA) neurotoxicity are shown. Experiments *in vitro* suggest that EAA neurotoxicity may have two components. The first component, mediated by excessive activation of non-NMDA (*N*-methyl-D-aspartate) receptors, is characterized by an influx of Na^+ followed by passive influx of Cl^- and H_2O, which may produce osmotic neuronal swelling. Acute events occur within hours of the exposure to EAA agonists. The second, more prominent component is produced by overactivation of NMDA receptors, which leads to a rise in the intracellular concentration of Ca^{++}. A sustained rise in intracellular Ca^{++} may trigger a biochemical cascade of events that lead to neuronal injury and death. Furthermore, activation of a subset of non-NMDA receptors coupled with polyphosphoinositide (PPI) hydrolysis also may elevate intracellular Ca^{++}. Excitatory amino acids released from synaptic terminals would further propagate neuronal injury. $[Ca^{++}]_i$, calcium concentration inside neuron. (From McDonald JW, Johnston MV. Physiological and pathophysiological roles of excitatory amino acids during central nervous system development. Brain Res Rev 1990; 15:41-70.)

BOX 10-6 Classification of Glutamate Receptors

N-Methyl-D-Aspartate (NMDA)–Type Receptors

- Inotropic receptor/channel complex

Non–NMDA-Type Receptors

- AMPA (alpha-amino-3-hydroxy-5-methyl-4-isoxazole-propionic acid) ionotropic receptors
- Kainate ionotropic receptors
- Metabotropic receptors

From Johnston MV. Cellular alterations associated with perinatal asphyxia. Clin Invest Med 1993; 16:122-32.

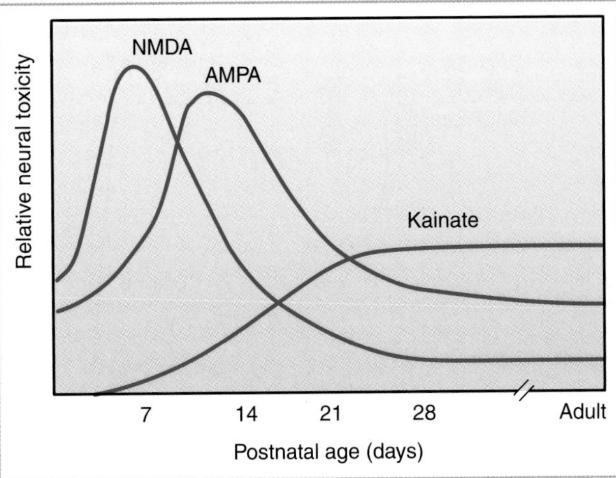

FIGURE 10-6 Relative neurotoxicity of three analogues of glutamate injected into the brain at different ages. Lines represent trends based on experimental work. AMPA, alpha-amino-3-hydroxy-5-methyl-4-isoxazole propionate; NMDA, *N*-methyl-D-aspartate. (From Johnston MV. Cellular alterations associated with perinatal asphyxia. Clin Invest Med 1993; 16:122-32.)

Clear gestational age–dependent changes occur in glutamate receptor subtype binding in the fetal brain; for example, a sharp increase in receptor density appears at mid-gestation. The changing density and distribution of these receptors may be related to the role of EAA pathways in synaptogenesis and may be responsible for the age-dependent selective vulnerability in the developing human fetal brain[180] Greenamyre et al.[181] demonstrated virtually no glutamatergic innervation of the globus pallidus (a portion of the basal ganglia) in adult humans but high concentrations in fetuses; a glutamate pathway may transiently exist in the globus pallidus during development and may play a role in the basal ganglia damage seen in some forms of cerebral palsy after intrauterine hypoxic-ischemic injury.

In addition to variations in EAA receptor distribution and density, the fetal brain may respond differently to anoxia than the adult brain. An increase in intracellular calcium levels appears to be one component of the final common pathway leading to irreversible neuronal injury.[182,183] The presence and function of glutamate receptor subtypes are undoubtedly important in the susceptibility of the fetal brain to glutamate-induced hypoxic-ischemic injury. For example, kainate, a potent neurotoxin in the adult brain, is relatively nontoxic in the immature brain, where its receptors follow the appearance of NMDA and AMPA receptors (Figure 10-6).[177] These receptors also serve a different function in the immature brain from that in the mature brain. For example, in the neocortex, striatum, and cerebellum of the rat, the rise in intracellular calcium level resulting from kainate/AMPA receptor activation is highest in the immature brain and markedly declines with age.[184]

The activation of EAA receptors can also lead to the intracellular production of nitric oxide and a subsequent exacerbation of neurotoxic processes (Figure 10-7).[177,185,186] The blockade of EAA receptors may help prevent hypoxic-ischemic neuronal injury during episodes of hypoxia in the fetus and neonate.[187-189] However, the clinical use of

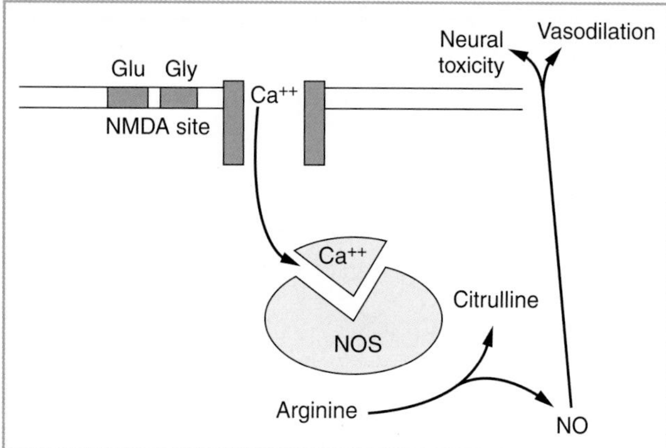

FIGURE 10-7 Proposed mechanism by which calcium entering neurons through excitatory amino acid channels stimulates production of the free-radical second messenger nitric oxide (NO). Nitric oxide can diffuse through membranes to cause vasodilation and neuronal toxicity. Glu, glucose; Gly, glycine; NMDA, *N*-methyl-D-aspartate; NOS, nitric oxide synthase. (From Johnston MV. Cellular alterations associated with perinatal asphyxia. Clin Invest Med 1993; 16:122-32.)

these drugs should be regarded as premature, because EAAs also have profound trophic effects on normal brain development[190,191]; thus any intervention in this process should be made with great caution.[192]

ENDOGENOUS FETAL NEUROPROTECTION

The fetus lives, moves, and grows in a low-oxygen environment; indeed, very high concentrations of oxygen may be toxic to fetal neurons. Nevertheless, immediately after birth, the neonate experiences a rapid increase in oxygen requirements that does not seem to be explained purely on the basis of increased metabolic needs. Some investigators have hypothesized that progesterone may suppress oxygen requirements or make fetal neurons more resistant to hypoxia *in utero*; when present in high concentrations, progesterone has general anesthetic and neuroprotective properties. Allopregnanolone, an endogenous metabolite of progesterone, appears to protect neurons against both NMDA-induced cell necrosis and apoptosis[193]; this finding is compatible with the observation that the inhibition of neurosteroid (e.g., allopregnanolone) synthesis exacerbates brain injury in fetal sheep exposed to asphyxial insults *in utero*.[194] Using microdialysis to measure allopregnanolone levels in the parietal cortex of fetal lambs subjected to umbilical cord occlusion, Nguyen et al.[195] found increased levels of allopregnanolone, but not pregnanolone, in the dialysate after hypoxia. An increase in allopregnanolone during hypoxic stress may be an adaptive mechanism that helps the brain tolerate brief episodes of hypoxemia.

Stein[196] reviewed the published studies of progesterone neuroprotection during pregnancy, menopause, and aging. Given the abundance of progesterone in viable pregnancies, it would seem unlikely that the administration of progesterone during pregnancy would confer additional protective fetal brain effects. However, there might be a role for administration of progesterone in preterm neonates. Specifically, progesterone could potentially enable the neonatal brain to tolerate lower oxygen tensions, allow "permissive hypoxemia," and possibly reduce the risk of oxygen toxicity and ventilator-associated barotrauma. Thus, administration of progesterone or allopregnanolone might someday be therapeutic in neonates.

OTHER CAUSES OF FETAL AND NEONATAL BRAIN INJURY

Drugs

Although most drugs cross the placenta and may affect the fetus, discussion in this chapter is limited to three commonly used drugs or types—alcohol, cocaine, and corticosteroids. **Fetal alcohol syndrome** is characterized by the triad of intrauterine growth restriction, craniofacial anomalies, and CNS abnormalities[197]; the heart, kidney, and musculoskeletal system may also be affected (see Chapter 53). The most common craniofacial abnormalities are microcephaly, short palpebral fissures, and midfacial hypoplasia. CNS effects consist of intellectual impairment and behavioral manifestations. During the early neonatal period, a withdrawal syndrome may occur that involves tremors, hypertonia, abdominal distention, irritability, and seizures. This syndrome can be distinguished from opioid withdrawal by the presence of abdominal distention (more common with alcohol withdrawal) and of yawning and diaphoresis (more common with opioid withdrawal).[198]

Smith et al.[199] reviewed the pathophysiologic effects of ethanol on the fetus. In rats, prenatal ethanol exposure results in a permanent reduction in the hippocampal neurons in offspring[200] and affects the composition of the glutamate receptor.[201] The glutamate receptors are important in the process of brain synaptogenesis; thus, fetal exposure to ethanol at crucial periods may disrupt normal development. Using long-term intrauterine microdialysis, Reynolds et al.[103] demonstrated that doses of ethanol that mimic binge ingestion are associated with paroxysmal increases in cortical glutamate concentrations.

Maternal cocaine abuse has increased dramatically and has numerous deleterious effects (see Chapter 53).[202] Cocaine may cause uteroplacental vasoconstriction, decreased uteroplacental perfusion, preterm labor, and placental abruption. In addition, cocaine may affect the fetal brain by causing severe cerebral vasoconstriction and subarachnoid and intraventricular hemorrhage (Figure 10-8).[202] Various teratogenic, developmental, and neurobehavioral disturbances in infants and children have been reported after *in utero* cocaine exposure (Table 10-2).[203-205]

Antenatal maternal corticosteroid administration has proven benefits for preterm neonates. The anti-inflammatory and maturational effects of corticosteroids (e.g., betamethasone) are well established. A single course of corticosteroids is recommended for all pregnant women between 24 and 34 weeks' gestation who are at risk for preterm delivery within 7 days.[206] However, the indiscriminant use of corticosteroids is controversial. In some animal and human studies,[207] antenatal and early neonatal administration of corticosteroids has been associated with higher rates of cerebral palsy and cognitive and psychiatric neurodevelopmental abnormalities.[208] In contrast, Watterberg et al.[209] reported improved developmental outcomes, and no difference in cerebral palsy rates, when low-dose

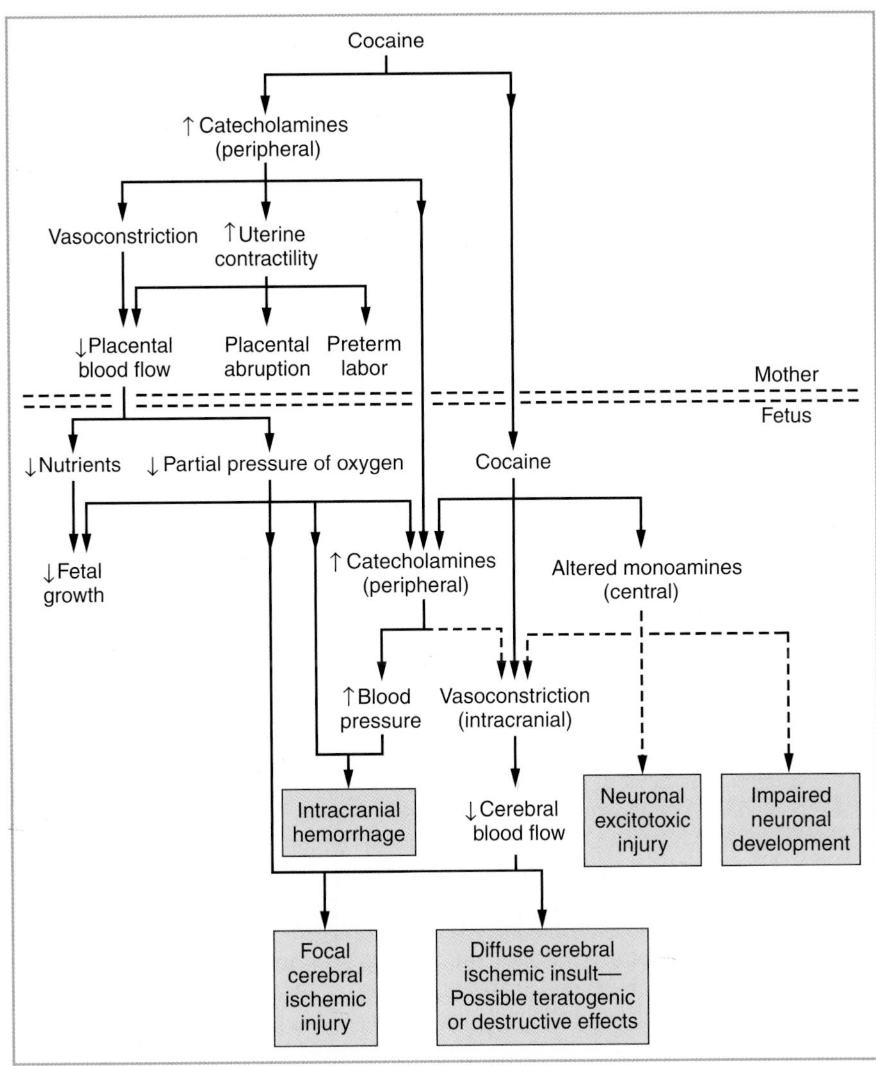

FIGURE 10-8 Deleterious effects of maternal cocaine use on fetuses. Effects that appear plausible on the basis of current information but whose confirmation requires more supporting evidence are indicated by *dotted arrows*. ↑, increased; ↓, decreased. (From Volpe JJ. Effect of cocaine use on the fetus. N Engl J Med 1992; 327:399-407.)

hydrocortisone was used for treatment of adrenal insufficiency in extremely LBW (ELBW) infants (less than 1000 g at delivery) receiving mechanical ventilation. The results should be interpreted with caution, because the study was terminated early because of greater gastrointestinal side effects in the corticosteroid group.

Maternal Trauma

Maternal trauma, the leading cause of nonobstetric maternal mortality, accounts for approximately 20% of maternal deaths (see Chapter 54).[210] Maternal trauma is an uncommon cause of fetal neurologic injury. A study from Western Australia noted an incidence of cerebral palsy of 2.6 per 1000 pregnant women who required hospitalization for trauma, compared with only 1.8 per 1000 who were hospitalized for another reason; however, this difference was not statistically significant.[211]

Mechanisms of fetal injury vary, but placental abruption, uterine rupture, and placental hypoperfusion due to maternal hypovolemia are more common than direct trauma. Placental abruption or fetal-maternal hemorrhage may cause delayed fetal injury, and consequently, serial examinations may be necessary. Although fetal head crush injuries may occur during motor vehicle accidents from compression between the seat belt and the maternal sacral promontory,[212] seat belts more commonly preserve maternal and fetal lives and should be worn appropriately during pregnancy (see Chapter 54).

Severe trauma does not necessarily mandate the performance of cesarean delivery. Late FHR decelerations may result from maternal hypovolemia, which may be relieved by volume replacement. The physiologic changes of pregnancy (e.g., uterine enlargement) may compromise cardiopulmonary resuscitation,[213] and aortocaval compression should be avoided at all times.

Fetal Trauma

The value of the elective performance of an episiotomy and use of outlet forceps to protect the preterm fetal head during vaginal delivery[214,215] is a matter of some dispute.[216] A successful outcome with the use of outlet forceps depends on operator skill, maternal anatomy and parity, gestational age, and the station of the fetal head.

The use of vacuum-assisted delivery has fluctuated in popularity. The availability of polymeric silicone (Silastic) cups has increased the frequency of this method of delivery.[217] The use of vacuum-assisted delivery in preterm infants is controversial because of an association with

TABLE 10-2 Disturbances in Human Brain Development Reported after Intrauterine Exposure to Cocaine

Event	Peak Gestational Period	Abnormality Reported after Cocaine Exposure
Neural tube formation	3-4 weeks	Myelomeningocele, encephalocele
Prosencephalic development	2-3 months	Agenesis of corpus callosum, agenesis of septum pellucidum, septo-optic dysplasia
Neuronal proliferation	3-4 months	Microcephaly
Neuronal migration	3-5 months	Schizencephaly, neuronal heterotopias
Neuronal differentiation	5 months (postnatal)	Abnormal cortical neuronal cytodifferentiation (preliminary)
Myelination	After birth	None

From Volpe JJ. Effect of cocaine use on the fetus. N Engl J Med 1992; 327:399-407.

cephalohematoma and a subsequent increase in hemolysis-induced neonatal jaundice[218] as well as a possible risk of intracranial hemorrhage.

Brachial plexus injuries (e.g., Erb's palsy) most often result from fetal macrosomia and shoulder dystocia (see Chapter 18). To avoid these injuries, the anesthesia provider may be asked to provide anesthesia to promote pelvic floor relaxation and facilitate delivery. In some cases, emergency cesarean delivery is required.

ANESTHESIA AND BRAIN INJURY

Anesthetic agents can have profound effects on brain metabolism and synaptic transmission[219-223] that could potentially improve the "oxygen margin of safety."[217] However, other effects of anesthetic agents (beyond their influence on brain metabolism) should also be considered. For example, although some agents (e.g., barbiturates) prolong the interval during which neurons can withstand anoxia *in vitro* and still regain synaptic activity,[224] these agents' systemic effects *in vivo* may result in hemodynamic alterations that the mother, but not the fetus, can tolerate.[98] In humans, there is a strong relationship among maternal blood pressure, uteroplacental perfusion, and fetal oxygenation. During administration of anesthesia in pregnant women, maternal blood pressure and oxygenation typically are tightly controlled; however, studies in small laboratory animals usually do not allow precise hemodynamic monitoring, and physiologic homeostasis may be altered in ways that are not readily apparent. Furthermore, there may be subtle interspecies differences in cerebral hypoxia-ischemia.[225] Nonetheless, some studies have demonstrated that nonpregnant rats given anesthetic agents, including volatile anesthetic agents, demonstrate less focal ischemic brain damage than awake controls.[226]

Some investigators have suggested that the protective effects of some drugs may occur through drug-induced hypothermia,[227] because even mild hypothermia (2° to 3° C) may be neuroprotective,[228] as demonstrated effectively in cardiac surgery. However, the neuroprotective effects of most anesthetic agents are likely to result from a complex combination of factors, including alterations in the release or activity of EAA neurotransmitters such as glutamate.[229] In experimental preparations, anesthetic agents (e.g., thiopental, ketamine, isoflurane, halothane, diethyl ether, and chloroform) have been observed to inhibit glutamate-induced responses.[230] Hyperpolarizing gamma-aminobutyric acid (GABA) receptor agonist drugs (e.g., benzodiazepines) may also antagonize the depolarizing effects of glutamate.[231,232]

Until recently, little information on the effects of anesthetic agents on the fetal brain was available. Myers and Myers[233] suggested that the maternal administration of sedative or anesthetic drugs may prevent or ameliorate the effects of fetal asphyxia at the time of delivery in the following ways: (1) decrease in fetal brain metabolism; (2) decrease in maternal stress response, which would tend to improve uteroplacental perfusion; (3) reduction in uterine contractility, which would increase uteroplacental perfusion; and (4) a limited increase in fetal glucose concentration, which would reduce fetal brain lactic acidosis from glycolysis. However, no published studies have determined which (if any) anesthetic drug or technique, when administered according to the recommended guidelines for good clinical practice, would be most likely to protect the fetal brain.

Various anesthetic agents may also have deleterious effects on fetal and neonatal brain development. In adults, anesthetic drugs may hasten some forms of Alzheimer's disease through the production of brain plaques and amyloid-β proteins. Under experimental conditions, anesthetic agents can kill brain cells or increase apoptotic processes in fetal and neonatal laboratory animals.[234] Ethanol, phencyclidine, isoflurane, nitrous oxide, benzodiazepines, propofol, ketamine, and even barbiturates have all been implicated in apoptotic neurodegeneration in developing rat brains.[235,236]

In clinical practice, however, the performance of surgery requires administration of anesthesia, the overall neurologic outcomes appear acceptable, and few alternatives exist.[237] More important, most of the animal evidence for neurotoxicity involved exposure to anesthetic agents for long durations, in large doses, and in the absence of surgical pain. These study conditions may not replicate the clinical situation, because the intended clinical effect of anesthesia (i.e., blunting of pain and surgical stress) may itself be beneficial to the developing brain. For example, Anand[238] demonstrated that repetitive neonatal pain in rat pups might lead to neuronal injury in cortical and subcortical brain regions with associated memory and other cognitive deficits; these negative effects were largely ameliorated with ketamine analgesia.

Overall, the following arguments support the continued use and safety of anesthetic agents in pregnant women and neonates:

- Major developmental differences exist among species; laboratory exposure in animals may not correlate with clinical exposure in humans, particularly because of significant differences across species in the timing of brain development.

- In experimental studies, the laboratory animals were typically exposed to large doses of anesthetic agents for prolonged periods.
- Most laboratory studies were performed in the absence of potentially harmful surgical stress, which is blunted or prevented by anesthesia.
- Clinical administration of anesthetic agents includes precise hemodynamic monitoring and maintenance of physiologic homeostasis, which may not be replicated in laboratory studies performed in small animals.

In a special article, Anand and Soriano[239] concluded, "Clinicians should administer anesthetic agents to newborn infants or pregnant mothers but avoid prolonged periods of anesthetic exposure . . . . Alleviation of pain and stress during the perinatal period should remain an essential clinical goal until further research defines the clinical importance of [experimental] results [observed in animals]." Likewise, the U.S. Food and Drug Administration (FDA), reviewing the published evidence of neurotoxic effects of anesthetic drugs on the developing brain in laboratory animals, acknowledged laboratory findings that warrant concern and further research, but they also acknowledged the lack of confirmatory data in humans.[240]

NEW THERAPIES

Perlman[241] has reviewed various strategies for treating hypoxic-ischemic neonatal injuries, including hypothermia, inflammatory mediator modulators, EAA receptor agonists and antagonists, free radical scavengers, and platelet-activating factor antagonists. These emerging therapeutic strategies stem from basic neuroscience research on brain development and the pathophysiology of ischemic injury.

Some investigators have described better outcomes after the use of **hypothermia** in neonates at risk for HIE. One group of investigators has described an experimental model of severe intrauterine hypoxia in preterm fetal sheep, in which asphyxia was produced by 25 minutes of complete umbilical cord occlusion.[242,243] Extradural head cooling from 39° to 29° C decreased the loss of striatal neurons and oligodendroglia; this finding was associated with improved basal ganglia function after ischemia.

These and other experimental results prompted a clinical trial of whole-body hypothermia for neonates with HIE.[244] Eligible infants were born at more than 36 weeks' gestation, had moderate or severe encephalopathy, and were admitted to the neonatal intensive care unit within 6 hours of birth. For infants in the hypothermia group, body temperature was lowered to 33.5° C for 72 hours. Death or moderate to severe disability at 18 to 22 months of age occurred in 44% of 102 infants in the hypothermia group, compared with 62% of 106 infants in the control group (risk ratio, 0.72; 95% CI, 0.54 to 0.95; $P = .01$). Although encouraging, these results are at odds with those from another large multicenter randomized trial.[245] In an editorial attempting to reconcile these opposing observations, several possible explanations were suggested.[246] Importantly, in the study that demonstrated no benefit, cooling began later and more time was required to achieve complete cooling, because head (not total body) cooling was employed. Moreover, the study that showed no benefit with hypothermia may have included babies who were so severely affected that no therapy would have been beneficial; this possibility highlights the importance of patient selection in these clinical trials. In the study that showed a benefit for hypothermia, no serious complications of therapy were reported; thus many institutions are selectively employing cooling for babies at risk. Improvements in selection criteria may ultimately clarify the role and efficacy of hypothermia in neonates at risk for HIE.

There is great interest in the naturally occurring process of **apoptosis,** also known as programmed cell death,[247,248] which is responsible for the purposeful killing of specific CNS cells. Apoptosis ensures that the number of surviving cells is appropriate and optimal. Glutamate receptor–mediated neuronal death may represent an inappropriate activation of apoptosis. Although the regulation of apoptosis is complex and incompletely understood, further discovery will be fundamental to significant progress in the prevention of cerebral palsy.

The role of white matter in the attenuation of hypoxic-ischemic brain damage (e.g., through uptake of EAAs or sequestration of potassium and hydrogen ions) is underappreciated,[249-251] and drugs that inhibit the release of EAAs or antagonize their receptors may be of benefit.[252] Multiple strategies may be necessary to inhibit the deleterious pathways initiated by brain ischemia and hypoxia.[253] The combination of oxygen free radical scavengers and calcium entry–blocking agents appears to have some efficacy in limiting postasphyxial injury in newborn sheep.[254] A "brain cocktail," consisting of free radical scavengers, modifiers of nitric oxide activity, metabolic inhibitors, calcium and iron chelators, and drugs that affect the EAA systems, may someday be administered to fetuses and neonates at risk for brain injury. Additional compounds that may inhibit CNS necrosis or apoptosis, either *in utero* or in the neonatal period, include agents that interrupt the inflammatory cascade, progesterone, and other steroids.

The ability to accurately predict which fetuses are at risk for neurologic injury, and when, is still rudimentary, because the most vulnerable periods of fetal development are still unknown and noninvasive fetal surveillance techniques are not very advanced. The ability to identify these "at risk" babies *in utero* is a necessary step in designing effective therapeutic regimens that interfere minimally with the normal trophic activities of the developing brain.

Meanwhile, the potential for anesthesia-related neurotoxicity will undoubtedly undergo continued scrutiny. In a comprehensive editorial[255] that accompanied several relevant publications,[256-262] McGowan and Davis made the following conclusions:

- Additional animal studies are needed to define molecular mechanisms, risks, and potential treatments for anesthetic-related neurotoxicity in the developing brain.
- Future studies should be relevant to human development and clinical practice.
- Human studies of adequate statistical power are needed to identify any evidence of injury from intrauterine exposure to anesthetic agents.

- Future studies should take advantage of advances in genomics and proteomics, and should target the identification of sensitive and specific biomarkers for neurocognitive injury.
- Some forms of developmental brain injury might be prevented or ameliorated by periprocedural therapy (e.g., anti-apoptotic agents such as melatonin).[255,263]

McGowan and Davis[255] affirmed the FDA's conclusion[240] that currently, "there [is] no scientific basis to recommend changes in clinical [anesthesia] practice." They noted that the "real enemy" includes "known and understood causes of brain injury and death," such as hypoxia and cardiovascular collapse. They cautioned, "[W]e must not let our enthusiasm for understanding the possible neurocognitive risks of anesthetics . . . obscure our awareness of this enemy or prevent us from alleviating pain."[255]

KEY POINTS

- Cerebral palsy is a nonprogressive disorder of the central nervous system that is present (but not always obvious) at birth and involves some impairment of motor function or posture. Intellectual disability may or may not be present.
- The term *birth asphyxia* should be used sparingly, if at all, in medical records. More descriptive terms that describe the newborn's tone, color, respiratory effort, and metabolic status should be used when possible.
- The incidence of cerebral palsy is approximately 2 per 1000 live births and has not decreased despite the widespread use of intrapartum fetal heart rate monitoring and a higher cesarean delivery rate.
- The false-positive rate for new-onset, persistent, late fetal heart rate decelerations as a predictor for the development of cerebral palsy is 99%.
- The Apgar score is a poor predictor of cerebral palsy.
- Spastic quadriplegia and, less commonly, dyskinesia are the only types of cerebral palsy associated with acute intrapartum hypoxic events.
- Intrapartum hypoxia sufficient to cause cerebral palsy is always accompanied by neonatal encephalopathy and seizures.
- Fetal compensatory responses to hypoxemia *in utero* include (1) a redistribution of fetal cardiac output, with increased blood flow to the brain, myocardium, and adrenal glands; (2) decreased fetal energy consumption as a result of decreased fetal breathing and body movements; and (3) maintenance of essential cellular processes at the expense of intrauterine fetal growth.
- Chorioamnionitis is associated with an increased risk for cerebral palsy. Epidural analgesia during labor is associated with an elevated maternal temperature (but not chorioamnionitis). More accurate diagnosis of chorioamnionitis may prevent unnecessary evaluations for sepsis in newborns of mothers with a small rise in temperature during labor.
- Excitatory amino acid neurotransmitters (e.g., glutamate) likely play an important role in hypoxic-ischemic brain injury *in utero*, and the intrauterine maturation of these transmitter systems may result in periods of susceptibility to hypoxic injury.
- The high levels of progesterone to which the fetus is exposed *in utero* may afford some endogenous fetal neuroprotection.
- No published data suggest that a given anesthetic drug or technique is more likely to protect fetal neurologic function (provided that the anesthetic technique is administered according to the recommended guidelines for good anesthesia practice).
- Better knowledge of the process and regulation of apoptosis (programmed neuronal cell death) may lead to the development of strategies to prevent irreversible fetal neurologic injury.

REFERENCES

1. Blumenthal I. Cerebral palsy: Medicolegal aspects. J R Soc Med 2001; 94:624-7.
2. The Definition and Classification of Cerebral Palsy. Dev Med Child Neurol 2007; 49(S109):1-44.
3. Nelson KB, Ellenberg JH. Apgar scores as predictors of chronic neurologic disability. Pediatrics 1981; 68:36-44.
4. Rosen MG, Dickinson JC. The incidence of cerebral palsy. Am J Obstet Gynecol 1992; 167:417-23.
5. Jarvis SN, Holloway JS, Hey EN. Increase in cerebral palsy in normal birth weight babies. Arch Dis Child 1985; 60:1113-21.
6. Nelson KB, Ellenberg JH. Antecedents of cerebral palsy. N Engl J Med 1986; 315:81-6.
7. Emond A, Golding J, Pecklam C. Cerebral palsy in two national cohort studies. Arch Dis Child 1989; 64:848-52.
8. Hagberg B, Hagberg G, Olow I, Von Wendt L. The changing panorama of cerebral palsy in Sweden. V. The birth period. 1979-82. Acta Pediatr Scand 1989; 78:283-90.
9. Holst K, Anderson E, Philip J, Henningen I. Antenatal and perinatal conditions correlated to handicap among 4-year-old children. Am J Perinatol 1989; 6:258-67.
10. Dowding VM, Barry C. Cerebral palsy: Changing patterns of birth weight and gestational age (1976/81). Irish Med J 1988; 812:25-8.
11. Stanley FJ, Watson L. The cerebral palsies in Western Australia: Trends, 1968 to 1981. Am J Obstet Gynecol 1988; 158:89-93.
12. Riikonen R, Raumavirta S, Sinivuori E, Seppala T. Changing pattern of cerebral palsy in the southwest region of Finland. Acta Pediatr Scand 1989; 78:581-7.
13. Torfs CP, Van den Berg BJ, Oechsli FW, Cummins S. Prenatal and perinatal factors in the etiology of cerebral palsy. J Pediatr 1990; 116:615-9.
14. Pharoah POD, Cooke T, Cooke RW, Rosenbloom I. Birth weight specific trends in cerebral palsy. Arch Dis Child 1990; 65:602-6.
15. Meberg A. Declining incidence of low birth weight: Impact on perinatal mortality and incidence of cerebral palsy. J Perinatal Med 1990; 18:195-200.
16. American College of Obstetricians and Gynecologists Committee on Obstetrics: Maternal and Fetal Medicine: Utility of umbilical cord blood acid-base assessment. ACOG Committee Opinion No. 91. Washington, DC, February 1991.
17. American College of Obstetricians and Gynecologists Committee on Obstetric Practice. Inappropriate use of the terms fetal distress and birth asphyxia. ACOG Committee Opinion No. 197. Washington, DC, February 1998. (Int J Gynaecol Obstet 1998; 61:309-10).

18. Myers RE. Two patterns of perinatal brain damage and their conditions of occurrence. Am J Obstet Gynecol 1972; 112:246-76.
19. Grant A, Joy M, O'Brien N, et al. Cerebral palsy among children born during the Dublin randomized trial of intrapartum monitoring. Lancet 1989; 2(8674):1233-6.
20. Freeman R. Intrapartum fetal monitoring: A disappointing story. N Engl J Med 1990; 322:624-6.
21. Hankins GDV, Erickson K, Zinberg S, et al. Neonatal encephalopathy and cerebral palsy: A knowledge survey of fellows of the American College of Obstetricians and Gynecologists. Obstet Gynecol 2003; 101:11-7.
22. MacDonald D, Grant A, Sheridan-Pereira M, et al. The Dublin randomized controlled trial of intrapartum fetal heart rate monitoring. Am J Obstet Gynecol 1985; 152:524-39.
23. Leveno KJ, Cunningham FG, Nelson S, et al. A prospective comparison of selective and universal electronic fetal monitoring in 34,995 pregnancies. N Engl J Med 1986; 315:615-9.
24. Schifrin BS, Dame L. Fetal heart rate patterns: Prediction of Apgar score. JAMA 1972; 219:1322-5.
25. Friedman EA. The obstetrician's dilemma: How much fetal monitoring and cesarean section is enough? N Engl J Med 1986; 315:641-3.
26. Rosen MG, Dickinson JC. The paradox of electronic fetal monitoring: More data may not enable us to predict or prevent infant neurologic morbidity. Am J Obstet Gynecol 1993; 168:745-51.
27. Freeman RK. Problems with intrapartum fetal heart rate monitoring interpretation and patient management. Obstet Gynecol 2002; 100:813-26.
28. Schifrin BS, Cohen WR. Medical legal issues in fetal monitoring. Clin Perinatol 2007; 34:329-43.
29. Cohen WR, Schifrin BS. Medical negligence lawsuits relating to labor and delivery. Clin Perinatol 2007; 34:345-60.
30. Towbin A. Obstetric malpractice litigation: The pathologist's view. Am J Obstet Gynecol 1986; 155:927-35.
31. American College of Obstetricians and Gynecologists. Shifting strategies in neurologic injury cases. ACOG Newsletter, November, 1991.
32. Bakketeig LS. Only a minor part of cerebral palsy cases begin in labour. BMJ 1999; 319:1016-7.
33. Blair E, Stanley FJ. Intrapartum asphyxia: A rare cause of cerebral palsy. J Pediatr 1988; 112:515-9.
34. Espinosa MI, Parer JT. Mechanisms of asphyxial brain damage, and possible pharmacological interventions, in the fetus. Am J Obstet Gynecol 1991; 164:1582-91.
35. MacLennan A. A template for defining a causal relation between acute intrapartum events and cerebral palsy: International consensus statement. BMJ 1999; 319:1054-9.
36. Nelson KB, Ellenberg JH. Antecedents of cerebral palsy. I. Univariate analysis of risks. Am J Dis Child 1985; 139:1031-8.
37. Nelson KB, Ellenberg JH. Antecedents of cerebral palsy: Multivariate analysis of risk. N Engl J Med 1986; 315:81-6.
38. Badawi N, Kurinczuk JJ, Keogh JM, et al. Intrapartum risk factors for neonatal encephalopathy: The Western Australia case-control study. BMJ 1998; 317:1554-8.
39. American College of Obstetricians and Gynecologists Taskforce on Neonatal Encephalopathy and Cerebral Palsy: Neonatal Encephalopathy and Cerebral Palsy: Defining the Pathogenesis and Pathophysiology. Washington, DC, American College of Obstetricians and Gynecologists, 2003.
40. Apgar V. A proposal for a new method of evaluation of the newborn infant. Anesth Analg 1953; 32:260-7.
41. Sykes GS, Johnson P, Ashworth F, et al. Do Apgar scores indicate asphyxia? Lancet 1982; 1(8270):494-6.
42. Marrin M, Paes BA. Birth asphyxia: Does the Apgar score have diagnostic value? Obstet Gynecol 1988; 72:120-3.
43. Catlin EA, Carpenter MW, Brann BS. The Apgar score revisited: Influence of gestational age. J Pediatr 1986; 109:865-8.
44. Wu TJ, Carlo WA; Neonatal Resuscitation Program. Neonatal resuscitation guidelines, 2000: Framework for practice. J Matern Fetal Neonatal Med 2002; 11:4-10.
45. Niermeyer S, Kattwinkel J, Van Reempts P, et al. International Guidelines for Neonatal Resuscitation: An excerpt from the Guidelines 2000 for Cardiopulmonary Resuscitation and Emergency Cardiovascular Care: International Consensus on Science. Contributors and Reviewers for the Neonatal Resuscitation Guidelines. Pediatrics 2000; 106:E29.
46. Helwig JT, Parer JT, Kilpatrick SJ, Laros RK. Umbilical cord blood acid-base state: What is normal? Am J Obstet Gynecol 1996; 174:1807-12.
47. Chiswick ML. Birth asphyxia and cerebral palsy. Int J Obstet Anesth 1992; 1:178-9.
48. Gilstrap LC III, Leveno KJ, Burris J, et al. Diagnosis of birth asphyxia on the basis of fetal pH, Apgar score, and newborn cerebral dysfunction. Am J Obstet Gynecol 1989; 161:825-30.
49. Hull J, Dodd K. What is birth asphyxia? Br J Obstet Gynaecol 1991; 98:953-5.
50. Fee SC, Malee K, Deddish R, et al. Severe acidosis and subsequent neurological status. Am J Obstet Gynecol 1990; 162:802-6.
51. Goodwin TM, Belai I, Hernandez P, et al. Asphyxial complications in the term newborn with severe umbilical acidemia. Am J Obstet Gynecol 1992; 167:1506-12.
52. Goldaber KG, Gilstrap LC, Leveno KJ, et al. Pathologic fetal acidemia. Obstet Gynecol 1991; 78:1103-7.
53. Low JA, Simpson LL, Ramsey DA. The clinical diagnosis of asphyxia responsible for brain damage in the human fetus. Am J Obstet Gynecol 1992; 167:11-5.
54. Low JA. Relationship of fetal asphyxia to neuropathology and deficits in children. Clin Invest Med 1993; 16:133-40.
55. Low JA, Pancham SR, Worthington D, Boston RW. Acid-base, lactate, and pyruvate characteristics of the normal obstetric patient and fetus during the intrapartum period. Am J Obstet Gynecol 1974; 120:862-7.
56. Low JA. The role of blood gas and acid-base assessment in the diagnosis of intrapartum fetal asphyxia. Am J Obstet Gynecol 1988; 159:1235-40.
57. Low JA, Wood SL, Killen HL, et al. Intrapartum asphyxia in the preterm fetus $<$ 2000 gm. Am J Obstet Gynecol 1990; 162:378-82.
58. Low JA, Galbraith RS, Muir DW, et al. Motor and cognitive deficits after intrapartum asphyxia in the mature fetus. Am J Obstet Gynecol 1988; 158:356-61.
59. Low JA, Galbraith RS, Muir DW, et al. Mortality and morbidity after intrapartum asphyxia in the preterm fetus. Obstet Gynecol 1992; 80:57-61.
60. Low JA, Panagiotopoulos C, Derrick EJ. Newborn complications after intrapartum asphyxia with metabolic acidosis in the term fetus. Am J Obstet Gynecol 1994; 170:1081-7.
61. Low JA, Panagiotopoulos C, Derrick EJ. Newborn complications after intrapartum asphyxia with metabolic acidosis in the preterm fetus. Am J Obstet Gynecol 1995; 172:805-10.
62. Low JA, Lindsay BG, Derrick EJ. Threshold of metabolic acidosis associated with newborn complications. Am J Obstet Gynecol 1997; 177:1391-4.
63. Nagel HTC, Vandenbussche FPHA, Oepkes D, et al. Follow-up of children born with an umbilical arterial blood pH $<$ 7. Am J Obstet Gynecol 1995; 173:1758-64.
64. Sehdev HM, Stamilio DM, Macones GA, et al. Predictive factors for neonatal morbidity in neonates with an umbilical arterial cord pH less than 7.00. Am J Obstet Gynecol 1997; 177:1030-4.
65. Gull I, Jaffa AJ, Oren M, et al. Acid accumulation during end-stage bradycardia in term fetuses: How long is too long? Br J Obstet Gynaecol 1996; 103:1096-101.
66. Ross MG, Gala R. Use of umbilical artery base excess: Algorithm for the timing of hypoxic injury. Am J Obstet Gynecol 2002; 187:1-9.
67. Phelan JP, Korst LM, Ahn MO, Martin GI. Neonatal nucleated red blood cell and lymphocyte counts in fetal brain injury. Obstet Gynecol 1998; 91:485-9.
68. Phelan JP, Ahn MO, Korst LM, Martin GI. Nucleated red blood cells: A marker for fetal asphyxia? Am J Obstet Gynecol 1995; 173:1380-4.
69. Korst LM, Phelan JP, Ahn MO, Martin GI. Nucleated red blood cells: An update on the marker for fetal asphyxia. Am J Obstet Gynecol 1996; 175:843-6.
70. Leikin E, Verma U, Klein S, Tejani N. Relationship between neonatal nucleated red blood cell counts and hypoxic-ischemic injury. Obstet Gynecol 1996; 87:439-43.

71. Murphy DJ. Placental infection and risk of cerebral palsy in very low birth weight infants. J Pediatr 1996; 129:776-7.
72. Grether JK, Nelson KB. Maternal infection and cerebral palsy in infants of normal birth weight. JAMA 1997; 278:207-11.
73. Silverstein F, Barks J, Hagan P, et al. Cytokines and perinatal brain injury. Neurochem Int 1997; 30:375-83.
74. Dammann O, Leviton A. Intrauterine infection, cytokines, and brain damage in the preterm newborn. Pediatr Res 1997; 42:1-8.
75. Dammann O, Leviton A. Does prepregnancy bacterial vaginosis increase a mother's risk of having a preterm infant with cerebral palsy? Dev Med Child Neurol 1997; 39:836-40.
76. Camann WR, Hortvet LA, Hughes N, et al. Maternal temperature regulation during extradural analgesia for labour. Br J Anaesth 1991; 67:565-8.
77. Fusi L, Steer PJ, Maresh MJA, Beard RW. Maternal pyrexia associated with the use of epidural analgesia in labour. Lancet 1989; 1(8649): 1250-2.
78. Gray D, Finucane BT. Epidurals and fever: Association or cause? Can Med Assoc J 1997; 157:511-2.
79. Lieberman E, Lang JM, Frigoletto F, et al. Epidural analgesia, intrapartum fever, and neonatal sepsis evaluation. Pediatrics 1997; 99:415-9.
80. Mayer DC, Chescheir NC, Spielman FJ. Increased intrapartum antibiotic administration associated with epidural analgesia in labor. Am J Perinatol 1997; 14:83-6.
81. Baud O, Ville Y, Zupan V, et al. Are neonatal brain lesions due to intrauterine infection related to mode of delivery? Br J Obstet Gynaecol 1998; 105:121-4.
82. Barkovich AJ, Sargent SK. Profound asphyxia in the premature infant: Imaging findings. Am J Neuroradiol 1995; 16:1837-46.
83. Barkovich AJ, Westmark K, Partridge C, et al. Perinatal asphyxia: MR findings in the first 10 days. Am J Neuroradiol 1995; 16:427-38.
84. Martin E, Barkovich AJ. Magnetic resonance imaging in perinatal asphyxia. Arch Dis Child 1995; 72:F62-70.
85. Sibony O, Stempfle N, Luton D, et al. In utero fetal cerebral intraparenchymal ischemia diagnosed by nuclear magnetic resonance. Dev Med Child Neurol 1998; 40:122-3.
86. Younkin DP. Magnetic resonance spectroscopy in hypoxic-ischemic encephalopathy. Clin Invest Med 1993; 16:115-21.
87. Huppi PS, Warfield S, Kikinis R, et al. Quantitative magnetic resonance imaging of brain development in premature and mature newborns. Ann Neurol 1998; 43:224-35.
88. Sugimoto T, Woo M, Nishida N, et al. When do brain abnormalities in cerebral palsy occur? An MRI study. Dev Med Child Neurol 1995; 37:285-92.
89. Okumura A, Kato T, Kuno K, et al. MRI findings in patients with spastic cerebral palsy. 2. Correlation with type of cerebral palsy. Dev Med Child Neurol 1997; 39:369-72.
90. Olsen P, Paakko E, Vainionpaa L, et al. Magnetic resonance imaging of periventricular leukomalacia and its clinical correlation in children. Ann Neurol 1997; 41:754-61.
91. Drobyshevsky A, Derrick M, Prasad PV, et al. Fetal brain magnetic resonance imaging response acutely to hypoxia-ischemia predicts postnatal outcome. Ann Neurol 2007; 61:307-14.
92. Fraser M, Bennet L, Helliwell R, et al. Regional specificity of magnetic resonance imaging and histopathology following cerebral ischemia in preterm fetal sheep. Reprod Sci 2007; 14:182-9.
93. Nanba Y, Matsui K, Aida N, et al. Magnetic resonance imaging regional T1 abnormalities at term accurately predict motor outcome in preterm infants. Pediatrics 2007; 120:e10-9.
94. Miller SP. Newborn brain injury: Looking back to the fetus. Ann Neurol 2007; 61:285-7.
95. Panigrahy A, Blüml S. Advances in magnetic resonance neuroimaging techniques in the evaluation of neonatal encephalopathy. Top Magn Reson Imaging 2007; 18:3-29.
96. Eken P, Jansen GH, Groenendaal F, et al. Intracranial lesions in the fullterm infant with hypoxic-ischaemic encephalopathy: Ultrasound and autopsy correlation. Neuropediatrics 1994; 25:301-7.
97. Raju TNK. Some animal models for the study of perinatal asphyxia. Biol Neonate 1992; 62:202-14.
98. Matsuda Y, Patrick J, Carmichael L, et al. Effects of sustained hypoxemia on the sheep fetus at midgestation: Endocrine, cardiovascular, and biophysical responses. Am J Obstet Gynecol 1992; 167:531-40.
99. Richardson BS, Carmichael L, Homan J, Patrick JE. Electrocortical activity, electroocular activity, and breathing movements in fetal sheep with prolonged and graded hypoxemia. Am J Obstet Gynecol 1992; 167:553-8.
100. Richardson BS, Patrick JE, Bousquet J, et al. Cerebral metabolism in fetal lamb after maternal infusion of ethanol. Am J Physiol 1985; 249:R505-9.
101. Hagberg H, Andersson P, Kjellmer I, et al. Extracellular overflow of glutamate, aspartate, GABA and taurine in the cortex and basal ganglia of fetal lambs during hypoxia-ischemia. Neurosci Lett 1987; 78:311-7.
102. Penning DH, Chestnut DH, Dexter F, et al. Glutamate release from the ovine fetal brain during maternal hemorrhage: A study using chronic in utero cerebral microdialysis. Anesthesiology 1995; 82:521-30.
103. Reynolds JD, Penning DH, Dexter F, et al. Dose-dependent effects of acute in vivo ethanol exposure on extracellular glutamate concentration in the cerebral cortex of the near-term fetal sheep. Alcohol Clin Exp Res 1995; 19:1447-53.
104. Richardson BS, Patrick JE, Abduljabbar H. Cerebral oxidative metabolism in the fetal lamb: Relationship to electrocortical state. Am J Obstet Gynecol 1985; 153:426-31.
105. Richardson B, Patrick J, Homan J, et al. Cerebral oxidative metabolism in fetal sheep with multiple-dose ethanol infusion. Am J Obstet Gynecol 1987; 157:1496-502.
106. Henderson JL, Reynolds JD, Dexter F, et al. Chronic hypoxemia causes extracellular glutamate concentration to increase in the cerebral cortex of the near-term fetal sheep. Brain Res Dev Brain Res 1998; 105:287-93.
107. Mallard EC, Gunn AJ, Williams CE, et al. Transient umbilical cord occlusion causes hippocampal damage in the fetal sheep. Am J Obstet Gynecol 1992; 167:1423-30.
108. Johnson G, Palahniuk R, Tweed W, et al. Regional cerebral blood flow changes during severe fetal asphyxia produced by slow partial umbilical cord compression. Am J Obstet Gynecol 1979; 135:48-52.
109. Clapp JF, Peress NS, Wesley M, Mann LI. Brain damage after intermittent partial cord occlusion in the chronically instrumented fetal lamb. Am J Obstet Gynecol 1988; 159:504-9.
110. Clapp JF, Mann LI, Peress NS, Szeto HH. Neuropathology in the chronic fetal lamb preparation: Structure-function correlates under different environmental conditions. Am J Obstet Gynecol 1981; 141:973-86.
111. Reynolds JD, Chestnut DH, Dexter F, et al. Magnesium sulfate adversely affects fetal lamb survival and blocks fetal cerebral blood flow response during maternal hemorrhage. Anesth Analg 1996; 83:493-9.
112. Hohimer AR, Chao CR, Bissonnette JM. The effect of combined hypoxemia and cephalic hypotension on fetal cerebral blood flow and metabolism. J Cereb Blood Flow Metab 1991; 11:99-105.
113. Robillard JE, Weitzman RE, Burmeister L, Smith FG. Developmental aspects of the renal response to hypoxemia in the lamb fetus. Circ Res 1981; 48:128-38.
114. Richardson BS. The fetal brain: Metabolic and circulatory responses to asphyxia. Clin Invest Med 1993; 16:103-14.
115. Lin BW, Globus MYT, Dietrich WD, et al. Differing neurochemical and morphological sequelae of global ischemia: Comparison of single-multiple and multiple-insult paradigms. J Neurochem 1992; 59:2213-23.
116. Mallard EC, Williams CE, Gunn AJ, et al. Frequent episodes of brief ischemia sensitize the fetal sheep brain to neuronal loss and induce striatal injury. Pediatr Res 1993; 33:61-5.
117. Richardson BS. Fetal adaptive responses to asphyxia. Clin Perinatol 1989; 16:595-611.
118. Edelstone DI. Fetal compensatory responses to reduced oxygen delivery. Semin Perinatol 1984; 8:184-91.

119. Gu W, Jones CT, Parer JT. Metabolic and cardiovascular effects on fetal sheep of sustained reduction of uterine blood flow. J Physiol 1985; 368:109-29.
120. Sieber FE, Smith DS, Traystman RJ, Wollman H. Glucose: A reevaluation of its intraoperative use. Anesthesiology 1987; 67:72-81.
121. Vannucci RC, Mujsce DJ. Effect of glucose on perinatal hypoxic-ischemic brain damage. Biol Neonate 1992; 62:215-24.
122. Blomstrand SB, Hrbek A, Karlsson K, et al. Does glucose administration affect the cerebral response to fetal asphyxia? Acta Obstet Gynecol Scand 1984; 63:345-53.
123. Hooper S. DNA synthesis is reduced in selected fetal tissue during prolonged hypoxemia. Am J Physiol 1991; 261:R508-14.
124. Rurak DW, Gruber NC. The effect of neuromuscular blockade on oxygen consumption and blood gases in the fetal lamb. Am J Obstet Gynecol 1983; 145:258-62.
125. Jensen A, Berger R. Fetal circulatory responses to oxygen lack. Brain Res Dev Brain Res 1991; 16:181-207.
126. Sheldon RE, Peeters LLH, Jones MD, et al. Redistribution of cardiac output and oxygen delivery in the hypoxic fetal lamb. Am J Obstet Gynecol 1979; 135:1071-8.
127. Jensen A, Hohmann M, Kunzel W. Dynamic changes in organ blood flow and oxygen consumption during acute asphyxia in fetal sheep. J Dev Physiol 1987; 9:543-59.
128. Penning DH, Grafe MR, Hammond R, et al. Neuropathology of the near-term and midgestation ovine fetal brain after sustained in utero hypoxemia. Am J Obstet Gynecol 1994; 170:1425-32.
129. Back SA, Riddle A, Hohimer AR. Role of instrumented fetal sheep preparations in defining the pathogenesis of human periventricular white-matter injury. J Child Neurol 2006; 21:582-9.
130. Dobbing J, Sands J. Comparative aspects of the brain growth spurt. Early Hum Dev 1979; 3:79-83.
131. Clancy B, Finlay BL, Darlington RB, Anand KJ. Extrapolating brain development from experimental species to humans. Neurotoxicology 2007; 28:931-7.
132. Battaglia FC, Meschia G. An Introduction to Fetal Physiology. Orlando, FL, Academic Press, 1986:257.
133. Derrick M, Luo NL, Bregman JC, et al. Preterm fetal hypoxia-ischemia causes hypertonia and motor deficits in the neonatal rabbit: A model for human cerebral palsy? J Neurosci 2004; 24:24-34.
134. Drobyshevsky A, Derrick M, Wyrwicz AM, et al. White matter injury correlates with hypertonia in an animal model of cerebral palsy. J Cereb Blood Flow Metab 2007; 27:270-81.
135. Derrick M, Drobyshevsky A, Ji X, Tan S. A model of cerebral palsy from fetal hypoxia-ischemia. Stroke 2007; 38(2 Suppl):731-5.
136. Schendel DE, Berg CJ, Yearginallsopp M, et al. Prenatal magnesium sulfate exposure and the risk for cerebral palsy or mental retardation among very low-birth-weight children aged 3 to 5 years. JAMA 1996; 276:1805-10.
137. Nelson KB, Grether JK. Can magnesium sulfate reduce the risk of cerebral palsy in very low birth weight infants? Pediatrics 1995; 95:263-9.
138. Mayor S. Prenatal magnesium sulphate cuts risk of cerebral palsy. BMJ 1996; 313:1505.
139. Nelson KB. Magnesium sulfate and risk of cerebral palsy in very low-birth-weight infants (editorial). JAMA 1996; 276:1843-4.
140. Rouse DJ, Hirtz DG, Thom E, et al. A randomized, controlled trial of magnesium sulfate for the prevention of cerebral palsy. N Engl J Med 2008; 359:895-905.
141. Collins M, Paneth N. Preeclampsia and cerebral palsy: Are they related? Dev Med Child Neurol 1998; 40:207-11.
142. Johnston MV. Neurotransmitters and vulnerability of the developing brain. Brain Dev 1995; 17:301-6.
143. de Haan HH, Alistair AJ, Williams CE, et al. Magnesium sulfate therapy during asphyxia in near-term fetal lambs does not compromise the fetus but does not reduce cerebral injury. Am J Obstet Gynecol 1997; 176:18-27.
144. Moon PF, Ramsay MM, Nathanielsz PW. Intravenous infusion of magnesium sulfate and regional redistribution of fetal blood flow during maternal hemorrhage in late gestation gravid ewes. Am J Obstet Gynecol 1999; 181:1486-94.
145. Sameshima H, Ota A, Ikenoue T. Pretreatment with magnesium sulfate protects against hypoxic-ischemic brain injury but postasphyxial treatment worsens brain damage in seven-day-old rats. Am J Obstet Gynecol 1999; 180:725-30.
146. Mittendorf R, Dambrosia J, Pryde PG, et al. Association between the use of antenatal magnesium sulfate in preterm labor and adverse health outcomes in infants. Am J Obstet Gynecol 2002; 186:1111-8.
147. Kirschbaum TH. Magnesium sulfate and prematurity. J Soc Gynecol Invest 2002; 9:58-9.
148. Farkouh LJ, Thorp JA, Jones PG, et al. Antenatal magnesium exposure and neonatal demise. Am J Obstet Gynecol 2001; 185:869-72.
149. Brann AW, Myers RE. Central nervous system findings in the newborn monkey following severe in utero partial asphyxia. Neurology 1975; 25:327-38.
150. Larroche JC. Fetal and perinatal brain damage. In Wigglesworth JS, Singer DB, editors. Textbook of Fetal and Perinatal Pathology. Boston, Blackwell Scientific, 1991:807-38.
151. Allan WC, Riviello JJ. Perinatal cerebrovascular disease in the neonate: Parenchymal ischemic lesions in term and preterm infants. Pediatr Clin North Am 1992; 39:621-50.
152. Volpe JJ. Hypoxic-ischemic encephalopathy: Neuropathology and pathogenesis. In Volpe JJ, editor. Neurology of the Newborn. 2nd edition. Philadelphia, WB Saunders, 1987:209-35.
153. Volpe JJ. Brain injury in the premature infant: Current concepts of pathogenesis and prevention. Biol Neonate 1992; 62:231-42.
154. Banker BQ, Larroche LJC. Periventricular leukomalacia of infancy: A form of neonatal anoxic encephalopathy. Arch Neurol 1962; 7:386-410.
155. Dubowitz LMS, Bydder GM, Mushin J. Developmental sequence of periventricular leukomalacia. Arch Dis Child 1985; 60:349-55.
156. DeReuck J. The human periventricular arterial blood supply and the anatomy of cerebral infarctions. Eur Neurol 1971; 5:321-34.
157. Nelson MDJ, Gonzalez-Gomez I, Gilles FH. The search for human telencephalic ventriculofugal arteries. Am J Neuroradiol 1991; 12:215-22.
158. Mayer PL, Kier EL. The controversy of the periventricular white matter circulation: A review of the anatomic literature. Am J Neuroradiol 1991; 12:223-8.
159. Ashwal S, Dale PS, Longo LD. Regional cerebral blood flow: Studies in the fetal lamb during hypoxia, hypercapnia, acidosis, and hypotension. Pediatr Res 1984; 18:1309-16.
160. Juurlink BHJ, Hertz L, Yager JY. Astrocyte maturation and susceptibility to ischaemia or substrate deprivation. Neuroreport 1992; 3:1135-7.
161. Choi DW. Excitotoxic cell death. J Neurobiol 1992; 23:1261-76.
162. Rothman SM, Olney JW. Glutamate and the pathophysiology of hypoxic-ischemic brain damage. Ann Neurol 1986; 19:105-11.
163. Fonnum F. Glutamate: A neurotransmitter in mammalian brain. J Neurochem 1984; 42:1-11.
164. Penning DH, Goh JW, Elbeheiry H, Brien JF. Effect of hypoxia on glutamate efflux and synaptic transmission in the guinea pig hippocampus. Brain Res 1993; 620:301-4.
165. Choi D. Glutamate neurotoxicity and diseases of the nervous system. Neuron 1988; 1:623-34.
166. Choi D. Cerebral hypoxia: Some new approaches and unanswered questions. J Neurosci 1990; 10:2493.
167. Choi D, Rothman S. The role of glutamate neurotoxicity in hypoxic-ischemic neuronal death. Ann Rev Neurosci 1990; 13:171-82.
168. Benveniste H. The excitotoxin hypothesis in relation to cerebral ischemia. Cerebrovasc Brain Metab Rev 1991; 3:213-45.
169. Nelson N, editor. Current Therapy in Neonatal-Perinatal Medicine. Toronto, BC Decker, 1990:276.
170. McDonald JW, Johnston MV. Physiological and pathophysiological roles of excitatory amino acids during central nervous system development. Brain Res Rev 1990; 15:41-70.
171. Fazekas JF, Alexander FAD, Himwich HE. Tolerance of the newborn to anoxia. Am J Physiol 1941; 134:281-7.

172. Kabat H. The greater resistance of very young animals to arrest of the brain circulation. Am J Physiol 1940; 130:588-99.
173. Glass HG, Snyder FF, Webster E. The rate of decline in resistance to anoxia of rabbits, dogs and guinea pigs from the onset of viability to adult life. Am J Physiol 1944; 140:609-15.
174. Silverstein FS, Torke L, Barks J, Johnston MV. Hypoxia-ischemia produces focal disruption of glutamate receptors in developing brain. Dev Brain Res 1987; 34:33-9.
175. Silverstein FS, Buchanan K, Johnston MV. Perinatal hypoxia-ischemia disrupts striatal high-affinity [3H]glutamate uptake into synaptosomes. J Neurochem 1986; 47:1614-9.
176. Penning DH, Patrick J, Jimmo S, Brien JF. Release of glutamate and gamma-aminobutyric acid in the ovine fetal hippocampus: Ontogeny and effect of hypoxia. J Dev Physiol 1991; 16:301-7.
177. Johnston MV. Cellular alterations associated with perinatal asphyxia. Clin Invest Med 1993; 16:122-32.
178. Gombos G, Levy O, Debarry J. Developmental changes of EAA metabotropic receptor activity in rat cerebellum. Neuroreport 1992; 3:877-80.
179. Ikonomidou C, Mosinger JL, Salles KS, et al. Sensitivity of the developing rat brain to hypobaric/ischemic damage parallels sensitivity to N-methyl-aspartate neurotoxicity. J Neurosci 1989; 9:2809-18.
180. Lee HS, Choi BH. Density and distribution of excitatory amino acid receptors in the developing human fetal brain: A quantitative autoradiographic study. Exp Neurol 1992; 118:284-90.
181. Greenamyre T, Penney JB, Young AB, et al. Evidence for transient perinatal glutamatergic innervation of globus pallidus. J Neurosci 1987; 7:1022-30.
182. Siesjo BK. Pathophysiology and treatment of focal cerebral ischemia. 1. Pathophysiology. J Neurosurg 1992; 77:169-84.
183. Siesjo BK. Pathophysiology and treatment of focal cerebral ischemia. 2. Mechanisms of damage and treatment. J Neurosurg 1992; 77:337-54.
184. Pellegrini-Giampietro DE, Bennett MVL, Zukin RS. Are C(2+)-permeable kainate/AMPA receptors more abundant in immature brain? Neurosci Lett 1992; 144:65-9.
185. Dawson VL, Dawson TM. Nitric oxide in neuronal degeneration. Proc Soc Exp Biol Med 1996; 211:33-40.
186. Dawson DA. Nitric oxide and focal cerebral ischemia: Multiplicity of actions and diverse outcome. Cerebrovasc Brain Metab Rev 1994; 6:299-324.
187. Olney JW, Ikonomidou C, Mosinger JL, Frierdich G. MK-801 prevents hypobaric-ischemic neuronal degeneration in infant rat brain. J Neurosci 1989; 9:1701-4.
188. McDonald JW, Silverstein FS, Johnston MV. MK-801 protects the neonatal brain from hypoxic-ischemic damage. Eur J Pharmacol 1987; 140:359-61.
189. Tan WKM, Williams CE, Gunn AJ, et al. Suppression of postischemic epileptiform activity with MK-801 improves neural outcome in fetal sheep. Ann Neurol 1992; 32:677-82.
190. Komuro H, Rakic P. Modulation of neuronal migration by NMDA receptors. Science 1993; 260:95-7.
191. Emerit MB, Riad M, Hamon M. Trophic effects of neurotransmitters during brain maturation. Biol Neonate 1992; 62:193-201.
192. Gluckman PD, Williams CE. Is the cure worse than the disease? Caveats in the move from laboratory to clinic. Dev Med Child Neurol 1992; 34:1015-8.
193. Lockhart EM, Warner DS, Pearlstein RD, et al. Allopregnanolone attenuates N-methyl-D-aspartate-induced excitotoxicity and apoptosis in the human NT2 cell line in culture. Neurosci Lett 2002; 328:33-6.
194. Yawno T, Yan EB, Walker DW, Hirst JJ. Inhibition of neurosteroid synthesis increases asphyxia-induced brain injury in the late gestation fetal sheep. Neuroscience 2007; 146:1726-33.
195. Nguyen PN, Yan EB, Castillo-Melendez M, et al. Increased allopregnanolone levels in the fetal sheep brain following umbilical cord occlusion. J Physiol 2004; 560(Pt 2):593-602.
196. Stein DG. The case for progesterone. Ann N Y Acad Sci 2005; 1052:152-69.
197. Clarren SK, Smith DW. The fetal alcohol syndrome. N Engl J Med 1978; 298:1063-7.
198. Cohen RS, Benitz WE, Stevenson DK. Fetal injury from drug abuse in pregnancy: Alcohol, narcotic, cocaine and phencyclidine. In Stevenson DK, Sunshine P, editors. Fetal and Neonatal Brain Injury: Mechanisms, Management, and the Risks of Practice. Philadelphia, BC Decker, 1989:57-64.
199. Smith GN, Patrick J, Sinervo KR, Brien JF. Effects of ethanol exposure on the embryo-fetus: Experimental considerations, mechanisms, and the role of prostaglandins. Can J Physiol Pharmacol 1990; 69:550-69.
200. Barnes DE, Walker DW. Prenatal ethanol exposure permanently reduces the number of pyramidal neurons in rat hippocampus. Dev Brain Res 1981; 1:333-40.
201. Snell LD, Tabakoff B, Hoffman PL. Radioligand binding to the N-methyl-D-aspartate receptor/ionophore complex: Alterations by ethanol in vitro and by chronic in vivo ethanol ingestion. Brain Res 1993; 602:91-8.
202. Volpe JJ. Effect of cocaine use on the fetus. N Engl J Med 1992; 327:399-407.
203. Cutler AR, Wilkerson AE, Gingras JL, Levin ED. Prenatal cocaine and/or nicotine exposure in rats: Preliminary findings on long-term cognitive outcome and genital development at birth. Neurotoxicol Teratol 1996; 18:635-43.
204. Richardson GA, Conroy ML, Day NL. Prenatal cocaine exposure: Effects on the development of school-age children. Neurotoxicol Teratol 1996; 18:627-34.
205. Martin JC, Barr HM, Martin DC, Streissguth AP. Neonatal neurobehavioral outcome following prenatal exposure to cocaine. Neurotoxicol Teratol 1996; 18:617-25.
206. Roberts D, Dalziel S. Antenatal corticosteroids for accelerating fetal lung maturation for women at risk of preterm birth. Cochrane Database Syst Rev 2006; (3):CD004454.
207. Smith GN, Kingdom JC, Penning DH, Matthews SG. Antenatal corticosteroids: Is more better? Lancet 2000; 355:251-2.
208. Baud O, Sola A. Corticosteroids in perinatal medicine: how to improve outcomes without affecting the developing brain? Semin Fetal Neonatal Med 2007; 12:273-9.
209. Watterberg KL, Shaffer ML, Mishefske MJ, et al. Growth and neurodevelopmental outcomes after early low-dose hydrocortisone treatment in extremely low birth weight infants. Pediatrics 2007; 120:40-8.
210. Smith CV, Phelan JP. Trauma in pregnancy. In Clark SL, Cotton DB, Hankins GDV, Phelan JP, editors. Critical Care Obstetrics. 2nd edition. Boston, Blackwell Scientific, 1991.
211. Gilles MT, Blair E, Watson L, et al. Trauma in pregnancy and cerebral palsy: Is there a link? Med J Aust 1996; 164:500-1.
212. Chetcuti P, Levene M. Seat belts: A potential hazard to the fetus. J Perinat Med 1987; 15:207-9.
213. Lee RV, Rodgers BD, White LM, Harvey RC. Cardiopulmonary resuscitation of pregnant women. Am J Med 1986; 81:311-8.
214. Bishop EH, Israel SL, Briscoe CC. Obstetric influences on the premature infant's first year of development: A report from the collaborative study of cerebral palsy. Obstet Gynecol 1965; 26:628.
215. Huff DL, Thurnau GR, Sheldon R. The outcome of protective forceps deliveries of 26-33 week infants (abstract). In Proceedings of the Annual Meeting of the Society of Perinatal Obstetricians. Orlando, FL, 1987.
216. Barrett JM, Boehm FH, Vaughn WK. The effect of type of delivery on neonatal outcome in singleton infants of birth weight of 1,000 g or less. JAMA 1983; 250:625-9.
217. Thomas RL, Ferguson JE, Repke JT. Complications of labor and delivery: Selected medical and surgical considerations. In Stevenson DK, Sunshine P, editors. Fetal and Neonatal Brain Injury: Mechanisms, Management, and the Risks of Practice. Philadelphia, BC Decker, 1989:34-45.
218. Broekhuizen FF, Washington JM, Johnson F. Vacuum extraction versus forceps delivery: Indications and complications, 1979 to 1984. Obstet Gynecol 1987; 69:338-42.

219. El-Beheiry H, Puil E. Anesthetic depression of excitatory synaptic transmission in neocortex. Exp Brain Res 1989; 77:87-93.
220. Puil E, El-Beheiry H. Anaesthetic suppression of transmitter actions in neocortex. Br J Pharmacol 1990; 101:61-6.
221. Charlesworth P, Pocock G, Richards CD. The action of anaesthetics on stimulus-secretion coupling and synaptic activity. Gen Pharmacol 1992; 23:977-84.
222. Elliott JR, Elliott AA, Harper AA, Winpenny JP. Effects of general anaesthetics on neuronal sodium and potassium channels. Gen Pharmacol 1992; 23:1005-11.
223. Krnjevic K. Cellular and synaptic actions of general anaesthetics. Gen Pharmacol 1992; 23:965-75.
224. Aitken PG, Schiff SJ. Barbiturate protection against hypoxic neuronal damage in vitro. J Neurosurg 1986; 65:230-2.
225. Ginsberg M, Busto R. Rodent models of cerebral ischemia. Stroke 1989; 20:1627-42.
226. Warner DS, Todd MM, Ludwig P, et al. Volatile anesthetics reduce focal ischemic brain damage in the rat. J Cereb Blood Flow Metab 1993; 13:S684.
227. Buchan A, Pulsinelli W. Hypothermia but not the N-methyl-D-aspartate antagonist, MK-801, attenuates neuronal damage in gerbils subjected to transient global ischemia. J Neurosci 1990; 10:311-6.
228. Ginsberg MD, Sternau LL, Globus MYT, et al. Therapeutic modulation of brain temperature: Relevance to ischemic brain injury. Cerebrovasc Brain Metab Rev 1992; 4:189-225.
229. Todd M, Warner D. A comfortable hypothesis reevaluated: Cerebral metabolic depression and brain protection during ischemia. Anesthesiology 1992; 76:161-4.
230. Carla V, Moroni F. General anaesthetics inhibit the responses induced by glutamate receptor agonists in the mouse cortex. Neurosci Lett 1992; 146:21-4.
231. Lyden PD, Hedges B. Protective effect of synaptic inhibition during cerebral ischemia in rats and rabbits. Stroke 1992; 23:1463-9.
232. Yatsu FM, Grotta JC. Protective effect of synaptic inhibition during cerebral ischemia in rats and rabbits (editorial comment). Stroke 1992; 23:1469-70.
233. Myers RE, Myers SE. Use of sedative, analgesic, and anesthetic drugs during labor and delivery: Bane or boon? Am J Obstet Gynecol 1979; 133:83-104.
234. Olney JW, Young C, Wozniak DF, et al. Do pediatric drugs cause developing neurons to commit suicide? Trends Pharmacol Sci 2004; 25:135-9.
235. Soriano SG, Anand KJ, Rovnaghi CR, Hickey PR. Of mice and men: Should we extrapolate rodent experimental data to the care of human neonates? Anesthesiology 2005; 102:866-8.
236. Bhutta AT, Venkatesan AK, Rovnaghi CR, Anand KJ. Anaesthetic neurotoxicity in rodents: Is the ketamine controversy real? Acta Paediatr 2007; 96:1554-6.
237. Todd MM. Anesthetic neurotoxicity: The collision between laboratory neuroscience and clinical medicine. Anesthesiology 2004; 101:272-3.
238. Anand KJ. Anesthetic neurotoxicity in newborns: Should we change clinical practice? Anesthesiology 2007; 107:2-4.
239. Anand KJ, Soriano SG. Anesthetic agents and the immature brain: Are these toxic or therapeutic? Anesthesiology 2004; 101:527-30.
240. Mellon RD, Simone AF, Rappaport BA. Use of anesthetic agents in neonates and young children. Anesth Analg 2007; 104:509-20.
241. Perlman JM. Intervention strategies for neonatal hypoxic-ischemic cerebral injury. Clin Ther 2006; 28:1353-65.
242. Bennet L, Roelfsema V, George S, et al. The effect of cerebral hypothermia on white and grey matter injury induced by severe hypoxia in preterm fetal sheep. J Physiol 2007; 578(Pt 2):491-506.
243. George S, Scotter J, Dean JM, et al. Induced cerebral hypothermia reduces post-hypoxic loss of phenotypic striatal neurons in preterm fetal sheep. Exp Neurol 2007; 203(1):137-47.
244. Shankaran S, Laptook AR, Ehrenkranz RA, et al. Whole-body hypothermia for neonates with hypoxic-ischemic encephalopathy. N Engl J Med 2005; 353:1574-84.
245. Gluckman PD, Wyatt JS, Azzopardi D, et al. Selective head cooling with mild systemic hypothermia after neonatal encephalopathy: Multicentre randomised trial. Lancet 2005; 365:663-70.
246. Papile LA. Systemic hypothermia—a "cool" therapy for neonatal hypoxic-ischemic encephalopathy. N Engl J Med 2005; 353:1619-20.
247. Choi DW, Lobner D, Dugan LL. Glutamate receptor-mediated neuronal death in the ischemic brain. In Hsu CY, editor. Ischemic Stroke: From Basic Mechanisms to New Drug Development. Basel, Switzerland, Karger, 1998:2-13.
248. Choi DW. At the scene of ischemic brain injury: Is PARP a perp? Nature Med 1997; 3:1073-4.
249. Swanson RA, Choi DW. Glial glycogen stores affect neuronal survival during glucose deprivation in vitro. J Cereb Blood Flow Metab 1993; 13:162-9.
250. Swanson RA. Astrocyte glutamate uptake during chemical hypoxia in vitro. Neurosci Lett 1992; 147:143-6.
251. Ransom BR. The pathophysiology of anoxic injury in central nervous system white matter. Stroke 1990; 21(Suppl III):III52-7.
252. Graham SH, Chen J, Sharp FR, Simon RP. Limiting ischemic injury by inhibition of excitatory amino acid release. J Cereb Blood Flow Metab 1993; 13:88-97.
253. Volpe JJ. Brain injury in the premature infant: From pathogenesis to prevention. Brain Dev 1997; 19:519-34.
254. Thiringer K, Hrbek A, Karlsson K, et al. Postasphyxial cerebral survival in newborn sheep after treatment with oxygen free radical scavengers and a calcium antagonist. Pediatr Res 1987; 22:62-6.
255. McGowan FX, Davis PJ. Anesthetic-related neurotoxity in the developing infant: Of mice, rats, monkeys and, possibly, humans. Anesth Analg 2008; 106:1599-602.
256. Loepke AW, McGowan FX Jr, Soriano SG. Con: The toxic effects of anesthetics in the developing brain: The clinical perspective. Anesth Analg 2008; 106:1664-9.
257. Jevtovic-Todorovic V, Olney JW. Pro: Anesthesia-induced developmental neuroapoptosis: Status of the evidence. Anesth Analg 2008; 106:1659-63.
258. Loepke AW, Soriano SG. An assessment of the effects of general anesthetics on developing brain structure and neurocognitive function. Anesth Analg 2008; 106:1681-707.
259. Wang C, Slikker W Jr. Strategies and experimental models for evaluating anesthetics: Effects on the developing nervous system. Anesth Analg 2008; 106:1643-58.
260. Sanders RD, Xu J, Ma D, Maze M. General anesthetics induce apoptotic neurodegeneration in the neonatal rat spinal cord. Anesth Analg 2008; 106:1708-11.
261. Degos V, Loron G, Mantz J, Gressens P. Neuroprotective strategies for the neonatal brain. Anesth Analg 2008; 106:1670-80.
262. Cattano D, Young C, Straiko MM, Olney JW. Subanesthetic doses of propofol induce neuroapoptosis in the infant mouse brain. Anesth Analg 2008; 106:1712-4.
263. Yon JH, Carter LB, Reiter J, Jevtovic-Todorovic V. Melatonin reduces the severity of anesthesia-induced apoptotic neurodegeneration in the developing rat brain. Neurobiol Dis 2006; 21:522-30.

Part IV

Foundations in Obstetric Anesthesia

As Simpson predicted, physicians used obstetric anesthesia sparingly until patients forced the issue. A major impetus came from early feminists. Suffragettes recognized that they could not participate fully in the economic and political life of the country unless they were healthy. For this reason they made obstetric care, including anesthesia, part of their campaign for political parity.

Early feminists had good reason to be concerned about obstetric care. Despite many improvements in medicine, maternal morbidity and mortality hardly changed between 1830 and 1930. Women were debilitated by the sequelae of poorly managed deliveries and exhausted by frequent pregnancies and management of large families. Accordingly, feminists sought care by obstetricians rather than by midwives, deliveries in hospitals rather than at home, and adequate time for recuperation before returning to their normal responsibilities. Other initiatives were construction of special maternity units, better instruction in obstetrics in medical schools, and training of more obstetricians.

They also campaigned for obstetric anesthesia. Feminists and physicians alike believed that the pain of childbirth, in and of itself, contributed to the disability of women later in life. To improve the quality and availability of anesthesia, feminists founded two organizations. The National Twilight Sleep Association began in the United States just before the beginning of World War I, and the National Birthday Trust Fund started in Great Britain in 1928.

Both organizations influenced the practice of obstetric anesthesia. Physicians explored new ways to manage the pain of childbirth, including use of rectal ether and intravenous opioids. They also performed many important studies on the use of regional anesthesia.

For obstetricians, regional anesthesia had several advantages. First, it appeared to be safe and easy to administer, a feature that was especially important because qualified anesthesiologists were in short supply. Second, regional anesthesia allowed obstetricians to make more liberal use of operative techniques for vaginal delivery (e.g., episiotomy, use of forceps), which were just coming into vogue. No less important, regional anesthesia appeared to satisfy the desires of women who wanted more comfortable deliveries. These motives prompted the use of various regional blocks, including presacral, paravertebral, spinal, lumbar epidural, and caudal epidural anesthesia. In conjunction with this clinical work, scientists studied the anatomy and physiology of uterine function and childbirth pain, including the neurologic pathways involved in the perception of childbirth pain. Our current practices of obstetric anesthesia, particularly the emphasis on regional anesthesia, are a direct outgrowth of scientific studies and clinical trials that began during this period.[1-4]

Donald Caton, M.D.

REFERENCES

1. Loudon I. Death in Childbirth: An International Study of Maternal Care and Maternal Mortality, 1800-1950. Oxford, Clarendon Press, 1992:187, 220-3, 172-233, 216-32.
2. Barnett R. "The future of the midwife depends on her power to relieve pain": The rise and fall of the Analgesia in Childbirth Bill (1949). Int J Obstet Anesth 2007; 16:35-9.
3. Lewis J. Mothers and maternal policies in the twentieth century. In Garcia J, Kilpatrick R, Richards M, editors. The Politics of Maternity Care: Services for Childbearing Women in Twentieth-Century Britain. Oxford, Clarendon Paperbacks, 1990:15-29.
4. Caton D. A century of spinals for childbirth. Int J Obstet Anesth 2000; 9:149-50.

Chapter 11

Patient Safety and Team Training

David J. Birnbach, M.D., M.P.H.
Eduardo Salas, Ph.D.

In 2000, the publication of the Institute of Medicine (IOM) report *To Err Is Human: Building a Safer Health Care System* was a seminal event for the health care system in the United States.[1] Prior to the publication of this report, many physicians and hospital administrators refused to acknowledge the frequent occurrence of preventable morbidity and mortality and the sad reality that our health care system was not adequately addressing the issue of patient safety. The IOM concluded that tens of thousands of patients were dying each year as a result of medical errors. In the past decade, numerous changes have been endorsed to improve patient safety; these include mandatory minimum nurse-to-patient ratios,[2] a reduction in duty hours for resident physicians,[3] mandatory time-outs before invasive procedures (to confirm patient identity and the procedure to be performed), and the use of simulation and teamwork training in the medical environment.[4,5] Data from high-risk organizations suggest that health care errors do not usually occur because of ill-trained medical personnel but rather result from systems that "set up" both the patient and health care provider. Wu[6] has aptly called these health care providers "second victims." This chapter reviews several modalities that can be used to improve patient safety and reduce the incidence and sequelae of medical errors on the labor and delivery unit.

PATIENT SAFETY

Traditional assessments of medical error have often blamed individuals and have failed to address the broader systems issues that allowed the error to occur. Newer approaches are based on an understanding that humans will make errors and encourage the creation of robust systems to prevent those errors from occurring or to minimize their effect on patients if they occur. This paradigm change has borrowed heavily from other high-risk industries, such as aviation.

The Swiss Cheese Model

Patients are typically not injured by a single event resulting from a single act of a careless individual. More often, an underlying systems problem made the error possible, and numerous individual actions are allowed to "fall through the cracks" of a system that does not "catch" them, resulting in error and harm. James Reason[7] described the "Swiss cheese" model of error (Figure 11-1), in which he explained how numerous contributing factors are responsible for the ultimate harm. Reason developed this model to illustrate how analyses of major accidents and catastrophic systems failures tend to reveal multiple, smaller failures that lead up to the actual adverse event. In Reason's model, each slice of cheese represents a safety barrier or precaution relevant to a particular hazard. For example, if the hazard were wrong-site surgery, slices of the cheese might include processes for identifying the right or left side on radiographic images, a protocol for signing the correct site when the surgeon and patient first meet, and a second protocol for reviewing the medical record and checking the previously marked site in the operating room. Each barrier has "holes"—hence, the term "Swiss cheese." For some serious events (e.g., operating on the wrong person), the holes will rarely align; however, even rare cases of preventable harm are unacceptable. Reason's model highlights the need to think of patient safety as a system of care—a set of organizational and cultural layers that influence and shape one another. Reason[8] has eloquently summarized the process as follows:

> *Rather than being the main instigators of an accident, operators tend to be the inheritors of system defects created by poor design, incorrect installation, faulty maintenance, and bad management decisions. Their part is usually that of adding the final garnish to a lethal brew whose ingredients have already been long in the cooking.*

Figure 11-2 illustrates the use of the Swiss cheese model to evaluate an actual "near-miss" case that involved the misidentification of an obstetric patient who nearly underwent the wrong procedure (a tubal ligation). It shows how

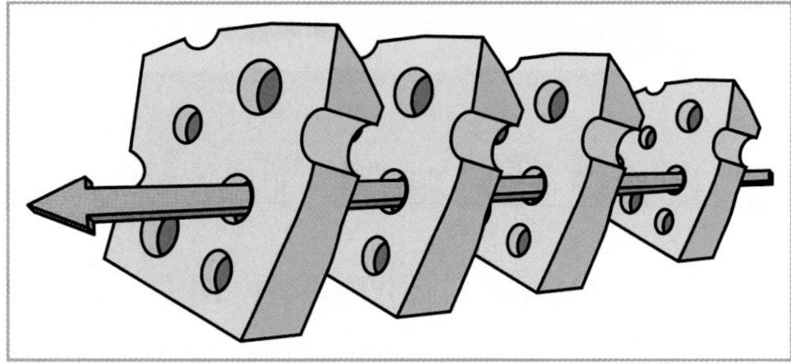

FIGURE 11-1 Swiss cheese model of organizational accidents. (From Reason JT. Human Error. Cambridge, UK, Cambridge University Press, 1990.)

the combination of numerous systems errors came very close to allowing the wrong procedure to be performed. The events unfolded as follows:

1. A nulliparous woman in active labor at term gestation arrived on the labor and delivery unit in severe pain. She spoke a foreign language and was poorly understood by the labor and delivery staff. No translator was called because her husband was helping with the translation.
2. Because the patient was in such severe pain, she hurriedly answered all the questions, and she answered several questions incorrectly. As per hospital policy (owing to HIPAA [Health Insurance Portability and Accountability Act of 1996] regulations), the husband was asked to leave the room while the history was taken, and therefore he was not present to assist with the translation.
3. Another patient on the labor and delivery unit had the same last name and a similar-sounding first name. The hospital protocol for this occurrence was not followed. Patient initials, not last names, were listed on the labor and delivery "board," so other staff were unaware of the fact that two patients had identical last names.
4. A nonreassuring fetal heart rate (FHR) tracing developed during the patient's labor, and she was scheduled to undergo urgent cesarean delivery. The obstetric resident physician informed the anesthesiologist of this decision

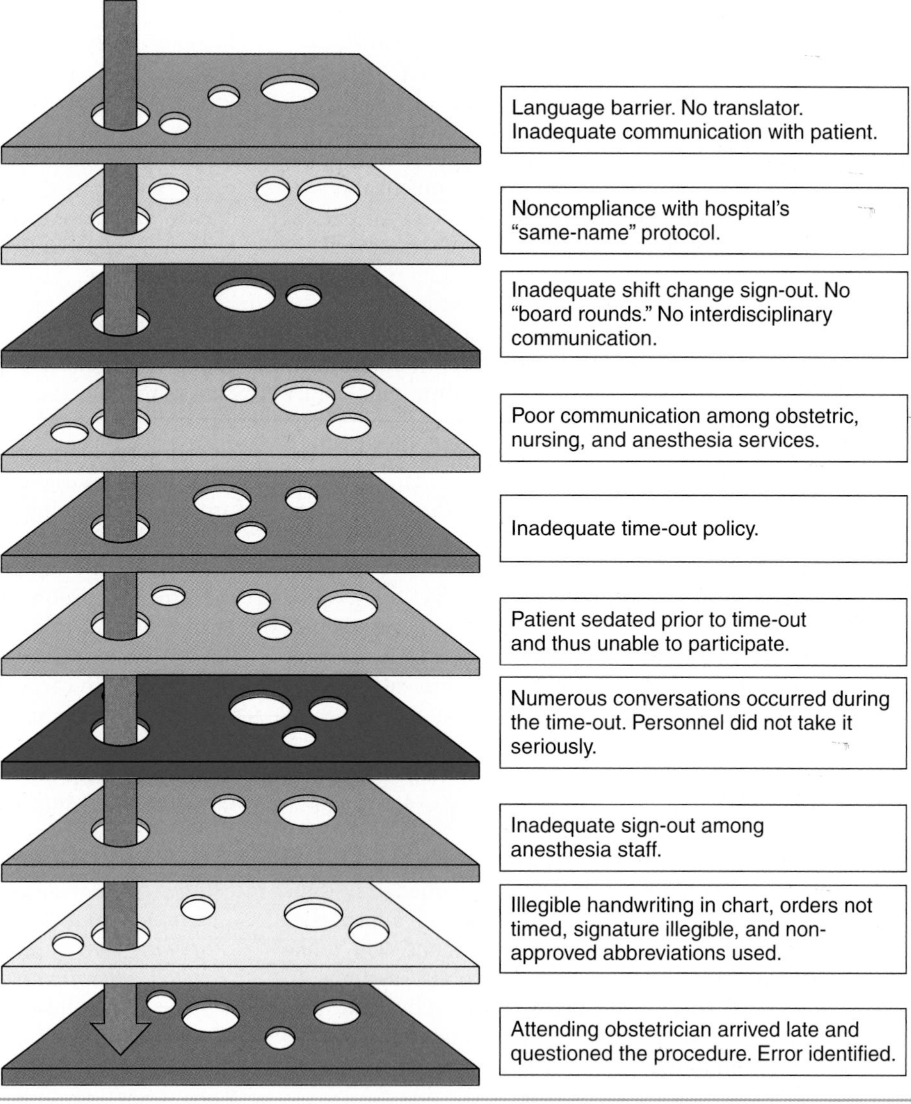

FIGURE 11-2 "Swiss cheese" diagram of a "near-miss" event, illustrating how numerous layers/barriers to harm were breached and this almost resulted in permanent harm (permanent sterility) to the patient. See text for explanation.

and, mistaking the two patients with identical names, informed staff that the patient would undergo a cesarean delivery *plus* a bilateral tubal ligation. Unlike the other patient with the same last name, the patient going to the operating room did not want or expect a tubal ligation.

5. The surgical case was delayed because of a shift change, and the obstetric residents urged the nurses to hurry. This behavior caused friction between the nurses and the obstetric residents, who did not work as a team. There were no "board rounds," and communication between labor and delivery staff and operating room staff was lacking.
6. On arrival in the operating room, the patient was anxious and crying. The anesthesiologist administered fentanyl 50 μg to calm the patient, and she became somnolent.
7. A time-out procedure was performed, but no one in the operating room took it seriously. The patient was asleep and did not participate. The attending obstetrician was not present. Conversations continued during the time-out procedure.
8. After the flawed time-out, all agreed that this patient was to undergo a primary cesarean delivery with tubal ligation. Her husband was not present during the time-out procedure, but he was brought to the room immediately afterward. The surgical procedure began.
9. The attending obstetrician arrived after the start of surgery and questioned the planned tubal ligation, not because he was aware of the other patient with the same last name, but because he was informed that this patient was nulliparous. Immediate investigation showed that this patient was *not* supposed to undergo a tubal ligation. A major error was narrowly averted.

Medical Errors

Today there is widespread interest in changing the health care culture in order to build safer systems, including ensuring the appropriate physical work environment, developing redundancies in safety procedures, allowing health care workers to report their mistakes (including "near misses") without fear of punishment, and providing mechanisms to learn from these experiences. Unfortunately, none of these steps will achieve the ultimate goal of patient safety without the support of physicians as well as hospital administrators. In addition, although they are vital to improving the current condition, these steps do not obviate the need for well-trained and well-rested physicians and nurses.[9]

The American College of Obstetricians and Gynecologists (ACOG) has stated that promotion of patient safety requires that all members of the health care team recognize that the potential for error exists and that teamwork and communication are the basis for fostering change and preventing errors.[10] The ACOG has recommended the following seven safety objectives:

1. Develop a commitment to encourage a culture of patient safety.
2. Implement recommended safe medication practices, including improved legibility of handwriting and avoidance of the use of nonstandard abbreviations.
3. Reduce the likelihood of surgical errors.
4. Improve communication.
5. Identify and resolve systems problems.
6. Establish a partnership with patients.
7. Make safety a priority in every aspect of practice.

Reports of medical errors causing morbidity and mortality are commonly found in the lay press. How should we, as anesthesia providers or obstetricians, define *error*? The IOM has defined **medical error** as a "failure of a planned action to be completed as intended, or the use of a wrong plan to achieve an aim."[1] Communication problems are consistently identified as a leading cause of medical errors in obstetrics,[11] and the Joint Commission (formerly the Joint Commission on the Accreditation of Health Care Organizations [JCAHO]) has said that the lack of effective communication is the primary cause of sentinel events (a **sentinel event** being "an unexpected occurrence involving death or serious physical or psychological injury, or the risk thereof").[12]

Progress in patient safety has not been as rapid as was once hoped. Leape and Berwick,[13] two pioneers in the field of patient safety, have suggested that the lack of progress after the release of the initial IOM report is due to the "culture of medicine." They believe that this culture is deeply rooted, both by custom and training, in autonomous individual performance.[13] We and others believe that systematic and appropriate use of medical simulation, along with other important changes in our health care system, will facilitate the necessary cultural change and lead to improved patient safety.

Labor and delivery units are not intrinsically safer than other health care environments, and most units still have many opportunities to change systems to optimize patient safety. Further, it has been suggested that the concept of patient safety in obstetrics is "not as strong as desirable for the provision of reliable health care."[14] In many units a punitive culture results in suppression of error reporting, lack of proper communication, and failure of appropriate feedback.[14] Obviously, this culture must change before we can significantly improve patient safety in obstetric practice.

TEAMS AND TEAMWORK

Health care should be considered a team activity. Teams take care of patients. Furthermore, health care teams operate in an environment characterized by heavy workload, acute stress, and high stakes for decision and action errors.[15] Individuals have limited capabilities. When the limitations are combined with organizational and environmental complexity, human error is virtually inevitable.[16] The labor and delivery unit is an exceedingly complex environment. In fact, safe intrapartum obstetric care requires intense, error-free vigilance with effective communication and teamwork among members of various clinical disciplines who, although working together, typically have never trained together. This group consists of obstetricians, midwives, anesthesia providers, nurses, and pediatricians.[17] The addition of trainees at all levels and in all disciplines enhances the potential for error in communication.

A **team** consists of two or more individuals who have specific roles, perform independent tasks, are adaptable, and share common goals. Salas et al.[18] have called **teamwork** a complex yet elegant phenomenon. It can be defined as a "set of interrelated behaviors, actions, cognitions and attitudes that facilitate the required task work that must be completed."[18] Lack of teamwork has been identified as a leading cause of adverse events in medicine. Team behavior and coordination, particularly communication or team information sharing, are critical for optimizing team performance.[19] Baker et al.[20] have stated that to work together effectively, team members must possess specific knowledge, skills, and attitudes (KSAs), including skill in monitoring one another's performance, knowledge of their own and their teammates' task responsibilities, and a positive disposition toward working in a team. These researchers have described characteristics of effective teams as team leadership, mutual performance monitoring, backup behavior, adaptability, shared mental models, communication, team/collective orientation, and mutual trust. Moreover, effective team performance in complex environments requires that team members hold a shared understanding of the task, their equipment, and their teammates.[21] Salas et al.[22] have defined the characteristics of effective teams, as highlighted in Table 11-1.

Teamwork is essential for safe patient care. The IOM has suggested that team training and implementation of team behaviors may improve patient safety.[23] Team training promotes the acquisition of adaptive behaviors, shared cognition, and relevant attitudes. It is an instructional strategy that ideally combines practice-based delivery methods with realistic events, guided by medical teamwork competencies (i.e., behaviors, cognitions, and/or attitudes). In a 2007 editorial, Murray and Enarson[24] stated that "when a crisis complicates patient care, teamwork among health care professionals is frequently strained, resulting in more frequent as well as more serious failures in managing critical events." This scenario occurs all too often on the labor and delivery unit.

TABLE 11-1 Characteristics of Effective Teams

Knowledge/Skills/ Attitudes	Characteristics of the Team
Leadership	Roles are clear but not overly rigid. Team members believe that leaders care about them.
Backup behavior	Members compensate for one another. Members provide feedback to one another.
Mutual performance monitoring	Members understand one another's roles.
Communication adaptability	Members communicate often and anticipate one another.
Mutual trust	Members trust one another's intentions.

Adapted from Salas E, Sims DE, Klein C. Cooperation and teamwork at work. In Spielberger CD, editor. Encyclopedia of Applied Physiology. San Diego, CA, Academic Press, 2004:499-505.

Team Leadership

There is a clear difference between the *leadership of individuals* and *team leadership*. A health care provider who is leading independent individuals will diagnose a problem, generate possible solutions, and implement the most appropriate solution. In contrast, team leadership does not involve autocratic "top-down" communication of solutions to team members but, rather, consists of defining team goals, setting expectations, coordinating activities, organizing team resources, and guiding the team to achieve the team's goals.[25]

Team leaders can improve team performance in many ways (e.g., by promoting coordination and cooperation). These individuals not only must be technically competent but also must be competent in leadership skills.[15] Anesthesiologists and other physicians often are not trained to be competent team leaders. Many of the necessary tasks can and must be learned during team training. Simulation may play a key role in this education. Team leadership training has been developed to successfully teach specific team leader behaviors, and the implementation of these programs has been shown to improve team performance.[18] Hackman[26] described successful team performance as consisting of the following three primary elements:

- Successful accomplishment of the team's goals.
- Satisfaction of team members with the team and commitment to the team's goals.
- The ability of the team to improve different facets of team effectiveness over time.

The Joint Commission has recommended a risk-reduction strategy for decreasing the incidence of perinatal injury and death. This strategy includes the implementation of team training and the performance of mock emergency drills for shoulder dystocia, emergency cesarean delivery, and maternal hemorrhage.[27] Several of the 2008 Joint Commission National Patient Safety Goals relate to error reduction on the labor and delivery unit. Departments of anesthesiology and obstetrics and gynecology should regularly review these goals (Box 11-1).[28] Hospitals are surveyed periodically to verify their compliance with these goals.

High-Reliability Organizations and Teams

Despite the inevitability of human error, some organizations that operate in complex environments are able to maintain an exceptionally safe workplace. These organizations, including the aviation and nuclear power industries, have been termed *high-reliability organizations* (HROs). Hospitals and other health care organizations can and should be HROs. Sundar et al.[29] defined high-reliability organizations as institutions in which individuals, working together in high-acuity situations and facing great potential for error and disastrous consequences, consistently deliver care with positive results and minimal errors. Teams that exhibit behaviors facilitating the characteristics and values held by the HRO may be defined as *high-reliability teams*

BOX 11-1 Key Joint Commission* National Patient Safety Goals

- Improve the accuracy of patient identification:
  - Use at least two patient identifiers when providing care.
  - Before the start of any invasive procedure, conduct a "time-out" to confirm the correct patient, procedure, and site.
- Improve the effectiveness of communication among caregivers:
  - Read-back verbal orders.
  - Standardize a list of abbreviations.
  - Measure, assess, and if appropriate, take action to improve timeliness of reporting and the receipt of critical test results.
  - Implement a standardized approach to hand-off communications.
- Improve the safety of using medications:
  - Standardize and limit the number of drug concentrations.
  - Identify and review a list of look-alike/sound-alike drugs used by the organization.
  - Label all medications.
- Reduce the risk of health care–associated infections:
  - Comply with Centers for Disease Control and Prevention (CDC) hand-hygiene guidelines.
- Accurately and completely reconcile medications across the continuum of care:
  - Implement a process for comparing the patient's current medications with those ordered for the patient.
  - Communicate a complete list of the patient's medications to the next provider.

*Summarized from the Joint Commission. National Patient Safety Goals, 2007 and 2008. Available at http://www.jointcommission.org/PatientSafety/NationalPatientSafetyGoals/07_npsgs_facts.htm/; and http://www.jointcommission.org/PatientSafety/NationalPatientSafetyGoals/08_hap_npsgs.htm

(HRTs). Wilson et al.[16] have defined five guidelines for HRTs, which must:

1. Use closed-loop communication and other forms of information exchange to promote shared situational awareness regarding factors internal and external to the team.
2. Develop shared mental models that allow team members to monitor other members' performance and offer backup assistance when needed.
3. Demonstrate a collective organization that enables members to be assertive, to take advantage of functional expertise, and to seek and value input from other team members.
4. Seek to recognize complexities of their task environment and accordingly develop plans that are adequate and promote flexibility.
5. Use semi-structured feedback mechanisms such as team self-correction to manage, and quickly learn from, errors.

Hunt et al.[30] defined the following characteristics associated with high-performing teams: situational awareness, leadership, followership, closed-loop communication, critical language, standardized practice, assertive communication, adaptive behaviors, and workload management. Salas et al.[31] have described an adaptive team performance framework that illustrates the relationship among variables, emerging states, and the multiple phases of the team adaptation cycle (Figure 11-3).

Cultural factors may play a significant role in team performance. According to Salas et al.,[22] these factors include **attitudes** (especially as they relate to previous experiences with teams) and **motivation**. Although it has been suggested that an individual team member's personality may be counterbalanced by others', Janis[32] concluded that openness, conscientiousness, and neuroticism are essential for individuals to succeed in command positions.

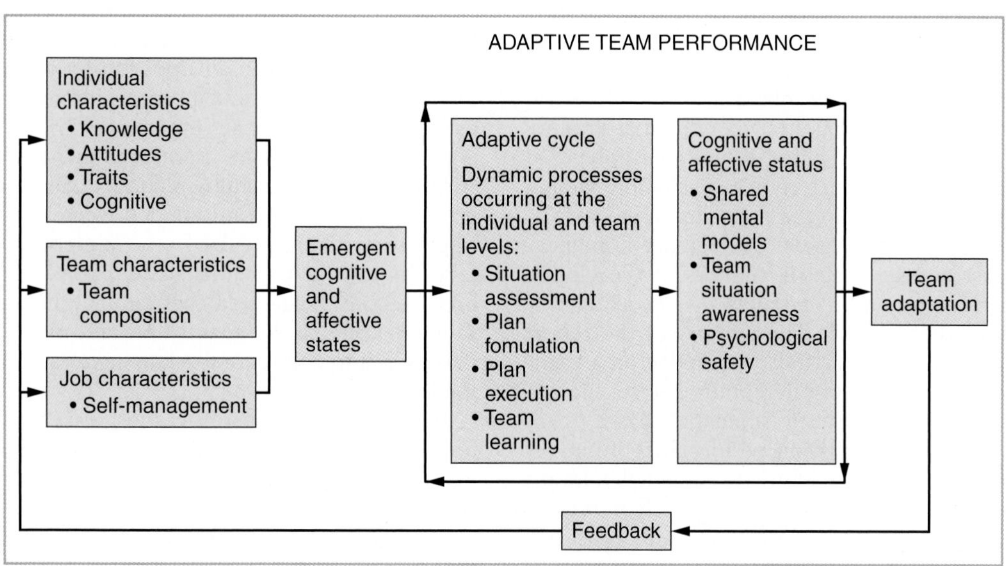

FIGURE 11-3 Adaptive team performance. (Adapted from Salas E, Rosen MA, Burke CS, et al. The making of a dream team: When expert teams do best. In Ericsson KA, Charness N, Feltovich RJ, Hoffman RR, editors. The Cambridge Handbook of Expertise and Expert Performance. Cambridge, UK, Cambridge University Press, 2006:439-56.)

Thomas et al.[33] conducted a qualitative assessment of teamwork and suggested that factors that influence the ability to work together could be divided into three categories: **provider characteristics** (personal attributes, reputation, expertise); **workplace factors** (staffing, work organization, work environment); and **group influences** (communication, relationships, and teamwork). Team members can address categories, at least in part, by working together in teams in a simulated environment that allows evaluation of teamwork and human performance. Lyndon[34] suggested that the application of human performance–based theory has demonstrated that "communication patterns, team function, workload, and coping mechanisms affect both individual and group ability to identify evolving problems and make appropriate management decisions in complex decision-making situations."[34]

Team Training

Patient safety is "predicated on trust, open communication, and effective interdisciplinary teamwork."[35] It is often the *interactions* among health care workers that determine whether a specific plan of care is effective or ineffective.[36] However, in the current environment, attending physicians, midwives, nurses, resident physicians, and medical and nursing students rarely learn or train to work as teams.

The Liaison Committee on Medical Education (LCME), which is jointly composed of members of the American Medical Association and the Association of American Medical Colleges, has affirmed the importance of teaching communications skills and teamwork. For example, LCME standard ED19 states that "there must be specific instruction in communication skills as they relate to professional responsibilities, including communication with patients, families, colleagues, and other health professionals."[37] Teamwork needs to be not only taught but also monitored. Box 11-2 summarizes best practices in team performance measurement in simulation-based training.

Why is teamwork training important for labor and delivery unit personnel? As stated previously, communication problems are consistently identified as a leading cause of medical error, and these problems can be addressed during team training. The 2000-2002 Confidential Enquiry into Maternal Deaths in the United Kingdom emphasized that "emergency drills for maternal resuscitation should be regularly practiced in clinical areas in all maternity units."[38] As an example, a review of competence in managing cardiac arrest among obstetric trainees in the United Kingdom documented a lack of knowledge about airway management and ventilation.[39] The authors of the report suggested that regular short periods of practice on a mannequin are necessary to facilitate retention of resuscitation skills.[39] Furthermore, research in simulation-based team training has shown that simulation performance improves when trainees have an opportunity to practice relevant competencies in a structured scenario and then receive diagnostic feedback on their individual and collective performance. This finding clearly indicates the importance of (1) guided practice of structured scenarios and (2) assessment of performance.

BOX 11-2 Summary of Best Practices in Team Performance Measurement

- Ground measures in theory:
  - Use theory to determine what variables to measure.
  - Capture aspects of **input→process→output** models of team performance.
- Design measures to meet specific learning outcomes.
- Clearly articulate the purpose of measurement.
- Design the measurement system to capture information necessary for making decisions about the learning outcomes.
- Capture competencies.
- Measure multiple levels of performance.
- Link measures to scenario events.
- Focus on observable behaviors.
- Incorporate multiple measures from different sources.
- Capture performance processes in addition to outcomes:
  - Obtain information not only about the end result, but also about how the team reached that performance outcome.
- Train observers and structure observation protocols.
- Facilitate post-training debriefing and training remediation.

Adapted from Rosen MA, Salas E, Wilson KA, et al. Measuring team performance in simulation-based training: Adopting best practices for healthcare. Simulation in Healthcare 2008; 3:33-41.

Simulation-Based Training in Obstetrics

Traditional medical and nursing education has relied on the treatment of real patients in actual clinical settings. Many educators now believe that the current availability of medical simulation and the knowledge gained from the science of team training may improve patient outcomes. Most medical and nursing schools have purchased simulators and are attempting to use them in undergraduate and graduate education.

Many researchers have suggested that drills are useful on the labor and delivery unit. Sorenson[40] stated that "mock emergency training is an opportunity for staff to learn to identify risk factors and prepare for interventions in the event of an obstetric emergency." According to the Agency for Healthcare Research and Quality (AHRQ),[41] "drills that are carefully planned can decrease medical errors by addressing unintended events that may result in injury to a patient arising from unintentional actions, mistakes in judgment, or inadequate plans of action." Gardner and Raemer[42] suggested that simulation is a practical and safe approach to the acquisition and maintenance of task-oriented and behavioral skills across the spectrum of medical specialties.

In the realm of obstetric anesthesia practice, investigators have demonstrated that simulation may be a useful tool for assessment of performance in a simulated emergency situation (e.g., failed intubation) when combined with practice and formal teaching.[43] Use of high-fidelity simulation for training in the management of perinatal emergencies improved the speed with which anesthesia providers responded to those emergencies and improved the quality

BOX 11-3 Advantages of Simulation for Research, Training, and Performance Assessment

- There is no risk to patients.
- Many scenarios can be presented, including uncommon but critical situations in which a rapid response is needed.
- Participants can see the results of their decisions and actions; errors can be allowed to occur and reach their conclusion. (In real life, a more capable clinician would be obligated to intervene.)
- Identical scenarios can be presented to different clinicians or teams.
- The underlying causes of the situation are known.
- With mannequin-based simulators, clinicians can use actual medical equipment, exposing limitations in the human-machine interface.
- With full recreations of actual clinical environments, complete interpersonal interactions with other clinical staff can be explored, and teamwork, leadership, and communication training can be provided.
- Intensive and intrusive recording of the simulation session is feasible, including audiotaping, videotaping, and even physiologic monitoring of participants. There are no issues of patient confidentiality; the recordings can be preserved for research, performance assessment, or accreditation.

Modified from Gaba DM. Anesthesiology as a model for patient safety in health care. BMJ 2000; 320:785-8.

of their care.[44] Johannsson et al.[45] suggested that simulation can be used as an educational tool to assist in transfer of knowledge, application of diagnostic skills, acquisition of surgical skills, emergency drill training, and team training. It is obvious that all of these factors are important components of care on the labor and delivery unit. Box 11-3 outlines the advantages of simulation for research, training, and performance assessment.

When an adverse perinatal outcome associated with an error occurs, it is likely that more than one individual will be involved and blamed.[46] Similarly, when an unexpected injury occurs to a mother or infant, several providers are typically involved, and often there is an issue with the "system" that allowed the error to occur. Obstetricians, midwives, anesthesia providers, pediatricians, labor nurses, and operating room staff all work together as part of this system. Therefore, optimal simulation exercises involve all these key "players" and evaluate not only their behaviors and communication skills but also problems within the system in which they work. Simulation of reality-based scenarios in the labor and delivery unit or operating room allows anesthesia providers, obstetricians, midwives, nurses, and pediatricians to practice their roles and communication skills. Hunt et al.[30] suggested that medical teams require practice in interaction and communication to be effective and efficient.

Simulations of perinatal events range from highly realistic scenarios using high-fidelity human simulators (typically located off-site) to low-tech simulations and drills that can be performed on the labor and delivery unit.[40] Simulated events commonly consist of maternal hemorrhage (antepartum as well as postpartum), failed intubation, failed neuraxial blockade, seizures, cardiac arrest, anaphylaxis, umbilical cord prolapse, and shoulder dystocia. Thompson et al.[47] reported that drills to practice management of eclampsia were successful in the identification of deficiencies in team preparation. These researchers concluded:

> *Repetition of drills in our unit has improved the care of simulated patients with eclampsia. In subsequent drills patient management has followed evidence-based practice, with an enhanced level of efficiency. Staff [are] summoned faster, the resuscitation process is better organized, and drugs are prepared and administered more quickly.*

Similarly, Crofts et al.[48] reported significant improvement in participants' knowledge after multidisciplinary obstetric emergency training.[48]

Simulated scenarios (structured to facilitate desired learning outcomes) can be designed to train nurses, obstetric and anesthesiology resident physicians, and students individually or as teams. Team training, however, should not be reserved for individuals in training; attending physicians may also benefit from participation. These drills not only enable various team members to practice articulating an appropriate plan during a crisis situation but also allow practice in communication among members of the operating room team and provide an opportunity for team members as well as administrators to identify areas that require further attention and improvement.

Maslovitz et al.[49] used simulation to identify five recurrent obstetric management mistakes, which are as follows:

- Delay in transporting a bleeding patient to the operating room.
- Unfamiliarity with prostaglandin administration to treat uterine atony.
- Poor cardiopulmonary resuscitation techniques.
- Inadequate documentation of shoulder dystocia (which is important for the legal defense of these cases).
- Delayed administration of blood products to treat disseminated intravascular coagulation.

The drills advocated for use by labor and delivery staff at the University of Miami Miller School of Medicine/Jackson Memorial Hospital are outlined in Box 11-4.

Simulation-based training must be implemented appropriately if it is to be effective. Salas et al.[5] suggested the following guidelines for appropriate implementation:

1. Understand the training needs and requirements.
2. Embed instructional features (such as performance measurement and feedback) within the simulation.
3. Craft the scenarios on the basis of expected/desired learning outcomes.
4. Create opportunities for assessing and diagnosing individual and/or team performance within the simulation.
5. Guide learning.
6. Focus on the cognitive and psychological fidelity of the simulation.

BOX 11-4 Drills Advocated for Use by Labor and Delivery Staff Undergoing Team Training*

- Profound fetal bradycardia
- Magnesium sulfate overdose
- Shoulder dystocia
- Maternal hemorrhage
- Failed intubation
- Anaphylaxis
- Amniotic fluid embolism
- Severe preeclampsia/eclampsia/HELLP (hemolysis, elevated liver enzymes, low platelet count) syndrome

*Used at the University of Miami Miller School of Medicine/ Jackson Memorial Hospital Center for Patient Safety.

7. Form a partnership between subject matter experts and learning experts.
8. Ensure the effectiveness of the training program.

Simulation exercises may also affect outcome by teaching improved communication to individuals and teams during transfer of a patient's care from one set of caregivers to another (i.e., so-called handovers or hand-offs). A survey from the United Kingdom found that handovers were rarely documented in writing and that 4% of obstetric units reported critical incidents after inadequate handovers in the preceding 12-month period.[50] (Some teaching physicians have questioned the wisdom of the mandatory reduction in resident duty hours by arguing that those reductions result in decreased continuity of care and more frequent hand-offs from one resident physician to another.) Sabir et al.[50] described the use of the SBAR (situation-background-assessment-recommendation) technique and the opportunity to practice sign-offs and handovers during drills.

Team Training in Obstetrics

As noted, teamwork is critical for the delivery of quality health care, especially in complex environments such as the labor and delivery unit. Awad et al.[51] reported that medical team training improved communication in the operating room, as assessed by team members using a validated scoring system. Why initiate team training on the obstetric service? The following case report by Sachs[52] illustrates the need. A healthy 38-year-old woman needed emergency cesarean delivery after a failed instrumental delivery. At surgery, the uterus was found to be ruptured and the fetus was stillborn. After unsuccessful attempts to repair the uterus, the patient underwent a cesarean hysterectomy and required massive transfusion and a 3-week hospital stay. Was anyone at fault? According to the root cause analysis, lack of teamwork on many levels played a significant role in this patient's protracted hospital course. In particular, Sachs[52] reported that communication was poor, and there was a lack of mutual performance cross-monitoring, inadequate conflict resolution, suboptimal situational awareness, and work overload.

CREW RESOURCE MANAGEMENT

Although relatively new to obstetrics, team drills have been used successfully in other areas of medicine, including anesthesia, intensive care, and emergency medicine, often using lessons learned from crew resource management (CRM) training. The human error factors in many aviation disasters are thought to involve failure of communication, decision-making, and leadership.[53] In the airline industry, CRM began as a program to train pilots to reduce error by making better use of human resources in the cockpit.[54] CRM training has led to safety and performance improvements beyond those produced by improvements in equipment and technology.[5,53]

CRM training is just one of many tools used by airlines to reduce human error. Other tools include the use of checklists, standardized maintenance, ability to report errors without fear of punitive retaliation, and use of simulator training. Not all of these tools, however, are easily adaptable to medicine. That said, Helmreich[55] identified several lessons learned from CRM that can be extrapolated to the practice of medicine. Helmreich believes that errors in competence require technical training and that errors in decision-making and communication require team training. Further, Helmreich[55] has suggested that adaptation of CRM to health care also requires the development of nonpunitive methods to collect information on errors so that this information can be used to evaluate and improve team performance. It has been suggested that elements of CRM that are useful in health care settings include briefings, conflict resolution procedures, and performance reviews.[18] Evidence suggests that operator attitudes about teamwork, hierarchy, errors, and stress affect performance among aviators working together in teams.[56] Evidence also suggests that these attitudes are relevant in the health care environment.[57]

Salas et al.[58] suggested that CRM training will not be effective or achieve its desired outcomes in health care without the following 12 prerequisites:

1. The physicians must be "on board."
2. The concept of teamwork becomes part of the "DNA" of the health care professional.
3. CRM is supplemented by other teamwork-focused training strategies.
4. The design, development, and delivery of CRM are scientifically rooted.
5. CRM training is designed systematically.
6. CRM is part of a learning organization's strategy to promote patient safety and quality care.
7. Teamwork is rewarded and reinforced by the health care provider.
8. CRM training is evaluated at multiple levels for specific outcomes.
9. CRM is supported by simulation or practice-based approaches.
10. The health care provider is "ready" to receive training.
11. The patient is part of the team.
12. The team training is recurrent.

Some health care providers benefit more than others from CRM training and learning. For example, one study noted that physicians with poorer performance at the beginning of CRM training showed greater improvement after training.[59]

DISRUPTIVE BEHAVIOR

Although miscommunication is common on the labor and delivery unit, some events are not caused by difficulties with communication but, rather, result from disruptive behavior on the part of one or more members of the team. It is estimated that 3% to 5% of physicians exhibit disruptive behavior.[60] Disruptive and intimidating behavior occurs frequently on labor and delivery units and is observed in personnel of diverse disciplines, including obstetricians, anesthesia providers, family physicians, pediatricians, nurses, midwives, and administrators. In one survey, disruptive behavior was reported on more than 60% of labor and delivery units that responded to a questionnaire.[61]

Disruptive behavior may consist of angry outbursts, rudeness, verbal attacks, physical threats, intimidation, noncompliance with policies, or sexual harassment. Disruptive behavior contributes to the nursing shortage and predisposes to "near misses" and adverse occurrences. This behavior does not always involve physicians. The occurrence of disruptive behavior among nursing staff, termed *horizontal hostility*, includes rudeness, verbal abuse, humiliating statements, unjustly critical statements, withholding of information, and gossip.[62] Disruptive behavior is not always effectively managed by the organization[61] and must be considered when simulation is used to improve team behaviors.

OPTIONS FOR SIMULATOR TRAINING IN OBSTETRICS

Both high-technology and low-technology approaches to simulation have been utilized for training labor and delivery staff.[40] Simulation centers often use high-fidelity simulation with interactive computerized mannequins in a realistic working environment (e.g., labor room or operating room) that contains a full complement of working equipment and staff.[63] The mannequin is quite realistic; it has a pulse, heart and breath sounds, ventilatory movements, and electrocardiogram and pulse oximetry tracings. All vital signs can be adjusted via computer control, as can the ability to intubate or ventilate.[63]

Not all simulation exercises and drills for obstetrics must be performed in high-fidelity simulators. Some authorities[64] have argued that classroom training is a better option, particularly given the high cost[65] and high level of resources necessary for high-fidelity simulation. The inability to arrange for staff of several disciplines to be absent from the labor and delivery unit simultaneously often precludes the use of high-technology simulation and may make on-site exercises more practical.[40]

On the other hand, Gaba[66] has countered that high-fidelity simulation need not be cost-prohibitive and that it provides the required realistic experience necessary for training in the management of complex real-life scenarios. In 2007, Morgan et al.[67] described an obstetric simulation model that allowed participation of trained surgeons (rather than actors playing the role of surgeons). This was the first published report of high-fidelity simulation of obstetric team performance, with obstetricians, anesthesia providers, and nurses involved in the hands-on management of obstetric crises.

Several options are available for teaching teamwork and crisis intervention in obstetrics. Multidisciplinary obstetric simulated emergency scenarios (MOSES), developed by the St. Bartholomew Hospital Group in the United Kingdom,[68] involves participation by obstetricians, anesthesia providers, and midwives in team training using a high-fidelity simulator. MedTeams was developed by the United States Armed Forces and Dynamics Research Corporation; originally employed in emergency departments,[53,69,70] it has now been used for team training in labor and delivery units.[17] The course consists of "train the trainer" sessions that focus on seven dimensions essential to teamwork. Behaviorally anchored rating scales (BARS) are used to assess various key behaviors.[55] A review of the program and the challenges of its implementation was published in 2006.[71]

Other evidence-based programs have emerged. TeamSTEPPS was developed by the U.S. Department of Defense (DOD) and the Agency for Healthcare Research and Quality as a team training and implementation toolkit.[72] The program is based on findings from the science of team performance; it is adaptable, medically relevant, and applicable to training on labor and delivery units.

The 2000-2002 report of the Confidential Enquiry into Maternal Deaths in the United Kingdom[38] recommended the MOET (Managing Obstetric Emergencies and Trauma) course. This 3-day course consists of lectures, skills training, workshops, and resuscitation stations. It is designed for both obstetricians and anesthesia providers and is offered by the Advanced Life Support Group, a registered medical education charity (http://www.alsg.org).

What is the evidence that team training and simulation reduce errors and improve patient safety and clinical outcomes? Morey et al.[53] reported that the MedTeams program reduced errors in the emergency department; they also observed a statistically significant improvement in team behaviors. The clinical error rate in providers who received MedTeams training dropped from 31% to 4%. Evidence suggests that medical simulation and team training improve teamwork and communication and allow recognition of potential areas of weakness in obstetric care. We believe that these are viable strategies to mitigate medical errors. Despite a somewhat short and unproven track record and a paucity of objective findings of improvement in patient safety and outcomes, many other researchers concur that team training is useful in the health care setting.[20,29,73] We agree with Pearlman et al.,[74] who stated:

> *We have the moral imperative as a specialty to fully engage in the identification of our own best practices, to advance safety research in obstetrics and gynecology, and to implement broadly those practices which are best.**

---

*Health care providers who want to learn more about the field of simulation might consider attending the annual meeting of the Society for Simulation in Healthcare. This multidisciplinary society represents a rapidly growing group of clinicians, educators, and researchers who utilize a variety of simulation techniques for education, testing, and research in healthcare (http://www.ssih.org/public/).

KEY POINTS

- Medical errors harm tens of thousands of patients each year.
- Human error is inevitable; therefore systems should be developed to prevent or "catch" errors before the patient is harmed.
- Poor communication among health care workers is the primary cause of sentinel events.
- Teamwork is essential to safe patient care, and team training may improve patient safety.
- Simulation-based training is an educational tool that may improve responses to obstetric emergencies.
- Adaptation of some elements of aviation crew resource management training may improve team performance in health care.
- Disruptive behavior interferes with safe patient care and is observed in physicians as well as other members of the health care team.

REFERENCES

1. Kohn LT, Corrigan JM, Donaldson MS, editors; Committee on Quality of Health Care in America, Institute of Medicine. To Err Is Human: Building a Safer Health Care System. Washington, DC, National Academy Press, 2000. Available at: http://www.nap.edu/catalog/9728.html/
2. Aiken LH, Clarke SP, Sloane DM, et al. Hospital nurse staffing and patient mortality, nurse burnout, and job dissatisfaction. JAMA 2002; 288:1987-93.
3. Landrigan CP, Rothschild JM, Cronin JW, et al. Effect of reducing interns' work hours on serious medical errors in intensive care units. N Engl J Med 2004; 351:1838-48.
4. Gaba DM. Anaesthesiology as a model for patient safety in health care. Br Med J 2000; 320:785-8.
5. Salas E, Wilson KA, Burke CS, Priest HA. Using simulation-based training to improve patient safety: What does it take? Jt Comm J Qual Patient Saf 2005; 31:363-71.
6. Wu AW. Medical error: The second victim. West J Med 2000; 172:358-9.
7. Reason J. Human error: Models and management. Br Med J 2000; 320:768-70.
8. Reason JT. Human Error. Cambridge, UK, Cambridge University Press, 1990.
9. Ong M, Bostrom A, Vidyarthi A, et al. House staff team workload and organization effects on patient outcomes in an academic general internal medicine inpatient service. Arch Intern Med 2007; 167:47-52.
10. American College of Obstetricians and Gynecologists Committee on Quality Improvement and Patient Safety. Patient safety in obstetrics and gynecology. ACOG Committee Opinion No. 286, October 2003. (Int J Gynaecol Obstet 2004; 86:121-3.)
11. Simpson KR, Knox GE. Adverse perinatal outcomes. Recognizing, understanding & preventing common accidents. AWHONN Lifelines 2003; 7:224-35.
12. Root cause of sentinel events. Joint Commission, 2008. Available at: http://www.jointcommission.org/SentinelEvents/Statistics/
13. Leape LL, Berwick DM. Five years after To Err Is Human: What have we learned? JAMA 2005; 293:2384-90.
14. Nabhan A, Ahmed-Tawfik MS. Understanding and attitudes towards patient safety concepts in obstetrics. Int J Gynaecol Obstet 2007; 98:212-6.
15. Salas E, Rosen MA, King H. Managing teams managing crises: Principles of teamwork to improve patient safety in the Emergency Room and beyond. Theoretical Issues in Ergonomics Science 2007; 8:381-94.
16. Wilson KA, Burke CS, Priest HA, Salas E. Promoting health care safety through training high reliability teams. Qual Saf Health Care 2005; 14:303-9.
17. Nielsen PE, Goldman MB, Mann S, et al. Effects of teamwork training on adverse outcomes and process of care in labor and delivery: A randomized controlled trial. Obstet Gynecol 2007; 109:48-55.
18. Salas E, Guthrie J, Wilson-Donnelly K, et al. Modeling team performance: The basic ingredients and research needs. In Rouse WB, Boff KR, editors. Organizational Simulation. Hoboken, NJ, Wiley-InterScience, 2005:185-216.
19. Blum RH, Raemer DB, Carroll JS, et al. A method for measuring the effectiveness of simulation-based team training for improving communication skills. Anesth Analg 2005; 100:1375-80.
20. Baker DP, Day R, Salas E. Teamwork as an essential component of high-reliability organizations. Health Serv Res 2006; 41:1576-98.
21. Salas E, Rosen MA, Burke CS, et al. Markers for enhancing team cognition in complex environments: The power of team performance diagnosis. Aviat Space Environ Med 2007; 78:B77-85.
22. Salas E, Sims D, Klein C. Cooperation and teamwork at work. In Spielberger C, editor. Encyclopedia of Applied Psychology. San Diego, CA, Academic Press, 2004:499-505.
23. Committee on Quality Healthcare in America, Institute of Medicine. Crossing the Quality Chasm: A New Health System for the 21st Century. 2001. Washington, DC, National Academy Press, 2001. Available at: http://www.nap.edu/catalog.php?record_id=10027#toc/
24. Murray D, Enarson C. Communication and teamwork: Essential to learn but difficult to measure (editorial). Anesthesiology 2007; 106:895-6.
25. Salas E, Wilson-Donnelly K, Sims D, et al. Teamwork training for patient safety: Best practices and guiding principles. In Carayon P, editor. Handbook of Human Factors and Ergonomics in Health Care and Patient Safety. Mahwah, NJ, Lawrence Erlbaum Associates, 2007.
26. Hackman JR. Groups that Work (and Those that Don't): Creating Conditions for Effective Teamwork. San Francisco, Jossey-Bass, 1990.
27. The Joint Commission. Preventing Infant Death and Injury during Delivery. Joint Commission, 2004. Sentinel Event Alert Issue #30. Available at: http://www.jointcommission.org/SentinelEvents/SentinelEventAlert/sea_30.htm/
28. Grunebaum A. Error reduction and quality assurance in obstetrics. Clin Perinatol 2007; 34:489-502.
29. Sundar E, Sundar S, Pawlowski J, et al. Crew resource management and team training. Anesthesiol Clin 2007; 25:283-300.
30. Hunt EA, Shilkofski NA, Stavroudis TA, Nelson KL. Simulation: Translation to improved team performance. Anesthesiol Clin 2007; 25:301-19.
31. Salas E, Rosen MA, Burke CS, et al. The making of a dream team: When expert teams do best. In Ericsson K, Charness N, Feltovich P, Hoffman R, editors. The Cambridge Handbook of Expertise and Expert Performance. Cambridge, UK, Cambridge University Press, 2006:439-56.
32. Janis IL. Crucial Decisions: Leadership in Policymaking and Crisis Management. New York, Free Press, 1989.
33. Thomas EJ, Sherwood GD, Mulhollem JL, et al. Working together in the neonatal intensive care unit: Provider perspectives. J Perinatol 2004; 24:552-9.
34. Lyndon A. Communication and teamwork in patient care: How much can we learn from aviation? J Obstet Gynecol Neonatal Nurs 2006; 35:538-46.
35. Simpson KR, James DC, Knox GE. Nurse-physician communication during labor and birth: Implications for patient safety. J Obstet Gynecol Neonatal Nurs 2006; 35:547-56.
36. Rosen M, Salas E, Wilson K, et al. Measuring team performance in simulation-based training: Adopting best practices for healthcare. Simulation in Healthcare 2008; 3:33-41.
37. Liaison Committee on Medical Education. Functions and Structure of a Medical School: Standards for Accreditation of Medical Education Programs Leading to the M.D. Degree. Chicago, LCME, 2007. Available at: http://www.lcme.org/functions2007jun.pdf/
38. Why Mothers Die: 2000-2002. The Sixth Report of the Confidential Enquiry into Maternal Deaths in the United Kingdom, National

Institute of Clinical Excellence. London, CEMACH, 2004. Available at: http://www.cemach.org.uk/Publications/Saving-Mothers-Lives-Report-2000-2002.aspx/

39. Morris S, Stacey M. Resuscitation in pregnancy. Br Med J 2003; 327:1277-9.
40. Sorensen SS. Emergency drills in obstetrics: Reducing risk of perinatal death or permanent injury. JONAS Healthc Law Ethics Regul 2007; 9:9-16.
41. Agency for Healthcare Research and Quality. Guide to Patient Safety Indicators. Washington, DC, AHRQ, 2007. Available from: http://www.qualityindicators.ahrq.gov/psi_download.htm/
42. Gardner R, Raemer DB. Simulation in obstetrics and gynecology. Obstet Gynecol Clin North Am 2008; 35:97-127.
43. Goodwin MW, French GW. Simulation as a training and assessment tool in the management of failed intubation in obstetrics. Int J Obstet Anesth 2001; 10:273-7.
44. Chopra V, Gesink BJ, de Jong J, et al. Does training on an anaesthesia simulator lead to improvement in performance? Br J Anaesth 1994; 73:293-7.
45. Johannsson H, Ayida G, Sadler C. Faking it? Simulation in the training of obstetricians and gynaecologists. Curr Opin Obstet Gynecol 2005; 17:557-61.
46. Furrow B. Medical mistakes: Tiptoeing toward safety. Houst J Health Law Policy 2003; 3:181-217.
47. Thompson S, Neal S, Clark V. Clinical risk management in obstetrics: Eclampsia drills. Br Med J 2004; 328:269-71.
48. Crofts JF, Ellis D, Draycott TJ, et al. Change in knowledge of midwives and obstetricians following obstetric emergency training: A randomised controlled trial of local hospital, simulation centre and teamwork training. Br J Obstet Gynecol 2007; 114:1534-41.
49. Maslovitz S, Barkai G, Lessing JB, et al. Recurrent obstetric management mistakes identified by simulation. Obstet Gynecol 2007; 109:1295-300.
50. Sabir N, Yentis SM, Holdcroft A. A national survey of obstetric anaesthetic handovers. Anaesthesia 2006; 61:376-80.
51. Awad SS, Fagan SP, Bellows C, et al. Bridging the communication gap in the operating room with medical team training. Am J Surg 2005; 190:770-4.
52. Sachs BP. A 38-year-old woman with fetal loss and hysterectomy. JAMA 2005; 294:833-40.
53. Morey JC, Simon R, Jay GD, et al. Error reduction and performance improvement in the emergency department through formal teamwork training: Evaluation results of the MedTeams project. Health Serv Res 2002; 37:1553-81.
54. Helmreich RL, Merritt AC, Wilhelm JA. The evolution of Crew Resource Management training in commercial aviation. Int J Aviat Psychol 1999; 9:19-32.
55. Helmreich RL. On error management: Lessons from aviation. Br Med J 2000; 320:781-5.
56. Bowers C, Jentsch F, Salas E, Braun C. Analyzing communication sequences for team training needs assessment. Human Factors 1998; 40:672-80.
57. Gaba D, Singer S, Sinaiko A, et al. Differences in safety climate between hospital personnel and naval aviators. Human Factors 2003; 45:173-85.
58. Salas E, Wilson K, Murphy CK, Baker D. What crew resource management training will not do for patient safety: unless . . . . J Patient Saf 2007; 3:62-4.
59. Alder J, Christen R, Zemp E, Bitzer J. Communication skills training in obstetrics and gynaecology: Whom should we train? Arch Gynecol Obstet 2007; 276:605-12.
60. Leape LL, Fromson JA. Problem doctors: Is there a system-level solution? Ann Intern Med 2006; 144:107-15.
61. Veltman LL. Disruptive behavior in obstetrics: A hidden threat to patient safety. Am J Obstet Gynecol 2007; 196:587. e1-4.
62. Thomas SP. Horizontal hostility. Am J Nurs 2003; 103:87-91.
63. Blackburn T, Sadler C. The role of human patient simulators in health-care training. Hosp Med 2003; 64:677-81.
64. Pratt S, Sachs B. Point Counterpoint: Team Training: Classroom Training vs. High Fidelity Simulation. Washington, DC, Agency for Healthcare Research and Quality, 2006. Available at: http://www.webmm.ahrq.gov/perspective.aspx?perspectiveID=21/
65. Kurrek MM, Devitt JH. The cost for construction and operation of a simulation centre. Can J Anaesth 1997; 44:1191-5.
66. Gaba DM. Two examples of how to evaluate the impact of new approaches to teaching. Anesthesiology 2002; 96:1-2.
67. Morgan PJ, Pittini R, Regehr G, et al. Evaluating teamwork in a simulated obstetric environment. Anesthesiology 2007; 106:907-15.
68. Freeth D, Ayida G, Berridge EJ, et al. MOSES: Multidisciplinary Obstetric Simulated Emergency Scenarios. J Interprof Care 2006; 20:552-4.
69. Risser DT, Rice MM, Salisbury ML, et al. The potential for improved teamwork to reduce medical errors in the emergency department. The MedTeams Research Consortium. Ann Emerg Med 1999; 34:373-83.
70. Simon R, Salisbury M, Wagner G. MedTeams: Teamwork advances emergency department effectiveness and reduces medical errors. Ambul Outreach 2000; 21-4.
71. Harris KT, Treanor CM, Salisbury ML. Improving patient safety with team coordination: Challenges and strategies of implementation. J Obstet Gynecol Neonatal Nurs 2006; 35:557-66.
72. Alonso A, Baker DP, Holtzman A, et al. Reducing medical error in the Military Health System: How can team training help? Human Resource Management Review 2006; 16:396-415.
73. Grogan EL, Stiles RA, France DJ, et al. The impact of aviation-based teamwork training on the attitudes of health-care professionals. J Am Coll Surg 2004; 199:843-8.
74. Pearlman MD. Patient safety in obstetrics and gynecology: An agenda for the future. Obstet Gynecol 2006; 108:1266-71.

Spinal, Epidural, and Caudal Anesthesia: Anatomy, Physiology, and Technique

Cynthia A. Wong, M.D.
Naveen Nathan, M.D.
David L. Brown, M.D.

Regional anesthesia is used extensively for obstetric patients. Of the estimated 4 million women that give birth in the United States each year, approximately 60% receive regional anesthesia. Of these, the overwhelming majority receive spinal or epidural analgesia or anesthesia. The purpose of this chapter is to review the anatomy, physiology, and techniques relevant to the administration of neuraxial anesthesia in obstetric patients. Technical features represent only one element of the successful use of spinal or epidural anesthesia. Conversely, sound medical judgment is of little benefit if a physician uses inadequate technique.

ANATOMY

Obstetric Pain Pathways

Pain during the first stage of labor results primarily from changes in the lower uterine segment and cervix. Pain is transmitted by visceral afferent nerve fibers that accompany the sympathetic nerves and enter the spinal cord at the T10 to L1 segments. During the late first stage and second stage of labor, pain results from distention of the pelvic floor, vagina, and perineum. Pelvic pain is transmitted by somatic nerve fibers, which enter the spinal cord at the S2 to S4 segments (Figure 12-1).

During cesarean delivery, additional nociceptive pathways are involved in the transmission of pain. Most cesarean deliveries are performed with a horizontal (e.g., Pfannenstiel) skin incision, which involves the infraumbilical T11 to T12 dermatomes. During surgery, stretching of the skin may involve dermatomes two to four levels higher. Intraperitoneal manipulation and dissection involve poorly localized visceral pain pathways. Visceral pain may be transmitted by pathways as high as the celiac plexus. Additional somatic pain impulses may occur as a result of diaphragmatic stimulation, because the intercostal nerves innervate a portion of the peripheral diaphragm.

Anatomic Changes of Pregnancy

The normal anatomic changes of pregnancy affect the use of neuraxial anesthesia techniques. Uterine enlargement and vena caval compression result in engorgement of the epidural veins. Unintentional intravascular cannulation and injection of local anesthetic are more common in pregnant patients than in nonpregnant patients. In addition, the vertebral foraminal veins, which are contiguous with the epidural veins, are enlarged and obstruct one of the pathways for anesthetic egress from the epidural space during administration of epidural anesthesia. The enlarged epidural veins also may displace cerebrospinal fluid (CSF) from the thoracolumbar region of the subarachnoid space, as does the

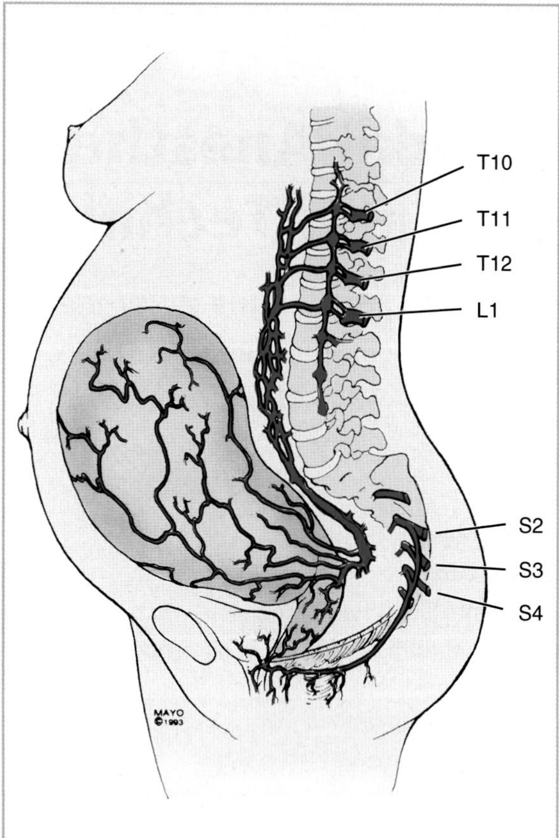

FIGURE 12-1 Pain pathways during labor and delivery. The afferent pain pathways from the cervix and uterus involve nerves that accompany sympathetic fibers and enter the neuraxis at T10 to L1. The pain pathways for the pelvic floor and perineum include the pudendal nerve fibers, which enter the neuraxis at S2 to S4.

greater intra-abdominal pressure of pregnancy; this displacement partly explains the lowered dose requirement for spinal anesthesia in pregnant women.[2] Subarachnoid dose requirements are also affected by the lower specific gravity of CSF in pregnant patients than in nonpregnant patients.[3]

The hormonal changes of pregnancy affect the perivertebral ligamentous structures, including the ligamentum flavum. The ligamentum flavum may feel less dense and "softer" in pregnant women than in nonpregnant patients; thus, feeling the passage of the epidural needle through the ligamentum flavum may be more difficult. It may also be more difficult for a pregnant woman to achieve flexion of the lumbar spine. Progressive accentuation of lumbar lordosis alters the relationship of surface anatomy to the vertebral column (Figure 12-2). At least three changes may occur. First, a pregnant woman's pelvis rotates on the long axis of the spinal column; thus, the line joining the iliac crests assumes a more cephalad relationship to the vertebral column (e.g., this imaginary line might cross the vertebral column at the L3 to L4 interspace rather than the L4 to L5 interspace). Second, there is less space between adjacent lumbar spinous processes during pregnancy. It may be more difficult to use the midline approach to identify the epidural or subarachnoid space in pregnant women. (Thus the often-heard comment, "She has a narrow interspace.") Third, magnetic resonance imaging has shown that the apex of the lumbar lordosis is shifted caudad during pregnancy, and the typical thoracic kyphosis in women is reduced during pregnancy.[4] These changes may influence the spread of intrathecal anesthetic solutions in supine patients (Figure 12-3). Finally, labor pain makes it more difficult for some women to assume and maintain an ideal position while the anesthesia provider performs neuraxial anesthesia.

Vertebral Anatomy

The administration of neuraxial anesthesia requires a complete understanding of the lumbar and sacral vertebral and perivertebral anatomy. Local anesthetics ultimately produce anesthesia through their effects on the spinal cord and nerve roots. The cephalad aspect of the spinal cord is continuous with the brainstem through the foramen magnum. In women of childbearing age, the spinal cord terminates as the conus medullaris at the level of the lower border of the first lumbar vertebral body. The conus medullaris is attached to the coccyx by means of a neural-fibrous band called the *filum terminale*, which is surrounded by the nerves of the lower lumbar and sacral roots, known as the

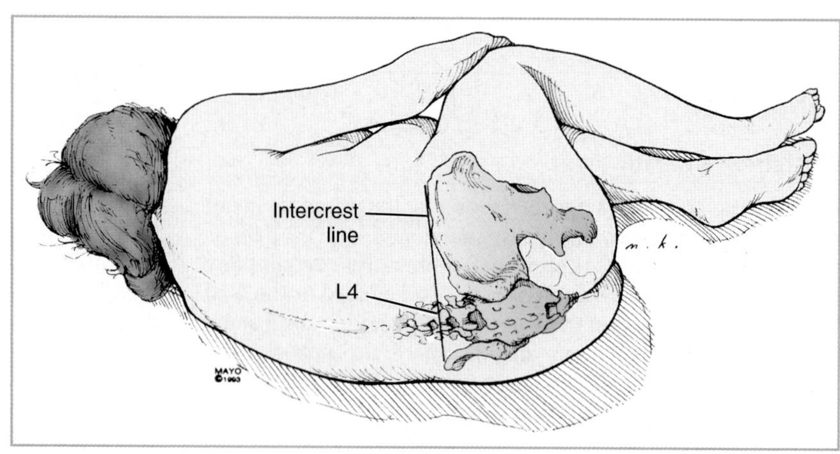

FIGURE 12-2 The surface anatomy used to estimate the lumbar vertebral level. In pregnant women, the interiliac crest line (Tuffier's line) may be slightly higher in relation to the lumbar vertebral axis because of the difficulty in flexing the lumbar spine.

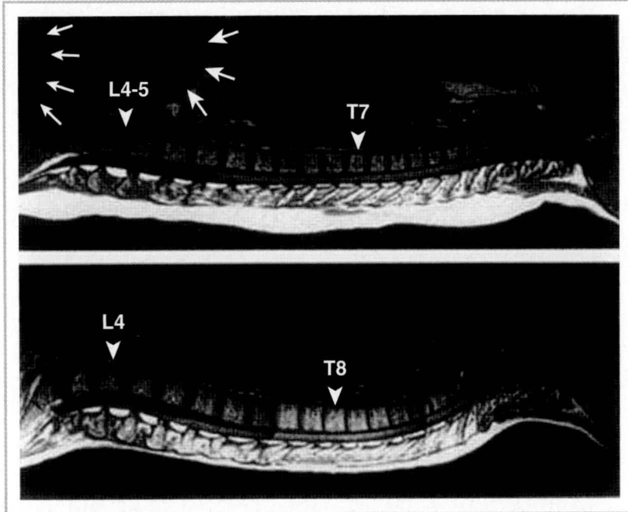

FIGURE 12-3 The curvature of the spinal column in the pregnant female (*top*) and nonpregnant female (*bottom*). The large and small *white arrows* indicate the uterus and fetal head, respectively. The apex of the lumbar lordosis moves caudad (*triangular arrow*), and the thoracic kyphosis is reduced and moves cephalad (*triangular arrow*) in the pregnant woman. (Reprinted with permission from Hirabayashi Y, Shimizu R, Fukuha H. Anatomical configuration of the spinal column in the supine position. II. Comparison of pregnant and non-pregnant women. Br J Anaesth 1995; 75:6-8.)

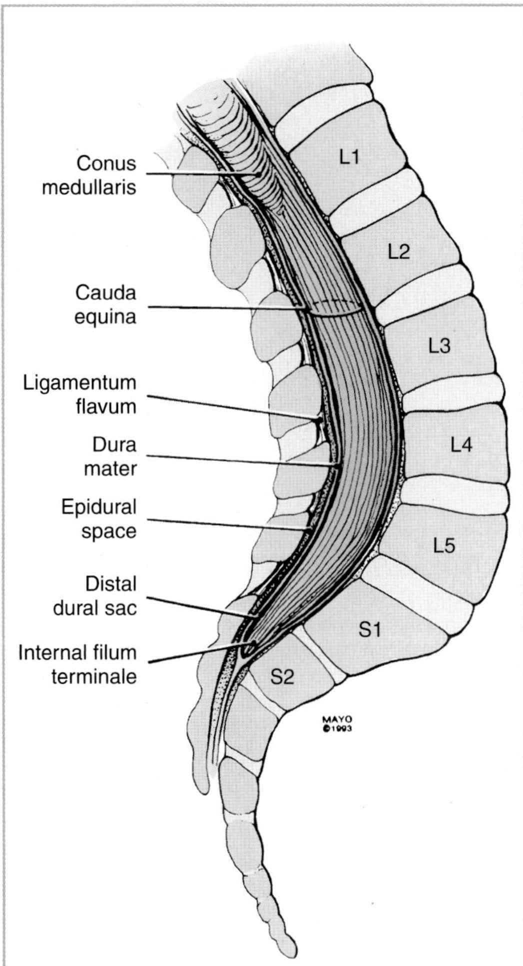

FIGURE 12-4 Distal centroneuraxis anatomy. In pregnant women, the spinal cord ends at the lower border of the first lumbar vertebral body. The subarachnoid space continues to the second sacral vertebral level.

cauda equina (Figure 12-4). Within the bony vertebral column are three membranes: the pia mater, the arachnoid mater, and the dura mater. The pia mater is a highly vascular membrane that closely invests the spinal cord and distally forms the filum terminale. The arachnoid mater is a delicate nonvascular membrane closely attached to the third and outermost layer, the dura. The subarachnoid space, located between the pia mater and arachnoid mater, contains (1) cerebrospinal fluid (CSF), (2) spinal nerves, (3) a trabecular network between the two membranes, (4) blood vessels that supply the spinal cord, and (5) lateral extensions of the pia mater—the dentate ligaments (these ligaments supply lateral support from the spinal cord to the dura mater). Although the spinal cord ends at the level of the bodies of L1 and L2 in most patients,[5] the subarachnoid space continues to the S2 level. At the end of the spinal cord, the cauda equina begins and continues to the level of S2.

The outermost membrane in the spinal canal is a longitudinally organized fibroelastic membrane called the *dura mater*. This layer is a direct extension of the cranial dura mater and extends from the foramen magnum to S2, where the filum terminale blends with the periosteum of the coccyx. A potential space (i.e., the subdural space) exists between the dura and the arachnoid mater. The dural border cells have lower collagen content and few cell junctions, allowing for easy shearing after needle penetration and fluid injection.[6] This "space" is not used intentionally by anesthesia providers. Unintentional subdural injection may explain some cases of failed spinal anesthesia; it may also explain the rare, slow-to-develop cases of high spinal anesthesia after the negative epidural test dose result and injection of additional local anesthetic.

Immediately external to the dura mater is the epidural space, which extends from the foramen magnum to the sacral hiatus. The posterior longitudinal ligaments form the anterior boundary of this space. The pedicles and intervertebral foramina form the lateral boundaries, and the ligamentum flavum forms the posterior boundary. The contents of the epidural space include nerve roots, fat, areolar tissue, lymphatics, and blood vessels, including the well-organized venous plexus of Batson. The epidural space is segmented and discontinuous; it is not the uniform cylindrical space many writers have described. As shown in Figure 12-5, the shape and contents of the epidural space vary with the level of cross section.[7]

Epiduroscopy and epidurography suggest the presence of a dorsal median connective tissue band in some individuals. Anatomic dissection and computerized tomographic epidurography have also suggested the presence of epidural space septa. This band (or these septa) may provide an explanation for unilateral or incomplete epidural anesthesia.[8] However, some investigators have suggested that the dorsal median band is an artifact of epidural space distention or an anatomic manifestation of the previously unappreciated epidural space segmentation.[9]

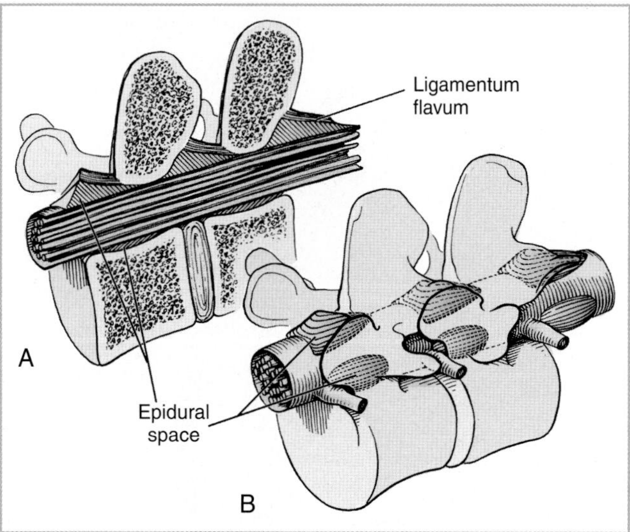

FIGURE 12-5 A, Sagittal section of the epidural space demonstrates that the contents of the epidural space depend on the level of the section. B, Three-dimensional drawing of the epidural space shows the discontinuity of the epidural contents. However, this potential space can be dilated by the injection of fluid into the epidural space. (Redrawn from the Mayo Foundation. From Stevens RA. Neuraxial blocks. In Brown DL, editor. Regional Anesthesia and Analgesia. Philadelphia, WB Saunders, 1976:323.)

The ligamentum flavum lies posterior to the epidural space. Historically some physicians have described the ligamentum flavum as a single ligament. In actuality, however, it is composed of two curvilinear ligaments that join in the middle and form an acute angle with a ventral opening (Figure 12-6).[9,10] The ligamentum flavum is not uniform from skull to sacrum; indeed, it is not uniform even within a single intervertebral space. The thickness of the

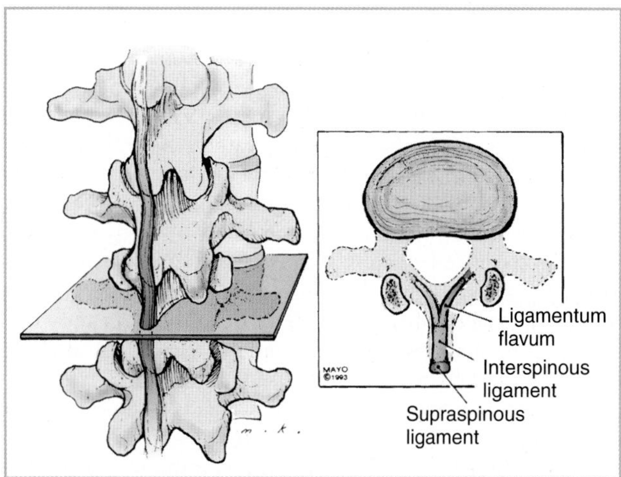

FIGURE 12-6 A horizontal section of the ligamentum flavum and associated neuraxis structures is shown next to an oblique parasagittal section of the lumbar vertebral neuraxis. The horizontal section illustrates the posterior ligamentous structures of the spinal column. The ligamentum flavum is composed of two leaves that meet in the midline at 90 degrees. The interspinous and supraspinous ligaments lie external to the posterior portion of the ligamentum flavum.

TABLE 12-1 Distance from the Skin to the Epidural Space in 1000 Parturients

Lumbar Interspace	Distance (cm) Median	5th Percentile	95th Percentile
L1-2	4.23	3.12	6.33
L2-3	4.86	3.29	7.32
L3-4	4.93	3.57	7.44
L4-5	4.78	3.25	6.75

From Harrison GR, Clowes NWB. The depth of the lumbar epidural space from the skin. Anaesthesia 1985; 40:685-7.

ligamentum flavum varies with vertebral level and position,[11] as does the distance between the skin and the epidural space (Table 12-1).[12,13] Hormonal changes may cause the ligamentum flavum to feel "softer" in pregnant women than in nonpregnant patients.

The lamina, the spinous processes of the vertebral bodies, and the interspinous ligaments lie posterior to the ligamentum flavum. Posterior to these structures are the supraspinous ligament (which extends from the external occipital protuberance to the coccyx), subcutaneous tissue, and skin (Figure 12-7).

Successful administration of caudal epidural anesthesia is complicated by widespread variations in sacral anatomy. Developmentally, the five sacral vertebrae fuse to form the sacrum. The sacral hiatus results from the failure of the laminae of S5, and usually part of S4, to fuse in the midline. The sacral hiatus is covered posteriorly by the posterior sacrococcygeal ligament, which is the functional counterpart to the ligamentum flavum. The shape of the bony defect varies from a narrow, slit-like opening to a wide-based, inverted "V." The sacral hiatus is absent in approximately 5% of all adult patients, and such an absence precludes the administration of caudal anesthesia.[14] The sacral hiatus is less likely to be absent in obstetric patients

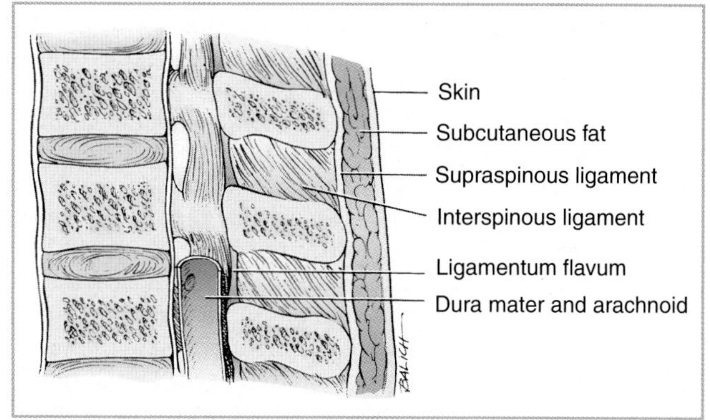

FIGURE 12-7 Midline sagittal anatomy of the vertebral column. When a needle is placed into the cerebrospinal fluid, it must pass through skin, subcutaneous fat, the supraspinous ligament, the interspinous ligament, the ligamentum flavum, the epidural space, and finally the dura mater and arachnoid.

than in older patients, because ossification of this opening seems to increase with age.

The interior of the sacrum contains the sacral canal, which in turn contains the terminal portion of the dural sac. The dural sac terminates cephalad to a line joining the posterior superior iliac spines at the level of the second sacral segment. The sacral canal also contains a venous plexus, which is part of the valveless internal vertebral venous plexus.

PHYSIOLOGY

Safe, successful administration of neuraxial anesthesia in pregnant women requires an understanding of the normal physiologic changes of pregnancy (see Chapter 2). Anesthesia providers, obstetricians, and nurses must appreciate the potential for aortocaval compression during spinal and epidural anesthesia. Only 10% of unanesthetized pregnant women manifest clinical evidence of the supine hypotension syndrome.[15,16] However, the sympathectomy and vasodilation that accompany neuraxial anesthesia cause women to be more susceptible to the effects of aortocaval compression. These undesirable hemodynamic changes can be mitigated by avoidance of aortocaval compression, particularly during the maintenance of spinal or epidural analgesia or anesthesia. Physicians and nurses should maintain left uterine displacement during labor or when performing a vaginal examination or placing a fetal scalp electrocardiogram (ECG) electrode or urethral catheter.

The greater oxygen consumption and diminished functional residual capacity associated with pregnancy result in a faster onset of hypoxemia during maternal apnea. Aortocaval compression hastens the onset of cardiovascular collapse during high/total spinal anesthesia, and resuscitation is more difficult. Anesthesia providers should administer spinal or epidural anesthesia only in a physical setting in which complications, such as unintentional intravenous or subarachnoid injection of local anesthetic, can be rapidly and efficiently managed. In cases of cardiovascular collapse, endotracheal intubation may be necessary to facilitate mechanical ventilation and oxygenation and to protect the lungs from aspiration of gastric contents. Equipment and supplies necessary for laryngoscopy, intubation, and mechanical ventilation should be immediately available.

Physiology of Neural Blockade

Hormonal changes, anatomic changes, and decreases in CSF specific gravity likely are responsible for the lower local anesthetic dose requirements during spinal anesthesia in pregnant women.[3,17] Local anesthetics produce conduction blockade primarily by blocking sodium channels in nerve membranes, thereby preventing the propagation of neural impulses. Differential blockade is manifested as differences in the extent of cephalad blockade of temperature discrimination and vasomotor tone, sensory loss to pinprick, sensory loss to touch, and motor function.[18] Temperature discrimination and vasomotor tone are blocked to the greatest extent (i.e., most cephalad level), and motor function to the least extent. During spinal anesthesia, local anesthetics act directly on neural tissue in the subarachnoid space. Regression of anesthesia can be explained by the simple vascular uptake of local anesthetic from the subarachnoid space and spinal cord.[19]

Epidural anesthesia has a much smaller zone of differential motor-sensory-sympathetic blockade; this difference suggests that the mechanism of epidural anesthesia must involve more than simple diffusion across the dura. For many years, nerve fiber size was presumed to be the primary determinant of susceptibility to local anesthetic blockade (i.e., smaller fibers are blocked more readily than larger fibers). However, later studies have shown that the length of nerve fiber exposed to local anesthetic is as important as the size of the nerve fiber. Fink[18] hypothesized that the length of nerve fiber exposed to local anesthetic affects the extent of the differential zone of motor and sensory blockade. With spinal anesthesia, the local anesthetic concentration required to block sufficient sodium channels to affect motor, sensory, and sympathetic function is less than that needed for the better-protected nerves found in the epidural space; thus, a wider band of differential blockade occurs during spinal anesthesia than during epidural anesthesia.

The understanding of the mechanisms of spinal and epidural anesthesia likely remains oversimplified. Nonetheless, it seems clear that spinal anesthesia results primarily from the effects of local anesthetic on the spinal cord, whereas epidural anesthesia results from the effects of local anesthetic on nerve tissue within both the epidural and subarachnoid spaces.

TECHNIQUE

Contraindications for neuraxial techniques include the following: (1) patient refusal or inability to cooperate; (2) increased intracranial pressure as a result of a mass lesion, which may predispose the patient to brainstem herniation after dural puncture; (3) skin or soft tissue infection at the site of needle puncture; (4) frank coagulopathy; (5) uncorrected maternal hypovolemia; and (6) inadequate training or experience in the technique. Whether mild or isolated abnormalities in tests of blood coagulation preclude the use of regional anesthesia is controversial. However, it is clear that the prophylactic administration of low-molecular-weight heparin is a clinical risk factor that mandates caution in the administration of neuraxial anesthesia.[20] The anesthesia provider should weigh the risks and benefits of neuraxial anesthesia for each patient.

Patient Position

Pregnant women have an exaggerated lumbar lordosis, and it is more difficult for them to flex the lumbar spine. However, most pregnant women are young, and youth usually allows sufficient flexibility to facilitate the insertion of a needle into the epidural or subarachnoid space. Whether the block is initiated in the lateral or sitting position is a matter of provider and patient preference. Most obstetric patients may assume the lateral decubitus position comfortably during the administration of spinal or epidural anesthesia; this position likely has less adverse effect on venous return and cardiac output than the sitting position and may allow easier fetal monitoring. Vincent and Chestnut[21] performed a study in which they observed that neither the sitting nor the lateral position was consistently superior with regard to patient comfort. However, pregnant women who preferred the left lateral decubitus position weighed less and had lower body mass indices than women who preferred the sitting position.

An assistant should be present to help the patient and monitor the fetus. If possible, the fetus should be monitored during, or at a minimum, immediately after all procedures. Equipment and drugs should be easily at hand and checked in advance of the procedure. Meticulous sterile technique includes thorough hand washing and the donning of a hat, mask, and sterile gloves by the anesthesia provider; the application of a skin disinfectant over a wide area of the lower back; and the use of a sterile barrier or drape. The donning of a sterile gown by the anesthesia provider is controversial.

When spinal or epidural anesthesia is performed with the patient in a lateral position, the patient's back should lie at, and parallel to, the edge of the bed, for at least two reasons. First, the edge is the most firm section of the mattress. If the patient lies away from the edge of the bed, the patient's weight will depress the mattress, and the anesthesia provider must work in a "downhill" direction. Second, this position allows anesthesia providers to keep their elbows flexed, facilitating control of fine hand and wrist muscle movements. The plane of the entire back should be perpendicular to the mattress. When asked to flex the lower back, patients typically roll the top shoulder forward, an action that rotates the spine (which is undesirable) but does not flex the lower back.

Similarly, patients positioned sitting should have their feet supported by a stool with the backs of their knees against the edge of the bed, a maneuver that helps position the patient's back closer to the anesthesia provider. The shoulders should be relaxed symmetrically over the hips and buttocks. Beds in obstetric units often break at the foot, and the split in the mattress encourages the patient's seat to slope downhill if she is straddling the mattress split; this position will cause spine rotation and may make the procedure more difficult.

The sitting position is likely associated with a higher incidence of orthostatic hypotension and syncope. However, the sitting position is preferred—and may be required—in obese parturients, in whom identification of the midline is significantly easier with the sitting position. Further, morbidly obese women may experience hypoxemia when placed in the lateral decubitus position. One study demonstrated a greater reduction in maternal cardiac output with maximal lumbar flexion in the lateral decubitus position than in the sitting position during identification of the epidural space.[22] The investigators in this study speculated that maximal lumbar flexion in the lateral decubitus position results in concealed aortocaval compression.

When spinal anesthesia is performed, the patient's posture relative to anesthetic baricity should be considered, as it influences the extent of blockade, the latency of blockade, and the incidence of hypotension. The incidence, timing, and extent of hypotension in the period immediately after initiation of the block depend on the type of block (i.e., spinal, epidural, or combined spinal-epidural), drug characteristics (e.g., baricity, concentration), patient position during the procedure, and patient position in the period following the procedure. For example, when spinal anesthesia is initiated with a hyperbaric solution for instrumental vaginal delivery, it often makes sense for the patient to be sitting to ensure the rapid onset of sacral anesthesia. Conversely, spinal anesthesia for cervical cerclage can be initiated in the steep lateral Trendelenburg position with a hypobaric anesthetic solution.

Posture has less influence on the spread of epidural anesthesia.[23-25] During epidural anesthesia, a unilateral block more likely results from the malposition of the catheter (or perhaps an anatomic barrier within the epidural space) than from patient position, particularly after a bolus injection. Norris et al.[25] observed that gravity did not augment the spread of anesthesia in patients receiving epidural anesthesia for cesarean delivery, and they concluded that posture does not need to be manipulated to ensure adequate bilateral epidural anesthesia. At least two studies have noted that the use of the sitting position is not necessary for the development of good sacral anesthesia when large volumes of epidural local anesthetic are given for cesarean delivery.[24,25] However, Reid and Thorburn[24] observed that use of the sitting position appeared to delay the spread of anesthesia to the midthoracic dermatomes. In comparison with the bolus administration of epidural local anesthetic, the extent of blockade may be more gravity dependent when the anesthetic is administered as a continuous infusion over a prolonged period.

Caudal anesthesia is used infrequently in modern obstetric anesthesia practice. However, there remain some circumstances in which a caudal technique is useful and/or advantageous. It is a good choice for the second stage of labor in selected patients in whom the lumbar epidural approach is hazardous or contraindicated (e.g., fusion or instrumentation of the lumbar spine). In most cases, caudal anesthesia can be successfully performed with the patient in a lateral decubitus position. Anatomic variation may require use of the knee-chest position in some patients.

ULTRASONOGRAPHIC GUIDANCE

Traditionally, surface anatomy visualization and palpation have been used to assess landmarks prior to initiation of the neuraxial procedure. Anesthesia providers are now beginning to use ultrasonography as a tool to help assess neuraxial anatomy. The use of ultrasonography has been shown to decrease both the number of attempts and the number of bony contacts.[26] In children, ultrasonography was shown to aid in verification of both local anesthetic spread and catheter placement.[27] Color Doppler has also been used to assess epidural vascularity in parturients,[28] and the skin–epidural space distance can be estimated.[26,29] Unlike for vascular access and peripheral nerve block techniques, ultrasonography for neuraxial techniques is not utilized in real time. Rather, it is a preprocedural tool to aid the operator in the assessment of needle insertion site, needle angle, and estimated depth of the epidural space.

A low-frequency (2- to 5-Hz) curvilinear probe allows visualization of neuraxial structures beneath the skin. The ultrasound beam can be used to identify first the spinous processes if these are not palpable, then the interspinous spaces, and finally, ligamentous structures. The ligamentum flavum and dura mater are dense tissues and will appear hyperechoic, like bone, whereas the less dense epidural and subarachnoid spaces will appear hypoechoic (Figure 12-8). Transverse and median longitudinal as well as paramedian longitudinal approaches have been documented. With the median longitudinal approach, the spinous process will produce a shadow

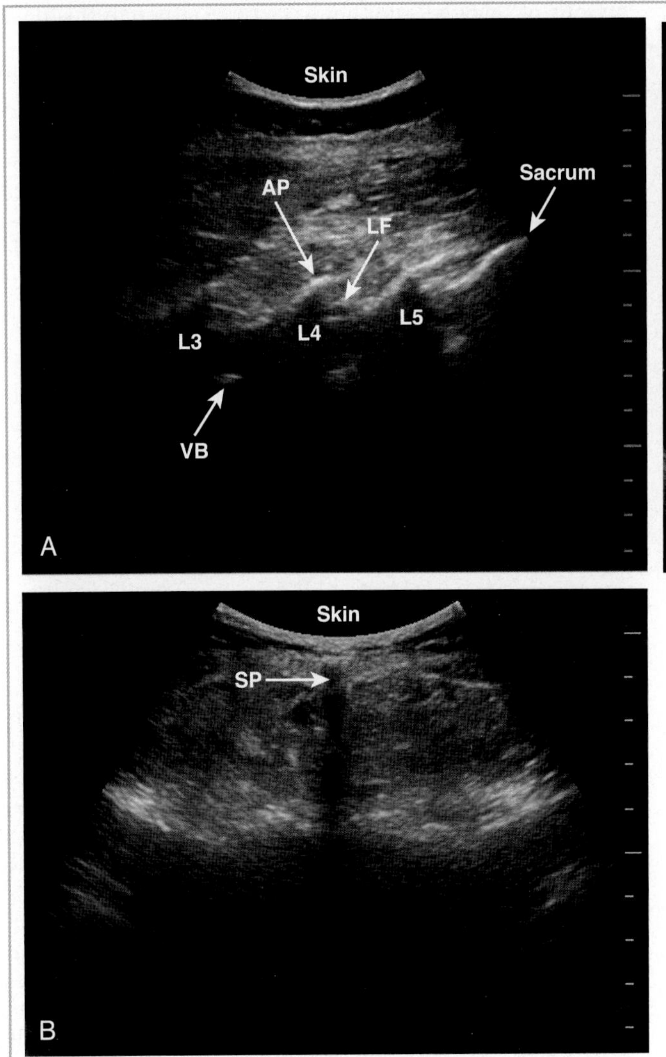

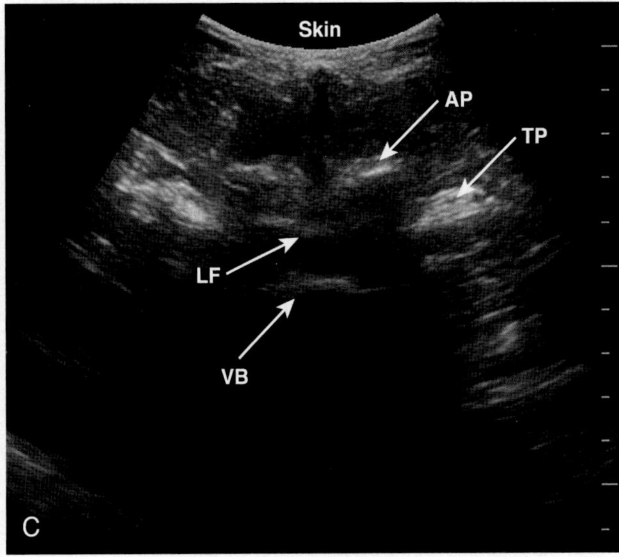

FIGURE 12-8 Ultrasonographic images of the lumbar spine obtained with use of a low-frequency curvilinear probe. **A,** Paramedian longitudinal plane. The typical "saw sign" is seen. The skin is at the top of the image. AP, articular process; LF, ligamentum flavum; VB, vertebral body. **B,** Transverse plane. The spinous process (SP) is seen as a hyperechoic signal immediately beneath the skin (top of image), generating a long vertical acoustic shadow. **C,** Transverse plane. The elements of the interspace include midline structures such as the ligamentum flavum and the vertebral body, and paramedian structures such as the transverse process (TP) and the articular process on each side. (Images courtesy of Jose Carvalho, M.D.)

when the beam is placed directly over it, thus reducing the ability to appreciate any ligaments beyond it.

Choice of Drug*

SPINAL ANESTHESIA

Anesthesia providers may give spinal anesthesia for cerclage, nonobstetric surgery during pregnancy, instrumental vaginal delivery, cesarean delivery, removal of a retained placenta, or postpartum tubal ligation. Spinal analgesia may be used for labor analgesia. Cesarean delivery represents the most common indication for spinal anesthesia in pregnant women. Most anesthesia providers administer a hyperbaric solution of local anesthetic for spinal anesthesia in obstetric patients. Use of a hyperbaric solution results in a faster onset of block and a higher maximum sensory level with a shorter duration of blockade.[30] The urgency and anticipated duration of surgery dictate the choice of local anesthetic agent. The most common choice in the United States is bupivacaine. Other agents include lidocaine and tetracaine. Ropivacaine and levobupivacaine may be used but are not approved for spinal administration in the United States, and levobupivacaine is not available in the United States. Lidocaine provides a short to intermediate duration of action. Bupivacaine, tetracaine, levobupivacaine, and ropivacaine provide intermediate to long durations of action.

Anesthesia providers often add an opioid to the local anesthetic to improve the quality of anesthesia, particularly with regard to visceral stimulation, and to provide postoperative analgesia.[31,32] The addition of an opioid to the local anesthetic decreases the incidence of intraoperative nausea and vomiting.[31] The short-acting, lipid-soluble opioids (i.e., fentanyl, sufentanil) contribute to intraoperative anesthesia, and morphine is often administered for postoperative analgesia. Epinephrine may be added to prolong block duration and perhaps improve block density. It was hoped that other adjuncts (e.g., clonidine, neostigmine) might allow for the administration of a lower dose of local anesthetic and thereby minimize sympatholytic side effects and hasten recovery. Side effects from these other adjuncts, however, have precluded their wide use in obstetric anesthesia practice (see Chapters 26 and 28).

EPIDURAL ANESTHESIA

Local anesthetic agents available for epidural administration in obstetric patients include 2-chloroprocaine, lidocaine,

*Chapter 13 contains a detailed discussion of anesthetic agents used for neuraxial anesthetic techniques.

mepivacaine, bupivacaine, ropivacaine, and etidocaine. Mepivacaine and etidocaine are used infrequently in obstetric anesthesia practice.

Bupivacaine remains the most popular local anesthetic for analgesia during labor and vaginal delivery because of its differential sensory blockade, long duration of action, low frequency of tachyphylaxis, and low cost. Anesthesia providers infrequently administer bupivacaine for cesarean delivery because of the risk of cardiac toxicity and maternal mortality after unintentional intravascular injection of the drug.

Ropivacaine has gained popularity as an agent for epidural analgesia and anesthesia because it may result in less cardiac toxicity and greater differential sensory blockade than bupivacaine.[33] **Levobupivacaine,** although not available in the United States, also has a more favorable safety profile than bupivacaine. Clinical trials have shown that ropivacaine and levobupivacaine have potency[34] and analgesic qualities similar to those of bupivacaine,[35,36] with the probable exception of less motor nerve block.[35,37]

Bupivacaine, ropivacaine, and levobupivacaine all have longer durations of action than lidocaine, and they may be preferred over shorter-acting agents when longer duration of anesthesia or analgesia is desirable. They are more commonly used for maintenance of epidural labor analgesia, whereas the shorter-acting agents are used for epidural surgical anesthesia. Despite some variation among reports, published clinical studies suggest no more than slight differences in onset and potency, and no differences in quality or duration of neural blockade, among the three drugs. However, bupivacaine is more cardiotoxic than the other agents *in vitro* and probably after unintentional intravascular administration.[38] It would seem prudent to use ropivacaine or levobupivacaine rather than bupivacaine when a bolus dose of a concentrated solution is being given. When administered as a low concentration infusion, improved safety has not been demonstrated with ropivacaine and levobupivacaine compared with bupivacaine.

The most popular choice of local anesthetic for epidural anesthesia for cesarean delivery is **2% lidocaine with epinephrine.** The addition of epinephrine (5 μg/mL) causes a modest prolongation of the block. The major advantage of epinephrine is that it improves the quality of epidural lidocaine anesthesia. Lam et al.[39] have shown that epidural labor analgesia can be extended to surgical anesthesia for cesarean delivery in 5.2 ± 1.5 minutes with the addition of bicarbonate and fentanyl to 2% lidocaine with epinephrine.

Many anesthesia providers reserve **2-chloroprocaine** for cases in which rapid extension of epidural anesthesia for vaginal delivery or urgent cesarean delivery is necessary. The onset of surgical anesthesia was several minutes faster with 2-chloroprocaine compared with lidocaine with freshly mixed epinephrine and sodium bicarbonate in the setting of urgent casarean delivery after epidural labor analgesia.[40] Therefore, when time is of the essence, 2-chloroprocaine is the drug of choice. Typically, in an emergency, a large volume of concentrated local anesthetic solution is injected quickly. An additional advantage of 2-chloroprocaine in this situation is that it is rapidly metabolized by plasma esterases. Therefore, the unintentional intravascular injection of a large volume of 2-chloroprocaine may be less likely to have serious adverse consequences. A potential disadvantage of 2-chloroprocaine is that it may interfere with the subsequent actions of opioids[41] and bupivacaine,[42] although this possibility is controversial.[43]

As in spinal anesthesia, epidural opioids work synergistically with local anesthetics. Fentanyl 50 to 100 μg or sufentanil 5 to 10 μg is frequently added to an amide local anesthetic for both labor analgesia (allowing a lower dose of local anesthetic and less motor block) and cesarean delivery (resulting in a denser block with better blockade of visceral stimulation). **Sodium bicarbonate** may be added to lidocaine[44] and 2-chloroprocaine[45] (1 mEq/10 mL local anesthetic) to decrease latency.

CAUDAL ANESTHESIA

The drugs used for caudal epidural anesthesia are identical to those used for lumbar epidural block. However, a much larger volume (e.g., 25 to 35 mL) of local anesthetic solution must be administered to extend a caudal block for cesarean delivery or labor analgesia. Such large volumes entail a greater risk of systemic local anesthetic toxicity.

Equipment and Needle and Catheter Placement

SPINAL ANESTHESIA

The first equipment decision involves determining whether to perform a single-shot or continuous technique. Continuous spinal anesthesia is not a new technique; indeed, some physicians gave continuous spinal anesthesia 50 years ago. Currently, a large-bore epidural needle and catheter must be used for continuous spinal anesthesia, because the U.S. Food and Drug Administration rescinded approval for the use of small-bore catheters in 1992.[46] Therefore, the risk of post–dural puncture headache is significant. This technique is useful after unintentional dural puncture with an epidural needle. In the morbidly obese patient, it may be easier to manipulate and advance a rigid epidural needle than a more flexible spinal needle; thus, the technique is useful for establishing continuous analgesia or anesthesia in this patient population, particularly when the need for anesthesia is urgent. However, for most obstetric patients, a single-shot technique is preferred for spinal anesthesia.

The primary equipment choice for spinal anesthesia concerns the type and size of the spinal needle. Cutting-bevel needles (e.g., Quincke) are rarely used in obstetric anesthesia practice today because of the unacceptably high incidence of post–dural puncture headache associated with their use.[47] Instead, non-cutting needles (e.g., Whitacre, Sprotte, Greene) are used almost exclusively (Figure 12-9). Some anesthesia providers refer to the Whitacre and Sprotte needles as "pencil-point needles." It is now believed that the pencil-point needles cause more trauma to the dura, which then results in a more intense inflammatory response than occurs with cutting-bevel needles. Presumably, the inflammation results in edematous closure of the dural defect.[48]

Needle size must also be determined. In general, the "ease-of-use" advantages associated with larger needles must be balanced against a lower incidence of post–dural puncture headache with smaller needles. For most anesthesia providers, the two curves cross at the use of a 25-gauge needle (i.e., with smaller needles, the technical difficulties increase enough to offset the small reduction in the incidence of post–dural puncture headache). However, anesthesia providers should make individual decisions based on

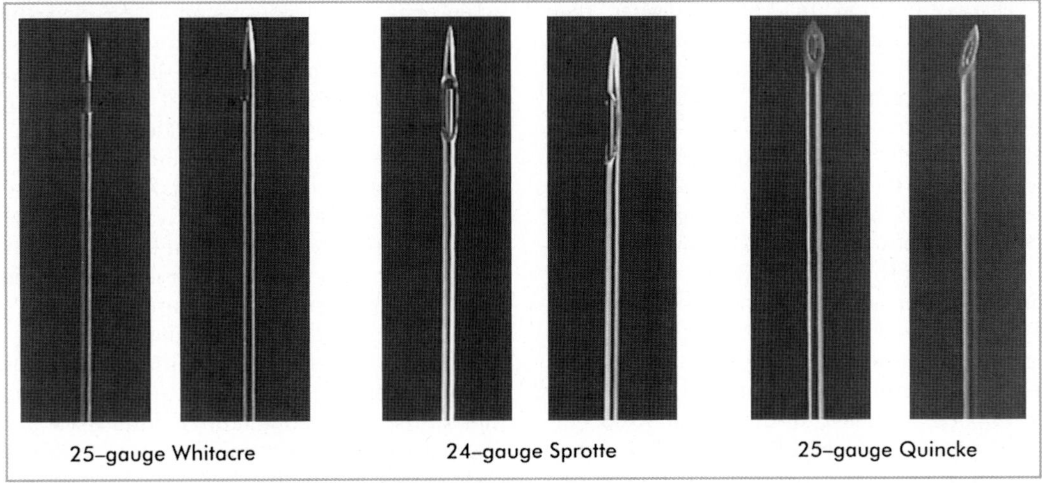

FIGURE 12-9 Spinal needle assortment often used in parturients. Each needle is shown in an open-bevel view and an oblique orientation. The Whitacre and Sprotte needles have cone-shaped bevels, whereas the Quincke has a cutting bevel. (Other sizes are available in some of these needle designs.)

their own skills, practice setting, and patient. The urgency of the procedure may also influence the choice of needle size. For example, a 27-gauge needle might be chosen for spinal anesthesia for an elective procedure, and a larger (e.g., 22-gauge) needle might be chosen when the subarachnoid space must be entered quickly because of severe fetal compromise.

With a small-gauge needle (i.e., 24-gauge or smaller), use of an introducer needle is preferable. The introducer needle allows for more accurate introduction of the spinal needle than is possible with use of a small-gauge spinal needle alone. The introducer needle also aids with skin puncture; it is often difficult to puncture the skin with non-cutting needles.

Either the midline or the paramedian approach can be used to enter the subarachnoid space. The **midline** approach requires the patient to reduce her lumbar lordosis to allow access to the subarachnoid space between adjacent spinous processes (usually L3 to L4, sometimes L4 to L5 or L2 to L3). The interspinous space may be identified with one (usually the thumb or index finger) or two fingers (usually the index and middle fingers) of the anesthesia provider's nondominant hand. The single finger "slides" along the skin in the midline from cephalad to caudad until it "settles" into an interspinous space. The two fingers identify the interspinous space by palpating the caudad border of the more cephalad spine. The fingers identify the midline by rolling in a medial-to-lateral direction (Figure 12-10). Next, the anesthesia provider injects local anesthetic intradermally and subcutaneously. The introducer needle is inserted into the substance of the interspinous ligament. It is helpful if the introducer needle is embedded in the interspinous ligament; therefore, obese patients may require a longer needle. The introducer needle should lie in the sagittal midline plane. It is then grasped and steadied with the fingers of the nondominant hand while the dominant hand holds the spinal needle like a dart. The fifth finger may be used as a tripod against the patient's back to prevent patient movement from causing

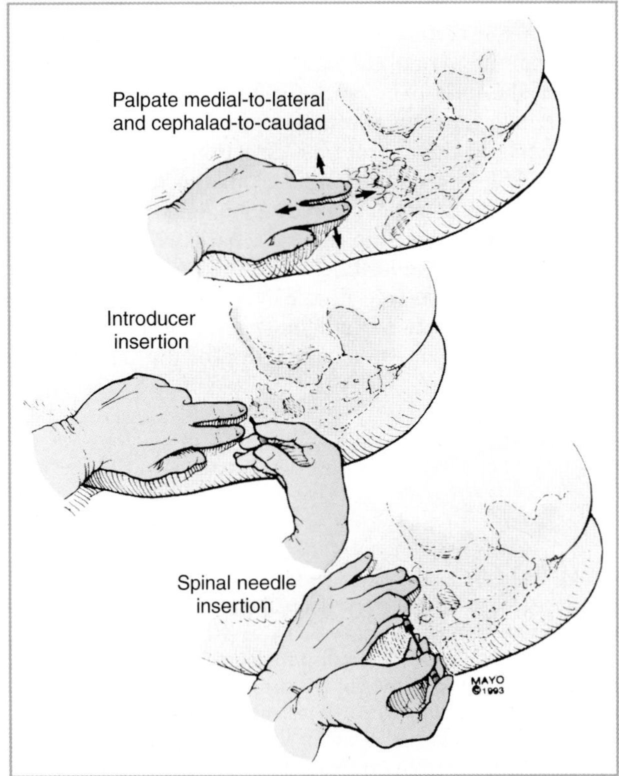

FIGURE 12-10 The midline approach for spinal needle insertion requires accurate identification of a lumbar interspinous space. The palpating fingers are rolled in a medial-to-lateral and cephalad-to-caudad direction; an introducer is then inserted through the interspinous space almost perpendicular to the lumbar spinous process. Once the introducer is seated in the interspinous ligament, the spinal needle is inserted; the needle is stabilized in a tripod fashion during insertion (much like a dart being thrown).

unintentional needle insertion to a level deeper than intended, and to "brake" the needle. As the needle passes through the ligamentum flavum and the dura, characteristic changes in resistance are noted. A "pop" is often perceived as the needle tip traverses the dura mater. The stylet is removed, and CSF should appear in the needle hub. If CSF does not appear, the stylet is replaced, and the needle is advanced a few millimeters and again checked for CSF flow. If CSF does not appear at this point and the needle is at an appropriate depth for the patient, the needle and introducer are withdrawn, and the process is repeated.

The most common reason for lack of CSF flow is insertion of the needle away from the midline. If the anesthesia provider achieves good anesthesia of the skin and subcutaneous tissues, correct use of the midline approach is almost painless. Significant pain suggests that the needle is directed away from the midline; indeed, a patient often indicates that the pain is localized to either the left or right side of the midline. In such cases, correct direction of the needle should be confirmed. Redirection of the needle often eliminates the patient's pain and results in the successful identification of the subarachnoid space.

Needle contact with bone also mandates redirection of the needle. If the needle is in the midline, the bone is either the cephalad or caudad spinous process, and the needle should be angled up or down in the sagittal midline plane. If the needle tip is angled off the midline or punctures the skin off the midline, the bone is probably the lamina of the vertebral arch. Needle contact with bone is usually painful. Again, the patient is often able to articulate whether she feels pain on the right or left side, or in the midline, allowing the anesthesia provider to make needle adjustments in the appropriate direction.

Once CSF is freely dripping from the needle hub, the dorsum of the provider's nondominant hand steadies the spinal needle against the patient's back while the syringe with local anesthetic is attached to the needle. After aspirating to ensure the free flow of CSF, the anesthesia provider injects the local anesthetic at a rate of approximately 0.2 mL per second. After completion of the injection, the anesthesia provider again aspirates approximately 0.2 mL of CSF and reinjects it into the subarachnoid space. This last step reconfirms the needle location and clears the needle of the remaining local anesthetic. The patient is then repositioned as appropriate.

For most patients, the midline approach is faster and less painful than the paramedian approach. The midline approach is also easier to teach than the paramedian approach, because it requires mental projection of the anatomy in only two planes, whereas the paramedian approach requires appreciation of a third plane and estimation of the depth of the subarachnoid space from the skin (Figure 12-11). Nevertheless, the **paramedian** approach is a useful technique that allows for the successful identification of the subarachnoid or epidural space in difficult cases. The paramedian approach does not require that the patient fully reduce her lumbar lordosis. This approach exploits the larger target that is available when the needle is inserted slightly off the midline.

A common error that is made with the paramedian approach is the insertion of the needle too far off the midline; the vertebral lamina then becomes a barrier to needle insertion. With the paramedian approach, the palpating fingers should again identify the caudad edge of the more cephalad spinous process. A skin wheal is raised 1 cm lateral and 1 cm caudad to this point; a longer needle is then used to infiltrate the deeper tissues in a cephalomedial plane. This step contrasts with the midline approach, in which the local anesthetic is not injected beyond the subcutaneous tissue. The spinal introducer is then inserted 10 to 15 degrees off the sagittal plane in a cephalomedial direction, and the spinal needle is advanced through the introducer needle toward the subarachnoid space. Another common error is to use an excessive cephalad angle with initial needle insertion. When the needle is inserted correctly and contacts bone, it is redirected slightly cephalad. If bone is again encountered, but at a deeper level, the slight stepwise increase in cephalad angulation is continued, and the needle is "walked" up and off the lamina. As with the midline approach, the characteristic feel of the ligamentum flavum and dura can be appreciated. The aim

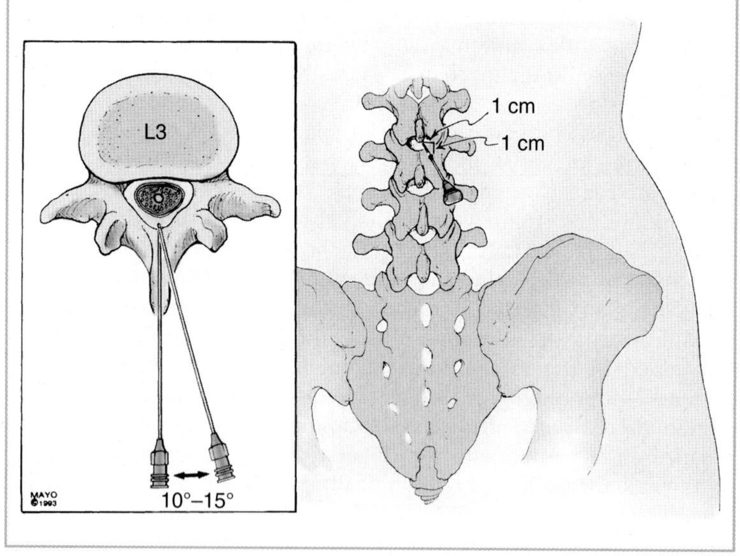

FIGURE 12-11 Vertebral anatomy of midline and paramedian approaches for spinal and epidural anesthesia. The midline approach requires anatomic projection in only two planes, sagittal and horizontal. The paramedian approach also requires consideration of the oblique plane. However, the paramedian approach requires less patient cooperation in reducing lumbar lordosis to allow for successful needle insertion. The paramedian needle insertion site is made 1 cm lateral and 1 cm caudad to the caudad edge of the more cephalad spinous process. The paramedian needle is inserted approximately 10 to 15 degrees off the sagittal plane (*inset*).

of the paramedian approach is to puncture the dura *in the midline*, even though the needle is inserted off the midline. Use of the paramedian approach requires insertion of a greater length of needle. Once CSF is obtained, the block is performed as it is with the midline approach.

The **Taylor** approach is a variation of the paramedian approach using the L5 to S1 interspace, which has the largest interlaminar space in the lumbosacral region. A 5-inch spinal needle is inserted in a cephalomedial plane from a site 1 cm medial and 1 cm caudad to the lowermost prominence of the posterior superior iliac spine. If bone is encountered on the first needle insertion, the needle is redirected in small steps cephalad to walk off the sacrum and into the subarachnoid space.

During the performance of any nerve block technique, needle advancement should stop if the patient complains of pain. If pain is the result of inadequate soft tissue anesthesia, additional local anesthetic should be injected. Pain or paresthesias may also result from needle contact with central nerves or the spinal cord. Patient perception of paresthesias during the initiation of spinal anesthesia may indicate that the needle tip is in the subarachnoid space. The anesthesia provider should remove the stylet and check for CSF. If the paresthesia has resolved, the local anesthetic may be injected. If the paresthesia persists, however, the needle should be withdrawn and repositioned. In any case, the anesthesia provider should never inject the local anesthetic if the patient is complaining of paresthesias or lancinating pain, either of which may signal injection into a nerve or the spinal cord.

EPIDURAL ANESTHESIA

Special equipment for epidural analgesia or anesthesia includes an epidural needle, an epidural catheter (for a continuous technique), and a loss-of-resistance syringe (for the loss-of-resistance technique to identify the epidural space). Single-shot epidural anesthesia is rarely used in obstetric practice, because the major advantage of epidural over spinal anesthesia is the ability to provide continuous anesthesia or analgesia without puncturing the dura with a large needle. Most anesthesia providers use the loss-of-resistance technique to identify the epidural space; therefore a syringe is necessary. An epidural needle with a lateral opening (e.g., Hustead, Tuohy) is most commonly used because it allows a catheter to be threaded through its orifice (Figure 12-12).

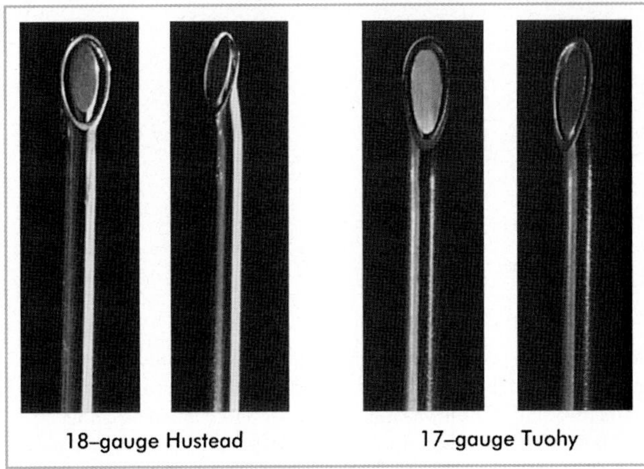

FIGURE 12-12 Epidural needles often used in parturients. Each needle is shown in an open-bevel view and an oblique orientation. The 18-gauge Hustead and 17-gauge Tuohy needles have lateral-facing openings, which direct epidural catheters to enter the epidural space more easily than if a single-shot Crawford needle design is used. (Other sizes and needle designs are available for obstetric epidural anesthesia.)

Several types of single-use, disposable epidural catheters are available. Catheters are made from plastic materials and differ as to the degree of "stiffness." Wire-embedded catheters are more flexible and are associated with a lower incidence of paresthesias and intravascular placement during catheter insertion.[49,50] The single-orifice catheter has one opening at its tip, whereas the multi-orifice catheter has a closed "bullet" tip with 3 lateral orifices between 0.5 and 1.5 cm from the tip (Figure 12-13). The proposed advantage of single-orifice, open-end catheters is that the injection of drugs is restricted to a single anatomic site. In theory, this arrangement should facilitate the detection of intravenous or subarachnoid placement of the catheter. Likewise, a theoretical disadvantage of multi-orifice, closed-end catheters is that local anesthetic may be injected into more than one anatomic site (e.g., both the epidural and subarachnoid spaces). A catheter initially placed in the epidural space can migrate into a vein or the subdural or subarachnoid space. Fortunately, this does not seem to be a common clinical problem. Regardless of the choice of catheter, aspiration should be performed before each dose of local anesthetic is injected.

An advantage of the multi-orifice catheter over the single-orifice catheter is the consistent ability to aspirate fluid (either blood or CSF) when the catheter is in a vessel or the subarachnoid space.[51] Multi-orifice catheters may lead to more even distribution of local anesthetic and a lower incidence of "patchy" or unilateral anesthesia when the anesthetic is injected as a bolus.[52] However, during an infusion into the epidural space, the solution exits only the most proximal hole,[53] and multi-orifice catheters thus behave like single-orifice catheters.

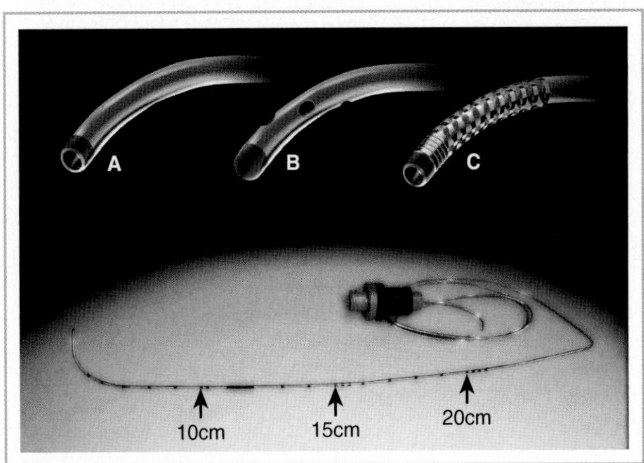

FIGURE 12-13 Epidural catheters. *A*, Single-orifice catheter; *B*, multi-orifice catheter with bullet tip; *C*, coiled wire reinforced catheter. *Bottom*, Epidural catheter with centimeter markings along distal end and Luer-Lok connector at proximal end. (Drawing by Naveen Nathan, M.D., Northwestern University Feinberg School of Medicine, Chicago, IL.)

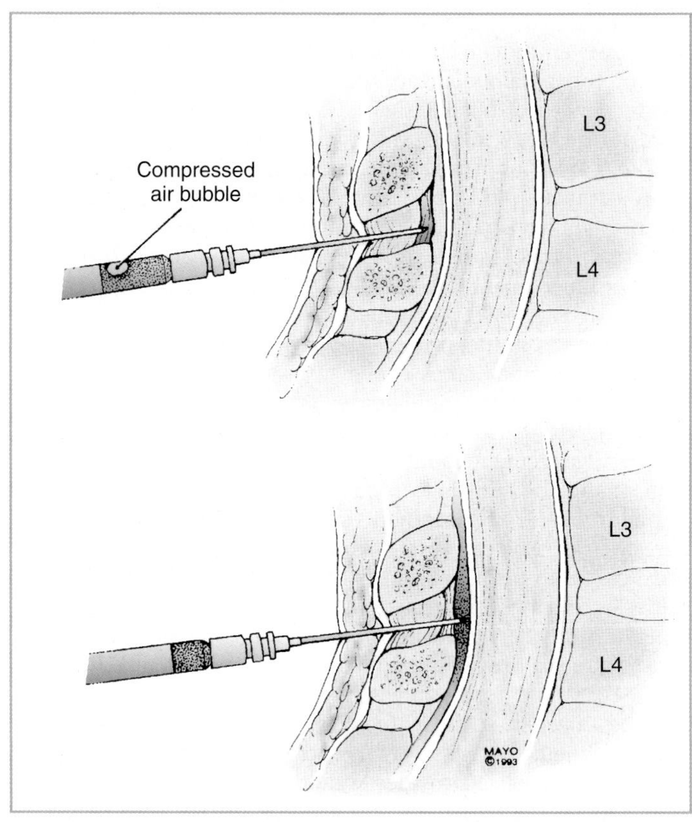

FIGURE 12-14 Loss-of-resistance technique for identifying the epidural space. The needle is first inserted into the interspinous ligament or ligamentum flavum, and a syringe containing an air bubble in saline is attached to the hub. After compression of the air bubble by pressure on the syringe-plunger, the needle is carefully advanced until a loss of resistance to syringe-plunger pressure is noted as the needle enters the epidural space.

Two methods are used to identify the epidural space during needle advancement: (1) hanging drop method and (2) loss-of-resistance method. The majority of anesthesia providers use the loss-of-resistance method (Figure 12-14). The traditional loss-of-resistance syringe is a finely ground glass syringe with a Luer-Lok connector. Plastic syringes are now available, and the choice is generally a matter of the anesthesia provider's preference. The syringe is filled with 2 to 4 mL of saline, air, or saline with a small air bubble. There is some controversy regarding the use of air versus saline for detecting the point of loss of resistance.[54] Saline causes some syringe plungers to stick and may be confused with CSF during initiation of combined spinal-epidural anesthesia. Conversely, injection of air into the epidural space may contribute to patchy anesthesia,[55] and unintentional pneumocephalus may increase the risk of post–dural puncture headache.[56] We prefer that the syringe contain both saline and a small (e.g., 0.25 mL) compressible bubble of air, although many anesthesia providers successfully use air.

Regardless of the technique used, success depends on correct placement of the needle tip within the ligamentum flavum. The needle should be advanced well into the interspinous ligament, or even into the ligamentum flavum, before the syringe is attached or before the hanging drop of solution is placed into the needle hub. This approach has at least three advantages. First, it encourages the anesthesia provider to use proprioception while directing and advancing the needle. Second, it shortens the time required for successful identification of the epidural space. Third, it lowers the likelihood of a false-positive loss of resistance. Undoubtedly, this false-positive identification of the epidural space is responsible for many cases of unsuccessful epidural anesthesia; it is even possible to insert a catheter between the interspinous ligament and the ligamentum flavum.

During advancement of the needle-syringe assembly, the needle should be moved toward the epidural space by the provider's nondominant hand while the thumb of the dominant hand applies constant pressure on the syringe plunger, thereby compressing the 0.25-mL air bubble. Alternatively, the intermittent, oscillating technique is typically employed when using loss of resistance to air. When the needle enters the epidural space, the pressure applied to the syringe plunger causes the solution or air to flow easily into the epidural space (see Figure 12-14).

In most obstetric cases, the anesthesia provider inserts a catheter and uses a continuous technique. The provider must decide whether to insert the catheter before or after the test and therapeutic doses of local anesthetic. Most practitioners insert the catheter before injecting local anesthetic, to allow for the slow, incremental injection of local anesthetic and the more controlled development of epidural anesthesia. However, there is little evidence that the incremental injection of local anesthetic through the catheter results in less significant hemodynamic change than incremental injection through the needle (followed by insertion of the catheter); also, injection through the needle may shorten the time to complete anesthesia or analgesia. Nonetheless, if the principal reason for using an epidural technique is the provision of continuous analgesia, it seems most practical to insert the catheter before injecting the therapeutic dose of local anesthetic so that correct catheter placement can be verified promptly. Alternatively, both techniques can be combined, in that a small dose of local anesthetic is injected through the needle and the remainder of the dose is injected through the catheter.

If the catheter is placed before the test and therapeutic doses of local anesthetic, it may be helpful to inject 5 to 10 mL of saline before threading the catheter, as this may reduce the incidence of epidural vein cannulation,[57,58] particularly when using stiffer epidural catheters. Rolbin et al.[59] noted that there was no advantage to the injection of 3 mL of fluid into the epidural space before insertion of the epidural catheter.

Six to eight centimeters of catheter are threaded into the epidural space before the epidural needle is removed. The catheter may then be pulled back until it is at the desired distance at the skin. Occasionally, the anesthesia provider will have difficulty advancing the catheter past the tip of the epidural needle. This difficulty may indicate that the epidural needle tip is not in the epidural space. However, if the provider is convinced that the needle is correctly placed, several maneuvers may facilitate catheter advancement. Often, having the patient take a deep breath allows catheter advancement. Saline may be injected through the epidural needle if this has not been done. Although some providers rotate the epidural needle in an attempt to successfully advance the catheter, we do not recommend this maneuver, because it may increase the risk of dural puncture. Instead, the epidural needle should be withdrawn 0.5 to 1 cm, and again advanced into the epidural space.

Many techniques are available for securing the epidural catheter at the skin entry site. If a catheter will be used for prolonged intrapartum or postoperative analgesia, care providers should be able to assess the skin surrounding the catheter. A transparent, sterile adhesive dressing applied over the catheter after application of skin adhesive generally works well, and the periphery of the dressing can be reinforced with tape. The position of the epidural catheter may change significantly with patient movement from the sitting-flexed to the sitting-upright or lateral decubitus position.[60] D'Angelo et al.[61] found that the risk of catheter dislodgement was higher when catheters were inserted 2 cm into the epidural space, but the risk of unilateral blockade was higher when catheters were inserted 6 to 8 cm. Therefore, if the catheter is to be used for a short period (e.g., cesarean delivery), it should be left 2 to 4 cm into the epidural space. In contrast, if the catheter will be used for many hours (e.g., labor), it should be left 4 to 6 cm into the space. To minimize catheter movement at the skin, the patient should be positioned sitting upright or in the lateral position before the catheter is secured.[60]

The potential for the contamination of local anesthetic solutions has prompted the use of micropore filters during the administration of continuous epidural anesthesia for labor. There is no evidence that filters decrease the rate of infection or of injection of undesirable foreign substances.[62] Additionally, filters may reduce the reliability of aspiration[63] and absorb local anesthetic solution, unless they are primed.[64] We believe that micropore filters have little utility in clinical obstetric anesthesia practice.

BOX 12-1 Advantages of Combined Spinal-Epidural Anesthetic Technique

Compared with Epidural Anesthesia

- Lower maternal, fetal, and neonatal plasma concentrations of anesthetic agents
- More rapid onset of analgesia and anesthesia
- More dense sensory blockade
- Complete early labor analgesia with opioid alone (no local anesthetic necessary)
- Lower failure rate

Compared with Spinal Anesthesia

- Technically easier in obese individuals: The epidural needle acts as an introducer for the spinal needle (it is easier to advance a rigid epidural needle).
- Ability to titrate anesthetic dose (Start with low subarachnoid dose, and titrate to effect using epidural injection.)
- Results in less hypotension
- Ability to extend the extent of neuroblockade (Spinal anesthesia for forceps delivery may be extended to epidural anesthesia for cesarean after failed forceps delivery.)
- Continuous technique: ability to extend duration of anesthesia

COMBINED SPINAL-EPIDURAL ANESTHESIA

Combined spinal-epidural (CSE) anesthesia combines the advantages and mitigates the disadvantages of single-shot spinal anesthesia and continuous epidural anesthesia (Box 12-1). Anesthesia is initiated with a subarachnoid injection of local anesthetic and maintained via an epidural catheter. It is useful for both cesarean delivery anesthesia and labor analgesia. The injection of the smaller dose of local anesthetic required for spinal (compared with epidural) anesthesia is inherently safer with regard to the possibility of unintentional intravascular injection. Additionally, the anesthesia provider can inject a local anesthetic dose that is lower than the ED_{95} (effective dose in 95% of cases) without fear of inadequate anesthesia. If surgical anesthesia is inadequate, the block can be "rescued" with epidural administration of local anesthetic. Lower intrathecal local anesthetic doses reduce the risk of maternal hypotension.[65] Compared with conventional epidural anesthesia for cesarean delivery, CSE anesthesia is associated with a more rapid onset of surgical anesthesia, less intraoperative pain and discomfort (e.g., a more dense block), better muscle relaxation, and less shivering and vomiting.[66]

During labor, CSE analgesia is associated with a faster onset of analgesia.[67] Studies differ as to whether CSE analgesia is associated with higher maternal satisfaction and fewer requests for supplemental analgesia. A 2007 systematic review comparing CSE analgesia with epidural labor analgesia concluded that onset was faster with the CSE technique but that there was no evidence for differences in maternal satisfaction, mode of delivery, ability to ambulate, or incidence of hypotension between the two techniques.[68] Several studies have found a lower incidence of failed *epidural* analgesia after the initiation of analgesia with a CSE technique.[69,70] Presumably, verification of the correct placement of the spinal needle by visualization of CSF increases the likelihood that the tip of the epidural needle is correctly placed in the epidural space.

A disadvantage of the CSE technique is that the correct placement of the epidural catheter in the epidural space cannot be verified until spinal anesthesia wanes. Therefore, if a functioning epidural catheter is important to the safe care of the mother and fetus (e.g., in the setting of a suspected difficult airway or nonreassuring fetal status), a CSE technique is not the technique of choice.

There are several techniques for CSE anesthesia.[71] The most popular is the needle-through-needle technique, in which the epidural needle is sited in the epidural space and serves as an introducer for the spinal needle. The spinal needle passes through the epidural needle to puncture the dura. After injection of the intrathecal dose, the spinal needle is removed and the epidural catheter is threaded through the epidural needle. An alternative technique uses two skin punctures and two different interspaces: The spinal needle and epidural needle and catheter are introduced sequentially in two different interspaces.

The needle-through-needle technique requires a long spinal needle. Typically, a small (25-gauge or smaller) non-cutting needle is used in order to minimize the risk of post–dural puncture headache. The tip of the spinal needle must protrude 12 to 17 mm beyond the tip of the epidural needle when the two needles are fully engaged (Figure 12-15). Failure to puncture the dura and visualize CSF occurred in 25% of patients when the spinal needle protruded 9 mm, compared with no patients when the needle protruded 17 mm.[72] A 127-mm spinal needle is commonly used with a standard 9-cm epidural needle. However, because of differences in hub configurations among needles, the two hubs may not "mesh," and spinal needle protrusion may vary with specific needle combinations. Alternatively, manufacturers now sell CSE needle "kits," in which the spinal needle is designed for a specific epidural needle. An additional small non–Luer-Lok syringe (1 to 3 mL) is required for the spinal dose.

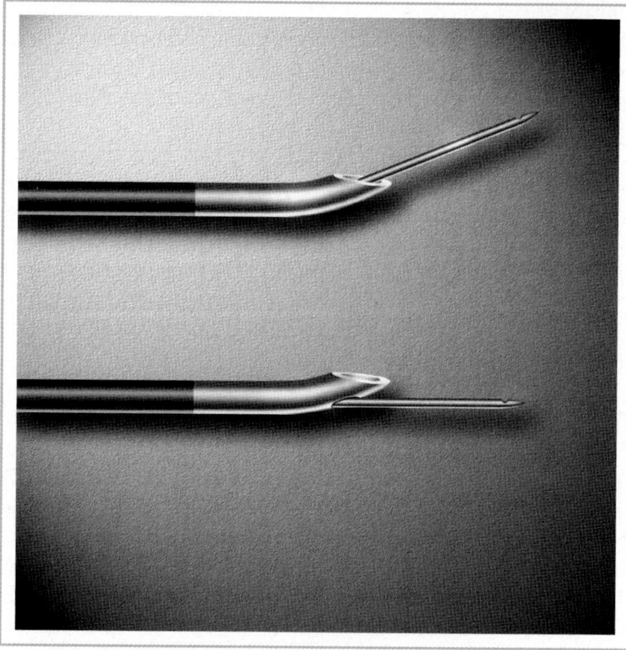

FIGURE 12-15 Combined spinal-epidural needle configuration. *Top*, Spinal needle exits the epidural needle through the normal epidural needle bevel. Because the epidural needle bevel opening faces sideways, the spinal needle exits the epidural needle at a slight angle to the long axis of the epidural needle. *Bottom*, Spinal needle exits the epidural needle through a special orifice. The axes of the spinal and epidural needles are aligned. The spinal needle must protrude from the tip of the epidural 12 to 17 mm when the hubs are engaged, or the ability to puncture the dura with the spinal needle is compromised. (Drawing by Naveen Nathan, M.D., Northwestern University Feinberg School of Medicine, Chicago, IL.)

CSE anesthesia is initiated much like epidural anesthesia. The epidural needle is sited in the epidural space (Figure 12-16). The spinal needle is introduced through the epidural needle with the anesthesia provider's dominant hand, while the nondominant hand is anchored against the patient's back to serve as a brake for further advancement of the spinal needle. The provider usually perceives the tip of the spinal needle passing the tip of the epidural needle as a slight increase in resistance. Spinal needle advancement should stop immediately after the anesthesia provider perceives the dural puncture "pop." Dural puncture is verified by visualization of CSF after removal of the spinal needle stylet. The provider's nondominant hand is anchored on the patient's back, and the spinal and epidural needle hubs are grasped together between the thumb and index finger of this hand. The dominant hand attaches the spinal syringe and injects the drug. We do not attempt to aspirate CSF, because it may not be possible to do so through long, small-bore needles and because attempted aspiration may result in movement of the spinal needle. After removal of the spinal syringe and needle as a unit, the epidural catheter is threaded in the usual fashion.

Failure to puncture the dura with the spinal needle may occur in several circumstances (Figure 12-17). The epidural needle tip may not be located in the epidural space, or the needle tip may be correctly placed, but the spinal needle may fail to puncture the dura or may not reach the dura because of the depth of the posterior epidural space. Alternatively, the epidural needle may be angled away from the midline or in a sagittal plane off the midline, and the spinal needle may traverse the lateral epidural space without puncturing the dura. In this latter circumstance, the anesthesia provider may elect to abandon the CSE technique and continue with epidural anesthesia (if convinced that the epidural needle tip is in the epidural space) or to reposition the epidural needle and reattempt the CSE technique.

CAUDAL ANESTHESIA

Equipment for caudal anesthesia is similar to that used for lumbar epidural techniques, except that a needle with a lateral-faced opening is not needed. A blunt-tipped needle is satisfactory even when a catheter is used, because the angle of needle insertion allows insertion of the catheter. Successful administration of caudal anesthesia requires the accurate identification of the sacral hiatus. The sacrococcygeal ligament (an extension of the ligamentum flavum) overlies the sacral hiatus between the sacral cornua. Identification of the posterior superior iliac spines facilitates

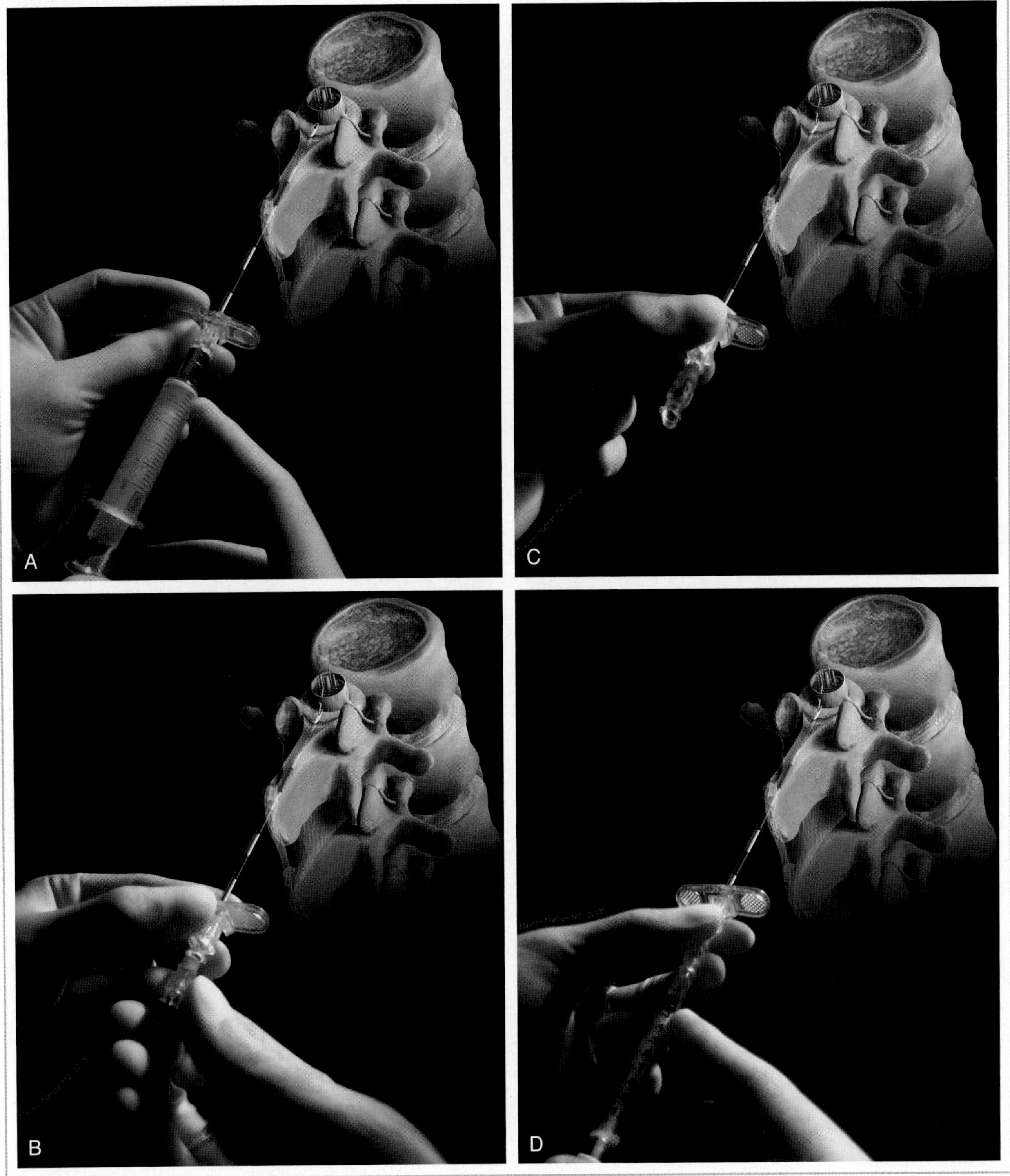

FIGURE 12-16 Needle-through-needle combined spinal-epidural technique. **A,** The epidural needle is sited in the epidural space. **B,** The long spinal needle is passed through the epidural needle and punctures the dura mater. **C,** The operator's nondominant hand stabilizes the spinal and epidural needles, and the spinal needle stylet is withdrawn. Cerebrospinal fluid is seen spontaneously dripping from the spinal needle. **D,** The syringe is attached to the spinal needle, and the intrathecal dose is injected.

Continued

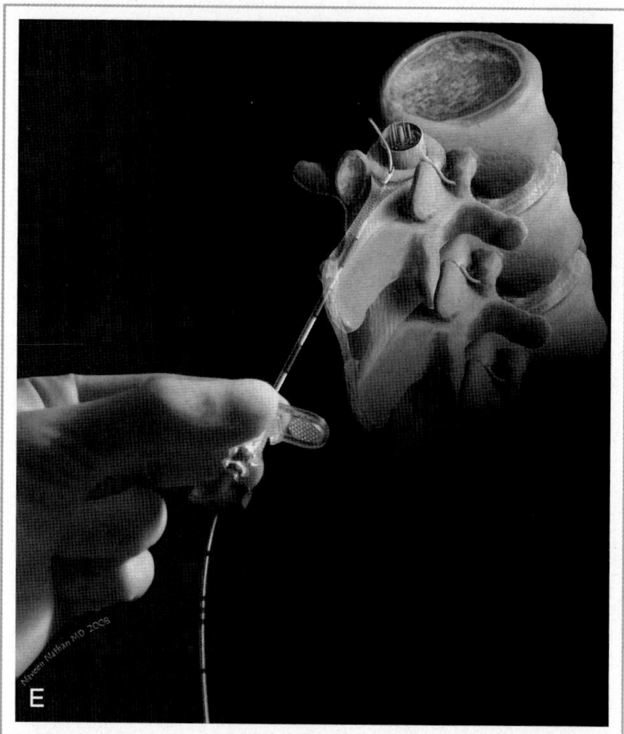

FIGURE 12-16 cont'd **E,** The spinal needle is withdrawn, and the epidural catheter is threaded through the epidural needle into the epidural space. (Drawing by Naveen Nathan, M.D., Northwestern University Feinberg School of Medicine, Chicago, IL.)

the identification of the sacral cornua; the location of the sacral hiatus is approximated by using the line between them as one side of an equilateral triangle (Figure 12-18). Once the sacral hiatus is identified, the palpating fingers are placed on the cornua, the skin is anesthetized, and the caudal needle is inserted with the hub at an angle approximately 45 degrees from the skin. A decrease in resistance is noted when the needle enters the caudal canal. The needle is advanced until it contacts bone (i.e., the dorsal aspect of the ventral plate of the sacrum). Next, the needle is withdrawn slightly and redirected so that the angle of insertion relative to the skin surface is decreased. In pregnant women, the final angle is approximately 15 degrees from a plane parallel to the sacrum.

Accurate placement of the caudal needle is verified primarily from the "feel" of the needle passing through the sacrococcygeal ligament. An additional maneuver may help providers with less experience to verify correct needle placement: Once the needle is believed to be within the caudal canal, 5 mL of saline is rapidly injected through the needle while the anesthesia provider's other hand is placed over the dorsum of the sacrum. If the needle is placed correctly, no mass or pressure wave is detected over the midline of the sacrum. Conversely, if the needle is malpositioned (often posterior to the caudal canal), a fluid mass or pressure wave is felt by the palpating hand.

The needle should be advanced only 1 to 2 cm into the caudal canal. Dural puncture or unintentional intravascular cannulation is more likely to occur with deeper insertion. A test dose similar to that used during administration of lumbar epidural anesthesia should be administered.

COMPLICATIONS OF NEURAXIAL TECHNIQUES

Unintentional Dural Puncture

Unintentional dural puncture with an epidural needle occurs at a rate of approximately 1.5% in the obstetric population.[73] Approximately 52% of women will experience a post–dural puncture headache after puncture with an epidural needle. Techniques to minimize the incidence of unintentional dural puncture include the following: (1) identification of the ligamentum flavum during epidural needle advancement; (2) understanding the likely depth of the epidural space in an individual patient; (3) advancement of the needle between contractions, when unexpected patient movement is less likely; (4) adequate control of the needle-syringe assembly during advancement of the needle; and (5) clearing the needle of clotted blood or bone plugs. Norris et al.[74] observed that post–dural puncture headache after unintentional dural puncture was less likely to result in headache if the epidural needle bevel faced lateral rather than cephalad. In contrast, Richardson et al.[75] found no difference between the two orientations. An *in vitro* study using cadaver dura found that fluid leakage rate through dural tears was not dependent on the orientation of the dura relative to the needle bevel.[76] We prefer to insert the epidural needle with the bevel oriented in a cephalad

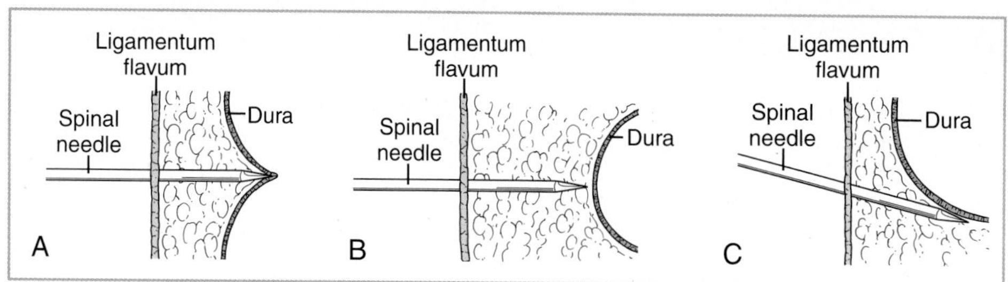

FIGURE 12-17 Reasons for failure of the combined spinal-epidural technique. **A,** The spinal needle tents the dura but does not puncture it. **B,** The spinal needle does not reach the dura. **C,** The spinal needle passes to the side of the dural sac. (Redrawn with permission from Riley ET, Hamilton CL, Ratner EF, Cohen SE. A comparison of the 24-gauge Sprotte and Gertie Marx spinal needles for combined spinal-epidural analgesia during labor. Anesthesiology 2002; 97:574.)

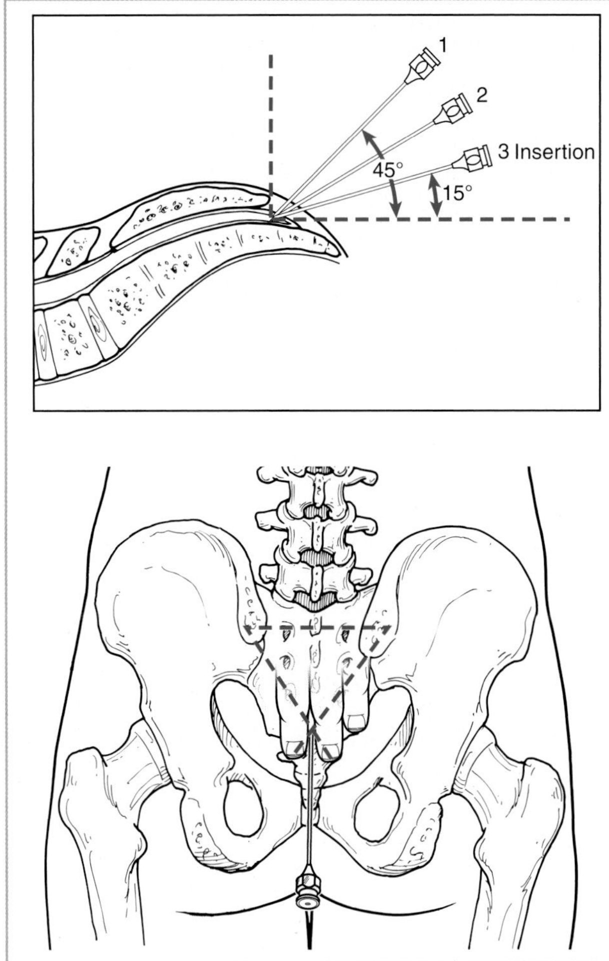

FIGURE 12-18 The location of the sacral hiatus for caudal anesthesia is facilitated by the identification of the posterior superior iliac spines. The posterior superior spines are marked, and a line drawn between them forms one edge of an equilateral triangle. If the triangle is completed as illustrated, the sacral hiatus should underlie the caudad tip of the equilateral triangle. *Inset,* Once the sacral hiatus is identified, the needle is inserted by insertion and withdrawal in a stepwise fashion from an initial 45-degree angle off the coronal plane. In pregnant women, the needle eventually enters the caudal canal at an angle approximately 15 degrees off the coronal plane. If the needle is placed properly, no subcutaneous "lump" develops after the injection of the local anesthetic solution. (Redrawn from Brown DL. Spinal, epidural, and caudal anesthesia. In Miller RD, editor. Miller's Anesthesia. 6th edition. Philadelphia, Churchill Livingstone, 2005:1653.)

direction so that there is no need to rotate the needle bevel within the epidural space. Cephalad bevel orientation also increases the likelihood of successful epidural anesthesia.[75,77]

The management of unintentional dural puncture depends on the clinical setting. One option is to site the epidural catheter within the subarachnoid space and to use a continuous spinal anesthetic technique. Evidence is conflicting as to whether the insertion of an epidural catheter through the dural puncture site decreases the incidence of post–dural puncture headache.[78-80] Continuous spinal anesthesia is an attractive option if identification of the epidural space has been difficult, or if the anticipated duration of epidural anesthesia or analgesia is relatively short (e.g., cesarean delivery, or vaginal delivery in parous women). The major disadvantage of an intrathecal catheter is the risk that it may be mistaken for an epidural catheter. Given that the local anesthetic dose required for epidural anesthesia is many times greater than that required for spinal anesthesia, unintentional administration of an epidural dose into the subarachnoid space will lead to total spinal anesthesia. Therefore, on a busy labor and delivery unit where multiple providers are giving anesthesia care, it may be safer to use an epidural catheter rather than an intrathecal catheter in women in whom prolonged analgesia is anticipated.

The new catheter should be placed in another lumbar interspace, if possible. Even if the second catheter is correctly placed in the epidural space, anesthesia providers must be wary of an unexpectedly high level of anesthesia after administration of usual doses of local anesthetic.[81,82] Leach and Smith[82] reported a patient who had an extensive block after unintentional dural puncture and subsequent epidural injection of bupivacaine. They presented radiologic evidence of the spread of local anesthetic from the epidural space to the subarachnoid space. The extent to which a dural tear affects the movement of substances from the epidural space to the subarachnoid space depends on the size of the hole, the lipophilicity of the drug (highly lipophilic drugs cross quickly regardless of the presence of a hole, whereas water-soluble drugs cross more quickly in the presence of a hole),[83] and whether the drug is administered into the epidural space as a bolus or an infusion.

Unfortunately, there is no reliable method to decrease the risk of post–dural puncture headache once dural puncture occurs. Obese patients appear to be at lower risk for the development of headache.[84] A prophylactic blood patch (injection of autologous blood before removal of the epidural catheter and before onset of a headache) does not reduce the risk of post–dural puncture headache.[85]

Unintentional Intravascular or Subarachnoid Injection

The unintentional injection of drugs into blood vessels or the subarachnoid space can lead to catastrophe. The incidence of intravascular catheter placement varies according to catheter type,[49] patient population,[86] and proper placement of the epidural needle tip in the midline. Pregnant women are at higher risk for unintentional intravenous cannulation. Because the unintentional intravascular or subarachnoid injection of large doses of local anesthetic can be life-threatening, several precautions should be taken to reduce the chances and risks of intravascular injection. These include aspiration before each injection, incremental administration of small amounts of drug, use of an infusion when appropriate, and administration of an epidural test dose.

EPIDURAL TEST DOSE

The purpose of the test dose is to help identify unintentional cannulation of a vein or the subarachnoid space. The test dose should contain a dose of local anesthetic and/or another marker sufficient to allow the recognition of intravenous or subarachnoid injection but not so large as to cause systemic toxicity or total spinal anesthesia. The most common intravascular test dose contains epinephrine, as recommended by Moore and Batra.[87] Intravenous injection of epinephrine 15 μg consistently causes a transient increase in heart rate during the first minute after injection in nonpregnant subjects.

The epinephrine test dose is not without detractors. Some anesthesia providers fear that intravenous injection of epinephrine may decrease uteroplacental perfusion and precipitate fetal compromise.[88-90] Counterarguments include the fact that changes in uterine blood flow after intravenous injection of epinephrine in pregnant laboratory animals were transient.[88] Similar transient declines in perfusion undoubtedly occur during normal uterine contractions, and the adverse maternal and fetal consequences of intravenous injection of a large therapeutic dose of local anesthetic would likely be more severe. There has been no report of adverse neonatal outcome after intravenous injection of an epinephrine-containing test dose.

The epinephrine test dose is less specific in laboring women because cyclic changes in maternal heart rate complicate interpretation of its effects.[91,92] For this reason, the test dose should be given immediately after a uterine contraction so there is less confusion as to whether tachycardia is caused by pain or intravenous epinephrine.[93] Another argument against routine use of a test dose is that aspiration of multi-orifice catheters is 98% sensitive in identifying their intravascular location.[51] Finally, because modern epidural labor analgesia involves the *infusion* of a *low* concentration of local anesthetic, unintentional intravascular administration is not likely to result in cardiovascular collapse.

Others argue that the epinephrine test dose still has a role in obstetric anesthesia practice.[94] Large volumes of a concentrated local anesthetic solution are still routinely administered for urgent cesarean delivery. Lee et al.[95] summarized injuries associated with regional anesthesia in the American Society of Anesthesiologists (ASA) Closed-Claims Database and identified unintentional intravascular injections as the second most common damaging event in obstetric claims. All events were associated with epidural or caudal anesthesia, and 75% resulted in cardiac arrest. Although a test dose was used in the majority of cases, only 30% of the test doses contained epinephrine.

Other methods of detecting intravascular injection are the injection of subtoxic doses of local anesthetic and the injection of isoproterenol,[96,97] a small volume of air,[98] or fentanyl[99,100] (Table 12-2).

It is imperative that the anesthesia provider take the time to look for evidence of intrathecal injection of local anesthetic. Intrathecal injection of lidocaine 30 to 45 mg or bupivacaine 5 to 7.5 mg is likely to produce objective evidence of spinal anesthesia within 5 minutes.[101,102] Asking the patient whether or not she can wiggle her toes several minutes after the test dose injection is not adequate. In one study, the presence of lower extremity warmth and impaired pinprick response was only 93% sensitive for intrathecal injection, whereas impaired leg raise 4 minutes after test dose injection had 100% sensitivity for intrathecal injection.[103]

Finally, every anesthesia provider should remember that no single test dose regimen can exclude every case of unintentional intravenous or subarachnoid injection.[104,105] Box 12-2 summarizes steps that may be taken to decrease the risk of unintentional intravenous or subarachnoid injection of local anesthetic.

TABLE 12-2 Test-Dose Regimens Designed to Identify Unintentional Intravascular Injection

Test Component*	Response
Epinephrine 15 μg[87]	15- to 20-bpm increase in heart rate
Isoproterenol 5 μg[96,97]	15- to 20-bpm increase in heart rate
Local anesthetic alone: Lidocaine 100 mg Bupivacaine 25 mg 2-Chloroprocaine 90 mg	Tinnitus, circumoral numbness, "dizziness"
Air 1 mL[98]	Mill-wheel murmur over right heart (use fetal Doppler probe to monitor)
Fentanyl 100 μg[99,100]	Dizziness, drowsiness

*Superscript numbers indicate references listed at the end of this chapter.

Inadequate Anesthesia

Pain during anesthesia represents a higher proportion of obstetric malpractice claims than of nonobstetric claims.[106] During labor, inadequate epidural analgesia may result from the inadequate extent of sensory blockade, nonuniform blockade, or inadequate density of blockade. When called to evaluate breakthrough pain, the anesthesia provider should first evaluate the extent of bilateral sensory blockade in *both the cephalad and caudad directions.* Particularly if labor is progressing quickly, the extent of sacral blockade may not be adequate. In this case, epidural injection of a large volume of local anesthetic may improve sacral blockade. In contrast, if the extent of sensory blockade is adequate but the patient is still experiencing pain, the

BOX 12-2 Steps to Decrease Risk of Unintentional Intravenous or Subarachnoid Injection of Local Anesthetic

- Lower the proximal end of the catheter below the site of insertion. Observe for the passive return of blood or cerebrospinal fluid.
- Aspirate before injecting each dose of local anesthetic.
- Give the test dose between uterine contractions.
- Use dilute solutions of local anesthetic during labor.
- Do not inject more than 5 mL of local anesthetic as a single bolus.
- Maintain verbal contact with the patient.
- If little or no block is produced after the injection of an appropriate dose of local anesthetic, assume that the local anesthetic was injected intravenously, and remove the catheter.

density of blockade may be insufficient. In this case, the provider should reestablish and maintain analgesia using a more concentrated solution of local anesthetic.

Total block failure usually results from failure to identify the epidural space correctly or from malposition of the catheter tip outside the epidural space (e.g., in a neuroforamen). A unilateral block may occur despite the use of good technique. Unilateral block can often be prevented by limiting the length of catheter within the epidural space to 3 cm or less. The problem with limited insertion of the catheter is that, in some patients, the catheter tends to migrate outward over time. (Patients undergoing surgery remain still; by contrast, laboring women change position frequently.) Obese women seem to be at higher risk for outward migration of the catheter tip. Prospective studies suggest that 4 to 6 cm is the optimal depth of epidural catheter insertion in laboring women.[60,61,107]

Whether or not catheter withdrawal in the setting of breakthrough pain is beneficial is not clear. Beilin et al.[108] compared catheter withdrawal followed by injection of local anesthetic with injection of local anesthetic without catheter withdrawal for the treatment of breakthrough pain. The ability to rescue analgesia was not different between the groups. Additionally, Gielen et al.[109] performed a radiologic study in which they observed no consistent relationship between catheter position and the asymmetric onset of sympathetic blockade. Unilateral or patchy sensory blockade likely results from the nonuniform distribution of local anesthetic solution in the epidural space.[110] Injection of a large volume of dilute local anesthetic solution into the epidural space usually corrects this problem, regardless of the location of the tip of the epidural catheter (provided it is actually in the epidural space). If analgesia cannot be rescued with a second injection, the catheter should be removed and replaced at another interspace.

The management of inadequate anesthesia is more problematic during cesarean delivery. Failure of spinal anesthesia may result from the maldistribution of local anesthetic within the subarachnoid space.[111,112] If inadequate spinal anesthesia is noted before incision, the anesthesia provider may perform a second spinal anesthetic procedure and give additional local anesthetic. However, in the ASA Closed-Claims Database, Drasner and Rigler[112] identified three cases of cauda equina syndrome complicating spinal anesthesia. In two cases, "failed spinal" anesthesia had occurred, followed by a repeat injection of local anesthetic. The researchers recommended that anesthesia providers determine the presence of anesthesia in the sacral dermatomes before giving additional local anesthetic into the subarachnoid space. Additionally, they stated that if CSF was aspirated during the original procedure, it should be assumed that local anesthetic was delivered into the subarachnoid space, and the total dose of local anesthetic be limited to the maximum dose a clinician would consider reasonable to administer in a single injection.[112] If partial blockade is present (even if it is limited to the sacral dermatomes), the second dose should be reduced accordingly. It may also be advisable to perform the second procedure at a different interspace or make other changes to the original procedure (e.g., alter the patient's position, use a local anesthetic with different baricity, or straighten the lumbosacral curvature).

If the patient complains of pain after incision, the anesthesia provider must decide between the administration of inhalation or intravenous analgesia and the administration of general anesthesia. Supplemental analgesia may be provided by giving 60% nitrous oxide in oxygen, small incremental boluses of ketamine (0.1 to 0.25 mg/kg), or small boluses of intravenous opioid. Supplemental infiltration of the wound with local anesthetic is sometimes helpful, especially when spinal anesthesia regresses near the end of an unexpectedly long operation. The anesthesia provider must ensure that the patient remains sufficiently alert to protect her airway. In most cases, severe pain unrelieved by modest doses of analgesic drug requires rapid-sequence induction of general anesthesia, followed by endotracheal intubation.

In some cases, inadequate epidural anesthesia results from failure to give a sufficient dose of local anesthetic or failure to wait a sufficient time after its administration. For example, after 0.5% bupivacaine is given epidurally, approximately 20 minutes must pass to achieve an adequate level of anesthesia, and additional local anesthetic may be needed to achieve an adequate density of blockade. In urgent cases or in cases with a "missed" segment, local infiltration with a local anesthetic often results in satisfactory anesthesia. Sometimes it is difficult to separate the beneficial effect of the local infiltration from the beneficial effect of waiting for the obstetrician to obtain, prepare, and inject the local anesthetic solution. Finally, the anesthesia provider should exercise caution when initiating spinal anesthesia after failure of epidural anesthesia because of a higher incidence of high spinal anesthesia in this setting.[113] Presumably, the large volume of local anesthetic within, or near, the epidural space results in decreased lumbar CSF volume, which predisposes to high spinal anesthesia. It may be advisable to reduce the dose of intrathecal local anesthetic, particularly in the presence of partial epidural blockade.

Equipment Problems

The frequency of major equipment malfunction is very low during the administration of neuraxial anesthesia. Most anesthesia providers in the United States use disposable needles, and the plastic needle hubs are attached to the needles' shafts with epoxy. Rarely, a needle breaks at the hub-shaft junction.[114] If a needle should break, the portion of the needle that remains in the patient should be removed, because it may migrate and cause injury.[115]

An epidural or spinal catheter may shear and break off if the catheter is withdrawn through a needle; thus an epidural or spinal catheter should never be withdrawn in this manner. Rather, if the catheter must be withdrawn, the needle and catheter should be withdrawn as a unit. It is also possible to break a catheter during attempts at removing it, although this is rare. If resistance to catheter removal is encountered, the patient should assume a position that reduces lumbar lordosis, thereby lessening the kinking of the catheter between perivertebral structures. If position change is not successful, the catheter should be taped under tension to the patient's back and left undisturbed for several hours. The catheter usually works its way out and is then easy to remove. Once the catheter has been removed successfully, it should be examined to ensure that it has been removed completely. Complete removal of the catheter should be documented in the medical record.

Rarely, catheters do break on removal. We favor aggressive attempts to remove broken *spinal* catheters. However, it may be unnecessary to remove broken *epidural* catheters; rather, in these circumstances, the patient can be informed of the complication and observed over time. The incidence of catheter migration or other delayed sequelae appears to be low. Computed tomography may help identify the precise location of a broken catheter, if necessary.[116]

During use, an epidural catheter occasionally becomes disconnected from the catheter connector. Options include replacing the epidural catheter or reconnecting the connector to the catheter. Langevin et al.[117] used an *in vitro* model to investigate whether microbial contamination precludes reconnection. They found that an area of the interior of the catheter distal to the disconnection may remain sterile for up to 8 hours if the fluid column within the catheter remains static (i.e., if "fluid does not move within the catheter when it is raised above the level of the patient"[117]). Therefore, they concluded that it *may* be safe to decontaminate the exterior of the catheter, cut the catheter with a sterile instrument, and reconnect it to a new sterile connector. However, given the potential catastrophic consequences of neuraxial infection, we recommend replacing the catheter. Also, wire-embedded catheters cannot be cut.

Resuscitation of the Obstetric Patient

Intravenous, spinal, or epidural injection of local anesthetic may rarely precipitate maternal cardiac arrest. If this event occurs before delivery, left uterine displacement must be maintained and aortocaval compression avoided during maternal resuscitation. Initially, the ABCs of resuscitation are important; these include (1) the establishment and protection of the patient's airway, (2) the provision of adequate ventilation, and (3) the restoration and maintenance of circulation.

The American Heart Association (AHA) has reviewed cardiopulmonary resuscitation in pregnant women.[118] The AHA guidelines state that standard algorithms and pharmacologic therapy should be used without modification for pregnancy. Left uterine displacement should be maintained during the resuscitation. If initial resuscitative efforts are unsuccessful, the obstetrician should consider emergency hysterotomy (cesarean delivery), because it may be impossible to resuscitate the mother until adequate venous return is restored. The decision to proceed with delivery depends on several factors, including gestational age, features of the cardiac arrest (e.g., duration of arrest and hypoxemia), and the professional setting (skills of surgeon, anesthesia provider, neonatologist, and presence of support personnel). If gestational age is less than 20 weeks, a hysterotomy may be performed to facilitate maternal resuscitation, but the fetus will not be viable. After 24 weeks' gestation, chances of survival for both the mother and baby may be improved with delivery. The resuscitation team leader should consider emergency delivery as soon as the arrest occurs, because best infant survival has been observed when delivery occurs within 5 minutes of the maternal arrest.[118] Hysterotomy should therefore begin within 4 minutes of the arrest.

KEY POINTS

- Physiologic changes of pregnancy alter neuraxial anatomy; alterations include accentuation of lumbar lordosis, a "softer" ligamentum flavum, and decreased space in the spinal canal due to vascular engorgement of epidural veins.
- Physiologic changes of pregnancy cause a more pronounced response to neuraxial anesthesia–induced sympathetic blockade than is seen in nonpregnant patients. These include higher baseline sympathetic tone and aortocaval compression.
- Pregnant women, particularly those with neuraxial blockade, should not be cared for in the supine position but rather in lateral tilt or in the full lateral position.
- Correct patient positioning, equipment, and technique are important to the success and safety of neuraxial techniques.
- The midline approach is faster and less painful than the paramedian approach to the epidural or subarachnoid space. However, the paramedian approach may allow for the successful identification of the subarachnoid or epidural space in difficult cases.
- Use of a non-cutting ("pencil-point") needle for spinal anesthesia reduces the incidence of post–dural puncture headache.
- Combined spinal-epidural (CSE) anesthesia has the advantages of both spinal anesthesia and epidural anesthesia.
- Approximately 20% to 30% less local anesthetic is required for epidural and spinal anesthesia in pregnant patients than in nonpregnant patients.
- Multiple techniques (e.g., test dose, aspiration, incremental dose injection) should be used to reduce the incidence and risk of unintentional subarachnoid or intravascular injection, because no one technique will completely exclude all cases of malpositioned needles or catheters.
- During maternal cardiac arrest, resuscitation follows normal guidelines but must be performed with the patient in a left lateral tilt position. Early consideration should be given to emergency hysterotomy and evacuation of the uterus.

REFERENCES

1. Bucklin BA, Hawkins JL, Anderson JR, Ullrich FA. Obstetric anesthesia workforce survey: Twenty-year update. Anesthesiology 2005; 103: 645-53.
2. Hogan QH, Prost R, Kulier A, et al. Magnetic resonance imaging of cerebrospinal fluid volume and the influence of body habitus and abdominal pressure. Anesthesiology 1996; 84:1341-9.
3. Richardson MG, Wissler RN. Density of lumbar cerebrospinal fluid in pregnant and nonpregnant humans. Anesthesiology 1996; 85:326-30.
4. Hirabayashi Y, Shimizu R, Fukuda H, et al. Anatomical configuration of the spinal column in the supine position. II. Comparison of pregnant and non-pregnant women. Br J Anaesth 1995; 75:6-8.

5. Reynolds F. Damage to the conus medullaris following spinal anaesthesia. Anaesthesia 2001; 56:238-47.
6. Haines DE, Harkey HL, al-Mefty O. The "subdural" space: A new look at an outdated concept. Neurosurgery 1993; 32:111-20.
7. Hogan QH. Epidural anatomy examined by cryomicrotome section. Influence of age, vertebral level, and disease. Reg Anesth 1996; 21: 395-406.
8. Savolaine ER, Pandya JB, Greenblatt SH, Conover SR. Anatomy of the human lumbar epidural space: New insights using CT-epidurography. Anesthesiology 1988; 68:217-20.
9. Hogan QH. Lumbar epidural anatomy: A new look by cryomicrotome section. Anesthesiology 1991; 75:767-75.
10. Zarzur E. Anatomic studies of the human ligamentum flavum. Anesth Analg 1984; 63:499-502.
11. Chung SS, Lee CS, Kim SH, et al. Effect of low back posture on the morphology of the spinal canal. Skeletal Radiol 2000; 29:217-23.
12. Harrison GR, Clowes NW. The depth of the lumbar epidural space from the skin. Anaesthesia 1985; 40:685-7.
13. Reynolds AF Jr, Roberts PA, Pollay M, Stratemeier PH. Quantitative anatomy of the thoracolumbar epidural space. Neurosurgery 1985; 17:905-7.
14. Senoglu N, Senoglu M, Oksuz H, et al. Landmarks of the sacral hiatus for caudal epidural block: An anatomical study. Br J Anaesth 2005; 95:692-5.
15. Marx GF. Aortocaval compression: Incidence and prevention. Bull N Y Acad Med 1974; 50:443-6.
16. Bieniarz J, Curuchet E, Crottogini JJ, et al. Aortocaval compression by the uterus in late human pregnancy. Am J Obstet Gynecol 1978; 100:203-17.
17. Datta S, Hurley RJ, Naulty JS, et al. Plasma and cerebrospinal fluid progesterone concentrations in pregnant and nonpregnant women. Anesth Analg 1986; 65:950-4.
18. Fink BR. Mechanisms of differential axial blockade in epidural and subarachnoid anesthesia. Anesthesiology 1989; 70:851-8.
19. Burm AG, van Kleef JW, Gladines MP, et al. Spinal anesthesia with hyperbaric lidocaine and bupivacaine: Effects of epinephrine on the plasma concentration profiles. Anesth Analg 1987; 66:1104-8.
20. Horlocker TT, Wedel DJ, Benzon H, et al. Regional anesthesia in the anticoagulated patient: Defining the risks (the second ASRA Consensus Conference on Neuraxial Anesthesia and Anticoagulation). Reg Anesth Pain Med 2003; 28:172-97.
21. Vincent RD, Chestnut DH. Which position is more comfortable for the parturient during identification of the epidural space? Int J Obstet Anesth 1991; 1:9-11.
22. Andrews PJ, Ackerman WE 3rd, Juneja MM. Aortocaval compression in the sitting and lateral decubitus positions during extradural catheter placement in the parturient. Can J Anaesth 1993; 40:320-4.
23. Norris MC, Leighton BL, DeSimone CA, Larijani GE. Lateral position and epidural anesthesia for cesarean section. Anesth Analg 1988; 67:788-90.
24. Reid JA, Thorburn J. Extradural bupivacaine or lignocaine anaesthesia for elective caesarean section: The role of maternal posture. Br J Anaesth 1988; 61:149-53.
25. Norris MC, Dewan DM. Effect of gravity on the spread of extradural anaesthesia for caesarean section. Br J Anaesth 1987; 59:338-41.
26. Grau T, Leipold RW, Conradi R, Martin E. Ultrasound control for presumed difficult epidural puncture. Acta Anaesthesiol Scand 2001; 45:766-71.
27. Willschke H, Marhofer P, Bosenberg A, et al. Epidural catheter placement in children: Comparing a novel approach using ultrasound guidance and a standard loss-of-resistance technique. Br J Anaesth 2006; 97:200-7.
28. Grau T, Leipold RW, Horter J, et al. Colour Doppler imaging of the interspinous and epidural space. Eur J Anaesthesiol 2001; 18:706-12.
29. Arzola C, Davies S, Rofaeel A, Carvalho JC. Ultrasound using the transverse approach to the lumbar spine provides reliable landmarks for labor epidurals. Anesth Analg 2007; 104:1188-92.
30. Khaw KS, Ngan Kee WD, Wong M, et al. Spinal ropivacaine for cesarean delivery: A comparison of hyperbaric and plain solutions. Anesth Analg 2002; 94:680-5.
31. Dahlgren G, Hulstrand C, Jakobsson J, et al. Intrathecal sufentanil, fentanyl, or placebo added to bupivacaine for Cesarean section. Anesth Analg 1997; 85:1288-93.
32. Choi DH, Ahn HJ, Kim MH. Bupivacaine-sparing effect of fentanyl in spinal anesthesia for cesarean delivery. Reg Anesth Pain Med 2000; 25:240-5.
33. Lyons G, Reynolds F. Toxicity and safety of epidural local anaesthetics. Int J Obstet Anesth 2001; 10:259-62.
34. Lyons G, Columb M, Wilson RC, Johnson RV. Epidural pain relief in labour: Potencies of levobupivacaine and racemic bupivacaine. Br J Anaesth 1998; 81:899-901.
35. Beilin Y, Guinn NR, Bernstein HH, et al. Local anesthetics and mode of delivery: Bupivacaine versus ropivacaine versus levobupivacaine. Anesth Analg 2007; 105:756-63.
36. Camorcia M, Capogna G. Epidural levobupivacaine, ropivacaine and bupivacaine in combination with sufentanil in early labour: A randomized trial. Eur J Anaesthesiol 2003; 20:636-9.
37. Lacassie HJ, Habib AS, Lacassie HP, Columb MO. Motor blocking minimum local anesthetic concentrations of bupivacaine, levobupivacaine, and ropivacaine in labor. Reg Anesth Pain Med 2007; 32:323-9.
38. Finucane BT. Ropivacaine cardiac toxicity—not as troublesome as bupivacaine. Can J Anaesth 2005; 52:449-53.
39. Lam DT, Ngan Kee WD, Khaw KS. Extension of epidural blockade in labour for emergency Caesarean section using 2% lidocaine with epinephrine and fentanyl, with or without alkalinisation. Anaesthesia 2001; 56:790-4.
40. Gaiser RR, Cheek TG, Gutsche BB. Epidural lidocaine versus 2-chloroprocaine for fetal distress requiring urgent Cesarean section. Int J Obstet Anesth 1994; 3:208-10.
41. Eisenach JC, Schlairet TJ, Dobson CE, Hood DH. Effect of prior anesthetic solution on epidural morphine analgesia. Anesth Analg 1991; 73:119-23.
42. Corke BC, Carlson CG, Dettbarn WD. The influence of 2-chloroprocaine on the subsequent analgesic potency of bupivacaine. Anesthesiology 1984; 60:25-7.
43. Hess PE, Snowman CE, Hahn CJ, et al. Chloroprocaine may not affect epidural morphine for postcesarean delivery analgesia. J Clin Anesth 2006; 18:29-33.
44. DiFazio CA, Carron H, Grosslight KR, et al. Comparison of pH-adjusted lidocaine solutions for epidural anesthesia. Anesth Analg 1986; 65:760-4.
45. Ackerman WE, Juneja MM, Denson DD, et al. The effect of pH and PCO_2 on epidural analgesia with 2% 2-chloroprocaine. Anesth Analg 1989; 68:593-8.
46. Benson JS. U.S. Food and Drug Administration safety alert: Cauda equina syndrome associated with use of small-bore catheters in continuous spinal anesthesia. AANA J 1992; 60:223.
47. Shutt LE, Valentine SJ, Wee MY, et al. Spinal anaesthesia for caesarean section: Comparison of 22-gauge and 25-gauge Whitacre needles with 26-gauge Quincke needles. Br J Anaesth 1992; 69:589-94.
48. Reina MA, de Leon-Casasola OA, Lopez A, et al. An in vitro study of dural lesions produced by 25-gauge Quincke and Whitacre needles evaluated by scanning electron microscopy. Reg Anesth Pain Med 2000; 25:393-402.
49. Banwell BR, Morley-Forster P, Krause R. Decreased incidence of complications in parturients with the Arrow (FlexTip Plus™) epidural catheter. Can J Anaesth 1998; 45:370-2.
50. Jaime F, Mandell GL, Vallejo MC, Ramanathan S. Uniport soft-tip, open-ended catheters versus multiport firm-tipped close-ended catheters for epidural labor analgesia: A quality assurance study. J Clin Anesth 2000; 12:89-93.
51. Norris MC, Ferrenbach D, Dalman H, et al. Does epinephrine improve the diagnostic accuracy of aspiration during labor epidural analgesia? Anesth Analg 1999; 88:1073-6.
52. D'Angelo R, Foss ML, Livesay CH. A comparison of multiport and uniport epidural catheters in laboring patients. Anesth Analg 1997; 84:1276-9.
53. Kaynar AM, Shankar KB. Epidural infusion: Continuous or bolus (letter)? Anesth Analg 1999; 89:534.

54. Shenouda PE, Cunningham BJ. Assessing the superiority of saline versus air for use in the epidural loss of resistance technique: A literature review. Reg Anesth Pain Med 2003; 28:48-53.
55. Beilin Y, Arnold I, Telfeyan C, et al. Quality of analgesia when air versus saline is used for identification of the epidural space in the parturient. Reg Anesth Pain Med 2000; 25:596-9.
56. Aida S, Taga K, Yamakura T, et al. Headache after attempted epidural block: The role of intrathecal air. Anesthesiology 1998; 88:76-81.
57. Verniquet AJ. Vessel puncture with epidural catheters: Experience in obstetric patients. Anaesthesia 1980; 35:660-2.
58. Mannion D, Walker R, Clayton K. Extradural vein puncture—an avoidable complication. Anaesthesia 1991; 46:585-7.
59. Rolbin SH, Halpern SH, Braude BM, et al. Fluid through the epidural needle does not reduce complications of epidural catheter insertion. Can J Anaesth 1990; 37:337-40.
60. Hamilton CL, Riley ET, Cohen SE. Changes in the position of epidural catheters associated with patient movement. Anesthesiology 1997; 86:778-84.
61. D'Angelo R, Berkebile BL, Gerancher JC. Prospective examination of epidural catheter insertion. Anesthesiology 1996; 84:88-93.
62. Tyagi A, Kumar R, Bhattacharya A, Sethi AK. Filters in anaesthesia and intensive care. Anaesth Intensive Care 2003; 31:418-33.
63. Charlton GA, Lawes EG. The effect of micropore filters on the aspiration test in epidural analgesia. Anaesthesia 1991; 46:573-5.
64. Westphal M, Hohage H, Buerkle H, et al. Adsorption of sufentanil to epidural filters and catheters. Eur J Anaesthesiol 2003; 20:124-6.
65. Van de Velde M, Van Schoubroeck D, Jani J, et al. Combined spinal-epidural anesthesia for cesarean delivery: Dose-dependent effects of hyperbaric bupivacaine on maternal hemodynamics. Anesth Analg 2006; 103:187-90.
66. Choi DH, Kim JA, Chung IS. Comparison of combined spinal epidural anesthesia and epidural anesthesia for cesarean section. Acta Anaesthesiol Scand 2000; 44:214-9.
67. Collis RE, Davies DW, Aveling W. Randomised comparison of combined spinal-epidural and standard epidural analgesia in labour. Lancet 1995; 345:1413-6.
68. Simmons S, Cyna A, Dennis A, Hughes D. Combined spinal-epidural versus epidural analgesia in labour. Cochrane Database Syst Rev 2007; (3):CD003401.
69. Norris MC. Are combined spinal-epidural catheters reliable? Int J Obstet Anesth 2000; 9:3-6.
70. Pan PH, Bogard TD, Owen MD. Incidence and characteristics of failures in obstetric neuraxial analgesia and anesthesia: A retrospective analysis of 19,259 deliveries. Int J Obstet Anesth 2004; 13:227-33.
71. Cook TM. Combined spinal-epidural techniques. Anaesthesia 2000; 55:42-64.
72. Riley ET, Hamilton CL, Ratner EF, Cohen SE. A comparison of the 24-gauge Sprotte and Gertie Marx spinal needles for combined spinal-epidural analgesia during labor. Anesthesiology 2002; 97:574-7.
73. Choi PT, Galinski SE, Takeuchi L, et al. PDPH is a common complication of neuraxial blockade in parturients: A meta-analysis of obstetrical studies. Can J Anaesth 2003; 50:460-9.
74. Norris MC, Leighton BL, DeSimone CA. Needle bevel direction and headache after inadvertent dural puncture. Anesthesiology 1989; 70:729-31.
75. Richardson MG, Wissler RN. The effects of needle bevel orientation during epidural catheter insertion in laboring parturients. Anesth Analg 1999; 88:352-6.
76. Angle PJ, Kronberg JE, Thompson DE, et al. Dural tissue trauma and cerebrospinal fluid leak after epidural needle puncture. Anesthesiology 2003; 99:1376-82.
77. Huffnagle SL, Norris MC, Arkoosh VA, et al. The influence of epidural needle bevel orientation on spread of sensory blockade in the laboring parturient. Anesth Analg 1998; 87:326-30.
78. Rutter SV, Shields F, Broadbent CR, et al. Management of accidental dural puncture in labour with intrathecal catheters: An analysis of 10 years' experience. Int J Obstet Anesth 2001; 10:177-81.
79. Paech M, Banks S, Gurrin L. An audit of accidental dural puncture during epidural insertion of a Tuohy needle in obstetric patients. Int J Obstet Anesth 2001; 10:162-7.
80. Ayad S, Demian Y, Narouze SN, Tetzlaff JE. Subarachnoid catheter placement after wet tap for analgesia in labor: Influence on the risk of headache in obstetric patients. Reg Anesth Pain Med 2003; 28:512-5.
81. Hodgkinson R. Total spinal block after epidural injection into an interspace adjacent to an inadvertent dural perforation. Anesthesiology 1981; 55:593-5.
82. Leach A, Smith GB. Subarachnoid spread of epidural local anaesthetic following dural puncture. Anaesthesia 1988; 43:671-4.
83. Bernards CM, Kopacz DJ, Michel MZ. Effect of needle puncture on morphine and lidocaine flux through the spinal meninges of the monkey in vitro: Implications for combined spinal-epidural anesthesia. Anesthesiology 1994; 80:853-8.
84. Faure E, Moreno R, Thisted R. Incidence of postdural puncture headache in morbidly obese parturients (letter). Reg Anesth 1994; 19:361-3.
85. Scavone BM, Wong CA, Sullivan JT, et al. Efficacy of a prophylactic epidural blood patch in preventing post dural puncture headache in parturients after inadvertent dural puncture. Anesthesiology 2004; 101:1422-7.
86. Bahar M, Chanimov M, Cohen ML, et al. The lateral recumbent head-down position decreases the incidence of epidural venous puncture during catheter insertion in obese parturients. Can J Anaesth 2004; 51:577-80.
87. Moore DC, Batra MS. The components of an effective test dose prior to epidural block. Anesthesiology 1981; 55:693-6.
88. Hood DD, Dewan DM, James FM 3rd. Maternal and fetal effects of epinephrine in gravid ewes. Anesthesiology 1986; 64:610-3.
89. Chestnut DH, Weiner CP, Martin JG, et al. Effect of intravenous epinephrine on uterine artery blood flow velocity in the pregnant guinea pig. Anesthesiology 1986; 65:633-6.
90. Leighton BL, Norris MC, Sosis M, et al. Limitations of epinephrine as a marker of intravascular injection in laboring women. Anesthesiology 1987; 66:688-91.
91. Cartwright PD, McCarroll SM, Antzaka C. Maternal heart rate changes with a plain epidural test dose. Anesthesiology 1986; 65:226-8.
92. Chestnut DH, Owen CL, Brown CK, et al. Does labor affect the variability of maternal heart rate during induction of epidural anesthesia? Anesthesiology 1988; 68:622-5.
93. Chadwick HS, Benedetti C, Ready LB, Williams V. Epinephrine-containing test doses—don't throw the baby out with the bath water. Anesthesiology 1987; 66:571.
94. Birnbach DJ, Chestnut DH. The epidural test dose in obstetric patients: Has it outlived its usefulness (editorial)? Anesth Analg 1999; 88:971-2.
95. Lee LA, Posner KL, Domino KB, et al. Injuries associated with regional anesthesia in the 1980s and 1990s: A closed claims analysis. Anesthesiology 2004; 101:143-52.
96. Leighton BL, DeSimone CA, Norris MC, Chayen B. Isoproterenol is an effective marker of intravenous injection in laboring women. Anesthesiology 1989; 71:206-9.
97. Marcus MA, Vertommen JD, Van Aken H, et al. Hemodynamic effects of intravenous isoproterenol versus saline in the parturient. Anesth Analg 1997; 84:1113-6.
98. Leighton BL, Norris MC, DeSimone CA, et al. The air test as a clinically useful indicator of intravenously placed epidural catheters. Anesthesiology 1990; 73:610-3.
99. Yoshii WY, Miller M, Rottman RL, et al. Fentanyl for epidural intravascular test dose in obstetrics. Reg Anesth 1993; 18:296-9.
100. Morris GF, Gore-Hickman W, Lang SA, Yip RW. Can parturients distinguish between intravenous and epidural fentanyl? Can J Anaesth 1994; 41:667-72.
101. Abraham RA, Harris AP, Maxwell LG, Kaplow S. The efficacy of 1.5% lidocaine with 7.5% dextrose and epinephrine as an epidural test dose for obstetrics. Anesthesiology 1986; 64:116-9.
102. Van Zundert A, Vaes L, Soetens M, et al. Every dose given in epidural analgesia for vaginal delivery can be a test dose. Anesthesiology 1987; 67:436-40.

103. Colonna-Romano P, Padolina R, Lingaraju N, Braitman LE. Diagnostic accuracy of an intrathecal test dose in epidural analgesia. Can J Anaesth 1994; 41:572-4.
104. Mulroy M, Glosten B. The epinephrine test dose in obstetrics: Note the limitations. Anesth Analg 1998; 86:923-5.
105. McLean BY, Rottman RL, Kotelko DM. Failure of multiple test doses and techniques to detect intravascular migration of an epidural catheter. Anesth Analg 1992; 74:454-6.
106. Chadwick HS, Posner K, Caplan RA, et al. A comparison of obstetric and nonobstetric anesthesia malpractice claims. Anesthesiology 1991; 74:242-9.
107. Beilin Y, Bernstein HH, Zucker-Pinchoff B. The optimal distance that a multiorifice epidural catheter should be threaded into the epidural space. Anesth Analg 1995; 81:301-4.
108. Beilin Y, Zahn J, Bernstein HH, et al. Treatment of incomplete analgesia after placement of an epidural catheter and administration of local anesthetic for women in labor. Anesthesiology 1998; 88:1502-6.
109. Gielen MJ, Slappendel R, Merx JL. Asymmetric onset of sympathetic blockade in epidural anaesthesia shows no relation to epidural catheter position. Acta Anaesthesiol Scand 1991; 35:81-4.
110. Hogan Q. Distribution of solution in the epidural space: Examination by cryomicrotome section. Reg Anesth Pain Med 2002; 27:150-6.
111. Rigler ML, Drasner K. Distribution of catheter-injected local anesthetic in a model of the subarachnoid space. Anesthesiology 1991; 75:684-92.
112. Drasner K, Rigler ML. Repeat injection after a "failed spinal": At times, a potentially unsafe practice (letter). Anesthesiology 1991; 75:713-4.
113. Furst SR, Reisner LS. Risk of high spinal anesthesia following failed epidural block for cesarean delivery. J Clin Anesth 1995; 7:71-4.
114. Schlake PT, Peleman RR, Winnie AP. Separation of the hub from the shaft of a disposable epidural needle. Anesthesiology 1988; 68:611-3.
115. Moore D. Complications of Regional Anesthesia. Springfield, IL, CC Thomas, 1955:242-6.
116. Moore DC, Artru AA, Kelly WA, Jenkins D. Use of computed tomography to locate a sheared epidural catheter. Anesth Analg 1987; 66:795-6.
117. Langevin PB, Gravenstein N, Langevin SO, Gulig PA. Epidural catheter reconnection: Safe and unsafe practice. Anesthesiology 1996; 85:883-8.
118. Cardiac arrest associated with pregnancy. Circulation 2005; 112:IV-150-3.

Local Anesthetics and Opioids

Alan C. Santos, M.D., M.P.H.
Brenda A. Bucklin, M.D.

Local anesthetics and opioids are often used for pain relief in obstetric practice. Local anesthetics may be used for infiltration anesthesia, peripheral (pudendal) nerve block, or neuraxial block, whereas opioids are administered both systemically and neuraxially. The physiologic changes that occur during pregnancy may affect the pharmacology of both local anesthetics and opioids. In turn, these analgesic drugs may have effects on the mother and the fetus.

LOCAL ANESTHETICS

Molecular Structure

All local anesthetic molecules except cocaine contain a desaturated carbon ring (aromatic portion) and a tertiary amine connected by an alkyl chain (Figure 13-1). The intermediate alkyl chain, by virtue of its ester or amide linkage, is the basis for the classification of local anesthetics as **amino-esters** (which are hydrolyzed by pseudocholinesterase) and **amino-amides** (which undergo hepatic microsomal metabolism) (Table 13-1). For the esters, the aromatic ring, which renders the molecule lipid soluble, is a derivative of benzoic acid. For the amides, the aromatic ring is a homologue of aniline. The tertiary-amine portion acts as a proton acceptor, which makes local anesthetics behave as weak bases. In its quaternary (i.e., "protonated") form, the terminal amine also is the water-soluble portion. The Henderson-Hasselbalch equation predicts the relative proportions of local anesthetic that exist in the ionized and un-ionized form. The higher the pK_B (base dissociation constant) relative to physiologic pH, the smaller the proportion of drug that exists in the un-ionized form. All amide local anesthetics (with the exception of lidocaine) exist as stereoisomers because of the presence of an asymmetric carbon adjacent to the terminal amine.

Clinical formulations of local anesthetics are prepared as hydrochloride salts to increase their solubility in water. These solutions are usually acidic (i.e., pH of 4 to 6) to enhance formation of the water-soluble quaternary amine and to prevent oxidation of the epinephrine present in epinephrine-containing solutions.

CHIRALITY

In 1984, the United States Food and Drug Administration (FDA) proscribed the use of the highest concentration of bupivacaine (0.75%) in pregnant women because of concerns about bupivacaine cardiotoxicity (see later). Subsequently, many anesthesiologists perceived a need for an alternative amide local anesthetic with the beneficial blocking properties of bupivacaine but a greater margin of safety. With the exception of lidocaine, amide local anesthetics are known as **chiral compounds** because they have a single asymmetric carbon adjacent to the amino group and thus exist in isomeric forms that are mirror images of each other. The direction in which the isomers rotate

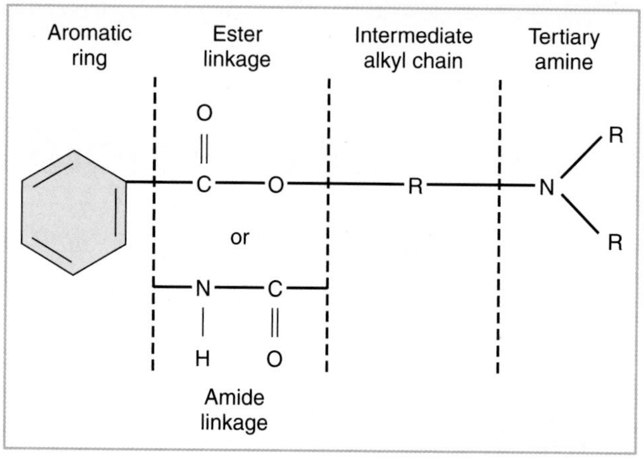

FIGURE 13-1 Structure of the molecule of a local anesthetic. R, alkyl group. (Modified from Santos AC, Pedersen H. Local anesthetics in obstetrics. In Petrie RH, editor. Perinatal Pharmacology. Cambridge, MA, Blackwell Scientific, 1989:373.)

polarized light distinguishes them as either dextrorotary (D) or levorotary (L) isomers. This distinction is important, because individual isomers of the same drug may have different biologic effects. As a rule, the levorotary isomer of a drug has greater vasoconstrictor activity and a longer duration of action but less potential for systemic toxicity than the dextrorotary form.[1]

The reduction in systemic toxicity observed with administration of the levorotary isomers may be both drug and concentration dependent. For example, one study in isolated guinea pig hearts noted that bupivacaine isomers lengthened atrioventricular conduction time more than ropivacaine isomers did. In contrast to other measured variables, "atrioventricular conduction time showed evident stereoselectivity" for bupivacaine at the lowest concentration studied (0.5 μM) but only at much higher concentrations for ropivacaine (greater than 30 μM).[2]

In the past, single-isomer formulations were costly to produce, and for that reason, local anesthetics used clinically have contained a racemic mixture of both the dextrorotary and levorotary forms of the drug. However, with improved techniques of selective extraction, two commercially available single-isomer formulations of local anesthetic are now available, ropivacaine and levobupivacaine. **Levobupivacaine** is the levorotary isomer of bupivacaine. **Ropivacaine** is a homologue of mepivacaine and bupivacaine, but unlike these other local anesthetics, it is formulated as a single levorotary isomer rather than as a racemic mixture. A propyl group on the pipechol ring distinguishes ropivacaine from bupivacaine (which has a butyl group) and mepivacaine (which has a methyl group).[3] Thus, it is not surprising that the physicochemical characteristics of ropivacaine are intermediate between those of mepivacaine and bupivacaine.

Mechanism of Action

At rest, the interior of a nerve cell is negatively charged in relation to its exterior. This resting potential of 60 to 90 mV exists because the concentration of sodium in the extracellular space greatly exceeds that in the intracellular space. The converse is true for potassium. Excitation results in the opening of membrane channels, which allows sodium ions to flow freely down their concentration gradient into the cell interior. Thus the electrical potential within the nerve cell becomes less negative until, at the critical threshold, rapid depolarization occurs. This depolarization is needed to initiate the same sequence of events in adjacent membrane segments and for propagation of the action potential. Thereafter, sodium channels close and the membrane once again becomes impermeable to the influx of sodium. The negative resting membrane potential is reestablished as sodium is removed from the cell by active transport. At the same time, potassium passively accumulates within the resting cell.

Interference with sodium-ion conductance appears to be the mechanism by which local anesthetics reversibly inhibit the propagation of the action potential. Four major theories attempt to explain this effect. The most prominent hypothesis is that the local anesthetic interacts with receptors in

TABLE 13-1 Physicochemical Characteristics and Fetal-Maternal (F/M) Blood Concentration Ratios at Delivery for Commonly Used Local Anesthetic Agents

	Molecular Weight (Base) (Da)	pK_B	Lipid Solubility*	% Protein Bound	F/M Ratio
Esters:					
2-Chloroprocaine	271	8.9	0.14	—	—
Tetracaine	264	8.6	4.1	—	—
Amides:					
Lidocaine	234	7.9	2.9	64	0.5-0.7
Mepivacaine	246	7.8	0.8	78	0.7
Etidocaine	276	7.7	141	94	0.2-0.3
Bupivacaine	288	8.2	28	96	0.2-0.4
Ropivacaine	274	8.0	3	90-95	0.2

*N-heptane/pH = 7.4 buffer.

Modified from Santos AC, Pedersen H. Local anesthetics in obstetrics. In Petrie RH, editor. Perinatal Pharmacology. Cambridge, MA, Blackwell Scientific, 1989:375.

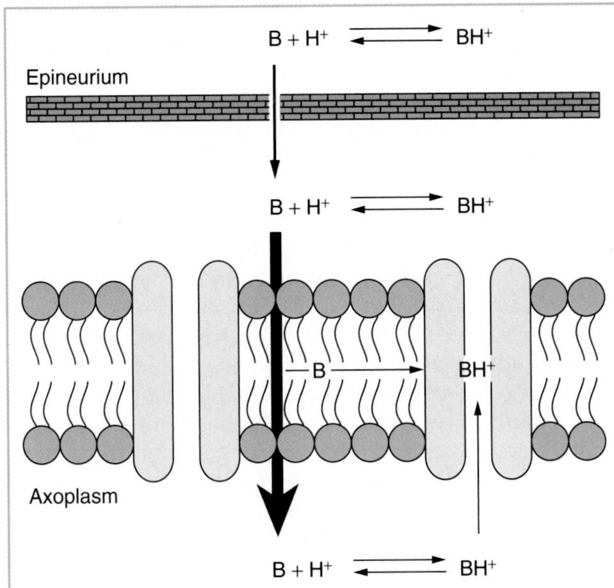

FIGURE 13-2 Local anesthetic access to the sodium channel. The uncharged molecule (B) diffuses most easily across the lipid membrane and interacts with the sodium channel at an intramembranous site. The charged molecule (BH^+) gains access to a specific receptor on the sodium channel in the intracellular space. (Modified from Carpenter RL, Mackey DC. Local anesthetics. In Barash PG, Cullen BF, Stoelting RK, editors. Clinical Anesthesia. Philadelphia, Lippincott, 1992:510.)

the nerve cell membrane that control channels involved in sodium conductance.[4] There may be more than one site at which local anesthetics bind to sodium-channel receptors (Figure 13-2).

The Meyer-Overton theory offers a second explanation for local anesthetic action. This hypothesis suggests that the lipid-soluble portion of the local anesthetic molecule expands the cell membrane and interferes with rapid sodium conductance. A third possibility is that local anesthetics may alter the membrane surface charge, a change that would inhibit propagation of the action potential. Fourth, local anesthetics may displace calcium from sites that control sodium conductance.

Both the un-ionized and ionized forms of a local anesthetic are involved in pharmacologic activity. The un-ionized base, which is lipid soluble, diffuses through the cell membrane, whereas the charged form is much more active in blocking the sodium channel.

Pharmacodynamics

Pregnant women typically require smaller doses of local anesthetic than do nonpregnant patients.[5] This difference has been attributed to enhanced spread of local anesthetic due to epidural venous engorgement. However, mechanical effects alone do not account for the observation that the spread of epidural analgesia in early pregnancy is similar to that in pregnant women at term.[5,6] In fact, pregnancy may also enhance neuronal sensitivity to local anesthetics. For example, pregnancy increases median nerve susceptibility to lidocaine.[7] *In vitro* studies demonstrated that the onset of neural blockade was faster, and lower concentrations of bupivacaine were required to block vagal fibers, in pregnant rabbits than in nonpregnant rabbits.[8]

Hormonal and biochemical changes may be responsible for the greater susceptibility to neural blockade during pregnancy. For example, one study demonstrated an enhanced effect of bupivacaine in isolated vagus fibers from nonpregnant, ovariectomized rabbits who had received long-term (4 days) but not short-term exposure to progesterone.[9] A higher pH and lower bicarbonate and total carbon dioxide content have been demonstrated in cerebrospinal fluid (CSF) from women undergoing cesarean delivery than in CSF from age-matched nonpregnant controls. A higher pH increases the proportion of local anesthetic that exists as the base form and facilitates diffusion of the drug across nerve membranes.[6]

Pharmacokinetics

Pregnancy is associated with progressive physiologic adaptations that may influence drug disposition (see Chapter 2). However, it is difficult to predict with certainty the effects of pregnancy on the pharmacokinetics of an individual drug.

2-CHLOROPROCAINE

2-Chloroprocaine is hydrolyzed rapidly by plasma pseudocholinesterase to chloroaminobenzoic acid and H_2O. The *in vitro* half-life of 2-chloroprocaine in sera from men is less than 15 seconds.[10] Although pregnancy is associated with a 30% to 40% decrease in pseudocholinesterase activity, the half-life of 2-chloroprocaine in maternal plasma *in vitro* is 11 to 21 seconds. After epidural injection, the half-life of 2-chloroprocaine in the mother ranges from 1.5 to 6.4 minutes.[11] The longer half-life after epidural administration results from continued absorption of the drug from the injection site. Administration of 2-chloroprocaine to patients with low pseudocholinesterase activity may result in prolonged local anesthetic effect and a greater potential for systemic toxicity.[12]

LIDOCAINE

The volume of the central compartment and the volume of distribution are greater in pregnant ewes than in nonpregnant ewes.[13,14] Bloedow et al.[14] observed that the total body clearance of lidocaine was similar in the two groups of animals. They concluded that the elimination half-life of lidocaine, which depends on the balance between volume of distribution and clearance, was longer in pregnant ewes.[14] In contrast, Santos et al.[13] concluded that the elimination half-life of lidocaine was similar in the two groups of sheep because the total body clearance of the drug was greater in pregnant animals than in nonpregnant animals. This discrepancy could result from differences in the complexity of the surgical preparation and the allowed recovery period. In pregnant women, the elimination half-life of lidocaine after epidural injection is approximately 114 minutes.[15]

Lidocaine is metabolized to two active compounds, monoethylglycinexylidide (MEGX) and glycinexylidide (GX). Monoethylglycinexylidide can be detected in maternal plasma within 10 to 20 minutes after neuraxial injection of lidocaine, whereas glycinexylidide can be detected within 1 hour of epidural injection but rarely after subarachnoid injection.[16,17] Urinary excretion of unchanged lidocaine is negligible in sheep (i.e., less than 2% of the administered dose) and is not affected by pregnancy.[13]

The physiologic changes that occur during pregnancy are progressive. However, little information is available about the pharmacokinetics of local anesthetics before term. In one study, total clearance of lidocaine was similar at 119 and 138 days' gestation in gravid ewes (term is 148 days).[18]

Lidocaine is predominantly bound to alpha-1-acid glycoprotein (AAG) in plasma.[19] Pregnancy leads to a decreased concentration of AAG; thus, the free plasma fraction of lidocaine is higher in term pregnant women than in nonpregnant controls.[19] The increase in the free fraction of lidocaine occurs early in gestation and is progressive.[20]

BUPIVACAINE

Bupivacaine is the most commonly used local anesthetic in obstetric anesthesia practice. At least two studies compared the pharmacokinetics of bupivacaine after epidural administration in pregnant and nonpregnant women.[21,22] The absorption rate, the area under the concentration-time curve, and the elimination half-life (12 to 13 hours) were similar in the two groups. The elimination half-life of bupivacaine after epidural administration is much longer than that reported after intravenous injection, largely because the drug is continuously absorbed over time from the epidural space.

After intravenous injection, the volume of distribution of bupivacaine is lower in pregnant sheep than in nonpregnant sheep.[18,23] In contrast, ovine pregnancy is associated with a greater volume of distribution of lidocaine.[13,14] The differences in gestational effects on the volume of distribution of the two local anesthetics may result from the greater binding of bupivacaine to plasma proteins during gestation (whereas the converse occurs with lidocaine).[23] In one study, urinary excretion of unchanged bupivacaine was not affected by pregnancy and was less than 1% of the administered dose.[21] Nonetheless, low concentrations of bupivacaine may be detected in the urine of pregnant women for as long as 3 days after delivery.[24]

Bupivacaine undergoes dealkylation in the liver to 2,6-pipecolyxylidide (PPX). After epidural injection of bupivacaine for cesarean delivery, PPX was detected in maternal plasma within 5 minutes and remained detectable for as long as 24 hours.[24] With the lower doses required for labor analgesia, PPX was found only if the block was maintained with multiple reinjections during a period that exceeded 4 hours.[25] Pregnancy may affect metabolism of bupivacaine.[21] For example, pregnant women have higher serum PPX concentrations, but the unconjugated 4-hydroxy metabolite is not produced in significant amounts. The reason for this finding is unclear but may be related to the effects of hormonal changes on hepatic enzyme systems. Both progesterone and estradiol are competitive inhibitors of microsomal oxidases, whereas reductive enzymes are induced by progesterone.[23]

Bupivacaine is bound extensively to AAG and albumin.[26] This protein binding is reduced during late pregnancy in humans.[27]

ROPIVACAINE

Pregnant sheep have a smaller volume of distribution and a slower clearance of ropivacaine than nonpregnant animals.[23] However, the relationship between volume of distribution and clearance is such that the elimination half-life is similar in pregnant and nonpregnant animals.

After intravenous injection in laboratory animals, the elimination half-life of ropivacaine is shorter than that of bupivacaine.[23,28] Similar findings have been described after intravenous injection in nonpregnant human volunteers.[29] The shorter elimination half-life of ropivacaine has been attributed to a faster clearance and a shorter mean residence time than those for bupivacaine.[23]

Peak plasma concentration (C_{max}) measurements after epidural administration of 0.5% ropivacaine and 0.5% bupivacaine for cesarean delivery are similar (1.3 μg/mL and 1.1 μg/mL, respectively).[30] The elimination half-life of ropivacaine is 5.2 ± 0.6 hours, which is shorter than that for bupivacaine, at 10.9 ± 1.1 hours. No difference in clearance between the two drugs has been noted.

Like bupivacaine, ropivacaine is metabolized by hepatic microsomal cytochrome P-450. The major metabolite is PPX, and minor metabolites are 3′- and 4′-hydroxy-ropivacaine.[31]

Ropivacaine is highly bound (approximately 92%) to plasma proteins but less so than bupivacaine (96%).[32] Indeed, at plasma concentrations occurring during epidural anesthesia for cesarean delivery, the free fraction of ropivacaine is almost twice that of bupivacaine.[30] In sheep, pregnancy is associated with a greater binding of ropivacaine (and bupivacaine) to plasma proteins.[23] In pregnant women undergoing epidural analgesia, the free fraction of ropivacaine decreases as the concentration of AAG increases, up to the point at which the receptors are saturated.[33] However, there is little correlation between the free fraction and umbilical cord blood levels of ropivacaine at delivery.[33]

EFFECT OF HISTAMINE (H_2)-RECEPTOR ANTAGONISTS

Histamine (H_2)-receptor antagonists (e.g., cimetidine, ranitidine, famotidine) are administered to increase gastric pH and reduce the parturient's risk of aspiration. Drug disposition may be affected by binding to hepatic cytochrome P-450, thereby reducing hepatic blood flow and renal clearance, especially with cimetidine. However, short-term administration of H_2-receptor antagonists does not alter the pharmacokinetics of amide local anesthetics in pregnant women.[34,35]

EFFECTS OF PREECLAMPSIA

Pathophysiologic changes associated with preeclampsia (e.g., reduced hepatic blood flow, abnormal liver function, decreased intravascular volume) may also affect maternal blood concentrations of local anesthetics (see Chapter 45). For example, Ramanathan et al.[36] found that total body clearance of lidocaine after epidural injection was significantly lower in preeclamptic women than in normotensive women; however, the elimination half-life of lidocaine was similar in the two groups. Nonetheless, decreased clearance may result in greater drug accumulation with repeated injections of lidocaine in women with preeclampsia. In contrast, long-acting amides have a relatively low hepatic extraction, and changes in liver blood flow with preeclampsia may have less effect on the metabolic clearance.

EFFECT OF DIURNAL VARIATION

Local anesthetic activity may exhibit chronobiology. For example, in one study, the duration of action of epidural bupivacaine was approximately 25% longer when it was administered between 7:00 AM and 7:00 PM than between 7:00 PM and 7:00 AM.[37]

Toxicity

Systemic absorption or intravascular injection of a local anesthetic may result in systemic toxicity. Toxicity most often involves the central nervous system (CNS), but cardiovascular toxicity also may occur. Less common are tissue toxicity and hypersensitivity reactions.

CENTRAL NERVOUS SYSTEM TOXICITY

The severity of CNS effects is proportional to the blood concentration of local anesthetic. This relationship is well described for lidocaine (Figure 13-3). Initially, the patient may complain of numbness of the tongue, tinnitus, or lightheadedness. At high plasma concentrations, convulsions occur because of a selective blockade of central inhibitory neurons that leads to increased CNS excitation.[38] At still higher concentrations, generalized CNS depression or coma may result from reversible blockade of both inhibitory and excitatory neuronal pathways. Finally, depression of the brainstem and cardiorespiratory centers may occur.

The relative toxicity of a local anesthetic correlates with its potency. For lidocaine, etidocaine, and bupivacaine, the ratio of the mean cumulative doses that cause convulsions in dogs is approximately 4:2:1, which is similar to their relative anesthetic potencies.[39] The same relative toxicity was demonstrated in human volunteers.[40] Local anesthetics may be ranked in order of decreasing CNS toxicity as follows: bupivacaine, tetracaine, etidocaine, lidocaine, mepivacaine, and 2-chloroprocaine.[41]

Other factors (e.g., the speed of injection) may affect CNS toxicity. In humans, the mean dose of etidocaine that elicited signs of CNS toxicity was lower during a 20-mg/min infusion than during a 10 mg/min infusion.[40] The seizure threshold also may be affected by metabolic factors. For example, in cats, an increase in $Paco_2$ or a decrease in pH results in a reduction in the seizure-dose threshold for local anesthetics. Respiratory acidosis may result in delivery of more drug to the brain; alternatively, respiratory acidosis may result in "ion trapping" of the local anesthetic and/or an increase in the unbound fraction of drug available for pharmacologic effect.[42-44]

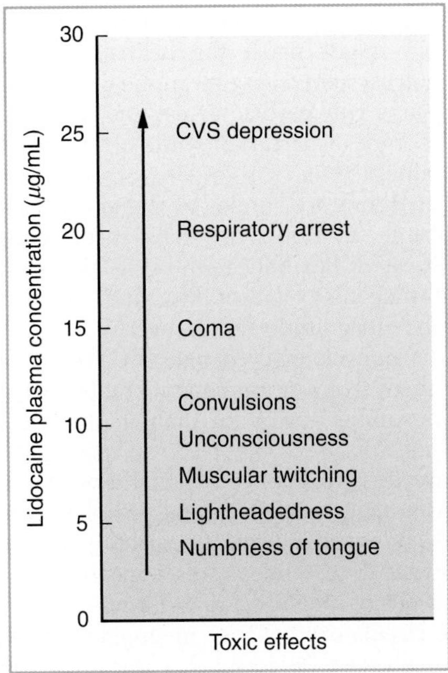

FIGURE 13-3 Signs and symptoms of systemic toxicity with increasing lidocaine concentrations. CVS, cardiovascular system. (Modified from Carpenter RL, Mackey DC. Local anesthetics. In Barash PG, Cullen BF, Stoelting RK, editors. Clinical Anesthesia. Philadelphia, Lippincott, 1992:527.)

CARDIOVASCULAR TOXICITY

The cardiovascular system is much more resistant than the CNS to the toxic effects of local anesthetics. Severe, direct cardiovascular depression is rare, especially in association with the use of lidocaine and mepivacaine. Prompt administration of oxygen and, if necessary, initiation of ventilatory and circulatory support usually prevent cardiac arrest after unintentional intravenous injection of these drugs.[45] Progressive depression of myocardial function and profound vasodilation occur only at extremely high plasma concentrations of lidocaine or mepivacaine.[45] In contrast, the more potent amide local anesthetics (i.e., bupivacaine, etidocaine) have a more narrow margin of safety, expressed as the ratio between the dose (or plasma concentration) required to produce cardiovascular collapse and the dose (or plasma concentration) required to produce convulsions.[45] A partial explanation is the fact that supraconvulsant doses of bupivacaine (but not of lidocaine or mepivacaine) precipitate lethal ventricular arrhythmias.[46-48] These arrhythmias may be caused by exaggerated electrophysiologic effects (e.g., depression of ventricular conduction) out of proportion to bupivacaine's anesthetic potency.[49]

Two theories have been proposed to explain why malignant ventricular arrhythmias occur with bupivacaine but not with lidocaine. Both bupivacaine and lidocaine rapidly block cardiac sodium channels during systole, but bupivacaine dissociates from these channels during diastole at a much slower rate than lidocaine.[49] Thus, at physiologic heart rates, the diastolic period is of sufficient duration for lidocaine to dissociate from sodium channels, whereas a bupivacaine block becomes intensified. This difference makes bupivacaine much more potent than lidocaine in depressing conduction and inducing reentrant-type ventricular arrhythmias. Alternatively, other investigators have suggested that high concentrations of local anesthetic in the brainstem may lead to systemic hypotension, bradycardia, and ventricular arrhythmias.[50] These effects occur more commonly with bupivacaine because of its high lipid solubility, which facilitates transfer across the blood-brain barrier. An echocardiographic study in anesthetized dogs suggested that bolus injection of bupivacaine results in systolic dysfunction, especially involving the right ventricle, which precedes the occurrence of arrhythmias.[51]

SYSTEMIC TOXICITY OF ROPIVACAINE AND LEVOBUPIVACAINE

In perfused preparations of myocardium, ropivacaine is intermediate between bupivacaine and lidocaine in its depressant effect on cardiac excitation and conduction as well as in its potential to induce reentrant-type ventricular arrhythmias.[32] In dogs, the margin of safety between convulsive or lethal doses and plasma concentrations of drug is greater for ropivacaine than for bupivacaine but less than that for lidocaine.[52] The arrhythmogenicity of ropivacaine in pigs also is intermediate between that of lidocaine and bupivacaine.[53] In sheep, the ratio of fatal doses of bupivacaine, ropivacaine, and lidocaine is 1:2:9.[54] Ropivacaine was found to cause fewer CNS symptoms and was 25% less toxic than bupivacaine (as defined by the doses and plasma concentrations that were tolerated) when administered to healthy male volunteers.[55]

Most studies comparing the systemic toxicity of ropivacaine and bupivacaine have used equal doses of each, and, therefore, cannot resolve the controversy as to whether ropivacaine truly is less cardiotoxic or merely less potent than bupivacaine. This issue would be of concern only if larger doses of ropivacaine than bupivacaine were required to produce comparable regional blocks. Indeed, one study suggested that the minimum local anesthetic concentration (MLAC) of ropivacaine in women undergoing epidural analgesia during labor is almost twice that for bupivacaine (see later).[56] If this suggestion is true, the need for a larger dose of ropivacaine could negate the expected benefits of its apparently wider margin of safety. Currently, this controversy remains unresolved. However, results from one laboratory study showed that ropivacaine produces less cardiotoxicity than bupivacaine, even when given at equipotent doses.[57]

Long-acting amide local anesthetics—even the newer drugs—are very potent and may cause cardiac arrest with a misplaced injection or relative overdose. Indeed, several cardiac arrests have been reported with the use of ropivacaine,[58,59] including one in a woman undergoing a cesarean delivery with epidural anesthesia.[60] In contrast to that induced by bupivacaine,[61] resuscitation from a cardiac arrest induced by ropivacaine may be successful more often than not.[58-60]

Evidence suggests that levobupivacaine causes fewer arrhythmias than the racemic drug. Valenzuela et al.[62] demonstrated that levobupivacaine caused less inhibition of inactivated sodium channels than either the dextrorotary or racemic drug. In comparison with dextrorotary and racemic bupivacaine, levobupivacaine resulted in less QRS widening and a lower frequency of malignant ventricular arrhythmias in isolated, perfused rabbit hearts.[63] Similarly, levobupivacaine produced less second-degree heart block and atrioventricular conduction delay than the other two forms of the drug in isolated perfused guinea pig hearts.[2]

In laboratory animals, the systemic toxicity of levobupivacaine is intermediate between that of bupivacaine and ropivacaine.[64] Unlike that of ropivacaine,[56] the MLAC of epidural levobupivacaine during labor is similar to that of bupivacaine.[65] Unfortunately, no single study has compared the MLAC of all three drugs. Altogether, published data and clinical experience suggest that any benefits from the reduction in risk of systemic toxicity with levobupivacaine are not obtained at the expense of efficacy. Like ropivacaine, levobupivacaine may cause cardiac arrest but is associated with a better response to resuscitation than racemic bupivacaine.[66]

EFFECTS OF PREGNANCY ON SYSTEMIC TOXICITY

Central Nervous System Toxicity

It is unclear whether pregnancy lowers the seizure threshold for amide local anesthetic agents. In one study, seizures occurred at lower doses of bupivacaine, levobupivacaine, and ropivacaine in pregnant ewes than in nonpregnant ewes.[64] However, the difference was small (10% to 15%) and probably of negligible clinical significance. In studies in sheep and rats, pregnancy did not reduce the doses required to cause convulsions after intravenous administration of mepivacaine, bupivacaine, or lidocaine.[48,67] Magnesium sulfate, which is frequently used in obstetric practice, does not affect the seizure-dose threshold of lidocaine.[68]

Cardiovascular Toxicity

In 1979, Albright[61] alerted anesthesiologists to several cases of sudden cardiovascular collapse after unintentional intravascular injection of bupivacaine and etidocaine in pregnant women. The fact that cardiac arrest occurred concurrently with or shortly after the onset of convulsions was especially disconcerting.[69] Most of these cases were fatal, and subsequent controversy centered on whether resuscitation was instituted promptly and effectively. Nonetheless, the FDA restricted the use of the highest concentration (0.75%) of bupivacaine in pregnant women.

Several physiologic changes that occur during pregnancy place the parturient at higher risk for refractory cardiac arrest. First, reduced functional residual capacity and higher metabolic rate increase the risk for and hasten the onset of hypoxemia during periods of hypoventilation or apnea. Second, aortocaval compression decreases the efficacy of closed-chest cardiac massage in the supine position.[70] Third, a large bolus of drug injected into an epidural vein might reach the heart rapidly through a dilated azygous system. However, none of these factors adequately explains why cardiac arrest and difficult resuscitation are very rare in parturients intoxicated with lidocaine or mepivacaine.[61,69]

Results of laboratory studies of the effects of pregnancy on bupivacaine cardiotoxicity have been contradictory. Pregnancy-related hormones enhance the cardiotoxicity and arrhythmogenicity of bupivacaine *in vitro*.[71,72] For example, the magnitude and severity of bupivacaine-induced electrophysiologic changes are greater in myocardium obtained from nonpregnant rabbits treated with progesterone or beta-estradiol than in myocardium from untreated controls.[71,72] The electrophysiologic effects of lidocaine are less pronounced than those of bupivacaine, even in hormonally treated animals. Studies conducted *in vivo* have been less conclusive. In earlier investigations, significantly lower doses and plasma concentrations of bupivacaine, but not of mepivacaine or lidocaine, were required to produce circulatory collapse in pregnant sheep than in nonpregnant sheep.[46-48] However, a study involving a larger number of sheep and more rigorous methods (e.g., randomization, blinding) failed to confirm that pregnancy enhances the cardiotoxicity of bupivacaine.[64]

Progesterone does not increase myocardial sensitivity to ropivacaine.[73] Likewise, pregnancy does not enhance the systemic toxicity of ropivacaine or levobupivacaine in sheep.[64]

Extrapolation of results of animal studies to obstetric anesthesia practice is difficult, for several reasons. First, in the aforementioned sheep studies, the drug was administered by constant-rate intravenous infusion. In contrast, in pregnant women intoxicated with bupivacaine, cardiac arrest occurred after unintended intravascular injection of a large bolus of drug. Second, a potential for bias existed in the animal studies because randomization and blinding were not used in all studies and some relied on historical controls.[46-48] Third, it is unclear whether resuscitation in the reported clinical cases was accompanied by prompt and effective relief of aortocaval compression.[70]

Nonetheless, bupivacaine remains a popular local anesthetic for obstetric anesthesia. In current practice, heightened vigilance, use of an appropriate test dose, and fractionation of the therapeutic dose have made epidural anesthesia a safe technique for use in obstetric patients. In a study of anesthesia-related maternal mortality, Hawkins et al.[74] noted that the number of maternal deaths resulting from local anesthetic toxicity decreased after 1984, the year that the FDA withdrew approval for the epidural administration of 0.75% bupivacaine in obstetric patients. In our judgment, adherence to the aforementioned clinical precautions—rather than the proscription against the epidural administration of 0.75% bupivacaine—has been responsible for the lower number of maternal deaths due to local anesthetic toxicity. Anesthesia providers should be aware that intravenous injection of 0.5% bupivacaine can also cause systemic local anesthetic toxicity.

The availability of single levorotary isomers of a local anesthetic may be advantageous because these drugs have a greater margin of safety than bupivacaine, with similar blocking properties, although at a higher cost. From the standpoint of systemic toxicity, the use of these isoforms may be more beneficial in parturients undergoing cesarean delivery, who require higher doses than administered for analgesia during labor. Nonetheless, a greater margin of safety with these new drugs should not be a substitute for proper technique.

TREATMENT OF SYSTEMIC TOXICITY

Meticulous attention to good technique and adherence to guidelines for maximum recommended dose are mandatory. (The use of a test dose to identify misplaced injections is discussed in other chapters.) Incremental injection of the therapeutic dose, careful observation of the patient, and monitoring of vital signs usually provide early warning of an impending reaction. In mild cases, discontinuation of the administration of drug, administration of supplemental oxygen, and maintenance of normal ventilation often limit the severity of the reaction. In patients who show signs of CNS excitation, a small dose of thiopental (50 mg) or diazepam (2.5 to 5 mg) may prevent convulsions. In one study, prophylactic administration of a benzodiazepine reduced both the incidence of convulsions and mortality in mice intoxicated with amide local anesthetics.[75]

If convulsions should occur, oxygenation and ventilation must be maintained to prevent hypoxemia, hypercarbia, and acidosis.[42,43,76] Patency of the airway must be restored. It may be necessary to suction the airway first in some patients. Management should consist of administration of 100% oxygen, application of cricoid pressure, and endotracheal intubation, if required. Convulsions may be terminated quickly with a small dose of thiopental or diazepam. Maternal circulation should be supported by maintenance of left uterine displacement and administration of a vasopressor as needed. Because a high plasma concentration of local anesthetic may cause myocardial depression and vasodilation, a mixed alpha- and beta-adrenergic agonist (e.g., ephedrine) may be preferable to a pure alpha agonist. Fortunately, convulsions induced by intravenous injection of a relatively small dose of local anesthetic are self-limited because of rapid redistribution of the drug.

Cardiac arrest should be treated according to the American Heart Association's Advanced Cardiac Life Support (ACLS) guidelines. In addition, the pelvis should be tilted leftward to prevent or relieve aortocaval compression, which would render cardiac massage ineffective. Prompt cesarean delivery of the infant may be necessary to restore maternal circulation.

Persistent hypotension and bradycardia after bupivacaine intoxication may require administration of high doses of epinephrine and atropine.[77] A study in dogs suggested that amrinone may be superior to epinephrine in improving cardiac contractility depressed by bupivacaine.[78] However, amrinone may worsen ventricular arrhythmias.[79] Bupivacaine-induced ventricular arrhythmias should not be treated with lidocaine, because local anesthetic toxicity is additive.

Currently there are no specific guidelines for the pharmacologic treatment of bupivacaine cardiotoxicity in parturients. Amiodarone is the preferred antiarrhythmic agent in the most current ACLS algorithm. However, there may be some limitations to the utility of amiodarone in the treatment of bupivacaine-induced ventricular arrhythmias. Amiodarone may block the same ion channels that are affected by bupivacaine. Further, amiodarone has a relatively slower onset of action than bretylium and lidocaine, and it can cause hypotension. Nonetheless, amiodarone has been successfully used to resuscitate laboratory animals intoxicated with bupivacaine,[80] and it now seems to be the drug of choice for treatment of bupivacaine-induced ventricular arrhythmias. Bupivacaine toxicity may result in a *torsades de pointes*–like arrhythmia, which may require rapid atrial pacing and administration of isoproterenol.[81] Prolonged resuscitation may be needed until myocardial washout of bupivacaine has occurred.[49]

In a 2006 case report, lipid emulsion was used to treat refractory cardiac arrest that resulted from bupivacaine toxicity.[82] Protocols for lipid rescue may be found online (http://www.lipidrescue.org). The salutary effect of lipid therapy may be related to the greater affinity of bupivacaine for the lipid and the dissociation of bupivacaine from the cardiac sodium channel or to the binding of plasma bupivacaine by the lipid fraction in the blood.

After maternal recovery, fetal condition should be assessed promptly. In theory, a delay in delivery may allow back-diffusion of local anesthetic from the fetus to the mother, which may be of benefit to the neonate by decreasing neonatal plasma bupivacaine levels. Laboratory studies have demonstrated this phenomenon after the administration of bupivacaine[83] but not lidocaine.[84]

TISSUE TOXICITY

Neurologic complications of regional anesthesia are rare and result mostly from direct neural trauma, infection, injection of toxic doses of local anesthetic, or the injection of the wrong drug.

Three decades ago, 2-chloroprocaine caused prolonged or permanent sensory and motor deficits after subarachnoid injection of a large dose intended for epidural block.[85] Studies comparing the neurotoxicity of 2-chloroprocaine with that of other local anesthetics have yielded conflicting results, most likely related to the use of different methodologies and different species.[86,87] It has been suggested that neurotoxicity was caused by sodium meta-bisulfite, an antioxidant present in the commercial formulation (Nesacaine-CE, Astra Pharmaceutical Products) used in the reported cases.[86] The pH of Nesacaine-CE was between 2.7 and 4.0. In CSF rendered more acidic by 2-chloroprocaine, meta-bisulfite generates sulfur dioxide, which is lipid soluble and can diffuse into the nerve cells.[88] Intracellular hydration of sulfur dioxide generates sulfurous acid, which may cause profound intracellular acidosis and irreversible damage.

Subsequently, the manufacturer released another preparation of 2-chloroprocaine (i.e., Nesacaine-MPF) which was free of bisulfite but contained ethylenediamine-tetraacetic acid (EDTA). This was followed by several reports of severe, incapacitating paralumbar pain and spasm associated with epidural injection of large volumes of drug.[89] The etiology is unclear, although chelation of calcium by disodium EDTA may result in a reduced tissue calcium concentration and local tetany of the affected muscles.

In a 2004 study, Taniguchi et al.[90] suggested that sodium bisulfite was the "scapegoat" for 2-chloroprocaine neurotoxicity. They concluded that neurologic deficits associated with unintentional intrathecal injection of 2-chloroprocaine likely resulted from a direct effect of the 2-chloroprocaine, not the sodium bisulfite.

The current preparation of 2-chloroprocaine that is marketed for epidural administration (Nesacaine-MPF) does not contain EDTA or other preservatives. It is packaged in colored vials to reduce the oxidation of the 2-chloroprocaine. Low-dose, preservative-free 2-chloroprocaine (30 to 60 mg) is now being studied as a possible alternative to lidocaine for spinal anesthesia.[91]

Lidocaine has been used for spinal anesthesia for more than 50 years, in thousands upon thousands of patients, with apparent safety. However, cauda equina syndrome, sacral nerve root deficits, or transient neurologic toxicity can occur after subarachnoid injection of lidocaine.[92,93] Neurotoxicity of local anesthetics is concentration dependent[94] and is not unique to lidocaine.[95,96] Some investigators have speculated that slow injection of local anesthetic through a spinal microcatheter results in maldistribution and pooling of high concentrations of hyperbaric lidocaine in the cauda equina area, resulting in neurotoxicity and cauda equina syndrome.[92,93]

Milder manifestations of neurotoxicity also may occur. As early as 1954, mild, transient neurologic symptoms were reported after spinal anesthesia with lidocaine.[97] Transient neurologic symptoms (TNS) (dysesthesia or low back pain radiating to the buttocks, thighs, and calves) have been observed in surgical patients even after conventional (i.e., single-shot) spinal anesthesia with hyperbaric 5% lidocaine.[93] In response to concerns that intrathecal injection of hyperbaric 5% lidocaine might be associated with TNS, in 1994 the FDA Advisory Committee on Anesthetic Drugs recommended that the injected drug concentration be reduced by dilution with an equal volume of either preservative-free saline or CSF. However, Pollock et al.[98] reported that there was no difference in the incidence of TNS when spinal lidocaine 50 mg was diluted to 2%, 1%, or 0.5% solutions before administration and that the overall incidence of TNS did not differ from that of historic controls given lidocaine 5%.

Interestingly, the exposure of frog sciatic nerve to lidocaine results in a progressive, irreversible loss of impulse activity beginning at a concentration of 1%.[94] The investigators in this study noted that "the range of lidocaine that produces such changes in mammalian nerve awaits determination."[94] Meanwhile, it seems prudent to take the following precautions[92,99]:

1. Dilute the commercial 5% lidocaine for intrathecal injection as recommended by the FDA.
2. Administer the lowest possible dose.
3. Avoid the use of hyperbaric lidocaine in clinical conditions (e.g., obesity) or situations (e.g., the lithotomy position) that may be associated with a higher incidence of TNS.

If pencil-point, side-hole spinal needles are used, the injection port should be directed cephalad. However, an epidemiologic survey did not implicate dose and needle bevel direction as factors that affect the risk of TNS.[99] A meta-analysis of randomized controlled trials comparing spinal lidocaine with other local anesthetics (bupivacaine, prilocaine, procaine, and mepivacaine) found that the relative risk (RR) for development of TNS was higher with lidocaine than with the other local anesthetic agents (RR, 4.35; 95% confidence interval [CI], 1.98 to 9.54).[100] It has not been conclusively proven that TNS are manifestations of neurotoxicity.

Pregnancy may be associated with a reduced risk of TNS. Studies suggest that the incidence of TNS following spinal anesthesia with lidocaine or bupivacaine is equally low (less than 3%) in women having cesarean delivery and those undergoing postpartum tubal ligation.[101,102] However, cervical cerclage is performed in the lithotomy position, and this may increase the risk of TNS with spinal lidocaine compared to bupivacaine in this patient population.[99]

ALLERGIC REACTIONS

True allergy to a local anesthetic is rare.[103] Further, anaphylactic and anaphylactoid reactions may be the result of additives such as methylparaben and meta-bisulfite.[104] Clinical criteria are important in the diagnosis, because there is often a delay in obtaining confirmatory laboratory data. The alleged allergy to a local anesthetic can be substantiated in only 15% of patients by a history of urticaria, bronchospasm, facial edema, and/or cardiovascular instability.[105] Adverse reactions (e.g., CNS and cardiovascular symptoms) may mimic hypersensitivity but may not actually be a result of hypersensitivity. These symptoms may be caused by hyperventilation or vasovagal syncope during injection of the drug, sympathetic stimulation (e.g., palpitations, tachycardia) from epinephrine, or edema related to the injection itself.

Some pregnant women claim to be allergic to "Novocaine" or "the caine" drugs. Obstetricians should refer such patients to an allergist and an anesthesiologist for appropriate evaluation well before the expected date of delivery. In many cases, a carefully obtained history excludes true hypersensitivity. Otherwise, an allergist may have to determine the type of reaction and the offending agent by means of skin tests, drug-specific basophil degranulation, and/or the radioallergosorbent test (RAST). The last two tests, although highly specific, are costly and time consuming and may not be available for all anesthetic agents. Intradermal skin testing, although less costly and easy to perform, is associated with a false-positive rate of 8% to 15%.[106]

Alternatively, subcutaneous provocative dose testing is a useful method for rapid identification of a safe local anesthetic for an individual patient.[105,106] It can be performed by any physician qualified to manage hypersensitivity reactions. Appropriate emergency equipment and drugs (e.g., epinephrine, H_1- and H_2-receptor antagonists) should be immediately available for resuscitation. Although not mentioned in many protocols, establishing intravenous access before testing seems prudent.[107]

The back and the ventral aspects of the forearm are the preferred sites for testing. Areas with abnormal skin coloration or dermographia should be avoided. A history of recent treatment with antihistamines, salicylates, or steroids may alter the test results.[108]

The following protocol has been proposed by Chandler et al.[106] (Table 13-2) and has been used successfully in at least one published case[107]: After a negative needle-prick test, increasing volumes of undiluted local anesthetic (typically 1% concentration) are injected subcutaneously at 15-minute intervals. In patients with an especially strong history of a severe reaction, the series may be preceded by injection of diluted solutions (e.g., a 1:100 solution, followed by a 1:10 solution). A fresh syringe and a 30-gauge needle should be used for each subsequent injection. Additional refinements may consist of the use of a negative control (e.g., normal saline) and a positive control of diluted histamine. A local anesthetic that is not in the same class as the drug in question should be tested; if an ester is suspected as the offending agent, testing should be performed with an amide agent, and vice versa. If possible, the drug tested should be suitable for local infiltration and for epidural and subarachnoid block.

The test is considered positive if there is a change in the patient's clinical status or if a skin wheal more than 10 mm in diameter, with or without a flare, arises within 10 minutes of injection and persists for at least 30 minutes.[108] If provocative dose testing is completed without a reaction, the local anesthetic used and the final dose given should be recorded; and the patient (and the referring physician) should be informed that her risk of an adverse reaction to subsequent administration of that drug and dose is no greater than that for the general population.[105-107]

Management of an Allergic Reaction

Pharmacologic therapy of a severe allergic reaction involves (1) inhibition of mediator synthesis and release; (2) reversal of the effects of these mediators on target organs; and (3) prevention of the recruitment of other inflammatory processes. In general, catecholamines, phosphodiesterase inhibitors, antihistamines, and corticosteroids have been used for this purpose (Box 13-1).[109] Higher doses of catecholamines may be required in a patient who has received sympathetic blockade. In addition, pregnancy itself decreases responsiveness to catecholamines.[110] Despite its potential adverse effect on uterine blood flow, epinephrine remains the cornerstone of therapy for allergic reactions. In one reported case, a mother was treated successfully with epinephrine 100 μg without any apparent adverse effects on the newborn.[111]

TABLE 13-2 A Protocol for Provocative Dose Testing with Local Anesthetics*

Step	Route	Volume (mL)	Dilution
1	Skin prick		Undiluted
2	Subcutaneous	0.1	Undiluted
3	Subcutaneous	0.5	Undiluted
4	Subcutaneous	1.0	Undiluted
5	Subcutaneous	2.0	Undiluted

*See text for initial dilutions in patients with a severe history of allergy.

From Chandler MJ, Grammer LC, Patterson R. Provocative challenge with local anesthetics in patients with a prior history of reaction. J Allergy Clin Immunol 1987; 79:885.

BOX 13-1 Management of Anaphylaxis

Initial Therapy

- Stop administration of antigen.
- Maintain airway with 100% oxygen.
- Discontinue all anesthetic agents.
- Start intravascular volume expansion: 2-4 L of crystalloid/colloid (25-50 mL/kg) to treat hypotension.
- Give epinephrine:
  - 5-10 μg intravenously for treatment of hypotension; titrate as needed
  - 0.5-1.0 mg intravenously for treatment of cardiovascular collapse

Secondary Treatments

- Catecholamine infusions (starting doses):
  - Epinephrine: 4-8 μg/min (0.05-0.1 μg/kg/min)
  - Norepinephrine: 4-8 μg/min (0.05-0.1 μg/kg/min)
  - Isoproterenol: 0.05-0.1 μg/min
- Antihistamines: 0.5-1.0 mg/kg of diphenhydramine
- Corticosteroids: 0.25-1.0 g of hydrocortisone; alternatively, 1-2 g (25 mg/kg) of methylprednisolone
- Bicarbonate: 0.5-1.0 mEq/kg in patients with persistent hypotension or acidosis
- Airway evaluation (before extubation)

From Levy JH. Anaphylactic Reactions in Anesthesia and Intensive Care. Stoneham, MA, Butterworth-Heinemann, 1992:162.

Effects on the Uterus and Placenta

UTERINE BLOOD FLOW

The association of paracervical block anesthesia with fetal bradycardia has been attributed to the high concentration of local anesthetic deposited in the vicinity of the uterine arteries.[112] Human uterine artery segments obtained at the time of cesarean hysterectomy constrict when exposed to high concentrations of lidocaine,[113] mepivacaine,[113] or bupivacaine.[114]

These findings also have been confirmed in laboratory animals. Fishburne et al.[115] observed a dose-related decrease in uterine blood flow during uterine arterial infusion of 2-chloroprocaine, lidocaine, or bupivacaine in gravid ewes. A 25% reduction in uterine blood flow occurred at the following calculated plasma concentrations of local anesthetic: bupivacaine, 7 μg/mL; 2-chloroprocaine, 11.5 μg/mL; and lidocaine, 19.5 μg/mL. However, when plasma local anesthetic concentrations mimic those that occur in ordinary clinical practice, local anesthetics have no adverse effect on uterine blood flow.[116-118] In pregnant ewes, uterine blood flow remained unchanged during an intravenous infusion of lidocaine or bupivacaine that resulted in plasma concentrations of 0.81 to 4.60 and 1.5 to 2.0 μg/mL, respectively.[116,118] Likewise, intravenous injection of 2-chloroprocaine, 0.67 and 1.34 mg/kg, did not reduce uterine blood flow velocity in pregnant guinea pigs.[117]

Pregnancy may enhance uterine vascular reactivity to local anesthetic agents. Isolated human uterine artery segments obtained from term parturients constrict at a lower lidocaine concentration than uterine artery segments from nonpregnant patients.[113,119] Uterine artery sensitivity to local anesthetics increases as early as the second trimester of pregnancy and may be related to an increase in estrogen levels.[113,115] However, these studies were performed before the recognition of the importance of intact vascular endothelium in the *in vitro* assessment of vascular tone.

The exact mechanism by which high concentrations of local anesthetics cause uterine artery vasoconstriction (while causing dilation in other vascular beds) is unclear. This vasoconstriction may result from modulation of calcium-channel regulation because verapamil and nifedipine ablate the response.[119] Alternatively, local anesthetics may affect cyclic nucleotides and alter the ionic content and contractility of uterine vascular smooth muscle.[120] Clinical experience with the use of local anesthetics supports the view that clinical concentrations of these drugs do not adversely affect the uterine vasculature.[121-127]

All local anesthetics can reduce uterine blood flow at plasma concentrations that greatly exceed those occurring during the routine practice of obstetric anesthesia.[115] There has been an added concern that the levorotary isomers of local anesthetics, which produce vasoconstriction at clinical doses,[128] may reduce uteroplacental perfusion and adversely affect fetal well-being. It is reassuring to note that ropivacaine, even at plasma concentrations that are almost two times greater than would be expected to occur during clinical use, does not reduce uterine blood flow or affect fetal heart rate, blood pressure, or acid-base measurements in pregnant sheep.[116] In humans, Doppler velocimetry studies have shown that ropivacaine has little effect on the uteroplacental or fetal circulation when it is administered to provide epidural anesthesia for cesarean delivery.[122] Similarly, clinically relevant plasma concentrations of levobupivacaine had no adverse effect on uterine blood flow.[116]

UMBILICAL BLOOD FLOW

Fetal well-being also depends on the adequacy of fetal perfusion of the placenta. The regulatory mechanisms that control flow through the umbilical vessels are poorly understood. Lidocaine does not affect spiral strips obtained from human umbilical artery segments at concentrations up to 5 μg/mL, but it produces relaxation in concentrations from 30 to 900 μg/mL.[129] Bupivacaine also does not constrict umbilical artery segments at clinically relevant concentrations of 0.3 and 1 μg/mL.[129] At higher concentrations, the effect of bupivacaine appears to be biphasic. Constriction occurs at concentrations of 5 to 25 μg/mL, and relaxation occurs at concentrations greater than 125 μg/mL.[129,130] Hypercarbia but not hypoxia lessens the contractile response of umbilical vessels to bupivacaine *in vitro*.[131]

Decreases in umbilical blood flow of as much as 43% accompany intravenous administration of lidocaine 4 mg/kg in pregnant sheep.[132] However, plasma concentrations of the drug were higher than would be expected with clinical use, and all ewes exhibited signs of CNS toxicity, which may reduce umbilical blood flow.

Advances in noninvasive Doppler imaging have facilitated clinical assessment of umbilical cord blood flow velocity. The ratio of the systolic (S) peak to the diastolic (D) trough of the umbilical artery waveform is used as a measure of vascular resistance. The S/D ratio in the umbilical artery decreases during normal pregnancy, and high ratios usually are associated with fetal compromise.[133] Local anesthetics administered for epidural anesthesia do not seem to adversely affect the umbilical artery S/D ratio.[134,135] In fact, during labor epidural analgesia with 1.5% lidocaine or 2% 2-chloroprocaine resulted in a decrease in the S/D ratio.[134,135] This favorable change may have resulted from pain relief. Other investigators have noted no appreciable change or a slight decrease in the S/D ratio after the epidural administration of amide local anesthetics for elective cesarean delivery.[122,126,136]

UTERINE TONE AND CONTRACTILITY

Changes in uterine tone and contractility may affect uteroplacental perfusion. Local anesthetics exert direct effects on uterine smooth muscle. One study reported that exposure to high concentrations of local anesthetic *in vitro* led to contraction of human myometrial segments obtained at the time of cesarean delivery.[137] These findings have been corroborated in laboratory animals.[138] Further, Belitzky et al.[139] observed that direct intramyometrial injection of 1% procaine resulted in uterine hyperstimulation and fetal compromise in pregnant women. In all of these reports, the myometrium was exposed to higher than normal concentrations of the drug. In other studies, however, intravenous infusion of lidocaine or bupivacaine that resulted in clinically relevant plasma concentrations did not affect uterine tone or uterine activity in pregnant ewes.[116,118]

Drug Interactions with 2-Chloroprocaine

Epidural 2-chloroprocaine may affect the efficacy of other drugs administered in the neuraxis. Previous administration of 2-chloroprocaine (even a test dose) may reduce the quality and duration of analgesia produced by subsequent epidural injection of morphine or fentanyl.[140,141] Several hypotheses have been proposed for this antagonism. The low pH of the 2-chloroprocaine solution may result in acidification of the epidural space and thus may favor formation of the poorly diffusible, charged form of the opioid. Second, it has been suggested that 2-chloroprocaine (or its metabolite, chloroaminobenzoic acid) may act as a specific μ-opioid receptor antagonist because a κ-opioid receptor agonist (e.g., butorphanol) is not antagonized by 2-chloroprocaine.[140] However, using an *in vitro* hippocampal slice model, Coda et al.[142] concluded that 2-chloroprocaine opioid antagonism did not appear to act through a μ-opioid receptor. Third, a "window" may be caused by the rapid regression of 2-chloroprocaine before the onset of analgesia with epidural morphine. This mechanism is supported by the results of a study[143] in which women who received spinal bupivacaine anesthesia for cesarean delivery were randomly assigned to receive either epidural morphine with 2-chloroprocaine or epidural morphine with saline-placebo. There was no difference in post–cesarean delivery epidural morphine analgesia between the two groups; presumably the spinal bupivacaine provided adequate analgesia until the onset of epidural morphine analgesia.[143]

2-Chloroprocaine also reduces the subsequent efficacy of bupivacaine.[144] Corke et al.[145] suggested that chloroaminobenzoic acid is responsible for this effect. Administration of buffered 2-chloroprocaine does not prevent the antagonism of epidural bupivacaine.[146]

Potency of Bupivacaine, Ropivacaine, and Levobupivacaine

The levorotary compounds ropivacaine and levobupivacaine were developed because of the concerns about the safety of high doses of bupivacaine. Many studies have addressed the question of relative potency among the three drugs. Ropivacaine is approximately 10 times less lipid soluble (*N*-heptane/buffer) than bupivacaine, a difference that is important for two reasons.[3] First, ropivacaine may penetrate more slowly into the large, heavily myelinated motor neurons, resulting in less motor block than occurs with bupivacaine. Second, the issue raises questions as to whether ropivacaine is equipotent to bupivacaine. Indeed, a higher dose of ropivacaine is required to produce a sensory and motor block comparable to that produced by bupivacaine after spinal injection.[147,148] Similarly, the MLAC of epidural ropivacaine is almost twice as great as that of epidural bupivacaine in laboring women.[56] Critics of the use of MLAC data argue that it provides no information on the shape and slope of the dose-effect relationship, which can vary with drug concentration, and further, that it provides no information on the effective clinical dose (ED_{95} [effective dose in 95% of cases]).[149]

In contrast to the MLAC of ropivacaine, the MLAC of epidural levobupivacaine during labor is similar to that of bupivacaine.[56,65] Unfortunately, no single study has compared the MLACs of all three drugs. Levobupivacaine may have a greater motor-sparing effect than bupivacaine when given for the initial intrathecal injection. For example, in one study, none of 37 women who received intrathecal levobupivacaine 2.5 mg (with sufentanil and epinephrine) had evidence of motor block.[150] In contrast, 13 of 38 (34%) women given intrathecal bupivacaine 2.5 mg demonstrated a Bromage grade 1 motor block.

In obstetric anesthesia practice, the clinical effects of epidural levobupivacaine and ropivacaine are indistinguishable from those of epidural bupivacaine for labor analgesia.[151] The choice of bupivacaine, levobupivacaine, or ropivacaine does not affect the method of delivery or neonatal condition.[151] For cesarean delivery, epidural levobupivacaine 0.5% is virtually identical to epidural bupivacaine 0.5%.[152] The levorotary isomers (ropivacaine and levobupivacaine) may provide a greater margin of safety when large volumes of a concentrated solution of local anesthetic are required (e.g., epidural anesthesia for cesarean delivery). However, there may be little advantage to using levobupivacaine or ropivacaine when dilute solutions are used for epidural labor analgesia or when a small dose is used for spinal anesthesia.

Placental Transfer

Most drugs, including local anesthetics, cross the placenta. The factors that influence the placental transfer of a drug include (1) the physicochemical characteristics of the drug, (2) the concentration of free drug in the maternal blood, (3) the permeability of the placenta, and (4) the hemodynamic events occurring within the fetal-maternal unit.

Local anesthetics cross placental membranes by a process of simple (i.e., passive) diffusion. The rate of transfer (not necessarily the amount) of a particular drug is described by the Fick equation, as follows:

$$Q/t = \frac{K \times A\ (C_m - C_f)}{D}$$

where Q/t is the rate of diffusion; K is the diffusion constant for the drug; A is the surface area available for transfer; C_m is free drug concentration in the maternal blood; C_f is the free drug concentration in the fetal blood; and D is the thickness of the trophoblastic epithelium. In general, K is affected by molecular size, lipid solubility, and the degree of ionization.

MOLECULAR SIZE

Compounds with a molecular weight of less than 500 Da cross the placenta easily, whereas drugs like digoxin, which have a molecular weight higher than 500 Da, have a slower rate of diffusion.[153] Molecular weights of local anesthetics range from 234 to 288 Da (see Table 13-1). These small differences in molecular weight should not affect the rate of placental transfer because the dissociation constant (K) is inversely proportional to the square root of the molecular weight.[154]

IONIZATION AND LIPID SOLUBILITY

The un-ionized molecule is more lipid soluble than the ionized moiety. Local anesthetics are weak bases; they have a relatively low degree of ionization and considerable lipid solubility at physiologic pH.

The relationship between pH and pK_B may affect drug accumulation in the fetus. For the amide local anesthetics, pK_B values are close enough to physiologic pH that changes

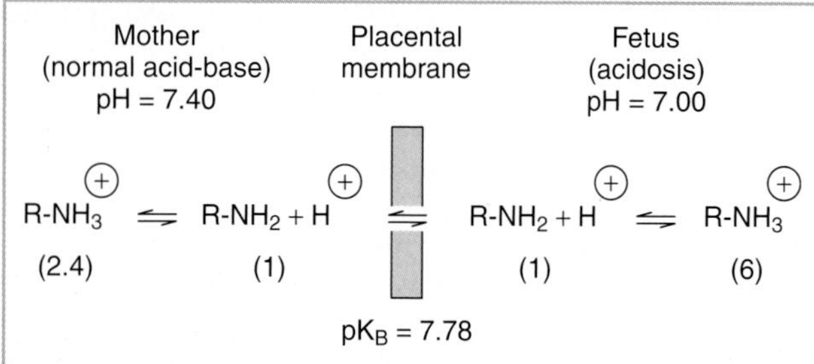

FIGURE 13-4 "Ion trapping" of a local anesthetic. The numbers in parentheses represent relative numbers of molecules. (From the American College of Obstetricians and Gynecologists. Obstet Gynecol 1976; 48:29.)

in fetal pH may alter the balance between ionized and un-ionized drug. In the acidotic fetus, a greater proportion of drug in the ionized form results in a larger total amount of local anesthetic in fetal plasma, because of "ion trapping" (Figure 13-4).[155-157] Elimination of lidocaine from fetal blood is slower in the asphyxiated fetus than in the non-asphyxiated fetus.[132] Accumulation of lidocaine may be greater in fetal tissues, where the pH is even lower than that in fetal blood.[157]

PROTEIN BINDING

Perhaps most confusing and least understood are the effects of protein binding on placental transfer. Amide local anesthetics are bound predominantly to AAG and to a much lesser extent to albumin.[19] The extent of protein binding varies among the local anesthetic agents (see Table 13-1). For a given local anesthetic, the proportion of free drug increases as blood concentration increases because of the saturation of binding sites. Binding of local anesthetics in the fetal plasma is approximately half that in the mother.[83,84]

The fetal-to-maternal (F/M) blood concentration ratios of amide local anesthetic agents are listed in Table 13-1. The lower F/M blood concentration ratios of highly protein-bound drugs (e.g., bupivacaine) have been attributed to their more restricted placental transfer compared with less protein-bound drugs (e.g., lidocaine). Indeed, the rate of bupivacaine transfer across rabbit placenta perfused *in situ* is lower than that of lidocaine transfer.[158,159] Some investigators have suggested that protein binding in the maternal plasma should not affect the diffusion of drugs across the placenta because the dissociation from plasma proteins is essentially instantaneous.[154,160] In more recent studies, the relatively low umbilical vein–to–maternal vein blood concentration ratio for bupivacaine has been attributed to differences in protein binding between maternal plasma and fetal plasma (Figure 13-5).[83,84,161,162] Let us assume that the total concentration of lidocaine or bupivacaine in the maternal plasma is 2 mg/L. Lidocaine and bupivacaine are approximately 50% and 90% bound to maternal plasma proteins, respectively. Thus, the free concentrations of drug available for placental transfer are 1.0 and 0.2 mg/L, respectively. At equilibrium, the concentration of free drug is equal on the two sides of the placenta. In the fetus, however, lidocaine and bupivacaine are approximately 25% and 50% bound to fetal plasma proteins, respectively. Thus the total lidocaine concentration in fetal plasma is 1.33 mg/L, resulting in an F/M ratio of 0.67; for bupivacaine, the corresponding values are 0.4 mg/L and 0.2.

Substantial accumulation of bupivacaine occurred in human fetuses whose mothers received the drug for epidural anesthesia.[24] After delivery, measurable plasma and urine concentrations persisted for as long as 3 days.[24] *In vitro* studies using a perfused human placental model have found that the placental transfer of ropivacaine is similar to that of bupivacaine.[163] Intravenous infusion of ropivacaine or bupivacaine to pregnant sheep results in steady-state maternal plasma concentrations of 1.5 to 1.6 μg/mL and fetal concentrations of approximately 0.28 μg/mL.[116] Tissue concentrations of ropivacaine in fetal heart, brain, liver, lung, kidneys, and adrenal glands were similar to those of bupivacaine.[116] Datta et al.[30] noted that the free fraction of ropivacaine at delivery was approximately twice that of bupivacaine in neonates whose mothers received the drug for epidural anesthesia during labor or cesarean delivery.

MATERNAL BLOOD CONCENTRATION OF DRUG

The maternal blood concentration of local anesthetic is determined by (1) the dose, (2) the site of administration, (3) metabolism and excretion, and (4) the effects of adjuvants such as epinephrine. For a given local anesthetic, the maternal blood concentration determines fetal drug

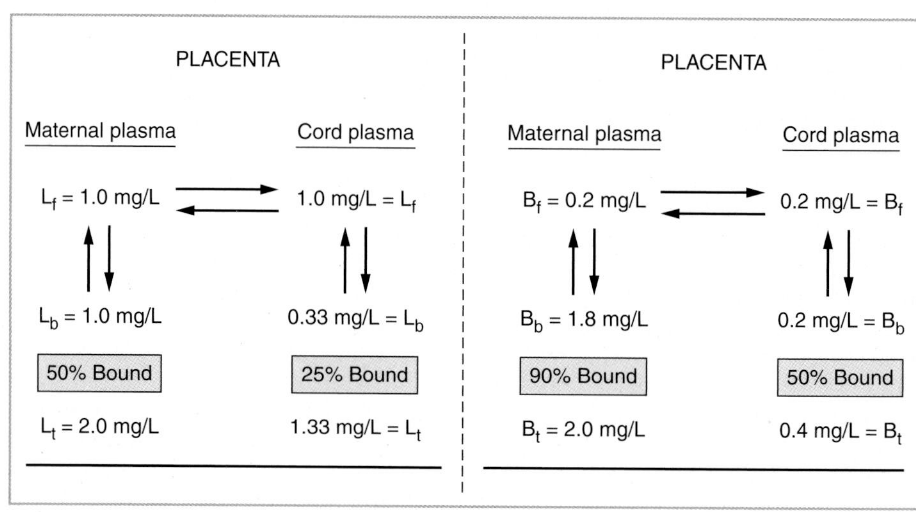

FIGURE 13-5 Demonstration of how distribution of local anesthetics across the placenta may be predicted from differences in drug protein binding in maternal and fetal plasma. *Left*, lidocaine (L); f, b, t, free, bound, and total drug concentrations, respectiviely. *Right*, bupivacaine (B). Lidocaine umbilical cord–to–maternal plasma ratio (F/M) = 0.67; bupivacaine F/M = 0.20. (From Tucker GT, Mather LE, Properties, absorption, and disposition of local anesthetic agents. In Cousins MJ, Bridenbaugh PO, editors. Neural Blockade in Clinical Anesthesia and Management of Pain. 2nd edition. Philadelphia, Lippincott, 1988:95.)

exposure and is the only variable of the Fick equation that may be influenced by the clinician.

Dose

In general, higher doses result in higher maternal and fetal blood concentrations. For example, Kuhnert et al.[17] found that doubling the dose of epidural lidocaine from 300 ± 195 mg to 595 ± 127 mg almost doubled the concentration in umbilical cord blood. The elimination half-life of amide local anesthetics is relatively long; thus, repeated epidural injection or continuous infusion of the drug may lead to accumulation in the maternal plasma. This statement does not apply to 2-chloroprocaine, however, which is rapidly hydrolyzed by pseudocholinesterase.[11]

Site of Administration

The rates of absorption and peak plasma concentrations depend on the vascularity at the site of administration. The peak plasma concentration of lidocaine is achieved within 9 to 10 minutes after paracervical block. In contrast, absorption from the lumbar epidural space, which is less vascular, occurs at a slower rate; the peak plasma concentration is not achieved until 25 to 40 minutes after administration.[17,164] Injection of local anesthetic into the caudal rather than the lumbar epidural space may result in higher blood levels because of the need for a higher drug volume to provide comparable anesthesia to that provided by lumbar epidural injection.[165]

In the past, it was thought that subarachnoid administration of a local anesthetic resulted in less systemic absorption than epidural administration. However, peak blood concentrations of lidocaine have been reported to be similar after subarachnoid and epidural administration.[166] In another study, subarachnoid administration of lidocaine 75 mg for cesarean delivery resulted in low but measurable fetal plasma concentrations of the drug.[16]

Epinephrine

Epinephrine is administered with a local anesthetic to enhance analgesia and delay the uptake of the drug from the site of administration. The latter action of epinephrine varies with the choice and concentration of local anesthetic as well as the concentration of epinephrine. The effect of epinephrine is greater when it is combined with lidocaine than when it is combined with mepivacaine or bupivacaine.[154,167] Even concentrations of epinephrine as low as 3.3 μg/mL (1:300,000) have been shown to be effective in reducing the plasma concentrations of lidocaine.[168]

In contrast, the addition of epinephrine to bupivacaine has transient effects. Reynolds and Taylor[169] observed that the addition of epinephrine 5 μg/mL (1:200,000) to bupivacaine resulted in decreased maternal plasma concentrations of drug only at 20 minutes after the first epidural injection and at 40 minutes after the second epidural injection in laboring women. In another study, the addition of epinephrine 3.3 μg/mL to 0.5% bupivacaine had no effect on maternal venous plasma concentrations of drug in laboring women.[170] Likewise, Reynolds et al.[171] observed no effect when they added epinephrine 5 μg/mL to bupivacaine during administration of epidural anesthesia for cesarean delivery.

The site of administration also may influence the effect of epinephrine on the absorption of individual drugs. For example, one group reported that the addition of epinephrine to bupivacaine resulted in a 50% decrease in maternal plasma concentrations of bupivacaine after paracervical block.[172] In another study, epinephrine did not alter absorption of lidocaine after subarachnoid injection.[173]

Studies of the effects of epinephrine on the placental transfer of local anesthetics have yielded contradictory results. In rabbits, epinephrine did not affect the F/M ratio of bupivacaine.[174] In pregnant women, the F/M ratio for bupivacaine has been found to be increased[169] or unchanged.[170,172,175] For mepivacaine, the F/M ratio has been found to be increased,[167] whereas for lidocaine it has variously been reported to be increased,[167,176] decreased,[168] or unchanged.[177]

PLACENTA

Maturation of the placenta may affect the rate of drug transfer. In pregnant mice, diazepam and its metabolites cross the placenta more rapidly in late pregnancy.[178] Uptake and metabolism of drugs by the placenta would be expected to reduce transfer to the fetus. However, placental drug uptake of local anesthetics is limited, and it is unlikely that this organ metabolizes the amide local anesthetic agents.[179] This may not be true for the ester local anesthetics. For example, cocaine is biotransformed when it is incubated with human placental microsomal fraction, presumably because of cholinesterase activity within the placenta.[180] Placental metabolism of para-aminobenzoic acid also has been demonstrated.[181]

Teratogenicity

The teratogenicity of anesthetics is not an issue during parturition, but local anesthetics often are used for procedures during the first trimester of pregnancy. *In vitro* studies have suggested that local anesthetics may have some adverse developmental effects. Even at low concentrations, these agents have caused reversible reduction of cell division in tissue culture.[182-187] However, structural anomalies have not been observed in intact animals.[188-190] Mid-pregnancy administration of lidocaine or mepivacaine in rats has been associated with behavioral changes in the offspring.[191,192]

Extrapolation of laboratory findings to humans is tenuous for several reasons. First, a drug may be teratogenic in one species but not in others. Second, a 1-hour drug exposure in a pregnant rat (with a gestation of 21 days) is excessive and not analogous to several hours of clinical anesthesia during human pregnancy. Third, the doses of local anesthetics used in animal studies greatly exceed those administered for clinical anesthesia. Indeed, a large, multicenter study demonstrated that the risk of congenital anomalies in humans was not increased by the administration of benzocaine, procaine, tetracaine, or lidocaine during early pregnancy.[193] However, a twofold increase in the incidence of congenital anomalies was noted in infants whose mothers had received mepivacaine. The small number of patients who received mepivacaine in this study (n = 82) and the fact that no adverse effects occurred with the use of other amide agents have raised doubts about the validity of this observation.[194]

Fetal and Neonatal Effects

PHARMACOKINETICS

Local anesthetics, once transferred across the placenta, are distributed in the fetus. Factors that influence tissue uptake of the drug include (1) fetal plasma protein binding, (2) lipid solubility, (3) the degree of ionization of the drug, and (4) hemodynamic changes that affect the distribution of fetal cardiac output. The fetal plasma protein-binding capacity of local anesthetics is approximately 50% that of maternal plasma.[83,84,195] Thus, at any given total plasma concentration of local anesthetic, there is greater availability of free drug in the fetus than in the mother.[83,84,195-197] Studies have examined the distribution of lidocaine in fetal tissues after an intravenous injection of the drug to animals.[18,198] The higher concentration of lidocaine in the liver, myocardium, and brain (compared with other fetal tissues) reflects rapid distribution of the drug to highly perfused tissues. The only organ in which lidocaine concentrations in the fetus have been found to exceed those in the mother is the liver. This finding is not surprising, given the high lipid content of the fetal liver and the fact that it receives most of the blood returning from the placenta by means of the umbilical vein.[198] Fetal acidosis and hypoxemia result in circulatory adaptations that increase blood flow to vital organs (e.g., brain, heart, adrenal glands).[199] The concentration of lidocaine in these organs is higher in asphyxiated fetuses than in healthy fetuses.[157,199]

Any drug that reaches the fetus undergoes metabolism and excretion. The term newborn has the hepatic enzymes necessary to metabolize local anesthetics.[16,17,200-204] Nonetheless, the elimination half-life of these drugs is longer in the neonate than in the adult.[202,204] The use of mepivacaine in obstetric epidural analgesia fell into disfavor after a report indicating that the elimination half-life of the drug in the newborn was approximately 9 hours, or three times as long as the neonatal half-life for lidocaine.[167] It is ironic that it later became known that the neonatal elimination half-life for bupivacaine may be as long as 14 hours.[205]

Morishima et al.[204] compared the pharmacokinetics of lidocaine among adult ewes and fetal and neonatal lambs. The metabolic (hepatic) clearance in the newborns was similar to that in adults, and renal clearance was greater than that in adults. Nonetheless, the elimination half-life was more prolonged in newborns. This latter finding has been attributed to a greater volume of distribution in the newborn. Thus, at any given time, a smaller fraction of lidocaine accumulated in the body is available for clearance by hepatic metabolism. The greater renal clearance noted in neonates is a result of decreased protein binding, which increases the proportion of drug available to the kidneys for excretion.

The elimination half-life of local anesthetics in the fetus is similar to that in the adult because, unlike the newborn, the fetus can excrete drug across the placenta back to the mother.[83,204] With bupivacaine, this transfer may occur even though the total plasma drug concentration in the mother may exceed that in the fetus.[83]

SYSTEMIC TOXICITY

In general, the newborn is more sensitive than the adult to the depressant effects of drugs. However, the seizure threshold for local anesthetics in the newborn appears to be similar to that in the adult.[206]

Morishima et al.[207] compared the relative CNS toxicity and cardiovascular toxicity of lidocaine in adult ewes and fetal and neonatal lambs. Greater doses (when calculated on a milligram-per-kilogram basis) were required to elicit toxic manifestations in the fetus and newborn than in the adult. However, the plasma concentrations of the drug associated with toxic manifestations were similar in the three groups of animals. The greater dose tolerated by fetuses than by newborns and adults was attributed to placental clearance of drug back to the mother and better maintenance of blood gas tensions during convulsions. In the newborn, a large volume of distribution is most likely responsible for the high doses of local anesthetic required to have toxic effects.

Studies of bupivacaine cardiotoxicity are inconsistent. *In vitro*, the sinoatrial node of newborn guinea pigs was found to be more sensitive than that of adults to the cardiodepressant effect of bupivacaine.[208] In contrast, newborn piglets (2 days old) demonstrated greater resistance than older animals to the arrhythmogenic and CNS effects of bupivacaine.[209]

FETAL HEART RATE

Changes in fetal heart rate (FHR) after administration of local anesthetics are most often related to indirect effects such as maternal hypotension and uterine hyperstimulation (tachysystole). Local anesthetics probably have little direct effect on FHR, except perhaps after paracervical block. Rather, labor itself may be the single most important factor that alters FHR patterns.[210] Transient changes in FHR variability and an increase in the incidence of periodic decelerations have been observed during administration of epidural analgesia in laboring women.[211-214] In contrast, in the absence of labor, FHR patterns are not affected even by the larger doses of local anesthetics required during administration of epidural anesthesia for cesarean delivery.[210] The FHR changes noted in laboring women were transient and did not affect the condition of their newborns.[211-214]

NEUROBEHAVIORAL TESTS

Neurobehavioral tests have been developed to detect subtle changes in organized behavior in the newborn. These tests include the Brazelton Neonatal Behavioral Assessment Scale (NBAS), the Early Neonatal Neurobehavioral Scale (ENNS), and the Neurologic and Adaptive Capacity Score (NACS). All are subjective and complex and lack specificity.

Other perinatal factors appear to have a more important effect on neonatal test performance than the choice of local anesthetic.[215] Indeed, neurobehavioral tests have been shown not to be a reliable measure of drug effect in the newborn.[216]

PRETERM FETUS AND NEWBORN

It has become axiomatic that the preterm infant is more vulnerable than the term infant to the effects of analgesic and anesthetic drugs. Causes of enhanced drug sensitivity in the preterm newborn that have been postulated are as follows: (1) less protein is available for drug binding, (2) higher levels of bilirubin are present and may compete with the drug for protein binding, (3) greater access of the drug to the CNS occurs because of a poorly developed blood-brain barrier, (4) the preterm infant has greater total body water and less fat content, and (5) the preterm infant has a diminished ability to metabolize and excrete drugs. Unfortunately, few systematic studies have determined the maternal and fetal pharmacokinetics and pharmacodynamics of drugs throughout gestation; nevertheless, these deficiencies of the preterm infant may not be as serious as we have been led to believe. Although the plasma albumin and AAG concentrations are lower in the preterm fetus, these factors primarily affect drugs that are highly bound to these proteins. Most local anesthetics, however, exhibit only low to moderate degrees of binding in fetal plasma.[83,84]

The placenta efficiently eliminates fetal bilirubin. Thus, the hyperbilirubinemia of prematurity normally occurs in the postpartum period. Bupivacaine has been implicated as a possible cause of neonatal jaundice.[217,218] High affinity of the drug for fetal erythrocyte membranes may lead to a decrease in filterability and deformability, which may render red blood cells more prone to hemolysis.[218] However, increased bilirubin production has not been demonstrated in newborns whose mothers received bupivacaine for epidural anesthesia during labor and delivery.[219]

Greater total body water in the preterm fetus results in a larger volume of distribution for drugs. Thus, to achieve equal blood concentrations, the immature fetus must receive a greater amount of drug transplacentally than the mature fetus.

The diminished ability to metabolize or excrete drugs associated with prematurity is certainly not a universal phenomenon. One study of the pharmacokinetics of lidocaine in preterm newborns noted that plasma clearance was similar to that in adults.[202]

During anesthesia for preterm labor, concerns about drug effects on the newborn are far less important than the prevention of asphyxia and trauma to the fetus. Indeed, healthy preterm fetal lambs tolerated clinically relevant plasma concentrations of lidocaine (e.g., approximately 1.5 μg/mL) as well as mature ones.[18,220]

ASPHYXIA

Circulatory adaptations important for fetal survival during asphyxia result in increased blood flow and oxygen delivery to vital organs (e.g., heart, brain, adrenal glands).[199] Little information exists about the effects of local anesthetics on these fetal responses. Adaptation to asphyxia was unaffected in mature fetal lambs exposed to lidocaine.[199] In contrast, lidocaine adversely affected asphyxiated preterm fetal lambs, which experienced a further deterioration of acid-base status and a reduction in cardiac output and blood flow to the brain and heart (Figure 13-6).[221] Also in asphyxiated preterm fetal lambs, exposure to bupivacaine reduced blood flow to vital organs; however, fetal heart rate, blood pressure, and acid-base measurements did not change.[222]

After performing an *in vitro* study using perfused human placentas, Johnson et al.[223] suggested that bupivacaine might be preferable to lidocaine in the presence of fetal acidosis because the greater maternal protein binding of bupivacaine may limit its placental transfer. However, this methodology does not consider the potential for greater fetal tissue uptake of bupivacaine (than of lidocaine) because of the fact that bupivacaine is more lipid soluble and more protein bound than lidocaine.

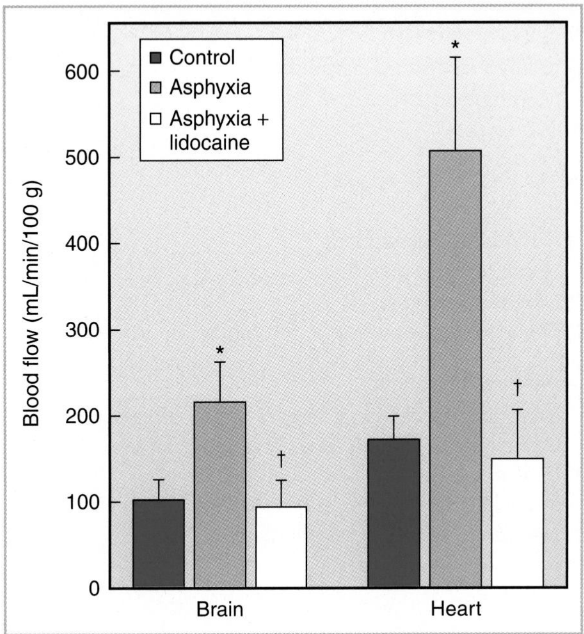

FIGURE 13-6 Blood flow to the brain and heart in the preterm fetal lamb before and during asphyxia and during exposure to lidocaine while asphyxiated (mean ± SEM). *Significantly different from control. †Significantly different from asphyxia. (Modified from Morishima HO, Pedersen H, Santos AC, et al. Adverse effects of maternally administered lidocaine on the asphyxiated preterm fetal lamb. Anesthesiology 1989; 71:110-5.)

In 1997, Santos et al.[222] reported that the effects of bupivacaine appeared less severe than those of lidocaine in asphyxiated preterm fetal lambs. However, the lidocaine data were generated in a separate experiment reported in 1989.[221] There are inherent limitations in a historical comparsion of two studies performed 8 years apart. Further, it is unclear whether these findings are applicable to humans because both lidocaine and bupivacaine have enjoyed a long history of safe use in obstetric anesthesia practice; prospective clinical studies are required before one drug can be recommended over the other.

OPIOIDS

Neuraxial opioid administration is unique in that it produces analgesia without loss of sensation or proprioception. Opioids are often co-administered with local anesthetic agents during intrapartum administration of neuraxial analgesia and anesthesia.

The term *opioid* refers to a series of compounds that are related to opium. These compounds may be classified as follows: (1) naturally occurring (e.g., morphine), (2) semisynthetic compounds (e.g., dihydromorphone), and (3) synthetic compounds (e.g., fentanyl) (Box 13-2). The only three naturally occurring opioids of clinical significance are morphine, codeine, and papaverine. These substances can be obtained from the poppy plant known botanically as *Papaver somniferum*. Development of synthetic drugs with morphine-like properties has led to development of the broad term *opioid*. These substances bind to several

BOX 13-2 Classification of Opioid Compounds

Naturally Occurring Compounds

- Morphine
- Codeine
- Papaverine
- Thebaine

Semisynthetic Compounds

- Heroin (diamorphine)
- Dihydromorphone
- Thebaine derivatives (e.g., etorphine, buprenorphine)

Synthetic Compounds

- Morphinan series (e.g., levorphanol, butorphanol)
- Diphenylpropylamine series (e.g., methadone)
- Benzomorphan series (e.g., pentazocine)
- Phenylpiperidine series (e.g., meperidine, fentanyl, sufentanil, alfentanil, remifentanil)

subpopulations of opioid receptors with resulting morphine-like effects. More than 30 years ago, identification of a dense concentration of opioid receptors in the dorsal horn of the spinal cord led to the use of neuraxial opioids as important adjuncts in obstetric anesthesia.

Molecular Structure

Naturally occurring opioids of significance can be divided into two distinct chemical classes, phenanthrenes (e.g., morphine) and benzylisoquinolines (e.g., papaverine) (Figure 13-7). The phenanthrenes are five-ring structures, and the benzylisoquinolines are three-ring structures. The semisynthetic opioids are morphine derivatives that have undergone relatively simple modification of the morphine molecule. For example, substitution of an ester for the hydroxyl group on carbon 6 of morphine results in hydromorphone (Figure 13-8). Synthetic opioids can be classified into the following four groups: (1) morphinan derivatives (e.g., levorphanol), (2) diphenyl or methadone derivatives (e.g., methadone, D-propoxyphene), (3) benzomorphan derivatives (phenazocine, pentazocine), and (4) phenylpiperidines (e.g., meperidine, fentanyl, sufentanil).

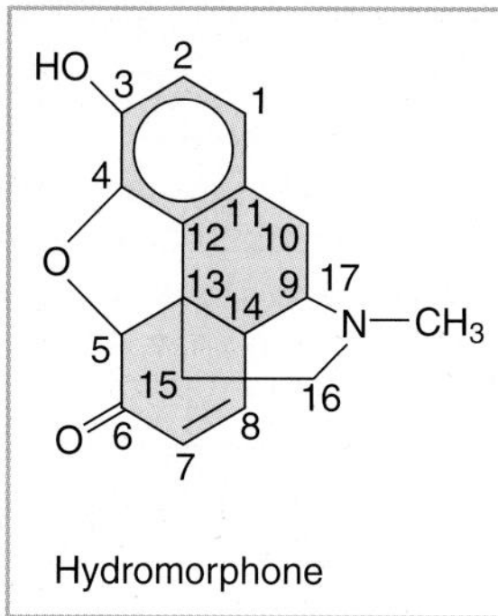

FIGURE 13-8 Semisynthetic opioids are morphine derivatives. For example, substitution of an ester for the hydroxyl group on carbon 6 of morphine results in hydromorphone.

Structurally, opioids are complex three-dimensional compounds that often exist as two optical isomers (e.g., morphine).[224] Usually the levorotary isomer is the only isomer capable of producing analgesia. Analgesic activity of the opioid compound depends on its stereochemical structure.[225] Even relatively minor molecular alterations (e.g., extent of ionization) can produce significant alterations in the pharmacologic activity of the opioid.

Morphine is the prototype opioid. It is a five-ring structure that conforms to a T shape.[226] Three of the rings lie in one plane, and the other two rings are perpendicular to the plane. This forms the basis for the T (Figure 13-9). Morphine demonstrates several other characteristics that are common to other opioids: (1) a tertiary, positively charged basic nitrogen; (2) a quaternary carbon that is separated from the basic nitrogen by an ethane chain and attached to a phenyl group; (3) a phenolic hydroxyl group (morphine derivatives) or a ketone group (meperidine); and (4) the presence of an aromatic ring.[226]

A phenylpiperidine structure (i.e., an aromatic ring attached to a six-member ring containing five carbons and one nitrogen) is also part of the morphine molecule and is present in some other opioids (e.g., fentanyl) (Figure 13-10).[226] Phenylalanine and tyrosine moieties are structural elements that are important to all opioids, including endogenous neurotransmitters and modulators.[227,228]

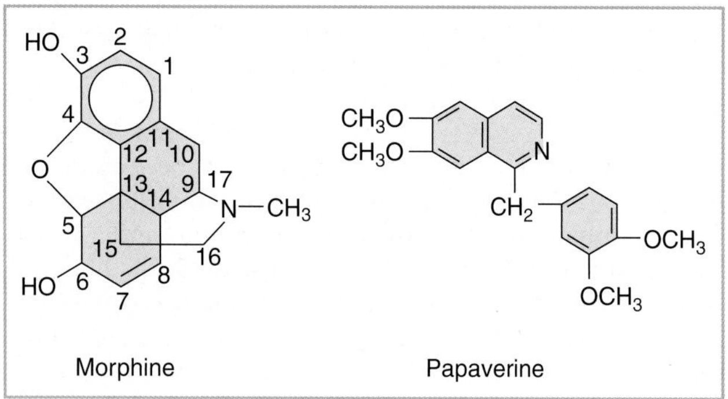

FIGURE 13-7 Naturally occurring opioids: phenanthrenes (e.g., morphine) and benzylisoquinolines (e.g., papaverine).

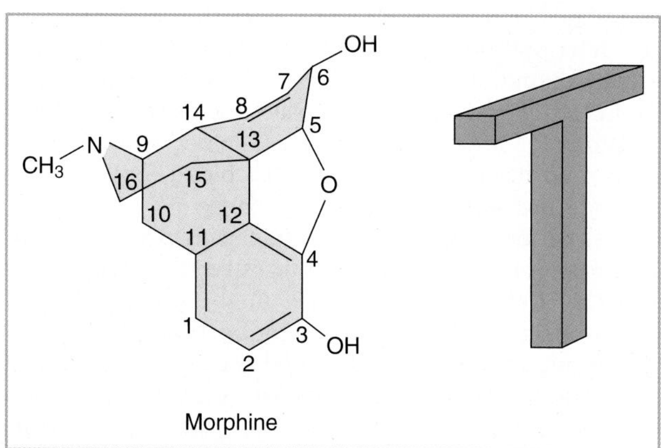

FIGURE 13-9 The T-shaped molecule of morphine.

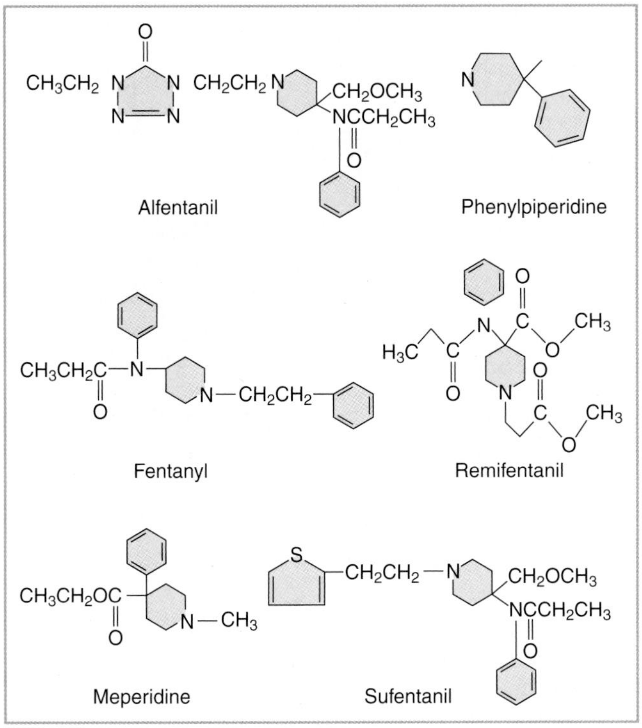

FIGURE 13-10 Chemical structures of phenylpiperidine, meperidine, and the 4-anilinopiperidine derivatives fentanyl, sufentanil, alfentanil, and remifentanil.

The poppy plant synthesizes morphine from two tyrosine molecules; many opioids contain a structure that is similar to alanine.[226]

Mechanism of Action

Since first described in 1979,[229] neuraxial opioid administration has become a mainstay in obstetric anesthesia practice. Clinical and laboratory research has focused on the mechanisms of synaptic transmission as well as assessment of opioids and neurotransmitters that modulate this transmission.

Pain perception involves a complex series of nociceptive transmissions that begin with stimulation of sensory nerves in the periphery, resulting in generation of action potentials within the spinal cord and synaptic transmission to other supraspinal sites.[230] Intraspinal administration of an opioid exploits the pharmacology of pain-modulating and pain-relieving systems that exist within the spinal cord (see Figure 20-10). In early studies, Yaksh[231] demonstrated that morphine could produce selective suppression of nociceptive processing without affecting motor function, sympathetic tone, or proprioception when it was administered to the superficial layers of the dorsal horn of the spinal cord. However, when small amounts of opioid were administered to the cortex, the effects on nociceptive processing were negligible. Collectively, this work demonstrated that small doses of opioid can be selectively administered to a receptor site (i.e., spinal cord) and produce profound analgesia. In contrast, systemic administration of a much larger dose of opioid results in activation of multiple central and peripheral receptors to produce analgesia, but with unwanted side effects.

All opioids produce analgesia by binding to G protein–coupled opioid receptors. Activation of opioid receptors subsequently inhibits both adenylate cyclase and voltage-gated calcium channels. Inhibition of these calcium channels inhibits the release of excitatory afferent neurotransmitters, including glutamate, substance P, and other tachykinins.[230] The result is inhibition of ascending nociceptive stimuli from the dorsal horn of the spinal cord.

Opioid receptors are nonuniformly distributed throughout the CNS. Although parenterally administered opioids most likely have both direct spinal and supraspinal effects, neuraxially administered opioids block the transmission of pain-related information by binding at presynaptic and postsynaptic receptor sites in the dorsal horn of the spinal cord (i.e., Rexed laminae I, II, V) (Figure 13-11). However, the rate and extent of neuraxial analgesia depend largely on the specific drug's physicochemical properties and ability to reach the opioid receptors in the spinal cord.

The following four broad classes of opioid receptors have been identified: (1) mu (μ) receptor for morphine type, (2) kappa (κ) receptor for ketocyclazocine type, (3) delta (δ) receptor, and (4) nociceptin/orphanin FQ (NOP) receptor.[232] Each receptor is encoded by a different gene and mediates a different physiologic effect (Table 13-3). Although all of these receptors may be involved with pain processing, the μ- or κ-opioid receptors have the most important clinical pharmacologic effects. Older studies also described a σ receptor; however, this receptor is now considered not to be an opioid receptor but rather a high-affinity binding site for phencyclidine and other related compounds.[233]

The distinct receptor subtypes have great significance in neuraxial opioid administration and drug development. Common pharmacologic effects (e.g., analgesia, respiratory depression) of morphine are mediated by μ-opioid receptors. Further, subclasses of μ-opioid receptors have been identified. Some specific functions have been ascribed to μ-opioid receptors, including mediation of respiratory depression and spinal opioid analgesia by μ_2 receptors, and production of supraspinal analgesia by μ_1 receptors.[234] Although subtype-specific μ agonists may have greater efficacy and less toxicity, no receptor-specific agents have been developed for clinical use.

Morphine also has effects at κ- and δ-opioid receptors when higher doses are administered. Responsible for analgesic, sedative, dysphoric, and diuretic effects,[235] κ receptors are located both within the CNS and peripherally.[236] Peripheral κ-opioid receptor agonists have been shown to modulate visceral pain, particularly in conditions that involve inflammation.[236]

The δ receptor is responsible for mediating some of the analgesic effects of the endogenous opioids (e.g., enkephalins, prodynorphan, proopioidmelanocortin, proorphanin, endomorphins) in the spinal cord.[237] Few of the opioids have effects at the δ receptor in clinically relevant doses, but if a μ agonist is administered in a high enough dose to treat an opioid-tolerant patient, the drug may be less selective and produce δ effects. The nociceptin/orphanin FQ receptor may also be involved in pain processing in spinal and supraspinal centers.[232]

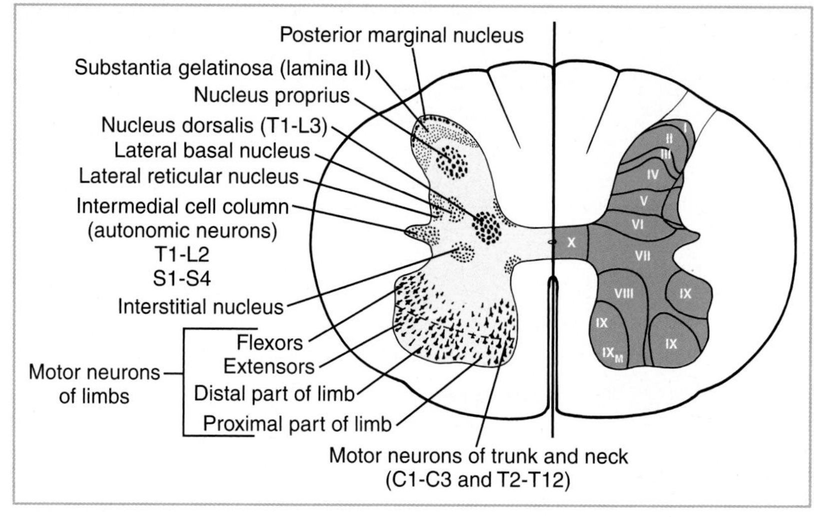

FIGURE 13-11 Architecture of the spinal cord, showing the gray matter nuclei (*left*) and Rexed laminae (*right*). (From Ross BK, Hughes SC. Epidural and spinal narcotic analgesia. Clin Obstet Gynecol 1987; 30:552-65.)

Pharmacokinetics and Pharmacodynamics

Many of the pharmacologic differences observed among neuraxially administered opioids depend on an opioid's ability to reach opioid receptors. An opioid's physicochemical properties, especially lipophilicity or hydrophilicity, largely determine the bioavailability of neuraxially administered opioids as well as the drug's ability to produce spinally mediated analgesia.

Before G protein–receptor activation can occur, the opioid must undergo a series of complex processes. Although several mechanisms have been proposed to explain the movement of opioids from the epidural space to the spinal cord, studies demonstrate that the only relevant mechanism is diffusion through the spinal meninges.[238-240] The opioid must traverse the dura and arachnoid membranes, diffuse through the CSF, and cross the pia membrane to reach the spinal cord (Figure 13-12). Once the drug reaches the surface of the spinal cord, it must diffuse through the white matter and then the gray matter in order to reach the site of action, the dorsal horn.[241] The rate and extent of opioid transfer to receptors

TABLE 13-3 Subtypes of Opioid Receptors

Receptor Type	Physiologic Response	Receptor Agonist
Mu (μ)	Analgesia Miosis Bradycardia Sedation Respiratory depression Decreased gastrointestinal transit	Morphine Fentanyl Sufentanil Meperidine
Kappa (κ)	Analgesia Sedation Respiratory depression Diuresis Psychotomimesis	Buprenorphine Pentazocine
Delta (δ)	Analgesia	Prodynorphin Endomorphins Enkephalins
Nociceptin/orphanin FQ (NOP)	Pain processing in spinal and supraspinal sites	

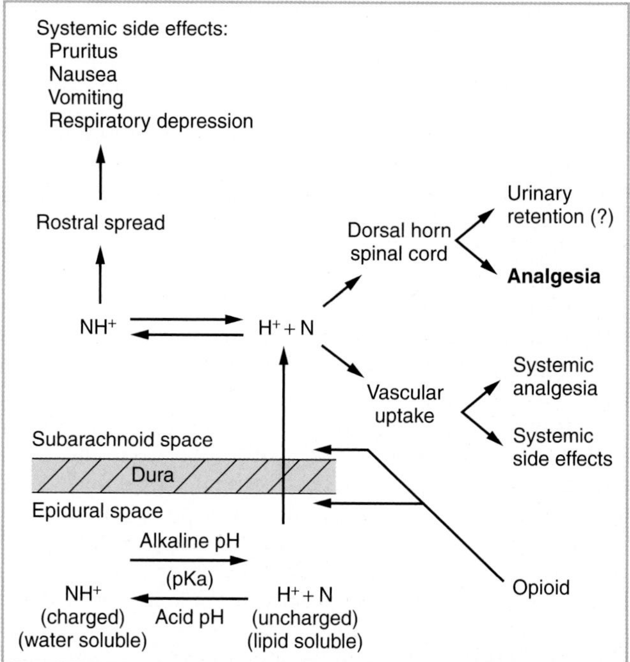

FIGURE 13-12 Epidural opioids traverse the dura and arachnoid membranes, diffuse through cerebrospinal fluid, and cross the pia membrane before reaching the spinal cord. Several factors, including physicochemical properties (e.g., pKa), affect the distribution of opioids within the neuraxis. (From Ross BK, Hughes SC. Epidural and spinal narcotic analgesia. Clin Obstet Gynecol 1987; 30:552-65.)

TABLE 13-4 Physicochemical Properties of Opioids Used for Neuraxial Analgesia

Opioid	Lipid Solubility*	pKa	Protein Binding (%)
Morphine	1.4	7.9	35
Meperidine	39	8.5	70
Diamorphine	280	7.8	40
Fentanyl	816	8.4	84
Sufentanil	1727	8.0	93

*Octanol-water partition coefficient.

Data from Camu F, Vanlersberghe C. Pharmacology of systemic analgesics. Best Pract Res Clin Anaesthesiol 2002; 16:475-88; and McLeod GA, Munishankar B, Columb MO. Is the clinical efficacy of epidural diamorphine concentration-dependent when used as analgesia for labour? Br J Anaesth 2005; 94:229-33.

largely depend on a drug's physicochemical properties, particularly lipid solubility, because competing processes (e.g., uptake into the epidural fat or systemic circulation) limit the agent's diffusion to opioid receptors. Greater lipid solubility of a drug results in more rapid onset of analgesia. For example, fentanyl is a highly lipid-soluble opioid (i.e., 600 times more lipid soluble than morphine); therefore, it has a more rapid onset of action than morphine (Table 13-4).

Latency, potency, and duration are also affected by other physicochemical properties, including molecular weight, pKa, and protein binding. For example, the lower the pKa, the greater the percentage of opioid existing in uncharged form (i.e., the anionic base) at a pH of 7.4. In the uncharged form, opioids penetrate the dura mater and dorsal horn more easily, resulting in a more rapid onset of analgesia.

The boundaries of the epidural space are the vertebral bodies, ligaments, and spinal meninges. Fat and the epidural venous plexus account for a large volume of the epidural space. The spinal meninges consist of the dura, arachnoid, and pia mater. Of these membranes, the arachnoid is the primary barrier for drug transfer from the epidural space to the spinal cord.[242] The arachnoid mater has multiple layers of overlapping cells that represent both a hydrophilic domain (consisting of extracellular and intracellular fluid) and a hydrophobic domain (the cell membranes).[240] In order for an opioid to navigate the arachnoid, it must diffuse through both domains before entering the CSF. Therefore, drugs of intermediate hydrophobicity move most readily across the arachnoid. Other physical characteristics of drugs (e.g., molecular weight) do not appear to play an important role in determining redistribution from the epidural space to the subarachnoid space.[240]

The efficacy of a drug also depends on its physicochemical properties, particularly lipid solubility. For example, the amount of drug that is sequestered in the epidural fat is entirely dependent on the drug's octanol-to-buffer distribution coefficient.[243] Consequently, lipophilic drugs (e.g., fentanyl) with a high octanol-to-buffer coefficient may never reach the arachnoid membrane and may partition in epidural fat. This lack of drug transfer across the meninges results in poor CSF bioavailability. To evaluate movement of opioids from the epidural to the subarachnoid space, Bernards et al.[243] used a porcine model to continuously sample opioid concentrations in the epidural and intrathecal spaces. Using microdialysis techniques, the investigators measured the redistribution of morphine, alfentanil, fentanyl, and sufentanil out of the epidural space. (These opioids were administered by epidural bolus injection.) Opioid concentrations were measured over time in the epidural space, subarachnoid space, systemic venous plasma, and epidural venous plasma. Results suggested that there was a strong linear relationship between lipid solubility and mean residence time, indicating that more lipid-soluble opioids spent a longer time in the epidural space. Consequently, these drugs partition themselves into the epidural fat with ongoing slow release back into the epidural space. Because of their long residence time in the epidural space, more lipid-soluble drugs are found in lower concentrations in the CSF (i.e., decreased bioavailability to opioid receptors in the dorsal horn).

Several human studies have evaluated whether epidurally administered fentanyl produces analgesia by a selective spinal mechanism or by systemic absorption and redistribution. Results of studies of lipophilic opioids (administered by epidural infusion) have suggested that low concentrations of lipophilic opioids are subject to rapid vascular uptake from the epidural space or sequestration in epidural fat, thereby limiting access to the spinal cord.[244-246] However, other studies have suggested the occurrence of a spinal effect when lipophilic opioids are administered by epidural bolus injection[247] or by epidural infusion of short duration.[248] Ginosar et al.[249] compared the analgesic effects of epidural bolus injection and epidural infusion of fentanyl in human volunteers. Study results suggested that epidural fentanyl infusion produced analgesia by uptake into the systemic circulation with redistribution to brain and peripheral opioid receptors. However, epidural bolus administration of fentanyl produced analgesia by selective spinal mechanisms. These results were consistent with previous reports that an epidural fentanyl bolus results in a larger amount of fentanyl in the epidural space than occurs at any time during an epidural infusion, leading to the greater availability of drug to activate opioid receptors in the dorsal horn of the spinal cord.

Although hydrophilic drugs (e.g., morphine) are subject to less systemic and epidural fat uptake than lipophilic drugs, the transfer of the former into the CSF is a somewhat inefficient process because they have difficulty in crossing the lipid bilayer of the arachnoid. However, despite these inefficiencies, morphine content in the spinal cord is significantly greater than lipophilic drug (e.g., fentanyl) content,[250] and morphine has much greater bioavailability in the spinal cord than do fentanyl and sufentanil.[243,250] In summary, although morphine clearly produces analgesia via a spinal mechanism, the extent of spinal analgesia produced by the neuraxial administration of fentanyl is less clear.

After a drug reaches the subarachnoid space, either by diffusion across the meninges or by direct injection into the CSF, its effects depend on its lipid solubility. All opioids produce at least some analgesia by spinal-specific mechanisms. Movement of these drugs within the CSF depends on their physicochemical properties. Drugs can diffuse within the CSF in either a cephalad or a caudad direction. Both morphine and fentanyl have been shown to move rapidly within the CSF.[251] Lipophilic drugs can also return to the epidural space by traversing previously mentioned structures.

Ummenhofer et al.[250] used a porcine model to investigate intrathecal administration of opioids. These investigators found that lipophilic opioids have a very large volume of distribution compared with hydrophilic drugs; the volume of distribution of sufentanil was 40 times greater that that of morphine. The reason is sufentanil's extreme lipid solubility, with the drug rapidly leaving the CSF and entering the epidural fat, from which it is absorbed systemically.[252]

The ultimate goal of neuraxial opioid administration is for the drug to penetrate the dorsal horn of the spinal cord and activate μ-opioid receptors. A drug's ability to move from the CSF to the dorsal horn depends on its physiochemical properties. Of the clinically relevant opioids, morphine has the most favorable physiochemical properties to allow penetration of the dorsal horn of the spinal cord (i.e., gray matter). Because of its extreme lipid solubility, sufentanil redistributes itself or partitions itself on the superficial layer (i.e., white matter) of the spinal cord.[250] Data suggest that the spinal bioavailability of the hydrophilic drugs (e.g., morphine, hydromorphone) is greater than that of hydrophobic opioids (e.g., fentanyl, sufentanil).

In summary, the onset and duration of analgesia as well as side effects produced by neuraxial opioid administration depend on the specific type of opioid receptor that is activated as well as on the dose, lipid solubility, and rate of movement and clearance of the opioid in the CSF.

Toxicity

Any agent that is injected into the epidural or subarachnoid space should be administered with caution owing to the potential for neurotoxicity and permanent neurologic damage. Although there is concern about injecting any type of medication into the neuraxis, the epidural space seems to be more forgiving than the subarachnoid space. In many cases, clinicians have injected medications that were not well tested in animal models. Yaksh and Collins[253] have urged careful administration of neuraxial drugs, stating that "studies in animals should precede human use of spinally administered drugs."

The most commonly administered neuraxial opioids in obstetric patients are preservative-free morphine, fentanyl, and sufentanil. Preservative-free morphine is commercially available for both epidural and intrathecal administration. To evaluate preservative-free morphine for potential neurotoxicity, Abouleish et al.[254] examined the short- and long-term effects of intrathecal morphine injection in monkeys. The meninges, nerve roots, and dorsal root ganglia were examined macroscopically and microscopically in both the study and the control groups. The researchers found no evidence of demyelination, arachnoiditis, or necrosis in either group.

Fentanyl is also available in a preservative-free form. Despite its widespread clinical use, few studies have assessed the histologic, physiologic, or clinical evidence of neurotoxicity with spinally administered fentanyl. One *in vitro* study evaluated the effects of fentanyl administration on nerve conduction.[255] Histopathologic studies of isolated rabbit vagus nerve axons did not show localized nerve damage after nerves were bathed in an isotonic solution of fentanyl. When axons were bathed in a hypotonic solution of fentanyl, permanent conduction deficits were noted. However, *in vivo*, relatively large doses of fentanyl would be required to create a hypotonic intrathecal environment.

Although no formal neurotoxicology studies have evaluated sufentanil administration in humans, there are no clinical reports of neurotoxicity despite its widespread use. In one study, sufentanil was administered to cats through an indwelling intrathecal catheter over 5 days.[256] Another study reported no evidence of abnormal morphologic effects with short- or long-term administration of sufentanil other than an inflammatory reaction secondary to catheter placement. Sabbe et al.[257] administered clinically relevant doses of intrathecal sufentanil to dogs over several weeks and reported no histopathologic changes. Rawal et al.[258] demonstrated dose-dependent spinal cord histopathologic changes after intrathecal administration of sufentanil (50 to 100 μg) every 6 hours for 72 hours. Because these doses are much larger than those used in clinical practice, these findings could reflect an artifact of experimental design (e.g., the frequent administration of a large-volume, hypotonic preparation).

Despite the paucity of data about possible neurotoxicity, both fentanyl and sufentanil are widely used in clinical practice. These drugs are not approved by the FDA for neuraxial use. However, there are no published reports of neurologic deficits after epidural or intrathecal administration of either agent in humans, and these drugs appear to be safe for neuraxial administration. Anesthesia providers should exercise extreme caution before injecting any untested agent into the spinal or epidural space, in order to prevent irritation or damage to neural structures.

Side Effects

Neuraxial opioid administration is associated with beneficial effects as well as potential complications and side effects. Intrathecal administration of relatively large doses of morphine is associated with a high incidence of side effects, including somnolence, nausea and vomiting, pruritus, and respiratory depression (Table 13-5). However, epidural injection and intrathecal injection of more lipid-soluble opioids have fewer side effects.

SENSORY CHANGES

An early study evaluating intrathecal sufentanil in laboring women reported sensory changes and hypotension, although no local anesthetics were administered.[259] Other investigators have reported high cervical sensory blockade associated with mental status changes, dysphagia, dyspnea, and automatisms after intrathecal sufentanil injection.[260-263] These symptoms are likely to be related to a dose-dependent opioid effect rather than neuraxial blockade–induced sympathectomy.[264] Further, these changes do not predict the quality or duration of analgesia or degree of hemodynamic change.[264] These sensory changes can be clinically significant, especially when they extend to the cervical dermatomes. Patients may feel that they cannot breathe or swallow, an effect that can be distressing.

TABLE 13-5 Incidence of Adverse Side Effects after Intrathecal Injection of 0.5 or 1.0 mg of Morphine*

	Incidence (%)		
Side Effect	Morphine 0.5 mg (n = 12)	Morphine 1 mg (n = 18)	Overall (n = 30)
Pruritus	58	94	80
Nausea/vomiting	50	56	53
Urinary retention	42	44	43
Drowsiness	33	50	43
Respiratory depression	0	6	3

*Modified from Abboud TK, Shnider SM, Dailey PA, et al. Intrathecal administration of hyperbaric morphine for the relief of pain in labour. Br J Anaesth 1984; 56:1351-60.

Fortunately, neither intrathecal sufentanil nor fentanyl affects the efferent limb of the nervous system, and motor function is not impaired. Patients should be reassured that their respiratory efforts are not impaired and that these symptoms will subside in 30 to 60 minutes. One report described the use of naloxone to treat the sensory changes associated with intrathecal sufentanil.[260]

NAUSEA AND VOMITING

Nausea and vomiting are common during labor and delivery. Intrapartum nausea and vomiting can occur from a variety of causes, including pregnancy, physiology of labor itself, pain associated with labor, and parenteral administration of an opioid that may have preceded the neuraxial opioid administration. Therefore, it is difficult to determine the incidence of nausea and vomiting as direct side effects of neuraxial analgesia. Although the mechanism of neuraxial opioid–mediated nausea is unclear, there are suggestions that it may be caused by modulation of afferent input to the area postrema (i.e., the chemoreceptor trigger zone) or at the nucleus of the tractus solitarius, a key relay station in the visceral sensory network.[265] Interestingly, nausea is more common after intrathecal administration of opioids to patients who have undergone cesarean delivery than in patients who received the same intrathecal regimen during labor and delivery. Norris et al.[266] reported that women receiving epidural or intrathecal opioid analgesia during labor had an incidence of nausea and vomiting of only 1.0% and 2.4%, respectively.

A number of treatments are available with minimal side effects. **Metoclopramide** 10 mg is very effective. One explanation for its efficacy is that it promotes gastric emptying. **Ondansetron** is also used in many centers for the treatment of opioid-induced nausea. In a study comparing transdermal scopolamine 1.5 mg, intravenous ondansetron 4 mg, and placebo, **scopolamine** was an effective prophylactic medication against nausea in parturients who received intrathecal morphine for postcesarean analgesia.[267] However, the use of scopolamine may be limited by bothersome side effects, including dry mouth, drowsiness, and blurred vision. Although **droperidol** is effective for the treatment of nausea, the FDA has issued a "black box" warning against its use because of concern about a higher risk for dysrhythmias in association with droperidol administration. In addition, pregnant patients may be especially vulnerable to the extrapyramidal side effects associated with droperidol administration.[268] More recently, intravenous **cyclizine** 50 mg was shown to be superior to **dexamethasone** 8 mg in reducing nausea following intrathecal morphine administration for cesarean delivery.[269]

PRURITUS

Pruritus is the most common side effect of neuraxial opioid administration.[259,270] Presentation is highly variable, but the incidence and severity seem to be dose dependent, especially with epidural opioid administration.[271] Onset of the pruritus occurs shortly after analgesia develops, and even small doses of intrathecal sufentanil may produce significant pruritus.[272] Some observers have noted a segmental pruritus, especially with lipophilic opioids. For example, patients often complain of perineal and truncal pruritus after intrathecal sufentanil injection.[259] Pruritus occurs more commonly with intrathecal opioid administration than with epidural administration (41.4% versus 1.3%, respectively).[266] The incidence and severity may be reduced by administration of a lower dose of opioid[273] or co-administration of the opioid with a local anesthetic.[274] Many patients do not complain about the pruritus and appear asymptomatic; however, when questioned, they acknowledge the problem.

Although the cause of opioid-induced pruritus is unknown, it appears to be unrelated to histamine release.[275] Some investigators have suggested that pruritus results from a perturbation of sensory input resulting from rostral spread of the opioid within the CSF to the trigeminal nucleus or subnucleus caudalis.[265,276] Itch-specific neuronal pathways may interact with pain pathways so that continuing activity of the pain-processing system suppresses activity in the spinal itch-processing neurons. Consequently, if pain is inhibited, pruritus can be unmasked (e.g., intrathecal morphine–induced pruritus). Pruritus can also be inhibited by pain (e.g., antipruritic effect of scratching).[277]

The serotoninergic system seems to contribute to modulation by providing a balance between nociception and antinociception in the network of pain-processing neurons.[278,279] The dorsal horn of the spinal cord and the spinal tract of the trigeminal nerve are abundant in 5-hydroxytryptamine-3 (5-HT_3) receptors. Because morphine is known to activate 5-HT_3 receptors by a mechanism independent of opioid receptors,[280] it is postulated that morphine may directly stimulate 5-HT_3 receptors and may cause intrathecal morphine–induced pruritus. Consequently, occupation of 5-HT_3 receptors by a 5-HT_3–receptor antagonist potentially prevents the pruritus.

Iatrou et al.[281] performed a randomized, double-blind, placebo-controlled study to evaluate the prophylactic effects of **ondansetron** and **dolasetron** in the treatment of intrathecal morphine–induced pruritus. Study results demonstrated that patients who received preemptive 5-HT_3–receptor antagonists reported significantly less pruritus and pruritus of less severity during the first 8 postoperative hours than patients who received placebo. The frequency of pruritus was reduced by 48% and 70% for ondansetron and dolasetron, respectively, compared with placebo. Although other studies have also demonstrated

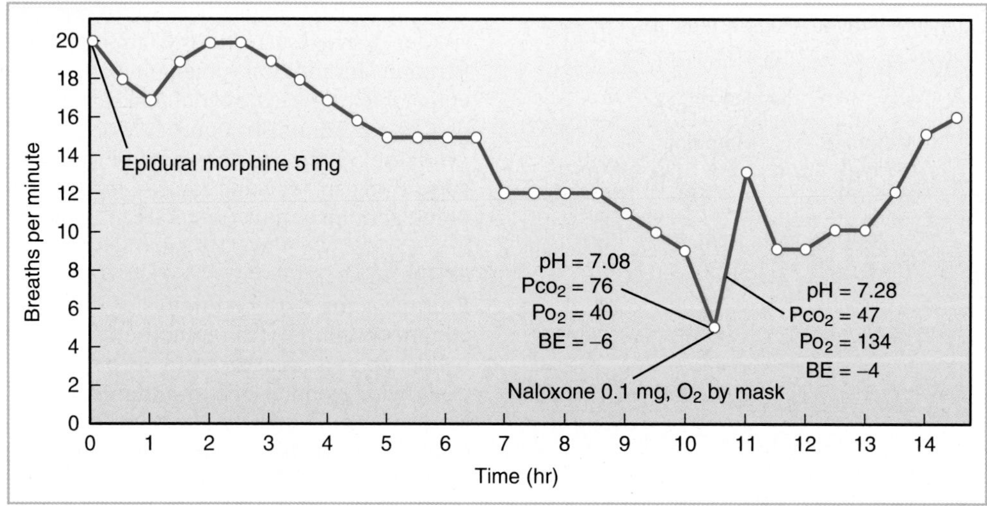

FIGURE 13-13 Respiratory rate of an obstetric patient who received 5 mg of morphine after cesarean delivery and who experienced delayed respiratory depression. (From Leicht CH, Hughes SC, Dailey PA, et al. Epidural morphine sulfate for analgesia after cesarean section: A prospective report of 1000 patients [abstract]. Anesthesiology 1986; 65:A366.)

efficacy in reduction of pruritus with 5-HT_3–receptor antagonists,[282-284] some studies have not,[285,286] suggesting that this treatment may not be effective with higher doses of morphine[285] or lipophilic opioids.[286]

Other treatments of intrathecal opioid–induced pruritus include administration of intravenous **naloxone** (40 to 80 μg) or **diphenhydramine** (25 mg). Despite the probability that the pruritus is unrelated to histamine release, there may be some benefit from the modest sedation that follows diphenhydramine administration. Administration of **nalbuphine** (2.5 to 5 mg intravenously[287,288] or 10 mg subcutaneously[287,289]) may also be helpful in reducing symptoms. The advantage of nalbuphine over naloxone is that it is less likely to reverse neuraxial opioid analgesia.[288] Intravenous **propofol** 10 mg has also been reported to relieve pruritus.[290,291] Regardless of the chosen treatment, pruritus can contribute significantly to patient dissatisfaction and should be treated promptly upon request.

HYPOTENSION

Decreased blood pressure was reported in early studies that evaluated intrathecal opioid administration.[259,264] Although hypotension occurs in 5% to 10% of parturients who receive intrathecal opioids,[259,264] the incidence is higher when a local anesthetic or clonidine is added to the opioid. Early reports suggested that hypotension was due to a sympathectomy, but later work suggests that hypotension results from pain relief[292] and decreased maternal levels of catecholamines, especially epinephrine.[293] Wang et al.[294] demonstrated that intrathecal opioids block the afferent information from A-delta and C-fibers to the spinal cord, but that efferent nerve impulses (e.g., sympathetic efferents) are not directly blocked. However, sympathetic blockade can be expected if either a local anesthetic or clonidine is administered intrathecally with the opioid.

RESPIRATORY DEPRESSION

All opioids can cause respiratory depression regardless of their route of administration. When opioids are administered either epidurally or intrathecally, the following factors affect the risk of respiratory depression: (1) choice of drug and its pharmacokinetics, (2) drug dose, and (3) concomitantly administered CNS depressants. The most important factor affecting the onset of respiratory depression induced by intrathecal opioids is lipid solubility.[295] When a lipophilic opioid (e.g., fentanyl, sufentanil) is administered, respiratory depression may occur within minutes because of rapid absorption of the opioid from the CSF to lipophilic tissues.[241] Its subsequent clearance and elimination are similar to those of the drug when intravenously injected. This means that the "time frame" for respiratory depression is short. Hydrophilic drugs (e.g., morphine, hydromorphone) are associated with delayed respiratory depression. This potentially serious side effect occurs because these hydrophilic opioids remain in the CSF for several hours. Although this characteristic improves the bioavailability of these opioids, rostral migration and absorption into the respiratory centers can produce respiratory depression 6 to 12 hours after injection (Figure 13-13).

The dose of opioid has also been shown to be an important factor in the occurrence of respiratory depression. The usual dose of intrathecal morphine for post–cesarean delivery analgesia is 0.1 to 0.2 mg. Not surprisingly, an early report of respiratory depression occurred after administration of intrathecal morphine 1 mg.[296] In a dose-response study, Palmer et al.[297] concluded that there was little justification for giving more than 0.1 mg of intrathecal morphine for post–cesarean delivery analgesia.

Although most cases of respiratory depression associated with sufentanil administration occur with larger doses, respiratory depression has also been reported with as little as 10 μg of intrathecal sufentanil administered for labor analgesia.[298,299] Larger doses (e.g., 15 μg) have not been found to produce better or more prolonged analgesia but do result in increased plasma opioid concentrations and a higher risk of respiratory depression. In a female volunteer study, Lu et al.[252] reported that doses of intrathecal sufentanil larger than 12.5 μg did not produce a proportionate increase in intensity or duration of analgesia. Similarly, there is little benefit to increasing the dose of intrathecal fentanyl beyond 25 μg when it is used as the sole agent for labor analgesia. These higher doses (i.e., more than 10 μg of sufentanil or more than 25 μg of fentanyl) should not be used in routine clinical practice.

Respiratory depression has been reported with as little as 100 μg of epidural fentanyl.[300] In a dose-response study of epidural morphine administration in post–cesarean delivery patients, investigators concluded that the quality of analgesia increases as the dose of epidural morphine increases to 3.75 mg but that increasing the dose to 5 mg does not improve analgesia.[301]

Several case reports have implicated previous parenteral administration of opioid as a contributing factor in respiratory arrest associated with intrathecal sufentanil administration in laboring women.[302,303] For example, Jaffee et al.[304] reported a case of apnea and unresponsiveness in a parturient who had received several doses of intravenous fentanyl in the 4 hours prior to intrathecal sufentanil administration. Although pregnancy-induced respiratory drive continues throughout labor and into the postpartum period and may provide some protection against respiratory depression, respiratory depression is the most serious side effect of neuraxial opioid administration.

Practice guidelines from the American Society of Anesthesiologists (ASA)[305] recommend that all patients who receive neuraxial opioids should be monitored for adequacy of **ventilation** (e.g., respiratory rate, depth of respiration), **oxygenation** (e.g., pulse oximetry when appropriate), and **level of consciousness**. In patients who receive a single neuraxial injection of a lipophilic opioid (e.g., fentanyl), continual monitoring should be performed for at least 2 hours after opioid administration. In patients who receive a single neuraxial injection of a hydrophilic opioid (e.g., morphine), monitoring should be performed hourly during the first 12 hours and then every 2 hours for the next 12 hours after opioid administration. For patients who receive a continuous infusion of a neuraxial opioid, monitoring should be performed hourly during the first 12 hours, every 2 hours for the next 12 hours, and then every 4 hours for the duration of the opioid infusion. In addition, the guidelines state that greater duration and intensity of monitoring and/or additional methods of monitoring may be indicated in patients at increased risk for respiratory depression (e.g., due to obesity, obstructive sleep apnea, concomitant administration of opioid analgesics by other routes).

URINARY RETENTION

Urinary retention is a bothersome side effect of intraspinal opioid administration. The incidence varies widely. It is more common with neuraxial opioid administration than with intramuscular or intravenous administration of equivalent doses. Urinary retention is unrelated to systemic absorption and is also dose independent. The onset of urinary retention appears to parallel the onset of analgesia. Evidence suggests that the rapid onset of this side effect is produced by relaxation of the detrusor muscle (Figure 13-14),[306] which most likely results from the sacral spinal action of opioids. Urinary retention can be treated with naloxone; however, because many parturients require catheterization for other reasons, urinary retention is often treated with bladder catheterization.

DELAYED GASTRIC EMPTYING

Labor may delay gastric emptying,[307] and opioids may further exacerbate this delay. Parenterally administered opioids are known to delay gastric emptying in laboring women.[308] However, clinically useful doses of epidural fentanyl have minimal effects on gastric emptying. In contrast, intrathecal administration of fentanyl produces greater delays in gastric emptying than epidural administration.[309]

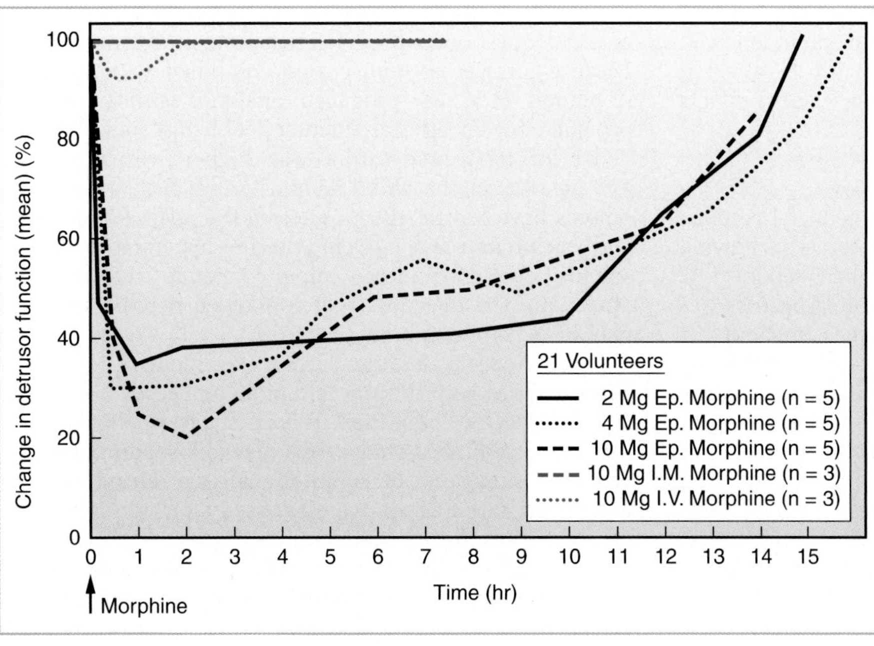

FIGURE 13-14 Urodynamic effects of epidural (Ep.), intramuscular (I.M.), and intravenous (I.V.) morphine administration in male volunteers. Depression of detrusor muscle function persisted for many hours after epidural morphine administration. This did not occur with parenteral opioids and may represent a local spinal cause (i.e., opioid receptors). (From Rawal N, Mollefors K, Axelsson K, et al. An experimental study of urodynamic effects of epidural morphine and of naloxone reversal. Anesth Analg 1983; 62:641-7.)

Delays in gastric emptying may increase the risk of nausea and vomiting and also increase the risk of aspiration if general anesthesia is necessary for emergency cesarean delivery.

RECRUDESCENCE OF HERPES SIMPLEX VIRUS INFECTIONS

Genital herpes infection (herpes simplex virus [HSV]) is the most common type of herpes viral infection during pregnancy[310]; however, oral HSV infections (common cold sore or fever blister) resulting from reactivation of latent HSV infection also occur during pregnancy. Some reports have suggested a relationship between intraspinal opioid administration and reactivation of oral herpes infection.[311,312] Some of the first reports of recurrent infections were noted in obstetric patients who received epidural morphine for post–cesarean delivery analgesia. Crone et al.[313] reported a 10% incidence of reactivation in patients who had received epidural morphine, compared with a 1% incidence in similar patients who did not receive epidural morphine. These observations have been confirmed in two prospective studies.[314,315] Two case reports have reported an association between intraspinal administration of fentanyl and meperidine and reactivation of oral herpes infection.[311,312]

Studies support a central mechanism. Viral reactivation is known to occur with exposure to ultraviolet light, immunosuppression, trauma, and fever. Proposed etiologies include (1) a skin trigger mechanism, whereby pruritus and scratching trigger reactivation[316]; (2) an altered immunologic response[317]; and (3) a ganglion trigger mechanism, whereby the intraspinal opioid spreads rostrally and binds to the trigeminal nerve.[318] The ganglion trigger mechanism involves an alteration of sensory modulation that results in reactivation. We are unaware of any serious maternal or neonatal complications that have resulted from neuraxial administration of an opioid and reactivation of oral herpes infection.

Placental Transfer and Fetal and Neonatal Effects

Neuraxial opioid administration may have a direct effect on the infant (i.e., respiratory depression at delivery) that results from systemic absorption of the opioid followed by transplacental transfer. The fetus may also be affected indirectly by opioid-related maternal side effects (i.e., hypoxemia, respiratory depression).

NEONATAL DEPRESSION

Systemic opioid absorption can result in neonatal respiratory depression, which is sometimes observed following systemic opioid administration during labor.[319,320] Neuraxial techniques may result in better Apgar scores and umbilical cord blood gas and pH measurements at delivery. Despite the rapid systemic uptake of intrathecally administered opioids, the technique involves administration of smaller doses of opioid.

Several studies have evaluated neonatal outcome after continuous maternal epidural infusion of opioids and local anesthetics.[321-323] Collectively, these studies have demonstrated that maternal epidural opioid administration by continuous infusion rarely results in drug accumulation and subsequent neonatal depression. However, Loftus et al.[324] evaluated placental transfer of sufentanil and fentanyl administered with bupivacaine during labor. There was a modest reduction in Neurologic and Adaptive Capacity Scores at 24 hours of age in babies whose mothers had received epidural fentanyl. Somewhat better scores were observed in babies whose mothers had received epidural sufentanil. Sufentanil was detected in only one umbilical arterial blood sample. More recently, Reynolds et al.[325] performed a systematic review of randomized and nonrandomized studies comparing epidural with systemic opioid analgesia. They reviewed 12 trials with a total study population of 2102 parturients. Epidural analgesia was associated with better umbilical cord blood acid-base measurements than systemic opioids, suggesting that placental exchange was well preserved despite maternal sympathetic blockade and effective analgesia. Although not all of the studies used neuraxial opioid infusions, the researchers suggested that replacement of systemic opioids with modest doses of neuraxial opioids not only produces superior analgesia but also may have a favorable effect on neonatal outcome.[325]

FETAL BRADYCARDIA

Although epidural or intrathecal opioid administration has little direct effect on FHR,[324,326,327] worrisome abnormalities such as late decelerations and fetal bradycardia have been observed after intrathecal lipophilic opioid administration. Several reports have described the abrupt onset of fetal bradycardia after intrathecal administration of fentanyl or sufentanil.[328-330] Clarke et al.[329] suggested that the bradycardia is an indirect effect of decreased circulating maternal epinephrine associated with the rapid onset of analgesia. Epinephrine has a tocolytic effect and causes uterine relaxation by stimulating $beta_2$-adrenergic receptors. Consequently, reduced epinephrine levels may lead to increased uterine tone. Because uteroplacental perfusion occurs during periods of uterine diastole (i.e., uterine relaxation), uterine hypertonus (tachysystole) may result in diminished uteroplacental perfusion and fetal hypoxia. Because norepinephrine is known to have uterine-stimulating effects,[331] the decrease in epinephrine concentration alongside an unchanged norepinephrine concentration may produce uterine hyperactivity and fetal compromise.

Other mechanisms may also be relevant. Van de Velde et al.[332] questioned the catecholamine imbalance theory, because intrathecal bupivacaine combined with low-dose sufentanil (1.5 μg) produced analgesia similar to that provided by intrathecal sufentanil (7.5 μg), but the incidence of fetal bradycardia was higher with sufentanil 7.5 μg. Russell et al.[333] demonstrated that intravenous opioids have central effects, altering the release of oxytocin and vasopressin and inducing uterine hyperactivity. Lipid-soluble opioids undergo rapid systemic redistribution after neuraxial injection; therefore, even neuraxial opioids may have central effects.

Initial reports indicated that the incidence of FHR abnormalities with intrathecal opioid analgesia was 15% to 20%.[259,334] One published report suggests that uterine hypertonus and fetal bradycardia may follow administration of either intrathecal or epidural analgesia during labor.[335] Fetal heart rate tracings were assessed after administration of either intrathecal sufentanil or epidural bupivacaine. There were no observed differences in the incidence of FHR abnormalities (i.e., recurrent late decelerations and/ or bradycardia) between groups (22% in the intrathecal sufentanil group versus 23% in the epidural bupivacaine group).[335] In contrast, Mardirosoff et al.[336] performed a systematic review of all randomized trials comparing intrathecal with nonintrathecal administration of opioids in laboring women. Twenty-four trials met criteria; the study population included 3513 women. The relative risk of FHR abnormalities in patients receiving spinal opioids was 1.81 (95% CI, 1.04 to 3.14). The risks of cesarean delivery for FHR abnormalities were similar in the two groups (6.0% for intrathecal administration versus 7.8% for other methods).

In a prospective study, Van de Velde et al.[332] investigated whether intrathecal sufentanil 7.5 μg produced more FHR abnormalities than either conventional epidural analgesia or intrathecal bupivacaine combined with sufentanil 1.5 μg. The high-dose sufentanil group had more FHR abnormalities (i.e., late decelerations, fetal bradycardia) but less hypotension than the low-dose sufentanil/bupivacaine group. The incidence of FHR abnormalities was similar in the low-dose sufentanil/bupivacaine and conventional epidural analgesia groups. The rates of cesarean delivery for FHR abnormalities were similar in the three groups. Although FHR abnormalities are worrisome, most published trials have not reported a higher risk of emergency cesarean delivery with intrathecal opioid analgesia.[332,336,337] However, Gambling et al.[338] reported more operative deliveries for nonreassuring fetal status after administration of intrathecal sufentanil 10 μg than with parenteral meperidine analgesia. The study's conclusions, however, were limited in that the two study groups differed in frequency of FHR assessment.

Given the potential risk of fetal bradycardia after neuraxial analgesia in laboring women, the FHR should be monitored during and after the initiation of epidural and intrathecal analgesia. FHR changes are usually transient and may be managed successfully with conservative measures, including (1) supplemental oxygen administration, (2) position changes to relieve aortocaval compression, (3) vasopressor therapy to treat hypotension, (4) discontinuation of oxytocin infusion, and (5) administration of a tocolytic agent for persistent uterine hypertonus (tachysystole).

In the past, intravenous or subcutaneous **terbutaline** was used to treat persistent uterine hypertonus. More recently, **nitroglycerin** has been used with some success. Nitroglycerin has several advantages over terbutaline. First, nitroglycerin has a short duration of action, and labor resumes shortly after the period of hypotonus. In addition, nitroglycerin rarely produces significant hypotension, and if hypotension occurs, it is easily treated. Several studies have evaluated nitroglycerin for the treatment of uterine hypertonus. Mercier et al.[339] described consistent success in treating FHR abnormalities resulting from uterine hypertonus after the administration of one or two doses of nitroglycerin (60 to 90 μg), and Bell[340] described the successful use of sublingual nitroglycerin (400 μg) in the treatment of uterine hypertonus. In contrast, Buhimschi et al.[341] observed that three doses of nitroglycerin spray (800 μg per dose) did not reduce uterine activity in laboring women. Therefore, if there is no response within 2 to 3 minutes of nitroglycerin administration, terbutaline 0.25 mg should be administered, and preparations should be made for emergency cesarean delivery if the fetal bradycardia does not resolve.

ADJUVANTS

Epinephrine

Epinephrine has a long history as a local anesthetic adjuvant. It is often added to epidural and spinal local anesthetic solutions to increase the duration of anesthesia, reduce peak plasma drug concentrations, improve block reliability, and intensify analgesia/anesthesia.[342-345] Despite these advantages, there have been concerns about epinephrine's effects on uterine blood flow and the maternal cardiovascular system. In addition, clinical and laboratory data have raised concerns about neurotoxicity with the addition of epinephrine to spinal lidocaine.[346,347]

Epinephrine prolongs the duration of epidural anesthesia by reducing uptake of local anesthetic into the systemic circulation through constriction of the epidural venous plexus. This effect helps maintain the concentration of local anesthetic at the site of injection. The efficacy of epinephrine depends on the specific local anesthetic as well as the site of injection. Epinephrine is more effective at prolonging the duration of short-acting local anesthetics (e.g., lidocaine, 2-chloroprocaine). During epidural administration, epinephrine has been shown to provide optimal vasoconstriction of lidocaine when it is added in a concentration of 5 μg/mL (1:200,000); this concentration of epinephrine nearly doubles the duration of epidural lidocaine anesthesia.[348] Epinephrine has not been shown to prolong the epidural anesthesia produced by bupivacaine and ropivacaine.[343] These local anesthetics have their own inherent vasoconstricting properties.

Epinephrine, when added at a concentration of 5 μg/mL, has been shown to reduce plasma concentrations of lidocaine and 2-chloroprocaine by 20% to 30%. However, plasma levels of ropivacaine are not reduced when epinephrine is added. Only modest decreases, of 10% to 20%, are observed with the addition of epinephrine to bupivacaine. Although epinephrine's effect on decreasing plasma levels of local anesthetic have been attributed to vasoconstriction resulting in reductions in blood flow and systemic absorption of local anesthetic in the epidural space, evidence suggests that reduced dural blood flow and increased hepatic clearance may contribute to lower plasma levels.[349]

Greater reliability and intensity of the block are also observed when epinephrine is added to epidurally administered local anesthetics. Epinephrine has intrinsic analgesic effects that are produced by stimulation of $alpha_2$-adrenergic receptors. These presynaptic adrenergic receptors are found at the terminals of primary afferent neurons. They can also be found centrally on neurons in superficial laminae of the spinal cord and in several brainstem nuclei.

In addition to the intrinsic analgesic effects of epinephrine, the inherent lipid solubility of each local anesthetic affects the degree of sensory blockade. Each local anesthetic has a lipid-to-water partition coefficient that determines the drug uptake between the aqueous and lipid phases within the spinal canal. The outcome of competition between these lipid and aqueous phases depends on the lipid solubility of the local anesthetic. If a local anesthetic is more lipid soluble, the advantage of adding epinephrine to the local anesthetic is less significant. For example, the lipid-to-water partition coefficient of lidocaine is 2.7. When epinephrine is added to lidocaine, there is marked improvement in the intensity of the block. However, since bupivacaine has a lipid-to-water partition coefficient 10 times greater than that of lidocaine, the effect of epinephrine on a bupivacaine block is less pronounced. Because ropivacaine has a lipid-to-water partition coefficient similar to that of lidocaine, epinephrine will intensify a ropivacaine block. However, the duration of the block remains unchanged.

In healthy fetuses, epidural administration of epinephrine does not affect umbilical cord blood flow. However, in fetuses with increased vascular resistance, epidural epinephrine administration can increase the umbilical artery S/D ratio.

Bicarbonate

The addition of sodium bicarbonate to a local anesthetic solution increases the pH closer to the pKa of the local anesthetic. This change increases the proportion of drug in un-ionized form that is available to penetrate the nerve sheath and membrane, thereby accelerating the onset of the block and decreasing the minimum concentration (C_m) required for conduction blockade.[350,351] Most studies have demonstrated that the addition of sodium bicarbonate to lidocaine, mepivacaine, bupivacaine, or 2-chloroprocaine hastens the onset of epidural blockade by as much as 10 minutes.[352-357] The speed of onset of a ropivacaine block does not seem to be affected by alkalinization, but as with the other local anesthetics, evidence suggests that alkalinization intensifies epidural ropivacaine anesthesia and improves spread to sacral dermatomes.[358] The effects of alkalinization are most pronounced in epinephrine-containing solutions, particularly commercially prepared epinephrine-containing formulations. These solutions are prepared at a lower pH, ranging from 3.2 to 4.2.[359] The lower pH of these solutions helps preserve the epinephrine but increases the latency of onset.

Sodium bicarbonate 1 mEq/mL (8.4%) may be freshly added to local anesthetic solutions shortly before use (Table 13-6). Alkalinization of bupivacaine must be performed carefully because the margin between satisfactory alkalinization and complete precipitation is very narrow. All local anesthetics have a tendency to precipitate, so solutions containing bicarbonate should be inspected for precipitation before being administered.

Hypotension occurs more frequently with epidural administration of an alkalinized local anesthetic than with administration of an unbuffered solution.[360] This likely results from an accelerated onset of sympathetic blockade. Carbonated salts of local anesthetics can also be administered for a rapid onset of epidural blockade. However, these drugs have limited availability. Like alkalinized local anesthetics, these preparations are more likely to produce hypotension.

TABLE 13-6 Alkalinization of Local Anesthetic Solutions

Local Anesthetic	Sodium Bicarbonate (mL)*
Lidocaine	1.0
Mepivacaine	1.0
Bupivacaine	0.1
2-Chloroprocaine	0.3

*Sodium bicarbonate 8.4% (1 mEq/mL) added to 10 mL local anesthetic solution. Suggested doses are from Horlocker T, Wedel D. Neuraxial anesthesia. In Longnecker D, Brown D, Newman M, Zapol W. Anesthesia. New York: McGraw-Hill, 2007:993.

Alpha$_2$-Adrenergic Agonists

Alpha$_2$-adrenergic agonists (e.g., **clonidine**) have been introduced as adjuvants to local anesthetic solutions after the demonstration of clonidine's safety and efficacy. The advantage of clonidine is its ability to provide analgesia without affecting sensation or producing motor blockade.[361] However, alpha$_2$-adrenergic agonists are known to produce hypotension by sympatho-inhibition at the level of the spinal cord as well as by effects on the brain itself.[362] In addition, alpha$_2$-adrenergic agonists produce dose-dependent sedation, which results from alpha$_2$-adrenergic stimulation in the locus ceruleus.[363]

Clonidine has been administered for labor as well as post–cesarean delivery analgesia. It exerts its effects by binding to alpha$_2$-adrenergic receptors located on primary afferent terminals of the spinal cord, substantia gelatinosa, and brainstem nuclei[364] as well as via a cholinergic mechanism.[365] Conduction blockade is produced by increases in potassium conductance and in acetylcholine and norepinephrine in the CSF, leading to decreased release of substance P and subsequent analgesia.[366]

Approximately 70% of alpha-adrenergic receptors on human myometrium are alpha$_2$-adrenergic receptors[367]; therefore, the potential effects of clonidine on labor and delivery have been evaluated. In an *in vitro* study, clonidine directly enhanced the frequency and amplitude of human myometrial contraction.[368] Alpha$_2$-adrenergic receptor stimulation in the uterus could theoretically enhance uterine contractions and decrease uterine blood flow.[362] Indeed, in animal studies, large doses of clonidine produced a decrease in FHR.[369] This effect probably resulted from direct fetal transfer of drug and from direct and indirect effects on baroreflexes. However, this effect is unlikely to occur with clinical doses of neuraxial clonidine.

INTRATHECAL CLONIDINE

Several studies have evaluated intrathecal clonidine administration in humans as an analgesic adjunct during labor and delivery. In one study, intrathecal clonidine was administered in doses of 100 to 200 μg as the sole drug. It produced excellent labor analgesia of short duration, but at the expense of profound sedation and hypotension.[370] Other studies have combined reduced doses of clonidine and local anesthetic and/or opioid to prolong analgesia, with more favorable effects. When more than 30 μg clonidine was administered with intrathecal sufentanil, the incidence of hypotension was greater than with sufentanil administration alone.[371] Duration of analgesia was prolonged from 97 to 125 minutes when clonidine was added. D'Angelo et al.[372] compared intrathecal bupivacaine-sufentanil with and without clonidine 50 μg. Labor analgesia was prolonged from 137 to 197 minutes when clonidine was added to intrathecal bupivacaine and sufentanil. No adverse effects were reported. Sia et al.[373] also added intrathecal clonidine (0 to 30 μg) to sufentanil and bupivacaine. The researchers reported better-quality and longer-lasting analgesia when intrathecal clonidine was added to sufentanil and bupivacaine, but with more hypotension and sedation. In contrast, when Paech et al.[374] added clonidine (0 to 45 μg) to intrathecal fentanyl and bupivacaine, the duration of spinal analgesia was unchanged, but there was a higher incidence of hypotension. Similarly, clonidine (30 μg) added to intrathecal ropivacaine and sufentanil resulted in longer duration of labor analgesia (122 versus 90 minutes).[375] However, more maternal hypotension and FHR abnormalities were noted, although Apgar scores and umbilical cord blood gas measurements were similar in the two groups.

In summary, it appears safe to add small doses of intrathecal clonidine (≤ 30 μg) to an opioid and bupivacaine to prolong labor analgesia. However, hypotension is a common side effect that must be treated promptly to avoid fetal compromise.

EPIDURAL CLONIDINE

Epidural administration of clonidine has also been evaluated for labor analgesia. Aveline et al.[376] demonstrated a 64% reduction in the MLAC of ropivacaine when clonidine 60 μg was added to epidural ropivacaine. However, clonidine administration was associated with a greater decrease in systolic blood pressure at 15 minutes as well as a higher incidence of sedation. The incidence of motor block or cesarean delivery was not increased. When hypotension was treated promptly, there were no fetal consequences. Landau et al.[377] noted prolonged analgesia and a local anesthetic–sparing effect when clonidine 75 μg was added to epidural ropivacaine. The researchers observed a decrease in motor block over time and no maternal sedation. However, fetal bradycardia was observed when hypotension developed. This occurred 20 to 120 minutes after epidural administration of clonidine. Apgar scores and umbilical cord blood gas measurements were unremarkable when the hypotension was treated promptly with ephedrine.

Clonidine (1.5 μg/mL) has also been added to bupivacaine for patient-controlled epidural analgesia.[378] This combination provided superior analgesia with lower bupivacaine requirements in comparison with bupivacaine plus fentanyl (2 μg/mL) but no clonidine. Similarly, Paech et al.[379] reported that the combination of epidural clonidine (22 to 45 μg/hr) with 0.0625% bupivacaine and fentanyl 2 μg/mL reduced the need for patient-controlled epidural boluses and improved pain relief during the first stage of labor.

Epidural clonidine has been administered for post–cesarean delivery analgesia. One study suggested that epidural clonidine (400 to 800 μg) provided postoperative analgesia, but a continuous infusion was required after 6 hours.[380] Others have demonstrated that clonidine (75 to 150 μg) lengthens the duration of postoperative analgesia without increasing the incidence of side effects.[381,382]

Despite the potential benefits of neuraxial clonidine, the routine use of this drug for obstetric analgesia is not recommended in the United States. The FDA has issued a "black box" warning against its use in obstetric patients because of concerns about hemodynamic instability after its use.

Neostigmine

Both nicotinic and muscarinic cholinergic receptors are present in the dorsal horn of the spinal cord. Neostigmine prevents breakdown of acetylcholine in the spinal cord. The acetylcholine then binds to muscarinic and nicotinic receptors of the spinal cord.[383-385] Stimulation of muscarinic receptors facilitates release of gamma-aminobutyric acid (GABA) in the dorsal horn of the spinal cord, resulting in analgesia.[365,386] Neostigmine and clonidine use a common pathway to produce analgesia mediated through acetylcholine release.

Several studies have evaluated the addition of neostigmine to intrathecal labor analgesics. Although results of these studies were inconsistent in terms of prolonging the duration of labor analgesia, all studies found that intrathecal administration of neostigmine produced severe nausea unresponsive to standard antiemetics.[387,388] These important gastrointestinal side effects limit its clinical use despite its ability to potentiate the analgesic effects of intrathecal opioids and clonidine.

Epidural neostigmine alone has limited efficacy. Neostigmine appears to be more effective at alleviating somatic pain than visceral pain.[389,390] Visceral afferents are located deep within the spinal cord. Because neostigmine has low lipid solubility, it has a limited ability to traverse biologic membranes. When it is administered without other agents, it is unable to reach these visceral afferents responsible for much of labor pain.[391] This accounts for the limited efficacy of neostigmine epidurally administered as the sole agent. However, when combined with epidural sufentanil or clonidine at the beginning of labor, neostigmine produces selective labor analgesia without side effects.[392,393] Large doses of neostigmine can potentially reduce uteroplacental blood flow by CNS activation and direct stimulation of uterine contractions.[394] Further studies are needed to evaluate neostigmine administration by continuous infusion for potential tachyphylaxis and side effects.[395] When administered for post–cesarean delivery analgesia, epidural neostigmine (75 to 300 μg) produced modest analgesia without nausea or vomiting.[396] It also allowed early mobilization but caused dose-independent sedation.

Although neostigmine is the only anticholinesterase that has been evaluated as a neuraxial analgesic in humans, other anticholinesterases may prove to be safe for neuraxial administration with fewer side effects. Neostigmine is not routinely used in clinical practice, and its neuraxial use is not approved by the FDA.

KEY POINTS

- Pregnancy enhances the effect of local anesthetic agents.
- Appropriate administration of epidural anesthesia does not adversely affect uterine tone or uterine or umbilical blood flow.
- Repeated epidural injections of lidocaine may result in a greater accumulation of drug in women with preeclampsia than in healthy pregnant women.
- Bupivacaine has greater cardiotoxicity than lidocaine because of its greater electrophysiologic effects, which predispose to ventricular arrhythmias.

- Single (levorotary) isomer formulations of amide local anesthetics, such as ropivacaine and levobupivacaine, have a lower potential for cardiotoxicity than racemic bupivacaine.
- Fetal acidosis results in a greater accumulation of amide local anesthetic in the fetus.
- Local anesthetics, as used clinically, are not teratogenic.
- The elimination half-life of amide local anesthetics is longer in the newborn than in the adult because the former has a greater volume of distribution.
- The fetus and newborn seem to be no more vulnerable to the toxic effects of local anesthetics than the adult.
- Neonatal neurobehavior depends on many factors other than the choice of local anesthetic.
- Alkalinization of a local anesthetic solution shortens the latency of neural blockade but increases the risk of hypotension during administration of epidural anesthesia.
- Neuraxial opioid administration produces analgesia without loss of sensation or proprioception.
- The combination of a neuraxial local anesthetic and an opioid increases block density and allows for administration of a lower total dose of local anesthetic and a lower incidence of side effects.
- Spinal bioavailability of the hydrophilic drugs (e.g., morphine, hydromorphone) is greater than that of hydrophobic (lipophilic) opioids (e.g., fentanyl, sufentanil).
- The most common side effects of neuraxial opioid administration are pruritus and nausea and vomiting. Fetal bradycardia and maternal respiratory depression are the most serious complications.

REFERENCES

1. Aberg G. Toxicological and local anesthetic effects of optically active isomers of two local anesthetic compounds. Acta Pharmacol Toxicol (Copenh) 1972; 31:273-86.
2. Graf BM, Abraham I, Eberbach N, et al. Differences in cardiotoxicity of bupivacaine and ropivacaine are the result of physicochemical and stereoselective properties. Anesthesiology 2002; 96:1427-34.
3. McClure JH. Ropivacaine. Br J Anaesth 1996; 76:300-7.
4. Strickartz G. The inhibition of sodium currents in the myelinated nerves by quaternary derivatives of lidocaine. J Gen Physiol 1973; 62:37-57.
5. Bromage PR. Continuous lumbar epidural analgesia for obstetrics. Can Med Assoc J 1961; 85:1136-40.
6. Fagraeus L, Urban BJ, Bromage PR. Spread of epidural analgesia in early pregnancy. Anesthesiology 1983; 58:184-7.
7. Butterworth JF IV, Walker FO, Lysak SZ. Pregnancy increases median nerve susceptibility of lidocaine. Anesthesiology 1990; 72:962-5.
8. Datta S, Lambert DH, Gregus J, et al. Differential sensitivities of mammalian nerve fibers during pregnancy. Anesth Analg 1983; 62:1070-2.
9. Bader AM, Datta S, Moller RA, Covino BG. Acute progesterone treatment has no effect on bupivacaine-induced conduction blockade in the isolated rabbit vagus nerve. Anesth Analg 1990; 71:545-8.
10. O'Brien JE, Abbey V, Hinsvark O, et al. Metabolism and measurement of chloroprocaine, an ester-type local anesthetic. J Pharm Sci 1979; 68:75-8.
11. Kuhnert BR, Kuhnert PM, Philipson EH, et al. The half-life of 2-chloroprocaine. Anesth Analg 1986; 65:273-8.
12. Monedero P, Hess P. High epidural block with chloroprocaine in a parturient with low pseudocholinesterase activity. Can J Anaesth 2001; 48:318-9.
13. Santos AC, Pedersen H, Morishima HO, et al. Pharmacokinetics of lidocaine in nonpregnant and pregnant ewes. Anesth Analg 1988; 67:1154-8.
14. Bloedow DC, Ralston DH, Hargrove JC. Lidocaine pharmacokinetics in pregnant and nonpregnant sheep. J Pharm Sci 1980; 69:32-7.
15. Downing JW, Johnson HV, Gonzalez HF, et al. The pharmacokinetics of epidural lidocaine and bupivacaine during cesarean section. Anesth Analg 1997; 84:527-32.
16. Kuhnert BR, Philipson EH, Pimental R, et al. Lidocaine disposition in mother, fetus, and neonate after spinal anesthesia. Anesth Analg 1986; 65:139-44.
17. Kuhnert BR, Knapp DR, Kuhnert PM, Prochaska AL. Maternal, fetal, and neonatal metabolism of lidocaine. Clin Pharmacol Ther 1979; 26:213-20.
18. Pedersen H, Santos AC, Morishima HO, et al. Does gestational age affect the pharmacokinetics and pharmacodynamics of lidocaine in mother and fetus? Anesthesiology 1988; 68:367-72.
19. Wood M, Wood AJJ. Changes in plasma drug binding and alpha1-acid glycoprotein in mother and newborn infant. Clin Pharmacol Ther 1981; 29:522-6.
20. Fragneto RY, Bader AM, Rosinia F, et al. Measurements of protein binding of lidocaine throughout pregnancy. Anesth Analg 1994; 79:295-7.
21. Pihlajamaki K, Kanto J, Lindberg R, et al. Extradural administration of bupivacaine: Pharmacokinetics and metabolism in pregnant and non-pregnant women. Br J Anaesth 1990; 64:556-62.
22. Tucker GT, Mather LE. Clinical pharmacokinetics of local anaesthetics. Clin Pharmacokinet 1979; 4:241-78.
23. Santos AC, Arthur GR, Lehning EJ, Finster M. Comparative pharmacokinetics of ropivacaine and bupivacaine in nonpregnant and pregnant ewes. Anesth Analg 1997; 85:87-93.
24. Kuhnert PM, Kuhnert BR, Stitts JM, Gross TL. The use of a selected ion monitoring technique to study the disposition of bupivacaine in mother, fetus, and neonate following epidural anesthesia for cesarean section. Anesthesiology 1981; 55:611-7.
25. Reynolds F, Taylor G. Maternal and neonatal blood concentrations of bupivacaine: A comparison with lignocaine during continuous extradural analgesia. Anaesthesia 1970; 25:14-23.
26. Mather LE, Thomas J. Bupivacaine binding to plasma protein fractions. J Pharm Pharmacol 1978; 30:653-4.
27. Wulf H, Munstedt P, Maier C. Plasma protein binding of bupivacaine in pregnant women at term. Acta Anaesthesiol Scand 1991; 35:129-33.
28. Arthur GR, Feldman HS, Covino BG. Comparative pharmacokinetics of bupivacaine and ropivacaine, a new amide local anesthetic. Anesth Analg 1988; 67:1053-8.
29. Lee A, Fagan D, Lamont M, et al. Disposition kinetics of ropivacaine in humans. Anesth Analg 1989; 69:736-8.
30. Datta S, Camann W, Bader A, VanderBurgh L. Clinical effects and maternal and fetal plasma concentrations of epidural ropivacaine versus bupivacaine for cesarean section. Anesthesiology 1995; 82:1346-52.
31. Oda Y, Furuichi K, Tanaka K, et al. Metabolism of a new local anesthetic, ropivacaine, by human hepatic cytochrome P450. Anesthesiology 1995; 82:214-20.
32. Moller R, Covino BG. Cardiac electrophysiologic properties of bupivacaine and lidocaine compared with those of ropivacaine, a new amide local anesthetic. Anesthesiology 1990; 72:322-9.
33. Porter JM, Kelleher N, Flynn R, Shorten GD. Epidural ropivacaine hydrochloride during labour: Protein binding, placental transfer and neonatal outcome. Anaesthesia 2001; 56:418-23.
34. Dailey PA, Hughes SC, Rosen MA, et al. Effect of cimetidine and ranitidine on lidocaine concentrations during epidural anesthesia for cesarean section. Anesthesiology 1988; 69:1013-7.
35. Brashear WT, Zuspan KJ, Lazebnik N, et al. Effect of ranitidine on bupivacaine disposition. Anesth Analg 1991; 72:369-76.

36. Ramanathan J, Bottorff M, Jeter JN, et al. The pharmacokinetics and maternal and neonatal effects of epidural lidocaine in preeclampsia. Anesth Analg 1986; 65:120-6.
37. Debon R, Chassard D, Duflo F, et al. Chronobiology of epidural ropivacaine: Variations in the duration of action related to the hour of administration. Anesthesiology 2002; 96:542-5.
38. de Jong RH, Robles R, Corbin RW. Central actions of lidocaine—transmission. Anesthesiology 1969; 30:19-23.
39. Liu PL, Feldman HS, Giasi R, et al. Comparative CNS toxicity of lidocaine, etidocaine, bupivacaine, and tetracaine in awake dogs following rapid intravenous administration. Anesth Analg 1983; 62:375-9.
40. Scott DB. Evaluation of the toxicity of local anaesthetic agents in man. Br J Anaesth 1975; 47:56-61.
41. Covino BG, Vassallo HG. Local Anesthetics: Mechanisms of Action and Clinical Use. New York, Grune & Stratton, 1976:126.
42. Englesson S. The influence of acid-base changes on central nervous system toxicity of local anaesthetic agents. I. An experimental study in cats. Acta Anaesthesiol Scand 1974; 18:79-87.
43. Englesson S, Grevsten S. The influence of acid-base changes on central nervous system toxicity of local anaesthetic agents. II. Acta Anaesthesiol Scand 1974; 18:88-103.
44. Burney RG, DiFazio CA, Foster JA. Effects of pH on protein binding of lidocaine. Anesth Analg 1978; 57:478-80.
45. de Jong RH, Ronfeld RA, DeRosa RA. Cardiovascular effects of convulsant and supraconvulsant doses of amide local anesthetics. Anesth Analg 1982; 61:3-9.
46. Morishima HO, Finster M, Arthur R, Covino BG. Pregnancy does not alter lidocaine toxicity. Am J Obstet Gynecol 1990; 162:320-4.
47. Santos AC, Pedersen H, Harmon TW, et al. Does pregnancy alter the systemic toxicity of local anesthetics? Anesthesiology 1989; 70:991-5.
48. Morishima HO, Pedersen H, Finster M, et al. Bupivacaine toxicity in pregnant and nonpregnant ewes. Anesthesiology 1985; 63:134-39.
49. Clarkson CW, Hondeghem LM. Mechanism for bupivacaine depression of cardiac conduction: Fast block of sodium channels during the action potential with slow recovery from block during diastole. Anesthesiology 1985; 62:396-405.
50. Thomas RD, Behbehani MM, Coyle DE, Denson DD. Cardiovascular toxicity of local anesthetics: An alternative hypothesis. Anesth Analg 1986; 65:444-50.
51. Coyle DE, Porembka DT, Sehlhorst CS, et al. Echocardiographic evaluation of bupivacaine cardiotoxicity. Anesth Analg 1994; 79:335-9.
52. Feldman HS, Covino BG. Comparative motor-blocking effects of bupivacaine and ropivacaine, a new amino amide local anesthetic, in the rat and dog. Anesth Analg 1988; 67:1047-52.
53. Reiz S, Haggmark S, Johansson G, Nath S. Cardiotoxicity of ropivacaine—a new amide local anaesthetic agent. Acta Anaesthesiol Scand 1989; 33:93-8.
54. Nancarrow C, Rutten AJ, Runciman WB, et al. Myocardial and cerebral drug concentrations and the mechanisms of death after fatal intravenous doses of lidocaine, bupivacaine, and ropivacaine in the sheep. Anesth Analg 1989; 69:276-83.
55. Scott DB, Lee A, Fagan D, et al. Acute toxicity of ropivacaine compared with that of bupivacaine. Anesth Analg 1989; 69:563-9.
56. Polley LS, Columb MO, Naughton NN, et al. Relative analgesic potencies of ropivacaine and bupivacaine for epidural analgesia in labor: Implications for therapeutic indexes. Anesthesiology 1999; 90:944-50.
57. Dony P, Dewinde V, Vanderick B, et al. The comparative toxicity of ropivacaine and bupivacaine at equipotent doses in rats. Anesth Analg 2000; 91:1489-92.
58. Chazalon P, Tourtier JP, Villevielle T, et al. Ropivacaine-induced cardiac arrest after peripheral nerve block: Successful resuscitation. Anesthesiology 2003; 99:1449-51.
59. Huet O, Eyrolle LJ, Mazoit JX, Ozier YM. Cardiac arrest after injection of ropivacaine for posterior lumbar plexus blockade. Anesthesiology 2003; 99:1451-3.
60. Yoshida M, Matsuda H, Fukuda I, Furuya K. Sudden cardiac arrest during cesarean section due to epidural anaesthesia using ropivacaine: A case report. Arch Gynecol Obstet 2008; 277:91-4.
61. Albright GA. Cardiac arrest following regional anesthesia with etidocaine or bupivacaine. Anesthesiology 1979; 51:285-7.
62. Valenzuela C, Snyders DJ, Bennett PB, et al. Stereoselective block of cardiac sodium channels by bupivacaine in guinea pig ventricular myocytes. Circulation 1995; 92:3014-24.
63. Mazoit JX, Boico O, Samii K. Myocardial uptake of bupivacaine. II. Pharmacokinetics and pharmacodynamics of bupivacaine enantiomers in the isolated perfused rabbit heart. Anesth Analg 1993; 77:477-82.
64. Santos AC, DeArmas PI. Systemic toxicity of levobupivacaine, bupivacaine, and ropivacaine during continuous intravenous infusion to nonpregnant and pregnant ewes. Anesthesiology 2001; 95:1256-64.
65. Lyons G, Columb M, Wilson RC, Johnson RV. Epidural pain relief in labour: Potencies of levobupivacaine and racemic bupivacaine. Br J Anaesth 1998; 81:899-901.
66. Foxall G, McCahon R, Lamb J, et al. Levobupivacaine-induced seizures and cardiovascular collapse treated with Intralipid. Anaesthesia 2007; 62:516-8.
67. Bucklin BA, Warner DS, Choi WW, et al. Pregnancy does not alter the threshold for lidocaine-induced seizures in the rat. Anesth Analg 1992; 74:57-61.
68. Kim YJ, McFarlane C, Warner DS, et al. The effects of plasma and brain magnesium concentrations on lidocaine-induced seizures in the rat. Anesth Analg 1996; 83:1223-8.
69. Marx GF. Cardiotoxicity of local anesthetics—the plot thickens. Anesthesiology 1984; 60:3-5.
70. Kasten GW, Martin ST. Resuscitation from bupivacaine-induced cardiovascular toxicity during partial inferior vena cava occlusion. Anesth Analg 1986; 65:341-4.
71. Moller RA, Datta S, Fox J, et al. Effects of progesterone on the cardiac electrophysiologic action of bupivacaine and lidocaine. Anesthesiology 1992; 76:604-8.
72. Moller RA, Datta S, Strichartz GR. Beta-estradiol acutely potentiates the depression of cardiac excitability by lidocaine and bupivacaine. J Cardiovasc Pharmacol 1999; 34:718-27.
73. Moller RA, Covino BG. Effect of progesterone on the cardiac electrophysiologic alterations produced by ropivacaine and bupivacaine. Anesthesiology 1992; 77:735-41.
74. Hawkins JL, Koonin LM, Palmer SK, Gibbs CP. Anesthesia-related deaths during obstetric delivery in the United States, 1979-1990. Anesthesiology 1997; 86:277-84.
75. de Jong RH, Bonin JD. Benzodiazepines protect mice from local anesthetic convulsions and deaths. Anesth Analg 1981; 60:385-9.
76. Rosen MA, Thigpen JW, Shnider SM, et al. Bupivacaine-induced cardiotoxicity in hypoxic and acidotic sheep. Anesth Analg 1985; 64:1089-96.
77. Feldman HS, Arthur GR, Pitkanen M, et al. Treatment of acute systemic toxicity after the rapid intravenous injection of ropivacaine and bupivacaine in the conscious dog. Anesth Analg 1991; 73:373-84.
78. Saitoh K, Hirabayashi Y, Shimizu R, Fukuda H. Amrinone is superior to epinephrine in reversing bupivacaine-induced cardiovascular depression in sevoflurane-anesthetized dogs. Anesthesiology 1995; 83:127-33.
79. Lindgren L, Randell T, Suzuki N, et al. The effect of amrinone on recovery from severe bupivacaine intoxication in pigs. Anesthesiology 1992; 77:309-15.
80. Haasio J, Pitkanen MT, Kytta J, Rosenberg PH. Treatment of bupivacaine-induced cardiac arrhythmias in hypoxic and hypercarbic pigs with amiodarone or bretylium. Reg Anesth 1990; 15:174-9.
81. Smith WM, Gallagher JJ. "Les torsades de pointes": An unusual ventricular arrhythmia. Ann Intern Med 1980; 93:578-84.
82. Rosenblatt MA, Abel M, Fischer GW, et al. Successful use of a 20% lipid emulsion to resuscitate a patient after a presumed bupivacaine-related cardiac arrest. Anesthesiology 2006; 105:217-8.
83. Kennedy RL, Miller RP, Bell JU, et al. Uptake and distribution of bupivacaine in fetal lambs. Anesthesiology 1986; 65:247-53.
84. Kennedy RL, Bell JU, Miller RP, et al. Uptake and distribution of lidocaine in fetal lambs. Anesthesiology 1990; 72:483-9.
85. Covino BG, Marx GF, Finster M, Zsigmond EK. Prolonged sensory/motor deficits following inadvertent spinal anesthesia (editorial). Anesth Analg 1980; 59:399-400.

86. Ready LB, Plumer MH, Haschke RH, et al. Neurotoxicity of intrathecal local anesthetics in rabbits. Anesthesiology 1985; 63:364-70.
87. Barsa J, Batra M, Fink BR, Sumi SM. A comparative in vivo study of local neurotoxicity of lidocaine, bupivacaine, 2-chloroprocaine, and a mixture of 2-chloroprocaine and bupivacaine. Anesth Analg 1982; 61:961-7.
88. Gissen AJ, Datta S, Lambert D. The chloroprocaine controversy. II. Is chloroprocaine neurotoxic? Reg Anesth 1984; 9:135-45.
89. Fibuch EE, Opper SE. Back pain following epidurally administered Nesacaine-MPF. Anesth Analg 1989; 69:113-5.
90. Taniguchi M, Bollen AW, Drasner K. Sodium bisulfite: Scapegoat for chloroprocaine neurotoxicity? Anesthesiology 2004; 100:85-91.
91. Yoos JR, Kopacz DJ. Spinal 2-chloroprocaine for surgery: An initial 10-month experience. Anesth Analg 2005; 100:553-8.
92. Rigler ML, Drasner K, Krejcie TC, et al. Cauda equina syndrome after continuous spinal anesthesia. Anesth Analg 1991; 72:275-81.
93. Schneider M, Ettlin T, Kaufmann M, et al. Transient neurologic toxicity after hyperbaric subarachnoid anesthesia with 5% lidocaine. Anesth Analg 1993; 76:1154-7.
94. Bainton CR, Strichartz GR. Concentration dependence of lidocaine-induced irreversible conduction loss in frog nerve. Anesthesiology 1994; 81:657-67.
95. Lambert LA, Lambert DH, Strichartz GR. Irreversible conduction block in isolated nerve by high concentrations of local anesthetics. Anesthesiology 1994; 80:1082-93.
96. Li DF, Bahar M, Cole G, Rosen M. Neurological toxicity of the subarachnoid infusion of bupivacaine, lignocaine or 2-chloroprocaine in the rat. Br J Anaesth 1985; 57:424-9.
97. Dripps RD, Vandam LD. Long-term follow-up of patients who received 10,098 spinal anesthetics: Failure to discover major neurological sequelae. J Am Med Assoc 1954; 156:1486-91.
98. Pollock JE, Liu SS, Neal JM, Stephenson CA. Dilution of spinal lidocaine does not alter the incidence of transient neurologic symptoms. Anesthesiology 1999; 90:445-50.
99. Freedman JM, Li DK, Drasner K, et al. Transient neurologic symptoms after spinal anesthesia: An epidemiologic study of 1,863 patients. Anesthesiology 1998; 89:633-41.
100. Zaric D, Christiansen C, Pace NL, Punjasawadwong Y. Transient neurologic symptoms after spinal anesthesia with lidocaine versus other local anesthetics: A systematic review of randomized, controlled trials. Anesth Analg 2005; 100:1811-6.
101. Aouad MT, Siddik SS, Jalbout MI, Baraka AS. Does pregnancy protect against intrathecal lidocaine-induced transient neurologic symptoms? Anesth Analg 2001; 92:401-4.
102. Philip J, Sharma SK, Gottumukkala VN, et al. Transient neurologic symptoms after spinal anesthesia with lidocaine in obstetric patients. Anesth Analg 2001; 92:405-9.
103. Brown DT, Beamish D, Wildsmith JA. Allergic reaction to an amide local anaesthetic. Br J Anaesth 1981; 53:435-7.
104. Simon RA. Adverse reactions to drug additives. J Allergy Clin Immunol 1984; 74:623-30.
105. Incaudo G, Shatz M, Patterson R. Administration of local anesthetics to patients with a history of prior history of reaction. J Allergy Clin Immunol 1978; 61:339-45.
106. Chandler MJ, Grammer LC, Patterson R. Provocative challenge with local anesthetics in patients with a prior history of reaction. J Allergy Clin Immunol 1987; 79:883-6.
107. Palmer CM, Voulgaropoulos D. Management of the parturient with a history of local anesthetic allergy. Anesth Analg 1993; 77:625-8.
108. Fisher M. Intradermal testing after anaphylactoid reaction to anaesthetic drugs: Practical aspects of performance and interpretation. Anaesth Intensive Care 1984; 12:115-20.
109. Levy J. Anaphylactic Reactions in Anesthesia and Intensive Care. Stoneham, MA, Butterworth-Heinemann, 1992:115.
110. Magness RR, Rosenfeld CR. Mechanisms for attenuated pressor responses to alpha-agonists in ovine pregnancy. Am J Obstet Gynecol 1988; 159:252-61.
111. Zucker-Pinchoff B, Ramanathan S. Anaphylactic reaction to epidural fentanyl. Anesthesiology 1989; 71:599-601.
112. Teramo K. Effects of obstetrical paracervical blockade on the fetus. Acta Obstet Gynecol Scand 1971; 16(:Suppl):1-55.
113. Cibils LA. Response of human uterine arteries to local anesthetics. Am J Obstet Gynecol 1976; 126:202-10.
114. Noren H, Lindblom B, Kallfelt B. Effects of bupivacaine and calcium antagonists on human uterine arteries in pregnant and non-pregnant women. Acta Anaesthesiol Scand 1991; 35:488-91.
115. Fishburne JI, Greiss FC, Hopkinson R, Rhyne AL. Responses of the gravid uterine vasculature to arterial levels of local anesthetic agents. Am J Obstet Gynecol 1979; 133:753-61.
116. Santos AC, Karpel B, Noble G. The placental transfer and fetal effects of levobupivacaine, racemic bupivacaine, and ropivacaine. Anesthesiology 1999; 90:1698-703.
117. Chestnut DH, Weiner CP, Herrig JE. The effect of intravenously administered 2-chloroprocaine upon uterine artery blood flow velocity in gravid guinea pigs. Anesthesiology 1989; 70:305-8.
118. Biehl D, Shnider SM, Levinson G, Callender K. The direct effects of circulating lidocaine on uterine blood flow and foetal well-being in the pregnant ewe. Can Anaesth Soc J 1977; 24:445-51.
119. Gintautas J, Kraynack B, Havasi G, et al. Responses of isolated uterine arteries to local anesthetic agents. Proc West Pharmacol Soc 1981; 24:191-2.
120. Gintautas J, Kraynack BJ, Warren PR, et al. Effects of adenine nucleotides on lidocaine induced contractions in isolated uterine artery. Proc West Pharmacol Soc 1980; 23:299-300.
121. Hollmen A, Jouppila R, Jouppila P, et al. Effect of extradural analgesia using bupivacaine and 2-chloroprocaine on intervillous blood flow during normal labor. Br J Anaesth 1982; 54:837-42.
122. Alahuhta S, Rasanen J, Jouppila P, et al. The effects of epidural ropivacaine and bupivacaine for cesarean section on uteroplacental and fetal circulation. Anesthesiology 1995; 83:23-32.
123. Alahuhta S, Rasanen J, Jouppila R, et al. Effects of extradural bupivacaine with adrenaline for caesarean section on uteroplacental and fetal circulation. Br J Anaesth 1991; 67:678-82.
124. Husemeyer RP, Crawley JC. Placental intervillous blood flow measured by inhaled ^{133}Xe clearance in relation to induction of epidural analgesia. Br J Obstet Gynaecol 1979; 86:426-31.
125. Huovinen K, Lehtovirta P, Forss M, et al. Changes in placental intervillous blood flow measured by the 133-xenon method during lumbar epidural block for elective caesarean section. Acta Anaesthesiol Scand 1979; 23:529-33.
126. Giles WB, Lah FX, Trudinger BJ. The effect of epidural anaesthesia for caesarean section on maternal uterine and fetal umbilical artery blood flow velocity waveforms. Br J Obstet Gynaecol 1987; 94:55-9.
127. Morrow RJ, Rolbin SH, Ritchie JW, Haley S. Epidural anaesthesia and blood flow velocity in mother and fetus. Can J Anaesth 1989; 36:519-22.
128. Kopacz DJ, Carpenter RL, Mackey DC. Effect of ropivacaine on cutaneous capillary blood flow in pigs. Anesthesiology 1989; 71:69-74.
129. Tuvemo T, Willdeck-Lund G. Smooth muscle effects of lidocaine, prilocaine, bupivacaine and etidocaine on the human umbilical artery. Acta Anaesthesiol Scand 1982; 26:104-7.
130. Noren H, Kallfelt B, Lindblom B. Influence of bupivacaine and morphine on human umbilical arteries and veins in vitro. Acta Obstet Gynecol Scand 1990; 69:87-91.
131. Halevy S, Rossner KL, Liu-Barnett M, et al. The response of umbilical vessels, with and without vascular endothelium, to local anesthesia in low Po_2 and hypercarbia. Reg Anesth 1995; 20:316-22.
132. Morishima HO, Heymann MA, Rudolph AM, et al. Transfer of lidocaine across the sheep placenta to the fetus: Hemodynamic and acid-base responses of the fetal lamb. Am J Obstet Gynecol 1975; 122:581-8.
133. Trudinger BJ, Giles WB, Cook CM. Uteroplacental blood flow velocity-time waveforms in normal and complicated pregnancy. Br J Obstet Gynaecol 1985; 92:39-45.
134. Marx GF, Elstein ID, Schuss M, et al. Effects of epidural block with lignocaine and lignocaine-adrenaline on umbilical artery velocity wave ratios. Br J Obstet Gynaecol 1990; 97:517-20.

135. Marx GF, Patel S, Berman JA, et al. Umbilical blood flow velocity waveforms in different maternal positions and with epidural analgesia. Obstet Gynecol 1986; 68:61-4.
136. Lindblad A, Marsal K, Vernersson E, Renck H. Fetal circulation during epidural analgesia for caesarean section. Br Med J (Clin Res Ed) 1984; 288:1329-30.
137. McGaughey HS, Corey EL, Eastwood D, Thornton WN. Effect of synthetic anesthetics on the spontaneous motility of human uterine muscle in vitro. Obstet Gynecol 1962; 19:233-40.
138. Morishima HO, Covino BG, Yeh MN, et al. Bradycardia in the fetal baboon following paracervical block anesthesia. Am J Obstet Gynecol 1981; 140:775-80.
139. Belitzky R, Delard LG, Novick LM. Oxytocic effect of intramyometrial injection of procaine in a pregnant woman. Am J Obstet Gynecol 1970; 107:973-5.
140. Camann WR, Hartigan PM, Gilbertson LI, et al. Chloroprocaine antagonism of epidural opioid analgesia: A receptor-specific phenomenon? Anesthesiology 1990; 73:860-3.
141. Grice SC, Eisenach JC, Dewan DM. Labor analgesia with epidural bupivacaine plus fentanyl: Enhancement with epinephrine and inhibition with 2-chloroprocaine. Anesthesiology 1990; 72:623-8.
142. Coda B, Bausch S, Haas M, Chavkin C. The hypothesis that antagonism of fentanyl analgesia by 2-chloroprocaine is mediated by direct action on opioid receptors. Reg Anesth 1997; 22:43-52.
143. Hess PE, Snowman CE, Hahn CJ, et al. Chloroprocaine may not affect epidural morphine for postcesarean delivery analgesia. J Clin Anesth 2006; 18:29-33.
144. Cohen SE, Thurlow A. Comparison of a chloroprocaine-bupivacaine mixture with chloroprocaine and bupivacaine used individually for obstetric epidural analgesia. Anesthesiology 1979; 51:288-92.
145. Corke BC, Carlson CG, Dettbarn WD. The influence of 2-chloroprocaine on the subsequent analgesic potency of bupivacaine. Anesthesiology 1984; 60:25-7.
146. Chestnut DH, Geiger M, Bates JN, Choi WW. The influence of pH-adjusted 2-chloroprocaine on the quality and duration of subsequent epidural bupivacaine analgesia during labor: A randomized, double-blind study. Anesthesiology 1989; 70:437-41.
147. van Kleef JW, Veering BT, Burm AG. Spinal anesthesia with ropivacaine: A double-blind study on the efficacy and safety of 0.5% and 0.75% solutions in patients undergoing minor lower limb surgery. Anesth Analg 1994; 78:1125-30.
148. Coppejans HC, Vercauteren MP. Low-dose combined spinal-epidural anesthesia for cesarean delivery: A comparison of three plain local anesthetics. Acta Anaesthesiol Belg 2006; 57:39-43.
149. D'Angelo R, James RL. Is ropivacaine less potent than bupivacaine? Anesthesiology 1999; 90:941-3.
150. Vercauteren MP, Hans G, De Decker K, Adriaensen HA. Levobupivacaine combined with sufentanil and epinephrine for intrathecal labor analgesia: A comparison with racemic bupivacaine. Anesth Analg 2001; 93:996-1000.
151. Beilin Y, Guinn NR, Bernstein HH, et al. Local anesthetics and mode of delivery: Bupivacaine versus ropivacaine versus levobupivacaine. Anesth Analg 2007; 105:756-63.
152. Bader AM, Tsen LC, Camann WR, et al. Clinical effects and maternal and fetal plasma concentrations of 0.5% epidural levobupivacaine versus bupivacaine for cesarean delivery. Anesthesiology 1999; 90:1596-601.
153. Mirkin BL. Maternal and fetal distribution of drugs in pregnancy. Clin Pharmacol Ther 1973; 14:643-7.
154. Tucker GT, Mather LE. Properties, absorption, and disposition of local anesthetic agents. In Cousins M, Bridenbaugh P, editors. Neural Blockade in Clinical Anesthesia and Management of Pain. 3rd edition. Philadelphia, Lippincott-Raven, 1998:55-96.
155. Brown WU Jr, Bell GC, Alper MH. Acidosis, local anesthetics, and the newborn. Obstet Gynecol 1976; 48:27-30.
156. Biehl D, Shnider SM, Levinson G, Callender K. Placental transfer of lidocaine: Effects of fetal acidosis. Anesthesiology 1978; 48:409-12.
157. Morishima HO, Covino BG. Toxicity and distribution of lidocaine in nonasphyxiated and asphyxiated baboon fetuses. Anesthesiology 1981; 54:182-6.
158. Hamshaw-Thomas A, Reynolds F. Placental transfer of bupivacaine, pethidine and lignocaine in the rabbit: Effect of umbilical flow rate and protein content. Br J Obstet Gynaecol 1985; 92:706-13.
159. Hamshaw-Thomas A, Rogerson N, Reynolds F. Transfer of bupivacaine, lignocaine and pethidine across the rabbit placenta: Influence of maternal protein binding and fetal flow. Placenta 1984; 5:61-70.
160. Vella LM, Knott C, Reynolds F. Transfer of fentanyl across the rabbit placenta: Effect of umbilical flow and concurrent drug administration. Br J Anaesth 1986; 58:49-54.
161. Petersen MC, Moore RG, Nation RL, McMeniman W. Relationship between the transplacental gradients of bupivacaine and alpha-1-acid glycoprotein. Br J Clin Pharmacol 1981; 12:859-62.
162. Thomas J, Long G, Moore G, Morgan D. Plasma protein binding and placental transfer of bupivacaine. Clin Pharmacol Ther 1976; 19:426-34.
163. Johnson RF, Cahana A, Olenick M, et al. A comparison of the placental transfer of ropivacaine versus bupivacaine. Anesth Analg 1999; 89:703-8.
164. Petrie RH, Paul WL, Miller FC, et al. Placental transfer of lidocaine following paracervical block. Am J Obstet Gynecol 1974; 120:791-801.
165. Mazze RI, Dunbar RW. Plasma lidocaine concentrations after caudal, lumbar epidural, axillary block, and intravenous regional anesthesia. Anesthesiology 1966; 27:574-9.
166. Giasi RM, D'Agostino E, Covino BG. Absorption of lidocaine following subarachnoid and epidural administration. Anesth Analg 1979; 58:360-3.
167. Brown WU, Bell GC, Lurie AO, et al. Newborn blood levels of lidocaine and mepivacaine in the first postnatal day following maternal epidural anesthesia. Anesthesiology 1975; 42:698-707.
168. Abboud TK, David S, Nagappala S, et al. Maternal, fetal, and neonatal effects of lidocaine with and without epinephrine for epidural anesthesia in obstetrics. Anesth Analg 1984; 63:973-9.
169. Reynolds F, Taylor G. Plasma concentrations of bupivacaine during continuous epidural analgesia in labour: The effect of adrenaline. Br J Anaesth 1971; 43:436-40.
170. Abboud TK, Sheik-ol-Eslam A, Yanagi T, et al. Safety of efficacy of epinephrine added to bupivacaine for lumbar epidural analgesia in obstetrics. Anesth Analg 1985; 64:585-91.
171. Reynolds F, Laishley R, Morgan B, Lee A. Effect of time and adrenaline on the feto-maternal distribution of bupivacaine. Br J Anaesth 1989; 62:509-14.
172. Beazley JM, Taylor G, Reynolds F. Placental transfer of bupivacaine after paracervical block. Obstet Gynecol 1972; 39:2-6.
173. Denson DD, Bridenbaugh PO, Turner PA, et al. Neural blockade and pharmacokinetics following subarachnoid lidocaine in the rhesus monkey. I. Effects of epinephrine. Anesth Analg 1982; 61:746-50.
174. Laishley RS, Carson RJ, Reynolds F. Effect of adrenaline on placental transfer of bupivacaine in the perfused in situ rabbit placenta. Br J Anaesth 1989; 63:439-73.
175. Abboud TK, Afrasiabi A, Zhu J, et al. Bupivacaine/butorphanol/epinephrine for epidural anesthesia in obstetrics: Maternal and neonatal effects. Reg Anesth 1989; 14:219-24.
176. Abboud TK, Kim KC, Noueihed R, et al. Epidural bupivacaine, chloroprocaine, or lidocaine for cesarean section—maternal and neonatal effects. Anesth Analg 1983; 62:914-9.
177. Thomas J, Climie CR, Long G, Nighjoy LE. The influence of adrenaline on the maternal plasma levels and placental transfer of lignocaine following lumbar epidural administration. Br J Anaesth 1969; 41:1029-34.
178. Idänpään-Heikkila JE, Taska RJ, Allen HA, Schoolar JC. Placental transfer of diazepam-^{14}C in mice, hamsters and monkeys. J Pharmacol Exp Ther 1971; 176:752-7.
179. Shnider SM, Way EL. The kinetics of transfer of lidocaine (Xylocaine) across the human placenta. Anesthesiology 1968; 29:944-50.
180. Roe DA, Little BB, Bawdon RE, Gilstrap LC 3rd. Metabolism of cocaine by human placentas: Implications for fetal exposure. Am J Obstet Gynecol 1990; 163:715-8.
181. Van Petten GR, Hirsch GH, Cherrington AD. Drug-metabolizing activity of the human placenta. Can J Biochem 1968; 46:1057-61.

182. Sturrock JE, Nunn JF. Cytotoxic effects of procaine, lignocaine and bupivacaine. Br J Anaesth 1979; 51:273-81.
183. Lee H, Bush KT, Nagele RG. Time-lapse photographic study of neural tube closure defects caused by Xylocaine in the chick. Teratology 1988; 37:263-9.
184. Lee H, Nagele RG. Neural tube defects caused by local anesthetics in early chick embryos. Teratology 1985; 31:119-27.
185. Anderson PL, Bamburg JR. Effects of local anesthetics on nerve growth in culture. Dev Neurosci 1981; 4:273-90.
186. O'Shea KS, Kaufman MH. Neural tube closure defects following in vitro exposure of mouse embryos to Xylocaine. J Exp Zool 1980; 214:235-8.
187. Stygall K, Mirsky R, Mowbray J. The effect of local anaesthetics and barbiturates on myogenesis and myotube integrity in rat skeletal muscle cultures. J Cell Sci 1979; 37:231-41.
188. Ramazzatto L, Curro F, Patterson J. Toxicological assessment of lidocaine in the pregnant rat. J Dent Res 1985; 64:1214-8.
189. Fujinaga M, Mazze RI. Reproductive and teratogenic effects of lidocaine in Sprague-Dawley rats. Anesthesiology 1986; 65:626-32.
190. Martin LV, Jurand A. The absence of teratogenic effects of some analgesics used in anaesthesia: Additional evidence from a mouse model. Anaesthesia 1992; 47:473-6.
191. Smith RF, Wharton GG, Kurtz SL, et al. Behavioral effects of mid-pregnancy administration of lidocaine and mepivacaine in the rat. Neurobehav Toxicol Teratol 1986; 8:61-8.
192. Smith RF, Kurkjian MF, Mattran KM, Kurtz SL. Behavioral effects of prenatal exposure to lidocaine in the rat: Effects of dosage and of gestational age at administration. Neurotoxicol Teratol 1989; 11:395-403.
193. Heinonen OP, Slone D, Shapiro S. Birth Defects and Drugs in Pregnancy. Littleton, MA, Publishing Sciences Group, 1977.
194. Friedman JM. Teratogen update: Anesthetic agents. Teratology 1988; 37:69-77.
195. Fletcher S, Carson R, Reynolds F, et al. Plasma total and free concentrations of bupivacaine and lignocaine in mother and fetus following epidural administration, singly or together. Int J Obstet Anesth 1992; 1:135-40.
196. Tucker GT, Boyes RN, Bridenbaugh PO, Moore DC. Binding of anilide-type local anesthetics in human plasma. II. Implications in vivo, with special reference to transplacental distribution. Anesthesiology 1970; 33:304-14.
197. Ehrnebo M, Agurell S, Jalling B, Boreus LO. Age differences in drug binding by plasma proteins: Studies on human foetuses, neonates and adults. Eur J Clin Pharmacol 1971; 3:189-93.
198. Finster M, Morishima HO, Boyes RN, Covino BG. The placental transfer of lidocaine and its uptake by fetal tissues. Anesthesiology 1972; 36:159-63.
199. Morishima HO, Santos AC, Pedersen H, et al. Effect of lidocaine on the asphyxial responses in the mature fetal lamb. Anesthesiology 1987; 66:502-7.
200. Meffin P, Long GJ, Thomas J. Clearance and metabolism of mepivacaine in the human neonate. Clin Pharmacol Ther 1973; 14:218-25.
201. Blankenbaker WL, DiFazio CA, Berry FA Jr. Lidocaine and its metabolites in the newborn. Anesthesiology 1975; 42:325-30.
202. Mihaly GW, Moore RG, Thomas J, et al. The pharmacokinetics and metabolism of the anilide local anaesthetics in neonates. I. Lignocaine. Eur J Clin Pharmacol 1978; 13:143-52.
203. Morgan D, McQuillan D, Thomas J. Pharmacokinetics and metabolism of the anilide local anaesthetics in neonates. II. Etidocaine. Eur J Clin Pharmacol 1978; 13:365-71.
204. Morishima HO, Finster M, Pedersen H, et al. Pharmacokinetics of lidocaine in fetal and neonatal lambs and adult sheep. Anesthesiology 1979; 50:431-6.
205. Lieberman BA, Rosenblatt DB, Belsey E, et al. The effects of maternally administered pethidine or epidural bupivacaine on the fetus and newborn. Br J Obstet Gynaecol 1979; 86:598-606.
206. Finster M, Poppers PJ, Sinclair JC, et al. Accidental intoxication of the fetus with local anesthetic drug during caudal anesthesia. Am J Obstet Gynecol 1965; 92:922-4.
207. Morishima HO, Pedersen H, Finster M, et al. Toxicity of lidocaine in adult, newborn, and fetal sheep. Anesthesiology 1981; 55:57-61.
208. Bosnjak ZJ, Stowe DF, Kampine JP. Comparison of lidocaine and bupivacaine depression of sinoatrial nodal activity during hypoxia and acidosis in adult and neonatal guinea pigs. Anesth Analg 1986; 65:911-7.
209. Badgwell JM, Heavner JE, Kytta J. Bupivacaine toxicity in young pigs is age-dependent and is affected by volatile anesthetics. Anesthesiology 1990; 73:297-303.
210. Loftus JR, Holbrook RH, Cohen SE. Fetal heart rate after epidural lidocaine and bupivacaine for elective cesarean section. Anesthesiology 1991; 75:406-12.
211. Boehm FH, Woodruff LF Jr, Growdon JH Jr. The effect of lumbar epidural anesthesia on fetal heart rate baseline variability. Anesth Analg 1975; 54:779-82.
212. Hehre FW, Hook R, Hon EH. Continuous lumbar peridural anesthesia in obstetrics. VI. The fetal effects of transplacental passage of local anesthetic agents. Anesth Analg 1969; 48:909-13.
213. Lavin JP, Samuels SV, Miodovnik M, et al. The effects of bupivacaine and chloroprocaine as local anesthetics for epidural anesthesia of fetal heart rate monitoring parameters. Am J Obstet Gynecol 1981; 141:717-22.
214. Abboud TK, Afrasiabi A, Sarkis F, et al. Continuous infusion epidural analgesia in parturients receiving bupivacaine, chloroprocaine, or lidocaine—maternal, fetal, and neonatal effects. Anesth Analg 1984; 63:421-8.
215. Kuhnert BR, Harrison MJ, Linn PL, Kuhnert PM. Effects of maternal epidural anesthesia on neonatal behavior. Anesth Analg 1984; 63:301-18.
216. Halpern SH, Littleford JA, Brockhurst NJ, et al. The neurologic and adaptive capacity score is not a reliable method of newborn evaluation. Anesthesiology 2001; 94:958-62.
217. Campbell N, Harvey D, Norman AP. Increased frequency of neonatal jaundice in a maternity hospital. Br Med J 1975; 2:548-52.
218. Clark DA, Landaw SA. Bupivacaine alters red blood cell properties: A possible explanation for neonatal jaundice associated with maternal anesthesia. Pediatr Res 1985; 19:341-3.
219. Gale R, Ferguson JE 2nd, Stevenson DK. Effect of epidural analgesia with bupivacaine hydrochloride on neonatal bilirubin production. Obstet Gynecol 1987; 70:692-5.
220. Smedstad KG, Morison DH, Harris WH, Pascoe P. Placental transfer of local anaesthetics in the premature sheep fetus. Int J Obstet Anesth 1993; 2:34-8.
221. Morishima HO, Pedersen H, Santos AC, et al. Adverse effects of maternally administered lidocaine on the asphyxiated preterm fetal lamb. Anesthesiology 1989; 71:110-5.
222. Santos AC, Yun EM, Bobby PD, et al. The effects of bupivacaine, L-nitro-L-arginine-methyl ester, and phenylephrine on cardiovascular adaptations to asphyxia in the preterm fetal lamb. Anesth Analg 1997; 85:1299-306.
223. Johnson RF, Herman NL, Johnson HV, et al. Effects of fetal pH on local anesthetic transfer across the human placenta. Anesthesiology 1996; 85:608-15.
224. Snyder SH. Opiate receptors and internal opiates. Sci Am 1977; 236:44-56.
225. Beckett AH. Analgesics and their antagonists: Some steric and chemical considerations. I. The dissociation constants of some tertiary amines and synthetic analgesics, the conformations of methadone-type compounds. J Pharm Pharmacol 1956; 8:848-59.
226. Thorpe DH. Opiate structure and activity—a guide to understanding the receptor. Anesth Analg 1984; 63:143-51.
227. Portoghese PS, Alreja BD, Larson DL. Allylprodine analogues as receptor probes: Evidence that phenolic and nonphenolic ligands interact with different subsites on identical opioid receptors. J Med Chem 1981; 24:782-7.
228. Gorin FA, Balasubramanian TM, Cicero TJ, et al. Novel analogues of enkephalin: Identification of functional groups required for biological activity. J Med Chem 1980; 23:1113-22.
229. Wang JK, Nauss LA, Thomas JE. Pain relief by intrathecally applied morphine in man. Anesthesiology 1979; 50:149-51.

230. Eisenach JC. Intraspinal analgesia in obstetrics. In Hughes SC, Levinson G, Rosen MA, editors. Shnider and Levinson's Anesthesia for Obstetrics. 2nd edition. Philadelphia, Lippincott Williams & Wilkins, 2001:149-54.
231. Yaksh TL. Spinal opiate analgesia: Characteristics and principles of action. Pain 1981; 11:293-346.
232. Mogil JS, Pasternak GW. The molecular and behavioral pharmacology of the orphanin FQ/nociceptin peptide and receptor family. Pharmacol Rev 2001; 53:381-415.
233. Atcheson R, Lambert DG. Update on opioid receptors. Br J Anaesth 1994; 73:132-4.
234. Pasternak GW. Multiple opiate receptors: Déjà vu all over again. Neuropharmacology 2004; 47(Suppl 1):312-23.
235. Stein C, Rosow CE. Analgesics: Receptor ligands and opiate narcotics. In Evers AS, Maze M, editors. Anesthetic Pharmacology: Physiologic Principles and Clinical Practice. Philadelphia, Churchill Livingstone, 2004:457-71.
236. Riviere PM. Peripheral kappa-opioid agonists for visceral pain. Br J Pharmacol 2004; 141:1331-4.
237. Porreca F, Heyman JS, Mosberg HI, et al. Role of mu and delta receptors in the supraspinal and spinal analgesic effects of [D-Pen2, D-Pen5]enkephalin in the mouse. J Pharmacol Exp Ther 1987; 241:393-400.
238. Bernards CM, Sorkin LS. Radicular artery blood flow does not redistribute fentanyl from the epidural space to the spinal cord. Anesthesiology 1994; 80:872-8.
239. Bernards CM, Hill HF. The spinal nerve root sleeve is not a preferred route for redistribution of drugs from the epidural space to the spinal cord. Anesthesiology 1991; 75:827-32.
240. Bernards CM, Hill HF. Physical and chemical properties of drug molecules governing their diffusion through the spinal meninges. Anesthesiology 1992; 77:750-6.
241. Bernards CM. Understanding the physiology and pharmacology of epidural and intrathecal opioids. Best Pract Res Clin Anaesthesiol 2002; 16:489-505.
242. Bernards CM, Hill HF. Morphine and alfentanil permeability through the spinal dura, arachnoid, and pia mater of dogs and monkeys. Anesthesiology 1990; 73:1214-9.
243. Bernards CM, Shen DD, Sterling ES, et al. Epidural, cerebrospinal fluid, and plasma pharmacokinetics of epidural opioids (part 1): Differences among opioids. Anesthesiology 2003; 99:455-65.
244. Coda BA, Brown MC, Schaffer RL, et al. A pharmacokinetic approach to resolving spinal and systemic contributions to epidural alfentanil analgesia and side-effects. Pain 1995; 62:329-37.
245. Coda BA, Brown MC, Risler L, et al. Equivalent analgesia and side effects during epidural and pharmacokinetically tailored intravenous infusion with matching plasma alfentanil concentration. Anesthesiology 1999; 90:98-108.
246. Miguel R, Barlow I, Morrell M, et al. A prospective, randomized, double-blind comparison of epidural and intravenous sufentanil infusions. Anesthesiology 1994; 81:346-52.
247. Liu SS, Gerancher JC, Bainton BG, et al. The effects of electrical stimulation at different frequencies on perception and pain in human volunteers: Epidural versus intravenous administration of fentanyl. Anesth Analg 1996; 82:98-102.
248. D'Angelo R, Gerancher JC, Eisenach JC, Raphael BL. Epidural fentanyl produces labor analgesia by a spinal mechanism. Anesthesiology 1998; 88:1519-23.
249. Ginosar Y, Riley ET, Angst MS. The site of action of epidural fentanyl in humans: The difference between infusion and bolus administration. Anesth Analg 2003; 97:1428-38.
250. Ummenhofer WC, Arends RH, Shen DD, Bernards CM. Comparative spinal distribution and clearance kinetics of intrathecally administered morphine, fentanyl, alfentanil, and sufentanil. Anesthesiology 2000; 92:739-53.
251. Eisenach JC, Hood DD, Curry R, Shafer SL. Cephalad movement of morphine and fentanyl in humans after intrathecal injection. Anesthesiology 2003; 99:166-73.
252. Lu JK, Schafer PG, Gardner TL, et al. The dose-response pharmacology of intrathecal sufentanil in female volunteers. Anesth Analg 1997; 85:372-9.
253. Yaksh TL, Collins JG. Studies in animals should precede human use of spinally administered drugs. Anesthesiology 1989; 70:4-6.
254. Abouleish E, Barmada MA, Nemoto EM, et al. Acute and chronic effects of intrathecal morphine in monkeys. Br J Anaesth 1981; 53:1027-32.
255. Power I, Brown DT, Wildsmith JA. The effect of fentanyl, meperidine and diamorphine on nerve conduction in vitro. Reg Anesth 1991; 16:204-8.
256. Yaksh TL, Noueihed RY, Durant PA. Studies of the pharmacology and pathology of intrathecally administered 4-anilinopiperidine analogues and morphine in the rat and cat. Anesthesiology 1986; 64:54-66.
257. Sabbe MB, Grafe MR, Mjanger E, et al. Spinal delivery of sufentanil, alfentanil, and morphine in dogs: Physiologic and toxicologic investigations. Anesthesiology 1994; 81:899-920.
258. Rawal N, Nuutinen L, Raj PP, et al. Behavioral and histopathologic effects following intrathecal administration of butorphanol, sufentanil, and nalbuphine in sheep. Anesthesiology 1991; 75:1025-34.
259. Cohen SE, Cherry CM, Holbrook RH Jr, et al. Intrathecal sufentanil for labor analgesia—sensory changes, side effects, and fetal heart rate changes. Anesth Analg 1993; 77:1155-60.
260. Scavone BM. Altered level of consciousness after combined spinal-epidural labor analgesia with intrathecal fentanyl and bupivacaine. Anesthesiology 2002; 96:1021-2.
261. Fragneto RY, Fisher A. Mental status change and aphasia after labor analgesia with intrathecal sufentanil/bupivacaine. Anesth Analg 2000; 90:1175-6.
262. Hamilton CL, Cohen SE. High sensory block after intrathecal sufentanil for labor analgesia. Anesthesiology 1995; 83:1118-21.
263. Currier DS, Levin KR, Campbell C. Dysphagia with intrathecal fentanyl. Anesthesiology 1997; 87:1570-1.
264. Riley ET, Ratner EF, Cohen SE. Intrathecal sufentanil for labor analgesia: Do sensory changes predict better analgesia and greater hypotension? Anesth Analg 1997; 84:346-51.
265. Bromage PR, Camporesi EM, Durant PA, Nielsen CH. Nonrespiratory side effects of epidural morphine. Anesth Analg 1982; 61:490-5.
266. Norris MC, Grieco WM, Borkowski M, et al. Complications of labor analgesia: Epidural versus combined spinal-epidural techniques. Anesth Analg 1994; 79:529-37.
267. Harnett MJ, O'Rourke N, Walsh M, et al. Transdermal scopolamine for prevention of intrathecal morphine–induced nausea and vomiting after cesarean delivery. Anesth Analg 2007; 105:764-9.
268. Thorpe SJ, Smith AF. A case of postoperative anxiety due to low dose droperidol used with patient-controlled analgesia. Int J Obstet Anesth 1996; 5:283-4.
269. Nortcliffe SA, Shah J, Buggy DJ. Prevention of postoperative nausea and vomiting after spinal morphine for Caesarean section: Comparison of cyclizine, dexamethasone and placebo. Br J Anaesth 2003; 90:665-70.
270. Abboud TK, Shnider SM, Dailey PA, et al. Intrathecal administration of hyperbaric morphine for the relief of pain in labour. Br J Anaesth 1984; 56:1351-60.
271. Lyons G, Columb M, Hawthorne L, Dresner M. Extradural pain relief in labour: Bupivacaine sparing by extradural fentanyl is dose dependent. Br J Anaesth 1997; 78:493-7.
272. Norris MC, Fogel ST, Holtmann B. Intrathecal sufentanil (5 vs. 10 microg) for labor analgesia: Efficacy and side effects. Reg Anesth Pain Med 1998; 23:252-7.
273. Bernard JM, Le Roux D, Barthe A, et al. The dose-range effects of sufentanil added to 0.125% bupivacaine on the quality of patient-controlled epidural analgesia during labor. Anesth Analg 2001; 92:184-8.
274. Asokumar B, Newman LM, McCarthy RJ, et al. Intrathecal bupivacaine reduces pruritus and prolongs duration of fentanyl analgesia during labor: A prospective, randomized controlled trial. Anesth Analg 1998; 87:1309-15.

275. Rawal N, Sjostrand U, Dahlstrom B. Postoperative pain relief by epidural morphine. Anesth Analg 1981; 60:726-31.
276. Hu JW, Dostrovsky JO, Sessle BJ. Functional properties of neurons in cat trigeminal subnucleus caudalis (medullary dorsal horn). I. Responses to oral-facial noxious and nonnoxious stimuli and projections to thalamus and subnucleus oralis. J Neurophysiol 1981; 45:173-92.
277. Ikoma A, Rukwied R, Stander S, et al. Neurophysiology of pruritus: Interaction of itch and pain. Arch Dermatol 2003; 139:1475-8.
278. Zeitz KP, Guy N, Malmberg AB, et al. The 5-HT_3 subtype of serotonin receptor contributes to nociceptive processing via a novel subset of myelinated and unmyelinated nociceptors. J Neurosci 2002; 22:1010-19.
279. Arcioni R, della Rocca M, Romano S, et al. Ondansetron inhibits the analgesic effects of tramadol: A possible 5-HT(3) spinal receptor involvement in acute pain in humans. Anesth Analg 2002; 94:1553-7.
280. Fan P. Nonopioid mechanism of morphine modulation of the activation of 5-hydroxytryptamine type 3 receptors. Mol Pharmacol 1995; 47:491-5.
281. Iatrou CA, Dragoumanis CK, Vogiatzaki TD, et al. Prophylactic intravenous ondansetron and dolasetron in intrathecal morphine-induced pruritus: A randomized, double-blinded, placebo-controlled study. Anesth Analg 2005; 101:1516-20.
282. Yeh HM, Chen LK, Lin CJ, et al. Prophylactic intravenous ondansetron reduces the incidence of intrathecal morphine-induced pruritus in patients undergoing cesarean delivery. Anesth Analg 2000; 91:172-5.
283. Charuluxananan S, Kyokong O, Somboonviboon W, et al. Nalbuphine versus ondansetron for prevention of intrathecal morphine-induced pruritus after cesarean delivery. Anesth Analg 2003; 96:1789-93.
284. Dimitriou V, Voyagis GS. Opioid-induced pruritus: Repeated vs single-dose ondansetron administration in preventing pruritus after intrathecal morphine. Br J Anaesth 1999; 83:822-3.
285. Yazigi A, Chalhoub V, Madi-Jebara S, et al. Prophylactic ondansetron is effective in the treatment of nausea and vomiting but not on pruritus after cesarean delivery with intrathecal sufentanil-morphine. J Clin Anesth 2002; 14:183-6.
286. Szarvas S, Chellapuri RS, Harmon DC, et al. A comparison of dexamethasone, ondansetron, and dexamethasone plus ondansetron as prophylactic antiemetic and antipruritic therapy in patients receiving intrathecal morphine for major orthopedic surgery. Anesth Analg 2003; 97:259-63.
287. Morgan PJ, Mehta S, Kapala DM. Nalbuphine pretreatment in cesarean section patients receiving epidural morphine. Reg Anesth 1991; 16:84-8.
288. Cohen SE, Ratner EF, Kreitzman TR, et al. Nalbuphine is better than naloxone for treatment of side effects after epidural morphine. Anesth Analg 1992; 75:747-52.
289. Davies GG, From R. A blinded study using nalbuphine for prevention of pruritus induced by epidural fentanyl. Anesthesiology 1988; 69:763-5.
290. Borgeat A, Wilder-Smith OH, Saiah M, Rifat K. Subhypnotic doses of propofol relieve pruritus induced by epidural and intrathecal morphine. Anesthesiology 1992; 76:510-2.
291. Saiah M, Borgeat A, Wilder-Smith OH, et al. Epidural-morphine-induced pruritus: Propofol versus naloxone. Anesth Analg 1994; 78:1110-3.
292. Riley ET, Walker D, Hamilton CL, Cohen SE. Intrathecal sufentanil for labor analgesia does not cause a sympathectomy. Anesthesiology 1997; 87:874-8.
293. Cascio M, Pygon B, Bernett C, Ramanathan S. Labour analgesia with intrathecal fentanyl decreases maternal stress. Can J Anaesth 1997; 44:605-9.
294. Wang C, Chakrabarti MK, Whitwam JG. Specific enhancement by fentanyl of the effects of intrathecal bupivacaine on nociceptive afferent but not on sympathetic efferent pathways in dogs. Anesthesiology 1993; 79:766-73.
295. Chaney MA. Side effects of intrathecal and epidural opioids. Can J Anaesth 1995; 42:891-903.
296. Glynn CJ, Mather LE, Cousins MJ, et al. Spinal narcotics and respiratory depression. Lancet 1979; 2:356-7.
297. Palmer CM, Emerson S, Volgoropolous D, Alves D. Dose-response relationship of intrathecal morphine for postcesarean analgesia. Anesthesiology 1999; 90:437-44.
298. Greenhalgh CA. Respiratory arrest in a parturient following intrathecal injection of sufentanil and bupivacaine. Anaesthesia 1996; 51:173-5.
299. Katsiris S, Williams S, Leighton BL, Halpern S. Respiratory arrest following intrathecal injection of sufentanil and bupivacaine in a parturient. Can J Anaesth 1998; 45:880-3.
300. Brockway MS, Noble DW, Sharwood-Smith GH, McClure JH. Profound respiratory depression after extradural fentanyl. Br J Anaesth 1990; 64:243-5.
301. Palmer CM, Nogami WM, Van Maren G, Alves DM. Postcesarean epidural morphine: A dose-response study. Anesth Analg 2000; 90:887-91.
302. Lu JK, Manullang TR, Staples MH, et al. Maternal respiratory arrests, severe hypotension, and fetal distress after administration of intrathecal sufentanil, and bupivacaine after intravenous fentanyl. Anesthesiology 1997; 87:170-2.
303. Ferouz F, Norris MC, Leighton BL. Risk of respiratory arrest after intrathecal sufentanil. Anesth Analg 1997; 85:1088-90.
304. Jaffee JB, Drease GE, Kelly T, Newman LM. Severe respiratory depression in the obstetric patient after intrathecal meperidine or sufentanil. Int J Obstet Anesth 1997; 6:182-4.
305. American Society of Anesthesiologists. ASA Practice Guidelines for the Prevention, Detection, and Management of Respiratory Depression Associated with Neuraxial Opioid Administration. Available at http://www.asahq.org/publicationsAndServices/practiceparam.htm/
306. Rawal N, Mollefors K, Axelsson K, et al. An experimental study of urodynamic effects of epidural morphine and of naloxone reversal. Anesth Analg 1983; 62:641-7.
307. Holdsworth JD. Relationship between stomach contents and analgesia in labour. Br J Anaesth 1978; 50:1145-8.
308. O'Sullivan GM, Sutton AJ, Thompson SA, et al. Noninvasive measurement of gastric emptying in obstetric patients. Anesth Analg 1987; 66:505-11.
309. Kelly MC, Carabine UA, Hill DA, Mirakhur RK. A comparison of the effect of intrathecal and extradural fentanyl on gastric emptying in laboring women. Anesth Analg 1997; 85:834-8.
310. Stagno S, Whitley RJ. Herpesvirus infections of pregnancy. Part II. Herpes simplex virus and varicella-zoster virus infections. N Engl J Med 1985; 313:1327-30.
311. Valley MA, Bourke DL, McKenzie AM. Recurrence of thoracic and labial herpes simplex virus infection in a patient receiving epidural fentanyl. Anesthesiology 1992; 76:1056-7.
312. Acalovschi I. Herpes simplex after spinal pethidine. Anaesthesia 1986; 41:1271-2.
313. Crone LA, Conly JM, Clark KM, et al. Recurrent herpes simplex virus labialis and the use of epidural morphine in obstetric patients. Anesth Analg 1988; 67:318-23.
314. Crone LA, Conly JM, Storgard C, et al. Herpes labialis in parturients receiving epidural morphine following cesarean section. Anesthesiology 1990; 73:208-13.
315. Boyle RK. Herpes simplex labialis after epidural or parenteral morphine: A randomized prospective trial in an Australian obstetric population. Anaesth Intensive Care 1995; 23:433-7.
316. Glaser R, Gotlieb-Stematsky T, editors. Human Herpes Virus Infections: Clinical Aspects. New York, M Dekker, 1982:1-40.
317. Gieraerts R, Navalgund A, Vaes L, et al. Increased incidence of itching and herpes simplex in patients given epidural morphine after cesarean section. Anesth Analg 1987; 66:1321-4.
318. Scott PV, Fischer HB. Spinal opiate analgesia and facial pruritus: A neural theory. Postgrad Med J 1982; 58:531-5.
319. Smith CV, Rayburn WF, Allen KV, et al. Influence of intravenous fentanyl on fetal biophysical parameters during labor. J Matern Fetal Med 1996; 5:89-92.

320. Rayburn WF, Smith CV, Parriott JE, Woods RE. Randomized comparison of meperidine and fentanyl during labor. Obstet Gynecol 1989; 74:604-6.
321. Bader AM, Fragneto R, Terui K, et al. Maternal and neonatal fentanyl and bupivacaine concentrations after epidural infusion during labor. Anesth Analg 1995; 81:829-32.
322. Porter J, Bonello E, Reynolds F. Effect of epidural fentanyl on neonatal respiration. Anesthesiology 1998; 89:79-85.
323. Elliott R. Continuous infusion epidural analgesia for obstetrics: Bupivacaine versus bupivacaine-fentanyl mixture. Can J Anaesth 1991; 38:303-10.
324. Loftus JR, Hill H, Cohen SE. Placental transfer and neonatal effects of epidural sufentanil and fentanyl administered with bupivacaine during labor. Anesthesiology 1995; 83:300-8.
325. Reynolds F, Sharma SK, Seed PT. Analgesia in labour and fetal acid-base balance: A meta-analysis comparing epidural with systemic opioid analgesia. Br J Obstet Gynaecol 2002; 109:1344-53.
326. Wilhite AO, Moore CH, Blass NH, Christmas JT. Plasma concentration profile of epidural alfentanil: Bolus followed by continuous infusion technique in the parturient: Effect of epidural alfentanil and fentanyl on fetal heart rate. Reg Anesth 1994; 19:164-8.
327. Viscomi CM, Hood DD, Melone PJ, Eisenach JC. Fetal heart rate variability after epidural fentanyl during labor. Anesth Analg 1990; 71:679-83.
328. Friedlander JD, Fox HE, Cain CF, et al. Fetal bradycardia and uterine hyperactivity following subarachnoid administration of fentanyl during labor. Reg Anesth 1997; 22:378-81.
329. Clarke VT, Smiley RM, Finster M. Uterine hyperactivity after intrathecal injection of fentanyl for analgesia during labor: A cause of fetal bradycardia? Anesthesiology 1994; 81:1083.
330. Kahn L, Hubert E. Combined spinal-epidural (CSE) analgesia, fetal bradycardia, and uterine hypertonus. Reg Anesth Pain Med 1998; 23:111-2.
331. Segal S, Csavoy AN, Datta S. The tocolytic effect of catecholamines in the gravid rat uterus. Anesth Analg 1998; 87:864-9.
332. Van de Velde M, Teunkens A, Hanssens M, et al. Intrathecal sufentanil and fetal heart rate abnormalities: A double-blind, double placebo-controlled trial comparing two forms of combined spinal-epidural analgesia with epidural analgesia in labor. Anesth Analg 2004; 98:1153-9.
333. Russell JA, Gosden RG, Humphreys EM, et al. Interruption of parturition in rats by morphine: A result of inhibition of oxytocin secretion. J Endocrinol 1989; 121:521-36.
334. Honet JE, Arkoosh VA, Norris MC, et al. Comparison among intrathecal fentanyl, meperidine, and sufentanil for labor analgesia. Anesth Analg 1992; 75:734-9.
335. Nielsen PE, Erickson JR, Abouleish EI, et al. Fetal heart rate changes after intrathecal sufentanil or epidural bupivacaine for labor analgesia: Incidence and clinical significance. Anesth Analg 1996; 83:742-6.
336. Mardirosoff C, Dumont L, Boulvain M, Tramer MR. Fetal bradycardia due to intrathecal opioids for labour analgesia: A systematic review. Br J Obstet Gynaecol 2002; 109:274-81.
337. Albright GA, Forster RM. Does combined spinal-epidural analgesia with subarachnoid sufentanil increase the incidence of emergency cesarean delivery? Reg Anesth 1997; 22:400-5.
338. Gambling DR, Sharma SK, Ramin SM, et al. A randomized study of combined spinal-epidural analgesia versus intravenous meperidine during labor: Impact on cesarean delivery rate. Anesthesiology 1998; 89:1336-44.
339. Mercier FJ, Dounas M, Bouaziz H, et al. Intravenous nitroglycerin to relieve intrapartum fetal distress related to uterine hyperactivity: A prospective observational study. Anesth Analg 1997; 84:1117-20.
340. Bell E. Nitroglycerin and uterine relaxation. Anesthesiology 1996; 85:683.
341. Buhimschi CS, Buhimschi IA, Malinow AM, Weiner CP. Effects of sublingual nitroglycerin on human uterine contractility during the active phase of labor. Am J Obstet Gynecol 2002; 187:235-8.
342. Burm AG, van Kleef JW, Gladines MP, et al. Epidural anesthesia with lidocaine and bupivacaine: Effects of epinephrine on the plasma concentration profiles. Anesth Analg 1986; 65:1281-4.
343. Lee BB, Ngan Kee WD, Plummer JL, et al. The effect of the addition of epinephrine on early systemic absorption of epidural ropivacaine in humans. Anesth Analg 2002; 95:1402-7.
344. Niemi G, Breivik H. Epinephrine markedly improves thoracic epidural analgesia produced by a small-dose infusion of ropivacaine, fentanyl, and epinephrine after major thoracic or abdominal surgery: A randomized, double-blinded crossover study with and without epinephrine. Anesth Analg 2002; 94:1598-605.
345. Sakura S, Sumi M, Morimoto N, Saito Y. The addition of epinephrine increases intensity of sensory block during epidural anesthesia with lidocaine. Reg Anesth Pain Med 1999; 24:541-6.
346. Hashimoto K, Hampl KF, Nakamura Y, et al. Epinephrine increases the neurotoxic potential of intrathecally administered lidocaine in the rat. Anesthesiology 2001; 94:876-81.
347. Gerancher JC. Cauda equina syndrome following a single spinal administration of 5% hyperbaric lidocaine through a 25-gauge Whitacre needle. Anesthesiology 1997; 87:687-9.
348. Liu SSHP. Local anesthetics. In Barash PGCB, Stoelting RF, editors. Clinical Anesthesia. Philadelphia, Lippincott-Raven, 2001:449-72.
349. Sharrock NE, Go G, Mineo R. Effect of i.v. low-dose adrenaline and phenylephrine infusions on plasma concentrations of bupivacaine after lumbar extradural anaesthesia in elderly patients. Br J Anaesth 1991; 67:694-8.
350. Gissen AJCB, Gregus J. Differential sensitivity of fast and slow fibres in mammalian nerve. IV. Effect of carbonation of local anesthetics. Reg Anesth 1985; 10:68-75.
351. Wong K, Strichartz GR, Raymond SA. On the mechanisms of potentiation of local anesthetics by bicarbonate buffer: Drug structure-activity studies on isolated peripheral nerve. Anesth Analg 1993; 76:131-43.
352. Capogna G, Celleno D, Laudano D, Giunta F. Alkalinization of local anesthetics: Which block, which local anesthetic? Reg Anesth 1995; 20:369-77.
353. DiFazio CA, Carron H, Grosslight KR, et al. Comparison of pH-adjusted lidocaine solutions for epidural anesthesia. Anesth Analg 1986; 65:760-4.
354. Capogna G, Celleno D, Varrassi G, et al. Epidural mepivacaine for cesarean section: Effects of a pH-adjusted solution. J Clin Anesth 1991; 3:211-4.
355. Ackerman WE, Juneja MM, Denson DD, et al. The effect of pH and PCO_2 on epidural analgesia with 2% 2-chloroprocaine. Anesth Analg 1989; 68:593-8.
356. Chestnut DH, Geiger M, Bates JN, Choi WW. The influence of pH-adjusted 2-chloroprocaine on the quality and duration of subsequent epidural bupivacaine analgesia during labor: A randomized, double-blind study. Anesthesiology 1989; 70:437-41.
357. Ackerman WE, Denson DD, Juneja MM, et al. Alkalinization of chloroprocaine for epidural anesthesia: Effects of pCO_2 at constant pH. Reg Anesth 1990; 15:89-93.
358. Ramos G, Pereira E, Simonetti MP. Does alkalinization of 0.75% ropivacaine promote a lumbar peridural block of higher quality? Reg Anesth Pain Med 2001; 26:357-62.
359. Berrada R, Chassard D, Bryssine S, et al. [In vitro effects of the alkalinization of 0.25% bupivacaine and 2% lidocaine]. Ann Fr Anesth Reanim 1994; 13:165-8.
360. Parnass SM, Curran MJ, Becker GL. Incidence of hypotension associated with epidural anesthesia using alkalinized and nonalkalinized lidocaine for cesarean section. Anesth Analg 1987; 66:1148-50.
361. Yaksh TL. Pharmacology of spinal adrenergic systems which modulate spinal nociceptive processing. Pharmacol Biochem Behav 1985; 22:845-58.
362. Eisenach JC, Tong CY. Site of hemodynamic effects of intrathecal alpha-2-adrenergic agonists. Anesthesiology 1991; 74:766-71.
363. Correa-Sales C, Rabin BC, Maze M. A hypnotic response to dexmedetomidine, an alpha 2 agonist, is mediated in the locus coeruleus in rats. Anesthesiology 1992; 76:948-52.

364. Gaumann DM, Brunet PC, Jirounek P. Hyperpolarizing afterpotentials in C fibers and local anesthetic effects of clonidine and lidocaine. Pharmacology 1994; 48:21-9.
365. Chiari A, Eisenach JC. Spinal anesthesia: Mechanisms, agents, methods, and safety. Reg Anesth Pain Med 1998; 23:357-62.
366. De Kock M, Eisenach J, Tong C, et al. Analgesic doses of intrathecal but not intravenous clonidine increase acetylcholine in cerebrospinal fluid in humans. Anesth Analg 1997; 84:800-13.
367. Jacobs MM, Hayashida D, Roberts JM. Human myometrial adrenergic receptors during pregnancy: Identification of the alpha-adrenergic receptor by [3H] dihydroergocryptine binding. Am J Obstet Gynecol 1985; 152:680-4.
368. Sia AT, Kwek K, Yeo GS. The in vitro effects of clonidine and dexmedetomidine on human myometrium. Int J Obstet Anesth 2005; 14:104-7.
369. Eisenach JC, Castro MI, Dewan DM, Rose JC. Epidural clonidine analgesia in obstetrics: Sheep studies. Anesthesiology 1989; 70:51-6.
370. Chiari A, Lorber C, Eisenach JC, et al. Analgesic and hemodynamic effects of intrathecal clonidine as the sole analgesic agent during first stage of labor: A dose-response study. Anesthesiology 1999; 91:388-96.
371. Mercier FJ, Dounas M, Bouaziz H, et al. The effect of adding a minidose of clonidine to intrathecal sufentanil for labor analgesia. Anesthesiology 1998; 89:594-601.
372. D'Angelo R, Evans E, Dean LA, et al. Spinal clonidine prolongs labor analgesia from spinal sufentanil and bupivacaine. Anesth Analg 1999; 88:573-6.
373. Sia AT. Optimal dose of intrathecal clonidine added to sufentanil plus bupivacaine for labour analgesia. Can J Anaesth 2000; 47:875-80.
374. Paech MJ, Banks SL, Gurrin LC, et al. A randomized, double-blinded trial of subarachnoid bupivacaine and fentanyl, with or without clonidine, for combined spinal/epidural analgesia during labor. Anesth Analg 2002; 95:1396-401.
375. Missant C, Teunkens A, Vandermeersch E, Van de Velde M. Intrathecal clonidine prolongs labour analgesia but worsens fetal outcome: A pilot study. Can J Anaesth 2004; 51:696-701.
376. Aveline C, El Metaoua S, Masmoudi A, et al. The effect of clonidine on the minimum local analgesic concentration of epidural ropivacaine during labor. Anesth Analg 2002; 95:735-40.
377. Landau R, Schiffer E, Morales M, et al. The dose-sparing effect of clonidine added to ropivacaine for labor epidural analgesia. Anesth Analg 2002; 95:728-34.
378. Kayacan N, Arici G, Karsli B, et al. Patient-controlled epidural analgesia in labour: The addition of fentanyl or clonidine to bupivacaine. Agri 2004; 16:59-66.
379. Paech MJ, Pavy TJ, Orlikowski CE, Evans SF. Patient-controlled epidural analgesia in labor: The addition of clonidine to bupivacaine-fentanyl. Reg Anesth Pain Med 2000; 25:34-40.
380. Mendez R, Eisenach JC, Kashtan K. Epidural clonidine analgesia after cesarean section. Anesthesiology 1990; 73:848-52.
381. Capogna G, Celleno D, Zangrillo A, et al. Addition of clonidine to epidural morphine enhances postoperative analgesia after cesarean delivery. Reg Anesth 1995; 20:57-61.
382. Massone ML, Lampugnani E, Calevo MG, et al. [The effects of a dose of epidural clonidine combined with intrathecal morphine for postoperative analgesia]. Minerva Anestesiol 1998; 64:289-96.
383. Seybold VS. Distribution of histaminergic, muscarinic and serotonergic binding sites in cat spinal cord with emphasis on the region surrounding the central canal. Brain Res 1985; 342:291-6.
384. Yaksh TL, Dirksen R, Harty GJ. Antinociceptive effects of intrathecally injected cholinomimetic drugs in the rat and cat. Eur J Pharmacol 1985; 117:81-8.
385. Bartolini A, Ghelardini C, Fantetti L, et al. Role of muscarinic receptor subtypes in central antinociception. Br J Pharmacol 1992; 105:77-82.
386. Baba H, Kohno T, Okamoto M, et al. Muscarinic facilitation of GABA release in substantia gelatinosa of the rat spinal dorsal horn. J Physiol 1998; 508(Pt 1):83-93.
387. Owen MD, Ozsarac O, Sahin S, et al. Low-dose clonidine and neostigmine prolong the duration of intrathecal bupivacaine-fentanyl for labor analgesia. Anesthesiology 2000; 92:361-6.
388. D'Angelo R, Dean LS, Meister GC, Nelson KE. Neostigmine combined with bupivacaine, clonidine, and sufentanil for spinal labor analgesia. Anesth Analg 2001; 93:1560-4.
389. Lauretti GR, Lima IC. The effects of intrathecal neostigmine on somatic and visceral pain: Improvement by association with a peripheral anticholinergic. Anesth Analg 1996; 82:617-20.
390. Lauretti GR, Mattos AL, Reis MP, Pereira NL. Combined intrathecal fentanyl and neostigmine: Therapy for postoperative abdominal hysterectomy pain relief. J Clin Anesth 1998; 10:291-6.
391. Lauretti GR, de Oliveira R, Reis MP, et al. Study of three different doses of epidural neostigmine coadministered with lidocaine for postoperative analgesia. Anesthesiology 1999; 90:1534-8.
392. Roelants F, Lavand'homme PM. Epidural neostigmine combined with sufentanil provides balanced and selective analgesia in early labor. Anesthesiology 2004; 101:439-44.
393. Roelants F, Lavand'homme PM, Mercier-Fuzier V. Epidural administration of neostigmine and clonidine to induce labor analgesia: Evaluation of efficacy and local anesthetic-sparing effect. Anesthesiology 2005; 102:1205-10.
394. Nelson KE, D'Angelo R, Foss ML, et al. Intrathecal neostigmine and sufentanil for early labor analgesia. Anesthesiology 1999; 91:1293-8.
395. Benhamou D. Are local anesthetics needed for local anesthesia? Anesthesiology 2004; 101:271-2.
396. Kaya FN, Sahin S, Owen MD, Eisenach JC. Epidural neostigmine produces analgesia but also sedation in women after cesarean delivery. Anesthesiology 2004; 100:381-5.

Part V

Anesthesia Before and During Pregnancy

During the early years of obstetric anesthesia, physicians were primarily concerned with its effect on neonatal respiration. Almost 25 years passed before some investigators began to suspect that anesthesia might cause other problems. In fact, it was the suspicion that chloroform caused icterus neonatorum that originally stimulated Paul Zweifel to study placental transmission.

Icterus neonatorum was not Zweifel's original interest. Under the guidance of Adolf Gusserow, one of the preeminent obstetricians in Europe, Zweifel had been studying glucose metabolism during pregnancy. In the course of his work, Zweifel unexpectedly found a reducing compound in the urine of infants whose mothers had received chloroform during labor. At first he suspected that the compound might be glucose, thinking that the metabolism of this compound had somehow been altered by chloroform. After further testing, however, he learned that the reducing substance was not glucose but chloroform itself.

Zweifel thought that chloroform, transmitted to the fetus during labor, might explain some cases of neonatal jaundice. By 1876 physicians already knew that chloroform affected the liver. To cause icterus neonatorum, sufficient quantities of the drug would have to traverse the placenta during the course of a normal labor; the rapidity of transfer was a point of contention among clinicians. To establish the possibility, Zweifel performed experiments that identified chloroform in fetal blood and urine.[1,2]

Zweifel later discounted chloroform as a cause of icterus neonatorum, and the issue was dropped. Another 75 years passed before physicians began to appreciate that drug exposure during pregnancy might have deleterious effects. Events that called attention to the problem included (1) sequelae from radiation exposure after the first use of the atomic bomb; (2) the skeletal deformities associated with the use of thalidomide, a drug once used to treat the nausea of early pregnancy; and (3) the high incidence of genital tumors among daughters of women who had been given diethylstilbestrol during pregnancy. By then the public had also been alerted through the publication of Rachel Carson's *Silent Spring*, which contained such graphic descriptions of the environmental effects of the indiscriminant use of insecticides. Physicians also knew more about embryology and toxicology, better techniques for testing drugs were available, procedures for collecting information were standardized, and information about complications was disseminated. Undoubtedly, greater public awareness of these developments contributed to the resurgence of natural childbirth after 1950.

Donald Caton, M.D.

REFERENCES

1. Zweifel P. Die Respiration des Fötus. Arch Gynäk 1876; 9:291-305.
2. Zweifel P. Der Uebergang von Chloroform und Salicylsäure in die Placenta. Arch Gynäk 1877; 12:235-7.

Chapter 14

Nonanesthetic Drugs during Pregnancy and Lactation

Jerome Yankowitz, M.D.

GENERAL TERATOLOGY

Teratology is the study of abnormal development or the study of birth defects. Multiple factors, including placental transfer, affect whether a particular exposure results in teratogenesis. The term *placental barrier* is a misnomer. The placenta allows many drugs and dietary substances to cross from mother to fetus. Several factors (e.g., lipid solubility, molecular weight, protein binding) affect the passage of drugs across the placenta. Lipid-soluble substances readily cross the placenta. Virtually all drugs cross the placenta to some extent, with the exception of large organic ions such as heparin and insulin.

To avoid unnecessary and potentially teratogenic exposures, patients should be educated about nonpharmacologic techniques to cope with tension, aches and pains, and viral illnesses during pregnancy. Drugs should be used only when necessary. The risk-to-benefit ratio should justify the use of any drug, and the minimum effective dose should be employed. Long-term effects of fetal drug exposure may not become apparent for many years. Therefore, physicians and patients should exercise caution in the use of any drug during pregnancy. On the other hand, the physician should ask the following question: What would be the appropriate treatment in the nonpregnant patient with the same condition? In most cases, the answer is the same as that for women who are pregnant.[1]

Sensitive serum pregnancy tests can diagnose pregnancy as early as one week after conception. Before drug therapy is started, a sensitive test should be used if there is any question about drug safety during a potential pregnancy.

In the United States, major malformations affect 2% to 3% of neonates.[2] Exogenous causes of birth defects (e.g., radiation, infections, maternal metabolic disorders, drugs, environmental chemicals) account for almost 10% of all birth defects and, therefore, affect only 0.2% to 0.3% of all births. Drug exposure explains only 2% to 3% of birth defects. Thus the majority of birth defects are of unknown etiology.

A *major malformation* is defined as one that is incompatible with survival (e.g., anencephaly), one that requires major surgery for correction (e.g., cleft palate, congenital heart disease), or one that causes mental retardation. If all minor malformations (e.g., ear tags, extra digits) are included, the incidence of congenital anomalies may be as high as 7% to 10%.

Drug teratogenicity is affected by species specificity, timing of exposure, dose, maternal physiology, embryology, and genetics. Drug teratogenicity is markedly species specific. For example, thalidomide produces phocomelia in primates but not in rodents. The timing of exposure is important. When administered between 35 and 37 days' gestation, thalidomide produces ear malformations; when administered between 41 and 44 days' gestation, it produces amelia or phocomelia. The dose of drug is also important. In most cases, administration of a low dose has no effect, whereas malformations may occur at intermediate doses and death at higher doses. Fetal death may allow organ-specific teratogenic activity to go unnoticed. Both the route and time of drug administration may affect outcome. Small doses administered over several days may have an effect different from that observed with the same total dose administered at one time. Sequential drug administration may induce the production of an enzyme that metabolizes the drug and thus results in less exposure. Constant exposure may destroy cells that would have catabolized the drug if it had been administered in periodic doses. Pregnancy-associated changes in maternal physiology may affect absorption, distribution, metabolism, and excretion. Placental transfer must also be considered. For example, warfarin derivatives easily cross the placenta and have teratogenic potential; in contrast, heparin does not cross the placenta.

Teratogen exposure in the first 2 weeks after conception is generally thought to be an all-or-nothing phenomenon (i.e., having either no effect or resulting in spontaneous fetal loss). Among women with a 28-day menstrual cycle, the classic period of susceptibility to teratogenic agents is during the period of organogenesis, which occurs primarily at 2½ to 8 weeks after conception (31 to 71 days, or 4 to 10 weeks, after the first day of the last menstrual period [LMP]) (Figure 14-1). After this period, embryonic development is characterized primarily by increasing organ size; thus, the principal effect of exposure consists of growth restriction and/or effects on the nervous system and gonadal tissue. For example, diethylstilbestrol (DES) exposure during the second trimester results in uterine anomalies that do not become apparent until after puberty. Fetal alcohol syndrome may occur with chronic exposure to alcohol during pregnancy. During organogenesis, each organ system has different critical periods of sensitivity. A teratogen can act by causing cell death, altering tissue growth (e.g., hyperplasia, hypoplasia, asynchronous growth), or interfering with cellular differentiation or other basic morphogenic processes.

The genotype of the mother and fetus can affect individual susceptibility to an agent. For example, fetuses with low levels of the enzyme epoxide hydrolase are more likely to manifest fetal hydantoin syndrome than those with normal levels of this enzyme.[3] Combinations of agents may produce different degrees of malformation and growth restriction from those of drugs administered individually. For example, fetuses whose mothers receive combination anticonvulsant therapy are at the highest risk for malformations, including neural tube defects and facial dysmorphic features.

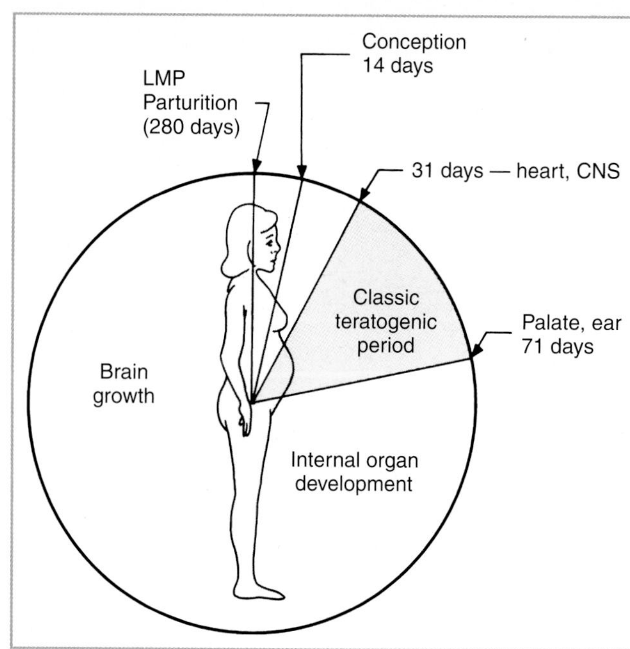

FIGURE 14-1 Gestational clock showing the classic teratogenic period. CNS, central nervous system; LMP, day of last menstrual period. (From Niebyl JR. Drug Use in Pregnancy. 2nd edition. Philadelphia, Lea & Febiger, 1988:2.)

U.S. Food and Drug Administration Categories

In 1979, the U.S. Food and Drug Administration (FDA) introduced a drug classification system to discourage nonessential use of medications during pregnancy (Box 14-1).

Unfortunately, maternal anxiety related to medication use can lead to unnecessary pregnancy terminations. Several characteristics of the FDA drug classification system contribute to public perception—and *misperception*—of the dangers of using medication during pregnancy. Although only 20 to 30 commonly used drugs are known teratogens, 7% of all the medications that are listed in the *Physicians' Desk Reference* are classified as category X.[4,5] All new medications are classified as category C, leading to an exaggerated impression of the danger of many medications.

The Teratology Society has suggested abandonment of the FDA classification scheme.[4] The FDA categories imply a progressive fetal risk from category A to X; however, the drugs in different categories may pose similar risks but may be listed in different categories on the basis of risk-to-benefit considerations. In addition, the categories create the impression that drugs within a category present similar risks, whereas the category definition permits inclusion (in the same category) of drugs that vary in type, degree, and extent of risk. When counseling patients or responding to queries from physicians, we prefer to avoid referring to the *Physicians' Desk Reference*. Rather, we use specific descriptions in teratogen databases to provide the best information available. Many resources are freely available online, in addition to the commercially available databases; they are listed in Table 14-1.

In 1997, the FDA held a public meeting to discuss labeling of drugs. There was consensus that the current

BOX 14-1 U.S. Food and Drug Administration Drug Classification System

Category A

Controlled studies have shown no risk. Adequate, well-controlled studies in pregnant women have failed to demonstrate a risk to the fetus in the first trimester (and there is no evidence of a risk in later trimesters), and the possibility of fetal harm appears remote.

Category B

No evidence of human fetal risk exists. Either animal reproduction studies have not demonstrated fetal risk but no controlled studies in pregnant women have been reported, or animal reproduction studies have shown an adverse effect (other than a decrease in fertility) that was not confirmed in controlled studies in women in the first trimester (and there is no evidence of risk in later trimesters).

Category C

Risk cannot be ruled out. Either studies in animals have revealed adverse effects on the fetus (teratogenic, embryocidal, or other) but no controlled studies in women have been reported, or studies in women and animals are not available. These drugs should be given only if the potential benefit justifies the potential risk to the fetus.

Category D

Positive evidence of human fetal risk exists. However, the benefits from use in pregnant women may be acceptable despite the risk (e.g., if the drug is needed for a life-threatening condition or for a serious disease for which safer drugs cannot be used or are ineffective).

Category X

Contraindicated in pregnancy. Studies in animals or human beings have demonstrated fetal abnormalities, or evidence exists of fetal risk based on human experience, or both, and the risk in pregnant women clearly outweighs any possible benefit. These drugs are contraindicated in women who are or may become pregnant.

Adapted from Friedman JM. Report of the Teratology Society Public Affairs Committee symposium on FDA classification of drugs. Teratology 1993; 48:5-6.

classification scheme is probably oversimplified and confusing, does not address the range of clinical situations or the range of possible effects, and should be replaced with narrative labeling. Subsequently a concept paper was presented that outlined a new model for labeling and included sections such as "clinical management statement," "summary risk assessment," and "discussion of data" for both pregnant and breast-feeding women.[6] This proposal has not yet been implemented. The FDA Office of Women's Health has created a pregnancy registry website, which lists a variety of registries that women who have used specific medications during pregnancy can consult (see Table 14-1).

DRUG USE DURING PREGNANCY

Anticonvulsants

All anticonvulsants cross the placenta. The fetal congenital anomaly rate in pregnant women with epilepsy who ingest anticonvulsant drugs is 4% to 8%; the background incidence for the general population is 2% to 3%.[7,8] A twofold higher risk of minor malformations also exists in this population.[8] Cleft lip with or without cleft palate and congenital heart disease are especially common. Administration of valproic acid or carbamazepine entails a 1% risk of neural tube defects and other malformations; thus, alpha-fetoprotein screening and targeted ultrasonography are appropriate for patients taking these agents. In addition, the offspring of epileptic women have a 2% to 3% incidence of epilepsy, which is five times that of the general population.

Holmes et al.[9] attempted to refute the unproven theory that women with epilepsy have a genetic propensity to have children with a higher risk of birth defects that is separate from the greater risk associated with the use of anticonvulsants. These investigators studied children of women who had a history of seizures but took no medications during the pregnancy. There was no difference in physical features or cognitive function between these children and a group of matched controls. This study was confounded by the inclusion of women with atypical seizure disorders (i.e., mild disease) in the seizure group, as evidenced by their lack of requirement for anticonvulsant drugs.

In a second study, Holmes et al.[10] screened 128,049 pregnant women at delivery to identify the following three groups of infants: (1) those exposed to anticonvulsant drugs; (2) those unexposed to anticonvulsant drugs but with a maternal history of seizures; and (3) those unexposed to anticonvulsant drugs with no maternal history of seizures (control group). The frequency of anticonvulsant embryopathy was higher in the 223 infants exposed to one anticonvulsant drug than in the 508 control infants (20.6% versus 8.5%, respectively; odds ratio [OR], 2.8; 95% confidence interval [CI], 1.1 to 9.7). The frequency was also higher in 93 infants exposed to two or more anticonvulsant drugs than in the controls (28.0% versus 8.5%; OR, 4.2; 95% CI, 1.1 to 5.1). The 98 infants whose mothers had a history of epilepsy but took no anticonvulsant drugs during pregnancy did not have a higher frequency of abnormalities than the control infants. The investigators concluded that "a distinctive pattern of physical abnormalities in infants of mothers with epilepsy is associated with the use of anticonvulsant drugs during pregnancy, rather than with epilepsy itself."

Possible causes of these congenital malformations include genetic differences in drug metabolism, the specific drugs themselves, and deficiency states (e.g., decreased folate levels) induced by the drugs. No congenital malformations appear to be unique to any one anticonvulsant. The characteristics of these syndromes are so similar that the broad term **fetal anticonvulsant syndrome** has been applied to almost every anticonvulsant drug. Fetal anticonvulsant syndrome consists primarily of orofacial, cardiovascular, and digital malformations.[11]

Among women taking **phenytoin,** there is a 2% to 5% risk of major congenital anomalies, primarily midline heart defects, orofacial clefts, and urogenital defects.[7] **Fetal hydantoin syndrome** is a constellation of minor anomalies,

TABLE 14-1 Web Resources for Additional Drug and Teratogen Information

Resource	URL
American Academy of Pediatrics: The Transfer of Drugs and Other Chemicals Into Human Milk	http://aappolicy.aappublications.org/cgi/reprint/pediatrics;108/3/776.pdf
The American Botanical Council	http://www.herbalgram.org
The American College of Obstetricians and Gynecologists	http://www.acog.org/departments/dept_notice.cfm?recno=20&bulletin=1538
Motherisk	http://www.motherisk.org
Organization of Teratology Information Specialists: Fact sheets on exposure during pregnancy to a variety of diseases, medications, and herbal remedies	http://otispregnancy.org/otis_fact_sheets.asp
The National Library of Medicine PubMed	http://www.ncbi.nlm.nih.gov/sites/entrez?db=pubmed
The National Institutes of Health National Center for Complementary and Alternative Medicine	http://nccam.nih.gov
The National Institutes of Health Office of Dietary Supplements	http://dietary-supplements.info.nih.gov
Perinatology.com: Drugs in Pregnancy and Breastfeeding	http://www.perinatology.com/exposures/druglist.htm
The Reproductive Toxicology Center*	http://www.reprotox.org
The Richard and Hinda Rosenthal Center for Complementary and Alternative Medicine	http://www.rosenthal.hs.columbia.edu
RxList: The Internet Drug Index	http://www.rxlist.com
SafeFetus.com	http://www.safefetus.com
University of Washington Clinical Teratology Web*	http://depts.washington.edu/~terisweb
U.S. FDA Office of Women's Health	http://www.fda.gov/womens/science.html#pregnancy; and http://www.fda.gov/womens/registries/registries.html

*Databases, including Reprotox, Reprotext, Teris, and Shepard's Catalog of Teratogenic Agents, can be purchased from these websites.

such as craniofacial abnormalities (short nose, flat nasal bridge, wide lips, hypertelorism, ptosis, epicanthal folds, low-set ears, and low hairline) and limb anomalies (distal digital hypoplasia, absent nails, and altered palmar crease). In addition, neonatal growth and performance delays have been documented. The risk of fetal hydantoin syndrome for the child of a woman taking phenytoin is approximately 10%.[10]

Phenytoin may act as a competitive inhibitor of the placental transport of vitamin K. This results in a decrease in fetal coagulation factors II, VII, IX, and X. In addition, phenytoin may induce fetal hepatic metabolism of the coagulation factors. The resulting reduction in fetal coagulation factors is associated with a higher risk of hemorrhagic disease in the newborn.[12] To help prevent this coagulopathy, some physicians advocate oral vitamin K supplementation (10 mg daily) for pregnant epileptic patients during the last month of pregnancy in addition to the parenteral administration of vitamin K to the neonate at birth.[13]

Several anticonvulsant medications have metabolites that typically are eliminated by the enzyme epoxide hydrolase. In one study, 19 women taking phenytoin underwent amniocentesis. All 4 of the women with low enzyme activity in amniocytes had affected fetuses. The 15 fetuses with normal amniocyte epoxide hydrolase activity did not have the characteristics of fetal hydantoin syndrome.[3]

Carbamazepine (Tegretol) is used to treat all types of seizure disorders, with the exception of petit mal epilepsy. It is most commonly used in the treatment of psychomotor (temporal lobe) epilepsy and grand mal epilepsy. In a prospective study involving 72 women with epilepsy who were taking carbamazepine, the incidence of congenital anomalies was higher in the 35 fetuses exposed only to this drug. There was an 11% incidence of craniofacial defects, a 26% incidence of fingernail hypoplasia, and a 20% incidence of developmental delay.[14] This constellation of fetal effects, named **fetal carbamazepine syndrome**, closely resembles the malformations seen in cases of fetal hydantoin syndrome. In addition, maternal carbamazepine exposure has been specifically associated with spina bifida. An analysis of all available data involving cohorts of pregnant women ingesting carbamazepine supports the conclusion that fetal exposure to this drug carries a 0.5% to 1% risk of spina bifida.[15]

Phenobarbital is used in the treatment of partial and generalized tonic-clonic seizures and status epilepticus.[16] Fetal exposure to phenobarbital has been associated with major malformations, such as congenital heart defects and orofacial clefting. **Fetal phenobarbital syndrome** is characterized by minor dysmorphic features similar to those seen with fetal hydantoin syndrome.[7] Fetal exposure to phenobarbital has also been associated with decreased intellectual and cognitive development in neonates and children. Maternal phenobarbital use during pregnancy can result in hemorrhagic disease of the newborn and neonatal withdrawal symptoms after delivery. The withdrawal symptoms consist mostly of irritability, begin at about 7 days of life, and usually last for approximately 2 to 6 weeks.[16]

Valproic acid (Depakene, Depakote) is used to treat absence and generalized tonic-clonic seizures. Infants exposed to valproic acid have a 1% to 2% risk of spina bifida. The neural tube defect tends to be lumbosacral. Fetal valproic acid exposure has also been associated with cardiac defects, orofacial clefting, and genitourinary anomalies. **Fetal valproate syndrome** has been described; it is characterized by dysmorphic features, including epicanthal folds, shallow orbits, hypertelorism, low-set ears, flat nasal bridge, upturned nasal tip, microcephaly, thin vermillion borders, downturned mouth, thin overlapping fingers and toes, and hyperconvex fingernails.[7]

Among the newer anticonvulsant drugs are felbamate, gabapentin, lamotrigine, oxcarbazepine, topiramate, tiagabine, and vigabatrin.[11] **Felbamate** was approved by the FDA for monotherapy, but later its use was severely restricted because of its association with aplastic anemia and hepatic failure. **Gabapentin** (Neurontin) was initially released in the United States as an adjunctive treatment for partial seizures and secondarily generated tonic-clonic seizures. This agent inhibits dopamine release in the central nervous system (CNS). **Lamotrigine** (Lamictal) appears to have efficacy comparable to that of carbamazepine in the monotherapy of partial epilepsy. An inhibitor of dihydrofolate reductase, lamotrigine decreases embryonic folate levels in experimental animals. This finding raises the concern that human use of lamotrigine may result in developmental toxicity. The manufacturer has established a registry to evaluate this possibility. A preliminary report from this registry has described a 6% rate of congenital malformations in fetuses exposed to this drug; this rate does not represent a clear increase in the baseline rate of malformations. However, there have not been sufficient numbers of fetal exposures to support any definite conclusions.[17-19]

Many patients who present to prenatal clinics are already taking these newer anticonvulsants. Patients should be counseled that although little information is available, no clear evidence of their teratogenicity exists. Some investigators have suggested avoiding the newer anticonvulsants until evidence of their safety is accumulated.[16]

Some women may be taking anticonvulsant drugs without having recently been reevaluated for their need to continue drug therapy. If a patient with idiopathic epilepsy has been seizure free for 2 years and has a normal electroencephalogram (EEG), the neurologist may try to withdraw the drug before pregnancy.[20]

If a patient first presents for care during pregnancy, most authorities agree that the benefits of anticonvulsant therapy during pregnancy outweigh the risks of discontinuing the drug. The blood level of the drug should be monitored to minimize the dose needed to ensure a therapeutic level of drug.

Isotretinoin (Accutane)

Isotretinoin is administered for the treatment of cystic acne. Isotretinoin is highly teratogenic. Lammer et al.[21] reported 21 infants with birth defects, 12 spontaneous abortions, 95 elective abortions, and 26 normal infants in 154 women who were taking isotretinoin during early pregnancy. Characteristic features of this embryopathy are CNS malformations, microtia or anotia, micrognathia, cleft palate, cardiac and great vessel defects, thymic abnormalities, and eye anomalies. Prospective studies suggest that the risk of congenital anomalies is approximately 25%, and an additional 25% of offspring have mental retardation.[22]

Unlike vitamin A, isotretinoin is not stored in tissue, and the drug is not detected in serum 5 days after ingestion. Therefore its use *before* pregnancy does not seem to be hazardous. The package insert for isotretinoin explains the extreme risk of teratogenic effects and clearly states that before a woman capable of childbearing initiates isotretinoin treatment, she must have two negative pregnancy test results and must commit to the use of two forms of contraception.

To combat the problem of birth defects in women taking isotretinoin, the FDA started the iPledge program. This was the most stringent attempt to verify that women were not pregnant when taking this medication. A study among Kaiser Permanente patients in southern California showed that only a minority of patients follow the suggestion to use two forms of birth control, thus increasing their risk of becoming pregnant while using this medication.[23] Later assessments have shown that failure to follow appropriate contraceptive guidelines while taking isotretinoin continues to be an international problem.[24]

Topical **tretinoin** (Retin-A) has not been associated with any teratogenic risk.

Tranquilizers

Results of human epidemiologic studies of the possible teratogenic effects of various tranquilizers, including **meprobamate** (Miltown) and **chlordiazepoxide** (Librium), are inconsistent. One report of nearly 400 patients found a 12% incidence of birth defects in the offspring of meprobamate users.[25] Another study of similar size did not identify any higher risk for malformations.[26] Similar data are available for chlordiazepoxide.[25,26]

Some studies have suggested that first-trimester exposure to **diazepam** increases the risk of cleft lip with or without cleft palate, neural tube defects, intestinal atresia, and limb defects.[27] Other reports have *not* suggested an increase in rate of congenital abnormalities after fetal exposure to **benzodiazepines**. In a case-control study of 611 infants with cleft lip or cleft palate and 2498 controls with other birth defects, no association between diazepam and cleft palate was found; after adjustment of the data for potential confounders, the odds ratios were 0.8 for cleft lip with or without cleft plate (95% CI, 0.4 to 1.7) and 0.8 for cleft palate alone (95% CI, 0.2 to 2.5).[28] One study found no difference in the incidence of congenital anomalies between 460 women exposed to benzodiazepines during pregnancy and 424 control women without such exposure (i.e., 3.1% versus 2.6%, respectively).[29] Nonetheless, in many clinical situations, the risk-to-benefit ratio does not justify the use of benzodiazepines during pregnancy. Perinatal use of diazepam has been associated with hypotonia, hypothermia, and respiratory depression.[30]

Lithium

In the International Registry of Lithium Babies, 25 of 217 (11.5%) infants exposed to lithium during the first trimester of pregnancy were malformed.[31] Eighteen infants had cardiovascular anomalies, and 6 had the rare Ebstein's anomaly, which occurs only once in 20,000 non-exposed pregnancies. Subsequent studies have suggested that ascertainment bias may have flawed the Registry; the reported risk of anomalies after lithium exposure is much less than that reported by the Registry.

In a cohort study linking the Swedish Birth Registry with the records of women with bipolar disorder, 59 infants were identified whose mothers had been treated with lithium early in pregnancy.[32] Four (6.8%) of the 59 infants exposed to lithium had congenital heart disease, compared with 2 (0.9%) of 228 infants not exposed to lithium (relative risk (RR), 7.7; 95% CI, 1.5 to 41.2). None of the infants had Ebstein's anomaly. In a prospective cohort study of 148 women treated with lithium during the first trimester and 148 controls not exposed to any known teratogen, there was no significant difference between groups in the incidence of major congenital anomalies or cardiac malformations,[33] although one lithium-exposed infant did have Ebstein's anomaly. The investigators concluded that lithium is not a major human teratogen, but they recommended that women exposed to lithium be offered ultrasonography and fetal echocardiography.[33] If the data are pooled, these two cohort studies do not suggest a statistically significant increase in risk of congenital malformations or cardiac malformations in women exposed to lithium during pregnancy. Although the risk for congenital malformations associated with intrauterine lithium exposure is likely to be lower than previously reported, an absence of risk cannot be assumed from the available data.

Two published cases associate polyhydramnios with maternal lithium treatment.[34,35] Nephrogenic diabetes insipidus has been reported in adults taking lithium; thus the presumed mechanism of polyhydramnios is fetal diabetes insipidus. Polyhydramnios may signal fetal lithium toxicity.

Pregnancy accelerates the excretion of lithium, so serum lithium levels should be monitored in pregnant women.[36] Perinatal effects of lithium include hypotonia, lethargy, and poor feeding in the infant. In addition, complications (e.g., goiter, hypothyroidism) similar to those seen in adults taking lithium have been noted in newborns.

Some authorities recommend discontinuation of lithium and substitution with another medication during pregnancy. However, the discontinuation of lithium is associated with a 70% chance of relapse of the affective disorder in one year, as opposed to a 20% risk of relapse with continuation of lithium therapy.[31]

Antidepressants

A summation of 14 studies assessing the effect of fetal exposure to **tricyclic antidepressants** evaluated 414 cases of first-trimester exposure.[37] When the study data were pooled or viewed individually, no significant association between fetal exposure to tricyclic antidepressants and congenital malformations was found.[37] In the Michigan Medicaid study, 467 newborns had been exposed to amitriptyline and 75 newborns had been exposed to imipramine during the first trimester; there was no association between tricyclic antidepressant use and congenital anomalies.[38]

The selective serotonin reuptake inhibitors (SSRIs) include **sertraline** (Zoloft), **paroxetine** (Paxil), **fluoxetine** (Prozac), and **citalopram** (Celexa). No higher risk of major malformations or developmental (language and behavior) abnormalities was identified with their use in earlier studies.[39-41] In a multicenter evaluation of birth defects, use of SSRIs was not associated with a higher risk of cardiac defects.[42] However, in analyses of the individual medications, sertraline was associated with an increased risk of septal defects (OR, 2.0; 95% CI, 1.2 to 4.0), and paroxetine with a higher risk of right ventricular outflow tract obstruction (OR, 3.3; 95% CI, 1.3 to 8.8). Sertraline was also associated with an increased risk of omphalocele, but this association was based on only three subjects. Another study found significantly higher risks for craniosynostosis, omphalocele, and anencephaly in association with exposure to SSRIs as a group; this study also found an association between paroxetine and right ventricular outflow tract lesions.[43]

A cohort study compared postnatal outcome for infants exposed to fluoxetine in late gestation (up to the time of delivery) with that for infants whose exposure was limited to the first trimester.[44] Infants exposed in the third trimester had a greater incidence of perinatal complications, including preterm delivery, admission to the special care nursery, poor neonatal adaptation, lower mean birth weight, and shorter body length.[44] A subsequent study suggested an association between the maternal use of SSRIs in late pregnancy and a higher risk of persistent pulmonary hypertension of the newborn.[45]

The American College of Obstetricians and Gynecologists (ACOG)[46] has recommended that use of paroxetine in pregnant women (and in women planning pregnancy) be avoided, if possible. In addition, they have suggested that fetal echocardiography should be considered in women who have used paroxetine during early pregnancy. Further, the ACOG has stated that treatment with all SSRIs should be individualized.[46]

Anticoagulants

Use of **warfarin** (Coumadin) in pregnancy can result in an embryopathy similar to the X-linked chondrodysplasia punctata (CDPX). The embryopathy can occur with fetal exposure between 6 and 12 weeks' gestation. Because deficiency of arylsulfatase E is responsible for the chondrodysplasia, the embryopathy may result from inhibition of arylsulfatase E by warfarin. The period between 6 and 9 weeks' gestation is especially critical. **Fetal warfarin syndrome** consists of nasal hypoplasia, depressed nasal bridge (often with a deep groove between the alae and nasal tip), stippled epiphyses, nail hypoplasia, mental retardation, and growth restriction. Second- and third-trimester exposures can result in other adverse fetal effects, including microcephaly, blindness, deafness, and growth restriction.

Hall et al.[47] reviewed all published cases of warfarin embryopathy through 1980. They identified 418 pregnancies complicated by warfarin use. One sixth of the live-born infants had abnormalities, one sixth of the pregnancies ended in stillbirth or spontaneous abortion, and the remaining two thirds had normal outcomes. Of the 45 pregnancies with only first-trimester exposure, 31 had some type of problem, including 22 abortions and 9 fetal malformations. For those with isolated second- or third-trimester exposure, the overall problem rate was 20% to 30%, but this rate was not further subdivided into losses and malformations. Three prospective studies of women exposed only in the second and third trimesters found that the incidence of malformations must be exceedingly low, as there was no evidence of fetal or neonatal CNS or eye abnormalities.[48] Some evidence suggests that a lower dose (less than 5 mg per day) has less teratogenic potential.[49]

Heparin is a large, water-soluble molecule that does not cross the placenta. Maternal administration of heparin does not have an adverse effect on the fetus, and heparin is the drug of choice for most pregnant women who require anticoagulation daily. Daily administration of 20,000 units of standard **unfractionated heparin** for more than 20 weeks may be associated with maternal bone demineralization.[50] Unfractionated heparin should be used for prolonged periods only when it is clearly necessary.

Low-molecular-weight heparin (LMWH) has some advantages over standard unfractionated heparin.[51] Like standard unfractionated heparin, LMWH does not cross the placenta. LMWH has a longer half-life, which typically allows once-daily dosing in nonpregnant patients. In addition, LMWH has a more predictable dose-response relationship in nonpregnant patients, which obviates monitoring. However, obstetric caregivers should be aware that pregnancy is associated with a higher volume of distribution and accelerated clearance of LMWH. Use of LMWH thromboprophylaxis during pregnancy requires adjustments in the dose of LMWH to accommodate for the changes in the pharmacokinetics of this drug that occur during pregnancy. For example, pregnant women may require twice-daily doses.[52]

Administration of LMWH poses a lower risk of heparin-induced thrombocytopenia than standard unfractionated heparin. Studies also suggest a lower risk of osteoporosis with LMWH. The cost of LMWH is higher than that of standard unfractionated heparin.

An isolated history of deep vein thrombosis does not necessarily justify full anticoagulation during pregnancy. Conservative measures, such as the use of elastic stockings and the avoidance of prolonged sitting or standing, should be considered.

In contrast, full anticoagulation is necessary in pregnant women with cardiac valve prostheses. Unfortunately, some reports have described catastrophic heparin failure and valve thrombosis leading to maternal and fetal morbidity and mortality. One report noted a 4.5-fold increase in the rate of valve thrombosis when heparin (rather than warfarin) was used, but in 8 of 12 cases there was evidence of suboptimal treatment.[53] Iturbe-Alessio et al.[54] studied 72 pregnant women with prosthetic heart valves. Among those who received warfarin, 25% to 30% had embryopathy, but there were cases of fatal prosthetic valve thromboses in the patients who received low-dose heparin. The investigators concluded that warfarin is a teratogen but that low-dose heparin is not appropriate for prophylaxis in patients with prosthetic heart valves.

In a systematic review of anticoagulation in pregnant women with mechanical heart valves, Chan et al.[55] evaluated outcomes with the following three anticoagulation regimens: (1) oral anticoagulants (most commonly warfarin) given throughout pregnancy; (2) heparin administered during the first trimester and then warfarin for the duration of pregnancy; and (3) heparin administered throughout pregnancy. The data demonstrated progressively higher rates of maternal death with regimens 1, 2, and 3 (i.e., 1.8%, 4.2%, and 15.0%, respectively). The use of warfarin throughout pregnancy was associated with warfarin embryopathy in 6.4% of live-born infants. The substitution of heparin at or before 6 weeks' gestation eliminated that risk.[55]

For women with prosthetic heart valves, the American College of Chest Physicians (ACCP)[52] has recommended use of one of the following three regimens: (1) administration of adjusted-dose, twice-daily LMWH throughout pregnancy; (2) aggressive adjusted-dose unfractionated heparin throughout pregnancy; or (3) administration of either unfractionated heparin or LMWH in the first trimester and then warfarin until the mid–third trimester, before resumption of heparin. In high-risk women with prosthetic heart valves, the AACP suggests the addition of low-dose aspirin to the anticoagulation regimen.[52]

Thyroid and Antithyroid Drugs

Drugs used to treat hyperthyroidism include propylthiouracil and methimazole. **Propylthiouracil** has been the mainstay of treatment. It can cause fetal and neonatal hypothyroidism and, rarely, goiter. The rate of congenital malformations is not higher among the infants of women treated with propylthiouracil.[56] **Methimazole** (Tapazole, Carbimazole), like propylthiouracil, is administered orally to treat hyperthyroidism. Aplasia cutis congenita of the scalp has been described among children whose mothers took methimazole during pregnancy.[57,58] On the other hand, the risk of a scalp defect appears to be small, because several large series found no cases of aplasia cutis.[59]

Radioactive iodine administered for thyroid ablation or diagnostic studies is not concentrated by the fetal thyroid until 10 to 12 weeks' gestation.[60] Thus inadvertent administration of either ^{131}I or ^{125}I near conception poses no specific risk to the fetal thyroid.

Women with hypothyroidism may require larger doses of **thyroxine** during pregnancy.[61] It is prudent to monitor thyroid function throughout pregnancy and to adjust the thyroxine dose to maintain a normal thyrotropin level, because there is some evidence of decreased intelligence in the offspring of women with subclinical maternal thyroid deficiency during pregnancy.[62]

Inotropic Agents

The inotropic agents include dopamine, dobutamine, isoproterenol, and digoxin. There are no reports of teratogenicity related to the use of dopamine or dobutamine during pregnancy. Among 31 women treated with isoproterenol during the first 4 months of pregnancy in the Collaborative Perinatal Project, there was no higher incidence of malformations.[63]

Digoxin is used to treat heart failure and cardiac arrhythmias. Physicians should monitor the maternal digoxin level to ensure a therapeutic level of drug during pregnancy. Among the infants of 142 women who were treated with digoxin during the first trimester, the frequency of congenital anomalies was no greater than expected.[64] The rate of anomalies was also not increased among the 52 women treated with cardiac glycosides in the first trimester or among the 129 women treated any time during pregnancy in the Collaborative Perinatal Project.[63]

Antihypertensive Drugs

Methyldopa and labetalol are often used to treat mild chronic hypertension during pregnancy. The drugs commonly used for treatment of severe hypertension in pregnancy are hydralazine, labetalol, sodium nitroprusside, nitroglycerin, calcium entry–blocking agents (including nicardipine and nifedipine), and beta-adrenergic receptor antagonists (including propranolol and atenolol).

METHYLDOPA

Methyldopa (Aldomet) has been widely used for the treatment of chronic hypertension during pregnancy. Postural hypotension may occur, but there is no evidence of teratogenicity or other adverse fetal effects.

HYDRALAZINE

Hydralazine (Apresoline) and labetalol are the preferred parenteral agents for treatment of severe hypertension during pregnancy. The frequency of congenital anomalies was not significantly increased among the children of 136 women treated with hydralazine during pregnancy in the Collaborative Perinatal Project.[65] However, only 8 of these women were treated in the first trimester. There is no evidence that hydralazine is teratogenic.

BETA-ADRENERGIC RECEPTOR ANTAGONISTS

There is no evidence that **propranolol** (Inderal) is teratogenic. Maternal administration of propranolol within 2 hours of delivery may result in neonatal bradycardia.[63] There is some evidence that maternal administration of propranolol may result in modest intrauterine growth restriction.[66] It seems prudent to use ultrasonography to assess intrauterine fetal growth in women receiving propranolol.

Atenolol (Tenormin) is a cardioselective beta-adrenergic receptor antagonist. In a large analysis of published trials involving beta-adrenergic receptor antagonist therapy, there was little or no information on teratogenicity for the multiple agents studied, including atenolol, labetalol, metoprolol, oxprenolol, pindolol, and propranolol.[67] Atenolol was associated with lower birth weight and a trend toward more frequent preterm delivery than with other antihypertensive drugs and with no therapy. These effects were more pronounced when the drug was administered earlier in pregnancy and for a long duration.[68] In one study, treatment of hypertension (mostly with atenolol) reduced the risk of severe hypertension and preterm labor.[69] In a randomized clinical trial, the same group observed that atenolol prevented preeclampsia but resulted in the birth of infants who weighed 440 g less than infants in the placebo group.[70]

LABETALOL

Labetalol (Normodyne, Trandate) is another commonly used agent for the treatment of severe hypertension. It is a nonselective beta-adrenergic receptor antagonist and postsynaptic $alpha_1$-receptor antagonist. Labetalol slows heart rate and decreases systemic vascular resistance. There are few data regarding the use of labetalol and the risk of congenital malformations. In one randomized double-blind trial of 152 women with hypertension, there were no malformations in either the treatment group or the placebo group, although the exposure to labetalol occurred in the second and third trimesters.[71]

ANGIOTENSIN-CONVERTING ENZYME INHIBITORS

The angiotensin-converting enzyme (ACE) inhibitors initially did not appear to be teratogenic when administered during the first trimester.[72] However, a 2007 study suggested an increase in the incidence of congenital anomalies, particularly cardiac and CNS defects, after first-trimester exposure to ACE inhibitors.[73] Some authorities contend that this study had major limitations.[74] Later in pregnancy, ACE inhibitors can cause fetal renal failure and oligohydramnios, which may result in fetal limb contractures, craniofacial deformities, and pulmonary hypoplasia.[75]

CALCIUM ENTRY–BLOCKING AGENTS

A case report noted the occurrence of myocardial infarction in a pregnant woman who was receiving nifedipine for treatment of preterm labor.[76] However, the overall maternal risk of nifedipine seems low, and it does not seem to cause an increase in the rate of malformations among exposed fetuses.[77]

Antiarrhythmia Drugs

Amiodarone (Cordarone) is structurally similar to thyroxine and contains 37% iodine by weight. In a review of the 64 reported pregnancies in which amiodarone was administered to the mothers, there was no clear increase in the incidence of malformations. However, 11 (17%) infants had evidence of hypothyroidism, and two (3%) neonates had goiter.[78,79] There was no clear effect on intelligence in the offspring, but there may be an association with a mild alteration of neurodevelopment.[79] This agent is used during pregnancy most often to treat fetal arrhythmias, and first-trimester exposure is rare.

There are scant data on **quinidine** (Duraquin, Quinaglute, Quinalan, Cardioquin, and Quinidex), **procainamide** (Pronestyl), **flecainide** (Tambocor), and **sotalol** (Beta-Cardone, Betapace), which are often also used to treat fetal arrhythmias.

Antineoplastic and Immunosuppressant Drugs

Azathioprine (Imuran) has been used successfully in pregnant women with systemic lupus erythematosus or renal transplants. There is no evidence of an increase in the incidence or distribution of anomalies among infants who are exposed to this drug *in utero*.[80,81]

Cyclosporin has been used for immunosuppression during pregnancy in renal transplant patients. No teratogenic effects have been reported.[82]

In human pregnancies, administration of **cyclophosphamide** during the first trimester has been associated with skeletal and palatal defects and with malformations of the limbs and eyes.[83] Administration of cyclophosphamide after the first trimester may be associated with low birth weight.

Chloroquine is safe in doses used as prophylaxis for malaria. One study noted no greater risk of birth defects in 169 infants exposed to 300 mg once weekly.[84] However, maternal administration of larger, therapeutic dosages (e.g., 250 to 500 mg/day) was associated with congenital abnormalities, including two cases of cochleovestibular paresis.[85]

Antiasthmatic Drugs

THEOPHYLLINE AND AMINOPHYLLINE

Both theophylline and aminophylline are safe for the treatment of asthma during pregnancy. No evidence of teratogenicity was found in 76 cases of fetal exposure to these agents in the Collaborative Perinatal Project,[86] although there was a slight increase over the expected rate of birth defects in the Michigan Medicaid study.[87]

EPINEPHRINE

Minor malformations have been reported after 3082 cases of exposure to a sympathomimetic amine, such as epinephrine, in the first trimester.[86] The most common sources of sympathomimetic amines were a variety of nonprescription preparations used to treat upper respiratory tract infections.

TERBUTALINE AND OTHER SHORT-ACTING BETA-SYMPATHOMIMETIC AGENTS

A Michigan Medicaid study with more than 1000 first-trimester exposures to short-acting beta-sympathomimetic agents (e.g., albuterol) and a smaller number of exposures to metaproterenol, terbutaline, and isoproterenol did not demonstrate any significant teratogenic risk in humans.[87]

CORTICOSTEROIDS

Inhaled corticosteroids provide effective therapy, but some of these drugs are absorbed systemically. All corticosteroids cross the placenta to some extent, but **prednisone** and **prednisolone** are inactivated by the placenta. After maternal administration of prednisone, the fetal concentration of active drug is less than 10% of that in the mother. Therefore, prednisone and prednisolone are the preferred systemic corticosteroids for treatment of maternal diseases such as asthma. Oral corticosteroid therapy has been associated with a 3.4-fold increase in the relative risk of cleft lip and palate.[88,89]

CROMOLYN SODIUM

A mast cell stabilizer, cromolyn sodium has been used for more than 25 years without a reported association with congenital defects.[87]

OTHER AGENTS

The **5-lipoxygenase** (5-LO) **inhibitors** and **leukotriene receptor antagonists** are newer agents. On the basis of limited data, these drugs do not appear to be teratogenic.[90]

Antiemetics

Two randomized, placebo-controlled trials have confirmed that **vitamin B_6** is effective therapy for nausea and vomiting during early pregnancy.[91,92] Thus vitamin B_6 should be the drug of choice for nausea and vomiting in pregnancy.[93] **Doxylamine** is available without a prescription as Unisom SleepTabs 25 mg, so patients can take a combination similar to the formerly marketed Bendectin. One 25-mg tablet of vitamin B_6 and one 25-mg tablet of doxylamine at bedtime, and half of each in the morning and again in the afternoon, is an effective combination. **Ginger** has also been shown to be an effective treatment for nausea and vomiting during pregnancy.[94,95]

TRIMETHOBENZAMIDE

Trimethobenzamide (Tigan) is an antinausea drug that is not classified as either an antihistamine or a phenothiazine. Data from a small number of patients are conflicting. In a Kaiser Health Plan study,[96] there was an increase in the incidence of congenital anomalies among 193 patients exposed to trimethobenzamide during pregnancy. However, the investigators observed no pattern of specific anomalies in these children and noted that some of the mothers also took other drugs. There was no evidence of an association between trimethobenzamide and congenital malformations in 340 patients in the Collaborative Perinatal Project.[97]

PHENOTHIAZINES

Chlorpromazine (Thorazine) and **promethazine** (Phenergan) effectively treat *hyperemesis gravidarum*. The most important side effect is drowsiness. Teratogenicity does not seem to be a problem with phenothiazines. In the Kaiser Health Plan study, 976 patients,[96] and in the Collaborative Perinatal Project, 1309 patients[97] were treated with phenothiazines, with no evidence of an association between these agents and congenital malformations.

METOCLOPRAMIDE

Metoclopramide (Reglan) is an alternative agent for the treatment of nausea and vomiting in pregnancy. In a Danish record linkage study,[98] the frequency of malformations was no greater than expected among the infants of 190 women who had been given a prescription for metoclopramide during the first trimester of pregnancy. Likewise, a multicenter study did not observe an increased incidence of anomalies with the use of this agent.[99]

ONDANSETRON

Ondansetron (Zofran) is similar in efficacy to promethazine for the treatment of hyperemesis gravidarum.[100] It is much more costly but less sedating than promethazine. There is no evidence that it has a teratogenic effect.[101]

Antihistamines

Some pregnant patients require treatment with antihistamines for allergies or other upper respiratory tract complaints such as the common cold. Patients should understand that these drugs represent symptomatic therapy for the common cold and have no influence on the course of the disease. Physicians should recommend other remedies, such as the use of a humidifier, rest, and fluids. If medication is necessary, patients should not use a combination of two drugs if one drug will suffice. If the patient has an allergy, an antihistamine alone may be all that is needed.

If the patient needs a decongestant, a topical nasal spray will involve less fetal exposure than systemic medication. One study suggested an association between **pseudoephedrine** and defects attributable to vascular disruption, including gastroschisis, small intestinal atresia, and hemifacial microsomia.[102] Physicians should discourage the use of nonprescription drugs for trivial indications because the long-term fetal effects of the chronic maternal use of these drugs are unknown.

Most sedating antihistamines are not associated with an increased malformation rate. These agents are chlorpheniramine, diphenhydramine, methapyrilene, thonzylamine, pyrilamine, tripelennamine, phenyltoloxamine, and buclizine.

Although there have been some conflicting reports about **brompheniramine,** a meta-analysis found no evidence to implicate it as a teratogen.[103] In the Boston Collaborative Program,[64] none of the sedating antihistamines was associated with malformations. Two combination products: **triprolidine with pseudoephedrine** (Actifed), and **phenylpropanolamine with chlorpheniramine** (Ornade) were not associated with malformations. In a cohort of 1502 San Diego women, antihistamines were not associated with congenital malformations.[104] This study involved 269 women exposed to **chlorpheniramine** (Chlor-Trimeton). **Azatadine** (Trinalin) was not found to be teratogenic among 127 Michigan Medicaid recipients.[38]

Limited safety information is available for the nonsedating antihistamines. In a cohort study, 114 women exposed to **astemizole** were matched with 114 women exposed to known nonteratogens (e.g., dental radiographs, acetaminophen).[105] There were two major malformations in the astemizole group, and two in the control group. (Astemizole has been withdrawn from the market in most countries because of concerns regarding uncommon but severe cardiac rhythm disturbances.) In a study of 39 women exposed to **cetirizine** (Zyrtec), the rate of malformations was no higher than in a control group.[106] This finding was replicated in a study performed through a teratogen information service.[107] There are no controlled human studies for **loratadine** (Claritin) or **fexofenadine** (Allegra).

Several antihistamines have primary indications not directly related to upper respiratory complaints: **Hydroxyzine** (Atarax, Vistaril) is used for treatment of pruritus, **meclizine** (Antivert) for dizziness, **diphenhydramine** (Benadryl) for sleep and pruritus, and **doxylamine** (a component of the former Bendectin) for treatment of nausea and vomiting of pregnancy. A meta-analysis of antihistamines used in early pregnancy mostly for nonrespiratory complaints found a protective effect against malformations (OR, 0.76; 95% CI, 0.60 to 0.94).[108] This apparent benefit may have resulted from an association between maternal nausea and good fetal outcomes rather than from a direct effect of antihistamines.

Antibiotics

Pregnant women are especially susceptible to vaginal yeast infections, and an antifungal agent may be necessary after antibiotic therapy. Therefore, antibiotics should be used only when clearly indicated.

PENICILLINS AND CEPHALOSPORINS

Use of penicillin derivatives (e.g., amoxicillin, ampicillin) appears to be safe during pregnancy. Use of the cephalosporins also appears to be safe. In a large case-control study, Czeizel et al.[109] found no teratogenic risk with the use of cephalosporins, primarily oral cephalexin.

ERYTHROMYCIN

An alternative to penicillin for the treatment of many diseases in pregnancy, erythromycin is used as a primary treatment for mycoplasmal and chlamydial infections. Although it is not generally thought to be a teratogen,[64,110] a few studies have questioned whether it might be associated with an increased risk of cardiac defects and pyloric stenosis.[111]

SULFONAMIDES

Sulfonamides compete with bilirubin for albumin-binding sites, and they may pose an increased risk of hyperbilirubinemia in the newborn. Thus they are not the first choice during the third trimester, especially if the mother is at risk for preterm labor.

Sulfasalazine is poorly absorbed after oral administration, so it is used for treatment of ulcerative colitis and Crohn's disease. Sulfasalazine crosses the placenta. The fetal concentration approximates the maternal concentration, although both are low. Neither kernicterus nor severe neonatal jaundice has been reported after maternal use of sulfasalazine, even when the drug was administered up to the time of delivery.[112]

TRIMETHOPRIM

Trimethoprim is often administered with sulfa for the treatment of a urinary tract infection. In 2296 Michigan Medicaid recipients, first-trimester trimethoprim exposure was associated with a slightly higher risk of birth defects, in particular cardiovascular anomalies.[38] Folic acid antagonists, which include trimethoprim, may increase the risk not only of neural tube defects but also of cardiovascular defects, oral clefts, and urinary tract defects.[113]

NITROFURANTOIN

No risk of birth defects has been noted after exposure to nitrofurantoin. However, this agent can induce hemolytic anemia in patients who are deficient in glucose-6-phosphate dehydrogenase. Because the newborn's red blood cells are deficient in reduced glutathione, the package insert for this agent warns against its use at term. However, there is no report of neonatal hemolytic anemia after intrauterine exposure.

TETRACYCLINES

First-trimester exposure to tetracycline or doxycycline does not appear to have a teratogenic effect.[114] However, tetracyclines bind to developing enamel and cause discoloration of the teeth. Tetracyclines affect deciduous teeth when administered between approximately 26 weeks of pregnancy and 6 months of age in the infant. They affect the permanent teeth only if administered to children between approximately 6 months and 5 years of age. In addition, tetracyclines deposit in developing osseous sites and inhibit bone growth beginning in the second trimester.[115] Physicians should prescribe alternative drugs during pregnancy.

AMINOGLYCOSIDES

No teratogenic effect was observed in 135 infants exposed to **streptomycin** in the first trimester. This agent crosses the placenta and in one study was found to cause ototoxicity in 3% to 11% of children of mothers who received prolonged streptomycin treatment for tuberculosis during pregnancy.[116] Similar ototoxicity has been seen after prolonged intrauterine exposure to **kanamycin**.

Physicians should limit the duration of therapy with aminoglycosides and should monitor maternal serum levels to minimize fetal exposure. Once-daily dosing (4 mg/kg intravenously) of **gentamicin** increases efficacy and decreases toxicity and cost.[117] It is not clear that gentamicin causes hearing loss in infants.[118] Aminoglycosides may also potentiate the neuromuscular weakness associated with the administration of magnesium sulfate or a nondepolarizing muscle relaxant.

QUINOLONES

The quinolones (e.g., ciprofloxacin, norfloxacin) have a high affinity for bone tissue and cartilage and may cause arthropathies in children. However, no malformations or musculoskeletal problems were noted in 38 infants exposed during the first trimester.[119] The manufacturer recommends against the use of this drug during pregnancy and in children.

METRONIDAZOLE

There is no apparent increase in the incidence of major congenital anomalies among the newborns of mothers treated with metronidazole (Flagyl) during early or late gestation.[120] One meta-analysis confirmed no teratogenic risk.[121] Metronidazole remains the most effective drug for trichomoniasis.

ACYCLOVIR AND OTHER ANTIVIRAL THERAPY

Administration of **acyclovir** (Zovirax) has resulted in no fetal abnormalities in 601 reported exposures.[122] The U.S. Centers for Disease Control and Prevention (CDC) recommends that pregnant women with disseminated infection (e.g., herpetic hepatitis, varicella pneumonia) be treated with acyclovir.

Zidovudine (AZT) has been studied because of its role in the treatment of acquired immunodeficiency syndrome (AIDS). In a prospective cohort study, children exposed to this agent during the perinatal period in the Pediatric AIDS Clinical Trials Group Protocol 076 (PACTG 076) were studied to a median age of 4.2 years. No adverse effects were observed.[123] Combination antiretroviral therapy has not been associated with major infant toxicity, even when the therapy was initiated in the first trimester of pregnancy.[124]

The Antiretroviral Pregnancy Registry was established in 1989 to detect any major teratogenic effect of the antiretroviral drugs. The registration process protects patient anonymity. The Registry depends on voluntary reporting of prenatal exposure to the antiretroviral drugs; therefore, drug-associated adverse events may not reflect true rates. Through July 2007, the Registry contained data for 6893 live-born children; of these, 2673 (38.8%) infants had first-trimester exposure to antiretroviral therapy.[125] The Registry includes reports of prenatal exposure (in all three trimesters of pregnancy) to almost all antiretroviral drugs, alone or in combination, with the exception of zalcitabine and delavirdine. Exposure to the last two drugs has been reported in the first and second trimesters. The number of pregnancy exposures to these various drugs has been rising, but in many cases, an assessment of the effects of individual drugs on the fetus is not possible. No evidence of teratogenicity has been reported.[126]

The four drugs currently approved for the control and prevention of influenza in the United States are amantadine, rimantadine, zanamivir, and oseltamivir. **Amantadine** and **rimantadine** are chemically related and demonstrate activity against influenza A but not influenza B viruses. **Zanamivir** and **oseltamivir** are neuraminidase inhibitors with activity against both influenza A and influenza B viruses. In a surveillance study of 333,000 live-born infants, 64 mothers had used amantadine during the first trimester.[127] Congenital anomalies were diagnosed in 5 of the children, although three such diagnoses had been expected. The CDC has stated that because of the unknown effects of influenza antiviral drugs on pregnant women and their fetuses, these four drugs should be used during pregnancy only if the potential benefit justifies the potential risk to the embryo or fetus.[128] These recommendations were reiterated for the 2007-2008 influenza season with regard to zanamivir and oseltamivir, the two agents active against that season's viruses.[129]

Mild Analgesics

Physicians should encourage patients to use nonpharmacologic remedies (e.g., locally applied heat, rest) for aches and pains during pregnancy.

ASPIRIN

There is no evidence of an overall increase in rates of congenital malformations with maternal use of aspirin during the first trimester. One review suggested a higher risk of gastroschisis.[130]

Aspirin causes permanent inhibition of prostaglandin synthetase in platelets. The drug inhibits platelet aggregation, and platelet function returns to normal only after the production of new platelets in the bone marrow. Thus aspirin may increase the risk of peripartum hemorrhage. One study noted platelet dysfunction in the newborn as late as 5 days after maternal ingestion of aspirin.[131]

Prostaglandins help maintain the patency of the ductus arteriosus *in utero*. Arcilla et al.[132] reported one case in which they suggested that the use of aspirin shortly before delivery caused closure of the ductus arteriosus *in utero*.

Low-dose aspirin may prevent fetal loss associated with autoimmune disease. In patients with antiphospholipid antibody syndrome, treatment with low-dose aspirin may help prevent pregnancy loss.[133] Low-dose aspirin does not significantly prolong the bleeding time.[134]

ACETAMINOPHEN

There is no known teratogenic risk associated with the use of acetaminophen (Tylenol, Datril).[64] Acetaminophen does not cause permanent inhibition of prostaglandin synthesis, and it does not prolong the bleeding time. Moreover, the usual maternal doses of acetaminophen do not result in neonatal toxicity. Thus, if a mild analgesic or antipyretic is required during pregnancy, acetaminophen is preferred over aspirin.

PROPOXYPHENE

Propoxyphene (Darvon) has no known teratogenic risk, and it may be prescribed during pregnancy. Because it has the potential for addiction, this agent should not be used for trivial indications. There are case reports of neonatal opioid-withdrawal symptoms in infants whose mothers were addicted to propoxyphene.[135]

CODEINE

No higher risk of malformations was observed in the infants of 563 mothers who used codeine during pregnancy in the Collaborative Perinatal Project.[63] Excessive antepartum use of codeine can cause maternal addiction and neonatal opioid-withdrawal symptoms.

INDOMETHACIN

Indomethacin is a nonsteroidal anti-inflammatory drug (NSAID) used in the treatment of disorders such as rheumatoid arthritis, ankylosing spondylitis, and osteoarthritis as well as in the treatment of preterm labor. Unlike aspirin, which causes an irreversible inhibition of the cyclooxygenase enzyme necessary for prostaglandin synthesis, indomethacin results in a competitive and reversible inhibition of this enzyme.

Oral administration of indomethacin may lead to intrauterine constriction of the ductus arteriosus, an effect that increases with advancing gestational age.[136] Its use for longer than 48 hours may cause oligohydramnios. No increased risk of teratogenicity has been reported with first-trimester use of this agent.[64]

OTHER NONSTEROIDAL ANTI-INFLAMMATORY DRUGS

No evidence of teratogenicity has been reported for other NSAIDs, including **ibuprofen** (Motrin, Advil), and **naproxen**[38] (Naprosyn), but limited information is available. Long-term use of these agents may lead to oligohydramnios. Also, constriction of the fetal ductus arteriosus or neonatal pulmonary hypertension may occur.

Caffeine

No evidence suggests that caffeine has any teratogenic effect in humans. A national registry study from Finland evaluated more than 700 malformations, including those of the CNS, cleft lip/palate, skeletal malformations, and congenital heart defects.[137] The investigators found no association with coffee consumption. Two large U.S. studies also found no relationship between coffee intake and congenital malformations.[138,139] Similarly, a Canadian study of 80,319 pregnancies found no increase in malformations related to coffee intake.[140]

Early uncontrolled studies suggested that heavy ingestion of caffeine was associated with an increased incidence of spontaneous abortion, low birth weight, preterm delivery, and stillbirth. However, these studies did not control for the use of tobacco and alcohol. In a subsequent study that did control for smoking, other habits, demographic characteristics, and medical history,[141] no relationship was found between heavy coffee consumption and low birth weight or preterm delivery. The retrospective data regarding caffeine and spontaneous abortion have not been widely accepted because of study bias.[141] Martin and Bracken[142] suggested that an increased incidence of growth-restricted term infants may occur in women who consume more than 300 mg of caffeine daily during pregnancy. One study indicated that the ingestion of caffeine might increase the risk of an early spontaneous abortion among nonsmoking women carrying fetuses with a normal karyotype.[143] Ingestion of at least 300 mg per day was required to increase the risk. Concomitant caffeine consumption and cigarette smoking may increase the risk of intrauterine growth restriction.[143] Maternal caffeine intake reduces iron absorption and may increase the risk of anemia.[144]

DRUG USE DURING LACTATION

Many drugs can be detected in breast milk at low concentrations that usually are not of clinical significance for the infant. The rate of drug transfer into breast milk depends on the lipid solubility, molecular weight, degree of ionization of the drug, level of protein binding, and presence or absence of active secretion. Nonionized molecules of small molecular weight (e.g., ethanol) are readily transferred into breast milk.

The amount of a drug that is detected in breast milk is a variable fraction of the maternal blood level, which is proportional to the oral maternal dose. The resulting dose usually is subtherapeutic for the infant. The average fetal dose is 1% to 2% of the maternal dose. Usually, this amount is so trivial that no adverse effects are noted. However, physicians and patients should be aware of the following disclaimers. First, in the case of toxic drugs, any exposure may be inappropriate. Second, the infant may be allergic to a drug consumed by the mother. Third, there may be unknown, long-term effects of even small doses of drugs. Fourth, if an increased dose of drug or decreased maternal renal function causes a high maternal blood concentration, a higher concentration of drug may be detected in breast milk. Finally, infants have immature enzyme systems and metabolic pathways, and some drugs are eliminated more slowly. The benefits of breast-feeding are well known, and the risk of drug exposure must be weighed against these benefits.

Lactation is not fully established during the first several days postpartum. The newborn infant receives only a small volume of colostrum, and little drug is excreted through milk at this time. Thus it is unlikely that analgesics or other drugs administered after vaginal or cesarean delivery adversely affect the newborn infant.

When a mother requires a daily dose of a drug during lactation, the minimum effective dose should be used. In general, medications should be taken after breast-feeding, and long-acting preparations should be avoided. If the infant nurses less frequently overnight, ingestion of a nighttime drug dose after nursing will decrease the infant's exposure.

The American Academy of Pediatrics (AAP)[145] has reviewed the use of drugs during lactation and has categorized the drugs as follows.

Cytotoxic Drugs that May Interfere with Cellular Metabolism of the Nursing Infant

Cytotoxic agents (e.g., cyclophosphamide, cyclosporine, doxorubicin, methotrexate) used for cancer chemotherapy may cause immunosuppression in the infant, although data on this issue are limited. There may also be an association with carcinogenesis. The potential risks of these drugs probably outweigh the benefits of continuing nursing.[145]

After oral administration to a lactating patient with choriocarcinoma, methotrexate was found in breast milk in low but detectable levels. Most mothers would elect to avoid any infant exposure to this drug, but in environments in which bottle-feeding is rarely practiced and presents practical and cultural difficulties, therapy with this drug would not appear to constitute a contraindication to breast-feeding.[146]

Drugs of Abuse for which Adverse Effects on the Breast-Feeding Infant Have Been Reported

Drugs of abuse such as **amphetamines, cocaine, heroin, marijuana,** and **phencyclidine** are all contraindicated during breast-feeding because they are hazardous to the nursing infant and to the health of the mother.[145]

Radioactive Compounds that Require Temporary Cessation of Breast-Feeding

If a breast-feeding woman must undergo a study or therapy using a radioactive compound, the AAP[145] suggests that consultation with a nuclear medicine physician take place so that the radionuclide with the shortest excretion time in breast milk can be used. The mother can attempt to store breast milk prior to the study. She should continue to pump her breasts to maintain milk production, but she should discard the milk produced during therapy. Radiopharmaceuticals require variable intervals of interruption of nursing to ensure that no radioactivity is detectable in the milk. Recommended intervals are as follows:

Gallium citrate (Ga 67): 2 weeks
Iodine 131 (^{131}I): 2 to 14 days
Radioactive sodium: 4 days
Technetium (Tc 99m): 15 hours to 3 days

The physician may reassure the patient by measuring the radioactivity of the milk before breast-feeding is resumed.

Drugs for which the Effects on Nursing Infants Are Unknown but May Be of Concern

The effects of the maternal administration of a large number of drugs on nursing infants are not known but may pose problems. This category comprises several classes of psychotropic drugs, **amiodarone** (which might affect the infant's thyroid function), **lamotrigine** (due to the potential for therapeutic plasma concentrations in the infant), **metoclopramide** (due to its antagonism of dopaminergic receptors, although no detrimental effects have been reported), and **metronidazole**.

PSYCHOTROPIC DRUGS

Psychotropic agents (e.g., antianxiety, antidepressant, and neuroleptic drugs) may be of concern when administered to nursing mothers. Maternal ingestion of these drugs results in milk-to-plasma concentration ratios of about 0.5. Many of these medications often have long half-lives, and the effect of even small doses on the developing nervous system is not known. If one of these agents must be used in a lactating woman, a relatively short-acting agent with inactive metabolites, such as oxazepam, lorazepam, orazepam, alprazolam, or midazolam, is recommended.[147] The infant should be monitored for sedation during maternal drug use, and for withdrawal symptoms after the medication is stopped or after discontinuation of breast-feeding.[148]

METRONIDAZOLE

During maternal metronidazole therapy, a single dose is preferred, and the mother may interrupt nursing for 12 to 24 hours to allow time for drug elimination.

Drugs that Have Been Associated with Significant Effects on Some Nursing Infants and Should Be Administered to Nursing Mothers with Caution

ATENOLOL

Atenolol has been associated with neonatal cyanosis and bradycardia.[145]

BROMOCRIPTINE

Bromocriptine is an ergot alkaloid derivative. It has an inhibitory effect on lactation. Bromocriptine is no longer approved for postpartum lactation suppression because of its association with puerperal seizures, stroke, and myocardial infarction.

ERGOTAMINE

Ergotamine, as used by breast-feeding mothers with migraine headache, has been associated with vomiting, diarrhea, and convulsions in infants. Therefore, ergotamine should be avoided during lactation. However, administration of an ergot alkaloid for the treatment of uterine atony does not contraindicate lactation.

LITHIUM

Breast milk levels of lithium are one third to one half maternal serum levels,[149,150] and infant serum levels during breast-feeding are much lower than fetal serum levels that occur when the mother takes lithium during pregnancy. The benefits of breast-feeding must be weighed against the theoretical effects of small amounts of the drug on the developing brain.

Maternal Medications Usually Compatible with Breast-Feeding

ANALGESICS, OPIOIDS, SEDATIVES, AND ANTICONVULSANTS

There is little transfer of **salicylates** into breast milk because these acids exist primarily in the ionized form. Following single oral doses, peak milk levels occur at approximately 3 hours with milk-to-plasma concentration ratios between 0.03 and 0.05.[151] Maternal ingestion of *high doses* (e.g., more than 16 tablets per day) may result in maternal and breast milk concentrations sufficiently high to affect platelet aggregation in the infant. The reduced clearance of salicylates by neonates may lead to drug accumulation and toxic effects, even when repeated exposures are small.[152] Because of these concerns, the World Health Organization (WHO) Working Group on Human Lactation has classified the salicylates as unsafe for use by nursing women.[153] The AAP Committee on Drugs[145] has stated that **aspirin** is "associated with significant effects on some nursing infants and should be administered to nursing mothers with caution," on the basis of a case report of a neonate in whom metabolic acidosis developed.[145]

No harmful effects of acetaminophen or the classic NSAIDs (e.g., indomethacin, ibuprofen) have been noted. The breast milk concentration of propoxyphene was half that of the maternal serum level in one patient who took propoxyphene in a suicide attempt.[154] Theoretically, a breast-feeding infant could receive up to 1 mg of propoxyphene per day if the mother were to consume the maximum dose.

In the past it was thought that opioid analgesics, sedatives, and anticonvulsants used by nursing mothers were highly unlikely to have adverse effects on breast-fed infants. Normal maternal doses of codeine, morphine, meperidine, carbamazepine, phenytoin, valproic acid, and magnesium sulfate do not have obvious adverse effects on most nursing infants.[7,145] The dose detectable in breast milk is approximately 1% to 2% of the mother's dose and is unlikely to have significant pharmacologic activity. In 2006, a full-term, 13-day-old infant died of an apparent morphine overdose. The mother was taking a modest dose of **codeine** for episiotomy pain. It was discovered that the mother was heterozygous for a CYP2D6*2A allele with CYP2D6*2×2 gene duplication, making her an ultra-rapid metabolizer of codeine. This condition resulted in a breast milk morphine concentration of 87 ng/mL, compared with the typical range of 1.9 to 20.5 ng/mL that would have been expected.[155] This case prompted the FDA[156] to release a Public Health Advisory advising caution in the use of codeine-containing medications by breast-feeding women. The FDA recommended that the lowest effective dose for the shortest necessary duration should be used, and that women should be taught how to recognize signs of high morphine levels in their infants. The number of ultra-rapid metabolizers is estimated to vary between 1 and 28 per 100 people.[156] Among analgesic drugs, ultra-rapid metabolism has been reported as a problem only with codeine, although the FDA[156] suggested that "it has the potential to affect other narcotics."

Studies have detected only small amounts of phenytoin, phenobarbital, and diazepam in breast milk.[157,158] However, infants eliminate phenobarbital and diazepam slowly, so these agents may accumulate. Women taking a barbiturate or a benzodiazepine should observe their infants for evidence of sedation and withdrawal.[8,145]

Cruikshank et al.[159] measured breast milk magnesium concentrations in 10 preeclamptic women who were receiving magnesium sulfate 1 g/hr intravenously for 24 hours after delivery. The mean breast milk magnesium concentration was 6.4 ± 0.4 mg/dL, compared with 4.8 ± 0.5 mg/dL in controls. Breast milk calcium concentrations were not affected by magnesium sulfate therapy.

ANTIBIOTICS AND OTHER ANTIMICROBIAL AGENTS

Penicillin and its derivatives are safe in nursing mothers. With the usual therapeutic doses of ampicillin, the milk-to-plasma concentration ratio is 0.2 or less, and no adverse effects are noted in nursing infants.[160] Theoretically, infant diarrhea or candidiasis might occur with prolonged therapy.

Dicloxacillin is 98% protein bound.[160] If this drug is used to treat a breast infection, very little drug is transferred into the breast milk, and nursing may continue.

Cephalosporins appear in trace amounts in breast milk. In one study, maternal administration of cefazolin (500 mg intramuscularly three times a day) resulted in nondetectable breast milk concentrations of drug.[161] Intravenous injection of 2 g of cefazolin resulted in a milk-to-plasma concentration ratio of 0.023; thus the infants were exposed to only 0.075% of the maternal dose.[161]

Tooth staining and delayed bone growth have not been reported in offspring after ingestion of tetracycline from a breast-feeding mother. The breast milk concentration of tetracycline is about half the maternal plasma concentration. However, tetracycline has a high affinity for both calcium and protein. Thus the amount of free tetracycline available for systemic absorption is too small to be clinically significant.

Sulfonamides displace bilirubin from binding sites on albumin, so these drugs are best avoided during the first 5 days of life or in mothers of preterm infants with hyperbilirubinemia. Otherwise, sulfonamides are not contraindicated during nursing. Sulfonamides appear in breast milk in small amounts. One study of sulfapyridine noted that the infant receives less than 1% of the maternal dose.[162] In another study, sulfasalazine was not detected in the breast milk of a mother taking this drug.[163] Sulfasalazine should be used with caution in a breast-feeding woman because it has been associated with a case of bloody diarrhea in an infant.[145]

Maternal administration of acyclovir does not contraindicate breast-feeding. If a mother takes 1 g/day, the infant probably receives less than 1 mg/day, a very low dose.[164] There are no reported adverse effects on infants of isoniazid administered to nursing mothers, and its use is considered compatible with breast-feeding.[145]

Other specific agents listed as compatible with breast-feeding include amoxicillin, aztreonam, ciprofloxacin, clindamycin, erythromycin, fluconazole, gentamicin, ketoconazole, nitrofurantoin, ofloxacin, rifampin, and ticarcillin.

ANTIHISTAMINES AND PHENOTHIAZINES

No harmful effects have been noted with maternal use of antihistamines or phenothiazines.[165] These drugs do not appear to affect the milk supply. However, women who are having trouble with their milk supply should avoid decongestants (i.e., vasoconstrictive agents).

THEOPHYLLINE AND OTHER ANTIASTHMATIC DRUGS

Maximum milk concentrations of theophylline are achieved between 1 and 3 hours after an oral dose. It has been calculated that the nursing infant receives less than 1% of the maternal dose. Such exposure appears to have no adverse effects.[145] Other asthma medications considered compatible with breast-feeding include terbutaline and metoprolol.[145]

ANTIHYPERTENSIVE DRUGS

One study detected no chlorothiazide in breast milk after a single 500-mg oral dose.[166] Miller et al.[167] reported a case in which daily ingestion of 50 mg of hydrochlorothiazide caused peak milk concentrations that were approximately 25% of maternal blood concentrations. These investigators did not detect any drug in the infant's serum, and the infant's electrolyte levels were normal.

A single 40-mg dose of propranolol results in breast milk drug concentrations that are less than 40% of peak maternal plasma concentrations.[168] In one study, a 30-day regimen of propranolol (240 mg/day) resulted in predose and 3-hour postdose breast milk concentrations of 26 ng/mL and 64 ng/mL, respectively. Thus, at a maternal dose of 240 mg/day, an infant ingesting 500 mL of milk per day would ingest a maximum dose of approximately 1% of the therapeutic dose for an infant, which is unlikely to cause any adverse effect.[169]

Atenolol is concentrated in breast milk at approximately three times the maternal plasma concentration.[170] However, after a peak-level feeding, the infant plasma concentration is less than 10 ng/mL, which is not associated with side effects in the infant. In addition, the total infant dose is only 1% of the maternal therapeutic dose. This agent should be used with caution in breast-feeding women because of its association with neonatal cyanosis and bradycardia.[145]

Breast milk clonidine concentrations are almost twice maternal serum concentrations. However, this exposure does not seem to have any adverse effects on the infant.[171]

ANTICOAGULANTS

Most mothers who require anticoagulation may continue to nurse their infants with no problems. **Heparin** does not cross into breast milk. Moreover, heparin is not active when administered orally.

Warfarin is 98% protein bound. Orme et al.,[172] who studied seven women taking warfarin (Coumadin) 5 to 12 mg/day, detected no warfarin in breast milk or infant plasma. Similarly, de Swiet and Lewis[173] found that warfarin appears in breast milk in insignificant quantities.

CORTICOSTEROIDS

Katz and Duncan[174] obtained breast milk 2 hours after an oral dose of 10 mg of prednisone in one nursing mother. They detected breast milk concentrations of prednisone and prednisolone that would be unlikely to result in any deleterious effect on the infant. McKenzie et al.[175] administered 5 mg of radioactive prednisolone to seven patients and found that 0.14% (a negligible quantity) of the radioactive label was secreted in the milk in the subsequent 60 hours. Thus breast-feeding is not contraindicated in mothers taking corticosteroids. Even at a maternal dosage of 80 mg/day, the nursing infant would ingest a dose equivalent to less than 10% of its endogenous cortisol production.[176]

DIGOXIN

After a maternal digoxin dose of 0.25 mg, peak breast milk concentrations of 0.6 to 1.0 ng/mL occur, and the milk-to-plasma concentration ratio at the 4-hour peak is between 0.8 and 0.9. Maternal protein binding limits infant drug exposure. In 24 hours an infant might receive approximately 1% of the maternal digoxin dose,[177] and no adverse effects have been reported in nursing infants of mothers taking this drug.

ORAL CONTRACEPTIVES

Some studies have suggested that the use of an estrogen-progestin oral contraceptive is associated with reductions in quantity of breast milk, duration of lactation, infant weight gain, and nitrogen and protein content in the milk.[178] However, most published studies evaluated the effect of the 50-μg estrogen preparations. Oral contraceptives cause less inhibition of lactation if the patient delays starting contraceptive therapy until 3 weeks after delivery.[179] Progestin-only contraceptives do not alter breast milk composition or volume. No long-term adverse effects on growth and development have been described in the children of mothers taking oral contraceptives.[145,179]

PROPYLTHIOURACIL

Only small amounts of propylthiouracil are found in breast milk. One study noted no change in thyroid function (including levels of thyroid-stimulating hormone) through 5 months of age in an infant exposed to maternal propylthiouracil.[180]

H_2-RECEPTOR ANTAGONISTS

In theory, H_2-receptor antagonists (e.g., ranitidine) might suppress gastric acidity or cause CNS stimulation in the infant, but these effects have not been confirmed in published studies. The AAP considers cimetidine to be compatible with breast-feeding.[145] Famotidine, nizatidine, and roxatidine are less concentrated in breast milk and may be preferable in nursing mothers.[181]

CAFFEINE

Moderate maternal intake of caffeine does not adversely affect an infant. One study noted that breast milk contains only 1% of the total maternal dose of caffeine.[182] If a mother drinks excessive amounts of coffee, caffeine might accumulate in the infant, and the infant might show signs of caffeine stimulation (e.g., irritability, poor sleeping pattern). Nursing mothers should limit their intake to a moderate level of caffeinated beverages (e.g., 2 to 3 cups per day).[145]

KEY POINTS

- The critical period of organ development extends from approximately day 31 to day 71 after the first day of the last menstrual period.
- Administration of anticonvulsants is associated with an increased risk of congenital anomalies, but monotherapy is associated with less risk than therapy with two or more drugs.
- Isotretinoin is highly teratogenic and should not be used during pregnancy.
- Heparin does not cross the placenta and is the anticoagulant of choice during pregnancy, except for women with prosthetic heart valves, who may receive warfarin after the first trimester.
- Angiotensin-converting enzyme inhibitors should be avoided during pregnancy because they cause fetal renal dysplasia and oligohydramnios.
- Only a small amount of prednisone crosses the placenta. Therefore prednisone is the preferred corticosteroid for most maternal diseases. In contrast, betamethasone and dexamethasone readily cross the placenta and are preferred when the obstetrician wants to accelerate fetal lung maturity.

- Most antibiotics are safe during pregnancy. Tetracyclines should be avoided because they cause tooth discoloration and inhibit bone growth in the fetus. Quinolones are contraindicated during pregnancy. Trimethoprim most likely should be avoided during the first trimester.
- Analgesic doses of aspirin increase the risk of peripartum hemorrhage.
- Lithium and ergotamine are best avoided during lactation.
- Most drugs are safe for use during lactation. Typically only 1% to 2% of the maternal dose appears in breast milk.

REFERENCES

1. Yankowitz J. Use of medications in pregnancy: General principles, teratology, and current developments. In Yankowitz J, Niebyl JR, editors. Drug Therapy in Pregnancy. 3rd edition. Philadelphia, Lippincott Williams & Wilkins, 2001.
2. Niebyl JR, Simpson JL. Drugs and environmental agents in pregnancy and lactation: Embryology, teratology, epidemiology. In Gabbe SG, Niebyl JR, Simpson JL, editors. Obstetrics: Normal and Problem Pregnancies. 5th edition. Philadelphia, Churchill Livingstone, 2007.
3. Buehler BA, Delimont D, van Waes M, Finnell RH. Prenatal prediction of risk of the fetal hydantoin syndrome. N Engl J Med 1990; 322:1567-72.
4. Teratology Society Public Affairs Committee. FDA classification of drugs for teratogenic risk. Teratology 1994; 49:446-7.
5. Friedman JM. Report of the Teratology Society Public Affairs Committee symposium on FDA classification of drugs. Teratology 1993; 48:5-6.
6. Doering PL, Boothby LA, Cheok M. Review of pregnancy labeling of prescription drugs: Is the current system adequate to inform of risks? Am J Obstet Gynecol 2002; 187:333-9.
7. Malone FD, D'Alton ME. Drugs in pregnancy: Anticonvulsants. Semin Perinatol 1997; 21:114-23.
8. Morrell MJ. Guidelines for the care of women with epilepsy. Neurology 1998; 51:S21-7.
9. Holmes LB, Rosenberger PB, Harvey EA, et al. Intelligence and physical features of children of women with epilepsy. Teratology 2000; 61:196-202.
10. Holmes LB, Harvey EA, Coull BA, et al. The teratogenicity of anticonvulsant drugs. N Engl J Med 2001; 344:1132-8.
11. Morrell MJ. The new antiepileptic drugs and women: Efficacy, reproductive health, pregnancy and fetal outcome. Epilepsia 1996; 37:S34-44.
12. Cornelissen M, Steegers-Theunissen R, Kollée L, et al. Increased incidence of neonatal vitamin K deficiency resulting from maternal anticonvulsant therapy. Am J Obstet Gynecol 1993; 168:923-8.
13. Cornelissen M, Steegers-Theunissen R, Kollée L, et al. Supplementation of vitamin K in pregnant women receiving anticonvulsant therapy prevents neonatal vitamin K deficiency. Am J Obstet Gynecol 1993; 168:884-8.
14. Jones KL, Lacro RV, Johnson KA, Adams J. Pattern of malformations in the children of women treated with carbamazepine during pregnancy. N Engl J Med 1989; 320:1661-6.
15. Rosa FW. Spina bifida in infants of women treated with carbamazepine during pregnancy. N Engl J Med 1991; 324:674-7.
16. Levy RH, Yerby MS. Effects of pregnancy on antiepileptic drug utilization. Epilepsia 1985; 26:S52-7.
17. Tennis P, Eldridge RR; International Lamotrigine Pregnancy Registry Scientific Advisory Committee. Preliminary results on pregnancy outcomes in women using lamotrigine. Epilepsia 2002; 43:1161-7.
18. Vajda FJ, Hitchcock A, Graham J, et al. Foetal malformations and seizure control: 52 months data of the Australian Pregnancy Registry. Eur J Neurol 2006; 13:645-54.
19. Shor S, Koren G, Nulman I. Teratogenicity of lamotrigine. Can Fam Physician 2007; 53:1007-9.
20. Kälviäinen R, Tomson T. Optimizing treatment of epilepsy during pregnancy. Neurology 2006; 67:S59-63.
21. Lammer EJ, Chen DT, Hoar RM, et al. Retinoic acid embryopathy. N Engl J Med 1985; 313:837-41.
22. Adams J. High incidence of intellectual deficits in 5-year-old children exposed to isotretinoin "in utero". Teratology 1990; 41:614.
23. Cheetham TC, Wagner RA, Chiu G, et al. A risk management program aimed at preventing fetal exposure to isotretinoin: Retrospective cohort study. J Am Acad Dermatol 2006; 55:442-8.
24. Garcia-Bournissen F, Tsur L, Goldstein LH, et al. Fetal exposure to isotretinoin—an international problem. Reprod Toxicol 2008; 25:124-8.
25. Milkovich L, van den Berg BJ. Effects of prenatal meprobamate and chlordiazepoxide hydrochloride on human embryonic and fetal development. N Engl J Med 1974; 291:1268-71.
26. Hartz SC, Heinonen OP, Shapiro S, et al. Antenatal exposure to meprobamate and chlordiazepoxide in relation to malformations, mental development, and childhood mortality. N Engl J Med 1975; 292:726-8.
27. Kjaer D, Horvath-Puhó E, Christensen J, et al. Use of phenytoin, phenobarbital, or diazepam during pregnancy and risk of congenital abnormalities: A case-time-control study. Pharmacoepidemiol Drug Saf 2007; 16:181-8.
28. Rosenberg L, Mitchell AA, Parsells JL, et al. Lack of relation of oral clefts to diazepam use during pregnancy. N Engl J Med 1983; 309:1282-5.
29. Ornoy A, Arnon J, Shechtman S, et al. Is benzodiazepine use during pregnancy really teratogenic? Reprod Toxicol 1998; 12:511-5.
30. Gillberg C. "Floppy infant syndrome" and maternal diazepam. Lancet 1977; 2(8031):244.
31. Linden S, Rich CL. The use of lithium during pregnancy and lactation. J Clin Psychiatry 1983; 44:358-61.
32. Källén B, Tandberg A. Lithium and pregnancy: A cohort study on manic-depressive women. Acta Psychiatr Scand 1983; 68:134-9.
33. Jacobson SJ, Jones K, Johnson K, et al. Prospective multicentre study of pregnancy outcome after lithium exposure during first trimester. Lancet 1992; 339:530-3.
34. Krause S, Ebbesen F, Lange AP. Polyhydramnios with maternal lithium treatment. Obstet Gynecol 1990; 75:504-6.
35. Ang MS, Thorp JA, Parisi VM. Maternal lithium therapy and polyhydramnios. Obstet Gynecol 1990; 76:517-9.
36. Schou M, Amdisen A, Streenstrup OR. Lithium and pregnancy. II. Hazards to women given lithium during pregnancy and delivery. Br Med J 1973; 2:137-8.
37. Altshuler LL, Cohen L, Szuba MP, et al. Pharmacologic management of psychiatric illness during pregnancy: Dilemmas and guidelines. Am J Psychiatry 1996; 153:592-606.
38. Briggs GG, Freeman RK, Yaffe SJ. Drugs in Pregnancy and Lactation. 7th edition. Philadelphia, Lippincott Williams & Wilkins, 2005.
39. Goldstein DJ, Corbin LA, Sundell KL. Effects of first-trimester fluoxetine exposure on the newborn. Obstet Gynecol 1997; 89:713-8.
40. Nulman I, Rovet J, Stewart DE, et al. Child development following exposure to tricyclic antidepressants or fluoxetine throughout fetal life: A prospective, controlled study. Am J Psychiatry 2002; 159:1889-95.
41. Hendrick V, Smith LM, Suri R, et al. Birth outcomes after prenatal exposure to antidepressant medication. Am J Obstet Gynecol 2003; 188:812-5.
42. Louik C, Lin AE, Werler MM, et al. First-trimester use of selective serotonin-reuptake inhibitors and the risk of birth defects. N Engl J Med 2007; 356:2675-83.
43. Alwan S, Reefhuis J, Rasmussen SA, et al. Use of selective serotonin-reuptake inhibitors in pregnancy and the risk of birth defects. N Engl J Med 2007; 356:2684-92.

44. Chambers CD, Johnson KA, Dick LM, et al. Birth outcomes in pregnant women taking fluoxetine. N Engl J Med 1996; 335:1010-5.
45. Chambers CD, Hernández-Diáz S, Van Marter LJ, et al. Selective serotonin-reuptake inhibitors and risk of persistent pulmonary hypertension of the newborn. N Engl J Med 2006; 354:579-87.
46. American College of Obstetricians and Gynecologists. Use of psychiatric medications during pregnancy and lactation. ACOG Practice Bulletin No. 87, November 2007. (Obstet Gynecol. 2007; 110:1179-98.)
47. Hall JG, Pauli RM, Wilson KM. Maternal and fetal sequelae of anticoagulation during pregnancy. Am J Med 1980; 68:122-40.
48. Jones KL, Smith DW. Smith's Recognizable Patterns of Human Malformation. 5th edition. Philadelphia, WB Saunders, 1997.
49. Vitale N, De Feo M, De Santo LS, et al. Dose-dependent fetal complications of warfarin in pregnant women with mechanical heart valves. J Am Coll Cardiol 1999; 33:1637-41.
50. Dahlman T, Lindvall N, Hellgren M. Osteopenia in pregnancy during long-term heparin treatment: A radiological study post partum. Br J Obstet Gynaecol 1990; 97:221-8.
51. American College of Obstetricians and Gynecologists. Thromboembolism in pregnancy. ACOG Practice Bulletin No. 19. Washington, DC, ACOG, August 2000.
52. Bates SM, Greer IA, Hirsh J, Ginsberg JS. Use of antithrombotic agents during pregnancy. The Seventh ACCP Conference on Antithrombotic and Thrombolytic Therapy. Chest 2004; 126:627S-44S.
53. Frewin R, Chisholm M. Anticoagulation of women with prosthetic heart valves during pregnancy. Br J Obstet Gynaecol 1998; 105:683-6.
54. Iturbe-Alessio I, Fonseca MC, Mutchinik O, et al. Risks of anticoagulant therapy in pregnant women with artificial heart valves. N Engl J Med 1986; 315:1390-3.
55. Chan WS, Anand S, Ginsberg JS. Anticoagulation of pregnant women with mechanical heart valves: A systematic review of the literature. Arch Intern Med 2000; 160:191-6.
56. Wing DA, Millar LK, Koonings PP, et al. A comparison of propylthiouracil versus methimazole in the treatment of hyperthyroidism in pregnancy. Am J Obstet Gynecol 1994; 170:90-5.
57. Martin-Denavit T, Edery P, Plauchu H, et al. Ectodermal abnormalities associated with methimazole intrauterine exposure. Am J Med Genet 2000; 94:338-40.
58. Vogt T, Stolz W, Landthaler M. Aplasia cutis congenita after exposure to methimazole: A causal relationship? Br J Dermatol 1995; 133:994-6.
59. Di Gianantonio E, Schaefer C, Mastroiacovo PP, et al. Adverse effects of prenatal methimazole exposure. Teratology 2001; 64:262-6.
60. Burrow GN. Thyroid diseases. In Burrow GN, Duffy TP, editors. Medical Complications during Pregnancy. Philadelphia, WB Saunders, 1999:135-61.
61. Alexander EK, Marqusee E, Lawrence J, et al. Timing and magnitude of increases in levothyroxine requirements during pregnancy in women with hypothyroidism. N Engl J Med 2004; 351:241-9.
62. Haddow JE, Palomaki GE, Allan WC, et al. Maternal thyroid deficiency during pregnancy and subsequent neuropsychological development of the child. N Engl J Med 1999; 341:549-55.
63. Heinonen OP, Slone D, Shapiro S. Birth Defects and Drugs in Pregnancy. Littleton, MA, Publishing Sciences Group, 1977:441.
64. Aselton P, Jick H, Milunsky A, et al. First-trimester drug use and congenital disorders. Obstet Gynecol 1985; 65:451-5.
65. Pruyn SC, Phelan JP, Buchanan GC. Long-term propranolol therapy in pregnancy: Maternal and fetal outcome. Am J Obstet Gynecol 1979; 135:485-9.
66. Redmond GP. Propranolol and fetal growth retardation. Semin Perinatol 1982; 6:142-7.
67. Magee LA, Bull SB, Koren G, Logan A. The generalizability of trial data; a comparison of β-blocker trial participants with a prospective cohort of women taking β-blockers in pregnancy. Eur J Obstet Gynecol Reprod Biol 2001; 94:205-10.
68. Lydakis C, Lip GY, Beevers M, Beevers DG. Atenolol and fetal growth in pregnancies complicated by hypertension. Am J Hypertens 1999; 12:541-7.
69. Easterling TR, Carr DB, Brateng D, et al. Treatment of hypertension in pregnancy: Effect of atenolol on maternal disease, preterm delivery, and fetal growth. Obstet Gynecol 2001; 98:427-33.
70. Easterling TR, Brateng D, Schmucker B, et al. Prevention of preeclampsia: A randomized trial of atenolol in hyperdynamic patients before onset of hypertension. Obstet Gynecol 1999; 93:725-33.
71. Pickles CJ, Symonds EM, Broughton Pipkin F. The fetal outcome in a randomized double-blind controlled trial of labetalol versus placebo in pregnancy-induced hypertension. Br J Obstet Gynaecol 1989; 96:38-43.
72. Burrows RF, Burrows EA. Assessing the teratogenic potential of angiotensin-converting enzyme inhibitors in pregnancy. Aust N Z J Obstet Gynaecol 1998; 38:306-11.
73. Cooper WO, Hernández-Diáz S, Arbogast PG, et al. Major congenital malformations after first-trimester exposure to ACE inhibitors. N Engl J Med 2006; 354:2443-51.
74. Ray JG, Vermeulen MJ, Koren G. Taking ACE inhibitors during early pregnancy: Is it safe? Can Fam Physician 2007; 53:1439-40.
75. Piper JM, Ray WA, Rosa FW. Pregnancy outcome following exposure to angiotensin-converting enzyme inhibitors. Obstet Gynecol 1992; 80:429-32.
76. Oei SG, Oei SK, Brölmann HA. Myocardial infarction during nifedipine therapy for preterm labor (letter). N Engl J Med 1999; 340:154.
77. Magee LA, Schick B, Donnenfeld AE, et al. The safety of calcium channel blockers in human pregnancy: A prospective, multicenter cohort study. Am J Obstet Gynecol 1996; 174:823-8.
78. Tan HL, Lie KI. Treatment of tachyarrhythmias during pregnancy and lactation. Eur Heart J 2001; 22:458-64.
79. Bartalena L, Bogazzi F, Braverman LE, Martino E. Effects of amiodarone administration during pregnancy on neonatal thyroid function and subsequent neurodevelopment. J Endocrinol Invest 2001; 24:116-30.
80. Källén B. The teratogenicity of antirheumatic drugs—what is the evidence? Scand J Rheumatol Suppl 1998; 107:119-24.
81. Polifka JE, Friedman JM. Teratogen update: Azathioprine and 6-mercaptopurine. Teratology 2002; 65:240-61.
82. Armenti VT, Moritz MJ, Davison JM. Drug safety issues in pregnancy following transplantation and immunosuppression: Effects and outcomes. Drug Saf 1998; 19:219-32.
83. Kirshon B, Wasserstrum N, Willis R, et al. Teratogenic effects of first-trimester cyclophosphamide therapy. Obstet Gynecol 1988; 72:462-4.
84. Wolfe MS, Cordero JF. Safety of chloroquine in chemosuppression of malaria during pregnancy. Br Med J (Clin Res Ed) 1985; 290:1466-7.
85. Hart CW, Naunton RF. The ototoxicity of chloroquine phosphate. Arch Otolaryngol 1964; 80:407-12.
86. Heinonen OP, Slone D, Shapiro S. Birth Defects and Drugs in Pregnancy. Littleton, MA, Publishing Sciences Group, 1977:367-70.
87. Rosa F. Databases in the assessment of the effect of drugs during pregnancy. J Allergy Clin Immunol 1999 Feb; 103:S360-1.
88. Park-Wyllie L, Mazzotta P, Pastuszak A, et al. Birth defects after maternal exposure to corticosteroids: Prospective cohort study and meta-analysis of epidemiological studies. Teratology 2000; 62:385-92.
89. Carmichael SL, Shaw GM. Maternal corticosteroid use and risk of selected congenital anomalies. Am J Med Genet 1999; 86:242-4.
90. Bakhireva LN, Jones KL, Schatz M, et al. Safety of leukotriene receptor antagonists in pregnancy. J Allergy Clin Immunol 2007; 119:618-25.
91. Sahakian V, Rouse D, Sipes S, et al. Vitamin B_6 is effective therapy for nausea and vomiting of pregnancy: A randomized, double-blind placebo-controlled study. Obstet Gynecol 1991; 78:33-6.
92. Vutyavanich T, Wongtrangan S, Ruangsri R. Pyridoxine for nausea and vomiting of pregnancy: A randomized, double-blind, placebo-controlled trial. Am J Obstet Gynecol 1995; 173:881-4.
93. American College of Obstetricians and Gynecologists. Nausea and vomiting of pregnancy. ACOG Practice Bulletin No. 52. Washington, DC, ACOG, April 2004.
94. Vutyavanich T, Kraisarin T, Ruangsri R. Ginger for nausea and vomiting in pregnancy: Randomized, double-masked, placebo-controlled trial. Obstet Gynecol 2001; 97:577-82.
95. Fischer-Rasmussen W, Kjaer SK, Dahl C, Asping U. Ginger treatment of hyperemesis gravidarum. Eur J Obstet Gynecol Reprod Biol 1991; 38:19-24.
96. Milkovich L, van den Berg BJ. An evaluation of the teratogenicity of certain antinauseant drugs. Am J Obstet Gynecol 1976; 125:244-8.

97. Heinonen OP, Slone D, Shapiro S. Birth Defects and Drugs in Pregnancy. Littleton, MA, Publishing Sciences Group, 1977:324.
98. Sørensen HT, Nielsen GL, Christensen K, et al. Birth outcome following maternal use of metoclopramide. Br J Clin Pharmacol 2000; 49:264-8.
99. Berkovitch M, Mazzota P, Greenberg R, et al. Metoclopramide for nausea and vomiting of pregnancy: A prospective multicenter international study. Am J Perinatol 2002; 19:311-6.
100. Sullivan CA, Johnson CA, Roach H, et al. A pilot study of intravenous ondansetron for hyperemesis gravidarum. Am J Obstet Gynecol 1996; 174:1565-8.
101. Einarson A, Maltepe C, Navioz Y, et al. The safety of ondansetron for nausea and vomiting of pregnancy: A prospective comparative study. Br J Obstet Gynaecol 2004; 111:940-3.
102. Werler MM. Teratogen update: Pseudoephedrine. Birth Defects Res A Clin Mol Teratol 2006; 76:445-52.
103. Seto A, Einarson T, Koren G. Evaluation of brompheniramine safety in pregnancy. Reprod Toxicol 1993; 7:393-5.
104. Schatz M, Zeiger RS, Harden K, et al. The safety of asthma and allergy medications during pregnancy. J Allergy Clin Immunol 1997; 100:301-6.
105. Pastuszak A, Schick B, D'Alimonte D, et al. The safety of astemizole in pregnancy. J Allergy Clin Immunol 1996; 98:748-50.
106. Einarson A, Bailey B, Jung G, et al. Prospective controlled study of hydroxyzine and cetirizine in pregnancy. Ann Allergy Asthma Immunol 1997; 78:183-6.
107. Paulus W, Schloemp S, Sterzik K, Stoz F. Pregnancy outcome after exposure to cetirizine/levocetirizine in the first trimester—a prospective controlled study. Reprod Toxicol 2004; 19:239-60.
108. Seto A, Einarson T, Koren G. Pregnancy outcome following first trimester exposure to antihistamines: Meta-analysis. Am J Perinatol 1997; 14:119-24.
109. Czeizel AE, Rockenbauer M, Sørensen HT, Olsen J. Use of cephalosporins during pregnancy and in the presence of congenital abnormalities: A population-based, case-control study. Am J Obstet Gynecol 2001; 184:1289-96.
110. Czeizel AE, Rockenbauer M, Sørensen HT, Olsen J. A population-based case-control teratologic study of oral erythromycin treatment during pregnancy. Reprod Toxicol 1999; 13:531-6.
111. Källén BA, Otterblad Olausson P, Danielsson BR. Is erythromycin therapy teratogenic in humans? Reprod Toxicol 2005; 20:209-14.
112. Järnerot G, Into-Malmberg MB, Esbjörner E. Placental transfer of sulphasalazine and sulphapyridine and some of its metabolites. Scand J Gastroenterol 1981; 16:693-7.
113. Hernández-Díaz S, Werler MM, Walker AM, Mitchell AA. Folic acid antagonists during pregnancy and the risk of birth defects. N Engl J Med 2000; 343:1608-14.
114. Czeizel AE, Rockenbauer M. Teratogenic study of doxycycline. Obstet Gynecol 1997; 89:524-8.
115. Tötterman LE, Saxén L. Incorporation of tetracycline into human foetal bones after maternal drug administration. Acta Obstet Gynecol Scand 1969; 48:542-9.
116. Robinson GC, Cambon KG. Hearing loss in infants of tuberculous mothers treated with streptomycin during pregnancy. N Engl J Med 1964; 271:949-51.
117. Mitra AG, Whitten MK, Laurent SL, Anderson WE. A randomized, prospective study comparing once-daily gentamicin versus thrice-daily gentamicin in the treatment of puerperal infection. Am J Obstet Gynecol 1997; 177:786-92.
118. Kirkwood A, Harris C, Timar N, Koren G. Is gentamicin ototoxic to the fetus? J Obstet Gynaecol Can 2007; 29:140-5.
119. Berkovitch M, Pastuszak A, Gazarian M, et al. Safety of the new quinolones in pregnancy. Obstet Gynecol 1994; 84:535-8.
120. Diav-Citrin O, Shechtman S, Gotteiner T, et al. Pregnancy outcome after gestational exposure to metronidazole: A prospective controlled cohort study. Teratology 2001; 63:186-92.
121. Burtin P, Taddio A, Ariburnu O, et al. Safety of metronidazole in pregnancy: A meta-analysis. Am J Obstet Gynecol 1995; 172:525-9.
122. Andrews EB, Yankaskas BC, Cordero JF, et al. Acyclovir in pregnancy registry: Six years' experience. The Acyclovir in Pregnancy Registry Advisory Committee. Obstet Gynecol 1992; 79:7-13.
123. Culnane M, Fowler M, Lee SS, et al. Lack of long-term effects of in utero exposure to zidovudine among uninfected children born to HIV-infected women. Pediatric AIDS Clinical Trials Group Protocol 219/076 Teams. JAMA 1999; 281:151-7.
124. McGowan JP, Crane M, Wiznia AA, Blum S. Combination antiretroviral therapy in human immunodeficiency virus-infected pregnant women. Obstet Gynecol 1999; 94:641-6.
125. The Antiretroviral Pregnancy Registry. The Antiretroviral Pregnancy Registry Interim Report. Kendle International, Inc. December, 2007. Available at http://www.apregistry.com/forms/interim_report.pdf/
126. Watts DH. Management of human immunodeficiency virus infection in pregnancy. N Engl J Med 2002; 346:1879-91.
127. Rosa F. Amantadine pregnancy experience (letter). Reprod Toxicol 1994; 8:531.
128. Bridges CB, Winquist AG, Fukuda K, et al. Prevention and control of influenza: Recommendations of the Advisory Committee on Immunization Practices (ACIP). MMWR Recomm Rep 2000; 49:1-38.
129. Fiore AE, Shay DK, Haber P, et al. Prevention and control of influenza: Recommendations of the Advisory Committee on Immunization Practices (ACIP). MMWR Recomm Rep 2007; 56:1-54.
130. Kozer E, Nikfar S, Costei A, et al. Aspirin consumption during the first trimester of pregnancy and congenital anomalies: A meta-analysis. Am J Obstet Gynecol 2002; 187:1623-30.
131. Stuart MJ, Gross SJ, Elrad H, Graeber JE. Effects of acetylsalicylic-acid ingestion on maternal and neonatal hemostasis. N Engl J Med 1982; 307:909-12.
132. Arcilla RA, Thilenius OG, Ranniger K. Congestive heart failure from suspected ductal closure in utero. J Pediatr 1969; 75:74-8.
133. Farquharson RG, Quenby S, Greaves M. Antiphospholipid syndrome in pregnancy: A randomized, controlled trial of treatment. Obstet Gynecol 2002; 100:408-13.
134. Williams HD, Howard R, O'Donnell N, Findley I. The effect of low dose aspirin on bleeding times. Anaesthesia 1993; 48:331-3.
135. Tyson HK. Neonatal withdrawal symptoms associated with maternal use of propoxyphene hydrochloride (Darvon). J Pediatr 1974; 85:684-5.
136. Moise KJ Jr. Effect of advancing gestational age on the frequency of fetal ductal constriction in association with maternal indomethacin use. Am J Obstet Gynecol 1993; 168:1350-3.
137. Kurppa K, Holmberg PC, Kuosma E, Saxén L. Coffee consumption during pregnancy and selected congenital malformations: A nationwide case-control study. Am J Public Health 1983; 73:1397-9.
138. Rosenberg L, Mitchell AA, Shapiro S, Slone D. Selected birth defects in relation to caffeine-containing beverages. JAMA 1982; 247:1429-32.
139. Linn S, Schoenbaum SC, Monson RR, et al. No association between coffee consumption and adverse outcomes of pregnancy. N Engl J Med 1982; 306:141-5.
140. McDonald AD, Armstrong BG, Sloan M. Cigarette, alcohol, and coffee consumption and congenital defects. Am J Public Health 1992; 82:91-3.
141. Infante-Rivard C, Fernández A, Gauthier R, et al. Fetal loss associated with caffeine intake before and during pregnancy. JAMA 1993; 270:2940-3.
142. Martin TR, Bracken MB. The association between low birth weight and caffeine consumption during pregnancy. Am J Epidemiol 1987; 126:813-21.
143. Beaulac-Baillargeon L, Desrosiers C. Caffeine-cigarette interaction on fetal growth. Am J Obstet Gynecol 1987; 157:1236-40.
144. Muñoz LM, Lönnerdal B, Keen CL, Dewey KG. Coffee consumption as a factor in iron deficiency anemia among pregnant women and their infants in Costa Rica. Am J Clin Nutr 1988; 48:645-51.
145. American Academy of Pediatrics Committee on Drugs. Transfer of drugs and other chemicals into human milk. Pediatrics 2001; 108:776-89.
146. Johns DG, Rutherford CD, Leighton PC, Vogel CL. Secretion of methotrexate into human milk. Am J Obstet Gynecol 1972; 112:978-80.

147. Chisholm CA, Kuller JA. A guide to the safety of CNS-active agents during breastfeeding. Drug Saf 1997; 17:127-42.
148. Allaire AD, Kuller JA. Psychotropic drugs in pregnancy and lactation. In Yankowitz J, Niebyl JR, eds. Drug Therapy in Pregnancy. 3rd edition. Philadelphia, Lippincott Williams & Wilkins, 2001.
149. Sykes PA, Quarrie J, Alexander FW. Lithium carbonate and breast-feeding. Br Med J 1976; 2:1299.
150. Schou M, Amdisen A. Lithium and pregnancy. III. Lithium ingestion by children breast-fed by women in lithium treatment. Br Med J 1973; 2:138.
151. Findlay JWA, DeAngelis RL, Kearney MF, et al. Analgesic drugs in breast milk and plasma. Clin Pharmacol Ther 1981; 29:625-33.
152. McNamara PJ, Burgio D, Yoo SD. Pharmacokinetics of acetaminophen, antipyrine, and salicylic acid in the lactating and nursing rabbit, with model predictions of milk to serum concentration ratios and neonatal dose. Toxicol Appl Pharmacol 1991; 109:149-60.
153. Bennet PN, editor. Drugs and Human Lactation: A Guide to the Content and Consequences of Drugs, Micronutrients, Radiopharmaceuticals, and Environmental and Occupational Chemicals in Human Milk. The WHO Working Group. New York, Elsevier, 1988:335-40.
154. Catz CS, Giacoia GP. Drugs and breast milk. Pediatr Clin North Am 1972; 19:151-66.
155. Koren G, Cairns J, Chitayat D, et al. Pharmacogenetics of morphine poisoning in a breastfed neonate of a codeine-prescribed mother. Lancet 2006; 368:704.
156. U.S. Food and Drug Administration, Center for Drug Evaluation and Research. FDA Public Health Advisory: Use of Codeine by Some Breastfeeding Mothers May Lead To Life-Threatening Side Effects in Nursing Babies. August 17, 2007. Available at http://www.fda.gov/cder/drug/advisory/codeine.htm/
157. Cole AP, Hailey DM. Diazepam and active metabolite in breast milk and their transfer to the neonate. Arch Dis Child 1975; 50:741-2.
158. Nau H, Rating D, Häuser I, et al. Placental transfer and pharmacokinetics of primidone and its metabolites phenobarbital, PEMA and hydroxyphenobarbital in neonates and infants of epileptic mothers. Eur J Clin Pharmacol 1980; 18:31-42.
159. Cruikshank DP, Varner MW, Pitkin RM. Breast milk magnesium and calcium concentrations following magnesium sulfate treatment. Am J Obstet Gynecol 1982; 143:685-8.
160. Wilson JT, Brown RD, Cherek DR, et al. Drug excretion in human breast milk: Principles, pharmacokinetics and projected consequences. Clin Pharmacokinet 1980; 5:1-66.
161. Yoshioka H, Cho K, Takimoto M, et al. Transfer of cefazolin into human milk. J Pediatr 1979; 94:151-2.
162. Berlin CM Jr, Yaffe SJ. Disposition of salicylazosulfapyridine (Azulfidine) and metabolites in human breast milk. Dev Pharmacol Ther 1980; 1:31-9.
163. Järnerot G, Into-Malmberg MB. Sulphasalazine treatment during breast feeding. Scand J Gastroenterol 1979; 14:869-71.
164. Meyer LJ, de Miranda P, Sheth N, Spruance S. Acyclovir in human breast milk. Am J Obstet Gynecol 1988; 158:586-8.
165. Lione A, Scialli AR. The developmental toxicity of the H_1 histamine antagonists. Reprod Toxicol 1996; 10:247-55.
166. Werthmann MW Jr, Krees SV. Excretion of chlorothiazide in human breast milk. J Pediatr 1972; 81:781-3.
167. Miller ME, Cohn RD, Burghart PH. Hydrochlorothiazide disposition in a mother and her breast-fed infant. J Pediatr 1982; 101:789-91.
168. Bauer JH, Pape B, Zajicek J, Groshong T. Propranolol in human plasma and breast milk. Am J Cardiol 1979; 43:860-2.
169. Anderson PO, Salter FJ. Propranolol therapy during pregnancy and lactation. Am J Cardiol 1976; 37:325.
170. White WB, Andreoli JW, Wong SH, Cohn RD. Atenolol in human plasma and breast milk. Obstet Gynecol 1984; 63:42S-4S.
171. Hartikainen-Sorri AL, Heikkinen JE, Koivisto M. Pharmacokinetics of clonidine during pregnancy and nursing. Obstet Gynecol 1987; 69:598-600.
172. Orme ME, Lewis PJ, de Swiet M, et al. May mothers given warfarin breast-feed their infants? Br Med J 1977; 1:1564-5.
173. de Swiet M, Lewis PJ. Excretion of anticoagulants in human milk. N Engl J Med 1977; 297:1471.
174. Katz FH, Duncan BR. Entry of prednisone into human milk. N Engl J Med 1975; 293:1154.
175. McKenzie SA, Seeley JA, Agnew JE. Secretion of prednisolone into breast milk. Arch Dis Child 1975; 50:894-6.
176. Ost L, Wettrell G, Björkhem I, Rane A. Prednisolone excretion in human milk. J Pediatr 1985; 106:1008-11.
177. Loughnan PM. Digoxin excretion in human breast milk. J Pediatr 1978; 92:1019-20.
178. Lönnerdal B, Forsum E, Hambraeus L. Effect of oral contraceptives on consumption and volume of breast milk. Am J Clin Nutr 1980; 33:816-24.
179. American Academy of Pediatrics Committee on Drugs. Breast-feeding and contraception. Pediatrics 1981; 68:138-40.
180. Kampmann JP, Johansen K, Hansen JM, Helweg J. Propylthiouracil in human milk: Revision of a dogma. Lancet 1980; 1(8171):736-7.
181. Anderson PO. Drug use during breast-feeding. Clin Pharm 1991; 10:594-624.
182. Berlin CM Jr, Denson HM, Daniel CH, Ward RM. Disposition of dietary caffeine in milk, saliva, and plasma of lactating women. Pediatrics 1984; 73:59-63.

Chapter 15

In Vitro Fertilization and Other Assisted Reproductive Technology

Lawrence C. Tsen, M.D.
Robert D. Vincent, Jr., M.D.

In 1978, Steptoe and Edwards[1] reported the first live birth of a baby produced from *in vitro* fertilization (IVF) techniques. Their case highlighted the laparoscopic recovery of a single oocyte just prior to ovulation in a natural menstrual cycle; after *in vitro* insemination, the resulting embryo was grown in culture media for 2.5 days to the eight-cell stage and was transferred to the uterine cavity (embryo transfer [ET]).

IVF techniques were initially developed as a treatment for infertility secondary to chronic tubal disease. Current indications for this emerging spectrum of new techniques, which as a group are referred to as assisted reproductive technology (ART), include (1) inadequate oocyte quality or number (donor oocyte therapy), irreparability or absence of the uterus (surrogate uterus programs), and significant co-morbidities (embryo cryopreservation) in women; (2) sperm deficiencies in men; and (3) certain genetic aberrations in couples.[2]

In 1981, Edwards[3] estimated that 15 to 20 babies would be born worldwide through the use of IVF and ET techniques. Advances in the science and international acceptance of ART procedures have resulted in a dramatic rise in the number of babies born; worldwide in the year 2000, an estimated 197,000 to 220,000 babies were born as a result of these techniques (Figure 15-1).[4] In the United States alone, the use of these cycles has also increased significantly (Figure 15-2); in 2005, the initiation of 134,260 ART cycles resulted in the birth of 52,041 neonates.[5]

Despite the application of ART procedures to more diverse and challenging etiologies of infertility, the probability of a live birth after a cycle of hormonal stimulation has increased from 6% in 1985 to 29% in 2005.[5] Attention to subtle differences in culture media as well as improvements in laboratory methods, retrieval routes, and transfer techniques are responsible for most of these better results.[6] Given the level of scrutiny and the rising costs (with limited insurance coverage) associated with ART (approximately $10,000 for each cycle that progresses to transfer),[7] it is prudent for anesthesia providers to be aware of the potential effects that anesthetic agents may have on gametes or embryos.

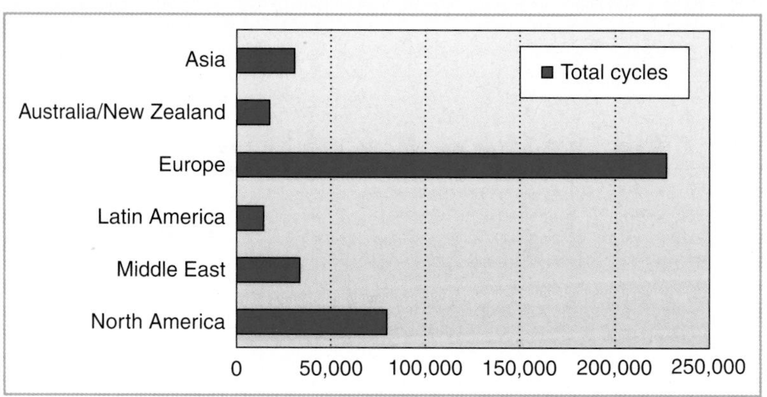

FIGURE 15-1 World figures for assisted reproductive technology performed by country for the year 2000. (Data from International Committee for Monitoring Assisted Reproductive Technology; Adamson GD, de Mouzon J, Lancaster P, Nygren KG, Sullivan E, Zegers-Hochschild. World collaborative report on *in vitro* fertilization, 2000. Fertil Steril 2006; 85:1586-622.)

ASSISTED REPRODUCTIVE TECHNOLOGY PROCEDURES

Hormonal Stimulation

Although the success of IVF was initially limited by the *single* preovulatory oocyte generated with each natural menstrual cycle,[1] the introduction of follicular hormonal stimulation has significantly increased the probability of a live birth through the retrieval of *multiple* oocytes per cycle. Hormonal regimens typically initiate a cycle with gonadotropin-releasing hormone agonist (GnRH-a) to induce pituitary and ovarian suppression, followed by follicle-stimulating hormone (FSH) and human menopausal gonadotropin (hMG) to encourage the development and growth of multiple ovarian follicles. Human chorionic gonadotropin (hCG) is later added to induce maturation and demargination of the oocyte from the follicular wall prior to retrieval. Although the goal of these regimens is the generation of 10 to 15 oocytes, superovulation can occur, resulting in the production of as many as 70 oocytes. All visible ovarian follicles are aspirated (see later), with each follicle usually containing a single oocyte.

Following oocyte retrieval, pituitary function is usually insufficient to provide adequate hormonal support to the growing corpus luteum. For this reason, parenteral progesterone is often provided daily until either the results of the pregnancy test are known or the first trimester of pregnancy is completed.

Oocyte Retrieval

Originally conducted with direct visualization of the ovarian follicles through pelvic laparoscopy,[1] the majority of oocyte retrievals are currently performed through a transvaginal approach with ultrasonographic guidance (Figure 15-3).[8] Laparoscopic oocyte retrieval is typically reserved for situations in which immediate tubal transfer is planned (i.e., gamete intrafallopian transfer [GIFT], zygote intrafallopian transfer [ZIFT]; see later).

Oocyte retrieval is performed approximately 34 to 36 hours after hCG administration. Retrieval must be performed promptly to prevent spontaneous ovulation from reducing the number of mature oocytes. With the use of a transvaginal ultrasound probe to visualize the ovary, mature follicles are punctured and aspirated with a needle introduced through the vaginal fornix. Oocytes are immediately washed in culture media and examined microscopically to determine their stage of meiosis. Oocytes are classified as postmature metaphase II, mature metaphase II, metaphase I, or prophase I on the basis of their nuclear, cytoplasmic, and extracellular composition.

In Vitro Fertilization

Although the term *in vitro fertilization* is often used synonymously with any aspect of ART, technically it applies only to the process of oocyte fertilization with spermatozoa in culture media. Following a microscopic examination,

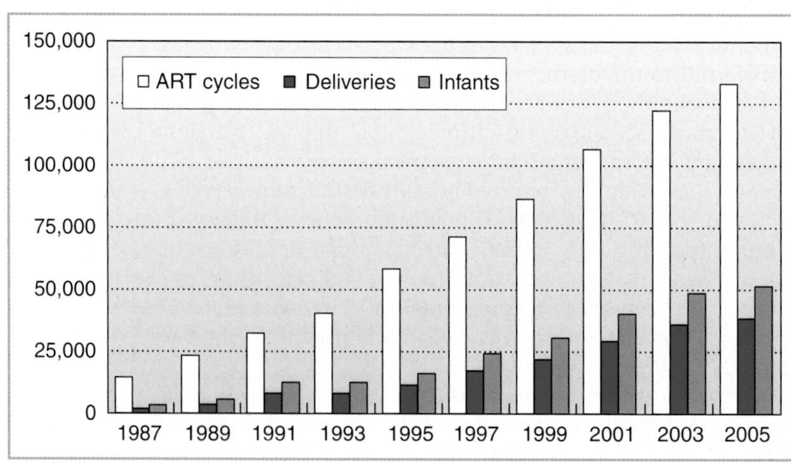

FIGURE 15-2 Numbers of assisted reproductive technology (ART) cycles performed, live-birth deliveries, and infants born using ART from 1987 through 2005, as reported to the Centers for Disease Control and Prevention, Division of Reproductive Health, and the Society for Assisted Reproductive Technology Registry. (Data from U.S. Department of Health and Human Services, Centers for Disease Control and Prevention, Division of Reproductive Health. 2005 Assisted Reproductive Technology [ART] Report. Atlanta, CDC/DRH, 2007.)

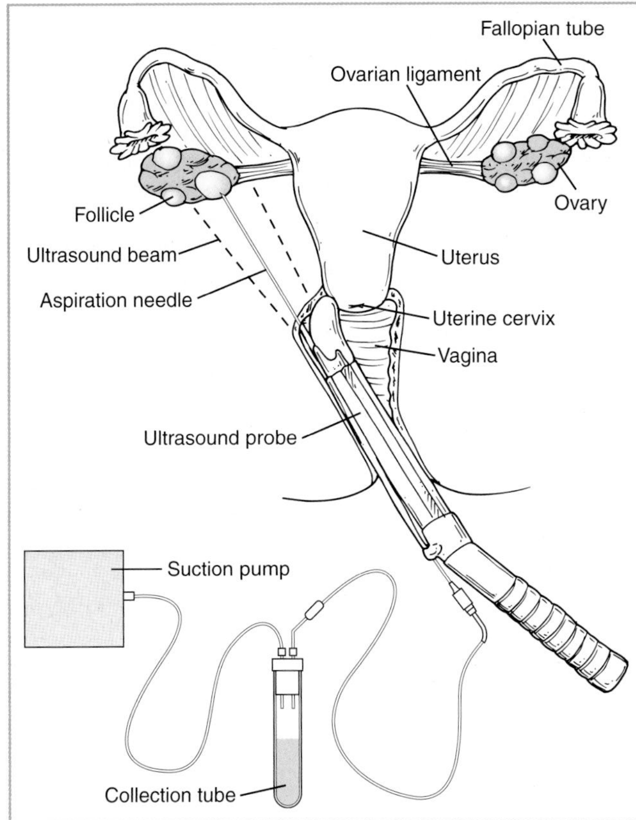

FIGURE 15-3 Transvaginal ultrasound-guided oocyte retrieval. The ultrasound probe is placed in the vagina and advanced into the posterior fornix. The needle, previously inserted through the needle guide, is advanced through the vaginal wall and ovarian capsule. (Redrawn from Steinbrook R. Egg donation and human embryonic stem-cell research. N Engl J Med 2006; 354:324-6. Copyright © 2006 Massachusetts Medical Society. All rights reserved.)

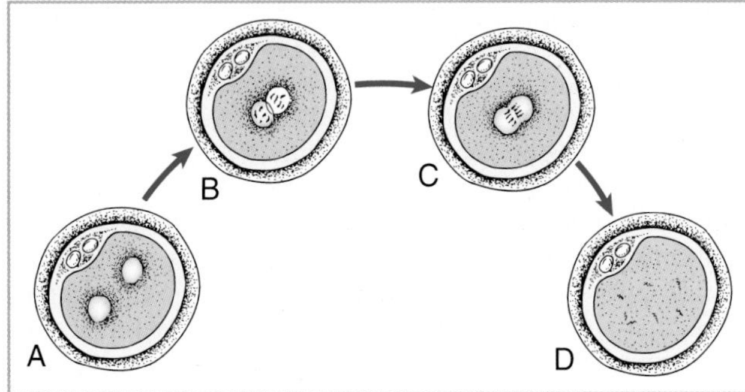

FIGURE 15-4 Pronuclear stage prezygote. **A,** At 8 to 10 hours after insemination, pronuclei are barely visible and may be spaced slightly apart. **B,** After 12 hours, pronuclei have migrated to the center of the cell and are clearly seen. **C,** At 20 to 22 hours, nuclear envelopes break down and pronuclei begin to fade from view. **D,** The one-cell zygote before the first cleavage. (Redrawn from Veeck LL. Atlas of the Human Oocyte and Early Conceptus. Baltimore, Williams & Wilkins, 1991:43.)

oocytes are incubated for approximately 4 to 6 hours in culture media that resembles human tubal fluid, and are then inseminated. The insemination process is sometimes delayed with immature oocytes (e.g., metaphase I) in an attempt to increase the probability of normal (i.e., monospermic) fertilization.

Approximately 16 to 20 hours after insemination, the oocytes are examined for evidence of fertilization (i.e., the presence of two pronuclei and two polar bodies in the perivitelline space) (Figure 15-4).[9] The advantages of IVF include the ability to document the process of fertilization and to use techniques to improve sperm motility or penetration (e.g., intracytoplasmic sperm injection). IVF followed by embryo transfer represents approximately 99% of the ART procedures used in the United States[5]; less than 1% occur via GIFT or ZIFT procedures (see later). Male factor infertility is present in approximately 35% of the couples seeking ART procedures, and intracytoplasmic sperm injection is currently used in more than 60% of the cases treated annually in the United States.[5]

Embryo Transfer

Embryos resulting from IVF may be transferred into the fallopian tubes (i.e., ZIFT) or the uterine cavity (IVF-ET). Most ET procedures are performed transcervically 3 to 5 days after retrieval, with the embryos transferred via a catheter. The advantages of transcervical ET are (1) simplicity—it does not require laparoscopy or anesthesia; (2) low cost, especially compared with laparoscopic intrafallopian transfer procedures; and (3) the ability to proceed without patent fallopian tube(s). The primary disadvantage of transcervical ET is that the probability of successful pregnancy is slightly less than that with an ET performed directly into the fallopian tubes (i.e., ZIFT). Embryos in excess of those required for transfer may be frozen in 1,2-propanediol or glycerol and stored for possible later transfer.

Gamete Intrafallopian Transfer

GIFT procedures consist of the transabdominal or transvaginal collection of oocytes followed by a microscopic inspection of the oocytes' quality and maturation in a laboratory adjacent to the operating room. Mature oocytes are aspirated into a transfer catheter with washed partner or donor sperm, and the contents (gametes) are injected into the distal 3 to 6 cm of one or both fallopian tubes. The catheter is subsequently inspected microscopically to verify that oocytes have not been retained. The GIFT procedure does not involve IVF, because fertilization occurs *in vivo* in the natural milieu of the fallopian tube.

Specific advantages of the GIFT procedure include (1) the convenience of oocyte retrieval and embryo transfer occurring within a single operative event; (2) the elimination of IVF; and (3) the fact that the embryos reach the uterine cavity at a potentially more appropriate (i.e., later) stage of development than with IVF-ET.[10] The primary disadvantage is that fertilization cannot be documented, an issue that may be critical when this capacity is in question (e.g., couples with male or immunologic factors). Normally, 50% to 70% of inseminated oocytes become fertilized[11]; however, lower fertilization rates are often observed in couples with severe male factor infertility or in women with antisperm antibodies. Other limitations are the required presence of at least one patent fallopian tube and the requirement for laparoscopic surgery.

Zygote Intrafallopian Transfer

ZIFT (also known as pronuclear stage transfer [PROST]) consists of oocyte retrieval followed by IVF. Approximately 16 to 20 hours after insemination, the oocytes are examined for the presence of two distinct pronuclei (i.e., the pronuclear stage; see Figure 15-4), which indicates that fertilization has occurred. The patient is anesthetized for laparoscopy, and pronuclear stage embryos (usually no more than four) are transferred through a catheter into the distal portion of a fallopian tube (as described for GIFT). Advantages of ZIFT include (1) the documentation of fertilization, (2) the avoidance of laparoscopy if fertilization is not successful (approximately 13% of inseminations),[5] (3) a shorter exposure to the laboratory environment than with IVF-ET, and (4) the potential for embryos to reach the uterine cavity at a more appropriate stage of development than with IVF-ET (i.e., approximately the fifth day after insemination). Its disadvantages and limitations include (1) the added inconvenience and cost of a two-stage procedure, (2) the requirement for laparoscopic surgery, and (3) the required presence of at least one patent fallopian tube.

SUCCESS OF ASSISTED REPRODUCTIVE TECHNOLOGY

The Society for Assisted Reproductive Technology (SART) and the American Society for Reproductive Medicine (ASRM) collaborate with the Centers for Disease Control and Prevention (CDC) to maintain a data registry and analyze the results of all ART cycles initiated during each calendar year in the United States.[5]

Maternal age is the dominant factor in determining the likelihood of a successful pregnancy after an ART procedure (Figure 15-5). For example, in 2005, 43.6% of IVF procedures without intracytoplasmic sperm injection in women younger than 35 years (in couples with no male factor infertility issues) led to the delivery of one or more infants.[5] By contrast, in a similar group of women older than 42 years who met optimal fertility criteria, only 5.4% of these procedures resulted in a live birth.

Although pregnancy and delivery rates have historically been higher for tubal transfers (i.e., GIFT, ZIFT) than for transcervical uterine transfers (IVF-ET), greater parity in these rates has developed in recent years.[5,11] The early postovulatory uterine environment has been postulated to be unfavorable to early embryo growth.[11] Tubal transfer procedures allow embryos 3 to 5 days to reach the uterine cavity, when the environment for implantation may be more receptive. Lower implantation rates after transcervical ET may also be explained by (1) adverse uterine effects produced by the transfer procedure, (2) uterine contractions expelling transfer fluid and embryos,[12] and (3) the absence of yet undiscovered tubal factors that promote early embryo growth and implantation.[11,13]

OBSTETRIC COMPLICATIONS

ART hormonal stimulation regimens are associated with increased coagulation and decreased fibrinolysis when evaluated by individual hemostatic markers and global assessment tools (i.e., thromboelastography).[14,15] These alterations are especially significant in the setting of the most common ovarian stimulation complication, a phenomenon termed *ovarian hyperstimulation syndrome* (OHSS). Mild cases of OHSS may manifest as abdominal discomfort, bilateral ovarian enlargement, and ascites, whereas severe cases may result in follicular rupture and hemorrhage, pleural effusion, hemoconcentration, oliguria, and thromboembolic events.[16-18] The anesthetic implications of OHSS include increased free drug concentrations (see later) and greater perioperative pain from higher follicle numbers. The fullest expression of the syndrome usually occurs after oocyte retrieval, particularly if the decision is made to proceed with an embryo transfer, which maintains exposure to endogenous and exogenous hormones. Rarely, an emergency laparoscopy or laparotomy is required for excision of a ruptured ovarian cyst or the release of an ovarian pedicle torsion.[18] Abdominal paracentesis and thoracentesis may be necessary before the induction of general anesthesia in patients with respiratory compromise due to massive ascites or pleural effusions.

Multiple-gestation pregnancies represented 32% of the deliveries that followed ART procedures in the United States in 2005.[5] Among these deliveries, 94% were twins and the remainder were a higher order. Transferring a higher number of embryos or oocytes increases both the

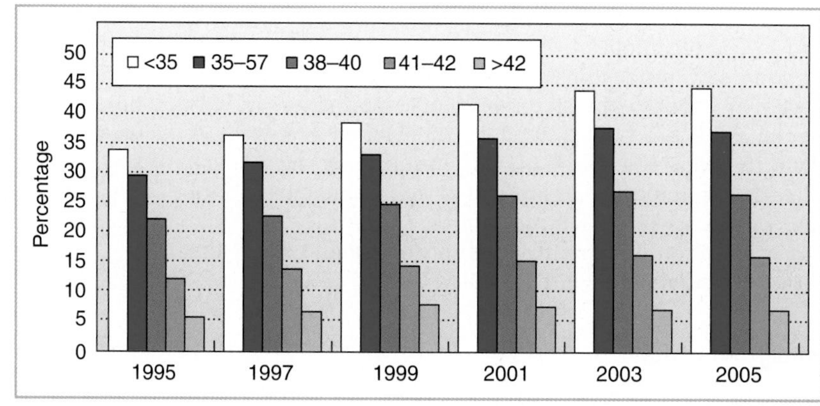

FIGURE 15-5 Percentage of transfers that resulted in live births with assisted reproductive technology (ART) cycles using fresh nondonor eggs or embryos, according to the women's age in the years from 1995 to 2005, as reported to the Centers for Disease Control and Prevention, Division of Reproductive Health, and the Society for Assisted Reproductive Technology Registry. (Data from U.S. Department of Health and Human Services, Centers for Disease Control and Prevention, Division of Reproductive Health. 2005 Assisted Reproductive Technology (ART) Report. Atlanta, CDC/DRH, 2007.)

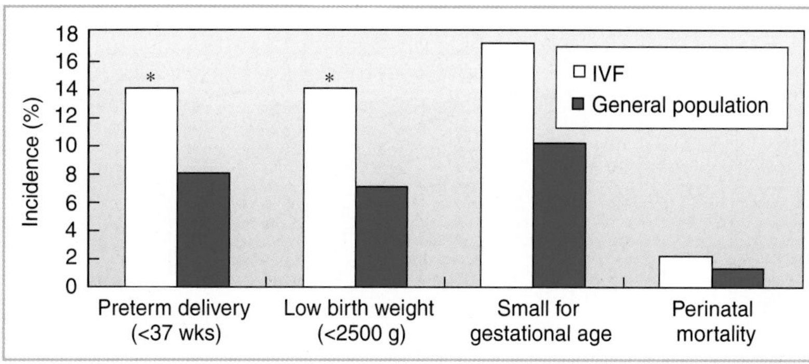

FIGURE 15-6 Outcomes associated with singleton *in vitro* fertilization (IVF) births compared with spontaneous pregnancies in the general population. *$P < .05$. (Modified from Cetin I, Cozzi V, Antonazzo P. Fetal development after assisted reproduction: A review. Placenta 2003; 24:S104-13.)

probability of a live birth and the likelihood of a multifetal pregnancy. Although many infertile couples consider a twin or triplet pregnancy preferable to a singleton pregnancy, maternal and perinatal morbidity and mortality for multiple-gestation pregnancies is at least double that for singleton-gestation pregnancies.[19] Further, overall medical costs escalate with each additional fetus. In 1997, Hidlebaugh et al.[20] observed mean obstetric and neonatal charges of approximately $9000, $20,000, and $153,000 for singleton, twin, and triplet deliveries, respectively, after IVF-ET. In an effort to reduce the incidence and sequelae of multifetal pregnancies, many ART programs and societies, and even some countries, have mandated a limit on the number of embryos or oocytes transferred.[21] Selective reductions of a triplet or higher-order gestation can be performed; however, some patients and physicians have moral and ethical objections to this option, despite the risk of high-order multifetal pregnancies.

Ectopic pregnancies occur more often with ART pregnancies than with natural pregnancies, primarily owing to the higher prevalence of tubal disease among infertility patients.[22] The transfer site (uterine versus tubal) per se does not appear to be a predisposing factor in the development of ectopic pregnancies; however, a greater number occur after uterine transfer, because women with bilateral tubal disease are not candidates for GIFT or ZIFT procedures. In approximately 10% of ectopic pregnancy cases, the ectopic embryo develops in conjunction with an ongoing intrauterine pregnancy and requires a termination or surgical removal within the first trimester.[22]

Preterm delivery, low birth-weight (LBW), and small-for-gestational-age (SGA) babies are more common with IVF pregnancies than with natural pregnancies.[23] This phenomenon persists even when the analysis is restricted to singleton gestations (Figure 15-6). The difference appears to be a result of infertility per se rather than the IVF procedures, because previously infertile women who conceive independent of IVF also are at greater risk for preterm delivery.[23]

EFFECTS OF ANESTHESIA ON REPRODUCTION

General Considerations

In 1987 Boyers et al.[24] reported that oocytes recovered by laparoscopic techniques in patients who had received general anesthesia (i.e., isoflurane or enflurane with 50% nitrous oxide and 50% oxygen) were less likely to be fertilized if the duration of the procedure was prolonged. Specifically, fertilization rates for the first- and last-recovered oocytes were 69% and 54%, respectively, when the difference in exposure time exceeded 5 minutes. The investigators advanced the following two plausible explanations for this difference: (1) the acidification of follicular fluid by intraperitoneal carbon dioxide and (2) the effects of anesthesia. This study prompted an assessment of anesthetic agents and techniques used during ART procedures.

Ideally, anesthetic techniques and agents used for ART procedures should not interfere with oocyte fertilization or early embryo development and implantation. Although anesthetic agents have been reported to interfere with some aspects of reproductive physiology in some species under certain conditions, the literature must be interpreted with caution. For example, one study concluded that oocyte cleavage rates were significantly lower with general anesthesia than with epidural anesthesia.[25] However, a laparoscopic (instead of transvaginal) retrieval method was utilized in the general anesthesia group, and carbon dioxide pneumoperitoneum may significantly decrease both follicular fluid pH and oocyte fertilization rates. Another report commented on the effects of different anesthetic techniques, but it did not disclose the actual anesthetic agents that were administered in the study.[26] In addition, conclusions based on animal data may not reflect the human experience owing to interspecies and assay method differences.[27]

Assessment of specific anesthetic drugs must also be interpreted in context; relevant factors include (1) the method of administration, (2) dose of anesthetic agents, (3) combination with other drugs, (4) timing of administration, and (5) duration of exposure. For example, local anesthetic agents yield dissimilar pharmacokinetic profiles when administered via paracervical, epidural, and intrathecal techniques. Anesthetic agents may also affect unfertilized oocytes and fertilized embryos differently; thus, studies of anesthetic agents used for a GIFT (prefertilization) procedure should not be directly compared with studies of agents used for a ZIFT (postfertilization) procedure. Finally, significantly higher free concentrations of certain agents (e.g., bupivacaine) exist during ART stimulation because of a decrease in plasma protein binding capacity.[28] Thus, when selecting anesthetic techniques or agents for an ART procedure, the clinician should weigh their known benefits (e.g., greater hemodynamic stability, less nausea, less psychomotor impairment) and hypothetical risks (e.g., lower delivery rates).

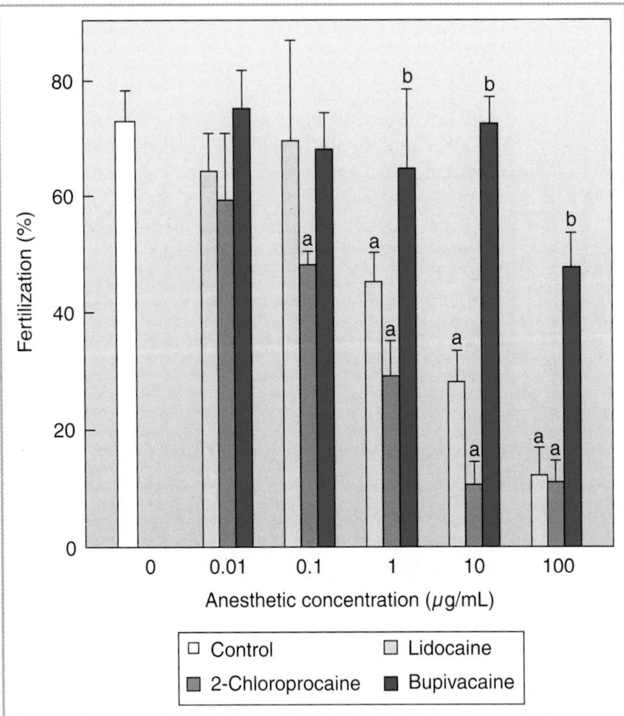

FIGURE 15-7 Fertilization of mouse oocytes at 48 hours (mean ± SD) for each anesthetic exposure group. a, *P* < .05 (anesthetics compared with control); b, *P* < .05 (lidocaine and 2-chloroprocaine compared with bupivacaine). (Modified from Schnell VL, Sacco AG, Savoy-Moore RT, et al. Effects of oocyte exposure to local anesthetics on *in vitro* fertilization and embryo development in th mouse. Reprod Toxicol 1992; 6:323-7, with kind permission from Elsevier Science, Ltd, Langford Lane, Kidlington OX51GB, UK.)

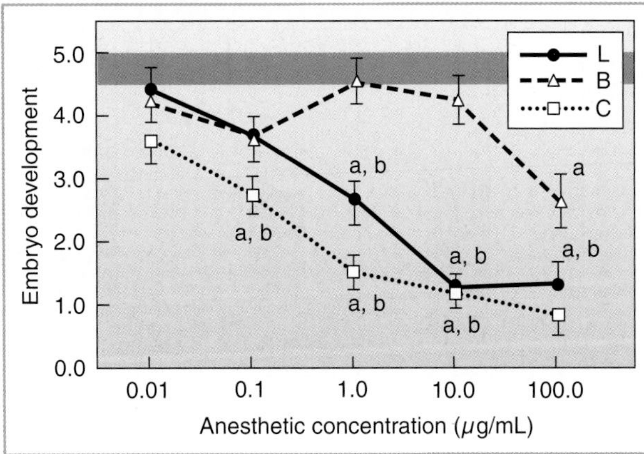

FIGURE 15-8 Embryo development scores (mean ± SD) at 72 hours as a function of anesthetic concentration. *Shaded area* represents embryo development score (4.75 ± 0.28) for the control mouse embryos. a, *P* < .01 (lidocaine [L], bupivacaine [B], and 2-chloroprocaine [C] compared with control); b, *P* < .01 (bupivacaine compared with lidocaine and 2-chloroprocaine). (Modified from Schnell VL, Sacco AG, Savoy-Moore RT, et al. Effects of oocyte exposure to local anesthetics on *in vitro* fertilization and embryo development in the mouse. Reprod Toxicol 1992; 6:323-7.)

Local Anesthetic Agents

In animal models, the effect of local anesthetic agents on reproductive physiology appears to be related to the agent, timing, and dose of exposure. Using mouse oocytes incubated for 30 minutes in culture media with known concentrations of lidocaine, bupivacaine, or 2-chloroprocaine, Schnell et al.[29] demonstrated that lidocaine and 2-chloroprocaine adversely affected both fertilization and embryo development at concentrations of 1.0 and 0.1 μg/mL, respectively (Figures 15-7 and 15-8). In contrast, bupivacaine produced adverse effects only at the highest concentration studied (100 μg/mL). Similarly, Del Valle et al.[30] demonstrated that after 48 hours of culture, 24% of mouse embryos exposed to lidocaine 10 μg/mL, in comparison with none in the control group, showed evidence of degeneration. Finally, Ahuja et al.[31] noted that hamster oocytes exposed to procaine or tetracaine demonstrated impaired zona reactions, potentially allowing additional sperm to enter the oocyte and create abnormal chromosomal numbers (polyploidy).

These *in vitro* findings may have limited clinical relevance, however, given the significantly lower anesthetic concentrations that occur in clinical practice and the washing and screening procedures that oocytes undergo prior to fertilization and transfer. Human trial data corroborate the minimal effect that local anesthetic agents have on oocytes or embryos during oocyte retrieval, GIFT, or ZIFT procedures. Wikland et al.[32] reported that the incidence of oocyte fertilization and clinical pregnancy was not reduced among women who received a modified paracervical block with lidocaine for transvaginal oocyte retrieval (Figure 15-9). Favorable pregnancy rates have also been reported after GIFT procedures performed during epidural lidocaine anesthesia.[25]

Opioids, Benzodiazepines, and Ketamine

Fentanyl, alfentanil, remifentanil, and meperidine do not appear to interfere with either fertilization or preimplantation embryo development in animal and human trials.[33,34] When given during oocyte retrieval, fentanyl and alfentanil were detected in extremely low (or nondectable) follicular fluid concentrations[35]; with alfentanil, a 10:1 ratio between serum and follicular fluid was observed 15 minutes after the initial bolus dose.[36] Morphine appears unique in terms of adverse effects; when sea urchin eggs were incubated in morphine (equivalent to a human dose of 50 mg), more than one sperm entered approximately 30% of the ooctyes.[37]

Midazolam administered systemically in preovulatory mice did not impair fertilization or embryo development *in vivo* or *in vitro*, even when given in doses up to 500 times those used clinically.[38] When used in small bolus or infusion doses for anxiolysis and sedation for ART in humans, midazolam has not been detected in follicular fluid and does not appear to be teratogenic.[39,40]

Ketamine 0.75 mg/kg, administered with midazolam 0.06 mg/kg, has been reported to be an acceptable alternative to general anesthesia with isoflurane.[41] Although the report was from a study with inadequate power, no differences in reproductive outcomes were observed.

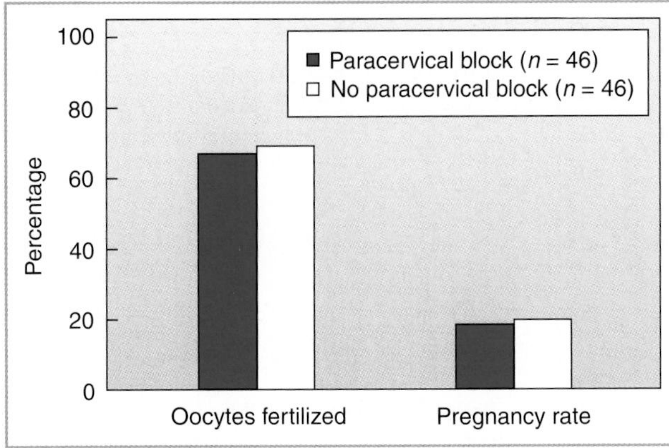

FIGURE 15-9 Fertilization and pregnancy rates after transvaginal oocyte retrieval with and without lidocaine paracervical block. Fertilization and cleavage rates did not differ in the two groups. (Modified from Wikland M, Evers H, Jakobsson AH, et al. The concentration of lidocaine in follicular fluid when used for paracervical block in a human IVF-ET programme. Hum Reprod 1990; 5:920-3.)

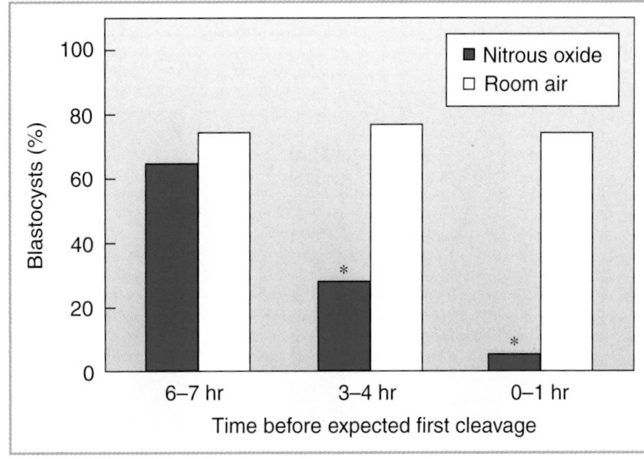

FIGURE 15-10 Developmental outcome of two-cell mouse embryos exposed to 60% nitrous oxide/40% oxygen for 30 minutes *in vitro*. Administration of nitrous oxide within 4 hours of anticipated cleavage decreased the percentage of embryos reaching the blastocyst stage. $^{*}P < .05$ compared with the room air (i.e., control) group. (Modified from Warren JR, Shaw B, Steinkampf MP. Effects of nitrous oxide on preimplantation mouse embryo cleavage and development. Biol Reprod 1990; 43:158-61.)

Propofol and Thiopental

The effect of propofol on reproductive outcomes is controversial; however, most animal and human trials suggest minimal effects on fertilization and early embryo development.[42-46] Although pharmacokinetic and pharmacodynamic studies have demonstrated a dose- and duration-dependent accumulation of propofol in the follicular fluid,[47,48] the threshold at which oocyte fertilization or early embryo development becomes impaired is unclear. Studies that correlate follicular fluid concentrations with reproductive outcome measures have observed no detrimental effects.[48,49] General anesthesia provided with propofol and a 50% oxygen-air mixture was associated with fertilization, embryo cleavage, and implantation rates similar to those associated with anesthesia provided by a mepivacaine paracervical block.[45] Moreover, sister chromatid exchange assays, a sensitive index of genotoxic effects, demonstrated no DNA damage—even through two metaphases—when hamster oocytes were exposed to very high concentrations of propofol (20 μg/mL).[50] Of interest, these concentrations are at least 40 times higher than those detected clinically in the follicular fluid of patients undergoing oocyte retrieval.[47,48] At least one study of GIFT procedures conducted with propofol for the induction and maintenance of general anesthesia demonstrated essentially no difference in outcomes from those with other forms of anesthesia.[43] However, these data conflict with results from another study that indicated a lower incidence of ongoing pregnancies among women given propofol–nitrous oxide anesthesia for ZIFT procedures than in a similar group given thiopental–nitrous oxide–isoflurane anesthesia.[51] Further investigation is necessary to elucidate the full effect of propofol on reproductive outcomes.

Both thiopental and thiamylal (5 mg/kg) can be detected in follicular fluid as early as 11 minutes after their administration for induction of general anesthesia in patients undergoing GIFT procedures.[52] No adverse reproductive effects have been observed with these agents, and when they were specifically compared with propofol (2.7 mg/kg) for GIFT procedures, no differences in clinical pregnancy rates were noted.[44]

Nitrous Oxide

Nitrous oxide reduces methionine synthetase activity, nonmethylated folate derivatives, and DNA synthesis in animals and humans.[53,54] Nitrous oxide also impairs the function of mitotic spindles in cell cultures.[55] Although Warren et al.[56] reported that two-cell mouse embryos exposed to nitrous oxide within 4 hours of the expected onset of cleavage were less likely to develop to the blastocyst stage (Figure 15-10), this difference had resolved by later stages of embryo development.[57]

Clinical studies of anesthesia for laparoscopic ART procedures support the administration of nitrous oxide during GIFT and ZIFT procedures.[43,51,58] In a multicenter study, Beilin et al.[43] observed a delivery rate of 35% among women given nitrous oxide for GIFT procedures, compared with 30% among women who did not receive nitrous oxide. In women undergoing oocyte retrieval, Handa-Tsutsui and Kodaka[59] reported lower target-controlled propofol doses with a 50% oxygen–nitrous oxide than with oxygen-air mixture, with no alterations in pregnancy rates, although the study was not adequately powered to specifically detect this difference.

Volatile Halogenated Agents

Volatile halogenated agents have been observed to depress DNA synthesis and mitosis in cell cultures.[60,61] Sturrock and Nunn[60] noted that volatile halogenated agents prevent cytoplasmic cleavage during mitosis, leading to a higher number of abnormal mitotic figures (e.g., tripolar and tetrapolar nuclear phases). Isoflurane adversely affects embryo development *in vitro*.[57,62] Warren et al.[62] reported that

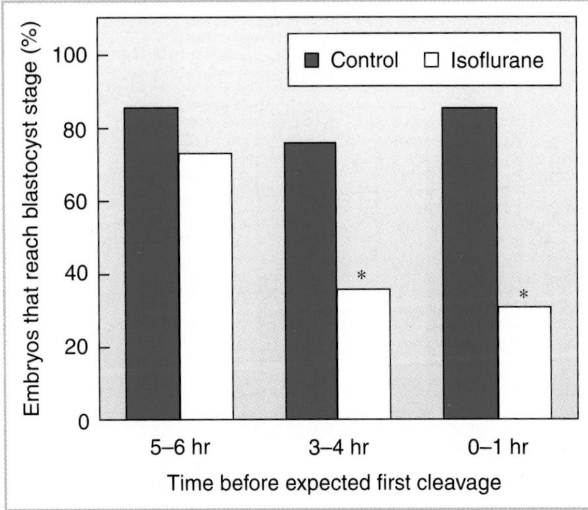

FIGURE 15-11 Developmental outcome of two-cell mouse embryos exposed *in vitro* to 3% isoflurane for 30 minutes at various times in relation to expected onset of the first cleavage *in vitro*. **P* < .01. (Modified from Warren JR, Shaw B, Steinkampf MP. Inhibition of preimplantation mouse embryo development by isoflurane. Am J Obstet Gynecol 1992; 166:693-8.)

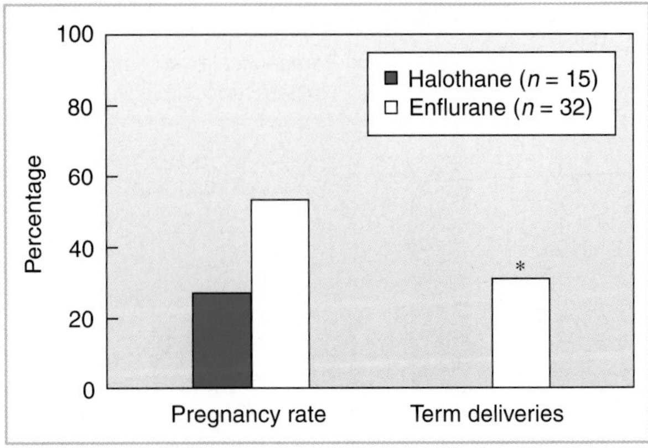

FIGURE 15-12 Pregnancy and term delivery rates after halothane and enflurane anesthesia for gamete intrafallopian transfer (GIFT). The percentage of term pregnancies after GIFT was greater after enflurane–nitrous oxide anesthesia than after halothane–nitrous oxide anesthesia. **P* < .05 compared with the halothane group. (Modified from Critchlow BM, Ibrahim Z, Pollard BJ. General anaesthesia for gamete intra-fallopian transfer. Eur J Anaesthesiol 1991; 8:381-4.)

two-cell mouse embryos exposed to 3% (but not 1.5%) isoflurane for 1 hour were less likely to develop to the blastocyst stage (Figure 15-11). As with their earlier study of embryos exposed to nitrous oxide, these researchers noted that the timing of anesthetic administration was critical. Developmental outcome was impaired only when isoflurane was given within 4 hours of the predicted onset of cleavage. It is questionable whether studies of two-cell mouse embryos are applicable to human oocytes and spermatozoa exposed during GIFT procedures or to one-cell embryos exposed during ZIFT procedures.

Volatile halogenated agents may also affect ART outcomes through an increase in prolactin levels. High prolactin levels have been associated with diminished oocyte development and uterine receptivity (see later); whether volatile halogenated agents can affect mature oocytes in the process of being retrieved, however, is questionable. Critchlow et al.[63] observed dramatic rises in plasma prolactin levels with an enflurane in nitrous oxide–oxygen technique for GIFT procedures, although these changes did not occur until 4 to 10 minutes after induction and did not affect follicular fluid prolactin levels or fertilization rates.

Volatile anesthetic agents have been compared in clinical studies. Fishel et al.[64] reported that pregnancy rates were significantly lower among women given halothane anesthesia for ET than in a similar group of women given enflurane; of interest, the anesthesia was administered in an attempt to decrease uterine activity during ET. Similarly, Critchlow et al.[63] reported lower pregnancy and delivery rates among women who received halothane for GIFT procedures than in women who received enflurane (Figure 15-12). General anesthesia with volatile halogenated agents has also been compared with conscious sedation. In a retrospective study with a sequential study design, Wilhelm et al.[33] noted lower pregnancy rates in patients undergoing oocyte retrieval with general anesthesia (i.e., isoflurane or propofol in combination with 60% nitrous oxide in oxygen) than in subsequent patients who received a remifentanil-based, monitored anesthesia care (MAC) technique. The investigators acknowledged that "the success rates of ART programs . . . improve over time, [and] it is possible that physician-related factors may have played a role in the improved success during the second (MAC) phase of [the] study."[33]

These data suggest that specific halogenated anesthetic agents can affect ART outcomes. Of note, the metabolic byproduct of sevoflurane, compound A, has been associated with genotoxic ovarian cell effects, although reproductive outcomes have not been assessed.[65] Therefore, caution is advised in the selection of a volatile halogenated agent, especially when the use of newer agents, such as sevoflurane, desflurane, and isodesox (a combination of 1% desflurane, 0.25% isoflurane, and 60% oxygen in nitrogen),[66] is contemplated, until further work has been done.

Antiemetic Agents

At least one study noted that droperidol and metoclopramide rapidly induce hyperprolactinemia with subsequent impairment of ovarian follicle maturation and corpus luteum function.[67] When these agents are given as a single dose immediately prior to oocyte retrieval, it is unlikely that the mature oocyte will be affected; however, if they are given on a routine basis after retrieval, the uterine receptivity to the embryo could be affected. Forman et al.[68] demonstrated that low plasma prolactin concentrations during ART procedures were associated with a higher incidence of pregnancy.

ANESTHETIC MANAGEMENT

Because most patients undergoing ART procedures are young and otherwise healthy, many institutions do not require preoperative laboratory studies, electrocardiograms, or chest radiographs for them. However, the application of

ART procedures to patients with a growing spectrum of pathologies, such as morbid obesity, cancer (with oocyte retrieval performed prior to chemotherapy or radiation therapy), and severe cardiac, pulmonary, or renal morbidities (with oocyte retrieval performed for ET in surrogate gestational carriers), has created special concerns that should be addressed individually.[69]

All patients should follow the fasting guidelines typically used for other patients undergoing ambulatory surgery. In patients with risk factors for pulmonary aspiration of gastric contents, a nonparticulate antacid should be given prior to the procedure. On occasion, a patient may not adhere to strict fasting guidelines, and although delay or cancellation of the procedure is an option, the decision should be made after careful analysis of the potential risks and benefits. If the window for maximal oocyte retrieval (34 to 36 hours after hCG administration) is missed, spontaneous ovulation with loss of oocytes can occur, invalidating the considerable effort and expense that have been incurred to that point. Moreover, if follicle aspiration is not performed, the patient would be at increased risk for OHSS, with its potential for significant morbidity. In contrast, the magnitude of risk for aspiration is difficult to quantify.

As with other ambulatory surgery cases, the ideal anesthetic technique results in effective pain relief with minimal postoperative nausea, sedation, pain, and psychomotor impairment.

Ultrasonographic-Guided Transvaginal Oocyte Retrieval

Although transvaginal oocyte retrievals can be performed under paracervical, spinal, epidural, and general anesthetic techniques, conscious sedation is the most commonly utilized technique.[70,71] It is usually adequate for surgical analgesia, but conscious sedation may need to progress to loss of consciousness (i.e., general anesthesia) to prevent patient movement at critical times; this problem has been observed in high-anxiety patients.[72] The need for additional pain relief should be anticipated when the needle penetrates the cul-de-sac and, later, each ovary. Of interest, one report noted a higher rate of hospital admission after oocyte retrieval, mostly secondary to intra-abdominal bleeding, when conscious sedation was used than when general anesthesia was used.[73] Self-administered inhalational analgesia with isodesox (see earlier) by face mask was associated with less effective analgesia and less patient satisfaction than physician-administered intravenous analgesia.[66]

Because paracervical anesthesia incompletely blocks sensation from the vaginal and ovarian pain fibers, additional analgesia is required, even when higher doses of local anesthetic are utilized.[74] Epidural and spinal techniques provide excellent pain relief with minimal oocyte exposure to anesthetic agents. Compared with sedation with propofol and mask-assisted ventilation with nitrous oxide, epidural bupivacaine anesthesia resulted in fewer complications, especially nausea and emesis.[75] Spinal anesthesia may be preferable to epidural anesthesia owing to the reduced anesthetic failure rate, lower systemic and follicular concentrations of anesthetic agent, and faster recovery profile.[76] Spinal administration of 1.5% hyperbaric lidocaine (60 mg) is associated with significantly shorter recovery times than spinal administration of 5% hyperbaric lidocaine (60 mg) in patients undergoing ART procedures.[77] The addition of intrathecal fentanyl 10 µg to lidocaine 45 mg improves postoperative analgesia for the first 24 hours, with no increase in time to urination, ambulation, and discharge, in comparison with intrathecal lidocaine alone.[78] Low-dose spinal bupivacaine has been evaluated for use in these patients, given the frequent association of spinal lidocaine with postoperative transient neurologic symptoms. However, the prolonged time to urination and discharge may prevent this agent from becoming a commonly used alternative.[79]

General anesthesia can be provided by total intravenous anesthesia using propofol (titrated) and fentanyl (50 to 100 µg), with midazolam (1 to 2 mg) as an optional premedication. With this option, most patients can be managed with spontaneous ventilation via high-flow oxygen mask and the use of carbon dioxide analysis.[40] (Individuals with significant risk factors for aspiration should undergo intubation with a cuffed endotracheal tube.) Anesthetics managed in this fashion have higher patient acceptance than conscious sedation, owing to better pain relief and less awareness during the surgical procedure.[40] Alternatively, endotracheal intubation and maintenance of anesthesia with a volatile halogenated agent has been utilized successfully; however, higher rates of nausea and emesis and more unplanned admissions have been observed with this technique than with a propofol, alfentanil, and air-oxygen mixture.[80]

Novel analgesic measures have been investigated during oocyte retrieval. One study evaluated electro-acupuncture as an alternative to intravenous alfentanil, although both groups also received a paracervical block, and the acupuncture group experienced higher degrees of preoperative stress and longer periods of discomfort during oocyte aspiration.[81]

Embryo Transfer

Described as relatively painless, transcervical embryo transfer procedures are most commonly performed without analgesia or anesthesia; however, on rare occasion, intravenous sedation or regional or general anesthesia may be requested. In contrast, transabdominal gamete or embryo transfer procedures (i.e., GIFT, ZIFT) are usually performed via laparoscopy under local, neuraxial, or general anesthesia. The anesthetic management for these procedures and the associated concerns with regard to the laparoscopic technique and the Trendelenburg position are described here. Major intraoperative complications associated with laparoscopy are rare but include gastric or intestinal perforation, hemorrhage, pneumothorax, pneumopericardium, mediastinal emphysema, gas embolism, and cardiac arrest.[82,83]

Pneumoperitoneum and the Trendelenburg Position

Carbon dioxide is the gas most commonly used to establish pneumoperitoneum. The high blood solubility of carbon dioxide facilitates absorption from the peritoneal cavity after laparoscopic surgery and may represent a life-saving property of the gas in the rare but potentially catastrophic event of gas embolization. For example, rapid intravenous injection of 5 to 10 mL/kg of carbon dioxide produces only transient (less than 1 minute) hypotension in anesthetized dogs (Figure 15-13),[84] whereas intravascular administration of a similar volume of a less soluble gas (e.g., helium, oxygen, nitrogen) is usually fatal.

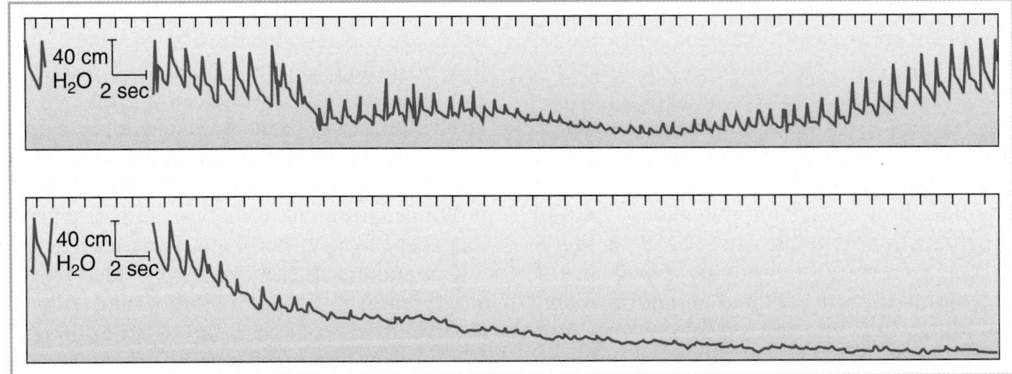

FIGURE 15-13 Arterial tracings after rapid intravenous injection of 7.5 mL/kg of carbon dioxide (*top*) and helium (*bottom*). Recovery occurs within 1 minute after the carbon dioxide injection, but complete cardiovascular collapse occurs after the helium injection. (Modified from Wolf JS, Carrier S, Stoller ML. Gas embolism: Helium is more lethal than carbon dioxide. J Laparoendosc Surg 1994; 4:173-7.)

Signs of embolization of large quantities of carbon dioxide (or any other gas) in anesthetized patients may include *hypo*capnia, hypotension, hypoxemia, ST-segment and T-wave changes, arrhythmias, and audible changes in the heart sounds.[85] Initial treatment of carbon dioxide embolism should include release of the pneumoperitoneum and pharmacologic support of the circulation. If initial resuscitation efforts are unsuccessful, aspiration of gas from the right atrium (using a multi-orifice central venous catheter) should be considered. Although the use of the left lateral recumbent position (Durant's maneuver) with or without head-down positioning has been suggested to facilitate removal of the postulated air lock from the right side of the heart,[86] laboratory evidence suggests that this maneuver may have a detrimental effect on cardiac function after venous gas embolism.[87]

Nearly as soluble in blood as carbon dioxide, nitrous oxide is associated with less peritoneal and diaphragmatic irritation[88] and has been suggested for the establishment of pneumoperitoneum in awake patients undergoing laparoscopy. A major disadvantage of nitrous oxide is its ability to support combustion, which could increase the possibility of an explosion if the surgeon uses electrocautery.

GIFT and ZIFT procedures are often performed with the patient in the Trendelenburg position to facilitate visualization of the fallopian tubes and other pelvic structures. Although their use is controversial, shoulder braces placed to prevent the patient from moving cephalad on the operating table should be positioned with padding against the acromioclavicular joints to prevent brachial plexus damage. The adduction of the patient's arms against her trunk has been suggested to reduce the risk of a brachial plexus injury, but the efficacy of this precaution is unproven.

Both pneumoperitoneum and the Trendelenburg position produce physiologic changes. Hemodynamic effects of moderate pneumoperitoneum (less than 20 mm Hg) in a patient in the Trendelenburg position include increased mean arterial and central venous pressures, increased systemic vascular resistance, and decreased stroke volume and cardiac output.[89] Heart rate usually does not change, but in some patients, pneumoperitoneum may elicit sinus bradycardia, heart block, or even cardiac arrest. Finally, pneumoperitoneum aggravates the respiratory effects of the Trendelenburg position (e.g., reduced chest wall compliance, increased venous admixture). Overall, most healthy patients easily tolerate the cardiovascular and pulmonary effects of intra-abdominal pressures lower than 20 mm Hg.

Laparoscopic-Assisted Reproductive Technology

The anesthetic plan for GIFT procedures is typically dictated by the method (i.e., transabdominal or transvaginal) of oocyte retrieval. Many ART programs harvest oocytes transabdominally during pelvic laparoscopy, the principal advantage being that the patient is positioned and anesthetized once for both the retrieval and transfer portions of the procedure. The major disadvantage of this technique is that oocytes are exposed to both carbon dioxide pneumoperitoneum and anesthetic agents. The induction of general anesthesia for GIFT procedures can be delayed until just before the skin incision in an effort to minimize unnecessary exposure to these agents. Induction is usually performed with intravenous propofol, lidocaine, fentanyl, and either succinylcholine or rocuronium. Following intubation, the anesthesia provider may decompress the patient's stomach with a suction catheter or Salem sump tube to reduce the risk of gastric perforation during instrumentation. Subsequently, a volatile halogenated agent in oxygen and air, with or without a short-acting muscle relaxant, is given to maintain anesthesia. The use of a propofol–nitrous oxide technique has been associated with less postoperative sedation, lower pain scores, and less emesis than an isoflurane–nitrous oxide technique.[51]

Alternatively, oocytes can be retrieved transvaginally and transferred—as ooctyes or embryos—laparoscopically. Of interest, this is the technique most commonly used with ZIFT procedures, whereby oocyte retrieval and IVF occur on the day prior to the ZIFT procedure. Advantages to the combined transvaginal/transabdominal approach include (1) the avoidance of laparoscopy in the 1% to 2% of cases in which oocyte quality or number is inadequate to justify proceeding with a tubal transfer,[3] and (2) the elimination of oocyte exposure to the carbon dioxide pneumoperitoneum. Disadvantages of this method include (1) the need to reposition the patient prior to laparoscopy and (2) a prolonged total operative time if performed on the same day (GIFT) or the need for a second procedure if performed on consecutive days (ZIFT).

A few patients prefer spinal or epidural anesthesia for GIFT procedures.[90,91] Healthy, nonobese patients have been reported to successfully undergo laparoscopic surgery in the Trendelenburg position with high thoracic (i.e., T2 to T4) spinal or epidural anesthesia.[90-93] Limiting intraperitoneal pressure to less than 10 mm Hg may facilitate the use of neuraxial anesthesia for these procedures. Obese women are not ideal candidates for neuraxial anesthesia in laparoscopic surgery.

Adequate analgesia for laparoscopic ART procedures has also been reported with the use of local anesthesia supplemented with intravenous sedation.[94-97] Padilla et al.[94] observed that the quality of intraoperative analgesia can be improved by limiting maximal intra-abdominal pressure to 8 to 10 mm Hg, reducing the rate of carbon dioxide insufflation to 1 L/min, and minimizing ovarian manipulation. The difficulty and pain frequently associated with cannulation of the fallopian tubes, however, may make local anesthesia an unwise choice for laparoscopic ART procedures. Waterstone et al.[95] noted that all 21 patients undergoing local anesthesia for laparoscopy experienced some discomfort when their fallopian tubes were mobilized. The use of local anesthesia should not be interpreted as being devoid of risk for serious complications (e.g., bradycardia, cardiac arrest). These life-threatening complications are rare, but the management and outcome are greatly assisted by individuals skilled in airway management and cardiopulmonary resuscitation.[98]

Postoperative Management

The incidence of anesthetic or surgical complications requiring hospital admission after ART procedures is low. Oskowitz et al.[73] reported admission rates after oocyte retrieval and GIFT procedures of 0.16% and 0.18%, respectively. The most common indications for hospitalization were hemoperitoneum and syncope after oocyte retrieval, and nausea, vomiting, and bowel injury after laparoscopic GIFT procedures. Incisional pain, diffuse abdominal pain, uterine cramping, and referred shoulder pain occur frequently after laparoscopy as a result of diaphragmatic irritation caused by retained intraperitoneal carbon dioxide. Although pain accompanied by nausea is usually a reasonable indication for the use of nonsteroidal anti-inflammatory drugs (NSAIDs), their use should be avoided because changes in the prostaglandin milieu can affect embryo implantation.[99,100] Instead, small doses of intravenous fentanyl (25 to 50 μg) or oral acetaminophen with codeine can be used to allay this discomfort.

Nausea and emesis can also occur; however, exposure to droperidol and metoclopramide should be limited (see earlier); treatment with nondopaminergic agents can be considered. Prior to discharge, patients should be able to drink and retain liquids, ambulate, and void. Patients undergoing anesthesia for an ART procedure should be called 24 hours after the procedure to allow assessment of recovery and potential complications.

FUTURE CONSIDERATIONS

The use of ART procedures has been extended to include patients within a broader range of ages and comorbidities. Check et al.[101] reported the successful delivery of infants through the use of donor oocytes, IVF, and ET in two postmenopausal women who were 51 years old; women in the seventh decade have also successfully delivered infants. Future studies should assess the short- and long-term maternal and perinatal consequences of ART procedures as well as the obstetric and anesthetic implications.[102]

Technical improvements in ultrasonography as well as fiberoptic methods of oocyte retrieval and fallopian tube cannulation could potentially make laparoscopic interventions less invasive or unnecessary. For example, small-diameter laparoscopes with optical views comparable to conventional instruments have allowed "mini-laparoscopic" procedures to be performed for GIFT procedures.[97] These alterations may allow for changes in anesthetic options.

The identification of agents and techniques that provide optimal analgesia or anesthesia with negligible impact on ART success is an important process to which anesthesia providers can and should contribute.

KEY POINTS

- Assisted reproductive technology (ART) includes techniques that are being applied to an increasingly diverse population of patients with a wide range of comorbidities.
- ART procedures usually involve a regimen of hormonal stimulation and oocyte retrieval followed by either *in vitro* fertilization with embryo transfer (IVF-ET) or gamete intrafallopian transfer (GIFT) procedures.
- Hormonal stimulation creates a number of oocytes for retrieval. On occasion, ovarian hyperstimulation syndrome can occur, with severe cases being associated with ascites, pleural effusion, hemoconcentration, oliguria, and thromboembolic events.
- Oocyte retrieval must be performed promptly, or ovulation will reduce the number of mature oocytes available for harvesting. Embryo transfer usually occurs transcervically; however, laparoscopic techniques (zygote intrafallopian transfer [ZIFT]) can be utilized.
- Conscious sedation, neuraxial anesthesia, and general anesthesia have all been used successfully to anesthetize women for ART procedures. Conscious sedation may have to progress to loss of consciousness (i.e., general anesthesia) to prevent patient movement at critical times during the procedure.
- Laboratory studies have suggested that local anesthetic agents, nitrous oxide, and the volatile halogenated agents interfere with some aspects of reproductive physiology *in vitro*. However, few clinical data show that brief administration of any contemporary anesthetic agent (except halothane) for an ART procedure adversely affects live-birth rates.
- The identification of agents and techniques that provide optimal analgesia or anesthesia with negligible impact on ART success is an important process to which anesthesia providers can and should contribute.

REFERENCES

1. Steptoe PC, Edwards RG. Birth after the reimplantation of a human embryo (letter). Lancet 1978; 2:366.
2. Toner JP. Progress we can be proud of: U.S. trends in assisted reproduction over the first 20 years. Fertil Steril 2002; 78:943-50.
3. Edwards RG. Test-tube babies. Nature 1981; 293:253-6.
4. International Committee for Monitoring Assisted Reproductive Technology; Adamson GD, de Mouzon J, Lancaster P, et al. World collaborative report on in vitro fertilization, 2000. Fertil Steril 2006; 85:1586-622.
5. U.S. Department of Health and Human Services, Centers for Disease Control and Prevention, Division of Reproductive Health. 2005 Assisted Reproductive Technology (ART) Report. Atlanta, CDC/DRH, 2007.
6. Cooke S, Quinn P, Kime L, et al. Improvement in early human embryo development using new formulation sequential stage-specific culture media. Fertil Steril 2002; 78:1254-60.
7. Jain T, Hornstein MD. Disparities in access to infertility services in a state with mandated insurance coverage. Fertil Steril 2005; 84:221-3.
8. Wikland M, Enk L, Hammarberg K, Nilsson L. Use of a vaginal transducer for oocyte retrieval in an IVF/ET program. J Clin Ultrasound 1987; 15:245-51.
9. Veeck LL. Atlas of the Human Oocyte and Early Conceptus. Baltimore, Williams & Wilkins, 1991:43.
10. Corson SL, Batzer F, Eisenberg E, et al. Early experience with the GIFT procedure. J Reprod Med 1986; 31:219-23.
11. Yovich JL, Yovich JM, Edirisinghe WR. The relative chance of pregnancy following tubal or uterine transfer procedures. Fertil Steril 1988; 48:858-64.
12. Schulman JD. Delayed expulsion of transfer fluid after IVF/ET (letter). Lancet 1986; 1(8471):44.
13. Abyholm T, Tanbo T, Henriksen T, Magnus O. Preliminary experience with embryo intrafallopian transfer (EIFT). Int J Fertil 1990; 35:339-42.
14. Magnani BJ, Tsen LC, Datta S, Bader AM. In-vitro fertilization: Do short-term changes in estrogen levels produce increased fibrinolysis? Am J Clin Pathol 1999; 112:485-91.
15. Harnett M, Bhavani-Shankar K, Datta S, Tsen LC. In-vitro fertilization induced alterations in coagulation and fibrinolysis as measured by thromboelastography. Anesth Analg 2002; 95:1063-6.
16. Dulitzky M, Cohen SB, Inbal A, et al. Increased prevalence of thrombophilia among women with severe ovarian hyperstimulation syndrome. Fertil Steril 2002; 77:463-7.
17. Bar-Hava I, Orvieto R, Dicker D, et al. A severe case of ovarian hyperstimulation: 65 liters of ascites aspirated in an on-going IVF-ET twin pregnancy. Gynecol Endocrinol 1995; 9:295-8.
18. Pryor RA, Wiczyk HP, O'Shea DL. Adnexal infarction after conservative surgical management of torsion of a hyperstimulated ovary. Fertil Steril 1995; 63:1344-6.
19. Schenker JG, Ezra Y. Complications of assisted reproductive techniques. Fertil Steril 1994; 61:411-22.
20. Hidlebaugh DA, Thompson IE, Berger MJ. Cost of assisted reproductive technology for a health maintenance organization. J Reprod Med 1997; 42:570-4.
21. Lieberman B, Ali R, Rangarajan S. Towards the elective replacement of a single embryo (eSET) in the United Kingdom. Hum Fertil (Camb) 2007; 10:123-7.
22. Cohen J. The efficiency and efficacy of IVF and GIFT. Hum Reprod 1991; 6:613-8.
23. Cetin I, Cozzi V, Antonazzo P. Fetal development after assisted reproduction: A review. Placenta 2003; 24:S104-13.
24. Boyers SP, Lavy G, Russell JB, DeCherney AH. A paired analysis of in vitro fertilization and cleavage rates of first-and last-recovered preovulatory human oocytes exposed to varying intervals of 100% CO_2 pneumoperitoneum and general anesthesia. Fertil Steril 1987; 48:969-74.
25. Lefebvre G, Vauthier D, Seebacher J, et al. In vitro fertilization: A comparative study of cleavage rates under epidural and general anesthesia—interest for gamete intrafallopian transfer. J In Vitro Fert Embryo Transf 1988; 5:305-6.
26. Lewin A, Margalioth EJ, Rabinowitz R, Schenker JG. Comparative study of ultrasonically guided percutaneous aspiration with local anesthesia and laparoscopic aspiration of follicles in an in vitro fertilization program. Am J Obstet Gynecol 1985; 151:621-5.
27. Davidson A, Vermesh M, Lobo RA, Paulson RJ. Mouse embryo culture as quality control for human in vitro fertilization: The one-cell versus the two-cell model. Fertil Steril 1988; 49:516-21.
28. Tsen LC, Datta S, Bader AM. Estrogen induced changes in protein binding of bupivacaine during in-vitro fertilization. Anesthesiology 1997; 87:879-83.
29. Schnell VL, Sacco AG, Savoy-Moore RT, et al. Effects of oocyte exposure to local anesthetics on in vitro fertilization and embryo development in the mouse. Reprod Toxicol 1992; 6:323-7.
30. Del Valle LJ, Orihuela PA. Cleavage and development in cultured preimplantation mouse embryos exposed to lidocaine. Reprod Toxicol 1996; 10:491-6.
31. Ahuja KK. In-vitro inhibition of the block to polyspermy of hamster eggs by tertiary amine local anaesthetics. J Reprod Fertil 1982; 65:15-22.
32. Wikland M, Evers H, Jakobsson AH, et al. The concentration of lidocaine in follicular fluid when used for paracervical block in a human IVF-ET programme. Hum Reprod 1990; 5:920-3.
33. Wilhelm W, Hammadeh ME, White PF, et al. General anesthesia versus monitored anesthesia care with remifentanil for assisted reproductive technologies: Effect on pregnancy rate. J Clin Anesth 2002; 14:1-5.
34. Chetkowski RJ, Nass TE. Isoflurane inhibits early mouse embryo development in vitro. Fertil Steril 1988; 49:171-3.
35. Bruce DL, Hinkley R, Norman PF. Fentanyl does not inhibit fertilization or early development of sea urchin eggs. Anesth Analg 1985; 64:498-500.
36. Shapira SC, Chrubasik S, Hoffmann A, et al. Use of alfentanil for in vitro fertilization oocyte retrieval. J Clin Anesth 1996; 8:282-5.
37. Cardasis C, Schuel H. The sea urchin egg as a model system to study the effects of narcotics on secretion. In Ford DH, Clouet DH, editors. Tissue Responses to Addictive Drugs. New York, Spectrum, 1976:631-40.
38. Swanson RF, Leavitt MG. Fertilization and mouse embryo development in the presence of midazolam. Anesth Analg 1992; 75:549-54.
39. Chopineau J, Bazin JE, Terrisse MP, et al. Assay for midazolam in liquor folliculi during in vitro fertilization under anesthesia. Clin Pharm 1993; 12:770-3.
40. Casati A, Valentini G, Zangrillo A, et al. Anaesthesia for ultrasound guided oocyte retrieval: Midazolam/remifentanil versus propofol/fentanyl regimens. Eur J Anaesthesiol 1999; 16:773-8.
41. Ben-Shlomo I, Moskovich R, Katz Y, Shalev E. Midazolam/ketamine sedative combination compared with fentanyl/propofol/isoflurane anaesthesia for oocyte retrieval. Hum Reprod 1999; 14:1757-9.
42. Rosenblatt MA, Bradford CN, Bodian CA, Grunfeld L. The effect of propofol-based sedation technique on cumulative embryo scores, clinical pregnancy rates, and implantation rates in patients undergoing embryo transfers with donor oocytes. J Clin Anesth 1997; 9:614-7.
43. Beilin Y, Bodian CA, Mukherjee T, et al. The use of propofol, nitrous oxide, or isoflurane does not affect the reproductive success rate following gamete intrafallopian transfer (GIFT): A multicenter pilot trial/survey. Anesthesiology 1999; 90:36-41.
44. Pierce ET, Smalky M, Alper MM, et al. Comparison of pregnancy rates following gamete intrafallopian transfer (GIFT) under general anesthesia with thiopental sodium or propofol. J Clin Anesth 1992; 4:394-8.
45. Christiaens F, Janssenswillen C, Van Steirteghem AC, et al. Comparison of assisted reproductive technology performance after oocyte retrieval under general anaesthesia (propofol) versus paracervical local anaesthetic block: A case-controlled study. Hum Reprod 1998; 13:2456-60.
46. Hein HA, Putman JM. Is propofol a proper proposition for reproductive procedures? J Clin Anesth 1997; 9:611-3.

47. Christiaens F, Janssenswillen C, Verborgh C, et al. Propofol concentrations in follicular fluid during general anaesthesia for transvaginal oocyte retrieval. Hum Reprod 1999; 14:345-8.
48. Ben-Shlomo I, Moskovich R, Golan J, et al. The effect of propofol anaesthesia on oocyte fertilization and early embryo quality. Hum Reprod 2000; 15:2197-9.
49. Imoedemhe DA, Sigue AB, Abdul Ghani I, et al. An evaluation of the effect of the anesthetic agent propofol (Diprivan) on the outcome of human in vitro fertilization. J Assist Reprod Genet 1992; 9:488-91.
50. Tomioka S, Nakajo N. No genotoxic effect of propofol in Chinese hamster ovary cells: Analysis by sister chromatid exchanges. Acta Anaesthesiol Scand 2000; 44:1261-5.
51. Vincent RD, Syrop CS, Van Voorhis BJ, et al. An evaluation of the effect of anesthetic technique on reproductive success after laparoscopic pronuclear stage transfer (PROST): Propofol-nitrous oxide versus isoflurane-nitrous oxide. Anesthesiology 1995; 82:352-8.
52. Endler GC, Stout M, Magyar DM, et al. Follicular fluid concentrations of thiopental and thiamylal during laparoscopy for oocyte retrieval. Fertil Steril 1987; 48:828-33.
53. Koblin DD, Waskell L, Watson JE, et al. Nitrous oxide inactivates methionine synthetase in human liver. Anesth Analg 1982; 61:75-8.
54. Baden JM, Serra M, Mazze RI. Inhibition of fetal methionine synthetase by nitrous oxide. Br J Anaesth 1984; 56:523-6.
55. Kieler J. The cytotoxic effect of nitrous oxide at different tensions. Acta Pharm Scand 1957; 13:301-8.
56. Warren JR, Shaw B, Steinkampf MP. Effects of nitrous oxide on preimplantation mouse embryo cleavage and development. Biol Reprod 1990; 43:158-61.
57. Chetkowski RJ, Nass TE. Isoflurane inhibits early mouse embryo development in vitro. Fertil Steril 1988; 49:171-3.
58. Rosen MA, Roizen MF, Eger EI, et al. The effect of nitrous oxide on in vitro fertilization success rate. Anesthesiology 1987; 67:42-4.
59. Handa-Tsutsui F, Kodaka M. Effect of nitrous oxide on propofol requirements during target-controlled infusion for oocyte retrieval. Int J Obstet Anesth 2007; 16:13-6.
60. Sturrock JE, Nunn JF. Mitosis in mammalian cells during exposure to anesthetics. Anesthesiology 1975; 43:21-33.
61. Nunn JF, Lovis JD, Kimball KL. Arrest of mitosis by halothane. Br J Anaesth 1971; 43:524-30.
62. Warren JR, Shaw B, Steinkampf MP. Inhibition of preimplantation mouse embryo development by isoflurane. Am J Obstet Gynecol 1992; 166:693-8.
63. Critchlow BM, Ibrahim Z, Pollard BJ. General anaesthesia for gamete intra-fallopian transfer. Eur J Anaesthesiol 1991; 8:381-4.
64. Fishel S, Webster J, Faratian B, Jackson P. General anesthesia for intrauterine placement of human conceptuses after in vitro fertilization. J In Vitro Fertil Embryo Transf 1987; 4:260-4.
65. Eger EI 2nd, Laster MJ, Winegar R, et al. Compound A induces sister chromatid exchanges in Chinese hamster ovary cells. Anesthesiology 1997; 86:918-22.
66. Thompson N, Murray S, MacLennan F, et al. A randomised controlled trial of intravenous versus inhalational analgesia during outpatient oocyte recovery. Anaesthesia 2000; 55:770-3.
67. Kauppila A, Leinonen P, Vihko R, Ylostalo P. Metoclopramide-induced hyperprolactinemia impairs ovarian follicle maturation and corpus luteum function in women. J Clin Endocrinol Metab 1982; 54:955-60.
68. Forman R, Fishel B, Edwards RG, Walters E. The influence of transient hyperprolactinemia on in vitro fertilization in humans. J Clin Endocrinol Metab 1984; 60:517-22.
69. Metzler E, Ginsburg E, Tsen LC. Use of assisted reproductive technologies and anesthesia in a patient with primary pulmonary hypertension. Fertil Steril 2004; 81:1684-7.
70. Ditkoff ECX, Plumb J, Selick A, Sauer MV. Anesthesia practices in the United States common to in vitro fertilization (IVF) centers. J Assist Reprod Genet 1997; 14:145-7.
71. Bokhari A, Pollard BJ. Anaesthesia for assisted conception: A survey of UK practice. Eur J Anaesthesiol 1999; 16:225-30.
72. Hong JY, Jee YS, Luthardt FW. Comparison of conscious sedation for oocyte retrieval between low-anxiety and high-anxiety patients. J Clin Anesth 2005; 17:549-53.
73. Oskowitz SP, Smalky M, Berger MJ, et al. Safety of a free standing surgical unit for the assisted reproductive technologies. Fertil Steril 1995; 63:874-9.
74. Ng EH, Tang OS, Chui DK, Ho PC. Comparison of two different doses of lignocaine used in paracervical block during oocyte collection in an IVF programme. Hum Reprod 2000; 15:2148-51.
75. Botta G, D'Angelo A, D'ari G, et al. Epidural anesthesia in an in vitro fertilization and embryo transfer program. J Assist Reprod Genet 1995; 12:187-90.
76. Endler GC, Magyar DM, Hayes MF, Moghiosi KS. Use of spinal anesthesia in laparoscopy for IVF. Fertil Steril 1985; 43:809.
77. Manica V, Bader AM, Fragneto G, et al. Anesthesia for in vitro fertilization: A comparison of 1.5% and 5% spinal lidocaine for ultrasonically guided oocyte retrieval. Anesth Analg 1993; 77:453-6.
78. Martin R, Tsen LC, Tseng G, Datta S. Comparison of 1.5% lidocaine with fentanyl with 1.5% lidocaine for in-vitro fertilization. Anesth Analg 1999; 88:523-6.
79. Tsen LC, Schultz R, Martin R, et al. Intrathecal low-dose bupivacaine vs. lidocaine for in-vitro fertilization procedures. Reg Anesth Pain Med 2001; 26:52-6.
80. Raftery S, Sherry E. Total intravenous anaesthesia with propofol and alfentanil protects against postoperative nausea and vomiting. Can J Anaesth 1992; 39:37-41.
81. Stener-Victorin E, Waldenstrom U, Nilsson L, et al. A prospective randomized study of electro-acupuncture versus alfentanil as anaesthesia during oocyte aspiration in in-vitro fertilization. Hum Reprod 1999; 14:2480-4.
82. Murphy AA. Diagnostic and operative laparoscopy. In Thompson JD, Rock JA, editors. TeLinde's Operative Gynecology. Philadelphia, JB Lippincott, 1992:361-84.
83. Doctor NH, Hussain Z. Bilateral pneumothorax associated with laparoscopy: A case report of a rare hazard and review of literature. Anaesthesia 1973; 28:75-81.
84. Wolf JS, Carrier S, Stoller ML. Gas embolism: Helium is more lethal than carbon dioxide. J Laparoendosc Surg 1994; 4:173-7.
85. Couture P, Boudreault D, Derouin M, et al. Venous carbon dioxide embolism in pigs: An evaluation of end-tidal carbon dioxide, transesophageal echocardiography, pulmonary artery pressure, and precordial auscultation monitoring modalities. Anesth Analg 1994; 79:867-73.
86. Durant TM, Long J, Oppenheimer MJ. Pulmonary (venous) air embolism. Am Heart J 1947; 33:269-81.
87. Geissler HJ, Allen SJ, Mehlhorn U, et al. Effect of body positioning after venous air embolism: An echocardiographic study. Anesthesiology 1997; 86:710-7.
88. Brown DR, Fishburn JI, Roberson VO, Hulka JF. Ventilatory and blood gas changes during laparoscopy with local anesthesia. Am J Obstet Gynecol 1976; 124:741-5.
89. McKenzie R, Wadhwa R, Bedger RC. Noninvasive measurement of cardiac output during laparoscopy. J Reprod Med 1980; 24:247-50.
90. Silva PD, Kang SB, Sloane KA. Gamete intrafallopian transfer with spinal anesthesia. Fertil Steril 1993; 59:841-3.
91. Chung PH, Yeko TR, Mayer JC, et al. Gamete intrafallopian transfer: Comparison of epidural vs. general anesthesia. J Reprod Med 1998; 43:681-6.
92. Burke RK. Spinal anesthesia for laparoscopy. A review of 1063 cases. J Reprod Med 1978; 21:59-62.
93. Ciofolo MJ, Clergue F, Seebacher J, et al. Ventilatory effects of laparoscopy under epidural anesthesia. Anesth Analg 1990; 70: 357-61.
94. Padilla SL, Smith RD, Dugan K, Zinder H. Laparoscopically assisted gamete intrafallopian transfer with local anesthesia. Fertil Steril 1996; 66:404-7.
95. Waterstone JJ, Bolton VN, Wren M, Parson JH. Laparoscopic zygote intrafallopian transfer using augmented local anesthesia. Fertil Steril 1992; 57:442-4.

96. Milki AA, Hardy RI, Danasouri IE, et al. Local anesthesia with conscious sedation for laparoscopic intrafallopian transfer. Fertil Steril 1992; 58:1240-2.
97. Pellicano M, Zullo F, Fiorentino A, et al. Conscious sedation versus general anaesthesia for minilaparoscopic gamete intra-fallopian transfer: A prospective randomized study. Hum Reprod 2001; 16:2295-7.
98. Ayestaran C, Matorras R, Gomez S, et al. Severe bradycardia and bradypnea following vaginal oocyte retrieval: A possible toxic effect of paracervical mepivacaine. Eur J Obstet Gynecol Reprod Biol 2000; 91:71-3.
99. von der Weiden RM, Helmerhorst FM, Keirse MJ. Influence of prostaglandins and platelet activating factor on implantation. Hum Reprod 1991; 6:436-42.
100. Marshburn PB, Shabanowitz RB, Clark MR. Immunohistochemical localization of prostaglandin H synthase in the embryo and uterus of the mouse from ovulation through implantation. Mol Reprod Dev 1990; 25:309-16.
101. Check JH, Nowroozi K, Barnea ER, et al. Successful delivery after age 50: A report of two cases as a result of oocyte donation. Obstet Gynecol 1993; 81:835-6.
102. Tsen LC. Anesthetic Risks of Oocyte Retrieval. In Giudice L, Santa E, Pool R, editors. The Medical Risks of Human Oocyte Donation for Stem Cell Research: Workshop Report. Washington, DC, National Academies Press, 2007.

Chapter 16

Problems of Early Pregnancy

Robert C. Chantigian, M.D.
Paula D. M. Chantigian, M.D., FACOG

Obstetric disease of early pregnancy may result in significant maternal morbidity and even mortality. Safe care of patients with obstetric disease involves a thorough understanding of the physiologic changes of early pregnancy as well as the specific issues associated with each pathologic condition. This chapter reviews specific obstetric problems of early pregnancy, including ectopic pregnancy, abortion, cervical insufficiency, and gestational trophoblastic disease.

PHYSIOLOGIC CHANGES OF EARLY PREGNANCY

Respiratory Changes

The respiratory system undergoes profound physiologic changes during early pregnancy.[1] Increased progesterone concentrations stimulate respiratory efforts by increasing the sensitivity of the respiratory center to carbon dioxide. The minute ventilation rises by at least 15% by 12 weeks' gestation and by 25% by 20 weeks' gestation. This rise in minute ventilation results from an increase in tidal volume (respiratory rate is unchanged) and exceeds that in oxygen consumption. The result is a respiratory alkalosis with maternal arterial partial pressure of carbon dioxide (Pa_{CO_2}) decreasing to 30 to 33 mm Hg by 10 to 12 weeks' gestation. Moreover, maternal arterial partial pressure of oxygen (Pa_{O_2}) rises to 106 to 108 mm Hg in the first trimester. Decreased bicarbonate concentration partially compensates for the modest respiratory alkalosis that results from the physiologic hyperventilation, leading to a maternal pH that is slightly above normal (i.e., approximately 7.44). There is little or no change in lung capacities during the first half of pregnancy. Women in early pregnancy who undergo mechanical ventilation require increased minute ventilation.

Cardiovascular Changes

The cardiovascular system also undergoes profound changes early in pregnancy.[1] Cardiac output increases 20% to 25% by 8 weeks' gestation and 35% to 40% by 20 weeks' gestation. Systemic vascular resistance (SVR) decreases 30% by 8 weeks' gestation. Maternal mean arterial pressure (MAP) decreases approximately 6 mm Hg at 16 to 24 weeks' gestation and returns to normal near term.

Aortocaval compression typically occurs after 18 to 20 weeks' gestation, at which time the uterine fundus reaches the umbilicus and is large enough to compress the aorta and vena cava whenever the patient assumes the supine position.[2] Use of the left uterine tilt position is rarely needed in early pregnancy. When the uterine size is equivalent to an 18- to 20-week gestation, left uterine tilt should be attained by elevating the right hip with a wedge or blankets. The need for left uterine tilt occurs earlier in gestation in the presence of multiple gestation, polyhydramnios, or gestational trophoblastic disease.

Blood volume increases throughout pregnancy; the average prepregnancy blood volume of 4350 mL (76 mL/kg) rises to 4700 mL (81 mL/kg) at 12 weeks' gestation, to 5500 mL (89 mL/kg) at 20 weeks' gestation, and to 6600 mL (97 mL/kg) at term. The increase in blood volume is primarily the result of greater plasma volume because red blood cell volume increases to a smaller degree (27 mL/kg).[3] Because pregnant women have an expanded blood volume, they typically tolerate a blood loss of 500 to 1500 mL during the first half of pregnancy. A blood loss of 500 to 1500 mL rarely requires blood transfusion, provided that the blood loss is replaced with an adequate volume of crystalloid or colloid.

Gastrointestinal Changes

During the first half of pregnancy, the physiologic changes of the gastrointestinal system are not clinically significant. Increased progesterone levels, however, may cause relaxation of lower esophageal sphincter tone as early as the first trimester. Fasting gastric volume is approximately 30 mL in both nonpregnant women and women in early pregnancy (i.e., 15 weeks' gestation). Metoclopramide 10 mg, administered intravenously 15 to 30 minutes before anesthesia, can reduce this volume by 50%.[4] In a study of 100 pregnant women undergoing general anesthesia by mask at 6 to 22 weeks' gestation, a pH electrode showed reflux of gastric contents into the esophagus in 17% of patients. Most episodes of reflux occurred in patients who experienced hiccups. Only 2% had regurgitation of gastric contents into the pharynx, and no patient demonstrated clinical evidence of pulmonary aspiration.[5]

General anesthesia may be safely administered by means of a mask or a laryngeal mask airway (LMA) by experienced anesthesia providers in selected obstetric patients during early pregnancy, without complication. Many anesthesia providers are comfortable managing an airway without intubation of the trachea until 18 to 20 weeks' gestation, when the uterus moves out of the pelvis. This movement leads to anatomic and intragastric pressure changes that contribute to gastroesophageal reflux. Some anesthesia providers prefer to intubate the trachea of pregnant women who require general anesthesia as early as 12 to 14 weeks' gestation, given that hormone changes leading to sphincter relaxation are present early in pregnancy. Patients who receive general anesthesia during the first half of pregnancy should be intubated if they are at increased risk of gastric content aspiration (e.g., history of gastroesophageal reflux, morbid obesity, food ingestion within 6 to 8 hours). Patients with a suspected difficult airway or a history of a difficult airway should also be intubated. Pharmacologic prophylaxis (e.g., sodium citrate, an H_2-receptor antagonist, and/or metoclopramide) is likely to further reduce the risk of aspiration pneumonia. Neuraxial anesthesia is associated with a lower risk of aspiration than general anesthesia.

Neurologic Changes

During early pregnancy, the nervous system is more sensitive to general and local anesthetic agents. The minimum alveolar concentration (MAC) is approximately 30% lower with halothane, enflurane, and isoflurane. Presumably, a reduction in MAC also occurs with desflurane and sevoflurane. The exact mechanism for the greater sensitivity in early pregnancy is unclear, but hormonal changes may play a role. Lower doses of these drugs should be considered.

ECTOPIC PREGNANCY

Ectopic pregnancy occurs when the fertilized ovum implants outside the endometrial lining of the uterus. Death, infertility, and recurrent ectopic pregnancy are possible sequelae. The frequency of ectopic pregnancy in the United States increased fourfold to fivefold between 1970 and 1992 but appears to have stabilized at a rate of approximately 16 per 1000 pregnancies.[6] A higher prevalence of associated risk factors, especially pelvic inflammatory disease (PID), as well as earlier diagnosis of previously unrecognized ectopic pregnancies may account for the reported increase.

Rupture of an ectopic pregnancy is the leading cause of pregnancy-related maternal death during the first trimester. Six percent of all pregnancy-related maternal deaths in the United States are due to ruptured ectopic pregnancies.[7,8] Most ectopic pregnancy–related maternal deaths result from hemorrhage (93%). Infection (2.5%), embolism (2.1%), and anesthetic complications (1.3%) are implicated in a minority of deaths.[9] More than 30% of women who have had an ectopic pregnancy subsequently suffer from infertility, and 5% to 23% have a second ectopic pregnancy.[10]

The case-fatality rate has dropped significantly from 35.5 deaths per 10,000 ectopic pregnancies in 1970 to 3.8 per 10,000 in 1989 in the United States,[11] and to 3.6 deaths per 10,000 ectopic pregnancies in the United Kingdom in 2002.[12] In some African and other developing countries, the case-fatality rates are 100 to 300 per 10,000 ectopic pregnancies.[6] A review of ectopic pregnancies in Michigan from 1985 through 1999 found that 18.7% of ectopic pregnancy deaths resulted from preventable medical errors. Three fourths of all nonpreventable ectopic deaths presented as sudden death.[8] Death from ectopic pregnancy occurs more often in teenagers, although ectopic pregnancy occurs up to three times more often in older women (35 to 44 years) than in younger women (15 to 24 years).[11] Reported ectopic pregnancy mortality rates are 3 to 18 times higher in African-American women than in white women in the United States.[8,9,11]

Factors that increase the risk of an ectopic pregnancy involve alterations in the normal fallopian tube transport system for the fertilized ovum. These factors include (1) prior ectopic pregnancy; (2) prior tubal surgery; (3) pelvic inflammation, especially *Chlamydia trachomatis* infection;

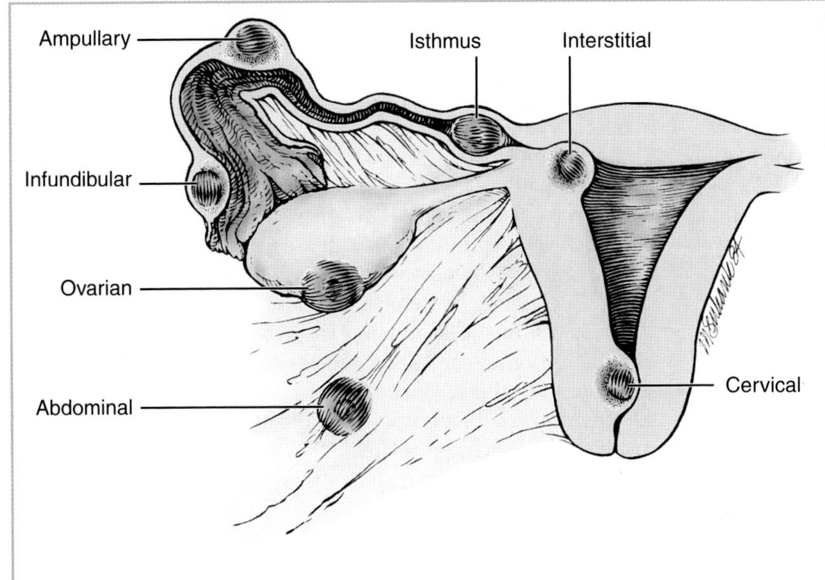

FIGURE 16-1 Potential location of ectopic pregnancies. The majority of ectopic pregnancies occur in the ampullary portion of the fallopian tube. (Modified from DeCherney AH, Seifer DB. Ectopic pregnancy. In Gabbe SG, Niebyl JR, Simpson JL, editors. Obstetrics: Normal and Problem Pregnancies. 2nd edition. New York, Churchill Livingstone, 1991:811.)

(4) congenital anatomic distortion such as that caused by exposure to diethylstilbestrol (DES) *in utero*; (5) previous pelvic or abdominal surgery; (6) use of a contraceptive intrauterine device (IUD), which may be associated with interstitial ectopic pregnancy; (7) delayed ovulation; (8) hormonal changes associated with ovulation induction or progestin-only oral contraceptives; (9) lifestyle choices (e.g., smoking, vaginal douching); (10) history of infertility; and (11) assisted reproductive technology (ART) procedures (e.g., zygote transfer into the fallopian tube or uterine cavity).[13] One third of patients with an ectopic pregnancy have no identifiable risk factors.[14]

The fertilized ovum can implant anywhere along the path of migration or in the abdominal cavity (Figure 16-1). Most ectopic pregnancies (98%) are **tubal** (infundibular or fimbrial, 6%; ampullary, 78%; isthmic, 12%; interstitial or cornual, 2%). The remaining 2% implant on the **cervix**, **vagina**, or **ovary** or elsewhere in the **abdomen**.[15] An increasing number of cesarean scar ectopic pregnancies are being reported.[16]

In patients who undergo ART procedures, ectopic pregnancies have been reported in approximately 2% of pregnancies.[13] Most of these pregnancies are tubal; however, approximately 6% are ovarian, abdominal, or cervical, and 12% to 15% are **heterotopic** (simultaneously intrauterine and extrauterine) pregnancies.[15]

Clinical Presentation

The clinical presentation of the patient with an ectopic pregnancy depends on the gestational age, the site of implantation, and the occurrence of significant hemorrhage. Prior to rupture, the signs and symptoms are often subtle. Classic clinical signs of impending rupture or a ruptured tubal pregnancy include abdominal or pelvic pain (95%), delayed menses (75% to 95%), and vaginal bleeding (60% to 80%).[17] Vaginal bleeding results from the breakdown and shedding of the decidual lining of the uterine wall, which is probably associated with decreased hormone production by the corpus luteum and inadequate human chorionic gonadotropin (hCG) production by the ectopic trophoblast. Pain often precedes vaginal bleeding. Patients with hemorrhage (with or without tubal rupture) may experience dizziness or syncope. They may have the urge to defecate because of the presence of blood in the cul-de-sac. Shoulder pain due to diaphragmatic irritation by intra-abdominal blood may be present.

Physical findings include abdominal tenderness with or without rebound (80% to 95%), a uterus that is smaller than expected for dates (30%), and a tender adnexal mass (30% to 50%). A bulging cul-de-sac suggests hemoperitoneum. With significant hemorrhage, orthostatic changes in blood pressure and heart rate or frank shock may occur. Some patients appear hemodynamically stable (e.g., normal blood pressure) despite a hemoperitoneum volume of 1000 to 1500 mL. Presumably, these patients have a slowly bleeding ectopic pregnancy and are able to compensate for the gradual blood loss.

Diagnosis

Pelvic pain with a positive pregnancy test result establishes the need to rule out an ectopic pregnancy. In a woman of reproductive age, the symptoms of ectopic pregnancy must be differentiated from (1) a threatened, inevitable, or incomplete abortion; (2) infection after attempted abortion; (3) pelvic inflammatory disease; (4) a degenerating fibroid; (5) appendicitis and other gastrointestinal diseases; (6) ovarian torsion; (7) a ruptured or bleeding ovarian cyst; (8) a trapped retroverted pregnant uterus; and (9) nephrolithiasis.

Current tests allow early diagnosis of ectopic pregnancy and prompt treatment, decreasing morbidity and mortality.[10,17] Diagnostic algorithms include the following guidelines:

1. Ultrasonography can reliably confirm only the presence of an intrauterine pregnancy. The ectopic pregnancy itself may be difficult to visualize.[18] **Transvaginal ultrasonography** is the current modality of choice because

it can detect an intrauterine gestational sac as soon as 21 days after conception (when beta-hCG concentrations are greater than 1400 mIU/mL with use of the International Reference Preparation [IRP] standard). **Transabdominal ultrasonography** visualizes an intrauterine pregnancy when the serum beta-hCG concentrations are higher than 6000 to 6500 mIU/mL IRP.[19]

2. Serial beta-hCG concentrations that decrease, plateau, or show a subnormal rise (less than 53% over 48 hours) usually indicate a nonviable pregnancy—either an ectopic pregnancy or an impending abortion.[20] With a spontaneous abortion, a decline in beta-hCG concentration of at least 21% to 35% should be seen over 2 days. A slower decline is suggestive of an ectopic pregnancy. Beta-hCG concentrations greater than 100,000 mIU/mL are usually associated with viable intrauterine pregnancies.[21]
3. A serum progesterone concentration higher than 25 ng/mL is usually associated with a viable pregnancy. A concentration less than or equal to 5 ng/mL usually indicates a nonviable pregnancy but cannot distinguish a spontaneous abortion from an ectopic pregnancy.[22] Most ectopic pregnancies are associated with progesterone levels between 5 and 25 ng/mL, a fact that limits the usefulness of this test.[23]
4. Uterine curettage can be performed when nonviability is established. Identification of trophoblastic villi confirms miscarriage of an intrauterine pregnancy. Absence of villi signals either a complete spontaneous abortion (confirmed by rapidly falling beta-hCG concentrations) or an ectopic pregnancy.

In the past, culdocentesis was used to aid in the diagnosis of hemoperitoneum and ectopic pregnancy. Although a positive culdocentesis result is highly predictive of hemoperitoneum, the advent of pelvic ultrasonography and rapid quantitative beta-hCG tests limits its value in the diagnosis of ectopic pregnancy.

Obstetric Management

Management options for ectopic pregnancy are expectant, medical, and surgical approaches. Management choice depends on the symptoms and diagnostic findings.

Expectant management may be used for selected asymptomatic patients with early tubal ectopic pregnancies and stable or decreasing beta-hCG levels. Successful resolution has been reported in approximately 50% of these selected patients.[6] If expectant management is unsuccessful, a medical or surgical approach is required.

Systemic, intramuscular, oral, and intragestational forms of chemotherapy have been used successfully in the **medical management** of ectopic pregnancy. Methotrexate, a folate antagonist that inhibits the growth of the trophoblastic cells of the placenta, is commonly used for this purpose. Early tubal pregnancies (i.e., no cardiac activity, a diameter less than 4 cm, and no evidence of tubal rupture or hemoperitoneum) have been successfully treated with single-dose methotrexate chemotherapy in 67% to 100% of selected patients.[24] Side effects include abdominal pain, vomiting, stomatitis, severe neutropenia, and pneumonitis. Unsuccessful resolution of the ectopic pregnancy requires surgical intervention.

Surgical management depends on the location of the pregnancy, the hemodynamic stability of the patient, the available equipment, and the surgeon's expertise. When a viable intrauterine pregnancy has been excluded, hemodynamically stable patients may first undergo dilation and uterine evacuation (D and E) to eliminate the possibility of an incomplete abortion. Subsequently, diagnostic laparoscopy is performed to confirm the diagnosis and locate the ectopic pregnancy. For tubal ectopic pregnancies, a salpingostomy, salpingotomy, or salpingectomy (usually partial) is performed by means of laparoscopy or laparotomy. To aid hemostasis during laparoscopic removal of the ectopic pregnancy, some obstetricians inject dilute vasopressin into the surface of the fallopian tube. This agent causes marked blanching of the tube and results in a relatively bloodless surgical field. If the vasopressin is accidentally injected intravenously, a marked rise in maternal blood pressure may occur.[25]

A laparotomy is indicated in cases in which the surgeon is not trained in operative laparoscopy, laparoscopic removal is anticipated to be difficult (e.g., tube diameter greater than 6 cm or an interstitial location of the ectopic pregnancy), or there is uncontrollable bleeding.[25] Hemodynamic instability should prompt the immediate performance of a laparotomy. These cases often require a partial or total salpingectomy. If a partial salpingectomy is performed, tubal repair may be performed primarily or during a second operation. The risk of persistent ectopic pregnancy may be higher after salpingostomy than after salpingectomy.[26]

Interstitial, cervical, cesarean scar, and abdominal ectopic pregnancies may present significant diagnostic and therapeutic challenges, resulting in delay of diagnosis and treatment. These pregnancies have the potential for massive hemorrhage due to significant disruption of organs and adjacent tissues. The desire to preserve fertility may result in higher blood loss as tissue and organ preservation are attempted.

Interstitial pregnancies often go unrecognized and may manifest as uterine wall rupture, massive hemorrhage, and shock. Conservative surgery (e.g., cornual resection) may be attempted, but hysterectomy may be required if uterine damage is severe.

Cervical pregnancies often result in massive hemorrhage because of the inability of the cervix to contract. In the past, most cervical pregnancies necessitated hysterectomy to control the hemorrhage. More current management options include (1) methotrexate therapy, (2) local excision, (3) cerclage and tamponade, (4) ligation of the hypogastric arteries or the cervical branches of the uterine arteries, and (5) angiographic embolization of the uterine arteries, followed by a D and E procedure.[27]

The incidence of **cesarean scar** ectopic pregnancies is rising; the current incidence is as high as 1 in 1800 pregnancies.[16,28,29] Jurkovic et al.[29] described two types of cesarean scar pregnancies, (1) implantation on the scar with enlargement into the uterine cavity and (2) implantation into a scar defect with growth into the myometrium. Depending on its progression, the former type of scar pregnancy may grow normally or may be treated medically. Scar implantation results in an increased risk of hemorrhage at delivery. Growth into the myometrium may lead to eventual rupture and bleeding in the first trimester;

prompt surgical intervention is preferred over medical management in this scenario.

In a review of 112 cases of cesarean scar ectopic pregnancies, Rotas et al.[28] found that approximately half occur in women with only one previous cesarean delivery. Many patients with such pregnancies present with vaginal bleeding, abdominal cramps, and/or lower abdominal pain. Up to one third of cases may be asymptomatic and diagnosed by ultrasonography. Management strategies include expectant management, dilation and curettage, wedge resection and repair of the implantation site, and medical management. The researchers concluded that both surgery and combined systemic and intragestational chemotherapy were successful in the treatment of cesarean scar ectopic pregnancies. Expectant management and dilation and curettage resulted in significant maternal morbidity.

Abdominal pregnancies are associated with a high incidence of maternal morbidity and a maternal mortality rate of 0.5% to 4.5%.[30,31] Diagnosis is difficult, being missed in as many as 1 of 9 cases.[30] Abdominal pain, vaginal bleeding, symptoms consistent with partial bowel obstruction, shock, or death may be the first indication of this unusual type of pregnancy.[32] Ultrasonography may aid in diagnosis but may miss the diagnosis in more than 50% of cases. Magnetic resonance imaging may prove to be a sensitive diagnostic tool.[32] Abdominal pregnancy is associated with decreased placental perfusion (which typically results in fetal growth restriction) and oligohydramnios (which often results in pulmonary hypoplasia and anatomic deformities). In 1993, Stevens[31] reviewed published cases of abdominal pregnancy since 1809 and found that 63% of infants survived when born after 30 weeks' gestation. Delayed delivery places the mother at risk for massive hemorrhage from premature separation of the placenta.

Management of an abdominal pregnancy consists of laparotomy and delivery of the fetus. Once the fetus is delivered, management of the placenta is controversial and fraught with hazard. Removal of the placenta is associated with massive hemorrhage; prolonged, complicated surgery (e.g., bowel resection); and increased maternal mortality. A decision to leave the placenta *in situ* results in a higher risk of infectious morbidity as well as a greater need for additional surgery.[31,32] The site of placental implantation and the ability to adequately ligate the blood supply often dictates the obstetrician's decision about management of the placenta.

Historically, **heterotopic** pregnancies were thought to occur in 1 in 30,000 spontaneous pregnancies.[33] With the advent of ART, the overall incidence of heterotopic pregnancy may be as high as 1 in 900.[34] In patients undergoing ART, 1% to 3% of pregnancies are heterotopic.[15] The difficulty in visualizing the entire fallopian tube on ultrasonography, combined with normal or slightly elevated beta-hCG measurements (i.e., low serum levels from the ectopic pregnancy combined with normal levels from the intrauterine pregnancy), make the early diagnosis of heterotopic pregnancy difficult.[35,36] This diagnosis should be suspected in cases in which clinical signs of an ectopic pregnancy and a confirmed intrauterine pregnancy coexist. In most cases the ectopic pregnancy is removed surgically. Alternatively, transvaginal ultrasonography-guided injection of potassium chloride into the ectopic pregnancy has been performed successfully, although as many as 55% of patients may require subsequent surgery.[37] The patient frequently sustains the normal intrauterine pregnancy to term.[34,35]

Patients with ectopic pregnancies who are Rh negative should receive $Rh_0(D)$ immune globulin.[24]

Anesthetic Management

Patients with an unruptured tubal pregnancy usually have a normal intravascular volume and little bleeding before and during surgery. The anesthetic and surgical risks are low. Laparoscopy or laparotomy can be performed safely with spinal, epidural, or general anesthesia (Box 16-1).[38] Most patients prefer general anesthesia. However, in motivated patients, neuraxial anesthesia with a sensory level of T2 to T4 is an alternative. If shoulder discomfort develops owing to the insufflation of carbon dioxide into the peritoneal cavity during laparoscopy, a modest dose of intravenous fentanyl (1 to 2 μg/kg) often relieves the referred diaphragmatic discomfort.

Ruptured ectopic pregnancy may be associated with significant preoperative blood loss. In a review of 300 consecutive surgically managed ectopic pregnancies, approximately 50% of patients had more than 500 mL, and 10% more than 1500 mL, of blood in the peritoneal cavity.[39] Estimation of preoperative blood loss is complicated by the fact that young women often maintain a normal blood pressure despite a markedly reduced circulating blood volume. General anesthesia is preferred in cases in which significant bleeding has occurred (e.g., ruptured tubal pregnancy) or is likely to occur (e.g., cervical, interstitial, cornual, cesarean scar, or abdominal ectopic pregnancy). Large-bore intravenous catheters should be placed as soon as possible. Several units of packed red blood cells should be immediately available. Intraoperative autologous blood transfusion can be used and may be especially useful in developing countries, where blood bank supplies are limited and women typically present late with significant hemoperitoneum and/or hypovolemic shock.[40] Invasive monitoring may be required in patients with hemodynamic instability. The desire to preserve fertility often results in higher blood loss as tissue and organ preservation are attempted.

ABORTION AND INTRAUTERINE FETAL DEMISE

Abortion refers to a pregnancy loss or termination, either before 20 weeks' gestation or when the fetus weighs less than 500 g. It can occur spontaneously or can be performed electively for personal or medical reasons. More than 839,000 elective abortions were reported in the United States in 2004, a rate of approximately 238 abortions per 1000 live births.[41] Most procedures were surgical (87% by curettage, 0.6% by intrauterine instillation of saline or prostaglandin), and approximately 10% were medical or nonsurgical abortions (most commonly with methotrexate and misoprostol, or mifepristone and misoprostol, performed before 8 weeks' gestation).

Hutchon[42] has suggested that physicians substitute the word *miscarriage* for the word *abortion* in cases of spontaneous early pregnancy loss. Further, he suggested

BOX 16-1 Suggested Anesthetic Techniques for Laparoscopy or Laparotomy for Patients with Ectopic Pregnancy

General Considerations

- Blood typing and antibody screening
- Aspiration prophylaxis if patient has a full stomach
- Routine noninvasive monitors (electrocardiogram, blood pressure cuff, pulse oximeter, temperature probe, and nerve stimulator [general anesthesia])
- One peripheral intravenous catheter with crystalloid solution
- Foley catheter
- If major bleeding has occurred or is expected to occur (e.g., ruptured tubal, interstitial, cervical, uterine scar, or abdominal ectopic pregnancy):
  - Two or more intravenous catheters
  - Typing and crossmatching of blood for several units of red blood cells
  - Consideration of invasive hemodynamic monitoring (e.g., arterial catheter, central venous pressure catheter)
  - Consideration of intraoperative cell salvage
- Neuraxial (spinal or epidural) anesthesia for hemodynamically stable patients with a low likelihood of significant hemorrhage (i.e., unruptured tubal pregnancy):
  - Prehydration with 1000 mL of crystalloid solution, supplemental oxygen, and minimal sedation with midazolam, opioid, and/or propofol

Spinal Anesthesia

- Single injection with a small-gauge spinal needle: bupivacaine 12 to 15 mg with fentanyl 25 μg, to achieve T2 to T4 sensory blockade

Epidural Anesthesia

- Placement of midlumbar epidural needle and catheter
- Lidocaine 2% with epinephrine 5 μg/mL (1:200,000), approximately 20 mL, and fentanyl 100 μg, injected incrementally, to achieve T2 to T4 sensory blockade

General Anesthesia

- Rapid-sequence induction with cricoid pressure if the patient has a good airway and has a full stomach
- Induction: thiopental or propofol (ketamine or etomidate should be considered if patient is hemodynamically unstable)
- Muscle relaxant for intubation and surgery
- Endotracheal intubation
- End-tidal carbon dioxide monitoring
- Maintenance: oxygen, nitrous oxide, opioid, and a volatile anesthetic agent or propofol infusion as tolerated
- Placement of an oral gastric tube, performance of suctioning, and removal of the tube
- Reversal of a muscle relaxant and extubation when the patient is awake and responds to verbal commands

that the word *miscarriage* may be modified with descriptive adjectives such as *threatened, incomplete*, and *complete*, and that the term *delayed miscarriage* replace the term *missed abortion*. In our judgment, either set of terms is acceptable.

Five percent of all pregnancy-related maternal deaths in the United States are associated with an elective or spontaneous abortion.[43] Death results from sepsis in approximately 36%, hemorrhage in approximately 20%, and embolism in approximately 16% of cases.[43] Of the 20 abortion-related maternal deaths in the United States in 2003, 10 were related to spontaneous abortion and 10 women died after legal abortions (6 after surgical procedures and 4 after medical or nonsurgical abortion procedures). There were no deaths reported after illegal abortions.[41]

Spontaneous abortion occurs in 10% to 15% of clinically recognized pregnancies; when subclinical pregnancies are also considered, the incidence of spontaneous pregnancy loss may be as high as 60%.[44,45] Although most spontaneous abortions manifest clinically at 8 to 14 weeks' gestation, ultrasonography suggests that fetal demise usually occurs before 8 weeks' gestation.[45] If the fetus is viable at 8 weeks' gestation, the incidence of subsequent fetal loss is only 3%.[45]

The etiology of spontaneous abortion varies among patients. Chromosomal abnormalities are responsible for at least 50% to 80% of all spontaneous abortions.[45,46] Other causes include (1) immunologic mechanisms, (2) maternal infections, (3) endocrine abnormalities (e.g., poorly controlled diabetes mellitus), (4) uterine anomalies, (5) incompetent cervix, (6) debilitating maternal disease, (7) trauma, and (8) possibly, environmental exposures (e.g., irradiation, smoking, certain drugs).[17,45,47]

Although some studies (conducted before scavenging of anesthetic gases was routine) suggested a higher incidence of spontaneous abortion among women who were exposed to trace concentrations of anesthetic agents in operating rooms,[48] reevaluation of these data demonstrated significant flaws in the study design, casting doubt on the original conclusions.[49] Later studies have shown no increased incidence of spontaneous abortion in women working in operating rooms.[50]

Clinical Presentation and Obstetric Management

The clinical presentation and management of a patient undergoing a spontaneous abortion vary. A **threatened abortion** is defined as uterine bleeding without cervical dilation before 20 weeks' gestation. Bleeding may be accompanied by cramping or backache. Once the diagnosis is confirmed, the patient's activities are restricted until symptoms resolve. Approximately 25% of pregnancies are complicated by a threatened abortion; approximately half of women affected go on to have a spontaneous abortion.[51]

An **inevitable abortion** is defined as cervical dilation or rupture of membranes without expulsion of the fetus or placenta. Spontaneous expulsion of the uterine contents usually occurs, but infection can be a complication.

A **complete abortion** is defined as a total, spontaneous expulsion of the fetus and placenta. Partial expulsion of the uterine contents (i.e., an **incomplete abortion**) is more common after 8 weeks' gestation.[52] Persistent bleeding and cramping after expulsion of tissue are signs of an incomplete abortion. An incomplete abortion usually requires a D and E procedure to remove any remaining fetal or placental tissue. Oxytocin and/or an ergot alkaloid (e.g., methylergonovine) increases uterine tone and may be administered intraoperatively and/or postoperatively to decrease the amount of uterine bleeding.

Fetal death may go unrecognized for several weeks in a patient with a **missed abortion**. Occasionally, coagulation defects such as disseminated intravascular coagulation (DIC) may complicate intrauterine fetal death; this possibility is more likely when the fetus dies at an advanced gestational age. If spontaneous expulsion of the uterine contents does not occur after a brief period of observation, evacuation of the uterus is indicated. Options are intravaginal or intracervical placement of a prostaglandin E_2 (PGE_2) preparation and a D and E procedure after laminaria placement. Side effects of prostaglandins include nausea, vomiting, diarrhea, and fever. Intra-amniotic instillation of hypertonic saline is not recommended in cases of intrauterine fetal death because coagulation defects may be induced or enhanced.[53]

Recurrent or **habitual abortion** refers to the occurrence of three or more consecutive spontaneous abortions in the same patient.

Obstetric Complications

Complications of a D and E procedure include cervical laceration, uterine perforation, hemorrhage, retained products of conception, and infection. The risk of these complications is increased in pregnancies that have progressed beyond the first trimester. Vasovagal events, postabortal syndrome (i.e., intrauterine blood clots with uterine atony, associated with lower abdominal pain, tachycardia, and diaphoresis), DIC, and unrecognized ectopic pregnancy can also occur. Management of uterine perforation may involve simple observation or immediate laparotomy with repair. Management depends on the suspected severity of injury to the uterus and adjacent structures.

Serious infection (e.g., **septic abortion**) complicates approximately 1 of 200,000 spontaneous abortions. Serious infection occurs more commonly after induced abortion, particularly illegal abortion.[51,54] Septic abortion causes significant morbidity and is life threatening. Blood cultures should be ordered, and broad-spectrum intravenous antibiotics should be promptly administered. Patients with hemodynamic instability may require invasive hemodynamic monitoring to guide fluid, blood, and vasoactive drug therapy. Lower genital tract or bowel injury should be excluded, and the uterus should be promptly reevacuated. On occasion, hysterectomy is necessary and may be lifesaving.

If the mother who aborts is Rh negative, $Rh_0(D)$ immune globulin (e.g., anti-D immune globulin) is administered to prevent Rh sensitization.[53] In the past, some obstetricians did not administer $Rh_0(D)$ immune globulin to Rh-negative women with threatened abortion. However, Von Stein et al.[55] demonstrated a positive Kleihauer-Betke test result (which indicates transplacental hemorrhage of fetal blood into the maternal circulation) in 11% of patients with threatened abortion. Therefore Rh-negative women with a threatened abortion should receive $Rh_0(D)$-immune globulin.

Women who suffer spontaneous abortion are at increased risk for depressive disorders during the 6 months after miscarriage.[56]

Anesthetic Management

Several anesthetic techniques are appropriate for a D and E procedure (Box 16-2). The choice depends on several factors (e.g., whether the cervix is dilated, the presence of significant blood loss, sepsis, full stomach, the emotional state of the patient). Dilation of the cervix is relatively painful, whereas suction and curettage are less painful. If the cervix is dilated, sedation with or without a paracervical block may suffice. Because spontaneous abortion is emotionally upsetting for many women, some patients prefer general anesthesia. If the cervix is not dilated, anesthesia is usually necessary. It may be accomplished with a paracervical block and sedation, or with spinal, epidural, or general anesthesia. Sensory blockade to T10 is necessary for neuraxial anesthesia.

Typically the cervix is already dilated in patients who have had significant preoperative bleeding. Rarely does a patient with a closed cervix have significant bleeding. In the presence of significant bleeding, restoration of intravascular volume before induction of anesthesia is appropriate. A paracervical block and sedation may then provide adequate analgesia. If a patient has significant discomfort after a paracervical block, general anesthesia is preferred. Substantial hemorrhage represents a relative contraindication to the use of spinal or epidural anesthesia. It is also probably best to avoid spinal or epidural anesthesia in patients with evidence of frank sepsis.

Propofol, thiopental, ketamine, or etomidate can be administered for the induction of general anesthesia. Ketamine may be an ideal agent for induction of general anesthesia in patients with significant bleeding. Large doses (1.5 to 2.0 mg/kg) of ketamine increase uterine tone,[57] which may be advantageous in patients who require evacuation of the uterus.

Drugs commonly administered for general anesthesia may influence blood loss during the procedure. The volatile anesthetic agents produce dose-dependent relaxation of uterine smooth muscle[58] and have been associated with increased uterine bleeding.[59,60] Two studies compared blood loss during elective first-trimester abortion in patients who received either propofol or isoflurane for maintenance of general anesthesia.[59,60] In both studies blood loss was greater in the isoflurane group. The differences in blood loss, however, may not be clinically significant in view of the blood volume expansion that occurs during pregnancy. Some obstetricians contend that relaxation of the uterus with a volatile anesthetic agent increases the risk of uterine perforation and prefer to avoid the administration of a volatile agent during D and E procedures.

General anesthesia is commonly maintained with oxygen, nitrous oxide, and an opioid (with or without a small dose of benzodiazepine). A propofol infusion or a low concentration (less than 0.5 MAC) of a volatile agent may be added. The volatile agent should be avoided or discontinued if there is any evidence of uterine atony. In most cases, oxytocin (20 U/L of crystalloid) is administered intravenously to increase uterine tone and decrease blood loss.

BOX 16-2 Suggested Anesthetic Techniques for Dilation and Uterine Evacuation for Spontaneous Abortion

General Considerations

- Blood typing and antibody screening or typing and crossmatching in patients with a large blood loss or those with advanced gestation
- Aspiration prophylaxis if patient has a full stomach
- Routine noninvasive monitors (electrocardiogram, blood pressure cuff, pulse oximeter, temperature probe, and nerve stimulator [general anesthesia])
- One peripheral intravenous catheter with crystalloid solution
- Neuraxial (spinal or epidural) anesthesia for hemodynamically stable patients without sepsis:
  - Prehydration with 1000 mL of crystalloid solution, supplemental oxygen, and minimal sedation with midazolam, opioid, and/or propofol
- Oxytocin and/or an ergot alkaloid available
- In patients with significant blood loss: observation of the patient on the operating table for evidence of hypotension for at least 5 minutes after the legs have been lowered from the lithotomy to the supine position

Monitored Anesthesia Care (Well Tolerated When the Cervix Is Dilated)

- Intravenous analgesia with fentanyl or alfentanil and sedation with midazolam or propofol
- Paracervical block if needed

Spinal Anesthesia

- Single injection with a small-gauge spinal needle: lidocaine 40 mg or bupivacaine 7.5 mg with fentanyl 20 μg, to achieve T8 to T10 sensory blockade

Epidural Anesthesia

- Placement of midlumbar epidural needle and catheter
- Lidocaine 2% with epinephrine 5 μg/mL, approximately 12 to 15 mL, and fentanyl 100 μg, injected incrementally, to achieve T8 to T10 cephalad to S4 caudad sensory blockade

General Anesthesia

- Rapid-sequence induction with cricoid pressure if the patient has a full stomach
- Induction: thiopental or propofol (ketamine or etomidate in cases of severe hemorrhage)
- Mask anesthesia or laryngeal mask airway during early pregnancy if stomach is empty and the patient is hemodynamically stable; otherwise endotracheal intubation with a muscle relaxant
- End-tidal carbon dioxide monitoring
- Maintenance: oxygen, nitrous oxide, an opioid, benzodiazepine, and/or a propofol infusion:
  - Low concentration ($<$ 0.5 MAC) of a volatile anesthetic agent may be added if there is little bleeding and no evidence of uterine atony
- Placement of an oral gastric tube (if trachea is intubated), performance of suctioning, and removal of tube
- Extubation when the patient is awake and responds to verbal commands

The D and E procedure is performed with the patient in the lithotomy position. After the procedure is completed, the patient's legs are lowered to the supine position. Hypotension may develop in patients who have lost a significant amount of blood during the procedure (especially if a spinal or epidural block was also performed).

CERVICAL INSUFFICIENCY OR INCOMPETENCE

An inherent or traumatic deficiency in the structure or function of the uterine cervix results in **cervical insufficiency or incompetence,** which is defined as the inability to sustain a pregnancy to full term. Cervical insufficiency is characterized by recurrent second-trimester pregnancy losses with (1) painless cervical dilation, (2) herniation followed by rupture of the fetal membranes, and (3) a short labor with delivery of a live, immature infant.

The true incidence of cervical insufficiency is difficult to determine owing to a lack of objective clinical findings and definitive diagnostic tests. The reported incidence of incompetent cervix varies from 1 in 100 to 1 in 2000.[61] The United States *National Vital Statistics Report* for 2004 cited a rate of 4.4 cervical cerclages performed per 1000 live births.[62] Lidegaard[63] reported an incidence of cervical incompetence of 4.6 women per 1000 births between 1980 and 1990 in Denmark.

Potential etiologies of cervical insufficiency include cervical trauma, congenital abnormalities, intrauterine infection, deficiencies in cervical collagen and elastin, and hormonal abnormalities.[64] A common cause of cervical insufficiency is trauma, occurring at the time of a previous vaginal delivery or a surgical procedure (e.g., dilation and curettage, conization of the cervix, partial amputation or resection of the cervix, cervical cauterization). Congenital abnormalities of the reproductive tract (e.g., unicornuate or bicornuate uterus) may be present in as many as 2% of patients with cervical insufficiency. Some anomalies may result from maternal exposure to diethylstilbestrol *in utero*. A study by Warren et al.[65] found that more than 25% of women with the diagnosis of cervical insufficiency have a positive family history of cervical insufficiency as well as a higher frequency of two genes associated with abnormalities of connective tissue, collagen, and extracellular matrix.

Diagnosis

Cervical insufficiency remains a clinical diagnosis. A definitive diagnosis is made when herniating fetal membranes are visualized or palpated through a partially dilated cervix during the second trimester of the current pregnancy. A characteristic history from a previous pregnancy allows the presumptive diagnosis of cervical insufficiency, once other causes of recurrent pregnancy loss are excluded. History suggestive of the diagnosis of cervical insufficiency consists of two or more second-trimester pregnancy losses, loss of each successive pregnancy at an earlier gestational age, painless cervical dilation to 4 to 6 cm, and cervical trauma or anomaly.[66] Uterine contractions, vaginal bleeding, or chorioamnionitis during a previous pregnancy suggests that other mechanisms are responsible for pregnancy loss.

Symptoms of cervical insufficiency include increased vaginal discharge, lower abdominal or back pressure or discomfort, vaginal fullness, and urinary frequency.

A higher risk of preterm birth has been associated with shortened cervical length at early gestational age.[67,68] Physical examination may reveal cervical shortening and/or cervical abnormalities. Serial ultrasonographic evaluations of cervical length and dilation should be considered in the early second trimester for pregnant women at high risk for cervical insufficiency, although clinical trials of this assessment modality have reported varying results.[66,69,70]

Obstetric Management

Management of cervical insufficiency is controversial, and large, well-controlled studies are lacking.[64] Despite the absence of conclusive evidence of its efficacy, many patients with a diagnosis of cervical insufficiency undergo surgical reinforcement of the cervix with a cervical cerclage. Berghella et al.,[71] performing a meta-analysis of studies, concluded that cerclage does not prevent preterm birth in all women and can actually be detrimental in multifetal pregnancies. However, the subgroup of women with a singleton pregnancy, a short cervix, and a history of cervical insufficiency may benefit from cerclage placement.[64,68]

The most commonly performed cerclage procedures are the modified **Shirodkar cerclage**[72] and the **McDonald cerclage**.[73] Both of these procedures are performed transvaginally. A ligature (e.g., polyester fiber [Mersilene] tape) is placed around the cervix at or near the level of the internal cervical os. In the more invasive modified Shirodkar procedure, the cervical mucosa is incised anteriorly and posteriorly, the bladder may be advanced, the ligature is placed submucosally and then tied, and the mucosal incisions are closed. The cervical mucosa is left intact with the McDonald cerclage; a purse-string ligature is placed around the cervix and then tied (Figure 16-2).[61] These two procedures result in comparable rates of fetal survival in patients with no history of prior cerclage.[74] In one study, better outcome (i.e., more advanced gestational age) was obtained when a Shirodkar cerclage was performed in patients who had a previous cerclage.[75]

Transvaginal cerclage can be performed in most patients with an incompetent cervix. However, if no substantial cervical tissue is present (e.g., severe cervical laceration, congenital or traumatic cervical shortening) or if a previous transvaginal cerclage has failed, a **transabdominal cerclage** may be performed.[76] The transabdominal cerclage can be performed before or during pregnancy. Although a posterior colpotomy and division of the transabdominal cerclage occasionally are performed in an attempt to allow vaginal delivery, most patients with transabdominal cerclage undergo cesarean delivery. The transabdominal cerclage can remain *in situ* if further pregnancies are desired, or it can be removed at the time of cesarean delivery.[77]

The efficacy of perioperative antibiotics, tocolytic drugs, and/or progesterone drugs has not been confirmed; obstetricians may choose to use one or more of these drugs.[66,75,77,78]

Contraindications to a cerclage procedure include preterm labor, vaginal bleeding, fetal anomalies, fetal death, rupture of membranes, placental abruption, and chorioamnionitis. Some obstetricians obtain specimens for culture of the amniotic fluid and/or cervix prior to placement of a cerclage.

A cerclage can be performed (1) **prophylactically** before or during pregnancy (interval or primary cerclage), (2) **therapeutically** when cervical changes are noted in the current pregnancy (secondary cerclage), or (3) **emergently** in patients with marked cervical changes, including membrane exposure to the vaginal milieu (tertiary cerclage).[79]

An interval cerclage may raise the risk of infertility and may not allow easy evacuation of the uterus in the case of a first-trimester spontaneous abortion. Because prophylactic cerclage is more effective than emergency cerclage (fetal survival is 78% to 87% versus 42% to 68%, respectively),[80,81] most obstetricians perform prophylactic cerclage in the at-risk patient at 12 to 18 weeks' gestation, once fetal viability is established. A cervical dilation of 2 cm or more is associated with a greater risk of premature rupture of membranes and/or preterm delivery.[75]

The greatest risk during the performance of emergency cerclage is rupture of the membranes. Several techniques have been described to facilitate replacement of the bulging fetal membranes into the uterus. Uterine relaxation is essential. One option is to administer a volatile anesthetic agent. Alternatively, a tocolytic drug (e.g., terbutaline)

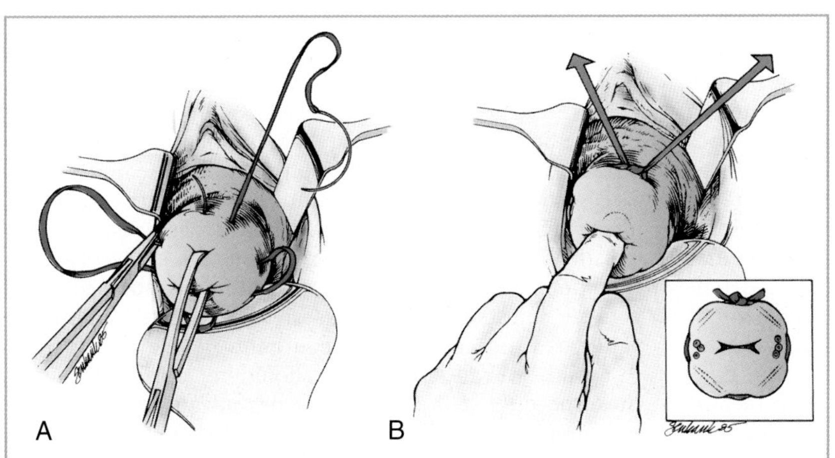

FIGURE 16-2 Placement of sutures for McDonald cervical cerclage. **A,** A double-headed polyester fiber (Mersilene) band with four "bites" is placed in the cervix, avoiding the vessels. **B,** The suture is placed high up on the cervix, close to the cervical-vaginal junction, approximately at the level of the internal os. (Modified from Iams JD. Preterm birth. In Gabbe SG, Niebyl JR, Simpson JL, editors. Obstetrics: Normal and Problem Pregnancies. 4th edition. New York, Churchill Livingstone, 2002:803.)

may be administered. Use of the steep Trendelenburg position allows for gravity assistance.

To assist in reduction of herniated membranes, some obstetricians fill the urinary bladder with sterile saline. Insertion of a 16-mm Foley catheter (with the tip removed) into the cervical canal with subsequent inflation of the balloon with 30 to 60 mL of saline has also been described.[82] The balloon is deflated and the catheter is removed at the end of the procedure.

Immediate complications of cervical cerclage include rupture of the fetal membranes, hemorrhage, and preterm labor. Delayed complications include infection, cervical stenosis secondary to scarring, and cervical lacerations and uterine rupture if labor proceeds with the cerclage in place. Rarely, sepsis may result in maternal mortality. Overall, patients who have had a cerclage have a higher rate of cesarean delivery. The Shirodkar procedure is associated with an almost twofold higher rate of cesarean delivery than McDonald cerclage (31% versus 17%, respectively).[75]

Anesthetic Management

Transvaginal cervical cerclage is usually performed with spinal, epidural, or general anesthesia (Box 16-3). The degree of cervical dilation may influence the choice of anesthesia. If the cervix is not dilated, spinal, epidural, or general anesthesia may be administered. McCulloch et al.[83] described the use of pudendal nerve block for performance of McDonald cerclage; however, pudendal block may not provide adequate anesthesia for many patients. Either spinal or epidural anesthesia is an excellent choice for performance of prophylactic cerclage. Spinal anesthesia results in a rapid, predictable onset of sacral anesthesia, which is desirable for these procedures. Sensory blockade from T10 through the sacral dermatomes is necessary, because both the cervix (L1 to T10) and vagina and perineum (S2 to S4) require anesthesia.

If the cervix is dilated—and especially if the fetal membranes are bulging—the choice of anesthesia is less straightforward. The advantages and disadvantages of each anesthetic technique must be weighed carefully. It is important to produce adequate analgesia for the mother and to prevent an increase in intra-abdominal and intrauterine pressure that may lead to further bulging and possible rupture of the fetal membranes, with subsequent fetal death. General anesthesia may be preferred in the patient with a dilated cervix and bulging fetal membranes. Administration of a volatile anesthetic agent such as isoflurane or sevoflurane relaxes uterine smooth muscle and results in a decrease in intrauterine pressure. A decrease in intrauterine pressure facilitates replacement of the bulging membranes and placement of the cerclage. On occasion, an amniocentesis may be performed before or during a cerclage procedure in an attempt to decrease intrauterine pressure and facilitate reduction of the fetal membranes. During induction and maintenance of general anesthesia, it is important to avoid endotracheal tube–induced coughing, which might raise intrauterine pressure. In addition, vomiting significantly raises intrauterine pressure. Administration of neuraxial anesthesia obviates the need for endotracheal intubation and the possibility of coughing on the endotracheal tube. However, some physicians worry that the acute dorsiflexion needed during initiation of the neuraxial blockade may raise intrauterine pressure.

BOX 16-3 Suggested Anesthetic Techniques for Transvaginal Cervical Cerclage

General Considerations

- Aspiration prophylaxis if patient has a full stomach
- Routine noninvasive monitors (electrocardiogram, blood pressure cuff, pulse oximeter, temperature probe, and nerve stimulator [for general anesthesia])
- One peripheral intravenous catheter with crystalloid solution
- Neuraxial anesthesia (spinal or epidural): prehydration with 1000 mL of crystalloid solution:
  - Supplemental oxygen and minimal sedation with midazolam, opioid, and/or propofol
- Left uterine displacement if the pregnancy is greater than 18 to 20 weeks' gestation
- Consideration of fetal heart rate (FHR) monitoring:
  - $<$ 24 weeks' gestation: FHR checked before and after procedure
  - $>$ 24 weeks' gestation: continuous FHR monitoring during and after the procedure

Spinal Anesthesia

- Single injection with a small-gauge spinal needle: lidocaine 40 mg or bupivacaine 7.5 mg with fentanyl 20 μg, to achieve T8 to T10 sensory blockade

Epidural Anesthesia

- Placement of midlumbar epidural needle and catheter
- Lidocaine 2% with epinephrine 5 μg/mL, approximately 12 to 15 mL, and fentanyl 100 μg, injected incrementally, to achieve T8 to T10 cephalad to S4 caudad sensory blockade

General Anesthesia (If Cervix Is Dilated and Uterine Relaxation Is Needed)

- Induction: thiopental or propofol
- Intubation preferable in patient with a full stomach or pregnancy greater than 18 to 20 weeks' gestation; otherwise, mask anesthesia or laryngeal mask airway acceptable
- End-tidal carbon dioxide monitoring
- Maintenance: oxygen, nitrous oxide, and a volatile anesthetic agent to provide uterine relaxation
- Avoidance of large increases in intra-abdominal and intrauterine pressures (e.g., patient coughing on endotracheal tube, vomiting)

Few clinical studies have compared obstetric outcomes after administration of neuraxial anesthesia and general anesthesia for cerclage. One retrospective study observed no difference in fetal outcome after administration of either general anesthesia (375 cases) or epidural anesthesia (114 cases) for cerclage procedures.[84]

Fetal heart rate monitoring should be considered during the procedure if the pregnancy has advanced enough for easy monitoring. In theory, it is possible that replacement of bulging membranes and closure of the cervix may raise intrauterine pressure with a subsequent reduction in placental blood flow. In this case, it would be reasonable to give a tocolytic agent to help reduce intrauterine pressure.

The transvaginal cerclage is removed at 37 to 38 weeks' gestation. The suture is removed earlier if rupture of membranes occurs or if labor begins. Removal of a McDonald cerclage often requires no anesthesia. Anesthesia (e.g., paracervical block, spinal anesthesia, epidural anesthesia) is usually necessary for removal of a Shirodkar cerclage. If the Shirodkar cerclage is epithelialized, some obstetricians elect to leave it intact and perform an elective cesarean delivery.

Labor often begins within a few hours or days after suture removal. If an epidural catheter was placed for cerclage removal, the epidural anesthetic can be allowed to regress while the patient is observed for evidence of cervical dilation and the onset of labor. When labor begins, the epidural labor analgesia can be initiated by means of the *in situ* catheter.

GESTATIONAL TROPHOBLASTIC DISEASE

In normal pregnancies, trophoblastic tissue forms the placenta. Abnormal trophoblastic proliferation results in gestational trophoblastic disease (GTD). The classification and terminology applied to GTD have varied and can be confusing. GTD can be divided into two main groups, **hydatidiform mole** and malignant **gestational trophoblastic neoplasia** (GTN). These two groups can be further classified both histologically and clinically (Box 16-4).

The reported incidence of hydatidiform mole varies. In the United States, hydatidiform mole is detected in 1 of 600 elective abortions and in 1 of 1500 pregnancies. Rates of 1 in 400 pregnancies are reported in Korea and Indonesia as well as among Native Americans.[85-87] Coexistence of a fetus with complete or partial molar components is extremely rare, occurring in 1 of 22,000 to 1 of 100,000 pregnancies.[87]

BOX 16-4 Classifications of Gestational Trophoblastic Disease

Histologic Classification

Hydatidiform mole:
- Complete
- Partial

Malignant gestational trophoblastic neoplasia (GTN):
- Postmolar GTN
  - Noninvasive trophoblastic proliferation
  - Invasive mole or chorioadenoma destruens
  - Gestational choriocarcinoma
  - Placental site trophoblastic tumor
- Gestational choriocarcinoma
- Placental site trophoblastic tumor

Clinical Classification

Hydatidiform mole:
- Complete
- Partial

Malignant gestational trophoblastic neoplasia (GTN):
- Nonmetastatic GTN
- Metastatic GTN:
  - Low risk
  - High risk
- Placental site trophoblastic tumor

Prior to 1970, most cases of GTN were fatal. Early diagnosis and effective chemotherapy have reduced the mortality of GTN to 0.1% in Britain and the Netherlands and to 1% in the United States.[85,88] Gestational trophoblastic disease caused 0.3% of all pregnancy-related maternal deaths in the United States between 1991 and 1999.[9] Risk factors for GTD include advanced maternal age, very young maternal age, history of previous molar pregnancy, and, possibly, nutritional factors.[89]

Etiology

Complete hydatidiform moles are derived solely from the paternal chromosomes. An ovum lacking its maternal chromosomal complement is fertilized most commonly by one sperm (46,XX androgenic) with reduplication, or by two sperm (dispermy, 46,XX or 46,XY androgenic). No fetus develops. Approximately 90% of hydatidiform moles are complete and are not associated with fetal tissue.[90]

Partial hydatidiform moles usually have complete trisomy with 69,XXX or 69,XXY. One set of haploid chromosomes are maternal, and there is either reduplication of the paternal donation after fertilization by a single sperm or dispermy. Partial moles are often focal and have associated fetal tissue. Patients with partial mole usually have a preoperative diagnosis of incomplete or missed abortion. Only 5% of partial moles are diagnosed before evacuation.[91]

Complete molar pregnancies have a higher rate of associated complications and a higher rate of subsequent malignant GTN than partial molar pregnancies. Approximately 20% of patients with complete molar pregnancy have postmolar nonmetastatic GTN (70% to 90%) or malignant GTN (10% to 30%) and require chemotherapy; in contrast, only 5% of patients with partial molar pregnancy require chemotherapy.[89,92-95]

Clinical Presentation and Diagnosis

HYDATIDIFORM MOLE

Clinically, patients with a complete molar pregnancy present with vaginal bleeding after delayed menses, suggestive of a threatened, missed, or incomplete abortion.[89,92,96] They may spontaneously pass hydropic vesicles. The absence of fetal cardiac activity, a uterus large for gestational age, and a marked elevation of beta-hCG concentration strongly suggest the diagnosis of hydatidiform mole. Large ovarian cysts, hyperemesis gravidarum, and early onset of pregnancy-induced hypertension (PIH) are also strongly suggestive of GTD. Ultrasonography may show characteristic multiechogenic regions that represent hydropic villi or hemorrhagic foci.

Increasingly, the diagnosis of hydatidiform mole is made after dilation and curettage for an incomplete abortion.[87] Baseline chest radiography and quantitative beta-hCG levels should be obtained promptly after surgery in such cases.

Molar pregnancies produce hCG in amounts proportional to the neoplastic volume.[96] Excessive uterine size is associated with a marked elevation of serum beta-hCG concentration (greater than 100,000 mIU/mL) secondary to a large tumor volume.

TABLE 16-1 Complications of Complete Molar Pregnancies

Complication	Incidence (%)
Excessive uterine size	30-53
Ovarian theca-lutein cysts (>6 cm)	4-50
Hyperemesis gravidarum	14-29
Pregnancy-induced hypertension	11-27
Anemia (hemoglobin <10 g/dL)	10-54
Hyperthyroidism	1-7
Trophoblastic emboli	2-7
Acute cardiopulmonary distress	6-27
Malignant sequelae (metastasis)	4-36
Other (renal, disseminated intravascular coagulation, infection)	Rare

Data from references 89, 92-96, 98-101.

Earlier diagnosis of molar pregnancy has diminished the incidence of medical complications. However, **excessive uterine size** occurs in up to half of patients with complete molar pregnancy and is associated with a higher incidence of medical complications. Medical complications occur in about 25% of patients with uterine size of more than 14 to 16 weeks' gestation; they include ovarian theca-lutein cysts, hyperemesis gravidarum, PIH, anemia, hyperthyroidism, DIC, and infection (sepsis) (Table 16-1).[86,87,89,92-96]

Ovarian theca-lutein cysts occur primarily in patients with extremely high serum beta-hCG concentrations (greater than 100,000 mIU/mL).[96] These cysts typically regress over 2 to 3 months; torsion, rupture, or infarction may rarely necessitate oophorectomy. Patients with theca-lutein cysts and a uterus more than 4 weeks larger than expected (for dates) have a 50% likelihood of development of postmolar GTN.[85]

Hyperemesis gravidarum can lead to significant electrolyte disturbances and volume depletion, all of which should be corrected before surgery.

PIH occurs in up to 27% of women with molar pregnancy. Most patients with PIH have an excessively large uterus.[95] The syndrome of PIH consists of hypertension with proteinuria, edema, and/or hyperreflexia. Although convulsions rarely occur in these patients,[96] prophylactic magnesium sulfate is administered. An antihypertensive agent (e.g., hydralazine, labetalol) is administered to reduce blood pressure. Gestational trophoblastic neoplasia should be strongly suspected in any patient who presents with PIH during early pregnancy.

Anemia frequently complicates a complete molar pregnancy. The visible vaginal bleeding may underestimate the total amount of hemorrhage. Occult bleeding into and around the tumor results in multiple hemorrhagic foci. Because blood loss may occur gradually, the patient may have a normal intravascular volume despite the presence of severe anemia. Transfusion is required in as many as 32% to 45% of patients.[92,94] Blood typing and antibody screening should be performed preoperatively.

Although it occurs infrequently, hyperthyroidism may result from a marked elevation of hCG,[97] which can have a thyrotropin-like effect. Alternatively, **hyperthyroidism** may result from some other thyrotropic substance produced by the neoplasm.[97] Anesthesia or surgery can precipitate thyroid storm (i.e., sinus tachycardia, atrial fibrillation, hyperthermia, cardiovascular collapse). A beta-adrenergic antagonist is administered to treat the cardiovascular effects of thyroid storm.

Acute cardiopulmonary distress has been observed after evacuation of molar pregnancy in as many as 27% of patients.[96,98-100] A higher risk of cardiopulmonary complications occurs in patients with a uterine size of 16 weeks or greater.[100,101] Signs and symptoms include chest pain, cough, tachycardia, tachypnea, hypoxemia, diffuse rales, and chest radiographic evidence of bilateral pulmonary infiltrates. **Trophoblastic embolization** is the etiology of cardiopulmonary distress in more than half the cases.[99,101] Other causes include (1) high-output cardiac failure from thyrotoxicosis, (2) pulmonary congestion from severe anemia, (3) PIH, (4) aspiration pneumonitis, and (5) iatrogenic fluid overload.[99,101] Symptoms usually develop within 12 hours of uterine evacuation.[99] Some patients require endotracheal intubation, mechanical ventilation, and invasive hemodynamic monitoring.[102] Symptoms usually subside within 72 hours; however, massive embolization[103] or adult respiratory distress syndrome[104] may result in death. If the patient survives trophoblastic embolization, **malignant sequelae** often develop.[89,99,104]

MALIGNANT GESTATIONAL TROPHOBLASTIC NEOPLASIA

Malignant gestational trophoblastic neoplasia can develop after any gestational event, including normal pregnancy, spontaneous or elective abortion, ectopic pregnancy, and molar pregnancy. Histologic forms of GTN that occur after molar pregnancies (postmolar GTN) include noninvasive trophoblastic proliferation, invasive mole (e.g., chorioadenoma destruens), gestational choriocarcinoma, and placental site trophoblastic tumor (PSTT). Diagnosis of postmolar GTN is made when beta-hCG levels plateau or rise.[86,87]

Signs and symptoms of malignant GTN after a nonmolar gestational event are very subtle and may delay diagnosis. A quantitative beta-hCG measurement should be performed in any patient with continued or abnormal vaginal bleeding 6 weeks after the end of gestation.

In any woman of reproductive age with metastatic disease from an unknown primary tumor, the diagnosis of gestational choriocarcinoma should be considered, given the fact that metastases of gestational choriocarcinoma can occur anywhere. The vagina, liver, lung, and brain are the most frequently involved sites.[86,87] Signs and symptoms are related to the affected site. Biopsy of metastases is rarely needed and can result in profuse bleeding. The diagnosis of metastatic GTN is suggested with a positive beta-hCG result and no pregnancy.[85-87]

With the exception of PSTT, the histologic pattern of GTN is less significant in determining clinical course and treatment response than are the stage and associated risk factors. The International Federation of Gynecology and Obstetrics updated the staging and risk-factor scoring systems for GTN in 2002 (Tables 16-2 and 16-3).[105] The identification of an individual patient's stage and risk-factor score is expressed by assigning a Roman numeral to the stage and an Arabic numeral to the risk-factor score, with the two numbers separated by a colon or a dash. Patients with a GTN risk factor score of 6 or less are considered low risk, and patients with a score of 7 or higher are considered

TABLE 16-2 International Federation of Gynecology and Obstetrics Staging of Gestational Trophoblastic Neoplasms*

Stage	Description
I	Gestational trophoblastic tumors confined strictly to the uterine corpus
II	Gestational trophoblastic tumors extending to the adnexa or vagina but limited to the genital structures
III	Gestational trophoblastic tumors extending to the lungs, with or without genital tract involvement
IV	All other metastatic sites

*The identification of an individual patient's stage and risk-factor score is expressed by assigning a Roman numeral to the stage and an Arabic numeral to the risk score, with the two numbers separated by a colon.

From Kohorn EI. Negotiating a staging and risk factor scoring system for gestational trophoblastic neoplasia: A progress report. J Reprod Med 2002; 47:445-50.

high risk. Single-agent chemotherapy is used to treat patients with low-risk GTN, and combination chemotherapy is used for those with high-risk GTN.[93] The rates of cure are nearly 100% for nonmetastatic GTN and 65% to 94% for metastatic GTN.[89,93,105] Hydatidiform mole with spontaneous resolution and PSTT are regarded as separate entities in the current staging and risk-scoring systems.

Obstetric Management

The following preoperative tests are recommended for patients with suspected hydatidiform mole: complete blood count with platelet count, clotting function studies, renal and liver function studies, blood typing and antibody screening, quantitative beta-hCG level, and chest radiography.[86,87] Prompt molar evacuation should be instituted, because a delay in uterine evacuation may raise the risk of complications. Once the patient is stabilized, suction curettage is performed to evacuate the uterus in patients who want to preserve fertility. Real-time ultrasonography may help the obstetrician perform a complete evacuation of the uterus in patients with excessive uterine size.[106] Hysterectomy is performed in patients who have completed childbearing. Hysterotomy and medical induction of labor are not recommended because they are associated with increased blood loss and a higher incidence of postmolar GTN.[86] Anti-D immune globulin should be administered to Rh-negative patients.

After uterine evacuation, the level of hCG should be measured weekly until it is undetectable for 3 weeks, then monthly for 6 months and every 2 months for another 6 months. Frequent pelvic examinations are performed while hCG levels remain high. Thorough evaluation of the patient with GTD includes screening for evidence of metastasis (e.g., vagina, liver, lung, brain) and other potential complications. Prevention of pregnancy is recommended for 12 months.[85]

Malignant GTN should be managed by an experienced team in a trophoblastic center to minimize mortality.[85-87,89] Chemotherapy is indicated in patients with (1) histologic evidence of invasive mole or choriocarcinoma; (2) a rise in beta-hCG levels of 10% or greater in three or more samples taken over at least 2 weeks; (3) a plateau of beta-hCG levels in four or more samples taken over 3 consecutive weeks; (4) persistence of measurable beta-hCG levels 6 months after molar evacuation; or (5) evidence of metastasis.[105] Some patients require delayed hysterectomy, thoracotomy for resection of pulmonary metastasis, and/or liver or brain irradiation.

TABLE 16-3 International Federation of Gynecology and Obstetrics Risk-Factor Scoring for Gestational Trophoblastic Neoplasms*

	Score			
Parameter	**0**	**1**	**2**	**4**
Age (yr)	—	≤ 39	> 39	—
Antecedent pregnancy	Hydatidiform mole	Abortion	—	Term pregnancy
Interval (mo) from index pregnancy	< 4	4-6	7-12	> 12
Pretreatment human chorionic gonadotropin (mIU/mL)	$< 10^3$	10^3-10^4	10^4-10^5	$> 10^5$
Largest tumor size, including uterus (cm)	—	3-4	5	—
Sites of metastasis	—	Spleen, kidney	Gastrointestinal tract	Brain, liver
Number of metastases identified	0	1-4	5-8	> 8
Previously failed chemotherapy	—	—	1 drug	≥ 2 drugs

*The identification of an individual patient's stage and risk-factor score is expressed by assigning a Roman numeral to the stage and an Arabic numeral to the risk score, with the two numbers separated by a colon.

Adapted from Kohorn EI. Negotiating a staging and risk factor scoring system for gestational trophoblastic neoplasia: A progress report. J Reprod Med 2002; 47:445-50.

Anesthetic Management

Preoperative assessment of the patient with a molar pregnancy consists of evaluation for specific complications of molar pregnancy, including hyperemesis gravidarum, PIH, anemia, and thyrotoxicosis. The presence of cardiopulmonary distress warrants the use of invasive hemodynamic monitoring before evacuation of the uterus.[89,99,101] Kohorn[101] recommended the preoperative assessment of arterial blood gas levels. Invasive arterial pressure and central venous pressure (CVP) or pulmonary artery catheter monitoring may also be indicated in the patient with hypoxemia, severe anemia, hemorrhage, severe PIH, hyperthyroidism, or a uterus of more than 16 weeks' size.[107] During evacuation of the uterus, blood loss may be substantial. Thus the anesthesia provider should establish adequate intravenous access (i.e., at least two large-gauge intravenous catheters), and blood products should be immediately available.

General anesthesia is preferred because of the potential for rapid, substantial blood loss during evacuation of the uterus (Box 16-5). Thiopental and propofol may cause marked hypotension in hypovolemic patients, and ketamine may result in marked tachycardia in hyperthyroid patients.[108] Thus etomidate is an excellent choice for patients with preoperative bleeding or preoperative evidence of hyperthyroidism. Maintenance of anesthesia should involve administration of oxygen, nitrous oxide, a benzodiazepine, and an opioid. It is best to avoid administration of a volatile anesthetic agent in most patients with molar pregnancy.[109]

Spinal anesthesia has been performed for a D and E procedure in a hyperthyroid patient with a hydatidiform mole, but careful attention to blood loss and the ability to rapidly transfuse the patient are essential.[110]

An intravenous oxytocin infusion (20 U/L of crystalloid) is begun either before[96,100] or during[89] uterine evacuation. Oxytocin helps the uterus contract, facilitating safe curettage and reducing blood loss. Some obstetricians have speculated that oxytocin may decrease trophoblastic embolization by constricting the uterine veins.[100] Postoperatively, the patient should be monitored closely for any evidence of uterine hemorrhage or cardiopulmonary distress.

BOX 16-5 Suggested Anesthetic Technique for Patients with Gestational Trophoblastic Neoplasm

Preoperative Evaluation

- Evaluation for complications of molar pregnancy
- Measurement of baseline arterial blood gas levels

General Anesthesia

- Routine noninvasive monitors (electrocardiogram, blood pressure cuff, pulse oximeter, temperature probe, and a nerve stimulator)
- Consideration of invasive hemodynamic monitoring in patients with hypoxemia, pregnancy-induced hypertension, severe anemia, hyperthyroidism, or a uterine size greater than 16 weeks' gestation
- Two large-gauge peripheral intravenous catheters
- Immediate availability of red blood cells
- Induction: etomidate
- Endotracheal intubation with muscle relaxant
- End-tidal carbon dioxide monitoring
- Maintenance: oxygen, nitrous oxide and an opioid, with or without a small dose of midazolam; avoidance of volatile anesthetic agents (due to increased risk of blood loss and uterine perforation)
- Oxytocin infusion (20 U/L) after cervical dilation or after partial uterine evacuation

HYPEREMESIS GRAVIDARUM

As many as 70% of women experience nausea and vomiting during pregnancy. These symptoms are often worse during the morning hours; ergo the term *morning sickness*. Symptoms typically improve or resolve by the end of the first trimester.

On rare occasions, pregnant women experience a persistent severe form of nausea and vomiting called *hyperemesis gravidarum*. These women demonstrate dehydration, ketonuria, nutritional compromise, weight loss, electrolyte abnormalities, and transient hepatic and renal dysfunction. Parenteral rehydration, correction of electrolyte abnormalities, pharmacologic antiemetic therapy, and, rarely, hyperalimentation are indicated.

Hyperemesis gravidarum may be associated with multiple gestation, thyrotoxicosis, and/or GTD. Other underlying diseases, such as hepatitis, cholecystitis, pancreatitis, pyelonephritis, and partial bowel obstruction, should be ruled out.

CORPUS LUTEUM CYSTS

Symptomatic corpus luteum cysts occasionally occur during early pregnancy. Typically, they resolve over several weeks. In some cases, hemorrhage or ovarian torsion necessitates ovarian cystectomy or oophorectomy. After the cyst is removed, the fetus usually is not affected, provided that supplemental progesterone is administered until 10 to 12 weeks' gestation.

KEY POINTS

- Aortocaval compression does not develop until the uterine fundus reaches the umbilicus (i.e., 18 to 20 weeks' gestation in a normal singleton pregnancy, or earlier in conditions with an enlarged uterus). Left uterine tilt should be initiated when the potential for aortocaval compression exists.
- General anesthesia may be administered by mask or laryngeal mask airway (LMA) for selected extra-abdominal procedures during the first 18 to 20 weeks of pregnancy, provided that the patient fulfills the criteria for an empty stomach and there is no difficulty with mask ventilation. Some anesthesiologists prefer to limit the use of mask anesthesia or the LMA to the first 12 to 14 weeks of pregnancy.

- During pregnancy, the nervous system is more sensitive to both local and general anesthetic agents. Lower doses of these drugs should be considered.
- Most ectopic pregnancies are located in one of the fallopian tubes. Ruptured tubal pregnancies, as well as interstitial, cervical, cesarean scar, and abdominal ectopic pregnancies, may result in substantial hemorrhage.
- The most painful part of a dilation and uterine evacuation procedure is the dilation of the cervix. If the cervix is already dilated, sedation (with or without paracervical block) often suffices. If the cervix is closed, either a paracervical block with sedation or neuraxial or general anesthesia may be necessary.
- Neuraxial anesthesia is an excellent choice for prophylactic cervical cerclage.
- In a patient who requires emergency cervical cerclage, it is important to prevent a marked increase in intra-abdominal and intrauterine pressures, which might cause rupture of bulging fetal membranes.
- The patient with a molar pregnancy may have hyperemesis gravidarum, pregnancy-induced hypertension, severe anemia, and/or hyperthyroidism. These complications are more common in patients with excessive uterine size.
- Signs and symptoms of acute cardiopulmonary distress develop after uterine evacuation in as many as 27% of patients with molar pregnancy.

REFERENCES

1. Crapo RO. Normal cardiopulmonary physiology during pregnancy. Clin Obstet Gynecol 1996; 39:3-16.
2. Marx GF. Aortocaval compression syndrome: Its 50-year history. Int J Obstet Anesth 1992; 1:60-4.
3. Lund CJ, Donovan JC. Blood volume during pregnancy: Significance of plasma and red cell volumes. Am J Obstet Gynecol 1967; 98:394-403.
4. Wyner J, Cohen SE. Gastric volume in early pregnancy: Effect of metoclopramide. Anesthesiology 1982; 57:209-12.
5. Vanner RG. Gastro-oesophageal reflux and regurgitation during general anaesthesia for termination of pregnancy. Int J Obstet Anesth 1992; 1:123-8.
6. Walker JJ. Ectopic pregnancy. Clin Obstet Gynecol 2007; 50:89-99.
7. Minino AM, Heron MP, Murphy SL, Kochanek KD. Deaths: Final data for 2004. Natl Vital Stat Rep 2007; 55:1-119.
8. Anderson FW, Hogan JG, Ansbacher R. Sudden death: Ectopic pregnancy mortality. Obstet Gynecol 2004; 103:1218-23.
9. Chang J, Elam-Evans LD, Berg CJ, et al. Pregnancy-related mortality surveillance—United States, 1991-1999. MMWR Surveill Summ 2003; 52:1-8.
10. Carson SA, Buster JE. Ectopic pregnancy. N Engl J Med 1993; 329:1174-81.
11. Goldner TE, Lawson HW, Xia Z, Atrash HK. Surveillance for ectopic pregnancy—United States, 1970-1989. MMWR CDC Surveill Summ 1993; 42:73-85.
12. Why Mothers Die: 2000-2002: The Sixth Report of the Confidential Enquiries into Maternal Deaths in the United Kingdom. National Institute of Clinical Excellence: Confidential Enquiry into Maternal and Child Health 2004. National Library Report No. 101245557. Available from: http://www.cemach.org.uk/Publications/Saving-Mothers-Lives-Report-2000-2002.aspx.
13. Clayton HB, Schieve LA, Peterson HB, et al. Ectopic pregnancy risk with assisted reproductive technology procedures. Obstet Gynecol 2006; 107:595-604.
14. Green LK, Kott M. Ectopic pregnancy: Clinical and pathological review of 150 cases. Tex Med 1988; 84:30-5.
15. Pisarska MD, Carson SA. Incidence and risk factors for ectopic pregnancy. Clin Obstet Gynecol 1999; 42:2-8.
16. Sowter MC, Farquhar CM. Ectopic pregnancy: An update. Curr Opin Obstet Gynecol 2004; 16:289-93.
17. Cunningham FG, Leveno KJ, Bloom SL, et al. William's Obstetrics. 22nd edition. New York, McGraw-Hill, 2005:253-72.
18. Levine D. Ectopic pregnancy. Radiology 2007; 245:385-97.
19. Fossum GT, Davajan V, Kletzky OA. Early detection of pregnancy with transvaginal ultrasound. Fertil Steril 1988; 49:788-91.
20. Seeber BE, Barnhart KT. Suspected ectopic pregnancy. Obstet Gynecol 2006; 107:399-413.
21. Stovall TG, Ling FW, Carson SA, Buster JE. Serum progesterone and uterine curettage in differential diagnosis of ectopic pregnancy. Fertil Steril 1992; 57:456-7.
22. McCord ML, Muram D, Buster JE, et al. Single serum progesterone as a screen for ectopic pregnancy: Exchanging specificity and sensitivity to obtain optimal test performance. Fertil Steril 1996; 66:513-6.
23. Gelder MS, Boots LR, Younger JB. Use of a single random serum progesterone value as a diagnostic aid for ectopic pregnancy. Fertil Steril 1991; 55:497-500.
24. Medical management of tubal pregnancy. ACOG Practice Bulletin No. 3. Washington, DC, ACOG, December 1998.
25. Pouly JL, Mahnes H, Mage G, et al. Conservative laparoscopic treatment of 321 ectopic pregnancies. Fertil Steril 1986; 46:1093-7.
26. Bangsgaard N, Lund CO, Ottesen B, Nilas L. Improved fertility following conservative surgical treatment of ectopic pregnancy. Br J Obstet Gynaecol 2003; 110:765-70.
27. Kirk E, Condous G, Haider Z, et al. The conservative management of cervical ectopic pregnancies. Ultrasound Obstet Gynecol 2006; 27:430-7.
28. Rotas MA, Haberman S, Levgur M. Cesarean scar ectopic pregnancies: Etiology, diagnosis, and management. Obstet Gynecol 2006; 107:1373-81.
29. Jurkovic D, Hillaby K, Woelfer B, et al. First-trimester diagnosis and management of pregnancies implanted into the lower uterine segment Cesarean section scar. Ultrasound Obstet Gynecol 2003; 21:220-7.
30. Atrash HK, Friede A, Hogue CJ. Abdominal pregnancy in the United States: Frequency and maternal mortality. Obstet Gynecol 1987; 69:333-7.
31. Stevens CA. Malformations and deformations in abdominal pregnancy. Am J Med Genet 1993; 47:1189-95.
32. Naim N, Ahmad S, Siraj HH, et al. Advanced abdominal pregnancy resulting from late uterine rupture. Obstet Gynecol 2008; 111:502-4.
33. Reece EA, Petrie RH, Sirmans MF, et al. Combined intrauterine and extrauterine gestations: A review. Am J Obstet Gynecol 1983; 146: 323-30.
34. Glassner MJ, Aron E, Eskin BA. Ovulation induction with clomiphene and the rise in heterotopic pregnancies: A report of two cases. J Reprod Med 1990; 35:175-8.
35. Barrenetxea G, Barinaga-Rementeria L, Lopez de Larruzea A, et al. Heterotopic pregnancy: Two cases and a comparative review. Fertil Steril 2007; 87:417. e9-15.
36. Lewin A, Simon A, Rabinowitz R, Schenker JG. Second-trimester heterotopic pregnancy after in vitro fertilization and embryo transfer: A case report and review of the literature. Int J Fertil 1991; 36:227-30.
37. Goldstein JS, Ratts VS, Philpott T, Dahan MH. Risk of surgery after use of potassium chloride for treatment of heterotopic pregnancy. Obstet Gynecol 2006; 107:506-8.
38. Chantigian RC, Chantigian PDM. Anesthesia for laparoscopy. In Corfman RS, Diamond MP, DeCherney A, editors. Complications of Laparoscopy and Hysteroscopy. 2nd edition. Boston, Blackwell Scientific Publications, 1997:5-13.

39. Brenner PF, Roy S, Mishell DR Jr. Ectopic pregnancy: A study of 300 consecutive surgically treated cases. JAMA 1980; 243:673-6.
40. Selo-Ojeme DO, Feyi-Waboso PA. Salvage autotransfusion versus homologous blood transfusion for ruptured ectopic pregnancy. Int J Gynaecol Obstet 2007; 96:108-11.
41. Strauss LT, Gamble SB, Parker WY, et al; Centers for Disease Control and Prevention (CDC). Abortion surveillance—United States 2004. MMWR Morb Mortal Wkly Rep 2007; 56:1-33.
42. Hutchon DJ. Understanding miscarriage or insensitive abortion: Time for more defined terminology? Am J Obstet Gynecol 1998; 179:397-8.
43. Berg CJ, Chang J, Callaghan WM, Whitehead SJ. Pregnancy-related mortality in the United States, 1991-1997. Obstet Gynecol 2003; 101: 289-96.
44. Wilcox AJ, Weinberg CR, O'Connor JF, et al. Incidence of early loss of pregnancy. N Engl J Med 1988; 319:189-94.
45. Simpson JL, Jauniaux ERM. Pregnancy loss. In Gabbe SG, Niebyl JR, Simpson JL, editors. Obstetrics: Normal and Problem Pregnancies. 5th edition. Philadelphia, Churchill Livingstone, 2005:629.
46. Strom CM, Ginsberg N, Applebaum M, et al. Analyses of 95 first-trimester spontaneous abortions by chorionic villus sampling and karyotype. J Assist Reprod Genet 1992; 9:458-61.
47. Cunningham FG, Leveno KJ, Bloom SL, et al. William's Obstetrics. 22nd edition. New York, McGraw-Hill, 2005:231-51.
48. Occupational disease among operating room personnel: A national study. Report of an Ad Hoc Committee on the Effect of Trace Anesthetics on the Health of Operating Room Personnel, American Society of Anesthesiologists. Anesthesiology 1974; 41:321-40.
49. Tannenbaum TN, Goldberg RJ. Exposure to anesthetic gases and reproductive outcome: A review of the epidemiologic literature. J Occup Med 1985; 27:659-68.
50. McGregor DG. Occupational exposure to trace concentrations of waste anesthetic gases. Mayo Clin Proc 2000; 75:273-7.
51. Stabile I. Spontaneous abortion: A clinical perspective. Female Patient 1992; 17:14-30.
52. McNeeley SG Jr. Early abortion. In Sciarra JJ, Dilts PV Jr, editors. Gynecology and Obstetrics, vol 2. Philadelphia, JB Lippincott, 1992:1-6.
53. Stubblefield PG. Pregnancy termination. In Gabbe SG, Niebyl JR, Simpson JL, editors. Obstetrics: Normal and Problem Pregnancies. 3rd edition. New York, Churchill Livingstone, 1996:1249-78.
54. Stubblefield PG, Grimes DA. Septic abortion. N Engl J Med 1994; 331:310-4.
55. Von Stein GA, Munsick RA, Stiver K, Ryder K. Fetomaternal hemorrhage in threatened abortion. Obstet Gynecol 1992; 79:383-6.
56. Neugebauer R, Kline J, Shrout P, et al. Major depressive disorder in the 6 months after miscarriage. JAMA 1997; 277:383-8.
57. Oats JN, Vasey DP, Waldron BA. Effects of ketamine on the pregnant uterus. Br J Anaesth 1979; 51:1163-6.
58. Munson ES, Embro WJ. Enflurane, isoflurane, and halothane and isolated human uterine muscle. Anesthesiology 1977; 46:11-4.
59. Hall JE, Ng WS, Smith S. Blood loss during first trimester termination of pregnancy: Comparison of two anaesthetic techniques. Br J Anaesth 1997; 78:172-4.
60. Kumarasinghe N, Harpin R, Stewart AW. Blood loss during suction termination of pregnancy with two different anaesthetic techniques. Anaesth Intensive Care 1997; 25:48-50.
61. Ludmir J, Owen J. Cervical incompetence. In Gabbe SG, Niebyl JR, Simpson JL, editors. Obstetrics: Normal and Problem Pregnancies. Philadelphia, Churchill Livingstone, 2007:650-64.
62. Martin JA, Menacker F. Expanded health data from the new birth certificate, 2004. Natl Vital Stat Rep 2007; 55:1-22.
63. Lidegaard O. Cervical incompetence and cerclage in Denmark, 1980-1990: A register based epidemiological survey. Acta Obstet Gynecol Scand 1994; 73:35-8.
64. Romero R, Espinoza J, Erez O, Hassan S. The role of cervical cerclage in obstetric practice: Can the patient who could benefit from this procedure be identified? Am J Obstet Gynecol 2006; 194:1-9.
65. Warren JE, Silver RM, Dalton J, et al. Collagen 1[alpha]1 and transforming growth factor-beta polymorphisms in women with cervical insufficiency. Obstet Gynecol 2007; 110:619-24.
66. American College of Obstetricians and Gynecologists. Cervical insufficiency. ACOG Practice Bulletin No. 48. Washington, DC, ACOG, 2003. (Obstet Gynecol 2003; 102:1091-9.)
67. Althuisius SM, Dekker GA, Hummel P, et al. Final results of the Cervical Incompetence Prevention Randomized Cerclage Trial (CIPRACT): Therapeutic cerclage with bed rest versus bed rest alone. Am J Obstet Gynecol 2001; 185:1106-12.
68. Berghella V, Roman A, Daskalakis C, et al. Gestational age at cervical length measurement and incidence of preterm birth. Obstet Gynecol 2007; 110:311-7.
69. Golan A, Barnan R, Wexler S, et al. Incompetence of the uterine cervix. Obstet Gynecol Surv 1989; 44:96-107.
70. Andrews WW, Copper R, Hauth JC, et al. Second-trimester cervical ultrasound: Associations with increased risk for recurrent early spontaneous delivery. Obstet Gynecol 2000; 95:222-6.
71. Berghella V, Odibo AO, To MS, et al. Cerclage for short cervix on ultrasound. Meta-analysis of trials using individual patient-level data. Obstet Gynecol 2005; 106:181-9.
72. Shirodkar VN. A new method of operative treatment for habitual abortions in the second trimester of pregnancy. Antiseptic 1955; 52:229-30.
73. McDonald IA. Suture of the cervix for inevitable miscarriage. J Obstet Gynaecol Br Emp 1957; 64:346-50.
74. Odibo AO, Berghella V, To MS, et al. Shirodkar versus McDonald cerclage for the prevention of preterm birth in women with short cervical length. Am J Perinatol 2007; 24:55-60.
75. Treadwell MC, Bronsteen RA, Bottoms SF. Prognostic factors and complication rates for cervical cerclage: A review of 482 cases. Am J Obstet Gynecol 1991; 165:555-8.
76. Zaveri V, Aghajafari F, Amankwah K, Hannah M. Abdominal versus vaginal cerclage after a failed transvaginal cerclage: A systematic review. Am J Obstet Gynecol 2002; 187:868-72.
77. Craig S, Fliegner JR. Treatment of cervical incompetence by transabdominal cervicoisthmic cerclage. Aust N Z J Obstet Gynaecol 1997; 37:407-11.
78. Berghella V, Seibel-Seamon J. Contemporary use of cervical cerclage. Clin Obstet Gynecol 2007; 50:468-77.
79. Secher NJ, McCormack CD, Weber T, et al. Cervical occlusion in women with cervical insufficiency: Protocol for a randomised, controlled trial with cerclage, with and without cervical occlusion. Br J Obstet Gynaecol 2007; 114:649, e1-6.
80. Harger JH. Comparison of success and morbidity in cervical cerclage procedures. Obstet Gynecol 1980; 56:543-8.
81. Magrina JF, Kempers RD, Williams TJ. Cervical cerclage: 20 years' experience at the Mayo Clinic. Minn Med 1983; 66:599-602.
82. Rust OA, Roberts WE. Does cerclage prevent preterm birth? Obstet Gynecol Clin North Am 2005; 32:441-56.
83. McCulloch B, Bergen S, Pielet B, et al. McDonald cerclage under pudendal nerve block. Am J Obstet Gynecol 1993; 168:499-502.
84. Crawford JS, Lewis M. Nitrous oxide in early human pregnancy. Anaesthesia 1986; 41:900-5.
85. Benedet JL, Bender H, Jones H, 3rd, et al. FIGO staging classifications and clinical practice guidelines in the management of gynecologic cancers. FIGO Committee on Gynecologic Oncology. Int J Gynaecol Obstet 2000; 70:209-62.
86. Soper JT. Gestational trophoblastic disease. Obstet Gynecol 2006; 108:176-87.
87. American College of Obstetricians and Gynecologists. Diagnosis and treatment of gestational trophoblastic disease. ACOG Practice Bulletin No. 53. (Obstet Gynecol 2004; 103:1365-77.)
88. Kohorn E. Practice bulletin No. 53—Diagnosis and treatment of gestational trophoblastic disease (letter). Obstet Gynecol 2004; 104:1422.
89. Soper JT, Lewis JL Jr, Hammond CB. Gestational trophoblastic disease. In Hoskins WJ, Perez CA, Young RC, editors. Principles and Practice of Gynecologic Oncology. 2nd edition. Philadelphia, Lippincott-Raven Publishers, 1997:1039-77.
90. Jones WB, Lauersen NH. Hydatidiform mole with coexistent fetus. Am J Obstet Gynecol 1975; 122:267-72.
91. Szulman AE, Surti U. The clinicopathologic profile of the partial hydatidiform mole. Obstet Gynecol 1982; 59:597-602.

92. Beischer NA, Bettinger HF, Fortune DW, Pepperell R. Hydatidiform mole and its complications in the state of Victoria. J Obstet Gynaecol Br Commonw 1970; 77:263-76.
93. Kohorn EI. Gestational trophoblastic neoplasia and evidence-based medicine. J Reprod Med 2002; 47:427-32.
94. Schlaerth JB, Morrow CP, Montz FJ, d'Ablaing G. Initial management of hydatidiform mole. Am J Obstet Gynecol 1988; 158:1299-1306.
95. Curry SL, Hammond CB, Tyrey L, et al. Hydatidiform mole: Diagnosis, management, and long-term followup of 347 patients. Obstet Gynecol 1975; 45:1-8.
96. Berkowitz RS, Goldstein DP. Diagnosis and management of the primary hydatidiform mole. Obstet Gynecol Clin North Am 1988; 15:491-503.
97. Amir SM, Osathanondh R, Berkowitz RS, Goldstein DP. Human chorionic gonadotropin and thyroid function in patients with hydatidiform mole. Am J Obstet Gynecol 1984; 150:723-8.
98. Hammond CB. Diagnosis and management of hydatidiform mole. Postgrad Obstet Gynecol 1982; 2:106.
99. Twiggs LB, Morrow CP, Schlaerth JB. Acute pulmonary complications of molar pregnancy. Am J Obstet Gynecol 1979; 135:189-94.
100. Cotton DB, Bernstein SG, Read JA, et al. Hemodynamic observations in evacuation of molar pregnancy. Am J Obstet Gynecol 1980; 138:6-10.
101. Kohorn EI. Clinical management and the neoplastic sequelae of trophoblastic embolization associated with hydatidiform mole. Obstet Gynecol Surv 1987; 42:484-8.
102. Natonson R, Shapiro BA, Harrison RA, Stanhope RC. Massive trophoblastic embolization and PEEP therapy. Anesthesiology 1979; 51:469-71.
103. Lipp RG, Kindschi JD, Schmitz R. Death from pulmonary embolism associated with hydatidiform mole. Am J Obstet Gynecol 1962; 83:1644-7.
104. Orr JW Jr, Austin JM, Hatch KD, et al. Acute pulmonary edema associated with molar pregnancies: A high-risk factor for development of persistent trophoblastic disease. Am J Obstet Gynecol 1980; 136:412-5.
105. Kohorn EI. Negotiating a staging and risk factor scoring system for gestational trophoblastic neoplasia: A progress report. J Reprod Med 2002; 47:445-50.
106. Evers JL, Schijf CP, Kenemans P, Martin CB Jr. Real-time ultrasound as an adjunct in the operative management of hydatidiform mole. Am J Obstet Gynecol 1981; 140:469-71.
107. Kim JM, Arakawa K, McCann V. Severe hyperthyroidism associated with hydatidiform mole. Anesthesiology 1976; 44:445-8.
108. Kaplan JA, Cooperman LH. Alarming reactions to ketamine in patients taking thyroid medication—treatment with propranolol. Anesthesiology 1971; 35:229-30.
109. Ackerman WE III. Anesthetic considerations for complicated hydatidiform molar pregnancies. Anesth Rev 1984; 11:20-4.
110. Solak M, Akturk G. Spinal anesthesia in a patient with hyperthyroidism due to hydatidiform mole. Anesth Analg 1993; 77:851-2.

Chapter 17

Nonobstetric Surgery during Pregnancy

Marc Van de Velde, M.D., Ph.D.

Estimates of the frequency of nonobstetric surgery performed during pregnancy range from 0.3% to 2.2%.[1-3] Thus, as many as 87,000 and 115,000 pregnant women in the United States and the European Union, respectively, may require a surgical or anesthetic intervention each year. These figures are likely to be an underestimate, because pregnancy may be unrecognized at the time of operation. In more recent studies, 0.3% of women undergoing ambulatory surgery, 2.6% of women undergoing laparoscopic sterilization, and 1.2% of adolescents scheduled for surgery have had positive pregnancy test results when they presented for surgery.[4-6] Universal pregnancy testing, however, has generally not been recommended.[6,7] If a patient's history suggests that she could be pregnant, specific questions regarding the possibility of pregnancy should precede pregnancy testing. In certain populations, however, medical history alone may be an unreliable means of excluding the possibility of pregnancy,[5,8] and routine testing may be an appropriate option.

Surgery may be necessary during any stage of pregnancy. Among 5405 Swedish women who had operations during pregnancy, 42% occurred during the first trimester, 35% during the second trimester, and 23% during the third trimester.[1] Laparoscopy for gynecologic indications was the most common first-trimester procedure (34%), whereas appendectomy was the most common procedure during the remainder of pregnancy. Indications may be pregnancy-related or non–pregnancy-related. Indications for pregnancy-related surgery include cervical incompetence and ovarian cysts. Also, fetal surgery is performed more often today than in the past (see Chapter 7). Indications for non–pregnancy-related surgery include acute abdominal disease (most commonly appendicitis and cholecystitis), trauma, and malignancies.

When caring for pregnant women undergoing nonobstetric surgery, anesthesia providers must ensure safe anesthesia for both mother and child. Standard anesthetic procedures may have to be modified to accommodate pregnancy-induced maternal physiologic changes and the presence of the fetus. The two latest reports of the Confidential Enquiries into Maternal and Child Health in the United Kingdom clearly demonstrate that even in early pregnancy mothers die from hemorrhage, sepsis, thromboembolism, and anesthesia.[9,10] Risks to the fetus include (1) the effects of the disease process itself or of related therapy; (2) the teratogenicity of anesthetic agents or other drugs administered during the perioperative period; (3) intraoperative perturbations of uteroplacental perfusion and/or fetal oxygenation; and (4) the risk of abortion or preterm delivery.

MATERNAL SAFETY: ALTERED MATERNAL PHYSIOLOGY

During pregnancy, profound changes in maternal physiology result from increased concentrations of various hormones, mechanical effects of the gravid uterus, greater metabolic demand, and the hemodynamic consequences of the low-pressure placental circulation. Hormonal changes are likely responsible for most of the changes that occur during the first trimester. Mechanical effects become apparent when the uterus emerges from the pelvis during the second half of gestation (see Chapter 2).

Respiratory System and Acid-Base Balance Changes

Alveolar ventilation increases 25% to 30% or more by the midpoint of pregnancy. This increase results in chronic respiratory alkalosis, with a $Paco_2$ of 28 to 32 mm Hg, a slightly alkaline pH (approximately 7.44), and decreased levels of bicarbonate and buffer base. Although oxygen consumption is increased, Pao_2 usually increases only slightly or remains within the normal range. Functional residual capacity (FRC) diminishes by approximately 20% as the uterus expands, resulting in decreased oxygen reserve and the potential for airway closure. When FRC is decreased further (e.g., from morbid obesity; perioperative intra-abdominal distention; placement of the patient in the supine, Trendelenburg, or lithotomy position; or induction of anesthesia), airway closure may be sufficient to cause hypoxemia.

Weight gain during pregnancy and capillary engorgement of the respiratory tract mucosa lead to more frequent problems with mask ventilation and endotracheal intubation. Failed intubation (a leading cause of anesthesia-related maternal death) is as much a risk during early pregnancy and nonobstetric surgery as it is during cesarean delivery.[9,10]

Decreased FRC, increased oxygen consumption, and diminished buffering capacity result in the rapid development of hypoxemia and acidosis during periods of hypoventilation or apnea. Moreover, induction of inhalation anesthesia occurs more rapidly during pregnancy because alveolar hyperventilation and decreased FRC allow faster equilibration of inhaled agents. In addition, induction of anesthesia is accelerated owing to the 30% to 40% decrease in the minimum alveolar concentration (MAC) for volatile anesthetic agents that occurs even during early gestation.[11,12] The anesthesia provider must be especially vigilant when administering subanesthetic concentrations of analgesic and anesthetic agents to the pregnant patient, in whom unconsciousness can occur quickly and unexpectedly.

Cardiovascular System Changes

Cardiac output increases by up to 50% during pregnancy because of increases in heart rate and stroke volume; both systemic and pulmonary vascular resistances decrease, but myocardial contractility is unaffected. Early in pregnancy (i.e., by 6 weeks' gestation), significant cardiovascular alterations are present.[13] By 8 weeks' gestation, 57% of the increase in cardiac output, 78% of the increase in stroke volume, and 90% of the decrease in systemic vascular resistance that are typically achieved by 24 weeks' gestation have occurred.[14]

During the second half of gestation, the weight of the uterus compresses the inferior vena cava when the mother lies supine; the compression reduces venous return and cardiac output by approximately 25% to 30%. Although upper extremity blood pressure may be maintained by compensatory vasoconstriction and tachycardia, uteroplacental perfusion is jeopardized whenever the mother lies supine. Frank hypotension may also occur when the pregnant woman lies supine, especially when neuraxial or general anesthesia attenuates or abolishes normal compensatory mechanisms. For these reasons, it is essential to displace the uterus laterally during any operation performed after 18 to 20 weeks' gestation. Vena caval compression also results in distention of the epidural venous plexus, which increases the likelihood of intravascular injection of local anesthetic during the administration of epidural anesthesia. The reduced capacity of the epidural space most likely contributes to the enhanced spread of small doses of epidural local anesthetic that occurs during pregnancy.

Changes in Blood Volume and Blood Constituents

Blood volume expands in the first trimester and increases 30% to 45% by term. Dilutional anemia occurs as a result of the smaller increase in red blood cell volume than in plasma volume. Although moderate blood loss is well tolerated during pregnancy, preexisting anemia decreases the patient's reserve when significant hemorrhage occurs. Pregnancy is associated with benign leukocytosis; consequently the white blood cell count is an unreliable indicator of infection. In general, pregnancy induces a hypercoagulable state, with increases in fibrinogen; factors VII, VIII, X, and XII; and fibrin degradation products. Pregnancy is associated with enhancement of platelet turnover, clotting, and fibrinolysis, and there is a wide range in the normal platelet count; thus pregnancy represents a state of accelerated but compensated intravascular coagulation.[15] Benign thrombocytopenia is present in approximately 1% of pregnant women. These patients, however, may still be hypercoagulable.[16] During the postoperative period, pregnant surgical patients are at high risk for thromboembolic complications; thus thromboembolism prophylaxis is recommended.[17]

Gastrointestinal System Changes

Incompetence of the lower esophageal sphincter and distortion of gastric and pyloric anatomy increase the risk of gastroesophageal reflux; thus the pregnant woman is at risk for regurgitation of gastric contents and aspiration pneumonitis. It is unclear at what stage during pregnancy this risk becomes significant. Although lower esophageal sphincter tone is impaired early in pregnancy (especially in patients with heartburn),[18] the mechanically induced factors do not become relevant until later in pregnancy. It seems prudent to consider any pregnant patient as having a higher risk for aspiration after 18 to 20 weeks' gestation, and some anesthesia providers contend that pregnant women are at risk for aspiration from the beginning of the second trimester onward.[18]

Altered Responses to Anesthesia

In addition to the decrease in MAC for inhaled anesthetic agents, thiopental requirements begin to decrease early in pregnancy.[19] In contrast, propofol requirements are not reduced during early pregnancy (Figure 17-1).[20] More extensive neural blockade is attained with epidural and spinal anesthesia in pregnant patients than in nonpregnant patients. Pregnancy also enhances the response to peripheral neural blockade.

Plasma cholinesterase levels decrease by approximately 25% from early in pregnancy until the seventh postpartum day. Fortunately, prolonged neuromuscular blockade with succinylcholine is uncommon, because the larger volume available for drug distribution offsets the impact of

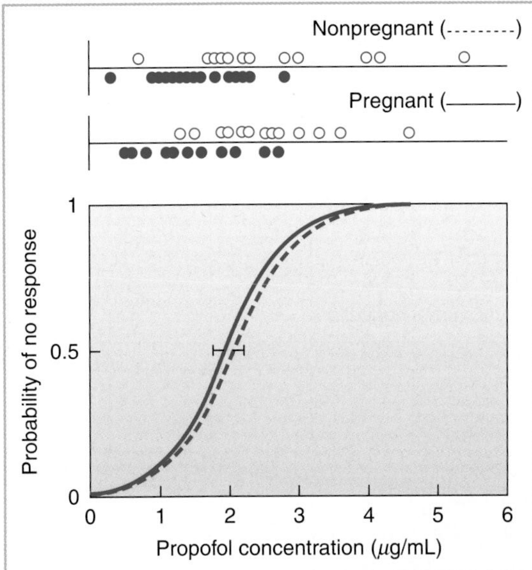

FIGURE 17-1 Relation between the serum propofol concentration and response to verbal command and tactile stimuli in nonpregnant (*top* on line graph; *dashed line* on bottom graph) and pregnant (*bottom* on line graph; *solid line* on bottom graph) women. The line graphs show the propofol serum concentration of every subject associated with a positive response (*open circles*) or negative response (*solid circles*). The concentration-effect curves were defined from the data shown in the upper diagrams of both groups using logistic regression. (Modified from Higuchi H, Adachi Y, Arimura S, et al. Early pregnancy does not reduce the C50 of propofol for loss of consciousness. Anesth Analg 2001; 93:1565-9.)

decreased drug hydrolysis.[21] Nevertheless, the dose of succinylcholine should be controlled carefully in the pregnant patient, and the anesthesia provider should monitor neuromuscular blockade with a nerve stimulator to ensure adequate reversal before extubation.

Decreased protein binding associated with low albumin concentrations during pregnancy may result in a larger fraction of unbound drug, with the potential for greater drug toxicity during pregnancy. Pregnant surgical patients may also require drugs that are used infrequently during pregnancy; little information may exist on the effects of pregnancy on the response to those drugs. Cautious administration of such agents is advisable, because their pharmacokinetic and pharmacodynamic profiles may differ from those in nonpregnant patients.

FETAL CONSIDERATIONS

Risk of Teratogenicity

Although maternal catastrophes that cause severe maternal hypoxia or hypotension pose the greatest risk to the fetus, considerable attention has focused on the role of anesthetic agents as abortifacients and teratogens. *Teratogenicity* has been defined as any significant postnatal change in function or form in an offspring after prenatal treatment. Concern about the potential harmful effects of anesthetic agents stems from their known effects on mammalian cells. These occur at clinical concentrations and include reversible decreases in cell motility, prolongation of DNA synthesis, and inhibition of cell division.[22] Despite these theoretical concerns, no data specifically link any of these cellular events with teratogenic changes. Unfortunately, prospective clinical studies of the teratogenic effects of anesthetic agents are impractical; such studies would require huge numbers of patients exposed to the drug under investigation. Therefore, investigations of anesthetic agents have taken one of the following directions: (1) studies of the reproductive effects of anesthetic agents in small animals, (2) epidemiologic surveys of operating room personnel constantly exposed to subanesthetic concentrations of inhalation agents, and (3) studies of pregnancy outcome in women who have undergone surgery while pregnant.

PRINCIPLES OF TERATOGENICITY

A number of important factors influence the teratogenic potential of a substance, including species susceptibility, dose of the substance, duration and timing of exposure, and genetic predisposition. Like other toxicologic phenomena, the effects of teratogens are dose dependent (Figure 17-2).[23] Most teratologists accept the principle

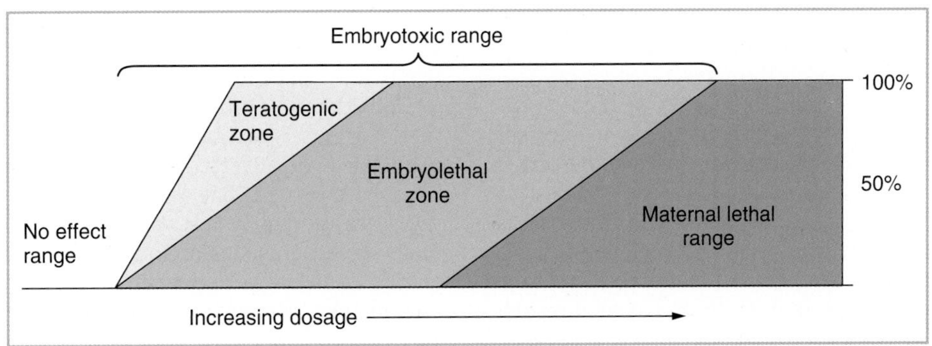

FIGURE 17-2 Toxic manifestations with increasing dosage of a teratogen. A no-effect range of dosage occurs below the threshold, at which embryotoxic effects abruptly appear. Teratogenesis and embryolethality often have similar thresholds and may increase at roughly parallel rates as dosage increases to a point at which all conceptuses are affected. Increasing dosage causes increased embryolethality, but teratogenicity appears to decrease, because many defective embryos die before term. A further increase in dosage reaches the maternal lethal range. (Modified from Wilson JG. Environment and Birth Defects. New York, Academic Press, 1973:31.)

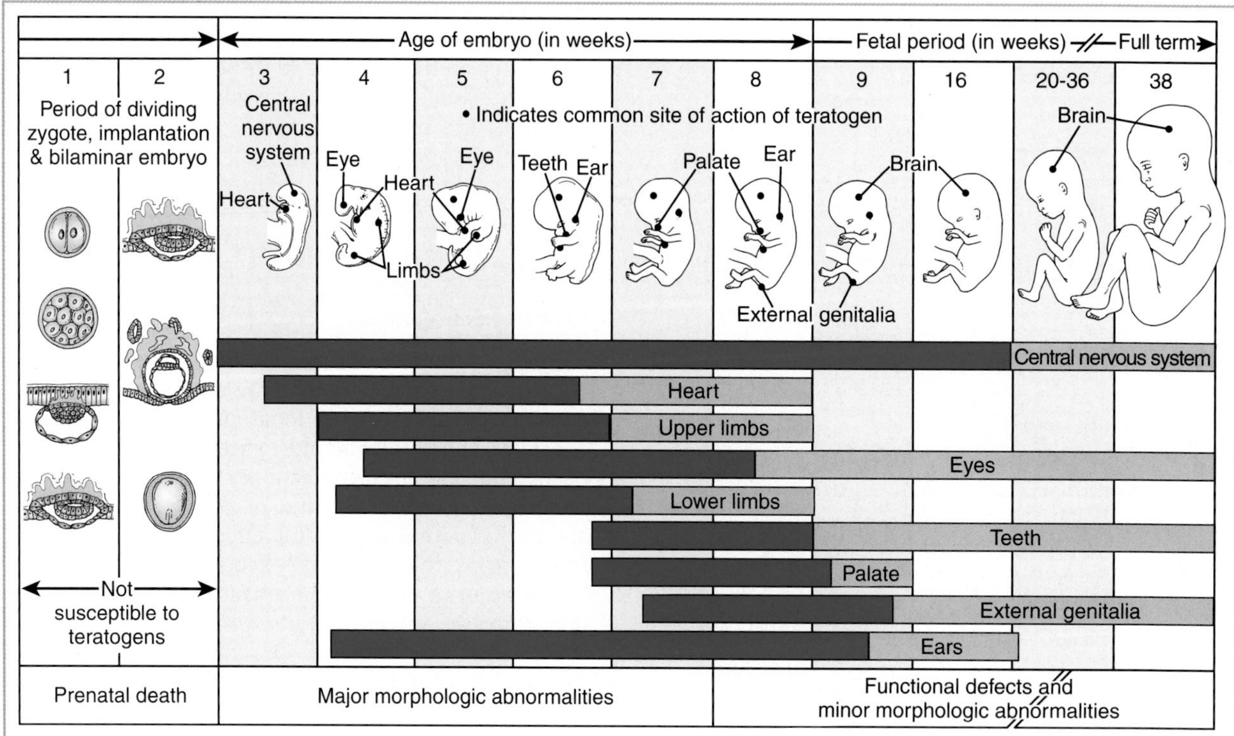

FIGURE 17-3 Critical periods in human development. During the first 2 weeks of development, the embryo typically is not susceptible to teratogens. During these predifferentiation stages, a substance either damages all or most cells of the embryo, resulting in its death, or damages only a few cells, allowing the embryo to recover without development of defects. The *dark bars* denote highly sensitive periods, whereas *light bars* indicate periods of lesser sensitivity. The ages shown refer to the actual ages of the embryo and fetus. Clinical estimates of gestational age represent intervals beginning with the first day of the last menstrual period. Because fertilization typically occurs 2 weeks after the first day of the last menstrual period, the reader should add 14 days to the ages shown here to convert to the estimated gestational ages that are used clinically. (Redrawn from Moore KL. The Developing Human. 4th edition. Philadelphia, WB Saunders, 1993:156.)

that any agent can be teratogenic in an animal provided that enough is given at the right time. Thus, the finding of teratogenesis of an agent after the single administration of a high dose or the long-term administration of a low dose does not imply that a single, short exposure (e.g., during a typical anesthetic) would incur similar risk. The interaction between dose and timing is also critical. A small dose of a teratogen may cause malformations or death in the susceptible early embryo, whereas much larger doses may prove harmless to the fetus,[23] as was shown with thalidomide. Most studies have used small animals (e.g., chick embryos, mice, rats), and their results cannot necessarily be extrapolated to other species, especially humans. Of the more than 2200 agents listed in *Shepard's Catalog of Teratogenic Agents*,[24] approximately 1200 are teratogenic in animals, but only about 30 of these are known to cause defects in humans.

Manifestations of teratogenicity include death, structural abnormality, growth restriction, and functional deficiency.[23] Depending on when it occurs, death is referred to as abortion, fetal death, or stillbirth in humans and as fetal resorption in animals. Structural abnormalities can lead to death if they are severe, although death may occur in the absence of congenital anomalies. Growth restriction is considered a manifestation of teratogenesis and may relate to multiple factors, including placental insufficiency and genetic and environmental factors. Functional deficiencies include a number of behavioral and learning abnormalities, the study of which is called *behavioral teratology*. The stage of gestation at which exposure occurs determines the target organs or tissues, the types of defects, and the severity of damage. Most structural abnormalities result from exposure during the period of organogenesis, which extends from approximately day 31 to day 71 after the first day of the last menstrual period. Figure 17-3 shows the critical stages of development and the related susceptibility of different organs to teratogens. Functional deficiencies are usually associated with exposure during late pregnancy or even after birth, because the central nervous system (CNS) continues to mature during this period.

Consideration of the possible teratogenicity of anesthetic agents must be viewed against the naturally high occurrence of adverse pregnancy outcomes. Roberts and Lowe[25] estimated that as many as 80% of human conceptions are ultimately lost; many are lost even before pregnancy is recognized. The incidence of congenital anomalies among humans is approximately 3%, most of which are unexplained. Indeed, exposure to drugs and environmental toxins accounts for only 2% to 3% of such defects (Table 17-1).[23] Shepard[24] has listed several criteria for determining that an agent is a human teratogen, including the following: (1) proven exposure to the agent at the critical time of development; (2) consistent findings in two or more high-quality epidemiologic studies; (3) careful delineation

TABLE 17-1 Etiology of Human Developmental Abnormalities

Causes of Developmental Defects in Humans	Percentage
Genetic transmission	20
Chromosomal aberration	3-5
Environmental causes:	
Radiation	<1
Infection	2-3
Maternal metabolic imbalance	1-2
Drugs and environmental chemicals	2-3
Unknown	65-70
Total	*100*

Modified from Wilson JG. Environmental and Birth Defects. New York, Academic Press, 1973:49.

of the clinical cases, ideally with the identification of a specific defect or syndrome; and (4) an association that "makes biological sense." Documentation of teratogenicity in experimental animals is important but not essential. The list of agents or factors that are proven human teratogens does not include anesthetic agents (which are listed as "unlikely teratogens") or any drug routinely used during the course of anesthesia (Box 17-1).

NONDRUG FACTORS ENCOUNTERED IN THE PERIOPERATIVE PERIOD

Anesthesia and surgery can cause derangements of maternal physiology that may result in hypoxia, hypercapnia, stress, and abnormalities of temperature and

BOX 17-1 Teratogenic Agents in Human Beings

Radiation

Atomic weapons, radioiodine, therapeutic uses

Infections

Cytomegalovirus, herpes virus hominis, parvovirus B-19, rubella virus, syphilis, toxoplasmosis, Venezuelan equine encephalitis virus

Maternal Metabolic Imbalance

Alcoholism, cretinism, diabetes, folic acid deficiency, hyperthermia, phenylketonuria, rheumatic disease and congenital heart block, virilizing tumors

Drugs and Chemicals

Aminopterin and methylaminopterin, androgenic hormones, busulphan, captopril, chlorobiphenyls, cocaine, coumarin anticoagulants, cyclophosphamide, diethylstilbestrol, diphenylhydantoin, enalapril, etretinate, iodides (goiter), lithium, mercury (organic), methimazole (scalp defects), penicillamine, 13-*cis*-retinoic acid (Accutane), tetracyclines, thalidomide, trimethadione, valproic acid

Modified from Shepard TH. Catalog of Teratogenic Agents. 7th edition. Baltimore, Johns Hopkins University Press, 1992.

carbohydrate metabolism. These states may be teratogenic themselves, or they may enhance the teratogenicity of other agents.[24,26-28] Severe hypoglycemia and prolonged hypoxia and hypercarbia have caused congenital anomalies in laboratory animals,[24,26,27] but there is no evidence to support teratogenicity after brief episodes in humans. The chronic hypoxemia experienced by mothers at high altitudes results in the delivery of infants with lower birth weights but with no increase in the rate of congenital defects.[24] Maternal stress and anxiety are teratogenic in animals,[28] but their significance as human teratogens remains questionable; supporting epidemiologic studies are lacking. Hypothermia is not teratogenic, whereas hyperthermia is teratogenic in both animals and humans.[24] Congenital anomalies, especially involving the CNS, have repeatedly been associated with maternal fever (higher than 38.9° C) during the first half of pregnancy. Embryonic oxidative stress from reactive oxygen species has been implicated as one of the mechanisms involved in teratogenicity of many agents.[29]

Ionizing radiation is also a human teratogen; potential adverse effects include an increased risk of malignant disease, genetic disease, congenital anomalies, and/or fetal death.[24,30] These effects are dose-related. The radiation dose of interest is the dose absorbed by the conceptus (not the mother). It is expressed as grays (Gy) or milligrays (mGy) (1 Gy = 100 rad). Potential adverse effects are results of the cumulative dose (i.e., background radiation and medical diagnostic radiation) during the whole of pregnancy. Background radiation during gestation is approximately 1.3 to 5.8 mGy.[30] There is no evidence that radiation exposure less than 50 mGy is associated with a teratogenic effect in either humans or animals.[30] The absorbed *fetal* dose for all conventional radiographic imaging procedures outside the abdomen and pelvis is negligible and is well below 50 mGy (Table 17-2). However, direct radiographic examination of the abdomen and pelvis (e.g., abdominal computed tomography) and abdominal imaging studies that include fluoroscopy (e.g., barium enema) may result in more significant fetal radiation exposure, with a dose that may approach 100 mGy.[30,31]

In contrast to the negligible risk of teratogenicity, observational studies suggest that there is a slightly higher risk of childhood cancer at radiation doses greater than or equal to 10 mGy.[31] The relative risk of childhood malignancy after maternal abdominal radiation exposure has been estimated to be 2.28 (95% confidence interval, 1.31 to 3.97).[30] Therefore, exposure to radiation should be minimized whenever possible during pregnancy. However, if the mother's condition necessitates diagnostic radiation and no other acceptable imaging modality is available, the benefits should be weighed against the risks. Radiation should not be withheld if the benefits to the mother (and, by extension, the fetus) are judged to outweigh the risks. In this case, the radiographer should take provisions to minimize the absorbed dose of radiation.

Diagnostic ultrasonography during pregnancy has long been considered to be devoid of embryotoxic effects. In animals, ultrasound intensities up to 20 W/cm^2 have been found to be safe.[32-34] However, when higher intensities (>30 W/cm^2) have been used, or when repeated exposure has occurred during early pregnancy, postnatal neurobehavioral effects have been described.[34,35] Ultrasound waves also increase the fetal temperature, and

TABLE 17-2 Fetal Radiation Exposure for Common Diagnostic Procedures

Procedure	Mean Exposure (mGy)	Maximum Exposure (mGy)
Conventional Radiographic Examination		
Abdomen	1.4	4.2
Chest	< 0.01	< 0.01
Intravenous urogram	1.7	10
Lumbar spine	1.7	10
Pelvis	1.1	4
Skull	< 0.01	< 0.01
Thoracic spine	< 0.01	< 0.01
Fluoroscopic Examination		
Barium meal (upper GI)	1.1	5.8
Barium enema	6.8	24
Computed Tomography		
Abdomen	8.0	49
Head	0.06	0.96
Chest	< 0.005	< 0.005
Lumbar spine	2.4	8.6
Pelvis	25	79

GI, gastrointestinal.

From Valentin J. Pregnancy and medical radiation. ICRP Publication 84. Ann ICRP 2000; 30:1-43.

hyperthermia is a known teratogen. Modern diagnostic ultrasound equipment is capable of inducing significant increases in temperature, especially when imaging is prolonged. Miller et al.[36] concluded that these temperature increments were within the range of temperatures that could be teratogenic. Epidemiologic human data are reassuring; however, it must be stressed that these epidemiologic studies were conducted in an era when ultrasound equipment was less potent and ultrasound-related increases in temperature were lower.

Some investigators have described teratogenic effects of magnetic resonance imaging (MRI) in rats.[37,38] However, later work in human fetal fibroblast cultures, exposed for a period of 24 hours to a magnetic field, demonstrated no effects on cell proliferation.[39] No adverse effects on pregnancy and neonatal outcome were noted in a small series of pregnant patients (n = 26) exposed to gadolinium (paramagnetic contrast medium).[40]

SYSTEMIC AGENTS

Animal Studies

Early studies documented teratogenicity after a variety of neurotropic agents (e.g., opioids, tricyclic antidepressants, phenothiazines, benzodiazepines, butyrophenones) were administered in high doses to rodents.[41-45] The fetuses exhibited a characteristic group of CNS malformations as well as skeletal abnormalities and growth restriction. In one study, fetal abnormalities were dose related with diamorphine, methadone, pentazocine, phenazocine, and propoxyphene, whereas no further increase in anomalies occurred above certain dose levels with morphine, hydromorphone, and meperidine.[41] Whether these investigations truly reflect the teratogenic potential of opioids is questionable, because the respiratory depression and impaired feeding that accompany large bolus injections of opioids may be teratogenic themselves. In a study designed to avoid such problems, Fujinaga and Mazze[46] maintained clinically relevant concentrations of morphine throughout most of pregnancy in rats by means of continuously implanted osmotic mini-pumps. Structural anomalies were not observed at any morphine dose, although fetal growth restriction was present, and mortality was increased among the offspring. Using the same methodology, Fujinaga et al.[47,48] found fentanyl, sufentanil, and alfentanil completely devoid of teratogenic effects. Additional animal studies have confirmed the absence of teratogenicity with other opioids.[49]

The many tranquilizers and anxiolytics taken by pregnant women have been investigated less systematically than the opioids. Animal studies have demonstrated structural or behavioral teratogenesis after exposure to some of the barbiturate, phenothiazine, and tricyclic antidepressant agents.[50-53] The reader is referred to standard teratology reference sources for animal data related to specific drugs.[24,54] The package insert provided by a drug's manufacturer typically describes unpublished in-house studies related to the drug's reproductive effects.

Disturbingly, information is now emerging that exposure of the immature brain to anesthetic agents such as propofol, thiopental, and ketamine can trigger significant brain cell apoptosis and cause functional learning deficits later in life.[55-57] These data were generated from studies in rodents. Whether this effect occurs in humans or other species remains to be determined. Some authorities have suggested that the observed changes may not represent a direct effect of the anesthetic agent but rather may reflect indirect causes such as hypoxia or hypoglycemia.[57]

Human Studies

Teratogenesis has not been associated with the use of any of the commonly used induction agents—including the barbiturates, ketamine, and the benzodiazepines—when they were administered in clinical doses during anesthesia.[24] Similarly, no evidence supports the teratogenicity of opioids in humans; there is no increase in the incidence of congenital anomalies among offspring of mothers who use morphine or methadone during pregnancy.[24,54]

Although human data relating to long-term tranquilizer therapy have raised questions about the possible teratogenicity of some agents, most studies have been retrospective and have suffered from a variety of methodologic flaws. Benzodiazepine therapy became controversial after several retrospective studies reported an association between maternal diazepam ingestion during the first trimester and infants with cleft palate, with or without cleft lip.[58,59] Subsequently, a number of investigations,[60,61] including one prospective study of 854 women who ingested diazepam during the first trimester,[61] did not demonstrate a higher risk associated with benzodiazepine therapy. Although the present consensus among teratologists is that diazepam is not a proven human teratogen,[24] it is appropriate to consider the risk-to-benefit ratio before initiating long-term benzodiazepine therapy during the first trimester. No evidence suggests that a single dose of a benzodiazepine (e.g., midazolam) during the course of anesthesia is harmful to the fetus.

LOCAL ANESTHETICS

Procaine, lidocaine, and bupivacaine cause reversible cytotoxic effects in cultures of hamster fibroblasts.[62] However, no evidence supports morphologic or behavioral teratogenicity associated with lidocaine administration in rats,[63,64] and no evidence supports teratogenicity associated with any local anesthetic used clinically in humans.[24] Maternal cocaine abuse is associated with adverse reproductive outcomes, including abnormal neonatal behavior and, in some reports, a higher incidence of congenital defects of the genitourinary and gastrointestinal tracts.[24] The greatest risk to the fetus most likely results from the high incidence of placental abruption associated with maternal cocaine use (see Chapter 53).

MUSCLE RELAXANTS

Testing muscle relaxants for teratogenicity using standard *in vivo* animal studies either is complicated by maternal respiratory depression and the need for mechanical ventilation (a complex undertaking in rats or mice) or requires the administration of very low doses of the drug. Fujinaga et al.[65] used the whole-embryo rat culture system to investigate the reproductive toxicity of high doses of D-tubocurarine, pancuronium, atracurium, and vecuronium. Although dose-dependent toxicity was manifested, these effects occurred only at concentrations 30-fold greater than those encountered in clinical practice. These findings are consistent with earlier studies demonstrating no toxicity with small doses of muscle relaxants.[66] Given that fetal blood concentrations of muscle relaxants are only 10% to 20% of maternal concentrations, these drugs appear to have a wide margin of safety when administered to the mother during organogenesis; whether their administration later in gestation has adverse effects is unclear. Prolonged disturbance of normal muscular activity by muscle relaxants has caused axial and limb deformities in the chick but has seldom been seen in other experimental animals. Although one case report described arthrogryposis (i.e., persistent joint flexure) in the infant of a woman with tetanus who received D-tubocurarine for 19 days beginning at 55 days' gestation, the patient also was hypoxic and received multiple other drugs.[67] Many women have received muscle relaxants for several days during late gestation without adverse effect on the neonate.

INHALATION ANESTHETICS

Animal Studies

Volatile Agents Many studies have shown that, under certain conditions, the volatile halogenated anesthetic agents can produce teratogenic changes in chicks or small rodents. Basford and Fink[68] observed skeletal abnormalities but no increase in fetal loss when rats were exposed *in utero* to 0.8% halothane for 12 hours on days 8 and 9 of pregnancy (i.e., the "critical period" in the 21-day rat gestation). Long-term exposure to subanesthetic concentrations of halothane caused fetal growth restriction in rats but no increase in the incidence of congenital anomalies,[69] whereas isoflurane had no adverse effects.[70]

More significant reproductive effects have occurred with greater exposures to anesthetic agents. Fetal skeletal abnormalities or death followed repeated or prolonged maternal exposure of mice to anesthetic concentrations of volatile anesthetic agents.[71,72] However, teratogenicity in these studies most likely was caused by the physiologic changes (e.g., profound hypothermia, hypoventilation) associated with anesthesia rather than by the anesthetic agent itself. Moreover, some strains of mice are especially likely to demonstrate anomalies such as cleft palate. Mazze et al.[73] exposed rats to 0.75 MAC of halothane, isoflurane, or enflurane, or 0.55 MAC of nitrous oxide, for 6 hours daily on 3 consecutive days at various stages of pregnancy. The animals remained conscious throughout the study, and normal feeding and sleep patterns were preserved. Under these conditions, no teratogenic effects were associated with any of the volatile agents. The only positive finding was a threefold increase in rate of fetal resorptions with nitrous oxide. No evidence has suggested reproductive toxicity with either sevoflurane or desflurane in clinical concentrations.

Nitrous Oxide In contrast to the volatile halogenated agents, nitrous oxide is a weak teratogen in rodents under certain conditions, even when normal homeostasis is maintained. Rats continually exposed to 50% to 70% nitrous oxide for 2 to 6 days (starting on day 8 of gestation) had an increased incidence of congenital abnormalities.[73-76] To exclude the possibility that adverse effects were a consequence of the anesthetic state, Lane et al.[77] exposed rats to 70% nitrous oxide or to a similar concentration of xenon (a slightly more potent anesthetic devoid of biochemical effects) for 24 hours on day 9 of gestation. Again, abnormalities occurred only in the nitrous oxide group. With the exception of one study in which extremely prolonged exposure to a low concentration of nitrous oxide had some minor effects,[78] at least 50% nitrous oxide has been required to consistently produce anomalies.[76] The threshold exposure time has not been rigorously determined, although exposure for at least 24 hours typically was necessary.

In vivo and embryo culture studies in rats have confirmed that nitrous oxide has several adverse reproductive effects, each of which results from exposure at a specific period of susceptibility.[79-82] Fetal resorptions occurred after exposure on days 8 and 11 of gestation, skeletal anomalies after exposure on day 8 or 9, and visceral anomalies (including *situs inversus*) only when exposure occurred on day 8 (Figure 17-4).[82]

Initially, teratogenicity associated with nitrous oxide was thought to result from its oxidation of vitamin B_{12}, which interferes with its function as a coenzyme for methionine synthase.[83] Transmethylation from methyltetrahydrofolate to homocysteine to produce tetrahydrofolate (THF) and methionine is catalyzed by methionine synthase (Figure 17-5). Thus, methionine synthase inhibition could cause a decrease in THF (with a resultant decrease in DNA synthesis) and lower methionine levels (with resultant impairment of methylation reactions). Nitrous oxide rapidly inactivates methionine synthase in both animals[84] and humans.[85] Prolonged human exposure to nitrous oxide leads to neurologic and hematologic symptoms, the latter probably resulting from diminished DNA synthesis.[83] The hematologic—but not the neurologic—changes are prevented by the co-administration of folinic acid (5-formyl THF) with nitrous oxide, with the goal of restoring DNA synthesis.

Considerable evidence indicates that methionine synthase inhibition and a consequent lack of THF are not

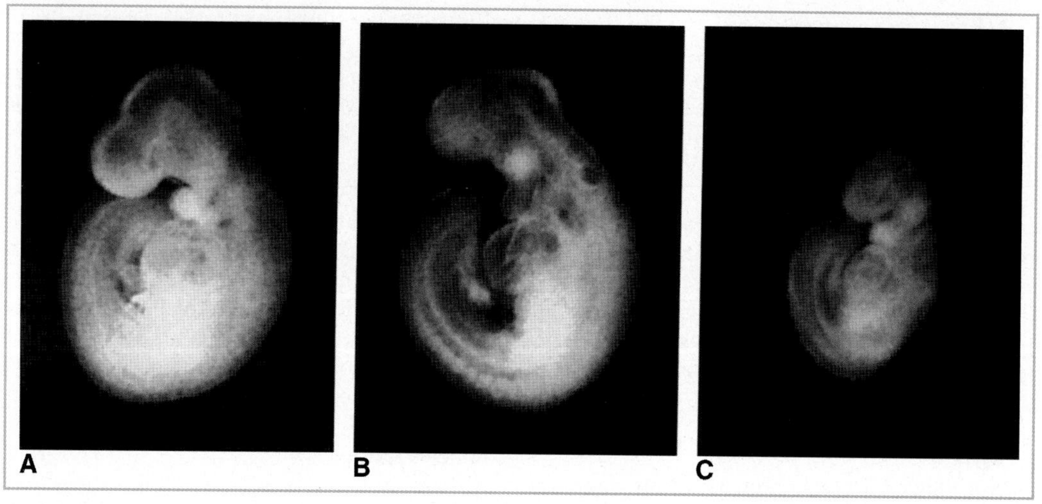

FIGURE 17-4 Effects of nitrous oxide on day 9 rat embryos grown in culture. **A,** Normal day 11 embryo. **B,** Day 11 embryo treated with 75% nitrous oxide for 24 hours from day 9. The embryo has a relatively small head compared with other parts of the body. **C,** Day 11 embryo similarly treated with 75% nitrous oxide on day 9. The embryo is smaller than normal and is severely malformed. (From Baden JM, Fujinaga M. Effects of nitrous oxide on day 9 rat embryos grown in culture. Br J Anaesth 1991; 66:500-3.)

solely responsible for the teratogenic effects of nitrous oxide. First, maximal inhibition of methionine synthase activity occurs at concentrations of nitrous oxide that are much lower than those required to produce teratogenic effects.[86] Second, folinic acid, which bypasses the effect of methionine synthase inhibition on THF formation, partially prevents only one of the structural abnormalities (i.e., minor skeletal defects) produced by nitrous oxide.[87] Third, the administration of isoflurane or halothane with nitrous oxide prevents almost all of the teratogenic effects but does not prevent the decrease in methionine synthase activity.[88,89] Fourth, studies using an *in vitro* whole-embryo rat culture system have shown that supplementation of nitrous oxide with methionine (but not with folinic acid) almost completely prevents growth restriction and all malformations with the exception of *situs inversus*.[90] Additional studies have implicated alpha$_1$-adrenergic receptor stimulation in the production of *situs inversus* by nitrous oxide.[81,91,92] Postulated mechanisms by which sympathetic stimulation might have adverse reproductive effects include a decrease in uterine blood flow and overstimulation of G protein–dependent membrane signal transduction pathways.[93] There is also evidence that nitrous oxide may cause neuronal apoptosis in rats.[94]

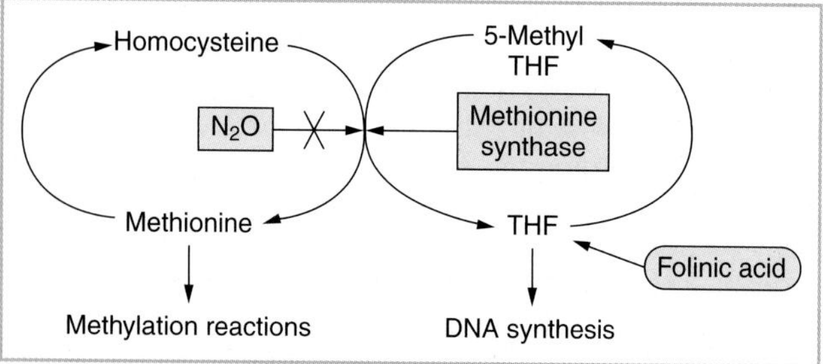

FIGURE 17-5 Pathway showing the inhibition of methionine synthase by nitrous oxide (N_2O) and its potential metabolic consequences (e.g., decreased DNA synthesis and impaired methylation reactions). THF, tetrahydrofolate. (Courtesy of M. Fujinaga, Palo Alto, CA.)

In summary, the evidence suggests that the etiology of nitrous oxide teratogenicity in rats is complex and multifactorial. Determination of the relative roles of methionine deficiency and sympathetic stimulation or other mechanisms awaits performance of further studies. Although nitrous oxide is considered a weak teratogen in rats and mice, reproductive effects occur only after prolonged exposure to high concentrations that are unlikely to be encountered in humans during clinical anesthesia. Whether nitrous oxide administration is associated with neuronal apoptosis and learning impairments in humans remains to be determined.

Human Studies

Occupational Exposure to Waste Anesthetic Agents Epidemiologic surveys dating from the 1960s and 1970s suggested that reproductive hazards (e.g., spontaneous abortion, congenital anomalies) were associated with operating room and dental surgery work.[95-99] These hazards were attributed to exposure to trace concentrations of anesthetic agents, principally nitrous oxide. Critical reviews of these studies questioned their conclusions. The reviewers noted that response bias, inappropriate control groups, lack of verification of medical data, and exposure to multiple environmental factors made definitive conclusions impossible.[100-102]

The most consistent risk associated with occupational exposure was spontaneous abortion, which carried a relative risk ratio of 1.3. The ratio for congenital anomalies (1.2) had borderline statistical significance.[100,102] These relative risks are well within the range that might be explained by bias or uncontrolled variables.[102] For example, the relative risk of second-trimester abortion among women who drink one or two alcoholic drinks per day is 1.98; this risk increases to 3.53 with more than three drinks daily.[103]

Similarly, cigarette smoking carries a relative risk of 1.8 for spontaneous abortion.[104]

Later studies have not confirmed an association between operating room work and higher reproductive risk.[105,106] Pregnancy outcomes were comparable in exposed and nonexposed operating room nurses when questionnaire information was matched with objective data obtained from medical records and registries of abortions, births, and congenital anomalies.[105] Similarly, in a 10-year prospective survey of all female physicians in the United Kingdom, Spence[106] found no differences in reproductive outcome when anesthesiologists were compared with other working female physicians. Although these studies may have missed a higher incidence of very early abortion, their data do not support a statistically demonstrable reproductive hazard resulting from operating room exposure to anesthetic agents.

It is possible that the higher waste levels of nitrous oxide encountered in dentists' offices pose a reproductive risk.[98,107,108] In 1980, Cohen et al.[98] reported a doubling of the spontaneous abortion rate among exposed female chair-side assistants and the wives of exposed male dentists. The incidence of birth defects among the children of exposed dental assistants was slightly higher than that for nonexposed assistants. However, the validity of this finding is doubtful; the incidence of anomalies among the offspring of nonexposed dentists was similar to that of the exposed assistants. Moreover, the expected dose-response relationship did not exist. Overall, the epidemiologic data do not support an increased risk of congenital anomalies with long-term exposure to nitrous oxide. Most recently, reduced fertility was reported among female dental assistants working with nitrous oxide in an unscavenged environment for more than 5 hours per week.[108] However, because the affected group consisted of only 19 individuals, it is difficult to draw firm conclusions from these data.

Studies of Operations Performed during Pregnancy In 1963, Smith[109] reviewed the obstetric records of 18,493 pregnant women. Sixty-seven (0.36%) had had an operation during pregnancy; only 10 procedures occurred during the first trimester. Fetal mortality was 11.2%, with the poorest survival occurring after operations for appendiceal abscess and cervical incompetence. In 1965, Shnider and Webster[110] examined the records of 9073 obstetric patients; 147 (1.6%) of this group had had operations during pregnancy. Preterm delivery followed operation in 8.8% of patients, and the incidences of perinatal mortality and low-birth-weight (LBW) infants were increased in patients who had surgery during pregnancy. Brodsky et al.[2] surveyed 12,929 pregnant dental assistants and wives of male dentists, 2% of whom had operations during gestation. Spontaneous abortions were more common in the surgical group than in the control group (8% versus 5.1% during the first trimester, and 6.9% versus 1.4% during the second trimester, respectively). None of these three studies reported a higher incidence of congenital anomalies among infants of women who underwent surgery during pregnancy. Two additional studies[111,112] that focused on the risks associated with nitrous oxide exposure during early pregnancy found no increase in the incidence of congenital abnormalities or spontaneous abortions.

Duncan et al.[113] used health insurance data to study the entire Manitoba, Canada, population between 1971 and 1978, matching 2565 women who had operations during pregnancy with similar controls who did not undergo surgery. Type of anesthesia was classified as nil (18%), general (57%), spinal/nerve block (2%), or local (24%). Although the incidence of congenital anomalies was similar in the surgical and control groups, spontaneous abortion was more common among women who had general anesthesia for surgery during the first or second trimester. This was true for both gynecologic procedures (relative risk [RR], 2.00) and nongynecologic procedures (RR, 1.58). Unfortunately, no conclusions regarding the relationship between anesthetic technique and fetal loss could be drawn, because most of the gynecologic and other major procedures were performed with general anesthesia. As in most studies, it is difficult to separate the effects of the anesthetic technique from those of the surgical procedure.

In the largest study to date, Mazze and Källén[1] linked data from three Swedish health care registries—the Medical Birth Registry, the Registry of Congenital Malformations, and the Hospital Discharge Registry—for the years 1973 to 1981. Among the population of 720,000 pregnant women, 5405 (0.75%) had nonobstetric surgery, including 2252 who had procedures during the first trimester. (Cervical cerclage was excluded from analysis.) Of the women who had surgery, 54% received general anesthesia, which included nitrous oxide in 97% of cases. The researchers examined the following adverse outcomes: (1) congenital anomalies, (2) stillbirths, (3) neonatal death within 7 days, and (4) LBW or very low-birth-weight (VLBW) infants. There was no difference between surgical and control patients with regard to the incidence of stillbirth or the overall incidence of congenital anomalies (Figure 17-6). Although the overall rate of anomalies among infants of women who had first-trimester operations was not higher, this group did have a higher-than-expected incidence of neural tube defects (6.0 observed versus

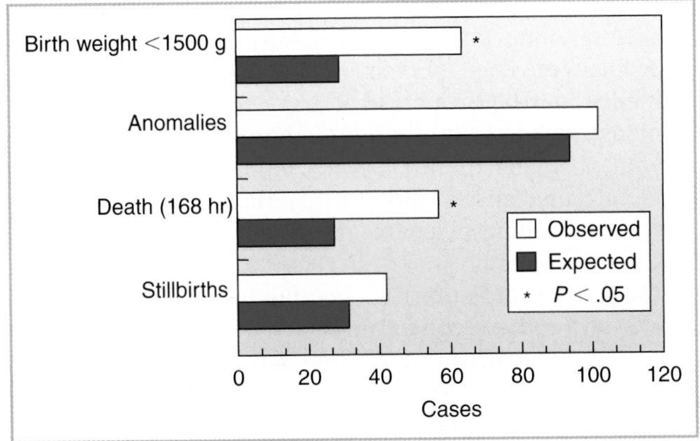

FIGURE 17-6 Total number of observed and expected adverse outcomes among women having nonobstetric operations during pregnancy. Incidences of infants with a birth weight of less than 1500 g and of infants born alive who died within 168 hours of birth were significantly increased. (Modified from Mazze RI, Källén B. Reproductive outcome after anesthesia and operation during pregnancy: A registry study of 5405 cases. Am J Obstet Gynecol 1989; 161:1178.)

2.5 expected).[114] Five of the 6 women whose infants had these defects were among the 572 women who had had surgery during gestational weeks 4 to 5, which is the period of neural tube formation; however, the researchers cautioned that this finding could have been a chance association.[114] However, if a true causal relationship exists between neural tube defects and anesthesia at this stage of gestation, it could represent an eightfold to ninefold increase in the risk for this anomaly (i.e., an absolute risk of almost 1%). Other positive findings were a higher incidence of LBW and VLBW infants in the surgical group, which resulted from both preterm delivery and intrauterine growth restriction.[1] A predictable consequence of preterm delivery was a higher number of deaths of live-born infants within the first 7 days of life. Finally, no anesthetic technique or operation was associated with a significantly higher number of adverse outcomes.

A case-control study of infants born in Atlanta between 1968 and 1980 gathered information regarding first-trimester exposure to general anesthesia from the mothers of 694 infants with major CNS defects and 2984 control mothers.[115] A striking association was found between general anesthesia exposure and hydrocephalus in conjunction with another major defect (the strongest association was with hydrocephalus and eye defects). Limitations of this study include its retrospective nature and a lack of information about the types of surgery, the anesthetic agents used, and the presence or absence of complications. The investigators cautioned that further studies are necessary to confirm their observations.

In summary, although anesthesia and surgery are associated with a higher incidence of abortion, intrauterine growth restriction, and perinatal mortality, these adverse outcomes can often be attributed to the procedure, the site of surgery (e.g., proximity to the uterus), and/or the underlying maternal condition. Evidence does not suggest that anesthesia results in an overall increase in congenital abnormalities, and there is no evidence of a clear relationship between outcome and type of anesthesia.

BEHAVIORAL TERATOLOGY

It is well known that some teratogens produce enduring behavioral abnormalities without any observable morphologic changes. The CNS may be especially sensitive to such influences during the period of major myelination, which in humans extends from the fourth intrauterine month to the second postnatal month. Several studies have shown that brief intrauterine exposure to halothane adversely affects postnatal learning behavior and causes CNS degeneration and decreased brain weight in rats.[116-118] The fetal nervous system in the rat is most susceptible to the effects of halothane during the second trimester.[116] Prenatal administration of systemic drugs—including barbiturates, meperidine, and promethazine—has also resulted in behavioral changes in animals,[119-121] whereas no effect has been noted with the administration of lidocaine.[64] Investigations of the effects of maternally administered analgesics at delivery have revealed transient, dose-related depression of newborn behavior.

Currently used general anesthetic agents act by one of two principal mechanisms, (1) the potentiation of gamma-aminobutyric acid $(GABA)_A$ receptors (as occurs with benzodiazepines, volatile halogenated agents, and barbiturates) or (2) the antagonism of *N*-methyl-D-aspartate (NMDA) receptors (as occurs with nitrous oxide and ketamine). More recent evidence suggests that drugs that act by either of these mechanisms induce widespread neuronal apoptosis in the developing rat brain when administered during the period of synaptogenesis (i.e., the brain growth-spurt period).[122-124] Jevtovic-Todorovic et al.[122] observed that the administration of a general anesthetic "cocktail" (midazolam, isoflurane, and nitrous oxide), in doses sufficient to maintain general anesthesia for 6 hours in 7-day-old infant rats, resulted in widespread apoptotic neurodegeneration in the developing brain, deficits in hippocampal synaptic function, and persistent memory/learning impairments. They concluded that these deficits are "subtle enough to be easily overlooked" but may persist into adolescence and adulthood.[122] Ikonomidou et al.[123] described neurodegeneration in rat pups after NMDA receptor antagonism. These data suggest that prolonged exposure to anesthetic agents at a critical period in brain development may accelerate the normal developmental process of apoptotic neurodegeneration, potentially resulting in prolonged behavioral deficits.[125] Thus the safety of providing anesthesia during early life has been questioned.[126]

The implications, if any, for the human fetus during the maternal administration of general anesthesia are unknown, as there are methodologic issues with these animal studies. Surgery may result not only in exposure to anesthetic agents but also in derangements in maternal physiology (e.g., hypoxia, stress, hypoglycemia) that can lead to apoptosis during the critical period of neuronal development.[127] Also, it should be noted that in experimental studies, the rats typically were exposed to large doses of anesthetic agents for prolonged periods. Hayashi et al.[128] demonstrated that a single dose of ketamine did not lead to apoptosis but that its repeated administration for several hours caused neuronal degeneration. It is also important to remember that painful stimuli per se can cause long-term behavioral changes.[129] Finally, the species model may be important. For example, McClain et al.[130] did not observe any histologic or functional effects of exposure to general anesthesia in fetal lambs. Anand and Soriano[126] concluded:

> *Clearer understanding of the mechanisms by which exposures to pain/stress or prolonged anesthesia in the perinatal period can alter the survival or development of immature neurons and glia may prevent some long-term neurobehavioral abnormalities in humans. In the meantime, clinicians should administer anesthetic agents to newborn infants or pregnant mothers but avoid prolonged periods of anesthetic exposure . . . . Alleviation of pain and stress during the perinatal period should remain an essential clinical goal until further research defines the clinical importance of [experimental] results [observed in animals].*

After a review of the data and a public hearing in March 2007, the Anesthetic and Life Support Drugs Advisory Committee of the U.S. Food and Drug Administration stated that currently "there are not adequate data to extrapolate the animal findings to humans."[131]

Fetal Effects of Anesthesia

MAINTENANCE OF FETAL WELL-BEING

The most serious fetal risk associated with maternal surgery during pregnancy is that of intrauterine asphyxia.

Because fetal oxygenation depends on maternal oxygenation, maintenance of normal maternal arterial oxygen tension, oxygen-carrying capacity, oxygen affinity, and uteroplacental perfusion are critical to fetal well-being.

Maternal and Fetal Oxygenation

Transient mild to moderate decreases in maternal $Pa{O_2}$ are well tolerated by the fetus, because fetal hemoglobin has a high affinity for oxygen. Severe maternal **hypoxemia** results in fetal hypoxia and, if persistent, may cause fetal death. Any complication that causes profound maternal hypoxemia (e.g., difficult intubation, esophageal intubation, pulmonary aspiration, total spinal anesthesia, systemic local anesthetic toxicity) is a potential threat to the fetus.

Studies of isolated human placental vessels have suggested that **hyperoxia** might cause uteroplacental vasoconstriction, with potential impairment of fetal oxygen delivery.[132] This fear has proved to be unfounded, because studies in pregnant women have demonstrated better fetal oxygenation with increasing maternal $Pa{O_2}$.[133] Fetal $Pa{O_2}$ never exceeds 60 mm Hg, even when maternal $Pa{O_2}$ increases to 600 mm Hg, because of a large maternal-fetal oxygen tension gradient. Thus, intrauterine retrolental fibroplasia and premature closure of the ductus arteriosus cannot result from high levels of maternal $Pa{O_2}$. McClain et al.[130] observed that the maternal administration of general anesthesia for 4 hours in gravid ewes produced an initial—but not sustained—increase in fetal systemic oxygenation, which was accompanied by a sustained increase in fetal cerebral oxygenation. The investigators hypothesized that the increase in fetal cerebral oxygenation resulted from greater cerebral perfusion, lower cerebral metabolic rate, or both. Histologic examination found no evidence of neurotoxicity.

Maternal Carbon Dioxide and Acid-Base Status

Maternal **hypercapnia** can cause fetal acidosis, because fetal $Pa{CO_2}$ correlates directly with maternal $Pa{CO_2}$. Although mild fetal respiratory acidosis is of little consequence, severe acidosis can cause fetal myocardial depression and hypotension. Maternal **hyperventilation** with low maternal $Pa{CO_2}$ and high pH can adversely affect fetal oxygenation by means of several mechanisms.[134-136] **Respiratory** or **metabolic alkalosis** can compromise maternal-fetal oxygen transfer by causing umbilical artery constriction[134] and by shifting the maternal oxyhemoglobin dissociation curve to the left.[135] In addition, hyperventilation, independent of changes in $Pa{CO_2}$, may reduce uterine blood flow and cause fetal acidosis.[136] This most likely is a consequence of mechanical ventilation, whereby increased intrathoracic pressure reduces venous return and cardiac output, which in turn decreases uteroplacental perfusion.

Thus, hyperventilation should be avoided in the pregnant surgical patient. Rather, the $Pa{CO_2}$ should be kept in the normal range for pregnancy.

Uteroplacental Perfusion

Maternal **hypotension** from any cause can jeopardize uteroplacental perfusion and cause fetal asphyxia. The most common causes of hypotension in the pregnant patient undergoing surgery include (1) deep levels of general anesthesia, (2) sympathectomy with high levels of spinal or epidural blockade, (3) aortocaval compression, (4) hemorrhage, and (5) hypovolemia. In monkeys, prolonged hypotension (i.e., systolic blood pressure less than 75 mm Hg) caused by deep halothane anesthesia resulted in fetal hypoxia, acidosis, and hypotension.[137] After experiencing as much as 5 hours of severe partial asphyxia *in utero* (pH < 7.00 for at least 1 hour), newborn monkeys were depressed and experienced seizures. Postnatal survival was poor, and pathologic brain changes included swelling, necrosis, and hemorrhage. The clinical course and neuropathologic findings in these animals resembled those in infants known to have suffered severe intrauterine asphyxia and who died within a few days of birth. Despite these alarming data, case reports have described good outcome following deliberate induction of moderate degrees of hypotension during pregnancy, usually to facilitate performance of a neurosurgical procedure.[138] Fetal and neonatal outcomes were unaffected when maternal systolic blood pressure was kept in the 70 to 80 mm Hg range, even when pressures as low as 50 mm Hg were briefly permitted. In such circumstances, the risk to the fetus must be balanced against the risk of uncontrolled maternal bleeding or stroke.

The multiple factors that influence uteroplacental blood flow are discussed in detail in Chapter 3. Of particular relevance to the pregnant surgical patient are drugs that cause uterine vasoconstriction. Preoperative anxiety and light anesthesia increase circulating catecholamines, possibly impairing uterine blood flow.[139] Drugs that cause uterine hypertonus (e.g., ketamine in early pregnancy in doses higher than 2 mg/kg,[140] toxic doses of local anesthetics[141]) may increase uterine vascular resistance, decreasing uteroplacental perfusion.

New evidence has challenged the historic view that the mixed-adrenergic agonist ephedrine is preferred to the alpha-adrenergic agonist phenylephrine for the treatment of hypotension during the administration of neuraxial anesthesia in obstetric patients.[142,143] A meta-analysis of randomized controlled trials comparing ephedrine with phenylephrine for the treatment of hypotension during spinal anesthesia for cesarean delivery resulted in the following conclusions: (1) there was no difference between phenylephrine and ephedrine for the prevention and treatment of maternal hypotension; (2) maternal bradycardia was more likely to occur with phenylephrine than with ephedrine; (3) women given phenylephrine had neonates with higher umbilical arterial blood pH measurements than those given ephedrine; and (4) there was no difference between the two vasopressors in the incidence of true fetal acidosis (i.e., umbilical arterial blood pH < 7.20).[142] Cooper et al.[143] randomly assigned 147 patients to receive phenylephrine, ephedrine, or both for the maintenance of maternal arterial pressure during spinal anesthesia for elective cesarean delivery. Fetal acidosis was more common in the women who received ephedrine. The investigators speculated that "increased fetal metabolic rate, secondary to ephedrine-induced beta-adrenergic stimulation, was the most likely mechanism for the increased incidence of fetal acidosis in the ephedrine group."[143] Clearly, the use of phenylephrine in pregnancy is acceptable; indeed, phenylephrine may be preferable to ephedrine for the treatment of maternal hypotension.

FETAL EFFECTS OF INHALATION AGENTS

The volatile halogenated anesthetic agents can affect the fetus directly (by depressing the fetal cardiovascular system or CNS) or indirectly (by causing maternal hypoxia or hypotension). Studies in gravid ewes have shown minimal fetal effects with maternal administration of moderate concentrations of a volatile agent.[144] Uterine perfusion was maintained during the inhalation of 1.0 and 1.5 MAC halothane or isoflurane, because uterine vasodilation compensated for small decreases in maternal blood pressure. Higher concentrations (e.g., 2.0 MAC) given for prolonged periods induced marked maternal hypotension. Consequently, reduced uteroplacental blood flow resulted in fetal hypoxia, diminished fetal cardiac output, and fetal acidosis.[144]

The effects of anesthesia on the stressed fetal lamb remain unclear. In one study, the administration of 1% halothane to the mothers of asphyxiated fetal lambs caused severe fetal hypotension, worsening of fetal acidosis, and decreases in cerebral blood flow and oxygen delivery.[145] In other studies, acidosis that was less severe or of a shorter duration was associated with the maintenance of fetal cardiac output and a preservation of the balance between oxygen supply and demand.[146-148] The protective compensatory mechanisms that exist during asphyxia may be abolished by high but not low concentrations of volatile agents.

The relevance of these data to the human mother undergoing surgery during pregnancy is not clear. Clinical experience does not support avoidance of volatile agents, provided that maternal hypotension is prevented. Indeed, the depressant effect of these agents on myometrial contractility may be beneficial. If intraoperative fetal heart rate (FHR) monitoring reveals signs of fetal compromise, it may be advisable to discontinue the volatile agent until the fetal condition improves.

FETAL EFFECTS OF SYSTEMIC DRUGS

Opioids and induction agents decrease FHR variability, possibly to a greater extent than the inhalation agents.[149-151] This finding most likely signals the presence of an anesthetized fetus and is not a cause for concern in the absence of maternal hypotension or other abnormalities. Fetal respiratory depression is relevant only if cesarean delivery is to be performed at the same time as the surgical procedure. Even then, high-dose opioid anesthesia need not be avoided when it is indicated for maternal reasons (e.g., anesthesia for patients with cardiac disease). The pediatrician should be informed of maternal drug administration so that preparations can be made to support neonatal respiration. Some data indicate that remifentanil may result in less neonatal depression than longer-acting opioids.[152]

Maternal administration of muscle relaxants and reversal agents typically has not proved to be problematic for the fetus. It has been suggested that rapid intravenous injection of an anticholinesterase agent might stimulate acetylcholine release, which might cause increased uterine tone and thus precipitate preterm labor.[153] Although this concern is unproven, slow administration of an anticholinesterase (after prior injection of an anticholinergic agent) is recommended. Atropine rapidly crosses the placenta and, when given in large doses, causes fetal tachycardia and loss of FHR variability.[154] Although neither atropine nor glycopyrrolate significantly affects FHR when standard clinical doses are administered,[155] glycopyrrolate is often recommended because it crosses the placenta less readily and may be a more effective antisialagogue. Although limited transplacental passage of neostigmine is expected, significant transfer occasionally may occur. One case report described mild fetal bradycardia when neostigmine was administered with glycopyrrolate during emergence from general anesthesia at 31 weeks' gestation.[156] This problem did not occur during the administration of a second general anesthetic to the same patient 4 days later, when atropine was administered with neostigmine, presumably because atropine undergoes greater placental transfer than glycopyrrolate. Because the effects of reversal agents are unpredictable, the monitoring of FHR during maternal drug administration is suggested.

Sodium nitroprusside and esmolol have been used during pregnancy to induce hypotension during surgical procedures. Standard doses of nitroprusside have proved to be safe for the fetus,[157] and the risk of fetal cyanide toxicity appears to be low, provided that tachyphylaxis does not occur and the total dose is limited. The use of esmolol during pregnancy remains controversial. Ostman et al.[158] observed minimal fetal effects after the administration of esmolol in gravid ewes, whereas Eisenach and Castro[159] reported significant decreases in FHR and blood pressure as well as a modest reduction in fetal $Pa{O_2}$. Fetal effects dissipated rapidly in the first study but persisted for 30 minutes or more in the second. Two case reports have described small decreases in FHR but no morbidity when esmolol was administered with nitroprusside during neurosurgical procedures.[160,161] In contrast, severe fetal compromise followed the administration of esmolol at 38 weeks' gestation to correct maternal supraventricular tachycardia.[162] Because fetal tachycardia preceded the onset of severe bradycardia in this case, the researchers speculated that fetal compromise resulted from reduced maternal cardiac output rather than fetal beta-adrenergic receptor blockade.

Prevention of Preterm Labor

Most epidemiologic studies of nonobstetric surgery during pregnancy have reported a higher incidence of abortion and preterm delivery.[1,110,111,163] It is unclear whether the surgery, manipulation of the uterus, or the underlying condition is responsible. In a study of 778 women who underwent appendectomy during pregnancy, Mazze and Källén[163] found that 22% of women who underwent surgery between 24 and 36 weeks' gestation delivered in the week after surgery. In the women in whom pregnancy continued beyond a week after surgery, there was no further increase in the rate of preterm birth. Although this study's database was unsuitable for determining the incidence of preterm delivery before 24 weeks' gestation, a similar increase appeared likely. Second-trimester procedures and operations that do not involve uterine manipulation carry the lowest risk for preterm labor.

Although the volatile agents depress myometrial irritability and theoretically are advantageous for abdominal procedures, evidence does not show that any one anesthetic agent or technique positively or negatively influences the risk of preterm labor. Published evidence does not support the routine use of prophylactic tocolytic agents.[164] Monitoring for uterine contractions may be performed intraoperatively with an external tocodynamometer (when technically feasible) and for several days postoperatively, allowing tocolytic therapy to be instituted, if appropriate. Additional surveillance is necessary in patients who receive potent postoperative analgesics, who may be unaware of mild uterine contractions. In the general pregnant population, increased risk for preterm labor and delivery can be predicted through the use of various methods, such as measurement of fetal fibronectin in cervicovaginal fluid and determination of cervical length using transvaginal ultrasonography.[165] A new class of tocolytic agents—oxytocin receptor antagonists (e.g., atosiban)—has been investigated.[166] Atosiban selectively blunts the calcium influx in the myometrium and thus inhibits myometrial contractility. Whether greater surveillance and early tocolytic therapy will reduce the risk of preterm delivery after surgery during pregnancy is not known.

PRACTICAL CONSIDERATIONS

Timing of Surgery

Elective surgery should not be performed during pregnancy. When possible, surgery should be avoided during the first trimester, especially during the period of organogenesis. The second trimester is the optimal time to perform surgery, because the risk of preterm labor is lowest at that time. Urgent operation is often indicated for abdominal emergencies, some malignancies, and neurosurgical and cardiac conditions. The management and timing of most acute surgical procedures should mimic that for nonpregnant patients.[167,168] The risk of perinatal loss is increased when maternal appendicitis is advanced.[168] Appendiceal perforation may be more common in pregnant patients than in nonpregnant patients because diagnostic difficulties may delay performance of surgery. Generalized peritonitis may also be more likely because increased steroid levels during pregnancy may suppress the normal inflammatory response and prevent the "walling off" of the appendix by the omentum.[168]

In the event of a serious maternal illness, the remote fetal risks associated with anesthesia and surgery are of secondary importance. The primary goal is to preserve the life of the mother. Hypothermia,[169] induced hypotension,[138] cardiopulmonary bypass,[170] and liver transplantation[171] have been associated with successful neonatal outcomes. The decision to perform simultaneous cesarean delivery depends on a number of factors, including the gestational age, the risk to the mother of a trial of labor at a later date, and the presence of intra-abdominal sepsis. Cesarean delivery may be performed immediately before the surgical procedure to avoid fetal risks associated with special patient positioning (e.g., the sitting or prone position),[172] prolonged anesthesia, major intraoperative blood loss, maternal hyperventilation, deliberate hypotension, or cardiopulmonary bypass.[170]

Abdominal Emergencies

Acute abdominal disease occurs in 1 in 500 to 1 in 635 pregnancies.[173,174] Accurate diagnosis, especially of an acute abdominal crisis (e.g, appendicitis, cholecystitis), can be very difficult during pregnancy.[168] Box 17-2 lists some of the conditions that must be considered in the differential diagnosis of abdominal pain during pregnancy. Nausea, vomiting, constipation, and abdominal distention are common symptoms of both normal pregnancy and abdominal pathology. Abdominal tenderness may be indistinguishable from ligamentous or uterine contraction pain. The expanding uterus makes a physical examination of the abdomen difficult. For example, the appendix rotates counterclockwise; thus, as term approaches, the tip typically lies over the right kidney (Figure 17-7).[175] Because the white blood cell count in normal pregnancy may reach 15,000/mm^3, it must be markedly elevated to be diagnostically helpful. Additional delay results from the reluctance to perform necessary imaging studies involving radiation. Mazze and Källén[163] reported the misdiagnosis of appendicitis during pregnancy in 36% of cases, with a lower rate

BOX 17-2 Nonobstetric Abdominal Crises in Pregnancy

Medical Conditions

- Abdominal crises due to systemic disease
  - Sickle cell disease
  - Diabetic ketoacidosis
  - Porphyria
- Renal disease
  - Glomerulonephritis
  - Pyelonephritis
- Pulmonary disease
  - Basal pneumonia with pleurisy
- Cholecystitis and pancreatitis (early, uncomplicated)
- Myocardial infarction, pericarditis
- Drug addiction (withdrawal symptoms)

Surgical Conditions

Gynecologic Problems

- Ovarian cyst/tumor
  - Rupture
  - Torsion
  - Hemorrhage
  - Infection
- Torsion of a fallopian tube
- Tubo-ovarian abscess
- Uterine myoma
  - Degeneration
  - Infection
  - Torsion

Nongynecologic Problems

- Acute appendicitis
- Acute cholecystitis and its complications
- Acute pancreatitis and its complications
- Intestinal obstruction
- Trauma with visceral injury or hemorrhage
- Vascular accidents (e.g., ruptured abdominal aneurysm)
- Peptic ulcer

Modified from Fainstat T, Bhat N. Surgical resolution of nonobstetric abdominal crises complicating pregnancy. In Baden JM, Brodsky JB, editors. The Pregnant Surgical Patient. Mount Kisko, NY, Futura Publishing, 1985:154.

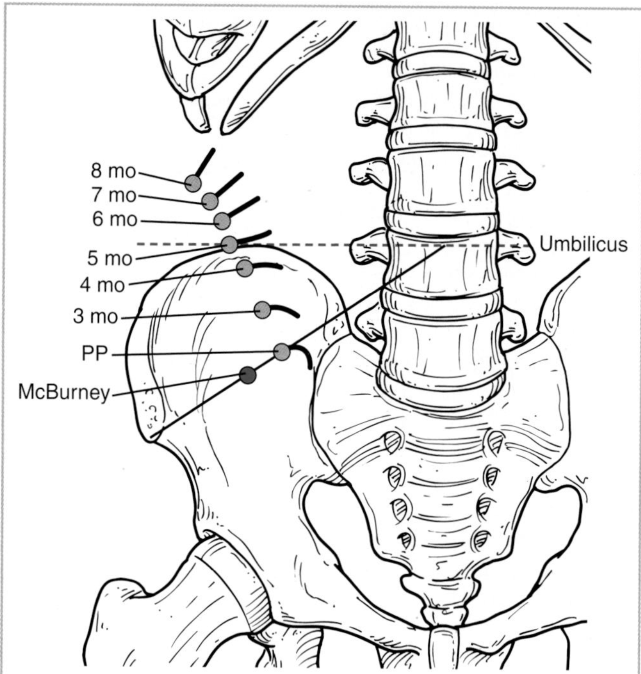

FIGURE 17-7 Changes in position and direction of the appendix during pregnancy. (Redrawn from Baer JL, Reis RA, Arens RA. Appendicitis in pregnancy with changes in position and axis of normal appendix in pregnancy. JAMA 1932; 98:1359.)

(23%) during the first trimester than during the last two trimesters (43%).

Often, the correct diagnosis is determined only at operation. The selection of the procedure and choice of incision are influenced by the stage of gestation, the nature of the surgical problem, the certainty of the probable diagnosis, and the experience of the surgeon. Laparoscopy is performed during pregnancy for both diagnostic and therapeutic indications with increasing frequency (see later). Laparotomy continues to be performed for many abdominal conditions that occur during the later stages of pregnancy.

Laparoscopy

Concerns exist about the effects of laparoscopy on fetal well-being, especially the risks of (1) uterine or fetal trauma; (2) fetal acidosis from absorbed carbon dioxide; and (3) decreased maternal cardiac output and uteroplacental perfusion resulting from an iatrogenic increase in intra-abdominal pressure. In some animal studies, maternal and fetal acidosis and tachycardia have occurred during intra-abdominal insufflation, perhaps because maternal ventilation was guided by measurements of end-tidal rather than arterial carbon dioxide levels.[176,177] A marked increase in Pa_{CO_2} to end-tidal CO_2 gradient developed during CO_2 insufflation in gravid ewes, suggesting that Pa_{CO_2} should be used to guide ventilation if maternal and fetal acidosis are to be avoided.[177] Uteroplacental perfusion decreased by 61% in one study in which gravid ewes were subjected to a CO_2 pneumoperitoneum at a pressure of 20 mm Hg (although there were no adverse fetal consequences).[178] It is unclear whether the severity of acidosis and decrement in uteroplacental perfusion are related to insufflation pressure.[177]

Many practitioners believe, however, that the potential benefits of laparoscopic surgery compared with open abdominal surgery outweigh the risks. Potential benefits include (1) shorter hospitalization, (2) less postoperative pain, (3) decreased risk of thromboembolic and wound complications, and (4) faster return to normal activities, including earlier return of normal gastrointestinal function, less uterine irritability, and decreased fetal depression.[179] Although rigorous studies comparing open abdominal surgery with laparoscopic procedures during pregnancy are lacking, it is clear that laparoscopy is being performed with growing frequency in pregnant women.[179-192] In a 1994 survey of laparoendoscopic surgeons, Reedy et al.[180] obtained data from 413 laparoscopic procedures performed during pregnancy and reviewed an additional 55 previously published cases. Among the procedures surveyed, 48% were cholecystectomies, 28% were adnexal operations, 16% were appendectomies, and 8% were diagnostic procedures. Thirty-two percent of operations were performed in the first trimester, 54% in the second, and 13% in the third.

Clinical studies and clinical experience suggest that the fetal effects of the CO_2 pneumoperitoneum and increased intra-abdominal pressure are limited. In one clinical study, there were no differences in the maternal pH, Pa_{CO_2} or arterial to end-tidal CO_2 pressure gradients before, during, or after termination of the pneumoperitoneum during laparoscopy.[193] Steinbrook and Bhavani-Shankar[194] used thoracic electrical bioimpedance cardiography to measure changes in cardiac output in four pregnant women undergoing laparoscopic cholecystectomy. They observed hemodynamic changes similar to those that typically occur during laparoscopic surgery in nonpregnant patients (i.e., decrease in cardiac index with concurrent increases in mean arterial pressure and systemic vascular resistance).

Reported clinical experiences with laparoscopy during pregnancy generally have been favorable; complications such as intraoperative perforation of the uterus with the Veress needle have occurred rarely.[180] Moreover, most investigators have reported no difference in maternal and fetal outcomes between laparoscopy and laparotomy and consider the former a safe procedure during pregnancy.[180-188,191,192] In contrast, Amos et al.[189] urged caution in a case-series study in which they reported fetal death after four of seven laparoscopic procedures. Therefore, because of concerns about the fetal effects of CO_2 pneumoperitoneum, some practitioners have suggested using a gasless laparoscopic technique.[195-198]

Careful surgical and anesthetic techniques are critical to avoid problems associated with pregnancy and the special hazards of laparoscopic surgery. The surgeon should be experienced with the technique, and the anesthesia provider must be aware of the accompanying cardiorespiratory changes. In 2007, the Society of American Gastrointestinal Endoscopic Surgeons[199] issued "Guidelines for Diagnosis, Treatment, and Use of Laparoscopy for Surgical Problems During Pregnancy" (Box 17-3). According to these guidelines, indications for laparoscopic surgery in pregnant patients do not differ from those for nonpregnant patients,

BOX 17-3 Suggested Guidelines for Laparoscopic Surgery during Pregnancy

- Indications for laparoscopic treatment of acute abdominal processes are the same as for nonpregnant patients.
- Laparoscopy can be safely performed during any trimester of pregnancy.
- Preoperative obstetric consultation should be obtained.
- Intermittent lower extremity pneumatic compression devices should be used intraoperatively and postoperatively to prevent venous stasis (i.e., as prophylaxis for deep vein thrombosis).
- The fetal heart rate and uterine tone should be monitored both preoperatively and postoperatively.
- End-tidal CO_2 should be monitored during surgery.
- Left uterine displacement should be maintained, in order to avoid aortocaval compression.
- An open (Hassan) technique, a Veress needle, or an optical trocar technique may be used to enter the abdomen.
- Low pneumoperitoneum pressures (between 10 and 15 mm Hg) should be used.
- Tocolytic agents should not be used prophylactically but should be considered when evidence of preterm labor is present.

Modified from Guidelines Committee of the Society of American Gastrointestinal and Endoscopic Surgeons, Yumi H. Guidelines for diagnosis, treatment, and use of laparoscopy for surgical problems during pregnancy. Surg Endosc 2008; 22:849-61.

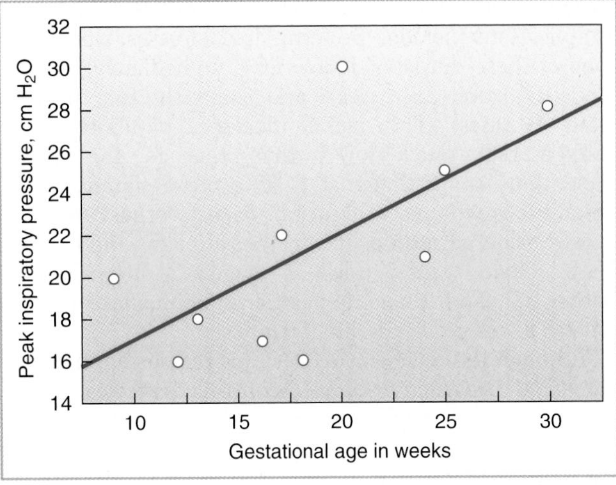

FIGURE 17-8 Peak inspiratory pressure during laparoscopic cholecystectomy during pregnancy as a function of gestational age. The best-fit line by linear regression is shown ($y = 12.1 + 0.5X$; $R^2 = 0.43$). Peak inspiratory pressure tends to increase with advancing gestation. (Modified from Steinbrook RA, Brooks DC, Datta S. Laparoscopic cholecystectomy during pregnancy. Surg Endosc 1996; 10:511-5.)

and the procedure may be performed during any trimester of pregnancy.

General anesthesia has been used in the vast majority of laparoscopic procedures, although the use of epidural anesthesia has also been described.[180] Steinbrook et al.[190] described their anesthetic technique for 10 cases of laparoscopic cholecystectomy during pregnancy. They administered general anesthesia with a rapid-sequence induction followed by endotracheal intubation and positive-pressure ventilation to maintain end-tidal CO_2 between 32 and 36 mm Hg. Anesthesia was maintained with a nondepolarizing muscle relaxant, an opioid, and a volatile halogenated agent, but nitrous oxide was avoided to prevent bowel distention and to allow administration of a higher concentration of inspired oxygen. The pneumoperitoneum resulted in increased peak airway pressure (Figure 17-8) and decreased total lung compliance, changes that were progressively greater with advancing gestation. Because the Trendelenburg position exacerbates these changes, further decreases in FRC and hypoxemia from airway closure may occur with this position. Hyperventilation, which may be necessary to maintain normal maternal Pa_{CO_2}, may reduce uteroplacental perfusion and affect fetal oxygenation. Hypotension may result from pneumoperitoneum, aortocaval compression, or use of the reverse Trendelenburg position, and a vasopressor may be needed to maintain maternal blood pressure during laparoscopy.[190] As with conventional surgery, fetal well-being is best preserved by keeping maternal oxygenation, acid-base status, and hemodynamic parameters within normal pregnancy limits. The FHR and uterine tone should be monitored both before and after surgery (see later).

Electroconvulsive Therapy

Psychiatric disease is an important cause of maternal morbidity and mortality during pregnancy.[10] The treatment of major psychiatric disorders during pregnancy is problematic, and optimal management remains controversial.[200] The risk of congenital malformations in the fetus exposed to psychotropic medications *in utero* must be balanced against the high rate of relapse that results from the discontinuation of psychotropic medications in pregnant women with mood disorders.[200] Because these medications are associated with a low but higher than normal risk of teratogenicity, the American Psychiatric Association has endorsed electroconvulsive therapy (ECT) as a treatment for major depression and bipolar disorders during all three trimesters of pregnancy.[201]

Published case reports represent the only available source of information about the effects of ECT during pregnancy. Miller[202] reviewed the details of 300 published cases of ECT during pregnancy between 1924 and 1991. ECT was begun in the first trimester in 14 (4.7%) cases, in the second trimester in 36 (12%) cases, and in the third trimester in 31 (10%) cases. In 219 (73%) cases the timing was not described. Complications were reported in 28 (9.3%) cases. The major complications included self-limited FHR abnormalities (5 cases), vaginal bleeding (5 cases), uterine contractions (2 cases), and abdominal pain (3 cases).

All neonates in these cases were born healthy. Additional complications included preterm labor (4 cases, although in none of these did labor follow ECT immediately), spontaneous abortion (5 cases), and stillbirth and neonatal death (3 cases). The overall incidence of abortion was 1.6%—a rate much lower than that in the general population—suggesting that ECT is not a significant risk factor for spontaneous abortion. Factors other than ECT were considered responsible for the stillbirths and neonatal deaths. There were 5 cases of congenital anomalies, but neither the pattern nor the number of anomalies suggested that ECT was a determining factor.

Although the review by Miller[202] is reassuring, there is a paucity of prospective or well-controlled studies. Pinette et al.[203] reported a case of cerebral infarction in a neonate whose mother had repeated ECT treatments during pregnancy. On the basis of this case and review of the available literature (and the paucity of well-designed studies), these investigators[203] as well as an editorialist[204] suggested that ECT should be used during pregnancy only when conventional medical treatment has failed.

Anesthetic agents commonly used during ECT are barbiturates, succinylcholine, and anticholinergics (e.g., glycopyrrolate); these agents have a long history of safe use during pregnancy. Ishikawa et al.[205] reported their management of a pregnant woman whose third ECT session was complicated by sustained uterine contractions (and fetal bradycardia) that were refractory to tocolytic therapy. During the sixth ECT session, general anesthesia was maintained with sevoflurane and oxygen, and uterine contractions were significantly diminished.[205]

Suggested guidelines for ECT during pregnancy are summarized in Box 17-4.[202,206] These include FHR and uterine monitoring, left uterine displacement, aspiration prophylaxis, and endotracheal intubation after the first trimester.

BOX 17-4 Suggested Guidelines for Electroconvulsive Therapy (ECT) during Pregnancy

- Preoperative obstetric consultation should be obtained.
- Tocodynamometry should be performed within 60 minutes of the procedure.
- Adequate hydration should be ensured.
- A nonparticulate antacid (0.3 M sodium citrate, 30 mL) should be administered within 20 minutes of ECT.
- Endotracheal intubation should be considered after the first trimester.
- Left uterine displacement should be maintained after 18 to 20 weeks' gestation.
- The fetal heart rate should be monitored before and after ECT.
- Uterine contractions and vaginal bleeding should be monitored after ECT.

Summarized from Miller LJ. Use of electroconvulsive therapy during pregnancy. Hosp Community Psychiatry 1994; 45:444-50; and Rabheru K. The use of electroconvulsive therapy in special patient populations. Can J Psychiatry 2001; 46:710-9.

Direct Current Cardioversion and Maternal Resuscitation

Palpitations are common during pregnancy. Furthermore, the incidence of cardiac disease in pregnancy is rising as patients with congenital cardiac disease survive to reproductive age and older women become pregnant. Direct current (DC) cardioversion may be necessary during pregnancy. It is safe in all stages of pregnancy. The electrical current that reaches the fetus is small.[207] Careful FHR monitoring during the procedure is required, as is left uterine displacement to avoid aortocaval compression. Endotracheal intubation is advisable after the first trimester.

If maternal cardiorespiratory arrest occurs during cardioversion or at any time during pregnancy, resuscitation should be initiated as for any nonpregnant patient.[208] Left uterine displacement should be maintained during resuscitation. If initial resuscitative efforts are unsuccessful, early performance of perimortem cesarean delivery should be considered, not only to save a viable fetus but also to improve the likelihood of successful resuscitation of the mother.

Fetal Monitoring during Surgery

Continuous FHR monitoring (using transabdominal Doppler ultrasonography) is feasible beginning at approximately 18 to 20 weeks' gestation.[209] However, technical problems may limit the use of continuous FHR monitoring between 18 and 22 weeks' gestation. Transabdominal monitoring may not be possible during abdominal procedures or when the mother is very obese; use of transvaginal Doppler ultrasonography may be considered in selected cases. The American College of Obstetricians and Gynecologists has stated that "the decision to use [intraoperative] fetal monitoring should be individualized, and each case warrants a team approach for optimal safety of the woman and her baby."[210]

FHR variability, which typically is a good indicator of fetal well-being, is present by 25 to 27 weeks' gestation. Changes in the baseline FHR and FHR variability caused by anesthetic agents or other drugs must be distinguished from changes that result from fetal hypoxia. Persistent severe fetal bradycardia typically indicates true fetal compromise.

Intraoperative FHR monitoring requires the presence of someone who can interpret the FHR tracing. In addition, a plan should be in place that addresses how to proceed in the event of persistent nonreassuring fetal status, including whether to perform emergency cesarean delivery. The greatest value of intraoperative FHR monitoring is that it allows for the optimization of the maternal condition if the fetus shows signs of compromise. In one case, for example, decreased FHR variability was associated with maternal hypoxia, and the pattern resolved when maternal oxygenation improved (Figure 17-9).[150] An unexplained change in FHR mandates the evaluation of maternal position, blood pressure, oxygenation, and acid-base status, and the inspection of the surgical site to ensure that neither surgeons nor retractors are impairing uterine perfusion.

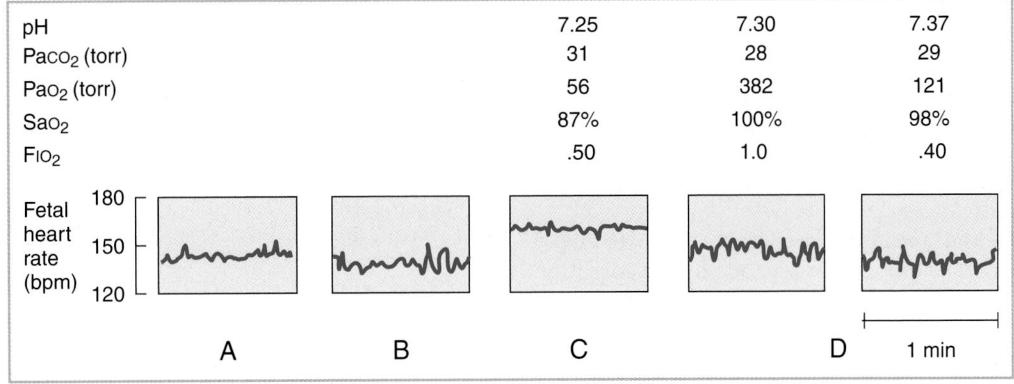

FIGURE 17-9 Serial samples of the fetal heart rate tracing and corresponding maternal arterial blood gas measurements in a patient undergoing eye surgery. **A** and **B,** Baseline fetal heart rate of 140 bpm with normal variability. **C,** Fetal tachycardia and decrease in variability during inadvertent maternal hypoxemia (maternal Pao_2 = 56 mm Hg). **D,** After correction of maternal ventilation, baseline fetal heart rate and variability return. (Redraw from Katz JD, Hook R, Barash PG. Fetal heart rate monitoring in pregnant patients undergoing surgery. Am J Obstet Gynecol 1976; 125:267.)

Anesthetic Management

PREOPERATIVE MANAGEMENT

Premedication may be necessary to allay maternal anxiety. Pregnant women are at increased risk for acid aspiration after 18 to 20 weeks' gestation (see earlier). Pharmacologic precautions against acid aspiration may include preanesthetic administration of a histamine (H_2) receptor antagonist, metoclopramide, and a clear nonparticulate antacid such as sodium citrate.

CHOICE OF ANESTHESIA

The choice of anesthesia should be guided by maternal indications and consideration of the site and nature of the surgery. No study has found an association between improved fetal outcome and any specific anesthetic technique, except for a single retrospective chart analysis in which the use of general anesthesia was associated with a significantly lower birth weight despite similar gestational age at delivery.[211] When possible, however, local or regional anesthesia (with the exception of paracervical block) is preferred, as it permits the administration of drugs with no laboratory or clinical evidence of teratogenesis. In addition, maternal respiratory complications occur less frequently with local and regional anesthetic techniques. These techniques are suitable for cervical cerclage and urologic or extremity procedures. Most abdominal operations require general anesthesia, because the incision typically extends to the upper abdomen. This situation may create an unacceptably high risk of aspiration in a pregnant patient with an unprotected airway.

PREVENTION OF AORTOCAVAL COMPRESSION

Beginning at 18 to 20 weeks' gestation, the pregnant patient should be transported on her side, and the uterus should be displaced leftward when she is positioned on the operating table.

MONITORING

Maternal monitoring should include noninvasive or invasive blood pressure measurement, electrocardiography, pulse oximetry, capnography, temperature monitoring, and the use of a peripheral nerve stimulator. The FHR and uterine activity should be monitored both before and after surgery. Intraoperative FHR monitoring may be considered when technically feasible, depending on the ease of monitoring, the type and site of surgery, and gestational age.

ANESTHETIC TECHNIQUE

General anesthesia mandates endotracheal intubation beginning at approximately 18 to 20 weeks' gestation, or earlier if gastrointestinal function is abnormal. Denitrogenation (i.e., preoxygenation) should precede the application of cricoid pressure, rapid-sequence induction, and endotracheal intubation. Drugs with a history of safe use during pregnancy include thiopental, morphine, fentanyl, succinylcholine, and the nondepolarizing muscle relaxants. Many obstetric anesthesia providers would now add propofol to this list of "safe" drugs.

A commonly used technique employs a high concentration of oxygen, a muscle relaxant, and an opioid and/or a moderate concentration of a volatile halogenated agent. Scientific evidence does not support avoidance of nitrous oxide during pregnancy,[212] particularly after the sixth week of gestation. Omission of nitrous oxide may increase fetal risk if inadequate anesthesia results or if a high dose of a volatile agent results in maternal hypotension. A cautious approach would restrict nitrous oxide administration to a concentration of 50% or less and would limit its use in extremely long operations. Hyperventilation should be avoided; rather, end-tidal CO_2 should be maintained in the normal range for pregnancy.

Rapid intravenous infusion of 1 L of crystalloid immediately before or during the initiation of spinal or epidural anesthesia seems prudent, although the anesthesia provider should not assume that this measure will prevent maternal hypotension. Some anesthesia providers would argue that colloids are more effective than crystalloid in preventing hypotension. Vasopressors should be available to treat hypotension if it occurs. Maternal hypotension should be treated aggressively. The usual precautions must be taken to guard against a high neuraxial blockade and systemic local anesthetic toxicity.

Regardless of the anesthetic technique, steps to avoid hypoxemia, hypotension, acidosis, and hyperventilation are the most critical elements of anesthetic management.

POSTOPERATIVE MANAGEMENT

The FHR and uterine activity should be monitored during recovery from anesthesia. Adequate analgesia should be ensured with systemic or neuraxial opioids, acetaminophen, or neural blockade. Nonsteroidal inflammatory agents (NSAIDs) may be used until the second half of pregnancy, at which time they should be used with caution. Prophylaxis against venous thrombosis should be considered, especially if patients are immobilized.

KEY POINTS

- A significant number of women undergo anesthesia and surgery during pregnancy for procedures unrelated to delivery.
- Maternal risks are associated with the anatomic and physiologic changes of pregnancy (e.g., difficult intubation, aspiration) and with the underlying maternal disease.
- The diagnosis of abdominal conditions often is delayed during pregnancy, increasing the risk of maternal and fetal morbidity.
- Maternal catastrophes involving severe hypoxia, hypotension, and acidosis pose the greatest acute risk to the fetus.
- Other fetal risks associated with surgery include fetal loss, preterm labor, growth restriction, and low birth weight. Clinical studies suggest that anesthesia and surgery during pregnancy do not increase the risk of congenital anomalies.
- It is unclear whether adverse fetal outcomes result from the anesthetic, the operation, or the underlying maternal disease.
- No anesthetic agent is a proven teratogen in humans, although some anesthetic agents, specifically nitrous oxide, are teratogenic in animals under certain conditions.
- Many anesthetic agents have been used for anesthesia during pregnancy, with no demonstrable differences in maternal or fetal outcome.
- The anesthetic management of the pregnant surgical patient should focus on the avoidance of hypoxemia, hypotension, acidosis, and hyperventilation.

REFERENCES

1. Mazze RI, Källén B. Reproductive outcome after anesthesia and operation during pregnancy: A registry study of 5405 cases. Am J Obstet Gynecol 1989; 161:1178-85.
2. Brodsky JB, Cohen EN, Brown BW, et al. Surgery during pregnancy and fetal outcome. Am J Obstet Gynecol 1980; 138:1165-7.
3. Shnider SM, Webster GM. Maternal and fetal hazards of surgery during pregnancy. Am J Obstet Gynecol 1965; 92:891-900.
4. Manley S, De Kelaita G, Joseph NJ. Preoperative pregnancy testing in ambulatory surgery. Anesthesiology 1995; 83:690-3.
5. Kasliwal A, Farquharson RG. Pregnancy testing prior to sterilisation. Br J Obstet Gynaecol 2000; 107:1407-9.
6. Azzam FJ, Padda GS, DeBoard JW, et al. Preoperative pregnancy testing in adolescents. Anesth Analg 1996; 82:4-7.
7. Anonymous. ASA practice advisory for preanesthesia evaluation. Anesthesiology 2002; 96:485-96.
8. Wheeler M, Coté CJ. Preoperative pregnancy testing in a tertiary care children's hospital: A medico-legal conundrum. J Clin Anesth 1999; 11:56-63.
9. The Confidential Inquiry into Maternal and Child Health. Why Mothers Die: 2000-2002. The Sixth Report of the Confidential Inquires into Maternal Death in the United Kingdom. London, CEMACH, 2005.
10. Lewis G, editor. The Confidential Inquiry into Maternal and Child Health, Saving Mothers' Lives: Reviewing maternal deaths to make motherhood safer: 2003-2005. The Seventh Report of the Confidential Inquiries into Maternal Death in the United Kingdom. London, CEMACH, 2007.
11. Gin T, Chan MTV. Decreased minimum alveolar concentration of isoflurane in pregnant humans. Anesthesiology 1994; 81:829-32.
12. Chan MTV, Mainland P, Gin T. Minimum alveolar concentrations of halothane and enflurane are decreased in early pregnancy. Anesthesiology 1996; 85:782-6.
13. Spaanderman ME, Meertens M, van Bussel M, et al. Cardiac output increases independently of basal metabolic rate in early human pregnancy. Am J Physiol Heart Circ Physiol 2000; 278:H1585-8.
14. Capeless EL, Clapp JF. Cardiovascular changes in early phase of pregnancy. Am J Obstet Gynecol 1989; 161:1449-53.
15. Gerbasi FR, Bottoms S, Farag A, et al. Increased intravascular coagulation associated with pregnancy. Obstet Gynecol 1990; 75:385-9.
16. Taniguchi S, Fukuda I, Minakawa M, et al. Emergency pulmonary embolectomy during the second trimester of pregnancy: Report of a case. Surg Today 2008; 38:59-61.
17. Duhl AJ, Paidas MJ, Ural SH, et al. Antithrombotic therapy and pregnancy: Consensus report and recommendations for prevention and treatment of venous thromboembolism and adverse pregnancy outcomes. Am J Obstet Gynecol 2007; 197:457.e1-21.
18. Brock-Utne JG, Dow TGB, Dimopoulos GE, et al. Gastric and lower oesophageal sphincter pressures early in pregnancy. Br J Anaesth 1981; 53:381-4.
19. Gin T, Mainland P, Chan MTV, et al. Decreased thiopental requirements in early pregnancy. Anesthesiology 1997; 86:73-8.
20. Higuchi H, Adachi Y, Arimura S, et al. Early pregnancy does not reduce the C50 of propofol for loss of consciousness. Anesth Analg 2001; 93:1565-9.
21. Leighton BL, Cheek TG, Gross JB, et al. Succinylcholine pharmacodynamics in peripartum patients. Anesthesiology 1986; 64:202-5.
22. Sturrock J, Nunn JF. Effects of halothane on DNA synthesis and the presynthetic phase (G_1) in dividing fibroblasts. Anesthesiology 1976; 45:413-20.
23. Wilson JG. Environment and Birth Defects. New York, Academic Press, 1973:1-82.
24. Shepard TH. Catalog of Teratogenic Agents. 7th edition. Baltimore, Johns Hopkins University Press, 1992.
25. Roberts CJ, Lowe CR. Where have all the conceptions gone? Lancet 1975; 1(7907):498-9.
26. Haring OM. Effects of prenatal hypoxia on the cardiovascular system in the rat. Arch Pathol 1965; 80:351-6.

27. Haring OM. Cardiac malformations in rats induced by exposure of the mother to carbon dioxide during pregnancy. Circ Res 1960; 8:1218-27.
28. Geber WF. Developmental effects of chronic maternal and audiovisual stress on the rat fetus. J Embryol Exp Morphol 1966; 16:1-16.
29. Ornoy A. Embryonic oxidative stress as a mechanism of teratogenesis with special emphasis on diabetic embryopathy. Reprod Toxicol 2007; 24:31-41.
30. Lowe SA. Diagnostic radiography in pregnancy: Risks and reality. Aust N Z J Obstet Gynaecol 2004; 44:191-6.
31. Valentin J. Pregnancy and medical radiation. ICRP Publication 84. Ann ICRP 2000; 30:1-43.
32. Fisher JE Jr, Acuff-Smith KD, Schilling MA, et al. Teratologic evaluation of rats prenatally exposed to pulsed-wave ultrasound. Teratology 1994; 49:150-5.
33. Child SZ, Carstensen EL, Gates AH, Hall WJ. Testing for teratogenicity of pulsed ultrasound in mice. Ultrasound Med Biol 1988; 14:493-8.
34. Vorhees CV, Acuff-Smith KD, Schilling MA, et al. Behavioral teratologic effects of prenatal exposure to continuous-wave ultrasound in unanaesthetized rats. Teratology 1994; 50:238-49.
35. Hande PM, Devi PU. Teratogenic effects of repeated exposures to X-rays and/or ultrasound in mice. Neurotoxicol Teratol 1995; 17:179-88.
36. Miller MW, Nyborgs WL, Dewey WC, et al. Hyperthermic teratogenicity, thermal dose and diagnostic ultrasound during pregnancy: Implications of new standards on tissue heating. Int J Hyperthermia 2002; 18:361-84.
37. Tyndall DA. MRI effects on craniofacial size and crown-rump length in C57BL/6J mice in 1.5T fields. Oral Surg Oral Med Oral Pathol 1993; 76:655-60.
38. Yip YP, Capriotti C, Talagala SL, Yip JW. Effects of exposure at 1.5T on early embryonic development of the chick. J Magn Reson Imaging 1994; 4:742-8.
39. Rodegerdts EA, Gronewaller EF, Kehlbach R, et al. In vitro evaluation of teratogenic effects by time-varying MR gradient fields on fetal human fibroblasts. J Magn Reson Imaging 2000; 12:150-6.
40. De Santis M, Straface G, Cavaliere AF, et al. Gadolinium preconceptional exposure: Pregnancy and neonatal outcome. Acta Obstet Gynecol 2007; 86:99-101.
41. Geber WF, Schramm LC. Congenital malformations of the central nervous system produced by narcotic analgesics in the hamster. Am J Obstet Gynecol 1975; 123:705-13.
42. Jurand A. Malformations of the central nervous system induced by neurotropic drugs in mouse embryos. Dev Growth Differentiation 1980; 22:61-78.
43. Harpel HS, Gautieri RF. Morphine induced fetal malformations. I. Exencephaly and axial skeletal fusion. J Pharm Sci 1968; 57:1590-7.
44. Jurand A, Martin LVH. Teratogenic potential of two neurotropic drugs, haloperidol and dextromoramide, tested on mouse embryos. Teratology 1990; 42:45-54.
45. Ciociola AA, Gautieri RF. Evaluation of the teratogenicity of morphine sulfate administered via a miniature implantable minipump. J Pharm Sci 1983; 72:742-5.
46. Fujinaga M, Mazze RI. Teratogenic and postnatal developmental studies of morphine in Sprague-Dawley rats. Teratology 1988; 38:401-10.
47. Fujinaga M, Stevenson JB, Mazze RI. Reproductive and teratogenic effects of fentanyl in Sprague-Dawley rats. Teratology 1986; 34:51-7.
48. Fujinaga M, Mazze RI, Jackson EC, et al. Reproductive and teratogenic effects of sufentanil and alfentanil in Sprague-Dawley rats. Anesth Analg 1988; 67:166-9.
49. Martin LVH, Jurand A. The absence of teratogenic effects of some analgesics used in anaesthesia. Anaesthesia 1992; 47:473-6.
50. McColl JD, Globus M, Robinson S. Drug induced skeletal malformations in the rat. Experientia 1963; 19:183-4.
51. Finnel RH, Shields HE, Taylor SM, et al. Strain differences in phenobarbital-induced teratogenesis in mice. Teratology 1987; 35:177-85.
52. Tonge SR. Permanent alterations in catecholamine concentrations in discrete areas of brain in the offspring of rats treated with methylamphetamine and chlorpromazine. Br J Pharmacol 1973; 47:425-7.
53. Robson JM, Sullivan FM. The production of foetal abnormalities in rabbits by imipramine. Lancet 1963; 1(7282):638-9.
54. Briggs GC, Freeman RK, Yaffe SJ. Drugs in Pregnancy and Lactation. 3rd edition. Baltimore, Williams & Wilkins, 1990.
55. Fredriksson A, Ponten E, Gordh T, Eriksson P. Neonatal exposure to a combination of N-methyl-D-aspartate and p-aminobutyric acid type A receptor anesthetic agents potentiates apoptotic neurodegeneration and persistent behavioral deficits. Anesthesiology 2007; 107:427-36.
56. Nikizad H, Yon JH, Carter LB, Jevtovic-Todorovic V. Early exposure to general anesthesia causes significant neuronal deletion in the developing rat brain. Ann N Y Acad Sci 2007; 1122:69-82.
57. Perouansky M. General anesthetics and long-term neurotoxicity. In Schuttler J, Schwilden H, editors. Modern Anesthetics: Handbook of Experimental Pharmacology. New York, Springer, 2008:143-57.
58. Safra MJ, Oakley GP. Association between cleft lip with or without cleft palate and prenatal exposure to diazepam. Lancet 1975; 2(7933):478-80.
59. Saxén I, Saxén L. Association between maternal intake of diazepam and oral clefts (letter). Lancet 1975; 2(7933):498.
60. Rosenberg L, Mitchell AA, Parsells JL, et al. Lack of correlation of oral clefts to diazepam use during pregnancy. N Engl J Med 1983; 309:1282-5.
61. Shiono PH, Mills JL. Oral clefts and diazepam use during pregnancy. N Engl J Med 1984; 311:919-20.
62. Sturrock JE, Nunn JF. Cytotoxic effects of procaine, lignocaine and bupivacaine. Br J Anaesth 1979; 51:273-81.
63. Fujinaga M, Mazze RI. Reproductive and teratogenic effects of lidocaine in Sprague-Dawley rats. Anesthesiology 1986; 65:626-32.
64. Teiling AKY, Mohammed AK, Minor BG, et al. Lack of effects of prenatal exposure to lidocaine on development of behavior in rats. Anesth Analg 1987; 66:533-41.
65. Fujinaga M, Baden JM, Mazze RI. Developmental toxicity of nondepolarizing muscle relaxants in cultured rat embryos. Anesthesiology 1992; 76:999-1003.
66. Jacobs RM. Failure of muscle relaxants to produce cleft palate in mice. Teratology 1971; 4:25-30.
67. Jago RH. Arthrogryposis following treatment of maternal tetanus with muscle relaxants. Arch Dis Child 1970; 45:227-9.
68. Basford A, Fink BR. Teratogenicity of halothane in the rat. Anesthesiology 1968; 29:1167-73.
69. Wharton RS, Mazze RI, Baden JM, et al. Fertility, reproduction and postnatal survival in mice chronically exposed to halothane. Anesthesiology 1978; 48:167-74.
70. Mazze RI. Fertility, reproduction, and postnatal survival in mice chronically exposed to isoflurane. Anesthesiology 1985; 63:663-7.
71. Wharton RS, Wilson AI, Mazze RI, et al. Fetal morphology in mice exposed to halothane. Anesthesiology 1979; 51:532-7.
72. Mazze RI, Wilson AI, Rice SA, et al. Fetal development in mice exposed to isoflurane. Teratology 1985; 32:339-45.
73. Mazze RI, Fujinaga M, Rice SA, et al. Reproductive and teratogenic effects of nitrous oxide, halothane, isoflurane, and enflurane in Sprague-Dawley rats. Anesthesiology 1986; 64:339-44.
74. Fink BR, Shepard TH, Blandau RJ. Teratogenic activity of nitrous oxide. Nature 1967; 214:146-8.
75. Bussard DA, Stoelting RK, Peterson C, et al. Fetal changes in hamsters anesthetized with nitrous oxide and halothane. Anesthesiology 1974; 41:275-8.
76. Mazze RI, Wilson AI, Rice SA, et al. Reproduction and fetal development in rats exposed to nitrous oxide. Teratology 1984; 30:259-65.
77. Lane GA, Nahrwold ML, Tait AR, et al. Anesthetics as teratogens: Nitrous oxide is teratogenic, xenon is not. Science 1980; 210:899-901.
78. Vieira E, Cleaton-Jones P, Austin JC. Effects of low concentrations of nitrous oxide on rat fetuses. Anesth Analg 1980; 59:175-7.
79. Fujinaga M, Baden JM, Mazze RI. Susceptible period of nitrous oxide teratogenicity in Sprague-Dawley rats. Teratology 1989; 40:439-44.
80. Fujinaga M, Baden JM, Shephard TH, et al. Nitrous oxide alters body laterality in rats. Teratology 1990; 41:131-5.
81. Fujinaga M, Baden JM. Critical period of rat development when sidedness of asymmetric body structures is determined. Teratology 1991; 44:453-62.

82. Baden JM, Fujinaga M. Effects of nitrous oxide on day 9 rat embryos grown in culture. Br J Anaesth 1991; 66:500-3.
83. Chanarin I. Cobalamins and nitrous oxide: A review. J Clin Pathol 1980; 33:909-16.
84. Koblin DD, Watson JE, Deady JE, et al. Inactivation of methionine synthetase by nitrous oxide in mice. Anesthesiology 1981; 54:318-24.
85. Koblin DD, Waskell L, Watson JE 2nd, et al. Nitrous oxide inactivates methionine synthetase in human liver. Anesth Analg 1982; 61:75-8.
86. Baden JM, Rice SA, Serra M, et al. Thymidine and methionine syntheses in pregnant rats exposed to nitrous oxide. Anesth Analg 1983; 62:738-41.
87. Keeling PA, Rocke DA, Nunn JF, et al. Folinic acid protection against nitrous oxide teratogenicity in the rat. Br J Anaesth 1986; 58:528-34.
88. Mazze RI, Fujinaga M, Baden JM. Halothane prevents nitrous oxide teratogenicity in Sprague-Dawley rats: Folinic acid does not. Teratology 1988; 38:121-7.
89. Fujinaga M, Baden JM, Yhap EO, et al. Reproductive and teratogenic effects of nitrous oxide, isoflurane, and their combination in Sprague-Dawley rats. Anesthesiology 1987; 67:960-4.
90. Fujinaga M, Baden JM. Methionine prevents nitrous oxide-induced teratogenicity in rat embryos grown in culture. Anesthesiology 1994; 81:184-9.
91. Fujinaga M, Baden JM. Evidence for an adrenergic mechanism in the control of body symmetry. Dev Biol 1991; 143:203-5.
92. Fujinaga M, Maze M, Hoffman BB, et al. Activation of alpha-1 adrenergic receptors modulates the control of left/right sidedness in rat embryos. Dev Biol 1992; 150:419-21.
93. Fujinaga M, Baden JM, Suto A, et al. Preventive effects of phenoxybenzamine on nitrous oxide-induced reproductive toxicity in Sprague-Dawley rats. Teratology 1991; 43:151-7.
94. Jevtovic-Todorovic V, Wozniak DF, Benshoff N, Olney JW. Commonly used anesthesia protocol causes neuronal suicide in the immature rat brain. Soc Neurosci Abstr 2001; 27:398.
95. Cohen EN, Belville JW, Brown BW. Anesthesia, pregnancy, and miscarriage: A study of operating room nurses and anesthetists. Anesthesiology 1971; 35:343-7.
96. Knill-Jones RP, Moir DD, Rodrigues LV, et al. Anaesthetic practice and pregnancy: Controlled survey of women anaesthetists in the United Kingdom. Lancet 1972; 2(7764):1326-8.
97. Cohen EN, Brown BW, Bruce DL, et al. Occupational disease among operating room personnel: A national study. Anesthesiology 1974; 41:321-40.
98. Cohen EN, Brown BW, Wu ML, et al. Occupational disease in dentistry and chronic exposure to trace anesthetic gases. J Am Dent Assoc 1980; 101:21-31.
99. Spence AA, Cohen EN, Brown BW. Occupational hazards for operating room-based physicians. JAMA 1977; 283:955-9.
100. Buring JE, Hennekens CH, Mayrent SL, et al. Health experiences of operating room personnel. Anesthesiology 1985; 62:325-30.
101. Tannenbaum TN, Goldberg RJ. Exposure to anesthetic gases and reproductive outcome. J Occup Med 1985; 27:659-68.
102. Mazze RI, Lecky JH. The health of operating room personnel (editorial). Anesthesiology 1985; 62:226-8.
103. Harlap S, Shiono PH. Alcohol, smoking, and incidence of spontaneous abortions in the first and second trimesters. Lancet 1980; 2(8187):173-6.
104. Kline J, Stein ZA, Susser M, et al. Smoking: A risk factor for spontaneous abortion. N Engl J Med 1977; 297:793-6.
105. Ericson HA, Källén B. Hospitalization for miscarriage and delivery outcome among Swedish nurses working in operating rooms, 1973-1978. Anesth Analg 1985; 64:981-8.
106. Spence AA. Environmental pollution by inhalation anaesthetics. Br J Anaesth 1987; 59:96-103.
107. Brodsky JB, Cohen EN. Health experiences of operating room personnel. Anesthesiology 1985; 63:461-3.
108. Rowland AS, Baird DD, Weinberger CR, et al. Reduced fertility among women employed as dental assistants exposed to high levels of nitrous oxide. N Engl J Med 1992; 327:993-7.
109. Smith BE. Fetal prognosis after anesthesia during gestation. Anesth Analg 1963; 42:521-6.
110. Shnider SM, Webster GM. Maternal and fetal hazards of surgery during pregnancy. Am J Obstet Gynecol 1965; 92:891-900.
111. Crawford JS, Lewis M. Nitrous oxide in early human pregnancy. Anaesthesia 1986; 41:900-5.
112. Aldridge IM, Tunstall ME. Nitrous oxide and the fetus: A review and the results of a retrospective study of 175 cases of anaesthesia for insertion of a Shirodkar suture. Br J Anaesth 1986; 58:1348-56.
113. Duncan PG, Pope WDB, Cohen MM, et al. Fetal risk of anesthesia and surgery during pregnancy. Anesthesiology 1986; 64:790-4.
114. Källén B, Mazze RI. Neural tube defects and first trimester operations. Teratology 1990; 41:717-20.
115. Sylvester GC, Khoury MJ, Lu X, et al. First trimester anesthesia exposure and the risk of central nervous system defects: A population-based case-control study. Am J Public Health 1994; 84:1757-60.
116. Smith RF, Bowman RE, Katz J. Behavioral effects of exposure to halothane during early development in the rat. Anesthesiology 1978; 49:319-23.
117. Levin ED, Bowman RE. Behavioral effects of chronic exposure to low concentrations of halothane during development in rats. Anesth Analg 1986; 65:653-9.
118. Chalon J, Hillman D, Gross S, et al. Intrauterine exposure to halothane increases murine postnatal autotolerance to halothane and reduces brain weight. Anesth Analg 1983; 62:565-7.
119. Armitage SG. The effects of barbiturates on the behavior of rat offspring as measured in learning and reasoning situations. J Comp Physiol Psychol 1952; 45:146-52.
120. Chalon J, Walpert L, Ramanathan S, et al. Meperidine-promethazine combination and learning function of mice and of their progeny. Can Anaesth Soc J 1982; 29:612-6.
121. Hoffeld DR, McNew J, Webster RL. Effect of tranquilizing drugs during pregnancy on activity of offspring. Nature 1968; 218:357-8.
122. Jevtovic-Todorovic V, Hartman RE, Izumi Y, et al. Early exposure to common anesthetic agents causes widespread neurodegeneration in the developing rat brain and persistent learning deficits. J Neurosci 2003; 23:876-82.
123. Ikonomidou C, Bosch F, Miksa M, et al. Blockade of NMDA receptors and apoptotic neurodegeneration in the developing brain. Science 1999; 283:70-4.
124. Ishimaru MJ, Ikonomidou C, Tenkova TI, et al. Distinguishing excitotoxic from apoptotic neurodegeneration in the developing rat brain. J Comp Neurol 1999; 408:461-76.
125. Kuan CY, Roth KA, Flavell RA, Rakic P. Mechanisms of programmed cell death in the developing brain. Trends Neurosci 2000; 23:291-7.
126. Anand KJS, Soriano SG. Anesthetic agents and the immature brain: Are these toxic or therapeutic agents? Anesthesiology 2004; 101:527-30.
127. Bhutta AT, Anand KJ. Vulnerability of the developing brain: Neuronal mechanisms. Clin Perinatol 2002; 29:357-72.
128. Hayashi H, Dikkes P, Soriano SG. Repeated administration of ketamine may lead to neuronal degeneration in the developing rat brain. Paediatr Anaesth 2002; 12:770-4.
129. Ruda MA, Ling QD, Hohmann AG, et al. Altered nociceptive neuronal circuits after neonatal peripheral inflammation. Science 2000; 289:628-31.
130. McClain RJ, Uemura K, de la Fuente SG, et al. General anesthesia improves fetal cerebral oxygenation without evidence of subsequent neuronal injury. J Cerebr Blood Flow Metab 2005; 25:1060-9.
131. U.S. Department of Health and Human Services, Food and Drug Administration, Center for Drug Evaluation and Research, Anesthetic and Life Support Drugs Advisory Committee. Meeting, Rockville, Maryland, March 29, 2007. Available at http://www.fda.gov/ohrms/dockets/ac/07/transcripts/2007-4285t1.pdf
132. Panigel M. Placental perfusion experiments. Am J Obstet Gynecol 1962; 84:1664-83.
133. Khazin AF, Hon EH, Hehre FW. Effects of maternal hyperoxia on the fetus. I. Oxygen tension. Am J Obstet Gynecol 1971; 109:628-37.

134. Motoyama EK, Rivard G, Acheson F, et al. The effect of changes in maternal pH and P_{CO_2} on the P_{O_2} of fetal lambs. Anesthesiology 1967; 28:891-903.
135. Kamban JR, Handte RE, Brown WU, et al. The effect of normal and preeclamptic pregnancies on the oxyhemoglobin dissociation curve. Anesthesiology 1986; 65:426-7.
136. Levinson G, Shnider SM, de Lorimier AA, et al. Effects of maternal hyperventilation on uterine blood flow and fetal oxygenation and acid-base status. Anesthesiology 1974; 40:340-7.
137. Brann AW, Myers RE. Central nervous system findings in the newborn monkey following severe in utero partial asphyxia. Neurology 1975; 25:327-38.
138. Newman B, Lam AM. Induced hypotension for clipping of a cerebral aneurysm during pregnancy. Anesth Analg 1986; 65:675-8.
139. Shnider SM, Wright RG, Levinson G, et al. Uterine blood flow and plasma norepinephrine changes during maternal stress in the pregnant ewe. Anesthesiology 1979; 50:524-7.
140. Oats JN, Vasey DP, Waldron BA. Effects of ketamine on the pregnant uterus. Br J Anaesth 1979; 51:1163-6.
141. Greiss FC, Still JG, Anderson SG. Effects of local anesthetic agents on the uterine vasculature and myometrium. Am J Obstet Gynecol 1976; 124:889-99.
142. Lee A, Ngan Kee WD, Gin T. A quantitative, systematic review of randomized controlled trials of ephedrine versus phenylephrine for the management of hypotension during spinal anesthesia for cesarean delivery. Anesth Analg 2002; 94:920-6.
143. Cooper DW, Carpenter M, Mowbray P, et al. Fetal and maternal effects of phenylephrine and ephedrine during spinal anesthesia for cesarean delivery. Anesthesiology 2002; 97:1582-90.
144. Palahniuk RJ, Shnider SM. Maternal and fetal cardiovascular and acid-base changes during halothane and isoflurane anesthesia in the pregnant ewe. Anesthesiology 1974; 41:462-72.
145. Palahniuk RJ, Doig GA, Johnson GN, et al. Maternal halothane anesthesia reduces cerebral blood flow in the acidotic sheep fetus. Anesth Analg 1980; 59:35-9.
146. Cheek DBC, Hughes SC, Dailey PA, et al. Effect of halothane on regional cerebral blood flow and cerebral metabolic oxygen consumption in the fetal lamb in utero. Anesthesiology 1987; 67:361-6.
147. Yarnell R, Biehl DR, Tweed WA, et al. The effect of halothane anaesthesia on the asphyxiated foetal lamb in utero. Can Anaesth Soc J 1983; 30:474-9.
148. Baker BW, Hughes SC, Shnider SM, et al. Maternal anesthesia and the stressed fetus: Effects of isoflurane on the asphyxiated fetal lamb. Anesthesiology 1990; 72:65-70.
149. Johnson ES, Colley PS. Effects of nitrous oxide and fentanyl anesthesia on fetal heart-rate variability intra- and postoperatively. Anesthesiology 1980; 52:429-30.
150. Liu PL, Warren TM, Ostheimer GW, et al. Foetal monitoring in parturients undergoing surgery unrelated to pregnancy. Can Anaesth Soc J 1985; 32:525-32.
151. Immer-Bansi A, Immer FF, Henle S, et al. Unnecessary emergency caesarean section due to silent CTG during anesthesia? Br J Anaesth 2001; 87:791-3.
152. Van de Velde M, Teunkens A, Kuypers M, et al. General anesthesia with target controlled infusion of propofol for planned caesarean section: Maternal and neonatal effects of a remifentanil-based technique. Int J Obstet Anesth 2004; 13:153-8.
153. McNall PG, Jafarnia MR. Management of myasthenia gravis in the obstetrical patient. Am J Obstet Gynecol 1965; 93:518-25.
154. Hellman LM, Johnson HL, Tolles WE, et al. Some factors affecting the fetal heart rate. Am J Obstet Gynecol 1961; 82:1055-64.
155. Abboud T, Raya J, Sadri S, et al. Fetal and maternal cardiovascular effects of atropine and glycopyrrolate. Anesth Analg 1983; 62:426-30.
156. Clark RB, Brown MA, Lattin DL. Neostigmine, atropine and glycopyrrolate: Does neostigmine cross the placenta? Anesthesiology 1996; 84:450-2.
157. Naulty J, Cefalo RC, Lewis PE. Fetal toxicity of nitroprusside in the pregnant ewe. Am J Obstet Gynecol 1981; 139:708-11.
158. Ostman PL, Chestnut DH, Robillard JE, et al. Transplacental passage and hemodynamic effects of esmolol in the gravid ewe. Anesthesiology 1988; 69:738-41.
159. Eisenach JC, Castro MI. Maternally administered esmolol produces beta-adrenergic blockade and hypoxemia in sheep. Anesthesiology 1989; 71:718-22.
160. Larson CP Jr, Shuer LM, Cohen SE. Maternally administered esmolol decreases fetal as well as maternal heart rate. J Clin Anesth 1990; 2:427-9.
161. Losasso TJ, Muzzi DA, Cucchiara RF. Response of fetal heart rate to maternal administration of esmolol. Anesthesiology 1991; 74:782-4.
162. Ducey JP, Knape KG. Maternal esmolol administration resulting in fetal distress and cesarean section in a term pregnancy. Anesthesiology 1992; 77:829-32.
163. Mazze RI, Källén B. Appendectomy during pregnancy: A Swedish registry study of 778 cases. Obstet Gynecol 1991; 77:835-40.
164. Ferguson JE II, Albright GA, Ueland K. Prevention of preterm labor following surgery. In Baden JM, Brodsky JB, editors. The Pregnant Surgical Patient. Mount Kisco, NY, Futura Publishing, 1985:223-46.
165. Groom KM. Pharmacological prevention of prematurity. Best Pract Res Clin Obstet Gynaecol 2007; 21:843-56.
166. Shim JY, Park YW, Yoon BH, et al. Multicentre, parallel group, randomised, single-blind study of the safety and efficacy of atosiban versus ritodrine in the treatment of acute preterm labour in Korean women. Br J Obstet Gynaecol 2006; 113:1228-34.
167. McKellar DP, Anderson CT, Boynton CJ, et al. Cholecystectomy during pregnancy without fetal loss. Surg Gynecol Obstet 1992; 174:465-8.
168. Cherry SH. The pregnant patient: Need for surgery unrelated to pregnancy. Mt Sinai J Med 1991; 58:81-4.
169. Stånge K, Halldin M. Hypothermia in pregnancy. Anesthesiology 1983; 58:460-1.
170. Strickland RA, Oliver WC, Chantigian RC, et al. Anesthesia, cardiopulmonary bypass, and the pregnant patient. Mayo Clin Proc 1991; 66:411-29.
171. Merritt WT, Dickstein R, Beattie C, et al. Liver transplantation during pregnancy: Anesthesia for two procedures in the same patient with successful outcome of pregnancy. Transplant Proc 1991; 23:1996-7.
172. Buckley TA, Yau GHM, Poon WS, et al. Caesarean section and ablation of a cerebral arterio-venous malformation. Anaesth Intensive Care 1990; 18:248-51.
173. Coleman NT, Trianfo VA, Rund DA. Nonobstetric emergencies in pregnancy: Trauma and surgical conditions. Am J Obstet Gynecol 1997; 177:497-502.
174. Augustin G, Majerovic M. Non-obstetrical acute abdomen during pregnancy. Eur J Obstet Gynecol Reprod Biol 2007; 131:4-12.
175. Babaknia A, Hossein P, Woodruff JD. Appendicitis during pregnancy. Obstet Gynecol 1977; 50:40-4.
176. Reynolds JD, Booth JV, de la Fuente S, et al. A review of laparoscopy for non-obstetric related surgery during pregnancy. Curr Surg 2003; 60:164-73.
177. Cruz AM, Southerland LC, Duke T, et al. Intraabdominal carbon dioxide insufflation in the pregnant ewe. Anesthesiology 1996; 85:1395-1402.
178. Barnard JM, Chaffin D, Droste S, et al. Fetal response to carbon dioxide peritoneum in the pregnant ewe. Obstet Gynecol 1995; 85:669-74.
179. Fatum M, Rojansky N. Laparoscopic surgery during pregnancy. Obstet Gynecol Surv 2001; 56:50-9.
180. Reedy MB, Galan HL, Richards WE. Laparoscopy during pregnancy: A survey of laparoendoscopic surgeons. J Reprod Med 1997; 42:33-8.
181. Reedy MB, Källén B, Kuehl TJ. Laparoscopy during pregnancy: A study of five fetal outcome parameters with use of the Swedish Health Registry. Am J Obstet Gynecol 1997; 177:673-9.
182. Affleck DG, Handrahan D, Egger MJ, et al. The laparoscopic management of appendicitis and cholelithiasis during pregnancy. Am J Surg 1999; 178:523-9.
183. Gouldman JW, Sticca RP, Rippon MB, et al. Laparoscopic cholecystectomy in pregnancy. Am Surg 1998; 64:93-7.

184. Tazuke SI, Nezhat FR, Nezhat CH, et al. Laparoscopic management of pelvic pathology during pregnancy. J Am Assoc Gynecol Laparosc 1997; 4:605-8.
185. Gurbuz AT, Peetz ME. The acute abdomen in the pregnant patient: Is there a role for laparoscopy? Surg Endosc 1997; 11:98-102.
186. Wishner JD, Zolfaghari D, Wohlgemuth SD, et al. Laparoscopic cholecystectomy in pregnancy: A report of 6 cases and review of the literature. Surg Endosc 1996; 10:314-8.
187. Lemaire BM, van Erp WF. Laparoscopic surgery during pregnancy. Surg Endosc 1997; 11:15-8.
188. Eichenberg BJ, Vanderlinden J, Miguel C, et al. Laparoscopic cholecystectomy in the third trimester of pregnancy. Am Surg 1996; 62:874-7.
189. Amos JD, Schorr SJ, Norman PF, et al. Laparoscopic surgery during pregnancy. Am J Surg 1996; 171:435-7.
190. Steinbrook RA, Brooks DC, Datta S. Laparoscopic cholecystectomy during pregnancy. Surg Endosc 1996; 10:511-6.
191. Moreno-Sanz C, Pascual-Pedreno A, Picazo-Yeste J, Seoane-Gonzalez JB. Laparoscopic appendectomy during pregnancy: Between personal experiences and scientific evidence. J Am Coll Surg 2007; 205:37-42.
192. Upadhyay A, Stanten S, Kazantsev G, et al. Laparoscopic management of a nonobstetric emergency in the third trimester of pregnancy. Surg Endosc 2007; 21:1344-8.
193. Bhavani-Shankar K, Steinbrook RA, Brooks DC, et al. Arterial to end-tidal carbon dioxide pressure difference during laparoscopic surgery in pregnancy. Anesthesiology 2000; 93:370-3.
194. Steinbrook RA, Bhavani-Shankar K. Hemodynamics during laparoscopic surgery in pregnancy. Anesth Analg 2001; 93:1570-1.
195. Tanaka H, Futamura N, Takubo S, et al. Gasless laparoscopy under epidural anesthesia for adnexal cysts during pregnancy. J Reprod Med 1999; 44:929-32.
196. Yamada H, Ohki H, Futimoto K, Okutsu Y. Laparoscopic ovarian cystectomy with abdominal lift during pregnancy under combined spinal-epidural anesthesia. Masui 2004; 53:1155-8.
197. Melgrati L, Damiani A, Gianalfredo F. Isobaric (gasless) laparoscopic myomectomy during pregnancy. J Min Invas Gynecol 2005; 12:379-81.
198. Damiani A, Melgrati L, Franzoni G, et al. Isobaric gasless laparoscopic myomectomy for removal of large uterine leiomyomas. Surg Endosc 2006; 20:1406-9.
199. Guidelines Committee of the Society of American Gastrointestinal and Endoscopic Surgeons, Yumi H. Guidelines for diagnosis, treatment, and use of laparoscopy for surgical problems during pregnancy. Surg Endosc 2008; 22:849-61.
200. Altshuler LL, Cohen L, Szuba MP, et al. Pharmacological management of psychiatric illness during pregnancy: Dilemmas and guidelines. Am J Psychiatry 1996; 153:592-605.
201. American Psychiatric Association; Task Force on ECT. The practice of ECT. Recommendations for treatment, training and privileging. Convuls Ther 1990; 6:85-120.
202. Miller LJ. Use of electroconvulsive therapy during pregnancy. Hosp Community Psychiatry 1994; 45:444-50.
203. Pinette MG, Santarpio C, Wax JR, Blackstone J. Electroconvulsive therapy in pregnancy. Obstet Gynecol 2007; 110:465-6.
204. Richards DS. Is electroconvulsive therapy in pregnancy safe? Obstet Gynecol 2007; 110:451-2.
205. Ishikawa T, Kawahara S, Saito T, et al. Anesthesia for electroconvulsive therapy during pregnancy: A case report. Masui 2001; 50:991-7.
206. Rabheru K. The use of electroconvulsive therapy in special patient populations. Can J Psychiatry 2001; 46:710-9.
207. Adamson DL, Nelson-Piercy C. Managing palpitations and arrhythmias during pregnancy. Heart 2007; 93:1630-6.
208. ECC Committee, Subcommittees and Task Forces of the American Heart Association. 2005 AHA Guidelines for Cardiopulmonary Resuscitation and Emergency Cardiovascular Care. Circulation 2005; 112:IV-150-3.
209. Biehl DR. Foetal monitoring during surgery unrelated to pregnancy. Can Anaesth Soc J 1985; 32:455-9.
210. American College of Obstetricians and Gynecologists Committee on Obstetric Practice. Nonobstetric Surgery in Pregnancy. ACOG Committee Opinion No. 284, 2003. (Obstet Gynecol 2003; 102:431.)
211. Jenkins TM, Mackey SF, Benzoni EM, et al. Non-obstetric surgery during gestation: Risk factors for lower birthweight. Aust N Z J Obstet Gynaecol 2003; 43:27-31.
212. Sanders RD, Weimann J, Maze M. Biologic effects of nitrous oxide. Anesthesiology 2008; 109:707-22.

Part VI

Labor and Vaginal Delivery

Medical and social connotations of pain have evolved through history. Since 1847 these interpretations often influenced obstetric anesthesia. During most of the nineteenth century, patients and physicians believed that an individual's physical sensitivity to pain varied with education, social standing, and acculturation. Like the princess in Hans Christian Andersen's fairy tale who could feel a pea through 40 mattresses, refined women experienced more pain than "savages." As American suffragette Elizabeth Cady Stanton observed, "[R]efined, genteel, civilized women have worse labor pain." Commenting on her own nearly painless delivery, Stanton once quipped, "Am I not almost a savage?" Upper class women often cited their sensitivity to pain as evidence of cultural superiority, and they used this fact to justify their need for obstetric anesthesia.[1]

As the nineteenth century came to a close, the social connotations of pain also changed. Many still maintained that civilized women experienced more pain than savages. On the other hand, "sensitivity" to pain now began to signify physical deterioration rather than cultural superiority. Thus one medical book published in 1882 ascribed painful labor to "the abuses of civilization, its dissipations, and the follies of fashion." Its author, an American obstetrician named Engelmann, suggested that the idle life of upper class women led to a "relaxed condition of the uterus and abdominal walls (and) a greater tendency to malposition." He suggested that the rigorous physical life of lower class women and "savages" prepared their bodies better for childbirth.[2]

Social and cultural interpretations of childbirth pain took yet another turn in 1943, with publication of the book *Revelation of Childbirth*. Its author, Grantly Dick-Read, subsequently republished his book in the United States with the title *Childbirth Without Fear*. It marked the beginning of the natural childbirth movement.

Dick-Read combined snippets of ideas from earlier concepts to formulate his own theory. He agreed with early nineteenth-century physiologists that savages have less pain than "modern women." Unlike Engelmann, Dick-Read attributed this sensitivity to cultural rather than physical factors. According to Dick-Read, modern women had painful deliveries only because the church and culture had taught them to expect it. He said that women should be reeducated and taught that childbirth is a natural physiologic process. He opined that women would then cease to fear childbirth and thereby have less pain. Dick-Read's method, the basis for childbirth education, was a prenatal program that toughened the body with exercise and prepared the mind with facts. In yet another variation, French obstetrician Fernand Lamaze substituted Pavlovian conditioning for Dick-Read's childbirth education.[3] With Dick-Read and Lamaze, many of the social concepts of childbirth pain came full circle.[4]

Donald Caton, M.D.

REFERENCES

1. Lawrence C. The nervous system and society in the Scottish enlightenment. In Barnes B, Shapin S, editors. Natural Order: Historical Studies of Scientific Culture. London, Sage Publications, 1979:19-40.
2. Engelmann GJ. Labor among Primitive Peoples: Showing the Development of the Obstetric Science of Today from the Natural and Instinctive Customs of all Races, Civilized and Savage, Past and Present. St. Louis, JH Chambers, 1882:130.
3. Dick-Read G. Revelation of Childbirth. London, Heinemann, 1943.
4. Caton D. Medical science and social values. Int J Obstet Anesth 2004; 13:167-73.

Chapter 18

Obstetric Management of Labor and Vaginal Delivery

Alan T. N. Tita, M.D., Ph.D.
Dwight J. Rouse, M.D., M.S.P.H.

THE PROCESS OF LABOR AND DELIVERY

Labor, which is also called *parturition*, is the process by which sufficiently frequent and strong uterine contractions cause thinning (i.e., effacement) and dilation of the cervix, thereby permitting passage of the fetus from the uterus through the birth canal.

Onset of Labor

TIMING

Fewer than 10% of pregnancies end on the expected date of delivery (EDD), although the majority of births occur within 7 days of the EDD. In the United States, approximately 13% of births occur preterm (before 37 weeks' gestation), and approximately 5% to 7% of pregnancies remain undelivered at 42 weeks' gestation (14 days after the EDD, known as post-term). These rates are lower for carefully dated pregnancies.

MECHANISM

The cause of the onset of labor in women—either term or preterm—remains unknown. In other mammalian species, a decline in serum progesterone concentration in association with a rise in estrogen concentration is followed by increases in prostaglandin production, oxytocin receptors, and myometrial gap junction formation. In sheep, the fetus apparently triggers parturition through a surge in fetal cortisol production. In women, progesterone concentrations do not fall before the onset of labor, and no surge in fetal cortisol secretion occurs. The laboring human uterus does manifest increases in prostaglandin production, oxytocin receptors, and myometrial gap junction formation.[1,2] As more is learned, it is likely that the apparent interspecies discrepancies will be resolved and that a unifying concept of the onset of mammalian labor will emerge. Preterm and post-term deliveries both constitute important obstetric problems, and when more is understood about the mechanism of the onset of labor, new approaches to preventing the preterm and post-term onset of parturition may evolve.

Stages of Labor

By convention, labor is divided into three stages. The first stage begins with the maternal perception of regular, painful uterine contractions and ends with the complete dilation of the cervix. Complete cervical dilation is the dilation necessary to allow movement of the fetus from the uterus into the vagina. At term gestation, 10 cm approximates complete cervical dilation. Preterm fetuses require less than 10 cm of cervical dilation. The second stage of labor begins with the complete dilation of the cervix and ends with the birth of the baby. The third stage begins with the birth of the baby and ends with the delivery of the placenta. The first stage of labor can be considered the cervical stage, the second stage the pelvic stage (reflecting the descent of the fetus through the pelvis), and the third stage the placental stage. Some authorities identify a fourth stage of labor, corresponding to the first postpartum hour, during which postpartum hemorrhage is most likely to occur.

Components of Labor and Delivery

When the events that occur during labor and vaginal delivery are considered, it is helpful to think about the following three

TABLE 18-1 Features Determined by Clinical Pelvimetry as Related to Pelvic Type

	Pelvic Type			
Suboptimal Features	**Gynecoid**	**Android**	**Anthropoid**	**Platypelloid**
Promontory reached (diagonal conjugate ≤ 12 cm)	−	±	−	+
Sacrum flat/forward (versus curved)	−	+	−	+
Spines prominent (found by medical student)	−	+	+	−
Sacrosciatic notch narrow (≤ 2 fingerbreadths)	−	+	−	−
Subpubic arch narrow (acute angle)	−	+	+	−

+, Present; −, absent; ±, variable.

From Zlatnik FJ. Normal labor and delivery and its conduct. In Scott JR, DiSaia PJ, Hammond CB, Spellacy WN, editors. Danforth's Obstetrics and Gynecology. 6th edition. Philadelphia, JB Lippincott, 1990;161-88.

components of the process: (1) the **powers** (uterine contractions and, in the second stage, the addition of voluntary maternal expulsive efforts); (2) the **passageway** (the bony pelvis and the soft tissues contained therein); and (3) the **passenger** (the fetus). The interaction of these three components determines the success or failure of the process.

THE POWERS

The uterus, which is a smooth muscle organ, contracts throughout gestation with variable frequency. The parturient verifies the onset of labor when she perceives regular, uncomfortable uterine contractions. In some women, the uterus remains relatively quiescent until the abrupt onset of labor. In others, the uterus contracts several times per hour for days without causing pain or even a clear perception of uterine contractions.

During labor, the frequency, duration, and intensity of uterine contractions increase. During early labor, the contractions may occur every 5 to 7 minutes, last 30 to 40 seconds, and develop intrauterine pressures (intensity) of 20 to 30 mm Hg above basal tone (10 to 15 mm Hg). Late in the first stage of labor, contractions typically occur every 2 to 2½ minutes, last 50 to 70 seconds, and are 40 to 60 mm Hg in intensity. This higher intensity reflects a more widespread propagation of the contractions, with the recruitment of more myometrial cells.

Retraction accompanies contraction as the myometrial cells shorten. The walls of the upper, contractile portion of the uterus thicken. Cervical dilation and effacement reflect the traction placed on the cervix by the contracting uterus. The passive lower uterine segment enlarges and becomes thinner as cervical tissue is pulled over the fetal presenting part by traction from the upper portion of the uterus. At the end of the first stage of labor, no cervix is palpable on vaginal examination. If there is no mechanical obstruction, additional uterine contractions force the fetus to descend through the birth canal. At this time, the parturient perceives an urge to defecate (reflecting pressure on the rectum). Her expulsive efforts add to the force of uterine contractions to hasten descent and shorten the second stage of labor.

THE PASSAGEWAY

The fetus must be of such size and conformation that there is no mechanical mismatch with the bony pelvis. At times, an ovarian or uterine tumor (e.g., leiomyoma), cervical cancer, or a vaginal septum may impede passage of the fetus through the birth canal, but these situations are unusual.

Four pelvic types have been described on the basis of the shape of the pelvic inlet (the plane bounded by the upper inner pubic symphysis, the linea terminalis of the iliac bones, and the sacral promontory) (Table 18-1).[3] The type and size of the pelvis constitute important predictors of the success of vaginal delivery.

The most common pelvic type and the one theoretically best suited for childbirth is the **gynecoid** pelvis. The flexed fetal head presents a circle to the bony pelvis; a pelvis with gynecoid features best accommodates this circle. The inlet is round or oval, with the transverse diameter only slightly greater than the anterior-posterior diameter. The pelvic sidewalls are straight and do not converge, the ischial spines are not prominent, the sacrum is hollow, and the subpubic arch is wide. The absence of prominent ischial spines is an important feature, because the distance between them—the transverse diameter of the midpelvis—is the narrowest pelvic dimension. The other pelvic types are less favorable for vaginal delivery.

Although radiographic pelvimetry provides much more information regarding pelvic dimensions and features than can be obtained by clinical pelvimetry alone, it has only a limited place in clinical management. In the absence of a history of pelvic fracture or musculoskeletal disease (e.g., a dwarfing condition), there are few circumstances in which the apparent pelvic anatomy precludes a trial of labor. A pelvis with smaller-than-average dimensions may be adequate for a particular fetus if the head is well-flexed, sufficient molding (i.e., overlapping of the unfused skull bones) has occurred, and the labor is strong; thus radiographic pelvimetry does not always predict the presence or absence of cephalopelvic disproportion.[4] Further, some risk is associated with radiographic pelvimetry. In addition to the potential for point mutations in the maternal oocytes and fetal germ cells, there is a small but apparently real increase in the incidence of malignancy and leukemia in children who were exposed to diagnostic radiation *in utero*. Some obstetricians use radiographic pelvimetry in cases of fetal breech presentation to assess whether fetal presentation, position, and lie are appropriate for vaginal delivery. The hope is to save a parturient from a long, futile labor

BOX 18-1 Positions of the Occiput in Early Labor, Listed in Order of Decreasing Frequency

- Left occiput transverse (LOT)
- Right occiput transverse (ROT)
- Left occiput anterior (LOA)
- Right occiput posterior (ROP)
- Right occiput anterior (ROA)
- Left occiput posterior (LOP)
- Occiput anterior (OA)
- Occiput posterior (OP)

and a hazardous delivery. Computed tomography is associated with less radiation exposure than traditional radiographic pelvimetry.

THE PASSENGER

Fetal size and the relationship of the fetus to the maternal pelvis affect labor progress. The **lie** of the fetus (the relationship of the long axis of the fetus to the long axis of the mother) can be transverse, oblique, or longitudinal. In the first two, vaginal delivery is impossible unless the fetus is very immature.

The **presentation** denotes that portion of the fetus overlying the pelvic inlet. The presentation may be cephalic, breech, or shoulder. Cephalic presentations are further subdivided into vertex, brow, or face presentations, according to the degree of flexion of the neck. In more than 95% of labors at term, the presentation is cephalic, and the fetal head is well flexed (i.e., vertex presentation).

The **position** of the fetus denotes the relationship of a specific presenting fetal bony point to the maternal pelvis. In vertex presentations, that bony point is the occiput. During vaginal examination, palpation of the sagittal suture and fontanels permits determination of the fetal position. Positions of the occiput in early labor are listed in Box 18-1. Other markers for position are the sacrum for breech presentation, the mentum for face presentation, and the acromion for shoulder presentation. (See Chapter 35 for a discussion of nonvertex presentations.)

THE MECHANISM OF LABOR

The *mechanism of labor* refers to the changes in fetal conformation and position (cardinal movements; Box 18-2) that occur during descent through the birth canal during the late first stage and the second stage of labor.

The first cardinal movement is **engagement,** which denotes passage of the biparietal diameter (BPD) (i.e., the widest transverse diameter of the fetal head) through the plane of the pelvic inlet. A direct clinical determination of engagement cannot be made, but obstetricians assume that engagement has occurred if the leading bony point of the fetal head is palpable at the level of the ischial spines. This is true because the distance between the leading bony point and the BPD is typically less than the distance between the ischial spines and the plane of the pelvic inlet. If the leading bony point is at the level of the spines, the vertex is said to be at zero station. If the leading bony point is 1 cm above the level of the spines, the station is designated as −1. Similarly, +1, +2, and +3 indicate that the leading bony point is 1, 2, and 3 cm below the ischial spines, respectively (Figure 18-1). At +5 station, delivery is imminent. *Station* refers to palpation of the leading bony point. Often marked edema of the scalp (e.g., caput succedaneum) occurs during labor. In such cases, the bony skull may be 2 to 3 cm higher than the scalp.

BOX 18-2 The Cardinal Movements of Labor

- Engagement
- Descent
- Flexion
- Internal rotation
- Extension
- External rotation
- Expulsion

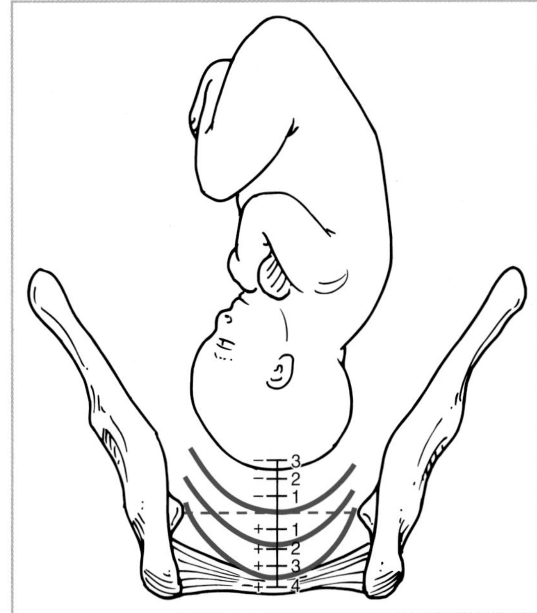

FIGURE 18-1 Stations of the fetal head. (Redrawn from Zlatnik FJ. Normal labor and delivery and its conduct. In Scott JR, DiSaia PJ, Hammond CB, Spellacy WN, editors. Danforth's Obstetrics and Gynecology. 7th edition. Philadelphia, JB Lippincott, 1994:116.)

The second cardinal movement is **descent,** although it is artificial to separate descent from the other movements because descent occurs throughout the birth process. The third cardinal movement is **flexion**. A very small fetus can negotiate the average maternal pelvis without increased flexion. However, under the usual circumstances at term, the force from above and resistance from below enhance flexion of the occiput (Figure 18-2).

The fourth cardinal movement is **internal rotation**. At the level of the midpelvis, the fetus meets the narrowest pelvic dimension, which is the transverse diameter between the ischial spines. Because the BPD of the fetal head is slightly smaller than the suboccipitobregmatic diameter, in most labors the vertex negotiates the midpelvis with the sagittal suture in an anterior-posterior direction. If this did not occur, a larger-than-necessary diameter

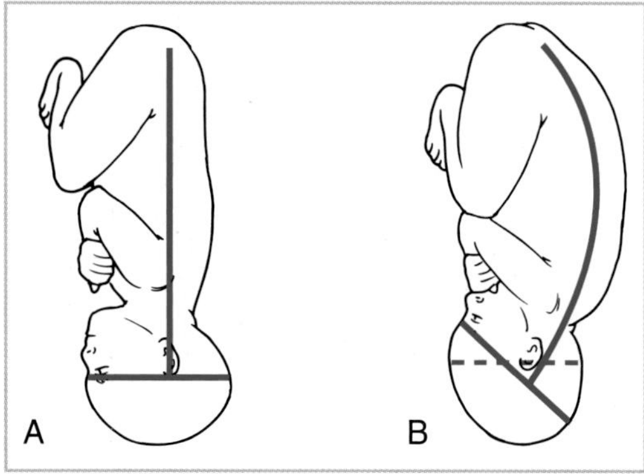

FIGURE 18-2 A, Relation of the head to the vertebral column before flexion. **B,** Relation of the head to the vertebral column after flexion. (Redrawn from Zlatnik FJ. Normal labor and delivery and its conduct. In Scott JR, DiSaia PJ, Hammond CB, Spellacy WN, editors. Danforth's Obstetrics and Gynecology. 6th edition. Philadelphia, JB Lippincott, 1990:174.)

would be forced to pass through the narrowest portion of the pelvis. Internal rotation describes the change in the position of the vertex from occiput transverse or oblique to anterior-posterior. The occiput tends to rotate to the roomiest part of the pelvis; thus, in gynecoid pelves, the fetus is delivered in an occiput anterior position.

The next cardinal movement is **extension,** which occurs as the fetal head delivers (Figure 18-3). Subsequently, the occiput rotates to the side of the back (**external rotation**) as the shoulders pass through the midpelvis in an oblique diameter. The anterior shoulder moves under the pubic symphysis. With gentle downward traction, it passes from the birth canal, and **expulsion** of the remainder of the fetus occurs.

This description recounts events in the typical gynecoid pelvis. Abnormalities of the pelvis affect the mechanism of labor in specific ways. In an **anthropoid** pelvis, the anterior-posterior diameter of the pelvic inlet exceeds the transverse diameter. Often internal rotation to the occiput posterior position rather than the occiput anterior position occurs. Because the pelvis is narrow transversely, further descent of the vertex occurs with the occiput in the posterior position. Delivery occurs with the occiput in the posterior position, or rotation to the occiput anterior position occurs just before delivery. In cases of persistent occiput posterior position, delivery occurs by flexion rather than extension of the fetal head (see Figure 18-3).

In **platypelloid** pelves, internal rotation may not take place. The widest diameter is the transverse diameter, and descent of the vertex may occur with the occiput in the transverse position; rotation to the occiput anterior position occurs only at delivery.

Clinical Course

ADMISSION

When a patient enters the labor and delivery unit, the first question that must be asked is, "Why?" Did she come because of regular, painful uterine contractions; decreased fetal activity; vaginal bleeding; ruptured membranes; or some other reason? If the tentative diagnosis is labor, is she at term?

The time of the onset of labor and the presumed status of the membranes should be determined. Observation of the patient's demeanor coupled with the assessment of cervical effacement and dilation will signal whether the patient is in early or advanced labor. Examination of the cervix is deferred in patients with vaginal bleeding in the second half of pregnancy, unless placenta previa has been ruled out, in order to avoid disruption and exacerbation of bleeding. To prevent infection, cervical examination may also be deferred in patients with premature rupture of membranes and no labor.

The obstetrician also directs attention to the second patient: the fetus. Abdominal examination is used to establish presentation and an estimate of fetal size. With most obstetric services, external electronic fetal heart rate (FHR) monitoring is used on admission to assess fetal condition. The baseline rate and variability and the presence or absence of accelerations and decelerations are of interest.

SUBSEQUENT CARE

The maternal vital signs and FHR are recorded periodically. In some obstetric services, continuous electronic FHR monitoring is used universally; with other services, it is monitored via intermittent auscultation in low-risk patients. Recording the FHR every 30 minutes in the first part of the first stage of labor, every 15 minutes in the latter part of the first stage, and every 5 minutes in the second stage is perfectly acceptable. During early labor, the patient may ambulate or assume any position of comfort on the labor bed or in a chair. During advanced labor, many women choose to lie down. Choices concerning analgesia or anesthesia are made according to the patient's wishes. Figure 18-4 shows a flow sheet (partogram) that may be useful for charting the course of labor.

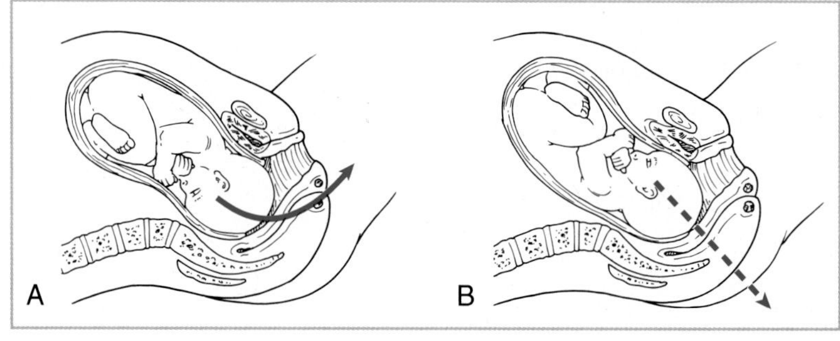

FIGURE 18-3 Vertex presentations. **A,** Occiput anterior position. **B,** Occiput posterior position. (Redrawn from Zlatnik FJ. Normal labor and delivery and its conduct. In Scott JR, DiSaia PJ, Hammond CB, Spellacy WN, editors. Danforth's Obstetrics and Gynecology. 6th edition. Philadelphia, JB Lippincott, 1990:174.)

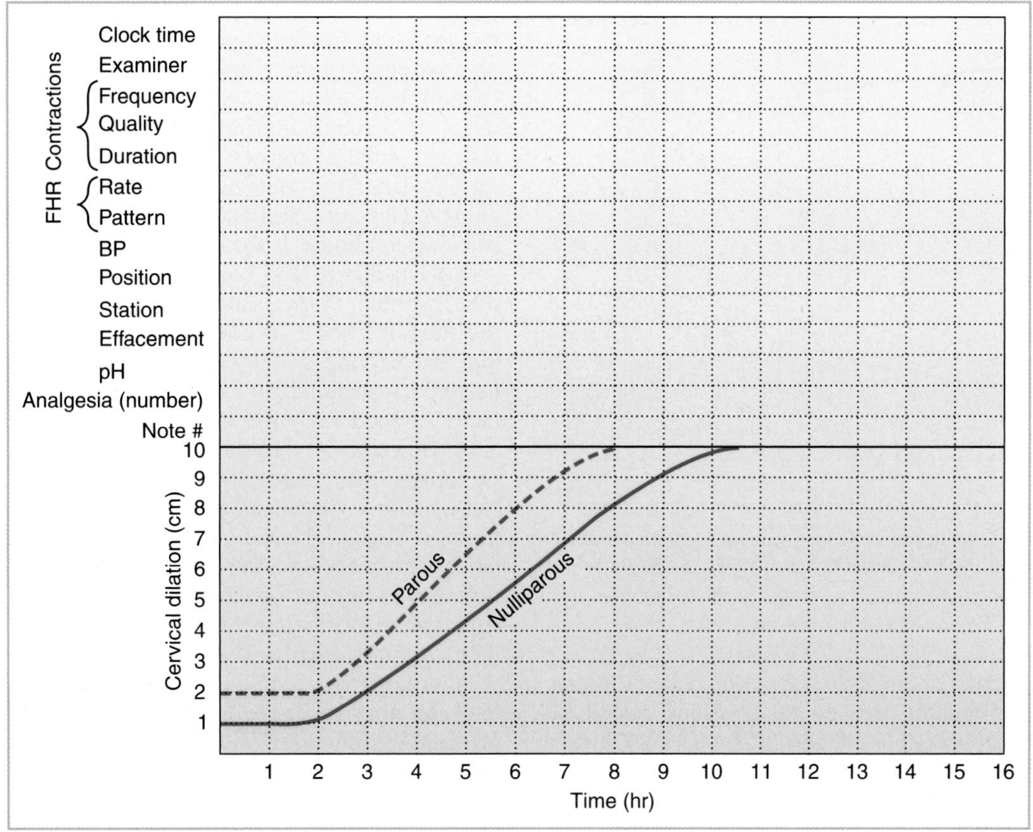

FIGURE 18-4 Flow sheet for charting labor progress. (From Zlatnik FJ. Normal labor and delivery and its conduct. BP, blood pressure. In Scott JR, DiSaia PJ, Hammond CB, Spellacy WN, editors. Danforth's Obstetrics and Gynecology. 7th edition. Philadelphia, JB Lippincott, 1994:107.)

During labor, those providing obstetric care must focus on the following two critical questions:

1. Is the fetus tolerating labor in a satisfactory fashion, or is there evidence of fetal compromise (see Chapter 8)?
2. Is the labor progress normal?

LABOR PROGRESS: THE FRIEDMAN CURVE

One of the central tasks of those providing intrapartum care is to determine whether labor is progressing normally and, if not, to determine the significance of the delay and what the response should be. Parity is an important determinant of labor length. (*Parity* refers to previous pregnancies of at least 20 weeks' gestation. A pregnant woman who is gravida 2, para 1 is pregnant for the second time, and her first pregnancy resulted in delivery after 20 weeks' gestation.)

A generation of obstetricians is indebted to Emanuel Friedman, whose landmark studies of labor provide a framework for judging labor progress. Friedman's approach was straightforward: He graphed cervical dilation on the *y*-axis and elapsed time on the *x*-axis for thousands of labors. He considered nulliparous and parous patients separately, and he determined the statistical limits of normal (Table 18-2).[5]

The curve of cervical dilation over time is S-shaped (Figure 18-5). Most authorities consider Friedman's most important contribution to be his separation of the latent

TABLE 18-2 Labor Length

Stage of Labor	Mean	Median	Mode	Limit
Nulliparous Women				
First stage (hr)	14.4	12.3	9.5	—
Latent phase (hr)	8.6	7.5	6.0	[20]
Active phase (hr)	4.9	4.0	3.0	12
Maximum slope (cm/hr)	3.0	2.7	1.5	[1.2]
Second stage (hr)	1.0	0.8	0.6	2.5
Parous Women				
First stage (hr)	7.7	6.5	5.1	—
Latent phase (hr)	5.3	4.5	3.5	[14]
Active phase (hr)	2.2	1.8	1.5	5.2
Maximum slope (cm/hr)	5.7	5.2	4.5	[1.5]
Second stage (hr)	0.2	0.2	0.1	0.8

Important limits are enclosed in boxes; see text for discussion.

Modified from Zlatnik FJ. Normal labor and delivery and its conduct. In Scott JR, DiSaia PJ, Hammond CB, Spellacy WN, editors. Danforth's Obstetrics and Gynecology. 6th edition. Philadelphia, JB Lippincott, 1990:161-88.

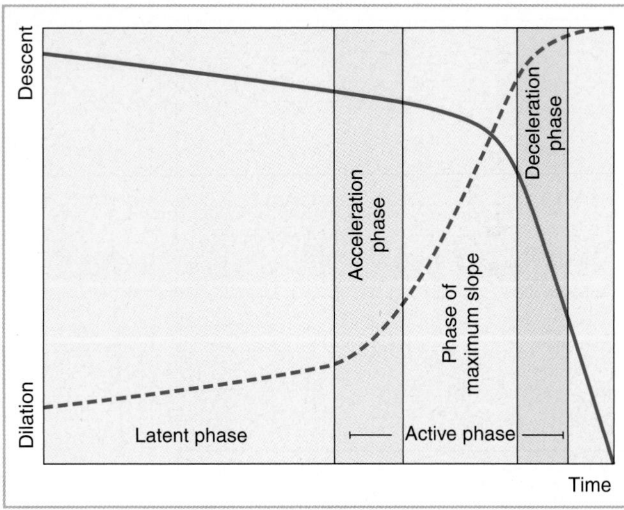

FIGURE 18-5 The Friedman curve. (From Friedman EA. Patterns of labor as indicators of risk. Clin Obstet Gynecol 1973; 16:172-83.)

phase from the active phase of the first stage of labor. Many hours of regular, painful uterine contractions may take place with little appreciable change in the cervix. During this latent (or preparatory) phase, the cervix may efface and become softer. Quite abruptly, the active (or dilation) phase begins, and regular increases in cervical dilation are expected over time. The transition from the latent to the active phase of the first stage of labor does not occur at an arbitrary cervical dilation but rather is known—in retrospect—by change in slope of the cervical dilation curve. Peisner and Rosen[6] evaluated the progress of labor for 1060 nulliparous women and 639 parous women. After excluding women with protracted or arrested labor, these researchers noted that 60% of the women had reached the latent-active phase transition by 4 cm of cervical dilation, and 89% by 5 cm.

A *nulliparous* woman may labor for 20 hours without achieving appreciable cervical dilation; 14 hours is the limit of the latent phase in the *parous* woman. Difficulty in assigning length to the latent phase lies not with its end (determined from the change in slope of the cervical dilation curve) but rather with its beginning. The onset of labor is self-reported by the parturient. The uterus contracts throughout gestation, and the level of prelabor uterine activity and its perception are variable. Often both the patient and the physician are uncertain as to exactly when labor started.

According to Friedman, in the active phase of the first stage of labor, a nulliparous woman's cervix should dilate at a rate of at least 1.2 cm per hour, and a parous woman's cervix should dilate at least 1.5 cm per hour. (The slopes of the dilation curves in Figure 18-5 represent the lower limits of normal.) If a woman's cervix fails to dilate at the appropriate rate during the active phase of labor, she is said to have **primary dysfunctional labor**. Graphically, her cervical dilation "falls off the curve." If cervical dilation ceases during a 2-hour period in the active phase of labor, **secondary arrest of dilation** has occurred. More contemporary studies have reported slower rates of cervical dilation and the absence of a deceleration phase.[7,8]

Abnormalities of the latent phase and active phase differ in associated factors, apparent etiologies, and significance. A prolonged latent phase is more likely if labor begins "before the cervix is ready."[5,9] Just as there is a wide range of prelabor uterine activity, so too is there a wide range of cervical softness, effacement, and dilation at the start of labor. In some women, appreciable cervical softening, effacement, and dilation take place in late pregnancy; thus, when clinical labor begins, the cervix may already be 3 to 4 cm dilated and completely effaced. Alternatively, in other women, there is no cervical effacement or dilation at the start of labor. Given these differences, it is not surprising that varying amounts of uterine contractile work are needed to cause dilation of the cervix. The most common factor associated with a prolonged latent phase is an "unripe" cervix at the start of labor. Some women with a prolonged latent phase are not in true labor at all but are in "false labor"; this diagnosis is made in retrospect. After hours of regular, painful contractions, uterine activity may cease without the occurrence of appreciable cervical dilation. Several hours or days later, the patient reappears in true labor. During the latent phase of labor, it is not known with certainty whether a woman is in true or false labor.

A prolonged latent phase alone is not associated with fetal compromise or cephalopelvic disproportion. However, primary dysfunctional labor and arrest of dilation during the active phase may indicate cephalopelvic disproportion.[5,10,11] Friedman's original work suggested that an arrest of dilation during the active phase was associated with the need for cesarean delivery nearly half of the time. Later studies suggest a lower percentage, but it is clear that women who experience active-phase arrest of dilation are more likely to require abdominal delivery than women with normal labor progress during the active phase. Friedman's analysis suggested that active-phase abnormalities pose a threat to the fetus, especially if they are combined with operative vaginal delivery.[12] A later study of women who delivered in the modern era of electronic FHR monitoring and decreased frequency of mid-forceps deliveries suggested that arrest disorders by themselves do not have adverse perinatal consequences.[11]

In summary, the prevailing view is that delays in the latent phase of the first stage of labor do not predict fetopelvic disproportion or the need for cesarean delivery, although data are conflicting.[13] In contrast, delays in the active phase do predict fetopelvic disproportion, although not with precision. Given current obstetric practice and fetal monitoring techniques, it is unlikely that first-stage labor abnormalities are intrinsically associated with neonatal depression at delivery.

AMNIOTOMY

The intact amnion serves as the vessel that contains the amniotic fluid and helps protect the uterine contents from the microbial flora of the vagina. The amniotic fluid provides mechanical protection for the fetus and umbilical cord and allows growth and movement.

In the absence of intervention, the membranes generally rupture at the onset of labor or near full cervical dilation. If the membranes are intact, should they be artificially ruptured during the course of labor? If so, when? Because there is concern about infection once the membranes are ruptured, the performance of an amniotomy commits the mother to delivery. For this reason, it should not be done during the latent phase of labor, unless: (1) there is an indication for effecting delivery and/or (2) the patient is close to her EDD, the cervix is favorable, and the physician can confidently predict that labor will progress easily.

Advantages of amniotomy during the active phase of the first stage of labor are that (1) the ruptured membranes permit the placement of a fetal electrocardiographic electrode, which can provide more consistent information than external FHR monitoring; (2) the amniotic fluid can be inspected for the presence or absence of meconium; and (3) amniotomy shortens the first stage of labor.[14,15] Disadvantages of amniotomy during the active phase of the first stage of labor are that it may result in increased scalp edema (i.e., caput succedaneum, which has no clinical significance) and that there may be a greater likelihood of variable decelerations of the FHR. If there is a nonvertex presentation or the vertex is high in the pelvis and not well applied to the cervix, amniotomy is deferred to decrease the risk of prolapse of the umbilical cord.

SECOND STAGE OF LABOR

When the cervix has been completely retracted to form the lower uterine segment and is therefore not palpable on vaginal examination, full or complete dilation has been achieved, and the second stage of labor begins. Strong uterine contractions coupled with voluntary expulsive efforts by the parturient cause the fetal presenting part to descend through the pelvis, resulting in delivery. At complete cervical dilation, there is frequently an increase in bloody show, the parturient may vomit, and, in the absence of anesthesia, she may complain that she needs to defecate. This sensation of needing to "bear down" encourages strong Valsalva maneuvers during uterine contractions. The effect of this sensation on the efficiency of "pushing" efforts during the second stage is reflected by the suggestion that the duration of the second stage of labor varies not only according to parity but also with the presence or absence of epidural analgesia.[16] A second stage longer than 2 hours may be considered prolonged for a nulliparous woman without epidural analgesia, but 3 hours are granted if the patient has epidural analgesia. For the parous patient the time limits are 1 and 2 hours, respectively.

The contemporary obstetrician is less concerned about the elapsed time during the second stage of labor than were earlier obstetricians. A generation ago, the teaching was that a long second stage meant trouble.[17] It often did, for at least two reasons. First, if cephalopelvic disproportion existed, the second stage was prolonged; this often resulted in a difficult operative vaginal delivery and serious fetal trauma. Second, umbilical cord compression may become severe with descent of the presenting part during the second stage of labor. If FHR monitoring was not performed conscientiously, considerable fetal/neonatal compromise could occur in association with delayed delivery. Although the cord arterial blood pH varies inversely with the length of the second stage of labor,[18] the contemporary view is that the second stage of labor does not need to be terminated at any arbitrary time provided that progress in descent continues and the FHR pattern is reassuring. Clearly it is inappropriate to perform a difficult forceps delivery or vacuum extraction simply because an arbitrary time limit has elapsed.[19]

If the parturient is allowed to choose her own positions during labor and delivery, she does not stay in one place.[20] Without instruction from birth attendants, the parturient frequently chooses to walk or sit in a chair during early labor. Late in the first stage, however, she often returns to the labor bed. During the second stage of labor, some women assume the squatting position, whereas others, with their legs supported by the nurse and the father of the baby, assume a semi-sitting position. The goal is to achieve a position in which the parturient's bearing-down efforts are most effective. The patient should avoid the supine position, which results in aortocaval compression. Aortocaval compression seems to be less severe with the patient in the semi-sitting position, and it is avoided altogether with the patient in the left lateral position. Indeed, it is perfectly acceptable for the patient to push and deliver while remaining in the left lateral position. A vaginal examination during a contraction may provide information as to which position is best for a particular individual.

As the fetal head distends the perineum shortly before delivery, an episiotomy may be performed. This incision extends either directly posteriorly from 6 o'clock (midline) or in a 45-degree angle to either side (mediolateral). The former causes less discomfort, is more anatomic, and is easier to repair than the latter. The mediolateral episiotomy's advantage is that extension through the anal sphincter and rectal mucosa is less likely to occur, but its major disadvantage is that it may cause severe postpartum pain. (If the patient has an epidural catheter, the anesthesia provider may give additional epidural local anesthetic or opioid to provide postpartum analgesia.)

The place of episiotomy in contemporary obstetrics is restricted.[21] In the past, episiotomy was advocated not only to shorten labor but also to protect the woman against the subsequent development of uterine prolapse, cystocele, and rectocele. An episiotomy hastens delivery, but only by a few minutes. Pelvic relaxation probably reflects the passage of the fetus through the levator sling rather than the presence or absence of an episiotomy at delivery. Tears involving the anal sphincter (third degree) and rectal mucosa (fourth degree) are more common after midline episiotomy than if episiotomy is not performed; in the absence of an episiotomy, however, anterior periurethral lacerations are almost inevitable. Although the latter rarely cause immediate problems, scientifically valid data on long-term outcome are lacking. Given the recognized association between midline episiotomies and third- and fourth-degree tears, the fact that these tears may be associated with long-term morbidity, and the failure to observe any benefits to routine episiotomy, more restrictive use of this incision is now recommended.[21,22] For example, an episiotomy may be indicated in some instances of operative vaginal delivery of a large infant, with suspected fetal compromise, or to manage shoulder dystocia.

THIRD STAGE OF LABOR

The third stage of labor begins with the delivery of the baby and ends with the delivery of the placenta. The placenta typically separates from the uterine wall within a few contractions after delivery of the baby, and expulsion follows a few minutes later. Signs of placental separation are listed in Box 18-3.

BOX 18-3 Signs of Placental Separation

- The uterus rises in the maternal abdomen.
- The shape of the uterus changes from discoid to globular.
- The umbilical cord lengthens.
- A gush of blood frequently occurs.

When the placenta has separated from the uterine wall, gentle traction on the umbilical cord, coupled with suprapubic pressure to elevate the uterus, serves to deliver the placenta and membranes. In the absence of excessive bleeding, the obstetrician waits for the signs of placental separation before attempting to deliver it. If traction is exerted on the umbilical cord before the placenta has separated, problems result. The least serious—but nonetheless embarrassing—complication involves separating the umbilical cord from the placenta. This tear in the cord leads to bleeding, which is of no concern because the blood is fetal-placental blood that would be discarded; however, the obstetrician's reputation for gentleness suffers as the detached segment of umbilical cord is held with the placenta remaining *in situ*. A much more serious problem is uterine inversion, which can occur in a case of fundal implantation of the placenta. If the placenta has not separated and the umbilical cord does not break, excessive traction turns the uterus inside out, resulting in severe hemorrhage (see Chapter 37).

If the placenta has not separated after 30 minutes or if significant bleeding occurs before 30 minutes, manual removal of the placenta is indicated. Although some obstetricians advocate performing this procedure with sedation or systemic analgesia, we prefer neuraxial or general anesthesia. Administration of sublingual or intravenous **nitroglycerin** or terbutaline may provide uterine relaxation, which facilitates manual removal of a retained placenta. The obstetrician's hand is then passed into the uterine cavity, and the edge of the placenta is identified. The hand is used as a trowel to separate the placenta from the uterine wall. If the obstetrician cannot easily develop a plane between the placenta and the uterine wall, the diagnosis of **placenta accreta** should be considered. Placenta accreta typically results in severe hemorrhage, which frequently mandates emergency hysterectomy (see Chapter 37).

After the placenta has been removed, uterotonic agents are administered to reduce bleeding. **Oxytocin** is given intravenously in a dilute solution (e.g., 20 units added to 1 L of intravenous fluid), or 10 units are given intramuscularly. Bolus intravenous injection of oxytocin can cause hypotension and should be avoided.[23]

If the uterus does not respond to oxytocin, other ecbolic agents can be tried. **Methylergonovine** (Methergine, 0.2 mg) has long been available for intramuscular administration. It contracts vascular smooth muscle and may cause hypertension. Methylergonovine should not be given intravenously except in cases of severe, life-threatening hemorrhage. In such cases, the physician should give the drug slowly and carefully monitor the maternal blood pressure.

15-Methylprostaglandin $F_{2\alpha}$ (carboprost, Hemabate) is a newer ecbolic agent. Given intramuscularly, 0.25 mg of 15-methylprostaglandin $F_{2\alpha}$ has been demonstrated to be an effective uterotonic agent when other drugs have failed.[24] It can also cause hypertension, but the hypertension is typically not as severe as that associated with administration of methylergonovine. More important, 15-methylprostaglandin $F_{2\alpha}$ may cause bronchospasm and is relatively contraindicated in patients with asthma.

Most obstetricians in the United States do not use ecbolic agents until the placenta has been delivered, whereas European obstetricians typically administer an ecbolic agent immediately after delivery of the infant or even with delivery of the anterior shoulder. The timing probably does not matter.[25] At most deliveries, the placenta is expelled soon after delivery of the baby. Immediately after the delivery of the placenta, if the obstetrician suspects an abnormality, the hand can be passed into the uterine cavity without causing undue discomfort. Within several minutes, however, the cervix and birth canal contract. Subsequent uterine exploration typically requires the administration of anesthesia.

FOURTH STAGE OF LABOR

Many obstetricians consider the first 60 minutes after delivery of the placenta to be the fourth stage of labor. Labor is completed, but this designation emphasizes that the patient must be watched carefully for bleeding. More than 90% of cases of postpartum hemorrhage result from uterine atony. If uterine atony is not identified during the first hour after delivery, it is unlikely to occur subsequently. The patient should be evaluated frequently to be certain that excessive bleeding is not occurring and that the uterus remains contracted. Considerable blood loss can occur in the presence of "normal" vital signs; a modest increment in additional blood loss can then be followed by profound shock. Uterine relaxation and excessive bleeding after delivery are initially treated with uterine massage and further ecbolic drug administration (see Chapter 37).

LABOR PROGRESS: FIVE MANAGEMENT QUESTIONS

The purpose of this section is to provide a personal, step-by-step approach to the management of the laboring woman by serially posing and answering the following five critical questions:

1. *Is the patient in labor?* If the answer is "Yes," certain factors must be considered before proceeding. Is the patient at term? If she is preterm, is she a candidate for tocolytic therapy? If the patient is at term, are there medical or obstetric conditions that affect management? Abnormal fetal size or presentation, twin gestation, preeclampsia, and vaginal bleeding are obstetric factors that may alter management of labor from the outset. If a singleton vertex presentation is identified in a patient without complications, the physician proceeds to the following question.
2. *Is the labor progress abnormal?* If progress is normal according to the Friedman curve, no problem exists. If progress is abnormal, the physician proceeds to the following question.
3. *Is the abnormality in the active phase?* An apparent prolongation of the latent phase may represent false labor. By itself, a prolonged latent phase does not predict

cephalopelvic disproportion or perinatal depression. Therefore, in the absence of some other indication for effecting delivery, the obstetrician should not administer oxytocin or perform amniotomy, which would involve committing the patient to a long labor with the risk of failure and the potential need for an unnecessary cesarean delivery. Long latent phases do increase patient anxiety and fatigue; reassurance is essential. At this point, ambulation and sedation are alternatives that may be selected on an individual basis, with input from the woman. If false labor has occurred, contractions will cease over time, or the patient will enter the active phase. If primary dysfunctional labor is the diagnosis or if a secondary arrest of dilation has occurred during the active phase, the physician is faced with an abnormality that may indicate cephalopelvic disproportion, a mechanical obstruction to delivery. The next question can then be asked.

4. *Is the fetus tolerating labor?* Although the FHR pattern should be monitored from admission until delivery, a delay in the active phase of labor calls for a reassessment. If the FHR pattern is nonreassuring, the physician should effect delivery. If not, the next question is asked.
5. *Does the pelvis appear to be adequate for this baby?* An active-phase delay indicates either insufficient uterine contractile effort to dilate the cervix or a mechanical obstruction to delivery. Obviously this is a critical issue, because the therapeutic alternatives are very different. If the pelvis is clinically small and/or the fetus is large and the labor seems strong (e.g., intense uterine contractions occurring every 2 minutes), the choice is cesarean delivery. If the fetopelvic relationship is favorable for vaginal delivery and the contractions are infrequent, the choice is intravenous oxytocin, amniotomy, or both. In the vast majority of cases, however, the obstetrician is uncertain as to whether oxytocin augmentation will result in successful vaginal delivery or whether cesarean delivery will ultimately be required despite oxytocin augmentation. Given the uncertainty about whether mechanical obstruction or insufficient uterine activity is the problem, the proper choice typically is to administer oxytocin to correct the latter, a decision that recognizes that, if the former is present, the attempt will ultimately fail. Data support longer periods of oxytocin augmentation for nonprogressive active-phase labor (at least 4 to 6 hours) provided the FHR pattern is reassuring.[26]

The benefit of intravenous oxytocin administration for labor arrest during the active phase of the first stage of labor is that the majority of the time it succeeds and cesarean delivery is avoided.[11] The risks of oxytocin stimulation are both maternal and fetal. If mechanical obstruction to delivery exists, greater uterine activity predisposes the patient to uterine rupture, which is one of the gravest obstetric complications. Multiparity and a scarred uterus are additional predisposing factors to uterine rupture.[27,28] Oxytocin has an antidiuretic effect, and in the past there were reports of water intoxication with seizures and even coma and death as iatrogenic complications of its use. In these cases, oxytocin was administered over many hours (often days) in electrolyte-free solutions, with little attention paid to maternal urinary output; infusion of electrolyte-containing solutions and close attention to the parturient's fluid balance should make this a theoretical rather than a practical concern. However, **uterine hyperstimulation** is a real concern when infusing oxytocin. The force generated during uterine contractions interrupts blood flow through the intervillous space, because placental perfusion occurs during periods of uterine relaxation, and uterine contractions can be regarded as episodes of "fetal breath-holding." If the contractions are occurring very frequently (e.g., at intervals less than 2 minutes apart), there may be insufficient time between contractions for placental gas exchange, the fetus may become hypoxemic, and fetal compromise may result. Continuous observation permits a timely diagnosis of uterine hyperstimulation. Decreasing the infusion rate or temporarily stopping the infusion promptly corrects the problem.

Currently, in the United States, oxytocin for stimulating or augmenting labor is given intravenously, typically by infusion pump. Continuous electronic FHR monitoring is used, and a physician or nurse constantly monitors the FHR pattern. Although the foregoing procedures are quite uniform from service to service, the selected doses of oxytocin are not.

The variability in protocols for oxytocin stimulation of labor reflects confusion in the literature.[27-32] The goal is to increase uterine activity efficiently to dilate the cervix without causing fetal compromise as a result of uterine hyperstimulation. However, the best way to do this is unclear. Recommended starting doses of oxytocin vary from 1 to 6 mU/min, and additional drug is administered until a satisfactory labor pattern is achieved. Dosage increments typically vary from 1 to 6 mU at intervals of 15 to 30 minutes. In a large randomized, double-blind study of oxytocin dosing, increasing the dose of oxytocin by 4.5 mU/min every 30 minutes resulted in a significantly shorter duration of labor than increasing it by 1.5 mU/min every 30 minutes, with no adverse maternal or fetal-neonatal effects.[33]

The Active Management of Labor

Dystocia, which is also called abnormal labor progress, is exceeded only by repeat cesarean delivery as an indication for abdominal delivery in the United States. Concern for the high cesarean delivery rate has created interest in the remarkable results achieved in the 1980s with the use of active management of labor at the National Maternity Hospital in Dublin, Ireland.[27,34] Components of the active management of labor include (1) a rigorous definition of labor, (2) early amniotomy, (3) constant nursing attendance, (4) the demand for continued progress in cervical dilation (1 cm or more per hour), (5) vigorous oxytocin stimulation for lack of progress, and (6) a "guarantee" that the parturient's stay in the labor unit will last no longer than 12 hours. In Dublin, these practices were associated with a cesarean birth rate of less than 5%; however, the rate has been higher in more recent years.

The introduction of the active management of labor in other obstetric services has been associated with lower cesarean delivery rates than those among historic controls. One randomized trial indicated that active management shortened labor, reduced the incidence of cesarean delivery for dystocia, and resulted in fewer maternal infectious complications without increasing maternal or neonatal morbidity.[35] Two other randomized trials confirmed shorter labors with active management but differed about its effect on the rate of cesarean delivery.[36,37]

SPECIAL SITUATIONS

Premature Rupture of Membranes

Premature rupture of the membranes (PROM) is defined as a rupture of the fetal membranes (i.e., the chorioamnion) before the onset of labor. It may occur preterm (before 37 weeks' gestation) or at term.

PRETERM PREMATURE RUPTURE OF MEMBRANES

The most significant complication of preterm PROM is preterm birth.[38] Although the length of the *latent period* (that interval between membrane rupture and the onset of labor) is inversely related to the length of gestation, only one in five women with preterm PROM have latent periods exceeding one week. Indeed, PROM is the precipitating factor in one third of preterm deliveries. Other risks of preterm PROM include chorioamnionitis and prolapse of the umbilical cord. If membrane rupture occurs during the second trimester and if the fetus experiences a long exposure to oligohydramnios, there is a risk of pulmonary hypoplasia and orthopedic deformities.

Current management of preterm PROM is conservative. After the diagnosis is confirmed by inspection and nitrazine and fern testing,[39] electronic FHR monitoring is used to identify variable decelerations that signal umbilical cord compression. The mother is also evaluated for fever and uterine tenderness, which may indicate chorioamnionitis. If these are absent, the clinician awaits the onset of labor or the subsequent development of infection. The adjunctive use of maternally administered corticosteroids to enhance fetal pulmonary maturity and/or antibiotics to prevent chorioamnionitis and delay the onset of labor is common.[40-42] Current evidence does not support the long-term use of tocolytic therapy to prolong pregnancy.[43] On many obstetric services, delivery is effected routinely at 34 weeks (a point beyond which the rate of severe neonatal morbidity and mortality is very low) or after documentation of fetal pulmonary maturity.

TERM PREMATURE RUPTURE OF MEMBRANES

Approximately 10% of term pregnancies are complicated by PROM; the natural history is summarized in Table 18-3.[44]

Although chorioamnionitis is more likely to occur preterm than at term with PROM, no clear relationship exists between the length of the latent period and chorioamnionitis in the preterm patient.[45] By contrast, chorioamnionitis at term is more likely if the latent period exceeds 24 hours. The relationship between prolonged latency and chorioamnionitis accounts for the usual practice in the United States of oxytocin induction of labor if the woman with PROM at term is not in labor by 6 to 12 hours after membrane rupture. Hannah et al.[46] conducted a trial comparing induction with expectant management in more than 5000 women with PROM at term; these investigators found similar rates of cesarean delivery and neonatal infection in the two groups. Oxytocin induction led to a lower rate of maternal infection than expectant management.

TABLE 18-3 Natural History of Premature Rupture of the Membranes at Term

Element	Percentage
Prevalence	10
Spontaneous labor within 24 hours	90
If cervix is unfavorable and no labor at 6 hours, percent laboring by 24 hours	60
Chorioamnionitis:	
Latent period < 24 hours	1-2
Latent period > 24 hours	5-10
Significant neonatal infection if chorioamnionitis is present	10

Modified from Zlatnik FJ. Management of premature rupture of membranes at term. Obset Gynecol Clin North Am 1992; 19:353-64

CHORIOAMNIONITIS

If chorioamnionitis develops, the uterus must be emptied. Intrapartum antibiotic administration improves the outcome for both mother and baby.[47] Ampicillin and gentamicin are often chosen to combat group B streptococcus and *Escherichia coli*, which are important neonatal pathogens. Because no relationship exists between the number of hours that chorioamnionitis has been present and perinatal outcome,[48-50] chorioamnionitis alone is not an indication for abdominal delivery. Antibiotics, oxytocin, and close observation of the mother and fetus are indicated.

Induction of Labor

Induction of labor can be defined as a surgical or medical intervention that leads to uterine contractions that progressively dilate the cervix. Because elective and indicated inductions differ in terms of eligibility criteria and the methods used, they are considered separately.

ELECTIVE INDUCTION

The rationale for elective induction of labor is convenience, both for the patient and for the physician. Because it is elective, the delivery should be easily accomplished, and the risks should approach zero. Requirements for elective induction of labor include (1) a parous patient, (2) a singleton vertex presentation, (3) a certain gestation of at least 39 weeks, (4) a favorable cervix, and (5) no contraindications to labor and vaginal delivery. The Bishop score (Table 18-4) helps quantitate the favorability of the cervix; the higher the score, the shorter the labor and the less likely induction will fail.[51] In Bishop's hands, a score of 9 or greater was not associated with failure. Friedman et al.[52] determined that the Bishop score primarily predicts the latent phase of labor. This finding is not surprising, because a high Bishop score indicates that the cervix is ready to dilate with uterine contractions (i.e., the cervix will soon enter the active phase). By contrast, a low score suggests that many hours of uterine contractions may be needed to soften and efface the cervix. When the components of the Bishop score are considered separately in terms of their effects on the latent phase, dilation is most critical. Effacement, station, and consistency are each half as important, and position has little effect.[52]

TABLE 18-4 The Bishop Cervix Score

Component	Score 0	1	2	3
Dilation (cm)	0	1-2	3-4	5+
Effacement (%)	0-30	40-50	60-70	80+
Station	−3	−2	−1/0	+1
Consistency	Firm	Medium	Soft	
Position	Posterior	Mid	Anterior	

From Bishop EH. Pelvic scoring for elective induction. Obstet Gynecol 1964; 24:266-8.

With a favorable cervix, elective induction is begun by performance of an amniotomy with or without concomitant oxytocin administration, which some obstetricians reserve for the patient who is not experiencing uterine contractions 4 to 6 hours after amniotomy. Amniotomy is typically performed early in the morning and is followed by delivery in the afternoon. Elective inductions have been criticized by some physicians because of the possibilities of induction failure and iatrogenic prematurity.[53] If candidates are selected with careful attention to the previously listed requirements, elective induction is both convenient and safe.

INDICATED INDUCTION

Indicated induction of labor is performed when delivery is indicated for maternal or fetal reasons and both mother and fetus can tolerate labor and vaginal delivery. Indicated inductions of labor often arise in the setting of a medical or obstetric complication such as diabetes mellitus, preeclampsia, intrauterine growth restriction, or the post-term pregnancy. By definition, the physician is dealing with a complicated pregnancy when performing an indicated induction of labor; therefore, close maternal and fetal monitoring is indicated. When considering the critical question whether induction should be undertaken, the obstetrician must weigh the perinatal risks of continued intrauterine versus extrauterine existence and must also consider the potential adverse maternal consequences of induction, including a higher risk of infection and/or cesarean delivery.

If the Bishop score is favorable, amniotomy alone suffices as a means of inducing labor. Often, however, the cervix is not favorable, and induction is typically accomplished with oxytocin administration combined with amniotomy. In some cases, if the cervix is unfavorable, oxytocin may be infused for one day, with the membranes intact. The infusion is stopped in the evening, and the patient is permitted to eat. The membranes are ruptured, and the oxytocin infusion is started again the following morning. Some obstetricians have advocated vaginal or cervical prostaglandins for the induction of labor; however, it is unclear that these agents offer an advantage over intravenous oxytocin for this purpose.[54]

When induction of labor is indicated in the setting of an unfavorable cervix, the obstetrician may attempt to raise the Bishop score ("ripen" the cervix) before beginning the induction. Both osmotic cervical dilators and pharmacologic techniques are effective in improving the Bishop score.[55,56] Typically these adjunctive measures are instituted the evening before the planned induction. A Foley catheter bulb may also be used for mechanical dilation. A common pharmacologic method involves the topical application of prostaglandin E_2, either in the vagina or in the cervical canal. **Prostaglandin E_2** has a local effect in the initiation of softening, effacement, and dilation of the cervix, and it also has an oxytocin-like effect on the myometrium. Women treated with prostaglandin E_2 commonly experience contractions and labor before amniotomy or oxytocin administration. The same is true for **misoprostol**, a prostaglandin E_1 analogue that is now widely used for cervical ripening and labor induction.[57]

Operative Vaginal Delivery

Cesarean delivery has become a too frequent solution to labor room problems. This safe operation is certainly preferable to the continuation of labor in the setting of genuine fetal compromise or to the performance of a difficult and traumatic vaginal delivery. Unfortunately, however, more traditional obstetric interventions (e.g., labor, additional labor, operative vaginal delivery) are often bypassed in favor of cesarean delivery, perhaps more for medicolegal than for medical concerns. The appropriate use of operative vaginal delivery techniques requires an accurate assessment of the situation, technical skills, and an honest and humble physician.

VERTEX PRESENTATION

Carefully selected and performed forceps or vacuum-assisted delivery shortens the second stage of labor in cases of nonreassuring fetal status, maternal illness or exhaustion, and/or undue prolongation of labor with little or no progress (Box 18-4). The station of the presenting vertex is critical to the safety of the procedure for mother and baby. The current American College of Obstetricians and Gynecologists classification permits a more rational approach to operative vaginal delivery than was available previously.[58,59]

For any operative vaginal delivery, adequate anesthesia is required. Outlet operative deliveries are perfectly safe for

BOX 18-4 Classification of Forceps Delivery

Outlet Forceps Delivery

- Scalp is visible.
- Skull has reached the pelvic floor, and head is on the perineum.
- Sagittal suture is in the anterior-posterior diameter or within 45 degrees (e.g., occiput anterior, left occiput anterior, right occiput posterior).

Low Forceps Delivery

- Station is +2 or greater.
- Hollow of the sacrum is filled.

Mid-forceps Delivery

- Vertex is engaged, but the station is 0 or +1.

both mother and fetus. The low station effectively rules out cephalopelvic disproportion, and little traction is required. Outlet operative deliveries shorten the second stage by only a few minutes. Sustained fetal bradycardia is a common indication for outlet operative delivery. An experienced physician may safely perform low-station operative deliveries in cases of fetal compromise or maternal illness or exhaustion. The higher the head, the harder the pull. Rotations increase the likelihood of vaginal tears.[59]

Midpelvic deliveries reflect a more complicated problem.[60,61] If the station is overestimated, the vertex may be barely engaged. The hollow of the sacrum is incompletely filled. Midpelvic deliveries should be regarded as "trials." The obstetrician must avoid excessive traction and must be willing to abandon the attempt in favor of cesarean delivery if vaginal delivery does not proceed easily.

Although operative vaginal delivery was traditionally accomplished with obstetric forceps, there has been interest in the soft plastic cup vacuum extractor.[62-65] Neither is uniformly better. The vacuum extractor is easier to apply, especially if the obstetrician is uncertain of the position of the occiput, and most likely it is associated with less maternal trauma. Forceps—but not the vacuum extractor—permits the correction of deflection or slight abnormalities of position that may impede progress. The vacuum extractor is more apt to slip off; whether this feature enhances safety is unknown. Neonatal results are comparable, but retinal hemorrhages, which are of unclear significance, are more likely with vacuum extraction. The obstetrician should be trained in both techniques and should individualize their use.

Persistent occiput-posterior positions often occur in anthropoid and android pelves. In modern obstetrics, the infants in most of these cases are delivered with the occiput posterior. Extension of the episiotomy is a common complication in this circumstance, which argues for the consideration of a mediolateral episiotomy.

Deep transverse arrests of the occiput were traditionally managed with rotation and delivery with Kielland's forceps. Current trainees typically have little experience with this instrument, and they are more likely to select the vacuum extractor in this circumstance.

NONVERTEX PRESENTATIONS

A persistent brow presentation or a transverse lie mandates cesarean delivery. Most face presentations and selected breech presentations can be safely delivered vaginally.[66] However, in response to a large international multicenter trial in which planned vaginal delivery was associated with worse perinatal outcomes than planned cesarean delivery,[67] the American College of Obstetricians and Gynecologists now recommends cesarean delivery for the persistent singleton breech presentation at term as the preferred mode for most physicians, particularly in light of diminishing experience in vaginal breech deliveries.[68]

FETAL DEATH

If fetal death has occurred, the obstetrician no longer has two patients, making maternal safety the only concern. Although placenta previa or absolute cephalopelvic disproportion may indicate cesarean delivery, the obstetrician is often more willing to choose a more complicated operative vaginal delivery than if the fetus were living.

BOX 18-5 Risk Factors for Shoulder Dystocia

- Fetal macrosomia
- Maternal diabetes mellitus
- Delayed active phase of labor
- Prolonged second stage of labor
- Operative vaginal delivery

Shoulder Dystocia

With vertex presentations, most mechanical difficulties are resolved with delivery of the head; once the head is delivered, the remainder of the fetus follows easily. In as many as 3% of vaginal deliveries, this is not the case. After the (often large) head is delivered, it seems to be "sucked" back into the perineum (the turtle sign). With maternal pushing and gentle traction, nothing happens. In this case, the anterior shoulder is trapped above the pubic symphysis. This serious complication is called *shoulder dystocia*. Recognition that shoulder dystocia exists is often followed by equanimity giving way to panic. If delivery is not accomplished soon, umbilical cord compression may result in asphyxia. Excessive traction on the fetal head may result in damage to the brachial plexus (e.g., Erb's palsy), which may be permanent or temporary. During the manipulations undertaken to effect delivery, a fracture of the clavicle or humerus may result.

Risk factors for shoulder dystocia are those that predict or reflect mechanical difficulty (Box 18-5).[69-72] Women with diabetes mellitus are predisposed to shoulder dystocia, not only because fetal macrosomia is more common but also because the fetus of a mother with diabetes has a shoulder circumference that is disproportionately large relative to head circumference. Desultory labor may be a harbinger of mechanical mismatch, and operative vaginal delivery can exacerbate the situation.

Appropriate management of shoulder dystocia begins with the recognition that there is sufficient time to deliver the baby safely. Neuraxial anesthesia is ideal but not essential. Extension of the episiotomy should be considered. The anterior shoulder is stuck behind the pubic symphysis. Although greater posterior room does not directly permit delivery, it does permit vaginal manipulations that may be necessary to effect delivery. Table 18-5 lists a personal plan of management for shoulder dystocia, but other choices are available.[69,72,73]

If suprapubic pressure (directed toward the floor) coupled with gentle traction on the head is not efficacious, the mother's thighs are removed from their supports and are hyperflexed alongside her abdomen. This maneuver (i.e., the McRoberts maneuver) elevates the symphysis in a cephalad direction and often frees the impacted shoulder and allows easy delivery. If the McRoberts maneuver is not successful, vaginal manipulations are undertaken to move the shoulders into an oblique position in the pelvis or to deliver the posterior arm. Despite previous assumptions to the contrary, vaginal delivery of the head does not necessarily commit one to vaginal birth of the baby. In the words of Yogi Berra, "It ain't over till it's over." Although we do not have personal experience with cephalic replacement (i.e., the Zavanelli maneuver), its potential use must be

TABLE 18-5 Management of Shoulder Dystocia

Maneuver	Desired Result
Suprapubic pressure	Anterior shoulder dislodged from above pubic symphysis
Hyperflexion of maternal thighs alongside abdomen (McRoberts maneuver)	Cephalad rotation of pubic symphysis
Intravaginal pressure on posterior shoulder	Anterior-posterior position of shoulders transformed to oblique position
Delivery of posterior arm	Once accomplished, added room permits delivery
Cephalic replacement (Zavenelli maneuver)	Cesarean delivery

kept in mind. If all measures have failed, the "tape is rewound," and the mechanism of labor is reversed. The position of the vertex is made occiput anterior, flexion is achieved, and the head is elevated, which may be facilitated by tocolysis (e.g., sublingual or intravenous nitroglycerin 100 μg, subcutaneous or intravenous terbutaline 0.25 mg, or general anesthesia with a volatile anesthetic agent). After the fetal head has been placed back into the vagina, prompt cesarean delivery is performed.[73]

Key Points

- The outcome of labor reflects the interaction of three components: the powers, the passageway, and the passenger.
- Assuming that the fetus is tolerating labor satisfactorily, the most important obstetric determination is whether the patient is in the latent or the active phase of the first stage of labor.
- Amniotomy shortens labor.
- Oxytocin is the most valuable obstetric drug, but there are conflicting opinions about the ideal dose regimen for induction and/or augmentation of labor.
- Expectant management is the standard choice for the very preterm patient with premature rupture of membranes; induction of labor is generally undertaken in patients exhibiting this condition at term.
- Elective induction of labor is an appropriate choice for a parous patient with a favorable cervix.
- The declining numbers of operative vaginal deliveries reflect medicolegal concerns rather than new scientific information.

REFERENCES

1. Casey ML, MacDonald PC. Biomedical processes in the initiation of parturition: Decidual activation. Clin Obstet Gynecol 1988; 31:533-52.
2. Garfield RE. Control of myometrial function in preterm versus term labor. Clin Obstet Gynecol 1984; 27:572-91.
3. Rouse DJ, St. John E. Normal labor, delivery, newborn care, and puerperium. In Scott JR, Gibbs RS, Karlan BY, Haney AF, editors. Danforth's Obstetrics and Gynecology. 9th edition. Philadelphia, Lippincott Williams & Wilkins, 2003:35-56.
4. Laube DW, Varner MW, Cruikshank DP. A prospective evaluation of x-ray pelvimetry. JAMA 1981; 246:2187-8.
5. Friedman EA. Labor: Clinical Evaluation and Management. 2nd edition. New York, Appleton-Century-Crofts, 1978.
6. Peisner DB, Rosen MG. Transition from latent to active labor. Obstet Gynecol 1986; 68:448-51.
7. Kelly G, Peaceman AM, Colangelo L, Rademaker A. Normal nulliparous labor: Are Friedman's definitions still relevant (abstract)? Am J Obstet Gynecol 2000; 182:S129.
8. Zhang J, Troendle J, Yancey M. Reassessing the labor curve in nulliparous women. Am J Obstet Gynecol 2002; 187:824-8.
9. Peisner DP, Rosen MG. Latent phase of labor in normal patients: A reassessment. Obstet Gynecol 1985; 66:644-8.
10. Bottoms SF, Sokol RJ, Rosen MG. Short arrest of cervical dilatation: A risk for maternal/fetal/infant morbidity. Am J Obstet Gynecol 1981; 140:108-13.
11. Bottoms SF, Hirsch VJ, Sokol RJ. Medical management of arrest disorders of labor: A current overview. Am J Obstet Gynecol 1987; 156:935-9.
12. Friedman EA. Patterns of labor as indicators of risk. Clin Obstet Gynecol 1973; 16:172-83.
13. Chelmow D, Kilpatrick SJ, Laros RK. Maternal and neonatal outcomes after prolonged latent phase. Obstet Gynecol 1993; 81:486-91.
14. Fraser WD, Marcoux S, Moutquin JM, et al. Effect of early amniotomy on the risk of dystocia in nulliparous women. N Engl J Med 1993; 328:1145-9.
15. Johnson N, Lilford R, Guthrie K, et al. Randomised trial comparing a policy of early with selective amniotomy in uncomplicated labour at term. Br J Gynaecol 1997; 104:340-6.
16. American College of Obstetricians and Gynecologists. Dystocia and the augmentation of labor. ACOG Practice Bulletin No. 49. Washington, DC, ACOG, December 2003. (Obstet Gynecol 2003; 102:1445-54.)
17. Hellman LM, Prystowsky H. The duration of the second stage of labor. Am J Obstet Gynaecol 1952; 63:1223-33.
18. Katz M, Lunenfeld E, Meizner I, et al. The effect of the duration of second stage of labour on the acid-base state of the fetus. Br J Obstet Gynaecol 1987; 94:425-30.
19. Altman MR, Lydon-Rochelle MT. Prolonged second stage of labor and risk of adverse maternal and perinatal outcomes: A systematic review. Birth 2006; 33:315-22.
20. Carlson JM, Diehl JA, Sachtleben-Murray M, et al. Maternal position during parturition in normal labor. Obstet Gynecol 1986; 68:443-7.
21. American College of Obstetricians and Gynecologists. Episiotomy: Clinical management guidelines for obstetrician-gynecologists. ACOG Practice Bulletin No. 71. Washington, DC, ACOG, April 2006. (Obstet Gynecol 2006; 107:957-62.)
22. Hartmann K, Viswanathan M, Palmieri R, et al. Outcomes of routine episiotomy: A systematic review. JAMA 2005; 293:2141-8.
23. Hendricks CH, Brenner WE. Cardiovascular effects of oxytocic drugs used postpartum. Am J Obstet Gynecol 1970; 108:751-9.
24. Hayashi RH, Castillo MS, Noah ML. Management of severe postpartum hemorrhage due to uterine atony using an analogue of prostaglandin F_2 alpha. Obstet Gynecol 1981; 58:426-9.
25. Jackson KW, Allbert JR, Schemmer GK, et al. A randomized controlled trial comparing oxytocin administration before and after placental delivery in the prevention of postpartum hemorrhage. Am J Obstet Gynecol 2001; 185:873-7.
26. Rouse DJ, Owen J, Savage KG, Hauth JC. Active phase labor arrest: Revisiting the two-hour minimum. Obstet Gynecol 2001; 98:550-4.

27. O'Driscoll K, Meagher D. Active Management of Labour: The Dublin Experience. 2nd edition. London, Baillière Tindall, 1986.
28. Satin AJ, Leveno KJ, Sherman ML, et al. High versus low dose oxytocin for labor stimulation. Obstet Gynecol 1992; 80:111-6.
29. Seitchik J, Castillo M. Oxytocin augmentation of dysfunctional labor. I. Clinical data. Am J Obstet Gynecol 1982; 144:899-905.
30. Xenakis EM, Langer O, Piper JM, et al. Low-dose versus high-dose oxytocin augmentation of labor: A randomized trial. Am J Obstet Gynecol 1995; 173:1874-8.
31. Satin AJ, Hankins GDV, Yeomans ER. A prospective study of two dosing regimens of oxytocin for the induction of labor in patients with unfavorable cervices. Am J Obstet Gynecol 1991; 165:980-4.
32. Blakemore KJ, Qin N, Petrie RH, Paine LL. A prospective comparison of hourly and quarter-hourly oxytocin dose increase intervals for the induction of labor at term. Obstet Gynecol 1990; 75:757-61.
33. Merrill DC, Zlatnik FJ. Randomized, double-masked comparison of oxytocin dosage in induction and augmentation of labor. Obstet Gynecol 1999; 94:455-63.
34. O'Driscoll K, Foley M, MacDonald D. Active management of labor as an alternative to cesarean section for dystocia. Obstet Gynecol 1984; 63:485-90.
35. Lopez-Zeno JA, Peaceman AM, Adashek JA, Socol ML. A controlled trial of a program for the active management of labor. N Engl J Med 1992; 326:450-4.
36. Frigoletto FD, Lieberman E, Lang JM, et al. A clinical trial of active management of labor. N Engl J Med 1995; 333:745-50.
37. Rogers R, Gilson GJ, Miller AC, et al. Active management of labor: Does it make a difference? Am J Obstet Gynecol 1997; 177:599-605.
38. Malee MP. Expectant and active management of preterm premature rupture of membranes. Obstet Gynecol Clin North Am 1992; 19:309-15.
39. American College of Obstetricians and Gynecologists. Premature rupture of membranes: Clinical management guidelines for obstetrician-gynecologists. ACOG Practice Bulletin No. 80. Washington, DC, ACOG, April 2007. (Obstet Gynecol 2007;109:1007-19.)
40. Mercer BM, Arheart KL. Antimicrobial therapy in expectant management of preterm premature rupture of the membranes. Lancet 1995; 346:1271-9.
41. Lovett SM, Weiss JD, Diogo MJ, et al. A prospective, double-blind, randomized, controlled clinical trial of ampicillin-sulbactam for preterm premature rupture of membranes in women receiving antenatal corticosteroid therapy. Am J Obstet Gynecol 1997; 176:1030-8.
42. Crowley P. Corticosteroids after preterm premature rupture of membranes. Obstet Gynecol Clin North Am 1992; 19:317-26.
43. Mercier BM. Is there a role for tocolytic therapy during conservative management of preterm premature rupture of membranes? Clin Obstet Gynecol 2007; 50:487-96.
44. Zlatnik FJ. Management of premature rupture of membranes at term. Obstet Gynecol Clin North Am 1992; 19:353-64.
45. Johnson JWC, Daikoku NH, Niebyl JR, et al. Premature rupture of the membranes and prolonged latency. Obstet Gynecol 1981; 57:547-56.
46. Hannah ME, Ohlsson A, Farine D, et al. Induction of labor compared with expectant management for prelabor rupture of the membranes at term. N Engl J Med 1996; 334:1005-10.
47. Gibbs RS, Dinsmoor MJ, Newton ER, Ramamurthy RS. A randomized trial of intrapartum versus immediate postpartum treatment of women with intra-amniotic infection. Obstet Gynecol 1988; 72:823-8.
48. Gibbs RS, Castillo MS, Rodgers PJ. Management of acute chorioamnionitis. Am J Obstet Gynecol 1980; 136:709-13.
49. Hauth JC, Gilstrap LC, Hankins GDV, Connor KD. Term maternal and neonatal complications of acute chorioamnionitis. Obstet Gynecol 1985; 66:59-62.
50. Rouse DJ, for the National Institute of Child Health Development and Maternal-Fetal Medicine Units Network. Maternal-Fetal Medicine Units Cesarean Registry: Fetal-neonatal outcome in relationship to chorioamnionitis and its duration (abstract). Am J Obstet Gynecol 2002; 187:S221.
51. Bishop EH. Pelvic scoring for elective induction. Obstet Gynecol 1964; 24:266-8.
52. Friedman EA, Niswander KR, Bayonet-Rivera NP, Sachtleben MR. Relation of prelabor evaluation to inducibility and the course of labor. Obstet Gynecol 1966; 28:495-501.
53. Rayburn WF, Zhang J. Rising rates of labor induction: Present concerns and future strategies. Obstet Gynecol 2002; 100:164-7.
54. American College of Obstetricians and Gynecologists. Induction of labor. ACOG Practice Bulletin No. 10. Washington, DC, ACOG, November 1999.
55. Cross WG, Pitkin RM. Laminaria as an adjunct in induction of labor. Obstet Gynecol 1978; 51:606-8.
56. Bernstein P. Prostaglandin E_2 gel for cervical ripening and labour induction: A multicentre placebo-controlled trial. Can Med Assoc J 1991; 145:1249-54.
57. Sanchez-Ramos L, Kaunitz AM, Wears RL, et al. Misoprostol for cervical ripening and labor induction: A meta-analysis. Obstet Gynecol 1997; 89:633-42.
58. American College of Obstetricians and Gynecologists. Operative vaginal delivery. ACOG Practice Bulletin No. 17. Washington, DC, ACOG, June 2000.
59. Hagadorn-Freathy AS, Yeomans ER, Hankins GDV. Validation of the 1988 ACOG forceps classification system. Obstet Gynecol 1991; 77:356-60.
60. Bashore RA, Phillips WH, Brinkman CR. A comparison of the morbidity of midforceps and cesarean delivery. Am J Obstet Gynecol 1990; 162:1428-34.
61. Robertson PA, Laros RK, Zhao RL. Neonatal and maternal outcome in low-pelvic and midpelvic operative deliveries. Am J Obstet Gynecol 1990; 162:1436-42.
62. Berkus MD, Ramamurthy RS, O'Connor PS, et al. Cohort study of Silastic obstetric vacuum cup deliveries. I. Safety of the instrument. Obstet Gynecol 1985; 66:503-9.
63. Dell DL, Sightler SE, Plauche WC. Soft cup vacuum extraction: A comparison of outlet delivery. Obstet Gynecol 1985; 66:624-8.
64. Broekhuizen FF, Washington JM, Johnson F, Hamilton PR. Vacuum extraction versus forceps delivery: Indications and complications, 1979-1984. Obstet Gynecol 1987; 69:338-42.
65. Williams MC, Knuppel RA, O'Brien WF, et al. A randomized comparison of assisted vaginal delivery by obstetric forceps and polyethylene vacuum cup. Obstet Gynecol 1991; 78:789-94.
66. Weiner CP. Vaginal breech delivery in the 1990s. Clin Obstet Gynecol 1992; 35:559-69.
67. Hannah ME, Hannah WJ, Hewson SA, et al., for the Term Breech Trial Collaborative Group. Planned caesarean section versus planned vaginal birth for breech presentation at term: A randomized multicentre trial. Lancet 2000; 356:1375-83.
68. American College of Obstetricians and Gynecologists. Mode of term singleton breech delivery. ACOG Committee Opinion No. 340. Washington, DC, ACOG, July 2006.
69. O'Leary JA, Leonetti HB. Shoulder dystocia: Prevention and treatment. Am J Obstet Gynecol 1990; 162:5-9.
70. Gross TL, Sokol RJ, Williams T, Thompson K. Shoulder dystocia: A fetal-physician risk. Am J Obstet Gynecol 1987; 156:1408-14.
71. Langer O, Berkus MD, Huff RW, Samueloff A. Shoulder dystocia: Should the fetus weighing 4000 grams be delivered by cesarean section? Am J Obstet Gynecol 1991; 165:831-7.
72. American College of Obstetricians and Gynecologists. Shoulder dystocia. Clinical management guidelines for obstetrician-gynecologists. ACOG Practice Bulletin No. 40. Washington, DC, ACOG, November 2002. (Obstet Gynecol 2002; 100:1045-1049.)
73. Sandberg EC. The Zavanelli maneuver extended: Progression of a revolutionary concept. Am J Obstet Gynecol 1988; 158:1347-52.

Vaginal Birth after Cesarean Delivery

David H. Chestnut, M.D.

In 1916, Edward Cragin[1] stated, "Once a cesarean, always a cesarean." This edict has had a profound effect on obstetric practice in the United States. The cesarean delivery rate rose from 5.5% of all deliveries in 1970 to 24.7% in 1988 (Figure 19-1). Much of the increase in the cesarean delivery rate resulted from performance of repeat cesarean deliveries.[2] In contemporary practice, elective repeat cesarean deliveries account for one third of all cesarean deliveries. Cesarean delivery is the most frequently performed major surgery in the United States.

For many years most U.S. physicians ignored Cragin's subsequent statement, "Many exceptions occur."[1] In 1981 the National Institute of Child Health and Human Development Conference on Childbirth concluded that vaginal birth after cesarean delivery (VBAC) is an appropriate option for many women.[3] Rosen et al.[4] modified Cragin's original dictum as follows: "Once a cesarean, a trial of labor should precede a second cesarean except in the most unusual circumstances." In 1988 and again in 1994, the American College of Obstetricians and Gynecologists (ACOG) [5] concluded, "The concept of routine repeat cesarean birth should be replaced by a specific decision process between the patient and the physician for a subsequent mode of delivery .... In the absence of a contraindication, a woman with one previous cesarean delivery with a lower uterine segment incision should be counseled and encouraged to undergo a trial of labor in her current pregnancy."

The VBAC rate increased from 2% in 1970 to 28% in 1995. This change in practice helped reduce the overall cesarean delivery rate from 24.7% in 1988 to 20.7% in 1996 (see Figure 19-1). However, in later years the safety of VBAC has undergone further scrutiny and criticism, and the VBAC rate has sharply declined.[6] The VBAC rate in the United States dropped from 28% in 1995 to 9% in 2004. Meanwhile, in 2006, the overall cesarean delivery rate rose to 31.1%, the highest rate ever recorded in this country.[7]

PRIMARY CESAREAN DELIVERY: CHOICE OF UTERINE INCISION

Obstetric practice in 1916 hardly resembled obstetric practice today. In 1916, only 1% to 2% of all infants were delivered by cesarean delivery. Most cesarean deliveries were performed in patients with a contracted bony pelvis, and obstetricians uniformly performed a classic uterine incision (i.e., a long vertical incision in the upper portion of the uterus) (Figure 19-2). A patient with a classic uterine incision is at high risk for catastrophic uterine rupture during a subsequent pregnancy. Such uterine rupture may occur before or during labor, and it often results in maternal and perinatal morbidity or mortality.

In 1922, De Lee and Cornell[8] advocated the performance of a vertical incision in the lower uterine segment. Unfortunately, low-vertical incisions rarely are confined to the lower uterine segment. Such incisions often extend to the body of the uterus, which does not heal as well as the lower uterine segment. Kerr[9] later advocated the performance of a low-transverse uterine incision (Figure 19-2). A low-transverse uterine incision results in less blood loss and is easier to repair than a classic uterine incision.[10] Further, a low-transverse uterine incision is more likely to heal satisfactorily and to maintain its integrity during a subsequent pregnancy. Thus, obstetricians prefer to make a low-transverse uterine incision during most cesarean deliveries.

Obstetricians reserve the low-vertical incision for patients whose lower uterine segment does not have enough width

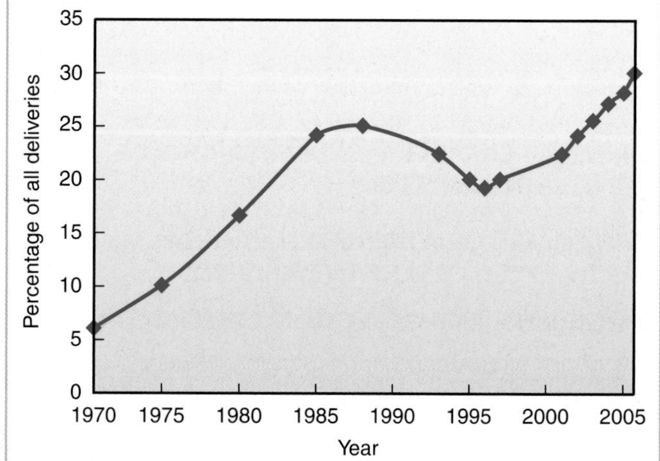

FIGURE 19-1 Incidence of cesarean delivery in the United States.

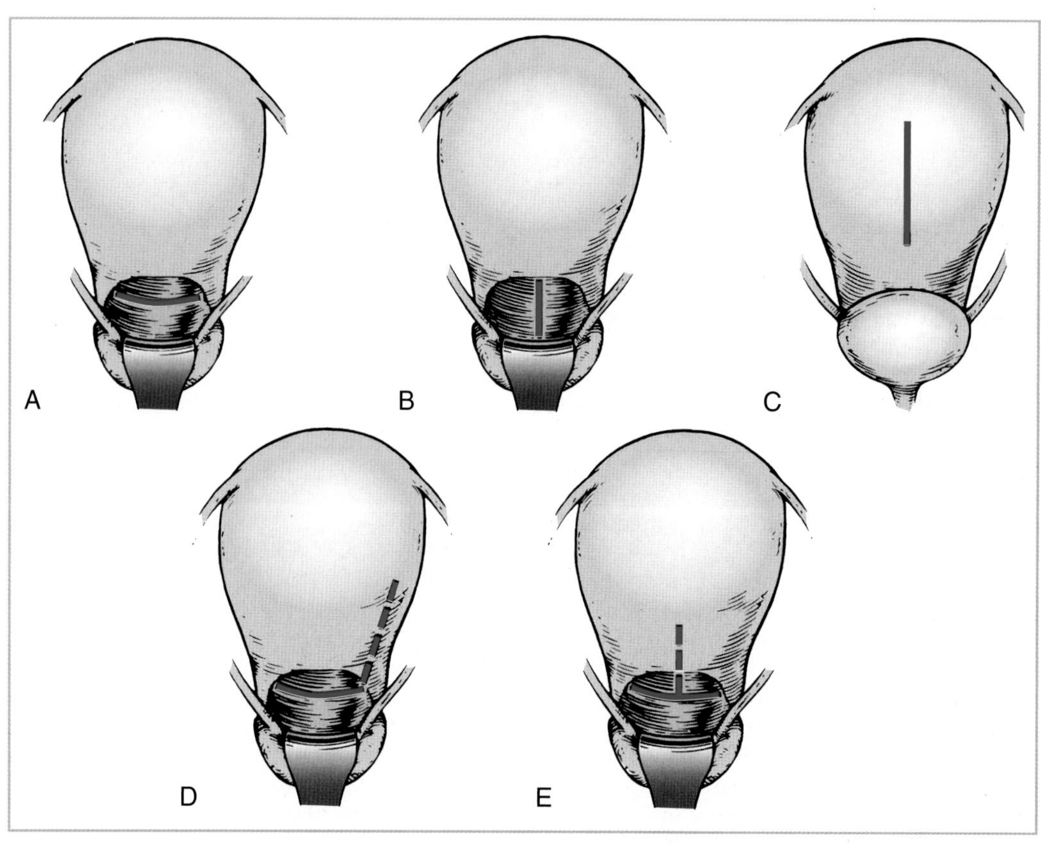

FIGURE 19-2 Uterine incisions for cesarean delivery. **A,** Low-transverse incision. The bladder is retracted downward, and the incision is made in the lower uterine segment, curving gently upward. If the lower segment is poorly developed, the incision also can curve sharply upward at each end to avoid extending into the ascending branches of the uterine arteries. **B,** Low-vertical incision. The incision is made vertically in the lower uterine segment after reflection of the bladder, with avoidance of extension into the bladder below. If more room is needed, the incision can be extended upward into the upper uterine segment. **C,** Classic incision. The incision is entirely within the upper uterine segment and can be at the level shown or in the fundus. **D,** J incision. If more room is needed when an initial transverse incision has been made, either end of the incision can be extended upward into the upper uterine segment and parallel to the ascending branch of the uterine artery. **E,** T incision. More room can be obtained in a transverse incision by an upward midline extension into the upper uterine segment. (From Landon MB. Cesarean delivery. In Gabbe SG, Niebyl JR, Simpson JL, editors. Obstetrics: Normal and Problem Pregnancies. 5th edition. Philadelphia, Churchill Livingstone Elsevier, 2007:493.)

to allow safe delivery. Preterm parturients may have a narrow lower uterine segment. In these patients, delivery through a transverse uterine incision may cause an extension of the incision into the vessels of the broad ligament. For example, a patient with preterm labor at 26 weeks' gestation may undergo cesarean delivery because of a breech presentation, and the obstetrician may perform a low-vertical incision to facilitate an atraumatic delivery of the fetal head.

Obstetricians rarely perform a classic uterine incision in modern obstetric practice. An obstetrician may perform a classic uterine incision when the need for extensive intrauterine manipulation of the fetus (e.g., delivery of a fetus with a transverse lie) is anticipated. Some obstetricians prefer a classic uterine incision in patients with an anterior placenta previa. In such cases, the performance of a classic incision allows the obstetrician to avoid cutting through the placenta, which might result in significant hemorrhage.

OUTCOMES OF ATTEMPTED VAGINAL BIRTH AFTER CESAREAN DELIVERY

A trial of labor is successful in 60% to 80% of women in whom a low-transverse uterine incision was made for a previous cesarean delivery.[11-15] Flamm et al.[11] performed a large multicenter study of VBAC. Among 5733 women who attempted VBAC, 4291 (75%) delivered vaginally. Some 10 of 5733 patients experienced uterine rupture, an incidence of 0.2%. There were no maternal deaths among the women who underwent a trial of labor, but there were two maternal deaths among the 9365 women who underwent elective repeat cesarean delivery.[11] Flamm et al.[12] subsequently performed another prospective multicenter study of VBAC. Of the 7229 patients, 5022 (70%) had a trial of labor and 2207 underwent elective repeat cesarean delivery. Some 3746 (75%) of the women who opted for a trial of labor delivered vaginally. The rate of uterine rupture was 0.8%. The incidence of postpartum transfusion, the incidence of postpartum fever, and the duration of hospitalization were significantly lower in the trial-of-labor group than in the elective repeat cesarean group. Likewise, in a meta-analysis of 31 studies, Rosen et al.[4] noted that maternal febrile morbidity was significantly lower among women who attempted VBAC than among those who underwent elective repeat cesarean delivery.

In contrast, McMahon et al.[16] performed a population-based longitudinal study of 6138 women in Nova Scotia who had previously undergone cesarean delivery and who delivered a single live infant between 1986 and 1992. Some 3249 women attempted VBAC, and 2889 women chose a repeat cesarean delivery. There was no difference between the two groups in the incidence of "minor complications" (e.g., puerperal fever, transfusion, wound infection). However, "major complications" (e.g., hysterectomy, uterine rupture, operative injury) were nearly twice as likely among women who attempted VBAC than among women who underwent elective repeat cesarean delivery.

Landon et al.[15] conducted a prospective 4-year observational study of all parturients with a singleton gestation and a prior cesarean delivery at 19 academic medical centers. Among the 17,898 women who attempted VBAC, 13,139 (73.4%) delivered vaginally. Symptomatic uterine rupture occurred in 124 (0.7%) women who underwent a trial of labor. The rate of endometritis was higher in women undergoing a trial of labor than in women undergoing elective repeat cesarean delivery (2.9% versus 1.8%), as was the rate of blood transfusion (1.7% versus 1.0%).[15]

Lydon-Rochelle et al.[17] conducted a population-based, retrospective cohort analysis of obstetric outcomes for all (i.e., 20,095) nulliparous women who gave birth to a live singleton infant by cesarean delivery in civilian hospitals in the State of Washington between 1987 and 1996 and who subsequently delivered a second singleton child during the same period. These investigators observed that spontaneous labor was associated with a tripling of the risk of uterine rupture (i.e., a uterine rupture rate of 5.2 per 1000 women who had spontaneous onset of labor versus 1.6 per 1000 women who underwent elective repeat cesarean delivery without labor). Further, the incidence of infant death was more than 10 times higher among the 91 women who experienced uterine rupture than among the 20,004 who did not (i.e., a 5.5% incidence of infant death versus a 0.5% incidence).[17]

In the study performed by McMahon et al.[16] there was no difference between the two groups in perinatal mortality or morbidity. However, two perinatal deaths occurred after uterine rupture in the trial-of-labor group. Landon et al.[15] observed that hypoxic-ischemic encephalopathy occurred in no infants whose mothers underwent elective repeat cesarean delivery and in 12 infants delivered at term whose mothers underwent a trial of labor ($P < .001$).

On the other hand, successful VBAC avoids the neonatal risks of elective cesarean delivery. Inappropriate assessment of fetal maturity occasionally leads to the delivery of a preterm infant. Thus, elective cesarean delivery results in some cases of iatrogenic neonatal respiratory distress.

ELIGIBILITY AND SELECTION CRITERIA

Most studies suggest a high likelihood of success with VBAC, even in women in whom the indication for previous cesarean delivery was dystocia or failure to progress in labor. Rosen and Dickinson[18] performed a meta-analysis of 29 studies of VBAC. Among patients whose previous cesarean deliveries were performed for dystocia or cephalopelvic disproportion, the average rate of successful vaginal delivery was 67%. Later studies have concluded that a history of previous vaginal delivery (including previous VBAC) is the greatest predictor for successful VBAC. No study has identified a reliable formula for predicting the success or failure of VBAC, but a history of dystocia, a need for induction of labor, and maternal obesity are associated with a lower likelihood of successful VBAC.[19-22]

The ACOG[14] has published the following revised selection criteria for the identification of candidates for VBAC:

- One previous low-transverse cesarean delivery
- Clinically adequate pelvis
- No other uterine scars or previous uterine rupture
- Immediate availability throughout active labor of a physician capable of monitoring labor and performing an emergency cesarean delivery
- Availability of an anesthesia provider and other personnel for performance of emergency cesarean delivery

The ACOG[14] also stated that it may be reasonable to offer a trial of labor to women in other specific obstetric circumstances.

History of More than One Cesarean Delivery

Earlier studies suggested that patients with more than one previous cesarean delivery may safely attempt VBAC.[11,23,24] However, Caughey et al.[25] observed that women with a history of two prior cesarean deliveries have an almost five-fold greater risk of uterine rupture during a trial of labor than women with only one previous cesarean delivery. However, women with a previous vaginal delivery followed by a cesarean delivery were only one-fourth as likely to sustain uterine rupture during a trial of labor.[25] Therefore, the ACOG[14] concluded that for women with two previous cesarean deliveries, only those with a prior vaginal delivery should be considered candidates for VBAC. In contrast, Landon et al.[26] performed a multicenter study that prompted them to question the basis for this precaution. They observed that a history of multiple cesarean deliveries was not associated with a higher risk of uterine rupture in women attempting VBAC than a history of a single previous cesarean delivery.

Previous Low-Vertical Incision

Some obstetricians allow a trial of labor after a previous low-vertical uterine incision, provided that there is documentation that the uterine incision was confined to the lower uterine segment. (Low-vertical uterine incisions often extend above the lower uterine segment, especially when performed in preterm patients.) Naef et al.[27] retrospectively reviewed outcomes for 174 women who attempted VBAC after a previous low-vertical cesarean delivery. Approximately 144 (83%) women delivered vaginally. Uterine rupture occurred in two (1.1%) of the patients. The researchers concluded that "the likelihood of successful outcome and the incidence of complications are comparable to those of published experience with a trial of labor after a previous low-segment transverse incision."[27] Adair et al.[28] made similar observations. The ACOG[14] has concluded that "women with a vertical incision within the lower uterine segment that does not extend into the fundus are candidates for VBAC."

Twin Gestation

Some obstetricians believe that uterine overdistention, which occurs with twin gestation, increases the risk of uterine rupture in patients with a history of previous cesarean delivery. Early reports suggested otherwise, but these studies were limited by the small number of patients.[29,30] Cahill et al.[31] performed a retrospective cohort study of 25,005 obstetric patients with at least one previous cesarean delivery, which included 535 patients with twin pregnancies. The investigators observed that women with twin gestations were less likely to attempt VBAC but were no more likely to have a failed VBAC or to experience major morbidity than women with singleton gestations.

Likewise, a report from the Maternal-Fetal Medicine Unit Cesarean Registry[32] included outcome measures for 186 women with a twin gestation who attempted VBAC. Some 120 (64.5%) women delivered vaginally. These researchers observed that women who attempted a trial of labor with twin gestation had no higher risk of transfusion, endometritis, intensive care unit admission, or uterine rupture than women choosing elective repeat cesarean delivery. They concluded that a trial of labor in women with a twin gestation after previous cesarean delivery does not appear to be associated with a higher risk of maternal morbidity.[32]

Ford et al.[33] examined outcomes for 6555 women with a twin gestation who delivered between 1993 and 2002. Among 1850 women who underwent a trial of labor, 836 (45.2%) delivered vaginally. The rate of uterine rupture was higher in the trial-of-labor group than in the elective cesarean delivery group (0.9% versus 0.1%, $P < .001$), but the rate of wound complications was lower in the trial-of-labor group (0.6% versus 1.3%, $P < .02$).

Unknown Uterine Scar

For some patients, there is no documentation of the type of incision performed during a previous cesarean delivery. Some obstetricians require documentation of the type of previous uterine incision before they allow a patient to attempt VBAC. At least two studies have concluded that a trial of labor does not significantly increase maternal or perinatal mortality in patients with an unknown uterine scar.[34,35] Perhaps this conclusion is true because most patients with an unknown uterine scar had a low-transverse uterine incision at previous cesarean delivery. Ultrasonography may help the obstetrician confirm the presence of a low-transverse uterine scar in the pregnant woman with an unknown uterine scar.[36]

Suspected Macrosomia

Flamm and Goings[37] evaluated obstetric outcome in 301 patients who attempted VBAC and whose infants weighed more than 4000 g at delivery. Among the 240 patients whose infants weighed between 4000 and 4500 g, 139 (58%) delivered vaginally. Among the 61 patients whose infants weighed more than 4500 g, 26 (43%) delivered vaginally. These researchers pooled their data with those of four other studies of VBAC in women with macrosomic infants. Among 807 women who attempted VBAC and delivered a macrosomic infant, 556 (69%) delivered vaginally. The researchers concluded that suspected fetal macrosomia does not contraindicate VBAC in nondiabetic pregnant women. (Diabetic women with fetal macrosomia have an increased risk for shoulder dystocia.) They emphasized that "care should be taken to ensure that crude estimates of 'macrosomia' are not used to discourage women with normal-size infants from pursuing vaginal birth after cesarean."[37]

In 1994 the ACOG[5] concluded that an estimated fetal weight of more than 4000 g does not contraindicate VBAC. However, in 1999, the ACOG included suspected macrosomia on the list of VBAC eligibility criteria that are controversial.[38] In 2004 the ACOG[14] noted that macrosomia is associated with a lower likelihood of successful VBAC but did not include a specific recommendation regarding VBAC in cases of suspected macrosomia. However, the ACOG cited one report observing that the rate of uterine rupture appears to be higher only in women without a previous vaginal delivery.[39] A report from the Maternal-Fetal Medicine Unit Cesarean Registry concluded that for women with a history of previous cesarean delivery for dystocia, a higher birth weight in a subsequent pregnancy (relative to the first pregnancy birth weight) diminishes the chances of successful VBAC.[40]

Gestation beyond 40 Weeks

At least three studies have concluded that awaiting spontaneous labor beyond 40 weeks' gestation decreases the likelihood of successful VBAC but that the risk of uterine rupture is not increased.[41-43] In one study of more than 1200 women attempting VBAC after 40 weeks' gestation, only induction of labor was associated with a higher risk of uterine rupture.[43]

Breech Presentation

Ophir et al.[44] reviewed their experience with 47 patients with breech presentation who attempted VBAC; 37 (79%) patients delivered vaginally. Sarno et al.[45] reported successful vaginal delivery in 13 (48%) of 27 patients with breech presentation who attempted VBAC. Breech presentation itself does not increase the risk of uterine rupture. In contemporary practice, most obstetricians do not allow a trial of labor in *any* patient with a breech presentation. Thus, most patients with breech presentation undergo elective cesarean delivery, with or without a history of previous cesarean delivery.

Size of Hospital

Most studies of VBAC have been conducted in university or tertiary care hospitals with in-house obstetricians, anesthesia providers, and operating room staff. The ACOG[38] has noted that "the safety of [a] trial of labor is less well documented in smaller community hospitals or facilities where resources may be more limited." In 1999 the ACOG issued a guideline stating that because uterine rupture may be catastrophic, VBAC should be attempted in institutions equipped to respond to emergencies with physicians *immediately* available to provide emergency care.[38]

The ACOG[46] has defended this guideline by noting that "VBAC is a completely elective procedure that allows for reasonable precautions in assuming this small but significant risk [of uterine rupture]." In contrast, other obstetric catastrophes (e.g., placental abruption, umbilical cord prolapse) cannot be predicted. The ACOG has also noted that "the operational definition of 'immediately available' personnel and facilities remains the purview of each local institution."[46] However, this requirement for the immediate availability of physicians and other personnel clearly represents a more stringent standard than the "readily available" requirement in other published guidelines for obstetric care.

Earlier, Zlatnik[47] made the following comments regarding performance of VBAC in a community hospital: "If a timely cesarean section cannot be performed in a community hospital, VBAC is out of the question, but the larger question is: Should obstetrics continue to be practiced there? Timely cesarean section is an essential option for all laboring women."

In contrast, the American Academy of Family Physicians (AAFP)[48] has published the following recommendations:

> *Women with one previous cesarean delivery with a low transverse incision are candidates for and should be offered a trial of labor (TOL) . . . . Trial of labor after cesarean (TOLAC) should not be restricted only to facilities with available surgical teams present throughout labor since there is no evidence that these additional resources result in improved outcomes. At the same time, it is clinically appropriate that a management plan for uterine rupture and other potential emergencies requiring rapid cesarean section should be documented for each woman undergoing TOLAC.*

The AAFP[48] has argued that the ACOG guidelines suggest that "one rare obstetrical catastrophe (e.g., uterine rupture) merits a level of resource that has not been recommended for other rare obstetrical catastrophes that may actually be more common." The AAFP has acknowledged that these other complications are "largely not predictable," whereas a TOLAC is a "planned event that may demand a different degree of preparedness." Nonetheless, they stated that their recommendations significantly differ from ACOG guidelines because they could find "no evidence to support a different level of care for TOLAC patients."[48]

In response, Dr. Gary Hankins, Chair of the ACOG Committee on Obstetric Practice, made the following statement:

> *It's very troubling when people who may not even be qualified to perform a cesarean section start issuing guidelines about the safety of this kind of thing. . . . Their argument is that the available data don't prove it's unsafe—they're not arguing that it is* safe*. . . . Our main concern is with having the best possible outcome for mother and baby. If women are given the true numbers about the bad outcomes that can be associated with VBAC, no woman is going to take the chance [of laboring without immediately available surgical support].*[49]

Contraindications

The ACOG[14] has listed the following contraindications to VBAC:

- Previous classic or T-shaped incision or extensive transfundal uterine surgery
- Previous uterine rupture
- Medical or obstetric complication that precludes vaginal delivery
- Inability to perform emergency cesarean delivery because of unavailable surgeon, anesthesia [provider], sufficient staff, or facility
- Two prior uterine scars and no vaginal deliveries

OTHER ISSUES

Why do most eligible patients choose to undergo elective repeat cesarean delivery? The low frequency of VBAC has resulted, in part, from both physician and patient preference. VBAC requires more physician effort than elective repeat cesarean delivery. Flamm et al.[11] stated, "Clearly, in any practice setting, it is easier for a physician to perform a scheduled 40-minute operation than to stay up all night with a laboring patient." In some cases, physician reimbursement is greater for elective repeat cesarean delivery than for VBAC, despite the fact that VBAC requires greater physician effort.

Stafford[50] reviewed the impact of nonclinical factors on the performance of repeat cesarean delivery in the State of California. He observed that "proprietary hospitals, with the greatest incentive to maximize reimbursement, had the highest repeat cesarean section rates." Nonteaching hospitals and hospitals with low-volume obstetric services had lower VBAC rates than teaching hospitals and hospitals with high-volume obstetric services. Likewise, Hueston and Rudy[51] found that women who undergo elective repeat cesarean delivery are more likely to have private insurance than women who attempt VBAC. Stafford[50] concluded, "Because a cesarean section is nearly twice as costly as a vaginal birth,... the higher repeat cesarean section rates associated with proprietary hospitals, non-teaching hospitals, and low-volume hospitals contribute to increased health care expenditures."

In contrast, Clark et al.,[52] after assessing both the direct and indirect costs of VBAC, concluded that "any economic savings for the healthcare system of a policy of trial of labor are at best marginal, even in a tertiary care center with a success rate for vaginal birth after cesarean of 70%." Further, they stated that "a policy of trial of labor does not result in any cost saving under most birthing circumstances encountered in the United States today."[52] The ACOG[38] had earlier acknowledged that "the difficulty in accessing the cost-benefit of VBAC is that the costs are not all incurred by one entity." The ACOG[14] has made the following conclusion:

> *A true analysis of the cost-effectiveness of VBAC should include hospital and physician costs, the method of reimbursement, potential professional liability expenses, and the probability that a woman will continue with childbearing after her first attempt at VBAC. Higher costs may be incurred by a hospital if a woman has a prolonged labor or has significant complications or if the newborn is admitted to a neonatal intensive care unit.*

Some women reject VBAC because they have experienced prolonged, painful labor during a previous pregnancy. They fear that they will again experience a prolonged, painful labor and ultimately need a repeat cesarean delivery. This fear is more common in women who have delivered in smaller hospitals without the availability of epidural analgesia during labor. Other women reject VBAC because they prefer to schedule the date of elective repeat cesarean delivery. (A scheduled, elective cesarean delivery allows the patient to arrange for a relative or friend to provide child care.) Kirk et al.[53] questioned 160 women regarding factors affecting their choice between VBAC and elective repeat cesarean delivery. These investigators concluded that "social exigencies appeared to play a more important role than an assessment of the medical risks in making these decisions." Similarly, Joseph et al.[54] observed that fear and inconvenience are the most common deterrents to VBAC. Finally, some women reject a trial of labor because of their concern about the adverse effects of labor and vaginal delivery on the maternal pelvic floor, with the risk of subsequent problems such as urinary and fecal incontinence.

Some insurance carriers previously required that eligible women with a history of previous cesarean delivery attempt VBAC in subsequent pregnancies. These carriers denied partial or full reimbursement to women who chose elective repeat cesarean delivery unless there was a medical reason to perform repeat cesarean delivery. The ACOG and others have agreed that hospitals and insurers should *not* mandate a trial of labor for pregnant women with a history of previous cesarean delivery.[55] The ACOG[14] has instead concluded, "After thorough counseling that weighs the individual benefits and risks of VBAC, the ultimate decision to attempt this procedure or undergo a repeat cesarean delivery should be made by the patient and her physician."

RISKS OF ATTEMPTED VAGINAL BIRTH AFTER CESAREAN DELIVERY

What is the risk of uterine rupture during VBAC? A lower uterine segment scar is relatively avascular, and massive hemorrhage rarely follows separation of a lower segment scar. In contrast, rupture of a classic uterine scar may result in massive intraperitoneal bleeding. Unfortunately, there is some inconsistency and confusion in reports of the incidence of asymptomatic uterine scar dehiscence as opposed to frank uterine rupture. **Uterine scar dehiscence** may be defined as a uterine wall defect that does not result in fetal compromise or excessive hemorrhage and that does not require emergency cesarean delivery or postpartum laparotomy. In contrast, **uterine rupture** is a uterine wall defect that results in fetal compromise, maternal hemorrhage, or both, sufficient to require cesarean delivery or postpartum laparotomy.[56] Using these definitions, Farmer et al.[56] noted that among 7598 patients who attempted VBAC at their hospital between 1983 and 1989, the incidence of uterine scar dehiscence was 0.7% and that of uterine rupture was 0.8%.

Some obstetricians have suggested that earlier studies underestimated the risks of VBAC. Scott[57] reported 12 women from Salt Lake City, Utah, who experienced clinically significant uterine rupture during attempted VBAC. Similarly, Jones et al.[58] reported eight women in Denver, Colorado, who experienced uterine rupture during attempted VBAC. There were no maternal deaths, but three women required obstetric hysterectomy. Four perinatal deaths and at least two cases of severe neurologic impairment occurred. Some of the women did not experience optimal obstetric management. For example, Scott's series included two women who labored at home.

Obstetricians understandably fear that they will be found liable if an adverse event occurs during attempted VBAC. In one case, a jury awarded a verdict of $98.5 million because of a delayed diagnosis of uterine rupture.[59] Phelan[60] cited another court decision that he predicted would have a "chilling effect on the future of VBAC." In this case, the fetal heart rate (FHR) was normal until it abruptly decreased to 80 beats per minute at a cervical dilation of 9 cm. The interval between the onset of the deceleration and emergency cesarean delivery was 27 minutes. At delivery, the fetal head was found in the left adnexa.

The mother required transfusion, and the child now suffers from developmental delay and cerebral palsy. The court found that the defendants were negligent in their failure to deliver the infant in a timely manner and to provide adequate informed consent. The court also concluded that "the ACOG 30-minute rule represented the maximum period of elapse" and did not represent the minimum standard of care. As a result of this verdict, Phelan[60] proposed the use of a VBAC consent form that includes the following statement: "I understand that if my uterus ruptures during my VBAC, there may not be sufficient time to operate and to prevent the death of or permanent brain injury to my baby." Flamm[61] responded that "widespread implementation of this or similar consent forms essentially would mean the end of VBAC." Flamm[61] also noted:

> *On a national level, giving up VBAC would mean performing an additional 100,000 cesareans every year. It is unlikely this huge number of operations could be performed without any serious complications and perhaps even some maternal deaths.*

In contrast, Greene[62] wrote a sobering editorial on the risks of VBAC. Observing that the study performed by Lydon-Rochelle et al.[17] was an observational study that reflected "broad experience in a wide range of clinical-practice settings," he stated that "there is no reason to believe that improvements in clinical care can substantially reduce the risks of uterine rupture and perinatal mortality." Greene[62] concluded his editorial as follows:

> *After a thorough discussion of the risks and benefits of attempting a vaginal delivery after cesarean section, a patient might ask, "But doctor, what is the safest thing for my baby?" Given the findings of Lydon-Rochelle et al., my unequivocal answer: elective repeated cesarean section.*

Later studies have provided conflicting data regarding maternal risk. In a systematic review of published studies of attempted VBAC, Guise et al.[63] observed no significant difference in the incidence of maternal death or hysterectomy between women attempting a trial of labor and those undergoing repeat cesarean delivery. Uterine rupture was more common in the women attempting a trial of labor, but the rates of asymptomatic uterine dehiscence did not differ. Wen et al.[64] performed a retrospective cohort study of 308,755 Canadian women with a history of previous cesarean delivery between 1988 and 2000. These investigators observed that the rates of uterine rupture (0.65%), transfusion (0.19%), and hysterectomy (0.10%) were significantly higher in the trial-of-labor group. However, the maternal in-hospital death rate was significantly lower in the trial-of-labor group (1.6 per 100,000) than in the elective cesarean delivery group (5.6 per 100,000). Cahill et al.[65] performed a multicenter cohort study in which they concluded that among the VBAC candidates who have had a prior vaginal delivery, those who attempt VBAC have a lower risk for overall major maternal morbidities, as well as maternal fever and transfusion, than women who choose repeat cesarean delivery. These investigators concluded that women who have had a prior vaginal delivery have "less composite maternal morbidity if they attempt VBAC compared with [those] undergoing an elective repeat cesarean delivery." Further, they concluded that a trial of labor is "a safer overall option for women who have had a prior vaginal birth."[65]

In an editorial, Pitkin[66] made the following statement regarding VBAC: "Many women with previous cesareans can be delivered vaginally, and thereby gain substantial advantage, but neither the decision for trial [of] labor nor management during that labor should be arrived at in a cavalier or superficial manner."

OBSTETRIC MANAGEMENT

Intravenous Access and Availability of Blood

It seems prudent to recommend the early establishment of intravenous access in women who attempt VBAC. Moreover, cross-matched blood should be readily available for these patients.

Fetal Heart Rate Monitoring

Continuous electronic FHR monitoring represents the best means of detecting uterine rupture.[67-69] Rodriguez et al.[68] reviewed 76 cases of uterine rupture at their hospital. A nonreassuring FHR pattern occurred in 59 of the 76 patients and was the most reliable sign of uterine rupture.

Intrauterine Pressure Monitoring

The intrauterine pressure catheter provides a quantitative measurement of uterine tone both during and between contractions. Some obstetricians contend that an intrauterine pressure catheter should be used in all patients who attempt VBAC, arguing that a loss of intrauterine pressure and cessation of labor will signal the occurrence of uterine rupture. In one study, 39 patients had an intrauterine pressure catheter at the time of uterine rupture. None of these patients experienced an apparent decrease in resting uterine tone or cessation of labor, but 4 patients experienced an increase in baseline uterine tone.[68] In these 4 patients, the increase in baseline uterine tone was associated with severe variable FHR decelerations that prompted immediate cesarean delivery. The authors concluded that the information obtained from the use of the intrauterine pressure catheter did not help obstetricians make the diagnosis of uterine rupture.[68]

Of course, obstetricians may use an intrauterine pressure catheter for other reasons in patients attempting VBAC. For example, it may be prudent to place an intrauterine pressure catheter in patients who receive oxytocin.

Use of Prostaglandins

Lydon-Rochelle et al.[17] observed a uterine rupture rate of 24.5 per 1000 women who attempted VBAC with prostaglandin-induced labor. The ACOG[14] noted that "there is considerable evidence that cervical ripening with prostaglandin preparations increases the likelihood of uterine rupture." The ACOG has concluded that "the use of prostaglandins for cervical ripening or induction of labor in most women with a previous cesarean delivery should be discouraged."[14] The ACOG[70] recently reaffirmed its position that "misoprostol should not be used in patients with a previous cesarean delivery or major uterine surgery."

Oxytocin Augmentation of Labor

Some obstetricians have long argued that the administration of oxytocin increases the likelihood of uterine rupture during VBAC. However, several studies have suggested that obstetricians may safely use oxytocin to augment labor in patients who attempt VBAC.[23,71,72] In a meta-analysis of 31 studies of VBAC, Rosen et al.[4] noted that the use of oxytocin did not increase the risk of uterine scar dehiscence or rupture during VBAC.

In contrast, in one large retrospective study of more than 20,000 women, uterine rupture was nearly five times more common among women undergoing induction of labor with oxytocin than in those who had an elective repeat cesarean delivery.[17] Zelop et al.[73] observed a higher rate of uterine rupture in women receiving oxytocin induction of labor for attempted VBAC than in similar women attempting VBAC with spontaneous labor. Further, the rate of uterine rupture was also higher in women receiving oxytocin for augmentation of labor, but the difference was not statistically significant. The ACOG[14] has noted that spontaneous labor is more likely than induction or augmentation of labor to result in successful VBAC.

ANESTHETIC MANAGEMENT

In the past, some obstetricians contended that epidural anesthesia might mask the pain of uterine scar separation or rupture and thereby delay the diagnosis of uterine scar dehiscence or rupture.[74-76] Plauché et al.[74] stated, "Regional anesthesia, such as epidural anesthesia, blunts the patient's perception of symptoms and the physician's ability to elicit signs of early uterine rupture." Others have argued that the sympathectomy associated with epidural anesthesia attenuates the maternal compensatory response to the hemorrhage associated with uterine rupture. For example, sympathectomy might prevent the compensatory tachycardia and vasoconstriction that occur during hemorrhage. However, consensus now exists that these concerns do not preclude administration of epidural analgesia, for several reasons.

First, pain, uterine tenderness, and tachycardia have low sensitivity as diagnostic symptoms and signs of lower uterine segment scar dehiscence or rupture. Some uterine scars separate painlessly. Many obstetricians have discovered an asymptomatic lower uterine segment scar dehiscence at the time of elective repeat cesarean delivery. Molloy et al.[77] reported eight cases of uterine rupture among 1781 patients who attempted VBAC. None of these 8 patients had abdominal pain, but all had FHR abnormalities. Johnson and Oriol[69] reviewed 14 studies of VBAC published between 1980 and 1989. Among 10,967 patients who attempted VBAC, 1623 patients received epidural anesthesia. Of those who experienced uterine rupture, 5 of 14 patients (35%) with epidural anesthesia experienced abdominal pain, compared with 4 of 23 patients (17%) without epidural anesthesia. FHR abnormalities represented the most common sign of uterine rupture among patients who did and did not receive epidural anesthesia. None of the investigators in these studies observed that epidural anesthesia delayed the diagnosis of uterine rupture.

Second, pain, uterine tenderness, and tachycardia have low specificity as diagnostic symptoms and signs of lower uterine segment scar dehiscence. Case et al.[78] reported 20 patients with a history of previous cesarean delivery in whom the indication for urgent repeat cesarean delivery was severe hypogastric pain, tenderness, or both. At surgery, they confirmed the presence of scar dehiscence in only one of the 20 patients. Eckstein et al.[79] suggested that the unexpected development of pain during previously successful epidural anesthesia might be indicative of uterine rupture. Crawford[80] referred to this phenomenon as the "epidural sieve." Others have described patients who received epidural anesthesia and subsequently complained of pain and tenderness secondary to uterine scar rupture.[81-84] I have provided anesthesia care for several patients in whom the first suggestion of scar separation was the sudden and unexpected development of "breakthrough pain" despite the continuous epidural infusion of bupivacaine. Thus, epidural analgesia may improve the specificity of abdominal pain as a symptom of uterine scar separation or rupture.

Third, most cases of lower uterine segment scar dehiscence do not lead to severe hemorrhage. In one report of six cases of uterine scar dehiscence or rupture, only one patient had intrapartum vaginal bleeding.[67] However, if significant bleeding should occur, epidural anesthesia may attenuate the maternal compensatory response to hemorrhage. Vincent et al.[85] observed that epidural anesthesia (median sensory level of T9) significantly worsened maternal hypotension, uterine blood flow, and fetal oxygenation during untreated hemorrhage (20 mL/kg) in gravid ewes. Intravascular volume replacement promptly eliminated the differences between groups in maternal mean arterial pressure, cardiac output, and fetal PaO_2. Maternal heart rate did not change significantly during hemorrhage in the control animals. However, there was a significant drop in maternal heart rate during hemorrhage in the animals that received epidural anesthesia.[85] Perhaps maternal bradycardia should prompt suspicion of maternal hemorrhage in patients undergoing VBAC with epidural anesthesia.

Fourth, several published series have reported the successful use of epidural analgesia in women undergoing VBAC.[11,23,35,56,67,80,86-88] There is little evidence that epidural analgesia either decreases the likelihood of vaginal delivery or adversely affects maternal or neonatal outcome in women who have uterine scar separation or rupture. Flamm et al.[89] reported a multicenter study of 1776 patients who attempted VBAC. Approximately 134 (74%) of 181 women who received epidural anesthesia delivered vaginally, compared with 1180 (74%) of 1595 women who did not receive epidural anesthesia. Phelan et al.[86] reported that among patients who received both oxytocin augmentation and epidural anesthesia, 69% delivered vaginally. This did not differ from the incidence of vaginal delivery among patients who received oxytocin without epidural anesthesia. Other investigators have reported results of smaller studies suggesting a lower rate of VBAC among patients who received epidural analgesia.[87,88] However, this effect was limited to patients who received oxytocin for the induction or augmentation of labor. These investigators concluded that epidural analgesia does *not* decrease the likelihood of successful VBAC.

Fifth, some obstetricians favor the use of epidural anesthesia because it facilitates postpartum uterine exploration to assess the integrity of the uterine scar. Meehan et al.[90] earlier supported routine palpation of the uterine scar. However, Meehan et al.[91] subsequently acknowledged that it is not necessary to repair all such defects. Many obstetricians manage asymptomatic uterine scar dehiscence with "expectant observation." Thus, they argue that routine palpation of the uterine scar is unnecessary after successful VBAC.[10]

Sixth, epidural analgesia provides rapid access to safe, surgical anesthesia if cesarean delivery or postpartum laparotomy should be required.[92]

Finally, it is inhumane to deny effective analgesia to women who attempt VBAC. Further, the ACOG[14] has concluded that "adequate pain relief may encourage more women to choose a trial of labor." Thus, the availability and use of epidural analgesia may decrease the incidence of unnecessary repeat cesarean delivery.

The ACOG[14] has concluded that VBAC does not contraindicate the use of epidural analgesia. In my judgment, the availability of epidural analgesia is an essential component of a successful VBAC program. It seems reasonable to provide analgesia—but not total anesthesia—during labor in patients attempting VBAC.

KEY POINTS

- Cesarean delivery is the most commonly performed major operation in the United States, and previous cesarean delivery is the most common indication.
- A trial of labor is successful in 60% to 80% of women in whom a low-transverse uterine incision was made during previous cesarean delivery.
- A previous vaginal delivery is the greatest predictor for successful vaginal birth after cesarean delivery (VBAC). A history of dystocia, the need for induction of labor, and/or maternal obesity are associated with a lower likelihood of successful VBAC.
- The American College of Obstetricians and Gynecologists has stated that physicians, anesthesia providers, and other personnel must be *immediately* available to provide emergency care for patients attempting VBAC.
- Hospitals and insurers should not mandate a trial of labor for pregnant women with a history of previous cesarean delivery.
- Continuous electronic FHR monitoring represents the best means of detecting uterine rupture.
- Women are more likely to attempt VBAC if they know that they will receive effective analgesia during labor.
- Epidural analgesia does not delay the diagnosis of uterine rupture or decrease the likelihood of successful VBAC.

REFERENCES

1. Cragin EB. Conservatism in obstetrics. New York Med J 1916; 104:1-3.
2. Taffel SM, Placek PJ, Liss T. Trends in the United States cesarean section rate and reasons for the 1980-85 rise. Am J Pub Health 1987; 77:955-9.
3. United States Department of Health and Human Services, Public Health Service, National Institutes of Health. Repeat cesarean birth. Cesarean childbirth. NIH Publication No. 82-2067. Washington DC, United States Government Printing Office, 1981:351-74.
4. Rosen MG, Dickinson JC, Westhoff CL. Vaginal birth after cesarean: A meta-analysis of morbidity and mortality. Obstet Gynecol 1991; 77:465-70.
5. American College of Obstetricians and Gynecologists Committee on Obstetric Practice. Vaginal delivery after a previous cesarean birth. ACOG Committee Opinion No. 143. Washington, DC, ACOG, October 1994.
6. Yeh J, Wactawiski-Wende J, Shelton JA, Reschke J. Temporal trend in the rates of trial of labor in low-risk pregnancies and their impact on the rates and success of vaginal birth after cesarean delivery. Am J Obstet Gynecol 2006; 194:144-52.
7. CDC National Center for Health Statistics. Teen birth rate rises for first time in 15 years. December 5, 2007. Available at: http://www.cdc.gov/nchs/pressroom/07newsreleases/teenbirth.htm/
8. De Lee JB, Cornell EL. Low cervical cesarean section (laparotrachelotomy). JAMA 1922; 79:109-12.
9. Kerr JMM. The technique of cesarean section, with special reference to the lower uterine segment incision. Am J Obstet Gynecol 1926; 12:729-34.
10. Landon MB. Cesarean delivery. In Gabbe SG, Niebyl JR, Simpson JL, editors. Obstetrics: Normal and Problem Pregnancies. 5th edition. Philadelphia, Churchill Livingstone Elsevier, 2007:486-520.
11. Flamm BL, Newman LA, Thomas SJ, et al. Vaginal birth after cesarean delivery: Results of a 5-year multicenter collaborative study. Obstet Gynecol 1990; 76:750-4.
12. Flamm BL, Goings JR, Liu Y, Wolde-Tsadik G. Elective repeat cesarean delivery versus trial of labor: A prospective multicenter study. Obstet Gynecol 1994; 83:927-32.
13. Miller DA, Diaz FG, Paul RH. Vaginal birth after cesarean: A 10-year experience. Obstet Gynecol 1994; 84:255-8.
14. American College of Obstetricians and Gynecologists. Vaginal birth after previous cesarean delivery. ACOG Practice Bulletin No. 54, Washington, DC, ACOG, July 2004.
15. Landon MB, Hauth JC, Leveno KJ, et al. Maternal and perinatal outcomes associated with a trial of labor after prior cesarean delivery. N Engl J Med 2004; 351:2581-9.
16. McMahon MJ, Luther ER, Bowes WA, Olshan AF. Comparison of a trial of labor with an elective second cesarean section. N Engl J Med 1996; 335:689-95.
17. Lydon-Rochelle M, Holt VL, Easterling TR, Martin DP. Risk of uterine rupture during labor among women with a prior cesarean delivery. N Engl J Med 2001; 345:3-8.
18. Rosen MG, Dickinson JC. Vaginal birth after cesarean: A meta-analysis of indicators for success. Obstet Gynecol 1990; 76:865-9.
19. Landon MB, Leindecker S, Spong CY, et al; National Institute of Child Health and Human Development Maternal-Fetal Medicine Units Network. The MFMU Cesarean Registry: Factors affecting the success of trial of labor after previous cesarean delivery. Am J Obstet Gynecol 2005; 193:1016-23.
20. Goodall PT, Ahn JT, Chapa JB, Hibbard JU. Obesity as a risk factor for failed trial of labor in patients with previous cesarean delivery. Am J Obstet Gynecol 2005; 192:1423-6.
21. Srinivas SK, Stamilio DM, Stevens EJ, et al. Predicting failure of a vaginal birth attempt after cesarean delivery. Obstet Gynecol 2007; 109:800-5.
22. Grobman WA, Lai Y, Landon MB, et al. Development of a nomogram for prediction of vaginal birth after cesarean delivery. Obstet Gynecol 2007; 109:806-12.

23. Phelan JP, Ahn MO, Diaz F, et al. Twice a cesarean, always a cesarean? Obstet Gynecol 1989; 73:161-5.
24. Asakura H, Myers SA. More than one previous cesarean delivery: A 5-year experience with 435 patients. Obstet Gynecol 1995; 85:924-9.
25. Caughey AB, Shipp TD, Repke JT, et al. Rate of uterine rupture during a trial of labor in women with one or two prior cesarean deliveries. Am J Obstet Gynecol 1999; 181:872-6.
26. Landon MB, Spong CY, Thom E, et al. Risk of uterine rupture during a trial labor in women with multiple and single prior cesarean delivery. Obstet Gynecol 2006; 108:12-20.
27. Naef RW, Ray MA, Chauhan SP, et al. Trial of labor after cesarean delivery with a lower-segment, vertical uterine incision: Is it safe? Am J Obstet Gynecol 1995; 172:1666-74.
28. Adair CD, Sanchez-Ramos L, Whitaker D, et al. Trial of labor in patients with a previous lower uterine vertical cesarean section. Am J Obstet Gynecol 1996; 174:966-70.
29. Strong TH, Phelan JP, Ahn MO, Sarno AP. Vaginal birth after cesarean delivery in the twin gestation. Am J Obstet Gynecol 1989; 161:29-33.
30. Miller DA, Mullin P, Hou D, Paul RH. Vaginal birth after cesarean section in twin gestation. Am J Obstet Gynecol 1996; 175:194-8.
31. Cahill A, Stamilio DM, Pare E, et al. Vaginal birth after cesarean (VBAC) attempt in twin pregnancies: Is it safe? Am J Obstet Gynecol 2005; 193:1050-5.
32. Varner MW, Leindecker S, Spong CY, et al. National Institute of Child Health and Human Development Maternal-Fetal Medicine Units Network. The Maternal-Fetal Medicine Unit Cesarean Registry: Trial of labor with a twin gestation. Am J Obstet Gynecol 2005; 193:135-40.
33. Ford AD, Bateman BT, Simpson LL. Vaginal birth after cesarean delivery in twin gestations: A large, nationwide sample of deliveries. Am J Obstet Gynecol 2006; 195:1138-42.
34. Beall M, Eglinton GS, Clark SL, Phelan JP. Vaginal delivery after cesarean section in women with unknown types of uterine scar. J Reprod Med 1984; 29:31-5.
35. Pruett KM, Kirshon B, Cotton DB. Unknown uterine scar and trial of labor. Am J Obstet Gynecol 1988; 159:807-10.
36. Lonky NM, Worthen N, Ross MG. Prediction of cesarean section scars with ultrasound imaging during pregnancy. J Ultrasound Med 1989; 8:15-9.
37. Flamm BL, Goings JR. Vaginal birth after cesarean section: Is suspected fetal macrosomia a contraindication? Obstet Gynecol 1989; 74:694-7.
38. American College of Obstetricians and Gynecologists. Vaginal birth after previous cesarean delivery. ACOG Clinical Management Guidelines for Obstetricians-Gynecologists No. 5. Washington, DC, ACOG, July 1999.
39. Elkousy MA, Sammel M, Stevens E, et al. The effect of birth weight on vaginal birth after cesarean delivery success rates. Am J Obstet Gynecol 2003; 188:824-30.
40. Peaceman AM, Gersnoviez R, Landon MB, et al. National Institute of Child Health and Human Development Maternal-Fetal Medicine Units Network. The MFMU Cesarean Registry: Impact of fetal size on trial of labor success for patients with previous cesarean for dystocia. Am J Obstet Gynecol 2006; 195:1127-31.
41. Coassolo KM, Stamilio DM, Pare E, et al. Safety and efficacy of vaginal birth after cesarean attempts at or beyond 40 weeks of gestation. Obstet Gynecol 2005; 106:700-6.
42. Yeh S, Huang X, Phelan JP. Postterm pregnancy after previous cesarean section. J Reprod Med 1984; 29:41-4.
43. Zelop CM, Shipp TD, Cohen A, et al. Trial of labor after 40 weeks' gestation in women with prior cesarean. Obstet Gynecol 2001; 97:391-3.
44. Ophir E, Oettinger M, Yagoda A, et al. Breech presentation after cesarean section: Always a section? Am J Obstet Gynecol 1989; 161:25-8.
45. Sarno AP, Phelan JP, Ahn MO, Strong TH. Vaginal birth after cesarean delivery: Trial of labor in women with breech presentation. J Reprod Med 1989; 34:831-3.
46. Anonymous. ACOG calls for "immediately available" VBAC services. ASA Newsl 1999; 63:21.
47. Zlatnik FJ. VBAC and the community hospital revisited. Iowa Perinat Lett 1989; 10:20.
48. The American Academy of Family Physicians. Trial of Labor after Cesarean (TOLAC), formerly Trial of Labor versus Elective Repeat Cesarean Section for the Woman with a Previous Cesarean Section. Leawood, KS, AAFP, March 2005. Available at: http://www.aafp.org/online/en/home/clinical/clinicalrecs/tolac.html
49. Sullivan MG. Family physicians' VBAC guideline raises concern. Ob Gyn News. September 1, 2005.
50. Stafford RS. The impact of nonclinical factors on repeat cesarean section. JAMA 1991; 265:59-63.
51. Hueston WJ, Rudy M. Factors predicting elective repeat cesarean delivery. Obstet Gynecol 1994; 83:741-4.
52. Clark SL, Scott JR, Porter TF, et al. Is vaginal birth after cesarean less expensive than repeat cesarean delivery? Am J Obstet Gynecol 2000; 182:599-602.
53. Kirk EP, Doyle KA, Leigh J, Garrard ML. Vaginal birth after cesarean or repeat cesarean section: Medical risks or social realities. Am J Obstet Gynecol 1990; 162:1398-405.
54. Joseph GF, Stedman CF, Robichaux AG. Vaginal birth after cesarean section: The impact of patient resistance to a trial of labor. Am J Obstet Gynecol 1991; 164:1441-7.
55. Sachs BP, Kobelin C, Castro MA, Frigoletto F. The risks of lowering the cesarean-delivery rate. N Engl J Med 1999; 340:54-7.
56. Farmer RM, Kirschbaum T, Potter D, et al. Uterine rupture during trial of labor after previous cesarean section. Am J Obstet Gynecol 1991; 165:995-1001.
57. Scott JR. Mandatory trial of labor after cesarean delivery: An alternative viewpoint. Obstet Gynecol 1991; 77:811-4.
58. Jones RO, Nagashima AW, Hartnett-Goodman MM, Goodlin RC. Rupture of low transverse cesarean scars during trial of labor. Obstet Gynecol 1991; 77:815-7.
59. Freeman G, editor. $98.5 million verdict in missed uterine rupture. OB-GYN Malpractice Prev 1996; 3:41-8.
60. Phelan JP. VBAC: Time to reconsider? OBG Management 1996; Nov:62-8.
61. Flamm BL. Once a cesarean, always a controversy. Obstet Gynecol 1997; 90:312-5.
62. Greene MF. Vaginal delivery after cesarean section: Is the risk acceptable (editorial)? N Engl J Med 2001; 345:54-5.
63. Guise JM, Berlin M, McDonagh M, et al. Safety of vaginal birth after cesarean: A systematic review. Obstet Gynecol 2004; 103:420-9.
64. Wen SW, Rusen ID, Walker M, et al. Comparison of maternal mortality and morbidity between trial of labor and elective cesarean section among women with previous cesarean delivery. Am J Obstet Gynecol 2004; 191:1263-9.
65. Cahill AG, Stamilio DM, Odibo AO, et al. Is vaginal birth after cesarean (VBAC) or elective repeat cesarean safer in women with a prior vaginal delivery? Am J Obstet Gynecol 2006; 195:1143-7.
66. Pitkin RM. Once a cesarean (editorial)? Obstet Gynecol 1991; 77:939.
67. Uppington J. Epidural analgesia and previous caesarean section. Anaesthesia 1983; 38:336-41.
68. Rodriguez MH, Masaki DI, Phelan JP, Diaz FG. Uterine rupture: Are intrauterine pressure catheters useful in the diagnosis? Am J Obstet Gynecol 1989; 161:666-9.
69. Johnson C, Oriol N. The role of epidural anesthesia in trial of labor. Reg Anesth 1990; 15:304-8.
70. American College of Obstetricians and Gynecologists, Committee on Obstetric Practice: Induction of labor for vaginal birth after cesarean delivery. ACOG Committee Opinion No. 342. Washington, DC, ACOG, August 2006.
71. Horenstein JM, Phelan JP. Previous cesarean section: The risks and benefits of oxytocin usage in a trial of labor. Am J Obstet Gynecol 1985; 151:564-9.

72. Flamm BL, Goings JR, Fuelberth NJ, et al. Oxytocin during labor after previous cesarean section: Results of a multicenter study. Obstet Gynecol 1987; 70:709-12.
73. Zelop CM, Shipp TD, Repke JT, et al. Uterine rupture during induced or augmented labor in gravid women with one prior cesarean delivery. Am J Obstet Gynecol 1999; 181:882-6.
74. Plauché WC, Von Almen W, Muller R. Catastrophic uterine rupture. Obstet Gynecol 1984; 64:792-7.
75. Abraham R, Sadovsky E. Delay in the diagnosis of rupture of the uterus due to epidural anesthesia in labor. Gynecol Obstet Invest 1992; 33:239-40.
76. Tehan B. Abolition of the extradural sieve by addition of fentanyl to extradural bupivacaine. Br J Anaesth 1992; 69:520-1.
77. Molloy BG, Sheil O, Duignan NM. Delivery after caesarean section: Review of 2176 consecutive cases. Br Med J 1987; 294:1645-7.
78. Case BD, Corcoran R, Jeffcoate N, Randle GH. Caesarean section and its place in modern obstetric practice. J Obstet Gynaecol Br Commonw 1971; 78:203-14.
79. Eckstein KL, Oberlander SG, Marx GF. Uterine rupture during extradural blockade. Can Anaesth Soc J 1973; 20:566-8.
80. Crawford JS. The epidural sieve and MBC (minimal blocking concentration): A hypothesis. Anaesthesia 1976; 31:1277-80.
81. Carlsson C, Nybell-Lindahl G, Ingemarsson I. Extradural block in patients who have previously undergone caesarean section. Br J Anaesth 1980; 52:827-30.
82. Rowbottom SJ, Tabrizian I. Epidural analgesia and uterine rupture during labour. Anaesth Intens Care 1994; 22:79-80.
83. Kelly MC, Hill DA, Wilson DB. Low dose epidural bupivacaine/fentanyl infusion does not mask uterine rupture. Int J Obstet Anesth 1997; 6:52-4.
84. Rowbottom SJ, Critchley LAH, Gin T. Uterine rupture and epidural analgesia during trial of labour. Anaesthesia 1997, 52:483-8.
85. Vincent RD, Chestnut DH, Sipes SL, et al. Epidural anesthesia worsens uterine blood flow and fetal oxygenation during hemorrhage in gravid ewes. Anesthesiology 1992; 76:799-806.
86. Phelan JP, Clark SL, Diaz F, Paul RH. Vaginal birth after cesarean. Am J Obstet Gynecol 1987; 157:1510-5.
87. Stovall TG, Shaver DC, Solomon SK, Anderson GD. Trial of labor in previous cesarean section patients, excluding classical cesarean sections. Obstet Gynecol 1987; 70:713-7.
88. Sakala EP, Kaye S, Murray RD, Munson LJ. Epidural analgesia: Effect on the likelihood of a successful trial of labor after cesarean section. J Reprod Med 1990; 35:886-90.
89. Flamm BL, Lim OW, Jones C, et al. Vaginal birth after cesarean section: Results of a multicenter study. Am J Obstet Gynecol 1988; 158:1079-84.
90. Meehan FP, Moolgaoker AS, Stallworthy J. Vaginal delivery under caudal analgesia after caesarean section and other major uterine surgery. Br Med J 1972; 2:740-2.
91. Meehan FP, Burke G, Kehoe JT, Magani IM. True rupture/scar dehiscence in delivery following prior section. Int J Gynecol Obstet 1990; 31:249-55.
92. Bucklin BA. Vaginal birth after cesarean delivery. Anesthesiology 2003; 99:1444-8.

Chapter 20

The Pain of Childbirth and Its Effect on the Mother and the Fetus

Peter H. Pan, M.D.
James C. Eisenach, M.D.

The gate control theory of pain, described more than 40 years ago by Melzack and Wall,[1] has revolutionized the understanding of the mechanisms responsible for pain and analgesia. Originally explained as the regulation of pain signals from the peripheral nerve to the spinal cord by the activity of other peripheral nerves, interneurons in the spinal cord, and central supraspinal centers (Figure 20-1), the theory has been refined with the concept of a neuromatrix, a remarkably dynamic system capable of undergoing rapid change.[2] Neural circuits and intraneural mechanisms regulate sensitivity at peripheral afferent terminals; along the conducting axons of peripheral nerves; in the spinal cord, pons, medulla, and thalamus; and at cortical sites of pain transmission and projection. For example, the peripheral application of capsaicin to the skin alters spinal gating mechanisms within 10 minutes, resulting in a light touch signal's being interpreted as burning pain.[3]

Despite research (initiated by the gate control theory) into the mechanisms and treatments for chronic pain, virtually no research on the neurophysiologic basis or therapies for labor pain has occurred. This discrepancy in focus has led to vastly different approaches to the treatment of patients with chronic versus obstetric pain. A patient with chronic pain typically undergoes a sophisticated physical assessment of sensory function[4]; is offered therapies, on the basis of the assessment, from nearly a dozen different classes of analgesics; and can benefit from the enormous resources expended by the pharmaceutical industry to introduce agents that act on novel receptors or enzymes. By contrast, a laboring woman receives no physical assessment of sensory function and is offered only a handful of systemic drugs that act primarily through the anatomic blockade of neural traffic. There is limited pharmaceutical industry interest in developing new drugs for the treatment of intrapartum pain, and therefore some observers consider labor pain to be an unmet medical need.[5]

This chapter examines this paradox in the approach to labor pain and reviews the basis for current therapy (anatomy), the basis for future therapy (neurophysiology), and the effects of labor pain on the mother and the baby.

EXISTENCE AND SEVERITY

The recognition and acceptance of chronic pain, which frequently lacks an obvious outward cause, contrasts with the recurrent denial of labor pain, which is accompanied by visible tissue injury. Dick-Read[6] suggested that labor is a natural process not considered painful by women in primitive cultures, which should be handled with education and preparation rather than through pain medications. Lamaze[7] popularized psychoprophylaxis as a method of birth preparation; this method now forms the basis for prepared childbirth training in the developed world. Although childbirth training acknowledges the existence of pain during labor, a number of individuals and scientific-thought leaders still consider labor pain to be minor and unimportant.

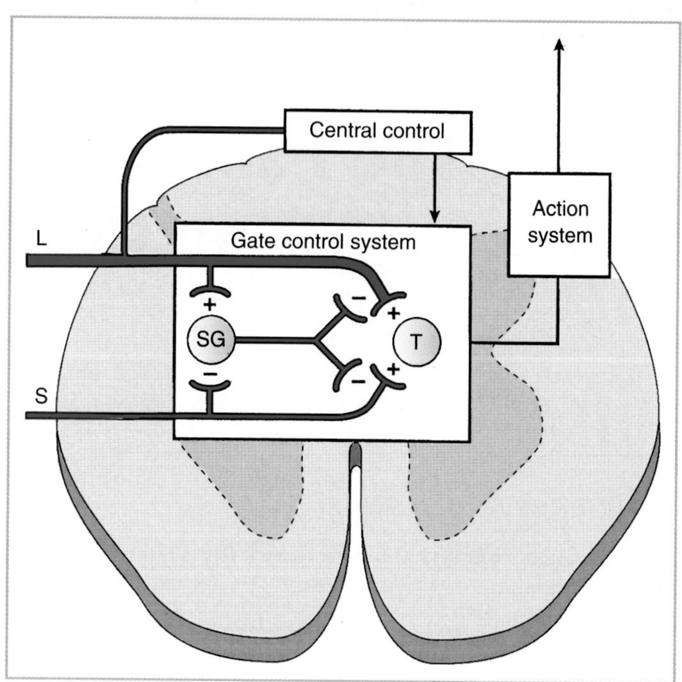

FIGURE 20-1 Gate control theory of pain. Activity in small-diameter afferents (S) stimulates transmission cells in the spinal cord (T), which send signals supraspinally and results in the perception of pain. Small-diameter afferents also inhibit cells in the spinal cord substantia gelatinosa (SG), the activity of which reduces excitatory input to T cells. Activity in large-diameter afferents (L) also stimulates T cells in a manner that is perceived as nonpainful and excites SG cells to "close the gate" and reduce S afferent activation of T cells. The gate mechanism is under regulation by central sites. (From Melzack R, Wall PD. Pain mechanisms: A new theory. Science 1965; 150:971-5.)

The severity of labor pain has been recognized previously. Melzack,[8] using a questionnaire developed to assess the intensity and emotional impact of pain, observed that among nulliparous women with no prepared childbirth training, labor pain was rated to be as painful as a digit amputation without anesthesia (Figure 20-2).[8] The Romans called delivery the *poena magna*—the "great pain" or "great punishment." More than 30 years before Melzack's quantification of pain, Javert and Hardy[9,10] trained subjects to reproduce the intensity of labor pain with the sensation of noxious heat applied to the skin from a radiant heat source. In these experiments, several women achieved "ceiling pain"—resulting in second-degree burns to the skin—when they attempted to match the intensity of uterine contraction pain.[9] Individual women also reported a close positive correlation between cervical dilation and pain intensity. Logistic regression analysis of the investigators' original data[9] indicates a high likelihood of severe pain as labor progresses, with a time course closely associated with cervical dilation (Figure 20-3). Other investigators have noted that uterine pressure during contractions accounts for more than 90% of the variability in labor pain intensity.[11] These observations are consistent with the conclusion that cervical distention is the primary cause of pain during the first stage of labor.

There is considerable variability in the rated intensity of pain during labor. Although 25% of women in one study reported labor pain to be minimal or mild, a nearly equal percentage considered the pain to be very severe or intolerable.[12] Nulliparous women rate labor pain as more severe than parous women; however, the differences are small and of questionable clinical relevance.[12] There is a correlation between the intensity of menses and labor pain, especially back discomfort,[12] although the reason for this relationship is unknown. It is possible that the rated intensity of labor pain reflects individual differences in the perception of all types of pain. A group of women who represented 10% of another study population and reported never having

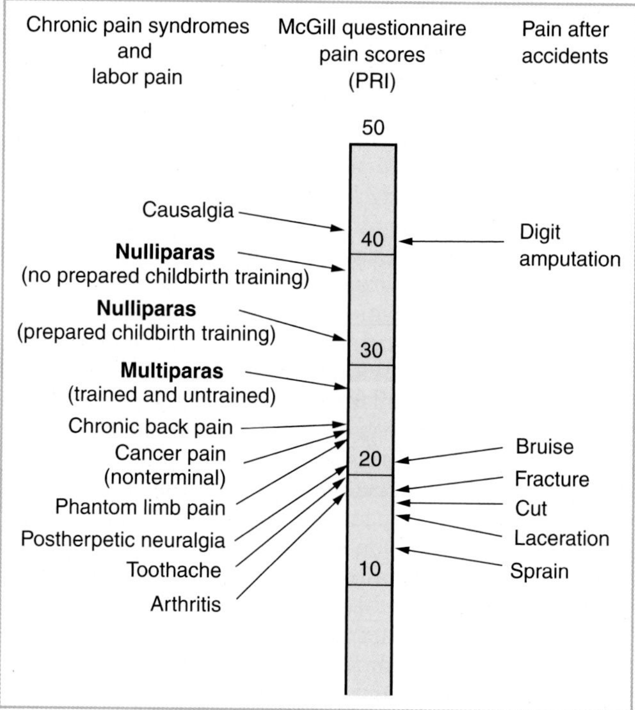

FIGURE 20-2 A comparison of pain scores obtained through the McGill Pain Questionnaire. Scores were collected from women in labor, patients in a general hospital clinic, and patients in the emergency department after accidents involving traumatic injury. Note the modest difference in pain scores between nulliparous women with and without prepared childbirth training. PRI, Pain rating index, which represents the sum of the rank values of all the words chosen from 20 sets of pain descriptors. (Modified from Melzack R. The myth of painless childbirth [The John J. Bonica Lecture]. Pain 1984; 19:321-37.)

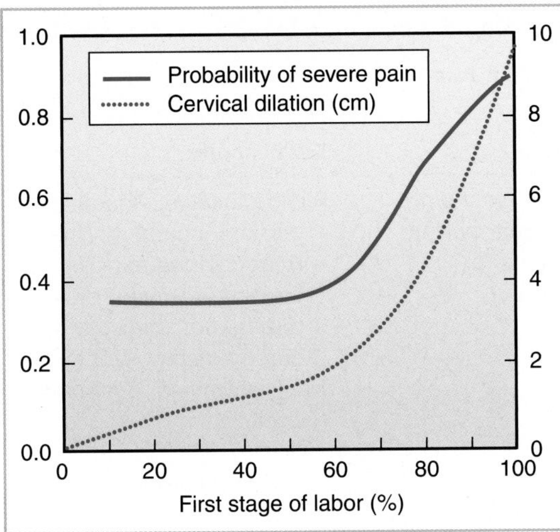

FIGURE 20-3 Likelihood of severe pain during labor. A significant minority of women (approximately one third) have severe pain (pain score > 6) in early labor, and the proportion of women with severe pain increases to nearly 90% later in labor, in close relationship with cervical dilation. (Data adapted from Hardy JD, Javert CT. Studies on pain: Measurements of pain intensity in childbirth. J Clin Invest 1949; 28:153-62.)

experienced pain before childbirth reported experiencing significantly less pain during labor and delivery than the women who had previously experienced pain.[13] In another study, the variability in the amount of pain reported after cesarean delivery could be predicted by the prior rating of pain intensity with a standardized noxious heat stimulus.[14]

The mechanism by which people perceive different levels of pain from the same stimulus remains unclear. A study involving brain imaging and a fixed acute noxious heat stimulus showed a strong correlation between verbal pain assessment and the level of activation of various cortical brain regions, especially the contralateral somatosensory cortex and anterior cingulate cortex.[15] The investigators also found that the degree of activation of the thalamus was essentially identical in all subjects, suggesting that differences in perceived pain resulted from modulation at suprathalamic levels rather than in the peripheral nerves or spinal cord. The situation in labor may be more complex. For example, a large genetic polymorphism regulates cytokine production and function as well as pregnancy outcome.[16] It is possible that interindividual differences in labor pain may partially reflect genetic differences in cytokine production or response.

In summary, although significant variability exists in the rated intensity of pain during labor and delivery, the majority of women experience more than minimal pain. The close correlation between cervical dilation and the rated severity of pain implies the existence of a causal relationship and increases the likelihood that a parturient will request analgesia as labor progresses.

PERSONAL SIGNIFICANCE AND MEANING

The International Association for the Study of Pain has defined pain as "an unpleasant sensory and emotional experience associated with actual or potential tissue damage, or described in terms of such damage."[17] Clearly, this reflects an intensity-discriminatory component and an emotional-cognitive component, with powerful interactions between the two. The focus of current interventions is heavily weighted toward the first component and assumes that labor pain is severe and in need of pharmacologic treatment. Largely ignored are coping strategies and the personal meaning of labor pain, which varies considerably among women.[18]

Although many women rate the pain of labor and delivery as severe, the terms used to more fully describe this pain reflect an emotional meaning. In a pioneering study of the quantification of pain from experimental dilation of the cervix, Bajaj et al.[19] compared pain descriptors in women in labor, those with experimental cervical dilation, those undergoing spontaneous abortion, and those with dysmenorrhea (Table 20-1). Women with dysmenorrhea used words that indicate suffering, such as "punishing" and "wretched," whereas those in labor did not. Some researchers have drawn parallels between the pain derived from mountain climbing, which is associated with a sense of euphoria, and the pain of labor.[18] As noted by one woman, "You mature and become a stronger personality when you've had a baby and have gone through the pain. I think that is the purpose of it, what the meaning of life is ... to protect our children, to be stronger."[20] However, other women have found no deeper meaning to the pain of labor or reasons why it should not be treated. Many conditions that involve pain (e.g., trauma, severe dental disease, cancer) are considered a "normal" part of human life without a spiritual meaning, thereby making labor pain unique.

In summary, there are large interindividual differences in how women experience the personal significance or meaning of labor pain. These different perceptions can lead to a long-term sense of failure and guilt when pharmacologic pain relief is provided or emotional trauma when it is withheld.

ANATOMIC BASIS

First Stage of Labor

Several lines of evidence suggest that the pain experienced during the first stage of labor is transduced by afferents with peripheral terminals in the cervix and lower uterine segment rather than the uterine body, as is often depicted (Figure 20-4). Uterine body afferents fire in response to distention, but in the absence of inflammation, uterine body distention has no or minimal effect on the behavior of laboratory animals.[21,22] These observations suggest that uterine body afferents may be an important site of chronic inflammatory disease and chronic pelvic pain but are much less relevant to acute obstetric and uterine cervical pain. In addition, afferents to the uterine body regress during normal pregnancy, whereas those to the cervix and lower uterine segment do not.[23] This denervation of the myometrium may protect against preterm labor by limiting alpha$_1$-adrenergic receptor stimulation by locally released norepinephrine. Javert and Hardy[9] reproduced the pain of uterine contractions in women during labor by manual

TABLE 20-1 Word Descriptors from the McGill Pain Questionnaire Used to Describe Pain from the Uterus and Cervix

Pain Descriptors	Type/Source of Pain: Balloon Distention of the Cervix*	Labor†	Abortion‡	Dysmenorrhea*
Sensory	Shooting, boring, sharp, hot, dull, taut	Throbbing, shooting, sharp, cramping, aching, taut	Cutting, cramping, tugging, pulling, aching	Pulsing, beating, shooting, pricking, boring, drilling, sharp, cutting, pinching, pressing, cramping, tugging, pulling, hot, stinging, dull, hurting, heavy, taut
Affective	—	Exhausting, tiring, frightening, grueling	Tiring	Tiring, sickening, punishing, wretched
Evaluative	Annoying	—	Intense	Annoying, intense
Miscellaneous	Drawing, squeezing	Tearing	Numb, squeezing	Piercing, drawing, squeezing, nagging

*Data from Bajaj P, Drewes AM, Gregersen H, et al. Controlled dilatation of the uterine cervix: An experimental visceral pain model. Pain 2002; 99:433-42.

†Data from Niven C, Gijsbers K. A study of labour pain using the McGill Pain Questionnaire. Soc Sci Med 1984; 19:1347-51.

‡Data from Wells N. Pain and distress during abortion. Health Care Women Int 1991; 12:293-302.

distention of the cervix. Bonica and Chadwick[24] later confirmed that women undergoing cesarean delivery under a local anesthetic field block experience pain from cervical distention (which mimics that of labor pain) but do not experience pain from uterine distention.[24]

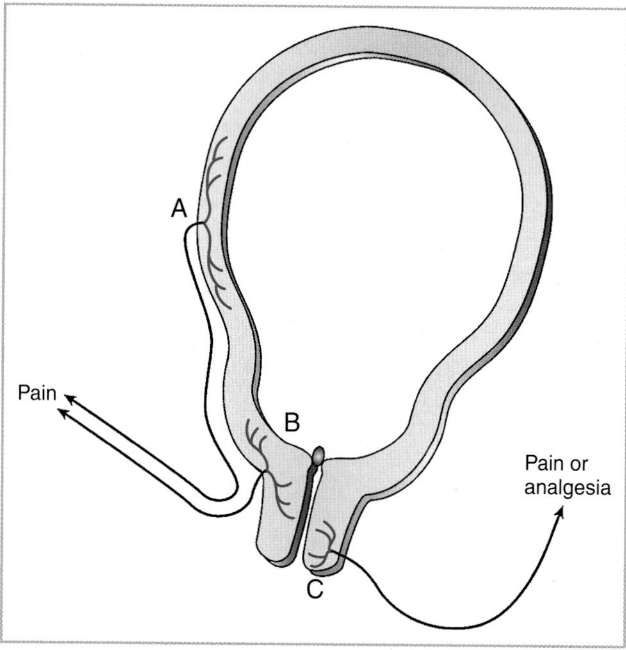

FIGURE 20-4 Uterocervical afferents activated during the first stage of labor. Uterine body afferents (A) partially regress during pregnancy and may contribute to the pain of the first stage of labor. However, the major input is from afferents in the lower uterine segment and endocervix (B). By contrast, at least in animals, the activation of afferents that innervate the vaginal surface of the cervix (C) result in analgesia, not pain, and they enter the spinal cord in sacral areas rather than at the site of referred pain in labor.

The uterine cervix has a dual innervation; afferents innervating the endocervix and lower uterine segment have cell bodies in thoracolumbar dorsal root ganglia (DRG), whereas afferents innervating the vaginal surface of the cervix and upper vagina have cell bodies in sacral DRG.[25] These two innervations result in different sensory input and referral of pain. Pelvic afferents that innervate the vaginal surface of the cervix are almost exclusively C fibers, with the majority containing the peptides substance P and calcitonin gene–related peptide (CGRP). These afferents express alpha and beta estrogen receptors and have an innervation pattern that is not affected by pregnancy.[26-28] Stimulation of the vaginal surface of the cervix in rats results in antinociception, lordosis, ovulation, and a hormonal state of pseudopregnancy, all of which are related to mating behaviors in this species.[29] In rats, these vaginal afferent terminals are activated only during delivery and not during labor, which suggests that they are not relevant to the pain of the first stage of labor.[30] By contrast, dilation of the endocervix in rats results in the activation of afferents entering the lower thoracic spinal cord and nociception rather than antinociception. These afferents, which are mostly or exclusively C fibers,[31] are activated during the first stage of labor, suggesting that they are relevant to pain during this period.

More than 75 years ago, experiments in dogs allowed Cleland[32] to identify T11 to T12 as the segmental level of entry into the spinal cord of afferents that transmit the pain of the first stage of labor. Because dysmenorrhea could be treated through the destruction of the superior or inferior hypogastric plexus,[33] Cleland reasoned that the sensory afferents and sympathetic efferents were likely intermingled; he subsequently demonstrated that the bilateral blockade of the lumbar paravertebral sympathetic chain could produce analgesia during the first stage of labor.[32] First-stage labor pain is transmitted by afferents that have cell bodies in T10 to L1 DRG and pass through the paracervical region, the hypogastric nerve and plexus, and the lumbar sympathetic chain (Figure 20-5).

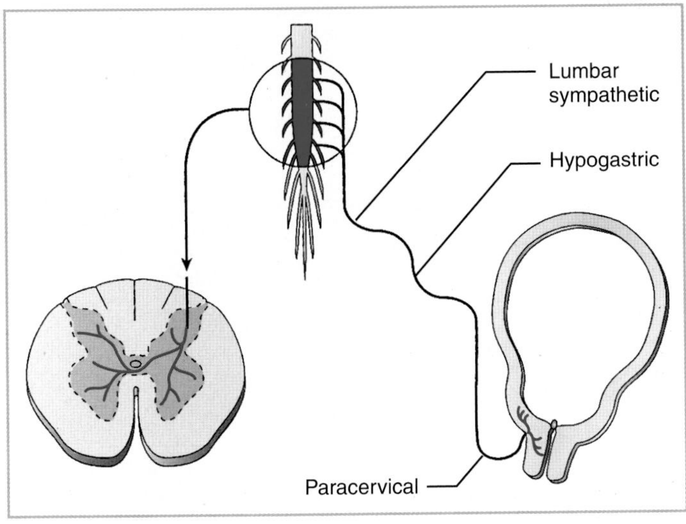

FIGURE 20-5 Pathways of the first stage of labor. Uterocervical afferents pass through the paracervical ganglion, the hypogastric nerve, and the lumbar sympathetic chain, entering the spinal cord in the T10 to L1 region. Unlike somatic afferents, these visceral afferents terminate in the deep dorsal horn and the ventral horn of the spinal cord and cross the midline to the contralateral side.

Classical teaching states that pain-transmitting C and A-delta nerve fibers enter the spinal cord through the dorsal roots and terminate in a dense network of synapses in the ipsilateral superficial laminae (I and II) of the dorsal horn, with minimal rostrocaudal extension of fibers. Whereas this characterization is true for somatic afferents, visceral C fiber afferents enter the cord primarily—but not exclusively—through the dorsal roots and terminate in a loose network of synapses in the superficial and deep dorsal horn and the ventral horn. These afferents also cross to the contralateral dorsal horn, with extensive rostrocaudal extension of fibers (see Figure 20-5). This anatomic distinction underlies the precise localization of somatic pain and the diffuse localization of visceral pain, which may cross the midline; it may also determine the potency or efficacy of drugs that must reach afferent terminals, such as intrathecal opioids. For example, the intrathecal doses of lipophilic agents, such as fentanyl and sufentanil, required to treat postcesarean (somatic) pain and labor (visceral) pain are similar, perhaps because these drugs can extensively penetrate the lipid-rich environment of the spinal cord. By contrast, a much larger intrathecal dose of a hydrophilic agent, such as morphine, is required to treat labor (visceral) pain than postcesarean (somatic) pain.

Pain-transmitting neurons in the spinal cord dorsal horn send axons to the contralateral ventral spinothalamic tract (stimulating thalamic neurons) with further projections to the somatosensory cortex, where pain is perceived. These spinal neurons also send axons through the spinoreticular and spinomesencephalic tracts to provide signals to the areas of vigilance (locus coeruleus, reticular formation), cardiorespiratory regulation (nucleus tractus solitarius, caudal medulla), and reflex descending inhibition (periaqueductal gray, locus coeruleus and subcoeruleus, nucleus raphe magnus, rostral medial medulla, cerebellum). Thalamic activation from painful stimuli results in the activation not only of the somatosensory cortex but also of areas of memory (prefrontal cortex), motor response (M1 motor cortex), and emotional response (insular cortex, anterior cingulate cortex) (Figure 20-6).

Brain imaging studies have yet to be performed in women in labor and in those undergoing experimental or therapeutic uterine cervical distention. Studies of patients undergoing esophageal distention suggest that visceral stimulation activates areas in the brain that are similar—but not identical—to those in patients undergoing somatic stimulation.[34] When stimuli are matched for levels of intensity, visceral stimulation is perceived to be more unpleasant than somatic stimulation. The region of the anterior cingulate cortex activated during visceral stimulation is more rostral than that activated during somatic stimulation and is immediately adjacent to a region activated by fear and distress.[34]

The anatomic basis for pain of the first stage of labor implies that amelioration of pain should occur after blockade of peripheral afferents (by paracervical, paravertebral sympathetic nerve, or epidural [T10 to L1 dermatome] block) or after blockade of spinal cord transmission (by intrathecal injection of a local anesthetic and/or opioid). In addition, the widespread distribution of visceral synapses in the spinal cord implies that intrathecally administered drugs (e.g., opioids) must have physicochemical properties that facilitate deep penetration into the cord to reach the terminals responsible for pain transmission.

Second Stage of Labor

Pain during the second stage of labor is transmitted by the same afferents activated during the first stage of labor but with additional afferents that innervate the cervix (vaginal surface), vagina, and perineum. These additional afferents course through the pudendal nerve DRG at S2 to S4, and are somatic in nature. Thus, the pain specific to the second stage of labor is precisely localized to the vagina and perineum and reflects distention, ischemia, and frank injury, either by stretching to the point of disruption or by surgical incision. Studies in animals have demonstrated that mechanical stimulation of the vaginal surface of the cervix and behaviors related to mating and ovulation result in an antinociceptive effect. Studies in nonpregnant women also indicate a minor analgesic effect of mechanical self-stimulation of the vaginal surface of the cervix[35]; this effect may result from the stimulation of C fibers, because in women with a high oral intake of capsaicin, the activity of such fibers is reduced.[36] The relevance of this minor effect

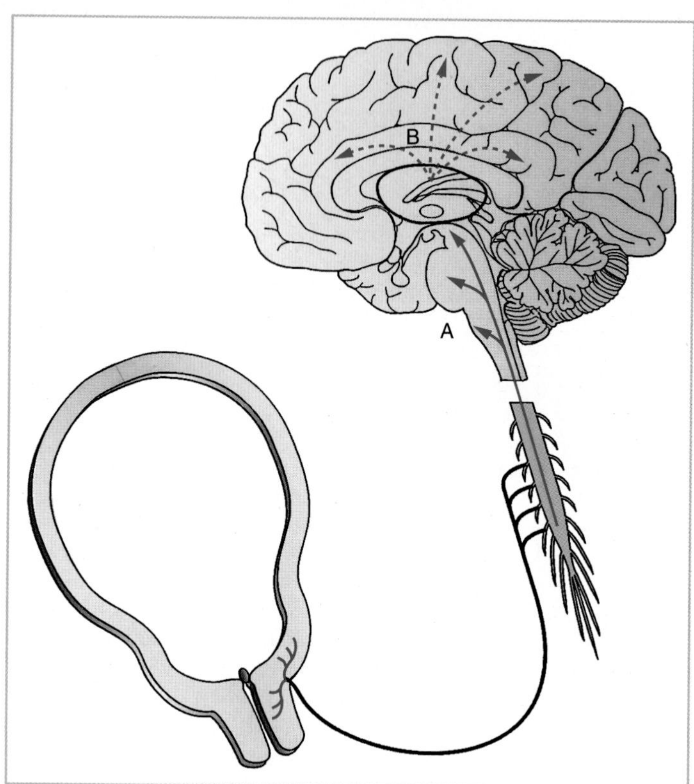

FIGURE 20-6 Supraspinal pain pathways activated by the pain of the first stage of labor. Ascending pathways project to the pons and the medulla (A), thereby activating centers of cardiorespiratory control and descending pathways as well as the thalamus (B), which in turn sends projections to anterior cingulate, motor, somatosensory, and limbic regions (*dotted lines*).

in reducing the pain of the second stage of labor is questionable and has not been examined; however, it does appear to provide evidence that noxious input during labor may activate endogenous analgesia (see later).

The anatomic basis for pain of the second stage of labor implies that analgesia can be obtained through a combination of methods used to treat the pain of the first stage with a pudendal nerve block or extension of the epidural blockade from T10 to S4.

NEUROPHYSIOLOGIC BASIS

Peripheral Afferent Terminals

Visceral nociceptors, such as those that transduce the pain of the first stage of labor, are activated by stretching and distention but, unlike somatic afferents, are not activated by cutting. With each uterine contraction, pressure is transmitted to distort and stretch the uterine cervix, thereby leading to the activation of these nerve terminals. How mechanical distention results in the depolarization of the nerve terminal and the generation of an action potential is not entirely known, but the following three mechanisms are likely:

1. A variety of ion channels respond to the distortion of the cell membrane, and one of them—brain sodium channel-1 (BNC-1) or acid-sensing ion channel-2 (ASIC-2)—is exclusively expressed in sensory afferents and might directly depolarize the nerve terminal by opening its channel when the membrane is distorted (Figure 20-7).[37]
2. Mechanical distortion may result in the acute release of a short-acting neurotransmitter that directly but transiently stimulates ion channel receptors on nerve terminals. Although this process has not yet been examined in the uterine cervix, studies have observed that stretching the bladder urothelium releases adenosine triphosphate, which directly stimulates a type of ligand-gated ion channel—P2X3—on sensory afferents in the bladder wall.[38] Because P2X3 receptors are widely expressed in C fibers,[39] this mechanism might be responsible for the pain that results from the acute distention of the uterine cervix.
3. Local ischemia during contractions may result in gated or spontaneous activity of other ion channels. Some of these ion channels—the ASIC family—respond directly to the low pH that occurs during ischemia,[40] whereas other classes of ion channels may be activated to open spontaneously. For example, the vanilloid receptor type 1 (VR-1) can be stimulated by capsaicin, the active ingredient in hot chili peppers. It is likely that VR-1 receptors (which also respond to noxious heat) are expressed on visceral afferent terminals, given that the application of

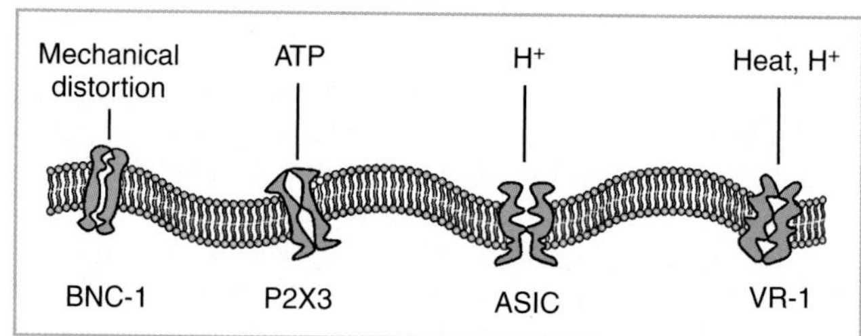

FIGURE 20-7 Afferent nerve endings contain multiple excitatory ligand-gated ion channels, including those that respond to mechanical distortion: BNC-1, brain sodium channel-1; ATP, adenosine triphosphate; P2X3, purinergic receptor; H^+, hydrogen ion; ASIC, acid-sensing ion channel; VR-1, vanilloid receptor type 1.

capsaicin or heat to the distal esophagus in humans results in pain.[41] VR-1 receptor–gated ion channels are not normally open in the absence of high temperature or capsaicin-like ligands; however, in the presence of low pH, the temperature response of these receptors shifts so that their channels open at body temperature.[42]

Uterine cervical afferents (including the C fibers that innervate the vaginal surface of the cervix) contain substance P, CGRP, and the enzyme nitric oxide synthase.[43] C fibers can be divided into two groups, (1) those that contain substance P and CGRP and respond to nerve growth factor through actions on tyrosine kinase A receptors and (2) those that contain somatostatin, instead of substance P and CGRP, and respond to glially derived growth factor through actions on a c-ret complex.[44] Some overlap exists between these rough classifications, and further definition of C fiber subtypes will likely occur as more markers and neuropeptides are examined. Other compounds commonly contained in C fiber terminals include glutamate, vasoactive intestinal peptide, and neuropeptide Y. The variable role of C fiber subtypes in the transmission of pain is also unclear. Given that somatostatin typically inhibits substance P release and pain transmission,[45,46] the net transmission of nociception at the spinal cord level may reflect a complex interaction between excitatory and inhibitory C fiber subtypes.

The peripheral afferent neurophysiology of pain during the first stage of labor suggests that the multiple ion channels that transduce the mechanical signal of cervical stretching to an electrical signal that generates the perception of pain, which are largely unexplored, may represent important new targets for local or systemic analgesic drug delivery. In addition, the understanding of the classification, function, and relevance to pain of different C fiber subtypes remains in its infancy. Research involving endocervical C fiber subtypes may identify new targets for the treatment of labor pain.

ROLE OF SENSITIZATION

Peripheral afferent terminals, like other parts of the sensory system, can change their properties in response to various conditions. Afferent terminals can be directly stimulated by the low pH associated with inflammation (Figure 20-8), and selective ligand-gated ion channels on these terminals can be stimulated by the release of bradykinin.[47] In addition, peripheral inflammation sensitizes afferent terminals by changing their properties; this process can result, over a short time, in a change in gene expression by these nerve fibers, thereby leading to a large amplification of pain signaling.

Although peripheral inflammation is most commonly associated with the pain that results from acute postoperative and chronic arthritic conditions, it may also play an essential role in labor pain. The cervical ripening process and labor itself both result from local synthesis and release of a variety of inflammatory products. The clinical implications of these inflammatory pathways include the application of inflammatory mediators (e.g., prostaglandin [PG] E_2) to prepare the cervix for labor induction and the administration of inflammatory mediator inhibitors (e.g., indomethacin) to stop preterm labor.

PGE_2 is an especially important sensitizing agent for uterine cervical afferents. In most species, the onset of labor is triggered by a sudden decrease in circulating estrogen concentrations. This decrease removes a tonic block on the expression of cyclooxygenase, leading to an increase in local production of prostaglandins, especially PGE_2.[48] PGE_2 is central to a variety of processes that are activated to allow ripening and dilation of the uterine cervix. During the 24 to 72 hours preceding the onset of labor, collagen in the cervix becomes disorganized owing to the activation of prostaglandin receptors and the activity of inflammatory cytokines (mostly interleukin-1 beta and tumor necrosis factor-α) and matrix metalloproteinases (especially types 2 and 9).[49,50] A series of studies in the rat paw have demonstrated that PGE_2 induces peripheral sensitization in a sex-independent manner by activation of protein kinase A[51] and nitric oxide synthase.[52]

Cytokines and growth factors are also released into the uterine cervix immediately before and during labor. The cytokine interleukin-1 beta enhances cyclooxygenase activity and substance P release in the DRG and

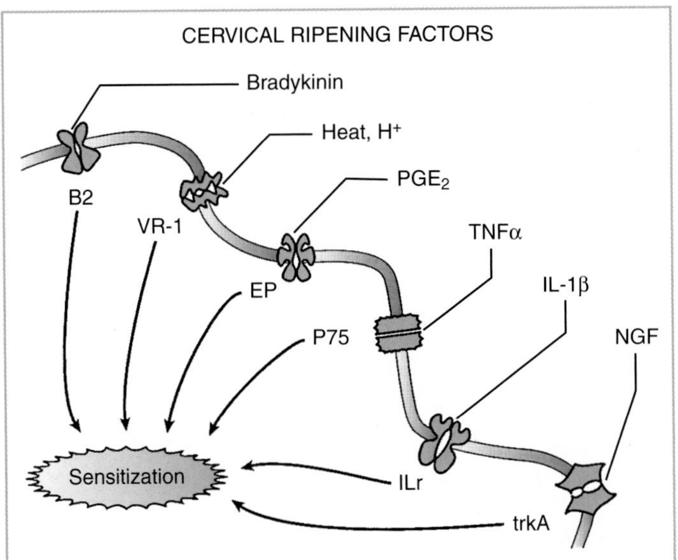

FIGURE 20-8 Effects of inflammation from cervical ripening on afferent terminals. A variety of factors—including bradykinin, heat and hydrogen ions, prostaglandins (including PGE_2), tumor necrosis factor-α (TNFα), interleukin-1 beta (IL-1β), and nerve growth factor (NGF)—act on their cognate receptors to sensitize nerve endings and amplify the perception and severity of pain from nerve stimulation. B_2, bradykinin-2 receptor; EP, prostaglandin E receptor; ILr, interleukin-1 receptor; p75, p75 TNFα receptor; trkA, tyrosine kinase A; VR-1, vanilloid receptor type 1.

spinal cord.[53,54] Tumor necrosis factor-α increases the spontaneous activity of afferent fibers[55] and enhances CGRP release and VR-1 receptor expression in DRG cells in culture.[56] Nerve growth factor also induces mechanical hypersensitivity.[57] These sensitizing substances (prostaglandins, cytokines, and growth factors) signal peripheral nerves in a manner that results in a host of changes in DRG cell number, peptide expression and release, receptor and ion channel expression, and biophysical properties. For example, inflammatory mediators alter the expression of sodium (Na^+) channel subtypes,[58,59] thereby resulting in more rapid, repetitive firing capability[60] and spontaneous afferent activity.[61]

Estrogen receptor signaling can dramatically affect the structure of the uterine cervix and possibly modulate pain responses. Long-term estrogen exposure sensitizes a subset of mechanosensitive afferents innervating the uterine cervix. The hypogastric afferents that innervate the uterine cervix are polymodal in nature and contain high-threshold (HT) and low-threshold (LT) fibers. Long-term estrogen exposure increases the spontaneous activities of both high- and low-threshold fibers, but only high-threshold fibers show greater responses to uterine cervical distention.[62] Long-term estrogen exposure also increases the proportion of hypogastric afferents innervating the uterine cervix, which express transient receptor potential vanilloid type 1 (TRPV-1). Capsaizepine, a TRPV-1 channel antagonist, reduces the hypogastric afferent responses to cervical distention in estrogen-treated animals, but not in ovariectomized animals without estrogen replacement.[63,64] These data suggest that the TRPV-1 receptor is important for estrogen-induced sensitization and amplification of pain responses to uterine cervical distention and that it may therefore represent a potential new target for preventing or treating such enhanced pain.

Implications of the peripheral sensitization of cervical afferents during labor are as follows:

1. Braxton-Hicks contractions, prior to the onset of this inflammatory process, may be as powerful as labor contractions but are painless.
2. Pain may increase with the progress of labor as a result of sensitization.
3. Inflammatory mediators may provide new targets to treat labor pain.

INHIBITORY RECEPTORS

Given the multiplicity of direct excitatory and sensitizing mechanisms on peripheral terminals, more plausible targets for peripheral pain treatment are the endogenous inhibitory receptors expressed on the afferent terminals (Figure 20-9). Opioid receptors have achieved the widest attention. Although μ-opioid receptors are expressed in some afferents in the setting of inflammation,[65] the efficacy of morphine provided by local instillation has proved disappointing[66] with the exception of an intra-articular injection.[67] Similarly, μ-opioid receptor agonists produce antinociception to uterine cervical distention through actions in the central nervous system but not in the periphery.[68]

κ-Opioid receptor agonists may effectively treat visceral pain owing to the presence of these receptors in visceral, but not somatic afferents, at least in the gastrointestinal tract.[69] κ-Opioid receptor agonists can also produce antinociception in response to uterine cervical distention through actions in the peripheral nervous system.[31,68] Pharmaceutical firms are developing drugs of this class that are restricted to the periphery, have few central side effects,[70,71] and presumably express little potential for placental transfer; potentially, such agents would be useful for labor analgesia. One of these new agents has been observed to effectively treat chronic visceral pain from pancreatitis in patients receiving poor analgesia from μ-opioid receptor agonists.[72]

Estrogen and progesterone can alter the analgesic response to opioids. In most cases involving somatic stimulation, tonic estrogen treatment reduces the efficacy of μ-opioid but not κ-opioid receptor agonists.[73] Further, κ-opioid receptor agonists have greater analgesic efficacy in women than in men.[74] In animals, tonic estrogen exposure reduces the inhibitory responses to uterine cervical distention by morphine but not to the κ-opioid receptor

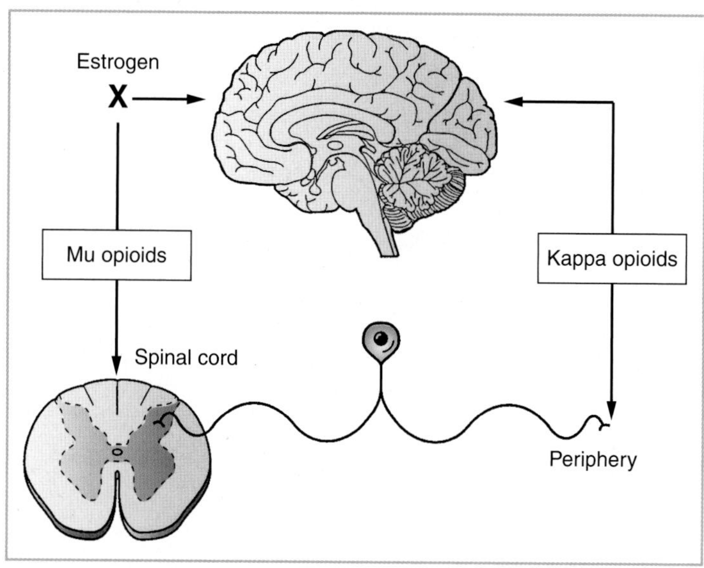

FIGURE 20-9 κ-Opioid receptor agonists act primarily at visceral afferent terminals in the periphery and in the supraspinal central nervous system to provide analgesia during the first stage of labor, whereas μ-opioid receptor agonists act in the spinal cord and the supraspinal central nervous system. Estrogens block the effect of μ-opioid receptor agonists at supraspinal sites.

agonist U-50488.[75] In contrast, the inhibitory action of *intrathecal* morphine against responses to uterine cervical distention is unaffected by tonic estrogen exposure,[76] which is consistent with the observation that intrathecal opioids relieve the pain of the first, but not second, stage of labor.

Implications of inhibitory receptors on afferent terminals are that κ- but not μ-opioid receptor agonists may produce pain relief through their actions in the periphery. Selective, peripherally restricted drugs are under development for the systemic treatment of visceral pain. In addition, estrogen-dependent inhibition of the supraspinal (but not the spinal) analgesic action of μ-opioid receptor agonists may underlie the limited analgesic effect produced by systemic opioids,[77] a finding that is in contrast to the efficacy of intrathecal opioids[78] in relieving the pain of the first stage of labor.

Peripheral Nerve Axons

The current approach to labor analgesia relies primarily on an understanding of the afferent axons and their level of entry into the spinal cord and on the administration of local anesthetics to block afferent traffic conduction. Traditionally axons have been considered conduits that allow for the propagation of action potentials by the transitory opening of Na^+ channels. More recent investigations have confirmed the existence of a variety of Na^+ channel subtypes and axons that modulate transmission through other ion channels.

Although a number of voltage-gated Na^+ channel subtypes exist, most studies have focused on three specific subtypes that are expressed in sensory afferents.[79] Two of these, NaV1.8 and NaV1.9, are relatively resistant to blockade by tetrodotoxin (TTX-R); NaV1.9 is often referred to as "persistent" owing to its very slow inactivation kinetics.[80] Inflammation and injury to nerves decrease the TTX-R current density in afferent cell bodies.[81] Some investigators have suggested that NaV1.8 is selectively trafficked to the periphery after injury and inflammation[81] and that a reduction of its expression reduces hypersensitivity.[82] Other investigators, using sucrose gap measurements of compound action potential, have demonstrated a shortened refractory period and a decrease in delayed depolarization after nerve injury[83,84] that are consistent with the greater expression of rapidly repriming tetrodotoxin-sensitive (TTX-S) channels and the decreased expression of kinetically slow TTX-R channels. To date, these studies have focused primarily on peripheral nerve injury models of chronic pain, and neither the subtypes nor their change during the cervical inflammation of labor have been studied.

Several pharmaceutical firms have discovery programs to produce Na^+ channel subtype–selective blockers that could improve both the safety and efficacy of the treatment of labor pain, because such agents would not interact with Na^+ channels in the brain, heart, or motor nerve fibers. Some investigators have observed that injection of the antidepressant amitriptyline, an agent known to block the NaV1.8 Na^+ channel, around the peripheral nerves provides a neural blockade twofold to fivefold longer than that provided by injection of long-acting local anesthetics.[85,86] Should studies prove the absence of toxicity, it is conceivable that amitriptyline, or other agents that interact with Na^+ channel subtypes, could be used for single-injection techniques (e.g., a paravertebral block) to produce prolonged labor analgesia.

Interactions within the large number of ion channels expressed on axons can alter neural conduction. An example is the transient refractory period caused by the membrane hyperpolarization that follows a short burst of nerve firing. This phenomenon results from the activation of the Na^+/K^+ exchange pump and dampens high-frequency nerve activity. The Na^+/K^+ exchange pump activity, in turn, can be reduced by a hyperpolarization-induced current termed I_h. Drugs that block the I_h current enhance the hyperpolarization caused by the Na^+/K^+ exchange pump and ultimately serve to reduce nerve traffic[87] and provide prolonged analgesia.[88] A second example is the desensitization of VR-1 receptors present on the axons of C fibers. The perineural injection of drugs that desensitize these receptors without first stimulating them avoids the induction of receptor-mediated acute pain, and instead produces very long periods of selective sensory analgesia without motor effects.[89] The mechanism by which VR-1 receptor desensitization alters the transmission of action potentials is under investigation.

Implications of the neurophysiology of axonal transmission of labor pain are that Na^+ channel subtype-selective agents—or those that affect other ion channels expressed on axons—may provide safer and more selective tools for regional analgesic techniques.

Spinal Cord

When action potentials invade the central terminals of C and A-delta fiber afferents in the spinal cord, voltage-gated calcium channels open and cause intracellular calcium concentrations to increase; this increase triggers a multistep process of neurotransmitter docking and fusion with the plasma membrane, which results in neurotransmitter release.[90] Inhibition of these calcium channels produces analgesia. Studies in animals suggest that at least one agent that affects the calcium channels, gabapentin, produces antinociception to visceral stimulation.[91]

A nociceptive stimulus can result in the release of multiple excitatory neurotransmitters, including amino acids (glutamate, aspartate) and peptides (especially substance P, CGRP, and neurokinin A) that interact with specific receptors on spinal cord neurons. Although the stimulation of neurokinin receptors is necessary for the perception of moderate to severe pain,[92] a complex and poorly understood interplay exists among these released neurotransmitters. For example, the response of a postsynaptic receptor to one neurotransmitter can modulate the response of a different receptor. The release of neurotransmitters from the afferent terminals may also be modulated by the firing frequency; as a consequence, factors that influence the firing frequency (e.g., the I_h current) can have a profound effect on the net stimulation observed in the spinal cord.

Neurotransmitter release at sensory afferent terminals is controlled by presynaptic receptors that act primarily by altering the flux of intracellular calcium when an action potential arrives. Some of these neurotransmitters are excitatory; for example, the action of acetylcholine on nicotinic acetylcholine receptors amplifies further neurotransmitter release.[93] Gamma-aminobutyric acid (GABA) is the key endogenous inhibitory neurotransmitter in the nervous system, and stimulation of GABA receptors significantly reduces the afferent terminal release of other neurotransmitters.[94] Multiple compounds produce analgesia by enhancing the release of GABA at afferent terminals in the spinal cord. The existence of excitatory and inhibitory systems can make the response to a neurotransmitter or an exogenously administered agent (such as a local anesthetic drug given intrathecally) difficult to predict. For example, acetylcholine can enhance or reduce the afferent terminal release of neurotransmitters by actions on nicotinic and muscarinic receptors, respectively.[95,96] The net effect of acetylcholine appears to be inhibitory, which is indicated by the analgesic effect of the cholinesterase inhibitor neostigmine administered intrathecally.[97]

The primary mechanism of action of the neurotransmitter enkephalin, which is released by spinal cord interneurons, and of norepinephrine, which is released by axons descending from pontine centers, is the inhibition of neurotransmitter release from primary afferent terminals. These substances act on μ-opioid and $alpha_2$-adrenergic receptors, respectively,[98,99] and may be responsible for some of the effects observed after the intrathecal administration of opioids and $alpha_2$-adrenergic agonists for the treatment of labor pain.

Amino acids and peptides released from sensory afferents stimulate a heterogeneous group of spinal cord neurons, including neurons that project to supraspinal structures, interneurons that modulate transmission at the afferent terminal itself (the "gate" of the control theory), and interneurons that stimulate motor and sympathetic nervous system reflexes. Large and sustained glutamate release from an intensely noxious stimulus can activate *N*-methyl-D-aspartate (NMDA) receptors, resulting in sustained depolarization and enhanced excitability of projection neurons (Figure 20-10).[100] Although the intrathecal injection of NMDA receptor antagonists (e.g., ketamine) has been restricted because of neurotoxicity concerns,[101] systemic infusion of magnesium sulfate has been observed to produce postoperative analgesia.[102] Magnesium is an endogenous inhibitory modulator of NMDA receptors, and it is conceivable that magnesium sulfate administered systemically for obstetric indications may have a minor effect on labor pain.

Prolonged and intense nociceptive stimuli can produce sensitization and amplification of pain signaling at the spinal cord level like the peripheral sensitization that occurs as a result of inflammation. Some of these processes are a direct consequence of receptors (e.g., NMDA receptors) that are activated only with highly intense and prolonged stimulation or by the long-term release of neurotranmitters that simultaneously activate the glutamate and substance P receptors on the same cell. Others reflect the synthesis and release of classic "inflammatory" substances by the spinal cord glial cells in response to prolonged afferent stimulation from nitric oxide and prostaglandins, especially PGE_2. Some nonsteroidal anti-inflammatory drugs (NSAIDs) produce analgesia by actions exclusively (e.g., acetaminophen) or primarily (e.g., aspirin) in the central nervous system (especially the spinal cord).[103]

Spinal sensitization processes represent a novel target for the treatment of labor pain. Over 75 years ago, Cleland[32] noted the presence of hypersensitivity to light touch on the skin of dermatomes T11 and T12 in laboring women, which likely represents the enhanced sensitivity of spinal cord neurons receiving both visceral input from the cervix and skin input at those levels.[104] When the visceral stimulation to these dermatomes was blocked by a paravertebral local anesthetic injection, Cleland[32] observed that the hypersensitivity was ablated; this observation is consistent with the later finding that ongoing C fiber input is required for hypersensitivity to occur.[105] Uterine cervical distention (UCD) results in a pattern of spinal cord neuronal activation similar to that witnessed during labor and delivery. In a study in rats reported by Tong et al.,[106] UCD significantly increased cFos immunoreactivity in the spinal cord from T12 to L2, with most of the cFos expression occurring in the deep dorsal horn and central canal regions. UCD-evoked cFos expression was prevented by prior infiltration of lidocaine into the cervix or by intrathecal administration of ketorolac (a cyclooxygenase [COX] inhibitor) in a dose-dependent manner.[106] Intrathecal administration of indomethacin (a nonspecific COX inhibitor) and the selective COX-2 inhibitor SC-58238 effectively ablated UCD-induced electromyographic activity without altering the hemodynamic response to UCD; by contrast, the selective COX-1 inhibitor SC-58360 was ineffective in ablating UCD-induced electromyographic activity, as was

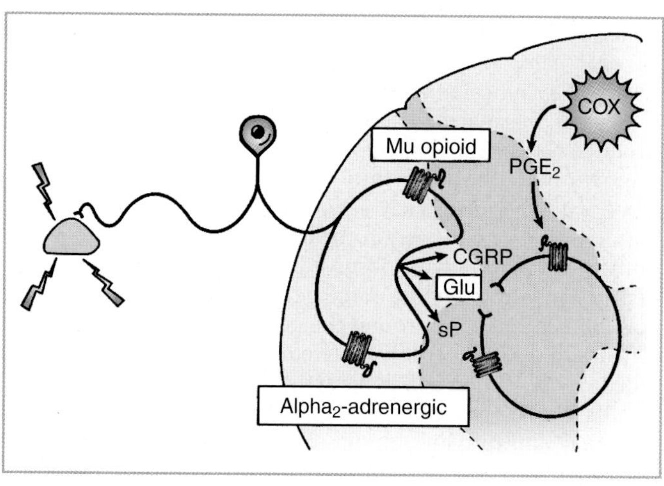

FIGURE 20-10 Pain transmission in the spinal cord. Excitatory transmission occurs directly by release of amino acids such as glutamate (Glu) and peptides (sP [substance P], CGRP [calcitonin gene–related peptide]) and indirectly via activation of enzymes such as cyclooxygenase (COX) in nearby glia, which synthesize prostaglandins, including prostaglandin E_2 (PGE_2). Inhibitory mechanisms are primarily presynaptic, μ-opioid and $alpha_2$-adrenergic receptors being the most common (or at least the most studied).

ketorolac, an agent with higher affinity for COX-1 than COX-2.[107] Together, these data suggest that targeting COX-2 is necessary to treat the acute visceral pain often associated with brief infrequent contractions in late pregnancy; therefore, intrathecal ketorolac would be predicted to be ineffective. However, in the setting of sustained, frequent, and repetitive contractions for a prolonged period (as occurs during active labor), intrathecal ketorolac might be effective. The intrathecal injection of ketorolac has been introduced into experimental human trials[108] and warrants examination as a potential modality for selective treatment of labor pain.

The neurophysiologic basis for labor pain in the spinal cord implies that purely inhibitory mechanisms (e.g., opioid and alpha$_2$-adrenergic receptors) can be mimicked by the intrathecal injection of agonists to these receptors; however, the administration of other agents (e.g., acetylcholine) in this location has less predictable results. Central sensitization mechanisms in the spinal cord most certainly occur during labor, and future treatments may target these mechanisms.

Ascending Projections

Spinal cord neurons project to multiple brainstem sites as well as the thalamus. More than 30 years ago, it was noted that descending systems—activated primarily by stimulation of the nucleus raphe magnus, the periaqueductal gray, and the locus coeruleus—could reduce pain transmission as described in the gate control theory.[109] Activation of descending pathways results in the spinal release of endogenous ligands for serotonergic, opioid, and alpha$_2$-adrenergic receptor–mediated analgesia. Spillover of neurotransmitters into the cerebrospinal fluid has been used as a measure of activation of these systems, and studies measuring these substances have shown no increase in enkephalin, but an increase in norepinephrine, in laboring women.[110] These descending systems can be activated by psychoprophylactic methods,[111] and agents that prolong or intensify the action of these ligands, such as enkephalinase inhibitors and blockers of monoamine reuptake, might further enhance analgesia.[112]

Brainstem activation by the pain of labor leads to other reflexes, such as increases in sympathetic nervous system activity and respiratory drive and, with prolonged activation, stimulation of descending pathways that amplify rather than reduce pain transmission at the spinal cord.[113,114] The circuitry and pharmacology of such pain-enhancing systems in the brainstem and their potential applications for treatment are under current investigation.

Our understanding of the areas of the brain activated during labor pain is limited, although studies of other types of experimental nociception in healthy volunteers indicate that visceral pain is considered more unpleasant than somatic pain; this difference reflects, in part, the greater activation of centers for negative emotions, including fear.[34] The perception of pain is greatly modulated in the brain; in normal volunteers, a simple noxious heat stimulus has been demonstrated to evoke a similar degree of thalamic activation in all subjects (i.e., the pain-signaling system from the periphery to the thalamus is similar), but greatly differing degrees of cortical activation.[15] The degree of cortical activation directly correlates with verbal assessments of pain intensity.[15] Although distraction methods do not alter the thalamic activation from noxious stimulation, a reduction in cortical activation and the report of pain have been observed,[115] supporting a suprathalamic mechanism of psychoprophylaxis in the reduction of pain.

The neurophysiologic basis of labor pain and ascending projections suggests the activation of multiple supraspinal sites. Some of these sites stimulate potentially detrimental cardiorespiratory reflexes. Other sites, which send descending projections that either reduce or enhance pain transmission in the spinal cord, may be targeted for the provision of analgesia. In addition, suprathalamic modulation of pain signals appears to account for the interindividual differences in pain perception and for the relative efficacy of psychoprophylaxis in reducing the intensity of reported pain.

EFFECT ON THE MOTHER

Obstetric Course

Several aspects of labor pain can affect the course of labor and delivery (Figure 20-11). Pain-induced increases in the activity of the sympathetic nervous system lead to higher plasma concentrations of catecholamines, especially epinephrine. The provision of labor analgesia reduces plasma concentrations of epinephrine and its associated beta-adrenergic tocolytic effects on the myometrium. This process may underlie the observations by some investigators who have noted, either anecdotally or under controlled conditions, a shift from dysfunctional to normal labor patterns in some women when analgesia is achieved with paravertebral[32,116] or epidural[117] blocks or with systemic meperidine analgesia.[118] The abrupt reduction in plasma epinephrine concentrations that follows the rapid onset of intrathecal opioid analgesia may result in an acute reduction of beta-adrenergic tocolysis and a transient period of uterine hyperstimulation; in some cases, these changes may lead to transient fetal stress and bradycardia.[119]

Ferguson's reflex involves neural input from ascending spinal tracts (especially from sacral sensory input) to the midbrain, thereby leading to enhanced oxytocin release. Although spontaneous labor and delivery occur in women with spinal cord injury (which disrupts this tract[120]), some investigators have argued that neuraxial analgesia can inhibit this reflex and prolong labor, especially the second stage. However, strong evidence for this does not exist. Some studies have noted a reduction in plasma oxytocin concentrations with epidural local anesthetic[121] or intrathecal opioid[122] analgesia, whereas others have not noted such a reduction.[123]

Papka and Shew[23] suggested that afferent terminals in the lower uterine segment and cervix might have an important secretory (efferent) function in the regulation of labor. Afferent terminals contain many substances that can *stimulate* (substance P, glutamate, vasoactive intestinal peptide) or *inhibit* (CGRP, nitric oxide) myometrial activity, and these substances can be released locally into the cervix and lower uterine segment when terminals are depolarized by contraction-related tissue distortion. In addition, depolarization of the afferent terminal can result in an action

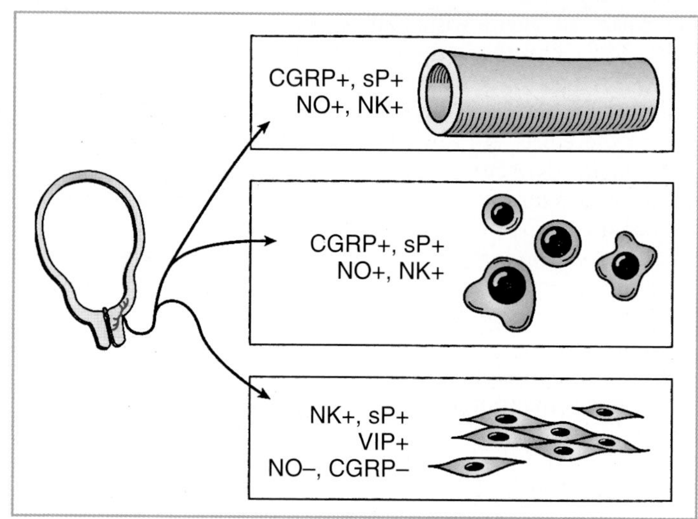

FIGURE 20-11 Aspects of pain that may affect the course of labor. In addition to indirect effects (e.g., beta-adrenergic tocolysis from increased secretion of epinephrine, greater release of oxytocin via Ferguson's reflex), depolarization of afferent terminals in the lower uterine segment and cervix can directly alter aspects of labor. Substances released by nerve terminals include those that increase local blood flow (CGRP [calcitonin gene–related peptide], sP [substance P], NO [nitric oxide], NK [neurokinin]), those that stimulate immune cell function, and those that stimulate (+) or inhibit (–) myometrial smooth muscle activity, including vasoactive intestinal peptide (VIP).

potential that, upon reaching a site of nerve branching, invades adjacent branches and travels distally to depolarize distant terminals of the same nerve. This axon reflex has long been recognized to occur in somatic nerves; owing to the more extensive arborizations believed to exist in visceral nerves, local stimulation should result in more widespread release of these transmitters. Therefore, it is tempting to speculate that these axon reflexes are more profoundly affected when local anesthetic is administered closer to the terminals associated with cervical dilation and labor (e.g., as occurs with paracervical and paravertebral blocks[116]) than occurs when local anesthetic is administered farther away from the terminals (e.g., with epidural block). This speculation would imply that the net effect of afferent terminal–released substances inhibits rather than accelerates labor.

In summary, neural stimulation through pain pathways leads to the release of substances that either increase (oxytocin) or inhibit (epinephrine) uterine activity and cervical dilation; therefore, the effect of analgesia on the course of labor can vary between and within individuals. In addition, axon reflexes can result in the release of neurotransmitters from afferents into the lower uterine segment and cervix; it is hoped that future investigation will determine whether the proximity of local anesthetic deposition affects the response of cervical dilation and labor.

Cardiac and Respiratory Effects

Labor exerts stresses on the cardiovascular and respiratory systems. The elevated plasma catecholamine concentrations observed during labor pain can increase maternal cardiac output and peripheral vascular resistance and decrease uteroplacental perfusion. Even transient stress is associated with dramatic increases in plasma concentrations of norepinephrine and subsequent decreases in uterine blood flow (Figure 20-12). Plasma epinephrine concentrations in women with painful labor are similar to those observed after intravenous administration of a bolus of epinephrine 15 μg[124]; intravenous bolus injection of 10 to 20 μg of epinephrine resulted in a significant (albeit transient) reduction in uterine blood flow in gravid ewes.[125] Effective neuraxial analgesia, provided by epidural local anesthetic[126] or intrathecal opioid administration,[127] significantly reduces (50%) maternal catecholamine concentrations. By contrast, neonatal catecholamine concentrations do not appear to be altered by maternal neuraxial anesthetic techniques; this relative independence of neonatal catecholamine responses may be important for the neonatal adaptation to extrauterine life.[128]

The intermittent pain of uterine contractions also stimulates the respiratory system and leads to periods of intermittent hyperventilation. In the absence of supplemental oxygen administration, compensatory periods of hypoventilation between contractions result in transient

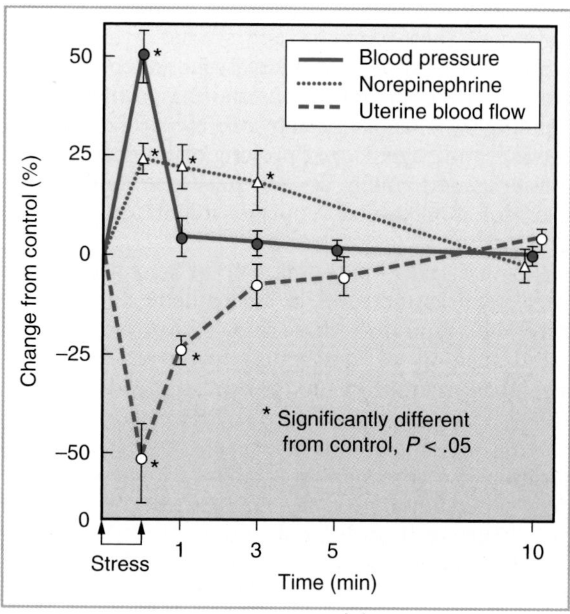

FIGURE 20-12 Effect of a painful stimulus on the hind leg on maternal blood pressure, norepinephrine concentrations, and uterine blood flow in gravid ewes. The increase in blood pressure was transient, but plasma norepinephrine concentrations remained elevated for several minutes; the elevation is reflected in the slow return of uterine blood flow to normal. (From Shnider SM, Wright RG, Levinson G, et al. Uterine blood flow and plasma norepinephrine changes during maternal stress in the pregnant ewe. Anesthesiology 1979; 50:524-7.)

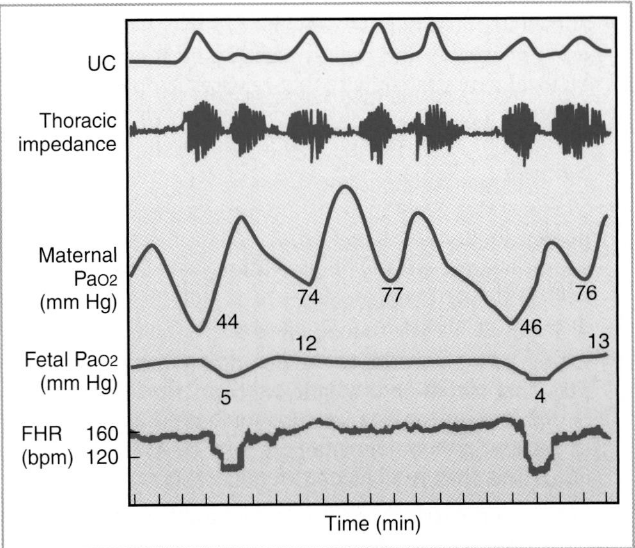

FIGURE 20-13 Maternal and fetal hypoxemia during hypoventilation between uterine contractions (UC), which are associated with maternal hyperventilation. (From Bonica JJ. Labour pain. In Wall PD, Melzack R, editors. Textbook of Pain. Churchill Livingstone, Edinburgh, 1984, as redrawn from Huch A, Huch R, Schneider H, Rooth GL. Continuous transcutaneous monitoring of fetal oxygen tension during labour. Br J Obstet Gynaecol 1977; 84[Suppl]:1-39.)

episodes of maternal, and even fetal, hypoxemia (Figure 20-13). Treatment of labor pain with epidural analgesia minimizes the increase in net minute ventilation and the accompanying rise in oxygen consumption.[129]

In general, the cardiovascular and respiratory system changes induced by labor pain are well tolerated by healthy parturients (with normal uteroplacental perfusion) and their fetuses. Some authors have concluded that these changes are of no concern or relevance in uncomplicated labor[18]; however, when maternal or fetal disease or compromise is observed, significant cardiopulmonary alterations may lead to maternal or fetal decompensation; effective analgesia may be especially important in such cases.

In summary, pain-induced activation of the sympathetic nervous system during labor is associated with cardiovascular and respiratory effects that may alter maternal and fetal well-being. The provision of effective neuraxial analgesia may mitigate many of these cardiopulmonary effects.

Psychological Effects

The meaning of labor pain is greatly influenced by psychosocial and environmental factors (as previously discussed) and varies considerably among women. Although the acceptance of labor analgesia has a minor overall effect on maternal satisfaction with the labor and delivery process,[130] individual women can be profoundly influenced. It has been suggested that women who understand the origin of their pain and view the labor and delivery process as positive and nonthreatening may undergo pain without suffering.[18] A small proportion (< 5%) of women who request and receive epidural labor analgesia describe a sense of deprivation because of missing the natural labor experience in its entirety[131]; some of these women may subsequently seek psychiatric counseling.[132]

By contrast, unrelieved severe labor pain can have psychological and physical consequences, including depression and negative thoughts about sexual relationships.[8,12] In a 5-year study in Sweden, 43 women requested elective cesarean delivery owing to a fear of labor and a vaginal delivery.[133] Some countries (e.g., Brazil) have an extremely high elective cesarean delivery rate (> 80%) among upper-class women because of their concerns about reduced sexual function after vaginal delivery. Frank psychotic reactions resembling post-traumatic stress disorder can occur after childbirth, although the incidence is rare (< 1%).[134]

Psychological effects of labor pain can occur in a small proportion of women. Psychological harm can be experienced through the provision or withholding of labor analgesia, underscoring the tremendous variability in the meaning of labor pain for different women.

Pain after Delivery

The experience and sequelae of childbirth can result in pain after delivery. Investigations into acute and chronic postpartum pain have reported a 7% incidence of perineal pain at 8 weeks after vaginal delivery[135,136]; in addition, a 48% incidence of punctate hyperalgesia at 48 hours and a 23% incidence of residual pain at 6 months have been observed after cesarean delivery.[137] Although there is significant interindividual variability with regard to acute postpartum pain,[138] the severity of acute postoperative pain in nonobstetric surgical patients has been correlated with the occurrence of chronic pain.[139] Whether the presence and severity of acute postpartum pain after either vaginal or cesarean delivery predicts the occurrence of chronic pain is under investigation. Retrospective studies suggest that cesarean delivery, particularly when performed under general anesthesia, is a risk factor for chronic pain.[140,141] Persistent or chronic pain may be particularly difficult for postpartum patients owing to the multiple stresses (e.g., care of the neonate) and sequelae encountered. An association between pain and depression exists, and depression is the most common complication after delivery, affecting approximately 13% of postpartum women.[142] Postpartum patients with depression are among those who frequently do not disclose depression even though they desire assistance.[143,144] Immediate and effective postpartum pain management (after both vaginal and cesarean deliveries) with adequate long-term follow-up may potentially prevent long-term morbidity and improve overall outcomes.

EFFECT ON THE FETUS

Because of the absence of direct neural connections from the mother to the fetus, maternal labor pain has no direct effects on the fetus. However, maternal labor pain can affect a number of systems that determine uteroplacental perfusion, as follows: (1) uterine contraction frequency and intensity, by the effect of pain on the release of oxytocin and epinephrine; (2) uterine artery vasoconstriction, by the effect of pain on the release of norepinephrine and epinephrine; and (3) maternal oxyhemoglobin desaturation, which may result from intermittent hyperventilation followed by hypoventilation, as discussed earlier. Although these effects are well tolerated in normal circumstances and are effectively blocked by analgesia, fetal well-being may be affected in situations of limited uteroplacental reserve.

SUMMARY

Pain during the first stage of labor results from the stimulation of visceral afferents that innervate the lower uterine segment and cervix, intermingle with sympathetic efferents, and enter the spinal cord at the T10 to L1 segments. Pain during the second stage of labor results from the additional stimulation of somatic afferents that innervate the vagina and perineum, travel within the pudendal nerve, and enter the spinal cord at the S2 to S4 segments. These pain signals are processed in the spinal cord and are transmitted to brainstem, midbrain, and thalamic sites, the last with projections to the cortex, resulting in the sensory-emotional experience of pain. Current obstetric anesthesia practice relies nearly exclusively on the blocking of pain transmission by deposition of local anesthetic—with or without adjuncts—along the afferent nerves from sites near the peripheral afferent terminals to sites near their central terminals.

The neurophysiology of visceral pain, especially in relation to labor pain, is currently under investigation, with considerable academic and pharmaceutical targeting of (1) the normal ionic transduction mechanisms and processes of sensitization in peripheral afferent terminals, (2) the mechanisms of inhibition available in the spinal cord and brainstem, and (3) the processes by which conscious distraction methods can be amplified and can relieve pain. Labor pain is an intensely variable and personal experience, and it is essential that the anesthesia provider play a flexible role within this context.

KEY POINTS

- Labor pain exists and is severe in many women, with a close correlation between cervical dilation and pain during the first stage.
- The first stage of labor involves visceral pain from the lower uterine segment and endocervix, which results in hypersensitivity to convergent somatic dermatomes. This pain is most likely amplified over time as a result of the sensitization of peripheral and central pain-signaling pathways. The second stage of labor results in somatic pain from the vagina and perineum and is briefer than the first stage.
- Afferent terminals transduce a mechanical process into electrical signals, which are probably amplified by the release of prostaglandins, cytokines, and growth factors into the cervix as part of the normal disruption of collagen that allows the cervix to soften and dilate.
- Pain transmission in the spinal cord is not hard wired; it is remarkably and rapidly plastic, and it is altered by local neuronal activity that releases μ-opioid receptor agonists and descending pathways that release $alpha_2$-adrenergic and serotonergic receptor agonists.
- There are large individual differences in pain perception, which likely reflect differences at suprathalamic sites. The activation of suprathalamic sites is the primary mechanism of action for distraction methods of analgesia.
- Labor pain alters the obstetric course and the maternal cardiac and respiratory function in a complex manner that normally is well tolerated, that can sometimes be detrimental to both mother and fetus, and that is alleviated by analgesia.
- Labor pain carries meaning in distinction from most other etiologies of severe pain. The treatment of labor pain should be applied within this context.
- Acute postpartum pain following either vaginal or cesarean delivery deserves attention and treatment; the factors or mechanisms responsible for the development of persistent or chronic postpartum pain are currently under investigation.

REFERENCES

1. Melzack R, Wall PD. Pain mechanisms: A new theory. Science 1965; 150:971-5.
2. Melzack R. From the gate to the neuromatrix. Pain 1999; Aug (Suppl 6):S121-6.
3. Simone DA, Baumann TK, LaMotte RH. Dose-dependent pain and mechanical hyperalgesia in humans after intradermal injection of capsaicin. Pain 1989; 38:99-107.
4. Woolf CJ, Max MB. Mechanism-based pain diagnosis: Issues for analgesic drug development. Anesthesiology 2001; 95:241-9.
5. Eisenach JC. The treatment of pain: Remaining challenges and future opportunities. Can J Anaesth 2002; 49:R1-3.
6. Dick-Read GP. Childbirth Without Fear: The Principles and Practice of Natural Childbirth. New York, Harper, 1953.
7. Lamaze F. Qu'est-ce que l'accouchement sans douleur par la méthode psychoprophylactique? Ses principes, sa réalisation, ses résultats. Paris, Savouret Connaitre, 1956.
8. Melzack R. The myth of painless childbirth (The John J. Bonica Lecture). Pain 1984; 19:321-37.
9. Javert CT, Hardy JD. Influence of analgesics on pain intensity during labor (with a note on "natural childbirth"). Anesthesiology 1951; 12:189-215.
10. Hardy JD, Javert CT. Studies on pain: Measurements of pain intensity in childbirth. J Clin Invest 1949; 28:153-62.
11. Algom D, Lubel S. Psychophysics in the field: Perception and memory for labor pain. Percept Psychophys 1994; 55:133-41.
12. Melzack R, Taenzer P, Feldman P, Kinch RA. Labour is still painful after prepared childbirth training. Can Med Assoc J 1981; 125:357-63.
13. Niven CA, Gijsbers KJ. Do low levels of labour pain reflect low sensitivity to noxious stimulation? Soc Sci Med 1989; 29:585-8.
14. Granot M, Lowenstein L, Yarnitsky D, et al. Postcesarean section pain prediction by preoperative experimental pain assessment. Anesthesiology 2003; 98:1422-6.
15. Coghill RC, McHaffie JG, Yen Y-F. Neural correlates of inter-individual differences in the subjective experience of pain. Proc Natl Acad Sci U S A 2003; 100:8538-42.
16. Reid JG, Simpson NA, Walker RG, et al. The carriage of pro-inflammatory cytokine gene polymorphisms in recurrent pregnancy loss. Am J Reprod Immunol 2001; 45:35-40.

17. Merskey H. Pain terms: A list with definitions and a note on usage. Recommended by the International Association for the Study of Pain (IASP) Subcommittee on Taxonomy. Pain 1979; 6:249-52.
18. Lowe NK. The nature of labor pain. Am J Obstet Gynecol 2002; 186:S16-24.
19. Bajaj P, Drewes AM, Gregersen H, et al. Controlled dilatation of the uterine cervix: An experimental visceral pain model. Pain 2002; 99:433-42.
20. Lundgren I, Dahlberg K. Women's experience of pain during childbirth. Midwifery 1998; 14:105-10.
21. Robbins A, Sato Y, Hotta H, Berkley KJ. Responses of hypogastric nerve afferent fibers to uterine distention in estrous or metestrous rats. Neurosci Lett 1990; 110:82-5.
22. Bradshaw HB, Temple JL, Wood E, Berkley KJ. Estrous variations in behavioral responses to vaginal and uterine distention in the rat. Pain 1999; 82:187-97.
23. Papka RE, Shew RL. Neural input to the uterus and influence on uterine contractility. In Garfield RE, Tabb TN, editors. Control of Uterine Contractility. London, CRC Press, Inc., 1993:375-99.
24. Bonica JJ, Chadwick HS. Labour pain. In Wall PD, Melzack R, editors. Textbook of Pain. 2nd edition. New York, Churchill Livingstone, 1989:482-99.
25. Berkley KJ, Robbins A, Sato Y. Functional differences between afferent fibers in the hypogastric and pelvic nerves innervating female reproductive organs in the rat. J Neurophysiol 1993; 69:533-44.
26. Papka RE, Storey-Workley M, Shughrue PJ, et al. Estrogen receptor-α and -β immunoreactivity and mRNA in neurons of sensory and autonomic ganglia and spinal cord. Cell Tissue Res 2001; 304: 193-214.
27. Papka RE, Storey-Workley M. Estrogen receptor-α and -β coexist in a subpopulation of sensory neurons of female rat dorsal root ganglia. Neurosci Lett 2002; 319:71-4.
28. Pokabla MJ, Dickerson IM, Papka RE. Calcitonin gene-related peptide-receptor component protein expression in the uterine cervix, lumbosacral spinal cord, and dorsal root ganglia. Peptides 2002; 23:507-14.
29. Komisaruk BR, Wallman J. Antinociceptive effects of vaginal stimulation in rats: Neurophysiological and behavioral studies. Brain Res 1977; 137:85-107.
30. Papka RE, Hafemeister J, Puder BA, et al. Estrogen receptor-α and neural circuits to the spinal cord during pregnancy. J Neurosci Res 2002; 70:808-16.
31. Sandner-Kiesling A, Pan HL, Chen SR, et al. Effect of kappa opioid agonists on visceral nociception induced by uterine cervical distention in rats. Pain 2002; 96:13-22.
32. Cleland JGP. Paravertebral anaesthesia in obstetrics. Surg Gynecol Obstet 1933; 57:51-62.
33. Cotte G. Sur le traitement des dysmenorrhées rébelles par la sympathectomie hypogastrique périarterielle ou la section du nerf présacre. Lyon Med 1925; LVI:153.
34. Strigo IA, Duncan GH, Boivin M, Bushnell MC. Differentiation of visceral and cutaneous pain in the human brain. J Neurophysiol 2003; 89:3294-303.
35. Whipple B, Komisaruk BR. Elevation of pain threshold by vaginal stimulation in women. Pain 1985; 21:357-67.
36. Whipple B, Martinez-Gomez M, Oliva-Zarate L, et al. Inverse relationship between intensity of vaginal self-stimulation-produced analgesia and level of chronic intake of a dietary source of capsaicin. Physiol Behav 1989; 46:247-52.
37. Lingueglia E, de Weille JR, Bassilana F, et al. A modulatory subunit of acid sensing ion channels in brain and dorsal root ganglion cells. J Biol Chem 1997; 272:29778-83.
38. Cockayne DA, Hamilton SG, Zhu QM, et al. Urinary bladder hyporeflexia and reduced pain-related behaviour in P2X3-deficient mice. Nature 2000; 407:1011-5.
39. Burnstock G. P2X receptors in sensory neurones. Br J Anaesth 2000; 84:476-88.
40. Waldmann R, Champigny G, Lingueglia E, et al. H(+)-gated cation channels. Ann N Y Acad Sci 1999; 868:67-76.
41. Drewes AM, Schipper KP, Dimcevski G, et al. Multimodal assessment of pain in the esophagus: A new experimental model. Am J Physiol Gastrointest Liver Physiol 2002; 283:G95-103.
42. Julius D, Basbaum AI. Molecular mechanisms of nociception. Nature 2001; 413:203-10.
43. Papka RE, McNeill DL, Thompson D, Schmidt HH. Nitric oxide nerves in the uterus are parasympathetic, sensory, and contain neuropeptides. Cell Tissue Res 1995; 279:339-49.
44. Bennett DL, Michael GJ, Ramachandran N, et al. A distinct subgroup of small DRG cells express GDNF receptor components and GDNF is protective for these neurons after nerve injury. J Neurosci 1998; 18:3059-72.
45. Kim SJ, Chung WH, Rhim H, et al. Postsynaptic action mechanism of somatostatin on the membrane excitability in spinal substantia gelatinosa neurons of juvenile rats. Neuroscience 2002; 114:1139-48.
46. Carlton SM, Du JH, Zhou ST, Coggeshall RE. Tonic control of peripheral cutaneous nociceptors by somatostatin receptors. J Neurosci 2001; 21:4042-9.
47. Linhart O, Obreja O, Kress M. The inflammatory mediators serotonin, prostaglandin E_2 and bradykinin evoke calcium influx in rat sensory neurons. Neuroscience 2003; 118:69-74.
48. Sato T, Michizu H, Hashizume K, Ito A. Hormonal regulation of PGE_2 and COX-2 production in rabbit uterine cervical fibroblasts. J Appl Physiol 2001; 90:1227-31.
49. Lyons CA, Beharry KD, Nishihara KC, et al. Regulation of matrix metalloproteinases (type IV collagenases) and their inhibitors in the virgin, timed pregnant, and postpartum rat uterus and cervix by prostaglandin E_2-cyclic adenosine monophosphate. Am J Obstet Gynecol 2002; 187:202-8.
50. Stygar D, Wang H, Vladic VS, et al. Increased level of matrix metalloproteinases 2 and 9 in the ripening process of the human cervix. Biol Reprod 2002; 67:889-94.
51. Aley KO, Levine JD. Role of protein kinase A in the maintenance of inflammatory pain. J Neurosci 1999; 19:2181-6.
52. Aley KO, McCarter G, Levine JD. Nitric oxide signaling in pain and nociceptor sensitization in the rat. J Neurosci 1998; 18: 7008-14.
53. Samad TA, Moore KA, Sapirstein A, et al. Interleukin-1beta-mediated induction of COX-2 in the CNS contributes to inflammatory pain hypersensitivity. Nature 2001; 410:471-5.
54. Inoue A, Ikoma K, Morioka N, et al. Interleukin-1beta induces substance P release from primary afferent neurons through the cyclooxygenase-2 system. J Neurochem 1999; 73:2206-13.
55. Leem J-G, Bove GM. Mid-axonal tumor necrosis factor-alpha induces ectopic activity in a subset of slowly conducting cutaneous and deep afferent neurons. J Pain 2002; 3:45-9.
56. Winston J, Toma H, Shenoy M, Pasricha PJ. Nerve growth factor regulates VR-1 mRNA levels in cultures of adult dorsal root ganglion neurons. Pain 2001; 89:181-6.
57. Rueff A, Dawson AJLR, Mendell LM. Characteristics of nerve growth factor induced hyperalgesia in adult rats: Dependence on enhanced bradykinin-1 receptor activity but not neurokinin-1 receptor activation. Pain 1996; 66:359-72.
58. Waxman SG, Kocsis JD, Black JA. Type III sodium channel mRNA is expressed in embryonic but not adult spinal sensory neurons, and is reexpressed following axotomy. J Neurophysiol 1994; 72:466-70.
59. Kim CH, Oh Y, Chung JM, Chung K. The changes in expression of three subtypes of TTX sensitive sodium channels in sensory neurons after spinal nerve ligation. Mol Brain Res 2001; 95:153-61.
60. Black JA, Cummins TR, Plumpton C, et al. Upregulation of a silent sodium channel after peripheral, but not central, nerve injury in DRG neurons. J Neurophysiol 1999; 82:2776-885.
61. Liu CN, Wall PD, Ben Dor E, et al. Tactile allodynia in the absence of C-fiber activation: Altered firing properties of DRG neurons following spinal nerve injury. Pain 2000; 85:503-21.
62. Baogang L, Eisenach JC, Tong C. Chronic estrogen sensitizes a subset of mechanosensitive afferents innervating the uterine cervix. J Neurophysiol 2005; 93:2167-73.

63. Yan T, Liu B, Du D, et al. Estrogen amplifies pain responses to uterine cervical distension in rats by altering transient receptor potential-1 function. Anesth Analg 2007; 104:1246-50.
64. Tong C, Conklin D, Clyne BB, et al. Uterine cervical afferents in throracolumbar dorsal root ganglia express transient receptor potential vanilloid type 1 channel and calcitonin gene-related peptide, but not P2X3 receptor and somatostatin. Anesthesiology 2006; 104:651-7.
65. Mousa SA, Zhang Q, Sitte N, et al. β-endorphin-containing memory-cells and μ-opioid receptors undergo transport to peripheral inflamed tissue. J Neuroimmunol 2001; 115:71-8.
66. Picard PR, Tramèr MR, McQuay HJ, Moore RA. Analgesic efficacy of peripheral opioids (all except intra-articular): A qualitative systematic review of randomised controlled trials. Pain 1997; 72:309-18.
67. Kalso E, Tramèr MR, Carroll D, et al. Pain relief from intra-articular morphine after knee surgery: A qualitative systematic review. Pain 1997; 71:127-34.
68. Sandner-Kiesling A, Eisenach JC. Pharmacology of opioid inhibition to noxious uterine cervical distention. Anesthesiology 2002; 97:966-71.
69. Sengupta JN, Su X, Gebhart GF. Kappa, but not μ or δ, opioids attenuate responses to distention of afferent fibers innervating the rat colon. Gastroenterology 1996; 111:968-80.
70. Gebhart GF, Su X, Joshi S, et al. Peripheral opioid modulation of visceral pain. Ann N Y Acad Sci 2000; 909:41-50.
71. Binder W, Walker JS. Effect of the peripherally selective kappa-opioid agonist, asimadoline, on adjuvant arthritis. Br J Pharmacol 1998; 124:647-54.
72. Eisenach JC, Carpenter R, Curry R. Analgesia from a peripherally active kappa-opioid receptor agonist in patients with chronic pancreatitis. Pain 2003; 101:89-95.
73. Cicero TJ, Nock B, O'Connor L, Meyer ER. Role of steroids in sex differences in morphine-induced analgesia: Activational and organizational effects. J Pharmacol Exp Ther 2002; 300:695-701.
74. Gear RW, Miaskowski C, Gordon NC, et al. Kappa-opioids produce significantly greater analgesia in women than in men. Nature Med 1996; 2:1248-50.
75. Sandner-Kiesling A, Eisenach JC. Estrogen reduces efficacy of μ- but not κ-opioid agonist inhibition in response to uterine cervical distention. Anesthesiology 2002; 96:375-9.
76. Shin SW, Eisenach JC. Intrathecal morphine reduces the visceromotor response to acute uterine cervical distention in an estrogen-independent manner. Anesthesiology 2003; 98:1467-71.
77. Olofsson C, Ekblom A, Ekman-Ordeberg G, et al. Lack of analgesic effect of systemically administered morphine or pethidine on labour pain. Br J Obstet Gynaecol 1996; 103:968-72.
78. Leighton BL, DeSimone CA, Norris MC, Ben-David B. Intrathecal narcotics for labor revisited: The combination of fentanyl and morphine intrathecally provides rapid onset of profound, prolonged analgesia. Anesth Analg 1989; 69:122-5.
79. Goldin AL, Barchi RL, Caldwell JH, et al. Nomenclature of voltage-gated sodium channels. Neuron 2000; 28:365-8.
80. Renganathan M, Cummins TR, Waxman SG. Nitric oxide blocks fast, slow, and persistent Na^+ channels in C-type DRG neurons by S-nitrosylation. J Neurophysiol 2002; 87:761-75.
81. Gold MS, Weinreich D, Kim CS, et al. NaV1.8 mediates neuropathic pain via redistribution in the axons of uninjured afferents (abstract). Soc Neurosci 2001; 55:6.
82. Lai J, Gold MS, Kim CS, et al. Inhibition of neuropathic pain by decreased expression of the tetrodotoxin-resistant sodium channel, NaV1.8. Pain 2002; 95:143-52.
83. Nonaka T, Honmou O, Sakai J, et al. Excitability changes of dorsal root axons following nerve injury: Implications for injury-induced changes in axonal Na(+) channels. Brain Res 2000; 859:280-5.
84. Sakai J, Honmou O, Kocsis JD, Hashi K. The delayed depolarization in rat cutaneous afferent axons is reduced following nerve transection and ligation, but not crush: Implications for injury-induced axonal Na^+ channel reorganization. Muscle Nerve 1998; 21:1040-7.
85. Gerner P, Mujtaba M, Sinnott CJ, Wang GK. Amitriptyline versus bupivacaine in rat sciatic nerve blockade. Anesthesiology 2001; 94:661-7.
86. Gerner P, Mujtaba M, Khan M, et al. N-phenylethyl amitriptyline in rat sciatic nerve blockade. Anesthesiology 2002; 96:1435-42.
87. Dalle C, Schneider M, Clergue F, et al. Inhibition of the Ih current in isolated peripheral nerve: A novel mode of peripheral antinociception? Muscle Nerve 2001; 24:254-61.
88. Chaplan SR, Guo HQ, Lee DH, et al. Neuronal hyperpolarization-activated pacemaker channels drive neuropathic pain. J Neurosci 2003; 23:1169-78.
89. Kissin I, Bright CA, Bradley EL. Selective and long-lasting neural blockade with resiniferatoxin prevents inflammatory pain hypersensitivity. Anesth Analg 2002; 94:1253-8.
90. Ludwig M, Sabatier N, Bull PM, et al. Intracellular calcium stores regulate activity-dependent neuropeptide release from dendrites. Nature 2002; 418:85-9.
91. Feng Y, Cui ML, Willis WD. Gabapentin markedly reduces acetic acid-induced visceral nociception. Anesthesiology 2003; 98:729-33.
92. Cao YQ, Mantyh PW, Carlson EJ, et al. Primary afferent tachykinins are required to experience moderate to intense pain. Nature 1998; 392:390-4.
93. Khan IM, Marsala M, Printz MP, et al. Intrathecal nicotinic agonist-elicited release of excitatory amino acids as measured by in vivo spinal microdialysis in rats. J Pharmacol Exp Ther 1996; 278:97-106.
94. Riley RC, Trafton JA, Chi SI, Basbaum AI. Presynaptic regulation of spinal cord tachykinin signaling via GABA-B but not GABA-A receptor activation. Neuroscience 2001; 103:725-37.
95. Li DP, Chen SR, Pan YZ, et al. Role of presynaptic muscarinic and GABA-B receptors in spinal glutamate release and cholinergic analgesia in rats. J Physiol 2002; 543:807-18.
96. Baba H, Kohno T, Okamoto M, et al. Muscarinic facilitation of GABA release in substantia gelatinosa of the rat spinal dorsal horn. J Physiol 1998; 508:83-93.
97. Lauretti GR, Hood DD, Eisenach JC, Pfeifer BL. A multi-center study of intrathecal neostigmine for analgesia following vaginal hysterectomy. Anesthesiology 1998; 89:913-8.
98. Lombard M-C, Besson J-M. Attempts to gauge the relative importance of pre- and postsynaptic effects of morphine on the transmission of noxious messages in the dorsal horn of the rat spinal cord. Pain 1989; 37:335-45.
99. Kuraishi Y, Hirota N, Sato Y, et al. Noradrenergic inhibition of the release of substance P from the primary afferents in the rabbit spinal dorsal horn. Brain Res 1985; 359:177-82.
100. Headley PM, Grillner S. Excitatory amino acids and synaptic transmission: The evidence for a physiological function. Trends Pharmacol Sci 1990; 11:205-11.
101. Karpinski N, Dunn J, Hansen L, Masliah E. Subpial vacuolar myelopathy after intrathecal ketamine: Report of a case. Pain 1997; 73:103-5.
102. Wilder-Smith CH, Knöpfli R, Wilder-Smith OHG. Perioperative magnesium infusion and postoperative pain. Acta Anaesthesiol Scand 1997; 41:1023-7.
103. Svensson CI, Yaksh TL. The spinal phospholipase-cyclooxygenase-prostanoid cascade in nociceptive processing. Annu Rev Pharmacol Toxicol 2002; 42:553-83.
104. Roza C, Laird JM, Cervero F. Spinal mechanisms underlying persistent pain and referred hyperalgesia in rats with an experimental ureteric stone. J Neurophysiol 1998; 79:1603-12.
105. Ossipov MH, Lopez Y, Nichols ML, et al. The loss of antinociceptive efficacy of spinal morphine in rats with nerve ligation injury is prevented by reducing spinal afferent drive. Neurosci Lett 1995; 199:87-90.
106. Tong C, Ma W, Shin S, James RL, Eisenach JC. Uterine cervical distention induces cFos expression in deep dorsal horn neurons of the rat spinal cord. Anesthesiology 2003; 99:205-11.
107. Du D, Eisenach JC, Ririe DG, Tong C. The antinociceptive effects of spinal cyclooxygenase inhibitors on uterine cervical distention. Brain Res 2004; 1024:130-6.
108. Eisenach JC, Curry R, Hood DD, Yaksh TL. Phase I safety assessment of intrathecal ketorolac. Pain 2002; 99:599-604.
109. Basbaum AI, Fields HL. Endogenous pain control mechanisms: Review and hypothesis. Ann Neurol 1978; 4:451-62.

110. Eisenach JC, Dobson CE, Inturrisi CE, et al. Effect of pregnancy and pain on cerebrospinal fluid immunoreactive enkephalins and norepinephrine in healthy humans. Pain 1990; 43:149-54.
111. Benedetti F, Arduino C, Amanzio M. Somatotopic activation of opioid systems by target-directed expectations of analgesia. J Neurosci 1999; 19:3639-48.
112. Millan MJ. The role of descending noradrenergic and serotoninergic pathways in the modulation of nociception: Focus on receptor multiplicity. In Dickenson A, Besson JM, editors. Handbook of Experimental Pharmacology: The Pharmacology of Pain. Berlin, Springer-Verlag, 1997:385-446.
113. Zhuo M, Sengupta JN, Gebhart GF. Biphasic modulation of spinal visceral nociceptive transmission from the rostroventral medial medulla in the rat. J Neurophysiol 2002; 87:2225-36.
114. Al Chaer ED, Traub RJ. Biological basis of visceral pain: Recent developments. Pain 2002; 96:221-5.
115. Jones AK, Kulkarni B, Derbyshire SW. Pain mechanisms and their disorders. Br Med Bull 2003; 65:83-93.
116. Leighton BL, Halpern SH, Wilson DB. Lumbar sympathetic blocks speed early and second stage induced labor in nulliparous women. Anesthesiology 1999; 90:1039-46.
117. Moir DD, Willocks J. Management of incoordinate uterine action under continuous epidural analgesia. BMJ 1967; 3:396-400.
118. Riffel HD, Nochimson DJ, Paul RH, Hon EH. Effects of meperidine and promethazine during labor. Obstet Gynecol 1973; 42:738-45.
119. Clarke VT, Smiley RM, Finster M. Uterine hyperactivity after intrathecal injection of fentanyl for analgesia during labor: A cause of fetal bradycardia. Anesthesiology 1994; 81:1083.
120. Hingson RA, Hellman LM. Anatomic and physiologic considerations. In Hingson RA, Hellman LM, editors. Anesthesia for Obstetrics. Philadelphia, JB Lippincott, 1956:74.
121. Rahm VA, Hallgren A, Hogberg H, et al. Plasma oxytocin levels in women during labor with or without epidural analgesia: A prospective study. Acta Obstet Gynecol Scand 2002; 81:1033-9.
122. Stocche RM, Klamt JG, Antunes-Rodrigues J, et al. Effects of intrathecal sufentanil on plasma oxytocin and cortisol concentrations in women during the first stage of labor. Reg Anesth Pain Med 2001; 26:545-50.
123. Scull TJ, Hemmings GT, Carli F, et al. Epidural analgesia in early labour blocks the stress response but uterine contractions remain unchanged. Can J Anaesth 1998; 45:626-30.
124. Leighton BL, Norris MC, Sosis M, et al. Limitations of epinephrine as a marker of intravascular injection in laboring women. Anesthesiology 1987; 66:688-91.
125. Hood DD, Dewan DM, James FM. Maternal and fetal effects of epinephrine in gravid ewes. Anesthesiology 1986; 64:610-3.
126. Shnider SM, Abboud TK, Artal R, et al. Maternal catecholamines decrease during labor after lumbar epidural anesthesia. Am J Obstet Gynecol 1983; 147:13-5.
127. Cascio M, Pygon B, Bernett C, Ramanathan S. Labour analgesia with intrathecal fentanyl decreases maternal stress. Can J Anaesth 1997; 44:605-19.
128. Jouppila R, Puolakka J, Kauppila A, Vuori J. Maternal and umbilical cord plasma noradrenaline concentrations during labour with and without segmental extradural analgesia, and during caesarean section. Br J Anaesth 1984; 56:251-4.
129. Hagerdal M, Morgan CW, Sumner AE, Gutsche BB. Minute ventilation during and oxygen consumption during labor with epidural analgesia. Anesthesiology 1983; 59:425-57.
130. Hodnett ED. Pain and women's satisfaction with the experience of childbirth: A systematic review. Am J Obstet Gynecol 2002; 186:S160-72.
131. Billewicz-Driemel AM, Milne MD. Long-term assessment of extradural analgesia for pain relief in labour. II. Sense of deprivation after extradural analgesia in labour: Relevant or not? Br J Anaesth 1976; 48:139-44.
132. Stewart DE. Psychiatric symptoms following attempted natural childbirth. Can Med Assoc J 1982; 127:713-6.
133. Ryding E. Psychosocial indications for cesarean section. Acta Obstet Gynecol Scand 1991; 70:47-9.
134. Ballard CG, Stanley AK. Post traumatic stress disorder after childbirth. Br J Psych 1995; 166:525-8.
135. Thompson JF, Roberts CL, Currie M, Ellwood DA. Prevalence and persistence of health problems after childbirth: Associations with parity and method of birth. Birth 2002; 29:83-94.
136. Macarthur AJ, Macarthur C. Incidence, severity, and determinants of perineal pain after vaginal delivery: A prospective cohort study. Am J Obstet Gynecol 2004; 191:1199-204.
137. Lavand'homme PM, Roelants F, Waterloos H, De Kock MF. Postoperative analgesic effects of continuous wound infiltration with diclofenac after cesarean delivery. Anesthesiology 2007; 106:1220-5.
138. Pan PH, Coghill R, Houle TT, et al. Multifactorial preoperative predictors for postcesarean section pain and analgesic requirement. Anesthesiology 2006; 104:417-25.
139. Kehlet H, Jensen TS, Woolf C. Persistent postsurgical pain: Risk factors and prevention. Lancet 2006; 367:1618-25.
140. Almeida EC, Nogueira AA, Candido dos Reis FJ, Rosa e Silva JC. Cesarean section as a cause of chronic pelvic pain. Int J Gynaecol Obstet 2002; 79:101-4.
141. Nikolajsen L, Sorensen HC, Jensen TS, Kehlet H. Chronic pain following Caesarean section. Acta Anaesthesiol Scand 2004; 48:111-6.
142. Wisner KL, Parry BL, Piontek CM. Clinical practice: Postpartum depression. N Engl J Med 2002; 337:194-9.
143. Brown S, Lumley J. Maternal health after childbirth: Results of an Australian population based survey. Br J Obstet Gynaecol 1998; 105:156-61.
144. Lydon-Rochelle MT, Holt VL, Martin DP. Delivery method and self-reported postpartum general health status among primiparous women. Paediatr Perinat Epidemiol 2001; 15:232-40.

Chapter 21

Childbirth Preparation and Nonpharmacologic Analgesia

Marie E. Minnich, M.D., M.M.M., M.B.A., C.P.E.

Pregnant women and their support person(s) obtain information about childbirth and analgesia from many sources, including obstetricians, childbirth preparation classes, lay periodicals, books and pamphlets, family, friends, and—increasingly—the Internet. Anesthesia providers should be familiar with this information. Patients' preparation and understanding or misunderstanding influence their birth experiences. Knowledge of the information and biases held by patients helps anesthesia providers in their interactions with pregnant women. Prepared childbirth training provides undeniable benefits to the pregnant woman and her support person. However, prepared childbirth training should not be equated with nonpharmacologic analgesia.[1] Some childbirth preparation instructors discourage the use of medications during labor and delivery, whereas others make a nonbiased presentation of the advantages and disadvantages of various analgesic techniques. The information contained in this chapter provides a basis for informed discussion of pain relief options among patients, nurses, obstetricians, and anesthesia providers.

PAIN PERCEPTION

Anesthesia providers are indebted to John Bonica and Ronald Melzack for their studies of the pain of childbirth. Investigators have used sophisticated questionnaires[2,3] and visual analog scales[4] to evaluate the maternal perception of pain during parturition. Melzack et al.[5,6] used the McGill Pain Questionnaire to measure the intensity of labor pain in nulliparous and parous women. They noted that labor pain is one of the most intense types of pain among those studied (see Figure 20-2). Parous women had lower pain scores than nulliparous women, but responses varied widely (Figures 21-1 and 21-2). Prepared childbirth training resulted in a modest decrease in the average pain score among nulliparous women, but it clearly did not eliminate pain in these women.[5,6]

CHILDBIRTH PREPARATION

History

The history of modern childbirth preparation began in the first half of the twentieth century; however, it is important to review earlier changes in obstetric practice to understand the perceived need for a new approach. Before the mid-nineteenth century, childbirth occurred at home in the company of family and friends. The specialty of obstetrics developed in an effort to decrease maternal mortality. Interventions initially developed for the management of complications became accepted and practiced as routine obstetric care. Physicians first administered anesthesia for childbirth during this period. The 1848 meeting of the American Medical Association included reports of the use of ether and chloroform in approximately 2000 obstetric cases.[7] The combination of morphine and scopolamine (i.e., twilight sleep) was introduced in the early twentieth century. These techniques were widely used, and influential

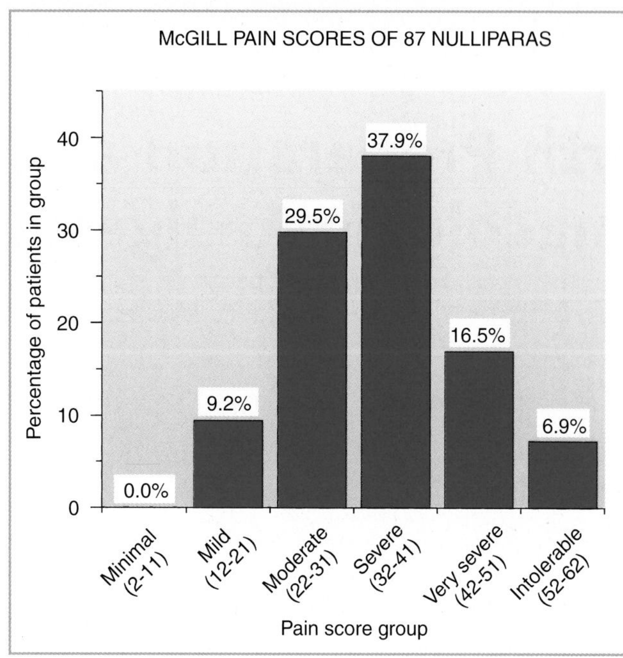

FIGURE 21-1 The severity of pain during labor as assessed by the McGill Pain Questionnaire for 87 nulliparous women. (Modified from Melzack R, Taezner P, Feldman P, Kinch RA. Labour is still painful after prepared childbirth training. Can Med Assoc J 1981; 125:357-63.)

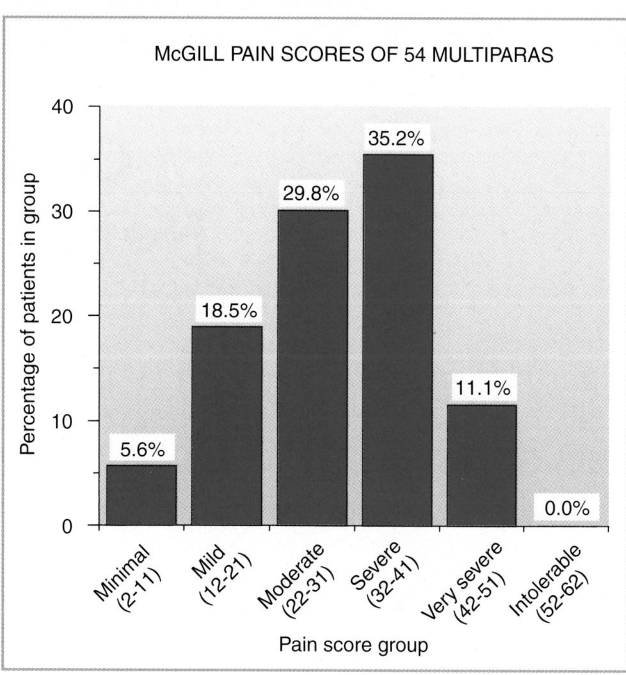

FIGURE 21-2 The severity of pain during labor as assessed by the McGill Pain Questionnaire for 54 parous women. (Modified from Melzack R, Taezner P, Feldman P, Kinch RA. Labour is still painful after prepared childbirth training. Can Med Assoc J 1981; 125:357-63.)

women demanded that they be made available to all parturients.[8] Together, these developments moved childbirth from the home and family unit to the hospital environment.[9] Despite their desire for analgesia/anesthesia for labor and delivery, women began to resent the fact that they were not active participants in childbirth.

Beck et al.[10] have written a detailed history of childbirth preparation. Dick-Read[11,12] reported the earliest method in his books, *Natural Childbirth* and *Childbirth Without Fear*. In his original publication, he asserted his belief that childbirth was not inherently painful. He opined that the pain of childbirth results from a "fear-tension-pain-syndrome." He believed—and taught—that antepartum instruction about muscle relaxation and elimination of fear would prevent labor pain. He later established antenatal classes that included groups of mothers and fathers. Some readers incorrectly concluded that he advocated a return to primitive obstetrics, but this was not the case. Review of his practice reveals that he used the available obstetric techniques—including analgesia, anesthesia, episiotomy, forceps, and abdominal delivery—as appropriate for the individual patient. However, he cautioned against the routine use of these procedures, and he encouraged active participation of mothers in the delivery of their infants. Unfortunately, he did not use the scientific method to validate his beliefs.

Although Dick-Read was the earliest proponent of natural childbirth, it was Fernand Lamaze[13] who introduced the Western world to psychoprophylaxis. His publications were based on techniques that he observed while traveling in Russia. Although his theories ostensibly were translations of teachings later published in the West by Velvovsky et al.,[14] they contained substantial differences and modifications. The "Lamaze method" became popular in the United States after Marjorie Karmel[15] described her childbirth experience under the care of Dr. Lamaze. Within a year of the publication of her popular book, the American Society for Psychoprophylaxis in Obstetrics was born. Lamaze and Karmel published their experience at a time when organizations such as the International Childbirth Education Association and the La Leche League were formed.[16] These organizations actively and aggressively encouraged a renewed emphasis on family-centered maternity care, and society was ripe for the ideas and theories promoted by these organizations. Women were ready to actively participate in childbirth and to have input in decisions about obstetric and anesthetic interventions. Childbirth preparation methods were taught and used extensively, despite a lack of scientific validation of their efficacy.

In 1975, Leboyer[17] described a modification of natural childbirth in his book, *Birth Without Violence*. He advocated childbirth in a dark, quiet room; gentle massage of the newborn without routine suctioning; and a warm bath soon after birth. He opined that these maneuvers result in a less shocking first-separation experience and a healthier, happier infancy and childhood. Although there are few controlled studies of this method, published observations do not support his claim of superiority.[18,19]

Physicians were the initial advocates of the various natural childbirth methods. Obstetricians had become increasingly aware that analgesic and anesthetic techniques were not harmless, and they supported the use of natural childbirth methods.[10] Subsequently, natural childbirth, like the methods of obstetric analgesia introduced earlier in the century, was actively promoted by lay groups rather

BOX 21-1 Goals of Childbirth Preparation

- Patient education about pregnancy, labor, and delivery
- Relaxation training
- Instruction in breathing techniques
- Participation of father/support person
- Early parental bonding

than physicians.[20] Lay publications, national advocacy groups, and formal instruction of patients accounted for the greater interest in psychoprophylaxis and other techniques associated with natural childbirth.

Goals and Advantages

The major goals of childbirth education that were initially promoted by Dick-Read are taught with little modification in formal childbirth preparation classes today. Most current classes credit Lamaze with the major components of childbirth preparation, even though Dick-Read was the first to promote patient education, relaxation training, breathing exercises, and paternal participation.[10] Box 21-1 describes the goals of current childbirth preparation classes. In addition, some instructors and training manuals claim other benefits of childbirth preparation (Box 21-2). Reviews by Beck and Hall[21] and Lindell[22] concluded that much of the research on the efficacy of childbirth education does not meet the fundamental requirements of the scientific method. Despite these shortcomings, childbirth preparation classes are widely available and attended.

Socioeconomic disparities exist in childbirth education class attendance.[23] In addition, the effect of childbirth education on attitude and childbirth experience depends in part on the social class to which the mother belongs. Most investigators have found that childbirth classes have a positive effect on the attitudes of both parents in all social classes, but this effect is more pronounced among "working class"[24] and indigent women[25]; this latter finding probably reflects the greater availability and use of other educational materials by middle- and upper-class women. Childbirth classes often are the only—or at least the primary—source of information for working class and indigent women.

Limitations

Limitations of the widespread application of psychoprophylaxis and other childbirth preparation methods remain. Proponents assume that these techniques are easily used during labor and delivery; however, Copstick et al.[26] concluded that this assumption is not valid. They found that patients were able to use the coping techniques in the early first stage of labor but that the successful use of the coping skills became less and less common as labor progressed. By the onset of the second stage, less than one third of mothers were able to use any of the breathing or postural techniques taught during their childbirth classes.[26] The method of preparation influences the ability of the pregnant woman to use the breathing and relaxation techniques. Bernardini et al.[27] observed that self-taught pregnant women are less likely to practice the techniques during the prenatal period or to use the techniques during labor.

Childbirth preparation classes may create false expectations. If a woman does not enjoy the "normal" delivery discussed during classes, she may experience a sense of failure or inferiority. Both Stewart[28] and Guzman Sanchez et al.[29] have discussed the psychological reactions of women who were unable to use psychoprophylaxis successfully during labor and delivery. In addition, several women have written about their disappointment with the dogmatic approach of their childbirth instructors; these women described instructors who rigidly defined the "correct" way to have a "proper" birth experience.[30,31]

BOX 21-2 Purported Benefits of Childbirth Preparation

- Greater maternal control and cooperation
- Decreased maternal anxiety
- Reduced maternal pain
- Decreased maternal need for analgesia/anesthesia
- Shorter labor
- Diminished maternal morbidity
- Less fetal stress/distress
- Strengthened family relationships as a result of the shared birth experience

Effects

Little scientific evidence supports the efficacy of childbirth preparation in mitigating labor pain. Psychology, nursing, obstetric, anesthesia, and lay journals provide extensive discussions of childbirth preparation, but most articles describe uncontrolled clinical experiences. Outcome studies often do not include a group of women who were randomly assigned to an untreated or a placebo-control group, and statistical analysis is often incomplete. Despite these shortcomings, supporters of childbirth preparation assume that it offers benefits for mother and child. Table 21-1 summarizes a few of the studies of Lamaze and other childbirth preparation techniques and their association with labor outcomes. The findings are not consistent. Some researchers have reported a *decreased* use of analgesics[32-35] or regional anesthesia,[32-36] shorter labor,[37] reduced performance of instrumental[32,34,36] and cesarean delivery,[36] and a lower incidence of nonreassuring fetal status,[36] whereas others have reported *no change* in the use of analgesics[36-40] or neuraxial analgesia,[38,39] length of labor,[34-36,38-41] performance of instrumental[38-40] and cesarean delivery,[34,38-40] or incidence of nonreassuring fetal status.[33,34,37,39] These diverse findings may reflect different patient populations, poor study design, or researcher bias.

To elucidate the effect of the coping techniques taught in childbirth classes, several investigators have attempted to quantify changes in pain threshold, pain perception, anxiety levels, and physiologic responses to standardized stimuli. Several studies have evaluated nonpregnant and nulliparous women in laboratory settings,[42-45] and another study evaluated pregnant women in the antepartum, intrapartum, and postpartum periods.[46] Conclusions varied according to the stimuli applied, the coping techniques studied, and the parameters analyzed. Together, these studies suggest that *practicing* these techniques facilitates their efficacy

TABLE 21-1 Effects of Childbirth Preparation

Study	Analgesic Use	Neuraxial Anesthesia	Length of Labor	Cesarean Delivery Rate	Instrumental Delivery Rate	Fetal Distress	Oxytocin Use
Patton et al.[39]	NC	NC	NC	NC	NC	NC	↑
Hetherington[32]	↓	↓	—	—	↓	—	—
Zax et al.[35]	↓	↓	NC	—	—	—	—
Scott & Rose[34]	↓	↓	NC	NC	↓	NC	NC
Hughey et al.[36]	NC	↓	NC	↓	↓	↓	NC
Sturrock & Johnson[40]	NC	—	NC	NC	NC	—	—
Brewin & Bradley[38]	NC	NC	NC	NC	NC	—	—
Delke et al.[37]	NC	—	↓	—	—	NC	NC
Rogers[33]	↓	—	—	—	—	NC	—

NC, No change; ↑, increased; ↓, decreased; —, not studied/reported.

and that newer cognitive techniques (e.g., systematic desensitization, sensory transformation) may be more effective than traditional Lamaze techniques of varied breathing patterns and relaxation. Further studies may help refine childbirth preparation to maximize the positive psychophysiologic effects.

NONPHARMACOLOGIC ANALGESIC TECHNIQUES

Nonpharmacologic analgesic techniques range from those that require minimal specialized equipment and training and are available to all patients to those that are offered only by institutions with the necessary equipment and personnel trained in their use (Box 21-3). Many studies have assessed nonpharmacologic methods of labor analgesia; however, most published studies have not fulfilled the requirements of the scientific method.[47-49] Several comprehensive reviews of alternative therapies for pain management during labor have been published,[47-49] providing a foundation for discussion with patients and obstetric providers. However, clinical evidence is insufficient to form the basis for an in-depth discussion of some of the more recent therapeutic suggestions, such as music therapy, aromatherapy, and chiropractic. These analgesic techniques may provide intangible benefits that are not easily documented by rigorous scientific method. Parturients may consider these benefits an integral and important part of their labor experience.

BOX 21-3 Nonpharmacologic Analgesic Techniques

Minimal Training/Equipment

- Emotional support
- Touch and massage
- Therapeutic use of heat and cold
- Hydrotherapy
- Vertical position

Specialized Training/Equipment

- Biofeedback
- Intradermal water injection
- Transcutaneous electrical nerve stimulation (TENS)
- Acupuncture
- Hypnosis

Continuous Labor Support

Some techniques that require minimum equipment and specialized training are taught as integral components of childbirth preparation classes. Continuous support during labor is essential to the process of a satisfying childbirth experience; typically, the parturient's husband or friend provides this support.[50,51] This support appears most helpful for the parturient who lives in a stable family unit. At least one study noted that husband participation was associated with decreased maternal anxiety and medication requirements.[51] Others have found that emotional support provided by unfamiliar trained individuals (e.g., doulas) also has a positive effect.[52-55] Several studies have evaluated the benefits of emotional support provided by doulas or other unrelated individuals on the length of labor,[52,53,55] oxytocin use,[53] requirements for analgesia and/or anesthesia,[52,53] incidence of operative delivery,[53] and maternal morbidity.[53,54] These studies all suggested that a patient's sense of isolation adversely affects her perception of labor. Further, the companionship of another woman who is not part of the medical establishment may reduce a parturient's anxiety more effectively than the companionship provided by her husband. In one study, women randomly assigned to receive intrapartum support from a friend or female relative (who was chosen by the parturient and trained as a doula) were more likely to have positive feelings about their delivery and had a higher rate of breast-feeding 6 to 8 weeks after delivery than women who were randomly assigned to receive usual care.[41]

A meta-analysis evaluated results from 16 studies that included more than 13,000 women who were randomly assigned to receive either continuous childbirth support or usual care (Table 21-2).[56] The pooled data suggested that women who received one-on-one support during labor were less likely to use neuraxial analgesia or receive any type of analgesia, were more likely to have a spontaneous vaginal delivery, and reported less dissatisfaction with the childbirth experience.[56] In addition, the mean duration

TABLE 21-2 Systematic Review: Continuous Labor Support versus Usual Care

Outcome	Number of Trials	Number of Subjects	Relative Risk*	95% Confidence Interval
Use of neuraxial analgesia	7	10,648	0.92	0.85 to 0.99
Use of any analgesia	12	11,651	0.89	0.82 to 0.96
Spontaneous vaginal delivery	15	13,357	1.07	1.04 to 1.12
Instrumental vaginal delivery	15	13,357	0.89	0.82 to 0.96
Cesarean delivery	16	13,391	0.91	0.83 to 0.99
Patient dissatisfaction with childbirth experience	6	9824	0.73	0.65 to 0.83
Duration of labor	10	10,922	−0.43 hr†	−0.83 to −0.04 hr

*For women who received continuous support

†Weighted mean difference

Data are summarized from Hodnett ED, Gates S, Hofmeyr GJ, Sakala C. Continuous support for women during childbirth. Cochrane Database Syst Rev 2007; (3):CD003766.

of labor was slightly shorter (approximately 26 minutes) in the women who received continuous support during labor. There were no differences in neonatal outcome.

These results are fascinating and have important implications for obstetric care. The patient populations studied represent special situations, and the results may not be reproduced in all populations. For example, a large randomized, controlled trial in a North American hospital (in which intrapartum medical intervention is routine) found no differences in the rate of cesarean delivery or other labor outcomes between women randomly assigned to receive continuous labor support from a specially trained nurse and women who received usual care.[57] In general, results from trials in North America do not appear as striking as those from Europe or Africa.[47] The aforementioned systematic review of continuous labor support suggested that benefits were greater when the support person was not a member of the hospital staff.[56] Further studies should compare different models of continuous childbirth support and should include outcomes such as cost analysis.[56] Meanwhile, all parturients should have access to emotional support, whether it is provided by the husband, a family member, a labor companion (e.g., doula), or professional hospital staff.

Touch and Massage

Various touch and massage techniques are discussed with women and their support persons during childbirth preparation classes. They include effleurage, counterpressure to alleviate back discomfort, light stroking, and merely a reassuring pat.[47] There has been minimal scientific study of the effects of touch and massage on labor progress and outcome[58-60]; nonetheless, touch and massage provide a comfort that is appreciated by women during labor. These measures may be used by the parturient, her support person, or the professional staff members providing intrapartum care.[59] The techniques are easily discontinued if the parturient desires. In some cases, touch and massage may reduce discomfort. More often, touch and massage transmit a sense of caring, which fosters a sense of security and well-being.

Therapeutic Use of Heat and Cold

Another simple technique for alleviating labor pain is the therapeutic use of temperature (hot or cold) applied to various regions of the body. Warm compresses may be placed on localized areas, or a warm blanket may cover the entire body. Alternatively, ice packs may be placed on the low back or perineum to decrease pain perception. The therapeutic use of heat and cold during labor has not been studied in a rigorously scientific manner. The use of superficial heat and cold for comfort is widespread (if not completely understood), and it has no discernible risk for the mother or the fetus.[47] Cold and heat should not be applied to anesthetized skin.

Hydrotherapy

Hydrotherapy may involve a simple shower or tub bath or may include the use of a whirlpool or large tub specially equipped for pregnant women. Purported benefits of hydrotherapy include decreased anxiety and pain and greater uterine contraction efficiency.[47] Results of randomized, controlled trials comparing water baths with usual care are inconsistent. For example, some studies have found no difference between groups in the use of pharmacologic analgesia,[61,62] whereas others have demonstrated a lower utilization in the water bath group.[63,64] A meta-analysis of eight published trials involving almost 3000 women concluded that there was a reduction in the use of neuraxial analgesia in women randomly assigned to water immersion compared with control subjects (odds ratio [OR], 0.84; 95% confidence interval [CI], 0.71 to 0.99).[65] There were no differences in rate of operative delivery or neonatal outcome, including infection. In summary, bathing, showering, and other hydrotherapy maneuvers are comfort measures with little risk to the mother and the infant, provided that appropriate monitoring continues during the immersion in water that is kept at body temperature.

Vertical Position

Several investigators have studied the effects of various positions on pain perception and labor outcome.

These positions are broadly categorized as *vertical* (e.g., sitting, standing, walking, squatting) or *horizontal* (e.g., supine, lateral). A systematic review summarized the results from 13 controlled trials of maternal posture during the first stage of labor.[66] In 7 trials in which women served as their own controls, women reported less pain in the standing and sitting positions than in the supine position. Six other trials randomly assigned women to either an experimental group who were encouraged to remain upright or a control group who remained supine or on the side. Women in the upright groups experienced less pain or no difference in pain when compared with the recumbent groups.

Ambulation in the presence of neuraxial analgesia does not appear to influence the outcome of labor.[67-69] In a prospective, randomized study, Bloom et al.[67] noted that walking did not shorten the duration of the first stage of labor or reduce the requirement for oxytocin augmentation, the use of analgesia, or the requirement for operative delivery. They concluded that "walking neither enhanced nor impaired active labor and was not harmful to the mothers or their infants."[67]

A number of studies have assessed maternal position during the second stage of labor. There is renewed interest in the squatting or modified squatting position and its greater comfort for some women during childbirth. Most authorities have noted that Western women have insufficient muscular strength and stamina to maintain an unsupported squatting position for any length of time.[70-72] Squatting does not appear to alter pelvic dimensions.[73] Gardosi et al.[70] designed and studied a birth cushion that allows a modified, supported squat, which resulted in a higher incidence of spontaneous delivery and a lower incidence of perineal tears. Others have yet to substantiate the results of this trial.

Some studies have evaluated the use of a birth chair to facilitate delivery in the sitting position.[74-76] These studies noted no difference in length of the second stage, mode of delivery, occurrence of perineal trauma, or Apgar scores in parturients who used a birth chair compared with those who did not. Of concern, two studies reported greater intrapartum blood loss and a higher incidence of postpartum hemorrhage in the birth-chair group.[75,76]

A systematic review of studies of maternal position in the second stage of labor in women without epidural anesthesia concluded that currently published trials are generally of poor quality.[77] Tentative results suggest that less severe pain and a lower rate of perineal trauma may be associated with giving birth in the upright position; however, blood loss may be greater. Although the investigators concluded that further study is required, many obstetricians and nurses believe that ambulation and the upright posture result in shorter labors that require less analgesia. An alternative explanation for the observation that ambulatory parturients appear to have a less painful and shorter labor is that shorter, less painful labor *allows* continued ambulation.

Other than the possibility of greater blood loss associated with the upright position during delivery, upright positions during most of labor are not associated with any harm to the mother or baby and may aid maternal comfort. It is unclear whether birthing cushions or stools confer any benefit to the mother or the baby.

Biofeedback

Biofeedback is a relaxation method that is used as an adjunct to the relaxation training taught in Lamaze classes and other childbirth education programs. Two biofeedback procedures may be applicable to the laboring woman: skin-conductance (autonomic) and electromyographic (voluntary muscle) relaxation. St. James-Roberts et al.[78] demonstrated that electromyographic but not skin-conductance biofeedback techniques could be taught effectively in Lamaze classes. They noted no difference in length of the first stage of labor, use of epidural analgesia, incidence of instrumental delivery, or Apgar scores among electromyographic, skin-conductance, and control groups. In a small study, Duchene[79] reported reduced pain perception during labor and delivery and a lower rate of epidural analgesia utilization (40% versus 70% for a control group) with electromyographic biofeedback; there was no difference between groups in Apgar scores. Biofeedback training does not appear to confer substantial benefit beyond that of traditional relaxation training taught in childbirth education classes.

Intradermal Water Injections

Intradermal or intracutaneous water injections are used to treat lower back pain, which is a common complaint during labor. The afferent nerve fibers that innervate the uterus and cervix, as well as the nerve fibers that innervate the lower back, all enter the spinal cord at the T10 through L1 spinal segments; therefore, a component of the pain may be referred pain. The technique consists of injecting 0.05 to 0.1 mL of sterile water, with an insulin or tuberculin syringe, at four sites on the lower back (i.e., over each posterior superior iliac spine, and at 1 cm medial and 3 cm caudad to the posterior superior iliac spine on both sides of the back, for a total of four injections) (Figure 21-3). The injections themselves are acutely painful for about 20 to 30 seconds, but as the injection pain fades, so does lower back pain.

Systematic reviews have summarized the four randomized controlled trials that compared intradermal water injections with placebo or standard care.[48,66] The results of these trials suggested that the intradermal injections are a simple method of reducing severe low back pain during labor without adverse effects on the mother and fetus. The analgesic effect appears to last for 45 to 120 minutes.[47] However, the performance of intradermal water injections does not appear to reduce the rate of utilization of other analgesic techniques.[48,66]

Transcutaneous Electrical Nerve Stimulation

Transcutaneous electrical nerve stimulation (TENS) involves the transmission of low-voltage electrical current to the skin via surface electrodes. It is most widely used for childbirth in Scandinavia and the United Kingdom.[47] A systematic review of eight trials in more than 700 women concluded that evidence for TENS-mediated reduction in pain during labor is weak.[80] Women who use TENS may be less likely to use other analgesic interventions; however, the systematic review suggested that the number needed to treat was 14.[80] There appears to be no effect on the

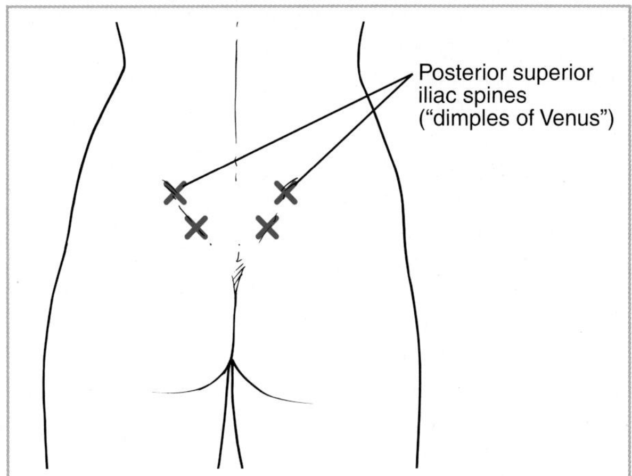

FIGURE 21-3 Placement of intradermal water blocks (x): Approximately 0.05 to 0.1 mL of sterile water is injected intradermally to form a small bleb over each posterior superior iliac spine and at 3 cm below and 1 cm medial to each spine on both sides of the back (i.e., for a total of four injections). The exact locations of the injections do not appear to be critical to the block success. (From Simkin P. Update on nonpharmacologic approaches to relieve labor pain and prevent suffering. J Midwifery Womens Health 2004; 49:489-504.)

duration of labor or the incidence of instrumental delivery. Pain perception was unchanged in most studies. In a later study, Chao et al.[81] evaluated the use of TENS at specific acupuncture points and observed a reduction in pain perception more commonly in the study group than in the control group.

Advantages of TENS are that it is easy to use and discontinue, is noninvasive, and has no demonstrable harmful effects on the fetus. The only stated disadvantage is the occasional interference with electronic fetal heart rate monitoring. Patients tend to rate the device as helpful, despite the fact that it does not reduce the use of additional analgesics. Widespread use of TENS does not seem warranted.

Acupuncture/Acupressure

Traditional Chinese medicine includes extensive use of acupuncture. Given that acupuncture can provide analgesia, there is interest in its use for intrapartum analgesia, although this is not a traditional use of the method. Early observational reports described conflicting results as to the efficacy of intrapartum acupuncture. Given the historic lack of use of acupuncture in obstetric patients, there is a lack of standardization of the acupuncture points to be stimulated.

Several randomized, controlled trials have compared "real" acupuncture to "false" or "minimal" acupuncture using shallow insertion of needles in non-acupuncture points,[82,83] whereas other investigators have used a control group that did not receive acupuncture.[84,85] Four randomized trials found that pain scores were lower in women randomly assigned to receive acupuncture treatment, as was the rate of use of other modes of analgesia (e.g., epidural and systemic meperidine).[82-85] These results suggest that acupuncture may hold promise for the treatment of labor pain.[82-85] Hantoushzadeh et al.[83] also observed a shorter duration of the active phase of labor and a reduction in use of oxytocin in the acupuncture group. No adverse maternal or fetal effects were identified.

A randomized, controlled trial of acupressure (treatment) compared with touch (control) at the SP6 acupoint found lower pain scores and a shorter duration of labor in the acupressure group.[86] A meta-analysis of three acupuncture trials concluded that acupuncture may hold promise for labor analgesia; however, larger studies are required for definitive conclusions.[87] All of the randomized, controlled acupuncture studies were performed outside the United States, in countries (primarily Scandinavian) in which the use of neuraxial labor analgesia is less widespread than in the United States. Also, the use of acupuncture requires trained personnel. (Scandinavian midwives have been trained to administer acupuncture.) For these reasons it is unlikely that either acupuncture or acupressure will gain widespread acceptance in the United States for intrapartum analgesia.

Hypnosis

The use of hypnosis for obstetric analgesia is not new.[88] Early proponents touted safety for the mother and the fetus, lower analgesic requirements, and shorter labor as the major advantages of intrapartum hypnosis. Whether hypnosis differs substantially from other childbirth preparation techniques is an unresolved controversy. Fee and Reilley[89] concluded that the breathing and relaxation exercises used in childbirth preparation do not represent a hypnotic trance; support for their conclusion is provided by the successful teaching of childbirth preparation exercises to women who are not susceptible to hypnosis. However, women susceptible to hypnosis may achieve a state much like a hypnotic trance when using the same exercises.

Instruction in the techniques of self-hypnosis before the onset of labor or, alternatively, availability of the hypnotist during labor is time consuming for the hypnotist. Proponents previously suggested that successful hypnosis training should begin early in the third trimester. Rock et al.[90] found that hypnosis could be introduced to untrained, nonvolunteer patients during labor. On average, this maneuver added approximately 45 minutes of care; however, all but 3 of 22 patients in the experimental group required additional analgesia. Some studies found that hypnosis did not decrease analgesic requirements,[91] but others noted that hypnosis resulted in lower analgesic requirements and a tendency toward less perineal trauma.[92]

Childbirth preparation and hypnosis seem to have similar effects on obstetric outcome. Harmon et al.[93] combined hypnosis and skill mastery with childbirth education. Experimental patients with a high susceptibility to hypnosis demonstrated less use of opioid, tranquilizer, and oxytocic medications; shorter first and second stages of labor; and a higher incidence of spontaneous delivery. Patients with a low susceptibility to hypnosis did not gain substantial advantage from the addition of hypnosis to the routine childbirth education provided for the control group.

In summary, hypnosis has at least the following three limitations: (1) antepartum training sessions are required, (2) trained hypnotherapists must be available during labor, and (3) it offers no clear benefit. Therefore hypnosis is unlikely to attain widespread use during childbirth.

IMPLICATIONS FOR ANESTHESIA PROVIDERS

Childbirth preparation classes and nonpharmacologic analgesic techniques are not comparable with regional analgesia/anesthesia for the relief of labor pain. Thus some might wonder whether it is important or useful for anesthesia providers to have knowledge of these techniques. If our only obligation to the obstetric patient is a technical one (i.e., to eliminate pain safely with the use of neuraxial anesthesia), knowledge of these techniques is, perhaps, superfluous. However, the practice of obstetric anesthesia should not be limited to the performance of pain-relieving procedures; our contributions to the care of the obstetric patient and her family should extend beyond the administration of neuraxial anesthesia.

Much has been written in professional and lay journals concerning the "proper" childbirth experience. Each patient's expectations of labor influence her childbirth experience. Yarrow[94] described the results of a nonscientific poll of 72,000 readers of *Parents Magazine*, which revealed that there is an undeniable movement toward more family-centered maternity care. Women currently view childbirth from the perspective of educated consumers; they expect to have choices and a level of control during childbirth. We may not always be comfortable with this situation, but it is a reality for modern obstetric practice. Our challenge is to provide safe, effective analgesia in a nonthreatening, "homelike" environment. We are not solely responsible for a patient's childbirth experience, but our interactions with the patient, her family, and her obstetrician will influence her perception of childbirth.

Anesthesia providers must become effective educators as well as health care providers. Patients should have realistic expectations about the pain of labor and the variability of individual labor patterns. They should be encouraged to define "success" as a positive childbirth experience regardless of the mode of delivery, use of analgesia and anesthesia, or other arbitrary definitions. An obstetrician advised prospective mothers:

> *If you do end up choosing some form of pain relief during labor, do not feel inadequate if a friend had her baby without assistance. Some labors are more intense than others. Ultimately, holding your baby in your arms is more important than the method you used to bring her into the world.*[95]

Anesthesia providers may effectively provide similar advice. Unfortunately, anesthesia providers usually have little involvement in prenatal education classes. Our active participation in childbirth education classes may help patients receive more accurate information about the risks and benefits of analgesia/anesthesia for labor, vaginal delivery, and cesarean delivery. Anesthesia providers can encourage childbirth instructors to prepare patients for the unexpected and to acknowledge that the commonly described "typical" labor may, in fact, be atypical. Well-informed patients are more likely to accept the interventions that may become necessary during labor. Women with medical or obstetric diseases that may increase anesthetic risk should be encouraged to discuss these problems with an anesthesia provider before the onset of labor; thus, we must develop procedures to facilitate antepartum consultation. In summary, the active participation of the anesthesia provider in childbirth education will lead women to perceive the anesthesia provider as an integral part of the obstetric care team.

Some nonpharmacologic analgesic techniques may have benefits other than decreased pain perception. For example, some obstetricians and nurses believe that ambulation and subsequent squatting (or use of a birth cushion) shortens labor and increases the rate of spontaneous vaginal delivery. Even if this belief proves not to be true, many women prefer to be mobile during labor and, at a minimum, to retain the ability to walk to the bathroom. We should attempt to develop and use analgesic techniques that take advantage of these relatively simple maneuvers. For example, the use of intrathecal opioids during early labor allows for continued ambulation and the use of showers and/or tubs. Some techniques of epidural analgesia allow sitting with support. Finally, epidural analgesia/anesthesia does not eliminate the beneficial effects of other comfort measures, such as massage, and continued emotional support from family and friends.

Whenever possible, anesthesia providers should provide safe anesthetic care that is compatible with reasonable patient expectations. Future studies on the efficacy of childbirth education, nonpharmacologic analgesic techniques, and neuraxial anesthetic techniques should evaluate the patient's overall experience and satisfaction rather than limit assessment to the usual measures of obstetric outcome.[96] In an editorial that accompanied the study by Bloom et al.,[67] Cefalo and Bowes[97] commented, "In the end, the nurses, midwives, and physicians who attend a woman with compassion, understanding, and professionalism are the most important factors in the management of any labor."

KEY POINTS

- Childbirth preparation does not eliminate the pain of labor or substantially reduce the use of analgesia/anesthesia, but it does decrease the anxiety associated with labor.
- Emotional support provided by doulas reduces the use of analgesics, the length of labor, and the incidence of operative deliveries in selected patient populations.
- Biofeedback, transcutaneous electrical nerve stimulation, acupuncture, and hypnosis may provide mild to moderate analgesic benefits for some patients.
- Intradermal water injections may provide effective treatment for low back pain during labor.
- Anesthesia providers should become active participants in childbirth education. We should encourage and facilitate the honest discussion of the risks and benefits of the analgesic/anesthetic techniques available at our hospitals.
- No nonpharmacologic technique consistently provides the quality of intrapartum pain relief that is provided by neuraxial analgesia.

REFERENCES

1. Ziemer MM. Does prepared childbirth mean pain relief? Top Clin Nurs 1980; 2:19-26.
2. Melzack R. The McGill Pain Questionnaire: Major properties and scoring methods. Pain 1975; 1:277-99.
3. Reading AE. A comparison of the McGill Pain Questionnaire in chronic and acute pain. Pain 1982; 13:185-92.
4. Scott J, Huskisson EC. Graphic representation of pain. Pain 1976; 2:175-84.
5. Melzack R. The myth of painless childbirth (The John J. Bonica Lecture). Pain 1984; 19:321-37.
6. Melzack R, Taenzer P, Feldman P, Kinch RA. Labour is still painful after prepared childbirth training. Can Med Assoc J 1981; 125:357-63.
7. Speert H. Obstetrics and Gynecology in America: A History. Baltimore, Waverly Press, 1980.
8. Wertz RW, Wertz DC. Lying-in: A History of Childbirth in America. New York, The Free Press, 1977.
9. Devitt N. The transition from home to hospital birth in the United States, 1930-1960. Birth Fam J 1977; 4:47-58.
10. Beck NC, Geden EA, Brouder GT. Preparation for labor: A historical perspective. Psychosom Med 1979; 41:243-58.
11. Dick-Read G. Childbirth Without Fear: The Principles and Practice of Natural Childbirth. New York, Harper & Brothers, 1944.
12. Dick-Read G. Natural Childbirth. London, Heinemann, 1933.
13. Lamaze F. Painless Childbirth: Psychoprophylactic Method. London, Burke, 1958.
14. Velvovsky IZ, Platonov K, Ploticher V, Shugom E. Painless Childbirth Through Psychoprophylaxis: Lectures for Obstetricians. Moscow, Foreign Languages Publishing House, 1960.
15. Karmel M. Thank You, Dr. Lamaze: A Mother's Experiences in Painless Childbirth. New York, Lippincott, 1959.
16. Karmel M. Thank You, Dr. Lamaze: A Mother's Experiences in Painless Childbirth. 2nd edition. New York, Harper & Row, 1981.
17. Leboyer F. Birth Without Violence. New York, Knopf, 1975.
18. Nelson NM, Enkin MW, Saigal S, et al. A randomized clinical trial of the Leboyer approach to childbirth. N Engl J Med 1980; 302:655-60.
19. Saigal S, Nelson NM, Bennett KJ, Enkin MW. Observations on the behavioral state of newborn infants during the first hour of life: A comparison of infants delivered by the Leboyer and conventional methods. Am J Obstet Gynecol 1981; 139:715-9.
20. Pitcock CD, Clark RB. From Fanny to Fernand: The development of consumerism in pain control during the birth process. Am J Obstet Gynecol 1992; 167:581-7.
21. Beck NC, Hall D. Natural childbirth: A review and analysis. Obstet Gynecol 1978; 52:371-9.
22. Lindell SG. Education for childbirth: A time for change. J Obstet Gynecol Neonat Nurs 1988; 17:108-12.
23. Lu MC, Prentice J, Yu SM, et al. Childbirth education classes: Sociodemographic disparities in attendance and the association of attendance with breastfeeding initiation. Matern Child Health J 2003; 7:87-93.
24. Nelson MK. The effect of childbirth preparation on women of different social classes. J Health Soc Behav 1982; 23:339-52.
25. Zacharias JF. Childbirth education classes: Effects on attitudes toward childbirth in high-risk indigent women. JOGN Nurs 1981; 10:265-7.
26. Copstick S, Hayes RW, Taylor KE, Morris NF. A test of a common assumption regarding the use of antenatal training during labour. J Psychosom Res 1985; 29:215-8.
27. Bernardini JY, Maloni JA, Stegman CE. Neuromuscular control of childbirth-prepared women during the first stage of labor. JOGN Nurs 1983; 12:105-11.
28. Stewart DE. Psychiatric symptoms following attempted natural childbirth. Can Med Assoc J 1982; 127:713-6.
29. Guzman Sanchez A, Segura Ortega L, Panduro Baron JG. Psychological reaction due to failure using the Lamaze method. Int J Gynaecol Obstet 1985; 23:343-6.
30. Behan M. Childbirth machismo. Parenting. 1988; April:53-7.
31. Crittendon D. Knock me out with a truck. Wall Street Journal, November 6, 1992: A14.
32. Hetherington SE. A controlled study of the effect of prepared childbirth classes on obstetric outcomes. Birth 1990; 17:86-90.
33. Rogers CH. Type of medications used in labor by Lamaze and non-Lamaze prepared subjects and the effect on newborn Apgar scores using analysis of variance: A thesis. Huntsville, University of Alabama (Huntsville), 1981:43.
34. Scott JR, Rose NB. Effect of psychoprophylaxis (Lamaze preparation) on labor and delivery in primiparas. N Engl J Med 1976; 294:1205-7.
35. Zax M, Sameroff AJ, Farnum JE. Childbirth education, maternal attitudes, and delivery. Am J Obstet Gynecol 1975; 123:185-90.
36. Hughey MJ, McElin TW, Young T. Maternal and fetal outcome of Lamaze-prepared patients. Obstet Gynecol 1978; 51:643-7.
37. Delke I, Minkoff H, Grunebaum A. Effect of Lamaze childbirth preparation on maternal plasma beta-endorphin immunoreactivity in active labor. Am J Perinatol 1985; 2:317-9.
38. Brewin C, Bradley C. Perceived control and the experience of childbirth. Br J Clin Psychol 1982; 21:263-9.
39. Patton LL, English EC, Hambleton JD. Childbirth preparation and outcomes of labor and delivery in primiparous women. J Fam Pract 1985; 20:375-8.
40. Sturrock WA, Johnson JA. The relationship between childbirth education classes and obstetric outcome. Birth 1990; 17:82-5.
41. Campbell D, Scott KD, Klaus MH, Falk M. Female relatives or friends trained as labor doulas: Outcomes at 6 to 8 weeks postpartum. Birth 2007; 34:220-7.
42. Geden E, Beck NC, Brouder G, et al. Self-report and psychophysiological effects of Lamaze preparation: An analogue of labor pain. Res Nurs Health 1985; 8:155-65.
43. Geden EA, Beck NC, Anderson JS, et al. Effects of cognitive and pharmacologic strategies on analogued labor pain. Nurs Res 1986; 35:301-6.
44. Manderino MA, Bzdek VM. Effects of modeling and information on reactions to pain: A childbirth-preparation analogue. Nurs Res 1984; 33:9-14.
45. Worthington EL Jr, Martin GA. A laboratory analysis of response to pain after training three Lamaze techniques. J Psychosom Res 1980; 24:109-16.
46. Whipple B, Josimovich JB, Komisaruk BR. Sensory thresholds during the antepartum, intrapartum and postpartum periods. Int J Nurs Stud 1990; 27:213-21.
47. Simkin P, Bolding A. Update on nonpharmacologic approaches to relieve labor pain and prevent suffering. J Midwifery Womens Health 2004; 49:489-504.
48. Huntley AL, Coon JT, Ernst E. Complementary and alternative medicine for labor pain: A systematic review. Am J Obstet Gynecol 2004; 191:36-44.
49. Gentz BA. Alternative therapies for the management of pain in labor and delivery. Clin Obstet Gynecol 2001; 44:704-32.
50. Bertsch TD, Nagishima-Whalen L, Dykeman S, et al. Labor support by first-time fathers: Direct observations. J Psychosom Obstet Gynecol 1990; 11:251-60.
51. Henneborn WJ, Cogan R. The effect of husband participation on reported pain and probability of medication during labor and birth. J Psychosom Res 1975; 19:215-22.
52. Hofmeyr GJ, Nikodem VC, Wolman WL, et al. Companionship to modify the clinical birth environment: Effects on progress and perceptions of labour, and breastfeeding. Br J Obstet Gynaecol 1991; 98:756-64.
53. Kennell J, Klaus M, McGrath S, et al. Continuous emotional support during labor in a US hospital: A randomized controlled trial. JAMA 1991; 265:2197-2201.
54. Klaus MH, Kennell JH, Robertson SS, Sosa R. Effects of social support during parturition on maternal and infant morbidity. Br Med J (Clin Res Ed) 1986; 293:585-7.
55. Campbell DA, Lake MF, Falk M, Backstrand JR. A randomized control trial of continuous support in labor by a lay doula. J Obstet Gynecol Neonatal Nurs 2006; 35:456-64.
56. Hodnett ED, Gates S, Hofmeyr GJ, Sakala C. Continuous support for women during childbirth. Cochrane Database Syst Rev 2007; (3): CD003766.

57. Hodnett ED, Lowe NK, Hannah ME, et al. Effectiveness of nurses as providers of birth labor support in North American hospitals: A randomized controlled trial. JAMA 2002; 288:1373-81.
58. Birch E. The experience of touch received during labor: Postpartum perceptions of therapeutic value. J Nurse Midwifery 1986; 31:270-6.
59. Chang MY, Wang SY, Chen CH. Effects of massage on pain and anxiety during labour: A randomized controlled trial in Taiwan. J Adv Nurs 2002; 38:68-73.
60. Penny KS. Postpartum perceptions of touch received during labor. Res Nurs Health 1979; 2:9-16.
61. Cammu H, Clasen K, Van Wettere L, Derde MP. 'To bathe or not to bathe' during the first stage of labor. Acta Obstet Gynecol Scand 1994; 73:468-72.
62. Eckert K, Turnbull D, MacLennan A. Immersion in water in the first stage of labor: A randomized controlled trial. Birth 2001; 28:84-93.
63. Rush J, Burlock S, Lambert K, et al. The effects of whirlpool baths in labor: A randomized, controlled trial. Birth 1996; 23:136-43.
64. Cluett ER, Pickering RM, Getliffe K, St George Saunders NJ. Randomised controlled trial of labouring in water compared with standard of augmentation for management of dystocia in first stage of labour. BMJ 2004; 328:314.
65. Cluett ER, Nikodem VC, McCandlish RE, Burns EE. Immersion in water in pregnancy, labour and birth. Cochrane Database Syst Rev 2004; (21):CD000111.
66. Simkin PP, O'Hara M. Nonpharmacologic relief of pain during labor: Systematic reviews of five methods. Am J Obstet Gynecol 2002; 186:S131-59.
67. Bloom SL, McIntire DD, Kelly MA, et al. Lack of effect of walking on labor and delivery. N Engl J Med 1998; 339:76-9.
68. Nageotte MP, Larson D, Rumney PJ, et al. Epidural analgesia compared with combined spinal-epidural analgesia during labor in nulliparous women. N Engl J Med 1997; 337:1715-9.
69. Collis RE, Harding SA, Morgan BM. Effect of maternal ambulation on labour with low-dose combined spinal-epidural analgesia. Anaesthesia 1999; 54:535-9.
70. Gardosi J, Hutson N, Lynch C. Randomised, controlled trial of squatting in the second stage of labour. Lancet 1989; 2(8654):74-7.
71. Gupta JK, Leal CB, Johnson N, Lilford RJ. Squatting in second stage of labour. Lancet 1989; 2(8662):561-2.
72. Johnson N, Johnson VA, Gupta JK. Maternal positions during labor. Obstet Gynecol Surv 1991; 46:428-34.
73. Gupta JK, Glanville JN, Johnson N, et al. The effect of squatting on pelvic dimensions. Eur J Obstet Gynecol Reprod Biol 1991; 42:19-22.
74. Shannahan MK, Cottrell BH. The effects of birth chair delivery on maternal perceptions. J Obstet Gynecol Neonatal Nurs 1989; 18:323-6.
75. Stewart P, Spiby H. A randomized study of the sitting position for delivery using a newly designed obstetric chair. Br J Obstet Gynaecol 1989; 96:327-33.
76. Waldenstrom U, Gottvall K. A randomized trial of birthing stool or conventional semirecumbent position for second-stage labor. Birth 1991; 18:5-10.
77. Gupta JK, Hofmeyr GJ. Position for women during second stage of labour. Cochrane Database Syst Rev. 2004; (1):CD002006.
78. St James-Roberts I, Chamberlain G, Haran FJ, Hutchinson CM. Use of electromyographic and skin-conductance biofeedback relaxation training to facilitate childbirth in primiparae. J Psychosom Res 1982; 26:455-62.
79. Duchene P. Effects of biofeedback on childbirth pain. J Pain Symptom Manage 1989; 4:117-23.
80. Carroll D, Tramer M, McQuay H, et al. Transcutaneous electrical nerve stimulation in labour pain: A systematic review. Br J Obstet Gynaecol 1997; 104:169-75.
81. Chao AS, Chao A, Wang TH, et al. Pain relief by applying transcutaneous electrical nerve stimulation (TENS) on acupuncture points during the first stage of labor: A randomized double-blind placebo-controlled trial. Pain 2007; 127:214-20.
82. Skilnand E, Fossen D, Heiberg E. Acupuncture in the management of pain in labor. Acta Obstet Gynecol Scand 2002; 81:943-8.
83. Hantoushzadeh S, Alhusseini N, Lebaschi AH. The effects of acupuncture during labour on nulliparous women: A randomised controlled trial. Aust N Z J Obstet Gynaecol 2007; 47:26-30.
84. Ramnero A, Hanson U, Kihlgren M. Acupuncture treatment during labour—a randomised controlled trial. Br J Obstet Gynaecol 2002; 109:637-44.
85. Nesheim BI, Kinge R, Berg B, et al. Acupuncture during labor can reduce the use of meperidine: A controlled clinical study. Clin J Pain 2003; 19:187-91.
86. Lee MK, Chang SB, Kang DH. Effects of SP6 acupressure on labor pain and length of delivery time in women during labor. J Altern Complement Med 2004; 10:959-65.
87. Smith CA, Collins CT, Cyna AM, Crowther CA. Complementary and alternative therapies for pain management in labour. Cochrane Database Syst Rev 2006; (4):CD003521.
88. August R. Hypnosis in Childbirth. New York, 1961.
89. Fee AF, Reilley RR. Hypnosis in obstetrics: A review of techniques. J Am Soc Psychosom Dent Med 1982; 29:17-29.
90. Rock NL, Shipley TE, Campbell C. Hypnosis with untrained, nonvolunteer patients in labor. Int J Clin Exp Hypn 1969; 17:25-36.
91. Freeman RM, Macaulay AJ, Eve L, et al. Randomised trial of self hypnosis for analgesia in labour. Br Med J (Clin Res Ed) 1986; 292:657-8.
92. Letts PJ, Baker PR, Ruderman J, Kennedy K. The use of hypnosis in labor and delivery: A preliminary study. J Womens Health Gend Based Med 1993; 2:335-41.
93. Harmon TM, Hynan MT, Tyre TE. Improved obstetric outcomes using hypnotic analgesia and skill mastery combined with childbirth education. J Consult Clin Psychol 1990; 58:525-30.
94. Yarrow L. Giving birth: 72,000 moms tell all. Parents 1992; 67:148-59.
95. Stevenson-Smith F, Salmon D. Pain relief during labor. Parents 1993; 68:127.
96. MacArthur C, Lewis M, Knox EG. Evaluation of obstetric analgesia and anaesthesia: Long-term maternal recollections. Int J Obstet Anesth 1993; 2:3-11.
97. Cefalo RC, Bowes WA Jr. Managing labor—never walk alone. N Engl J Med 1998; 339:117-8.

Chapter 22

Systemic Analgesia: Parenteral and Inhalational Agents

Roshan Fernando, FRCA
Tanya Jones, M.B.Ch.B., MRCP, FRCA

Systemic drugs have been used to diminish the pain of childbirth since 1847, when James Young Simpson used diethyl ether to anesthetize a parturient with a deformed pelvis. A heightened awareness of neonatal effects and the greater desire of women to actively participate in childbirth have prompted physicians to abandon heavy sedation during labor and also to discontinue the administration of general anesthesia during uncomplicated vaginal delivery. Epidural and spinal analgesia provide effective maternal pain relief with few adverse effects on the infant. These techniques have replaced systemic drugs as the preferred method of intrapartum analgesia for many parturients.

Epidural analgesia is now used more commonly than parenteral analgesia in laboring women in the United States. Bucklin et al.[1] published the results of a survey of obstetric anesthesia practice in the United States in 2001 and compared the results with those of similar surveys in 1981 and 1992. They noted an increase in the use of neuraxial techniques for labor analgesia, with labor epidural analgesia rates of 34% to 61% depending on the size of the labor and delivery unit. Of interest, the survey identified greater availability of neuraxial anesthesia in smaller facilities than in previous years. The researchers also noted a corresponding decrease in the number of women who received parenteral drugs for labor analgesia (i.e., between 34% and 42% in 2001 versus 50% in 1981).

In the United Kingdom, the NHS Maternity Statistics of 2005-2006[2] showed that a third of parturients received neuraxial techniques during labor and delivery. A 1997 Canadian survey by Breen et al.[3] found that epidural analgesia was available in 93% of the community-based practices and in 97% of the university-based practices.

The use of systemic analgesia, however, remains common practice in many institutions in many parts of the world, for several reasons. Many women labor and deliver in environments where safe neuraxial labor analgesia is not available. Some women decline neuraxial analgesia or choose to receive systemic analgesia in the early stages of labor. Finally, some women may have a medical condition that contraindicates neuraxial procedures (e.g., coagulopathy) or contributes to a technically difficult or impossible procedure (e.g., lumbar spine surgery).

PARENTERAL OPIOID ANALGESIA

Opioids are the most widely used systemic medications for labor analgesia. Use of these drugs does not require specialized equipment or personnel. Opioid analgesia allows the parturient to better tolerate the pain of labor, but systemic opioids typically do not provide complete analgesia. Systemic opioids have become less popular because of their frequency of maternal side effects (e.g., nausea, vomiting, delayed gastric emptying, dysphoria, drowsiness, hypoventilation) and potential for adverse neonatal effects.

Although systemic opioids have long been used for labor analgesia, little scientific evidence suggests that one drug is intrinsically better than another for this purpose; most often the selection of an opioid is based on institutional tradition and/or personal preference (Table 22-1). The efficacy of systemic opioid analgesia and the incidence of side effects are largely dose dependent rather than drug dependent.

Because of their lipid solubility and low molecular weight (less than 500 daltons), all opioids easily cross the placenta by diffusion and are associated with risk of neonatal respiratory depression and neurobehavioral changes. Metabolism and elimination of drugs are slower in neonates than in adults, and opioids may also have effects *in utero*. The blood-brain barrier is less well developed in the fetus and neonate than in the adult. Opioids may cause decreased

TABLE 22-1 Systemic Opioids for Labor Analgesia

Drug	Usual Dose	Onset	Duration (hr)	Comments
Meperidine	25-50 mg IV 50-100 mg IM	5-10 min IV 40-45 min IM	2-3	Has an active metabolite with a long half-life Maximal neonatal depression 1-4 hr after dose
Morphine	2-5 mg IV 5-10 mg IM	3-5 min IV 20-40 min IM	3-4	More neonatal respiratory depression than meperidine Has an active metabolite
Diamorphine	5-7.5 mg IV/IM	5-10 min IM	90 min	Morphine pro-drug More euphoria, less nausea than with morphine
Fentanyl	25-50 μg IV 100 μg IM	2-3 min IV 10 min IM	30-60 min	Usually administered as an infusion or by PCA Accumulates during an infusion Less neonatal depression than with meperidine
Nalbuphine	10-20 mg IV/IM	2-3 min IV 15 min IM/SQ	3-6	Opioid agonist/antagonist Ceiling effect on respiratory depression Lower neonatal neurobehavioral scores than with meperidine
Butorphanol	1-2 mg IV/IM	5-10 min IV 10-30 min IM	3-4	Opioid agonist/antagonist Ceiling effect on respiratory depression
Meptazinol	100 mg IM	15 min IM	2-3	Partial opioid agonist Less sedation and respiratory depression than with other opioids
Pentazocine	20-40 mg IV/IM	2-3 min IV 5-20 min IM/SQ	2-3	Opioid agonist/antagonist Psychomimetic effects possible
Tramadol	50-100 mg IV/IM	10 min IM	2-3	Less efficacy than with meperidine More side effects than meperidine

IM, intramuscular; IV, intravenous; PCA, patient-controlled analgesia; SQ, subcutaneous.

variability of the fetal heart rate (FHR); however, this change usually does not reflect a worsening of fetal oxygenation or acid-base status. The likelihood of neonatal respiratory depression depends on the dose and timing of opioid administration. Even in the absence of obvious neonatal depression at birth, subtle changes in neonatal neurobehavior may be present for several days.[4] The long-term clinical significance of these changes, however, is unclear. Reynolds et al.[5] performed a meta-analysis of studies comparing epidural analgesia with systemic opioid analgesia using meperidine, butorphanol, or fentanyl. The researchers concluded that lumbar epidural analgesia was associated with better neonatal acid-base status. A multicenter randomized controlled trial comparing patient-controlled analgesia (PCA) using a parenteral opioid with patient-controlled epidural analgesia (PCEA) using a local anesthetic combined with an opioid demonstrated an increased need for active neonatal resuscitation in the parenteral opioid group (52% versus 31%).[6]

Opioids may be administered as intermittent bolus doses or as PCA. Bolus doses are used more commonly, but newer synthetic opioids may be more suitable for PCA.

INTERMITTENT BOLUS PARENTERAL OPIOID ANALGESIA

Opioids may be given intermittently via subcutaneous, intramuscular, or intravenous administration. The route and timing of administration influence maternal uptake and placental transfer. Subcutaneous and intramuscular injections have the advantage of simplicity but are painful. Absorption varies with the site of injection, and injection is followed by a delay in the onset of analgesia; thus subcutaneous or intramuscular injection leads to analgesia of variable onset, quality, and duration. Advantages of intravenous administration are (1) less variability in the peak plasma concentration of drug; (2) faster onset of analgesia; and (3) the ability to titrate dose to effect. Thus the intravenous route is generally preferred.

Meperidine

Meperidine (pethidine) is the most commonly used opioid for labor analgesia worldwide. Eighty-four percent of labor and delivery units in the United Kingdom prescribe meperidine for labor analgesia.[7] The usual dose is 100 mg intramuscularly, and this dose may be repeated once (4 hours later). Onset of analgesia occurs in 45 minutes, with a 2- to 3-hour duration. Familiarity, ease of administration, low cost, and lack of evidence that alternative opioids show any benefit over meperidine encourage its widespread use.

There have been significant doubts as to the efficacy of meperidine. Some studies have demonstrated that less than 20% of women obtain satisfactory pain relief[8]; however, the first randomized, placebo-controlled, double-blind study of intramuscular meperidine (100 mg) for labor analgesia identified some benefit.[9] The study was terminated prematurely when interim analysis revealed that meperidine provided significantly greater reduction in visual analog scale (VAS) pain scores than placebo. The analgesic effect was modest, however, with a median change in VAS pain score of 11 mm (95% CI of 2 to 26 mm, using a 100-mm scale) at 30 minutes.

Maternal, fetal, and neonatal side effects are ongoing concerns with meperidine administration. Maternal nausea, vomiting, and sedation are common. Fetal and neonatal effects relate to the pharmacokinetic properties of meperidine. A synthetic opioid that readily crosses the placenta by passive diffusion, meperidine equilibrates between the maternal and fetal compartments within 6 minutes.[10] Decreased FHR variability occurs 25 to 40 minutes after administration and resolves within an hour.[11] Maternal half-life is 2.5 to 3 hours, but neonatal half-life is prolonged, at 18 to 23 hours.[12]

Meperidine is metabolized in the liver to produce normeperidine, a pharmacologically active metabolite that is a potent respiratory depressant. Normeperidine crosses the placenta. Additional normeperidine is formed as a result of fetal and neonatal metabolism of meperidine that has crossed the placenta. Normeperidine has a half-life of 60 hours in the neonate.[13]

Neonatal complications relate to the total dose of meperidine and the dose-delivery interval. Maximal fetal uptake of meperidine occurs 2 to 3 hours after maternal intramuscular administration, and studies have shown that infants born within this interval have an increased risk of respiratory depression.[14,15] Normeperidine accumulates after multiple doses or after a prolonged dose-delivery interval[16] and may be associated with altered neonatal neurobehavior, including reductions in duration of wakefulness and attentiveness, and impaired breast-feeding.[16-20]

The effect of meperidine on the progress of labor is contentious. Some obstetricians argue that it may prolong the latent phase of labor, but others administer meperidine to shorten the length of the first stage of labor in cases of dystocia. Sosa et al.[21] concluded that meperidine does not benefit labor in women with dystocia and should not be used for this indication because of the greater risk of adverse neonatal outcome compared with placebo.

Morphine

Several decades ago, morphine was administered in combination with scopolamine to provide “twilight sleep” during childbirth. Good analgesia was obtained at the expense of excessive maternal sedation and neonatal depression. Currently morphine is prescribed infrequently in labor but can be given at intramuscular doses of 5 to 10 mg or intravenous doses of 2 to 5 mg. The onset time is 20 to 40 minutes and 3 to 5 minutes, respectively, and the duration of analgesia is 3 to 4 hours.[22]

Morphine is metabolized by conjugation to morphine-3-glucuronide, the major inactive metabolite, and is excreted in the urine with 66% clearance in 6 hours.[23,24] Morphine-6-glucuronide, an active metabolite, is produced in smaller amounts. It has significant analgesic properties but is also a respiratory depressant.[25,26] Morphine rapidly crosses the placenta, and a fetal-to-maternal plasma concentration ratio of 0.96 is observed at 5 minutes.[27] The elimination half-life is longer in neonates than in adults. The propensity for drug to cross the blood-brain barrier appears to be higher in the fetus than in the adult brain. Like other opioids, morphine decreases FHR variability. Pregnancy alters morphine pharmacokinetics. Greater plasma clearance, shorter elimination half-life, and earlier peak metabolite levels occur in pregnant women than in nonpregnant women. In theory, these characteristics should reduce fetal exposure. Indeed, one study observed no cases of neonatal depression, prompting the researchers to suggest that morphine use in labor should be reevaluated.[23]

Oloffson et al.[28] assessed the analgesic efficacy of intravenous morphine during labor (0.05 mg/kg every third contraction to a maximum dose of 0.2 mg/kg) and found clinically insignificant reductions in pain intensity. These investigators also compared intravenous morphine (up to 0.15 mg/kg) with intravenous meperidine (up to 1.5 mg/kg) and found that high pain scores were maintained in both groups despite high levels of sedation.[29]

Way et al.[30] showed that intramuscular morphine given to newborns caused greater respiratory depression than an equipotent dose of meperidine when response to CO_2 was measured. The investigators attributed this observation to a greater permeability of the neonatal brain to morphine.

Diamorphine

Diamorphine (3,6-diacetylmorphine, heroin) is a synthetic derivative of morphine used for labor analgesia in the United Kingdom. It has been reported to provide rapid, effective analgesia with more euphoria and less nausea and vomiting than morphine. It is used in 34% of labor and delivery units in the United Kingdom, and in some areas of the country, diamorphine is used more frequently than meperidine.[7]

Diamorphine is rapidly metabolized to 6-mono-acetylmorphine via hydrolytic ester cleavage.[31] This metabolite is more lipid soluble than morphine, a feature that accounts for the greater speed of onset. The metabolite 6-mono-acetylmorphine is responsible for a significant proportion of analgesic activity. It also crosses the placenta and is associated with respiratory depression. Further breakdown to morphine occurs, which is followed by conjugation in the liver.[32] A typical intramuscular dose of diamorphine is 5 to 7.5 mg. Higher doses have been linked to neonatal respiratory depression.[33]

Rawal et al.[33] investigated the effects of a single dose of diamorphine on free morphine concentrations in the umbilical cord at delivery. After intramuscular administration of diamorphine 7.5 mg, there was evidence of rapid fetal exposure to morphine and a significant negative correlation between the dose-delivery interval and umbilical cord blood morphine levels. There was a nonsignificant correlation between higher morphine concentrations and lower 1-minute Apgar scores (and the need for neonatal resuscitation). This finding suggests that infants born shortly after maternal diamorphine administration are at greater risk for depression.

Fairlie et al.,[34] comparing intramuscular meperidine (150 mg) with diamorphine (7.5 mg), found that significantly more women in the meperidine group reported no or poor pain relief at 60 minutes. The trial was small, but the results suggested that at the administered doses, diamorphine conferred some benefit over meperidine with regard to maternal side effects (notably vomiting) and neonatal condition as assessed by 1-minute Apgar scores. However, a large proportion of women in the two groups required second-line analgesia, suggesting poor efficacy for both drugs.

Fentanyl

Fentanyl is a highly lipid-soluble, highly protein-bound synthetic opioid with analgesic potency 100 times that of morphine and 800 times that of meperidine. Its rapid onset (peak effect at 3 to 4 minutes), short duration of action, and lack of active metabolites make it attractive for labor analgesia. Large doses of fentanyl may accumulate, however, and the context-sensitive half-life ($T_{1/2}$) of fentanyl (the time for the plasma concentration to decrease by 50% after cessation of an infusion that has achieved a steady-state plasma concentration) increases with infusion duration.

Fentanyl readily crosses the placenta, but the average umbilical-to-maternal concentration ratio remains low at 0.31. Eisele et al.[35] found intravenous fentanyl 1 μg/kg provided good analgesia with no appreciable hemodynamic effect and no adverse effects on Apgar scores, fetal acid-base status, or neurobehavioral scores at 2 and 24 hours. Rayburn et al.[36] administered intravenous fentanyl 50 to 100 μg as often as once per hour at maternal request during labor. All patients experienced transient analgesia (duration of 45 minutes) and sedation. Reduced FHR variability occurred, but there was no difference in Apgar scores, respiratory depression, or Neurologic and Adaptive Capacity Scores (NACS) at 2 to 4 hours or 24 hours between infants whose mothers received fentanyl and those whose mothers did not. Rayburn et al.[37] also compared intravenous fentanyl (50 to 100 μg every hour) with an equi-analgesic dose of meperidine (25 to 50 mg every 2 to 3 hours). The researchers found less sedation, vomiting, and neonatal naloxone administration with fentanyl, but they observed no difference between groups in NACS. The two groups had similarly high pain scores, suggesting that both drugs have poor analgesic efficacy.

Nalbuphine

Nalbuphine is a mixed agonist-antagonist opioid analgesic. Nalbuphine and morphine are of similar potency and result in respiratory depression at equi-analgesic doses. However, nalbuphine demonstrates a ceiling effect for respiratory depression with increasing doses. Maximal respiratory depression occurs with a 30-mg dose in the average adult. Nalbuphine appears to be more effective in women than in men. Concerns that it may have an anti-analgesic affect led to the withdrawal of nalbuphine in the United Kingdom in 2003.

The usual dose is 10 to 20 mg every 4 to 6 hours. The onset of analgesia occurs within 2 to 3 minutes of intravenous administration and within 15 minutes of intramuscular or subcutaneous administration. The duration of analgesia ranges from 3 to 6 hours.

Wilson et al.[38] performed a randomized, double-blind comparison of intramuscular nalbuphine 20 mg and meperidine 100 mg for labor analgesia. Nalbuphine was associated with less nausea and vomiting but more maternal sedation. Analgesia was comparable in the two groups. Neonatal neurobehavioral scores at 2 to 4 hours were lower in the nalbuphine group, but there was no difference at 24 hours. The mean umbilical vein-to-maternal concentration ratio was higher for nalbuphine (mean ± SEM, 0.78 ± 0.03) than meperidine (0.61 ± 0.02).

Nicolle et al.[39] evaluated transplacental transfer of nalbuphine and neonatal pharmacokinetics. They found a high fetal-to-maternal ratio (0.74), which did not correlate with the maternal dose. The estimated neonatal half-life was 4.1 hours, which is greater than the adult half-life and, more importantly, greater than the half-life of naloxone. Reduction in FHR variability occurred in 54% of fetuses, lasting 10 to 35 minutes. Analgesia was rated as effective by 54% of parturients.

Giannina et al.[40] compared the effects of nalbuphine and meperidine on intrapartum FHR tracings. Nalbuphine significantly reduced both the number of accelerations and FHR variability. Meperidine had little significant effect. Case reports of a variety of suboptimal FHR changes have been reported after maternal administration of nalbuphine.

Butorphanol

Butorphanol is an opioid with agonist-antagonist properties that resemble those of pentazocine. It is five times as potent as morphine and 40 times as potent as meperidine.[41,42] The typical dose during labor is 1 to 2 mg intravenously or intramuscularly. Ninety-five percent of butorphanol is metabolized in the liver to inactive metabolites. Excretion is primarily renal. Butorphanol and morphine result in similar respiratory depression at equi-analgesic doses, but as occurs with nalbuphine, a ceiling effect is noted with butorphanol. Butorphanol 2 mg produces respiratory depression similar to that with morphine 10 mg or meperidine 70 mg. However, butorphanol 4 mg results in less respiratory depression than morphine 20 mg or meperidine 140 mg.[41,42]

Maduska and Hajghassemali[43] compared intramuscular butorphanol (1 to 2 mg) with meperidine (40 to 80 mg) and found similar efficacy of labor analgesia. They noted rapid placental transfer of butorphanol, with a mean umbilical vein-to-maternal concentration ratio of 0.84 at 30 to 210 minutes after injection (similar to meperidine). No differences in FHR tracings, Apgar scores, time to sustained respiration, or umbilical cord blood gas measurements were found.

Similarly, Hodgkinson et al.[44] performed a double-blind assessment of intravenous butorphanol (1 or 2 mg) and meperidine (40 or 80 mg) for labor analgesia. Both drugs provided adequate maternal pain relief, but there were fewer maternal side effects (e.g., nausea, vomiting, dizziness) in the women who received butorphanol. There was no difference between groups in Apgar scores or neonatal neurobehavioral scores. Finally, Quilligan et al.,[45] in a double-blind comparison of intravenous butorphanol (1 or 2 mg) and meperidine (40 or 80 mg) during labor, noted better analgesia at 30 minutes and 1 hour after the administration of butorphanol. There was no difference in Apgar scores between the two groups of infants.

Nelson and Eisenach[46] investigated the possible synergistic effect of giving both intravenous butorphanol and meperidine; they compared the administration of both drugs with administration of either drug alone. All three treatment groups showed a similar reduction in pain intensity (25% to 35%), and there was no difference among groups in maternal side effects or Apgar scores. The investigators concluded that there was no therapeutic benefit to combining the two drugs.

Butorphanol offers analgesia with some sedation, an effect similar to that of the combination of meperidine and a phenothiazine. It has a short half-life and inactive metabolites. These properties, combined with a ceiling effect on maternal respiratory depression and favorable neurobehavioral outcomes in the neonate, make butorphanol a useful agent for labor analgesia.

Meptazinol

Meptazinol is a partial opioid agonist specific to μ_1-opioid receptors. It has a rapid onset (i.e., 15 minutes after intramuscular administration), and a duration of action similar to that of meperidine. The usual intramuscular dose is 100 mg. Its partial agonist activity is thought to result in less sedation, respiratory depression, and risk of dependence than the activity of other opioid agonists.[47]

Meptazinol is metabolized by glucuronidation in the liver, a process that is more mature in neonates than the metabolic pathway for meperidine. A theoretical advantage of meptazinol is that its rapid elimination may minimize the risk of neonatal depression. The neonatal half-life is 3.4 hours, and the adult half-life is 2.2 hours.[48]

Nicholas and Robson[49] compared intramuscular meptazinol 100 mg with meperidine 100 mg in a large randomized, blinded study. They demonstrated significantly better pain relief at 45 and 60 minutes and a trend toward fewer side effects with meptazinol than with meperidine (28% versus 35%). Use of meptazinol was associated with a higher rate of 1-minute Apgar scores greater than 7. Otherwise, there was no significant difference between groups in neonatal outcome.

Morrison et al.[50] did not find much benefit for meptazinol over meperidine in a large study of 1100 patients. Pain scores were similar for the two treatment groups at 60 minutes after intramuscular administration. Drowsiness was significantly less pronounced with meptazinol than with meperidine, but the incidence of vomiting was higher. FHR changes and neonatal outcomes (i.e., need for resuscitation, Apgar scores, suckling ability) were not different in the two groups. The overall use of naloxone was similar in the groups, but if the dose-delivery interval exceeded 180 minutes, significantly more neonates in the meperidine group required naloxone.

De Boer et al.[51] assessed blood gas and acid-base measurements in neonates following maternal intramuscular administration of meptazinol (1.5 mg/kg) or meperidine (1.5 mg/kg) during labor. Capillary blood gas measurements at 10 minutes of life showed significantly lower pH and higher Pa_{CO_2} in the meperidine group, although this difference resolved by 60 minutes. These findings suggest that meptazinol has less depressant effect on neonatal respiration.

In summary, meptazinol may have some benefit over meperidine in neonatal outcome, but it is not as widely used. The cost of meptazinol is considerably higher than that of meperidine. Meptazinol is not available in the United States.

Pentazocine

Pentazocine is a synthetic opioid with both agonist and weak antagonist properties. Pentazocine 30 to 60 mg is equipotent to morphine 10 mg. Peak analgesia occurs within 10 minutes after intravenous administration of pentazocine, whereas peak plasma levels occur 15 to 60 minutes after intramuscular administration.[52] A ceiling effect for respiratory depression occurs at doses of 40 to 60 mg. Clinical studies have demonstrated that single injections of meperidine 100 mg and pentazocine 40 to 45 mg produce similar degrees of neonatal respiratory depression. However, repeated maternal doses of pentazocine do not increase neonatal respiratory depression proportionately, whereas the respiratory depression with repeated doses of meperidine is cumulative.[53,54] Psychomimetic effects may occur with standard doses of pentazocine, but they occur more frequently after larger doses. The potential for psychomimetic side effects has limited the popularity of pentazocine in obstetrics.

Tramadol

An atypical, weak, synthetic opioid, tramadol has low μ-opioid receptor affinity but also exerts gamma-aminobutyric acid–ergic (GABA-ergic), noradrenergic, and serotonergic effects. Its potency is approximately 10% that of morphine. It causes no clinically significant respiratory depression at usual doses. Onset of analgesia occurs within 10 minutes of the intramuscular administration of tramadol 100 mg, and the duration of analgesia is approximately 2 hours. Tramadol has an elimination half-life of 6 hours. It is metabolized by the liver to an active metabolite, O-desmethyltramadol (M1), which has an elimination half-life of 9 hours.[55]

Claahsen-van der Grinten et al.[56] demonstrated high placental permeability for tramadol, with an umbilical vein-to-maternal concentration ratio of 0.97. Neonates possess complete hepatic capacity for metabolism of tramadol to its active metabolite M1. The elimination profile of M1 suggests a terminal half-life of 85 hours because of its requirement for renal elimination, which is an immature process in neonates. Neonatal outcome, assessed by Apgar score and NACS, was within normal limits and showed no correlation to tramadol or M1 concentrations. The single neonate who required naloxone, however, had the highest plasma concentration of tramadol.

Keskin et al.[57] compared intramuscular tramadol 100 mg with meperidine 100 mg for labor analgesia. Pain scores at 30 and 60 minutes were significantly lower in the meperidine group, and tramadol was associated with a higher incidence of nausea. There was no significant difference between groups in neonatal outcome, but more infants in the tramadol group required oxygen for respiratory distress and hypoxemia. The investigators concluded that meperidine provided superior analgesia to tramadol and was associated with a better side-effect profile.

PATIENT-CONTROLLED OPIOID ANALGESIA

Patient-controlled analgesia (PCA) is widely used in the management of postoperative pain. Although continuous intravenous infusion of opioids has been used for at least four decades, the growing popularity of PCA for postoperative analgesia has prompted the use of this technique for labor analgesia. A 2007 survey of United Kingdom practice showed that 49% of labor and delivery units offered PCA for labor analgesia.[58] Purported advantages of PCA are (1) superior pain relief with lower doses of drug; (2) less risk of maternal respiratory depression (compared with bolus intravenous administration); (3) less placental transfer of drug; (4) less need for antiemetic agents; and (5) higher patient satisfaction.[59] More frequent administration of small doses of drug should achieve a more stable plasma drug concentration and a more consistent analgesic effect.[59]

TABLE 22-2 Opioids Used for Intravenous Patient-Controlled Analgesia during Labor

Drug	Patient-Controlled Dose	Lockout Interval (min)
Meperidine	10-15 mg	8-20
Nalbuphine	1-3 mg	6-10
Fentanyl	10-25 μg	5-12
Remifentanil (bolus only)	0.4-0.5 μg/kg	2-3
Remifentanil (background infusion with bolus dose)	Infusion rate: 0.05 μg/kg/min Bolus dose: 0.25 μg/kg	2-3

PCA for labor is not without limitations. Despite frequent administration, small doses of opioid may not always be effective for the fluctuating intensity of labor pain, especially in the late first stage or second stage of labor.[59] Moreover, the risk to the fetus and neonate remains unclear; studies have used variable methods of neonatal assessment. Variable doses and lockout intervals have been used, including PCA with and without a continuous infusion. Meperidine, nalbuphine, fentanyl, and more recently, remifentanil, have been the opioids most commonly used for PCA. The most appropriate drug, dose, and dosing schedule have not, however, been defined (Table 22-2).

PCA offers an attractive alternative for labor analgesia in hospitals in which neuraxial anesthesia is unavailable or when it is contraindicated or unsuccessful. The mother can tailor the administration of analgesia to her individual needs. Although PCA may result in higher patient satisfaction than other methods of systemic opioid administration, most studies have not demonstrated reduced drug use or improved analgesia with PCA than with intravenous administration of an opioid by the obstetric nurse.

Meperidine

Isenor and Penny-McGillivray[60] compared intermittent intramuscular boluses of meperidine (50 to 100 mg every 2 hours) and meperidine PCA (background infusion 60 mg/hr; PCA bolus 25 mg, up to a maximum dose of 200 mg). Women in the PCA group received more meperidine and had lower pain scores than women in the control group.

However, even when controlling for dose, pain scores were lower in the PCA group. There was no difference in maternal side effects, FHR tracings, or Apgar scores between treatment groups in this small study.

Meperidine PCA may have disadvantages when compared with PCA using shorter-acting opioids. Volikas and Male[61] compared meperidine PCA (bolus 10 mg, lockout interval 5 minutes) with remifentanil PCA (bolus 0.5 μg/kg, lockout interval 2 minutes). The study was terminated after enrollment of 17 subjects because of concern about poor Apgar scores in the meperidine group (median 1- and 5-minute scores of 5.5 and 7.5, respectively). Blair et al.[62] also compared meperidine PCA (bolus 15 mg, lockout interval 10 minutes) with remifentanil PCA (bolus 40 μg, lockout interval 2 minutes). Visual analog pain scores were similar in the two groups, but NACS were significantly lower in the meperidine group.

Morphine and Diamorphine

There is concern that the use of morphine PCA for labor analgesia might result in the accumulation of the active metabolite, morphine-6-glucuronide, thus leading to an increased incidence of neonatal adverse events. No published studies have compared morphine PCA with intermittent bolus administration of morphine in laboring women. In one study, diamorphine PCA was associated with higher pain scores and lower satisfaction scores than intermittent intramuscular administration of diamorphine during labor.[63] Neither morphine nor diamorphine is used frequently for labor PCA.

Fentanyl

The pharmacokinetic profile of fentanyl (i.e., rapid onset, high potency, short duration, absence of active metabolites) makes it particularly suitable for PCA during labor and delivery. It is one of the most commonly used opioids for labor PCA. In the United Kingdom it is used in 26% of the units that offer PCA during labor.[58]

Rayburn et al.[64] compared fentanyl PCA (bolus 10 μg, lockout interval 12 minutes) to intermittent intravenous fentanyl (50 to 100 μg every hour) and found similar levels of analgesia and sedation in the two groups. Both groups had incomplete analgesia during late labor. Neonatal Apgar scores, naloxone requirements, and neurobehavioral scores were comparable. Morley-Forster and Weberpals [65] found a 44% incidence of moderate neonatal depression (1-minute Apgar score less than 6) in a retrospective review of 32 neonates whose mothers had received fentanyl PCA during labor. The total dose of fentanyl was significantly higher in the mothers of neonates who required naloxone than in those who did not (mean ± SD: 770 ± 233 μg versus 298 ± 287 μg, respectively).

Alfentanil

Alfentanil, a fentanyl derivative, is approximately 10 times less potent than fentanyl. It is less lipophilic and more protein bound. Its low volume of distribution and low pKa result in a rapid onset (within 1 minute), a short duration of action, and rapid clearance (elimination half-life of 90 minutes). Furthermore, its context-sensitive half-life is shorter than that of fentanyl. However, it has been associated with greater neonatal depression than meperidine PCA.[66] Morley-Forster et al.[67] compared alfentanil PCA (bolus 200 μg, lockout interval 5 minutes, basal infusion 200 μg/hr) to fentanyl PCA (bolus 20 μg, lockout interval 5 minutes, basal infusion 20 μg/hr). Alfentanil failed to provide adequate analgesia late in labor, when compared to fentanyl. There were no significant differences in maternal side effects or neonatal outcome. The authors concluded that alfentanil PCA was less effective than fentanyl at the prescribed doses and lockout intervals.

Nalbuphine

In one study patient satisfaction was increased with nalbuphine PCA (bolus 1 mg, lockout interval 6 to 10 minutes) compared to intermittent intravenous bolus administration (10 to 20 mg every 4 to 6 hours).[68] Analgesia and Apgar scores were similar between groups, and no neonates required naloxone.

Frank et al.[69] concluded that nalbuphine PCA (bolus 3 mg, lockout interval 10 minutes) provided better analgesia than meperidine PCA (bolus 15 mg, lockout interval 10 minutes). Maternal sedation scores were similar, and there was no difference in neonatal outcome as assessed by Apgar scores, time to sustained respiration, or neurobehavioral assessment at 6 to 10 hours after delivery.

Remifentanil

Remifentanil is an ultra-short acting synthetic μ_1-opioid receptor agonist. It has a rapid onset of action (brain-blood equilibration occurs in 1.2 to 1.4 minutes) and is rapidly metabolized by plasma and tissue esterases to an inactive metabolite.[70] The context-sensitive half-life is 3.5 minutes, irrespective of the duration of infusion. The effective analgesic half-life is 6 minutes, thus allowing effective analgesia for consecutive uterine contractions.[71] Plasma concentrations in pregnant patients are approximately half those found in nonpregnant patients. This difference may be due to the greater volume of distribution (larger blood volume and reduced protein binding), higher clearance (increased cardiac output and renal perfusion), and higher esterase activity in pregnant women. Remifentanil rapidly crosses the placenta; the umbilical vein-to-maternal concentration ratio is 0.85. However, the umbilical artery-to-vein concentration ratio is 0.29, demonstrating that the drug is rapidly redistributed and metabolized by the fetus.[72]

Remifentanil was introduced into obstetric analgesia practice a decade ago. Because of its pharmacokinetic profile, this agent has advantages over other opioids for labor PCA. Thirty-three percent of United Kingdom labor and delivery units that offer PCA are now using remifentanil.[58] This percentage is likely to increase as confidence with PCA remifentanil grows.

The efficacy of remifentanil has been assessed in comparison with that of many other analgesics. Thurlow et al.[73] compared remifentanil PCA (bolus 20 μg, lockout interval 3 minutes) to the most commonly used opioid analgesic, intramuscular meperidine 100 mg. Significantly lower pain scores were found in the remifentanil group (median pain score 48/100 versus 72/100, $P = .004$). Maternal side effects included mild sedation and more episodes of Sa_{O_2} less than 94% in the remifentanil group, but also less nausea and vomiting. No significant difference in neonatal Apgar scores was found. Volmanen et al.[74] performed a double-blind crossover trial (subjects used both analgesics in random order) comparing remifentanil PCA (bolus 0.4 μg/kg, lockout interval 1 minute) with 50% nitrous oxide analgesia. Pain scores were significantly lower with remifentanil, and there was no difference in maternal side effects except sedation with remifentanil.

Efficacy is related to remifentanil dose and the administration regimen. Remifentanil can be administered as a bolus with a lockout interval, as a continuous infusion, or as a combination of the two. Volikas et al.[75] found that a PCA bolus of 0.5 μg/kg with a lockout interval of 2 minutes was effective in 86% of subjects, and this regimen was associated with acceptable levels of maternal side effects and minimal neonatal side effects. The median effective remifentanil bolus dose was 0.4 μg/kg (0.2 to 0.8 μg/kg).[76] This was associated with numeric pain scores of approximately 3 to 5 (0 to 10 scale). However, Sa_{O_2} below 94% occurred in 10 of 17 subjects. Volmanen et al.[74] have suggested that pain scores are improved if the remifentanil PCA bolus dose is titrated to patient request rather than being fixed. This approach allows for interindividual variability in response to pain as well as in response to the escalation in pain intensity throughout the course of labor. With the bolus titration technique, median pain intensity difference was −4.2, compared with −1.5 for use of a fixed bolus dose of 0.4 μg/kg.[74,76]

Balki et al.[77] attempted to establish the ideal PCA remifentanil regimen by comparing a group who received a fixed bolus dose with a titratable background infusion and a group who received a fixed background infusion with a titratable bolus dose. The starting point was a background infusion of 0.025 μg/kg/min with a bolus dose of 0.25 μg/kg and a lockout interval of 2 minutes. Either the background infusion rate or the bolus dose was increased in a stepwise manner on patient request to a maximum infusion of 0.1 μg/kg/min or a maximum bolus dose of 1 μg/kg. Mean pain and satisfaction scores were similar in the two groups, as were the cumulative remifentanil doses. Only 1 of 20 study subjects eventually requested epidural analgesia. Neonatal side effects were similar, with only one infant having a 1-minute Apgar score less than 9. However, the incidence of maternal side effects was significantly higher in the escalating bolus group than in the escalating infusion group; they included drowsiness (100% versus 30%, respectively) and frequency of Sa_{O_2} below 95% (60% versus 40%). The researchers therefore advocated the use of a titrated background infusion (range 0.025 to 0.1 μg/kg/min) with a constant PCA bolus dose (0.25 μg/kg) and a lockout interval of 2 minutes.

Opioid doses are commonly restricted by the fear of side effects, often resulting in administration of ineffective doses. Volikas et al.[75] investigated the maternal and neonatal effects of remifentanil PCA (bolus 0.5 μg/kg, lockout interval 2 minutes) in 50 women. Drowsiness was the most common problem (44%), although drowsy women remained arousable to voice. There was no change from baseline in the incidence of nausea, and there was no evidence of cardiovascular instability. Five women had a decrease in heart rate greater than 15%, but none required intervention. No muscle rigidity or hypoventilation occurred, and the lowest recorded Sa_{O_2} was 93%. FHR changes occurred in 10 women 20 minutes after initiation of PCA, but again, none required intervention. Median 1- and 5-minute Apgar scores were 9 and 9, respectively, and umbilical cord blood gas measurements and neonatal neurologic examinations were within normal limits.

The encouraging results with remifentanil PCA led to the hypothesis that it may provide analgesia comparable to epidural analgesia. In a randomized, double-blind trial, Volmanen et al.[78] compared a titrated remifentanil PCA (mean effective bolus 0.5 μg/kg [range 0.3 to 0.7 μg/kg], lockout interval 1 minute) to lumbar epidural analgesia (20 mL of levobupivacaine 0.625 mg/mL and fentanyl 2 μg/mL). Median cervical dilation at initiation of analgesia was 4 cm. Twenty-six percent of women in the remifentanil group and 52% in the epidural group reported acceptable pain scores. Some women in the remifentanil group were reluctant to increase their doses further to achieve lower pain scores because of concern about sedation. Fifty-four percent of the remifentanil group required supplemental oxygen, an effect related to doses greater than 0.5 μg/kg. There was no difference between groups in fetal and neonatal outcomes. The investigators concluded that epidural analgesia is superior to "optimal" PCA.

In the United Kingdom, remifentanil is currently the most commonly used opioid for labor PCA.[58] It is not specifically approved for this use either in the United States or the United Kingdom. Remifentanil PCA requires strict adherence to local guidelines for safe practice (Box 22-1).

BOX 22-1 Guidelines for Patient-Controlled Anesthesia (PCA) with Remifentanil*

Eligibility

- Informed consent
- No opioids in the previous 4 hours
- Dedicated intravenous cannula for remifentanil administration

PCA Protocol

- PCA bolus: 40 μg
- Lockout interval: 2 min

Continuous Observations

- Sa_{O_2} (pulse oximetry)
- Nursing supervision: One-on-one

30-Minute Observations

- Respiratory rate
- Sedation score
- Pain score

Indications for Contacting the Anesthesia Provider

- Excessive sedation score (not arousable to voice)
- Respiratory rate < 8 breaths/min
- Sa_{O_2} < 90% while breathing room air

*Sample guidelines adapted from those used by the Ulster Community and Hospitals Trust, Ulster, United Kingdom. Labor nurses must establish competency in the use of remifentanil PCA prior to providing care.

Labor nurses undergo a period of supervised practice with remifentanil PCA until they are deemed competent. One-on-one nursing care is essential. Women must not have received other opioids in the previous 4 hours, and they are fully informed of side effects, including a 10% chance of requiring supplemental oxygen. A dedicated intravenous cannula is used solely for the PCA infusion. Continuous pulse oximetry is established, and sedation scores are recorded every 30 minutes. Clear triggers for contacting the anesthesia service are defined.

In summary, the analgesic efficacy of remifentanil has been demonstrated. Optimal PCA may require dose titration and escalation as labor progresses. Currently, the results of a number of studies suggest that remifentanil PCA has an acceptable safety profile for parturients and neonates but its use requires careful monitoring and one-on-one nursing care because of the potential for adverse maternal events.

OPIOID ANTAGONISTS

Naloxone is the opioid antagonist of choice for reversing the neonatal effects of maternal opioid administration. There is no neonatal benefit to the maternal administration of naloxone during labor or just before delivery. This practice antagonizes maternal analgesia during labor and delivery, without decreasing opioid-related maternal side effects[79]; at best, it provides uncertain and/or incomplete reversal of the depressive effects on the neonate. When maternal administration of an opioid is anticipated to lead to neonatal respiratory depression, it is best to administer naloxone directly to the newborn.

Naloxone reverses opioid depression of newborn minute ventilation and increases the slope of the CO_2-response curve in infants affected by the maternal administration of an opioid.[80] The recommended dose is 0.1 mg/kg of a 1 mg/mL or 0.4 mg/mL solution. Administration of naloxone is not recommended during the primary steps of neonatal resuscitation, but it may be performed if respiratory depression continues after positive-pressure ventilation has restored normal heart rate *and* color and the mother received an opioid within the previous 4 hours.[81] The preferred route of administration is intravenous. If intravenous access is not available, intramuscular administration is acceptable, although absorption may be delayed with this route. Endotracheal administration of naloxone is not recommended.[81] Naloxone may precipitate a withdrawal reaction in the newborn of the opioid-dependent mother.

OPIOID ADJUNCTS AND SEDATIVES

Many drugs have been used as adjuncts to parenteral opioid analgesia. Most of them cause sedation and neonatal depression and are now used infrequently, because neuraxial or opioid PCA techniques achieve adequate analgesia more safely.

Barbiturates are sedative agents and have no analgesic effect. They are lipid soluble, rapidly cross the placenta, and are detectable in fetal blood. Barbiturate administration entails a risk of neonatal depression, especially if combined with systemic use of analgesics.

Phenothiazines may be used in combination with opioids to provide sedation and reduce nausea and vomiting. They rapidly cross the placenta and reduce FHR variability, but there is no evidence of neonatal respiratory depression. Neurobehavioral outcomes after the maternal administration of these agents have not been studied carefully. Phenothiazines may cause unacceptable hypotension from alpha-adrenergic receptor blockade. Intravenous or intramuscular **promethazine** (25 to 50 mg) may produce profound sedation, although this is associated with mild respiratory stimulation, which may counteract opioid-induced respiratory depression. Promethazine appears in fetal blood 1 to 2 minutes after maternal intravenous administration and equilibrates within 15 minutes.[82] **Propiomazine** is a mild respiratory depressant that may further depress maternal ventilation when co-administered with opioids. It has a faster onset and a shorter duration than promethazine. Only two studies have suggested that phenothiazines may potentiate the effect of meperidine.[83,84]

Metoclopramide is used to reduce nausea and vomiting and increase gastric emptying. It is nonsedating. Vella et al.[85] observed that administration of metoclopramide reduced requirements for nitrous oxide during labor. Similarly, women who received both meperidine and metoclopramide had slightly better pain scores than women who received meperidine alone.

Benzodiazepines have been used for sedation in obstetric patients but are associated with significant side effects. Diazepam rapidly crosses the placenta and accumulates in the fetus at concentrations that may exceed maternal concentrations. It has a long elimination half-life (24 to 48 hours) and an active metabolite with an elimination half-life of 51 to 120 hours.[86] Administration of **diazepam** during labor has been associated with neonatal hypotonicity and respiratory depression. It impairs neonatal thermoregulation and the stress response.[87] These effects may be dose related.

Lorazepam has a shorter half-life than diazepam (12 hours) and is metabolized to an inactive glucuronide. McAuley et al.[88] gave lorazepam 2 mg or placebo prior to administration of meperidine 100 mg for labor analgesia. Analgesia was better in the group receiving lorazepam, but these patients also experienced a nonsignificant increase in respiratory depression. Neurobehavioral scores were similar. Amnesia was common with lorazepam.

Midazolam has a rapid onset and a short duration of action, with inactive metabolites. It has been shown to cross the placenta, and at high doses used for induction of general anesthesia, this agent causes neonatal hypotonia. Midazolam is a potent amnesic, a characteristic that may be undesirable for the childbirth experience.

Ketamine is a phencyclidine derivative. Small doses administered intravenously or intramuscularly provide a dissociative state of analgesia with or without amnesia; larger doses (1 mg/kg) are used to induce general anesthesia. Ketamine is best avoided in preeclamptic patients because it causes sympathetic nervous system stimulation and may exacerbate hypertension; however, it may be the induction agent of choice for patients with hypovolemia or asthma. Small doses of ketamine do not cause neonatal depression; high doses have been associated with low Apgar scores and abnormal neonatal muscle tone.[89]

Intravenous ketamine has a rapid onset (30 seconds) and a short duration of action (3 to 5 minutes). Ketamine may provide effective analgesia just before vaginal delivery in parturients without regional anesthesia or may be used as an adjunctive agent in parturients with unsatisfactory regional anesthesia. A 10- to 20-mg dose may be repeated at intervals of 2 to 5 minutes, while not exceeding a total dose of 1 mg/kg during a 30-minute period. When used in this manner, ketamine is associated with a low incidence of maternal hallucinations; however, amnesia is common. The anesthesia provider must maintain continual verbal contact with the patient. It is critical that the patient remain awake and able to protect her airway.

INHALATION ANALGESIA

In the United States, the use of inhalation analgesia for labor is uncommon. Although many of the inhaled anesthetic agents used in surgery have been tried for pain relief in childbirth, only **nitrous oxide** remains in regular use. There has also been interest in sevoflurane as a labor analgesic. In Canada, nitrous oxide is used in 77% to 86% of facilities,[3] and in the United Kingdom, nitrous oxide mixed 1:1 with oxygen (**Entonox**) is used in 100% of labor and delivery units and may be administered by unsupervised labor nurses.[7]

Nitrous Oxide

Intermittent inhalation of nitrous oxide can provide analgesia for labor, but it does not completely eliminate the pain of uterine contractions. In recent years, the efficacy of Entonox for labor analgesia has been questioned. Several studies of intrapartum analgesia have noted that 30% to 40% of mothers report little or no benefit from Entonox.[90] Other investigators argue that, when properly timed, inhalation of 50% nitrous oxide provides significant pain relief in as many as half of parturients.[91] To achieve substantial pain relief with nitrous oxide, maternal cooperation is required. There must be an analgesic concentration of nitrous oxide in the blood (and thus the brain) at the peak of the uterine contraction. The patient is encouraged to breathe the mixture of 50% nitrous oxide in oxygen from the very beginning of the contraction and to continue until the end of the contraction. Nitrous oxide does not interfere with uterine activity.[92]

Suitable equipment must be available to provide safe and satisfactory inhalation analgesia with nitrous oxide. An apparatus that limits the concentration of nitrous oxide (e.g., a nitrous oxide/oxygen blender or a premixed 1:1 cylinder) is required, and it must be checked periodically to prevent the unintentional administration of a high concentration of nitrous oxide and a hypoxic concentration of gas. Inhalation may occur through a mask or a mouthpiece with a one-way valve to limit pollution of the labor suite with unscavenged gases.

Environmental pollution from unscavenged nitrous oxide may be significant.[93] It is unclear whether regular occupational exposure to subanesthetic concentrations of nitrous oxide results in significant health risks for health care workers.[94] Overall, epidemiologic data do not suggest the presence of higher reproductive risk in health care workers exposed to nitrous oxide in the work environment (see Chapter 17).

Some physicians have expressed concern about the possibility of diffusion hypoxia after the administration of a nitrous oxide/oxygen mixture, which may lead to hypoxemia during labor. Carstoniu et al.[95] compared parturients breathing 50% nitrous oxide in oxygen with a similar group of women breathing compressed air. The maternal Sa_{O_2} measurements between contractions were slightly higher in the nitrous oxide/oxygen group than in the compressed air group. Unfortunately, there was no difference between the two groups in mean pain scores. By contrast, other physicians have observed episodes of maternal hypoxemia with the use of nitrous oxide analgesia during labor.[96] Some studies have also suggested that the combined use of nitrous oxide and opioids increases the risk of maternal hypoxemia during labor.[97,98] Physicians, midwives, and nurses must be aware of the additive effects of inhalation agents and systemic opioids and/or sedatives that lead to the increased potential for hypoxemia.

With the intermittent inhalation of nitrous oxide, accumulation over time is negligible, and the neonate eliminates most of the gas within minutes of birth, principally via the lungs. Used in this way, nitrous oxide does not depress neonatal respiration or affect neonatal neurobehavior.[99] If neonatal respiratory depression occurs, the infant should be ventilated with 100% oxygen, which rapidly eliminates nitrous oxide.

Volatile Halogenated Agents

All volatile halogenated agents cause dose-related relaxation of uterine smooth muscle. The concentration of sevoflurane required to decrease the myometrial contractile response by 50% (ED_{50}) has varied from 0.8 to 1.0 minimum alveolar concentration (MAC)[100,101] to 1.72 MAC[102] in studies performed *in vitro*. Similarly, the ED_{50} of desflurane has ranged from approximately 0.9 MAC[101] to 1.4 MAC.[100,102] In contrast, in a study in which isoflurane was compared with other anesthetics, the ED_{50} of isoflurane (2.4 MAC) was significantly higher than that for sevoflurane, desflurane, and halothane.[102] Whether or not this finding means that isoflurane is less likely to be associated with uterine atony in clinical practice requires further study. In general, when uterine tone is desirable (e.g., after delivery), volatile anesthetic concentrations higher than 0.5 MAC are not recommended, and intravenous oxytocin should be administered concurrently.

Abboud et al.[103] compared administration of 0.25% to 1.25% **enflurane** in oxygen with administration of 30% to 60% nitrous oxide during the second stage of labor. Approximately 89% of the enflurane group and 76% of the nitrous oxide group rated their analgesia as satisfactory. The rates of amnesia were similar (7% and 10%). There were no differences in blood loss, Apgar scores, or umbilical cord blood gas measurements.

Isoflurane alone[104] as well as isoflurane-Entonox mixtures have been compared to Entonox alone[103,105,106] for labor analgesia. Ross et al.[106] compared 0.25% isoflurane mixed with Entonox and Entonox alone in 221 parturients. A demand valve was used with premixed gas cylinders. No mother became unduly sedated, and there was no increased rate of need for neonatal resuscitation except in infants whose mothers had received systemic opioids. Blood loss was no greater than expected. The rate of intolerance to the odor was 8%. Fourteen percent of subjects eventually requested epidural analgesia. The same investigators have assessed the clinical safety of the cylinder system to verify clinically acceptable performance.[107]

Desflurane is associated with rapid onset and recovery. Abboud et al.[108] found similar analgesia scores when comparing 1% to 4% desflurane in oxygen with 30% to 60% nitrous oxide; however, the amnesia rate was 23%. Neonatal outcomes were similar in the two groups.

Sevoflurane is the volatile halogenated agent most commonly used for inhalation induction of general anesthesia. It has short onset and offset of action, but it is less irritating and has a less unpleasant odor than the other volatile agents. Toscano et al.[109] performed a small safety and feasibility study of 50 parturients breathing intermittent 2% to 3% sevoflurane in oxygen/air via a compact anesthesia system. They aimed for an end-tidal sevoflurane concentration of 1% to 1.5% at the peak of uterine contractions. The mean (± SD) pain score was significantly lower during the times when parturients inhaled sevoflurane compared with times without inhalation of sevoflurane (3.3 ± 1.5 versus 8.7 ± 1.0, respectively, on a scale of 0 to 10). Oxygen desaturation and loss of consciousness did not occur, blood loss was unremarkable, FHR tracings were unchanged, and the median 1-minute Apgar score was 9.

After determining that 0.8% sevoflurane was the optimal concentration for labor analgesia,[110] Yeo et al.[111] compared 0.8% sevoflurane with Entonox in 32 parturients using a double-crossover study design. Two subjects could not tolerate the odor of sevoflurane, and 5 requested epidural analgesia during the Entonox phase. Median pain relief scores (100-mm scale) were significantly higher for sevoflurane (67 mm [interquartile range 55 to 74 mm]) than for Entonox (51 mm [interquartile range 41 to 70 mm]). There were no other adverse events—SaO_2 less than 98%, apnea, or change in end-tidal CO_2—although subjects experienced more subjective sleepiness with sevoflurane. The investigators concluded that sevoflurane can provide useful analgesia for labor and is superior to Entonox.

Routine use of inhalation analgesia may be limited by the need for specialized equipment, concern for environmental pollution, and the potential for maternal amnesia and loss of protective airway reflexes. Although sedation occurs during intermittent use of volatile anesthetic agents, profound sedation to the extent that airway reflexes are jeopardized has not been reported. Further research and refinement of intermittent inhalation of a volatile agent for labor analgesia may allow use of this technique for women in whom neuraxial anesthesia is contraindicated. Among the volatile agents, sevoflurane appears to be best suited for inhalation labor analgesia.

KEY POINTS

- Systemic analgesia is commonly used in laboring women around the world.
- All opioid analgesic drugs rapidly cross the placenta and cause a transient reduction in fetal heart rate variability.
- Meperidine is most commonly administered as an intermittent bolus. Its active metabolite is associated with neonatal respiratory depression and neurobehavioral changes.
- There is little evidence that any individual opioid confers significant benefit over meperidine when administered as a bolus.
- Babies whose mothers received systemic opioid analgesia are more likely to exhibit neonatal depression than those whose mothers received no analgesia or neuraxial analgesia during labor.
- Patient-controlled analgesia (PCA) with remifentanil provides good analgesia and has minimal effect on neonatal outcome. Remifentanil PCA requires intensive monitoring because of the risk of maternal sedation and the potential for serious complications.
- Inhalation analgesia is used during labor in some countries outside the United States. Nitrous oxide may provide some analgesia.
- Initial studies of intermittent sevoflurane analgesia are promising, but larger studies are needed to assess the incidence of maternal compromise.

REFERENCES

1. Bucklin BA, Hawkins JL, Anderson JR, Ullrich FA. Obstetric anesthesia workforce survey: Twenty-year update. Anesthesiology 2005; 103:645-53.
2. United Kingdom National Health Service, The Information Centre for Health and Social Care. NHS Maternity Statistics, England: 2005-06. Available at http://www.ic.nhs.uk/webfiles/publications/maternity 0506/NHSMaternityStatsEngland200506_fullpublication%20V3.pdf/
3. Breen TW, McNeil T, Dierenfield L. Obstetric anesthesia practice in Canada. Can J Anaesth 2000; 47:1230-42.
4. Spielman FJ. Systemic analgesics during labor. Clin Obstet Gynecol 1987; 30:495-504.
5. Reynolds F, Sharma SK, Seed PT. Analgesia in labour and fetal acid-base balance: A meta-analysis comparing epidural with systemic opioid analgesia. Br J Obstet Gynaecol 2002; 109:1344-53.
6. Halpern SH, Muir H, Breen TW, et al. A multicenter randomized controlled trial comparing patient-controlled epidural with intravenous analgesia for pain relief in labor. Anesth Analg 2004; 99:1532-8.
7. Tuckey JP, Prout RE, Wee MY. Prescribing intramuscular opioids for labour analgesia in consultant-led maternity units: A survey of UK practice. Int J Obstet Anesth 2008; 17:3-8.
8. Ranta P, Jouppila P, Spalding M, et al. Parturients' assessment of water blocks, pethidine, nitrous oxide, paracervical and epidural blocks in labour. Int J Obstet Anesth 1994; 3:193-8.
9. Tsui MH, Ngan Kee WD, Ng FF, Lau TK. A double blinded randomised placebo-controlled study of intramuscular pethidine for pain relief in the first stage of labour. Br J Obstet Gynaecol 2004; 111:648-55.
10. Shnider SM, Way WL, Lord MJ. Rate of appearance and disappearance of meperidine in fetal blood after administration of narcotic to the mother (abstract). Anesthesiology 1966; 27:227-8.
11. Kariniemi V, Ammala P. Effects of intramuscular pethidine on fetal heart rate variability during labour. Br J Obstet Gynaecol 1981; 88:718-20.
12. Kuhnert BR, Kuhnert PM, Tu AS, et al. Meperidine and normeperidine levels following meperidine administration during labor. I. Mother. Am J Obstet Gynecol 1979; 133:904-8.
13. Caldwell J, Wakile LA, Notarianni LJ, et al. Maternal and neonatal disposition of pethidine in childbirth—a study using quantitative gas chromatography-mass spectrometry. Life Sci 1978; 22:589-96.

14. Shnider SM, Moya F. Effects of meperidine on the newborn infant. Am J Obstet Gynecol 1964; 89:1009-15.
15. Kuhnert BR, Kuhnert PM, Tu AS, Lin DC. Meperidine and normeperidine levels following meperidine administration during labor. II. Fetus and neonate. Am J Obstet Gynecol 1979; 133:909-14.
16. Belfrage P, Boreus LO, Hartvig P, et al. Neonatal depression after obstetrical analgesia with pethidine: The role of the injection-delivery time interval and of the plasma concentrations of pethidine and norpethidine. Acta Obstet Gynecol Scand 1981; 60:43-9.
17. Hodgkinson R, Bhatt M, Wang CN. Double-blind comparison of the neurobehaviour of neonates following the administration of different doses of meperidine to the mother. Can Anaesth Soc J 1978; 25:405-11.
18. Belsey EM, Rosenblatt DB, Lieberman BA, et al. The influence of maternal analgesia on neonatal behaviour. I. Pethidine. Br J Obstet Gynaecol 1981; 88:398-406.
19. Kuhnert BR, Linn PL, Kennard MJ, Kuhnert PM. Effects of low doses of meperidine on neonatal behavior. Anesth Analg 1985; 64:335-42.
20. Nissen E, Widstrom AM, Lilja G, et al. Effects of routinely given pethidine during labour on infants' developing breastfeeding behaviour: Effects of dose-delivery time interval and various concentrations of pethidine/norpethidine in cord plasma. Acta Paediatr 1997; 86:201-8.
21. Sosa CG, Balaguer E, Alonso JG, et al. Meperidine for dystocia during the first stage of labor: A randomized controlled trial. Am J Obstet Gynecol 2004; 191:1212-8.
22. Stoelting RK. Opioid agonists and antagonists. In Stoelting RK, editor. Pharmacology and Physiology in Anesthetic Practice. 2nd edition. Philadelphia, JB Lippincott, 1991:74-82.
23. Gerdin E, Salmonson T, Lindberg B, Rane A. Maternal kinetics of morphine during labour. J Perinat Med 1990; 18:479-87.
24. Brunk SF, Delle M. Morphine metabolism in man. Clin Pharmacol Ther 1974; 16:51-7.
25. Osborne R, Thompson P, Joel S, et al. The analgesic activity of morphine-6-glucuronide. Br J Clin Pharmacol 1992; 34:130-8.
26. Peat SJ, Hanna MH, Woodham M, et al. Morphine-6-glucuronide: Effects on ventilation in normal volunteers. Pain 1991; 45:101-4.
27. Gerdin E, Rane A, Lindberg B. Transplacental transfer of morphine in man. J Perinat Med 1990; 18:305-12.
28. Olofsson C, Ekblom A, Ekman-Ordeberg G, et al. Analgesic efficacy of intravenous morphine in labour pain: A reappraisal. Int J Obstet Anesth 1996; 5:176-80.
29. Olofsson C, Ekblom A, Ekman-Ordeberg G, et al. Lack of analgesic effect of systemically administered morphine or pethidine on labour pain. Br J Obstet Gynaecol 1996; 103:968-72.
30. Way WL, Costley EC, Leongway E. Respiratory sensitivity of the newborn infant to meperidine and morphine. Clin Pharmacol Ther 1965; 6:454-61.
31. Boerner U. The metabolism of morphine and heroin in man. Drug Metab Rev 1975; 4:39-73.
32. Barrett DA, Barker DP, Rutter N, et al. Morphine, morphine-6-glucuronide and morphine-3-glucuronide pharmacokinetics in newborn infants receiving diamorphine infusions. Br J Clin Pharmacol 1996; 41:531-7.
33. Rawal N, Tomlinson AJ, Gibson GJ, Sheehan TM. Umbilical cord plasma concentrations of free morphine following single-dose diamorphine analgesia and their relationship to dose-delivery time interval, Apgar scores and neonatal respiration. Eur J Obstet Gynecol Reprod Biol 2007; 133:30-3.
34. Fairlie FM, Marshall L, Walker JJ, Elbourne D. Intramuscular opioids for maternal pain relief in labour: A randomised controlled trial comparing pethidine with diamorphine. Br J Obstet Gynaecol 1999; 106:1181-7.
35. Eisele JH, Wright R, Rogge P. Newborn and maternal fentanyl levels at cesarean section (abstract). Anesth Analg 1982; 61:179-80.
36. Rayburn W, Rathke A, Leuschen MP, et al. Fentanyl citrate analgesia during labor. Am J Obstet Gynecol 1989; 161:202-6.
37. Rayburn WF, Smith CV, Parriott JE, Woods RE. Randomized comparison of meperidine and fentanyl during labor. Obstet Gynecol 1989; 74:604-6.
38. Wilson CM, McClean E, Moore J, Dundee JW. A double-blind comparison of intramuscular pethidine and nalbuphine in labour. Anaesthesia 1986; 41:1207-13.
39. Nicolle E, Devillier P, Delanoy B, et al. Therapeutic monitoring of nalbuphine: Transplacental transfer and estimated pharmacokinetics in the neonate. Eur J Clin Pharmacol 1996; 49:485-9.
40. Giannina G, Guzman ER, Lai YL, et al. Comparison of the effects of meperidine and nalbuphine on intrapartum fetal heart rate tracings. Obstet Gynecol 1995; 86:441-5.
41. Nagashima H, Karamanian A, Malovany R, et al. Respiratory and circulatory effects of intravenous butorphanol and morphine. Clin Pharmacol Ther 1976; 19:738-45.
42. Kallos T, Caruso FS. Respiratory effects of butorphanol and pethidine. Anaesthesia 1979; 34:633-7.
43. Maduska AL, Hajghassemali M. A double-blind comparison of butorphanol and meperidine in labour: Maternal pain relief and effect on the newborn. Can Anaesth Soc J 1978; 25:398-404.
44. Hodgkinson R, Huff RW, Hayashi RH, Husain FJ. Double-blind comparison of maternal analgesia and neonatal neurobehaviour following intravenous butorphanol and meperidine. J Int Med Res 1979; 7:224-30.
45. Quilligan EJ, Keegan KA, Donahue MJ. Double-blind comparison of intravenously injected butorphanol and meperidine in parturients. Int J Gynaecol Obstet 1980; 18:363-7.
46. Nelson KE, Eisenach JC. Intravenous butorphanol, meperidine, and their combination relieve pain and distress in women in labor. Anesthesiology 2005; 102:1008-13.
47. Holmes B, Ward A. Meptazinol: A review of its pharmacodynamic and pharmacokinetic properties and therapeutic efficacy. Drugs 1985; 30:285-312.
48. Franklin RA, Frost T, Robson PJ, Jackson MB. Preliminary studies on the disposition of meptazinol in the neonate. Br J Clin Pharmacol 1981; 12:88-90.
49. Nicholas AD, Robson PJ. Double-blind comparison of meptazinol and pethidine in labour. Br J Obstet Gynaecol 1982; 89:318-22.
50. Morrison CE, Dutton D, Howie H, Gilmour H. Pethidine compared with meptazinol during labour: A prospective randomised double-blind study in 1100 patients. Anaesthesia 1987; 42:7-14.
51. de Boer FC, Shortland D, Simpson RL, et al. A comparison of the effects of maternally administered meptazinol and pethidine on neonatal acid-base status. Br J Obstet Gynaecol 1987; 94:256-61.
52. Jaffe JH, Martin WR. Opioids with mixed actions: Partial agonists. In Gilman AG, Rall TW, Nies AS, Taylor P, editors. Goodman and Gilman's The Pharmacological Basis of Therapeutics. 8th edition. New York, Pergamon Press, 1990:512-4.
53. Moore J, Ball HG. A sequential study of intravenous analgesic treatment during labour. Br J Anaesth 1974; 46:365-72.
54. Refstad SO, Lindbaek E. Ventilatory depression of the newborn of women receiving pethidine or pentazocine: A double-blind comparative trial. Br J Anaesth 1980; 52:265-71.
55. Lee CR, McTavish D, Sorkin EM. Tramadol: A preliminary review of its pharmacodynamic and pharmacokinetic properties, and therapeutic potential in acute and chronic pain states. Drugs 1993; 46:313-40.
56. Claahsen-van der Grinten HL, Verbruggen I, van den Berg PP, et al. Different pharmacokinetics of tramadol in mothers treated for labour pain and in their neonates. Eur J Clin Pharmacol 2005; 61:523-9.
57. Keskin HL, Keskin EA, Avsar AF, et al. Pethidine versus tramadol for pain relief during labor. Int J Gynaecol Obstet 2003; 82:11-6.
58. Saravanakumar K, Garstang JS, Hasan K. Intravenous patient-controlled analgesia for labour: A survey of UK practice. Int J Obstet Anesth 2007; 16:221-5.
59. McIntosh DG, Rayburn WF. Patient-controlled analgesia in obstetrics and gynecology. Obstet Gynecol 1991; 78:1129-35.
60. Isenor L, Penny-MacGillivray T. Intravenous meperidine infusion for obstetric analgesia. J Obstet Gynecol Neonatal Nurs 1993; 22:349-56.
61. Volikas I, Male D. A comparison of pethidine and remifentanil patient-controlled analgesia in labour. Int J Obstet Anesth 2001; 10:86-90.

62. Blair JM, Dobson GT, Hill DA, et al. Patient controlled analgesia for labour: A comparison of remifentanil with pethidine. Anaesthesia 2005; 60:22-7.
63. McInnes RJ, Hillan E, Clark D, Gilmour H. Diamorphine for pain relief in labour: A randomised controlled trial comparing intramuscular injection and patient-controlled analgesia. Br J Obstet Gynaecol 2004; 111:1081-9.
64. Rayburn WF, Smith CV, Leuschen MP, et al. Comparison of patient-controlled and nurse-administered analgesia using intravenous fentanyl during labor. Anesthesiol Rev 1991; 18:31-6.
65. Morley-Forster PK, Weberpals J. Neonatal effects of patient-controlled analgesia using fentanyl in labor. Int J Obstet Anesth 1998; 7:103-7.
66. Shannon KT, Ramanathan S. Systemic medication for labor analgesia. Obstet Pain Manage 1995; 2:1-6.
67. Morley-Forster PK, Reid DW, Vandeberghe H. A comparison of patient-controlled analgesia fentanyl and alfentanil for labour analgesia. Can J Anaesth 2000; 47:113-9.
68. Podlas J, Breland BD. Patient-controlled analgesia with nalbuphine during labor. Obstet Gynecol 1987; 70:202-4.
69. Frank M, McAteer EJ, Cattermole R, et al. Nalbuphine for obstetric analgesia: A comparison of nalbuphine with pethidine for pain relief in labour when administered by patient-controlled analgesia (PCA). Anaesthesia 1987; 42:697-703.
70. Egan TD, Minto CF, Hermann DJ, et al. Remifentanil versus alfentanil: Comparative pharmacokinetics and pharmacodynamics in healthy adult male volunteers. Anesthesiology 1996; 84:821-33.
71. Glass SA, Hardman D, Kamiyama Y, et al. Preliminary pharmacokinetics and pharmacodynamics of an ultra-short-acting opioid: Remifentanil (GI87084B). Anesth Analg 1993; 77:1031-40.
72. Kan RE, Hughes SC, Rosen MA, et al. Intravenous remifentanil: Placental transfer, maternal and neonatal effects. Anesthesiology 1998; 88:1467-74.
73. Thurlow JA, Laxton CH, Dick A, et al. Remifentanil by patient-controlled analgesia compared with intramuscular meperidine for pain relief in labour. Br J Anaesth 2002; 88:374-8.
74. Volmanen P, Akural E, Raudaskoski T, et al. Comparison of remifentanil and nitrous oxide in labour analgesia. Acta Anaesthesiol Scand 2005; 49:453-8.
75. Volikas I, Butwick A, Wilkinson C, et al. Maternal and neonatal side-effects of remifentanil patient-controlled analgesia in labour. Br J Anaesth 2005; 95:504-9.
76. Volmanen P, Akural EI, Raudaskoski T, Alahuhta S. Remifentanil in obstetric analgesia: A dose-finding study. Anesth Analg 2002; 94:913-7.
77. Balki M, Kasodekar S, Dhumne S, et al. Remifentanil patient-controlled analgesia for labour: Optimizing drug delivery regimens. Can J Anaesth 2007; 54:626-33.
78. Volmanen P, Sarvela J, Akural EI, et al. Intravenous remifentanil vs. epidural levobupivacaine with fentanyl for pain relief in early labour: A randomised, controlled, double-blinded study. Acta Anaesthesiol Scand 2008; 52:249-55.
79. Girvan CB, Moore J, Dundee JW. Pethidine compared with pethidine-naloxone administered during labour: A study of analgesic treatment by a sequential method. Br J Anaesth 1976; 48:563-9.
80. Gerhardt T, Bancalari E, Cohen H, Rocha LF. Use of naloxone to reverse narcotic respiratory depression in the newborn infant. J Pediatr 1977; 90:1009-12.
81. Anonymous. Neonatal resuscitation guidelines. Circulation 2005; 112:IV188-95.
82. Clark RB, Seifen AB. Systemic medication during labor and delivery. Obstet Gynecol Annu 1983; 12:165-97.
83. Powe CE, Kiem IM, Fromhagen C, Cavanagh D. Propiomazine hydrochloride in obstetrical analgesia: A controlled study of 520 patients. JAMA 1962; 181:290-4.
84. Ullery JC, Bair JR. Maternal-fetal effects of propiomazine-meperidine analgesia. Am J Obstet Gynecol 1962; 84:1051-6.
85. Vella L, Francis D, Houlton P, Reynolds F. Comparison of the antiemetics metoclopramide and promethazine in labour. Br Med J (Clin Res Ed) 1985; 290:1173-5.
86. Mandelli M, Tognoni G, Garattini S. Clinical pharmacokinetics of diazepam. Clin Pharmacokinet 1978; 3:72-91.
87. McElhatton PR. The effects of benzodiazepine use during pregnancy and lactation. Reprod Toxicol 1994; 8:461-75.
88. McAuley DM, O'Neill MP, Moore J, Dundee JW. Lorazepam premedication for labour. Br J Obstet Gynaecol 1982; 89:149-54.
89. Akamatsu TJ, Bonica JJ, Rehmet R, et al. Experiences with the use of ketamine for parturition. I. Primary anesthetic for vaginal delivery. Anesth Analg 1974; 53:284-7.
90. Yentis SM. The use of Entonox for labour pain should be abandoned. Int J Obstet Anesth 2001; 10:25-7.
91. Rosen M. Recent advances in pain relief in childbirth. I. Inhalation and systemic analgesia. Br J Anaesth 1971; 43:837-48.
92. Marx GF, Katsnelson T. The introduction of nitrous oxide analgesia into obstetrics. Obstet Gynecol 1992; 80:715-8.
93. Mills GH, Singh D, Longan M, et al. Nitrous oxide exposure on the labour ward. Int J Obstet Anesth 1996; 5:160-4.
94. Bernow J, Bjordal J, Wiklund KE. Pollution of delivery ward air by nitrous oxide: Effects of various modes of room ventilation, excess and close scavenging. Acta Anaesthesiol Scand 1984; 28:119-23.
95. Carstoniu J, Levytam S, Norman P, et al. Nitrous oxide in early labor: Safety and analgesic efficacy assessed by a double-blind, placebo-controlled study. Anesthesiology 1994; 80:30-5.
96. Lucas DN, Siemaszko O, Yentis SM. Maternal hypoxaemia associated with the use of Entonox in labour. Int J Obstet Anesth 2000; 9:270-2.
97. Deckardt R, Fembacher PM, Schneider KT, Graeff H. Maternal arterial oxygen saturation during labor and delivery: Pain-dependent alterations and effects on the newborn. Obstet Gynecol 1987; 70:21-5.
98. Irestedt L. Current status for nitrous oxide for obstetric pain relief. Acta Anaesthesiol Scand 1994; 38:771-2.
99. Stefani SJ, Hughes SC, Schnider SM, et al. Neonatal neurobehavioral effects of inhalation analgesia for vaginal delivery. Anesthesiology 1982; 56:351-5.
100. Yildiz K, Dogru K, Dalgic H, et al. Inhibitory effects of desflurane and sevoflurane on oxytocin-induced contractions of isolated pregnant human myometrium. Acta Anaesthesiol Scand 2005; 49:1355-9.
101. Turner RJ, Lambros M, Kenway L, Gatt SP. The in-vitro effects of sevoflurane and desflurane on the contractility of pregnant human uterine muscle. Int J Obstet Anesth 2002; 11:246-51.
102. Yoo KY, Lee JC, Yoon MH, et al. The effects of volatile anesthetics on spontaneous contractility of isolated human pregnant uterine muscle: A comparison among sevoflurane, desflurane, isoflurane, and halothane. Anesth Analg 2006; 103:443-7.
103. Abboud TK, Shnider SM, Wright RG, et al. Enflurane analgesia in obstetrics. Anesth Analg 1981; 60:133-7.
104. McLeod DD, Ramayya GP, Tunstall ME. Self-administered isoflurane in labour: A comparative study with Entonox. Anaesthesia 1985; 40:424-6.
105. Arora S, Tunstall M, Ross J. Self-administered mixture of Entonox and isoflurane in labour. Int J Obstet Anesth 1992; 1:199-202.
106. Ross JA, Tunstall ME, Campbell DM, Lemon JS. The use of 0.25% isoflurane premixed in 50% nitrous oxide and oxygen for pain relief in labour. Anaesthesia 1999; 54:1166-72.
107. Ross JA, Tunstall ME. Simulated use of premixed 0.25% isoflurane in 50% nitrous oxide and 50% oxygen. Br J Anaesth 2002; 89:820-4.
108. Abboud TK, Swart F, Zhu J, et al. Desflurane analgesia for vaginal delivery. Acta Anaesthesiol Scand 1995; 39:259-61.
109. Toscano A, Pancaro C, Giovannoni S, et al. Sevoflurane analgesia in obstetrics: A pilot study. Int J Obstet Anesth 2003; 12:79-82.
110. Yeo ST, Holdcroft A, Yentis SM, Stewart A. Analgesia with sevoflurane during labour. I. Determination of the optimum concentration. Br J Anaesth 2007; 98:105-9.
111. Yeo ST, Holdcroft A, Yentis SM, et al. Analgesia with sevoflurane during labour. II. Sevoflurane compared with Entonox for labour analgesia. Br J Anaesth 2007; 98:110-5.

Chapter 23

Epidural and Spinal Analgesia/Anesthesia for Labor and Vaginal Delivery

Cynthia A. Wong, M.D.

Epidural analgesia and spinal analgesia are the most effective methods of intrapartum pain relief in contemporary clinical practice.[1,2] During the first stage of labor, pain results primarily from distention of the lower uterine segment and cervix. Painful impulses are transmitted by means of visceral afferent nerve fibers, which accompany sympathetic nerve fibers and enter the spinal cord at the 10th, 11th, and 12th thoracic and 1st lumbar spinal segments. As labor progresses and the fetus descends in the birth canal, distention of the vagina and perineum results in painful impulses that are transmitted via the pudendal nerve to the second, third, and fourth sacral spinal

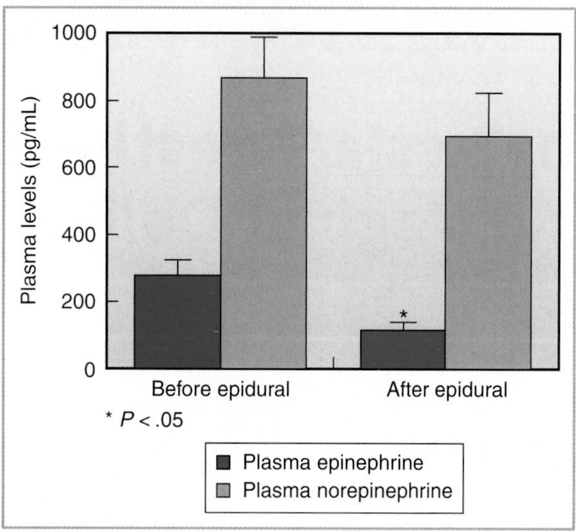

FIGURE 23-1 Influence of epidural analgesia on maternal plasma concentrations of catecholamines during labor. *$P < .05$ compared with before epidural. (Modified from Shnider SM, Abboud TK, Artal R, et al. Maternal catecholamines decrease during labor after lumbar epidural anesthesia. Am J Obstet Gynecol 1983; 147:13-5.)

segments. Neuraxial analgesia is the only form of analgesia that provides complete analgesia for both stages of labor. During the first stage of labor, visceral pain impulses entering the spinal cord at T10 to L1 must be blocked. During the late first stage of labor and the second stage of labor, somatic impulses entering the spinal cord from S2 to S4 must also be blocked (see Chapter 20).

In a survey of 1000 consecutive women who chose a variety of analgesic techniques for labor and vaginal delivery (including nonpharmacologic methods, transcutaneous electrical nerve stimulation, intramuscular meperidine, inhalation of nitrous oxide, epidural analgesia, and a combination of these techniques), pain relief and overall satisfaction with the birth experience were greater in patients who received epidural analgesia.[2] Similarly, randomized studies that have compared epidural analgesia with systemic opioids and/or inhalation analgesia (i.e., nitrous oxide) have shown that pain scores are lower and patients are more satisfied with neuraxial analgesia.[3-7]

The provision of analgesia for labor may result in other benefits. Effective epidural analgesia reduces maternal plasma concentrations of catecholamines (Figure 23-1).[8] Decreased alpha- and beta-adrenergic receptor stimulation may result in better uteroplacental perfusion and more effective uterine activity.[9,10] Painful uterine contractions result in maternal hyperventilation. The hyperventilation, in turn, leads to maternal respiratory alkalosis, a leftward shift of the oxyhemoglobin dissociation curve, increased maternal hemoglobin affinity for oxygen, and reduced oxygen delivery to the fetus.[11] Hypocarbia also leads to hypoventilation between contractions, which can cause a decrease in maternal Pa_{O_2}. Effective epidural analgesia blunts this "hyperventilation-hypoventilation" cycle.[12] Finally, the presence of an epidural catheter and effective epidural *analgesia* facilitate the rapid initiation of epidural *anesthesia* for emergency cesarean delivery. Neuraxial anesthesia for cesarean delivery is associated with greater overall maternal safety than emergency administration of general anesthesia.[13]

Neuraxial analgesia is not used by all laboring women, although surveys of obstetric anesthesia practice in the United States have shown that the use of neuraxial analgesia has grown over the past three decades.[14] In 1981, 22% of laboring women who delivered in U.S. hospitals with more than 1500 deliveries per year chose epidural analgesia. By 2001, 77% of women chose to receive neuraxial (epidural, spinal, or combined spinal-epidural) analgesia.[14] In the United Kingdom, the National Health Service Maternity Statistics for 2005-2006 show that one third of parturients chose neuraxial analgesia during childbirth.[15]

The availability of skilled anesthesia providers influences the neuraxial analgesia rate.[14,16] Other factors include the information and advice provided to pregnant women by obstetricians, nurses, and childbirth education instructors. Obstetric complications,[2] as well as the personal and cultural expectations of a laboring woman, also have an effect on the childbirth experience and the use of neuraxial analgesia (see Chapters 20 and 21).

In contemporary clinical practice, health care costs have assumed significant importance. Studies published between 2000 and 2002 estimated that the incremental cost to society for providing epidural labor analgesia was $260 to $340 per parturient.[17,18] A major problem with such analyses is the difficulty of determining the total value of neuraxial analgesia. For example, the ability to rapidly convert epidural analgesia to surgical anesthesia may also have value.

Ideally, the anesthesia provider should tailor the analgesic technique to meet the individual parturient's needs. Factors that should be considered in formulating an analgesic plan for individual parturients include coexisting maternal disease, the airway examination, fetal status, stage of labor, and anticipated risk for operative delivery. The risks and benefits of the various epidural and spinal analgesic techniques should be assessed for each parturient. Good technique requires thoughtful preparation and meticulous attention to detail to ensure maternal and fetal safety.

The ideal labor analgesic technique is safe for both the mother and the baby, does not interfere with the progress of labor and delivery, and provides flexibility in response to changing conditions. In addition, the ideal technique provides consistent pain relief, has a long duration of action, minimizes undesirable side effects (e.g., motor block), and minimizes ongoing demands on the anesthesia provider's time. No single technique or anesthetic agent is ideal for all parturients during labor. Updated practice guidelines for obstetric anesthesia were published by the American Society of Anesthesiologists (ASA) in 2007 (see Appendix B).[19] All obstetric anesthesia providers should review these guidelines. This chapter considers specific neuraxial techniques for labor analgesia, including their advantages, disadvantages, side effects, and complications.

PREPARATION FOR NEURAXIAL ANALGESIA

Indications and Contraindications

Epidural analgesia is indicated to treat the pain experienced by a woman in labor. In 2006 the American College of

Obstetricians and Gynecologists (ACOG),[20] and in 2007 the ASA,[21] reaffirmed the earlier, jointly published opinion stating that "in the absence of a medical contraindication, maternal request is a sufficient medical indication for pain relief during labor" and that "decisions regarding analgesia should be closely coordinated among the obstetrician, the anesthesiologist, the patient, and skilled support personnel." Neuraxial analgesia is an appropriate treatment for the pain of labor, including early labor (defined as regular uterine contractions that cause progressive effacement and dilation of the uterine cervix). Randomized controlled trials[6,7,22-24] and a meta-analysis[25] have confirmed that initiation of neuraxial analgesia in early labor does not increase the risk of cesarean delivery (see later).

Epidural analgesia may facilitate an atraumatic vaginal breech delivery, the vaginal delivery of twin infants, and vaginal delivery of a preterm infant (see Chapters 34 and 35). By providing effective pain relief, epidural analgesia facilitates blood pressure control in preeclamptic women (see Chapter 45). Epidural analgesia also blunts the hemodynamic effects of uterine contractions (e.g., sudden increase in preload) and the associated pain response (tachycardia, increased systemic vascular resistance, hypertension, hyperventilation) in patients with other medical complications (e.g., mitral stenosis, spinal cord injury, intracranial neurovascular disease, asthma; see Chapters 41, 49, and 52).

Box 23-1 lists the contraindications to administration of epidural or spinal analgesia. Some anesthesiologists have suggested that the presence of systemic maternal infection or preexisting neurologic disease is a relative contraindication. However, most cases of systemic infection (especially if properly treated) or neurologic disease do not contraindicate the administration of neuraxial analgesia (see Chapters 36 and 49). It is also controversial whether mild or isolated abnormalities in tests of blood coagulation preclude the use of epidural analgesia (see Chapter 43). The anesthesia provider should consider the risks and benefits of neuraxial analgesia for each patient individually.

Thorough preparation for neuraxial labor analgesia involves several steps (Box 23-2). These include (1) a review of the parturient's obstetric history; (2) a focused preanesthetic evaluation that includes maternal obstetric, anesthetic, and health history; and (3) a brief physical examination (i.e., vital signs, airway, heart, lungs, and back).[19] Routine measurement of a platelet count is not necessary; however, assessment of the platelet count and other laboratory measurements may be indicated in some patients.[19] Also, routine intrapartum blood typing and screening or crossmatching are not necessary in healthy parturients, although consideration should be given to sending a blood sample to the blood bank (to facilitate the rapid availability of blood products in case of emergency need).[19] For parturients at increased risk for hemorrhage, intrapartum typing and screening or crossmatching should be performed. Fetal well-being should be assessed by a skilled provider, and equipment (including resuscitation equipment) should be checked by the anesthesia provider. Informed consent should be obtained. Early and ongoing communication between the obstetric and anesthesia providers, nursing staff, and other members of the multidisciplinary team are encouraged.

BOX 23-1 Contraindications to Epidural and Spinal Analgesia

- Patient refusal or inability to cooperate
- Increased intracranial pressure secondary to a mass lesion
- Skin or soft tissue infection at the site of needle placement
- Frank coagulopathy
- Uncorrected maternal hypovolemia (e.g., hemorrhage)
- Inadequate training in or experience with the technique

BOX 23-2 Checklist: Preparation for Neuraxial Labor Analgesia

1. Communicate (early) with the obstetric provider:
   - Review parturient's obstetric history.
2. Perform focused preanesthetic evaluation:
   - Review maternal obstetric, anesthetic, and health history.
   - Perform targeted physical examination (vital signs, airway, heart, lungs, back).
3. Review relevant laboratory measurements and imaging studies.
4. Consider need for blood typing and screening or crossmatching.
5. Formulate analgesia plan.
6. Obtain informed consent.
7. Perform equipment check:
   - Check routine equipment.
   - Check emergency resuscitation equipment.
8. Obtain peripheral intravenous access.
9. Apply maternal monitors (blood pressure, heart rate, pulse oximetry).
10. Monitor fetal heart rate.
11. Perform a team time-out.

Types of Neuraxial Analgesia

The technical aspects of neuraxial anesthetic/analgesic techniques are discussed in detail in Chapter 12. These techniques include continuous epidural, combined spinal-epidural, and caudal analgesia and continuous and single-shot spinal analgesia. Continuous epidural and combined spinal-epidural analgesia are the most common techniques utilized for neuraxial labor analgesia. There are advantages and disadvantages to each technique (Table 23-1).

EPIDURAL ANALGESIA

Continuous lumbar epidural analgesia has been the mainstay of neuraxial labor analgesia for many years. Placement of an epidural catheter allows analgesia to be maintained until after delivery. No dural puncture is required. The presence of a catheter and effective analgesia allow the conversion to epidural *anesthesia* if cesarean delivery should be necessary. Injection of a local anesthetic in the lumbar epidural space allows spread of the anesthetic solution both cephalad and caudad. Neuroblockade of the T10 to L1 spinal cord segments is necessary to relieve the pain of uterine contractions and cervical dilation, whereas blockade of the S2 to S4 spinal cord segments is necessary to block the pain of vaginal and perineal distention.

TABLE 23-1 Advantages and Disadvantages of Neuraxial Analgesia Techniques for Labor

Neuraxial Technique	Advantages	Disadvantages
Continuous epidural	Continuous analgesia No dural puncture required Ability to extend analgesia to anesthesia for cesarean delivery	Slow onset of analgesia Larger drug doses required, when compared with spinal techniques: Greater risk of maternal systemic toxicity Greater fetal drug exposure
Combined spinal-epidural	Continuous analgesia Low doses of local anesthetic and opioid Rapid onset of analgesia Rapid onset of sacral analgesia Ability to extend analgesia to anesthesia for cesarean delivery Complete analgesia with opioid alone Decreased incidence of failed epidural analgesia	Delayed verification of functioning epidural catheter Higher incidence of pruritus Possible higher risk of fetal bradycardia
Continuous spinal	Continuous analgesia Low doses of local anesthetic and opioid Rapid onset of analgesia Ability to extend analgesia to anesthesia for cesarean delivery	Large dural puncture increases risk of post–dural puncture headache Possibility of overdose and total spinal anesthesia if the spinal catheter is mistaken for an epidural catheter
Continuous caudal	Continuous analgesia Avoids need to access spinal canal through a lumbar interspace in patients with previous lumbar spine surgery	Requires large volumes/doses of drugs May be technically more difficult than other neuraxial techniques Possible higher risk of infection than with other neuraxial techniques Risk of inadvertent fetal injection
Single-shot spinal	Technically simple Rapid onset of analgesia Immediate sacral analgesia Low drug doses	Limited duration of analgesia

Analgesia is initiated by bolus injection of drug(s) through the epidural needle, catheter, or both. Analgesia is maintained with intermittent bolus injections or a continuous epidural infusion. The catheter is removed after delivery when there is no further need for analgesia or anesthesia.

COMBINED SPINAL-EPIDURAL ANALGESIA

Combined spinal-epidural (CSE) analgesia has become increasingly popular in the past decade. Onset of complete analgesia is significantly faster than with epidural techniques (2 to 5 minutes versus 10 to 15 minutes, respectively).[26] In a meta-analysis of comparisons of the onset of epidural with CSE analgesia in 285 parturients,[26] the weighted mean difference in onset was −5.6 minutes (95% confidence interval [CI], −6.6 to −4.6). More women with spinal analgesia than with epidural analgesia had effective analgesia at 10 minutes (relative risk [RR], 2.0; 95% CI, 1.5 to 2.6). In particular, the onset of sacral analgesia is significantly slower after the initiation of lumbar epidural analgesia than after the initiation of spinal analgesia. It may take several hours of lumbar epidural infusion, or several bolus injections of local anesthetic into the lumbar epidural space, to achieve sacral analgesia. Rapid onset of sacral analgesia is advantageous in the parturient in whom analgesia is initiated late in the first stage of labor or in a parous parturient with rapid progress of labor. Spinal analgesia requires a significantly lower amount of drug(s) to attain effective analgesia than does epidural analgesia; therefore, the risk of systemic toxicity is decreased. In addition, there is less systemic absorption of spinal anesthetic agents into the maternal circulation, so maternal and fetal plasma drug concentrations are lower with spinal analgesia than with epidural analgesia.

An additional advantage of spinal analgesia is that complete analgesia for early labor can be accomplished with the intrathecal injection of a lipid-soluble opioid without the addition of a local anesthetic. Thus motor blockade is avoided and the risk of hypotension is lower.[27] This method is ideal for patients who wish to ambulate or for those with preload-dependent conditions such as stenotic heart lesions. Finally, use of the CSE technique may lower the incidence of failure of epidural analgesia (e.g., a nonfunctioning epidural catheter).[28,29]

CSE analgesia has several undesirable side effects. Dural puncture is required to initiate CSE analgesia, although puncture with a small-gauge pencil-point needle does not appear to increase the risk of post–dural puncture headache.[26] A more serious concern, however, is that dural puncture during labor may be a risk factor for postpartum neuraxial infection, a rare but potentially life-threatening complication (see Chapter 32).

The incidence of pruritus is higher with intrathecal opioid administration than with epidural opioid administration.[26] Another potential drawback of CSE analgesia is that it is not clear for 1 to 2 hours after initiation of analgesia whether the epidural catheter is properly sited in the epidural space. Thus, CSE analgesia may not be the technique of choice if a functioning epidural catheter is critical to the safe care of the patient (e.g., a mother with an anticipated difficult airway or a worrisome fetal heart rate [FHR] tracing).

The most common CSE technique for labor analgesia is the needle-through-needle technique in a midlumbar interspinous space. Analgesia is maintained via the epidural catheter, as with traditional epidural analgesia.

CONTINUOUS SPINAL ANALGESIA

Continuous spinal analgesia is used occasionally for labor analgesia but is not practical for most parturients. Because the available catheters (essentially epidural catheters) require use of a large-gauge introducer needle, the technique is associated with an unacceptably high incidence of post–dural puncture headache. However, continuous spinal analgesia is a management option in patients with unintentional dural puncture. Continuous spinal *analgesia* can readily be converted to surgical *anesthesia* if necessary.

CAUDAL ANALGESIA

Continuous caudal epidural analgesia is used infrequently in modern obstetric anesthesia practice. It is technically more difficult to place a caudal catheter than a lumbar epidural catheter. Large volumes of anesthetic solution are required to extend neuroblockade to the low thoracic spinal segments, resulting in higher maternal plasma concentrations of drug. There is a risk of needle/catheter misplacement and direct injection into the fetus. However, this technique is useful for parturients in whom access to the lumbar spinal canal is not possible (e.g., because of a fused lumbar spine).

SINGLE-SHOT TECHNIQUES

In general, single-shot techniques (spinal, lumbar epidural, or caudal) are not useful for most laboring patients because of their limited duration of action. These techniques may be indicated for parturients who require analgesia or anesthesia shortly before anticipated vaginal delivery or in settings in which continuous epidural analgesia is not possible.[30]

Informed Consent

Informed consent should include a frank discussion about anesthetic procedures and risks. Surveys of postpartum women have demonstrated that most parturients want to know the possible complications of epidural analgesia, even those that are rare.[31,32] It is best to relay this information before the onset of labor (e.g., during antenatal classes),[33] or early in the intrapartum period, although doing so is not always feasible. Some anesthesia providers fear that distressed, desperate, or sedated parturients may not understand the discussion of anesthetic procedures. However, adequacy of consent can be demonstrated not only by documentation of information provided to the patient but also by the lack of patient objection to a procedure and the cooperation provided by the patient during the procedure.[34]

BOX 23-3 Suggested Resuscitation Equipment and Drugs That Should Be Available During Administration of Neuraxial Analgesia

Drugs
- Sedative-hypnotic agents (thiopental, propofol, ketamine, midazolam)
- Succinylcholine
- Ephedrine
- Epinephrine
- Phenylephrine
- Atropine
- Calcium chloride
- Sodium bicarbonate
- Naloxone

Equipment
- Oxygen source
- Suction source with tubing and catheters
- Self-inflating bag and mask for positive-pressure ventilation
- Face masks
- Oral airways
- Laryngoscope and assorted blades
- Endotracheal tubes with stylet
- Eschmann stylet (bougie)
- Qualitative carbon dioxide detector
- Intravenous catheters, tubing, and fluid
- Syringes and needles

We do not find it difficult to explain the procedure and the risks of epidural analgesia to a laboring woman. The preanesthetic evaluation allows the physician to communicate a sense of concern and to demonstrate a commitment to the patient's care. Most laboring women understand the need for informed consent, and they appreciate the opportunity to participate in decisions about their care.

Equipment

Resuscitation equipment, drugs, and supplies must be immediately available for the management of serious complications of epidural analgesia (e.g., hypotension, total spinal anesthesia, systemic local anesthetic toxicity) (Box 23-3).[19] Emergency airway equipment should be checked before the administration of neuraxial analgesia.

Monitors

During the initiation of neuraxial analgesia, we monitor all patients with an automatic blood pressure cuff and a pulse oximeter to facilitate continuous assessment of the maternal heart rate and oxygenation. Maternal blood pressure is measured every 1 to 2½ minutes after the administration of the test and therapeutic doses of local anesthetic for approximately 15 to 20 minutes, or until the mother is hemodynamically stable. Subsequently (during maintenance of neuraxial analgesia), maternal blood pressure is measured every 15 to 30 minutes, or more frequently if hypotension ensues. Continuous pulse oximetry during maintenance analgesia is used in selected patients (e.g., patients with obstructive sleep apnea or cardiovascular disease). Rarely, invasive hemodynamic monitoring is necessary.

BOX 23-4 Assessment of Motor Block

- **Complete:** patient unable to move feet or knees
- **Almost complete:** patient able to move feet only
- **Partial:** patient just able to move knees
- **None:** patient capable of full flexion of knees and feet

Adapted from Bromage PR. Epidural Analgesia. Philadelphia, WB Saunders, 1978:144.

The sensory level of analgesia and the intensity of motor block are assessed after the administration of the test and therapeutic doses of local anesthetic. Subsequently, sensory level and motor block are assessed every several hours (Box 23-4).

When possible, we monitor the FHR continuously during initiation of neuraxial analgesia. The ASA Task Force on Obstetric Anesthesia[19] has stated:

> *The fetal heart rate should be monitored by a qualified individual before and after administration of regional analgesia for labor. The Task Force recognizes that* continuous *electronic recording of the fetal heart rate may not be necessary in every clinical setting and may not be possible during initiation of neuraxial anesthesia.*

The ACOG has provided no specific guidelines regarding the use of FHR monitoring during neuraxial analgesia.[35]

The anesthesia provider cannot predict when hypotension will occur during the administration of neuraxial anesthesia. In addition, there is concern that intrathecal opioid administration is associated with a higher incidence of nonreassuring FHR patterns than non-intrathecal opioid neuraxial techniques (see later).[36] Thus we believe that continuous electronic FHR monitoring should be performed both during (if possible) and after the administration of neuraxial analgesia in all laboring women. In some cases, the mother's position or maternal obesity precludes the use of an external Doppler device to monitor the FHR. In such cases (especially when there is concern regarding fetal well-being), it is helpful for the obstetric provider to place a fetal scalp electrode to monitor the FHR.

Intravenous Hydration

Placement of an intravenous catheter (preferably 18-gauge or larger) and correction of hypovolemia with intravenous hydration are necessary before the initiation of neuraxial analgesia to prevent hypotension that can result from sympathetic blockade. Most anesthesia providers administer approximately 500 mL of lactated Ringer's solution (without dextrose), although the ASA Task Force on Obstetric Anesthesia has stated that a fixed volume of intravenous fluid is not required before neuraxial analgesia is initiated.[19] Severe hypotension is less likely with the contemporary practice of administering a dilute solution of local anesthetic for epidural analgesia or an intrathecal opioid for spinal analgesia. However, deterioration in FHR patterns has been observed when the fluid preload was omitted.[37] Studies of intravenous hydration and spinal *anesthesia* for cesarean delivery suggest that administering the fluid at the time of initiation of anesthesia (co-load) is more effective in preventing hypotension than administering the fluid ahead of time (preload).[38] We continue to give a 500-mL fluid bolus at the time of initiation of labor analgesia in laboring women at Northwestern Memorial Hospital. Rarely, hydration should be guided by the measurement of central venous or pulmonary artery pressure. Fluid administration should be judicious in patients at risk for pulmonary edema (e.g., women with severe preeclampsia).

Lactated Ringer's solution (without dextrose) is the most commonly used intravenous fluid in laboring women, for both bolus administration and maintenance infusion. Data are conflicting as to whether the maintenance intravenous infusion of dextrose-containing fluid during labor is associated with a lower incidence of umbilical cord acidemia.[39,40] However, anesthesia and obstetric providers should avoid the *bolus* administration of dextrose-containing solutions in laboring women.

Maternal Positioning

Either the lateral decubitus or the sitting position can be used during initiation of neuraxial analgesia (see Chapter 12). The lateral position has the following advantages over the sitting position: (1) orthostatic hypotension is less likely, (2) the position often facilitates continuous FHR monitoring during placement of the epidural catheter, and (3) some patients find it more comfortable.[41] One study demonstrated a greater reduction in maternal cardiac output with maximal lumbar flexion in the lateral decubitus position than in the sitting position during identification of the epidural space in laboring women.[42] The researchers speculated that maximal lumbar flexion in the lateral decubitus position results in concealed aortocaval compression. In contrast, they suggested that the uterus falls forward (and thus does not cause aortocaval compression) when the patient assumes the sitting flexed position. They recommended that "the tight fetal curl position be avoided," especially when the patient assumes the lateral decubitus position for identification of the epidural or intrathecal space.[42]

In obese women, the sitting position is often advantageous. It may provide better respiratory mechanics, facilitate the identification of the midline and bony landmarks, and improve maternal comfort during placement of the epidural catheter.[41] Maternal position during placement of the epidural catheter does not seem to affect the incidence of unintentional dural puncture. However, adoption of the lateral recumbent head-down position for epidural catheter placement may reduce the incidence of epidural venous puncture.[43]

Aortocaval compression must be avoided at all times. The gravid uterus can occlude the inferior vena cava and aorta when the parturient assumes the supine position.[44-46] This position may cause maternal hypotension[47,48] and reduce uteroplacental perfusion,[49] even in the absence of anesthesia. Increased venous tone in the lower extremities helps overcome partial occlusion of the inferior vena cava in unanesthetized pregnant women. If maternal hydration is inadequate and if aortocaval compression is not avoided, the onset of anesthesia-induced sympathetic blockade will result in decreased venous return, cardiac output, and uteroplacental perfusion.[46] The avoidance of aortocaval compression is essential to maintain normal cardiac output and uteroplacental perfusion.[46,47]

Some anesthesiologists contend that maternal position after epidural catheter placement affects the efficacy of epidural analgesia, although this is a matter of some dispute (see later). Beilin et al.[50] observed that the placement of the laboring woman in the supine position with a 30-degree leftward tilt was associated with better epidural analgesia than maintenance of the left lateral decubitus position. In contrast, Preston et al.[51] observed no difference in analgesia and a significantly higher incidence of fetal bradycardia with the supine wedged position than with the full lateral position.

BOX 23-5 Suggested Procedure for Initiation of Epidural Labor Analgesia

1. Complete the "preparation for neuraxial analgesia" checklist (see Box 23-2).
2. Position patient with the help of an assistant (lateral decubitus or sitting).
3. Initiate maternal blood pressure, maternal pulse oximetry, and fetal heart rate monitoring.
4. Give an intravenous fluid bolus (500 mL of lactated Ringer's solution).
5. Site epidural catheter in epidural space with use of sterile technique.
6. Administer an epidural test dose (see Table 23-2).
7. If result of the test dose is negative, secure epidural catheter and position patient in the lateral position.
8. Administer 5 to 15 mL of epidural local anesthetic, in 5-mL increments (usually a low concentration of a local anesthetic combined with a lipid-soluble opioid [see Table 23-3]).
9. Monitor maternal blood pressure every 1 to 2½ minutes for 15 to 20 minutes, or until the parturient is hemodynamically stable.
10. Assess pain score and extent of sensory blockade (both cephalad and caudad).
11. Initiate maintenance epidural analgesia (see Table 23-6).

INITIATION OF EPIDURAL ANALGESIA

A procedure for initiating epidural labor analgesia is outlined in Box 23-5. Usually, the epidural space is identified and the epidural catheter is sited in the epidural space. A test dose is administered to rule out intrathecal or intravascular placement of the epidural catheter. After a negative test dose result, epidural analgesia is established with the incremental injection of a local anesthetic, usually in combination with a lipid-soluble opioid. Maternal vital signs are monitored and clinical analgesia is verified.

Epidural Test Dose

Epidural catheter placement may be complicated by blood vessel or dural puncture with the needle or catheter. To prevent possible local anesthetic toxicity and high or total spinal anesthesia, the anesthesia provider must recognize the unintentional intravenous or subarachnoid placement of the needle or catheter. The purpose of the test dose is to allow early recognition of a malpositioned catheter. The ideal test dose must be readily available, safe, and effective. Its use should have a high sensitivity (i.e., low false-negative rate) and a high specificity (i.e., low false-positive rate). The intravascular and intrathecal test doses may be combined (a single injection to test for both intravascular and subarachnoid placement) or administered separately. A negative response to an epidural test dose does not guarantee the correct placement of the epidural catheter in the epidural space, nor does it guarantee that the catheter is not malpositioned in a blood vessel or the subarachnoid space. Rather, it *decreases the likelihood* that the catheter tip is in a blood vessel or the subarachnoid space.

INTRAVASCULAR TEST DOSE

The ideal method for excluding intravenous placement of the catheter is controversial. Blood vessel puncture (indicated by aspiration of blood or blood-tinged fluid through the epidural catheter) occurs in 9% to 20% of obstetric patients,[52,53] and intravenous placement of an epidural catheter occurs in approximately 7% to 8.5% of obstetric patients.[54] Failure to recognize intravenous placement of the epidural catheter and subsequent intravenous injection of a large dose of local anesthetic may lead to systemic local anesthetic toxicity, with central nervous system (CNS) symptoms, seizures, cardiovascular collapse, and death.[55]

The intravascular test dose typically contains epinephrine 15 μg.* In normal volunteers, intravenous injection of epinephrine 15 μg (3 mL of a 1:200,000 solution) reliably causes tachycardia.[56,57] An increase in heart rate of 20 beats per minute (bpm) within 45 seconds was 100% sensitive and specific for intravascular injection in unpremedicated patients.[56] An increase in systolic blood pressure of between 15 and 25 mm Hg was also observed. Some anesthesiologists have expressed concerns about the use of an epinephrine-containing test dose in laboring women. Intravenous epinephrine may cause a transient decline in uterine blood flow as a result of alpha-adrenergic receptor–mediated constriction of the uterine arteries (Figure 23-2).[58-60] However, this decrease in uterine blood flow is transient and comparable to the decrease that occurs during a uterine contraction. Youngstrom et al.[61] noted that this intravenous dose of epinephrine did not worsen fetal condition in acidotic fetal lambs. In healthy parturients, any transient effect of epinephrine on uterine blood flow likely represents a less severe insult than systemic local anesthetic toxicity. An epinephrine-containing test dose, however, may not be appropriate in parturients with severe hypertension or uteroplacental insufficiency.

*The Joint Commission has recommended that health care providers substitute "mcg" for "μg" as an abbreviation for micrograms (http://www.aapmr.org/hpl/pracguide/jcahosymbols.htm). The Joint Commission contends that the abbreviation "μg" may be mistaken for "mg" (milligrams), which would result in a 1000-fold overdose. On the other hand, most scholarly publications have continued to use the abbreviation "μg." The editors have chosen to retain the use of the abbreviation "μg" throughout this text. However, the editors recommend the use of the abbreviation "mcg" in clinical practice, especially with handwritten orders.

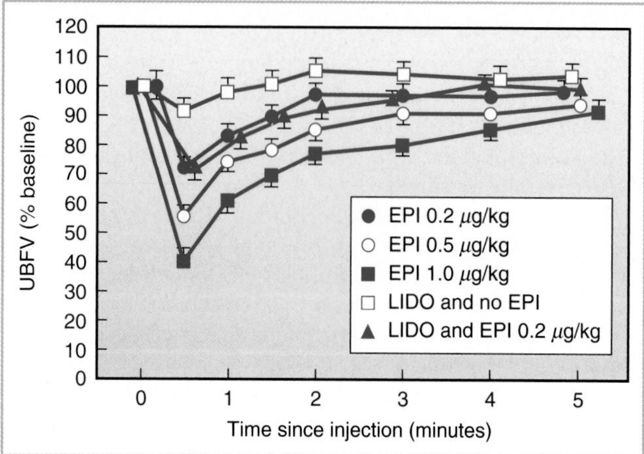

FIGURE 23-2 The effect of intravenous epinephrine (EPI), lidocaine (LIDO), and lidocaine with epinephrine on uterine artery blood flow velocity (UBFV) in the pregnant guinea pig. The dose of lidocaine was 0.4 mg/kg. Values are presented as mean ± SEM percentage of baseline. (From Chestnut DH, Weiner CP, Martin JG, et al. Effect of intravenous epinephrine on uterine artery blood flow velocity in the pregnant guinea pig. Anesthesiology 1986; 65:633-6.)

Some anesthesiologists argue that the epinephrine-containing test dose lacks *specificity* in laboring women. The maternal tachycardic response to intravenous injection of epinephrine cannot always be distinguished from other causes of tachycardia (e.g., pain during a uterine contraction) (Figure 23-3).[62,63] Cartwright et al.[63] noted that 12% of laboring women had an increase in heart rate of at least 30 bpm after epidural injection of 3 mL of 0.5% bupivacaine without epinephrine. A study in laboring women compared the intravenous injection of epinephrine (10 to 15 μg) with that of saline; the sensitivity was 100%, the area under the receiver operator curve was 0.91 to 0.93, and the negative predictive value was 100%.[64] However, the positive predictive value was 55% to 73%. The results suggested that if a positive heart rate response to an epinephrine-containing test dose occurs in 20% of patients, 5% to 9% of epidural catheters would be identified incorrectly as intravascular and removed unnecessarily. Colonna-Romano and Nagaraj[65] concluded that the intravenous injection of an epinephrine-containing test dose results in "a sudden and fast acceleration in maternal heart rate within one minute." Thus, careful assessment of the rate of increase in maternal heart rate may help distinguish a contraction-induced increase in heart rate from the effect of intravenously injected epinephrine, thereby improving the specificity of the epinephrine test.[65] It is unclear whether such an assessment is clinically practical or will actually reduce the incidence of false-positive results.[66]

Additionally, some anesthesiologists argue that the epinephrine-containing test dose lacks *sensitivity* (the ability to elicit a predictable increase in heart rate when the catheter is intravascular). An increase in maternal heart rate of 25 bpm occurring within 2 minutes of drug injection and lasting at least 15 seconds was observed in only 5 of 10 laboring women who received intravenous epinephrine 15 μg (Figure 23-4).[67] Detection of intravenous epinephrine injection was improved when the authors retrospectively defined a positive maternal tachycardic response as a 10-bpm increase in the maximum maternal heart rate observed in the 2-minute period preceding the epinephrine injection. Others have confirmed that these revised criteria improve the sensitivity of the epinephrine-containing test dose in laboring women.[64]

The usefulness of an epinephrine-containing test dose also improves if additional information is obtained. For example, investigators administered intravenous bupivacaine 12.5 mg with epinephrine 12.5 μg or saline to

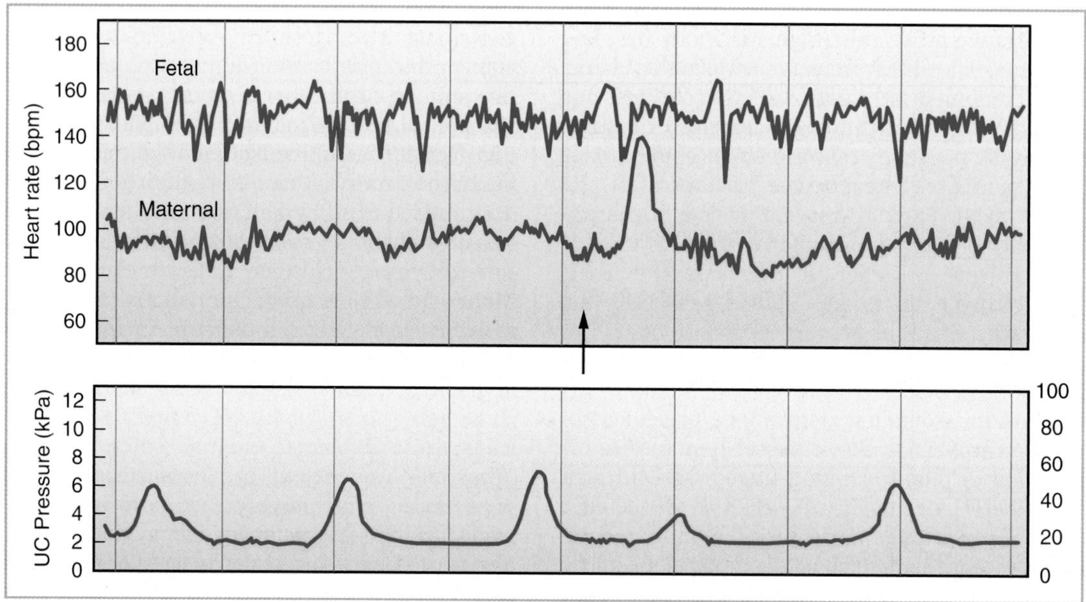

FIGURE 23-3 Heart rate of a laboring patient (maternal heart rate [MHR]), fetal heart rate, and uterine contractions (UC) are shown. This tracing was obtained with the use of an FHR monitor with dual heart rate capacity. Note the variability of the MHR with uterine contractions. An intravenous injection of bupivacaine 12.5 mg and epinephrine 12.5 μg was given (*arrow*). Note the marked increase in MHR in response to intravenous injection of the test dose. The maternal tachycardia had a duration of approximately 40 seconds. (From Van Zundert AA, Vaes LE, De Wolf AM. ECG monitoring of mother and fetus during epidural anesthesia. Anesthesiology 1987; 66:584-5.)

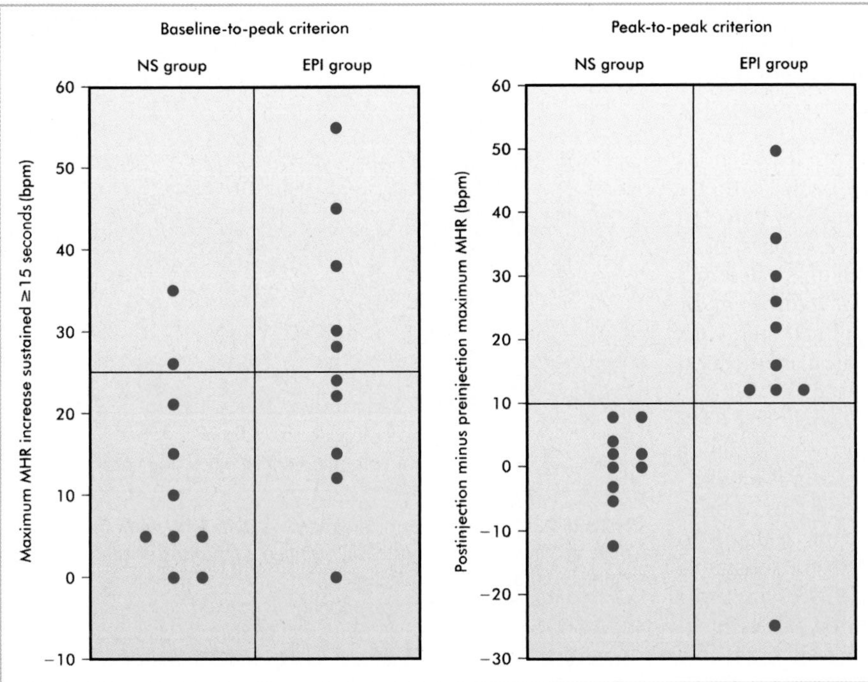

FIGURE 23-4 Maximum maternal heart rate (MHR) changes after intravenous injection of 15 µg of epinephrine (EPI group) or saline (NS group). Baseline-to-peak criterion for a positive heart rate response to epinephrine was prospectively defined as an increase in heart rate of more than 25 bpm above that at the time of epinephrine injection, which occurred within 120 seconds of drug injection. Peak-to-peak criterion for a positive heart rate response was retrospectively defined as an increase in heart rate of more than 10 bpm during the 2 minutes after the injection as compared with the maximum MHR recorded during the 2 minutes preceding the injection. (From Leighton BL, Norris MC, Sosis M, et al. Limitations of epinephrine as a marker of intravascular injection in laboring women. Anesthesiology 1987; 66:688-91.)

laboring women.[68] They correctly identified the test solution in 39 of 40 women when they assessed maternal heart rate, blood pressure, uterine contractions, the timing of the injection, the presence of analgesia, and subjective signs and symptoms of intravascular injection (e.g., palpitations, lightheadedness, dizziness). The tachycardic response to intravenous epinephrine is not a reliable indicator of intravascular injection in patients who have received a beta-adrenergic receptor antagonist.[56]

Other means of identifying intravascular placement of an epidural catheter have been proposed and may be clinically useful in specific patients (Table 23-2). Intravenous administration of isoproterenol 5 µg consistently results in tachycardia in pregnant women.[69,70] Data from animals[60,71] and noninvasive measurements in parturients[70] suggest that isoproterenol is devoid of the adverse effects of epinephrine on uterine blood flow, and limited neurotoxicity evaluations have not revealed adverse effects.[71] Marcus et al.[72] randomly assigned 80 laboring women to receive bupivacaine 0.125% with sufentanil 7.5 µg and either epinephrine 12.5 µg or isoproterenol 5 µg; the investigators observed no clinical evidence of neurotoxicity. However, isoproterenol

TABLE 23-2 Epidural Test Dose Regimens*

Test Dose Components	Positive Intravascular Test Dose	Positive Intrathecal Test Dose
Combined Intrathecal and Intravenous Test Dose:		
Lidocaine 1.5% with epinephrine 5 µg/mL (1:200,000): 3 mL Bupivacaine 0.25% with epinephrine 5 µg/mL (1:200,000): 3 mL	Increase in heart rate of 20 bpm within 1 minute	Motor blockade at 3-5 minutes†
Intravenous Test Dose:		
Lidocaine 100 mg Bupivacaine 25 mg 2-Chloroprocaine 100 mg	Tinnitus, circumoral numbness, "dizziness"	
Fentanyl 100 µg	Dizziness, drowsiness	
Air 1 mL	Change in Doppler heart sounds over right side of heart	
Intrathecal Test Dose:		
Lidocaine 40-60 mg Bupivacaine 7.5 mg		Motor blockade at 3-5 minutes†

*Test doses may be less sensitive in premedicated patients, patients treated with a beta-adrenergic receptor antagonist, pregnant patients, and anesthetized patients.

†Weakness in hip flexion.

Modified from Yilmaz M, Wong CA. Technique of neuraxial anesthesia. In Wong CA, editor. Spinal and Epidural Anesthesia. New York, McGraw-Hill, 2007:27-73.

has not been approved for epidural or intrathecal administration. Given the lack of adequate information regarding potential neurotoxicity, we do not recommend the use of isoproterenol as an epidural test dose.

Leighton et al.[73] have advocated the use of air as an objective marker of intravascular injection. Intravenous injection of 1 or 2 mL of air through a single-orifice catheter consistently produces changes in heart sounds as detected by the use of precordial Doppler ultrasonography.[73] (The external FHR monitor can be used for this purpose.) False-negative results may occur when small volumes of air are injected through a multi-orifice epidural catheter; thus the air test is not a reliable test for intravascular injection when multi-orifice epidural catheters are used.[74]

Local anesthetic–induced symptoms of subclinical CNS toxicity have also been evaluated as a means of recognizing the unintentional intravenous injection of epidural medications. Colonna-Romano et al.[75] administered intravenous saline, lidocaine 100 mg, or 2-chloroprocaine 100 mg to laboring women. Observers blinded as to which substance was administered recorded the presence of CNS symptoms (i.e., dizziness, tinnitus, funny taste) after intravenous injection of local anesthetic. Lidocaine 100 mg was a reliable marker of intravenous injection when the symptoms of tinnitus and funny taste were considered (sensitivity 100%; specificity 81%). 2-Chloroprocaine was less reliable (sensitivity 81% to 94%; specificity 69% to 81%). In a volunteer study, a dose of 1.5 mg/kg of 2-chloroprocaine was necessary to produce a probability of 90% that the subject would report symptoms of intravenous injection.[76]

Administration of fentanyl 100 μg has been described as a test for intravenous injection.[77] Morris et al.[78] evaluated the accuracy and reliability of the fentanyl test dose in a double-blind study in which either intravenous or epidural fentanyl 100 μg was administered to parturients, and the investigators sought evidence of the occurrence of sedation, dizziness, euphoria, and/or analgesia. Dizziness was the most reliable symptom of intravenous fentanyl injection, with a sensitivity of 92% and a specificity of 92%.

Some situations reduce the reliability of subjective symptoms as a signal of intravenous injection of a drug. Tests that rely on the self-reporting of subjective symptoms require clear communication with the patient and thus are less useful when the anesthesia provider and patient speak different languages. Patient exhaustion and/or prior opioid administration also may affect the reliability of the test.

Lastly, the epidural catheter design and speed of injection may affect the reliability of the epidural test dose. An epinephrine-containing test dose should be injected rapidly; otherwise rapid redistribution and metabolism of the drug decrease the actual dose administered to chronoreceptors. Multi-orifice epidural catheters have three potential sites of exit for injected fluid or air, and the orifices may lie within two different body compartments. If injected too slowly, air or fluid preferentially exits the proximal orifice. The speed of injection used in clinical practice typically exceeds that required to ensure that fluid will exit all three orifices. In contrast, air must be injected at a much greater speed to ensure that it exits all three orifices; this speed is not practical for clinical use. The distal orifice is both the most difficult to test and the one most likely to be positioned outside the epidural space.[79]

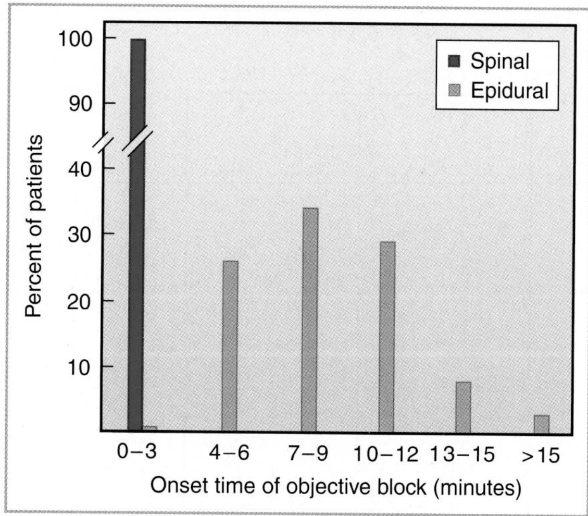

FIGURE 23-5 Percentage of pregnant patients who demonstrated objective evidence of anesthesia (defined as the loss of sensation to pinprick) after epidural injection of 2 to 3 mL of hyperbaric 1.5% lidocaine with 1:200,000 epinephrine *(light teal bars)* (n = 250) or after intrathecal injection of 2 mL of hyperbaric 1.5% lidocaine with 1:200,000 epinephrine *(dark teal bar)* (n = 15). (From Abraham RA, Harris AP, Maxwell LG, et al. The efficacy of 1.5% lidocaine with 7.5% dextrose and epinephrine as an epidural test dose for obstetrics. Anesthesiology 1986; 64:116-9.)

INTRATHECAL TEST DOSE

The intrathecal test dose should allow easy identification of subarachnoid (intrathecal) placement of the catheter without causing high or total spinal anesthesia and hemodynamic compromise. Bupivacaine (7.5 mg) and lidocaine (45 to 60 mg) are the local anesthetics most often used for an intrathecal test dose (see Table 23-2) (Figure 23-5).[80,81] In a study of older, nonpregnant patients receiving continuous spinal anesthesia for surgery, Colonna-Romano et al.[81] used plain lidocaine 45 mg plus epinephrine 15 μg and assessed patient perception of lower extremity warmth and heaviness, sensory loss to pinprick, and ability to perform a straight-leg raise. Patients usually perceived warmth in their legs within 1 minute of the intrathecal injection; however, impaired straight-leg raise 4 minutes after an intrathecal test dose injection was the only test that had a sensitivity of 100% for intrathecal injection. The application of these data to pregnant patients is unclear.

Richardson et al.[82] described the rapid onset (1 to 3 minutes) of high levels of spinal anesthesia with motor block and hypotension in five parturients who had received a test dose of plain lidocaine 45 mg plus epinephrine 15 μg. This solution is slightly hypobaric relative to cerebrospinal fluid (CSF) at body temperature; thus the upright posture of these parturients during the injection may have contributed to the high levels of spinal anesthesia. The anesthesia provider must recognize the possible range of responses to the dose of local anesthetic used to assess the position of an epidural catheter and should perform a careful assessment of sensory, motor, and sympathetic function 3 to 5 minutes after administration of the test dose before concluding that the intrathecal test dose result is negative. Ropivacaine 15 mg is *not* a useful intrathecal test dose because the slow onset of motor blockade precludes timely diagnosis of intrathecal injection.[83] 2-Chloroprocaine is the only local anesthetic that can be used as a single, combined intravascular and intrathecal test dose; in most patients, 100 mg results in dense, but not total spinal anesthesia after intrathecal injection and produces systemic signs of subclinical toxicity (tinnitus, funny taste) after intravascular injection.

The epidural injection of local anesthetic for the purpose of ruling out intrathecal or intravascular catheter placement augments *epidural* analgesia and should be considered in the calculation of the initial therapeutic dose of local anesthetic. Several groups of investigators demonstrated that the test dose enhanced the density of epidural blockade and adversely affected the ability to ambulate. A test dose containing lidocaine 45 mg/epinephrine 15 μg adversely affected the ability to ambulate when injected immediately before initiation of epidural analgesia with 0.125% bupivacaine (18.75 mg) with sufentanil (10 μg).[84] Similarly, the same test dose interfered with ambulation when administered immediately after the intrathecal injection of bupivacaine 2.5 mg and fentanyl 25 μg.[85] Finally, a lidocaine 60 mg/epinephrine 15 μg test dose adversely affected the ability to ambulate in women who received neostigmine 500 μg with sufentanil 10 μg for initiation of analgesia.[86]

TECHNIQUES TO MINIMIZE LOCAL ANESTHETIC TOXICITY

No perfect test dose exists. Some anesthesia providers elect not to administer a test dose because it contributes to motor blockade.[84,85] In addition, aspiration of a *multi-orifice* epidural catheter for blood has 98% sensitivity for detection of an intravascular location.[87] Inadvertent intravascular injection of a solution containing a low concentration of local anesthetic is unlikely to result in serious morbidity. However, this conclusion depends heavily on the use of small doses of local anesthetic.[88] Laboring women may need large doses of local anesthetic for operative delivery. In some cases, large doses are administered quickly (without incremental injection) for emergency cesarean delivery. The anesthesia provider wants to determine as soon as possible that the epidural catheter is correctly positioned within the epidural space. Even if no morbidity results, it is inconvenient for both the patient and the anesthesia provider to have to repeat the procedure and replace the catheter once the drape has been removed and the patient has been repositioned. The epinephrine-containing test dose provides an objective marker of intravascular injection that has stood the test of time. Thus, we typically give a test dose that contains either bupivacaine 7.5 mg or lidocaine 45 to 60 mg with 15 μg of epinephrine. No matter whether a test dose is injected, drugs should be injected incrementally into the epidural space, because no test is 100% sensitive, and catheters may migrate during use. Each incremental dose should be treated as a "test dose" (i.e., the dose should be small enough that it will not cause systemic toxicity if unintentionally injected intravascularly or total spinal anesthesia if injected intrathecally). Pregnant women are very difficult to resuscitate from local anesthetic cardiovascular toxicity.[55]

Steps to minimize the possibility of local anesthetic toxicity are summarized in Box 12-2. They include observation for passive return of CSF or blood (by lowering the proximal end of the epidural catheter below the insertion site), administration of the test dose between contractions, aspiration before each dose, incremental dose administration, maintaining verbal contact with the patient, and assessment for an appropriate level and density of sensory and motor blockade (which indicates correct placement of the catheter in the epidural space).

Choice of Drugs

The ideal analgesic drug for labor would provide rapid onset of effective analgesia with minimal motor blockade, minimal risk of maternal toxicity, and negligible effect on uterine activity and uteroplacental perfusion. It would undergo limited transplacental transfer and thus have minimal direct effect on the fetus. Finally, this ideal agent would have a long duration of action. Although this perfect analgesic drug does not exist, the combination of a local anesthetic with an opioid allows us to approach this goal.

Traditionally, local anesthetics were administered to block both the visceral pain of labor (lower uterine segment distention and cervical dilation) and the somatic pain (descent of the fetus in the birth canal). Three decades ago, investigators identified dense concentrations of opiate receptors in the dorsal horn of the spinal cord.[89] The application of small doses of an opioid to these receptor sites generates a specific and profound opioid response.[89] The introduction of neuraxial opioids to the armamentarium of the obstetric anesthesia provider moved us closer to the prediction made by Benjamin Rush in 1805: "A medicine would be discovered which should suspend sensibility altogether and leave irritability or powers of motion unimpaired."[90] Intrathecal opioids effectively relieve the visceral pain of the early first stage of labor, although they must be combined with a local anesthetic to effectively relieve the somatic pain of the late first stage and the second stage of labor. The combination of a local anesthetic with a lipid-soluble opioid allows for the use of lower doses of each agent, thus minimizing undesirable side effects. For example, when used alone without an opioid, the local anesthetic dose required for effective epidural analgesia is associated with an unacceptably high incidence of motor blockade. Similarly, used alone, high doses of epidural opioid are required for satisfactory analgesia during early labor, and such doses are associated with significant systemic absorption and systemic side effects. The addition of an opioid to the local anesthetic also shortens latency,[91] an important aspect of labor analgesia, especially with the use of long-acting (and therefore, long-latency) local anesthetics. Thus contemporary epidural labor analgesia practice most often incorporates low doses of a long-acting local anesthetic combined with a lipid-soluble opioid.

LOCAL ANESTHETICS

Bupivacaine

The amide local anesthetic bupivacaine is the local anesthetic most commonly used for epidural labor analgesia. Bupivacaine is highly protein bound, a feature that limits transplacental transfer. The umbilical vein–to–maternal vein concentration ratio is approximately 0.3.[92] After epidural administration of bupivacaine (without opioid) during labor, the patient first perceives pain relief within approximately 8 to 10 minutes,[93] but approximately 20 minutes are required to achieve the peak effect. Duration of analgesia is approximately 90 minutes. Bupivacaine 6.25 to 12.5 mg (10 to 20 mL of a 0.0625% solution, or 5 to 10 mL of a 0.125% solution) combined with fentanyl or sufentanil is adequate to initiate labor analgesia in most parturients (Table 23-3).

TABLE 23-3 Drugs Used for the Initiation of Epidural and Spinal Labor Analgesia

Drug	Epidural Analgesia*	Spinal Analgesia
Local Anesthetics†		
Bupivacaine	0.0625%-0.125%	1.25-2.5 mg
Ropivacaine	0.08%-0.2%	2.5-4.5 mg
Levobupivacaine	0.0625%-0.125%	2.5-4.5 mg
Lidocaine‡	0.75%-1.0%	NA
Opioids†		
Fentanyl	50-100 μg	15-25 μg
Sufentanil	5-10 μg	1.5-5 μg
Morphine‡	NA	0.125-0.25 mg

NA, not applicable.

*The volume required to initiate epidural labor analgesia is 5-20 mL of local anesthetic solution.

†The local anesthetic dose/concentration and the fentanyl or sufentanil dose are reduced if the drugs are combined, or if a local anesthetic–containing epidural test dose is administered before the initial therapeutic dose.

‡Lidocaine and morphine are not commonly used for labor analgesia because of their short duration of action (lidocaine) and long latency (morphine).

TABLE 23-4 Comparison of Epidural Bupivacaine 0.25% and 0.125%: Minimum Effective Volume and Dose

Parameter	Bupivacaine 0.125% (w/v)‡	Bupivacaine 0.25% (w/v)‡
MLAV*		
Up-down analysis (mL)	13.6 (12.4-14.8)	9.2 (6.9-11.5)
Probit analysis (mL)	13.5 (11.4-15.9)	8.6 (7.2-10.3)
MLAD†		
Up-down analysis (mg)	17.0 (15.5-18.5)	23.1 (17.2-28.9)
Probit analysis (mg)	16.8 (14.2-19.9)	21.5 (17.9-25.7)

*Minimum local anesthetic volume (median effective volume) at a fixed concentration.

†Minimum local anesthetic dose (median effective dose) at a fixed concentration (w/v = weight/volume).

‡95% confidence intervals shown in parentheses, which were calculated using up-down sequential and probit analysis.

Modified from Lyons GR, Kocarev MG, Wilson RC, Columb MO. A comparison of minimum local anesthetic volumes and doses of epidural bupivacaine (0.125% w/v and 0.25% w/v) for analgesia in labor. Anesth Analg 2007; 104:412-5.

The potency of local anesthetics for neuraxial labor analgesia is often assessed by determining the minimum local anesthetic concentration (MLAC). MLAC is the median effective concentration of local anesthetic solution when administered as a 20-mL bolus. It is lower both for women in early labor[94] and when the local anesthetic is combined with a lipid-soluble opioid.[95]

It is important to consider both the local anesthetic *dose* and *concentration* for initiation and maintenance of epidural analgesia. Christiaens et al.[96] randomly assigned parturients to receive epidural bupivacaine 20 mg diluted in 4 mL, 10 mL, or 20 mL (0.5%, 0.2%, and 0.1% solutions, respectively). Analgesia was superior in the 10-mL and 20-mL groups to that in the 4-mL group, and duration of analgesia was longest in the 20-mL group. Lyons et al.[97] compared the minimum local anesthetic volume (MLAV) and minimum local anesthetic dose (MLAD) for 0.125% and 0.25% bupivacaine for epidural labor analgesia. Bupivacaine 0.125% produced analgesia equivalent to that provided by bupivacaine 0.25%, with a 50% increase in required volume and a 25% reduction in dose (Table 23-4). Stated differently, a dose-sparing effect is achieved by administering a 0.125% solution of bupivacaine rather than a 0.25% solution. These data suggest that epidural analgesia and safety are improved with the use of low concentration–high volume local anesthetic solutions.

Ropivacaine

Ropivacaine, an amide local anesthetic, is similar to bupivacaine in structure and pharmacodynamics.[98] It is a homologue of bupivacaine and mepivacaine, but unlike these other local anesthetics, it is formulated as a single-levorotary enantiomer rather than a racemic mixture (see Chapter 13). Studies *in vitro* and *in vivo* have shown that ropivacaine is less cardiodepressant and arrhythmogenic than bupivacaine when equal doses are compared.[99,100] Studies of pregnant sheep have demonstrated that clinically relevant plasma concentrations of ropivacaine do not adversely affect uterine blood flow.[101] Ropivacaine is cleared more rapidly than bupivacaine after intravenous administration in both pregnant and nonpregnant sheep. Consequently, a larger dose of drug—but not a higher plasma concentration—is required to produce systemic toxicity.[102] These findings suggest that ropivacaine has a greater margin of safety than bupivacaine if unintentional intravenous injection occurs in pregnant women. However, many early investigations assumed that ropivacaine and bupivacaine are equipotent; subsequent studies have demonstrated that ropivacaine is 40% less potent than bupivacaine.[103,104] When ropivacaine concentrations are adjusted for this difference in potency, there is a less clear advantage for ropivacaine in terms of the risk of systemic toxicity.[103] In reality, systemic toxicity is not a major concern with the contemporary administration of a dilute solution of local anesthetic for epidural labor analgesia.

Several studies that compared equal concentrations of ropivacaine and bupivacaine given by patient-controlled epidural analgesia (PCEA) have not found any significant difference in clinical efficacy between the two local anesthetics.[105-109] Other studies that adjusted for the potency difference and compared equipotent concentrations (e.g., 0.0625% bupivacaine versus 0.1% ropivacaine) also found no difference in clinical efficacy.[110,111] It is important to recognize that potency is an unchanging property of a drug, whereas clinical efficacy is influenced by multiple variables. For example, ropivacaine has a longer duration of analgesia than bupivacaine,[103] which may offset its lesser potency when it is administered by continuous epidural infusion.

Early clinical studies suggested that ropivacaine is associated with less motor block than bupivacaine[112,113]; avoidance of motor blockade is a desirable characteristic of a local anesthetic used for epidural analgesia during labor. However, these studies also compared equal concentrations of ropivacaine and bupivacaine, and the observed lower degree of motor blockade may reflect the lesser potency of ropivacaine. A study of the relative motor-blocking potencies of epidural ropivacaine and bupivacaine showed that ropivacaine was less potent than bupivacaine in terms of motor blockade,[114] a finding that corresponded to the relative analgesic potencies of the two drugs.[103,104] The differences in potency of motor blockade may not be relevant with the use of low concentrations of local anesthetic. Several clinical studies[105,109,115] and a well-conducted meta-analysis of studies comparing epidural ropivacaine and bupivacaine[116] did not demonstrate an advantage for ropivacaine in terms of outcome of labor (see later), although the incidence of motor blockade was less in the ropivacaine groups.[109,115,116]

It is difficult to justify the higher cost of ropivacaine without evidence of clear patient benefit. There is no definitive evidence of greater patient safety or lower risk of instrumental vaginal delivery when ropivacaine is used to provide epidural analgesia in laboring women, and there is no significant difference between ropivacaine and bupivacaine in obstetric or neonatal outcome.[116] In contrast, ropivacaine offers greater patient safety in settings in which high concentrations and greater volumes of drugs are administered (e.g., brachial plexus blockade or epidural anesthesia for cesarean delivery).[117]

Like bupivacaine, ropivacaine is often combined with fentanyl or sufentanil for labor analgesia. Ropivacaine concentrations used to initiate epidural analgesia range from 0.08% to 0.2% (see Table 23-3). Higher concentrations are used if the drug is administered without an opioid.

Levobupivacaine

Levobupivacaine is the purified levorotary enantiomer of racemic bupivacaine. It is not available in the United States. Both preclinical and clinical studies have suggested that, like ropivacaine, levobupivacaine has less potential for cardiotoxicity than bupivacaine when equal concentrations of the two drugs are compared.[118,119] Toxicity can be properly evaluated, however, only when equipotent concentrations of drug are compared. Levobupivacaine has been compared with bupivacaine in laboring women and has been found to be essentially equipotent to bupivacaine with a potency ratio of 0.98 (95% CI, 0.67 to 1.41).[120] Other studies have suggested that levobupivacaine and ropivacaine have similar potency.[121,122] When considered together, these observations are confusing, given the clear evidence that ropivacaine is less potent than bupivacaine. In an MLAC study that compared motor blockade with use of bupivacaine, levobupivacaine, and ropivacaine in laboring women,[114] bupivacaine was more potent than ropivacaine. The study was insufficiently powered to allow a difference between bupivacaine and levobupivacaine, or levobupivacaine and ropivacaine, to be found, although a separate study did identify a difference in motor-blocking potency between bupivacaine and levobupivacaine.[123] Beilin et al.[109] compared epidural bupivacaine, ropivacaine, and levobupivacaine (0.0625% with fentanyl 2 μg/mL) for labor analgesia. There were no differences among groups in obstetric outcomes, although the incidence of motor blockade was lower in the ropivacaine and levobupivacaine groups. Therefore, although epidural bupivacaine is more potent than ropivacaine for both sensory and motor blockade during labor, and may be more potent than levobupivacaine, there do not appear to be any clinical advantages of one drug over the other two drugs for labor analgesia.

Lidocaine

Lidocaine is an amide local anesthetic with a duration of action intermediate between those of bupivacaine and 2-chloroprocaine. During labor, the administration of a 0.75% to 1.5% solution of lidocaine typically provides satisfactory analgesia, but it may not provide analgesia comparable to that provided by bupivacaine.[124]

Lidocaine is not commonly used for initiation or maintenance of epidural labor analgesia, in part because of its shorter duration of action in comparison with bupivacaine, ropivacaine, and levobupivacaine. Lidocaine is less protein bound than these other amide local anesthetics, and at delivery, the umbilical vein–to–maternal vein lidocaine concentration ratio is approximately twice that of bupivacaine.[125,126] Early studies discouraged the epidural administration of lidocaine in pregnant women because epidural lidocaine was associated with abnormal neonatal neurobehavioral findings.[127] Subsequently, several larger, carefully controlled studies have demonstrated that the epidural administration of lidocaine, bupivacaine, and 2-chloroprocaine have similar neonatal outcomes.[128,129] Although some investigators have observed subtle differences in neurobehavior between infants exposed to lidocaine and those exposed to other local anesthetics, these differences are within the inherent variability of the examinations and are not clinically significant. Other factors (e.g., mode of delivery) appear to be much more important determinants of neonatal condition.

2-Chloroprocaine

An ester local anesthetic, 2-chloroprocaine has a rapid onset of action. Epidural administration of 5 to 10 mL of 2% 2-chloroprocaine provides effective analgesia for approximately 40 minutes. The short duration of action limits its usefulness during labor. In addition, the epidural administration of 2-chloroprocaine may adversely affect the efficacy of subsequently administered epidural bupivacaine and opioids,[130,131] although it is unclear whether the mechanism is related to pharmacokinetic or pharmacodynamic properties of the drug.[132] In obstetric practice, 2-chloroprocaine is most commonly used for extension of epidural labor analgesia for instrumental vaginal delivery (see later) or emergency cesarean delivery (see Chapter 26).

OPIOIDS

Lipid-Soluble Opioids: Fentanyl and Sufentanil

Morphine was one of the first opioids to be studied for labor analgesia. However, because of its long latency, side effects, and inconsistent analgesia, morphine has largely been replaced by the lipid-soluble opioids **fentanyl** and **sufentanil** (see Chapter 13). The lipid-soluble agents have a rapid onset of action. Permeability (of the dura-arachnoid) is not a rate-limiting factor, and increasing the concentration gradient (through administration of a larger dose) facilitates faster entry into the spinal cord. The high lipid solubility of these agents also results in a shorter duration of action and greater systemic absorption than seen with water-soluble drugs.

Some investigators have suggested that the improved analgesia results from a supraspinal action rather than a primary spinal action. However, several studies have refuted this theory, including studies of epidural opioid administration by bolus[133] and continuous infusion.[134] Vella et al.[133] observed that the initiation of epidural analgesia with 0.25% bupivacaine with *epidural* fentanyl 80 μg resulted in more rapid, complete, and prolonged analgesia than *intravenous* fentanyl 80 μg, even though plasma fentanyl concentrations were higher in the intravenous group. Similarly, D'Angelo et al.[134] demonstrated that a continuous epidural infusion but not an intravenous infusion of fentanyl reduced epidural bupivacaine requirements in laboring women. Polley et al.[135] determined that the MLAC of epidural bupivacaine administered as a 20-mL *bolus* in laboring women was reduced from 0.064% to 0.034% when epidural rather than intravenous fentanyl was co-administered with bupivacaine. Finally, Ginosar et al.[136] determined that the MLAC of bupivacaine administered by *continuous epidural infusion* during labor was lower by a factor of three when it was co-administered with an epidural (rather than intravenous) fentanyl infusion. These studies strongly suggest that during labor, epidural fentanyl provides analgesia primarily through a spinal site of action.

The addition of a lipid-soluble opioid to a local anesthetic for epidural labor analgesia decreases latency, prolongs the duration of analgesia, improves the quality of analgesia, and decreases the overall local anesthetic dose. The addition of an opioid allows the anesthesia provider to give a more dilute solution of local anesthetic to provide excellent analgesia during labor.[137-139] For example, Reynolds and O'Sullivan[140] showed that epidural bupivacaine 10 mg combined with fentanyl 100 μg was more effective for the treatment of breakthrough pain, and had a faster onset and longer duration of action than either bupivacaine 25 mg or fentanyl 100 μg administered alone. Epidural fentanyl and sufentanil decrease epidural bupivacaine requirements during labor in a dose-dependent fashion.[95,141] In similar studies. Lyons et al.[141] showed that the MLAC of bupivacaine decreased with the addition of epidural fentanyl in a dose-dependent manner (Figure 23-6), and Polley et al.[95] showed that the MLAC of bupivacaine was decreased with the addition of sufentanil. The reduction in MLAC by the addition of fentanyl or sufentanil is observed with levobupivacaine,[142,143] ropivacaine,[143,144] and 2-chloroprocaine[145] as well as bupivacaine.

The dose-sparing effects of fentanyl and sufentanil are also evident when the drugs are combined with a low-concentration solution of bupivacaine used for the maintenance of analgesia throughout labor. For example, the total bupivacaine dose (mean ± SD) was 34 ± 17 mg in laboring women who received 0.125% bupivacaine/epinephrine 1.25 μg/mL with sufentanil, compared with 42 ± 19 mg in those who received bupivacaine/epinephrine without sufentanil.[146] Similarly, in women randomly assigned to receive bupivacaine/epinephrine with or without fentanyl 100 μg, the total bupivacaine dose was 55 mg or 110 mg, respectively.[147] Advantages of a lower total dose of local anesthetic include (1) decreased risk of systemic local anesthetic toxicity, (2) decreased risk of high or total spinal anesthesia, (3) decreased plasma concentrations of local anesthetic in the fetus and neonate, and (4) decreased intensity of motor blockade.

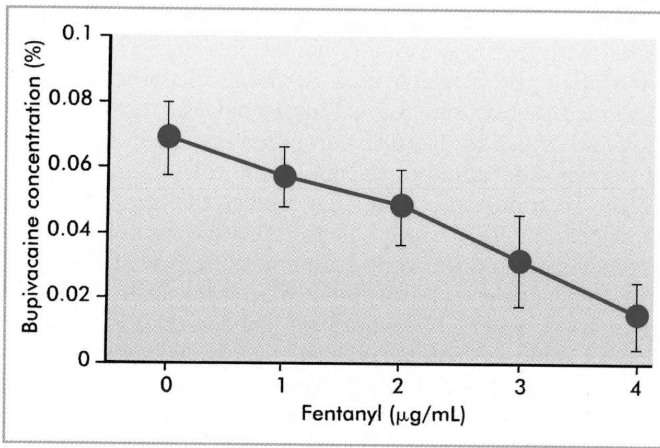

FIGURE 23-6 The effect of epidural fentanyl on the minimum local anesthetic concentration (defined as the effective concentration in 50% of subjects [EC_{50}]) for epidural bupivacaine analgesia during labor. Data are expressed as median concentrations with 95% confidence intervals. (Data from Lyons G, Columb M, Hawthorne L, Dresner M. Extradural pain relief in labour: Bupivacaine sparing by extradural fentanyl is dose dependent. Br J Anaesth 1997; 78:493-6.)

The addition of fentanyl or sufentanil to bupivacaine for the initiation of epidural analgesia hastens the onset of effective analgesia and prolongs the duration of analgesia.[146-148] Onset of analgesia was 10.3 ± 3.8 minutes in women randomly assigned to receive bupivacaine 12.5 mg without sufentanil, whereas it was 8.7 ± 2.6 minutes in women who received bupivacaine combined with sufentanil 7.5 μg.[148] Duration of analgesia was longer in the sufentanil group (131 minutes, versus 86 minutes without sufentanil).[148] The addition of fentanyl 100 μg to 0.125% bupivacaine prolonged the mean duration of analgesia from 55 minutes to 106 minutes.[147]

The quality of analgesia is also better with the addition of an opioid to the local anesthetic.[146-148] For example, 86% of women rated their analgesia as excellent after epidural analgesia was initiated with bupivacaine combined with sufentanil, compared with 50% of those who received bupivacaine without sufentanil.[148] The percentage of women who experienced no or short periods of pain during the first stage of labor was 94% in women who received sufentanil and 76% in women who did not.[146] After initiation of analgesia with 0.125% bupivacaine with epinephrine 1.25 μg/mL, 43% of women randomly assigned to receive epidural fentanyl 100 μg rated their analgesia as excellent, compared with 6% in a control group that did not receive fentanyl.[147]

In clinical practice, either fentanyl or sufentanil is frequently combined with a low-concentration, long-acting amide local anesthetic to initiate epidural labor analgesia. In theory, any of three lipid-soluble opioids—fentanyl, sufentanil, and alfentanil—may be combined with a local anesthetic to provide effective epidural analgesia. Loftus et al.[149] evaluated the addition of either fentanyl (75-μg bolus followed by a continuous epidural infusion of 1.5 μg/mL) or sufentanil (15-μg bolus followed by a continuous epidural infusion of 0.25 μg/mL) to 0.25% bupivacaine (12-mL bolus followed by an epidural infusion of a 0.125% solution at 10 mL/hr). The researchers made the following observations:

1. Although they administered fentanyl and sufentanil in a ratio of 5.7:1, the ratio of fentanyl to sufentanil in maternal venous plasma was 27:1. This finding suggests that higher plasma concentrations of drug result from a given dose of fentanyl than from an equivalent dose of sufentanil.
2. The umbilical vein–to–maternal vein concentration ratios were 0.37 for fentanyl and 0.81 for sufentanil. When viewed in isolation, these data would suggest that placental transfer of sufentanil is greater than that of fentanyl.
3. Fentanyl was detected in most umbilical artery blood samples, whereas sufentanil was detected in only one of nine samples.
4. Neonatal outcome was uniformly good, as determined by Apgar scores and umbilical cord blood gas and pH measurements. However, the 24-hour Neurologic and Adaptive Capacity Scores (NACS) were somewhat lower in the fentanyl group. It is unclear whether these differences were clinically significant.
5. Pain scores were similar in the two groups, except for better pain scores in the sufentanil group at 20 and 120 minutes.

Epidural sufentanil administration results in low concentrations in the fetal circulation because of the drug's high lipid solubility and large volume of distribution. When epidural sufentanil is absorbed systemically, it has a larger volume of distribution than that of fentanyl. Therefore, epidural sufentanil administration results in a relatively lower plasma concentration of drug. When transferred across the placenta, sufentanil has a larger volume of distribution and a correspondingly lower fetal plasma concentration of drug in comparison with fentanyl. (This remains true even though the umbilical vein–to–maternal vein concentration ratio for sufentanil is higher than that for fentanyl.) The somewhat better analgesia provided by sufentanil probably results from its greater potency (i.e., greater affinity for opioid receptors) and its greater lipid solubility (which results in better penetration into the spinal cord).

In the United States, fentanyl is more commonly used because historically it has had a lower acquisition cost than sufentanil. Additionally, the concentration of the commercially available sufentanil preparation (50 μg/mL) may make drug errors more likely with sufentanil than with fentanyl because sufentanil doses significantly lower than 50 μg are used for initiation of epidural analgesia.

Epidural fentanyl alone provides *moderate* analgesia in early labor,[91] but the dose needed to provide complete analgesia is accompanied by significant side effects (e.g., pruritus, nausea, maternal sedation, perhaps neonatal depression). In addition, epidural administration of an opioid alone provides inadequate analgesia during the later first stage of labor as well as during the second stage. In a study comparing sufentanil alone, sufentanil with bupivacaine, and bupivacaine alone,[150] women randomly assigned to the sufentanil (30 μg) group experienced satisfactory analgesia after the initial dose, but not after subsequent doses. However, the initial dose was administered after an epidural test dose that contained lidocaine 60 mg. Therefore, in clinical practice, epidural fentanyl and sufentanil are usually administered with a local anesthetic for the initiation of analgesia (at a minimum, with a local anesthetic–containing epidural test dose).

There are few rigorous *dose-response* studies of epidural fentanyl or sufentanil combined with bupivacaine for initiation of epidural labor analgesia. Herman et al.[151] randomly assigned 100 laboring women with a cervical dilation of 5 cm or less to receive 0.125% bupivacaine 10 mL, combined with fentanyl 0 to 100 μg (in 25-μg increments) or sufentanil 0 to 25 μg (in 5-μg increments), injected after a negative epidural test dose (bupivacaine 7.5 mg with epinephrine 15 μg). Using a log-probit dose-response analysis, these researchers calculated the effective dose in 95% of subjects (ED_{95}) to be 50 μg for fentanyl and 8 μg for sufentanil; these figures equate to a sufentanil-to-fentanyl potency ratio of 6.3:1. Capogna et al.[152] sought to determine the minimum effective analgesic dose (ED_{50}) of epidural fentanyl and sufentanil alone (no local anesthetic) for the initiation of epidural analgesia in nulliparous women with a cervical dilation between 2 and 4 cm. The ED_{50} of fentanyl was 124 μg (95% CI, 118 to 131) and the ED_{50} of sufentanil was 21 μg (95% CI, 20 to 22), with a potency ratio of 5.9:1. The potency ratio in volunteers subjected to an electrical stimulus was approximately 5:1.[153] Taken together, these data suggest that the potency ratio of sufentanil to fentanyl administered into the epidural space is approximately 6:1.

Two studies found that the diluent volume (2 to 20 mL) did not affect the onset and duration of epidural labor analgesia when fentanyl was injected into the epidural space after the injection of a local anesthetic solution.[154,155]

Several studies have directly compared the administration of epidural fentanyl or sufentanil combined with a local anesthetic for the initiation of labor analgesia. There were no differences in analgesia in women in early labor randomly assigned to receive fentanyl 100 μg or sufentanil 20 μg immediately following a lidocaine 45 mg/epinephrine 15 μg test dose.[156] In contrast, a second study demonstrated slightly better analgesia 20 minutes after injection of 0.125% bupivacaine (15 mg) with sufentanil 15 μg than after the same dose of bupivacaine with fentanyl 75 μg.[149]

Several studies have compared bupivacaine combined with fentanyl 50 μg and 100 μg. No differences in the onset, duration, and quality of analgesia were noted in Asian women randomly assigned to receive 0.125% bupivacaine (10 mg) combined with either 50 or 100 μg of fentanyl.[139] In contrast, when 0.125% bupivacaine (15 mg) with epinephrine 15 μg was administered to laboring Italian women with either 50 or 100 μg of fentanyl, there was no difference in the onset or duration of analgesia, but more women in the 100-μg group had excellent analgesia.[147]

There were no differences in latency, duration of analgesia, and quality of analgesia when analgesia was induced with 0.125% bupivacaine (12.5 mg)/epinephrine 12.5 μg and either 7.5 or 15 μg of sufentanil.[148] Similarly, after injection of a lidocaine 60-mg/epinephrine 15-μg test dose, another study found no differences in latency and quality of analgesia among epidural sufentanil doses of 5, 10, 20, 30, 40, and 50 μg.[157] However, the duration of analgesia was longer after the higher doses of sufentanil.

The range of fentanyl and sufentanil doses used for the initiation of epidural labor analgesia is shown in Table 23-3. In clinical practice the dose is varied according to several factors, including stage of labor, parity, presence of ruptured membranes, and whether the opioid is administered in combination with a local anesthetic. One study reported that the ED_{50} of epidural sufentanil was higher in women undergoing prostaglandin induction of labor than in women with spontaneous labor.[158] Doses at the lower end of the dose range are appropriate for nulliparous women, for women in early labor, or when the opioid is co-administered with a local anesthetic.

Higher doses are associated with a higher incidence of maternal side effects and potential for neonatal depression (see later). The major maternal side effect of epidural fentanyl and sufentanil for labor analgesia is pruritus. In general, neonatal outcomes do not appear to be adversely affected by the addition of fentanyl or sufentanil to a local anesthetic for epidural analgesia. In fact, the combination of drugs allows lower doses of both drugs to be administered, resulting in lower concentrations of both drugs in the neonate.

Other Opioids

Morphine was one of the first opioids used for labor analgesia. Hughes et al.[159] compared analgesia using epidural administration of morphine (2.0, 5.0, and 7.5 mg) with that using epidural bupivacaine 0.5%. Morphine was effective in 7 of 11 parturients until the end of the first stage of labor, but all parturients required bupivacaine for adequate analgesia during the second stage of labor. Subsequently investigators combined morphine with bupivacaine and noted a longer duration of analgesia compared with that for bupivacaine alone.[160] However, the inconsistent analgesia, long latency (30 to 60 minutes), and high incidence of side effects of morphine (which continued after delivery), along with the introduction of lipid-soluble opioids and epidural infusion pumps into clinical practice, have made the use of epidural morphine for labor analgesia largely obsolete.

Several studies described the use of **alfentanil** with bupivacaine for labor analgesia.[161,162] Alfentanil has lower lipid solubility than both fentanyl and sufentanil. To our knowledge, no study has compared alfentanil with fentanyl or sufentanil for epidural labor analgesia. However, there is no reason to believe that alfentanil would have any advantages over those agents.

Several groups of investigators have reported the use of epidural **hydromorphone** for labor analgesia.[163-165] The lipid solubility of hydromorphone lies between those of morphine and fentanyl but is closer to that of morphine.[166] In a large prospective observational study, effective labor analgesia was obtained by initiating analgesia with 0.25% bupivacaine (20 to 25 mg) with epinephrine (40 to 50 μg), followed by hydromorphone 100 μg.[163] However, Mhyre[165] observed that effective labor analgesia could not be provided by 0.035% bupivacaine (7 mg) with hydromorphone 100 to 110 μg. In another trial, parturients were randomly assigned to receive epidural hydromorphone 300 μg or saline-control immediately after the initiation of analgesia with lidocaine 45 mg, epinephrine 15 μg, and fentanyl 100 μg.[164] Durations of analgesia and side effects were similar in the two groups. At the current time, further investigation is required before hydromorphone can be recommended for epidural labor analgesia.

Meperidine may be used effectively alone (without a local anesthetic), in part because it possesses local anesthetic properties.[167] When given during labor, epidural meperidine 100 mg provides analgesia similar to that provided by 0.25% bupivacaine, with less motor blockade. However, this dose of epidural meperidine produces more sedation, nausea, and pruritus than epidural bupivacaine. Handley and Perkins[168] observed that the addition of meperidine 25 mg to 0.125%, 0.187%, or 0.25% bupivacaine (10 mL) provided adequate analgesia for the first stage of labor. The use of the more concentrated solutions (i.e., 0.187% and 0.25% bupivacaine) did not enhance the quality or duration of analgesia but did shorten latency (10 to 20 minutes versus 20 to 30 minutes for the less concentrated solution). Epidural administration of meperidine effectively prevents or treats the shivering that often occurs during labor.[169] Investigators from Saudi Arabia randomly allocated women to receive 0.1% bupivacaine with meperidine 1 mg/mL or fentanyl 2 μg/mL.[170] No differences were noted between groups in analgesic characteristics, except that women in the meperidine group had a higher incidence of nausea and vomiting. Currently there is no evidence that meperidine alone or in combination with bupivacaine has any advantages over a combination of a long-acting amide local anesthetic and a lipid-soluble opioid.

Butorphanol is a lipid-soluble opioid agonist-antagonist, with weak μ-receptor and strong κ-receptor activity. Because κ receptors appear to be involved in the modulation of visceral pain, κ-receptor agonists should be useful agents for the relief of labor pain, which has a significant visceral component (see Chapter 20).[160,171,172] Somnolence is the most prominent side effect of epidural butorphanol. The addition of butorphanol 1, 2, or 3 mg to 0.25% bupivacaine (25 mg) shortened latency and prolonged the duration of analgesia in comparison with epidural bupivacaine alone in one study.[171] The investigators concluded that the optimal dose of butorphanol was 2 mg. Of concern was the observation of a transient sinusoidal FHR pattern in the 3-mg group that was not unlike that seen after the intravenous administration of butorphanol.[172] However, there was no difference among groups in Apgar scores, umbilical cord blood gas and pH measurements, or neurobehavioral scores. Similarly, Abboud et al.[160] observed that the addition of butorphanol 1 or 2 mg to 0.25% bupivacaine resulted in better quality and longer duration of analgesia than the epidural administration of bupivacaine alone, without maternal or neonatal side effects. However, some anesthesia providers have noted that the epidural administration of butorphanol results in somnolence and occasional dysphoria, which are side effects of κ-receptor stimulation. Additional studies that include both maternal psychometric assessment and an assessment of neonatal outcome are needed.

Diamorphine (heroin) is available for epidural analgesia in the United Kingdom. Using isobolographic analysis, McLeod et al.[173] concluded that the combination of diamorphine and levobupivacaine is additive when used for first-stage labor analgesia. Several studies from the United Kingdom have reported diamorphine doses between 250 and 500 μg/hr (i.e., diamorphine 25 to 50 μg/mL

TABLE 23-5 Adjuvants to Neuraxial Labor Analgesia

	Epidural Analgesia		Spinal Analgesia
Adjuvant Drug	**Initiation Bolus Dose**	**Maintenance Infusion Dose***	**Initiation Bolus Dose**
Epinephrine	25-75 μg†	25-50 μg/hr†	2.25-200 μg
Clonidine	75-120 μg	19-37 μg/hr	15-30 μg
Neostigmine	500 μg (0.5 mg)	ND	NR
Morphine	NA	NA	0.1-0.25 mg

NA, not applicable; ND, no data; NR, not recommended.

*Usually co-administered with a low-concentration local anesthetic infusion (e.g., bupivacaine < 0.08%), 10-20 mL/hr.

†Usually administered in a 1:800,000 to 1:200,000 solution (1.25-5 μg/mL) with a local anesthetic and/or opioid.

combined with a low concentration of bupivacaine).[161,174] Whether diamorphine offers any advantages over fentanyl or sufentanil has not been studied. It is not available for clinical administration in the United States.

ADJUVANTS

Although the contemporary mainstay of epidural labor analgesia includes administration of a long-acting amide local anesthetic combined with a lipid-soluble opioid, other drugs may be added as adjuvants. Adjuvants may prolong the duration of analgesia or decrease the required anesthetic dose, thus reducing the risk of specific side effects.

Epinephrine

Some anesthesia providers add a low dose of epinephrine (1.25 to 5 μg/mL [1:800,000 to 1:200,000]) to the local anesthetic solution (Table 23-5). The addition of epinephrine shortens the latency and prolongs the duration of analgesia of epidural bupivacaine analgesia.[93,175] The MLAC of bupivacaine with epinephrine (66 μg) is 29% lower than that of bupivacaine without epinephrine,[176] perhaps as a result of the stimulation of alpha-adrenergic receptors in the spinal cord.

The addition of epinephrine to the local anesthetic has a variable effect on the systemic uptake of the local anesthetic in obstetric patients.[177-179] The systemic absorption of epinephrine may increase maternal heart rate and may also transiently decrease uterine activity as a result of beta-adrenergic receptor stimulation.[93,180,181] However, some studies have shown that the addition of epinephrine to either bupivacaine or lidocaine does not result in longer labor than the epidural administration of bupivacaine or lidocaine without epinephrine[180,182] or levobupivacaine-sufentanil without epinephrine.[183] Epidural administration of an epinephrine-containing local anesthetic solution does not adversely affect intervillous blood flow[184] or neonatal outcome.[175,177,183] One disadvantage of the use of epinephrine is that it increases the intensity of motor blockade.[182,183] The addition of epinephrine may improve the efficacy of epidural opioids,[185] but the enhanced effect is insufficient to make use of epidural opioids (without local anesthetic) an attractive regimen for the duration of labor. The addition of another drug to the local anesthetic solution may also increase the risk of drug error and contamination. For these reasons, we do not routinely administer epinephrine-containing local anesthetic solutions during labor. However, other anesthesia providers have a different view, and some consider epinephrine a useful adjuvant, especially when added to a very dilute solution of local anesthetic with an opioid.

Clonidine

Analgesia is enhanced by the direct stimulation of alpha$_2$-adrenergic receptors and the inhibition of neurotransmitter release in the dorsal horn of the spinal cord (see Chapter 20). Epidural administration of clonidine alone provides modest analgesia. Studies have evaluated the epidural administration of clonidine, an alpha$_2$-adrenergic receptor agonist, as an adjuvant to a local anesthetic alone,[186,187] to local anesthetic and opioid combinations,[188-190] to fentanyl,[191] and to neostigmine (see later).[192] Clonidine 60 μg, but not 30 μg, decreased the MLAC of ropivacaine by approximately two thirds.[193] Unlike epinephrine, clonidine does not increase the motor blockade that results from the epidural administration of a local anesthetic, but it does potentiate both the quality and duration of analgesia.[186-190] In a "black box" warning on the package insert, the manufacturer of Duraclon (the epidural clonidine formulation approved by the U.S. Food and Drug Administration) recommends against its use in obstetric patients because of the risk of hypotension[188,189,193] and bradycardia. Most studies, however, have found that the hypotension is readily amenable to treatment. An additional side effect is maternal sedation.[189,190,193] High doses (> 150 μg) may be associated with FHR changes,[188] although no adverse fetal affects have been observed with lower doses.

We currently do not recommend epidural clonidine administration for routine epidural labor analgesia. However, it may be indicated in the rare patient in whom other epidural analgesics are contraindicated.

Neostigmine

Neostigmine prevents the breakdown of acetylcholine within the spinal cord. Acetylcholine binds to muscarinic receptors, leading to a reduction in neurotransmitter release and subsequent analgesia. Roelants et al.[194] randomly assigned parturients to receive either epidural ropivacaine (20 mg) alone, or epidural neostigmine (4 μg/kg) combined with ropivacaine 10 mg, with or without sufentanil 10 μg. Motor blockade was less dense in the neostigmine group; however, the magnitude and duration of analgesia were less than in the ropivacaine/sufentanil group. Neostigmine is hydrophilic, and the researchers hypothesized that only a small portion of the epidural dose penetrates the spinal cord.[194] In a subsequent study the same researchers compared epidural sufentanil 20 μg with sufentanil 10 μg combined with neostigmine 250, 500, or 750 μg.[195] Neostigmine 250 μg with sufentanil was ineffective, but both 500 and 750 μg of neostigmine produced effective analgesia similar in duration to that with sufentanil alone. Because a synergistic antinociceptive effect of spinal alpha$_2$-adrenergic agonists and cholinesterase inhibitors is suggested by animal[196] and human volunteer studies,[197] the researchers also investigated neostigmine combined with clonidine.[192] The combination of clonidine 75 μg with neostigmine 500 or 750 μg provided acceptable analgesia (visual analog pain score $< 30/100$ in 30 minutes) in approximately 80% of parturients. No significant adverse maternal or neonatal effects were observed in any of the studies. Further studies are required to determine the role of epidural neostigmine for routine labor analgesia.

SUMMARY

The advantages of the addition of an opioid to an epidural solution of local anesthetic are as follows: (1) lower total dose of anesthetic, (2) decreased motor blockade, (3) reduced shivering, and (4) greater patient satisfaction. Some anesthesia providers contend that local anesthetic–opioid techniques result in a lower risk of hypotension, but this belief is unproven. Other adjuvants (e.g., epinephrine, clonidine, neostigmine) may prove useful in selected patients, but they currently do not offer any significant advantages to low-dose local anesthetic/lipid-soluble opioid combinations.

INITIATION OF SPINAL ANESTHESIA

Initiation of neuraxial analgesia with the intrathecal injection of an opioid, or an opioid combined with a local anesthetic, results in rapid onset of analgesia with a low dose of drug(s). The intrathecal injection is usually performed as part of a CSE analgesic technique and usually consists of a lipid-soluble opioid alone (fentanyl or sufentanil), or a combination of an opioid and a long-acting amide local anesthetic (see Table 23-3). Intrathecal opioids can provide complete analgesia during early labor when the pain stimuli are primarily visceral. Onset of analgesia occurs within 5 minutes[198] and lasts 70 to 120 minutes.[199-201] An intrathecal local anesthetic without an opioid is not commonly used for labor analgesia. Doses high enough to provide analgesia are associated with significant motor blockade, and lower doses either do not provide satisfactory analgesia or are associated with an unacceptably short duration of action.[202,203] A lipid-soluble opioid is combined with a local anesthetic (bupivacaine, ropivacaine, or levobupivacaine) when sacral analgesia is necessary for complete analgesia (e.g., initiation of analgesia during the active first stage or the second stage of labor). Studies in animal models support a synergistic action between spinal local anesthetics and opioids.[204,205] Like the combination of an epidural local anesthetic with an opioid, the combination of an intrathecal opioid with a local anesthetic results in better quality and longer duration of analgesia[27,206] as well as lower dose requirement for both drugs.[202,203,207]

Choice of Drugs

OPIOIDS

Fentanyl and Sufentanil

The two opioids most commonly used for initiation of spinal labor analgesia are **fentanyl** and **sufentanil**. When administered alone in early labor, intrathecal fentanyl and sufentanil provide complete analgesia without a sympathectomy or motor blockade. This is a particularly useful technique for patients in whom a sudden decrease in preload (secondary to neuraxial local anesthetic–induced sympathectomy) might not be well tolerated (e.g., patients with a stenotic heart lesion).

Studies suggest that the ED_{50} of intrathecal fentanyl varies from 5.5 to 18 μg.[199,201,208] These published results may differ because of differences in patient population (e.g., parity), cervical dilation at initiation of analgesia, and definition of successful analgesia. Herman et al.[208] determined that the ED_{95} of intrathecal fentanyl for parturients of mixed parity in early labor (cervical dilation ≤ 5 cm) was 17.4 μg (95% CI, 13.8 to 27.1) (Figure 23-7). The duration of analgesia is dose dependent but plateaus at approximately 80 to 120 minutes after administration of 15 to 25 μg of fentanyl (Figure 23-8).[199] There does not appear to be any reason to administer doses higher than 25 μg, because side effects (i.e., pruritus, respiratory depression) are also dose dependent.[199,208]

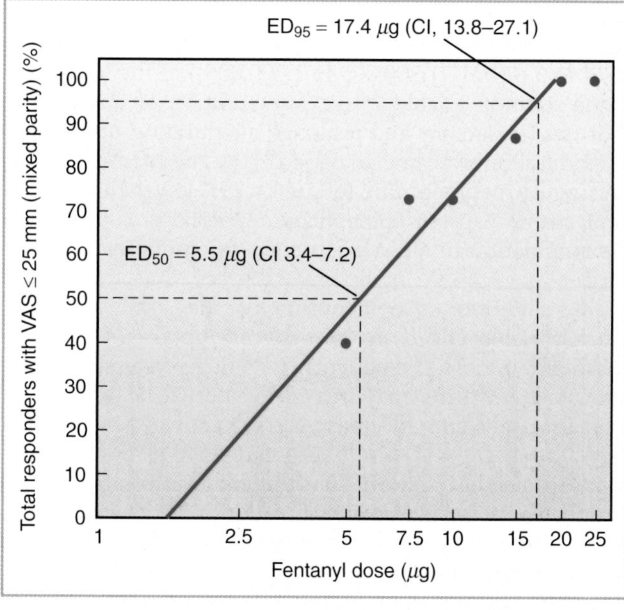

FIGURE 23-7 Dose-response relationship of intrathecal fentanyl in parturients in early labor (≤ 5 cm cervical dilation). The percent response for each dose (plotted on a common log scale) reflects the number of patients with adequate analgesia (visual analog scale [VAS] pain score $\leq 25/100$ mm). The intrathecal fentanyl doses, 5, 7.5, 10, 15, and 20 μg, fell on the steep slope of the dose-response curve (between 40% and 100% responders). These data were used to construct the regression line to derive the 50% and 95% effective doses (ED_{50} and ED_{95}, respectively) by observation. Each data point represents n = 15. CI, 95% confidence interval. (From Herman NL, Choi KC, Affleck AJ, et al. Analgesia, pruritus, and ventilation exhibit a dose-response relationship in parturients receiving intrathecal fentanyl during labor. Anesth Analg 1999; 89:378-83.)

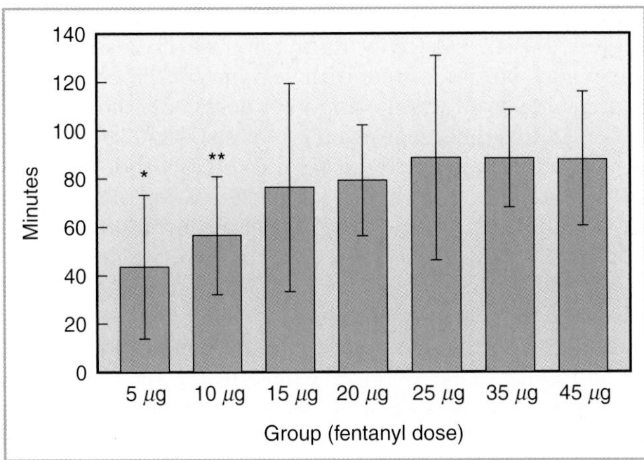

FIGURE 23-8 Duration of intrathecal fentanyl analgesia (mean ± SD) among nulliparous women in active labor who received 5, 10, 15, 20, 25, 35, or 45 μg. Duration of analgesia (time from intrathecal dose to first request for additional analgesia) differed significantly among the groups (analysis of variance [ANOVA], $P < .005$). *$P < .05$ versus groups 15 through 45 μg; **$P < 0.05$ versus groups 25 through 45 μg. (From Palmer CM, Cork RC, Hays R, et al. The dose-response relationship of intrathecal fentanyl for labor analgesia. Anesthesiology 1998; 88:355-61.)

The ED_{50} of intrathecal sufentanil varies from 1.8 to 4.1 μg,[200,209-211] and the ED_{95} is approximately 8 to 10 μg.[200,211] The relative potency ratio of intrathecal sufentanil to fentanyl for labor analgesia is 4.4:1.[201] When the drugs were administered at twice the ED_{50} (fentanyl 36 μg, sufentanil 8 μg), the duration of sufentanil analgesia was 25 minutes longer than that of fentanyl analgesia (104 versus 79 minutes), although the incidence of side effects was no different.[201]

Typically, an intrathecal opioid injection for labor analgesia is administered as part of a CSE technique. Maintenance epidural analgesia (with either a continuous epidural infusion or PCEA) is usually initiated soon after initiation of spinal analgesia. Therefore, the duration of intrathecal analgesia is relatively less important. Nelson et al.[201] concluded, and we concur, that the longer duration of sufentanil analgesia in comparison with fentanyl analgesia does not necessarily justify the former's use. Other factors, such as cost and the greater risk of a drug dose error with sufentanil (because of its greater potency), should be considered. In some European countries sufentanil is available in a dilute concentration (5 μg/mL), possibly making it easier and safer to use.

Intrathecal fentanyl (or sufentanil) is often co-administered with an amide local anesthetic (see later), most commonly bupivacaine. The addition of a local anesthetic to intrathecal fentanyl or sufentanil markedly decreases the dose of opioid necessary to produce analgesia. Wong et al.[202] randomly assigned parous women to receive intrathecal bupivacaine 2.5 mg and intrathecal sufentanil 0, 2.5, 5, 7.5, or 10 μg, followed by a standard epidural test dose. There were no differences among the sufentanil groups in quality and duration of analgesia, although the severity of pruritus was dose dependent. These results suggest that a sufentanil dose as small as 2.5 μg is effective when combined with bupivacaine 2.5 mg. In current clinical practice, it is common to combine bupivacaine 2.5 mg with sufentanil 1.5 to 2 μg.[212] Stocks at al.[206] demonstrated that three different doses of intrathecal fentanyl (5, 15, and 25 μg) led to similar reductions in the ED_{50} of intrathecal bupivacaine, although both the duration of analgesia and the incidence of pruritus were dose dependent. As with sufentanil, the dose of intrathecal fentanyl is usually reduced when combined with bupivacaine. Intrathecal fentanyl 10 to 15 μg, combined with bupivacaine 2.5 mg, provides effective analgesia for most parturients.

Other Opioids

Early studies demonstrated that the intrathecal administration of 0.5 to 2 mg of **morphine** reliably produced analgesia during the first stage of labor, but the analgesia was less reliable during the second stage of labor and during instrumental vaginal delivery.[213,214] However, intrathecal administration of these relatively large doses of morphine resulted in a high incidence of side effects, including somnolence, nausea and vomiting, pruritus, and respiratory depression. In addition, the onset of analgesia is slower with intrathecal morphine than with lipid-soluble opioids, and the long duration of action may be a disadvantage (i.e., the parturient may deliver before the regression of side effects). Abouleish[215] reported a case of life-threatening respiratory depression 1 hour after delivery and 7 hours after the administration of 1 mg of hyperbaric intrathecal morphine.

Low-dose morphine ($\leq$0.25 mg) (see Table 23-5), however, has been successfully combined with intrathecal bupivacaine and fentanyl; the combination resulted in a short latency of onset and a prolonged duration of analgesia.[30,216-218] This combination of drugs may be particularly useful in settings in which continuous epidural infusion techniques are impractical.[30] A combination of intrathecal bupivacaine 2.5 mg, fentanyl 25 μg, and morphine 0.25 mg has reliably provided acceptable analgesia.[30] When used as part of a CSE technique, the addition of intrathecal morphine to bupivacaine and fentanyl resulted in less breakthrough pain during labor[216-218] as well as decreased analgesic use in the first 24 hours postpartum in comparison with intrathecal bupivacaine and fentanyl without morphine.[216,217] The incidence of intrapartum side effects was similar[216,218]; however, the morphine group had a higher incidence of postpartum nausea (17%, versus 0% for no morphine).[216]

An alternative drug is **meperidine**. Meperidine is unique among the opioids in that it possesses weak local anesthetic properties,[167] and it has been used in large doses (e.g., 1 mg/kg) as the sole agent to provide spinal anesthesia for surgical procedures.[219] Intrathecal administration of meperidine (10 to 20 mg) results in effective labor analgesia within 2 to 12 minutes, with a duration of 1 to 3 hours. Honet et al.[220] compared the efficacy of intrathecal meperidine 10 mg, fentanyl 10 μg, and sufentanil 5 μg in 65 laboring women. The three drugs were similar in onset of analgesia (less than 5 minutes) and duration of effective analgesia (80 to 100 minutes). However, the meperidine group had significantly lower pain scores after cervical dilation had progressed beyond 6 cm. As labor advances, the nature of pain becomes increasingly somatic; only meperidine also functions as a spinal anesthetic. This fact helps explain why meperidine may provide more effective analgesia during advanced labor, including the second stage. Booth et al.[221] observed that intrathecal meperidine was associated with a significantly higher incidence of nausea and vomiting than a combination of fentanyl and bupivacaine for labor analgesia. Therefore, intrathecal meperidine does not seem to offer any advantages over bupivacaine-fentanyl for routine intrathecal analgesia, although it may be useful for the rare patient with a contraindication to bupivacaine-fentanyl administration. The usual dose of meperidine for labor analgesia is 10 to 20 mg.

In the United Kingdom, some anesthesia providers have advocated the intrathecal administration of **diamorphine** (heroin) for labor analgesia, although it is not commonly used for this purpose. This drug is unavailable for clinical use in the United States. Kestin et al.[222] observed that the intrathecal administration of diamorphine (0.2 to 0.5 mg) provided good to excellent analgesia in 90% of laboring women. The mean duration of analgesia was approximately 100 minutes. However, 75% of patients had pruritus, nausea, and vomiting. In contrast, Vaughan et al.[223] randomly assigned parturients to receive intrathecal bupivacaine 2.5 mg with either fentanyl 25 μg or diamorphine 0.25 mg. Duration of analgesia was longer in the diamorphine group, but the incidence of side effects was low in both groups.

LOCAL ANESTHETICS

In the late first stage and the second stage of labor, a local anesthetic must be added to the opioid in order to block somatic stimuli from the vagina and perineum caused by descent of the fetus. The local anesthetic works synergistically with the opioid, so lower doses of both drugs can be used.[202,206,224] **Bupivacaine** is most commonly combined with fentanyl or sufentanil. The ED_{95} of bupivacaine was 3.3 mg when combined with sufentanil 1.5 μg,[212] and 1.66 mg when combined with fentanyl 15 μg.[225] Intrathecal bupivacaine doses between 1.25 and 2.5 mg are commonly used (see Table 23-3). Levobupivacaine and ropivacaine are not approved for intrathecal use in the United States. They are less potent than bupivacaine for intrathecal labor analgesia (Figure 23-9).[212,226] Common doses are shown in Table 23-3.

Controversy exists as to whether the lower incidence and degree of motor blockade associated with ropivacaine and levobupivacaine[109,226] are a result of their inherent difference in potency or of greater sensory-motor separation with the S-enantiomer drugs.[212] Camorcia et al.[226] have suggested that, especially during intrathecal use, ropivacaine may be associated with less motor blockade than bupivacaine, even when equipotent doses are administered. However, this difference, even if it exists, is unlikely to have any clinical significance during intrathecal labor analgesia because all local anesthetics administered for this purpose are administered in low doses that lead to minimal motor blockade.

Baricity of Intrathecal Solution

The local anesthetic/opioid solutions commonly injected for intrathecal labor analgesia have lower specific gravity relative to that of CSF and hence are hypobaric.[227] The extent of cephalad sensory blockade is higher for spinal analgesia initiated with the parturient in the sitting position than in the lateral position.[228] Adding dextrose to the solution (opioid alone or opioid with local anesthetic) to make the solution hyperbaric results in less extensive sensory blockade but also in inadequate analgesia.[229-231] It is probably necessary for the opioid to penetrate the spinal cord rather than just the nerve roots; therefore, injection of a hyperbaric solution of opioid and local anesthetic below the level of the spinal cord may lead to inadequate analgesia, even though the local anesthetic provides sensory blockade to the T10 dermatome.

INTRATHECAL ADJUVANTS

Several drugs have been investigated as adjuvants to local anesthetics, opioids, or combinations of local anesthetics and opioids for intrathecal labor analgesia (see Table 23-5). In one study, the addition of **clonidine** 30 μg to sufentanil (2.5 to 5 μg) prolonged the duration of analgesia from 104 to 145 minutes without motor block.[232] Other investigators have had similar results when clonidine was combined with sufentanil,[233] bupivacaine/ropivacaine and sufentanil,[234,235] and neostigmine.[236] Intrathecal clonidine alone also provides labor analgesia.[237] Unfortunately, a disadvantage of clonidine is the high incidence of maternal hypotension and sedation as well as FHR abnormalities. The slightly longer duration of analgesia provided by the addition of clonidine to bupivacaine and sufentanil is not an advantage when maintenance analgesia is provided by a continuous epidural infusion. Therefore, at present, intrathecal clonidine

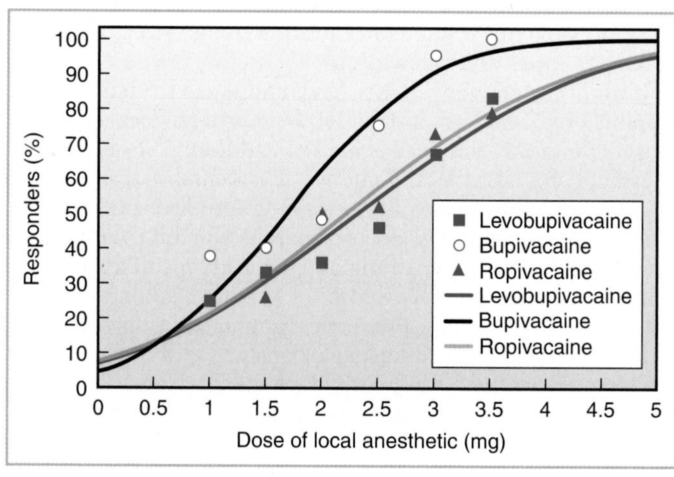

FIGURE 23-9 Predicted (*lines*) and observed (*symbols*) dose-response of intrathecal bupivacaine, levobupivacaine, and ropivacaine combined with sufentanil 1.5 μg in 450 laboring women. The dose-response curves were constructed with the use of a probit regression model. The curves were compared with use of likelihood ratio tests. No difference was observed between ropivacaine and levobupivacaine. Significant differences were observed between bupivacaine and ropivacaine ($P = .003$) and bupivacaine and levobupivacaine ($P < .001$). (From Van de Velde M, Dreelinck R, Dubois J, et al. Determination of the full dose-response relation of intrathecal bupivacaine, levobupivacaine, and ropivacaine, combined with sufentanil, for labor analgesia. Anesthesiology 2007; 106:149-56.)

cannot be recommended for routine intrathecal labor analgesia, although it might be considered in parturients with contraindications to the use of other drugs.

Adding intrathecal **neostigmine** to sufentanil, bupivacaine/sufentanil, or clonidine has been found to potentiate the analgesia and prolong its duration.[236,238] However, intrathecal neostigmine was associated with a markedly higher incidence of severe nausea that was unresponsive to standard antiemetics.[236,238] Therefore, neostigmine cannot be recommended as an adjuvant for intrathecal labor analgesia.

Analgesia is prolonged by 15 to 40 minutes when **epinephrine** is added to intrathecal bupivacaine-opioid compared with bupivacaine-opioid without epinephrine.[239-241] Even an epinephrine dose as low as 2.25 μg prolonged analgesia by 15 minutes.[240] However, epinephrine 200 μg combined with bupivacaine 2.5 mg and sufentanil 10 μg resulted in a significant incidence of motor blockade,[239] and epinephrine doses between 12.5 and 100 μg prolonged analgesia without any difference in the quality of analgesia.[241]

In summary, no adjuvant studied to date prolongs the duration of fentanyl or sufentanil/bupivacaine analgesia long enough to avoid the use of maintenance epidural analgesia for most parturients, and no adjuvant reduces or eliminates the side effects associated with the analgesic drugs used clinically. Therefore, it makes little sense to routinely add adjuvant drugs, because they are associated with higher cost, higher rate or severity of side effects, and, probably, an increased risk for drug error.

TABLE 23-6 Anesthetic Solutions for Maintenance of Epidural Analgesia: Continuous Infusion or Patient-Controlled Epidural Analgesia*

Drug†	Concentration
Local Anesthetics	
Bupivacaine	0.05-0.125%
Ropivacaine	0.08-0.2%
Lidocaine‡	0.5-1.0%
Opioids	
Fentanyl	1.5-3 μg/mL
Sufentanil	0.2-0.33 μg/mL

*Local anesthetic is most often combined with an opioid.

†Continuous infusions are usually administered at a rate of 8-15 mL/hr into the lumbar epidural space.

‡Lidocaine is not usually used for maintenance of epidural analgesia because of its relatively short duration of analgesia.

MAINTENANCE OF ANALGESIA

Epidural Analgesia

Painful labor lasts several hours in most parturients; therefore, a single intrathecal or epidural injection of local anesthetic and/or opioid typically does not provide adequate analgesia for the duration of labor. Supplemental doses are needed to maintain analgesia in most women. Neuraxial analgesia is maintained with the intermittent or continuous administration of analgesics, usually a combination of a long-acting amide local anesthetic and a lipid-soluble opioid. By far the most common technique is administration of drugs via a catheter into the epidural space. It is occasionally advantageous to administer drugs via a catheter into the subarachnoid space.

DRUGS FOR THE MAINTENANCE OF EPIDURAL ANALGESIA

In the past, epidural labor analgesia was maintained with the intermittent or continuous injection of a neuraxial local anesthetic alone. Currently, most anesthesia providers maintain analgesia with a combination of a low-dose, long-acting amide local anesthetic and a lipid-soluble opioid (Table 23-6). In practice, neither lidocaine nor 2-chloroprocaine is used for maintenance of analgesia. Both have too short a duration of action, and analgesia regresses rapidly. There is no evidence that any one of the three long-acting local anesthetics (bupivacaine, ropivacaine, levobupivacaine) has any advantages in terms of clinical outcomes over the other two.[109,116] Fentanyl is more often detected in umbilical artery blood samples than sufentanil (as discussed earlier)[149]; however, neonatal outcomes are good following maintenance epidural analgesia with either drug.

As with the induction dose, the combination of a local anesthetic with a lipid-soluble opioid for maintenance of analgesia allows administration of a lower total dose of local anesthetic. This approach improves safety and leads to less motor blockade and greater patient satisfaction. Chestnut et al.[137] demonstrated that maintenance of epidural analgesia by a continuous infusion of 0.0625% bupivacaine with fentanyl 2 μg/mL resulted in comparable maternal and neonatal outcomes, with a lower incidence of motor blockade, compared with maintenance of analgesia by a continuous epidural infusion of 0.125% bupivacaine alone. When administered as intermittent epidural boluses for the maintenance of analgesia, the addition of sufentanil to bupivacaine resulted in better quality analgesia and decreased motor blockade at delivery.[148]

In contemporary clinical practice, the bupivacaine concentration of maintenance bupivacaine/opioid solutions ranges from 0.05% to 0.125%. Hess et al.[242] retrospectively analyzed the use of three solutions at their institution: bupivacaine 0.125% and bupivacaine 0.0625%, both with fentanyl 2 μg/mL, administered at 8 to 12 mL/hr, and bupivacaine 0.04% with fentanyl 1.7 μg/mL and epinephrine 1.7 μg/mL. There were more interventions for breakthrough pain in the two low-concentration groups, and more interventions for hypotension and motor blockade in the high-concentration group. Beilin et al.[243] initiated analgesia with intrathecal bupivacaine/fentanyl and an epidural test dose, and then randomly assigned women to receive maintenance epidural analgesia with bupivacaine 0.125%, bupivacaine 0.0625%, or bupivacaine 0.04% with epinephrine 1.7 μg/mL, all with fentanyl 2 μg/mL, or saline alone at 10 mL/hr. The time to request for supplemental analgesia was longest in the bupivacaine 0.125% group; however, this group also had a higher incidence of motor blockade than the other groups. Therefore, in order to avoid motor blockade, it would seem reasonable to use a bupivacaine concentration less than 0.125%, especially if it is administered via continuous epidural infusion (see later).

The dose responses for fentanyl and sufentanil combined with a local anesthetic for the maintenance of epidural analgesia have not been well studied. The concentration range of fentanyl used in clinical practice is 1.5 to 3 μg/mL, and that of sufentanil, 0.2 to 0.33 μg/mL. The optimal opioid concentration probably varies according to the local anesthetic concentration, the mode of drug delivery (i.e., bolus versus infusion), presence of epinephrine, and the stage of labor, among other factors. Bader et al.[244] infused epidural bupivacaine 0.125% with fentanyl 2 μg/mL at 10 mL/hr for 1 to 15 hours. Maternal and neonatal fentanyl concentrations, and their ratio, remained constant over the infusion period, and no adverse maternal or neonatal outcomes were noted. Porter et al.[245] compared neonatal outcomes in women randomly assigned to receive epidural bupivacaine with fentanyl 2.5 μg/mL or bupivacaine alone to maintain analgesia. There were no differences between groups in measures of neonatal well-being at birth or 24 hours after delivery.

Bernard et al.[246] combined sufentanil 0, 0.078, 0.156, 0.312, or 0.468 μg/mL with bupivacaine 0.125% and epinephrine 1.25 μg/mL. Each solution was administered as a 12-mL bolus via PCEA. Sufentanil concentrations lower than 0.156 μg/mL did not provide adequate analgesia for the second stage of labor, and higher doses were associated with an increased incidence of pruritus. Loftus et al.[149] compared bupivacaine with sufentanil 0.25 μg/mL or fentanyl 1.5 μg/mL as a continuous epidural infusion at 10 mL/hr. The fentanyl group had slightly lower 24-hour NACS than the sufentanil group.

ADMINISTRATION TECHNIQUES

Intermittent Bolus

With the intermittent bolus technique, epidural analgesia is maintained by administration of an additional therapeutic bolus dose of local anesthetic when analgesia begins to wane. When the patient begins to experience recurrent pain, the anesthesia provider assesses the pain relative to the stage of labor and the extent of sensory blockade, and then administers another epidural bolus of local anesthetic.

The spread and quality of analgesia may change with repeated lumbar epidural injections of local anesthetic. After several injections, blockade of the sacral segments, intense motor blockade, or both may develop.[182] Analgesia is usually reestablished with the bolus injection of 8 to 12 mL of a local anesthetic/opioid solution. The sensory level and the intensity of motor blockade should be assessed and recorded before and after each bolus injection of local anesthetic.

This intermittent bolus technique has several disadvantages, the most salient of which is that pain relief is constantly interrupted by the regression of analgesia. The patient must notify the labor nurse or midwife that she is again uncomfortable and request additional analgesia. In the United States, labor nurses are not allowed to administer additional epidural analgesia[247]; therefore, the nurse must call the anesthesia provider, resulting in unavoidable delays in administration of additional analgesia and additional pain for the patient.

Continuous Infusion

Administration of a continuous epidural infusion of a dilute solution of local anesthetic combined with an opioid is a popular technique for the maintenance of epidural analgesia during labor. The potential benefits of continuous epidural infusion include the maintenance of a stable level of analgesia and a less frequent need for bolus doses of local anesthetic, which may reduce the risk of systemic local anesthetic toxicity. An additional advantage is a decreased workload for the anesthesia provider.

Published studies have suggested that the continuous epidural infusion and intermittent bolus injection techniques have comparable safety. Studies comparing intermittent bolus injections with continuous infusion were performed before the era of neuraxial opioid administration; thus, the studies used concentrations of bupivacaine (0.125% to 0.25%) higher than those typically used in contemporary practice. In theory, maintenance of a constant level of anesthesia should promote maternal hemodynamic stability and improve fetal and neonatal outcome. Only one published study has suggested a trend toward less frequent hypotension and a lower incidence of abnormal FHR patterns during the continuous epidural infusion of bupivacaine than with intermittent bolus injections of bupivacaine; however, neonatal outcomes were similar with the two techniques.[248]

Controlled trials of intrapartum epidural analgesia maintained by either intermittent bolus injection or continuous infusion of bupivacaine have consistently demonstrated that women require fewer bolus injections administered by the anesthesia provider (i.e., fewer episodes of breakthrough pain) with the continuous infusion technique.[248-250] The continuous infusion technique lengthens the time between bolus injections and leads to greater patient satisfaction.[250,251] This is advantageous in a busy obstetric anesthesia practice, in which an anesthesia provider is not always available to give an additional bolus dose of local anesthetic immediately after the onset of recurrent pain.

Most studies suggest that the continuous epidural infusion technique leads to the administration of a larger total dose of bupivacaine,[249-252] but such a dose does not seem to result in higher maternal venous or umbilical venous bupivacaine concentrations at delivery.[250,252] The continuous epidural infusion of bupivacaine often achieves satisfactory perineal analgesia, obviating the need for a bolus dose of local anesthetic at delivery. Unfortunately, a prolonged epidural infusion of 0.125% bupivacaine at 10 to 14 mL/hr may cause significant motor blockade.[128,248,249,251,252] Titrating the dose of bupivacaine to meet the individual needs of each patient (rather than administering the same dose to all patients), as well as reducing the total mass of bupivacaine by lowering the local anesthetic concentration and adding an opioid, helps minimize motor blockade while providing effective analgesia.

Migration of the epidural catheter into the subarachnoid, subdural, or intravenous space can occur with either the intermittent bolus injection or continuous infusion technique. If the epidural catheter should migrate into a vein during the continuous epidural infusion of a dilute solution of local anesthetic, it is unlikely that the patient will have symptoms of local anesthetic toxicity; rather, the level of anesthesia will regress. For this reason, the anesthesia provider should suspect the intravenous migration of an epidural catheter when a patient unexpectedly complains of pain during maintenance of analgesia during a continuous epidural infusion.

Migration of the epidural catheter into the subdural or subarachnoid space during an infusion should result in the slow ascent of the level of anesthesia and a greater density of motor blockade. These observations apply to the epidural infusion of a 0.125% solution of bupivacaine at a modest rate (e.g., 10 to 15 mL/hr). The continuous infusion of a more concentrated solution or the use of a more rapid rate of infusion most likely narrows the margin of safety.

Patient-Controlled Epidural Analgesia

The method of delivering the anesthetic solution into the epidural space influences the density of neuroblockade. Given the same concentration of local anesthetic, analgesia maintained by infusion results in greater drug utilization, a higher degree of motor blockade,[249,253] and a higher incidence of instrumental vaginal delivery than intermittent boluses.[252] However, intermittent manual bolus administration by the anesthesia provider results in more breakthrough pain, less patient satisfaction, and more work for the anesthesia provider. Patient-controlled epidural analgesia (PCEA) is a method of delivering anesthetic solution to the epidural space that overcomes these disadvantages. Since its first description in 1988 by Gambling et al.,[254] many studies have consistently found that the analgesia with PCEA is comparable to that with continuous infusion techniques, patient satisfaction is equal or better,[255] the incidence of motor blockade is equal or less,[256-258] local anesthetic consumption is reduced,[253,256,258-261] there is less need for anesthesia provider intervention,[253,255,257] and there are no differences in obstetric or neonatal outcomes.[253,255-260] PCEA can be used with or without a background infusion.

Van der Vyver et al.[262] summarized the results of nine randomized controlled trials (n = 640) comparing PCEA (without a background infusion) with continuous epidural infusion analgesia. There were fewer anesthetic interventions in the PCEA group, which received less bupivacaine and had a lower incidence of motor blockade (Figure 23-10).

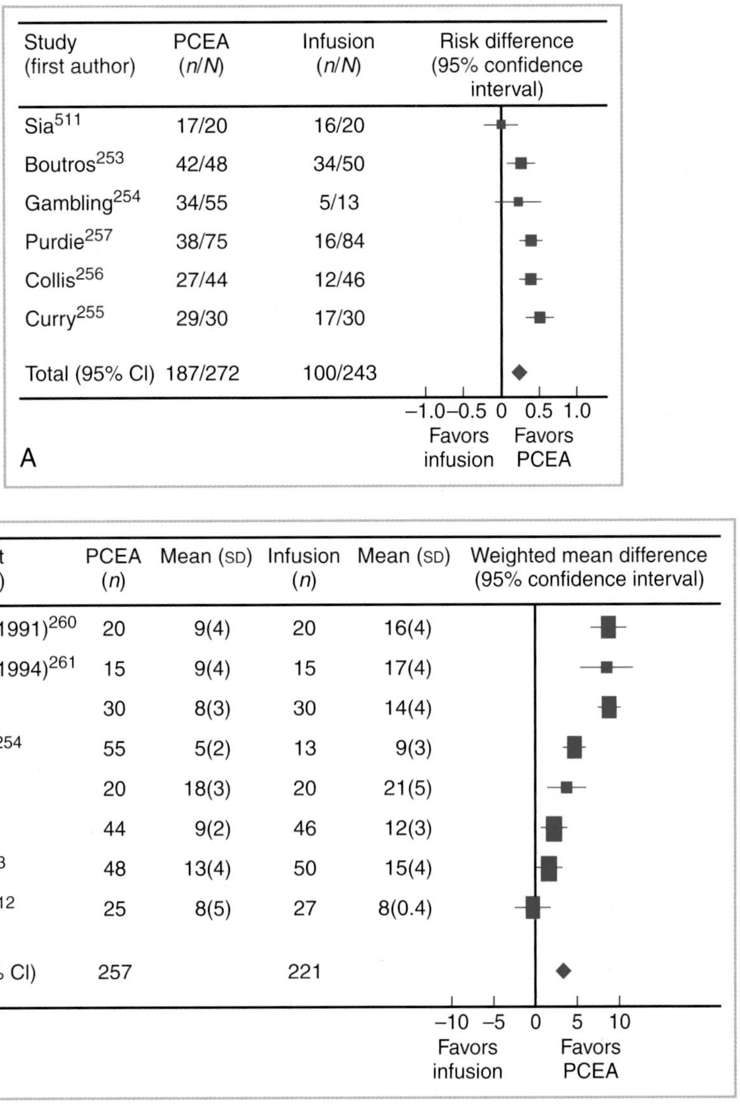

Study (first author)	PCEA (*n*/*N*)	Infusion (*n*/*N*)	Risk difference (95% confidence interval)
Sia[511]	17/20	16/20	
Boutros[253]	42/48	34/50	
Gambling[254]	34/55	5/13	
Purdie[257]	38/75	16/84	
Collis[256]	27/44	12/46	
Curry[255]	29/30	17/30	
Total (95% CI)	187/272	100/243	

−1.0 −0.5 0 0.5 1.0
Favors infusion — Favors PCEA

A

Study (first author [yr])	PCEA (*n*)	Mean (SD)	Infusion (*n*)	Mean (SD)	Weighted mean difference (95% confidence interval)
Ferrante (1991)[260]	20	9(4)	20	16(4)	
Ferrante (1994)[261]	15	9(4)	15	17(4)	
Curry[255]	30	8(3)	30	14(4)	
Gambling[254]	55	5(2)	13	9(3)	
Sia[511]	20	18(3)	20	21(5)	
Collis[256]	44	9(2)	46	12(3)	
Boutros[253]	48	13(4)	50	15(4)	
Smedvig[512]	25	8(5)	27	8(0.4)	
Total (95% CI)	257		221		

−10 −5 0 5 10
Favors infusion — Favors PCEA

B

FIGURE 23-10 Meta-analysis of patient-controlled epidural analgesia (PCEA) without background infusion compared with continuous epidural infusion for maintenance of analgesia. **A,** The number of patients requiring no unscheduled interventions by the anesthesia provider was lower in the PCEA group (risk difference 27%; 95% confidence interval [CI], 18 to 36). **B,** The dose of local anesthetic (mg/hr) was lower in the PCEA group (weighted mean difference, −3.9 mg; 95% CI, −5.4 to −2.4). (From van der Vyver M, Halpern S, Joseph G. Patient-controlled epidural analgesia versus continuous infusion for labour analgesia: A meta-analysis. Br J Anaesth 2002; 89:459-65.)

TABLE 23-7 Sample Patient-Controlled Epidural Analgesia (PCEA) Settings*

PCEA Technique	Basal Infusion Rate (mL/hr)	Bolus Dose (mL)	Lockout Interval (min)
Without background infusion	0	8-12	10-20
With background infusion	4-8	5-8	10-15

*Anesthetic solutions are shown in Table 23-6.

Data are conflicting as to whether PCEA should include a background infusion.[261,263-268] Most studies have reported background infusions of 3 to 4 mL/hr. Bupivacaine consumption is higher in PCEA with a background infusion than in a pure PCEA technique without a background infusion.[266] A meta-analysis of five studies[261,264,265,267,268] reported in the ASA Practice Guidelines for Obstetric Anesthesia[19] concluded that a background infusion provides better analgesia than pure PCEA without a background infusion (odds ratio [OR], 3.3; 95% CI, 1.9 to 5.9). In a review, Halpern[269] concluded that a background infusion improves analgesia and results in fewer unscheduled interventions by the anesthesia provider. There is no evidence that the higher bupivacaine dose associated with a background infusion increases motor blockade or has adverse effects on obstetric outcome. A typical background infusion provides one third to one half of the total hourly dose.

A wide variety of PCEA regimens have been described (Table 23-7).[259,270-273] The anesthesia provider can manipulate the infusion solution (local anesthesia/opioid concentration), patient-controlled bolus volume, lockout interval, background infusion rate, and maximum allowable dose per hour. Patient-controlled bolus doses from 2 to 20 mL and lockout intervals from 5 to 30 minutes have been reported[259,270-273]; most studies have evaluated patient-controlled bolus doses of 4 to 12 mL. No study has found any differences in unscheduled provider interventions when investigators manipulated the patient-controlled bolus dose and lockout interval. There are no published reports of toxicity with larger bolus volumes, although the study populations were too small to allow determination of safety. These studies, taken together, suggest that there is no ideal bolus dose or lockout interval for labor PCEA.

Various local anesthetic concentrations have also been studied. No studies have reported any differences in analgesia efficacy. Use of more concentrated local anesthetic solutions resulted in higher local anesthetic consumption[274-276] and greater motor blockade than use of less concentrated solutions.[274,277] Thus, as with continuous infusion epidural analgesia, administration of a dilute local anesthetic solution combined with an opioid results in less local anesthetic consumption and motor blockade without a reduction in analgesia efficacy.

In summary, solutions used for PCEA are identical to those used for continuous epidural infusion analgesia (see Table 23-6). We suggest that larger bolus volumes be used if PCEA is administered without a background infusion. Early PCEA studies investigated higher-concentration local anesthetic solutions (i.e., 0.125% to 0.25% bupivacaine), smaller bolus volumes (≤ 5 mL), and low background infusion rates (3 to 5 mL/hr). Given the more recent data supporting the efficacy of more dilute concentration local anesthetic solutions administered in higher volumes into the epidural space, it appears reasonable to apply this principle to PCEA. The safety of large-volume boluses (> 10 mL) has not been determined.

Timed Intermittent Bolus Injection

Bolus administration of a local anesthetic into the epidural space results in better analgesia than continuous epidural infusion. Likewise, larger volumes of a less concentrated anesthetic solution provide better analgesia than smaller volumes of a more concentrated solution. Presumably, distribution of anesthetic solution in the epidural space is better when larger volumes are administered under high pressure.[278] Several studies have demonstrated that timed (automated) intermittent boluses (5 to 10 mL every 30 to 60 minutes) administered via a programmable pump result in improved patient satisfaction, less drug use, longer duration of analgesia, and less breakthrough pain than a continuous infusion of the same mass of drug per unit of time.[279-283] For example, Wong et al.[279] randomly assigned patients to receive either a continuous infusion of a dilute bupivacaine/fentanyl solution at 12 mL/hr, or 6 mL of the same solution delivered as an automated bolus every 30 minutes. Similarly, Sia et al.[283] randomly assigned patients to receive either a continuous infusion of a ropivacaine/fentanyl solution at 5 mL/hr or 5 mL of the same solution delivered as an automated bolus every hour. All patients in both studies were allowed PCEA for the treatment of breakthrough pain. The total dose of local anesthetic was smaller in the automated bolus groups than in the continuous infusion groups. This technique was associated with less breakthrough pain requiring provider intervention and greater patient satisfaction.[279,280] Although currently not available, commercial pumps that allow easy utilization of this mode of anesthetic solution delivery are being developed.

PATIENT MONITORING DURING MAINTENANCE EPIDURAL ANALGESIA

The use of a continuous epidural infusion technique or PCEA does not abolish the need for frequent assessment of the patient. The anesthesia provider should assess the patient every several hours. Assessment should involve determining the quality of analgesia and progress of labor, recording the sensory level and intensity of motor block, and reviewing maternal blood pressure measurements and FHR tracings for the previous hour. An inappropriately high level of anesthesia signals the administration of an excessive dose of local anesthetic or subdural or subarachnoid migration of the catheter. A low level of anesthesia may signal intravenous migration of the catheter, movement of the catheter outside the epidural space, or administration of an inadequate dose of local anesthetic.

EQUIPMENT

Anesthesia providers should consider the safety of their equipment when choosing a maintenance technique. The use of an infusion pump identical to that used for the intravenous administration of other drugs increases the chance that a nurse or physician will inject oxytocin, magnesium sulfate, or another drug into the epidural space unintentionally. Thus we recommend the use of an infusion pump that is used exclusively for epidural analgesia and that differs from the pumps used for intravenous drug and fluid administration. The pump should be easy to use, reliable, adjustable, and sturdy. PCEA pumps should differ from patient-controlled intravenous analgesia (PCIA) pumps. The PCEA "buttons" should be labeled with instructions that only the patient (not medical providers or family members) should push the button. If possible, pumps should be (pre)programmed with maximum safe limits to prevent errors in pump programming.

The anesthesia provider should use infusion tubing (which connects the pump to the epidural catheter) that is unique for the epidural administration of drugs. Some tubing is color-coded. The presence of an injection side-port increases the likelihood of unintentional epidural administration of the wrong drug; thus we recommend the use of tubing that does not have an injection side-port. A less desirable alternative is to wrap tape over the injection side-port on the tubing. In any case, the epidural catheter and tubing should be clearly labeled with the word "epidural."

Each labor unit must have a clear policy as to who may administer and adjust epidural infusion parameters. Anesthesia personnel should be responsible for changes in the content or rate of the infusion and the volume of bolus doses. In the presence of maternal distress or fetal bradycardia, the nurse or obstetrician may discontinue the epidural infusion, but the anesthesia provider should be notified immediately.

Solutions for maintenance of neuraxial analgesia, consisting of dilute local anesthetic and opioid, require careful preparation, as these solutions are not commercially available. We recommend that a hospital pharmacist prepare the solution, preferably in a sterile environment. Anesthesia providers may prepare the solutions with strict attention to sterile technique. Preservative-free drugs and saline should be used to prepare the solutions. Solution contents should always be double-checked by the anesthesia provider before analgesia is initiated.

Spinal Analgesia

Placement of a catheter in the subarachnoid space allows the anesthesia provider to administer continuous spinal analgesia by intermittent bolus injection or continuous infusion of a local anesthetic combined with an opioid. Continuous spinal analgesia is an option when unintentional dural puncture has occurred (see later). The technique has been described for use in patients in whom placement of an epidural catheter is difficult (e.g., in patients with morbid obesity or abnormal vertebral anatomy, such as kyphoscoliosis[284,285]) or in patients with severe cardiac disease who require careful titration of analgesia.[286,287]

Reports of this technique usually describe the use of a standard epidural catheter placed through an 18- or 19-gauge epidural needle. In order to reduce the risk of post–dural puncture headache, very small (e.g., 28- to 32-gauge) catheters were developed for insertion through small (e.g., 22- to 26-gauge) spinal needles. Unfortunately, several cases of cauda equina syndrome (associated with the use of spinal microcatheters during surgery in nonpregnant patients) prompted the U.S. Food and Drug Administration to remove these microcatheters from the market in 1992.[288] The etiology of these neurologic deficits is unclear. Some anesthesiologists have suggested that neurologic injury may result from the maldistribution of local anesthetic within the subarachnoid space.[289] The very slow rate of injection through a caudally directed microcatheter may lead to pooling of local anesthetic solution in the terminal part of the dural sac. If the local anesthetic solution is hyperbaric, the neighboring elements of the cauda equina experience prolonged exposure to a high concentration of local anesthetic and a hyperglycemic, hyperosmotic marinade (e.g., 550 to 800 mOsm). Permanent neural damage may occur from the combination of tissue dehydration and a toxic concentration of local anesthetic. It is unclear whether this complication is unique to the use of microcatheters.

Arkoosh et al.[290] reported a randomized multicenter study comparing continuous spinal labor analgesia (via a 28-gauge catheter) with continuous epidural analgesia. The incidence of neurologic complications was not different between the two groups, and patients in the spinal group had better early analgesia, less motor blockade, and better patient satisfaction. The incidence of post–dural puncture headache also was not different between the two groups (spinal 9%, epidural 4%; $P = .10$); however, the spinal catheter was associated with a higher incidence of technical difficulties and catheter failures. The researchers concluded that larger studies are needed to determine the safety of the spinal catheter, which is not marketed in the United States.

Continuous spinal analgesia can be initiated with the same drug combination and dose used to initiate CSE analgesia (see Table 23-3). For maintenance of analgesia, we administer our standard epidural solution (0.06% bupivacaine with fentanyl 2 μg/mL) at an initial rate of 2 mL/hr. The infusion is then titrated to patient needs. We prefer to use our standard PCEA pumps for the continuous infusion, with the PCEA function disabled. This approach allows the anesthesia provider to administer a small (1 to 3 mL) bolus from the infusion bag without disconnecting the spinal catheter from the infusion tubing. Opening the infusion system to air may increase the risk of contamination and drug error. The catheter and pump should be clearly labeled so that all care providers know that the catheter is a spinal, not an epidural, catheter.

Patient-controlled spinal analgesia for labor has been described.[291] Continuous spinal analgesia with opioids has also been described for patients with obstructive cardiac lesions.[286,287] If intrathecal local anesthetics are used for intrapartum analgesia, the sensory level and the intensity of motor blockade should be monitored. Moreover, the anesthesia provider must be prepared to treat hypotension and other complications associated with high spinal anesthesia.

Ambulatory "Walking" Analgesia

The term "walking" or "mobile" epidural analgesia was first coined to describe low-dose CSE opioid analgesia because motor function was maintained and the ability to walk was not impaired.[292] However, the term is more accurately applied to any neuraxial analgesic technique that allows safe ambulation. Initial studies using clinical testing to assess sensory and motor impairment and dorsal column function produced conflicting results. After initiation of epidural analgesia with 15 mL of 0.1% bupivacaine/fentanyl 2 μg/mL, Buggy et al.[293] demonstrated that 66% of women had altered proprioception and 38% had impaired vibration sense. In contrast, Parry et al.[294] found that dorsal column function was impaired in only 7% of laboring women who received low-dose epidural or CSE analgesia. The same group of investigators then used computerized dynamic posturography to assess balance in nonpregnant women, term pregnant women not in labor, and laboring women after initiation of CSE analgesia with bupivacaine 2.5 mg and fentanyl 5 μg.[295] Pregnancy significantly affected balance function, but initiation of CSE analgesia did not further impair function. However, further supplementation of analgesia with the epidural injection of 10 mL of 0.1% bupivacaine/fentanyl 2 μg/mL in a subgroup of patients resulted in impaired balance function. The investigators concluded that the results support the safety of allowing ambulation after low-dose CSE analgesia, but further studies are required to understand the relative contributions of dorsal column function, proprioception, and lower limb motor strength to overall balance and ability to ambulate.[295]

Several studies have shown that an epidural test dose containing lidocaine 45 mg and epinephrine 15 μg adversely affects the ability to ambulate after initiation of CSE or low-dose epidural analgesia.[84,85]

The concept of the "walking epidural" is popular in the lay press; however, many women, once comfortable, prefer to sleep rather than ambulate. The ability to walk to the toilet or sit in a chair at the bedside, however, remains desirable to many laboring women. Although ambulation per se has not been shown to positively or negatively affect the progress or outcome of labor, dense motor blockade may adversely affect the spontaneous vaginal delivery rate (see later). Thus, the intent of the "walking epidural"—minimization of motor blockade—should be the goal of the anesthesia provider, whether or not the patient wishes to ambulate.

Safe ambulation during labor requires several safeguards (Box 23-6). Prior to ambulation, orthostatic blood pressure and heart rate should be measured, and motor function and balance must be assessed. The patient should never ambulate alone.

BOX 23-6 Criteria for Ambulation during Labor with Neuraxial Analgesia

- Reassuring fetal status
- Engagement of fetal presenting part
- Stable orthostatic vital signs (asymptomatic and within 10% of baseline)
- Ability to perform bilateral straight-leg raises in bed against resistance
- Ability to step up on a step stool with either leg taking the first step, without assistance
- Satisfactory trial of walking accompanied by a nurse or midwife
- Patient must be accompanied by a companion at all times
- Intermittent fetal heart rate monitoring (every 15 minutes)

ANALGESIA/ANESTHESIA FOR VAGINAL DELIVERY

During the second stage of labor, pain results from distention of the pelvic floor, vagina, and perineum. Pain impulses are transmitted to the spinal cord by means of somatic nerve fibers that enter the cord at S2 to S4. These somatic nerve fibers are larger than the visceral afferent nerve fibers that transmit the pain of the first stage of labor. Blockade of these larger nerve fibers may require administration of a more concentrated solution and/or a greater volume of local anesthetic than is required during the first stage of labor[94]; this need often creates a dilemma for the anesthesia provider. Administration of a more concentrated solution of local anesthetic results in more intense motor blockade at a time when maternal expulsive efforts are helpful.

The continuous epidural infusion of bupivacaine often leads to the gradual development of sacral analgesia. Likewise, several lumbar epidural injections of local anesthetic (given every 60 to 90 minutes) may result in sacral analgesia.[182] If analgesia is not adequate for the second stage of labor, the anesthesia provider can give additional doses of local anesthetic to augment perineal analgesia (Box 23-7). Some anesthesia providers contend that the use of the sitting position helps facilitate the onset of perineal analgesia. Published studies suggest that maternal position does not consistently affect the spread of local anesthetic in the epidural space[296,297]; rather, the administration of a larger volume of local anesthetic solution facilitates the onset of sacral analgesia.[298] Unfortunately, the larger volume also results in a higher (i.e., more cephalad) sensory

BOX 23-7 Anesthesia for Vaginal Delivery

Lumbar Epidural Catheter

- Supplement existing analgesia with 5 to 10 mL of 1% or 2% lidocaine or with 5 to 10 mL of 2% or 3% 2-chloroprocaine.

Spinal Anesthesia

- Intrathecal injection of hyperbaric bupivacaine 6 to 8 mg or hyperbaric lidocaine 25 to 50 mg.
- Administer a larger dose for a "trial of forceps" in case cesarean delivery is necessary.

Combined Spinal-Epidural Anesthesia

- Intrathecal injection of bupivacaine 2.5 to 5 mg with fentanyl 15 to 25 μg.
- Follow with administration of additional drug(s) via epidural catheter if anesthesia is inadequate.

level of analgesia, so the patient should be observed for evidence of hemodynamic or respiratory compromise.

Dense anesthesia is often required for delivery, especially if the obstetrician performs an episiotomy or a forceps or vacuum-extraction delivery. After administration of a test dose (3 mL of the local anesthetic solution), we administer 5 to 10 mL of 1% to 2% lidocaine or 2% to 3% 2-chloroprocaine. We inject this "delivery dose" when the fetal head is visible on the perineum during pushing or when the obstetrician has decided to proceed with instrumental vaginal delivery. The anesthesia provider should monitor the maternal blood pressure carefully, especially if excessive blood loss occurs in a patient with extensive anesthesia.

Occasionally a parturient tolerates the pain of labor until late in the first stage (i.e., more than 8 cm cervical dilation) and then requests analgesia. Advanced labor does not preclude initiation of neuraxial analgesia, especially in a nulliparous woman, in whom the second stage of labor may last 2 to 3 hours. However, initiation of lumbar epidural analgesia in the late first stage of labor often results in inadequate sacral analgesia unless large volumes of a concentrated local anesthetic solution are administered. This leads to higher cephalad sensory blockade than necessary and dense motor blockade. Another option is to administer CSE analgesia. The advantages of this technique are that it provides a rapid onset of spinal analgesia with sacral coverage for advanced labor and that it includes the placement of an epidural catheter. Additional local anesthetics can be administered through the epidural catheter if the extent or duration of spinal analgesia is inadequate. One disadvantage is that the correct placement of the epidural catheter in the epidural space cannot be verified until intrathecal analgesia regresses. For this reason, we do not advocate the CSE technique in the parturient with morbid obesity, a potentially difficult airway, or a nonreassuring FHR pattern; in such women, it is essential to verify epidural catheter position at the time of placement to avoid the risks of general anesthesia should urgent cesarean delivery be necessary.

A caudal epidural catheter, which facilitates the onset of sacral analgesia, is an option for analgesia late in labor. Caudal analgesia was the first form of neuraxial analgesia used during labor. However, caudal analgesia is used infrequently in modern obstetric anesthesia practice. Sacral analgesia adequate for labor and delivery can be achieved with an injection of 12 to 15 mL of 0.25% bupivacaine, 1.0% to 1.5% lidocaine, or 2% 2-chloroprocaine.

Single-shot spinal anesthesia for vaginal delivery may be indicated in a patient who does not have epidural anesthesia and who requires perineal anesthesia. A so-called saddle block can be administered to achieve blockade of the sacral spinal segments; a small dose of a hyperbaric local anesthetic solution is adequate for this purpose. A saddle block may be advantageous in the patient with a preterm fetus or a vaginal breech presentation. In these cases, dense perineal relaxation may facilitate an atraumatic vaginal delivery. A saddle block performed with the patient in the sitting position with hyperbaric anesthetic solution provides excellent anesthesia for an outlet/low forceps delivery. A higher level (T10) of anesthesia often is required for a midforceps delivery.

Clear communication between the obstetrician and anesthesia provider is essential. If the obstetrician is certain that the application of forceps (or vacuum extraction) will result in a successful delivery, a saddle block will likely provide satisfactory anesthesia. However, in some cases, the obstetrician will perform a *trial* of forceps. We alter our technique when giving spinal anesthesia for a trial of forceps. If the trial fails, cesarean delivery must follow. In some cases, we give a dose of local anesthetic appropriate for cesarean delivery (e.g., 1.6 mL of hyperbaric 0.75% bupivacaine). Alternatively, a saddle block can be administered via the CSE technique. If spinal anesthesia is inadequate for the planned procedure, additional local anesthetic can be given through the epidural catheter.

SIDE EFFECTS OF NEURAXIAL ANALGESIA

Hypotension

Neuraxial anesthesia–induced sympathetic blockade leads to peripheral vasodilation and increased venous capacitance. Increased venous capacitance results in reduced venous return to the heart, which may lead to decreased maternal blood pressure and cardiac output. Hypotension is often defined as a 20% to 30% drop in systolic blood pressure (compared with baseline) or a systolic blood pressure less than 100 mm Hg. Modest hypotension rarely has adverse consequences in young, nonpregnant patients. However, during pregnancy, uteroplacental perfusion depends on the maintenance of normal maternal blood pressure. Uncorrected hypotension results in decreased uteroplacental perfusion. If hypotension is severe and prolonged, hypoxia and acidosis will develop in the fetus. Blood pressure should be monitored frequently (every 2 to 3 minutes) after initiation of analgesia, until stable blood pressure is ascertained.

The incidence of hypotension after initiation of neuraxial analgesia *during labor* is approximately 10%.[26] Kinsella and Black[299] reported that maternal position and the position of the blood pressure cuff markedly influence the measured blood pressure. With laboring patients in the full lateral position, they found the mean difference in systolic blood pressure between the dependent and upper arm to be 10 mm Hg; the mean difference in diastolic pressure was 14 mm Hg. Therefore, the incidence of hypotension may vary with the position of both the patient and the blood pressure cuff.

A meta-analysis of studies comparing low-dose epidural analgesia with CSE analgesia found no difference in the incidence of hypotension between the two techniques.[26]

The prevention of hypotension includes avoidance of aortocaval compression. Preston et al.[51] noted a higher incidence of severe FHR decelerations in women placed in the supine-lateral tilt than in those in the full lateral position after initiation of epidural analgesia. In contrast, Beilin et al.[50] found no difference in maternal blood pressure and FHR decelerations between the two positions.

Traditionally, intravenous "prehydration" with 0.5 to 1.5 L of crystalloid solution has been used to reduce the incidence and severity of hypotension following the initiation of neuraxial labor analgesia. However, several randomized controlled trials have shown that the incidence of hypotension after prehydration with 0.5 to 1.0 L of fluid is no lower than that after no prehydration.[37,300] Dyer et al.[38] showed that rapid intravenous crystalloid administration initiated *at the time of* intrathecal injection (co-load) resulted in a significantly lower incidence of hypotension than crystalloid administration *prior to* the initiation of neuroblockade (preload) in patients undergoing spinal *anesthesia* for elective cesarean delivery. Whether the co-load technique would reduce the incidence and severity of hypotension after the initiation of neuraxial *analgesia* in *laboring* women has not been studied. In our practice, we administer approximately 0.5 L of intravenous crystalloid at the time of initiation of neuraxial labor analgesia.

The incidence of neuraxial analgesia/anesthesia–induced hypotension is lower in laboring women than in nonlaboring women who receive neuraxial anesthesia for elective cesarean delivery. The hypotension is usually easily treated. Treatment includes the administration of additional intravenous crystalloid and the placement of the mother in the full lateral (and Trendelenburg) position. If these measures do not result in the prompt restoration of blood pressure, if hypotension is severe, or if a nonreassuring FHR pattern is noted, the anesthesia provider should administer an intravenous vasopressor. Traditionally, ephedrine 5 to 10 mg has been administered; however, studies in women undergoing spinal anesthesia for elective cesarean delivery have shown that phenylephrine is equally efficacious in restoring blood pressure and is associated with higher umbilical arterial blood pH measurements at birth.[301] No differences in neonatal outcome have been noted. Because there is no evidence that the choice of vasopressor influences maternal or neonatal outcome, the use of either drug is acceptable. Phenylephrine may be more appropriate for women with tachycardia, whereas ephedrine may be more appropriate for women with bradycardia. The FHR should be monitored continuously, and treatment should be more aggressive if worrisome patterns are noted or if the mother is symptomatic (e.g., presence of presyncope or nausea). Ephedrine crosses the placenta and may increase both FHR and FHR variability (e.g., saltatory FHR pattern).[302,303]

Several studies have described a drop in blood pressure after intrathecal opioid administration in laboring women.[198,304] Initially some investigators concluded that intrathecal opioids exerted a local anesthetic effect, which resulted in a sympathectomy. However, subsequent studies have demonstrated that the decreased blood pressure results from pain relief rather than from a sympathectomy.[305] Sympathetic blockade can be expected if either a local anesthetic or clonidine is administered intrathecally with the opioid.

Data are conflicting as to whether there is a dose-response relationship between hypotension and intrathecal local anesthetics when these drugs are administered in low doses for labor analgesia. Palmer et al.[306] found no difference in blood pressure in women randomly assigned to receive intrathecal fentanyl combined with either 1.25 or 2.5 mg of bupivacaine. In contrast, Lee et al.[307] noted a greater drop in blood pressure at 10 minutes in women who received bupivacaine 2.5 mg than in women who received 1.25 mg. Because 1.25 mg is less than the ED_{95} for bupivacaine (when combined with fentanyl)[225] and there is no apparent advantage to combining bupivacaine 1.25 mg with fentanyl over using fentanyl alone,[308] it does not make sense to reduce the dose of intrathecal bupivacaine with the goal of decreasing the incidence and severity of hypotension.

Pruritus

Pruritus is the most common side effect of epidural or intrathecal opioid administration.[157,304] Intrathecal opioid administration is associated with a higher incidence and severity of pruritus than epidural opioid administration (41.4% versus 1.3% in one study[309]). The incidence of pruritus after intrathecal opioid administration is close to 100% in some studies, although the need for treatment is much lower.[202] The incidence and severity of pruritus are dose dependent for both epidural[141] and spinal[202,208] opioid administration. The co-administration of local anesthetic decreases the incidence of pruritus,[224] whereas the co-administration of epinephrine may worsen pruritus.[310]

The cause of the pruritus is poorly understood, but it appears to be unrelated to histamine release. Pruritus may be caused by a perturbation of sensory input that results from rostral spread of the opioid within the CSF to the level of the trigeminal nucleus in the medullary dorsal horn.[311] A disruption of sensory modulation is consistent with the observation that a similar pattern of pruritus is seen in medical conditions in which sensory modulation is disturbed (e.g., diabetic neuropathy, multiple sclerosis).[312] There is growing evidence that neuraxial opioid–induced pruritus is mediated through central μ-opioid receptors.[311,313] It is possible that neuraxial opioids also cause itching by antagonizing central inhibitory neurotransmitters (e.g., gamma-aminobutyric acid [GABA] and glycine) or by interaction with central 5-HT_3 receptors.[311,313] These receptors are concentrated in areas of the CNS with high μ-opioid receptor density (e.g., trigeminal nerve nucleus and dorsal horn of the spinal cord). The observation that the intrathecal administration of a lipid-soluble opioid (e.g., sufentanil) results in segmental pruritus is unproven. For example, patients often complain of perineal and truncal pruritus after intrathecal sufentanil administration.[224,304] In contrast, patients more often complain of facial pruritus after intrathecal morphine administration. Intrathecal bupivacaine may lower the incidence of truncal pruritus by direct neuronal blockade or modulation of the μ-opioid receptor.[224]

Few studies have addressed the *treatment* of established pruritus. The most effective treatment is a centrally acting μ-opioid agonist (e.g., naloxone or naltrexone) or a partial agonist-antagonist such as nalbuphine (Table 23-8). However, the use of these agents in a bolus or continuous infusion may reverse the analgesia. Antihistamines (e.g., diphenhydramine) are often prescribed but are usually ineffective because the mechanism of pruritus is not related

TABLE 23-8 Treatment of Neuraxial Opioid–Induced Pruritus

Drug	Dose
Naloxone	40-80 μg intravenous bolus 1-2 μg/kg/hr continuous intravenous infusion
Nalbuphine	2.5-5 mg intravenous bolus
Naltrexone	6 mg per os (by mouth)

to histamine release. Any observed effect of diphenhydramine is probably related to its sedating effects.

A number of drugs have been investigated for *prophylaxis* against neuraxial opioid–induced pruritus, primarily coincident with neuraxial morphine administration. Some investigators have described the effectiveness of prophylactic ondansetron in reducing the incidence of intrathecal opioid-induced pruritus,[314,315] whereas others have found ondansetron to be ineffective.[316,317] Similarly, some investigators have found that subhypnotic doses of propofol (10 to 20 mg) decrease the incidence of pruritus after neuraxial opioid administration,[318] and others have found propofol to be ineffective.[319]

We do not routinely administer prophylaxis for the pruritus associated with neuraxial administration of opioids for labor analgesia. The pruritus is typically self-limiting; the severity of pruritus usually diminishes markedly in the first hour after opioid administration, and most women do not require treatment. For moderate to severe pruritus that requires treatment, we usually administer **nalbuphine** 2.5 mg, and repeat the dose in 10 to 15 minutes if no improvement is noted. The advantage of nalbuphine is that it is less likely to reverse the intrathecal or epidural opioid analgesia.[320]

Nausea and Vomiting

Nausea and vomiting occur frequently during labor. It is difficult to determine the incidence of nausea and vomiting directly related to epidural and intrathecal opioid administration. Nausea and vomiting may also be related to neuraxial analgesia–induced hypotension. Maternal blood pressure should be measured when the patient complains of nausea in the presence of neuroblockade. Other causes of nausea and vomiting during labor are pregnancy itself, pain, opioid-induced delay of gastric emptying (see later), and systemic opioids, which are sometimes administered before intrathecal or epidural opioids. In one study, the incidences of nausea (7% versus 44%) and vomiting (2% versus 17%) were significantly lower in women randomly assigned to receive intrathecal fentanyl than in those assigned to receive systemic hydromorphone analgesia in early labor.[7]

The etiology of neuraxial opioid–associated nausea is unclear, but it may be caused by the modulation of afferent input at the area postrema (i.e., the chemoreceptor trigger zone) or at the nucleus of the tractus solitarius, which is a key relay station in the visceral sensory network.[321] Of interest, nausea is less common after epidural or intrathecal opioid administration during labor than after the administration of the same drugs for post–cesarean delivery analgesia. Norris et al.[309] noted that women who received epidural or intrathecal opioid analgesia during labor had an incidence of nausea of only 1.0% or 2.4%, respectively.

Although the incidence of nausea is low, treatment should be available. No studies, however, have specifically addressed the *treatment* of neuraxial analgesia-associated nausea and vomiting during labor. **Metoclopramide, ondansetron,** and **droperidol** have been used *prophylactically* in women who received neuraxial morphine for analgesia after cesarean delivery or nonobstetric surgery. Used in low doses, these agents have few significant side effects. When administered intravenously, metoclopramide should be administered slowly (over several minutes) in order to minimize extrapyramidal side effects.[322] A partial explanation for metoclopramide's efficacy may be its action in promoting gastric emptying. The package insert for droperidol contains a "black box" warning because of concern that the administration of this agent may increase the risk of severe cardiac dysrhythmias (secondary to prolongation of the QT interval and *torsades de pointes*). The warning suggests that patients be monitored for dysrhythmias for several hours after droperidol administration. Because maternal electrocardiographic monitoring is rarely undertaken in healthy parturients, the drug is now rarely used by obstetric anesthesia providers.

Fever

Clinical studies have noted a gradual rise in core temperature over several hours in laboring women receiving epidural analgesia that was not observed in women receiving no analgesia, inhaled nitrous oxide, or parenteral opioids.[323-326] The increase in core temperature is typically small (less than 1.0° C, with a maximum temperature of approximately 38° C) and is greatest in women who labor in rooms with relatively warm ambient temperatures (i.e., 23° to 29° C).[326] In a retrospective study, Herbst et al.[327] identified the use of epidural analgesia as a risk factor for intrapartum fever, along with prolonged labor and a prolonged interval between rupture of membranes and delivery. In another retrospective study, the incidence of fever (temperature > 38° C) was 15% in women who had epidural analgesia, compared with 1% in those who did not (adjusted OR, 14.5; 95% CI, 6.3 to 33.2).[324]

There are several reasons why temperatures may be higher in women who receive epidural analgesia. These women already may have longer labor and may therefore be at higher risk for infection, such as chorioamnionitis; thus the lack of random allocation to analgesic technique in these reports introduces the potential for selection bias. Alternatively, epidural analgesia may alter maternal temperature regulation; thus a greater core temperature is "tolerated" in the presence of an epidural block. In volunteer subjects, epidural analgesia raises the threshold for thermoregulatory sweating and, presumably by means of sympathectomy, can prevent sweating and evaporative heat loss in the part of the body affected by the block.[328] Consequently, laboring patients with epidural analgesia who are in a warm environment would likely have a small rise in core temperature.

The significance of these small temperature changes is unclear, but increases in fetal temperature and FHR can occur, and it may be difficult to distinguish this temperature change from one indicating infection. One retrospective, nonrandomized study found a higher rate of neonatal sepsis evaluations among infants of women who had received epidural analgesia during labor.[324] Subsequent retrospective reviews have found that epidural analgesia during labor is associated with more neonatal sepsis evaluations but not with a higher incidence of neonatal sepsis.[329,330] The overall high rate of neonatal sepsis evaluations among these otherwise healthy populations suggests that the criteria used for sepsis evaluations are inappropriate and need to be reevaluated.

Nulliparity and dysfunctional labor, two situations in which epidural analgesia is often employed, are also associated with maternal fever.[331] In a prospective cohort study of 99 women who requested labor analgesia,[332] 22% became febrile at some time before delivery. The absolute mean temperature rise was 0.72° C. In the women who remained afebrile there was no temperature rise in the first 4 hours after initiation of analgesia, whereas in the subset of women who became febrile, temperature increases were significant within the first hour after initiation of analgesia. The researchers concluded that most women do not become febrile after epidural analgesia and that, therefore, it is unlikely that a perturbation in thermoregulation induced by epidural analgesia is the cause of epidural analgesia–associated fever. In a randomized controlled trial, prophylactic methylprednisolone during labor reduced the incidence of fever in women with epidural analgesia, suggesting that the etiology may be related to inflammation.[333]

In summary, the preponderance of evidence suggests that epidural analgesia is associated with an increased risk of maternal fever during labor. The mechanism is unclear, but recent findings suggest that it may be related to inflammation. Because of the growing evidence that maternal inflammation and infection, which manifests as fever, can be detrimental to the fetal brain, anesthesia providers should not dismiss this apparent physiologic effect as a mere curiosity. When maternal fever occurs, good clinical practice dictates that efforts be made to lower maternal temperature and identify and treat a presumed maternal infection. (See Chapter 36 for a more complete discussion of this subject.)

Shivering

A number of factors, including hormonal factors, likely influence thermoregulatory response during labor and delivery. Shivering is frequently observed during labor and may occur more commonly after epidural analgesia.[334] Panzer et al.[335] performed an observational study of shivering during labor. Before delivery 18% of women shivered, and 15% of these episodes were associated with normothermia and vasodilation, suggesting a nonthermoregulatory cause of the shivering. After delivery, shivering was observed in 16% of women, and in 28% of them, it was nonthermoregulatory. There was no difference in the incidence of shivering between women who chose epidural (bupivacaine/fentanyl) analgesia and those who chose systemic meperidine analgesia. The addition of an opioid to the local anesthetic solution may affect the shivering response.[169,336] At least one study has suggested that the epidural administration of epinephrine increases shivering[336]; the etiology of this response is unknown.

Urinary Retention

Urinary retention is a troublesome side effect of neuraxial anesthesia/analgesia. The bladder and urethral sphincters receive sympathetic innervation from the low thoracic/high lumbar sympathetic fibers, and parasympathetic innervation from sacral fibers. Neuraxial local anesthetics cause urinary retention through blockade of sacral nerve roots. Efferent and afferent nerve traffic via the S2, S3, and S4 nerve roots controls the detrusor muscle (responsible for urine storage and micturition) and internal and external sphincter function. Intrathecal opioids cause dose-dependent suppression of detrusor muscle contractility and decreased urge sensation via inhibition of sacral parasympathetic nervous system outflow.[321,337] The onset of urinary retention appears to parallel the onset of analgesia.

It is difficult to determine the magnitude of this problem during labor, because parturients often require catheterization for other reasons. Postpartum bladder dysfunction was observed in 14% of women who had a normal spontaneous vaginal delivery and in 38% of women who underwent instrumental vaginal delivery, all without epidural analgesia.[338]

Several observational studies suggest that there is a higher risk of intrapartum and postpartum urinary retention in women who receive epidural labor analgesia than in those who receive non-epidural or no analgesia.[339,340] Whether this higher risk reflects a cause-and-effect relationship or patient selection bias is not clear. The difference in bladder function appears to be short-lived; differences between groups in one study had resolved by postpartum day 1.[339] In patients in two studies who were randomly assigned to receive epidural analgesia with or without an opioid, there was no difference between groups in the incidence of intrapartum[341] or postpartum[340] urinary retention.

Parturients should be regularly observed during labor for evidence of bladder distention, especially if they complain of suprapubic pain during contractions. The differential diagnosis of breakthrough pain during neuraxial labor analgesia should include bladder distention. Personal observation suggests that many women can void in the presence of low-dose neuroblockade if placed on a bedpan or escorted to the toilet, even if they do not perceive a full bladder. Inability to void and bladder distention should prompt catheterization to empty the bladder.

Recrudescence of Herpes Simplex Virus

The seroprevalence of herpes simplex virus (HSV) among pregnant women was 72% in the period 1999-2002.[342] HSV type 1 (HSV-1) is typically found in the trigeminal ganglia and causes orofacial lesions, whereas HSV-2 is more commonly found in the lumbosacral ganglia. However, either of these viruses can infect any region of the body.

The common cold sore or fever blister is a manifestation of the reactivation of latent infection. Reactivation can occur after exposure to ultraviolet light, fever, immunosuppression, or trauma. Prospective randomized studies have demonstrated a higher incidence of postpartum *oral* HSV reactivation in women randomly assigned to receive neuraxial (epidural,[343,344] intrathecal[345]) morphine than among women assigned to receive systemic morphine for post–cesarean delivery analgesia. Case reports have associated intraspinal administration of meperidine and fentanyl with the subsequent recurrence of HSV infection.[346,347]

To our knowledge, postcesarean reactivation of HSV infection after neuraxial opioid administration has not resulted in clinically significant maternal or neonatal complications. In addition, we are unaware of any study that has determined whether epidural or intrathecal opioid administration during labor increases the incidence of recurrent oral HSV infection after vaginal delivery. Therefore, we do not withhold neuraxial opioids during labor in women with a history of oral herpes.

Delayed Gastric Emptying

Labor may result in delayed gastric emptying, which may be exacerbated by opioid administration.[348] Intravenous or intramuscular opioid administration results in delayed gastric emptying in laboring women. Studies suggest that epidural fentanyl combined with bupivacaine and administered as part of a continuous epidural infusion does not result in delayed gastric emptying compared with infusion of bupivacaine alone[349,350]; however, delayed gastric emptying may occur with epidural fentanyl administered as a bolus (50 to 100 μg)[351,352] or with a *prolonged* infusion.[349] In another study, intrathecal fentanyl 25 μg resulted in delayed gastric emptying compared with epidural fentanyl 50 μg plus bupivacaine or bupivacaine alone.[353] Delayed gastric emptying may predispose a patient to nausea and vomiting. In addition, it may result in a greater volume of gastric contents, which—in theory—might be problematic in patients who require induction of general anesthesia for emergency cesarean delivery.

COMPLICATIONS OF NEURAXIAL ANALGESIA

Inadequate Analgesia

The reported failure rate for neuraxial analgesia varies according to the definition of "failure."[29,354,355] In survey studies the rate of epidural catheter replacement has ranged from 5% to 13%.[29,354,355] Successful location of the epidural space is not always possible, and satisfactory analgesia does not always occur, even when the epidural space has been identified correctly. Factors such as patient age and weight, the specific technique, the type of epidural catheter, and the skill of the anesthesia provider are associated with the rate of failure of neuraxial analgesia.[29,355] Failure to provide adequate analgesia not only results in a dissatisfying experience for the patient but may also lead to litigation.[356] The risk of failed anesthesia and the potential need to place a second epidural catheter should be discussed with the patient during the preanesthetic evaluation, before placement of the first epidural catheter.

Pan et al.[29] used quality assurance data to retrospectively assess the failure rate for more than 12,000 neuraxial procedures performed for labor analgesia over a 3-year period (Table 23-9). The overall failure rate of 12% included procedures resulting in no or inadequate analgesia, unintentional dural puncture with an epidural needle or catheter, intravenous cannulation with the epidural catheter, or replacement of the catheter for any reason. After initial adequate analgesia, 6.8% of the catheters were replaced, although eventually 98.8% of women received adequate pain relief. The rate of failed analgesia was significantly lower after CSE than after epidural analgesia (10% versus 14%, respectively; $P < .001$).

Typically, failed analgesia after injection of intrathecal or epidural anesthetics results in no neuroblockade, unilateral blockade or missed segments, or inadequate density of neuroblockade. Patient complaints of pain should prompt timely evaluation and treatment (Box 23-8). The progress of labor should be assessed (expectations and treatment

TABLE 23-9 Characteristics of Neuraxial Analgesia Failures*

Characteristic	Rate According to Type of Analgesia (%)			*P* value
	Epidural (n = 7849)	Combined Spinal-Epidural (n = 4741)	Total (n = 12,590)	
Overall failure rate	14	10	12	< .001
Initial Catheter Failure				
Intravenous catheter	7	5	6	< .001
Recognized dural puncture†	1.4	0.8	1.2	< .002
Other Failure				
No cerebrospinal fluid or spinal analgesia	NA	2.4	NA	
Inadequate analgesia with epidural catheter	8.4	4.2	6.8	< .001
Catheter replacement for inadequate analgesia‡	7.1	3.2	5.6	< .001
Multiple replacements of epidural catheter	1.9	0.7	1.5	< .001

*Retrospective audit of all neuraxial analgesic procedures for labor analgesia at a single teaching institution over a 3-year period. Most of the procedures were performed by residents.

†Dural puncture with epidural needle or catheter.

‡Epidural catheter initially functional, but replaced during the course of labor.

Modified from Pan PH, Bogard TD, Owen MD. Incidence and characteristics of failures in obstetric neuraxial analgesia and anesthesia: A retrospective analysis of 19,259 deliveries. Int J Obstet Anesth 2004; 13:227-33.

BOX 23-8 Assessment and Management of Inadequate Neuraxial Analgesia

- Assess progress of labor:
  - Rule out other causes of pain (distended bladder, ruptured uterus).
- Perform an honest evaluation of the anesthetic:
  - Is the catheter really in the epidural space?
  - If in doubt, replace the catheter.
- If the catheter is in the epidural space, but the extent of neuroblockade is inadequate (does not extend from T10 to S4, as is required for late labor):
  - Inject a dilute solution of local anesthetic (5 to 15 mL), with or without an opioid.
  - Alter maintenance technique (e.g., increase volume, decrease concentration).
  - If this maneuver is unsuccessful, replace the catheter.
- If catheter is in the epidural space, but the block is asymmetric:
  - Inject a dilute solution of local anesthetic (5 to 15 mL), with or without an opioid.
  - Alter maintenance technique (e.g., increase volume, decrease concentration).
  - Place the less blocked side in the dependent position.
  - If this maneuver is unsuccessful, replace the catheter.
- If the catheter is in the epidural space, but the patient has breakthrough pain despite adequate extent of neuroblockade:
  - Inject a more concentrated solution of local anesthetic, with or without an opioid.
  - Alter maintenance technique (e.g., increase concentration of local anesthetic).

may be different for patients with cervical dilation of 2 cm and 10 cm), and the patient should be queried as to the nature of the pain. The bladder should be checked and emptied if distended. The position of the epidural catheter at the skin should be checked to rule out the possibility of catheter migration out of the epidural space.

The extent of neuroblockade should be assessed with a cold or sharp stimulus that starts over the lateral thighs (dermatomal level at which the tip of the epidural catheter is sited) and moves both *cephalad* and *caudad* on both sides. Inexperienced anesthesia providers often fail to check for the presence of sacral blockade. In the case of no neuroblockade, the procedure should be repeated and the epidural catheter should be replaced. If the extent of neuroblockade is inadequate (in either the cephalad or caudad direction), or if there is unilateral blockade or missed segments, the injection of a large volume (5 to 15 mL) of a dilute local anesthetic solution (e.g., 0.0625% to 0.125% bupivacaine) may result in satisfactory analgesia. A lipid-soluble opioid may be added to the solution. An advantage of using a more dilute solution of local anesthetic is the ability to increase the volume administered to ensure adequate spread of analgesia.

Some anesthesia providers advocate pulling the epidural catheter out 1 to 2 cm before administering the bolus injection. Beilin et al.[357] investigated this practice by randomly assigning women with incomplete analgesia to one of two treatments, (1) immediate injection of 0.25% bupivacaine 5 mL or (2) withdrawal of the (multi-orifice) epidural catheter 1 cm followed by injection of the same dose of bupivacaine. There was no difference in the ability to rescue analgesia between the two treatments (74% versus 77%, respectively).

Maternal position has only a small effect on the development of an asymmetric block.[358,359] Husemeyer and White[358] gave 10 mL of epidural 1.5% lidocaine to pregnant women who were in the lateral position; they observed greater spread (two to three spinal segments) of anesthesia on the dependent side. In contrast, others have observed that posture has little influence on the spread of local anesthetic within the epidural space.[297,360] It is likely that the position of the epidural catheter in relation to other epidural space structures (e.g., connective tissue, fatty tissue, blood vessels) affects the spread and quality of analgesia to a greater extent than maternal position. Anatomic barriers (e.g., a longitudinal connective tissue band between the dura and ligamentum flavum) or placement of the catheter tip in the anterior epidural space or paravertebral space may explain some cases of single nerve root, unilateral, or asymmetric blockade.[361-364]

Pain often becomes more intense as labor progresses. An epidural block that was adequate at 4-cm cervical dilation may not be adequate at 8-cm cervical dilation. The anesthesia provider should be aware of the progress of the patient's labor when assessing inadequate analgesia. The patient may need a larger dose of local anesthetic; a 5- to 15-mL bolus of 0.125% bupivacaine or a 5- to 10-mL bolus of 0.25% bupivacaine is often adequate. Alternatively, an opioid may be added to the solution of local anesthetic. This addition is especially helpful if the patient is experiencing back pain because the fetus is in the occiput posterior position. Inadequate analgesia may result from migration of the epidural catheter into a vein or movement of the catheter outside of the epidural space. Before giving a bolus dose of local anesthetic, the anesthesia provider should give a test dose to exclude intravenous migration of the catheter. The response to the bolus dose should be assessed, and the catheter should be replaced (with the patient's consent) if satisfactory analgesia is not obtained.

Unintentional Dural Puncture

In a meta-analysis of 13 studies that involved more than 300,000 obstetric patients, Choi et al.[365] determined that the rate of unintentional dural puncture with an epidural needle or catheter was 1.5% (95% CI 1.5% to 1.5%) (see Chapter 31). Dural puncture may be detected at the time of insertion of the epidural needle or after placement of the catheter. If dural puncture is detected with the epidural needle, the anesthesia provider has two primary options. He or she may elect to remove the needle and place an epidural catheter at another interspace; if CSE analgesia was planned, the intrathecal dose may be injected through the epidural needle before it is removed and resited at a different interspace. Alternatively, the anesthesia provider may place a catheter in the subarachnoid space and administer continuous spinal analgesia for labor and delivery. This latter technique is particularly advantageous for patients at high risk for repeat dural puncture or in cases in which it may be difficult to enter either the epidural or subarachnoid space successfully at an alternative interspace (e.g., in obese women or in patients with abnormal anatomy of the lumbar spine). It is very important to append a label that clearly identifies the catheter as a spinal catheter to decrease the risk of injecting an epidural dose of local anesthetic into the subarachnoid space. All providers on the labor and delivery unit, including nurses, midwives, and other anesthesia providers, must be made aware of the intrathecal catheter.

Resiting the epidural catheter in a different interspace eliminates the problem of mistaking an intrathecal catheter for an epidural catheter. However, local anesthetic or opioid injected through the epidural catheter may pass through the dural puncture site and into the subarachnoid space, resulting in unexpectedly high neuroblockade.[366] This complication is more likely to occur with the bolus injection of local anesthetic than with an epidural infusion of local anesthetic.

If dural puncture is not recognized until CSF is aspirated from the catheter, or if administration of the test dose results in spinal anesthesia, the anesthesia provider has the following two options: (1) replace the epidural catheter at an alternative interspace or (2) provide continuous spinal analgesia through the existing catheter.

Respiratory Depression

The administration of opioids by any route entails risk of respiratory depression. Factors that affect the risk of respiratory depression after neuraxial opioid administration include the choice and dose of drug, and its interaction with systemically administered opioids and other CNS depressants (see Chapter 13). The most important factor affecting the onset of respiratory depression is the lipid solubility of the drug.[321] In general, if respiratory depression is going to occur, it will do so within 2 hours of the injection of a lipid-soluble opioid such as fentanyl or sufentanil. When a lipid-soluble opioid gains access to the CSF, it is quickly absorbed by lipophilic body tissues. Subsequent clearance and elimination are similar to those associated with intravenous injection of the same drug. Thus, with spinal or epidural injection of a lipid-soluble opioid, the "time window" for respiratory depression is short. Conversely, with a hydrophilic drug such as morphine, the onset of respiratory depression is delayed. Once a hydrophilic drug such as morphine enters the CSF, it tends to stay in the CSF. Rostral migration and absorption into the respiratory centers occur over several hours, so respiratory depression may not occur until 6 to 12 hours after injection of the drug (see Figure 13-13).

The dose of opioid is a major determinant of the risk of respiratory depression.[208] Herman et al.[208] observed an increase in end-tidal CO_2 concentration with intrathecal fentanyl doses of 15 μg or higher. The time of maximum end-tidal CO_2 was approximately 30 minutes after the intrathecal injection. Respiratory arrest has been reported after intrathecal sufentanil 10 μg in parturients.[367,368] A risk factor for respiratory depression is previous parenteral opioid administration. Several reports have implicated prior intravenous opioid administration as a contributing factor to the respiratory arrest that occurred after intrathecal sufentanil administration in laboring women.[367,368] For this reason, we refrain from administering a bolus dose of epidural or spinal opioid to women who have recently received systemic opioid analgesia.

Intravascular Injection of Local Anesthetic

The incidence of fatal systemic toxic reactions to local anesthetics appears to have declined since 1984.[13] In a prospective audit from the United Kingdom of more than 145,000 obstetric epidural procedures, the incidence of intravascular injection was 1 in 5000 (Table 23-10). Bupivacaine 0.75% is no longer used for epidural anesthesia in obstetric patients. Ropivacaine and levobupivacaine have replaced bupivacaine when high concentrations are required for operative epidural anesthesia, and low concentrations of local anesthetic are now routinely used for labor analgesia. Nonetheless, systemic local anesthetic toxicity remains a serious potential complication during the administration of epidural anesthesia in obstetric patients.

Intravenous injection of a large dose of local anesthetic causes CNS symptoms (e.g., restlessness, dizziness, tinnitus, perioral paresthesia, difficulty speaking, seizures, loss of consciousness). Cardiovascular effects may progress from increased blood pressure (as a result of sympathetic stimulation) to bradycardia, depressed ventricular function, and ventricular tachycardia and fibrillation. Bupivacaine cardiotoxicity may be fatal in pregnant women.[55]

Box 23-9 lists steps for the management of the unintentional intravascular injection of local anesthetic (see Chapter 13). They include treatment of convulsions, supporting oxygenation and ventilation, and initiating advanced cardiac life support, if indicated.[369] Amiodarone should be administered for the treatment of life-threatening ventricular arrhythmias. Early delivery of the infant should be considered, because it may improve the likelihood of successful resuscitation.

Several reports have described intravenous administration of lipid emulsion for successful resuscitation of patients

TABLE 23-10 Incidence of Unintentional Intravascular, Intrathecal, and Subdural Injections during Attempted Epidural Labor Analgesia*

Event	Incidence	Rate (%)†
Intravascular injection	1:5000	0.020 (0.014-0.029)
Intrathecal injection	1:2900	0.035 (0.027-0.046)
Subdural injection	1:4200	0.025 (0.017-0.033)
High/total spinal anesthesia	1:16,200	0.006 (0.003-0.012)

*Prospective data collection of 145,550 epidural procedures for obstetric patients in 14 maternity units in the South West Thames Region (United Kingdom) over a 17-year period.

†95% confidence intervals shown in parentheses.

Modified from Jenkins JG. Some immediate serious complications of obstetric analgesia and anaesthesia: A prospective study of 145,550 epidurals. Int J Obstet Anesth 2005; 14:37-42.

BOX 23-9 Management of Unintentional Intravenous Injection of Local Anesthetic

- Be aware that hypoxemia and acidosis develop rapidly during a seizure. Stop the seizure with a barbiturate or benzodiazepine.
- Administer 100% oxygen to maintain maternal oxygenation.
- Use positive-pressure ventilation if necessary. Endotracheal intubation will facilitate support of ventilation and help protect the airway, but do not delay administration of oxygen in order to intubate the trachea.
- Prevent maternal respiratory and metabolic acidosis.
- Avoid aortocaval compression.
- Monitor maternal vital signs and fetal heart rate.
- Support maternal blood pressure with fluids and vasopressors.
- Initiate advanced cardiac life support if necessary.
- Prepare for emergency delivery. Consider cesarean delivery of the infant if the mother is not resuscitated within 4 minutes, as it may facilitate successful resuscitation of the mother.
- Consider intravenous bolus administration of 20% lipid emulsion, approximately 1.5 mL/kg (100 mL in an adult). This can be followed by a continuous intravenous infusion at 0.25 to 0.5 mL/kg/min for 10 minutes or longer.[370,510]

BOX 23-10 Management of Total Spinal Anesthesia

- High spinal anesthesia may occur several minutes after the unintentional intrathecal injection of local anesthetic or as a result of overdose of epidural local anesthetic. Communication with the patient is important. Agitation, dyspnea, difficulty speaking, and profound hypotension may herald the onset of total spinal anesthesia.
- Avoid aortocaval compression.
- Administer 100% oxygen.
- Provide positive-pressure ventilation, preferably through an endotracheal tube.
- Monitor maternal vital signs, electrocardiogram, and fetal heart rate.
- Support maternal circulation with intravenous fluids and vasopressors as needed. Do not hesitate to give epinephrine if needed.
- Maintain verbal communication with the mother or administer a small dose of a sedative-hypnotic agent. Total spinal anesthesia does not signal brain anesthesia. Patients may lose consciousness and stop breathing because of hypoperfusion of the brain and brainstem, not brain anesthesia.

who have suffered systemic local anesthetic toxicity refractory to standard resuscitative measures.[370] The mechanism requires further elucidation, but the lipid may be acting as a preferential lipid sink. The risks are unclear, but case reports have described intravenous administration of a bolus dose of approximately 1.5 mL/kg (100 mL in an adult) of 20% lipid emulsion, followed by a continuous intravenous infusion of 0.25 to 0.5 mL/kg/min for 10 minutes or longer.[370]

High Neuroblockade or Total Spinal Anesthesia

An unexpectedly high level of anesthesia may result from one of several situations. First, high (or total) spinal blockade may occur after the unintentional and unrecognized placement of the epidural catheter in either the subarachnoid or subdural space and injection of an epidural dose of local anesthetic through that catheter. Second, the epidural catheter may migrate into the subarachnoid or subdural space during the course of labor and delivery. Finally, high spinal blockade may result from an overdose of local anesthetic in the epidural space. Crawford[366] reported 6 cases of high or total spinal anesthesia in a series of nearly 27,000 cases of lumbar epidural anesthesia administered during labor (an incidence of approximately 1 in 4500). Paech et al.[354] reported 8 cases of unexpectedly high neuroblockade in a series of 10,995 epidural blocks in obstetric patients (an incidence of approximately 1 in 1400). Two patients required intubation and mechanical ventilation. Jenkins[371] reported an incidence of 1 in 16,200 procedures (see Table 23-10).

Aspiration alone, particularly through a single-orifice catheter, is an inadequate method of excluding subarachnoid placement of the catheter. Administration of an appropriate test dose and careful assessment of the patient's response to the test dose should minimize the chance of unintentional injection of a large dose of local anesthetic into the subarachnoid space.

High or total spinal anesthesia results in agitation, profound hypotension, dyspnea, the inability to speak, and loss of consciousness. Loss of consciousness usually results from hypoperfusion of the brain and brainstem, not from brain anesthesia. Evidence of spinal anesthesia may be apparent shortly after intrathecal injection of a local anesthetic, but the maximal spread may not be evident for several minutes. This delay underscores the need for the anesthesia provider to carefully assess the effects of both the test and therapeutic doses of local anesthetic. If total spinal anesthesia should occur, the anesthesia provider must be prepared to maintain oxygenation, ventilation, and circulation (Box 23-10). Immediate management consists of avoidance of aortocaval compression, ventilation with 100% oxygen, endotracheal intubation, and administration of intravenous fluids and vasopressors to support the blood pressure as needed. The FHR should be monitored continuously.

Extensive neuroblockade may also result from subdural injection of a local anesthetic.[372-374] A subdural injection may be difficult to diagnose because onset is later than that with an intrathecal injection and more closely resembles that associated with epidural neuroblockade.

The subdural space is a potential space between the dura mater and the arachnoid mater. A retrospective review of 2182 lumbar epidural injections for pain management found that clinical signs of subdural catheter placement occurred in approximately 0.82% of patients.[372]

TABLE 23-11 Clinical Features of Epidural, Subdural, and Spinal Blocks

	Epidural Block	Subdural Block	Spinal Block
Onset time	Slow	Intermediate	Rapid
Spread	As expected	Higher than expected; may extend intracranially, but sacral sparing is common	Higher than expected; may extend intracranially, and a sacral block is typically present
Nature of block	Segmental	Patchy	Dense
Motor block	Minimal	Minimal	Dense
Hypotension	Less than spinal, and dependent on the extent of the block	Intermediate between spinal and epidural, and dependent on the extent of the block	Likely

Subdural injection of local anesthetic typically results in unexpectedly high (but patchy) blockade with an onset time that is intermediate between that of spinal anesthesia and epidural anesthesia (i.e., 10 to 20 minutes) (Table 23-11). Cranial spread is more extensive than caudal spread of the local anesthetic, so sacral analgesia typically is absent. The block may involve the cranial nerves. (The subdural space, unlike the epidural space, extends intracranially.) Thus, apnea and unconsciousness can occur during a subdural block. Horner's syndrome has been reported.[373] A subdural block usually results in less intense motor blockade than the blockade that occurs with high or total spinal anesthesia. This difference may reflect the limited spread of the local anesthetic within the subdural space, which helps spare the anterior motor fibers.[374] Subdural block results in less severe hypotension than that with high or total spinal anesthesia, most likely because subdural injection leads to less sympathetic blockade than spinal anesthesia. The unpredictable spread of local anesthetic, the slower onset of maximal spread (in comparison with spinal anesthesia), the patchy nature of the block, and the sacral sparing make it difficult to use a subdural catheter safely during labor and delivery. If we suspect that a catheter is positioned within the subdural space, we replace it with an epidural catheter.

Unexpectedly high neuroblockade may result from the migration of an epidural catheter into the subdural or subarachnoid space.[374] It is unclear how a soft epidural catheter can penetrate the dura. Disposable epidural needles are sharp, and insertion of the needle into the epidural space may result in an unrecognized nick in the dura, which may represent a site for delayed migration of the catheter into the subdural or subarachnoid space. Subdural or subarachnoid injection of local anesthetic also may occur if a multi-orifice catheter is used, of which one orifice is located within the epidural space and another within the subdural or subarachnoid space. In this situation, the force of injection determines the ultimate destination of the local anesthetic. Thus, each bolus injection of local anesthetic should serve as a test dose. During the continuous infusion with a local anesthetic, a gradual increase in the level of anesthesia and intensity of motor blockade may herald the intrathecal infusion of the local anesthetic solution.

Extensive Motor Blockade

Clinically significant motor block may occur after repeated bolus doses[182] or after many hours of a continuous infusion of local anesthetic.[375] The administration of bupivacaine with epinephrine results in a greater likelihood of dense motor blockade than the administration of bupivacaine alone.[182] Extensive motor blockade is often bothersome for the patient, and it may impair maternal expulsive efforts during the second stage of labor and increase the likelihood of instrumental vaginal delivery (see later). Some obstetricians argue that pelvic floor relaxation prevents rotation of the fetal head and increases the likelihood of an abnormal position of the vertex at delivery.

If intense motor blockade develops during the continuous epidural infusion of local anesthetic, the infusion can be discontinued for a short period (e.g., 30 minutes). Subsequently, the infusion can be restarted at a reduced rate or with a more dilute solution of local anesthetic. Extensive motor blockade does not occur with administration of a very dilute solution of local anesthetic combined with an opioid.

Prolonged Neuroblockade

Rarely, the duration of neuraxial analgesia/anesthesia exceeds the time expected. Most cases of unexpectedly prolonged neuroblockade follow the epidural administration of a high concentration of local anesthetic with epinephrine.[376] Abnormal neurologic findings after the administration of neuraxial anesthesia should prompt the anesthesia provider to look for evidence of peripheral nerve injury or an epidural hematoma (see Chapter 32). Factors that argue against the presence of an epidural hematoma include (1) the absence of back pain, (2) a unilateral block, and (3) regression (rather than progression) of the symptoms. Peripheral nerve injuries typically result in a neurologic deficit in the distribution of a specific peripheral nerve. Neurologic or neurosurgical consultation and immediate imaging studies should be obtained if there is any question about the etiology of prolonged anesthesia. Avoiding the use of a high concentration of local anesthetic should help minimize the incidence of prolonged neuroblockade during and after labor and vaginal delivery.

Sensory Changes

In one of the early studies of intrathecal opioid administration during labor, Cohen et al.[304] observed sensory changes in women who received intrathecal sufentanil. Subsequent studies have demonstrated that these sensory changes do not result from a local anesthetic effect of sufentanil. Sensory changes do not predict the quality or duration of analgesia or the extent of hemodynamic change.[377] Further, intrathecal sufentanil does not cause a sympathectomy.[305] Wang et al.[378] have provided the best explanation for these sensory changes. They showed that intrathecal opioids block the afferent information from A-delta and C fibers to the spinal cord but that efferent nerve impulses are unaffected. These sensory changes can be clinically significant, especially when they extend to the cervical dermatomes. In such cases, patients may feel that they cannot breathe or swallow, a sensation that can be quite distressing. Fortunately, neither intrathecal sufentanil nor fentanyl affects the efferent limb of the nervous system and so does not impair motor function. Affected patients should be reassured that respiratory efforts are not compromised and that these symptoms will subside in 30 to 60 minutes.[379,380]

In addition to sensory changes, two case reports have described mental status changes, aphasia, and automatisms after the intrathecal injection of fentanyl[381] and sufentanil.[382] These symptoms seem to be related to an opioid effect. In one case, the symptoms were partially reversed by naloxone.[381]

Back Pain

Approximately 50% of women complain of back pain during pregnancy and the puerperium.[383] The most significant risk factors for postpartum back pain are antepartum back pain and inability to reduce weight to prepregnancy levels.[383-385] MacArthur et al.[386,387] earlier suggested that the administration of epidural analgesia increases the risk of postpartum back pain. Data collected from a retrospective review of 11,701 case records and patient questionnaires (mailed 1 to 9 years after delivery) demonstrated a significant association between the use of intrapartum epidural analgesia and persistent postpartum back pain.[386] However, retrospective studies suffer not only from patient recall bias (i.e., patients with a problem are much more likely to complete and return the questionnaire) but also from selection bias in the epidural and nonepidural groups. Patients who select epidural analgesia for labor may have obstetric, orthopedic, social, or other unidentified factors that predispose them to postpartum back pain.

In an attempt to assess anesthetic factors that might contribute to postpartum backache (e.g., motor blockade), Russell et al.[385] randomly assigned laboring women requesting epidural analgesia to receive either bupivacaine alone or bupivacaine plus an opioid. Despite the expected differences in motor blockade, the incidence of backache did not differ between the two anesthetic groups (bupivacaine alone, 39%; bupivacaine plus an opioid, 30%). In addition, the incidence of backache in both epidural groups was similar to that found in a nonrandomized control group of women who labored without epidural analgesia (31%).

Prospective reports have not shown a significant relationship between the use of epidural analgesia and long-term backache. Breen et al.[384] observed no difference in the incidence of postpartum backache among women who delivered vaginally with or without epidural analgesia. Finally, Loughnan et al.[388] enrolled 310 women in a randomized controlled trial that compared epidural bupivacaine to systemic meperidine analgesia. The primary outcome was back pain 6 months after delivery. There was no difference between the two groups in the incidence of backache (epidural 48%, meperidine 50%). Similarly, another randomized controlled trial of epidural versus nonepidural analgesia found no difference in the incidence of backache at 3 and 12 months,[389] and several years[390] after delivery.

A prospective Canadian study assessed the relationship between postpartum backache and patient-selected intrapartum analgesia.[391] The rate of low back pain was greater in the epidural group (53%) than in the nonepidural group (43%) on the first postpartum day, but the rates were similar on postpartum day 7 and at 6 weeks and 1 year.[392] These investigators suggested that the higher incidence of backache immediately after delivery may have resulted from tissue trauma during epidural needle placement.

In summary, prospective studies have consistently shown that no causal relationship exists between epidural analgesia and the development of long-term postpartum backache. Short-term backache (several days) may be related to local tissue trauma at the site of skin puncture.

Pelvic Floor Injury

Few studies have evaluated the possible effects of epidural analgesia on postpartum pelvic floor function. In a case-matched study of 140 nulliparous women, Sartore et al.[393] observed no significant difference in the incidence of stress urinary incontinence, anal incontinence, or vaginal prolapse 3 months after vaginal delivery between those women who did and those who did not receive epidural analgesia. Any factor that might increase the likelihood of instrumental vaginal delivery might be expected to increase the risk of pelvic floor injury and subsequent pelvic floor dysfunction (see later). However, to our knowledge, there is no evidence that epidural analgesia per se predisposes to pelvic floor injury. Further studies in this area—with longer periods of follow-up—would be of interest to both physicians and patients.

EFFECTS OF NEURAXIAL ANALGESIA ON THE PROGRESS OF LABOR

Neuraxial analgesia during labor is associated with a prolonged labor and operative delivery. (The term *operative delivery* refers to both cesarean delivery and instrumental vaginal delivery [e.g., forceps delivery or vacuum extraction]). Controversy has existed as to whether there is a cause-and-effect relationship between the use of these analgesic techniques and prolonged labor or operative delivery. The understanding of this subject has been limited by the difficulty of performing controlled trials in which parturients are randomly assigned to neuraxial analgesia or a control group. Ideally, if one wants to study the effect of neuraxial analgesia on the progress and outcome of labor, the control group would receive no analgesia. However, such a study is not ethical, and even if it were and women volunteered to participate in it, the crossover rate would probably be high, and the data consequently would not be interpretable. Therefore, controlled trials have randomly assigned parturients to receive neuraxial analgesia or an alternative form of pain relief, usually with systemic opioids. However, even when the control group receives some type of analgesia, the crossover rate may be high because the quality of neuraxial analgesia is markedly superior to that of all other modes of labor analgesia.[4]

The difficulty in performing and interpreting the results of labor analgesia trials was aptly described by Noble et al.,[394] who assessed obstetric outcome in 245 patients randomly assigned to receive either epidural analgesia or "conventional" analgesia (i.e., meperidine, nitrous oxide, or no analgesia). The investigators made the following comments:

> *Of 245 selected patients, 43 had to be removed from the trial after labor ensued.... Most of the patients removed from the non-epidural group were apparently experiencing severe pain; they were usually primigravidae whose baby presented in the occipito-posterior position.... The majority of patients removed from the epidural group were apparently normal and usually multigravidas; their labors were so rapid it was not possible to arrange for an epidural block.*[394]

In other words, patients at low risk for operative delivery were excluded from the epidural group, and patients at high risk were excluded from the non-epidural group. Nonetheless, there was only one cesarean delivery in the epidural group, compared with three in the control group. The investigators' candid comments illustrate that, even when a prospective, randomized study is performed, it is difficult to maintain conditions that allow for the comparison of women at equal risk for abnormal labor and operative delivery.

Another concern is the external validity of these studies. Women who agree to participate in research trials may be inherently different from women who refuse to participate. Many women make a decision regarding labor analgesia well before the onset of labor and are unwilling to let chance randomization determine the type of labor analgesia. Thus, the study results may not be generalizable to the general obstetric population.

Ironically, the effect of systemic opioids on the progress and outcome of labor has not been well studied. Furthermore, there may be differences among the opioids.[395,396] Finally, neuraxial analgesia is not a generic procedure. Conclusions about the effect of one technique on the progress of labor may not be applicable to other techniques.

Additional factors prevent rigorous scientific study of this issue. Ideally a randomized controlled trial should be double-blinded. This is not possible for studies that compare neuraxial analgesia with another mode of analgesia, because of the marked difference in the quality of analgesia. Therefore, the potential for bias on the part of the parturient, nurses, and anesthesia and obstetric providers is substantial. Additionally, a number of factors are known to affect or to be associated with the progress and outcome of labor, including parity, artificial rupture of membranes, use of oxytocin, and payer status; these should be controlled in well-conducted studies.

One factor known to markedly influence the outcome of labor is the obstetric provider. Neuhoff et al.[397] retrospectively reviewed the records of 607 nulliparous women at term gestation and compared mode of delivery in "clinic" patients (whose care was given primarily by residents) and private patients (whose care was provided primarily by private obstetricians). Approximately 42% of patients received epidural analgesia during labor. Five percent of patients in the clinic group and 17% of patients in the private group underwent cesarean delivery ($P < .001$). More striking was the difference between groups in the incidence of cesarean delivery for dystocia (0.5% versus 13.7%, respectively; $P < .001$).

Similarly, Guillemette and Fraser[398] observed marked obstetrician variation in cesarean delivery rates, despite similarities in the use of oxytocin and epidural analgesia. Fraser et al.[399] observed a temporal variation in the incidence of cesarean delivery. The incidence peaked in the evening, which was consistent with the hypothesis that it was more convenient for the obstetrician to operate at this time. De Regt et al.[400] suggested that private physicians may be more concerned about adverse outcomes and potential litigation than resident physicians.

Retrospective studies are difficult to interpret because they suffer from selection bias. In some cases, distinguishing between anesthesia administered for pain relief during labor and anesthesia administered in preparation for operative delivery is difficult. Moreover, women at higher risk for prolonged labor and operative delivery are more likely to request and receive epidural analgesia during labor than women who have a rapid, uncomplicated labor.[401] Wuitchik et al.[401] observed a relationship between pain and cognitive activity during early labor and the subsequent progress of labor in 115 healthy nulliparous women. During the latent phase, higher levels of pain were predictive of longer latent and active phases of labor. Those women who reported "horrible" or "excruciating" pain during the latent phase were more than twice as likely to require instrumental delivery as women who only had "discomfort." In addition, women who reported "distress" rather than "coping" had a fivefold higher incidence of abnormal FHR patterns, and a fourfold higher requirement for assistance from pediatricians during neonatal resuscitation.

Greater pain intensity during labor appears to be a risk factor for operative delivery. This fact will significantly bias observational studies of labor analgesia because women with greater pain intensity request analgesia, specifically neuraxial analgesia, at a higher rate than women with less intense pain. Alexander et al.[402] performed a secondary analysis of data from a randomized controlled trial in which one group of laboring women received patient-controlled intravenous meperidine analgesia (PCIA). The rate of cesarean delivery was 14% in women who self-administered 50 mg/hr or more of meperidine, compared with 1.4% in women who self-administered less than 50 mg/hr. In a retrospective study of factors that predict operative delivery in laboring women, Hess et al.[403] found that the cesarean delivery rate in women who had more breakthrough pain during low-dose bupivacaine/fentanyl epidural analgesia was more than twice as high as the rate in women with less breakthrough pain (OR 2.62; 95% CI, 2.01 to 3.43) (Figure 23-11).

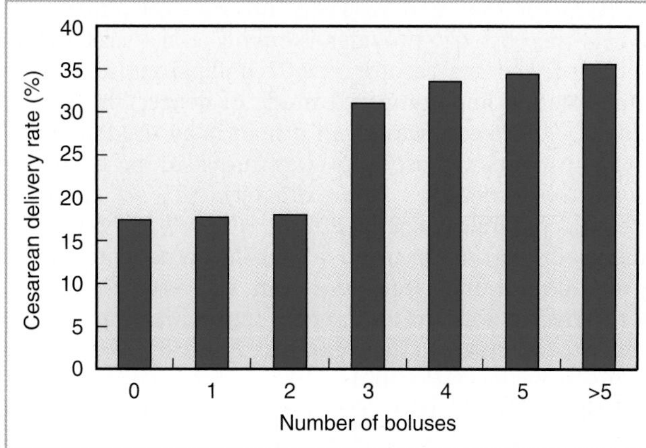

FIGURE 23-11 The rate of cesarean delivery as a function of the number of incidents of breakthrough pain during epidural analgesia maintained with a continuous infusion of low-dose bupivacaine or bupivacaine-fentanyl. The need for supplemental bolus analgesia was considered a marker for breakthrough pain. The rate of cesarean delivery was more than twice as high in women who required three or more supplemental bolus doses than in women who required two or fewer bolus doses (odds ratio, 2.62; 95% confidence interval, 2.01 to 3.43). (From Hess PE, Pratt SD, Soni AK, et al. Association between severe labor pain and cesarean delivery. Anesth Analg 2000; 90:881-6.)

Taken together, these studies suggest that the early onset of severe pain and the requirement of high doses of analgesic agents predict higher risks for abnormal labor, FHR abnormalities, and operative delivery. These findings may explain the observed association between neuraxial analgesia and operative delivery.

Cesarean Delivery Rate

RANDOMIZED CONTROLLED TRIALS

A number of randomized controlled trials have studied the effect of neuraxial (primarily epidural) and systemic opioid (primarily meperidine) analgesia on the cesarean delivery rate.[3-5,389,404-416] These trials differ in a number of ways, as follows: (1) the population studied (e.g., nulliparous women or women of mixed parity); (2) onset of labor (spontaneous labor alone or a mix of spontaneous and induced labors); (3) type of neuraxial analgesia; (4) density of neuraxial analgesia; (5) route of administration of systemic analgesia (although all the studies included meperidine with or without an adjuvant); (6) the crossover rate; and (7) management of labor (e.g., active management of labor, including electronic FHR monitoring, artificial rupture of membranes, and oxytocin infusion).

All but one of these studies found no difference in the rate of cesarean delivery between women randomly assigned to receive either neuraxial or systemic opioid analgesia. In a study of 93 indigent nulliparous women reported by Thorp et al.,[5] 12 (25%) of women in the epidural group—versus 1 (2%) woman in the meperidine group—-underwent cesarean delivery. The cesarean delivery rate in the epidural group was significantly higher, and that in the meperidine group significantly lower, than the historical norm (15%) for the institution in which the study was performed. This anomalous outcome, coupled with the fact that the investigators in the study assumed responsibility for decisions about the method of delivery, suggests that bias in the decision to perform cesarean delivery cannot be eliminated. In addition, other factors known to influence the outcome of labor (timing and dose of oxytocin, rupture of membranes) were not standardized for the two groups.

Four prospective, randomized trials were performed at the University of Texas Southwestern Medical Center, Parkland Hospital, in Dallas.[4,407,410,412] This institution is unique among many others that have performed randomized trials, in that the population is composed largely of indigent women whose labor is managed by the same group of resident physicians and midwives, supervised by the same core group of attending obstetricians. In the first study, 1330 women of mixed parity were randomly assigned to receive either epidural bupivacaine/fentanyl or intravenous meperidine for labor analgesia.[4] Approximately one third of the women did not receive the assigned treatment. The cesarean delivery rates were 9.0% in women who received epidural analgesia and 3.9% in women who received intravenous meperidine. However, the investigators did not report an intent-to-treat analysis of these data; thus it was unclear whether there was a higher incidence of cesarean delivery in the women randomly assigned to the epidural analgesia group. Subsequently, the investigators published a re-analysis of the data that included an intent-to-treat analysis (Table 23-12).[417] The cesarean delivery rate in both groups was 6%. These analyses support the conclusion that women who choose epidural analgesia have an inherent risk factor(s) for cesarean delivery and that the administration of neuraxial analgesia per se does not alter this risk.

TABLE 23-12 Parkland Hospital Randomized Controlled Trial of Epidural versus Systemic Opioid Analgesia and Rate of Cesarean Delivery: Actual Treatment versus Intent-to-Treat Analysis*

	Cesarean Delivery Rate (%)	
Analysis	**Epidural Analgesia (n = 664)**	**Systemic Opioid Analgesia (n = 666)**
Actual treatment†	9.0	3.9‡
Intent-to-treat	6	6

*In the systemic opioid group, 103 women requested and received epidural analgesia because opioid analgesia was inadequate. The initial analysis was published in 1995. The intent-to-treat analysis of the same data was published in 2000.

†The protocol violation rate was 35%.

‡$P < .05$ compared with epidural analgesia group.

Data from Ramin SM, Gambling DR, Lucas MJ, et al. Randomized trial of epidural versus intravenous analgesia during labor. Obstet Gynecol 1995; 86:783-9; and Sharma SK, Leveno KJ. Update: Epidural analgesia does not increase cesarean births. Curr Anesthesiol Rep 2000; 2:18-24.

In an attempt to lower the rate of crossover by providing better analgesia to the control (meperidine) group, the Parkland investigators performed another study in which meperidine was administered by PCIA.[407] A significant number of women in both groups did not receive their assigned treatment, although the reason in all cases was rapid labor. Only 5 of 357 women randomly assigned to the meperidine group crossed over to receive epidural analgesia. Using an intent-to-treat analysis, the investigators observed no difference between the groups in the incidence of cesarean delivery (4% in the epidural group and 5% in the PCIA group). There was no difference between the two groups in neonatal outcome, except that more babies in the PCIA group received naloxone to reverse respiratory depression at birth.

Only one randomized trial has compared CSE and systemic opioid analgesia.[410] In this large study (n = 1223), patients of mixed parity were randomly assigned to receive CSE analgesia (intrathecal sufentanil 10 μg, followed by epidural bupivacaine with fentanyl at the second request for analgesia) or intravenous meperidine (50 mg every hour on request). Approximately 60% of patients complied with the protocol. An intent-to-treat analysis showed that there was no difference between groups in the rate of cesarean delivery (CSE 6%, systemic opioid 5.5%).

The studies comparing neuraxial with systemic opioid analgesia have been systematically reviewed in several meta-analyses.[418,419] The latest meta-analysis covered outcomes for 6701 women from 17 studies (Figure 23-12).[418] The odds ratio for cesarean delivery in women randomly assigned to receive neuraxial analgesia compared with those assigned to receive systemic opioid analgesia was 1.03 (95% CI, 0.86 to 1.22).[418] In an individual patient meta-analysis of the studies performed at Parkland Hospital (n = 4465),[419] the odds ratio was 1.04 (95% CI, 0.81 to 1.34).

Mode and Density of Neuraxial Analgesia and Effect on Cesarean Delivery Rate

If neuraxial analgesia adversely affects the outcome of labor, one would expect to observe a dose-response effect.[418] The COMET study randomly assigned more than 1000 parturients to one of three groups: (1) "high-dose" epidural analgesia (traditional epidural analgesia with bupivacaine 0.25%); (2) "low-dose" epidural analgesia (bupivacaine 0.1%/fentanyl 2 μg/mL bolus, followed by a continuous epidural infusion); and (3) "low-dose" CSE analgesia (intrathecal bupivacaine/fentanyl followed by intermittent boluses of epidural bupivacaine 0.1%/fentanyl 2 μg/mL).[420] There was no difference in cesarean delivery rates among groups (Figure 23-13). Similarly, several other studies comparing traditional epidural analgesia using bupivacaine 0.25% with low-dose CSE techniques found no difference between groups in the cesarean delivery rate.[421-423] The results of these studies suggest that "high-dose" neuraxial analgesia does not entail a higher risk for cesarean delivery than "low-dose" techniques; in other words, no dose-response effect has been observed.

There is no evidence that CSE analgesia influences the mode of delivery, when compared to epidural analgesia alone. Large randomized controlled trials comparing CSE analgesia with epidural analgesia alone have found no difference between groups in the rate of cesarean delivery.[420-422,424]

IMPACT STUDIES

Some physicians have questioned whether prospective, randomized studies provide an accurate representation of the effect of neuraxial analgesia on the mode of delivery in actual clinical practice. They have suggested the possibility that prospective studies may introduce a Hawthorne effect (which may be defined as the appearance or disappearance of a phenomenon on initiation of a study to confirm or exclude its existence.) An alternative study design is to assess obstetric outcome immediately before and after a sentinel event, such as the introduction of an epidural analgesia service in a given hospital. The results of these studies may be generalizable to the general population because patients have not chosen to participate in a study. It also eliminates the problem of treatment group crossover because epidural analgesia was not available in the control period. One limitation of this study design is that it assumes that there were no other changes in obstetric management in the "after" period.

In 1999 Yancey et al.[425] published an impact study using data from the Tripler Army Hospital in Hawaii. Because of relative homogeneity in socioeconomic status, universal access to health care, and the availability of dedicated health care providers in the population served by this hospital, its rate of cesarean delivery may not be subject to influences common to other hospitals. Prior to 1993 the rate of epidural analgesia was less than 1% at Tripler Army Hospital. In 1993 a policy change within the U.S. Department of Defense mandated on-demand availability of neuraxial labor analgesia in military hospitals. At Tripler Army Hospital the rate of epidural labor analgesia rose from less than 1% to approximately 80% in a 1-year period (Figure 23-14). The rate of cesarean delivery in nulliparous women in spontaneous labor remained unchanged during the same period (19.0% versus 19.4%, respectively).

Obstetricians in the United States have long admired the low rate of cesarean delivery at the National Maternity Hospital in Dublin, Ireland. Obstetricians at this hospital were the first physicians to advocate the active management of labor. Some obstetricians in the United States have suggested that the low cesarean delivery rate in Dublin resulted in part from the infrequent use of epidural analgesia during labor. Impey et al.[426] compared obstetric outcome for the first 1000 nulliparous women (term gestation, singleton fetus, cephalic presentation, spontaneous labor) who delivered at the National Maternity Hospital in 1987 with the outcome for a similar group of women who delivered in 1992 and 1994. The epidural analgesia rate rose from 10% in 1987 to 45% in 1992 and 57% in 1994. In each of these 3 years, 82% of women underwent spontaneous vaginal delivery. The cesarean delivery rate was 4% in 1987, 5% in 1992, and 4% in 1994 (P = NS) (Figure 23-15). The investigators concluded that the consistency of the operative delivery rates in each of 3 years with very different epidural rates suggests that epidural analgesia does not increase the cesarean delivery rate.

Socol et al.[427] evaluated the impact of three initiatives to reduce the cesarean delivery rate in their hospital. First, they strongly encouraged a trial of labor and vaginal birth after cesarean delivery. Second, after the 1988 calendar year, they circulated data showing the cesarean delivery rate of every obstetrician to each attending physician. Third, they

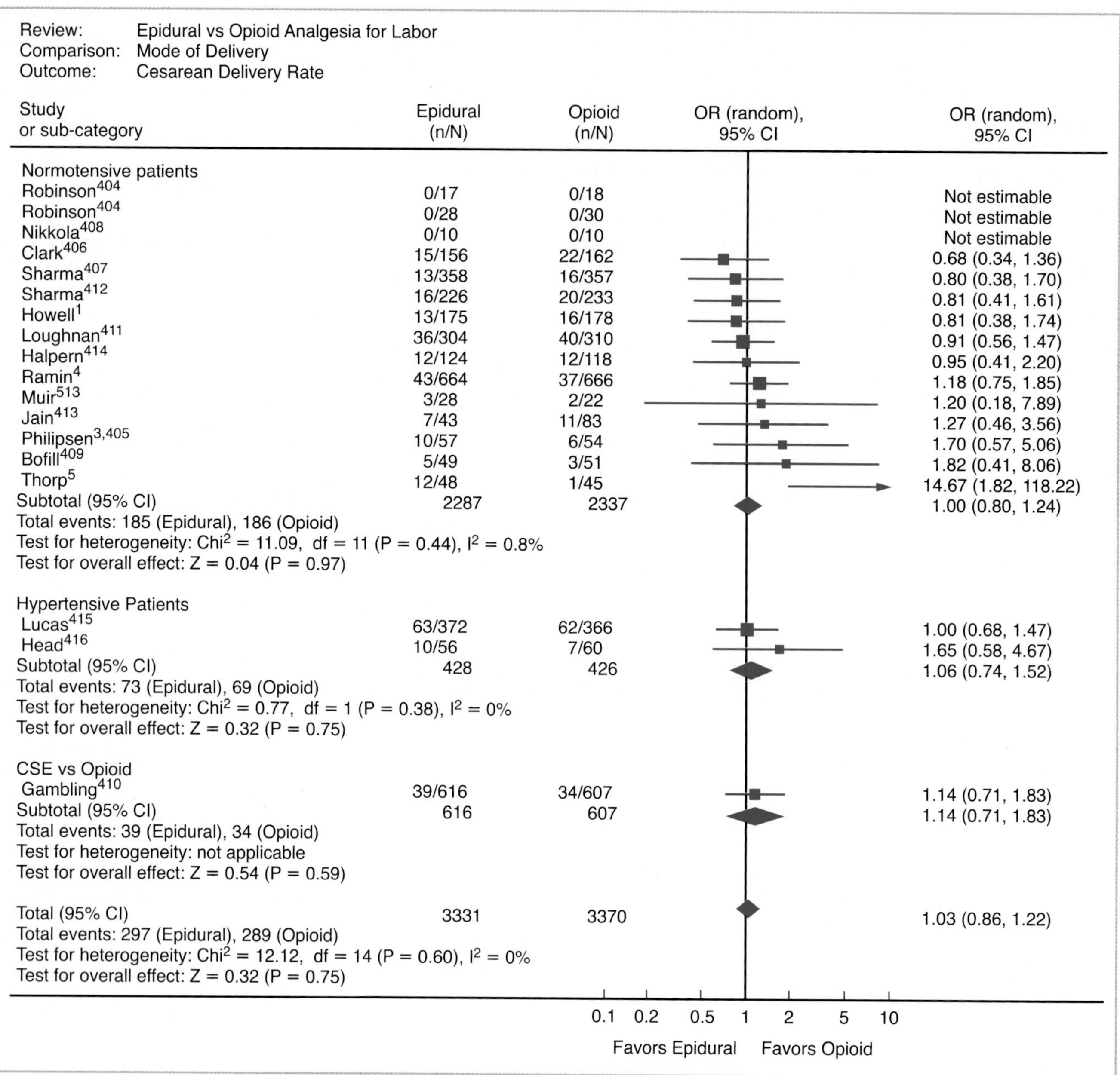

FIGURE 23-12 Meta-analysis of cesarean delivery rate in women randomly assigned to undergo neuraxial or systemic opioid analgesia. The number of women who had a cesarean delivery, the odds ratio (OR), and 95% confidence interval (CI) of the odds ratio (random effects model) are shown for each study. The size of the *teal box* is proportional to the weight of the study in the meta-analysis. The scale is logarithmic. For studies with no cesarean deliveries the OR could not be calculated. N, total number of patients in the epidural or opioid group; n, number of events (cesarean delivery) in the spinal or opioid group; CSE, combined spinal-epidural. (Modified from Halpern SH, Leighton BL. Epidural analgesia and the progress of labor. In Halpern SH, Douglas MJ, editors. Evidence-Based Obstetric Anesthesia. Oxford, UK, Blackwell, 2005:10-22.)

recommended the active management of labor as the preferred method of labor management for term nulliparous women. The rates of total, primary, and repeat cesarean deliveries dropped from 27%, 18%, and 9% in 1986 to 17%, 11%, and 6%, respectively, in 1991 ($P < .001$ for all three comparisons). Meanwhile, the use of epidural analgesia rose from 28% in 1986 to 48% in 1991 ($P < .001$). There was no change in the incidence of instrumental vaginal delivery (13% in 1986 versus 13% in 1991).

A number of other impact studies have found no association between neuraxial analgesia and cesarean delivery.[425,428-431] In a meta-analysis, Segal et al.[432] identified nine impact studies involving a total of 37,753 patients. These researchers found no increase in the rate of cesarean delivery with the increase in availability of epidural analgesia (Figure 23-16). Thus, the before-after impact studies support the results of randomized controlled trials—namely, that neuraxial analgesia does not cause an increase in the cesarean delivery rate.

Several studies have assessed whether there is a relationship between an individual obstetrician's cesarean delivery rate and the rate of epidural analgesia for his or her

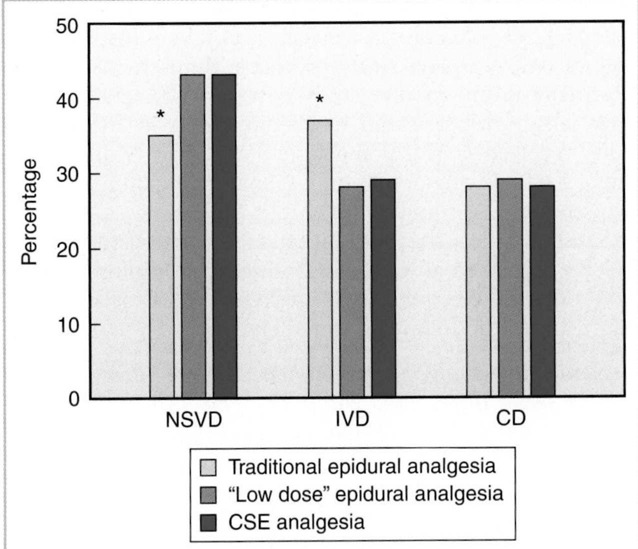

FIGURE 23-13 Outcome of labor in the COMET study. Parturients were randomly assigned to traditional epidural analgesia or to one of two "low-dose" neuraxial techniques (see text). There was no difference among groups in the cesarean delivery (CD) rate. *Women who received traditional epidural analgesia had a higher rate of instrumental vaginal delivery (IVD) than those who received either "low-dose" technique ($P = .04$). CSE, combined spinal-epidural; NSVD, normal spontaneous vaginal delivery. (Data from Comparative Obstetric Mobile Epidural Trial Study Group UK. Effect of low-dose mobile versus traditional epidural techniques on mode of delivery: A randomised controlled trial. Lancet 2001; 358:19-23.)

patients.[433,434] For example, Lagrew et al.[433] divided obstetricians into two groups according to whether their individual cesarean delivery rates were more than 15% (the control group) or less than 15% (the target group). Obstetricians in the target group used epidural analgesia more often than obstetricians in the control group. In other words, the target group of obstetricians was able to achieve a lower cesarean delivery rate despite their greater use of epidural analgesia.

TIMING OF INITIATION OF NEURAXIAL ANALGESIA

Review of observational data suggests an association between cesarean delivery and the initiation of neuraxial analgesia during early labor (often defined as a cervical dilation less than 4 to 5 cm).[5,422,435] For example, in a retrospective study of 1917 nulliparous women, the rate of cesarean delivery was twice as high in women who received neuraxial analgesia at a cervical dilation less than 4 cm than in those in whom neuraxial analgesia was initiated at a cervical dilation of 4 cm or more (18.9% versus 8.9%, respectively).[435] As a result of these data, for many years the ACOG suggested that women delay requesting epidural analgesia, "when feasible, until the cervix is dilated to 4 to 5 cm."[436] However, as with the cause-and-effect question raised by the association of neuraxial labor analgesia and cesarean delivery, the question arises as to whether the early initiation of neuraxial labor analgesia *causes* a higher risk of cesarean delivery or whether the request for, and administration of, early labor analgesia is a marker for some other risk factor(s) for cesarean delivery.

A number of randomized controlled trials have addressed the question of whether initiation of neuraxial analgesia during early labor adversely affects the mode of delivery.[6,7,22-24] All except one small study[24] compared early labor neuraxial analgesia with systemic opioid analgesia, which was followed by neuraxial analgesia when cervical dilation reached 4 to 5 cm. (The control group in the Luxman et al.[24] study received no analgesia). Chestnut et al. randomly assigned nulliparous women who were in spontaneous labor[6] or were receiving oxytocin[23] to receive early epidural analgesia or early intravenous nalbuphine analgesia followed by epidural analgesia when cervical dilation reached 5 cm. There was no difference between groups in the cesarean delivery rate. However, the median cervical dilation at the time of initiation of analgesia was 3.5 cm[23] and 4 cm[6] in the two studies. Many women, particularly

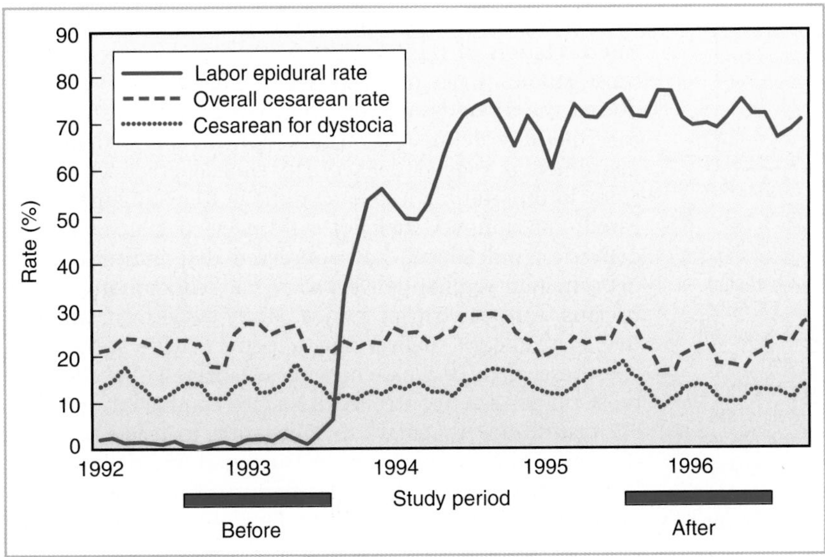

FIGURE 23-14 Epidural analgesia and cesarean delivery rates for nulliparous women who delivered at Tripler Army Medical Center for the years 1992 to 1996. (From Zhang J, Yancey MK, Klebanoff MA, et al. Does epidural analgesia prolong labor and increase risk of cesarean delivery? A natural experiment. Am J Obstet Gynecol 2001; 185:128-34.)

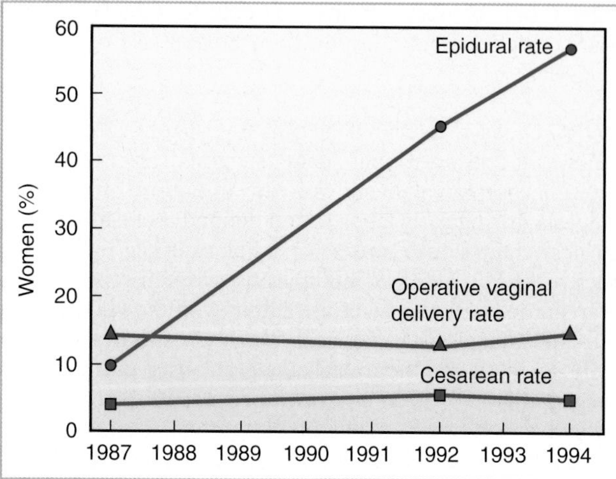

FIGURE 23-15 Epidural analgesia and cesarean and instrumental vaginal delivery rates for 1000 consecutive nulliparous women in spontaneous labor at term during three different years at the National Maternity Hospital in Dublin, Ireland. (From Impey L, MacQuillan K, Robson M. Epidural analgesia need not increase operative delivery rates. Am J Obstet Gynecol 2000; 182:358-63.)

those with premature rupture of membranes and those undergoing induction of labor, request analgesia when cervical dilation is less than 3 to 4 cm.

Subsequently, Wong et al.[7] and Ohel et al.[22] reported randomized trials comparing early labor neuraxial analgesia with systemic opioid analgesia in which the median cervical dilation at initiation of analgesia was 2 cm. As in the previous studies, there was no difference between the two groups in rate of cesarean delivery or in rate of instrumental vaginal delivery. The study protocols differed in that the treatment group in one study received *CSE* analgesia in early labor,[7] whereas the treatment group in the second study received *epidural* analgesia alone.[22] In addition, the use of oxytocin augmentation was markedly different in the two studies (94%[7] and 29%[22]).

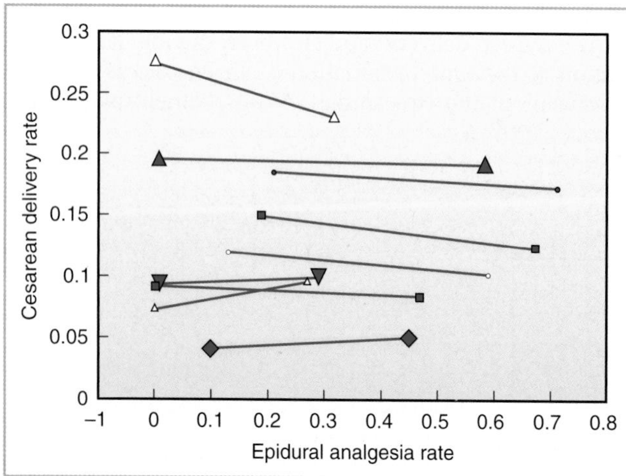

FIGURE 23-16 Rates of cesarean delivery during periods of higher and lower availability of epidural analgesia in 9 studies (n = 37,753) subjected to meta-analysis. Each pair of symbols shows data from one investigation (the left symbol is the epidural analgesia rate and cesarean rate during the period of low epidural availability, and the right symbol is the epidural analgesia rate and cesarean delivery rate during the period of high epidural availability). The size of the plot symbol is proportional to the number of patients in the analysis. (From Segal S, Su M, Gilbert P. The effect of a rapid change in availability of epidural analgesia on the cesarean delivery rate: A meta-analysis. Am J Obstet Gynecol 2000; 183:974-8.)

Subsequent to the publication of the later studies, the ACOG published an updated Committee Opinion entitled *Analgesia and Cesarean Delivery Rates*.[20] This revised opinion includes the following statement:

> *Neuraxial analgesia techniques are the most effective and least depressant treatments for labor pain. The American College of Obstetricians and Gynecologists previously recommended that practitioners delay initiating epidural analgesia in nulliparous women until the cervical dilation reached 4-5 cm. However, more recent studies have shown that epidural analgesia does not increase the risks of cesarean delivery. The choice of analgesic technique, agent, and dosage is based on many factors, including patient preference, medical status, and contraindications. The fear of unnecessary cesarean delivery should not influence the method of pain relief that women can choose during labor.*

A 2007 meta-analysis of eight randomized controlled trials and cohort studies of early labor versus late labor initiation of neuraxial analgesia (n = 3320) supported this recommendation. The researchers concluded that early initiation of neuraxial analgesia does not increase the rate of cesarean delivery (OR, 1.00; 95% CI, 0.82 to 1.23) (Figure 23-17).[25] In addition, the neonates born to women randomly assigned to early systemic opioid analgesia had lower umbilical arterial blood pH measurements and were more likely to receive naloxone after delivery.

Instrumental Vaginal Delivery Rate

Observational data associate neuraxial labor analgesia with a higher rate of instrumental (forceps or vacuum extraction) vaginal delivery. The effect of neuraxial analgesia on mode of vaginal delivery has not been assessed as a primary outcome in randomized controlled trials, although it has been assessed as a secondary outcome in multiple trials. Interpretation of these results is clouded by the fact that most studies have not assessed the quality of analgesia during the second stage of labor. Further, most investigators did not define the criteria for the performance of instrumental vaginal delivery. In clinical practice, and in study interpretation, it is often difficult to distinguish "indicated" instrumental deliveries from elective instrumental deliveries. Indeed, we have observed that indications for instrumental vaginal delivery vary markedly among obstetricians. An obstetrician is more likely to perform an elective instrumental delivery in a patient with satisfactory anesthesia than in a patient without analgesia. In addition, most randomized controlled trials are conducted in teaching institutions that have an obligation to teach obstetric residents how to perform instrumental vaginal delivery. Instrumental vaginal deliveries performed for the purpose of teaching are more likely to be done in women with adequate analgesia.

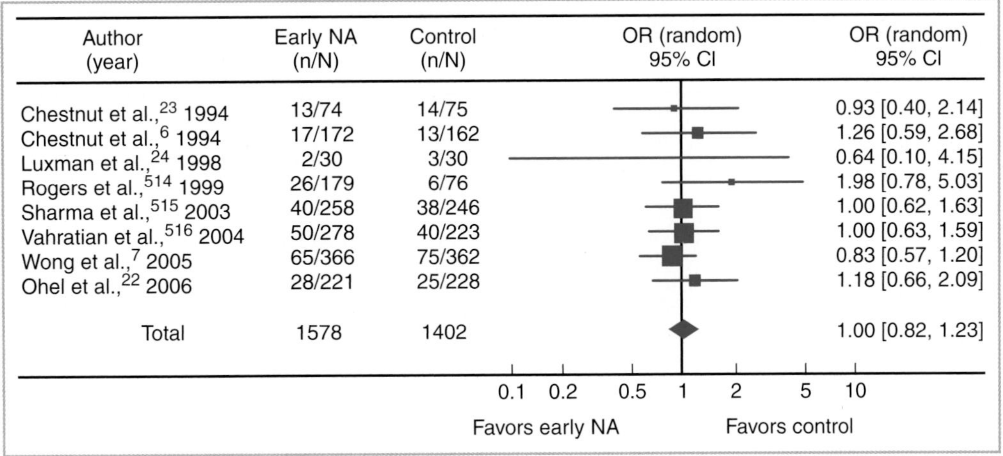

FIGURE 23-17 Meta-analysis of rates of cesarean delivery for individual studies comparing early-labor initiation of neuraxial analgesia with control (initiation of neuraxial analgesia at a cervical dilation of 4 to 5 cm). The size of the *teal box* at the point estimate for each study is proportional to the number of patients in the study. The *diamond* represents the point estimate of the pooled odds ratio, and the length of the *diamond* is proportional to the confidence interval. N, total number of patients in the treatment or control group; n, number of events (cesarean delivery) in the treatment or control group; NA, neuraxial analgesia. (From Marucci M, Cinnella G, Perchiazzi G, et al. Patient-requested neuraxial analgesia for labor: Impact on rates of cesarean and instrumental vaginal delivery. Anesthesiology 2007; 106:1035-45.)

Multiple randomized, controlled studies comparing epidural analgesia with systemic opioid analgesia have assessed the rate of instrumental vaginal delivery as a secondary outcome variable. Most systematic reviews have concluded that epidural analgesia is associated with a higher risk for instrumental vaginal delivery than systemic analgesia.[418,419] For example, in the latest meta-analysis of 16 studies, by Halpern and Leighton,[418] the odds ratio for instrumental vaginal delivery in women randomly assigned to receive epidural analgesia was 1.92 (95% CI, 1.52 to 2.42) (Figure 23-18). Similarly, in the individual patient meta-analysis reported by Sharma et al.,[419] the adjusted odds ratio was 1.86 (95% CI, 1.43 to 2.40).

In contrast to these studies, many of the impact studies observed no difference in the instrumental vaginal delivery rate between the control and study periods.[425,426,430,437] For example, despite a rise in the epidural analgesia rate from 1% to almost 80% at Tripler Army Hospital, the rate of instrumental vaginal delivery did not change (11.1% versus 11.9%).[425] Similarly, despite a more than fivefold increase in the epidural rate at the National Maternity Hospital in Dublin (see earlier), the instrumental vaginal delivery rate remained unchanged (see Figure 23-15). A systematic review of seven impact studies[432] involving more than 28,000 patients did not identify a difference in instrumental vaginal delivery rates between periods of low and periods of high epidural analgesia rates (mean change 0.76%; 95% CI, −1.2 to 2.8).

Obstetricians and anesthesiologists have suggested that multiple factors (e.g., station and position of the fetal vertex, maternal pain and the urge to bear down, and neuraxial analgesia–induced motor blockade) may contribute to the outcome of the second stage of labor. The contribution of these factors to the mode of vaginal delivery, and their interactions, are not well understood and have not been well controlled in many studies.

Several studies have specifically assessed the effect of maintenance of neuraxial analgesia until delivery with regard to the duration and outcome of the second stage of labor.[375,438-442] Chestnut et al.[375] randomly assigned women already receiving epidural analgesia at 8 cm of cervical dilation to receive a continuous epidural infusion of 0.75% lidocaine or saline until delivery. There was no difference between groups in the rate of instrumental vaginal delivery, but women in the lidocaine group as well as the saline group had inadequate second-stage analgesia. In a similar study in which patients were randomly assigned to receive epidural bupivacaine 0.125% or saline (control),[439] second-stage analgesia was clearly better in the bupivacaine group than in the control group, but the rate of instrumental vaginal delivery was nearly double (52% versus 27%, respectively; $P < .05$), and the duration of the second stage was longer. In a third study, second-stage analgesia was maintained with 0.0625% bupivacaine with fentanyl 2 μg/mL or saline-placebo.[438] There was no difference between groups in the instrumental vaginal delivery rate, but analgesia was only marginally better in the treatment group.

The effect of neuraxial analgesia on the outcome of the second stage of labor may be influenced by the density of neuraxial analgesia. High concentrations of epidural local anesthetic may cause maternal motor blockade, leading to relaxation of pelvic floor musculature, which in turn may interfere with fetal rotation during descent. Abdominal muscle relaxation may decrease the effectiveness of maternal expulsive efforts. The effects of specific analgesic techniques, concentration of local anesthetic, total dose of local anesthetic, and degree of motor blockade on the risk of instrumental vaginal delivery are overlapping and difficult to study. For example, some studies suggest that administration of epidural analgesia using higher concentrations of bupivacaine is associated with a higher risk of instrumental vaginal delivery than that using lower concentrations.[420,422,423,443] James et al.[443] randomly assigned parturients to receive intermittent epidural bupivacaine 0.25% or bupivacaine 0.1% with fentanyl 2 μg/mL. The severity of

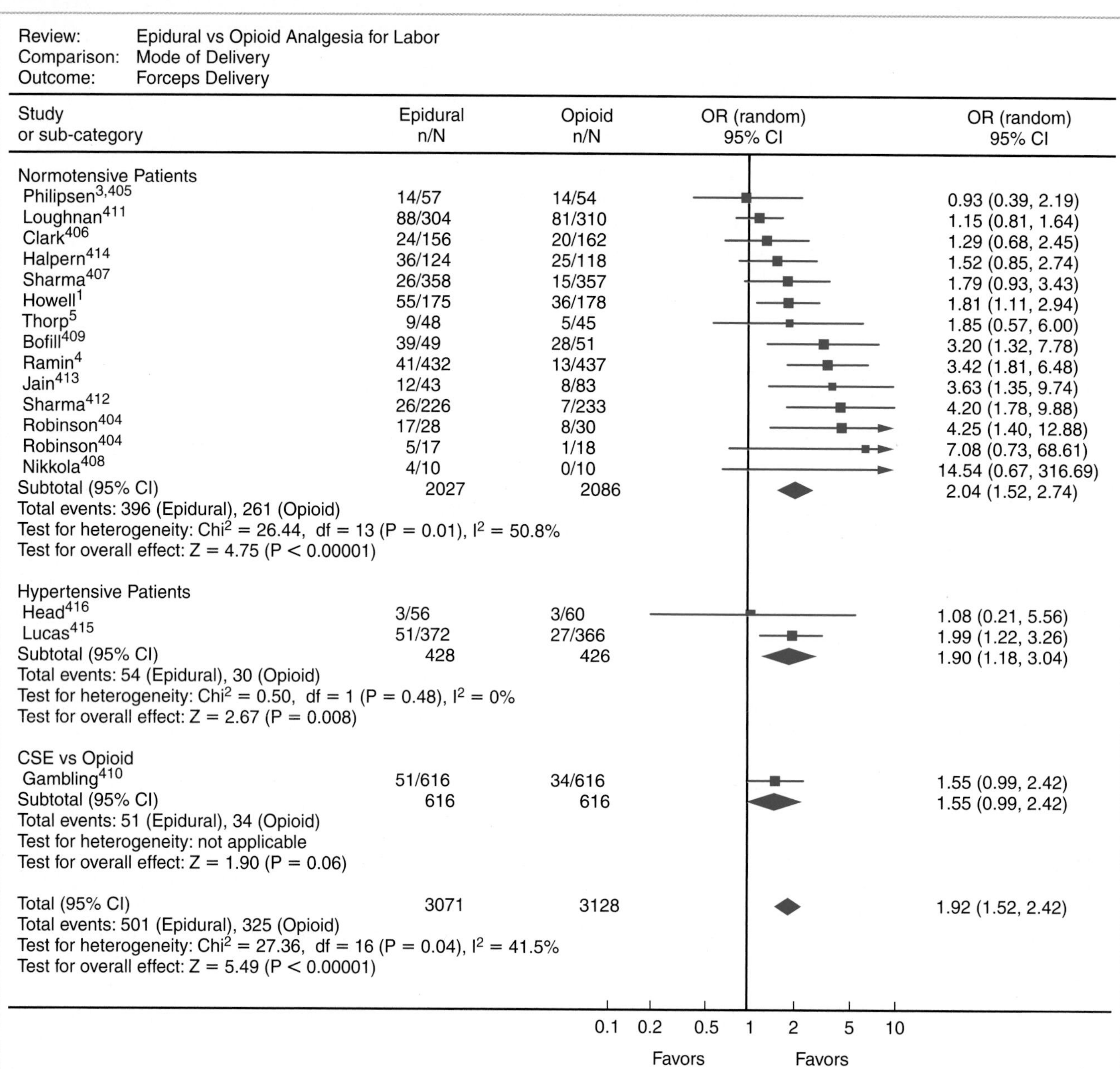

FIGURE 23-18 Meta-analysis of instrumental vaginal delivery rate in women randomly assigned to neuraxial or systemic opioid analgesia. The number of women who had instrumental vaginal delivery, the odds ratio (OR), and the 95% confidence interval (CI) of the odds ratio (random effects model) are shown for each study. The size of each *teal box* is proportional to the weight of the study in the meta-analysis. The scale is logarithmic. N, total number of patients in the epidural or opioid group; n, number of events (instrumental vaginal delivery) in the epidural or opioid group. (From Halpern SH, Leighton BL. Epidural analgesia and the progress of labor. In Halpern SH, Douglas MJ, editors. Evidence-Based Obstetric Anesthesia. Oxford, UK, Blackwell, 2005:10-22.)

motor blockade and the incidence of instrumental vaginal delivery were less in the low-dose group (6% versus 24% for high-dose; P = .03). Similarly, in a much larger study that compared CSE (low-dose) with traditional high-dose epidural analgesia, the rate of instrumental vaginal delivery was lower in the CSE group.[422] In another large study, Olofsson et al.[423] noted a lower instrumental vaginal delivery rate in women randomly assigned to "low-dose" bupivacaine 0.125% with sufentanil than in those receiving "high-dose" bupivacaine 0.25% with epinephrine.

In contrast, Collis et al.[421] observed no difference in mode of delivery between women randomly assigned to receive either a high-dose or a low-dose neuraxial technique. Even more confusing, the COMET investigators reported a lower rate of instrumental vaginal delivery in the two groups of women randomly assigned to receive either the low-dose epidural or CSE technique than in the group that received 0.25% bupivacaine (see earlier discussion and Figure 23-13).[420] However, the total bupivacaine *dose* in the traditional "high-dose" epidural group did not actually differ from that in the "low-dose" epidural group because the former was administered by intermittent injection and the latter by continuous infusion. In contrast, the total bupivacaine dose was significantly lower in the CSE group.

In general, the dose of bupivacaine is significantly lower if epidural analgesia is maintained with an intermittent bolus technique rather than a continuous infusion technique (see earlier). Most investigators have noted a difference in motor blockade between the two techniques; higher total bupivacaine doses (i.e., continuous infusion techniques) are associated with a greater degree of motor blockade. However, the relationship between motor blockade and instrumental vaginal delivery is inconsistent. Smedstad and Morison[252] reported a higher incidence of instrumental vaginal delivery when bupivacaine 0.25% was administered as a continuous epidural infusion than as intermittent bolus injections. In contrast, the COMET investigators observed no difference in the instrumental vaginal delivery rate in the two groups who received "low-dose" bupivacaine/fentanyl, one by infusion and the other by intermittent bolus.[420] Similarly, in a meta-analysis of PCEA (without background infusion) compared with continuous epidural infusion analgesia,[262] the dose of bupivacaine and degree of motor blockade were significantly lower in the PCEA group, but the rates of instrumental vaginal delivery did not differ.

It is possible that the inconsistent results can be explained by the actual absolute differences in bupivacaine dose and motor blockade. For example, the differences in dose and motor blockade may have clinically significant adverse effects on the outcome of the second stage of labor if bupivacaine 0.25% is compared with bupivacaine 0.125%, but not if bupivacaine 0.125% is compared with bupivacaine 0.0625%.

Motor blockade may increase the risk of malrotation of the fetal vertex. Robinson et al.[444] and LeRay et al.[445] observed a higher incidence of occiput malposition at delivery in patients who received epidural analgesia before engagement of the fetal head. In contrast, Yancey et al.[446] and Sheiner et al.[447] noted that the administration of on-demand epidural analgesia did not increase the frequency of malposition of the fetal head at delivery; the incidence of instrumental vaginal delivery was not related to fetal station at initiation of analgesia. In a prospective cohort study using ultrasonography, Lieberman et al.[448] reported that fetal position changed frequently during labor but that epidural analgesia was associated with a higher incidence of occiput posterior position at delivery (13% versus 3%, $P < .002$). However, these results should be interpreted with caution as women were not randomly assigned to the treatment group. Factors that cause women to request analgesia when the fetal head is high may also be independent risk factors for instrumental vaginal delivery.

In an editorial, Chestnut[449] concluded that *effective* second-stage analgesia increases the risk of instrumental vaginal delivery. Minimizing the risk of instrumental vaginal delivery while maximizing analgesia is both an art and a science and requires the attention of the anesthesia provider to the individual needs of the patient. A single analgesic technique or single dose/concentration of drug(s) is not likely to have optimal results for everyone. In our opinion, the best technique incorporates the use of PCEA with a low-rate background infusion (4 to 8 mL/hr) using a dilute solution of local anesthetic combined with an opioid. Use of a dilute local anesthetic solution without PCEA leads to inadequate analgesia for many women. Increasing the infusion dose improves analgesia and reduces the workload for the anesthesia provider but will result in overly dense analgesia for some patients, thus increasing the risk for instrumental vaginal delivery.

Why should anesthesia providers give attention to the effects of analgesia on the method of vaginal delivery? A properly performed outlet- or low-forceps delivery does not increase the risk of adverse neonatal outcome.[450-453] However, a difficult midforceps delivery likely increases neonatal risk.[451-454] Instrumental delivery also results in a higher risk of maternal trauma (e.g., third- and fourth-degree vaginal lacerations, which are associated with a small but not negligible risk of rectovaginal fistula). Robinson et al.[455] observed that epidural analgesia was associated with an increased rate of severe perineal trauma because of the more frequent use of instrumental vaginal delivery and episiotomy in nulliparous patients who received epidural analgesia. In contrast, several large observational studies suggest that epidural analgesia is associated with a decreased risk of anal sphincter laceration in nulliparous women.[456,457] Regardless of the presence or magnitude of the risks of maternal or neonatal injury, many women want to minimize the likelihood of operative delivery, and they perceive that a higher risk of instrumental vaginal delivery is undesirable.

Duration of Labor

FIRST STAGE OF LABOR

The effect of neuraxial labor analgesia on the duration of the first stage of labor was addressed as a secondary outcome variable in many of the randomized controlled trials. A meta-analysis[418] of nine studies found no difference in the duration of the first stage of labor between women who were randomly assigned to receive epidural analgesia and those assigned to receive systemic opioid analgesia (Table 23-13). There was significant heterogeneity in the outcome because of the mixed parity of the patient populations and differences among studies in the definition of the duration of the first stage of labor. In contrast, the individual meta-analysis of the Parkland Hospital data showed a significant prolongation of the first stage of labor (approximately 0.5 hour) in nulliparous women who were randomly assigned to receive epidural analgesia.[419]

Wong et al.[7] and Ohel et al.[22] assessed duration of labor as a secondary outcome in their randomized controlled trials of the initiation of neuraxial analgesia during early labor. Both groups of investigators determined that the duration of the first stage of labor was significantly *shorter* in women randomly assigned to receive early labor neuraxial analgesia than in those assigned to receive systemic opioid analgesia (Figure 23-19).

Determining the duration of labor requires that investigators document start and end times. The definition of the start time varies among studies but is usually consistent between groups within a study. The end of the first stage of labor is defined as the time of full (10 cm) cervical dilation. This point can be determined only with manual cervical examination. Most studies do not mandate regular

TABLE 23-13 Meta-Analyses of the Duration of the First and Second Stages of Labor

		First Stage of Labor			Second Stage of Labor		
Meta-analysis	**N**	**Neuraxial**	**Systemic Opioid**	***P* Value**	**Neuraxial**	**Systemic Opioid**	***P* Value**
Halpern & Leighton (2005)[418]	2200* 2550†	WMD 24 min (95% CI, 4, 54)		0.09	WMD 16 min (95% CI, 10, 23)		<.001
Sharma et al (2004)[419]	2703	8.1 ± 5 hr	7.5 ± 5 hr	0.01	60 ± 56 min	47 ± 57 min	<.001

WMD, weighted mean difference. CI, confidence interval;

*First stage of labor.

†Second stage of labor.

Data from Halpern SH, Leighton BL. Epidural analgesia and the progress of labor. In Halpern SH, Douglas MJ, editors. Evidence-Based Obstetric Anesthesia. Oxford, Blackwell, 2005:10-22; and Sharma SK, McIntire DD, Wiley J, Leveno KJ: Labor analgesia and cesarean delivery: An individual patient meta-analysis of nulliparous women. Anesthesiology 2004; 100:142-8.

cervical examinations by study protocol, or if they do, the intervals are fairly large (e.g., 1 to 2 hours). Clinically, full cervical dilation is diagnosed when a cervical examination is performed because the patient complains of rectal pressure. It is likely that women with effective epidural analgesia will complain of rectal pressure at a later time (and lower fetal station) than women with systemic opioid analgesia. In other words, the patient may be fully dilated for a significant time before cervical examination verifies full cervical dilation. This difference serves to artificially prolong the duration of the first stage of labor in the epidural group,

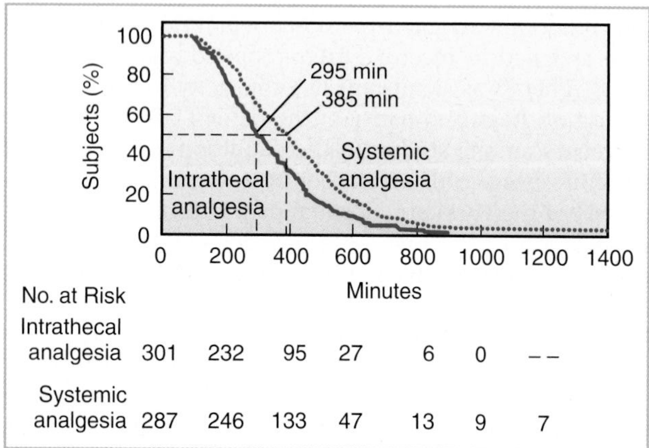

FIGURE 23-19 Kaplan-Meier survival analysis of duration of labor (proportion of undelivered women) in which time zero is the time of first request for labor analgesia in women randomly assigned to either early intrathecal analgesia (cervical dilation < 4 cm) or systemic opioid analgesia followed by late neuraxial analgesia (cervical dilation ≥ 4 cm). The duration of the first stage of labor (minutes) was significantly shorter in the intrathecal group than in the systemic opioid group (median difference, −90 minutes; 95% confidence interval, −123 to −35; *P* <.001). (From Wong CA, Scavone BM, Peaceman AM, et al. The risk of cesarean delivery with neuraxial analgesia given early versus late in labor. N Engl J Med 2005; 352:655-65.)

although it shortens the apparent duration of the second stage of labor.

Other factors may also influence the duration of the first stage of labor. Some clinicians have noted enhanced uterine activity in some patients for approximately 30 minutes after the initiation of neuraxial analgesia, whereas uterine activity appears to be reduced in other patients. Schellenberg[458] suggested that aortocaval compression is responsible for the transient decrease in uterine activity that occurs after the administration of epidural anesthesia in some patients. He concluded that this effect does not occur if aortocaval compression is avoided. Cheek et al.[459] noted that uterine activity decreased after the intravenous infusion of 1 L of crystalloid solution, but not after infusion of 0.5 L or maintenance fluid alone. There was no decrease in uterine activity after the administration of epidural anesthesia. Zamora et al.[460] made similar observations. Miller et al.[461] hypothesized that a fluid bolus might inhibit antidiuretic hormone (vasopressin) release from the posterior pituitary gland. Since this organ also releases oxytocin, the production of that hormone might also be transiently suppressed; this possible decrease in oxytocin release may partially explain the transient changes in uterine contractility observed in association with epidural analgesia.

In a prospective but nonrandomized study, Rahm et al.[462] observed that epidural analgesia (bupivacaine with sufentanil) was associated with lower plasma oxytocin levels at 60 minutes after initiation of analgesia than in healthy controls who did not receive epidural analgesia. Behrens et al.[463] noted that epidural analgesia during the first stage of labor significantly reduced the release of prostaglandin $F_{2\alpha}$ and "impede[d] the normal progressive increase in uterine activity." In contrast, Nielsen et al.[464] measured upper and lower uterine segment intrauterine pressures for 50 minutes before and after the administration of epidural bupivacaine analgesia in 11 nulliparous women during spontaneous labor. The investigators observed no significant difference in the number of contractions before and after epidural analgesia. There was greater intrauterine pressure in the upper uterine segment than in the lower segment (consistent with fundal dominance) both before and after initiation of epidural analgesia. Further, fundal dominance was higher after epidural analgesia than in the pre-analgesia period.

Increased uterine activity after the initiation of neuraxial analgesia has been hypothesized to be an indirect effect of neuraxial analgesia (see later).[465] Initiation of neuraxial analgesia is associated with an acute decrease in the maternal plasma concentration of circulating epinephrine.[8] Epinephrine is a tocolytic, and the acute decrease in maternal concentration may result in greater uterine activity. This may be an explanation for the salutary effect on the progress of labor that is observed in some women with dysfunctional labor after the initiation of neuraxial analgesia[466] or in women who are extremely anxious.[467]

The epidural administration of a local anesthetic with epinephrine is followed by systemic absorption of both drugs. Some physicians have expressed concern that the epinephrine may exert a systemic beta-adrenergic tocolytic effect and slow labor. Early studies, which used large doses of epinephrine, suggested that the caudal epidural administration of local anesthetic with epinephrine prolonged the first stage of labor and increased the number of patients who required oxytocin augmentation of labor.[468] Subsequently, most studies have suggested that the addition of epinephrine 1.25 to 5 µg/mL (1:800,000 to 1:200,000) to the local anesthetic solution does not affect the progress of labor or method of delivery.[93,130,175,177,180,469]

There is no evidence that the specific local anesthetic or opioid used for neuraxial analgesia directly or indirectly affects the duration of labor.[128,470] In a randomized controlled trial, Tsen et al.[471] observed a higher rate of cervical dilation in women who received CSE analgesia than in those who received epidural analgesia. However, randomized controlled trials comparing CSE with epidural analgesia have not found a difference in the duration of labor between the two techniques.[420-422,424]

In summary, neuraxial analgesia appears to have a variable effect on the duration of labor. It may shorten labor in some women and lengthen it in others. However, analgesia-related prolongation of the first stage of labor, if it occurs, has not been shown to have adverse maternal or neonatal effects and is probably of minimal clinical significance.

SECOND STAGE OF LABOR

There is little doubt that effective neuraxial analgesia prolongs the second stage of labor. Meta-analyses of randomized controlled trials comparing neuraxial with systemic opioid analgesia support this clinical observation (see Table 23-13).[418,419] The mean duration of the second stage is approximately 15 minutes longer in women randomly assigned to receive neuraxial analgesia than in women assigned to receive systemic opioid analgesia. Some studies have suggested that a prolonged second stage of labor results in progressive fetal acidosis.[472] In the past, few obstetricians allowed the second stage to progress beyond 2 hours. Most contemporary studies have suggested that a delay in the second stage is not harmful to the infant or mother provided that (1) electronic FHR monitoring confirms the absence of nonreassuring fetal status, (2) the mother is well hydrated and has adequate analgesia, and (3) there is ongoing progress in the descent of the fetal head.[473-475] The ACOG has defined a *prolonged second stage* in nulliparous women as lasting more than 3 hours with neuraxial analgesia and more than 2 hours without neuraxial analgesia; for parous women, it is more than 2 hours in those with neuraxial analgesia and more than 1 hour in those without neuraxial analgesia.[476]

Kadar et al.[477] concluded that for most patients, little benefit is gained from allowing the second stage of labor to exceed 3 hours. Paterson et al.[478] evaluated the second stage of labor in 25,069 women who delivered infants of at least 37 weeks' gestation, with a vertex presentation, after the spontaneous onset of labor. The researchers concluded that for parous women without epidural analgesia, the likelihood of spontaneous vaginal delivery after 1 hour in the second stage was low, but in parous women with epidural analgesia and in all nulliparous women, there was no clear cutoff point for expectation of spontaneous delivery. The ACOG has stated that if progress is being made, the duration of the second stage alone does not mandate intervention.[476] The decision as to whether to perform an operative delivery in the second stage or allow continued observation should be made on the basis of clinical assessment of the woman and the fetus and the skill and training of the obstetrician.

Second-Stage Management: Immediate versus "Delayed" Pushing

Many women are asked to begin "pushing" as soon as full cervical dilation has been confirmed, regardless of the fetal station. Some practitioners have suggested that "delayed" pushing might result in less maternal exhaustion and better maternal and fetal outcomes. Several studies have sought to determine whether immediate or delayed pushing for women with epidural analgesia during the second stage of labor affects labor duration and outcome.[479-483] Data are conflicting. In a large randomized multicenter controlled trial ($n = 1862$),[482] nulliparous women were randomly assigned to immediate or delayed pushing (up to 2 hours after full cervical dilation). Spontaneous vaginal delivery occurred more frequently in the delayed pushing group (57.5% versus 52.7% for immediate pushing; RR, 1.09; 95% CI, 1.00 to 1.18), and the risk of rotational mid-forceps delivery was significantly lower in this group. The overall duration of the second stage of labor was longer in the delayed pushing group (187 versus 123 minutes for immediate pushing; $P < .001$), although the duration of pushing was shorter. There were no significant differences in neonatal outcome.

A meta-analysis of nine randomized controlled trials involving approximately 3000 women concluded that delayed pushing did not change the rate of instrumental vaginal delivery (RR, 0.92; 95% CI, 0.84 to 1.01) (Figure 23-20) or the rate of second-stage cesarean delivery but did result in a lower incidence of rotational or midpelvic instrumental deliveries (RR, 0.69; 95% CI, 0.55 to 0.87).[484] The total duration of the second stage was longer with delayed pushing, but there were no differences in neonatal outcomes.

Although there do not appear to be any major advantages to delayed pushing, it does not seem reasonable to ask the mother to push from a high fetal station. We are commonly asked to decrease or discontinue neuraxial analgesia because the mother does not feel the urge to push when she is fully dilated. However, women with effective neuraxial

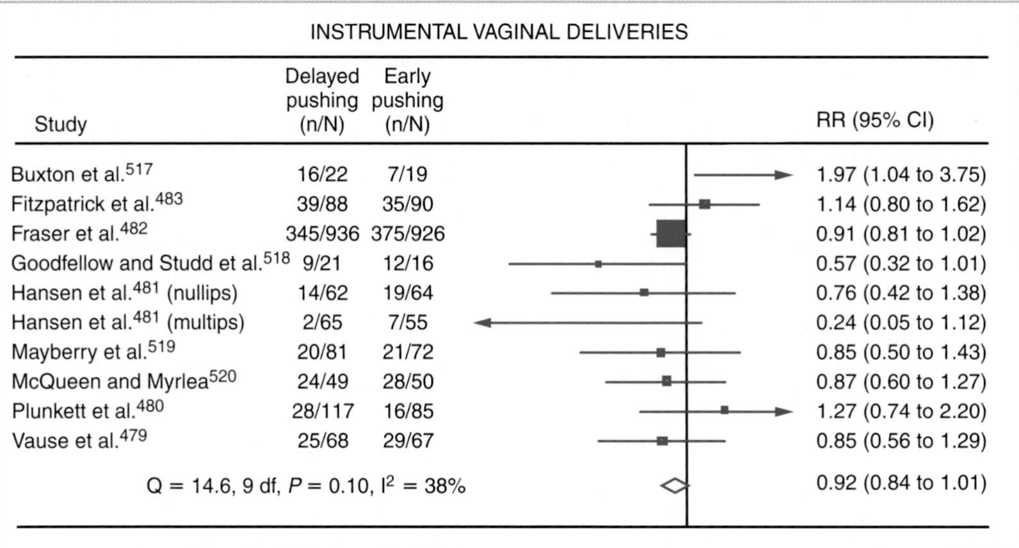

FIGURE 23-20 Meta-analysis of the effect of delayed versus early pushing on the rate of instrumental vaginal delivery among women with neuraxial analgesia. The size of the *teal box* at the point estimate for each study is proportional to the number of patients in the study. The *diamond* represents the point estimate of the pooled odds ratio, and the length of the diamond is proportional to the confidence interval. N, total number of patients in the treatment or control group; n, number of events (instrumental vaginal delivery) in the treatment or control group; RR, relative risk; CI, confidence interval. (From Roberts CL, Torvaldsen S, Cameron CA, Olive E. Delayed versus early pushing in women with epidural analgesia: A systemic review and meta-analysis. Br J Obstet Gynaecol 2004; 111:1333-40.)

analgesia do not feel the urge to push at a high fetal station. The density of neuraxial analgesia should not be decreased until the fetus has descended and the mother still does not feel the urge to push. In this case the maintenance dose may be reduced. Discontinuing the maintenance of analgesia is rarely indicated because analgesia/anesthesia may be difficult to reestablish if the need for operative delivery arises.

THIRD STAGE

Rosaeg et al.[485] retrospectively reviewed the outcomes of 7468 women who underwent vaginal delivery at their hospital between 1996 and 1999. Epidural analgesia was not associated with a prolonged third stage of labor. The duration of the third stage of labor was shorter in women who received epidural analgesia and subsequently required manual removal of the placenta. The researchers suggested that epidural analgesia "provided a 'permissive' role"—in other words, epidural analgesia likely facilitated and/or encouraged earlier intervention by the obstetrician.

Other Factors and Progress of Labor

OXYTOCIN

Active management of labor has been advocated as a way to lower the rate of cesarean delivery, shorten the duration of labor, and decrease maternal complications (e.g., chorioamnionitis).[486,487] The components of the active management of labor include strict criteria for the diagnosis of labor, early amniotomy, prompt intervention with high-dose oxytocin for the treatment of inefficient uterine contractions, and one-on-one nursing care.

In randomized controlled trials comparing the effects of neuraxial with systemic opioid analgesia on the outcome of labor, women receiving neuraxial opioids have been noted to have a higher rate of oxytocin augmentation.[419,488] Kotaska et al.[489] have questioned the external validity of these randomized controlled trials because of oxytocin management. In a search of the medical literature, they identified 16 randomized controlled trials. Eight of the 16 trials included descriptions of labor management and these trials were included in the analysis. Seven of the 8 trials described active management of labor and found no difference in the mode of delivery between groups. Only one of 8 trials described the use of low-dose oxytocin and reported a markedly higher rate of cesarean delivery in the neuraxial analgesia group. Kotaska et al.[489] concluded that epidural analgesia in the setting of low-dose oxytocin probably increases the rate of cesarean delivery. The researchers were correct in stating that the role of oxytocin in neuraxial analgesia outcome studies has not been well controlled. However, their conclusion that epidural analgesia in the setting of low-dose oxytocin probably causes an increase in the rate of cesarean delivery is highly flawed because the researchers did not include the 8 studies in their analysis that did not describe the management of labor. In all probability the management of labor in these studies was not active (e.g., did not include high-dose oxytocin administration), or this would have been described. Additionally, although the researchers did not identify the excluded studies, other systematic reviews have identified the study by Thorp et al.[5] as the only randomized controlled trial in which the rate of cesarean delivery was higher in the epidural group than in the systemic opioid group. Therefore, the excluded studies were probably negative studies, thus highly skewing the analysis.

Randomized controlled trials comparing early with late initiation of neuraxial analgesia have utilized markedly different oxytocin protocols, yet all have concluded that early initiation of neuraxial analgesia does not have an adverse effect on the outcome of labor. For example, one trial by Chestnut et al.[6] included women in spontaneous labor without prior or planned administration of oxytocin. Approximately 35% of all patients in the study eventually received oxytocin, but the rates of oxytocin augmentation of labor did not differ between groups. The second study performed by this group involved only women who were undergoing oxytocin induction or augmentation of labor (100% oxytocin rate), yet the results were the same.[23] In the study of early CSE analgesia by Wong et al.,[7] the oxytocin utilization rate was high in both groups (approximately 93%). However, the maximum oxytocin infusion rate in the control (early systemic opioid) group was significantly *higher* than that in the early CSE group even though the median duration of labor was 90 minutes shorter in the CSE group. In the study of early epidural analgesia by Ohel et al.,[22] the oxytocin utilization rate in both groups was much lower (approximately 29%); however, as in the study by Wong et al.,[7] the duration of labor was significantly shorter in the early neuraxial analgesia group. Taken together, the results of these studies do not support the hypothesis that oxytocin played a major role in the outcomes.

The ACOG supports the use of oxytocin for the treatment of dystocia or arrest of labor in the first or second stage, whether or not the patient is receiving neuraxial analgesia.[476]

AMBULATION

Observational studies suggest that ambulation may be associated with less pain and a shorter duration of labor.[490] However, randomized controlled trials comparing ambulation with bed rest during the first stage of labor in women with neuraxial analgesia have not demonstrated any advantages of ambulation with regard to the progress or outcome of labor.[422,491-494] Nageotte et al.[422] randomly assigned 505 nulliparous women to CSE analgesia either with or without ambulation. There was no difference between groups in the mode of delivery or duration of labor. These results agree with those of a meta-analysis of five randomized controlled trials involving 1161 women.[495] In addition, there were no differences between groups in the use of oxytocin augmentation, satisfaction with analgesia, or Apgar scores. No adverse effects were reported. These results agree with those of trials comparing ambulation and bed rest in women without neuraxial analgesia.[496]

EFFECTS OF NEURAXIAL ANALGESIA ON THE FETUS AND NEONATE

Neuraxial analgesia may affect the fetus directly, indirectly, or both. First, systemic absorption of the anesthetic agents may be followed by transplacental transfer of the drug, which has a direct effect on the fetus. Second, the effects of neuraxial blockade on the mother may affect the fetus indirectly. Effects of local anesthetics and opioids on the fetus and neonate are discussed in detail in Chapter 13.

Direct Effects

Direct fetal effects include intrapartum effects on the FHR as well as possible respiratory depression after delivery. The determinants of maternal plasma drug concentration, transfer across the placenta, and effects on the neonate are discussed in Chapters 4 and 13. Determinants of maternal plasma drug concentration include dose, site of administration, metabolism and excretion of the drug, and the presence of adjuvants (e.g., epinephrine). Factors that influence placental transfer include maternal and fetal placental perfusion, the physiochemical characteristics of the drug, concentration of the free drug in maternal plasma, and permeability of the placenta. Most anesthetic and analgesic drugs, including local anesthetics and opioids, readily cross the placenta.

FETAL HEART RATE

Effects of local anesthetics and opioids on FHR may be direct and indirect (see earlier)[465,470,497]; however, there is little evidence for a direct effect when these drugs are administered as components of neuraxial analgesia. Transient changes in FHR variability and periodic decelerations have been observed during epidural labor analgesia with bupivacaine and other local anesthetics.[470,498,499] These FHR decelerations were not associated with maternal hypotension. However, Loftus et al.[500] did not observe FHR decelerations in women who received epidural bupivacaine for elective cesarean delivery, despite the use of larger doses of bupivacaine and the occurrence of more extensive sympathetic blockade in comparison with epidural labor analgesia. Of interest, one study noted that the administration of either epidural bupivacaine or intrathecal sufentanil was followed by a similar incidence of FHR decelerations (23% and 22%, respectively) in laboring women.[501] Other studies have not observed a higher incidence of FHR decelerations after the epidural administration of bupivacaine during labor.[502] Further, the reports of FHR decelerations after bupivacaine did not demonstrate adverse neonatal outcome; thus the significance of these decelerations is unclear. There are no published data on the relationship between the concentration of bupivacaine used for intrapartum epidural analgesia and the incidence of FHR decelerations. Altogether, these data suggest that epidural local anesthetics have minimal, if any, direct effect on FHR.

Similarly, neuraxial opioid administration has little direct effect on the FHR.[149,503,504] In contrast, in one study systemic meperidine labor analgesia was associated with a greater reduction of FHR variability and fewer FHR accelerations than epidural bupivacaine analgesia.[505] Spinal administration of local anesthetics and opioids results in lower maternal plasma concentrations of drug(s) than epidural administration and is therefore even less likely to cause a direct fetal effect.

NEONATAL DEPRESSION

Systemic absorption of local anesthetic or opioid may have neonatal effects. This occurs more often after the systemic administration of opioid for labor analgesia.[4,506] The neonatal depressant effects of drugs administered to the mother in the intrapartum period are usually assessed with neurobehavioral testing. Unfortunately, these tests are quite subjective and lack specificity. Additionally, scientifically rigorous studies are lacking, and most of the local anesthetic studies were performed in the era when high-dose epidural analgesia was common; these studies found that local anesthetics administered as components of epidural analgesia sometimes had minor, transient effects on neonatal behavior.[128,470,507]

When given by continuous epidural infusion, epidural opioid administration rarely results in accumulation of the drug and subsequent neonatal respiratory depression.[138,146,149,157,244,245] Bader et al.[244] noted that a continuous epidural infusion of 0.125% bupivacaine with fentanyl 2 μg/mL over a period of 1 to 15 hours did not result in significant fetal drug accumulation or adverse neonatal effects. (In this study, the maximal cumulative dose of fentanyl was 300 μg.) Porter et al.[245] reported no adverse effect of fentanyl on neurobehavorial scores or other indices of fetal welfare when patients received an epidural infusion of 0.0625% bupivacaine with or without fentanyl 2.5 μg/mL. The mean ± SD maternal dose of fentanyl was 183 ± 75 μg (range, 53 to 400 μg). Loftus et al.[149] observed only a modest reduction in NACS at 24 hours in babies whose mothers had received epidural fentanyl during labor. Babies exposed to sufentanil during labor had somewhat higher NACS at 24 hours. Sufentanil was detected in the umbilical arterial blood in only one of nine samples (see earlier). Vertommen et al.[146] observed no difference in Apgar scores or NACS in neonates whose mothers were randomly assigned to receive epidural sufentanil (up to 30 μg) during the course of labor and a control group that did not receive sufentanil.[146] Maternal sufentanil levels were below the sensitivity of the assay (0.1 ng/mL) after an epidural bolus of 10 μg.[157]

Intrathecal administration of an opioid during labor has even fewer direct effects on the fetus than epidural administration. Smaller doses of opioid are administered, and less drug is absorbed systemically.

Indirect Effects

The indirect fetal effects of epidural and intrathecal opioids may be more significant than the direct effects. Obviously, if the mother has severe respiratory depression and hypoxemia, fetal hypoxemia and hypoxia will follow.[368] More common is the occurrence of fetal bradycardia after initiation of neuraxial analgesia. The presumed etiology is that the rapid onset of analgesia results in decreased plasma concentrations of catecholamines.[465] Epinephrine causes uterine relaxation by stimulating beta$_2$-adrenergic uterine receptors. A reduced circulating concentration of epinephrine may result in increased uterine tone. Because uteroplacental perfusion occurs during periods of uterine diastole (i.e., uterine relaxation), uterine hypertonus (tachysystole) may result in decreased uteroplacental perfusion and fetal hypoxia.

Published observations suggest that uterine tachysystole and fetal bradycardia may follow the administration of either intrathecal or epidural analgesia during labor. Nielsen et al.[501] assessed FHR tracings after the administration of either intrathecal sufentanil or epidural bupivacaine during labor. They observed no difference in the incidence of FHR abnormalities (i.e., recurrent late decelerations and/or bradycardia: 22% in the intrathecal sufentanil group versus 23% in the epidural bupivacaine group).

Fortunately, fetal bradycardia after labor analgesia does not appear to increase the overall risk for adverse outcome. Albright and Forster[508] retrospectively reviewed outcomes for 2560 women who delivered at their hospital between March 1995 and April 1996. Approximately half of the patients received CSE analgesia (10 to 15 μg of intrathecal sufentanil), and the other half received either systemic opioids or no medication. There was no difference between the two groups in the incidence of emergency cesarean delivery (1.3% versus 1.4%, respectively). Mardirosoff et al.[36] performed a systematic review of reports of randomized comparisons of intrathecal opioid analgesia with any non-intrathecal opioid regimen in laboring women. The investigators noted that intrathecal opioid analgesia appeared to lead to a significant increase in the risk of fetal bradycardia (OR, 1.8; 95% CI, 1.0 to 3.1). However, the risk of cesarean delivery for FHR abnormalities was similar in the two groups (6.0% versus 7.8%, respectively). Van de Velde et al.[509] randomly assigned laboring women to one of the following three treatment regimens: intrathecal sufentanil 7.5 μg, intrathecal sufentanil 1.5 μg/bupivacaine 2.5 mg/epinephrine 2.5 μg, and epidural bupivacaine 12.5 mg/sufentanil 7.5 μg/epinephrine 12.5 μg. Although the incidence of FHR abnormalities was higher in the high-dose intrathecal sufentanil group, there was no difference among groups in the need for emergency cesarean delivery.

Given the risk of fetal bradycardia with neuraxial analgesia in laboring women, the FHR should be monitored during and after the administration of either epidural or intrathecal analgesia. Treatment of fetal bradycardia includes (1) relief of aortocaval compression; (2) discontinuation of intravenous oxytocin; (3) administration of supplemental oxygen; (4) treatment of maternal hypotension, if present; and (5) fetal scalp stimulation. Persistent uterine tachysystole should also prompt the administration of a tocolytic drug (e.g., terbutaline or nitroglycerin).

CONCLUSIONS AND RECOMMENDATIONS

Philosophy of Labor Analgesia

An unacceptably high number of women involuntarily experience severe pain during labor. As noted by the ASA and the ACOG, "There is no other circumstance where it is considered acceptable for a person to experience severe pain, amenable to safe intervention, while under a physician's care."[20,21] Unfortunately, labor represents one of the few circumstances in which the provision of effective analgesia is alleged to interfere with the parturient's and obstetrician's goal (e.g., spontaneous vaginal delivery). Dense neuraxial anesthesia may adversely affect the progress of labor in some patients. Indeed, given the complicated neurohumoral and mechanical processes involved in childbirth, it would be unreasonable to expect that neuroblockade of the lower half of the body would *not* have an effect on this process, whether positive or negative. However, maternal-fetal factors and obstetric management—not the use of neuraxial analgesia—are the most important determinants of the outcome of labor. Anesthesia providers should identify those methods of analgesia that provide the most effective pain relief without unduly increasing the risk of obstetric intervention. Operative delivery increases the risk of maternal morbidity and mortality and is more expensive than spontaneous vaginal delivery. Randomized trials suggest that the contemporary use of neuraxial analgesia does not increase the cesarean delivery rate but may adversely influence the instrumental vaginal delivery rate.[418] Further, neuraxial analgesia may occasionally, either directly or indirectly, have adverse—usually temporary—effects on the fetus.

Despite these risks, many women opt for neuraxial analgesia because no other method of labor analgesia provides its benefits (almost complete analgesia), and the risks are acceptably low. Even no analgesia may be more hazardous to some women than neuraxial analgesia (e.g., patients with an anticipated difficult airway or those at high risk for emergency cesarean delivery). Therefore, it is the duty of the anesthesia provider to provide appropriate (albeit not always total) pain relief during the first and second stages of labor. Analgesia should be tailored to the individual patient's labor, medical condition, preferences, and goals. Most women strongly dislike dense motor blockade, and many prefer to maintain some sensation of uterine contractions and perineal pressure, especially during the second stage of labor. However, a few women may accept the probable increase in risk of instrumental vaginal delivery in exchange for dense analgesia.

A Practical Guide to Neuraxial Labor Analgesia

INITIATION OF ANALGESIA

Neuraxial labor analgesia may be initiated with either the intrathecal (CSE) or the epidural injection of analgesic/anesthetic agents. The decision regarding the specific technique and choice of drugs and doses is individualized for each parturient. Parity, stage and phase of labor, use of intravenous oxytocin, and the presence of any coexisting disease(s), as well as the status of the fetus, are all considered in the decision.

In healthy *nulliparous* women in *early* labor (less than 4 to 5 cm cervical dilation), we often initiate CSE analgesia with an intrathecal opioid alone (e.g., fentanyl 25 μg or sufentanil 5 μg), followed by placement of an epidural catheter and administration of a standard lidocaine 45 mg/epinephrine 15 μg epidural test dose. Some anesthesia providers initiate intrathecal analgesia with both an opioid and a local anesthetic. The addition of a local anesthetic is unnecessary for achieving complete spinal analgesia during early labor; it likely increases the risk of hypotension and may result in motor blockade in some patients, particularly if it is followed by injection of an epidural test dose that contains a local anesthetic. However, the intrathecal administration of both an opioid and a local anesthetic achieves a longer duration of analgesia and lower incidence and severity of pruritus than intrathecal injection of an opioid alone.

Alternatively, epidural analgesia can be initiated with injection of a low-concentration local anesthetic solution (bupivacaine 0.0625% to 0.125%) combined with an opioid (fentanyl 50 to 100 μg). The epidural catheter is sited and a standard epidural test dose is injected, followed by administration of 5 to 15 mL of the local anesthetic/opioid solution, injected in 5-mL increments. Five to 10 mL provides satisfactory analgesia for most nulliparous women in early labor; injection of 15 mL may be necessary if a dilute solution (e.g., 0.0625% bupivacaine) is used.

We typically give an epinephrine-containing test dose before initiation of epidural analgesia in laboring women. Some anesthesia providers elect to omit the epidural test dose when initiating epidural labor analgesia, particularly if a woman wishes to ambulate in early labor. The omission of the epidural test dose requires that the therapeutic dose of local anesthetic be injected slowly, incrementally, and cautiously, because the therapeutic dose functions as the test dose. These precautions should be followed with all bolus injections of local anesthetic through an epidural catheter.

For *nulliparous* women in the active phase of the first stage of labor, we usually initiate CSE analgesia with the intrathecal injection of an opioid combined with a local anesthetic (fentanyl 15 μg and bupivacaine 2.5 mg). Alternatively, epidural analgesia can be initiated with a local anesthetic (bupivacaine 0.125%) combined with an opioid (fentanyl 100 μg). Women in active labor may require a higher total volume of epidural local anesthetic solution (15 to 20 mL) than women in early labor (5 to 15 mL) as well as a higher local anesthetic concentration (e.g., 0.125% rather than 0.0625% bupivacaine).

Labor typically progresses at a faster rate in *parous* women, who often require a more rapid onset of analgesia and more extensive neuroblockade than nulliparous women when neuraxial analgesia is initiated at the same cervical dilation. Therefore, in healthy parous women we usually initiate CSE analgesia with an intrathecal opioid combined with a local anesthetic, regardless of the stage and phase of labor. Alternatively, epidural analgesia is initiated with bupivacaine 0.125% combined with fentanyl 100 μg.

CSE analgesia with both a local anesthetic and an opioid is particularly advantageous for parous women in the late active phase of the first stage of labor and in all women in whom neuraxial analgesia is initiated in the second stage of labor. Sacral neuroblockade is required for complete analgesia during the second stage of labor; this neuroblockade is difficult to accomplish in a timely fashion with an initial (*de novo*) lumbar epidural injection of analgesic/anesthetic agents. (For initiation of lumbar epidural anesthesia in late labor, the injection of a large volume [$\geq$ 20 mL] of local anesthetic solution may be required to achieve sacral analgesia, and this injection often results in a mid- or high-thoracic neuroblockade that is more extensive than desired. Therefore, when initiating neuraxial analgesia in late labor, we prefer to use a CSE technique.)

MAINTENANCE OF ANALGESIA

We typically initiate maintenance epidural analgesia soon after the initiation of analgesia (within 15 to 30 minutes) rather than wait for the neuroblockade to regress. There are several advantages to this technique. Most women experience seamless analgesia (i.e., there is no window of pain as the initial block regresses). The workload for the anesthesia provider is lessened, as he or she can set up and initiate the epidural infusion while monitoring the patient for hypotension after initiation of neuroblockade.

Finally, an epidural bolus of local anesthetic is not required to reestablish or extend neuroblockade, possibly enhancing safety.

Analgesia is typically maintained with a dilute solution of an amide local anesthetic and an opioid, administered by continuous infusion or PCEA. We prefer PCEA because it allows patient titration of neuroblockade and entails less risk of breakthrough pain. Patient satisfaction is better and the workload for the anesthesia provider is decreased. At our institution, the PCEA infusion pump parameters are the same for all laboring women, so there are fewer errors in pump setup. However, when a continuous infusion is used without PCEA to maintain analgesia, it may be necessary to titrate the continuous infusion rate to individual patient needs. For example, women in early labor require less drug to maintain analgesia (6 to 10 mL/hr), whereas women in more advanced labor may require a higher infusion rate (8 to 15 mL/hr). Similarly, a parous patient may require a higher infusion rate than a nulliparous patient, even though analgesia is initiated at the same stage of labor.

Some parturients experience breakthrough pain. After evaluating the nature of the pain, the extent of neuroblockade, and the progress of labor, we usually treat breakthrough pain with a bolus epidural injection of bupivacaine 0.125%, 10 to 15 mL, administered in 5-mL increments. The patient may benefit from additional instruction about the optimal use of PCEA. Occasionally, we may elect to use a more concentrated local anesthetic solution (e.g., bupivacaine 0.25%), particularly in the presence of an abnormal fetal position or dysfunctional labor. In this case, the concentration of the maintenance solution may also need to be increased.

This maintenance technique usually results in satisfactory perineal analgesia for delivery. Occasionally, women with epidural analgesia require additional (more dense) analgesia for delivery, particularly if an instrumental vaginal delivery is planned. In this case, we often administer 5 to 12 mL of 1% to 2% lidocaine or 2% to 3% 2-chloroprocaine. This usually results in satisfactory sacral anesthesia in a patient with preexisting epidural labor analgesia.

There is no single correct way to provide neuraxial labor analgesia, although for particular patients and specific clinical conditions, some methods may have advantages over others. Frequent communication with members of the obstetric team (obstetricians, midwives, and nurses) is essential to the safe and satisfactory provision of neuraxial labor analgesia. In addition, within each labor and delivery unit, consistency among anesthesia providers in their choice of techniques, specific drugs, and drug doses/concentrations is likely to result in less error and higher satisfaction among other caregivers and patients.

KEY POINTS

- Neuraxial analgesia is the most effective form of intrapartum analgesia currently available.
- In most cases, maternal request for pain relief represents a sufficient indication for the administration of neuraxial analgesia.
- The safe administration of neuraxial analgesia requires a thorough (albeit directed) preanesthetic evaluation and the immediate availability of appropriate resuscitation equipment.
- The administration of the epidural test dose should allow the anesthesia provider to recognize most cases of unintentional intravascular or intrathecal placement of the epidural catheter. All therapeutic doses of local anesthetic should be administered incrementally.
- Bupivacaine is the local anesthetic most often used for epidural analgesia during labor. Ropivacaine and levobupivacaine are satisfactory (although more expensive) alternatives. Most anesthesia providers reserve 2-chloroprocaine and lidocaine for cases that require the rapid extension of epidural anesthesia for vaginal or cesarean delivery.
- The addition of a lipid-soluble opioid to a neuraxial local anesthetic allows the anesthesia provider to provide excellent analgesia while reducing the total dose of local anesthetic and minimizing the side effects of each agent. Perhaps the major advantage of this technique is that the severity of motor block can be minimized during labor.
- The lipid-soluble opioids have largely supplanted morphine for neuraxial administration during labor.
- Intrathecal opioids alone may provide complete analgesia during the early first stage of labor. Epidural opioids without local anesthetics do not provide complete analgesia during labor.
- Administration of a local anesthetic (with or without an opioid) is necessary to provide complete neuraxial analgesia for the late first stage and the second stage of labor. Although a neuraxial local anesthetic alone can provide complete analgesia, the required dose is often associated with an undesirably dense degree of motor blockade.
- Hypotension is a common side effect of neuraxial analgesia. Prophylaxis and treatment involve the avoidance of aortocaval compression and the administration of a vasopressor as needed. The administration of an intravenous fluid "preload" does not significantly decrease the incidence of hypotension in euvolemic patients.
- Other potential side effects of neuraxial analgesia include pruritus, shivering, urinary retention, delayed gastric emptying, maternal fever, and fetal heart rate changes.
- Complications of neuraxial analgesia include inadequate analgesia, unintentional dural puncture, respiratory depression, unintentional intravenous injection, and extensive or total spinal anesthesia.
- The presence of severe pain during early labor—and/or an increase in local anesthetic/opioid dose requirements—may signal a higher risk for prolonged labor and operative delivery.

- Neuraxial labor analgesia is not associated with a higher rate of cesarean delivery than systemic opioid analgesia.
- Initiation of neuraxial analgesia in early labor (cervical dilation less than 4 to 5 cm) does not increase the rate of cesarean delivery or prolong the duration of labor.
- Effective neuraxial analgesia likely results in a modest prolongation of the second stage of labor. Controversy exists as to whether there is a cause-and-effect relationship between neuraxial labor analgesia and the rate of instrumental vaginal delivery. Dense neuroblockade (e.g., presence of significant motor blockade) and complete analgesia during the second stage of labor probably increase the rate of instrumental vaginal delivery. It seems intuitive that neuraxial analgesia with a dilute solution of local anesthetic and opioid is less likely to adversely affect the progress of labor.
- Neuraxial analgesia during labor is not a generic procedure. The procedure should be tailored to individual patient needs. Conclusions about the effect of one technique on the progress of labor may not be applicable to other techniques.
- Maternal-fetal factors and obstetric management—not the use of neuraxial analgesia—are the most important determinants of the cesarean delivery rate.

REFERENCES

1. Howell CJ, Chalmers I. A review of prospectively controlled comparisons of epidural with non-epidural forms of pain relief during labour. Int J Obstet Anesth 1992; 1:93-110.
2. Paech MJ. The King Edward Memorial Hospital 1,000 mother survey of methods of pain relief in labour. Anaesth Intensive Care 1991; 19:393-9.
3. Philipsen T, Jensen N-H. Epidural block or parenteral pethidine as analgesic in labour: A randomized study concerning progress in labour and instrumental deliveries. Eur J Obstet Gynecol Reprod Biol 1989; 30:27-33.
4. Ramin SM, Gambling DR, Lucas MJ, et al. Randomized trial of epidural versus intravenous analgesia during labor. Obstet Gynecol 1995; 86:783-9.
5. Thorp JA, Hu DH, Albin RM, et al. The effect of intrapartum epidural analgesia on nulliparous labor: A randomized, controlled, prospective trial. Am J Obstet Gynecol 1993; 169:851-8.
6. Chestnut DH, McGrath JM, Vincent RD, et al. Does early administration of epidural analgesia affect obstetric outcome in nulliparous women who are in spontaneous labor? Anesthesiology 1994; 80:1201-8.
7. Wong CA, Scavone BM, Peaceman AM, et al. The risk of cesarean delivery with neuraxial analgesia given early versus late in labor. N Engl J Med 2005; 352:655-65.
8. Shnider SM, Abboud TK, Artal R, et al. Maternal catecholamines decrease during labor after lumbar epidural anesthesia. Am J Obstet Gynecol 1983; 147:13-5.
9. Lederman RP, Lederman E, Work B, McCann DS. Anxiety and epinephrine in multiparous labor: Relationship to duration of labor and fetal heart rate pattern. Am J Obstet Gynecol 1985; 153:870-7.
10. Jouppila R, Hollmen A. The effect of segmental epidural analgesia on maternal and foetal acid-base balance, lactate, serum potassium and creatine phosphokinase during labour. Acta Anaesthiol Scand 1976; 20:259-68.
11. Levinson G, Shnider SM, deLorimier AA, Steffenson JL. Effects of maternal hyperventilation on uterine blood flow and fetal oxygenation and acid-base status. Anesthesiology 1974; 40:340-7.
12. Peabody JH. Transcutaneous oxygen measurement to evaluate drug effects. Clin Perinatol 1979; 6:109-21.
13. Hawkins JL, Koonin LM, Palmer SK, Gibbs CP. Anesthesia-related deaths during obstetric delivery in the United States, 1979-1990. Anesthesiology 1997; 86:277-84.
14. Bucklin BA, Hawkins JL, Anderson JR, Ullrich FA. Obstetric anesthesia workforce survey: Twenty-year update. Anesthesiology 2005; 103:645-53.
15. United Kingdom National Health Service, The Information Centre for Health and Social Care. NHS Maternity Statistics, England: 2005-06. Available at http://www.ic.nhs.uk/statistics-and-data-collections/hospital-care/maternity/nhs-maternity-statistics-2005-06/
16. Davies MW, Harrison JC, Ryan TD. Current practice of epidural analgesia during normal labour: A survey of maternity units in the United Kingdom. Anaesthesia 1993; 48:63-5.
17. Huang C, Macario A. Economic considerations related to providing adequate pain relief for women in labour: Comparison of epidural and intravenous analgesia. Pharmacoeconomics 2002; 20:305-18.
18. Macario A, Scibetta WC, Navarro J, Riley E. Analgesia for labor pain: A cost model. Anesthesiology 2000; 92:841-50.
19. American Society of Anesthesiologists Task Force on Obstetric Anesthesia. Practice guidelines for obstetric anesthesia. Anesthesiology 2007; 106:843-63.
20. American College of Obstetricians and Gynecologists Committee on Obstetric Practice. Analgesia and cesarean delivery rates. ACOG Committee Opinion No. 339. Washington, DC, ACOG, June 2006. (Obstet Gynecol 2006; 107:1487.)
21. American Society of Anesthesiologists. Statement on pain relief during labor. 1999 (reaffirmed 2007). Available at http://www.asahq.org/publicationsAndServices/standards/47.pdf/
22. Ohel G, Gonen R, Vaida S, et al. Early versus late initiation of epidural analgesia in labor: Does it increase the risk of cesarean section? A randomized trial. Am J Obstet Gynecol 2006; 194:600-5.
23. Chestnut DH, Vincent RD, McGrath JM, et al. Does early administration of epidural analgesia affect obstetric outcome in nulliparous women who are receiving intravenous oxytocin? Anesthesiology 1994; 90:1193-1200.
24. Luxman D, Wolman I, Groutz A, et al. The effect of early epidural block administration on the progression and outcome of labor. Int J Obstet Anesth 1998; 7:161-4.
25. Marucci M, Cinnella G, Perchiazzi G, et al. Patient-requested neuraxial analgesia for labor: Impact on rates of cesarean and instrumental vaginal delivery. Anesthesiology 2007; 106:1035-45.
26. Simmons SW, Cyna AM, Dennis AT, Hughes D. Combined spinal-epidural versus epidural analgesia in labour. Cochrane Database Syst Rev 2007; (3):CD003401.
27. Campbell DC, Camann WR, Datta S. The addition of bupivacaine to intrathecal sufentanil for labor analgesia. Anesth Analg 1995; 81:305-9.
28. Norris MC. Are combined spinal-epidural catheters reliable? Int J Obstet Anesth 2000; 9:3-6.
29. Pan PH, Bogard TD, Owen MD. Incidence and characteristics of failures in obstetric neuraxial analgesia and anesthesia: A retrospective analysis of 19,259 deliveries. Int J Obstet Anesth 2004; 13:227-33.
30. Minty RG, Kelly L, Minty A, Hammett DC. Single-dose intrathecal analgesia to control labour pain: Is it a useful alternative to epidural analgesia? Can Fam Physician 2007; 53:437-42.
31. Bethune L, Harper N, Lucas DN, et al. Complications of obstetric regional analgesia: How much information is enough? Int J Obstet Anesth 2004; 13:30-4.
32. Jackson A, Henry R, Avery N, et al. Informed consent for labour epidurals: What labouring women want to know. Can J Anaesth 2000; 47:1068-73.

33. Swan HD, Borshoff DC. Informed consent—recall of risk information following epidural analgesia in labour. Anaesth Intensive Care 1994; 22:139-41.
34. Knapp RM. Legal view of informed consent for anesthesia during labor. Anesthesiology 1990; 72:211.
35. American College of Obstetricians and Gynecologists. Intrapartum fetal heart rate monitoring. ACOG Practice Bulletin No. 70. Washington, DC, ACOG, December 2005. (Obstet Gynecol 2005; 106:1453-60.)
36. Mardirosoff C, Dumont L, Boulvain M, Tramer MR. Fetal bradycardia due to intrathecal opioids for labour analgesia: A systematic review. Br J Obstet Gynaecol 2002; 109:274-81.
37. Kinsella SM, Pirlet M, Mills MS, et al. Randomized study of intravenous fluid preload before epidural analgesia during labour. Br J Anaesth 2000; 85:311-3.
38. Dyer RA, Farina Z, Joubert IA, et al. Crystalloid preload versus rapid crystalloid administration after induction of spinal anaesthesia (coload) for elective caesarean section. Anaesth Intensive Care 2004; 32:351-7.
39. Fisher AJ, Huddleston JF. Intrapartum maternal glucose infusion reduces umbilical cord acidemia. Am J Obstet Gynecol 1997; 177:765-9.
40. Cerri V, Tarantini M, Zuliani G, et al. Intravenous glucose infusion in labor does not affect maternal and fetal acid-base balance. J Matern Fetal Med 2000; 9:204-8.
41. Vincent RD, Chestnut DH. Which position is more comfortable for the parturient during identification of the epidural space? Int J Obstet Anesth 1991; 1:9-11.
42. Andrews PJ, Ackerman WE 3rd, Juneja MM. Aortocaval compression in the sitting and lateral decubitus positions during extradural catheter placement in the parturient. Can J Anaesth 1993; 40:320-4.
43. Bahar M, Chanimov M, Cohen ML, et al. Lateral recumbent head-down posture for epidural catheter insertion reduces intravascular injection. Can J Anaesth 2001; 48:48-53.
44. Bieniarz J, Curuchet E, Crottogini JJ, et al. Aortocaval compression by the uterus in late human pregnancy. Am J Obstet Gynecol 1978; 100:203-17.
45. Kerr MG, Scott DB, Samuel E. Studies of the inferior vena cava in late pregnancy. Br Med J 1964; 1(5382):532-3.
46. Scott DB. Inferior vena caval occlusion in late pregnancy and its importance in anaesthesia. Br J Anaesth 1968; 40:120-8.
47. Eckstein KL, Marx GF. Aortocaval compression and uterine displacement. Anesthesiology 1974; 40:92-6.
48. Marx GF, Husain FJ, Shiau HF. Brachial and femoral blood pressures during the prenatal period. Am J Obstet Gynecol 1980; 136:11-3.
49. Ellington C, Katz VL, Watson WJ, Spielman FJ. The effect of lateral tilt on maternal and fetal hemodynamic variables. Obstet Gynecol 1991; 77:201-3.
50. Beilin Y, Abramovitz SE, Zahn J, et al. Improved epidural analgesia in the parturient in the 30 degree tilt position. Can J Anaesth 2000; 47:1176-81.
51. Preston R, Crosby ET, Kotarba D, et al. Maternal positioning affects fetal heart rate changes after epidural analgesia for labour. Can J Anaesth 1993; 40:1136-41.
52. Mannion D, Walker R, Clayton K. Extradural vein puncture—an avoidable complication. Anaesthesia 1991; 46:585-7.
53. Verniquet AJ. Vessel puncture with epidural catheters: Experience in obstetric patients. Anaesthesia 1980; 35:660-2.
54. Mulroy MF, Norris MC, Liu SS. Safety steps for epidural injection of local anesthetics: Review of the literature and recommendations. Anesth Analg 1997; 85:1346-56.
55. Albright GA. Cardiac arrest following regional anesthesia with etidocaine or bupivacaine. Anesthesiology 1979; 51:285-7.
56. Guinard JP, Mulroy MF, Carpenter RL, Knopes KD. Test doses: Optimal epinephrine content with and without acute beta-adrenergic blockade. Anesthesiology 1990; 73:386-92.
57. Moore DC, Batra MS. The components of an effective test dose prior to epidural block. Anesthesiology 1981; 55:693-6.
58. Hood DD, Dewan DM, James FM 3rd. Maternal and fetal effects of epinephrine in gravid ewes. Anesthesiology 1986; 64:610-3.
59. Chestnut DH, Weiner CP, Martin JG, et al. Effect of intravenous epinephrine on uterine artery blood flow velocity in the pregnant guinea pig. Anesthesiology 1986; 65:633-6.
60. Marcus MA, Vertommen JD, Van Aken H, Wouters PF. Hemodynamic effects of intravenous isoproterenol versus epinephrine in the chronic maternal-fetal sheep preparation. Anesth Analg 1996; 82:1023-6.
61. Youngstrom P, Hoyt M, Veille JC, et al. Effects of intravenous test dose epinephrine on fetal sheep during acute fetal stress and acidosis. Reg Anesth 1990; 15:237-41.
62. Chestnut DH, Owen CL, Brown CK, et al. Does labor affect the variability of maternal heart rate during induction of epidural anesthesia? Anesthesiology 1988; 68:622-5.
63. Cartwright PD, McCarroll SM, Antzaka C. Maternal heart rate changes with a plain epidural test dose. Anesthesiology 1986; 65:226-8.
64. Colonna-Romano P, Lingaraju N, Godfrey SD, Braitman LE. Epidural test dose and intravascular injection in obstetrics: Sensitivity, specificity, and lowest effective dose. Anesth Analg 1992; 75:372-6.
65. Colonna-Romano P, Nagaraj L. Tests to evaluate intravenous placement of epidural catheters in laboring women: A prospective clinical study. Anesth Analg 1998; 86:985-8.
66. Mulroy M, Glosten B. The epinephrine test dose in obstetrics: Note the limitations. Anesth Analg 1998; 86:923-5.
67. Leighton BL, Norris MC, Sosis M, et al. Limitations of epinephrine as a marker of intravascular injection in laboring women. Anesthesiology 1987; 66:688-91.
68. Gieraerts R, Van Zundert A, De Wolf A, Vaes L. Ten ml bupivacaine 0.125% with 12.5 micrograms epinephrine is a reliable epidural test dose to detect inadvertent intravascular injection in obstetric patients: A double-blind study. Acta Anaesthesiol Scand 1992; 36:656-9.
69. Leighton BL, DeSimone CA, Norris MC, Chayen B. Isoproterenol is an effective marker of intravenous injection in laboring women. Anesthesiology 1989; 71:206-9.
70. Marcus MA, Vertommen JD, Van Aken H, et al. Hemodynamic effects of intravenous isoproterenol versus saline in the parturient. Anesth Analg 1997; 84:1113-6.
71. Norris MC, Arkoosh VA, Knobler R. Maternal and fetal effects of isoproterenol in the gravid ewe. Anesth Analg 1997; 85:389-94.
72. Marcus MA, Vertommen JD, Van Aken H, et al. The effects of adding isoproterenol to 0.125% bupivacaine on the quality and duration of epidural analgesia in laboring parturients. Anesth Analg 1998; 86:749-52.
73. Leighton BL, Norris MC, DeSimone CA, et al. The air test as a clinically useful indicator of intravenously placed epidural catheters. Anesthesiology 1990; 73:610-3.
74. Leighton BL, Topkis WG, Gross JB, et al. Multiport epidural catheters: Does the air test work? Anesthesiology 2000; 92:1617-20.
75. Colonna-Romano P, Lingaraju N, Braitman LE. Epidural test dose: Lidocaine 100 mg, not chloroprocaine, is a symptomatic marker of i.v. injection in labouring parturients. Can J Anaesth 1993; 40:714-7.
76. Rathmell JP, Viscomi CM, Ashikaga T. Detection of intravascular epidural catheters using 2-chloroprocaine: Influence of local anesthetic dose and nalbuphine premedication. Reg Anesth 1997; 22:113-8.
77. Yoshii WY, Miller M, Rottman RL, et al. Fentanyl for epidural intravascular test dose in obstetrics. Reg Anesth 1993; 18:296-9.
78. Morris GF, Gore-Hickman W, Lang SA, Yip RW. Can parturients distinguish between intravenous and epidural fentanyl? Can J Anaesth 1994; 41:667-72.
79. Power I, Thorburn J. Differential flow from multihole epidural catheters. Anaesthesia 1988; 43:876-8.
80. Abraham RA, Harris AP, Maxwell LG, Kaplow S. The efficacy of 1.5% lidocaine with 7.5% dextrose and epinephrine as an epidural test dose for obstetrics. Anesthesiology 1986; 64:116-9.
81. Colonna-Romano P, Padolina R, Lingaraju N, Braitman LE. Diagnostic accuracy of an intrathecal test dose in epidural analgesia. Can J Anaesth 1994; 41:572-4.
82. Richardson MG, Lee AC, Wissler RN. High spinal anesthesia after epidural test dose administration in five obstetric patients. Reg Anesth 1996; 21:119-23.

83. Ngan Kee WD, Khaw KS, Lee BB, et al. The limitations of ropivacaine with epinephrine as an epidural test dose in parturients. Anesth Analg 2001; 92:1529-31.
84. Cohen SE, Yeh JY, Riley ET, Vogel TM. Walking with labor epidural analgesia: The impact of bupivacaine concentration and a lidocaine-epinephrine test dose. Anesthesiology 2000; 92:387-92.
85. Calimaran AL, Strauss-Hoder TP, Wang WY, et al. The effect of epidural test dose on motor function after a combined spinal-epidural technique for labor analgesia. Anesth Analg 2003; 96:1167-72.
86. Roelants F, Mercier-Fuzier V, Lavand'homme PM. The effect of a lidocaine test dose on analgesia and mobility after an epidural combination of neostigmine and sufentanil in early labor. Anesth Analg 2006; 103:1534-9.
87. Norris MC, Ferrenbach D, Dalman H, et al. Does epinephrine improve the diagnostic accuracy of aspiration during labor epidural analgesia? Anesth Analg 1999; 88:1073-6.
88. Birnbach DJ, Chestnut DH. The epidural test dose in obstetric patients: Has it outlived its usefulness (editorial)? Anesth Analg 1999; 88:971-2.
89. Pert CB, Kuhar MJ, Snyder SH. Opiate receptor: Autoradiographic localization in rat brain. Proc Natl Acad Sci U S A 1976; 73:3729-33.
90. Rush B. Medical Inquiries and Observations. Vol 4. 2nd edition. Philadelphia, T&G Palmer, 1805:356.
91. Justins DM, Francis D, Houlton PG, Reynolds F. A controlled trial of extradural fentanyl in labour. Br J Anaesth 1982; 54:409-14.
92. Belfrage P, Berlin A, Raabe N, Thalme B. Lumbar epidural analgesia with bupivacaine in labor. Drug concentration in maternal and neonatal blood at birth and during the first day of life. Am J Obstet Gynecol 1975; 123:839-44.
93. Eisenach JC, Grice SC, Dewan DM. Epinephrine enhances analgesia produced by epidural bupivacaine during labor. Anesth Analg 1987; 66:447-51.
94. Capogna G, Celleno D, Lyons G, et al. Minimum local analgesia concentration of extradural bupivacaine increases with progression of labor. Br J Anaesth 1998; 80:11-3.
95. Polley LS, Columb MO, Wagner DS, Naughton NN. Dose-dependent reduction of the minimum local analgesic concentration of bupivacaine by sufentanil for epidural analgesia in labor. Anesthesiology 1998; 89:626-32.
96. Christiaens F, Verborgh C, Dierick A, Camu F. Effects of diluent volume of a single dose of epidural bupivacaine in parturients during the first stage of labor. Reg Anesth Pain Med 1998; 23:134-41.
97. Lyons GR, Kocarev MG, Wilson RC, Columb MO. A comparison of minimum local anesthetic volumes and doses of epidural bupivacaine (0.125% w/v and 0.25% w/v) for analgesia in labor. Anesth Analg 2007; 104:412-5.
98. Katz JA, Bridenbaugh PO, Knarr DC, et al. Pharmacodynamics and pharmacokinetics of epidural ropivacaine in humans. Anesth Analg 1990; 70:16-21.
99. Santos AC, Arthur GR, Pedersen H, et al. Systemic toxicity of ropivacaine during ovine pregnancy. Anesthesiology 1991; 75:137-41.
100. Moller R, Covino BG. Cardiac electrophysiologic properties of bupivacaine and lidocaine compared with those of ropivacaine, a new amide local anesthetic. Anesthesiology 1990; 72:322-9.
101. Santos AC, Arthur GR, Roberts DJ, et al. Effect of ropivacaine and bupivacaine on uterine blood flow in pregnant ewes. Anesth Analg 1992; 74:62-7.
102. Santos AC, Arthur GR, Wlody D, et al. Comparative systemic toxicity of ropivacaine and bupivacaine in nonpregnant and pregnant ewes. Anesthesiology 1995; 82:734-40.
103. Polley LS, Columb MO, Naughton NN, et al. Relative analgesic potencies of ropivacaine and bupivacaine for epidural analgesia in labor: Implications for therapeutic indexes. Anesthesiology 1999; 90:944-50.
104. Capogna G, Celleno D, Fusco P, et al. Relative potencies of bupivacaine and ropivacaine for analgesia in labour. Br J Anaesth 1999; 82:371-3.
105. Owen MD, D'Angelo R, Gerancher JC, et al. 0.125% ropivacaine is similar to 0.125% bupivacaine for labor analgesia using patient-controlled epidural infusion. Anesth Analg 1998; 86:527-31.
106. Meister GC, D'Angelo R, Owen M, et al. A comparison of epidural analgesia with 0.125% ropivacaine with fentanyl versus 0.125% bupivacaine with fentanyl during labor. Anesth Analg 2000; 90:632-7.
107. Owen MD, Thomas JA, Smith T, et al. Ropivacaine 0.075% and bupivacaine 0.075% with fentanyl 2 microg/mL are equivalent for labor epidural analgesia. Anesth Analg 2002; 94:179-83.
108. Chua NP, Sia AT, Ocampo CE. Parturient-controlled epidural analgesia during labour: Bupivacaine vs. ropivacaine. Anaesthesia 2001; 56:1169-73.
109. Beilin Y, Guinn NR, Bernstein HH, et al. Local anesthetics and mode of delivery: Bupivacaine versus ropivacaine versus levobupivacaine. Anesth Analg 2007; 105:756-63.
110. Parpaglioni R, Capogna G, Celleno D. A comparison between low-dose ropivacaine and bupivacaine at equianalgesic concentrations for epidural analgesia during the first stage of labor. Int J Obstet Anesth 2000; 9:83-6.
111. Fernandez-Guisasola J, Serrano ML, Cobo B, et al. A comparison of 0.0625% bupivacaine with fentanyl and 0.1% ropivacaine with fentanyl for continuous epidural labor analgesia. Anesth Analg 2001; 92:1261-5.
112. Brockway MS, Bannister J, McClure JH, et al. Comparison of extradural ropivacaine and bupivacaine. Br J Anaesth 1991; 66:31-7.
113. Griffin RP, Reynolds F. Extradural anaesthesia for caesarean section: A double-blind comparison of 0.5% ropivacaine with 0.5% bupivacaine. Br J Anaesth 1995; 74:512-6.
114. Lacassie HJ, Habib AS, Lacassie HP, Columb MO. Motor blocking minimum local anesthetic concentrations of bupivacaine, levobupivacaine, and ropivacaine in labor. Reg Anesth Pain Med 2007; 32:323-9.
115. Halpern SH, Breen TW, Campbell DC, et al. A multicenter, randomized, controlled trial comparing bupivacaine with ropivacaine for labor analgesia. Anesthesiology 2003; 98:1431-5.
116. Halpern SH, Walsh V. Epidural ropivacaine versus bupivacaine for labor: A meta-analysis. Anesth Analg 2003; 96:1473-9.
117. Yoshida M, Matsuda H, Fukuda I, Furuya K. Sudden cardiac arrest during cesarean section due to epidural anaesthesia using ropivacaine: A case report. Arch Gynecol Obstet 2008; 277:91-4.
118. Bardsley H, Gristwood R, Baker H, et al. A comparison of the cardiovascular effects of levobupivacaine and rac-bupivacaine following intravenous administration to healthy volunteers. Br J Clin Pharmacol 1998; 46:245-9.
119. Vanhoutte F, Vereecke J, Verbeke N, Carmeliet E. Stereoselective effects of the enantiomers of bupivacaine on the electrophysiological properties of the guinea-pig papillary muscle. Br J Pharmacol 1991; 103:1275-81.
120. Lyons G, Columb M, Wilson RC, Johnson RV. Epidural pain relief in labour: Potencies of levobupivacaine and racemic bupivacaine. Br J Anaesth 1998; 81:899-901.
121. Polley LS, Columb MO, Naughton NN, et al. Relative analgesic potencies of levobupivacaine and ropivacaine for epidural analgesia in labor. Anesthesiology 2003; 99:1354-8.
122. Benhamou D, Ghosh C, Mercier FJ. A randomized sequential allocation study to determine the minimum effective analgesic concentration of levobupivacaine and ropivacaine in patients receiving epidural analgesia for labor. Anesthesiology 2003; 99:1383-6.
123. Lacassie HJ, Columb MO. The relative motor blocking potencies of bupivacaine and levobupivacaine in labor. Anesth Analg 2003; 97:1509-13.
124. Milaszkiewicz R, Payne N, Loughnan B, et al. Continuous extradural infusion of lignocaine 0.75% vs bupivacaine 0.125% in primiparae: Quality of analgesia and influence on labour. Anaesthesia 1992; 47:1042-6.
125. Kennedy RL, Bell JU, Miller RP, et al. Uptake and distribution of lidocaine in fetal lambs. Anesthesiology 1990; 72:483-9.

126. Biehl D, Shnider SM, Levinson G, Callender K. Placental transfer of lidocaine: Effects of fetal acidosis. Anesthesiology 1978; 48:409-12.
127. Scanlon JW, Brown WU Jr, Weiss JB, Alper MH. Neurobehavioral responses of newborn infants after maternal epidural anesthesia. Anesthesiology 1974; 40:121-8.
128. Abboud TK, Afrasiabi A, Sarkis F, et al. Continuous infusion epidural analgesia in parturients receiving bupivacaine, chloroprocaine, or lidocaine—maternal, fetal, and neonatal effects. Anesth Analg 1984; 63:421-8.
129. Kuhnert BR, Harrison MJ, Linn PL, Kuhnert PM. Effects of maternal epidural anesthesia on neonatal behavior. Anesth Analg 1984; 63:301-8.
130. Grice SC, Eisenach JC, Dewan DM. Labor analgesia with epidural bupivacaine plus fentanyl: Enhancement with epinephrine and inhibition with 2-chloroprocaine. Anesthesiology 1990; 72:623-8.
131. Corke BC, Carlson CG, Dettbarn WD. The influence of 2-chloroprocaine on the subsequent analgesic potency of bupivacaine. Anesthesiology 1984; 60:25-7.
132. Hess PE, Snowman CE, Hahn CJ, et al. Chloroprocaine may not affect epidural morphine for postcesarean delivery analgesia. J Clin Anesth 2006; 18:29-33.
133. Vella LM, Willatts DG, Knott C, et al. Epidural fentanyl in labour: An evaluation of the systemic contribution to analgesia. Anaesthesia 1985; 40:741-7.
134. D'Angelo R, Gerancher JC, Eisenach JC, Raphael BL. Epidural fentanyl produces labor analgesia by a spinal mechanism. Anesthesiology 1998; 88:1519-23.
135. Polley LS, Columb MO, Naughton NN, et al. Effect of intravenous versus epidural fentanyl on the minimum local analgesic concentration of epidural bupivacaine in labor. Anesthesiology 2000; 93:122-8.
136. Ginosar Y, Columb MO, Cohen SE, et al. The site of action of epidural fentanyl infusions in the presence of local anesthetics: A minimum local analgesic concentration infusion study in nulliparous labor. Anesth Analg 2003; 97:1439-45.
137. Chestnut DH, Owen CL, Bates JN, et al. Continuous infusion epidural analgesia during labor: A randomized, double-blind comparison of 0.0625% bupivacaine/0.0002% fentanyl versus 0.125% bupivacaine. Anesthesiology 1988; 68:754-9.
138. Elliott RD. Continuous infusion epidural analgesia for obstetrics: Bupivacaine versus bupivacaine-fentanyl mixture. Can J Anaesth 1991; 38:303-10.
139. Yau G, Gregory MA, Gin T, et al. The addition of fentanyl to epidural bupivacaine in first stage labour. Anaesth Intensive Care 1990; 18:532-5.
140. Reynolds F, O'Sullivan G. Epidural fentanyl and perineal pain in labour. Anaesthesia 1989; 44:341-4.
141. Lyons G, Columb M, Hawthorne L, Dresner M. Extradural pain relief in labour: Bupivacaine sparing by extradural fentanyl is dose dependent. Br J Anaesth 1997; 78:493-7.
142. Robinson AP, Lyons GR, Wilson RC, et al. Levobupivacaine for epidural analgesia in labor: The sparing effect of epidural fentanyl. Anesth Analg 2001; 92:410-4.
143. Buyse I, Stockman W, Columb M, et al. Effect of sufentanil on minimum local analgesic concentrations of epidural bupivacaine, ropivacaine and levobupivacaine in nullipara in early labour. Int J Obstet Anesth 2007; 16:22-8.
144. Palm S, Gertzen W, Ledowski T, et al. Minimum local analgesic dose of plain ropivacaine vs. ropivacaine combined with sufentanil during epidural analgesia for labour. Anaesthesia 2001; 56:526-9.
145. Polley LS, Columb MO, Lyons G, Nair SA. The effect of epidural fentanyl on the minimum local analgesic concentration of epidural chloroprocaine in labor. Anesth Analg 1996; 83:987-90.
146. Vertommen JD, Vandermeulen E, Van Aken H, et al. The effects of the addition of sufentanil to 0.125% bupivacaine on the quality of analgesia during labor and on the incidence of instrumental deliveries. Anesthesiology 1991; 74:809-14.
147. Celleno D, Capogna G. Epidural fentanyl plus bupivacaine 0.125 per cent for labour: Analgesic effects. Can J Anaesth 1988; 35:375-8.
148. van Steenberge A, Debroux HC, Noorduin H. Extradural bupivacaine with sufentanil for vaginal delivery: A double-blind trial. Br J Anaesth 1987; 59:1518-22.
149. Loftus JR, Hill H, Cohen SE. Placental transfer and neonatal effects of epidural sufentanil and fentanyl administered with bupivacaine during labor. Anesthesiology 1995; 83:300-8.
150. Steinberg RB, Dunn SM, Dixon DE, et al. Comparison of sufentanil, bupivacaine, and their combination for epidural analgesia in obstetrics. Reg Anesth 1992; 17:131-8.
151. Herman NL, Sheu KL, Van Decar TK, et al. Determination of the analgesic dose-response relationship for epidural fentanyl and sufentanil with bupivacaine 0.125% in laboring patients. J Clin Anesth 1998; 10:670-7.
152. Capogna G, Camorcia M, Columb MO. Minimum analgesic doses of fentanyl and sufentanil for epidural analgesia in the first stage of labor. Anesth Analg 2003; 96:1178-82.
153. Coda BA, Brown MC, Schaffer R, et al. Pharmacology of epidural fentanyl, alfentanil, and sufentanil in volunteers. Anesthesiology 1994; 81:1149-61.
154. Connelly NR, Parker RK, Pedersen T, et al. Diluent volume for epidural fentanyl and its effect on analgesia in early labor. Anesth Analg 2003; 96:1799-804.
155. Lirzin JD, Jacquinot P, Jorrot JC, et al. Effect of diluting fentanyl on epidural bupivacaine during labor analgesia. Reg Anesth 1989; 14:279-81.
156. Connelly NR, Parker RK, Vallurupalli V, et al. Comparison of epidural fentanyl versus epidural sufentanil for analgesia in ambulatory patients in early labor. Anesth Analg 2000; 91:374-8.
157. Steinberg RB, Powell G, Hu XH, Dunn SM. Epidural sufentanil for analgesia for labor and delivery. Reg Anesth 1989; 14:225-8.
158. Capogna G, Parpaglioni R, Lyons G, et al. Minimum analgesic dose of epidural sufentanil for first-stage labor analgesia: A comparison between spontaneous and prostaglandin-induced labors in nulliparous women. Anesthesiology 2001; 94:740-4.
159. Hughes SC, Rosen MA, Shnider SM, et al. Maternal and neonatal effects of epidural morphine for labor and delivery. Anesth Analg 1984; 63:319-24.
160. Abboud TK, Afrasiabi A, Zhu J, et al. Epidural morphine or butorphanol augments bupivacaine analgesia during labor. Reg Anesth 1989; 14:115-20.
161. Hill DA, McCarthy G, Bali IM. Epidural infusion of alfentanil or diamorphine with bupivacaine in labour—a dose finding study. Anaesthesia 1995; 50:415-9.
162. Cooper RA, Devlin E, Boyd TH, Bali IM. Epidural analgesia for labour using a continuous infusion of bupivacaine and alfentanil. Eur J Anaesthesiol 1993; 10:183-7.
163. Sinatra RS, Eige S, Chung JH, et al. Continuous epidural infusion of 0.05% bupivacaine plus hydromorphone for labor analgesia: An observational assessment in 1830 parturients. Anesth Analg 2002; 94:1310-1.
164. Parker RK, Connelly NR, Lucas T, et al. The addition of hydromorphone to epidural fentanyl does not affect analgesia in early labour. Can J Anaesth 2002; 49:600-4.
165. Mhyre JM. Strategies to induce labor analgesia with epidural hydromorphone. Int J Obstet Anesth 2008; 17:81-2.
166. Liu S, Carpenter R. Lipid solubility and epidural opioid efficacy (letter). Anesthesiology 1995; 83:427-8.
167. Jaffe RA, Rowe MA. A comparison of the local anesthetic effects of meperidine, fentanyl, and sufentanil on dorsal root axons. Anesth Analg 1996; 83:776-81.
168. Handley G, Perkins G. The addition of pethidine to epidural bupivacaine in labour—effect of changing bupivacaine strength. Anaesth Intensive Care 1992; 20:151-5.
169. Brownridge P. Shivering related to epidural blockade with bupivacaine in labour, and the influence of epidural pethidine. Anaesth Intensive Care 1986; 14:412-7.
170. Massad IM, Khadra MM, Alkazaleh FA, et al. Bupivacaine with meperidine versus bupivacaine with fentanyl for continuous epidural labor analgesia. Saudi Med J 2007; 28:904-8.

171. Hunt CO, Naulty JS, Malinow AM, et al. Epidural butorphanol-bupivacaine for analgesia during labor and delivery. Anesth Analg 1989; 68:323-7.
172. Hatjis CG, Meis PJ. Sinusoidal fetal heart rate pattern associated with butorphanol administration. Obstet Gynecol 1986; 67:377-80.
173. McLeod GA, Munishankar B, Columb MO. An isobolographic analysis of diamorphine and levobupivacaine for epidural analgesia in early labour. Br J Anaesth 2007; 98:497-502.
174. Lowson SM, Eggers KA, Warwick JP, et al. Epidural infusions of bupivacaine and diamorphine in labour. Anaesthesia 1995; 50:420-2.
175. Abboud TK, Sheik-ol-Eslam A, Yanagi T, et al. Safety of efficacy of epinephrine added to bupivacaine for lumbar epidural analgesia in obstetrics. Anesth Analg 1985; 64:585-91.
176. Polley LS, Columb MO, Naughton NN, et al. Effect of epidural epinephrine on the minimum local analgesic concentration of epidural bupivacaine in labor. Anesthesiology 2002; 96:1123-8.
177. Abboud TK, David S, Nagappala S, et al. Maternal, fetal, and neonatal effects of lidocaine with and without epinephrine for epidural anesthesia in obstetrics. Anesth Analg 1984; 63:973-9.
178. Reynolds F, Taylor G. Plasma concentrations of bupivacaine during continuous epidural analgesia in labour: The effect of adrenaline. Br J Anaesth 1971; 43:436-40.
179. Reynolds F, Laishley R, Morgan B, Lee A. Effect of time and adrenaline on the feto-maternal distribution of bupivacaine. Br J Anaesth 1989; 62:509-14.
180. Craft JB Jr, Epstein BS, Coakley CS. Effect of lidocaine with epinephrine versus lidocaine (plain) on induced labor. Anesth Analg 1972; 51:243-6.
181. Matadial L, Cibils LA. The effect of epidural anesthesia on uterine activity and blood pressure. Am J Obstet Gynecol 1976; 125:846-54.
182. Yarnell RW, Ewing DA, Tierney E, Smith MH. Sacralization of epidural block with repeated doses of 0.25% bupivacaine during labor. Reg Anesth 1990; 15:275-9.
183. Soetens FM, Soetens MA, Vercauteren MP. Levobupivacaine-sufentanil with or without epinephrine during epidural labor analgesia. Anesth Analg 2006; 103:182-6.
184. Albright GA, Jouppila R, Hollmen AI, et al. Epinephrine does not alter human intervillous blood flow during epidural anesthesia. Anesthesiology 1981; 54:131-5.
185. Skjoldebrand A, Garle M, Gustafsson LL, et al. Extradural pethidine with and without adrenaline during labour: Wide variation in effect. Br J Anaesth 1982; 54:415-20.
186. Landau R, Schiffer E, Morales M, et al. The dose-sparing effect of clonidine added to ropivacaine for labor epidural analgesia. Anesth Analg 2002; 95:728-34.
187. Tremlett MR, Kelly PJ, Parkins J, et al. Low-dose clonidine infusion during labour. Br J Anaesth 1999; 83:257-61.
188. Chassard D, Mathon L, Dailler F, et al. Extradural clonidine combined with sufentanil and 0.0625% bupivacaine for analgesia in labour. Br J Anaesth 1996; 77:458-62.
189. Paech MJ, Pavy TJ, Orlikowski CE, Evans SF. Patient-controlled epidural analgesia in labor: The addition of clonidine to bupivacaine-fentanyl. Reg Anesth Pain Med 2000; 25:34-40.
190. Claes B, Soetens M, Van Zundert A, Datta S. Clonidine added to bupivacaine-epinephrine-sufentanil improves epidural analgesia during childbirth. Reg Anesth Pain Med 1998; 23:540-7.
191. Buggy DJ, MacDowell C. Extradural analgesia with clonidine and fentanyl compared with 0.25% bupivacaine in the first stage of labour. Br J Anaesth 1996; 76:319-21.
192. Roelants F, Lavand'homme PM, Mercier-Fuzier V. Epidural administration of neostigmine and clonidine to induce labor analgesia: Evaluation of efficacy and local anesthetic-sparing effect. Anesthesiology 2005; 102:1205-10.
193. Aveline C, El Metaoua S, Masmoudi A, et al. The effect of clonidine on the minimum local analgesic concentration of epidural ropivacaine during labor. Anesth Analg 2002; 95:735-40.
194. Roelants F, Rizzo M, Lavand'homme P. The effect of epidural neostigmine combined with ropivacaine and sufentanil on neuraxial analgesia during labor. Anesth Analg 2003; 96:1161-6.
195. Roelants F, Lavand'homme PM. Epidural neostigmine combined with sufentanil provides balanced and selective analgesia in early labor. Anesthesiology 2004; 101:439-44.
196. Naguib M, Yaksh TL. Antinociceptive effects of spinal cholinesterase inhibition and isobolographic analysis of the interaction with mu and alpha 2 receptor systems. Anesthesiology 1994; 80:1338-48.
197. Hood DD, Mallak KA, Eisenach JC, Tong C. Interaction between intrathecal neostigmine and epidural clonidine in human volunteers. Anesthesiology 1996; 85:315-25.
198. D'Angelo RD, Anderson MT, Phillip J, Eisenach JC. Intrathecal sufentanil compared to epidural bupivacaine for labor analgesia. Anesthesiology 1994; 80:1209-15.
199. Palmer CM, Cork RC, Hays R, et al. The dose-response relation of intrathecal fentanyl for labor analgesia. Anesthesiology 1998; 88:355-61.
200. Herman NL, Calicott R, Van Decar TK, et al. Determination of the dose-response relationship for intrathecal sufentanil in laboring patients. Anesth Analg 1997; 84:1256-61.
201. Nelson KE, Rauch T, Terebuh V, D'Angelo R. A comparison of intrathecal fentanyl and sufentanil for labor analgesia. Anesthesiology 2002; 96:1070-3.
202. Wong CA, Scavone BM, Loffredi M, et al. The dose-response of intrathecal sufentanil added to bupivacaine for labor analgesia. Anesthesiology 2000; 92:1553-8.
203. Wong CA, Scavone BM, Slavenas JP, et al. Efficacy and side effect profile of varying doses of intrathecal fentanyl added to bupivacaine for labor analgesia. Int J Obstet Anesth 2004; 13:19-24.
204. Saito Y, Kaneko M, Kirihara Y, et al. Interaction of intrathecally infused morphine and lidocaine in rats (part I): Synergistic antinociceptive effects. Anesthesiology 1998; 89:1455-63.
205. Penning JP, Yaksh TL. Interaction of intrathecal morphine with bupivacaine and lidocaine in the rat. Anesthesiology 1992; 77:1186-2000.
206. Stocks GM, Hallworth SP, Fernando R, et al. Minimum local analgesic dose of intrathecal bupivacaine in labor and the effect of intrathecal fentanyl. Anesthesiology 2001; 94:593-8.
207. Sia AT, Chong JL, Chiu JW. Combination of intrathecal sufentanil 10 mcg plus bupivacaine 2.5 mg for labor analgesia: Is half the dose enough? Anesth Analg 1999; 88:362-6.
208. Herman NL, Choi KC, Affleck PJ, et al. Analgesia, pruritus, and ventilation exhibit a dose-response relationship in parturients receiving intrathecal fentanyl during labor. Anesth Analg 1999; 89:378-83.
209. Nelson KE, D'Angelo R, Foss ML, et al. Intrathecal neostigmine and sufentanil for early labor analgesia. Anesthesiology 1999; 91:1293-8.
210. Arkoosh VA, Cooper M, Norris MC, et al. Intrathecal sufentanil dose response in nulliparous patients. Anesthesiology 1998; 89:364-70.
211. Camann W, Abouleish A, Eisenach J, et al. Intrathecal sufentanil and epidural bupivacaine for labor analgesia: Dose-response of individual agents and in combination. Reg Anesth Pain Med 1998; 23:457-62.
212. Van de Velde M, Dreelinck R, Dubois J, et al. Determination of the full dose-response relation of intrathecal bupivacaine, levobupivacaine, and ropivacaine, combined with sufentanil, for labor analgesia. Anesthesiology 2007; 106:149-56.
213. Baraka A, Noueihid R, Hajj S. Intrathecal injection of morphine for obstetric analgesia. Anesthesiology 1981; 54:136-40.
214. Abboud TK, Shnider SM, Dailey PA, et al. Intrathecal administration of hyperbaric morphine for the relief of pain in labour. Br J Anaesth 1984; 56:1351-60.
215. Abouleish E. Apnoea associated with the intrathecal administration of morphine in obstetrics: A case report. Br J Anaesth 1988; 60:592-4.
216. Vasudevan A, Snowman CE, Sundar S, et al. Intrathecal morphine reduces breakthrough pain during labour epidural analgesia. Br J Anaesth 2007; 98:241-5.
217. Hess PE, Vasudevan A, Snowman C, Pratt SD. Small dose bupivacaine-fentanyl spinal analgesia combined with morphine for labor. Anesth Analg 2003; 97:247-52.
218. Yeh HM, Chen LK, Shyu MK, et al. The addition of morphine prolongs fentanyl-bupivacaine spinal analgesia for the relief of labor pain. Anesth Analg 2001; 92:665-8.

219. Kafle SK. Intrathecal meperidine for elective caesarean section: A comparison with lidocaine. Can J Anaesth 1993; 40:718-21.
220. Honet JE, Arkoosh VA, Norris MC, et al. Comparison among intrathecal fentanyl, meperidine, and sufentanil for labor analgesia. Anesth Analg 1992; 75:734-9.
221. Booth JV, Lindsay DR, Olufolabi AJ, et al. Subarachnoid meperidine (Pethidine) causes significant nausea and vomiting during labor. Anesthesiology 2000; 93:418-21.
222. Kestin IG, Madden AP, Mulvein JT, Goodman NW. Analgesia for labour and delivery using incremental diamorphine and bupivacaine via a 32-gauge intrathecal catheter. Br J Anaesth 1992; 68:244-7.
223. Vaughan DJ, Ahmad N, Lillywhite NK, et al. Choice of opioid for initiation of combined spinal-epidural analgesia in labour—fentanyl or diamorphine. Br J Anaesth 2001; 86:567-9.
224. Asokumar B, Newman LM, McCarthy RJ, et al. Intrathecal bupivacaine reduces pruritus and prolongs duration of fentanyl analgesia during labor: A prospective, randomized controlled trial. Anesth Analg 1998; 87:1309-15.
225. Whitty R, Goldszmidt E, Parkes RK, Carvalho JC. Determination of the ED_{95} for intrathecal plain bupivacaine combined with fentanyl in active labor. Int J Obstet Anesth 2007; 16:341-5.
226. Camorcia M, Capogna G, Columb MO. Minimum local analgesic doses of ropivacaine, levobupivacaine, and bupivacaine for intrathecal labor analgesia. Anesthesiology 2005; 102:646-50.
227. Richardson MG, Wissler RN. Densities of dextrose-free intrathecal local anesthetics, opioids, and combinations measured at 37 degrees C. Anesth Analg 1997; 84:95-9.
228. Richardson MG, Thakur R, Abramowicz JS, Wissler RN. Maternal posture influences the extent of sensory block produced by intrathecal dextrose-free bupivacaine with fentanyl for labor analgesia. Anesth Analg 1996; 83:1229-33.
229. Ferouz F, Norris MC, Arkoosh VA, et al. Baricity, needle direction, and intrathecal sufentanil labor analgesia. Anesthesiology 1997; 86:592-8.
230. Gage JC, D'Angelo R, Miller R, Eisenach JC. Does dextrose affect analgesia or the side effects of intrathecal sufentanil? Anesth Analg 1997; 85:826-30.
231. Rofaeel A, Lilker S, Fallah S, et al. Intrathecal plain vs hyperbaric bupivacaine for labour analgesia: Efficacy and side effects. Can J Anaesth 2007; 54:15-20.
232. Gautier PE, De Kock M, Fanard L, et al. Intrathecal clonidine combined with sufentanil for labor analgesia. Anesthesiology 1998; 88:651-6.
233. Mercier FJ, Dounas M, Bouaziz H, et al. The effect of adding a minidose of clonidine to intrathecal sufentanil for labor analgesia. Anesthesiology 1998; 89:594-601.
234. Missant C, Teunkens A, Vandermeersch E, Van de Velde M. Intrathecal clonidine prolongs labour analgesia but worsens fetal outcome: A pilot study. Can J Anaesth 2004; 51:696-701.
235. Sia AT. Optimal dose of intrathecal clonidine added to sufentanil plus bupivacaine for labour analgesia. Can J Anaesth 2000; 47:875-80.
236. D'Angelo R, Dean LS, Meister GC, Nelson KE. Neostigmine combined with bupivacaine, clonidine, and sufentanil for spinal labor analgesia. Anesth Analg 2001; 93:1560-4.
237. Chiari A, Lorber C, Eisenach JC, et al. Analgesic and hemodynamic effects of intrathecal clonidine as the sole analgesic agent during first stage of labor: A dose-response study. Anesthesiology 1999; 91:388-96.
238. Owen MD, Ozsarac O, Sahin S, et al. Low-dose clonidine and neostigmine prolong the duration of intrathecal bupivacaine-fentanyl for labor analgesia. Anesthesiology 2000; 92:361-6.
239. Campbell DC, Banner R, Crone LA, et al. Addition of epinephrine to intrathecal bupivacaine and sufentanil for ambulatory labor analgesia. Anesthesiology 1997; 86:525-31.
240. Vercauteren MP, Jacobs S, Jacquemyn Y, Adriaensen HA. Intrathecal labor analgesia with bupivacaine and sufentanil: The effect of adding epinephrine 2.25 microg to epinephrine. Reg Anesth Pain Med 2001; 26:473-7.
241. Gurbet A, Turker G, Kose DO, Uckunkaya N. Intrathecal epinephrine in combined spinal-epidural analgesia for labor: Dose-response relationship for epinephrine added to a local anesthetic-opioid combination. Int J Obstet Anesth 2005; 14:121-5.
242. Hess PE, Pratt SD, Oriol NE. An analysis of the need for anesthetic interventions with differing concentrations of labor epidural bupivacaine: An observational study. Int J Obstet Anesth 2006; 15:195-200.
243. Beilin Y, Nair A, Arnold I, et al. A comparison of epidural infusions in the combined spinal/epidural technique for labor analgesia. Anesth Analg 2002; 94:927-32.
244. Bader AM, Fragneto R, Terui K, et al. Maternal and neonatal fentanyl and bupivacaine concentration after epidural infusion during labor. Anesth Analg 1995; 81:829-32.
245. Porter J, Bonello E, Reynolds F. Effect of epidural fentanyl on neonatal respiration. Anesthesiology 1998; 89:79-85.
246. Bernard JM, Le Roux D, Barthe A, et al. The dose-range effects of sufentanil added to 0.125% bupivacaine on the quality of patient-controlled epidural analgesia during labor. Anesth Analg 2001; 92:184-8.
247. Association of Women's Health Obstetric and Neonatal Nurses. Role of the registered nurse (RN) in the care of the pregnant woman receiving analgesia/anesthesia by catheter techniques (epidural, intrathecal, spinal, PCEA catheters). 2007. Available at http://www.awhonn.org/awhonn/content.do?name=05_HealthPolicyLegislation/5H_PositionStatements.htm/
248. Lamont RF, Pinney D, Rodgers P, Bryant TN. Continuous versus intermittent epidural analgesia. Anaesthesia 1989; 44:893-6.
249. Bogod DG, Rosen M, Rees GA. Extradural infusion of 0.125% bupivacaine at 10 mL/hr to women during labor. Br J Anaesth 1987; 59:325-30.
250. Li DF, Rees GAD, Rosen M. Continuous extradural infusion of 0.0625% or 0.125% bupivacaine for pain relief in primigravid labour. Br J Anaesth 1985; 57:264-70.
251. Hicks JA, Jenkins JG, Newton MC, Findley IL. Continuous epidural infusion of 0.075% bupivacaine for pain relief in labour. Anaesthesia 1988; 43:289-92.
252. Smedstad KG, Morison DH. A comparative study of continuous and intermittent epidural analgesia for labour and delivery. Can J Anaesth 1988; 35:234-41.
253. Boutros A, Blary S, Bronchard R, Bonnet F. Comparison of intermittent epidural bolus, continuous epidural infusion and patient controlled-epidural analgesia during labor. Int J Obstet Anesth 1999; 8:236-41.
254. Gambling DR, Yu P, Cole C, et al. A comparative study of patient controlled epidural analgesia (PCEA) and continuous infusion epidural analgesia (CIEA) during labour. Can J Anaesth 1988; 35:249-54.
255. Curry PD, Pacsoo C, Heap DG. Patient-controlled epidural analgesia in obstetric anaesthetic practice. Pain 1994; 57:125-8.
256. Collis RE, Plaat FS, Morgan BM. Comparison of midwife top-ups, continuous infusion and patient-controlled epidural analgesia for maintaining mobility after a low-dose combined spinal-epidural. Br J Anaesth 1999; 82:233-6.
257. Purdie J, Reid J, Thorburn J, Asbury AJ. Continuous extradural analgesia: Comparisons of midwife top-ups, continuous infusions and patient controlled administration. Br J Anaesth 1992; 68:580-4.
258. Tan S, Reid J, Thorburn J. Extradural analgesia in labour: Complications of three techniques of administration. Br J Anaesth 1994; 73:619-23.
259. Gambling DR, Huber CJ, Berkowitz J, et al. Patient-controlled epidural analgesia in labour: Varying bolus dose and lockout interval. Can J Anaesth 1993; 40:211-7.
260. Ferrante FM, Lu L, Jamison SB, Datta S. Patient-controlled epidural analgesia: Demand dosing. Anesth Analg 1991; 73:547-52.
261. Ferrante FM, Rosinia FA, Gordon C, Datta S. The role of continuous background infusions in patient-controlled epidural analgesia for labor and delivery. Anesth Analg 1994; 79:80-4.
262. van der Vyver M, Halpern S, Joseph G. Patient-controlled epidural analgesia versus continuous infusion for labour analgesia: A meta-analysis. Br J Anaesth 2002; 89:459-65.

263. Paech MJ. Patient-controlled epidural analgesia in labour—is a continuous infusion of benefit? Anaesth Intensive Care 1992; 20:15-20.
264. Petry J, Vercauteren M, Van Mol I, et al. Epidural PCA with bupivacaine 0.125%, sufentanil 0.75 microgram and epinephrine 1/800.000 for labor analgesia: Is a background infusion beneficial? Acta Anaesthesiol Belg 2000; 51:163-6.
265. Boselli E, Debon R, Cimino Y, et al. Background infusion is not beneficial during labor patient-controlled analgesia with 0.1% ropivacaine plus 0.5 microg/ml sufentanil. Anesthesiology 2004; 100:968-72.
266. Vallejo MC, Ramesh V, Phelps AL, Sah N. Epidural labor analgesia: Continuous infusion versus patient-controlled epidural analgesia with background infusion versus without a background infusion. J Pain 2007; 8:970-5.
267. Missant C, Teunkenst A, Vandermeersch E, Van de Velde M. Patient-controlled epidural analgesia following combined spinal-epidural analgesia in labour: The effects of adding a continuous epidural infusion. Anaesth Intensive Care 2005; 33:452-6.
268. Bremerich DH, Waibel HJ, Mierdl S, et al. Comparison of continuous background infusion plus demand dose and demand-only parturient-controlled epidural analgesia (PCEA) using ropivacaine combined with sufentanil for labor and delivery. Int J Obstet Anesth 2005; 14:114-20.
269. Halpern S. Recent advances in patient-controlled epidural analgesia for labour. Curr Opin Anaesthesiol 2005; 18:247-51.
270. Siddik-Sayyid SM, Aouad MT, Jalbout MI, et al. Comparison of three modes of patient-controlled epidural analgesia during labour. Eur J Anaesthesiol 2005; 22:30-4.
271. Stratmann G, Gambling DR, Moeller-Bertram T, et al. A randomized comparison of a five-minute versus fifteen-minute lockout interval for PCEA during labor. Int J Obstet Anesth 2005; 14:200-7.
272. Carvalho B, Cohen SE, Giarrusso K, et al. "Ultra-light" patient-controlled epidural analgesia during labor: Effects of varying regimens on analgesia and physician workload. Int J Obstet Anesth 2005; 14:223-9.
273. Bernard JM, Le Roux D, Frouin J. Ropivacaine and fentanyl concentrations in patient-controlled epidural analgesia during labor: A volume-range study. Anesth Analg 2003; 97:1800-7.
274. Gogarten W, Van de Velde M, Soetens F, et al. A multicentre trial comparing different concentrations of ropivacaine plus sufentanil with bupivacaine plus sufentanil for patient-controlled epidural analgesia in labour. Eur J Anaesthesiol 2004; 21:38-45.
275. Boselli E, Debon R, Duflo F, et al. Ropivacaine 0.15% plus sufentanil 0.5 microg/mL and ropivacaine 0.10% plus sufentanil 0.5 microg/mL are equivalent for patient-controlled epidural analgesia for labor. Anesth Analg 2003; 96:1173-7.
276. Nikkola E, Laara A, Hinkka S, et al. Patient-controlled epidural analgesia in labor does not always improve maternal satisfaction. Acta Obstet Gynecol Scand 2006; 85:188-94.
277. Sia AT, Ruban P, Chong JL, Wong K. Motor blockade is reduced with ropivacaine 0.125% for parturient-controlled epidural analgesia during labour. Can J Anaesth 1999; 46:1019-23.
278. Hogan Q. Distribution of solution in the epidural space: Examination by cryomicrotome section. Reg Anesth Pain Med 2002; 27:150-6.
279. Wong CA, Ratliff JT, Sullivan JT, et al. A randomized comparison of programmed intermittent epidural bolus with continuous epidural infusion for labor analgesia. Anesth Analg 2006; 102:904-9.
280. Lim Y, Sia AT, Ocampo C. Automated regular boluses for epidural analgesia: A comparison with continuous infusion. Int J Obstet Anesth 2005; 14:305-9.
281. Chua SM, Sia AT. Automated intermittent epidural boluses improve analgesia induced by intrathecal fentanyl during labour. Can J Anaesth 2004; 51:581-5.
282. Fettes PD, Moore CS, Whiteside JB, et al. Intermittent vs continuous administration of epidural ropivacaine with fentanyl for analgesia during labour. Br J Anaesth 2006; 97:359-64.
283. Sia AT, Lim Y, Ocampo C. A comparison of a basal infusion with automated mandatory boluses in parturient-controlled epidural analgesia during labor. Anesth Analg 2007; 104:673-8.
284. Moran DH, Johnson MD. Continuous spinal anesthesia with combined hyperbaric and isobaric bupivacaine in a patient with scoliosis. Anesth Analg 1990; 70:445-7.
285. Milligan KR, Carp H. Continuous spinal anaesthesia for caesarean section in the morbidly obese. Int J Obstet Anesth 1992; 1:111-3.
286. Van de Velde M, Budts W, Vandermeersch E, Spitz B. Continuous spinal analgesia for labor pain in a parturient with aortic stenosis. Int J Obstet Anesth 2003; 12:51-4.
287. Okutomi T, Kikuchi S, Amano K, et al. Continuous spinal analgesia for labor and delivery in a parturient with hypertrophic obstructive cardiomyopathy. Acta Anaesthesiol Scand 2002; 46:329-31.
288. Rigler MI, Drasner K, Krejcie TC, et al. Cauda equina syndrome after continuous spinal anesthesia. Anesth Analg 1991; 72:275-281.
289. Rigler ML, Drasner K. Distribution of catheter-injected local anesthetic in a model of the subarachnoid space. Anesthesiology 1991; 75:684-92.
290. Arkoosh VA, Palmer CM, Yun EM, et al. A randomized, double-masked, multicenter comparison of the safety of continuous intrathecal labor analgesia using a 28-gauge catheter versus continuous epidural labor analgesia. Anesthesiology 2008; 108:286-98.
291. Pavy TJ. Patient-controlled spinal analgesia for labour and cesarean delivery. Anaesth Intensive Care 2001; 29:58-61.
292. Collis RE, Baxandall ML, Srikantharajah ID, et al. Combined spinal-epidural analgesia with ability to walk throughout labour. Lancet 1993; 341:767-8.
293. Buggy D, Hughes N, Gardiner J. Posterior column sensory impairment during ambulatory extradural analgesia in labour. Br J Anaesth 1994; 73:540-2.
294. Parry MG, Fernando R, Bawa GPS, Poulton BB. Dorsal column function after epidural and spinal blockade: Implications for the safety of walking following low-dose regional analgesia for labour. Anaesthesia 1998; 53:382-7.
295. Davies J, Fernando R, McLeod A, et al. Postural stability following ambulatory regional analgesia for labor. Anesthesiology 2002; 97:1576-81.
296. Merry AF, Cross JA, Mayadeo SV, Wild CJ. Posture and the spread of extradural analgesia in labour. Br J Anaesth 1983; 55:303-7.
297. Park WY, Hagins FM, Massengale MD, Macnamara TE. The sitting position and anesthetic spread in the epidural space. Anesth Analg 1984; 63:863-4.
298. Erdemir HA, Soper LE, Sweet RB. Studies of factors affecting peridural anesthesia. Anesth Analg 1965; 44:400-4.
299. Kinsella SM, Black AM. Reporting of 'hypotension' after epidural analgesia during labour: Effect of choice of arm and timing of baseline readings. Anaesthesia 1998; 53:131-5.
300. Kubli M, Shennan AH, Seed PT, O'Sullivan G. A randomised controlled trial of fluid pre-loading before low dose epidural analgesia for labour. Int J Obstet Anesth 2003; 12:256-60.
301. Lee A, Ngan Kee WD, Gin T. A quantitative, systematic review of randomized controlled trials of ephedrine versus phenylephrine for the management of hypotension during spinal anesthesia for cesarean delivery. Anesth Analg 2002; 94:920-6.
302. Hughes SC, Ward MG, Levinson G, et al. Placental transfer of ephedrine does not affect neonatal outcome. Anesthesiology 1985; 63:217-9.
303. Wright RG, Shnider SM, Levinson G, et al. The effect of maternal administration of ephedrine on fetal heart rate and variability. Obstet Gynecol 1981; 57:734-8.
304. Cohen SE, Cherry CM, Holbrook RH, Jr., et al. Intrathecal sufentanil for labor analgesia—sensory changes, side effects, and fetal heart rate changes. Anesth Analg 1993; 77:1155-60.
305. Riley ET, Walker D, Hamilton CL, Cohen SE. Intrathecal sufentanil for labor analgesia does not cause a sympathectomy. Anesthesiology 1997; 87:874-8.
306. Palmer CM, Van Maren G, Nogami WM, Alves D. Bupivacaine augments intrathecal fentanyl for labor analgesia. Anesthesiology 1999; 91:84-9.
307. Lee BB, Ngan Kee WD, Hung VYS, Wong ELY. Combined spinal-epidural analgesia in labour: Comparison of two doses of intrathecal bupivacaine with fentanyl. Br J Anaesth 1999; 83:868-71.
308. Lim EH, Sia AT, Wong K, Tan HM. Addition of bupivacaine 1.25 mg to fentanyl confers no advantage over fentanyl alone for intrathecal analgesia in early labor. Can J Anaesth 2002; 49:57-61.

309. Norris MC, Grieco WM, Borkowski M, et al. Complications of labor analgesia: Epidural versus combined spinal-epidural techniques. Anesth Analg 1994; 79:529-37.
310. Douglas MJ, Kim JH, Ross PL, McMorland GH. The effect of epinephrine in local anaesthetic on epidural morphine-induced pruritus. Can Anaesth Soc J 1986; 33:737-40.
311. Waxler B, Dadabhoy ZP, Stojiljkovic L, Rabito SF. Primer of postoperative pruritus for anesthesiologists. Anesthesiology 2005; 103:168-78.
312. Scott PV, Fischer HB. Spinal opiate analgesia and facial pruritus: A neural theory. Postgrad Med J 1982; 58:531-5.
313. Ganesh A, Maxwell LG. Pathophysiology and management of opioid-induced pruritus. Drugs 2007; 67:2323-33.
314. Charuluxananan S, Kyokong O, Somboonviboon W, et al. Nalbuphine versus ondansetron for prevention of intrathecal morphine-induced pruritus after cesarean delivery. Anesth Analg 2003; 96:1789-93.
315. Yeh HM, Chen LK, Lin CJ, et al. Prophylactic intravenous ondansetron reduces the incidence of intrathecal morphine-induced pruritus in patients undergoing cesarean delivery. Anesth Analg 2000; 91:172-5.
316. Sarvela PJ, Halonen PM, Soikkeli AI, et al. Ondansetron and tropisetron do not prevent intraspinal morphine- and fentanyl-induced pruritus in elective cesarean delivery. Acta Anaesthesiol Scand 2006; 50:239-44.
317. Wells J, Paech MJ, Evans SF. Intrathecal fentanyl-induced pruritus during labour: The effect of prophylactic ondansetron. Int J Obstet Anesth 2004; 13:35-9.
318. Horta ML, Morejon LC, da Cruz AW, et al. Study of the prophylactic effect of droperidol, alizapride, propofol and promethazine on spinal morphine-induced pruritus. Br J Anaesth 2006; 96:796-800.
319. Warwick JP, Kearns CF, Scott WE. The effect of subhypnotic doses of propofol on the incidence of pruritus after intrathecal morphine for caesarean section. Anaesthesia 1997; 52:270-5.
320. Cohen SE, Ratner EF, Kreitzman TR, et al. Nalbuphine is better than naloxone for treatment of side effects after epidural morphine. Anesth Analg 1992; 75:747-52.
321. Chaney MA. Side effects of intrathecal and epidural opioids. Can J Anaesth 1995; 42:891-903.
322. Bateman DN, Rawlins MD, Simpson JM. Extrapyramidal reactions with metoclopramide. Br Med J (Clin Res Ed) 1985; 291:930-2.
323. Camann WR, Hortvet LA, Hughes N, et al. Maternal temperature regulation during extradural analgesia for labour. Br J Anaesth 1991; 67:565-8.
324. Lieberman E, Lang JM, Frigoletto F Jr, et al. Epidural analgesia, intrapartum fever, and neonatal sepsis evaluation. Pediatrics 1997; 99:415-9.
325. Fusi L, Steer PJ, Maresh MJ, Beard RW. Maternal pyrexia associated with the use of epidural analgesia in labour. Lancet 1989; 1(8649):1250-2.
326. Macaulay JH, Bond K, Steer PJ. Epidural analgesia in labor and fetal hyperthermia. Obstet Gynecol 1992; 80:665-9.
327. Herbst A, Wolner-Hanssen P, Ingemarsson I. Risk factors for fever in labor. Obstet Gynecol 1995; 86:790-4.
328. Glosten B, Savage M, Rooke GA, Brengelmann GL. Epidural anesthesia and the thermoregulatory responses to hyperthermia—preliminary observations in volunteer subjects. Acta Anaesthesiol Scand 1998; 42:442-6.
329. Goetzl L, Cohen A, Frigoletto F Jr, et al. Maternal epidural use and neonatal sepsis evaluation in afebrile mothers. Pediatrics 2001; 108:1099-102.
330. Yancey MK, Zhang J, Schwarz J, et al. Labor epidural analgesia and intrapartum maternal hyperthermia. Obstet Gynecol 2001; 98:763-70.
331. Philip J, Alexander JM, Sharma SK, et al. Epidural analgesia during labor and maternal fever. Anesthesiology 1999; 90:1271-5.
332. Goetzl L, Rivers J, Zighelboim I, et al. Intrapartum epidural analgesia and maternal temperature regulation. Obstet Gynecol 2007; 109:687-90.
333. Goetzl L, Zighelboim I, Badell M, et al. Maternal corticosteroids to prevent intrauterine exposure to hyperthermia and inflammation: A randomized, double-blind, placebo-controlled trial. Am J Obstet Gynecol 2006; 195:1031-7.
334. Kapusta L, Confino E, Ismajovich B, et al. The effect of epidural analgesia on maternal thermoregulation in labor. Int J Gynaecol Obstet 1985; 23:185-9.
335. Panzer O, Ghazanfari N, Sessler DI, et al. Shivering and shivering-like tremor during labor with and without epidural analgesia. Anesthesiology 1999; 90:1609-16.
336. Shehabi Y, Gatt S, Buckman T, Isert P. Effect of adrenaline, fentanyl and warming of injectate on shivering following extradural analgesia in labour. Anaesth Intensive Care 1990; 18:31-7.
337. Kuipers PW, Kamphuis ET, van Venrooij GE, et al. Intrathecal opioids and lower urinary tract function: A urodynamic evaluation. Anesthesiology 2004; 100:1497-503.
338. Grove LH. Backache, headache and bladder dysfunction after delivery. Br J Anaesth 1973; 45:1147-9.
339. Weiniger CF, Wand S, Nadjari M, et al. Post-void residual volume in labor: A prospective study comparing parturients with and without epidural analgesia. Acta Anaesthesiol Scand 2006; 50:1297-303.
340. Olofsson CI, Ekblom AO, Ekman-Ordeberg GE, Irestedt LE. Post-partum urinary retention: A comparison between two methods of epidural analgesia. Eur J Obstet Gynecol Reprod Biol 1997; 71:31-4.
341. Evron S, Muzikant G, Rigini N, et al. Patient-controlled epidural analgesia: The role of epidural fentanyl in peripartum urinary retention. Int J Obstet Anesth 2006; 15:206-11.
342. Kriebs JM. Understanding herpes simplex virus: Transmission, diagnosis, and considerations in pregnancy management. J Midwifery Womens Health 2008; 53:202-8.
343. Crone LA, Conly JM, Storgard C, et al. Herpes labialis in parturients receiving epidural morphine following cesarean section. Anesthesiology 1990; 73:208-13.
344. Boyle RK. Herpes simplex labialis after epidural or parenteral morphine: A randomized prospective trial in an Australian obstetric population. Anaesth Intensive Care 1995; 23:433-7.
345. Davies PW, Vallejo MC, Shannon KT, et al. Oral herpes simplex reactivation after intrathecal morphine: A prospective randomized trial in an obstetric population. Anesth Analg 2005; 100:1472-6.
346. Valley MA, Bourke DL, McKenzie AM. Recurrence of thoracic and labial herpes simplex virus infection in a patient receiving epidural fentanyl. Anesthesiology 1992; 76:1056-7.
347. Acalovschi I. Herpes simplex after spinal pethidine (letter). Anaesthesia 1986; 41:1271-2.
348. Holdsworth JD. Relationship between stomach contents and analgesia in labour. Br J Anaesth 1978; 50:1145-8.
349. Porter JS, Bonello E, Reynolds F. The influence of epidural administration of fentanyl infusion on gastric emptying in labour. Anaesthesia 1997; 52:1151-6.
350. Zimmermann DL. Adding fentanyl 0.0002% to epidural bupivacaine 0.125% does not delay gastric emptying in laboring patients. Anesth Analg 1996; 82:612-6.
351. Ewah B, Yau K, King M, et al. Effect of epidural opioids on gastric emptying in labour. Int J Obstet Anesth 1993; 2:125-8.
352. Wright PMC, Allen RW, Moore J, Donnelly JP. Gastric emptying during lumbar extradural analgesia in labor: Effect of fentanyl supplementation. Br J Anaesth 1992; 68:248-51.
353. Kelly MC, Carabine UA, Hill DA, Mirakhur RK. A comparison of the effect of intrathecal and extradural fentanyl on gastric emptying in laboring women. Anesth Analg 1997; 85:834-8.
354. Paech MJ, Godkin R, Webster GS. Complications of obstetric epidural analgesia and anaesthesia: A prospective analysis of 10,995 cases. Int J Obstet Anesth 1998; 7:5-11.
355. Eappen S, Blinn A, Segal S. Incidence of epidural catheter replacement in parturients: A retrospective chart review. Int J Obstet Anesth 1998; 7:220-5.
356. Chadwick HS. An analysis of obstetric anesthesia cases from the American Society of Anesthesiologists closed claims project database. Int J Obstet Anesth 1996; 5:258-63.

357. Beilin Y, Zahn J, Bernstein HH, et al. Treatment of incomplete analgesia after placement of an epidural catheter and administration of local anesthetic for women in labor. Anesthesiology 1998; 88:1502-6.
358. Husemeyer RP, White DC. Lumbar extradural injection pressures in pregnant women: An investigation of relationships between rate of infection, injection pressures and extent of analgesia. Br J Anaesth 1980; 52:55-60.
359. Apostolou GA, Zarmakoupis PK, Mastrokostopoulos GT. Spread of epidural anesthesia and the lateral position. Anesth Analg 1981; 60:584-6.
360. Norris MC, Leighton BL, DeSimone CA, Larijani GE. Lateral position and epidural anesthesia for cesarean section. Anesth Analg 1988; 67:788-90.
361. Savolaine ER, Pandya JB, Greenblatt SH, Conover SR. Anatomy of the human lumbar epidural space: New insights using CT-epidurography. Anesthesiology 1988; 68:217-20.
362. Asato F, Goto F. Radiographic findings of unilateral epidural block. Anesth Analg 1996; 83:519-22.
363. Blomberg RG, Olsson SS. The lumbar epidural space in patients examined with epiduroscopy. Anesth Analg 1989; 68:157-60.
364. McCrae AF, Whitfield A, McClure JH. Repeated unilateral epidural blockade. Anaesthesia 1992; 47:859-61.
365. Choi PT, Galinski SE, Takeuchi L, et al. PDPH is a common complication of neuraxial blockade in parturients: A meta-analysis of obstetrical studies. Can J Anaesth 2003; 50:460-9.
366. Crawford JS. Some maternal complications of epidural analgesia for labour. Anaesthesia 1985; 40:1219-25.
367. Lu JK, Manullang TR, Staples MH, et al. Maternal respiratory arrests, severe hypotension, and fetal distress after administration of intrathecal sufentanil and bupivacaine after intravenous fentanyl. Anesthesiology 1997; 87:170-2.
368. Ferouz F, Norris MC, Leighton BL. Risk of respiratory arrest after intrathecal sufentanil. Anesth Analg 1997; 85:1088-90.
369. American Heart Association. Cardiac arrest associated with pregnancy. Circulation 2005; 112:IV150-3.
370. Turner-Lawrence DE, Kerns IW. Intravenous fat emulsion: A potential novel antidote. J Med Toxicol 2008; 4:109-14.
371. Jenkins JG. Some immediate serious complications of obstetric epidural analgesia and anaesthesia: A prospective study of 145,550 epidurals. Int J Obstet Anesth 2005; 14:37-42.
372. Lubenow T, Keh-Wong E, Kristof K, et al. Inadvertent subdural injection: A complication of an epidural block. Anesth Analg 1988; 67:175-9.
373. Rodriguez J, Barcena M, Taboada-Muniz M, Alvarez J. Horner syndrome after unintended subdural block: A report of 2 cases. J Clin Anesth 2005; 17:473-7.
374. Abouleish E, Goldstein M. Migration of an extradural catheter into the subdural space: A case report. Br J Anaesth 1986; 58:1194-7.
375. Chestnut DH, Bates JN, Choi WW. Continuous infusion epidural analgesia with lidocaine: Efficacy and influence during the second stage of labor. Obstet Gynecol 1987; 69:323-7.
376. Cuerden C, Buley R, Downing JW. Delayed recovery after epidural block in labour: A report of four cases. Anaesthesia 1977; 32:773-6.
377. Riley ET, Ratner EF, Cohen SE. Intrathecal sufentanil for labor analgesia: Do sensory changes predict better analgesia and greater hypotension? Anesth Analg 1997; 84:346-51.
378. Wang C, Chakrabarti MK, Whitwam JG. Specific enhancement by fentanyl of the effects of intrathecal bupivacaine on nociceptive afferent but not on sympathetic efferent pathways in dogs. Anesthesiology 1993; 79:766-73.
379. Hamilton CL, Cohen SE. High sensory block after intrathecal sufentanil for labor analgesia. Anesthesiology 1995; 83:1118-21.
380. Abu Abdou W, Aveline C, Bonnet F. Two additional cases of excessive extension of sensory blockade after intrathecal sufentanil for labor analgesia. Int J Obstet Anesth 2000; 9:48-50.
381. Scavone BM. Altered level of consciousness after combined spinal-epidural labor analgesia with intrathecal fentanyl and bupivacaine. Anesthesiology 2002; 96:1021-2.
382. Fragneto RY, Fisher A. Mental status change and aphasia after labor analgesia with intrathecal sufentanil/bupivacaine. Anesth Analg 2000; 90:1175-6.
383. To WW, Wong MW. Factors associated with back pain symptoms in pregnancy and the persistence of pain 2 years after pregnancy. Acta Obstet Gynecol Scand 2003; 82:1086-91.
384. Breen TW, Ransil BJ, Groves PA, Oriol NE. Factors associated with back pain after childbirth. Anesthesiology 1994; 81:29-34.
385. Russell R, Dundas R, Reynolds F. Long term backache after childbirth: Prospective search for causative factors. Br Med J 1996; 312:1384-8.
386. MacArthur C, Lewis M, Knox EG, Crawford JS. Epidural anaesthesia and long term backache after childbirth. Br Med J 1990; 301:9-12.
387. MacArthur C, Lewis M, Knox EG. Investigation of long term problems after obstetric epidural anaesthesia. Br Med J 1992; 304:1279-82.
388. Loughnan BA, Carli F, Romney M, et al. Epidural analgesia and backache: A randomized controlled comparison with intramuscular meperidine for analgesia during labour. Br J Anaesth 2002; 89:466-72.
389. Howell CJ, Kidd C, Roberts W, et al. A randomised controlled trial of epidural compared with non-epidural analgesia in labour. Br J Obstet Gynaecol 2001; 108:27-33.
390. Howell CJ, Dean T, Lucking L, et al. Randomised study of long term outcome after epidural versus non-epidural analgesia during labour. Br Med J 2002; 325:357.
391. Macarthur A, Macarthur C, Weeks S. Epidural anesthesia and low back pain after delivery: A prospective cohort study. Br Med J 1995; 311:1336-9.
392. Macarthur AJ, Macarthur C, Weeks SK. Is epidural anesthesia in labor associated with chronic low back pain? A prospective cohort study. Anesth Analg 1997; 85:1066-70.
393. Sartore A, Pregazzi R, Bortoli P, et al. Effects of epidural analgesia during labor on pelvic floor function after vaginal delivery. Acta Obstet Gynecol Scand 2003; 82:143-6.
394. Noble AD, Craft IL, Bootes JA, et al. Continuous lumbar epidural analgesia using bupivacaine: A study of the fetus and newborn child. J Obstet Gynaecol Br Commonw 1971; 78:559-63.
395. Sivalingam T, Pleuvry BJ. Actions of morphine, pethidine and pentazocine on the oestrus and pregnant rat uterus in vitro. Br J Anaesth 1985; 57:430-3.
396. Yoo KY, Lee J, Kim HS, Jeong SW. The effects of opioids on isolated human pregnant uterine muscles. Anesth Analg 2001; 92:1006-9.
397. Neuhoff D, Burke MS, Porreco RP. Cesarean birth for failed progress in labor. Obstet Gynecol 1989; 73:915-20.
398. Guillemette J, Fraser WD. Differences between obstetricians in caesarean section rates and the management of labour. Br J Obstet Gynaecol 1992; 99:105-8.
399. Fraser W, Usher RH, McLean FH, et al. Temporal variation in rates of cesarean section for dystocia: Does "convenience" play a role? Am J Obstet Gynecol 1987; 156:300-4.
400. de Regt RH, Minkoff HL, Feldman J, Schwarz RH. Relation of private or clinic care to the cesarean birth rate. N Engl J Med 1986; 315:619-24.
401. Wuitchik M, Bakal D, Lipshitz J. The clinical significance of pain and cognitive activity in latent labor. Obstet Gynecol 1989; 73:35-42.
402. Alexander JM, Sharma SK, McIntire DD, et al. Intensity of labor pain and cesarean delivery. Anesth Analg 2001; 92:1524-8.
403. Hess PE, Pratt SD, Soni AK, et al. An association between severe labor pain and cesarean delivery. Anesth Analg 2000; 90:881-6.
404. Robinson JO, Rosen M, Evans JM, et al. Maternal opinion about analgesia for labour: A controlled trial between epidural block and intramuscular pethidine combined with inhalation. Anaesthesia 1980; 35:1173-81.
405. Philipsen T, Jensen NH. Maternal opinion about analgesia in labour and delivery: A comparison of epidural blockade and intramuscular pethidine. Eur J Obstet Gynecol Reprod Biol 1990; 34:205-10.
406. Clark A, Carr D, Loyd G, et al. The influence of epidural analgesia on cesarean delivery rates: A randomized, prospective clinical trial. Am J Obstet Gynecol 1998; 179:1527-33.
407. Sharma SK, Sidawi JE, Ramin SM, et al. Cesarean delivery: A randomized trial of epidural versus patient-controlled meperidine analgesia during labor. Anesthesiology 1997; 87:487-94.

408. Nikkola EM, Ekblad UU, Kerno PO, et al. Intravenous fentanyl PCA during labour. Can J Anaesth 1997; 44:1248-55.
409. Bofill JA, Vincent RD, Ross EL, et al. Nulliparous active labor, epidural analgesia, and cesarean delivery for dystocia. Am J Obstet Gynecol 1997; 177:1465-70.
410. Gambling DR, Sharma SK, Ramin SM, et al. A randomized study of combined spinal-epidural analgesia versus intravenous meperidine during labor: Impact on cesarean delivery rate. Anesthesiology 1998; 89:1336-44.
411. Loughnan BA, Carli F, Romney M, et al. Randomized controlled comparison of epidural bupivacaine versus pethidine for analgesia in labour. Br J Anaesth 2000; 84:715-9.
412. Sharma SK, Alexander JM, Messick G, et al. Cesarean delivery: A randomized trial of epidural analgesia versus intravenous meperidine analgesia during labor in nulliparous women. Anesthesiology 2002; 96:546-51.
413. Jain S, Arya VK, Gopalan S, Jain V. Analgesic efficacy of intramuscular opioids versus epidural analgesia in labor. Int J Gynaecol Obstet 2003; 83:19-27.
414. Halpern SH, Muir H, Breen TW, et al. A multicenter randomized controlled trial comparing patient-controlled epidural with intravenous analgesia for pain relief in labor. Anesth Analg 2004; 99:1532-8.
415. Lucas MJ, Sharma SK, McIntire DD, et al. A randomized trial of labor analgesia in women with pregnancy-induced hypertension. Am J Obstet Gynecol 2001; 185:970-5.
416. Head BB, Owen J, Vincent RD Jr, et al. A randomized trial of intrapartum analgesia in women with severe preeclampsia. Obstet Gynecol 2002; 99:452-7.
417. Sharma SK, Leveno KJ. Update: Epidural analgesia does not increase cesarean births. Curr Anesthesiol Rep 2000; 2:18-24.
418. Halpern SH, Leighton BL. Epidural analgesia and the progress of labor. In Halpern SH, Douglas MJ, editors. Evidence-based Obstetric Anesthesia. Oxford, Blackwell, 2005:10-22.
419. Sharma SK, McIntire DD, Wiley J, Leveno KJ. Labor analgesia and cesarean delivery: An individual patient meta-analysis of nulliparous women. Anesthesiology 2004; 100:142-8.
420. Comparative Obstetric Mobile Epidural Trial (COMET) Study Group UK. Effect of low-dose mobile versus traditional epidural techniques on mode of delivery: A randomised controlled trial. Lancet 2001; 358:19-23.
421. Collis RE, Davies DW, Aveling W. Randomised comparison of combined spinal-epidural and standard epidural analgesia in labour. Lancet 1995; 345:1413-6.
422. Nageotte MP, Larson D, Rumney PJ, et al. Epidural analgesia compared with combined spinal-epidural analgesia during labor in nulliparous women. N Engl J Med 1997; 337:1715-9.
423. Olofsson C, Ekblom A, Ekman-Ordeberg G, Irestedt L. Obstetric outcome following epidural analgesia with bupivacaine-adrenaline 0.25% or bupivacaine 0.125% with sufentanil—a prospective randomized controlled study in 1000 parturients. Acta Anaesthesiol Scand 1998; 42:284-92.
424. Norris MC, Fogel ST, Conway-Long C. Combined spinal-epidural versus epidural labor analgesia. Anesthesiology 2001; 95:913-20.
425. Yancey MK, Pierce B, Schweitzer D, Daniels D. Observations on labor epidural analgesia and operative delivery rates. Am J Obstet Gynecol 1999; 180:353-9.
426. Impey L, MacQuillan K, Robson M. Epidural analgesia need not increase operative delivery rates. Am J Obstet Gynecol 2000; 182:358-63.
427. Socol ML, Garcia PM, Peaceman AM, Dooley SL. Reducing cesarean births at a primarily private university hospital. Am J Obstet Gynecol 1993; 168:1748-58.
428. Johnson S, Rosenfield JA. The effect of epidural anesthesia on the length of labor. J Fam Pract 1995; 40:244-7.
429. Gribble RK, Meier PR. Effect of epidural analgesia on the primary cesarean rate. Obstet Gynecol 1991; 78:231-4.
430. Lyon DS, Knuckles G, Whitaker E, Salgado S. The effect of instituting an elective labor epidural program on the operative delivery rate. Obstet Gynecol 1997; 90:135-41.
431. Fogel ST, Shyken JM, Leighton BL, et al. Epidural labor analgesia and the incidence of Cesarean delivery for dystocia. Anesth Analg 1998; 87:119-23.
432. Segal S, Su M, Gilbert P. The effect of a rapid change in availability of epidural analgesia on the cesarean delivery rate: A meta-analysis. Am J Obstet Gynecol 2000; 183:974-8.
433. Lagrew DC Jr, Adashek JA. Lowering the cesarean section rate in a private hospital: Comparison of individual physicians' rates, risk factors, and outcomes. Am J Obstet Gynecol 1998; 178:1207-14.
434. Segal S, Blatman R, Doble M, Datta S. The influence of the obstetrician in the relationship between epidural analgesia and cesarean section for dystocia. Anesthesiology 1999; 91:90-6.
435. Seyb ST, Berka RJ, Socol ML, Dooley SL. Risk of cesarean delivery with elective induction of labor at term in nulliparous women. Obstet Gynecol 1999; 94:600-7.
436. American College of Obstetricians and Gynecologists. Obstetric analgesia and anesthesia. ACOG Practice Bulletin No. 36. Washington, DC, July 2002. (Obstet Gynecol, 2002; 100:177-91.)
437. Zhang J, Yancey MK, Klebanoff MA, et al. Does epidural analgesia prolong labor and increase risk of cesarean delivery? A natural experiment. Am J Obstet Gynecol 2001; 185:128-34.
438. Chestnut DH, Laszewski LJ, Pollack KL, et al. Continuous epidural infusion of 0.0625% bupivacaine-0.0002% fentanyl during the second stage of labor. Anesthesiology 1990; 72:613-8.
439. Chestnut DH, Vandewalker GE, Owen CL, et al. The influence of continuous epidural bupivacaine analgesia on the second stage of labor and method of delivery in nulliparous women. Anesthesiology 1987; 66:774-80.
440. Phillips KC, Thomas TA. Second stage of labour with or without extradural analgesia. Anaesthesia 1983; 38:972-6.
441. Johnsrud ML, Dale PO, Lovland B. Benefits of continuous infusion epidural analgesia throughout vaginal delivery. Acta Obstet Gynecol Scand 1988; 67:355-8.
442. Luxman D, Wolman I, Niv D, et al. Effect of second-stage 0.25% epidural bupivacaine on the outcome of labor. Gynecol Obstet Invest 1996; 42:167-70.
443. James KS, McGrady E, Quasim I, Patrick A. Comparison of epidural bolus administration of 0.25% bupivacaine and 0.1% bupivacaine with 0.0002% fentanyl for analgesia during labour. Br J Anaesth 1998; 81:501-10.
444. Robinson CA, Macones GA, Roth NW, Morgan MA. Does station of the fetal head at epidural placement affect the position of the fetal vertex at delivery? Am J Obstet Gynecol 1996; 175:991-4.
445. Le Ray C, Carayol M, Jaquemin S, et al. Is epidural analgesia a risk factor for occiput posterior or transverse positions during labour? Eur J Obstet Gynecol Reprod Biol 2005; 123:22-6.
446. Yancey MK, Zhang J, Schweitzer DL, et al. Epidural analgesia and fetal head malposition at vaginal delivery. Obstet Gynecol 2001; 97:608-12.
447. Sheiner E, Sheiner EK, Segal D, et al. Does the station of the fetal head during epidural analgesia affect labor and delivery? Int J Gynaecol Obstet 1999; 64:43-7.
448. Lieberman E, Davidson K, Lee-Parritz A, Shearer E. Changes in fetal position during labor and their association with epidural analgesia. Obstet Gynecol 2005; 105:974-82.
449. Chestnut DH. Epidural anesthesia and instrumental vaginal delivery. Anesthesiology 1991; 74:805-8.
450. Livnat EJ, Fejgin M, Scommegna A, et al. Neonatal acid-base balance in spontaneous and instrumental vaginal deliveries. Obstet Gynecol 1978; 52:549-51.
451. McBride WG, Black BP, Brown CJ, et al. Method of delivery and developmental outcome at five years of age. Med J Aust 1979; 1:301-4.
452. Friedman EA, Sachtleben-Murray MR, Dahrouge D, Neff RK. Long-term effects of labor and delivery on offspring: A matched-pair analysis. Am J Obstet Gynecol 1984; 150:941-5.
453. Gilstrap LC 3rd, Hauth JC, Schiano S, Connor KD. Neonatal acidosis and method of delivery. Obstet Gynecol 1984; 63:681-5.
454. Dierker LJ Jr, Rosen MG, Thompson K, Lynn P. Midforceps deliveries: Long-term outcome of infants. Am J Obstet Gynecol 1986; 154:764-8.

455. Robinson JN, Norwitz ER, Cohen AP, et al. Episiotomy, operative vaginal delivery, and significant perinatal trauma in nulliparous women. Am J Obstet Gynecol 1999; 181:1180-4.
456. Baumann P, Hammoud AO, McNeeley SG, et al. Factors associated with anal sphincter laceration in 40,923 primiparous women. Int Urogynecol J Pelvic Floor Dysfunct 2007; 18:985-90.
457. Dahl C, Kjolhede P. Obstetric anal sphincter rupture in older primiparous women: A case-control study. Acta Obstet Gynecol Scand 2006; 85:1252-8.
458. Schellenberg JC. Uterine activity during lumbar epidural analgesia with bupivacaine. Am J Obstet Gynecol 1977; 127:26-31.
459. Cheek TG, Samuels P, Miller F, et al. Normal saline i.v. fluid load decreases uterine activity in active labour. Br J Anaesth 1996; 77:632-5.
460. Zamora JE, Rosaeg OP, Lindsay MP, Crossan ML. Haemodynamic consequences and uterine contractions following 0.5 or 1.0 litre crystalloid infusion before obstetric epidural analgesia. Can J Anaesth 1996; 43:347-52.
461. Miller AC, DeVore JS, Eisler EA. Effects of anesthesia on uterine activity and labor. In Shnider SM, Levinson G, editors. Anesthesia for Obstetrics. 3rd edition. Baltimore, Williams & Wilkins, 1993:53-69.
462. Rahm VA, Hallgren A, Hogberg H, et al. Plasma oxytocin levels in women during labor with or without epidural analgesia: A prospective study. Acta Obstet Gynecol Scand 2002; 81:1033-9.
463. Behrens O, Goeschen K, Luck HJ, Fuchs AR. Effects of lumbar epidural analgesia on prostaglandin F_2 alpha release and oxytocin secretion during labor. Prostaglandins 1993; 45:285-96.
464. Nielsen PE, Abouleish E, Meyer BA, Parisi VM. Effect of epidural analgesia on fundal dominance during spontaneous active-phase nulliparous labor. Anesthesiology 1996; 84:540-4.
465. Clarke VT, Smiley RM, Finster M. Uterine hyperactivity after intrathecal injection of fentanyl for analgesia during labor: A cause of fetal bradycardia? Anesthesiology 1994; 81:1083.
466. Moir DD, Willocks J. Management of incoordinate uterine action under continuous epidural analgesia. Br Med J 1967; 3:396-400.
467. Lederman RP, Lederman E, Work BA Jr, McCann DS. The relationship of maternal anxiety, plasma catecholamines, and plasma cortisol to progress in labor. Am J Obstet Gynecol 1978; 132:495-500.
468. Gunther RE, Bauman J. Obstetrical caudal anesthesia. I. A randomized study comparing 1 per cent mepivacaine with 1 per cent lidocaine plus epinephrine. Anesthesiology 1969; 31:5-19.
469. Yau G, Gregory MA, Gin T, Oh TE. Obstetric epidural analgesia with mixtures of bupivacaine, adrenaline and fentanyl. Anaesthesia 1990; 45:1020-3.
470. Abboud TK, Khoo SS, Miller F, et al. Maternal, fetal, and neonatal responses after epidural anesthesia with bupivacaine, 2-chloroprocaine, or lidocaine. Anesth Analg 1982; 61:638-44.
471. Tsen LC, Thue B, Datta S, Segal S. Is combined spinal-epidural analgesia associated with more rapid cervical dilation in nulliparous patients when compared with conventional epidural analgesia? Anesthesiology 1999; 91:920-5.
472. Katz M, Lunenfeld E, Meizner I, et al. The effect of the duration of the second stage of labour on the acid-base state of the fetus. Br J Obstet Gynaecol 1987; 94:425-30.
473. Saunders NS, Paterson CM, Wadsworth J. Neonatal and maternal morbidity in relation to the length of the second stage of labour. Br J Obstet Gynaecol 1992; 99:381-5.
474. Derham RJ, Crowhurst J, Crowther C. The second stage of labour: Durational dilemmas. Aust N Z J Obstet Gynaecol 1991; 31:31-6.
475. Menticoglou SM, Manning F, Harman C, Morrison I. Perinatal outcome in relation to second-stage duration. Am J Obstet Gynecol 1995; 173:906-12.
476. American College of Obstetricians and Gynecologists. Dystocia and augmentation of labor. ACOG Practice Bulletin No. 49. Washington, DC, December 2003. (Obstet Gynecol 2003; 102:1445-54.)
477. Kadar N, Cruddas M, Campbell S. Estimating the probability of spontaneous delivery conditional on time spent in the second stage. Br J Obstet Gynaecol 1986; 93:568-76.
478. Paterson CM, Saunders NS, Wadsworth J. The characteristics of the second stage of labour in 25,069 singleton deliveries in the North West Thames Health Region, 1988. Br J Obstet Gynaecol 1992; 99:377-80.
479. Vause S, Congdon HM, Thornton JG. Immediate and delayed pushing in the second stage of labor for nulliparous women with epidural analgesia: A randomized controlled trial. Br J Obstet Gynaecol 1998; 105:186-8.
480. Plunkett BA, Lin A, Wong CA, et al. Management of the second stage of labor in nulliparas with continuous epidural analgesia. Obstet Gynecol 2003; 102:109-14.
481. Hansen SL, Clark SL, Foster JC. Active pushing versus passive fetal descent in the second stage of labor: A randomized controlled trial. Obstet Gynecol 2002; 99:29-34.
482. Fraser WD, Marcoux S, Krauss I, et al. Multicenter, randomized, controlled trial of delayed pushing for nulliparous women in the second stage of labor with continuous epidural analgesia. The PEOPLE (Pushing Early or Pushing Late with Epidural) Study Group. Am J Obstet Gynecol 2000; 182:1165-72.
483. Fitzpatrick M, Harkin R, McQuillan K, et al. A randomised clinical trial comparing the effects of delayed versus immediate pushing with epidural analgesia on mode of delivery and faecal continence. Br J Obstet Gynaecol 2002; 109:1359-65.
484. Roberts CL, Torvaldsen S, Cameron CA, Olive E. Delayed versus early pushing in women with epidural analgesia: A systematic review and meta-analysis. Br J Obstet Gynaecol 2004; 111:1133-40.
485. Rosaeg OP, Campbell N, Crossan ML. Epidural analgesia does not prolong the third stage of labour. Can J Anaesth 2002; 49:490-2.
486. Lopez-Zeno JA, Peaceman AM, Adashek JA, Socol ML. A controlled trial of a program for the active management of labor. N Engl J Med 1992; 326:450-4.
487. O'Driscoll K, Meagher D, Boylan P. Active Management of Labor. 3rd edition. London, Mosby-Year Book, 1993.
488. Leighton BL, Halpern SH. The effects of epidural analgesia on labor, maternal, and neonatal outcomes: A systematic review. Am J Obstet Gynecol 2002; 186:S69-77.
489. Kotaska AJ, Klein MC, Liston RM. Epidural analgesia associated with low-dose oxytocin augmentation increases cesarean births: A critical look at the external validity of randomized trials. Am J Obstet Gynecol 2006; 194:809-14.
490. Lupe PJ, Gross TL. Maternal upright posture and mobility in labor—a review. Obstet Gynecol 1986; 67:727-34.
491. Collis RE, Harding SA, Morgan BM. Effect of maternal ambulation on labour with low-dose combined spinal-epidural analgesia. Anaesthesia 1999; 54:535-9.
492. Frenea S, Chirossel C, Rodriguez R, et al. The effects of prolonged ambulation on labor with epidural analgesia. Anesth Analg 2004; 98:224-9.
493. Karraz MA. Ambulatory epidural anesthesia and the duration of labor. Int J Gynaecol Obstet 2003; 80:117-22.
494. Vallejo MC, Firestone LL, Mandell GL, et al. Effect of epidural analgesia with ambulation on labor duration. Anesthesiology 2001; 95:857-61.
495. Roberts CL, Algert CS, Olive E. Impact of first-stage ambulation on mode of delivery among women with epidural analgesia. Aust N Z J Obstet Gynaecol 2004; 44:489-94.
496. Bloom SL, McIntire DD, Kelly MA, et al. Lack of effect of walking on labor and delivery. N Engl J Med 1998; 339:76-9.
497. Eddleston JM, Maresh M, Horsman EL, Young H. Comparison of the maternal and fetal effects associated with intermittent or continuous infusion of extradural analgesia. Br J Anaesth 1992; 69:154-158.
498. Lavin JP, Samuels SV, Miodovnik M, et al. The effects of bupivacaine and chloroprocaine as local anesthetics for epidural anesthesia of fetal heart rate monitoring parameters. Am J Obstet Gynecol 1981; 141:717-22.
499. Boehm FH, Woodruff LF Jr, Growdon JH Jr. The effect of lumbar epidural anesthesia on fetal heart rate baseline variability. Anesth Analg 1975; 54:779-82.
500. Loftus JR, Holbrook RH, Cohen SE. Fetal heart rate after epidural lidocaine and bupivacaine for elective cesarean section. Anesthesiology 1991; 75:406-12.

501. Nielsen PE, Erickson JR, Abouleish EI, et al. Fetal heart rate changes after intrathecal sufentanil or epidural bupivacaine for labor analgesia: Incidence and clinical significance. Anesth Analg 1996; 83:742-6.

502. Pello LC, Rosevear SK, Dawes GS, et al. Computerized fetal heart rate analysis in labor. Obstet Gynecol 1991; 78:602-10.

503. Viscomi CM, Hood DD, Melone PJ, Eisenach JC. Fetal heart rate variability after epidural fentanyl during labor. Anesth Analg 1990; 71:679-83.

504. Wilhite AO, Moore CH, Blass NH, Christmas JT. Plasma concentration profile of epidural alfentanil: Bolus followed by continuous infusion technique in the parturient: Effect of epidural alfentanil and fentanyl on fetal heart rate. Reg Anesth 1994; 19:164-8.

505. Hill JB, Alexander JM, Sharma SK, et al. A comparison of the effects of epidural and meperidine analgesia during labor on fetal heart rate. Obstet Gynecol 2003; 102:333-7.

506. Smith CV, Rayburn WF, Allen KV, et al. Influence of intravenous fentanyl on fetal biophysical parameters during labor. J Matern Fetal Med 1996; 5:89-92.

507. Scanlon JW, Ostheimer GW, Lurie AO, et al. Neurobehavioral responses and drug concentrations in newborns after maternal epidural anesthesia with bupivacaine. Anesthesiology 1976; 45:400-5.

508. Albright GA, Forster RM. Does combined spinal-epidural analgesia with subarachnoid sufentanil increase the incidence of emergency cesarean delivery? Reg Anesth 1997; 22:400-5.

509. Van de Velde M, Teunkens A, Hanssens M, et al. Intrathecal sufentanil and fetal heart rate abnormalities: A double-blind, double placebo-controlled trial comparing two forms of combined spinal epidural analgesia with epidural analgesia in labor. Anesth Analg 2004; 98:1153-9.

510. Weinberg G. LipidRescue for cardiac resuscitation. Available at www.lipidrescue.org/

511. Sia AT, Chong JL. Epidural 0.2% ropivacaine for labour analgesia: Parturient-controlled or continuous infusion? Anaesth Intensive Care 1999; 27:154-8.

512. Smedvig JP, Soreide E, Gjessing L. Ropivacaine 1 mg/mL plus fentanyl 2 µg/mL for epidural analgesia during labor: Is mode of administration important? Acta Anaesthesiol Scand 2001; 45:595-9.

513. Muir HA, Shukla R, Liston R, Writer D. Randomized trial of labour analgesia. A pilot study to compare patient-controlled intravenous analgesia with patient-controlled epidural analgesia to determine if analgesia method affects delivery outcome (abstract). Can J Anaesth 1996; 43:A60.

514. Rogers R, Gilson G, Kammerer-Doak D. Epidural analgesia and active management of labor and mode of delivery. Obstet Gynecol 1999; 93:995-8.

515. Sharma SK, Alexander JM, Wiley J, Leveno KJ. Effects of epidural analgesia in early labor on cesarean delivery. Anesthesiology 2003; 98(Suppl 1):34.

516. Vahratian A, Zhang J, Hasling J, et al. The effect of early epidural versus early intravenous analgesia use on labor progression: A natural experiment. Am J Obstet Gynecol 2004; 191:259-65.

517. Buxton EJ, Redmon CWE, Obhrai M. Delayed pushing with lumbar epidural in labor—does it increase the incidence of spontaneous delivery? J Obstet Gynaecol 1988; 8:258-61.

518. Goodfellow CF, Studd C. The reduction in forceps in primigravidae with epidural analgesia—a controlled trial. Br J Clin Pract 1979; 33:287-8.

519. Mayberry LJ, Hammer R, Kelly C, et al. Use of delayed pushing with epidural anesthesia: Findings from a randomized, controlled trial. J Perinatol 1999; 19:26-30.

520. McQueen J, Myrlea L. Lumbar epidural analgesia in labor. Br Med J 1977; 1:640-1.

Chapter 24

Alternative Regional Anesthetic Techniques: Paracervical Block, Lumbar Sympathetic Block, Pudendal Nerve Block, and Perineal Infiltration

David H. Chestnut, M.D.

Epidural analgesia/anesthesia and spinal analgesia/anesthesia are the most flexible analgesic techniques available for obstetric patients. The anesthesia provider may use an epidural or a spinal technique to provide effective analgesia during the first and/or second stage of labor. Subsequently, the epidural or spinal technique may be used to achieve profound anesthesia for either vaginal or cesarean delivery. Unfortunately, some maternal conditions (e.g., coagulopathy, hemorrhage) contraindicate the administration of epidural and spinal analgesia. Many parturients do not have access to epidural or spinal analgesia, and others do not want it. The purpose of this chapter is to discuss alternative regional anesthetic techniques for labor and vaginal delivery.

PARACERVICAL BLOCK

During the first stage of labor, pain results primarily from dilation of the cervix and distention of the lower uterine segment and upper vagina. Pain impulses are transmitted from the upper vagina, cervix, and lower uterine segment by visceral afferent nerve fibers that join the sympathetic chain at L2 to L3 and enter the spinal cord at T10 to L1. Some obstetricians perform paracervical block to provide analgesia during the first stage of labor. The goal is to block transmission through the paracervical ganglion—also known as *Frankenhäuser's ganglion*—which lies immediately lateral and posterior to the cervicouterine junction.

Paracervical block does not adversely affect the progress of labor. Further, it provides analgesia without the annoying sensory and motor blockade that may result from epidural and spinal anesthesia. The paracervical technique does not block somatic sensory fibers from the lower vagina, vulva, and perineum. Thus, it does not relieve the pain caused by distention of these structures during the late first stage and second stage of labor. Contemporary experience suggests that paracervical block results in good to excellent analgesia during the first stage of labor in 50% to 75% of parturients. One study noted that paracervical block provided better analgesia in nulliparous women than in parous women, probably because paracervical block does not provide effective analgesia for the sudden and rapid descent of the presenting part that often occurs in parous women.[1]

In 1981, approximately 5% of obstetric patients in the United States received paracervical block.[2] Approximately 12% of parturients received paracervical block during labor in Sweden between 1983 and 1986,[3] and in some parts of Scandinavia it remains the most commonly used form of regional analgesia during labor. In the United States, the decline in the popularity of paracervical block has resulted from both fear of fetal complications and the greater popularity of epidural and spinal anesthetic techniques.

American and European medical journals have reported more than 50 perinatal deaths associated with paracervical block.[4-7] As early as 1963, Nyirjesy et al.[4] stated, "We feel that the high incidence of infant complications found in this study warrants the discontinuation of the obstetric use of paracervical block in our own practice." In 1986, Shnider[8] opined that paracervical block during labor "should be largely abandoned." Subsequently, he recommended that this technique be avoided in cases of uteroplacental insufficiency or preexisting fetal compromise. He acknowledged that "there may be exceptions if other anesthetic techniques are contraindicated or pose a greater hazard to the mother or fetus."[7] As recently as 2001, 2% to 3% of parturients in the United States received paracervical block during labor.[9]

Some obstetricians argue that in the absence of fetal bradycardia, paracervical block has few adverse effects on the infant. Jensen et al.[10] randomly assigned 117 nulliparous women to receive either paracervical block with 12 mL of 0.25% bupivacaine or 75 mg of intramuscular meperidine. Women in the paracervical block group had significantly better analgesia than women in the meperidine group at 20, 40, and 60 minutes. During the first 60 minutes, pain relief was complete or acceptable in 78% of the women in the paracervical block group but in only 31% of the women in the meperidine group. Two fetuses in the paracervical block group and one in the meperidine group had transient bradycardia. A total of 6 infants in the paracervical block group and 16 infants in the meperidine group ($P < .05$) had fetal/neonatal depression, which the investigators defined as an umbilical arterial blood pH of 7.15 or less and/or a 1-minute Apgar score of 7 or less.[10]

Kangas-Saarela et al.[11] compared neonatal neurobehavioral responses in 10 infants whose mothers received bupivacaine paracervical block with those in 12 infants whose mothers received no analgesia. The investigators performed paracervical block while each patient lay in a left lateral position, and they limited the depth of the injection into the vaginal mucosa to 3 mm or less. They observed no significant differences between groups in neurobehavioral responses at 3 hours, 1 day, 2 days, or 4 to 5 days after delivery. These investigators concluded that properly performed paracervical block does not adversely affect newborn behavior or neurologic function.[11]

Technique

Paracervical block is performed with the patient in a modified lithotomy position. The uterus should be displaced leftward during performance of the block; this displacement may be accomplished by placing a folded pillow beneath the patient's right buttock. The physician uses a needle guide to define and limit the depth of the injection and to reduce the risk of vaginal or fetal injury. The physician introduces the needle and needle guide into the vagina with the left hand for the left side of the pelvis and with the right hand for the right side (Figure 24-1). The needle and needle guide are introduced into the left or right lateral vaginal fornix, near the cervix, at the 4 o'clock or 8 o'clock position. The needle is advanced through the vaginal mucosa to a depth of 2 to 3 mm.[12] The physician should aspirate before each injection of local anesthetic. A total of 5 to 10 mL of local anesthetic, without epinephrine, is injected on each side.[13] Some obstetricians recommend giving incremental doses of local anesthetic on each side (e.g., 2.5 to 5 mL of local anesthetic between the 3 and 4 o'clock positions, followed by 2.5 to 5 mL between the 4 and 5 o'clock positions).[12,14,15]

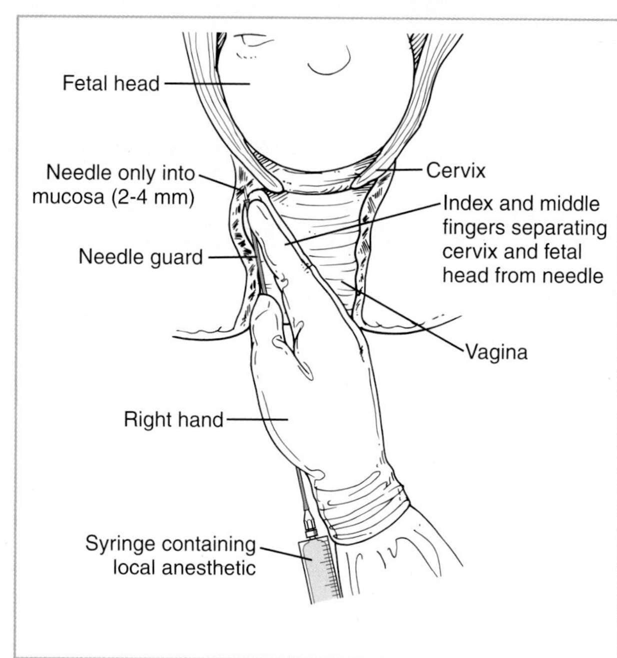

FIGURE 24-1 Technique of paracervical block. Notice the position of the hand and fingers in relation to the cervix and fetal head. No undue pressure is applied at the vaginal fornix by the fingers or the needle guide, and the needle is inserted to a shallow depth. (Redrawn from Abouleish E. Pain Control in Obstetrics. New York, JB Lippincott, 1977:344.)

After injecting the local anesthetic in either the left or right lateral vaginal fornix, the physician should wait 5 to 10 minutes and observe the fetal heart rate (FHR) before injecting the local anesthetic on the other side.[15] Some obstetricians do not endorse this recommendation. Van Dorsten et al.[16] randomly assigned 42 healthy parturients at term to either of two methods of paracervical block. The study group experienced a 10-minute interval between injections of local anesthetic on the left and right sides of the vagina. The control group had almost simultaneous injections on the left and right sides. No cases of fetal bradycardia occurred in either group. The investigators concluded that patient selection and lateral positioning after the block have a more important role in the prevention of post–paracervical block fetal bradycardia than spacing the injections of local anesthetic. However, because they studied only 42 patients and had no cases of fetal bradycardia in either group, they could not exclude the possibility that incremental injection might reduce the incidence of fetal bradycardia in a larger series of patients.

Choice of Local Anesthetic

The physician should administer small volumes of a dilute solution of local anesthetic. There is no reason to inject more than 10 mL of local anesthetic on each side. Further, there is no indication for the use of concentrated solutions, such as 2% lidocaine, 0.5% bupivacaine, or 3%

2-chloroprocaine. Nieminen and Puolakka[17] observed that paracervical block with 10 mL of 0.125% bupivacaine (5 mL on each side) provided analgesia similar to that provided by 10 mL of 0.25% bupivacaine.

The choice of local anesthetic is controversial. The North American manufacturers of bupivacaine have stated that bupivacaine is contraindicated for the performance of paracervical block. In contrast, many European obstetricians—especially those in Finland—have expressed a preference for bupivacaine for this procedure. Bupivacaine has greater cardiotoxicity than other local anesthetic agents, and some investigators have suggested that its use leads to a higher incidence of fetal bradycardia or adverse outcome than use of other local anesthetics for paracervical block. In a review of 50 cases of perinatal death associated with paracervical block, Teramo[6] found that the local anesthetic was bupivacaine in at least 29 of the 50 cases.

Palomaki et al.[18] hypothesized that levobupivacaine might result in a lower incidence of post–paracervical block fetal bradycardia than racemic bupivacaine. In a randomized double-blind study of 397 laboring women, paracervical block was performed with 10 mL of either 0.25% levobupivacaine or 0.25% racemic bupivacaine. The incidence of transient FHR abnormalities was 10.4% in the levobupivacaine group and 12.8% in the racemic bupivacaine group, and that of fetal bradycardia was 2.6% in the levobupivacaine group and 3.8% in the racemic bupivacaine group (P = NS).

Some physicians have suggested that 2-chloroprocaine is the local anesthetic of choice for paracervical block. Published studies suggest but do not prove that post–paracervical block fetal bradycardia occurs less frequently with 2-chloroprocaine than with amide local anesthetics.[14,19-21] Weiss et al.[19] performed a double-blind study in which 60 patients were randomly assigned to receive 20 mL of either 2% 2-chloroprocaine or 1% lidocaine for paracervical block. Bradycardia occurred in 1 of the 29 fetuses in the 2-chloroprocaine group, compared with 5 of 31 fetuses in the lidocaine group (P = .14). LeFevre[21] retrospectively observed that fetal bradycardia occurred after 2 (6%) of 33 paracervical blocks performed with 2-chloroprocaine versus 44 (12%) of 361 paracervical blocks performed with mepivacaine (P = 0.29).

2-Chloroprocaine undergoes rapid enzymatic hydrolysis. Thus it has the shortest intravascular half-life among the local anesthetics used clinically. This rapid metabolism seems advantageous in the event of unintentional intravascular or fetal injection. Philipson et al.[20] performed paracervical block with 10 mL of 1% 2-chloroprocaine in 16 healthy parturients. At delivery, only trace concentrations of 2-chloroprocaine were detected in 1 (6%) of the maternal blood samples and 4 (25%) of the umbilical cord venous blood samples. The investigators concluded:

> *In all of the studies of paracervical block with 2-chloroprocaine, there were no cases in which the abnormal fetal heart rate patterns were associated with depressed neonates. This is in contrast to the studies with amide local anesthetics and may be explained by the rapid enzymatic inactivation of 2-chloroprocaine.*[20]

Some obstetricians dislike 2-chloroprocaine because of its relatively short duration of action. However, in one study the mean duration of analgesia was 40 minutes after paracervical administration of either 2-chloroprocaine or lidocaine.[19] Philipson and Kuhnert[22] suggested that if paracervical block with 2-chloroprocaine has a shorter duration than the amide local anesthetics, "frequent contact with the anesthetist or obstetrician provides opportunities for additional support and reassurance of the patient."

BOX 24-1 Maternal Complications of Paracervical Block

- Vasovagal syncope
- Laceration of the vaginal mucosa
- Systemic local anesthetic toxicity
- Parametrial hematoma
- Postpartum neuropathy
- Paracervical, retropsoal, or subgluteal abscess

Maternal Complications

Maternal complications of paracervical block are uncommon but may be serious (Box 24-1).[23-26] Systemic local anesthetic toxicity may result from direct intravascular injection or rapid systemic absorption of the local anesthetic. Postpartum neuropathy may follow direct sacral plexus trauma, or it may result from hematoma formation. Retropsoal and subgluteal abscesses are rare but may result in major maternal morbidity or mortality.[25,26]

Fetal Complications

In some cases, fetal injury results from direct injection of local anesthetic into the fetal scalp during paracervical block.[7,27] Fetal scalp injection of 10 or 20 mL of local anesthetic undoubtedly causes systemic local anesthetic toxicity, which may result in fetal death. Fetal scalp injection seems more likely to occur when the obstetrician performs paracervical block in the presence of advanced (i.e., more than 8 cm) cervical dilation.

Bradycardia is the most common fetal complication. Fetal bradycardia typically develops within 2 to 10 minutes after the injection of local anesthetic. Most cases resolve within 5 to 10 minutes, but some cases of bradycardia persist for as long as 30 minutes. Published studies have noted an incidence of bradycardia that varies between 0 and 70%.[15,21,28-34] These figures represent extremes on either side of the true incidence of this complication. Some studies have overstated the problem by defining bradycardia as a baseline FHR of less than 120 bpm. (A baseline FHR of 110 bpm does not necessarily indicate fetal compromise.) Experienced obstetricians clearly do not encounter clinically significant fetal bradycardia after 70% of their paracervical blocks. It is equally clear that the incidence of clinically significant fetal bradycardia is not zero, and it is difficult to teach this technique without placing some fetuses at risk. In a review of four randomized controlled trials published between 1975 and 2000, Rosen[34] estimated that the incidence of post–paracervical block fetal bradycardia is 15%.

Shnider et al.[30] reported that fetal bradycardia occurred after 24% of 845 paracervical blocks administered to 705 patients with either 1% mepivacaine, 1% lidocaine, or 1% propitocaine. Neonatal depression occurred significantly more often in infants who had FHR changes after paracervical block than in a control group or in a group of infants with no FHR changes after paracervical block. In contrast, Carlsson et al.[31] performed 523 paracervical blocks with 0.125% or 0.25% bupivacaine in 469 women. Of the total, 9 (1.9%) fetuses had bradycardia, but all 9 of these neonates had a 5-minute Apgar score of 9 or 10.

Goins[32] noted that fetal bradycardia occurred in 24 (13%) of 182 patients who received paracervical block with 20 mL of 1% mepivacaine between 1988 and 1990. He compared neonatal outcome for these patients with neonatal outcome for 343 patients who received other analgesic/anesthetic techniques. There was a slightly higher incidence of low Apgar scores at 1 minute and 5 minutes in the paracervical block group, but the difference was not statistically significant. LeFevre[21] observed fetal bradycardia after 46 (11%) of 408 paracervical blocks. Fetal bradycardia was more common in those patients with nonreassuring FHR tracings before the performance of paracervical block.

ETIOLOGY OF FETAL BRADYCARDIA

The etiology of fetal bradycardia after paracervical block is unclear. Investigators have offered at least four theories that might explain the etiology of fetal bradycardia, as discussed here.

Reflex Bradycardia

Manipulation of the fetal head, the uterus, or the uterine blood vessels during performance of the block may cause reflex fetal bradycardia.[29]

Direct Fetal Central Nervous System and Myocardial Depression

The performance of paracervical block results in the injection of large volumes of local anesthetic close to the uteroplacental circulation. Local anesthetic rapidly crosses the placenta[35] and may cause fetal central nervous system (CNS) depression, myocardial depression, and/or umbilical vasoconstriction. Puolakka et al.[36] observed that the most common abnormality after paracervical block was the disappearance of FHR accelerations. They speculated that FHR changes result from rapid transplacental passage of local anesthetic into the fetal circulation, followed by a direct toxic effect of the local anesthetic on the FHR regulatory centers.

Some investigators have suggested that fetal bradycardia results from a direct toxic effect of the local anesthetic on the fetal heart.[37,38] Shnider et al.[37] reported that in four cases of fetal bradycardia, mepivacaine concentrations in fetal scalp blood were higher than peak concentrations in maternal arterial blood. Asling et al.[38] made similar observations in six of seven cases of fetal bradycardia. They suggested that local anesthetic reaches the fetus by a more direct route than maternal systemic absorption, and they speculated that high fetal concentrations of local anesthetic result from local anesthetic diffusion across the uterine arteries. This would lead to local anesthetic concentrations in intervillous blood that are higher than concentrations in maternal brachial arterial blood. High fetal concentrations would then occur from the passive diffusion of local anesthetic across the placenta.

High fetal concentrations of local anesthetic also may result from fetal acidosis and ion trapping.[39,40] Local anesthetics are weak bases, and if acidosis develops in a fetus, increasing amounts of local anesthetic will cross the placenta regardless of the site of maternal injection. It is also possible that the obstetrician may directly inject local anesthetic into uterine blood vessels.

Most studies have noted that local anesthetic concentrations in the fetus are consistently lower than those in the mother after paracervical block.[13] Further, fetal bradycardia has not consistently occurred in documented cases of fetal local anesthetic toxicity. Freeman et al.[41] injected 300 mg of mepivacaine directly into the fetal scalps of two anencephalic fetuses. The QRS complex widened, the P-R interval lengthened, and both fetuses died, but fetal bradycardia did not occur before fetal death. In contrast, the investigators observed no widening of the QRS complex or lengthening of the P-R interval in normal fetuses demonstrating bradycardia after paracervical block. Rather, the fetal electrocardiogram (ECG) changes were consistent with sinoatrial node suppression with a wandering atrial pacemaker. The investigators concluded that a mechanism other than direct fetal myocardial depression is responsible for fetal bradycardia after paracervical block.

Increased Uterine Activity

Increased uterine activity results in decreased uteroplacental perfusion. Fishburne et al.[42] noted that direct uterine arterial injection of bupivacaine consistently caused a significant increase in uterine tone in gravid ewes. Uterine arterial injection of 2-chloroprocaine did not affect myometrial tone, whereas injection of lidocaine had an intermediate effect.

Myometrial injection of a local anesthetic also may cause greater uterine activity. Morishima et al.[43] performed paracervical block with either lidocaine or 2-chloroprocaine in pregnant baboons with normal and acidotic fetuses. A transient increase in uterine activity and a significant reduction in uterine blood flow occurred after paracervical block in 73% of the mothers. Approximately 33% of the normal fetuses and all of the acidotic fetuses had bradycardia after paracervical block. The acidotic fetuses had more severe bradycardia, greater hypoxemia, and slower recovery of oxygenation compared with fetuses that were well oxygenated before paracervical block. The researchers concluded that post–paracervical block fetal bradycardia is in part a result of greater uterine activity, diminished uteroplacental perfusion, and decreased oxygen delivery to the fetus. They also concluded that paracervical block should be avoided in the presence of fetal compromise.

Uterine and/or Umbilical Artery Vasoconstriction

The deposition of local anesthetic in close proximity to the uterine arteries may cause uterine artery vasoconstriction, with a subsequent drop in uteroplacental perfusion. At least two studies noted that lidocaine and mepivacaine caused vasoconstriction of human uterine arteries *in vitro*.[44,45] (These studies were performed before recognition of the importance of intact endothelium during investigation of vascular smooth muscle response.) Similarly, Norén et al.[46,47] noted that bupivacaine caused concentration-dependent contraction of uterine arterial smooth muscle from rats and pregnant women. The calcium entry–blocking drugs verapamil and nifedipine decreased the vascular smooth muscle contraction caused by bupivacaine.

The researchers concluded that the use of bupivacaine for paracervical block may cause uterine artery vasoconstriction, especially when the bupivacaine is injected close to the uterine arteries. Further, they suggested that the administration of a calcium entry–blocking drug may successfully eliminate this vasoconstrictive effect of bupivacaine. (Although these studies were performed in 1991, the researchers did not mention whether they preserved, removed, or even observed the presence of the vascular endothelium. The presence of vascular endothelium may alter the response of vascular smooth muscle to local anesthetics.[48])

Greiss et al.[49] observed that intra-aortic injection of lidocaine or mepivacaine led to decreased uterine blood flow in gravid ewes. Similarly, Fishburne et al.[42] noted that direct uterine arterial injection of lidocaine, bupivacaine, or 2-chloroprocaine reduced uterine blood flow in gravid ewes. They concluded that only paracervical block "would be expected to produce the high, sustained uterine arterial concentrations of anesthetic drugs that cause the significant reductions in uterine blood flow which we now feel are the etiology of fetal bradycardia."[42] In a later study, Manninen et al.[50] observed that paracervical injection of 10 mL of 0.25% bupivacaine led to an increase in the uterine artery pulsatility index (PI)—an estimate of uterine vascular resistance—in healthy nulliparous women, suggesting that paracervical block may result in uterine artery vasoconstriction.

In contrast, Puolakka et al.[36] used xenon 133 (^{133}Xe) to measure intervillous blood flow before and after the performance of paracervical block with 10 mL of 0.25% bupivacaine in 10 parturients. They observed no decrease in mean intervillous blood flow in these patients. Further, they noted minimal change in intervillous blood flow in the three patients who had fetal bradycardia after paracervical block. Using Doppler ultrasonography, Räsänen and Jouppila[51] observed no significant change in either uterine or umbilical artery PI after the performance of paracervical block with 10 mL of 0.25% bupivacaine in 12 healthy parturients. However, fetal bradycardia occurred in two patients, and in those two cases, a marked increase in umbilical artery PI occurred.

Baxi et al.[52] performed paracervical block with 20 mL of 1% lidocaine in 10 pregnant patients. They observed a decrease in fetal transcutaneous Po_2 5 minutes after injecting lidocaine in each of the 10 patients. There was a maximum decline in transcutaneous Po_2 at 11.5 minutes, and transcutaneous Po_2 returned to baseline by approximately 31 minutes. Some but not all of the patients had increased uterine activity after paracervical block. In contrast, Jacobs et al.[53] observed a consistent, sustained decrease in fetal transcutaneous Po_2 after only 1 of 10 paracervical blocks performed with 10 mL of 0.25% bupivacaine. These investigators attributed their good results to the following precautions: (1) performance of paracervical block only in healthy mothers with normal pregnancies; (2) administration of a small dose of bupivacaine; (3) a limited depth of injection; (4) administration of bupivacaine in four incremental injections (i.e., two injections on each side); and (5) use of the left lateral position immediately after performance of the block. In a later study, Kaita et al.[54] observed that paracervical injection of 10 mL of 0.25% bupivacaine in 10 healthy parturients resulted in a slight (clinically insignificant) increase in fetal Sao_2 as measured by fetal pulse oximetry.

Summary

Most observers currently believe that post–paracervical block bradycardia results from reduced uteroplacental and/or fetoplacental perfusion. Reduction in uteroplacental perfusion may occur because of increased uterine activity and/or a direct vasoconstrictive effect of the local anesthetic. Likewise, decreased umbilical cord blood flow may result from increased uterine activity and/or umbilical cord vasoconstriction. Regardless of the etiology, the severity and duration of fetal bradycardia correlate with the incidence of fetal acidosis and subsequent neonatal depression. Freeman et al.[41] reported a significant drop in pH and a rise in base deficit only in fetuses with bradycardia of longer than 10 minutes' duration. In an observational study of paracervical block and nalbuphine analgesia during labor, Levy et al.[55] observed no association between paracervical block and low umbilical artery blood pH at delivery.

Physician Complications

The performance of paracervical block requires the physician to make several blind needle punctures within the vagina. The needle guide does not consistently protect the physician from a needle-stick injury. Thus the performance of paracervical block may entail the risk of physician exposure to human immunodeficiency virus (HIV) or another virus.

Recommendations

It is difficult for me to offer enthusiasm for the performance of paracervical block in contemporary obstetric practice. Nonetheless, there likely remain some circumstances in which paracervical block is an appropriate technique. I offer the following recommendations for safe practice:

1. Perform paracervical block only in healthy parturients at term who have no evidence of uteroplacental insufficiency or fetal compromise.
2. Continuously monitor the FHR and uterine activity before, during, and after performance of paracervical block. Perform paracervical block only in patients with a reassuring FHR tracing. An obvious exception would be a patient whose fetus has an anomaly incompatible with life (e.g., anencephaly).
3. Do not perform paracervical block when the cervix is dilated 8 cm or more.
4. Establish intravenous access before performing paracervical block.
5. Maintain left uterine displacement while performing the block.
6. Limit the depth of injection to approximately 3 mm.
7. Aspirate before each injection of local anesthetic.
8. After injecting the local anesthetic on one side, wait 5 to 10 minutes and observe the FHR before injecting the local anesthetic on the other side.
9. Administer small volumes of a dilute solution of local anesthetic; 2-chloroprocaine is the agent of choice.

10. Avoid the administration of epinephrine-containing local anesthetic solutions.
11. Monitor the mother's blood pressure after performance of the block. Maintain normal maternal blood pressure.
12. If fetal bradycardia should occur, try to achieve fetal resuscitation *in utero*. Discontinue oxytocin, administer supplemental oxygen, and ensure that the patient is on her left side. Perform operative delivery if the fetal bradycardia persists beyond 10 minutes.

LUMBAR SYMPATHETIC BLOCK

In 1933, Cleland[56] demonstrated that lower uterine and cervical visceral afferent sensory fibers join the sympathetic chain at L2 to L3. Subsequently, lumbar sympathetic block was used as an effective—if not popular—method of first-stage analgesia in some hospitals.[57-60] Like paracervical block, paravertebral lumbar sympathetic block interrupts the transmission of pain impulses from the cervix and lower uterine segment to the spinal cord. Lumbar sympathetic block provides analgesia during the first stage of labor but does not relieve pain during the second stage.[61] It provides analgesia comparable to that provided by paracervical block but with less risk of fetal bradycardia.

Lumbar sympathetic block may have a favorable effect on the progress of labor. Hunter[62] reported that lumbar sympathetic block accelerated labor in 20 of 39 patients with a normal uterine contractile pattern before performance of the block. (Indeed, some of the patients in that study had a 5- to 15-minute period of uterine hypertonus after the block.) Further, he observed that lumbar sympathetic block converted an abnormal uterine contractile pattern to a normal pattern in 14 of 19 patients. He concluded that lumbar sympathetic block represents "one of the most reliable methods reported to actively convert an abnormal labor pattern to a normal pattern."[62] In a later study, Leighton et al.[63] randomly assigned 39 healthy nulliparous women at term to receive either epidural analgesia or lumbar sympathetic block. The women who received lumbar sympathetic block had a more rapid rate of cervical dilation during the first 2 hours of analgesia, a shorter second stage of labor, and a nonsignificant trend toward a lower incidence of cesarean delivery for dystocia. However, there was no difference between the groups in the rate of cervical dilation during the active phase of the first stage of labor.

Anesthesiologists may successfully perform lumbar sympathetic block when a history of previous back surgery precludes the successful administration of epidural anesthesia.[64] Some anesthesiologists offer lumbar sympathetic block to prepared childbirth enthusiasts who desire first-stage analgesia without any motor block or loss of perineal sensation. Meguiar and Wheeler[65] stated that the primary usefulness of lumbar sympathetic block is "in cases where continuous lumbar epidural analgesia is refused or contraindicated." They administered 20 mL of 0.5% bupivacaine with 1:200,000 epinephrine to 40 nulliparous women. Among these women, 38 experienced good analgesia, and 28 delivered before resolution of the block. Pain recurred before delivery in the remaining 12 women; the mean duration of analgesia was 283 ± 103 minutes among these patients.[65] Leighton et al.[63] administered the same dose of bupivacaine, but they observed a shorter duration of analgesia than that observed by Meguiar and Wheeler.[65]

During the last three decades, lumbar sympathetic block has all but disappeared from obstetric anesthesia practice in the United States, for several reasons. Anesthesiologists may minimize motor block during epidural analgesia by giving dilute solutions of local anesthetic, with or without an opioid. For those few patients who want to retain full perineal sensation, anesthesiologists may give an opioid alone, either intrathecally or epidurally. Thus there are few patients for whom lumbar sympathetic block holds unique advantages. Further, the procedure often is painful, and few anesthesiologists have acquired and maintained proficiency in performing lumbar sympathetic block in obstetric patients.

Lumbar sympathetic block remains an attractive technique in a small number of patients.[64] Alternatively, Nair and Henry[66] described the performance of bilateral paravertebral block for women in whom epidural analgesia is contraindicated.

Technique

With the patient in the sitting position, a 10-cm, 22-gauge needle is used to identify the transverse process on one side of the second lumbar vertebra. The needle is then withdrawn, redirected, and advanced another 5 cm so that the tip of the needle is at the anterolateral surface of the vertebral column, just anterior to the medial attachment of the psoas muscle. It is possible to place the needle within a blood vessel or the subarachnoid space; thus the anesthesiologist must aspirate before injecting the local anesthetic. Two 5-mL increments of a dilute solution of local anesthetic (with or without epinephrine) are then injected, and the procedure is repeated on the opposite side of the vertebral column.

Complications

Modest hypotension occurs in 5% to 15% of patients.[62,63,65] The incidence of hypotension can be reduced by giving 500 mL of lactated Ringer's solution intravenously before performing the block. Less common maternal complications are systemic local anesthetic toxicity, total spinal anesthesia, retroperitoneal hematoma, Horner's syndrome,[67] and post–dural puncture headache (PDPH).[68]

Fetal complications are unlikely unless hypotension or increased uterine activity results in decreased uteroplacental perfusion.

PUDENDAL NERVE BLOCK

During the second stage of labor, pain results from distention of the lower vagina, vulva, and perineum. The pudendal nerve, which includes somatic nerve fibers from the anterior primary divisions of the second, third, and fourth sacral nerves, represents the primary source of sensory innervation for the lower vagina, vulva, and perineum. The pudendal nerve also provides motor innervation to the perineal muscles and to the external anal sphincter.

In 1916, King[69] reported the use of pudendal nerve block for vaginal delivery. This procedure did not become popular until 1953 and 1954, when Klink[70] and Kohl[71] described the anatomy and reported modified techniques. Obstetricians often perform pudendal nerve block in patients without epidural or spinal anesthesia. The goal is to block the pudendal nerve distal to its formation by the anterior divisions of S2 to S4 but proximal to its division into its terminal branches (i.e., dorsal nerve of the clitoris, perineal nerve, and inferior hemorrhoidal nerve). Pudendal nerve block may provide satisfactory anesthesia for spontaneous vaginal delivery and perhaps for outlet-forceps delivery, but it provides inadequate anesthesia for mid-forceps delivery, postpartum examination and repair of the upper vagina and cervix, and manual exploration of the uterine cavity.[72]

Efficacy and Timing

The efficacy of pudendal nerve block varies according to the experience of the obstetrician. Unilateral or bilateral failure is common. Thus obstetricians typically perform simultaneous infiltration of the perineum, especially if the performance of pudendal nerve block is delayed until delivery. Scudamore and Yates[73] reported bilateral success rates of approximately 50% after use of the transvaginal route and of approximately 25% after use of the transperineal route. They concluded:

> *The term "pudendal block" is often a misnomer . . . If this limitation were more widely appreciated, then many mothers would be spared the unnecessary pain which is caused when relatively complicated procedures are attempted under inadequate anesthesia.*[73]

In the United States, most obstetricians perform pudendal nerve block immediately before delivery. This practice reflects their concern that perineal anesthesia prolongs the second stage of labor. An advantage to early pudendal nerve block is that the obstetrician may repeat the block on one or both sides if it should fail, provided that the maximum safe dose of local anesthetic is not exceeded. European obstetricians seem more willing to perform pudendal nerve block at the onset of the second stage of labor. Langhoff-Roos and Lindmark[74] administered pudendal nerve block before or just after complete cervical dilation in 551 (64%) of 865 women. In a nonrandomized study, Zador et al.[75] evaluated obstetric outcome in 24 patients who received pudendal nerve block when the cervix was completely dilated and in 24 patients who did not receive pudendal block. Pudendal nerve block slightly prolonged the second stage of labor, but it did not increase the incidence of instrumental vaginal delivery.[75]

It is barbaric to withhold analgesia during the second stage of labor. Obstetricians need not delay the administration of pudendal nerve block until delivery. Rather, for those patients without epidural or spinal analgesia, it seems appropriate to perform pudendal nerve block when the patient complains of vaginal and perineal pain. A 2004 study suggested that pudendal nerve block does not provide reliable analgesia during the second stage of labor but has greater efficacy for episiotomy and repair.[76] In a randomized, double-blind, placebo-controlled study, Aissaoui et al.[77] recently observed that unilateral, nerve stimulator–guided pudendal nerve block with ropivacaine was associated with decreased pain and less need for supplemental analgesia during the first 48 hours after performance of mediolateral episiotomy at vaginal delivery.

Technique

The transvaginal approach is more popular than the transperineal approach in the United States. The obstetrician uses a needle guide (either the Iowa trumpet or the Kobak needle guide) to prevent injury to the vagina and fetus. In contrast to the technique for paracervical block, the needle must protrude 1.0 to 1.5 cm beyond the needle guide to allow adequate penetration for injection of the local anesthetic. The obstetrician introduces the needle and needle guide into the vagina with the left hand for the left side of the pelvis and with the right hand for the right side (Figure 24-2). The needle is introduced through the vaginal mucosa and sacrospinous ligament, just medial and posterior to the ischial spine. The pudendal artery lies in close proximity to the pudendal nerve; thus the obstetrician must aspirate before and during the injection of local anesthetic. The obstetrician typically injects 7 to 10 mL of local anesthetic solution on each side. (Some obstetricians inject 3 mL of local anesthetic just above the

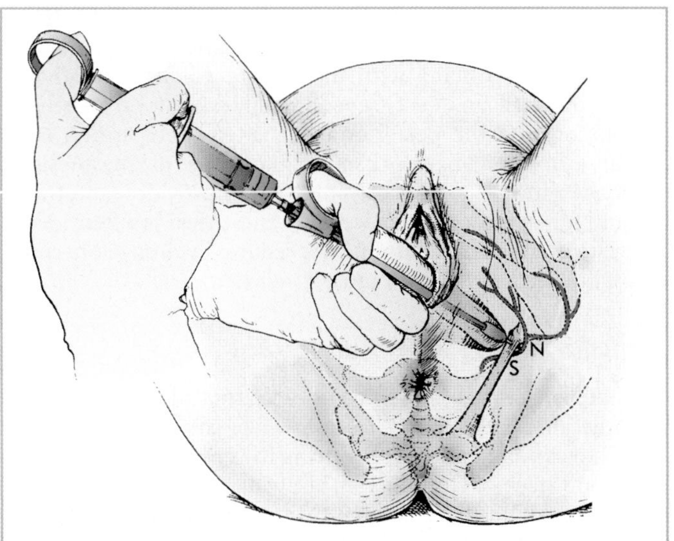

FIGURE 24-2 Local infiltration of the pudendal nerve. Transvaginal technique showing the needle extended beyond the needle guard and passing through the sacrospinous ligament (S) to reach the pudendal nerve (N). (From Cunningham FG, MacDonald PC, Gant NF, et al. Williams Obstetrics. 20th edition. Stamford, CT, Appleton and Lange, 1997:389.)

ischial spine on each side.[78]) The obstetrician should pay attention to the total dose of local anesthetic given, especially when repetitive pudendal nerve blocks or both pudendal nerve block and perineal infiltration are performed.

Choice of Local Anesthetic

Rapid maternal absorption of the local anesthetic occurs after the performance of pudendal nerve block.[75,78] Zador et al.[75] detected measurable concentrations of lidocaine in maternal venous and fetal scalp capillary blood samples within 5 minutes of the injection of 20 mL of 1% lidocaine. They detected peak concentrations between 10 and 20 minutes after injection. Kuhnert et al.[79] reported that after pudendal nerve block, neonatal urine concentrations of lidocaine and its metabolites were similar to those measured in neonatal urine after epidural administration of lidocaine.

Some physicians favor the administration of 2-chloroprocaine. Its rapid onset of action provides an advantage when pudendal nerve block is performed immediately before delivery. Its rapid metabolism and short intravascular half-life lower the likelihood of maternal or fetal systemic toxicity. 2-Chloroprocaine has the disadvantage of a short duration of action. However, if the obstetrician performs pudendal nerve block with 2-chloroprocaine at the onset of the second stage of labor, the block can be repeated as needed. When the block is performed immediately before delivery, the brief duration of action of 2-chloroprocaine is not a disadvantage for the experienced obstetrician.

Merkow et al.[80] evaluated neonatal neurobehavior in infants whose mothers received 30 mL of 0.5% bupivacaine, 1% mepivacaine, or 3% 2-chloroprocaine for pudendal nerve block and perineal infiltration before delivery. Neonatal response to pinprick at 4 hours was better in the mepivacaine group; otherwise there were no significant differences among groups in neurobehavioral scores at 4 and 24 hours after delivery.

Regardless of the choice of local anesthetic, there is no indication for the administration of a concentrated solution. For example, it is unnecessary, and perhaps dangerous, to give 0.5% bupivacaine, 2% lidocaine, or 3% 2-chloroprocaine. Rather, the obstetrician should use 2% 2-chloroprocaine or 1% lidocaine.

Some obstetricians contend that the addition of epinephrine to the local anesthetic solution improves the quality of pudendal nerve block. Langhoff-Roos and Lindmark[74] reported a randomized, double-blind study of 865 patients who received pudendal nerve block with 16 mL of 1% mepivacaine, 1% mepivacaine with epinephrine, or 0.25% bupivacaine. Mepivacaine with epinephrine provided effective anesthesia more often and also caused a greater "loss of the urge to bear down" than did the other two local anesthetic solutions. However, there was no significant difference among groups in the duration of the second stage or the incidence of instrumental vaginal delivery. Schierup et al.[81] randomly assigned 151 patients to receive pudendal nerve block with 20 mL of 1% mepivacaine either with or without epinephrine. The addition of epinephrine did not improve the quality of anesthesia. The results showed that 64 of 75 patients (85%) in the epinephrine group and 69 of 76 patients (91%) in the no-epinephrine group had excellent or good pain relief. The addition of epinephrine slightly prolonged the interval between pudendal nerve block administration and delivery. Maternal venous blood mepivacaine concentrations were slightly higher in the no-epinephrine group, but there was no difference between groups in umbilical cord blood concentrations of mepivacaine.

BOX 24-2 Maternal Complications of Pudendal Nerve Block

- Laceration of the vaginal mucosa
- Systemic local anesthetic toxicity
- Vaginal, ischiorectal, or retroperitoneal hematoma
- Retropsoal or subgluteal abscess

Complications

Maternal complications of pudendal nerve block are uncommon but may be serious (Box 24-2). Systemic local anesthetic toxicity may result from either direct intravascular injection or systemic absorption of an excessive dose of local anesthetic. Toxicity may occur if the obstetrician exceeds the safe dose of local anesthetic during repetitive injections performed to obtain a successful block. Vaginal, ischiorectal, and retroperitoneal hematomas may result from trauma to the pudendal artery.[82] These hematomas are typically small and rarely require operative intervention. Subgluteal and retropsoal abscesses are rare but can result in significant morbidity or mortality.[25,26]

Fetal complications are rare. The primary fetal complications result from fetal trauma and/or direct fetal injection of local anesthetic.[7]

As with paracervical block, the performance of pudendal nerve block requires the obstetrician to make several blind needle punctures within the vagina. The needle guide does not uniformly protect the physician from a needle-stick injury. Thus performance of pudendal nerve block may entail a risk of physician exposure to HIV or another virus.

PERINEAL INFILTRATION

Perineal infiltration is perhaps the most common local anesthetic technique used for vaginal delivery. Given the frequent failure of pudendal nerve block, obstetricians often perform pudendal nerve block and perineal infiltration simultaneously. Perineal infiltration also may be required in patients with incomplete epidural anesthesia. The obstetrician injects several milliliters of local anesthetic solution into the posterior fourchette. There are no large nerve fibers to be blocked, so the onset of anesthesia is rapid. However, perineal infiltration provides anesthesia only for episiotomy and repair. Anesthesia is often inadequate even for these limited procedures. Moreover, perineal infiltration provides no muscle relaxation.

Choice of Local Anesthetic

Philipson et al.[83] evaluated the pharmacokinetics of lidocaine after perineal infiltration. They gave 1% or 2% lidocaine without epinephrine during the crowning phase of the second stage of labor in 15 healthy parturients. The mean ± SD dose of lidocaine was 79 ± 3 mg, and the mean drug-to-delivery interval was 7.8 ± 7.0 minutes. The investigators detected lidocaine in maternal plasma as early as 1 minute after injection. Peak maternal plasma concentrations of lidocaine occurred between 3 and 15 minutes after injection. Despite the administration of small doses of lidocaine and the short drug-to-delivery intervals, there was rapid placental transfer of significant amounts of lidocaine. The mean fetal-to-maternal lidocaine concentration ratio of 1.32 was significantly higher than the ratio reported after administration of lidocaine for paracervical block, pudendal nerve block, or epidural anesthesia for vaginal or cesarean delivery. There was a significant correlation between the fetal-to-maternal lidocaine concentration ratio and the length of the second stage of labor. These investigators speculated that fetal tissue acidosis increased the fetal-to-maternal lidocaine ratio after perineal infiltration in this study. Finally, they noted the persistence of lidocaine and its pharmacologically active metabolites for at least 48 hours after delivery.[83]

Subsequently, Philipson et al.[84] evaluated the placental transfer of 2-chloroprocaine after perineal administration of 1% or 2% 2-chloroprocaine to 17 women shortly before delivery. The mean ± SD dose of 2-chloroprocaine was 81.8 ± 27.0 mg, and the mean drug-to-delivery interval was 6.7 ± 4.3 minutes. Perineal infiltration of 2-chloroprocaine provided adequate anesthesia for episiotomy repair except in two patients who required additional local anesthetic for repair of fourth-degree lacerations. The investigators did not detect 2-chloroprocaine in maternal plasma after infiltration or at delivery. Further, they detected 2-chloroprocaine at delivery in only one umbilical cord venous blood sample, and no 2-chloroprocaine in neonatal plasma. In contrast, they consistently detected the drug's metabolite, chloroaminobenzoic acid, in maternal plasma, umbilical cord venous plasma, and neonatal urine. The fetal-to-maternal ratio of chloroaminobenzoic acid (0.80) was similar to that reported after the administration of 2-chloroprocaine for paracervical block and epidural anesthesia for cesarean delivery. The investigators suggested that very little, if any, unchanged 2-chloroprocaine reaches the fetus after perineal infiltration. They concluded that 2-chloroprocaine may be preferable to lidocaine for antepartum perineal infiltration.[84]

Complications

The obstetrician must take care to avoid injecting the local anesthetic into the fetal scalp. Kim et al.[85] reported a case of newborn lidocaine toxicity after maternal perineal infiltration of 6 mL of 1% lidocaine before vaginal delivery. Similarly, DePraeter et al.[86] reported a case of neonatal lidocaine toxicity in a newborn whose mother received perineal infiltration with 10 mL of 2% lidocaine 4 minutes before delivery. In both cases, the infants were initially vigorous but required endotracheal intubation 15 minutes after delivery. No lidocaine was detected in umbilical cord blood, but neonatal blood samples revealed concentrations of 14 μg/mL at 2 hours and 13.8 μg/mL at 6.5 hours. Small scalp puncture wounds suggested that the lidocaine toxicity resulted from direct fetal scalp injection. Pignotti et al.[87] reported two cases of neonatal local anesthetic toxicity. In one case, lidocaine and prilocaine cream had been applied to the maternal perineum. In the second case, 10 mL of 2% mepivacaine had been injected into the perineum. Both infants required endotracheal intubation and mechanical ventilation, but in both cases, neurodevelopmental outcome was normal at 12 months of age. Kim et al.[85] suggested that the presence of a molded head in the occiput posterior position may predispose to unintentional direct injection of the fetal scalp. These cases support the recommendation of 2-chloroprocaine for perineal infiltration.

KEY POINTS

- Paracervical block and lumbar sympathetic block may provide effective analgesia for the first stage of labor. Neither technique relieves pain during the second stage.
- Fetal bradycardia is the most worrisome complication of paracervical block.
- Paracervical block is contraindicated in patients with uteroplacental insufficiency or preexisting fetal compromise.
- For patients without epidural or spinal anesthesia, it is appropriate to perform pudendal nerve block when the patient complains of pelvic floor pain.
- Pudendal nerve block may provide satisfactory anesthesia for spontaneous vaginal delivery and outlet-forceps delivery, but it provides inadequate anesthesia for mid-forceps delivery, postpartum repair of the cervix, and manual exploration of the uterine cavity.
- Perineal infiltration provides anesthesia only for episiotomy and repair.
- It is unnecessary—and perhaps dangerous—to give concentrated solutions of local anesthetic for paracervical block, pudendal nerve block, or perineal infiltration.
- Some cases of fetal injury result from direct fetal scalp injection of local anesthetic during attempted paracervical block, pudendal nerve block, or perineal infiltration.
- 2-Chloroprocaine is most likely the safest choice of local anesthetic for paracervical block, pudendal nerve block, and perineal infiltration.
- The performance of either paracervical block or pudendal nerve block requires the obstetrician to make several blind needle punctures within the vagina. Thus there is a risk of physician needle-stick injury during the performance of either procedure.

REFERENCES

1. Palomaki O, Huhtala H, Kirkinen P. What determines the analgesic effect of paracervical block? Acta Obstet Gynecol Scand 2005; 84:962-6.
2. Gibbs CP, Krischer J, Peckham BM, et al. Obstetric anesthesia: A national survey. Anesthesiology 1986; 65:298-306.
3. Gerdin E, Cnattingius S. The use of obstetric analgesia in Sweden 1983-1986. Br J Obstet Gynaecol 1990; 97:789-96.
4. Nyirjesy I, Hawks BL, Hebert JE, et al. Hazards of the use of paracervical block anesthesia in obstetrics. Am J Obstet Gynecol 1963; 87:231-5.
5. Rosefsky JB, Petersiel ME. Perinatal deaths associated with mepivacaine paracervical-block anesthesia in labor. N Engl J Med 1968; 278:530-3.

6. Teramo K. Effects of obstetrical paracervical blockade on the fetus. Acta Obstet Gynecol Scand 1971; 16(Suppl):1-55.
7. Shnider SM, Levinson G, Ralston DH. Regional anesthesia for labor and delivery. In Shnider SM, Levinson G, editors. Anesthesia for Obstetrics. 3rd edition. Baltimore, Williams & Wilkins, 1993:135-53.
8. Shnider SM. Criticizes paracervical block for analgesia during labor. Ob Gyn News 1986; Apr.
9. Bucklin BA, Hawkins JL, Anderson JR, Ullrich FA. Obstetric anesthesia workforce survey: Twenty-year update. Anesthesiology 2005; 103:645-53.
10. Jensen F, Qvist I, Brocks V, et al. Submucous paracervical blockade compared with intramuscular meperidine as analgesia during labor: A double-blind study. Obstet Gynecol 1984; 64:724-7.
11. Kangas-Saarela T, Jouppila R, Puolakka J, et al. The effect of bupivacaine paracervical block on the neurobehavioural responses of newborn infants. Acta Anaesthesiol Scand 1988; 32:566-70.
12. Jägerhorn M. Paracervical block in obstetrics: An improved injection method. Acta Obstet Gynecol Scand 1975; 54:9-27.
13. Cibils LA, Santonja-Lucas JJ. Clinical significance of fetal heart rate patterns during labor. III. Effect of block paracervical anesthesia. Am J Obstet Gynecol 1978; 130:73-100.
14. Freeman DW, Arnold NI. Paracervical block with low doses of chloroprocaine: Fetal and maternal effects. JAMA 1975; 231:56-7.
15. King JC, Sherline DM. Paracervical and pudendal block. Clin Obstet Gynecol 1981; 24:587-95.
16. Van Dorsten JP, Miller FC, Yeh SY. Spacing the injection interval with paracervical block: A randomized study. Obstet Gynecol 1981; 58:696-702.
17. Nieminen K, Puolakka J. Effective obstetric paracervical block with reduced dose of bupivacaine. Acta Obstet Gynecol Scand 1997; 76:50-4.
18. Palomaki O, Huhtala H, Kirkinen P. A comparative study of the safety of 0.25% levobupivacaine and 0.25% racemic bupivacaine for paracervical block in the first stage of labor. Acta Obstet Gynecol Scand 2005; 84:956-61.
19. Weiss RR, Halevy S, Almonte RO, et al. Comparison of lidocaine and 2-chloroprocaine in paracervical block: Clinical effects and drug concentrations in mother and child. Anesth Analg 1983; 62: 168-73.
20. Philipson EH, Kuhnert BR, Syracuse CB, et al. Intrapartum paracervical block anesthesia with 2-chloroprocaine. Am J Obstet Gynecol 1983; 146:16-22.
21. LeFevre ML. Fetal heart rate pattern and postparacervical fetal bradycardia. Obstet Gynecol 1984; 64:343-6.
22. Philipson EH, Kuhnert BR. Letter to the editor. Acta Obstet Gynecol Scand 1984; 63:187.
23. Gaylord TG, Pearson JW. Neuropathy following paracervical block in the obstetric patient. Obstet Gynecol 1982; 60:521-5.
24. Mercado AO, Naz JF, Ataya KM. Postabortal paracervical abscess as a complication of paracervical block anesthesia. J Reprod Med 1989; 34:247-9.
25. Hibbard LT, Snyder EN, McVann RM. Subgluteal and retropsoal infection in obstetric practice. Obstet Gynecol 1972; 39:137-50.
26. Svancarek W, Chirino O, Schaefer G, Blythe JG. Retropsoas and subgluteal abscesses following paracervical and pudendal anesthesia. JAMA 1977; 237:892-4.
27. Chase D, Brady JP. Ventricular tachycardia in a neonate with mepivacaine toxicity. J Pediatr 1977; 90:127-9.
28. Teramo K, Widholm O. Studies of effect of anaesthetics on foetus. I. Effect of paracervical block with mepivacaine upon foetal acid-base values. Acta Obstet Gynecol Scand 1967; 46(Suppl 2):1-39.
29. Rogers RE. Fetal bradycardia associated with paracervical block anesthesia in labor. Am J Obstet Gynecol 1970; 106:913-6.
30. Shnider SM, Asling JH, Holl JW, Margolis AJ. Paracervical block anesthesia in obstetrics. I. Fetal complications and neonatal morbidity. Am J Obstet Gynecol 1970; 107:619-25.
31. Carlsson BM, Johansson M, Westin B. Fetal heart rate pattern before and after paracervical anesthesia: A prospective study. Acta Obstet Gynecol Scand 1987; 66:391-5.
32. Goins JR. Experience with mepivacaine paracervical block in an obstetric private practice. Am J Obstet Gynecol 1992; 167:342-5.
33. Ranta P, Jouppila P, Spalding M, et al. Paracervical block: A viable alternative for labor pain relief? Acta Obstet Gynecol Scand 1995; 74:122-6.
34. Rosen MA. Paracervical block for labor analgesia: A brief historic review. Am J Obstet Gynecol 2002; 186:S127-30.
35. Gordon HR. Fetal bradycardia after paracervical block: Correlation with fetal and maternal blood levels of local anesthetic (mepivacaine). N Engl J Med 1968; 279:910-4.
36. Puolakka J, Jouppila R, Jouppila P, Puukka M. Maternal and fetal effects of low-dosage bupivacaine paracervical block. J Perinat Med 1984; 12:75-84.
37. Shnider SM, Asling JH, Margolis AJ, et al. High fetal blood levels of mepivacaine and fetal bradycardia (letter). N Engl J Med 1968; 279:947-8.
38. Asling JH, Shnider SM, Margolis AJ, et al. Paracervical block anesthesia in obstetrics. II. Etiology of fetal bradycardia following paracervical block anesthesia. Am J Obstet Gynecol 1970; 107:626-34.
39. Brown WU, Bell GC, Alper MH. Acidosis, local anesthetics, and the newborn. Obstet Gynecol 1976; 48:27-30.
40. Biehl D, Shnider SM, Levinson G, Callender K. Placental transfer of lidocaine: Effects of fetal acidosis. Anesthesiology 1978; 48:409-12.
41. Freeman RK, Gutierrez NA, Ray ML, et al. Fetal cardiac response to paracervical block anesthesia. Part I. Am J Obstet Gynecol 1972; 113:583-91.
42. Fishburne JI, Greiss FC, Hopkinson R, Rhyne AL. Responses of the gravid uterine vasculature to arterial levels of local anesthetic agents. Am J Obstet Gynecol 1979; 133:753-61.
43. Morishima HO, Covino BG, Yeh MN, et al. Bradycardia in the fetal baboon following paracervical block anesthesia. Am J Obstet Gynecol 1981; 140:775-80.
44. Cibils LA. Response of human uterine arteries to local anesthetics. Am J Obstet Gynecol 1976; 126:202-10.
45. Gibbs CP, Noel SC. Response of arterial segments from gravid human uterus to multiple concentrations of lignocaine. Br J Anaesth 1977; 49:409-12.
46. Norén H, Lindblom B, Källfelt B. Effects of bupivacaine and calcium antagonists on the rat uterine artery. Acta Anesthesiol Scand 1991; 35:77-80.
47. Norén H, Lindblom B, Källfelt B. Effects of bupivacaine and calcium antagonists on human uterine arteries in pregnant and non-pregnant women. Acta Anaesthesiol Scand 1991; 35:488-91.
48. Halevy S, Freese KJ, Liu-Barnett M, Altura BM. Endothelium-dependent local anesthetics action on umbilical vessels. FASEB J 1991; 5:A1421.
49. Greiss FC, Still JG, Anderson SG. Effects of local anesthetic agents on the uterine vasculature and myometrium. Am J Obstet Gynecol 1976; 124:889-99.
50. Manninen T, Aantaa R, Salonen M, et al. A comparison of the hemodynamic effects of paracervical block and epidural anesthesia for labor analgesia. Acta Anaesthesiol Scand 2000; 44:441-5.
51. Räsänen J, Jouppila P. Does a paracervical block with bupivacaine change vascular resistance in uterine and umbilical arteries? J Perinat Med 1994; 22:301-8.
52. Baxi LV, Petrie RH, James LS. Human fetal oxygenation following paracervical block. Am J Obstet Gynecol 1979; 135:1109-12.
53. Jacobs R, Stalnacke B, Lindberg B, Rooth G. Human fetal transcutaneous Po_2 during paracervical block. J Perinat Med 1982; 10:209-14.
54. Kaita TM, Nikkola EM, Rantala MI, et al. Fetal oxygen saturation during epidural and paracervical analgesia. Acta Obstet Gynecol Scand 2000; 79:336-40.
55. Levy BT, Bergus GR, Hartz A, et al. Is paracervical block safe and effective? A prospective study of its association with neonatal umbilical artery pH values. J Fam Pract 1999; 48:778-84.
56. Cleland JGP. Paravertebral anaesthesia in obstetrics: Experimental and clinical basis. Surg Gynecol Obstet 1933; 57:51-62.
57. Shumacker HB, Manahan CP, Hellman LM. Sympathetic anesthesia in labor. Am J Obstet Gynecol 1943; 45:129.

58. Jarvis SM. Paravertebral sympathetic nerve block: A method for the safe and painless conduct of labor. Am J Obstet Gynecol 1944; 47:335-42.
59. Reich AM. Paravertebral lumbar sympathetic block in labor: A report on 500 deliveries by a fractional procedure producing continuous conduction anesthesia. Am J Obstet Gynecol 1951; 61: 1263-76.
60. Cleland JGP. Continuous peridural and caudal analgesia in obstetrics. Analg Anesth 1949; 28:61-76.
61. Bonica JJ. Principles and Practice of Obstetric Analgesia and Anesthesia. Philadelphia, FA Davis, 1967:520-6.
62. Hunter CA. Uterine motility studies during labor: Observations on bilateral sympathetic nerve block in the normal and abnormal first stage of labor. Am J Obstet Gynecol 1963; 85:681-6.
63. Leighton BL, Halpern SH, Wilson DB. Lumbar sympathetic blocks speed early and second stage induced labor in nulliparous women. Anesthesiology 1999; 90:1039-46.
64. Suelto MD, Shaw DB. Labor analgesia with paravertebral lumbar sympathetic block. Reg Anesth Pain Med 1999; 4:179-81.
65. Meguiar RV, Wheeler AS. Lumbar sympathetic block with bupivacaine: Analgesia for labor. Anesth Analg 1978; 57:486-90.
66. Nair V, Henry R. Bilateral paravertebral block: A satisfactory alternative for labour analgesia. Can J Anesth 2001; 48:179-84.
67. Wills MH, Korbon GA, Arasi R. Horner's syndrome resulting from a lumbar sympathetic block. Anesthesiology 1988; 68:613-4.
68. Artuso JD, Stevens RA, Lineberry PJ. Postdural puncture headache after lumbar sympathetic block: A report of two cases. Regional Anesth 1991; 16:288-91.
69. King R. Perineal anesthesia in labor. Surg Gynecol Obstet 1916; 23:615-8.
70. Klink EW. Perineal nerve block: An anatomic and clinical study in the female. Obstet Gynecol 1953; 1:137-46.
71. Kohl GC. New method of pudendal nerve block. Northwest Med 1954; 53:1012-3.
72. Hutchins CJ. Spinal analgesia for instrumental delivery: A comparison with pudendal nerve block. Anaesthesia 1980; 35:376-7.
73. Scudamore JH, Yates MJ. Pudendal block—a misnomer? Lancet 1966; 1(7427):23-4.
74. Langhoff-Roos J, Lindmark G. Analgesia and maternal side effects of pudendal block at delivery: A comparison of three local anesthetics. Acta Obstet Gynecol Scand 1985; 64:269-73.
75. Zador G, Lindmark G, Nilsson BA. Pudendal block in normal vaginal deliveries. Acta Obstet Gynecol Scand Suppl 1974; 34:51-64.
76. Pace MC, Aurilio C, Bulletti C, et al. Subarachnoid analgesia in advanced labor: A comparison of subarachnoid analgesia and pudendal block in advanced labor. Analgesic quality and obstetric outcome. Ann N Y Acad Sci 2004; 1034:356-63.
77. Aissaoui Y, Bruyere R, Mustapha H, et al. A randomized controlled trial of pudendal nerve block for pain relief after episiotomy. Anesth Analg 2008; 107:625-9.
78. Cunningham FG, Leveno KL, Bloom SL, et al. Williams Obstetrics. 22nd edition. New York, McGraw-Hill, 2005:478-9.
79. Kuhnert BR, Knapp DR, Kuhnert PM, Prochaska AL. Maternal, fetal, and neonatal metabolism of lidocaine. Clin Pharmacol Ther 1979; 26:213-20.
80. Merkow AJ, McGuinness GA, Erenberg A, Kennedy RL. The neonatal neurobehavioral effects of bupivacaine, mepivacaine, and 2-chloroprocaine used for pudendal block. Anesthesiology 1980; 52:309-12.
81. Schierup L, Schmidt JF, Jensen AT, Rye BAO. Pudendal block in vaginal deliveries: Mepivacaine with and without epinephrine. Acta Obstet Gynecol Scand 1988; 67:195-7.
82. Kurzel RB, Au AH, Rooholamini SA. Retroperitoneal hematoma as a complication of pudendal block: Diagnosis made by computed tomography. West J Med 1996; 164:523-5.
83. Philipson EH, Kuhnert BR, Syracuse CD. Maternal, fetal, and neonatal lidocaine levels following local perineal infiltration. Am J Obstet Gynecol 1984; 149:403-7.
84. Philipson EH, Kuhnert BR, Syracuse CD. 2-Chloroprocaine for local perineal infiltration. Am J Obstet Gynecol 1987; 157:1275-8.
85. Kim WY, Pomerance JJ, Miller AA. Lidocaine intoxication in a newborn following local anesthesia for episiotomy. Pediatrics 1979; 64:643-5.
86. DePraeter C, Vanhaesebrouch P, De Praeter N, Govaert P. Episiotomy and neonatal lidocaine intoxication (letter). Eur J Pediatr 1991; 150:685-6.
87. Pignotti MS, Indolfi G, Ciuti R, Donzelli G. Perinatal asphyxia and inadvertent neonatal intoxication from local anaesthetics given to the mother during labor. BMJ 2005; 350:34-5.

Chapter 25

Postpartum Tubal Sterilization

Joy L. Hawkins, M.D.

Many parous women choose tubal ligation for permanent contraception. Half of tubal ligation procedures are performed postpartum (more than 350,000 annually in the United States), and half as interval ambulatory procedures.[1] The purpose of this chapter is to discuss the considerations and controversies regarding the administration of anesthesia for postpartum tubal ligation.

AMERICAN SOCIETY OF ANESTHESIOLOGISTS GUIDELINES

The American Society of Anesthesiologists (ASA) has published "Practice Guidelines for Obstetric Anesthesia,"[2] which includes a discussion of postpartum tubal ligation (see Appendix B at the end of the text). The ASA Task Force recommendations can be summarized as follows:

1. For postpartum tubal ligation, the patient should have no oral intake of solid foods within 6 to 8 hours of the surgery, depending on the type of food ingested (e.g., fat content).
2. Aspiration prophylaxis should be considered.
3. Both the timing of the procedure and the decision to use a specific anesthetic technique (i.e., neuraxial versus general) should be individualized on the basis of anesthetic risk factors, obstetric risk factors (e.g., blood loss), and patient preferences.
4. Neuraxial techniques are preferred to general anesthesia for most postpartum tubal ligations. The anesthesia provider should be aware that gastric emptying is delayed in patients who have received opioids during labor and that an epidural catheter placed for labor may be more likely to fail with longer post-delivery intervals.
5. If a postpartum tubal ligation is to be performed before the patient is discharged from the hospital, the procedure should not be attempted at a time when it might compromise other aspects of patient care on the labor and delivery unit.[2]

SURGICAL CONSIDERATIONS

Tubal sterilization can be performed satisfactorily at any time, but the early postpartum period has several advantages for women who have had uncomplicated vaginal delivery,[3] as follows: (1) the patient avoids the cost and inconvenience of a second hospital visit; (2) the uterine fundus remains near the umbilicus for several days postpartum, allowing easy access to the fallopian tubes; and (3) rates of serious complications (e.g., bowel laceration, vascular injury) may be lower during minilaparotomy than during laparoscopy.[4]

There are at least two potential disadvantages to immediate postpartum sterilization. First, parous women are at increased risk for uterine atony and postpartum hemorrhage. (This risk decreases substantially 12 hours after delivery.) Second, immediate surgery results in sterilization before assessment of the newborn is complete. Postpartum tubal ligation is not wise if the patient is ambivalent about permanent sterilization. Women who undergo postpartum sterilization may have a higher probability of regret than women who undergo interval sterilization.[5]

Several techniques are used for postpartum tubal sterilization (Figure 25-1).[6] The failure rate for puerperal sterilization is lower than that of most interval procedures, and is lowest (approximately 0.75%) if some form of tubal resection occurs.[7] With the Irving procedure, the obstetrician buries the cut ends of the tubes in the myometrium

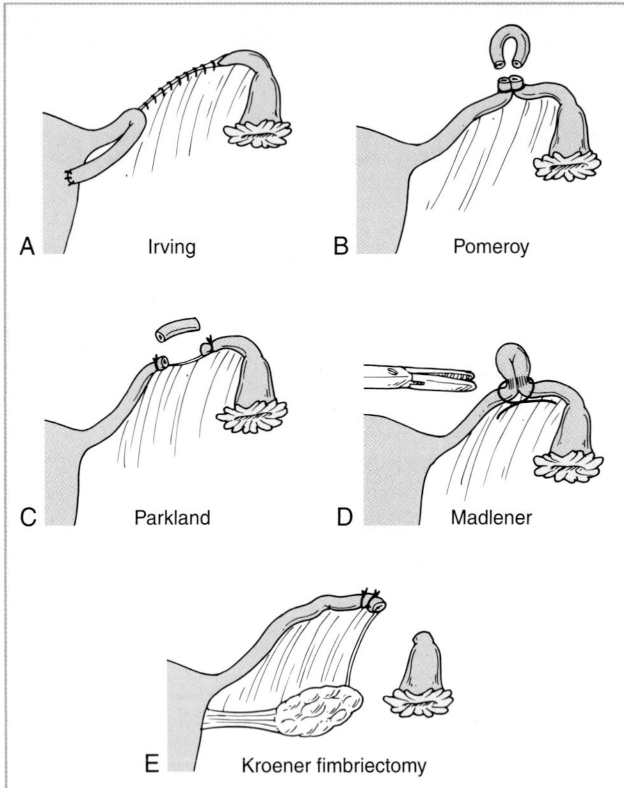

FIGURE 25-1 Techniques for tubal sterilization. **A,** Irving procedure. The medial cut end of the oviduct is buried in the myometrium posteriorly, and the distal cut end is buried in the mesosalpinx. **B,** Pomeroy procedure. A loop of oviduct is ligated, and the knuckle of tube above the ligature is excised. **C,** Parkland procedure. A mid-segment of tube is separated from the mesosalpinx at an avascular site, and the separated tubal segment is ligated proximally and distally and then excised. **D,** Madlener procedure. A knuckle of oviduct is crushed and then ligated without resection; this technique has an unacceptably high failure rate of approximately 7%. **E,** Kroener procedure. The tube is ligated across the ampulla, and the distal portion of the ampulla, including all of the fimbriae, is resected; some studies have reported an unacceptably high failure rate with this technique. (Redrawn from Cunningham FG, MacDonald PC, Gant NF, et al. Williams Obstetrics. 20th edition. Stamford, CT, Appleton & Lange, 1997:1376.)

and mesosalpinx. This technique is least likely to fail, but it requires more extensive exposure and increases the risk of hemorrhage. The Pomeroy procedure is simplest. The surgeon ligates a loop of oviduct and excises the loop above the suture. With the Parkland procedure, the obstetrician ligates the tube proximally and distally and then excises the mid-segment. The last two methods are most commonly performed during postpartum tubal ligations. Regardless of the technique, the obstetrician should document that fimbriae are present to preclude ligation of another structure such as the round ligament. The excised portions are typically sent to a pathologist for verification.

NONMEDICAL ISSUES

Nonmedical issues affect decisions regarding the timing of tubal sterilization. The obstetrician must obtain and document informed consent for surgery.[8] Tubal ligation should be considered an irreversible procedure. Therefore most obstetricians require a discussion with the patient before labor and delivery. Physicians should be aware of state laws or insurance regulations that may require a specific interval between obtaining consent and performing sterilization procedures. Regulations often do not allow the woman to give consent while in labor or immediately after delivery. For example, the Medicaid reimbursement program includes the following requirements for sterilization[9]:

- The patient must be at least 21 years of age and mentally competent when consent is obtained.
- Informed consent may not be obtained while the patient is in labor or during childbirth.
- Consent may not be obtained while the patient is undergoing an abortion or under the influence of alcohol or other substances.
- A total of 30 days must pass between the date the consent is signed and the date the procedure is performed. (Exceptions to the 30-day waiting period can be made for preterm delivery or emergency abdominal surgery.)
- Consent is valid for only 180 days.

In some cases the obstetrician may schedule a patient for a postpartum tubal ligation because of a fear that the patient will not return for interval tubal sterilization 6 weeks after delivery. Concerns about patient compliance should not prompt the performance of postpartum tubal ligation in patients with significant medical or obstetric complications.

PREOPERATIVE EVALUATION

The patient scheduled for postpartum tubal ligation requires a thorough preoperative evaluation, and a reevaluation should be performed even if the patient is known to the anesthesia providers as a result of the provision of labor analgesia. A cursory evaluation should not be performed simply because the patient is young and healthy. Patients with pregnancy-induced hypertension may safely receive neuraxial or general anesthesia for postpartum tubal ligation provided that there is no evidence of pulmonary edema, oliguria, or thrombocytopenia.[10]

Physicians and nurses often underestimate blood loss during delivery.[11] Excessive blood loss from uterine atony is not uncommon in parous women. The possibility of orthostatic changes in blood pressure and heart rate should be excluded, especially if an immediate postpartum procedure is to be performed. At the University of Colorado, for surgery performed the day after delivery, we determine the patient's hematocrit several hours after delivery (to allow for equilibration) and compare it with the antepartum measurement. We do not obtain a hematocrit measurement before an immediate postpartum tubal sterilization (performed less than 8 hours after delivery), provided that the antepartum hematocrit was acceptable, there are no orthostatic vital sign changes, and there was no evidence of excessive blood loss during delivery.

No absolute value of hematocrit requires a delay of surgery, but physical signs of hemodynamic instability or laboratory evidence of excessive blood loss should prompt postponement of the procedure until 6 to 8 weeks postpartum. Fever may signal the presence of endometritis or urinary tract infection and also may require postponement of surgery until a later date. Finally, the condition of the neonate should be confirmed before surgery to exclude any unexpected problems.

Often mothers are concerned that medications administered during surgery might affect their ability to breast-feed or that these medications might harm the neonate. Any drug present in the mother's blood will be present in breast milk, with the concentration depending on factors such as protein binding, lipid solubility, and extent of ionization.[12] Typically the amount of drug present in breast milk is small. Opioids, barbiturates, and propofol administered during anesthesia are excreted in insignificant amounts. (See Chapter 14 for a detailed discussion of interactions between drugs and breast-feeding.)

RISK OF ASPIRATION

Historically, anesthesia providers have considered maternal aspiration the major risk associated with anesthesia for postpartum tubal ligation, although the evidence for this belief is scant and conflicting.[13] A review of anesthesia-related maternal mortality found no maternal deaths associated with aspiration during postpartum tubal ligation, despite the tracking of deaths for 1 year after delivery.[14] However, several factors may put the pregnant woman at increased risk for aspiration. Some but not all of these factors are resolved at delivery. The placenta is the primary site of progesterone production, and progesterone concentrations fall rapidly after the delivery of the placenta (Figure 25-2).[15,16] Typically, progesterone concentrations decline within 2 hours of delivery, and by 24 hours postpartum, progesterone concentrations are similar to those found during the luteal phase of the menstrual cycle.

Two important questions to address during the preanesthetic evaluation are as follows: (1) What is the duration of the fast for solids? (2) Were parenteral opioids administered during labor?

Gastric Emptying

Several studies have assessed gastric emptying in pregnant and postpartum women. O'Sullivan et al.[17] used an epigastric impedance technique to compare gastric emptying times for solids and liquids in women during the third trimester of pregnancy, in women during the first hour postpartum, and in nonpregnant controls. The investigators observed that the overall rate of emptying was lower in the postpartum patients than in pregnant or nonpregnant patients. When patients who had received opioids in labor were separated from those who had not, the investigators found that rates of gastric emptying for women who had not received opioids were similar to those for nonpregnant controls. They concluded that the rate of gastric emptying in postpartum women is delayed only if opioids have been administered during labor.

Other studies have used the paracetamol (acetaminophen) absorption technique to assess gastric emptying. Gin et al.[18] studied women on the first and third days after delivery and at 6 weeks postpartum. They found comparable times to peak concentration of paracetamol in all three groups. These researchers concluded that gastric emptying was no different in the immediate postpartum period from that 6 weeks later, and they recommended that "the approach to prophylaxis against acid aspiration should be more consistent between nonpregnant and postpartum patients."[18] Whitehead et al.[19] observed no

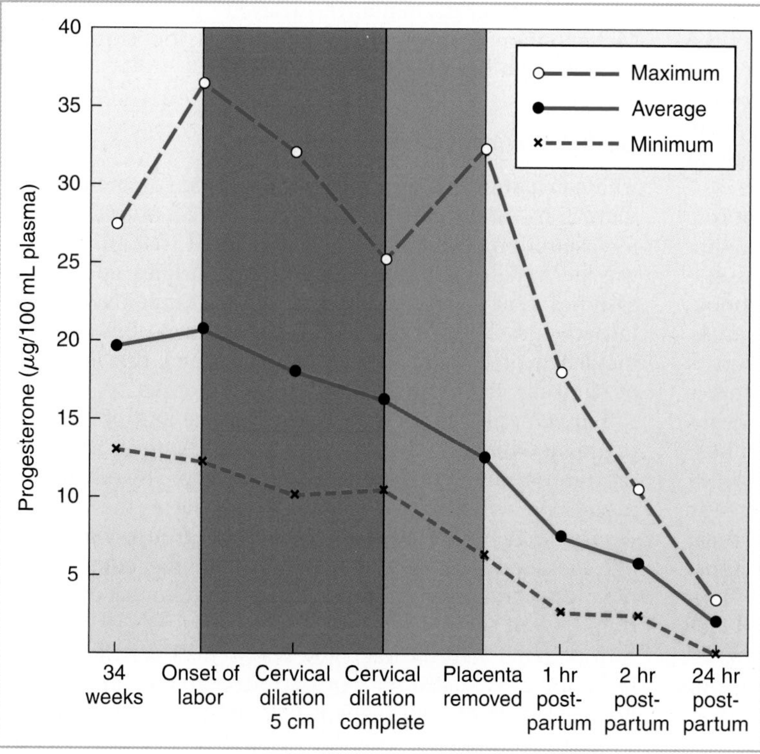

FIGURE 25-2 Average progesterone concentrations with the highest and lowest measurements of 13 pregnant women at given intervals. The *dark* and *medium shaded boxes* represent the intrapartum interval. (Modified from Llauro JL, Runnebaum B, Zander J. Progesterone in human peripheral blood before, during and after labor. Am J Obstet Gynecol 1968; 101:871.)

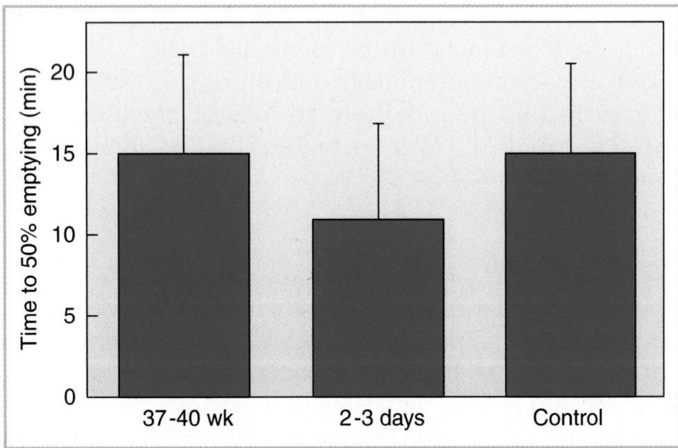

FIGURE 25-3 Mean (SEM) times to 50% gastric emptying (minutes) as determined with applied potential tomography. No significant differences were noted among term pregnant, postpartum, and nonpregnant control women. (From Sandhar BK, Elliott RH, Windram I, Rowbotham DJ. Peripartum changes in gastric emptying. Anaesthesia 1992; 47:197.)

significant delay in gastric emptying during the first, second, or third trimesters of pregnancy or between 18 and 48 hours postpartum in comparison with gastric emptying in nonpregnant controls. However, they observed that gastric emptying was significantly delayed during the first 2 hours after vaginal delivery. (At least 4 of the 17 women studied had received intramuscular meperidine during labor.) The researchers did not measure gastric emptying between 2 and 18 hours postpartum. They concluded, "The presence of delayed gastric emptying in the immediate (within 2 hours) postpartum period confirms that strict precautions against acid aspiration . . . should be provided to mothers who are newly delivered and requiring anaesthesia."[19]

Sandhar et al.[20] used applied potential tomography to measure gastric emptying in 10 patients at term gestation, 2 to 3 days postpartum, and 6 weeks postpartum (the 6-week measurement served as each woman's control value). All measurements were made after administration of an H_2-receptor antagonist. The times to 50% emptying after ingestion of 400 mL of water were not different in the three periods of testing (Figure 25-3).

Wong et al.[21] assessed gastric emptying in nonlaboring pregnant women at term gestation, after ingestion of either 50 or 300 mL of water, with two techniques: (1) serial assessment of acetaminophen absorption and (2) serial ultrasonography to determine gastric antrum cross-sectional areas. Gastric emptying was significantly faster after ingestion of 300 mL of water, consistent with the observation that a liquid meal may actually accelerate gastric emptying. Repeating the study in obese women had similar results.[22] Kubli et al.[23] compared the effects of isotonic "sport drinks" with those of water on residual gastric volume in women in early labor. Women who received the sport drinks had similar gastric volumes and a similar incidence of vomiting to those in women who received water, but the ingestion of sport drinks prevented the rise in ketone production that occurred in the control (water) group. Altogether, these studies suggest that gastric emptying of clear liquids is not delayed during pregnancy, early labor, or the postpartum period unless an opioid has been administered.

In contrast, Jayaram et al.[24] found that 39% of postpartum patients, but not nonpregnant patients presenting for gynecologic surgery, had solid food particles in the stomach, as demonstrated by ultrasonography. Four hours after a standardized meal, 95% of postpartum women—compared with only 19% of nonpregnant subjects—still had solid food particles in the stomach. Prior administration of an opioid did not seem to be a risk factor for delayed gastric emptying in this study. Scrutton et al.[25] randomly assigned 94 women presenting in early labor to receive either a light diet or water only during labor. The mothers who ate a light diet had significantly larger gastric antrum cross-sectional areas (determined by ultrasonography) and were twice as likely to vomit at or around delivery as those who had water only. Also, the volumes vomited were significantly larger in the women who ate a light diet.

In summary, the preponderance of evidence suggests that (1) administration of an opioid during labor increases the likelihood of delayed gastric emptying during the early postpartum period; (2) gastric emptying of *solids* is delayed during labor in all parturients; and (3) gastric emptying of clear liquids is probably *not* delayed unless parenteral opioids were administered. There are few data on gastric emptying during the first 8 hours postpartum.

During the preoperative assessment of any woman scheduled for postpartum tubal ligation, the anesthesia provider should determine when the patient last consumed solids and whether opioids were administered by any route. Systemic absorption of an opioid occurs after epidural administration. However, published studies have provided conflicting results about the effect of epidural opioid administration on gastric emptying. Wright et al.[26] observed that epidural administration of 10 mL of 0.375% bupivacaine with fentanyl 100 μg caused a modest prolongation of gastric emptying during labor in comparison with epidural administration of bupivacaine alone. However, Kelly et al.[27] found that intrathecal, but not epidural, administration of fentanyl delayed gastric emptying. Metoclopramide may not accelerate gastric emptying in patients who have received an opioid.

Gastric Volume and pH

The conventional wisdom is that a gastric volume of more than 25 mL and a gastric pH of less than 2.5 are risk factors for aspiration pneumonitis. Coté[28] noted that this dogma was derived from unpublished animal studies and that it assumes that every milliliter of gastric fluid is directed into the trachea. A marked disparity exists between the incidence of patients labeled "at risk" and the incidence of clinically significant aspiration pneumonitis.

Blouw et al.[29] measured gastric volume and pH in nonpregnant women undergoing gynecologic surgery and postpartum women 9 to 42 hours after delivery. The researchers found no significant difference between the groups. Approximately 75% of women in each group had gastric pH measurements less than 2.5. When the combination of volume and pH was used to determine the risk of aspiration, 64% of the control patients but only 33% of postpartum patients were at risk. The researchers concluded that 8 hours after delivery, postpartum patients are not at greater risk than nonpregnant patients undergoing elective surgery. They did not examine patients earlier than 8 hours

TABLE 25-1 Gastric Volume and pH at Intervals after Delivery

	Gastric Volume > 25 mL (%)	pH < 2.5 (%)	At Risk* (%)
Group 1 (1-8 hr)	73	100	73
Group 2 (9-23 hr)	40	100	40
Group 3 (24-45 hr)	73	80	67
Group 4 (control)	67	80	60

*Gastric contents with pH < 2.5 and volume > 25 mL.

From James CF, Gibbs CP, Banner T. Postpartum perioperative risk of aspiration pneumonia. Anesthesiology 1984; 61:757-8.

after delivery. In addition, they acknowledged that a large number of patients in both groups were at risk.

James et al.[30] attempted to determine the "safe" interval (i.e., the interval that lowers the risk of aspiration) after delivery. They compared gastric volume and pH in postpartum women 1 to 8 hours, 9 to 23 hours, and 24 to 45 hours after delivery with those in a control group of nonpregnant women undergoing elective surgery. There were no significant differences between the group of patients undergoing elective surgery and any of the postpartum groups (Table 25-1). Approximately 60% of all patients were considered "at risk" for aspiration pneumonitis. The investigators concluded that there was no difference in the risk for sequelae if aspiration should occur, but they speculated that hormonal changes or mechanical factors might make aspiration more likely during the postpartum period.

Finally, Lam et al.[31] administered 150 mL of water to 50 women 2 to 3 hours before tubal ligation scheduled to be performed 1 to 5 days postpartum. Another 50 postpartum women and 50 nonpregnant women fasted after midnight. The researchers found no differences in gastric pH or volume among the postpartum-water group, the postpartum-fasted group, and the group of nonpregnant controls undergoing elective surgery.

In conclusion, there is little evidence that postpartum women are at greater risk for aspiration than patients undergoing elective surgery solely on the basis of pregnancy-induced changes in gastric pH and volume.

Gastroesophageal Reflux

Women in the third trimester of pregnancy have decreased lower esophageal barrier pressures compared with nonpregnant controls.[32] Those with symptoms of heartburn have even lower pressures and a higher incidence of gastric reflux. Vanner and Goodman[33] asked parturients to swallow a pH electrode to measure lower esophageal pH at term and on the second postpartum day. Patients were placed in four positions—supine with tilt, left lateral, right lateral, and lithotomy—and were then asked to perform a Valsalva and other maneuvers to promote reflux. A total of 17 of 25 patients had reflux at term, whereas only 5 of 25 had reflux after delivery. The investigators concluded that the incidence of reflux returns toward normal by the second day after delivery. However, this conclusion is arguable, given the fact that the investigators did not define *normal* by determining the incidence of reflux before or 6 to 8 weeks after pregnancy.

Summary

No data indicate that the postpartum patient's safety is enhanced by delaying surgery or is compromised by proceeding with surgery immediately after delivery. This situation has led to confusion and inconsistency in the development of policies for the performance of postpartum tubal ligation.[34] No waiting interval guarantees that the postpartum patient is free of risk for aspiration. It is probably prudent to use some form of aspiration prophylaxis in all patients undergoing postpartum tubal ligation. However, significant aspiration pneumonitis is so rare that it will be difficult to document cost-effectiveness and decreased rates of morbidity and mortality from the use of these measures. H_2-receptor antagonists and antacids do not reduce the possibility of regurgitation and aspiration, but they may make the consequences less severe. Metoclopramide may decrease the incidence of reflux by increasing lower esophageal sphincter tone.[32] None of these medications can guarantee that gastric contents will not enter the lungs. Aspiration is best prevented by an experienced anesthesia provider using careful airway management and/or with the use of neuraxial anesthetic techniques.

Performance of an immediate postpartum tubal ligation (within 8 hours of delivery) may diminish both the length of the hospital stay and hospital costs.[35] In this era of health care cost containment, any decision to postpone surgery that requires an extra day of hospitalization must be evaluated carefully. Anesthesia providers and obstetricians have questioned the need to wait 8 or more hours after delivery if gastric emptying time and gastric volume and pH are no different in the postpartum patient from those in nonpregnant women. Reasons given for an 8-hour delay are as follows. First, women may remain at increased risk for gastroesophageal reflux immediately after delivery. Second, delays in gastric emptying due to the antepartum administration of opioids will resolve during this period. Third, an 8-hour delay allows the administration of aspiration prophylaxis drugs, although they might also be given during labor. Fourth, maximal hemodynamic stress and potential instability occur immediately postpartum, when central blood volume suddenly increases because of contraction of the evacuated uterus, relief of aortocaval compression, and loss of the low-resistance placental circuit; indeed, the patient with cardiovascular disease is at greatest risk for hemodynamic decompensation immediately postpartum. Fifth, if there are concerns about excessive blood loss at delivery, an 8-hour delay allows the physician to assess serial hemodynamic measurements (including the presence or absence of orthostatic changes), obtain an equilibrated postpartum hematocrit measurement, and, if necessary, restore intravascular volume. Sixth, delay allows a more thorough evaluation of the infant. Finally, delay allows the woman more time to assess her decision.

In summary, we perform immediate postpartum tubal ligation in patients in whom a functioning epidural catheter is in place. We give these patients an H_2-receptor antagonist and metoclopramide intravenously during labor, and we administer a clear (nonparticulate) antacid after delivery, just before taking the patient to the operating room. In other patients who do not want (or are unable to receive) epidural analgesia for labor, we give an H_2-receptor antagonist and metoclopramide intravenously after delivery and wait at least 2 hours for maximal effect. This is an elective procedure, and all patients should be prevented from consuming solid food for 8 hours, as are nonpregnant patients undergoing elective surgery. Before surgery we monitor blood loss and assess orthostatic vital signs. We then give a clear antacid just before the patient goes to the operating room. Most of these patients (without preexisting epidural analgesia) receive spinal anesthesia for postpartum tubal ligation. However, we are willing to provide general anesthesia using rapid-sequence induction with cricoid pressure.

ANESTHETIC MANAGEMENT

Local, general, or neuraxial anesthesia may be used successfully for postpartum tubal sterilization. Physiology remains altered in the postpartum patient and requires some modification in anesthetic technique. It seems reasonable to give all postpartum patients some form of aspiration prophylaxis. This may include a clear (nonparticulate) antacid, an H_2-receptor antagonist, and/or metoclopramide to increase lower esophageal sphincter tone and hasten gastric emptying. Metoclopramide also may prevent emesis during and after surgery. Patients with additional risk factors for aspiration (e.g., morbid obesity, diabetes mellitus) warrant prophylaxis with all three classes of drugs.

Local Anesthesia

Local anesthesia is used for more than 75% of tubal sterilizations worldwide, although neuraxial anesthesia is administered for postpartum tubal sterilization most often in the United States.[3] Several reports have documented the efficacy and safety of local anesthesia for postpartum or laparoscopic tubal ligation in the hospital operating room, a freestanding outpatient facility, or the obstetrician's office. An anesthesiologist may or may not be involved. Cruikshank et al.[36] described the use of intraperitoneal lidocaine for postpartum tubal ligation. After intravenous administration of diazepam, lidocaine 100 mg was used to infiltrate the skin and subcutaneous tissue. The peritoneum was entered, and lidocaine 400 mg (80 mL of 0.5% solution) was instilled into the peritoneal cavity. A Pomeroy tubal ligation was performed 5 minutes later. All patients had complete peritoneal anesthesia, and all patients stated that they would have the same procedure again. None recalled any pain or discomfort 24 hours later. There were no signs of lidocaine toxicity in any patient, and the maximum lidocaine blood level obtained was 5.3 µg/mL. Surgeons rated the conditions excellent.

Poindexter et al.[37] described almost 3000 laparoscopic tubal sterilization procedures performed with local anesthesia in an ambulatory surgical facility. After intravenous sedation with midazolam (5 to 10 mg) and fentanyl (50 to 100 µg), the skin was infiltrated with 10 mL of 0.5% bupivacaine. After insertion of the trocar, the abdomen was insufflated with nitrous oxide. Each tube was sprayed with 5 mL of 0.5% bupivacaine, and a polymeric silicone (Silastic) ring was applied. Patients were discharged home after approximately 1 hour in the post-anesthesia care unit (PACU). The investigators reported a technical failure rate of 0.14% and no unintended laparotomies or intraoperative complications. Surgical time was reduced by 33% and cost by 68% to 85% in comparison with procedures performed with use of general anesthesia. The investigators presented no data regarding patient satisfaction, and they made no comment about the use of pulse oximetry or blood pressure monitors. Four percent of patients, however, required supplemental oxygen "for adequate tissue perfusion." This study was done in the 1980s, before many ambulatory surgery facilities had institutional guidelines for sedation.

General Anesthesia

Much of the impetus for performing sterilization procedures with use of local anesthesia came from two reports in 1983 indicating that morbidity and mortality were much higher when general anesthesia was used. The first report involved 3500 interval (not postpartum) laparoscopic tubal sterilizations at nine university medical centers.[38] Among all patients, the risk of intraoperative or postoperative complications was 1.75%, but the risk was five times higher with general anesthesia than with local anesthesia. (In this report, local anesthesia consisted of local, epidural, and spinal anesthesia.) The reason(s) for the difference was unclear. In the second report, the U.S. Centers for Disease Control and Prevention examined deaths attributed to tubal sterilization procedures from 1977 to 1981.[39] They included both immediate postpartum laparotomies and interval laparoscopic procedures. Of the 29 deaths, 11 followed complications of general anesthesia and were caused by hypoventilation or cardiorespiratory arrest. Aspiration was not reported as a cause of death. Of the 6 patients whose deaths were definitely attributed to hypoventilation, none had been intubated, and 5 of the 11 deaths attributed to general anesthesia occurred during postpartum laparotomy. Of these, only 1 woman had been intubated; all others underwent mask ventilation. The investigators concluded, "It appears that for tubal sterilization, like abortion, the greatest risk of death is that associated with the anesthesia used during the procedure."[39]

In the 25 years since those reports, appropriate airway management with endotracheal intubation has become standard practice. Adequate monitoring of ventilation—through adherence to ASA standards for basic anesthesia monitoring—should help prevent morbidity and mortality associated with general anesthesia. At the University of Colorado, we perform a rapid-sequence induction (with cricoid pressure) and intubate all patients who receive general anesthesia for postpartum tubal ligation.

Volatile anesthetic agents cause uterine relaxation, and could potentially increase the risk for postpartum hemorrhage if administered to women in the immediate postpartum period. Therefore, the question has been raised as to whether the anesthesia provider should use an inhalation or an intravenous technique to maintain general anesthesia for postpartum tubal ligation. Marx et al.[40] measured postpartum uterine activity and the response to oxytocin with different concentrations of halothane or enflurane (Figure 25-4). Impairment of spontaneous uterine

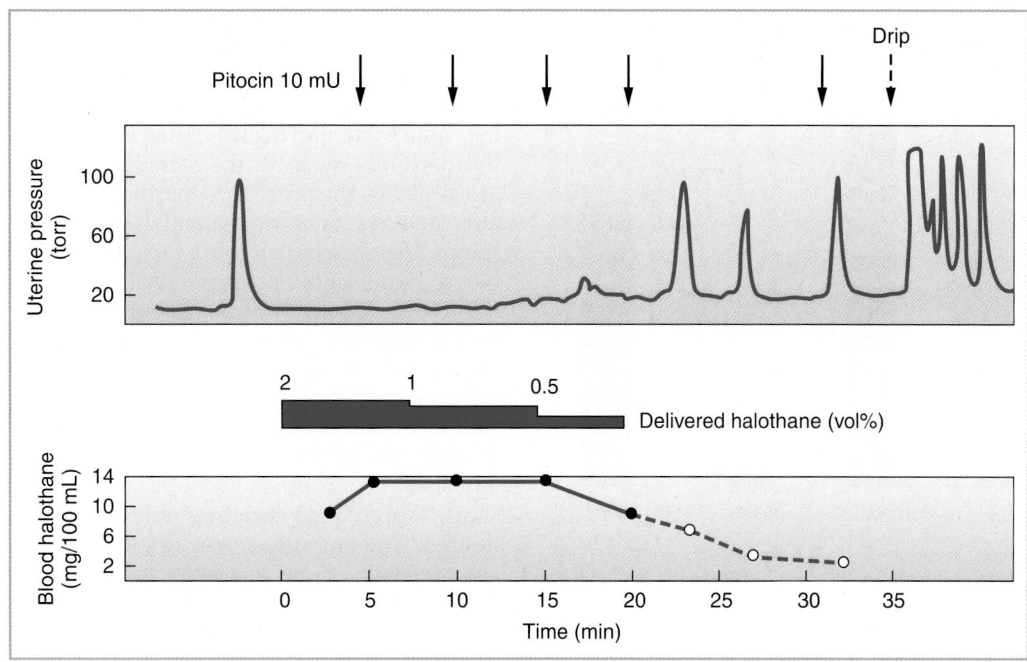

FIGURE 25-4 Halothane anesthesia blocked the normal response to oxytocin when arterial blood levels exceeded 10.5 mg/100 mL or approximately 0.8 minimum alveolar concentration (MAC). (Modified from Marx GF, Kim YI, Lin CC, et al. Postpartum uterine pressures under halothane or enflurane anesthesia. Obstet Gynecol 1978; 51:697.)

activity occurred at 0.5 minimum alveolar concentration (MAC) of both agents, and loss of the response to oxytocin occurred near 1.0 MAC. Spontaneous contractions reappeared when anesthetic concentrations were reduced below these levels. Parous women are at risk for postpartum uterine atony, and administration of a high concentration of a volatile halogenated agent may precipitate postpartum hemorrhage. The anesthesia provider should not give a high concentration of a volatile halogenated agent during the postpartum period.

Two studies have determined the MAC of isoflurane during the postpartum period. Chan et al.[41] found a positive correlation between MAC and the length of time after delivery, with nonpregnant values achieved by 72 hours postpartum. Zhou et al.[42] determined that isoflurane MAC was approximately 0.75% in the first 12 hours postpartum and 1.04% in patients who were 12 to 24 hours postpartum. No significant difference in MAC existed between the latter group and a control group of nonpregnant gynecologic patients. Together these results demonstrate that the reduced MAC observed during pregnancy persists for a variable period between 12 and 36 hours postpartum.

Propofol has some advantages (e.g., rapid awakening, decreased incidence of emesis) that make it attractive for short sterilization procedures. When propofol was used for induction and maintenance of anesthesia for cesarean delivery, breast milk samples obtained at 4 and 8 hours postpartum had a low concentration of the drug, suggesting negligible neonatal exposure to propofol.[43] Use of sodium thiopental for induction of anesthesia also results in negligible neonatal exposure during subsequent breast-feeding.

Alterations occur in the activity of both depolarizing and nondepolarizing muscle relaxants during the postpartum period. Evans and Wroe[44] described the changes in plasma cholinesterase activity during pregnancy. A rapid fall in activity occurred during the first trimester. This low level of activity was maintained until delivery and was followed by an even lower level of activity during the first week postpartum. Ganga et al.[45] found that a lower dose of succinylcholine was required to achieve 80% twitch suppression in postpartum women than in nonpregnant women. Time to recovery also was prolonged and correlated with lower cholinesterase activity in the postpartum patients. Leighton et al.[46] studied four groups of patients: nonpregnant, nonpregnant using oral contraceptives, term pregnant, and postpartum women. Cholinesterase activity was significantly lower in both term pregnant and postpartum women. Recovery time was 25% longer in the postpartum patients than in other groups (685 seconds versus approximately 500 seconds). Although a 3-minute prolongation of paralysis may not seem clinically significant, it could be important if airway difficulties occur.[46] Metoclopramide prolongs neuromuscular block with succinylcholine by 135% to 228% because of its inhibition of plasma cholinesterase.[47] Ranitidine does not affect either plasma cholinesterase activity or the duration of action of succinylcholine.[48]

Several studies have evaluated the use of the nondepolarizing muscle relaxants rocuronium, mivacurium, vecuronium, atracurium, and cisatracurium in postpartum patients. The duration of action of rocuronium is prolonged by approximately 25% in postpartum patients,[49] and that of mivacurium by approximately 20%.[50] In postpartum patients the duration of action of vecuronium is prolonged by more than 50%.[51] In contrast, the duration of action for atracurium is unchanged (Figure 25-5),[52] and that of cisatracurium is significantly shorter, in the postpartum period.[53]

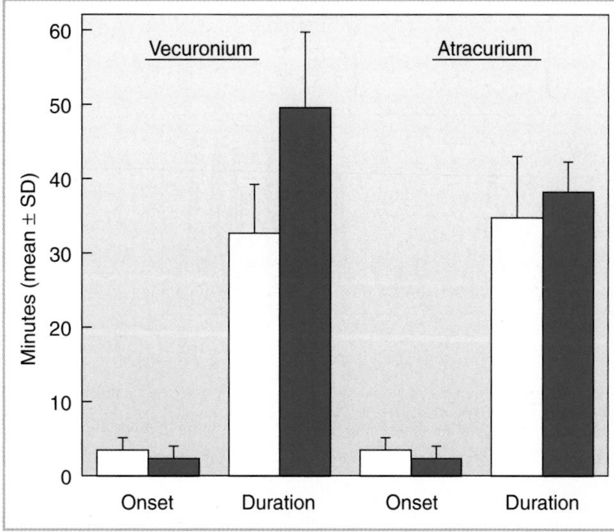

FIGURE 25-5 Onset and duration of action of vecuronium (0.1 mg/kg) and atracurium (0.5 mg/kg) in postpartum (*dark teal bar*) and nonpregnant control (*white bar*) patients. $P < .001$ for duration of vecuronium in postpartum compared with nonpregnant patients. (Modified from Khuenl-Brady KS, Koller J, Mair P, et al. Comparison of vecuronium- and atracurium-induced neuromuscular blockade in postpartum and nonpregnant patients. Anesth Analg 1991; 72:110-3.)

Prolongation of neuromuscular blockade could be clinically significant during a short procedure. Khuenl-Brady et al.[52] suggested that a relative decrease in hepatic blood flow and/or competition between vecuronium and steroid hormones for hepatic uptake may interfere with the hepatic clearance of vecuronium in postpartum women. Alternatively, Gin et al.[54] concluded that the duration of action for rocuronium is not prolonged in postpartum women if lean body mass—rather than total body weight—is used to calculate dose. These researchers speculated that the prolonged duration noted earlier[49] might be explained by relative drug overdose if the dose of rocuronium is based on the patient's temporarily increased body weight.[54]

Neuraxial Anesthesia

Spinal and epidural anesthesia both provide excellent operating conditions for postpartum tubal ligation. Airway obstruction, hypoventilation, and aspiration are much less likely during and after neuraxial anesthesia. A sensory level of T4 is needed to block visceral pain during exposure and manipulation of the fallopian tubes. The choice between spinal and epidural anesthesia is a matter of personal preference for the patient and the anesthesia provider.

EPIDURAL ANESTHESIA

When the performance of postpartum tubal ligation is anticipated in a parous patient, I encourage administration of epidural analgesia for labor and delivery. The epidural anesthetic can be extended for immediate postpartum tubal ligation if appropriate. I avoid administration of parenteral opioids during labor if immediate postpartum tubal ligation is planned. Immediate postpartum tubal ligation may save the patient the cost and inconvenience of an extra day in the hospital, allow her to eat shortly after delivery (and surgery), and enable her to avoid the apprehension of undergoing a surgical procedure the following day. The avoidance of opioids helps maintain normal gastric emptying, which should decrease the risk of aspiration during postpartum surgery. If the patient is stable and personnel are available, the procedure may be performed immediately after delivery, after the patient is moved to the operating room. The obstetrician must exclude excessive intrapartum blood loss[11] and document that the patient has given informed consent. Additional intravenous crystalloid may be administered, an epidural test dose is given to rule out intrathecal or intravascular migration of the epidural catheter, and the sensory level is extended with a concentration of local anesthetic suitable for surgical anesthesia. A short-acting local anesthetic (e.g., 3% 2-chloroprocaine) is usually appropriate because the procedure is quite short. Appropriate sedative drugs also may be given, if desired. The anesthesia provider should be cautious about giving sedative drugs that may cause prolonged postpartum amnesia. Most women want to remember their first several hours of contact with their newborn. In some cases, peripartum administration of a benzodiazepine may cause retrograde amnesia, and the patient may not recall childbirth.[55]

If surgery is not performed immediately, the catheter may be left in place for later postpartum tubal ligation. Several studies have evaluated the efficacy of using a previously placed epidural catheter for a tubal ligation performed several hours after delivery. Vincent and Reid[56] found that the mean delivery-to-surgery interval was shorter in patients with adequate epidural anesthesia than in those without adequate anesthesia (10.6 versus 14.8 hours, respectively). The chance of successful epidural anesthesia was greatest if the catheter was used within 4 hours of delivery. Lawlor et al.[57] reported an overall 87% success rate (using an indwelling epidural catheter for postpartum tubal ligation), but they observed no difference in the catheter placement–to-surgery interval between the successful epidural and failed epidural groups (21.4 versus 20.5 hours, respectively). In this study each epidural catheter was threaded 4 to 7.5 cm into the epidural space. Similarly, Goodman and Dumas[58] reported an overall success rate of 92% with the use of indwelling epidural catheters for postpartum tubal ligation. The success rate was 93% among patients who underwent surgery less than 24 hours after delivery and 80% among the 10 patients who underwent surgery more than 24 hours after delivery (Figure 25-6). This difference was not significant; however, the study was insufficiently powered to allow identification of a difference of this magnitude. Clinical experience suggests that if the anesthesia provider uses an epidural catheter placed for labor, the risk of anesthesia failure may be greater if surgery is delayed more than 10 hours after delivery. To ensure maximal success when using a multi-orifice catheter, the anesthesia provider should thread the catheter 4 to 6 cm into the epidural space and have the patient assume a de-flexed position before taping the catheter to the skin.[59,60]

SPINAL ANESTHESIA

Spinal anesthesia for postpartum tubal ligation has several advantages over epidural anesthesia. Epidural anesthesia requires the use of large volumes of local anesthetic and

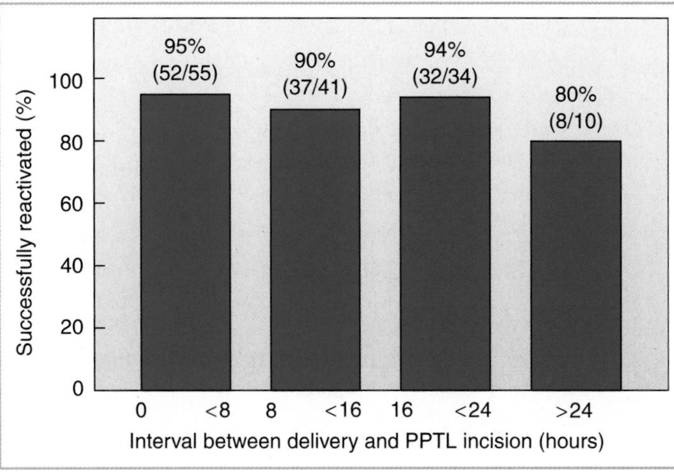

FIGURE 25-6 Rate of successful reactivation of epidural catheters for various intervals between delivery and the incision for postpartum tubal ligation (PPTL). There was no difference among groups in the success rate. (From Goodman EJ, Dumas SD. The rate of successful reactivation of labor epidural catheters for postpartum tubal ligation surgery. Regional Anesth Pain Med 1998; 23:258-61.)

thereby introduces the risk of intravascular injection and cardiotoxicity.[61] Epidural anesthesia also is time consuming; the induction of epidural anesthesia may require more time than the tubal ligation itself. Spinal anesthesia is simple to perform, is rapid in onset, and provides dense sensory and motor block. In one study, spinal anesthesia for postpartum tubal ligation was associated with lower professional fees and operating room charges than attempted reactivation of an epidural catheter placed during labor.[62] The ability to reinject a catheter intraoperatively is not necessary for a short procedure such as postpartum tubal ligation, and there is no need for prolonged postoperative analgesia. The risk of post–dural puncture headache is low if small-gauge (25- or 27-gauge) pencil-point or noncutting spinal needles are used. Indeed, some anesthesiologists have suggested that the incidence of post–dural puncture headache in obstetric patients is no different after spinal anesthesia with a 25-gauge Whitacre needle from that after planned epidural anesthesia (Table 25-2).

Local anesthetic requirements for spinal and epidural anesthesia are decreased during pregnancy, but studies have demonstrated a return to nonpregnant requirements by 36 hours postpartum. Assali and Prystowsky[63] demonstrated a return to nonpregnant requirements by 36 to 48 hours postpartum. Abouleish[64] prospectively compared the dose of spinal bupivacaine required for cesarean delivery with that required for postpartum tubal ligation. He noted that 30% more bupivacaine was required to achieve a T4 dermatomal anesthesia level in women who underwent operation 8 to 24 hours after delivery. The reason for the rapid decrease in sensitivity to local anesthetics is unclear but may be related to the rapid fall in progesterone levels after delivery of the placenta.

TABLE 25-2 Risk of Post–Dural Puncture Headache (PDPH) after Spinal and Epidural Anesthesia in Obstetric Patients

Needle Used*	Number of Anesthetics	Incidence of PDPH (%)
26 g Quincke	2256	5.2
27 g Quincke	852	2.7
25 g Whitacre	1000	1.2
17 g Epidural	21,578	1.3

*Quincke needles have a cutting bevel. Whitacre needles have a pencil-point tip. There was a significant difference in the incidence of post–dural puncture headache between the Quincke needle and the epidural needle ($P < .05$), but not between the Whitacre needle and the epidural needle.

Modified from Lambert DH, Hurley RJ, Hertwig L, Datta S. Role of needle gauge tip configuration in the production of lumbar puncture headache. Reg Anesth 1997; 22:66-72.

Datta et al.[65] examined plasma and cerebrospinal fluid (CSF) progesterone concentrations and spinal lidocaine requirements in nonpregnant, term pregnant, and postpartum women 12 to 18 hours after delivery. Plasma progesterone levels in pregnant women were 60 times higher than those in nonpregnant women but only seven times higher than those in postpartum women. CSF progesterone concentrations were eight times higher in term pregnant women and three times higher in postpartum women than in nonpregnant women. Intrathecal lidocaine requirements were similar in pregnant and postpartum patients, even though plasma and CSF progesterone concentrations were lower in the postpartum women. The investigators suggested "that a minimum level of progesterone in the CSF and/or plasma is necessary for this heightened local anesthetic activity" associated with progesterone. Together these studies suggest that local anesthetic requirements return to nonpregnant levels 12 to 36 hours after delivery.[63-65]

Huffnagle et al.[66] gave hyperbaric subarachnoid lidocaine 75 mg to postpartum women to determine whether age, weight, height, body mass index, vertebral column length, or time from delivery to initiation of the block correlated with the spread of sensory block. Only patient height had a weak positive correlation, and it accounted for less than 15% of the variance in height of the block. Because of the large variation in the spread of sensory block among patients of the same height, the investigators concluded that there was little use in adjusting the dose of local anesthetic on the basis of height.

Many anesthesia providers have discontinued the use of hyperbaric lidocaine for spinal anesthesia because of concern about transient neurologic symptoms (TNS). In a randomized controlled trial, Philip et al.[67] compared spinal administration of hyperbaric 5% lidocaine with that of hyperbaric 0.75% bupivacaine for postpartum tubal ligation. They observed a 3% incidence of transient neurologic symptoms with the use of lidocaine, compared with a 7% incidence with the use of bupivacaine, a nonsignificant difference. In an editorial accompanying their report, Schneider and Birnbach[68] acknowledged that "there are no very short-acting hyperbaric spinal local anesthetics that have taken the place of lidocaine for these short procedures, and many believe that spinal bupivacaine lasts too long to be a reasonable choice of anesthetic for a procedure that will last less than 20 min." However, they concluded, "Because pregnant patients represent a population that lies to the extreme in terms of the criteria for safety and lack of morbidity, we believe that for the present, there is still insufficient safety evidence to suggest that spinal hyperbaric 5% lidocaine be routinely used in obstetrics." In a dose-response study, Huffnagle et al.[69] found that hyperbaric bupivacaine 7.5 mg injected intrathecally in the lateral position provided adequate surgical anesthesia for postpartum tubal ligation with "a minimum duration of motor block and recovery time."

Postpartum women seem to be at lower risk for hypotension during spinal anesthesia than pregnant women. Abouleish[64] gave ephedrine to correct maternal hypotension in 83% of pregnant women who received spinal bupivacaine anesthesia for cesarean delivery. In contrast, only 7% of postpartum women who received spinal anesthesia for tubal ligation required ephedrine. Pregnant women undergo an autotransfusion immediately after delivery. The greater intravascular volume and the lack of aortocaval compression may help protect postpartum patients from hypotension during spinal anesthesia. Sharma et al.[70] compared the use of crystalloid with the use of 6% hetastarch for the prevention of hypotension during spinal anesthesia for postpartum tubal ligation. They observed a 52% incidence of hypotension in the crystalloid group and a 16% incidence in the hetastarch group. However, they acknowledged that the higher expense of colloid might not be justifiable. Suelto et al.,[71] comparing normotensive and hypertensive patients who received hyperbaric lidocaine for postpartum tubal ligation, found no difference in the use or dose of ephedrine for treatment of hypotension.

Preservative-free intrathecal meperidine can be used as an alternative to local anesthetic for postpartum tubal ligation. The typical dose is 1 mg per kg prepregnant weight (50 to 80 mg) for cesarean delivery or tubal ligation. With an onset time of 3 to 5 minutes and duration of 30 to 60 minutes, meperidine compares favorably with 5% lidocaine. In a study that compared lidocaine 70 mg with meperidine 60 mg for postpartum tubal ligation, patients who received meperidine had more pruritus but longer postoperative analgesia (448 versus 83 minutes, respectively).[72] There was no difference between groups in rates of nausea, hemoglobin desaturation, or patient satisfaction. Intrathecal meperidine may be an alternative to lidocaine for postpartum tubal ligation.

Box 25-1 summarizes a personal approach to anesthetic management for postpartum tubal ligation.

BOX 25-1 Anesthetic Management for Postpartum Tubal Ligation

Intrapartum Management

- Encourage use of epidural analgesia.
- Avoid administration of parenteral opioids.
- Keep patient on *nil per os* (NPO) status except for clear liquids.
- Give aspiration prophylaxis if the procedure is to be performed immediately after delivery.

Timing of Surgery

- Consider performing surgery immediately postpartum if the patient is hemodynamically stable and has received aspiration prophylaxis.
- An epidural catheter placed for labor may provide more reliable anesthesia if used within 10 hours of delivery.

Epidural Anesthesia

- Requires a T4 sensory level of anesthesia.
- After a negative epidural test dose result, consider using 3% 2-chloroprocaine unless a longer procedure is planned.
- If a catheter placed during labor is used, beware of a higher risk of failure if the delivery-to-surgery interval is prolonged.
- Give fentanyl 50 to 100 μg via the epidural catheter for intraoperative and postoperative analgesia.

Spinal Anesthesia

- Requires a T4 sensory level of anesthesia.
- It is the preferred technique for delayed postpartum tubal ligation or for immediate surgery in patients who did not have epidural labor analgesia or in whom epidural analgesia during labor and delivery was inadequate.
- Use a small-gauge, noncutting, pencil-point spinal needle.
- Give lidocaine 75 mg with fentanyl 10 to 25 μg, or bupivacaine 7.5 mg with fentanyl 10 to 25 μg.

General Anesthesia

- Perform a rapid-sequence induction with cricoid pressure.
- Intubate the trachea and control ventilation.
- Avoid high concentrations (> 1.0 minimal alveolar concentration [MAC]) of a volatile anesthetic agent.
- Monitor neuromuscular blockade if a nondepolarizing muscle relaxant is used.

POSTOPERATIVE ANALGESIA

Postpartum tubal ligation produces modest postoperative pain of short duration. Patients typically receive one dose of parenteral opioid postoperatively, followed by oral analgesics. Optimal analgesia encourages early ambulation, interaction with the neonate, and early discharge from the hospital. An oral nonsteroidal anti-inflammatory drug (NSAID) such as ibuprofen may be given to supplement other analgesics. When epinephrine 0.2 mg was added to lidocaine with fentanyl 10 μg for spinal anesthesia, the duration of complete and effective analgesia was prolonged and the incidence of pruritus was decreased; however, the time to complete motor recovery was prolonged.[73] Habib et al.[74] reported that adding intrathecal morphine 0.05 mg to intrathecal bupivacaine and fentanyl for postpartum tubal ligation resulted in less intense pain at rest and with movement at 4 hours after surgery than with saline control. However, patients who received morphine had more vomiting and pruritus. Despite side effects, patients who received morphine were significantly more satisfied. Similarly, in a comparison of epidural morphine 2 mg, 3 mg, or 4 mg with saline control, Marcus et al.[75] found that epidural morphine 2 mg provided better analgesia without increasing the need to treat side effects, in comparison with a regimen of oral opioids and NSAIDs without epidural morphine. Although effective, spinal and epidural morphine analgesia should be used with caution because patients who receive it may be discharged soon after postpartum tubal ligation, before the risk period for delayed respiratory depression has ended.

Local anesthetic infiltration of the mesosalpinx with bupivacaine or topical application of a local anesthetic to the fallopian tubes significantly decreases opioid requirements postoperatively.[76] These are simple, rapid techniques that can be used by the obstetrician. Wittels et al.[77] reported that multimodal therapy after spinal or epidural anesthesia, consisting of intravenous ketorolac 60 mg, intravenous metoclopramide 10 mg, and infiltration of the incised skin, fallopian tubes, and mesosalpinx with 0.5% bupivacaine, prevented pain, nausea, and painful uterine cramping in both the immediate postoperative period and for 7 days after postpartum tubal ligation in 9 of 10 patients. The manufacturer of ketorolac has stated that the agent is contraindicated in nursing mothers because of the possible adverse effects of prostaglandin synthetase inhibitors on neonates. In contrast, the American Academy of Pediatrics considers ketorolac to be compatible with breast-feeding.[78]

KEY POINTS

- Postpartum tubal sterilization is an elective procedure. No data indicate that the postpartum patient's safety is enhanced by a delay of surgery or compromised by the performance of tubal ligation immediately after delivery.
- Postpartum sterilization offers the advantages of convenience for the patient and technical simplicity for the surgeon.
- Postpartum patients do not have lower gastric pH or higher gastric volumes than nonpregnant patients undergoing elective surgery. Some studies suggest that gastric emptying is delayed postpartum only if the patient has received an opioid analgesic during labor.
- The incidence of gastroesophageal reflux returns toward normal by the second postpartum day.
- Modern anesthetic drugs do not appear in breast milk in amounts that affect the neonate.
- The duration of succinylcholine-, rocuronium-, mivacurium-, and vecuronium-induced neuromuscular blockade is prolonged during the postpartum period. In contrast, the duration of action for atracurium is unchanged, and that of cisatracurium is shorter.
- An epidural catheter placed for labor may be used for postpartum tubal ligation, but the risk of anesthesia failure may be greater if surgery is delayed more than 10 hours after delivery.
- Spinal anesthesia is preferred for delayed postpartum tubal ligation, regardless of whether an epidural catheter was placed for labor anesthesia.
- The local anesthetic dose for spinal anesthesia returns to nonpregnant requirements by 12 to 36 hours postpartum.
- Postoperative multimodal analgesia improves maternal mobilization and infant bonding, and facilitates earlier hospital discharge.

REFERENCES

1. Westhoff C, Davis A. Tubal sterilization: Focus on the U.S. experience. Fertil Steril 2000; 73:913-22.
2. Practice Guidelines for Obstetric Anesthesia. An updated report by the American Society of Anesthesiologists Task Force on Obstetric Anesthesia. Anesthesiology 2007; 106:843-63.
3. Pati S, Cullins V. Female sterilization, evidence. Obstet Gynecol Clin North Am 2000; 27:859-99.
4. World Health Organization, Task Force on Female Sterilization, Special Programme of Research, Development and Research Training in Human Reproduction. Minilaparotomy or laparoscopy for sterilization: A multicenter, multinational randomized study. Am J Obstet Gynecol 1982; 143:645-52.
5. Hillis SC, Marchbanks PA, Tylor LR, et al. Poststerilization regret: Findings from the United States collaborative review of sterilization. Obstet Gynecol 1999; 93:889-94.
6. Cunningham FG, Hauth JC, Leveno KJ, et al. Williams Obstetrics. 22nd edition. New York, McGraw-Hill, 2005:752-3.
7. Peterson HB, Zhisen X, Hughes JM, et al. The risk of pregnancy after tubal sterilization: Findings from the U.S. Collaborative Review of Sterilization. Am J Obstet Gynecol 1996; 174:1161-70.
8. American College of Obstetricians and Gynecologists Committee on Technical Bulletins. Sterilization. ACOG Technical Bulletin No. 222. Washington, DC, ACOG, 1996.
9. Medicaid. Sterilizations, hysterectomies and abortions. Consent form, Form 499-A, MED-178 (rev 11/85). Available at: http://hlunix.hl.state.ut.us/medicaid/pdfs/forms/sterilizationconsent.pdf
10. Vincent RD, Martin RQ. Postpartum tubal ligation after pregnancy complicated by preeclampsia or gestational hypertension. Obstet Gynecol 1996; 88:119-22.
11. Toledo P, McCarthy RJ, Hewlett BJ, et al. The accuracy of blood loss estimation after simulated vaginal delivery. Anesth Analg 2007; 105:1736-40.
12. Ito S. Drug therapy: Drug therapy for breast-feeding women. N Engl J Med 2000; 343:118-25.
13. Bucklin BA, Smith CV. Postpartum tubal ligation: Safety, timing, and other implications for anesthesia. Anesth Analg 1999; 89:1269-74.
14. Hawkins JL. Anesthesia-related maternal mortality. Clin Obstet Gynecol 2003; 46:679-87.

15. Deshpande GN, Turner AK, Sommerville IF. Plasma progesterone and pregnanediol in human pregnancy, during labour and post-partum. J Obstet Gynaecol Br Emp 1960; 67:954-61.
16. Llauro JL, Runnebaum B, Zander J. Progesterone in human peripheral blood before, during and after labor. Am J Obstet Gynecol 1968; 101:867-73.
17. O'Sullivan GM, Sutton AJ, Thompson SA, et al. Noninvasive measurement of gastric emptying in obstetric patients. Anesth Analg 1987; 66:505-11.
18. Gin T, Cho AMW, Lew JKL, et al. Gastric emptying in the postpartum period. Anaesth Intens Care 1991; 19:521-4.
19. Whitehead EM, Smith M, Dean Y, O'Sullivan G. An evaluation of gastric emptying times in pregnancy and the puerperium. Anaesthesia 1993; 48:53-7.
20. Sandhar BK, Elliott RH, Windram I, Rowbotham DJ. Peripartum changes in gastric emptying. Anaesthesia 1992; 47:196-8.
21. Wong CA, Loffredi M, Ganchiff JN, et al. Gastric emptying of water in term pregnancy. Anesthesiology 2002; 96:1395-1400.
22. Wong CA, McCarthy RJ, Fitzgerald PC, et al. Gastric emptying of water in obese pregnant women at term. Anesth Analg 2007; 105:751-5.
23. Kubli M, Scrutton MJ, Seed PT, et al. An evaluation of isotonic "sport drinks" during labor. Anesth Analg 2002; 94:404-8.
24. Jayaram A, Bowen MP, Deshpande S, Carp HM. Ultrasound examination of the stomach contents of women in the postpartum period. Anesth Analg 1997; 84:522-6.
25. Scrutton MJ, Metcalfe GA, Lowy C, et al. Eating in labour: A randomized controlled trial assessing the risks and benefits. Anaesthesia 1999; 54:329-34.
26. Wright PMC, Allen RW, Moore J, Donnelly JP. Gastric emptying during lumbar extradural analgesia in labor: Effect of fentanyl supplementation. Br J Anaesth 1992; 68:248-51.
27. Kelly MC, Carabine UA, Hill DA, Mirakhur RK. A comparison of the effect of intrathecal and extradural fentanyl on gastric emptying in laboring women. Anesth Analg 1997; 85:834-6.
28. Coté CJ. Aspiration: An overrated risk in elective patients. In Stoelting RK, Barash PG, Gallagher TJ, editors. Advances in Anesthesia. St. Louis, Mosby, 1992:5-6.
29. Blouw R, Scatliff J, Craig DB, Palahniuk RJ. Gastric volume and pH in postpartum patients. Anesthesiology 1976; 45:456-7.
30. James CF, Gibbs CP, Banner T. Postpartum perioperative risk of aspiration pneumonia. Anesthesiology 1984; 61:756-9.
31. Lam KK, So HY, Gin T. Gastric pH and volume after oral fluids in the postpartum patient. Can J Anaesth 1993; 40:218-21.
32. Brock-Utne JG, Dow TGB, Welman S, et al. The effect of metoclopramide on the lower oesophageal sphincter in late pregnancy. Anaesth Intens Care 1978; 6:26-9.
33. Vanner RG, Goodman NW. Gastro-oesophageal reflux in pregnancy at term and after delivery. Anaesthesia 1989; 44:808-11.
34. Bogod DG. The postpartum stomach: When is it safe (editorial)? Anaesthesia 1994; 49:1-2.
35. Barton ACH, Spielman FJ, Onder R, Mayer DC. Timing of postpartum sterilization: Complications and cost-savings of early tubal ligations. Anesthesiology 1996; 85:A896.
36. Cruikshank DP, Laube DW, DeBacker LJ. Intraperitoneal lidocaine anesthesia for postpartum tubal ligation. Obstet Gynecol 1973; 42:127-30.
37. Poindexter AN, Abdul-Malak M, Fast JE. Laparoscopic tubal sterilization under local anesthesia. Obstet Gynecol 1990; 75:5-8.
38. DeStefano F, Greenspan JR, Dicker RC, et al. Complications of interval laparoscopic tubal sterilization. Obstet Gynecol 1983; 61:153-8.
39. Peterson HB, DeStefano F, Rubin GL, et al. Deaths attributable to tubal sterilization in the United States, 1977 to 1981. Am J Obstet Gynecol 1983; 146:131-6.
40. Marx GF, Kim YI, Lin CC, et al. Postpartum uterine pressures under halothane or enflurane anesthesia. Obstet Gynecol 1978; 51:695-8.
41. Chan MTV, Gin T. Postpartum changes in the minimum alveolar concentration of isoflurane. Anesthesiology 1995; 82:1360-3.
42. Zhou HH, Norman P, DeLima LGR, Mehta M, Bass D. The minimum alveolar concentration of isoflurane in patients undergoing bilateral tubal ligation in the postpartum period. Anesthesiology 1995; 82:1364-8.
43. Dailland P, Cockshott ID, Lorzin JD, et al. Intravenous propofol during cesarean delivery: Placental transfer, concentrations in breast milk, and neonatal effects: A preliminary study. Anesthesiology 1989; 71:827-34.
44. Evans RT, Wroe JM. Plasma cholinesterase changes during pregnancy. Anaesthesia 1980; 35:651-4.
45. Ganga CC, Heyduk JV, Marx GF, Sklar GS. A comparison of the response to suxamethonium in postpartum and gynaecological patients. Anaesthesia 1982; 37:903-6.
46. Leighton BL, Cheek TG, Gross JB, et al. Succinylcholine pharmacodynamics in peripartum patients. Anesthesiology 1986; 64:202-5.
47. Kao YJ, Turner DR. Prolongation of succinylcholine block by metoclopramide. Anesthesiology 1989; 70:905-8.
48. Woodworth GE, Sears DH, Grove TM, et al. The effect of cimetidine and ranitidine on the duration of action of succinylcholine. Anesth Analg 1989; 68:295-7.
49. Puhringer FK, Spart HJ, Mitterschiffthaler G, et al. Extended duration of action of rocuronium in postpartum patients. Anesth Analg 1997; 84:352-4.
50. Gin T, Derrick JL, Chan MTV, et al. Postpartum patients have slightly prolonged neuromuscular block after mivacurium. Anesth Analg 1998; 86:82-5.
51. Hawkins JL, Adenwala J, Camp C, Joyce TH. The effect of H_2-receptor antagonist premedication on the duration of vecuronium-induced neuromuscular blockade in postpartum patients. Anesthesiology 1989; 71:175-7.
52. Khuenl-Brady KS, Koller J, Mair P, et al. Comparison of vecuronium and atracurium-induced neuromuscular blockade in postpartum and nonpregnant patients. Anesth Analg 1991; 72:110-3.
53. Pan PH, Moore C. Comparison of cisatracurium-induced neuromuscular blockade between immediate postpartum and nonpregnant patients. J Clin Anesth 2001; 13:112-7.
54. Gin T, Chan MTV, Chan KL, et al. Prolonged neuromuscular block after rocuronium in postpartum patients. Anesth Analg 2002; 94:686-9.
55. Camann W, Cohen MB, Ostheimer GW. Is midazolam desirable for sedation in parturients (letter)? Anesthesiology 1986; 65:441.
56. Vincent RD, Reid RW. Epidural anesthesia for postpartum tubal ligation using epidural catheters placed during labor. J Clin Anesth 1993; 5:289-91.
57. Lawlor M, Weiner M, Fantauzzi M, Johnson C. Efficacy of epidural anesthesia for post-partum tubal ligation utilizing indwelling labor epidural catheters. Reg Anesth 1994; 19:54.
58. Goodman EJ, Dumas SD. The rate of successful reactivation of labor epidural catheters for postpartum tubal ligation surgery. Reg Anesth Pain Med 1998; 23:258-61.
59. Beilin Y, Bernstein HH, Zucker-Pinchoff B. The optimal distance that a multiorifice epidural catheter should be threaded into the epidural space. Anesth Analg 1995; 81:301-4.
60. Hamilton CL, Riley ET, Cohen SE. Changes in the position of epidural catheters associated with patient movement. Anesthesiology 1997; 86:778-84.
61. Abouleish EI, Elias M, Nelson C. Ropivacaine-induced seizure after extradural anaesthesia. Br J Anaesth 1998; 80:843-4.
62. Viscomi CM, Rathmell JP. Labor epidural catheter reactivation or spinal anesthesia for delayed postpartum tubal ligation: A cost comparison. J Clin Anesth 1995; 7:380-3.
63. Assali NS, Prystowsky H. Studies on autonomic blockade. I. Comparison between the effects of tetraethylammonium chloride (TEAC) and high selective spinal anesthesia on blood pressure of normal and toxemic pregnancy. J Clin Invest 1950; 29:1354-66.
64. Abouleish EI. Postpartum tubal ligation requires more bupivacaine for spinal anesthesia than does cesarean section. Anesth Analg 1986; 65:897-900.

65. Datta S, Hurley RJ, Naulty JS, et al. Plasma and cerebrospinal fluid progesterone concentrations in pregnant and nonpregnant women. Anesth Analg 1986; 65:950-4.
66. Huffnagle S, Norris MC, Leighton BL, et al. Do patient variables influence the subarachnoid spread of hyperbaric lidocaine in the postpartum patient? Reg Anesth 1994; 19:330-4.
67. Philip J, Sharma SK, Gottumukkala VNR, et al. Transient neurologic symptoms after spinal anesthesia with lidocaine in obstetric patients. Anesth Analg 2001; 92:405-9.
68. Schneider MC, Birnbach DJ. Lidocaine neurotoxicity in the obstetric patient: Is the water safe? Anesth Analg 2001; 92:287-90.
69. Huffnagle SL, Norris MC, Huffnagle HJ, et al. Intrathecal hyperbaric bupivacaine dose response in postpartum tubal ligation patients. Reg Anesth Pain Med 2002; 27:284-8.
70. Sharma SK, Gajraj NM, Sidawi JE. Prevention of hypotension during spinal anesthesia: A comparison of intravascular administration of hetastarch versus lactated Ringer's solution. Anesth Analg 1997; 84:111-4.
71. Suelto MD, Vincent RD, Larmon JE, et al. Spinal anesthesia for postpartum tubal ligation after pregnancy complicated by preeclampsia or gestational hypertension. Reg Anesth Pain Med 2000; 25:170-3.
72. Norris MC, Honet JE, Leighton BL, et al. A comparison of meperidine and lidocaine for spinal anesthesia for postpartum tubal ligation. Reg Anesth 1996; 21:84-8.
73. Malinow AM, Mokriski BLK, Nomura MK, et al. Effect of epinephrine on intrathecal fentanyl analgesia in patients undergoing postpartum tubal ligation. Anesthesiology 1990; 73:381-5.
74. Habib AS, Muir HA, White WD, et al. Intrathecal morphine for analgesia after postpartum bilateral tubal ligation. Anesth Analg 2005; 100:239-43.
75. Marcus RL, Wong CA, Lehor A, et al. Postoperative epidural morphine for postpartum tubal ligation analgesia. Anesth Analg 2005; 101:876-81.
76. Alexander CD, Wetchler BV, Thompson RE. Bupivacaine infiltration of the mesosalpinx in ambulatory surgical laparoscopic tubal sterilization. Can J Anaesth 1987; 34:362-5.
77. Wittels B, Faure EAM, Chavez R, et al. Effective analgesia after bilateral tubal ligation. Anesth Analg 1998; 87:619-23.
78. American Academy of Pediatrics Committee on Drugs. The transfer of drugs and other chemicals into human milk. Pediatrics 2001; 108:776-89.

Part VII

Cesarean Delivery

During most of the nineteenth century, physicians performed very few cesarean deliveries because the mortality rate was so high. For example, in his case books, John Snow mentions more than 90 patients anesthetized for vaginal delivery, but not one cesarean delivery.[1] The procedure was reserved for desperate situations. One physician quipped that a woman had a better chance of surviving an abdominal delivery if she performed the surgery herself, or if her abdomen were accidentally ripped open by the horn of a bull.[2]

Hemorrhage and infection caused most deaths. The use of anesthesia allowed surgeons to develop techniques to deal with these problems. Italian surgeon Eduardo Porro made the first important innovation in 1876. To limit hemorrhage he excised the uterus after delivering the child. Others had left the uterine incision open in the belief that it would heal better. In 1882, German surgeon Max Sänger advised closing the uterus with sutures, thereby obviating the need for a hysterectomy. Sänger, benefiting from the advances in bacteriology, also devised techniques to limit the risk of infection.[3]

In 1910, J. Whitridge Williams of John Hopkins still called cesarean delivery a "dangerous procedure" despite the fact that the maternal mortality rate had fallen to 10%. He performed it only for the most severe cases of contracted pelvis.[2,4] In fact, Williams warned that a cesarean delivery "should never be performed when the child is dead or in serious danger." Even in 1970, cesarean delivery rates remained below 7% in the United States, and at less than 2% in many European countries.[5]

With few agents to choose from, anesthetic techniques for cesarean delivery also evolved slowly. Regional anesthesia was not available before 1900. Ether and chloroform were the only two potent agents available for general anesthesia until the addition of cyclopropane. Until curare was introduced to clinical practice, use of these agents necessitated achieving an anesthetic depth sufficient to obtain abdominal relaxation.

Only in the past five decades have there been incentives to develop better anesthetic techniques for cesarean delivery. First, obstetricians began to perform cesarean delivery more often to deal with fetal and maternal problems. Second, physicians developed a better understanding of the physiology of pregnancy, especially the nature of risks associated with anesthesia. Third, anesthesiologists and obstetricians began to place greater emphasis on the well-being of the neonate, a change that required the development of anesthetic techniques that would protect the mother but have the least possible effect on the child.

Donald Caton, M.D.

REFERENCES

1. Ellis RH, editor. The Case Books of Dr. John Snow. Med Hist Suppl 1994:14.
2. Williams JW. Obstetrics: A Textbook for the Use of Students and Practitioners. New York, D. Appleton and Company, 1907:400-11.
3. O'Dowd M, Philipp EE. The History of Obstetrics and Gynaecology New York, Parthenon Publishing, 1994:157-65.
4. Loudon I. Death in Childbirth: An International Study of Maternal Care and Maternal Mortality, 1800-1850. New York, Oxford University Press, 1992:132-9.
5. Hellman LM, Pritchard JA, Wynn RM. Williams Obstetrics. New York, Appleton-Century-Crofts, 1971:1007-167.

Chapter 26

Anesthesia for Cesarean Delivery

Lawrence C. Tsen, M.D.

HISTORY

Cesarean delivery is defined as the birth of an infant through incisions in the abdomen (laparotomy) and uterus (hysterotomy). Although the technique is commonly associated with the manner in which the Roman Emperor Julius Caesar (100 BC) was purportedly born, medical historians have found evidence of the continued presence of Caesar's mother in his life at a time when such operations were invariably fatal.[1] The term *cesarean section* is commonly used; however, the Latin words *caedere* and *sectio* both imply *to cut*, and modern linguists argue that use of both words is redundant. Consequently, *cesarean delivery* is the preferred term.

Morbidity and mortality, most often associated with hemorrhage and infection, limited the use of cesarean delivery until the twentieth century, when advances in aseptic, surgical, and anesthetic techniques improved the safety for both mother and baby. Today, cesarean delivery accounts for more than 30% of all births and is the most common surgical procedure performed in the United States, with more than 1 million performed each year[2]; in other

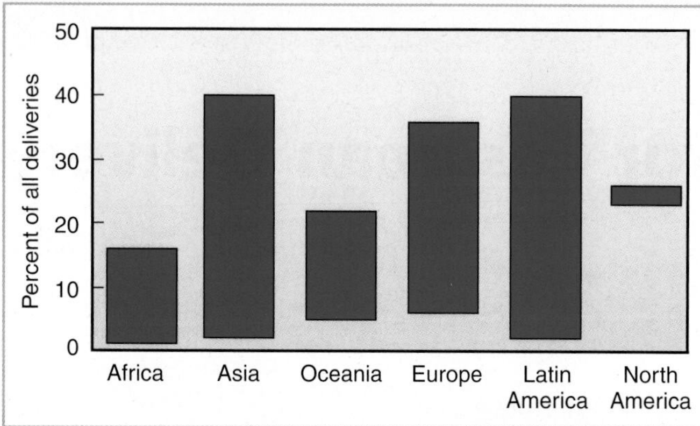

FIGURE 26-1 The range of cesarean delivery rates by world region as collected in surveys or vital registration system reports. (Data adapted from Betran AP, Merialdi M, Lauer JA, et al. Rates of caesarean section: Analysis of global, regional and national estimates. Paediatr Perinat Epidemiol 2007; 21:98-113.)

developed countries the cesarean delivery rate varies between 15% and more than 30%.[3] Since 1970, a progressive increase in the cesarean delivery rate has been observed worldwide (Figure 26-1). Maternal, obstetric, fetal, medicolegal, and social factors are largely responsible for this trend (Box 26-1). There is significant variation in cesarean delivery rates among institutions and obstetricians in the United States.[4]

INDICATIONS

The common indications for cesarean delivery include dystocia, malpresentation, nonreassuring fetal status, previous cesarean delivery, and maternal request (Box 26-2). A prior cesarean delivery does not require performance of cesarean delivery in a subsequent pregnancy. A trial of labor after cesarean (TOLAC), which if successful is called a vaginal birth after cesarean (VBAC), is an alternative option that has declined in use (Figure 26-2) (see Chapter 19).

BOX 26-1 Factors Contributing to the Increasing Cesarean Delivery Rate

Maternal Factors
- Increasing proportion of deliveries in nulliparous women
- Delayed childbearing and increasing maternal age
- Increasing prevalence of obesity

Obstetric Factors
- Increasing use of labor induction
- Fewer vaginal breech deliveries
- Fewer instrumental vaginal deliveries
- Fewer attempts at trial of labor after cesarean delivery
- Increasing availability of cesarean delivery in developing nations

Fetal Factors
- Increasing incidence of fetal macrosomia
- Increasing incidence of multiple gestation
- *Ex utero* intrapartum treatment (EXIT) procedures

Practice Environment Factors
- Concern for malpractice litigation
- Increased use of electronic fetal heart rate monitoring
- Concern for pelvic floor injury associated with vaginal birth
- Desire for scheduled procedures (convenience)

BOX 26-2 Indications for Cesarean Delivery

Maternal
- Antepartum or intrapartum hemorrhage
- Arrest of labor
- Breech presentation
- Chorioamnionitis
- Deteriorating maternal condition (e.g., severe preeclampsia)
- Dystocia
- Failure of induction of labor
- Genital herpes (active lesions)
- High-order multiple gestation (or twin gestation in which twin A has a breech presentation)
- Maternal request
- Placenta previa
- Placental abruption
- Previous myomectomy
- Prior classic uterine incision
- Uterine rupture

Fetal
- Breech presentation or other malpresentation
- Fetal intolerance of labor
- Macrosomia
- Nonreassuring fetal status
- Prolapsed umbilical cord

Obstetrician
- Desire to avoid difficult forceps or vacuum delivery

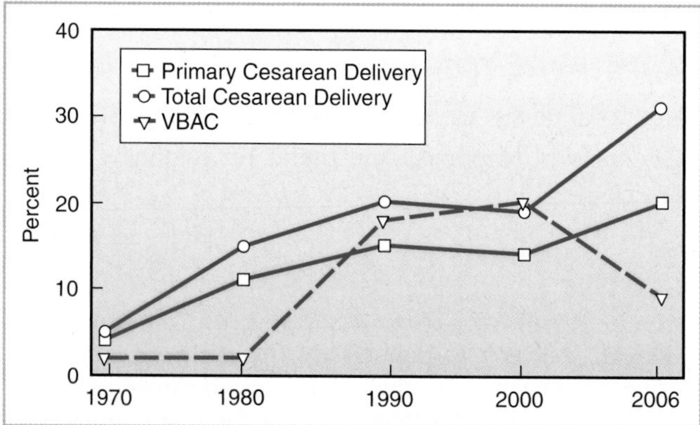

FIGURE 26-2 Rates of primary cesarean delivery, total cesarean delivery, and vaginal birth after cesarean delivery in the United States, 1970 to 2006. VBAC, vaginal birth after cesarean delivery. (Data for 1970-1988 from the National Hospital Discharge Survey; data for 1989-2006 from the National Vital Statistics System, Centers for Disease Control and Prevention. Available at http://www.cdc.gov)

OPERATIVE TECHNIQUE

The technical aspects of performing a cesarean delivery are comparable worldwide, with minor variations.[2] A midline vertical *abdominal* incision allows rapid access and greater surgical exposure; however, the horizontal suprapubic (Pfannenstiel) incision offers better cosmesis and wound strength. Similarly, a low transverse *uterine* incision allows for a low incidence of uterine dehiscence or rupture in subsequent pregnancies as well as a reduction in the risks of infection, blood loss, and bowel and omental adhesions in comparison with a vertical uterine incision. Vertical uterine incisions are most often used in the following situations: (1) when the lower uterine segment is underdeveloped (before 34 weeks' gestation), (2) in delivery of a preterm infant in a woman who has not labored, and (3) in selected patients with multiple gestation and/or malpresentation. In some cases, a vertical uterine incision is performed high on the anterior uterine wall (i.e., classic incision), especially in the patient with a low-lying anterior placenta previa or when a cesarean hysterectomy is planned.

Uterine exteriorization following delivery facilitates visualization and repair of the uterine incision, particularly when the incision has been extended laterally. Although the effect of exteriorization on blood loss and febrile morbidity remains controversial,[5] higher rates of intraoperative nausea, emesis, and venous air embolism as well as postoperative pain have been observed.[6-8]

MORBIDITY AND MORTALITY

Complications of cesarean delivery include hemorrhage, infection, thromboembolism, ureteral and bladder injury, abdominal pain, uterine rupture in subsequent pregnancies, and death (Box 26-3).[9,10] Nonelective cesarean delivery is associated with a greater risk of maternal morbidity than elective cesarean delivery; a 2008 study of all deliveries in Finland indicated that the rates of severe maternal morbidity were 5.2, 12.1, and 27.2 per 1000 vaginal, elective cesarean, and nonelective cesarean deliveries, respectively.[11]

Maternal mortality has decreased during the past 70 years. Since 1937, when maternal mortality for nulliparous women undergoing cesarean delivery in the United States was 6%, the risk of death associated with the procedure has decreased by a factor of nearly 1000 owing to the availability of blood transfusions, antibiotics, safer anesthetic techniques, and critical care units.[12] Maternal morbidity and mortality vary widely from country to country. In most developed nations, the rate of maternal death associated with all cesarean deliveries remains higher than that associated with vaginal deliveries.[3,13-15] The risk of maternal death for a planned, elective primary cesarean delivery may not differ from that associated with a planned vaginal delivery, but performance of cesarean delivery places the mother at higher risk for morbidity (and perhaps mortality) in subsequent pregnancies and cesarean deliveries.[16]

Clark et al.[13] identified the causes of maternal death in a retrospective study of 1.5 million deliveries that occurred between 2000 and 2006 within a health care network composed of primary, secondary, and tertiary level hospitals in 20 states (Table 26-1). Only 15% of maternal deaths were related to preexisting medical conditions; most deaths occurred in women classified as being at low risk at the beginning of pregnancy. The investigators concluded that 17 deaths (18%) could have been prevented by provision of more appropriate medical care. (Causality was determined by evaluating whether the maternal death could have been avoided with the use of an alternate route of delivery, with the assumption that all other details remained the same prior to delivery.) The preventable deaths were associated with postpartum hemorrhage (8), preeclampsia (5), medication error (3), and infection (1). Cesarean delivery was determined to be directly responsible for maternal death in 4 cases, including hemorrhage from surgical vascular injury in 3 cases and sepsis from surgical injury to the bowel in the fourth. Deaths associated with, but not directly caused by, cesarean delivery were associated with perimortem procedures or caused by thromboembolic phenomena; of the 9 patients who died from thromboembolic phenomena, none had received peripartum thromboprophylaxis via pharmacologic therapy or pneumatic compression devices. The investigators concluded that cesarean delivery per se was only rarely the causative factor in maternal death; in the majority of cases, the death was related to the indication for the cesarean delivery rather than the operative procedure. Nonetheless, these investigators also concluded that the risk of death *caused* by cesarean delivery is approximately 10 times higher than that for vaginal birth and likely could be reduced with the implementation of universal perioperative thromboprophylaxis.

Neonatal morbidity, in particular respiratory system morbidity (thus potentially resulting in the anesthesia provider's involvement in neonatal resuscitation), is increased by performance of elective cesarean delivery.[17] Patterns and rates of neonatal mortality are similar to those of maternal mortality; the higher neonatal mortality rates observed following cesarean delivery most likely reflect the conditions that prompt nonelective cesarean delivery.[18]

BOX 26-3 Complications of Cesarean Delivery

Anesthetic Complications

Hemorrhage
- Uterine atony
- Uterine lacerations
- Broad ligament hematoma

Infection
- Endometritis
- Wound infection

Postoperative Complications
- Cardiovascular: venous thromboembolism
- Gastrointestinal: ileus, adhesions, injury
- Genitourinary: bladder or ureteral injury
- Respiratory: atelectasis, aspiration
- Chronic pain

Future Pregnancy Risks
- Placenta previa
- Placenta accreta
- Uterine rupture
- Obstetric hysterectomy

TABLE 26-1 Relationship between Route of Delivery and Maternal Death

		Association of Delivery Route with Maternal Death*		Causal Relationship of Delivery Route with Maternal Death†	
Delivery Type	**Number of Procedures**	**Number of Deaths**	**Frequency of Death (per 100,000 Procedures)**	**Number of Deaths**	**Frequency of Death (per 100,000 Procedures)**
Vaginal	1,003,173	17	1.7	2	0.2
Primary cesarean	282,632	46	16.3	7	2.5
Repeat cesarean	175,465	12	7.4	2	1.1
Total cesarean	458,097	58	12.7	9	2.0
Not delivered/dilation and curettage	NA	20	NA	NA	NA
Total	1,461,270	95	6.5‡	20	1.4

NA, not applicable.

***Association relationships:** For vaginal birth versus total cesarean, vaginal birth versus primary cesarean, and vaginal birth versus repeat cesarean, $P < .001$. For primary cesarean versus repeat cesarean, $P = .01$.

†**Causal relationships:** For vaginal birth versus total cesarean and vaginal birth versus primary cesarean, $P < .001$. For vaginal birth versus repeat cesarean, $P = 0.12$. For primary cesarean versus repeat cesarean, $P = .50$. For vaginal birth versus primary, repeat, and total cesarean delivery, excluding pulmonary embolism deaths preventable with universal prophylaxis, $P = .07$, $P = .38$, and $P = .08$, respectively.

‡Deaths per 100,000 pregnancies.

Adapted from data in Clark SL, Belfort MA, Dildy GA, et al. Maternal death in the 21st century: Causes, prevention, and relationship to cesarean delivery. Am J Obstet Gynecol 2008; 199:36.e1-5.

PREVENTION OF CESAREAN DELIVERY

Neuraxial labor analgesic techniques were earlier thought to increase the cesarean delivery rate; however, randomized controlled trials and sentinel event studies have indicated that epidural analgesia is not associated with a higher cesarean delivery rate than systemic opioid analgesia (see Chapter 23).[19,20] Moreover, the combined spinal-epidural (CSE) technique for labor analgesia (despite its association with fetal bradycardia) does not result in an increase in the total cesarean delivery rate.[21-23] On the other hand, some cesarean deliveries may be avoided through the provision of (1) adequate labor analgesia, including analgesia for trial of labor after cesarean delivery and instrumental vaginal delivery; (2) analgesia for external cephalic version; and (3) intrauterine resuscitation, including pharmacologic uterine relaxation in cases of uterine tachysystole.

Maternal Labor Analgesia

The National Institutes of Health consensus statement on cesarean delivery on maternal request emphatically concluded that "maternal request for cesarean delivery should not be motivated by unavailability of effective [labor] pain management."[24] It is of concern that a survey of 1300 hospitals indicated that as recently as 2001, 6% to 12% of hospitals in the United States did not provide any form of labor analgesia.[25] Although the rate of provision of labor analgesia, especially in the form of neuraxial techniques, has increased during the past three decades,[25] there are still institutions, of all sizes, where cesarean deliveries are performed because of maternal discomfort.

Adequate maternal analgesia is also important for instrumental (forceps, vacuum) vaginal deliveries, which although declining in frequency, require sufficient maternal analgesia and relaxation for the application of instruments. Neuraxial techniques can provide sufficient analgesia for these obstetric procedures (see Chapter 23).

External Cephalic Version

External cephalic version (ECV) is the procedure by which manual external pressure is applied to the maternal abdomen to change the fetal presentation from breech to cephalic. ECV is usually performed between 36 and 39 weeks' gestation.[26,27] The provision of analgesia or anesthesia may improve the success of an ECV of a fetus with a breech presentation (see Chapter 35).

Neuraxial analgesia is often requested for a repeat attempt of ECV after prior attempts have failed. Thus, the ECV attempts that are uncomplicated and straightforward are often performed without the assistance of neuraxial analgesia, whereas in the more difficult cases, which have lower success rates, neuraxial analgesia/anesthesia is used. In two studies, when repeat ECV was attempted with the addition of epidural anesthesia 1 to 3 weeks after the initial attempt, low success rates (i.e., 40% and 56%, respectively) were observed.[28,29] By contrast, a third study reported that when repeat ECV was attempted with the addition of epidural anesthesia immediately after the first failed attempt at 37 weeks' gestation, success rates were very high (89%).[30]

The effect of tocolytic agents on ECV success rates remains controversial; however, both the American College of Obstetricians and Gynecologists (ACOG)[27] and a review of randomized and quasi-randomized trials[31] support their use, especially in nulliparous women. Fernandez et al.[32] demonstrated that use of tocolytic agents (e.g., beta-adrenergic agonists) is associated with a higher ECV success rate than use of placebo (52% versus 27%, respectively). Some evidence suggests that nitroglycerin may improve the ECV success rate,[30,33] but further studies are needed.

Schorr et al.[34] randomly assigned patients (all of whom received a tocolytic agent) to undergo ECV with or without epidural analgesia (2% lidocaine with epinephrine to achieve analgesia at the T6 sensory level). The overall success rate of ECV was higher in the epidural group (69% versus 32%, respectively), and more successful ECVs occurred in this group on the first attempt. Abdominal delivery was ultimately performed in 79% of the patients in the control group but in only 34% in the epidural group.

Intrauterine Resuscitation

Evidence of intrapartum fetal compromise (nonreassuring fetal status) should prompt the obstetrician and the anesthesia provider to attempt intrauterine fetal resuscitation (Box 26-4).

In cases of uterine tachysystole or hypertonus,[35,36] the administration of nitroglycerin (50 to 100 μg intravenously [IV]) may provide a rapid onset (40 to 50 seconds) of uterine relaxation. Nitroglycerin provides uterine relaxation via a direct action on uterine smooth muscle mediated by nitric oxide production.[37] Although the use of nitroglycerin has not been uniformly demonstrated to be superior to placebo for the promotion of uterine relaxation,[38] a number of reports have indicated its value in cases requiring acute tocolysis.[39] Nitroglycerin does not provide total relaxation of the cervix because the majority (85%) of cervical fibers are fibrous in origin.[40]

PREPARATION FOR ANESTHESIA

The anesthetic management of cesarean delivery is linked with the obstetric indications for operative delivery. Past medical, surgical, and obstetric history, the presence or absence of labor, the urgency of the case, and the resources available should be considered by the anesthesia provider preparing to administer anesthesia for cesarean delivery.

BOX 26-4 Obstetric Management of Nonreassuring Fetal Status

- Optimize maternal position:
  - To avoid or relieve aortocaval compression.
  - To relieve umbilical cord compression.
- Administer supplemental oxygen.
- Maintain maternal circulation:
  - Perform rapid intravenous administration of a non–dextrose-containing, balanced salt solution.
  - Treat hypotension with either ephedrine or phenylephrine.
- Discontinue oxytocin.
- Consider administration of a tocolytic agent for treatment of uterine tachysystole or hypertonus.

Preanesthetic Evaluation

All women admitted for labor and delivery are potential candidates for the emergency administration of anesthesia, and an anesthesia provider ideally should evaluate every woman shortly after admission. Optimally, for high-risk patients, preanesthesia consultation should occur in the late second or early third trimester, even if a vaginal delivery is planned. This practice offers the opportunity to provide patients with information, solicit further consultations, optimize medical conditions, and discuss plans and preparations for the upcoming delivery.[41,42] Early communication among the members of the multidisciplinary team is encouraged.[43] In some cases, the urgent nature of the situation allows limited time for evaluation before induction of anesthesia and commencement of surgery; nonetheless, essential information must be obtained, and risks and benefits of anesthetic management decisions should be discussed.

A focused preanesthetic history and physical examination includes (1) a review of maternal health and anesthetic history, relevant obstetric history, allergies, and baseline blood pressure and heart rate measurements; and (2) performance of an airway, heart, and lung examination consistent with the American Society of Anesthesiologists (ASA) guidelines.[43,44]

Informed Consent

Recognized by the courts as early as the eighteenth century, the concept of *informed medical consent* was defined in 1957 as a requirement that the physician explain to the patient the "risks, benefits, and alternatives" of a procedure.[45] The ethical issues in obtaining consent from the obstetric patient can be challenging because of the clinical situations encountered, such as (1) the pain and stress of labor; (2) birth plans (in which the patient dictates in advance those interventions that are "acceptable" and "not acceptable"); (3) rapidly changing maternal and fetal status, often requiring emergency care; and (4) fetal considerations, which may involve the presence or absence of extrauterine viability and the definition of independent moral status (i.e., the existence of fetal rights equal to those of the mother). Discussion of this last issue may invoke theological, moral, ethical, and philosophical arguments (see Chapter 33).

Informed consent has the following three elements: threshold, information, and consent (Box 26-5).[46]

THRESHOLD ELEMENTS

Threshold elements include the ability of the patient to meet the basic definition of **competence,** which refers to the patient's legal authority to make a decision about her health care. Although some cognitive functions may be compromised by the effects of pain, exhaustion, and analgesic drugs,[47] evidence suggests that most laboring women retain the **capacity** to hear and comprehend information during the consent process.[45]

INFORMATION ELEMENTS

Information elements include the patient's being informed about the material risks of a planned procedure in language that the patient understands. In part, the difficulty with

BOX 26-5 Elements of Informed Consent

Threshold Elements

- Patient is competent to provide consent (i.e., refers to the patient's legal authority to make decisions regarding her health care).

Information Elements

- Provider discloses information about material risks.
- Patient understands information.

Consent Elements

- Provider offers information in a noncoercive manner.
- Patient gives authorization voluntarily.

Information from Barkham M, Peters G, Pace N. Ethical and medico-legal aspects of obstetric anaesthesia. Anaesth Intensive Care Med 2005; 6:127-129.

obtaining informed consent for anesthesia lies in determining the incidence of anesthesia-related morbidity and mortality. Jenkins and Baker[48] surveyed published rates of anesthesia-related morbidity and mortality and compared them with risks associated with daily living, in order to provide contextual comparisons for patients. The investigators concluded that the perception (by surgeons, anesthesia providers, and the public) that anesthesia is generally safe is somewhat optimistic and that discussions of risk should include a more educated and realistic disclosure.

A second difficulty is determining what risks require disclosure. White and Baldwin[49] stated:

> *Anesthesia is by nature a practical specialty; every procedure [is] performed carrying a range of risks, which may be minor or major in consequence, common or rare in incidence, causal or incidental to the harm sustained (if any), convenient or inconvenient in timing, expected or unexpected, relative or absolute, operator-dependent or any combination of the above. In addition, there are significant difficulties in communicating risk, caused by patient perceptions, anaesthetist perceptions and the doctor-patient interaction, and complicated by the range of communication methods (numerical, verbal, or descriptive).*

A survey conducted among obstetric anesthesia providers in the United Kingdom and Ireland found a general consensus that the following neuraxial anesthetic risk factors should be disclosed: (1) the possibility of intraoperative discomfort and a failed/partial blockade, (2) the potential need to convert to general anesthesia, (3) the presence of weak legs, (4) hypotension, and (5) the occurrence of an unintentional dural puncture (with the use of an epidural technique).[50] Backache and urinary retention were considered "optional" for discussion, and the risk for paraplegia was considered unworthy of mention unless the patient specifically asked about it.[50]

Among obstetric patients, the desire for risk disclosure varies. Bethune et al.[51] reported a significant range (between 1:1 and 1:1,000,000,000) in the level of risk of complications of epidural analgesia at which pregnant women wish to be informed. Overall, pregnant women appear to want more rather than less information regarding the risks of anesthetic interventions.[52,53]

CONSENT ELEMENTS

In obtaining consent, care must be taken to preserve patient autonomy by providing information in a noncoercive, nonmanipulative manner (i.e., avoiding a paternalistic or maternalistic approach). Barkham et al.[46] observed that there are occasions when noncoercive forms of influence may be appropriate, and reasoned argument can be used to persuade patients of the merits of a particular course of action. For example, a woman requesting general anesthesia for an elective cesarean delivery may reconsider her choice after rational persuasion.

In many cases, the course of action most appropriate for maternal health is also beneficial to the fetus. In some cases, however, the best interests of the mother may conflict with the best interests of the fetus. For example, emergency cesarean delivery with general anesthesia is often performed primarily for the benefit of the fetus but may involve a higher risk to the mother than a nonemergency procedure performed with neuraxial anesthesia. This conflict in relative risks and benefits will most likely be accentuated in the future as intrauterine fetal surgery becomes more common.

INFORMED REFUSAL

The National Institute of Clinical Excellence (NICE) is a part of the National Health Service in the United Kingdom. NICE guidelines for cesarean delivery state that "after providing the pregnant woman with evidence-based information and in a manner that respects the woman's dignity, privacy, views, and culture whilst taking into consideration the clinical situation . . . , a competent pregnant woman is entitled to refuse treatment, even when the treatment would clearly benefit her or her baby's health. Refusal of treatment needs to be one of the woman's options."[54] Although compliance with maternal requests is the usual course of action, a court-based decision is sometimes made on behalf of the unborn infant (see Chapter 33).

The concept of informed refusal can also be invoked by the anesthesia provider when a patient's or obstetrician's request (e.g., general anesthesia in a morbidly obese patient with a difficult airway) conflicts with the clinician's experience and knowledge of acceptable risks and benefits.[55]

Overall, anesthesia providers are encouraged to (1) engage in, rather than withhold, a discussion of anesthetic risks; (2) recognize their own biases that may influence the presentation of risks; (3) understand how the perception of risks is modified by the situation; and (4) provide contextual explanation of risks, to help place potential complications in perspective.[56] When recognized as an opportunity to foster a closer patient-physician relationship and greater involvement of the patient in her care, rather than simply as a tool to avoid litigation, informed consent can help guide the decision-making associated with anesthesia care.[56]

Blood Products

Peripartum hemorrhage remains a leading cause of maternal mortality worldwide (see Chapters 37 and 39).[57] There is little difference in blood loss between an uncomplicated elective cesarean delivery and an uncomplicated planned vaginal birth[58]; however, a cesarean delivery performed during labor is associated with greater blood loss.[59] Risk factors for peripartum hemorrhage are listed in Box 26-6.

BOX 26-6 Selected Risk Factors for Peripartum Hemorrhage

- Abnormal placentation
- Advanced maternal age
- Anticoagulation
- Bleeding disorder
- Chorioamnionitis
- Fetal demise
- Fetal malpresentation
- General anesthesia
- Increased parity/grand multiparity
- Instrumental vaginal delivery
- Internal trauma (e.g., curettage, internal version)
- Oxytocin augmentation of labor
- Placental abruption
- Precipitous delivery
- Preeclampsia (thrombocytopenia, coagulopathy)
- Premature rupture of membranes
- Previous uterine surgery (cesarean delivery, myomectomy)
- Prolonged labor
- Retained placenta
- Tocolytic therapy
- Trauma (blunt or penetrating)
- Uterine distention (e.g., macrosomia, multiple gestation, polyhydramnios)
- Uterine leiomyoma

Preparation for obstetric hemorrhage includes (1) reviewing the patient's history for anemia or risk factors for hemorrhage (e.g., placenta previa, prior uterine surgery, possible placenta accreta); (2) consulting with the obstetric team regarding the presence of additional risk factors; (3) reviewing reports of ultrasonographic or magnetic resonance images of placentation; (4) obtaining a blood sample for a type and screen or cross-match; (5) contacting the blood bank to ensure the availability of blood products; (6) obtaining and checking the necessary equipment (blood filters and warmers, infusion pumps and tubing, compatible fluids and medications, and standard clinical laboratory collection tubes [to check hemoglobin, electrolytes, coagulation factors]); and (7) consulting with a hematologist or interventional radiologist in selected cases (Box 26-7).

Currently, there is a lack of consensus as to which patients require a blood type and screen, and which patients require a cross-match.[43] The maternal history (previous transfusion, existence of known antibodies) and anticipated hemorrhagic complications as well as local institutional policies should guide decision-making. In certain high-risk cases (e.g., suspected placenta accreta), blood products (i.e., 2 to 4 units of packed red blood cells) should be physically present in the operating room prior to surgical incision, if possible.[60]

If an interventional radiologist plans to place prophylactic intravascular balloon occlusion catheters before surgery, and if neuraxial anesthesia is planned, the anesthesia

BOX 26-7 Suggested Resources for Obstetric Anesthesia

Monitors
- Electrocardiogram
- Noninvasive blood pressure
- Pulse oximetry
- Capnography
- Oxygen and volatile agent analyzers
- Ventilator (with appropriate pressure and disconnection sensors/alarms)
- Peripheral nerve stimulator

For Potential Hemorrhage
- Large-bore intravenous catheters
- Fluid warmer
- Forced-air body warmer
- Availability of blood bank resources
- Equipment for infusing intravenous fluids and blood products rapidly (e.g., hand-squeezed fluid chambers, hand-inflated pressure bags, automatic infusion devices)

For Routine Airway Management
- Laryngoscope and assorted blades
- Oral airways of assorted sizes
- Endotracheal tubes of assorted sizes (6.5 and 7.0 mm) with stylets
- Oxygen source
- Suction source with tubing and catheters
- Self-inflating bag and mask for positive-pressure ventilation
- Medications for blood pressure support, hypnosis, and muscle relaxation
- Carbon dioxide detector
- Pulse oximeter

For Difficult Airway Management
- Rigid laryngoscope blades of alternative design and size from those routinely used
- Laryngeal mask airway
- Endotracheal tube guides (e.g., semirigid stylets with or without hollow cores for jet ventilation, light wands, and forceps designed to manipulate the distal portion of the endotracheal tube)
- Retrograde intubation equipment
- At least one device suitable for emergency nonsurgical airway ventilation (e.g., hollow jet ventilation stylet with a transtracheal jet ventilator; supraglottic airway device, such as a Combitube [Sheridan Catheter Corporation, Argyle, NY] or intubating LMA [Fastrach LMA, LMA North America, San Diego, CA])
- Fiberoptic intubation equipment
- Equipment suitable for emergency surgical airway access (e.g., cricothyrotomy)
- Topical anesthetics and vasoconstrictors

Adapted from the American Society of Anesthesiologists Task Force on Obstetric Anesthesia. Practice guidelines for obstetric anesthesia. Anesthesiology 2007; 106:843-63. (The full text of the practice guidelines is published as Appendix B at the end of this text.)

provider should consider placing an epidural catheter prior to placement of the balloon catheters (see later).[61]

Monitoring

Attention should be given to the availability and proper functioning of equipment and monitors for the provision of anesthesia and the management of potential complications (e.g., failed intubation, cardiopulmonary arrest).[43] Equipment should be checked on a daily basis and serviced at recommended intervals. The equipment and facilities available in the labor and delivery operating room suite should be comparable to those available in the main operating room.[43]

Basic monitoring consists of maternal pulse oximetry, electrocardiogram (ECG), and noninvasive blood pressure monitoring* as well as fetal heart rate (FHR) monitoring.

Automated blood pressure monitors that use oscillometric methods produce lower systolic and diastolic blood pressures.[65] Forearm, wrist, and finger blood pressure monitors have been developed but have not yet undergone adequate validation. In general, locations distal to the heart tend to increase and decrease systolic and diastolic blood pressures, respectively.[64] Invasive hemodynamic monitoring should be considered in women with severe cardiac disease, refractory hypertension, pulmonary edema, or unexplained oliguria.[63]

ECG abnormalities are often observed in late pregnancy and are believed to be due to hyperdynamic circulation, circulating catecholamines, and/or altered estrogen and progesterone concentration ratios. During cesarean delivery with neuraxial anesthesia, ECG changes have a reported incidence of 25% to 60%.[66,67] The significance of the ECG findings as an indicator of cardiac pathology remains controversial; however, measurement of cardiac troponin indicates that only a very small minority of parturients experience myocardial ischemia.[68] The monitoring of additional ECG leads improves the sensitivity of detecting ischemic events; monitoring leads II, V4, and V5 can result in a sensitivity of 96%.[69] In a prospective study of 254 healthy women undergoing cesarean delivery with spinal anesthesia, Shen et al.[70] determined the incidence of first- and second-degree atrioventricular block (3.5% for each), severe bradycardia (< 50 beats/min; 6.7%), and multiple premature ventricular contractions (1.2%). The investigators speculated that a relative increase in parasympathetic activity occurred as a result of spinal blockade of cardiac sympathetic activity. Most of the dysrhythmias were transient and resolved spontaneously.

Monitors that process the electroencephalogram to indicate the depth of anesthesia have received only limited evaluation in women undergoing cesarean delivery.[71] Whether these monitors will provide benefit in the assessment of depth of anesthesia (and perhaps reduce the incidence of intraoperative awareness) during general anesthesia for cesarean delivery is unclear (see later).[72]

An indwelling urinary catheter is used in almost all women undergoing cesarean delivery.[73] A urinary catheter helps avoid overdistention of the bladder during and after surgery. In cases of hypovolemia and/or oliguria, a collection system that allows precise measurement of urine volume should be used.

An evaluation of the FHR tracing by a qualified individual may be useful before and after administration of anesthesia.[43] The ACOG[74] has stated that the decision to monitor the fetus either by electronic FHR monitoring or by ultrasonography prior to a *scheduled (elective)* cesarean delivery should be individualized, because data are insufficient to determine the value of monitoring before elective cesarean delivery in patients without risk factors. The presence of fetal heart activity should be documented prior to surgery.[74] In contrast, the NICE guidelines state that the FHR should be recorded during the initiation of the neuraxial technique and until the abdominal skin preparation has begun.[54]

In most cases of *emergency* cesarean delivery, a previously placed fetal scalp (or buttock) ECG lead can be used to monitor the FHR before, during, and after the initiation of anesthesia. Typically the fetal scalp electrode is removed when the drapes are applied to the abdomen, but in some cases the scalp electrode may be left in place until just before delivery, when the circulating nurse reaches under the drapes to disconnect the ECG lead.

In cases of emergency cesarean delivery, continuous FHR monitoring is useful for at least three reasons. First, the FHR abnormality often resolves; in some cases, the obstetrician will then forgo the performance of a cesarean delivery. In other cases, the obstetrician may continue with plans to perform a cesarean delivery, but continuous FHR monitoring may facilitate the administration of neuraxial anesthesia. For example, an improved FHR tracing allows the anesthesia provider to wait for an extension of adequate epidural anesthesia. Alternatively, an improved FHR tracing allows the anesthesia provider to administer spinal anesthesia. Second, continuous FHR monitoring may guide management in cases of failed intubation. If intubation fails and there is no evidence of fetal compromise, both the anesthesia provider and the obstetrician will have greater confidence in a decision to awaken the patient and proceed with an alternative anesthetic technique. By contrast, if there is evidence of ongoing fetal compromise, the anesthesia provider may decide to provide general anesthesia by means of a face mask or laryngeal mask airway, and the obstetrician may proceed with cesarean delivery (see Chapter 30). Third, intraoperative FHR monitoring allows the obstetrician to modify the surgical technique according to the urgency of delivery.

Medication Availability and Storage

The necessary drugs, including vasopressors, emergency medications, and drugs used for the provision of general and neuraxial anesthesia, should be readily available. The Joint Commission[75] mandates that all medications should

*Outside the operating room, and before the onset of labor, maternal blood pressure is ideally measured using a manual sphygmomanometer with an appropriately sized cuff (a bladder length that is 80%, and a width that is at least 46% of the arm circumference)[62] after a rest period of 10 minutes or more, with the pregnant woman sitting or lying on her left side with her arm at the level of the right atrium.[63,64] The onset (phase 1) and disappearance (phase 5) of Korotkoff sounds correspond to systolic and diastolic pressures, respectively.[64]

be secured. Currently, only Schedule II controlled substances as classified by the Drug Enforcement Agency[76] need to be secured in a "substantially constructed locked cabinet." Other drugs and products, including anesthetic medications, should be "reasonably secure" but not necessarily locked. These drugs include the Schedule III drug thiopental, as well as succinylcholine and vasopressor agents. The Joint Commission has defined "reasonably secure" as storage in areas not readily accessible or easily removed by the public. Federal law requires that all hospitals receiving Medicare funding adhere to conditions of participation, which state that "drugs and biologicals must be kept in a secure area, and locked when appropriate."[77] This rule applies to noncontrolled substances.

Equipment

Labor and delivery units may be adjacent to or remote from the operating rooms. In some facilities, the unit is located on a separate floor but shares a common operating room facility (used for other surgical procedures), whereas in others, it is a geographically separate, self-contained unit with its own operating room facilities. Regardless of location, the equipment, facilities, and support personnel available in the labor and delivery operating room should be comparable to those available in the main operating room.[43] In addition, personnel and equipment should be available to care for obstetric patients recovering from major neuraxial or general anesthesia.

Resources for the conduct and support of neuraxial anesthesia and general anesthesia should include those necessary for the basic delivery of anesthesia and airway management as well as those required to manage complications (e.g., failed intubation). The *immediate* availability of these resources is particularly important, given the frequency and urgency of the anesthesia care provided. Consideration should be given to having some of the equipment and supplies immediately available in one location or in a cart (e.g., difficult airway cart, massive hemorrhage cart, malignant hyperthermia box) specifically located on the labor and delivery unit. Equipment and supplies should be checked on a frequent and regular basis. Securing special-situation equipment and supplies in a cart with a single-use breakthrough plastic tie helps ensure that the cart is kept in a fully stocked state.

Aspiration Prophylaxis

The patient should be asked about oral intake, although insufficient evidence exists regarding the relationship between recent ingestion and subsequent aspiration pneumonitis (see Chapter 29). Gastric emptying of clear liquids during pregnancy occurs relatively quickly; the residual content of the stomach (as measured by the cross-sectional area of the gastric antrum 60 minutes after the ingestion of 300 mL of water) does not appear to be different from baseline fasting levels in either lean or obese nonlaboring pregnant women.[78,79] Moreover, when measured by serial gastric ultrasonographic examinations and acetaminophen absorption, the gastric emptying half-time of 300 mL of water is shorter than that of 50 mL of water in healthy, nonlaboring, nonobese pregnant women (24 ± 6 versus 33 ± 8 minutes, respectively).[79]

The uncomplicated patient undergoing *elective* cesarean delivery may drink modest amounts of clear liquids up to 2 hours before induction of anesthesia.[43] Examples of clear liquids are water, fruit juices without pulp, carbonated beverages, clear tea, black coffee, and sports drinks. The volume of liquid ingested is less important than the absence of particulate matter. Patients with additional risk factors for aspiration (e.g., morbid obesity, diabetes, difficult airway), or laboring patients at increased risk for cesarean delivery (e.g., nonreassuring FHR pattern) may have further restrictions of oral intake, determined on a case-by-case basis.[43]

Ingestion of solid foods should be avoided in laboring patients and patients undergoing elective surgery (e.g., scheduled cesarean delivery or postpartum tubal ligation). A fasting period for solids of 6 to 8 hours, depending on the fat content of the food, has been recommended.[43]

A nonparticulate antacid (0.3 M **sodium citrate**) increases gastric pH without affecting gastric volume.[80] Administration of sodium citrate is believed to decrease the risk of damage to the respiratory epithelium if aspiration should occur.[81] However, greater nausea has been reported with sodium citrate than with administration of a histamine H_2-receptor antagonist (famotidine).[82] **H_2-receptor antagonists (ranitidine, famotidine)** reduce secretion of gastric acid. **Metoclopramide** is a promotility agent that hastens gastric emptying and also increases lower esophageal sphincter tone.[83,84] Metoclopramide has the additional advantage of being an antiemetic agent. **Omeprazole,** a proton pump inhibitor, achieves a higher gastric pH than ranitidine,[85,86] although ranitidine combined with sodium citrate is more cost effective.[87] Intravenously administered H_2-receptor antagonists and metoclopramide require at least 30 to 40 minutes to effectively reduce gastric acid.

Prophylactic Antibiotics

Both the incidence and severity of postcesarean infections, especially endometritis, are reduced with the use of antibiotic prophylaxis. Prophylactic antibiotics (i.e., administered *either* before abdominal incision *or* immediately after umbilical cord clamping) are beneficial in both elective (nonlaboring) and nonelective (laboring) cesarean deliveries. A 60% decrease in the incidence of endometritis, a 25% to 65% decrease in the incidence of wound infection, and fewer episodes of fever and urinary tract infections have been demonstrated after prophylactic administration of antibiotics.[88-90]

The ACOG[90] has recommended the administration of narrow-spectrum antibiotics (e.g., a first-generation cephalosporin) for prophylaxis. The optimal timing of antibiotic administration (before skin incision versus after clamping of the umbilical cord) and the potential value of more broad-spectrum antibiotics have been assessed. Heretofore, prophylactic antibiotics typically have been administered after cord clamping, because of concern that fetal antibiotic exposure might mask a nascent infection and/or increase the likelihood of a neonatal sepsis evaluation. However, a 2008 meta-analysis concluded that pre-incision antibiotic prophylaxis reduces the incidence of post–cesarean delivery endometritis and total maternal infectious morbidity, without evidence of adverse neonatal effects.[91] Moreover, although earlier studies suggested that ampicillin and first-generation cephalosporins are similar in efficacy to more broad-spectrum agents,[88-90] more recent trials have suggested that there is benefit associated with extended-spectrum antibiotic prophylaxis that includes the addition of an agent covering other organisms such as *Ureaplasma*.[92] In the presence of an active or presumed infection, use of an extended-spectrum antibiotic regimen is recommended. Currently it is acceptable to administer prophylactic antibiotics either before skin incision or after cord clamping.

Aseptic Technique

In the early nineteenth century, Ignác Semmelweis observed that puerperal fever, known as "childbed fever," was most likely transmitted when the first stage of labor was prolonged and multiple individuals performed vaginal examinations with contaminated hands. The institution of hand hygiene has caused a significant reduction in maternal and neonatal infectious morbidity.

Epidural abscess and meningitis have been reported as complications of neuraxial procedures in obstetric patients (see Chapter 32). These cases have prompted questions regarding the best solution for disinfecting the skin[93] and the most appropriate dressings to apply at the neuraxial catheter insertion site (see Chapters 12 and 32). During the performance of neuraxial techniques, there is wide variation in aseptic practices. Regrettably, some anesthesia providers do not wear a face mask, whereas others wear a gown in addition to a face mask and hat.[94] Moreover, a "rapid-sequence spinal" has been described for use in emergency cesarean delivery cases in which the use of draping is omitted[95]; many obstetric anesthesia providers would argue that this practice is unwise.

Although there appear to be limited (if any) clinical consequences of the subtle changes in circulating immunoglobulin levels in pregnancy,[96] obstetric anesthesia providers should always give careful attention to aseptic technique, especially during performance of a neuraxial technique. Proper sterile technique consists of wearing a face mask, giving careful attention to hand hygiene, and donning sterile gloves before initiating neuraxial blockade.

Attention should also be given to the careful preparation of anesthetic drugs during administration of either general or neuraxial anesthesia. Propofol and other agents can support bacterial growth.[97] An increasing number of institutions use premixed solutions of local anesthetic and opioid (prepared under aseptic conditions in the hospital pharmacy) during administration of neuraxial anesthesia.

Intravenous Access and Fluid Management

The establishment of functional intravenous access is of critical importance to the successful outcome of many situations in obstetric anesthesia practice. According to the Hagen-Poiseuille equation, the infusion rate of a catheter is directly related to the pressure gradient of the fluid and the fourth power of the catheter's radius, and inversely related to the viscosity of the fluid and the catheter's length. Because the size of the catheter, more than the size of the vein, dictates the flow rate, the use of a short, larger-diameter catheter, such as a 16- or 18-gauge catheter, is associated with the best flow.[98]

In general, a smaller but functional catheter is more important than a larger catheter that is unreliable, requires frequent manipulation, or is nonfunctional. Volume and blood resuscitation can be satisfactorily achieved using 20- and 22-gauge catheters (without evidence of greater red blood cell destruction) with the use of dilution, pressurization, or both.[99] Occasionally, when peripheral venous access is problematic or when multiple blood products are required, the anesthesia provider may choose to insert a central venous catheter; the placement difficulties and complications of such an approach during pregnancy should be considered.[100]

Although the administration of intravenous fluids may decrease the frequency of neuraxial anesthesia–associated hypotension, initiation of anesthesia should not be delayed in order to administer a fixed volume of fluid.[43] This statement is especially true in the case of an emergency cesarean delivery, in which the life and health of the mother and the infant are best preserved with timely delivery. Vasopressors can be used for both prophylaxis and treatment of hypotension. The type of fluid (crystalloid, colloid) and the volume, rate, and timing of administration are relevant factors in the prevention and treatment of hypotension.[101] In most situations, a balanced salt solution such as lactated Ringer's solution is acceptable. Blood products are most often administered with normal saline. Crystalloid or colloid solutions that contain calcium or glucose should not be administered with blood products, because of the risks of clotting (due to reversal of the citrate anticoagulant) and clumping of red blood cells, respectively.

Traditionally, 1 to 1.5 L of crystalloid solution has been administered intravenously (as "prehydration") to prevent or reduce the incidence and severity of hypotension during neuraxial anesthesia for cesarean delivery. However, prehydration with crystalloid does not reliably prevent neuraxial anesthesia–induced hypotension. Dyer et al.[102] observed that rapid intravenous crystalloid administration (20 mL/kg) initiated *at the time of* intrathecal injection (co-load) was as effective at preventing intraoperative hypotension as administration of crystalloid *prior* to the initiation of neuroblockade (preload); the required dose of ephedrine prior to delivery was lower in the co-load group.

We typically initiate a rapid infusion of warmed lactated Ringer's solution as we begin to position the patient for administration of neuraxial anesthesia. We administer approximately 1 L of solution while we initiate anesthesia. For patients at higher risk for hypotension or the consequences of hypotension, we often administer a colloid solution shortly before the initiation of anesthesia. Thereafter, the choice of fluid and rate of fluid administration are titrated to individual patient needs.

Supplemental Medications for Anxiety

To avoid anterograde and retrograde amnesia, benzodiazepines are typically avoided during awake cesarean delivery.[103] However, in women with severe anxiety, the use of low doses of intravenous midazolam or an opioid may facilitate performance of a neuraxial technique or the induction of general anesthesia. Such anxiolysis may be particularly valuable in the setting of an emergency cesarean delivery, in which greater feelings of distress have been related to the development of post-traumatic stress disorder.[104]

Positioning

After 20 weeks' gestation, all pregnant women should be positioned with left uterine displacement to minimize aortocaval compression. The **supine hypotensive syndrome,** which is caused by compression of the aorta and inferior vena cava by the gravid uterus, can manifest as pallor, tachycardia, sweating, nausea, hypotension, and dizziness.[105,106] Uteroplacental blood flow is compromised by decreased venous return and cardiac output, increased uterine venous pressure, and compression of the aorta or common iliac arteries.

The full lateral position minimizes aortocaval compression, but obviously that position does not allow performance of cesarean delivery. In most cases the extent of **left uterine displacement** (with a pelvic wedge or table tilt) may be reduced to 15 degrees to facilitate performance of surgery. Both the aorta and the inferior vena cava remain compressed with 15 degrees of lateral tilt[107]; thus a minority of women may still exhibit supine hypotension in the lateral tilt position. Not surprisingly, the fetal effects mirror the maternal cardiovascular effects; change of the mother's position from left lateral to supine may result in a decrease in maternal blood pressure and abnormal uterine artery flow velocity waveforms.[108] Anesthesia providers should recognize that (1) visual estimates of lateral tilt may be in error,[109] (2) individual susceptibility to aortocaval compression varies,[110] and (3) in symptomatic women, increasing the extent of left uterine displacement may be beneficial. A minimum left lateral tilt of 15 degrees should be employed.[111]

The use of a slight (10 degrees) **head-up position** may help reduce the incidence of hypotension after initiation of hyperbaric spinal anesthesia.[112] Use of the so-called ramp position can be particularly valuable in morbidly obese patients, not only to improve oxygenation but also to improve the laryngoscopic view of the glottis if general anesthesia should be necessary[113]; this can be accomplished with blankets or commercially available devices (see Chapters 30 and 50). If blankets are used to create the ramp position, they should be stacked rather than interlaced, to allow for rapid readjustment of the head and neck position if necessary. Ideal positioning leads to the horizontal alignment between the external auditory meatus and the sternal notch; this position (1) aligns the oral, pharyngeal, and tracheal axes ("sniffing position") and (2) facilitates insertion of the laryngoscope blade (see Chapter 30).[113,114]

Theoretically, the **Trendelenburg (head-down) position** may augment venous return and increase cardiac output. The value of this approach in *preventing* hypotension during neuraxial anesthesia has been questioned. After the initiation of hyperbaric spinal anesthesia, the Trendelenburg position has been reported to result in more cephalad spread of anesthesia in one study,[115] but not in others.[116,117] However, this position had no effect on the incidence of hypotension after administration of hyperbaric spinal anesthesia.[115,117]

The optimal position for insertion of a neuraxial needle (or catheter) may depend on clinical circumstances and the preferences and skills of the anesthesia provider. Whether the use of the **lateral** or the **sitting position** is best for routine initiation of neuraxial anesthesia is controversial.[118,119] Advocates of the lateral position cite a reduction of vagal reflexes, which can otherwise result in dizziness, perspiration, pallor, bradycardia, and hypotension.[120] Moreover, the lateral position may allow better uteroplacental blood flow than the sitting position. Using technetium Tc 99m–radiolabeled isotopes in pregnant women in the third trimester, Suonio et al.[121] observed a 23% reduction in uteroplacental blood flow when pregnant patients moved from the left lateral recumbent to the sitting position. In contrast, Andrews et al.[122] observed a greater decrease in cardiac output in parturients in the left lateral position than in those in the sitting position during initiation of epidural analgesia.

Some parturients find the lateral position more comfortable during administration of neuraxial anesthesia[123]; this position may also limit side-to-side and front-to-back patient motion during needle insertion. Moreover, because uterine compression of the vena cava diverts blood into the epidural venous plexus,[124] the use of the lateral position can reduce hydrostatic pressure and return the engorged epidural venous plexus to its size in the nonpregnant state.[125] Bahar et al.[126,127] observed that fewer needle/catheter replacements occurred for needle- or catheter-induced venous trauma when epidural procedures were performed in the lateral recumbent head-down position than in either the sitting or the lateral recumbent horizontal position in both obese and nonobese parturients.

The lateral position may also be of value during epidural needle placement because it minimizes the prominence of the dural sac. On the other hand, a bulging dural sac might be preferable during administration of spinal anesthesia. Magnetic resonance imaging and computed tomography studies have indicated that the cross-sectional area and the anteroposterior diameter of the dural sac at the L3 to L4, L4 to L5, and L5 to S1 levels are significantly influenced by posture.[128] Lumbar cerebrospinal fluid (CSF) pressure is lower and dural sac cross-sectional area smaller in the recumbent position than in the upright position.[128] Bulging of the lumbar dural sac—particularly in the sitting position—may decrease the force required to create a dural puncture with a Tuohy epidural needle, but this possibility is unproven.

In a randomized controlled trial, Yun et al.[129] observed that the severity and duration of hypotension were greater, as was the requirement for ephedrine to treat hypotension, in women randomly assigned to receive CSE anesthesia (hyperbaric spinal bupivacaine with fentanyl) in the sitting position than in those in the lateral position.

The sitting position offers some advantages, especially during neuraxial needle placement in obese parturients.[119] The distance from the skin to the epidural space is shorter in the sitting position.[130] Anesthesia trainees often prefer to perform neuraxial techniques with the patient in the sitting position. In addition, some anesthesia providers contend that the sitting position allows faster performance of neuraxial anesthesia techniques, an advantage when delivery is urgent. However, anesthesia providers should practice and be comfortable with the placement of needles for neuraxial techniques in both the sitting position and the lateral position. The sitting position cannot be used to initiate neuraxial anesthesia in some situations (e.g., fetal head entrapment, umbilical cord prolapse, footling breech presentation).[118]

Supplemental Oxygen

The routine administration of supplemental oxygen during elective cesarean delivery with neuraxial anesthesia has been a common practice since publication of the seminal report by Fox and Houle.[131] Later evidence suggests that routine oxygen administration may be unnecessary and ineffective,[132] and may even be detrimental.[133] The use of a fractional inspired concentration of oxygen (F_{IO_2}) of 0.35 to 0.4 (which cannot be obtained by nasal cannulae or a simple face mask with a flow rate less than 6 L/min[134]) does not improve fetal oxygenation during labor or elective cesarean delivery. Although respiratory function can deteriorate in parturients receiving neuraxial anesthesia,[135,136] maternal or fetal hypoxia does not normally occur when parturients breathe room air.[136] An F_{IO_2} of 0.6 in nonlaboring women undergoing elective cesarean delivery with spinal anesthesia increases the umbilical venous oxygen content by only 12%; an increase in oxygen content is not observed when the uterine incision-to-delivery (U-D) interval exceeds 180 seconds.[137]

Supplemental oxygen has both beneficial and detrimental effects. Through normal biologic processes, oxygen is converted to reactive oxygen species, including free radicals. The reactive oxygen species cause lipid peroxidation, alteration of cellular enzymatic functions, and destruction of genetic material[138]; these adverse effects occur with the restoration of perfusion after a period of ischemia (i.e., ischemia-reperfusion injury).[139-141] Uterine contractions during labor can be regarded as a series of repeated ischemia-reperfusion events. Reactive oxygen species are present during hyperoxia (causing such disorders as neonatal retinopathy and bronchopulmonary dysplasia) and in the setting of prolonged labor, oligohydramnios, intermittent umbilical cord compression, and/or fetal compromise.[139,140,142] Hyperoxia in these settings (i.e., during the period of reperfusion following ischemia) results in a higher level of lipid peroxidation.[133,140]

Term (but not preterm) fetuses may be able to withstand the adverse effects of these reactive oxygen species through a compensatory increase in antioxidants during labor.[143,144] Antioxidants, the defense against reactive oxygen species, consist of enzymatic inactivators (superoxide dismutase, catalase, peroxidase) and scavengers (ascorbate, glutathione, transferrin, lactoferrin, ceruloplasmin). The activity of these compensatory mechanisms and their relationships to gestational age and labor suggest that the highest risk for ischemia-reperfusion injury occurs in preterm fetuses prior to the onset of labor.[133,144]

The use of a very high F_{IO_2} improves oxygen delivery to hypoxic fetuses for a limited period (approximately 10 minutes); beyond this time, continued hyperoxia, especially in the setting of restored perfusion, increases reactive oxygen species, placental vasoconstriction, and fetal acidosis.[145,146] A lower F_{IO_2} may be of benefit in some situations. When asphyxiated infants are immediately resuscitated at birth with air instead of 100% oxygen, better short-term outcomes have been observed[147]; this finding may be a result of the shift in the balance between beneficial oxygenation and detrimental free radicals.

In summary, no significant improvement in maternal-fetal oxygen transfer occurs until very high levels of maternal F_{IO_2} are used. At these levels, the resulting hyperoxia creates reactive oxygen species. Preterm fetuses in nonlaboring mothers are the population at highest risk for hyperoxia-induced injury. Nonetheless, the emergency cesarean delivery of the compromised fetus *should* include maternal administration of a high F_{IO_2}. The greater maternal oxygen consumption and reduced fetal oxygen delivery associated with uterine contractions may exacerbate the fetal compromise; in these situations, supplemental oxygen potentially augments fetal oxygenation and, perhaps, reduces the severity of fetal hypoxia. However, diminishing fetal benefit appears to occur after 10 minutes.

All women who are at risk for requiring general anesthesia for emergency cesarean delivery should receive an F_{IO_2} of 1.0 after transfer to the operating table. Denitrogenation should always be performed; if it is not, the mother is at risk for hypoxemia, in turn putting the fetus at risk. When general anesthesia is administered in a patient with fetal compromise, the mother should receive an F_{IO_2} of 1.0 before and immediately after induction of anesthesia, even though the subsequent increases in umbilical venous and arterial oxygen content are not dramatic.

The value of supplemental maternal oxygen during *elective* cesarean delivery of a noncompromised fetus is questionable. The only reason some obstetric anesthesia providers place nasal cannulae in patients undergoing elective cesarean delivery with neuraxial anesthesia is to facilitate the monitoring of expired carbon dioxide (to monitor the parturient's ventilation).

ANESTHETIC TECHNIQUE

Providing anesthesia to the parturient is a dynamic, multistep process (Table 26-2). The most appropriate anesthetic technique for cesarean delivery depends on maternal, fetal, and obstetric factors (Table 26-3). The urgency and anticipated duration of the operation play an important role in the selection of an anesthetic technique.

In cases of dire fetal compromise, the anesthesia provider may need to perform a preanesthetic evaluation simultaneously with other tasks (i.e., establishing intravenous access and placing a blood pressure cuff, pulse oximeter probe, and ECG electrodes). Regardless of the urgency, the anesthesia provider should not compromise maternal safety by failing to obtain critical information about previous medical and anesthetic history, allergies, and the airway. Effective communication with the obstetric team is critical to establish the degree of urgency, which helps guide decisions regarding anesthetic management. Further, contemporary standards for patient safety require that all members of the surgical team participate in a pre–cesarean delivery "time-out" to verify (1) the correct patient identity, position, and operative site; (2) agreement on the procedure to be performed; and (3) the availability of special equipment, if needed.

In cases of emergency cesarean delivery, the emotional needs of the infant's mother and father are also important. Parental distress often occurs in this setting. The anesthesia provider is often the best person to reassure an anxious mother and her husband or support person. All members of the obstetric care team should remember that unnecessary chaos need not accompany urgency.

TABLE 26-2 Provision of Anesthesia for Cesarean Delivery*

Phase	Issues	Specific Concerns
Preparation	Preanesthetic evaluation	History and physical examination Indicated laboratory measurements Imaging studies
	Oral intake	No clear liquids and solid foods for 2 hours and 6-8 hours, respectively, prior to elective surgery, in absence of comorbid conditions
	Communication with obstetric team	Indication(s) for cesarean delivery, including extent of urgency Anticipated surgical complications
	Informed consent	Threshold, information, and consent elements Informed refusal
	Blood products	Risk factors Baseline hematocrit Blood type and screen or cross-match Equipment for rapid transfusion
	Monitoring	Pulse oximetry, electrocardiogram, blood pressure, fetal heart rate, urinary catheter Consider electroencephalographic (bispectral index) monitoring during general anesthesia (controversial) Invasive monitoring in selected patients
	Medication availability	Anesthetic (vasopressors, general and neuraxial anesthetic drugs) Obstetric (uterotonic agents) Emergency (advanced cardiac life support, malignant hyperthermia)
	Equipment availability	Anesthesia, airway management
	Aspiration prophylaxis	Fasting guidelines, nonparticulate antacid, histamine H_2-receptor antagonist, metoclopramide
	Prophylactic antibiotics†	Either before incision or after cord clamping
	Intravenous access and fluid management	16- or 18-gauge intravenous catheter Fluid type, volume, and rate
	Supplemental medications	Consider anxiolysis for severe anxiety
	Positioning	Lateral or sitting position for neuraxial needle/catheter placement Left uterine displacement, slight head up for surgery "Sniffing" position if general anesthesia is planned
	Supplemental oxygen	Preoxygenation/denitrogenation required before general anesthesia Of unclear benefit during neuraxial anesthesia for elective delivery of a noncompromised fetus
Selection of anesthetic technique	Neuraxial	Adequate sacral and cephalad spread (T4) and density of neuroblockade Prevention or treatment of hypotension
	General	Airway management Prevention of awareness and recall Prevention of anesthesia-associated uterine atony
	Local	Usually a supplement for inadequate neuraxial anesthesia Can facilitate emergency delivery in absence of an anesthesia provider Rarely provides satisfactory anesthesia as a primary technique
Recovery	Oral intake	Fluids and foods allowed within 4 to 8 hours of surgery, in absence of complications
	Removal of urinary catheter	Typically within 24 hours
	Postoperative assessment and discharge	Hemodynamic stability Resolution of neuroblockade Effective analgesia Recognition and treatment of surgical and anesthetic complications

*Procedures, techniques, and drugs may need to be modified for individual patients and circumstances.

†Evidence now suggests that administration of prophylactic antibiotics *before* incision (rather than after cord clamping) reduces the incidence of post–cesarean delivery endometritis and total maternal infectious morbidity.[88]

TABLE 26-3 Selection of Anesthetic Technique for Cesarean Delivery

Indication(s)	Comments/Examples
For Neuraxial Anesthesia*	
Maternal desire to witness birth and/or avoid general anesthesia	Most common maternal preference
Risk factors for difficult airway or aspiration	Physical examination predicts possible difficult airway History of difficult intubation High body mass index (obesity) History of gastroesophageal reflux (common in pregnancy)
Presence of comorbid conditions	Malignant hyperthermia history Pulmonary disease
General anesthesia intolerance or failure	History of significant side effects with general anesthesia Attempted general anesthesia with failed intubation; patient awakened
Other benefits	Plan for neuraxial analgesia after surgery Reduced fetal drug exposure Reduced blood loss Allows presence of husband or support person
For General Anesthesia*	
Maternal refusal or failure to cooperate with neuraxial technique	Strong maternal preference, in the absence of factors that predict a difficult airway Severe psychiatric disorder Severe developmental delay Severe emotional immaturity or lability
Presence of comorbid conditions that contraindicate a neuraxial technique	Coagulopathy Local infection at neuraxial insertion site Sepsis Severe uncorrected hypovolemia (e.g., hemorrhage from placenta previa or uterine rupture) Intracranial mass with increased intracranial pressure Known allergy to local anesthetic (rare)
Insufficient time to induce neuraxial anesthesia for urgent delivery	Umbilical cord prolapse with persistent fetal bradycardia
Failure of neuraxial technique	Multiple needle placement failures Missed spinal segments Persistent intraoperative pain that is not treated successfully
Fetal issues	Planned *ex utero* intrapartum treatment (EXIT) procedure

*Many indications for or contraindications to specific anesthesia techniques are relative, and the choice of anesthetic must be tailored to individual circumstances.

Neuraxial versus General Anesthesia

Overall, neuraxial (epidural, spinal, CSE) techniques are the preferred method of providing anesthesia for cesarean delivery, and specific benefits and risks of each technique dictate the eventual choice. In contemporary practice, neuraxial anesthesia is administered to some patients who would have received general anesthesia in the past. For example, umbilical cord prolapse, placenta previa, and severe preeclampsia (assuming an acceptable platelet count) are no longer considered absolute indications for general anesthesia; in some cases a prolapsed umbilical cord can be decompressed, and if fetal status is reassuring, a neuraxial technique can be used. In an analysis of obstetric anesthesia trends in the United States between 1981 and 2001, a progressive increase was noted in the use of neuraxial anesthesia, especially spinal anesthesia, for both elective and emergency cesarean deliveries (Figure 26-3).[25] Neuraxial anesthesia has been used for more than 80% of cesarean deliveries since 1992. Similar increases have occurred in the United Kingdom and in other developed as well as developing countries.[148]

The greater use of neuraxial anesthesia for cesarean delivery has been attributed to several factors, including (1) the growing use of epidural techniques for labor analgesia, (2) an awareness of the possibility that an *in situ* epidural catheter (even if not used during labor) may decrease the necessity for general anesthesia in an urgent situation, (3) improvement in the quality of neuraxial anesthesia with the addition of an opioid to the local anesthetic, (4) appreciation of the risks of airway complications during general anesthesia in parturients, (5) the desire for limited neonatal drug transfer, and (6) the ability of the mother to remain awake to experience childbirth and to have her husband or support person present in the operating room.

Maternal *mortality* following general anesthesia has been a primary motivator for the transition toward greater use of neuraxial anesthesia for cesarean delivery. Hawkins et al.[149] compared the anesthesia-related maternal mortality rate

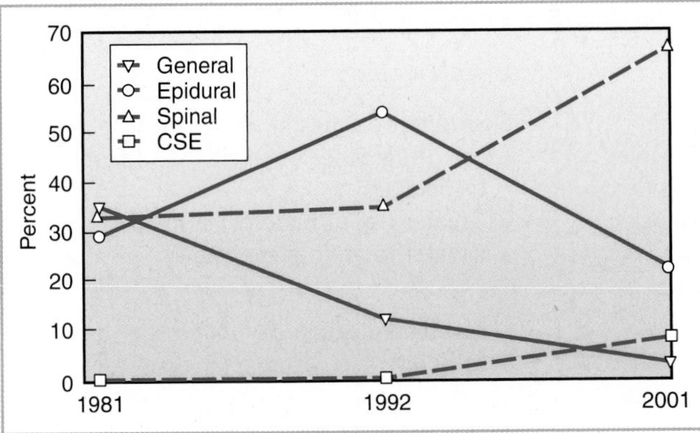

FIGURE 26-3 Rates of types of anesthesia for cesarean delivery in the United States. Data from random sample of hospitals in the United States stratified by geographic region and number of births per year. Data shown represent hospitals in stratum I (> 1500 births/year), and are presented as percentages of cesarean births by anesthesia type. CSE, combined spinal-epidural anesthesia. Data from 2001 represent anesthetic technique selected for elective cesarean delivery. (Data adapted from Bucklin BA, Hawkins JL, Anderson JR, Ullrich FA. Obstetric anesthesia workforce survey: Twenty-year update. Anesthesiology 2005; 103:645-53.)

from 1979 to 1984 with that for the period from 1985 to 1990 in the United States. The estimated case-fatality risk ratio for general versus neuraxial anesthesia was as high as 16.7 in the years 1985 to 1990; however, a similar analysis by the same group of investigators observed a nonsignificant risk ratio of 1.7 in the years 1991 to 2002.[150] Of interest, these data may overstate the relative risk of general anesthesia, because this form of anesthesia is used principally when neuraxial anesthetic techniques are contraindicated for medical reasons or time constraints[151,152]; these data also suggest that the relative risk associated with neuraxial anesthesia has increased. However, this change may reflect the growing acceptance of performing neuraxial techniques in parturients with comorbidities (e.g., obesity, severe preeclampsia, cardiac disease).

Maternal *morbidity* is also lower with the use of neuraxial anesthesia techniques than with general anesthesia. In a systematic review of randomized and quasi-randomized controlled trials comparing major maternal and neonatal outcomes with the use of neuraxial anesthesia and general anesthesia for cesarean delivery, Afolabi et al.[153] found less maternal blood loss and shivering but more nausea in the neuraxial group. The "perception" of pain was greater in the neuraxial group, but the time elapsed prior to the first postoperative request for analgesia was longer. Prospective audits of post–cesarean delivery outcomes have indicated that in the first postoperative week, patients who received neuraxial anesthesia had less pain, gastrointestinal stasis, coughing, fever, and depression and were able to breastfeed and ambulate more quickly than patients who received general anesthesia.[154]

Differences in neonatal outcomes among different anesthetic techniques are not as clear. Apgar and neonatal neurobehavioral scores are relatively insensitive measures of neonatal well-being, and umbilical cord blood gas and pH measurements may reflect the reason for the cesarean delivery rather than differences in anesthetic techniques' effect on fetal well-being. In a meta-analysis, lower umbilical cord blood pH measurements were associated with spinal, but not epidural anesthesia when compared with general anesthesia.[155] However, the study included both randomized and nonrandomized trials and both elective and nonelective procedures. In a systematic review of randomized trials in which the indication for cesarean delivery was not urgent, no differences in umbilical arterial blood pH measurements were found.[153]

Overview of Neuraxial Anesthetic Techniques

Table 26-4 outlines the advantages and disadvantages of the various neuraxial anesthetic techniques for cesarean delivery. With all neuraxial techniques, an adequate sensory level of anesthesia is necessary to minimize maternal pain and avoid the urgent need for administration of general anesthesia. Because motor nerve fibers are typically larger and more difficult to block, the complete absence of hip flexion and ankle dorsiflexion most likely indicates that a functional sensory and sympathetic block is also present in a similar (primarily lumbosacral) distribution. However, because afferent nerves innervating abdominal and pelvic organs accompany sympathetic fibers that ascend and descend in the sympathetic trunk (T5 to L1), a sensory block that extends rostrally from the sacral dermatomes to T4 should be the goal for cesarean delivery anesthesia.

The manner in which the level of sensory blockade is assessed has implications for the success of a neuraxial technique. The different methods of assessing the extent of sensory blockade (i.e., light touch, pinprick, cold) may suggest levels of blockade that differ by several spinal segments. Russell[156] prospectively demonstrated a differential sensitivity to neuraxial blockade in women undergoing cesarean delivery; pinprick evaluation identified a dermatomal level of blockade that was several segments more rostral than that identified by light touch. A subsequent study of spinal anesthesia in parturients undergoing cesarean delivery indicated that although sensory blockade to light touch differed from sensory blockade to pinprick or cold sensation by 0 to 11 spinal segments, no constant relationship between these levels could be determined.[157] The investigators concluded that a T6 blockade to touch would likely provide a pain-free cesarean delivery for most women.

In a survey performed in the United Kingdom, the majority of anesthesiologists used the absence of cold temperature sensation to a T4 level to indicate an adequate blockade height for cesarean delivery.[158] Sensory examination should move caudad to cephalad in the midaxillary line on the lower extremities but can be performed in the midclavicular line on the torso. The time at which an adequate block is achieved, as well as the cephalad and caudad extent of the block, should be documented on the anesthetic record.

Because the undersurface of the diaphragm (C3 to C5) and the vagus nerve may be stimulated by surgical manipulation during cesarean delivery,[159] maternal discomfort and other symptoms (e.g., nausea and vomiting) may occur despite a T4 level of blockade. Neuraxial or systemic opioids help prevent or alleviate these symptoms.

Spinal Anesthesia

Spinal anesthesia is a simple and reliable technique that allows visual confirmation of correct needle placement

TABLE 26-4 Advantages and Disadvantages of Neuraxial Anesthetic Techniques for Cesarean Delivery

Neuraxial Technique	Advantages	Disadvantages
Epidural	No dural puncture required Can use *in situ* catheter placed for earlier administration of labor analgesia Ability to titrate extent of sensory blockade Continuous intraoperative anesthesia Continuous postoperative analgesia	Slow onset of anesthesia Larger drug doses required than for spinal techniques: • Greater risk of maternal systemic toxicity • Greater fetal drug exposure
Combined spinal-epidural	May be technically easier than spinal anesthesia in obese patients Low doses of local anesthetic and opioid Rapid onset of dense lumbosacral and thoracic anesthesia Ability to titrate extent of sensory blockade Continuous intraoperative anesthesia Continuous postoperative analgesia	Delayed verification of functioning epidural catheter
Continuous spinal	Low doses of local anesthetic and opioid Rapid onset of dense anesthesia Ability to titrate extent of sensory blockade Continuous intraoperative anesthesia	Large dural puncture increases risk of post–dural puncture headache Possibility of overdose and total spinal anesthesia if the spinal catheter is mistaken for an epidural catheter
Single-shot spinal	Technically simple Low doses of local anesthetic and opioid Rapid onset of dense lumbosacral and thoracic anesthesia	Limited duration of anesthesia Limited ability to titrate extent of sensory blockade

(by visualization of CSF) and is technically easier to perform than an epidural technique. Spinal anesthesia provides a rapid onset of dense neuroblockade that is typically more profound than that provided with an epidural technique, resulting in a reduced need for supplemental intravenous analgesics or conversion to general anesthesia.[160-162] Only a small amount of local anesthetic is needed to establish a functional spinal blockade; therefore spinal anesthesia is associated with negligible maternal risk for systemic local anesthetic toxicity and with minimal drug transfer to the fetus.[163] Given these advantages, spinal anesthesia is now the most commonly used anesthetic technique for cesarean delivery.[25,148] Spinal anesthesia is also accompanied by a predictable and relatively prompt recovery that allows patients to quickly recover in the postanesthesia care unit (PACU); in some settings, such a recovery may represent a cost savings to the institution.[160]

Spinal anesthesia is usually administered as a single-injection procedure ("single-shot" technique) through a non-cutting, pencil-point needle that is 24-gauge or smaller. A number of different needle designs are available[164]; the size and design of the needle tip affect the incidence and severity of post–dural puncture headache (PDPH) (see Chapter 31).

The spinal technique should be performed at the L3 to L4 interspace or below (see Chapter 12). This space is used to avoid the potential for spinal cord trauma; although the spinal cord ends at L1 in most adults, it extends to the L2 to L3 interspace in a small minority. However, anesthesia providers tend to misidentify the location of the needle insertion site on the spinal column, and the needle may be introduced at a higher level than intended.

On occasion, a continuous spinal anesthetic technique is used, particularly in the setting of an unintentional dural puncture with an epidural needle. Intentional continuous spinal anesthesia may be desirable in certain settings, when the reliability of a spinal technique and the ability to precisely titrate the initiation and duration of anesthesia are strongly desired (e.g., a morbidly obese patient with a difficult airway). Although microcatheters (27- to 32-gauge) were used to provide spinal analgesia and anesthesia in the 1980s, these catheters were withdrawn from the market by the U.S. Food and Drug Administration (FDA) because of concerns about cauda equina syndrome; the catheters are still being used in Europe, particularly in Germany. Arkoosh et al.[165] published a labor analgesia study in which continuous spinal analgesia with a 28-gauge spinal microcatheter was compared with epidural analgesia; they noted that the incidence of neurologic complications was less than 1% with the use of the 28-gauge catheter. Technical difficulties and catheter failures were more common with the microcatheter than with a 20-gauge epidural catheter. Currently the administration of continuous spinal anesthesia requires the use of a 17- or 18-gauge epidural needle and a 19- or 20-gauge catheter; this technique is associated with a high incidence of post–dural puncture headache.

LOCAL ANESTHETIC AGENTS

The choice of local anesthetic agent (and adjuvants) used to provide spinal anesthesia depends on the expected duration of the surgery, the postoperative analgesia plan, and the preferences of the anesthesia provider. For cesarean delivery, the local anesthetic agent of choice is typically **bupivacaine** (Table 26-5). In the United States, spinal bupivacaine is formulated as a 0.75% solution in dextrose 8.25%. Intrathecal administration of bupivacaine results in a dense block of long duration.

TABLE 26-5 Drugs Used for Spinal Anesthesia for Cesarean Delivery

Drug	Dose Range	Duration (min)*
Local Anesthetics		
Lidocaine	60-80 mg	45-75
Bupivacaine	7.5-15 mg	60-120
Levobupivacaine	7.5-15 mg	60-120
Ropivacaine	15-25 mg	60-120
Opioids		
Fentanyl	10-25 µg	180-240
Sufentanil	2.5-5 µg	180-240
Morphine	0.1-0.2 mg	720-1440
Meperidine†	60-70 mg	60
Adjuvant Drugs		
Epinephrine‡	0.1-0.2 mg	—

*For the local anesthetics, the duration is defined as the time to two-segment regression. For the opioids, the duration is defined as the period of analgesia (or time to first request for a supplemental analgesic drug).

†Meperidine has both local anesthetic and opioid properties and can provide surgical anesthesia without the addition of a local anesthetic. The dose indicated represents meperidine used without local anesthetic.

‡The addition of epinephrine may augment the duration of local anesthetics by 15 to 20 minutes.

The dose of intrathecal bupivacaine that has been successfully used for cesarean delivery ranges from 4.5 to 15 mg. In general, pregnant patients require smaller doses of spinal local anesthetic than nonpregnant patients. Reasons include (1) a smaller CSF volume in pregnancy, (2) cephalad movement of hyperbaric local anesthetic in the supine pregnant patient, and (3) greater sensitivity of nerve fibers to the local anesthetic during pregnancy.[166] Overall, the mass of local anesthetic, rather than the concentration or volume, is thought to influence the spread of the resulting blockade[167]; however, the specific influence of the dose and baricity on the efficacy of the block is controversial. The necessary dose may be influenced by other factors, such as co-administration of neuraxial opioids and surgical technique. (Exteriorization of the uterus during closure of the uterus is more stimulating than closure *in situ.*) Carvalho et al.[168] determined that the effective dose for 95% of recipients (ED_{95}) for plain bupivacaine with fentanyl 10 µg* and morphine 0.2 mg in women undergoing cesarean delivery was 13 mg, whereas the effective dose for 50% of recipients (ED_{50}) was 7.25 mg. By contrast, Sarvela et al.[169] demonstrated that spinal hyperbaric or plain bupivacaine 9 mg with fentanyl 20 µg provided satisfactory anesthesia to all but one of 76 subjects. Anesthesia characteristics and hemodynamic changes were similar in the hyperbaric and plain bupivacaine groups; more than 50% of patients in both groups required vasopressor support.

Vercauteren et al.[170] demonstrated that hyperbaric bupivacaine 6.6 mg with sufentanil 3.3 µg provided better anesthesia and less hypotension than a similar dose of plain bupivacaine. Ben-David et al.[171] reported that reducing the dose of plain bupivacaine from 10 to 5 mg decreased the incidence of hypotension and nausea; however, these findings were obscured by the variable use of opioids in the low-dose group. Finally, Bryson et al.[172] compared plain bupivacaine 4.5 mg with hyperbaric bupivacaine 12 mg (both with fentanyl 50 µg and morphine 0.2 mg); they observed similar cephalad sensory levels (C8), incidence of hypotension (approximately 75%), side effects, and rates of patient satisfaction with the two approaches. Five of 27 (19%) patients in the bupivacaine 4.5-mg group and 1 of 25 (4%) patients in the 12-mg group required supplemental analgesia; no conversions to general anesthesia occurred. Altogether, these data indicate that lower anesthetic doses *can* be used; whether they *should* be used is controversial. The anesthesia provider should consider whether adjuvant drugs will be used and whether the risks of giving supplemental analgesia or conversion to general anesthesia that are associated with low doses of bupivacaine outweigh the potential benefits (i.e., less hypotension, faster recovery).

For a single-shot spinal technique, most clinicians use a dose of bupivacaine between 10 and 15 mg, in combination with an opioid. Studies of hyperbaric bupivacaine (12 to 15 mg) have determined that the patient's age, height, weight, body mass, and vertebral column length do not affect the resulting neuraxial blockade.[173,174] The use of the larger dose (15 mg) results in a longer duration of surgical anesthesia; however, cervical sensory blockade is achieved more frequently (Figure 26-4). In patients with extremes of height (less than 5 feet [152 cm], or more than 6 feet [183 cm]), some anesthesia providers alter the dose of local anesthetic. The baricity of the local anesthetic *does* affect the extent of spread of blockade. When the cephalad spread of hyperbaric local anesthetic is desired, the patient can be placed in a slight head-down position.

Ropivacaine is approximately 40% less potent than bupivacaine following spinal injection in nonpregnant individuals.[175] Ogun et al.[176] assessed plain spinal ropivacaine 0.5% and bupivacaine 0.5%, both administered with morphine 0.15 mg; ropivacaine was associated with a slower onset, less hypotension, and faster recovery. Khaw et al.[177] randomly assigned 72 patients undergoing elective cesarean delivery to receive CSE anesthesia with plain spinal ropivacaine 10, 15, 20, or 25 mg; the ED_{50} and ED_{95} were 16.7 mg and 26.8 mg, respectively. Subsequently, the same investigators demonstrated that hyperbaric spinal ropivacaine 25 mg produced a more rapid block with faster recovery and fewer requirements for supplemental epidural anesthesia than the same dose of plain ropivacaine in women undergoing cesarean delivery with spinal anesthesia.[178] Gautier et al.[179] randomly assigned 90 parturients to receive bupivacaine 8 mg, levobupivacaine 8 mg, or ropivacaine 12 mg

*The Joint Commission has recommended that health care providers substitute mcg for µg as an abbreviation for micrograms (http://www.aapmr.org/hpl/pracguide/jachosymbols.htm). The Joint Commission contends that the abbreviation µg may be mistaken for mg (milligrams), which would result in a 1000-fold overdose. On the other hand, most scholarly publications have continued to use the abbreviation µg. The editors have chosen to retain the use of the abbreviation µg throughout this text. However, the editors recommend the use of the abbreviation mcg in clinical practice, especially with handwritten orders.

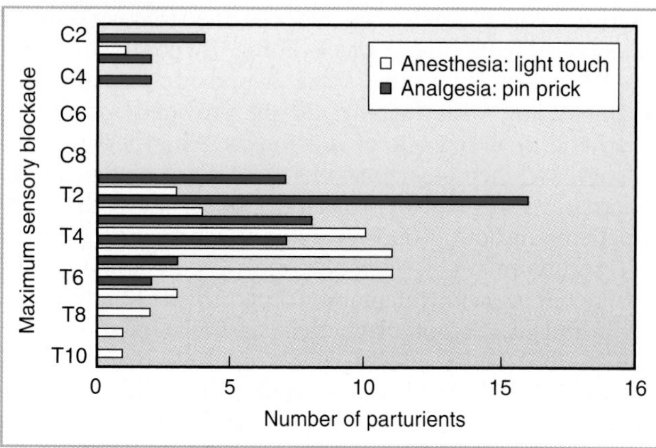

FIGURE 26-4 Maximum cephalad sensory level for analgesia or anesthesia in 52 term parturients after spinal injection of hyperbaric bupivacaine 15 mg with morphine 0.15 mg. (Adapted from Norris MC. Patient variables and the subarachnoid spread of hyperbaric bupivacaine in the term patient. Anesthesiology 1990; 72:478-82.)

(all with sufentanil 2.5 μg); they observed effective anesthesia in 97%, 80%, and 87% of patients, respectively. The duration of levobupivacaine and ropivacaine sensory and motor blockade was shorter than that with bupivacaine blockade.[179]

For spinal anesthesia, the value of ropivacaine and levobupivacaine is questionable. Given the small doses administered, a reduction in risk for systemic local anesthetic toxicity is not a consideration. Further, it is not clear that ropivacaine produces spinal anesthesia of similar quality to that provided by bupivacaine. Neither ropivacaine nor levobupivacaine is approved by the FDA for intrathecal administration. Thus, in the United States, bupivacaine remains the predominant agent for spinal anesthesia for cesarean delivery.

In some institutions where the obstetricians can reliably perform cesarean delivery in less than 45 minutes, hyperbaric **lidocaine** (60 to 80 mg) is used. The use of hyperbaric lidocaine for spinal anesthesia remains controversial because of concerns about transient neurologic symptoms (see Chapters 13 and 32).

Adjuvant Agents

Adjuvant medications contribute to spinal anesthesia by different mechanisms from those of local anesthetics. For cesarean delivery, adjuvant agents improve the quality of intraoperative anesthesia, prolong postoperative analgesia, and reduce the dose, and therefore the side effects, of local anesthetics. Opioids, dextrose, and epinephrine are commonly used adjuvants; neostigmine and clonidine are two agents undergoing clinical investigation.

Preservative-free **morphine** is the most commonly used adjuvant in many countries, except in the United Kingdom, where diamorphine is available. Both agents are effective in providing prolonged (12 to 24 hours) post–cesarean delivery analgesia (see Chapter 28). Spinal morphine produces significant analgesia with acceptable side-effect profiles when given in doses ranging from 0.1 to 0.25 mg. Palmer et al.[180] conducted a dose-response study of the addition of morphine to hyperbaric bupivacaine 12.75 mg; after surgery, patients could access intravenous morphine via patient-controlled analgesia (PCA). A spinal morphine dose of 0.1 mg was found to be optimal, producing post–cesarean delivery analgesia comparable to that provided by doses as high as 0.5 mg, but with less severe pruritus. Whereas the occurrence of pruritus appeared to be dose related, this relationship was not observed with nausea and vomiting. Patient satisfaction appears higher with neuraxial administration of morphine than with intermittent intravenous or intramuscular opioid administration, which can result in delayed analgesia of variable quality.[181]

Delayed respiratory depression can occur with the rostral spread of subarachnoid morphine; monitoring protocols should be in place to observe for this complication, particularly in high-risk patients (e.g., those with sleep apnea, obesity). In a retrospective study of 1915 parturients receiving spinal morphine 0.15 mg for cesarean delivery, 5 patients (0.26%) experienced bradypnea, and 1 patient (0.052%) required naloxone.[182] Overall, very few cases of respiratory depression with spinal morphine (0.1 to 0.2 mg) have been reported in pregnant women undergoing cesarean delivery[183,184]; however, the definition of respiratory depression has varied among studies, making comparisons difficult. Clinicians should be aware that the duration of action of naloxone is approximately 90 minutes[185]; therefore, the respiratory depressant effect of many opioids would be expected to outlast the duration of naloxone's antagonism. Additional doses or a continuous infusion of naloxone should be considered when necessary.

Diamorphine, which is typically used in spinal doses of 0.3 mg to 0.4 mg, is reported to have less severe side effects than morphine. Saravanan et al.[186] observed that the minimum dose of intrathecal diamorphine required to prevent intraoperative supplementation of spinal anesthesia with bupivacaine 12.5 mg was 0.4 mg.

Dahl et al.[183] performed a systematic review of spinal **fentanyl,** administered in doses ranging from 2.5 to 60 μg to augment spinal anesthesia for cesarean delivery. Pruritus, nausea, and vomiting were significantly reduced when doses lower than 35 μg were administered, in comparison with doses of 40 to 60 μg. However, requests for supplemental analgesia were significantly lower only in patients receiving doses of fentanyl 40 μg or greater. Other investigators have observed that spinal fentanyl in doses as low as 6.25 μg improves the quality and duration of cesarean delivery anesthesia.[187] Moreover, in a study of healthy parturients, spinal fentanyl 20 μg was superior to intravenous ondansetron 4 mg for the prevention of perioperative nausea (but not vomiting) during spinal anesthesia for cesarean delivery; the investigators attributed these findings to a possible reduction in visceral stimulation.[188] Spinal doses of fentanyl 10 to 25 μg are commonly used for cesarean delivery anesthesia.[183,189]

Spinal **sufentanil** 2.5 to 20 μg has been used with bupivacaine for cesarean delivery. In a study of 37 parturients undergoing elective cesarean delivery with sufentanil 0, 10, 15, or 20 μg added to hyperbaric bupivacaine 10.5 mg, Courtney et al.[190] found better quality and longer duration of analgesia in all sufentanil groups than in control groups, with similar Apgar scores, umbilical cord blood gas measurements, and Early Neonatal Neurobehavioral Scale

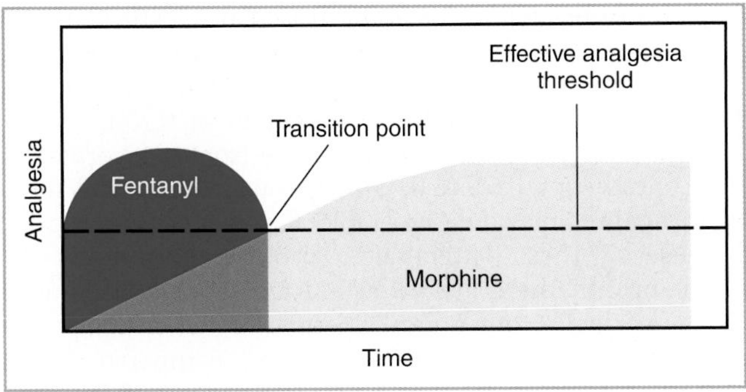

FIGURE 26-5 Schematic illustration of the pharmacokinetic and pharmacodynamic activities resulting from the neuraxial administration of a lipid-soluble opioid (e.g., fentanyl) and a water-soluble opioid (e.g., morphine) for analgesia. The transition point varies according to the opioid drugs and doses administered. For most commonly used opioids, this transition point occurs in the postoperative period.

(ENNS) scores. No cases of respiratory depression occurred. Braga Ade et al.[191] randomly assigned parturients to receive hyperbaric bupivacaine 12.5 mg with sufentanil 0, 2.5, 5, or 7.5 µg. Analgesia lasted longer with sufentanil 5 and 7.5 µg, and pruritus and somnolence were more pronounced with 7.5 µg. Thus there appears to be little justification for giving a dose of sufentanil greater than 5 µg in this setting.

The administration of both a lipid-soluble opioid and a water-soluble opioid takes advantage of the fast onset of the lipid-soluble agent and the prolonged duration of the water-soluble agent (Figure 26-5). Investigators have expressed concern that more rapid-acting, lipid-soluble agents (e.g., fentanyl, sufentanil) would diminish the response (i.e., cause acute opioid tolerance) to more water-soluble agents (e.g., morphine); however, this possibility is controversial. Cooper et al.[192] observed that spinal fentanyl 25 µg or saline added to plain bupivacaine 10 mg resulted in no difference in intravenous PCA morphine consumption within the first 6 hours after cesarean delivery; between 6 and 23 hours, there was a 63% increase in morphine utilization in the group that received fentanyl. By contrast, in a study of 37 women undergoing cesarean delivery with fentanyl 0, 5, 10, or 25 µg combined with hyperbaric bupivacaine 12 mg and morphine 0.2 mg, Giarrusso et al.[193] did not find a difference among groups in postoperative intravenous PCA morphine consumption. It is likely that the spinal morphine administration in the second study affected the outcome. We recommend the combined administration of a lipid-soluble opioid (with a short latency) and a water-soluble opioid (with a long duration of action) when spinal anesthesia is used for cesarean delivery.

Most spinal local anesthetics are prepared in **dextrose** to make the agents hyperbaric. *Baricity* is defined as the density of the local anesthetic divided by the density of CSF measured at the same temperature. The density of CSF is reduced in pregnancy.[194]

Intrathecal administration of an alpha-adrenergic agonist, combined with a local anesthetic, increases the density of sensory and motor blockade and may prolong the duration of blockade and contribute to post–cesarean delivery analgesia. Abouleish[195] observed that intrathecal **epinephrine** 0.1 to 0.2 mg, when combined with hyperbaric bupivacaine, improved the quality of intraoperative analgesia and prolonged both sensory and motor blockade by approximately 15% in comparison with bupivacaine alone.[195]

Spinal **clonidine,** in doses of 60 to 150 µg, improves intraoperative analgesia and decreases shivering in women undergoing cesarean delivery; however, it has been associated with hypotension and sedation.[196] This agent is not used commonly in the United States, although it may be considered in specific circumstances (e.g., when neuraxial opioid analgesia is contraindicated). The FDA has issued a "black box" warning against its use in obstetric patients because of concerns about hemodynamic instability.

In women undergoing cesarean delivery, spinal **neostigmine** in doses up to 100 µg significantly reduced postoperative pain with no effect on FHR or Apgar scores; however, 100% of patients who received 100 µg complained of nausea.[197] In a dose-response investigation in nonpregnant volunteers, spinal doses of neostigmine as low as 6.25 µg have been associated with a high incidence of side effects, including prolonged motor blockade, nausea, and vomiting.[198] In a study of spinal neostigmine 75 µg combined with hyperbaric bupivacaine in women undergoing abdominal hysterectomy, there was no difference in the incidence of hypotension or bradycardia between women randomly assigned to receive neostigmine and those receiving saline.[199] Collectively, these studies suggest that the high incidence of nausea associated with intrathecal neostigmine will likely limit its clinical utility.

At many institutions, including our own, the spinal agents and doses are standardized so that all anesthesia providers can obtain consistent results during the provision of spinal anesthesia for cesarean delivery. Such standardization enables the anesthesia providers and nursing staff to anticipate predictable recovery characteristics and also facilitates recognition of—and response to—profiles that are not within the norm. In addition, drug and dose standardization results in fewer errors. At our institution, spinal anesthesia for cesarean delivery is provided with 0.75% hyperbaric bupivacaine 12 mg, fentanyl 10 µg, and morphine 0.2 mg. Administration of these doses of fentanyl and morphine allows administration of the same volume (0.2 mL) of each agent (fentanyl 50 µg/mL, morphine 1 mg/mL), thereby helping to prevent dosing errors. Furthermore, the opioids are drawn up in a tuberculin syringe to improve measurement accuracy.

Epidural Anesthesia

The use of epidural anesthesia for nonelective cesarean delivery has increased, primarily as a result of the greater use of epidural analgesia during labor. Conversely, the use of epidural anesthesia for *elective* cesarean delivery, and the overall use of epidural anesthesia (see Figure 26-3), is becoming less common, in part because the resulting block is less reliable than that with spinal anesthesia, and the CSE technique offers the benefits of both the fast onset of spinal anesthesia and the placement of an epidural catheter for subsequent augmentation or prolongation of anesthesia if needed. Although medications used in the spinal and epidural spaces are identical, epidural local anesthetic and opioid doses are 5 to 10 times greater than doses given intrathecally. Local anesthetic administered epidurally must penetrate the nerve roots that traverse the space. Moreover, the epidural space has greater capacity than the intrathecal space and subsequently requires a greater volume of local anesthetic to ensure adequate spread. The epidural space also contains a venous plexus that becomes progressively more engorged during pregnancy; thus greater systemic absorption of agents also occurs with epidural administration.

Advantages of the epidural technique include a slower onset of sympathetic blockade, which may allow compensatory mechanisms to attenuate the occurrence and severity of hypotension. A catheter-based technique also allows titration of the level, density, and duration of anesthesia. Continuous post–cesarean delivery analgesia can also be provided through an epidural catheter.

LOCAL ANESTHETIC AGENTS

The most common local anesthetic used for the initiation and maintenance of epidural anesthesia for cesarean delivery is 2% **lidocaine with epinephrine** (Table 26-6). The epidural administration of lidocaine in concentrations less than 2%, or without the addition of epinephrine (which independently augments the analgesia through alpha-adrenergic receptor blockade), may result in anesthesia that is inadequate for surgery.[200]

Surgical anesthesia can be produced with epidural administration of 0.5% **bupivacaine**; however, the slow onset of neuroblockade and the risk of cardiovascular sequelae from unintentional intravascular injection (or systemic absorption) limit the contemporary use of this agent. (The risk of cardiovascular sequelae resulted in a proscription against the epidural administration of 0.75% bupivacaine in obstetric patients.) The single-isomer, levorotatory local anesthetics, 0.5% to 0.75% **ropivacaine** and 0.5% **levobupivacaine,** may be preferable to racemic bupivacaine because of their better safety profiles. Except for the safety profile, there are no significant clinical advantages to these single-isomer local anesthetics when equipotent doses are administered. Bader et al.[201] compared 30 mL of epidural 0.5% levobupivacaine with racemic 0.5% bupivacaine in women undergoing elective cesarean delivery; they observed no differences in the block onset or resolution, signal-averaged ECG results, complications, or maternal and fetal plasma pharmacokinetic profiles between the treatment groups. Following administration of 25 mL of 0.5% levobupivacaine or 0.5% racemic bupivacaine for epidural anesthesia in women undergoing cesarean delivery, Faccenda et al.[202] observed no difference in onset, spread, or duration of sensory block between the agents, although levobupivacaine produced lower limb motor blockade of longer duration but less intensity. Datta et al.[203] demonstrated that the onset, duration, and regression of sensory blockade with 0.5% ropivacaine was similar to that provided by 0.5% bupivacaine, although a faster onset and longer duration of motor blockade was observed with bupivacaine. The free concentrations of ropivacaine were approximately twice those of bupivacaine in both maternal and neonatal blood at delivery; however, these measurements were less than the concentrations shown to be toxic in animals.

TABLE 26-6 Drugs Used for Epidural Anesthesia for Cesarean Delivery

Drug	Dose Range*	Duration (min)†
Local Anesthetics		
Lidocaine 2% with epinephrine 5 μg/mL	300-500 mg	75-100
2-Chloroprocaine 3%	450-750 mg	40-50
Bupivacaine 0.5%	75-125 mg	120-180
Ropivacaine 0.5%	75-125 mg	120-180
Opioids		
Fentanyl	50-100 μg	120-240
Sufentanil	10-20 μg	120-240
Morphine	3-4 mg	720-1440
Meperidine	50-75 mg	240-720

*Both the mass and volume of local anesthetic affect the extent and quality of anesthesia. The usual volume of local anesthetic solution administered into the epidural space at the indicated concentrations is 15 to 25 mL. More mass/volume is required for initiating epidural anesthesia *de novo*; conversely, less is required if epidural labor analgesia is being extended to surgical anesthesia.

†For the local anesthetics, the duration is defined as the time to two-segment regression. For the opioids, the duration is defined as the period of analgesia (or time to first request for a supplemental analgesic drug).

2-Chloroprocaine 3% has the most rapid onset and the shortest duration of action of available local anesthetics given epidurally, and it is an excellent choice for emergency cesarean delivery, for which the dose is administered rapidly. In this setting, even if unintentional intravenous administration of drug were to occur, the sequelae would likely be less severe than the response to intravenous administration of an amide local anesthetic agent. Administration of 2-chloroprocaine has been associated with neurologic sequelae and paralumbar muscle spasms and pain; the neurologic sequelae were thought to be associated with the antioxidant sodium bisulfite, and the muscle pain was thought to result from calcium chelation by the preservative EDTA. Current preparations of 2-chloroprocaine do not contain either the antioxidant or a preservative (see Chapter 13). Epidural administration of 2-chloroprocaine may be associated with a rapid onset of hypotension and a reduction in the clinical efficacy of subsequently administered epidural opioids or local anesthetics. These side effects limit the use of 2-chloroprocaine to those situations in which the rapid onset of anesthesia is paramount.

ADJUVANT AGENTS

As with spinal anesthesia, adjuvant medications are utilized for their intrinsic properties and to reduce the dose and side effects of local anesthetic agents. For cesarean delivery, the use of adjuvants improves the intraoperative quality of anesthesia and prolongs postoperative analgesia, with an associated reduction in motor blockade.

Whereas some anesthesia providers administer an epidural opioid with the initial therapeutic dose of local anesthetic, others delay opioid administration until after the umbilical cord is clamped to prevent transfer of opioid to the fetus (see Chapter 28). The onset of analgesia is dictated by complex pharmacokinetics; however, the lipid-soluble drugs (e.g., fentanyl, sufentanil) have greater availability, more rapid onset, and more rapid clearance than the more water-soluble opioids.[204]

Epidural administration of the hydrophilic drug **morphine** provides prolonged post–cesarean delivery analgesia. In a dose-response study of epidural morphine 1.25, 2.5, 3.75, and 5 mg, Palmer et al.[205] found 3.75 mg to be an optimal dose beyond which postcesarean analgesia (as measured by PCA morphine demands) was no better. Although Duale et al.[184] demonstrated that epidural morphine 2 mg resulted in better post–cesarean delivery analgesia than intrathecal morphine 0.075 mg, it appears that nonequipotent doses were used. Sarvela et al.,[206] comparing epidural morphine (3 mg) to spinal morphine (0.1 mg and 0.2 mg), observed that analgesia progressed from greatest to least in the following order: spinal 0.2 mg, epidural 3 mg, and spinal 0.1 mg; pruritus and nausea were observed with increasing frequency in the opposite order.

An extended-release formulation of morphine (DepoDur) has been developed to provide prolonged epidural analgesia. Carvalho et al.[207] evaluated epidural administration of 5, 10, and 15 mg of extended-release morphine; the 10- and 15-mg doses provided analgesia for 48 hours after cesarean delivery, with no significant side effects. The same investigators compared conventional preservative-free epidural morphine 4 mg with the extended-release epidural morphine 10 mg for post–cesarean delivery analgesia[208]; lower pain scores and fewer requests for supplemental analgesia were observed in the extended-release group over the first 48 hours after surgery. No differences in nausea, pruritus, or sedation scores were observed. A disadvantage of the extended-release preparation is that it cannot be co-administered with a local anesthetic. (Some evidence suggests that the local anesthetic may alter the sustained-release effect derived from the lipid-vesicle preparation.) The package insert for DepoDur states that local anesthetics other than a 3-mL test dose of lidocaine are not permitted, and that if the 3-mL test dose is used, the epidural catheter should be flushed with 1 mL of saline and 15 minutes should be allowed to elapse before epidural administration of the extended-release morphine. The only practical method of using extended-release morphine for post–cesarean delivery analgesia is to administer it as part of a CSE technique (i.e., using spinal anesthesia for intraoperative anesthesia and providing postoperative analgesia with epidural administration of the extended-release morphine).

In the United Kingdom, epidural **diamorphine** (2.5 mg) represents an alternative regimen for providing prolonged post–cesarean delivery analgesia.[209]

The bolus administration of epidural **fentanyl** (50 to 100 μg) results in activity at both spinal and supraspinal sites of action[210] and improves the quality of anesthesia during cesarean delivery.[211,212] The optimal dose of fentanyl has not been determined for patients undergoing cesarean delivery; however, Eichenberger et al.[213] observed a segmental effect of epidural fentanyl on the characteristics of muscle pain after epidural administration of 100 μg, but not 50 μg, in nonpregnant patients. Although some anesthesia providers delay the epidural administration of opioids until after the umbilical cord is clamped, the administration of fentanyl with the initial therapeutic dose of local anesthetic improves intraoperative anesthesia and, in doses between 50 and 100 μg, does not appear to adversely affect the neonate.[214]

Epidural **sufentanil** (10 to 20 μg), when added to 0.5% bupivacaine with epinephrine 5 μg/mL, provides significantly better intraoperative anesthesia and longer postoperative analgesia than bupivacaine and epinephrine alone, with minimal maternal side effects and no adverse neonatal effects.[215,216] Epidural sufentanil is approximately five times as potent as epidural fentanyl, but when equipotent doses are administered, no differences between the agents in onset, quality, or duration of analgesia have been observed.[215,216]

Epidural **clonidine** (75 to 200 μg) combined with morphine or fentanyl reduces the requirement for post–cesarean delivery morphine analgesia.[217,218] Eisenach et al.[217] demonstrated an additive rather than synergistic effect of epidural clonidine and fentanyl in producing post–cesarean delivery analgesia. Common side effects include hypotension and sedation. Currently epidural clonidine has only one specific neuraxial indication (intractable cancer pain), and the package insert has a "black box" FDA warning stating that "epidural clonidine is not recommended for obstetrical, postpartum and perioperative pain management."

Epidural **neostigmine** produces a modest amount of post–cesarean delivery analgesia when given after umbilical cord clamping. Kaya et al.[219] investigated the administration of 75, 150, or 300 μg of epidural neostigmine in women undergoing elective cesarean delivery. An increase in intraoperative shivering and sedation was observed in the 300-μg group only; by contrast, a dose-independent reduction in postoperative pain and sedation was observed in all groups.

Epinephrine is frequently added to the local anesthetic agent to minimize systemic absorption and the peak blood level of local anesthetic, increase the density of sensory and motor blockade, and prolong the duration of anesthesia.[220-222] Bernards et al.[223] observed that the pharmacokinetic effects of epinephrine co-administered with an opioid vary with the opioid and the sampling site. In the lumbar epidural space, epinephrine lengthened the mean residence time of morphine but shortened that of fentanyl and sufentanil. The epidural administration of epinephrine in preeclamptic women is controversial (see Chapter 45).[224] Animal and clinical studies suggest that epidural epinephrine 0.1 mg does not decrease uterine blood flow.[225-227] Alahuhta et al.[228] used maternal Doppler ultrasonography and fetal M-mode echocardiography to evaluate the hemodynamic effects of the addition of epidural epinephrine (approximately 5 μg/mL) to bupivacaine; maternal diastolic pressure, but not systolic pressure or uterine blood flow, was decreased with the addition of epinephrine.

Epinephrine in doses of 2.5 or 5 μg/mL (i.e., 1:400,000 or 1:200,000) can be administered epidurally. The addition of epinephrine to a solution of plain local anesthetic just prior to administration results in a solution that has a higher pH than commercially prepared epinephrine-containing products, which use (low-pH) antioxidants to preserve the efficacy of the epinephrine.

The addition of **sodium bicarbonate** results in a solution with more local anesthetic molecules in a non-ionized state, which hastens the onset and augments the quality of the local anesthetic blockade, particularly if sodium bicarbonate is added to a low-pH solution (see later).

Combined Spinal-Epidural Anesthesia

The combined CSE technique incorporates the rapid and predictable onset of a spinal blockade with the ability to augment anesthesia by injection of additional drug through the epidural catheter.[229-231] In 1981, Brownridge[229] reported the first use of the CSE technique for cesarean delivery through separate spinal and epidural needles introduced at different interspaces. Carrie and O'Sullivan[230] subsequently reported the needle-through-needle technique via a single interspace for cesarean delivery; this has become the more popular technique. Davies et al.[231] compared CSE with epidural anesthesia alone for elective cesarean delivery and reported more rapid onset, greater motor blockade, and lower pain scores at delivery in the CSE group; they observed no difference in the incidence of maternal hypotension, nausea, headache, the use of supplemental analgesics, or overall patient satisfaction.

The advantage of the CSE technique is more fully realized when the duration of surgery is prolonged or when the anesthesia provider wants to use the epidural catheter to provide postoperative analgesia. Other applications of this technique include (1) use of the epidural needle as an introducer for a longer spinal needle when attempts with a traditional introducer and spinal needle have failed, and (2) use of the spinal needle to determine what lies within the path of the advancing epidural needle, a maneuver that may prevent a dural puncture with the larger epidural needle.

Conventional doses (e.g., 12 mg) of hyperbaric bupivacaine are most often used to provide CSE anesthesia for cesarean delivery; however, a satisfactory block has been reported with plain bupivacaine drug doses as low as 4.5 mg.[172] Although the use of lower amounts of local anesthetic is enabled by the presence of the epidural catheter (because additional agents can be administered if discomfort occurs), the CSE technique may inherently provide a different block with the same dose of medication from that provided by a single-shot spinal technique. Goy et al.[232] demonstrated that the median effective doses of intrathecal hyperbaric bupivacaine (to achieve a T6 sensory level of anesthesia for 60 minutes in men undergoing surgery) for the CSE and spinal techniques were 9.18 mg and 11.37 mg, respectively. The investigators speculated that the use of the loss-of-resistance to air (during introduction of the epidural needle) could result in a reduction in lumbar CSF volume. Lumbar CSF volume is inversely related to the peak sensory level during spinal blockade. Ithnin et al.[233] observed median sensory levels of C6 and T3 with the CSE and spinal techniques, respectively, following administration of bupivacaine 10 mg in parturients undergoing an *elective* cesarean delivery. The loss-of-resistance to air was performed with 2 mL, and the epidural catheter was not inserted. The investigators speculated that the loss of negative pressure in the epidural space (which occurs with the introduction of the epidural needle) may be responsible for the differences observed with the CSE versus spinal technique. By contrast, using the same anesthetic techniques to provide cesarean delivery anesthesia in *laboring* women, investigators from the same institution found no differences in block characteristics between the two techniques.[234] The reason for these different results are unclear.

The *sequential* CSE technique uses a lower dose of spinal bupivacaine (7.5 to 10 mg) followed by incremental injection of local anesthetic through the epidural catheter to achieve a T4 level of anesthesia.[235,236] The purported advantage of this approach is a lower incidence of hypotension. With the sequential CSE technique, Thoren et al.[236] observed a more gradual onset of hypotension and a lower initial anesthesia level with the spinal dose (T7 and T4 with the CSE and spinal technique, respectively); however, all parturients in the CSE group required additional doses of local anesthetic through the epidural catheter. The sequential CSE technique may be of particular advantage in certain high-risk parturients (e.g., significant cardiac disease) in whom avoidance of severe hypotension can be vital.

Another CSE technique is the *extradural volume extension* (EVE) technique.[235,237] Intrathecal administration of a small dose of local anesthetic is followed by the administration of saline through the epidural catheter. In a review of this technique, McNaught and Stocks[235] observed a higher cephalad spread of 1 to 4 dermatomal segments. However, the effect of EVE may depend on the initial spinal dose, the time interval between spinal and epidural dosing, the amount of epidural volume, and the outcomes measured. Kucukguclu et al.[237] found no clinical differences when 10 mL of epidural saline was administered within 5 minutes of hyperbaric versus isobaric 0.5% bupivacaine 8 to 9 mg with fentanyl 20 μg.

Potential drawbacks of CSE techniques include an untested epidural catheter and hypotension. Yun et al.[129] reported greater severity and duration of hypotension when the CSE technique was administered in the sitting position than in the lateral decubitus position. The hypotension may be related to the delay in moving the patient from the sitting to the supine (with leftward tilt) position. Alternatively, greater hypotension may result from a higher level of sympathetic blockade with the CSE technique.

Extension of Epidural Labor Analgesia

The extension of epidural labor *analgesia* to surgical *anesthesia* sufficient for cesarean delivery can be accomplished with one of several local anesthetic agents. The selection of agent often depends on the urgency of the case. Extension of epidural analgesia can be initiated as preparations are being made to move the patient from the labor room to the operating room.

Lucas et al.[238] compared the extension of existing labor epidural analgesia with 0.5% bupivacaine, with 2% lidocaine with epinephrine 5 μg/mL (1:200,000), and with a 50:50 combination of the two solutions; they observed no difference among groups in the time required to obtain a bilateral loss to cold sensation at T4. Bjornestad et al.[239] observed no significant difference in onset of anesthesia between epidural administration of 3% 2-chloroprocaine and that of 2% lidocaine with freshly added epinephrine 5 μg/mL; median onset was 8 minutes (range of 4 to 13 minutes) in the 2-chloroprocaine group and 5 minutes (range 2 to 22 minutes) in the lidocaine group. The investigators concluded that in view of the time taken for preparation of the lidocaine with epinephrine solution, administration of "a pre-prepared solution, such as 2-chloroprocaine, may be preferred."[239] Of interest, 30% and 20% of patients in the 2-chloroprocaine and lidocaine groups, respectively, required intravenous alfentanil for supplementation of anesthesia.

Alkalinization of the local anesthetic solution not only increases the speed of onset but also improves the quality and prolongs the duration of neuroblockade.[240] Alkalinization shifts more of the local anesthetic molecules to the non-ionized lipid-soluble form, which allows the local anesthetic to pass more easily through the bilipid neuronal membrane surrounding the sodium channel. Although this phenomenon can be demonstrated for all local anesthetics, alkalinization is most often performed with local anesthetic agents of short and medium duration (e.g., 2-chloroprocaine, lidocaine). Typically 1 mL of 8.4% sodium bicarbonate (1 mEq/mL) is added to 10 mL of lidocaine or 2-chloroprocaine. Longer-acting agents (e.g., bupivacaine, ropivacaine, levobupivacaine) easily precipitate with the addition of sodium bicarbonate. Precipitation occurs with the addition of less than 0.2 mEq of bicarbonate to 20 mL of 0.5% bupivacaine.[241] Alkalinization exerts the greatest effect when the combination is freshly prepared; however, the mixture is relatively stable. Tuleu et al.[242] evaluated the stability of pH-adjusted lidocaine with epinephrine, prepared with 2 mEq of sodium bicarbonate added to 20 mL of 2% lidocaine and epinephrine 0.1 mg. Although the local anesthetic activity was unchanged, the epinephrine showed evidence of partial degradation at 6 hours.

Lam et al.[240] evaluated the extension of a T10 level of epidural labor analgesia with the addition of 1.2 mL of 8.4% sodium bicarbonate (or saline) to 12 mL of premixed 2% lidocaine with epinephrine 5 μg/mL (1:200,000) and fentanyl 75 μg (Figure 26-6). The mean times to attain a T6 anesthesia level with and without bicarbonate were 5.2 minutes and 9.7 minutes, respectively. Gaiser et al.[243] evaluated the addition of 2 mL of 8.4% sodium bicarbonate to 23 mL of either 1.5% lidocaine with epinephrine 5 μg/mL (1:200,000) or 3% 2-chloroprocaine; the mean onset time to extend the T10 analgesia level to a surgical level of anesthesia was 4.4 minutes for lidocaine and 3.1 minutes for 2-chloroprocaine. Malhotra and Yentis[244] evaluated the use of 20 mL of 0.5% levobupivacaine, with and without fentanyl 75 μg, to extend a T9 labor analgesia level to a T4 sensory level. The onset time did not differ between groups, averaging 10 to 11 minutes.

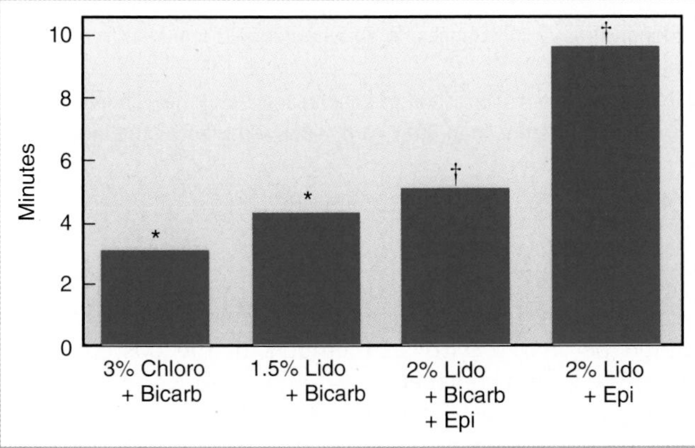

FIGURE 26-6 Onset time for extension of existing labor analgesia blockade (T10 sensory level) with different local anesthetic preparations. Results between the two studies cannot be directly compared due to differences in labor analgesia regimens, different sensory testing methods and target levels, and presence of epidural opioids. The 2% lidocaine with epinephrine solution was premixed. The epinephrine dose was 5 μg/mL. Chloro, 2-chloroprocaine; Bicarb, bicarbonate; Lido, lidocaine; Epi, epinephrine 5 μg/mL. ***To T4 sensory level.** (Data adapted from Gaiser RR, Cheek TG, Gutsche BB. Epidural lidocaine versus 2-chloroprocaine for fetal distress requiring urgent cesarean section. Int J Obstet Anesth 1994; 3:208-10.). **†To T6 sensory level.** (Data adapted from Lam DT, Ngan Kee WD, Khaw KS. Extension of epidural blockade in labour for emergency Caesarean section using 2% lidocaine with epinephrine and fentanyl, with or without alkalinisation. Anaesthesia 2001; 56:790-4.)

Extension of a T10 level of *analgesia* to a T4 level of *anesthesia* typically requires a volume of approximately 15 to 20 mL of local anesthetic with one or more adjuvants. At our institution the extension of epidural labor analgesia begins with assessment of the quality of analgesia. For emergency cesarean delivery, we often initiate the extension of epidural anesthesia in the labor room by giving 5 to 10 mL of alkalinized 2% lidocaine (with epinephrine) or 3% 2-chloroprocaine. The sensory blockade is assessed after transfer of the patient to the operating room; if the blockade is bilateral and moving in a cephalad direction, an additional 5 to 10 mL is administered to bring the sensory level to T4. The use of this fractionated dosing schedule offers several advantages, including: (1) greater hemodynamic stability during patient transfer; (2) assessment of the evolving sensory level prior to administration of the full dose of local anesthetic; (3) minimization of dural sac compression,[245] which enables a less difficult and safer conversion to spinal anesthesia if extension of epidural anesthesia is not successful; and (4) early sensory blockade at the incision site, so that surgery can be initiated in emergency cases prior to establishment of a full T4 sensory level. We acknowledge that the extension of epidural analgesia to epidural anesthesia in the labor room is controversial.[246] Some anesthesia providers delay epidural administration of additional local anesthetic until the patient has arrived in the operating room.

General Anesthesia

Although neuraxial techniques are typically preferred when anesthesia is provided for cesarean delivery, there are some clinical situations in which the administration of general anesthesia is considered the most appropriate option (see Table 26-3). In addition, general anesthesia offers an advantage in cases in which uterine relaxation would be beneficial (e.g., cesarean delivery as part of an *ex utero* intrapartum treatment [EXIT] procedure).

The basic elements for preparation and care of the obstetric patient undergoing cesarean delivery also apply to the patient undergoing general anesthesia (Box 26-8; see Table 26-2). The preanesthetic evaluation should focus on assessment of physical characteristics (e.g., airway) and comorbidities. The consent process should feature the risks associated with airway management, aspiration, and awareness. The importance of a careful airway evaluation cannot be overemphasized; pregnancy-induced changes in the upper airway may be exacerbated during labor. Kodali et al.[247] used acoustic reflectometry to

BOX 26-8 General Anesthesia for Cesarean Delivery*

1. Discuss the operative plan with the multidisciplinary team.
2. Perform preanesthetic assessment and obtain informed consent.
3. Prepare necessary medications and equipment.
4. Place patient supine with left uterine displacement.
5. Secure 16- or 18-gauge intravenous access. Send blood specimen for baseline laboratory measurements; consider type and screen (or cross-match) if risk factors for peripartum hemorrhage are present.
6. Give metoclopramide 10 mg and/or ranitidine 30 mg intravenously more than 30 minutes before induction, if possible.
7. Give a nonparticulate antacid orally less than 30 minutes before induction.†
8. Administer antibiotic prophylaxis (either before incision or after cord clamping).‡
9. Initiate monitoring.
10. Perform a team "time-out"; to verify patient identity, position, and operative site; procedure to be performed; and availability of special equipment, if needed.
11. Provide 100% oxygen with a tight-fitting face mask for 3 minutes or longer, when possible, for denitrogenation/preoxygenation. Otherwise, instruct the patient to take 4 to 8 vital-capacity breaths immediately before induction of anesthesia.
12. After the abdomen has been prepared and operative drapes are in place, verify that the surgeon and assistant are ready to begin surgery.
13. Initiate rapid-sequence induction:
    a. Cricoid pressure 10 N while awake; increase to 30 N after loss of consciousness.
    b. Thiopental 4 to 5 mg/kg and succinylcholine 1 to 1.5 mg/kg; wait 30 to 40 seconds.#
14. Perform endotracheal intubation. Confirm correct placement of endotracheal tube.
15. Provide maintenance of anesthesia:
    a. Use isoflurane, sevoflurane, or desflurane (approximately 1 MAC) in 100% oxygen, or oxygen/nitrous oxide (up to 50%).
    b. Treat hypotension (e.g., phenylephrine, ephedrine).
    c. If additional muscle relaxant (e.g., rocuronium, vecuronium) is necessary, titrate dose according to response to peripheral nerve stimulator.
16. Observe delivery of baby.
17. Begin a continuous infusion of oxytocin; consider other uterotonic agents (e.g., methylergonovine, 15-methyl prostaglandin $F_{2\alpha}$, misoprostol) if uterine tone is inadequate. Monitor blood loss and respond as necessary.
18. Adjust maintenance technique after delivery of the infant:
    a. Administer a reduced concentration of a volatile halogenated agent (0.5 to 0.75 MAC).
    b. Supplement anesthesia with nitrous oxide and an intravenous opioid.
    c. Give attention to risk of awareness and recall. Consider administration of a benzodiazepine (e.g., midazolam).
19. Perform extubation when neuromuscular blockade is fully reversed and the patient is awake and responds to commands.
20. Evaluate postoperative issues (e.g., pain, nausea).

IV, intravenously; MAC, minimal alveolar concentration.

*The events and sequence of events may need to be modified and tailored to individual circumstances. In an emergency, some tasks may have to be performed simultaneously.

†Some anesthesiologists suggest that sodium citrate should be administered within 20 minutes of induction of general anesthesia (see Chapter 29).

‡Recent evidence suggests that administration of prophylactic antibiotics *before* incision (rather than after cord clamping) reduces the incidence of post–cesarean delivery endometritis and total maternal infectious morbidity.[91]

#Drugs and doses may have to be modified for individual patients and circumstances.

determine that soft tissue mucosal edema in both the oral (incisor teeth to oropharyngeal junction) and pharyngeal (oropharyngeal junction to the glottis) tissue increases during labor; these changes occurred over an average labor duration of 11 hours, of which 75 minutes was in the second stage, and resulted in worsening of the initial prelabor airway classification. Failed intubation, failed ventilation and oxygenation, and pulmonary aspiration of gastric contents remain leading anesthesia-related causes of maternal death. If the airway evaluation suggests the possibility of a difficult intubation, consideration should be given to the placement of a neuraxial catheter during early labor, even if it is not used to provide labor analgesia.[43]

PREPARATION

All pregnant patients requiring surgical anesthesia should be considered at risk for pulmonary aspiration of gastric contents (see Chapter 29). Attempts should be made to minimize both the risk of maternal aspiration and the risk of pulmonary injury if aspiration occurs. Fasting policies should be shared with all members of the obstetric care team. We administer metoclopramide 10 mg and ranitidine 50 mg intravenously between 30 and 60 minutes before induction of general anesthesia, to diminish gastric volume and gastric acid secretion, respectively.[248,249] A clear, nonparticulate antacid (sodium citrate 30 mL) should also be administered to neutralize gastric acid, especially in an emergency situation, for which metoclopramide and ranitidine may not have been administered in a timely manner.

If the patient has airway characteristics that herald a difficult mask ventilation or intubation, preparations should be made to perform an awake endotracheal intubation (see Chapter 30). Preparations include administering an antisialagogue (e.g., glycopyrrolate), judicious sedation (e.g., midazolam), and topical airway anesthesia (e.g., aerosolized lidocaine). Glossopharyngeal and laryngeal nerve blocks may also be considered.

The patient should be placed supine with left uterine displacement. The head, neck, and shoulders should be optimally positioned for airway management (i.e., the sniffing position). Routine monitoring should be established, including ECG, pulse oximetry, blood pressure, and capnography. Preoxygenation (denitrogenation) with 100% oxygen should be performed to delay the onset of hypoxemia during apnea; this hypoxemia occurs more rapidly due to the pregnancy-induced decrease in functional residual capacity and increase in oxygen consumption. Ideally, preoxygenation is accomplished by 3 minutes of tidal-volume breathing with a tight-fitting face mask.[250,251] Although 4 maximal deep breaths over 30 seconds (4 DB/30 sec) with an FIO_2 of 1.0 can achieve a similar PaO_2, the same protection against rapid oxyhemoglobin desaturation is not afforded due to differences in tissue and venous compartment oxygen reserves.[250,251] The method of 8 deep breaths over 1 minute (8 DB/1 min) appears to provide better protection from oxyhemoglobin desaturation during apnea than the 4 DB/30 sec method.[252]

In contrast to most surgical procedures, the patient's abdomen is prepared and draped prior to induction of general anesthesia in order to minimize fetal exposure to general anesthesia. After the surgical drapes have been applied and the operating personnel are ready at the tableside, the surgeon should be instructed to delay the incision until the anesthesia provider confirms correct placement of the endotracheal tube and gives verbal instructions to proceed with surgery.

INDUCTION

A rapid-sequence induction is initiated with denitrogenation/preoxygenation followed by administration of an induction agent and paralysis; mask ventilation is not performed, to prevent unintentional insufflation of the stomach. Initially, an assistant should apply 10 newtons (N) of force on the cricoid cartilage, which is increased to 30 N after loss of consciousness; application of the full amount of force while the patient is still awake can provoke active retching and regurgitation. The higher force is continued until correct placement of the endotracheal tube is confirmed. In some cases, the brief release of cricoid pressure may be necessary for successful intubation; often the benefit of release outweighs the risk of regurgitation. Cricoid pressure should then be reapplied until the correct endotracheal tube position is confirmed.

The induction agent of choice is **thiopental** (4 to 5 mg/kg), but **propofol** (2 to 2.8 mg/kg) can also be used. Propofol, in a dose sufficient for induction and to prevent maternal awareness (2.5 mg/kg), depresses the infant more than thiopental. In the presence of hemodynamic instability, **ketamine** (1 to 1.5 mg/kg) or **etomidate** (0.3 mg/kg) should be substituted for thiopental. Paralysis is achieved by **succinylcholine** (1 to 1.5 mg/kg) in approximately 30 to 40 seconds; fasciculations are an unreliable sign, and a peripheral nerve stimulator can be used to confirm neuromuscular blockade. Administration of a defasciculating dose of a nondepolarizing muscle relaxant is *not* recommended, as it may delay the onset of neuromuscular blockade with succinylcholine. Moreover, Cook et al.[253] demonstrated that d-tubocurarine 0.05 mg/kg given prior to succinylcholine 1.5 mg/kg did not reduce the severity of fasciculations or postoperative muscle pain in women undergoing cesarean delivery. Pregnancy also appears to be associated with less severe fasciculations and less succinylcholine-induced muscle pain.[254]

Rocuronium (0.6 to 1 mg/kg) may provide intubating conditions similar to those with succinylcholine for cesarean delivery,[255,256] and is a viable alternative in situations in which succinylcholine should be avoided (e.g., malignant hyperthermia, myotonic dystrophy, spastic paraparesis).[257] The use of a priming preinduction dose of a nondepolarizing muscle relaxant is not recommended during pregnancy, because it may result in complete paralysis and increase the risk of aspiration.[258] In addition, the activity of nondepolarizing muscle relaxants is enhanced in patients receiving magnesium sulfate.[259]

A smaller-diameter cuffed endotracheal tube (i.e., 6.5 or 7.0 mm) should be used; the use of a flexible stylet within the endotracheal tube optimizes the first attempt at intubation. Tissue trauma and airway edema may occur with repeated attempts at intubation. Correct endotracheal tube placement should be confirmed by auscultation in both axillae and over the stomach to detect inadvertent endobronchial and esophageal intubation, respectively. Expired end-tidal carbon dioxide may be detected transiently with an esophageal intubation[260]; thus the anesthesia provider should observe ongoing evidence of a normal capnographic tracing and adequate maternal oxyhemoglobin saturation as well as bilateral thoracic movement and breath sounds. If doubts persist, the anesthesia provider can perform direct laryngoscopy or fiberoptic bronchoscopy to confirm the correct placement of the endotracheal tube in the trachea. If incorrect endotracheal tube placement is promptly recognized, extubation (with continued cricoid pressure) will often allow another attempt without the need for additional muscle relaxant.

Failed endotracheal intubation should invoke the difficult airway algorithm and a call for assistance (see Chapter 30). Options include (1) allowing the patient to awaken, (2) using alternative techniques to place an endotracheal tube, and (3) using alternative airway devices. The laryngeal mask airway (LMA) does not prevent pulmonary soiling with gastric contents as efficiently as an endotracheal tube, but it can be a lifesaving device in situations of failed intubation. Han et al.[261] reported clinically effective airway management with a simple LMA, which was placed successfully on the first attempt in 98% of 1067 healthy parturients undergoing elective cesarean delivery with general anesthesia. Cricoid pressure was maintained throughout the cesarean delivery, and no adverse sequelae occurred. A number of variations to the original LMA have been developed (see Chapter 30). Emergency airway equipment should be immediately available in all obstetric operating rooms.[43]

MAINTENANCE

The goals for anesthetic maintenance include (1) adequate maternal and fetal oxygenation, with maintenance of normocapnia for pregnancy; (2) appropriate depth of anesthesia to promote maternal comfort and a quiescent surgical field and to prevent awareness and recall; (3) minimal effects on uterine tone after delivery; and (4) minimal adverse effects on the neonate.

Fetal oxygenation appears maximal when a maternal FIO_2 of 1.0 is used[262]; however, in the absence of fetal compromise, an FIO_2 of 0.3 appears to provide sufficient oxygenation while minimizing the production of oxygen free radicals (as discussed earlier). Although maternal arterial and umbilical venous blood oxygen content is increased with a greater FIO_2, no differences in 1- or 5-minute Apgar or neurobehavioral scores have been observed with the higher FIO_2.[263,264] As a consequence, in the absence of fetal compromise, inspired oxygen concentrations should be guided by pulse oximetry rather than provision of an arbitrarily set level of FIO_2.

Maternal ventilation should maintain normocapnia, which at term gestation is approximately 30 to 32 mm Hg. Excessive ventilation can cause uteroplacental vasoconstriction and a leftward shift of the oxyhemoglobin dissociation curve, which may result in compromised fetal oxygenation.[265] On the other hand, hypercapnia can lead to maternal tachycardia and is also undesirable.

Initially, high fresh-gas flows should be used to ensure an adequate end-tidal concentration of the volatile halogenated agent. No specific volatile halogenated agent has been demonstrated to be superior to another. The anesthetic requirements for volatile halogenated agents are diminished 25% to 40% during pregnancy.[266] End-tidal levels of halogenated agent greater than 1 to 1.5 times the minimum alveolar concentration (MAC) may reduce the effect of oxytocin on uterine tone and lead to greater blood loss after delivery.[267] To prevent intraoperative awareness, a bispectral index (BIS) measurement less than 60 has been suggested, which typically requires more than 0.75 MAC of a volatile halogenated agent combined with 50% nitrous oxide.[268] However, the value of the bispectral index in reducing the incidence of awareness and recall during administration of general anesthesia for cesarean delivery is unproven and unclear.

In clinical practice, approximately 1.0 MAC of a volatile halogenated agent is typically administered between intubation and delivery, and the concentration of the volatile agent is then reduced to 0.5 to 0.75 MAC after delivery. Nitrous oxide is often administered and titrated as necessary; a concentration of 50% nitrous oxide in oxygen allows a reduction in the concentration of the volatile halogenated agent and thus decreases the influence of the volatile agent on uterine tone. The anesthesia provider may also consider administration of a benzodiazepine (e.g., midazolam) after delivery to reduce the risk of maternal awareness.

Given the stretching of the abdominal wall that occurs during pregnancy, additional neuromuscular blockade is often unnecessary, provided that the mother has an adequate depth of anesthesia (with administration of both a volatile agent and an opioid). If necessary, a small dose of a short-acting nondepolarizing agent (or an infusion of succinylcholine) can be administered. A peripheral nerve stimulator should be used to monitor the maternal response.

Comparison of neonatal outcomes following general anesthesia and epidural anesthesia for cesarean delivery suggests the occurrence of small, transient differences; however, with both techniques, a U-D interval longer than 180 seconds can result in lower Apgar scores and greater fetal acidosis.[137] (This result most likely reflects difficulty in delivering the baby rather than a direct effect of the anesthetic agents.) General anesthetic agents can redistribute from the neonatal fat to the circulation, however, and lead to secondary depression of neonatal ventilatory effort; thus the presence of a pediatrician (or another neonatal provider) is advisable until a normal ventilatory pattern is observed.

EMERGENCE AND EXTUBATION

When the patient awakens, extubation should be undertaken with the patient in a semirecumbent position. The patient should demonstrate purposeful response to verbal commands and return of protective airway reflexes. If repeated airway manipulation, massive hemorrhage, or emergency hysterectomy has occurred, delayed extubation and/or transfer to an intensive care unit (ICU) can be considered.

PHARMACOLOGY

Thiopental

Historically the barbiturates (e.g., thiopental [thiopentone], methohexital, thiamylal) have been the induction agents most commonly used for cesarean delivery. Extensive published data have confirmed the safety and efficacy of thiopental for induction of anesthesia in patients undergoing cesarean delivery at various gestational ages. Thiopental 4 mg/kg provides a rapid and reliable induction of anesthesia. As a negative inotrope and vasodilator, thiopental can cause decreased cardiac output and blood pressure,[269] which may result in significant hypotension in hypovolemic patients. Some investigators have attempted to minimize this effect by using a lower dose of thiopental in combination with ketamine or propofol, with varying success.

Thiopental rapidly crosses the placenta. In 11 healthy subjects who underwent induction of general anesthesia with thiopental, the mean umbilical artery–to–umbilical vein (UA/UV) ratio was 0.87 with an induction-to-delivery (I-D) interval that ranged from 8 to 22 minutes.[270] The equilibration of thiopental occurs relatively rapidly in the fetus; however, fetal brain concentrations rarely exceed the threshold required for neonatal depression. With a maternal induction dose of 4 mg/kg, umbilical vein concentrations of thiopental are well below the arterial plasma concentrations necessary to produce anesthesia in adults.[271] However, with large induction doses (8 mg/kg), thiopental can produce significant neonatal depression.[272]

The following theories have been proposed to explain the clinical occurrence of an unconscious mother but an awake neonate: (1) preferential uptake of thiopental by the fetal liver, which is the first organ perfused by blood coming from the umbilical vein[272]; (2) the higher relative water content of the fetal brain[273]; (3) rapid redistribution of the drug into the maternal tissues, which causes a rapid reduction in the maternal-to-fetal concentration gradient; (4) nonhomogeneity of blood flow in the intervillous space; and (5) progressive dilution by admixture with the various components of the fetal circulation.[274] Because of this rapid equilibration of thiopental and the low fetal brain concentration of thiopental, there is no advantage in delaying delivery until thiopental concentrations decline. There is no evidence that thiopental causes adverse fetal effects when the I-D time is prolonged.

Propofol

Propofol is an intravenous induction agent with a rapid onset, rapid recovery, and favorable side-effect profile, which includes a low incidence of nausea and vomiting.

Induction with propofol can result in pain on injection, and a reduction in maternal blood pressure and cardiac output.[275] The pharmacokinetics of propofol are similar in pregnant and nonpregnant women, except for a more rapid clearance observed during pregnancy, which may partially reflect drug removal through blood loss and the delivery of the infant and placenta.[276]

When given as an intravenous bolus, by continuous infusion, or both, propofol rapidly crosses the placenta and results in an umbilical vein–to–maternal vein (UV/MV) ratio of approximately 0.7.[277,278] Celleno et al.[279] randomly assigned 40 mothers undergoing cesarean delivery with general anesthesia to receive either propofol 2.8 mg/kg or thiopental 5 mg/kg for induction; they observed significantly lower Apgar and neurobehavioral scores in the propofol group. The I-D and U-D intervals in the two groups were nearly identical. Five infants exposed to propofol had profound muscular hypotonus at birth and at 5 minutes, and one newborn was somnolent. Other studies have found no effect of propofol on neurobehavioral scores or the time to sustained spontaneous respiration with induction bolus doses of propofol 2.5 mg/kg or with infusion doses less than 6 mg/kg/hr.[276,280] However, higher doses of propofol (9 mg/kg/hr) have been correlated with a low Neurologic and Adaptive Capacity Score (NACS).[281]

Compared with thiopental, propofol results in a greater incidence of maternal hypotension,[282,283] which may more effectively attenuate the response to laryngoscopy and intubation[284,285] at the risk of reduced uteroplacental blood flow. Moreover, in women undergoing cesarean delivery, Celleno et al.[283] demonstrated that propofol 2.4 mg/kg, in comparison with thiopental 5 mg/kg, resulted in electroencephalographic patterns consistent with a lighter depth of anesthesia, which was confirmed by the presence of clinical signs of light anesthesia in 50% of the patients. Other studies have not observed significant hypotension after the administration of propofol (2 to 2.8 mg/kg) or lower umbilical blood gas and pH measurements than after administration of thiopental (4 to 5 mg/kg)[280,286] or thiamylal (3 to 4 mg/kg).[287] However, one report noted a transient but severe episode of maternal bradycardia after administration of propofol followed by succinylcholine for rapid-sequence induction.[288] This effect has also been demonstrated in pregnant ewes; one animal experienced severe bradycardia that led to a sinus arrest.[289]

In a study of nonpregnant women, the interaction of propofol and ketamine was found to be additive at hypnotic and anesthetic endpoints; the cardiostimulant effects of ketamine appear to offset the cardiodepressant effects of propofol.[290]

Propofol is more expensive than thiopental, provides a vehicle for bacterial growth, has undergone less investigation in pregnant women (especially preterm parturients), is painful on administration, and may lead to a higher incidence of adverse maternal and neonatal effects. Thus, propofol does not offer a significant benefit over thiopental for the induction of general anesthesia for cesarean delivery.

Ketamine

The sympathomimetic properties of ketamine make it an ideal induction agent in the setting of an urgent cesarean delivery in a patient with hypotension or an acute exacerbation of asthma.[291] Ketamine is an analgesic, hypnotic, and amnestic agent associated with minimal respiratory depression; it is often used to supplement a neuraxial technique that may not be providing optimal anesthesia.[292] Ketamine's effect is likely related to antagonism of the *N*-methyl-D-aspartate (NMDA) receptor.

An induction dose of ketamine 1 mg/kg is associated with an increase in blood pressure immediately after induction, and a further increase is observed after laryngoscopy and intubation.[293] Such an increase can be desirable in the bleeding hypotensive patient but should be avoided in the parturient with hypertension (e.g., preeclampsia). However, in patients with severe hypovolemia, ketamine may cause direct myocardial depression, decreased cardiac output, and hypotension.[294]

Laboratory animal studies suggest that the use of ketamine is not associated with a reduction in uterine blood flow.[295-297] Ketamine is associated with dose-dependent increases in uterine tone, but a single induction dose does not increase uterine tone at term gestation.[298] Using an induction dose of ketamine 0.7 mg/kg, Craft et al.[296] observed a 39% increase in resting uterine tone with no effect on uterine blood flow in gravid ewes.

Ketamine rapidly crosses the placenta. No neonatal depression is observed with doses less than 1 mg/kg.[299,300] At higher doses, low Apgar scores, neonatal respiratory depression, and neonatal muscular hypertonicity have been reported.[301,302] Apgar scores and umbilical cord blood gas and pH measurements at delivery with ketamine are similar to those with thiopental.[284,303,304] A ketamine S+ isomer has been developed and approved for clinical use. In chronically instrumented pregnant sheep, Strumper et al.[295] found that the effects of the isomer were similar to those of the racemic mixture in terms of maternal and fetal hemodynamics and uterine perfusion; however, the isomer was associated with a smaller increase in maternal and fetal P_{CO_2} than that seen with racemic ketamine in spontaneously breathing animals.

The emergence delirium and hallucinations experienced with ketamine, particularly in the unpremedicated patient, have limited the adoption of this drug as a routine induction agent for cesarean delivery.[305] If ketamine is used, a benzodiazepine should be administered to decrease the incidence of these psychomimetic effects.[306] Maternal awareness may still occur following an induction dose of ketamine 1 to 1.5 mg/kg,[307] but the incidence is lower than with thiopental 4 mg/kg or a mixture of ketamine 0.5 mg/kg and thiopental 2 mg/kg.[304] The incidence of maternal awareness can also be diminished with the co-administration of a benzodiazepine.

When used to maintain general anesthesia with 50% nitrous oxide in oxygen for cesarean delivery, a continuous infusion of ketamine (70 μg/kg/minute) was followed by a higher incidence of factual recall and postoperative pain than seen with a volatile anesthetic technique.[308] Ngan Kee et al.[303] found that patients who received ketamine 1 mg/kg (prior to maintenance of anesthesia with nitrous oxide and isoflurane) alone for induction had lower postoperative consumption of morphine than patients who received thiopental 4 mg/kg for induction. Some investigators have suggested that lower doses of ketamine (0.5 to 0.7 mg/kg) combined with thiopental or propofol may be preferable to the administration of any one individual agent. There appears to be limited advantage to this approach with thiopental in terms of maternal recall, maternal hemodynamic status, and neonatal neurobehavioral scores.[309,310]

Etomidate

Etomidate is an intravenous induction agent that produces a rapid onset of anesthesia with minimal effects on cardiorespiratory function. This property makes it ideal for parturients who are hemodynamically unstable or who would not tolerate hemodynamic aberrations well (e.g., patients with severe cardiac disease).[311] With an induction dose of 0.2 to 0.3 mg/kg, etomidate undergoes rapid hydrolysis, thereby allowing rapid recovery.[312] Intravenous administration of etomidate may cause pain and involuntary muscle movements in unpremedicated patients; etomidate is also associated with nausea and vomiting, potential activation of seizures in patients with an epileptogenic foci, and an impaired glucocorticoid response to stress.[313]

Etomidate crosses the placenta rapidly; however, large variations in the UV/MV ratio (0.04 to 0.5) have been reported.[312,314] Downing et al.[315] observed that an induction dose of etomidate 0.3 mg/kg was associated with better neonatal acid-base measurements and overall clinical condition than with thiopental 3.5 mg/kg. A transient (less than 6 hours) reduction in neonatal cortisol production has been observed when an induction dose of etomidate is used for cesarean delivery[316,317]; however, the clinical relevance of this finding is unclear.

Midazolam

Midazolam is a short-acting, water-soluble benzodiazepine that has few adverse hemodynamic effects and provides hypnosis and amnesia. Although most commonly used as a premedicant prior to anesthesia, midazolam can be used as an induction agent for cesarean delivery. Crawford et al.[318,319] observed that induction with either midazolam 0.3 mg/kg or thiopental 4 mg/kg resulted in similar maternal hemodynamic responses and Apgar scores. By contrast, Bland et al.[320] reported that midazolam 0.2 mg/kg for induction of anesthesia resulted in a greater incidence of low Apgar scores and longer time to spontaneous respiration in the neonates than thiopental 3.5 mg/kg. Umbilical cord blood gas measurements did not differ between the two groups; however, the infants exposed to midazolam had lower neurobehavioral scores, body temperature, general body tone, and arm recoil. These differences did not persist at 4 hours after delivery. There are few indications for the use of midazolam for the induction of general anesthesia for cesarean delivery; it should be used only when there are relative or absolute contraindications to the use of other agents.

Muscle Relaxants

Muscle relaxants are commonly used before delivery to provide optimal intubation and operating conditions. Most muscle relaxants are highly ionized with low lipid solubility; thus they do not undergo significant placental transfer.

The depolarizing agent **succinylcholine** (1 to 1.5 mg/kg) is the muscle relaxant of choice for most parturients undergoing rapid-sequence induction for general anesthesia. Maternal administration provides adequate intubating conditions within approximately 45 seconds of intravenous administration. Succinylcholine is a highly ionized and water-soluble molecule, and only small amounts cross the placenta. Although high doses of succinylcholine (2 to 3 mg/kg) can result in detectable levels in umbilical cord blood, very large doses (10 mg/kg) are required to lead to placental transfer sufficient to cause neonatal muscle weakness.[321]

Succinylcholine is rapidly metabolized by plasma pseudocholinesterase, the concentration of which is decreased during pregnancy; however, in most patients this effect is offset by the pregnancy-induced increase in volume of distribution. Thus, recovery from succinylcholine is not prolonged, unless the patient has extremely low levels of pseudocholinesterase[322] or atypical pseudocholinesterase.[323] The administration of metoclopramide may also prolong succinylcholine-induced neuromuscular blockade, perhaps by inhibiting plasma pseudocholinesterase[324]; this effect is rarely (if ever) clinically significant. The return of neuromuscular function should be confirmed before additional doses of muscle relaxant are given.

Rocuronium is a suitable alternative to succinylcholine when a nondepolarizing agent is preferred for rapid-sequence induction (e.g., history of malignant hyperthermia). Abouleish et al.[325] observed that rocuronium (0.6 mg/kg) administered with an induction dose of thiopental (4 to 6 mg/kg) provided good to excellent intubating conditions in pregnant women in 79 seconds, and maximal intubating conditions in 98 seconds. Rocuronium did not adversely affect neonatal Apgar scores, acid-base measurements, time to sustained respiration, or neurobehavioral scores. Neuromuscular blockade was reversed satisfactorily at the end of cesarean delivery. Magorian et al.[326] demonstrated that rocuronium 1.2 mg/kg resulted in an onset of paralysis similar to that provided by succinylcholine (55 seconds), but it had a significantly longer clinical duration of action.

Vecuronium 0.1 mg/kg may be administered when the use of succinylcholine is contraindicated; however, its onset of action is significantly slower than that of rocuronium (144 seconds).[326] Hawkins et al.[327] evaluated the use of two methods of vecuronium administration for rapid-sequence induction of anesthesia for elective cesarean delivery. One group of women received vecuronium 0.01 mg/kg as a priming dose prior to administration of 0.1 mg/kg 4 to 6 minutes later; the other group received 0.2 mg/kg as a single bolus. The onset time for both groups (177 seconds and 175 seconds, respectively) was much longer than that for succinylcholine; moreover, the duration of blockade was prolonged (73 minutes in the priming group and 115 minutes in the bolus group). The same group performed a separate study in women undergoing postpartum tubal ligation; the duration of action of vecuronium (57 minutes) was significantly longer in these women than in nonpregnant controls (35 minutes).[328] Vecuronium crossed the placenta in small amounts; however, neonatal outcome, as assessed by Apgar scores and NACS, does not appear to be adversely affected.[329]

Atracurium is a less desirable agent for rapid-sequence induction because the high dose required for a rapid onset of action may result in significant histamine release, which may cause hypotension. The isomer **cisatracurium** does not have these undesirable side effects, but its relatively slow onset makes it less than optimal.[330]

Regardless of the choice of agent, laryngoscopy and intubation should not be attempted until adequate muscle relaxation has occurred. The use of a nerve stimulator allows an objective assessment of the onset and duration of the neuromuscular blockade. Residual neuromuscular blockade can be reversed with neostigmine and glycopyrrolate. To diminish the risk of aspiration, the anesthesia provider should confirm that the patient responds appropriately to verbal commands prior to extubation.

Nitrous Oxide

Nitrous oxide is an inhalational agent commonly used in the setting of a cesarean delivery because of its minimal effects on maternal blood pressure and uterine tone. The use of nitrous oxide allows for a reduction in the concentration of the volatile halogenated agent. (High concentrations of a volatile halogenated agent decrease uterine tone.) Administration of 50% nitrous oxide in oxygen *without* another anesthetic agent does not provide complete anesthesia and can result in maternal awareness in 12% to 26% of cases.[331,332]

Nitrous oxide is transferred rapidly across the placenta, where the fetal tissue uptake reduces the fetal arterial concentration for the first 20 minutes. Karasawa et al.[333] evaluated the relationship between duration of exposure to nitrous oxide 67% and the resulting umbilical vein–to–maternal artery (UV/MA) nitrous oxide concentration ratios; they observed different ratios according to duration of exposure: 2 to 9 minutes (0.37), 9 to 14 minutes (0.61), and 14 to 50 minutes (0.70). Apgar scores at 1 minute inversely correlated with duration of anesthesia, an effect observed in other studies.[334] The use of a lower concentration (e.g., 50%) of nitrous oxide may reduce but not eliminate these neonatal effects. Piggott et al.[262] randomly assigned parturients undergoing general anesthesia to receive either 100% oxygen or 50% nitrous oxide in oxygen, both supplemented by isoflurane (1.5 MAC for the first 5 minutes and 1.0 MAC thereafter). Neonates exposed to nitrous oxide required more resuscitation, although no significant differences were observed in Apgar scores.

Volatile Halogenated Agents

Volatile halogenated agents are perhaps the most commonly used agents for maintaining general anesthesia for cesarean delivery. Volatile halogenated agents produce central nervous system and cardiovascular effects in a dose-dependent manner; of particular concern for the obstetric patient are the resulting decreases in blood pressure (which may result in reduced uterine blood flow) and uterine tone. The uptake and delivery of a volatile halogenated agent is determined by inspired partial pressure, blood flow, and the blood/gas/tissue partition coefficient. The alveolar partial pressure of volatile agents during pregnancy follows known patterns of equilibration; the following commonly used agents are listed in order of more rapid to slower equilibration: nitrous oxide, desflurane, sevoflurane, and isoflurane. Volatile halogenated agents cross the placenta rapidly and equilibrate quickly with fetal tissues.[335] Some neonatal depression can occur. This is typically not a clinical issue when volatile anesthetic agents are used for emergency cesarean delivery, because the delivery usually occurs before much of the volatile agent crosses the placenta (particularly if uteroplacental insufficiency is the reason for emergency delivery). Also, the maternal hemodynamic response to laryngoscopy and intubation typically offsets any hypotension that might result from administration of a volatile halogenated agent before delivery.

Munson and Embro[336] evaluated three concentrations (0.5, 1.0, and 1.5 MAC) of isoflurane, enflurane, and halothane in an *in vitro* study of gravid and nongravid uterine myometrial strips; the amount of depression of uterine contractile activity was dose-related for each agent and was similar for the three agents. In a similar study, Dogru et al.[337] evaluated the effect of 0.5, 1.0, and 2.0 MAC of desflurane and sevoflurane on gravid uterine myometrial strips; a dose-dependent decrease in uterine contractions was observed. Importantly, the duration, amplitude, and frequency of oxytocin-induced uterine contractions were affected in a dose-dependent manner and were completely inhibited at 2 MAC.[337] The same group of investigators also reported that 1 MAC of desflurane inhibits the amplitude of oxytocin-induced myometrial contractions to a lesser extent than sevoflurane[338] and that pregnant myometrium is more sensitive than nonpregnant myometrium to the inhibitory effects of volatile halogenated agents.[339] These effects may influence maternal blood loss after delivery.[340]

Lower amounts of volatile halogenated agents are required during pregnancy. Gin et al.[341] demonstrated a 28% lower MAC for isoflurane in pregnant women at 8 to 12 weeks' gestation than in nonpregnant women. The same group of investigators found a 27% and 30% decrease in MAC of halothane and enflurane, respectively.[342] These findings were correlated with an increase in progesterone level. In an animal model, Datta et al.[343] demonstrated that long-term administration of progesterone was associated with a reduction in the MAC of halothane. Chan and Gin[344] observed that the reduction in MAC persists for 24 to 36 hours postpartum, with a gradual increase to normal values by 72 hours.

Local Anesthesia

As a method used primarily for supplementation of neuraxial anesthesia, the infiltration of local anesthesia can also be utilized to facilitate an emergency cesarean delivery. This latter technique has been well described and is used predominantly in developing countries, where contemporary anesthesia techniques may not be readily available. Few contemporary obstetricians are familiar or proficient with this technique in developed countries.

The success of local infiltration depends on the obstetrician's making a midline abdominal incision, avoiding use of retractors, and not exteriorizing the uterus. In settings in which an anesthesia provider might not be readily available, the obstetrician might begin surgery with the aid of local infiltration; following delivery of the infant, the achievement of temporary hemostasis, and the arrival of the anesthesia provider, surgery may be completed once general anesthesia has been induced.

Local infiltration is performed in sequential steps as the operation progresses (Box 26-9).[345] The use of 0.5% lidocaine with epinephrine is recommended; the use of a more concentrated solution is likely to result in systemic toxicity. A 25-gauge spinal needle is used to make the intracutaneous injection; the needle is inserted just below the umbilicus and is directed in the midline toward the symphysis pubis. Approximately 10 mL of local anesthetic is required to

BOX 26-9 Local Infiltration Anesthesia for Cesarean Delivery

1. Professional support person with patient
2. Infiltration with 0.5% lidocaine with epinephrine (total dose should not exceed 500 mg)
3. Intracutaneous injection in the midline from the umbilicus to the symphysis pubis
4. Subcutaneous injection
5. Incision down to the rectus fascia
6. Rectus fascia blockade
7. Parietal peritoneum infiltration and incision
8. Visceral peritoneum infiltration and incision
9. Paracervical injection
10. Uterine incision and delivery
11. Administration of general endotracheal anesthesia for uterine repair and abdominal closure, if needed

create a skin wheal that extends from the symphysis pubis to the umbilicus. The subcutaneous injection is also performed for the full length of the planned incision with approximately 10 to 20 mL of local anesthetic. Ideally, the obstetrician should then wait for 3 to 4 minutes to allow the local anesthetic agent to exert its effect before making the skin incision.

A vertical skin incision is made between the umbilicus and the symphysis pubis and is extended down to the rectus fascia. The obstetrician then infiltrates local anesthetic into the rectus fascia and rectus muscles by making three to five laterally directed injections on each side. The needle should be passed between the rectus sheath at an angle of 10 to 15 degrees and a depth of 3 to 5 cm; aspiration is performed, and 2 to 3 mL of local anesthetic is injected at each site with an additional 1 mL injected with needle withdrawal. The obstetrician should also make oblique injections at the upper and lower poles of the incision. The local anesthetic will spread freely in the rectus sheath, but it takes 4 to 5 minutes for anesthesia to be complete. The suprapubic area must also be generously infiltrated to ensure blockade of the branches of the iliohypogastric nerve. The disadvantage of the rectus sheath block is the large volume (40 to 50 mL) of local anesthetic required; a less effective alternative that requires less volume and time is to raise a longitudinal paramedian wheal in the rectus fascia on each side of the midline and to infiltrate the suprapubic region.

The obstetrician then extends the incision through the rectus sheath, and the peritoneum is grasped with forceps clamps. If the patient has pain, the parietal peritoneum may be infiltrated with 5 to 10 mL of local anesthetic and then incised. The visceral peritoneum overlying the area of the uterine incision is injected with 10 mL of local anesthetic, and is then incised and reflected appropriately. Paracervical infiltration with 5 to 10 mL of local anesthetic may block pain impulses from the uterus and cervix.

A uterine incision is made, and the infant is delivered. The surgeon must avoid forceful retraction and blunt dissection of tissue planes, and uterine manipulation should be kept to a minimum. A support person at the head of the table who can provide coaching and reassurance to the mother is invaluable.

The major disadvantages of local infiltration anesthesia are patient discomfort and the potential for systemic local anesthetic toxicity, given that as much as 100 mL of local anesthetic solution is required. The latter disadvantage may be especially problematic in the absence of a skilled anesthesia provider to assist with maternal resuscitation. Another disadvantage is the amount of time required for maximal anesthesia to develop; maternal discomfort often accompanies an urgent delivery performed with this form of anesthesia. Finally, local infiltration does not provide satisfactory operating conditions in the event of a surgical complication (e.g., uterine laceration, broad ligament hematoma).

Cesarean delivery with use of local infiltration, if successful, has the advantages of preserving maternal cardiovascular stability and a patent airway while allowing the initiation of surgery in emergency cases. However, the technique is frequently associated with incomplete maternal anesthesia, which subsequently presents significant management issues, because the surgical procedure has commenced, positioning options are limited, and the consequences of the operative procedure (e.g., hemorrhage) may require immediate attention.

RECOVERY FROM ANESTHESIA

Cesarean delivery represents a major abdominal surgical procedure with significant anatomic, physiologic, and hormonal sequelae, even when it is performed electively without complications in a healthy parturient. The risk of adverse outcomes is greater in the presence of significant maternal comorbidity or in the setting of surgical complications (e.g., massive blood loss, cesarean hysterectomy).[346]

Cohen et al.[347] evaluated revised PACU discharge criteria in their tertiary care center for patients who received neuraxial anesthesia for cesarean delivery. They suggested that the majority of patients undergoing cesarean delivery could meet revised discharge criteria (i.e., presence of a normal level of consciousness, stable vital signs, adequate analgesia, and ability to flex the knees) within 60 minutes, a period that would shorten the average duration of PACU stay and result in cost savings. However, 26% to 36% of patients remained in the PACU for up to 180 minutes because of pain, sedation, nausea and vomiting, pruritus, prolonged neuroblockade, and/or drug treatment. In addition, 16% to 22% remained in the PACU for up to 210 minutes for cardiovascular (e.g., bleeding, hypertension, hypotension, tachycardia) or respiratory events. Moreover, the study did not include the most seriously ill or highest-risk patients, who were transferred directly to an ICU.

The National Sentinel Caesarean Section Audit in the United Kingdom reported that 10% of women undergoing cesarean delivery required admission to a high-dependency unit.[348] Moreover, 3.5% of these women required subsequent transfer to an ICU. Preexisting comorbid conditions accounted for the majority (80%) of these ICU admissions; a smaller fraction were due to the medical emergency (e.g., uterine rupture, placental abruption) that prompted the cesarean delivery.[348] Although ICU admission is uncommon in obstetric patients, it occurs more frequently (approximately 9 per 1000 patients) after cesarean delivery.[348]

Of concern, inadequate postoperative care has been cited as a recurring factor in maternal deaths (see Chapter 39). The ASA Practice Guidelines for Obstetric Anesthesia state that "appropriate equipment and personnel should be available to care for obstetric patients recovering from major neuraxial or general anesthesia."[43] Similarly, the National Obstetric Anaesthetic Service Guidelines from the United Kingdom state that postoperative care of the patient undergoing cesarean delivery should meet the same standard of care as required for any postoperative patient.[349] More specifically, these guidelines state:

> *After caesarean (delivery), women should be observed on a one-to-one basis by a properly trained member of staff until they have regained airway control and cardiorespiratory stability and are able to communicate. After recovery from anaesthesia, observations (respiratory rate, heart rate, blood pressure, pain and sedation) should be continued every half hour for two hours and hourly thereafter provided that the observations are stable or satisfactory. If these observations are not stable, more frequent observations and medical review are recommended.*[349]

Oral Intake

Mangesi and Hofmeyr[350] performed a systematic review of six randomized clinical trials comparing early with delayed oral intake of fluids and foods after cesarean delivery; they found that the early consumption (within 4 to 8 hours) was associated with a shorter time to return of bowel sounds and a shorter hospital stay. No differences were reported in nausea and vomiting, abdominal distention, time to bowel activity, paralytic ileus, or need for analgesia. The NICE guidelines state that "women who are recovering well and who do not have complications . . . can eat and drink when they feel hungry or thirsty."[54]

Removal of Urinary Catheter

There are no differences in the incidence of urinary retention after general anesthesia and epidural anesthesia following cesarean delivery.[351] Risk factors for postpartum urinary retention after cesarean delivery include the use of postoperative opioid analgesia (particularly when given via an epidural catheter), multiple gestation, and a low body mass index.[352] Most urinary catheters are removed either immediately following cesarean delivery or within 24 hours; there are no differences between these two options in regard to postoperative urinary retention, dysuria, urgency, fever, positive microscopy, or length of hospital stay.[353]

Postoperative Assessment and Discharge

The anesthesia provider should assess for recovery of motor and sensory function if a neuraxial technique was administered. Women should be reassured that breast-feeding is safe, even after general anesthesia, and that postoperative analgesics have a favorable safety profile. Early mobility and ambulation should be encouraged.

ANESTHETIC COMPLICATIONS

Awareness and Recall

The following factors contribute to the risk of maternal awareness during general anesthesia for cesarean delivery: (1) the avoidance of sedative premedications, (2) the deliberate use of a low concentration of a volatile halogenated agent, (3) the use of muscle relaxants, (4) the reduction in dose of anesthetic agents during hypotension or hemorrhage, (5) the presence of a partial neuraxial blockade in parturients requiring conversion to general anesthesia, and (6) the (mistaken) assumption that high baseline sympathetic tone is responsible for intraoperative tachycardia in parturients.

Concern about neonatal depression and uterine atony associated with volatile halogenated agents has led to administration of relatively low doses of these agents. Administration of a barbiturate induction agent followed by nitrous oxide 50% in oxygen resulted in maternal awareness in 12% to 26% of cases.[331,332] Using an isolated forearm technique, King et al.[354] assessed 30 women undergoing cesarean delivery with thiopental 250 mg, succinylcholine infusion, and 0.5% halothane in 50% nitrous oxide; the majority of patients signaled pain in the first minute. The incidence of recall with this anesthetic regimen was approximately 1%.[355] The use of higher concentrations of a volatile halogenated agent has subsequently become a more common practice, leading to a lower incidence of maternal awareness.[356] However, the result of increasing the depth of maternal anesthesia is that neonates born to women who receive general anesthesia tend to have lower Apgar and neurobehavioral scores, particularly when the I-D interval exceeds 8 minutes.[357]

The optimal doses and concentrations of anesthetic agents to prevent awareness remain unclear, in part because of the difficulty in assessing awareness. Studies have evaluated several tools for assessment of depth of maternal anesthesia, including the electroencephalogram,[304] brainstem auditory evoked potentials, and the bispectral index.[71,358-360] Unfortunately these options are often not suitable for the emergency conditions under which most general anesthetics for cesarean delivery are administered. The bispectral index is an empirically derived electroencephalographic parameter that measures the hypnotic component of anesthesia; values below 60 are thought to be associated with a low probability of intraoperative recall and awareness.[361] However, there are insufficient data validating this threshold in pregnant women.

Yeo et al.[359] evaluated 20 women undergoing cesarean delivery and noted that an end-tidal concentration of 1% sevoflurane (approximately 0.5 MAC) with 50% nitrous oxide resulted in a range of bispectral index values between 52 and 70; no patient experienced intraoperative dreams, recall, or awareness. Using a similar regimen, Yoo et al.[358] demonstrated that bispectral index values were lower during general anesthesia in women who were in labor prior to cesarean delivery than in nonlaboring women; the nonlaboring group did not reliably have values less than 60, and the mean value at tracheal intubation was 64 ± 10. Ittichaikulthol et al.[360] found that mean bispectral index values in women undergoing cesarean delivery with 3% and 4.5% desflurane in 50% nitrous oxide were 62 ± 8 and 49 ± 12, respectively.

Although pregnancy diminishes anesthetic requirements by 25% to 40%,[266] administration of 0.5 MAC of a volatile halogenated agent may not reliably provide adequate depth of anesthesia to consistently prevent maternal awareness. Lyons and Macdonald[356] have recommended larger induction doses of barbiturate (e.g., thiopental 5 to 7 mg/kg instead of 3 to 4 mg/kg), isoflurane 1% prior to delivery, and the administration of an opioid and isoflurane 0.5% after the delivery. Intravenous techniques that may reduce the risk of maternal awareness include the administration of repeat doses of thiopental,[362] the use of ketamine,[307] or a combination of the two agents.[309,310] Midazolam 0.075 mg/kg provides 30 to 60 minutes of anterograde amnesia when given to women undergoing elective cesarean delivery under epidural anesthesia.[363] Infusion of propofol 8 mg/kg/hr with 67% nitrous oxide has also been used with satisfactory amnestic effect.[71]

Further investigation into the anesthetic regimens and monitoring necessary to prevent awareness and recall in women undergoing cesarean delivery is needed. These studies should incorporate the growing data on gender- and pregnancy-related differences in pharmacokinetics and pharmacodynamics[364,365] and should be adequately powered to assess the incidence of recall. The psychological morbidity associated with awareness should not be underestimated.

Paradoxically, the issue of recall is not limited to the administration of general anesthesia. In women undergoing cesarean delivery with a neuraxial technique who desire treatment for anxiety, the administration of anxiolytic or hypnotic agents may result in a lack of recall of delivery, which is typically undesirable.

Dyspnea

Following the administration of a neuraxial technique, the patient may complain of dyspnea. The most common cause of this complaint is hypotension (causing hypoperfusion of the brainstem); therefore the complaint of difficulty in breathing should prompt immediate assessment of blood pressure and treatment, if appropriate. Other causes of dyspnea are the blunting of thoracic proprioception, the partial blockade of abdominal and intercostal muscles, and the recumbent position, which increases the pressure of the abdominal contents against the diaphragm. Despite these changes, significant respiratory compromise is unlikely, because the neuraxial blockade rarely affects the cervical nerves that control the diaphragm.

If the patient loses the ability to vocalize, give a strong hand grip, and/or maintain normal oxyhemoglobin saturation (e.g., symptoms suggestive of high spinal anesthesia), a rapid-sequence induction with cricoid pressure and placement of an endotracheal tube can be performed to maintain ventilation and prevent pulmonary soiling with gastrointestinal contents.

Hypotension

Hypotension is a common sequela of neuraxial anesthetic techniques and, when severe and sustained, can lead to impairment of uteroplacental perfusion, resulting in fetal hypoxia, acidosis, and neonatal depression or injury.[366] Severe maternal hypotension can also have adverse maternal outcomes, including unconsciousness, pulmonary aspiration, apnea, and cardiac arrest.

The definition of maternal hypotension is controversial; however, many investigators accept the following definition: (1) a decrease in systolic blood pressure of more than 20% to 30% from baseline measurements or (2) a systolic blood pressure lower than 100 mm Hg.[367] Neuraxial anesthetic techniques produce hypotension through blockade of sympathetic nerve fibers, which control vascular smooth muscle tone. Preganglionic sympathetic fiber blockade primarily causes an increase in venous capacitance, which shifts a major portion of blood volume into the splanchnic bed and the lower extremities, thereby reducing venous return to the heart; it also decreases the resistance in arterial pre- and postcapillary resistance vessels. The rate and extent of the sympathetic involvement, and subsequently the severity of hypotension, are determined by the onset and spread of the neuraxial blockade[368]; therefore, hypotension may be less common with epidural anesthesia than with spinal anesthesia because of the slower onset of neuroblockade. The delayed onset of hypotension with epidural anesthesia may also allow earlier treatment before hypotension becomes severe.

RISK FACTORS FOR HYPOTENSION

A number of studies have attempted to identify pregnant women at increased risk for development of hypotension. Of interest, women with severe preeclampsia[369] or in established labor appear less likely to experience hypotension during administration of spinal anesthesia for cesarean delivery.

Using a modified orthostatic challenge (i.e., "tilt test"), Kinsella and Norris[370] were unable to establish a correlation in the observed change in blood pressure or heart rate with hypotension after spinal anesthesia. Similarly, Frolich and Caton[371] could not establish a correlation between orthostatic blood pressure and heart rate changes and the hypotension that developed after spinal anesthesia; however, the investigators found that patients with a baseline heart rate higher than 90 beats/min had a 83% chance (positive predictive value) of experiencing marked hypotension (decrease in blood pressure greater than 30%), whereas patients with a baseline heart rate lower than 90 beats/min had a 75% chance (negative predictive value) of *not* experiencing marked hypotension.

Dahlgren et al.[372] hypothesized that the response of pregnant women to a preoperative *supine stress test* would predict the occurrence of maternal symptoms, a need for ephedrine, or a decrease in blood pressure below 80 mm Hg during administration of spinal anesthesia for cesarean delivery. The supine stress test was considered positive if it was associated with (1) an increase in maternal heart rate greater than 10 beats/min, (2) a decrease in systolic blood pressure of more than 15 mm Hg, or (3) signs and symptoms related to the supine position (e.g., nausea, dizziness). These investigators found that the preoperative stress test had a sensitivity of 69% and a specificity of 92% in identifying those who would have hypotension.

Investigators have used other methods, including assessment of heart rate variability[373-375] and noninvasive measurements of systemic vascular resistance (e.g., thoracic impedance[376]) in an attempt to identify parturients at risk for hypotension during administration of neuraxial anesthesia for cesarean delivery, but these methods require further refinement before being introduced into clinical practice. A new minimally invasive technique for hemodynamic monitoring, LiDCO plus (LiDCO, London), uses two proprietary algorithms—a continuous arterial waveform analysis system, PulseCO, coupled to a single-point lithium indicator dilution calibration system, LiDCO—to determine cardiac output. This device may shift the focus from blood pressure to cardiac output as a key hemodynamic variable before and during administration of neuraxial anesthesia for cesarean delivery. Published experience with this device in pregnant women is limited; one group has evaluated women with severe preeclampsia undergoing spinal anesthesia for cesarean delivery.[377,378]

To date, predicting which parturients will have hypotension following neuraxial anesthesia for cesarean delivery has not proven feasible clinically; the reason may be the myriad of factors that control the physiologic and hormonal changes and hemodynamic responses that occur during pregnancy.

PREVENTION OF HYPOTENSION

A number of strategies have been used, with variable success, in an attempt to prevent hypotension following spinal anesthesia for cesarean delivery, including left uterine displacement, prehydration to expand blood volume, vasopressor administration, and leg elevation or wrapping. In a systematic review of 75 randomized controlled trials (which involved a total of 4624 women and 49 comparisons of different methods of prophylaxis), Cyna et al.[367] concluded that the following interventions reduced the incidence of hypotension: (1) preload with crystalloid 20 mL/kg versus control, (2) preload with colloid versus crystalloid, (3) prophylaxis with ephedrine versus control, and (4) lower limb compression devices versus control. The investigators also concluded that colloids were more effective than crystalloids, which in turn were more effective than no fluids; no differences were detected for different doses, rates, or methods of administering colloids or crystalloids. Ueyama et al.[379] demonstrated that the administration of 1.5 L of lactated Ringer's solution, 0.5 L of hydroxyethyl starch solution (HES) 6%, or 1 L of HES 6% prior to spinal anesthesia for cesarean delivery was associated with an incidence of hypotension (systolic blood pressure less than 100 mm Hg and less than 80% of baseline) of 75%, 58%, and 17%, respectively. Moreover, only 28% of lactated Ringer's solution and 100% of HES remained in the intravascular space at 30 minutes; this finding underscores the importance of the timing of preanesthesia fluid administration and resulting effects on cardiac output (Figure 26-7). Of interest, the rapid administration of 1500 to 2000 mL of fluid can cause a release of atrial natriuretic peptide, which can cause vasodilation and can reduce sensitivity to vasoconstrictors.[380]

Ephedrine, phenylephrine, and dopamine are more effective than placebo or crystalloid in preventing hypotension; by contrast, no differences have been observed between the use of angiotensin or glycopyrrolate and that of placebo. A meta-analysis concluded that ephedrine was superior to placebo in the prevention of hypotension for women receiving spinal anesthesia for cesarean delivery.[381] However, a 32% to 55% incidence of hypotension still occurred in the ephedrine group. Ephedrine doses higher than 10 mg may provide more effective prophylaxis, but reactive hypertension and fetal metabolic acidosis can occur with higher doses.

Ngan Kee et al.[382] reduced the incidence of spinal anesthesia–associated hypotension to almost zero (1.9%)

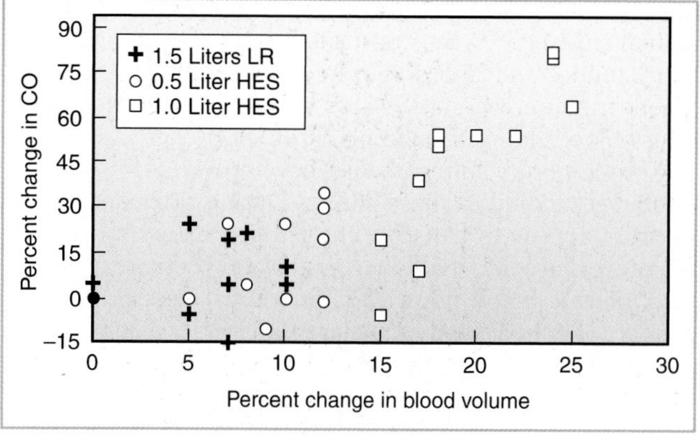

FIGURE 26-7 The relationship between the changes (%) in blood volume and cardiac output after volume preload in parturients undergoing spinal anesthesia. Cardiac output (CO) estimated with indocyanine green pulse spectrophotometry methodology. HES, hydroxyethyl starch solution; LR, lactated Ringer's solution. (Adapted from Ueyama H, He Y, Tanigami H, et al. Effects of crystalloid and colloid preload on blood volume in the parturient undergoing spinal anesthesia for elective cesarean section. Anesthesiology 1999; 91:1571-6.)

by combining a rapid crystalloid co-load (initiated at the time of intrathecal injection) with a prophylactic phenylephrine infusion (beginning at 100 µg/min); the incidence of hypotension was 28% in the women who received phenylephrine without the co-load. No difference in neonatal outcome was observed.

Physical methods to prevent hypotension include the use of lower limb compression bandages or inflatable boots. Moreover, pneumatic compression devices help prevent thromboembolic complications.

In their meta-analysis, Cyna et al.[367] did not confirm that the use of left uterine displacement reduces the occurrence of maternal hypotension during cesarean delivery. In part, their conclusion stems from the inclusion in their study of two randomized controlled trials that found the lateral position did not reduce the incidence of hypotension during administration of spinal anesthesia for *emergency* cesarean delivery. This situation most likely reflects the variable occurrence of supine hypotensive syndrome, which does not uniformly occur in all pregnant women. On the other hand, adequate left uterine displacement improves umbilical arterial blood pH measurements and neonatal outcomes, highlighting the fact that maternal blood pressure, measured at the level of the brachial artery, may not always predict uteroplacental perfusion. It is not known *a priori* who will experience hypotension; more important, diminished uterine blood flow may occur in the presence or absence of maternal hypotension. Thus the use of left uterine displacement is mandatory during anesthesia for cesarean delivery.

TREATMENT OF HYPOTENSION

The ideal treatment for hypotension would be reliable, titratable, easy to use, and devoid of maternal and fetal side effects. More than 30 years ago, ephedrine, a mixed alpha- and beta-adrenergic receptor agonist, emerged as the leading choice for the treatment of hypotension on the basis of studies demonstrating its efficacy and apparent superiority (over other agents) in protecting and/or restoring uterine blood flow in gravid ewes and other pregnant animal models.[383] By contrast, other agents, including metaraminol and phenylephrine, while restoring maternal blood pressure, were associated with a decrease in uterine artery blood flow and fetal pH.[383]

Contemporary animal studies have provided a mechanistic understanding of these effects. During pregnancy vasopressors appear to constrict the femoral artery more than the uterine artery, which increases blood pressure and protects uterine blood flow. This differential pressor effect is greater for ephedrine than metaraminol.[384] A second mechanism appears to be the upregulation of nitric oxide synthase (NOS) in the uterine artery during pregnancy.[385] The presence of NOS potentially makes this artery less sensitive to vasopressors; this effect may be further augmented by ephedrine, a drug noted to independently cause the release of NOS.

In a quantitative systematic review, Lee et al.[386] noted that the use of ephedrine for treatment of maternal hypotension during administration of spinal anesthesia for cesarean delivery was associated with lower umbilical cord blood pH measurements than the use of phenylephrine. These somewhat surprising clinical results (which differ from results in animal studies) may reflect interspecies differences in vascular smooth muscle physiology, control of blood flow, and drug metabolism. Also, these results may reflect the fetal effect of ephedrine given to the mother. Cooper et al.[387] developed a measurement index by subtracting the umbilical artery P_{CO_2} from the umbilical vein P_{CO_2} to determine the amount of CO_2 generated by the fetus; the index correlated with the use of ephedrine, suggesting that the fetal metabolic production of CO_2 was enhanced in the group whose mothers received ephedrine.

Administration of ephedrine may lead to tachyphylaxis. Also, the tachycardia caused by ephedrine's beta-adrenergic activity may be distressing to the patient. On the other hand, when administered as a sole agent, phenylephrine may cause maternal bradycardia.

The combined prophylactic intravenous infusion of ephedrine and phenylephrine has been demonstrated to result in better maternal hemodynamics and neonatal acid-base status than with administration of ephedrine alone.[388] The use of an infusion pump and the need for frequent adjustments in pump settings can be cumbersome, especially in comparison with the more commonly used bolus administration of vasopressors. The efficacy of a bolus administration of *both* vasopressors in preventing and treating hypotension associated with spinal anesthesia has been evaluated[389]; however, a dose combination that reliably prevents hypotension has not yet been identified. Methods under investigation include a closed-loop feedback computer-controlled infusion of phenylephrine for maintaining blood pressure during spinal anesthesia.[390]

The utilization of phenylephrine as a sole agent or as an adjuvant to ephedrine appears to have clinical value. The NICE guidelines state that phenylephrine and ephedrine are equally effective as vasopressors.[54] Given the efficacy of phenylephrine in the treatment of hypotension and the better umbilical cord blood acid-base measurements associated with its use in clinical studies, many anesthesia providers now use phenylephrine as a first-line agent for the prevention and treatment of maternal hypotension.[391] Regardless of the vasopressor agent selected to treat hypotension, therapy should be administered as soon as the blood pressure begins to fall, rather than after the occurrence of clinically significant hypotension.[392] Ephedrine is usually administered intravenously in bolus doses of 5 to 10 mg. Phenylephrine may be administered intravenously in bolus doses of 50 to 100 µg, or by continuous infusion beginning at 100 µg/min.[393]

Failure of Neuraxial Blockade

A "failed" neuraxial block can be defined as neuroblockade insufficient in extent, density, or duration to provide anesthesia for cesarean delivery. Approximately 4% to 13% of epidural anesthetics and 0.5% to 4% of spinal anesthetics fail to provide sufficient anesthesia for the initiation or completion of cesarean delivery.[162,394] Epidural techniques are more often associated with failure, given the fact that the catheter is often placed during early labor, and over time the catheter may migrate out of the epidural space. Factors that may correlate with failed extension of labor epidural anesthesia for cesarean delivery include a higher number of bolus doses for the provision of labor analgesia, patient characteristics (e.g., obesity, distance from the skin to the epidural space), and the time elapsed between placement of the catheter and cesarean delivery.

The causes of failure of neuraxial techniques include anatomic, technical, and obstetric factors. Steps to reduce the likelihood of epidural block failure include meticulous attention to technical detail, the administration of a solution that contains both a local anesthetic and an opioid, and a better understanding of the characteristics of epidural versus spinal blockade. Moreover, the patient should be prepared to expect the sensation of deep pressure and movement, yet be reassured that reports of discomfort or pain will be addressed promptly. Initiation of surgery should be delayed until adequate thoracic and sacral sensory blockade has been achieved; on rare occasions, in the setting of an urgent procedure for which a developing epidural block is present at T10 but has yet to achieve a T4 level, surgery can commence with the understanding that adjuvant treatments or alternative forms of anesthesia may be required.

Evaluation of intraoperative pain requires (1) determination of the location and extent of discomfort, (2) evaluation of the level of anesthesia, (3) assessment of the current status of the surgery (e.g., incision, delivery, uterine repair, skin closure), and (4) assessment of the presence of confounding factors (e.g., hemorrhage, anxiety). Shoulder pain can originate from irritation of the diaphragm and is mediated by the phrenic nerve (C3 to C5); prolonged abduction and extension of the arms can also cause discomfort. Additional discomfort can occur from visceral stimulation such as uterine manipulation, which often involves the greater splanchnic nerve (T5 to T10). Inadequate anesthesia can result from regression of the block from a cephalad or caudad direction.

Management should commence with acknowledgement of the discomfort. If no block exists and time allows, neuraxial anesthesia can be repeated; however, emergency situations may require administration of general anesthesia. If an inadequate, partial block exists in an elective situation, either the surgery can be postponed (to allow resolution of the partial block), or a second neuraxial technique may be performed *with caution*. The performance of a spinal technique in the setting of a partial but failed epidural or spinal anesthetic technique is controversial. In this setting, intrathecal administration of a standard intrathecal dose of bupivacaine may result in a high spinal block. Moreover, radiographic evidence suggests that the dural sac is compressed by prior epidural drug administration.[395] Thus, when performing a spinal anesthetic technique after failed epidural or spinal anesthesia, the anesthesia provider should consider (1) reducing the dose of bupivacaine (with the chosen dose depending on the extent of existing neuroblockade); (2) placing the patient in a semisitting (Fowler's) position to limit cephalad spread of the local anesthetic; (3) using a CSE technique with a small intrathecal dose of local anesthetic, and if necessary, titrating the sensory level with additional drugs administered through the epidural catheter; and (4) intentionally placing an epidural catheter into the intrathecal space for administration of continuous spinal anesthesia. This last strategy may be especially useful in obese patients, in whom the technical difficulty of the neuraxial approach may otherwise limit success.

If discomfort is reported after the start of surgery, it is often helpful to ask the surgeons to halt the operation while an assessment is made. If an epidural catheter is in place, an alkalinized local anesthetic with an opioid (e.g., 3% 2-chloroprocaine with fentanyl) should be administered. The density of epidural anesthesia may be improved by "repainting the fence." An additional dose of local anesthetic (20% to 30% of the initial dose [e.g., 4 to 7 mL]) is administered approximately 20 minutes after the initial dose. This second dose serves to improve the density of neuroblockade without extending the sensory level. Some anesthesia providers routinely administer this supplemental dose, without waiting for a patient's complaint of breakthrough pain.

Intravenous administration of an opioid (fentanyl), inhalation of nitrous oxide (40% to 50% in oxygen), or intravenous anxiolysis (midazolam) may be helpful for the treatment of breakthrough pain. Severe pain may require intravenous ketamine in 5- to 10-mg increments, with the understanding that significant sedation, loss of consciousness, and psychomimetic and amnestic effects may occur. The obstetrician can infiltrate the wound or instill the peritoneal cavity with local anesthetic; however, at this point, the induction of general anesthesia with endotracheal intubation is often necessary.

If the anesthesia provider anticipates that the duration of the surgical procedure will be longer than the predicted duration of epidural or CSE anesthesia, additional local anesthetic (with or without an opioid) should be administered *before* anticipated regression of neuroblockade (see Table 26-6). The usual dose to maintain neuroblockade is half of the initial dose.

High Neuraxial Blockade

It is not uncommon for the parturient to report mild dyspnea or reduced ability to cough, especially if the neuraxial blockade has achieved a T2 level. If impaired phonation, unconsciousness, respiratory depression, or significant impairment of ventilation occurs, administration of general anesthesia should be performed. High neuraxial blockade may also result in cardiovascular sequelae, including bradycardia and hypotension.

High neuraxial block can be caused by several mechanisms, including an exaggerated spread of spinal or epidural drugs and unintentional intrathecal or subdural administration of an "epidural dose" of local anesthetic.

Nausea and Vomiting

Nausea and vomiting are regulated by the chemoreceptor trigger zone and the vomiting center, which are located in the area postrema and the medullary lateral reticular formation, respectively. The vomiting center receives impulses from the vagal sensory fibers in the gastrointestinal tract, the semicircular canals and ampullae (labyrinth) of the inner ear, higher cortical centers, the chemoreceptor trigger zone, and intracranial pressure receptors. Impulses from these structures are influenced by dopaminergic, muscarinic, tryptaminergic, histaminic, and opioid receptors, which are subsequently the targets for antiemetic agents. Efferent impulses from the vomiting center are transmitted through the vagus, phrenic, and spinal nerves to the abdominal muscles, which causes the physical act of vomiting.

PREOPERATIVE NAUSEA AND VOMITING

Nausea and vomiting may occur separately or in combination and are not uncommon during pregnancy. Rapidly increasing blood levels of chorionic gonadotropin, estrogens, or both appear to have a relationship with hyperemesis during pregnancy.[396] When vomiting is sufficiently severe to produce weight loss, dehydration, acidosis from starvation, alkalosis from loss of hydrochloric acid in vomitus, and hypokalemia, it is referred to as *hyperemesis gravidarum*. This disorder most commonly occurs in early pregnancy, but as many as 10% of pregnant women have nausea and vomiting that persist beyond 22 weeks' gestation.[397] Severe and persistent hyperemesis may result in maternal morbidity.[398]

The presence of delayed gastric emptying during labor and administration of opioids are risk factors for nausea and vomiting before cesarean delivery.

INTRAOPERATIVE NAUSEA AND VOMITING

Intraoperative nausea and vomiting associated with cesarean delivery can be variable in incidence and presentation, depending on preexisting symptoms, on anesthetic and obstetric techniques, and on preventive and therapeutic measures taken.[399] The incidence of nausea may be as high as 80%, particularly when the anesthesia provider specifically assesses for the presence of intraoperative symptoms; symptoms occur more often with exteriorization of the uterus.[6] Anesthetic causes of intraoperative nausea and vomiting include hypotension and increased vagal activity; nonanesthetic causes include surgical stimuli, bleeding, medications (e.g., uterotonic agents, antibiotics), and motion at the end of surgery.[399] Many of these elements occur simultaneously.

Hypotension is among the most common sequelae associated with the administration of neuraxial anesthesia. Centrally, hypotension may lead to cerebral and brainstem hypoperfusion, which results in stimulation of the medullary vomiting center. Peripherally, hypotension may cause gut ischemia with release of emetogenic substances (e.g., serotonin) from the intestine.[400] Strict maintenance of intraoperative blood pressure can reduce the occurrence of emesis; Datta et al.[392] observed that the incidence of intraoperative nausea and vomiting was 66% when the blood pressure decreased more than 30% from baseline, but was less than 10% when blood pressure was maintained at baseline with ephedrine. Similarly, Ngan Kee et al.[393] demonstrated progressive increases in intraoperative nausea and vomiting when blood pressure control with an infusion of phenylephrine was less aggressive; the incidence of nausea and vomiting was 4% when blood pressure was maintained at 100% of baseline, 16% when maintained at 90% of baseline, and 40% when maintained at 80% of baseline during spinal anesthesia for cesarean delivery.

Uterotonic agents may also contribute to intraoperative nausea and vomiting. Ergot alkaloids may cause nausea and vomiting by interacting with dopaminergic and serotoninergic receptors. Oxytocin causes nausea and vomiting primarily as a result of the hypotension produced through release of nitric oxide and atrial natriuretic peptide.[401] A 29% incidence of nausea and a 9% incidence of vomiting have been reported with an intravenous bolus of oxytocin 5 U during elective cesarean delivery with neuraxial anesthesia.[402] Administration of 15-methyl prostaglandin $F_{2\alpha}$ (Hemabate) causes nausea through the stimulation of smooth muscles of the gastrointestinal tract; a 10% incidence of nausea and vomiting has been observed after administration of 250 μg intramuscularly.[399]

Surgical stimuli, including exteriorization of the uterus, intra-abdominal manipulation, and peritoneal traction, can cause visceral pain and subsequent nausea through the stimulation of vagal fibers and activation of the vomiting center; despite high levels of thoracic sensory block obtained for cesarean delivery anesthesia, visceral pain may still occur, particularly after the neuraxial administration of a local anesthetic alone.[403] The administration of neuraxial opioids reduces visceral pain–induced nausea and vomiting.[183] Neuraxial fentanyl both improves the quality of neuraxial anesthesia and decreases intraoperative nausea; the minimal effective doses are 6.25 μg given intrathecally and 50 μg given epidurally, respectively.

POSTOPERATIVE NAUSEA AND VOMITING

Risk factors for postoperative nausea and vomiting have not been specifically studied in obstetric patients; however, studies have identified risk factors in nonobstetric patients receiving general or neuraxial anesthesia (Box 26-10).[404,405] Apfel et al.[405] identified the following four highly predictive factors for postoperative nausea and vomiting in nonobstetric patients after general anesthesia, which may have relevance in the pregnant population: (1) female gender, (2) history of motion sickness or postoperative nausea and vomiting, (3) nonsmoking status, and (4) the use of perioperative opioids. If none, one, two, three, or four of these risk factors were present, the incidence of postoperative nausea and vomiting was 10% for the presence of no risk factors, 21% for one, 39% for two, 61% for three, and 79% for four. A subset of pregnant women may have a lower threshold for nausea and vomiting associated with motion.[406] Changes in position and transfer to and on the stretcher may stimulate afferent neural pathways that trigger emesis. Because histamine H_1 and muscarinic cholinergic pathways play a primary role in this response, antihistamine and anticholinergic agents should play a first-line role in treatment.[406] Postoperative nausea and vomiting may be related to postoperative ileus, which in turn is influenced by the effect of opioids on the gastrointestinal tract, the activation of the sympathetic nervous system, the occurrence of intestinal wall inflammation, and the presence of volume overload or edema.[407]

BOX 26-10 Risk Factors for Nausea and Vomiting

General Anesthesia–Related Factors
- Female gender
- History of motion sickness or postoperative nausea and vomiting
- Nonsmoking status
- Use of perioperative opioids

Spinal Anesthesia–Related Factors
- Block height of T5 or higher
- History of motion sickness
- Hypotension
- Omission of neuraxial opioids

Information from Gan TJ. Risk factors for postoperative nausea and vomiting. Anesth Analg 2006; 102:1884-98; and Apfel CC, Laara E, Koivuranta M, et al. A simplified risk score for predicting postoperative nausea and vomiting: Conclusions from cross-validations between two centers. Anesthesiology 1999; 91:693-700.

PROPHYLAXIS AND TREATMENT OF NAUSEA AND VOMITING

Preventing maternal hypotension may be the best means of preventing nausea and vomiting. Several options exist for the pharmacologic prophylaxis of nausea and vomiting, and several different classes of drugs are available (Table 26-7). Although various algorithms have been developed to prevent postoperative nausea and vomiting, primarily targeting the nonpregnant patient population, none has been universally successful.[408] However, the prophylactic use of these agents either before or after cord clamping during cesarean delivery with neuraxial anesthesia has been demonstrated to be highly effective. Balki and Carvalho[399] suggested an algorithm consisting of metoclopramide as a first-line agent, dimenhydrinate as a second-line agent, and ondansetron or granisetron as a third-line agent. Multimodal therapies may eventually prove the most effective.

Metoclopramide is the agent most frequently given owing to its favorable prokinetic effects. Common side effects include dizziness, drowsiness, and fatigue; rarer side effects include extrapyramidal reactions and acute dystonias. Lussos et al.[409] reported a significant decrease in the incidence of intraoperative nausea (from 81% to 14%) and vomiting (from 43% to 5%) with the administration of metoclopramide 10 mg prior to spinal anesthesia for cesarean delivery. Chestnut et al.[410] noted a reduction of nausea (from 36% to 12%) and of vomiting (from 15% to 0%) with the administration of metoclopramide 0.15 mg/kg after cord clamping in patients undergoing cesarean delivery with epidural anesthesia.

Abouleish et al.[411] found that **ondansetron** was more effective than placebo during cesarean delivery with spinal anesthesia. Pan and Moore[412] observed that when given

TABLE 26-7 Agents for Prevention of Nausea and Vomiting in Women Undergoing Cesarean Delivery with Neuraxial Anesthesia*

Drug	Dose	Optimal or Recommended Timing	Comments
Dexamethasone	4-8 mg IV	Unknown for patients undergoing cesarean delivery†	Delayed onset of action; used infrequently in patients undergoing cesarean delivery
Dimenhydrinate‡	25-50 mg IV	Unknown for patients undergoing cesarean delivery	Antihistamine
Dolasetron	12.5 mg IV	After cord clamping	Serotonin antagonist; not effective in the single published randomized controlled trial
Droperidol	0.625-1.25 mg IV	End of surgery	Butyrophenone with a package insert that contains an FDA "black box" warning regarding prolongation of corrected QT interval on electrocardiogram
Ephedrine‡	0.5 mg/kg IM	End of surgery	Vasopressor
Granisetron	40 μg/kg IV	After cord clamping	Serotonin antagonist
Metoclopramide	10 mg IV	Prior to surgery or after cord clamping	Benzamide
Ondansetron	4 mg IV	After cord clamping	Serotonin antagonist
Scopolamine	1.5-mg transdermal patch	Unknown	Muscarinic antagonist

IM, intramuscularly; IV, intravenously.

*If nausea and vomiting occur despite prophylaxis, the anesthesia provider should consider administration of a drug from a different pharmacologic class. There is no evidence that a second administration of the same drug within 6 hours provides additional benefit.

†Studies in nonobstetric patients suggest that administration of dexamethasone at induction of anesthesia results in better efficacy, but the optimal timing in obstetric patients is unclear.

‡Has not been studied in patients undergoing cesarean delivery with neuraxial anesthesia; however, this drug has proved effective for prophylaxis of postoperative nausea and vomiting in studies of nonobstetric patients after administration of general anesthesia.

after cord clamping, ondansetron 4 mg was more effective than metoclopramide 10 mg in preventing nausea (26% versus 51%) but not vomiting (15% versus 18%). In an animal toxicology study that was followed by a human clinical trial, Han et al.[413] demonstrated no histologic changes in spinal cord tissues after *epidural* administration of ondansetron in rats; moreover, in 80 women undergoing elective cesarean delivery with CSE anesthesia, the incidence of postoperative nausea was lower with epidural infusion of ondansetron 8 mg than with intravenous infusion of ondansetron 8 mg at 24 hours (25% versus 45%) and at 48 hours (10% versus 35%). Future investigations are needed to validate the safety of the neuraxial administration of ondansetron.

The administration of a **transdermal scopolamine** 1.5 mg patch after cord clamping was found to be effective in the prevention of nausea and vomiting during spinal anesthesia for cesarean delivery. However, the use of scopolamine was associated with side effects such as dry mouth and blurry vision.[414]

Alternative therapies may play a role in preventing or treating perioperative nausea and vomiting. Several studies have found a favorable effect of **acupressure** on the P6 acupoint (on the inner aspect of the wrist).[415,416] Compared with placebo, acupressure has been observed to result in a lower incidence of nausea (36% and 15%, respectively) and vomiting (17% and 9%, respectively).[417] One study demonstrated that acupressure was comparable to metoclopramide in decreasing nausea, but not vomiting, during cesarean delivery.[418] Other investigators have also found that acupressure reduces nausea but does not prevent emesis during cesarean delivery with spinal anesthesia.[419]

One study found that the administration of **supplemental oxygen** (FIO_2 of 0.7) between cord clamping and the end of cesarean delivery with neuraxial anesthesia was not associated with a lower incidence of nausea and vomiting than the administration of room air.[420] This finding contrasted to the findings in nonpregnant populations, in whom supplemental oxygen (FIO_2 of 0.8) given intraoperatively and continued 2 hours postoperatively was as effective as intravenous ondansetron 8 mg (administered with an FIO_2 of 0.3) in reducing postoperative nausea and vomiting.[421]

Administration of subhypnotic doses of **propofol** (1 mg/kg/hr), given after cord clamping in women undergoing cesarean delivery with spinal anesthesia, was found to be comparable in efficacy to droperidol 1.25 mg and metoclopramide 10 mg.[422] The majority of patients remained awake, with some being drowsy but not asleep or excessively sedated. The efficacy of propofol has been attributed to direct antiemetic properties as well as weak serotonin receptor antagonism.[423] The same investigators found that the subhypnotic dose of propofol (1 mg/kg/hr) was more effective at preventing nausea, retching, and vomiting when **dexamethasone** 8 mg was added.[424]

Perioperative Pain

In contrast to surveys performed in the general surgical patient population, in which patients have revealed a primary concern for postoperative nausea and vomiting, a survey performed in obstetric patients during their expectant parent class indicated that pain during and after cesarean delivery was their greatest concern.[425] Pain during cesarean delivery is the most common successful obstetric claim made during litigation in the United Kingdom. It is also a common cause of complaint in the American Society of Anesthesiologists Closed-Claims Project database (see Chapter 33).

A preoperative discussion about pain and discomfort can help allay patient concerns. The anesthesia provider should (1) explain that there may be some deep pressure, pain, or discomfort during cesarean delivery performed with a neuraxial technique; (2) reassure the patient that the anesthesia provider will be present throughout the operation to administer additional analgesics or general anesthesia if necessary; (3) ensure and document adequacy of neuraxial blockade prior to the start of surgery; (4) communicate with the patient frequently during the procedure, specifically about pain or discomfort; and (5) treat pain when it arises, in agreement with the patient's wishes. During the postoperative visit, the anesthesia provider should address any issues that may have arisen during or after surgery.

The anesthetic technique for the cesarean delivery may be altered because of postoperative pain management considerations. For example, an epidural catheter–based technique may be optimal for the patient with a significant pain history (e.g., sickle cell vaso-occlusive crises, chronic pain syndromes, drug-seeking behavior).

By directly activating spinal and supraspinal opioid receptors, epidurally and spinally administered opioids blunt nociceptive input and produce analgesia of greater intensity than parenterally or intramuscularly administered doses.[210] A number of opioids have been utilized in the epidural and spinal spaces; however, morphine has emerged as the leading agent for post–cesarean delivery analgesia, owing to its long duration of action and low cost. When morphine is administered intrathecally or epidurally, doses of 0.1 mg and 3.75 mg, respectively, appear to provide optimal analgesia after cesarean delivery.[180,205] Neuraxial morphine has a peak analgesic effect at 60 to 90 minutes but continues to provide effective analgesia for up to 24 hours.[205] A sustained-release epidural morphine preparation has been developed that can provide up to 48 hours of post–cesarean delivery analgesia[207,208]; however, it cannot be co-administered with a local anesthetic (as discussed earlier). Intravenous infusion of naloxone, an opioid antagonist, reduces the severity but not the incidence of pruritus after epidural morphine administration.[426]

Some evidence suggests that the local anesthetic selected for epidural anesthesia may influence the efficacy of epidural morphine, although this remains a matter of some dispute.[427] The prior epidural administration of 2-chloroprocaine may adversely affect the subsequent efficacy of epidural morphine analgesia.[428] The mechanism by which 2-chloroprocaine affects the efficacy of opioids, as well as local anesthetics, is unknown. Use of 2-chloroprocaine should be limited to emergency situations in which rapid augmentation of epidural anesthesia is desired.

Adverse effects of neuraxial morphine include pruritus, nausea and vomiting, urinary retention, and delayed respiratory depression (see Chapter 28). Frequent evaluations (hourly for the first 12 hours, and then every 2 hours for another 12 hours) should be conducted. Postpartum women who are morbidly obese or have preexisting respiratory issues (sleep apnea) are at greater risk of respiratory depression. Patients receiving the new extended-release preparation of morphine should be monitored for at least 48 hours for evidence of respiratory depression.

Postoperative pain may have at least two components, somatic and visceral. A multimodal approach seems to provide the most effective post–cesarean delivery analgesia. Such an approach often includes administration of a nonsteroidal anti-inflammatory drug (NSAID). Concerns have been expressed regarding possible adverse effects (platelet dysfunction, uterine atony), but these agents are widely used. Some investigators have expressed concern about the use of NSAIDs in nursing mothers, but the American Academy of Pediatrics[429] has stated that ibuprofen and ketorolac are compatible with breast-feeding.

Pruritus

The administration of opioids can cause pruritus. The incidence is as high as 30% to 100%, and pruritus is more commonly observed when opioids are administered intrathecally than epidurally. Pruritus is typically self-limited and may be generalized or localized to regions of the nose, face, and chest. Opioid-induced pruritus appears to be influenced by the particular combination of local anesthetic and opioid; of interest, the addition of epinephrine to an opioid–local anesthetic solution appears to augment the pruritus.[430] This side effect does not represent an allergic reaction to the neuraxial opioid. If flushing, urticaria, rhinitis, bronchoconstriction, or cardiac symptoms also occur, allergic reaction to another drug should be considered.

The cause of neuraxial opioid–induced pruritus is not known, although multiple theories have been proposed. They include μ-opioid receptor stimulation at the medullary dorsal horn, antagonism of inhibitory transmitters, and activation of an "itch center" in the central nervous system.[431] Pharmacologic prophylaxis or treatment of pruritus may include an opioid antagonist, an opioid agonist/antagonist, droperidol, a serotonin antagonist (e.g., ondansetron), and/or a subhypnotic dose of propofol (Table 26-8).[431] Yeh et al.[432] observed that ondansetron significantly reduced the incidence of intrathecal morphine–induced pruritus. Although opioid antagonists, such as naltrexone and naloxone, and partial agonist/antagonists, such as nalbuphine, are probably the most effective treatments for pruritus, the use of any of these agents, either as a single dose or in continuous intravenous infusion, may also reverse analgesia. Antihistamines are often prescribed but are largely ineffective because the mechanism of pruritus is not related to histamine release.

TABLE 26-8 Agents for Prevention or Treatment of Pruritus in Women Undergoing Cesarean Delivery

Drug Class	Drug and Dose	Comments
Opioid antagonists	Naloxone infusion 1-2 μg/kg/hr IV	May reverse analgesia
	Naltrexone 6-9 mg PO	
Opioid agonist/antagonist	Nalbuphine 2.5-5 mg IV	
Sedative/hypnotic agent	Propofol 10-20 mg IV	Subhypnotic dose with conflicting evidence regarding efficacy in treating pruritus
Serotonin antagonist	Ondansetron 0.1 mg/kg IV	Conflicting evidence regarding efficacy in treating pruritus
Butyrophenone	Droperidol 1.25 mg IV	Package insert contains an FDA "black box" warning regarding prolongation of corrected QT interval on electrocardiogram

IV, intravenously; PO, orally.

Shivering

Intraoperative and postoperative shivering may also have several etiologies and treatments; intravenous meperidine 25 mg, clonidine 150 μg, doxapram 100 mg, ketanserin 10 mg, and alfentanil 250 μg have all been reported to be effective. Meperidine appears to be the most consistently effective agent.[433]

OBSTETRIC COMPLICATIONS

Postpartum Hemorrhage

A leading cause of maternal and fetal morbidity and mortality worldwide, mild to moderate obstetric hemorrhage can be masked by pregnancy-related physiologic changes. Underestimation of blood loss and inadequate resuscitation remain common problems.

Failure of the uterus to contract following delivery accounts for most cases of postpartum hemorrhage and remains a leading cause of postpartum hysterectomy and blood transfusion. Approximately 600 to 700 mL of blood flows through the placental intervillous spaces each minute; thus obstetric hemorrhage can rapidly result in maternal shock. Uterine atony occurs more commonly after cesarean delivery than after vaginal delivery, perhaps as a reflection of the condition(s) that prompted the cesarean delivery or possibly because surgery disrupts the normal postpartum response to uterotonic hormones and pharmacologic agents. Causes of uterine atony include (1) high parity, (2) an overdistended uterus (multiple gestation, macrosomia, polyhydramnios), (3) prolonged labor (augmented by oxytocin), (4) chorioamnionitis, (5) abnormalities in placentation (placenta accreta, increta, or percreta), (6) retained placental tissue, and (7) poor perfusion of the uterine myometrium (e.g., with hypotension).

Initial efforts to control uterine atony include uterine massage and intravenous **oxytocin**. Postpartum oxytocin is administered in a wide range of doses and timing patterns (e.g., before or after delivery of the placenta). The use of an intravenous oxytocin infusion at a rate of 200 mU/min (20 U/L of a balanced salt solution at a rate of 10 mL/min) for several minutes until the uterus remains firmly contracted and bleeding is controlled has been recommended[434]; the infusion rate may then be reduced to 1 to 2 mL/min until the mother is ready for transfer from the PACU to the postpartum unit. The timing of oxytocin administration varies with individual practice; however, when it is given immediately after the delivery of the infant's shoulders (or the full body of the infant), but before delivery of the placenta, decreased blood loss has been observed.[434]

The administration of oxytocin as a rapid intravenous bolus may cause significant hypotension and even cardiovascular collapse.[435-437] These events result from a direct relaxing effect on the vascular smooth muscle, which leads to decreased systemic vascular resistance, hypotension, and tachycardia.[436] Tachycardia may result from a direct effect on specific oxytocic receptors in the myocardium, thereby affecting atrioventricular conduction and myocardial repolarization.[436] Other side effects of oxytocin include chest pain, signs suggestive of myocardial ischemia, and anaphylaxis.[438] However, it is unclear whether these effects are dose related; a randomized trial comparing oxytocin infusion regimens of 20 U/L and 160 U/L demonstrated no difference between the two regimens in the incidence of hypotension.[439] Oxytocin can also cause water intoxication, given the agent's structural similarity to vasopressin; when severe, this effect can lead to hyponatremia, confusion, convulsions, and coma.

The effect of oxytocin on uterine tone seems to be dose related; however, its efficacy likely depends on the number of oxytocin receptors in the uterus. Pregnancy causes a 180-fold increase in the concentration of oxytocin receptors; a significant proportion of this increase occurs just before the onset of labor.[440]

If oxytocin proves ineffective, the ergot alkaloid derivative **methylergonovine** (0.2 mg) can be given intramuscularly to provide a uterotonic effect within 10 minutes that lasts 3 to 6 hours. Intravenous administration (in small divided doses) should be performed only *with great caution*, because intense vasoconstriction may lead to acute hypertension, seizures, cerebrovascular accident, retinal detachment, and myocardial arrest[441]; this possibility is of special concern in patients with preeclampsia or cardiac disease. Methylergonovine also has additive hemodynamic effects when given with sympathomimetic agents, such as ephedrine and phenylephrine. Nausea and vomiting are common side effects, which most likely reflect a direct central nervous system effect. The co-administration of oxytocin and ergometrine has been demonstrated to improve uterine contractions (as measured by the requirement for additional uterotonic agents); however, the need for blood transfusion and the symptoms of nausea and vomiting were greater with the oxytocin-ergometrine combination.[442]

Uterine sensitivity to prostaglandins increases with advancing gestation. **15-Methyl prostaglandin $F_{2\alpha}$** (Hemabate) causes a dose-dependent increase in the force and the frequency of uterine contractions. The initial recommended dose is 250 μg given intramuscularly; this dose can be repeated if necessary at 15- to 90-minute intervals up to a maximum of 8 doses.[443] Whether 15-methyl-prostaglandin $F_{2\alpha}$ is more effective than oxytocin is controversial[444]; however, it clearly has a role in the treatment of refractory uterine atony.[445] In approximately 20% of women, the following side effects occur (listed in descending order of frequency): diarrhea, hypertension, vomiting, fever, flushing, and tachycardia.[445] Bronchospasm, pulmonary vasoconstriction, and oxyhemoglobin desaturation can also occur.[446]

Rectal administration of **prostaglandin E_1 (misoprostol)** has a rapid onset of action and may be effective in women with no response to parenteral oxytocic agents. A systematic review of misoprostol (given orally or sublingually at a dose of 600 μg) found that this agent is not preferable to conventional injectable uterotonic agents but that it might be associated with fewer blood transfusions (depending on other components of management).[447] A side effect of misoprostol is hyperthermia.

PREPARATION FOR BLOOD LOSS

When risk factors for hemorrhage are identified, several preparatory steps can be considered. **Iron supplementation** and use of **recombinant human erythropoietin** are effective therapies for producing red blood cells, particularly in patients with preexisting anemia, renal failure, and/or reasons for preoperative donation of autologous blood.[448] Antepartum erythropoietin administration may be of value in pregnant women at high risk for hemorrhage; however, additional investigation is needed to determine the optimal dosing, goals of therapy, and side-effect profiles. Hypertension, a problem associated with the use of erythropoietin in patients with renal failure, is a relevant concern during pregnancy. Although normal pregnancy is associated with a twofold to fourfold rise in maternal erythropoietin levels, isolated studies of the effect of erythropoietin on placental vessels suggest that dose-dependent vasoconstriction occurs.[449] Observation of high erythropoietin levels in hypertensive and preeclamptic parturients has fueled speculation that erythropoietin participates in the humoral mechanisms responsible for preeclampsia and intrauterine growth restriction.[450] A hyperglycosylated analogue of recombinant human erythropoietin (darbepoetin) has a threefold longer terminal half-life and results in a more rapid and greater erythropoietic response than recombinant human erythropoietin. This novel protein may be useful in the setting of anticipated or actual obstetric hemorrhage if concerns about its adverse effects are alleviated.[448]

The efficacy of preoperative **autologous blood donation** is limited by the maximum life span of stored blood; collection can start no sooner than 6 weeks before a planned delivery, with an average unit collection interval of 3 to 7 days. This method may be of some use in a woman with maternal antibodies to red cell antigens. The technique seems safe but has limited applicability and efficacy in obstetric patients (see Chapter 37).

Acute normovolemic hemodilution has the advantage of reducing the risk of administrative errors and bacterial contamination and allowing the infusion of whole blood replete with functional coagulation factors and platelets. This technique may reduce the need for transfusion in selected patients, and it may be acceptable to Jehovah's Witness patients at increased risk for blood loss during cesarean delivery.

The use of **intraoperative red blood cell salvage** in obstetric patients is controversial but is gaining greater acceptance.[451,452] In the past obstetric anesthesia providers have expressed concern that intraoperative cell salvage might precipitate amniotic fluid embolism (anaphylactoid syndrome of pregnancy). Allam et al.[451] noted that "existing cell salvage systems differ in their ability to clear contaminants and all require the addition of a leucocyte depletion filter." The cell salvage process does not remove all fetal red cells and hemoglobin, and maternal isoimmunization may occur.[452] Intraoperative cell salvage may be used to prevent morbidity and mortality in parturients who refuse homologous blood or in cases of intractable hemorrhage that may overwhelm blood bank supplies (see Chapter 37).[43]

Future resuscitation strategies during pregnancy may include synthetic hemoglobin solutions, which have demonstrated favorable characteristics in pregnant sheep.[453]

RESPONSE TO BLOOD LOSS

Underestimation of blood loss and inadequate resuscitation are common problems in the management of obstetric hemorrhage. Rapid volume replacement is more important to maintain tissue perfusion and oxygenation than the type of fluid given, although colloids and blood products should be considered early, along with a request for assistance, establishment of a second large-bore intravenous catheter, and use of pressurized transfusion equipment. Many institutions require performance of a blood type and screen for parturients at high risk for hemorrhage undergoing a vaginal delivery, and in all parturients undergoing cesarean delivery. The immediate availability of two to four units of cross-matched packed red blood cells should be considered when the potential for significant blood loss appears imminent, such as in suspected placenta accreta. In situations in which the need for emergency blood transfusion precedes the availability of cross-matched blood, type-specific (or type O, Rh-negative blood) should be administered. Continued blood loss and hemodynamic instability despite transfusion of packed red blood cells is often an indication for placement of an arterial line and invasive central monitoring; however, restoration of circulating volume takes precedence. Urine output, heart rate, and blood pressure assessments can assist in the rapid evaluation of the adequacy of volume resuscitation.

Fortunately, most pregnant women are healthy and tolerate modest blood loss well. Also, concerns about uteroplacental perfusion and fetal oxygenation are no longer present after delivery of the infant. The ASA Task Force on Blood Component Therapy[454] has concluded that transfusion of packed red blood cells is rarely indicated when the hemoglobin concentration is greater than 10 g/dL, and is almost always indicated when the hemoglobin concentration is less than 6 g/dL. Transfusion of platelets is rarely indicated unless the platelet count is less than 50,000/mm^3 (unless platelet dysfunction and microvascular bleeding are present), and replacement of fibrinogen is rarely indicated unless the fibrinogen concentration is less than 80 to 100 mg/dL in the presence of microvascular bleeding.

The prophylactic placement of **intravascular balloon occlusion catheters** has facilitated the timely control of obstetric bleeding in some parturients at high risk for hemorrhage.[455] O'Rourke et al.[456] described three cases of women with placental implantation abnormalities who underwent selective uterine artery balloon catheter placement and in whom subsequent cesarean delivery was performed in the interventional radiology suite. Interventional radiologists may also be asked to assist in the management of acute hemorrhage, although the lack of immediately available equipment and personnel may compromise success.

When uterine bleeding occurs postpartum, the use of **uterine tamponade balloon catheters** has been demonstrated to tamponade and potentially treat intrauterine sources of bleeding and allow time to correct coagulopathy.[457] The Sengstaken-Blakemore esophageal balloon catheter is inserted into the uterus and filled with 70 to 300 mL of warm saline until the distended balloon is palpable in the abdomen; if significant bleeding continues into the cervix or the gastric lumen of the catheter, a surgical intervention is performed. In a series of 16 cases of intractable postpartum hemorrhage, 14 (87.5%) responded to the tamponade and did not require surgery. The use of a Foley catheter in a similar manner has been suggested, but the amount of fluid is limited to 150 mL, which may not be as effective.[458] A new tamponade obstetric hemorrhage balloon (SOS Bakri Tamponade Balloon Catheter, Cook Ob/Gyn, Spence, IN) may have efficacy in some cases.[459]

A relatively new approach for treatment of postpartum hemorrhage is the use of **human recombinant factor VIIa** (rFVIIa), a vitamin K–dependent protein licensed by the FDA for the treatment of bleeding episodes in patients who have hemophilia A or B with inhibitors to factor VIII or factor IX. Off-label administration of rFVIIa has resulted in an almost complete reversal of severe bleeding refractory to standard hematologic or hemostatic support in a variety of animal and human trials and case reports; the successful treatment of severe postpartum hemorrhage with disseminated intravascular coagulation (DIC) unresponsive to medical or surgical treatments has been reported.[460] Administration of rFVIIa works by promoting clotting primarily through the extrinsic (tissue factor) pathway; however, coagulation factors in the intrinsic pathway are also activated.[461] Given as an intravenous dose of 60 to 100 μg/kg, rFVIIa has been observed to have a clinical effect within 10 minutes in some cases, a half-life of approximately 2 hours, and side effects consisting primarily of hypertension, hypotension, bradycardia, and renal dysfunction. Observational trials in the setting of traumatic injury are being performed, but to date there have been no large randomized studies of rFVIIa in obstetric patients.

Obstetric Hysterectomy

The incidence of cesarean hysterectomy and emergency postpartum hysterectomy ranges from 0.03% to 0.33% in different hospital settings and countries.[462] Frequently performed in the setting of life-threatening hemorrhage, cesarean hysterectomy is related to a number of factors, including placental disorders (e.g., placenta previa, placenta accreta), uterine disorders (e.g., rupture, atony), infection, intrauterine fetal death, and DIC. Moreover, El-Sayed et al.[463] found a higher incidence of postpartum hemorrhage and hysterectomy in parturients in whom a trial of labor failed after a previous cesarean delivery. Recent studies have indicated that placenta accreta has replaced uterine atony as the most common indication for emergency postpartum hysterectomy.[462,464,465] Improvements in ultrasonography, color flow Doppler ultrasonography, and magnetic resonance imaging have allowed earlier identification of some women with placenta accreta; however, limitations in diagnostic sensitivity and specificity exist.[466]

Cesarean hysterectomy is considered a high-risk procedure owing to the vascularity and size of the uterus and the distorted anatomic relationships. Bladder and ureteral injuries are common. Prior to performance of hysterectomy, various conservative medical and surgical treatment modalities may be attempted (see Chapter 37).[467] The ligation or embolization of major and collateral uterine vessels with the assistance of an interventional radiologist is becoming more common, particularly in tertiary care settings.[61,468]

The amount of blood loss depends in part on whether the hysterectomy is elective or an emergency. In a prospective review of all obstetric hysterectomies at five university hospitals, Chestnut et al.[469] found an average blood loss of 1319 mL and 2526 mL in 25 elective and 21 emergency cases, respectively, with an average replacement of 1.6 units and 6.6 units of blood, respectively. In a more recent study, Briery et al.[470] performed a multicenter retrospective review of operative and postpartum outcomes in 30 elective and 35 emergency cesarean hysterectomies; the average blood loss for elective and emergency cases was 1963 ± 1180 mL versus 2597 ± 1369 mL, with 33% and 66% of the patients requiring blood transfusion, respectively.

The anesthesia provider should consult with the obstetric team to discuss risk factors and the planned course of management. Preparations for the management of potentially massive blood loss should be made. If prophylactic intravascular balloon catheter placement is planned, some anesthesia providers place an epidural catheter before the procedure for the following reasons[61]: (1) once the balloon catheter is placed, flexion of the hips (during positioning for a neuraxial anesthetic technique) is discouraged, as it may result in balloon dislodgement or occlusion and subsequent thrombosis; (2) epidural anesthesia seems preferable to the use of local anesthesia with sedation for balloon catheter placement; (3) during balloon catheter placement, small amounts of heparin are sometimes used, and it seems preferable to have the epidural catheter in place prior to anticoagulation; and (4) should untoward events (e.g., fetal compromise, vessel rupture) occur during the procedure, the epidural catheter allows for rapid extension of anesthesia for cesarean delivery.

An elective cesarean hysterectomy or a cesarean delivery in which the patient is at high risk for emergency hysterectomy is not a contraindication to a neuraxial anesthetic technique, although a catheter-based technique is recommended. Moreover, the occurrence of an emergency cesarean hysterectomy does not necessitate immediate conversion to general anesthesia. Consideration should be given to (1) maternal history (e.g., number of prior abdominal operative procedures, which may lead to more scarring and adhesions); (2) the risk factors present (e.g., extent of placentation abnormality, coagulation status); (3) the potential difficulty of conversion to general anesthesia if required (e.g., presence of difficult airway, level of assistance available); and (4) the desires of the patient and the obstetric team. Chestnut et al.[469] observed in their review that none of the 12 patients who received continuous epidural anesthesia for cesarean delivery (8 patients from the elective group and 4 from the emergency group) required intraoperative induction of general anesthesia for hysterectomy. In addition, there was no evidence that epidural anesthesia significantly affected blood loss, crystalloid replacement, or requirement for transfusion.

Following cesarean hysterectomy, particularly if it is accompanied by significant blood loss, observation of the patient in an ICU setting should be considered.[465] In a report of 117 emergency peripartum hysterectomies, Zelop et al.[464] noted the presence of respiratory complications and DIC in 21% and 27% of the patients, respectively.

Thromboembolic Events

Thromboembolic events, which constitute a leading cause of maternal death in the United States and the United Kingdom, are related to maternal age, obesity, and smoking.[471] A number of prophylactic interventions have been evaluated; however, the trials have been too small to provide robust results.[472,473] Recommended thromboprophylaxis measures include hydration, early mobilization, pneumatic compression devices,[13] and, in high-risk patients, pharmacologic prophylaxis (see Chapter 38). At least one major health care system has decided to implement a policy of universal use of **pneumatic compression devices** for all women undergoing cesarean delivery in that system.[13]

KEY POINTS

- Cesarean delivery is the most common surgical procedure performed in the United States. The rate of cesarean delivery is increasing worldwide.
- Some cesarean deliveries might be avoided through the provision of satisfactory neuraxial analgesia for labor (including a trial of labor after cesarean delivery), instrumental vaginal delivery, and external cephalic version.
- Gastric emptying is unchanged during pregnancy. The parturient without complications may drink modest amounts of clear liquids up to 2 hours before induction of anesthesia for *elective* cesarean delivery. The fasting period for solids should be 6 to 8 hours. Slower digestion is observed for foods with high fat content.
- A histamine H_2-antagonist or a proton pump inhibitor may be given intravenously to increase gastric fluid pH, and intravenous metoclopramide may be given to both accelerate gastric emptying and increase lower esophageal sphincter tone. If possible, these agents should be administered *more than* 30 minutes before induction of general anesthesia. Oral sodium citrate, which also increases gastric fluid pH, should be administered *less than* 30 minutes before induction.
- Antibiotic prophylaxis, given *either* before abdominal incision *or* immediately after umbilical cord clamping, but before conclusion of surgery, decreases the risk of maternal infectious complications after cesarean delivery.
- Although the use of intravenous fluids may reduce the frequency of maternal hypotension, initiation of neuraxial anesthesia should not be delayed in order to administer a fixed volume of fluid.
- The value of supplemental maternal oxygen during neuraxial anesthesia for the elective cesarean delivery of a noncompromised fetus is questionable.
- Left uterine displacement is essential during cesarean delivery, regardless of the anesthetic technique.
- The estimated case-fatality risk ratio for general versus neuraxial anesthesia has been as high as 16.7 in the years 1985 to 1990; however, in the latest analysis, covering the years 1991 to 2002, a nonsignificant risk ratio of 1.7 was observed.
- Umbilical cord prolapse (without fetal bradycardia), placenta previa, and severe preeclampsia (in a patient with an acceptable platelet count) are no longer considered absolute indications for general anesthesia.
- The anesthesia provider should practice and be comfortable with the initiation of neuraxial techniques in patients in both the sitting and lateral positions, because there are obstetric situations in which the sitting position is relatively or absolutely contraindicated.
- The combined spinal-epidural technique offers the benefits of both spinal and epidural anesthesia while minimizing the disadvantages of either technique alone. Advantages include the fast onset of dense anesthesia with a small dose of local anesthetic and the ability to provide prolonged anesthesia and continuous postoperative analgesia.
- Alkalinization of the local anesthetic solution not only increases the speed of onset but also improves the quality and prolongs the duration of neuroblockade. Administration of 3% 2-chloroprocaine with 8.4% sodium bicarbonate (10 mL of 3% 2-chloroprocaine mixed with 1 mL [1 mEq] of bicarbonate) allows the fastest onset of epidural anesthesia.
- Cricoid pressure to prevent passive regurgitation during induction of general anesthesia should be initiated with 10 newtons (N) of force on the cricoid cartilage, and increased to 30 N once the patient loses consciousness.
- When choosing the concentration of a volatile halogenated agent to maintain general anesthesia, the anesthesia provider must consider the reduced MAC of pregnancy as well as the potential for

maternal awareness and the uterine relaxation caused by these agents.

- Either phenylephrine or ephedrine may be used for the prevention and treatment of maternal hypotension during neuraxial or general anesthesia for cesarean delivery.
- Underestimation of blood loss and inadequate intravascular volume resuscitation during peripartum hemorrhage are common occurrences that contribute to maternal morbidity and mortality.
- Poor postoperative care of women undergoing cesarean delivery has been cited as a recurring factor in maternal deaths.

REFERENCES

1. Todman D. A history of caesarean section: From ancient world to the modern era. Aust N Z J Obstet Gynaecol 2007; 47:357-61.
2. Berghella V, Baxter JK, Chauhan SP. Evidence-based surgery for cesarean delivery. Am J Obstet Gynecol 2005; 193:1607-17.
3. Betran AP, Merialdi M, Lauer JA, et al. Rates of caesarean section: Analysis of global, regional and national estimates. Paediatr Perinat Epidemiol 2007; 21:98-113.
4. Clark SL, Belfort MA, Hankins GD, et al. Variation in the rates of operative delivery in the United States. Am J Obstet Gynecol 2007; 196:526. e1-5.
5. Jacobs-Jokhan D, Hofmeyr G. Extra-abdominal versus intra-abdominal repair of the uterine incision at caesarean section. Cochrane Database Syst Rev 2004; (4):CD000085.
6. Siddiqui M, Goldszmidt E, Fallah S, et al. Complications of exteriorized compared with in situ uterine repair at cesarean delivery under spinal anesthesia: A randomized controlled trial. Obstet Gynecol 2007; 110:570-5.
7. Epps SN, Robbins AJ, Marx GF. Complete recovery after near-fatal venous air embolism during cesarean section. Int J Obstet Anesth 1998; 7:131-3.
8. Nafisi S. Influence of uterine exteriorization versus in situ repair on post-Cesarean maternal pain: A randomized trial. Int J Obstet Anesth 2007; 16:135-8.
9. Belizan JM, Althabe F, Cafferata ML. Health consequences of the increasing caesarean section rates. Epidemiology 2007; 18:485-6.
10. Leung GM, Ho LM, Tin KY, et al. Health care consequences of cesarean birth during the first 18 months of life. Epidemiology 2007; 18:479-84.
11. Pallasmaa N, Ekblad U, Gissler M. Severe maternal morbidity and the mode of delivery. Acta Obstet Gynecol Scand 2008; 87:662-8.
12. Ecker JL, Frigoletto FD Jr. Cesarean delivery and the risk-benefit calculus. N Engl J Med 2007; 356:885-8.
13. Clark SL, Belfort MA, Dildy GA, et al. Maternal death in the 21st century: Causes, prevention, and relationship to cesarean delivery. Am J Obstet Gynecol 2008; 199:36. e1-5.
14. Vadnais M, Sachs B. Maternal mortality with cesarean delivery: A literature review. Semin Perinatol 2006; 30:242-6.
15. Deneux-Tharaux C, Carmona E, Bouvier-Colle MH, et al. Postpartum maternal mortality and cesarean delivery. Obstet Gynecol 2006; 108:541-8.
16. Visco AG, Viswanathan M, Lohr KN, et al. Cesarean delivery on maternal request: Maternal and neonatal outcomes. Obstet Gynecol 2006; 108:1517-29.
17. Hansen AK, Wisborg K, Uldbjerg N, et al. Risk of respiratory morbidity in term infants delivered by elective caesarean section: Cohort study. Br Med J 2008; 336:85-7.
18. MacDorman MF, Declercq E, Menacker F, et al. Infant and neonatal mortality for primary cesarean and vaginal births to women with "no indicated risk," United States, 1998-2001 birth cohorts. Birth 2006; 33:175-82.
19. Halpern SH, Leighton BL, Ohlsson A, et al. Effect of epidural versus parenteral opioid analgesia on the progress of labor: A meta-analysis. JAMA 1998; 280:2105-10.
20. Segal S, Su M, Gilbert P. The effect of a rapid change in availability of epidural analgesia on the cesarean delivery rate: A meta-analysis. Am J Obstet Gynecol 2000; 183:974-8.
21. Albright GA, Forster RM. Does combined spinal-epidural analgesia with subarachnoid sufentanil increase the incidence of emergency cesarean delivery? Reg Anesth 1997; 22:400-5.
22. Van de Velde M, Teunkens A, Hanssens M, et al. Intrathecal sufentanil and fetal heart rate abnormalities: A double-blind, double placebo-controlled trial comparing two forms of combined spinal-epidural analgesia with epidural analgesia in labor. Anesth Analg 2004; 98:1153-9.
23. Gambling DR, Sharma SK, Ramin SM, et al. A randomized study of combined spinal-epidural analgesia versus intravenous meperidine during labor: Impact on cesarean delivery rate. Anesthesiology 1998; 89:1336-44.
24. National Institutes of Health state-of-the-science conference statement: Cesarean delivery on maternal request, March 27-29, 2006. Obstet Gynecol 2006; 107:1386-97.
25. Bucklin BA, Hawkins JL, Anderson JR, et al. Obstetric anesthesia workforce survey: Twenty-year update. Anesthesiology 2005; 103:645-53.
26. Sanchez-Ramos L, Wells TL, Adair CD, et al. Route of breech delivery and maternal and neonatal outcomes. Int J Gynaecol Obstet 2001; 73:7-14.
27. American College of Obstetricians and Gynecologists. External cephalic version. ACOG Practice Bulletin No. 13. Washington, DC, ACOG, February 2000.
28. Rozenberg P, Goffinet F, de Spirlet M, et al. External cephalic version with epidural anaesthesia after failure of a first trial with beta-mimetics. Br J Obstet Gynaecol 2000; 107:406-10.
29. Neiger R, Hennessy MD, Patel M. Reattempting failed external cephalic version under epidural anesthesia. Am J Obstet Gynecol 1998; 179:1136-9.
30. Cherayil G, Feinberg B, Robinson J, et al. Central neuraxial blockade promotes external cephalic version success after a failed attempt. Anesth Analg 2002; 94:1589-92.
31. Hofmeyr GJ, Kulier R. Cephalic version by postural management for breech presentation. Cochrane Database Syst Rev 2000; (3): CD000051.
32. Fernandez CO, Bloom SL, Smulian JC, et al. A randomized placebo-controlled evaluation of terbutaline for external cephalic version. Obstet Gynecol 1997; 90:775-9.
33. Yanny H, Johanson R, Balwin KJ, et al. Double-blind randomised controlled trial of glyceryl trinitrate spray for external cephalic version. Br J Obstet Gynaecol 2000; 107:562-4.
34. Schorr SJ, Speights SE, Ross EL, et al. A randomized trial of epidural anesthesia to improve external cephalic version success. Am J Obstet Gynecol 1997; 177:1133-7.
35. Friedlander JD, Fox HE, Cain CF, et al. Fetal bradycardia and uterine hyperactivity following subarachnoid administration of fentanyl during labor. Reg Anesth 1997; 22:378-81.
36. Kahn L, Hubert E. Combined spinal-epidural (CSE) analgesia, fetal bradycardia, and uterine hypertonus. Reg Anesth Pain Med 1998; 23:111-2.
37. Ekerhovd E, Brannstrom M, Weijdegard B, et al. Nitric oxide synthases in the human cervix at term pregnancy and effects of nitric oxide on cervical smooth muscle contractility. Am J Obstet Gynecol 2000; 183:610-6.
38. Morgan PJ, Kung R, Tarshis J. Nitroglycerin as a uterine relaxant: A systematic review. J Obstet Gynaecol Can 2002; 24:403-9.
39. Chandraharan E, Arulkumaran S. Acute tocolysis. Curr Opin Obstet Gynecol 2005; 17:151-6.

40. Mercier FJ, Benhamou D. Nitroglycerin for fetal head entrapment during vaginal breech delivery? Anesth Analg 1995; 81:654-5.
41. Rosaeg OP, Yarnell RW, Lindsay MP. The obstetrical anaesthesia assessment clinic: A review of six years experience. Can J Anaesth 1993; 40:346-56.
42. Rai MR, Lua SH, Popat M, et al. Antenatal anaesthetic assessment of high-risk pregnancy: A survey of UK practice. Int J Obstet Anesth 2005; 14:219-22.
43. American Society of Anesthesiologists Task Force on Obstetric Anesthesia. Practice guidelines for obstetric anesthesia. Anesthesiology 2007; 106:843-63.
44. American Society of Anesthesiologists Task Force on Preanesthesia Evaluation. Practice advisory for preanesthesia evaluation. Anesthesiology 2002; 96:485-96.
45. Hoehner PJ. Ethical aspects of informed consent in obstetric anesthesia—new challenges and solutions. J Clin Anesth 2003; 15:587-600.
46. Barkham M, Peters G, Pace N. Ethical and medico-legal aspects of obstetric anaesthesia. Anaesth Intensive Care Med 2005; 6:127-9.
47. Worthington R. Ethical dichotomies and methods of seeking consent. Anaesthesia 2004; 59:525-7.
48. Jenkins K, Baker AB. Consent and anaesthetic risk. Anaesthesia 2003; 58:962-84.
49. White SM, Baldwin TJ. Consent for anaesthesia. Anaesthesia 2003; 58:760-74.
50. Lanigan C, Reynolds F. Risk information supplied by obstetric anaesthetists in Britain and Ireland to mothers awaiting elective caesarean section. Int J Obstet Anesth 1995; 4:7-13.
51. Bethune L, Harper N, Lucas DN, et al. Complications of obstetric regional analgesia: How much information is enough? Int J Obstet Anesth 2004; 13:30-4.
52. Kelly GD, Blunt C, Moore PA, et al. Consent for regional anaesthesia in the United Kingdom: What is material risk? Int J Obstet Anesth 2004; 13:71-4.
53. Plaat F, McGlennan A. Women in the 21st century deserve more information: Disclosure of material risk in obstetric anaesthesia. Int J Obstet Anesth 2004; 13:69-70.
54. Wee MY, Brown H, Reynolds F. The National Institute of Clinical Excellence (NICE) guidelines for caesarean sections: Implications for the anaesthetist. Int J Obstet Anesth 2005; 14:147-58.
55. Meyer JH Jr. Informed consent, informed refusal, and informed choices. Am J Obstet Gynecol 2003; 189:319-26.
56. Tsen LC. Gerard W. Ostheimer "What's New in Obstetric Anesthesia" Lecture. Anesthesiology 2005; 102:672-9.
57. Kominiarek MA, Kilpatrick SJ. Postpartum hemorrhage: A recurring pregnancy complication. Semin Perinatol 2007; 31:159-66.
58. Hannah ME, Hannah WJ, Hewson SA, et al. Planned caesarean section versus planned vaginal birth for breech presentation at term: A randomised multicentre trial. Term Breech Trial Collaborative Group. Lancet 2000; 356:1375-83.
59. Stones RW, Paterson CM, Saunders NJ. Risk factors for major obstetric haemorrhage. Eur J Obstet Gynecol Reprod Biol 1993; 48:15-8.
60. Shevell T, Malone FD. Management of obstetric hemorrhage. Semin Perinatol 2003; 27:86-104.
61. Harnett MJ, Carabuena JM, Tsen LC, et al. Anesthesia for interventional radiology in parturients at risk of major hemorrhage at cesarean section delivery. Anesth Analg 2006; 103:1329-30.
62. Pickering TG, Hall JE, Appel L, et al. Response to recommendations for blood pressure measurement in human and experimental animals. Part 1: Blood pressure measurement in humans and miscuffing: A problem with new guidelines. Addendum. Hypertension 2006; 48.e5-6.
63. American College of Obstetricians and Gynecologists. Diagnosis and management of preeclampsia and eclampsia. ACOG Practice Bulletin No. 33. Washington, DC, ACOG, January 2002. (Obstet Gynecol 2002; 99:159-67.)
64. Pickering TG, Hall JE, Appel LJ, et al. Recommendations for blood pressure measurement in humans and experimental animals. Part 1: Blood pressure measurement in humans. A statement for professionals from the Subcommittee of Professional and Public Education of the American Heart Association Council on High Blood Pressure Research. Circulation 2005; 111:697-716.
65. Quinn M. Automated blood pressure measurement devices: A potential source of morbidity in preeclampsia? Am J Obstet Gynecol 1994; 170:1303-7.
66. Zakowski MI, Ramanathan S, Baratta JB, et al. Electrocardiographic changes during cesarean section: A cause for concern? Anesth Analg 1993; 76:162-7.
67. Palmer CM, Norris MC, Giudici MC, et al. Incidence of electrocardiographic changes during cesarean delivery under regional anesthesia. Anesth Analg 1990; 70:36-43.
68. Moran C, Ni Bhuinneain M, Geary M, et al. Myocardial ischaemia in normal patients undergoing elective Caesarean section: A peripartum assessment. Anaesthesia 2001; 56:1051-8.
69. London MJ, Hollenberg M, Wong MG, et al. Intraoperative myocardial ischemia: Localization by continuous 12-lead electrocardiography. Anesthesiology 1988; 69:232-41.
70. Shen CL, Ho YY, Hung YC, et al. Arrhythmias during spinal anesthesia for Cesarean section. Can J Anaesth 2000; 47:393-7.
71. Tsai PS, Huang CJ, Hung YC, et al. Effects on the Bispectral Index during elective caesarean section: A comparison of propofol and isoflurane. Acta Anaesthesiol Sin 2001; 39:17-22.
72. Dahaba AA. Different conditions that could result in the Bispectral Index indicating an incorrect hypnotic state. Anesth Analg 2005; 101:765-73.
73. Tully L, Gates S, Brocklehurst P, et al. Surgical techniques used during caesarean section operations: Results of a national survey of practice in the UK. Eur J Obstet Gynecol Reprod Biol 2002; 102:120-6.
74. American College of Obstetricians and Gynecologists Committee on Obstetric Practice. Fetal monitoring prior to scheduled cesarean delivery. ACOG Committee Opinion No. 382. Washington, DC, ACOG, October 2007. (Obstet Gynecol 2007; 110:961.)
75. http://www.jointcommission.org/accreditationprograms/ambulatory care/standards/
76. U.S. Drug Enforcement Administration. Drug Scheduling. Available at http://www.usdoj.gov/dea/pubs/scheduling.html/
77. Department of Health and Human Services, Center for Medicare and Medicaid Services. Hospital Conditions of Participation. CMS-3122F, 72 FR 68672. Baltimore, MD. November 27, 2006.
78. Wong CA, McCarthy RJ, Fitzgerald PC, et al. Gastric emptying of water in obese pregnant women at term. Anesth Analg 2007; 105:751-5.
79. Wong CA, Loffredi M, Ganchiff JN, et al. Gastric emptying of water in term pregnancy. Anesthesiology 2002; 96:1395-400.
80. Dewan DM, Floyd HM, Thistlewood JM, et al. Sodium citrate pretreatment in elective cesarean section patients. Anesth Analg 1985; 64:34-7.
81. James CF, Gibbs CP. An evaluation of sodium citrate solutions. Anesth Analg 1983; 62:241.
82. Kjaer K, Comerford M, Kondilis L, et al. Oral sodium citrate increases nausea amongst elective Cesarean delivery patients. Can J Anaesth 2006; 53:776-80.
83. Cohen SE, Jasson J, Talafre ML. Does metoclopramide decrease the volume of gastric contents in patients undergoing cesarean section? Anesthesiology 1984; 61:604-7.
84. Murphy DF, Nally B, Gardiner J, et al. Effect of metoclopramide on gastric emptying before elective and emergency caesarean section. Br J Anaesth 1984; 56:1113-6.
85. Ewart MC, Yau G, Gin T, et al. A comparison of the effects of omeprazole and ranitidine on gastric secretion in women undergoing elective caesarean section. Anaesthesia 1990; 45:527-30.
86. Tripathi A, Somwanshi M, Singh B, et al. A comparison of intravenous ranitidine and omeprazole on gastric volume and pH in women undergoing emergency caesarean section. Can J Anaesth 1995; 42:797-800.
87. Yau G, Kan AF, Gin T, et al. A comparison of omeprazole and ranitidine for prophylaxis against aspiration pneumonitis in emergency caesarean section. Anaesthesia 1992; 47:101-4.
88. Hopkins L, Smaill F. Antibiotic prophylaxis regimens and drugs for cesarean section. Cochrane Database Syst Rev 2000; (2):CD001136.

89. Smaill F, Hofmeyr GJ. Antibiotic prophylaxis for cesarean section. Cochrane Database Syst Rev 2002; (3):CD000933.
90. American College of Obstetricians and Gynecologists. Prophylactic antibiotics in labor and delivery. ACOG Practice Bulletin No. 47. Washington, DC, ACOG, October 2003. (Obstet Gynecol 2003; 102:875-82.)
91. Costantine MM, Rahman M, Ghulmiyah L, et al. Timing of perioperative antibiotics for cesarean delivery: A metaanalysis. Am J Obstet Gynecol 2008; 199:301. e1-6.
92. Tita AT, Hauth JC, Grimes A, et al. Decreasing incidence of postcesarean endometritis with extended-spectrum antibiotic prophylaxis. Obstet Gynecol 2008; 111:51-6.
93. Birnbach DJ, Meadows W, Stein DJ, et al. Comparison of povidone iodine and DuraPrep, an iodophor-in-isopropyl alcohol solution, for skin disinfection prior to epidural catheter insertion in parturients. Anesthesiology 2003; 98:164-9.
94. Reynolds F. Neurological infections after neuraxial anesthesia. Anesthesiol Clin 2008; 26:23-52.
95. Scrutton M, Kinsella SM. The immediate caesarean section: Rapid-sequence spinal and risk of infection. Int J Obstet Anesth 2003; 12:143-4.
96. Stirrat G. Clinical Physiology in Pregnancy. In Hytten F, Chamberlain G, editors. Clinical Physiology in Obstetrics. London, Blackwell, 1991:101.
97. Seeberger MD, Staender S, Oertli D, et al. Efficacy of specific aseptic precautions for preventing propofol-related infections: Analysis by a quality-assurance programme using the explicit outcome method. J Hosp Infect 1998; 39:67-70.
98. Scott DA, Fox JA, Cnaan A, et al. Resistance to fluid flow in veins. J Clin Monit 1996; 12:331-7.
99. de la Roche MR, Gauthier L. Rapid transfusion of packed red blood cells: Effects of dilution, pressure, and catheter size. Ann Emerg Med 1993; 22:1551-5.
100. Ogura JM, Francois KE, Perlow JH, et al. Complications associated with peripherally inserted central catheter use during pregnancy. Am J Obstet Gynecol 2003; 188:1223-5.
101. Hepner D, Tsen LC. Fluid management in obstetrics. In Hahn R, Prough DS, Svensen CH, editors. Perioperative Fluid Therapy. New York, Informa Healthcare, 2007:405-22.
102. Dyer RA, Farina Z, Joubert IA, et al. Crystalloid preload versus rapid crystalloid administration after induction of spinal anaesthesia (coload) for elective caesarean section. Anaesth Intensive Care 2004; 32:351-7.
103. Takano M, Takano Y, Sato I. [The effect of midazolam on the memory during cesarean section and the modulation by flumazenil]. Masui 1999; 48:73-5.
104. Olde E, van der Hart O, Kleber R, et al. Posttraumatic stress following childbirth: A review. Clin Psychol Rev 2006; 26:1-16.
105. Kinsella SM, Lohmann G. Supine hypotensive syndrome. Obstet Gynecol 1994; 83:774-88.
106. Marx GF, Bassell GM. Hazards of the supine position in pregnancy. Clin Obstet Gynaecol 1982; 9:255-71.
107. Kinsella SM. Lateral tilt for pregnant women: Why 15 degrees? Anaesthesia 2003; 58:835-6.
108. Pirhonen JP, Erkkola RU. Uterine and umbilical flow velocity waveforms in the supine hypertensive syndrome. Obstet Gynecol 1990; 76:176-9.
109. Jones SJ, Kinsella SM, Donald FA. Comparison of measured and estimated angles of table tilt at Caesarean section. Br J Anaesth 2003; 90:86-7.
110. Morgan DJ, Paull JD, Toh CT, et al. Aortocaval compression and plasma concentrations of thiopentone at caesarean section. Br J Anaesth 1984; 56:349-54.
111. Mendonca C, Griffiths J, Ateleanu B, et al. Hypotension following combined spinal-epidural anaesthesia for Caesarean section: Left lateral position vs. tilted supine position. Anaesthesia 2003; 58: 428-31.
112. Loke GP, Chan EH, Sia AT. The effect of 10 degrees head-up tilt in the right lateral position on the systemic blood pressure after subarachnoid block for Caesarean section. Anaesthesia 2002; 57:169-72.
113. Brodsky JB, Lemmens HJM, Brock-Utne JG, Saidman LJ. Anesthetic considerations for bariatric surgery: Proper positioning is important for laryngoscopy. Anesth Analg 2002; 96:1841-2.
114. Mhyre JM. Anesthetic management for the morbidly obese pregnant woman. Int Anesthesiol Clin 2007; 45:51-70.
115. Miyabe M, Namiki A. The effect of head-down tilt on arterial blood pressure after spinal anesthesia. Anesth Analg 1993; 76:549-52.
116. Miyabe M, Sato S. The effect of head-down tilt position on arterial blood pressure after spinal anesthesia for cesarean delivery. Reg Anesth 1997; 22:239-42.
117. Sinclair CJ, Scott DB, Edstrom HH. Effect of the Trendelenburg position on spinal anaesthesia with hyperbaric bupivacaine. Br J Anaesth 1982; 54:497-500.
118. Tsen LC. Neuraxial techniques for labor analgesia should be placed in the lateral position. Int J Obstet Anesth 2008; 17:146-9.
119. Polley LS. Neuraxial techniques for labor analgesia should be placed in the lateral position. Int J Obstet Anesth 2008; 17:149-52.
120. Jones AY, Dean E. Body position change and its effect on hemodynamic and metabolic status. Heart Lung 2004; 33:281-90.
121. Suonio S, Simpanen AL, Olkkonen H, et al. Effect of the left lateral recumbent position compared with the supine and upright positions on placental blood flow in normal late pregnancy. Ann Clin Res 1976; 8:22-6.
122. Andrews PJ, Ackerman WE, Juneja MM. Aortocaval compression in the sitting and lateral decubitus positions during extradural catheter placement in the parturient. Can J Anaesth 1993; 40:320-4.
123. Vincent RD, Chestnut DH. Which position is more comfortable for the parturient during identification of the epidural space? Int J Obstet Anesth 1991; 1:9-11.
124. Igarashi T, Hirabayashi Y, Shimizu R, et al. The fiberscopic findings of the epidural space in pregnant women. Anesthesiology 2000; 92:1631-6.
125. Hirabayashi Y, Shimizu R, Fukuda H, et al. Effects of the pregnant uterus on the extradural venous plexus in the supine and lateral positions, as determined by magnetic resonance imaging. Br J Anaesth 1997; 78:317-9.
126. Bahar M, Chanimov M, Cohen ML, et al. The lateral recumbent head-down position decreases the incidence of epidural venous puncture during catheter insertion in obese parturients. Can J Anaesth 2004; 51:577-80.
127. Bahar M, Chanimov M, Cohen ML, et al. Lateral recumbent head-down posture for epidural catheter insertion reduces intravascular injection. Can J Anaesth 2001; 48:48-53.
128. Hirasawa Y, Bashir WA, Smith FW, et al. Postural changes of the dural sac in the lumbar spines of asymptomatic individuals using positional stand-up magnetic resonance imaging. Spine 2007; 32: E136-40.
129. Yun EM, Marx GF, Santos AC. The effects of maternal position during induction of combined spinal-epidural anesthesia for cesarean delivery. Anesth Analg 1998; 87:614-8.
130. Hamza J, Smida M, Benhamou D, Cohen SE. Parturient's posture during epidural puncture affects the distance from skin to epidural space. J Clin Anesth 1995; 7:1-4.
131. Fox GS, Houle GL. Acid-base studies in elective caesarean sections during epidural and general anaesthesia. Can Anaesth Soc J 1971; 18:60-71.
132. Cogliano MS, Graham AC, Clark VA. Supplementary oxygen administration for elective Caesarean section under spinal anaesthesia. Anaesthesia 2002; 57:66-9.
133. Khaw KS, Wang CC, Ngan Kee WD, et al. Effects of high inspired oxygen fraction during elective caesarean section under spinal anaesthesia on maternal and fetal oxygenation and lipid peroxidation. Br J Anaesth 2002; 88:18-23.
134. Ryerson EG, Block AJ. Oxygen as a drug. In Burton GG, Hodgkin JE, Ward JJ, editors. Respiratory Care: A Guide to Clinical Practice. 3rd edition. Philadelphia, JB Lippincott, 1991:319-39.
135. Harrop-Griffiths AW, Ravalia A, Browne DA, et al. Regional anaesthesia and cough effectiveness: A study in patients undergoing caesarean section. Anaesthesia 1991; 46:11-3.

136. Kelly MC, Fitzpatrick KT, Hill DA. Respiratory effects of spinal anaesthesia for caesarean section. Anaesthesia 1996; 51:1120-2.
137. Khaw KS, Ngan Kee WD, Lee A, et al. Supplementary oxygen for elective Caesarean section under spinal anaesthesia: Useful in prolonged uterine incision-to-delivery interval? Br J Anaesth 2004; 92:518-22.
138. McCord JM. The evolution of free radicals and oxidative stress. Am J Med 2000; 108:652-9.
139. Rogers MS, Murray HG, Wang CC, et al. Oxidative stress in the fetal lamb brain following intermittent umbilical cord occlusion: A path analysis. Br J Obstet Gynaecol 2001; 108:1283-90.
140. Rogers MS, Wang W, Mongelli M, et al. Lipid peroxidation in cord blood at birth: A marker of fetal hypoxia during labour. Gynecol Obstet Invest 1997; 44:229-33.
141. Thiel M, Chouker A, Ohta A, et al. Oxygenation inhibits the physiological tissue-protecting mechanism and thereby exacerbates acute inflammatory lung injury. PLoS Biol 2005; 3:e174.
142. Qin Y, Wang CC, Kuhn H, et al. Determinants of umbilical cord arterial 8-iso-prostaglandin F2alpha concentrations. Br J Obstet Gynaecol 2000; 107:973-81.
143. Yamada T, Yoneyama Y, Sawa R, et al. Effects of maternal oxygen supplementation on fetal oxygenation and lipid peroxidation following a single umbilical cord occlusion in fetal goats. J Nippon Med Sch 2003; 70:165-71.
144. Buhimschi IA, Buhimschi CS, Pupkin M, et al. Beneficial impact of term labor: Nonenzymatic antioxidant reserve in the human fetus. Am J Obstet Gynecol 2003; 189:181-8.
145. Thorp JA, Trobough T, Evans R, et al. The effect of maternal oxygen administration during the second stage of labor on umbilical cord blood gas values: A randomized controlled prospective trial. Am J Obstet Gynecol 1995; 172:465-74.
146. Khazin AF, Hon EH, Hehre FW. Effects of maternal hyperoxia on the fetus. I. Oxygen tension. Am J Obstet Gynecol 1971; 109:628-37.
147. Vento M, Asensi M, Sastre J, et al. Resuscitation with room air instead of 100% oxygen prevents oxidative stress in moderately asphyxiated term neonates. Pediatrics 2001; 107:642-7.
148. Shibli KU, Russell IF. A survey of anaesthetic techniques used for caesarean section in the UK in 1997. Int J Obstet Anesth 2000; 9:160-7.
149. Hawkins JL, Koonin LM, Palmer SK, et al. Anesthesia-related deaths during obstetric delivery in the United States, 1979-1990. Anesthesiology 1997; 86:277-84.
150. Hawkins JL, Chang J, Palmer SK. Anesthesia-related maternal mortality in the United States, 1997-2002 (abstract). Oral presentation at the 40th Annual Meeting of the Society for Obstetric Anesthesia and Perinatology, Chicago, Apr 30-May 4, 2008.
151. Chestnut DH. Anesthesia and maternal mortality. Anesthesiology 1997; 86:273-6.
152. Tsen LC, Pitner R, Camann WR. General anesthesia for cesarean section at a tertiary care hospital 1990-1995: Indications and implications. Int J Obstet Anesth 1998; 7:147-52.
153. Afolabi BB, Lesi FE, Merah NA. Regional versus general anaesthesia for caesarean section. Cochrane Database Syst Rev 2006; (4):CD004350.
154. Morgan BM, Aulakh JM, Barker JP, et al. Anaesthetic morbidity following caesarean section under epidural or general anaesthesia. Lancet 1984; 1(8372):328-30.
155. Reynolds F, Seed PT. Anaesthesia for Caesarean section and neonatal acid-base status: A meta-analysis. Anaesthesia 2005; 60:636-53.
156. Russell IF. Levels of anaesthesia and intraoperative pain at caesarean section under regional block. Int J Obstet Anesth 1995; 4:71-7.
157. Russell IF. A comparison of cold, pinprick and touch for assessing the level of spinal block at caesarean section. Int J Obstet Anesth 2004; 13:146-52.
158. Bourne TM, deMelo AE, Bastianpillai BA, et al. A survey of how British obstetric anaesthetists test regional anaesthesia before caesarean section. Anaesthesia 1997; 52:901-3.
159. Burns SM, Barclay PM. Regional anaesthesia for Caesarean section. Curr Anaesth Crit Care 2000; 11:73-9.
160. Riley ET, Cohen SE, Macario A, et al. Spinal versus epidural anesthesia for cesarean section: A comparison of time efficiency, costs, charges, and complications. Anesth Analg 1995; 80:709-12.
161. Garry M, Davies S. Failure of regional blockade for caesarean section. Int J Obstet Anesth 2002; 11:9-12.
162. Pan PH, Bogard TD, Owen MD. Incidence and characteristics of failures in obstetric neuraxial analgesia and anesthesia: A retrospective analysis of 19,259 deliveries. Int J Obstet Anesth 2004; 13:227-33.
163. Kuhnert BR, Philipson EH, Pimental R, et al. Lidocaine disposition in mother, fetus, and neonate after spinal anesthesia. Anesth Analg 1986; 65:139-44.
164. Tsen LC, Hepner DL. Needles used for spinal anesthesia. Expert Rev Med Devices 2006; 3:499-508.
165. Arkoosh VA, Palmer CM, Yun EM, et al. A randomized, double-masked, multicenter comparison of the safety of continuous intrathecal labor analgesia using a 28-gauge catheter versus continuous epidural labor analgesia. Anesthesiology 2008; 108:286-98.
166. Kestin IG. Spinal anaesthesia in obstetrics. Br J Anaesth 1991; 66:596-607.
167. Greene NM. Distribution of local anesthetic solutions within the subarachnoid space. Anesth Analg 1985; 64:715-30.
168. Carvalho B, Durbin M, Drover DR, et al. The ED_{50} and ED_{95} of intrathecal isobaric bupivacaine with opioids for cesarean delivery. Anesthesiology 2005; 103:606-12.
169. Sarvela PJ, Halonen PM, Korttila KT. Comparison of 9 mg of intrathecal plain and hyperbaric bupivacaine both with fentanyl for cesarean delivery. Anesth Analg 1999; 89:1257-62.
170. Vercauteren MP, Coppejans HC, Hoffmann VH, et al. Small-dose hyperbaric versus plain bupivacaine during spinal anesthesia for cesarean section. Anesth Analg 1998; 86:989-93.
171. Ben-David B, Miller G, Gavriel R, et al. Low-dose bupivacaine-fentanyl spinal anesthesia for cesarean delivery. Reg Anesth Pain Med 2000; 25:235-9.
172. Bryson GL, Macneil R, Jeyaraj LM, et al. Small dose spinal bupivacaine for Cesarean delivery does not reduce hypotension but accelerates motor recovery. Can J Anaesth 2007; 54:531-7.
173. Norris MC. Height, weight, and the spread of subarachnoid hyperbaric bupivacaine in the term parturient. Anesth Analg 1988; 67:555-8.
174. Hartwell BL, Aglio LS, Hauch MA, et al. Vertebral column length and spread of hyperbaric subarachnoid bupivacaine in the term parturient. Reg Anesth 1991; 16:17-9.
175. McDonald SB, Liu SS, Kopacz DJ, et al. Hyperbaric spinal ropivacaine: A comparison to bupivacaine in volunteers. Anesthesiology 1999; 90:971-7.
176. Ogun CO, Kirgiz EN, Duman A, et al. Comparison of intrathecal isobaric bupivacaine-morphine and ropivacaine-morphine for Caesarean delivery. Br J Anaesth 2003; 90:659-64.
177. Khaw KS, Ngan Kee WD, Wong EL, et al. Spinal ropivacaine for cesarean section: A dose-finding study. Anesthesiology 2001; 95:1346-50.
178. Khaw KS, Ngan Kee WD, Wong M, et al. Spinal ropivacaine for cesarean delivery: A comparison of hyperbaric and plain solutions. Anesth Analg 2002; 94:680-5.
179. Gautier P, De Kock M, Huberty L, et al. Comparison of the effects of intrathecal ropivacaine, levobupivacaine, and bupivacaine for Caesarean section. Br J Anaesth 2003; 91:684-9.
180. Palmer CM, Emerson S, Volgoropolous D, et al. Dose-response relationship of intrathecal morphine for postcesarean analgesia. Anesthesiology 1999; 90:437-44.
181. Swart M, Sewell J, Thomas D. Intrathecal morphine for caesarean section: An assessment of pain relief, satisfaction and side-effects. Anaesthesia 1997; 52:373-7.
182. Kato R, Shimamoto H, Terui K, et al. Delayed respiratory depression associated with 0.15 mg intrathecal morphine for cesarean section: A review of 1915 cases. J Anesth 2008; 22:112-6.
183. Dahl JB, Jeppesen IS, Jorgensen H, et al. Intraoperative and postoperative analgesic efficacy and adverse effects of intrathecal opioids in

patients undergoing cesarean section with spinal anesthesia: A qualitative and quantitative systematic review of randomized controlled trials. Anesthesiology 1999; 91:1919-27.
184. Duale C, Frey C, Bolandard F, et al. Epidural versus intrathecal morphine for postoperative analgesia after Caesarean section. Br J Anaesth 2003; 91:690-4.
185. Kaufman RD, Gabathuler ML, Bellville JW. Potency, duration of action and pA2 in man of intravenous naloxone measured by reversal of morphine-depressed respiration. J Pharmacol Exp Ther 1981; 219:156-62.
186. Saravanan S, Robinson AP, Qayoum Dar A, et al. Minimum dose of intrathecal diamorphine required to prevent intraoperative supplementation of spinal anaesthesia for Caesarean section. Br J Anaesth 2003; 91:368-72.
187. Hunt CO, Naulty JS, Bader AM, et al. Perioperative analgesia with subarachnoid fentanyl-bupivacaine for cesarean delivery. Anesthesiology 1989; 71:535-40.
188. Manullang TR, Viscomi CM, Pace NL. Intrathecal fentanyl is superior to intravenous ondansetron for the prevention of perioperative nausea during cesarean delivery with spinal anesthesia. Anesth Analg 2000; 90:1162-6.
189. Shende D, Cooper GM, Bowden MI. The influence of intrathecal fentanyl on the characteristics of subarachnoid block for caesarean section. Anaesthesia 1998; 53:706-10.
190. Courtney MA, Bader AM, Hartwell B, et al. Perioperative analgesia with subarachnoid sufentanil administration. Reg Anesth 1992; 17:274-8.
191. Braga Ade F, Braga FS, Potério GM, et al. Sufentanil added to hyperbaric bupivacaine for subarachnoid block in Caesarean section. Eur J Anaesthesiol 2003; 20:631-5.
192. Cooper DW, Lindsay SL, Ryall DM, et al. Does intrathecal fentanyl produce acute cross-tolerance to i.v. morphine? Br J Anaesth 1997; 78:311-3.
193. Giarrusso KA, Mirikitani E, Carvalho B, et al. Does intrathecal fentanyl induce acute tolerance to opioids? Anesthesiology 2002; 96: A1042.
194. Lui AC, Polis TZ, Cicutti NJ. Densities of cerebrospinal fluid and spinal anaesthetic solutions in surgical patients at body temperature. Can J Anaesth 1998; 45:297-303.
195. Abouleish EI. Epinephrine improves the quality of spinal hyperbaric bupivacaine for cesarean section. Anesth Analg 1987; 66:395-400.
196. Roelants F. The use of neuraxial adjuvant drugs (neostigmine, clonidine) in obstetrics. Curr Opin Anaesthesiol 2006; 19:233-7.
197. Kruskowski J, Hood D, Eisenach J, et al. Intrathecal neostigmine for post-cesarean section analgesia: Dose response. Anesth Analg 1997; 84:1269-75.
198. Liu SS, Hodgson PS, Moore JM, et al. Dose-response effects of spinal neostigmine added to bupivacaine spinal anesthesia in volunteers. Anesthesiology 1999; 90:710-7.
199. Lauretti GR, Reis MP. Subarachnoid neostigmine does not affect blood pressure or heart rate during bupivacaine spinal anesthesia. Reg Anesth 1996; 21:586-91.
200. Sakura S, Sumi M, Kushizaki H, et al. Concentration of lidocaine affects intensity of sensory block during lumbar epidural anesthesia. Anesth Analg 1999; 88:123-7.
201. Bader AM, Tsen LC, Camann WR, et al. Clinical effects and maternal and fetal plasma concentrations of 0.5% epidural levobupivacaine versus bupivacaine for cesarean delivery. Anesthesiology 1999; 90:1596-601.
202. Faccenda KA, Simpson AM, Henderson DJ, et al. A comparison of levobupivacaine 0.5% and racemic bupivacaine 0.5% for extradural anesthesia for caesarean section. Reg Anesth Pain Med 2003; 28:394-400.
203. Datta S, Camann W, Bader A, et al. Clinical effects and maternal and fetal plasma concentrations of epidural ropivacaine versus bupivacaine for cesarean section. Anesthesiology 1995; 82:1346-52.
204. Bernards CM, Shen DD, Sterling ES, et al. Epidural, cerebrospinal fluid, and plasma pharmacokinetics of epidural opioids (part 1): Differences among opioids. Anesthesiology 2003; 99:455-65.
205. Palmer CM, Nogami WM, Van Maren G, et al. Postcesarean epidural morphine: A dose-response study. Anesth Analg 2000; 90:887-91.
206. Sarvela J, Halonen P, Soikkeli A, et al. A double-blinded, randomized comparison of intrathecal and epidural morphine for elective cesarean delivery. Anesth Analg 2002; 95:436-40.
207. Carvalho B, Riley E, Cohen SE, et al. Single-dose, sustained-release epidural morphine in the management of postoperative pain after elective cesarean delivery: Results of a multicenter randomized controlled study. Anesth Analg 2005; 100:1150-8.
208. Carvalho B, Roland LM, Chu LF, et al. Single-dose, extended-release epidural morphine (DepoDur) compared to conventional epidural morphine for post-cesarean pain. Anesth Analg 2007; 105:176-83.
209. Hallworth SP, Fernando R, Bell R, et al. Comparison of intrathecal and epidural diamorphine for elective caesarean section using a combined spinal-epidural technique. Br J Anaesth 1999; 82:228-32.
210. Ginosar Y, Riley ET, Angst MS. The site of action of epidural fentanyl in humans: The difference between infusion and bolus administration. Anesth Analg 2003; 97:1428-38.
211. Gaffud MP, Bansal P, Lawton C, et al. Surgical analgesia for cesarean delivery with epidural bupivacaine and fentanyl. Anesthesiology 1986; 65:331-4.
212. Helbo-Hansen HS, Bang U, Lindholm P, et al. Maternal effects of adding epidural fentanyl to 0.5% bupivacaine for caesarean section. Int J Obstet Anesth 1993; 2:21-6.
213. Eichenberger U, Giani C, Petersen-Felix S, et al. Lumbar epidural fentanyl: Segmental spread and effect on temporal summation and muscle pain. Br J Anaesth 2003; 90:467-73.
214. Helbo-Hansen HS, Bang U, Lindholm P, et al. Neonatal effects of adding epidural fentanyl to 0.5% bupivacaine for caesarean section. Int J Obstet Anesth 1993; 2:27-33.
215. Madej TH, Strunin L. Comparison of epidural fentanyl with sufentanil: Analgesia and side effects after a single bolus dose during elective caesarean section. Anaesthesia 1987; 42:1156-61.
216. Grass JA, Sakima NT, Schmidt R, et al. A randomized, double-blind, dose-response comparison of epidural fentanyl versus sufentanil analgesia after cesarean section. Anesth Analg 1997; 85:365-71.
217. Eisenach JC, D'Angelo R, Taylor C, Hood DD. An isobolographic study of epidural clonidine and fentanyl after cesarean section. Anesth Analg 1994; 79:285-90.
218. Capogna G, Celleno D, Zangrillo A. Addition of clonidine to epidural morphine enhances postoperative analgesia after cesarean delivery. Reg Anesth 1995; 20:57-61.
219. Kaya FN, Sahin S, Owen MD, et al. Epidural neostigmine produces analgesia but also sedation in women after cesarean delivery. Anesthesiology 2004; 100:381-5.
220. Sakura S, Sumi M, Morimoto N, Saito Y. The addition of epinephrine increases intensity of sensory block during epidural anesthesia with lidocaine. Reg Anesth Pain Med 1999; 24:541-6.
221. Mather LE, Tucker GT, Murphy TM, et al. The effects of adding adrenaline to etidocaine and lignocaine in extradural anaesthesia. II: Pharmacokinetics. Br J Anaesth 1976; 48:989-94.
222. Murphy TM, Mather LE, Stanton-Hicks M, et al. The effects of adding adrenaline to etidocaine and lignocaine in extradural anaesthesia. I: Block characteristics and cardiovascular effects. Br J Anaesth 1976; 48:893-8.
223. Bernards CM, Shen DD, Sterling ES, et al. Epidural, cerebrospinal fluid, and plasma pharmacokinetics of epidural opioids. Part II: Effect of epinephrine. Anesthesiology 2003; 99:466-75.
224. Hadzic A, Vloka J, Patel N, et al. Hypertensive crisis after a successful placement of an epidural anesthetic in a hypertensive parturient: Case report. Reg Anesth 1995; 20:156-8.
225. Albright GA, Jouppila R, Hollmen AI, et al. Epinephrine does not alter human intervillous blood flow during epidural anesthesia. Anesthesiology 1981; 54:131-5.
226. Skjoldebrand A, Eklund J, Lunell NO, et al. The effect on uteroplacental blood flow of epidural anaesthesia containing adrenaline for caesarean section. Acta Anaesthesiol Scand 1990; 34:85-9.
227. Marx GF, Elstein ID, Schuss M, et al. Effects of epidural block with lignocaine and lignocaine-adrenaline on umbilical artery velocity wave ratios. Br J Obstet Gynaecol 1990; 97:517-20.

228. Alahuhta S, Rasanen J, Jouppila R, et al. Effects of extradural bupivacaine with adrenaline for caesarean section on uteroplacental and fetal circulation. Br J Anaesth 1991; 67:678-82.
229. Brownridge P. Epidural and subarachnoid analgesia for elective caesarean section. Anaesthesia 1981; 36:70.
230. Carrie LE, O'Sullivan G. Subarachnoid bupivacaine 0.5% for caesarean section. Eur J Anaesthesiol 1984; 1:275-83.
231. Davies SJ, Paech MJ, Welch H, et al. Maternal experience during epidural or combined spinal-epidural anesthesia for cesarean section: A prospective, randomized trial. Anesth Analg 1997; 85:607-13.
232. Goy RW, Chee-Seng Y, Sia AT, et al. The median effective dose of intrathecal hyperbaric bupivacaine is larger in the single-shot spinal as compared with the combined spinal-epidural technique. Anesth Analg 2005; 100:1499-502.
233. Ithnin F, Lim Y, Sia AT, et al. Combined spinal epidural causes higher level of block than equivalent single-shot spinal anesthesia in elective cesarean patients. Anesth Analg 2006; 102:577-80.
234. Lim Y, Teoh W, Sia AT. Combined spinal-epidural does not cause a higher sensory block than single-shot spinal technique for cesarean delivery in laboring women. Anesth Analg 2006; 103:1540-2.
235. McNaught AF, Stocks GM. Epidural volume extension and low-dose sequential combined spinal-epidural blockade: Two ways to reduce spinal dose requirement for caesarean section. Int J Obstet Anesth 2007; 16:346-53.
236. Thoren T, Holmstrom B, Rawal N, et al. Sequential combined spinal-epidural block versus spinal block for cesarean section: Effects on maternal hypotension and neurobehavioral function of the newborn. Anesth Analg 1994; 78:1087-92.
237. Kucukguclu S, Unlugenc H, Gunenc F, et al. The influence of epidural volume extension on spinal block with hyperbaric or plain bupivacaine for Caesarean delivery. Eur J Anaesthesiol 2008; 25:307-13.
238. Lucas DN, Ciccone GK, Yentis SM. Extending low-dose epidural analgesia for emergency Caesarean section: A comparison of three solutions. Anaesthesia 1999; 54:1173-7.
239. Bjornestad E, Iversen OL, Raeder J. Similar onset time of 2-chloroprocaine and lidocaine + epinephrine for epidural anesthesia for elective Cesarean section. Acta Anaesthesiol Scand 2006; 50:358-63.
240. Lam DT, Ngan Kee WD, Khaw KS. Extension of epidural blockade in labour for emergency Caesarean section using 2% lidocaine with epinephrine and fentanyl, with or without alkalinisation. Anaesthesia 2001; 56:790-4.
241. Peterfreund RA, Datta S, Ostheimer GW. pH adjustment of local anesthetic solutions with sodium bicarbonate: Laboratory evaluation of alkalinization and precipitation. Reg Anesth 1989; 14:265-70.
242. Tuleu C, Allam J, Gill H, et al. Short term stability of pH-adjusted lidocaine-adrenaline epidural solution used for emergency caesarean section. Int J Obstet Anesth 2008; 17:118-22.
243. Gaiser RR, Cheek TG, Adams HK, et al. Epidural lidocaine for cesarean delivery of the distressed fetus. Int J Obstet Anesth 1998; 7:27-31.
244. Malhotra S, Yentis SM. Extending low-dose epidural analgesia in labour for emergency Caesarean section—a comparison of levobupivacaine with or without fentanyl. Anaesthesia 2007; 62:667-71.
245. Higuchi H, Adachi Y, Kazama T. Effects of epidural saline injection on cerebrospinal fluid volume and velocity waveform: A magnetic resonance imaging study. Anesthesiology 2005; 102:285-92.
246. Regan KJ, O'Sullivan G. The extension of epidural blockade for emergency Caesarean section: A survey of current UK practice. Anaesthesia 2008; 63:136-42.
247. Kodali BS, Chandrasekhar S, Bulich LN, et al. Airway changes during labor and delivery. Anesthesiology 2008; 108:357-62.
248. Rao TL, Madhavareddy S, Chinthagada M, et al. Metoclopramide and cimetidine to reduce gastric fluid pH and volume. Anesth Analg 1984; 63:1014-6.
249. Rout CC, Rocke DA, Gouws E. Intravenous ranitidine reduces the risk of acid aspiration of gastric contents at emergency cesarean section. Anesth Analg 1993; 76:156-61.
250. Gagnon C, Fortier LP, Donati F. When a leak is unavoidable, preoxygenation is equally ineffective with vital capacity or tidal volume breathing. Can J Anaesth 2006; 53:86-91.
251. Gambee AM, Hertzka RE, Fisher DM. Preoxygenation techniques: Comparison of three minutes and four breaths. Anesth Analg 1987; 66:468-70.
252. Soro DM, Belda Nacher FJ, Aguilar AG, et al. [Preoxygenation for anesthesia]. Rev Esp Anestesiol Reanim 2004; 51:322-7.
253. Cook WP, Schultetus RR, Caton D. A comparison of d-tubocurarine pretreatment and no pretreatment in obstetric patients. Anesth Analg 1987; 66:756-60.
254. Thind GS, Bryson TH. Single dose suxamethonium and muscle pain in pregnancy. Br J Anaesth 1983; 55:743-5.
255. Abu-Halaweh SA, Massad IM, Abu-Ali HM, et al. Rapid sequence induction and intubation with 1 mg/kg rocuronium bromide in cesarean section: Comparison with suxamethonium. Saudi Med J 2007; 28:1393-6.
256. Baraka AS, Sayyid SS, Assaf BA. Thiopental-rocuronium versus ketamine-rocuronium for rapid-sequence intubation in parturients undergoing cesarean section. Anesth Analg 1997; 84:1104-7.
257. McIver T, Jolley D, Pescod D. General anaesthesia and Caesarean section for a patient with hereditary spastic paraparesis (Strumpell's disease). Int J Obstet Anesth 2007; 16:190-1.
258. Cherala S, Eddie D, Halpern M, et al. Priming with vecuronium in obstetrics. Anaesthesia 1987; 42:1021.
259. Guay J, Grenier Y, Varin F. Clinical pharmacokinetics of neuromuscular relaxants in pregnancy. Clin Pharmacokinet 1998; 34:483.
260. Bhavani-Shankar K, Moseley H, Kumar AY, Delph Y. Capnometry and anaesthesia. Can J Anaesth 1992; 39:617-32.
261. Han TH, Brimacombe J, Lee EJ, et al. The laryngeal mask airway is effective (and probably safe) in selected healthy parturients for elective Cesarean section: A prospective study of 1067 cases. Can J Anaesth 2001; 48:1117-21.
262. Piggott SE, Bogod DG, Rosen M, et al. Isoflurane with either 100% oxygen or 50% nitrous oxide in oxygen for caesarean section. Br J Anaesth 1990; 65:325-9.
263. Matthews P, Dann WL, Cartwright DP, Taylor E. Inspired oxygen concentration during general anesthesia for caesarean section. Eur J Anaesthesiol 1989; 6:295-301.
264. Parpaglioni R, Capogna G, Celleno D, Fusco P. Intraoperative fetal oxygen saturation during Caesarean section: General anaesthesia using sevoflurane with either 100% oxygen or 50% nitrous oxide in oxygen. Eur J Anaesthesiol 2002; 19:115-8.
265. Levinson G, Shnider SM, DeLorimier AA, et al. Effects of maternal hyperventilation on uterine blood flow and fetal oxygenation and acid-base status. Anesthesiology 1974; 40:340-7.
266. Palahniuk RJ, Shnider SM, Eger EI. Pregnancy decreases the requirement for inhaled anesthetic agents. Anesthesiology 1974; 41:82-3.
267. Lertakyamanee J, Chinachoti T, Tritrakarn T, et al. Comparison of general and regional anesthesia for cesarean section: Success rate, blood loss and satisfaction from a randomized trial. J Med Assoc Thai 1999; 82:672-80.
268. Chin KJ, Yeo SW. A BIS-guided study of sevoflurane requirements for adequate depth of anaesthesia in Caesarean section. Anaesthesia 2004; 59:1064-8.
269. Horwitz LD. Effects of intravenous anesthetic agents on left ventricular function in dogs. Am J Physiol 1977; 232:H44-8.
270. Morgan DJ, Blackman GL, Paull JD, et al. Pharmacokinetics and plasma binding of thiopental. II: Studies at cesarean section. Anesthesiology 1981; 54:474-80.
271. Kosaka Y, Takahashi T, Mark LC. Intravenous thiobarbiturate anesthesia for cesarean section. Anesthesiology 1969; 31:489-506.
272. Finster M, Morishima HO, Mark LC, et al. Tissue thiopental concentrations in the fetus and newborn. Anesthesiology 1972; 36:155-8.
273. Flowers CE. The placental transmission of barbiturates and thiobarbiturates and their pharmacological action on the mother and the infant. Am J Obstet Gynecol 1959; 78:730-42.
274. Born GV, Dawes GS, Mott JC, et al. Changes in the heart and lungs at birth. Cold Spring Harb Symp Quant Biol 1954; 19:102-8.
275. Skues MA, Prys-Roberts C. The pharmacology of propofol. J Clin Anesth 1989; 1:387-400.

276. Gin T, Gregory MA, Chan K, et al. Pharmacokinetics of propofol in women undergoing elective caesarean section. Br J Anaesth 1990; 64:148-53.
277. Gin T, Gregory MA, Chan K, et al. Maternal and fetal levels of propofol at caesarean section. Anaesth Intensive Care 1990; 18:180-4.
278. Dailland P, Cockshott ID, Lirzin JD, et al. Intravenous propofol during cesarean section: Placental transfer, concentrations in breast milk, and neonatal effects: A preliminary study. Anesthesiology 1989; 71:827-34.
279. Celleno D, Capogna G, Tomassetti M, et al. Neurobehavioural effects of propofol on the neonate following elective caesarean section. Br J Anaesth 1989; 62:649-54.
280. Yau G, Gin T, Ewart MC, et al. Propofol for induction and maintenance of anaesthesia at caesarean section: A comparison with thiopentone/enflurane. Anaesthesia 1991; 46:20-3.
281. Gregory MA, Gin T, Yau G, et al. Propofol infusion anaesthesia for caesarean section. Can J Anaesth 1990; 37:514-20.
282. Grounds RM, Twigley AJ, Carli F, et al. The haemodynamic effects of intravenous induction: Comparison of the effects of thiopentone and propofol. Anaesthesia 1985; 40:735-40.
283. Celleno D, Capogna G, Emanuelli M, et al. Which induction drug for cesarean section? A comparison of thiopental sodium, propofol, and midazolam. J Clin Anesth 1993; 5:284-8.
284. Peltz B, Sinclair DM. Induction agents for Caesarean section: A comparison of thiopentone and ketamine. Anaesthesia 1973; 28:37-42.
285. Gin T, Gregory MA, Oh TE. The haemodynamic effects of propofol and thiopentone for induction of caesarean section. Anaesth Intensive Care 1990; 18:175-9.
286. Moore J, Bill KM, Flynn RJ, et al. A comparison between propofol and thiopentone as induction agents in obstetric anaesthesia. Anaesthesia 1989; 44:753-7.
287. Abboud TK, Zhu J, Richardson M, et al. Intravenous propofol vs thiamylal-isoflurane for caesarean section: Comparative maternal and neonatal effects. Acta Anaesthesiol Scand 1995; 39:205-9.
288. Baraka A. Severe bradycardia following propofol-suxamethonium sequence. Br J Anaesth 1988; 61:482-3.
289. Alon E, Ball RH, Gillie MH, et al. Effects of propofol and thiopental on maternal and fetal cardiovascular and acid-base variables in the pregnant ewe. Anesthesiology 1993; 78:562-76.
290. Hui TW, Short TG, Hong W, et al. Additive interactions between propofol and ketamine when used for anesthesia induction in female patients. Anesthesiology 1995; 82:641-8.
291. Corssen G, Gutierrez J, Reves JG, et al. Ketamine in the anesthetic management of asthmatic patients. Anesth Analg 1972; 51:588-96.
292. Erdemir H, Huber FC, Corssen G. Dissociative anesthesia with ketamine: A suitable adjunct to epidural anesthesia. Anesth Analg 1970; 49:623-7.
293. McDonald JS, Mateo CV, Reed EC. Modified nitrous oxide or ketamine hydrochloride for cesarean section. Anesth Analg 1972; 51:975-83.
294. Horwitz LD. Effects of intravenous anesthetic agents on left ventricular function in dogs. Am J Physiol 1997; 232:H44-8.
295. Strumper D, Gogarten W, Durieux ME, et al. The effects of S+-ketamine and racemic ketamine on uterine blood flow in chronically instrumented pregnant sheep. Anesth Analg 2004; 98:497-502.
296. Craft JB, Coaldrake LA, Yonekura ML, et al. Ketamine, catecholamines, and uterine tone in pregnant ewes. Am J Obstet Gynecol 1983; 146:429-34.
297. Levinson G, Shnider SM, Gildea JE, et al. Maternal and foetal cardiovascular and acid-base changes during ketamine anaesthesia in pregnant ewes. Br J Anaesth 1973; 45:1111-5.
298. Oats JN, Vasey DP, Waldron BA. Effects of ketamine on the pregnant uterus. Br J Anaesth 1979; 51:1163-6.
299. Little B, Chang T, Chucot L, et al. Study of ketamine as an obstetric anesthetic agent. Am J Obstet Gynecol 1972; 113:247-60.
300. Janeczko GF, el-Etr AA, Younes S. Low-dose ketamine anesthesia for obstetrical delivery. Anesth Analg 1974; 53:828-31.
301. Downing JW, Mahomedy MC, Jeal DE, et al. Anaesthesia for Caesarean section with ketamine. Anaesthesia 1976; 31:883-92.
302. Eng M, Bonica JJ, Akamatsu TJ, et al. Respiratory depression in newborn monkeys at Caesarean section following ketamine administration. Br J Anaesth 1975; 47:917-21.
303. Ngan Kee WD, Khaw KS, Ma ML, et al. Postoperative analgesic requirement after cesarean section: A comparison of anesthetic induction with ketamine or thiopental. Anesth Analg 1997; 85:1294-8.
304. Gaitini L, Vaida S, Collins G, et al. Awareness detection during caesarean section under general anaesthesia using EEG spectrum analysis. Can J Anaesth 1995; 42:377-81.
305. Bovill JG, Coppel DL, Dundee JW, et al. Current status of ketamine anaesthesia. Lancet 1971; 1(7712):1285-8.
306. Dich-Nielsen J, Holasek J. Ketamine as induction agent for caesarean section. Acta Anaesthesiol Scand 1982; 26:139-42.
307. Baraka A, Louis F, Dalleh R. Maternal awareness and neonatal outcome after ketamine induction of anaesthesia for Caesarean section. Can J Anaesth 1990; 37:641-4.
308. Mankowitz E, Downing JW, Brock-Utne JG, et al. Total intravenous anaesthesia using low-dose ketamine infusion for caesarean section. A comparison with a standard inhalation anaesthetic technique. S Afr Med J 1984; 65:246-50.
309. Krissel J, Dick WF, Leyser KH, et al. Thiopentone, thiopentone/ketamine, and ketamine for induction of anaesthesia in caesarean section. Eur J Anaesthesiol 1994; 11:115-22.
310. Schultetus RR, Hill CR, Dharamraj CM, et al. Wakefulness during cesarean section after anesthetic induction with ketamine, thiopental, or ketamine and thiopental combined. Anesth Analg 1986; 65:723-8.
311. Orme RM, Grange CS, Ainsworth QP, et al. General anaesthesia using remifentanil for caesarean section in parturients with critical aortic stenosis: A series of four cases. Int J Obstet Anesth 2004; 13:183-7.
312. Esener Z, Sarihasan B, Guven H, et al. Thiopentone and etomidate concentrations in maternal and umbilical plasma, and in colostrum. Br J Anaesth 1992; 69:586-8.
313. Bergen JM, Smith DC. A review of etomidate for rapid sequence intubation in the emergency department. J Emerg Med 1997; 15:221-30.
314. Gregory MA, Davidson DG. Plasma etomidate levels in mother and fetus. Anaesthesia 1991; 46:716-8.
315. Downing JW, Buley RJ, Brock-Utne JG, et al. Etomidate for induction of anaesthesia at caesarean section: Comparison with thiopentone. Br J Anaesth 1979; 51:135-40.
316. Crozier TA, Flamm C, Speer CP, et al. Effects of etomidate on the adrenocortical and metabolic adaptation of the neonate. Br J Anaesth 1993; 70:47-53.
317. Reddy BK, Pizer B, Bull PT. Neonatal serum cortisol suppression by etomidate compared with thiopentone, for elective caesarean section. Eur J Anaesthesiol 1988; 5:171-6.
318. Crawford ME, Carl P, Bach V, et al. A randomized comparison between midazolam and thiopental for elective cesarean section anesthesia. I. Mothers. Anesth Analg 1989; 68:229-33.
319. Ravlo O, Carl P, Crawford ME, et al. A randomized comparison between midazolam and thiopental for elective cesarean section anesthesia: II. Neonates. Anesth Analg 1989; 68:234-7.
320. Bland BA, Lawes EG, Duncan PW, et al. Comparison of midazolam and thiopental for rapid sequence anesthetic induction for elective cesarean section. Anesth Analg 1987; 66:1165-8.
321. Kvisselgaard N, Moya F. Investigation of placental thresholds to succinylcholine. Anesthesiology 1961; 22:7-10.
322. Shnider SM. Serum cholinesterase activity during pregnancy, labor and the puerperium. Anesthesiology 1965; 26:335-9.
323. Baraka A, Haroun S, Bassili M, et al. Response of the newborn to succinylcholine injection in homozygotic atypical mothers. Anesthesiology 1975; 43:115-6.
324. Kao YJ, Turner DR. Prolongation of succinylcholine block by metoclopramide. Anesthesiology 1989; 70:905-8.
325. Abouleish E, Abboud T, Lechevalier T, et al. Rocuronium (Org 9426) for caesarean section. Br J Anaesth 1994; 73:336-41.
326. Magorian T, Flannery KB, Miller RD. Comparison of rocuronium, succinylcholine, and vecuronium for rapid-sequence induction of anesthesia in adult patients. Anesthesiology 1993; 79:913-8.

327. Hawkins JL, Johnson TD, Kubicek MA, et al. Vecuronium for rapid-sequence intubation for cesarean section. Anesth Analg 1990; 71:185-90.
328. Hawkins JL, Adenwala J, Camp C, et al. The effect of H_2-receptor antagonist premedication on the duration of vecuronium-induced neuromuscular blockade in postpartum patients. Anesthesiology 1989; 71:175-7.
329. Dailey PA, Fisher DM, Shnider SM, et al. Pharmacokinetics, placental transfer, and neonatal effects of vecuronium and pancuronium administered during cesarean section. Anesthesiology 1984; 60:569-74.
330. Eikermann M, Peters J. Nerve stimulation at 0.15 Hz when compared to 0.1 Hz speeds the onset of action of cisatracurium and rocuronium. Acta Anaesthesiol Scand 2000; 44:170-4.
331. Warren TM, Datta S, Ostheimer GW, et al. Comparison of the maternal and neonatal effects of halothane, enflurane, and isoflurane for cesarean delivery. Anesth Analg 1983; 62:516-20.
332. Crawford JS. Awareness during operative obstetrics under general anaesthesia. Br J Anaesth 1971; 43:179-82.
333. Karasawa F, Takita A, Fukuda I, et al. Nitrous oxide concentrations in maternal and fetal blood during caesarean section. Eur J Anaesthesiol 2003; 20:555-9.
334. Palahniuk RJ, Cumming M. Foetal deterioration following thiopentone-nitrous oxide anaesthesia in the pregnant ewe. Can Anaesth Soc J 1977; 24:361-70.
335. Dwyer R, Fee JP, Moore J. Uptake of halothane and isoflurane by mother and baby during caesarean section. Br J Anaesth 1995; 74:379-83.
336. Munson ES, Embro WJ. Enflurane, isoflurane, and halothane and isolated human uterine muscle. Anesthesiology 1977; 46:11-4.
337. Dogru K, Yildiz K, Dalgic H, et al. Inhibitory effects of desflurane and sevoflurane on contractions of isolated gravid rat myometrium under oxytocin stimulation. Acta Anaesthesiol Scand 2003; 47:472-4.
338. Yildiz K, Dogru K, Dalgic H, et al. Inhibitory effects of desflurane and sevoflurane on oxytocin-induced contractions of isolated pregnant human myometrium. Acta Anaesthesiol Scand 2005; 49:1355-9.
339. Gultekin H, Yildiz K, Sezer Z, et al. Comparing the relaxing effects of desflurane and sevoflurane on oxytocin-induced contractions of isolated myometrium in both pregnant and nonpregnant rats. Adv Ther 2006; 23:39-46.
340. Ghaly RG, Flynn RJ, Moore J. Isoflurane as an alternative to halothane for caesarean section. Anaesthesia 1988; 43:5-7.
341. Gin T, Chan MT. Decreased minimum alveolar concentration of isoflurane in pregnant humans. Anesthesiology 1994; 81:829-32.
342. Chan MT, Mainland P, Gin T. Minimum alveolar concentration of halothane and enflurane are decreased in early pregnancy. Anesthesiology 1996; 85:782-6.
343. Datta S, Migliozzi RP, Flanagan HL, et al. Chronically administered progesterone decreases halothane requirements in rabbits. Anesth Analg 1989; 68:46-50.
344. Chan MT, Gin T. Postpartum changes in the minimum alveolar concentration of isoflurane. Anesthesiology 1995; 82:1360-3.
345. Bonica JJ. Local-regional analgesia for abdominal delivery. In Bonica JJ, editor. Obstetric Analgesia and Anesthesia. Philadelphia, FA Davis, 1967:527-38.
346. Waterstone M, Bewley S, Wolfe C. Incidence and predictors of severe obstetric morbidity: Case-control study. BMJ 2001; 322:1089-93.
347. Cohen SE, Hamilton CL, Riley ET, et al. Obstetric postanesthesia care unit stays: Reevaluation of discharge criteria after regional anesthesia. Anesthesiology 1998; 89:1559-65.
348. Thomas J, Paranjothy S. The National Sentinel Caesarean Section Audit Report: Clinical Effectiveness Support Unit of the Royal College of Obstetricians and Gynaecologists. London, RCOG, 2001.
349. Guidelines for Obstetric Anaesthesia Services. London, Association of Anaesthetists of Great Britain and Ireland and Obstetric Anaesthetists' Association, 1998.
350. Mangesi L, Hofmeyr GJ. Early compared with delayed oral fluids and food after caesarean section. Cochrane Database Syst Rev 2002; (3):CD003516.
351. Sharma KK, Mahmood TA, Smith NC. The short term effect of obstetric anaesthesia on bladder function. J Obstet Gynaecol 1994; 14:254-64.
352. Liang CC, Chang SD, Chang YL, et al. Postpartum urinary retention after cesarean delivery. Int J Gynaecol Obstet 2007; 99:229-32.
353. Onile TG, Kuti O, Orji EO, et al. A prospective randomized clinical trial of urethral catheter removal following elective cesarean delivery. Int J Gynaecol Obstet 2008; 102:267-70.
354. King H, Ashley S, Brathwaite D, et al. Adequacy of general anesthesia for cesarean section. Anesth Analg 1993; 77:84-8.
355. Moir DD. Anaesthesia for Caesarean section: An evaluation of a method using low concentrations of halothane and 50 per cent of oxygen. Br J Anaesth 1970; 42:136-42.
356. Lyons G, Macdonald R. Awareness during caesarean section. Anaesthesia 1991; 46:62-4.
357. Datta S, Ostheimer GW, Weiss JB, et al. Neonatal effect of prolonged anesthetic induction for cesarean section. Obstet Gynecol 1981; 58:331-5.
358. Yoo KY, Jeong CW, Kang MW, et al. Bispectral index values during sevoflurane-nitrous oxide general anesthesia in women undergoing cesarean delivery: A comparison between women with and without prior labor. Anesth Analg 2008; 106:1827-32.
359. Yeo SN, Lo WK. Bispectral Index in assessment of adequacy of general anaesthesia for lower segment caesarean section. Anaesth Intensive Care 2002; 30:36-40.
360. Ittichaikulthol W, Sriswasdi S, Prachanpanich N, et al. Bispectral Index in assessment of 3% and 4.5% desflurane in 50% N_2O for caesarean section. J Med Assoc Thai 2007; 90:1546-50.
361. Glass PS, Bloom M, Kearse L, et al. Bispectral analysis measures sedation and memory effects of propofol, midazolam, isoflurane, and alfentanil in healthy volunteers. Anesthesiology 1997; 86:836-47.
362. Mark LC, Poppers PJ. The dilemma of general anesthesia for cesarean section: Adequate fetal oxygenation vs. maternal awareness during operation. Anesthesiology 1982; 56:405-6.
363. Kanto J, Aaltonen L, Erkkola R, et al. Pharmacokinetics and sedative effect of midazolam in connection with caesarean section performed under epidural analgesia. Acta Anaesthesiol Scand 1984; 28:116-8.
364. Dahan A, Kest B, Waxman AR, Sarton E. Sex-specific responses to opiates: Animal and human studies. Anesth Analg 2008; 107:83-95.
365. Hoymork SC, Raeder J. Why do women wake up faster than men from propofol anaesthesia? Br J Anaesth 2005; 95:627-33.
366. Corke BC, Datta S, Ostheimer GW, et al. Spinal anaesthesia for Caesarean section: The influence of hypotension on neonatal outcome. Anaesthesia 1982; 37:658-62.
367. Cyna AM, Andrew M, Emmett RS, et al. Techniques for preventing hypotension during spinal anaesthesia for caesarean section. Cochrane Database Syst Rev 2006; (4):CD002251.
368. Mark JB, Steele SM. Cardiovascular effects of spinal anesthesia. Int Anesthesiol Clin 1989; 27:31-9.
369. Aya AGM, Mangin R, Vialles N, et al. Patients with severe preeclampsia experience less hypotension during spinal anesthesia for elective cesarean delivery than healthy parturients: A prospective cohort comparison. Anesth Analg 2003; 97:867-72.
370. Kinsella SM, Norris MC. Advance prediction of hypotension at cesarean delivery under spinal anesthesia. Int J Obstet Anesth 1996; 5:3-7.
371. Frolich MA, Caton D. Baseline heart rate may predict hypotension after spinal anesthesia in prehydrated obstetrical patients. Can J Anaesth 2002; 49:185-9.
372. Dahlgren G, Granath F, Wessel H, et al. Prediction of hypotension during spinal anesthesia for Cesarean section and its relation to the effect of crystalloid or colloid preload. Int J Obstet Anesth 2007; 16:128-34.
373. Chamchad D, Arkoosh VA, Horrow JC, et al. Using heart rate variability to stratify risk of obstetric patients undergoing spinal anesthesia. Anesth Analg 2004; 99:1818-21.
374. Hanss R, Ohnesorge H, Kaufmann M, et al. Changes in heart rate variability may reflect sympatholysis during spinal anaesthesia. Acta Anaesthesiol Scand 2007; 51:1297-304.

375. Hanss R, Bein B, Ledowski T, et al. Heart rate variability predicts severe hypotension after spinal anesthesia for elective cesarean delivery. Anesthesiology 2005; 102:1086-93.
376. Ouzounian JG, Masaki DI, Abboud TK, et al. Systemic vascular resistance index determined by thoracic electrical bioimpedance predicts the risk for maternal hypotension during regional anesthesia for cesarean delivery. Am J Obstet Gynecol 1996; 174:1019-25.
377. Dyer RA, Piercy JL, Reed AR, et al. Hemodynamic changes associated with spinal anesthesia for cesarean delivery in severe preeclampsia. Anesthesiology 2008; 108:802-11.
378. Langesaeter E. Is it more informative to focus on cardiac output than blood pressure during spinal anesthesia for cesarean delivery in women with severe preeclampsia? Anesthesiology 2008; 108: 771-2.
379. Ueyama H, He YL, Tanigami H, et al. Effects of crystalloid and colloid preload on blood volume in the parturient undergoing spinal anesthesia for elective Cesarean section. Anesthesiology 1999; 91: 1571-6.
380. Pouta AM, Karinen J, Vuolteenaho OJ, et al. Effect of intravenous fluid preload on vasoactive peptide secretion during Caesarean section under spinal anaesthesia. Anaesthesia 1996; 51:128-32.
381. Lee A, Ngan Kee WD, Gin T. A dose-response meta-analysis of prophylactic intravenous ephedrine for the prevention of hypotension during spinal anesthesia for elective cesarean delivery. Anesth Analg 2004; 98:483-90.
382. Ngan Kee WD, Khaw KS, Ng FF. Prevention of hypotension during spinal anesthesia for cesarean delivery: An effective technique using combination of phenylephrine infusion and crystalloid cohydration. Anesthesiology 2005; 103:744-50.
383. Ralston DH, Shnider SM, DeLorimier AA. Effects of equipotent ephedrine, metaraminol, mephentermine, and methoxamine on uterine blood flow in the pregnant ewe. Anesthesiology 1974; 40:354-70.
384. Tong C, Eisenach JC. The vascular mechanism of ephedrine's beneficial effect on uterine perfusion during pregnancy. Anesthesiology 1992; 76:792-8.
385. Li P, Tong C, Eisenach JC. Pregnancy and ephedrine increase the release of nitric oxide in ovine uterine arteries. Anesth Analg 1996; 82:288-93.
386. Lee A, Ngan Kee WD, Gin T. A quantitative, systematic review of randomized controlled trials of ephedrine versus phenylephrine for the management of hypotension during spinal anesthesia for cesarean delivery. Anesth Analg 2002; 94:920-6.
387. Cooper DW, Carpenter M, Mowbray P, et al. Fetal and maternal effects of phenylephrine and ephedrine during spinal anesthesia for cesarean delivery. Anesthesiology 2002; 97:1582-90.
388. Mercier FJ, Riley ET, Frederickson WL, et al. Phenylephrine added to prophylactic ephedrine infusion during spinal anesthesia for elective cesarean section. Anesthesiology 2001; 95:668-74.
389. Loughrey JP, Yao N, Datta S, et al. Hemodynamic effects of spinal anesthesia and simultaneous intravenous bolus of combined phenylephrine and ephedrine versus ephedrine for cesarean delivery. Int J Obstet Anesth 2005; 14:43-7.
390. Ngan Kee WD, Tam YH, Khaw KS, et al. Closed-loop feedback computer-controlled infusion of phenylephrine for maintaining blood pressure during spinal anaesthesia for caesarean section: A preliminary descriptive study. Anaesthesia 2007; 62:1251-6.
391. Riley ET. Spinal anaesthesia for Caesarean delivery: Keep the pressure up and don't spare the vasoconstrictors. Br J Anaesth 2004; 92:459-61.
392. Datta S, Alper MH, Ostheimer GW, et al. Method of ephedrine administration and nausea and hypotension during spinal anesthesia for cesarean section. Anesthesiology 1982; 56:68-70.
393. Ngan Kee WD, Khaw KS, Ng FF. Comparison of phenylephrine infusion regimens for maintaining maternal blood pressure during spinal anaesthesia for Caesarean section. Br J Anaesth 2004; 92:469-74.
394. Eappen S, Blinn A, Segal S. Incidence of epidural catheter replacement in parturients: A retrospective chart review. Int J Obstet Anesth 1998; 7:220-5.
395. Higuchi H, Adachi Y, Kazama T. Effects of epidural saline injection on cerebrospinal fluid volume and velocity waveform: A magnetic resonance imaging study. Anesthesiology 2005; 102:285-92.
396. Goodwin TM, Hershman JM, Cole L. Increased concentration of the free beta-subunit of human chorionic gonadotropin in hyperemesis gravidarum. Acta Obstet Gynecol Scand 1994; 73:770-2.
397. Lacroix R, Eason E, Melzack R. Nausea and vomiting during pregnancy: A prospective study of its frequency, intensity, and patterns of change. Am J Obstet Gynecol 2000; 182:931-7.
398. Holmgren C, Aagaard-Tillery KM, Silver RM, et al. Hyperemesis in pregnancy: An evaluation of treatment strategies with maternal and neonatal outcomes. Am J Obstet Gynecol 2008; 198:56. e1-4.
399. Balki M, Carvalho JC. Intraoperative nausea and vomiting during cesarean section under regional anesthesia. Int J Obstet Anesth 2005; 14:230-41.
400. Borgeat A, Ekatodramis G, Schenker CA. Postoperative nausea and vomiting in regional anesthesia: A review. Anesthesiology 2003; 98:530-47.
401. Pinder AJ, Dresner M, Calow C, et al. Haemodynamic changes caused by oxytocin during caesarean section under spinal anaesthesia. Int J Obstet Anesth 2002; 11:156-9.
402. Dansereau J, Joshi AK, Helewa ME, et al. Double-blind comparison of carbetocin versus oxytocin in prevention of uterine atony after cesarean section. Am J Obstet Gynecol 1999; 180:670-6.
403. Alahuhta S, Kangas-Saarela T, Hollmen AI, et al. Visceral pain during caesarean section under spinal and epidural anaesthesia with bupivacaine. Acta Anaesthesiol Scand 1990; 34:95-8.
404. Gan TJ. Risk factors for postoperative nausea and vomiting. Anesth Analg 2006; 102:1884-98.
405. Apfel CC, Laara E, Koivuranta M, et al. A simplified risk score for predicting postoperative nausea and vomiting: Conclusions from cross-validations between two centers. Anesthesiology 1999; 91:693-700.
406. Goodwin TM. Nausea and vomiting of pregnancy: An obstetric syndrome. Am J Obstet Gynecol 2002; 186:S184-9.
407. Kreis ME. Postoperative nausea and vomiting. Auton Neurosci 2006; 129:86-91.
408. Kranke P, Eberhart LH, Gan TJ, et al. Algorithms for the prevention of postoperative nausea and vomiting: An efficacy and efficiency simulation. Eur J Anaesthesiol 2007; 24:856-67.
409. Lussos SA, Bader AM, Thornhill ML, et al. The antiemetic efficacy and safety of prophylactic metoclopramide for elective cesarean delivery during spinal anesthesia. Reg Anesth 1992; 17:126-30.
410. Chestnut DH, Vandewalker GE, Owen CL, et al. Administration of metoclopramide for prevention of nausea and vomiting during epidural anesthesia for elective cesarean section. Anesthesiology 1987; 66:563-6.
411. Abouleish EI, Rashid S, Haque S, et al. Ondansetron versus placebo for the control of nausea and vomiting during Caesarean section under spinal anaesthesia. Anaesthesia 1999; 54:479-82.
412. Pan PH, Moore CH. Comparing the efficacy of prophylactic metoclopramide, ondansetron, and placebo in cesarean section patients given epidural anesthesia. J Clin Anesth 2001; 13:430-5.
413. Han DW, Hong SW, Kwon JY, et al. Epidural ondansetron is more effective to prevent postoperative pruritus and nausea than intravenous ondansetron in elective cesarean delivery. Acta Obstet Gynecol Scand 2007; 86:683-7.
414. Harnett MJ, O'Rourke N, Walsh M, et al. Transdermal scopolamine for prevention of intrathecal morphine-induced nausea and vomiting after cesarean delivery. Anesth Analg 2007; 105:764-9.
415. Duggal KN, Douglas MJ, Peteru EA, et al. Acupressure for intrathecal narcotic-induced nausea and vomiting after caesarean section. Int J Obstet Anesth 1998; 7:231-6.
416. Ho CM, Hseu SS, Tsai SK, et al. Effect of P-6 acupressure on prevention of nausea and vomiting after epidural morphine for post-cesarean section pain relief. Acta Anaesthesiol Scand 1996; 40:372-5.
417. Harmon D, Ryan M, Kelly A, et al. Acupressure and prevention of nausea and vomiting during and after spinal anaesthesia for caesarean section. Br J Anaesth 2000; 84:463-7.

418. Stein DJ, Birnbach DJ, Danzer BI, et al. Acupressure versus intravenous metoclopramide to prevent nausea and vomiting during spinal anesthesia for cesarean section. Anesth Analg 1997; 84:342-5.
419. Ho CM, Tsai HJ, Chan KH, et al. P6 acupressure does not prevent emesis during spinal anesthesia for cesarean delivery. Anesth Analg 2006; 102:900-3.
420. Phillips TW Jr, Broussard DM, Sumrall WD, et al. Intraoperative oxygen administration does not reduce the incidence or severity of nausea or vomiting associated with neuraxial anesthesia for cesarean delivery. Anesth Analg 2007; 105:1113-7.
421. Goll V, Akca O, Greif R, et al. Ondansetron is no more effective than supplemental intraoperative oxygen for prevention of postoperative nausea and vomiting. Anesth Analg 2001; 92:112-7.
422. Numazaki M, Fujii Y. Subhypnotic dose of propofol for the prevention of nausea and vomiting during spinal anaesthesia for caesarean section. Anaesth Intensive Care 2000; 28:262-5.
423. Numazaki M, Fujii Y. Reduction of emetic symptoms during cesarean delivery with antiemetics: Propofol at subhypnotic dose versus traditional antiemetics. J Clin Anesth 2003; 15:423-7.
424. Fujii Y, Numazaki M. Randomized, double-blind comparison of subhypnotic-dose propofol alone and combined with dexamethasone for emesis in parturients undergoing cesarean delivery. Clin Ther 2004; 26:1286-91.
425. Carvalho B, Cohen SE, Lipman SS, et al. Patient preferences for anesthesia outcomes associated with cesarean delivery. Anesth Analg 2005; 101:1182-7.
426. Thind GS, Wells JC, Wilkes RG. The effects of continuous intravenous naloxone on epidural morphine analgesia. Anaesthesia 1986; 41:582-5.
427. Hess PE, Snowman CE, Hahn CJ, et al. Chloroprocaine may not affect epidural morphine for postcesarean delivery analgesia. J Clin Anesth 2006; 18:29-33.
428. Karambelkar DJ, Ramanathan S. 2-Chloroprocaine antagonism of epidural morphine analgesia. Acta Anaesthesiol Scand 1997; 41:774-8.
429. American Academy of Pediatrics Committee on Drugs. The transfer of drugs and other chemicals into human milk. Pediatrics 2001; 108:776-89.
430. Douglas MJ, Kim JH, Ross PL, et al. The effect of epinephrine in local anaesthetic on epidural morphine-induced pruritus. Can Anaesth Soc J 1986; 33:737-40.
431. Szarvas S, Harmon D, Murphy D. Neuraxial opioid-induced pruritus: A review. J Clin Anesth 2003; 15:234-9.
432. Yeh HM, Chen LK, Lin CJ, et al. Prophylactic intravenous ondansetron reduces the incidence of intrathecal morphine-induced pruritus in patients undergoing cesarean delivery. Anesth Analg 2000; 91:172-5.
433. Kranke P, Eberhart LH, Rower N, Tramer MR. Pharmacological treatment of postoperative shivering: A quantitative systematic review of randomized controlled trials. Anesth Analg 2002; 94:453-60.
434. Cunningham FG, Leveno KJ, Bloom SL, et al. Williams Obstetrics. 22nd edition. New York, McGraw-Hill, 2005:587-606.
435. Bolton TJ, Randall K, Yentis SM. Effect of the Confidential Enquiries into Maternal Deaths on the use of Syntocinon at Caesarean section in the UK. Anaesthesia 2003; 58:277-9.
436. Svanström MC, Biber B, Hanes M, et al. Signs of myocardial ischaemia after injection of oxytocin: A randomized double-blind comparison of oxytocin and methylergometrine during Caesarean section. Br J Anaesth 2008; 100:683-9.
437. Archer TL, Knape K, Liles D, et al. The hemodynamics of oxytocin and other vasoactive agents during neuraxial anesthesia for cesarean delivery: Findings in six cases. Int J Obstet Anesth 2008; 17:247-54.
438. Ogata J, Minami K. Synthetic oxytocin and latex allergy. Br J Anaesth 2007; 98:845-6.
439. Munn MB, Owen JV. Comparison of two oxytocin regimens to prevent uterine atony at cesarean delivery: A randomized controlled trial. Obstet Gynecol 2001; 98:386-90.
440. Zingg HH. Vasopressin and oxytocin receptors. Baillieres Clin Endocrinol Metab 1996; 10:75-96.
441. Abouleish E. Postpartum hypertension and convulsion after oxytocic drugs. Anesth Analg 1976; 55:813-5.
442. Balki M, Dhumne S, Kasodekar S, et al. Oxytocin-ergometrine co-administration does not reduce blood loss at caesarean delivery for labour arrest. Br J Obstet Gynaecol 2008; 115:579-84.
443. Cunningham FG, Leveno KJ, Bloom SL, et al. Williams Obstetrics. 22nd edition. New York, McGraw-Hill, 2005:809-54.
444. Chou MM, MacKenzie IZ. A prospective, double-blind, randomized comparison of prophylactic intramyometrial 15-methyl prostaglandin F2 alpha, 125 micrograms, and intravenous oxytocin, 20 units, for the control of blood loss at elective cesarean section. Am J Obstet Gynecol 1994; 171:1356-60.
445. Oleen MA, Mariano JP. Controlling refractory atonic postpartum hemorrhage with Hemabate sterile solution. Am J Obstet Gynecol 1990; 162:205-8.
446. Hankins GD, Berryman GK, Scott RT, et al. Maternal arterial desaturation with 15-methyl prostaglandin F2 alpha for uterine atony. Obstet Gynecol 1988; 72:367-70.
447. Gülmezoglu AM, Forna F, Villar J, et al. Prostaglandins for preventing postpartum haemorrhage. Cochrane Database Syst Rev 2007; (3):CD000494.
448. de Souza A, Permezel M, Anderson M, et al. Antenatal erythropoietin and intra-operative cell salvage in a Jehovah's Witness with placenta praevia. Br J Obstet Gynaecol 2003; 110:524-6.
449. Resch BE, Gaspar R, Sonkodi S, et al. Vasoactive effects of erythropoietin on human placental blood vessels in vitro. Am J Obstet Gynecol 2003; 188:993-6.
450. Teramo KA, Hiilesmaa VK, Schwartz R, et al. Amniotic fluid and cord plasma erythropoietin levels in pregnancies complicated by preeclampsia, pregnancy-induced hypertension and chronic hypertension. J Perinat Med 2004; 32:240-7.
451. Allam J, Cox M, Yentis SM. Cell salvage in obstetrics. Int J Obstet Anesth 2008; 17:37-45.
452. Sullivan I, Faulds J, Ralph C. Contamination of salvaged maternal blood by amniotic fluid and fetal red cells during elective caesarean section. Br J Anaesth 2008; 101:225-9.
453. Posner LP, Moon PF, Bliss SP, et al. Colloid osmotic pressure after hemorrhage and replenishment with Oxyglobin Solution, hetastarch, or whole blood in pregnant sheep. Vet Anaesth Analg 2003; 30:30-6.
454. American Society of Anesthesiologists Task Force on Blood Component Therapy. Practice guidelines for blood component therapy. Anesthesiology 1996; 84:732-47.
455. Hansch E, Chitkara U, McAlpine J, et al. Pelvic arterial embolization for control of obstetric hemorrhage: A five-year experience. Am J Obstet Gynecol 1999; 180:1454-60.
456. O'Rourke N, McElrath T, Baum R, et al. Cesarean delivery in the interventional radiology suite: A novel approach to obstetric hemostasis. Anesth Analg 2007; 104:1193-4.
457. Condous GS, Arulkumaran S, Symonds I, et al. The "tamponade test" in the management of massive postpartum hemorrhage. Obstet Gynecol 2003; 101:767-72.
458. Marcovici I, Scoccia B. Postpartum hemorrhage and intrauterine balloon tamponade: A report of three cases. J Reprod Med 1999; 44:122-6.
459. Sinha SM. The "tamponade test" in the management of massive postpartum hemorrhage. Obstet Gynecol 2003; 102:641.
460. Bouwmeester FW, Jonkhoff AR, Verheijen RH, et al. Successful treatment of life-threatening postpartum hemorrhage with recombinant activated factor VII. Obstet Gynecol 2003; 101:1174-6.
461. Branch DW, Rodgers GM. Recombinant activated factor VII: A new weapon in the fight against hemorrhage. Obstet Gynecol 2003; 101:1155-6.
462. Daskalakis G, Anastasakis E, Papantoniou N, et al. Emergency obstetric hysterectomy. Acta Obstet Gynecol Scand 2007; 86:223-7.
463. El-Sayed YY, Watkins MM, Fix M, et al. Perinatal outcomes after successful and failed trials of labor after cesarean delivery. Am J Obstet Gynecol 2007; 196:583.e1-5.
464. Zelop CM, Harlow BL, Frigoletto FD Jr, et al. Emergency peripartum hysterectomy. Am J Obstet Gynecol 1993; 168:1443-8.

465. Glaze S, Ekwalanga P, Roberts G, et al. Peripartum hysterectomy: 1999 to 2006. Obstet Gynecol 2008; 111:732-8.
466. Comstock CH, Love JJ Jr, Bronsteen RA, et al. Sonographic detection of placenta accreta in the second and third trimesters of pregnancy. Am J Obstet Gynecol 2004; 190:1135-40.
467. American College of Obstetricians and Gynecologists. Postpartum hemorrhage. ACOG Educational Bulletin No. 243. Washington, DC, ACOG, January 1998. (Int J Gynaecol Obstet 1998; 61:79-86.)
468. Fuller AJ, Carvalho B, Brummel C, et al. Epidural anesthesia for elective cesarean delivery with intraoperative arterial occlusion balloon catheter placement. Anesth Analg 2006; 102:585-7.
469. Chestnut DH, Dewan DM, Redick LF, et al. Anesthetic management for obstetric hysterectomy: A multi-institutional study. Anesthesiology 1989; 70:607-10.
470. Briery CM, Rose CH, Hudson WT, et al. Planned vs emergent cesarean hysterectomy. Am J Obstet Gynecol 2007; 197:154. e1-5.
471. Simpson EL, Lawrenson RA, Nightingale AL, et al. Venous thromboembolism in pregnancy and the puerperium: Incidence and additional risk factors from a London perinatal database. Br J Obstet Gynaecol 2001; 108:56-60.
472. Gates S, Brocklehurst P, Davis LJ. Prophylaxis for venous thromboembolic disease in pregnancy and the early postnatal period. Cochrane Database Syst Rev 2002; (2):CD001689.
473. Gates S, Brocklehurst P, Ayers S, et al. Thromboprophylaxis and pregnancy: Two randomized controlled pilot trials that used low-molecular-weight heparin. Am J Obstet Gynecol 2004; 191:1296-303.

Postoperative Analgesia: Systemic and Local Techniques

David Hepner, M.D.
Sunil Eappen, M.D.

Optimal postcesarean analgesia allows early ambulation and is associated with minimal side effects such as sedation and nausea. Many women undergoing cesarean delivery in developed countries currently receive neuraxial opioids for postcesarean analgesia.[1] Neuraxial opioids are highly effective, but many patients require additional analgesics for ongoing pain control[2]; also, patients who receive general anesthesia typically require systemic analgesics for postoperative analgesia. A paucity of studies has specifically examined the mechanisms and sequelae of postcesarean pain. This chapter reviews and summarizes the data on the use of systemic and local techniques for postoperative analgesia in obstetric patients.

PAIN PATHWAYS

The skin, abdominal wall, and uterine incisions for cesarean delivery generate postoperative pain. Although most cesarean deliveries are performed with a low horizontal Pfannenstiel skin incision, an infraumbilical midline vertical incision may be used when an expedited delivery is required.[3,4] Whether the severity of postoperative pain from the two types of incisions differs has not been robustly evaluated; however, it is logical to expect that the smaller number of sensory dermatomes involved in a transverse skin incision (T11 to T12) may result in less pain than a vertical incision (T10 to L1).

Whether skin and visceral nociception are transmitted by different nerve fiber subgroups or discharge patterns is controversial.[5,6] The uterine (visceral) afferent fibers stimulated by pressure and vasoconstriction primarily include C fibers with some A-delta fibers. By contrast, the majority of afferent fibers that relay nociceptive stimuli from the skin are A-delta fibers. Postoperative pain results from **direct trauma** to nerve endings and subsequent **inflammation** induced by tissue injury.[7,8] These components may yield different sensations of pain that might benefit from different types of therapy. In clinical practice, analgesic agents are administered to treat both types of pain simultaneously. Although multimodal therapy has long been advocated for postoperative pain in nonobstetric patients,[9] the same strategy has only recently been advocated for the provision of postcesarean analgesia.[10-12]

PSYCHOLOGICAL FACTORS

Pain is a subjective experience with physiologic, cognitive, cultural, social, and emotional factors. Observations from studies performed in nonobstetric patients may not be directly applicable to obstetric patients undergoing cesarean delivery. Postpartum pain may be modulated by the unique hormonal and emotional changes of pregnancy; stress, anxiety, and depression can accompany postpartum sleep disturbances and the responsibilities of providing care for a newborn infant.[13]

Preoperative anxiety and **postoperative depression** affect the use of—and satisfaction with—postoperative analgesic techniques. Higher preoperative anxiety scores are associated with greater intravenous morphine bolus demands in patients receiving patient-controlled analgesia (PCA) after abdominal hysterectomy.[14] Postoperative depression is also associated with higher opioid requirements.[14] To assess the contribution of anxiety to postoperative pain, Egan et al.[15] utilized two separate patient-controlled pumps in women who had undergone abdominal hysterectomy. One pump contained either midazolam or a placebo; patients were instructed to use this pump when they felt anxious, tense, or worried. The other pump contained morphine; patients were instructed to use this pump when they felt pain. Patients in the midazolam group had lower visual analog anxiety scores, but there was no difference between groups in the overall severity of pain or amount of PCA morphine used. The low dose of midazolam (0.125-mg bolus with a lockout interval of 8 minutes) may have accounted for the lack of effect on the pain scores. Nevertheless, careful assessment of and attention to postoperative anxiety are essential for the optimal management of postoperative pain. In addition, preoperative patient education about PCA is associated with an improvement in postoperative analgesia.[14]

PREDICTORS OF PAIN

A few investigations have evaluated preoperative predictors of the severity of pain and the requirements for analgesia after cesarean delivery.[13,16] In one study, the **magnitude estimation of suprathreshold heat pain stimuli,** but not the determination of the heat pain threshold, identified patients who were more likely to experience severe postcesarean pain at rest and during activity.[16] The investigators in this study suggested that suprathreshold painful stimuli "more closely mimic the postcesarean clinical pain experience ... at a level between threshold and tolerance."[16] Another study demonstrated that the evaluation of the **thermal pain threshold** predicted pain with activity, overall pain, and analgesic requirements after cesarean delivery; these observations may be explained, in part, by the investigators' evaluation of pain thresholds both at the dermatomes specifically involved in the generation of postcesarean pain and at the more traditional evaluation site on the volar surface of the forearm.[13]

Patient expectations of postcesarean pain have also been associated with pain at rest but not during activity; however, preexisting pain during pregnancy is not a predictor of postcesarean pain.[13] Preoperative increases in blood pressure, which may reflect patient anxiety, have also been strongly correlated with overall pain.[14] Preoperative anxiety, as measured by State Trait and Anxiety Inventory (STAI), was found to be an important predictor of postcesarean analgesic requirements.[13]

The experience of pain appears to be associated with **genetic variability of the μ-opioid receptor**.[17-19] Landau et al.[17] demonstrated a 19% frequency of the G118 allele of the μ-opioid receptor in a diverse obstetric population. The G118 allele has been associated with higher pressure pain thresholds, and also with lower heat pain ratings in men but higher heat pain ratings in women.[20] In women homozygous for the G118 allele, a greater use of PCA morphine has been observed after total abdominal hysterectomy.[18,19] Investigators have suggested that the presence of the G118 allele may promote μ-opioid receptor receptivity and binding affinity for beta-endorphin, an endogenous opioid that activates the receptor.[21] Furthermore, beta-endorphin is more potent in signal transduction in the presence of this allele.[21] Someday anesthesia providers may be able to identify which patients will experience greater postcesarean pain and have greater analgesic requirements.

THE JOINT COMMISSION MANDATE

In January 2001, The Joint Commission (formerly known as the Joint Commission on the Accreditation of Healthcare Organizations [JCAHO]) announced new standards requiring the appropriate assessment and management of pain in hospitalized patients.[22,23] The Joint Commission emphasized the need to assess pain in a standardized manner, including the use of an 11-point visual analog pain scale (i.e., a scale of 0 to 10, in which 0 represents no pain and 10 represents severe pain). The Joint Commission stated that appropriate pain management leads to faster clinical recovery with a shorter hospital stay and a lower likelihood of readmission. The Joint Commission has encouraged a **multidisciplinary, multimodal approach** to pain management; physicians, nurses, pharmacists, and other health care providers should be involved in postoperative pain management.

ANALGESIC AGENTS

Opioids

Opioids bind to pre- and post-synaptic receptors in the central nervous system (CNS), particularly the brainstem and spinal cord.[24] When bound to these receptors, opioids inhibit adenylate cyclase activity, resulting in the suppression of spontaneous and evoked responses. Furthermore, opioids interfere with the release of neurotransmitters, including acetylcholine, dopamine, norepinephrine, and substance P, and prevent the transmembrane transport of calcium ions.[24] Opioids are classified according to their chemical structure (Table 27-1).

The analgesic effect of opioids can vary significantly among patients, with up to a fivefold difference in the maximum blood drug concentrations still associated with pain (MCP).[25] The MCP decreases over time after a surgical procedure. The goal of opioid administration is to achieve a minimum effective analgesic concentration (MEAC) with minimal side effects.[26] Because the MEAC, like the MCP, varies greatly among patients, an **individualized approach** to pain control is required. There are no maximum allowable doses for specific opioids, so the primary limiting factor in this individualized approach is the occurrence of side effects (Table 27-2).

Patients with hepatic or renal dysfunction (which may occur with severe preeclampsia), obstructive sleep apnea, or morbid obesity are particularly susceptible to the respiratory depressant effects of opioids. It is important to monitor the respiratory rate and sedation level of a patient before giving an additional dose or adjusting the bolus dose that the patient can self-administer; patients who have never received opioids may be especially prone to the occurrence

TABLE 27-1 Commonly Used Opioids Classified According to Chemical Structure

Classification	Opioid
Phenanthrenes	Codeine Hydrocodone Hydromorphone Levorphanol Morphine Oxycodone Oxymorphone
Phenylpiperidines	Fentanyl Meperidine Sufentanil
Diphenylheptanes	Methadone Propoxyphene

Table courtesy of the Dana Farber Cancer Institute Pain and Palliative Care Program and the Brigham and Women's Hospital Pain Committee. Modified with permission from Bridget C. Fowler, Pharm. D., Clinical Pharmacy Manager, Dana Farber Cancer Institute.

of side effects. After adjusting the dose, the physician must document the respiratory rate and pattern, sedation level, and analgesic response. The use of a multimodal analgesic approach helps provide adequate analgesia while limiting opioid-related side effects (see later).

In the past, opioids were commonly administered intramuscularly or subcutaneously; these simple routes of administration do not require the postoperative return of bowel activity or the use of sophisticated equipment.[27] Intramuscular and subcutaneous medications are inexpensive, easy to administer, and associated with a long history of safety. Disadvantages of this approach include the need for repeated painful injections, a delayed (and sometimes erratic) absorption of drug, and an inconsistent analgesic response due to variations in plasma opioid concentrations.[27]

Bloomfield et al.[28] evaluated the analgesic efficacy and potency of the use of two oral controlled-released morphine preparations after cesarean delivery beginning on the second or third postoperative day. Overall, the 90-mg dose of MS Contin was more effective than the 30- or 90-mg doses of Oramorph SR and the 30-mg dose of MS Contin. Side effects (primarily drowsiness) were mild to moderate and dose related, with a similar incidence observed at equipotent doses.[28] The administration of oral preparations of opioids as the sole analgesic modality for postcesarean analgesia has been investigated[29,30]; advantages of this approach are cost-effectiveness, facilitation of early mobility by discontinuation of the intravenous catheter and other equipment, and, perhaps, greater patient satisfaction.

A **multimodal regimen** that includes oral **nonsteroidal anti-inflammatory drugs (NSAIDs)** may be more effective than opioids alone. Jakobi et al.[29] compared the oral administration of the NSAID **dipyrone** 1 g as needed (prn) and a rescue oral dose of immediate-release morphine 30 mg with the same dose of morphine given prn and a rescue dose of dipyrone. Only one of 109 patients in the dipyrone group crossed over to the morphine group for the second analgesia request, whereas 18 of 90 (20%) patients in the morphine group crossed over to the dipyrone group. Among the patients who left the morphine group, the primary reasons for change were insufficient analgesia and complaints of drowsiness. Patients who remained in their assigned groups reported high satisfaction scores, with only 30% requesting additional analgesia after the first 24 hours following cesarean delivery. Dipyrone is no longer marketed in the United States and much of Europe because of the rare, but serious adverse effects, including agranulocytosis, aplastic anemia, thrombocytopenic purpura, and hemolytic anemia.[31,32] The use of dipyrone is justified primarily in the treatment of severe pain in developing countries where suitable alternatives are not readily available.[33]

Regardless of whether opioids are administered alone or in combination with NSAIDs, it may be important to administer analgesics at fixed intervals rather than on a prn basis. Jakobi et al.[30] assessed patient satisfaction and pain scores with an oral NSAID (**ibuprofen** 400 mg), when given at regular fixed intervals or on patient demand. The patients in the fixed-interval group received their first dose of ibuprofen 3 hours after cesarean delivery; by contrast, the first request for analgesia in the prn group occurred more than 5 hours after surgery. Although the rates of use of rescue (oral morphine) analgesia were not significantly different in the two groups (18.5% in the fixed-interval group and 25% in the on-demand group), higher overall patient satisfaction and significantly lower pain scores were found in the fixed-interval group.[30] These and other data suggest that patients do not always ask for analgesia despite being in pain. Thus, there may be a benefit in giving analgesic agents early and at fixed intervals, especially in the first 12 to 24 hours after cesarean delivery.

The American Society of Anesthesiologists (ASA) Practice Guidelines for Obstetric Anesthesia recommend the use of neuraxial opioids over the use of intermittent intravenous or intramuscular administration of opioids for postcesarean analgesia.[34] (The guidelines acknowledge that the literature is insufficient to enable comparison of the efficacy of neuraxial opioids with that of intravenous PCA.[34]) However, some institutions may not have the capability to monitor postoperative patients receiving neuraxial opioids. In these circumstances, intravenous PCA is a commonly used and viable alternative to neuraxial opioids.[35]

Meperidine PCA has been utilized with intravenous and epidural routes of administration. The two routes of administration have similar onsets of analgesia, but higher pain scores with rest and movement, greater sedation, and lower patient satisfaction have been observed with the intravenous route.[36] Moreover, plasma meperidine and normeperidine concentrations are almost double when the intravenous route is used.[36] Similarly, another study that compared intravenous with epidural **fentanyl** after cesarean delivery reported higher pain scores and greater fentanyl consumption with the intravenous route; nonetheless, patient satisfaction ratings were similar in the two groups.[37] Another study compared intravenous with epidural hydromorphone after cesarean delivery.[38] Hydromorphone requirements were threefold to fourfold higher in the intravenous group. The two groups had similar pain and sedation scores, but patients in the intravenous group had greater drowsiness and less pruritus.[38]

TABLE 27-2 Management of Opioid Side Effects*

Adverse Effect(s)	Management Considerations
Allergic reaction	True immunoglobulin E–mediated allergic reactions are rare. Anaphylactoid-type signs and symptoms (e.g., hypotension, bronchoconstriction) are usually secondary to mast cell activation and subsequent histamine release. Selection of another opioid class is usually necessary only in the event of a documented true allergic reaction (e.g., rash, hives, difficulty breathing).
Confusion, delirium, hallucinations	Reduce dose, use a different opioid, and/or give neuroleptic therapy (e.g., haloperidol) or olanzapine.
Constipation	Consider prophylaxis when opioid therapy is initiated. Include a mild stimulant laxative (senna) ± stool softener (docusate salts at night or twice daily) as prophylaxis. Consider adding lactulose or Miralax when necessary. In patients allowed no oral intake, consider intravenous metoclopramide.
Myoclonic jerking	Reduce dose, use a different opioid, and/or treat with clonazepam or baclofen.
Nausea/vomiting	Tolerance may develop. It may be helpful to administer one antiemetic on a fixed schedule for a few days in patients with a prior history of opioid-associated nausea and vomiting. Otherwise, the following treatment can be given on an as-needed basis: metoclopramide, ondansetron, prochlorperazine, promethazine, or a scopolamine patch.
Pruritus	Pruritus in the absence of rash is a central μ receptor–related phenomenon (not related to histamine). It is best treated with nalbuphine intravenously as needed and not with an antihistamine. For refractory pruritus, consider changing opioids.
Respiratory depression	Withhold opioid, use tactile and verbal stimulation, and implement supportive measures. Assist ventilation with bag-valve mask and supplemental oxygen if patient cannot be aroused. Give dilute naloxone (0.4 mg in 9 mL normal saline, or 40 μg/mL) in 1- to 2-mL increments at 2- to 3-minute intervals until a response is observed. Naloxone's half-life is shorter than that of most of the opioid agonists, and respiratory depression may recur. Be alert for the need to re-administer a bolus dose of naloxone, or consider use of a naloxone infusion.
Sedation	Tolerance typically develops. First withhold sedatives and anxiolytics; then consider withholding the opioid or reduce the dose. If sedation is persistent, consider a central nervous system stimulant such as caffeine, methylphenidate, or dextroamphetamine.

*Nonopioid analgesic options should be considered to limit opioid-related side effects. All adverse events should be carefully evaluated to rule out other potential causes.

Table courtesy of the Dana Farber Cancer Institute Pain and Palliative Care Program and the Brigham and Women's Hospital Pain Committee. Modified with permission from Bridget C. Fowler, Pharm. D., Clinical Pharmacy Manager, Dana Farber Cancer Institute.

Despite the improved analgesia provided by neuraxial opioids, some studies of postcesarean analgesia have demonstrated greater patient satisfaction with intravenous PCA than with single-dose epidural or intramuscular opioids.[39] This situation may reflect a more immediate response to patient-controlled bolus doses of opioid and an improved ability to titrate the level of analgesia and side effects (e.g., pruritus). However, in the majority of studies comparing intravenous with epidural PCA after cesarean delivery, the epidural route has been associated with lower pain scores, decreased total opioid consumption, and lower plasma opioid levels.[37,39] The epidural administration of morphine has also been associated with better postcesarean analgesia and side-effect profiles than that resulting from intravenous morphine.[40]

The ASA Task Force on Acute Pain Management supports the use of intravenous PCA rather than intramuscular opioid techniques for postoperative analgesia.[35] Intravenous meperidine PCA is associated with better postcesarean analgesia and less sedation than intramuscular meperidine.[41] Another study observed that patients receiving intramuscular meperidine experienced a longer delay in sitting, walking, and drinking after cesarean delivery than patients receiving intravenous meperidine PCA.[42] Studies utilizing other opioids have reported similar findings. Perez-Woods et al.[43] found that intravenous **morphine** PCA was associated with better analgesia and earlier ambulation, less sedation, and greater patient satisfaction than intramuscular morphine. In this study, a larger amount of morphine was used in the intravenous PCA group; however, a secondary hypothesis that more analgesia would lead to better respiratory function (i.e., vital capacity) was not demonstrated. Eisenach et al.[39] and Harrison et al.[44] compared outcomes for intravenous morphine PCA and intramuscular morphine for postcesarean analgesia. Although one trial demonstrated better analgesia, greater opioid use, and better patient satisfaction in the intravenous PCA group,[39] the other trial demonstrated no differences in quality of analgesia, opioid use, or length of hospital stay.[44] Both studies demonstrated a nonsignificant trend toward more pruritus in the intravenous PCA group but no overall differences between groups in the incidence of side effects.

Several meta-analyses have evaluated studies that compared **intravenous PCA** with other modalities for postoperative analgesia in patients who had undergone a variety of procedures, including cesarean delivery. One meta-analysis of 15 trials comparing the outcomes of intravenous PCA with those of intramuscular opioids demonstrated better analgesia and greater patient satisfaction with intravenous PCA.[45] There were no significant differences between groups in the occurrence of side effects, and trends toward less opioid use and shorter length of hospital stay in the intravenous PCA group were nonsignificant. None of these studies utilized a continuous basal (background) infusion with intravenous PCA. Another meta-analysis showed that intravenous PCA, compared with intramuscular, subcutaneous, or continuous intravenous opioid administration, resulted in better analgesia with no differences in opioid consumption or side effects.[46] A later Cochrane meta-analysis comparing intravenous PCA with conventional nurse-administered opioid analgesia demonstrated better postoperative analgesia and greater patient satisfaction with intravenous PCA.[47] However, the use of intravenous PCA was associated with greater opioid use and a higher incidence of pruritus but not of other side effects.[47] Potential reasons for the different results observed include the use of different opioids (although approximately 70% of the studies used morphine),[46] varied dosing regimens (e.g., dose, lockout interval, maximum allowable dose), variations in the timing of pain assessments, and the use of different analgesic end points. Also, differences in therapies for breakthrough pain, nausea, and pruritus may have affected the results.

In a study comparing intravenous morphine PCA with fentanyl PCA (without a background infusion) after cesarean delivery using general anesthesia, both opioids provided effective analgesia with no differences in patient satisfaction or side effects.[48] However, a higher number of patients in the fentanyl group required dose adjustments and supplemental analgesics to achieve satisfactory analgesia. This difference is likely a result of the shorter duration of action of intravenous fentanyl.

Intravenous morphine PCA has also been compared with intravenous meperidine PCA, as well as with intramuscular morphine and meperidine, for postcesarean analgesia.[49] Intravenous morphine PCA was associated with lower morphine consumption than intramuscular morphine, but with no difference in the quality of analgesia. By contrast, intravenous meperidine PCA was associated with greater drug consumption and better analgesia than intramuscular meperidine. Overall, intravenous morphine PCA and intramuscular morphine were more effective than intravenous meperidine PCA for pain control. Sinatra et al.,[50] who evaluated intravenous morphine, meperidine, and oxymorphone PCA at equipotent dosages without a background infusion for postcesarean delivery analgesia, demonstrated no differences among groups in overall opioid use. Although there were no differences among groups in analgesia at rest, more patients in the meperidine group had pain with movement. Oxymorphone had a faster onset of action but resulted in more nausea and vomiting. Patients in the morphine group experienced more sedation and pruritus. The investigators concluded that both oxymorphone and meperidine are useful alternatives to morphine for postcesarean intravenous PCA. However, the American College of Obstetricians and Gynecologists (ACOG)[51] now discourages the use of meperidine for this indication owing to the accumulation of the metabolite normeperidine in the neonate, which may worsen neurobehavioral scores. Wittels et al.[52] observed that nursing infants whose mothers received intravenous meperidine PCA for postcesarean analgesia had greater **neurobehavioral depression** than nursing infants exposed to morphine PCA.

Overall, factors that should affect the choice of opioid are speed of onset, duration of action, overall efficacy, and the type and frequency of side effects (Table 27-3). Should side effects prevent adequate analgesia, other opioids or nonopioid adjuvants should be used. Patient preferences based on past experiences and desired analgesia should also be considered.

In December 2004, The Joint Commission[53] issued a Sentinel Event Alert on PCA "by proxy" (i.e., when other individuals, including family members, become involved in drug administration). The Joint Commission acknowledged that PCA is a safe and effective method of controlling pain when used as prescribed; however, serious adverse events, including oversedation, respiratory depression, and death, can result when analgesia is delivered "by proxy." The Joint Commission[53] made the following recommendations: (1) develop criteria for selecting appropriate candidates for PCA, (2) carefully monitor patients, (3) teach patients and family members about the proper use of PCA and the dangers of others' pressing the button for the patient, (4) alert staff to the dangers of administering a dose outside a prescribed protocol, and (5) consider placing warning tags on all PCA delivery pendants stating, "Only the patient should press this button."

Health professionals who use PCA should (1) be able to evaluate candidates for PCA (e.g., mental state, level of consciousness, patient understanding); (2) know drug selection, dosing schedules, lockout periods, and infusion devices; (3) be able to provide patient education on pain management and the use of PCA; (4) understand when to alter PCA settings and when to give or withhold additional (rescue) doses of medications; and (5) be able to respond to side effects and adverse events.

A number of PCA variables must be considered, including drug choice, incremental dose, maximum dose, and lockout interval (Table 27-4). Owen et al.[25,54-56] performed a number of investigations with PCA in patients undergoing abdominal surgery. In an assessment of PCA morphine (demand bolus dose of 0.5, 1, or 2 mg with a 5-minute lockout interval), more patients in the 0.5-mg group had inadequate pain relief, whereas those in the 2-mg group had more side effects, including respiratory depression

TABLE 27-3 Opioid Characteristics

Agonist	Route	Onset (min)	Peak Effect (min)	Duration of Effect (hr)
Morphine	IV	5-10	10-30	3-5
	Oral	15-60	90-120	4
Codeine	IM	10-30	90-120	4-6
	Oral	30-45	60	3-4
Hydromorphone	IV	5-20	15-30	3-4
	Oral	15-30	90-120	4-6
Oxycodone	IV	—	—	—
	Oral	15-30	30-60	4-6
Methadone	IV	10-20	60-120	4-6
	Oral	30-60	90-120	4-12
Fentanyl	IV	< 1	5-7	0.75-2+
	Oral	—	—	—
Oxymorphone	IV	5-10	30-60	3-6
	Oral	60 (meaningful relief)	—	4-6

IM, intramuscular; IV, intravenous.

Table courtesy of the Dana Farber Cancer Institute Pain and Palliative Care Program and the Brigham and Women's Hospital Pain Committee. Modified with permission from Bridget C. Fowler, Pharm.D., Clinical Pharmacy Manager, Dana Farber Cancer Institute.

(respiratory rate less than 10 breaths/min).[54] These results correlated with the total dose of self-administered morphine. Although the role of the lockout interval was not addressed in this study, the investigators suggested that inadequate analgesia could be produced by lockout intervals that were too long or demand doses that were too small. By contrast, larger doses or shorter lockout intervals might lead to more opioid-related side effects. Therefore, longer lockout intervals typically require larger bolus doses, whereas smaller bolus doses typically require shorter lockout intervals.

Although patients who experience inadequate analgesia would be expected to make more PCA demands, this is often not the case.[54] It has been suggested that patients may expect a greater analgesic effect, are discouraged by an inadequate effect, or wait for a delayed effect.[54]

TABLE 27-4 General PCA Dosing in Opioid-Naive Patients

Drug	Morphine	Hydromorphone	Fentanyl
Concentration	5 mg/mL	1 mg/mL	10 μg/mL
PCA bolus dose	1-1.5 mg	0.2 mg	20 μg
Lockout interval (minutes)	7	7	7
4-hour dose limit	Calculated by settings	Calculated by settings	Calculated by settings
Typical PCA dose change	0.5 mg	0.1 mg	5 μg
Rescue doses	2 mg IV q 5 min (up to 3 doses)	0.3 mg IV q 5 min (up to 3 doses)	25 μg IV q 5 min (up to 3 doses)
Remarks	Relatively contraindicated in patients with impaired renal function	More potent than morphine	Shorter clinical effect

Recorded as: PCA bolus dose/lockout interval/4-hour limit/continuous infusion rate. A continuous background infusion is typically avoided except in selected cases (e.g., opioid tolerance).

IV, intravenous.

Table courtesy of the Dana Farber Cancer Institute Pain and Palliative Care Program and the Brigham and Women's Hospital Pain Committee. Modified with permission from Bridget C. Fowler, Pharm.D., Clinical Pharmacy Manager, Dana Farber Cancer Institute.

Additionally, patients may be afraid to administer too much opioid. For these reasons, a hydrophilic opioid (e.g., morphine) may be preferred over a lipophilic opioid (e.g., fentanyl) despite its longer latency and lower potency.

The amount of opioid delivered in a **continuous basal (background) infusion** may or may not alter the analgesic efficacy of patient-controlled bolus doses. One study compared PCA bolus doses of morphine (0.4, 0.7, or 1.0 mg combined with a continuous infusion of morphine at 1.5 mg/hr) following gynecologic surgery.[56] The number of demand bolus doses and the quality of analgesia did not vary among groups despite the overall higher use of morphine in the group that received the largest bolus dose. In addition, there were no differences among groups in patient satisfaction or side effects. In an earlier study, Owen et al.[55] observed that despite provision of additional morphine through a continuous infusion (1.5 mg/hr), there was no difference between groups in the dose of self-administered morphine. Moreover, the quality of analgesia was similar in the two groups despite a twofold higher total morphine dose in the group receiving a continuous infusion.

Controversy exists regarding the use of a continuous basal infusion during administration of intravenous opioid PCA. Continuous basal infusions are often avoided in opioid-naive patients because of concern about the risks of oversedation and respiratory depression.[8] However, the ASA Task Force on Acute Pain Management concluded that PCA with a continuous background infusion improves the quality of analgesia without increasing the incidence of nausea, vomiting, pruritus, or sedation.[35] Although acknowledging that higher morphine consumption might predispose patients to respiratory depression, the Task Force concluded that the literature was insufficient to draw a causal relationship between respiratory depression and the use of a continuous background infusion. Nonetheless, the Task Force concluded that special caution should be used when a continuous infusion is used owing to the potential for adverse effects from opioid accumulation.[35] The American Pain Society has also urged caution in the use of a continuous basal infusion in opioid-naive patients receiving intravenous opioid PCA.[57]

Sinatra et al.[58] evaluated the role of morphine and oxymorphone administered with and without a continuous infusion for postcesarean analgesia. Patients receiving a continuous infusion received a dose of morphine or oxymorphone (0.6 mg/hr or 0.1 mg/hr, respectively) equivalent to a third of the bolus dose used (1.8 mg or 0.3 mg, respectively). Patients who received a continuous opioid infusion had less pain with movement; however, only those in the oxymorphone group had decreased pain at rest. The continuous infusion group demonstrated a higher incidence of nausea and vomiting. No differences in overall drug use or patient satisfaction were found.

Studies of patients undergoing gynecologic surgery do not support the use of a continuous background infusion to provide better postoperative analgesia. Parker et al.[59] evaluated 230 women who had undergone an abdominal hysterectomy; one group received a demand bolus dose of morphine (1 to 2 mg), and the other three groups received a continuous infusion of morphine (0.5, 1, or 2 mg/hr) in addition to the demand bolus dose.[59] No differences in the demand or delivered doses per hour, pain scores, or overall morphine consumption were observed, except that an overall higher use of morphine occurred in the 2 mg/hr group than in the demand bolus–only group. A subsequent study by the same investigators in a similar patient population compared a group receiving an intravenous PCA morphine (2 mg) regimen with a group receiving the same intravenous PCA regimen and a nighttime continuous infusion of morphine (1 mg/hr).[60] There were no differences between groups in postoperative pain, sleep patterns, demand or delivered bolus doses per hour, opioid consumption, or recovery from surgery. The investigators cautioned that the use of a continuous infusion resulted in six errors during the programming of the device and that three patients required discontinuation of the continuous infusion because of significant oxygen desaturation.[60]

When intravenous PCA is used for postoperative analgesia, guidelines for safe administration should be employed and documented. At many institutions (including our own), two registered nurses must verify all pump settings when they are entered or changed and during communications associated with all patient transfers or nurse shift changes. The amount of opioid administered is recorded from the pump every 2 hours and when a drug cartridge is changed. The PCA settings (drug, demand dose, lockout interval, 4-hour limit, and the continuous infusion rate, if used) are documented on a flow sheet. Any changes in PCA settings are clearly documented. In our institution, the use of a continuous background infusion is discouraged except in patients who were taking opioids preoperatively or in patients in whom nonstandard dosing requirements have already been demonstrated.

With the use of PCA, the ratio of patient demands to bolus doses delivered appears to be a good measure of analgesia and is strongly correlated with pain scores.[61] A high ratio is likely to reflect patient misunderstanding or inadequate analgesia, but a ratio close to 1 signifies adequate pain relief. Patients utilize PCA bolus demands for different reasons, including worsening pain at rest, pain with movement or coughing, and anticipation of an activity that is likely to produce pain.[56] A continuous background infusion may be most beneficial for resting pain, because a therapeutic plasma concentration of opioid might (theoretically) be maintained. However, inadequate analgesia can most likely be improved by an increase in the demand bolus dose, a shorter lockout interval, or a change of opioid. Patients should also be encouraged to use demand bolus doses before movement or activity.

Some investigators have advocated the use of **oral analgesics** rather than intravenous PCA for postcesarean pain (as discussed earlier).[28-30] Davis et al.[62] compared **oral oxycodone/acetaminophen** (5/325 mg) starting immediately after completion of cesarean delivery and at fixed intervals (every 3 hours) with intravenous morphine PCA (1 mg/hr continuous infusion and 1-mg bolus dose with a lockout interval of 6 minutes) for the first 12 hours after cesarean delivery. After 12 hours, all patients made the transition to oral oxycodone/acetaminophen on a prn basis (i.e., 1 to 2 tablets every 4 hours prn). The investigators demonstrated that pain scores were lower with oral analgesia than with intravenous PCA at 6 hours (3.2 versus 4.1, respectively) and at 24 hours after the procedure (2.9 versus 4.1, respectively). Nausea and drowsiness were more common in the PCA group at 6 hours, and nausea was more common in the oral analgesia group at 24 hours. No patients in either group opted to cross over to the other group, and less than 10% of patients required rescue medication. Unfortunately, a number of variables were not disclosed, including baseline pain scores, the use of analgesia prior to the start of intravenous PCA, and the limits on the dose of morphine. In addition, because the overall dose of intravenous morphine utilized was not reported, it is difficult to assess whether this route of analgesia was adequate or understood by the patients. Furthermore, all patients received intravenous ketorolac 30 mg at the end of surgery followed by an intravenous dose of 15 mg every 6 hours for the first 24 hours; this multimodal approach may have affected the results. Finally, patients were allowed oral fluids and food immediately after delivery, an approach seldom used in many institutions. In patients tolerating oral intake after elective cesarean delivery and receiving intravenous ketorolac at fixed intervals, it appears that oral oxycodone/acetaminophen is a useful alternative to intravenous morphine PCA for postoperative analgesia. This approach may be attractive to women who do not desire to be attached to an intravenous PCA device or who have a history of severe postoperative nausea or vomiting attributed to intravenous opioids.

A commonly neglected but important guideline is the achievement of adequate analgesia and the initiation of intravenous PCA *before* the patient is discharged from the postanesthesia care unit (PACU). Although there is significant variation in individual perception of pain and response to analgesia, the assessment of pain scores can assist in evaluating the adequacy of analgesia. In a study of postoperative patients (the surgical procedures were not disclosed) following general anesthesia, Aubrun et al.[63] demonstrated that the relationship between visual analog pain scores (VAPS, on a scale of 0 to 100) and morphine requirements was represented by a sigmoid curve; they observed one plateau below a score of 40 and another plateau above a score of 80. Although patients with a VAPS of 70 or higher were considered to have severe pain and required a larger total dose of morphine to obtain a VAPS lower than 50, a smaller total dose of morphine was required to reduce a VAPS of 50 to a score of 30 or less.[63,64] This study suggests that pain scores are slow to change when severe pain exists but that the scores decline rapidly once pain begins to improve. Other investigators have identified relevant VAPS thresholds associated with changes in intravenous PCA dose requirements after intra-abdominal surgery as 30 or less, 31 to 70, and more than 70.[65] Only 4% of patients with a VAPS of 30 or less requested an increase in analgesic dose, whereas 80% of patients with a VAPS higher than 70 requested a higher dose. Among patients with a VAPS between 31 and 70, those whose scores improved at least 10 points were less likely to request additional analgesia than those with little change or an increase in VAPS.[65] Thus, a patient's perception of pain improvement may depend, in part, on her initial pain score. Paradoxically, another study of nonobstetric patients undergoing oral surgery observed that "a relatively greater degree of pain relief was considered desirable as the initial hypothetical pain intensity became less."[66]

Severe pain most likely antagonizes the sedative and respiratory depressant side effects of opioids, a possibility that becomes increasingly important in patients requesting higher doses of opioids. Therefore, a transition from an opioid-only to a multimodal, balanced analgesia approach should be employed to optimize pain control and minimize opioid-related side effects. The morbidity associated with high doses of opioids should invoke the application of algorithms for pain assessment, management, and monitoring. At many institutions (including our own), postcesarean patients are assessed every 4 hours for respiratory rate and quality, oxygen saturation, pain score, and sedation level. Patients are asked whether their level of pain relief is acceptable, and if not, an adjustment of analgesic dose is performed and documented. The pain score is reassessed within 15 to 30 minutes before additional interventions are made. High-risk patients, including those with hepatic or renal dysfunction, obstructive sleep apnea, and morbid obesity, are assessed every 2 hours for 12 hours after initiation of intravenous PCA therapy and then every 4 hours if the respiratory rate is 8 breaths/min or higher, oxygenation is stable, and sedation level is minimal. Patients are assessed every 30 minutes for the first hour after the intravenous PCA dose is increased, and thereafter, if pain relief is adequate and the clinical condition is unchanged, every 4 hours as previously described.

Acute postoperative pain is limited in duration, so a plan should be devised for the transition from intravenous opioids to oral agents. An oral opioid dose equi-analgesic to at least half the prior daily intravenous dose can be given for the first 2 days, which can subsequently be reduced by 25% every 2 days until the total dose in oral morphine equivalents is 30 mg/day. The drug may be discontinued after 2 days on the 30 mg/day dose. If the patient experiences more pain, the dose of opioid may be increased. Table 27-5 lists the equi-analgesic doses for the most commonly used opioids.

The postcesarean use of intranasal fentanyl, which is rapidly absorbed and has pharmacokinetics similar to those with intravenous administration, has been described.

TABLE 27-5 Opioid Equi-analgesic Doses

Drug	Oral/Per Rectum (mg)	Subcutaneous/ Intravenous (mg)
Morphine	30	10
Oxycodone	20	N/A
Hydrocodone	20	N/A
Hydromorphone	7.5	1.5
Fentanyl	N/A A 25-μg/hr transdermal patch is equi-analgesic to ≈50 mg of oral morphine per day	0.1 (i.e., 100 μg)
Oxymorphone	10	1

N/A, not applicable.

Table courtesy of the Dana Farber Cancer Institute Pain and Palliative Care Program and the Brigham and Women's Hospital Pain Committee. Modified with permission from Bridget C. Fowler, Pharm. D., Clinical Pharmacy Manager, Dana Farber Cancer Institute.

Wong et al.[67] provided postcesarean patient-controlled intranasal analgesia (PCINA) with fentanyl (4.5-μg dose, 3-minute lockout, maximum dose of 90 μg/hr) and compared it with intramuscular morphine (10 mg prn every 4 hours). Rescue analgesia was provided with intravenous morphine if the pain score was higher than 5 (on a scale of 0 to 10). The intranasal fentanyl and intramuscular morphine groups had mean pain scores of 4.5 and 5.1, respectively, and greater use of rescue doses was observed in the intramuscular morphine group. No significant side effects occurred in either group. Although these results were not statistically significant owing to the small sample size (n = 21), the investigators suggested that intranasal fentanyl may become a viable alternative to intramuscular morphine because of the ease of administration, efficacy, and high patient satisfaction. Additional studies are needed to determine the optimal dose and side-effect profile of fentanyl administered as patient-controlled intranasal analgesia.[67]

Nonsteroidal Anti-inflammatory Drugs

NSAIDs have become a standard adjuvant in the management of moderate to severe postoperative pain.[68-71] These agents provide analgesia and suppress inflammation by inhibiting cyclooxygenase, an enzyme that enhances the conversion of arachidonic acid to prostaglandins and thromboxane. Although the exact mechanism of action involved in the analgesic effect of NSAIDs remains unclear, the decrease in prostaglandin synthesis is believed responsible. Unfortunately, the inhibition of prostaglandin synthesis may also result in gastric and renal toxicity as well as platelet inhibition. A number of NSAIDs have been evaluated as adjuncts for postcesarean analgesia, including ketorolac, diclofenac, and ibuprofen administered parenterally, orally, and rectally. These drugs may be particularly effective in combating the inflammatory components of pain emanating from the uterus as well as the nociceptive components originating from the incision site.

A single **indomethacin** 50-mg rectal suppository has been demonstrated to reduce opioid requirements by more than 25% after cesarean delivery with neuraxial anesthesia.[72] Similarly, in 24 women randomly assigned to receive (or not receive) a single **diclofenac** 100-mg rectal suppository, a 33% reduction in patient-controlled epidural analgesia (ropivacaine 0.2% with fentanyl 2 μg/mL) dose requirements was observed. However, pain and satisfaction scores did not differ between the two groups.[73] Other investigations with rectal indomethacin and diclofenac and intramuscular diclofenac have also demonstrated an "opioid-sparing" effect (i.e., allowed the use of lower amounts of opioid) and consequently a reduction in opioid-related side effects in the postcesarean setting.[74-79] Diclofenac may be synergistic with morphine at high doses,[80] and it reliably reduces opioid requirements after cesarean delivery.[81-83]

Repeated oral doses of NSAIDs have followed the use of rectal NSAIDs and neuraxial opioids for postcesarean analgesia, with good effect. In one study, the use of rectal **naproxen** 500 mg at the conclusion of cesarean delivery (performed with a spinal anesthetic that included morphine 0.2 mg), followed by oral naproxen sodium 550 mg every 12 hours for 6 doses, reduced both incisional pain at 36 hours and overall opioid consumption.[84] Thus, even in the setting of neuraxial morphine administration, this study supports the immediate and repeated use of NSAIDs for postcesarean analgesia for at least 48 hours.

As the only NSAID available for intravenous administration in the United States, **ketorolac** is a commonly used adjuvant for the treatment of postoperative pain and has been demonstrated to enhance opioid analgesia after both nonobstetric and obstetric surgery.[85,86] An oral dose of ketorolac 10 mg has been shown to be superior to aspirin 650 mg for treatment of moderate to severe postpartum uterine pain.[87] Ketorolac 15 mg, given as an intravenous bolus 20 minutes before induction of general anesthesia for elective cesarean delivery, has been demonstrated to result in smaller increases in heart rate and systolic blood pressure, lower plasma cortisol concentrations, lower pain scores at rest and movement for the first 2 postoperative hours, and a longer time to first request for analgesia.[88] An intramuscular dose of ketorolac 30 mg has been shown to greatly improve the efficacy of epidural morphine 2 mg after cesarean delivery without potentiating its adverse effects.[89] Pavy et al.[90] observed that the use of intravenous ketorolac (15-mg bolus after delivery, continuous infusion of 105 mg over 24 hours starting in the postanesthesia care unit) produced a 30% dose reduction in patient-controlled epidural meperidine requirements, but without significant improvements in analgesia, opioid-related side effects, or patient outcome.

Administration of small intravenous doses of ketorolac (15 to 30 mg) for short periods (24 hours) is unlikely to have the side effects typically associated with long-term use of NSAIDs, such as renal and gastrointestinal toxicity and postoperative bleeding. The NSAID indomethacin is an effective tocolytic agent[91]; however, there is no evidence that NSAIDs cause postpartum uterine atony. The onset of postpartum hypertension has been reported in a series of 6 patients taking NSAIDs.[92] The exact mechanism of NSAID-induced hypertension is unknown but has been hypothesized to result from the inhibition of vasodilatory prostaglandins, retention of sodium, or enhanced production of endothelin-1.[93] Until a more complete assessment of the mechanism of NSAID-induced hypertension is published, physicians should exercise caution in the administration of these agents to women with preexisting or pregnancy-associated renal or hypertensive disease.

The **instillation of NSAIDs** directly into the surgical incision exploits the knowledge that hyperalgesia can occur after tissue damage and can potentially be modulated peripherally.[94] A systematic review investigating the evidence for a peripheral analgesic effect of NSAID wound instillation observed inconclusive results in nonobstetric patients.[95] By contrast, Lavand'homme et al.[96] demonstrated that continuous wound infiltration with diclofenac (300 mg in 240 mL) for 48 hours after cesarean delivery resulted in significantly lower morphine use during the first 2 days postpartum than the same diclofenac dose administered intravenously. Moreover, these investigators demonstrated that a diclofenac infusion at the surgical incision provided analgesia similar to that provided by a ropivacaine infusion at the surgical incision combined with intravenous diclofenac.[96] Rates of punctate hyperalgesia at the wound site at 24 and 48 hours and residual pain at 1 and 6 months after cesarean delivery did not differ among the treatment groups.

In summary, NSAIDs provide effective analgesia for moderate to severe postoperative pain and should be incorporated into the multimodal therapy used after cesarean delivery.[97,98] Administration of NSAIDs in patients receiving intravenous morphine PCA results in a 30% to 50% reduction in morphine consumption.[99] A meta-analysis of randomized controlled trials demonstrated that administration of NSAIDs in patients receiving intravenous morphine PCA resulted in a 30% reduction in the relative risk of nausea and vomiting and a 29% reduction in the relative risk of sedation.[99]

Cyclooxygenase-2 Inhibitors

The potential side effects of nonselective NSAIDs, including gastrointestinal bleeding and uterine atony, coupled with maternal concern about neonatal transfer via breast milk (see later), has prompted interest in the use of selective cyclooxygenase-2 (COX-2) inhibitors. Cyclooxygenase exists in at least two isoforms, COX-1 and COX-2, with COX-2 activity being expressed by the cytokine activity associated with inflammation and pain. Therapies directed at modulating the COX-2 isoform should minimize the undesirable gastrointestinal, renal, and antiplatelet effects mediated by COX-1 inhibition.[100-103] Although the manufacturers' voluntary withdrawal of two COX-2 inhibitors (valdecoxib and rofecoxib) from the market because of serious cardiovascular events in at-risk patients has diminished much of the early interest in this class of drugs, **celecoxib** remains available but is under U.S. Food and Drug Administration (FDA) scrutiny.

A number of studies have demonstrated comparable postoperative analgesia for selective COX-2 inhibitors and nonspecific NSAIDs in nonobstetric patients.[103-106] However, limited data suggest that these agents may not represent a useful adjuvant for postcesarean analgesia. Carvalho et al.[107] evaluated the analgesic and opioid-sparing effects of **valdecoxib** following cesarean delivery; parturients received spinal anesthesia with intrathecal morphine 0.1 mg, and were randomly assigned to receive either valdecoxib 20 mg or placebo twice daily for the first 3 postoperative days. There were no differences between groups in the time to first analgesic request, pain scores, morphine consumption, need for supplemental analgesia, side effects, or patient satisfaction. Currently, there is no evidence to justify the use of selective COX-2 inhibitors as part of multimodal therapy for postcesarean pain.

Acetaminophen

A number of studies have demonstrated that acetaminophen can provide a substantial opioid-sparing effect after surgery.[108,109] Although self-administration of acetaminophen combined with oral morphine and diclofenac has been used successfully to improve satisfaction with analgesia in obstetric patients, it is important that explicit instructions and dose limits be communicated.[110] However, some evidence suggests that acetaminophen may have limited utility in providing relief of the pain of uterine cramping. Rectal acetaminophen 1 g, given immediately after cervical dilation and vacuum aspiration, neither enhanced opioid analgesia nor decreased opioid use after elective termination of pregnancy.[111]

Propacetamol, the parenteral prodrug of acetaminophen with 100% bioavailability, has also been shown to have a significant opioid-sparing effect, to decrease pain scores, and to limit the duration of PCA opioid use after orthopedic surgery.[108,112] Advantages of this drug may include a combined central and peripheral site of action. Centrally, propacetamol is believed to inhibit prostaglandin synthetase in the brain and activate the spinal serotoninergic system[80]; peripherally, propacetamol may have anti-inflammatory effects. However, Siddik et al.[80] found no evidence of better analgesia or greater opioid-sparing effect with the administration of propacetamol 2 g every 6 hours when the medication was given immediately following cesarean delivery and continued for the first 24 hours postoperatively. Furthermore, the use of propacetamol did not provide an additive benefit to rectal diclofenac 100 mg every 8 hours in this setting.[80] It is possible that the visceral pain associated with postcesarean uterine contractions may not be responsive to this treatment modality. A meta-analysis concluded that acetaminophen reduces morphine consumption by less than 10 mg in 24 hours, and does not lower the incidence of side effects after major surgery.[113]

In parturients who require surgical repair of lacerations incurred at vaginal delivery, NSAIDs appear to provide superior analgesia compared with acetaminophen. Peter et al.[114] compared a group of patients taking ibuprofen 400 mg with another group taking acetaminophen 600 mg with codeine 60 mg and caffeine 15 mg after repair of an episiotomy or a third- or fourth-degree laceration.[114] Ibuprofen provided analgesia similar to that provided by acetaminophen with codeine and caffeine, with fewer side effects. In many institutions, NSAIDs alone (oral ibuprofen 600 mg) are used to supplement neuraxial opioid analgesia after cesarean delivery, with intravenous ketorolac given in the presence of significant ongoing discomfort. Oxycodone alone, instead of oxycodone with acetaminophen, can be used for ongoing discomfort; acetaminophen is of limited value for uterine pain and adds the risk of liver toxicity when total daily doses greater than 4 g are taken. In summary, although acetaminophen has long been used to supplement opioid analgesia postpartum, additional studies are needed to validate its use for the provision of postcesarean analgesia.

Local Anesthetics

Because of their analgesic properties and minimal adverse effects, local anesthetic drugs have become increasingly popular in the treatment of surgical pain.[115,116] Local anesthetics temporarily block sodium channels, thereby preventing the initiation and propagation of nerve impulses and pain transduction. The use of **local anesthetic infiltration** around the surgical incision has not been uniformly accepted owing to conflicting results of its use in clinical studies. Studies in general and gynecologic surgery patients have demonstrated better analgesia with reduced use of opioids when local anesthetic instillation into the surgical wound was employed[117-119]; these findings contrast with the results of earlier studies.[120] This contrast may reflect differences in study design, including the earlier use of single-dose regimens that would not be expected to alter long-term analgesic requirements.

Studies comparing local anesthetic infiltration with placebo for postcesarean analgesia have had mixed results.

Trotter et al.[121] observed no reduction in pain scores or 24-hour morphine requirements after injection of 20 mL of 0.5% bupivacaine into the incision-site subcutaneous tissue after elective cesarean delivery. Furthermore, Pavy et al.[122] showed that a single preoperative skin infiltration of 30 mL of 0.5% bupivacaine provided no improvement in pain scores for the first 3 days after cesarean delivery; the results of this study may have been confounded by the use of intrathecal morphine for postcesarean analgesia.

Later studies have shown a positive analgesic effect for the use of **continuous incisional infusion of local anesthetic** after cesarean delivery. Ranta et al.[123] showed that intermittent subfascial infusion with 10 mL of 0.25% levobupivacaine (via a 22-gauge catheter placed at the incision site) provided postcesarean analgesia and patient satisfaction similar to that provided by intermittent epidural bolus doses of 10 mL of 0.125% levobupivacaine. Although lower pain scores and decreased local anesthetic consumption were observed in the epidural group for the first 4 hours postoperatively, pain scores were similar in the two groups thereafter, with comparable use of rescue opioids for the first 3 days postoperatively and a very low side-effect profile. Fredman et al.[124] evaluated the postcesarean efficacy of the instillation of 0.2% ropivacaine or an equal volume of sterile water via a multi-orifice 20-gauge epidural catheter placed above the fascia of the skin incision site. Fewer patients in the ropivacaine instillation group received rescue analgesics; moreover, although pain scores at rest were no different in the two groups, pain scores with coughing and leg raising were significantly lower in the ropivacaine instillation group. Givens et al.[125] used an elastomer pump connected to two 20-gauge latex infusion catheters (placed in the subcutaneous space at the incision site) to infuse 0.25% bupivacaine or normal saline at 4 mL/hr for 48 hours after cesarean delivery. (The subcutaneous tissue was infiltrated with 25 mL of the assigned solution before the continuous infusion was started.) Patients who received the bupivacaine infusion had lower cumulative doses of morphine, but there was no difference between groups in pain scores at any time.

A systematic review of randomized controlled trials (involving both obstetric and nonobstetric patients) found that continuous infusion of local anesthetic through catheters placed at the incisional site led to an improvement in analgesia and patient satisfaction and reductions in opioid use, side effects, and duration of hospital stay in comparison with administration of systemic opioids alone.[126] In light of their efficacy, technical simplicity, and low side-effect profile, instillation catheters placed at the incisional site should be used more frequently for postcesarean analgesia, particularly in patients receiving general anesthesia and in those with opioid sensitivities.[10,98,123] In these patients, either a continuous or a patient-controlled infusion of local anesthetic through a peri-incisional catheter appears to provide better analgesia than parenteral opioids alone and reduces the requirement for rescue opioids for at least 24 hours. It is unclear whether local anesthetic wound instillation enhances analgesia in patients who have received long-acting central neuraxial opioids.

Early studies of **ilioinguinal nerve block** suggested that this technique has limited efficacy for postcesarean analgesia. Bell et al.[127] subsequently observed that multilevel **iliohypogastric-ilioinguinal nerve block** reduced the use of morphine PCA but did not reduce the occurrence of opioid-related side effects after cesarean delivery. In a later study, Gucev et al.[128] reported three cases of the successful use of bilateral, ultrasound-guided, continuous ilioinguinal-iliohypogastric nerve block for postcesarean analgesia. These patients also received oral ibuprofen 600 mg every 6 hours. McDonnell et al.[129] observed that **transversus abdominis plane block** provided analgesia that was superior to that provided by placebo, when administered as part of a multimodal analgesic regimen that included oral acetaminophen (1 g every 6 hours), rectal diclofenac (100 mg every 18 hours), and intravenous morphine PCA after cesarean delivery. It is unclear whether these techniques offer any advantages over continuous infusion of local anesthetic at the incision site.

Alpha$_2$-Adrenergic Receptor Agonists

Clonidine and **dexmedetomidine** are alpha$_2$-adrenergic receptor agonists that modulate pain in the primary afferent nerve terminals and the superficial layers of the spinal cord.[130] Although most of the available data for postcesarean analgesia originated from the neuraxial use of clonidine (see Chapter 28), the intravenous administration of dexmedetomidine has now been approved. The intravenous infusion of dexmedetomidine has resulted in greater analgesia and use of smaller doses of opioid during the postoperative period,[131] although the routine use of this medication for postcesarean analgesia has yet to be evaluated. A potential undesirable side effect of dexmedetomidine is somnolence, which could impair breast-feeding and early ambulation after cesarean delivery.[132] Future studies should address the use of low doses of alpha$_2$-adrenergic receptor agonists, especially because of their relative maintenance of oxygenation and respiratory rate.

Magnesium Sulfate

Magnesium sulfate, the drug of choice for seizure prophylaxis in preeclamptic women, may also be used to reduce postcesarean pain. Magnesium is an *N*-methyl-D-aspartate (NMDA) receptor antagonist and may be involved in pain modulation at the level of the spinal cord. Animal studies and clinical trials in nonobstetric patients suggest that the use of magnesium is associated with an improvement in analgesia and a reduction in use of rescue pain medications.[133-136] However, in patients undergoing cesarean delivery who received either an intravenous infusion of magnesium sulfate at two different doses (50 mg/kg loading dose and then 2 g/hr, or 25 mg/kg loading dose and then 1 g/hr) or a placebo, no alterations in pain scores (at rest and with movement) or cumulative meperidine requirements were observed at multiple time points up to 48 hours postpartum.[137] A systematic review of randomized trials of the postoperative administration of magnesium sulfate observed that less than half of the studies demonstrated favorable effects on postoperative pain intensity or analgesic dose requirements.[138]

Gabapentin

Gabapentin is an anticonvulsant that binds to the presynaptic voltage-gated calcium channels, which are upregulated in the dorsal root ganglia and spinal cord after surgical trauma. By inhibiting calcium influx, gabapentin prevents the release of excitatory neurotransmitters (e.g., substance P, calcitonin gene–related peptide) from the primary afferent nerve fibers in the pain pathway.[139] A meta-analysis of the perioperative use of gabapentin demonstrated improved analgesia with an opioid-sparing effect following an oral dose (300 to 1200 mg) administered within the 4 hours preceding surgery.[140] Gabapentin use was associated with sedation and anxiolysis, but no differences in rates of lightheadedness, dizziness, nausea, or vomiting. A later meta-analysis[141] as well as a systematic review of randomized controlled trials[142] demonstrated similar results, with the addition of a lower incidence of vomiting and pruritus with the use of gabapentin. None of these studies or meta-analyses assessed outcome in patients undergoing cesarean delivery; moreover, to date there are no reported cases of gabapentin use for postcesarean analgesia.

Ketamine and Dextromethorphan

Ketamine, a noncompetitive NMDA antagonist, is a phencyclidine derivative that provides potent analgesia at subanesthetic doses. This analgesia is presumed to be due to an interaction between ketamine and opioid receptors in the CNS, where it may act as an antagonist and block spinal nociceptive reflexes.[143] In the setting of an elective cesarean delivery performed with spinal bupivacaine anesthesia, patients were randomly assigned to receive either intrathecal fentanyl 10 μg or a continuous intravenous infusion of ketamine (0.15 mg/kg), which was started after administration of spinal anesthesia and continued throughout the procedure.[144] Patients in the ketamine group experienced a longer time to first request for analgesia, lower postoperative pain scores, and lower analgesic requirements in the first 24 hours, but not thereafter. A subsequent meta-analysis of the perioperative use of ketamine for postoperative analgesia demonstrated improved analgesia with an opioid-sparing effect for the first 24 hours and a decreased incidence of nausea and vomiting.[145]

Some investigators have suggested that ketamine may have a preemptive effect.[144] The goal of **preemptive analgesia** is to prevent the establishment of central sensitization, which amplifies postoperative pain.[146] In patients with inadequate analgesia prior to a noxious stimulus, post-injury analgesia may have a reduced effect because central sensitization has already been established. Prevention of **postinjury hypersensitivity** also requires the analgesia to be maintained throughout the procedure and postoperatively to prevent inflammatory changes that might lead to central sensitization. In summary, preemptive analgesia must (1) occur before the injury, (2) be adequate to prevent central sensitization, and (3) be maintained postoperatively to prevent the inflammatory changes associated with postinjury hypersensitivity.[146]

The inability to prevent central sensitization may explain why another NMDA acid antagonist, **dextromethorphan,** has not been as effective as ketamine. When oral dextromethorphan 60 mg was given to patients undergoing cesarean delivery with use of spinal anesthesia and intrathecal morphine 0.05, 0.1, or 0.2 mg, there was no improvement in postoperative pain scores despite a lower incidence of nausea and vomiting.[147] A systematic review of the perioperative use of dextromethorphan failed to lead to a valid meta-analysis because of substantial differences in the methodology and reporting among the trials; the investigators of this effort concluded that "the consistency of the potential opioid-sparing and pain-reducing effect [of dextromethorphan] must be questioned."[148]

NONPHARMACOLOGIC INTERVENTIONS

Nonpharmacologic interventions, including transcutaneous and percutaneous electrical nerve stimulation (TENS and PENS), acupuncture, and massage, have gained popularity because of the belief that they may provide effective analgesia with minimal side effects. These interventions have been used with variable success during labor (see Chapter 21).[149,150] **Transcutaneous electrical nerve stimulation** has been reported to reduce postoperative opioid requirements significantly in nonobstetric patients.[151-154] In one prospective, randomized study of women undergoing gynecologic surgery or cesarean delivery, PCA morphine requirements were reduced by 50% to 80% in women who received electrical stimulation via **percutaneous intradermal electrodes** placed on each side of the lower abdominal surgical incision.[155] In another study in patients undergoing gynecologic surgery, transcutaneous electrical nerve stimulation at a dermatome corresponding to the surgical incision site led to improved analgesia, a reduced duration of PCA use, and a lower incidence of postoperative complications such as pruritus, nausea, and dizziness.[156] Although the exact mechanism of action is unclear, there is some evidence that electrical stimulation stimulates the release of proenkephalin-derived peptides that act at the μ-opioid receptor.[157-160]

Reports of the use of complementary and alternative medicines in obstetric and gynecologic patients have had mixed results.[149,150,161] Although many studies have been criticized for being unclear regarding hypothesis, description of methods, and results or conclusions, it should be possible to conduct prospective, randomized studies with suitable controls to measure the efficacy and the risk-to-benefit ratio of complementary and alternative medicine interventions.[156] The value of these therapies in multimodal analgesic techniques is unclear.

MULTIMODAL ANALGESIA

The goals for postcesarean analgesia are to provide adequate pain relief, encourage early ambulation, enable the care of the newborn, and minimize side-effect profiles in both the mother and the baby. The use of a multimodal approach to analgesia, which employs a number of different agents that work through different mechanisms and minimizes the reliance on opioids, seems feasible and attractive. Although current data primarily support the multimodal approach in nonobstetric patients, a growing number of studies seem to justify this approach for postcesarean analgesia.[10] Meta-analyses of randomized trials evaluating multimodal therapy with acetaminophen, NSAIDs, or selective COX-2 inhibitors for postoperative pain have shown that all of these agents have a morphine-sparing effect.[162] However, only NSAIDs (in combination with morphine) reduced pain intensity and the incidence of morphine-related side effects. Neither acetaminophen nor selective COX-2 inhibitors affected the incidence of nausea, vomiting, or sedation. Physicians should consider the instillation of local anesthetic at the surgical incision site as part of multimodal therapy, particularly in selected patients who have sensitivities to opioids or who did not receive neuraxial opioids. Future studies are likely to focus on outcomes other than analgesia, including quality of life and recovery issues as well as patient satisfaction.[163]

BREAST-FEEDING ISSUES

The American Academy of Pediatrics (AAP) strongly supports breast-feeding because of its benefits to the infant, mother, and society, which include reductions in infant mortality and morbidity due to infectious diseases and immune-mediated disorders (e.g., insulin-dependent diabetes mellitus).[164,165] Nonpregnant breast-feeding women are more likely than pregnant women to take medications, including analgesics such as NSAIDs and acetaminophen.[166] However, patients may discontinue breast-feeding when taking these analgesic medications because of incomplete or incorrect concerns regarding neonatal health.[167] The AAP Committee on Drugs recommends that physicians take the following steps before prescribing medications to breast-feeding women: (1) determination of the reasons for the medication, (2) identification of the safest available medication in a particular category, and (3) measurement of blood concentrations of drug in those neonates for whom the drug presents a significant risk.[168] The AAP has also suggested that the best time for the mother to take a medication is immediately after breast-feeding or just before the infant takes a nap.[168]

The two most important items needed to determine the potential neonatal risks of maternal drug administration are the amount of medication excreted in breast milk and the therapeutic effect of that medication when given to the infant.[165] Some investigators have arbitrarily defined a breast milk concentration lower than 10% of the therapeutic infant plasma concentration (or a breast milk dose less than 10% of the weight-normalized maternal dose) as a safe level of exposure. In breast-feeding infants, the estimated *absolute infant drug dose* is calculated by multiplying the average infant breast milk intake (0.151 kg/day) by the average concentration of the drug in the milk (area under the pharmacokinetic curve). The absolute infant drug dose is then expressed as a percentage of the maternal dose, normalized by weight (mg/kg/day), to yield the *relative infant dose*.[169-171] For example, the maternal administration of methadone (10 to 80 mg), a synthetic opioid that is often used for treatment of moderate to severe pain and/or drug detoxification and maintenance therapy in patients with opioid addiction, has been found to result in infant drug levels consistent with an analgesic dose.[165,172] By contrast, other investigators have concluded that maternal doses up to 80 mg/day lead to minimal exposure in breast milk.[173] A conservative approach would measure blood levels in those infants whose mothers are taking more than 20 mg/day and either discontinue the drug, modify the dose, or change to a different analgesic drug if the level reaches an analgesic dose or if side effects attributed to the medication are detected in the infant. Short-term administration of other potent medications commonly used for sedation and analgesia (e.g., midazolam, propofol, fentanyl) has been found to result in breast milk doses less than 1.25% of the weight-normalized maternal dose.[174]

Although acetaminophen and NSAIDs are considered safe to take during breast-feeding, high-dose **aspirin** has been associated with a case of neonatal metabolic acidosis. The AAP regards aspirin as a medication that may be associated with adverse effects in some nursing infants and recommends that aspirin should be given with caution; the AAP further recommends that measurement of infant plasma salicylate concentrations be considered.[168]

Although **indomethacin** is an NSAID usually compatible with breast-feeding, some have cautioned against its use because of case reports of neonatal seizures and nephrotoxicity.[175] Furthermore, although maternally administered **naproxen** is transported minimally into breast milk and its use is considered safe during lactation, it has been associated with a case of neonatal anemia, rectal bleeding, and hematuria.[176] Therefore, both indomethacin and naproxen should be used with caution during breast-feeding, especially when suitable, effective alternatives such as ibuprofen are available.

Ketorolac is often used when there is the need to give a NSAID intravenously, despite an FDA "black box" warning on the package insert against its use in laboring and nursing mothers. The warning reflected concerns related to the potential adverse effects on the fetal circulation, the uterus, or the neonate.[177] Regardless, the AAP has endorsed its safety and use in breast-feeding mothers.[168] Wischnik et al.[178] studied the transfer of ketorolac into breast milk in 10 women given oral doses of 10 mg four times daily for 2 days. The maternal plasma concentrations were within established ranges for ketorolac; the peak breast milk levels were 8 ng/mL with a milk-to-plasma ratio of 0.015 to 0.037. On a weight-adjusted basis, the potential infant exposure was between 0.16% and 0.40% of the total daily maternal dose.[178]

Meperidine administration has been associated with neonatal neurobehavioral depression[51] and should be avoided during lactation.[52] Morphine and hydromorphone are alternatives to meperidine for PCA. Investigators have noted that breast milk **oxycodone** levels could be as high as 10% of the therapeutic dose in infants.[165] In a study of 50 breast-feeding mothers after a cesarean delivery, rectal oxycodone 30 mg was given at the end of surgery, followed by oral oxycodone 10 mg every 2 hours prn. Patients received total doses of oxycodone between 30 and 90 mg in the first 24 hours after delivery, resulting in a milk-to-plasma ratio of 3.2:1; this ratio suggests the presence of a very high amount of oxycodone in the breast milk with the possibility of the neonate's receiving more than 10% of the therapeutic infant dose.[179] However, as explained by Ito,[165] this ratio is misleading because it represents only the amount of the medication in the breast milk and not the true level of infant exposure. The infant's exposure also depends on the neonatal intake of milk and on the amount of absorption and rate of clearance of the drug in the infant. As a result, only one neonate in the oral oxycodone study had detectable levels, allowing the researchers to conclude that the infant risk is minimal because low volumes of breast milk are ingested early after delivery.[179]

Furthermore, the amount of colostrum secreted the first few days after cesarean delivery is small.[175]

Acetaminophen and hydrocodone are often administered together for treatment of postoperative pain during lactation; hydrocodone concentrations of 3.1% to 3.7% of the maternal weight-adjusted dose have been measured in the breast milk.[180]

Acetaminophen and codeine are often used together for treatment of mild to moderate postoperative pain in the early postpartum period. Low infant plasma levels of codeine and its metabolite morphine were found after the ingestion of moderate doses of codeine (as many as four 60-mg doses).[181] Typically the dose detected in breast milk is approximately 1% to 2% of the mother's dose and is low enough to have no significant pharmacologic activity in most infants; however, the death of a full-term, 13-day-old neonate from an apparent morphine overdose from breast milk ingestion has been reported.[182] The mother was taking a modest dose of acetaminophen with codeine for episiotomy pain. It was discovered that the mother was heterozygous for a CYP2D6*2A allele with CYP2D6*2×2 gene duplication, making her an ultrarapid metabolizer of codeine. Codeine is metabolized to morphine, which in this situation resulted in a breast milk morphine concentration of 87 ng/mL, compared with the typical range of 1.9 to 20.5 ng/mL. In response, the FDA released a Public Health Advisory recommending caution in the use of codeine-containing medications by breast-feeding women.[183] The FDA recommended that the lowest effective dose for the shortest necessary duration should be used. Moreover, the FDA recommended that women be instructed in how to recognize signs of high morphine levels in their infants. In the presence of neonatal side effects, physicians should consider administration of naloxone and performance of genotype analysis.[182-184] The incidence of ultrarapid metabolizers of codeine is estimated to vary between 1 and 28 per 100 people.[183]

Studies of **gabapentin** have demonstrated a breast milk concentration of 1.3% to 3.8% of the weight-normalized dose received by the mother.[185,186] Investigations of the COX-2 inhibitor **celecoxib** have demonstrated breast milk concentrations of 0.23% to 0.3% of the weight-adjusted maternal dose.[171,187] There are no studies of the breast milk concentrations of maternally administered ketamine. Other maternal medications compatible with breast-feeding include lidocaine, sumatriptan, and magnesium sulfate. Because the use of moderate amounts of **caffeine** appears to be safe and there is no contraindication to the use of short-acting barbiturates during lactation,[168,188] the use of butalbital 50 mg/acetaminophen 325 to 500 mg/caffeine 40 mg (Fioricet) for the treatment of postoperative headaches, including post–dural puncture headache, is not contraindicated.

KEY POINTS

- Postcesarean pain is produced by direct trauma to nerve endings and/or subsequent inflammation induced by tissue injury.
- The experience of pain appears to be associated with genetic variability of the μ-opioid receptor.
- Results from studies of postoperative analgesia in nonobstetric patients may not be directly applicable to pregnant women undergoing cesarean delivery.
- Postpartum pain may be modulated by the unique hormonal and emotional changes of pregnancy. In addition, stress, anxiety, and depression may accompany postpartum sleep disturbances and the responsibilities of providing care for a newborn infant.
- Opioids are the most common systemic medications administered for postcesarean analgesia. Adverse effects associated with opioids, which often limit their utility, include respiratory depression, sedation, constipation, nausea and vomiting, urinary retention, and pruritus.
- Factors that should affect the choice of opioid are the speed of onset, duration of action, and overall efficacy of the agent, and the type and frequency of its side effects.
- There are no maximum allowable doses for specific opioids; therefore, the main limiting factor in an individualized approach to pain control is the side effects associated with their use.
- Optimal postcesarean analgesia consists of a multidisciplinary approach that should involve physicians, nurses, pharmacists, and other health care providers.
- There may be a benefit to giving oral analgesic drugs early in the postoperative period and on a fixed, rather than patient request (prn) interval.
- Multimodal techniques provide effective postcesarean analgesia by acting on different pain pathways. In addition, multimodal analgesia achieves better analgesia while limiting side effects. One multimodal strategy might consist of the continuous instillation of local anesthetic at the surgical incision site, the administration of a nonsteroidal anti-inflammatory drug, and intravenous opioid patient-controlled anesthesia.
- The two most important items necessary to determine the potential neonatal risks of maternal drug administration are an estimate of the amount of medication excreted in breast milk and the therapeutic effect of that medication when given to the infant.

REFERENCES

1. Faboya A, Uncles D. Postcesarean delivery pain management: Multimodal approach. Int J Obstet Anesth 2007; 16:185-6.
2. Kan RK, Lew E, Yeo SW, Thomas E. General anesthesia for cesarean section in a Singapore maternity hospital: A retrospective survey. Int J Obstet Anesth 2004; 13:221-6.
3. Cunningham FG, Grant NF, Leveno KJ, et al. Williams Obstetrics. 21st edition. New York, McGraw-Hill, 2001:483-564.
4. Ayers JW, Morley GW. Surgical incision for cesarean section. Obstet Gynecol 1987; 70:706-8.

5. Meyer RA, Ringkamp M, Campbell JN, Raja SN. Peripheral mechanisms of cutaneous nociception. In McMahon SB, Koltzenburg M, editors. Wall and Melzack's Textbook of Pain. 5th edition. Philadelphia, Churchill Livingstone, 2005:3-34.
6. Raja SN, Dougherty PM. Reversing tissue injury-induced plastic changes in the spinal cord: The search for the magic bullet. Reg Anesth Pain Med 2000; 25:441-4.
7. Woolf CJ. Pain: Moving from symptom control toward mechanism-specific pharmacologic management. Ann Intern Med 2004; 140:441-51.
8. Leung AY. Postoperative pain management in obstetric anesthesia—new challenges and solutions. J Clin Anesth 2004; 16:57-65.
9. Jin F, Chung F. Multimodal analgesia for postoperative pain control. J Clin Anesth 2001; 13:524-39.
10. Pan PH. Post cesarean delivery pain management: Multimodal approach. Int J Obstet Anesth 2006; 15:185-8.
11. Rosaeg OP, Lui AC, Cicutti NJ, et al. Peri-operative multimodal pain therapy for caesarean section: Analgesia and fitness for discharge. Can J Anaesth 1997; 44:803-9.
12. Halpern SH, Walsh VL. Multimodal therapy for post-cesarean delivery pain. Reg Anesth Pain Med 2001; 26:298-300.
13. Pan PH, Coghill R, Houle TT, et al. Multifactorial preoperative predictors for postcesarean section pain and analgesic requirement. Anesthesiology 2006; 104:417-25.
14. Jamison RN, Taft K, O'Hara JP, Ferrante FM. Psychosocial and pharmacologic predictors of satisfaction with intravenous patient-controlled analgesia. Anesth Analg 1993; 77:121-5.
15. Egan KJ, Ready LB, Nessly M, Greer BE. Self-administration of midazolam for postoperative anxiety: A double blinded study. Pain 1992; 49:3-8.
16. Granot M, Lowenstein L, Yarnitsky D, et al. Postcesarean section pain prediction by preoperative experimental pain assessment. Anesthesiology 2003; 98:1422-6.
17. Landau R, Cahana A, Smiley RM, et al. Genetic variability of mu-opioid receptor in an obstetric population. Anesthesiology 2004; 100:1030-3.
18. Landau R. One size does not fit all: Genetic variability of mu-opioid receptor and postoperative morphine consumption. Anesthesiology 2006; 105:235-7.
19. Chou WY, Wang CH, Liu PH, et al. Human opioid receptor A118G polymorphism affects intravenous patient-controlled analgesia morphine consumption after total abdominal hysterectomy. Anesthesiology 2006; 105:334-7.
20. Fillingim RB, Kaplan L, Staud R, et al. The A118G single nucleotide polymorphism of the mu-opioid receptor gene (OPRM1) is associated with pressure pain sensitivity in humans. J Pain 2005; 6:159-67.
21. Bond C, LaForge KS, Tian M, et al. Single-nucleotide polymorphism in the human mu opioid receptor gene alters beta-endorphin binding and activity: Possible implications for opiate addiction. Proc Natl Acad Sci U S A 1998; 95:9608-13.
22. Lanser P, Gesell S. Pain management: The fifth vital sign. Healthc Benchmarks 2001; 8:62, 68-70.
23. Phillips DM. JCAHO pain management standards are unveiled. Joint Commission on Accreditation of Healthcare Organizations. JAMA 2000; 284:428-9.
24. Stoelting RK, Hillier SC. Opioid agonists and antagonists. In Pharmacology and Physiology in Anesthetic Practice. 4th edition. Philadelphia, Lippincott Williams & Wilkins 2006:87-117.
25. Owen H, Brose WG, Plummer JL, Mather LE. Variables of patient-controlled analgesia. 3. Test of an infusion-demand system using alfentanil. Anaesthesia 1990; 45:452-5.
26. Mather LE, Owen H. The scientific basis of patient-controlled analgesia. Anaesth Intensive Care 1988; 16:427-36.
27. Gadsden J, Hart S, Santos AC. Post-cesarean delivery analgesia. Anesth Analg 2005; 101:S62-9.
28. Bloomfield SS, Cissell GB, Mitchell J, et al. Analgesic efficacy and potency of two oral controlled-release morphine preparations. Clin Pharmacol Ther 1993; 53:469-78.
29. Jakobi P, Weiner Z, Solt I, et al. Oral analgesia in the treatment of post-cesarean pain. Eur J Obstet Gynecol Reprod Biol 2000; 93:61-4.
30. Jakobi P, Solt I, Tamir A, Zimmer EZ. Over-the-counter oral analgesia for postcesarean pain. Am J Obstet Gynecol 2002; 187:1066-9.
31. Weintraub A, Mankuta D. Dipyrone-induced oligohydramnios and ductus arteriosus restriction. Isr Med Assoc J 2006; 8:722-3.
32. Bar-Oz B, Clementi M, Di Giantonio E, et al. Metamizole (dipyrone, optalgin) in pregnancy, is it safe? A prospective comparative study. Eur J Obstet Gynecol Reprod Biol 2005; 119:176-9.
33. Edwards JE, McQuay HJ. Dipyrone and agranulocytosis: What is the risk? Lancet 2002; 360:1438.
34. American Society of Anesthesiologists Task Force on Obstetric Anesthesia. Practice guidelines for obstetric anesthesia. Anesthesiology 2007; 106:843-63.
35. American Society of Anesthesiologists Task Force on Acute Pain Management. Practice guidelines for acute pain management in the perioperative setting. Anesthesiology 2004; 100:1573-81.
36. Paech MJ, Moore JS, Evans SF. Meperidine for patient-controlled analgesia after cesarean section: Intravenous versus epidural administration. Anesthesiology 1994; 80:1268-76.
37. Ngan Kee WD, Lam KK, Chen PP, Gin T. Comparison of patient-controlled epidural analgesia with patient-controlled intravenous analgesia using pethidine or fentanyl. Anaesth Intensive Care 1997; 25:126-32.
38. Parker RK, White PF. Epidural patient-controlled analgesia: An alternative to intravenous patient-controlled analgesia for pain relief after cesarean delivery. Anesth Analg 1992; 75:245-51.
39. Eisenach JC, Grice SC, Dewan DM. Patient-controlled analgesia following cesarean section: A comparison with epidural and intramuscular narcotics. Anesthesiology 1988; 68:444-8.
40. Cade L, Ashley J, Ross AW. Comparison of epidural and intravenous opioid analgesia after elective caesarean section. Anaesth Intensive Care 1992; 20:41-5.
41. Rayburn WF, Geranis BJ, Ramadei CA, et al. Patient-controlled analgesia for post-cesarean section pain. Obstet Gynecol 1988; 72:136-9.
42. Cohen SE, Subak LL, Brose WG, Halpern J. Analgesia after cesarean delivery: Patient evaluations and costs of five opioid techniques. Reg Anesth 1991; 16:141-9.
43. Perez-Woods R, Grohar JC, Skaredoff M, et al. Pain control after cesarean birth: Efficacy of patient-controlled analgesia vs. traditional therapy (IM morphine). J Perinatol 1991; 11:174-81.
44. Harrison DM, Sinatra R, Morgese L, Chung JH. Epidural narcotic and patient-controlled analgesia for post-cesarean section pain relief. Anesthesiology 1988; 68:454-7.
45. Ballantyne JC, Carr DB, Chalmers TC, et al. Postoperative patient-controlled analgesia: Meta-analyses of initial randomized control trials. J Clin Anesth 1993; 5:182-93.
46. Walder B, Schafer M, Henzi I, Tramer MR. Efficacy and safety of patient-controlled opioid analgesia for acute postoperative pain: A quantitative systematic review. Acta Anaesthesiol Scand 2001; 45:795-804.
47. Hudcova J, McNicol E, Quah C, et al. Patient controlled opioid analgesia versus conventional opioid analgesia for postoperative pain. Cochrane Database Syst Rev 2006; (4):CD003348.
48. Howell PR, Gambling DR, Pavy T, et al. Patient-controlled analgesia following caesarean section under general anaesthesia: A comparison of fentanyl with morphine. Can J Anaesth 1995; 42:41-5.
49. Yost NP, Bloom SL, Sibley MK, et al. A hospital-sponsored quality improvement study of pain management after cesarean delivery. Am J Obstet Gynecol 2004; 190:1341-6.
50. Sinatra RS, Lodge K, Sibert K, et al. A comparison of morphine, meperidine, and oxymorphone as utilized in patient-controlled analgesia following cesarean delivery. Anesthesiology 1989; 70:585-90.
51. American College of Obstetricians and Gynecologists. Obstetric analgesia and anesthesia. ACOG Practice Bulletin No. 36. Washington, DC, July 2002. (Obstet Gynecol 2002; 100:177-91).
52. Wittels B, Glosten B, Faure EAM, et al. Postcesarean analgesia with both epidural morphine and intravenous patient-controlled analgesia: Neurobehavioral outcomes among nursing neonates. Anesth Analg 1997; 85:600-6.

53. JCAHO alert gives new recommendations for PCA. Hosp Peer Rev 2005; 30:24-5.
54. Owen H, Plummer JL, Armstrong I, et al. Variables of patient-controlled analgesia. 1. Bolus size. Anaesthesia 1989; 44:7-10.
55. Owen H, Szekely SM, Plummer JL, et al. Variables of patient-controlled analgesia. 2. Concurrent infusion. Anaesthesia 1989; 44:11-3.
56. Owen H, Kluger MT, Plummer JL. Variables of patient-controlled analgesia. 4. The relevance of bolus dose size to supplement a background infusion. Anaesthesia 1990; 45:619-22.
57. American Pain Society. Principles of Analgesic Use in the Treatment of Acute Pain and Cancer Pain. 5th edition. Glenview, IL, American Pain Society, 2003.
58. Sinatra R, Chung KS, Silverman DG, et al. An evaluation of morphine and oxymorphone administered via patient-controlled analgesia (PCA) or PCA plus basal infusion in postcesarean-delivery patients. Anesthesiology 1989; 71:502-7.
59. Parker RK, Holtmann B, White PF. Patient-controlled analgesia: Does a concurrent opioid infusion improve pain management after surgery? JAMA 1991; 266:1947-52.
60. Parker RK, Holtmann B, White PF. Effects of a nighttime opioid infusion with PCA therapy on patient comfort and analgesic requirements after abdominal hysterectomy. Anesthesiology 1992; 76:362-7.
61. McCoy EP, Furness G, Wright PM. Patient-controlled analgesia with and without background infusion: Analgesia assessed using the demand:delivery ratio. Anaesthesia 1993; 48:256-60.
62. Davis KM, Esposito MA, Meyer BA. Oral analgesia compared with intravenous patient-controlled analgesia for pain after cesarean delivery: A randomized controlled trial. Am J Obstet Gynecol 2006; 194:967-71.
63. Aubrun F, Langeron O, Quesnel C, et al. Relationships between measurement of pain using visual analog score and morphine requirements during postoperative intravenous morphine titration. Anesthesiology 2003; 98:1415-21.
64. Berde CB, Brennan TJ, Raja SN. Opioids: More to learn, improvements to be made. Anesthesiology 2003; 98:1309-12.
65. Bodian CA, Freedman G, Hossain S, et al. The visual analog scale for pain: Clinical significance in postoperative patients. Anesthesiology 2001; 95:1356-61.
66. Campbell WI, Patterson CC. Quantifying meaningful changes in pain. Anaesthesia 1998; 53:121-5.
67. Wong P, Chadwick FD, Karovits J. Intranasal fentanyl for postoperative analgesia after elective Caesarean section. Anaesthesia 2003; 58:818-9.
68. Reasbeck PG, Rice ML, Reasbeck JC. Double-blind controlled trial of indomethacin as an adjunct to narcotic analgesia after major abdominal surgery. Lancet 1982; 2(8290):115-8.
69. Engel C, Kristensen SS, Axel C, et al. Indomethacin and the stress response to hysterectomy. Acta Anaesthesiol Scand 1989; 33:540-4.
70. Harrison RF, Devitt M. Indomethacin and ethamsylate alone and in combination for the relief of post episiotomy pain. Ir J Med Sci 1992; 161:493-7.
71. Crocker S, Paech M. Preoperative rectal indomethacin for analgesia after laparoscopic sterilisation. Anaesth Intensive Care 1992; 20:337-40.
72. Ambrose FP. A retrospective study of the effect of postoperative indomethacin rectal suppositories on the need for narcotic analgesia in patients who had a cesarean delivery while they were under regional anesthesia. Am J Obstet Gynecol 2001; 184:1544-7.
73. Lim NL, Lo WK, Chong JL, Pan AX. Single dose diclofenac suppository reduces post-Cesarean PCEA requirements. Can J Anaesth 2001; 48:383-6.
74. Pavy TJ, Gambling DR, Merrick PM, Douglas MJ. Rectal indomethacin potentiates spinal morphine analgesia after caesarean delivery. Anaesth Intensive Care 1995; 23:555-9.
75. Dennis AR, Leeson-Payne CG, Hobbs GU. Analgesia after caesarean section: The use of rectal diclofenac as an adjunct to spinal morphine. Anaesthesia 1995; 50:297-9.
76. Olofsson CI, Legeby MH, Nygards EB, Ostman KM. Diclofenac in the treatment of pain after caesarean delivery: An opioid-saving strategy. Eur J Obstet Gynecol Reprod Biol 2000; 88:143-6.
77. Luthman J, Kay NH, White JB. The morphine sparing effect of diclofenac sodium following caesarean section under spinal anaesthesia. Int J Obstet Anesth 1994; 3:82-6.
78. Cardoso MM, Carvalho JC, Amaro AR, et al. Small doses of intrathecal morphine combined with systemic diclofenac for postoperative pain control after cesarean delivery. Anesth Analg 1998; 86:538-41.
79. Bush DJ, Lyons G, MacDonald R. Diclofenac for analgesia after caesarean section. Anaesthesia 1992; 47:1075-7.
80. Siddik SM, Aouad MT, Jalbout MI, et al. Diclofenac and/or propacetamol for postoperative pain management after cesarean delivery in patients receiving patient controlled analgesia morphine. Reg Anesth Pain Med 2001; 26:310-5.
81. Al-Waili NS. Efficacy and safety of repeated postoperative administration of intramuscular diclofenac sodium in the treatment of post-cesarean section pain: A double-blind study. Arch Med Res 2001; 32:148-54.
82. Wilder-Smith CH, Hill L, Dyer RA, et al. Postoperative sensitization and pain after cesarean delivery and the effects of single IM doses of tramadol and diclofenac alone and in combination. Anesth Analg 2003; 97:526-33.
83. Dahl V, Hagen IE, Sveen AM, et al. High-dose diclofenac for postoperative analgesia after elective caesarean section in regional anaesthesia. Int J Obstet Anesth 2002; 11:91-4.
84. Angle PJ, Halpern SH, Leighton BL, et al. A randomized controlled trial examining the effect of naproxen on analgesia during the second day after cesarean delivery. Anesth Analg 2002; 95:741-5.
85. O'Hara DA, Fanciullo G, Hubbard L, et al. Evaluation of the safety and efficacy of ketorolac versus morphine by patient-controlled analgesia for postoperative pain. Pharmacotherapy 1997; 17:891-9.
86. Lowder JL, Shackelford DP, Holbert D, Beste TM. A randomized, controlled trial to compare ketorolac tromethamine versus placebo after cesarean section to reduce pain and narcotic usage. Am J Obstet Gynecol 2003; 189:1559-62.
87. Bloomfield SS, Mitchell J, Cissell GB, et al. Ketorolac versus aspirin for postpartum uterine pain. Pharmacotherapy 1986; 6:247-52.
88. El-Tahan MR, Warda OM, Yasseen AM, et al. A randomized study of the effects of preoperative ketorolac on general anaesthesia for caesarean section. Int J Obstet Anesth 2007; 16:214-20.
89. Tzeng JI, Mok MS. Combination of intramuscular ketorolac and low dose epidural morphine for the relief of post-caesarean pain. Ann Acad Med Singapore 1994; 23:10-3.
90. Pavy TJ, Paech MJ, Evans SF. The effect of intravenous ketorolac on opioid requirement and pain after cesarean delivery. Anesth Analg 2001; 92:1010-4.
91. Giles W, Bisits A. The present and future of tocolysis. Best Pract Res Clin Obstet Gynaecol 2007; 21:857-68.
92. Makris A, Thornton C, Hennessy A. Postpartum hypertension and nonsteroidal analgesia. Am J Obstet Gynecol 2004; 190:577-8.
93. Curhan GC, Willett WC, Rosner B, Stampfer MJ. Frequency of analgesic use and risk of hypertension in younger women. Arch Intern Med 2002; 162:2204-8.
94. Burian M, Geisslinger G. COX-dependent mechanisms involved in the antinociceptive action of NSAIDs at central and peripheral sites. Pharmacol Ther 2005; 107:139-54.
95. Romsing J, Moiniche S, Ostergaard D, Dahl JB. Local infiltration with NSAIDs for postoperative analgesia: Evidence for a peripheral analgesic action. Acta Anaesthesiol Scand 2000; 44:672-83.
96. Lavand'homme PM, Roelants F, Waterloos H, De Kock MF. Postoperative analgesic effects of continuous wound infiltration with diclofenac after elective cesarean delivery. Anesthesiology 2007; 106:1220-5.
97. Dahl JB, Kehlet H. Non-steroidal anti-inflammatory drugs: Rationale for use in severe postoperative pain. Br J Anaesth 1991; 66:703-12.
98. Wee MY, Brown H, Reynolds F. The National Institute of Clinical Excellence (NICE) guidelines for caesarean sections: Implications for the anaesthetist. Int J Obstet Anesth 2005; 14:147-58.

99. Marret E, Kurdi O, Zufferey P, Bonnet F. Effects of nonsteroidal antiinflammatory drugs on patient-controlled analgesia morphine side effects: Meta-analysis of randomized controlled trials. Anesthesiology 2005; 102:1249-60.
100. Urban MK. COX-2 specific inhibitors offer improved advantages over traditional NSAIDs. Orthopedics 2000; 23:S761-4.
101. Meli R, Antonelli E, Cirino G. Analgesia and cyclo-oxygenase inhibitors. Dig Liver Dis 2001; 33(Suppl 2):S8-11.
102. Masferrer JL, Isakson PC, Seibert K. Cyclooxygenase-2 inhibitors: A new class of anti-inflammatory agents that spare the gastrointestinal tract. Gastroenterol Clin North Am 1996; 25:363-72.
103. Fenton C, Keating GM, Wagstaff AJ. Valdecoxib: A review of its use in the management of osteoarthritis, rheumatoid arthritis, dysmenorrhoea and acute pain. Drugs 2004; 64:1231-61.
104. Sinatra R. Role of COX-2 inhibitors in the evolution of acute pain management. J Pain Symptom Manage 2002; 24:S18-27.
105. Desjardins PJ, Shu VS, Recker DP, et al. A single preoperative oral dose of valdecoxib, a new cyclooxygenase-2 specific inhibitor, relieves post-oral surgery or bunionectomy pain. Anesthesiology 2002; 97:565-73.
106. Gan TJ, Joshi GP, Zhao SZ, et al. Presurgical intravenous parecoxib sodium and follow-up oral valdecoxib for pain management after laparoscopic cholecystectomy surgery reduces opioid requirements and opioid-related adverse effects. Acta Anaesthesiol Scand 2004; 48:1194-207.
107. Carvalho B, Chu L, Fuller A, et al. Valdecoxib for postoperative pain management after cesarean delivery: A randomized, double-blind, placebo-controlled study. Anesth Analg 2006; 103:664-70.
108. Schug SA, Sidebotham DA, McGuinnety M, et al. Acetaminophen as an adjunct to morphine by patient-controlled analgesia in the management of acute postoperative pain. Anesth Analg 1998; 87:368-72.
109. Moore A, Collins S, Carroll D, McQuay H. Paracetamol with and without codeine in acute pain: A quantitative systematic review. Pain 1997; 70:193-201.
110. Snell P, Hicks C. An exploratory study in the UK of the effectiveness of three different pain management regimens for post-caesarean section women. Midwifery 2006; 22:249-61.
111. Hein A, Jakobsson J, Ryberg G. Paracetamol 1 g given rectally at the end of minor gynaecological surgery is not efficacious in reducing postoperative pain. Acta Anaesthesiol Scand 1999; 43:248-51.
112. Peduto VA, Ballabio M, Stefanini S. Efficacy of propacetamol in the treatment of postoperative pain: Morphine-sparing effect in orthopedic surgery. Italian Collaborative Group on Propacetamol. Acta Anaesthesiol Scand 1998; 42:293-8.
113. Remy C, Marret E, Bonnet F. Effects of acetaminophen on morphine side-effects and consumption after major surgery: Meta-analysis of randomized controlled trials. Br J Anaesth 2005; 94:505-13.
114. Peter EA, Janssen PA, Grange CS, Douglas MJ. Ibuprofen versus acetaminophen with codeine for the relief of perineal pain after childbirth: A randomized controlled trial. Can Med Assoc J 2001; 165:1203-9.
115. Kehlet H, Dahl JB. The value of "multimodal" or "balanced analgesia" in postoperative pain treatment. Anesth Analg 1993; 77:1048-56.
116. Dahl JB, Moiniche S, Kehlet H. Wound infiltration with local anaesthetics for postoperative pain relief. Acta Anaesthesiol Scand 1994; 38:7-14.
117. Rawal N. Incisional and intra-articular infusions. Best Pract Res Clin Anaesthesiol 2002; 16:321-43.
118. Vintar N, Pozlep G, Rawal N, et al. Incisional self-administration of bupivacaine or ropivacaine provides effective analgesia after inguinal hernia repair. Can J Anaesth 2002; 49:481-6.
119. Zohar E, Fredman B, Phillipov A, et al. The analgesic efficacy of patient-controlled bupivacaine wound instillation after total abdominal hysterectomy with bilateral salpingo-oophorectomy. Anesth Analg 2001; 93:482-7.
120. Moiniche S, Mikkelsen S, Wetterslev J, Dahl JB. A qualitative systematic review of incisional local anaesthesia for postoperative pain relief after abdominal operations. Br J Anaesth 1998; 81:377-83.
121. Trotter TN, Hayes-Gregson P, Robinson S, et al. Wound infiltration of local anaesthetic after lower segment caesarean section. Anaesthesia 1991; 46:404-7.
122. Pavy TJ, Gambling DR, Kliffer AP, et al. Effect of preoperative skin infiltration with 0.5% bupivacaine on postoperative pain following cesarean section under spinal anesthesia. Int J Obstet Anesth 1994; 3:199-202.
123. Ranta PO, Ala-Kokko TI, Kukkonen JE, et al. Incisional and epidural analgesia after caesarean delivery: A prospective, placebo-controlled, randomised clinical study. Int J Obstet Anesth 2006; 15:189-94.
124. Fredman B, Shapiro A, Zohar E, et al. The analgesic efficacy of patient-controlled ropivacaine instillation after Cesarean delivery. Anesth Analg 2000; 91:1436-40.
125. Givens VA, Lipscomb GH, Meyer NL. A randomized trial of postoperative wound irrigation with local anesthetic for pain after cesarean delivery. Am J Obstet Gynecol 2002; 186:1188-91.
126. Liu SS, Richman JM, Thirlby RC, Wu CL. Efficacy of continuous wound catheters delivering local anesthetic for postoperative analgesia: A quantitative and qualitative systematic review of randomized controlled trials. J Am Coll Surg 2006; 203:914-32.
127. Bell EA, Jones BP, Olufolabi AJ, et al. Iliohypogastric-ilioinguinal peripheral nerve block for post-cesarean delivery analgesia decreases morphine use but not opioid-related side effects. Can J Anesth 2002; 49:694-700.
128. Gucev G, Yasui GM, Chang TY, Lee J. Bilateral ultrasound-guided continuous ilioinguinal-iliohypogastric block for pain relief after cesarean delivery. Anesth Analg 2008; 106:1220-2.
129. McDonnell JG, Curly G, Carney J, et al. The analgesic efficacy of transversus abdominis plane block after cesarean delivery: A randomized controlled trial. Anesth Analg 2008; 106:186-91.
130. Unnerstall JR, Kopajtic TA, Kuhar MJ. Distribution of alpha-2-agonist binding sites in the rat and human central nervous system: Analysis of some functional, anatomic correlates of the pharmacologic effects of clonidine and related adrenergic agents. Brain Res 1984; 319:69-101.
131. Arain SR, Ruehlow RM, Uhrich TD, Ebert TJ. The efficacy of dexmedetomidine versus morphine for postoperative analgesia after major inpatient surgery. Anesth Analg 2004; 98:153-8.
132. Hall JE, Uhrich TD, Barney JA, et al. Sedative, amnestic, and analgesic properties of small-dose dexmedetomidine infusions. Anesth Analg 2000; 90:699-705.
133. Xiao WH, Bennett GJ. Magnesium suppresses neuropathic pain responses in rats via a spinal site of action. Brain Res 1994; 666:168-72.
134. Levaux C, Bonhomme V, Dewandre PY, et al. Effect of intra-operative magnesium sulphate on pain relief and patient comfort after major lumbar orthopaedic surgery. Anaesthesia 2003; 58:131-5.
135. Unlugenc H, Gunduz M, Ozalevli M, Akman H. A comparative study on the analgesic effect of tramadol, tramadol plus magnesium, and tramadol plus ketamine for postoperative pain management after major abdominal surgery. Acta Anaesthesiol Scand 2002; 46:1025-30.
136. Bhatia A, Kashyap L, Pawar DK, Trikha A. Effect of intraoperative magnesium infusion on perioperative analgesia in open cholecystectomy. J Clin Anesth 2004; 16:262-5.
137. Paech MJ, Magann EF, Doherty DA, et al. Does magnesium sulfate reduce the short- and long-term requirements for pain relief after caesarean delivery? A double-blind placebo-controlled trial. Am J Obstet Gynecol 2006; 194:1596-602.
138. Lysakowski C, Dumont L, Czarnetzki C, Tramer MR. Magnesium as an adjuvant to postoperative analgesia: A systematic review of randomized trials. Anesth Analg 2007; 104:1532-9.
139. Tiippana EM, Hamunen K, Kontinen VK, Kalso E. Do surgical patients benefit from perioperative gabapentin/pregabalin? A systematic review of efficacy and safety. Anesth Analg 2007; 104:1545-56.
140. Hurley RW, Cohen SP, Williams KA, et al. The analgesic effects of perioperative gabapentin on postoperative pain: A meta-analysis. Reg Anesth Pain Med 2006; 31:237-47.
141. Peng PW, Wijeysundera DN, Li CC. Use of gabapentin for perioperative pain control—a meta-analysis. Pain Res Manag 2007; 12:85-92.
142. Ho KY, Gan TJ, Habib AS. Gabapentin and postoperative pain—a systematic review of randomized controlled trials. Pain 2006; 126:91-101.

143. Stoelting RK, Hillier SC. Nonbarbiturate induction drugs. In Pharmacology and Physiology in Anesthetic Practice. 4th edition. Philadelphia, Lippincott Williams & Wilkins, 2006:155-78.
144. Sen S, Ozmert G, Aydin ON, et al. The persisting analgesic effect of low-dose intravenous ketamine after spinal anaesthesia for caesarean section. Eur J Anaesthesiol 2005; 22:518-23.
145. Bell RF, Dahl JB, Moore RA, Kalso E. Perioperative ketamine for acute postoperative pain. Cochrane Database Syst Rev 2006; (1):CD004603.
146. Hepner DL. Preemptive analgesia: What does it really mean? Anesthesiology 2000; 93:1368.
147. Choi DM, Kliffer AP, Douglas MJ. Dextromethorphan and intrathecal morphine for analgesia after Caesarean section under spinal anaesthesia. Br J Anaesth 2003; 90:653-8.
148. Duedahl TH, Romsing J, Moiniche S, Dahl JB. A qualitative systematic review of peri-operative dextromethorphan in post-operative pain. Acta Anaesthesiol Scand 2006; 50:1-13.
149. Chez RA, Jonas WB. Complementary and alternative medicine. Part I. Clinical studies in obstetrics. Obstet Gynecol Surv 1997; 52:704-8.
150. Umeh BU. Sacral acupuncture for pain relief in labour: Initial clinical experience in Nigerian women. Acupunct Electrother Res 1986; 11:147-51.
151. Wang B, Tang J, White PF, et al. Effect of the intensity of transcutaneous acupoint electrical stimulation on the postoperative analgesic requirement. Anesth Analg 1997; 85:406-13.
152. Chen L, Tang J, White PF, et al. The effect of location of transcutaneous electrical nerve stimulation on postoperative opioid analgesic requirement: Acupoint versus nonacupoint stimulation. Anesth Analg 1998; 87:1129-34.
153. Ali J, Yaffe CS, Serrette C. The effect of transcutaneous electric nerve stimulation on postoperative pain and pulmonary function. Surgery 1981; 89:507-12.
154. Benedetti F, Amanzio M, Casadio C, et al. Control of postoperative pain by transcutaneous electrical nerve stimulation after thoracic operations. Ann Thorac Surg 1997; 63:773-6.
155. Evron S, Schenker JG, Olshwang D, et al. Postoperative analgesia by percutaneous electrical stimulation in gynecology and obstetrics. Eur J Obstet Gynecol Reprod Biol 1981; 12:305-13.
156. Hamza MA, White PF, Ahmed HE, Ghoname EA. Effect of the frequency of transcutaneous electrical nerve stimulation on the postoperative opioid analgesic requirement and recovery profile. Anesthesiology 1999; 91:1232-8.
157. Han JS, Chen XH, Sun SL, et al. Effect of low- and high-frequency TENS on Met-enkephalin-Arg-Phe and dynorphin A immunoreactivity in human lumbar CSF. Pain 1991; 47:295-8.
158. Han JS, Xie GX, Goldstein A. Analgesia induced by intrathecal injection of dynorphin B in the rat. Life Sciences 1984; 34:1573-9.
159. Han JS, Xie GX, Ding XZ, Fan SC. High and low frequency electroacupuncture analgesia are mediated by different opioid peptides. Pain 1984; 2:471-4.
160. Chen XH, Han JS. All three types of opioid receptors in the spinal cord are important for 2/15 Hz electroacupuncture analgesia. Eur J Pharmacol 1992; 211:203-10.
161. Chez RA, Jonas WB. Complementary and alternative medicine. Part II. Clinical studies in gynecology. Obstet Gynecol Surv 1997; 52:709-16.
162. Elia N, Lysakowski C, Tramer MR. Does multimodal analgesia with acetaminophen, nonsteroidal antiinflammatory drugs, or selective cyclooxygenase-2 inhibitors and patient-controlled analgesia morphine offer advantages over morphine alone? Meta-analyses of randomized trials. Anesthesiology 2005; 103:1296-304.
163. Liu SS, Wu CL. The effect of analgesic technique on postoperative patient-reported outcomes including analgesia: A systematic review. Anesth Analg 2007; 105:789-808.
164. Gartner LM, Morton J, Lawrence RA, et al. Breastfeeding and the use of human milk. Pediatrics 2005; 115:496-506.
165. Ito S. Drug therapy for breast-feeding women. N Engl J Med 2000; 343:118-26.
166. Stultz EE, Stokes JL, Shaffer ML, et al. Extent of medication use in breastfeeding women. Breastfeed Med 2007; 2:145-51.
167. Della-Giustina K, Chow G. Medications in pregnancy and lactation. Emerg Med Clin North Am 2003; 21:585-613.
168. American Academy of Pediatrics Committee on Drugs. Transfer of drugs and other chemicals into human milk. Pediatrics 2001; 108:776-89.
169. Bennett PN. Use of the monographs on drugs. In Bennett P, editor. Drugs and Human Lactation. Amsterdam, Elsevier, 1996:67-74.
170. Hale TW. Maternal medications during breastfeeding. Clin Obstet Gynecol 2004; 47:696-711.
171. Hale TW, McDonald R, Boger J. Transfer of celecoxib into human milk. J Hum Lact 2004; 20:397-403.
172. Blinick G, Inturrisi CE, Jerez E, Wallach RC. Methadone assays in pregnant women and progeny. Am J Obstet Gynecol 1975; 121:617-21.
173. Wojnar-Horton RE, Kristensen JH, Yapp P, et al. Methadone distribution and excretion into breast milk of clients in a methadone maintenance programme. Br J Clin Pharmacol 1997; 44:543-7.
174. Nitsun M, Szokol JW, Saleh HJ, et al. Pharmacokinetics of midazolam, propofol, and fentanyl transfer to human breast milk. Clin Pharmacol Ther 2006; 79:549-57.
175. Rathmell JP, Viscomi CM, Ashburn MA. Management of nonobstetric pain during pregnancy and lactation. Anesth Analg 1997; 85:1074-87.
176. Fidalgo I, Correa R, Gomez Carrasco JA, Martinez Quiroga F. Acute anemia, rectorrhagia and hematuria caused by ingestion of naproxen. An Esp Pediatr 1989; 30:317-9.
177. Ketorolac Product Insert. Nutley, NJ, Roche Pharmaceuticals, 2002.
178. Wischnik A, Manth SM, Lloyd J, et al. The excretion of ketorolac tromethamine into breast milk after multiple oral dosing. Eur J Clin Pharmacol 1989; 36:521-4.
179. Seaton S, Reeves M, McLean S. Oxycodone as a component of multimodal analgesia for lactating mothers after Caesarean section: Relationships between maternal plasma, breast milk and neonatal plasma levels. Aust N Z J Obstet Gynaecol 2007; 47:181-5.
180. Anderson PO, Sauberan JB, Lane JR, Rossi SS. Hydrocodone excretion into breast milk: The first two reported cases. Breastfeed Med 2007; 2:10-4.
181. Meny RG, Naumburg EG, Alger LS, et al. Codeine and the breastfed neonate. J Hum Lact 1993; 9:237-40.
182. Koren G, Cairns J, Chitayat D, et al. Pharmacogenetics of morphine poisoning in a breastfed neonate of a codeine-prescribed mother. Lancet 2006; 368:704.
183. US Food and Drug Administration Center for Drug Evaluation and Research. FDA Public Health Advisory. Use of Codeine by Some Breastfeeding Mothers May Lead to Life-Threatening Side Effects in Nursing Babies. August 17, 2007. Available at http://www.fda.gov/cder/drug/advisory/codeine.htm/
184. Madadi P, Koren G, Cairns J, et al. Safety of codeine during breastfeeding: Fatal morphine poisoning in the breastfed neonate of a mother prescribed codeine. Can Fam Physician 2007; 53:33-5.
185. Kristensen JH, Ilett KF, Hackett LP, Kohan R. Gabapentin and breastfeeding: A case report. J Hum Lact 2006; 22:426-8.
186. Ohman I, Vitols S, Tomson T. Pharmacokinetics of gabapentin during delivery, in the neonatal period, and lactation: Does a fetal accumulation occur during pregnancy? Epilepsia 2005; 46:1621-4.
187. Gardiner SJ, Doogue MP, Zhang M, Begg EJ. Quantification of infant exposure to celecoxib through breast milk. Br J Clin Pharmacol 2006; 61:101-4.
188. Borgatta L, Jenny RW, Gruss L, et al. Clinical significance of methohexital, meperidine, and diazepam in breast milk. J Clin Pharmacol 1997; 37:186-92.

Chapter 28

Postoperative Analgesia: Epidural and Spinal Techniques

Brendan Carvalho, M.B.B.Ch., FRCA
Alexander Butwick, M.B.B.S., FRCA

More than 1 million cesarean deliveries, accounting for more than 30% of all births, are performed each year in the United States.[1] The cesarean delivery rate in developed countries continues to rise as a result of changing patterns in obstetric practice and maternal requests for this mode of delivery.[1,2] Postoperative pain after cesarean delivery can be moderate to severe and is equivalent to that reported after abdominal hysterectomy.[3] Management of postoperative pain is frequently substandard, with 30% to 80% of patients experiencing moderate to severe postoperative pain.[4,5] In an effort to improve pain management in the United States, The Joint Commission (formerly known as The Joint Commission on Accreditation of Healthcare Organizations) has stated that postoperative pain should be the "fifth vital sign." The Joint Commission also proposed the goal of having patients experience uniformly low postoperative pain scores of less than 3 (as measured by a numerical pain scale [0 to 10] at rest and with movement, with the worst pain being a score of 10). In the United Kingdom, the Royal College of Anaesthetists[6] has proposed the following standards for adequate postcesarean analgesia:

1. More than 90% of women should have a pain score of less than 3 out of 10 (as measured by a numerical pain scale [0 to 10], with the worst pain being a score of 10).
2. More than 90% of women should be satisfied with their pain management.[6]

TABLE 28-1 Women's Ranking and Relative Value of Potential Anesthesia Outcomes Prior to Cesarean Delivery*

Outcome	Rank†	Relative Value‡
Pain during cesarean	8.4 ± 2.2	27 ± 18
Pain after cesarean	8.3 ± 1.8	18 ± 10
Vomiting	7.8 ± 1.5	12 ± 7
Nausea	6.8 ± 1.7	11 ± 7
Cramping	6.0 ± 1.9	10 ± 8
Itching	5.6 ± 2.1	9 ± 8
Shivering	4.6 ± 1.7	6 ± 6
Anxiety	4.1 ± 1.9	5 ± 4
Somnolence	2.9 ± 1.4	3 ± 3
Normal	1	0

*Data are mean ± standard deviation.

†Rank = 1 to 10 from the most desirable (1) to the least desirable (10) outcome.

‡Relative value = dollar value patients would pay to avoid an outcome (e.g., they would pay $27 of a theoretical $100 to avoid pain during cesarean delivery).

From Carvalho B, Cohen SE, Lipman SS, et al. Patient preferences for anesthesia outcomes associated with cesarean delivery. Anesth Analg 2005; 101:1182-7.

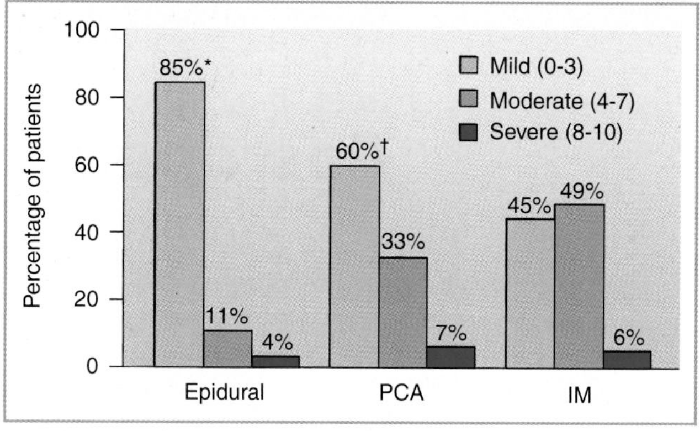

FIGURE 28-1 Percentage of patients recovering from cesarean delivery and treated with either epidural analgesia, intravenous patient-controlled analgesia (PCA), or intramuscular (IM) administration of morphine and reporting mild, moderate, or severe discomfort during a 24-hour study period. *$P < .05$, epidural versus PCA and IM; †P = NS, PCA versus IM. (From Harrison DM, Sinatra RS, Morgese L, et al. Epidural narcotic and PCA for postcesarean section pain relief. Anesthesiology 1988; 68:454-7.)

A 2007 study suggested that these goals for postcesarean analgesia and maternal satisfaction are frequently not attained.[7] Pain associated with cesarean delivery is the most important concern for expectant mothers prior to delivery (Table 28-1).[8] Effective pain management should be highlighted as an essential element of postoperative care.

NEURAXIAL TECHNIQUES FOR CESAREAN DELIVERY

In the United States and the United Kingdom, most cesarean deliveries are performed with neuraxial anesthesia (spinal, epidural, or combined spinal-epidural [CSE] techniques).[9,10] The use of noncutting spinal needles (e.g., Sprotte, Whitacre) is associated with a low incidence of post–dural puncture headache and has increased the percentage of cesarean deliveries performed with spinal anesthesia.[10] Spinal anesthesia has been shown to be more cost effective than epidural anesthesia for cesarean delivery, because needle placement is technically less challenging and adequate surgical anesthesia is achieved more rapidly.[11] Nonetheless, both epidural and spinal techniques are commonly utilized in modern obstetric anesthesia practice. A meta-analysis found no differences between the two techniques with regard to failure rate, additional requests for intraoperative analgesia, conversion to general anesthesia, maternal satisfaction, postoperative analgesia requirements, or neonatal outcomes.[12]

A workforce survey in the United States demonstrated that the majority of laboring women receive epidural analgesia.[9] If a patient receiving epidural analgesia during labor subsequently requires a cesarean delivery, most anesthesia providers would choose to administer medications through the epidural catheter to achieve adequate surgical anesthesia.[9,10] The CSE technique incorporates the rapid administration and onset of spinal anesthesia with placement of an epidural catheter to permit administration of additional agents, if necessary. After surgery, patients with an epidural catheter *in situ* may benefit from intermittent bolus injection or continuous epidural infusion of local anesthetic with opioid for postoperative analgesia.

Administration of neuraxial opioids has become a popular means of augmenting intraoperative anesthesia and optimizing postoperative analgesia. A meta-analysis of studies involving a broad population of patients undergoing a variety of surgical procedures confirmed that opioids delivered by either patient-controlled epidural analgesia or continous epidural infusion provide postoperative pain relief that is superior to that provided by intravenous patient-controlled analgesia (PCA).[13] Similar results have been reported in studies comparing intrathecal and epidural opioids with intravenous opioid PCA or intramuscular opioids after cesarean delivery (Figure 28-1).[14-17]

Although neuraxial opioids provide superior postcesarean analgesia to that provided by systemic opioids, some opioid-related side effects (e.g., pruritus) commonly occur with this mode of administration.[14,17,18] Both higher[18,19] and lower[20,21] maternal satisfaction scores have been reported with neuraxial versus systemic opioid administration for postcesarean analgesia. This dichotomy in maternal satisfaction may relate to the degree of analgesia versus side effects (e.g., pruritus, nausea and vomiting) experienced.

BENEFITS OF POSTOPERATIVE ANALGESIA

Reduced Complications and Improved Outcome

In selected high-risk patients undergoing nonobstetric surgery, the use of neuraxial anesthetic/analgesic techniques may confer physiologic benefits that decrease perioperative complications and improve postoperative outcomes.[22-24] The potential benefits include a lower rate of perioperative cardiovascular complications, a lower incidence of pulmonary infection and pulmonary embolism, an earlier return of gastrointestinal function, fewer coagulation disturbances, and a reduction in inflammatory and stress-induced responses to surgery.[22-24] Although studies and meta-analyses have consistently shown a reduction in postoperative pain with neuraxial analgesia, less consistent results have been demonstrated in other postoperative outcome measures.[22]

Neuraxial opioids currently represent the "gold standard" for providing effective postcesarean analgesia. Most patients undergoing cesarean delivery are young, healthy, and at low risk for serious perioperative morbidity and mortality. For this patient population, the benefits of neuraxial analgesia include better postoperative analgesia, increased functional ability, earlier ambulation, and earlier return of bowel function.[25-28] However, differences in postcesarean complication rates with the use of neuraxial versus systemic opioid analgesia have not been definitively demonstrated.[25,29]

Surgical trauma and postoperative immobility are associated with an increased risk of postoperative deep vein thrombosis and pulmonary embolism. In addition, the risk of venous thromboembolism is sixfold higher in pregnant women and 10-fold higher in puerperal women than in nonpregnant women of similar age.[30] In theory, early ambulation and avoidance of prolonged immobility may reduce the risk of postpartum thrombosis and pulmonary embolism. Effective postoperative analgesia after neuraxial anesthesia can reduce pain on movement, thereby facilitating deep breathing, coughing, and early ambulation. These beneficial effects might lower the incidence of pulmonary complications (i.e., atelectasis, pneumonia) after cesarean delivery.

Neuraxial analgesic techniques may be more likely to reduce perioperative morbidity in high-risk obstetric patients. Women with severe preeclampsia, cardiovascular disease, and morbid obesity may benefit from the reduction in cardiovascular stress and improved pulmonary function associated with effective postcesarean analgesia.[31,32] Rawal et al.[32] compared the efficacy of intramuscular versus epidural morphine in 30 nonpregnant, morbidly obese patients after abdominal surgery. Patients in the epidural morphine group were more alert, ambulated more quickly, recovered bowel function earlier, and had fewer pulmonary complications.

Investigators have found that a continuous epidural infusion (CEI) of an opioid with a dilute solution of local anesthetic attenuates coagulation abnormalities, hemodynamic fluctuation, and stress hormone responses in nonpregnant patients.[33-35] Some studies have suggested that opioid-based, patient-controlled epidural analgesia (PCEA) may improve postoperative outcome.[36-38] Patients treated with PCEA meperidine following cesarean delivery ambulated more quickly and experienced an earlier return of gastrointestinal function than similar patients who received intravenous meperidine PCA.[36]

Breast-feeding and Interactions with the Newborn

Maternal-infant bonding may be impeded by incisional pain after cesarean delivery. Postoperative epidural analgesia may indirectly improve the mother's ability to breast-feed and interact with her newborn infant after cesarean delivery.[39,40] Ambulation, breast-feeding, early maternal-infant bonding, and neonatal care may be hampered by the side effects (e.g., sedation, dysphoria, nausea and vomiting) associated with systemic administration of opioids.[41] In addition, nursing mothers are frequently concerned about neonatal exposure to analgesic drugs through breast milk.[8,42,43] Although only a small percentage (1% to 3%) of maternal opioid doses is transferred in breast milk to the neonate, large systemic maternal doses may result in neonatal neurobehavioral depression (especially with meperidine)[44] and potentially interfere with breast-feeding success.[39,45]

CHRONIC POSTOPERATIVE PAIN

Chronic postoperative pain (incisional pain that persists 12 weeks or more after surgery) is well described following various types of surgery, including amputation, inguinal herniorrhaphy, cholecystectomy, mastectomy, and thoracotomy.[46,47] The incidence varies (10% to 50%) with different surgical procedures and patient populations.[46,47]

Chronic incisional and pelvic pain have been described after cesarean delivery.[48-50] A retrospective questionnaire study of 244 patients found that 12% of the 220 respondents reported persistent incisional pain at 10 months after cesarean delivery.[49] A prospective study by Lavand'homme et al.[48] found that 15% of patients reported incisional pain at 6 months. A similar incidence of persistent pain after cesarean delivery has been reported in other studies.[51] In contrast, a study involving more than 2500 women found a lower incidence of chronic pain after cesarean delivery (9% at 8 weeks and 2% at 6 months), with no difference between patients who underwent a cesarean and those who had a vaginal delivery.[52] Regardless, even a low incidence of persistent pain has a significant social impact owing to the large number of women undergoing cesarean delivery each year.[1,2]

Many psychosocial and pathophysiologic factors may increase the likelihood of chronic postoperative pain.[46,47] Severe acute postoperative pain is one of the most prominent risk factors.[46,49] The development of chronic pain after surgery has been associated with central sensitization, hyperalgesia, and allodynia. Measures to attenuate or prevent pain sensitization may reduce the likelihood of development of chronic postoperative pain. Studies have shown that the use of perioperative neuraxial blockade may prevent central sensitization and chronic pain following colonic surgery.[53,54] De Kock et al.[54] postulated that intrathecal clonidine, administered prior to colonic surgery, had anti-hyperalgesic effects and resulted in less residual pain at 6 months than placebo. Lavand'homme et al.[53] reported that the co-administration of a multimodal antihyperalgesic regimen (intravenous ketamine and epidural analgesia [bupivacaine, sufentanil, clonidine]) was associated with a lower incidence of residual pain 1 year after colonic surgery than the use of conventional intravenous analgesia during and after surgery. Additional studies are needed to provide a better understanding of the mechanisms involved in the development of persistent pain after cesarean delivery. Additional research is also needed to assess whether the use of unimodal or multimodal analgesic and antihyperalgesic treatments can reduce the occurrence of persistent pain after cesarean delivery.[46,55]

PHARMACOLOGY OF NEURAXIAL OPIOIDS

Prior to 1974, investigators speculated that the analgesic effect of opioids was due to pain modulation at supraspinal centers or increased activation of descending inhibitory pathways, without a direct effect at the spinal cord. The identification of endogenous opioid peptides, specific opioid binding sites, and opioid receptor subtypes has helped to clarify the site and mechanism of action of opioids within the central nervous system (CNS) (Figure 28-2).[56-59] The discovery that opioid receptors are localized within discrete areas in the CNS (lamina II of the dorsal horn) suggested that exogenous opioids could be administered neuraxially to produce nociception.[60] Opioids administered to superficial layers of the dorsal horn produced selective analgesia of prolonged duration without affecting motor function, sympathetic tone, or proprioception.[61] In addition, the analgesia provided by intraspinal opioids suggested that many of the unwanted side effects of intraspinal local anesthetic administration could be avoided.[62] In 1979, Wang et al.[63] published the first report of intraspinal opioid administration in humans. Intrathecal morphine (0.5 to 1 mg) produced complete pain relief for 12 to 24 hours in six of eight patients suffering from intractable cancer pain, with no evidence of sedation, respiratory depression, or impairment of motor function. Subsequently, researchers and clinicians have validated the analgesic efficacy of neuraxial opioids.

Pharmacokinetics and Pharmacodynamics

CENTRAL NERVOUS SYSTEM PENETRATION

Opioids administered epidurally must penetrate the dura, pia, and arachnoid membranes in order to reach the dorsal horn and activate the spinal opioid receptors. The arachnoid layer is the primary barrier to drug transfer into the spinal cord.[64] Movement through this layer is passive and depends on the physicochemical properties of the opioid. Drugs penetrating this arachnoid layer must first move into a lipid bilayer membrane, then traverse the hydrophilic cell itself, and finally partition into the other cell membrane before entering the cerebrospinal fluid (CSF). Opioid penetration of spinal tissue is proportional to the drug's lipid solubility. Opioids that are highly lipid soluble (e.g., sufentanil, fentanyl) are unable to cross the hydrophilic cell, whereas those that are hydrophilic have difficulty crossing the lipid membrane.[65] Highly lipid-soluble drugs have poor CSF bioavailablility because of (1) poor penetration through the arachnoid layer, (2) rapid absorption and sequestration by epidural fat, and (3) high vascular uptake by epidural veins.

Some investigators have questioned the neuraxial specificity of lipophilic opioids given epidurally and have suggested that the primary analgesic effect occurs via vascular uptake, systemic absorption, and redistribution of the drug to supraspinal sites.[66-72] Earlier studies suggested that parenteral fentanyl provides analgesia equivalent to that provided by epidural fentanyl.[72,73] Investigators postulated that systemic absorption of fentanyl from the epidural space resulted in the subsequent analgesic effect.[72,73] Ionescu et al.[74] reported that plasma levels of sufentanil were

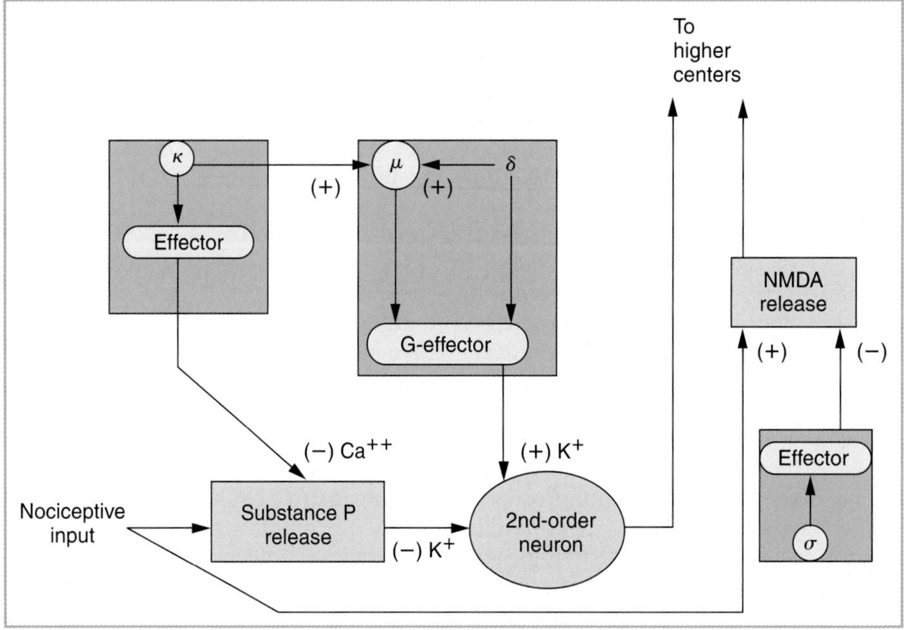

FIGURE 28-2 Overview of opioid receptor subtypes mediating spinal analgesia. Ligand-specific binding at mu (μ) and delta (δ) subtypes result in receptor conformational changes and activation (coupling) of guanosine nucleotide effector proteins. G-effector activation inhibits adenylate cyclase, resulting in decreased cyclic adenosine monophosphate (cAMP) synthesis, increased K^+ conductance, and neuronal hyperpolarization. Kappa (κ)-receptor binding activates an uncharacteristic effector protein, which decreases the Ca^{++} flux required for substance P release. Sigma (σ)-receptor subtypes modulate pain at supraspinal sites by inhibiting *N*-methyl-D-aspartate (NMDA) release. The μ and δ receptors may exist as a complex within the same cell. Activation of δ and κ subtypes may enhance μ receptor–mediated analgesia. Ca^{++}, calcium; K^+, potassium; (+), increases; (−), decreases. (From Sinatra RS, Hord AH, Ginsberg B, Preble LM, editors. Acute Pain: Mechanisms and Management. St Louis, Mosby, 1992:3.)

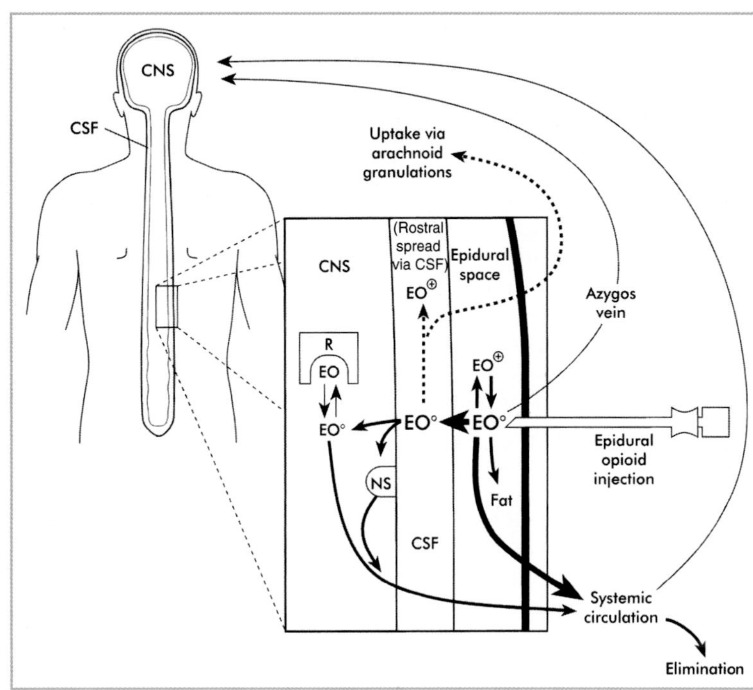

FIGURE 28-3 Factors that influence dural penetration, cerebrospinal fluid (CSF) sequestration, and vascular clearance of epidurally administered opioids. The major portion of epidurally administered opioids (EO) is absorbed by epidural and spinal blood vessels or dissolved into epidural fat. Molecules taken up by the epidural plexus and azygos system may recirculate to supraspinal centers and mediate central opioid effects. A smaller percentage of uncharged opioid molecules (EO^0) traverse the dura and enter the CSF. Lipophilic opioids rapidly exit the CSF and penetrate into spinal tissue. As with intrathecal dosing, the majority of these molecules either are trapped within lipid membranes (nonspecific binding sites [NS]) or are rapidly removed by the spinal vasculature. A small fraction of molecules bind to and activate opioid receptors (R). Hydrophilic opioids penetrate pia-arachnoid membranes and spinal tissue slowly. A larger proportion of these molecules remain sequestered in CSF and are slowly transported rostrally. This CSF depot permits gradual spinal uptake, greater dermatomal spread, and a prolonged duration of activity. CNS, central nervous system; EO^+, charged epidurally administered opioid molecules. (From Sinatra RS. Pharmacokinetics and pharmacodynamics of spinal opioids. In Sinatra RS, Hord AH, Ginsberg B, Preble LM, editors. Acute Pain: Mechanisms and Management. St Louis, Mosby, 1992:106.)

comparable throughout a 3-hour sampling interval after epidural or intravenous injection. In contrast, more recent evidence suggests that epidural fentanyl provides postcesarean analgesia via a spinal mechanism.[75-77] Cohen et al.,[78] comparing a continuous infusion of intravenous fentanyl with epidural fentanyl after cesarean delivery, reported improved analgesia and less supplemental analgesic consumption despite lower plasma fentanyl levels with epidural administration. There is evidence that bolus administration of lipophilic opioids has both spinal and supraspinal effects in obstetric patients.[75-77] After the administration of an epidural bolus of sufentanil 50 µg,* CSF concentrations of sufentanil were 140 times greater than those found in plasma; however, the amount detected in cisternal CSF was only 5% of that measured in lumbar CSF.[79]

Hydrophilic morphine has a higher CSF bioavailability, with better penetration into the CSF and less systemic absorption. A bolus dose of epidural morphine 6 mg results in peak plasma concentration of 34 ng/mL at 15 minutes after administration, and a peak CSF concentration of approximately 1000 ng/mL at 1 hour.[70] Following epidural administration, a poor correlation between the analgesic effect and plasma levels of morphine has been observed, indicating a predominantly spinal location of action.[80,81]

*The Joint Commission has recommended that health care providers substitute "mcg" for "µg" as an abbreviation for micrograms (http://www.aapmr.org/hpl/pracguide/jcahosymbols.htm). The Joint Commission contends that the abbreviation "µg" may be mistaken for "mg" (milligrams), which would result in a 1000-fold overdose. On the other hand, most scholarly publications have continued to use the abbreviation µg. The editors have chosen to retain the use of the abbreviation µg throughout this text. However, the editors recommend the use of the abbreviation mcg in clinical practice, especially with hand-written orders.

Intrathecal administration allows for injection of the drug directly into the CSF. This is a more efficient method of delivering opioid to spinal cord receptors. A bolus dose of intrathecal morphine 0.5 mg results in a CSF concentration higher than 10,000 ng/mL, with barely detectable plasma concentrations.[82]

DISTRIBUTION AND MOVEMENT OF OPIOIDS WITHIN THE CENTRAL NERVOUS SYSTEM

The movement and distribution of opioids within the CNS has been described as follows (Figure 28-3):

1. **Movement into the spinal cord (white and gray matter)**. Lipophilic agents (e.g., fentanyl) are taken up by the white matter with much greater affinity than hydrophilic agents (e.g., morphine), and less drug will reach the dorsal horn in the gray matter.[64,65,83]
2. **Movement into the epidural space (and subsequently epidural fat or veins)**. Lipophilic agents are more likely to move from the CSF into the epidural space and to be absorbed and transported by the systemic circulation to the CNS.
3. **Rostral spread in the CSF to the brainstem**. Rostral spread is determined by CSF drug bioavailability and the drug concentration gradient; hydrophilic opioids (e.g, morphine) are associated with more rostral spread.[79,84]

Although opioid dose, volume of injectate, and degree of ionization are important variables, lipid solubility plays the key role in determining the onset of analgesia, the dermatomal spread, and the duration of activity (Table 28-2).[67,85] Highly lipid-soluble opioids penetrate the spinal cord more rapidly and have a quicker **onset of action** than more ionized water-soluble agents. The **duration of activity** is affected by the rate of clearance of the drug from the sites of activity. Lipid-soluble opioids are rapidly absorbed from the epidural space, whereas hydrophilic agents remain in the

TABLE 28-2 Spinal Opioid Physiochemistry and Pharmacodynamics

Opioid	Molecular Weight	Lipid Solubility*	Parenteral Potency	pKa	μ-Receptor Affinity	Dissociation Kinetics	Potency Gain (Epidural vs. IV or SC)	Onset of Analgesia	Duration of Analgesia
Morphine	285	1.4	1	7.9	Moderate	Slow	10	Delayed	Prolonged
Meperidine	247	39	0.1	8.5	Moderate	Moderate	2-3	Rapid	Intermediate
Methadone	309	116	2	9.3	High	Slow	2-3	Rapid	Intermediate
Hydromorphone	285	25	10	—	High	Slow	5	Rapid	Prolonged
Alfentanil	417	129	25	6.5	High	Very rapid	1-2	Very rapid	Short
Fentanyl	336	816	80	8.4	High	Rapid	1-2	Very rapid	Short
Sufentanil	386	1727	800	8.0	Very high	Moderate	1-1.5	Very rapid	Short

IV, Intravenous; SC, subcutaneous.

*Octanol-water partition coefficient at pH of 7.4

CSF and spinal tissues for a longer time (see Figure 28-3).[67,85] Sufentanil is more lipid soluble than fentanyl; however, sufentanil has a greater μ-receptor affinity, resulting in a comparatively longer duration of analgesia after neuraxial administration.

Intrathecal and epidural opioids often produce analgesia of greater intensity than similar doses administered parenterally. The gain in potency is inversely proportional to the lipid solubility of the agent used. Hydrophilic opioids exhibit the greatest gain in potency; the potency ratio for intrathecal to systemic morphine is approximately 1:100.[85,86]

EPIDURAL OPIOIDS

The provision of cesarean delivery anesthesia using an epidural catheter (placed during labor or as part of a CSE technique) has prompted an extensive evaluation of epidural opioids to facilitate intraoperative and postoperative analgesia (Table 28-3).

Morphine

Preservative-free morphine received U.S. Food and Drug Administration (FDA) approval for neuraxial administration in 1984, and subsequently epidural morphine administration has been widely investigated and extensively utilized.[87] Epidural administration of morphine provides superior postcesarean analgesia to that provided by intravenous or intramuscular morphine.[14-16,21]

SINGLE-DOSE REGIMENS FOR POSTCESAREAN ANALGESIA

In a prospective dose-response study, Palmer et al.[88] observed that postcesarean analgesia (measured by intravenous PCA use) improved as the dose of epidural morphine

TABLE 28-3 Epidural Opioids for Cesarean Delivery

Drug(s)	Dose	Onset (min)	Peak Effect (min)	Duration (hr)	Advantages	Disadvantages
Morphine	2-4 mg	30-60	60-90	12-24	Long duration	Delayed onset Side effect profile Potential for delayed respiratory depression
Fentanyl	50-100 μg	5	20	2-3	Rapid onset	Short duration
Sufentanil	10-25 μg	5	15-20	2-4	Rapid onset	Short duration
Meperidine	25-50 mg	15	30	4-6	Rapid onset	Nausea and vomiting
Hydromorphone	0.4-1 mg	15	45-60	10-20	Intermediate onset and duration	Side effect profile similar to that of morphine
Morphine/fentanyl	3 mg/50 μg	10	15	12-24	Rapid onset Long duration Fewer side effects than morphine 5-mg dose	
Morphine/sufentanil	3 mg/10 μg	5	15	12-24	Rapid onset Long duration Fewer side effects than morphine 5-mg dose	

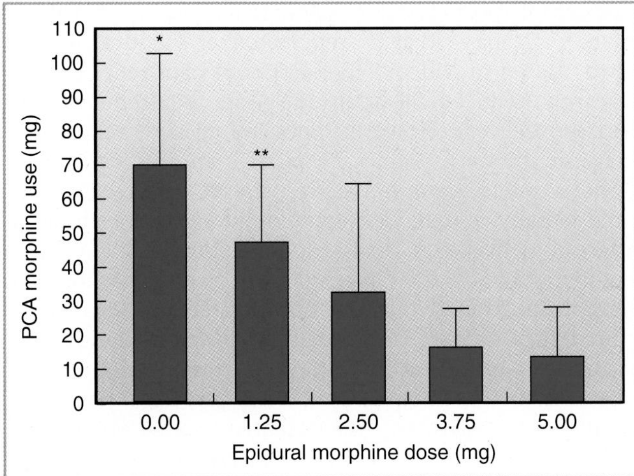

FIGURE 28-4 Total 24-hour patient-controlled analgesia (PCA) morphine use. Data are mean ± 95% confidence interval. Groups were significantly different ($P < .001$). *Group 0.0 mg was significantly different from groups 2.5, 3.75, and 5.0 mg. **Group 1.25 mg was significantly different from groups 3.75 and 5.0 mg. (From Palmer CM, Nogami WM, Van Maren G, Alves DM. Postcesarean epidural morphine: A dose-response study. Anesth Analg 2000; 90:887-91.)

increased from 0 to 3.75 mg. A further increase in dose (to 5 mg) did not significantly improve analgesia or reduce the amount of supplemental intravenous PCA morphine used in the first 24 postoperative hours (Figure 28-4).[88] Chumpathong et al.[89] did not observe any difference in pain relief, patient satisfaction, or side effects in women receiving epidural morphine 2.5, 3, or 4 mg for postcesarean analgesia. Rosen et al.[90] found that epidural morphine 5 mg and 7.5 mg provided similar analgesic efficacy, as opposed to a 2-mg dose, which provided ineffective analgesia. Epidural morphine 3 mg was recommended by Fuller et al.[91] after a large retrospective study of postcesarean analgesia.

In contemporary clinical practice, doses of epidural morphine 2 to 4 mg are most commonly utilized. Lower doses may not provide effective analgesia, and women may require additional supplemental analgesia,[88,90] whereas higher doses may increase opioid-related side effects without improving analgesia.

In theory, a low-dose, continuous infusion of morphine after cesarean delivery might result in lower initial peak CSF concentrations and subsequently reduce the incidence of side effects. Leicht et al.[92] found superior pain relief and less nausea and vomiting with a bolus dose of epidural morphine 2.5 mg followed by a continuous epidural infusion of 0.5 mg/hr in comparison with a bolus dose of 5 mg. The long duration of epidural morphine analgesia prompts many clinicians to remove the epidural catheter after bolus administration. However, some investigators have proposed that the epidural catheter should be left *in situ* to allow administration of additional doses.[93] Zakowski et al.[93] reported that only 36% of patients who received two doses (at the time of delivery and at 24 hours postoperatively) of epidural morphine 5 mg required supplemental analgesics, compared with 76% of patients who received one dose of 5 mg at the time of delivery.

ONSET AND DURATION

After epidural administration, plasma morphine concentrations are similar to those observed after intramuscular injection. Epidural morphine has a relatively slow onset of action, as a result of its low lipid solubility and slower penetration into spinal tissue.[67-69,85] The peak analgesic effect is observed 60 to 90 minutes after epidural administration.[70] Nonetheless, we prefer to delay epidural morphine administration until immediately after delivery of the infant, or later if maternal hemodynamic instability warrants further delay.

Morphine has a prolonged duration of analgesia, and analgesic efficacy typically persists long after plasma concentrations have declined to subtherapeutic levels.[67,70,85] Epidural morphine provides pain relief for approximately 24 hours after cesarean delivery[27,89-91]; however, there is wide variation in analgesic duration and efficacy among patients. Within the narrow range of doses studied, investigators have not demonstrated a correlation between the dose of morphine and the duration of analgesia.[88,89,91]

The volume of the diluent does not appear to affect the pharmacokinetics or clinical activity of epidural morphine. The quality and duration of analgesia, the need for supplemental analgesics, and the incidence of side effects were similar when epidural morphine 4 mg was administered with 2, 10, and 20 mL of sterile saline.[94]

The choice of local anesthetic used for epidural anesthesia may affect the subsequent efficacy of epidural morphine.[95] Some parturients who received 2-chloroprocaine as the primary local anesthetic agent for cesarean delivery have experienced unexpectedly poor postoperative analgesia (typically lasting less than 4 hours).[95,96] In contrast, Hess et al.[97] observed no difference in pain scores, side effects, or the need for supplemental analgesics when epidural morphine 3 mg was administered after administration of preservative-free 3% 2-chloroprocaine or placebo; however, the epidural agents were administered 30 minutes after a CSE technique that included an intrathecal dose of hyperbaric bupivacaine 11.25 mg and fentanyl 25 μg in women undergoing elective cesarean delivery. The occurrence of inadequate analgesia may therefore be related to the relatively rapid regression of 2-chloroprocaine anesthesia and the delay to peak effect of epidural morphine, rather than the postulated μ-receptor antagonism of 2-chloroprocaine.[95,97,98]

EPIDURAL VERSUS INTRATHECAL ADMINISTRATION

A number of studies have compared the postcesarean analgesic efficacy of epidural administration and intrathecal administration of opioids.[12,99,100] Equipotent doses have been evaluated, with use of a conversion ratio of 20:1 to 30:1 between epidural and intrathecal administration. Sarvela et al.[100] compared epidural morphine 3 mg with intrathecal morphine 0.1 mg and 0.2 mg; they found that the two routes of administration provided analgesia with similar efficacy and equal duration after cesarean delivery (Figure 28-5). Duale et al.[99] found modest improvements in pain scores and less morphine consumption with epidural morphine 2 mg than with intrathecal morphine 0.075 mg. In both studies, the incidence of side effects (e.g., sedation, pruritus, nausea and vomiting) was not significantly different for epidural administration and intrathecal administration.[99,100] Inadvertent subdural or intrathecal

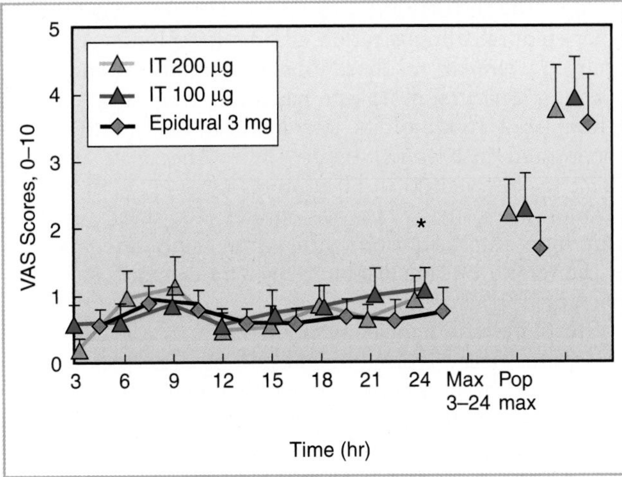

FIGURE 28-5 Visual analog scale (VAS) scores of postoperative pain during the first 24 hours at 3-hour intervals. The maximal pain score for each patient during the first 24 hours at rest (max 3-24) and the maximal pain score when moving (pop max), expressed as means and 95% error bars in the three groups: epidural 3 mg, intrathecal (IT) 100 µg, and intrathecal (IT) 200 µg. *$P < .05$. (From Sarvela J, Halonen P, Soikkeli A, Korttila K. A double-blinded, randomized comparison of intrathecal and epidural morphine for elective cesarean delivery. Anesth Analg 2002; 95:436-40.)

administration of a dose intended for epidural administration can lead to profound sedation and respiratory depression, requiring opioid reversal and intensive care monitoring with possible ventilatory support.[101] A meta-analysis concluded that both epidural and intrathecal techniques provide effective postcesarean analgesia, with neither technique being superior in terms of analgesic efficacy.[12]

Fentanyl

Fentanyl is not FDA-approved for neuraxial administration, but it is very commonly administered "off-label" for postcesarean analgesia. Commercial preparations of fentanyl contain no preservatives. They are suitable for epidural or intrathecal administration and have an excellent safety record. Grass et al.[102] reported that the 50% and 95% effective doses (ED_{50} and ED_{95}, respectively) of epidural fentanyl to reduce postcesarean pain scores to less than 10 mm (visual analog scale 0 to 100 mm) were 33 µg and 92 µg, respectively. Epidural fentanyl doses of 1 µg/kg have also been suggested to optimize *intra*operative analgesia[103]; in clinical practice, doses of 50 to 100 µg are given in isolation or combination with epidural morphine. Adverse neonatal effects should be considered if fentanyl is administered before delivery; with high doses, it may be prudent to delay administration until the umbilical cord has been clamped.

The slow onset of action of morphine limits its ability to provide optimal intraoperative analgesia, and more lipophilic opioids (e.g., fentanyl) with a faster onset of analgesia are more appropriate for supplementation of intraoperative analgesia (see Table 28-2).[85,104,105] Although single-dose epidural fentanyl improves intraoperative analgesia, no meaningful postoperative pain relief occurs beyond 4 hours.[106] Naulty et al.[107] reported that epidural fentanyl 50 to 100 µg provided 4 to 5 hours of pain relief and significantly reduced 24-hour analgesic requirements after cesarean delivery. However, Sevarino et al.[108] reported an analgesic duration of only 90 minutes and no reduction in 24-hour opioid requirements in patients who received epidural fentanyl 100 µg with epidural lidocaine anesthesia for cesarean delivery. A dose-response study using epidural fentanyl 25, 50, 100, and 200 µg (with lidocaine and epinephrine) found that the duration of analgesia ranged from 1 to 2 hours.[102] These discrepancies in the duration of analgesia can likely be attributed to the use of different local anesthetics in these studies. Bupivacaine has a long duration of action and may potentiate spinal opioid analgesia by altering opioid receptor conformation and facilitating opioid binding.[109,110] Prior epidural administration of 2-chloroprocaine may reduce the subsequent duration of epidural fentanyl analgesia. This effect does not appear to be a pH-dependent phenomenon and may reflect µ-receptor antagonism caused by 2-chloroprocaine.[98]

Lipophilic opioids do not spread rostrally in CSF to any great extent and tend to have limited dermatomal spread.[67,85] Birnbach et al.[111] found that the onset and duration of analgesia provided by epidural fentanyl 50 µg could be improved by increasing the volume of normal saline in the epidural injectate (Figure 28-6); this finding contrasts with observations associated with epidural morphine (see earlier).

Local anesthetics may have a synergistic effect with epidurally administered opioids. The concurrent administration of local anesthetic reduces epidural fentanyl dose requirements after cesarean delivery.[112] Epidural fentanyl, administered either as a single dose or as a continuous or patient-controlled infusion, generally has fewer side effects

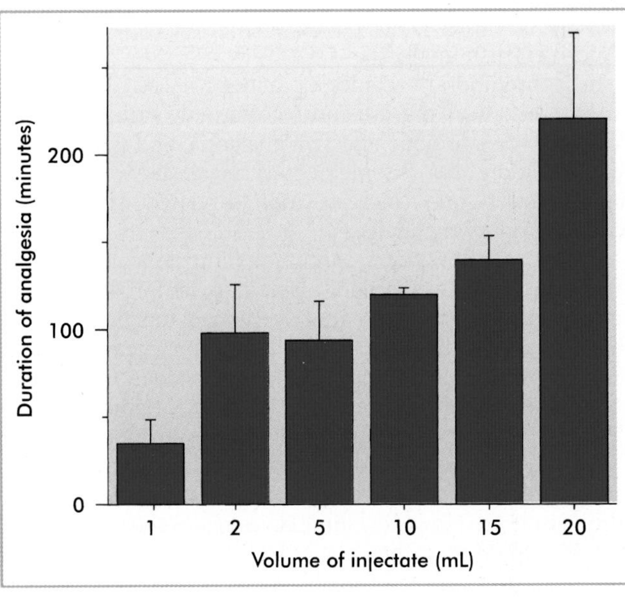

FIGURE 28-6 Duration of postcesarean analgesia provided by epidural fentanyl 50 µg administered in different volumes of normal saline. (From Birnbach DJ, Johnson MD, Arcario T, et al. Effect of diluent volume on analgesia produced by epidural fentanyl. Anesth Analg 1989; 68:808-10.)

than epidural morphine.[71,107,108] Some investigators have suggested that the administration of epidural fentanyl before incision may provide preemptive analgesia that improves postoperative analgesia.[103]

Sufentanil

Epidural sufentanil is a lipid-soluble opioid that provides a rapid onset of effective postcesarean analgesia. In patients recovering from cesarean delivery, the potency ratio of epidural sufentanil to epidural fentanyl is approximately 5:1.[102] No differences in onset, quality, or duration of analgesia were found following epidural administration of equianalgesic doses of sufentanil and fentanyl.[102] Like fentanyl, epidural sufentanil does not provide postoperative analgesia of significant duration. Rosen et al.[113] compared postcesarean epidural morphine 5 mg with epidural sufentanil 30, 45, or 60 μg. Although most patients who received sufentanil reported pain relief within 15 minutes, the duration of analgesia was 4 to 5 hours, in contrast to the 26 hours of analgesia with epidural morphine.[113] The duration of analgesia is dose dependent; an epidural bolus of sufentanil 25 μg produced less than 2 hours of analgesia, whereas 60 μg provided 5 hours of pain relief.[102,113]

The rapid onset and short duration of action of sufentanil are desirable characteristics for continuous epidural infusion. The vascular uptake of epidural sufentanil is significant, and plasma concentrations increase progressively. However, no data exist to establish dose limits for epidural sufentanil administration in this setting.

Meperidine

Epidural meperidine has been used for postcesarean analgesia, and it has local anesthetic properties (in contrast to other opioids). Two clinical trials compared the safety and efficacy of epidural meperidine 50 mg and intramuscular meperidine 100 mg in patients following cesarean delivery.[114,115] Epidural meperidine provided a faster onset of analgesia with a duration (2 to 4 hours) similar to that provided by intramuscular meperidine. Paech[116] evaluated the quality of analgesia and side effects produced by a single epidural bolus of meperidine 50 mg or fentanyl 100 μg. The onset of pain relief was slightly faster with fentanyl; however, the duration of analgesia was longer with meperidine. Ngan Kee et al.[117,118] compared different doses of epidural meperidine (12.5, 25, 50, 75, and 100 mg) as well as varying volumes of diluent. The investigators concluded that meperidine 25 mg diluted in 5 mL of saline is superior to 12.5 mg, and that doses greater than 50 mg offered no improvement in the quality or duration of analgesia. Epidural meperidine is not associated with marked hemodynamic effects, which are more commonly observed after intrathecal administration.[119]

Other Epidural Opioids

HYDROMORPHONE

Hydromorphone is a hydroxylated derivative of morphine with a lipid solubility intermediate between that of morphine and meperidine.[120] The quality of epidural hydromorphone analgesia after cesarean delivery appears to be similar to that observed with epidural morphine; however, its onset is faster, and its duration is somewhat shorter.[121-123] Evidence suggests a potency ratio of 3:1 to 5:1 between epidural morphine and epidural hydromorphone.[120]

Chestnut et al.[123] evaluated postcesarean analgesia with epidural hydromorphone 1 mg. Most patients reported good or excellent pain relief, and the mean time to first request for supplemental analgesia was 13 hours. Dougherty et al.[121] reported that epidural hydromorphone 1.5 mg provided 18 hours of postcesarean analgesia and could be prolonged to 24 hours with the addition of epinephrine. Henderson et al.[122] observed 19 hours of postcesarean analgesia with epidural hydromorphone 1 mg. The incidence of pruritus was high in the two latter studies.[121,122] However, Halpern et al.[124] found no overall differences in quality of analgesia or severity of side effects in patients undergoing cesarean delivery with epidural hydromorphone 0.6 mg or epidural morphine 3 mg. Pruritus was more pronounced in the hydromorphone group in the first 6 hours, but the incidence was higher in the morphine group at 18 hours. A Cochrane review suggests little difference in analgesic efficacy and side effects between morphine and hydromorphone administered epidurally.[125]

DIAMORPHINE

Diamorphine is a lipid-soluble derivative of morphine that is commonly administered neuraxially in the United Kingdom.[126] The lipid solubility of diamorphine provides rapid-onset analgesia, and its principal metabolite (morphine) facilitates a prolonged duration of analgesia.[127] Epidural diamorphine 5 mg provides rapid onset and effective postcesarean analgesia.[128,129] Roulson et al.[130] found that epidural diamorphine 2.5 mg provided postcesarean analgesia for 16 hours. Other investigators have found the duration of postcesarean analgesia provided by epidural diamorphine to be 6 to 12 hours.[128,129,131] In the United Kingdom, the National Institute of Clinical Excellence (NICE) suggests a dose of epidural diamorphine of 2.5 to 5 mg for postcesarean analgesia.[127]

BUTORPHANOL

The mixed agonist-antagonist opioid butorphanol offers two theoretical advantages when administered epidurally: (1) modulation of visceral nociception due to selective κ-opioid receptor activity and (2) a ceiling effect for respiratory depression even if opioid molecules spread rostrally to the brainstem.[57] Unfortunately, significant sedation often occurs as a result of vascular uptake and activation of supraspinal κ-opioid receptors.[132] Although epidural butorphanol 2 to 4 mg provides up to 8 hours of postcesarean analgesia,[133,134] a dose-dependent increase in sedation occurs. Camann et al.[135] found that epidural butorphanol 2 mg offered few advantages over a similar dose given intravenously. In addition to excessive maternal somnolence, there is concern about the neurologic safety of epidural butorphanol, which is based on observations after repeated intrathecal injections in animals.[136,137] Epidural butorphanol is *not* recommended for postcesarean analgesia because of its potential neurotoxicity, and it is not FDA approved for neuraxial use.

NALBUPHINE

Nalbuphine is a semisynthetic opioid with higher lipid solubility than morphine. *In vitro* studies have shown that moderate agonist activity occurs at κ-opioid receptors, and antagonist activity occurs at μ-opioid receptors. In animal models, neuraxial nalbuphine provides effective analgesia. The rapid onset and intermediate duration of action of nalbuphine are consistent with its lipid solubility and rapid clearance.[138] However, Camann et al.[139] found that in doses ranging from 10 to 30 mg, epidural nalbuphine provided minimal analgesia and significant somnolence after cesarean delivery. The addition of nalbuphine 0.02 to 0.08 mg/mL to an epidural infusion of hydromorphone 0.075 mg/mL did not improve analgesia after cesarean delivery.[140]

Epidural Opioid Combinations

Theoretically, the epidural administration of a lipophilic opioid combined with morphine should provide analgesia of rapid onset and prolonged duration. The use of lipophilic opioids administered intrathecally (e.g., fentanyl 15 μg) or epidurally (e.g., fentanyl 100 μg in combination with epidural morphine 3.5 mg) improves analgesia and reduces nausea and vomiting *during* cesarean delivery.[141,142] Some investigators have expressed concern that opioid interactions might reduce analgesic efficacy after epidural administration. It has been observed that the intraoperative administration of epidural fentanyl may decrease the subsequent efficacy of epidural morphine analgesia after cesarean delivery.[14] Neuraxial fentanyl might initiate acute tolerance or might affect the pharmacokinetic and receptor-binding characteristics of morphine. However, these concerns have not been confirmed in subsequent studies.[142,143] In another study, epidural fentanyl (administered immediately after delivery of the infant) improved the quality of intraoperative analgesia without worsening epidural morphine analgesia after cesarean delivery.[142]

Dottrens et al.[144] compared a single epidural dose of either morphine 4 mg, sufentanil 50 μg, or morphine 2 mg with sufentanil 25 μg. The addition of sufentanil to epidural morphine provided a more rapid onset, but similar duration, of pain relief than morphine alone.[144] Morphine alone or in combination with sufentanil provided analgesia of significantly longer duration than sufentanil alone (Figure 28-7). Sinatra et al.[145] were unable to show any potentiation when epidural sufentanil 30 μg was added to morphine 3 mg, and the duration of this combination was shorter than that of epidural morphine 5 mg alone. The addition of a lipophilic opioid to epidural morphine is popular clinically and may improve intraoperative analgesia; however, the dose of morphine should not be reduced because postoperative analgesia may be compromised.

Studies evaluating the combination of butorphanol and morphine have provided conflicting results.[146-148] Lawhorn et al.[147] found that the combination of epidural morphine 4 mg and butorphanol 3 mg provided a duration of analgesia similar to that provided by epidural morphine alone. Wittels et al.[146] noted that patients who received epidural butorphanol 3 mg with morphine 4 mg reported superior pain control, a lower incidence of pruritus, and greater satisfaction during the first 12 hours after cesarean delivery than patients who received morphine alone. In contrast, Gambling et al.[148] observed no significant differences in pain, satisfaction, nausea, or pruritus when epidural butorphanol (1, 2, or 3 mg) was added to morphine 3 mg; however, butorphanol administration resulted in significantly higher somnolence scores.

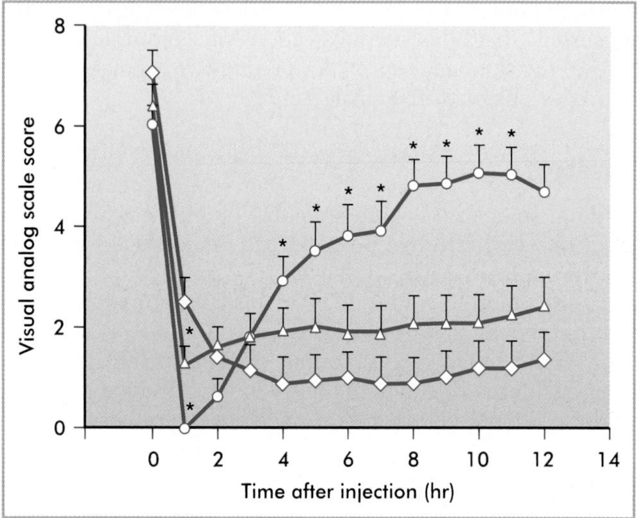

FIGURE 28-7 Pain as measured by visual analog scale before and after epidural administration of morphine 4 mg (◇), sufentanil 50 μg (○), or the combination of morphine 2 mg and sufentanil 25 μg (△). *$P < .05$ in comparison with time-matched data points for epidural morphine administration. (From Dottrens M, Rifat K, Morel DR. Comparison of extradural administration of sufentanil, morphine and sufentanil-morphine combination after caesarean section. Br J Anaesth 1992; 69:9-12.)

Patient-Controlled Epidural Analgesia

The use of continuous epidural analgesia is a popular means of providing postoperative analgesia in nonobstetric patients undergoing thoracic or upper abdominal surgery. Werawatganon et al.[149] found that epidural analgesia was associated with lower pain scores than intravenous opioid PCA for up to 72 hours after intra-abdominal surgery. These improved analgesic outcomes have been corroborated in reviews of studies that compared epidural analgesia with intravenous PCA following nonobstetric surgery.[5,13]

Several studies have suggested that PCEA, using fentanyl and bupivacaine, provides better analgesia than CEI.[150,151] Other potential advantages of PCEA over CEI are lower total doses of local anesthetic, fewer nursing and physician interventions, improved patient autonomy, and better patient satisfaction.[152] A systematic review of studies comparing PCEA, CEI, and intravenous PCA suggested that CEI provides significantly better analgesia than PCEA in nonobstetric patients.[13] However, marked heterogeneity between the studies prevented an accurate comparative analysis, and whether the observed differences are clinically significant is questionable.

The pharmacologic profile of epidural morphine, with its prolonged latency and risk for delayed respiratory depression, makes it unsuitable for PCEA use. Thus, more lipophilic drugs have been more widely evaluated for PCEA after cesarean delivery (Table 28-4).

Previous investigations have compared **meperidine** PCEA with other routes of parenteral administration (PCA, intramuscular). Yarnell et al.[36] reported that PCEA meperidine provided better postcesarean analgesia than

TABLE 28-4 Comparative Studies Investigating Opioid-Containing, Patient-Controlled Epidural Analgesia (PCEA) Regimens for Postcesarean Analgesia

Comparison(s)*	PCEA Dosing Regimen	Pain Scores	Mean Total 24-Hour Opioid Usage
PCEA vs. Intramuscular Opioids			
Meperidine PCEA vs. meperidine IM (100 mg, q 3-4 hours)[36]	B = 10 mg LO = 20 minutes BI = 10 mg/hr	PCEA group lower VAS (3-24 hours)	625 mg vs. 485 mg (PCEA versus IM; $P < .05$)
PCEA vs. Epidural Opioid			
Meperidine PCEA vs. epidural morphine (B = 4 mg)[154]	B = 15 mg LO = 10 minutes No BI	VAS lower at 2 hours; higher at 8, 10, 24 hours in PCEA group	PCEA = 192 mg (NA for epidural morphine)
Fentanyl PCEA vs. epidural morphine (B = 3 mg)[158]	B = 50 μg LO = 5 minutes (max 100 μg/hr)	No differences in pain outcome measurements	PCEA = 680 μg
PCEA vs. PCA			
Meperidine PCEA vs. meperidine PCA (B = 20 mg; LO = 5 minutes)[153]	B = 20 mg LO = 5 minutes No BI	PCEA lower VAS (2-24 hours)	NA
Meperidine PCEA vs. PCA; fentanyl PCEA vs. PCA (4 groups: cross-over study)[156]	Meperidine PCEA/PCA: B = 20 mg LO = 6 minutes No BI Fentanyl PCEA/PCA: B = 40 μg LO = 6 minutes No BI	Meperidine PCEA vs. PCA: lower VAS Meperidine vs. fentanyl: no difference in VAS (PCEA and PCA)	NA
Hydromorphone PCEA vs. PCA (B = 0.15 mg, LO = 10 minutes)[159]	Hydromorphone PCEA: Loading dose = 0.225-0.9 mg B = 0.15 mg LO = 30 minutes	No differences in pain VAS	PCEA 1.8-2.1 mg vs. PCA 7.6 mg
PCEA vs. PCEA			
Meperidine PCEA vs. fentanyl PCEA[157]	Meperidine PCEA: B = 25 mg LO = 20 minutes No BI Fentanyl PCEA: B = 50 μg LO = 20 minutes	No differences in pain VAS	NA
Three groups: Bupivacaine 0.1% PCEA Fentanyl PCEA 4 μg/mL Bupivacaine 0.1% + fentanyl PCEA 4 μg/mL[37]	All PCEA regimens: B = 5 mL LO = 10 minutes	No differences in pain VAS on coughing	NA

B, bolus; BI, background infusion; IM, intramuscular injection; LO, lockout interval; NA, data not available; PCA, intravenous patient-controlled analgesia; PCEA, patient-controlled epidural analgesia; VAS = visual analog score.
*Superscript numbers indicate chapter references.
†Both groups received 0.01% bupivacaine + epinephrine 0.5 μg/mL.

Continued

TABLE 28-4 Comparative Studies Investigating Opioid-Containing, Patient-Controlled Epidural Analgesia (PCEA) Regimens for Postcesarean Analgesia—cont'd

Comparison(s)*	PCEA Dosing Regimen	Pain Scores	Mean Total 24-Hour Opioid Usage
Four groups: Hydromorphone PCEA Hydromorphone PCEA + BI Hydromorphone + 0.08% bupivacaine PCEA Hydromorphone + 0.08% bupivacaine PCEA + combination BI[38]	All PCEA regimens: B = 2 mL LO = 30 minutes Hydromorphone BI = 0.0375 mg/hr Combination BI = hydromorphone 0.0375 mg/hr + bupivacaine 0.04 mg/hr	No differences in pain VAS	NA
Sufentanil PCEA 0.8 μg/mL vs. fentanyl PCEA 2 μg/mL[† 160]	All PCEA regimens: B = 3 mL LO = 15 minutes BI = 16 mL/hr	No differences in pain VAS	NA

intermittent intramuscular meperidine. Patients receiving PCEA were also able to ambulate and nurse their infants earlier. Paech et al.[153] performed a crossover study to compare PCEA with PCA meperidine for the first 24 hours after cesarean delivery; patients were randomly assigned to either PCEA or PCA for 12 hours before crossing over to the other route of drug administration for 12 hours. The PCEA and PCA meperidine protocols in this study were identical (20-mg bolus, 5-minute lockout). Patients receiving meperidine PCEA had lower pain scores at rest and with coughing than patients receiving intravenous PCA in both arms of the study. Other studies have compared PCEA meperidine with other opioids for postcesarean analgesia. Fanshawe[154] compared PCEA meperidine with single-dose epidural morphine. Postoperative pain scores were significantly lower with PCEA meperidine at 2 hours but were higher at 6, 8, and 24 hours. The investigators speculated that the variability in analgesic outcomes could have resulted from a suboptimal PCEA meperidine bolus dose of 15 mg. Other studies have suggested that a meperidine bolus dose of 25 mg would be better suited for PCEA use (analgesic onset 12 minutes, median duration 165 minutes).[118,155] Ngan Kee et al.[156] and Goh et al.[157] used different crossover study designs to investigate the analgesic effects of meperidine and fentanyl using intravenous PCA and PCEA modalities. The analgesic outcome results from the two studies were mixed.

Fentanyl PCEA (50-μg bolus, 5-minute lockout, maximum dose 100 μg/hr) has been shown to produce similar analgesia and less pruritus when compared to epidural morphine 3 mg.[158] Cooper et al.[37] postulated that the combination of epidural fentanyl with local anesthetic (fentanyl 2 μg/mL with 0.05% bupivacaine) would provide better analgesia than that provided by a single-drug regimen (fentanyl 4 μg/mL or 0.1% bupivacaine PCEA). The combination-drug regimen was associated with lower pain scores at rest and significantly lower total drug requirements. However, no significant differences in pain scores during coughing were reported among the three groups (Figure 28-8).

The efficacy of **hydromorphone** (single drug and combination) PCEA regimens after cesarean delivery has been investigated (see Table 28-3).[38,140,159] Parker and White[159] compared hydromorphone PCEA with intravenous PCA. Although no significant differences in pain scores were found between the two treatment groups, the investigators found that patients who received hydromorphone PCEA received less opioid in the first 24 hours, had less pruritus, and had a more rapid return of bowel function. In a follow-up study, these investigators assessed hydromorphone PCEA in combination with either 0.08% bupivacaine or a background hydromorphone infusion (0.0375 mg/hr).[38] No differences in pain scores, PCEA usage, or 24-hour PCEA requirements were noted, and the combination of PCEA with a background infusion was associated

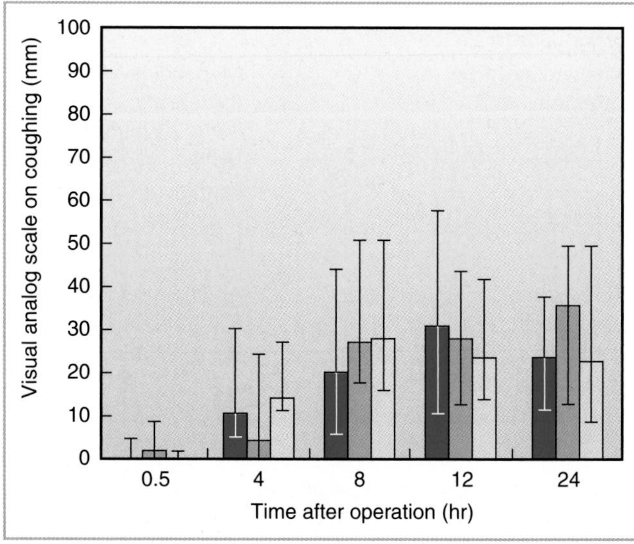

FIGURE 28-8 Pain scores on a visual analog scale for coughing. Median score and interquartile range for groups who received epidural bupivacaine *(dark teal bars)*, fentanyl *(medium teal bars)*, and bupivacaine plus fentanyl *(light teal bars)*. (From Cooper DW, Ryall DM, McHardy FE, et al. Patient-controlled extradural analgesia with bupivacaine, fentanyl, or a mixture of both, after caesarean section. Br J Anaesth 1996; 76:611-5.)

with significantly more lower extremity sensory deficits (e.g., numbness).

Parker et al.[140] assessed how varying concentrations of epidural **nalbuphine** may alter the analgesic efficacy and side-effect profile of hydromorphone PCEA. The investigators found that higher doses of nalbuphine were associated with a partial reversal of analgesia, more pruritus, less nausea, and decreased urinary retention.

PCEA **sufentanil** has been assessed in a few comparative studies of postcesarean analgesia.[160,161] Cohen et al.[160] compared fentanyl and sufentanil PCEA following cesarean delivery. The PCEA regimen in each group included 0.01% bupivacaine and epinephrine 0.5 μg/mL. Pain scores and side effects (nausea, pruritus, and sedation) were similar in the two groups; however, vomiting occurred more commonly in the sufentanil group. Vercauteren et al.[161] compared sufentanil PCEA (bolus 5 μg, lockout 10 minutes) with an identical PCEA regimen and a background infusion of sufentanil 4 μg/hr.[161] Pain was significantly lower at 6 hours in the group receiving PCEA with a background infusion, although no other differences in analgesia were reported between 6 and 24 hours. The overall incidence and severity of sedation were higher in the background infusion group.

Integrating different epidural regimens (PCEA with CEI) may be beneficial in optimizing postoperative analgesia. In a study assessing analgesia after intra-abdominal surgery, patients receiving fentanyl PCEA with bupivacaine CEI reported pain scores similar to those in patients receiving a bupivacaine-fentanyl CEI; the total fentanyl requirements were lower in the PCEA group.[162]

Further work is necessary to evaluate PCEA regimens that optimize analgesic efficacy, yet maintain adequate patient mobility and ambulation after surgery. It remains unclear whether single- or combination-drug regimens are preferable or whether a background infusion optimizes analgesia for patients receiving PCEA.

Although CEI or PCEA can provide satisfactory postoperative analgesia, these techniques diminish maternal mobility, increase costs, and potentially increase the risk of catheter-related complications (e.g., hematoma, infection) in comparison with single-dose administration of neuraxial morphine.[163] In addition, epidural catheter movement commonly occurs with ambulation and ultimately can result in ineffective postoperative analgesia.[41] These disadvantages associated with epidural catheter–based techniques (CEI and PCEA) have limited their popularity for provision of postcesarean analgesia, compared with single bolus doses of intrathecal or epidural morphine.

Extended-Release Epidural Morphine

Extended-release epidural morphine (EREM) (DepoDur) is an FDA-approved drug that delivers standard morphine sulfate via DepoFoam (Pacira Pharmaceuticals, Inc., San Diego, California). DepoFoam is a drug-delivery system composed of multivesicular lipid particles containing nonconcentric aqueous chambers that encapsulate the active drug.[164,165] These naturally occurring lipids are broken down by erosion and reorganization, resulting in a sustained release of morphine for up to 48 hours after epidural administration of a single dose.[165,166]

Two studies have evaluated the analgesic efficacy of EREM for postcesarean analgesia.[26,27] Both studies concluded that patients in the EREM groups reported lower pain scores and lower requirements for supplemental analgesia over 48 hours than patients in the standard epidural morphine groups.[26,27] In the first study, overall supplemental opioid use was approximately 50% less in the EREM 10-mg and 15-mg groups than in the standard epidural morphine 5-mg group (Figure 28-9).[26] A follow-up study, which allowed concomitant administration of a nonsteroidal anti-inflammatory drug (NSAID) in both groups, compared a single dose of EREM 10 mg with standard epidural morphine 4 mg after cesarean delivery. The investigators found that analgesic consumption was 60% less in women in the EREM group than in women in the standard epidural morphine group.[27] Patients who received EREM also had better and more prolonged pain control both at rest and with movement (Figure 28-10). Other studies have documented the analgesic efficacy of EREM following hip and knee arthroplasty and lower abdominal surgery.[167-169]

In the two postcesarean studies, there were no significant differences in the occurrence of nausea, pruritus, or sedation between the EREM and standard epidural morphine groups.[26,27] No respiratory depression or hypoxic events were observed in either study. However, it is likely that the study groups were too small for accurate evaluation of

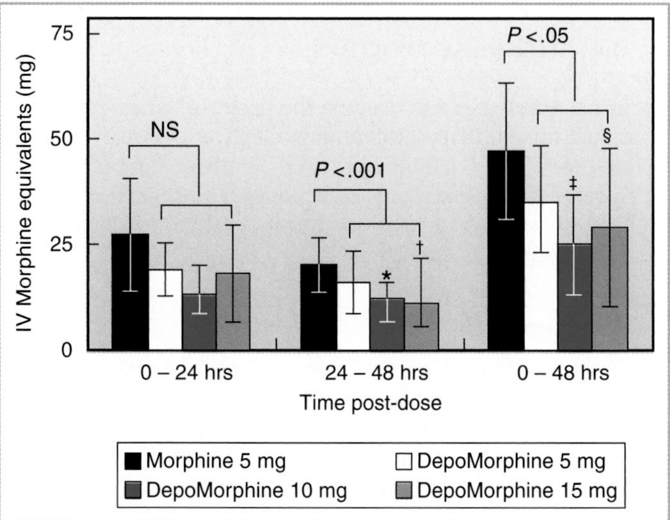

FIGURE 28-9 Use of supplemental opioid analgesics (in morphine mg-equivalents) during the 48 hours after the study dose. IV, intravenous. $^{*}P = .0134$; $^{\dagger}P = .0001$; $^{\ddagger}P = .0108$; $^{\S}P = .0065$. (Modified from Carvalho B, Riley E, Cohen SE, et al. Single-dose, sustained-release epidural morphine in the management of postoperative pain after elective cesarean delivery: Results of a multicenter randomized controlled study. Anesth Analg 2005; 100:1150-8.)

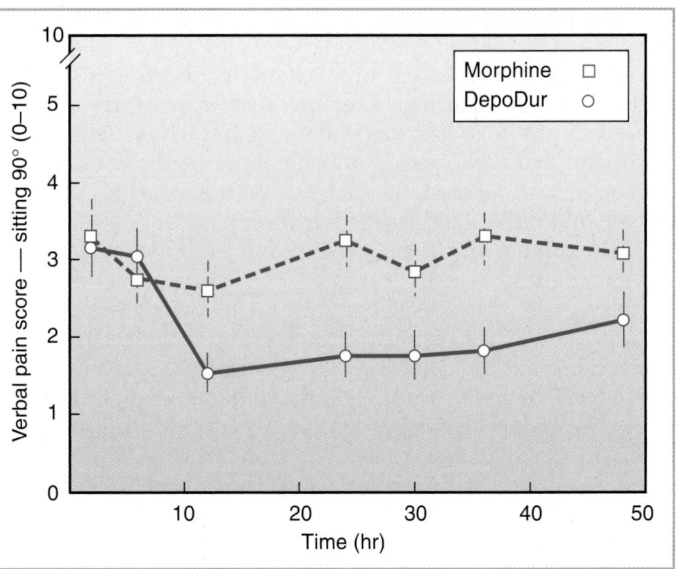

FIGURE 28-10 Pain intensity over time (verbal rating scale for pain [VRSP] 0-10) during activity (sitting up 90°) plotted as means with standard deviations; $P = .003$ for extended-release epidural morphine (DepoDur) group versus the conventional morphine group. (From Carvalho B, Roland LM, Chu LF, et al. Single-dose, extended-release epidural morphine (DepoDur) compared to conventional epidural morphine for post-cesarean pain. Anesth Analg 2007; 105:176-83.)

side-effect profiles. Pooled data from EREM studies for nonobstetric surgery suggest that EREM is associated with more side effects than standard epidural morphine, especially with higher doses.[165,170] Further research is needed to assess the side-effect and safety profile of EREM in obstetric patients.

The greatest concern with all opioids, including EREM, is respiratory depression. Although adverse respiratory events associated with opioid use are more common in the setting of patient debilitation, age greater than 65 years, obesity, and compromised respiratory function (e.g., obstructive sleep apnea), the last two patient characteristics are not uncommon in the obstetric population. Monitoring capabilities, resuscitative equipment, and opioid antagonists should be immediately available. When EREM is given correctly in the epidural space, monitoring should be continued for up to 48 hours. Inadvertent intrathecal EREM administration may result in profound and prolonged opioid-related side effects and a greater potential for respiratory depression. Although single-dose EREM may reduce the need for additional doses of opioid, it requires more prolonged monitoring and introduces unique challenges for nursing care.[171]

Currently there is insufficient clinical evidence to advocate a change in the planned anesthetic technique (from a spinal to an epidural or CSE technique) *solely* for the purpose of EREM administration in patients undergoing cesarean delivery. However, many clinicians already use CSE techniques for elective cesarean delivery in selected patients (when the duration of the cesarean delivery is expected to extend beyond that provided by spinal anesthesia). In addition, many cesarean deliveries are performed in women in whom epidural catheters have been placed previously, during labor. Therefore, it is possible that EREM may be an attractive option for clinicians who plan to use or insert an epidural catheter for cesarean delivery. However, caution should be exercised when the administration of EREM follows administration of any epidural local anesthetic; early pharmacokinetic studies suggested a potential physicochemical interaction between EREM and epidural local anesthetics, which could negate the *sustained-release* effect derived from the DepoFoam. However, Gambling et al.[172] demonstrated no differences in the pharmacokinetic and pharmacodynamic profiles of EREM when administered 15, 30, and 60 minutes after epidural bupivacaine 0.25%. Until further data are obtained, the guidance contained in the package insert should be followed: "Local anesthetics other than a 3-mL test dose of lidocaine are not permitted. If the 3-mL test dose is utilized, wait 15 minutes and then flush the epidural catheter with 1 mL of saline before administration of EREM."[173]

In summary, EREM provides effective postoperative pain relief and reduces the need for supplemental analgesics in comparison with standard epidural morphine for up to 48 hours after cesarean delivery.[26,27] This analgesic advantage must be weighed against potential disadvantages associated with EREM administration. The role of EREM for post-cesarean analgesia remains unclear[170]; however, selective use may be beneficial in a subset of patients with significant analgesic needs. In such cases, a single dose of EREM 6 to 10 mg is recommended after the infant is delivered (and the umbilical cord is clamped), as an alternative to standard epidural morphine.

INTRATHECAL OPIOIDS

Spinal anesthesia has become the preferred anesthetic technique for patients undergoing elective cesarean delivery in the United States and the United Kingdom.[9,10,174] Intrathecal opioids are commonly administered with a local anesthetic to improve intraoperative and postoperative analgesia (Table 28-5).

Morphine

The potency differences between intrathecal and epidural opioids account for the smaller doses of intrathecal opioid used for cesarean delivery; intrathecal morphine 0.075 to 0.2 mg has been found to be equivalent to epidural morphine 2 to 3 mg.[99,100] Initial reports of increased side effects with intrathecal administration likely resulted from the use

TABLE 28-5 Intrathecal Opioids for Cesarean Delivery

Drug	Dose	Onset (min)	Peak Effect (min)	Duration (hr)	Advantages	Disadvantages
Morphine	0.075-0.2 mg	30-60	60-90	12-28	Long duration	Side-effect profile Potential for delayed respiratory depression
Fentanyl	10-25 μg	5	10	2-3	Rapid onset	Minimal postoperative analgesia Short duration Pruritus
Sufentanil	2.5-5 μg	5	10	2-4	Rapid onset	Minimal postoperative analgesia Short duration Pruritus
Meperidine	10 mg	10-15	15-20	4-5	Rapid onset	Minimal postoperative analgesia Nausea and vomiting

of very high doses (2 to 10 mg). The analgesic efficacy, duration of action, and side-effect profile of intrathecal morphine are similar to that of epidural morphine in patients undergoing cesarean delivery (see earlier).[99,100,175]

ONSET AND DURATION

Intrathecal morphine administration may result in a faster onset of analgesia than epidural morphine, but it still requires 45 to 60 minutes to achieve a peak effect. The duration of analgesia is similar to the duration after epidural administration (14 to 36 hours).[19,20,85,99,100,175-178] A systematic review found that the median time to first analgesic request was 27 hours (range, 11 to 29 hours) following intrathecal morphine administration for postcesarean analgesia (Figure 28-11).[20] The duration of analgesia may be dose dependent.[20,176] Abboud et al.[176] observed that postcesarean analgesia increased from 19 to 28 hours with intrathecal morphine 0.1 and 0.25 mg, respectively.

DOSAGE

Several studies have attempted to determine the optimal dose of intrathecal morphine for postcesarean analgesia. Palmer et al.[179] compared postcesarean intravenous PCA morphine use after doses of intrathecal morphine ranging from 0.025 to 0.5 mg. The investigators found no significant difference in PCA morphine use between the intrathecal morphine 0.075-mg and 0.5-mg groups despite the higher dose in the latter group.[179] They concluded that there was little justification for using a dose of intrathecal morphine higher than 0.1 mg for postcesarean analgesia. Milner et al.[180] noted that intrathecal morphine 0.1 mg and 0.2 mg produced comparable analgesia but that the lower dose led to less nausea and vomiting. Yang et al.[181] showed that intrathecal morphine 0.1 mg provided similar postcesarean analgesia with fewer side effects in comparison with 0.25 mg. Uchiyama et al.[182] performed a dose-response study with intrathecal morphine 0, 0.05, 0.1, and 0.2 mg. They observed that 0.1 mg and 0.2 mg provided comparable and effective postcesarean analgesia for 28 hours; the 0.05-mg dose was less effective. Lower postoperative analgesic requirements were observed in all study groups than in the control group; however, the incidence of side effects was greater with the 0.2-mg dose. The investigators concluded that intrathecal morphine 0.1 mg is the optimal dose for postcesarean analgesia. In a separate study, Gerancher et al.[183] estimated that the ED_{50} of intrathecal morphine for postcesarean analgesia was 0.02 ± 0.05 mg, although significant variation in dose requirements was observed among the study subjects. A systematic review recommended 0.1 mg as the intrathecal morphine dose of choice (see Figure 28-11).[20]

Several studies have compared the analgesic efficacy and side-effect profile of intrathecal morphine with those of PCEA after cesarean delivery. A study comparing intrathecal morphine 0.15 mg with PCEA 0.06% bupivacaine and sufentanil 1 μg/mL found superior analgesia and less side effects with the PCEA regimen.[163] Paech et al.[184] compared intrathecal morphine 0.2 mg with PCEA meperidine for postcesarean analgesia. In this latter study, patients in the morphine group reported lower pain scores but also had a higher incidence of pruritus, nausea, and drowsiness.

In summary, the intrathecal administration of a small dose of morphine (0.075 to 0.2 mg) provides effective analgesia for 14 to 36 hours after cesarean delivery. Larger doses may increase side effects without conferring additional analgesic benefit, and smaller doses may reduce the duration of analgesia and increase the need for supplemental analgesics. Because of the variability in patient response to intrathecal morphine, some patients may experience inadequate postoperative analgesia and/or opioid-related side effects.

Fentanyl

Intrathecal fentanyl improves intraoperative analgesia (especially during uterine exteriorization), reduces intraoperative nausea and vomiting, and provides a better postoperative transition to other pain medications during recovery from spinal anesthesia.[185-188] However, intrathecal fentanyl provides limited postoperative analgesia, with a median time to first request for additional analgesia of 4 hours (range, 2 to 13 hours) (see Figure 28-11).[20] The analgesic

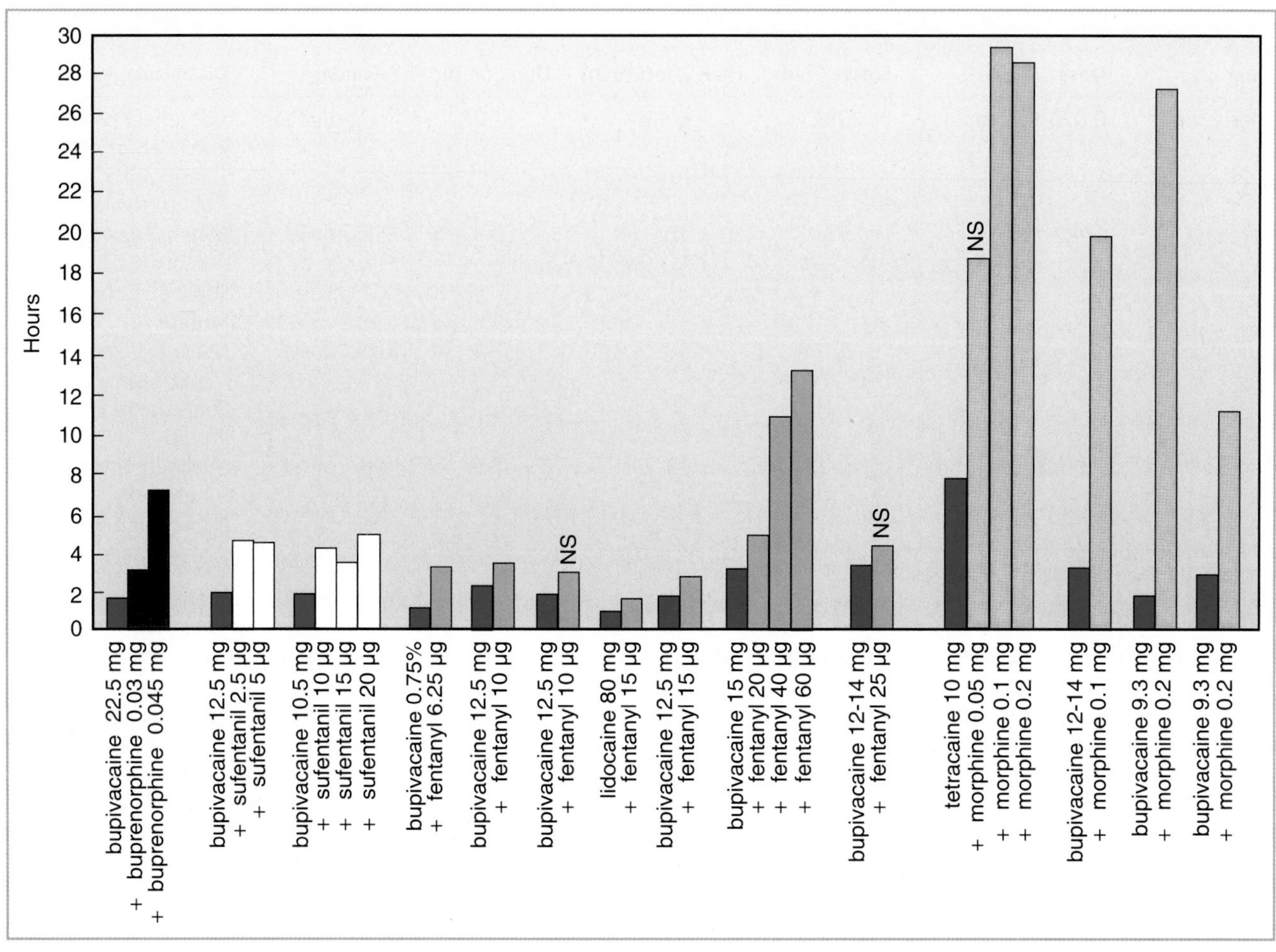

FIGURE 28-11 Time to first administration (in hours) of postoperative supplemental analgesics in patients receiving spinal anesthesia with local anesthetic alone (*dark teal bars*) or local anesthetic combined with buprenorphine, sufentanil, fentanyl, or morphine in varying doses (*various bars*). *NS*, No significant difference from control. (From Dahl JB, Jeppesen IS, Jorgensen H, et al. Intraoperative and postoperative analgesic efficacy and adverse effects of intrathecal opioids in patients undergoing cesarean section with spinal anesthesia. Anesthesiology 1999; 91:1919-27.)

effects, duration of analgesia, and side effects after intrathecal fentanyl are dose related.[20,185,187] Belzarena et al.[185] found that intrathecal fentanyl provided analgesia for a duration of 305 to 787 minutes (with 0.25 and 0.75 μg/kg, respectively). However, patients who received the higher dose experienced decreased respiratory rates and a high incidence of side effects (e.g., pruritus, nausea). Dahlgren et al.[187] reported that intrathecal fentanyl 10 μg added to bupivacaine improved the mean time of effective analgesia from 121 to 181 minutes. Hunt et al.[189] compared a range of intrathecal fentanyl doses (2.5 to 50 μg) in combination with intrathecal bupivacaine for cesarean delivery. Intrathecal fentanyl doses larger than 6.25 μg were associated with better intraoperative analgesia and longer time to first request for additional analgesia than administration of bupivacaine alone (72 versus 192 minutes, respectively).[189] Chu et al.[190] found that fentanyl doses of 12.5 to 15 μg were required to increase the duration of effective analgesia.

Although fentanyl may reduce intraoperative pain and provide immediate postoperative analgesia, intrathecal fentanyl (10 to 25 μg) provides limited postcesarean analgesia (2 to 4 hours) and does not decrease subsequent postoperative analgesic requirements.[20,178]

Sufentanil

Sufentanil has a short onset of action, which may improve intraoperative analgesia. However, its pharmacokinetic properties limit the duration of effective postcesarean analgesia after intrathecal administration.[20] Courtney et al.[191] found that intrathecal sufentanil 10, 15, or 20 μg resulted in a mean duration of postcesarean analgesia of approximately 3 hours. More than 90% of patients reported pruritus, but only one patient required treatment. Dahlgren et al.[187] compared the safety and efficacy of the co-administration of sufentanil 2.5 or 5 μg, fentanyl 10 μg, or placebo with hyperbaric bupivacaine 12.5 mg for cesarean delivery. The duration of effective analgesia was longer with the opioids, particularly in the sufentanil groups; sufentanil 5 μg provided the longest duration of analgesia but also the highest incidence of pruritus. Patients receiving intrathecal sufentanil had lower requirements for intraoperative antiemetics and postoperative intravenous morphine.[187] Braga Ade et al.,[192] comparing intrathecal sufentanil 2.5, 5, and 7.5 μg, found that 5 μg and 7.5 μg provided more effective postcesarean analgesia than was observed in the control group (no intrathecal opioids); however, pruritus was higher with sufentanil, especially with the 7.5-μg dose.

Karaman et al.[193] found that intrathecal sufentanil 5 μg delayed the time to first analgesic request to 6 hours, compared with 20 hours for intrathecal morphine 0.2 mg.

Other Intrathecal Opioids

MEPERIDINE

Intrathecal meperidine reduces the intensity of pain associated with the regression of spinal anesthesia and provides postoperative analgesia of intermediate duration (4 to 5 hours).[194,195] Yu et al.[196] found that the addition of meperidine 10 mg to hyperbaric bupivacaine 10 mg prolonged the duration of postcesarean analgesia (234 minutes in the meperidine group versus 125 minutes in a placebo group). However, the incidence of intraoperative nausea and vomiting was greater in the meperidine group.

Unlike other opioids, meperidine has local anesthetic qualities. Some anesthesia providers have administered intrathecal 5% meperidine (1 mg/kg) as the sole anesthetic agent for cesarean delivery under spinal anesthesia. However, surgical anesthesia was unreliable, with a mean anesthetic duration of 41 ± 15 minutes.[194,195]

DIAMORPHINE

Diamorphine has several physicochemical properties that are of value in providing intrathecal analgesia. A high lipophilicity (octanol-water coefficient 280) results in a rapid onset of analgesia, and diamorphine's active metabolite (morphine) provides a prolonged duration of analgesia.

Kelly et al.[197] compared intrathecal diamorphine 0.125, 0.250, and 0.375 mg for cesarean delivery. The 0.25-mg and 0.375-mg doses provided effective postcesarean analgesia; the occurrence of both vomiting and pruritus was dose-related. Stacey et al.[198] reported that the duration of analgesia was dose dependent and found that intrathecal diamorphine 1 mg provided 10 hours of postcesarean analgesia, compared with 7 hours for 0.5 mg. The rapid onset of diamorphine is a potential advantage in the provision of intraoperative as well as postoperative analgesia.[199,200] Saravanan et al.[201] concluded that the ED_{95} for intrathecal diamorphine to prevent intraoperative discomfort was 0.4 mg.

Husaini et al.[202] observed that intrathecal diamorphine 0.2 mg and intrathecal morphine 0.2 mg provided similar postcesarean analgesia as measured by postoperative intravenous PCA morphine requirements. However, the patients who received intrathecal morphine had a higher incidence of pruritus and drowsiness. Hallworth et al.[203] reported that *intrathecal* diamorphine 0.25 mg produced the same duration and quality of postcesarean analgesia as *epidural* diamorphine 5 mg, with less nausea and vomiting.

Diamorphine has been commonly utilized in the United Kingdom, but it is not available for clinical use in the United States. In the United Kingdom, the National Institute of Clinical Excellence (NICE) suggests an intrathecal diamorphine dose of 0.3 to 0.4 mg for postcesarean analgesia.[127]

NALBUPHINE

Culebras et al.[204] compared intrathecal morphine 0.2 mg with intrathecal nalbuphine (0.2, 0.8, or 1.6 mg) for postcesarean analgesia. Intrathecal nalbuphine 0.8 mg provided good intraoperative and early postoperative analgesia without side effects. However, intrathecal morphine provided significantly longer postoperative analgesia. In an editorial accompanying its publication, the study was criticized because safety and neurotoxicity of nalbuphine had not been adequately assessed.[138]

Intrathecal Opioid Combinations

Intrathecal administration of morphine in combination with a lipophilic opioid (e.g., fentanyl, sufentanil) may offer some advantages. Intrathecal morphine has a delayed onset, and therefore lipophilic opioids with a rapid onset may improve intraoperative analgesia and reduce the intensity of pain associated with the regression of spinal anesthesia. Chung et al.[205] found that the combination of intrathecal meperidine 10 mg and morphine 0.15 mg provided better intraoperative analgesia, less need for supplemental analgesia, and higher satisfaction than intrathecal morphine alone during cesarean delivery.

Some studies have suggested that intrathecal morphine may be less effective when concurrently administered with intrathecal fentanyl.[206,207] Lee et al.[206] observed that patients who received both intrathecal fentanyl 20 μg and morphine 0.2 mg had more pain than those who received intrathecal morphine only. The investigators suggested that the intrathecal morphine was not effective because it was not binding to the spinal opioid receptors that were occupied by the intrathecal fentanyl.[206] Cooper et al.[207] reported that patients who received intrathecal fentanyl 25 μg with bupivacaine had higher postoperative intravenous morphine PCA requirements than patients who received bupivacaine alone. The investigators postulated that this phenomenon was due to acute spinal opioid tolerance. However, Giarrusso et al.[208] found that postoperative analgesia requirements did not change with the addition of increasing doses of intrathecal fentanyl (5, 10, or 25 μg) to intrathecal morphine 0.2 mg for cesarean delivery. Sibilla et al.[178] found that the intrathecal combination of fentanyl 25 μg with morphine 0.1 mg provided similar postoperative analgesia to that provided by intrathecal morphine alone. Many anesthesia providers currently administer both intrathecal morphine and fentanyl when giving spinal anesthesia for cesarean delivery; the co-administration of intrathecal fentanyl does *not* appear to compromise the postoperative analgesia provided by intrathecal morphine.

Maternal Safety and Neonatal Effects

Careful evaluation of the potential adverse effects of neuraxial pharmacologic agents is necessary prior to clinical administration of those agents.[209] In obstetric patients, adverse maternal effects (e.g., neurotoxicity, altered uteroplacental perfusion) as well as potential adverse neonatal effects should be assessed. Although many agents are used routinely and safely in clinical practice, not all are licensed for neuraxial administration in the United States.

MATERNAL SAFETY

Neurotoxicity (safety) studies that have been conducted for morphine, fentanyl, sufentanil, meperidine, clonidine, and neostigmine suggest that these agents are safe for neuraxial administration.[210-213] Morphine is approved by the FDA for neuraxial administration.[211,212] Although unlicensed for neuraxial administration, fentanyl and sufentanil have been used for many years without evidence of neurotoxicity. Studies in sheep have reported potential neurotoxicity with intrathecal butorphanol.[136] Culebras et al.[204] demonstrated potential toxic interactions with the co-administration of nalbuphine and local anesthetics. However, Rawal et al.[136] evaluated the behavioral and histopathologic effects of butorphanol, sufentanil, and nalbuphine after intrathecal administration in sheep, and found that nalbuphine caused the least evidence of neural tissue damage.

Clinicians should avoid neuraxial administration of any agent before adequate evaluation for potential neurotoxicity has been completed.[214-216] Drugs and diluents that are proven safe for parenteral use may have adverse effects when administered intrathecally. Despite these valid concerns, a number of opioid analgesics have been administered intrathecally to healthy obstetric patients without adequate investigation of their safety profile in animal and clinical volunteer studies.[216]

Preservatives that are added to many commercial preparations may be hazardous if administered neuraxially. Examples are sodium (meta)bisulfite and disodium ethylenediaminetetraacetic acid (EDTA), which are known to incite inflammatory and fibrotic changes in pia-arachnoid and spinal tissue following intrathecal administration. Dezocine has been shown to cause neuropathologic changes in dog spinal cord.[217] Similarly, glycine, a preservative added to remifentanil preparations, is contraindicated for neuraxial use.

NEONATAL EFFECTS

All opioids have the potential for placental transfer and neonatal effects. Minimal neonatal effects have been found after the administration of epidural morphine 2 to 7.5 mg for cesarean delivery.[218] However, it may be preferable to administer neuraxial opioids after cord clamping to avoid placental transfer. Lipophilic opioids are associated with greater systemic uptake; if indicated (e.g., intraoperative pain during cesarean delivery), the smallest necessary dose should be administered. Courtney et al.[191] found that intrathecal sufentanil (10, 15, or 20 μg) did not affect neonatal outcome as assessed by umbilical cord blood gas measurements and Apgar and neurobehavioral scores. Intrathecal opioids are associated with less neonatal drug transfer than epidural or intravenous opioid administration, given that smaller doses are used for intrathecal administration.[219]

SIDE EFFECTS OF NEURAXIAL OPIOIDS

Respiratory Depression

PHARMACOKINETICS AND PHARMACODYNAMICS

Neuraxial opioids can depress the respiratory centers in the brainstem via direct and/or indirect mechanisms (Table 28-6).[67,69,84,85,220-222] Respiratory depression after neuraxial morphine administration is biphasic.[223] Early respiratory depression can occur 30 to 90 minutes after epidural morphine administration (owing to systemic vascular absorption),[85] whereas delayed respiratory depression can occur 6 to 18 hours after epidural or intrathecal morphine (owing to rostral spread in CSF and slow penetration into the brainstem).[104] In contrast, lipophilic opioids (e.g., fentanyl, sufentanil) do not cause delayed respiratory depression but may cause early-onset respiratory depression, typically within 30 minutes, because of significant vascular uptake and rostral spread in CSF, and, potentially, direct transit in epidural veins.[220,221]

TABLE 28-6 Neuraxial Opioids and the Principal Mechanisms of Action Leading to Respiratory Depression

Mechanism	Lipophilic Opioids (e.g., fentanyl)	Hydrophilic Opioids (e.g., morphine)
Vascular uptake (by the epidural or subarachnoid venous plexuses and circulation) to the respiratory center in the brainstem	+++	+
Rostral spread via direct perimedullary vascular channels	++	+
Dural penetration of opioids	+	++
Rostral spread via the aqueous cerebrospinal fluid to the brainstem	+	+++

The + symbols denote the relative importance of the mechanism for the type of opioid.

Data from references 67,68,191-193.

INCIDENCE

Although rare, respiratory depression represents a significant concern with the epidural or intrathecal administration of opioids. Data from closed medical claims include at least 16 cases of respiratory depression involving neuraxial opioids; well over half of the patients in these cases died or suffered permanent brain damage.[224] Nonobstetric studies have reported an incidence of respiratory depression after neuraxial opioid administration of 0.01% to 7%[225,226]; however, these numbers are derived from large retrospective observational studies, which may underestimate the true incidence. Moreover, no standard definition exists for the diagnosis of respiratory depression.[227] Low respiratory rate, hypercarbia, low Sp_{O_2}, sedation, depressed ventilatory response to hypoxia or hypercarbia, and treatment with naloxone have all been used as indicators of respiratory depression.

MORPHINE

The incidence of postcesarean respiratory depression with morphine given epidurally (2 to 5 mg) or intrathecally (0.1 to 0.2 mg) ranges from 0.07% to 0.9%.[91,176,228-230] No studies have reported serious morbidity, although some patients have required naloxone administration.[91,228] Early reports suggested that intrathecal morphine was more likely to cause delayed respiratory depression than epidural morphine.[85] However, this likely reflected the higher intrathecal morphine doses (1 to 10 mg) used in early clinical studies.[231] Subsequently, smaller doses of intrathecal morphine were found to provide effective analgesia with a low risk of clinically significant respiratory depression. Abboud et al.[176] evaluated CO_2 responses for 24 hours after intrathecal morphine 0.1 or 0.25 mg and those after subcutaneous morphine 8 mg. Neither intrathecal dose affected CO_2 response or minute ventilation, whereas both measurements were depressed after subcutaneous morphine administration.

EXTENDED-RELEASE EPIDURAL MORPHINE

Two studies noted that EREM provided prolonged postcesarean analgesia without significant respiratory depression.[26,27] However, the small sample sizes did not allow an accurate assessment of the risk or incidence of respiratory depression. Respiratory depression has been reported with larger EREM doses (15 to 30 mg) administered for patients undergoing hip and knee arthroplasty and lower abdominal surgery.[167-169] The dose-related incidence of respiratory depression ranged from 2% to 16%, with 8% to 21% of patients requiring naloxone to reverse opioid-related adverse effects.[167-169] However, patients in these studies were older, had more comorbidities, and often received general anesthesia for surgery. EREM use should be carefully considered prior to its administration in high-risk obstetric patients (e.g., obesity, obstructive sleep apnea, coadministration of magnesium sulfate). Single-dose EREM may reduce the need for supplemental analgesia, but more prolonged monitoring and nursing education are required.[171]

LIPOPHILIC OPIOIDS

The incidence of respiratory depression after neuraxial administration of a lipophilic agent in obstetric patients is unknown. In one case, respiratory depression occurred 25 minutes after spinal anesthesia with intrathecal fentanyl 15 μg, and required reversal with naloxone.[232] Respiratory depression has been described after administration of epidural fentanyl 90 to 100 μg for cesarean delivery.[233,234] Cohen et al.[221] reported that epidural sufentanil 30 to 50 μg depressed the ventilatory response to CO_2 after cesarean delivery, although overt respiratory depression did not occur. Plasma levels of sufentanil in this study peaked at 10 to 15 minutes, and the highest sedation scores and depression of CO_2 response occurred 45 minutes after administration. Another group reported that epidural fentanyl 100 μg or sufentanil 10 to 50 μg added to lidocaine for cesarean delivery caused significant changes in respiratory rate and end-tidal CO_2.[235] In another study, intrathecal fentanyl 20 μg, added to bupivacaine for cesarean delivery, improved the quality of anesthesia but did not cause deterioration in peak expiratory flow rate or vital capacity.[236]

PREVENTION

Identify Patients at Risk

Risk factors for respiratory depression include advanced age, obesity, cardiopulmonary disease, obstructive sleep apnea, and preoperative opioid tolerance.[225] Most obstetric patients are relatively young and healthy and rarely present with significant pulmonary disease or other risk factors for respiratory depression. However, opioid-induced respiratory depression occasionally occurs in healthy patients who receive standard doses of neuraxial opioid,[224] and vigilance is needed to prevent this rare but hazardous complication (Table 28-7).[224,237]

TABLE 28-7 Recommendations to Reduce the Risk of Respiratory Depression after Neuraxial Administration of Opioids

Principle	Recommendation(s)	Clinical Example(s)
Prevention	Identify high-risk patients	• Patients with obesity or sleep apnea or who are receiving magnesium or sedatives
	Limit neuraxial morphine dose	• Intrathecal morphine 0.075 to 0.2 mg • Epidural morphine 2 to 4 mg
Detection	Appropriate monitoring of:	
	• Level of consciousness	• Clinical signs, sedation scores
	• Adequacy of ventilation	• Respiratory rate, end-tidal CO_2 level
	• Adequacy of oxygenation	• Pulse oximetry, blood gas levels
	Monitoring continued for duration of effect	• Fentanyl/sufentanil—4 hours • Morphine—24 hours • Extended-release epidural morphine—48 hours
Treatment	Implementation of clinical protocols for detecting and treating respiratory depression	
	Nursing and physician education	

Obese patients are likely to be at higher risk for postcesarean respiratory depression after neuraxial morphine administration. In one study of 856 patients who underwent cesarean delivery, respiratory depression was observed in 8 obese patients who had received intrathecal morphine.[177] A history and physical examination (directed at identification of sleep apnea and coexisting diseases) should be performed prior to neuraxial administration of opioids. Hypermagnesemia can cause respiratory depression, and extra vigilance is needed for preeclamptic women who are receiving magnesium sulfate for seizure prophylaxis. Caution should be exercised when other opioids or sedative drugs (e.g., diphenhydramine) are administered, as these agents may increase the risk of respiratory depression.[224] Multiple sets of orders that prescribe parenteral or oral opioids to treat breakthrough pain can pose a particular hazard to patients who have received neuraxial opioids.

Limit Opioid Dose

Historically, the incidence of respiratory depression was more common in patients receiving doses of neuraxial opioid greater than those currently used in modern practice. For cesarean delivery, neuraxial morphine appears to have a limit or "ceiling" in terms of analgesic efficacy. More specifically, effective doses of intrathecal and epidural morphine are 0.075 to 0.2 mg[20,179] and 2 to 4 mg,[88] respectively. Higher doses of neuraxial morphine may increase side effects without significant improvement or prolongation of analgesia.[179,238]

MONITORING, DETECTION, AND TREATMENT

Monitor Respiration and Understand the Limitations of Monitoring Techniques

A closed-claims analysis showed that 56% of respiratory events after neuraxial opioids could have been prevented.[224] The American Society of Anesthesiologists (ASA) has approved guidelines that address the prevention, detection, and management of respiratory depression associated with neuraxial opioid administration.[225] However, these guidelines do not specifically address obstetric patients.

Opioid effects on respiration include reduced minute ventilation (decrease in respiratory rate, tidal volume, or both), decreased response to hypoxia, and a rightward shift and depression of the CO_2 response.[239] All patients receiving neuraxial opioids should be monitored for adequacy of ventilation, oxygenation, and level of consciousness. Unfortunately, current monitoring technology and clinical observation practices have limitations.[224] Intermittent evaluation of **clinical signs** (respiratory rate, level of sedation, pupil size) are often unreliable predictors of respiratory depression.[224,240] The respiratory rate of patients with sleep apnea may be misleading, because chest wall movement may occur without ventilation because of airway obstruction.[224] **Pulse oximetry** has poor sensitivity in detecting hypoventilation and hypercarbia, especially when supplemental oxygen is administered. Greater surveillance is warranted in patients at high risk for respiratory depression who are receiving supplemental oxygen. Brief episodes of desaturation are common up to 24 hours after cesarean delivery; in one study, 71% of post–cesarean delivery patients had one or more episodes of Spo_2 values less than 85% after epidural morphine 5 mg.[241] Continuous pulse oximetry is often inconvenient owing to motion-artifact alarms that may affect sleep and nursing care. **Apnea monitors,** also frequently associated with false alarms, do not detect hypoventilation. **End-tidal CO_2 monitoring** in patients who are not intubated has significant limitations and is not universally available.

Continuous pulse oximetry, although appropriate for the obstetric patient with risk factors such as obesity, may be unnecessary in healthy post–cesarean delivery patients receiving small doses of neuraxial opioid (e.g., intrathecal morphine $\leq$0.2 mg, epidural morphine $\leq$4 mg).[224] Intermittent respiratory monitoring may miss transient episodes of desaturation and bradypnea, because respiratory depression typically progresses slowly and is often preceded by increasing maternal sedation.[242] Hourly assessments and vigilant nursing observations of respiratory effort, respiratory rate, and somnolence are probably adequate in low-risk obstetric patients.[91,243,244] Nursing staff should be adequately trained in detecting and treating opioid-induced respiratory depression, and an anesthesia provider should be readily available to manage complications that may arise.

Monitor Respiration for an Appropriate Duration

CO_2 responsiveness was depressed for up to 24 hours after cesarean delivery after administration of epidural morphine 5 mg.[133] Therefore it is prudent to continue respiratory monitoring on the basis of the expected duration of action of the opioid being used. Patients receiving a continuous infusion of neuraxial opioid should be monitored during the infusion and for the expected residual duration of action after cessation of the infusion. Patients receiving EREM should be monitored for 48 hours.[170,225] The ASA recommends that respiratory monitoring after neuraxial morphine administration should occur at least every hour for the first 12 hours, then every 2 hours for the next 12 hours (and every 4 hours for another 24 hours after EREM administration).[225]

Early-onset respiratory depression associated with lipophilic opioids usually occurs within 30 minutes of administration and is likely to occur in a high-visibility, controlled setting (e.g., operating or labor room). The ASA recommends that respiratory monitoring after administration of neuraxial fentanyl should continue for a minimum of 2 hours. However, it is prudent to continue monitoring for at least 3 to 4 hours, because delayed respiratory depression has occurred after administration of lipophilic opioids. Brockway et al.[233] reported respiratory depression 100 minutes after epidural fentanyl 100 μg for cesarean delivery. In another study of ventilatory changes after epidural fentanyl 200 μg, the investigators found that ventilatory function returned to baseline in 180 minutes.[220]

Treat Respiratory Depression

Physicians and nursing staff must be educated to prevent, recognize, and treat respiratory depression. Treatment protocols and mechanisms to ensure a rapid response to respiratory events are recommended. The patient who displays altered level of consciousness, bradypnea, or hypoxemia should receive continuous supplemental oxygen until she is alert with no respiratory depression or hypoxemia. However, the routine use of supplemental oxygen is not advised because of the associated risk of prolonged apnea as well as limitations in the sensitivity of pulse oximetry to detect hypoventilation.[224] An intravenous bolus dose of naloxone is indicated in patients with profound somnolence and respiratory depression that does not respond to arousal; continued observation is necessary in these patients, as the opioid may have a longer duration of action than the naloxone (half-life = 43 to 90 minutes). If naloxone fails to reverse severe respiratory depression or arrest, prompt mask ventilation and/or endotracheal intubation should be performed. An intravenous infusion of naloxone should be maintained for as long as the patient remains symptomatic; often the naloxone infusion can be titrated to treat respiratory depression without significantly reducing the quality of neuraxial analgesia.[245-247] The routine administration of prophylactic naloxone is not recommended.[244] Patients already using continuous positive airway pressure devices should continue to do so postpartum.

SUMMARY

The analgesic benefits derived from neuraxial opioids far outweigh the risks of respiratory depression that these agents pose. Neuraxial opioids are not associated with a higher risk of respiratory depression than parenteral opioids. Clinically significant respiratory depression may occur in rare cases after cesarean delivery and can lead to significant morbidity or mortality.[224] "At-risk" patients should be identified before surgery, and adequate monitoring should be in place to assess respiratory function and sedation in the postoperative period. Care providers should be adequately educated and trained to recognize and manage respiratory depression in postcesarean patients receiving neuraxial opioids.

Nausea and Vomiting

Nausea and vomiting are common complaints following cesarean delivery, and the etiology of these symptoms is likely to be multifactorial. A 2005 review highlighted the anesthetic and nonanesthetic causes of intraoperative nausea and vomiting (IONV) (Table 28-8).[248] It is unclear whether patients are at increased risk for postoperative nausea and vomiting (PONV) if these symptoms occur intraoperatively. Neuraxial opioids may increase the risk of PONV after cesarean delivery. Nausea results either from the rostral spread of opioid in the CSF to the brainstem or from vascular uptake and delivery to the vomiting center and chemoreceptor trigger zone.[104,249] However, Palmer et al.[179] found no difference in PONV between intrathecal morphine (0.025 to 0.5 mg) and placebo, nor a relationship of PONV with morphine dose. A similar study by the same group found no difference in severity of PONV in patients receiving increasing doses of epidural morphine 1.25 to 5 mg.[88] Importantly, neither study was powered to investigate PONV as a primary outcome measure.

TABLE 28-8 Causes, Preventive Measures, and Treatment Measures for Intraoperative Nausea and Vomiting during Cesarean Delivery

Causes	Prevention/Treatment
Anesthetic Causes	
Hypotension	Left uterine displacement, adequate preload, vasopressors
Neuraxial opioids	Use optimal doses
Parenteral opioids	Avoid or use minimum effective doses
Increased vagal activity	Use vagolytics
Nonanesthetic Causes	
Surgical manipulation	Avoid excessive manipulation
Motion	Avoid vigorous movements
Uterotonic agents	Titrate to clinical effect with adequate doses

Modified from Balki M, Carvalho JCA. Intraoperative nausea and vomiting during cesarean section under regional anesthesia. Int J Obstet Anesth 2005; 14:230-41.

Many studies have investigated different regimens to reduce PONV in patients receiving neuraxial opioids for cesarean delivery. However, the lack of standardization of PONV outcome measures in these studies hinders the ability to interpret comparative data. In addition, studies have not assessed risk-stratification or predictive models for PONV in patients receiving neuraxial opioids for cesarean delivery.

INDIVIDUAL ANTIEMETIC AGENTS

Older-generation antiemetics, such as metoclopramide and droperidol, have been commonly used to prevent or treat neuraxial opioid-induced emesis. **Metoclopramide** 10 mg has been shown to decrease early PONV, after intraoperative intravenous fentanyl and epidural morphine administration.[250] Metoclopramide, which antagonizes dopamine receptors in the chemoreceptor trigger zone, is often administered preoperatively owing to its favorable prokinetic properties and an associated reduction in rates of IONV and PONV in patients receiving spinal anesthesia.[251] **Droperidol** is a buterophenone that also antagonizes dopaminergic (D_2) receptors in the chemoreceptor trigger zone. Prophylactic administration of droperidol 0.5 mg to 2.5 mg has been shown to decrease early PONV after spinal anesthesia without neuraxial opioids[252] and with epidural morphine 2 mg, respectively.[253] Sedation and drowsiness may occur with droperidol, although their appearance does not appear to be a dose-related phenomenon. However, droperidol has been less widely used by anesthesia providers since the FDA issued a "black box" warning in 2001 associating administration of droperidol with QT prolongation and an increased risk of development of *torsades de pointes*. The use of a transdermal **scopolamine** patch may also lower the incidence of nausea and vomiting, especially during the first 10 hours after cesarean delivery.[254] Transdermal scopolamine has a latency period of 3 to 4 hours, which limits its ability to treat early PONV, and it also has a number of commonly reported side effects, including dry mouth, visual disturbances, dizziness, and agitation.

Serotonin (5-HT_3) receptor antagonists have been used for prophylactic and therapeutic treatment of PONV. These drugs specifically bind to 5-HT_3 receptors in the chemoreceptor trigger zone and at vagal afferents in the gastrointestinal tract. Prophylactic administration of **ondansetron** 4 to 8 mg has been shown to have a better antiemetic profile in the first 24 hours (compared with placebo) after intrathecal and epidural opioid administration (Figure 28-12).[255,256] **Granisetron** has been investigated in two studies of antiemetic prophylaxis in patients receiving spinal anesthesia without neuraxial opioids for cesarean delivery.[257,258] Less PONV was reported with use of granisetron 40 to 80 μg/kg in comparison with placebo,[257] and with use of granisetron 3 mg compared with either metoclopramide 10 mg or droperidol 1.25 mg.[258]

The corticosteroid **dexamethasone** has been successful in treating and preventing emesis after chemotherapy, and subsequently it has become more popular as an antiemetic agent in anesthesia practice. Corticosteroids have various effects in the CNS, including the regulation of transmitter levels, receptor densities, and neuronal configurations.[259] Corticosteroid receptors have been identified in areas important to the signal processing of nausea and vomiting,

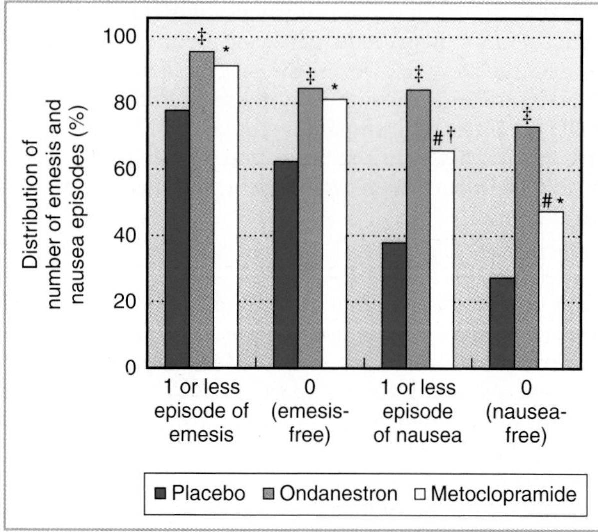

FIGURE 28-12 Postoperative nausea and emesis in patients undergoing cesarean delivery with epidural anesthesia (2% lidocaine with epinephrine and fentanyl). Values are given as percentages. #Group metoclopramide versus ondansetron; $P < .05$. *Group metoclopramide versus placebo; $P < .05$. †Group metoclopramide versus placebo; $P < .005$. ‡Group ondansetron versus placebo; $P < .005$. (Data from Pan PH, Moore CM. Comparing the efficacy of prophylactic metoclopramide, ondansetron, and placebo in cesarean section patients given epidural anesthesia. J Clin Anesth 2001; 13:430-5.)

including the nucleus of the solitary tract, the nucleus of raphe, and the area postrema. Tzeng et al.[259] reported similar efficacy in the prevention of PONV with intravenous dexamethasone 8 mg compared with droperidol 1.25 mg. Wang et al.[260] suggested that dexamethasone 5 mg is the minimum effective dose for preventing PONV. In these studies, patients received epidural morphine 3 mg. However, a later study showed that **cyclizine** 50 mg was associated with significantly fewer episodes of PONV (0 to 12 hours after cesarean delivery) than dexamethasone 8 mg after intrathecal opioid (fentanyl and morphine) administration.[261]

COMBINATION ANTIEMETIC REGIMENS

Few studies have compared the effects of individual with those of combination antiemetic regimens. Administration of drugs acting at two different receptor sites may improve antiemetic efficacy through synergism.[262] Drug combinations may also facilitate a concomitant reduction in drug doses. Wu et al.[263] reported lower rates of PONV after intrathecal morphine administration with use of a combination of dexamethasone 8 mg and droperidol 0.625 mg than with use of dexamethasone 8 mg or droperidol 1.25 mg alone.

NONPHARMACOLOGIC TECHNIQUES

A number of studies have investigated the prophylactic use of **acupressure** (through wrist bands with a plastic bead placed bilaterally on the P-6 [HG-6] acupoint) in reducing PONV after neuraxial anesthesia for cesarean delivery. Ho et al.[264] reported significantly less PONV with acupressure in cesarean delivery patients who received epidural morphine (3-mg increments, 8 mg average total dose) in the postanesthesia care unit. A similar effect was seen in a study of patients who received intrathecal morphine 0.2 mg.[265] However, other studies investigating prophylactic acupressure prior to spinal anesthesia reported no reduction in PONV in patients who received intrathecal morphine 0.25 mg and fentanyl 10 μg[266] or in patients who did not receive neuraxial opioids.[267]

Pruritus

Pruritus is a common side effect of neuraxial opioid administration in obstetric patients. A retrospective review of 4880 cesarean delivery patients who received epidural morphine 2 to 5 mg observed that 58% reported pruritus.[91] However, patients receiving spinal anesthesia for cesarean delivery rank pain, nausea, and vomiting as more undesirable than pruritus (see Table 28-1).[8] The incidence and severity of pruritus are likely to vary according to the opioid dose, location of deposition (more common after intrathecal administration), and method of assessment.[268] Approximately 40% of patients reporting pruritus after receiving epidural morphine request treatment.[91,269,270]

Pruritus can manifest in the dermatomal distribution of neuraxial opioid spread as well as nonspecific areas of the head and neck.[271] These effects typically occur within a few hours of opioid administration.[249] Although opioid-induced histamine release from mast cells is well described, there does not appear to be a causative association between this process and pruritus, because plasma opioid and histamine levels are clinically insignificant at the time of symptom presentation (3 to 6 hours after intraspinal morphine administration).[85,104,272] In addition, sufentanil and fentanyl can produce pruritus but do not stimulate histamine release. At present, the mechanisms of spinal and epidural opioid-induced pruritus remain unclear. Postulated theories of causation include (1) direct or indirect excitatory effects on peripheral opioid receptors; (2) cephalad migration of the opioid within the CSF to the trigeminal nucleus (which contains the subnucleus caudalis, integrates facial sensory input, and exhibits high opioid receptor density); and (3) excitatory effects on dorsal or ventral horn neurons.[272,273] Pregnant patients may be more susceptible as a result of possible estrogenic interactions with opioid receptors.[274]

DRUG THERAPY

There is no consensus for treatment of neuraxial opioid–induced pruritus following cesarean delivery.[275] Historically, **antihistamines** have been a popular first choice for treatment. However, the efficacy of these agents should be questioned for patients receiving neuraxial opioids that do not cause histamine release (e.g., fentanyl, sufentanil). One study demonstrated that diphenhydramine was less effective than nalbuphine (higher itching scores and more treatment failures) after administration of intrathecal morphine 0.2 mg.[276]

Opioid antagonists are commonly employed to treat opioid-related pruritus. The efficacy of opioid antagonists depends, in part, on the drug-opioid receptor interaction (antagonist versus mixed agonist-antagonist). Studies comparing opioid antagonists have revealed mixed results in treating pruritus. Cohen et al.[270] compared naloxone (0.2 mg, with a maximum of three doses) with nalbuphine (5 mg, with a maximum of three doses) after administration of epidural morphine 5 mg for postcesarean analgesia. Nalbuphine significantly reduced the severity of pruritus after 30 minutes, and fewer patients in the nalbuphine group required additional doses for treatment of persistent pruritus. Somrat et al.[277] suggested that smaller doses of nalbuphine (2 to 3 mg) could adequately treat moderate or severe pruritus after intrathecal morphine administration.

Pretreatment with opioid antagonists has also been investigated as a method of reducing the incidence of opioid-induced pruritus. Morgan et al.[278] reported that pretreatment with nalbuphine (20 mg, at skin closure) with subsequent postoperative administration (40 mg, in divided doses) was ineffective in reducing pruritus in patients receiving epidural morphine. Similarly, pretreatment with subcutaneous naloxone (0.4 mg) did not significantly reduce the incidence of pruritus in patients receiving intrathecal fentanyl and morphine for elective cesarean delivery.[279] Naloxone may be more efficacious as an infusion, and Luthman et al.[280] reported reductions in the severity and incidence of pruritus using a naloxone infusion (0.1 mg/hr) after cesarean delivery. Naloxone and nalbuphine in patient-controlled bolus doses, combined with a background infusion, have also been found to reduce the incidence of pruritus in post–cesarean delivery patients who received epidural morphine 5 mg.[269] Abboud et al.[281] observed that the use of the long-acting opioid antagonist naltrexone (9 mg, administered orally) was associated with a lower incidence of pruritus after cesarean delivery in patients who received epidural morphine 4 mg, but these investigators also noted a significant increase in the incidence of unsatisfactory analgesia. A similar trend was reported with a 6-mg dose of oral naltrexone following administration of intrathecal morphine 0.25 mg.[282]

The effects of neuraxially administered opioid antagonists have also been investigated. Jeon et al.[283] reported less pruritus in patients receiving epidural naloxone (1.2 mg over 48 hours) with epidural 0.1% bupivacaine and morphine (6 mg over 48 hours) than in a control group not receiving naloxone. Similarly, Culebras et al.[204] investigated the effects of three different doses of intrathecal nalbuphine (0.2, 0.8, and 1.6 mg). They reported a significantly lower incidence of pruritus in all of the nalbuphine groups than in a control group receiving intrathecal morphine; however, the duration of analgesia was significantly shorter in the nalbuphine groups. Studies in animals and nonobstetric patients have suggested no adverse neurologic effects following neuraxial administration of opioid antagonists. However, the use of experimental drugs and drugs not approved for neuraxial administration continues to raise concerns due to potential neurotoxic adverse effects. Thus, neuraxial administration of these drugs for the prevention and treatment of opioid-induced pruritus and other side effects is limited. Further work is necessary to validate the optimal dose for each opioid antagonist, relative to specific routes of administration (intravenous, subcutaneous, neuraxial), for preventing and treating pruritus while avoiding reversal of the analgesia provided by neuraxial opioids.

NSAIDs are often incorporated into multimodal analgesic regimens for patients undergoing cesarean delivery. Some investigators have postulated that prostaglandins are involved in the etiology of pruritus after intraspinal opioid administration, owing to their ability to enhance C-fiber transmission to the CNS and release histamine.[284] However, there is limited evidence that NSAIDs reduce the occurrence of opioid-induced pruritus. A study evaluating the effect of oral celecoxib 200 mg after intrathecal morphine 0.3 mg reported no significant difference in the severity of pruritus or the need for rescue medications between the treatment group and a placebo group.[285]

Propofol has been reported to relieve pruritus caused by neuraxial opioids in nonobstetric patients.[286] The antipruritic effect of propofol has been proposed to occur as a result of inhibitory effects on posterior horn transmission rather than specific antagonism of the opioid receptors.[286] However, this effect has not been observed in obstetric patients who received subhypnotic doses of propofol (10 to 20 mg) for treatment of intrathecal morphine–induced pruritus.[287,288] Furthermore, a separate comparative study demonstrated that intravenous nalbuphine 3 mg is superior to propofol 20 mg for treating pruritus after administration of intrathecal morphine.[289]

The use of **5-HT$_3$ receptor antagonists** may represent an alternative method of treating opioid-induced pruritus. Direct stimulation of 5-HT$_3$ receptors, found in the dorsal horn of the spinal cord and in the nucleus of the spinal tract of the trigeminal nerve in the medulla, may occur after subarachnoid administration of opioids. **Ondansetron** 4 to 8 mg was more effective than placebo in reducing the incidence of pruritus following intrathecal administration of morphine 0.15 to 0.2 mg.[290,291] However, other studies comparing ondansetron 8 mg with placebo found no significant reduction in pruritus after intrathecal administration of morphine (0.1 to 0.2 mg) alone[292] or in combination with a lipophilic opioid (sufentanil or fentanyl).[255,293] The antipruritic effects associated with 5-HT$_3$ receptor antagonists (prophylactic or therapeutic) may depend on the dose, lipophilicity, and duration of action of the intrathecal opioid.[294] A study of epidurally administered ondansetron (8 mg over 2 days), in patients who received epidural ropivacaine 0.3% and morphine after cesarean delivery, demonstrated a reduction in the incidence of pruritus.[295] The investigators also performed an animal study that assessed potential neurotoxic effects of intrathecal ondansetron in rats, and no neurotoxic sequelae were found on histologic examination. However, further research is needed before the use of neuraxial 5-HT$_3$ antagonists can be regarded as a viable therapeutic option.

Urinary Retention

It is unclear whether the residual effects of neuraxial opioids affect the recovery of urinary function (and occurrence of urinary retention) after removal of the urethral catheter following cesarean delivery. The nonspecific definition of postpartum urinary retention following cesarean delivery makes an assessment of the potential effects of neuraxial opioids on urinary function difficult. Postpartum urinary retention has been previously described as "no spontaneous voiding within 6 hours of removal of an indwelling catheter (more than 24 hours after cesarean delivery)."[296] Some authorities advocate a diagnosis based on clinical diagnostic features (e.g., "the sudden inability to void") or post-void residual bladder volume (PVRV). However, there is marked variability in defining "significant" PVRV values (40 to 500 mL) associated with postpartum urinary retention.[297]

The mechanisms by which neuraxial opioids affect specific components of micturition (urge sensation, detrusor and sphincter function) are not fully understood, although spinal and supraspinal sites of action are likely to be involved. Kuipers et al.[298] performed urodynamic studies on healthy male volunteers receiving intrathecal sufentanil and morphine. Both opioids caused dose-dependent decreases in detrusor contractility and the "urgency to void." Patients receiving intrathecal sufentanil had earlier recovery of lower urinary tract function than those receiving intrathecal morphine.[298] Intrathecal local anesthetics (bupivacaine and lidocaine) have been shown to cause complete absence of detrusor contractility and urge sensation until the dermatomal block regresses to S2 to S3, with no partial recovery until this regression has occurred.[299]

Evron et al.[300] performed an observational study investigating the effects of epidural morphine and methadone in 120 women undergoing cesarean delivery. The rates of urinary retention and catheterization were highest in the morphine group (50% and 57%, respectively).[300] Other risk factors for postcesarean urinary retention include low body mass index (BMI) and multiparity.[301]

Hypothermia and Shivering

Perioperative and postoperative hypothermia and shivering are commonly observed in patients undergoing neuraxial anesthesia for cesarean delivery, and are caused by a number of inter-related processes. The true incidence of core hypothermia and shivering in this setting is unclear; however, results from earlier studies suggest that these complications may occur in up to 66% and 85% of patients, respectively.[302,303] Core-to-periphery heat redistribution is the major cause of core hypothermia following spinal or epidural anesthesia and is due to the effects of sympathetic and motor nerve blockade.[304] A study in healthy volunteers reported that core temperature can decrease 0.8° ± 0.3° C in the first hour of anesthesia.[305] Neuraxial anesthesia also impairs centrally mediated thermoregulatory control, lowers the vasoconstriction and shivering thresholds, and promotes greater environmental heat loss than metabolic heat production.[306-308]

The onset and the severity of hypothermia and shivering vary according to the individual anesthetic technique, the anesthetic agents administered, and baseline thermal status of the patient. Saito et al.[309] found that spinal anesthesia reduces initial core temperature more rapidly than epidural anesthesia during cesarean delivery. Interestingly, although there was no difference in the incidence of shivering between groups, the severity of shivering was significantly less in the spinal anesthesia group.[309] The more intense sensory block observed with spinal anesthesia inhibits central thermoregulatory control more than epidural anesthesia, which can affect shivering thresholds and intensity.[310]

The effect of neuraxial opioids on thermoregulation and shivering in patients undergoing cesarean delivery is not fully understood. Patients receiving intrathecal morphine 0.15 mg had a greater degree of hypothermia than patients receiving no intrathecal opioid.[311] However, intrathecal administration of both fentanyl and morphine is associated with a lower incidence of shivering than single-dose intrathecal morphine alone.[312] Furthermore, Hong and Lee[313] reported that intrathecal meperidine 10 mg produced fewer and less intense shivering episodes than intrathecal morphine 0.1 and 0.2 mg. Core hypothermia occurred to a similar extent in all study groups. The effect of epidural opioids on thermoregulation may be more consistent, with a number of studies reporting a reduction in the incidence and severity of shivering after epidural meperidine, butorphanol, fentanyl, and sufentanil.[314-317]

Preoperative patient warming using forced-air warming has been shown to reduce the incidence of perioperative and postoperative core hypothermia and shivering in patients undergoing cesarean delivery with *epidural* anesthesia.[318] However, a subsequent study found that perioperative forced-air warming does *not* prevent maternal hypothermia after cesarean delivery with *spinal* anesthesia.[302] It is likely that forced-air warming cannot compensate for the initial rapid drop in core temperature (from heat redistribution) following spinal anesthesia. It is unclear whether multimodal warming techniques may reduce the incidence of hypothermia and shivering after neuraxial anesthesia in this setting.

NEURAXIAL NONOPIOID ANALGESIC ADJUVANTS

The addition of neuraxial nonopioid adjuvants to local anesthetic agents may improve the quality of both intraoperative and postcesarean analgesia. Nonopioid neuraxial adjuvants have different sites and mechanisms of actions, and interactions between neuraxial opioids and nonopioid adjuvants may be additive or synergistic. Other potential advantages of neuraxial drug combinations include (1) a reduction in dose of individual drugs (with subsequent reductions in dose-dependent side effects) and (2) a reduction in postoperative opioid requirements and opioid-related side effects.[319]

Alpha-Adrenergic Agonists

The alpha$_2$-adrenergic agonists bind to presynaptic and postsynaptic alpha$_2$ receptors at peripheral, spinal (dorsal horn), and brainstem sites. Epidural and intrathecal alpha$_2$-adrenergic agonists provide analgesia by mimicking the activity of the descending noradrenergic system.[320,321] This process subsequently leads to norepinephrine release, which in turn modulates pain processing in the dorsal horn by inhibiting the release of substance P and increasing acetylcholine levels to produce analgesia.[322,323] **Clonidine,** an alpha$_2$-adrenergic agonist, causes a more potent analgesic response when administered neuraxially than when administered systemically. Clonidine is also associated with more profound sensory and motor block when administered with epidural local anesthetics and acts synergistically or additively with intraspinal opioids.[319,323] Pregnancy may enhance the analgesic effects of alpha$_2$-adrenergic agonists.[324]

Initial clinical studies of **epidural clonidine** 700 to 900 μg demonstrated a rapid onset of analgesia (within 20 minutes) lasting approximately 5 hours.[325] Mendez et al.[326] compared the analgesic efficacy of low-dose clonidine (400 μg bolus) with that of high-dose clonidine (800 μg bolus) followed by an epidural clonidine infusion at 10 or 20 μg/hr after cesarean delivery. The investigators found

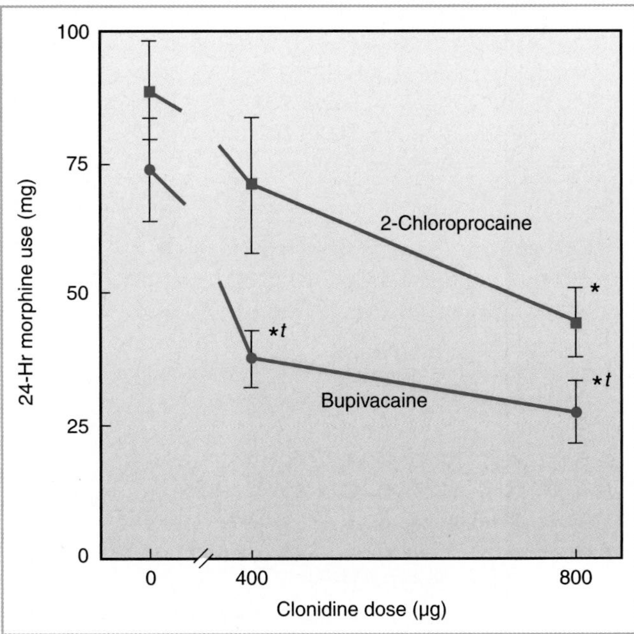

FIGURE 28-13 Twenty-four-hour morphine use after epidural injection of clonidine in women receiving intraoperative anesthesia from 2-chloroprocaine (■) or bupivacaine (•). * $P < .05$ vs. saline control. $^{t}P < .05$ vs. 2-chloroprocaine group. (From Huntoon M, Eisenach JC, Boese P. Epidural clonidine after cesarean section. Appropriate dose and effect of prior local anesthetic. Anesthesiology 1992; 76:187-93.)

the efficacy of analgesia, as measured by additional morphine requirements, to be dose dependent in the first 6 hours. Furthermore, dose-dependent sedation and motor block were observed in the first 3 hours postoperatively. These time-dependent side effects could lead to delays in the discharge of the patient from the postanesthesia care unit. Huntoon et al.[327] reported similar postcesarean analgesia in patients receiving epidural clonidine 400 or 800 μg following epidural bupivacaine anesthesia. The same effect was not observed in separate groups that received epidural 2-chloroprocaine anesthesia; absent or reduced postcesarean analgesia was observed with epidural clonidine 400 or 800 μg, respectively, a finding that may have been due to the calcium chelator (disodium ethylenediaminetetraacetic acid [EDTA]) present in the 2-chloroprocaine solution (Figure 28-13). These investigators also evaluated the effect of a postoperative epidural clonidine infusion (40 μg/hr). Postcesarean analgesia was sustained in patients who received epidural bupivacaine; in the 2-chloroprocaine group, analgesia was prolonged only in patients who received epidural clonidine 800 μg.[327]

Few studies have compared epidural clonidine with other opioids. Narchi et al.[328] found that postcesarean pain scores were lower after individual bolus doses of epidural clonidine 150 to 300 μg than with intramuscular morphine 10 mg in the first 3 hours after cesarean delivery. However, the investigators reported that clonidine 300 μg was paradoxically associated with higher pain scores and significant episodes of obstructive apnea with desaturation ($Spo_2 \leq 90\%$) in comparison with clonidine 150 μg.

Several studies have investigated epidural clonidine in combination with other epidural opioids for optimizing postcesarean analgesia. An isobolographic evaluation of epidural clonidine (in doses ranging from 50 to 400 μg) plus fentanyl (15 to 135 μg) did not demonstrate synergy between clonidine and fentanyl in patients recovering from cesarean delivery.[329] Results of this study suggest that these two drugs interact in an additive rather than a synergistic manner in humans. However, marked variability in drug response and failure of high doses to produce complete analgesia limited the accuracy of dose-response and ED_{50} analyses. Capogna et al.[330] observed that the addition of clonidine 75 to 150 μg to epidural morphine 2 mg significantly lengthened the duration of postcesarean analgesia without increasing the incidence of side effects. Vercauteren et al.[331] compared three different PCEA regimens with an epidural background infusion (sufentanil 2 μg/mL; sufentanil 2 μg/mL + epinephrine 2.5 μg/mL; sufentanil 2 μg/mL + clonidine 3 μg/mL) in patients who had undergone cesarean delivery. Although 24-hour sufentanil consumption was lowest in the clonidine admixture group, there were no significant differences among groups with regard to pain scores (at 10 or 24 hours), sedation, or hypotension.

A number of studies have evaluated the potential role of **intrathecal clonidine** for postcesarean analgesia. Filos et al.[332] observed that patients undergoing general anesthesia for cesarean delivery, who were randomly assigned to receive intrathecal clonidine 150 μg 45 minutes after extubation, experienced earlier onset of analgesia (within 20 minutes), lower maximal pain scores at 90 minutes, and more prolonged analgesia (> 6 hours) than patients who received intrathecal saline (control). Patients in the clonidine group had higher sedation scores, a greater maximal decrease in mean arterial pressure, and more complaints of dry mouth than the control group. The same investigators used a similar study design in a follow-up study comparing different doses of intrathecal clonidine (150, 300, or 450 μg).[333] The investigators observed that both the onset and duration of analgesia and sedation were dose dependent. A significant reduction in mean arterial pressure (21% compared with baseline) was observed in the group receiving clonidine 150 μg. On the basis of results from previous animal studies,[334] the investigators speculated that intrathecal clonidine may have a biphasic hemodynamic effect and concluded that intrathecal doses between 150 and 450 μg may provide hemodynamic stability. Later studies have evaluated postoperative analgesia in patients receiving intrathecal clonidine *before* surgery. Van Tuijl et al.[335] assessed postcesarean analgesia in patients receiving either intrathecal clonidine 75 μg combined with bupivacaine or bupivacaine alone. Early (1 to 2 hours) postoperative analgesia was improved with clonidine; however, no difference was found in 24-hour morphine consumption between the groups.

Studies of intrathecal opioids in combination with clonidine have investigated the contribution of each drug to the subsequent analgesia and side-effect profile. Benhamou et al.[336] evaluated the addition of intrathecal clonidine 75 μg ± fentanyl 12.5 μg with hyperbaric bupivacaine in patients undergoing cesarean delivery. Patients receiving the clonidine-fentanyl combination reported less intraoperative pain and more prolonged postcesarean analgesia (time to first analgesia request 215 minutes) than those receiving bupivacaine-clonidine and bupivacaine alone (183 and 137 minutes, respectively).

However, significantly higher rates of pruritus and sedation were reported for the clonidine-fentanyl group. Paech et al.[337] performed a six-arm study assessing postcesarean analgesia after intrathecal bupivacaine 12.5 mg with fentanyl 15 μg immediately followed by one of the following regimens: clonidine 150 μg; morphine 0.1 mg; and morphine 0.1 mg + clonidine 30, 60, 90 or 150 μg). The investigators concluded that the morphine-clonidine regimens provided optimal postcesarean analgesia with significantly lower pain scores at rest and with coughing in the first 4 hours. The minimum effective intrathecal dose of clonidine was 30 to 60 μg when combined with bupivacaine, fentanyl 15 μg, and morphine 0.1 mg. However, a significant increase in intraoperative sedation was observed in all groups receiving clonidine.

In summary, neuraxial clonidine does not offer substantial improvement in analgesia over that with neuraxial opioids and cannot currrently be recommended as an adjunct for postcesarean analgesia. Epidural clonidine (150 to 800 μg) may improve postcesarean analgesia in combination with epidural opioids. Intrathecal clonidine (75 to 450 μg) has modest efficacy and a relatively short duration of action. However, epidural or intrathecal clonidine administration is associated with adverse side effects (sedation, hypotension) that limit the use of this agent by those routes in the postcesarean setting.

No published studies have assessed the administration of neuraxial **dexmedetomidine** in pregnant patients. A study in patients undergoing bladder surgery who received spinal anesthesia with bupivacaine and clonidine 30 μg or dexmedetomidine 3 μg found similar sensory and motor block duration, with no hemodynamic compromise or sedation.[338] However, when dexmedetomidine was applied to strips of pregnant human myometrium *in vitro*, significant increases in uterine contractility were observed.[339]

Neostigmine

By interfering with the breakdown of acetylcholine, neostigmine indirectly stimulates spinal nicotinic and muscarinic receptors and the release of nitric oxide. The resulting analgesia is most likely due to central and peripheral alterations in pain modulation and transmission. Initial studies of intrathecal neostigmine in animals and human volunteers have demonstrated analgesic effects without neurotoxic effects.[209,340-342] However, despite the production of dose-dependent analgesia, intrathecal neostigmine at doses greater than 25 μg also produces nausea that is resistant to traditional antiemetic treatment (droperidol, ondansetron) and cholinergic antagonists.[342]

Krukowski et al.[343] reported that escalating doses of intrathecal neostigmine (10 to 100 μg) improved analgesia in a dose-independent manner when given after epidural anesthesia for cesarean delivery. The reduction in morphine requirements lasted up to 10 hours. The incidence of nausea varied from 50% to 100%. Chung et al.[344] showed that the postoperative analgesia provided by intrathecal neostigmine 25 μg was similar to that observed with intrathecal morphine 0.1 mg. Moreover, the investigators observed that the combination of neostigmine 12.5 μg with morphine 0.05 mg prolonged the analgesia in an additive (rather than a synergistic) manner, and had fewer side effects than observed with either drug alone in higher doses

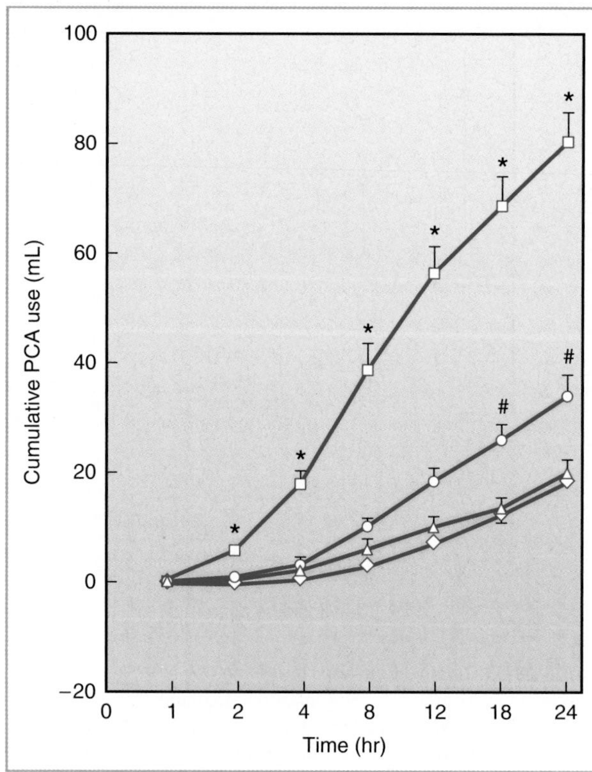

FIGURE 28-14 Cumulative patient-controlled analgesia (PCA) consumption after the administration of intrathecal saline (□), neostigmine 25 μg (○), morphine 0.1 mg (△), or the combination of neostigmine 12.5 μg and morphine 0.05 mg (◇) with hyperbaric bupivacaine 12 mg. Intravenous PCA was started with fentanyl 500 μg and ketorolac 150 mg in a total volume of 100 mL. The PCA device was set to deliver a bolus of 5 mL (i.e., fentanyl 25 μg and ketorolac 7.5 mg), with a lockout interval of 10 minutes and no basal infusion. Each value represents the mean ± SE. $^{*}P < .05$ versus the other three groups; $^{\#}P < .05$ versus the combination group. (From Chung CJ, Kim JS, Park HS, Chin YJ. The efficacy of intrathecal neostigmine, intrathecal morphine, and their combination for post-cesarean section analgesia. Anesth Analg 1998; 87:341-6.)

(Figure 28-14). Pan et al.[345] compared analgesic outcomes after intrathecal bupivacaine given either alone or in combination with intrathecal neostigmine 50 μg, intrathecal clonidine 150 μg, or a neostigmine-clonidine combination (same doses of each). Although patients in the clonidine-neostigmine group had lower pain scores in the first 10 postoperative hours, they experienced more significant side effects, including a prolongation of motor block, a higher incidence of hypotension, and a higher incidence (with greater severity) of nausea and vomiting.

Kaya et al.[346] assessed analgesic efficacy of epidural administration of neostigmine following cesarean delivery. They used a CSE technique with intrathecal bupivacaine 8 mg and fentanyl 10 μg. Patients subsequently received epidural neostigmine doses of 75, 150, or 300 μg after delivery. The investigators reported modest, short-lived, and dose-independent reductions in postoperative pain in the neostigmine groups.[346] In addition, no differences among groups in 24-hour morphine consumption after surgery were observed.

The dose-dependent side effects of intrathecal neostigmine limit its use as a single neuraxial adjunct for post-cesarean analgesia. Intrathecal neostigmine 12.5 to 25 μg may be used in combination regimens to improve analgesia and reduce side effects. The use of epidural neostigmine is not currently recommended until additional studies substantiate greater postcesarean analgesic benefits with fewer side effects.

N-Methyl-D-Aspartic Acid Antagonists

KETAMINE

Anesthetic and subanesthetic doses of ketamine have analgesic properties as a result of noncompetitive antagonism of N-methyl-D-aspartate (NMDA) receptors. Animal studies suggest that NMDA receptor blockade can prevent opioid tolerance and reduce the progressive increase in action potential discharge known as the "wind-up phenomenon."[347-349] Limited data exist for the role of neuraxial ketamine, an NMDA antagonist, in the provision of postcesarean analgesia.

In patients undergoing cesarean delivery randomly assigned to receive intrathecal bupivacaine alone or in combination with S(+) ketamine 0.05 mg/kg or fentanyl 25 μg,[350] significantly prolonged analgesia of better quality was observed in the fentanyl group. No significant differences in side effects were observed between the ketamine and fentanyl groups.[350] It is unclear whether the S(+) or R(−) isomers of ketamine have analgesic advantages over the racemate. Currently, the use of intrathecal ketamine does not appear to offer an analgesic benefit for postcesarean analgesia; moreover, neurotoxic concerns exist with both preservative-containing and preservative-free ketamine.[351]

Two systematic reviews have evaluated postoperative analgesia with perioperative epidural ketamine administration in patients undergoing nonobstetric surgery.[352,353] Subramaniam et al.[352] analyzed results from eight studies comparing a combination of epidural ketamine and opioids with epidural opioids alone. Although marked heterogeneity was observed between studies, the pain scores at rest were moderately lower in groups receiving epidural ketamine. In contrast, no overall difference between the groups was observed in pain scores with movement. A Cochrane review also reported marked heterogeneity and mixed analgesic outcomes in studies assessing preoperative and postoperative epidural administration of ketamine.[353] To date, no published studies have evaluated perioperative epidural ketamine administration in patients undergoing cesarean delivery. In a study of patients undergoing gynecologic surgery, Kawana et al.[354] noted that low-dose epidural ketamine (4, 6, or 8 mg) provided inferior analgesia compared with epidural morphine 3 mg.

Zohar et al.[355] assessed the analgesic effects of postcesarean wound instillation with ketamine as an adjunct to spinal bupivacaine anesthesia without opioids. A suprafascial catheter was placed intraoperatively and was connected to a PCA device containing either plain 0.125% bupivacaine or 0.125% bupivacaine with ketamine (1 mg/mL). The postoperative analgesic efficacy was poor in both groups, and no between-group differences were found in the use of rescue medication doses in the first 24 hours.

Sen et al.[356] evaluated the role of a preincisional, subanesthetic, intravenous bolus of ketamine in patients undergoing cesarean delivery; patients were randomly assigned to receive intrathecal bupivacaine 15 mg, bupivacaine 15 mg with fentanyl 10 μg, or bupivacaine 15 mg with intravenous ketamine 0.15 mg/kg. The patients receiving ketamine had the longest time to first request for postoperative analgesia, the lowest pain scores in the first 180 minutes, and the lowest 24-hour analgesic requirements.

Epidural ketamine provides limited postcesarean analgesia and cannot be recommended for patients undergoing cesarean delivery. Further research is needed to evaluate the role of epidural and intrathecal ketamine as part of a multimodal regimen for postcesarean analgesia.

MAGNESIUM

Magnesium is an NMDA antagonist that may alter pain signaling following nociceptive stimulation. No published studies have assessed the effects of neuraxial administration of magnesium sulfate in patients undergoing cesarean delivery. Buvanendran et al.[357] found that intrathecal magnesium sulfate 50 mg added to intrathecal fentanyl 25 μg resulted in only modest prolongation of the duration of labor analgesia (75 versus 60 minutes), with no differences in side effects. Intrathecal magnesium sulfate 50 mg has been shown to prolong the duration of spinal anesthesia in patients undergoing nonobstetric surgery with bupivacaine and fentanyl spinal anesthesia.[358] Arcioni et al.[359] randomly assigned 120 patients undergoing orthopedic surgery to receive spinal anesthesia (levobupivacaine with sufentanil) only or spinal anesthesia combined with (1) intrathecal magnesium sulfate (94.5 mg); (2) epidural magnesium sulfate infusion (100 mg/hr) postoperatively; or (3) combined intrathecal and epidural administration of magnesium sulfate. The investigators determined that magnesium was associated with a significant reduction (decrease of 38%, 49%, or 69% in the three magnesium groups, respectively) in morphine consumption at 36 hours postoperatively compared with spinal anesthesia alone. No differences in side effects were found.

Intravenous magnesium sulfate, given in either a "low-dose" regimen (25 mg/kg bolus and a 24-hour infusion at 1 g/hr) or a "high-dose" regimen (50 mg/kg bolus and a 24-hour infusion at 2 g/hr), was evaluated in patients undergoing spinal anesthesia for cesarean delivery.[360] No differences in sequential pain scores or cumulative opioid consumption were found up to 48 hours postoperatively. Some investigators have postulated that the blood-brain barrier may affect the rate of transfer of Mg^{2+} into the CSF, a possibility that may explain why CSF Mg^{2+} concentrations do not directly reflect plasma concentrations.[359]

In summary, intrathecal administration of magnesium has modest analgesic effects with no apparent maternal side effects after cesarean delivery. Parenteral administration of magnesium sulfate has mixed results in terms of postoperative analgesic efficacy.

Epinephrine

Robertson et al.[71] reported that epidural epinephrine 25 μg prolonged the duration of analgesia with epidural fentanyl 100 μg, but increased the incidence of pruritus. Similar improvements in duration of analgesia have been observed when epinephrine (5 to 30 μg/mL) was combined with either epidural diamorphine or sufentanil; however, the rate of side effects, including vomiting requiring treatment, was increased.[129,361] In contrast, McMorland et al.[362] found that epidural epinephrine did not enhance the efficacy of postcesarean analgesia provided by epidural sufentanil.

In a study assessing postoperative outcome measures for PCEA, patients receiving 0.01% bupivacaine with epinephrine and fentanyl reported better analgesia than those receiving either fentanyl or fentanyl-epinephrine.[112] No significant differences in side effects were reported between PCEA regimens with and without epinephrine. In another study, no improvement in analgesia and no reduction in opioid consumption was found with the addition of epinephrine 5 μg/mL to PCEA meperidine 5 mg/mL.[363] Patients in the epinephrine group reported more nausea at 2 and 24 hours as well as higher pruritus scores at 2 hours than the no-epinephrine group. The investigators attributed the epinephrine-associated increase in side effects to enhanced transfer of meperidine into the CSF.

Studies of epidural 2% lidocaine or 0.5% bupivacaine with epinephrine (5 μg/mL) have not demonstrated any detrimental effects of epinephrine on umbilical artery flow-velocity waveforms, uteroplacental or fetal vascular resistance, fetal myocardial function, or fetal heart rate.[364,365]

The use of intrathecal epinephrine as an adjuvant to local anesthetics, with or without opioids, has been evaluated in a number of studies. The addition of epinephrine 200 μg to hyperbaric spinal bupivacaine improved perioperative analgesia, but was associated with longer duration of residual sensory and motor block.[366] In a separate study, a combined intrathecal regimen of epinephrine 200 μg with morphine 0.2 mg did not significantly improve postoperative analgesia compared to intrathecal morphine 0.2 mg alone.[367] Zakowski et al.[368] found earlier and higher peak plasma bupivacaine concentrations with the addition of spinal epinephrine 200 μg to spinal bupivacaine in patients undergoing cesarean delivery. The investigators postulated that epinephrine might have a vasodilatory or biphasic action on certain vascular beds. Interestingly, the study also reported the absorption profile of morphine and bupivacaine in the presence of epinephrine. Peak plasma concentrations of unconjugated morphine and bupivacaine occurred at 3 hours and 15 minutes, respectively.[368]

In summary, the use of epidural epinephrine (2.5 to 30 μg/mL) seems to prolong the duration of analgesia with epidural opioids, but may increase opioid-related side effects. The use of intrathecal epinephrine 200 μg does not seem to enhance neuraxial opioid analgesia and is associated with prolonged sensory and motor block.

Newer Agents

In the future, some newer agents and adjuvants may enhance postoperative pain management strategies in patients receiving neuraxial anesthesia for cesarean delivery.[368] **Adenosine** (and adenosine analogues) may have antinociceptive effects that involve spinal adenosine A_1 receptors.[370] Intrathecal adenosine may enhance the effect of intrathecal clonidine, ketamine, and morphine. However, two later studies did not demonstrate improved analgesia with intrathecal administration of adenosine in patients undergoing hysterectomy.[371,372]

A direct relationship may exist between central K^+ channels and antinociception. Several animal studies have investigated **K^+ channel openers** (nicorandil, sildenafil) given by the intrathecal[373] or epidural[374] route. These drugs may also enhance the analgesic effects of neuraxial opioids and alpha$_2$-adrenergic agonists.

Intrathecal **midazolam** produces analgesia by acting on $GABA_A$ receptors and reducing spinal cord excitability. One study demonstrated that intrathecal midazolam enhanced the analgesic effect of intrathecal fentanyl during labor.[375] The impact of multimodal regimens that include intrathecal midazolam on postcesarean analgesia remains unclear.

Several neuraxially administered drugs have been shown to produce antinociceptive effects by altering calcium channel conductance at the spinal level. Intrathecal **gabapentin** reduced incision-induced allodynia in rats,[376,377] and epidural **verapamil** lowered postoperative opioid consumption following lower abdominal surgery.[378] **Ziconotide,** a selective, neuronal N-type voltage-sensitive calcium entry–blocking agent, has been shown to have analgesic effects after intrathecal administration.[369]

Before recommendations can be made about the potential use of new adjuncts, neurotoxicity studies must be performed to ensure these agents' safety for neuraxial administration. In addition, studies assessing analgesic efficacy, side effects, and toxicity must demonstrate that these agents result in significant improvement over the neuraxial local anesthetic and opioid regimens used in current clinical practice.

FUTURE APPLICATIONS

Despite the advances and improvements in pain management with the application of neuraxial techniques, the quality and duration of postcesarean analgesia is often substandard. A multimodal approach to treatment of postcesarean pain is currently recommended to optimize analgesia.[28,41,55,379] Multimodal strategies, including neuraxial opioids, postoperative NSAIDs, and acetaminophen, can facilitate a reduction in the dose of opioids with a concomitant diminution in dose-dependent side effects. However, the majority of women still request rescue analgesia and report opioid-related side effects after cesarean delivery.[27,99]

The future development of novel analgesics will almost certainly improve our current practice of providing postcesarean analgesia. Newer developments have focused on novel drug delivery systems to optimize and prolong the efficacy of current systemic and neuraxial analgesic techniques. For example, depot preparations permit slow, sustained release of a drug, thereby extending its duration of activity and potentially reducing side effects.[27,165]

The incidence and severity of postcesarean pain and side effects can be quite variable. Predictive models (using multifactorial forms of assessment) may identify women who are at risk for significant postoperative pain. Relevant data might be used to derive patient-specific analgesic requirements for the perioperative and postoperative periods. Later studies have shown that simple preoperative assessment using quantitative sensory tests (thermal stimuli[380,381] and pressure pain tolerance[382]) can predict postoperative pain and analgesic consumption. Use of a multifactorial predictive model[383] (physical and psychological somatization and anxiety tests) might further improve the ability to predict postcesarean pain. Our ability to predict analgesic requirements may also be improved with advances in pharmacogenomics.[384] At present, the use of neuraxial morphine, combined with multimodal analgesia (NSAIDs, acetaminophen, and oral opioids) is recommended to ensure optimal postcesarean analgesia.

KEY POINTS

- Epidural or intrathecal administration of opioids provides better postoperative pain relief than systemic administration.
- Effective postoperative analgesia provided by neuraxial techniques confers many physiologic benefits and may improve postoperative maternal and neonatal outcomes after cesarean delivery.
- Neuraxial administration of a hydrophilic opioid (e.g., morphine) has a delayed onset of analgesia owing to slow penetration of drug into the spinal cord, but results in a prolonged duration of action (14 to 36 hours) because of high bioavailability in the cerebrospinal fluid and minimal absorption into the systemic circulation.
- Neuraxial administration of a lipophilic opioid (e.g., fentanyl, sufentanil) has a rapid onset of analgesia owing to rapid spinal tissue penetration of drug. Thus neuraxial administration of lipophilic opioids may improve intraoperative analgesia. However, these agents are also rapidly absorbed systemically and consequently have a limited duration of activity (2 to 4 hours) after cesarean delivery.
- In clinical practice, single-dose epidural (2 to 4 mg) or intrathecal (0.075 to 0.2 mg) administration of morphine is most commonly utilized. Lower doses may not provide effective postoperative analgesia, so administration of additional analgesics may be required. Higher doses may increase opioid-related side effects without improving analgesia.
- Epidural administration and intrathecal administration of morphine provide similar analgesic efficacy and result in comparable opioid-related side effects.
- Patient-controlled epidural analgesia (PCEA) regimens with lipophilic opioids (e.g., meperidine, fentanyl, sufentanil) may improve postcesarean analgesia and maternal satisfaction. No consensus currently exists regarding optimal PCEA regimens (e.g., opioid ± local anesthetic; demand bolus ± background infusion). The disadvantages associated with PCEA (reduced maternal mobility, higher cost, additional nursing workload, and potential catheter-related complications) have led to less use of this method in the postcesarean setting in comparison with single-bolus doses of neuraxial morphine.
- Delayed respiratory depression is rare after neuraxial morphine administration for cesarean delivery, but when it occurs, it may result in maternal morbidity or mortality. "At-risk" patients should be identified prior to cesarean delivery, and adequate monitoring should be in place to assess respiratory function and sedation in the postoperative period.
- Pruritus, nausea, and vomiting are common postoperative side effects of neuraxial opioid administration. Opioid antagonists (e.g., nalbuphine 2 to 5 mg) are effective in managing opioid-related pruritus; 5-HT_3 antagonists are useful in treating nausea and vomiting. Combination regimens may be more effective than individual antiemetic agents in treating nausea and vomiting.
- Nonopioid adjuncts (e.g., α_2-agonists, anticholinesterases) may be considered as alternatives to, or in combination with, neuraxial opioids. However, these adjuncts are associated with modest analgesic benefits and significant side effects.

REFERENCES

1. Hamilton BE, Martin JA, Ventura SJ. Births: Preliminary Data for 2005. Hyattsville, MD, National Center for Health Statistics. Available at www.cdc.gov/nchs/products/pubs/pubd/hestats/prelimbirths05/prelimbirths05.htm/
2. Martin JA, Hamilton BE, Menacker F, et al. Preliminary births for 2004: Infant and maternal health. Hyattsville, MD, National Center for Health Statistics. Available at www.cdc.gov/nchs/products/pubs/pubd/hestats/prelimbirths04/prelimbirths04health.htm/
3. Fassoulaki A, Gatzou V, Petropoulos G, Siafaka I. Spread of subarachnoid block, intraoperative local anaesthetic requirements and postoperative analgesic requirements in Caesarean section and total abdominal hysterectomy. Br J Anaesth 2004; 93:678-82.
4. Apfelbaum JL, Chen C, Mehta SS, Gan TJ. Postoperative pain experience: Results from a national survey suggest postoperative pain continues to be undermanaged. Anesth Analg 2003; 97:534-40.
5. Dolin SJ, Cashman JN, Bland JM. Effectiveness of acute postoperative pain management. I. Evidence from published data. Br J Anaesth 2002; 89:409-23.
6. Kinsella M, ed. Obstetric Services. Section 8.9: Pain relief after caesarean section. In Raising the Standard: A Compendium of Audit Recipes. 2nd edition. London, Royal College of Anaesthetists, 2006. Available at http://www.rcoa.ac.uk/docs/arb-section8.pdf/
7. Wrench IJ, Sanghera S, Pinder A, et al. Dose response to intrathecal diamorphine for elective caesarean section and compliance with a national audit standard. Int J Obstet Anesth 2007; 16:17-21.
8. Carvalho B, Cohen SE, Lipman SS, et al. Patient preferences for anesthesia outcomes associated with cesarean delivery. Anesth Analg 2005; 101:1182-7.
9. Bucklin BA, Hawkins JL, Anderson JR, Ullrich FA. Obstetric anesthesia workforce survey: Twenty-year update. Anesthesiology 2005; 103:645-53.
10. Jenkins JG, Khan MM. Anaesthesia for caesarean section: A survey in a UK region from 1992 to 2002. Anaesthesia 2003; 58:1114-8.
11. Riley ET, Cohen SE, Macario A, et al. Spinal versus epidural anesthesia for cesarean section: A comparison of time efficiency, costs, charges, and complications. Anesth Analg 1995; 80:709-12.
12. Ng K, Parsons J, Cyna AM, Middleton P. Spinal versus epidural anaesthesia for caesarean section. Cochrane Database Syst Rev 2004; (2):CD003765.

13. Wu CL, Cohen SR, Richman JM, et al. Efficacy of postoperative patient-controlled and continuous infusion epidural analgesia versus intravenous patient-controlled analgesia with opioids: A meta-analysis. Anesthesiology 2005; 103:1079-88.
14. Cohen SE, Subak LL, Brose WG, Halpern J. Analgesia after cesarean delivery: Patient evaluations and costs of five opioid techniques. Reg Anesth 1991; 16:141-9.
15. Lim Y, Jha S, Sia AT, Rawal N. Morphine for post-caesarean section analgesia: Intrathecal, epidural or intravenous? Singapore Med J 2005; 46:392-6.
16. Harrison DM, Sinatra R, Morgese L, Chung JH. Epidural narcotic and patient-controlled analgesia for post-cesarean section pain relief. Anesthesiology 1988; 68:454-7.
17. Cade L, Ashley J, Ross AW. Comparison of epidural and intravenous opioid analgesia after elective caesarean section. Anaesth Intensive Care 1992; 20:41-5.
18. Terajima K, Onodera H, Kobayashi M, et al. Efficacy of intrathecal morphine for analgesia following elective cesarean section: Comparison with previous delivery. J Nippon Med Sch 2003; 70:327-33.
19. Swart M, Sewell J, Thomas D. Intrathecal morphine for caesarean section: An assessment of pain relief, satisfaction and side-effects. Anaesthesia 1997; 52:373-7.
20. Dahl JB, Jeppesen IS, Jorgensen H, et al. Intraoperative and postoperative analgesic efficacy and adverse effects of intrathecal opioids in patients undergoing cesarean section with spinal anesthesia: A qualitative and quantitative systematic review of randomized controlled trials. Anesthesiology 1999; 91:1919-27.
21. Eisenach JC, Grice SC, Dewan DM. Patient-controlled analgesia following cesarean section: A comparison with epidural and intramuscular narcotics. Anesthesiology 1988; 68:444-8.
22. Tziavrangos E, Schug SA. Regional anaesthesia and perioperative outcome. Curr Opin Anaesthesiol 2006; 19:521-5.
23. Guay J. The benefits of adding epidural analgesia to general anesthesia: A metaanalysis. J Anesth 2006; 20:335-40.
24. Richman JM, Wu CL. Epidural analgesia for postoperative pain. Anesthesiol Clin North Am 2005; 23:125-40.
25. Cohen SE, Woods WA. The role of epidural morphine in the post-cesarean patient: Efficacy and effects on bonding. Anesthesiology 1983; 58:500-4.
26. Carvalho B, Riley E, Cohen SE, et al. Single-dose, sustained-release epidural morphine in the management of postoperative pain after elective cesarean delivery: Results of a multicenter randomized controlled study. Anesth Analg 2005; 100:1150-8.
27. Carvalho B, Roland LM, Chu LF, et al. Single-dose, extended-release epidural morphine (DepoDur) compared to conventional epidural morphine for post-cesarean pain. Anesth Analg 2007; 105:176-83.
28. Rosaeg OP, Lui AC, Cicutti NJ, et al. Peri-operative multimodal pain therapy for caesarean section: Analgesia and fitness for discharge. Can J Anaesth 1997; 44:803-9.
29. Stenkamp SJ, Easterling TR, Chadwick HS. Effect of epidural and intrathecal morphine on the length of hospital stay after cesarean section. Anesth Analg 1989; 68:66-9.
30. Kujovich JL. Hormones and pregnancy: Thromboembolic risks for women. Br J Haematol 2004; 126:443-54.
31. Ramanathan J, Coleman P, Sibai B. Anesthetic modification of hemodynamic and neuroendocrine stress responses to cesarean delivery in women with severe preeclampsia. Anesth Analg 1991; 73:772-9.
32. Rawal N, Sjostrand U, Christoffersson E, et al. Comparison of intramuscular and epidural morphine for postoperative analgesia in the grossly obese: Influence on postoperative ambulation and pulmonary function. Anesth Analg 1984; 63:583-92.
33. Tuman KJ, McCarthy RJ, March RJ, et al. Effects of epidural anesthesia and analgesia on coagulation and outcome after major vascular surgery. Anesth Analg 1991; 73:696-704.
34. Yeager MP, Glass DD, Neff RK, Brinck-Johnsen T. Epidural anesthesia and analgesia in high-risk surgical patients. Anesthesiology 1987; 66:729-36.
35. Armitage EN: Postoperative pain—prevention or relief? Br J Anaesth 1989; 63:136-8.
36. Yarnell RW, Polis T, Reid GN, et al. Patient-controlled analgesia with epidural meperidine after elective cesarean section. Reg Anesth 1992; 17:329-33.
37. Cooper DW, Ryall DM, McHardy FE, et al. Patient-controlled extradural analgesia with bupivacaine, fentanyl, or a mixture of both, after Caesarean section. Br J Anaesth 1996; 76:611-5.
38. Parker RK, Sawaki Y, White PF. Epidural patient-controlled analgesia: Influence of bupivacaine and hydromorphone basal infusion on pain control after cesarean delivery. Anesth Analg 1992; 75:740-6.
39. Hirose M, Hara Y, Hosokawa T, Tanaka Y. The effect of postoperative analgesia with continuous epidural bupivacaine after cesarean section on the amount of breast feeding and infant weight gain. Anesth Analg 1996; 82:1166-9.
40. Wittels B, Toledano A. The effects of epidural morphine and epidural butorphanol on maternal outcomes after cesarean delivery. Anesth Analg 1995; 81:1317-8.
41. Pan PH. Post cesarean delivery pain management: Multimodal approach. Int J Obstet Anesth 2006; 15:185-8.
42. Hale TW. Anesthetic medications in breastfeeding mothers. J Hum Lact 1999; 15:185-94.
43. Spigset O. Anaesthetic agents and excretion in breast milk. Acta Anaesthesiol Scand 1994; 38:94-103.
44. Wittels B, Glosten B, Faure EA, et al. Postcesarean analgesia with both epidural morphine and intravenous patient-controlled analgesia: Neurobehavioral outcomes among nursing neonates. Anesth Analg 1997; 85:600-6.
45. Wittels B, Scott DT, Sinatra RS. Exogenous opioids in human breast milk and acute neonatal neurobehavior: A preliminary study. Anesthesiology 1990; 73:864-9.
46. Perkins FM, Kehlet H. Chronic pain as an outcome of surgery: A review of predictive factors. Anesthesiology 2000; 93:1123-33.
47. Kehlet H, Jensen TS, Woolf CJ. Persistent postsurgical pain: Risk factors and prevention. Lancet 2006; 367:1618-25.
48. Lavand'homme PM, Roelants F, Vanderbeck B, Alluin L. Risk to develop chronic pain after elective cesarean delivery in young healthy parturients. Anesthesiology 2005; 102:A18.
49. Nikolajsen L, Sorensen HC, Jensen TS, Kehlet H. Chronic pain following Caesarean section. Acta Anaesthesiol Scand 2004; 48:111-6.
50. Almeida EC, Nogueira AA, Candido dos Reis FJ, Rosa e Silva JC. Cesarean section as a cause of chronic pelvic pain. Int J Gynaecol Obstet 2002; 79:101-4.
51. Lavand'homme PM, Roelants F, Waterloos H, De Kock MF. Postoperative analgesic effects of continuous wound infiltration with diclofenac after elective cesarean delivery. Anesthesiology 2007; 106:1220-5.
52. Pan PH, Smiley R, Houle T, et al. Chronic pain after delivery—is it different between vaginal and operative delivery? Anesthesiology 2007; 106:A-28.
53. Lavand'homme P, De Kock M, Waterloos H. Intraoperative epidural analgesia combined with ketamine provides effective preventive analgesia in patients undergoing major digestive surgery. Anesthesiology 2005; 103:813-20.
54. De Kock M, Lavand'homme P, Waterloos H. The short-lasting analgesia and long-term antihyperalgesic effect of intrathecal clonidine in patients undergoing colonic surgery. Anesth Analg 2005; 101:566-72.
55. Lavand'homme P. Postcesarean analgesia: Effective strategies and association with chronic pain. Curr Opin Anaesthesiol 2006; 19:244-8.
56. Atweh SF, Kuhar MJ. Autoradiographic localization of opiate receptors in rat brain. I. Spinal cord and lower medulla. Brain Res 1977; 124:53-67.
57. Schmauss C, Yaksh TL. In vivo studies on spinal opiate receptor systems mediating antinociception. II. Pharmacological profiles suggesting a differential association of mu, delta and kappa receptors with visceral chemical and cutaneous thermal stimuli in the rat. J Pharmacol Exp Ther 1984; 228:1-12.
58. Kitahata LM, Kosaka Y, Taub A, et al. Lamina-specific suppression of dorsal-horn unit activity by morphine sulfate. Anesthesiology 1974; 41:39-48.

59. Yaksh TL, Reddy SV. Studies in the primate on the analgetic effects associated with intrathecal actions of opiates, alpha-adrenergic agonists and baclofen. Anesthesiology 1981; 54:451-67.
60. Nishio Y, Sinatra RS, Kitahata LM, Collins JG. Spinal cord distribution of 3H-morphine after intrathecal administration: Relationship to analgesia. Anesth Analg 1989; 69:323-7.
61. Cousins MJ, Mather LE, Glynn CJ, et al. Selective spinal analgesia. Lancet 1979; 1(8126):1141-2.
62. Yaksh TL. Spinal opiate analgesia: Characteristics and principles of action. Pain 1981; 11:293-346.
63. Wang JK, Nauss LA, Thomas JE. Pain relief by intrathecally applied morphine in man. Anesthesiology 1979; 50:149-51.
64. Bernards CM, Hill HF. Morphine and alfentanil permeability through the spinal dura, arachnoid, and pia mater of dogs and monkeys. Anesthesiology 1990; 73:1214-9.
65. Bernards CM, Hill HF. Physical and chemical properties of drug molecules governing their diffusion through the spinal meninges. Anesthesiology 1992; 77:750-6.
66. George MJ. The site of action of epidurally administered opioids and its relevance to postoperative pain management. Anaesthesia 2006; 61:659-64.
67. Gourlay GK, Cherry DA, Plummer JL, et al. The influence of drug polarity on the absorption of opioid drugs into CSF and subsequent cephalad migration following lumbar epidural administration: Application to morphine and pethidine. Pain 1987; 31:297-305.
68. Bernards CM, Shen DD, Sterling ES, et al. Epidural, cerebrospinal fluid, and plasma pharmacokinetics of epidural opioids (part 2): Effect of epinephrine. Anesthesiology 2003; 99:466-75.
69. Bernards CM, Shen DD, Sterling ES, et al. Epidural, cerebrospinal fluid, and plasma pharmacokinetics of epidural opioids (part 1): Differences among opioids. Anesthesiology 2003; 99:455-65.
70. Nordberg G, Hedner T, Mellstrand T, Dahlstrom B. Pharmacokinetic aspects of epidural morphine analgesia. Anesthesiology 1983; 58:545-51.
71. Robertson K, Douglas MJ, McMorland GH. Epidural fentanyl, with and without epinephrine for post-Caesarean section analgesia. Can Anaesth Soc J 1985; 32:502-5.
72. Glass PS, Estok P, Ginsberg B, et al. Use of patient-controlled analgesia to compare the efficacy of epidural to intravenous fentanyl administration. Anesth Analg 1992; 74:345-51.
73. Ellis DJ, Millar WL, Reisner LS. A randomized double-blind comparison of epidural versus intravenous fentanyl infusion for analgesia after cesarean section. Anesthesiology 1990; 72:981-6.
74. Ionescu TI, Taverne RH, Houweling PL, et al. Pharmacokinetic study of extradural and intrathecal sufentanil anaesthesia for major surgery. Br J Anaesth 1991; 66:458-64.
75. D'Angelo R, Gerancher JC, Eisenach JC, Raphael BL. Epidural fentanyl produces labor analgesia by a spinal mechanism. Anesthesiology 1998; 88:1519-23.
76. Liu SS, Gerancher JC, Bainton BG, et al. The effects of electrical stimulation at different frequencies on perception and pain in human volunteers: Epidural versus intravenous administration of fentanyl. Anesth Analg 1996; 82:98-102.
77. Ginosar Y, Riley ET, Angst MS. The site of action of epidural fentanyl in humans: The difference between infusion and bolus administration. Anesth Analg 2003; 97:1428-38.
78. Cohen S, Pantuck CB, Amar D, et al. The primary action of epidural fentanyl after cesarean delivery is via a spinal mechanism. Anesth Analg 2002; 94:674-9.
79. Stevens RA, Petty RH, Hill HF, et al. Redistribution of sufentanil to cerebrospinal fluid and systemic circulation after epidural administration in dogs. Anesth Analg 1993; 76:323-7.
80. Youngstrom PC, Cowan RI, Sutheimer C, et al. Pain relief and plasma concentrations from epidural and intramuscular morphine in post-cesarean patients. Anesthesiology 1982; 57:404-9.
81. Weddel SJ, Ritter RR. Serum levels following epidural administration of morphine and correlation with relief of postsurgical pain. Anesthesiology 1981; 54:210-4.
82. Nordberg G, Hedner T, Mellstrand T, Dahlstrom B. Pharmacokinetic aspects of intrathecal morphine analgesia. Anesthesiology 1984; 60:448-54.
83. Ummenhofer WC, Arends RH, Shen DD, Bernards CM. Comparative spinal distribution and clearance kinetics of intrathecally administered morphine, fentanyl, alfentanil, and sufentanil. Anesthesiology 2000; 92:739-53.
84. Gourlay GK, Murphy TM, Plummer JL, et al. Pharmacokinetics of fentanyl in lumbar and cervical CSF following lumbar epidural and intravenous administration. Pain 1989; 38:253-9.
85. Cousins MJ, Mather LE. Intrathecal and epidural administration of opioids. Anesthesiology 1984; 61:276-310.
86. van den Hoogen RH, Colpaert FC. Epidural and subcutaneous morphine, meperidine (pethidine), fentanyl and sufentanil in the rat: Analgesia and other in vivo pharmacologic effects. Anesthesiology 1987; 66:186-94.
87. Brill S, Gurman GM, Fisher A. A history of neuraxial administration of local analgesics and opioids. Eur J Anaesthesiol 2003; 20:682-9.
88. Palmer CM, Nogami WM, Van Maren G, Alves DM. Postcesarean epidural morphine: A dose-response study. Anesth Analg 2000; 90:887-91.
89. Chumpathong S, Santawat U, Saunya P, et al. Comparison of different doses of epidural morphine for pain relief following cesarean section. J Med Assoc Thai 2002; 85(Suppl 3):S956-62.
90. Rosen MA, Hughes SC, Shnider SM, et al. Epidural morphine for the relief of postoperative pain after cesarean delivery. Anesth Analg 1983; 62:666-72.
91. Fuller JG, McMorland GH, Douglas MJ, Palmer L. Epidural morphine for analgesia after caesarean section: A report of 4880 patients. Can J Anaesth 1990; 37:636-40.
92. Leicht CH, Durkan WJ, Fians DH. Postoperative analgesia with epidural morphine: Single bolus vs. Daymate elastomeric continuous infusion technique (abstract). Anesthesiology 1990; 73:A931.
93. Zakowski MI, Ramanathan S, Turndorf H. A two-dose epidural morphine regimen for cesarean section patients: Therapeutic efficacy. Acta Anaesthesiol Scand 1992; 36:698-701.
94. Asantila R, Eklund P, Rosenberg PH. Epidural analgesia with 4 mg of morphine following caesarean section: Effect of injected volume. Acta Anaesthesiol Scand 1993; 37:764-7.
95. Eisenach JC, Schlairet TJ, Dobson CE, Hood DH. Effect of prior anesthetic solution on epidural morphine analgesia. Anesth Analg 1991; 73:119-23.
96. Karambelkar DJ, Ramanathan S. 2-Chloroprocaine antagonism of epidural morphine analgesia. Acta Anaesthesiol Scand 1997; 41:774-8.
97. Hess PE, Snowman CE, Hahn CJ, et al. Chloroprocaine may not affect epidural morphine for postcesarean delivery analgesia. J Clin Anesth 2006; 18:29-33.
98. Camann WR, Hartigan PM, Gilbertson LI, et al. Chloroprocaine antagonism of epidural opioid analgesia: A receptor-specific phenomenon? Anesthesiology 1990; 73:860-3.
99. Duale C, Frey C, Bolandard F, et al. Epidural versus intrathecal morphine for postoperative analgesia after Caesarean section. Br J Anaesth 2003; 91:690-4.
100. Sarvela J, Halonen P, Soikkeli A, Korttila K. A double-blinded, randomized comparison of intrathecal and epidural morphine for elective cesarean delivery. Anesth Analg 2002; 95:436-40.
101. Chadwick HS, Bernards CM, Kovarik DW, Tomlin JJ. Subdural injection of morphine for analgesia following cesarean section: A report of three cases. Anesthesiology 1992; 77:590-4.
102. Grass JA, Sakima NT, Schmidt R, et al. A randomized, double-blind, dose-response comparison of epidural fentanyl versus sufentanil analgesia after cesarean section. Anesth Analg 1997; 85:365-71.
103. Preston PG, Rosen MA, Hughes SC, et al. Epidural anesthesia with fentanyl and lidocaine for cesarean section: Maternal effects and neonatal outcome. Anesthesiology 1988; 68:938-43.
104. Bromage PR, Camporesi EM, Durant PA, Nielsen CH. Rostral spread of epidural morphine. Anesthesiology 1982; 56:431-6.
105. Wolfe MJ, Nicholas AD. Selective epidural analgesia. Lancet 1979; 2(8134):150-1.

106. King MJ, Bowden MI, Cooper GM. Epidural fentanyl and 0.5% bupivacaine for elective caesarean section. Anaesthesia 1990; 45:285-8.
107. Naulty JS, Datta S, Ostheimer GW, et al. Epidural fentanyl for post-cesarean delivery pain management. Anesthesiology 1985; 63:694-8.
108. Sevarino FB, McFarlane C, Sinatra RS. Epidural fentanyl does not influence intravenous PCA requirements in the post-caesarean patient. Can J Anaesth 1991; 38:450-3.
109. Tejwani GA, Rattan AK, McDonald JS. Role of spinal opioid receptors in the antinociceptive interactions between intrathecal morphine and bupivacaine. Anesth Analg 1992; 74:726-34.
110. Penning JP, Yaksh TL. Interaction of intrathecal morphine with bupivacaine and lidocaine in the rat. Anesthesiology 1992; 77:1186-2000.
111. Birnbach DJ, Johnson MD, Arcario T, et al. Effect of diluent volume on analgesia produced by epidural fentanyl. Anesth Analg 1989; 68:808-10.
112. Cohen S, Lowenwirt I, Pantuck CB, et al. Bupivacaine 0.01% and/or epinephrine 0.5 microg/ml improve epidural fentanyl analgesia after cesarean section. Anesthesiology 1998; 89:1354-61.
113. Rosen MA, Dailey PA, Hughes SC, et al. Epidural sufentanil for postoperative analgesia after cesarean section. Anesthesiology 1988; 68:448-54.
114. Perriss BW, Latham BV, Wilson IH. Analgesia following extradural and i.m. pethidine in post-caesarean section patients. Br J Anaesth 1990; 64:355-7.
115. Brownridge P, Frewin DB. A comparative study of techniques of postoperative analgesia following caesarean section and lower abdominal surgery. Anaesth Intensive Care 1985; 13:123-30.
116. Paech MJ. Epidural pethidine or fentanyl during caesarean section: A double-blind comparison. Anaesth Intensive Care 1989; 17:157-65.
117. Ngan Kee WD, Lam KK, Chen PP, Gin T. Epidural meperidine after cesarean section: The effect of diluent volume. Anesth Analg 1997; 85:380-4.
118. Ngan Kee WD, Lam KK, Chen PP, Gin T. Epidural meperidine after cesarean section: A dose-response study. Anesthesiology 1996; 85:289-94.
119. Khaw KS, Ngan Kee WD, Critchley LA. Epidural meperidine does not cause hemodynamic changes in the term parturient. Can J Anaesth 2000; 47:155-9.
120. de Leon-Casasola OA, Lema MJ. Postoperative epidural opioid analgesia: What are the choices? Anesth Analg 1996; 83:867-75.
121. Dougherty TB, Baysinger CL, Henenberger JC, Gooding DJ. Epidural hydromorphone with and without epinephrine for post-operative analgesia after cesarean delivery. Anesth Analg 1989; 68:318-22.
122. Henderson SK, Matthew EB, Cohen H, Avram MJ. Epidural hydromorphone: A double-blind comparison with intramuscular hydromorphone for postcesarean section analgesia. Anesthesiology 1987; 66:825-30.
123. Chestnut DH, Choi WW, Isbell TJ. Epidural hydromorphone for postcesarean analgesia. Obstet Gynecol 1986; 68:65-9.
124. Halpern SH, Arellano R, Preston R, et al. Epidural morphine vs hydromorphone in post-caesarean section patients. Can J Anaesth 1996; 43:595-8.
125. Quigley C. Hydromorphone for acute and chronic pain. Cochrane Database Syst Rev 2002; (1):CD003447.
126. Rawal N, Allvin R. Acute pain services in Europe: A 17-nation survey of 105 hospitals. The EuroPain Acute Pain Working Party. Eur J Anaesthesiol 1998; 15:354-63.
127. Wee MY, Brown H, Reynolds F. The National Institute of Clinical Excellence (NICE) guidelines for caesarean sections: Implications for the anaesthetist. Int J Obstet Anesth 2005; 14:147-58.
128. Haynes SR, Davidson I, Allsop JR, Dutton DA. Comparison of epidural methadone with epidural diamorphine for analgesia following caesarean section. Acta Anaesthesiol Scand 1993; 37:375-80.
129. Semple AJ, Macrae DJ, Munishankarappa S, et al. Effect of the addition of adrenaline to extradural diamorphine analgesia after caesarean section. Br J Anaesth 1988; 60:632-8.
130. Roulson CJ, Bennett J, Shaw M, Carli F. Effect of extradural diamorphine on analgesia after caesarean section under subarachnoid block. Br J Anaesth 1993; 71:810-3.
131. Macrae DJ, Munishankrappa S, Burrow LM, et al. Double-blind comparison of the efficacy of extradural diamorphine, extradural phenoperidine and i.m. diamorphine following caesarean section. Br J Anaesth 1987; 59:354-9.
132. Martin WR, Eades CG, Fraser HF, Wikler A. Use of hindlimb reflexes of the chronic spinal dog for comparing analgesics. J Pharmacol Exp Ther 1964; 144:8-11.
133. Abboud TK, Moore M, Zhu J, et al. Epidural butorphanol or morphine for the relief of post-cesarean section pain: Ventilatory responses to carbon dioxide. Anesth Analg 1987; 66:887-93.
134. Palacios QT, Jones MM, Hawkins JL, et al. Post-caesarean section analgesia: A comparison of epidural butorphanol and morphine. Can J Anaesth 1991; 38:24-30.
135. Camann WR, Loferski BL, Fanciullo GJ, et al. Does epidural administration of butorphanol offer any clinical advantage over the intravenous route? A double-blind, placebo-controlled trial. Anesthesiology 1992; 76:216-20.
136. Rawal N, Nuutinen L, Raj PP, et al. Behavioral and histopathologic effects following intrathecal administration of butorphanol, sufentanil, and nalbuphine in sheep. Anesthesiology 1991; 75:1025-34.
137. Eisenach J. Opioid antagonist adjuncts to epidural morphine for postcesarean analgesia: Maternal outcomes. Anesth Analg 1994; 79:611-2.
138. Yaksh T, Birnbach DJ. Intrathecal nalbuphine after cesarean delivery: Are we ready? Anesth Analg 2000; 91:505-8.
139. Camann WR, Hurley RH, Gilbertson LI, et al. Epidural nalbuphine for analgesia following caesarean delivery: Dose-response and effect of local anaesthetic choice. Can J Anaesth 1991; 38:728-32.
140. Parker RK, Holtmann B, White PF. Patient-controlled epidural analgesia: Interactions between nalbuphine and hydromorphone. Anesth Analg 1997; 84:757-63.
141. Palmer CM, Voulgaropoulos D, Alves D. Subarachnoid fentanyl augments lidocaine spinal anesthesia for cesarean delivery. Reg Anesth 1995; 20:389-94.
142. Vincent RD Jr, Chestnut DH, Choi WW, et al. Does epidural fentanyl decrease the efficacy of epidural morphine after cesarean delivery? Anesth Analg 1992; 74:658-63.
143. Cooper DW, Garcia E, Mowbray P, Millar MA. Patient-controlled epidural fentanyl following spinal fentanyl at Caesarean section. Anaesthesia 2002; 57:266-70.
144. Dottrens M, Rifat K, Morel DR. Comparison of extradural administration of sufentanil, morphine and sufentanil-morphine combination after caesarean section. Br J Anaesth 1992; 69:9-12.
145. Sinatra RS, Sevarino FB, Chung JH, et al. Comparison of epidurally administered sufentanil, morphine, and sufentanil-morphine combination for postoperative analgesia. Anesth Analg 1991; 72:522-7.
146. Wittels B, Glosten B, Faure EA, et al. Opioid antagonist adjuncts to epidural morphine for postcesarean analgesia: Maternal outcomes. Anesth Analg 1993; 77:925-32.
147. Lawhorn CD, McNitt JD, Fibuch EE, et al. Epidural morphine with butorphanol for postoperative analgesia after cesarean delivery. Anesth Analg 1991; 72:53-7.
148. Gambling DR, Howell P, Huber C, Kozak S. Epidural butorphanol does not reduce side effects from epidural morphine after cesarean birth. Anesth Analg 1994; 78:1099-104.
149. Werawatganon T, Charuluxanun S. Patient controlled intravenous opioid analgesia versus continuous epidural analgesia for pain after intra-abdominal surgery. Cochrane Database Syst Rev 2005; (1):CD004088.
150. Lubenow TR, Tanck EN, Hopkins EM, et al. Comparison of patient-assisted epidural analgesia with continuous-infusion epidural analgesia for postoperative patients. Reg Anesth 1994; 19:206-11.
151. Nightingale JJ, Knight MV, Higgins B, Dean T. Randomized, double-blind comparison of patient-controlled epidural infusion vs nurse-administered epidural infusion for postoperative analgesia in patients undergoing colonic resection. Br J Anaesth 2007; 98:380-4.
152. Liu SS, Allen HW, Olsson GL. Patient-controlled epidural analgesia with bupivacaine and fentanyl on hospital wards: Prospective experience with 1,030 surgical patients. Anesthesiology 1998; 88:688-95.

153. Paech MJ, Moore JS, Evans SF. Meperidine for patient-controlled analgesia after cesarean section: Intravenous versus epidural administration. Anesthesiology 1994; 80:1268-76.
154. Fanshawe MP. A comparison of patient-controlled epidural pethidine versus single-dose epidural morphine for analgesia after caesarean section. Anaesth Intensive Care 1999; 27:610-4.
155. Ngan Kee WD. Epidural pethidine: Pharmacology and clinical experience. Anaesth Intensive Care 1998; 26:247-55.
156. Ngan Kee WD, Lam KK, Chen PP, Gin T. Comparison of patient-controlled epidural analgesia with patient-controlled intravenous analgesia using pethidine or fentanyl. Anaesth Intensive Care 1997; 25:126-32.
157. Goh JL, Evans SF, Pavy TJ. Patient-controlled epidural analgesia following caesarean delivery: A comparison of pethidine and fentanyl. Anaesth Intensive Care 1996; 24:45-50.
158. Yu PY, Gambling DR. A comparative study of patient-controlled epidural fentanyl and single-dose epidural morphine for post-caesarean analgesia. Can J Anaesth 1993; 40:416-20.
159. Parker RK, White PF. Epidural patient-controlled analgesia: An alternative to intravenous patient-controlled analgesia for pain relief after cesarean delivery. Anesth Analg 1992; 75:245-51.
160. Cohen S, Amar D, Pantuck CB, et al. Postcesarean delivery epidural patient-controlled analgesia: Fentanyl or sufentanil? Anesthesiology 1993; 78:486-91.
161. Vercauteren MP, Coppejans HC, ten Broecke PW, et al. Epidural sufentanil for postoperative patient-controlled analgesia (PCA) with or without background infusion: A double-blind comparison. Anesth Analg 1995; 80:76-80.
162. Boudreault D, Brasseur L, Samii K, Lemoing JP. Comparison of continuous epidural bupivacaine infusion plus either continuous epidural infusion or patient-controlled epidural injection of fentanyl for postoperative analgesia. Anesth Analg 1991; 73:132-7.
163. Vercauteren M, Vereecken K, La Malfa M, et al. Cost-effectiveness of analgesia after Caesarean section: A comparison of intrathecal morphine and epidural PCA. Acta Anaesthesiol Scand 2002; 46:85-9.
164. Howell SB. Clinical applications of a novel sustained-release injectable drug delivery system: DepoFoam technology. Cancer J 2001; 7:219-27.
165. Angst MS, Drover DR. Pharmacology of drugs formulated with DepoFoam: A sustained release drug delivery system for parenteral administration using multivesicular liposome technology. Clin Pharmacokinet 2006; 45:1153-76.
166. Mantripragada S. A lipid based depot (DepoFoam technology) for sustained release drug delivery. Prog Lipid Res 2002; 41:392-406.
167. Gambling D, Hughes T, Martin G, et al. A comparison of DepoDur, a novel, single-dose extended-release epidural morphine, with standard epidural morphine for pain relief after lower abdominal surgery. Anesth Analg 2005; 100:1065-74.
168. Viscusi ER, Martin G, Hartrick CT, et al. Forty-eight hours of postoperative pain relief after total hip arthroplasty with a novel, extended-release epidural morphine formulation. Anesthesiology 2005; 102:1014-22.
169. Hartrick CT, Martin G, Kantor G, et al. Evaluation of a single-dose, extended-release epidural morphine formulation for pain after knee arthroplasty. J Bone Joint Surg Am 2006; 88:273-81.
170. Nagle PC, Gerancher JC. DepoDur (extended-release epidural morphine): A review of an old drug in a new vehicle. Tech Reg Anesth Pain Manag 2007; 11:9-18.
171. Keck S, Glennon C, Ginsberg B. DepoDur extended-release epidural morphine: Reshaping postoperative care: What perioperative nurses need to know. Orthop Nurs 2007; 26:86-93.
172. Gambling D, Hughes T, Gould E, Manvelian G. A pharmacokinetic and pharmacodynamic study of a single dose of epidural DepoDur following epidural bupivacaine: A randomized controlled trial in patients undergoing lower abdominal surgery. Reg Anesth Pain Med 2006; 30:A29.
173. Package insert, DepoDur. San Diego, CA, Pacira Pharmaceuticals, Inc. 2007-02.
174. Hawkins JL, Gibbs CP, Orleans M, et al. Obstetric anesthesia work force survey, 1981 versus 1992. Anesthesiology 1997; 87:135-43.
175. Chadwick HS, Ready LB. Intrathecal and epidural morphine sulfate for post-cesarean analgesia—a clinical comparison. Anesthesiology 1988; 68:925-9.
176. Abboud TK, Dror A, Mosaad P, et al. Mini-dose intrathecal morphine for the relief of post-cesarean section pain: Safety, efficacy, and ventilatory responses to carbon dioxide. Anesth Analg 1988; 67:137-43.
177. Abouleish E, Rawal N, Rashad MN. The addition of 0.2 mg subarachnoid morphine to hyperbaric bupivacaine for cesarean delivery: A prospective study of 856 cases. Reg Anesth 1991; 16:137-40.
178. Sibilla C, Albertazz P, Zatelli R, Martinello R. Perioperative analgesia for caesarean section: Comparison of intrathecal morphine and fentanyl alone or in combination. Int J Obstet Anesth 1997; 6:43-8.
179. Palmer CM, Emerson S, Volgoropolous D, Alves D. Dose-response relationship of intrathecal morphine for postcesarean analgesia. Anesthesiology 1999; 90:437-44.
180. Milner AR, Bogod DG, Harwood RJ. Intrathecal administration of morphine for elective Caesarean section: A comparison between 0.1 mg and 0.2 mg. Anaesthesia 1996; 51:871-3.
181. Yang T, Breen TW, Archer D, Fick G. Comparison of 0.25 mg and 0.1 mg intrathecal morphine for analgesia after Cesarean section. Can J Anaesth 1999; 46:856-60.
182. Uchiyama A, Nakano S, Ueyama H, et al. Low dose intrathecal morphine and pain relief following caesarean section. Int J Obstet Anesth 1994; 3:87-91.
183. Gerancher JC, Floyd H, Eisenach J. Determination of an effective dose of intrathecal morphine for pain relief after cesarean delivery. Anesth Analg 1999; 88:346-51.
184. Paech MJ, Pavy TJ, Orlikowski CE, et al. Postoperative intraspinal opioid analgesia after caesarean section: A randomised comparison of subarachnoid morphine and epidural pethidine. Int J Obstet Anesth 2000; 9:238-45.
185. Belzarena SD. Clinical effects of intrathecally administered fentanyl in patients undergoing cesarean section. Anesth Analg 1992; 74:653-7.
186. Yee I, Carstoniu J, Halpern S, Pittini R. A comparison of two doses of epidural fentanyl during caesarean section. Can J Anaesth 1993; 40:722-5.
187. Dahlgren G, Hultstrand C, Jakobsson J, et al. Intrathecal sufentanil, fentanyl, or placebo added to bupivacaine for cesarean section. Anesth Analg 1997; 85:1288-93.
188. Siddik-Sayyid SM, Aouad MT, Jalbout MI, et al. Intrathecal versus intravenous fentanyl for supplementation of subarachnoid block during cesarean delivery. Anesth Analg 2002; 95:209-13.
189. Hunt CO, Naulty JS, Bader AM, et al. Perioperative analgesia with subarachnoid fentanyl-bupivacaine for cesarean delivery. Anesthesiology 1989; 71:535-40.
190. Chu CC, Shu SS, Lin SM, et al. The effect of intrathecal bupivacaine with combined fentanyl in cesarean section. Acta Anaesthesiol Sin 1995; 33:149-54.
191. Courtney MA, Bader AM, Hartwell B, et al. Perioperative analgesia with subarachnoid sufentanil administration. Reg Anesth 1992; 17:274-8.
192. Braga Ade F, Braga FS, Poterio GM, et al. Sufentanil added to hyperbaric bupivacaine for subarachnoid block in Caesarean section. Eur J Anaesthesiol 2003; 20:631-5.
193. Karaman S, Kocabas S, Uyar M, et al. The effects of sufentanil or morphine added to hyperbaric bupivacaine in spinal anaesthesia for caesarean section. Eur J Anaesthesiol 2006; 23:285-91.
194. Kafle SK. Intrathecal meperidine for elective caesarean section: A comparison with lidocaine. Can J Anaesth 1993; 40:718-21.
195. Nguyen Thi TV, Orliaguet G, Ngu TH, Bonnet F. Spinal anesthesia with meperidine as the sole agent for cesarean delivery. Reg Anesth 1994; 19:386-9.
196. Yu SC, Ngan Kee WD, Kwan AS. Addition of meperidine to bupivacaine for spinal anaesthesia for Caesarean section. Br J Anaesth 2002; 88:379-83.

197. Kelly MC, Carabine UA, Mirakhur RK. Intrathecal diamorphine for analgesia after caesarean section: A dose finding study and assessment of side-effects. Anaesthesia 1998; 53:231-7.
198. Stacey R, Jones R, Kar G, Poon A. High-dose intrathecal diamorphine for analgesia after Caesarean section. Anaesthesia 2001; 56:54-60.
199. Cowan CM, Kendall JB, Barclay PM, Wilkes RG. Comparison of intrathecal fentanyl and diamorphine in addition to bupivacaine for caesarean section under spinal anaesthesia. Br J Anaesth 2002; 89:452-8.
200. Lane S, Evans P, Arfeen Z, Misra U. A comparison of intrathecal fentanyl and diamorphine as adjuncts in spinal anaesthesia for Caesarean section. Anaesthesia 2005; 60:453-7.
201. Saravanan S, Robinson AP, Qayoum Dar A, et al. Minimum dose of intrathecal diamorphine required to prevent intraoperative supplementation of spinal anaesthesia for Caesarean section. Br J Anaesth 2003; 91:368-72.
202. Husaini SW, Russell IF. Intrathecal diamorphine compared with morphine for postoperative analgesia after caesarean section under spinal anaesthesia. Br J Anaesth 1998; 81:135-9.
203. Hallworth SP, Fernando R, Bell R, et al. Comparison of intrathecal and epidural diamorphine for elective caesarean section using a combined spinal-epidural technique. Br J Anaesth 1999; 82:228-32.
204. Culebras X, Gaggero G, Zatloukal J, et al. Advantages of intrathecal nalbuphine, compared with intrathecal morphine, after cesarean delivery: An evaluation of postoperative analgesia and adverse effects. Anesth Analg 2000; 91:601-5.
205. Chung JH, Sinatra RS, Sevarino FB, Fermo L. Subarachnoid meperidine-morphine combination: An effective perioperative analgesic adjunct for cesarean delivery. Reg Anesth 1997; 22:119-24.
206. Lee SHR, Herman NL, Leighton BL. Does IT fentanyl affect IT morphine analgesia after cesarean delivery (abstract)? Anesthesiology 2000; 92:A77.
207. Cooper DW, Lindsay SL, Ryall DM, et al. Does intrathecal fentanyl produce acute cross-tolerance to i.v. morphine? Br J Anaesth 1997; 78:311-3.
208. Giarrusso K, Mirikitani E, Carvalho B, et al. Does intrathecal fentanyl induce acute tolerance to opioids? Anesthesiology 2002; 97:A1042.
209. Eisenach JC, James FM, Gordh T, Yaksh TL. New epidural drugs: Primum non nocere. Anesth Analg 1998; 87:1211-2.
210. Yaksh TL, Grafe MR, Malkmus S, et al. Studies on the safety of chronically administered intrathecal neostigmine methylsulfate in rats and dogs. Anesthesiology 1995; 82:412-27.
211. Yaksh TL, Rathbun M, Jage J, et al. Pharmacology and toxicology of chronically infused epidural clonidine HCl in dogs. Fundam Appl Toxicol 1994; 23:319-35.
212. Sabbe MB, Grafe MR, Mjanger E, et al. Spinal delivery of sufentanil, alfentanil, and morphine in dogs: Physiologic and toxicologic investigations. Anesthesiology 1994; 81:899-920.
213. Abouleish E, Barmada MA, Nemoto EM, et al. Acute and chronic effects of intrathecal morphine in monkeys. Br J Anaesth 1981; 53:1027-32.
214. Hodgson PS, Neal JM, Pollock JE, Liu SS. The neurotoxicity of drugs given intrathecally (spinal). Anesth Analg 1999; 88:797-809.
215. Eisenach JC, Yaksh TL. Safety in numbers: How do we study toxicity of spinal analgesics? Anesthesiology 2002; 97:1047-9.
216. Yaksh TL, Collins JG. Studies in animals should precede human use of spinally administered drugs. Anesthesiology 1989; 70:4-6.
217. Coombs DW, Colburn RW, Allen CD, et al. Toxicity of chronic spinal analgesia in a canine model: Neuropathologic observations with dezocine lactate. Reg Anesth 1990; 15:94-102.
218. Hughes SC, Rosen MA, Shnider SM, et al. Maternal and neonatal effects of epidural morphine for labor and delivery. Anesth Analg 1984; 63:319-24.
219. Baraka A, Noueihid R, Hajj S. Intrathecal injection of morphine for obstetric analgesia. Anesthesiology 1981; 54:136-40.
220. Negre I, Gueneron JP, Ecoffey C, et al. Ventilatory response to carbon dioxide after intramuscular and epidural fentanyl. Anesth Analg 1987; 66:707-10.
221. Cohen SE, Labaille T, Benhamou D, Levron JC. Respiratory effects of epidural sufentanil after cesarean section. Anesth Analg 1992; 74:677-82.
222. Bernards CM. Recent insights into the pharmacokinetics of spinal opioids and the relevance to opioid selection. Curr Opin Anaesthesiol 2004; 17:441-7.
223. Kafer ER, Brown JT, Scott D, et al. Biphasic depression of ventilatory responses to CO_2 following epidural morphine. Anesthesiology 1983; 58:418-27.
224. Weinger M. Dangers of postoperative opioids: APSF workshop and white paper address prevention of postoperative respiratory complications. APSF Newsl 2007; 21:61-8.
225. Horlocker TS. Practice guidelines for the prevention, detection and management of respiratory depression associated with neuraxial opioid administration: Preliminary report by ASA Task Force on Neuraxial Anesthesia. ASA Newsl 2007; 71:24-6.
226. Shapiro A, Zohar E, Zaslansky R, et al. The frequency and timing of respiratory depression in 1524 postoperative patients treated with systemic or neuraxial morphine. J Clin Anesth 2005; 17:537-42.
227. Ko S, Goldstein DH, VanDenKerkhof EG. Definitions of "respiratory depression" with intrathecal morphine postoperative analgesia: A review of the literature. Can J Anaesth 2003; 50:679-88.
228. Leicht CH, Hughes SC, Dailey PA, et al. Epidural morphine sulfate for analgesia after cesarean section: A prospective report of 1000 patients. Anesthesiology 1986; 65:A366.
229. Kotelko DM, Dailey PA, Shnider SM, et al. Epidural morphine analgesia after cesarean delivery. Obstet Gynecol 1984; 63:409-13.
230. McMorland GH, Douglas MJ. Epidural morphine for postoperative analgesia. Can Anaesth Soc J 1986; 33:115-6.
231. Etches RC, Sandler AN, Daley MD. Respiratory depression and spinal opioids. Can J Anaesth 1989; 36:165-85.
232. Palmer CM. Early respiratory depression following intrathecal fentanyl-morphine combination. Anesthesiology 1991; 74:1153-5.
233. Brockway MS, Noble DW, Sharwood-Smith GH, McClure JH. Profound respiratory depression after extradural fentanyl. Br J Anaesth 1990; 64:243-5.
234. Noble DW, Morrison LM, Brockway MS, McClure JH. Adrenaline, fentanyl or adrenaline and fentanyl as adjuncts to bupivacaine for extradural anaesthesia in elective caesarean section. Br J Anaesth 1991; 66:645-50.
235. Madej TH, Strunin L. Comparison of epidural fentanyl with sufentanil: Analgesia and side effects after a single bolus dose during elective caesarean section. Anaesthesia 1987; 42:1156-61.
236. Arai YC, Ogata J, Fukunaga K, et al. The effect of intrathecal fentanyl added to hyperbaric bupivacaine on maternal respiratory function during Cesarean section. Acta Anaesthesiol Scand 2006; 50:364-7.
237. Hughes SC. Respiratory depression following intraspinal narcotics: Expect it! Int J Obstet Anesth 1997; 6:145-6.
238. Albright GA, Forster RM. The safety and efficacy of combined spinal and epidural analgesia/anesthesia (6,002 blocks) in a community hospital. Reg Anesth Pain Med 1999; 24:117-25.
239. Etches RC, Sandler AN, Daley MD. Respiratory depression and spinal opioids. Can J Anaesth 1989; 36:165-85.
240. Bailey PL, Rhondeau S, Schafer PG, et al. Dose-response pharmacology of intrathecal morphine in human volunteers. Anesthesiology 1993; 79:49-59.
241. Brose WG, Cohen SE. Oxyhemoglobin saturation following cesarean section in patients receiving epidural morphine, PCA, or IM meperidine analgesia. Anesthesiology 1989; 70:948-53.
242. Carvalho B. Respiratory depression after neuraxial opioids in the obstetric setting. Anesth Analg 2008; 107:956-61.
243. Celleno D, Capogna G, Sebastiani M, et al. Epidural analgesia during and after cesarean delivery: Comparison of five opioids. Reg Anesth 1991; 16:79-83.
244. Ready LB, Loper KA, Nessly M, Wild L. Postoperative epidural morphine is safe on surgical wards. Anesthesiology 1991; 75:452-6.

245. Johnson A, Bengtsson M, Soderlind K, Lofstrom JB. Influence of intrathecal morphine and naloxone intervention on postoperative ventilatory regulation in elderly patients. Acta Anaesthesiol Scand 1992; 36:436-44.
246. Thind GS, Wells JC, Wilkes RG. The effects of continuous intravenous naloxone on epidural morphine analgesia. Anaesthesia 1986; 41:582-5.
247. Cannesson M, Nargues N, Bryssine B, et al. Intrathecal morphine overdose during combined spinal-epidural block for Caesarean delivery. Br J Anaesth 2002; 89:925-7.
248. Balki M, Carvalho JC. Intraoperative nausea and vomiting during cesarean section under regional anesthesia. Int J Obstet Anesth 2005; 14:230-41.
249. Chaney MA. Side effects of intrathecal and epidural opioids. Can J Anaesth 1995; 42:891-903.
250. Chestnut DH, Vandewalker GE, Owen CL, et al. Administration of metoclopramide for prevention of nausea and vomiting during epidural anesthesia for elective cesarean section. Anesthesiology 1987; 66:563-6.
251. Lussos SA, Bader AM, Thornhill ML, Datta S. The antiemetic efficacy and safety of prophylactic metoclopramide for elective cesarean delivery during spinal anesthesia. Reg Anesth 1992; 17:126-30.
252. Mandell GL, Dewan DM, Howard G, Floyd HM. The effectiveness of low dose droperidol in controlling nausea and vomiting during epidural anesthesia for cesarean section. Int J Obstet Anesth 1992; 1:65-8.
253. Sanansilp V, Areewatana S, Tonsukchai N. Droperidol and the side effects of epidural morphine after cesarean section. Anesth Analg 1998; 86:532-7.
254. Kotelko DM, Rottman RL, Wright WC, et al. Transdermal scopolamine decreases nausea and vomiting following cesarean section in patients receiving epidural morphine. Anesthesiology 1989; 71:675-8.
255. Yazigi A, Chalhoub V, Madi-Jebara S, et al. Prophylactic ondansetron is effective in the treatment of nausea and vomiting but not on pruritus after cesarean delivery with intrathecal sufentanil-morphine. J Clin Anesth 2002; 14:183-6.
256. Pan PH, Moore CH. Comparing the efficacy of prophylactic metoclopramide, ondansetron, and placebo in cesarean section patients given epidural anesthesia. J Clin Anesth 2001; 13:430-5.
257. Fujii Y, Tanaka H, Toyooka H. Granisetron prevents nausea and vomiting during spinal anaesthesia for caesarean section. Acta Anaesthesiol Scand 1998; 42:312-5.
258. Fujii Y, Tanaka H, Toyooka H. Prevention of nausea and vomiting with granisetron, droperidol and metoclopramide during and after spinal anaesthesia for caesarean section: A randomized, double-blind, placebo-controlled trial. Acta Anaesthesiol Scand 1998; 42:921-5.
259. Tzeng JI, Wang JJ, Ho ST, et al. Dexamethasone for prophylaxis of nausea and vomiting after epidural morphine for post-Caesarean section analgesia: Comparison of droperidol and saline. Br J Anaesth 2000; 85:865-8.
260. Wang JJ, Ho ST, Wong CS, et al. Dexamethasone prophylaxis of nausea and vomiting after epidural morphine for post-Cesarean analgesia. Can J Anaesth 2001; 48:185-90.
261. Nortcliffe SA, Shah J, Buggy DJ. Prevention of postoperative nausea and vomiting after spinal morphine for Caesarean section: Comparison of cyclizine, dexamethasone and placebo. Br J Anaesth 2003; 90:665-70.
262. Heffernan AM, Rowbotham DJ. Postoperative nausea and vomiting—time for balanced antiemesis? Br J Anaesth 2000; 85:675-7.
263. Wu JI, Lo Y, Chia YY, et al. Prevention of postoperative nausea and vomiting after intrathecal morphine for Cesarean section: A randomized comparison of dexamethasone, droperidol, and a combination. Int J Obstet Anesth 2007; 16:122-7.
264. Ho CM, Hseu SS, Tsai SK, Lee TY. Effect of P-6 acupressure on prevention of nausea and vomiting after epidural morphine for post-cesarean section pain relief. Acta Anaesthesiol Scand 1996; 40:372-5.
265. Harmon D, Ryan M, Kelly A, Bowen M. Acupressure and prevention of nausea and vomiting during and after spinal anaesthesia for caesarean section. Br J Anaesth 2000; 84:463-7.
266. Duggal KN, Douglas MJ, Peteru EA, Merrick PM. Acupressure for intrathecal narcotic-induced nausea and vomiting after caesarean section. Int J Obstet Anesth 1998; 7:231-6.
267. Ho CM, Tsai HJ, Chan KH, Tsai SK. P6 acupressure does not prevent emesis during spinal anesthesia for cesarean delivery. Anesth Analg 2006; 102:900-3.
268. Slappendel R, Weber EW, Benraad B, et al. Itching after intrathecal morphine: Incidence and treatment. Eur J Anaesthesiol 2000; 17:616-21.
269. Kendrick WD, Woods AM, Daly MY, et al. Naloxone versus nalbuphine infusion for prophylaxis of epidural morphine-induced pruritus. Anesth Analg 1996; 82:641-7.
270. Cohen SE, Ratner EF, Kreitzman TR, et al. Nalbuphine is better than naloxone for treatment of side effects after epidural morphine. Anesth Analg 1992; 75:747-52.
271. Morgan M. The rational use of intrathecal and extradural opioids. Br J Anaesth 1989; 63:165-88.
272. Scott PV, Fischer HB. Intraspinal opiates and itching: A new reflex? Br Med J (Clin Res Ed) 1982; 284:1015-6.
273. Ballantyne JC, Loach AB, Carr DB. Itching after epidural and spinal opiates. Pain 1988; 33:149-60.
274. LaBella FS, Kim RS, Templeton J. Opiate receptor binding activity of 17-alpha estrogenic steroids. Life Sci 1978; 23:1797-804.
275. Kjellberg F, Tramer MR. Pharmacological control of opioid-induced pruritus: A quantitative systematic review of randomized trials. Eur J Anaesthesiol 2001; 18:346-57.
276. Alhashemi JA, Crosby ET, Grodecki W, et al. Treatment of intrathecal morphine-induced pruritus following caesarean section. Can J Anaesth 1997; 44:1060-5.
277. Somrat C, Oranuch K, Ketchada U, et al. Optimal dose of nalbuphine for treatment of intrathecal-morphine induced pruritus after caesarean section. J Obstet Gynaecol Res 1999; 25:209-13.
278. Morgan PJ, Mehta S, Kapala DM. Nalbuphine pretreatment in cesarean section patients receiving epidural morphine. Reg Anesth 1991; 16:84-8.
279. Lockington PF, Fa'aea P. Subcutaneous naloxone for the prevention of intrathecal morphine induced pruritus in elective Caesarean delivery. Anaesthesia 2007; 62:672-6.
280. Luthman JA, Kay NH, White JB. Intrathecal morphine for post caesarean section analgesia: Does naloxone reduce the incidence of pruritus? Int J Obstet Anesth 1992; 1:191-4.
281. Abboud TK, Afrasiabi A, Davidson J, et al. Prophylactic oral naltrexone with epidural morphine: Effect on adverse reactions and ventilatory responses to carbon dioxide. Anesthesiology 1990; 72:233-7.
282. Abboud TK, Lee K, Zhu J, et al. Prophylactic oral naltrexone with intrathecal morphine for cesarean section: Effects on adverse reactions and analgesia. Anesth Analg 1990; 71:367-70.
283. Jeon Y, Hwang J, Kang J, et al. Effects of epidural naloxone on pruritus induced by epidural morphine: A randomized controlled trial. Int J Obstet Anesth 2005; 14:22-5.
284. Colbert S, O'Hanlon DM, Galvin S, et al. The effect of rectal diclofenac on pruritus in patients receiving intrathecal morphine. Anaesthesia 1999; 54:948-52.
285. Lee LH, Irwin MG, Lim J, Wong CK. The effect of celecoxib on intrathecal morphine-induced pruritus in patients undergoing Caesarean section. Anaesthesia 2004; 59:876-80.
286. Borgeat A, Wilder-Smith OH, Saiah M, Rifat K. Subhypnotic doses of propofol relieve pruritus induced by epidural and intrathecal morphine. Anesthesiology 1992; 76:510-2.
287. Beilin Y, Bernstein HH, Zucker-Pinchoff B, et al. Subhypnotic doses of propofol do not relieve pruritus induced by intrathecal morphine after cesarean section. Anesth Analg 1998; 86:310-3.
288. Warwick JP, Kearns CF, Scott WE. The effect of subhypnotic doses of propofol on the incidence of pruritus after intrathecal morphine for caesarean section. Anaesthesia 1997; 52:270-5.

289. Charuluxananan S, Kyokong O, Somboonviboon W, et al. Nalbuphine versus propofol for treatment of intrathecal morphine-induced pruritus after cesarean delivery. Anesth Analg 2001; 93:162-5.
290. Charuluxananan S, Kyokong O, Somboonviboon W, et al. Nalbuphine versus ondansetron for prevention of intrathecal morphine-induced pruritus after cesarean delivery. Anesth Analg 2003; 96:1789-93.
291. Yeh HM, Chen LK, Lin CJ, et al. Prophylactic intravenous ondansetron reduces the incidence of intrathecal morphine-induced pruritus in patients undergoing cesarean delivery. Anesth Analg 2000; 91:172-5.
292. Siddik-Sayyid SM, Aouad MT, Taha SK, et al. Does ondansetron or granisetron prevent subarachnoid morphine-induced pruritus after cesarean delivery? Anesth Analg 2007; 104:421-4.
293. Sarvela PJ, Halonen PM, Soikkeli AI, et al. Ondansetron and tropisetron do not prevent intraspinal morphine- and fentanyl-induced pruritus in elective cesarean delivery. Acta Anaesthesiol Scand 2006; 50:239-44.
294. Yazigi A, Chalhoub V, Madi-Jebara S, Haddad F. Ondansetron for prevention of intrathecal opioids-induced pruritus, nausea and vomiting after cesarean delivery. Anesth Analg 2004; 98:264.
295. Han DW, Hong SW, Kwon JY, et al. Epidural ondansetron is more effective to prevent postoperative pruritus and nausea than intravenous ondansetron in elective cesarean delivery. Acta Obstet Gynecol Scand 2007; 86:683-7.
296. Kermans G, Wyndaele JJ, Thiery M, De Sy W. Puerperal urinary retention. Acta Urol Belg 1986; 54:376-85.
297. Yip SK, Sahota D, Pang MW, Chang A. Postpartum urinary retention. Acta Obstet Gynecol Scand 2004; 83:881-91.
298. Kuipers PW, Kamphuis ET, van Venrooij GE, et al. Intrathecal opioids and lower urinary tract function: A urodynamic evaluation. Anesthesiology 2004; 100:1497-503.
299. Kamphuis ET, Ionescu TI, Kuipers PW, et al. Recovery of storage and emptying functions of the urinary bladder after spinal anesthesia with lidocaine and with bupivacaine in men. Anesthesiology 1998; 88:310-6.
300. Evron S, Samueloff A, Simon A, et al. Urinary function during epidural analgesia with methadone and morphine in post-cesarean section patients. Pain 1985; 23:135-44.
301. Liang CC, Chang SD, Chang YL, et al. Postpartum urinary retention after cesarean delivery. Int J Gynaecol Obstet 2007; 99:229-32.
302. Butwick AJ, Lipman SS, Carvalho B. Intraoperative forced-air warming during cesarean delivery under spinal anesthesia does not prevent maternal hypothermia. Anesth Analg 2007; 105:1413-9.
303. Roy JD, Girard M, Drolet P. Intrathecal meperidine decreases shivering during cesarean delivery under spinal anesthesia. Anesth Analg 2004; 98:230-4.
304. Sessler DI. Perioperative heat balance. Anesthesiology 2000; 92:578-96.
305. Matsukawa T, Sessler DI, Christensen R, et al. Heat flow and distribution during epidural anesthesia. Anesthesiology 1995; 83:961-7.
306. Emerick TH, Ozaki M, Sessler DI, et al. Epidural anesthesia increases apparent leg temperature and decreases the shivering threshold. Anesthesiology 1994; 81:289-98.
307. Ozaki M, Kurz A, Sessler DI, et al. Thermoregulatory thresholds during epidural and spinal anesthesia. Anesthesiology 1994; 81:282-8.
308. Kurz A, Sessler DI, Schroeder M, Kurz M. Thermoregulatory response thresholds during spinal anesthesia. Anesth Analg 1993; 77:721-6.
309. Saito T, Sessler DI, Fujita K, et al. Thermoregulatory effects of spinal and epidural anesthesia during cesarean delivery. Reg Anesth Pain Med 1998; 23:418-23.
310. Leslie K, Sessler DI. Reduction in the shivering threshold is proportional to spinal block height. Anesthesiology 1996; 84:1327-31.
311. Hui CK, Huang CH, Lin CJ, et al. A randomised double-blind controlled study evaluating the hypothermic effect of 150 microg morphine during spinal anaesthesia for Caesarean section. Anaesthesia 2006; 61:29-31.
312. Techanivate A, Rodanant O, Tachawattanawisal W, Somsiri T. Intrathecal fentanyl for prevention of shivering in cesarean section. J Med Assoc Thai 2005; 88:1214-21.
313. Hong JY, Lee IH. Comparison of the effects of intrathecal morphine and pethidine on shivering after Caesarean delivery under combined-spinal epidural anaesthesia. Anaesthesia 2005; 60:1168-72.
314. Macintyre PE, Pavlin EG, Dwersteg JF. Effect of meperidine on oxygen consumption, carbon dioxide production, and respiratory gas exchange in postanesthesia shivering. Anesth Analg 1987; 66:751-5.
315. Juneja M, Ackerman WE, Heine MF, et al. Butorphanol for the relief of shivering associated with extradural anesthesia in parturients. J Clin Anesth 1992; 4:390-3.
316. Sevarino FB, Johnson MD, Lema MJ, et al. The effect of epidural sufentanil on shivering and body temperature in the parturient. Anesth Analg 1989; 68:530-3.
317. Sutherland J, Seaton H, Lowry C. The influence of epidural pethidine on shivering during lower segment caesarean section under epidural anaesthesia. Anaesth Intensive Care 1991; 19:228-32.
318. Horn EP, Schroeder F, Gottschalk A, et al. Active warming during cesarean delivery. Anesth Analg 2002; 94:409-14.
319. Walker SM, Goudas LC, Cousins MJ, Carr DB. Combination spinal analgesic chemotherapy: A systematic review. Anesth Analg 2002; 95:674-715.
320. Kitahata LM. Spinal analgesia with morphine and clonidine. Anesth Analg 1989; 68:191-3.
321. Taiwo YO, Fabian A, Pazoles CJ, Fields HL. Potentiation of morphine antinociception by monoamine reuptake inhibitors in the rat spinal cord. Pain 1985; 21:329-37.
322. Kuraishi Y, Hirota N, Sato Y, et al. Noradrenergic inhibition of the release of substance P from the primary afferents in the rabbit spinal dorsal horn. Brain Res 1985; 359:177-82.
323. Eisenach JC, De Kock M, Klimscha W. Alpha(2)-adrenergic agonists for regional anesthesia: A clinical review of clonidine (1984-1995). Anesthesiology 1996; 85:655-74.
324. Iwasaki H, Collins JG, Saito Y, et al. Low-dose clonidine enhances pregnancy-induced analgesia to visceral but not somatic stimuli in rats. Anesth Analg 1991; 72:325-9.
325. Eisenach JC, Lysak SZ, Viscomi CM. Epidural clonidine analgesia following surgery: Phase I. Anesthesiology 1989; 71:640-6.
326. Mendez R, Eisenach JC, Kashtan K. Epidural clonidine analgesia after cesarean section. Anesthesiology 1990; 73:848-52.
327. Huntoon M, Eisenach JC, Boese P. Epidural clonidine after cesarean section: Appropriate dose and effect of prior local anesthetic. Anesthesiology 1992; 76:187-93.
328. Narchi P, Benhamou D, Hamza J, Bouaziz H. Ventilatory effects of epidural clonidine during the first 3 hours after caesarean section. Acta Anaesthesiol Scand 1992; 36:791-5.
329. Eisenach JC, D'Angelo R, Taylor C, Hood DD. An isobolographic study of epidural clonidine and fentanyl after cesarean section. Anesth Analg 1994; 79:285-90.
330. Capogna G, Celleno D, Zangrillo A, et al. Addition of clonidine to epidural morphine enhances postoperative analgesia after cesarean delivery. Reg Anesth 1995; 20:57-61.
331. Vercauteren MP, Vandeput DM, Meert TF, Adriaensen HA. Patient-controlled epidural analgesia with sufentanil following caesarean section: The effect of adrenaline and clonidine admixture. Anaesthesia 1994; 49:767-71.
332. Filos KS, Goudas LC, Patroni O, Polyzou V. Intrathecal clonidine as a sole analgesic for pain relief after cesarean section. Anesthesiology 1992; 77:267-74.
333. Filos KS, Goudas LC, Patroni O, Polyzou V. Hemodynamic and analgesic profile after intrathecal clonidine in humans: A dose-response study. Anesthesiology 1994; 81:591-601.
334. Castro MI, Eisenach JC. Pharmacokinetics and dynamics of intravenous, intrathecal, and epidural clonidine in sheep. Anesthesiology 1989; 71:418-25.
335. van Tuijl I, van Klei WA, van der Werff DB, Kalkman CJ. The effect of addition of intrathecal clonidine to hyperbaric bupivacaine on

postoperative pain and morphine requirements after Caesarean section: A randomized controlled trial. Br J Anaesth 2006; 97:365-70.
336. Benhamou D, Thorin D, Brichant JF, et al. Intrathecal clonidine and fentanyl with hyperbaric bupivacaine improves analgesia during cesarean section. Anesth Analg 1998; 87:609-13.
337. Paech MJ, Pavy TJ, Orlikowski CE, et al. Postcesarean analgesia with spinal morphine, clonidine, or their combination. Anesth Analg 2004; 98:1460-6.
338. Ala-Kokko TI, Pienimaki P, Lampela E, et al. Transfer of clonidine and dexmedetomidine across the isolated perfused human placenta. Acta Anaesthesiol Scand 1997; 41:313-9.
339. Sia AT, Kwek K, Yeo GS. The in vitro effects of clonidine and dexmedetomidine on human myometrium. Int J Obstet Anesth 2005; 14:104-7.
340. Bouaziz H, Tong C, Eisenach JC. Postoperative analgesia from intrathecal neostigmine in sheep. Anesth Analg 1995; 80:1140-4.
341. Hood DD, Eisenach JC, Tong C, et al. Cardiorespiratory and spinal cord blood flow effects of intrathecal neostigmine methylsulfate, clonidine, and their combination in sheep. Anesthesiology 1995; 82:428-35.
342. Hood DD, Eisenach JC, Tuttle R. Phase I safety assessment of intrathecal neostigmine methylsulfate in humans. Anesthesiology 1995; 82:331-43.
343. Krukowski JA, Hood DD, Eisenach JC, et al. Intrathecal neostigmine for post-cesarean section analgesia: Dose response. Anesth Analg 1997; 84:1269-75.
344. Chung CJ, Kim JS, Park HS, Chin YJ. The efficacy of intrathecal neostigmine, intrathecal morphine, and their combination for post-cesarean section analgesia. Anesth Analg 1998; 87:341-6.
345. Pan PM, Huang CT, Wei TT, Mok MS. Enhancement of analgesic effect of intrathecal neostigmine and clonidine on bupivacaine spinal anesthesia. Reg Anesth Pain Med 1998; 23:49-56.
346. Kaya FN, Sahin S, Owen MD, Eisenach JC. Epidural neostigmine produces analgesia but also sedation in women after cesarean delivery. Anesthesiology 2004; 100:381-5.
347. Woolf CJ, Salter MW. Neuronal plasticity: Increasing the gain in pain. Science 2000; 288:1765-9.
348. Price DD, Mayer DJ, Mao J, Caruso FS. NMDA-receptor antagonists and opioid receptor interactions as related to analgesia and tolerance. J Pain Symptom Manage 2000; 19:S7-11.
349. Mao J. Opioid-induced abnormal pain sensitivity: Implications in clinical opioid therapy. Pain 2002; 100:213-7.
350. Unlugenc H, Ozalevli M, Gunes Y, et al. A double-blind comparison of intrathecal S(+) ketamine and fentanyl combined with bupivacaine 0.5% for Caesarean delivery. Eur J Anaesthesiol 2006; 23:1018-24.
351. Schmid RL, Sandler AN, Katz J. Use and efficacy of low-dose ketamine in the management of acute postoperative pain: A review of current techniques and outcomes. Pain 1999; 82:111-25.
352. Subramaniam K, Subramaniam B, Steinbrook RA. Ketamine as adjuvant analgesic to opioids: A quantitative and qualitative systematic review. Anesth Analg 2004; 99:482-95.
353. Bell RF, Dahl JB, Moore RA, Kalso E. Perioperative ketamine for acute postoperative pain. Cochrane Database Syst Rev 2006; (1):CD004603.
354. Kawana Y, Sato H, Shimada H, et al. Epidural ketamine for postoperative pain relief after gynecologic operations: A double-blind study and comparison with epidural morphine. Anesth Analg 1987; 66:735-8.
355. Zohar E, Shapiro A, Eidinov A, et al. Postcesarean analgesia: The efficacy of bupivacaine wound instillation with and without supplemental diclofenac. J Clin Anesth 2006; 18:415-21.
356. Sen S, Ozmert G, Aydin ON, et al. The persisting analgesic effect of low-dose intravenous ketamine after spinal anaesthesia for caesarean section. Eur J Anaesthesiol 2005; 22:518-23.
357. Buvanendran A, McCarthy RJ, Kroin JS, et al. Intrathecal magnesium prolongs fentanyl analgesia: A prospective, randomized, controlled trial. Anesth Analg 2002; 95:661-6.
358. Ozalevli M, Cetin TO, Unlugenc H, et al. The effect of adding intrathecal magnesium sulphate to bupivacaine-fentanyl spinal anaesthesia. Acta Anaesthesiol Scand 2005; 49:1514-9.
359. Arcioni R, Palmisani S, Tigano S, et al. Combined intrathecal and epidural magnesium sulfate supplementation of spinal anesthesia to reduce post-operative analgesic requirements: A prospective, randomized, double-blind, controlled trial in patients undergoing major orthopedic surgery. Acta Anaesthesiol Scand 2007; 51:482-9.
360. Paech MJ, Magann EF, Doherty DA, et al. Does magnesium sulfate reduce the short- and long-term requirements for pain relief after caesarean delivery? A double-blind placebo-controlled trial. Am J Obstet Gynecol 2006; 194:1596-602.
361. Leicht CH, Kelleher AJ, Robinson DE, Dickerson SE. Prolongation of postoperative epidural sufentanil analgesia with epinephrine. Anesth Analg 1990; 70:323-5.
362. McMorland GH, Douglas MJ, Kim JH, et al. Epidural sufentanil for post-caesarean section analgesia: Lack of benefit of epinephrine. Can J Anaesth 1990; 37:432-7.
363. Ngan Kee WD, Khaw KS, Ma ML. The effect of the addition of adrenaline to pethidine for patient-controlled epidural analgesia after caesarean section. Anaesthesia 1998; 53:1012-6.
364. McLintic AJ, Danskin FH, Reid JA, Thorburn J. Effect of adrenaline on extradural anaesthesia, plasma lignocaine concentrations and the feto-placental unit during elective caesarean section. Br J Anaesth 1991; 67:683-9.
365. Alahuhta S, Rasanen J, Jouppila R, et al. Effects of extradural bupivacaine with adrenaline for caesarean section on uteroplacental and fetal circulation. Br J Anaesth 1991; 67:678-82.
366. Abouleish EI. Epinephrine improves the quality of spinal hyperbaric bupivacaine for cesarean section. Anesth Analg 1987; 66:395-400.
367. Abouleish E, Rawal N, Tobon-Randall B, et al. A clinical and laboratory study to compare the addition of 0.2 mg of morphine, 0.2 mg of epinephrine, or their combination to hyperbaric bupivacaine for spinal anesthesia in cesarean section. Anesth Analg 1993; 77:457-62.
368. Zakowski MI, Ramanathan S, Sharnick S, Turndorf H. Uptake and distribution of bupivacaine and morphine after intrathecal administration in parturients: Effects of epinephrine. Anesth Analg 1992; 74:664-9.
369. Schug SA, Saunders D, Kurowski I, Paech MJ. Neuraxial drug administration: A review of treatment options for anaesthesia and analgesia. CNS Drugs 2006; 20:917-33.
370. Gan TJ, Habib AS. Adenosine as a non-opioid analgesic in the perioperative setting. Anesth Analg 2007; 105:487-94.
371. Rane K, Sollevi A, Segerdahl M. Intrathecal adenosine administration in abdominal hysterectomy lacks analgesic effect. Acta Anaesthesiol Scand 2000; 44:868-72.
372. Sharma M, Mohta M, Chawla R. Efficacy of intrathecal adenosine for postoperative pain relief. Eur J Anaesthesiol 2006; 23:449-53.
373. Araiza-Saldana CI, Reyes-Garcia G, Bermudez-Ocana DY, et al. Effect of diabetes on the mechanisms of intrathecal antinociception of sildenafil in rats. Eur J Pharmacol 2005; 527:60-70.
374. Asano T, Dohi S, Iida H. Antinociceptive action of epidural K^+(ATP) channel openers via interaction with morphine and an alpha(2)-adrenergic agonist in rats. Anesth Analg 2000; 90:1146-51.
375. Tucker AP, Mezzatesta J, Nadeson R, Goodchild CS. Intrathecal midazolam. II. Combination with intrathecal fentanyl for labor pain. Anesth Analg 2004; 98:1521-7.
376. Cheng JK, Chen CC, Yang JR, Chiou LC. The antiallodynic action target of intrathecal gabapentin: Ca^{2+} channels, KATP channels or *N*-methyl-D-aspartic acid receptors? Anesth Analg 2006; 102:182-7.
377. Cheng JK, Lai YJ, Chen CC, et al. Magnesium chloride and ruthenium red attenuate the antiallodynic effect of intrathecal gabapentin in a rat model of postoperative pain. Anesthesiology 2003; 98:1472-9.
378. Choe H, Kim JS, Ko SH, et al. Epidural verapamil reduces analgesic consumption after lower abdominal surgery. Anesth Analg 1998; 86:786-90.

379. Elia N, Lysakowski C, Tramer MR. Does multimodal analgesia with acetaminophen, nonsteroidal antiinflammatory drugs, or selective cyclooxygenase-2 inhibitors and patient-controlled analgesia morphine offer advantages over morphine alone? Meta-analyses of randomized trials. Anesthesiology 2005; 103:1296-304.
380. Granot M, Lowenstein L, Yarnitsky D, et al. Postcesarean section pain prediction by preoperative experimental pain assessment. Anesthesiology 2003; 98:1422-6.
381. Strulov L, Zimmer EZ, Granot M, et al. Pain catastrophizing, response to experimental heat stimuli, and post-cesarean section pain. J Pain 2007; 8:273-9.
382. Hsu YW, Somma J, Hung YC, et al. Predicting postoperative pain by preoperative pressure pain assessment. Anesthesiology 2005; 103:613-8.
383. Pan PH, Coghill R, Houle TT, et al. Multifactorial preoperative predictors for postcesarean section pain and analgesic requirement. Anesthesiology 2006; 104:417-25.
384. Landau R. Pharmacogenetics: Implications for obstetric anesthesia. Int J Obstet Anesth 2005; 14:316-23.

Part VIII

Anesthetic Complications

James Young Simpson introduced anesthesia to obstetrics when the practice of medicine was in a period of great flux. As late as 1820, most Western medical schools were still practicing a form of medicine derived from the teachings of Galen, a second-century Greek physician. According to Galenic principles, all disease originated from an imbalance among the four elements (earth, air, fire, and water), hydraulic pressures, or electrical forces. Treatment consisted of the time-honored measures of purging, bleeding, cupping, or the administration of stimulants or depressants. Simpson, Meigs, Channing, and all the others involved in the early debate about obstetric anesthesia learned this style of practice as students.

Within a few years of their graduation, Galenic forms of medicine had been discredited and had disappeared. In its place Laennec, Louis, and other French physicians developed principles of medical theory and practice that we use today—physical diagnosis, statistical analysis, physiology, pathology, and chemistry.[1]

Thus the introduction of anesthesia represented a significant challenge. Physicians who had once been taught to treat the pain of childbirth with bloodletting could now use ether or chloroform. They recognized the therapeutic potential of the drugs, but they also recognized their dangers and questioned their safety and effects on labor and the newborn.[2]

Evaluating the risks of anesthesia was quite different from recognizing the problems. In 1850, pharmacology was in its infancy, and medical physiology, pathology, and biochemistry were not very well developed. There was no tradition for drug testing that Simpson and Meigs could model. Their inexperience with medical science was reflected in their response to obstetric anesthesia. For example, seeking a better agent to replace ether, Simpson simply tried a series of compounds on himself and his friends until he stumbled upon one that worked—-chloroform. Within a month he had administered chloroform to a patient and had published a paper. He conducted no animal studies or clinical trials, collected no data, and performed no statistical analyses of his results. His claims were reviewed by no clinical board or governmental agency, and he had no reason to fear a malpractice suit. Such an approach led to a rapid dissemination of new ideas, but it took years before anyone identified the problems associated with the new remedy, much less sorted them out. Accordingly, after the introduction of obstetric anesthesia, more than half a century passed before physicians began to develop the tools that they needed to understand the problems associated with the use of ether and chloroform.[3]

Donald Caton, M.D.

REFERENCES

1. Temkin O. Galenism: Rise and Decline of a Medical Philosophy. Ithaca, NY, Cornell University Press, 1973.
2. Rosenberg CE. The therapeutic revolution: Medicine, meaning, and social change in nineteenth-century America. In Vogel MJ, Rosenberg CE, editors. The Therapeutic Revolution: Essays in the Social History of American Medicine. Philadelphia, University of Pennsylvania Press, 1979:3-26.
3. Newman C. The Evolution of Medical Education in the Nineteenth Century. New York, Oxford University Press, 1957.

Chapter 29

Aspiration: Risk, Prophylaxis, and Treatment

Geraldine O'Sullivan, M.D., FRCA
M. Shankar Hari, M.D., FRCA

HISTORY

In 1848, Sir James Simpson first suggested aspiration as a cause of death during anesthesia. Hannah Greener, a 15-year-old given chloroform for a toenail extraction, became cyanotic and "sputtered" during the anesthetic. A "rattling in her throat" then developed, and she soon expired. Her physician administered water and brandy by mouth. Simpson[1] contended that it was the aspiration of water and brandy, and not the adverse effects from the chloroform, that caused her death. In 1940, an obstetrician published a report of 15 cases of aspiration, 14 of which occurred in mothers receiving inhalation anesthesia for a vaginal or cesarean delivery.[2] Among the 14 obstetric cases, 5 mothers died.

Subsequently, Curtis Mendelson's landmark paper described a series of animal experiments that clearly described the clinical course and pathology of pulmonary acid aspiration.[3] In the same paper, Mendelson also audited 44,016 deliveries at the New York Lying-In Hospital between 1932 and 1945. He identified 66 (0.15%) cases of aspiration, in 45 of which the aspirated material was recorded; 40 mothers aspirated liquid, and the remaining 5 aspirated solid food. Importantly, no mothers died from acid aspiration, but two mothers died from asphyxiation caused by the aspiration of solid food. At this time general anesthesia usually involved the inhalation of ether, often, as Mendelson observed, by "a new and inexperienced intern." Mendelson therefore advocated (1) the withholding of food during labor, (2) the greater use of regional anesthesia, (3) the administration of antacids, (4) the emptying of the stomach before administration of general anesthesia, and (5) the competent administration of general anesthesia. This advice became the foundation of obstetric anesthesia practice during subsequent decades.

INCIDENCE, MORBIDITY, AND MORTALITY

Maternal mortality from pulmonary aspiration of gastric contents has declined to almost negligible levels in the past three decades (Figure 29-1).[4-6] This decline can probably be attributed to the following factors: (1) the greater use of neuraxial anesthesia; (2) the use of antacids, histamine (H_2)-receptor antagonists, and/or proton pump

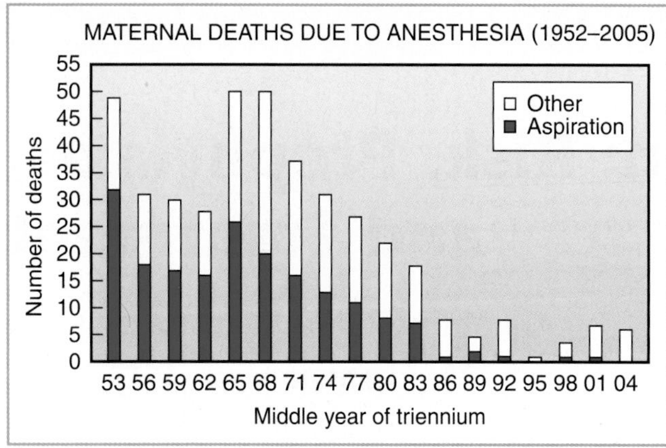

FIGURE 29-1 Maternal mortality from anesthesia and pulmonary aspiration, 1952-2005. (Compiled from data from references 4-6.)

inhibitors; (3) the use of a rapid-sequence induction of general anesthesia; (4) an improvement in the training of anesthesia providers; and (5) the establishment and enforcement of *nil per os* (NPO) policies. Arguably the common use of neuraxial analgesic/anesthetic techniques, both during labor and for cesarean delivery, is the single most important factor in this remarkable decline in maternal mortality.

The reported incidence of aspiration pneumonitis depends on the criteria used for making the diagnosis. The relative risk of aspiration in pregnant versus nonpregnant women can be best estimated from comparisons within single study populations. Olsson et al.[7] reported an overall incidence of aspiration of 1 in 2131 in the general population undergoing anesthesia and 1 in 661 in women undergoing cesarean delivery (i.e., a threefold higher aspiration risk). In two other surveys related to aspiration (one a retrospective review of 172,334 consecutive patients undergoing general anesthesia, and the other a review of 133 cases of aspiration from the Australian Anaesthetic Incident Monitoring Study [AIMS]), there were no cases of pulmonary aspiration in women undergoing either elective or emergency cesarean delivery.[8,9] However, in both studies, emergency surgery was a significant predisposing factor for aspiration; this finding may be relevant for the practice of obstetric anesthesia, given that many obstetric surgical procedures are performed on an urgent or emergency basis. The Australian study also implicated obesity as a significant risk factor for aspiration; others have noted that obesity is associated with an increased risk of maternal mortality.[5,6]

Morbidity and mortality associated with aspiration vary according to (1) the physical status of the patient, (2) the type and volume of aspirate, (3) the therapy administered, and (4) the criteria used for making the diagnosis. Since 1952, the Department of Health in the United Kingdom has published detailed triennial reports on all maternal deaths. Data from these reports, which are now entitled *Confidential Enquiry into Maternal and Child Health* (CEMACH), indicate that death from pulmonary aspiration in obstetrics is vanishingly rare (see Figure 29-1).[4-6] In the last three reports, which cover the period from 1997 to 2005, there were two maternal deaths from aspiration, one in an obese parturient and the other in a mother who required anesthesia 3 days after delivery. Although the number of anesthetics administered to mothers during this 9-year period is unknown, there were 6,335,090 deliveries, indicating that the mortality rate from aspiration was less than 1 in 3.2 million deliveries. Data on pulmonary aspiration in obstetrics in the United States are difficult to evaluate; despite the establishment of an ongoing National Pregnancy Mortality Surveillance System by the Centers for Disease Control and Prevention (CDC), it remains difficult to obtain adequate and detailed information about every maternal death. Prior to 1990, aspiration was the most common cause of anesthesia-related maternal death in the United States. In 1991 through 1997, problems associated with airway management, sometimes complicated by aspiration, had become the most significant cause of anesthesia-related maternal death.[10] In a review of all forensic cases referred for autopsy in South Carolina between January 1989 and December 2003, there were no anesthesia-related maternal deaths and no maternal deaths from pulmonary aspiration.[11] In general, mortality statistics are a poor predictor of maternal morbidity. Because several studies have indicated that perioperative aspiration can be associated with significant morbidity in obstetric patients,[12,13] all possible measures must still be taken to prevent pulmonary aspiration in obstetric patients.

GASTROESOPHAGEAL ANATOMY AND PHYSIOLOGY

Esophagus

In the adult, the esophagus is approximately 25 cm long, and the esophagogastric junction is approximately 40 cm from the incisor teeth. In humans, the proximal one third of the esophagus is composed of striated muscle, but the distal end contains only smooth muscle. At both ends are muscular sphincters that are normally closed. The cricopharyngeal or upper esophageal sphincter prevents the entry of air into the esophagus during respiration, and the gastroesophageal or lower esophageal sphincter prevents the reflux of gastric contents. The lower esophageal sphincter is characterized anatomically and manometrically as a 3-cm zone of specialized muscle that maintains tonic activity. The end-expiratory pressure in the sphincter is 8 to 20 mm Hg above the end-expiratory gastric pressure. The lower esophageal sphincter is kept in place by the phreno-esophageal ligament, which inserts into the esophagus approximately 3 cm above the diaphragmatic opening (Figure 29-2). The lower esophageal sphincter is not always closed; transient relaxations occur, accounting for the gastroesophageal reflux that normal subjects experience.[14]

Gastrointestinal Motility

Differences in fasting and fed patterns of gut motility are now firmly established. During fasting, the main component of peristalsis is the migrating motor complex (MMC).[15] Each MMC cycle is approximately 90 to 120 minutes in duration and is composed of four phases. Phase I has little or no electrical spike activity and thus no measurable contractions; phase II has intermittent

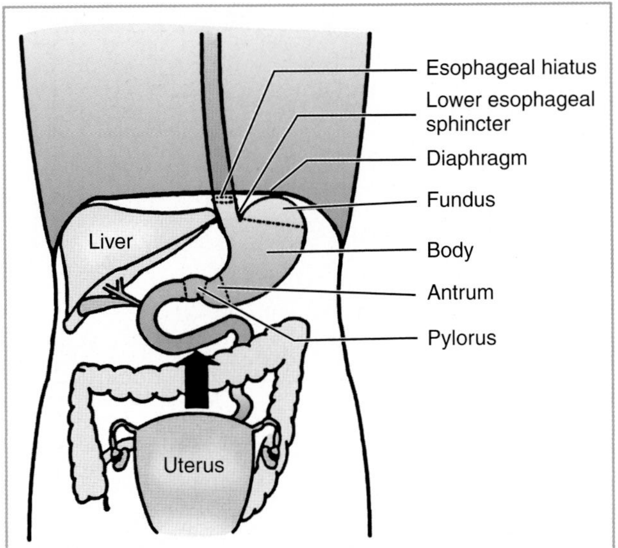

FIGURE 29-2 The stomach and its relationship to the diaphragm. The stomach consists of a fundus, body, antrum, and pylorus. The function of the lower esophageal sphincter depends on the chronic contraction of circular muscle fibers, the wrapping of the esophagus by the crus of the diaphragm at the esophageal hiatus, and the length of the esophagus exposed to intra-abdominal pressure. The gravid uterus may encroach on the stomach and alter the effectiveness of the lower esophageal sphincter.

spike activity; phase III has spikes of large amplitude and is associated with strong contractile activity; and phase IV is a brief period of intermittent activity leading back to phase I. The MMC first appears in the lower esophageal sphincter and stomach, followed by the duodenum, and finally the terminal ileum, at which time a new cycle begins in the lower esophageal sphincter and stomach. The phase of the MMC at the time of administration of certain drugs can affect absorption and thereby the onset of therapeutic effect.[16] Eating abolishes the MMC and induces a pattern of intermittent spike activity that appears similar to that in phase II. The duration of the fed pattern is determined both by the calorie content and the type of nutrients in the meal.

The stomach, through the processes of receptive relaxation and gastric accommodation, can accept 1.0 to 1.5 L of food before intragastric pressure begins to increase. The contraction waves that propel food into the small intestine begin in the antrum of the stomach. The pylorus closes midway through the contraction wave, allowing some fluid to exit into the duodenum, but causing the remaining fluid to move retrograde toward the body of the stomach.[17] The jet of fluid that exits the pylorus primarily contains liquid and fine particles. Large particles that lag behind are caught in the retrograde flow of fluid, which assists in breaking up these particles. Therefore, the way in which individual components of a meal pass through the stomach depends on the particle size and the viscosity of the suspension. Small particles and fluids exit the stomach faster than larger particles.[17] The outlet of the stomach—the pylorus—takes advantage of both its chronic tone and anatomic position to limit outflow. The pylorus is higher than the most dependent portion of the stomach in both the supine and standing positions.[17]

Gastric Secretion

In one day, the stomach produces as much as 1500 mL of highly acidic fluid containing the proteolytic enzyme pepsin.[18] Normal individuals can produce a peak acid output of 38 mmol/hr.[19] Acid is secreted at a low basal rate of approximately 10% of maximal output, even when the stomach is empty.[19,20] There is diurnal variation in this basal rate of gastric acid secretion, with the lowest and highest outputs occurring in the morning and evening, respectively.

The stomach lining has two types of glands, pyloric and oxyntic. The **pyloric glands** contain chief cells, which secrete pepsinogen, the precursor for pepsin. The **oxyntic glands** contain the oxyntic cells, which secrete hydrochloric acid. Water molecules and carbon dioxide in the oxyntic cells combine to form carbonic acid, which dissociates into hydrogen ions and bicarbonate. The bicarbonate leaves the cell for the blood stream, and the hydrogen ions are actively exchanged for the potassium ions in the canaliculi connecting with the lumen of the oxyntic gland. The secretions of the oxyntic cell can contain a hydrochloric acid concentration of as much as 160 mmol/L (pH of 0.8).[18] Proton pump inhibitors (PPIs) block the hydrogen ion pump on the canaliculi to decrease acid production.[21]

The pylorus contains G cells, which secrete **gastrin** into the blood stream when stimulated by the vagus nerve, stomach distention, tactile stimuli, or chemical stimuli (e.g., amino acids, certain peptides). Gastrin combines with gastrin receptors on the oxyntic cell to stimulate the secretion of hydrochloric acid. **Acetylcholine** binds to muscarinic (M_1) receptors on the oxyntic cell to cause an increase in intracellular calcium ion concentration, which results in hydrochloric acid secretion. **Histamine** potentiates the effects of both acetylcholine and gastrin by combining with H_2 receptors on the oxyntic cell to increase the intracellular cyclic adenosine monophosphate (cAMP) concentration, leading to a dramatic increase in the production of acid.[18] H_2-receptor antagonists (e.g., ranitidine, famotidine) prevent histamine's potentiation of acid production (Figure 29-3).

Ingestion of Food

When a meal is eaten, the mechanisms that control the secretion of gastric juice and the motility and emptying of the stomach interact in a complex manner to coordinate the functions of the stomach. The response to eating is divided into three phases: cephalic, gastric, and intestinal. Chewing, tasting, and smelling cause an increase in the vagal stimulation of the stomach, which in turn increases gastric acid production. This represents the **cephalic phase** of digestion.[18] In this phase, gastric acid output increases to approximately 55% of peak output.[22] The **gastric phase** begins with the release of gastrin. Gastric acid secretion depends on antral distention, vagal activity, gastrin concentrations, and the composition of the meal.[20,22,23] Gastric acid secretion during a mixed-composition meal increases to approximately 80% of peak acid output.[19] The **intestinal phase** begins with the movement of food into the small intestine and is largely inhibitory. Hormones (e.g., gastrin, cholecystokinin, secretin) and an enterogastric reflex further modulate gastric acid secretion and motility depending on the composition and volume of the food in the

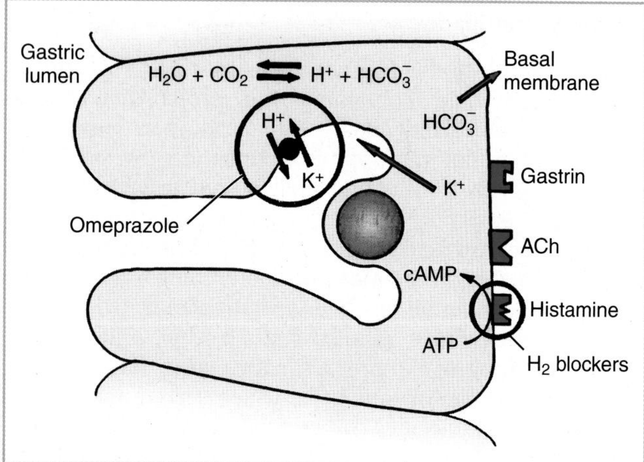

FIGURE 29-3 The oxyntic cell produces hydrogen ions that are secreted into the gastric lumen and bicarbonate ions that are secreted into the blood stream. H_2-receptor antagonists (e.g., ranitidine, famotidine) and proton pump inhibitors act on the oxyntic cell to reduce gastric acid secretion. Omeprazole blocks the active transport of the hydrogen ions into the gastric lumen. H_2-receptor antagonists block the histamine receptor on the basal membrane to decrease hydrogen ion production in the oxyntic cell. ACh, acetylcholine; ATP, adenosine triphosphate; cAMP, cyclic adenosine monophosphate; CO_2, carbon dioxide; H^+, hydrogen ion; HCO_3^-, bicarbonate; H_2O, water; K^+, potassium.

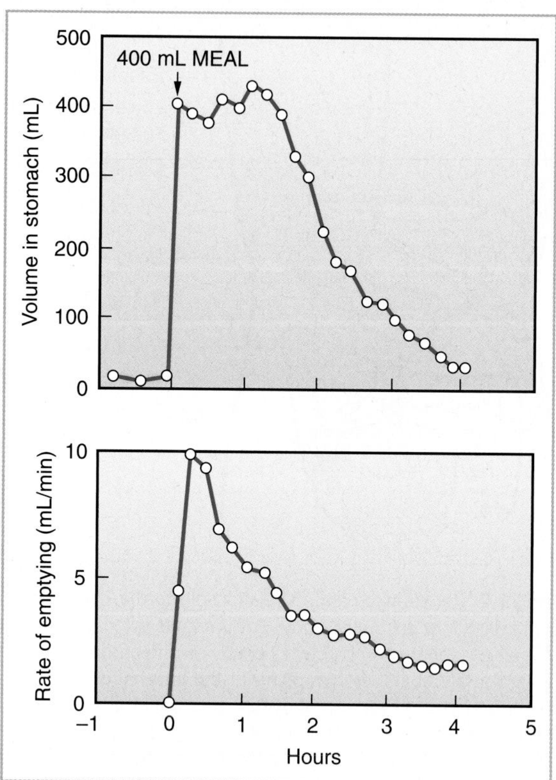

FIGURE 29-4 Volume of gastric contents and rate of gastric emptying in a subject eating a 400-mL meal of steak, bread, and vanilla ice cream. (From Malagelada JR, Longstreth GF, Summerskill WHJ, et al. Measurements of gastric functions during digestion of ordinary solid meals in man. Gastroenterology 1976; 70:203-10.)

duodenum.[18] This inhibition of gastric emptying by food in the duodenum enables the duodenal contents to be processed before more material is delivered from the stomach.

After the ingestion of a meal, gastric emptying depends on (1) the pre-meal volume, (2) the volume ingested, (3) the composition of the meal, (4) the size of the solids, (5) the amount of gastric secretion, (6) the physical characteristics of the stomach contents entering the duodenum, and (7) patient position.[18,20,24,25] A mixture of liquids and solids passes through the stomach much more slowly than liquids alone. Gastric emptying of a meal is slowed by high lipid content, high caloric load, and large particle size.[20,26,27] Thus, predicting an exact time for the passage of liquids and solids through the stomach is very difficult. For non-nutrient liquids (e.g., normal saline), the gastric volume decreases exponentially with respect to time.[24] In one study,[25] 90% of a 150-mL saline meal given to fasting adults in the sitting position passed through the stomach in a median time of 14 minutes; however, in adults in the left lateral position, the median time for gastric emptying was 28 minutes. In another study, 100% of a 500-mL saline meal given to fasting adults passed through the stomach within 2 hours, as determined by a polyethylene glycol marker.[20] However, despite complete emptying of the saline test meal, the mean residual gastric volume at the end of 2 hours was 46 mL; this was due to greater secretion of gastric acid. Progressively less complete gastric emptying and higher mean residual gastric contents were observed with meals containing amino acids, glucose, and glucose with fat.[20] These studies indicate that the volume and composition of the test meal, as well as the resulting gastric secretions, strongly affect gastric emptying and residual gastric content. For example, the subject described in Figure 29-4 responded to the test meal by secreting 800 mL of gastric juice, and consequently the volume in the stomach remained high for almost 2 hours despite early, rapid emptying.[28]

Effects of Pregnancy on Gastric Function

Gastroesophageal reflux, resulting in heartburn, is a common complication of late pregnancy. Pregnancy compromises the integrity of the lower esophageal sphincter. It alters the anatomic relationship of the esophagus to the diaphragm and stomach, raises intragastric pressure, and in some women limits the ability of the lower esophageal sphincter to increase its tone.[29-32] Progesterone, which relaxes smooth muscle, probably accounts for the inability of the lower esophageal sphincter to increase its tone.[33] Lower esophageal pH monitoring in pregnant women at term has shown a higher incidence of reflux than in nonpregnant controls, even in women who are asymptomatic. Therefore, at term gestation, the pregnant woman who requires anesthesia should be regarded as having an incompetent lower esophageal sphincter. These physiologic changes return to their pre-pregnancy levels by 48 hours after delivery.[31]

Serial studies assessing **gastric acidity** during pregnancy have proved difficult to perform because pregnant women do not usually wish to repeatedly swallow nasogastric tubes for research purposes. However, in the most comprehensive study of gastric acid secretion during pregnancy, basal and histamine-augmented gastric acid secretion was measured in 10 controls and 30 pregnant women equally distributed throughout the three trimesters of pregnancy.[34] No significant differences in basal gastric acid secretion were seen between the pregnant and nonpregnant women. However, when the mothers were divided into groups according to gestational age, the mean rate of gastric acid secretion was reduced during the second trimester. The maximal response to histamine was significantly lower in women in the first and second trimesters than in women who were either not pregnant or in the third trimester of pregnancy.[34]

Assessment of **gastric emptying** during pregnancy and labor presents technical and ethical challenges, and a variety of techniques have been used (Table 29-1).[35-59] Pregnancy does not significantly alter the rate of gastric emptying.[39] In addition, gastric emptying is not delayed in either obese or nonobese parturients who ingest 300 mL of water after an overnight fast.[58,59] Gastric emptying appears to be normal in early labor but becomes delayed as labor advances.[40,41] The cause of the delay in gastric emptying during advanced labor is unclear. Pain is known to delay gastric emptying, but even when labor pain is abolished with epidural analgesia using a local anesthetic alone, the delay still occurs.[41] Parenteral opioids cause a significant delay in gastric emptying, as do bolus doses of epidural and intrathecal opioids.[40,49,51,55,56] Continuous epidural infusion of low-dose local anesthetic with fentanyl does not appear to delay gastric emptying until the total dose of fentanyl exceeds 100 μg.[56]

Plasma concentrations of the gastrointestinal hormone motilin are decreased during pregnancy.[60] Studies have shown either no change[30,32,61] or an increase[62] in the plasma concentrations of gastrin.

RISK FACTORS FOR ASPIRATION PNEUMONITIS

Mendelson[3] divided aspiration pneumonitis into two types, liquid and solid. Whereas the aspiration of solids could result in asphyxiation, Mendelson demonstrated that the sequelae from the aspiration of liquids were more severe clinically and pathologically when the liquid was highly acidic (Figure 29-5). His observations, together with the results from other investigations,[63-71] allow the speculation that the morbidity and mortality of aspiration depends on the following three variables: (1) the chemical nature of the aspirate, (2) the physical nature of the aspirate, and (3) the volume of the aspirate. Aspirates with a pH less than 2.5 cause an ongoing granulocytic reaction beyond the acute phase.[65] Aspiration of particulate material can engender a clinical picture with severity equal to or greater than that caused by the aspiration of acidic liquid.[69] Aspiration of small volumes of neutral liquid results in a very low rate of mortality. However, aspiration of large volumes of neutral liquid results in a high mortality rate, presumably as a result of the disruption of surfactant by a large volume of liquid or from a mechanism similar to that seen in "near drowning."[71]

Historically, anesthesia providers have considered a nonparticulate gastric fluid with a pH less than 2.5 and a gastric volume greater than 25 mL (i.e., 0.4 mL/kg) as risk factors for aspiration pneumonitis.[63,68,70] No human studies have directly addressed the relationship between preoperative fasting, gastric acidity, or gastric volume and the risk of pulmonary aspiration during anesthesia.[72,73] A reasonable scientific basis appears to exist for the use of a gastric pH of less than 2.5 as a risk factor. In animal experiments, the risk of aspiration pneumonitis clearly increased with decreasing pH of the tracheal aspirate.[63,71] Awe et al.[63] illustrated this concept in their graph of Pa_{O_2} versus time for aspirates of varying pH (see Figure 29-5).

Animal studies have also demonstrated that an increase in the volume of tracheal aspirate is associated with a higher risk of aspiration pneumonitis.[71] However, the volume of aspirated material associated with this risk has been disputed. The commonly accepted volume of 0.4 mL/kg (approximately 25 mL in a 70-kg adult) originated from an experiment in a single rhesus monkey in which 0.4 mL/kg of an acidic liquid was administered into the right mainstem bronchus and resulted in the animal's death.[70] The investigators made the assumption that this entire volume, if contained in the stomach, could be aspirated. However, Raidoo et al.[74] demonstrated variability in the response of juvenile monkeys to different volumes of an acidic tracheal aspirate. Death was seen with aspirate volumes of 0.8 mL/kg and 1.0 mL/kg, but not with volumes of 0.4 mL/kg and 0.6 mL/kg. Likewise, Plourde and Hardy[75] refuted the assumption that all the gastric contents would be aspirated and demonstrated that gastric volumes of 0.4 mL/kg did not increase the risk of aspiration. Hence the gastric volume that puts a patient at risk for aspiration pneumonitis has not been determined. However, a reasonable goal of any prophylactic therapy would be a gastric pH greater than 2.5 and a gastric volume as low as possible.

PATHOPHYSIOLOGY

Aspiration pneumonitis (Mendelson's syndrome) is a chemical injury to the tracheobronchial tree and alveoli caused by the inhalation of sterile acidic gastric contents, whereas **aspiration pneumonia** may be regarded as an infectious process of the respiratory tract caused by the inhalation of oropharyngeal secretions that are colonized by pathogenic bacteria. Aspiration of gastric contents could therefore result in acid injury to the lung with or without bacterial and particulate matter–related effects.

Aspiration of acidic liquid injures the alveolar epithelium and results in an alveolar exudate composed of edema, albumin, fibrin, cellular debris, and red blood cells,[3,65,68,69] whereas the aspiration of neutral, nonparticulate liquid leads to an alveolar exudate with minimal damage to the alveolus. The phospholipid and apoprotein composition of the surfactant changes, exerting a negative effect on the surface-active properties of the surfactant.[76] This effect leads to an increase in intra-alveolar water and protein content and a loss of lung volume, resulting in a decrease in pulmonary compliance and intrapulmonary shunting of blood. The cellular debris and bronchial denuding cause bronchial obstruction. The exudative pulmonary edema, bronchial obstruction, reduced lung compliance, and shunting result in hypoxemia, increased pulmonary vascular resistance, and increased work of breathing. After the direct

TABLE 29-1 Studies of Gastric Emptying during Pregnancy and Labor

Method of Assessment	Study*	Study Period and Subjects	Gastric Emptying
Radiographic	Hirsheimer et al. (1938)[35]	Labor (10 subjects)	Delay in 2 subjects
	La Salvia et al. (1950)[36]	Third trimester and labor	Third trimester: no delay Third trimester + opioids: marked delay Labor: slight delay Labor + opioids: marked delay
	Crawford (1956)[37]	Labor (12 subjects)	Delay in 1 subject
Large-volume test meal	Hunt & Murray (1958)[38]	Serial study Small numbers Second and third trimesters, postpartum	No change
Double-sampling test meal	Davison et al. (1970)[39]	Third trimester and labor	Labor: delay, with altered pattern of emptying
Epigastric impedance	O'Sullivan et al. (1987)[42]	Nonpregnant controls, third trimester, 60 minutes postpartum	No delay
Applied potential tomography	Sandar et al. (1992)[48]	Sequential study 10 mothers: 37-40 weeks' gestation, 2-3 days postpartum, 6 weeks postpartum	No delay
Acetaminophen absorption	Nimmo et al. (1975)[40]	Labor with intramuscular opioids Postpartum 2-5 days	Labor: No delay Labor + opioids: marked delay Postpartum: no delay
	Nimmo et al. (1977)[41]	Labor	Labor: slight delay Labor + epidural analgesia (no opioid): slight delay
	Simpson et al. (1988)[43]	Nonpregnant controls, 8-11 weeks' gestation, 12-14 weeks' gestation	8-11 weeks: no delay 12-14 weeks: delay
	Macfie et al. (1991)[44]	Nonpregnant controls, first, second, and third trimesters	No delay in any trimester
	Geddes et al. (1991)[45]	Postcesarean delivery Epidural fentanyl 100 μg	Delay
	Gin et al. (1991)[46]	Postpartum: day 1 and day 3, 6 weeks	No delay
	Wright et al. (1992)[49]	Labor with epidural bolus: (1) bupivacaine 0.375%; (2) bupivacaine 0.375% + fentanyl 100 μg	Epidural opioids: delay
	Whitehead et al. (1993)[50]	Nonpregnant controls, first, second, and third trimesters Postpartum: 2, 18-24, and 24-48 hours	Pregnancy: No change Postpartum: 2 hours: delay 18-24 hours: no delay 24-48 hours: no delay
	Ewah et al. (1993)[51]	Labor with epidural infusion: (1) bupivacaine 0.25%; (2) bupivacaine 0.25% + fentanyl 50 or 100 μg, or diamorphine 2.5 or 5 mg	Epidural opioids: delay
	Levy et al. (1994)[52]	Nonpregnant controls, 8-12 weeks' gestation	Delay
	Stanley et al. (1995)[53]	Second and third trimesters and 8 weeks postpartum	No delay

*Superscript numbers indicate citation references at the end of the chapter.

TABLE 29-1—cont'd Studies of Gastric Emptying during Pregnancy and Labor

Method of Assessment	Study*	Study Period and Subjects	Gastric Emptying
	Zimmerman et al. (1996)[54]	Labor with epidural infusion: (1) bupivacaine 0.125%; (2) bupivacaine 0.125% + fentanyl 2 μg/mL	No delay
	Porter et al. (1997)[55]	Labor with epidural infusion: (1) bupivacaine 0.125%; (2) bupivacaine 0.125% + fentanyl 2.5 μg/mL	Epidural fentanyl total: <100 μg: no delay >100 μg: delay
	Kelly et al. (1997)[56]	Labor with neuraxial bolus: (1) epidural bupivacaine 0.375%; (2) epidural bupivacaine 0.25% + fentanyl 50 μg; (3) intrathecal bupivacaine 2.5 mg + fentanyl 25 μg	Epidural fentanyl: no delay Intrathecal fentanyl: delay
Real-time ultrasonography	Carp et al. (1992)[47]	Nonpregnant controls, third trimester	No delay
	Chiloiro et al. (2001)[57]	Serial study in 11 women: first and third trimesters, 4-6 months postpartum	No delay
Real-time ultrasonography and acetaminophen absorption	Wong et al. (2002)[58]	Third trimester Crossover study	50 mL or 300 mL water: no delay Faster gastric emptying with 300 mL
	Wong et al. (2007)[59]	10 obese parturients Third trimester Crossover study	50 mL or 300 mL water: no delay

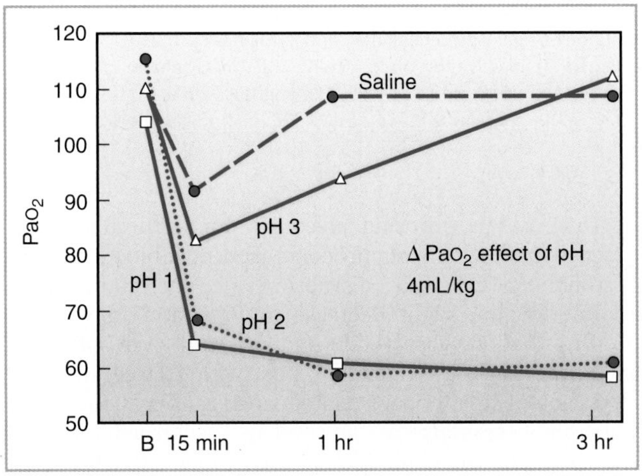

FIGURE 29-5 Relationship between acidity and Pao_2. In this study, 4 mL/kg of fluid of varying pH was instilled into the tracheas of dogs. The severity of the hypoxemia correlated with the pH of the aspirate. A maximal decrease in Pao_2 occurred with aspirates with a pH of less than 2.5. B, baseline. (From Awe WC, Fletcher WS, Jacob SW. The pathophysiology of aspiration pneumonitis. Surgery 1966; 60:232-9.)

acid-mediated injury of the respiratory tract, an intense inflammatory response ensues from macrophage activation and secretion of cytokines, interleukin-1 (IL-1), IL-6, IL-8, and IL-10, and tumor necrosis factor-α.[77] These inflammatory mediators lead to the chemotaxis, accumulation, and activation of neutrophils in the alveolar exudate, upregulation of adhesion molecules within the pulmonary vasculature, and activation of the complement pathways. The neutrophils subsequently release oxidants, proteases, leukotrienes, and other proinflammatory molecules.[77] Amplification of these inflammatory processes may result in the development of acute lung injury (ALI) or acute respiratory distress syndrome (ARDS) (Figure 29-6).[76,77]

The acidic contents of the stomach prevent the growth of bacteria under normal conditions. However, gastric contents may become colonized with pathogenic gram-negative bacteria in patients receiving antacid therapy or with enteral feeding tubes, gastroparesis, or intestinal obstruction. The bacterial content adds to the inflammatory response to acid aspiration.[78]

Aspiration of particulate matter in the supine position most commonly involves injury to the posterior segments of the upper lobe and the apical segments of the lower lobe; aspiration in the semirecumbent or upright position typically leads to injury to the lower lobe. The right lower lobe is the most common site of aspiration injury owing to the

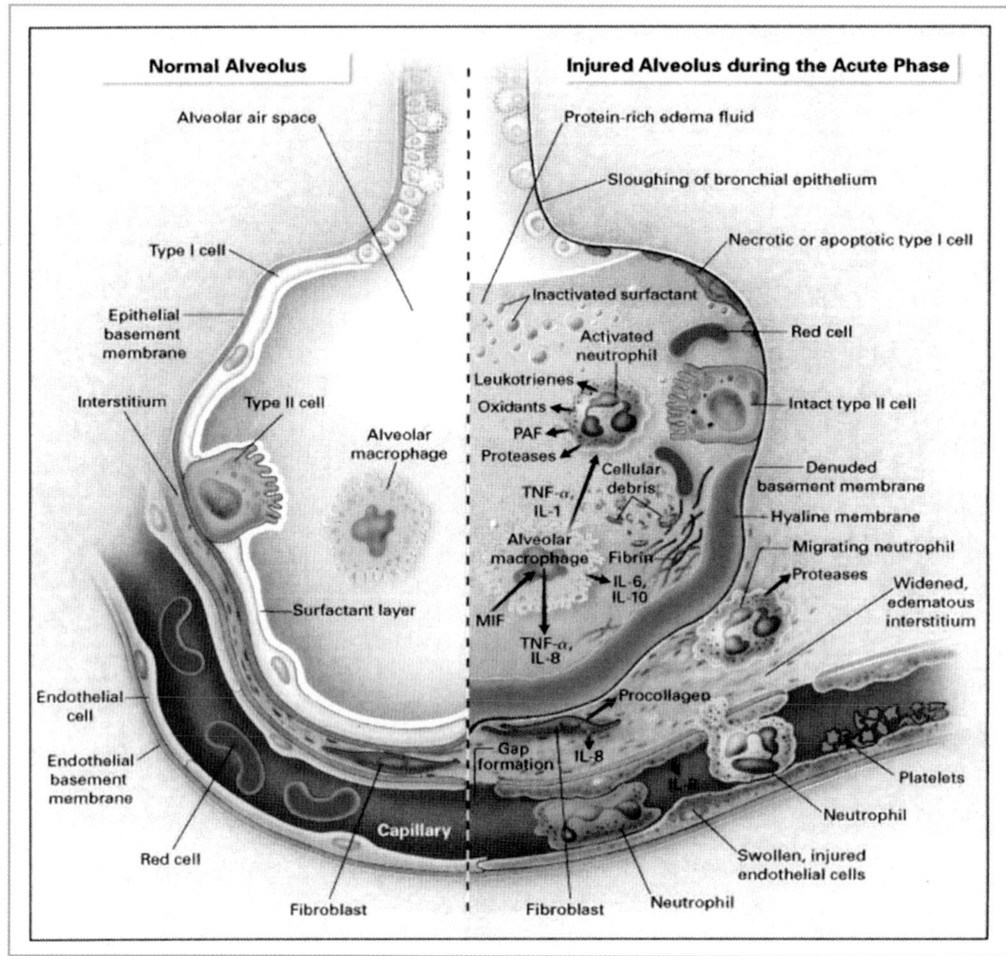

FIGURE 29-6 The normal alveolus (*left*) and the injured alveolus in the acute phase of acute lung injury and the acute respiratory distress syndrome (*right*). In the acute phase of the syndrome, there is sloughing of both the bronchial and alveolar epithelial cells, with the formation of protein-rich hyaline membranes on the denuded basement membrane. Neutrophils are shown adhering to the injured capillary endothelium and marginating through the interstitium into the air space, which is filled with protein-rich edema fluid. In the air space, an alveolar macrophage is secreting cytokines, interleukins 1, 6, 8, and 10 (IL-1, IL-6, IL-8, and IL-10), and tumor necrosis factor-α (TNF-α), which act locally to stimulate chemotaxis and activate neutrophils. Macrophages also secrete other cytokines, including IL-1, IL-6, and IL-10. Interleukin-1 can also stimulate the production of an extracellular matrix by fibroblasts. Neutrophils can release oxidants, proteases, leukotrienes, and other proinflammatory molecules, such as platelet-activating factor (PAF). A number of anti-inflammatory mediators are also present in the alveolar milieu, including interleukin-1-receptor antagonist, soluble tumor necrosis factor receptor, autoantibodies against interleukin-8, and cytokines such as IL-10 and IL-11 (not shown). The influx of protein-rich edema fluid into the alveolus has led to the inactivation of surfactant. MIF, macrophage inhibitory factor. (From Ware L, Mathay M. The acute respiratory distress syndrome. N Engl J Med 2000; 342:1334-49.)

larger and more vertical architecture of the right (versus left) mainstem bronchus. Obstruction of the bronchus or bronchioles results in bronchial denudation and collapse of the bronchopulmonary segments. Persistent or unresolved collapse can lead to lung abscesses and cavitation.[78]

After the acute period previously described, the process resolves through the proliferation and differentiation of surviving type II pneumocytes in the alveolar epithelial cells.[77,79] The type II pneumocytes actively transport sodium out of the alveolus, and water follows passively. Soluble proteins are removed by paracellular diffusion and endocytosis, and insoluble proteins are removed by macrophages. Neutrophils are removed by programmed cell death and subsequent phagocytosis by macrophages. Type II pneumocytes gradually restore the normal composition of the surfactant. In a subset of patients with ARDS, the injury progresses to a fibrosing alveolitis—an accumulation of mesenchymal cells, their products, and new blood vessels.

Bronchospasm and disruption of surfactant likely account for the slight decrease in Pa_{O_2} and increase in shunting that are observed.[65] Aspiration of large solid particles may cause atelectasis by obstructing large airways.[3] Aspiration of smaller particulate matter causes an exudative neutrophilic response at the level of the bronchioles and alveolar ducts; the clinical picture is similar after the aspiration of acidic liquid.[65,66,69]

CLINICAL COURSE

In most cases of aspiration during anesthesia, the anesthesia provider witnesses regurgitation of gastric contents

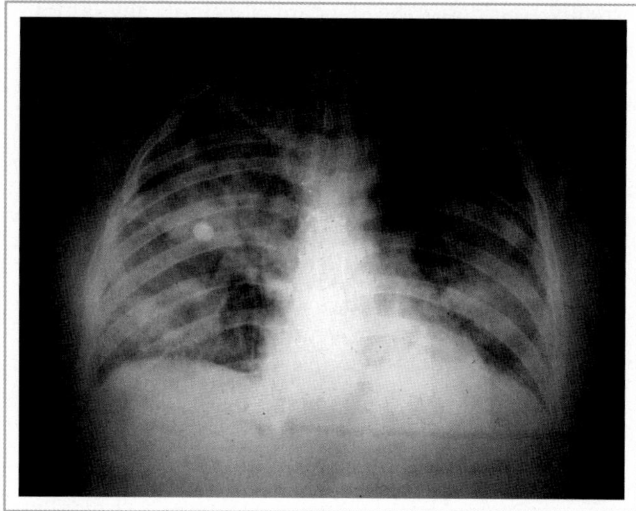

FIGURE 29-7 Radiographic changes following pulmonary aspiration of gastric contents in pregnancy.

into the hypopharynx.[3] Patients who aspirate while breathing spontaneously have a brief period of breath-holding followed by tachypnea, tachycardia, and a slight respiratory acidosis. Significant aspiration always results in some hypoxemia caused by greater shunting and frequent bronchospasm.

Approximately 85% to 90% of patients who aspirate gastric contents demonstrate an abnormality on chest radiographs.[64,80] Because these chest radiographic findings may lag behind clinical signs by as much as 12 to 24 hours, the initial radiograph may appear normal.[80] In mild cases, alveolar infiltrates are seen in the dependent portions of the lungs. Severe aspiration results in diffuse bilateral infiltrates without signs of heart failure (i.e., engorged pulmonary vasculature and/or enlarged cardiac silhouette) (Figure 29-7).

These symptoms and signs may progress to satisfy the American-European Consensus Conference criteria for ALI or ARDS, which are as follows[81]:

- Clinical: acute onset of respiratory distress
- Biochemical: Pa_{O_2}/F_{IO_2} ratio less than 300 for ALI or less than 200 for ARDS
- Radiographic: bilateral diffuse fluffy alveolar infiltrates

TREATMENT

Management of Aspiration

Management principles include rigid bronchoscopy, appropriate use of antibiotics, and management of hypoxemia with continuous positive airway pressure (CPAP) in nonintubated patients. Common treatments that lack evidence to support their use are the administration of corticosteroids and lung lavage with saline and bicarbonate.[78]

RIGID BRONCHOSCOPY AND LAVAGE

Suction of the upper airway followed by endotracheal intubation and suction of the primary bronchi commonly precedes rigid bronchoscopy. Rigid bronchoscopy is useful in removing large food particles that cause airway obstruction. Lung lavage with saline or bicarbonate does *not* reduce the parenchymal damage caused by acid aspiration and can worsen preexisting hypoxemia.[78]

ANTIBIOTICS

Prophylactic antibiotics are *not* efficacious in aspiration and may lead to the development of infection with resistant organisms. Infection is not a component of acute pulmonary aspiration of sterile gastric contents.[78] Antibiotics should be administered only in the presence of clinical findings that suggest infection (e.g., fever, worsening infiltrates on chest radiographs, leukocytosis, positive result of Gram stain of sputum, clinical deterioration).

In patients who are intubated, a nondirected bronchoalveolar lavage sample can be sent for laboratory analysis. Tracheal sputum samples may be insufficient to identify a bacterial pathogen, and some authorities recommend sampling of the lower respiratory tract with a protected specimen brush.[78]

Empiric antibiotic therapy is appropriate in patients with suspected bacterial colonization of gastric contents. The "at risk" group (see earlier) includes patients who have gastroparesis or bowel obstruction and those who are receiving enteral feedings or antacid therapy. Empiric antibiotic therapy is also appropriate in patients with aspiration pneumonitis that fails to resolve within 48 hours. The choice of antibiotic depends on the observed local patterns of antibiotic resistance. The target pathogens are gram-positive organisms (e.g., *Streptococcus pneumoniae, Staphylococcus aureus, Haemophilus influenzae*) and some gram-negative organisms (e.g., Enterobacteriaceae) when the diagnosis is made less than 48 hours after hospital admission (i.e., community-acquired pneumonia). *Pseudomonas aeruginosa* is a common pathogen in cases of nosocomial (hospital-acquired) aspiration pneumonia. Anaerobes are no longer believed to be present in the majority of cases.[78] Pharmacologic therapy should be altered when specific pathogens and their antibiotic sensitivities are determined.

TREATMENT OF HYPOXEMIA

Exudation of fluid into the alveoli, decreased surface activity of surfactant, and atelectasis all result in intrapulmonary shunting and hypoxemia. The administration of CPAP in patients breathing spontaneously or the administration of positive end-expiratory pressure (PEEP) in patients undergoing mechanical ventilation restores functional residual capacity, reduces pulmonary shunting, and reverses hypoxemia.

CORTICOSTEROID USE

Despite the use of corticosteroids for decades in the management of aspiration pneumonitis, animal and human studies have failed to demonstrate a beneficial effect on pulmonary function, lung injury, alveolar-capillary permeability, or clinical outcomes after acid aspiration.[78] Thus, the administration of corticosteroids for aspiration pneumonitis cannot be recommended.

Management of Respiratory Failure

Pulmonary aspiration can result in the intrapulmonary processes consistent with ALI and ARDS. The basic tenets of management of ALI and ARDS include the use of "lung-protective" ventilation strategies, the judicious management of fluids, and the application of basic critical care algorithms.

MECHANICAL VENTILATION

Mechanical ventilation can be effective while avoiding alveolar overdistention and elevated transpulmonary pressures. Such "lung-protective" strategies have been demonstrated to correlate with improved outcomes in a prospective multicenter trial of management of "early" ARDS, which compared the use of initial tidal volumes and plateau airway pressures of 6 mL/kg and 30 cm H_2O or less with the use of 12 mL/kg and 50 cm H_2O or less, respectively.[82] The trial was stopped after the fourth interim analysis because of significantly lower mortality in the low tidal volume and plateau pressure group (31% versus 40%; $P < .007$). The low tidal volume group had significantly lower plasma IL-6 levels than the group that received the more traditional tidal volume of 12 mL/kg. The greater activation of inflammatory processes in the high tidal volume group is thought to be a result of alveoli distention injuries or the opening and closing of the alveoli in atelectatic lung tissue.[82]

POSITIVE END-EXPIRATORY PRESSURE

The National Heart, Lung, and Blood Institute's ARDS Clinical Trials Network research group[83] conducted a prospective clinical trial (N = 549 patients) that compared the effects of low and intermediate PEEP levels set according to predetermined combinations of PEEP and FIO_2, in the setting of the lung-protective mechanical ventilation strategy (see earlier). There were no significant differences in hospital mortality (24.9% versus 27.5%, respectively) or days to unassisted breathing (14.5 days versus 13.8 days, respectively) between the two groups. The investigators concluded that in patients with ALI/ARDS who receive lung-protective mechanical ventilation, clinical outcomes are "similar whether lower or higher PEEP levels are used."[83]

FLUID MANAGEMENT

The ARDS Clinical Trials Network research group[84] also reported a randomized controlled trial of 1000 patients with ARDS in which conservative and liberal fluid resuscitation strategies were compared. The group that received conservative fluid management, which was guided by central venous pressure and/or pulmonary capillary wedge pressure measurements, had much lower net fluid balance, better lung function, and a shorter duration of mechanical ventilation and intensive care; in addition, no increase in nonpulmonary organ failures, prevalence of shock, or need for dialysis was observed in this group.

BASIC CRITICAL CARE ALGORITHMS

To minimize the risk of sepsis, central venous catheters and other invasive hemodynamic monitors should be removed as early as is clinically feasible. Aseptic precautions should be utilized during care, and infections should be treated with antibiotics specific to the bacterial pathogen for 3 to 7 days. Whether tight and rigorous glycemic control should be employed is controversial; however, occasional withdrawal of sedation and the use of prophylaxis for gastrointestinal bleeding and thromboembolic events are currently considered the standard of care in any critically ill patient.[85]

CORTICOSTEROID USE

Recovery from ALI/ARDS depends on the functional resolution of the underlying pulmonary disorder, which may follow one of two courses: (1) rapid improvement in lung function with an uncomplicated recovery, or (2) slow improvements in lung function, oxygenation, and ventilation with prolonged weaning and recovery.

As with the response to pulmonary aspiration (see earlier), the use of corticosteroids does *not* appear to improve lung function or recovery in patients with ALI or ARDS. Bernard et al.[86] gave methylprednisolone 30 mg/kg every 6 hours for 24 hours to patients with early ARDS; these investigators observed no evidence of reversal of ARDS and no evidence of a reduction in mortality. A multicenter randomized trial conducted over 6 years also did not show a survival benefit with methylprednisolone treatment aimed at lung healing in patients with ARDS lasting for more than 7 days (i.e., "late" ARDS). In addition, among patients who began receiving corticosteroids 2 or more weeks after the onset of ARDS, mortality was four times higher at 60 days than in the placebo group. The corticosteroid group also had a higher incidence of persistent muscular weakness.[87]

PROPHYLAXIS

Pregnant women undergoing cesarean delivery or other surgical procedures are at increased risk for aspiration pneumonitis and should receive pharmacologic prophylaxis. The risk of failed intubation is 3 to 11 times greater in pregnant patients than in nonpregnant patients.[88,89] Airway edema, breast enlargement, obesity, and the high rate of emergency surgery all contribute to the risk of failed intubation in pregnant women (see Chapter 30). Aspiration pneumonitis is often associated with difficult or failed intubation during the induction of general anesthesia. In a survey conducted by the Society for Obstetric Anesthesia and Perinatology, difficult or failed intubation occurred in 14 of 19 cases of aspiration associated with intubation.[90] Warner et al.[8] documented that the risk of aspiration during emergence from anesthesia is almost as high as that during induction of anesthesia. Thus the prophylactic regimen must provide protection during both induction of—and emergence from—general anesthesia.

Because the incidence of aspiration pneumonitis is low, the efficacy of prophylactic regimens is measured by their ability to alter gastric pH and volume. Approximately 30% to 43% of pregnant women have a fasting gastric volume greater than 25 mL and a gastric fluid pH less than 2.5.[91,92] However, the percentage of term pregnant patients at risk may not differ from that of patients undergoing elective abortion, postpartum sterilization, or gynecologic surgery (Table 29-2).[93-95] Gastric volume and acidity at term gestation are similar to gastric volume and acidity during early pregnancy, during the postpartum period, and in nonpregnant patients.[91-98] Decreased lower esophageal sphincter tone and a higher risk of difficult intubation are the primary

TABLE 29-2 Prevalence of Fasting Gastric Findings in Various Populations (%)

Population*	pH < 2.5	Volume > 25 mL	pH < 2.5 and Volume > 25 mL
Pregnant[90-92]	57-80	51-54	31-43
Nonpregnant[92-94]	75-95	45-67	45-60
Postpartum[93-95]	54-93	61	60
Children[96,97]	93-100	64-78	64-77
Obese, nonpregnant[98]	88	86	75

*Superscript numbers indicate citation references at the end of the chapter.

factors that increase the risk of aspiration during pregnancy and the immediate postpartum period.

Preoperative Oral Fluid Administration

Multiple studies have described no increase in gastric volume or acidity after the oral administration of 150 mL of fluid (e.g., coffee, tea, water, other clear liquids, orange juice without pulp) in nonpregnant adults 2 hours before elective surgery.[99,100] All of these patients fasted overnight and should have had a low gastric volume when the test meal was given. Similarly, other studies have demonstrated that unrestricted intake of clear fluids up to 2 hours before anesthesia has no adverse effect on gastric volume and pH in pediatric patients.[100] However, ingestion of milk and orange juice containing pulp increases gastric volume.[99] Lewis and Crawford[101] noted that in patients undergoing elective cesarean delivery, those who consumed a meal of both tea and toast 2 to 4 hours preoperatively had an increase in gastric volume and a decrease in gastric pH in comparison with a control group of patients. Consumption of tea without toast resulted in an increase in gastric volume but it did not alter gastric pH. Particulate material was aspirated from the stomachs of 2 of the 11 patients who consumed both tea and toast. The investigators did not state the volume of tea consumed by these patients.

In addition, when gastric emptying of both 50 mL and 300 mL of water was assessed in nonlaboring pregnant women at term, the gastric emptying half-time for 300 mL was significantly shorter than that for 50 mL.[58] When a similar study was conducted in obese nonlaboring pregnant women at term (mean prepregnancy body mass index = 41 ± 9 kg/m^2), the gastric emptying time for 300 mL was not longer than that for 50 mL.[59] This finding suggests that the American Society of Anesthesiologists (ASA) Guidelines for Obstetric Anesthesia,[73] which state that "the uncomplicated patient undergoing elective cesarean delivery may have modest amounts of clear liquids up to 2 hours before induction of anesthesia," could also be applied to healthy, *obese* pregnant women presenting for elective surgery. However, factors other than the rate of gastric emptying can influence the rate of pulmonary aspiration, particularly in obese subjects. Obesity is associated with a higher incidence of gastroesophageal reflux and difficulty with airway management (both intraoperatively and postoperatively). In addition, the cesarean delivery rate is higher and the success rate of vaginal birth after cesarean (VBAC) is lower in obese parturients.[102,103]

Choice of Anesthesia

The Obstetric Anesthesia Work Force Survey demonstrated that the use of neuraxial anesthesia for cesarean delivery rose dramatically from 1981 to 2001, with the use of general anesthesia accounting for less than 5% of elective procedures.[104] A review of procedures performed at a large tertiary care obstetric facility showed that from 1990 to 1995 the use of general anesthesia for cesarean delivery decreased from 7.2% to 3.6%. The yearly incidence of difficult intubation ranged from 1.3% to 16.3%, with one maternal death resulting from a failed intubation.[105] Hawkins et al.[10] reported 67 maternal deaths resulting from complications of general anesthesia and 33 maternal deaths resulting from complications of neuraxial anesthesia in the United States for the years 1979 to 1990. Approximately 73% of general anesthesia–related maternal deaths were due to airway problems, primarily failed intubation, and/or aspiration. In contrast, deaths from neuraxial anesthesia began to decline in the mid-1980s, coincident with the withdrawal of 0.75% bupivacaine from the market, an increased awareness of local anesthetic toxicity, and the more consistent use of epidural test doses.[10] For the years 1985 to 1990, Hawkins et al.[10] estimated that the risk of maternal death was 16.7 times greater with general anesthesia than with neuraxial anesthesia for cesarean delivery. However, in more recent years, this relative risk ratio has decreased (see Chapter 30).

Assessment of these data should be tempered by the recognition that general anesthesia is often reserved for pregnant patients at greater risk for complications from anesthesia. For example, the general anesthesia group undoubtedly included a disproportionate number of women who required emergency cesarean delivery for maternal and/or fetal indications (e.g., uterine rupture, placental abruption). The increased use of neuraxial anesthesia for operative obstetrics has resulted in part from the greater use of epidural analgesia during labor. An additional reason for the decreased use of general anesthesia is the perception that administration of neuraxial anesthesia reduces/eliminates the risk of failed intubation and aspiration. In the United Kingdom, many of the anesthesia-related maternal deaths were associated with the use of general anesthesia, suggesting a better safety profile with neuraxial anesthesia for cesarean delivery.[4-6]

Antacids

The ASA Practice Guidelines for Obstetric Anesthesia state, "Before surgical procedures (i.e., cesarean delivery, postpartum tubal ligation) practitioners should consider the timely administration of nonparticulate antacids, H_2-receptor antagonists, and/or metoclopramide for aspiration prophylaxis."[73] Particulate antacids should not be used as prophylaxis; when aspirated they cause pulmonary shunting and hypoxemia similar in magnitude to those caused by acid aspiration and greater than those caused by saline, alkalinized saline, or sodium citrate.[106] Nonparticulate antacids (e.g., 0.3 M sodium citrate, Bicitra, Alka-Seltzer effervescent) should be used, and their efficacy depends on the baseline gastric volume and acidity.[107,108] A total of 30 mL of sodium citrate neutralizes 255 mL of hydrochloric acid with a pH of 1.0. The effective duration of action of sodium citrate is variable and depends on the rate of gastric emptying.[109,110] O'Sullivan and Bullingham[109,110] used radiotelemetry pH pills to perform noninvasive assessments of the efficacy of sodium citrate in pregnant women. After the administration of 15 mL of sodium citrate to women in the third trimester of pregnancy, the time that the pH remained greater than 3.0 was less than 30 minutes.[109] When the same study was repeated in laboring women,[110] the time that the pH remained higher than 3.0 was 57 minutes in subjects who had received no analgesia and 166 minutes in those who had received meperidine. Nonparticulate antacids should be administered within 20 minutes of the induction of general anesthesia, particularly if the procedure is an emergency and there is insufficient time for a co-administered H_2-receptor antagonist to be effective.

Histamine H_2-Receptor Antagonists

The ASA Task Force on Obstetric Anesthesia concluded that H_2-receptor antagonists are efficacious in reducing gastric acidity and volume.[73] H_2-receptor antagonists block histamine receptors on the oxyntic cell and thus diminish gastric acid production, leading to a slight reduction in gastric volume in the fasting patient.[111] When given intravenously, an H_2-receptor antagonist begins to take effect in as little as 30 minutes, but 60 to 90 minutes is required for maximal effect.[111,112] After oral administration, gastric pH is higher than 2.5 in approximately 60% of patients at 60 minutes, and in 90% at 90 minutes.[111,112] The duration of action is sufficiently long to cover emergence from general anesthesia for a cesarean delivery.

Cimetidine (given in doses of 200 to 400 mg intravenously, intramuscularly, or orally) reduces gastric acidity within 60 to 90 minutes.[111,112] Therapeutic plasma concentrations are sustained for approximately 4 hours. Cimetidine may decrease the rate of plasma clearance of certain drugs, including some local anesthetics (e.g., lidocaine), by binding to the cytochrome P-450 system in the hepatocyte and by reducing hepatic blood flow.[113] Feely et al.[114] observed that long-term administration of cimetidine results in higher plasma lidocaine concentrations and a higher risk of toxicity during an intravenous infusion of lidocaine. Cimetidine crosses the placenta, but it does not appear to have harmful effects.[115] Because arrhythmias and cardiac arrest have been reported with the rapid intravenous administration of cimetidine,[116] a slower rate of intravenous administration or the use of an oral route is recommended. The use of cimetidine in obstetric anesthesia has largely been replaced by the use of ranitidine.

Ranitidine, a chemically substituted amino-alkyl furan, has been evaluated after the administration of an intravenous or intramuscular dose of 50 to 100 mg or an oral dose of 150 mg.[117-119] These studies have noted that the administration of ranitidine results in a gastric pH greater than 2.5 within 1 hour and sustained therapeutic concentrations for approximately 8 hours.[117-119] Ranitidine does not have any major interaction with the cytochrome P-450 system[120] and does not alter plasma local anesthetic concentrations after epidural administration of lidocaine or bupivacaine.[121]

Nizatidine (given in doses of 150 to 300 mg orally) and **famotidine** (given in doses of 20 to 40 mg orally or intravenously) are alternative H_2-receptor antagonists.[122,123] Both have a duration of action of greater than 10 hours and do not interfere with the metabolism of other drugs by the cytochrome P-450 system.[122,123]

Tramadol, a synthetic 4-phenyl-piperidine analogue of codeine with a low affinity for μ-opioid receptors, has the additional ability to inhibit type 3 muscarinic receptors that mediate gastric gland secretion and smooth muscle contraction. In one study, 60 healthy parturients, undergoing elective cesarean delivery under general anesthesia, were randomly assigned to receive either intramuscular tramadol 100 mg or famotidine 20 mg 1 hour before surgery. The median (range) gastric fluid pH after induction of anesthesia was 6.4 (1.7 to 7.2) in the tramadol group and 6.3 (1.9 to 8.1) in the famotidine group. Two patients in each group had a gastric volume greater than 0.4 mL/kg with a pH less than 2.5. Parturients in the tramadol group had better pain scores and used less analgesia during the first 24 hours after delivery. Neonatal well-being was similar in the two groups.[124] Further investigation is required before such a novel method of antacid prophylaxis is adopted into everyday clinical practice.

Proton Pump Inhibitors

Omeprazole (20 to 40 mg orally) and **lansoprazole** (15 to 30 mg orally) are substituted benzimidazoles that inhibit the hydrogen ion pump on the gastric surface of the oxyntic cell.[21,125-127] Purported advantages of PPIs are a long duration of action, low toxicity, and the potential for low maternal and fetal blood concentrations at the time of delivery. For elective surgery, the efficacy of prophylaxis with a PPI is similar to that achieved with an H_2-receptor antagonist. For emergency cesarean delivery, studies have demonstrated that H_2-receptor antagonists and PPIs, administered intravenously, are equally effective adjuncts to sodium citrate for reducing gastric acidity and volume.[125]

Metoclopramide

Metoclopramide is a procainamide derivative that is a cholinergic agonist peripherally and a dopamine receptor antagonist centrally. An intravenous dose of metoclopramide 10 mg increases lower esophageal sphincter tone and reduces gastric volume by increasing gastric peristalsis. Metoclopramide can have a significant effect on gastric volume in as little as 15 minutes.[90] Unfortunately, prior administration of an opioid or atropine antagonizes the effect of metoclopramide.[128] Extrapyramidal effects represent a major side effect of metoclopramide.

Metoclopramide crosses the placenta, but studies have reported no significant effects on the fetus or neonate.[129]

A Cochrane review of antacid prophylaxis concluded that there was no evidence to support the routine administration of drugs to women in normal labor to reduce the incidence of pulmonary aspiration or Mendelson's syndrome.[130] This conclusion reflects the low incidence of pulmonary aspiration of gastric contents and the absence of high-quality studies of antacid prophylaxis, rather than the presence of studies demonstrating negative results; the Cochrane review cited only three studies, published in 1971, 1980, and 1984. One study assessed the use of metoclopramide and perphenazine in women receiving meperidine in labor, and the other two studies focused on the use of particulate antacids. An audit of acid aspiration prophylaxis during labor in the United Kingdom showed a decreasing number of institutions with policies to administer routine antacid prophylaxis to all laboring women. However, many institutions attempted to identify women at high risk for an emergency cesarean delivery, to whom they gave oral ranitidine 150 mg at 6-hour intervals throughout labor.[131]

Sellick Maneuver

Sellick demonstrated that the occlusion of the esophagus by cricoid pressure in cadavers prevented the flow of barium from the stomach to the pharynx. He also reported the successful use of this maneuver in 26 cases to prevent the passive regurgitation of gastric contents into the airway.[132] For proper application of cricoid pressure, the head should be fully extended; it may help to have a trained assistant place a hand behind the patient's neck, so that the cervical vertebrae and esophagus are brought forward, making it easier to occlude the latter. The trained assistant should place the thumb and middle finger on either side of the cricoid cartilage; no more than light pressure should be applied while the patient is awake, to prevent coughing, straining, retching, and esophageal rupture. After denitrogenation (preoxygenation) and administration of induction agents, an increasingly firm downward pressure is applied to the cricoid cartilage as loss of consciousness occurs. Full application of cricoid pressure requires a force of 30 Newtons (N), with one N being the unit of force required to accelerate a mass of one kilogram one meter per second squared. (Force cannot be represented by weight alone, but as a practical clinical conversion to guide the amount of force to apply, 10 N is approximately equivalent to 1 kg.) Vanner and Pryle[133] demonstrated that 30 N of cricoid force prevented regurgitation of saline in cadavers with esophageal pressures as high as 40 mm Hg. They recommended a modest cricoid force before loss of consciousness, increasing to 30 N after loss of consciousness; their data suggested that such pressure should be sufficient to prevent passive regurgitation of esophageal contents during induction of general anesthesia in most patients.[134,135] Cricoid pressure is maintained until the endotracheal tube cuff is inflated and endotracheal tube position is confirmed.

The value of cricoid pressure has been questioned. Use of cricoid pressure is based on the premise that the esophagus lies directly posterior to the cricoid cartilage and can be effectively occluded; both of these assumptions may not be true. Magnetic resonance imaging of 22 healthy volunteers of mixed gender noted that the resting position of the esophagus was lateral relative to the cricoid cartilage in 53% of the subjects without cricoid pressure and in 91% with cricoid pressure. In addition, cricoid pressure displaced the esophagus relative to its initial resting position to the left and right in 68% and 21% of the subjects, respectively (Figure 29-8). Furthermore, cricoid pressure displaced the airway relative to the vertebral body midline in 67% of the subjects. Although the maneuver was performed on awake subjects, this study suggests that cricoid pressure may lead to airway displacement and does not reliably produce midline esophageal compression; both of these factors may limit the protective effect of the maneuver in protecting against passive reflux and make the intubation process more difficult.[136] Randomized controlled trials have yet to be conducted to assess the efficacy and value of the use of cricoid pressure.[137]

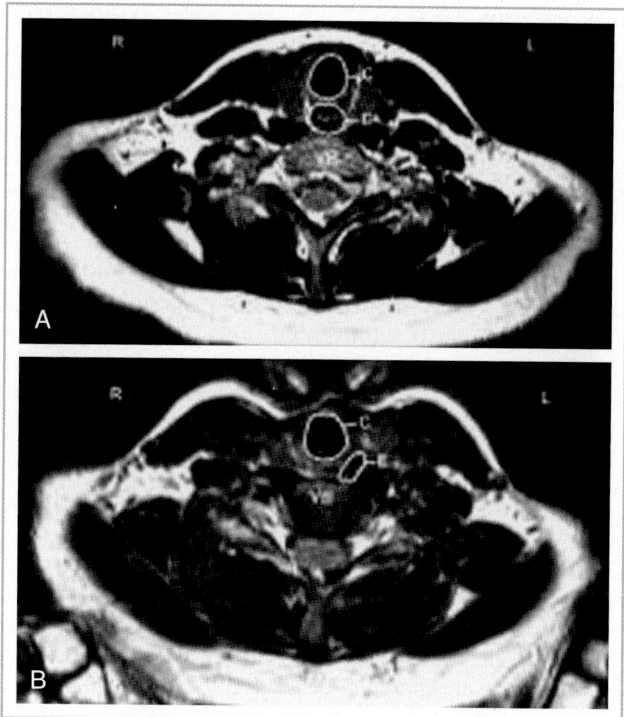

FIGURE 29-8 Magnetic resonance images of the neck without cricoid pressure (**A**) and of the same subject demonstrating 12.1 mm of lateral esophageal displacement to the left with application of cricoid pressure (**B**). C, cricoid cartilage; E, esophagus; VB, vertebral body.

RECOMMENDATIONS FOR CESAREAN DELIVERY

When possible, all mothers should be encouraged to have neuraxial anesthesia for cesarean delivery. Mothers with a potentially difficult airway, and who require general anesthesia, should undergo an awake fiberoptic intubation. For **elective cesarean delivery,** a suitable antacid regimen may include the oral administration of an H_2-receptor antagonist (e.g., ranitidine 150 mg or famotidine 20 mg) or a PPI (omeprazole 40 mg) at bedtime and again 60 to 90 minutes before the induction of anesthesia. (The patient may take the preoperative dose with water.) Some practitioners also give metoclopramide 10 mg orally at the same time as the H_2-receptor antagonist or intravenously at least 15 minutes before the induction of anesthesia. Administration of metoclopramide not only increases lower esophageal sphincter tone and accelerates gastric emptying but also decreases the incidence of nausea and vomiting during the administration of neuraxial anesthesia for cesarean delivery.[138]

For **emergency cesarean delivery with the patient under general anesthesia,** 30 mL of sodium citrate should be administered just after transfer of the patient to the operating room. This timing is important because sodium citrate has a relatively short duration of action, except in those mothers in whom gastric emptying has been delayed by the administration of an opioid. In addition, ranitidine 50 mg (or omeprazole 40 mg) and metoclopramide 10 mg should be given intravenously when time allows. Administration of these drugs may not reduce gastric volume or acidity at the time of intubation, but will decrease the risk of aspiration at the time of extubation. Some units administer an H_2-receptor antagonist orally every 6 hours during labor to all mothers considered to be at risk for an operative delivery.

The evidence that H_2-receptor antagonists or PPIs reduce maternal morbidity and mortality has not been conclusively demonstrated; however, increasing the pH and reducing the volume of gastric contents should assist in limiting damage if pulmonary aspiration occurs. Although further studies are necessary to validate the efficacy of cricoid pressure in preventing passive regurgitation, its use as part of a rapid-sequence induction technique remains standard practice.

ORAL INTAKE DURING LABOR

Women in the third trimester of pregnancy exhibit a state of "accelerated starvation" if denied food and drink.[139] Fasting results in the production of ketones, primarily beta-hydroxybutyrate and acetoacetic acid, and the nonesterified fatty acids from which they are derived. These changes are exacerbated by the metabolic demands of labor and delivery. Consequently some obstetricians and nurse-midwives have suggested that maternal oral intake policies should be liberalized during labor.[140,141] It is argued that allowing mothers to eat and drink during labor prevents ketosis and dehydration and subsequently improves obstetric outcome. The widespread use of neuraxial analgesia has resulted in a reduction in the use of systemic opioids for labor analgesia[104]; thus fewer women may be at risk for opioid-induced delays in gastric emptying (with its inherent potential for aspiration). This trend has increased the demand to liberalize NPO policies during labor.

A randomized controlled trial of intravenous hydration with lactated Ringer's solution, 125 mL/hr versus 250 mL/hr, on the progress of labor demonstrated that the frequency of labor lasting more than 12 hours was significantly higher in the 125 mL/hr group (20/78 [26%] versus 12/91 [13%]; $P = .047$).[142] Differences in the use of oxytocin and the route of delivery did not reach statistical significance. The investigators concluded that inadequate hydration during labor may be a contributing factor to dysfunctional labor. If further investigations validate these results, and in consideration of the limited duration of intravenous fluids in the intravascular space during pregnancy,[143] some practitioners have suggested that hydration should be maintained by an oral route and that the volume consumed should be dictated by maternal thirst.

A prospective randomized study examined the effect of a light diet on the maternal metabolic profile, the residual gastric volume, and the outcome of labor.[144] Women presenting in early uncomplicated labor at term were stratified by parity and randomly assigned to receive either a light diet or water only. The results showed that mothers who consumed a light diet did not have the increase in beta-hydroxybutyrate and nonesterified acid levels seen in the mothers who consumed water only. However, the gastric volumes as measured by ultrasonography were significantly larger in those who had eaten, as were the incidence of vomiting and the volume of the vomitus. Thus, mothers who consume a light diet during labor are at greater risk of aspiration if general anesthesia is required.

The same study design was used in another group of mothers, but isotonic "sport drinks" were administered instead of solid food.[145] It was found that isotonic "sport drinks" reduced ketosis without increasing intragastric volume, and the incidence of vomiting and the volume of the vomitus were similar in the two groups. However, in both studies the mean volume of the vomitus in all of the groups was more than 100 mL. No difference in labor outcome was seen in either study, but the numbers were too small to allow statistical evaluation of obstetric outcomes.

A recent randomized controlled study[146] evaluated the effect of food intake during labor on obstetric outcome. A total of 2443 low-risk nulliparous women in labor were randomly assigned to either an "eating" or a "water only" group. Intention-to-treat analysis was performed on the data. No significant differences were found in (1) the normal vaginal delivery rate, (2) the instrumental vaginal delivery rate, (3) the cesarean delivery rate, or (4) the incidence of vomiting (Figure 29-9). Similarly, there was no difference between groups in the duration of labor; the geometric mean (GM) labor duration was 597 minutes in

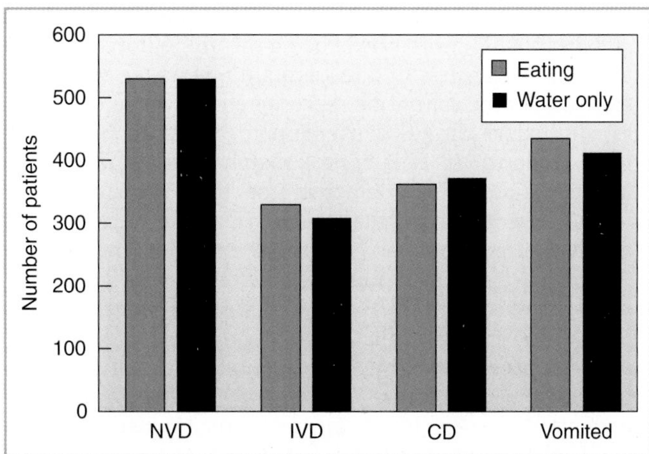

FIGURE 29-9 The effect of eating during labor on maternal obstetric outcome. CD, cesarean delivery; IVD, instrumental vaginal delivery; NVD, normal vaginal delivery. (Data from O'Sullivan G, Liu B, Hart D, et al. A randomized controlled trial to evaluate the effect of food intake during labour on obstetric outcome. 2008; submitted for publication.)

the "eating" group and 612 minutes in the "water only" group (ratio of GM, 0.975; 95% confidence interval, 0.927 to 1.025).[146]

Maternal death from Mendelson's syndrome is now extremely rare, and its decline probably owes more to the widespread use of neuraxial anesthesia than to NPO policies. Regardless, some benefits have been attributed to the use of oral or intravenous hydration during labor. Rigid NPO policies are therefore no longer appropriate on the labor and delivery unit, and mothers should be allowed to alleviate thirst during labor by consuming ice chips and clear fluids (e.g., isotonic sports drinks, fruit juices without pulp, black tea and coffee). In some high-risk pregnancies, it will remain appropriate to achieve hydration by an intravenous route, and such cases must be managed individually. Although countries with a more liberal attitude to eating during labor (Holland, United Kingdom, Australia) have not witnessed a higher incidence of maternal deaths from pulmonary aspiration, current evidence suggests that solid or semisolid meals should be avoided once a mother is in active labor or has received opioid-containing analgesics.

KEY POINTS

- Airway problems associated with the use of general anesthesia now represent the most common cause of anesthesia-related maternal deaths.
- Reduced lower esophageal sphincter tone and a higher risk of difficult intubation are the primary factors that increase the risk for aspiration during pregnancy and the immediate postpartum period.
- Although pulmonary aspiration of gastric contents is rare in contemporary obstetric anesthesia practice, fatal aspiration may occur during difficult or failed intubation at cesarean delivery.
- The most effective way to decrease the risk of aspiration is to avoid the administration of general anesthesia.
- The mother undergoing elective cesarean delivery should fast from solid food. Preoperative prophylaxis should include a nonparticulate antacid and may include an H_2-receptor antagonist or a proton pump inhibitor.
- Administration of a clear antacid effectively increases gastric pH. A clear antacid is preferred because aspiration of a particulate antacid results in pulmonary parenchymal damage similar to the damage that occurs after the aspiration of gastric acid.
- Hypoxemia is the hallmark of aspiration pneumonitis. Mechanical ventilation with positive end-expiratory pressure is the most effective treatment for severe hypoxemia. "Lung-protective" ventilation strategies (i.e., lower tidal volumes and inspiratory pressures) should be employed.
- The oral intake of clear fluids may be allowed during labor.
- Eating during labor results in larger residual gastric volumes, a higher incidence of vomiting, and a greater volume of vomitus. Eating does not improve obstetric outcomes.

REFERENCES

1. Simpson JY. Remarks on the alleged case of death from the action of chloroform. Lancet 1848; 1:175.
2. Hall CC. Aspiration pneumonitis: An obstetric hazard. JAMA 1940; 114:728-33.
3. Mendelson CL. The aspiration of stomach contents into the lungs during obstetric anesthesia. Am J Obstet Gynecol 1946; 52:191-205.
4. Lewis G, Drife J. Why Mothers Die 1997-1999: The Confidential Enquiries into Maternal Deaths in the United Kingdom. London, RCOG Press, 2001.
5. Why Mothers Die 2000-2002. Report on Confidential Enquiries into Maternal and Child Health. London, RCOG Press, 2004.
6. Lewis G, editor. Confidential Enquiry into Maternal and Child Health (CEMACH). Saving Mothers' Lives: Reviewing (Maternal) Deaths to Make Motherhood Safer 2003-2005. The Seventh Report on Confidential Enquiries into Maternal Deaths in the United Kingdom. London, CEMACH, 2007.
7. Olsson GL, Hallen B, Hambraeus-Jonzon K. Aspiration during anaesthesia: A computer-aided study of 185,358 anaesthetics. Acta Anaesthesiol Scand 1986; 30:84-92.
8. Warner MA, Warner ME, Weber JG. Clinical significance of pulmonary aspiration during the perioperative period. Anesthesiology 1993; 78:56-62.
9. Kluger MT, Short TG. Aspiration during anaesthesia: A review of 133 cases from the Australian Anaesthetic Incident Monitoring Study (AIMS). Anaesthesia 1999; 54:19-26.
10. Hawkins JL, Koonin LM, Palmer SK, Gibbs CP. Anesthesia-related deaths during obstetric delivery in the United States, 1979-1990. Anesthesiology 1997; 86:277-84.
11. Christiansen LR, Collins KA. Pregnancy-associated deaths: A 15 year retrospective study and overall review of maternal pathophysiology. Am J Forensic Med Pathol 2006; 27:11-9.
12. Soreide E, Bjornestad E, Steen PA. An audit of perioperative aspiration pneumonitis in gynaecological and obstetric patients. Acta Anaesthesiol Scand 1996; 40:14-9.
13. Catanzarite V, Willms D, Wong D, et al. Acute respiratory distress syndrome in pregnancy and the puerperium: Causes, courses and outcome. Obstet Gynecol 2001; 97:760-4.
14. Dodds WJ, Dent J, Hogan WJ, et al. Mechanisms of gastroesophageal reflux in patients with reflux esophagitis. N Engl J Med 1982; 307:1547-52.
15. Code CF, Marlett JA. The interdigestive myo-electric complex of the stomach and small bowel of dogs. J Physiol (Lond) 1975; 246:289-309.
16. Schurizek BA, Kraglund K, Andreasen F, et al. Gastrointestinal motility and gastric pH and emptying following ingestion of diazepam. Br J Anaesth 1988; 61:712-9.
17. Meyer JH. Motility of the stomach and gastroduodenal junction. In Johnson LR, editor. Physiology of the Gastrointestinal Tract. New York, Raven Press, 1987:613-29.
18. Brooks FP. Physiology of the stomach. In Berk JE, editor. Gastroenterology. Philadelphia, WB Saunders, 1985:874-940.
19. Feldman M, Richardson CT. Total 24-hour gastric acid secretion in patients with duodenal ulcer: Comparison with normal subjects and effects of cimetidine and parietal cell vagotomy. Gastroenterology 1986; 90:540-4.
20. Richardson CT, Walsh JH, Hicks MI, et al. Studies on the mechanisms of food-stimulated gastric acid secretion in normal human subjects. J Clin Invest 1976; 58:623-31.
21. Ewart MC, Yau G, Gin T, et al. A comparison of the effects of omeprazole and ranitidine on gastric secretion in women undergoing elective caesarean section. Anaesthesia 1990; 45:527-30.
22. Mayer G, Arnold R, Feurle G, et al. Influence of feeding and sham feeding upon serum gastrin and gastric acid secretion in control subjects and duodenal ulcer patients. Scand J Gastroenterol 1974; 9:703-10.
23. Bergegardh S, Olbe L. Gastric acid response to antrum distention in man. Scand J Gastroenterol 1975; 10:171-6.

24. Hunt JN, MacDonald I. The influence of volume on gastric emptying. J Physiol (London) 1954; 126:459-74.
25. Anvari M, Horowitz M, Fraser R, et al. Effect of posture on gastric emptying of nonnutrient liquid and antropyloroduodenal motility. Am J Physiol 1995; 268:G868-71.
26. Jian R, Vigneron N, Najean Y, et al. Gastric emptying and intragastric distribution of lipids in man: New scintigraphic method of study. Dig Dis Sci 1982; 27:705-11.
27. Collins PJ, Horowitz M, Maddox A, et al. Effects of increasing solid component size of a mixed solid/liquid meal on solid and liquid gastric emptying. Am J Physiol 1996; 271:G549-54.
28. Malagelada JR, Longstreth GF, Summerskill WHJ, et al. Measurements of gastric functions during digestion of ordinary solid meals in man. Gastroenterology 1976; 70:203-10.
29. Lind JF, Smith AM, McIver DK, et al. Heartburn in pregnancy: A manometric study. Can Med Assoc J 1968; 98:571-4.
30. Hey VMF, Cowley DJ, Ganguli PC, et al. Gastro-oesophageal reflux in late pregnancy. Anaesthesia 1977; 32:372-7.
31. Vanner RG, Goodman NW. Gastro-oesophageal reflux in pregnancy at term and after delivery. Anaesthesia 1989; 44:808-11.
32. Van Thiel DH, Gavaler JS, Joshi SN, et al. Heartburn of pregnancy. Gastroenterology 1977; 72:666-8.
33. Van Thiel DH, Gavaler JS, Stremple J. Lower esophageal sphincter pressure in women using sequential oral contraceptives. Gastroenterology 1976; 71:232-4.
34. Murray FA, Erskine JP, Fielding J. Gastric secretion in pregnancy. Br J Obstet Gynaecol 1957; 64:373-81.
35. Hirsheimer A, January DA, Daversa JJ. An X-ray study of gastric function during labor. Am J Obstet Gynecol 1938; 36:671-3.
36. La Salvia LA, Steffen EA. Delayed gastric emptying in labor. Am J Obstet Gynecol 1950; 59:1075-81.
37. Crawford JS. Some aspects of obstetric anesthesia. Br J Anaesth 1956; 28:201-8.
38. Hunt JN, Murray FA. Gastric function in pregnancy. Br J Obstet Gynaecol 1958; 65:78-83.
39. Davison JS, Davison MC, Hay DM. Gastric emptying in late pregnancy. Br J Obstet Gynaecol 1970; 77:37-41.
40. Nimmo WS, Wilson J, Prescott LF. Narcotic analgesics and delayed gastric emptying during labour. Lancet 1975; 1(7912):890-3.
41. Nimmo WS, Wilson J, Prescott LF. Further studies of gastric emptying during labour. Anaesthesia 1977; 32:100-1.
42. O'Sullivan G, Sutton AJ, Thompson SA, et al. Noninvasive measurement of gastric emptying in obstetric patients. Anesth Analg 1987; 66:505-9.
43. Simpson JH, Stakes AF, Miller M. Pregnancy delays paracetamol absorption and gastric emptying in patients undergoing surgery. Br J Anaesth 1988; 60:24-7.
44. Macfie AG, Magides AD, Richmond MN, Reilly CS. Gastric emptying in pregnancy. Br J Anaesth 1991; 54-7.
45. Geddes SM, Thorburn J, Logan RW. Gastric emptying following caesarean section and the effect of epidural fentanyl. Anaesthesia 1991; 46:1016-8.
46. Gin T, Cho AMW, Lew JKL, et al. Gastric emptying in the postpartum period. Anaesth Intensive Care 1991; 19:521-4.
47. Carp H, Jayaram A, Stoll M. Ultrasound examination of the stomach contents of parturients. Anesth Analg 1992; 74:683-7.
48. Sandar BK, Elliott RH, Windram I, Rowbotham DJ. Peripartum changes in gastric emptying. Anaesthesia 1992; 74:683-7.
49. Wright PM, Allen RW, Moore J, et al. Gastric emptying during lumbar extradural analgesia in labour: Effect of fentanyl supplementation. Br J Anaesth 1992; 68:248-51.
50. Whitehead E, Smith M, Dean Y, O'Sullivan G. An evaluation of gastric emptying times in pregnancy and the puerperium. Anaesthesia 1993; 49:53-7.
51. Ewah B, Yau K, King M, et al. Effect of epidural opioids on gastric emptying in labour. Int J Obstet Anesth 1993; 2:125-8.
52. Levy DM, Williams OA, Magides AD, Reilly CS. Gastric emptying is delayed at 8-12 weeks' gestation. Br J Anaesth 1994; 73:237-8.
53. Stanley K, Magides A, Arnot M, et al. Delayed gastric emptying as a factor in delayed postprandial glycaemic response in pregnancy. Br J Obstet Gynaecol 1995; 102:288-91.
54. Zimmerman DL, Breen TW, Fick G. Adding fentanyl 0.0002% to epidural bupivacaine 0.125% does not delay gastric emptying in laboring parturients. Anesth Analg 1996; 82:612-6.
55. Porter JS, Bonello E, Reynolds F. The influence of epidural administration of fentanyl infusion on gastric emptying in labour. Anaesthesia 1997; 52:1151-6.
56. Kelly MC, Carabine UA, Hill DA, Mirakhur RK. A comparison of the effect of intrathecal and extradural fentanyl on gastric emptying in laboring women. Anesth Analg 1997; 85:834-8.
57. Chiloiro M, Darconza G, Piccoli E, et al. Gastric emptying and orocecal transit time in pregnancy. J Gastroenterol 2001; 36:538-43.
58. Wong CA, Loffredi M, Ganchiff JN, et al. Gastric emptying of water in term pregnancy. Anesthesiology 2002; 96:1395-400.
59. Wong CA, McCarthy RJ, Fitzgerald PC, et al. Gastric emptying of water in obese pregnant women at term. Anesth Analg 2007; 105:751-5.
60. Christofides ND, Ghatei MA, Bloom SR, et al. Decreased plasma motilin concentrations in pregnancy. Br Med J 1982; 285:1453.
61. O'Sullivan G, Sear JW, Bullingham RES, et al. The effect of magnesium trisilicate mixture, metoclopramide and ranitidine on gastric pH, volume and serum gastrin. Anaesthesia 1985; 40:246-53.
62. Attia RR, Ebeid AM, Fischer JE, et al. Maternal fetal and placental gastrin concentrations. Anaesthesia 1982; 37:18.
63. Awe WC, Fletcher WS, Jacob SW. The pathophysiology of aspiration pneumonitis. Surgery 1966; 60:232-9.
64. LeFrock JL, Clark TS, Davies B, Klainer AS. Aspiration pneumonia: A ten-year review. Am Surg 1979; 45:305-13.
65. Teabeaut JR. Aspiration of gastric contents: An experimental study. Am J Pathol 1951; 28:51-67.
66. Hamelberg W, Bosomworth PP. Aspiration pneumonitis: Experimental studies and clinical observations. Anesth Analg 1964; 43:669-77.
67. Exarhos ND, Logan WD, Abbott OA, et al. The importance of pH and volume in tracheobronchial aspiration. Dis Chest 1965; 47:167-9.
68. Roberts RB, Shirley MA. Reducing the risk of acid aspiration during cesarean section. Anesth Analg 1974; 53:859-68.
69. Schwartz DJ, Wynne JW, Gibbs CP, et al. The pulmonary consequences of aspiration of gastric contents at pH values greater than 2.5. Am Rev Respir Dis 1980; 121:119-26.
70. Roberts RB, Shirley MA. Antacid therapy in obstetrics (letter). Anesthesiology 1980; 53:83.
71. James CF, Modell JH, Gibbs CP, et al. Pulmonary aspiration: Effects of volume and pH in the rat. Anesth Analg 1984; 63:665-8.
72. American Society of Anesthesiologists Task Force on Preoperative Fasting. Practice guidelines for preoperative fasting and the use of pharmacologic agents to reduce the risk of pulmonary aspiration: Application to healthy patients undergoing elective procedures. Anesthesiology 1999; 90:896-905.
73. American Society of Anesthesiologists Task Force on Obstetric Anesthesia. Practice guidelines for obstetric anesthesia. Anesthesiology 2007; 106:843-63.
74. Raidoo DM, Rocke DA, Brock-Utne JG, et al. Critical volume for pulmonary acid aspiration: Reappraisal in a primate model. Br J Anaesth 1990; 65:248-50.
75. Plourde G, Hardy JF. Aspiration pneumonia: Assessing the risk of regurgitation in the cat. Can Anaesth Soc J 1986; 33:345-8.
76. Gunther A, Ruppert C, Schmidt R, et al. Surfactant alteration and replacement in acute respiratory distress syndrome. Respir Res 2001; 2:353-64.
77. Matthay MA. Conference summary: Acute lung injury. Chest 1999; 116:119-26S.
78. Marik PE. Aspiration pneumonitis and aspiration pneumonia. N Engl J Med 2001; 344:665-71.
79. Ware LB, Matthay MA. The acute respiratory distress syndrome. N Engl J Med 2000; 342:1334-49.
80. Landay MJ, Christensen EE, Bynum LJ. Pulmonary manifestations of acute aspiration of gastric contents. AJR Am J Roentgenol 1978; 131:587-92.

81. Bernard GR, Artigas A, Brigham KL, et al. The American-European Consensus Conference on ARDS: Definitions, mechanisms, relevant outcomes, and clinical trial coordination. Am J Respir Crit Care Med 1994; 149:818-24.
82. The Acute Respiratory Distress Syndrome Network. Ventilation with lower tidal volumes as compared with traditional tidal volumes for acute lung injury and the acute respiratory distress syndrome. N Engl J Med 2000; 342:1301-8.
83. Brower RG, Lanken PN, MacIntyre N, et al. National Heart, Lung, and Blood Institute ARDS Clinical Trials Network. Higher versus lower positive end-expiratory pressures in patients with the acute respiratory distress syndrome. N Engl J Med 2004; 351:327-36.
84. The National Heart, Lung, and Blood Institute Acute Respiratory Distress Syndrome (ARDS) Clinical Trials Network. Comparison of two fluid-management strategies in acute lung injury. N Engl J Med 2006; 354:2564-75.
85. Takala J, Dellinger RP, Koskinen K, et al. Development and simultaneous application of multiple care protocols in critical care: A multicenter feasibility study. Int Care Med 2008; 34:1401-10.
86. Bernard GR, Luce JM, Sprung CL, et al. High-dose corticosteroids in patients with the adult respiratory distress syndrome. N Engl J Med 1987; 317:1565-70.
87. The National Heart, Lung, and Blood Institute Acute Respiratory Distress Syndrome (ARDS) Clinical Trials Network. Efficacy and safety of corticosteroids for persistent acute respiratory distress syndrome. N Engl J Med 2006; 354:1671-84.
88. Lyons G. Failed intubation: Six years' experience in a teaching maternity unit. Anaesthesia 1985; 40:759-62.
89. Rocke DA, Murray WB, Rout CC, et al. Relative risk analysis of factors associated with difficult intubation in obstetric anesthesia. Anesthesiology 1992; 77:67-73.
90. Gibbs CP, Rolbin SH, Norman P. Cause and prevention of maternal aspiration (letter). Anesthesiology 1984; 61:111-2.
91. Cohen SE, Jasson J, Talafre ML, et al. Does metoclopramide decrease the volume of gastric contents in patients undergoing cesarean section? Anesthesiology 1984; 61:604-7.
92. McCaughey W, Howe JP, Moore J, et al. Cimetidine in elective caesarean section: Effect on gastric acidity. Anaesthesia 1981; 36:167-72.
93. Wyner J, Cohen SE. Gastric volume in early pregnancy: Effect of metoclopramide. Anesthesiology 1982; 57:209-12.
94. Blouw R, Scatliff J, Craig DB, et al. Gastric volume and pH in postpartum patients. Anesthesiology 1976; 45:456-7.
95. James CF, Gibbs CP, Banner T. Postpartum perioperative risk of aspiration pneumonia. Anesthesiology 1984; 61:756-9.
96. Rennie AL, Richard JA, Milne MK, et al. Postpartum sterilization: An anaesthetic hazard? Anaesthesia 1979; 34:267-9.
97. Cote CJ, Goudsouzian NG, Liu LM, et al. Assessment of risk factors related to the acid aspiration syndrome in pediatric patients: Gastric pH and residual volume. Anesthesiology 1982; 56:70-72.
98. Vaughan RW, Bauer S, Wise L. Volume and pH of gastric juice in obese patients. Anesthesiology 1975; 43:686-9.
99. Kallar SK, Everett LL. Potential risks and preventive measures for pulmonary aspiration: New concepts in preoperative fasting guidelines. Anesth Analg 1993; 77:171-82.
100. Agarwal A, Chari P, Singh H. Fluid deprivation before operation: The effect of a small drink. Anaesthesia 1989; 44:632-4.
101. Lewis M, Crawford JS. Can one risk fasting the obstetric patient for less than 4 hours? Br J Anaesth 1987; 59:312-4.
102. Barau G, Robillard P-Y, Hulsey TC, et al. Linear association between maternal pre-pregnancy body mass index and risk of caesarean section in term deliveries. Br J Obstet Gynaecol 2006; 113:1173-7.
103. Durnwald CP, Ehrenberg HM, Mercer BM. The impact of maternal obesity and weight gain on vaginal birth after cesarean section success. Am J Obstet Gynecol 2004; 191:954-7.
104. Bucklin B, Hawkins JL, Anderson JR, Ullrich FA. Obstetric anesthesia work force survey: Twenty-year update. Anesthesiology 2005; 103:645-53.
105. Tsen LC, Pitner R, Camann WR. General anesthesia for cesarean section at a tertiary care hospital 1990-1995: Indications and implications. Int J Obstet Anesth 1998; 7:147-52.
106. Gibbs CP, Schwartz DJ, Wynne JW, et al. Antacid pulmonary aspiration in the dog. Anesthesiology 1979; 51:380-5.
107. Gibbs CP, Spohr L, Schmidt D. The effectiveness of sodium citrate as an antacid. Anesthesiology 1982; 57:44-6.
108. Chen CT, Toung TJ, Haupt HM, et al. Evaluation of the efficacy of Alka-Seltzer Effervescent in gastric acid neutralization. Anesth Analg 1984; 63:325-9.
109. O'Sullivan GM, Bullingham RES. The assessment of gastric acidity and antacid effect in pregnant women by a noninvasive radiotelemetry technique. Br J Obstet Gynaecol 1984; 91:973-8.
110. O'Sullivan GM, Bullingham RES. Noninvasive assessment of antacid effect during labor. Anesth Analg 1985; 64:95-100.
111. Coombs DW, Hooper D, Colton T. Acid-aspiration prophylaxis by use of preoperative oral administration of cimetidine. Anesthesiology 1979; 51:352-6.
112. Johnston JR, McCaughey W, Moore J, et al. Cimetidine as an oral antacid before elective Caesarean section. Anaesthesia 1982; 37:26-32.
113. Somogyi A, Gugler R. Drug interactions with cimetidine. Clin Pharmacokinet 1982; 7:23-41.
114. Feely J, Wilkinson GR, McAllister CB, et al. Increased toxicity and reduced clearance of lidocaine by cimetidine. Ann Intern Med 1982; 96:592-4.
115. Howe JP, McGowan WA, Moore J, et al. The placental transfer of cimetidine. Anaesthesia 1981; 36:371-5.
116. Lineberger AS, Sprague DH, Battaglini JW. Sinus arrest associated with cimetidine. Anesth Analg 1985; 64:554-6.
117. Dammann HG, Muller P, Simon B. Parenteral ranitidine: Onset and duration of action. Br J Anaesth 1982; 54:1235-6.
118. Francis RN, Kwik RS. Oral ranitidine for prophylaxis against Mendelson's syndrome. Anesth Analg 1982; 61:130-2.
119. Maile CJ, Francis RN. Pre-operative ranitidine: Effect of a single intravenous dose on pH and volume of gastric aspirate. Anaesthesia 1983; 38:324-6.
120. Kirch W, Hoensch H, Janisch HD. Interactions and non-interactions with ranitidine. Clin Pharmacokinet 1984; 9:493-510.
121. Dailey PA, Hughes SC, Rosen MA, et al. Effect of cimetidine and ranitidine on lidocaine concentrations during epidural anesthesia for cesarean section. Anesthesiology 1988; 69:1013-7.
122. Pattichis K, Louca LL. Histamine, histamine H_2-receptor antagonists, gastric acid secretion and ulcers: An overview. Drug Metab Drug Interact 1995; 12:1-36.
123. Howden CW, Tytgat GN. The tolerability and safety profile of famotidine. Clin Ther 1996; 18:36-54.
124. Elhakim M, Abd El-Megid W, Metry A, et al. Analgesic and antacid properties of i.m. tramadol given before cesarean section under general anesthesia. Br J Anaesth 2005; 95:811-5.
125. Yau G, Kan AF, Gin T, et al. A comparison of omeprazole and ranitidine for prophylaxis against aspiration pneumonitis in emergency caesarean section. Anaesthesia 1992; 47:101-4.
126. Blum RA, Shi H, Karol MD, et al. The comparative effects of lansoprazole, omeprazole, and ranitidine in suppressing gastric acid secretion. Clin Ther 1997; 19:1013-23.
127. Levack ID, Bowie RA, Braid DP, et al. Comparison of the effect of two dose schedules of oral omeprazole with oral ranitidine on gastric aspirate pH and volume in patients undergoing elective surgery. Br J Anaesth 1996; 76:567-9.
128. Hey VM, Ostick DG, Mazumder JK, et al. Pethidine, metoclopramide and the gastro-oesophageal sphincter: A study in healthy volunteers. Anaesthesia 1981; 36:173-6.
129. Bylsma-Howell M, Riggs KW, McMorland GH, et al. Placental transport of metoclopramide: Assessment of maternal and neonatal effects. Can Anaesth Soc J 1983; 30:487-92.
130. Gyte GM, Richens Y. Routine prophylactic drugs in normal labour for reducing gastric aspiration and its effects. Cochrane Database Syst Rev 2006;(3):CD005298.

131. Calthorpe N, Lewis M. Acid aspiration prophylaxis in labour: A survey of UK obstetric units. Int J Obstet Anesth 2005; 14:300-4.
132. Sellick BA. Cricoid pressure to control regurgitation of stomach contents during induction of anaesthesia. Lancet 1961; 1(7199):404-6.
133. Vanner RG, Pryle BJ. Regurgitation and oesophageal rupture with cricoid pressure: A cadaver study. Anaesthesia 1992; 47:732-5.
134. Vanner RG, O'Dwyer JP, Pryle BJ, Reynolds F. Upper oesophageal sphincter pressure and the effect of cricoid pressure. Anaesthesia 1992; 47:95-100.
135. Vanner RG, Pryle BJ, O'Dwyer JP, Reynolds F. Upper oesophageal sphincter pressure and the intravenous induction of anaesthesia. Anaesthesia 1992; 47:371-5.
136. Smith KJ, Dobranowski J, Yip G, et al. Cricoid pressure displaces the esophagus: An observational study using magnetic resonance imaging. Anesthesiology 2003; 99:60-4.
137. Maltby JR, Beriault MT. Science, pseudoscience and Sellick. Can J Anesth 2002; 49:443-6.
138. Lussos SA, Bader AM, Thornhill ML, Datta S. The antiemetic efficacy and safety of prophylactic metoclopramide for elective cesarean section delivery during spinal anesthesia. Reg Anesth 1992; 17:126-30.
139. Metzger BE, Vileisis RA, Ramikar V, et al. "Accelerated starvation" and the skipped breakfast in late normal pregnancy. Lancet 1982; 1(8272):588-92.
140. Elkington KW. At the water's edge: Where obstetrics and anesthesia meet. Obstet Gynecol 1991; 77:304-8.
141. O'Sullivan G, Shennan A. Labour—a gastronomic experience! Int J Obstet Anesth 2002; 11:1-3.
142. Garite TJ, Weeks J, Peters-Phair K, et al. A randomized control trial of the effect of increased intravenous hydration on the course of labor in nulliparous women. Am J Obstet Gynecol 2000; 183:1544-8.
143. Ueyama H, He Y, Tanigami H, et al. Effects of crystalloid and colloid preload on blood volume in the parturient undergoing spinal anesthesia for elective cesarean section. Anesthesiology 1999; 91:1571-6.
144. Scrutton MJ, Metcalfe GA, Lowy C, et al. Eating in labour. Anaesthesia 1999; 54:329-34.
145. Kubli M, Scrutton MJ, Seed PT, et al. An evaluation of isotonic "sport drinks" during labor. Anesth Analg 2002; 94:404-8.
146. O'Sullivan G, Liu B, Hart D, et al. A randomized controlled trial to evaluate the effect of food intake during labour on obstetric outcome. 2008; submitted for publication.

Chapter 30

The Difficult Airway: Risks, Prophylaxis, and Management

John A. Thomas, M.D.
Carin A. Hagberg, M.D.

RISKS

Incidence and Epidemiology

For more than two decades, anesthesiologists have articulated the need for guidelines and training specific to the management of the obstetric airway.[1] This concern appears to be even more relevant today.[2-4] Despite numerous advances in airway equipment and an overall reduction in anesthesia-related maternal mortality, the incidence of failed intubation in the obstetric population has remained stable at approximately 1 in 300,[4] an occurrence that is nearly 8 times that observed in the general surgical population (1 in 2330).[5]

Several writers have warned that a higher incidence of failed intubation in obstetric patients should be expected in the future.[4,6-9] One reason for this concern is that the significant increase in the use of neuraxial analgesic and anesthetic techniques has limited opportunities to teach and practice the skills necessary for obstetric airway management. Another reason is a change in the demographics of the obstetric population. The prevalence of obesity is rising at an alarming rate in both developed and developing countries worldwide, and obesity is associated with an increased risk of airway management problems during pregnancy.[10] In addition, anesthesia providers today provide care for older parturients with more comorbidities, in part as a result of delayed childbearing and the use of assisted reproductive technologies (see Chapter 15); these comorbid conditions may exacerbate the effects of hypoxemia, hypercarbia, and acidosis during a delayed or failed intubation. One editorial implored the obstetric anesthesia community to become more aggressive in encouraging research and in developing clinical protocols that specifically address airway issues in the obstetric population.[11]

The American Society of Anesthesiologists (ASA) Difficult Airway Algorithm[12] represents a vital clinical tool with which every obstetric anesthesia provider should be familiar. Further, a specialized obstetric airway algorithm should consider the evolving anatomic and physiologic alterations that occur during pregnancy, labor, and delivery. This chapter addresses the management of both anticipated and unanticipated cases of a difficult airway in obstetric patients.

Maternal Morbidity and Mortality

Airway complications remain the leading cause of anesthesia-related mortality, with many deaths attributed to substandard care.[13-16] In the United States, anesthetic complications represent the seventh leading cause of maternal mortality—after embolic disorders, hemorrhage, hypertensive disorders, infection, cardiac disease, and cerebrovascular accidents.[17] General anesthesia is associated with a greater risk of maternal mortality than neuraxial anesthetic techniques.[18] Hawkins et al.[18] estimated that the case-fatality risk ratio for general versus neuraxial anesthesia was as high as 16.7 in the years 1985 to 1990; a more recent analysis by the same investigators suggested a nonsignificant relative risk of 1.7 in the years 1997 to 2002.[19] These data may overstate the risk of general anesthesia, because this form of anesthesia is used principally when neuraxial anesthetic techniques are contraindicated for medical reasons or time constraints.[20] Of concern, in contrast to the decline in case-fatality rates for general anesthesia over the last two decades, Hawkins et al.[19] recently reported an increase in case-fatality rates for neuraxial anesthesia.

Airway complications are prominent in the majority of cases of maternal mortality attributed to general anesthesia.[18] The incidence of *fatal* failed intubation in the obstetric population has been estimated to be 13 times higher than that in the general surgical population[21]; the overwhelming majority of these fatalities have occurred in the setting of an emergency cesarean delivery.[22]

These trends must be evaluated in the context of contemporary obstetric practice, which has witnessed a growing demand for cesarean delivery. In the United States, more than 30% of all deliveries are cesarean deliveries.[23] Because some of these cesarean deliveries are performed as emergencies and/or in patients with contraindications to neuraxial anesthetic techniques, the overall number of cases performed with general anesthesia and, as a consequence, the number of parturients found to have a difficult airway, will most likely increase, particularly because of the changing body habitus of parturients. The incidence of obesity is increasing at an alarming rate in both developed and developing countries worldwide.[24] It is estimated that more than 30% of parturients in North America and the United Kingdom are obese (body mass index [BMI] > 30 kg/m^2).[24] The potential airway complications associated with obesity are discussed in two reviews of maternal mortality in Michigan.[25,26] From 1972 to 1984, anesthesia complications were the primary cause of death in 15 cases; 80% of these parturients were obese, and 80% of the cases involved emergency surgery.[25] A similar review of maternal deaths from 1985 to 2003 identified eight anesthesia-related maternal deaths, in which six of the parturients were obese[26]; of interest, all of the anesthesia-related deaths that resulted from airway obstruction or hypoventilation occurred during emergence and recovery rather than during induction and intubation. Furthermore, system errors played a role in the majority of the maternal deaths.[26]

Not surprisingly, difficulties in airway management may have medicolegal implications. The single largest class of injury-related claims in the ASA Closed-Claims database comprises respiratory events, and the majority have been judged to involve substandard management.[13,27] Most of the cases also involved inadequate ventilation, esophageal intubation, and/or difficult intubation. Clearly, the potential for morbidity and mortality associated with airway management remains a significant concern for the obstetric anesthesia provider.

Definition and Classification

A **difficult airway** can be defined in several ways. Most commonly this term refers to the difficulty in placing an endotracheal tube (ETT) through the vocal cords with the use of direct laryngoscopy. However, it can also include difficulty in providing mask ventilation. The degree of difficulty with either direct laryngoscopy or mask ventilation can vary significantly. A difficult intubation is often defined by the alterations in management associated with failure to secure a successful ETT placement (e.g., change in positioning, use of different laryngoscope blades, multiple attempts by more than one experienced anesthesia provider, posterior cephalad displacement of the larynx by external pressure).

Impossible mask ventilation can be defined as the inability to provide positive-pressure ventilation despite (1) repositioning of the head and neck, (2) lifting of the jaw anteriorly, (3) use of an oral and/or nasal airway, and (4) use of a two-person technique, in which one anesthesia provider positions the head and holds the mask against the face with two hands while an assistant squeezes the reservoir bag.

In obstetric patients, airway difficulties are frequently unexpected and have a reported incidence of 7.9%,[28] which is more than three times the incidence witnessed in the nonobstetric population.[29] Although the incidence of difficult or impossible mask ventilation has not been reported in the obstetric population, a range from 0.02% to as high as 15.5% has been estimated in the general surgical population. Kheterpal et al.[30] reviewed 22,600 attempts at mask ventilation and found that ventilation was difficult or impossible in 0.37% of cases. In another study of 576 patients in which direct laryngoscopy was graded as difficult, Yildiz et al.[31] found the incidence of difficult mask ventilation to be 15.5%.

Difficulties with intubation and mask ventilation can exist independently of each other; a patient who can be easily ventilated by mask may be difficult to intubate, and vice versa. In addition, multiple attempts at intubation can lead to trauma, airway swelling, and a deterioration in the ability to provide mask ventilation. Therefore, it is prudent for the anesthesia provider to limit the number of intubation attempts, keeping in mind the primary goals of oxygenation and ventilation.

Physiologic and Anatomic Changes of Pregnancy

The physiologic and anatomic changes of pregnancy may contribute to the difficulty observed in the management of the maternal airway (Box 30-1).

BOX 30-1 Risk Factors for Airway Complications during Pregnancy

- Airway edema
- Decreased functional residual capacity
- Increased oxygen consumption
- Weight gain
- Enlarged breasts
- Full dentition
- Decreased lower esophageal sphincter tone
- Decreased gastric emptying during labor

AIRWAY EDEMA

Higher levels of estrogen and an increase in maternal blood volume contribute to the development of capillary engorgement, mucosal edema, and tissue friability in the airway, including the nasal and oral pharynx, larynx, and trachea.[32-35] Such changes most likely account for the difficulty with nasal breathing, the voice changes, and the potential for nasal bleeding observed during pregnancy.[14] Because of these alterations, the tissues are more easily traumatized during airway instrumentation (e.g., intubation, nasogastric tube placement), which in turn may result in significant bleeding. In addition, enlargement of the tongue may make its displacement into the mandibular space by the laryngoscope blade more difficult.[36] Furthermore, edema can distort the anatomy of the larynx, decrease the size of the laryngeal opening, and necessitate the use of a smaller ETT to minimize trauma and facilitate easier passage of the ETT into the trachea.[37]

Airway edema can be significantly worsened by preeclampsia, respiratory tract infection, expulsive efforts during the second stage of labor, and/or excessive administration of fluids.[32] Using acoustic reflectometry, Kodali et al.[38] observed that labor and delivery were associated with a decrease in upper airway volume (presumably a result of an increase in soft tissue mucosal edema) of both the oral component (from incisor teeth to oropharyngeal junction) and the pharyngeal component (from oropharyngeal junction to glottis). In addition, these investigators demonstrated that the initial prelabor airway classification worsened during labor and delivery in a significant number of parturients. Swelling and edema in the face, neck, and tongue can also lead to acute airway compromise.[35,37]

RESPIRATORY AND METABOLIC CHANGES

The metabolic requirements for oxygen are greater during pregnancy (see Chapter 2). The pain and stress response associated with labor further increase these requirements. The anatomic alterations of pregnancy compromise the pregnant woman's ability to meet the greater oxygen demands. For example, the gravid uterus pushes the diaphragm cephalad, resulting in diminished lung volumes; a 15% to 30% reduction in expiratory reserve volume and functional residual capacity (FRC) occurs during pregnancy.[22,37] The decrease in FRC can lead to small airway closure during normal tidal-volume breathing, particularly if the patient is placed in the supine or Trendelenburg position or has a high BMI.

In the supine position, the gravid uterus may compress the inferior vena cava, leading to a decrease in venous return, cardiac output, and uterine blood flow. In approximately 15% of parturients, a pronounced supine hypotensive syndrome may occur, as evidenced by hypotension, pallor, sweating, nausea, vomiting, and changes in cerebration.[37]

These factors predispose pregnant women to rapid arterial oxyhemoglobin desaturation and hypoxemia during periods of hypoventilation or apnea. Adequate denitrogenation (i.e., administration of 100% oxygen, or so-called preoxygenation) is essential prior to rapid-sequence induction of general anesthesia. Elevating the head of the bed and providing 3 to 5 minutes of denitrogenation (when time allows) maximizes PaO_2 and provides a greater margin of safety during apnea.[39] Computer modeling of the rate of arterial oxyhemoglobin desaturation in fully preoxygenated patients (fractional alveolar concentration of oxygen [FAO_2] = 0.87) suggests that this process occurs significantly more rapidly in moderately ill and obese patients than in normal healthy adults (Figure 30-1).[40] Using computer simulation, McClelland et al.[41] likewise observed reduced tolerance for apnea in pregnancy. The desaturation that occurs during apnea in a term parturient in the supine or Trendelenburg position mimics the desaturation that occurs in morbidly obese patients and is a result of the increased oxygen consumption and decreased FRC in pregnant women. Most important, if ventilation is impossible, the time to severe, life-threatening hypoxemia is significantly shorter than the time needed to recover from apnea produced by administration of succinylcholine 1 mg/kg.[40,41]

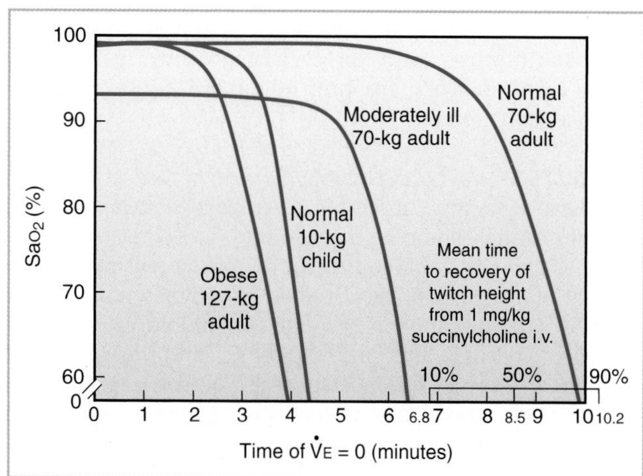

FIGURE 30-1 Time to hemoglobin desaturation (initial FAO_2 = 0.87). SaO_2 versus time of apnea for various types of patients. (From Benumof JL, Dagg R, Benumof R. Critical hemoglobin desaturation will occur before return to an unparalyzed state following 1 mg/kg intravenous succinylcholine. Anesthesiology 1997; 87:979-82.)

WEIGHT GAIN

Pregnancy results in significant increases in fat deposition, blood and interstitial fluid volume, and uterine and fetal mass. Overall, most women gain 15 kg or more during pregnancy. This weight gain may predispose to both difficult and impossible mask ventilation and difficult endotracheal intubation.[24,30,42] The likelihood of encountering a difficult airway is increased in parturients with a high BMI as a result of the baseline anatomy and pregnancy- and labor-related changes to the airway. In addition, obese parturients have a higher risk for emergency cesarean delivery.[43] Obesity can result in further reductions in FRC and diaphragm excursion; the impact of these alterations is compounded by the greater metabolic demands associated with obesity, which results in increased oxygen consumption and more rapid oxyhemoglobin desaturation during periods of apnea.

BREAST TISSUE ENLARGEMENT

A potentially significant impediment to intubation during pregnancy is the enlargement of breast tissue. In the supine position, significantly enlarged breasts can interfere with proper placement of a laryngoscope blade and inhibit laryngoscope manipulation to improve the visualization of the larynx.[14] This problem may be minimized by (1) properly positioning the patient in a semi-upright position through the placement of blankets or commercially available positioning devices under the shoulders, neck, and occiput (the sniffing position helps avoid the problems that occur when the laryngoscope handle is in the same horizontal plane as the breasts); (2) using a short-handled laryngoscope; (3) directing the distal end of the laryngoscope handle laterally toward the shoulder on insertion of the blade into the mouth, with redirection toward the midline once inserted; (4) inserting the laryngoscope blade without the handle attached, and then attaching the handle once the blade is moved into the midline; (5) using a pediatric laryngoscope handle attached to an adult-sized blade[44,45]; and/or (6) fixing the breasts with tape in a lateral and caudal direction away from the airway field.

FULL DENTITION

Full dentition is typically present in young pregnant women and can interfere with direct laryngoscopy, particularly if the front incisors are protruding or the thyromental distance is decreased.

GASTROESOPHAGEAL CHANGES

During pregnancy, progesterone mediates relaxation of gastrointestinal smooth muscle and a decrease in the lower esophageal sphincter tone, thereby increasing the frequency of gastroesophageal reflux. Labor may also lead to delayed gastric emptying.[46,47] Further inhibition of gastric emptying occurs after the systemic administration of opioids, and some evidence suggests that neuraxial opioid administration may also delay gastric emptying during labor.[48,49] In addition, the enlarged uterus anatomically distorts the gastroesophageal junction, further increasing the risk of lower esophageal sphincter incompetence.[14,22,32,37] As a consequence and particularly after 20 weeks' gestation, when the uterus emerges from the pelvis into the abdomen, pregnant women should be considered at risk for regurgitation and aspiration of gastric contents (see Chapter 29).

AIRWAY ASSESSMENT

The majority of airway disasters occur because the potential management difficulty was not appreciated or anticipated.[14] Although it is estimated that as many as 90% of cases of difficult airway could have been predicted,[50] a prospective study of 1200 patients found that only 51% of the difficult intubations were anticipated.[51] Moreover, the opportunity to assess the maternal airway in a nonurgent manner is frequently missed, particularly in patients undergoing nonelective cesarean delivery. In a prospective observational study, Morgan et al.[52] found that the need for emergency cesarean delivery could be anticipated in 87% of cases. Such cases represent an opportunity to assess for physical characteristics associated with a difficult airway and to appropriately counsel the patient regarding the placement of a prophylactic epidural catheter to facilitate the avoidance of airway manipulation if the need for cesarean delivery occurs.[53] Early performance of a few simple bedside assessments (e.g., Mallampati class, thyromental distance, atlanto-occipital extension, mandibular protrusion) has value in determining potential airway difficulty (see later). Consideration of patient conditions, such as obesity and preeclampsia, may enhance the predictive value of these assessments.[28]

Multivariable Assessment of Airway Difficulty

Frerk[54] prospectively assessed the use of the Mallampati classification combined with an evaluation of the thyromental distance in 244 nonpregnant patients, and found that this approach had a 98% specificity and 80% sensitivity in predicting airway difficulty. Lewis et al.[55] assessed the combination of the Mallampati classification with an evaluation of the depth of the mandibular space. These investigators evaluated 214 consecutive patients and used a statistical method to calculate a performance index (PI), which was then used to calculate sensitivity, specificity, positive and negative predictive values, and probability of difficulty with intubation. They determined that most of the difficult intubations could be predicted, but approximately half of those predicted to be difficult were easy.

Wilson et al.[56] studied various combinations of the following five risk factors for airway difficulty: patient's weight, head and neck movement, jaw movement, and the presence or absence of a receding mandible or prominent incisor teeth. One of three levels of severity was assigned for each risk factor, and a predictive index (i.e., the Wilson Risk Sum) was created. Seventy-five percent of the cases associated with difficult laryngoscopy could be predicted with this approach, whereas in 12% of the cases, the airway was falsely predicted to be difficult. Oates et al.[57] found the Wilson Risk Sum to be less likely than the Mallampati classification to overestimate airway difficulty.

Rocke et al.[28] prospectively studied 1500 parturients presenting for elective or emergency cesarean delivery under general anesthesia. These investigators found that a higher Mallampati score and/or the presence of a short neck, protruding incisors, or a receding mandible increased the relative risk for intubation difficulty (Table 30-1).

Tse et al.[58] evaluated a combination of the Mallampati classification, thyromental distance, and head extension in

TABLE 30-1 Relative Risk Factors Associated with Difficult Tracheal Intubation*

Risk Factors	Relative Risk (95% Confidence Intervals)
Mallampati class:	
II	3.23 (1.70-6.13)
III	7.58 (4.07-14.12)
IV	11.30 (5.03-25.38)
Short neck	5.01 (2.40-10.45)
Receding mandible	9.71 (1.91-49.32)
Protruding maxillary incisors	8.0 (1.50-42.50)

*Compared with a risk of 1.0 for patients with an uncomplicated Mallampati class I airway.

From Rocke DA, Murray WB, Rout CC, Gouws E. Relative risk analysis of factors associated with difficult intubation in obstetric anesthesia. Anesthesiology 1992; 77:67-73.

predicting intubation difficulty in 471 nonpregnant patients. Alone or in different combinations, these variables lacked sensitivity in predicting a difficult airway but had a high level of specificity in identifying easy intubations. In a large prospective analysis of more than 10,000 consecutive surgical patients, el-Ganzouri et al.[59] used a multivariate model to stratify risk of intubation difficulty. Their criteria were mouth opening, thyromental distance, neck movement, mandibular protrusion, body weight, the Mallampati classification, and the presence of a difficult intubation history. All seven criteria were independent predictors of difficulty with visualization at laryngoscopy; in addition, a risk index derived from several of the criteria was superior to the Mallampati classification alone in predicting difficult visualization.

Kheterpal et al.[30] examined risk factors for difficult or impossible mask ventilation and subsequent difficult intubation in more than 22,000 cases. Independent predictors for impossible mask ventilation and difficult intubation were limited or severely limited mandibular protrusion, abnormal neck anatomy, the presence of sleep apnea, a history of snoring, and a BMI of 30 kg/m^2 or higher.

In a study of 1502 patients that excluded those undergoing otolaryngologic, obstetric, and emergency surgery, Langeron et al.[42] identified criteria that were associated with difficult mask ventilation, which was defined as the inability of an unassisted anesthesia provider to maintain Sp_{O_2} above 92% or to prevent or reverse signs of inadequate ventilation with positive-pressure mask ventilation in a patient undergoing general anesthesia. The investigators observed a 5% overall incidence of difficult mask ventilation, with five criteria (age > 55 years, BMI > 26 kg/m^2, lack of teeth, presence of a beard, history of snoring) noted to be independent risk factors; the presence of any two of these criteria indicated a high likelihood of difficult mask ventilation (sensitivity 72%, specificity 73%). Lower rates of difficult mask ventilation, ranging from 0.08% to 4%, have been reported in other prospective studies[29,59]; the absence of a standardized definition for difficult mask ventilation may explain, in part, the variation in the reported incidence of this problem.

The ASA Practice Guidelines for Management of the Difficult Airway outline the essential components for preoperative assessment of the airway.[12] The assessment includes 11 components that together help determine the index of suspicion for difficulty with intubation (Table 30-2). One individual test is rarely adequate to predict difficulty in airway management accurately. Four of the most common airway examinations utilized in clinical practice are discussed in more detail below.

Mallampati Classification

Multiple investigators have identified a significant correlation between the ability to visualize the oropharyngeal structures and the ease with which laryngoscopy and intubation can be achieved.[5,28,60,61] The Mallampati classification provides a rough assessment of the size of the tongue relative to the size of the oropharyngeal cavity. Mallampati et al.[61] originally hypothesized that if the base of the tongue were large enough to obscure the visualization of the tonsillar pillars and uvula, subsequent attempts at laryngoscopy and intubation would be more difficult. Samsoon and Young[5] later modified the Mallampati classification to add a fourth classification, and subsequently they validated a correlation between their modified Mallampati classification and difficulty with visualization at laryngoscopy. The modified Mallampati classification (Figure 30-2), the most common airway assessment tool in contemporary anesthesia practice, is defined as follows:

- Class I: visualization of soft palate, uvula, and tonsillar pillars
- Class II: visualization of soft palate and base of uvula
- Class III: visualization of soft palate only
- Class IV: visualization of hard palate only

The Mallampati test should be performed with the examiner using a light source at eye level with the patient. The patient should be sitting upright with her head in a neutral position. The patient is instructed to open her mouth as wide as possible and to protrude her tongue as far as possible *without* phonation. The airway is then classified on the basis of the pharyngeal structures that can be visualized.[61]

Cormack and Lehane[60] developed a grading system for the structures visualized with laryngoscopy and found a significant correlation with the Mallampati class. Their grading system is defined as follows (Figure 30-3):

- Grade I: Most of the laryngeal aperture is visualized.
- Grade II: Only the posterior portion of the laryngeal aperture can be visualized.
- Grade III: Only the epiglottis can be seen; no portion of the glottis is visualized.
- Grade IV: Even the epiglottis cannot be seen.

A grade III or IV laryngoscopic view is associated with difficulty in the placement of an ETT, whereas intubation is usually easy with a grade I or II view. Most Mallampati class I findings are associated with a grade I laryngoscopic view; similarly, a Mallampati class III or IV airway is more likely to have a grade III or IV laryngoscopic view. Cormack and Lehane[60] also suggested that a grade III laryngoscopic view is the "main cause of trouble" in the airway management of

TABLE 30-2 Preoperative Airway Examination, Minimal Acceptable/Desirable Values/Endpoints, and Significance of the Airway Examination

Preoperative Airway Examination	Minimal Acceptable/Desirable Values/Endpoints	Significance of the Airway Examination
1. Length of incisors	Qualitative/relative	Long incisors misalign the oral axis from the pharyngeal axis (creating a sharper angle between the two axes)
2. Involuntary anterior overriding of maxillary teeth on the mandibular teeth	No overriding of maxillary teeth on the mandibular teeth	Same as for long incisors
3. Voluntary protrusion of the mandibular teeth anterior to the maxillary teeth	Anterior protrusion of the mandibular teeth relative to the maxillary teeth	Test of temporomandibular joint function; a positive result means that a good view of the larynx with conventional laryngoscopy is likely
4. Inter-incisor distance	> 3 cm	A positive result (> 3 cm) means that the 2-cm-deep flange on a Macintosh blade can be easily inserted without hitting the teeth
5. Oropharyngeal class (visibility of the uvala)	≤ Class II	A positive result (≤ class II) means that the tongue is reasonably small in relation to the size of the oropharyngeal cavity and will be relatively easy to retract out of the line of sight
6. Configuration of the palate	Should not appear very narrow and/or highly arched	A narrow palate decreases the oropharyngeal volume and the ability to continue to visualize the larynx when both the laryngoscope and endotracheal tube are in the mouth
7. Mandibular space length (thyromental distance)	≥ 5 cm, or ≥ 3 ordinary-sized fingerbreadths	A positive result means that the larynx is reasonably posterior relative to the other upper airway structures, leading to a favorable line of sight
8. Mandibular space compliance	Qualitative palpation of normal resilience/softness	A laryngoscope retracts the tongue into the mandibular space. The compliance of the mandibular space determines the ability of the mandibular space to accept the tongue and create a favorable line of sight
9. Length of neck	Qualitative; a quantitative index is not yet available	A short neck reduces the ability to align the upper airway axes
10. Thickness of neck	Qualitative; a quantitative index is not yet available	A thick neck reduces the ability to align the upper airway axes
11. Range of motion of head and neck	Neck flexed 35 degrees on the chest, and head extended 80 degrees on the neck (i.e., the sniffing position)	The sniffing position aligns the oral, pharyngeal, and laryngeal axes to create a favorable line of sight

From the American Society of Anesthesiologists Task Force on Management of the Difficult Airway. Practice guidelines for management of the difficult airway. Anesthesiology 2003; 98:1269-77.

obstetric patients, and they recommended that this view should be used during simulation as a way for trainees to practice.

The Mallampati classification is often used as an assessment of possible intubation difficulty in obstetric patients. Of concern, Mallampati scores seem to increase with gestational age and weight gain during pregnancy; a 34% increase in the number of Mallampati class IV airways was observed in a cohort of 242 pregnant examined initially at 12 weeks' gestation and reassessed at 38 weeks' gestation.[62] Higher Mallampati scores have also been observed during the course of labor, particularly with a prolonged second stage.[38,63]

Several investigators have reported significant false-negative[64-66] and false-positive[65,67] results when the Mallampati classification is used; Mallampati classifications of II or III are associated with a range of laryngoscopic views from I to IV.[64-67] Several reasons have been proposed for this poor predictive value, including (1) the use of phonation (saying "ah") during the examination, which can falsely improve visualization; (2) placement of the patient in an improper position (i.e., supine instead of seated); (3) involuntary arching of the tongue, which may obscure visualization; and (4) the interobserver variability in interpretation.[64] As a consequence, the Mallampati classification should be used in combination with other evaluations to improve the overall sensitivity and specificity of the preanesthesia airway assessment.[65]

Atlanto-occipital Joint Extension

Adequate atlanto-occipital joint extension is needed to achieve the *sniffing* or Magill position,[68,69] which aligns the oral, pharyngeal, and laryngeal axes. This position

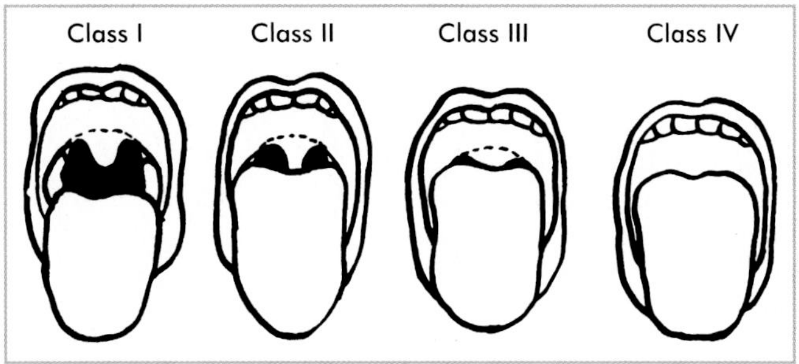

FIGURE 30-2 Modified Mallampati classification of the oropharynx. Classification of the upper airway in terms of the size of the tongue and the pharyngeal structures that are visible with the mouth open. In class I, the soft palate, fauces, uvula, and anterior and posterior tonsillar pillars can be seen. In class II, all of the preceding features can be seen except the tonsillar pillars, which are hidden by the tongue. In class III, only the soft palate and the base of the uvula can be seen. In class IV, not even the uvula can be visualized. (From Mallampati SR, Gatt SP, Gugino LD, et al. A clinical sign to predict difficult tracheal intubation: A prospective study. Can J Anaesth 1985; 32:429-34.)

allows for easier displacement of the tongue during laryngoscopy and better visualization of the larynx.[70] Atlanto-occipital joint extension can be evaluated by having the patient seated in a neutral face-forward position with her head erect and then maximally extended backward. Decreased atlanto-occipital joint extension can be expressed as a fraction of normal extension, which is 35 degrees (Figure 30-4).[37,71] A reduction in atlanto-occipital joint extension of 12 degrees (33%) or more correlates with intubation difficulty; complete joint immobility significantly compromises the laryngoscopic view of the larynx.[71] The accuracy and validity of the atlanto-occipital joint extension assessment have been questioned, and like many other clinical examinations, this assessment is subject to wide inter-observer variability.

Thyromental Distance

The size or depth of the mandibular space is another important indicator of intubation difficulty.[14,55,72,73] During laryngoscopy, the tongue is normally displaced into the mandibular space, which lies just anterior to the larynx. The size of this space can be estimated by measuring, either with a ruler or fingerbreadths, the thyromental

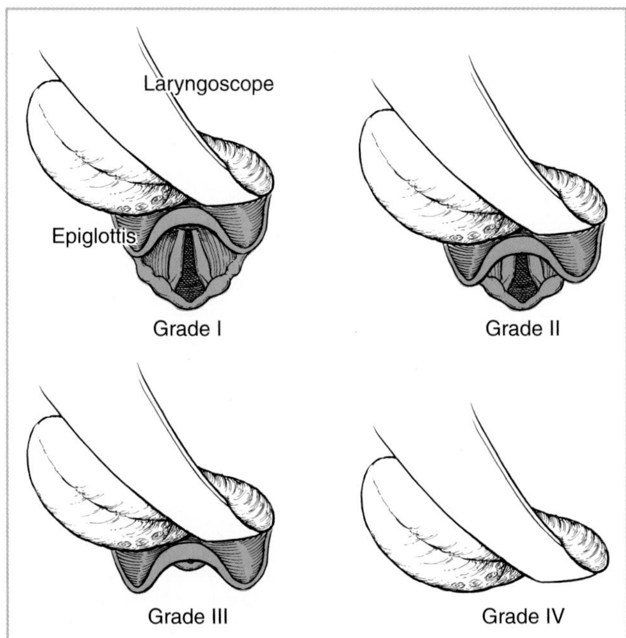

FIGURE 30-3 Cormack and Lehane laryngoscopic view grades. Grade I is visualization of the entire laryngeal aperture. Grade II is visualization of only the posterior portion of the laryngeal aperture. Grade III is visualization of only the epiglottis. Grade IV is visualization of only the soft palate. (From Cormack RS, Lehane J. Difficult tracheal intubation in obstetrics. Anaesthesia 1984; 39:1105-11.)

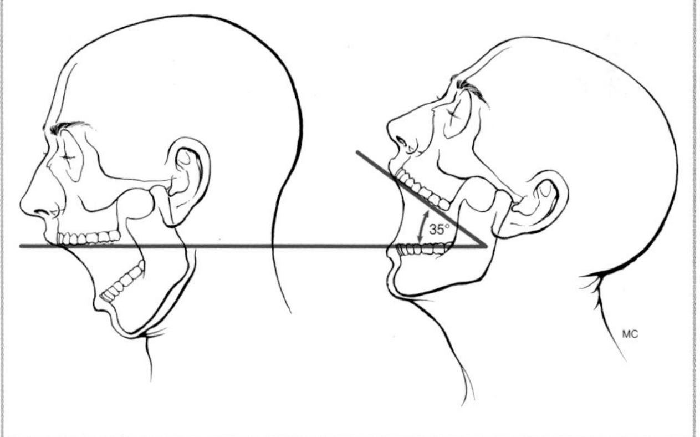

FIGURE 30-4 Clinical method for quantifying atlanto-occipital joint extension. When the head is held erect and faces forward, the plane of the occlusal surface of the upper teeth is horizontal and parallel to the floor. When the atlanto-occipital joint is extended, the occlusal surface of the upper teeth form an angle with the plane parallel to the floor. The angle between the erect and the extended planes of the occlusal surface of the upper teeth quantifies the atlanto-occipital joint extension. A normal person can produce 35 degrees of atlanto-occipital joint extension. (From Bellhouse CP, Dore C. Criteria for estimating likelihood of difficulty of endotracheal intubation with Macintosh laryngoscope. Anaesth Intensive Care 1988; 16:329-37.)

distance (from the chin to the notch of the thyroid cartilage) and/or the horizontal length of the mandible. A thyromental distance of more than 6.5 cm and a horizontal mandible length of more than 9 cm, without any other abnormalities, indicates that intubation by direct laryngoscopy should be easy. By contrast, a thyromental distance less than 6 cm suggests that direct laryngoscopy may be difficult.[14] An inverse correlation exists between the Mallampati classification and both the thyromental distance and the horizontal length of the mandible.[74,75] An assessment of the ratio of the patient's height (cm) to thyromental distance (RHTMD) has been proposed as having a better predictive value than thyromental distance alone. In Caucasian men and women, an RHTMD value of 25 or more was found to predict a poor laryngoscopic view.[76] In women undergoing cesarean delivery in Iran, an RHTMD value of 21.24 or more predicted difficult laryngoscopy.[77] Whether thyromental distance or RHTMD is altered during pregnancy or with variations in ethnicity warrants further investigation.

Anatomically, if the mandibular space is small and unable to accommodate the soft tissues displaced by the laryngoscope blade, few alterations will improve the line of vision during direct laryngoscopy (Figure 30-5).[71] When the mandibular space is small, the larynx lies relatively anterior, and the tongue must be pulled forward maximally and compressed into a smaller compartment to expose the larynx.

Mandibular Protrusion Test

The patient's ability to extend the mandibular teeth anteriorly beyond the line of the maxillary teeth may predict adequate visualization of the larynx during direct laryngoscopy. Calder et al.[78] performed a mandibular protrusion test (or upper lip bite test) in 253 patients prior to surgery (Figure 30-6). Patients were asked to protrude the mandible as far as possible, and the amount of protrusion was then assigned one of three classes: class A if the lower incisors could be protruded anterior to the upper incisors, class B if the lower incisors could be brought into line with the edge of the upper incisors but not anterior to them, and class C if the lower incisors could not be brought in line with the

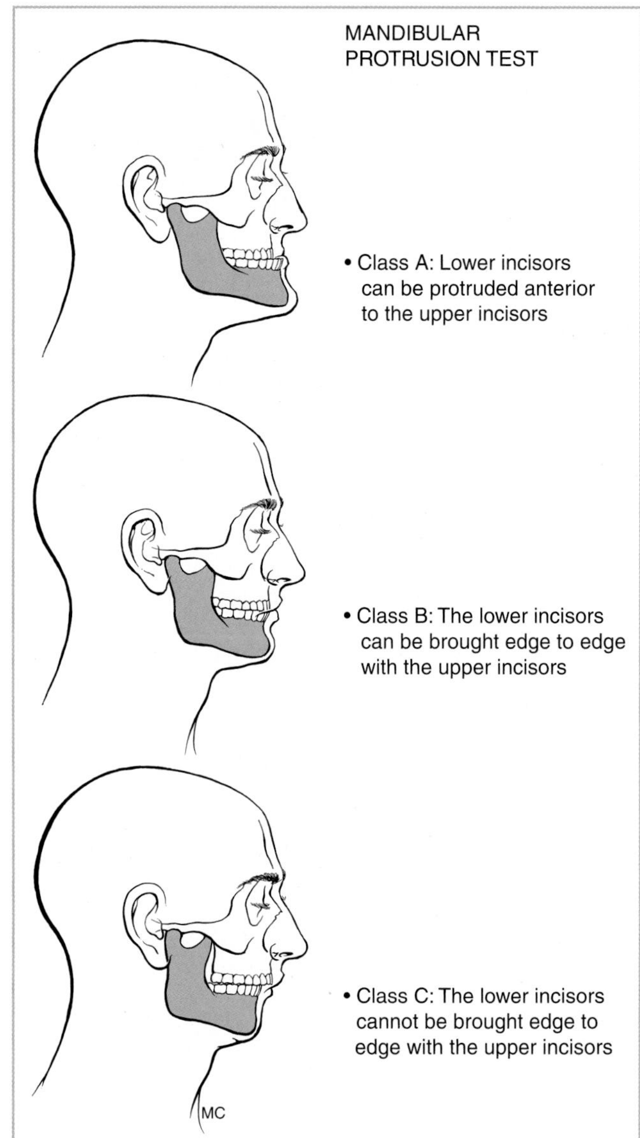

FIGURE 30-6 Mandibular protrusion test. Three classifications are based on the test, which is also referred to as the upper lip bite test. (Redrawn from Munnur U, de Boisblanc B, Suresh MS. Airway problems in pregnancy. Crit Care Med 2005; 33:S259-68.)

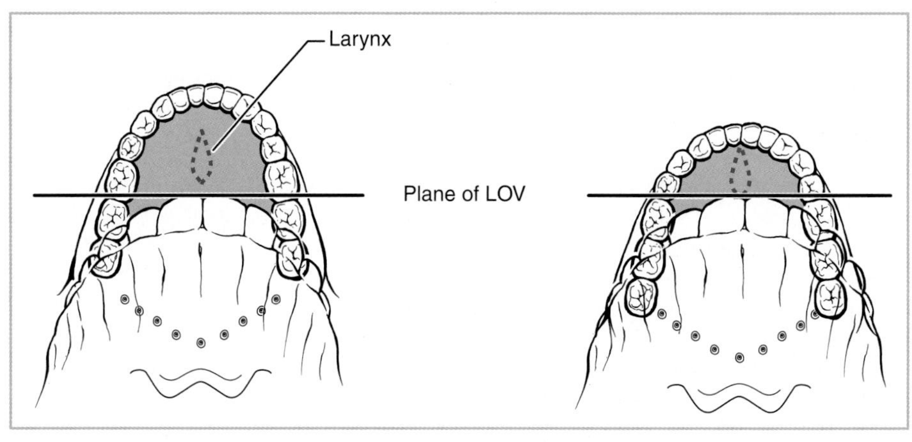

FIGURE 30-5 The mandibular space. The mandibular space (*shaded area*) is the area bounded by the plane of the line of vision (LOV) and the part of the mandibular arch in front of this plane. (From Bellhouse CP, Doré C. Criteria for estimating likelihood of difficulty of endotracheal intubation with Macintosh laryngoscope. Anaesth Intensive Care 1988; 16:329-37.)

upper incisors. Class C mandibular protrusion was always associated with a difficult laryngoscopy. In contrast, a class A mandibular protrusion was a good predictor for easy laryngoscopy. An external prospective evaluation of the reliability and validity of the upper lip bite test showed that the interobserver reliability was better than with the modified Mallampati classification.[79] Nonetheless, the test could not be performed on edentulous patients (11% of 1425 patients), and the investigators concluded that, like the modified Mallampati classification, the upper lip bite test was a poor predictor when used as a single screening test for difficulty of visualization of the larynx.

Other Factors

MORBID OBESITY

The prevalence of obesity is rapidly increasing in both developed and developing countries worldwide. Obesity is associated with higher maternal mortality.[11,24-26,80] Patients with morbid obesity have a significantly higher risk of cesarean delivery, failed epidural anesthesia, pulmonary aspiration of gastric contents, and maternal death from airway complications than parturients with normal BMI.[24-26,80] Hood et al.[43] found that difficult intubation occurred in 35% of morbidly obese parturients (> 300 lbs) compared with 0% of a control group. In a meta-analysis of bedside screening tests, Shiga et al.[65] reported that the incidence of difficult intubation was much greater in obese patients than in patients of normal weight. Several studies have also suggested that a high Mallampati score has a greater positive predictive value for difficult intubation in obese patients than in patients of normal weight.[64,81,82] Brodsky et al.[83] found that a high Mallampati score (class III or IV) in combination with a large neck circumference (when measured at the level of the thyroid cartilage) increases the potential for difficult laryngoscopy and intubation; using a logistic regression model, they found the probability of a difficult intubation to be approximately 5% and 35% with neck circumferences of 40 cm and 60 cm, respectively.

Gonzalez et al.[84] also observed that an increased neck circumference and a Mallampati score of III or IV were associated with a difficult intubation in obese patients (BMI > 30 kg/m^2). Increased BMI alone has also been identified as an independent risk factor for difficult or impossible mask ventilation.[30,42] Furthermore, individuals with high BMI not infrequently have obstructive sleep apnea, which has been independently correlated with a higher risk for aspiration and other postoperative complications.[85] These findings put obese parturients in a high-risk category for airway complications.

PREECLAMPSIA

Parturients with preeclampsia tend to retain extravascular fluid, exhibit low plasma oncotic pressure, and have greater endothelial cell permeability, all of which predispose to significant tissue edema.[14,86] Excessive fluid overload and/or retention can quickly lead to airway edema, tongue swelling, and upper airway narrowing in these patients; in severe cases, edema can result in acute airway compromise.[87] Visible swelling of the head, neck, or tongue in preeclamptic patients may indicate significant airway edema that can subsequently lead to sudden and complete airway obstruction. In addition, preeclamptic women can have thrombocytopenia and coagulation abnormalities.[14,32,88] Upper airway bleeding may occur with repeat attempts at intubation.

Therefore, avoidance of airway manipulation is encouraged in women with severe preeclampsia. Severe preeclampsia is an indication for a prophylactic or early epidural catheter placement, assuming the platelet count and coagulation status are acceptable.

TEAMWORK

The responsibility for appropriate management of an obstetric patient with a potentially difficult airway should not fall entirely on the anesthesia team. A coordinated and multidisciplinary approach by the anesthesia provider, obstetrician, neonatologist, and nursing teams promotes the highest level of care for high-risk parturients. Early and open communication among team members can help limit the need for crisis-induced decisions. The American College of Obstetricians and Gynecologists (ACOG) has recommended that members of the obstetric team alert the anesthesia team any time they become aware of potential general anesthesia risk factors.[89] The ACOG has also acknowledged that early placement of an epidural catheter should be considered during labor in such patients. Educating obstetricians on the potential risk factors and problems associated with general anesthesia is critical. In addition, when a patient is identified as having a potentially difficult airway, this information should be shared with all members of the team, and recommendations for anesthetic management should be articulated. Obstetricians should be aware that early administration of neuraxial anesthesia is often desirable in these patients and that a neuraxial anesthetic technique may be the safest option for both mother and baby, even in the presence of fetal compromise.

Summary

Assessment of Mallampati classification, atlanto-occipital extension, thyromental distance, and mandibular protrusion are four useful examinations for predicting difficulty with laryngoscopy.[12,14,37,55] However, because no single test is sufficient to identify a patient with a difficult airway, anesthesia providers should perform a complete airway evaluation in obstetric patients, as outlined in the ASA Practice Guidelines (see Table 30-2).[12] A preanesthesia evaluation may identify risk factors for difficulty with mask ventilation, laryngoscopy, intubation, and/or performance of a surgical airway. In some cases, the history may supply information (e.g., prior failed intubation, history of head and neck surgery, oropharyngeal pathology) that is likely to affect airway management. Other associated risk factors (e.g., obesity, preeclampsia) can be identified and may influence the anesthetic preparation and management. Early identification allows for time to (1) discuss the risks and benefits of various procedures with the patient, (2) discuss options and concerns with the obstetric team, (3) establish a functional neuraxial anesthetic technique, and/or (4) plan and prepare for possible airway interventions, such as an awake intubation.

PROPHYLAXIS

Use of Neuraxial Analgesic Techniques during Labor

The widespread acceptance and use of neuraxial analgesic techniques for obstetric patients has improved maternal and fetal outcomes in a number of ways. First, it has significantly reduced the need for general anesthesia and airway manipulation by providing a mechanism by which anesthesia for cesarean delivery can be delivered in a safe and predictable manner. Second, it has led to advances in the delivery of neuraxial anesthesia, thereby making these techniques more safe.[2,18] Such advances include (1) administration of an epidural test dose, (2) use of a dilute solution of local anesthetic for epidural analgesia, (3) administration of the therapeutic dose of local anesthetic in incremental boluses through an epidural catheter, (4) maintenance of adequate left uterine displacement to prevent aortocaval compression, and (5) prompt and aggressive treatment of hypotension.

Third, the widespread use of neuraxial techniques has led to a greater acceptance of early or prophylactic placement of an epidural catheter in high-risk parturients. A *prophylactic* epidural catheter is one that is placed and tested with a small dose of local anesthetic; analgesia is not established until active labor occurs, the patient requests analgesia, and/or an operative delivery is required. Such a catheter provides a readily available conduit for providing neuraxial analgesia or anesthesia, especially if rapid onset (e.g., an emergency operative delivery) is desirable. Early epidural catheter placement also allows the procedure to take place in a controlled setting and allows time for catheter manipulation and replacement, if necessary, before further pathophysiologic changes (e.g., decrease in platelet count, worsening airway edema) occur.

Preparation for General Anesthesia

ASPIRATION PROPHYLAXIS

All pregnant patients requiring surgical anesthesia should be considered at risk for pulmonary aspiration of gastric contents. The anatomic and physiologic changes of pregnancy and labor (e.g., reduced lower esophageal sphincter tone, delayed gastric emptying) increase the risk of aspiration (see Chapter 29). Failed or difficult intubation is also associated with aspiration.[18,32,89] Therefore, given that a failed neuraxial anesthetic may require conversion to general anesthesia, some form of pharmacologic prophylaxis to alter gastric pH should be administered to all parturients requiring surgical intervention whether or not they receive general or neuraxial anesthesia.

Oral administration of a clear nonparticulate antacid is the most common method of pharmacologic aspiration prophylaxis in obstetric patients.[90] Sodium citrate (0.3 M) 30 mL should be administered within 30 minutes of induction of anesthesia to ensure optimal neutralization of stomach acid.[91,92] This regimen effectively increases gastric pH above 2.5, which should reduce the risk of pulmonary injury if aspiration occurs. H_2-receptor antagonists are also effective in reducing the release of gastric acid, but require at least 40 to 60 minutes to be effective if administered intravenously.[93] Because ranitidine has a sustained therapeutic effect for approximately 8 hours, the higher gastric fluid pH should be sustained during emergence from anesthesia and extubation, when the risk of aspiration is again present.[93,94]

Metoclopramide promotes gastric emptying and also increases lower esophageal sphincter tone, helping to counteract the physiologic relaxation of the lower esophageal sphincter that occurs with pregnancy.[95,96] Historically, metoclopramide has been commonly used in parturients, particularly in conjunction with a nonparticulate antacid, to decrease aspiration risk. However, the effectiveness of metoclopramide is decreased when it is administered in conjunction with opioids.[97] Proton pump inhibitors (e.g., omeprazole) may also reduce gastric acid secretion[94,98] but require 40 minutes or more to produce the desired effect.[99]

Rapid-sequence induction and application of cricoid pressure are standard procedures during the induction of general anesthesia in parturients. Administration of an induction agent (e.g., sodium thiopental, propofol), followed immediately by succinylcholine (1.0 to 1.5 mg/kg) and the prompt placement of a cuffed ETT, avoids the use of mask ventilation, which may inadvertently insufflate the stomach.

Sellick[100] described cricoid pressure as a means to prevent regurgitated gastric contents from entering the posterior pharynx and subsequently passing into the lungs; the maneuver also prevents excessive amounts of air from entering the stomach during positive-pressure mask ventilation. The cricoid cartilage forms a complete ring, and the upper end of the esophagus can be compressed between the body of the fifth cervical vertebrae and the posterior part of the cricoid cartilage. An effective esophageal barrier to fluid from the stomach can be achieved by applying 10 newtons (N) of downward pressure to the cricoid cartilage in the awake supine patient, and increasing it to 30 N after the patient loses consciousness (see Chapter 29).[101-103] A limited amount of cricoid pressure (10 N) is used initially to avoid retching and regurgitation in the awake patient.

The anesthesia provider (or assistant) may easily identify the cricoid cartilage by moving his or her fingers cephalad (along the trachea) from the sternal notch to a distinctive wide cartilage that is palpated just inferior to the thyroid cartilage. Downward pressure on the cricoid cartilage is typically maintained by an assistant with the thumb and index finger.[100,103,104] Some investigators have recommended a "bimanual" technique, in which the assistant's other hand is placed behind the patient's neck for additional stabilization.[105,106] This double-handed technique also helps extend the atlanto-occipital joint and may improve intubating conditions. Although some authorities have advocated the use of a bimanual technique, others have rejected its routine use.[107,108] Which method of applying cricoid pressure is more effective and interferes less with intubation remains controversial. Cricoid pressure should be continued until the correct placement of the ETT has been confirmed. If difficulty arises with intubation, cricoid pressure can be continued during rescue mask ventilation, with the acknowledgment that firm cricoid pressure may distort the anatomy and lead to difficulty with airway management.[109,110] Successful visualization of the larynx or placement of a rescue device (e.g., laryngeal mask airway [see later]) may require brief release of cricoid pressure (Figure 30-7).[111-113]

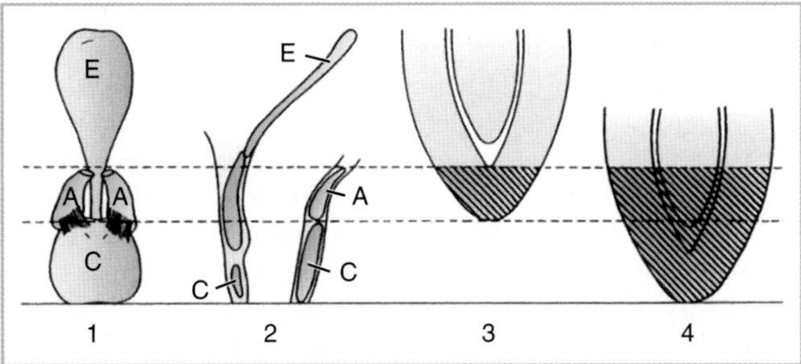

FIGURE 30-7 The level of the distal part of the laryngeal mask airway (LMA). The *hatched area* indicates the distal part of the LMA that occupies the hypopharynx. **1,** Posterior view of the larynx. **2,** Lateral view of the larynx. **3,** Position of the tip of the LMA when cricoid pressure is applied. When cricoid pressure is applied before placement, the LMA, in theory, might be wedged in the hypopharynx but is more likely to occupy the space behind the arytenoid cartilages. The LMA is positioned at least 2 cm more proximal than usual. **4,** Position of the LMA when no cricoid pressure is applied. When the LMA is placed correctly, the distal tip is at the distal end of C5 (fifth cervical vertebra), and the distal part of the LMA should fully occupy the hypopharynx and the pharyngeal space behind both the arytenoid and cricoid cartilages. A, arytenoid cartilages; C, cricoid cartilage; E, epiglottis. (From Asai T, Barclay K, Power I, et al. Cricoid pressure and the LMA: Efficacy and interpretation (letter). Br J Anaesth 1994; 73:863-5.)

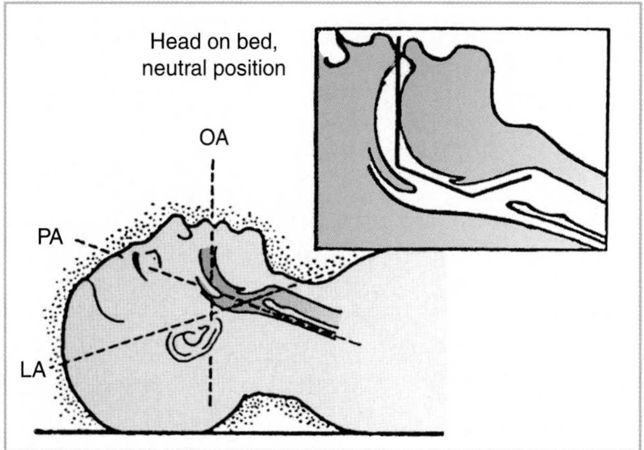

FIGURE 30-8 The alignment of the oral axis (OA), pharyngeal axis (PA), and laryngeal axis (LA) is shown. With the head in the neutral position, there is marked nonalignment of the OA, PA, and LA. (From Benumof JL. Conventional [laryngoscopic] orotracheal and nasotracheal intubation [single-lumen type]. In Benumof JL, editor. Clinical Procedures in Anesthesia and Intensive Care. Philadelphia, JB Lippincott, 1991:115-48.)

PATIENT POSITIONING

Correctly positioning the patient on the operating room table to maximize the chances for a successful intubation is a critical step that is often overlooked. Proper positioning is perhaps the most important factor for ensuring a successful direct laryngoscopy and endotracheal intubation, particularly in the obese parturient. The optimal view of the larynx by direct laryngoscopy is achieved by aligning the oral, pharyngeal, and laryngeal axes (Figures 30-8 and 30-9). The neck should be slightly flexed and elevated to bring the laryngeal axis in line with the pharyngeal axis. In an obese parturient, the head, neck, and upper back should be elevated to facilitate neck flexion; this positioning can usually be achieved by placing pads or blankets under the shoulders and upper back or through the use of commercially available wedge-shaped positioning cushions (Figure 30-10). The head must then be extended at the atlanto-occipital joint to place the patient in the sniffing or Magill position and align the oral axis with the pharyngeal and laryngeal axes. The operating room table should also be elevated to a height at which the laryngoscopist is most comfortable, and space at the head of the bed should be created to allow the anesthesia team to have complete access to the patient. Left uterine displacement, which is essential to prevent aortocaval compression, can be

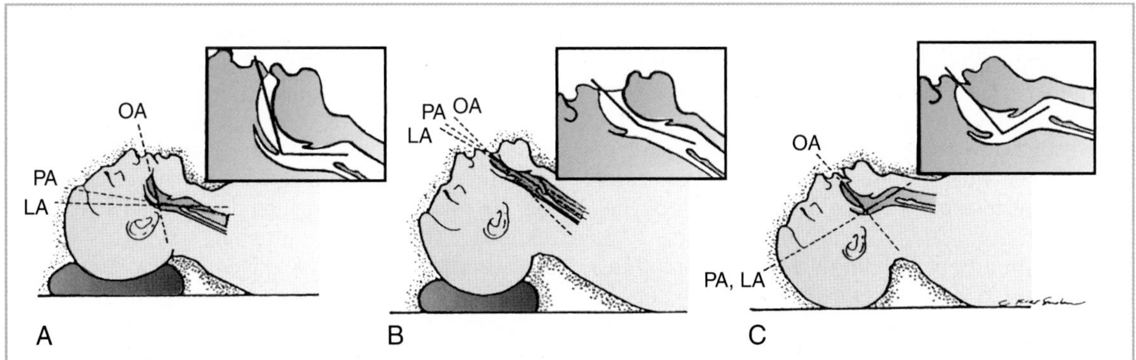

FIGURE 30-9 As the head position changes from neutral, the continuity of the oral axis (OA), pharyngeal axis (PA), and laryngeal axis (LA) changes within the upper airway. **A,** The head is resting on a large pad that flexes the neck on the chest and aligns the LA with the PA (the neutral position). **B,** The head is resting on a pad (which flexes the neck on the chest) and concomitant extension of the head on the neck can be seen, which brings all three axes into alignment (the sniffing position). **C,** Extension of the head on the neck without concomitant elevation of the head on a pad, which results in nonalignment of the PA and LA with the OA. (From Benumof JL. Conventional [laryngoscopic] orotracheal and nasotracheal intubation [single-lumen type]. In Benumof JL, editor. Clinical Procedures in Anesthesia and Intensive Care. Philadelphia, JB Lippincott, 1991:115-48.)

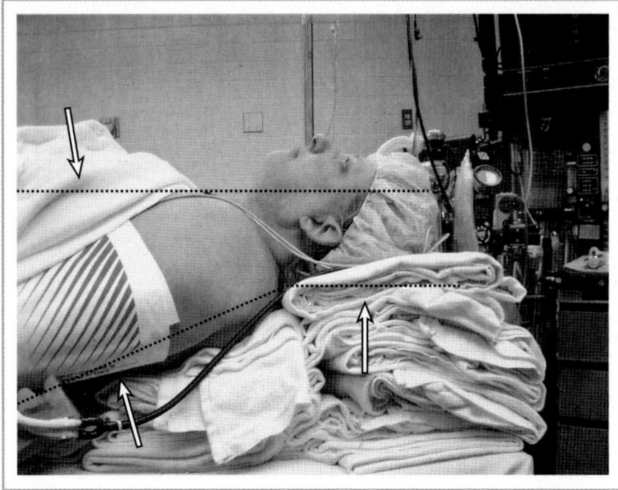

FIGURE 30-10 A morbidly obese patient will be in an optimal position for direct laryngoscopy when an imaginary horizontal line can be drawn from the sternal notch through (or slightly anterior to) the external auditory meatus. To achieve this, the upper back and shoulders should be significantly elevated with pads or blankets to allow the head to be extended at the atlanto-occipital joint. Additional blankets should be used to support the head in this position.

achieved by tilting the operating room table 15 degrees to the left or by placing a wedge under the patient's right buttock. Prevention of aortocaval compression helps preserve cardiac output and uteroplacental blood flow during general anesthesia.

DENITROGENATION (PREOXYGENATION)

Following the induction of general anesthesia, oxyhemoglobin desaturation occurs after a shorter duration of apnea in pregnant women than in nonpregnant patients. During apnea the body's continuing requirements for oxygen are supplied primarily by the FRC. In pregnancy, oxygen requirements are increased and the FRC is decreased, so that oxyhemoglobin desaturation ensues much more rapidly. Therefore, denitrogenation (preoxygenation) of the FRC becomes more important as a mechanism to increase oxygen content and maximize the time before desaturation occurs. A number of techniques have been evaluated for their efficacy in denitrogenating the lungs.

Several investigators have used the partial pressure of oxygen in arterial blood (Pa_{O_2}) as an indirect estimate of the time that may elapse prior to the occurrence of oxyhemoglobin desaturation.[114-116] Some investigators have found that 3 to 5 minutes of normal tidal-volume breathing at a fractional inspired oxygen concentration (F_{IO_2}) of 1.0 resulted in a Pa_{O_2} similar to that after the use of four maximal deep breaths (vital capacity breaths with maximal inspiration and expiration) over 30 seconds (4 DB/30 sec).[114-116] Norris and Dewan,[115] studying pregnant women undergoing rapid-sequence induction of general anesthesia for cesarean delivery, reported similar Pa_{O_2} measurements after the 4 DB/30 sec method and a 3-minute period of preoxygenation. Unfortunately, these results have led to the misconception that the 4 DB/30 sec method affords the same protection against oxyhemoglobin desaturation as the traditional method of 3 to 5 minutes of tidal-volume breathing.[117] However, several studies have refuted this assumption.[118-120] In these studies, preoxygenation with the 4 DB/30 sec method was followed by more rapid desaturation than the traditional method. This occurrence likely reflects the fact that more than 30 seconds are needed to maximize oxygen storage in the tissue and vascular compartments of the body, which also helps explain the longer period of apnea that can be tolerated after 3 to 5 minutes of preoxygenation. During apnea, the time before the onset of arterial oxyhemoglobin desaturation depends on (1) the amount of oxygen stored in the lungs, tissue, and intravascular space; (2) the mixed venous oxyhemoglobin saturation; and (3) the presence or absence of intrapulmonary shunting.[121] Each of these factors plays a role in the more rapid rate of desaturation seen during apnea in children, obese individuals, postoperative patients, and pregnant women.[121]

In a comparison of two techniques of preoxygenation, Rapaport et al.[122] compared 8 deep breaths over 1 minute (8 DB/1 min) with 3 minutes of tidal-volume breathing in obese patients (BMI > 40 kg/m^2). The investigators evaluated end-tidal fractional oxygen concentration (F_{ETO_2}) and the time to oxyhemoglobin desaturation from 100% to 95% ($T_{95\%}$) during apnea. The investigators concluded that the two techniques resulted in similar F_{ETO_2} and $T_{95\%}$ values; however, the implications of hyperventilation and decreased end-tidal CO_2 witnessed in the 8 DB/1 min group were not evaluated. Likewise, Chiron et al.[120] demonstrated that both 3 minutes of tidal-volume breathing and the 8 DB/1 min technique provided more effective preoxygenation in pregnant volunteers at 36 to 38 weeks' gestation than the 4 DB/30 sec method. The 8 DB/1 min method of preoxygenation appears to provide better protection from desaturation during apnea than the 4 DB/30 sec method.[121]

It is wise to apply a tight-fitting face mask and administer oxygen ($F_{IO_2} = 1.0$) as soon as the patient is moved onto the operating table; doing so helps achieve denitrogenation while other preparations are being made. Denitrogenation is more than 95% complete after 3 minutes when the patient breaths through a circle system with a fresh gas flow of 4 L/min or higher and no leak.[119] In the presence of large tidal volumes and a high respiratory rate, the time required for preoxygenation can be very short. However, if tidal volumes are diminished or the respiratory rate is low, a longer duration (i.e., 3 to 5 minutes) of preoxygenation is necessary. In urgent situations, such as an emergency cesarean delivery for significant hemorrhage, the patient should be instructed to take eight deep breaths (8 DB/1 min) to extend the safe interval before oxyhemoglobin desaturation occurs. In extreme situations, when little or no time is available, a 4 deep breath method (4 DB/30 sec) is a rapid way to raise Pa_{O_2} and obtain some protection against oxyhemoglobin desaturation during apnea.

CART AND EQUIPMENT FOR DIFFICULT AIRWAY

A well-stocked difficult airway cart, easily accessible from both the operating room and the labor floor, is essential for every obstetric anesthesia service. The cart should contain a range of laryngoscope blade sizes and styles, smaller-diameter ETTs and stylets, and various alternative devices for securing an airway (i.e., laryngeal mask airway, gum elastic bougie, light wand, needle cricothyrotomy kit). This cart, or an entirely separate cart, should contain fiberoptic equipment, local anesthetic agents for providing topical anesthesia of the airway, and a light source. A cart and laryngoscope that can accommodate a peripheral visual monitor (i.e., a television monitor) is preferable so that more than one provider can visualize the airway field; this capability can be critical for those assisting with external pressure or manipulation to help improve the view of the larynx.

MANAGEMENT

The approach to the difficult airway in the obstetric patient depends on the situation as well as the skills of the anesthesia provider. Figure 30-11 outlines a suggested approach to management of the anticipated difficult airway. In the case of an unanticipated or unrecognized difficult airway, an algorithm should be employed to ensure oxygenation and ventilation. In some cases the simultaneous provision of care for two patients—the mother and the unborn child—may alter the algorithm used for managing the unexpected difficult airway (see later).[21,32,123,124] Lack of forethought and planning can lead to poor decision-making in crisis situations.

Neuraxial Anesthesia

In patients with an anticipated difficult airway undergoing an urgent cesarean delivery and without a previously placed epidural catheter, a neuraxial anesthetic technique (e.g., single-shot spinal anesthesia, combined spinal-epidural anesthesia) may still be preferable to the time-consuming performance of awake fiberoptic intubation. A continuous spinal anesthesia technique offers an alternative that allows for incremental injection of local anesthetic to achieve a desired level and density of anesthesia more quickly than a continuous epidural technique. Because this technique often relies on equipment typically used for placing an epidural catheter (i.e., a 19- or 20-gauge catheter inserted through a 17- or 18-gauge Touhy needle), its use is associated with a significant risk of post–dural puncture headache (see Chapter 31).

Despite optimal planning and execution, a neuraxial anesthesia technique may occasionally fail to provide a surgical blockade of adequate density or duration.[20,32,37,123,125] Therefore, plans for securing the airway must always be considered, and standard airway equipment, as well as alternative devices, should be readily available.

In cases in which extreme difficulty with the airway is expected or known to exist, extra precautions must be taken. An awake intubation should be a primary consideration, and preparations should be made for positioning the patient for optimal intubation conditions and ensuring immediate access to ancillary airway devices, including a means of providing transtracheal jet ventilation. In some cases, acquiring the standby assistance of a surgeon skilled in establishing a surgical airway may be desirable.

Awake Intubation before General Anesthesia

Performing an awake intubation may be the safest option for the patient with an anticipated difficult airway, particularly when a very difficult or impossible mask ventilation is anticipated.[125] The primary advantage to this approach is that the patient maintains her own ventilation through a natural airway (i.e., muscle tone and a partial gag or cough reflex remain intact). Induction of general anesthesia with paralysis can distort the airway anatomy by allowing soft tissue relaxation and movement of the larynx in an anterior direction; this airway distortion can subsequently make attempts at laryngoscopy more difficult. Disadvantages of an awake intubation are patient discomfort and anxiety as well as the time-consuming and often difficult nature of the procedure, particularly for those practitioners who have limited experience with the technique.[32]

A successful awake intubation requires adequate preparation; several steps must be performed for the procedure to go smoothly.[126] An antisialogogue (e.g., glycopyrrolate) should be administered before administration of a

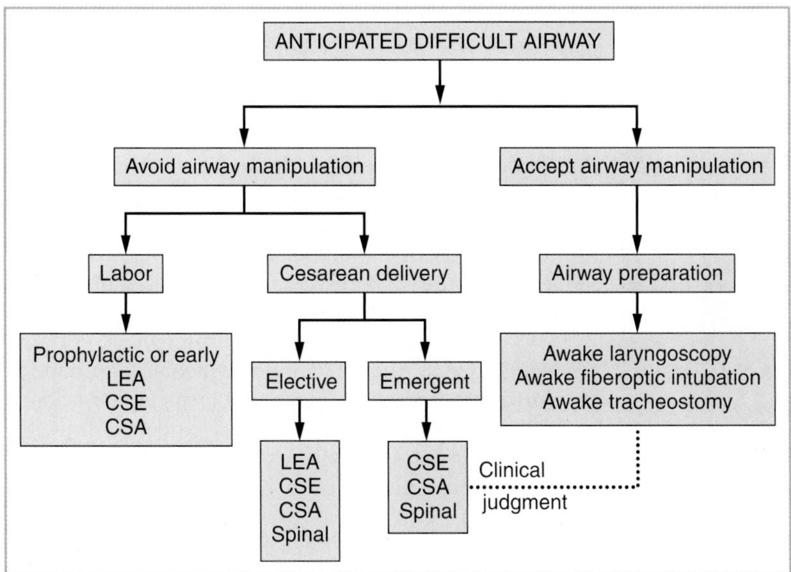

FIGURE 30-11 Algorithm for anticipated difficult airway. This algorithm is not intended to provide comprehensive guidance that addresses every contingency. Rather, it should help anesthesia providers consider the various options that are available. Management should be individualized, and the anesthesia provider's clinical skills and judgment should guide decision-making. For additional information, the reader is referred to the American Society of Anesthesiologists practice guidelines.[12,53] CSA, continuous spinal analgesia or anesthesia technique; CSE, combined spinal-epidural technique; LEA, lumbar epidural analgesia or anesthesia technique; spinal, spinal anesthesia technique.

topical anesthetic. Standard monitoring—pulse oximetry, capnography, continuous electrocardiography (ECG), and blood pressure monitoring—is an absolute necessity. Supplemental oxygen should be administered. The equipment necessary to suction the airway should be immediately available. Sedation with small amounts of a benzodiazepine (e.g., midazolam) should be titrated to the needs of the individual patient; the maintenance of continuous verbal contact is an optimal method for avoiding oversedation.[125,126]

Adequate topical anesthesia of the upper airway is critical to a successful procedure and can be achieved using aerosolized 2% or 4% lidocaine.[126] An easy way to administer topical lidocaine is to use a standard nebulizer with a wall oxygen source (Figure 30-12). Atomization of 2% or 4% lidocaine is another very simple and effective method of providing topical airway anesthesia. Several commercially provided devices are available, such as the Mucosal Atomization Device (Wolfe Tory Medical, Inc., Salt Lake City, UT).

The lingual branch of the glossopharyngeal nerve, which innervates the submucosal pressure receptors at the base of the tongue, can be blocked directly with the bilateral administration of approximately 3 mL of 1% lidocaine just under the mucosa at the base of the anterior tonsillar pillars. The value or necessity of this block during performance of awake intubation in obstetric patients is controversial.[127]

Laryngeal and tracheal sensation can be minimized with blockade of the internal branch of the superior laryngeal nerve and the transtracheal administration of lidocaine, respectively. Blockade of the superior laryngeal nerve may be performed by locating the greater cornu of the hyoid bone, advancing a small-bore needle until the bone is contacted, walking the needle off the edge of the bone into the thyrohyoid membrane, and injecting approximately 3 mL of 1% lidocaine. The technique is then repeated on the other side. An alternative way to anesthetize the airway both above and below the level of the vocal cords is by advancing a fiberoptic laryngoscope to the glottis and injecting lidocaine through the side-port; the lidocaine then exits at the tip of the laryngoscope.

Regardless of which anesthetizing technique(s) is used, it is often difficult to achieve complete airway anesthesia.

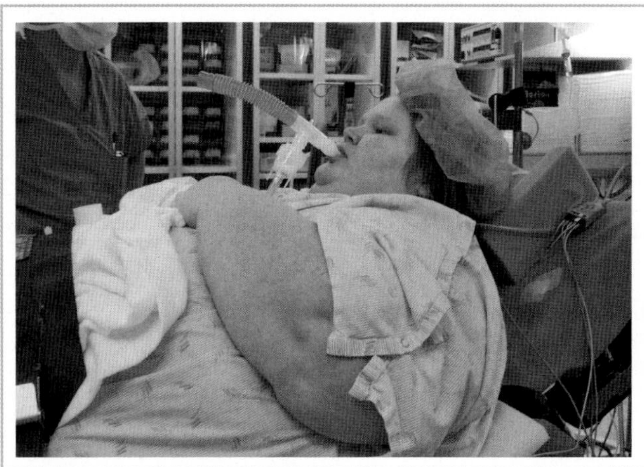

FIGURE 30-12 Technique for providing topical anesthesia of the airway with aerosolized lidocaine.

Total airway anesthesia also raises the concern that the patient's ability to protect her airway may be compromised, especially if sedation is excessive. Thus there is some controversy as to the appropriate use and extent of local anesthesia for awake intubation in a patient with a presumed full stomach. It seems intuitive that total airway anesthesia might pose a risk for aspiration, and some anesthesiologists have recommended preservation of some element of the cough reflex during awake intubation. Others contend, however, that effective airway anesthesia is essential to successful awake intubation. The key to minimizing the risk of aspiration is avoidance of oversedation. Nonetheless, administration of aspiration prophylaxis is advised, and the patient should be monitored for possible reflux or emesis.

Fiberoptic laryngoscopy is the most common method of facilitating awake intubation. Fiberoptic laryngoscopy is less stimulating than direct laryngoscopy and can be performed either orally or nasally. (However, nasal trauma may cause significant nasal bleeding in pregnant women.) The major impediments to successful fiberoptic laryngoscopy are significant amounts of blood or secretions and lack of patient preparation and cooperation. Another common problem occurs when the right arytenoid cartilage or right vocal cord obstructs the ETT as it is passed off the fiberoptic bronchoscope. This problem is corrected by withdrawing the ETT slightly and then rotating it 90 degrees counterclockwise so that the bevel tip and Murphy eye are at the 12 o'clock position.

Direct laryngoscopy results in more noxious stimulation than fiberoptic laryngoscopy, but well prepared and highly motivated patients may tolerate direct laryngoscopy surprisingly well. Other techniques for awake intubation (e.g., blind nasal intubation, retrograde intubation) are performed infrequently in obstetric patients.

Video Fiberoptic Laryngoscopy

Video-assisted fiberoptic laryngoscopes have become available and may prove to be useful in managing the difficult airway in obstetric patients[128]; these devices can be used if conventional laryngoscopy is—or is anticipated to be—difficult. The GlideScope video laryngoscope (Verathon Inc., Bothell, WA) has been shown to provide a better view of the larynx than that provided by standard direct laryngoscopy.[128] Use of the GlideScope has a high rate of successful intubation and has been associated with faster intubation times than the intubating laryngeal mask airway.[129] In addition, this device may be used for awake intubation or to assist fiberoptic intubation.[130,131] However, several reports have described pharyngeal and palatal injury with use of the GlideScope.[132-136] Other video-assisted fiberoptic laryngoscope systems have also been reported to be useful in the management of the difficult airway, including the Direct Coupler Interface video laryngoscope[137] (Karl Storz Endoscopy, Tuttlingen, Germany/Culver City, CA), the McGrath videolaryngoscope[138] (LMA North America, San Diego, CA), the Airway Scope (AWS-S100)[139] (Pentax, Tokyo, Japan), and the TruView EVO2 laryngoscope[140] (a Macintosh-type blade with an attached optical lens; Truphatek International Ltd., Netanya, Israel; distributed by Rusch Inc., Research Triangle Park, NC). These devices may prove useful for difficult intubation in obstetric patients.

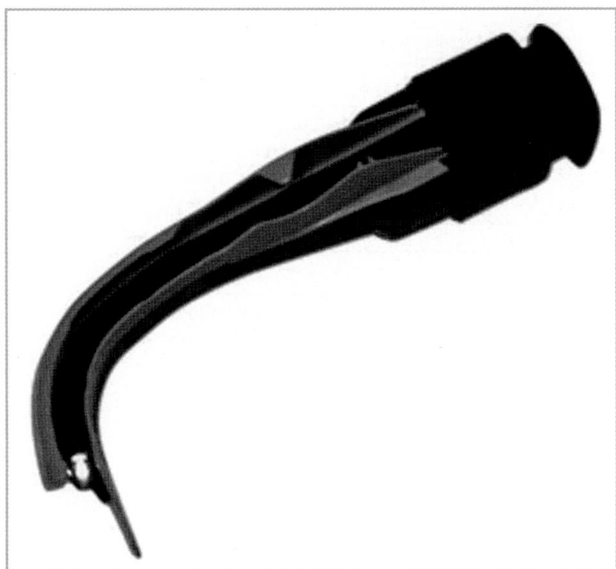

FIGURE 30-13 The Airtraq optical laryngoscope (King Systems Corporation, Noblesville, IN). A disposable indirect laryngoscope that provides a magnified angular view of the larynx and adjacent structures. The device features two separate channels, an optical channel for viewing and a guiding channel for passage of the endotracheal tube. The device also has a low-temperature light for visualization.

The Airtraq (King Systems Corporation, Noblesville, IN) is a new disposable indirect laryngoscope that has been used in patients with a normal airway and also with simulated difficult airways (Figure 30-13). Dhonneur et al.[141] reported the successful use of the Airtraq for endotracheal intubation in two morbidly obese patients undergoing emergency cesarean delivery. The investigators developed a difficult airway algorithm in which the Airtraq was to be used in parturients as a rescue device when endotracheal intubation failed after 2 minutes of direct laryngoscopy. During a 6-month period, 69 parturients underwent emergency cesarean delivery under general anesthesia, of whom 2 required the Airtraq. The investigators suggested that the Airtraq might be an acceptable primary airway management device in cases of emergency cesarean delivery in parturients with an anticipated difficult airway.

Surgery Standby or Awake Tracheostomy

It is possible to perform an awake tracheostomy with local anesthesia, and this technique may be required in some situations in which airway management is anticipated to be extremely difficult and possibly dangerous.[126,142,143] In these cases, particularly if there is known pathology of the airway, it may be prudent to request that a surgical team proficient in emergency surgical airway management be immediately available during the administration of anesthesia for cesarean delivery.

Local Anesthesia for Cesarean Delivery

Rarely the infiltration of local anesthesia may be utilized as a *primary* anesthetic technique for emergency cesarean delivery in the patient with an anticipated difficult airway, primarily in cases in which extreme urgency mandates delivery before the airway can be safely secured. (In addition, local infiltration may be an appropriate anesthetic technique for the rare parturient who is *in extremis*.) This technique, which has been well described, is utilized primarily in developing countries, where contemporary anesthetic techniques may not be readily available.[144-146] Few obstetricians today are familiar or proficient with this technique, but some resident training programs still provide instruction on its use.[14] A large volume (i.e., 75 to 100 mL) of a dilute solution of local anesthetic agent (e.g., 0.5% lidocaine) is often required. Administration of such a large volume of local anesthetic agent entails a risk of systemic local anesthetic toxicity.

In some cases it is possible to perform the entire procedure with local infiltration, provided that the obstetrician makes a midline abdominal incision, makes minimal use of retractors, and does not exteriorize the uterus. Alternatively, the obstetrician might begin surgery and deliver the infant with the aid of local infiltration. Temporary hemostasis may be achieved until the airway is secured, and surgery may be completed after the induction of general anesthesia.

Cesarean delivery performed with local infiltration, if successful, has the advantages of preserving maternal hemodynamic stability and a natural airway while allowing emergency delivery of the infant. However, the technique requires a skilled and patient obstetrician. Maternal anesthesia is typically incomplete and often inadequate, a fact that subsequently presents significant management issues, given that the abdomen has been opened, positioning options are limited, and the consequences of the surgical procedure (e.g., hemorrhage) may require immediate attention.

THE UNANTICIPATED DIFFICULT AIRWAY

Despite attempts to adequately assess parturients preoperatively, cases of unanticipated difficulty with airway management may occur (Figure 30-14).[21] Whether because of an unrecognized anatomic variation, airway edema from preeclampsia, airway changes during labor, or some other unanticipated cause, such patients may undergo induction of general anesthesia without the preanesthesia recognition of potential problems. Initial management consists of repositioning the patient to achieve the proper sniffing position. Use of a different laryngoscope blade, a gum elastic bougie (Eschmann stylet), and/or a smaller-diameter ETT should also be considered. In experienced hands, laryngoscopy attempts should be limited to no more than three, and the second or third attempt should be performed only in those cases in which a portion of the laryngeal anatomy is visible (grade III or better). If a grade IV laryngoscopic view is identified with the initial laryngoscopy attempt, the anesthesia provider should immediately focus attention on ensuring adequate oxygenation and ventilation of the mother.[125,143,147]

Maintenance of maternal and fetal oxygenation is always the first priority. Mask ventilation should be attempted with maintenance of cricoid pressure, and assistance should be requested. Placement of an oral airway may also be helpful. If difficulty is encountered, a two-person mask technique should be employed, with one person firmly holding the mask in place with two hands while providing a jaw lift as

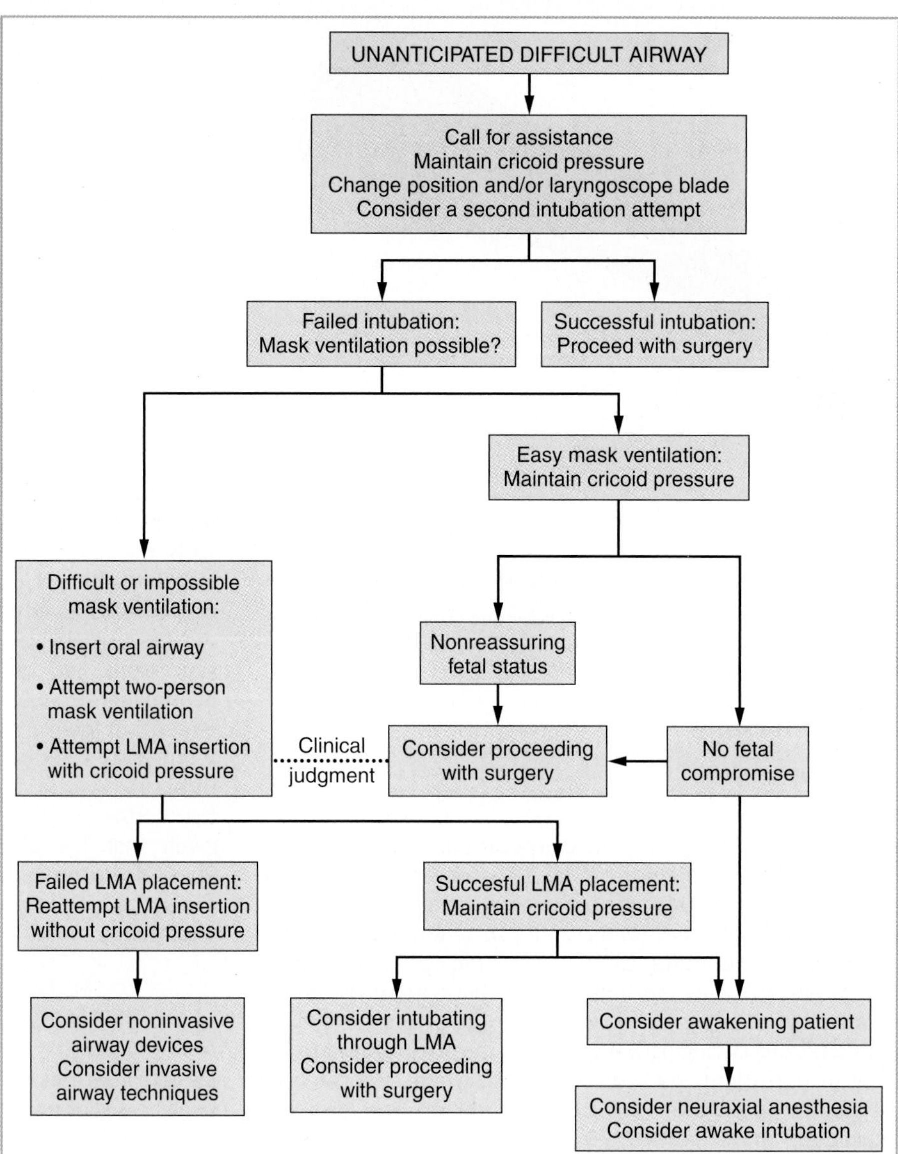

FIGURE 30-14 Unanticipated difficult airway algorithm. This algorithm is not intended to provide comprehensive guidance that addresses every contingency. Rather, it should help anesthesia providers consider the various options that are available. Management should be individualized, and the anesthesia provider's clinical skills and judgment should guide decision-making. For additional information, the reader is referred to the American Society of Anesthesiologists practice guidelines.[12,53] LMA, laryngeal mask airway.

the second person squeezes the reservoir bag.[14,21] Consideration should be given to awakening the mother, if possible, and utilizing a different anesthetic technique if her oxyhemoglobin saturation can be maintained.[125] Once mask ventilation is attempted, several scenarios may arise, which are discussed below.

Cannot Intubate but Can Ventilate

In the "cannot intubate but can ventilate" scenario, the maternal and fetal status should be assessed in consultation with the obstetrician. If the mother and the fetus are not considered to be in any immediate jeopardy, the most conservative (and often the most prudent) course is to awaken the mother, especially when another skilled anesthesia provider is not immediately available to provide assistance.[14,21,125] Once this is accomplished, other anesthetic options, such as an awake intubation or a neuraxial anesthetic technique, should be contemplated. Alternatively, the anesthesia provider may consider proceeding with surgery; however, this option represents an elective commitment to the possibility of mask airway failure, more airway manipulation, and a risk of progression to a "cannot ventilate" scenario.

If the mother is considered to be in immediate jeopardy secondary to hemorrhage (e.g., uterine rupture, placental abruption), it may be necessary to proceed with cesarean delivery to optimize outcome for both the mother and the baby. Significant angst and controversy often accompany decision-making in the management of a stable mother with evidence of life-threatening fetal compromise (e.g., fetal bradycardia as a result of a prolapsed umbilical cord). In such cases, if mask ventilation is easy and adequate, the risk/benefit ratio of proceeding with an unsecured airway and an increased risk of aspiration should be weighed against the benefits of prompt delivery of the infant. In cases where the maternal risk of aspiration is considered low and mask ventilation is easy, it may be reasonable to continue mask ventilation and avoid further intubation attempts. It is unclear as to whether continued mask ventilation or repeated intubation attempts represents the greater risk to the mother; even insertion of a laryngeal mask airway may further traumatize the airway or precipitate regurgitation.[125]

The anesthesia provider should carefully consider the maternal risks of proceeding with cesarean delivery in a mother with an unsecured and unprotected airway, especially when no urgency exists and/or in patients in whom mask ventilation is difficult. Some obstetric anesthesiologists argue that even a nonreassuring (but non-life-threatening) fetal heart rate tracing does not always justify proceeding with cesarean delivery under general anesthesia in a patient with an unsecured airway. On the other hand, in some of these cases, proceeding with cesarean delivery (via mask ventilation or with a laryngeal mask airway) may be a better option than awakening the patient, especially in patients in whom neuraxial techniques are contraindicated. In these cases, the importance of open and honest communication between the obstetric and anesthesia teams cannot be overemphasized (see Chapter 33).

Cannot Intubate and Cannot Ventilate

In the "cannot intubate and cannot ventilate" scenario, the first objective remains the maintenance of maternal and fetal oxygenation. If partial ventilation exists and succinylcholine has been given, it may be possible to allow the neuromuscular blockade to resolve and spontaneous ventilation to return. Assistance should be summoned, and if attempted mask ventilation fails, the head and neck should be repositioned, and an attempt at two-person mask ventilation should be made. If these efforts fail, the following emergency rescue options are available: (1) insertion of a laryngeal mask airway, (2) insertion of an alternative supralaryngeal airway device (e.g., laryngeal tube), (3) needle cricothyrotomy with transtracheal jet ventilation, and (4) emergency cricothyrotomy or tracheostomy. Should these noninvasive or invasive airway devices and methods prove successful, the risks and benefits of proceeding with surgery should be discussed among team members; both maternal and fetal health should be considered. A 14- or 16-gauge catheter placed by needle cricothyroidotomy is inherently unstable; ideally a more definitive airway should be established before surgery is commenced (see later).[14,21,125]

Laryngeal Mask Airway

The introduction of the laryngeal mask airway (LMA) into anesthesia practice was a significant advance in airway management that has resulted in a major alteration of the ASA Difficult Airway Algorithm.[12] The insertion of an LMA in an obstetric patient who can easily be ventilated by face mask is somewhat controversial, because little additional ventilation benefit is obtained, and the placement of an LMA can induce vomiting and aspiration in this setting.[126] However, in any situation in which conventional mask ventilation is difficult or impossible, the LMA is the rescue device of choice.

The LMA has many advantages, most notably its ease of use and a very high initial success rate.[148] Moreover, the LMA need not be perfectly positioned over the larynx to allow adequate ventilation. When assessed by flexible fiberoptic endoscopy, radiography, and magnetic resonance imaging, the placement of the LMA around the larynx is variable[148]; however, 94% to 99% of patients with an LMA have little or no difficulty with ventilation.

In a prospective study, an LMA was inserted by experienced users in 1067 healthy parturients undergoing *elective* cesarean delivery under general anesthesia.[149] The investigators demonstrated that a clinically effective and acceptable airway was obtained on the first attempt in 98% of the patients, and on the second or third attempt in an additional 1%. Fewer than 1% of patients required intubation for failure to obtain satisfactory LMA placement within 90 seconds, Spo_2 less than 94%, or end-tidal CO_2 greater than 45 mm Hg. Moreover, the airway management (which was accomplished with the LMA, maintenance of cricoid pressure until delivery, and mechanical tidal-volume ventilation of 8 to 12 mL/kg), was associated with no episodes of hypoxemia ($Spo_2 < 90\%$), regurgitation, aspiration, laryngospasm, bronchospasm, or gastric insufflation. The investigators concluded that in experienced hands, an LMA is effective and "probably safe" for ventilation and the administration of a volatile anesthetic agent for general anesthesia in selected healthy patients undergoing elective cesarean delivery.[149]

A number of reports have described the use of an LMA as a rescue device for obstetric patients in whom conventional methods of securing the airway have failed.[150-155] Moreover, an LMA can act as a conduit for intubation and can facilitate fiberoptic intubation with a bronchoscope[156]; the success rate of fiberoptic intubation performed in this manner has approached 100% in some studies.[148]

Despite these benefits, the LMA has been associated with the following disadvantages: (1) placement can induce vomiting; (2) aspiration of gastric contents is not prevented; (3) improper positioning can lead to gastric insufflation; (4) multiple insertion attempts may be required for proper placement, which may result in airway trauma; and (5) use of positive-pressure ventilation may be limited.[125] In approximately 0.4% to 0.6% of patients with normal airway findings, the placement of an LMA leads to inadequate clinical ventilation[125]; reasons for this outcome have been reported to include (1) backfolding of the distal cuff, (2) occlusion of the glottis by the distal cuff, (3) complete downfolding of the epiglottis, and (4) 90- to 180-degree rotation of the mask around its long axis.[125]

Several variations in the original classic LMA design have become available. The most useful of these in a difficult airway situation in the parturient are the Fastrach LMA (LMA North America, San Diego, CA) and the ProSeal LMA (LMA North America). The Fastrach or intubating LMA was designed specifically to act as a conduit for blind tracheal intubation, but it also can be combined with fiberoptic bronchoscopy (Figure 30-15).[157,158] Both reusable and disposable versions are available. When properly placed, the intubating LMA allows ventilation similar to that with the original LMA; however, a more rigid J-shaped design improves the alignment of the mask over the glottic opening and better accommodates a special soft-tipped ETT for blind intubation. This special silicone ETT minimizes the risk of airway trauma and is available in diameter sizes 6.0 to 8.0 mm. In addition, the intubating LMA has an epiglottis elevator bar at its distal end that acts to lift the epiglottis anteriorly as the ETT exits the intubating LMA into the glottis.[159] When a fiberoptic bronchoscope is used with an intubating LMA, the ETT should be introduced far enough to partially elevate the epiglottis

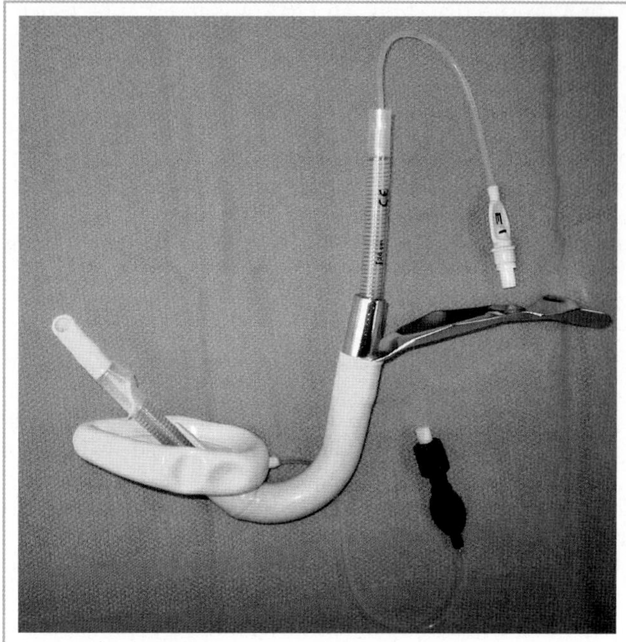

FIGURE 30-15 Intubating laryngeal mask airway (LMA). This device features a more rigid J-shaped design than the conventional LMA to facilitate the alignment of the mask over the glottic opening and better accommodate a special soft-tipped endotracheal tube for blind intubation.

elevator bar because it can damage or hamper the passage of the fiberoptic scope into the trachea. A variation of the intubating LMA, the Air-Q LMA (Mercury Medical, Clearwater, FL) has a different mask tip, a keyhole-shaped airway outlet, and a removable circuit connector that accommodates an 8.5-mm ETT (Figure 30-16). To date, there have been no published reports of the use of this device in parturients.

The ProSeal LMA has a specialized high-volume/low-pressure cuff that allows the device to achieve a better fit over the glottis (Figure 30-17).[160] This allows the use of higher ventilation pressures (up to 30 to 40 cm H_2O) with less air leakage around the cuff and a lower risk of air entry into the stomach. The ProSeal LMA also contains a specialized drainage tube that bypasses the bowl of the LMA and prevents gastric fluid from entering the glottic area. Additionally, a gastric tube can be passed down this gastric lumen to empty (or decompress) the stomach; it has been shown to be effective in venting both passive and active regurgitation.[161,162]

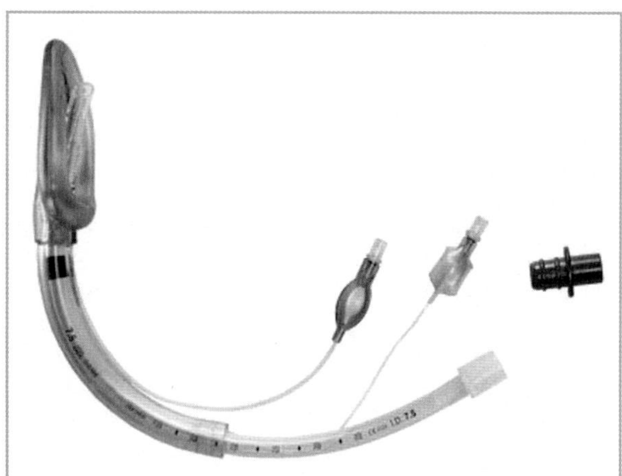

FIGURE 30-16 The Air-Q LMA (laryngeal mask airway) (Mercury Medical, Clearwater, FL). This intubating LMA device features a unique mask tip, a keyhole-shaped airway outlet that elevates the epiglottis, and a removable circuit connector that accommodates an 8.5-mm endotracheal tube (ETT). The LMA depicted has an ETT within its lumen.

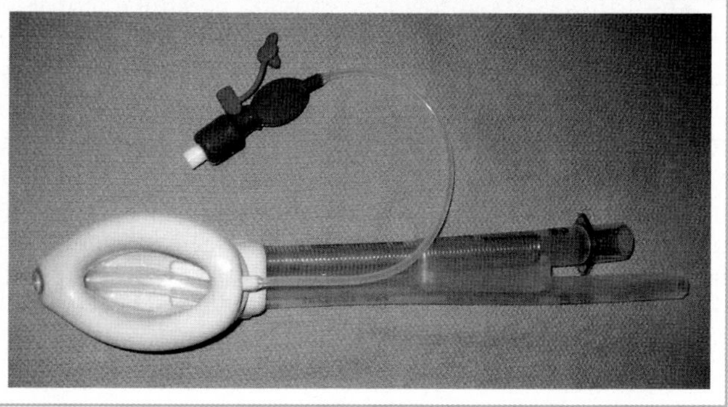

FIGURE 30-17 The ProSeal LMA (laryngeal mask airway) (LMA North America, San Diego, CA). This LMA device has a specialized high-volume/low-pressure cuff, which allows glottis coverage that enables the use of higher ventilation pressures (up to 30-40 cm H_2O) with less air leakage around the cuff and a lower risk of entry of air into the stomach. The ProSeal LMA also contains a specialized drainage tube that bypasses the bowl of the LMA and prevents gastric fluid from entering the glottic area. A gastric tube can be passed down this drainage lumen to assist in emptying the stomach contents.

Evans et al.[163] assessed insertion characteristics, airway seal pressures, hemodynamic responses to insertion, ease of gastric tube placement, gastric insufflation, and postoperative discomfort associated with the use of the ProSeal LMA in 300 anesthetized adults. The investigators concluded that the ProSeal is a reliable supralaryngeal airway device that can provide an effective glottic seal in both paralyzed and nonparalyzed patients. They also demonstrated easy passage of a gastric tube, minimal hemodynamic responses to insertion, and an acceptable incidence of sore throat. Cook et al.[164] randomly assigned 180 nonparalyzed anesthetized patients to undergo placement of either the ProSeal or the original, "classic" LMA. The investigators found that the ProSeal more reliably allowed positive-pressure ventilation; this feature, combined with the ability to vent regurgitant material, may make it an attractive choice for obstetric patients.

The ProSeal LMA has been utilized effectively in parturients for rescue after failed intubation, for postoperative respiratory support, and during electroconvulsive therapy in a woman at 20 to 22 weeks' gestation.[165] One potential disadvantage of the device is that the drainage tube traversing the bowl of the LMA might make passage of an ETT more difficult.[166]

THE LARYNGEAL MASK AIRWAY AND CRICOID PRESSURE

With the possible exception of the ProSeal, an LMA does not protect against aspiration, and its placement may precipitate regurgitation in a lightly anesthetized patient.[167] Therefore, it is generally recommended that continuous cricoid pressure be maintained after the placement of an

LMA in obstetric patients. Although a properly placed LMA does not appear to compromise the effectiveness of cricoid pressure,[168] the use of cricoid pressure can inhibit proper insertion of the LMA and, in some cases, may make correct insertion impossible (see Figure 30-7).[111,112,169-172] The application of cricoid pressure can prevent the tip of the LMA from fully occupying the hypopharynx behind the arytenoid and cricoid cartilages. Therefore, if difficulty with insertion of an LMA is encountered during an obstetric airway emergency, consideration should be given to releasing cricoid pressure temporarily while a second attempt is made to insert an LMA.[170] The risk of hypoxia from failed LMA placement is most likely greater than the small risk of aspiration due to the temporary release of cricoid pressure. Several authors have reported that this maneuver increases the chances of a successful LMA placement. Once the LMA is in place, cricoid pressure can be reapplied and should not prohibit adequate ventilation.[168] However, in some patients, reapplication of cricoid pressure may decrease tidal volumes during positive-pressure ventilation through an LMA.[173] Difficult ventilation after placement of an LMA should raise suspicion of overzealous administration of cricoid pressure; in such cases, a reduction in the force of cricoid pressure typically allows adequate ventilation.

THE LARYNGEAL MASK AIRWAY AS A CONDUIT FOR INTUBATION

Intubation through an LMA can be achieved blindly, especially with an intubating LMA, or with the assistance of a fiberoptic bronchoscope. Before this maneuver is begun, the risks and benefits of an intubation attempt must be weighed.[174] Intubation attempts should never supersede or compromise active ventilation; however, in certain situations, such as a patient at significant risk for aspiration or when current ventilation is marginal, securing the airway with an ETT may take precedence. The use of a fiberoptic bronchoscope through the LMA has been reported to be nearly 100% successful.[148] A 6-mm internal diameter (ID) cuffed ETT may be passed over the fiberoptic bronchoscope and through the shaft of a size 3 or 4 LMA; of note, a nasal RAE tube (Nellcor, Boulder, CO) is a suitable match for this purpose owing to its adequate length and widespread availability. A 7-mm ID cuffed ETT may be passed in a similar manner through the shaft of a size 5 LMA. If a larger ETT is desired, a smaller ETT should be placed, followed by passage of an airway exchange catheter; the LMA and ETT are then withdrawn, and a new ETT is placed over the exchange catheter.

When a fiberoptic bronchoscope is passed through an LMA, the bronchoscope should be placed through a self-sealing diaphragm of an elbow adapter attached to the ETT and the airway circuit to allow continuous ventilation (Figure 30-18). The space available for ventilation around a 4-mm outer diameter (OD) fiberoptic bronchoscope placed within a 6-mm ID ETT is equivalent to that available with a 4.5-mm ID ETT.[126,151] A fiberoptic bronchoscope also can be placed through the lumen of an Aintree Exchange Catheter (Cook Critical Care, Bloomington, IN) and passed through a size 3 LMA. The LMA subsequently can be removed over the catheter, followed by the placement of an ETT.

Laryngeal Tube and Combitube

The laryngeal tube (VBM Medizintechnik, Sulz, Germany, and King Systems Corporation, Noblesville, IN) is another supraglottic airway device introduced into clinical practice.[175-177] Laryngeal tubes are manufactured from either silicone or polyvinylchloride (PVC) and have ventilation apertures between a proximal oropharyngeal cuff and a distal esophageal cuff. The laryngeal tube is inserted into the oropharynx until resistance is met, which should result in positioning of the ventilation apertures directly above the glottic opening. These devices are reported to provide seal pressures similar to those with the ProSeal LMA (e.g., 40 cm H_2O), and insertion times and success rates comparable to those with the LMA.[178,179] The Laryngeal Tube-S (LTS) contains a second lumen that can be used for drainage of the stomach.[180] The LTS has been used successfully after a failed intubation and ventilation in a patient undergoing emergency cesarean delivery.[181]

The esophageal-tracheal Combitube (ETC) (Sheridan Catheter Corporation, Argyle, NY) is a plastic, twin-lumen tube with an outer diameter of 13 mm. One lumen has an open distal end and thus resembles an ETT (i.e., the tracheal lumen), and the other (esophageal) lumen has a closed distal end. A 100-mL proximal pharyngeal balloon is located on the ETC, so that when the ETC is properly positioned, the pharyngeal balloon fills the space between the base of the tongue and the soft palate. The inflated proximal balloon serves to seal the oral and nasal cavities. Just distal to the pharyngeal balloon but proximal to the level of the larynx are eight perforations in the esophageal lumen. A smaller, 15-mL distal cuff (similar to an ETT cuff) serves to seal either the esophagus or trachea when inflated. The ETC is inserted with or without the aid of a laryngoscope, but its insertion does not require visualization of the larynx. (In the usual clinical context, the larynx cannot be visualized). The ETC usually (96% of the time) enters the esophagus, and the patient can be ventilated by means of the esophageal lumen perforations. If the ETC enters the trachea, the patient can be ventilated directly through the tracheal lumen. In terms of ability to ventilate the patient, it does not matter whether the ETC enters the trachea or the esophagus. Adequate ventilation can be provided, assuming the anesthesia provider correctly identifies which lumen should be used for ventilation purposes.

The ETC allows adequate ventilation while preventing aspiration of gastric contents. Use of the ETC has resulted in adequate ventilation and oxygenation under diverse clinical conditions (e.g., failed intubation during surgery, cardiopulmonary resuscitation, respiratory failure in the intensive care unit). In the esophageal position, the unused tracheal lumen can be connected to a suction device for aspiration of gastric fluids. Exchange of the ETC for an ETT should be considered if long-term ventilation is anticipated or required.

Use of the ETC in the out-of-hospital setting has been associated with a notable incidence of serious complications, including upper airway bleeding, esophageal laceration and perforation, and mediastinitis.[182] Although a lower incidence of serious complications would be expected in the more controlled operating room environment (with an anesthesiologist using a laryngoscope to facilitate placement of the ETC), the stiffness and the anterior curvature of

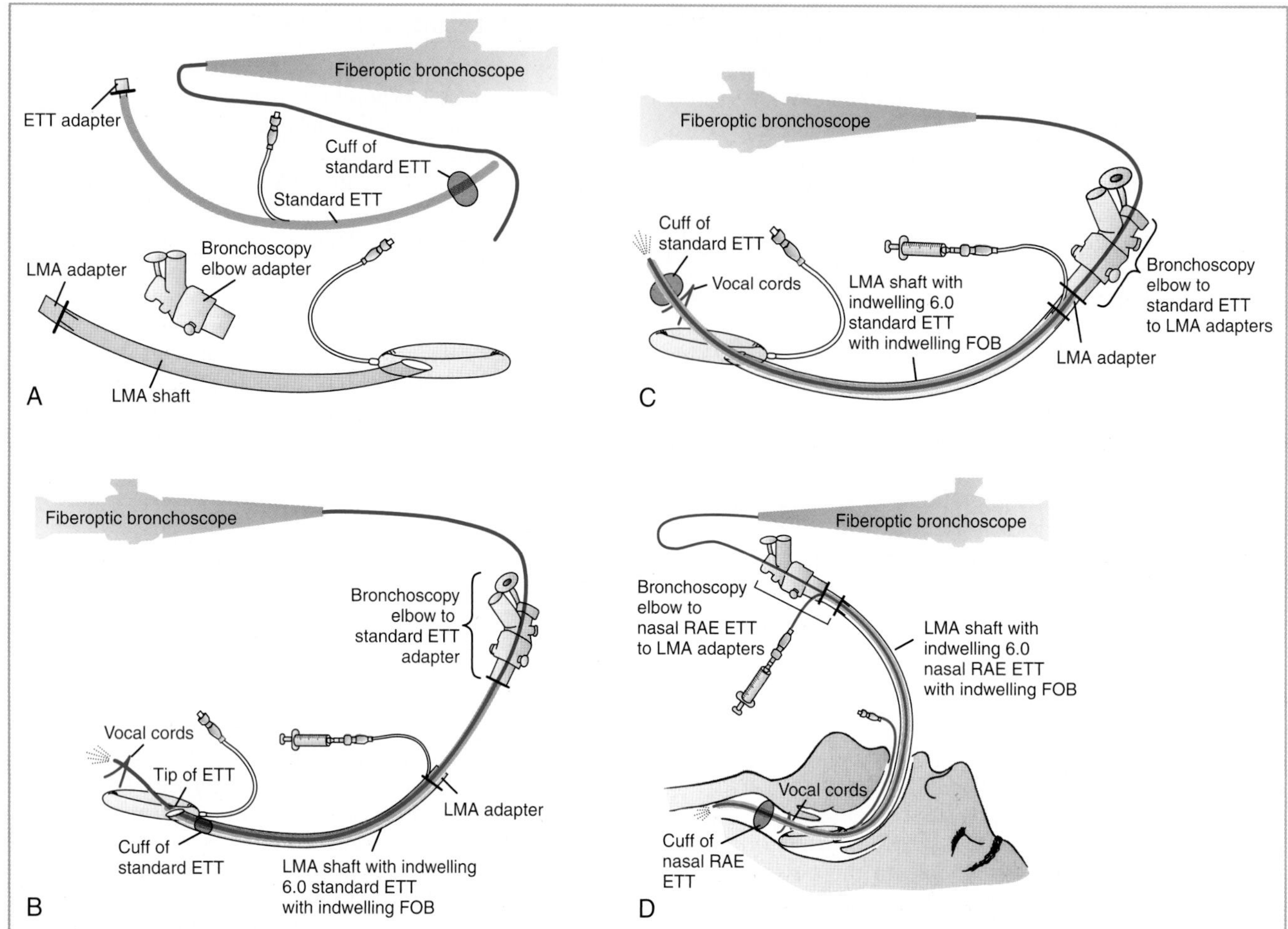

FIGURE 30-18 Schematic diagram showing that a patient can be continuously ventilated during fiberoptic tracheal intubation through use of the laryngeal mask airway (LMA) as a conduit for both the endotracheal tube (ETT) and the fiberoptic bronchoscope (FOB). In **A** and **B,** a standard 28-cm-long ETT is shown. A 6-mm inner diameter nasal RAE tube may also be used. **A,** Components of the continuous ventilation system. **B,** With passage of the tip of a cuffed 6-mm inner diameter ETT to the level of the grille on the LMA and a 4-mm outer diameter FOB through the self-sealing diaphragm of a bronchoscopy elbow adapter, ventilation can occur around the FOB but within the lumen of the ETT; the deflated cuff of the ETT inside the shaft of the LMA makes an airtight seal and permits positive-pressure ventilation. **C,** Once the FOB is passed well into the trachea, the 6-mm inner diameter ETT is pushed over the FOB into the trachea until the adapter of the ETT is near the adapter of the LMA (nasal RAE tube, Nellcor, Boulder, CO) or is flush up against the adapter of the LMA (standard ETT). The preformed curvature of the nasal RAE tube presents no problem with insertion if the outside of the tube is adequately lubricated. **D,** Schematic of **C,** with superimposed upper airway anatomy.

the ETC, as well as the potential for balloon overinflation, still represent potential sources of airway and esophageal injury.[182]

Transtracheal Jet Ventilation

Despite the use of advanced airway management techniques and devices, inadequate oxygenation and ventilation still occur. In these situations, the use of needle cricothyrotomy and subsequent transtracheal jet ventilation (TTJV) can be life sustaining for both the mother and the fetus. In most cases the percutaneous placement of a 14- or 16-gauge intravenous catheter through the cricothyroid membrane and into the trachea can be done quickly and with relatively few risks. Needle cricothyrotomy is faster and carries significantly fewer risks than emergency tracheostomy.[183,184] The catheter should be attached to a small syringe, and after needle insertion into the trachea, air should be freely aspirated and then the catheter introduced. Once in place, the catheter should be held firmly, so that it does not become kinked or dislodged while performing jet ventilation; when possible, one person should be assigned to perform this duty. Air should be aspirated again from the catheter to confirm tracheal placement, and then the hub of the catheter should be connected to a TTJV system (several commercial systems are available) and a high-pressure oxygen source (approximately 20 to 50 pounds per square inch [psi]); this amount of pressure is required to deliver oxygen through the tubing and high- resistance catheter.[14] Central oxygen sources, such as a wall source, must be downregulated to avoid barotrauma to the lungs.[183]

Most TTJV systems have an inline regulator that allows the pressure to be controlled to between 0 and 50 psi. A pressure of 20 to 30 psi is adequate to provide appropriate tidal volumes (V_T) and minute ventilation (V_E) for the majority of patients. During TTJV, it is critical that the operator allow time for exhalation of inspired gas to avoid hyperinflation of the lungs, potential air trapping, and barotrauma. Moreover, the airway should be kept patent by some means (nasal/oral airway, jaw thrust) to

BOX 30-2 Considerations for Minimizing the Risk of Barotrauma during Transtracheal Jet Ventilation (TTJV)

Clinical Considerations for Minimizing Barotrauma	Rationale
1. Reaspirate/reconfirm free flow of air through the catheter prior to TTJV.	1. Ensures correct placement of catheter in tracheal lumen after initial identification of tracheal lumen.
2. Use a preassembled, commercially made TTJV system that has an additional inline pressure regulator (0-50 psi).	2. Obtains the quality assurance associated with a commercial product and the ability to downregulate standard wall gas pressure to a lower level (see #3).
3. Preset the additional inline regulator at 25 to 30 psi. Setting can be increased incrementally by 5 to 10 psi at a time if necessary.	3. Minimizes risk of barotrauma and, with a 14- to 16-gauge catheter, maintains efficacy.
4. Use a 0.5-second inspiratory time.	4. Minimizes risk of barotrauma and, with a 14- to 16-gauge catheter, maintains efficacy.
5. Ensure maximal upper airway patency by *continuously* maintaining bilateral jaw thrust and by placing oropharyngeal and nasopharyngeal airways.	5. Exhalation occurs *only* through a patent upper airway.

facilitate exhalation.[14,183] Box 30-2 lists several important clinical considerations involved in minimizing the risks of barotrauma (e.g., subcutaneous air, pneumomediastinum, pneumothorax) during TTJV.[185-187] There are numerous reports of the use of TTJV as a means to prevent hypoxia during life-threatening airway emergencies[184,188-190] and as a temporizing measure before a more definitive surgical airway can be established.

EXTUBATION OF THE PATIENT WITH A DIFFICULT AIRWAY

In cases in which intubation was difficult, consideration should be given to the possibility of airway compromise after extubation. This issue is particularly important in obstetric patients who are obese, have a history of obstructive sleep apnea, received a large amount of fluid and/or blood products, had a lengthy surgical procedure, and/or have a disease process that may increase the risk of development of airway edema (e.g., preeclampsia).[191,192] These concerns are highlighted by the number of anesthetic deaths in parturients involving airway obstruction or hypoventilation, the majority of which occurred during emergence from anesthesia, following extubation, or in the postanesthesia period.[26] Patients considered to be at risk for postoperative airway obstruction or hypoventilation should be monitored appropriately with continuous pulse oximetry and dedicated nursing care.

Predicting Difficulty with Extubation

Studies attempting to clearly identify risk factors that can reliably predict difficulty with extubation have been inconclusive.[193-195] Demling et al.[194] prospectively examined the use of standard criteria for extubation in 700 consecutive surgical intensive care unit (ICU) patients and could not identify any good predictors for extubation failure. Many practitioners use the **leak test** in patients with the potential for airway edema as a method of evaluating whether the airway caliber is sufficient for ventilation; however, its routine use remains controversial.[196-198] One performs the test by deflating the ETT cuff, occluding the proximal end of the ETT, and evaluating whether the patient can spontaneously ventilate around the ETT. Although several investigators have reported that this is a useful test that predicts successful extubation, this finding has not been uniformly demonstrated.[196-198] In one evaluation of the leak test in 72 spontaneously breathing ICU patients, the presence of a cuff leak indicated that extubation was likely to be successful.[199] In another study, however, a negative leak test result did not indicate that extubation would uniformly fail.[200] The researchers recommended that in patients with no cuff leak, extubation should be carried out only in the presence of experienced personnel who can manage the potentially difficult airway and re-intubation. Ideally, extubation should be performed in a controlled setting and after a full assessment of the patient (i.e., ability to follow commands, appropriate level of consciousness).

Use of Airway Exchange Catheters and Other Preventive Measures

The placement of an airway exchange catheter (AEC) through an ETT can add a measure of safety to the extubation process.[201,202] After removal of the ETT, the AEC can be used to (1) re-intubate by providing a conduit to the airway (i.e., an ETT can be placed over the exchange catheter into the trachea); (2) provide oxygen via its central lumen either for passive oxygenation or jet ventilation; and (3) intermittently measure P_{ECO_2} from the trachea.[202] There are many commercially available AECs (Cook Critical Care [Bloomington, IN], Sheridan Catheter Corporation [Argyle, NY], and CardioMed Supplies [Gormley, Ontario, Canada]). Many of the AECs are manufactured especially for the purposes just described, with appropriate markings for centimeter depth, and are available in a variety of sizes. Some of these products have a removable, malleable stylet that allows the clinician to shape the AEC and use it as an intubating stylet. AECs with larger diameters enable greater re-intubation success and allow easier intraluminal ventilation; however, spontaneous breathing around the AEC is more difficult. Successful re-intubation can be enhanced by the use of a smaller ETT and rotation of the ETT 90 degrees during insertion to facilitate passage of the bevel through the vocal cords.[202]

In all patients, with or without a difficult airway, routine measures should be applied prior to extubation. All tubes (e.g., ETT, nasogastric) should be suctioned, and the oropharynx and nasopharynx cleared of any excess secretions or blood. Laryngospasm after extubation is often precipitated by the presence of secretions.[203] As with the procedure used prior to intubation, the patient should be given 100% oxygen for at least 3 to 5 minutes to provide adequate denitrogenation and oxygenation. The lungs are then inflated to near total capacity just prior to deflation of the ETT cuff and extubation; this technique causes the patient to cough, owing to the high expiratory flow generated during the elastic recoil of the lungs, thus clearing secretions from the vocal cords and airway.

KEY POINTS

- The potential morbidity and mortality associated with airway management in the parturient remain a significant concern to the obstetric anesthesia provider.
- Physiologic and anatomic changes associated with pregnancy (e.g., airway edema, respiratory and metabolic changes, weight gain, enlarged breasts, risk of gastroesophageal reflux) can further contribute to difficulty with airway management.
- Predicting potential airway difficulties can be accomplished with simple bedside assessments, including assessment of Mallampati class, thyromental distance, atlanto-occipital extension, and the ability to protrude the mandible.
- Prophylactic or early administration of epidural analgesia in high-risk parturients, including those who are morbidly obese or have an anticipated difficult airway, should be encouraged.
- Pharmacologic aspiration prophylaxis should be administered to all parturients requiring surgical intervention regardless of whether they receive neuraxial or general anesthesia.
- Correctly positioning the patient on the operating room table in order to maximize the chance of a successful intubation is a critical step that is often overlooked.
- Securing an airway while the patient remains awake may be the safest route that can be taken in a patient whose airway is expected to be difficult.
- The maintenance of maternal and fetal oxygenation should be the primary goal in the management of an unanticipated difficult airway.
- In any situation in which conventional mask ventilation is difficult or impossible, the laryngeal mask airway is the rescue device of choice.
- Needle cricothyrotomy and subsequent transtracheal jet ventilation can be life sustaining when other means have failed to achieve adequate oxygenation.
- In parturients with a history of a difficult intubation or who exhibit risk factors for a difficult airway, caution should be employed with both intubation and extubation.
- There should be open communication with the obstetric team regarding parturients with comorbid conditions, including potential airway concerns. Management decisions should incorporate multidisciplinary communication and cooperation.

REFERENCES

1. Tunstall ME. Failed intubation in the parturient. Can J Anaesth 1989; 36:611-3.
2. Tsen LC, Pitner R, Camann WR. General anesthesia for cesarean section at a tertiary care hospital 1990-1995: Indications and implications. Int J Obstet Anesth 1998; 7:147-52.
3. Panni MK, Camann WR, Tsen LC. Resident training in obstetric anesthesia in the United States. Int J Obstet Anesth 2006; 15:284-9.
4. Russell R. Failed intubation in obstetrics: A self-fulfilling prophecy. Int J Obstet Anesth 2006; 16:1-3.
5. Samsoon GL, Young JR. Difficult tracheal intubation: A retrospective study. Anaesthesia 1987; 42:487-90.
6. Cormack RS, Lehane JR. Intubation training in the real world: A defence of the Northwick Park drill. Anaesthesia 2007; 62:975-8.
7. Barnardo PD, Jenkins JG. Failed tracheal intubation in obstetrics: A 6-year review in a UK region. Anaesthesia 2000; 55:690-4.
8. Hawthorne L, Wilson R, Lyons G, Dresner M. Failed intubation revisited: 17-yr experience in a teaching maternity unit. Br J Anaesth 1996; 76:680-4.
9. Rahman K, Jenkins JG. Failed tracheal intubation in obstetrics: No more frequent but still managed badly. Anaesthesia 2005; 60: 168-71.
10. Cooper GM, McClure JH. Maternal deaths from anaesthesia: An extract from *Why Mothers Die 2000-2002*, the Confidential Enquiries into Maternal Deaths in the United Kingdom. Chapter 9: Anaesthesia. Br J Anaesth 2005; 94:417-23.
11. D'Angelo R. Anesthesia-related maternal mortality: A pat on the back or a call to arms? Anesthesiology 2007; 106:1082-4.
12. American Society of Anesthesiologists Task Force on Management of the Difficult Airway. Practice guidelines for management of the difficult airway. Anesthesiology 2003; 98:1269-77.
13. Caplan RA, Posner KL, Ward RJ, Cheney FW. Adverse respiratory events in anesthesia: A closed claims analysis. Anesthesiology 1990; 72:828-33.
14. Munnur U, de Boisblanc B, Suresh MS. Airway problems in pregnancy. Crit Care Med 2005; 33:S259-68.
15. Clutton-Brock T. Maternal deaths from anaesthesia: An extract from *Why Mothers Die 2000-2002*, the Confidential Enquiries into Maternal Deaths in the United Kingdom. Chapter 17: Trends in intensive care. Br J Anaesth 2005; 94:424-9.
16. Enohumah KO, Imarengiaye CO. Factors associated with anaesthesia-related maternal mortality in a tertiary hospital in Nigeria. Acta Anaesthesiol Scand 2006; 50:206-10.
17. Hawkins JL. Anesthesia-related maternal mortality. Clin Obstet Gynecol 2003; 46:679-87.
18. Hawkins JL, Koonin LM, Palmer SK. Anesthesia-related deaths during obstetric delivery in the United States, 1979-1990. Anesthesiology 1997; 86:277-84.
19. Hawkins JL, Chang J, Palmer SK, et al. Anesthesia-related maternal mortality in the United States, 1997-2002 (abstract). Oral presentation at the 2008 Annual Meeting of the Society for Obstetric Anesthesia and Perinatology, Chicago, IL, April 30-May 4, 2008.
20. Chestnut DH. Anesthesia and maternal mortality. Anesthesiology 1997; 86:273-6.
21. Suresh MS. Difficult airway in the parturient. Probl Anesth 2001; 13:88-99.
22. Dennehy KC, Pian-Smith MC. Airway management of the parturient. Int Anesthesiol Clin 2000; 38:147-59.
23. Hamilton BE, Martin JA, Ventura SJ. Births: Preliminary data for 2005. Natl Vital Stat Rep 2006; 55:1-18.
24. Saravanakumar K, Rao SG, Cooper GM. The challenges of obesity and obstetric anaesthesia. Curr Opin Obstet Gynecol 2006; 18:631-5.
25. Endler GC, Mariona FG, Sokol RJ, Stevenson LB. Anesthesia-related maternal mortality in Michigan, 1972 to 1984. Am J Obstet Gynecol 1988; 159:187-93.
26. Mhyre JM, Riesner MN, Polley LS, Naughton NN. A series of anesthesia-related maternal deaths in Michigan, 1985-2003. Anesthesiology 2007; 106:1096-104.

27. Cheney FW. The American Society of Anesthesiologists Closed Claims Project: What have we learned, how has it affected practice, and how will it affect practice in the future? Anesthesiology 1999; 91:552-6.
28. Rocke DA, Murray WB, Rout CC, Gouws E. Relative risk analysis of factors associated with difficult intubation in obstetric anesthesia. Anesthesiology 1992; 77:67-73.
29. Rose DK, Cohen MM. The airway: Problems and predictions in 18,500 patients. Can J Anaesth 1994; 41:372-83.
30. Kheterpal S, Han R, Tremper KK, et al. Incidence and predictors of difficult and impossible mask ventilation. Anesthesiology 2006; 105:885-91.
31. Yildiz TS, Solak M, Toker K. The incidence and risk factors of difficult mask ventilation. J Anesth 2005; 19:7-11.
32. Ezri T, Szmuk P, Evron S, et al. Difficult airway in obstetric anesthesia: A review. Obstet Gynecol Surv 2001; 56:631-41.
33. Brock-Utne JG, Downing JW, Seedat F. Laryngeal oedema associated with pre-eclamptic toxaemia. Anaesthesia 1977; 32:556-8.
34. Jouppila R, Jouppila P, Hollmen A. Laryngeal edema as an obstetric anesthesia complication: Case reports. Acta Anaesthesiol Scand 1980; 24:97-8.
35. Brimacombe J. Acute pharyngolaryngeal oedema and pre-eclamptic toxaemia. Anaesth Intensive Care 1992; 20:97-8.
36. Boliston TA. Difficult tracheal intubation in obstetrics. Anaesthesia 1985; 40:389.
37. Munnur U, Suresh MS. Airway problems in pregnancy. Crit Care Clin 2004; 20:617-42.
38. Kodali BS, Chandrasekhar S, Bulich LN, et al. Airway changes during labor and delivery. Anesthesiology 2008; 108:357-62.
39. Dixon BJ, Dixon JB, Carden JR, et al. Preoxygenation is more effective in the 25 degrees head-up position than in the supine position in severely obese patients: A randomized controlled study. Anesthesiology 2005; 102:1110-5.
40. Benumof JL, Dagg R, Benumof R. Critical hemoglobin desaturation will occur before return to an unparalyzed state following 1 mg/kg intravenous succinylcholine. Anesthesiology 1997; 87:979-82.
41. McClelland SH, Bogod DG, Hardman JG. Apnoea in pregnancy: An investigation using physiological modelling. Anaesthesia 2008; 63:264-9.
42. Langeron O, Masso E, Huraux C, et al. Prediction of difficult mask ventilation. Anesthesiology 2000; 92:1229-36.
43. Hood DD, Dewan DM. Anesthetic and obstetric outcome in morbidly obese parturients. Anesthesiology 1993; 79:1210-8.
44. Datta S, Briwa J. Modified laryngoscope for endotracheal intubation of obese patients. Anesth Analg 1981; 60:120-1.
45. Kay NH. Mammomegaly and intubation. Anaesthesia 1982; 37:221.
46. Carp H, Jayaram A, Stoll M. Ultrasound examination of the stomach contents of parturients. Anesth Analg 1992; 74:683-7.
47. Brownridge P. The nature and consequences of childbirth pain. Eur J Obstet Gynecol Reprod Biol 1995; 59(Suppl):S9-15.
48. Kelly MC, Carabine UA, Hill DA, Mirakhur RK. A comparison of the effect of intrathecal and extradural fentanyl on gastric emptying in laboring women. Anesth Analg 1997; 85:834-8.
49. Wright PM, Allen RW, Moore J, Donnelly JP. Gastric emptying during lumbar extradural analgesia in labour: Effect of fentanyl supplementation. Br J Anaesth 1992; 68:248-51.
50. Sia RL, Edens ET. How to avoid problems when using the fibre-optic bronchoscope for difficult intubation. Anaesthesia 1981; 36:74-5.
51. Management of difficult intubation. In Latto IP, Rosen M, editors. Difficulties in Tracheal Intubation. London, Bailliere Tindall, 1985: 99-141.
52. Morgan BM, Magni V, Goroszenuik T. Anaesthesia for emergency caesarean section. Br J Obstet Gynaecol 1990; 97:420-4.
53. American Society of Anesthesiologists Task Force on Obstetric Anesthesia. Practice guidelines for obstetric anesthesia: An updated report by the American Society of Anesthesiologists Task Force on Obstetric Anesthesia. Anesthesiology 2007; 106:843-63.
54. Frerk CM. Predicting difficult intubation. Anaesthesia 1991; 46:1005-8.
55. Lewis M, Keramati S, Benumof JL, Berry CC. What is the best way to determine oropharyngeal classification and mandibular space length to predict difficult laryngoscopy? Anesthesiology 1994; 81:69-75.
56. Wilson ME, Spiegelhalter D, Robertson JA, Lesser P. Predicting difficult intubation. Br J Anaesth 1988; 61:211-6.
57. Oates JD, Macleod AD, Oates PD, et al. Comparison of two methods for predicting difficult intubation. Br J Anaesth 1991; 66:305-9.
58. Tse JC, Rimm EB, Hussain A. Predicting difficult endotracheal intubation in surgical patients scheduled for general anesthesia: A prospective blind study. Anesth Analg 1995; 81:254-8.
59. el-Ganzouri AR, McCarthy RJ, Tuman KJ, et al. Preoperative airway assessment: Predictive value of a multivariate risk index. Anesth Analg 1996; 82:1197-204.
60. Cormack RS, Lehane J. Difficult tracheal intubation in obstetrics. Anaesthesia 1984; 39:1105-11.
61. Mallampati SR, Gatt SP, Gugino LD, et al. A clinical sign to predict difficult tracheal intubation: A prospective study. Can Anaesth Soc J 1985; 32:429-34.
62. Pilkington S, Carli F, Dakin MJ, et al. Increase in Mallampati score during pregnancy. Br J Anaesth 1995; 74:638-42.
63. Farcon EL, Kim MH, Marx GF. Changing Mallampati score during labour. Can J Anaesth 1994; 41:50-1.
64. Wilson ME, John R. Problems with the Mallampati sign. Anaesthesia 1990; 45:486-7.
65. Shiga T, Wajima Z, Inoue T, Sakamoto A. Predicting difficult intubation in apparently normal patients: A meta-analysis of bedside screening test performance. Anesthesiology 2005; 103:429-37.
66. Charters P, Perera S, Horton WA. Visibility of pharyngeal structures as a predictor of difficult intubation. Anaesthesia 1987; 42:1115.
67. Cohen SM, Laurito CE, Segil LJ. Examination of the hypopharynx predicts ease of laryngoscopic visualization and subsequent intubation: A prospective study of 665 patients. J Clin Anesth 1992; 4:310-4.
68. Magill IW. Technique in endotracheal anaesthesia. Br Med J 1930; 2:817-20.
69. Salem MR, Mathrubhutham M, Bennett EJ. Current concepts: Difficult intubation—critical appraisal. N Engl J Med 1976; 295:879-81.
70. Asai T, Marfin AG, Thompson J, et al. Ease of insertion of the laryngeal tube during manual-in-line neck stabilisation. Anaesthesia 2004; 59:1163-6.
71. Bellhouse CP, Doré C. Criteria for estimating likelihood of difficulty of endotracheal intubation with the Macintosh laryngoscope. Anaesth Intensive Care 1988; 16:329-37.
72. Savva D. Prediction of difficult tracheal intubation. Br J Anaesth 1994; 73:149-53.
73. Al Ramadhani S, Mohamed LA, Rocke DA, Gouws E. Sternomental distance as the sole predictor of difficult laryngoscopy in obstetric anaesthesia. Br J Anaesth 1996; 77:312-6.
74. Patil VU, Stehling LC, Zauder HL. Techniques of Endotracheal Intubation: Fiberoptic Endoscopy in Anaesthesia. Chicago, Year Book Medical Publishers, 2007:79.
75. Cohen SM, Laurito CE, Segil LJ. Oral exam to predict difficult intubations: A large prospective study (abstract). Anesthesiology 1989; 42:A937.
76. Schmitt HJ, Kirmse M, Radespiel-Troger M. Ratio of patient's height to thyromental distance improves prediction of difficult laryngoscopy. Anaesth Intensive Care 2002; 30:763-5.
77. Honarmand A, Safavi MR. Prediction of difficult laryngoscopy in obstetric patients scheduled for Caesarean delivery. Eur J Anaesthesiol 2008; 25:714-20.
78. Calder I, Calder J, Crockard HA. Difficult direct laryngoscopy in patients with cervical spine disease. Anaesthesia 1995; 50:756-63.
79. Eberhart LH, Arndt C, Cierpka T, et al. The reliability and validity of the upper lip bite test compared with the Mallampati classification to predict difficult laryngoscopy: An external prospective evaluation. Anesth Analg 2005; 101:284-9.
80. Vallejo MC. Anesthetic management of the morbidly obese parturient. Curr Opin Anaesthesiol 2007; 20:175-80.
81. Juvin P, Lavaut E, Dupont H, et al. Difficult tracheal intubation is more common in obese than in lean patients. Anesth Analg 2003; 97:595-600.

82. Voyagis GS, Kyriakis KP, Dimitriou V, Vrettou I. Value of oropharyngeal Mallampati classification in predicting difficult laryngoscopy among obese patients. Eur J Anaesthesiol 1998; 15:330-4.
83. Brodsky JB, Lemmens HJ, Brock-Utne JG, et al. Morbid obesity and tracheal intubation. Anesth Analg 2002; 94:732-6.
84. Gonzalez H, Minville V, Delanoue K, et al. The importance of increased neck circumference to intubation difficulties in obese patients. Anesth Analg 2008; 106:1132-6.
85. Hiremath AS, Hillman DR, James AL, et al. Relationship between difficult tracheal intubation and obstructive sleep apnoea. Br J Anaesth 1998; 80:606-11.
86. Izci B, Riha RL, Martin SE, et al. The upper airway in pregnancy and pre-eclampsia. Am J Respir Crit Care Med 2003; 167:137-40.
87. Rocke DA, Scoones GP. Rapidly progressive laryngeal oedema associated with pregnancy-aggravated hypertension. Anaesthesia 1992; 47:141-3.
88. Rasmussen GE, Malinow AM. Toward reducing maternal mortality: The problem airway in obstetrics. Int Anesthesiol Clin 1994; 32:83-101.
89. American College of Obstetricians and Gynecologists Committee on Obstetrics. Anesthesia for emergency deliveries: Maternal and fetal medicine. ACOG Committee Opinion No. 104. Washington, DC, ACOG, March 1992. (Int J Gynaecol Obstet 1992; 39:148.)
90. Burgess RW, Crowhurst JA. Acid aspiration prophylaxis in Australian obstetric hospitals—a survey. Anaesth Intensive Care 1989; 17:492-5.
91. Dewan DM, Floyd HM, Thistlewood JM, et al. Sodium citrate pretreatment in elective cesarean section patients. Anesth Analg 1985; 64:34-7.
92. O'Sullivan GM, Bullingham RE. Does twice the volume of antacid have twice the effect in pregnant women at term? Anesth Analg 1984; 63:752-6.
93. Rout CC, Rocke DA, Gouws E. Intravenous ranitidine reduces the risk of acid aspiration of gastric contents at emergency cesarean section. Anesth Analg 1993; 76:156-61.
94. Yau G, Kan AF, Gin T, Oh TE. A comparison of omeprazole and ranitidine for prophylaxis against aspiration pneumonitis in emergency caesarean section. Anaesthesia 1992; 47:101-4.
95. Rao TL, Madhavareddy S, Chinthagada M, El Etr AA. Metoclopramide and cimetidine to reduce gastric fluid pH and volume. Anesth Analg 1984; 63:1014-6.
96. Brock-Utne JG, Dow TG, Welman S, et al. The effect of metoclopramide on the lower oesophageal sphincter in late pregnancy. Anaesth Intensive Care 1978; 6:26-9.
97. McNeill MJ, Ho ET, Kenny GN. Effect of i.v. metoclopramide on gastric emptying after opioid premedication. Br J Anaesth 1990; 64:450-2.
98. Gin T, Ewart MC, Yau G, Oh TE. Effect of oral omeprazole on intragastric pH and volume in women undergoing elective caesarean section. Br J Anaesth 1990; 65:616-9.
99. Rocke DA, Rout CC, Gouws E. Intravenous administration of the proton pump inhibitor omeprazole reduces the risk of acid aspiration at emergency cesarean section. Anesth Analg 1994; 78:1093-8.
100. Sellick BA. Cricoid pressure to control regurgitation of stomach contents during induction of anaesthesia. Lancet 1961; 2(7199):404-6.
101. Vanner RG, Pryle BJ. Regurgitation and oesophageal rupture with cricoid pressure: A cadaver study. Anaesthesia 1992; 47:732-5.
102. Herman NL, Carter B, Van Decar TK. Cricoid pressure: Teaching the recommended level. Anesth Analg 1996; 83:859-63.
103. Wraight WJ, Chamney AR, Howells TH. The determination of an effective cricoid pressure. Anaesthesia 1983; 38:461-6.
104. Howells TH, Chamney AR, Wraight WJ, Simons RS. The application of cricoid pressure: An assessment and a survey of its practice. Anaesthesia 1983; 38:457-60.
105. Yentis SM. The effects of single-handed and bimanual cricoid pressure on the view at laryngoscopy. Anaesthesia 1997; 52:332-5.
106. Levitan RM, Kinkle WC, Levin WJ, Everett WW. Laryngeal view during laryngoscopy: A randomized trial comparing cricoid pressure, backward-upward-rightward pressure, and bimanual laryngoscopy. Ann Emerg Med 2006; 47:548-55.
107. Vanner RG, Clarke P, Moore WJ, Raftery S. The effect of cricoid pressure and neck support on the view at laryngoscopy. Anaesthesia 1997; 52:896-900.
108. Cook TM. Cricoid pressure: Are two hands better than one? Anaesthesia 1996; 51:365-8.
109. Hartsilver EL, Vanner RG. Airway obstruction with cricoid pressure. Anaesthesia 2000; 55:208-11.
110. Ellis DY, Harris T, Zideman D. Cricoid pressure in emergency department rapid sequence tracheal intubations: A risk-benefit analysis. Ann Emerg Med 2007; 50:653-65.
111. Aoyama K, Takenaka I, Sata T, Shigematsu A. Cricoid pressure impedes positioning and ventilation through the laryngeal mask airway. Can J Anaesth 1996; 43:1035-40.
112. Brimacombe J, White A, Berry A. Effect of cricoid pressure on ease of insertion of the laryngeal mask airway. Br J Anaesth 1993; 71:800-2.
113. Li CW, Xue FS, Xu YC, et al. Cricoid pressure impedes insertion of, and ventilation through, the ProSeal laryngeal mask airway in anesthetized, paralyzed patients. Anesth Analg 2007; 104:1195-8.
114. Gold MI, Duarte I, Muravchick S. Arterial oxygenation in conscious patients after 5 minutes and after 30 seconds of oxygen breathing. Anesth Analg 1981; 60:313-5.
115. Norris MC, Dewan DM. Preoxygenation for cesarean section: A comparison of two techniques. Anesthesiology 1985; 62:827-9.
116. Goldberg ME, Norris MC, Larijani GE, et al. Preoxygenation in the morbidly obese: A comparison of two techniques. Anesth Analg 1989; 68:520-2.
117. Benumof JL: Preoxygenation: Best method for both efficacy and efficiency. Anesthesiology 1999; 91:603-5.
118. Gambee AM, Hertzka RE, Fisher DM. Preoxygenation techniques: Comparison of three minutes and four breaths. Anesth Analg 1987; 66:468-70.
119. Gagnon C, Fortier LP, Donati F. When a leak is unavoidable, preoxygenation is equally ineffective with vital capacity or tidal volume breathing. Can J Anaesth 2006; 53:86-91.
120. Chiron B, Laffon M, Ferrandiere M, et al. Standard preoxygenation technique versus two rapid techniques in pregnant patients. Int J Obstet Anesth 2004; 13:11-4.
121. Soro Domingo M, Belda Nácher FJ, Aguilar Aguilar G, et al. [Preoxygenation for anesthesia]. Rev Esp Anestesiol Reanim 2004; 51:322-7.
122. Rapaport S, Joannes-Boyau O, Bazin R, Janvier G. [Comparison of eight deep breaths and tidal volume breathing preoxygenation techniques in morbid obese patients]. Ann Fr Anesth Reanim 2004; 23:1155-9.
123. Lewin SB, Cheek TG, Deutschman CS. Airway management in the obstetric patient. Crit Care Clin 2000; 16:505-13.
124. Harmer M. Difficult and failed intubation in obstetrics. Int J Obstet Anesth 1997; 6:25-31.
125. Kuczkowski KM, Reisner LS, Benumof JL. Airway problems and new solutions for the obstetric patient. J Clin Anesth 2003; 15:552-63.
126. Benumof JL. Management of the difficult adult airway: With special emphasis on awake tracheal intubation. Anesthesiology 1991; 75:1087-110.
127. Sitzman BT, Rich GF, Rockwell JJ, et al. Local anesthetic administration for awake direct laryngoscopy: Are glossopharyngeal nerve blocks superior? Anesthesiology 1997; 86:34-40.
128. Sun DA, Warriner CB, Parsons DG, et al. The GlideScope® Video Laryngoscope: Randomized clinical trial in 200 patients. Br J Anaesth 2005; 94:381-4.
129. Fun WL, Lim Y, Teoh WH. Comparison of the GlideScope video laryngoscope vs. the intubating laryngeal mask for females with normal airways. Eur J Anaesthesiol 2007; 24:486-91.
130. Jones PM, Harle CC. Avoiding awake intubation by performing awake GlideScope® laryngoscopy in the preoperative holding area. Can J Anaesth 2006; 53:1264-5.
131. Moore MS, Wong AB. GlideScope intubation assisted by fiberoptic scope. Anesthesiology 2007; 106:885.
132. Cross P, Cytryn J, Cheng KK. Perforation of the soft palate using the GlideScope videolaryngoscope. Can J Anaesth 2007; 54:588-9.

133. Hirabayashi Y. Pharyngeal injury related to GlideScope videolaryngoscope. Otolaryngol Head Neck Surg 2007; 137:175-6.
134. Chin KJ, Arango MF, Paez AF, Turkstra TP. Palatal injury associated with the GlideScope. Anaesth Intensive Care 2007; 35:449-50.
135. Malik AM, Frogel JK. Anterior tonsillar pillar perforation during GlideScope video laryngoscopy. Anesth Analg 2007; 104:1610-1.
136. Hsu WT, Hsu SC, Lee YL, et al. Penetrating injury of the soft palate during GlideScope intubation. Anesth Analg 2007; 104:1609-10.
137. Hagberg CA, Vogt-Harenkamp CC, Iannucci DG. Successful airway management of a patient with a known difficult airway with the Direct Coupler Interface Video Laryngoscope. J Clin Anesth 2007; 19:629-31.
138. Shippey B, Ray D, McKeown D. Use of the McGrath videolaryngoscope in the management of difficult and failed tracheal intubation. Br J Anaesth 2008; 100:116-9.
139. Hirabayashi Y, Seo N. Use of a new videolaryngoscope (Airway Scope) in the management of difficult airway. J Anesth 2007; 21:445-6.
140. Matsumoto S, Asai T, Shingu K. Truview video laryngoscope in patients with difficult airways. Anesth Analg 2006; 103:492-3.
141. Dhonneur G, Ndoko S, Amathieu R, et al. Tracheal intubation using the Airtraq in morbid obese patients undergoing emergency cesarean delivery. Anesthesiology 2007; 106:629-30.
142. Benumof JL. Management of the difficult airway. Ann Acad Med Singapore 1994; 23:589-91.
143. Burtner DD, Goodman M. Anesthetic and operative management of potential upper airway obstruction. Arch Otolaryngol 1978; 104:657-61.
144. Ranney B, Stanage WF. Advantages of local anesthesia for cesarean section. Obstet Gynecol 1975; 45:163-7.
145. Busby T. Local anesthesia for cesarean section. Am J Obstet Gynecol 1963; 87:399-404.
146. Cooper MG, Feeney EM, Joseph M, McGuinness JJ. Local anaesthetic infiltration for caesarean section. Anaesth Intensive Care 1989; 17:198-201.
147. Benumof JL. The unanticipated difficult airway. Can J Anaesth 1999; 46:510-1.
148. Benumof JL. Laryngeal mask airway and the ASA difficult airway algorithm. Anesthesiology 1996; 84:686-99.
149. Han TH, Brimacombe J, Lee EJ, Yang HS. The laryngeal mask airway is effective (and probably safe) in selected healthy parturients for elective Cesarean section: A prospective study of 1067 cases. Can J Anaesth 2001; 48:1117-21.
150. Chadwick IS, Vohra A. Anaesthesia for emergency caesarean section using the Brain laryngeal airway. Anaesthesia 1989; 44:261-2.
151. McClune S, Regan M, Moore J. Laryngeal mask airway for caesarean section. Anaesthesia 1990; 45:227-8.
152. McCrirrick A. The laryngeal mask airway for failed intubation at caesarean section. Anaesth Intensive Care 1991; 19:135.
153. Priscu V, Priscu L, Soroker D. Laryngeal mask for failed intubation in emergency caesarean section. Can J Anaesth 1992; 39:893.
154. Storey J. The laryngeal mask for failed intubation at caesarean section. Anaesth Intensive Care 1992; 20:118-9.
155. Bailey SG, Kitching AJ. The laryngeal mask airway in failed obstetric tracheal intubation. Int J Obstet Anesth 2005; 14:270-1.
156. Zagnoev M, McCloskey J, Martin T. Fiberoptic intubation via the laryngeal mask airway. Anesth Analg 1994; 78:813-4.
157. Joo HS, Rose DK. The intubating laryngeal mask airway with and without fiberoptic guidance. Anesth Analg 1999; 88:662-6.
158. Kamiya I, Satomoto M, Tokunaga M, et al. [Intubation in a patient with lingual tonsil hypertrophy using an intubating laryngeal mask airway in combination with fiberoptic intubation]. Masui 2002; 51:523-5.
159. Brain AIJ, Verghese C. LMA-Fastrach Instruction Manual. Irvine, CA, ProSeal Automedics, Inc, 1998.
160. Brimacombe J, Keller C. The ProSeal laryngeal mask airway: A randomized, crossover study with the standard laryngeal mask airway in paralyzed, anesthetized patients. Anesthesiology 2000; 93:104-9.
161. Evans NR, Gardner SV, James MF. ProSeal laryngeal mask protects against aspiration of fluid in the pharynx. Br J Anaesth 2002; 88:584-7.
162. Keller C, Brimacombe J, Kleinsasser A, Loeckinger A. Does the ProSeal laryngeal mask airway prevent aspiration of regurgitated fluid? Anesth Analg 2000; 91:1017-20.
163. Evans NR, Gardner SV, James MF, et al. The ProSeal laryngeal mask: Results of a descriptive trial with experience of 300 cases. Br J Anaesth 2002; 88:534-9.
164. Cook TM, Nolan JP, Verghese C, et al. Randomized crossover comparison of the ProSeal with the classic laryngeal mask airway in unparalysed anaesthetized patients. Br J Anaesth 2002; 88: 527-33.
165. Brown NI, Mack PF, Mitera DM, Dhar P. Use of the ProSeal laryngeal mask airway in a pregnant patient with a difficult airway during electroconvulsive therapy. Br J Anaesth 2003; 91:752-4.
166. Matioc A, Arndt GA. Intubation using the ProSeal laryngeal mask airway and a Cook airway exchange catheter set. Can J Anaesth 2001; 48:932.
167. Asai T, Appadurai I. LMA for failed intubation. Can J Anaesth 1993; 40:802.
168. Strang TI. Does the laryngeal mask airway compromise cricoid pressure? Anaesthesia 1992; 47:829-31.
169. Asai T, Barclay K, Power I, Vaughan RS. Cricoid pressure impedes placement of the laryngeal mask airway. Br J Anaesth 1995; 74:521-5.
170. Brimacombe J, Berry A. LMA for failed intubation. Can J Anaesth 1993; 40:802-3.
171. Ansermino JM, Blogg CE. Cricoid pressure may prevent insertion of the laryngeal mask airway. Br J Anaesth 1992; 69:465-7.
172. Harry RM, Nolan JP. The use of cricoid pressure with the intubating laryngeal mask. Anaesthesia 1999; 54:656-9.
173. Asai T, Barclay K, McBeth C, Vaughan RS. Cricoid pressure applied after placement of the laryngeal mask prevents gastric insufflation but inhibits ventilation. Br J Anaesth 1996; 75:772-6.
174. Benumof JL. Laryngeal mask airway: Indications and contraindications. Anesthesiology 1992; 77:843-6.
175. Asai T, Shingu K. The laryngeal tube. Br J Anaesth 2005; 95:729-36.
176. Agro F, Cataldo R, Alfano A, Galli B. A new prototype for airway management in an emergency: The Laryngeal Tube. Resuscitation 1999; 41:284-6.
177. Genzwuerker HV, Hilker T, Hohner E, Kuhnert-Frey B. The laryngeal tube: A new adjunct for airway management. Prehosp Emerg Care 2000; 4:168-72.
178. Figueredo E, Martinez M, Pintanel T. A comparison of the ProSeal laryngeal mask and the laryngeal tube in spontaneously breathing anesthetized patients. Anesth Analg 2003; 96:600-5.
179. Langlois C, Pean D, Testa S, et al. [The LTD laryngeal tube: A new single-use airway device]. Ann Fr Anesth Reanim 2007; 26:197-201.
180. Genzwürker H, Finteis T, Hinkelbein J, Ellinger K. [First clinical experiences with the new LTS: A laryngeal tube with an oesophageal drain]. Anaesthetist 2003; 52:697-702.
181. Zand F, Amini A. Use of the laryngeal tube-S for airway management and prevention of aspiration after a failed tracheal intubation in a parturient. Anesthesiology 2005; 102:481-3.
182. Vezina MC, Trepanier CA, Nicole PC, Lessard MR. Complications associated with the Esophageal-Tracheal Combitube in the pre-hospital setting. Can J Anaesth 2007; 54:124-8.
183. Benumof JL, Scheller MS. The importance of transtracheal jet ventilation in the management of the difficult airway. Anesthesiology 1989; 71:769-78.
184. McLellan I, Gordon P, Khawaja S, Thomas A. Percutaneous transtracheal high frequency jet ventilation as an aid to difficult intubation. Can J Anaesth 1988; 35:404-5.
185. Bellemain A, Ghimouz A, Goater P, et al. [Bilateral tension pneumothorax after retrieval of transtracheal jet ventilation catheter]. Ann Fr Anesth Reanim 2006; 25:401-3.
186. Cook TM, Bigwood B, Cranshaw J. A complication of transtracheal jet ventilation and use of the Aintree intubation catheter during airway resuscitation. Anaesthesia 2006; 61:692-7.
187. Craft TM, Chambers PH, Ward ME, Goat VA. Two cases of barotrauma associated with transtracheal jet ventilation. Br J Anaesth 1990; 64:524-7.

188. Chandradeva K, Palin C, Ghosh SM, Pinches SC. Percutaneous transtracheal jet ventilation as a guide to tracheal intubation in severe upper airway obstruction from supraglottic oedema. Br J Anaesth 2005; 94:683-6.
189. McHugh R, Kumar M, Sprung J, Bourke D. Transtracheal jet ventilation in management of the difficult airway. Anaesth Intensive Care 2007; 35:406-8.
190. Patel RG. Percutaneous transtracheal jet ventilation: A safe, quick, and temporary way to provide oxygenation and ventilation when conventional methods are unsuccessful. Chest 1999; 116:1689-94.
191. de La Chapelle A, Benoit S, Bouregba M, et al. The treatment of severe pulmonary edema induced by beta adrenergic agonist tocolytic therapy with continuous positive airway pressure delivered by face mask. Anesth Analg 2002; 94:1593-4.
192. Rout CC. Anaesthesia and analgesia for the critically ill parturient. Best Pract Res Clin Obstet Gynaecol 2001; 15:507-22.
193. Caroleo S, Agnello F, Abdallah K, et al. Weaning from mechanical ventilation: An open issue. Minerva Anestesiol 2007; 73:417-27.
194. Demling RH, Read T, Lind LJ, Flanagan HL. Incidence and morbidity of extubation failure in surgical intensive care patients. Crit Care Med 1988; 16:573-7.
195. Tahvanainen J, Salmenpera M, Nikki P. Extubation criteria after weaning from intermittent mandatory ventilation and continuous positive airway pressure. Crit Care Med 1983; 11:702-7.
196. Chung YH, Chao TY, Chiu CT, Lin MC. The cuff-leak test is a simple tool to verify severe laryngeal edema in patients undergoing long-term mechanical ventilation. Crit Care Med 2006; 34:409-14.
197. Ding LW, Wang HC, Wu HD, et al. Laryngeal ultrasound: A useful method in predicting post-extubation stridor. A pilot study. Eur Respir J 2006; 27:384-9.
198. Kriner EJ, Shafazand S, Colice GL. The endotracheal tube cuff-leak test as a predictor for postextubation stridor. Respir Care 2005; 50:1632-8.
199. Adderley RJ, Mullins GC. When to extubate the croup patient: The "leak" test. Can J Anaesth 1987; 34:304-6.
200. Fisher MM, Raper RF. The "cuff-leak" test for extubation. Anaesthesia 1992; 47:10-2.
201. Benumof JL. Airway exchange catheters: Simple concept, potentially great danger. Anesthesiology 1999; 91:342-4.
202. Benumof JL. Airway exchange catheters for safe extubation: The clinical and scientific details that make the concept work. Chest 1997; 111:1483-6.
203. Visvanathan T, Kluger MT, Webb RK, Westhorpe RN. Crisis management during anaesthesia: Laryngospasm. Qual Saf Health Care 2005; 14:e3.

Chapter 31

Postpartum Headache

Alison Macarthur, B.M.Sc., M.D., M.Sc., FRCPC

Postpartum headache is the complaint of cephalic, neck, or shoulder pain occurring during the first 6 weeks after delivery. The overall incidence of postpartum headache has not been determined in a prospective study. However, information is available from a prospective evaluation of women during the first week postpartum[1] and from a prospectively collected database that recorded symptoms during pregnancy and the first week after delivery.[2] Among 985 women in the prospective evaluation, the incidence of headache in the first week postpartum was 38.7%.[1] The median time from delivery to onset of symptoms was 2 days, and the median duration of headache was 4 hours. Benhamou et al.[2] examined information collected on pregnant women who delivered at their institution during a 2-year period; exclusion criteria included recognized dural puncture, preterm delivery, multiple gestation, and/or elective cesarean delivery. Headache was reported by 12% of 1058 patients who had epidural anesthesia without dural puncture and by 15% of 140 patients who delivered without epidural anesthesia.

Post–dural puncture headache (PDPH) is one of the most common postpartum complications of neuraxial anesthesia. However, physicians and nurses should be aware that dural puncture is only one of many causes of postpartum headache (Table 31-1). Difficult diagnostic problems may require the opinion of a neurologist. The purpose of this chapter is to discuss the differential diagnosis of postpartum headache and of PDPH in particular.

DIFFERENTIAL DIAGNOSIS

The classification of headaches follows the International Classification of Headache Disorders (ICHD), created in 1988 by the Headache Classification Committee of the International Headache Society. This classification system, which has been updated (ICHD-II), identifies two broad categories of headaches, primary and secondary (Box 31-1).[3] Primary headaches include migraine, tension-type headache, cluster headache, and other trigeminal autonomic cephalgias. Secondary headaches are attributable to specific underlying pathology. Primary headaches are 20 times more common than secondary headaches among women in the first postpartum week.[1]

After delivery, women frequently suffer from headache. A retrospective study reviewed 5 years of hospital records to identify women who had postpartum headaches between 24 hours and 6 weeks after delivery.[4] Ninety-five women met these criteria, and although the incidence could not be calculated, the study did identify some important features of postpartum headache. Most women (82%) were still in the hospital at the time of onset of the headache. The demographics of the study population largely reflected the general population; the mean age was 25 years, 87% of the women had received some type of neuraxial analgesia/anesthesia, and 29% had a cesarean delivery.

Primary Headaches

The postpartum patient can present with a recurrence of her known primary disorder or with the first manifestation of a primary condition. Patients with a history of headache disorders typically are diagnosed with one of four major types of primary headaches. The most common postpartum headaches are tension-type and migrainous headaches, which account for almost two thirds of headaches during this period.[1,2] **Tension-type headaches** are often circumferential and constricting, can be associated with scalp tenderness, and are usually of mild to moderate severity.

MIGRAINE

Migrainous headaches (or migraines) are defined as recurring cranial pain lasting 4 to 72 hours, often with typical features such as pulsating pain in a unilateral location,

TABLE 31-1 Differential Diagnosis of Postpartum Headache

Headache Etiology	Percentage of Postpartum Headaches*	Primary Symptoms/Signs	Diagnostic Modality
Tension headache	39	Mild to moderate headache, lasting 30 minutes to 7 days Often bilateral, nonpulsating, and not aggravated by physical activity	History and physical examination
Migraine	11-34	Recurrent moderate to severe headache, lasting 4 to 72 hours Often unilateral, pulsating, and aggravated by physical activity Associated with nausea, photophobia, and phonophobia	History and physical examination
Musculoskeletal	11-15	Mild to moderate headache accompanied by neck and/or shoulder pain	History and physical examination
Preeclampsia/Eclampsia	8-24	Hypertension and/or HELLP (hemolysis, elevated liver enzymes, low platelet count) syndrome Headache often bilateral, pulsating and aggravated by physical activity	History and physical examination Laboratory evaluation (alanine aminotransferase [ALT], aspartate transaminase [AST], uric acid, platelet count, urine protein)
Post–dural puncture headache	5-16	Headache within 5 days of dural puncture Worsens within 15 minutes of sitting or standing Associated with neck stiffness, tinnitus, photophobia, and nausea	History and physical examination Possible MRI
Cortical vein thrombosis	3	Nonspecific headache that may have a postural component Often accompanied by focal neurologic signs and seizures	History and physical examination CT or MRI Possible angiography
Subarachnoid hemorrhage	1	Abrupt onset of an intense and incapacitating headache Often unilateral Accompanied by nausea, nuchal rigidity, and altered consciousness	History and physical examination CT without contrast or MRI (FLAIR sequence)
Posterior reversible (leuko)encephalopathy (PRES) syndrome	Unknown	Severe and diffuse headache with an acute or gradual onset Possible focal neurologic deficits and seizures	History and physical examination MRI
Brain tumor	Unknown	Progressive and often localized headache Often worse in the morning Aggravated by coughing/straining	History and physical examination CT or MRI
Subdural hematoma	Unknown	Headache usually without typical features Often overshadowed by focal neurologic signs and/or altered consciousness	History and physical examination CT or MRI
Cerebral infarction/ ischemia	Unknown	Moderate headache accompanied by focal neurologic signs and/or altered consciousness	History and physical examination CT or MRI (showing angiographic "string of beads" appearance)

CSF, cerebrospinal fluid; CT, computed tomography; MRI, magnetic resonance imaging; FLAIR, fluid-attenuated inversion recovery.

*Estimated from Goldszmidt E, Kern R, Chaput A, Macarthur A. The incidence and etiology of postpartum headaches: A prospective cohort study. Can J Anaesth 2005;52:971-7; and Stella CL, Jodicke CD, How HY, et al. Postpartum headache: Is your work-up complete? Am J Obstet Gynecol 2007;196:318.e1-7.

TABLE 31-1—cont'd Differential Diagnosis of Postpartum Headache

Headache Etiology	Percentage of Postpartum Headaches*	Primary Symptoms/Signs	Diagnostic Modality
Pseudotumor cerebri/ Benign intracranial hypertension	Unknown	Progressive nonpulsating headache Aggravated by coughing/straining Associated with increased CSF pressure and normal CSF chemistry	History and physical examination Lumbar puncture
Spontaneous intracranial hypotension	Unknown	No history of dural trauma Diffuse, dull headache worsening within 15 minutes of sitting or standing Associated with neck stiffness, nausea, tinnitus, and photophobia CSF opening pressure < 60 mm H_2O in the sitting position	History and physical examination Lumbar puncture Radioisotope cisternography CT myelography
Sinusitis	Unknown	Frontal headache with accompanying pain in the face Development of headache coincides with nasal obstruction Purulent nasal discharge, anosmia, and fever	History and physical examination Nasal endoscopy CT or MRI
Meningitis	Unknown	Headache is most frequent symptom Often diffuse Intensity increases with time Associated with nausea, photophobia, phonophobia, general malaise, and fever	History and physical examination Lumbar puncture
Pneumocephalus	Unknown	Frontal headache Often an abrupt onset immediately following dural puncture Symptoms can worsen with upright posture	History and physical examination CT
Caffeine withdrawal	Unknown	Onset of headache within 24 hours of cessation of regular caffeine consumption[†] Often bilateral and pulsating Relieved within 1 hour of ingestion of caffeine 100 mg	History and physical examination
Lactation headache	Unknown	Mild to moderate headache associated temporally with onset of breast-feeding or with breast engorgement	History and physical examination

[†]The ICHD-II criteria state that caffeine-withdrawal headache occurs upon cessation of ≥ 200 mg daily caffeine consumption for more than 2 weeks.[3] However, others have suggested that caffeine-withdrawal headache may occur after as little as 3 days' exposure to 300 mg/day, or 7 days' exposure to 100 mg/day.[39]

nausea, and photophobia.[3] Headache with aura is a subtype of migraine that is characterized by focal neurologic symptoms preceding the headache. The prevalence of migraine is approximately 17% in the female population (three times more common than the prevalence in the male population) and is more common in patients between 30 and 50 years of age.[5] Pregnancy has an ameliorating effect on migraine frequency in the majority of sufferers. However, symptoms may recur soon after delivery, with reports of 34% recurrence within the first week postpartum and 55% within the first month.[6] Generally the symptoms are similar to their typical pattern, although often milder and less often unilateral. It is rare for a migraine to manifest for the first time during the postpartum period. There appears to be an association between migraine and preeclampsia, which may reflect an underlying predisposition to cerebral ischemic injury.[7]

Secondary Headaches

A common secondary headache in the postpartum period is the musculoskeletal headache, exacerbated by the maternal physical exertion of labor and associated sleep deprivation. This headache has accompanying neck and shoulder pain

BOX 31-1 International Classification of Headache Disorders (ICHD-II) Classification

Primary

- Migraine
- Tension-type headache
- Cluster headache and other trigeminal autonomic cephalgias
- Other primary headaches

Secondary

- Headache attributed to:
  - Head and/or neck trauma
  - Cranial or cervical vascular disorder
  - Nonvascular intracranial disorder
  - A substance or its withdrawal
  - Infection
  - Disorder of homeostasis
  - Disorder of the cranial structures (e.g., eyes, ears, nose, sinuses, teeth, mouth)
  - Psychiatric disorder
- Cranial neuralgias and central causes of facial pain
- Other headache, cranial neuralgia, central or primary facial pain

Modified from Headache Classification Committee of the International Headache Society. The international classification of headache disorders. Cephalalgia 2004; 24(Suppl 1):1-160.

without a history of dural puncture. Approximately 11% of postpartum headaches are diagnosed as musculoskeletal.[1] Other causes of secondary headache are discussed in the following paragraphs.

HYPERTENSION

Gestational hypertension is commonly associated with headache. Eclampsia is a form of hypertensive encephalopathy characterized by headache, visual disturbances, nausea, vomiting, seizures, stupor, and sometimes coma. Seizures may occur in the absence of severe hypertension. Headache is a serious premonitory sign, being present in over 50% of women in whom eclampsia develops.[8] Eclampsia first manifests postpartum in 11% to 44% of affected women.[8] Other hypertensive disorders, with or without superimposed preeclampsia, may also cause postpartum headache and lead to encephalopathy.

POSTERIOR REVERSIBLE LEUKOENCEPHALOPATHY SYNDROME

Posterior reversible (leuko)encephalopathy syndrome (PRES) was described in 1996 following recognition of a consistent symptom presentation in a diverse group of patients. Conditions associated with PRES include preeclampsia, uremia, hemolytic-uremic syndrome, and exposure to immunosuppressant drugs.[9] Approximately 25% of cases of PRES occur in pregnant patients. PRES symptoms include headache, seizures, altered mental status, visual changes, and, occasionally, focal neurologic deficits.[10]

The neuroradiologic features of PRES include symmetric areas of cerebral edema, predominantly involving the white matter regions of the posterior circulation (i.e., occipital lobes, posterior parietal, and temporal lobes) (Figure 31-1). The pathophysiology of PRES is similar to that of hypertensive encephalopathy, in that altered cerebrovascular regulation causes loss of blood-brain barrier integrity. The accompanying vasogenic edema can be reversed by prompt recognition and supportive therapy (i.e., cessation of provocative medications, aggressive treatment of hypertension, seizure prophylaxis). However, irreversible cytotoxic edema with permanent neurologic damage can occur if the initial disorder is not diagnosed early. This syndrome often manifests in the postpartum period, usually in conjunction with preeclampsia.[11-15] Diagnosis may be delayed if other potential causes of headache are also present (e.g., dural puncture).[13,14] Typical features that distinguish PRES from other postpartum headaches include seizures and focal neurologic deficits, such as temporary loss of vision.

SUBARACHNOID HEMORRHAGE

The incidence of subarachnoid hemorrhage is increased during pregnancy, being estimated at approximately 20 per 100,000 deliveries. It usually occurs in patients with a cerebral aneurysm, arteriovenous malformation, or hypertensive encephalopathy.[16] The classic presentation consists of the sudden onset of a severe headache that is unlike any previous headache. Pregnancy may increase the risk of bleeding because of increased blood volume and hormonal changes that affect arterial integrity. Other factors associated with subarachnoid hemorrhage during pregnancy include cigarette smoking, genetic diseases (e.g., polycystic kidney disease), and nulliparity. Suspicion of subarachnoid hemorrhage necessitates urgent investigation by computed tomography (CT), because nonsurgical therapies (e.g., endovascular ablation) are available and long-term sequelae can be minimized.

CORTICAL VEIN THROMBOSIS

The incidence of cerebral cortical vein thrombosis is increased in pregnancy, and is estimated to be 10 to 20 per 100,000 deliveries in developed countries.[17] The incidence appears higher in developing countries (e.g., 450 per 100,000 deliveries in India). Often it is difficult to distinguish cortical vein thrombosis from PDPH, because the headache of cortical vein thrombosis may have a postural component. Preceding dural puncture has been reported in several cases,[18-20] and it has been hypothesized that the reductions in cerebrospinal fluid (CSF) pressure and cerebral vasodilation that accompany dural puncture predispose to thrombosis development. Associated features include focal neurologic signs, seizures, and coma. Cerebral infarction may ensue if diagnosis is delayed. Diagnosis is best confirmed by magnetic resonance imaging (MRI), because CT appears to identify only a third of cases.[21] Treatment of cortical vein thrombosis largely is symptomatic, with the aim of preventing seizures. Some studies have suggested that anticoagulation therapy may improve outcome; however, additional data are needed.[22,23]

CEREBRAL INFARCTION/ISCHEMIA

Cerebral arterial insufficiency is one cause of stroke in pregnancy, with an estimated incidence of 19 per 100,000 deliveries.[24] Approximately half of the events occur in the peripartum period, and the clinical presentation often

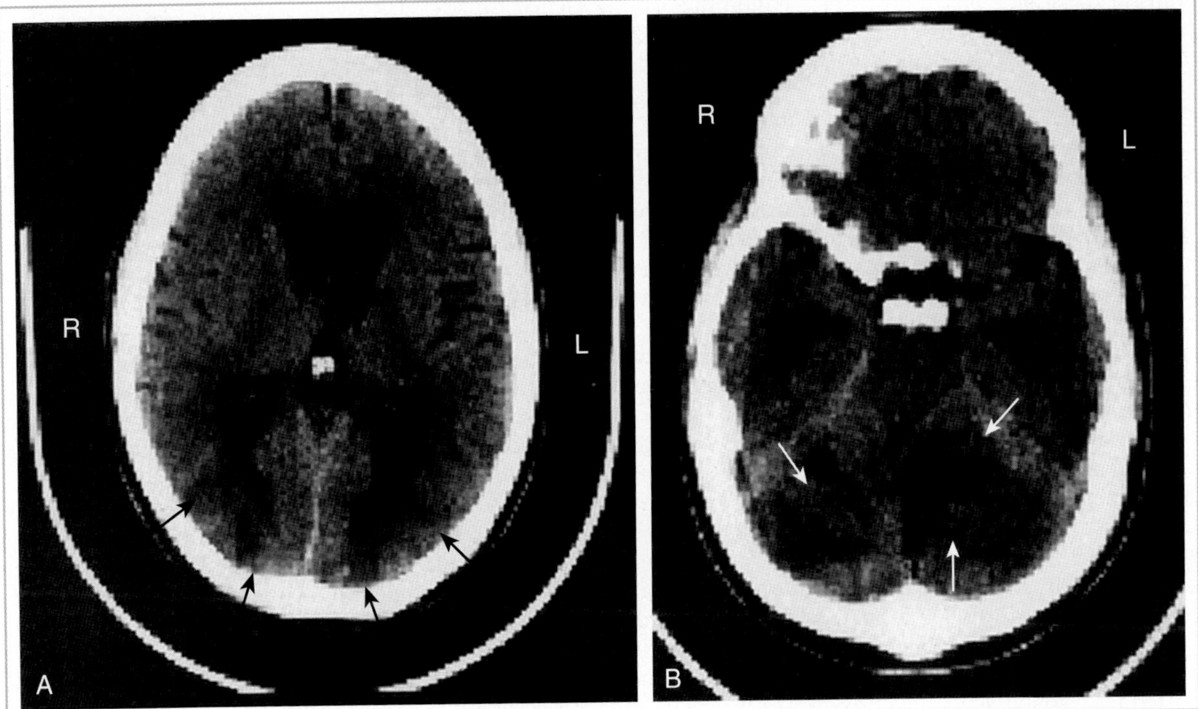

FIGURE 31-1 Posterior reversible (leuko)encephalopathy syndrome (PRES). **A,** Areas of hypodensity in the parieto-occipital white matter (*black arrows*). **B,** Abnormal hypodensity is also seen in the cerebellum (*white arrows*), with the abnormality larger on the left (L) than the right (R). (From Hinchey J, Chaves C, Appignani B, et al. A reversible posterior leukoencephalopathy syndrome. N Engl J Med 1996; 334:494-500.)

comprises a sudden onset of headache, vomiting, seizures, and focal neurologic deficits. Postpartum cerebral angiopathy has been detected with the aid of cerebral angiography, in which a characteristic "arterial beading" indicative of arterial spasm is evident. Several case reports have described the delayed diagnosis of cerebral infarction because providers assumed a diagnosis of PDPH.[25,26] The key feature was a *nonpostural* headache. Initial CT and MRI findings are often normal, and intracranial Doppler or angiographic investigations may be necessary to diagnose ischemia or infarct.

SUBDURAL HEMATOMA

In rare instances, dural puncture is associated with the subsequent development of a subdural hematoma. In several case reports, the identification of the subdural hematoma was preceded by symptoms of a PDPH.[27-29] Dural puncture results in leakage of CSF and decreased intracranial pressure (ICP). Presumably, the reduction in ICP causes stress on bridging cerebral vessels, thereby precipitating bleeding. Neurologic signs of subdural hematoma are variable but include evidence of increased ICP (e.g., headache, somnolence, vomiting, confusion) and focal abnormalities.

PNEUMOCEPHALUS

The subdural or subarachnoid injection of air used for identification of the epidural space may be associated with the sudden onset of severe headache, sometimes accompanied by neck pain, back pain, or changes in mental status.[30] Headache symptoms can mimic those of PDPH, in that they are worse in the sitting position and may be relieved by lying down. Radiologic studies confirm the presence of intracranial air, and the headache typically resolves over the first week.

MENINGITIS

The severe headache of meningitis typically manifests within the first several postpartum days (see Chapter 32). It is accompanied by fever, nuchal rigidity, and the presence of Kernig and Brudzinski signs. Lethargy, confusion, vomiting, seizures, and a rash may also occur. Usual pathogens include streptococci of the viridans type.[31] The diagnosis is confirmed by examination and culture of the CSF.

PSEUDOTUMOR CEREBRI/BENIGN INTRACRANIAL HYPERTENSION

Parturients with pseudotumor cerebri (i.e., increased ICP in the absence of a mass lesion) present with headache and visual disturbances, usually in the antepartum period. The features of the postpartum headache of pseudotumor cerebri mimic the usual chronic headache symptoms experienced by the patient. The diagnosis largely is one of exclusion (see Chapter 49). Treatment involves reduction of CSF pressure through the use of glucocorticoids, carbonic-anhydrase inhibitors, diuretics, or serial lumbar punctures.

BRAIN TUMOR

Intracranial tumors may manifest as postpartum headache.[32-34] Headache that is dull rather than throbbing in character may be an early symptom of a brain tumor. Nausea, vomiting, seizures, and/or focal neurologic signs may be present. Neurologic examination may reveal evidence of increased ICP. Case reports suggest that atypical presentation of headache, either with persisting headache symptoms in the supine position or exacerbation following epidural blood patch, should prompt further neuroradiologic investigations.[32-34]

SPONTANEOUS INTRACRANIAL HYPOTENSION

Spontaneous intracranial hypotension develops because of CSF leakage secondary to dural tears. The tears usually occur at the thoracic spinal level and are not associated with prior neuraxial procedures.[35] Diagnosis requires radioisotope cisternography and CT myelography, which may also identify the level of the leak. Presentation of this disorder is identical to that of PDPH, as the pathophysiology is the same. The only difference is the lack of a prior neuraxial procedure in spontaneous intracranial hypotension. One case report has described the development of a postural headache 4 days after a spontaneous vaginal delivery without neuraxial anesthesia.[36] The patient was found to have a cervical-thoracic dural leak.

SINUSITIS

Headache caused by inflamed paranasal sinuses is associated with purulent nasal discharge and, occasionally, fever. Pain may be unilateral or bilateral, depending on the extent of the disease, and the skin over the affected sinus may be tender. Frontal sinus infection causes headache in the frontal region. Ethmoidal and sphenoidal sinus infections cause periorbital pain, and maxillary sinus infection may cause diffuse facial discomfort. The sinuses fill overnight, and pain typically is worse on awakening. Pain improves in the upright position, which assists drainage.[37]

CAFFEINE WITHDRAWAL

The withdrawal of caffeine may lead to headache, increased fatigue, and anxiety. Caffeine withdrawal headaches have been reported in the postoperative period[38] and may occur after as little as 3 days' exposure to 300 mg/day or 7 days' exposure to 100 mg/day of caffeine.[39] Normal-sized caffeinated drinks usually contain 50 to 100 mg of caffeine per serving. Women often decrease their caffeine intake in the puerperium, and although caffeine withdrawal headache has not been confirmed as a cause of postpartum headache, the diagnosis should be considered.

LACTATION HEADACHE

Askmark and Lundberg[40] reported episodes of intense headache during periods of breast-feeding in a woman known to suffer from migraine. Onset of headaches occurred within the first few minutes of breast-feeding, and the headaches resolved after cessation of nursing. The headaches were associated with an increase in plasma vasopressin concentration. Headaches have also been described in women with breast engorgement who either have elected not to breast-feed or have reduced the frequency of breast-feeding.[41]

POST–DURAL PUNCTURE HEADACHE

Incidence

Post–dural puncture headache (PDPH) may occur after intentional dural puncture with a spinal needle or unintentional dural puncture with an epidural or other needle.

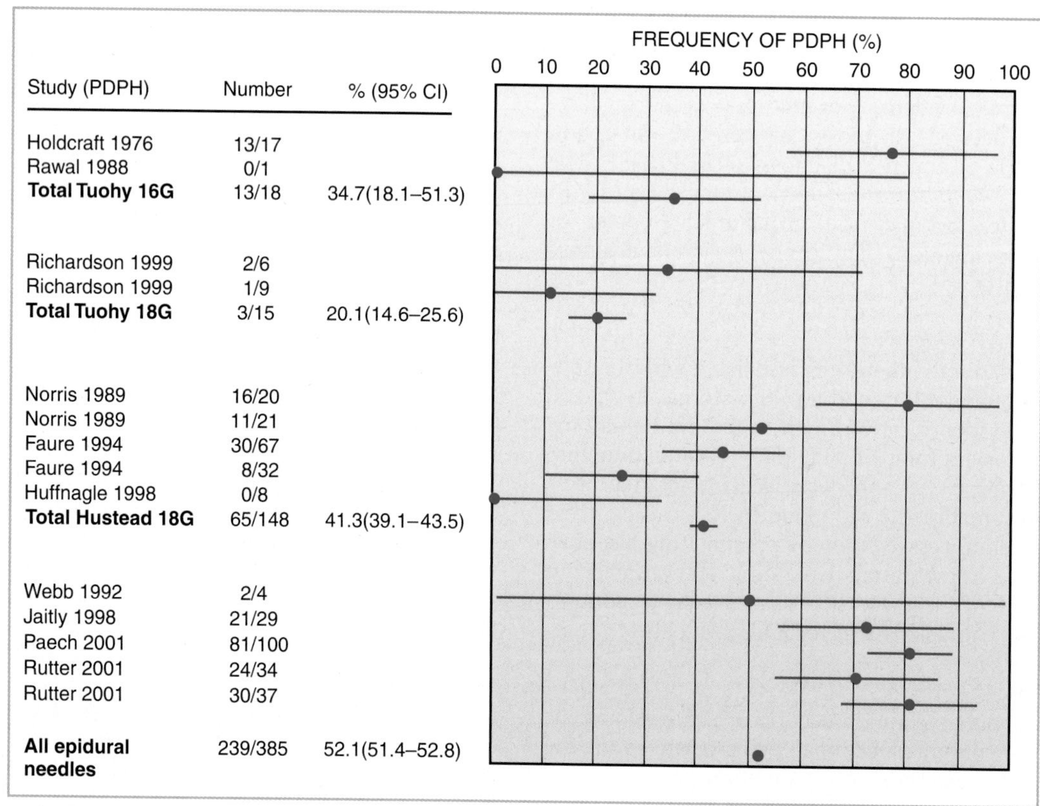

FIGURE 31-2 Meta-analysis of post–dural puncture headache (PDPH) frequency for epidural needles in the obstetric population. The *dots* represent the percentages of patients experiencing the event. The *horizontal lines* represent the 95% confidence interval (CI). (From Choi PT, Galinski SE, Takeuchi L, et al. PDPH is a common complication of neuraxial blockade in parturients: A meta-analysis of obstetric studies. Can J Anaesth 2003; 50:460-9.)

A meta-analysis of studies of PDPH in obstetric patients (n = 328,769) calculated a pooled risk of unintentional dural puncture with any epidural needle of 1.5% (95% confidence interval [CI], 1.5% to 1.5%).[42] Following a dural puncture with an epidural needle, the risk of PDPH was 52.1% (95% CI, 51.4% to 52.8%) (Figure 31-2). The rate of PDPH after dural puncture with spinal needles ranged between 1.5% and 11.2%, depending on the needle size and type of needle (see later) (Table 31-2). Although PDPH is often considered a "minor" complication of dural puncture, it was the cause of 14% of obstetric claims in the American Society of Anesthesiologists (ASA) Closed-Claims Project database (see Chapter 33).

Symptoms

Patients typically experience headache pain in the frontal and occipital regions. Pain often radiates to the neck, which may be "stiff." Some women have a mild headache that permits full ambulation. In others, pain is severe and incapacitating. Symptoms are worse in the upright position and are usually relieved in the horizontal position. Abdominal compression may relieve pain in some patients. The ICHD-II defines PDPH as occurring within 15 minutes of a patient's moving to an upright position (sitting or standing) and resolving within 15 minutes of the patient's moving to the supine position.[3]

The ICHD-II criteria for PDPH require one of the following symptoms to be present: neck stiffness, tinnitus, hypacusis, photophobia, and nausea. Lybecker et al.[43] reported the incidence of these symptoms in a prospective study of 75 nonobstetric patients with PDPH (Table 31-3). Cranial nerve palsy, thought to be secondary to nerve traction due to low CSF volume, is occasionally associated with PDPH. The sixth cranial nerve is most susceptible to traction during its long intracranial course. The traction results in failure of the involved eye to abduct, and patients may have diplopia. Hearing loss is usually in the low-frequency range and is related to reduction of CSF pressure and alteration of hair cell position in the inner ear.[44] The risk of hearing loss appears to be higher with advanced age (more than 40 years) and dural puncture with larger-gauge needles.

Rarer symptoms associated with PDPH include seizures, abdominal pain, and diarrhea. Shearer et al.[45] reported postpartum seizures in eight women with severe PDPH without convincing evidence of preexisting hypertension. Cerebral vasospasm was thought to be the etiologic factor. Vercauteren et al.[46] described a woman who had received epidural analgesia and experienced postpartum seizures with a severe headache. The CSF was blood-stained, but a CT scan showed no source of hemorrhage. This patient improved dramatically after the performance of a blood patch. A 20-year-old man experienced PDPH after administration of spinal anesthesia with a 25-gauge Quincke needle.[47] Twelve days after the anesthetic administration, he experienced abdominal pain and diarrhea, which persisted despite the lack of evidence of mucosal or organic disease. One month following spinal anesthesia, an epidural blood patch procedure was performed, which resulted in prompt resolution of headache and gastrointestinal symptoms. The investigators speculated that this patient had noninfectious arachnoiditis with lumbosacral root involvement, which resulted in visceral hyperalgesia and dysfunction.

TABLE 31-2 Frequency of Post–Dural Puncture Headache in Obstetric Patients According to Spinal Needle Design

Needle Design	Gauge	n/N	Frequency of PDPH (%)*	95% Confidence Interval
Quincke†	24	15/238	11.2	10.2-12.2
	25	90/1624	6.3	6.3-6.3
	26	139/2467	5.6	5.6-5.7
	27	28/1007	2.9	2.8-3.0
Atraucan‡	26	16/350	4.6	2.6-7.3
Whitacre†	22	1/68	1.5	1.2-2.8
	25	103/6366	2.2	2.2-2.2
	27	10/668	1.7	1.6-1.8
Sprotte†	24	57/1767	3.5	3.5-3.5
Polymedic†	25	22/292	6.6	5.9-7.4
BD†	26	205/2560	5.8	5.6-5.9

n, number of headaches; N, total number of procedures; PDPH, post–dural puncture headache.

*Meta-analysis of estimated pooled event rate using a random effects model.

†Data from reference 42.

‡Data from references 71-73.

Onset and Duration

Headache typically occurs on the first or second day after dural puncture; by ICHD-II criteria, it must appear within 5 days of dural puncture.[3] Ninety-five percent of PDPH headaches last less than a week. The National Obstetric Anaesthetic Database project of the Obstetric Anaesthetists' Association of the United Kingdom demonstrated that 75% of 975 women with PDPH suffered from headache-associated difficulty in performing the activities of daily living.[48] Rarely, symptoms may persist for months or even years.[49]

TABLE 31-3 Symptoms Associated with Post–Dural Puncture Headache

Symptom	Incidence (%)
Nausea	60
Vomiting	24
Neck stiffness	43
Ocular*	13
Auditory†	12

*Ocular symptoms include photophobia, diplopia, and difficulty in accommodation.

†Auditory symptoms include hearing loss, hypacusis, and tinnitus.

Data from Lybecker H, Djernes M, Schmidt JF. Postdural puncture headache (PDPH): Onset, duration, severity, and associated symptoms. An analysis of 75 consecutive patients with PDPH. Acta Anaesthesiol Scand 1995;39:605-12.

Imaging

Imaging investigations are not routinely recommended for the postpartum patient with a PDPH unless the symptoms suggest other diagnoses and the diagnosis of PDPH is in doubt. Contrast-enhanced MRI is the method of choice to study the meninges and has revealed characteristic findings of PDPH.[50,51] These findings include marked, diffuse contrast enhancement with thickening of the dura mater, occasional extradural fluid collections, and enhancement and expansion of the superior sagittal sinus. The enlarged venous sinus may represent compensatory venous expansion in response to low CSF pressure.[51]

Pathophysiology

Debate continues regarding the precise etiology of PDPH symptoms. The original theory was that pain-sensitive nerve fibers were stimulated by a downward shift of the brain secondary to a loss of CSF volume. German surgeon August Bier[52] is credited with the first description of PDPH after his pioneering work on spinal anesthesia with cocaine. Bier and an assistant performed spinal anesthesia on each other, using blows to the shin with an iron hammer and application of a burning cigar to the skin to demonstrate sensory blockade.[52] Both experienced severe PDPH. The assistant forced himself to work the next day, but Bier stayed home for 9 days. Bier suggested that the PDPH might be caused by CSF loss. Today there is no doubt that leakage of CSF initiates the syndrome. Kunkle et al.[53] consistently produced PDPH by draining 20 mL of CSF from volunteers. Symptoms were relieved immediately by subarachnoid injection of saline to restore initial CSF pressure.

Total CSF volume is estimated to be 150 mL, and the production rate is approximately 0.35 mL/min, or a daily production rate of 500 mL. The rate of CSF leakage through a dural hole may exceed the rate of CSF production. If this occurs, low CSF pressure results in a loss of the cushioning effect provided by intracranial fluid.

CSF pressure during labor is normal between contractions but increases significantly during *painful* contractions and expulsive efforts.[54] Effective epidural analgesia attenuates this increase in CSF pressure. In a study of postpartum epidural space pressures following unintentional dural puncture in five women, epidural space pressures were normal preceding the development of headache.[55] However, with development of headache symptoms, the mean epidural pressure measurements were found to be decreased significantly.

Not all parturients with PDPH have decreased CSF pressure, and not all parturients with a significant CSF leak experience symptoms.[56] The pain of PDPH may be caused, in part, by an increase in cerebral blood flow (and cerebral vasodilation) as a consequence of low CSF pressure or volume. This phenomenon has been observed in animals.[57,58] The inverse relationship between intracranial blood volume and CSF volume reflects the body's effort to maintain a constant intracranial volume.[59] The lumbar CSF compartment is a dynamic structure that acts as a reservoir for intracranial CSF volume adjustment. The occurrence of cerebral vasodilation may explain the relief of headache symptoms with vasoconstrictors such as caffeine, theophylline, and sumatriptan.

Risk Factors

In a classic study of 10,098 spinal anesthetic procedures published in 1956, Vandam and Dripps[60] noted three demographic factors associated with PDPH: age, gender, and pregnancy. The analysis did not allow determination as to whether these factors were independent risk factors. Subsequently, other risk factors for development of PDPH have been identified.

AGE

Extensive evidence supports the observation that PDPH is uncommon in patients older than 60 years and is most common in patients younger than 40 years. In the elderly, the dura may be inelastic and less likely to gape after puncture. CSF leakage may be impeded by adhesions and calcification. The cerebrovascular system also may be less reactive in older patients. Further, this group is less active physically, and older patients may be less likely to complain.

GENDER

Vandam and Dripps[60] observed a twofold higher incidence of PDPH in women than in men (14% versus 7%, respectively). This difference may be related to differences in cerebral vascular reactivity, because it is well known that migraine occurs predominantly in females and is influenced by hormonal changes. Women may have enhanced vascular reactivity, or perhaps changes in cerebral blood flow are more likely to produce pain in women than in men. A meta-analysis of randomized clinical trials identified a twofold higher risk for PDPH in nonpregnant females than in males.[61]

VAGINAL DELIVERY

Vandam and Dripps[60] also observed a high incidence of PDPH (22%) after vaginal delivery. This higher incidence may be a result of the mechanical consequences of expulsive efforts during the second stage of labor and/or postpartum hormonal changes in cerebrovascular reactivity. Expulsive efforts during the second stage of labor may increase CSF leakage. This possibility has prompted some physicians to restrict maternal pushing after unintentional dural puncture and to use forceps to shorten the second stage of labor. In a 20-year retrospective review of 460 parturients who experienced unintentional dural puncture during labor at the Birmingham Maternity Hospital in the United Kingdom, Stride and Cooper[62] did not identify a lower incidence of PDPH in women who underwent prophylactic forceps delivery than in those who had spontaneous vaginal delivery. In contrast, in a retrospective review of the records of 33 laboring women who had experienced unintentional dural puncture, Angle et al.[63] found that women who were allowed to push were much more likely to experience PDPH (relative risk, 7.4; 95% CI, 1.1 to 48.2) and also were more likely to require an epidural blood patch.

MORBID OBESITY

Some evidence suggests that morbidly obese patients are less susceptible to PDPH and are also less likely to receive an epidural blood patch for treatment of PDPH,[64] suggesting either a reduced severity of PDPH or anesthesia provider reticence to perform an epidural blood patch in this patient population. Possible but unproven explanations for the lower incidence and severity of PDPH in obese patients include increased abdominal pressure (which may reduce the extent of CSF leak) and/or reduced physical activity of these patients. Other confounding factors, such as differences in the mode of delivery (higher rate of cesarean delivery) and neuraxial opioid administration, may also play a role.

AIR TRAVEL

PDPH has been reported during air travel after spinal anesthesia.[65] Presumably, the headache is precipitated by a change in the gradient between the subarachnoid space and the epidural space due to decreased atmospheric pressure.

HISTORY OF PREVIOUS POST–DURAL PUNCTURE HEADACHE

A history of PDPH after previous spinal anesthesia is associated with the development of PDPH with subsequent spinal anesthesia.[66] A cohort of nonobstetric women with a history of previous spinal anesthesia were monitored prospectively after a second spinal anesthesia procedure. Those with a previous history of PDPH were 2.3 times more likely (95% CI, 1.0 to 5.1) to have a second PDPH than women without a history of headache (24.2% versus 10.6%, respectively).[66] This finding suggests that certain individuals are predisposed to the development of PDPH.

MULTIPLE DURAL PUNCTURES

Seeberger et al.[67] found that multiple dural punctures significantly increased the risk for PDPH. Surgical patients who received a second spinal injection owing to failure of the initial spinal injection had a 4.2% incidence of PDPH, compared with a 1.6% incidence among patients who had a single dural puncture.

NEURAXIAL ANESTHETIC TECHNIQUE

Technical factors related to the neuraxial technique influence the incidence of PDPH.

Epidural Needle Size/Design

The high rate of PDPH following unintentional dural puncture with an epidural needle has led investigators to alter the epidural needle design or size in an attempt to reduce headache incidence or severity. Data on the success of this endeavor are conflicting. In an *in vitro* study using cadaver dura, no differences were found in fluid leak rate among punctures made with Hustead, Tuohy, Crawford, and Sprotte epidural needles.[68] In contrast, in an *in vivo* study, Morley-Forster et al.[69] observed a lower incidence of PDPH with use of an 18-gauge Sprotte needle than with use of the standard 17-gauge Tuohy needle, despite there being no difference in the unintentional dural puncture rate. A pilot study has examined the utility of a 19-gauge Tuohy needle with a 23-gauge epidural catheter.[70]

Spinal Needle Design

Historically the beveled, cutting-tip Quincke needle (Figure 31-3) has been the most widely used needle for dural puncture for both diagnostic and anesthetic purposes (see Chapter 12). A modification of the Quincke needle, the Atraucan needle, has a cutting tip and a double bevel, which are intended to cut a small dural hole and then dilate it.[71] Clinical experience with the Atraucan needle has been generally good,[71,72] although studies appear to suggest that the use of this needle is associated with a higher risk of PDPH than the use of a noncutting, pencil-point needle (see Table 31-2).[73]

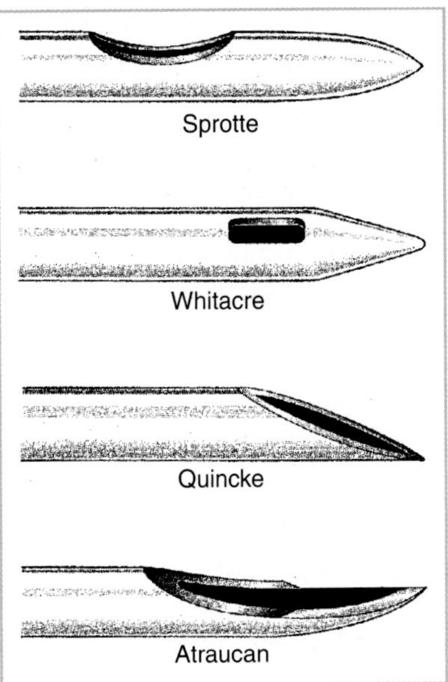

FIGURE 31-3 Designs of spinal needle tips (not to scale).

In 1951, Hart and Whitacre[74] introduced a solid-tipped, pencil-point spinal needle with a lateral injection port, which is now known as the Whitacre design (see Figure 31-3). They believed that their needle would stretch and separate rather than cut the dural fibers, resulting in a lower incidence of PDPH. Currently, both 25- and 27-gauge Whitacre needles are very popular, and studies have confirmed the anticipated low incidence of PDPH.[42] A randomized comparison of 27-gauge Quincke and pencil-point needles found a significantly lower incidence of PDPH in the pencil-point needle group.[75,76] *In vitro* evidence suggests that the rate of fluid leak is lower through the dural puncture site after use of a pencil-point needle than after use of a beveled needle.[77]

With the recognition that pencil-point spinal needle tips reduce the incidence of PDPH, other tip designs have appeared. In 1987, Sprotte et al.[78] reported experience with the use of a needle that was designed to reduce the risk of neural and dural trauma (see Figure 31-3). The Sprotte needle has a solid oval tip and a longer orifice than the Whitacre needle. The incidence of PDPH was 0.02% with its use in a heterogeneous population of almost 35,000 patients.[78] Subsequent studies have shown that the incidence of PDPH with the Sprotte needle is lower than that with Quincke needles of smaller gauge (see Table 31-2).[42] Other noncutting needle products are the Gertie Marx needle and the Polymedic needle.

Spinal Needle Size

With the Quincke needle, the incidence and severity of PDPH are directly related to the size of the needle. The incidence of PDPH appears to be lower with a 27-gauge needle than with 25- and 26-gauge needles (see Table 31-2). A similar relationship may exist with pencil-point needles. When needles smaller than 27-gauge are used, the incidence of PDPH is very low, but technical problems with needle insertion and failure to produce adequate anesthesia are more common.[79] Locating the epidural space before insertion of the spinal needle (e.g., using the epidural needle as an introducer needle) may improve the rate of success with fine-gauge needles.

The current popularity of spinal anesthesia in obstetric patients is largely a result of new needle technology, which has led to a reduction in the incidence of PDPH. Because of the morbidity associated with PDPH, every effort should be made to use a needle associated with a low incidence of PDPH (e.g., a small-gauge, noncutting needle). There are times when urgency or body habitus dictates the use of a larger needle, but there is seldom justification for using a Quincke needle larger than 27-gauge.

Direction of Bevel of the Quincke Needle

Studies have confirmed that puncturing the dura mater with the Quincke needle bevel parallel to the long axis of the spine is associated with an incidence of PDPH 70% lower than that associated with a perpendicular orientation.[80] An early study by Franksson and Gordh[81] demonstrated that orientation of the bevel of a Quincke spinal needle parallel to the long axis of the spine produced less dural trauma than occurred when the bevel was inserted perpendicularly. These investigators thought that the dural fibers were predominantly longitudinal in direction. Electron microscopy has shown that the dural structure is far more complex than originally was supposed. Fink and Walker[82] noted that the dura consists of multidirectional interlacing collagen fibers and both transverse and longitudinal elastic fibers. They suggested that the insertion of the needle with the bevel parallel to the long axis of the spine most likely results in less tension on the dural hole, and therefore, a smaller aperture with less CSF leak. *In vitro* studies of bevel orientation and fluid leak have provided conflicting results.[83,84] However, despite confusing anatomic evidence, clinical experience strongly supports insertion of the Quincke needle with the bevel parallel to the long axis of the spine.

Direction of the Bevel of the Tuohy Needle

Norris et al.[85] examined two groups of women who received epidural anesthesia with a Tuohy needle. In one group the needle was inserted with the bevel perpendicular to the long axis of the spine. In the other group the needle entered the epidural space with the bevel parallel to the long axis and was rotated 90 degrees before insertion of the catheter. The investigators observed a lower incidence of PDPH in the latter group. However, some anesthesia providers argue that rotation of the needle within the epidural space may increase the risk of unintentional dural puncture. Richardson and Wissler[86] randomly assigned laboring patients to a cephalad or lateral orientation of the Tuohy bevel during epidural needle insertion. The needle was not rotated before insertion of the epidural catheter. There was no difference in dural puncture rates, but catheter insertion was easier with a cephalad orientation of the bevel.[86]

Midline or Paramedian Approach

There is conflicting evidence as to whether the spinal needle approach affects the incidence of PDPH. Hatfalvi[87] reported no cases of PDPH in a retrospective survey of 4465 spinal anesthesia procedures. This investigator used a paramedian approach with a 20-gauge Quincke needle, and the skin was punctured 3 cm from the midline. He suggested that tangential dural puncture creates a dural flap and prevents PDPH. In contrast, Viitanen et al.,[88] prospectively monitoring obstetric patients after administration of single-shot spinal analgesia for labor (27-gauge Quincke needle), observed PDPH in 3 of 85 (3.5%) patients in whom the midline approach was used, compared with 15 of 127 (11.8%) patients in whom the paramedian approach was used. Using a rigid paper cylinder model of the dura, Kempen and Mocek[89] studied midline and paramedian punctures with a 22-gauge Quincke needle in different orientations. With midline punctures, all entry and exit holes were of uniform size regardless of bevel orientation, and no dural flaps were seen. After paramedian punctures, flaps formed when the needle bevel faced the cylinder surface with a near-tangential angle of perforation.

Skin Preparation

In a nonrandomized, nonblinded study reported in a letter, Gurmarnik[90] found that the removal of dried povidone-iodine from the skin before placement of the spinal needle was associated with a lower incidence of PDPH (6% versus 0%). This investigator recommended removal of the povidone-iodine before insertion of the spinal needle, and suggested that chemical meningismus resulting from povidone-iodine introduced into the intrathecal space by the spinal needle contributed to PDPH. This finding has not been confirmed by other investigators. (*Editors' Note:* We do not recommend removal of povidone-iodine before initiating neuraxial analgesia, because povidone-iodine works by desiccating bacteria, and removing the povidone-iodine reduces its antibacterial effect.)

Air versus Saline Method of Locating the Epidural Space

The method of locating the epidural space may influence the incidence of PDPH.[91] Many anesthesia providers have adopted the loss-of-resistance-to-saline technique in the belief that it is associated with a lower incidence of unintentional dural puncture and PDPH than the use of air.[62,92] However, the data are inconsistent, and not all studies have found a difference.[92-94] In a study of epidural steroid injections (at all spinal levels) in a pain clinic, a single practitioner performed more than 3700 procedures, alternating weekly between use of the loss-of-resistance to air and saline methods.[95] There was no difference between groups in the incidence of unintentional dural puncture. Although the incidence of postprocedure headache was lower in the saline group, the definition of headache was not rigorous, and it was not possible to differentiate between headache from pneumocephalus and classic PDPH.[95]

Choice of Local Anesthetic Drug for Spinal Anesthesia

Naulty et al.[96] reported that the use of bupivacaine-glucose or lidocaine-glucose for spinal anesthesia was associated with a higher incidence of PDPH than use of tetracaine-procaine. They postulated that osmotic, cerebral (meningeal) irritant and/or cerebrovascular effects of the glucose could be responsible for these findings.

Continuous Spinal Anesthesia

A multicenter trial published in 2008 reexamined the safety and utility of 28-gauge microcatheters for spinal labor analgesia.[97] There was no difference in the incidence of

PDPH (9% versus 4%, respectively) or epidural blood patch (5% versus 2%, respectively), between women randomly assigned to receive an intrathecal catheter and those who received an epidural catheter; however, the study was insufficiently powered to assess these outcomes. Spinal microcatheters currently are not commercially available in North America.

Combined Spinal-Epidural Anesthesia

Combined spinal-epidural (CSE) analgesia/anesthesia is widely used for labor analgesia and, to a lesser extent, for cesarean delivery. Intuitively, it seems that the incidence of PDPH should be identical to that after single-shot spinal anesthesia with the same size and type of needle. Many anesthesia providers believe that the intentional dural puncture with the CSE technique is associated with a higher incidence of PDPH than epidural anesthesia alone. However, the available evidence, primarily from observational studies, suggests that the risk of PDPH is not increased with the CSE technique.[98-100] PDPH rates for the CSE technique in these three studies were 1.7%, 0.43%, and 1.4%, respectively, compared with 1.6%, 0.45%, and 0.8% for the epidural technique.[98-100] Initial placement of the epidural needle facilitates precise dural puncture, and the subsequent increase in epidural space pressure after the epidural injection of local anesthetic may reduce CSF leakage. If the anesthesia provider is in doubt about correct epidural needle placement, a needle-through-needle dural puncture might resolve the issue and prevent unintentional dural puncture with a large-gauge epidural needle.

Complications

The immediate problems associated with PDPH include (1) the inability to perform the activities of daily living, such as providing care for the newborn; (2) an extended duration (almost one full day) of hospitalization; and (3) a higher number of emergency room visits, with almost 40% of patients returning for at least one visit.[101] Although these complications are very bothersome to the patient, they are short-lived and do not result in long-term morbidity. However, rare but serious complications may occur after dural puncture and PDPH.

Zeidan et al.[102] reviewed the published reports of **subdural hematoma** after dural puncture. They found that subdural hematoma was associated with new neurologic symptoms in addition to changing headache characteristics. The proposed mechanism of subdural hematoma development is ongoing intracranial hypotension leading to caudal movement of the brain and rupture of fragile, bridging subdural veins. These cases have been managed with an epidural blood patch as well as with neurosurgical decompression.

Dural sinus thrombosis has been documented after unintentional dural puncture and treatment of PDPH with an epidural blood patch.[18-20] Responsible factors may be cerebral venous dilation (associated with decreased ICP) and the hypercoagulability that occurs during pregnancy. Therapy may include anticoagulation.

Diplopia or **hearing loss** after dural puncture, secondary to cranial nerve dysfunction, may be permanent, even after successful treatment of the PDPH with an epidural blood patch. A review of 95 cases of neurapraxia or axonotmesis of the ocular cranial nerves concluded that symptoms may last from 2 weeks to 8 months but that almost 90% of patients recover.[103]

Two surveys from a single institution have attempted to estimate long-term morbidity arising from unintentional dural puncture or spinal anesthesia in obstetric patients.[104,105] Women delivering between 1978 and 1985,[104] and between 1991 and 1996,[105] were asked to recall symptoms beginning after their deliveries, including back pain and headache. The responses of women with unintentional dural puncture or PDPH following spinal anesthesia were compared with those of women who had uneventful procedures. The first study found that 18% of women with unintentional dural puncture had complaints of frequent headaches or neck ache, compared with only 7% of women experiencing uneventful neuraxial procedures.[104] The later study did not confirm a higher risk of headache with prior unintentional dural puncture but, instead, found a higher rate of backache symptoms.[105] These results have not been confirmed in a prospective study or by other investigators and likely suffer from the limitations of surveys that rely on patient recall.

Prevention

A 2005 survey of British obstetric anesthetists identified the frequency of practices and maneuvers that many believe will reduce the likelihood of a PDPH after unintentional dural puncture with an epidural needle.[106] These include encouraging postpartum fluid intake (91%) and regular analgesia administration (83%), and placement of an intrathecal catheter (15%) at the time of the unintentional dural puncture. Older practices, such as avoiding pushing during the second stage, restricting postpartum mobility, and prophylactic epidural administration of saline or autologous blood, appear to be declining in use.

POSTURE

In a Cochrane systematic review, Sudlow and Warlow[107] reviewed the evidence for reducing the incidence of PDPH by use of bed rest rather than early mobilization (usually within 6 hours of dural puncture). The review included the only randomized trial of obstetric patients, and results were consistent for all patient types; there was no benefit for bed rest over early mobilization (PDPH incidence 31% versus 27%, respectively). It is important to encourage early ambulation during the puerperium. Pregnant women are hypercoagulable and at higher risk for deep vein thrombosis and pulmonary embolism, and immobility increases this risk (see Chapter 38).

HYDRATION

Despite the widespread practice of encouraging women to increase oral fluid intake after unintentional dural puncture, there is little evidence that greater hydration prevents PDPH. The Cochrane review identified only one randomized trial of 100 nonobstetric patients.[107] There was no difference in the incidence of PDPH in patients randomly assigned to receive either 3 L or 1.5 L of fluid per day.

ABDOMINAL BINDER

In a 1975 study, the use of a tight abdominal binder placed immediately after delivery and continued until discharge home apparently was successful in reducing the incidence of PDPH.[108] The study included parturients who received single-shot spinal anesthesia through 22-gauge cutting needles, which are more likely to lead to PDPH than modern-day spinal needles. However, the applicability of this technique to prevent PDPH after unintentional dural puncture with an epidural needle has not been evaluated. Abdominal binders are seldom used today.

CAFFEINE

Two clinical trials in nonobstetric patients have evaluated the efficacy of oral caffeine to prevent PDPH, but neither study showed a reduction in the incidence of headache.[109] At this time, prophylactic caffeine is not advocated for prevention of PDPH.

INTRASPINAL OPIOIDS

Earlier studies suggested that prophylactic neuraxial administration of a hydrophilic or lipophilic opioid does not reduce the incidence of PDPH after spinal anesthesia or unintentional dural puncture.[110,111] However, in a randomized blinded trial published in 2008, 50 obstetric patients with unintentional dural puncture and subsequent epidural analgesia received epidural morphine 3 mg or saline-placebo after delivery and again at 24 hours before removal of the epidural catheter.[112] The incidence of PDPH was 48% in the saline-placebo group and 12% in the morphine group. Although no complications were reported, we would caution against routine administration of epidural morphine in these circumstances until this finding is confirmed and further safety studies are undertaken. The movement of morphine across the dura is increased by the presence of a large-gauge needle puncture,[113] possibly increasing the risk of respiratory depression.

INTRATHECAL CATHETER

Placing a 19- or 20-gauge epidural catheter into the intrathecal space after an unintentional dural puncture with an epidural needle has become an increasingly popular technique.[93,106,114-118] The immediate benefits of an intrathecal catheter are reliable, low-dose labor analgesia and rapid-onset surgical anesthesia should it be required. Some authorities have speculated that the intrathecal catheter may reduce the immediate CSF leak into the epidural space by mechanical obstruction and induce an inflammatory fibrous reaction in the dura, which facilitates closure of the puncture site after removal of the catheter. Currently available studies are mostly retrospective and observational and lack rigorous outcome definitions and follow-up. Data from these studies are conflicting but suggest that intrathecal catheters do not significantly reduce the incidence of PDPH unless they are left in place for 24 hours after delivery (Table 31-4). The safety of this practice has not been well studied. Randomized clinical trials to assess the effect of intrathecal catheters on the incidence of PDPH are desirable but would likely require multicenter participation owing to the infrequent occurrence of unintentional dural puncture.

PROPHYLACTIC EPIDURAL/INTRATHECAL SALINE

Trivedi et al.[119] randomly assigned patients with unintentional dural puncture to receive a prophylactic epidural saline bolus (40 to 60 mL) or a prophylactic epidural blood patch (15 mL) given just prior to epidural catheter removal, or conservative therapy without a saline bolus or blood. The incidence of PDPH was no different between the saline and control groups (88% versus 67%, respectively). Shah[120] studied 17 patients who received an epidural saline infusion (at a rate of approximately 40 mL/hr) for 24 to 36 hours after unintentional dural puncture. Four patients complained of severe interscapular pain, which resolved when the infusion rate was reduced. Severe PDPH developed in 47% of patients after the infusion was stopped. Despite these discouraging results, prophylactic epidural saline infusions continue to be popular in some centers. The saline infusion should not be initiated, however, until residual local anesthetic effects have resolved.

In a nonrandomized, nonblinded study of patients with unintentional dural puncture, Charsley and Abram[121]

TABLE 31-4 Rate of Post–Dural Puncture Headache after Unintentional Dural Puncture and Prophylactic Intrathecal Catheter Placement

Study*	Study Design	Spinal Catheter, n/N (%)	No Spinal Catheter, n/N (%)
Norris & Leighton[114]	Retrospective cohort; catheter left in place for 2 hr	19/35 (54)	11/21 (52)
Cohen et al.[115]	Retrospective cohort:		5/15 (33)
	Catheter discontinued immediately after delivery	8/17 (47)	
	Catheter left in place for 24 hr	0/13 (0)†	
Dennehy & Rosaeg[116]	Case series; catheter left in place for 13-19 hr	0/3 (0)	—
Paech[93]	Prospective cohort; catheter discontinued immediately after delivery	21/24 (87)	60/76 (79)
Rutter et al.[117]	Retrospective cohort; catheter left in place for unknown duration	24/34 (71)	30/37 (81)
Ayad et al.[118]	Retrospective cohort:		34/37 (92)
	Catheter discontinued immediately after delivery	18/35 (51)†	
	Catheter left in place for 24 hr	2/31 (6)†	

*Superscript numbers indicate reference citations at the end of the chapter.

†Different than no-catheter, $P < .05$.

No epidural blood patch procedures were performed. CT scans showed or suggested infarction in two of these subjects. The investigators stated that before the occurrence of these three cases, ACTH had been used regularly to treat PDPH in their institution but that subsequently they had discontinued the administration of ACTH as a therapy for PDPH. No conclusion can be drawn about the possible contribution of ACTH therapy to the observed seizure activity. With the evidence to date, it appears that ACTH therapy cannot be recommended as first-line treatment of PDPH but may be considered for cases that are not amenable to epidural blood patch therapy.

Miscellaneous Medications

Other agents evaluated for their effectiveness in reducing PDPH symptoms are gabapentin, methylergonovine, and hydrocortisone. Perhaps the most compelling evidence is for the use of intravenous hydrocortisone (200-mg loading dose followed by 100 mg three times daily for 2 days).[151] Noyan Ashraf et al.[151] evaluated 60 parturients who experienced PDPH after spinal anesthesia and were randomly assigned to receive intravenous hydrocortisone or conventional therapy, which consisted of bed rest, hydration, and scheduled acetaminophen with meperidine. Patients who received hydrocortisone had a 50% reduction in headache severity as assessed by VAS scores at 6 to 48 hours. A criticism of this study is the lack of blinding of the study participants, which may have influenced their perception of headache pain.

Use of gabapentin or methylergonovine has been reported only in case series. Efficacy and side effects (maternal and neonatal) are unclear.[152,153] All three drugs require further study before they can be recommended for therapy of PDPH.

EPIDURAL MORPHINE

Eldor et al.[154] reported six nonobstetric patients who received epidural morphine 3.5 to 4.5 mg to relieve the symptoms of PDPH. However, this therapy should be used with caution because epidural morphine injected in the presence of a large dural puncture site may pass readily into the CSF and predispose to respiratory depression.

EPIDURAL/INTRATHECAL SALINE

The use of epidural or intrathecal fluids to treat PDPH preceded epidural blood patch therapy. Intrathecal injection of fluid was first described by Jacobaeus et al.[155] in 1923, and epidural injection of saline was first described by Rice and Dabbs[156] in 1950. These first reports were described in conjunction with research attempting to understand the pathophysiology of PDPH, and they demonstrated transient elevation of CSF pressure after fluid injection. Subsequently there has been sporadic interest in the injection of fluids (other than blood) into the neuraxial space to treat PDPH.

Usubiaga et al.[157] reported the injection of 10 to 30 mL of saline through a lumbar epidural catheter in 11 patients with PDPH after spinal anesthesia in whom 48 hours of conservative therapy failed. Immediate relief of headache was observed in 10 patients, and the relief was permanent in 8 patients. However, the investigators did not comment whether other therapies (e.g., supine posture, abdominal binder, analgesics) were continued. In a quasi-randomized trial, 43 parturients with PDPH after unintentional dural puncture during an epidural procedure or after spinal anesthesia with a 25-gauge needle were assigned to receive a 30-mL epidural saline bolus in the lumbar region or a 10-mL lumbar epidural blood patch.[158] Forty-two patients had dramatic relief of their symptoms in the first hour following the intervention; however 12 of the 21 (57%) patients who received saline had recurrence of the PDPH in the next 24 hours.

Prolonged epidural saline infusion may provide better therapy for PDPH symptoms than therapy with a single bolus.[159,160] Two case reports described the use of epidural saline infusion for parturients with an unintentional dural puncture, whose PDPH symptoms returned after epidural blood patch therapy. The rate of infusion (15 to 25 mL/hr) was limited by the onset of pain in the back, legs, and eyes. A comparative study of epidural saline bolus versus infusion to treat PDPH is needed to determine whether either modality continued over 24 hours would provide better results than conservative therapy. This option might be considered for patients who have a contraindication to epidural blood patch therapy.

EPIDURAL BLOOD PATCH

Efficacy

The epidural blood patch procedure, regarded by many as the gold standard therapy for PDPH, was first described by Gormley[161] in 1960. He reported relief of PDPH symptoms in seven patients after epidural administration of 2 to 3 mL of blood. However, this report was largely ignored until 1970, when DiGiovanni and Dunbar[162] described the immediate and permanent cure of PDPH in 41 of 45 patients in whom 10 mL of autologous blood was injected into the epidural space. Their success led to the widespread adoption of this technique for the relief of PDPH. An excellent review of the history of PDPH and the development of the blood patch was written by Harrington.[163]

In early case series, the reported success rate of epidural blood patch therapy for PDPH was between 89% and 91%.[162,164] Subsequent studies have not confirmed this high rate of success. Taivainen et al.[165] studied 81 patients with PDPH after spinal needle puncture. Initially symptoms were relieved in 88% to 96% of patients; however, a permanent cure was achieved in only 61%. Safa-Tisseront et al.[166] reviewed the experience with blood patch therapy at their institution over a 12-year period (n = 504, including 78 obstetric patients). Complete relief of PDPH was obtained in 75%, partial relief occurred in 18%, and treatment failed in 7% of patients. The investigators noted a significantly higher failure rate of blood patch after large-gauge needle puncture of the dura. The difference in early reports and more modern audits of PDPH and epidural blood patch therapy success may be related to differences in the duration of follow-up, or perhaps to other differences in management after blood patch therapy, such as delayed mobilization.

In studies limited to obstetric patients, the published success rates of the epidural blood patch have been even less encouraging. Stride and Cooper[62] noted complete and permanent relief of PDPH in 64% of patients after one blood patch procedure. Williams et al.[94] reported that only 33% of their patients obtained complete and permanent relief from the first blood patch. Banks et al.[167] prospectively monitored 100 patients with unintentional dural puncture. Fifty-eight patients received a therapeutic blood patch; the treatment completely failed in 3 patients, and 17 patients had recurrence of moderate or severe headache requiring further therapy. These observational studies also describe the use of repeated epidural blood patch procedures for parturients with a recurrence of PDPH.

A 2002 Cochrane systematic review[124] identified only one small randomized trial[168] evaluating the efficacy of epidural blood patch therapy. This trial involved 12 heterogeneous patients with PDPH who were randomly assigned to undergo epidural blood patch therapy with 10 to 20 mL of blood or a sham patch procedure. Five of 6 patients receiving a blood patch had complete relief of headache symptoms at 24 hours, and none of the sham procedure patients did. Subsequently two additional randomized trials have been reported.[169,170] Sandesc et al.[169] reported 32 obstetric and nonobstetric patients who had PDPH symptoms for a minimum of 24 hours, who were randomly assigned to receive either conservative therapy or an epidural blood patch. The primary outcome was headache VAS scores at 2 and 24 hours. At 2 hours the mean VAS score for the conservative therapy group was 8.2 ± 1.4 cm compared with 1.0 ± 0.18 cm for the group receiving a blood patch ($P < .001$). This difference remained evident at 24 hours. In the largest trial to date, 40 subjects who had PDPH for 1 to 7 days were randomly assigned to receive either conservative therapy or an epidural blood patch using 15 to 20 mL of autologous blood.[170] The primary outcome was headache 24 hours after intervention, but patients were followed up for 1 week after therapy. The incidence of headache at 24 hours was 58% in the blood patch group compared with 90% in the conservative therapy group (relative risk, 0.64; 95% CI, 0.43 to 0.96). At 1 week the difference widened, with 16% incidence of headache in the blood patch group versus 86% in the conservative group. In summary, administration of an autologous epidural blood patch, while not perfect, often dramatically relieves this debilitating condition, and at present, it is the therapy with the greatest likelihood of success.

The optimal volume of injected blood remains controversial. Better results have been obtained with injection of 20 mL of blood than with the smaller volumes used by Gormley and DiGiovanni.[161,162] Szeinfeld et al.[171] used a gamma camera to observe the epidural spread of technetium-labeled red blood cells during and after epidural blood patch. They injected blood until pain occurred in the back, buttocks, or legs. The mean ± SD volume injected was 14.8 ± 1.7 mL of blood, and the mean ± SD spread was 9.0 ± 2.0 spinal segments. Blood spread more readily in the cephalad than in the caudad direction. Blood patch relieved headache in all 10 patients. The investigators concluded that 12 to 15 mL of blood should be a sufficient patch volume for most patients. Taivainen et al.[165] found that injection of a "height-adjusted" volume of blood (minimum of 10 mL to a maximum of 15 mL) conferred no advantage over a standard 10-mL injection. Most anesthesia providers inject 10 to 20 mL of blood.

Beards et al.[172] performed MRI studies after the performance of epidural blood patches (18 to 20 mL) in five patients. They noted that the injected blood spread over three to five segments in a predominantly cephalad direction. All patients had an extensive hematoma in the subcutaneous fat, and some also had displacement of nerve roots and/or evidence of intrathecal blood. A thick layer of mature clot had formed by 7 hours, which had broken up into smaller clots by 18 hours. These findings may help explain the back pain and occasional nerve root pain that occur after blood patch.

In another MRI study, Vakharia et al.[50] noted compression of the thecal sac and a mean spread over 4.6 segments after the injection of 20 mL of blood (Figure 31-4). Djurhuus et al.[173] employed CT epidurography in four patients immediately and 24 hours after an 18-mL blood patch. Initial images showed adherence of clot to the dura in three patients as well as dural compression in two patients, but there was no evidence of compression at 24 hours.

Using a goat model, DiGiovanni et al.[174] examined the microscopic appearance of the dura as late as 6 months after dural puncture. Some study animals received a 2-mL blood patch in addition to dural puncture. The investigators concluded that the blood patch acted as a gelatinous tampon that produced no harmful tissue reaction.

The mechanism of epidural blood patch for relief of PDPH is unclear. Pain relief is often rapid, but CSF volume is not restored immediately. Thus, there must be another explanation for the immediate relief of headache besides "patching" of the dural puncture. Carrie[175] hypothesized that epidural injection of blood increases lumbar CSF pressure, an action that restores intracranial CSF pressure and decreases symptoms. Increased CSF pressure also may result in reflex cerebral vasoconstriction. Coombs and Hooper[176] demonstrated that epidural blood patch therapy resulted in a threefold increase in lumbar CSF pressure. Further, they noted that 15 minutes later, lumbar CSF pressure was sustained at more than 70% of the peak pressure observed after the injection of blood. Kroin et al.[177] observed that epidural injection of blood in rats caused a sustained increase in CSF pressure throughout a 4-hour study period.

MRI and CT studies have shown that the epidural blood is largely resorbed or broken up 18 to 24 hours after the procedure.[172,173] It is unlikely that the increase in CSF pressure is sustained or that the blood acts as a mechanical plug to block CSF leak for a prolonged duration. The blood applied to the hole in the dura may initiate an inflammatory reaction that facilitates puncture site repair and closure. It is possible, and even likely, that an epidural blood patch ameliorates PDPH by several mechanisms.

Timing

The optimal timing for administration of a blood patch has not been studied adequately. Observational studies suggest that failure is more likely if the blood patch is performed within 24 hours of the dural puncture.[166,178] It is unclear, however, whether this observation is a result of selection bias. Early-onset PDPH (often resulting from dural puncture with a large-gauge needle) is likely to be more severe and more difficult to treat. Alternatively, a large CSF leak may displace the clot. Partial healing of the dura may have already occurred if a blood patch procedure is delayed, a possibility that may explain the better outcome of a delayed patch procedure.

Technique for Blood Patch

The anesthesia provider should thoroughly explain the risks and benefits of the blood patch procedure to the patient,

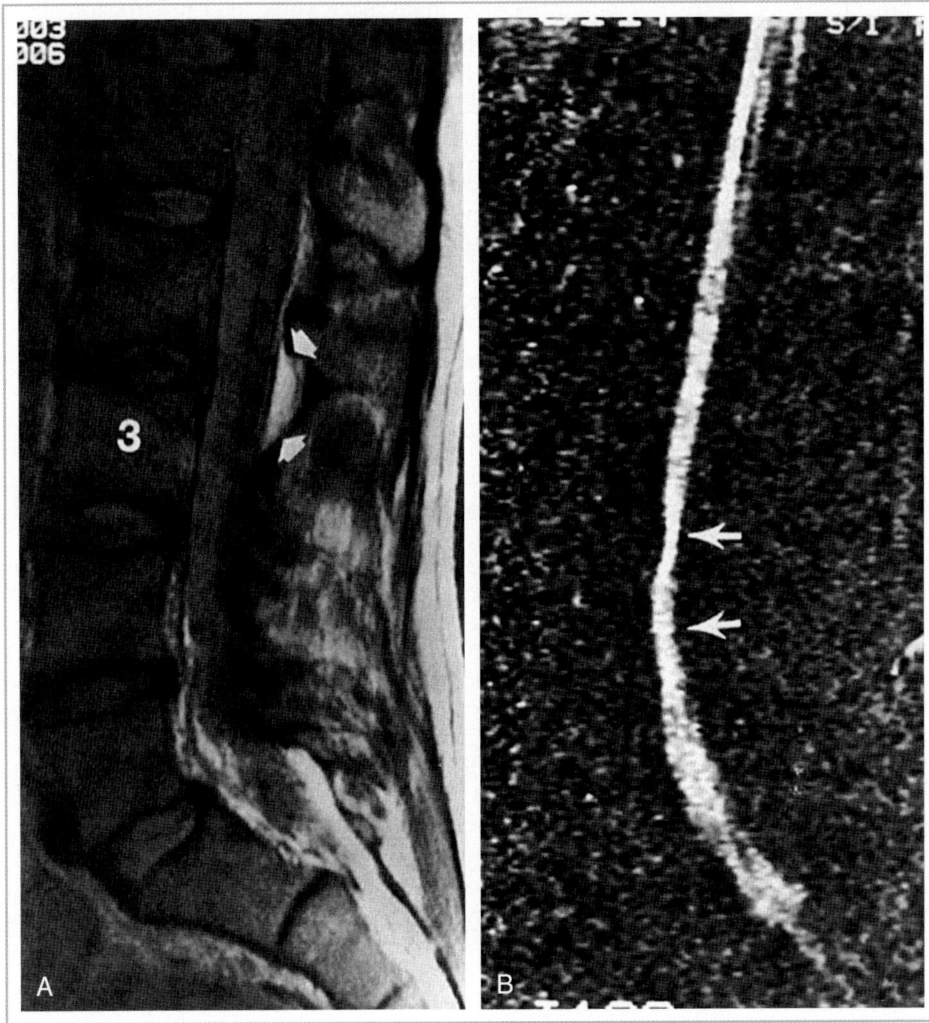

FIGURE 31-4 **A,** Pre–blood patch magnetic resonance imaging using sagittal spin-echo proton density. The dural puncture has been performed at L2 to L3, which local static fluid collection (*arrows*) affirms; "3" denotes L3 vertebral body. **B,** Post–blood patch magnetic resonance imaging of cerebrospinal fluid flow in systole shows the long length of the compression of the thecal sac posteriorly (*arrows*). (From Vakharia SB, Thomas PS, Rosenbaum AE, et al. Magnetic resonance imaging of cerebrospinal fluid leak and tamponade effect of blood patch in postdural puncture headache. Anesth Analg 1997;84:585-90.)

and the patient should give written informed consent for the procedure. An epidural blood patch can be accomplished on an outpatient basis. Contraindications to the administration of an epidural blood patch are related to complications of placing a needle in the central neuraxis or the administration of blood into the epidural space; they include (1) known coagulopathy, (2) local cutaneous infection or untreated systemic infection, (3) increased ICP due to a space-occupying lesion, and (4) patient refusal. Transient bradycardia has been observed after administration of an epidural blood patch,[179] and some anesthesia providers may choose to establish intravenous access and monitor the electrocardiogram (ECG) in selected patients.

The blood patch procedure should employ sterility measures equivalent to those used in the performance of any neuraxial procedure. The lateral position is more comfortable than the sitting position for patients with severe PDPH. If the anesthesia provider is uncertain about the location of the dural puncture, the more caudad interspace should be chosen. The epidural space is identified in the usual manner. Using meticulous sterile technique (including skin preparation and draping, and donning of a mask and sterile gloves), an assistant withdraws the desired volume of blood into a syringe, usually 10 to 20 mL. This autologous blood is injected slowly through the epidural needle, but the injection is terminated if severe back, leg, or neck pain or pressure occurs. Sometimes slowing the injection rate leads to resolution of the back pain. Blood patch procedures can be administered to Jehovah's Witness patients with a technique designed to keep blood in continuity with the circulation.[180]

Occasionally, a few drops of CSF are encountered upon entry of the needle into the epidural space, leading to doubt about correct needle placement. In this situation a small test dose of a local anesthetic agent may be administered, sufficient to cause a rapid onset of spinal anesthesia if the needle tip is in the intrathecal space. If no neuroblockade occurs, a blood patch can be performed.

After the procedure the patient should rest quietly in the horizontal position for 1 to 2 hours.[181] Subsequently the patient may resume ambulation, but she should avoid vigorous physical activity for several days. It would be wise for the patient to avoid the Valsalva maneuver and heavy lifting. A stool softener should be prescribed. Most patients report almost instantaneous relief of headache symptoms but may continue to have neck and back fullness over the next 24 hours. Patients should be counseled to immediately report fever, severe back pain, or radiating lower extremity pain. The anesthesia provider should contact the patient daily for several days after the blood patch procedure.

The blood patch procedure may be repeated if the first one fails to relieve pain. Often the second procedure is successful. The diagnosis should be reconsidered if headache persists after two failed blood patch procedures. A neurology consultation is desirable when a PDPH fails to respond to two blood patch procedures, and should definitely be requested if there is any doubt about the diagnosis. Imaging of the head should be considered to exclude other causes of headache.

Complications of Blood Patch Procedures

Ong et al.[182] reported that the success of neuraxial anesthesia/analgesia was impaired in women with a prior history of unintentional dural puncture with or without epidural blood patch therapy. However, this conclusion has been refuted by follow-up studies in both obstetric[183] and nonobstetric patients.[184] In both of these retrospective studies, a history of blood patch therapy had no apparent effect on the quality of subsequent epidural anesthesia. Loughrey et al.[185] described a patient who experienced PDPH after diagnostic lumbar puncture at term gestation. A blood patch was administered and the headache was relieved, but 6 hours later, urgent cesarean delivery was required. Spinal anesthesia was administered via the same intervertebral space as the blood patch procedure. The anesthetic course and postoperative period were uneventful, and the patient had no recurrence of headache.

Although epidural blood patch therapy is the most reliable method of relieving PDPH symptoms, adverse outcomes are associated with the procedure. These adverse events can be categorized into two broad groups, infectious/hematologic and neurologic.

Infectious/Hematologic Complications Conventional wisdom holds that the patient should be afebrile at the time of a blood patch procedure. Many anesthesia providers believe that it is wise to avoid the epidural injection of blood in the presence of systemic infection. Meningitis has been reported after a blood patch.[186] After conservative measures have failed, the optimal treatment of a febrile patient with severe, persistent PDPH is controversial. Epidural infusion of saline involves the use of an indwelling epidural catheter for many hours, which may also be undesirable in a febrile patient. A patch using dextran-40 may be an alternative in febrile patients, but further experience in healthy patients is needed before this technique can be recommended. The presence of high fever or other evidence of sepsis contraindicates the performance of a blood patch procedure. However, we do not believe that a low-grade fever of known etiology is an absolute contraindication to epidural blood patch therapy, provided that the patient is receiving appropriate antibiotic therapy. Management should be individualized, and the known benefits of blood patch therapy should be weighed against the unknown risk of infection.

The risk of epidural blood patch therapy in the presence of human immunodeficiency virus (HIV) infection has been debated (see Chapter 44). However, the central nervous system is infected with HIV at the time of primary infection; therefore, it seems unlikely that injection of autologous blood into the epidural space would alter progression of the disease. There are published reports of the successful use of epidural blood patch therapy, without sequelae, in patients who have acquired immunodeficiency syndrome (AIDS) or who are HIV-positive.[187,188]

The incidence of cancer during pregnancy is increasing secondary to advancing maternal age. The development of PDPH in this population has raised a theoretical concern about seeding the neuraxial space with neoplastic cells if a blood patch is performed. This concern should be discussed with the patient and her oncologist before the procedure. Bucklin et al.[189] reported the conservative management of a woman with acute leukemia and PDPH; the investigators discussed the therapeutic options for this immunocompromised patient. The use of epidural fibrin glue was reported in a nonobstetric patient with metastatic breast cancer and PDPH,[190] whereas a blood patch procedure was performed for PDPH in a young women with rhabdomyosarcoma.[191]

Neurologic Complications Serious or permanent problems after epidural blood patch therapy are rare. Diaz et al.[192] wrote an excellent review of case reports of adverse neurologic complications after epidural blood patch procedures. These authors identified 26 reports published between 1966 and 2004 and stratified the complications into neurologic, neurovascular, or inflammatory events. The events occurring in obstetric patients included lumbovertebral symptoms (defined as low back pain with neurologic impairment of the lower extremities), subdural hematoma, arachnoiditis, radicular back pain, pneumocephalus, seizures, and acute meningeal irritation. Compression complications (i.e., lumbovertebral syndrome, subdural hematoma, cauda equina syndrome) were associated with a larger blood patch volume (mean of 35 mL) than the non-compression complications (17 mL). Cranial nerve palsy symptoms that were present prior to the blood patch procedure did not uniformly resolve. The delay in administering the blood patch may have been a significant factor. Two patients who were treated within 4 days of the onset of PDPH recovered within 6 weeks, whereas three patients treated on days 9 to 11 had palsy that persisted for 3 to 4 months. Two obstetric patients experienced new cranial nerve palsies (involving cranial nerve VII), which manifested as facial weakness after administration of an epidural blood patch.[192]

Abouleish et al.[164] reported the results of the long-term evaluation of 118 patients who had received an epidural blood patch. Back pain was the most common complication; it occurred during the first 48 hours in 35% of patients and persisted in 16% of patients, with a mean duration of 27 days. These investigators also noted some cases of neck pain, lower extremity radicular pain, and transient temperature elevation.

The development of an inflammatory reaction to epidural blood can cause acute arachnoiditis, an entity that can manifest several days after the successful cure of a PDPH with a blood patch.[193] This phenomenon is believed to be secondary to free radical damage to spinal nerve roots in the intrathecal space after hemoglobin degradation. There are case reports of obstetric patients presenting with this entity and requiring analgesic therapy for prolonged periods.[194] The diagnosis is made from a presenting history of severe back pain, often with radicular pain, and characteristic MRI findings such as nerve root clumping in the intrathecal space and adhesions between nerve roots.

The occurrence of new neurologic symptoms after an epidural blood patch procedure should prompt consideration of the presence of other intracranial pathology. Such symptoms may include (1) mental deterioration due to increased ICP from an intracranial tumor and (2) seizures due to late-onset eclampsia.[26,32,195]

Diaz[196] described a woman in whom permanent paraparesis and cauda equina syndrome developed after an epidural blood patch with 30 mL of blood injected slowly and without symptoms. Low back pain and leg pain developed after the blood patch procedure, and later the patient also experienced incontinence. Twelve days after the procedure, a subdural hematoma at L2 to L4 was diagnosed and surgically treated. Six months later the patient still had significant symptoms. Although a larger volume of blood than usual was injected, the technique appears to have been within normal practice standards. Other long-term sequelae reported in obstetric patients include a postpartum cerebral ischemic event after two epidural blood patch procedures that resulted in permanent hemianopsia[197] and a calcified epidural blood patch leading to chronic back pain.[198]

Dextran/Gelatin Patch

Dextran-40 and gelatin-based solutions, including Gelfoam and Plasmion, have been substituted for blood in epidural patches.[130,199,200] These were chosen as alternatives to blood owing to relative contraindications to injection of blood. The use of alternative solutions appears to be more common in countries outside North America. In an observational study of 56 patients, Barrios-Alarcon et al.[201] reported that epidural administration of 20 to 30 mL of dextran-40 was safe and effective for the relief of PDPH; all headaches were relieved permanently. The only side effect was a transient discomfort or burning sensation at the time of injection in 6 patients. Some physicians have treated intractable PDPH successfully by administering a dextran-40 patch followed by epidural infusion of dextran at 3 mL/hr for 5 to 12 hours.[202,203]

Information on the neurotoxicity of these materials is scant.[204] Chanimov et al.[204] did not identify neurotoxicity after infusion of dextran-40 or polygeline (a gelatin powder) into the rat intrathecal space. However, further information is needed before these materials can be widely adopted for epidural patches. From MRI studies of patients with blood patches, we can anticipate that some dextran will enter the subarachnoid space. The small but definite risk of anaphylaxis after the injection of dextran also must be considered, although the risk appears minimal with dextran-40.

Fibrin Sealant Patch

Fibrin sealant is composed of fibrinogen and thrombin. Several commercial products are prepared from human pooled plasma. Products may also contain antifibrinolytics, such as animal aprotinin.[205] When injected, these products form a firm, nonretractable fibrin clot. Epidural injection of fibrin glue in rats produces a sustained increase in CSF pressure comparable to the increase that occurs after injection of blood.[176] Fibrin sealant has been evaluated for its effectiveness in preventing dural leaks after spinal surgery.[206] Epidural fibrin glue patch procedures have been used successfully to treat recurrent PDPH,[207] spontaneous intracranial hypotension,[208] and CSF leak after long-term intrathecal catheterization.[209] In the future, fibrin glue may have a role in patients with intractable PDPH, but further study is required before it can be recommended for routine use.

Surgery

There are rare reports of curative surgical closure of a dural rent for intractable PDPH. In one case, the interval between dural puncture and surgery was 5 years.[210]

SUMMARY OF TREATMENT

The parturient with PDPH should be actively managed with scheduled analgesics, and she should receive psychological support as she cares for her newborn and manages her symptoms. If the headache is severe, the physician may either try caffeine or proceed directly to epidural blood patch. Epidural administration of fluids other than blood, such as saline or dextran, typically is not first-line therapy but may be considered when there are contraindications to the epidural injection of autologous blood. The accuracy of PDPH diagnosis must always be considered when atypical symptoms are present or when therapy fails.

Unanswered Questions

Important information about PDPH is still lacking. A large, detailed prospective study of PDPH, with and without blood patch therapy, with a long follow-up period (e.g., 1 year) is needed in obstetric patients. What are the long-term effects of both PDPH and blood patch therapy? How common are residual back pain, neurologic symptoms, and auditory/visual symptoms, and do they interfere with everyday life? Answers to these questions are needed to enable anesthesia providers to give patients reliable information, establish a sound basis for informed consent, and administer the best possible care. The Obstetric Anaesthetists' Association and the Association of Anaesthetists of Great Britain and Ireland[211] have recommended that each facility providing obstetric anesthesia services have institution-specific protocols for the management of PDPH, in order to facilitate the identification of parturients with this complication and to provide consistent care.

KEY POINTS

- Dural puncture is only one of many causes of postpartum headache, although many are quick to blame postpartum headaches on dural puncture. A detailed history and physical examination along with indicated neuroimaging in selected cases should ensure diagnostic accuracy.
- A patient with post–dural puncture headache experiences an exacerbation of symptoms when she moves from the horizontal to the upright position, possibly owing to decreased intracranial pressure and secondary cerebral vasodilation, which affect pain-sensitive intracranial structures.
- Anesthesia providers should use small-gauge ($\leq$ 24-gauge), noncutting (pencil-point) spinal needles whenever possible to decrease the risk of post–dural puncture headache.

- The initial therapy for post–dural puncture headache consists of psychological support, bed rest in the horizontal position, and scheduled oral analgesics. Although dehydration should be avoided, no evidence supports a role for vigorous hydration for prophylaxis or therapy of post–dural puncture headache.
- The "gold standard" for therapy of post–dural puncture headache is autologous epidural blood patch. A second blood patch procedure may be performed—and typically is successful—if the first one fails. If the second procedure fails, alternative diagnoses should be excluded. Other therapies have not proved as effective and safe as the epidural blood patch for treatment of post–dural puncture headache.

REFERENCES

1. Goldszmidt E, Kern R, Chaput A, Macarthur A. The incidence and etiology of postpartum headaches: A prospective cohort study. Can J Anaesth 2005; 52:971-7.
2. Benhamou D, Hamza J, Ducot B. Post partum headache after epidural analgesia without dural puncture. Int J Obstet Anesth 1995; 4:17-20.
3. Headache Classification Committee of the International Headache Society. The international classification of headache disorders. Cephalalgia 2004; 24(Suppl 1):1-160.
4. Stella CL, Jodicke CD, How HY, et al. Postpartum headache: Is your work-up complete? Am J Obstet Gynecol 2007; 196:318. e1-7.
5. Lipton RB, Scher AI, Kolodner K, et al. Migraine in the United States: Epidemiology and patterns of health care use. Neurology 2002; 58:885-94.
6. Sances G, Granella F, Nappi RE, et al. Course of migraine during pregnancy and postpartum: A prospective study. Cephalalgia 2003; 23:197-205.
7. Adeney KL, Williams MA. Migraine headaches and preeclampsia: An epidemiologic review. Headache 2006; 46:794-803.
8. Sibai BM. Diagnosis, prevention, and management of eclampsia. Obstet Gynecol 2005; 105:402-10.
9. Hinchey J, Chaves C, Appignani B, et al. A reversible posterior leukoencephalopathy syndrome. N Engl J Med 1996; 334:494-500.
10. Pande AR, Ando K, Ishikura R, et al. Clinicoradiological factors influencing the reversibility of posterior reversible encephalopathy syndrome: A multicenter study. Radiat Med 2006; 24:659-68.
11. Crosby ET, Preston R. Obstetrical anaesthesia for a parturient with preeclampsia, HELLP syndrome and acute cortical blindness. Can J Anaesth 1998; 45:452-9.
12. Prout RE, Tuckey JP, Giffen NJ. Reversible posterior leukoencephalopathy syndrome in a peripartum patient. Int J Obstet Anesth 2007; 16:74-6.
13. Torrillo TM, Bronster DJ, Beilin Y. Delayed diagnosis of posterior reversible encephalopathy syndrome (PRES) in a parturient with preeclampsia after inadvertent dural puncture. Int J Obstet Anesth 2007; 16:171-4.
14. Ho CM, Chan KH. Posterior reversible encephalopathy syndrome with vasospasm in a postpartum woman after postdural puncture headache following spinal anesthesia. Anesth Analg 2007; 105:770-2.
15. Long TR, Hein BD, Brown MJ, et al. Posterior reversible encephalopathy syndrome during pregnancy: Seizures in a previously healthy parturient. J Clin Anesth 2007; 19:145-8.
16. Selo-Ojeme DO, Marshman LA, Ikomi A, et al. Aneurysmal subarachnoid haemorrhage in pregnancy. Eur J Obstet Gynecol Reprod Biol 2004; 116:131-43.
17. Lockhart EM, Baysinger CL. Intracranial venous thrombosis in the parturient. Anesthesiology 2007; 107:652-8.
18. Borum SE, Naul LG, McLeskey CH. Postpartum dural venous sinus thrombosis after postdural puncture headache and epidural blood patch. Anesthesiology 1997; 86:487-90.
19. Stocks GM, Wooller DJ, Young JM, Fernando R. Postpartum headache after epidural blood patch: Investigation and diagnosis. Br J Anaesth 2000; 84:407-10.
20. Gewirtz EC, Costin M, Marx GF. Cortical vein thrombosis may mimic postdural puncture headache. Reg Anesth 1987; 12:188-90.
21. Bousser MG. Cerebral venous thrombosis: Diagnosis and management. J Neurol 2000; 247:252-8.
22. de Bruijn SF, Stam J. Randomized, placebo-controlled trial of anticoagulant treatment with low-molecular-weight heparin for cerebral sinus thrombosis. Stroke 1999; 30:484-8.
23. Ferro JM, Canhao P. Acute treatment of cerebral venous and dural sinus thrombosis. Curr Treat Options Neurol 2008; 10:126-37.
24. Jaigobin C, Silver FL. Stroke and pregnancy. Stroke 2000; 31:2948-51.
25. Konstantinopoulos PA, Mousa S, Khairallah R, Mtanos G. Postpartum cerebral angiopathy: An important diagnostic consideration in the postpartum period. Am J Obstet Gynecol 2004; 191:375-7.
26. Nicol GL, Millns JP. Cerebellar infarction as a cause of post-partum headache. Int J Obstet Anesth 2002; 11:306-9.
27. Kardash K, Morrow F, Beique F. Seizures after epidural blood patch with undiagnosed subdural hematoma. Reg Anesth Pain Med 2002; 27:433-6.
28. Vaughan DJ, Stirrup CA, Robinson PN. Cranial subdural haematoma associated with dural puncture in labour. Br J Anaesth 2000; 84:518-20.
29. Davies JM, Murphy A, Smith M, O'Sullivan G. Subdural haematoma after dural puncture headache treated by epidural blood patch. Br J Anaesth 2001; 86:720-3.
30. Smarkusky L, DeCarvalho H, Bermudez A, Gonzalez-Quintero VH. Acute onset headache complicating labor epidural caused by intrapartum pneumocephalus. Obstet Gynecol 2006; 108:795-8.
31. Reynolds F. Neurological infections after neuraxial anesthesia. Anesthesiol Clin 2008; 26:23-52, v.
32. Eede HV, Hoffmann VL, Vercauteren MP. Post-delivery postural headache: Not always a classical post-dural puncture headache. Acta Anaesthesiol Scand 2007; 51:763-5.
33. Dutton DA. A 'postspinal headache' associated with incidental intracranial pathology. Anaesthesia 1991; 46:1044-6.
34. Alfery DD, Marsh ML, Shapiro HM. Post-spinal headache or intracranial tumor after obstetric anesthesia. Anesthesiology 1979; 51:92-4.
35. Mokri B. Headaches caused by decreased intracranial pressure: Diagnosis and management. Curr Opin Neurol 2003; 16:319-26.
36. Albayram S, Tuzgen S, Gunduz A, et al. Spontaneous intracranial hypotension after labor without spinal intervention. Eur J Neurol 2008; 15:91-3.
37. Sobol SE, Frenkiel S, Nachtigal D, et al. Clinical manifestations of sinonasal pathology during pregnancy. J Otolaryngol 2001; 30:24-8.
38. Weber JG, Klindworth JT, Arnold JJ, et al. Prophylactic intravenous administration of caffeine and recovery after ambulatory surgical procedures. Mayo Clin Proc 1997; 72:621-6.
39. Shapiro RE. Caffeine and headaches. Neurol Sci 2007; 28(Suppl 2):S179-83.
40. Askmark H, Lundberg PO. Lactation headache—a new form of headache? Cephalalgia 1989; 9:119-22.
41. Thorley V. Lactational headache: A lactation consultant's diary. J Hum Lact 1997; 13:51-3.
42. Choi PT, Galinski SE, Takeuchi L, et al. PDPH is a common complication of neuraxial blockade in parturients: A meta-analysis of obstetrical studies. Can J Anaesth 2003; 50:460-9.
43. Lybecker H, Djernes M, Schmidt JF. Postdural puncture headache (PDPH): Onset, duration, severity, and associated symptoms: An analysis of 75 consecutive patients with PDPH. Acta Anaesthesiol Scand 1995; 39:605-12.
44. Ok G, Tok D, Erbuyun K, et al. Hearing loss does not occur in young patients undergoing spinal anesthesia. Reg Anesth Pain Med 2004; 29:430-3.

45. Shearer VE, Jhaveri HS, Cunningham FG. Puerperal seizures after post-dural puncture headache. Obstet Gynecol 1995; 85:255-60.
46. Vercauteren MP, Vundelinckx GJ, Hanegreefs GH. Postpartum headache, seizures and bloodstained CSF: A possible complication of dural puncture? Intensive Care Med 1988; 14:176-7.
47. Yang CP, Lee CH, Borel CO, et al. Postdural puncture headache with abdominal pain and diarrhea. Anesth Analg 2005; 100:879-81.
48. Chan TM, Ahmed E, Yentis SM, Holdcroft A. Postpartum headaches: Summary report of the National Obstetric Anaesthetic Database (NOAD) 1999. Int J Obstet Anesth 2003; 12:107-12.
49. Klepstad P. Relief of postural post dural puncture headache by an epidural blood patch 12 months after dural puncture. Acta Anaesthesiol Scand 1999; 43:964-6.
50. Vakharia SB, Thomas PS, Rosenbaum AE, et al. Magnetic resonance imaging of cerebrospinal fluid leak and tamponade effect of blood patch in postdural puncture headache. Anesth Analg 1997; 84:585-90.
51. Bakshi R, Mechtler LL, Kamran S, et al. MRI findings in lumbar puncture headache syndrome: Abnormal dural-meningeal and dural venous sinus enhancement. Clin Imaging 1999; 23:73-6.
52. Bier A. Versuche ueber cocainisirung des rueckenmarkes. Dtsch Zeitschr Chir 1899; 51:361-9.
53. Kunkle K, Ray B, Wolff H. Experimental studies on headache: Analysis of the headache associated with changes in intracranial pressure. Arch Neurol Psychiatry 1943; 49:323-58.
54. Marx GF, Zemaitis MT, Orkin LR. Cerebrospinal fluid pressures during labor and obstetrical anesthesia. Anesthesiology 1961; 22:348-54.
55. Shah JL. Epidural pressure and postdural puncture headache in the parturient. Int J Obstet Anesth 1993; 2:187-9.
56. Benzon HT, Wong CA. Postdural puncture headache: Mechanisms, treatment, and prevention. Reg Anesth Pain Med 2001; 26:293-5.
57. Hattingh J, McCalden TA. Cerebrovascular effects of cerebrospinal fluid removal. S Afr Med J 1978; 54:780-1.
58. Boezaart AP. Effects of cerebrospinal fluid loss and epidural blood patch on cerebral blood flow in swine. Reg Anesth Pain Med 2001; 26:401-6.
59. Grant R, Condon B, Patterson J, et al. Changes in cranial CSF volume during hypercapnia and hypocapnia. J Neurol Neurosurg Psychiatry 1989; 52:218-22.
60. Vandam LD, Dripps RD. Long-term follow-up of patients who received 10,098 spinal anesthetics: Syndrome of decreased intracranial pressure (headache and ocular and auditory difficulties). J Am Med Assoc 1956; 161:586-91.
61. Wu CL, Rowlingson AJ, Cohen SR, et al. Gender and post-dural puncture headache. Anesthesiology 2006; 105:613-8.
62. Stride PC, Cooper GM. Dural taps revisited: A 20-year survey from Birmingham Maternity Hospital. Anaesthesia 1993; 48:247-55.
63. Angle P, Thompson D, Halpern S, Wilson DB. Second stage pushing correlates with headache after unintentional dural puncture in parturients. Can J Anaesth 1999; 46:861-6.
64. Faure E, Moreno R, Thisted R. Incidence of postdural puncture headache in morbidly obese parturients. Reg Anesth 1994; 19:361-3.
65. Panadero A, Bravo P, Garcia-Pedrajas F. Postdural puncture headache and air travel after spinal anesthesia with a 24-gauge Sprotte needle. Reg Anesth 1995; 20:463-4.
66. Amorim JA, Valenca MM. Postdural puncture headache is a risk factor for new postdural puncture headache. Cephalalgia 2008; 28:5-8.
67. Seeberger MD, Kaufmann M, Staender S, et al. Repeated dural punctures increase the incidence of postdural puncture headache. Anesth Analg 1996; 82:302-5.
68. Angle PJ, Kronberg JE, Thompson DE, et al. Dural tissue trauma and cerebrospinal fluid leak after epidural needle puncture: Effect of needle design, angle, and bevel orientation. Anesthesiology 2003; 99:1376-82.
69. Morley-Forster PK, Singh S, Angle P, et al. The effect of epidural needle type on postdural puncture headache: A randomized trial. Can J Anaesth 2006; 53:572-8.
70. Angle PJ, Hussain K, Morgan A, et al. High quality labour analgesia using small gauge epidural needles and catheters. Can J Anaesth 2006; 53:263-7.
71. Sharma SK, Gambling DR, Joshi GP, et al. Comparison of 26-gauge Atraucan and 25-gauge Whitacre needles: Insertion characteristics and complications. Can J Anaesth 1995; 42:706-10.
72. Pan PH, Fragneto R, Moore C, Ross V. Incidence of postdural puncture headache and backache, and success rate of dural puncture: Comparison of two spinal needle designs. South Med J 2004; 97:359-63.
73. Vallejo MC, Mandell GL, Sabo DP, Ramanathan S. Postdural puncture headache: A randomized comparison of five spinal needles in obstetric patients. Anesth Analg 2000; 91:916-20.
74. Hart JR, Whitacre RJ. Pencil-point needle in prevention of postspinal headache. JAMA 1951; 147:657-8.
75. Santanen U, Rautoma P, Luurila H, et al. Comparison of 27-gauge (0.41-mm) Whitacre and Quincke spinal needles with respect to post-dural puncture headache and non-dural puncture headache. Acta Anaesthesiol Scand 2004; 48:474-9.
76. Corbey MP, Bach AB, Lech K, Frorup AM. Grading of severity of postdural puncture headache after 27-gauge Quincke and Whitacre needles. Acta Anaesthesiol Scand 1997; 41:779-84.
77. Westbrook JL, Uncles DR, Sitzman BT, Carrie LE. Comparison of the force required for dural puncture with different spinal needles and subsequent leakage of cerebrospinal fluid. Anesth Analg 1994; 79:769-72.
78. Sprotte G, Schedel R, Pajunk H, Pajunk H. An "atraumatic" universal needle for single-shot regional anesthesia: Clinical results and a 6-year trial in over 30,000 regional anesthesias. Reg Anaesth 1987; 10:104-8.
79. Lesser P, Bembridge M, Lyons G, Macdonald R. An evaluation of a 30-gauge needle for spinal anaesthesia for caesarean section. Anaesthesia 1990; 45:767-8.
80. Richman JM, Joe EM, Cohen SR, et al. Bevel direction and postdural puncture headache: A meta-analysis. Neurologist 2006; 12:224-8.
81. Franksson C, Gordh T. Headache after spinal anesthesia and a technique for lessening its frequency. Acta Chir Scand 1946; 94:443-54.
82. Fink BR, Walker S. Orientation of fibers in human dorsal lumbar dura mater in relation to lumbar puncture. Anesth Analg 1989; 69:768-72.
83. Cruickshank RH, Hopkinson JM. Fluid flow through dural puncture sites: An in vitro comparison of needle point types. Anaesthesia 1989; 44:415-8.
84. Ready LB, Cuplin S, Haschke RH, Nessly M. Spinal needle determinants of rate of transdural fluid leak. Anesth Analg 1989; 69:457-60.
85. Norris MC, Leighton BL, DeSimone CA. Needle bevel direction and headache after inadvertent dural puncture. Anesthesiology 1989; 70:729-31.
86. Richardson MG, Wissler RN. The effects of needle bevel orientation during epidural catheter insertion in laboring parturients. Anesth Analg 1999; 88:352-6.
87. Hatfalvi BI. Postulated mechanisms for postdural puncture headache and review of laboratory models: Clinical experience. Reg Anesth 1995; 20:329-36.
88. Viitanen H, Porthan L, Viitanen M, et al. Postpartum neurologic symptoms following single-shot spinal block for labour analgesia. Acta Anaesthesiol Scand 2005; 49:1015-22.
89. Kempen PM, Mocek CK. Bevel direction, dura geometry, and hole size in membrane puncture: Laboratory report. Reg Anesth 1997; 22:267-72.
90. Gurmarnik S. Skin preparation and spinal headache. Anaesthesia 1988; 43:1057-8.
91. Russell R, Douglas J. Controversies: Loss of resistance to saline is better than air for obstetric epidurals. Int J Obstet Anesth 2001; 10:302-6.
92. Gleeson CM, Reynolds F. Accidental dural puncture rates in UK obstetric practice. Int J Obstet Anesth 1998; 7:242-6.
93. Paech M, Banks S, Gurrin L. An audit of accidental dural puncture during epidural insertion of a Tuohy needle in obstetric patients. Int J Obstet Anesth 2001; 10:162-7.
94. Williams EJ, Beaulieu P, Fawcett WJ, Jenkins JG. Efficacy of epidural blood patch in the obstetric population. Int J Obstet Anesth 1999; 8:105-9.
95. Aida S, Taga K, Yamakura T, et al. Headache after attempted epidural block: The role of intrathecal air. Anesthesiology 1998; 88:76-81.

96. Naulty JS, Hertwig L, Hunt CO, et al. Influence of local anesthetic solution on postdural puncture headache. Anesthesiology 1990; 72:450-4.
97. Arkoosh VA, Palmer CM, Yun EM, et al. A randomized, double-masked, multicenter comparison of the safety of continuous intrathecal labor analgesia using a 28-gauge catheter versus continuous epidural labor analgesia. Anesthesiology 2008; 108:286-98.
98. Norris MC, Fogel ST, Conway-Long C. Combined spinal-epidural versus epidural labor analgesia. Anesthesiology 2001; 95:913-20.
99. van de Velde M, Teunkens A, Hanssens M, et al. Post dural puncture headache following combined spinal-epidural or epidural anaesthesia in obstetric patients. Anaesth Intensive Care 2001; 29:595-9.
100. Miro M, Guasch E, Gilsanz F. Comparison of epidural analgesia with combined spinal-epidural analgesia for labor: A retrospective study of 6497 cases. Int J Obstet Anesth 2008; 17:15-9.
101. Angle P, Tang SL, Thompson D, Szalai JP. Expectant management of postdural puncture headache increases hospital length of stay and emergency room visits. Can J Anaesth 2005; 52:397-402.
102. Zeidan A, Farhat O, Maaliki H, Baraka A. Does postdural puncture headache left untreated lead to subdural hematoma? Case report and review of the literature. Int J Obstet Anesth 2006; 15:50-8.
103. Nishio I, Williams BA, Williams JP. Diplopia: A complication of dural puncture. Anesthesiology 2004; 100:158-64.
104. MacArthur C, Lewis M, Knox EG. Accidental dural puncture in obstetric patients and long term symptoms. Br Med J 1993; 306:883-5.
105. Jeskins GD, Moore PA, Cooper GM, Lewis M. Long-term morbidity following dural puncture in an obstetric population. Int J Obstet Anesth 2001; 10:17-24.
106. Baraz R, Collis RE. The management of accidental dural puncture during labour epidural analgesia: A survey of UK practice. Anaesthesia 2005; 60:673-9.
107. Sudlow C, Warlow C. Posture and fluids for preventing post-dural puncture headache. Cochrane Database Syst Rev 2002; CD001790.
108. Mosavy SH, Shafei M. Prevention of headache consequent upon dural puncture in obstetric patient. Anaesthesia 1975; 30:807-9.
109. Halker RB, Demaerschalk BM, Wellik KE, et al. Caffeine for the prevention and treatment of postdural puncture headache: Debunking the myth. Neurologist 2007; 13:323-7.
110. Devcic A, Sprung J, Patel S, et al. PDPH in obstetric anesthesia: Comparison of 24-gauge Sprotte and 25-gauge Quincke needles and effect of subarachnoid administration of fentanyl. Reg Anesth 1993; 18:222-5.
111. Abboud TK, Zhu J, Reyes A, et al. Effect of subarachnoid morphine on the incidence of spinal headache. Reg Anesth 1992; 17:34-6.
112. Al-Metwalli RR. Epidural morphine injections for prevention of post dural puncture headache. Anaesthesia 2008; 63:847-50.
113. Bernards CM, Kopacz DJ, Michel MZ. Effect of needle puncture on morphine and lidocaine flux through the spinal meninges of the monkey in vitro: Implications for combined spinal-epidural anesthesia. Anesthesiology 1994; 80:853-8.
114. Norris MC, Leighton BL. Continuous spinal anesthesia after unintentional dural puncture in parturients. Reg Anesth 1990; 15:285-7.
115. Cohen S, Amar D, Pantuck EJ, et al. Decreased incidence of headache after accidental dural puncture in caesarean delivery patients receiving continuous postoperative intrathecal analgesia. Acta Anaesthesiol Scand 1994; 38:716-8.
116. Dennehy KC, Rosaeg OP. Intrathecal catheter insertion during labour reduces the risk of post-dural puncture headache. Can J Anaesth 1998; 45:42-5.
117. Rutter SV, Shields F, Broadbent CR, et al. Management of accidental dural puncture in labour with intrathecal catheters: An analysis of 10 years' experience. Int J Obstet Anesth 2001; 10:177-81.
118. Ayad S, Demian Y, Narouze SN, Tetzlaff JE. Subarachnoid catheter placement after wet tap for analgesia in labor: Influence on the risk of headache in obstetric patients. Reg Anesth Pain Med 2003; 28:512-5.
119. Trivedi NS, Eddi D, Shevde K. Headache prevention following accidental dural puncture in obstetric patients. J Clin Anesth 1993; 5:42-5.
120. Shah JL. Epidural pressure during infusion of saline in the parturient. Int J Obstet Anesth 1993; 2:190-2.
121. Charsley MM, Abram SE. The injection of intrathecal normal saline reduces the severity of postdural puncture headache. Reg Anesth Pain Med 2001; 26:301-5.
122. Colonna-Romano P, Shapiro BE. Unintentional dural puncture and prophylactic epidural blood patch in obstetrics. Anesth Analg 1989; 69:522-3.
123. Ackerman W, Juneja M, Kaczorowski D. Prophylactic epidural blood patch for the prevention of postdural puncture headache in the parturient. Anesthesiol Rev 1990; 17:45-9.
124. Sudlow C, Warlow C. Epidural blood patching for preventing and treating post-dural puncture headache. Cochrane Database Syst Rev 2002; (2):CD001791.
125. Scavone BM, Wong CA, Sullivan JT, et al. Efficacy of a prophylactic epidural blood patch in preventing post dural puncture headache in parturients after inadvertent dural puncture. Anesthesiology 2004; 101:1422-7.
126. Allen DL, Berenguer JV, White JB. A potential complication of early blood patching following inadvertent dural puncture. Int J Obstet Anesth 1993; 2:202-3.
127. Tobias MD, Pilla MA, Rogers C, Jobes DR. Lidocaine inhibits blood coagulation: Implications for epidural blood patch. Anesth Analg 1996; 82:766-9.
128. Leivers D. Total spinal anesthesia following early prophylactic epidural blood patch. Anesthesiology 1990; 73:1287-9.
129. Aldrete JA, Brown TL. Intrathecal hematoma and arachnoiditis after prophylactic blood patch through a catheter. Anesth Analg 1997; 84:233-4.
130. Salvador L, Carrero E, Castillo J, et al. Prevention of post dural puncture headache with epidural-administered dextran 40. Reg Anesth 1992; 17:357-8.
131. Magides AD. A personal view of postdural puncture headache. Anaesthesia 1991; 46:694.
132. Weir EC. The sharp end of the dural puncture. Br Med J 2000; 320:127.
133. Costigan SN, Sprigge JS. Dural puncture: The patients' perspective: A patient survey of cases at a DGH maternity unit 1983-1993. Acta Anaesthesiol Scand 1996; 40:710-4.
134. Berger CW, Crosby ET, Grodecki W. North American survey of the management of dural puncture occurring during labour epidural analgesia. Can J Anaesth 1998; 45:110-4.
135. Camann WR, Murray RS, Mushlin PS, Lambert DH. Effects of oral caffeine on postdural puncture headache: A double-blind, placebo-controlled trial. Anesth Analg 1990; 70:181-4.
136. Mathew RJ, Wilson WH. Caffeine induced changes in cerebral circulation. Stroke 1985; 16:814-7.
137. Cohen SM, Laurito CE, Curran MJ. Grand mal seizure in a postpartum patient following intravenous infusion of caffeine sodium benzoate to treat persistent headache. J Clin Anesth 1992; 4:48-51.
138. Bolton VE, Leicht CH, Scanlon TS. Postpartum seizure after epidural blood patch and intravenous caffeine sodium benzoate. Anesthesiology 1989; 70:146-9.
139. Paech M. Unexpected postpartum seizures associated with post-dural puncture headache treated with caffeine. Int J Obstet Anesth 1996; 5:43-6.
140. McSwiney M, Phillips J. Post dural puncture headache. Acta Anaesthesiol Scand 1995; 39:990-5.
141. Ryu JE. Effect of maternal caffeine consumption on heart rate and sleep time of breast-fed infants. Dev Pharmacol Ther 1985; 8:355-63.
142. Feuerstein TJ, Zeides A. Theophylline relieves headache following lumbar puncture: Placebo-controlled, double-blind pilot study. Klin Wochenschr 1986; 64:216-8.
143. Carp H, Singh PJ, Vadhera R, Jayaram A. Effects of the serotonin-receptor agonist sumatriptan on postdural puncture headache: Report of six cases. Anesth Analg 1994; 79:180-2.
144. Connelly NR, Parker RK, Rahimi A, Gibson CS. Sumatriptan in patients with postdural puncture headache. Headache 2000; 40:316-9.
145. Foster P. ACTH treatment for post-lumbar puncture headache. Br J Anaesth 1994; 73:429.

146. Kshatri AM, Foster PA. Adrenocorticotropic hormone infusion as a novel treatment for postdural puncture headache. Reg Anesth 1997; 22:432-4.
147. Gupta S, Agrawal A. Postdural puncture headache and ACTH. J Clin Anesth 1997; 9:258.
148. Carter BL, Pasupuleti R. Use of intravenous cosyntropin in the treatment of postdural puncture headache. Anesthesiology 2000; 92:272-4.
149. Rucklidge MW, Yentis SM, Paech MJ. Synacthen Depot for the treatment of postdural puncture headache. Anaesthesia 2004; 59:138-41.
150. Oliver CD, White SA. Unexplained fitting in three parturients suffering from postdural puncture headache. Br J Anaesth 2002; 89:782-5.
151. Noyan Ashraf MA, Sadeghi A, Azarbakht Z, et al. Evaluation of intravenous hydrocortisone in reducing headache after spinal anesthesia: A double blind controlled clinical study. Middle East J Anesthesiol 2007; 19:415-22.
152. Hakim S, Khan RM, Maroof M, et al. Methylergonovine maleate (Methergine) relieves postdural puncture headache in obstetric patients. Acta Obstet Gynecol Scand 2005; 84:100.
153. Lin YT, Sheen MJ, Huang ST, et al. Gabapentin relieves post-dural puncture headache—a report of two cases. Acta Anaesthesiol Taiwan 2007; 45:47-51.
154. Eldor J, Guedj P, Cotev S. Epidural morphine injections for the treatment of postspinal headache. Can J Anaesth 1990; 37:710-1.
155. Jacobaeus HC, Frumerie K. About the leakage of spinal fluid after lumbar puncture and its treatment. Acta Med Scand 1923; 58:102-8.
156. Rice GG, Dabbs CH. The use of peridural and subarachnoid injections of saline in the treatment of severe postspinal headache. Anesthesiology 1950; 11:17-23.
157. Usubiaga JE, Subiaga LE, Brea LM, Goyena R. Effect of saline injections on epidural and subarachnoid space pressures and relation to postspinal anesthesia headache. Anesth Analg 1967; 46:293-6.
158. Bart AJ, Wheeler AS. Comparison of epidural saline placement and epidural blood patch in the treatment of post-lumbar-puncture headache. Anesthesiology 1978; 48:221-3.
159. Stevens RA, Jorgensen N. Successful treatment of dural puncture headache with epidural saline infusion after failure of epidural blood patch. Case report. Acta Anaesthesiol Scand 1988; 32:429-31.
160. Baysinger CL, Menk EJ, Harte E, Middaugh R. The successful treatment of dural puncture headache after failed epidural blood patch. Anesth Analg 1986; 65:1242-4.
161. Gormley JB. Treatment of postspinal headache. Anesthesiology 1960; 21:565-6.
162. DiGiovanni AJ, Dunbar BS. Epidural injections of autologous blood for postlumbar-puncture headache. Anesth Analg 1970; 49:268-71.
163. Harrington BE. Postdural puncture headache and the development of the epidural blood patch. Reg Anesth Pain Med 2004; 29:136-63.
164. Abouleish E, Vega S, Blendinger I, Tio TO. Long-term follow-up of epidural blood patch. Anesth Analg 1975; 54:459-63.
165. Taivainen T, Pitkanen M, Tuominen M, Rosenberg PH. Efficacy of epidural blood patch for postdural puncture headache. Acta Anaesthesiol Scand 1993; 37:702-5.
166. Safa-Tisseront V, Thormann F, Malassine P, et al. Effectiveness of epidural blood patch in the management of post-dural puncture headache. Anesthesiology 2001; 95:334-9.
167. Banks S, Paech M, Gurrin L. An audit of epidural blood patch after accidental dural puncture with a Tuohy needle in obstetric patients. Int J Obstet Anesth 2001; 10:172-6.
168. Seebacher J, Ribeiro V, LeGuillou JL, et al. Epidural blood patch in the treatment of post dural puncture headache: A double blind study. Headache 1989; 29:630-2.
169. Sandesc D, Lupei MI, Sirbu C, et al. Conventional treatment or epidural blood patch for the treatment of different etiologies of post dural puncture headache. Acta Anaesthesiol Belg 2005; 56:265-9.
170. van Kooten F, Oedit R, Bakker SL, Dippel DW. Epidural blood patch in post dural puncture headache: A randomised, observer-blind, controlled clinical trial. J Neurol Neurosurg Psychiatry 2008; 79:553-8.
171. Szeinfeld M, Ihmeidan IH, Moser MM, et al. Epidural blood patch: Evaluation of the volume and spread of blood injected into the epidural space. Anesthesiology 1986; 64:820-2.
172. Beards SC, Jackson A, Griffiths AG, Horsman EL. Magnetic resonance imaging of extradural blood patches: Appearances from 30 min to 18 h. Br J Anaesth 1993; 71:182-8.
173. Djurhuus H, Rasmussen M, Jensen EH. Epidural blood patch illustrated by CT-epidurography. Acta Anaesthesiol Scand 1995; 39:613-7.
174. DiGiovanni AJ, Galbert MW, Wahle WM. Epidural injection of autologous blood for postlumbar-puncture headache. II. Additional clinical experiences and laboratory investigation. Anesth Analg 1972; 51:226-32.
175. Carrie LE. Epidural blood patch: Why the rapid response? Anesth Analg 1991; 72:129-130.
176. Coombs DW, Hooper D. Subarachnoid pressure with epidural blood patch. Reg Anesth 1979; 4:3-6.
177. Kroin JS, Nagalla SK, Buvanendran A, et al. The mechanisms of intracranial pressure modulation by epidural blood and other injectates in a postdural puncture rat model. Anesth Analg 2002; 95: 423-9.
178. Loeser EA, Hill GE, Bennett GM, Sederberg JH. Time vs. success rate for epidural blood patch. Anesthesiology 1978; 49:147-8.
179. Andrews PJ, Ackerman WE, Juneja M, et al. Transient bradycardia associated with extradural blood patch after inadvertent dural puncture in parturients. Br J Anaesth 1992; 69:401-3.
180. Brimacombe J, Clarke G, Craig L. Epidural blood patch in the Jehovah's Witness. Anaesth Intensive Care 1994; 22:319.
181. Martin R, Jourdain S, Clairoux M, Tetrault JP. Duration of decubitus position after epidural blood patch. Can J Anaesth 1994; 41:23-5.
182. Ong BY, Graham CR, Ringaert KR, et al. Impaired epidural analgesia after dural puncture with and without subsequent blood patch. Anesth Analg 1990; 70:76-9.
183. Blanche R, Eisenach JC, Tuttle R, Dewan DM. Previous wet tap does not reduce success rate of labor epidural analgesia. Anesth Analg 1994; 79:291-4.
184. Hebl JR, Horlocker TT, Chantigian RC, Schroeder DR. Epidural anesthesia and analgesia are not impaired after dural puncture with or without epidural blood patch. Anesth Analg 1999; 89:390-4.
185. Loughrey JP, Eappen S, Tsen LC. Spinal anesthesia for cesarean delivery shortly after an epidural blood patch. Anesth Analg 2003; 96:545-7.
186. Harding SA, Collis RE, Morgan BM. Meningitis after combined spinal-extradural anaesthesia in obstetrics. Br J Anaesth 1994; 73:545-7.
187. Tom DJ, Gulevich SJ, Shapiro HM, et al. Epidural blood patch in the HIV-positive patient: Review of clinical experience. San Diego HIV Neurobehavioral Research Center. Anesthesiology 1992; 76:943-7.
188. Parris WC. Post-dural puncture headache and epidural blood patch in an AIDS patient. J Clin Anesth 1997; 9:87-8.
189. Bucklin BA, Tinker JH, Smith CV. Clinical dilemma: A patient with postdural puncture headache and acute leukemia. Anesth Analg 1999; 88:166-7.
190. Decramer I, Fuzier V, Franchitto N, Samii K. Is use of epidural fibrin glue patch in patients with metastatic cancer appropriate? Eur J Anaesthesiol 2005; 22:724-5.
191. Scher CS, Amar D, Wollner N. Extradural blood patch for post-lumbar puncture headaches in cancer patients. Can J Anaesth 1992; 39:203-4.
192. Diaz JH, Weed JT. Correlation of adverse neurological outcomes with increasing volumes and delayed administration of autologous epidural blood patches for postdural puncture headaches. Pain Pract 2005; 5:216-22.
193. Rice I, Wee MY, Thomson K. Obstetric epidurals and chronic adhesive arachnoiditis. Br J Anaesth 2004; 92:109-20.
194. Kalina P, Craigo P, Weingarten T. Intrathecal injection of epidural blood patch: A case report and review of the literature. Emerg Radiol 2004; 11:56-9.

195. Marfurt D, Lyrer P, Ruttimann U, et al. Recurrent post-partum seizures after epidural blood patch. Br J Anaesth 2003; 90:247-50.
196. Diaz JH. Permanent paraparesis and cauda equina syndrome after epidural blood patch for postdural puncture headache. Anesthesiology 2002; 96:1515-7.
197. Mercieri M, Mercieri A, Paolini S, et al. Postpartum cerebral ischaemia after accidental dural puncture and epidural blood patch. Br J Anaesth 2003; 90:98-100.
198. Willner D, Weissman C, Shamir MY. Chronic back pain secondary to a calcified epidural blood patch. Anesthesiology 2008; 108:535-7.
199. Ambesh SP, Kumar A, Bajaj A. Epidural gelatin (Gelfoam) patch treatment for post dural puncture headache. Anaesth Intensive Care 1991; 19:444-7.
200. Chiron B, Laffon M, Ferrandiere M, Pittet JF. Postdural puncture headache in a parturient with sickle cell disease: Use of an epidural colloid patch. Can J Anaesth 2003; 50:812-4.
201. Barrios-Alarcon J, Aldrete JA, Paragas-Tapia D. Relief of post-lumbar puncture headache with epidural dextran 40: A preliminary report. Reg Anesth 1989; 14:78-80.
202. Reynvoet ME, Cosaert PA, Desmet MF, Plasschaert SM. Epidural dextran 40 patch for postdural puncture headache. Anaesthesia 1997; 52:886-8.
203. Aldrete JA. Persistent post-dural-puncture headache treated with epidural infusion of dextran. Headache 1994; 34:265-7.
204. Chanimov M, Berman S, Cohen ML, et al. Dextran 40 (Rheomacrodex) or polygeline (Haemaccel) as an epidural patch for post dural puncture headache: A neurotoxicity study in a rat model of dextran 40 and polygeline injected intrathecally. Eur J Anaesthesiol 2006; 23:776-80.
205. Spotnitz WD, Burks S. Hemostats, sealants, and adhesives: Components of the surgical toolbox. Transfusion (Paris) 2008; 48:1502-16.
206. Nakamura H, Matsuyama Y, Yoshihara H, et al. The effect of autologous fibrin tissue adhesive on postoperative cerebrospinal fluid leak in spinal cord surgery: A randomized controlled trial. Spine 2005; 30:E347-51.
207. Crul BJ, Gerritse BM, van Dongen RT, Schoonderwaldt HC. Epidural fibrin glue injection stops persistent postdural puncture headache. Anesthesiology 1999; 91:576-7.
208. Kamada M, Fujita Y, Ishii R, Endoh S. Spontaneous intracranial hypotension successfully treated by epidural patching with fibrin glue. Headache 2000; 40:844-7.
209. Gerritse BM, van Dongen RT, Crul BJ. Epidural fibrin glue injection stops persistent cerebrospinal fluid leak during long-term intrathecal catheterization. Anesth Analg 1997; 84:1140-1.
210. Harrington H, Tyler HR, Welch K. Surgical treatment of post-lumbar puncture dural CSF leak causing chronic headache: Case report. J Neurosurg 1982; 57:703-7.
211. Obstetric Anaesthetists' Association and the Association of Anaesthetists of Great Britain and Ireland. OAA-AAGBI guidelines for obstetric anesthetic services revised edition 2005. May 2005. Available at www.oaa-anaes.ac.uk/assets/_managed/editor/File/PDF/Publications/obstetric-guidelines.pdf/

Chapter 32

Neurologic Complications of Pregnancy and Neuraxial Anesthesia

Felicity Reynolds, M.D., M.B., B.S., FRCA, FRCOG (ad eundem)

Neurologic complications of childbirth may be associated with neuraxial analgesia and anesthesia or may result from childbirth itself. Complications of neuraxial anesthesia may be immediate (e.g., motor blockade, unexpectedly high or prolonged blockade, seizures after unintentional intravenous injection of local anesthetic), or they may be prolonged or delayed (sequelae). Immediate complications of neuraxial anesthesia are described in Chapter 23; this chapter is concerned with neurologic sequelae.

Although neurologic disorders following childbirth are more likely to have obstetric than anesthetic causes, neuraxial anesthesia is all too often blamed. For example, Tubridy and Redmond[1] described seven women referred with neurologic symptoms, all of which had been attributed to epidural analgesia. The women suffered from brachial neuritis, peroneal neuropathy, femoral neuropathy, neck strain, and leg symptoms for which there was no obvious physical cause. In such circumstances, a careful history and neurologic examination, together with diagnostic aids such as electromyography, nerve conduction studies, and imaging techniques, can localize the lesion and differentiate obstetric from anesthesia-related causes. For example, it should be possible to distinguish by simple clinical means between a mononeuropathy, which is likely to have an obstetric cause, and a radiculopathy resulting from neuraxial blockade. Accurate and prompt diagnosis is essential.

THE INCIDENCE OF NEUROLOGIC SEQUELAE

Patients frequently ask obstetricians and anesthesia providers about the incidence of complications of neuraxial anesthesia, but even if accurate data were available, the question has no true answer. The incidence of neurologic complications varies widely according to local practice and the skill and training of the practitioners. Some old surveys are based on accurate local records, but the data relate to a time when obstetric and anesthetic practices, equipment, and drugs were less safe and sophisticated than they are today. The incidence of serious complications is now too low to be estimated accurately on a local basis. Nonetheless, anesthesia providers have a duty to inform patients of the complications associated with a proposed procedure and are expected to give some figure for the level of risk, however meaningless such an estimate may be.

Obstetric Surveys

Between 1935 and 1965 the reported incidence of neurologic deficits in obstetric patients ranged from 1 in 2100 to 1 in 6400.[2-5] During this period, long labor and difficult rotational forceps delivery were commonplace, and neuraxial anesthesia was relatively unusual. Many surveys have subsequently attempted to assess the incidence of neurologic complications of neuraxial anesthesia, although they have many sources of error (Box 32-1).

BOX 32-1 Limitations of Surveys of Neurologic Sequelae of Neuraxial Anesthesia in Obstetrics

- Poor response rate
- Positive reporting bias
- Absence of controls without neuraxial anesthesia
- Greater attention given to those who received neuraxial anesthesia
- Inadequate investigation and lack of accurate diagnosis
- Variable skill and care of obstetric and anesthetic providers
- Older surveys relate to outdated obstetric and anesthetic practices
- Lack of statistical power to assess incidence of rare disorders
- Inaccurate counting of numerator and denominator
- Likelihood of missing cases that arise after hospital discharge

Some of the more recent surveys are listed in Table 32-1. Earlier surveys were ably reviewed by Loo et al.[6] in 2000. In one of them, Ong et al.[7] reviewed the charts of all women who delivered in Winnipeg over a 9-year period and interviewed all those who received anesthesia. All neurologic deficits in this series were transient, with none lasting more than 72 hours. The incidence of neurologic symptoms was similar after epidural anesthesia and general anesthesia, but symptoms were more likely to be reported by women who received any form of anesthesia than by those who received none. This latter fact is not surprising because only women who received anesthesia were interviewed. Indeed, the survey identified 45 cases of neurologic deficit; only 10 had been noted in the hospital record, suggesting that many deficits may have been missed in the patients who did not receive anesthesia. Moreover, modern statistical methods such as logistic regression analysis were not used to tease out the influence of prolonged labor and traumatic delivery, which the investigators noted as possible causative factors.

In a large retrospective survey of long-term symptoms, women who delivered in one hospital in Birmingham, United Kingdom, were asked to recall events 2 to 9 years after delivery.[8] The two main problems with this survey were a response rate of 39% and the fact that all those (and only those) who received epidural analgesia had been interviewed intensively about their symptoms immediately postpartum, thereby enhancing subsequent recall in this subset of the population. Logistic regression analysis demonstrated a link between epidural analgesia and many symptoms, including tingling and numbness. However, these symptoms were much more common in the arms than in the legs, calling into question any causative link with neuraxial anesthesia. No major neurologic sequelae were detected.

Scott and Hibbard[9] conducted a retrospective British survey of more than 500,000 epidural procedures administered between 1982 and 1986, which detected a number of serious sequelae, including one epidural abscess, one hematoma, and one anterior spinal artery syndrome, but many of the diagnoses were presumptive.[9] This survey probably failed to detect many minor lesions, but it was followed by a smaller prospective survey by Scott et al.,[10] which included some spinal procedures and involved a self-selected group of respondents. The investigators found no major neurologic disorders but a more believable number of what were termed *mononeuropathies*.

A French survey based on a questionnaire covering the years 1988 to 1993, and sent to all hospitals with maternity units, recorded one cranial subdural hematoma but no cases of epidural abscess or hematoma, out of 288,351 obstetric epidural procedures.[11] Seven deaths were reported. Complications of spinal anesthesia were not included in this survey.

Both the Scott surveys[9,10] and the French inquiry[11] overlooked the need for a control group of patients who did not receive neuraxial analgesia/anesthesia. The study by Holdcroft et al.[12] avoided this pitfall; the denominator consisted of all 48,066 women who delivered in one region over a year, and every effort was made to detect genuine neurologic symptoms in the community. Because the women themselves were not sent questionnaires, however, the response rate could not be estimated. The investigators judged that only one case of paresthesia, without physical signs, could be attributed to epidural analgesia, and none to spinal anesthesia. Peripheral nerve damage was more common. The most serious was one case of footdrop in a woman who had spontaneous delivery of a large baby with inhalation analgesia only.

With the greater popularity of spinal anesthesia, concern about the growing numbers of reports of paresthesias and possible root trauma led Holloway et al.[13] to conduct a retrospective U.K. national survey of spinal and combined spinal-epidural (CSE) anesthesia in the 1990s. No difference in frequency of neuropathy was detected between Whitacre and Sprotte needles or between single-shot spinal and CSE techniques. Imprecise diagnoses made it difficult to differentiate anesthetic from coincidental causes, but after eliminating obvious obstetric or peripheral nerve palsies while otherwise erring on the pessimistic side, the investigators estimated that the incidence of neurologic sequelae was approximately 1 in 1000, including two cases of conus damage, one case of meningitis, and the rest minor root palsies. A retrospective local audit of CSE labor analgesia from the United States found no cases with serious sequelae or permanent neurologic injury.[14]

Two thorough local audit reports of immediate postpartum symptoms provided somewhat contrasting findings. One from Perth, Australia,[15] involved prospective recording of complications in 10,995 women who received epidural analgesia, but it regrettably did not include a control group. The investigators detected only a single lasting neurologic problem. Although they termed the injury a traumatic mononeuropathy, it was apparently a radiculopathy, because it was attributed to a traumatic epidural procedure.

The second report, from Leeds, United Kingdom, involved 3991 women delivered in one year.[16] Twenty-one women presenting with symptoms after neuraxial blockade were matched with 21 asymptomatic control patients who had also received neuraxial blockade and 21 who had not.[16] Only 1 woman who had not had a neuraxial block presented with symptoms, and she was found to have footdrop after a vacuum extraction. Typical peripheral neuropathies occurred among those who delivered vaginally;

TABLE 32-1 Surveys of Neurologic Complications of Childbirth and Neuraxial Blockade in Obstetrics

Study*	Type of Study	Population	Numbers of Neurologic Deficits (Incidence)
Ong et al., 1987[7]	Chart review of all patients, interview of those receiving anesthesia in one center (1975-83)	23,827 deliveries	45 (1/530) all transient
		12,964 inhalation or no analgesia	5 (1/2593)
		9403 epidural procedures	34 (1/277)
		1460 general anesthetics	6 (1/243)
Scott & Hibbard, 1990[9]	Retrospective multicenter review, no control group (1982-86)	505,000 epidural procedures	47 (1/10,745) 1 anterior spinal artery syndrome, 1 epidural abscess, 1 epidural hematoma (unconfirmed), 38 mononeuropathies, 5 cranial nerve palsies, 1 subdural hematoma
MacArthur et al., 1992[8]	Questionnaire sent in 1987 to mothers delivering in one center (1978-85)	11,701 women (39% response rate)	Tingling/paresthesias:
		4766 epidural procedures	143 upper limb, 23 lower limb
		6935 no epidural procedures	150 upper limb, 3 lower limb
Palot et al., 1994[11]	Questionnaire listing possible complications sent to hospitals with obstetric units, no control group (1988-93)	288,351 epidural procedures	92 (1/3134) 1 cranial subdural hematoma, 88 temporary radiculopathy (1/3277), 3 meningitis (1/96,117); (also reported negligence cases: 1 sciatic nerve palsy, 1 intracranial hematoma)
Scott & Tunstall, 1995[10]	Prospective multicenter review, no controls (1990-91)		46 total neuropathies
		108,133 epidural procedures	38 (1/2846)
		14,856 spinal procedures	8 (1/1857)
Holdcroft et al., 1995[12]	Regional community and hospital-based prospective audit (1991-92)	48,066 deliveries	10 new neurologic complications (1/4807)
		34,430 no neuraxial procedures	1 footdrop, 1 cervical nerve lesion (1/17,215)
		13,007 epidural procedures	1 paresthesia of nerve root distribution (1/13,007) *(Disorders unrelated to anesthesia: 2 cranial nerve palsies, 1 hypotensive cord damage, 5 peripheral nerve lesions)*
		629 spinal procedures	0 complications
Paech et al., 1998[15]	Prospective local audit, no controls (1989-94)	10,995 epidural procedures	1 traumatic "mononeuropathy" (1/10,995)
Albright & Forster, 1999[14]	Retrospective local audit, no control group, follow-up unspecified	4164 CSE procedures	No permanent nerve injury, no epidural abscess or hematoma
Holloway et al., 2000[13]	Retrospective multicenter audit, elastic time frame, no control group	29,698 spinal procedures	4 unrelated to anesthesia (3 meralgia paresthetica, 1 peroneal neuropathy). 10 ?root damage, 1 conus damage, 22 uncertain; (overall incidence ?1/986)
		12,254 CSE procedures	5 unrelated to anesthesia (1 femoral neuropathy, 2 footdrop, 2 paresthesia). 6 root damage, 1 meningitis, 1 conus damage, 6 uncertain (overall incidence ?1/901)

CSE, combined spinal-epidural.

*Superscript numbers indicate reference citations at the end of this chapter.

Continued

TABLE 32-1—cont'd Surveys of Neurologic Complications of Childbirth and Neuraxial Blockade in Obstetrics

Study*	Type of Study	Population	Numbers of Neurologic Deficits (Incidence)
Dar et al., 2002[16]	Prospective local audit of immediate symptoms (1998-99)	1376 vaginal deliveries without anesthesia (random sample of 21 examined + 1 complaint)	4 peripheral neuropathy, 1 footdrop, 2 vague (1/3)
		2615 neuraxial procedures (all followed up):	21 neurologic symptoms:
		1782 vaginal deliveries	7 peripheral neuropathies, 1 footdrop, 3 vague (1/162)
		833 cesarean deliveries	8 numb areas, 2 vague (1/83)
Auroy et al., 2002[18]	Prospective multicenter survey	297,328 epidural procedures	0 complications
		5640 spinal procedures	2 "peripheral neuropathy"
Moen et al., 2004[19]	National postal survey and search of administrative files, no controls (1990-99)	205,000 epidural procedures	1 epidural hematoma (HELLP), 1 epidural abscess, 2 cord damage, 2 intracranial subdural hematoma, 1 abducent nerve palsy (1/29,286)
		50,000 spinal procedures	1 spinal hematoma (HELLP), 1 cord damage (1/25,000)

HELLP, hemolysis, elevated liver enzymes, low platelets.

sacral numbness was most commonly detected after cesarean delivery. All changes were transient, and none could be attributed to neuraxial anesthesia. Similar neurologic deficits were detected among the randomly selected, asymptomatic 21 control patients who had had no anesthetic intervention. In contrast, negligible deficits could be detected among the 21 asymptomatic control women who *had* had an anesthetic intervention. These results demonstrate that minor neurologic deficits are to be found postpartum quite frequently if sought, but that women who have not had an anesthetic intervention are less likely to complain.

A prospective survey among 6057 women who delivered in one year in Chicago[17] does not feature in Table 32-1, because the patients were not grouped by type of analgesia, but the findings of this survey corroborate those of the Leeds study.[16] The incidence of lower limb nerve injuries was approximately 1%: 24 lateral femoral cutaneous nerve, 22 femoral nerve, 3 peroneal nerve, 3 lumbosacral plexus, 2 sciatic nerve, 3 obturator nerve, and 5 radicular injuries.[17] Significant risk factors identified by logistic regression analysis included nulliparity and a prolonged second stage of labor, but not neuraxial anesthesia.

In a nationwide 10-month prospective French survey, only two so-called peripheral neuropathies and no major sequelae were detected among 5640 spinal and 29,732 epidural procedures in obstetric patients.[18] In contrast, in a retrospective Swedish national survey covering the years 1990 to 1999, Moen et al.[19] reported nine serious sequelae among an estimated 200,000 epidural and 50,000 spinal procedures in parturients.

An attempt was made to conflate the findings of various surveys in order to derive a consensus incidence of neurologic injury after obstetric epidural block.[20] Unfortunately, this study took no account of the now widespread use of spinal and CSE techniques, denominators were calculated inaccurately, and the findings of surveys were not always interpreted correctly. (For example, cranial subdural hematoma was counted as a spinal hematoma.) Therefore, reliable information cannot be derived from this publication.

Several conclusions can be drawn from these surveys. Despite an increased cesarean delivery rate, obstetric palsies (albeit now more short-lived) still occur, and the reported frequency of neurologic sequelae depends on how hard one seeks them. The risk of transient mild deficits after childbirth may be quite high.[16,17] A true figure for anesthetic complications cannot be calculated even from accurate surveys because (1) the diagnosis is rarely firm; (2) definitions, severity, and duration are often ill-defined; and (3) anesthesia provider skills vary. Table 32-1 demonstrates a variation in incidence of neurologic sequelae from 1 in 3 for mild symptoms with no neuraxial block[16] to 1 in 30,000 for epidural analgesia.[19] Moreover, bias is created when more attention is paid postpartum to patients who have received neuraxial blockade than to those who have not.

Nonobstetric Surveys

Modern surveys of neurologic complications of spinal and epidural anesthesia among nonobstetric populations may yield more reliable results, but still lack sensitivity to detect all potential problems and are commonly conducted in a relatively elderly and sick population. Moreover, the occurrence of case clusters gives the lie to the existence of a "true" incidence of complications.[19] The surveys by Auroy et al.[18] and Moen et al.[19] both had mixed obstetric/nonobstetric populations and found a higher incidence of serious sequelae in nonobstetric than in obstetric patients. It is therefore not valid to extrapolate findings from one population to the other. The reported risk of neurologic problems varies greatly with the patient population, local practice and skill, completeness of detection, and inclusion criteria. Therefore, it is meaningless to attempt to put any firm figure on the risk of neurologic complications after neuraxial anesthesia.

PERIPHERAL NERVE PALSIES

Peripheral nerve palsies may arise from compression in the pelvis by the fetal head, or from more distal compression, the signs of which may be overlooked in the presence of neuraxial anesthesia. In contemporary obstetric practice, cesarean delivery is usually preferred to prolonged labor and difficult high- or mid-forceps delivery. Therefore, the incidence of pelvic nerve trauma and compression should be lower than in years past. Surveys have shown that although obstetric palsies still occur,[13,16,17] most are short-lived and less disabling than hitherto.[2-5] Footdrop, however, is still reported,[21] even in the developed world, in cases in which the effort to avoid cesarean delivery leads to vaginal delivery of a disproportionately large baby.[13,16] Abnormal presentation, persistent occiput posterior position, fetal macrosomia, breakthrough pain during epidural labor analgesia, a prolonged second stage of labor, difficult instrumental delivery, and prolonged use of the lithotomy position may be risk factors for postpartum neuropathy.

Neuraxial blockade is often blamed for obstetric palsy, but reference to the distribution of spinal dermatomes and peripheral nerve sensory innervation clearly demonstrates the distinction between the two lesions (Figure 32-1). Spinal nerve root lesions are also manifested by weakness that involves several lower extremity joints and movements (Figure 32-2).

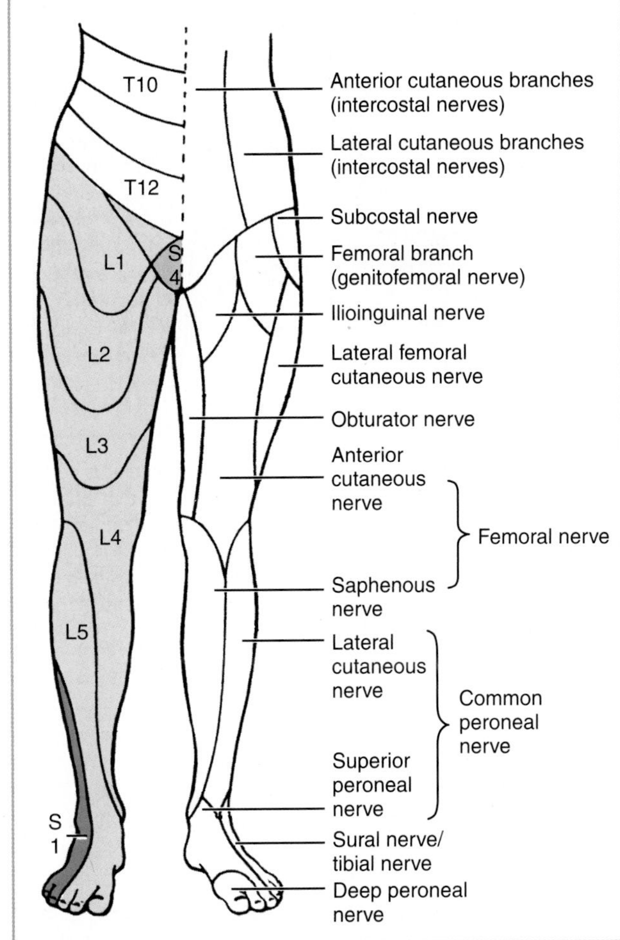

FIGURE 32-1 The segmental (*right leg*) and peripheral (*left leg*) sensory nerve distributions useful in distinguishing central from peripheral nerve injury. (From Redick LF. Maternal perinatal nerve palsies. Postgrad Obstet Gynecol 1992; 12:1-6.)

		L1	L2	L3	L4	L5	S1	S2	S3	S4
Hip	Flexion	■	■	■	░					
	Extension				■	■	■	■		
	Abduction					■	■			
	Adduction		■	■	■					
	Medial rotation	■	■	■	■	■	■			
	Lateral rotation					■	■	■		
Knee	Flexion		░	░	░	■	■	■		
	Extension		■	■	■					
Ankle	Dorsiflexion				■	■				
	Plantar flexion						■	■		
Big toe dorsiflexion					■	■	■			
Levator ani								■	■	■
Coccygeus										■

FIGURE 32-2 The spinal segments involved in the movements of joints in the leg. *Lighter shading* denotes a minor contribution. (From Russell R. Assessment of motor blockade during epidural analgesia in labour. Int J Obstet Anesth 1992; 4:230-4.)

Compression of the Lumbosacral Trunk

Compression of the lumbosacral trunk is probably the most common cause of postpartum footdrop. In addition to weakness that predominantly affects ankle dorsiflexion (footdrop), compression of the lumbosacral trunk produces sensory disturbance mainly involving the L5 dermatome (see Figure 32-1). This palsy most often results from some cephalopelvic disproportion and is therefore typically seen after prolonged labor and difficult vaginal delivery.[2-5,12,17] The fetal head, usually the brow, may compress the lumbosacral trunk as it crosses the pelvic brim and descends in front of the ala of the sacrum (Figure 32-3).

Obturator Nerve Palsy

The obturator nerve is susceptible to compressive injury as it crosses the brim of the pelvis or within the obturator canal (see Figure 32-3). The mother may complain of pain when the damage occurs, followed by weakness of hip adduction and internal rotation, with sensory disturbance over the upper inner thigh (see Figure 32-1). Cases are occasionally reported among parturients[22]; three were detected in a prospective study by Wong et al.[17] Because the nerve would appear to be in a vulnerable position, it may be that the correct diagnosis is often missed.

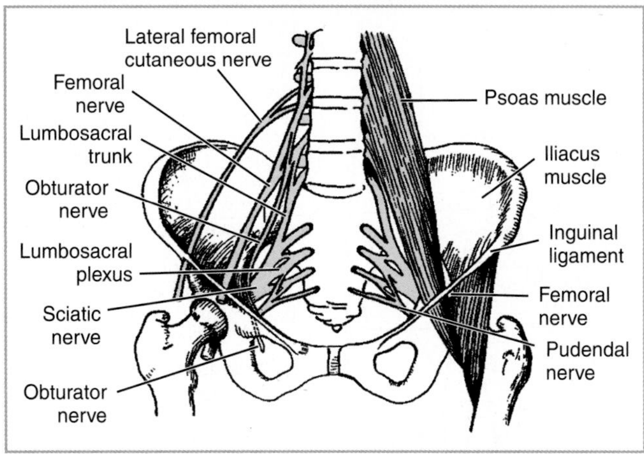

FIGURE 32-3 The lumbosacral trunk (L4 to L5) and obturator nerve (L2 to L4) are vulnerable to pressure as they cross the pelvic brim, particularly in cases of cephalopelvic disproportion. The femoral (L2 to L4) and lateral femoral cutaneous (L2 to L3) nerves are particularly vulnerable in the lithotomy position, where they pass beneath the inguinal ligament. (Adapted from Cole JT. Maternal obstetric paralysis. Am J Obstet Gynecol 1946; 52:374.)

Femoral Nerve Palsy

Femoral nerve palsy is more commonly diagnosed than lumbosacral trunk and obturator nerve palsies.[17] Approximately one third of the postpartum palsies detected by Wong et al.[17] were femoral nerve palsies. Dar et al.[16] detected five cases in their small population, although the symptoms were transient. The femoral nerve is vulnerable to stretch injury as it passes beneath the inguinal ligament. Damage may result from prolonged flexion, abduction, and external rotation of the hips during the second stage of labor, and also following procedures conducted in an excessive lithotomy position.[23] Therefore the hips should never remain continuously flexed during the second stage of labor. In a true femoral neuropathy, the nerve supply to the iliopsoas muscle is spared, so that some hip flexion is still possible. The patient with a femoral neuropathy may walk satisfactorily on a level surface but may be unable to climb stairs; the patellar reflex is diminished or absent.

Meralgia Paresthetica

Meralgia paresthetica is a neuropathy of the lateral femoral cutaneous nerve, a purely sensory nerve also known as the lateral cutaneous nerve of the thigh. First described more than 100 years ago, meralgia paresthetica is probably the most commonly encountered neuropathy in any survey related to childbirth (see Table 32-1).[13,16,17] It may arise both during pregnancy, typically at about 30 weeks' gestation, and intrapartum,[17,24] in association with increasing intra-abdominal pressure. It may recur during successive pregnancies. The most likely cause is entrapment of the nerve as it passes around the anterior superior iliac spine beneath or through the inguinal ligament,[25] where its vulnerability is increased by a large intra-abdominal mass or by retractors used during pelvic surgery. The compressive effect of edema may also contribute, as it does in the higher incidence during pregnancy of carpal tunnel syndrome and, possibly, Bell's palsy.[26] Meralgia paresthetica manifests as numbness, tingling, burning, or other paresthesias affecting the anterolateral aspect of the thigh. The distribution is quite unlike that of a nerve root lesion (see Figure 32-1), yet the disturbance is commonly attributed to neuraxial blockade by those ignorant of neuroanatomy. The condition can be expected to resolve after childbirth; transient pain may be relieved by local infiltration analgesia.

Sciatic Nerve Palsy

Sciatic nerve palsy is not commonly mentioned in surveys or generally recognized as a complication of childbirth, possibly because it is mistaken for a lesion of the lumbosacral trunk. Although it was first described in 1944,[27] its occurrence following childbirth was overlooked until 1996, when it was described in two parturients who had cesarean deliveries.[28] One woman with a breech presentation was thin and was kept sitting in one position while her leg numbness was wrongly attributed to epidural blockade. The other woman was obese with a nonengaged fetal head; she suffered a period of hypotension during preparation for elective cesarean delivery using epidural anesthesia. Both women experienced (1) loss of sensation, with subsequent dysesthesia below the knee, with sparing of the medial side; and (2) loss of movement below the knee, which recovered more quickly than the sensory changes. Both had intact posterior cutaneous nerve and gluteal function, implying that the damage was distal to the lumbosacral plexus, where the gluteal nerves branch off the sciatic nerve (Figure 32-4). Had these women undergone vaginal delivery, and had they received less conscientious evaluation, their lesions would probably have been attributed to nerve root or plexus damage. Subsequently, three cases were detected by Wong et al.,[17] and three more cases have been described following cesarean delivery[29-31] (one associated with hypotension), in which compression of the sciatic nerve by a hip wedge was implicated. Despite the peripheral location of the lesions, neuraxial anesthesia cannot be entirely exonerated, because the symptoms of nerve compression, which otherwise would have prompted a change of position, were overlooked or wrongly attributed to sensory blockade.

Peroneal Nerve Palsy

The common peroneal nerve is vulnerable to compression as it passes around the head of the fibula below the knee. It may also be susceptible to damage while it still forms part of the sciatic nerve as it leaves the pelvis. Peroneal nerve palsy may be caused by prolonged squatting, sometimes popular in "natural childbirth," by excessive knee flexion for any reason, by compression of the lateral side of the knee against any hard object, and by prolonged use of the lithotomy position.[32] When the peroneal nerve is damaged at the knee, there is sensory impairment on the anterolateral calf and the dorsum of the foot; footdrop may be profound, with steppage gait and weak ankle eversion, but plantar flexion and inversion at the ankle are preserved.

Anesthesia providers cannot be wholly absolved from responsibility for peripheral neuropathies, and adverse

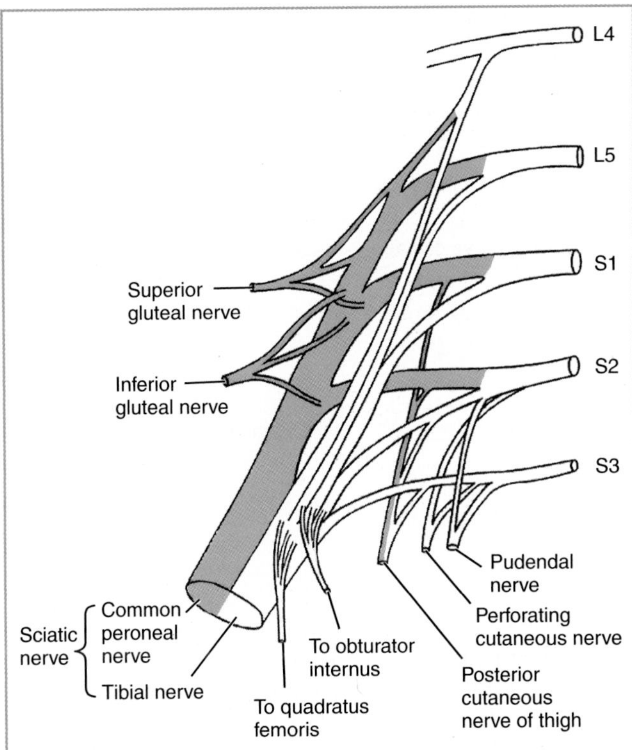

FIGURE 32-4 The sacral plexus. The dorsal divisions of the anterior primary rami are shaded. (From Silva M, Mallinson C, Reynolds F. Sciatic nerve palsy following childbirth. Anaesthesia 1996; 51:1144-8.)

factors can be minimized by attention to simple rules (Box 32-2). One group of patients, those with hereditary neuropathy with liability to pressure palsy, requires particular attention. In these women even relatively brief periods of immobility or pressure on any one site must be avoided.[33,34]

BOX 32-2 Safeguards to Minimize Peripheral Nerve Compression

- Be watchful for patient positioning that contributes to nerve compression, particularly with neuraxial blockade.
- Avoid prolonged use of the lithotomy position; regularly reduce hip flexion and abduction.
- Avoid prolonged positioning that may cause compression of the sciatic or peroneal nerve.
- Place the hip wedge under the bony pelvis rather than the buttock.
- Use low-dose local anesthetic/opioid combinations during labor to minimize numbness and allow maximum mobility.
- Encourage the parturient to change position regularly.
- Ensure that those caring for women receiving low-dose local anesthetic/opioid combinations understand that numbness or weakness may be signs of nerve compression; such symptoms should prompt an immediate change of position.

POSTPARTUM BLADDER DYSFUNCTION

There are several mechanisms by which bladder function may be disturbed postpartum (Figure 32-5). In theory, neuraxial blockade (1) may provoke the need for bladder catheterization with increased risk of infection, (2) may allow bladder distention to go undetected, and (3) on very rare occasions, may be associated with cauda equina syndrome (see later). However, several studies of bladder function have found no association with neuraxial analgesia[35,36] or only a weak correlation between epidural analgesia and an increased residual volume in the immediate postpartum period.[37] In contrast, a prolonged second stage of labor, instrumental delivery, and perineal damage have been identified as significant factors for postpartum bladder dysfunction.[35-37] Not surprisingly, in the previously described large survey of long-term symptoms after childbirth conducted in Birmingham, United Kingdom, no association was found between epidural analgesia and stress incontinence or urinary frequency.[38] By far the most common cause of bladder dysfunction appears to be non-neurologic. Nevertheless, it must be part of the anesthesia provider's responsibility to ensure that the bladder does not become overdistended either intrapartum or postpartum.

CENTRAL NERVOUS SYSTEM LESIONS

Lesions of the central nervous system (CNS) after childbirth have complex etiologies (Figure 32-6). The etiologies may be classified as **traumatic** (to nervous tissue, meninges, or blood vessels), **infective, ischemic,** or **chemical** (to nervous tissue or meninges). Anesthesia providers should bear in mind that even central lesions may have causes other than neuraxial block, the most obvious being a prolapsed intervertebral disc. Serious iatrogenic complications are remarkably rare; by far the most common are related to dural puncture.[11]

Neurologic Sequelae of Dural Puncture

The subject of post–dural puncture headache is discussed in detail in Chapter 31. There are several other causes of severe postpartum headache, some of which have serious neurologic implications. Postpartum headache requires diagnosis first and foremost, followed by treatment that is curative rather than palliative.

Cortical vein and venous sinus thrombosis are more common than expected because of the hypercoagulable state of the blood after delivery.[39-41] Cortical vein thrombosis has been associated with dural puncture and post–dural puncture headache.[39,41] Headaches caused by meningitis, venous sinus thrombosis, preeclampsia, hypertensive encephalopathy, subdural hematoma, internal carotid artery dissection, and posterior reversible encephalopathy syndrome may cause difficulty in diagnosis, particularly if they occur after epidural bolus injection, unintentional dural puncture, or administration of an epidural blood patch.[39-46] Seizures may occur in patients with eclampsia, hypertensive encephalopathy, meningitis, or pneumocephalus but may also follow dural puncture or performance of an epidural blood patch.[42,47-51]

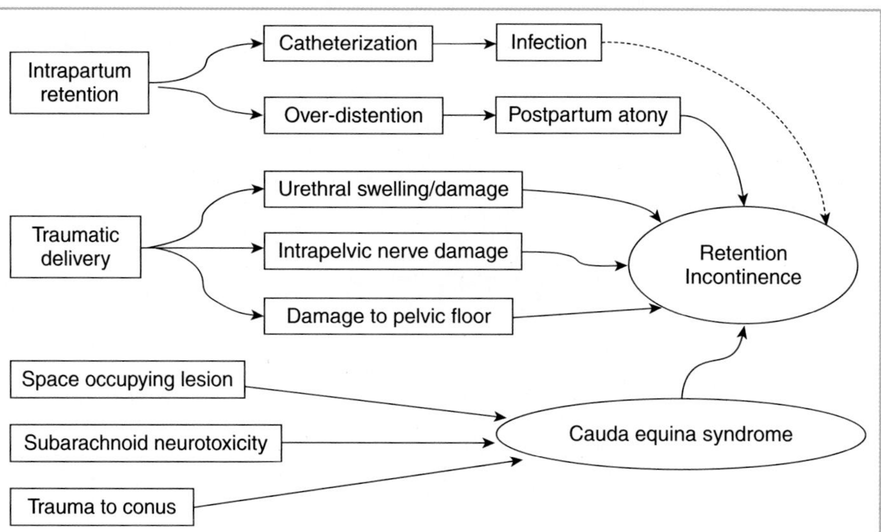

FIGURE 32-5 Mechanisms by which bladder function may be disturbed after parturition.

It is commonly assumed that headache after dural puncture will resolve spontaneously over time, but unfortunately, a dural leak can persist and may occasionally have more serious consequences, including cranial nerve palsy and subdural hematoma. Neglected cerebrospinal fluid (CSF) leak has also been known to induce medullary and tentorial coning.[52] Although serious problems are more likely to occur from unintentional dural puncture with a large epidural needle and a neglected headache, they may occasionally follow deliberate dural puncture with a small-gauge spinal needle.[52]

CRANIAL NERVE PALSY

Major loss of CSF, usually following unintentional dural puncture with a large needle, may cause a number of cranial nerve palsies. Because of its long course within the cranium, the **abducent nerve** is the most vulnerable. Recovery may be delayed even after an epidural blood patch.[53-55] Facial nerve palsy may require weeks to recover.[54,56-58] Eighth cranial nerve dysfunction requires a prompt epidural blood patch; otherwise tinnitus may become permanent.[59,60] Visual field defects have been reported and may also become permanent.[61] Trigeminal nerve dysfunction is usually a transient effect of high spinal blockade.

CRANIAL SUBDURAL HEMATOMA

More seriously, reduced CSF pressure may cause rupture of bridge meningeal veins and result in cranial subdural hematoma, a potentially fatal condition that has been reported sporadically over many years.[43,52] In 2000, Loo et al.[6]

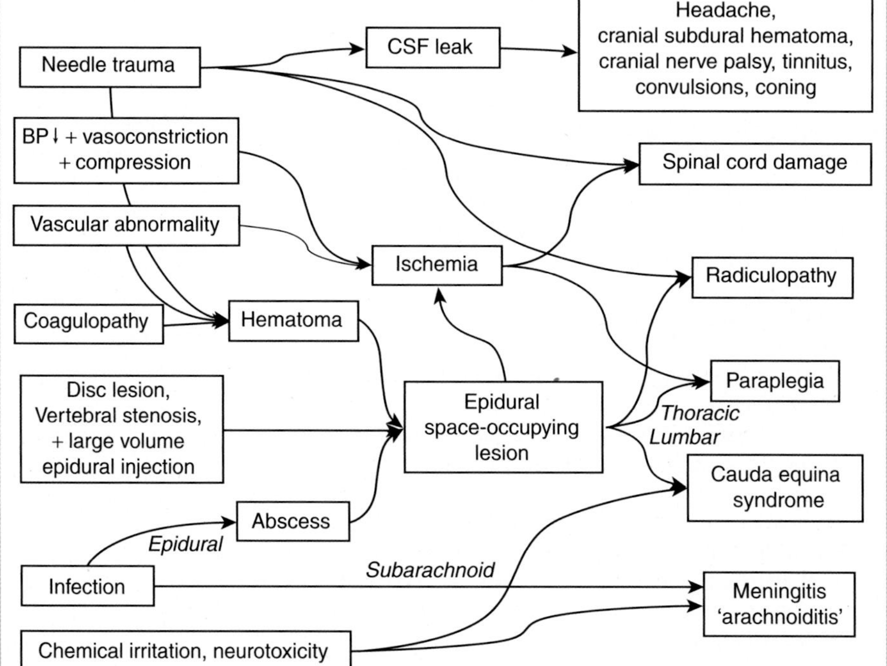

FIGURE 32-6 Mechanisms by which lesions of the central nervous system may arise in parturients.

identified eight obstetric cases, and more have been reported since.[62-66] Although commonly believed to result only from neglect of a dural puncture with a large needle or a cutting spinal needle, subdural hematoma requiring craniotomy has been reported after puncture with a small-gauge, pencil-point spinal needle[63] and after an unintentional dural puncture that had been treated with an epidural blood patch.[64] Whenever headache persists after dural puncture and treatment with an epidural blood patch (particularly if the headache is accompanied by altered consciousness, seizures, or other focal neurologic findings), magnetic resonance imaging (MRI) is warranted to exclude subdural hematoma, which may be fatal without urgent surgery.

One case of cranial *epidural* hematoma arose after spinal anesthesia for removal of the placenta; the hematoma occurred after a seizure.[67] Nothing was as it seemed, however; the seizure was not eclamptic, but rather epileptic, and the hematoma was not a result of spinal anesthesia.

Trauma to Nerve Roots and the Spinal Cord

Insertion of a spinal needle or epidural catheter is not infrequently accompanied by paresthesia that is sometimes painful. Although a flexible catheter is unlikely to do lasting damage to a nerve root in the epidural space, nerve roots in the subarachnoid space are more vulnerable.

TRAUMA ASSOCIATED WITH ATTEMPTED EPIDURAL CATHETER INSERTION

Epidural catheters may injure nerve roots either because they are inappropriately rigid[68] or because an undue length is threaded and ensnares a root.[69] A catheter seemingly threaded into the epidural space may lodge in an intervertebral foramen or even pass into the paravertebral space. In rare instances the epidural catheter and the artery of Adamkiewicz may share the same foramen. If the epidural catheter is stiff enough to compress the artery within the unyielding foramen, the blood supply to the spinal cord may be impaired. This is a possible cause of anterior spinal artery syndrome. Clinical reports indicate that the condition resolves rapidly and completely if the catheter is withdrawn before permanent damage has occurred.[70,71]

Injury to the spinal cord may result from attempted identification of the epidural space in the presence of undetected spina bifida occulta or a tethered cord,[72,73] or as a result of an unsteady grip or uncontrolled advancement of the epidural needle. Insertion of an epidural catheter in an anesthetized patient greatly increases the risk of spinal cord damage, and catastrophic injury may occur with injection of fluid into the substance of the spinal cord.[74,75]

TRAUMA ASSOCIATED WITH SPINAL ANESTHESIA

Insertion of a spinal needle below the level of the spinal cord sometimes causes brief radiating pain or paresthesia, which may be associated with persistent paresthesia in the same dermatomal distribution. Prolonged symptoms involving more than one spinal segment suggest damage to the spinal cord itself. Damage to the terminal portion of the cord (the conus medullaris) without intracord injection has also been reported in healthy conscious parturients receiving spinal or CSE anesthesia using a pencil-point needle.[13,19,76,77] Typically the patient complains of pain on needle insertion before any fluid is injected, often followed by the normal appearance of CSF from the needle hub, easy injection of the local anesthetic agent, and a normal onset of neural blockade. On recovery, there is unilateral numbness, which is succeeded by pain and paresthesia in the L5 to S1 distribution and footdrop, and in some cases urinary symptoms; sensory symptoms may last for months or years. The MRI appearance is one of a small syrinx or hematoma within the conus at the level of the body of T12 on the same side as the pain on insertion and subsequent leg symptoms (Figure 32-7).[77] In the majority of cases, the anesthesia provider believed the interspace selected was L2-L3. In one patient who subsequently died from other causes, hematomyelia was confirmed at autopsy.[78]

These injuries may have occurred for the following reasons:

- Anesthesia providers, accustomed to siting epidural needles and catheters, had forgotten the precautions necessary to avoid contact with the spinal cord during dural puncture. Moreover, the option to use an *upper* lumbar interspace was sanctioned by some reputable textbooks.[79]
- Identification of lumbar interspaces is far from accurate. Two studies have shown that it is common to select a space that is higher than assumed by one, two, or even more segments (Figure 32-8).[80,81] Anesthesia providers, who rarely use radiologic verification, have little opportunity for feedback to improve their skill in interspace identification.
- Although the spinal cord typically ends level with the lower body of L1 or the L1-L2 interspace, the length varies (Figure 32-9).[82] From the L1-L2 interspace, the needle tip can easily reach the conus in 27% of men and 43% of women.[83]
- The standard method of identifying lumbar interspaces involves the use of Tuffier's line, the imaginary line joining the two iliac crests. This method can be inaccurate, however, particularly in obese or pregnant women (Figure 32-10). Moreover, even when accurately assessed, Tuffier's line is an inconstant landmark.[84] Although typically at the level of the L4 spinous process, it may lie anywhere between the L3-L4 and L5-S1 interspaces. Other means of identifying the interspace, such as counting down from C7 or finding the vertebra that is attached to the 12th rib, are tedious and of little help in obese patients.
- Pencil-point spinal needles must be advanced further than cutting needles before the orifice is within the subarachnoid space, at which point the tip may impinge on the spinal cord.

Medical students and residents are usually instructed to select the L4-L5 interspace for diagnostic lumbar puncture, but anesthesia providers have been more liberal in their approach.[79] Given the inaccuracy of identification of lumbar interspaces and the variability of the position of the conus, it is both logical and prudent to insert a spinal needle below the spinous process of L3, or at least into a lower lumbar interspace, especially in women. Box 32-3 gives a summary of problems and precautions in identifying lumbar interspaces and avoiding damage to the conus medullaris.

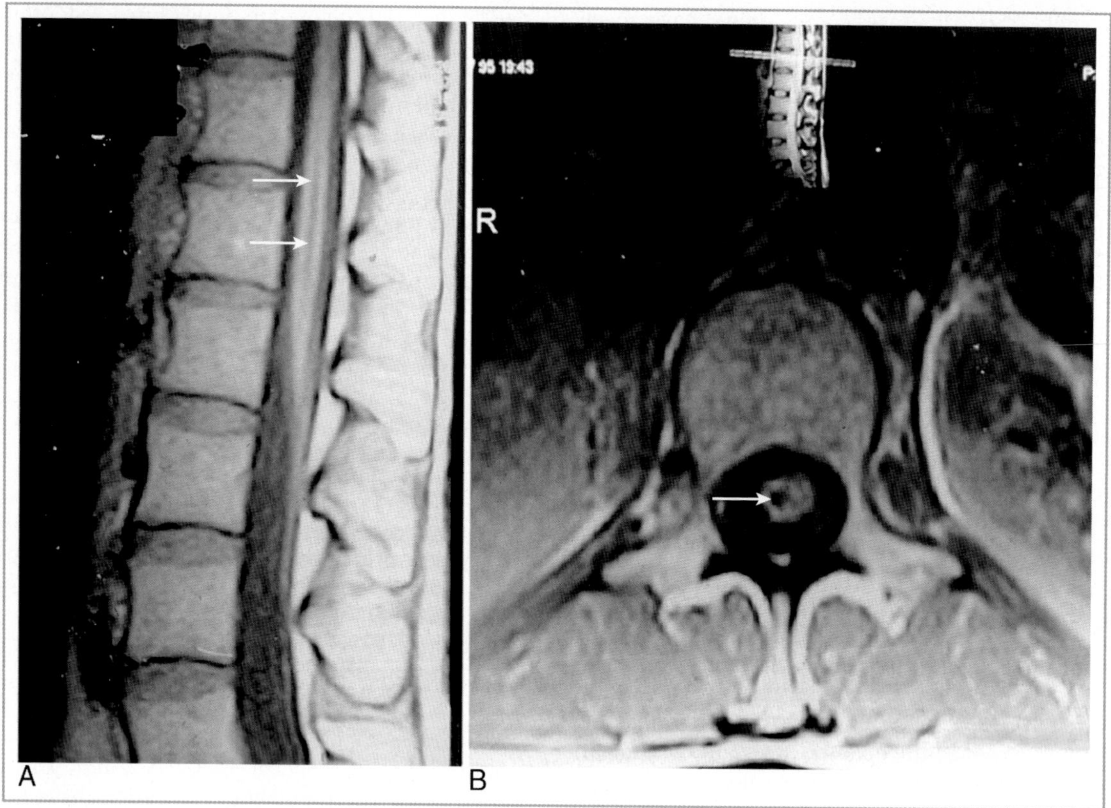

FIGURE 32-7 **A** and **B**, Magnetic resonance images of a conus medullaris lesion (*arrows*). (From Reynolds F. Damage to the conus medullaris following spinal anaesthesia. Anaesthesia 2001; 56:238-47.)

Space-Occupying Lesions of the Vertebral Canal

Space-occupying lesions of the vertebral canal include intraspinal hematomas (epidural or subdural), epidural abscess, and intraspinal tumors, any of which, within the rigid confines of the bony spinal canal, can cause dangerous compression of nervous tissue and its blood supply. Urgent laminectomy is required to avoid permanent neurologic damage. Delayed recognition and treatment (more than 6 to 12 hours after onset of symptoms) may have a catastrophic outcome and grave medicolegal consequences.

Preexisting vertebral stenosis or lumbar disc protrusion may exacerbate nervous tissue compression or mimic a

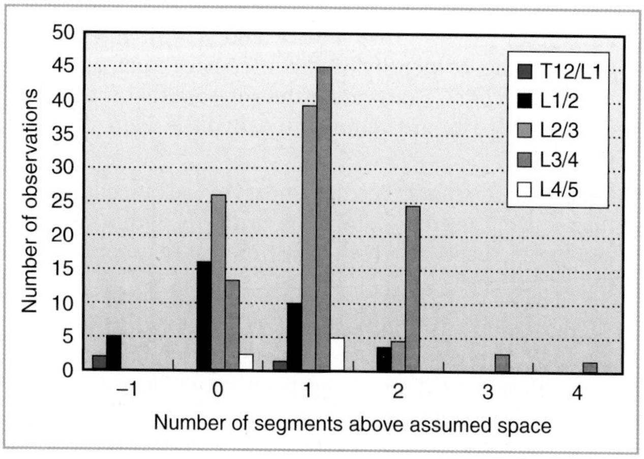

FIGURE 32-8 Identification of lumbar interspaces by Oxford anesthetists. The horizontal axis shows the position of the actual interspace, identified on magnetic resonance imaging, relative to the assumed space, in 200 observations. (Data from Broadbent CR, Maxwell WB, Ferrie R, et al. Ability of anaesthetists to identify a marked lumbar interspace. Anaesthesia 2000; 55:1122-6.)

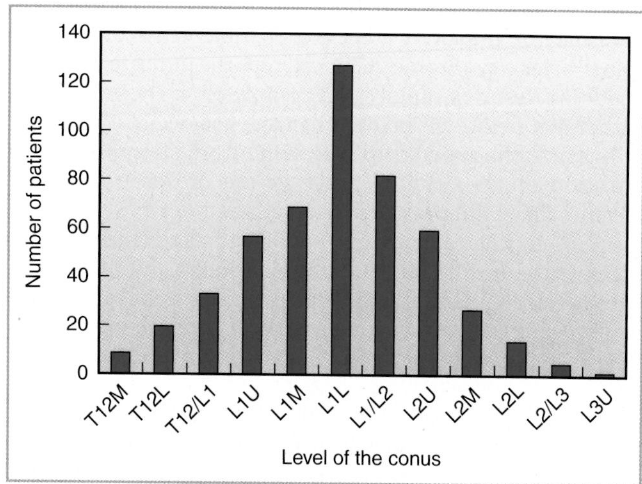

FIGURE 32-9 Variation in the level of the tip of the conus medullaris assessed by magnetic resonance imaging of the lumbar spine among 504 consecutive adults. L, lower third of vertebral body listed; M, middle third of vertebral body listed; T12/L1, interspace between T12 and L1; U, upper third of vertebral body listed. (Data derived from Saifuddin A, Burnett SJ, White J. The variation of position of the conus medullaris in an adult population: A magnetic resonance imaging study. Spine 1998; 23:1452-6.)

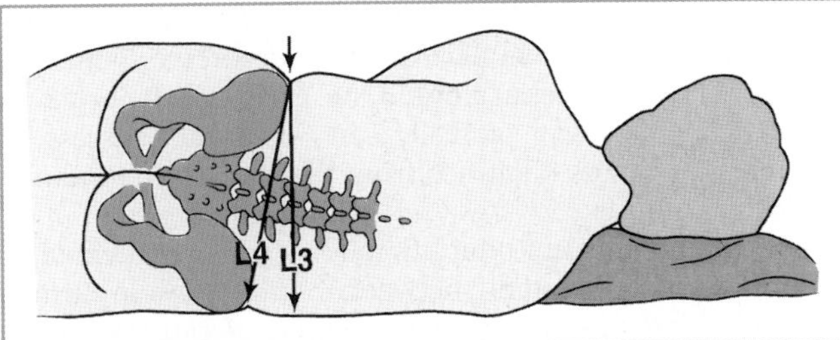

FIGURE 32-10 Error that may arise if Tuffier's line is judged in a pregnant patient in the lateral position, when a line is drawn perpendicularly from the upper iliac crest rather than through both iliac crests. In pregnant patients at term, the hips may have a greater width than the shoulders. The resulting cephalad pelvic tilt may lead to an error in the cephalad direction.

space-occupying lesion. Patients may be symptom-free until the balance is tipped by injection of a large volume into the epidural space.[85-87] The neurologic deficit that may arise from a compressive lesion depends on the vertebral level; lower thoracic lesions are associated with leg weakness or paraplegia, and lumbar lesions are associated with cauda equina syndrome, including urinary retention and incontinence. Back pain (often radiating to the legs) is a common feature.

EPIDURAL HEMATOMA

Epidural hematoma causing neurologic deficit typically arises in an elderly patient with arterial disease; it is very rare in obstetric patients, despite the engorgement and possible fragility of epidural veins during pregnancy. One case, without confirmatory details, was reported in a retrospective survey of 505,000 obstetric epidural procedures.[9] Five surveys that involved 717,814 obstetric epidural procedures identified no cases,[10-12,15,18] although in the last Swedish national survey there were two cases, both in patients with HELLP (hemolysis, elevated liver enzymes, low platelets) syndrome.[19] Loo et al.[6] identified three published cases of epidural hematoma in the *absence* of neuraxial anesthesia in obstetric patients, and more cases have subsequently been reported.[88] Any estimate of the incidence of epidural hematoma in the nonobstetric surgical population is equally unreliable, because it depends on how assiduously neuraxial blockade is avoided in the presence of coagulopathy[18,19,89,90] and also on the incidence of vessel puncture, which in turn is affected by the skill of the anesthesia provider. Risk factors identified from comprehensive reviews of case reports include (1) difficult or traumatic epidural needle/catheter placement, (2) coagulopathy or therapeutic anticoagulation, (3) spinal deformity, and (4) spinal tumor.[90-93] Antiplatelet therapy does not appear to increase the incidence of neurologic dysfunction after neuraxial anesthesia.[94]

Both coagulopathy and vessel damage are necessary to produce a hematoma large enough to cause a neurologic deficit in the parturient. It should be remembered that trauma can arise not only during insertion but also on removal of the epidural catheter. Epidural catheters have been placed with impunity in parturients with thrombocytopenia,[95-97] although the frequency of vessel trauma among these patients was not regularly recorded. One important factor in minimizing the occurrence of spinal epidural hematoma in parturients may be the normally hypercoagulable status of their blood. Another is the ease with which a large volume of anticoagulated blood may flow out of the unrestricting intervertebral foramina in young patients. Injected blood is known to disappear from the epidural space rapidly in the parturient.[98] In the performance of an epidural blood patch, 20 mL of blood is commonly injected with impunity. Though compressive symptoms may be experienced with a volume larger than 20 mL, they do not normally presage any neurologic deficit in obstetric patients.

In addition to the two reported cases of epidural hematoma in patients with HELLP syndrome,[19] the only case report of authenticated epidural hematoma with neurologic sequelae in a parturient occurred in association with coagulopathy resulting from cholestasis.[99] Coagulation status was not investigated before insertion of the epidural catheter. A small epidural hematoma was found on MRI in a parturient with neurofibromatosis who experienced urinary incontinence after multiple traumatic attempts at epidural catheter insertion, accidental dural puncture, and CSE anesthesia, but the symptoms resolved spontaneously.[93] A preeclamptic patient with thrombocytopenia suffered a persistent lower limb deficit after a traumatic epidural catheter insertion using the loss-of-resistance-to-air technique.[100] Laminectomy revealed multiple bubbles and a 4-mL blood clot, the exact site of which was not stated.

SUBDURAL HEMATOMA

Spinal subdural hematoma has been reported in obstetric patients, one in association with an ependymoma,[92] and another in a woman with preeclampsia, known vessel puncture, and mild coagulopathy.[101] Both patients developed cauda equina syndrome. Dural puncture (with or without arachnoid puncture) is a prerequisite for subdural hematoma. On the other hand, coagulopathy may *not* be a prerequisite, because the extravasated blood is confined to the

BOX 32-3 Points to Remember to Reduce Risk of Damage to the Conus Medullaris during Spinal Anesthesia

- The conus reaches L2 in 27% of men but in 43% of women.
- Tuffier's line is not in a constant position relative to the spine.
- The interspace chosen is usually higher than supposed.
- The spinal needle should not knowingly be inserted above the L3 spinous process.
- Pencil-point spinal needles have at least 1 mm of "blind tip" beyond the orifice.
- Spinal needles must be advanced with gentleness and control.
- Advancement of the spinal needle should be halted immediately, and the stylet removed to check for CSF, if entry of the needle tip into the subarachnoid space is suspected.
- The procedure should be abandoned if the patient is unable to cooperate.

subdural space and may compress adjacent nerve roots more readily than in the capacious epidural space.

If neuraxial blockade is found to have been conducted in the presence of risk factors for spinal hematoma, it is an essential responsibility of the anesthesia provider to examine the lower extremities after delivery, to confirm and document the return of normal motor and sensory function, and to request subsequent checks by the nursing staff. Severe back pain, a significant delay in normal recovery, or deterioration of lower extremity or bladder function signals the need for emergency imaging of the spine. If intraspinal compression is confirmed by MRI, a neurosurgical opinion must be urgently sought.

The dangers of neuraxial anesthesia in the presence of coagulopathy and anticoagulant treatment are also discussed in Chapters 38 and 43.

Infection

Neuraxial infection (epidural abscess and meningitis) was identified as the most common cause of neuraxial injury in obstetric cases in the American Society of Anesthesiologists Closed-Claims database between 1980 and 1999.[102] Infections that have been reported include epidural abscess, epidural-related infection, and meningitis.

EPIDURAL ABSCESS

Epidural abscess, though rare, is considerably more frequently reported in obstetric patients than epidural hematoma. One case was detected in the retrospective survey of 505,000 obstetric epidural procedures,[9] one among 205,000 procedures in the latest national Swedish survey,[19] and none among the remaining surveys summarized in Table 32-1. A conflation of the findings of 10 surveys yielded an incidence of 1 in 302,757 obstetric epidural procedures.[103] The incidence among surgical patients has been reported as 10-fold[19] to 100-fold[104] higher. Most cases arose after prolonged epidural catheterization in elderly and immunocompromised patients. Epidural abscess arising spontaneously in the puerperium has also been reported.[6]

Sixteen case reports of epidural abscess after epidural catheterization in obstetric patients[105-120] have been tabulated elsewhere.[103] All cases occurred after epidural catheterization, three as part of CSE anesthesia. None followed spinal anesthesia alone. One case was reported as meningitis but was actually an epidural abscess.[118] Possible risk factors identified from these cases are outlined in Table 32-2.

An epidural abscess typically follows prolonged epidural catheterization, reportedly between 1 and 4 days in obstetric cases. The shortest recorded period of catheterization to be followed by epidural abscess was 6.5 hours, in a patient with evidence of venous trauma during placement of the epidural catheter.[109] Other possible etiologic factors are epidural administration of opioid *without* local anesthetic,[107,114,115] traumatic or difficult insertion of the catheter,[114] and diabetes or immunosuppression from any cause.[104,114] Inflammation at the epidural catheter entry point may presage epidural space infection.[113,115] Blood in the epidural space is a potential nidus for infection but only rarely appears to be a factor.[109] In light of these reports it may be prudent to avoid prolonged epidural catheterization in the patient with other risk factors for infection.

Some practitioners have suggested that administration of an epidural blood patch necessitates prior blood culture. However, a Medline search carried out in October 2008 for *epidural abscess* AND *epidural blood patch* did not yield any cases, and the only recorded instance of an infected blood patch is one that appears to have entered the subcutaneous fat (see later).

Clinical Presentation

Symptoms of epidural abscess typically start between 4 and 10 days after removal of the epidural catheter. Severe backache (with local tenderness) and fever, with or without radiating or root pain, are the presenting features. The catheter entry point may be inflamed with some fluid leak, and a hematology screen typically reveals a leukocytosis and an increased C-reactive protein level. Fever, neck stiffness, headache, and signs of inflammation serve to differentiate epidural abscess from hematoma. These signs and symptoms should prompt MRI, which may allow early diagnosis before the onset of neurologic changes (Figure 32-11).[121] Untreated, symptoms may progress to leg weakness,

TABLE 32-2 Possible Etiologic Factors for Epidural Abscess and Meningitis

Factor	Epidural Abscess	Meningitis
• Entry point	• Through the catheter or along its tissue track	• Blood, via the dural puncture
• Usual causative organism	• *Staphylococcus aureus*	• Viridans-type streptococcus
• Possible source of infection	• Patient's skin, tracking along the catheter entry point • Epidural equipment contaminated by operator's skin • Body fluids in the bed • Injectate without racemic local anesthetic	• Anesthesia provider's oropharyngeal cavity • Talking without a mask • Blood-borne • Vagina
• Risk factors	• Prolonged catheterization • Poor aseptic technique • Multiple attempts at insertion, or traumatic insertion • Lying in a wet contaminated bed • Immunocompromise: steroids, diabetes, AIDS	• Dural puncture • Labor • Anesthesia provider not wearing a mask • Vaginal infection • Bacteremia • Immunocompromise?

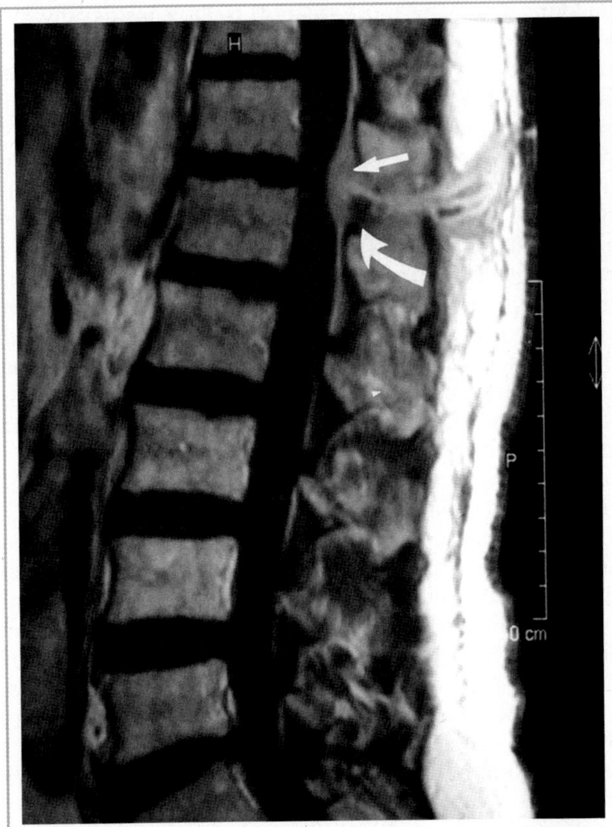

FIGURE 32-11 Epidural abscess. Midsagittal T1-weighted magnetic resonance image of the lumbar and lower thoracic region, after intravenous gadolinium DTPA. Note the dorsal epidural mass located at T12-L1 (*arrows*), convex anteriorly but not compressing the conus. Normal epidural fat is flat anteriorly. (From Royakers AANM, Willigers H, van der Ven AJ, et al. Catheter-related epidural abscesses—don't wait for neurological deficits. Acta Anaesthesiol Scand 2002; 46:611-5.)

paresthesias, bladder dysfunction, and other evidence of cauda equina syndrome. Blood culture may identify the organism before or without surgical drainage. Diagnostic lumbar puncture is contraindicated.

Etiology

Staphylococcus aureus is the most common causative organism in cases of epidural abscess, with the occasional streptococcus and pseudomonas. The skin appears to be the most likely source of infection.[6] The few reported cases of epidural abscess caused by β-hemolytic streptococci[108,112] may have stemmed from vaginal infection and hematogenous spread.

The skin is commonly colonized by *Staphylococcus epidermidis* and other weakly pathogenic bacteria, and occasionally by *S. aureus*. The highest concentration of colonies is found in the hair follicles,[122] where organisms may be protected from briefly applied disinfectants. Infectious organisms from the skin can reach deeper tissue planes via needle tracks and implanted epidural catheters to create localized abscesses in the paraspinal or epidural spaces. Despite all aseptic precautions, some level of detectable bacterial colonization of the epidural catheter is very common, but robust host defenses normally prevent infection. When defenses are weak and infection containment breaks down, epidural abscess formation begins.

The potential for the parturient's bed to be contaminated with amniotic fluid and excrement has prompted the use of occlusive dressings. A meta-analysis of studies comparing transparent occlusive dressings with gauze dressings for peripheral *intravenous* catheters found that the risk of infection was greater with occlusive dressings[123]; however, the American Society of Regional Anesthesia and Pain Medicine (ASRA) has concluded that there is currently not enough evidence to recommend one type of dressing over another.[124]

Most local anesthetics, such as racemic bupivacaine and lidocaine, have an antibacterial effect in concentrations administered for neuraxial anesthesia, although the antibacterial effect of the pure L-isomers levobupivacaine and ropivacaine is weaker than that of racemic preparations.[125-128]

Management

As with spinal hematoma, once neurologic signs are present, early diagnosis with prompt laminectomy is essential to recovery. The prognosis is improved if the abscess is evacuated before neurologic signs develop. In the presence of mild symptoms without neurologic changes, successful conservative treatment with antibiotics has been reported.[110] Successful percutaneous needle drainage of epidural abscesses has also been reported,[129] although only laminectomy can ensure that all loculations are drained under direct vision. Prompt identification of the infectious organism(s) and directed antibiotic therapy are mandatory. Antibiotic treatment should be continued for 2 to 4 weeks.[121]

EPIDURAL-RELATED INFECTION

Inflammation at the site of catheter insertion, along the track and adjacent to, but not involving the epidural space, has also been described. Paraspinal abscess after epidural analgesia,[130-133] and discitis after spinal blockade[134] have been reported in obstetric patients. Catheter-site inflammation is relatively common with prolonged postoperative epidural analgesia.[135,136] One report described both a subdural abscess after CSE anesthesia and infection in the subcutaneous tissues following an apparently misplaced epidural blood patch.[137]

A variety of organisms have been associated with epidural-related infections.[103] All such conditions are associated with back pain and signs of inflammation and pose a threat of spread to the epidural space. Moreover, paraspinal abscess may itself be associated with neurologic deficit.[132,133]

MENINGITIS

Although not frequently mentioned in surveys, post-spinal meningitis has become a cause for concern[138] and is an important serious neurologic complication of neuraxial labor analgesia. It was suspected in two cases in the prospective survey of 108,133 epidural procedures and 14,865 spinal anesthetic procedures by Scott and Tunstall,[10] although the specific type of anesthesia was not stated. Palot et al.[11] reported three cases of meningitis among 288,351 obstetric epidural procedures but did not state whether they followed dural puncture. One case was identified in a survey of spinal and CSE anesthesia

(1/42,000 procedures).[13] No case of meningitis was reported among the other surveys summarized in Table 32-1. A recent review found published reports of 38 cases in obstetric patients[50,118,138-162] (summarized in Table 32-3) and an incidence derived from surveys of spinal and CSE anesthesia of 1 in 39,000.[103]

Etiology and Risk Factors

Risk factors and sources of infection are summarized in Table 32-2. Although community-acquired meningitis is caused by *Neisseria meningitidis*, *Streptococcus pneumoniae*, or *Haemophilus influenzae*, post-spinal meningitis is most commonly caused by streptococci of the viridans type (*salivarius, sanguis, uberis*).[6,19,103,138] These organisms are found in the upper airway and the vagina. *Pseudomonas meningitidis* has also been reported.[144] Neither *Pseudomonas* nor *Streptococcus viridans* is normally virulent; they do not, for example, cause wound infection, but they thrive in a watery medium and flourish if introduced into CSF. In several reported cases no organisms were grown on culture, and chemical meningitis was diagnosed. In most cases, however, there were features of bacterial meningitis, including low CSF glucose concentration. It must be remembered that streptococci of the viridans type do not grow readily in conventional culture media.[138]

Dural puncture is probably a prerequisite for iatrogenic meningitis. A retrospective review of surgical patients in one hospital in Brazil found three cases among 38,128 spinal anesthetics (1/12,709) and none among 12,822 patients receiving other types of anesthesia.[163] In normal circumstances the blood-brain barrier (the endothelial lining of the capillaries, which are continuous with tight junctions and no pinocytotic vesicles) protects the CNS against weakly pathogenic bacteria. The dura mater should not be confused with the blood-brain barrier, but dural puncture is commonly associated with vascular trauma,[164] which allows blood to enter the CSF. Among the 38 published cases of puerperal meningitis for which details are available (see Table 32-3), 32 occurred after known dural puncture.

Among the six cases that followed apparently uncomplicated epidural analgesia, one was viral and may have been a chance event,[153] one was probably an epidural abscess,[157] and two were blood-borne from vaginal infection due to group B streptococcus.[145,149] One case, sadly fatal, followed multiple attempts at epidural catheter insertion.[143] Does uncomplicated epidural catheterization itself increase the risk of puerperal meningitis? Although epidural analgesia is used more commonly than spinal analgesia during labor, case reports of meningitis after spinal analgesia far outnumber those after epidural analgesia.

Is epidural analgesia meningitis purely coincidental? If so, one would expect meningitis to be reported following vaginal delivery without neuraxial blockade. A Medline search (1970 to 2007) that combined *meningitis* with *puerperium* or *labor* or *labor and delivery* found mention of neonatal meningitis but no reports of maternal meningitis without neuraxial anesthesia. In one survey from Iowa, among 73 women with β-hemolytic streptococcal infections in the puerperium, the only one who suffered meningitis had received spinal anesthesia.[165] Women with other types of streptococcal infection were not investigated. A search of 30 years of maternal mortality reports from the United Kingdom (involving more than 20 million births) revealed (1) fulminating streptococcal septicemia without overt meningitis as a repeated cause of death, (2) one case of *Escherichia coli* meningitis in the 1979 to 1981 report, (3) one case of pneumococcal meningitis in mid-pregnancy, (4) one case of group A streptococcal meningitis in a patient with spina bifida, and (5) one case of purulent meningitis after spinal anesthesia for cesarean delivery in a sick patient in the 1997 to 1999 report.[161] It appears that vaginal delivery, even with genital tract sepsis, but without neuraxial anesthesia, is not a risk factor for meningitis, unless meningitis is regarded as a chance finding and never reported. Therefore a causative relationship between epidural catheterization and meningitis after vaginal delivery cannot be excluded and may be attributed to unrecognized dural puncture, which may occur during multiple attempts at epidural catheter insertion or even with apparently uncomplicated catheter insertion.

Labor may also be a risk factor for meningitis. The great majority of parturients with nosocomial meningitis had labored (see Table 32-3). In the latest survey from Sweden, where spinal and CSE anesthesia are rarely used during labor, meningitis was found only among surgical patients.[19] Meningitis appears surprisingly rare when spinal anesthesia is used for elective cesarean delivery. This finding is remarkable, given that spinal anesthesia is used so commonly for this purpose. Moreover, the five exceptions were among six unusual cases in Sri Lanka, which resulted from *Aspergillus* contamination of syringes that had been donated after the 2005 tsunami and stored in an unsuitable warehouse at 41° C and 75% humidity.[159]

The possible reasons why meningitis is reported more commonly in laboring women than among those undergoing elective cesarean delivery are as follows:

1. The vagina may be colonized by streptococci, and vaginal delivery is commonly followed by mild bacteremia. Thus labor, with its potential for vaginal trauma, is clearly an important risk factor. Unlike vaginal delivery, elective cesarean delivery is not normally associated with streptococcal bacteremia.
2. For cesarean delivery, spinal anesthesia is administered in the operating room, which is a cleaner environment than the labor and delivery room.
3. The anesthesia provider is more likely to wear a mask in the operating room.
4. The nonlaboring patient is not thrashing about in a (possibly) contaminated bed.
5. An antibiotic is usually administered immediately before or after cesarean delivery.

Infection at a remote site may also be a risk factor for meningitis. Bacteremia has been detected in approximately 8% of women with chorioamnionitis,[166] although two small studies found no evidence of spinal infection among 12 women with bacteremia who received epidural blockade without antibiotic treatment.[167,168] Although such negative findings are reassuring, they are not conclusive and do not apply to spinal anesthesia. Human immunodeficiency virus (HIV) infection and acquired immunodeficiency syndrome (AIDS) should not be regarded as contraindications to neuraxial analgesia, in view of the early presence of the virus within the CNS (see Chapter 44).[169] Performing an epidural

TABLE 32-3 Case Reports of Post–Dural Puncture Meningitis among Obstetric Patients

Background (Total No. Cases)	Report*	Number of Cases	Organism and Comments
Spinal analgesia in labor (9 cases)	Gibbons, 1969[148]	3	No growth, "chemical meningitis" CSF findings suggested bacterial etiology
	Phillips, 1970[155]	1	No growth CSF findings suggested bacterial etiology
	Corbett & Rosenstein, 1971[144]	3	*Pseudomonas aeruginosa* Nonsterile technique
	Newton et al., 1994[154]	1	*Streptococcus salivarius*
	Lurie et al., 1999[152]	1	*Streptococcus viridans*
Spinal anesthesia for cesarean delivery (11 cases)	Bugedo et al., 1991[141]	1	Signs of bacterial meningitis Labor status unknown
	Lee & Parry, 1991[151]	1	No growth CSF findings suggested bacterial etiology In labor Three attempts at spinal anesthesia
	Stallard & Barry, 1995[160]	1	No growth CSF findings suggested bacterial etiology Three attempts at epidural for neuraxial labor analgesia Spinal anesthesia in same interspace
	Donnelly et al., 1998[146]	1	No growth CSF findings suggested bacterial etiology Membranes ruptured
	Thomas & Cooper, 2001[161]	1	Preeclampsia Labor status unknown Patient died
	Rodrigo et al., 2007[159]	6	*Aspergillus* equipment contamination 5 cases from elective cesarean deliveries, 1 during labor 3 patients died
Spinal anesthesia for retained placenta (1 case)	Roberts & Petts, 1990[158]	1	No growth CSF findings suggested bacterial etiology
CSE analgesia in labor (7 cases)	Harding et al., 1994[150]	2	No growth CSF findings suggested bacterial etiology
	Cascio & Heath, 1996[142]	1	*S. salivarius* (dismissed as contaminant)
	Bouhemad et al., 1998[140]	1	*S. salivarius*
	Duflo et al., 1998[147]	1	*S. viridans*
	Pinder & Dresner, 2003[156]	1	*Neisseria meningitidis* (?chance event)
	Vernis et al., 2004[162]	1	One case in the course of a randomized trial
Unintentional dural puncture during epidural analgesia in labor (3 cases)	Berga & Trierweiler, 1989[139]	1	*Streptococcus sanguis*
	Sansome et al., 1991[50]	1	No growth CSF findings equivocal
	Baer, 2006[138]	1	*Staphylococcus simulans* and *S. salivarius* Patient died
"Uncomplicated" epidural analgesia in labor (6 cases)	Neumark et al., 1980[153]	1	Coxsackie B virus (?chance event)
	Ready & Helfer, 1989[157]	2	1 *Streptococcus uberis* 1 *Streptococcus faecalis* (epidural inflammation)

CSE, combined spinal-epidural anesthesia; CSF, cerebrospinal fluid.

*Superscript numbers indicate reference citations at the end of the chapter.

Continued

TABLE 32-3—cont'd Case Reports of Post–Dural Puncture Meningitis among Obstetric Patients

Background (Total No. Cases)	Report*	Number of Cases	Organism and Comments
"Uncomplicated" epidural analgesia in labor (6 cases) *(continued)*	Davis et al., 1993[145]	1	Group B streptococcus
	Goldstein et al., 1996[149]		
	Choy, 2000[143]	1	Group B streptococcus
		1	No growth CSF findings suggested bacterial etiology Two attempts at epidural analgesia Patient died
Total: 38 cases	32 known dural punctures 5 elective cesarean deliveries, remainder in labor 6 deaths		

blood patch in the presence of bacteremia is also a theoretical risk for both meningitis and abscess, but neither has been reported in this context. Chapter 36 discusses neuraxial analgesia in the presence of maternal fever in detail.

Other risk factors for meningitis include faulty technique, in particular failure to wear a mask (see later). Manual removal of the placenta is a postulated risk factor for meningitis, and one such case has been reported,[158] although given the popularity of spinal anesthesia for this procedure, one would perhaps expect a higher frequency. It has been postulated that use of the CSE technique, with the presence of a foreign body next to a dural hole, may increase the risk of meningitis.

Clinical Presentation and Management

Fever, headache, photophobia, nausea, vomiting, and neck stiffness are typical symptoms of meningitis, and when they are accompanied by confusion, drowsiness, and Kernig's sign (i.e., inability to straighten the knee when the hip is flexed), meningitis should be strongly suspected. The onset may be 12 hours to a few days after delivery. Diagnostic lumbar puncture shows increased CSF pressure, increases in protein level and white blood cell count (mainly polymorphonuclear leukocytes in patients with bacterial meningitis), and a CSF glucose concentration that is lower than that in the blood. Because of the nature of the *S. viridans* group, culture on plates rather than in broth may have negative results, particularly if antibiotics have been given, or the growth may be assumed to be a contaminant.[138] Treatment with an appropriate antibiotic should not await the microbiology results and should result in full recovery.[6] Vancomycin and third-generation cephalosporins have been recommended as first-line treatment.[163] The treatment regimen should be adjusted according to results of culture and sensitivity testing.

PREVENTION OF INTRASPINAL INFECTION AFTER NEURAXIAL ANESTHESIA

Measures to prevent intraspinal infection are summarized in Box 32-4. Means of preventing meningitis and epidural abscess are not identical, because abscess usually follows epidural catheterization and is commonly caused by *S. aureus*, which enters via the skin, whereas meningitis classically follows dural puncture, is caused by vaginal or nasal organisms, may be blood-borne, and is usually caused by streptococcus and never by *S. aureus.*

Because adverse outcomes are rare, the use of sterile precautions can rarely be supported by evidence from randomized trials. Sterile technique tends to be a matter of

BOX 32-4 Procedures to Decrease the Risk of Infection after Neuraxial Anesthesia

- Avoid dural puncture unless indicated:
  - During labor.
  - In the presence of known genital tract infection.
- Wear an effective mask; wear a new mask for each patient.
- Remove hand jewelry and watches, and wash hands with an alcohol-based scrub solution.
- In the United Kingdom, a gown is worn for epidural catheter insertion.
- Don sterile gloves in a sterile manner.
- Paint the patient's skin with chlorhexidine in alcohol solution, following the package instructions, and allow the skin to dry after application.
- Make sure the back is securely draped.
- Avoid contaminating any equipment that is used in the procedure, and minimize touching parts of the equipment that will enter the patient.
- Apply a suitable dressing to the catheter entry point.
- Use a bacterial filter with an indwelling epidural or spinal catheter if the catheter will remain in place longer than several days.
- Do not leave an epidural catheter *in situ* after delivery if:
  - The dura has been punctured during labor.
  - Multiple attempts at insertion were made.
  - There is any evidence of sepsis.
  - Immunosuppression is present for any reason.
- If there is concern about sepsis or contamination, administer appropriate antibiotics.

local and individual habit, but the components of good sterile technique should be guided by common sense and the best available indirect evidence. It is notable that in many case reports of neuraxial infection, sterile precautions used in initiating neuraxial blockade receive no mention.

Face Mask

Several surveys indicate widespread disregard of surgical masks for infection control during neuraxial block administration.[163,170,171] Among case reports of nosocomial meningitis, a mask was not mentioned[139,157] or was not worn[145,154] ("as it is of doubtful value"[151] or because it "contributes little to prevent infection during spinal or epidural anesthesia,"[152] or is not considered part of "full aseptic technique"[145]).

Confusion has arisen because randomized trials have demonstrated that the omission of masks in the operating room does not increase the occurrence of wound infection.[172] This is not surprising, however, because organisms from the upper airway do not cause wound infection, although they certainly do cause nosocomial meningitis. The effect of wearing a mask in the prevention of such rare complications cannot readily be ascertained by a randomized controlled trial. Nevertheless, it has not been difficult to demonstrate the obvious value of masks in reducing the dispersion of bacteria from the mouth and nose.[173,174] The ASRA recommends, and the U.S. Centers for Disease Control and Prevention (CDC) requires, that anesthesia providers wear a mask during administration of neuraxial analgesia/anesthesia.[124,175] Masks must be of good quality, preferably fiberglass and not simply woven linen or paper, and they should be changed for each patient.[163]

Sterile Gown

Though undeniably part of "full aseptic precautions" employed by surgeons, a sterile gown is rarely worn for spinal needle placement. For insertion of epidural catheters, anesthesia providers in the United Kingdom commonly wear gowns, although this is not the typical practice in the United States and France.[176] The value of wearing a gown is not supported by good evidence, but it can only be safer than not doing so. When an epidural catheter is being inserted by a novice who is not wearing a gown, the catheter may inadvertently come into contact with the skin of the provider's upper arm or the unsterile clothing on his or her body. This occurrence may facilitate entry, via the catheter, of skin organisms that may cause epidural abscess.

Sterilizing the Skin

Evidence from laboratory and clinical studies shows that 2% chlorhexidine in 70% alcohol consistently outperforms povidone-iodine for skin disinfection.[103,122,135,177] Alcohol provides the rapid onset, and chlorhexidine provides the longer duration of action. Moreover, open bottles of povidone-iodine may be contaminated with various bacterial rods and skin flora,[178] attesting to its feeble antibacterial effect. DuraPrep (3M, St. Paul, MN) is a skin disinfectant that contains an iodophor combined with isopropyl alcohol. Birnbach et al.[179] observed that it was superior to povidone-iodine for skin disinfection before epidural catheter insertion in parturients. The alcohol provides rapid antisepsis and may prolong the effect of the iodophor. When placed on the skin, the solution may form a film of disinfectant that resists washing.[179]

Neither chlorhexidine nor iodine is licensed for skin sterilization before neuraxial block administration. However, the CDC guidelines for skin preparation for surgery and for central venous and arterial catheterization recommend the use of chlorhexidine.[180] The ASRA convened a Practice Advisory Council on Infection Complications Associated with Regional Anesthesia in 2004. In its report, the Council stated that "alcohol-based chlorhexidine solutions should be considered the antiseptic of choice before regional anesthetic techniques."[124]

Maintaining Sterility of the Epidural Catheter, Its Contents, and the Entry Point

The entry point of the epidural catheter clearly needs to be protected from contamination by a suitable dressing.[103,124] For prolonged analgesia, racemic bupivacaine may be safer than an opioid alone or the pure L-isomers of local anesthetics, either of which may permit bacterial growth in the solution.[125-128] There is no evidence to support or discourage the use of a bacterial filter during a short-term (several days) epidural infusion.[124] Prolonged catheterization is best avoided after dural puncture, whether unintentional or deliberate, and when sepsis or immunocompromise is present or suspected.

Vascular Disorders

ISCHEMIC INJURY TO THE SPINAL CORD

Ischemic injury to the spinal cord is typically seen in elderly patients after epidural or spinal anesthesia, often with an epinephrine-containing solution, and indeed after general anesthesia with accompanying hypotension. It is rare in the obstetric population, in whom arterial disease is unusual and hypotension is treated aggressively.

The blood supply to the spinal cord depends on a single anterior spinal artery and bilateral posterior spinal arteries. The arteries arise from the circle of Willis and receive reinforcements during their descent in the spinal canal. The posterior spinal arteries receive regular contributions from radicular arteries, but the single anterior spinal artery, which supplies the anterior two thirds of the spinal cord, receives only sporadic reinforcement. **Anterior spinal artery syndrome,** which may result from arterial compression or hypotension, is characterized by a predominantly motor deficit, with or without loss of pain and temperature sensation, but with sparing of vibration and joint sensations, which are transmitted in the posterior columns. The condition has been reported among obstetric patients with particular risk factors (see later).[6,9,181] One report described a series of accidents[182]: A parous woman received epidural analgesia with lidocaine, then bupivacaine with epinephrine, followed by 2-chloroprocaine when she required urgent cesarean delivery. Hypotension due to blood loss from a placenta previa *and* a ruptured uterus was followed by typical irreversible anterior spinal artery syndrome. Hypotension due to blood loss is likely to cause a greater degree of ischemia than that due to vasodilation, and the use of epinephrine may have contributed to the adverse outcome in this case.

Chemical Injury

THE EPIDURAL SPACE

The epidural space is remarkably tolerant of foreign and potentially neurotoxic substances because of two protective factors. First, vascular uptake and outward flow via the intervertebral foramina remove a large proportion of drugs deposited in the epidural space. Second, nerve roots within the epidural space are protected by a cuff of dura and arachnoid as well as pia mater. Severe neuraxial damage occurs only when these defenses are overwhelmed either by gross overdose or if there is unintentional contamination of the subarachnoid space. There are many case reports of unintentional epidural injection of the wrong substance, including the following:

1. **Thiopental**. Vascular uptake has led to transient somnolence or light anesthesia, but no permanent sequelae.
2. **Vasopressors (ephedrine** and **metaraminol)**. Epidural administration resulted in severe hypertension.[183]
3. **Potassium chloride**. At least four well-documented cases have been reported.[184,185] All the patients had profound motor and sensory block with pain or depolarizing spasms. Only one, who received the largest epidural dose (15 mL of 11.25% KCl), remained permanently paraplegic.[185]
4. **Other potentially noxious substances**. Administration of an unknown substance, possibly paraldehyde, given in error as an epidural bolus injection during labor, resulted in permanent painful quadriplegia and the largest monetary award for damages in Great Britain at that time.[186] Unintentional misconnections of intravenous and epidural infusion systems have led to large-volume epidural infusions of potentially harmful substances, including total parenteral nutrition solutions with a high osmolality[187] and ranitidine in a phenol-containing solution.[188] Fortunately, in most cases of this type of drug error, neurologic sequelae have not been reported.

In summary, with a few exceptions, the epidural space appears to be merely an exotic means of systemic administration of analgesia/anesthesia. Nevertheless, the possibility of occult dural puncture means that unintentional administration of a potentially neurotoxic substance (e.g., traces of alcohol, antioxidant, or preservative) may migrate into the subarachnoid space. Vigilance and systems to avoid these errors are mandatory.

THE SUBARACHNOID SPACE

The subarachnoid space, having direct communication with intracranial structures, presents a greater risk than the epidural space for adverse outcome after unintentional injection of toxic substances. Intrathecal potassium does not merely maim, it can kill.[189] Irritant solutions may also cause neurotoxicity and arachnoiditis.

Nerve roots within the subarachnoid space are highly vulnerable to chemical damage, particularly the sacral roots, which are poorly myelinated. Therefore, neurotoxicity associated with intrathecal injection classically produces **cauda equina syndrome**. For example, in 1937, 14 cases of severe cauda equina syndrome were reported after spinal anesthesia using a solution called "heavy duracaine," a mixture, in 15% ethanol, of procaine, glycerin, and gliadin or gum acacia, which presumably was added in an attempt to prolong the action of procaine.[190] In the 1940s and 1950s in the United Kingdom, the spinal injection of 10 mL of hypo-osmolar dibucaine was associated with paraplegia, but whether the paraplegia resulted from disturbance of the intrathecal milieu or contamination with phenol is argued.

BOX 32-5 Risk Factors for Chemical Damage to the Cauda Equina

- Poor subarachnoid dispersion of local anesthetic:
  - Block failure, followed by a repeat injection
  - Fine-gauge or pencil-point needle
  - Spinal microcatheter
  - Continuous infusion
  - Hyperbaric anesthetic solution
  - Lithotomy position
- Unintentional intrathecal injection of a large volume intended for the epidural space
- Incorrect formulation, with unsuitable preservative or antioxidant
- Intrathecal **lidocaine,** particularly 5% (also tetracaine or dibucaine?)

In later reports, cauda equina syndrome has occurred in association with intrathecal injection of less obviously noxious spinal agents. Cases of cauda equina syndrome have followed continuous or single-shot spinal anesthesia, usually with 5% hyperbaric lidocaine, but also with tetracaine and dibucaine.[191,192] Cases have also followed unintentional intrathecal administration of 2% lidocaine intended for the epidural space.[193,194]

Various risk factors for neurotoxic damage have been identified (Box 32-5). There is ample evidence to suggest that the danger is diminished if bupivacaine rather than another local anesthetic agent is used,[195] although cauda equina syndrome has also been reported in an elderly man after apparently uneventful intrathecal administration of bupivacaine.[196] In all cases, other causes of neurologic deficit (trauma, ischemia, infection, compression, contamination, and adverse positioning) were absent.

Drasner[197] has concluded that spinal lidocaine appears to have a vanishing therapeutic index, and its continued use in the spinal space would appear to have little logic.[198] (*Editors' Note:* Unfortunately, a short-acting local anesthetic alternative is not readily available. Some anesthesia providers in the United States continue to give modest doses of spinal lidocaine for short procedures.) Hyperbaric lidocaine is not available in either Australia or the United Kingdom.

Conus damage and *cauda equina syndrome* may appear similar. Although conus damage may involve upper motor neuron signs, these are not always present, and both conditions may have unilateral or bilateral features.[77] However, the causation is different. Whereas conus damage may result from ischemia or trauma, cauda equina syndrome typically results from compression within the lumbar spinal canal or from chemical damage.

TRANSIENT NEUROLOGIC SYNDROME

Transient neurologic syndrome (also called transient radicular irritation) is not associated with any detectable neurologic deficit, but the distribution of the pain in the back, buttocks, and thighs mirrors the distribution of nerve

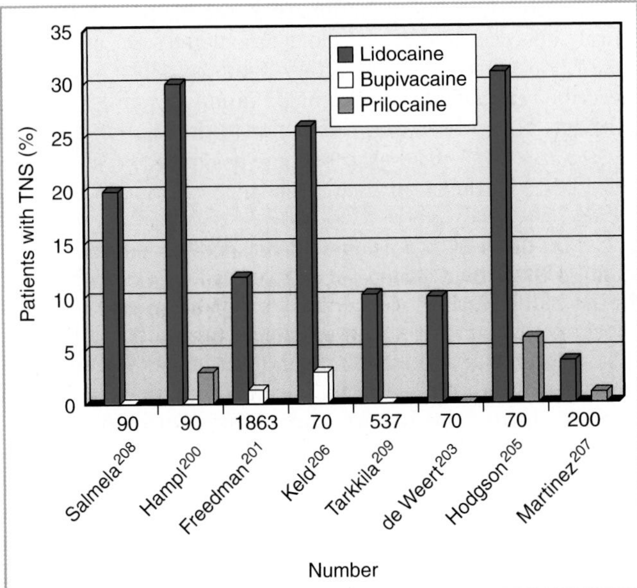

FIGURE 32-12 Proportions of patients reporting transient neurologic symptoms (TNS) after spinal anesthesia. The trials selected are those in which lidocaine was compared with bupivacaine and/or prilocaine, except that by Hodgson et al.,[205] which compared procaine. *Note zero values on the floor of the chart.* The total numbers of patients in the trials are shown on a line below the *x*-axis.

damage in cauda equina syndrome sufficiently to support the theory that the nerves are indeed irritated by a noxious intrathecal injection. Moreover, the risk factors for cauda equina syndrome and transient neurologic syndrome appear to be similar (see Box 32-5). Transient neurologic syndrome has occurred after intrathecal administration of 2% as well as 5% lidocaine.[199,200] Early mobility has been proposed as both a risk factor[201] and a protective factor.[202] The incidence of transient neurologic syndrome varies greatly among studies,[201,203-209] but the preponderance of evidence suggests that, as with cauda equina syndrome, bupivacaine is relatively blameless (Figure 32-12). Parturients are not exempt from transient neurologic symptoms, although they may be at lower risk than other surgical patients.[210-214]

ARACHNOIDITIS

Arachnoiditis is a disastrous condition, often with a delayed onset of permanent paraplegia. It has not been described in any surveys of neurologic sequelae of obstetric neuraxial blockade. Among parturients, chronic adhesive arachnoiditis of chemical origin has arisen after unintentional intrathecal injection of a large dose of 2-chloroprocaine with antioxidant and preservative intended for the epidural space,[215] whereas seven cases occurring after epidural analgesia for childbirth with 2% lidocaine, probably with preservative, were described in a single report from Miami.[216] Six cases were reported among Italian surgical patients following apparently standard epidural anesthesia with bupivacaine and/or mepivacaine, usually with epinephrine.[217] The local anesthetic agents, however, were obtained from multidose vials containing parabens as preservative, and the glass syringes used for loss-of-resistance identification of the epidural space had been washed in detergent. With earlier publications it is not always possible to distinguish the cause of paraplegia, but arachnoiditis seems to appear in clusters, suggesting that there may have been shortcomings in anesthetic technique.

Vulnerable Patients

Various conditions may render some women more vulnerable than normal to neurologic injury precipitated by neuraxial anesthesia. The following discussion of conditions is not exhaustive.

VERTEBRAL ABNORMALITY

Skeletal abnormalities involving the spine, including congenital anomaly, trauma, and back surgery, can make epidural or spinal needle insertion difficult. Patients with spina bifida are at risk for accidental dural puncture and nerve root damage unless the needle is inserted above the defect. Those with tethered cord syndrome are at risk for cord damage if spinal or epidural needle insertion is attempted at a vertebral level that would normally be expected to be below the conus.[72] In my judgment, tethered cord should be regarded as an absolute contraindication to neuraxial blockade. (*Editors' Note:* Other anesthesiologists believe that neuraxial procedures may be performed in selected patients with tethered cord syndrome [see Chapter 48].)

Pressure from spinal stenosis or prolapsed intervertebral disc, coupled with a large-volume epidural injection, may result in spinal cord compression and neurologic deficit.[85-87]

VASCULAR ABNORMALITIES

Vascular disease and malformation are risk factors for spinal cord ischemia, hematoma, and compression. The major supply to the lumbar enlargement of the spinal cord is the artery of Adamkiewicz, a unilateral structure that typically arises from the lower thoracic or upper lumbar portion of the aorta between T9 and L2. Compression of this single vessel may therefore jeopardize the blood supply to the lower cord in susceptible individuals (as discussed earlier). In 15% of individuals, a secondary blood supply to the spinal cord that ascends from the internal iliac arteries[218] assumes a major role. These ascending arteries lie close to the lumbosacral trunk and are, in theory, vulnerable to pressure from the fetal head or damage by obstetric instrumentation, thus causing conus ischemia.

An **arteriovenous malformation** is an obvious cause for concern for the obstetric anesthesia provider.[219] Small arterial feeders from a segmental intercostal artery supply dilated serpiginous epidural veins that may extend over many segments of the spinal canal.[220] The resulting hemangioma raises the pressure on epidural veins and reduces spinal cord blood flow. Oxygen delivery to local tissues is reduced, and the risk of spinal hematoma or ischemic damage and compression is increased. Pregnancy and epidural analgesia have been known to precipitate paraplegia in previously asymptomatic patients[220,221]; aortocaval compression, a large blood volume, and a large epidural injection (which may cause severe pain) all increase epidural pressure.

The preanesthesia examination should include inspection of the back for cutaneous angiomata or macular areas of skin discoloration, which may suggest the presence of an underlying spinal angioma at the same segmental level. Because spinal cord capillary flow is compromised in the drainage area of an arteriovenous malformation, systemic arterial pressure should be kept close to normal throughout the peripartum period, regardless of the anesthetic technique.

SPINAL TUMOR

Epidural blockade has been reported to precipitate neurologic symptoms in the presence of previously undiagnosed spinal tumors. Hitherto undiagnosed ependymoma has been associated with a spinal subdural hematoma manifesting 4 days after delivery with epidural analgesia[92] and with extreme pain precipitated by epidural analgesia.[222] Similar problems have been reported in surgical patients found to have spinal metastases.[223]

COAGULOPATHY OR ANTICOAGULATION

The risk of neuraxial procedures in patients with a preexisting coagulopathy or anticoagulation therapy are discussed earlier in this chapter and also in Chapters 38 and 43.

IMMUNOCOMPROMISE

The majority of cases of epidural infection that have been reported in surveys involve elderly patients with immunocompromise.[19,104] This topic is covered in an excellent review.[224] It is advisable to avoid prolonged epidural catheterization in immunocompromised patients.

PREEXISTING NEUROLOGIC DISORDER

Relapse rates in patients with multiple sclerosis are increased after delivery, and the fear is that neuraxial blockade will be blamed.[225] It has been postulated that spinal anesthesia may worsen demyelinating conditions, although surveys are inconclusive.[226] If affected nerve roots are indeed at higher risk from neurotoxicity, epidural anesthesia may be safer than spinal anesthesia. Indeed, some anesthesia providers prefer epidural or even general anesthesia over spinal anesthesia in women with multiple sclerosis. It is clearly important to document neurologic status and to discuss relapse rates with the mother before and after any anesthetic intervention.

Patients with hereditary neuropathy with liability to pressure palsy are particularly sensitive to compression neuropathy during the course of labor and delivery (as discussed earlier).[33,34]

It is postulated that patients with preexisting peripheral neuropathies may be more susceptible to nerve injury when exposed to a second insult, the so-called *double crush phenomenon*.[226] To explore whether neuraxial anesthesia represented such an insult, Hebl et al.[226] reviewed the charts of 567 patients with peripheral neuropathies who had spinal or epidural blockade, including 12 obstetric patients. There were two instances of worsening neurologic status, both in elderly diabetic patients. There were no control patients, but clearly, if there is a risk that neuraxial anesthesia will exacerbate a neuropathy, it is very small.

DIABETES

Diabetic patients are vulnerable to neurologic injury for three reasons. They are susceptible to infection, they may have vascular disease, and they may have a peripheral neuropathy. Diabetic patients are at increased risk for epidural abscess, either catheter-associated or spontaneous.[19,104] Anterior spinal artery syndrome has also been described in diabetic parturients,[181] and worsening neuropathy has been observed in diabetic surgical patients.[226]

FOLLOW-UP AND RISK MANAGEMENT

High-risk women should be referred to the obstetric anesthesia clinic during pregnancy, so that an anesthesia provider can obtain a thorough history, examine the patient, organize consultations or imaging studies as needed, and plan the anesthetic strategy. The recommended points to explore during the history and physical examination are summarized in Boxes 32-6 and 32-7.

In addition to minimizing risk by adopting good and safe practices, vigilance must be extended to the postpartum period to detect, diagnose, and treat any disorders that may arise. Early hospital discharge presents a problem in the detection of post–dural puncture headache and space-occupying lesions, both of which require assessment and treatment, the latter on an urgent basis. It is important that those caring for postpartum women are taught to look for signs of neurologic pathology and that such women, once home, know how to recognize postanesthesia symptoms and to contact an anesthesia provider if they experience them.

Diagnosis of Possible Neurologic Injury

Through simple clinical examination coupled with knowledge of basic neuroanatomy outlined in this chapter, it is usually possible to distinguish peripheral from central lesions. Preanesthesia history and physical examination may reveal some helpful clues, and any preexisting signs or deficits documented in the record will narrow the search or even provide an immediate answer. The history and physical examination should seek to establish whether the complaint is genuine and to determine its site and cause.

The basic physical examination outlined in Box 32-7 should be repeated, and the results should be compared

BOX 32-6 Issues to Explore in the Preanesthesia History

- Allergies or recreational drugs?
- Diabetes or cardiovascular disorder?
- Previous spinal or epidural anesthetics? What was the outcome?
- Preexisting neurologic signs or symptoms (e.g., sciatica, leg weakness)?
- Skeletal abnormality or back surgery?
- History of trauma or automobile accident, and if so, is it under litigation?
- Anticoagulant medication?
- Recent history of bleeding gums after dental hygiene (common in late pregnancy and not relevant as an isolated sign) or bruising?
- Recent infection, including vaginal infection or skin infection involving the back?
- Possibility of immunocompromise?

BOX 32-7 Preanesthesia Neurologic Examination

- If there is a question of neurologic disorder, examine the lower limbs:
  - Sensation to pinprick or ice, and vibration sense using a tuning fork
  - Knee and ankle tendon reflexes and Babinski reflex
  - Motor power of hips, knees, and ankles
- Examine the back for:
  - Signs of infection (e.g., pustules or rash)
  - Nevi, suggesting arteriovenous malformation
  - Midline hair tuft or fat pad, suggesting dysraphism (e.g., spina bifida occulta)
  - Scoliosis
  - In the presence of severe scoliosis or extensive back surgery, is there an easily palpable sacral hiatus as an alternative to the lumbar epidural space?
- Look for signs of bleeding diathesis
- Document:
  - The history and physical findings
  - Abnormalities and treatment decisions
  - Differences of opinion
  - The reasons an anesthetic is administered despite the presence of a relative contraindication

with the preanesthesia findings. Fever and leukocytosis indicate an infective cause. Severe back pain and localized tenderness suggest epidural abscess, and pain radiating to the legs or buttocks is a late and urgent sign of spinal cord or cauda equina compression. Headache, fever, and neck stiffness suggest meningitis. Viral or other community-acquired types of meningitis may coincide with pregnancy, but the responsible organisms differ from those causing nosocomial infection.

MRI has revolutionized the speed and precision with which intraspinal lesions can be identified, and gadolinium enhancement further improves its sensitivity. MRI cannot distinguish clearly between blood and other fluid, although the distinction can usually be made on other grounds. In the presence of meningitis, MRI with gadolinium enhancement shows swelling of the cord and punctate areas of increased density, reflecting inflammatory cell infiltrates. Arteriovenous malformations of the cord or dura also may be visible, and the enlarged veins draining them may be seen as serpiginous signal voids.

KEY POINTS

- Maternal obstetric palsy may arise from (1) the process of childbirth, (2) preexisting maternal disease that predisposes to peripartum palsy, (3) coincidental pathology, or (4) neurologic injury directly attributable to the anesthetic.
- Intrapartum nerve compression may go unnoticed during neuraxial analgesia/anesthesia; therefore neurologic status should be regularly assessed, and the patient should be encouraged to change positions.
- Postpartum neurologic deficit is less likely to have anesthetic than other causes. Transient postpartum peripheral palsy is common. Nevertheless, there is a widespread tendency to attribute neurologic deficits to neuraxial anesthesia.
- Careful examination and knowledge of anatomy can usually suggest whether the lesion is central or peripheral.
- Meticulous technique, vigilance, and frequent observation of the patient are keystones to avoiding complications.
- Proper sterile technique involves wearing a mask, handwashing, and donning sterile gloves before initiating neuraxial blockade.
- Good epidural needle insertion technique should minimize the risk of accidental dural puncture. Post–dural puncture headache, should it occur, must never be neglected.
- Risk of trauma to the spinal cord may be minimized by choosing a lower lumbar interspace (below L3) for insertion of the spinal needle.
- The risk of neuraxial infection may be decreased by avoiding dural puncture during labor in a patient with systemic or vaginal infection.
- Mistakes in drug administration must be avoided by obsessive and careful reading of drug labels.
- The results of the history and physical examination, the rationale behind the chosen anesthetic procedure, and the details of all procedures should be thoroughly documented.
- Rapid diagnosis and treatment are essential to minimizing permanent neurologic sequelae. Compressive intraspinal lesions require urgent laminectomy within 6 to 12 hours of the onset of symptoms.
- Early hospital discharge creates the need for a safety net to detect neurologic complications arising after the return home. Patients should be informed about the presenting symptoms of rare but potentially catastrophic complications of neuraxial anesthesia.

REFERENCES

1. Tubridy N, Redmond JM. Neurological symptoms attributed to epidural analgesia in labour: An observational study of seven cases. Br J Obstet Gynaecol 1996; 103:832-3.
2. Tillman A. Traumatic neuritis in the puerperium. Am J Obstet Gynecol 1935; 29:660-6.
3. Chalmers JA. Traumatic neuritis of the puerperium. J Obstet Gynaecol Br Emp 1949; 56:205-16.
4. Hill EC. Maternal obstetric paralysis. Am J Obstet Gynecol 1962; 83:1452-60.
5. Murray RR. Maternal obstetrical paralysis. Am J Obstet Gynecol 1964; 88:399-403.
6. Loo CC, Dahlgren G, Irestedt L. Neurological complications in obstetric regional anaesthesia. Int J Obstet Anesth 2000; 9:99-124.
7. Ong BY, Cohen MM, Esmail A, et al. Paresthesias and motor dysfunction after labor and delivery. Anesth Analg 1987; 66:18-22.
8. MacArthur C, Lewis M, Knox EG. Investigation of long term problems after obstetric epidural anaesthesia. Br Med J 1992; 304:1279-82.
9. Scott DB, Hibbard BM. Serious non-fatal complications associated with extradural block in obstetric practice. Br J Anaesth 1990; 64:537-41.

10. Scott DB, Tunstall ME. Serious complications associated with epidural/spinal blockade in obstetrics: A two-year prospective study. Int J Obstet Anesth 1995; 4:133-9.
11. Palot M, Visseaux H, Botmans C, Pire JC. Epidemiology of complications of obstetrical epidural analgesia. Cah Anesthesiol 1994; 42:229-33.
12. Holdcroft A, Gibberd FB, Hargrove RL, et al. Neurological complications associated with pregnancy. Br J Anaesth 1995; 75:522-6.
13. Holloway J, Seed PT, O'Sullivan G, Reynolds F. Paraesthesiae and nerve damage following combined spinal-epidural and spinal anaesthesia: A pilot survey. Int J Obstet Anesth 2000; 9:151-5.
14. Albright GA, Forster RM. The safety and efficacy of combined spinal and epidural analgesia/anesthesia (6,002 blocks) in a community hospital. Reg Anesth Pain Med 1999; 24:117-25.
15. Paech MJ, Godkin R, Webster S. Complications of obstetric epidural analgesia and anaesthesia: A prospective analysis of 10,995 cases. Int J Obstet Anesth 1998; 7:5-11.
16. Dar AQ, Robinson AP, Lyons G. Postpartum neurological symptoms following regional blockade: A prospective study with case controls. Int J Obstet Anesth 2002; 11:85-90.
17. Wong CA, Scavone BM, Dugan S, et al. Incidence of postpartum lumbosacral spine and lower extremity nerve injuries. Obstet Gynecol 2003; 101:279-88.
18. Auroy Y, Benhamou D, Bargues L, et al. Major complications of regional anesthesia in France: The SOS Regional Anesthesia Hotline Service. Anesthesiology 2002; 97:1274-80.
19. Moen V, Dahlgren N, Irestedt L. Severe neurological complications after central neuraxial blockades in Sweden, 1990-1999. Anesthesiology 2004; 101:950-9.
20. Ruppen W, Derry S, McQuay H, Moore RA. Incidence of epidural hematoma, infection, and neurologic injury in obstetric patients with epidural analgesia/anesthesia. Anesthesiology 2006; 105:394-9.
21. Gedefaw M, Darge K. Postpartum foot drop: A report of four cases. Trop Doct 2003; 33:52-3.
22. Haas DM, Meadows RS, Cottrell R, Stone WJ. Postpartum obturator neurapraxia: A case report. J Reprod Med 2003; 48:469-70.
23. Gherman RB, Ouzounian JG, Incerpi MH, Goodwin TM. Symphyseal separation and transient femoral neuropathy associated with the McRoberts' maneuver. Am J Obstet Gynecol 1998; 178:609-10.
24. Peters G, Larner AJ. Meralgia paresthetica following gynecologic and obstetric surgery. Int J Gynaecol Obstet 2006; 95:42-3.
25. Van Diver T, Camann W. Meralgia paresthetica in the parturient. Int J Obstet Anesth 1995; 4:109-12.
26. Farrar D, Raoof N. Bell's palsy, childbirth and epidural analgesia. Int J Obstet Anesth 2001; 10:68-70.
27. O'Connell JE. Maternal obstetrical paralysis. Surg Gynecol Obstet 1944; 79:374-82.
28. Silva M, Mallinson C, Reynolds F. Sciatic nerve palsy following childbirth. Anaesthesia 1996; 51:1144-8.
29. Umo-Etuk J, Yentis SM. Sciatic nerve injury and caesarean section. Anaesthesia 1997; 52:605-6.
30. Roy S, Levine AB, Herbison GJ, Jacobs SR. Intraoperative positioning during cesarean as a cause of sciatic neuropathy. Obstet Gynecol 2002; 99:652-3.
31. Postaci A, Karabeyoglu I, Erdogan G, et al. A case of sciatic neuropathy after caesarean section under spinal anaesthesia. Int J Obstet Anesth 2006; 15:317-9.
32. Babayev M, Bodack MP, Creatura C. Common peroneal neuropathy secondary to squatting during childbirth. Obstet Gynecol 1998; 91:830-2.
33. Lepski GR, Alderson JD. Epidural analgesia in labour for a patient with hereditary neuropathy with liability to pressure palsy. Int J Obstet Anesth 2001; 10:198-201.
34. Peters G, Hinds NP. Inherited neuropathy can cause postpartum foot drop. Anesth Analg 2005; 100:547-8.
35. Chien P, Khan K, Agustsson P. The determinants of residual bladder volume following spontaneous vaginal delivery. J Obstet Gynecol 1996; 16:146-50.
36. Weissman A, Grisaru D, Shenhav M, et al. Postpartum surveillance of urinary retention by ultrasonography: The effect of epidural analgesia. Ultrasound Obstet Gynecol 1995; 6:130-4.
37. Liang C-C, Wong S-Y, Tsay P-T. The effect of epidural analgesia on postpartum urinary retention in women who deliver vaginally. Int J Gynaecol Obstet 2002; 11:164-9.
38. MacArthur C, Lewis M, Knox EG. Health after childbirth. Br J Obstet Gynaecol 1991; 98:1193-5.
39. Borum SE, Naul LG, McLeskey CH. Postpartum dural venous sinus thrombosis after postdural puncture headache and epidural blood patch. Anesthesiology 1997; 86:487-90.
40. Ravindran RS, Zandstra GC, Viegas OJ. Postpartum headache following regional analgesia: A symptom of cerebral venous thrombosis. Can J Anaesth 1989; 36:705-7.
41. Katzin LW, Levine M, Singhal AB. Dural puncture headache, postpartum angiopathy, pre-eclampsia and cortical vein thrombosis after an uncomplicated pregnancy. Cephalalgia 2007; 27:461-4.
42. Ariola SE, Russo TO, Marx GF. Postdural puncture headache or incipient eclampsia? Int J Obstet Anesth 1991; 1:33-4.
43. Diemunsch P, Balabaud VP, Petiau C, et al. Bilateral subdural hematoma following epidural anesthesia. Can J Anaesth 1998; 45:328-31.
44. Shah JL. Severe headache following an epidural 'top-up'. Int J Obstet Anesth 1991; 1:29-31.
45. Torrillo TM, Bronster DJ, Beilin Y. Delayed diagnosis of posterior reversible encephalopathy syndrome (PRES) in a parturient with pre-eclampsia after inadvertent dural puncture. Int J Obstet Anesth 2007; 16:171-4.
46. Waidelich JM, Bullough AS, Mhyre JM. Internal carotid artery dissection: An unusual cause of postpartum headache. Int J Obstet Anesth 2008; 17:61-5.
47. Marfurt D, Lyrer P, Ruttimann U, et al. Recurrent post-partum seizures after epidural blood patch. Br J Anaesth 2003; 90:247-50.
48. Oliver CD, White SA. Unexplained fitting in three parturients suffering from postdural puncture headache. Br J Anaesth 2002; 89:782-5.
49. Rodrigo P, Garcia JM, Ailagas J. General convulsive crisis related to pneumocephalus after inadvertent dural puncture in an obstetric patient. Rev Esp Anestesiol Reanim 1997; 44:247-9.
50. Sansome AJ, Barnes GR, Barrett RF. An unusual presentation of meningitis as a consequence of inadvertent dural puncture. Int J Obstet Anesth 1991; 1:35-7.
51. Shearer VE, Jhaveri HS, Cunningham FG. Puerperal seizures after post-dural puncture headache. Obstet Gynecol 1995; 85:255-60.
52. Reynolds F. Dural puncture and headache. Br Med J 1993; 306:874-6.
53. Chohan U, Khan M, Saeed Uz Z. Abducent nerve palsy in a parturient with a 25-gauge Sprotte needle. Int J Obstet Anesth 2003; 12:235-6.
54. Dunbar SA, Katz NP. Failure of delayed epidural blood patching to correct persistent cranial nerve palsies. Anesth Analg 1994; 79:806-7.
55. Heyman HJ, Salem MR, Klimov I. Persistent sixth cranial nerve paresis following blood patch for postdural puncture headache. Anesth Analg 1982; 61:948-9.
56. Carrero EJ, Agusti M, Fabregas N, et al. Unilateral trigeminal and facial nerve palsies associated with epidural analgesia in labour. Can J Anaesth 1998; 45:893-7.
57. Lowe DM, McCullough AM. Seventh nerve palsy after extradural blood patch. Br J Anaesth 1990; 65:721-2.
58. Perez M, Olmos M, Garrido FJ. Facial nerve paralysis after epidural blood patch. Reg Anesth 1993; 18:196-8.
59. Martin-Hirsch DP, Martin-Hirsch PL. Vestibulocochlear dysfunction following epidural anaesthesia in labour. Br J Clin Pract 1994; 48:340-1.
60. Viale M, Narchi P, Veyrac P, Benhamou D. Chronic tinnitus and hearing loss caused by cerebrospinal fluid leak treated with success with peridural blood patch: Apropos of 2 cases. Ann Otolaryngol Chir Cervicofac 1996; 113:175-7.
61. Weitz SR, Drasner K. Spontaneous intracranial hypotension: A series. Anesthesiology 1996; 85:923-5.
62. Akpek EA, Karaaslan D, Erol E, et al. Chronic subdural haematoma following caesarean section under spinal anaesthesia. Anaesth Intensive Care 1999; 27:206-8.

63. Cantais E, Benhamou D, Petit D, Palmier B. Acute subdural hematoma following spinal anesthesia with a very small spinal needle. Anesthesiology 2000; 93:1354-6.
64. Davies JM, Murphy A, Smith M, O'Sullivan G. Subdural haematoma after dural puncture headache treated by epidural blood patch. Br J Anaesth 2001; 86:720-3.
65. Kardash K, Morrow F, Beique F. Seizures after epidural blood patch with undiagnosed subdural hematoma. Reg Anesth Pain Med 2002; 27:433-6.
66. Kayacan N, Arici G, Karsli B, Erman M. Acute subdural haematoma after accidental dural puncture during epidural anaesthesia. Int J Obstet Anesth 2004; 13:47-9.
67. Ayorinde BT, Mushambi MC. Extradural haematoma in a patient following manual removal of the placenta under spinal anaesthesia: Was the spinal to blame? Int J Obstet Anesth 2002; 11:216-8.
68. Yoshii W, Rottman R, Rosenblatt R. Epidural catheter induced traumatic radiculopathy in obstetrics: One center's experience. Reg Anesth 1994; 19:132-5.
69. Loo C, Cheong K. Monoplegia following obstetric epidural anaesthesia. Ann Acad Med Singapore 1997; 26:232-4.
70. Ben-David B, Vaida S, Collins G, et al. Transient paraplegia secondary to an epidural catheter. Anesth Analg 1994; 79:598-600.
71. Richardson J, Bedder M. Transient anterior spinal cord syndrome with continuous postoperative epidural analgesia. Anesthesiology 1990; 72:764-6.
72. Reynolds F. Litigation in obstetric regional anaesthesia. In Zurdert AV, editor. Highlights in Pain Therapy and Regional Anaesthesia. Barcelona, Publicidad Permanyer, 1996:39-43.
73. Warder DE, Oakes WJ. Tethered cord syndrome: The low-lying and normally positioned conus. Neurosurgery 1994; 34:597-600.
74. Bromage PR, Benumof JL. Paraplegia following intracord injection during attempted epidural anesthesia under general anesthesia. Reg Anesth Pain Med 1998; 23:104-7.
75. Katz N, Hurley R. Epidural anesthesia complicated by fluid collection within the spinal cord. Anesth Analg 1993; 77:1064-5.
76. Rajakulendran Y, Rahman S, Venkat N. Long-term neurological complication following traumatic damage to the spinal cord with a 25-gauge Whitacre spinal needle. Int J Obstet Anesth 1999; 8:62-6.
77. Reynolds F. Damage to the conus medullaris following spinal anaesthesia. Anaesthesia 2001; 56:238-47.
78. Greaves JD. Serious spinal cord injury due to haematomyelia caused by spinal anaesthesia in a patient treated with low-dose heparin. Anaesthesia 1997; 52:150-4.
79. Reynolds F. Logic in the safe practice of spinal anaesthesia. Anaesthesia 2000; 55:1045-6.
80. Broadbent CR, Maxwell WB, Ferrie R, et al. Ability of anaesthetists to identify a marked lumbar interspace. Anaesthesia 2000; 55:1122-6.
81. Van Gessel EF, Forster A, Gamulin Z. Continuous spinal anesthesia: Where do spinal catheters go? Anesth Analg 1993; 76:1004-7.
82. Saifuddin A, Burnett SJ, White J. The variation of position of the conus medullaris in an adult population: A magnetic resonance imaging study. Spine 1998; 23:1452-6.
83. Thomson A. Fifth Annual Report of the Committee of Collective Investigation of the Anatomical Society of Great Britain and Ireland for the Year 1893-94. J Anat Physiol 1894; 29:35-60.
84. Render CA. The reproducibility of the iliac crest as a marker of lumbar spine level. Anaesthesia 1996; 51:1070-1.
85. Ballin NC. Paraplegia following epidural analgesia. Anaesthesia 1981; 36:952-3.
86. Chaudhari LS, Kop BR, Dhruva AJ. Paraplegia and epidural analgesia. Anaesthesia 1978; 33:722-5.
87. Forster MR, Nimmo GR, Brown AG. Prolapsed intervertebral disc after epidural analgesia in labour. Anaesthesia 1996; 51:773-5.
88. Bose S, Ali Z, Rath GP, Prabhakar H. Spontaneous spinal epidural haematoma: A rare cause of quadriplegia in the post-partum period. Br J Anaesth 2007; 99:855-7.
89. Haljamae H. Thromboprophylaxis, coagulation disorders, and regional anaesthesia. Acta Anaesthesiol Scand 1996; 40:1024-40.
90. Vandermeulen EP, Van Aken H, Vermylen J. Anticoagulants and spinal-epidural anesthesia. Anesth Analg 1994; 79:1165-77.
91. Esler MD, Durbridge J, Kirby S. Epidural haematoma after dural puncture in a parturient with neurofibromatosis. Br J Anaesth 2001; 87:932-4.
92. Roscoe MW, Barrington TW. Acute spinal subdural hematoma: A case report and review of literature. Spine 1984; 9:672-5.
93. Wulf H. Epidural anaesthesia and spinal haematoma. Can J Anaesth 1996; 43:1260-71.
94. Horlocker TT, Wedel DJ, Schroeder DR, et al. Preoperative antiplatelet therapy does not increase the risk of spinal hematoma associated with regional anesthesia. Anesth Analg 1995; 80:303-9.
95. Beilin Y, Zahn J, Comerford M. Safe epidural analgesia in thirty parturients with platelet counts between 69,000 and 98,000 mm(−3). Anesth Analg 1997; 85:385-8.
96. Hew-Wing P, Rolbin SH, Hew E, Amato D. Epidural anaesthesia and thrombocytopenia. Anaesthesia 1989; 44:775-7.
97. Rasmus KT, Rottman RL, Kotelko DM, et al. Unrecognized thrombocytopenia and regional anesthesia in parturients: A retrospective review. Obstet Gynecol 1989; 73:943-6.
98. Beards SC, Jackson A, Griffiths AG, Horsman EL. Magnetic resonance imaging of extradural blood patches: Appearances from 30 min to 18 h. Br J Anaesth 1993; 71:182-8.
99. Yarnell RW, D'Alton ME. Epidural hematoma complicating cholestasis of pregnancy. Curr Opin Obstet Gynecol 1996; 8:239-42.
100. Yuen TS, Kua JS, Tan IK. Spinal haematoma following epidural anaesthesia in a patient with eclampsia. Anaesthesia 1999; 54:350-4.
101. Lao TT, Halpern SH, MacDonald D, Huh C. Spinal subdural haematoma in a parturient after attempted epidural anaesthesia. Can J Anaesth 1993; 40:340-5.
102. Lee LA, Posner KL, Domino KB, et al. Injuries associated with regional anesthesia in the 1980s and 1990s: A closed claims analysis. Anesthesiology 2004; 101:143-52.
103. Reynolds F. Neurological infections after neuraxial anesthesia. Anesthesiol Clin 2008; 26:23-52.
104. Wang LP, Hauerberg J, Schmidt JF. Incidence of spinal epidural abscess after epidural analgesia: A national 1-year survey. Anesthesiology 1999; 91:1928-36.
105. Borum SE, McLeskey CH, Williamson JB, et al. Epidural abscess after obstetric epidural analgesia. Anesthesiology 1995; 82:1523-6.
106. Chiang HL, Chia YY, Chen YS, et al. Epidural abscess in an obstetric patient with patient-controlled epidural analgesia—a case report. Int J Obstet Anesth 2005; 14:242-5.
107. Collier CB, Gatt SP. Epidural abscess in an obstetric patient. Anaesth Intensive Care 1999; 27:662-6.
108. Crawford JS. Pathology in the extradural space. Br J Anaesth 1975; 47:412-5.
109. Dhillon AR, Russell IF. Epidural abscess in association with obstetric epidural analgesia. Int J Obstet Anesth 1997; 6:118-21.
110. Dysart RH, Balakrishnan V. Conservative management of extradural abscess complicating spinal-extradural anaesthesia for caesarean section. Br J Anaesth 1997; 78:591-3.
111. Evans PR, Misra U. Poor outcome following epidural abscess complicating epidural analgesia for labour. Eur J Obstet Gynecol Reprod Biol 2003; 109:102-5.
112. Jenkin G, Woolley IJ, Brown GV, Richards MJ. Postpartum epidural abscess due to group B *Streptococcus*. Clin Infect Dis 1997; 25:1249.
113. Kindler C, Seeberger M, Siegemund M, Schneider M. Extradural abscess complicating lumbar extradural anaesthesia and analgesia in an obstetric patient. Acta Anaesthesiol Scand 1996; 40:858-61.
114. Ngan Kee WD, Jones MR, Thomas P, Worth RJ. Extradural abscess complicating extradural anaesthesia for caesarean section. Br J Anaesth 1992; 69:647-52.
115. Rathmell JP, Garahan MB, Alsofrom GF. Epidural abscess following epidural analgesia. Reg Anesth Pain Med 2000; 25:79-82.
116. Rohrbach M, Plotz J. Epidural abscess following delivery with peridural analgesia: The question of prevention. Anaesthesist 2001; 50:411-5.

117. Schroeder TH, Krueger WA, Neeser E, et al. Spinal epidural abscess—a rare complication after epidural analgesia for labour and delivery. Br J Anaesth 2004; 92:896-8.
118. Trautmann M, Lepper PM, Schmitz FJ. Three cases of bacterial meningitis after spinal and epidural anesthesia. Eur J Clin Microbiol Infect Dis 2002; 21:43-5.
119. Unseld H, Eisinger I. Epidural abscess following repeated epidural catheter placement for delivery. Anaesthesist 2000; 49:960-3.
120. Veiga Sanchez AR. Vertebral osteomyelitis and epidural abscess after epidural anesthesia for a cesarean section. Rev Esp Anestesiol Reanim 2004; 51:44-6.
121. Royakkers AA, Willigers H, van der Ven AJ, et al. Catheter-related epidural abscesses—don't wait for neurological deficits. Acta Anaesthesiol Scand 2002; 46:611-5.
122. Sato S, Sakuragi T, Dan K. Human skin flora as a potential source of epidural abscess. Anesthesiology 1996; 85:1276-82.
123. Hoffmann KK, Weber DJ, Samsa GP, Rutala WA. Transparent polyurethane film as an intravenous catheter dressing: A meta-analysis of the infection risks. JAMA 1992; 267:2072-6.
124. Hebl JR. The importance and implications of aseptic techniques during regional anesthesia. Reg Anesth Pain Med 2006; 31:311-23.
125. Goodman EJ, Jacobs MR, Bajaksouzian S, et al. Clinically significant concentrations of local anesthetics inhibit *Staphylococcus aureus* in vitro. Int J Obstet Anesth 2002; 11:95-9.
126. Hodson M, Gajraj R, Scott NB. A comparison of the antibacterial activity of levobupivacaine vs. bupivacaine: An in vitro study with bacteria implicated in epidural infection. Anaesthesia 1999; 54: 699-702.
127. Pere P, Lindgren L, Vaara M. Poor antibacterial effect of ropivacaine: Comparison with bupivacaine. Anesthesiology 1999; 91:884-6.
128. Zaidi S, Healy TE. A comparison of the antibacterial properties of six local analgesic agents. Anaesthesia 1977; 32:69-70.
129. Tabo E, Ohkuma Y, Kimura S, et al. Successful percutaneous drainage of epidural abscess with epidural needle and catheter. Anesthesiology 1994; 80:1393-5.
130. Hill JS, Hughes EW, Robertson PA. A *Staphylococcus aureus* paraspinal abscess associated with epidural analgesia in labour. Anaesthesia 2001; 56:873-8.
131. Huang YY, Zuo Z, Yuan HB, et al. A paraspinal abscess following spinal anaesthesia for caesarean section and patient-controlled epidural analgesia for postoperative pain. Int J Obstet Anesth 2005; 14:252-5.
132. Kinahan AM, Douglas MJ. Piriformis pyomyositis mimicking epidural abscess in a parturient. Can J Anaesth 1995; 42:240-5.
133. Raj V, Foy J. Paraspinal abscess associated with epidural in labour. Anaesth Intensive Care 1998; 26:424-6.
134. Bajwa ZH, Ho C, Grush A, et al. Discitis associated with pregnancy and spinal anesthesia. Anesth Analg 2002; 94:415-6.
135. Cameron CM, Scott DA, McDonald WM, Davies MJ. A review of neuraxial epidural morbidity: Experience of more than 8,000 cases at a single teaching hospital. Anesthesiology 2007; 106:997-1002.
136. Cohen S, Uzum N, Alptekin B. Aseptic precautions for inserting an epidural catheter. Anaesthesia 2003; 58:930.
137. Collis RE, Harries SE. A subdural abscess and infected blood patch complicating regional analgesia for labour. Int J Obstet Anesth 2005; 14:246-51.
138. Baer ET. Post-dural puncture bacterial meningitis. Anesthesiology 2006; 105:381-93.
139. Berga S, Trierweiler MW. Bacterial meningitis following epidural anesthesia for vaginal delivery: A case report. Obstet Gynecol 1989; 74:437-9.
140. Bouhemad B, Dounas M, Mercier FJ, Benhamou D. Bacterial meningitis following combined spinal-epidural analgesia for labour. Anaesthesia 1998; 53:292-5.
141. Bugedo G, Valenzuela J, Munoz H. Aseptic meningitis following spinal anesthesia: Report of a case. Rev Med Chil 1991; 119:440-2.
142. Cascio M, Heath G. Meningitis following a combined spinal-epidural technique in a labouring term parturient. Can J Anaesth 1996; 43:399-402.
143. Choy JC. Mortality from peripartum meningitis. Anaesth Intensive Care 2000; 28:328-30.
144. Corbett JJ, Rosenstein BJ. *Pseudomonas* meningitis related to spinal anesthesia: Report of three cases with a common source of infection. Neurology 1971; 21:946-50.
145. Davis L, Hargreaves C, Robinson PN. Postpartum meningitis. Anaesthesia 1993; 48:788-9.
146. Donnelly T, Koper M, Mallaiah S. Meningitis following spinal anaesthesia—a coincidental infection? Int J Obstet Anesth 1998; 7:170-2.
147. Duflo F, Allaouchiche B, Mathon L, Chassard D. [Bacterial meningitis following combined obstetric spinal and peridural anesthesia]. Ann Fr Anesth Reanim 1998; 17:1286.
148. Gibbons R. Chemical meningitis following spinal anesthesia. JAMA 1969; 210:900-2.
149. Goldstein MJ, Parker RL, Dewan DM. Status epilepticus amauroticus secondary to meningitis as a cause of postpartum cortical blindness. Reg Anesth 1996; 21:595-8.
150. Harding SA, Collis RE, Morgan BM. Meningitis after combined spinal-extradural anaesthesia in obstetrics. Br J Anaesth 1994; 73:545-7.
151. Lee JJ, Parry H. Bacterial meningitis following spinal anaesthesia for caesarean section. Br J Anaesth 1991; 66:383-86.
152. Lurie S, Feinstein M, Heifetz C, Mamet Y. Iatrogenic bacterial meningitis after spinal anesthesia for pain relief during labor. J Clin Anesth 1999; 11:438-9.
153. Neumark J, Feichtinger W, Gassner A. Epidural block in obstetrics followed by aseptic meningoencephalitis. Anesthesiology 1980; 52:518-9.
154. Newton JA Jr, Lesnik IK, Kennedy CA. *Streptococcus salivarius* meningitis following spinal anesthesia. Clin Infect Dis 1994; 18:840-1.
155. Phillips O. Aseptic meningitis following spinal anesthesia. Anesth Analg 1970; 49:866-71.
156. Pinder AJ, Dresner M. Meningococcal meningitis after combined spinal-epidural analgesia. Int J Obstet Anesth 2003; 12:183-7.
157. Ready LB, Helfer D. Bacterial meningitis in parturients after epidural anesthesia. Anesthesiology 1989; 71:988-90.
158. Roberts SP, Petts HV. Meningitis after obstetric spinal anaesthesia. Anaesthesia 1990; 45:376-7.
159. Rodrigo N, Perera KN, Ranwala R, et al. *Aspergillus* meningitis following spinal anaesthesia for caesarean section in Colombo, Sri Lanka. Int J Obstet Anesth 2007; 16:256-60.
160. Stallard N, Barry P. Another complication of the combined extradural-subarachnoid technique. Br J Anaesth 1995; 75:370-1.
161. Thomas T, Cooper G. Confidential enquiries into maternal deaths in the United Kingdom. In Press R, editor. Why Mothers Die: 1997-1999. London, RCOG Press, 2001:147.
162. Vernis L, Duale C, Storme B, et al. Perispinal analgesia for labour followed by patient-controlled infusion with bupivacaine and sufentanil: Combined spinal-epidural vs. epidural analgesia alone. Eur J Anaesthesiol 2004; 21:186-92.
163. Videira RL, Ruiz-Neto PP, Brandao Neto M. Post spinal meningitis and asepsis. Acta Anaesthesiol Scand 2002; 46:639-46.
164. Knowles PR, Randall NP, Lockhart AS. Vascular trauma associated with routine spinal anaesthesia. Anaesthesia 1999; 54:647-50.
165. White C, Koontz F. Hemolytic streptococcus infections in postpartum patients. Obstet Gynecol 1973; 41:27-32.
166. Gibbs RS, Castillo MS, Rodgers PJ. Management of acute chorioamnionitis. Am J Obstet Gynecol 1980; 136:709-13.
167. Bader AM, Gilbertson L, Kirz L, Datta S. Regional anesthesia in women with chorioamnionitis. Reg Anesth 1992; 17:84-6.
168. Goodman EJ, DeHorta E, Taguiam JM. Safety of spinal and epidural anesthesia in parturients with chorioamnionitis. Reg Anesth 1996; 21:436-41.
169. Gershon RY, Manning-Williams D. Anesthesia and the HIV infected parturient: A retrospective study. Int J Obstet Anesth 1997; 6:76-81.
170. Panikkar KK, Yentis SM. Wearing of masks for obstetric regional anaesthesia: A postal survey. Anaesthesia 1996; 51:398-400.
171. Sellors JE, Cyna AM, Simmons SW. Aseptic precautions for inserting an epidural catheter: A survey of obstetric anaesthetists. Anaesthesia 2002; 57:593-6.

172. Tunevall T. Postoperative wound infections and surgical face masks: A controlled study. World J Surg 1992; 16:147-8.
173. McLure HA, Talboys CA, Yentis SM, Azadian BS. Surgical face masks and downward dispersal of bacteria. Anaesthesia 1998; 53:624-6.
174. Phillips B, Fergusson S, Armstrong P, Wildsmith J. Surgical facemasks are effective in reducing bacterial contamination caused by dispersal from the upper airway. Br J Anaesth 1992; 69:407-8.
175. Siegel JD, Rhinehart E, Jackson M, Chiarello L, and the Healthcare Infection Control Practices Advisory Committee. 2007 Guideline for Isolation Precautions: Preventing Transmission of Infectious Agents in Healthcare Settings, June 2007. Atlanta, US Department of Health and Human Services, Centers for Disease Control and Prevention, Public Health Service, 2007. Available at www.cdc.gov/ncidod/dhqp/gl_isolation.html/
176. Benhamou B, Mercier FJ, Dounas M. Hospital policy for prevention of infection after neuraxial blocks in obstetrics. Int J Obstet Anesth 2002; 11:265-9.
177. Sakuragi T, Yanagisawa K, Dan K. Bactericidal activity of skin disinfectants on methicillin-resistant *Staphylococcus aureus*. Anesth Analg 1995; 81:555-8.
178. Birnbach DJ, Stein DJ, Murray O, et al. Povidone-iodine and skin disinfection before initiation of epidural anesthesia. Anesthesiology 1998; 88:668-72.
179. Birnbach DJ, Meadows W, Stein DJ, et al. Comparison of povidone-iodine and DuraPrep, an iodophor-in-isopropyl alcohol solution, for skin disinfection prior to epidural catheter insertion in parturients. Anesthesiology 2003; 98:164-9.
180. Centers for Disease Control and Prevention. Guidelines for the prevention of intravascular catheter-related infections. MMWR 2002; 51(No.RR-10):1-36.
181. Eastwood DW. Anterior spinal artery syndrome after epidural anesthesia in a pregnant diabetic patient with scleredema. Anesth Analg 1991; 73:90-1.
182. Ackerman WE, Juneja MM, Knapp RK. Maternal paraparesis after epidural anesthesia and cesarean section. South Med J 1990; 83:695-7.
183. Savage R, Beattie C. Inadvertent epidural administration of metaraminol. Anaesthesia 2004; 59:624-5.
184. Lin D, Becker K, Shapiro HM. Neurologic changes following epidural injection of potassium chloride and diazepam: A case report with laboratory correlations. Anesthesiology 1986; 65:210-2.
185. Shanker KB, Palkar NV, Nishkala R. Paraplegia following epidural potassium chloride. Anaesthesia 1985; 40:45-7.
186. Brahams D. Record award for personal injuries sustained as a result of negligent administration of epidural anaesthetic. Lancet 1982; 1(8264):159.
187. Patel PC, Sharif AM, Farnando PU. Accidental infusion of total parenteral nutrition solution through an epidural catheter. Anaesthesia 1984; 39:383-4.
188. McGuinness JP, Cantees KK. Epidural injection of a phenol-containing ranitidine preparation. Anesthesiology 1990; 73:553-5.
189. Meel B. Inadvertent intrathecal administration of potassium chloride during routine spinal anesthesia: Case report. Am J Forensic Med Pathol 1998; 19:255-7.
190. Ferguson F, Watkins K. Paralysis of the bladder and associated neurological sequelae of spinal anaesthesia (cauda equina syndrome). Br J Surg 1937; 25:735-52.
191. Rigler ML, Drasner K, Krejcie TC, et al. Cauda equina syndrome after continuous spinal anesthesia. Anesth Analg 1991; 72:275-81.
192. Yamauchi Y, Nomoto Y. Irreversible damage to the cauda equina following repeated intrathecal injection of hyperbaric dibucaine. J Anesth 2002; 16:176-8.
193. Cheng AC. Intended epidural anesthesia as possible cause of cauda equina syndrome. Anesth Analg 1994; 78:157-9.
194. Drasner K, Rigler ML, Sessler DI, Stoller ML. Cauda equina syndrome following intended epidural anesthesia. Anesthesiology 1992; 77:582-5.
195. Loo CC, Irestedt L. Cauda equina syndrome after spinal anaesthesia with hyperbaric 5% lignocaine: A review of six cases of cauda equina syndrome reported to the Swedish Pharmaceutical Insurance 1993-1997. Acta Anaesthesiol Scand 1999; 43:371-9.
196. Chabbouh T, Lentschener C, Zuber M, et al. Persistent cauda equina syndrome with no identifiable facilitating condition after an uneventful single spinal administration of 0.5% hyperbaric bupivacaine. Anesth Analg 2006; 101:1847-8.
197. Drasner K. Local anesthetic neurotoxicity: Clinical injury and strategies that may minimize risk. Reg Anesth Pain Med 2002; 27:576-80.
198. Pollock JE. Transient neurologic symptoms: Etiology, risk factors, and management. Reg Anesth Pain Med 2002; 27:581-6.
199. Fenerty J, Sonner J, Sakura S, Drasner K. Transient radicular pain following spinal anesthesia: Review of the literature and report of a case involving 2% lidocaine. Int J Obstet Anesth 1996; 5:32-5.
200. Hampl KF, Heinzmann-Wiedmer S, Luginbuehl I, et al. Transient neurologic symptoms after spinal anesthesia: A lower incidence with prilocaine and bupivacaine than with lidocaine. Anesthesiology 1998; 88:629-33.
201. Freedman JM, Li DK, Drasner K, et al. Transient neurologic symptoms after spinal anesthesia: An epidemiologic study of 1,863 patients. Anesthesiology 1998; 89:633-41.
202. Viitanen H, Porthan L, Viitanen M, et al. Postpartum neurologic symptoms following single-shot spinal block for labour analgesia. Acta Anaesthesiol Scand 2005; 49:1015-22.
203. de Weert K, Traksel M, Gielen M, et al. The incidence of transient neurological symptoms after spinal anaesthesia with lidocaine compared to prilocaine. Anaesthesia 2000; 55:1020-4.
204. Hiller A, Rosenberg PH. Transient neurological symptoms after spinal anaesthesia with 4% mepivacaine and 0.5% bupivacaine. Br J Anaesth 1997; 79:301-5.
205. Hodgson P, Liu S, Batra M. Procaine compared with lidocaine for incidence of transient neurologic symptoms. Reg Anesth Pain Med 2000; 25:215-7.
206. Keld DB, Hein L, Dalgaard M, et al. The incidence of transient neurologic symptoms (TNS) after spinal anaesthesia in patients undergoing surgery in the supine position. Hyperbaric lidocaine 5% versus hyperbaric bupivacaine 0.5%. Acta Anaesthesiol Scand 2000; 44:285-90.
207. Martinez-Bourio R, Arzuaga M, Quintana JM, et al. Incidence of transient neurologic symptoms after hyperbaric subarachnoid anesthesia with 5% lidocaine and 5% prilocaine. Anesthesiology 1998; 88:624-8.
208. Salmela L, Aromaa U. Transient radicular irritation after spinal anesthesia induced with hyperbaric solutions of cerebrospinal fluid-diluted lidocaine 50 mg/ml or mepivacaine 40 mg/ml or bupivacaine 5 mg/ml. Acta Anaesthesiol Scand 1998; 42:765-9.
209. Tarkkila P, Huhtala J, Tuominen M. Transient radicular irritation after spinal anaesthesia with hyperbaric 5% lignocaine. Br J Anaesth 1995; 74:328-9.
210. Wong CA, Slavenas P. The incidence of transient radicular irritation after spinal anesthesia in obstetric patients. Reg Anesth Pain Med 1999; 24:55-8.
211. Newman LM, Iyer NR, Tuman KJ. Transient radicular irritation after hyperbaric lidocaine spinal anesthesia in parturients. Int J Obstet Anesth 1997; 6:132-4.
212. Philip J, Sharma SK, Gottumukkala VN, et al. Transient neurologic symptoms after spinal anesthesia with lidocaine in obstetric patients. Anesth Analg 2001; 92:405-9.
213. Rorarius M, Suominen P, Haanpaa M, et al. Neurologic sequelae after caesarean section. Acta Anaesthesiol Scand 2001; 45:34-41.
214. Aouad MT, Siddik SS, Jalbout MI, Baraka AS. Does pregnancy protect against intrathecal lidocaine-induced transient neurologic symptoms? Anesth Analg 2001; 92:401-4.
215. Reisner LS, Hochman BN, Plumer MH. Persistent neurologic deficit and adhesive arachnoiditis following intrathecal 2-chloroprocaine injection. Anesth Analg 1980; 59:452-4.
216. Sklar EM, Quencer RM, Green BA, et al. Complications of epidural anesthesia: MR appearance of abnormalities. Radiology 1991; 181: 549-54.

217. Sghirlanzoni A, Marazzi R, Pareyson D, et al. Epidural anaesthesia and spinal arachnoiditis. Anaesthesia 1989; 44:317-21.
218. Lazorthes G, Poulhes J, Bastide G. La vascularization de la moelle épinière (étude anatomique et physiologique). Rev Neurol 1962; 106:535-7.
219. Ong BY, Littleford J, Segstro R, et al. Spinal anaesthesia for Caesarean section in a patient with a cervical arteriovenous malformation. Can J Anaesth 1996; 43:1052-8.
220. Hirsch NP, Child CS, Wijetilleka SA. Paraplegia caused by spinal angioma—possible association with epidural analgesia. Anesth Analg 1985; 64:937-40.
221. Liu CL, Yang DJ. Paraplegia due to vertebral hemangioma during pregnancy: A case report. Spine 1988; 13:107-8.
222. Martin HB, Gibbons JJ, Bucholz RD. An unusual presentation of spinal cord tumor after epidural anesthesia. Anesth Analg 1992; 75:844-6.
223. Kararmaz A, Turhanoglu A, Arslan H, et al. Paraplegia associated with combined spinal-epidural anaesthesia caused by preoperatively unrecognized spinal vertebral metastasis. Acta Anaesthesiol Scand 2002; 46:1165-7.
224. Horlocker TT, Wedel DJ. Regional anesthesia in the immunocompromised patient. Reg Anesth Pain Med 2006; 31:334-45.
225. Drake E, Drake M, Bird J, Russell R. Obstetric regional blocks for women with multiple sclerosis: A survey of UK experience. Int J Obstet Anesth 2006; 15:115-23.
226. Hebl JR, Kopp SL, Schroeder DR, Horlocker TT. Neurologic complications after neuraxial anesthesia or analgesia in patients with preexisting peripheral sensorimotor neuropathy or diabetic polyneuropathy. Anesth Analg 2006; 103:1294-9.

Chapter 33

Medicolegal Issues in Obstetric Anesthesia

Mark S. Williams, M.D., M.B.A., J.D.
Joanna M. Davies, M.B.B.S., FRCA
Brian K. Ross, M.D., Ph.D.

For most women and their families, the childbirth experience is one of celebration. Expectations are high, and there is great disappointment when the outcome is less than expected. Obstetric anesthesia providers have a unique and challenging role. Some women view anesthesia for labor as nonessential or undesirable, yet many of these women ultimately request and/or need anesthesia services. In contrast, most women have high expectations about both the availability and the quality of anesthesia services for labor and vaginal or cesarean delivery. Pregnant women and their families may have misconceptions regarding anesthesia options, procedures, and risks. They may be influenced by the biases and anxieties of their family and friends. Further, the process of obtaining informed consent may be problematic in patients who are experiencing severe pain during active labor. These and other factors may affect a patient's decision to seek legal remedies for real or perceived injuries or other adverse events.

The financial and emotional costs of litigation are significant and affect both patients and health care providers. Patients and their families must adjust to the reality of the adverse outcome as well as to the overwhelming (and in some cases ongoing) financial costs. All medicolegal claims (both with and without merit) raise the cost of liability premiums, encourage the practice of defensive medicine, and increase the cost of health care services. Further, fear of litigation may have an adverse effect on the availability of health care services. Ultimately, society bears the cost of litigation.

Anesthesia providers should be aware of basic medicolegal issues and should proactively embrace risk management strategies that minimize both patient dissatisfaction and the legal consequences of an unanticipated adverse outcome.

LAWSUITS INVOLVING CLAIMS AGAINST HEALTH CARE PROVIDERS

Importance of Effective Communication

There is a growing awareness of the need for more effective communication among caregivers, patients, and their families. Communication lapses have been identified as problems in the areas of informed consent, patient satisfaction, patient safety, and explanation of unanticipated adverse outcomes. It has been suggested that the most common cause of malpractice suits is failed communication with patients and their families.[1] The expanding cultural diversity of patients has prompted the development of formal programs that foster improved communication between caregivers and patients.[2] Institutions and providers should actively pursue improvements in communication.

Theories of Liability

Every physician has a duty to provide professional services that are consistent with a minimum level of competence. This is an objective standard based on the physician's qualifications, level of expertise, and the circumstances of the particular case.[3] The failure to meet this objective standard of care may give rise to a cause of action for medical negligence. The standard of care for medical practice is dynamic and changes as the profession adopts new treatments and approaches for patient care. Therefore, changes in accepted medical practice may create additional professional obligations and, in turn, additional legal responsibilities for physicians.

Although the specific medical malpractice laws vary from state to state, several different causes of action may be brought against a physician. Patients may sue for injuries resulting from the provision of health care by using one or more of three different theories (or causes of action): (1) medical malpractice, (2) breach of contractual promise that injury would not occur, and (3) lack of informed consent.[4] Plaintiffs (patients) commonly file lawsuits that allege improper care on the basis of more than one of these theories (e.g., alleging both a violation of the standard of care and a lack of informed consent for the medical treatment rendered). Medical malpractice may involve a failure to make the diagnosis, failure to obtain informed consent, surgical errors, drug prescription and administration errors, and other mistakes. For a plaintiff to prevail with regard to a medical malpractice claim, he or she must prove that the injury resulted from the failure of the health care provider to follow the accepted standard of care. The standard of care may be defined as "that degree of care, skill, and learning expected of a reasonably prudent health care provider at that time in the profession or class to which he belongs . . . acting in the same or similar circumstances."[5] This objective standard is applied to the particular facts of the plaintiff's situation in a malpractice action.

A mistake or a bad result does not necessarily denote negligence. Similarly, unless a physician contracts otherwise with the patient (i.e., makes a promise of a specific outcome), the provision of medical care alone does not warrant or guarantee that an illness or disease will be cured. A physician is liable for a misjudgment or mistake only when it is proved to have occurred through a failure to act in accordance with the care and skill of a reasonably prudent practitioner.

Claims of medical malpractice must be filed within a certain period after the alleged incident of medical malpractice. Most jurisdictions in the United States have enacted **statutes of limitations** that are specifically applicable to malpractice claims. Recognizing that a significant time may elapse before symptoms or injury manifest, many states have established **discovery rules** that apply to situations in which the patient has no way of knowing that the injury was caused by wrongdoing or negligence.[5] One example of an unknown injury is sterility that is discovered only when the patient attempts to conceive. Another example is the Rh-negative mother who delivers an Rh-positive child and does not receive anti-RhD antibody therapy (RhoGAM). Such an injury would be apparent only when the mother has another child with Rh-positive blood. Other exceptions to—or extensions of—the statutes of limitations might involve situations of fraudulent concealment, an undiscovered foreign object, situations involving long-term continuous treatment, and issues involving infants or minors.

Establishing Medical Malpractice

In most malpractice cases, the following four elements are required for proving medical negligence:

1. **Duty**. It must be shown that a duty to provide care existed (i.e., a health care provider–patient relationship existed). This may apply to situations in which the provider renders medical advice over the telephone to a patient never seen in the office or through a "curbside" consult with another physician.
2. **Breach**. It must be shown that the health care provider failed to meet his or her duty to provide reasonable care (i.e., the health care provider was negligent).
3. **Injury**. It must be shown that the patient experienced an injury that resulted in damages.
4. **Proximate cause**. It must be shown that the negligence of the health care provider proximately caused the patient's injury (i.e., there must be a sufficiently direct connection between the negligence of the health care provider and the injury experienced by the patient).[5]

If any one of these elements is missing, the plaintiff cannot establish medical malpractice. The plaintiff has the burden of proof to establish each of these elements by a "preponderance of the evidence." This quantum of proof means that a proposition is more probably true than not true (i.e., greater than 50% certainty).

If the malpractice claim involves the issue of whether a physician used a proper method of treatment, the plaintiff must use expert testimony to establish that the defendant physician violated the standard of care and that such violation probably caused the plaintiff's injury.[7] Expert testimony to establish how a reasonably prudent health care practitioner would act under similar circumstances typically must be provided by an expert with the same educational background and training as the defendant physician.

In certain cases, the plaintiff may not be required to present expert testimony to prove negligence, and the burden of proof may shift to the defendant. This represents the doctrine of *res ipsa loquitur* (i.e., the thing speaks for itself). This doctrine has the following three conditions: (1) the injury ordinarily does not occur in the absence of negligence, (2) the injury must be caused by an agency or instrumentality within the exclusive control of the defendant, and (3) the injury must not have been a result of any voluntary action or contribution on the part of the plaintiff.[3] Claims involving injuries sustained during administration of anesthesia (e.g., misplaced surgical instruments) have been made under this doctrine.[7,8] Nerve injury cases have been described as "custom made" for *res ipsa loquitur*.[9]

Establishing Lack of Informed Consent

Lack of informed consent is a common cause of action in medical malpractice claims. Within the context of the physician-patient relationship, the **doctrine of informed consent** is based in English common law, by which doctors could be charged with the tort of *battery* if they had not gained the consent of their patient prior to the performance of surgery or another procedure. In the United States, the New York Court of Appeals established the legal principle of informed consent in 1914.[10] In this case the plaintiff, Mary Schloendorff, was admitted to a New York hospital and consented to examination under ether anesthesia to determine whether a fibroid tumor was malignant, but she withheld consent for its removal. The physician examined the tumor, found it to be malignant, and removed it—in disregard of the patient's wishes. The Court found that this operation constituted medical battery. Writing on behalf of the Court, Justice Benjamin Cardozo wrote, "Every human being of adult years and sound mind has a right to determine what shall be done with his own body; and a surgeon who performs an operation without his patient's consent commits an assault for which he is liable in damages. This is true except in cases of emergency where the patient is unconscious and where it is necessary to operate before consent can be obtained."[10]

This principle remains embedded in modern medical ethics and has been adopted by most state legislatures in the form of informed consent statutes. To establish negligence for failure to obtain informed consent, a plaintiff must prove (1) the existence of a material and reasonably foreseeable risk unknown to the patient, (2) a failure of the physician to inform the plaintiff of that risk, (3) that disclosure of the risk would have led a reasonable patient in the plaintiff's position to reject the medical procedure or choose a different course of treatment, and (4) a causal connection between the failure to inform the plaintiff of the risk and the injury resulting from the occurrence of the nondisclosed risk.[11]

Expert testimony is typically required to establish at least some of the elements of an informed consent claim, especially the materiality of the risk. However, expert testimony is not essential if an issue falls within the general knowledge of lay persons or if the doctor failed to give the patient *any* information about the risks involved, because a lay person can conclude that in the absence of any information, informed consent is not possible.

The obligation to obtain informed consent lies with the physician.[12] Ordinarily, the hospital or other organization has no independent duty to obtain a patient's informed consent. Likewise, a consultant physician who advises the treating physician has no such duty. A referring physician is not required to obtain informed consent unless he or she actually participates in or controls the subsequent treatment by the other physician.[13]

There are differences of opinion as to the perspective to be embraced when a physician is disclosing the nature and likelihood of a given risk. Specifically, should it arise from the patient's or the physician's point of view? Theoretically, both would desire the same scope of disclosure. Often, the pivotal issue is the determination of which party's viewpoint should dictate the standard for judging the physician's conduct.[14] Most jurisdictions use a "reasonable person" or "prudent patient" standard. Under this rule, a physician is expected to disclose to the patient in lay terms all material information that a prudent or reasonable patient would consider significant to making his or her decision.[15] This approach concerns itself with the patient's needs, rather than the physician's judgment; this approach follows the rationale that the physician should neither impose his or her values on the patient nor substitute his or her level of risk aversion for that of the patient.[16] Under this standard, the jury determines whether a reasonable person in the plaintiff's position would have considered the risk significant in making his or her decision. The issue is not what a particular patient would want to know but rather what a reasonable person in the patient's condition would want to know, taking into account factors such as the individual's medical condition, age, and risk factors.[17] This objective standard protects physicians from potentially self-serving testimony of plaintiffs, who inevitably assert that they would have refused a given procedure if they had been properly informed of the risk.

The materiality of risk is an issue under this "reasonable" or "prudent" patient standard. It is generally accepted that a physician is not required to present every possible risk of a proposed treatment. If the probability of its occurrence is practically nonexistent, then the risk, no matter how severe, is not material. Conversely, even a small risk of occurrence may be significant to a patient's decision if the potential consequences could be severe.[18] Disputes concerning the proper scope of disclosure tend to center on whether the risk was foreseeable or remote.

Some jurisdictions adhere to the *professional* standard of disclosure. This approach assumes the perspective of the physician and is concerned with what information a reasonable practitioner would share with a patient under the same or similar circumstances.[19]

Even in circumstances in which the health care providers acknowledge their failure to provide important information to the patient or the patient's legally authorized surrogate decision-maker, the jury is still asked to decide whether the patient or the patient's decision-maker would have consented to such a course of treatment despite the risk. For example, in *Barth v. Rock*, a 5-year-old patient suffered a cardiac arrest (and eventual death) after receiving general anesthesia by mask with sodium thiopental, nitrous oxide, and a succinylcholine infusion for open reduction of an arm fracture. Both the surgeon and the nurse anesthetist admitted that they failed to inform the minor patient's parents about the risks of general anesthesia. The appellate court held that the jury should have been instructed that, as a matter of law, there was no informed consent; the jury then should have decided whether the parents would have consented to the anesthesia had they been adequately informed of the risks.[20]

If a plaintiff establishes the four elements for a cause of action based on lack of informed consent, the burden shifts to the physician to establish a defense that justifies why the material information was not provided (e.g., the insignificant nature of the risk) or why disclosure would not have altered the chosen course of treatment. In addition, the health care providers may claim that the case was a medical emergency. State laws generally supply a defense of "implied consent" for provision of necessary emergency treatment when the patient is unable to provide his or her own consent and no legally authorized surrogate decision-maker is immediately available.[21] If the health care providers' treatment was authorized under a medical emergency, the providers should carefully document their determination of same. The documentation in the patient's medical record should contain a description of the patient's presenting condition, its immediacy, its magnitude, and the nature of the immediate threat of harm to the patient. It is advisable for at least two health care providers to document this information, because the documentation would support their actions if a lack-of-informed-consent lawsuit were filed. The "emergency treatment" rule is limited in two respects. First, the patient must require immediate care to preserve life or health. Second, the physician may provide only the care that is reasonable in light of the patient's condition.

THE LITIGATION PROCESS

It is helpful for health care providers to have a basic understanding of sources of law, how lawsuits are initiated, and typical steps in the litigation process.

Sources of Law

Legal authority has multiple sources, including federal and state constitutions, federal and state statutes, federal and state regulations, and federal and state case law. **Constitutions** are the fundamental laws of a nation or state, which establish the role of government in relation to the governed. Constitutions act as philosophical touchstones for the society, from which other ideas may be drawn. One example is the "right to privacy" established in case law, which flows from the constitutional recognition of individual liberty.[22] **Statutes** are the laws written and enacted by elected officials in legislative bodies. **Regulations** are written by government agencies as permitted by statutory delegation. Although regulations have the force and effect of law, they must be consistent with their enabling legislation. **Case law** refers to written opinions or decisions of judges that arise from individual lawsuits. Case law that may be cited as legal authority (precedent) is limited to cases at the appellate court level (i.e., cases appealed from trial court decisions). The vast majority of lawsuits settle before trial, and only a small percentage of trial court decisions result in appeal; thus case law reflects a very small portion of actual litigation. Like medicine, the practice of law is dynamic and changes as new legislation and regulations are adopted or new case law is created. In addition, any one or several of these sources of law may be relevant to a particular case.

When creating new laws or applying the law in deciding the proper result for a particular case, a legislative body or a court may also consider other information about standards for health care providers' conduct. For example, the court may give strong weight to the Joint Commission standards and find that a provider acting in accordance with Joint Commission requirements was adhering to his or her professional obligations.[23] In writing legislation or court decisions, lawmakers also may defer to standards and practice guidelines adopted by professional organizations, such as the American Society of Anesthesiologists (ASA). The adoption of professional standards and practice guidelines strengthens the influence of professional organizations in the lawmaking process because lawmakers often are willing to defer to professional organizations' statements on standards of care and professional ethics.

Attorneys and courts have employed clinical guidelines for both inculpatory and exculpatory purposes in malpractice litigation (see later). The evidentiary weight placed on adherence or nonadherence to clinical pathways and practice guidelines varies from state to state but may be significant. There is evidence that deviations from evidence-based guidelines may increase a practitioner's liability risk, whereas adherence to such guidelines serves to reduce this risk.[24]

Initiation of a Lawsuit

Medical malpractice lawsuits are typically initiated when a plaintiff files a **Complaint** with the court. Some states have enacted statutes that impose certain conditions (including notification of the defendant physician) before a complaint is filed.[25] The physician receives notice of the legal action when he or she is served with a copy of the **Summons** and the Complaint. In the Complaint, the plaintiff alleges the facts giving rise to the cause(s) of action against the physician. The Complaint requires a written **Answer** to be filed (by the attorney representing the physician) with the court within a specified period. If a timely Answer is not filed, a default judgment may be entered against the physician (i.e., a judgment is allowed because *no response* may be treated as *no defense* against the allegations).

In civil actions against health care providers, plaintiffs are frequently motivated to sue for an award of monetary damages. Medical malpractice lawsuits may involve multiple defendants, such as the treating physician, the hospital, manufacturers of health care equipment, and pharmaceutical companies. Defense counsel evaluates its client's potential liability exposure (i.e., any aspect of care arguably not meeting the standard of care). Both plaintiff counsel and defense counsel weigh the perceived risks if the case proceeds to trial and then determine how much they think the case is worth. The valuation of a case may include more than the estimated dollar value; it may also include considerations such as setting a potential precedent or maintaining a business relationship.

Discovery

Discovery refers to the early phase of litigation after a lawsuit is initiated. During this phase, the litigants on both sides research the strengths and weakness of their cases by obtaining and examining medical records, reviewing medical literature, and interviewing and deposing witnesses, including the plaintiff(s), the treating health care provider(s), and potential expert witnesses.

During discovery, certain methods of gathering information are generally used. The methods include interrogatories and depositions. **Interrogatories** are written questions that are served on one party from an opposing party. Interrogatories must be answered in writing, under oath, within a prescribed period. Failure to respond as required may result in the court's issuing sanctions against the nonresponding party. **Depositions** involve testimony given under oath that is recorded by a court reporter. In a deposition taken for the purpose of discovery, the attorneys representing all opposing litigants participate and ask questions of the witness. The purposes of discovery depositions are (1) to obtain facts and other evidence, (2) to encourage the other side to commit to a position "on the record" (i.e., in preserved testimony), (3) to discover the names of other potential witnesses, (4) to assess how strong a witness the deposed individual may make, (5) to limit facts and issues for the lawsuit, (6) to encourage the other side to make admissions against its own interests in the lawsuit, and (7) to evaluate the case for its dollar (or other) value and potential for settlement.

Trial

A trial typically consists of (1) jury selection, (2) opening statements, (3) plaintiff's trial testimony, (4) defendant's trial testimony, (5) closing arguments, (6) jury instructions given by the judge, and (7) delivery of the jury's verdict. There also may be post-verdict proceedings and motions. The lawyers for all parties file briefs with the court in advance of the trial to outline the case for the trial judge. The lawyers also prepare and argue over the content of jury instructions, seeking the best language to support their theories of the case. The judge decides which jury instructions will be given and reads them to the jurors immediately prior to jury deliberation. Attorneys commonly file motions about significant trial proceedings, such as the scope of admissible evidence. The trial judge rules on these motions outside the presence of the jury.

A jury verdict does not necessarily end the case. If a verdict in favor of the plaintiff(s) is reached, defense counsel may file a motion (1) asking the court to set aside the verdict and grant a new trial, (2) asking the court to change the verdict and enter a judgment in the defendant's favor, or (3) asking for a reduction in the amount of damages awarded to the plaintiff(s). Defense counsel also may seek to reopen settlement negotiations or may choose to appeal the case. The plaintiff(s) may take similar post-verdict steps if the jury renders a verdict in favor of the defendant(s).

The vast majority of medical malpractice cases never go to trial. A 1991 study showed that only 2% of persons injured by physicians' negligence ever file a lawsuit.[26] Subsequently, only 10% of all medical malpractice claims go to trial.[27] Settlement negotiations result in the disposal of many cases. Other cases are withdrawn by plaintiffs or are dismissed by the court on legal grounds such as **summary judgment,** whereby a judge may rule that a plaintiff's case is legally insufficient. Defendants win approximately 71% of medical malpractice claims.[27]

In seeking to minimize the often lengthy and costly litigation process, some states have turned to various types of alternative dispute resolution to resolve claims against health care providers. The state of Washington has passed legislation that requires that all causes of action for damages arising from injury resulting from health care be subject to mandatory mediation prior to trial.[28]

INFORMED CONSENT

Process and Documentation

A patient's right of self-determination lies at the root of informed consent. A patient can make an informed decision only after (1) a discussion of the diagnosis and the indications for the procedure or therapy; (2) disclosure of material risks, benefits, and alternatives; and (3) provision of an opportunity for questions and answers. This process is neither accomplished nor affirmed solely by having the patient's or the patient surrogate's signature on a document asserting informed consent. Evidence of this process and the physician's involvement in the process may be found among office notes, informational aids shared with patients, hospital notes, and signed forms acknowledging informed consent.

The necessity of having a specific process is not only an ethical obligation but also a requirement of various state and federal agencies. For example, the U.S. Centers for Medicare and Medicaid Services (CMS) have *Conditions of Participation* that define the requirements that facilities must satisfy in order to participate in the Medicare and Medicaid programs.[29] Specifically, the *Patients' Rights Conditions of Participation* contain the following interpretive guidelines: "Hospitals must utilize an informed consent process that assures patients or their representatives are given the information and disclosure needed to make an informed decision about whether to consent to a procedure, intervention, or type of care that requires consent."[29] Further, the interpretive guidelines for the CMS *Surgical Services Conditions of Participation* specifically state the following:

> *The primary purpose of the informed consent process is to ensure that the patient, or the patient's representative, is provided information necessary to enable him/her to evaluate a proposed surgery before agreeing to the surgery. Typically, this information would include potential short and longer term risks and benefits to the patient of the proposed intervention, including the likelihood of each, based on the available clinical evidence, as informed by the responsible practitioner's professional judgment. Informed consent must be obtained, and the informed consent form must be placed in the patient's medical record, prior to surgery, except in the case of emergency surgery.*[30]

The interpretive guidelines note that there is no specific requirement for informed consent governing anesthesia services but also state that "given that surgical procedures generally entail the use of anesthesia, hospitals may wish to consider specifically extending their informed consent policies to include obtaining informed consent for the anesthesia component of the surgical procedure."[30]

Because patients have pursued nontraditional sources of medical information (i.e., Internet-based sources) and have become increasingly engaged in the health care decision-making process, additional aids in the informed consent process have been proposed. Studies have demonstrated that standard counseling often results in inadequate decision quality.[31] In addition, patients may have unrealistic expectations of a treatment's risks and benefits, and clinicians are often poor judges of patients' values; consequently there may be overuse of treatments that informed patients would not choose or value.[32] Thus, the aim of a decision-making aid is to improve both the quality of informed consent and to reduce unnecessary practice variations by (1) providing facts about the condition, options, outcomes, and risks; (2) clarifying patients' evaluations of the outcomes that are most meaningful to them; and (3) guiding patients in the steps of deliberation and communication so that a choice can be made that reflects their informed values. These decision-making aids may be utilized by practitioners and/or patients in either individual or group settings and might be delivered in a variety of formats, such as print, video, the Internet, and interactive devices.[32] In essence, this approach attempts to address the weaknesses in both the "reasonable patient" and the "professional standard" approaches to disclosure, and becomes even more valuable as the diversity of practitioners and patients expands. Anesthesia providers might find this approach particularly valuable in preparing patients who are scheduled for elective obstetric or gynecologic procedures.

Formal documentation of informed consent has other advantages. Adequate documentation helps health care providers defend their actions if patients subsequently challenge their consent for health care. In some jurisdictions, a valid consent form signed by the patient may provide a direct means of defense and actually shift the burden of proof to the plaintiff who wishes to make a claim of lack of informed consent.[33] Some large medical liability insurance providers have strongly recommended that the clinician responsible for providing anesthesia care should obtain a separate written consent.[34] Further, some organizations have recommended not only that an anesthesia-specific form should be used but also that practitioners should highlight specific risks that may be present.[35] A separate anesthesia consent form that highlights specific risks demonstrates a meaningful effort to engage patients in a full discussion of relevant issues, and may help establish the basis of a potential defense against a medical malpractice claim.

In discussing anesthetic options for a given procedure, anesthesia providers should consider several aspects, including the best options given the skill set of the provider, the comorbidities of the patient, and the preferences of the surgeon. In a review of anesthesia consent procedures, O'Leary and McGraw[36] recommended that an explanation of the relevant risks and benefits of alternative techniques as well as the likelihood and details of a backup plan should be included in informed consent. The investigators recommended that anesthesia providers adopt a separate, written consent for the administration of anesthesia services. A form that clearly delineates common risks but allows documentation of patient-specific risks should be used. Ideally, the anesthesia provider should obtain the consent and should not rely upon other professionals who are not competent to explain the risks and benefits of anesthesia options.[36]

Capacity to Consent/Mental Competence

Physicians are bound by ethics and required by law to obtain a patient's informed consent before initiating treatment. This premise assumes that a patient is competent and/or has the capacity to successfully participate in this process. **Competence** generally refers to the patients' legal authority to make decisions about their health care. Adult patients, typically 18 years of age or older, are presumed to be legally competent to make such decisions unless otherwise determined by a court of law. **Capacity** typically focuses on the clinical situation surrounding the informed consent process. For example, an otherwise normal patient who has been given sedation may be legally competent but temporarily incapacitated and therefore unable to give informed consent.[37] The determination as to whether a patient has the capacity to provide informed consent generally is a professional judgment made by the treating health care provider. However, if a court has made a judgment regarding a patient's capacity to make such decisions, the health care provider(s) should obtain a copy of the court order, because it may delineate whether the patient is considered able to make his or her own health care decisions. For example, a guardianship is a type of court proceeding that may have an impact on the informed consent process. If a patient has a legal guardian with the authority to make health care decisions on behalf of the patient, that guardian should be consulted about the patient's care and is the person legally authorized to provide consent. A failure to recognize a lack of capacity may expose a physician to liability for treating a patient without valid informed consent.

The legal standards for decision-making capacity vary among jurisdictions but generally encompass the following criteria: The patient must be able to (1) understand the relevant information, (2) appreciate the situation and its consequences, (3) reason about treatment options, and (4) communicate a choice.[38] When the patient is unable to do so, surrogate decision-makers may be sought. In emergency situations, physicians can provide necessary care under the presumption that a reasonable person would have consented to the anticipated treatment.[39] Most states have laws that delineate who is legally authorized to provide consent for health care decisions on behalf of an incapacitated individual. State laws vary, but they typically provide a list of persons (in order of priority) who may give consent. These laws assume that legal relatives are the most appropriate surrogate decision-makers. However, the competent patient is free to select any competent adult to act as his or her health care decision-maker by executing a **Durable Power of Attorney for Health Care,** which appoints that person as his or her agent. For example, Washington state law authorizes the following persons to make decisions for an incapacitated patient, in order of priority: guardian, holder of Durable Power of

Attorney, spouse, adult children, parents, and adult brothers and sisters.[20] Health care providers are required to make reasonable efforts to locate a person in the highest possible category to provide consent. If there are two or more persons in the same category (e.g., adult children), then the medical treatment decision must be unanimous among those persons. These surrogate decision-makers generally are required to make "substituted judgment" decisions on behalf of the patient (i.e., they are obligated to decide as they believe the patient would, not as they may prefer). If what the patient would want under the circumstances is unknown, then the surrogate must make a decision consistent with the patient's "best interests."[40] The surrogate decision-maker has the authority to provide consent for medical treatment, including nontreatment.

Minor Patients

Existing laws regarding the ability of minors to provide their own consent for medical care may be understood as a patchwork quilt. Statutes and case law differ from state to state. There are three ways in which a minor may be deemed able to give his or her own consent for medical care: (1) by state law that permits the minor to consent for the specific type of care, (2) by a clinical determination made by the health care providers that the minor is mature and emancipated for consent purposes, and (3) by a judicial determination of emancipation.

Parental involvement in a minor's health care decisions is usually desirable. For most health care decisions, a parent is required to provide consent for medical treatment of a minor patient.[41] On the other hand, many minors will not take advantage of some available medical services if they are required to involve their parents.[42] The list of services for which minors can legally give consent has recently expanded to include (1) sexual and reproductive health care, (2) mental health services, and (3) alcohol and drug abuse treatment. The majority of states also permit minor parents to make important health care decisions regarding their own children.

In most states, consent laws apply to minors 12 years of age and older. For example, 25 states and the District of Columbia allow minors (12 years of age and older) to consent to contraceptive services. All states and the District of Columbia allow minors to consent to treatment for sexually transmitted infections. Thirty states and the District of Columbia allow minor parents to consent to medical care for their children. For some medical treatment, including contraception and obstetric care, case law has generally held that minors have rights of privacy and autonomy that are fundamental and equivalent to the rights of adults.[43] The issue of abortion presents a more complex issue, with the courts often taking a compromise position between (1) affording minors the right to make their own decisions regarding the continuation of pregnancy and (2) according parents or guardians unchallenged authority to determine that a pregnancy will be continued to term.[44] Currently, two states and the District of Columbia explicitly allow minors to consent to abortion services, while 22 states require at least one parent's consent to a minor's abortion, and 11 states require prior notification of at least one parent. Two states, Oklahoma and Utah, require both notification and consent. Seven states have parental involvement laws that are currently enjoined, and six states have no relevant policy or case law.[42]

In addition to statutes and case law regarding a minor's ability to provide consent, there also exists a broader legal concept—the **emancipated or mature minor doctrine**.[45,46] This doctrine allows health care providers to determine whether a minor is emancipated for providing medical consent. Case law may not give a precise definition of an emancipated minor, but it may list criteria that health care providers should consider. Such criteria may include the minor's age, maturity, intelligence, training, experience, economic independence, and freedom from parental control. When a minor is deemed emancipated for medical consent, the health care provider should document the objective facts that support the emancipation decision, consistent with institutional policies and/or other legal guidance.

Some states have adopted emancipation statutes that permit minors to file for emancipation status in court.[47] Typically a minor is required to be a minimum age to file for emancipation. Once the court grants emancipation status, a minor generally has the right to give informed consent for health care. A signed copy of the court's emancipation order should be placed in the patient's medical record.

Emancipation per se does not alter the requirement that a patient provide informed consent for medical treatment, including nontreatment. Emancipation status affords the minor patient rights (for providing consent) that are equal to those of an adult patient. The emancipated minor (like any adult patient) must have the ability to weigh the risks and the benefits of the proposed treatment or nontreatment.

In summary, health care providers typically should obtain consent from the minor's parents before providing nonemergency treatment unless the minor is emancipated (by either a clinical or judicial determination) or the minor is permitted by statute to give consent to the type of health care sought.

Consent for Labor Analgesia

It is common practice for surgical patients to sign a preoperative consent form, which often includes a statement giving consent for anesthesia. The situation in obstetrics is somewhat different in that not all laboring women require operative delivery. Several years ago, an unpublished survey of obstetric centers in the greater Seattle, Washington, area revealed that approximately half of the institutions did not require a signed consent form for obstetric procedures other than cesarean delivery. At many of these institutions, a separate written consent signed by the patient is not obtained before administration of anesthesia. A 1995 survey of obstetric anesthesiologists in the United States and United Kingdom indicated that 52% of U.S. anesthesiologists (but only 15% of U.K. anesthetists) obtain a separate written consent for epidural analgesia during labor.[48]

Some health care facilities and organizations have begun using a consent form for obstetric and anesthetic procedures that may be desired or necessary during labor and delivery. The process of reviewing and signing the consent form provides a specific opportunity for the patient to ask questions. It also furnishes additional documentation that consent was obtained. The combined form has the additional advantage of not requiring the patient to sign multiple medicolegal documents. Although a signed consent form is not necessary, it should be standard practice for anesthesia providers to document that verbal informed consent was obtained before administration of anesthesia.

Ideally, the anesthesia provider will discuss anesthetic options before the patient is in severe pain and distress. Unfortunately, the anesthesia provider often first encounters the patient when she is in severe pain. Although the provider may tailor the consent process to the circumstances, the presence of maternal pain and distress does not obviate the need for a frank discussion of the risks of anesthesia as well as the alternatives. A survey of Canadian women revealed their strong preference to be informed of all possible complications of epidural anesthesia, especially serious ones, even when the risk was quite low.[49] This study and others have emphasized that parturients desire to have these discussions as early in labor as possible.

Gerancher et al.[50] performed a study to evaluate the ability of laboring women to recall the details of a preanesthesia discussion and to determine whether verbal consent alone or a combination of verbal and written consent provided better recall. The investigators randomly assigned 113 laboring women to one of two groups, those from whom verbal consent alone was obtained and those from whom verbal consent plus written consent was obtained. The verbal-plus-written consent group had significantly higher recall scores (90 ± 2) than the verbal-only group (80 ± 2). Only two women (both in the verbal group) believed that they were unable (because of either inadequate information or situational stress) to give valid consent. The investigators concluded that "the high recall scores achieved by the women in both groups suggest that the majority of laboring women are at least as mentally and physically competent to give consent as preoperative cardiac patients."[50]

Clark et al.[51] randomly assigned hospital inpatients to receive either an oral anesthesia discussion alone or both an oral anesthesia discussion and a preprinted anesthesia consent form. In contrast to the results of Gerancher et al.,[50] these investigators found that "patients remembered less of the information concerning anesthetic risks discussed during the preoperative interview if they received a preprinted, risk-specific anesthesia consent form at the beginning of the interview."[51] They speculated that "patients who see an anesthesia consent form for the first time during the preoperative interview may try to read and listen simultaneously and with their attention divided, may remember less of the preoperative discussion."[51]

Anesthesia providers have expressed concern about the adequacy of the informed consent process when women are experiencing the severe pain of active labor. A 2005 study evaluated whether labor pain and neuraxial fentanyl administration affect the intellectual function of laboring women.[52] The Mini-Mental Status Examination (MMSE) was used to evaluate orientation, registration, attention, calculation, recall, and language both before and after initiation of analgesia in 41 laboring women. There was no difference in MMSE scores before and after administration of neuraxial analgesia.[52]

In summary, it seems reasonable for the patient to provide her signature as evidence of her consent, if her condition permits. This consent can be furnished on a separate anesthesia consent form or as part of a consent form for all obstetric care, including anesthesia. A signed consent form is preferable, but it should be standard practice for the anesthesia provider to explain the intended procedure, risks, and alternatives, and to document this discussion in the medical record.

REFUSAL OF CARE

Documentation

Competent adult patients may refuse medical treatment, including life-saving care.[41] Health care providers generally determine whether a patient is capable of making medical treatment choices (see earlier discussion). In theory, the health care providers' clinical judgment about a patient's capacity to provide informed consent is the same regardless of whether the patient approves or disapproves the treatment plan. In practice, however, these situations are often handled differently. When a patient consents to the recommended medical treatment, minimal scrutiny of his or her decision-making capacity is typically made. However, when a patient refuses potentially life-saving treatment, a higher level of scrutiny is applied to the patient's ability to understand and make a choice for nontreatment. Determination of a patient's capacity to give informed consent is typically a clinical judgment. State law may provide some definitions as to when a person may not be competent.

If a patient refuses potentially life-saving treatment, the health care providers should carefully assess the patient's capacity to provide informed consent. It may be advisable to obtain a psychiatric consultation as part of this clinical determination. It is important to document the determination of capacity and the objective facts supporting the decision. If a patient is deemed able to provide consent, he or she is able to either choose or reject the recommended treatment plan. Institutional policies may require the patient (or health care provider if the patient refuses) to sign an "Against Medical Advice" form for a non–medically approved discharge. If a patient is deemed unable to consent, the health care providers should obtain consent from a legally authorized surrogate decision-maker on the patient's behalf. If an incompetent patient needs emergency medical care, it may be provided consistent with an "emergency exception" (as discussed earlier).

Conflicts Arising out of the Maternal-Fetal Relationship

Almost all pregnant women consider the welfare of their unborn child to be of utmost importance. However, there may be two situations in which maternal and fetal interests appear divergent or, potentially, in conflict. The first situation occurs when a pregnant woman refuses a diagnostic procedure, a medical treatment, or a surgical procedure that is intended to enhance or preserve fetal well-being. The second situation arises when the pregnant woman's behavior may be harmful to the fetus.[53] Physicians who care for pregnant women may confront challenging dilemmas when their patients reject medical recommendations, use illegal drugs, or engage in other behaviors that may adversely affect fetal well-being.

Appellate court decisions typically have held that a pregnant woman's decisions regarding medical treatment take precedence over the presumed fetal consequences of the maternal decisions.[54] One case illustrates the evolution of this judicial approach. Angela Carder was a 26-year-old married woman who had had cancer since age 13. At 25 weeks' gestation she was admitted to George Washington University Hospital, where a massive tumor was found in her lung. Her physicians determined that she would die within a short time. Her husband, her mother, and her physician agreed with her expressed wishes to be kept comfortable during her dying process. Ultimately, the hospital sought judicial review of this course of action. The hospital asked whether a surgical delivery should be authorized to save the potentially viable fetus. The situation was presented to a judge, who authorized an emergency cesarean delivery without first ascertaining (using the principle of substituted judgment) the patient's wishes. A cesarean delivery was performed without full consideration of the patient's wishes, the infant died approximately 2 hours after delivery, and the mother died 2 days later.

This case spawned extensive debate as to whether coercive intervention to protect the fetus is ever morally and legally justifiable.[46,55] With the assistance of the American Civil Liberties Union, Angela's parents sued the hospital, two administrators, and 33 physicians for claims including battery, false imprisonment, discrimination, and medical malpractice. These civil lawsuits were settled after several years of litigation, and as part of this process, the hospital adopted a written policy concerning decision-making for pregnant patients.[56] The court later reversed its initial decision authorizing the surgical delivery and ultimately issued an opinion setting forth the legal principles that should govern the doctor–pregnant patient relationship.[57] The court stated, "In virtually all cases the question of what is to be done is to be decided by the patient—the pregnant woman—on behalf of herself and the fetus. If the patient is incompetent . . . her decision must be ascertained through substituted judgment."[57] In affirming that the patient's wishes, once ascertained, must be followed in "virtually all cases" unless there are "truly extraordinary or compelling reasons to override them," the court did not foreclose the possibility of exceptions to this rule.[57]

Many contemporary medical ethicists agree that a pregnant woman's informed refusal of medical intervention should prevail as long as she has the capacity to make medical decisions.[58] Newer legislation and some high-profile legal cases (some involving criminal prosecution) have challenged this notion and have raised the question of whether there are circumstances in which a pregnant woman's rights to informed consent and bodily integrity may be subordinated to protect her unborn child. In 2004 Amber Rowland, a woman who had given birth vaginally to six children (with birth weights up to 12 pounds), was told by her treating physicians at a Pennsylvania hospital that she should undergo a cesarean delivery on the basis of an ultrasonographic examination that suggested an estimated birth weight of 13 pounds. When she refused, the hospital obtained a court order for a "medically necessary" cesarean delivery. She and her husband left the hospital against medical advice and went to another facility, where she uneventfully delivered a healthy 11-pound daughter.[59]

Other cases have focused on the pregnant woman's potentially harmful behavior. In 1991 Regina McKnight, who was pregnant at the time, began using cocaine after her mother's death. She had a stillbirth, and the state of South Carolina charged her with homicide by child abuse, claiming that her drug use caused the stillbirth. She became the first South Carolina woman to be convicted of this crime, for what both the defense and prosecution agreed was an unintentional stillbirth, and she spent nearly 8 years in jail. In 2008, the South Carolina Supreme Court unanimously reversed her conviction on the grounds that she did not receive a fair trial, primarily on the basis that her attorney failed to challenge the science that was used to convict her.[60]

Also in 2008, the Southern Poverty Law Center, along with 25 medical, public health, and health advocacy groups, filed an *amicus curiae* brief against the prosecution of pregnant women in Covington County, Alabama, subsequent to the following event. Shekelia Ward delivered an infant on January 8, 2008. Both she and her newborn infant tested positive for cocaine during their hospital stay, and the facility reported it to authorities for possible child abuse.[61] The following day she was arrested, imprisoned, and charged with a felony—chemical endangerment of a child. The state statute at issue was passed by the Alabama legislature in 2006, for the purpose of prosecuting parents who exposed children to the toxins associated with methamphetamine production; the statute did not mention pregnant women or their unborn babies.[62]

These statutes reflect the concept that a fetus can and should be treated as separable and legally, philosophically, and essentially independent from the mother.[54] The refinement of techniques of intrauterine fetal imaging, testing, and treatment prompted the view that fetuses are independent patients who can be treated directly while *in utero*.[63] The prominence of some ethical models that have asserted that physicians have moral obligations to fetal patients separate from their obligations to pregnant women also contributed to these developments.[64] Finally, a number of laws (primarily passed at the state level) were enacted with the aim of defining fetal rights separate from a pregnant woman's rights.

In response, in 2005 the American College of Obstetricians and Gynecologists (ACOG) Committee on Ethics issued a statement entitled *Maternal Decision Making, Ethics, and the Law*.[54] The ACOG emphasized a conceptual model that revolves around a central theme of a unique and essential connection between the pregnant woman and her fetus rather than the "two-patient" model embraced by some. The ACOG identified several reasons why coercive and punitive approaches to the behavior of pregnant women are neither prudent or justifiable,[54] and made the following recommendations (abbreviated):

- "In caring for pregnant women, practitioners should recognize that in the majority of cases, the interests of the pregnant woman and her fetus converge rather than diverge."
- "Pregnant women's autonomous decisions should be respected, and concerns about fetal well-being should be discussed in the context of medical evidence and understood within the context of each woman's broad social network, cultural beliefs, and values."

- "Pregnant women should not be punished for adverse perinatal outcomes."
- "Policy makers, legislators and physicians should work together to find constructive and evidence-based ways to address the needs of women with alcohol and other substance abuse problems."[54]

The American Medical Association (AMA) has taken a similar position, stating that (1) drug addiction is a disease amenable to treatment rather than a criminal activity and (2) there is a pressing need for maternal drug treatment and supportive child protective services.[65] Any legislation that criminalizes maternal drug addiction or requires physicians to function as agents of law enforcement will be opposed by the AMA.[65]

During the past two decades, practitioners have only infrequently resorted to court-ordered interventions against the wishes of the pregnant woman. In overturning the previous court's decision in the Angela Carder case (see earlier), the Washington, D.C., Court of Appeals noted that if a pregnant woman makes an informed decision, "her wishes will control in virtually all cases."[57] The court added, "We do not foreclose the possibility that a conflicting state interest may be so compelling that the patient's wishes must yield, but we anticipate that such cases will be extremely rare and truly exceptional."[57]

Medical ethicists and practitioners agree that clear communication and patient education represent the best means to address maternal-fetal conflict. Failing resolution, a 1999 ACOG opinion offered the following three options: (1) respect the patient's autonomy and not proceed with the recommended intervention regardless of the consequences, (2) offer the patient the option of obtaining medical care from another individual before conditions become emergent, and (3) request that the court issue an order to permit the recommended treatment.[66] In 2004 the ACOG addressed the situation in which health care providers may consider this last option (i.e., legal intervention against a pregnant woman).[67] Specifically, the ACOG stated that the following criteria should be satisfied: (1) "there is a high probability of serious harm to the fetus in respecting the patient's decision"; (2) "there is a high probability that the recommended treatment will prevent or substantially reduce harm to the fetus"; (3) "there are no comparably effective, less intrusive options to prevent harm to the fetus"; and (4) "there is a high probability that the recommended treatment [will] also benefit the pregnant woman or that the risks to the pregnant woman are relatively small."[67]

The ACOG opinions assume the presence of competency and informed consent. Thus, if a pregnant patient is believed to be incompetent and incapable of providing informed consent, the health care providers may not be required to respect the patient's refusal of care. Moreover, if the patient is deemed incompetent and/or a medical emergency exists, care may be provided with consent from a legally authorized surrogate decision-maker or as an "emergency exception."

In summary, two approaches are available to the practitioner dealing with maternal-fetal conflict. One approach is to honor a competent pregnant patient's refusal of care. The other approach (which appears least favored by many medical ethicists and the ACOG) is to seek judicial authorization of treatment, which overrides a competent pregnant woman's refusal of care.[68]

In honoring a competent patient's desires to refuse treatment, the health care providers should carefully document the woman's competency and ability to provide informed consent. Every attempt should be made to counsel her to follow the treatment recommendations. Documentation should include how, when, and what information was provided to the patient and the patient's husband and family regarding the significant risks to both the patient and the unborn child if the recommended care were not provided. If time permits, the treatment options should be reevaluated with the patient at frequent intervals, with detailed documentation in the patient's medical record. Additionally, legal counsel for the health care providers and medical facility may wish to prepare an "assumption of risk" form for the patient (and, if possible, her husband) to sign. This form represents another level of documentation (beyond the detailed notes in the patient's medical record) demonstrating that the patient was fully informed about the risks associated with her refusal of treatment and that she voluntarily elected to accept those risks. However, such a release signed by the parents may not protect the physician and medical facility from a claim brought on behalf of the child who suffers an injury as a result of nonintervention. In some cases the court has found that physicians have a duty to provide care to the unborn child.[69,70]

Patient "assumption of risk" does not release a health care provider from his or her obligations to provide other treatment within the accepted standard of care. For example, in *Shorter v. Drury*, a case that involved a patient's refusal of blood transfusion because of religious preferences, the court upheld the validity of an "assumption of risk" (i.e., release) that relieved the physician from liability for compliance with the patient's refusal of blood transfusion before and after surgery, but nonetheless held him partially responsible for her death because of his negligent performance of the surgery.[71]

Before deciding whether to seek court review, health care providers should identify what issue they want the court to resolve. Is it whether the pregnant woman is competent? Is it whether there is a superior state interest in preserving the life of the viable fetus and/or the pregnant woman despite the (competent) patient's desire to refuse recommended care? Health care providers also should consider whether a court is the proper forum for resolving those issues, or whether another forum (e.g., an institutional ethics committee) may be a better choice. If a patient care dilemma is put before a judge, the health care providers give up a large amount of control over the disposition of the case. Nonetheless, if a patient's competency is at issue and there is adequate time, court review to settle the patient's competency may be beneficial and is supported by both the ACOG guidelines[67] and the *In re: A.C.* decision.[57] It is beneficial to obtain authorization for the provision of medically recommended care without waiting until the situation becomes an emergency. If the patient is deemed incompetent, the court may either appoint a surrogate decision-maker or directly authorize (by court order) the provision of medically indicated care.

In the case of a mentally ill pregnant patient, a referral to mental health authorities may be necessary to obtain authorization to keep her hospitalized. Several years ago, the University of Washington obtained a court order authorizing a recommended cesarean delivery for a mentally ill woman who was unable to provide consent and who was estranged from her family, who were her legally authorized surrogate decision-makers. This type of judicial resolution differs from a request for a court order to compel treatment over the objections of a competent patient.

DISCLOSURE OF UNANTICIPATED OUTCOMES AND MEDICAL ERRORS

In 1999, the Institute of Medicine (IOM) estimated that preventable medical errors in the hospital setting kill 44,000 to 98,000 patients each year.[72] In December 2006, the Institute for Healthcare Improvement (IHI) initiated the 5 Million Lives Campaign.[73] The IHI estimates that 15 million incidents of harm occur in U.S. hospitals each year (40,000 per day).

Most practitioners strive to provide the highest quality of care, but even in the current practice environment (with its growing focus on patient safety), unintended consequences—including patient injury and death—do occur. Unfortunately, most physicians remain largely unprepared to engage patients and their families in a timely, truthful, and candid manner in the aftermath of such events. In 1984, David Hilfiker wrote candidly of a life-altering mistake that he had made as a family physician treating a young woman in a small town in Minnesota.[74] Hilfiker was caring for a young woman named Barb Daily whom they both believed to be pregnant. He had delivered Barb and Russ Daily's first child, Heather, 2 years earlier, and he had been a friend of the couple for some years. After several months of care, her serial urine pregnancy test results remained negative and her uterus was only slightly enlarged. Concluding that she may have experienced a missed abortion, Hilfiker scheduled her for a dilation and curettage. The procedure was performed but it became apparent that the diagnosis was incorrect and the procedure had been carried out with a live fetus. In his reflections on the event, Hilfiker wrote of a physician's expectations of perfection, the lack of training in dealing with unexpected outcomes and mistakes, and the damaging effects of these conditions on physicians.[74]

Disclosure of errors and unanticipated outcomes is a key component in the national patient safety movement. It is also an ethical mandate and a regulatory requirement. The ethical imperative is captured in the following passage from the *Charter on Medical Professionalism*, published by the American Board of Internal Medicine (ABIM) Foundation:

> *Physicians should also acknowledge that in health care, medical errors that injure patients do sometimes occur. Whenever patients are injured as a consequence of medical care, patients should be informed promptly because failure to do so seriously compromises patient and societal trust. Reporting and analyzing medical mistakes provide the basis for appropriate prevention and improvement strategies and for appropriate compensation for injured parties.*[75]

The AMA's *Code of Medical Ethics* contains the following statement: "It is a fundamental ethical requirement that a physician should at all times deal honestly and openly with patients. . . . Concern regarding legal liability, which might result following truthful disclosure, should not affect the physician's honesty with a patient."[76] The Joint Commission standard RI.2.90 requires that "patients and, when appropriate, their families, are informed about the outcomes of care, treatment, and services that have been provided, including unanticipated outcomes."[77] Many states require reporting of medical errors, and some have legislated "apology" laws that encourage practitioners to be empathetic and honest with patients by allowing certain statements of sympathy to be made without fear of admitting medical liability.[78]

Physicians and other health care providers should undergo disclosure training to help them provide prompt and honest communication with patients and families and to help manage the risks of legal liability. Many untoward outcomes do not represent malpractice; they may simply reflect risks or complications of procedures that may or may not have been adequately discussed with patients and their families before the procedure or treatment. Adequate informed consent is an essential element of an effective disclosure program. Iatrogenic injuries, obvious mistakes, wrong-site surgeries, medication errors, and similar events that harm the patient should clearly be disclosed. A failure to disclose such an error may lead the patient (or the attorney) to conclude that health care providers made a deliberate effort to "cover up" the error. Furthermore, nondisclosure after such an event can lead to a charge of fraud. In most situations in which a provider conceals an error, the law provides that the statute of limitations "clock" for filing a malpractice claim does not begin to run until the fraudulent concealment is discovered.

Progressive medical liability insurance providers have recognized the ethical need for—and value of—promoting responsible disclosure policies. Although some physicians might believe that malpractice insurance carriers would discourage their clients from admitting mistakes to patients, this is not typically the case. For example, at least one major liability insurance provider has encouraged its clients to go directly to the patient and disclose the mistake, but the provider also recommends that clients consult the company to get help in planning the process; this company contends that it is better to maintain a good relationship with the patient by being genuinely caring and honest.[79]

The process of disclosure is a complex but necessary activity in the event of an unanticipated outcome or harmful medical error. Disclosure is ethically and legally the proper choice, and the overall goal is to promote trust of the medical profession and, ultimately, to improve patient safety and clinical outcomes. We recommend that practitioners and their organizations develop programs and policies in anticipation of such events. Assistance in the development of these procedures is available from a number of organizations, including some malpractice insurance providers.[78]

LIABILITY PROFILES IN OBSTETRIC ANESTHESIA: THE AMERICAN SOCIETY OF ANESTHESIOLOGISTS CLOSED-CLAIMS PROJECT

In 1985 the ASA Committee on Professional Liability began an ongoing study of insurance company liability claims involving anesthesiologists. Cases that are closed (i.e., no longer active) are reviewed by practicing anesthesiologists, abstracted, double-checked by the ASA Closed-Claims Committee, and entered into a computer database. In 1991 the first analysis of obstetric anesthesia claims was published, based on a total database of 1541 claims.[80] Another comprehensive analysis of the obstetric anesthesia claims was published in 1996 when the database contained 3533 claims.[81] As of December 2003, some 6894 claims (excluding those for dental injuries) from more than 35 insurance companies across the country had been reviewed and entered into the ASA Closed-Claims Project database. The analysis reported in this chapter focuses specifically on the 850 obstetric claims in the ASA Closed-Claims database as of December 2003.

It is important to recognize the limitations of this kind of study. A closed-claims study cannot determine the incidence of a complication, for a number of reasons. First, the denominator is unknown. That is to say, neither the total number of anesthetics given each year in each category nor the actual number of injuries per year is known. Second, not all injuries lead to claims of malpractice, and the anesthesiologist may not be named in a claim resulting from an anesthesia-related injury. This latter category may constitute a significant population of patients, which may make the relationship between cause and injury impossible to construct.[82] Conversely, anesthesiologists may be named in claims in which there was no anesthesia-related adverse event.

The claims that have been reviewed are not a random sample of such data. However, given the large number of participating insurance carriers, they are likely to be broadly representative of liability claims involving obstetric anesthesia care in the United States.

Despite the significant limitations of closed-claims studies, such efforts do provide information that cannot be obtained in other ways. For example, claims involving obstetric anesthesia care can be compared with those from other types of anesthesia practice to determine whether different patterns of injury and outcome emerge. We can ask such questions as: What injuries are most common in obstetric anesthesia claims? What is the relationship between the type of anesthesia and the presumed injury? What are the precipitating events that lead to the injuries? How do payment rates compare between obstetric and nonobstetric claims?

Approximately 12% of the 6894 claims in the ASA Closed-Claims Project database as of 2003 involved anesthesia care for patients undergoing vaginal or cesarean delivery. Of these obstetric claims, 66% involved cesarean delivery. The anesthesia workforce surveys conducted in 1981, 1992, and 2001 revealed a significant increase in the proportion of cesarean deliveries performed with neuraxial anesthesia and a corresponding decrease in those performed with general anesthesia.[83] An analysis of the ASA Closed-Claims Project database illustrates a similar trend in the claims for cases involving neuraxial and general anesthesia for cesarean delivery (Figure 33-1).

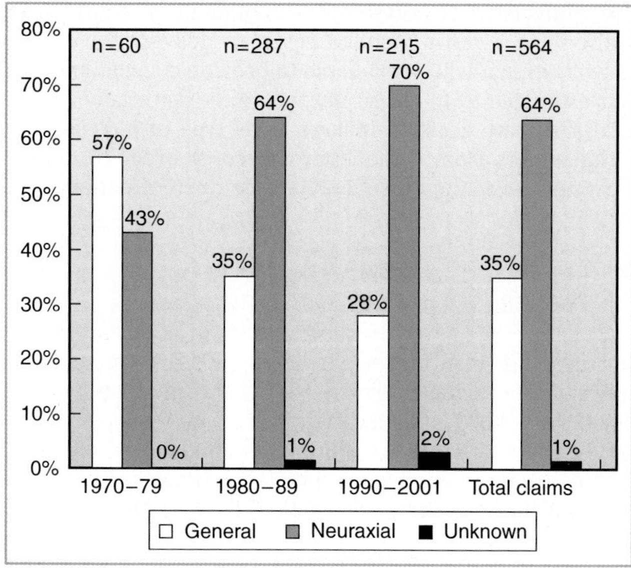

FIGURE 33-1 The percentage of claims in which the anesthetic technique for cesarean delivery was either general, neuraxial (regional), or unknown. Data are shown as the percentage of the total number of claims for the years indicated. (Data from the American Society of Anesthesiologists Closed-Claims Project database, n = 6894, December 2003.)

Anesthesia-Related Injuries

Table 33-1 lists all obstetric injuries or complications that had a frequency of 3% or greater in the ASA Closed-Claims database, as well as the type of anesthesia that resulted in the injury. **Maternal death** and **neonatal brain damage** were the most common injuries. A significantly greater proportion of the maternal deaths involved general anesthesia. Since the 1970s the proportion of maternal deaths in the ASA Closed-Claims database involving neuraxial anesthesia has declined, whereas the proportion of deaths involving general anesthesia has remained relatively constant (K. Posner, personal communication, 2007). As the number of women receiving general anesthesia for cesarean delivery decreases, this group of patients may be disproportionately represented by the highest-risk patients.[84]

The reports of neonatal brain damage also varied according to the type of anesthesia, with a significantly higher proportion of claims associated with general anesthesia. Determining whether a causal link exists between the anesthetic care (negligent or otherwise) and the injury to the newborn is often difficult. A closer analysis of newborn brain damage cases in the 1990s found that anesthesia care may have contributed to adverse neonatal outcome in less than a third of cases, but that in over half of these cases, some delay in anesthesia care was alleged.[85] By comparison, a causal relationship was thought probable between anesthesia and injury in 65% of all obstetric claims (maternal and neonatal) and 66% of all nonobstetric claims. The payment rate was 47% in the claims involving neonatal brain damage, which is lower than the payment rate in all obstetric (51%) and nonobstetric (58%) liability claims.

Some injuries (e.g., headache, pain during anesthesia, back pain) were almost exclusively associated with neuraxial anesthetic techniques. Most claims involving pain during anesthesia were associated with cesarean delivery (see Table 33-1). This fact may indicate that inadequate analgesia for labor and vaginal delivery is rarely a source of liability risk, whereas women expect to have satisfactory anesthesia during cesarean delivery, as do patients undergoing other

TABLE 33-1 Most Common Injuries in Obstetric Anesthesia Claims*

		Type of Anesthesia		Type of Delivery	
Injury	**Obstetric Claims (n = 850)**	**Neuraxial Anesthesia (n = 615)**	**General Anesthesia (n = 218)**	**Cesarean (n = 564)**	**Vaginal (n = 286)**
Maternal death	15% (131)	8% (51)†	36% (79)	20% (110)†	7% (21)
Neonatal brain damage	18% (152)	15% (95)†	26% (57)	20% (111)	16% (46)
Headache	14% (116)	19% (114)†	1% (2)	9% (52)†	22% (64)
Maternal nerve damage	15% (125)	20% (120) †	2% (5)	12% (68)†	20% (57)
Pain during anesthesia	7% (62)	9% (57)†	2% (4)	10% (56)†	2% (6)
Back pain	9% (75)	12% (75)†	0% (0)	5% (29)†	16% (46)
Maternal brain damage	6% (53)	5% (31)	9% (20)	7% (42)‡	4% (11)
Emotional distress	8% (64)	8% (50)	6% (14)	8% (47)	6% (17)
Neonatal death	6% (50)	5% (30)‡	9% (20)	7% (42)	5% (13)
Aspiration pneumonitis	3% (27)	1% (5)†	10% (22)	4% (22)	2% (5)

*The most common injuries in the obstetric group of claims are shown as % (n). Percentages are based on the total number of claims in each group. Some claims indicated more than one injury and are represented more than once. Claims involving brain damage apply only to patients who were alive when the claims were closed. In some claims, the type of anesthesia was not recorded; thus the total *n* for the anesthesia claims is 833 rather than 850.

†$P < .01$.

‡$P < .05$.

Data from the American Society of Anesthesiologists Closed-Claims Project database, n = 6894, December 2003.

types of surgery. It is also interesting that headache and back pain are relatively more common in the claims involving vaginal delivery. This finding may be, in part, a result of factors unique to labor and vaginal delivery (e.g., back strain from assumption of unnatural positions during anesthesia, bearing down during the second stage of labor).[86,87]

Table 33-2 lists the most common injuries identified after eliminating those involving only the newborn. This distinction allows comparison of the profiles of maternal injury with those among the nonobstetric population. The most striking finding is that the maternal claims contain a much higher proportion of relatively minor injuries, such as headache, pain during anesthesia, back pain, and emotional distress (37%), than the nonobstetric claims (8%). Obstetric patients may be at greater risk for some of these complications.[88] For example, the popularity of neuraxial anesthetic techniques in obstetrics combined with the greater risk for post–dural puncture headache in young women may account for the greater number of headache claims in the obstetric group. Pain during anesthesia is almost always associated with cesarean delivery conducted with neuraxial anesthesia. Some of these claims may have resulted from the anesthesia providers' reluctance to convert to general anesthesia because of the risk of aspiration or difficult intubation. In some cases, claims may have resulted from other factors, such as unrealistic expectations and general dissatisfaction with the care provided.

TABLE 33-2 Maternal Injuries Compared with Similar Injuries in Nonobstetric Claims*

Injury	Maternal Injury Claims (n = 850)	Nonobstetric Injury Claims (n = 6032)
Death	16% (131)†	31% (1852)
Headache	14% (116)†	2% (115)
Nerve damage	15% (125)†	19% (1148)
Pain during anesthesia	7% (62)†	1% (51)
Back pain	9% (75)†	2% (110)
Brain damage	6% (53)†	10% (628)
Emotional distress	8% (64)†	4% (224)
Aspiration pneumonitis	3% (27)	2% (138)

*The most common maternal injuries in the obstetric anesthesia claims are shown as % (n). Percentages are based on the total number of claims in each group. Some claims, especially those with a fatal outcome, had more than one injury and are represented more than once. Claims involving brain damage apply only to patients who were alive when the claims were closed.

†$P < .01$.

Data from the American Society of Anesthesiologists Closed-Claims Project database, n = 6894, December 2003.

Precipitating Events Leading to Injuries

Perhaps even more important than knowledge of the injuries and complications that may result in claims is an

TABLE 33-3 Most Common Precipitating Events in Obstetric Anesthesia Claims Compared with Nonobstetric Claims*

Event	Nonobstetric Claims (n = 6032)	Obstetric Claims (n = 850)	Type of Obstetric Anesthesia	
			Neuraxial (n = 615)	General (n = 218)
Respiratory system–related:	24% (1429)†	12% (98)	2% (13)†	39% (85)
Difficult intubation	6% (332)	5% (39)	0% (0)†	18% (39)
Aspiration	2% (122)	2% (20)	0% (1)†	9% (19)
Esophageal intubation	3% (200)†	1% (10)	0% (0)†	5% (10)
Inadequate ventilation/ oxygenation	6% (354)†	2% (13)	1% (7)	3% (6)
Bronchospasm	1% (59)	1% (7)	0% (2)	2% (5)
Premature extubation	2% (111)†	0% (4)	0% (0)‡	2% (4)
Airway obstruction	2% (125)†	0% (3)	0% (2)	0% (1)
Inadequate F_{IO_2}	0% (5)	0% (2)	0% (1)	0% (1)
Block-related:	12% (708)†	40% (341)	55% (341)†	0% (0)
Cardiac arrest	2% (92)‡	3% (26)	4% (26)†	0% (0)
High spinal/epidural	1% (40)†	4% (33)	5% (33)†	0% (0)
Inadequate analgesia	<1% (15)†	7% (57)	9% (57)†	0% (0)
Equipment problems	11% (657)†	2% (13)	1% (6)	3% (7)
Cardiovascular system	13% (764)†	5% (39)	3% (19)‡	8% (17)
Wrong drug/dose	6% (363)†	3% (26)	3% (16)	5% (10)

*The most common damaging events in the obstetric claims are shown as % (n). Percentages are based on the total number of claims in each group. Specific precipitating events were not identified in all claims. In claims indicating more than one damaging event, only the most significant event is listed. Columns do not sum to 100% because minor events are not listed. Statistical comparisons are made between obstetric and equivalent nonobstetric claims as well as between obstetric neuraxial (regional) and obstetric general anesthetics.

†$P < .01$.

‡$P < .05$.

Data from the American Society of Anesthesiologists Closed-Claims Project database, n = 6894, December 2003.

understanding of the precipitating events that lead to the injuries (Table 33-3). Critical events involving the respiratory system are the most common events in the nonobstetric claims and in obstetric claims involving general anesthesia. The literature supports the observation that difficult tracheal intubation and pulmonary aspiration are more likely in pregnant than in nonpregnant patients undergoing general anesthesia.[89,90] Difficult intubation was the precipitating event in 39 (5%) of the obstetric claims, and pulmonary aspiration in 20 (2%). Except for one case of aspiration, which occurred during neuraxial anesthesia, general anesthesia was the primary anesthetic technique in these cases. Many of the cases of aspiration occurred during difficult endotracheal intubation or after an esophageal intubation. In several cases general anesthesia was given by mask either as the technique of choice or following failed intubation, and in three cases aspiration was noted to have occurred during the induction of general anesthesia without cricoid pressure. In four cases, patients suffered postoperative respiratory complications resulting from premature extubation, inadequate monitoring in the recovery area or intensive care unit, hypoventilation, and/or airway obstruction.

Several reports have suggested that difficult intubation and pulmonary aspiration are the leading causes of anesthesia-related maternal death.[85,90] Interestingly, a study of anesthesia-related maternal deaths in Michigan between 1985 and 2003 found that no deaths occurred during induction of general anesthesia.[91] All causes of airway obstruction or hypoventilation occurred during emergence and recovery, often when monitoring was inadequate.[91]

Together, these data reemphasize that (1) all obstetric patients are at risk for airway complications (e.g., difficult intubation, aspiration); (2) anesthesia providers should be familiar with protocols such as the ASA difficult airway algorithm; (3) equipment should be immediately available for the management of patients in whom endotracheal intubation proves difficult; and (4) obstetric patients require the same standard of postanesthesia care as nonobstetric patients (see ASA "Guidelines for Regional Anesthesia in Obstetrics" [see Appendix A]).

Obesity increases the risk for both obstetric[92,93] and anesthetic[93,94] complications in pregnant women (see Chapter 50). In the ASA Closed-Claims Project database, damaging events related to the respiratory system were significantly more common in the claims involving obese parturients (18%) than in the claims involving nonobese parturients (8%) ($P < .05$). However, the rates of other injuries were not significantly different in obese and nonobese parturients.[81]

With the increasing use of neuraxial anesthesia for both vaginal and cesarean deliveries, it is not surprising that neuraxial blockade–related events are the most common precipitating events in the obstetric population, accounting for a significantly greater proportion of cases than that found in the nonobstetric files. The use of an effective test dose, the incremental injection of the therapeutic dose of local anesthetic, and the proscription against the epidural injection of

0.75% bupivacaine in pregnant women have undoubtedly contributed to a reduction in the risk of serious adverse outcomes associated with epidural anesthesia in obstetric patients.[84] However, the database includes several claims for neuraxial anesthesia–associated cardiac arrest (predominantly secondary to inadvertent intrathecal injection of drug) and for high spinal or epidural blockade. Neuraxial anesthesia is also associated with a higher rate of claims for inadequate analgesia/anesthesia during cesarean delivery.

Some obstetric patients are reluctant to accept neuraxial anesthesia because of the fear of nerve injury. Fortunately such injuries are uncommon. However, nerve injury was the second most common complication among the maternal injury claims (see Table 33-2), and it was the most common maternal injury in obstetric claims from 1990 through 2003.[85] Unfortunately, in many nerve injuries it is almost impossible to differentiate between an anesthetic cause and an obstetric cause. An ASA Closed-Claims analysis of injuries associated with neuraxial anesthesia in the 1980s and 1990s found that a significantly greater proportion of obstetric claims were associated with temporary and low-severity injuries when compared with nonobstetric claims.[88] Epidural abscess accounted for a greater proportion and epidural hematoma accounted for a significantly smaller proportion of obstetric neuraxial complications in comparison with nonobstetric claims. If claims for epidural abscess and meningitis were combined, infection was the leading cause (46%) of obstetric complications of neuraxial anesthesia.[88]

Payments

The practice of obstetrics is associated with high medicolegal risk. The obstetric anesthesia provider may also be named in a malpractice suit in an attempt to increase payments beyond policy limits. This belief is reinforced by well-publicized cases involving huge monetary awards. However, the ASA Closed-Claims Project provides a somewhat different perspective. For the purposes of this discussion, a payment is considered to be any expenditure by the insurance carrier in the form of a settlement or award. Obstetric claims constitute 12% of the ASA Closed-Claims database. Similarly, the obstetric claims account for 11% of the total number of payments made and for 14% of the total number of dollars expended in payments. Clearly, the payments for obstetric claims were not disproportionately frequent or large. Table 33-4 provides additional payment information. For claims in which payments were made, the median payment was higher in the obstetric group. This fact is not surprising, considering that there are two patients at risk in obstetric anesthesia cases, and both the mother and her infant are younger than the average age of patients in the nonobstetric files. Although the obstetric claims contained a lower proportion of deaths (either maternal or newborn), there was a greater proportion of brain injuries (either maternal or newborn) than in the nonobstetric claims. Such injuries typically result in higher payments for projected lifelong care requirements.

Lessons Learned

The obstetric anesthesia claims reveal a risk profile that differs from that of the nonobstetric anesthesia claims. Predictably, problems involving airway management, especially difficult intubation and pulmonary aspiration, are disproportionately represented in the obstetric claims. The incidence of systemic local anesthetic toxicity has diminished. However, the database continues to receive information on claims for severe adverse outcome resulting from neuraxial anesthesia–associated cardiac arrest (primarily due to inadvertent and unrecognized intrathecal injection of drug). The data suggest that we need to continue our efforts to reduce the risks of major complications of both general and neuraxial anesthesia. However, the large number of claims for pain during neuraxial anesthesia for cesarean delivery suggests that general anesthesia should not be delayed or avoided if a patient has inadequate anesthesia from neuraxial blockade.

Unfortunately, anesthesia providers are frequently named in lawsuits involving "bad baby" outcomes, despite growing evidence that cerebral palsy is associated with birth asphyxia in only 6% to 8% of cases, and even in these children, prevention may not be possible.[95] In 2003, an ACOG task force published criteria to help define the causal relationship between acute intrapartum events and cerebral palsy (see Chapter 10).[96] Potentially preventable anesthetic causes of newborn injury include delays in

TABLE 33-4 Payment Data for Obstetric Anesthesia Claims Compared with Nonobstetric Anesthesia Claims*

	Nonobstetric Claims (n = 6032)	Obstetric Claims (n = 850)	Type of Obstetric Anesthesia: Neuraxial (n = 615)	Type of Obstetric Anesthesia: General (n = 218)
No payment made	42% (2330)†	49% (383)	55% (307)†	34% (70)
Payment made	58% (3180)†	51% (393)	45% (248)†	66% (136)
Median payment ($)	205,875	285,000	155,445	817,188
Range ($)	43 to 44,950,000	771 to 19,780,000	771 to 13,180,000	1623 to 19,780,000

*Payment frequency, shown as % (n), and dollar amounts (adjusted to 2007 values). Percentages are based on the total number of claims in each group with payment data. Statistical comparisons are made between obstetric and nonobstetric claims and between claims involving obstetric neuraxial and obstetric general anesthetics. Claims with missing payment data were excluded from calculations of median payment and range.

†$P < .01$.

Data from the American Society of Anesthesiologists Closed-Claims Project database, n = 6894, December 2003.

anesthetic care and poor communication between the obstetrician and the anesthesiologist.[85]

Perhaps the most surprising finding of the analysis of the obstetric cases in the ASA Closed-Claims database is the large proportion of relatively minor injuries in the obstetric claims. This proportion markedly contrasts with that in the nonobstetric claims, suggesting that efforts to reduce the incidence of major injuries will not solve the medical malpractice problem in obstetric anesthesia. Clearly, factors other than major injury must motivate patients to bring a claim. It is overly simplistic to equate lawsuits with injury. A 1991 study found that the proportion of patients harmed by negligent care who actually file a claim is only 2%.[80] However, a lawsuit does not occur unless someone perceives that he or she or a loved one has been wronged. One of the unique advantages of closed-claims studies is that they reflect the consumer perspective.

To some extent the large proportion of relatively minor injuries in the obstetric claims may reflect a higher incidence of such problems among obstetric patients. However, it is clear that many of these patients were unhappy with the care provided and believed that they had been ignored or mistreated. It has been suggested that malpractice litigation serves the purposes not only of reparation of injury and deterrence of substandard care but also of emotional vindication.[97,98] Anesthesia providers should give attention to conducting themselves in such a manner that patients will not be motivated to bring suit for an unexpected outcome.[99] The importance of establishing good rapport with patients cannot be overemphasized. Whenever possible, anesthesia providers should involve themselves in the prenatal education process. A careful preanesthesia evaluation is very important and should occur as early in labor as possible. Special care should be taken to provide patients with realistic expectations and knowledge of potential major and minor risks associated with anesthetic procedures.

PROFESSIONAL PRACTICE STANDARDS

One beneficial effect of closed-claims analyses has been greater attention to steps to minimize the occurrence of severe adverse outcomes. On the basis of an analysis of malpractice claims in 1985, the Harvard University–affiliated medical institutions adopted a set of minimal monitoring standards within their system. Since that time the malpractice losses (normalized for the number of anesthetics given) have declined by more than 50%.[100] In 1986 the ASA became the first professional medical society to promulgate professional standards of care. The introduction of the ASA "Standards for Basic Intra-Operative Monitoring" was accompanied by a drop in the number of anesthesia-related liability claims. Although it is difficult to prove a cause-and-effect relationship between the introduction of these standards and fewer claims and payments, the arguments seem compelling.[100] Better monitoring, especially the greater use of pulse oximetry and capnography, has undoubtedly contributed to the decrease in severe complications and associated large awards.[101,102]

The ASA also has directed its efforts at improving obstetric anesthesia care in this country through a variety of position statements. In 1986 the ASA House of Delegates and the ACOG approved a joint statement entitled "Optimal Goals for Anesthesia Care in Obstetrics" (see Appendix C). This policy-oriented document (which was revised in 2000 and revised again in 2008) recognized the need for (1) appropriately trained physicians to provide anesthesia care when necessary, (2) a qualified obstetrician to be readily available during the administration of anesthesia, and (3) equipment, facilities, and support personnel for labor and delivery units equal to those provided in the surgical suite. The document served as the basis for the ASA "Standards for Conduction Anesthesia in Obstetrics," which was approved by the ASA House of Delegates in 1988. Unfortunately, unlike the widely acclaimed "Standards for Basic Intra-Operative Monitoring," these obstetric anesthesia practice standards generated immediate and widespread controversy. In part, this controversy occurred because the standards had implications with regard to nursing, obstetric, and pediatric practices and were considered too restrictive and too difficult to meet, especially for smaller or rural obstetric facilities. Consequently, in 1991, the document was revised and renamed "Guidelines for Regional Anesthesia in Obstetrics"; it was last amended in 2007 (see Appendix A).

In October 1998, the ASA House of Delegates approved a document developed by the ASA Task Force on Obstetric Anesthesia. This evidence-based document, titled "Practice Guidelines for Obstetric Anesthesia," is more clinically oriented than the aforementioned guidelines and was last amended in 2007 (see Appendix B).[103] It synthesizes a large body of published studies "to enhance the quality of anesthesia care for obstetric patients, reduce the incidence and severity of anesthesia-related complications, and increase patient satisfaction."[103] The document provides systematic analyses and meta-analyses of specific anesthetic techniques and practices, along with general recommendations.

It is hoped that these practice guidelines will positively affect the quality of care and the liability profiles in obstetric anesthesia practice. Practice guidelines suggest a standard of care and are based on both evidence and expert opinion. As such they often are used as evidence in cases of medical malpractice. Such documents can be used for exculpatory purposes (i.e., to exonerate a defendant physician) or as inculpatory evidence (i.e., to implicate a defendant physician). A two-part study surveyed 960 randomly selected malpractice attorneys and 259 open and closed claims involving obstetric and anesthetic cases from two malpractice insurance companies.[104] The claims were opened during a 2-year period (1990 to 1992). Practice guidelines played a pivotal role in 17 cases. In 12 cases they were used as inculpatory evidence, and in 4 cases as exculpatory evidence. (In 1 case the use of practice guidelines could not be classified.) Similarly, the surveyed attorneys responded that guidelines were used to implicate malpractice more than twice as often as they were used to defend against a claim of malpractice (54% versus 23%, respectively). The ACOG guidelines were used most commonly in these claims, and the ASA guidelines were used rarely. The investigators in this study speculated that the simplicity and clarity of the ASA guidelines may make compliance easier. Clearly, practice guidelines may act as a double-edged sword in medical litigation. Nonetheless, guidelines may reduce litigation expenses by dissuading plaintiffs' attorneys from pursuing cases in which guidelines have been met or by encouraging early settlement in cases in which guidelines were not followed without good reason.

POTENTIAL RISK MANAGEMENT PROBLEM AREAS

Obstetric anesthesia is often an unpredictable, difficult, and high-stress environment for the anesthesia provider. Compared with the operating room environment, the typical obstetric service is less familiar and more chaotic. The role and responsibility of the anesthesia provider is less clearly defined. Anesthesia services may be urgently requested in a situation in which there is little information available about the patient and the patient is unable or unwilling to answer questions. Laboring women are typically not sedated or calm when they request neuraxial analgesia. Rather, women in active labor may be uncooperative and even combative during the administration of neuraxial analgesia. The anesthesia provider may need to provide care for multiple patients simultaneously and may need to entrust some monitoring responsibilities to nurses and midwives. Sometimes the choice of labor analgesia is dictated by other people, and anesthesia providers may feel that they are little more than technicians. Perhaps it is not surprising that many anesthesia providers are uncomfortable in this environment and prefer to minimize their liability and discomfort by limiting their time practicing obstetric anesthesia.

Unique to obstetric anesthesia is the presence of the patient's husband, boyfriend, or other support person during anesthesia care. In the past it was considered a privilege for a husband or relative to be present during a cesarean delivery, and often there were preconditions such as documentation of attendance at prenatal classes. Today, in many obstetric centers, it is taken for granted that one or more support persons will be present for virtually any type of delivery. Undoubtedly, this trend has resulted in part from a sincere desire to provide a more family-centered experience. A second motivation may be to attract patients in a competitive, market-oriented environment.

We are not aware of specific case law regarding the issues involving support persons. However, the topic does raise a number of risk management questions. What are the parturient's rights with regard to having support personnel present during labor and delivery? What are the rights of the institution and health care providers? The presence of a support person often helps reassure and calm the parturient, but this is not always true. In some cases the presence of a support person can adversely affect patient care. Melzack[105] found that women have higher pain scores during labor when their husbands are present. Many anesthesia providers are not accustomed to having lay observers present during anesthesia procedures. Their presence can distract the anesthesia provider's attention and adversely affect judgment and performance. It is helpful, especially in obstetrics, for the anesthesia provider to develop a close physician-patient relationship. The presence of a support person often distracts the patient's attention away from the conversation and activities of the anesthesia provider. In some cases this distraction is helpful, but in others it interferes with the provision of anesthesia care.

The support person may also be at risk of unanticipated injury.[106] We are aware of a number of instances in which a father suffered an injury as a consequence of a vasovagal episode. In one case the father dropped the newborn infant on the floor as he lost consciousness. The potential for liability is self-evident.

In some cases, support persons may request that they be present during the delivery even when the patient receives general anesthesia. At the University of Washington, we do not allow support persons in the operating room during administration of general anesthesia. Even under the best of circumstances, the presence of such a person makes it more difficult for the anesthesia provider to give full attention to the patient. Routine anesthesia practices and procedures during general anesthesia may be frightening and misunderstood by laypersons. No matter how well intentioned and well prepared the support person, the sight of a loved one who is unresponsive, intubated, and mechanically ventilated can be traumatic emotionally. (*Editors' Note:* We are aware of hospitals in which the support person is allowed to enter the operating room after intubation, provided that the patient is stable and no maternal complications are anticipated. The support person sits beyond the foot of the operating table and is unable to see the face of the patient. The circulating nurse assumes responsibility for the support person. The support person leaves the operating room when the pediatrician exits with the infant.)

Physicians and hospitals also should consider policies on the use of audio/video equipment in the delivery room. Clearly all patients have a right to refuse to be photographed, filmed, or videotaped. However, a woman often wants a photographic record or videotape of events surrounding her delivery. Such a record can provide dramatic documentation of unfortunate interactions or suboptimal medical care. Courts typically allow videotapes to be entered into evidence and permit videotapes to be edited reasonably.[107] The visual impact of delivery room events can have a profound effect on a jury, regardless of whether the videotape has been edited to the advantage of the plaintiff. After the presentation of such evidence, it may be difficult to persuade a jury of the appropriateness of treatment.

A survey of 35 members of the American College of Legal Medicine identified nine cases in which an obstetric videotape was used as evidence.[107] In response to such cases, some hospitals have instituted policies to limit the use of video equipment in their labor and delivery suites. Such policies may antagonize patients and prompt them to seek care elsewhere. A balanced approach may be the best solution; that is, it may be reasonable to allow use of video equipment but to establish clear, fair, and unambiguous policies for its use. The policies must be understood by all members of the staff and should be made known to patients and their families, preferably before the patient is admitted to the hospital. Prenatal classes can serve as a means to disseminate such information. One approach is to have informational material and/or specific consent forms for patients and their families. Another option is to combine such policy statements with a "hold harmless" waiver for the support person. Although none of these measures can eliminate the potential liability risks associated with these issues, they may serve to educate patients and their families about their rights and about hospital policies and procedures.

KEY POINTS

- Effective communication with the patient and her family is an important component of obstetric anesthesia practice.
- Honest, caring, and comprehensive discussion with the patient before the administration of anesthesia meets legal and ethical standards for obtaining informed consent, improves the image of the anesthesia provider, and reduces the likelihood of dissatisfaction and possible litigation after unanticipated complications.
- Informed consent may be either verbal or both verbal and written. Written consent provides documentation that the consent process has occurred. If possible, it is best to obtain consent early in labor, before the onset of severe labor pain.
- Refusal of care by a pregnant patient may raise unique legal and ethical concerns. In such situations, the woman's competency or ability to make an informed medical decision may be an issue. When the patient is competent, the health care providers should attempt to resolve treatment conflicts through additional patient education and discussion. In general, a pregnant woman's informed refusal of medical intervention should prevail as long as she has the capacity to make medical decisions. Rarely, it may be advisable to seek a court order to resolve competency and/or medical treatment issues.
- Critical events involving the respiratory system were the most common precipitating events related to adverse outcome in both nonobstetric claims and obstetric claims involving general anesthesia in the American Society of Anesthesiologists (ASA) Closed-Claims Project database. Failed intubation and pulmonary aspiration are more common during administration of general anesthesia in pregnant women than in nonpregnant women.
- Obstetric claims involve a much higher proportion of relatively minor injuries (e.g., headache, pain during anesthesia, back pain, emotional distress) than nonobstetric claims.
- The careful use of an effective test dose, the incremental injection of the therapeutic dose of local anesthetic, and the proscription against the epidural injection of 0.75% bupivacaine in pregnant women appear to have reduced the incidence of major complications during the administration of epidural anesthesia in obstetric patients.
- Potentially preventable anesthetic causes of newborn injury include delays in anesthetic care and poor communication between the obstetrician and the anesthesiologist.
- Guidelines for obstetric anesthesia practice have been published by the ASA, and a joint statement has been published by the ASA and the American College of Obstetricians and Gynecologists.

REFERENCES

1. Eastaugh SR. Reducing litigation costs through better patient communication. Physician Exec 2004; 30:36-8.
2. The Joint Commission. "What did the doctor say?" Improving health literacy to protect patient safety. 2007. Available at http://www.jointcommission.org/NewsRoom/PressKits/Health_Literacy/
3. Furrow BR. Liability and Quality Issues in Health Care. 4th edition. St. Paul, MN, West Group, 2001:139-48, 163-6.
4. Rev. Code Wash. (ARCW) § 7.70.030 (Lexis 2003).
5. Rev. Code Wash. (ARCW) § 7.70.040 (Lexis 2003).
6. Tennessee: *Shadrick v. Coker*, 963 S.W.2d 726, 733 (Tenn. 1998).
7. *Miller v. Jacoby*. 145 Wash. 2d 65, 33 P.3d 68 (2001).
8. *Brown v. Dahl*. 41 Wash. App. 565, 705 P.2d 781 (1985).
9. Cheney FW. Perioperative ulnar nerve injury: A continuing medical and liability problem. ASA Newsl June 1998; 62. Available at http://www.asahq.org/index.htm/
10. *Schloendorff v. Society of New York Hospital*, 211 NY 125 (1914).
11. Alabama: *Phelps v. Dempsey*, 656 So.2d 377, 380 (Ala. 1995), *rehearing denied* 700 So.2d 1340 (Ala. 1997).
12. *Auler v. Van Natta*, 686 N.E.2d 172, 175-176 (Ind. App. 1997).
13. *O'Neal v. Hammer*, 87 Hawaii 183, 953 P.2d 561, 568 (1998).
14. *Carr v. Strode*, 904 P.2d 489, 498 (Hawaii 1995).
15. District of Columbia Circuit: *Canterbury v. Spence*, 464 F.2d 772, (D.C. Cir.) *cert denied* 409 U.S. 1064 (1972).
16. *Matthies v. Mastromonaco*, 160 N.J. 26, 39, 733 A.2d 456, 463 (1999).
17. Washington: *Backlund v. University of Wash.*, 137 Wash.2d 651, 667, 975 P.2d 950, 959 (1999).
18. *Martin by Scoptur v. Richards*, 531 N.W.2d 70, 75 (Wis. 1995).
19. Alabama: *Otwell v. Bryant*, 497 So.2d 111, 118 (Ala. 1986).
20. *Barth v. Rock*, 36 Wn. App. 400, 674 P.2d 1265 (1984), rev. denied, 101 Wn.2d 1014 (1984).
21. Rev. Code Wash. (ARCW) § 7.70.050 (Lexis 2003).
22. *Roe v Wade*, 410 U.S. 113, 93 S. Ct. 705, 35 L. Ed. 2d 147 (1973).
23. *Woe v. Coumo*, 729 F.2d 96 (2nd Cir 1984).
24. Ransom SB, Studdert DM, Dombrowski MP, et al. Reduced medicolegal risk by compliance with obstetric clinical pathways: A case-control study. Obstet Gynecol 2003; 101:751-5.
25. Florida. Fla. Stat. Ann. § 768.57(2).
26. Localio AR, Lawthers AG, Brennan TA, et al. Relation between malpractice claims and adverse events due to negligence: Results of the Harvard Medical Practice Study III. N Engl J Med 1991; 325:245-51.
27. Ostrom BJ, Rottman D, Hanson RA. What are tort awards really like? The untold story from the state courts. Williamsburg, VA, National Center for State Courts, 1992:77-81.
28. Rev. Code Wash. (ARCW) § 7.70.100 (Lexis 2003).
29. 42 CFR § 482.13(b)(2).
30. 42 CFR §482.51(b)(2).
31. O'Connor AM, Stacey D, Entwistle V, et al. Decision aids for people facing health treatment or screening decisions. Cochrane Database Syst Rev 2003; (2):CD001431.
32. O'Connor AM, Wennberg JE, Legare F, et al. Toward the 'tipping point': Decision aids and informed patient choice. Health Aff (Millwood) 2007; 26:716-25.
33. Rev. Code Wash. (ARCW) § 7.70.060 (Lexis 2003).
34. Controlled Risk Insurance Company/Risk Management Foundation. Informed consent. 2008. Available at http://www.rmf.harvard.edu/high-risk-areas/surgery/informed-consent/index.aspx/
35. Sanford S. Informed consent: The verdict is in. ASA Newsl 2006; 70:7.
36. O'Leary CE, McGraw RS. Informed consent requires active communication. Anesth Patient Safety Foundation Newsletter 2008; 23:4-5.
37. Appelbaum PS. Clinical practice: Assessment of patients' competence to consent to treatment. N Engl J Med 2007; 357:1834-40.
38. Grisso T, Appelbaum PS. Assessing Competence to Consent to Treatment: A Guide for Physicians and Other Health Care Professionals. New York, Oxford University Press, 1998:224.
39. Berg JW, Appelbaum PS, Lidz CW, Parker L. Informed Consent: Legal Theory and Clinical Practice. 2nd edition. New York, Oxford University Press, 2001:41-74.

40. Rev. Code Wash. (ARCW) § 7.70.065 (Lexis 2003).
41. Rosovsky FA: Consent to Treatment: A Practical Guide. 3rd edition. Gaithersburg, MD, Aspen, 2001.
42. Guttmacher Institute. State policies in brief: An overview of minors' consent law. August 2008. Available at http://www.guttmacher.org/statecenter/spibs/spib_OMCL.pdf/
43. *State v. Koome*, 84 Wash.2d 901, 530 P.2d 260 (1975).
44. Katz KD. The pregnant child's right to self-determination. Albany Law Rev 1999; 62:1119-45.
45. Holder AR. Minors' rights to consent to medical care. JAMA 1987; 257:3400-2.
46. Annas GJ. The Rights of Patients: The Basic ACLU Guide to Patient Rights. 2nd edition. Totowa, NJ, Humana Press, 1992:110-4, 127-130.
47. Hawkins LA. Living will statutes: A minor oversight. Virginia Law Review 1992; 78:1581-615.
48. Bush DJ. A comparison of informed consent for obstetric anaesthesia in the USA and the UK. Int J Obstet Anesth 1995; 4:1-6.
49. Pattee C, Ballantyne M, Milne B. Epidural analgesia for labour and delivery: Informed consent issues. Can J Anaesth 1997; 44:918-23.
50. Gerancher JC, Grice SC, Dewan DM, Eisenach J. An evaluation of informed consent prior to epidural analgesia for labor and delivery. Int J Obstet Anesth 2000; 9:168-73.
51. Clark SK, Leighton BL, Seltzer JL. A risk-specific anesthesia consent form may hinder the informed consent process. J Clin Anesth 1991; 3:11-3.
52. Siddiqui MN, Siddiqui S, Ranasinghe S, et al. Does labor pain and labor epidural analgesia impair decision capabilities of parturients? The Internet Journal of Anesthesiology 2005; 10. Available at http://www.ispub.com/ostia/index.php?xmlFilePath=journals/ija/vol10n1/labor.xml/
53. American College of Obstetricians and Gynecologists. Ethics in Obstetrics and Gynecology. 2nd edition. Washington DC, ACOG, 2004.
54. American College of Obstetricians and Gynecologists Committee on Ethics. Maternal decision making, ethics, and the law. ACOG Committee Opinion No. 321. Washington, DC, ACOG, November 2005. (Obstet Gynecol 2005; 106:1127-37.)
55. Neale H. Mother's rights prevail: In re A.C. and the status of forced obstetrical intervention in the District of Columbia. J Health Hosp Law 1990; 23:208-13.
56. Mishkin DB, Povar GJ. Decision making with pregnant patients: A policy born of experience. Joint Comm J Qual Improv 1993; 89:80-4.
57. *In re: A.C.*, 573 A.2d 1235, 1237 (D.C. App. 1990).
58. Annas GJ. Protecting the liberty of pregnant patients. N Engl J Med 1987; 316:1213-4.
59. CBS News. Debate revived on mother's rights. May 19, 2004. Available at http://www.cbsnews.com/stories/2004/05/19/health/main618535.shtml?source=search_story/
60. Drug Policy Alliance Network. South Carolina Supreme Court reverses 20-year homicide conviction of Regina McKnight. May 12, 2008. Available at http://www.drugpolicy.org/news/pressroom/pressrelease/pr051208.cfm/
61. ABC 33/40 News. New Alabama law being used to prosecute drug-using moms. Feb 14, 2008. Available at www.abc3340.com/news/stories/0208/496076.html/
62. Alabama, Ala. Stat. Ann § 26-15-3.2.
63. Bianchi DW, Crombleholme TM, D'Alton ME. Fetology: Diagnosis and Management of the Fetal Patient. New York, McGraw-Hill, 2000.
64. McCullough L, Chervenak F. Ethics in Obstetrics and Gynecology. New York, Oxford University Press, 1994.
65. American Medical Association Policy H-420.970: Treatment versus criminalization – Physician role in drug addiction during pregnancy. Available at http://www.ama-assn.org/apps/pf_new/pf_online/
66. American College of Obstetricians and Gynecologists Committee on Ethics. Patient choice and the maternal-fetal relationship. ACOG Committee Opinion No. 214. Washington, DC, ACOG, April 1999 (Int J Gynaecol Obstet 1999; 65:213-215.)
67. American College of Obstetricians and Gynecologists Committee on Ethics. Ethics in Obstetrics and Gynecology. 2nd edition. Washington DC, American College of Obstetricians and Gynecologists, 2004:34-6.
68. Jonsen AR, Siegler M, Winslade WJ. Clinical Ethics: A Practical Approach to Ethical Decisions in Clinical Medicine. 3rd edition. New York, McGraw-Hill, 1992:177-8.
69. *Moen v. Hanson*, 85 Wash.2d 597, 537 P.2d 266 (1975).
70. *Harbeson v. Parke-Davis, Inc.*, 98 Wash.2d 460, 656 P.2d 483 (1983).
71. *Shorter v. Drury*, 103 Wash.2d, 695 P.2d 116 (1985).
72. Institute of Medicine. To Err Is Human: Building A Safer Health System. Washington, DC, National Academies Press, 1999.
73. McCannon C, Hackbarth A, Griffin F. Miles to go: An introduction to the 5 million lives campaign. Jt Comm J Qual Patient Saf 2007; 33:477-84.
74. Hilfiker D. Facing our mistakes. N Engl J Med 1984; 310:118-22.
75. American Board of Internal Medicine Foundation. Medical professionalism in the new millennium: A physician charter. 2004. Available at http://www.abimfoundation.org/professionalism/pdf_charter/ABIM_Charter_Ins.pdf.
76. American Medical Association. AMA code of medical ethics. Date accessed: August 5, 2008. Available at http://www.ama-assn.org/ama/pub/category/2498.html/
77. The Joint Commission. Standard RI.2.90. Available at http://www.jointcommission.org/Standards/
78. SorryWorks! Coalition. SorryWorks! 2006. Available at http://www.sorryworks.net/
79. Millar S, Kayes C. Keeping your patients and yourselves out of litigious situations. Available at http://www.magmutual.com/mmic/articles/2004_10_23_litigious.pdf/
80. Chadwick HS, Posner K, Caplan RA, et al. A comparison of obstetric and nonobstetric anesthesia malpractice claims. Anesthesiology 1991; 74:242-9.
81. Chadwick HS. An analysis of obstetric anesthesia cases from the American Society of Anesthesiologists closed claims project database. Int J Obstet Anesth 1996; 5:258-63.
82. Edbril SD, Lagasse RS. Relationship between malpractice litigation and human errors. Anesthesiology 1999; 91:848-55.
83. Bucklin BA, Hawkins JL, Anderson JR, Ullrich FA. Obstetric anesthesia workforce survey: Twenty-year update. Anesthesiology 2005; 103:645-53.
84. Hawkins JL, Koonin LM, Palmer SK, Gibbs CP. Anesthesia-related deaths during obstetric delivery in the United States, 1979-1990. Anesthesiology 1997; 86:277-84.
85. Davies JM, Posner KL, Lee LA, et al. Liability associated with obstetric anesthesia: A closed claims analysis. Anesthesiology 2009; 110:131-9.
86. Okell RW, Sprigge JS. Unintentional dural puncture: A survey of recognition and management. Anaesthesia 1987; 42:1110-3.
87. MacArthur C, Lewis M, Knox EG, Crawford JS. Epidural anaesthesia and long-term backache after childbirth. Br Med J 1990; 301:9-12.
88. Lee LA, Posner KL, Domino KB, et al. Injuries associated with regional anesthesia in the 1980s and 1990s. Anesthesiology 2004; 101:143-52.
89. Soreide E, Bjornestad E, Steen PA. An audit of perioperative aspiration pneumonitis in gynaecological and obstetric patients. Acta Anaesthesiol Scand 1996; 40:14-9.
90. Hawkins JL. Anesthesia-related maternal mortality. Clin Obstet Gynecol 2003; 46:679-87.
91. Mhyre JM, Riesner MN, Polley LS, Naughton NN. A series of anesthesia-related maternal deaths in Michigan, 1985-2003. Anesthesiology 2007; 106:1096-104.
92. Driul L, Cacciaguerra G, Citossi A, et al. Prepregnancy body mass index and adverse pregnancy outcomes. Arch Gynecol Obstet 2008; 278:23-6.
93. Hood DD, Dewan DM. Anesthetic and obstetric outcome in morbidly obese parturients. Anesthesiology 1993; 79:1210-8.
94. Saravanakumar K, Rao SG, Cooper GM. The challenges of obesity and obstetric anesthesia. Curr Opin Obstet Gynecol 2006; 18:631-5.
95. Reddihough DS, Collins KJ. The epidemiology and causes of cerebral palsy. Aust J Physiother 2003; 49:7-12.

96. Hankins GD, Speer M. Defining the pathogenesis and pathophysiology of neonatal encephalopathy and cerebral palsy. Obstet Gynecol 2003; 102:628-36.
97. Meyers AR. 'Lumping it': The hidden denominator of the medical malpractice crisis. Am J Public Health 1987; 77:1544-8.
98. Hickson GB, Clayton EW, Githens PB, Sloan FA. Factors that prompted families to file medical malpractice claims following perinatal injuries. JAMA 1992; 267:1359-63.
99. Palmer SK, Gibbs CP. Risk management in obstetric anesthesia. Int Anesthesiol Clin 1989; 27:188-99.
100. Holzer JF. The advent of clinical standards for professional liability. QRB Qual Rev Bull 1990; 16:71-9.
101. Eichhorn JH. Prevention of intraoperative anesthesia accidents and related severe injury through safety monitoring. Anesthesiology 1989; 70:572-7.
102. Tinker JH, Dull DL, Caplan RA, et al. Role of monitoring devices in prevention of anesthetic mishaps: A closed claims analysis. Anesthesiology 1989; 71:541-6.
103. Practice guidelines for obstetric anesthesia. An updated report by the American Society of Anesthesiologists Task Force on Obstetric Anesthesia. Anesthesiology 2007; 106:843-63.
104. Hyams AL, Brandenburg JA, Lipsitz SR, et al. Practice guidelines and malpractice litigation: A two-way street. Ann Intern Med 1995; 122:450-5.
105. Melzack R. The myth of painless childbirth (the John J. Bonica lecture). Pain 1984; 19:321-37.
106. DeVore JS, Asrani R. Paternal fractured skull as a complication of obstetric anesthesia. Anesthesiology 1978; 48:386.
107. Eitel DR, Yankowitz J, Ely JW. Legal implications of birth videos. J Fam Pract 1998; 46:251-6.

Part IX

Obstetric Complications

The philosophy of obstetric management changed in the early decades of the twentieth century, and this change had a profound effect on the use of obstetric anesthesia. Until 1900, obstetricians considered childbirth a physiologic process best left to proceed without interference by physician or midwife. They criticized "meddlesome practices" for normal deliveries. Then a new generation of obstetricians, concerned about the high rate of complications associated with routine deliveries, began to advocate more active management of childbirth. They envisioned the practice of obstetrics as a form of preventive medicine. Leaders of this movement, such as Joseph DeLee of Chicago, became strong advocates for the routine use of episiotomy, forceps delivery, and manual removal of the placenta. Of course, these measures also necessitated greater use of anesthesia.[1]

DeLee acknowledged that his method "interferes much with Nature's process," but he felt justified. With conservative management, he said, a dismal outcome was so common that he "often wondered whether Nature did not deliberately intend women should be used up in the process of reproduction, in a manner analogous to that of the salmon, which dies after spawning. Perhaps laceration, prolapse and all the evils are, in fact, natural to labor and therefore normal. ... If you adopt this view, I have no ground to stand on, but, if you believe that a woman after delivery should be as healthy, as well as anatomically perfect as she was before, and that the child should be undamaged, then you will have to agree with me that labor is pathogenic, because experience has proved such ideal results exceedingly rare."[2] Other physicians agreed with DeLee. Austin Flint asked how a "process that kills thousands of women each year, leaves a quarter of all cases more or less invalidate, is attended by severe pain and tearing of tissues, and kills three to seven percent of all babies, can be called a normal or physiologic function?"[3]

The change in the philosophy of obstetric management was further stimulated by early feminists. In the United States, but especially in Great Britain, feminists formed a coalition with obstetricians to improve teaching, build new facilities, and fund better care for women in hospitals. They also demanded better anesthesia coverage and even funded research to develop new anesthetic techniques. In response to this movement, physicians developed many new techniques for laboring patients. Many of the anesthetic methods now favored for normal deliveries are a direct outgrowth of public support for innovation and improvement that began during this time.

Donald Caton, M.D.

REFERENCES

1. Leavitt W. Joseph B. DeLee and the practice of preventive obstetrics. Am J Public Health 1988; 78:1353-9.
2. DeLee JB. The prophylactic forceps operation. Am J Obstet Gynecol 1920; 1:34-44.
3. Flint A. Responsibility of the medical profession in further reducing maternal mortality. Am J Obstet Gynecol 1925; 19:864-6.

Chapter 34

Preterm Labor and Delivery

Holly A. Muir, M.D., FRCPC
Cynthia A. Wong, M.D.

Preterm delivery is defined as delivery before 37 weeks' gestation. It is estimated to occur in 12% to 13% of all pregnancies in the United States and in 5% to 9% of pregnancies in other developed countries.[1] It is responsible for 75% to 80% of all neonatal deaths and considerable neonatal morbidity.[1,2] Birth statistics in the United States reveal a 20% increase in the preterm delivery rate between 1990 and 2005 (from 10.6% to 12.7%) (Figure 34-1)[3] and a 30% increase since 1981.[4] The societal economic burden associated with preterm birth in the United States was at least $26.2 billion in 2005.[4] More detailed review of almost 1.3 million deliveries in 12 states in 2005 suggests that the current rate of preterm delivery is approximately 13.1%.[5] The rate was highest in non-Hispanic blacks (18.5%) and in women older than 40 years (17%) or younger than 20 years (15%).[5,6] The increase in preterm births has been associated with a significant increase in cesarean delivery rates, especially among the late preterm births, thus increasing the need for anesthesia services for these deliveries.[7]

In *Healthy People 2010*, published in 2000, the U.S. Department of Health and Human Services acknowledged the magnitude of this problem and announced its desire to reduce the incidence of preterm birth from 11.6% to 7.6% or less over the next decade.[8] Unfortunately, just the opposite has occurred: the rate has increased to approximately 13%.

This issue is not confined to the United States; the World Health Organization (WHO) and other nongovernmental organizations have identified this as a health issue near crisis. WHO uses low birth weight as an indicator of early gestation because true gestational age at delivery is often not known. Worldwide, the incidence of low birth weight, defined as a birth weight less than 2500 g, is 15.5 per 1000 births.[9] Africa and Asia have the highest incidence of low birth weight, at 14.3 and 18.3 per 1000, respectively. In contrast, in Europe and North America the incidence of low birth weight is 6.4 and 7.7 per 1000, respectively.[9] These data parallel infant mortality rates, which are similarly very high in the developing nations, particularly the sub-Saharan African countries. The United States has a higher infant mortality rate than Europe (6 versus 3 per 1000 births, respectively), which also reflects the higher U.S. preterm birth rate.[10]

In a report published in 2006, the Institute of Medicine recommended that investigators focus on (1) better definition of the problem; (2) treatment to prevent preterm birth and the treatment of children born preterm; (3) identification of the causes of preterm birth, including identification of modifiable risk factors and the reasons for disparity among different ethnic, racial, and socioeconomic groups; and (4) development of policies and public programs that can be used to reduce the rate of preterm birth.[4]

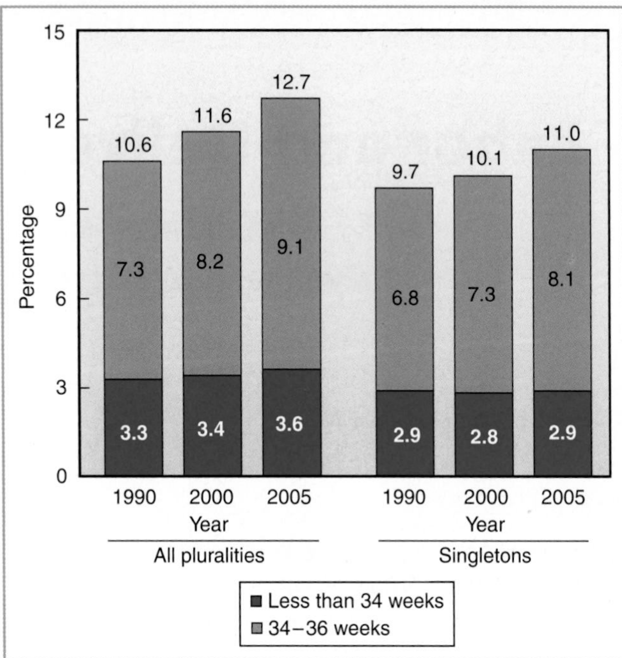

FIGURE 34-1 Preterm birth rates for all births and for singletons only: United States, 1990, 2000, and 2005. (From Martin JA, Hamilton BE, Sutton PD, et al. Births: Final data for 2005. Natl Vital Stat Rep 2007; 56:1-103.)

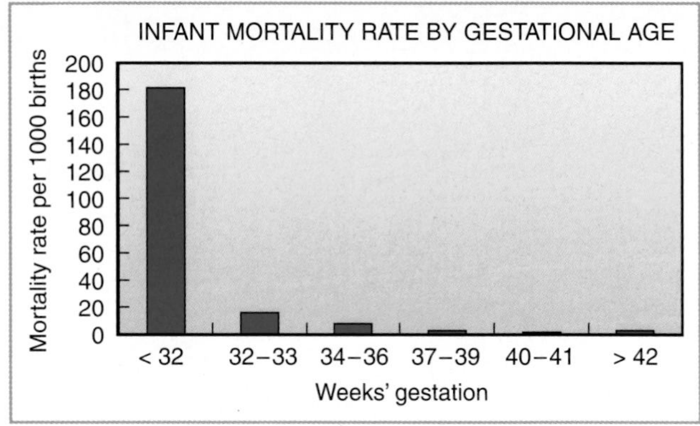

FIGURE 34-2 Neonatal mortality rate by gestational age at birth: United States, 2004. (From Centers for Disease Control and Prevention, National Center for Health Statistics. Available at http://www.cdc.gov/nchs/VitalStats.htm)

In addition, significant attention is currently being focused on the role of genetic contributions to preterm birth.[11]

DEFINITIONS

A preterm infant is defined as one delivered between 20 and 37 weeks after the first day of the last menstrual period (i.e., at least 3 weeks before the expected date of term delivery). Gestational age often is unknown or difficult to determine in small neonates. Some of these infants are small for gestational age (SGA) rather than preterm. An infant who weighs less than 2500 g at birth is considered a low-birth-weight (LBW) infant, regardless of gestational age. Likewise, an infant who weighs less than 1500 g at birth is considered a very low-birth-weight (VLBW) infant, and an infant who weighs less than 1000 g at birth is considered an extremely low-birth-weight (ELBW) infant.

NEONATAL MORTALITY

The survival rate among neonates increases as the birth weight and/or gestational age increases (Figures 34-2 and 34-3; Table 34-1). During the past three decades, there has been a significant improvement in the survival rate in every VLBW subgroup, with the greatest improvement occurring in the subgroup with a birth weight between 750 and 1000 g.[12,13] Infants with a birth weight of less than 750 g continue to have a high mortality rate. Emphasis on neonatal outcomes has focused on intact survival rather than mortality. In a cohort of neonates delivered between 1997 and 2002, the mortality rate was 45% for infants weighing between 501 and 750 g, 12% for those between 751 and 1000 g, and 6% for those between 1001 and 1250 g.[2] After data are controlled for gestational age and weight, male infants have a higher mortality than female infants.[14]

The rate of neonatal survival now exceeds 90% for infants born after 30 weeks' gestation, and a neonatal survival rate near 100% can be expected for infants born after 32 weeks' gestation. Greater attention is now given to infants born before 32 weeks' gestation. These represent approximately 1% to 2% of all deliveries and 30% to 40% of all preterm deliveries. However, this cohort of patients accounts for 60% of all cases of perinatal mortality, 50% of cases of long-term neurologic morbidity, and 40% of the estimated 6600 cases of cerebral palsy diagnosed each year.[2,15]

A retrospective cohort study assessed the survival and cost of pregnancies delivered at 24 to 26 weeks' gestation.[16] Neonatal survival was 43%, 74%, and 83% at 24, 25, and 26 weeks' gestation, respectively. The majority of women received antenatal corticosteroids, and the majority of neonates received exogenous surfactant. This study suggested that the greatest gain in survival is achieved by prolonging gestation beyond 24 weeks' gestation. A delay in delivery of even 1 week leads to significantly better outcome and reduced cost. A similar study examining a cohort born between 1998 and 2002 showed a survival rate of 0% at 21 completed weeks' gestation; the survival rate rose steadily to 75% at 25 completed weeks' gestation (see Table 34-1).[14]

Infants born at the threshold of viability (22 to 24 weeks' gestation) continue to be at the greatest risk for poor outcome. The Vermont Oxford Network collected data from more than 650 neonatal intensive care units in the United States and abroad.[17] Among infants born between 1996 and 2000 with a birth weight of 401 to 500 g and a mean gestational age of 23.2 weeks, mortality was 83%. Most survivors had some level of serious short-term medical complications and long-term disability.[17] In another large cohort, the EPICure study reported outcomes for all infants born at 20 to 25 weeks' gestation over a 10-month period in

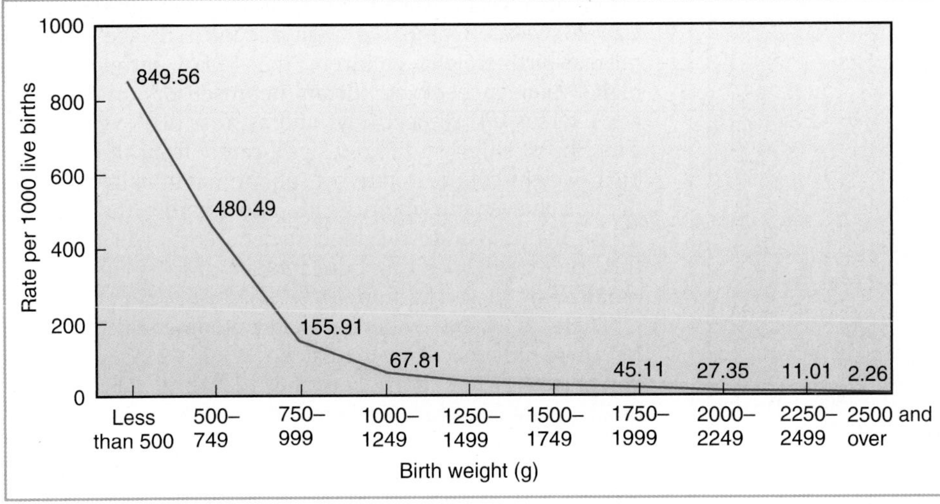

FIGURE 34-3 Infant mortality rates by birth weight: United States, 2004. (From Mathews TJ, MacDorman MF. Infant mortality statistics from the 2004 period linked birth/infant death data set. Natl Vital Stat Rep 2007; 55:1-32.)

1995 in the United Kingdom and Ireland.[18] Of 4004 infants, 811 (20%) received intensive care, and 39% of those survived to discharge. It is estimated that 2% to 5% of VLBW infants who survive to hospital discharge die within 2 years because of medical complications of prematurity.[2]

NEONATAL MORBIDITY

Approximately 90% of preterm births occur between 30 and 36 weeks' gestation. Morbidity is the primary concern at this gestational age. A significant reduction in morbidity from respiratory distress syndrome (RDS) occurs by extending an otherwise uncomplicated pregnancy until 36 weeks' gestation. The incidence of high-grade (III or IV) intraventricular hemorrhage (IVH) diminishes rapidly after 27 weeks' gestation, and grade III or IV hemorrhages are very rare after 32 weeks' gestation. Likewise, neonatal morbidity from patent ductus arteriosus and necrotizing enterocolitis diminishes significantly after 32 weeks' gestation.[12,19,20] Data from the National Institute of Child Health and Development (NICHD) Neonatal Research Network sites from 1997 through 2002 indicate that survival without complications (bronchopulmonary dysplasia, severe IVH, necrotizing enterocolitis, or a combination of these disorders) ranged from 20% for infants with a birth weight between 501 and 750 g to 89% for those with a birth weight between 1251 and 1500 g (Figure 34-4).[2]

TABLE 34-1 Newborn Deaths by Gestational Age

Completed Weeks' Gestation	Percentage of Deaths*
21	100
22	79
23	70
24	50
25	25
26	20
27	10
28	8
29	5
30	3
31	5
32	7
33	5
34-42	5

*Death rate before discharge by gestational age among infants born in the National Institute of Child Health and Human Development (NICHD) Neonatal Research Network Centers in 1995 and 1996.

Data from Lemons JA, Bauer CR, Oh W, et al. Very low birth weight outcomes of the National Institute of Child Health and Human Development Neonatal Research Network, January 1995 through December 1996. NICHD Neonatal Research Network. Pediatrics 2001; 107:E1.

The economic costs of the care of surviving preterm infants (especially VLBW infants) can be enormous. In 2003, preterm infants accounted for approximately $18.1 billion in health care costs, representing half of the total hospital cost for newborn care in the United States.[2] In a 2006 report, the Institute of Medicine estimated that the societal economic burden associated with preterm birth in the United States was at least $26.2 billion in 2005, or $51,600 per infant born preterm.[4] These figures will continue to rise with both the escalating cost of health care and the rising rate of preterm delivery.

Piecuch et al.[21] reported data for a cohort of 138 nonanomalous infants delivered between 24 and 26 weeks' gestation between 1990 and 1994. The incidence of cerebral palsy did not differ significantly among the three groups born at 24, 25, and 26 weeks' gestation (11%, 20%, and 11%, respectively). However, the incidence of normal cognitive outcome rose with increasing gestational age at birth (28%, 47%, and 71% at 24, 25, and 26 weeks' gestation, respectively).

The EPICure study group assessed the association between extreme preterm delivery and long-term physical and mental disability in a cohort of infants delivered between 22 and 25 weeks' gestation during a 10-month period in 1995.[22] They noted rates of severe disability of

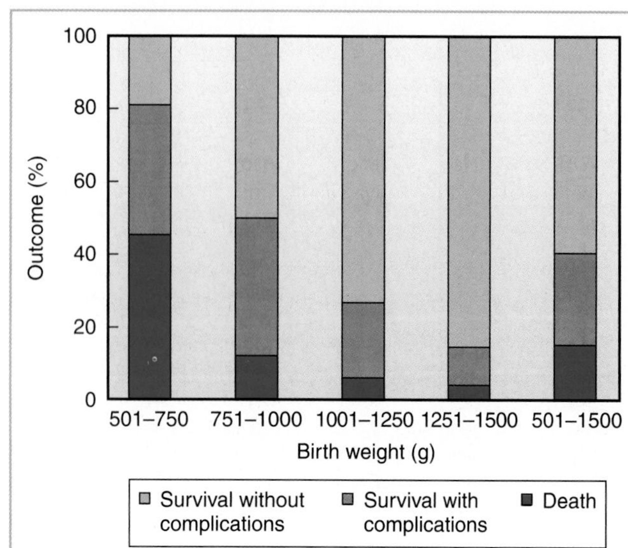

FIGURE 34-4 Short-term outcomes of very low-birth-weight infants according to birth-weight group. Complications include bronchopulmonary dysplasia, severe intraventricular hemorrhage, and necrotizing enterocolitis). (From Eichenwald EC, Stark AR. Management of outcomes of very low birth weight. N Engl J Med 2008; 358:1700-11. Copyright © 2005 Massachusetts Medical Society. All rights reserved.)

54%, 52%, and 45% among infants delivered at 23, 24, and 25 weeks' gestation, respectively. In a later cohort of infants, born between 1997 and 2002, the rates of severe disability were 33%, 21%, and 12% for infants delivered at 23, 24, and 25 weeks' gestation, respectively.[23] A 6-year follow-up to the EPICure study cohort showed persistent severe disability in 25%, 29%, and 18% of infants born at 23, 24, and 25 weeks' gestation, respectively.[24]

Hack et al.[20] monitored a cohort of ELBW infants born between 1992 and 1995 until they were 8 years old. The mean birth weight was 810 g, and gestational age at delivery was 26 weeks. Compared with a cohort of age-matched normal-birth-weight children, the ELBW group had a higher incidence of significant neurosensory impairment (16% versus 0%, respectively) and asthma (21% versus 9%). The ELBW children differed significantly from the normal-birth-weight cohort in rates of suboptimal intelligence, academic achievement, motor skills, and adaptive functioning. These data illustrate the high societal costs of supporting the long-term medical, educational, and other services required by these children.

There is some evidence that outcome is improving for these infants. Wilson-Costello et al.[19] examined outcomes for infants born between 1982 and 2002 with a birth weight between 500 and 999 g. The rate of survival to 20 months of age rose significantly during this time (Table 34-2). Significant changes in therapy included the introduction of maternal antenatal corticosteroid and neonatal exogenous surfactant administration. Neurodevelopmental outcomes at 20 months of age, including the incidence of cerebral palsy, blindness, and deafness, also improved. Of interest (and concern) was the noted lack of improvement in cognitive testing results, which the researchers were unable to explain.[19]

PRETERM LABOR

Risk Factors

Box 34-1 lists factors associated with preterm labor.[25-27] These associations do not necessarily indicate cause-and-effect relationships. Significant risk factors include a history of previous preterm delivery, non-Hispanic black race (irrespective of socioeconomic status), and multiple gestation. One of the most important risk factors is a history of previous preterm delivery, suggesting a possible genetic contribution to the etiology of this condition.

The process of normal parturition involves anatomic, physiologic, and biochemical changes that lead to (1)

TABLE 34-2 Improved Outcomes for Extremely Low-Birth-Weight Infants, 1982 to 2002*

	1982-1989 (N = 496)	1990-1999 (N = 749)	2000-2002 (N = 233)	*P* Value
Use of therapies (%):				
Antenatal corticosteroid therapy	0	41	78	<.001
Surfactant therapy	1	62	82	<.001
Outcomes (%):				
Death within 48 hr of birth	67	58	57	.06
Survival to 20 months of age	49	68	71	<.001
Cerebral palsy†	8	13	5	.01
Blindness†	5	1	1	.003
Deafness†	3	6	1	.003
Bayley mental development index (mean ± SD)	86.4 ± 20	84.0 ± 19	85.9 ± 20	.28

*Data are from extremely low-birth-weight (500 to 999 g) infants born at a single perinatal center between 1982 and 2002. Mean birth weight among the three groups ranged from 750 to 762 g, and mean gestational age from 25.5 to 25.8 weeks.

†At age 20 months.

Data from Wilson-Costello D, Friedman H, Minich N, et al. Improved neurodevelopmental outcomes for extremely low birth weight infants in 2000-2002. Pediatrics 2007; 119:37-45.

BOX 34-1 Factors Associated with Preterm Labor

Demographic Characteristics
- Non-white race
- Extremes of age (< 17 or > 35 years)
- Low socioeconomic status
- Low prepregnancy body mass index
- History of preterm delivery
- Interpregnancy interval < 6 months
- Abnormal uterine anatomy (e.g., myomas)
- Abnormal cervical anatomy
- Trauma
- Abdominal surgery during pregnancy
- Acute or chronic systemic disease

Behavioral Factors
- Physically strenuous work (controversial)
- Psychological stress (controversial)
- Tobacco use
- Substance abuse

Obstetric Factors
- Vaginal bleeding
- Infection (systemic, genital tract, periodontal)
- Cervical length/incompetent cervix
- Multiple gestation
- Assisted reproductive technologies*
- Preterm premature rupture of membranes
- Abnormal fetal placentation
- Polyhydramnios

Fetal Factors
- Genetic abnormalities
- Fetal death

*Independent of multiple gestation.

Data from references 1, 27, and 28.

greater uterine contractility, (2) cervical ripening, and (3) membrane/decidual activation.[28,29] The fetus also appears to play a role in parturition. It is hypothesized that the mature fetal hypothalamus secretes more corticotropin-releasing hormone (CRH), which in turn stimulates fetal adrenal production of adrenocorticotropic hormone (ACTH) and cortisol.[28] Preterm birth results from the pathologic activation of one or more of these components (Figure 34-5).[30] The causes of preterm birth are thought to be related to premature rupture of membranes (PROM) in 30% of cases, maternal or fetal indications for early delivery in 20% to 25% of cases, and spontaneous preterm labor without a clear etiology in 40% to 45% of cases.[31] As the understanding of the mechanism(s) for the initiation of labor at term improves, a better understanding of the various etiologies of preterm labor should also develop. It is evident that preterm labor is a syndrome with multiple causes influenced by a number of genetic, biologic, biophysical, psychosocial, and environmental factors. It is unlikely that any one mechanism underlies preterm labor and delivery.

Two emerging factors of interest are the influences of **infection** and **uterine distention** on initiation of myometrial contractility. Infection is thought to be present in up to 40% of preterm deliveries.[1] Commonly identified organisms include *Ureaplasma urealyticum*, *Bacteroides* species, *Neisseria gonorrhoeae*, *Chlamydia trachomatis*, group B streptococci, *Staphylococcus aureus*, *Treponema pallidum*, and enteropharyngeal bacteria.[32-34] Untreated acute pyelonephritis is also associated with preterm labor. Although approximately 50% of preterm deliveries occur in women with no apparent risk factors, subclinical infection may precipitate preterm labor in some of these cases.[33] Positive results of amniotic fluid cultures and products of infection (e.g., C-reactive protein[35]) are present in some patients who present with preterm labor.[1] Studies of prostaglandins, their metabolites, and cytokines suggest a biochemical mechanism for preterm labor in the presence of infection.[1]

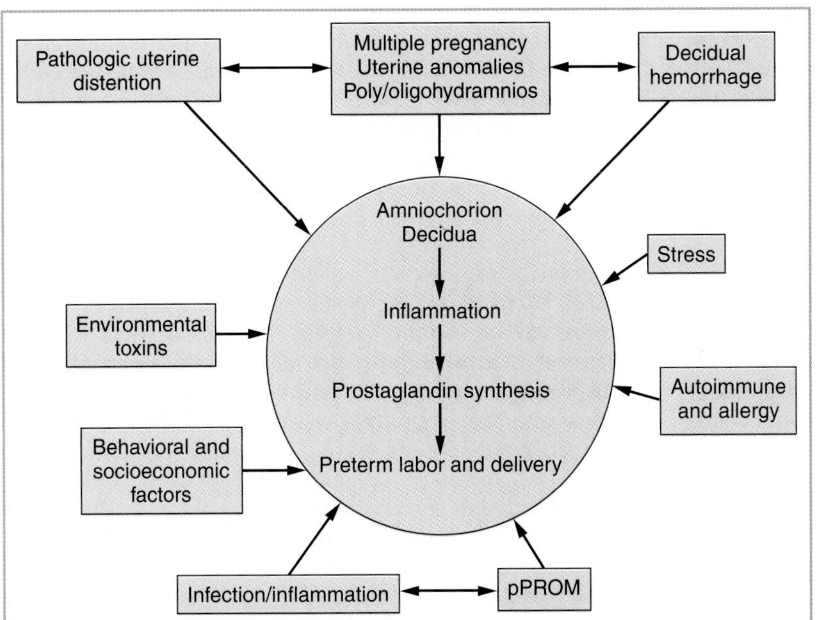

FIGURE 34-5 Major etiologic factors in preterm birth, including activation of the maternal or fetal hypothalamic-pituitary axis (stress), inflammation, decidual hemorrhage, and pathologic distention of the myometrium. The pathways are not mutually exclusive and may overlap, and they share a common biochemical pathway. pPROM, preterm premature rupture of membranes. (From Menon R. Spontaneous preterm birth, a clinical dilemma: Etiologic, pathophysiologic and genetic heterogeneities and racial disparity. Acta Obstet Gynecol Scand 2008; 87:590-600.)

A growing body of literature suggests an association between **periodontal disease** and preterm delivery,[36-38] which may be related to the association between periodontal disease and systemic infection. Prostaglandins and cytokines are produced in the presence of periodontal disease and may affect the maternal-fetal nutritional, hormonal, and immunologic systems. A 2006 systematic analysis of 25 studies demonstrated an association between periodontal disease and both preterm delivery and very preterm delivery.[36] It also suggested a relationship between treatment of periodontal disease and a reduction in preterm delivery. However, the investigators concluded that evidence supporting this association is weak and further rigorous scientific study is required.[36,37]

The past three decades have witnessed a significant rise in the incidence of **multiple gestation** (19.3 per 1000 live births in 1980 versus 33.8 per 1000 in 2005).[3] The twin birth rate has increased by 70% since 1980, and the triplet and higher-order multiple birth rate rose by over 400% between 1980 and 1998.[3] This trend is due, in part, to the significant increase in the use of **assisted reproductive technologies** (ARTs).[39] Multiple gestations account for 17% of all preterm births.[40] ART pregnancies are also associated with a substantial increase in risk for preterm delivery, even for singleton pregnancies.[41] A 2004 meta-analysis of 15 studies, which compared outcomes for 12,283 ART singleton pregnancies with those for 1.9 million spontaneously conceived singleton pregnancies, demonstrated a higher risk of preterm delivery and a higher risk of delivery of LBW, VLBW, and/or SGA infants among the ART pregnancies.[41] Placenta previa, gestational diabetes, preeclampsia, and neonatal intensive care unit admission were also more prevalent in the ART group.[41]

As many as 20% to 25% of all preterm deliveries do not follow preterm labor or preterm PROM. The obstetrician may perform elective delivery for maternal or fetal indications, such as severe preeclampsia or a nonreassuring fetal heart rate (FHR) pattern. Unfortunately, some cases of RDS are iatrogenic (i.e., the obstetrician may unnecessarily perform an elective repeat cesarean delivery in a preterm patient).

An association between maternal **obesity** and *indicated* preterm delivery has been observed.[42,43] Preterm PROM and preterm delivery in obese women are associated with an increase in neonatal mortality and may be associated with a higher risk of chorioamnionitis.[43] Given the current obesity epidemic, an ongoing increase in the absolute number of preterm births in obese pregnant women may be anticipated.

Prediction and Prevention of Preterm Labor

The ability to prevent spontaneous preterm birth necessitates the ability to identify women at risk for preterm labor and to intervene prophylactically to prevent preterm labor as well the ability to treat preterm labor once it occurs. Several methods of predicting preterm birth have been proposed, including home uterine activity monitoring, salivary estriol measurement, screening for bacterial vaginosis, fetal fibronectin screening, and cervical ultrasonography.[44]

The use of **home uterine activity monitoring** (HUAM) to identify women at risk for preterm labor has been investigated in a number of randomized controlled trials of variable quality.[44] Dyson et al.[45] randomly assigned 2422 women with risk factors for preterm labor, including multiple gestation, to weekly contact with a nurse, daily contact with a nurse, or daily contact with a nurse combined with HUAM. Daily nurse contact, with or without HUAM, did not result in better outcomes than weekly nurse contact. The American College of Obstetricians and Gynecologists (ACOG) has stated that "data are insufficient to support a benefit from HUAM in preventing preterm birth."[44]

Salivary estriol levels have been assessed as a marker for risk of preterm delivery in several studies.[46,47] In humans a surge in maternal estriol levels occurs approximately 3 weeks before delivery. Although elevated estriol levels are predictive of a higher risk for spontaneous preterm birth, the specificity is too low to make the test clinically useful.[44] Other biochemical markers of risk for preterm delivery, including cytokines, alpha-fetoprotein, CRH, and C-reactive protein, have also been investigated.[48] None has proved sufficiently sensitive when used alone to be clinically useful. Sensitivity is increased when these markers are combined.[48,49]

Fetal fibronectin (fFN) is a basement membrane glycoprotein produced by the fetal membranes. It functions as an adhesive protein of the placental membranes to the decidua.[50] fFN is normally absent from vaginal secretions from 20 weeks' gestation until near term. Detection of elevated levels of fFN is associated with an increased risk of preterm delivery. It is hypothesized that the presence of fFN is a marker of choriodecidual disruption. A study from the Maternal-Fetal Medicine Units Network documented that a positive fFN test result at 22 to 24 weeks' gestation had a sensitivity of 63% in predicting preterm labor before 28 weeks' gestation.[51] If fFN is absent (i.e., a negative result), the risk of preterm delivery within 1 or 2 weeks is less than 1%.[52] The high negative predictive value of this test may make it a useful tool to rule out impending delivery in *symptomatic* women; however, currently there is no role for the test in screening low-risk asymptomatic women.[44]

Short cervical length, as assessed by transvaginal ultrasonography, is associated with a greater risk of preterm labor (Figure 34-6).[53] In a 2006 systematic analysis, Kagan et al.[54] concluded that assessment of cervical length may be useful in *symptomatic* women in order to predict imminent delivery. However, like fFN testing and other screening tools, routine determination of cervical length in asymptomatic or low-risk patients is not recommended because of its poor positive predictive value.[44] Ultrasonographic examinations may be considered in women with historical risk factors for cervical insufficiency, beginning at 16 to 20 weeks' gestation.[55]

Bacterial vaginosis is a syndrome in which the normal vaginal bacterial milieu is disrupted and replaced by an overgrowth of certain bacteria. It is associated with an increased risk of preterm delivery.[56] Data are conflicting as to whether screening for and treating bacterial vaginosis reduces the risk of preterm delivery.[57-60] The ACOG currently does not support routine screening and treatment of bacterial vaginosis in pregnancy.[44] However, some clinicians believe that there is benefit to antibiotic treatment if used early in pregnancy in women with high-grade bacterial vaginosis.[61] On the other hand, the results of several studies suggest that metronidazole may be associated with an *increased* risk of preterm delivery.[62,63]

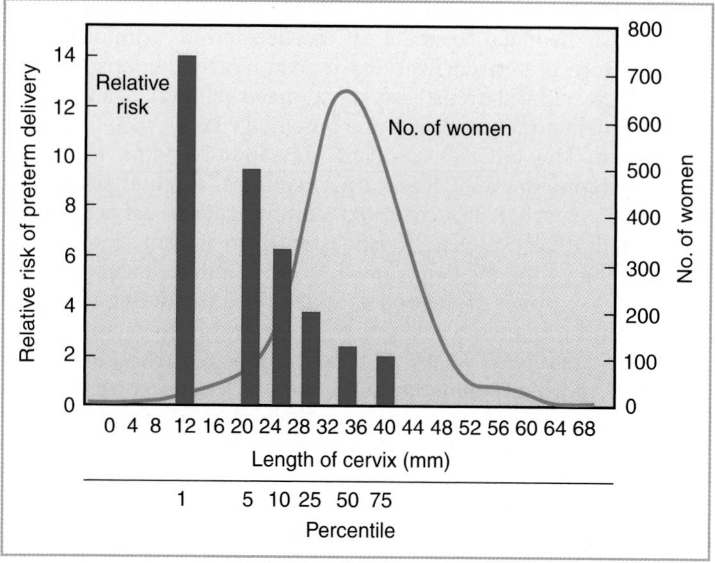

FIGURE 34-6 Relative risk of preterm delivery (before 35 weeks' gestation) as a function of cervical length at 24 weeks' gestation (*bars*) and the distribution of cervical length at 24 weeks' gestation (*solid line*). The risks among women with cervical length at or below the 1st, 5th, 10th, 25th, 50th, and 75th percentiles were compared with the risk among women with cervical length above the 75th percentile. (From Iams JD, Goldenberg RL, Meis PJ, et al. The length of the cervix and the risk of spontaneous premature delivery. N Engl J Med 1996; 334:567-72. Copyright © 2005 Massachusetts Medical Society. All rights reserved.)

PREVENTION OF PRETERM LABOR

Antenatal screening for risk factors for preterm labor and delivery is of value only if interventions are available that decrease the risk of preterm delivery and improve neonatal outcome.[44] Unfortunately, few if any interventions have been shown to definitively improve this outcome. Interventions that have been studied include detection and suppression of uterine contractions, antimicrobial therapy (as discussed earlier), prophylactic cervical cerclage (see Chapter 16), maternal nutritional supplements, reduction in maternal stress, and hormonal therapy.[28] It is not surprising that most of these simple interventions have not been shown to alter outcome, given that preterm labor is increasingly understood to be a complex syndrome with multiple, overlapping etiologies.[28]

The ACOG[55] has recommended that elective (prophylactic) **cervical cerclage** be restricted to women with a history of three or more unexplained second-trimester pregnancy losses or preterm deliveries. The results of currently available studies are inconclusive and do not support performance of cervical cerclage to treat cervical insufficiency after fetal viability (24 weeks' gestation).[55,64]

Data also do *not* support the administration of **prophylactic antibiotics** in asymptomatic women at risk for preterm labor.[65] Neither is there evidence to support the prophylactic use of **beta-adrenergic agonists** to prevent preterm labor in high-risk women.[66] In contrast, evidence suggests that **progesterone** therapy may be effective in reducing the rate of preterm birth in some patient populations. The Maternal-Fetal Medicine Units Network published a randomized controlled trial comparing prophylactic intramuscular 17-alpha-hydroxyprogesterone caproate (250 mg once a week until delivery or 36 weeks' gestation) with placebo administered to women with a history of spontaneous preterm delivery beginning at 16 to 20 weeks' gestation.[67] The risk of delivery before 37 weeks' gestation was reduced in the progesterone group (relative risk [RR], 0.66; 95% confidence interval [CI], 0.54 to 0.81). Similarly, in a study published in 2003, da Fonseca et al.[68] demonstrated a decreased risk of preterm delivery (< 34 weeks' gestation) in high-risk women randomly assigned to receive either vaginal progesterone (100 mg daily) or placebo. The authors of a systematic review of 11 randomized controlled trials (n = 2425) also concluded that progesterone was associated with a significant reduction in preterm births in women with a history of spontaneous preterm delivery.[69] However, there is currently insufficient evidence of improved neonatal outcome with the use of progesterone.[69] Additionally, the optimal type, timing, and dose of progesterone have not been determined. Studies of the potential long-term effects of this therapy on childhood development are ongoing.

Progesterone therapy has also been studied in other populations at risk for preterm delivery. It was not shown to be beneficial to women at risk for preterm delivery because of multiple gestation.[70] In one study, progesterone was associated with a lower risk of preterm delivery among women with a very short cervix who were randomly assigned to receive either progesterone or placebo.[71]

Diagnosis

Often it is difficult to determine whether a woman is in early preterm labor or in false labor. Criteria for the diagnosis of preterm labor include (1) gestational age between 20 and 37 weeks, (2) at least four documented uterine contractions in 20 minutes or eight in 60 minutes, and (3) documented change in cervical dilation or effacement, cervical dilation of 2 cm, or cervical effacement of 80% or more.[72] Several investigators have noted that the absence of fetal breathing movements (as seen during real-time ultrasonography) is predictive of imminent delivery (within 48 hours).[73]

Assessment and Therapy

Initial assessment of the patient with possible preterm labor includes physical examination, FHR monitoring, and ultrasonographic evaluation. Only 20% of women evaluated for preterm labor have preterm delivery.[74] Acute conditions associated with preterm labor should be sought, including infection and placental abruption. Maternal physical

examination may include a sterile speculum examination to exclude preterm PROM. In many women, uterine contractions cease spontaneously. In the past, clinicians assumed that intravenous hydration was a necessary component of therapy. However, there is no evidence that hydration leads to better outcome than bed rest alone in euvolemic patients.[75] Ultrasonographic evaluation is noninvasive and can be performed on admission to estimate gestational age and fetal weight. If necessary, amniocentesis can be performed to determine fetal lung maturity and to look for evidence of infection.

Once the diagnosis of preterm labor is established, the obstetrician must decide whether to begin tocolytic therapy. Tocolytic therapy for established preterm labor does not prolong pregnancy beyond 2 to 7 days.[26] In some cases, however, there are benefits to a short course of tocolytic therapy, even if the patient delivers soon thereafter. Tocolytic therapy may facilitate transfer of the patient from a small community hospital to a tertiary care facility that can provide optimal care for the preterm neonate. Moreover, a short course of tocolytic therapy may delay delivery for 24 to 48 hours, allowing maternal administration of a corticosteroid to accelerate fetal lung maturity and administration of antibiotic therapy to prevent neonatal group B streptococcal infection.

Criteria for the use of tocolytic therapy include (1) gestational age between 20 and 34 weeks, (2) reassuring fetal status, and (3) no clinical signs of infection. The potential benefits of delaying delivery of the preterm infant (i.e., decreased neonatal morbidity and mortality) must be weighed against the maternal and fetal risks (i.e., maternal and/or fetal sepsis, maternal side effects of tocolytic drugs, deterioration of a compromised fetus). Box 34-2 lists contraindications to the inhibition of labor.

Controversy continues regarding the use of tocolytic therapy in patients with preterm PROM. Historically, obstetricians have worried that tocolytic therapy might increase the risk for maternal and/or fetal infection in these patients. It also seems logical that tocolytic therapy is less effective in patients with preterm PROM. Prospective, randomized studies have shown that tocolytic therapy does not improve neonatal outcome compared with conservative expectant management in patients with preterm PROM.[76] However, Weiner et al.[77] suggested that tocolytic therapy may have some benefit in patients with preterm PROM before 28 weeks' gestation. The most recent ACOG guidelines on preterm PROM do not make a definitive recommendation for or against the use of tocolytic agents in patients with preterm PROM who are having contractions.[78]

BOX 34-2 Contraindications to Tocolytic Therapy for Preterm Labor

- Fetal death
- Fetal anomalies incompatible with life
- Nonreassuring fetal status
- Chorioamnionitis/fever of unknown origin
- Severe hemorrhage
- Severe chronic and/or pregnancy-induced hypertension

ANTENATAL ADMINISTRATION OF CORTICOSTEROIDS

The neonatal benefits of corticosteroid administration before preterm delivery have been clearly demonstrated in large clinical trials. For most maternal/fetal dyads, these benefits often outweigh the potential risks of tocolytic therapy. The NICHD Neonatal Research Network evaluated outcome for 11,718 preterm infants delivered after antenatal maternal corticosteroid administration between 1988 and 1992. Antenatal corticosteroid treatment significantly reduced the incidence of RDS, IVH, and neonatal death in all subgroups of the population studied (including male and female infants, black and white infants, and infants delivered before 30 weeks' gestation).[79] The reduction in neonatal morbidity and mortality from antenatal corticosteroid administration is additive to the reduction observed with the use of neonatal surfactant alone.[80]

Although there is little controversy about the efficacy of a single course of antenatal corticosteroids, there remains debate over the use of multiple courses of corticosteroids for women who remain undelivered 7 days after the initial dose of corticosteroids. A 2001 review[81] and a National Institutes of Health (NIH) consensus panel statement[82] did not recommend multiple courses of corticosteroids; however, both documents cited some evidence of their possible benefit. These documents also identified possible risks, including a higher incidence of neonatal infection and potentially deleterious effects on neuronal and organ growth.[81,82] A large study performed by the Maternal-Fetal Medicine Units Network randomly assigned women at risk for preterm delivery between 23 and 32 weeks' gestation to receive either a single course or repeated (weekly) courses of antenatal corticosteroids.[83] Weekly corticosteroid administration did not significantly reduce the composite primary morbidity outcome but did significantly reduce the need for neonatal surfactant, mechanical ventilation, and continuous positive airway pressure (CPAP), as well as the incidence of pneumothorax. On the other hand, weekly corticosteroid administration was associated with an increase in the delivery of SGA infants, and there was a significant reduction in birth weight in the infants whose mothers received four or more courses of corticosteroids. Follow-up of these children between ages 2 and 3 years found no differences in physical or neurocognitive outcomes in children exposed to repeated courses and those exposed to single courses of antenatal corticosteroid administration.[84] The current consensus is to limit corticosteroid therapy to a single course of betamethasone or dexamethasone when there is a significant risk of preterm delivery between 24 and 34 weeks' gestation (Table 34-3).[82]

Questions have been posed about differences in efficacy between dexamethasone and betamethasone. A well-conducted but small trial comparing the two drugs found that the rates of most adverse fetal outcomes (e.g., RDS, neonatal sepsis, necrotizing enterocolitis) were no different between the two groups, although dexamethasone was associated with a lower rate of IVH.[85]

ANTIBIOTIC THERAPY

Empiric trials of antibiotic therapy have had conflicting results in patients with preterm labor and intact membranes. The results of a large multicenter randomized controlled trial[86] and a meta-analysis[87] did *not* support the use of prophylactic antibiotic therapy in the management of

TABLE 34-3 Antenatal Corticosteroid Therapy

Drug	Dose and Route	Frequency/ Duration
Betamethasone	12 mg IM	Every 24 hr × 2
Dexamethasone	6 mg IM	Every 12 hr × 4

IM, intramuscular.

From National Institutes of Health Consensus Development Panel. Antenatal corticosteroids revisited: Repeat courses—National Institutes of Health Consensus Development Conference Statement, August 17-18, 2000. Obstet Gynecol 2001; 98:144-50.

preterm labor in patients with intact membranes. The ACOG does not recommend empiric antibiotic therapy in this population.[26]

In contrast, in patients with preterm PROM, randomized controlled trials and a meta-analysis have concluded that antimicrobial therapy prolongs pregnancy and reduces both maternal and neonatal morbidity.[88,89] The ACOG recommends a 7-day course of antimicrobial therapy with intravenous ampicillin and erythromycin (48 hours), followed by oral amoxicillin and erythromycin (5 days) for the expectant management of preterm PROM remote from term.[78]

SELECTION OF TOCOLYTIC AGENTS

Once the obstetrician has decided to begin tocolytic therapy, an appropriate agent must be selected (Table 34-4). (Each specific class of tocolytic agent is discussed in detail later in this chapter.) A number of tocolytic agents have passed in and out of favor, some because of intolerable side effects and others after the scientific community reviewed their efficacy. Ethanol is an example of a tocolytic agent that has been abandoned because of intolerable side effects. An analysis comparing the four classes of tocolytic agents currently in use (beta-adrenergic agonists, calcium entry–blocking agents, magnesium sulfate, and nonsteroidal anti-inflammatory drugs [NSAIDs]) concluded that all showed some evidence of prolongation

TABLE 34-4 Tocolytic Drugs for Preterm Labor

Drug	Contraindications	Maternal Side Effects	Fetal/Neonatal Side Effects
Calcium entry–blocking agents	Cardiac disease Renal disease (use with caution) Maternal hypotension Concomitant magnesium sulfate therapy	Transient hypotension, flushing, headache, dizziness, nausea	None identified
Cyclooxygenase inhibitors (NSAIDs)	Significant renal or hepatic impairment Active peptic ulcer disease Coagulation disorders or thrombocytopenia NSAID-sensitive asthma Other NSAID sensitivities	Nausea, heartburn	Constriction of the ductus arteriosus, pulmonary hypertension, reversible renal dysfunction (leading to oligohydramnios), IVH,* hyperbilirubinemia, necrotizing enterocolitis*
Beta-adrenergic receptor agonists	Cardiac dysrhythmias Poorly controlled thyroid disease Poorly controlled diabetes mellitus	*Cardiopulmonary*: dysrhythmias, pulmonary edema, myocardial ischemia, hypotension, tachycardia *Metabolic*: hyperglycemia, hyperinsulinemia, hypokalemia, antidiuresis, altered thyroid function *Other*: tremor, palpitations, nervousness, nausea/vomiting, fever, hallucinations	*Fetal*: tachycardia, hyperinsulinemia, hyperglycemia, myocardial and septal hypertrophy, myocardial ischemia *Neonatal*: tachycardia, hypoglycemia, hypocalcemia, hyperbilirubinemia, hypotension, IVH
Magnesium sulfate	Myasthenia gravis Myotonic dystrophy	Flushing, lethargy, headache, muscle weakness, diplopia, dry mouth, pulmonary edema, cardiac arrest	Lethargy, hypotonia, respiratory depression, demineralization (prolonged use)

NSAIDs, nonsteroidal anti-inflammatory drugs; IVH, intraventricular hemorrhage.

*Data are conflicting as to whether cyclooxygenase inhibitors increase risk.

Modified from Hearne AE, Nagey DA. Therapeutic agents in preterm labor: Tocolytic agents. Clin Obstet Gynecol 2000; 43:787-801.

of pregnancy, but the analysis found no evidence of a beneficial effect on neonatal morbidity or mortality.[90] Although controversial, a more recent analysis suggests that magnesium sulfate is not efficacious and may cause harm.[91] No study has demonstrated superiority of one agent over another, but beta-adrenergic agonists appear to pose the greatest risk of harm to the mother.[90]

PHYSIOLOGY OF UTERINE CONTRACTIONS

The contractile elements in myometrial smooth muscle consist of thick (myosin) and thin (actin) filaments that interact and slide past one another, generating the contractile force for uterine contractions. The myometrium has pacemaker cells with spontaneous contractile ability, which spread activity throughout the rest of the uterus by means of gap junctions between myometrial cells. Myometrial contractions are preceded by a rise in intracellular calcium concentration through the influx of calcium across the sarcolemma and/or release from internal stores such as the sarcoplasmic reticulum. Hormones and neurotransmitters may play a role in the regulation of uterine activity by causing agonist-induced entry of calcium or other ions by means of receptor-controlled channels and the release of calcium from internal stores.[92]

The rise in intracellular calcium results in the formation of a complex between calcium and calmodulin (a regulatory enzyme), which activates myosin light-chain kinase (MLCK). Activated MLCK then phosphorylates the light-chain subunit of myosin, allowing actin to bind to myosin and activate myosin adenosine triphosphatase. Adenosine triphosphate (ATP) is then hydrolyzed, and muscle shortening or contraction results. Relaxation of smooth muscle results from a reduction in the intracellular calcium concentration and/or dephosphorylation of the myosin light chain by myosin light-chain phosphatase. Increases in intracellular cyclic adenosine monophosphate (cAMP) also can result in muscle relaxation by two mechanisms, (1) activation of a cAMP-dependent protein kinase, which decreases the activity of MLCK; and (2) a reduction of the intracellular calcium concentration.

The control of labor and the processes for signaling its onset are complex and incompletely understood. During pregnancy, the uterus remains in a state of functional quiescence as a result of the activity of various inhibitors, including progesterone, prostacyclin, relaxin, nitric oxide, parathyroid hormone–related peptide, CRH, human placental lactogen, calcitonin gene–related peptide, adrenomedullin, and vasoactive intestinal peptide (Figure 34-7).[34] Before term the uterus goes through an activation phase in response to uterotropins, including estrogen. This activation phase is characterized by (1) greater expression of a series of contraction-associated proteins (including myometrial receptors for prostaglandins and oxytocin), (2) activation of certain ion channels, and (3) an increase in connexin-43 concentration. Once activated the uterus can be stimulated to contract by the action of uterotonins such as oxytocin and prostaglandins E_2 and $F_{2\alpha}$. A parturition cascade likely removes the mechanisms that have maintained uterine quiescence and recruits factors that promote uterine activity.

Once the uterus has been "activated," endocrine, paracrine, and autocrine factors from the fetoplacental unit initiate a change in the pattern of uterine activity from irregular to regular contractions. Evidence from animal

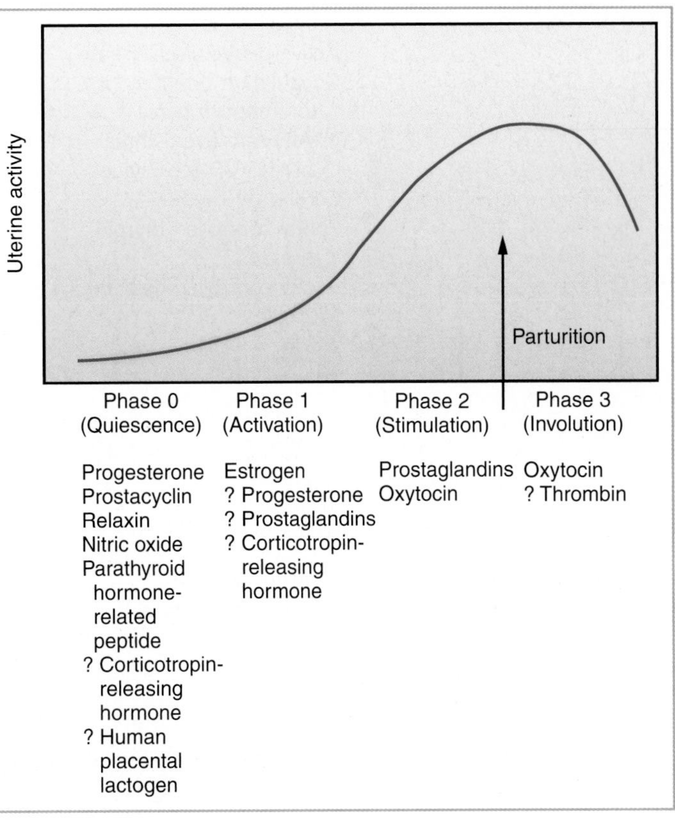

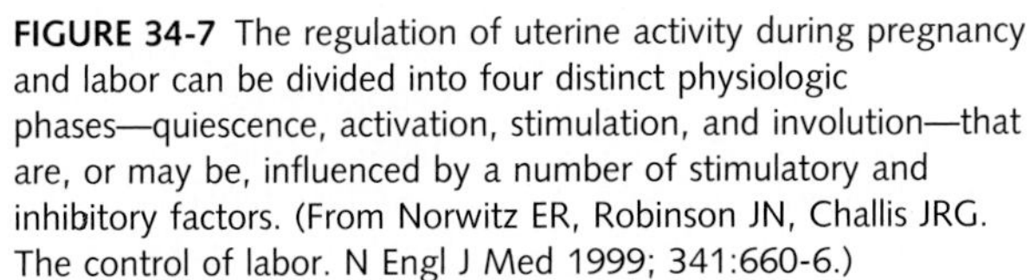

FIGURE 34-7 The regulation of uterine activity during pregnancy and labor can be divided into four distinct physiologic phases—quiescence, activation, stimulation, and involution—that are, or may be, influenced by a number of stimulatory and inhibitory factors. (From Norwitz ER, Robinson JN, Challis JRG. The control of labor. N Engl J Med 1999; 341:660-6.)

models suggests that the fetus may coordinate this change in activity through (1) its influence on the production of placental steroid hormones, (2) mechanical distention of the uterus, and (3) secretion of neurohypophyseal hormones and other stimulators of prostaglandin synthesis. The final common pathway for labor in all species is thought to be the activation of the fetal hypothalamic-pituitary-adrenal axis.[34] Of interest, however, is the observation that spontaneous labor occurs in women with an anencephalic fetus (with no residual pituitary/adrenal function), suggesting that intact neurohypophyseal function is not a prerequisite for the onset of human labor.[93]

Preterm labor may result from a loss of inhibitory factors on uterine quiescence or may represent a short-circuiting of the normal parturition cascade through the overproduction of a critical factor. As the understanding of the physiology of uterine activity increases, the approach to both predicting and treating preterm labor will become more focused. Multimodal therapy may become a standard, given that evidence now suggests that labor is initiated by the interaction of multiple factors.

Significant attention has focused on the role of progesterone in parturition. In nonhuman mammals, the onset of labor is associated with progesterone withdrawal.[93] Although the understanding of its role in human labor remains incomplete, a number of isoforms of the progesterone receptor (PGR) have been identified. One isoform, PGR-B may play a role in quiescence, whereas PGR-A may act to initiate functional progesterone withdrawal. PGR-A receptors are increasingly expressed with the onset of labor. In concert with the increase in PGR-A relative to PGR-B, an increase in estrogen receptor transcripts is observed. This change may lead to an increase in estrogen responsiveness. A third isoform, PGR-C, may also contribute to antagonism of uterine quiescence. Through a complex interplay of co-regulators such as cAMP, progesterone receptors seem to be responsible for both uterine quiescence and the stimulation of the onset of labor.[93]

Gap junctions facilitate the propagation of electrical impulses and movement of small molecules between cells. Gap junction protein alpha-1 (GJA1, or connexin-43) is one of the main protein components of myometrial gap junctions. The appearance of gap junctions in myometrium is thought to herald the onset of labor.[93] GJA1 expression is stimulated by estradiol and is inhibited by progesterone. Microarray studies of human myometrium (i.e., preterm myometrium, term myometrium not in labor, term myometrium in labor) have added to the knowledge of the genetic modulation that occurs during pregnancy and labor.[94] Differential expression of 118 genes has been identified. A process of remodeling and maturation of the uterus, and the differential expression of the genes that regulate this process, are evident throughout gestation. Further work is needed to fully elucidate the signaling pathways that contribute to human labor.[94]

EFFICACY OF TOCOLYTIC THERAPY

There is general consensus that tocolytic therapy for the treatment of preterm labor offers only limited benefit and does not reduce the rate of preterm birth.[26] Meta-analysis suggests that **calcium entry–blocking agents** such as nifedipine are as efficacious as beta-adrenergic agonists, with fewer maternal and fetal side effects.[95] However, nifedipine has not been compared with placebo. The mechanism of action is thought to be inhibition of voltage-dependent calcium channels, which results in decreased calcium influx into smooth muscle cells, as well as decreased release of intracellular calcium stores into the myoplasm.

The **beta-adrenergic receptor agonists** (e.g., ritodrine, terbutaline) have been widely used as tocolytic agents for many years but are falling out of favor. Ritodrine is no longer marketed in the United States. Beta-adrenergic agonists relax smooth muscle via $beta_2$-adrenergic receptor stimulation. A 2004 meta-analysis included 17 studies, 11 of which compared beta-adrenergic agonists with placebo.[96] Use of beta-adrenergic agonists reduced the number of women who delivered within 48 hours, but there was no decrease in the number of births within 7 days or in perinatal death or neonatal morbidity. Tocolysis was significantly associated with adverse maternal side effects (see Table 34-4). The authors concluded that there were too few data to support the use of any one beta-adrenergic agonist over the others. Other tocolytic agents (e.g., nifedipine, oxytocin antagonists) are equally efficacious with fewer side effects.[95,97]

Prostaglandins are mediators in the final pathways of uterine contraction. They increase intracellular calcium concentrations, increase activation of MLCK, and promote gap junction formation.[28] A 2005 meta-analysis of 13 trials found that **cyclooxygenase inhibition** results in a decreased rate of preterm delivery.[98] The nonselective cyclooxygenase inhibitor indomethacin has been most often studied. Serious maternal side effects are uncommon, but data are inadequate for assessment of this agent's fetal safety. Fetal concerns include a possible risk of constriction of the ductus arteriosus, oligohydramnios (due to renal dysfunction), and pulmonary hypertension.

The **oxytocin receptor antagonist** atosiban has received attention as a tocolytic agent. Although available in Europe, the drug was not approved by the U.S. Food and Drug Administration because of a higher rate of fetal deaths in the atosiban arm of a randomized controlled trial.[99] However, this finding was likely due to an imbalance in the number of women less than 26 weeks' gestation who were randomly assigned to receive atosiban. A 2005 meta-analysis concluded that atosiban did not achieve a lower rate of preterm birth than placebo or beta-adrenergic agonists. In contrast, several small, randomized controlled trials comparing atosiban with nifedipine have suggested that the drugs are equally efficacious for acute tocolysis.[100,101]

Magnesium sulfate has been used in the past as a tocolytic agent. A 2002 meta-analysis of nine high-quality randomized controlled trials that compared magnesium with placebo concluded that magnesium is ineffective in delaying or preventing preterm birth.[91]

The **nitric oxide donor** nitroglycerin has also been studied. A meta-analysis suggested that nitroglycerin does not delay delivery or improve neonatal outcome in comparison with placebo or other tocolytic agents.[102]

In summary, there is no clear "first-line" tocolytic drug.[26] Combining tocolytics increases the risk of side effects and is not routinely recommended. There is no evidence that maintenance treatment with tocolytic agents, after completion of acute treatment, alters outcome.[26]

THE PRETERM INFANT

Physiology

The healthy term fetus tolerates the stress of labor and delivery well. The preterm fetus (especially if less than 30 weeks' gestation or less than 1500 g in weight) is physiologically less well adapted to withstand this stress.[103] Some (but not all) studies have suggested that the incidence of intrapartum acidosis and asphyxia is greater in the preterm fetus than in the mature fetus.[104] The preterm fetus has lower hemoglobin concentration and oxygen-carrying capacity than a term fetus.[103] Of interest, these characteristics do not result in higher risk for intrapartum fetal neurologic injury.

Short-term problems associated with VLBW infants include RDS, bronchopulmonary dysplasia, hyperbilirubinemia, necrotizing enterocolitis, IVH, perinatal infection, retinopathy of prematurity, patent ductus arteriosus, pulmonary hypertension, water and electrolyte imbalances, acid-base disturbances, anemia, and hypoglycemia.[2] Long-term problems include bronchopulmonary dysplasia, reactive airway disease, failure to thrive, cerebral palsy, neurodevelopmental delay, hearing loss, blindness, pulmonary hypertension, hypertension as an adult, and impaired glucose regulation.[2] Progress in medical care has contributed to greater survival of preterm infants; however, disability in survivors remains high.

Method of Delivery

The ideal method of delivery for the preterm infant (especially the VLBW infant) remains controversial. Some studies have suggested that the preterm fetus is at higher risk for acidosis during labor and delivery,[104] and the preterm infant is at higher risk for IVH. Therefore obstetric management includes FHR monitoring and efforts to minimize trauma during delivery.

Evidence does not support a conclusion that routine cesarean delivery of VLBW infants improves outcome. Malloy et al.[105] analyzed birth and death certificate information from Missouri for the years 1980 to 1984. The cesarean delivery rate for VLBW infants (500 to 1499 g) rose from 24% to 44%. During the same period, the cesarean delivery rate increased from 21% to 26% for infants weighing 1500 to 2499 g and from 14% to 18% for infants weighing 2500 g or more. The first-day death rates were significantly higher among the smallest infants (weighing 500 to 749 g) that were delivered vaginally than among those delivered by cesarean (59% and 33%, respectively). However, the mortality rates for the two methods of delivery for these infants did not differ after the first 6 days of life. There was no association between the method of delivery and first-day death rates for infants weighing between 750 and 1500 g. The investigators concluded that the use of cesarean delivery did not improve overall survival for VLBW infants.

Malloy et al.[106] later reviewed the incidence of IVH and neonatal mortality in 1765 VLBW infants admitted to seven neonatal intensive care units between 1987 and 1988. After adjusting the data for gestational age and other maternal and fetal factors, these investigators concluded that cesarean delivery did not lower the risk of either mortality or IVH for infants who weighed less than 1500 g at birth. A systematic review of six randomized controlled trials comparing elective with selective cesarean delivery for preterm infants (n = 122) found no difference in outcomes between the groups, although the confidence intervals were wide because of the small number of patients involved in the analysis.[107] A retrospective analysis of 2466 VLBW preterm births in the state of Washington between 1994 and 2003 was unable to demonstrate any benefit of cesarean delivery for improving survival.[108] A modest diminution in the odds of IVH was noted in the cesarean delivery group.

Preterm cesarean delivery may increase maternal risk in subsequent pregnancies. In an observational study that involved 26,454 women with previous cesarean delivery, the Maternal-Fetal Medicine Units Network noted that women with a prior *preterm* cesarean delivery were at higher risk for uterine rupture than women with a prior *term* cesarean delivery (odds ratio, 1.6; 95% CI, 1.01 to 2.50; $P = .043$).[109]

Most obstetricians perform cesarean delivery for the delivery of VLBW infants with a breech presentation, although better outcomes have not been well documented.[105,106,110,111] Head entrapment behind an incompletely dilated cervix is more common in preterm fetuses with a breech presentation because the head is somewhat larger than the wedge formed by the buttocks and thighs. Similarly, cesarean delivery has been recommended for LBW twins in whom twin A has a nonvertex presentation, although there are no prospective, controlled studies to support this practice.[112] The management of preterm twins (when twin A is vertex and twin B is nonvertex) is more controversial; there are no good prospective data. On the basis of extensive observational data, however, Chervenak et al.[112] recommended that external cephalic version or total breech extraction of twin B is a reasonable plan if the estimated fetal weight is more than 2000 g. However, if the estimated fetal weight is less than 2000 g, the authors recommended that cesarean delivery be performed after failed external version. Given that the rate of planned vaginal delivery of a singleton fetus with a breech presentation (either preterm or at term) has markedly declined in the United States (see Chapter 35), it is likely that most preterm breech infants, whether singletons or multiples, will be delivered by cesarean.

The survival rate remains low for infants with a birth weight of 500 to 750 g. In these cases, obstetricians must decide whether to recommend cesarean delivery in cases of nonreassuring fetal status or breech presentation. The neonatologist is frequently asked to speak with the patient about the infant's risk of morbidity and mortality so that the patient can make an informed decision about the method of delivery. Regardless of the mode of delivery, if resuscitation is planned, additional support personnel (ideally a neonatologist and a neonatal resuscitation team) should be prepared and present for the delivery.

Ethical Issues

The antenatal maternal administration of corticosteroids, the application of advanced neonatal ventilation techniques, the use of neonatal surfactant therapy, and the use of extracorporeal membrane oxygenation (ECMO) have reduced mortality and morbidity for preterm neonates. A clear association exists between the likelihood of survival and advanced gestational age; however, the relationship is more difficult to define at the lower extremes of extrauterine viability. Further, questions remain regarding the risk of long-term morbidity for these infants. These uncertainties often lead to controversy about the decision to resuscitate (or not resuscitate) a preterm infant. Obstetricians tend to be more pessimistic than neonatologists regarding the prognosis for these infants. Obstetricians may underestimate survival rates for neonates born between 23 and 29 weeks' gestation by as much as 25% to 30%.[113] This situation is further complicated by the lack of precision in estimation of gestational age and birth weight,[114] as well as by concerns about long-term neurologic and neurodevelopmental abnormalities in infants with a birth weight less than 1000 g.[21]

Parents, obstetricians, and neonatologists must be involved in the decision-making process. For an infant of 25 weeks' or more gestation with no known anomalies, the decision to offer full resuscitation and support is typically straightforward. Controversy and conflict may arise in decisions about infants born at 22 to 24 weeks' gestation. Many ethicists recommend assessment of the "best interests" of the patient. However, it is often difficult to define the "best interests" of the patient in these situations. Some even argue (incorrectly in our view) that ELBW infants should not be granted personhood because they may lack advanced brain function. Other questions relate to the extent of acceptable pain and suffering for these newborn infants as well as the definition of an "acceptable" outcome. However, most ethicists agree that it is preferable to withdraw therapy, when appropriate, rather than withhold it.

Anesthesia providers may find themselves in the middle of these ethical dilemmas if they are practicing in a location wherein the anesthesia provider is responsible for neonatal resuscitation. Unfortunately no firm guidelines exist—but some basic principles can be applied. First, the parents have a critical role in the decision-making process. Second, it is difficult to make decisions about withholding therapy without adequate data. Third, discussion of these issues should be held before delivery, not in the moment of crisis. The ACOG[110] has published general recommendations about the care of infants on the threshold of viability but has not made specific recommendations for neonatal resuscitation on the basis of gestational age. However, the Canadian Paediatric Society and the Society of Obstetricians and Gynaecologists of Canada have issued relatively specific recommendations.[115] For an infant at 22 to 23 weeks' gestation, they suggest that resuscitation efforts be initiated only if uncertainty about gestational age exists or fully informed parents request that resuscitation be performed. For an infant at 23 to 24 weeks' gestation, resuscitation can be offered as long as parents are informed of the need to reassess this decision at critical intervals and possibly withdraw therapy. For an infant at 25 weeks' gestation, they recommend full resuscitation in the absence of lethal anomalies.[115] The American Heart Association and the American Academy of Pediatrics have stated that, with few exceptions, resuscitation is not indicated if the infant is delivered at less than 23 completed weeks' gestation or with a weight less than 400 g.[116] Revised neonatal resuscitation guidelines address the ethical issues of noninitiation or discontinuation of resuscitation in the delivery room.[23,116] In some cases, a trial of therapy may be appropriate, but such a trial does not always mandate continued support.

Fetal Heart Rate Monitoring

Most obstetricians use continuous electronic FHR monitoring once preterm labor becomes established. Preterm gestation may complicate the interpretation of FHR patterns. Preterm fetuses may have decreased variability, and the baseline FHR is higher in preterm fetuses (especially those at less than 34 weeks' gestation) than in term fetuses.[117] The presence of chorioamnionitis or the use of beta-adrenergic agonist therapy also can confound the interpretation of the FHR tracing.

The value of continuous electronic FHR monitoring over intermittent auscultation of the FHR remains controversial. Luthy et al.[118] performed a randomized trial comparing continuous electronic FHR monitoring (with selective fetal blood gas assessment) with periodic auscultation of the FHR during preterm labor in women with fetuses weighing between 700 and 1750 g. There was no significant difference between groups in the incidence of cesarean delivery, low 5-minute Apgar scores, intrapartum acidosis, intracranial hemorrhage, or perinatal death. At 18 months of age, the incidence of cerebral palsy was significantly higher in the electronic FHR group than in the intermittent auscultation group (20% versus 8%, respectively).[119]

ANESTHETIC MANAGEMENT

Anesthesia providers often participate in the care of preterm parturients. Many of these women request neuraxial analgesia for labor and vaginal delivery. Such patients also have a higher incidence of cesarean delivery, often in situations of nonreassuring fetal status, which necessitates urgent administration of anesthesia.

Conventional wisdom holds that the preterm fetus is more vulnerable than the term fetus to the depressant effects of analgesic and anesthetic drugs for the following reasons: (1) less protein available for drug binding, leading to a reduction in protein-drug affinity; (2) higher levels of bilirubin, which may compete with the drug for protein binding; (3) greater drug access to the central nervous system (CNS) because of the presence of an incomplete blood-brain barrier; (4) decreased ability to metabolize and excrete drugs; and (5) a higher incidence of acidosis during labor and delivery.[104,120] However, few controlled studies have documented the maternal and fetal pharmacokinetics and pharmacodynamics of anesthetic agents throughout gestation. The preterm fetus may be less vulnerable to the depressant effects of local anesthetics than originally thought. The human fetal liver cytochrome P-450 system is present as early as the 14th week of gestation and has the capability to oxidize several drugs.[121,122]

Teramo et al.[123] noted that the amount of lidocaine necessary to produce seizure activity in preterm fetal lambs was greater than that required in older fetal lambs. These investigators also observed that the cardiovascular response to lidocaine (i.e., increases in blood pressure and heart rate) was less severe in fetuses with a younger gestational age. Pedersen et al.[124] evaluated the effects of gestational age on the pharmacokinetics and pharmacodynamics of lidocaine in gravid ewes and fetal lambs. They studied two groups of animals, preterm (119 ± 1 days' gestation or 0.8 of term pregnancy) and near-term (138 ± 1 days' gestation or 0.95 of term pregnancy). They administered an intravenous infusion of lidocaine to obtain a maternal steady-state plasma concentration of 2 μg/mL. Transplacental transfer of lidocaine did not adversely affect fetal cardiac output, organ blood flow, or blood gas and acid-base measurements in either group. Tissue uptake of lidocaine was similar in the two groups of fetal lambs, except that it was greater in the lungs and liver of the term fetuses. The investigators concluded that there was no significant difference in the pharmacokinetics and pharmacodynamics of lidocaine between the two gestational ages studied.[124]

Smedstad et al.[125] also concluded that there was no difference in fetal blood pressure, heart rate, or blood gas measurements in response to maternal intravenous infusion of lidocaine or bupivacaine between early preterm (119 days' gestation) and late preterm (132 days' gestation) fetal lambs. In addition, the plasma concentrations of bupivacaine and lidocaine and the fetal-to-maternal ratios of both drugs were similar in the two groups of fetuses.

None of these studies evaluated the effects of anesthetic agents on the acidotic preterm fetus. Asphyxia may increase the risk of adverse effects by causing the following changes in the fetal environment: (1) reduced plasma protein-binding capacity (which increases the proportion of free drug available)[126]; (2) greater maternal-fetal hydrogen ion difference, which causes "ion trapping" of weak bases (e.g., amide local anesthetics, opioids) on the fetal side of the circulation[127]; (3) greater blood-brain barrier permeability[128]; and (4) enhanced susceptibility to the myocardial depressant effects of local anesthetics.[129,130]

Morishima et al.[129] subjected a group of preterm fetal lambs (0.8 of term gestation) to asphyxia by causing partial occlusion of the umbilical cord. They subsequently administered either lidocaine or saline-control intravenously to the gravid ewes for 180 minutes. The maternal and fetal steady-state plasma lidocaine concentrations were 2.32 ± 0.12 and 1.23 ± 0.17 μg/mL, respectively. (These concentrations are similar to those that occur during epidural anesthesia in humans.) Umbilical cord occlusion resulted in the typical fetal compensatory response to hypoxia (i.e., decreased FHR and increased blood flow to the fetal brain, heart, and adrenal glands). Maternal administration of saline-control did not result in additional deterioration of the fetus. However, maternal administration of lidocaine resulted in a significant increase in Pa_{CO_2}, and decreases in pH, mean arterial pressure (MAP), and blood flow to the brain, myocardium, and adrenal glands. Thus lidocaine attenuated the normal fetal compensatory response to asphyxia.

In an earlier study, the same investigators observed that lidocaine did not affect the fetal compensatory response to asphyxia in term fetuses.[130] They concluded that "the immature fetus loses its cardiovascular adaptation to asphyxia when exposed to clinically acceptable plasma concentrations of lidocaine obtained transplacentally from the mother."[130] Limitations of this study include (1) a failure to compare the fetal response to lidocaine with the response to other anesthetic, analgesic, or sedative drugs and (2) consideration of only the effects of a steady-state concentration of lidocaine in the presence of asphyxia. That is, the investigators did not evaluate the potential benefits derived from epidural anesthesia, such as reduced maternal concentrations of catecholamines and the ability of epidural anesthesia to facilitate a controlled, atraumatic delivery of the preterm infant.

Bupivacaine has a low fetal-to-maternal plasma concentration ratio because of its relatively high (96%) maternal protein binding; therefore the potential for fetal toxicity seems minimal.[120] Studies of the effects of bupivacaine on the compensatory response to asphyxia in the preterm fetal lamb have demonstrated results similar to those seen with lidocaine. Santos et al.[131] observed that bupivacaine abolished the compensatory increase in blood flow to vital organs in asphyxiated preterm fetal lambs. However, bupivacaine did not affect fetal heart rate, blood pressure, or acid-base measurements. The investigators suggested that these changes were less severe than those seen with lidocaine in their earlier study.[129,131]

Ropivacaine and bupivacaine have almost identical dissociation constants (pK_B of 8.0 and 8.2, respectively), but ropivacaine's protein binding is slightly less than that for bupivacaine (92% versus 96%, respectively), and it is substantially less lipid soluble than bupivacaine.[132] These differences may affect maternal and fetal free plasma concentrations of drug. Investigators have documented higher maternal and fetal plasma concentrations with ropivacaine than with bupivacaine.[133,134] Studies suggest that ropivacaine is less cardiotoxic than bupivacaine. However, no study has evaluated the effect of ropivacaine on the fetal compensatory response to hypoxia.

2-Chloroprocaine also is a good choice of local anesthetic in preterm patients because it is rapidly metabolized in both the maternal plasma and fetal plasma.[135] Further, placental transfer of 2-chloroprocaine is not increased by fetal acidosis.[136]

Vaginal Delivery

Specific anesthetic requirements for vaginal delivery of the preterm infant include (1) inhibition of inappropriate expulsive efforts before complete cervical dilation, especially with a breech presentation; (2) avoidance of precipitous delivery, which can result in rapid decompression of the infant's head and increase the risk of intracranial hemorrhage; and (3) provision of a relaxed pelvic floor and perineum to facilitate a smooth, controlled delivery of the infant's head, which is especially important with a breech delivery. There is no evidence that "prophylactic" forceps delivery to protect the infant's head results in a better outcome.[28]

Neither pudendal nerve block nor local infiltration of the perineum provides profound relaxation of the levator ani and bulbocavernosus muscles. Continuous lumbar epidural analgesia is the technique of choice during labor and vaginal delivery. If delivery appears imminent, a low level of spinal anesthesia ("saddle block") may be a good choice. Epidural analgesia also decreases the likelihood of premature maternal expulsive efforts and precipitous delivery of the vulnerable, preterm fetal head. In cases of preterm fetal breech presentation, it is essential that the mother not push the breech fetus through a partially dilated cervix.

Epidural analgesia decreases maternal concentrations of catecholamines, and in some patients, it may improve uteroplacental perfusion in the absence of hypotension.[137] No prospective, controlled studies have evaluated the effect of epidural anesthesia on outcome for the preterm infant; however, many obstetricians consider neuraxial analgesia an essential component of an optimal preterm delivery. One retrospective multicenter study compared outcome for preterm infants whose mothers received anesthesia with that for preterm infants whose mothers received no anesthesia.[138] The perinatal death rate for preterm infants was 446 per 1000 when no anesthesia was given, compared with 157 per 1000 when anesthesia was used.

The timing of the administration of neuraxial analgesia in preterm parturients may be problematic for several reasons. First, women in preterm labor often have a prolonged latent phase of labor because of the administration of tocolytic agents for several hours or days. Second, when tocolysis fails, the patient may be in advanced labor, and delivery may be imminent. Third, a cervical dilation of only 6 or 7 cm (rather than 10 cm) may be sufficient to allow delivery of the small preterm infant. We recommend early placement of an epidural catheter in patients at high risk for failure of tocolysis. In some cases, it may be appropriate to establish epidural analgesia while the obstetrician continues efforts to stop labor. In these cases, preterm labor may cease after administration of epidural analgesia, and the anesthesia provider may allow analgesia to regress and even remove the catheter. We consider it preferable to have an occasional patient cease preterm labor after administration of epidural analgesia rather than to have too many patients deliver precipitously without adequate anesthesia. Moreover, early induction of epidural analgesia facilitates the use of neuraxial anesthesia for emergency cesarean delivery. Although the obstetrician may attempt tocolysis, there is a high likelihood that tocolysis will fail and that the patient will require urgent or emergency delivery.

Combined spinal-epidural (CSE) analgesia has gained popularity. For preterm patients, the advantages of CSE analgesia include its rapid onset and a reduction in the total dose of drug(s) needed to provide analgesia. However, these advantages should be weighed against the disadvantages of CSE analgesia. Some studies suggest that there is a higher incidence of transient fetal bradycardia after intrathecal opioid administration (see Chapter 23). This bradycardia does not seem to increase the overall risk of adverse outcome in term infants,[139] but no study has evaluated outcome in preterm infants. Further, when the CSE technique is used, there is a delay in confirmation of correct placement of the epidural catheter in the epidural space. This delay may be a problem if urgent cesarean delivery must be performed before the location and function of the epidural catheter have been confirmed. Finally, some investigators have expressed concern that CSE analgesia is associated with an increased incidence of meningitis.[140] The published reports of meningitis following CSE analgesia may represent publication bias resulting from the identification of complications associated with a relatively new technique. Nonetheless, given the association between infection (e.g., chorioamnionitis) and preterm labor, some anesthesia providers worry that use of the CSE technique may result in an increased risk of meningitis in preterm patients. At present, this concern represents speculation.

Cesarean Delivery

Administration of general anesthesia is similar to that for parturients at term (see Chapter 26). Most anesthetic agents that are used for induction and maintenance of general anesthesia cross the placenta and may further depress the already compromised preterm infant. If cesarean delivery is necessary, conventional wisdom holds that it is preferable to give either epidural anesthesia or spinal anesthesia to avoid the depressant effects of agents given for general anesthesia. Rolbin et al.[141] observed that preterm infants exposed to epidural anesthesia for cesarean delivery had higher 1- and 5-minute Apgar scores than similar infants exposed to general anesthesia. However, some cases of dire maternal distress or fetal bradycardia require the administration of general anesthesia.

Many have considered the maternal administration of supplemental oxygen during cesarean delivery essential, regardless of the choice of anesthetic technique. Recent studies, however, have questioned this practice. Fetal or neonatal hyperoxia may lead to production of oxygen free radicals that ultimately may result in neuronal damage.[142] Investigators have not been able to demonstrate any clear improvement in neonatal outcome with supplemental oxygen administration, even after a prolonged uterine incision-to-delivery interval, a circumstance thought to increase the risk of neonatal depression.[143,144] Currently it is not clear whether the maternal administration of supplemental oxygen adversely affects neonatal outcome.

Disturbingly, information is now emerging that exposure of the immature brain to anesthetic agents such as propofol, thiopental, ketamine, and inhalation agents can trigger significant brain cell apoptosis and cause functional learning deficits later in life.[145,146] These data were generated from studies in rodents, and times of exposure to anesthetic agents were much longer than those typical for cesarean delivery in humans. Whether clinical exposure to anesthetic agents results in significant brain cell apoptosis in humans remains to be determined (see Chapters 10 and 17).

Similar concern has focused on the risk of altered fetal cerebral blood flow during general anesthesia. In the fetal sheep model, investigators were unable to demonstrate any evidence for loss of cerebral autoregulation in the preterm fetus exposed to isoflurane despite a drop in fetal MAP and pH and an increase in fetal Pa_{CO_2} over time.[147]

INTERACTIONS BETWEEN TOCOLYTIC THERAPY AND ANESTHESIA

Indications for Anesthesia during and after Tocolytic Therapy

There are several situations in which obstetric patients require analgesia or anesthesia during or after tocolytic therapy. First, failure of tocolysis often occurs. In this case, the patient may desire pain relief during labor and vaginal delivery or may require anesthesia for cesarean delivery. Second, some obstetricians give a tocolytic agent before and during the performance of cervical cerclage. Third, some obstetricians advocate the bolus injection of a tocolytic agent to facilitate fetal resuscitation in cases of FHR abnormalities. Uteroplacental perfusion occurs during uterine diastole. Therefore relaxation of the uterus should result in better uteroplacental perfusion. Fourth, many obstetricians administer tocolysis for attempted external cephalic version, and some obstetricians and patients request neuraxial analgesia or anesthesia for this procedure.

Calcium Entry–Blocking Agents

Calcium entry–blocking drugs are capable of inhibiting uterine contractions. Among these drugs, **nifedipine** has undergone the most extensive evaluation as a tocolytic agent. Nifedipine has fewer effects on cardiac conduction, more specific effects on myometrial contractility, and less effect on serum electrolytes than the other calcium entry–blocking drugs. Maternal side effects are typically mild.[95,148] Meta-analyses of randomized comparisons of nifedipine with beta-adrenergic agonists have concluded that nifedipine is more effective than beta-adrenergic agonists in delaying delivery at least 48 hours, is more likely to result in a prolongation of pregnancy beyond 34 weeks' gestation, and is associated with fewer side effects and better neonatal outcome (i.e., fewer cases of neonatal RDS).[95,149]

Many obstetricians have suggested that calcium entry–blocking drugs should become first-line therapy in the treatment of preterm labor because of their low incidence of significant maternal and fetal side effects. However, these agents have not been compared with placebo in a randomized controlled trial. Typical nifedipine dose regimens for preterm labor are listed in Table 34-5.

MECHANISM OF ACTION

Calcium entry–blocking drugs act by blocking the aqueous voltage-dependent cell membrane channels that are selective for calcium. They also act by preventing calcium release from the sarcoplasmic reticulum. The net result is a decrease in available intracellular calcium, which inhibits MLCK activity. This inhibition leads to decreased actin-myosin interaction, which results in relaxation of smooth muscle (including myometrial smooth muscle).[150,151]

SIDE EFFECTS

Nifedipine has fewer side effects than beta-adrenergic agents. Hypotension is the most common side effect. Other side effects include headache, flushing, dizziness, and nausea.[152] Most effects are mild, but pulmonary edema[153] and myocardial infarction[154] have been reported after calcium entry–blocking agent therapy for preterm labor.

Early animal studies noted that nifedipine and nicardipine decreased uterine blood flow (UBF) and resulted in fetal hypoxemia and acidosis.[155,156] However, two clinical studies have suggested that short-term administration of nifedipine does not adversely affect the uteroplacental or fetal circulation.[157,158]

ANESTHETIC MANAGEMENT

Although nifedipine has fewer effects on cardiac conduction than some of the other calcium entry–blocking agents, it has the potential to cause vasodilation, hypotension, myocardial depression, and conduction defects when used in combination with one of the volatile halogenated anesthetic agents.[159] One report noted that administration of both nifedipine and magnesium sulfate caused neuromuscular blockade in a preeclamptic patient at 28 weeks' gestation.[160] Postpartum hemorrhage may result from postpartum uterine atony that is unresponsive to oxytocin and prostaglandin $F_{2\alpha}$.[161] It seems prudent to establish large-bore intravenous access in these patients and to ensure the ready availability of blood products.

Cyclooxygenase Inhibitors

Effective tocolytic agents that are easily administered orally or rectally, cyclooxygenase inhibitors (also known as prostaglandin synthetase inhibitors or NSAIDs) are well tolerated by the mother.[98] **Indomethacin** is the prototype cyclooxygenase inhibitor used for tocolysis. Both **sulindac** and **ketorolac** have also been evaluated and found to be effective. Ketorolac may offer the advantage of intravenous administration.[162] Sulindac is reported to have fewer fetal side effects, possibly because its active metabolite crosses the placenta less readily than the native drug.[163,164] Typical NSAID doses used for tocolysis are listed in Table 34-5.

MECHANISM OF ACTION

NSAIDs inhibit cyclooxygenase and thus prevent the synthesis of prostaglandins from the precursor, arachidonic acid. Prostaglandins E_2 and $F_{2\alpha}$ play an important role in the stimulation of uterine contractions by increasing

TABLE 34-5 Tocolytic Dose Regimens for Preterm Labor

Drug	Initiation Dose	Maintenance Dose
Nifedipine	20-30 mg PO or SL	10-20 mg every 4-6 hr
Cyclooxygenase inhibitors (NSAIDs)*:		
Indomethacin	50-100 mg PO or per rectum	25-50 mg every 4 hr
Ketorolac	60 mg IM	30 mg every 6 hr
Sulindac	200 mg PO	200 mg every 12 hr
Terbutaline†	0.25 mg SQ	0.25 mg every 20 min to 3 hr
Magnesium sulfate	4-6 g IV bolus over 20 min	2-4 g/hr continuous IV infusion

NSAIDs, nonsteroidal anti-inflammatory drugs; IV, intravenously; PO, per os (orally); SL, sublingually; IM, intramuscularly; SQ, subcutaneously.

*NSAID administration should be limited to 48 to 72 hours and restricted to gestations less than 32 weeks.

†Terbutaline is given until uterine quiescence occurs or maternal heart rate reaches 120 bpm.

Data from references 28 and 148.

intracellular calcium and activation of MLCK, and promoting gap junction formation.[28] During parturition, blood and amniotic fluid prostaglandin concentrations rise. Increased concentrations of prostaglandin metabolites have been measured in patients who present with preterm labor.[27,165]

SIDE EFFECTS

Maternal side effects from indomethacin are minimal when it is used for tocolytic therapy. Indomethacin does not alter maternal heart rate or blood pressure. The most common complaints are nausea and heartburn.[166] Inhibition of cyclooxygenase results in decreased production of thromboxane A_2 and abnormal platelet aggregation. In contrast to aspirin, which permanently inhibits cyclooxygenase and therefore inhibits platelet aggregation for the lifetime of the platelet (7 to 10 days), indomethacin and other NSAIDs reversibly inhibit cyclooxygenase; thus their effect on platelet function is only transient.[167]

Maternal administration of an NSAID may cause premature closure of the ductus arteriosus *in utero* and result in persistent fetal circulation after delivery. Indomethacin is often used to promote closure of the ductus arteriosus in the preterm neonate.[166] Moise et al.[168] used fetal echocardiography to evaluate the fetal response to short-term (less than 72 hours) indomethacin therapy. They observed evidence of transient ductal constriction in 7 of 14 fetuses between 26 and 31 weeks' gestation. Tricuspid regurgitation was also noted in three fetuses. These changes were reversed within 24 hours of discontinuation of indomethacin.

Clinical studies suggest that indomethacin is less likely to cause intrauterine closure of the ductus arteriosus at earlier gestational ages.[166,169-171] Studies suggest that adverse neonatal effects (including closure of the ductus arteriosus) are unlikely if indomethacin is used in short courses (e.g., 24 to 48 hours).[166,170,171] For example, Moise[171] retrospectively analyzed fetal echocardiograms performed in 44 patients with preterm labor or polyhydramnios who were treated with indomethacin. The frequency of ductal constriction was relatively low (approximately 5% to 10%) until 32 weeks' gestation, when it rose to approximately 50%. Vermillion et al.[170] concluded that ductal constriction can occur at any gestational age but that it is reversible with early identification followed by timely discontinuation of indomethacin therapy.

Long-term indomethacin administration may result in fetal oligohydramnios secondary to decreased fetal urine output.[148] Kirshon et al.[173] noted reduced fetal urine output after short-term[172] and long-term (15 to 28 days) maternal administration of indomethacin for tocolytic therapy. Amniotic fluid volume reaccumulated within 1 week after the discontinuation of indomethacin. Indomethacin may be used to treat polyhydramnios in selected cases. One mechanism that has been proposed to explain the decrease in fetal urine output is an enhanced antidiuretic hormone effect after inhibition of cyclooxygenase.[174] Wurtzel[175] evaluated renal function during the first 10 postnatal days in 14 preterm infants exposed to indomethacin *in utero* and in 10 control infants. This investigator found that maternal administration of indomethacin did not significantly alter neonatal renal function.

Data are conflicting as to whether maternal NSAID administration increases the risk of other adverse neonatal outcomes, including IVH and necrotizing enterocolitis. Authors of a 2005 meta-analysis concluded that maternal administration of indomethacin at less than 34 weeks' gestation did not lead to an increased risk of adverse events.[176] However, they cautioned that there was significant heterogeneity in study design that makes it difficult to draw definitive conclusions.

The current recommendation for use of cyclooxygenase inhibitors is to limit the course of therapy to less than 72 hours. This approach may delay delivery and allow maternal administration of corticosteroids to accelerate fetal lung maturity.

ANESTHETIC MANAGEMENT

The effects of indomethacin on platelet function are transient. In the past, some anesthesia providers obtained a bleeding time measurement in patients who had recently received an NSAID for tocolysis. Several large studies have demonstrated the safety of epidural and spinal anesthesia in patients receiving low-dose aspirin or one of a variety of NSAIDs.[177-179] The Second Consensus Conference on Neuraxial Anesthesia and Anticoagulation (sponsored by the American Society of Regional Anesthesia and Pain Medicine) concluded that NSAID therapy is not a contraindication to administration of neuraxial anesthesia.[180]

CYCLOOXYGENASE-2–SPECIFIC INHIBITORS

Prostaglandins and nitric oxide are intimately involved with cervical ripening. Both cyclooxygenase-1 (COX-1) and cyclooxygenase-2 (COX-2) are present in the uterus during pregnancy.[181] Although the expression of COX-1 remains constant throughout gestation, there is an exponential rise in COX-2 throughout gestation in the fetal membranes, chorion-decidua, and myometrium, especially immediately before the onset of labor.[181] Prostaglandin synthesis in fetal membranes is inhibited by COX-2–specific inhibitors, but not COX-1–specific inhibitors.

NSAIDs differ in their relative specificities for COX-1 and COX-2 inhibition. In animal models, administration of a COX-2 inhibitor was effective in delaying the onset of labor.[182] On the basis of the different roles of the COX isoforms in the ductus and kidneys, investigators hoped that COX-2–selective drugs might have a more favorable side-effect profile when used for the treatment of preterm labor.[181] Sulindac is seven times more COX-2 selective than indomethacin, and nimesulide may be even more selective for COX-2.[181] Initial studies in humans demonstrated encouraging results with the use of nimesulide for the treatment of preterm labor.[183] However, oligohydramnios was reported in 54% of 44 women treated with nimesulide between 17 and 32 weeks' gestation.[184] More disturbing have been reports of neonatal renal failure[185] and renal dysgenesis.[186] Clearly, treatment of preterm labor with COX-2–selective agents is associated with potential serious fetal side effects. Whether these are due to the COX-1 or COX-2 effects of these agents is not clear.[181]

Beta-Adrenergic Agonists

In the past **ritodrine** and **terbutaline** were commonly used beta-adrenergic tocolytic agents; however, their use has declined in the past decade. **Salbutamol** and other beta-adrenergic agents have also been studied. Ritodrine is no longer available in the United States. Maternal side effects continue to be a limiting factor in their use.[96] All beta-adrenergic tocolytic drugs have both $beta_1$-receptor and $beta_2$-receptor effects, but in different proportions. $Beta_2$ receptors are found in smooth muscle (uterus, blood vessels, bronchi, intestine, detrusor, and spleen capsule), adipose tissue, liver, skeletal muscle, pancreas, and salivary glands. Ritodrine and terbutaline are relatively selective for $beta_2$ receptors; stimulation of these receptors in the myometrium results in relaxation of uterine smooth muscle. Unfortunately, other undesired $beta_2$ effects (vasodilation, glycogenolysis) and $beta_1$ effects still occur. $Beta_1$ receptors are located predominantly in the heart and adipose tissue. $Beta_1$-receptor stimulation has clinically significant cardiovascular side effects, such as increased maternal heart rate and cardiac output.[187]

MECHANISM OF ACTION

Beta-adrenergic agents interact with $beta_2$-receptor sites on the outer membrane of uterine myometrial cells, activating the enzyme adenyl cyclase. This enzyme catalyzes the conversion of ATP to cAMP, causing a rise in the intracellular concentration of cAMP. The higher cAMP concentration decreases the available intracellular concentration of calcium and inhibits MLCK activity. This inhibition in turn decreases the interaction between actin and myosin, resulting in myometrial relaxation.[148]

TREATMENT REGIMEN

Before beginning tocolytic therapy with a beta-adrenergic agent, the obstetrician should determine baseline maternal vital signs and weight and should exclude significant cardiovascular or pulmonary disease. In the past, some physicians recommended the performance of a baseline electrocardiogram (ECG).[188] Although it seems prudent to avoid beta-adrenergic therapy in a patient with cardiovascular disease, a screening ECG rarely affects management; therefore, many obstetricians no longer obtain a baseline ECG before giving beta-adrenergic tocolytic therapy in healthy preterm patients.

If uterine activity persists, the obstetrician may substitute an alternative tocolytic agent for the beta-adrenergic agonist. Prolonged administration of a beta-adrenergic tocolytic agent is ineffective, in part because prolonged administration results in downregulation (or desensitization) of the myometrial $beta_2$ receptors.[189] There is no evidence that a continuous infusion of terbutaline alters outcome.[190]

SIDE EFFECTS

The administration of beta-adrenergic tocolytic therapy may have the following troublesome maternal side effects: (1) hypotension; (2) tachycardia, with or without cardiac arrhythmias and myocardial ischemia; (3) pulmonary edema; (4) hyperglycemia; and (5) hypokalemia.[148] The incidence of these side effects is unclear. Earlier studies reported an incidence of 2% to 9%.[191,192] However, Perry et al.[193] performed a retrospective review of outcome for 8709 patients who had received a low-dose, continuous infusion of terbutaline. These investigators noted adverse cardiopulmonary effects in only 47 of 8709 patients, an incidence of 0.54%.

Hypotension and Tachycardia

The frequency and severity of cardiovascular side effects are dose related and can be minimized by limiting the dose of the beta-adrenergic agent. Stimulation of the $beta_1$ receptors on the myocardium has direct inotropic and chronotropic effects.[188] To a lesser extent, stimulation of $beta_2$-receptor sites in the vascular beds causes vasodilation, diastolic hypotension, and a reflex compensatory increase in heart rate, stroke volume, and cardiac output. Palpitations and chest pain or tightness are common complaints during beta-adrenergic therapy. Cardiac arrhythmias, primarily supraventricular tachycardia, and myocardial ischemia have been reported.[188] ECG changes such as ST-segment depression and T-wave flattening or inversion may occur; these changes typically resolve after the discontinuation of beta-adrenergic therapy.[194] It is unclear whether these ECG changes represent myocardial ischemia.

Pulmonary Edema

Pulmonary edema is a life-threatening complication of beta-adrenergic tocolytic therapy. Earlier reports estimated that pulmonary edema occurred in as many as 5% of patients who received beta-adrenergic tocolytic therapy.[195] Later studies suggested a lower incidence of pulmonary edema during beta-adrenergic therapy.[193]

In several case reports, pulmonary edema developed within 24 to 72 hours after the start of beta-adrenergic therapy.[191,196] Earlier reports suggested an association between the concurrent use of corticosteroids (e.g., dexamethasone, betamethasone) and the development of pulmonary edema in patients receiving beta-adrenergic therapy.[191,196] However, these steroids have little mineralocorticoid activity, and pulmonary edema has occurred in patients who did not receive a corticosteroid. Philipsen et al.[197] concluded that corticosteroid therapy is not a risk factor for the development of pulmonary edema during ritodrine therapy.

The underlying mechanism for the development of pulmonary edema during beta-adrenergic therapy remains unclear. Some investigators have speculated that beta-adrenergic therapy precipitates myocardial failure, and others have suggested that the pulmonary edema is noncardiogenic (i.e., due to increased pulmonary vascular permeability).[191,198] Several studies have found no evidence of myocardial failure in patients receiving beta-adrenergic therapy.[199,200]

Plasma volume expansion leading to volume overload during beta-adrenergic therapy has also been proposed as the principal mechanism for pulmonary edema.[201] Fluid overload during beta-adrenergic therapy may occur as a result of intravenous overhydration and/or as a result of fluid and sodium retention secondary to increases in renin and antidiuretic hormone activity from beta-adrenergic receptor stimulation.[201]

Kleinman et al.[187] studied the circulatory and renal effects of ritodrine infusion with three different types of intravenous hydration in gravid ewes. The investigators suggested that the central hemodynamic effects of beta-adrenergic receptor stimulation place an added overload on the circulatory system during pregnancy (which is already associated with increased cardiac output and plasma volume). In addition, they suggested that the antidiuretic and antinatriuretic effects of beta-adrenergic therapy lead to fluid retention and further circulatory overload.

The result is enhancement of fluid diffusion from the pulmonary vasculature to the pulmonary interstitium.

Other investigators have noted that concurrent administration of an intravenous saline solution with a beta-adrenergic agent may increase the risk for development of pulmonary edema. Philipsen et al.[197] found that intravenous infusion of isotonic sodium chloride caused retention of more fluid than infusion of glucose solution, and patients in the saline group were more likely to experience pulmonary congestion that required treatment. In pregnant baboons there was more fluid and sodium retention when ritodrine was administered with lactated Ringer's solution than when lactated Ringer's solution was given alone.[202] Although colloid oncotic pressure diminished in both groups, the ritodrine-treated group had a colloid oncotic pressure–to–pulmonary artery pressure gradient that favored net movement of water from the pulmonary vasculature to the pulmonary interstitium.

Normal-to-low pulmonary capillary wedge pressures (PCWPs) have been reported in patients who experienced pulmonary edema during beta-adrenergic therapy,[203] suggesting a noncardiogenic mechanism (i.e., increased pulmonary vascular permeability) for the development of pulmonary edema. Women with preterm labor and concurrent infection may be at greater risk for development of pulmonary edema during beta-adrenergic tocolysis.[188,192] Infection may increase pulmonary vascular permeability through the release of endotoxin and may lead to noncardiogenic pulmonary edema.[204]

Regardless of the etiology, the hypoxemia that accompanies beta-adrenergic therapy–related pulmonary edema may seem disproportionate to the severity of edema seen on a chest radiograph. Conover et al.[205] demonstrated in dogs that ritodrine significantly inhibits hypoxic pulmonary vasoconstriction; such inhibition may worsen the hypoxemia that accompanies pulmonary edema during beta-adrenergic therapy.

Total intake and output, daily weights, and serial hematocrit determinations should be monitored carefully during beta-adrenergic therapy. The choice of intravenous fluid may influence the extent of fluid retention and the development of metabolic changes.[206] Isotonic solutions (e.g., normal saline) increase the severity of sodium and fluid retention, and dextrose-containing solutions increase the likelihood of hyperglycemia and hypokalemia. One option is to give the beta-adrenergic agent with a solution of 0.45% sodium chloride without dextrose. It seems reasonable to limit total fluid intake to 1.5 to 2.5 L every 24 hours.

Limiting the dose of the beta-adrenergic agent also should lessen the risk of pulmonary edema. Little tocolytic efficacy is gained by administering more beta-adrenergic agent than that necessary to increase maternal heart rate by 20% to 30%. Patients receiving beta-adrenergic tocolysis should be monitored closely for signs of pulmonary edema. Pulse oximetry facilitates detection of early changes in oxygenation in patients receiving beta-adrenergic tocolysis.

If pulmonary edema develops, the beta-adrenergic agent should be discontinued immediately, supplemental oxygen should be administered, fluids should be restricted, and a diuretic agent should be administered. Most patients show response to these simple measures. Rarely, patients with severe, persistent hypoxemia require invasive hemodynamic monitoring, endotracheal intubation, and mechanical ventilation.

Hyperglycemia

Plasma glucose levels rise rapidly after the initiation of beta-adrenergic therapy.[198] Insulin release, most likely mediated by direct beta-adrenergic receptor stimulation of the maternal pancreas, occurs before the rise in glucose levels, and parallels the level of hyperglycemia. Glucose levels return to baseline within 24 hours of initiation of therapy, and supplemental insulin typically is not necessary in nondiabetic patients.[207] The use of a beta-adrenergic agent in insulin-dependent diabetic patients is controversial.[198,208] Hyperglycemia and ketoacidosis typically can be avoided with careful monitoring of plasma glucose concentrations and concurrent intravenous insulin infusion.[208]

Hypokalemia

Hypokalemia most likely results from insulin-mediated transport of potassium and glucose from the extracellular space to the intracellular space. Urinary excretion of potassium is not increased, so total body potassium levels remain unchanged,[198] and correction is not necessary. Serum potassium concentrations typically return to normal within 24 hours of starting beta-adrenergic therapy, and no adverse effects associated with hypokalemia have been reported.[148,198]

Hyperkalemia

Several reports have documented a rebound hyperkalemia after treatment with ritodrine.[209-211] The patients in these reports had received supplemental potassium for treatment of hypokalemia prior to discontinuation of the beta-adrenergic agent, followed by general anesthesia (with and without succinylcholine). Thus, anesthesia providers should exercise caution when administering general anesthesia immediately after cessation of beta-adrenergic therapy, especially if the patient received supplemental potassium for treatment of hypokalemia during beta-adrenergic therapy.

Other Maternal Side Effects

Other uncommon maternal side effects reported with the use of beta-adrenergic agents are elevations in serum transaminase levels,[212] paralytic ileus,[213] cerebral vasospasm in patients with a previous history of migraine,[214] and respiratory arrest due to increased muscle weakness in a patient with myasthenia gravis.[215]

Fetal Side Effects

Placental transfer of beta-adrenergic agents is rapid. Increased FHR, which is presumed to be a result of direct stimulation of fetal myocardial $beta_1$ receptors, may be seen. Neonatal hypoglycemia may occur as a result of maternal hyperglycemia and hyperinsulinemia.[148,216] Retrospective studies have not demonstrated any long-term adverse fetal/neonatal effects of beta-adrenergic therapy.[217,218] Although some studies have shown transient echocardiographic evidence of reduced fetal myocardial contractility after prolonged beta-adrenergic tocolysis,[219,220] no long-term, adverse effect on the fetal and neonatal heart has been noted.[221]

ANESTHETIC MANAGEMENT

It would seem ideal to delay administration of anesthesia until maternal tachycardia subsides. A delay of 15 minutes often results in slowing of the maternal heart rate. However, advanced labor, an abnormal presentation, and/or nonreassuring fetal status often require emergency administration of anesthesia. Published reports of anesthetic management after administration of a beta-adrenergic agent are scarce.[222-227] Ravindran et al.[224] reported one case each of intraoperative pulmonary edema, sinus tachycardia, and ventricular arrhythmia during general anesthesia in patients who had received terbutaline therapy immediately before or 15 minutes after the induction of anesthesia. These investigators recommended that induction of general anesthesia be delayed at least 10 minutes after discontinuation of the beta-adrenergic agent.

Shin and Kim[227] retrospectively observed that maternal hypotension was more common when induction of anesthesia occurred within 30 minutes of the discontinuation of ritodrine than when induction was delayed more than 30 minutes. Chestnut et al.[228] performed a controlled study to determine whether administration of ritodrine worsens maternal hypotension during epidural anesthesia in gravid ewes. Prior administration of ritodrine did not worsen maternal hypotension during epidural lidocaine anesthesia in gravid ewes. The investigators suggested that "the inotropic and chronotropic activity of ritodrine helped maintain maternal cardiac output and uterine blood flow during epidural anesthesia.[228]

Theoretically, induction of epidural analgesia or anesthesia after beta-adrenergic therapy may cause less hemodynamic compromise than spinal anesthesia because of the slower onset of sympathetic blockade. However, this theory remains unproven. Patients receiving beta-adrenergic therapy are at risk for development of pulmonary edema (as discussed earlier). Therefore aggressive hydration should be avoided before and during the induction of anesthesia in these patients. We first administer a modest fluid bolus (e.g., 250 to 500 mL of lactated Ringer's solution) and then slowly induce epidural anesthesia. Additional intravenous crystalloid and a vasopressor can be administered to maintain normal maternal blood pressure. Until recently, ephedrine, a mixed alpha- and beta-adrenergic agonist, had been the vasopressor of choice for treatment of hypotension in obstetric practice because of its protective effect on UBF in gravid ewes.[229] Historically, anesthesia providers have believed that ephedrine's beta-receptor activity increases cardiac output, compensating for its alpha-receptor–mediated uterine vasoconstriction. Chestnut et al.[230,231] hypothesized that in a patient already receiving a beta-adrenergic agonist, any vasopressor effect of ephedrine should result from alpha-receptor stimulation. The accompanying uterine vasoconstriction subsequently would result in decreased UBF. However, one study reported that ephedrine restored uterine blood flow velocity (UBFV) during hemorrhagic hypotension in gravid guinea pigs subjected to terbutaline infusion (Figure 34-8).[230] In a subsequent study, ephedrine preserved UBFV during ritodrine infusion in normovolemic gravid guinea pigs.[231] Both epinephrine and phenylephrine decreased UBFV, whereas mephentermine resulted in an intermediate response. These studies suggest that ephedrine does not depend solely on beta-adrenergic stimulation to increase cardiac output.

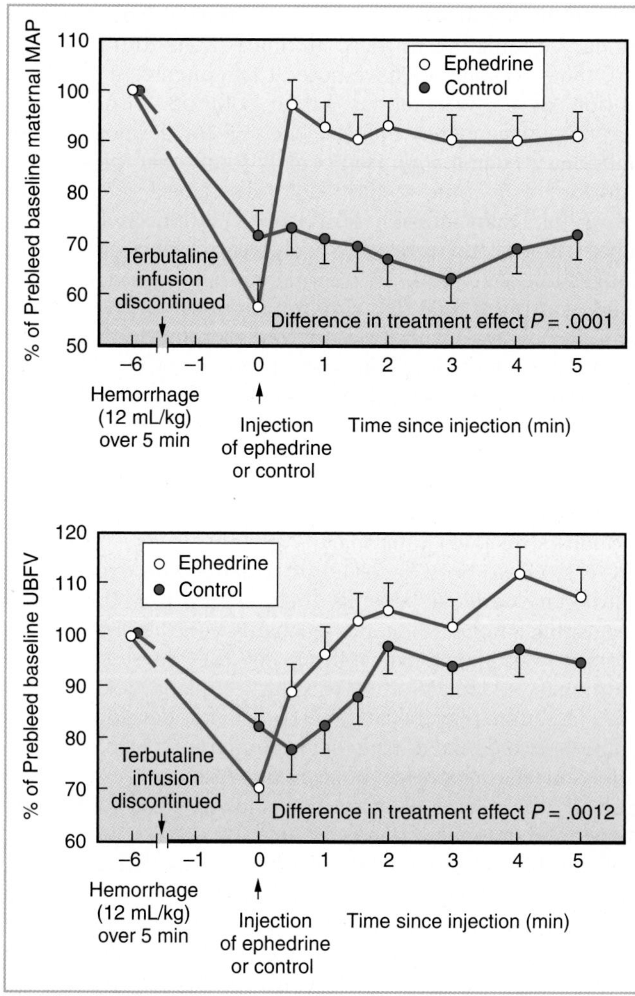

FIGURE 34-8 Response over time of maternal mean arterial pressure (MAP) and uterine artery blood flow velocity (UBFV) after hemorrhage and intravenous administration of ephedrine, 1.0 mg/kg, or control (saline, 0.2 mL) in gravid guinea pigs subjected to terbutaline infusion. All values are expressed as mean (± SEM) percentage of the prebleed baseline value. (From Chestnut DH, Weiner CP, Wang JP, et al. The effect of ephedrine upon uterine artery blood flow velocity in the pregnant guinea pig subjected to terbutaline infusion and acute hemorrhage. Anesthesiology 1987; 66:508-12.)

McGrath et al.[232] evaluated the use of ephedrine and phenylephrine for the treatment of hypotension during ritodrine infusion and epidural anesthesia in gravid ewes. Ephedrine restored UBF, whereas phenylephrine led to a significant decrease in UBF and an increase in uterine vascular resistance. Although the results of these studies suggest that ephedrine remains a satisfactory choice of vasopressor in patients who have recently received beta-adrenergic therapy, caution should be exercised in the extrapolation of animal study results to humans.

Data from *healthy, term* women undergoing spinal anesthesia for cesarean delivery suggest that phenylephrine is a safe alternative to ephedrine for the treatment of hypotension.[233,234] A randomized clinical trial comparing ephedrine, phenylephrine, and a combination of phenylephrine and ephedrine noted a higher incidence of fetal acidosis in infants whose mothers had received ephedrine during administration of spinal anesthesia for elective cesarean delivery.[234] The investigators speculated that "increased fetal metabolic rate, secondary to ephedrine-induced beta-adrenergic stimulation, was the most likely mechanism for the increased incidence of fetal acidosis in the ephedrine group."[234] The use of phenylephrine has not been studied in preterm pregnant women who have recently undergone beta-adrenergic tocolytic therapy. However, clinical experience suggests that phenylephrine can be safely administered for treatment of maternal hypotension during neuraxial anesthesia, and a growing number of obstetric anesthesiologists argue that phenylephrine is now the preferred vasopressor for treatment of maternal hypotension, especially when there is concern that ephedrine may worsen maternal tachycardia or precipitate arrhythmia.

If general anesthesia is required in a patient who has recently received beta-adrenergic tocolysis, agents that might exacerbate maternal tachycardia (e.g., atropine, glycopyrrolate, pancuronium) should be avoided. Residual maternal tachycardia may make it more difficult to assess volume status and depth of anesthesia. Halothane—which sensitizes the myocardium to catecholamine-induced arrhythmias—should not be used. Hyperventilation should be avoided, because it may exacerbate hypokalemia and potentiate the hyperpolarization of the cell membrane. In nonpregnant patients, Slater et al.[235] found that terbutaline pretreatment shortened the onset time and recovery of succinylcholine-induced neuromuscular blockade. It seems prudent to monitor neuromuscular function with a peripheral nerve stimulator during general anesthesia.

Obstetricians continue to question the efficacy of beta-adrenergic tocolytic therapy. Nonetheless, anesthesia providers are likely to continue to encounter occasional patients who require urgent administration of anesthesia shortly after administration of a beta-adrenergic agent. Research has now identified a beta$_3$-adrenergic receptor (ADRβ3), which may have functional effects on myometrial contractility.[236] Studies have confirmed the presence of this receptor on human myometrium near term. It may have resistance to long-term agonist-induced desensitization. Whether beta$_3$-adrenergic receptor agonists will have a better safety profile than the beta$_2$-adrenergic receptor agonists in current use remains to be elucidated.

Oxytocin Antagonists

Atosiban (1-deamino-2-D-Tyr-[OEt]-4-Thr-8-Orn-vasotocin/oxytocin) is an oxytocin antagonist. It is a competitive inhibitor of oxytocin that binds to both myometrial and decidual receptors. It does not alter the subsequent sensitivity of the myometrium to oxytocin.[237] Clinically this feature represents a major advantage; it should reduce the risk of postpartum uterine atony and hemorrhage.

Phase II and III studies have shown that atosiban is an effective tocolytic agent.[99,238-242] It has few maternal side effects, undergoes minimal placental transfer, and does not increase maternal blood loss at delivery.[99,238] Studies have suggested that atosiban has efficacy similar to that of beta-adrenergic agonists in obtaining and maintaining uterine quiescence.[241,242] However, a meta-analysis of studies comparing atosiban with either placebo or beta-adrenergic agonists did not demonstrate that atosiban resulted in a reduction in preterm birth or improved neonatal outcome,[243] although side effects were fewer with atosiban. The U.S. Food and Drug Administration has not approved atosiban for use in the United States because of a higher rate of perinatal deaths in the atosiban arm of the study that it reviewed.[99]

There are no data on the interaction between atosiban and anesthetic agents. However, given the hemodynamic profile of this agent, one would not expect significant interactions. This agent is in widespread clinical use in Europe.

Magnesium Sulfate

Although magnesium sulfate has been used for tocolysis in the treatment of preterm labor for a number of years, there is little scientific evidence to support its use for this purpose.[91,244] Extracellular magnesium functions as a competitive antagonist of calcium either at the motor end plate or cell membrane, thus reducing calcium influx into the myocyte.[28,148] It also competes with calcium for low-affinity calcium-binding sites on the outside of the sarcoplasmic reticulum membrane and prevents the rise in free intracellular calcium concentration. Hypermagnesemia results in abnormal neuromuscular function. Magnesium also decreases the release of acetylcholine at the neuromuscular junction and the sensitivity of the end plate to acetylcholine.

SIDE EFFECTS

Most studies have reported that magnesium sulfate results in less frequent and less severe cardiovascular side effects in unstressed patients than the beta-adrenergic tocolytic agents.[245-247] Nonetheless, magnesium sulfate may have side effects similar to those that occur during beta-adrenergic tocolytic therapy. Chest pain and tightness, palpitations, nausea, transient hypotension, blurred vision, sedation, and pulmonary edema have been reported.[246,247] Hypermagnesemia may attenuate the normal compensatory responses to hemorrhage in the mother and fetus.[248,249]

Magnesium is eliminated almost entirely by renal excretion. Therefore patients with abnormal renal function should be monitored carefully if they receive magnesium sulfate. Fortunately, most patients who receive magnesium sulfate for tocolytic therapy have normal renal function. Therefore magnesium toxicity occurs less frequently during tocolytic therapy than during the administration of magnesium sulfate for seizure prophylaxis in preeclamptic women.

There is significant controversy as to whether magnesium administered to mothers prior to delivery positively or negatively affects perinatal outcome. Several studies found an increased risk of perinatal death in women randomly assigned to receive magnesium sulfate,[250,251] as did a meta-analysis of studies comparing magnesium with other tocolytic agents.[91] However, other investigators found no difference in perinatal mortality in women who received magnesium.[252] A retrospective trial suggested that children of women who received antenatal magnesium sulfate for the treatment of preterm labor or preeclampsia had a lower risk of cerebral palsy.[253] A retrospective case-control study suggested that antenatal exposure to a high cumulative tocolytic dose (> 48 g) of magnesium sulfate was associated with a significant increase in perinatal mortality among neonates weighing 700 to 1249 g at delivery.[254] In contrast, a large retrospective analysis of data from 12,876 deliveries from 100 tertiary care centers did not identify any evidence of increased mortality in the neonates exposed to magnesium sulfate.[255] A multicenter trial published in 2008[256] randomized 2241 women between 24 and 31 weeks' gestation who were at imminent risk of delivery to receive magnesium therapy or placebo. The combined risk of moderate/severe cerebral palsy or death was not different between groups; however, the rate of cerebral palsy was reduced among survivors in the magnesium group.[256]

Review of these studies suggests that high cumulative doses of magnesium sulfate may be deleterious to the fetus.[257,258] Unfortunately, doses suggested to be detrimental (> 50 g) are similar to those used for tocolysis in the management of preterm labor. There is speculation and some evidence that "low-dose" magnesium sulfate may have some neuroprotective effect and may decrease the incidence of cerebral palsy in preterm infants.[257,258] However, given the weak evidence for the efficacy of magnesium sulfate as a tocolytic agent for arrest of preterm labor, and the ongoing controversy about possible adverse effects on perinatal mortality rates when magnesium sulfate is used at doses necessary to induce uterine quiescence, a move is under way to abandon the use of magnesium sulfate as a tocolytic agent.[244] Whether or not lower magnesium sulfate doses administered before delivery of preterm infants will result in improved outcome remains to be determined.

ANESTHETIC MANAGEMENT

It has been suggested that magnesium sulfate should be discontinued before the administration of epidural anesthesia because magnesium may increase the likelihood of hypotension through its generalized vasodilating properties. Vincent et al.[259] observed that magnesium sulfate reduced maternal MAP but not UBF or fetal oxygenation during epidural lidocaine anesthesia in gravid ewes. This study suggests that hypermagnesemia may increase the likelihood of modest hypotension during neuraxial anesthesia in normotensive parturients.

Magnesium attenuates the release of acetylcholine at the neuromuscular junction, reduces the sensitivity of the end plate to acetylcholine, and decreases the excitability of the muscle membrane. The drug potentiates the action of both depolarizing and nondepolarizing muscle relaxants.[260] A defasciculating dose of a nondepolarizing muscle relaxant should not be given before administration of succinylcholine in hypermagnesemic women. A standard intubating dose of muscle relaxant (e.g., succinylcholine 1 mg/kg) should be used because the extent of potentiation by magnesium sulfate is variable.[261] However, a lower dose of a nondepolarizing muscle relaxant should be administered during the maintenance of anesthesia. We have observed that patients who have received prolonged magnesium sulfate therapy are especially sensitive to nondepolarizing muscle relaxants. Neuromuscular blockade should be monitored with a peripheral nerve stimulator.

Parturients receiving magnesium sulfate often appear sedated. Thompson et al.[262] evaluated the anesthetic effects of magnesium sulfate and ritodrine on the minimum alveolar concentration (MAC) of halothane in pregnant and nonpregnant rats. They reported a 20% decrease in MAC with serum magnesium levels of 7 to 11 mg/dL. A more detailed discussion of magnesium sulfate and its interactions with anesthetic agents is found in Chapter 45.

INVESTIGATIONAL TOCOLYTIC AGENTS

Nitric Oxide Donors

For several years, anesthesia providers have used nitroglycerin in situations in which a rapid onset of profound uterine relaxation is desired (e.g., uterine hyperstimulation [tachysystole], fetal head entrapment, internal version and extraction of the second twin, uterine inversion, retained placenta).[263] Nitroglycerin acts as a nitric oxide donor, and it is a potent smooth muscle relaxant. This effect is mediated, in part, by activation of guanylate cyclase, which results in an increase in intracellular cyclic guanosine monophosphate (cGMP). The increased cGMP activates cGMP-dependent protein kinase, which inhibits the influx of calcium from the extracellular space and the release of calcium from intracellular stores. The protein kinase also activates the calcium pump, thereby increasing calcium extrusion across the plasma membrane and calcium reuptake by the sarcoplasmic reticulum.[264] Nitric oxide can also relax human myometrium by other pathways, such as direct activation of calcium-activated potassium channels.[264-266] Nitric oxide may be responsible for the normal vascular adaptation to pregnancy, and disturbances in this system may lead to preeclampsia (see Chapter 45).

Nitric oxide is synthesized from L-arginine by nitric oxide synthase (NOS). The constitutive isoforms of NOS found in endothelial cells and neurons depend on calcium for their activity. The inducible forms (iNOS) are calcium-independent, can synthesize nitric oxide at very high rates, and are present in the myometrium and placenta.[264] The ability of the myometrium to synthesize nitric oxide—as well as its sensitivity to nitric oxide—varies during and after pregnancy, labor, and delivery. There appears to be reduced production of, and sensitivity to, nitric oxide within the myometrium during labor than in late gestation.[266] Nitric oxide of placental origin may play a role in maintaining uterine quiescence, because placental nitric oxide activity decreases near term.[266] A downregulation of uteroplacental nitric oxide activity may initiate labor.

Uterine muscle sensitivity to nitric oxide is much lower than that of vascular smooth muscle, so large amounts of nitric oxide would be required to inhibit uterine contractions. At these doses, one might expect to see significant hemodynamic side effects. Studies in laboring sheep have demonstrated that nitroglycerin effectively inhibits spontaneous uterine contractions and results in a modest reduction in maternal blood pressure without having an adverse effect on fetal circulation, oxygenation, or acid-base status.[267,268] Bootstaylor et al.[268] suggested that "intravenous nitroglycerin has an excellent margin of safety and possibly could be used as a uterine tocolytic agent." However, a clinical study observed that sublingual administration of nitroglycerin (three doses of 800 μg, administered 10 minutes apart) did not reduce uterine activity or tone in healthy laboring women at term, despite reducing maternal MAP approximately 20%.[269]

A 2002 meta-analysis of five studies (n = 466) found insufficient evidence to support the use of nitric oxide donors for treatment of preterm labor compared to placebo or other tocolytic agents.[102] A randomized controlled trial published in 2004 compared a nitroglycerin patch with beta-adrenergic therapy for treatment of preterm labor.[270]

Patients in the nitroglycerin group required rescue therapy more often, and there was no difference between the treatment groups in gestational age at delivery. In contrast, a Canadian group of investigators found transdermal nitroglycerin to be significantly more efficacious than placebo when used to treat preterm labor in patients presenting before 28 weeks' gestation.[271] Given the different results of these trials, further study is merited before any conclusions on efficacy of this agent can be made.

KEY POINTS

- Despite improved antenatal care, the incidence of preterm delivery in the United States has not decreased and is now higher than 13%.
- Preterm birth is a leading cause of neonatal mortality. Survivors have a high incidence of disability.
- Preterm labor is the cause of most preterm births.
- Treatment with tocolytic therapy may prolong labor by 2 to 7 days and (1) facilitate transfer of the patient from a small community hospital to a tertiary care facility; (2) delay delivery to allow maternal administration of a corticosteroid to accelerate fetal lung maturity; and (3) facilitate fetal resuscitation *in utero* in cases of nonreassuring fetal status. Long-term tocolytic therapy does not improve neonatal outcome.
- Nifedipine and indomethacin are widely used to treat preterm labor in the United States. The oxytocin antagonist atosiban is widely used in Europe. Magnesium sulfate has been widely used in the United States but may be falling out of favor because of failure to demonstrate efficacy and concerns about higher perinatal mortality in association with its use (especially with administration of large cumulative doses). Terbutaline is associated with a high incidence of maternal and fetal side effects.
- During labor and delivery, the preterm fetus is at greater risk for acidosis and has a higher incidence of intracranial hemorrhage.
- Specific anesthesia requirements for vaginal delivery of the preterm infant include (1) inhibition of inappropriate maternal expulsive efforts before complete cervical dilation, especially in patients with a breech presentation; (2) prevention of precipitous delivery, which can result in rapid decompression of the infant's head and increase the risk of intracranial hemorrhage; and (3) provision of a relaxed pelvic floor and perineum to facilitate a smooth, controlled delivery of the more vulnerable, preterm infant's head.
- Side effects of beta-adrenergic tocolytic therapy include (1) hypotension; (2) tachycardia, with or without cardiac arrhythmias and myocardial ischemia; (3) pulmonary edema; (4) hyperglycemia; and (5) hypokalemia. Pulmonary edema is the most serious complication, and it may be life threatening.
- Prior administration of a beta-adrenergic tocolytic agent does not contraindicate the administration of neuraxial anesthesia.
- Cyclooxygenase inhibitors reversibly inhibit cyclooxygenase, resulting in a transient effect on platelet function. However, their use does not necessitate the assessment of platelet or coagulation function before administration of neuraxial analgesia/anesthesia in a patient whose only risk factor is recent ingestion of a cyclooxygenase inhibitor.
- Studies of new agents for the treatment of preterm labor are in progress. Advancement in the understanding of the physiology of labor will help guide future directions for therapy. The ideal therapy will likely target multiple mechanisms involved in the physiology of labor and will have minimal adverse effects on the mother and fetus.

REFERENCES

1. Goldenberg RL, Culhane JF, Iams JD, Romero R. Epidemiology and causes of preterm birth. Lancet 2008; 371:75-84.
2. Eichenwald EC, Stark AR. Management and outcomes of very low birth weight. N Engl J Med 2008; 358:1700-11.
3. Martin JA, Hamilton BE, Sutton PD, et al. Births: Final data for 2005. Natl Vital Stat Rep 2007; 56:1-103.
4. Institute of Medicine. Preterm birth: Causes, consequences, and prevention. Washington, DC, Institute of Medicine, 2006. Available at http://www.iom.edu/CMS/3740/25471/35813.aspx/
5. Menacker F, Martin JA. Expanded health data from the new birth certificate, 2005. Natl Vital Stat Rep 2008; 56:1-24.
6. Callaghan WM, MacDorman MF, Rasmussen SA, et al. The contribution of preterm birth to infant mortality rates in the United States. Pediatrics 2006; 118:1566-73.
7. Bettegowda V, Dias T, Davidoff M, et al. The relationship between cesarean delivery and gestational age among US singleton births. Clin Perinatol 2008; 25:309-23.
8. U.S. Department of Health and Human Services, Office of Disease Prevention and Health Promotion. Healthy People 2010. Washington, DC, US Department of Health and Human Services, 2000.
9. Wardlaw T, Zupan J, Ahman E. Low Birthweight: Country, Regional and Global Estimates. New York, UNICEF, 2004. Available at http://www.unicef.org/publications/files/low_birthweight_from_EY.pdf/
10. The state of the world's children 2007: Women and children: The double dividend of gender equality. New York, UNICEF, 2007. Available at http://www.unicef.org/sowc07/
11. Plunkett J, Muglia LJ. Genetic contributions to preterm birth: Implications from epidemiological and genetic association studies. Ann Med 2008; 40:167-95.
12. Wilson-Costello D, Friedman H, Minich N, et al. Improved survival rates with increased neurodevelopmental disability for extremely low birth weight infants in the 1990s. Pediatrics 2005; 115:997-1003.
13. Riley K, Roth S, Sellwood M, Wyatt JS. Survival and neurodevelopmental morbidity at 1 year of age following extremely preterm delivery over a 20-year period: A single centre cohort study. Acta Paediatr 2008; 97:159-65.
14. Lemons JA, Bauer CR, Oh W, et al. Very low birth weight outcomes of the National Institute of Child Health and Human Development Neonatal Research Network, January 1995 through December 1996. NICHD Neonatal Research Network. Pediatrics 2001; 107:E1.

15. Hack M, Fanaroff AA. Outcomes of children of extremely low birth-weight and gestational age in the 1990s. Semin Neonatol 2000; 5:89-106.
16. Kilpatrick SJ, Schlueter MA, Piecuch R, et al. Outcome of infants born at 24-26 weeks' gestation. I. Survival and cost. Obstet Gynecol 1997; 90:803-8.
17. Lucey JF, Rowan CA, Shiono P, et al. Fetal infants: The fate of 4172 infants with birth weights of 401 to 500 grams—the Vermont Oxford Network experience (1996-2000). Pediatrics 2004; 113:1559-66.
18. Costeloe K, Hennessy E, Gibson AT, et al. The EPICure study: Outcomes to discharge from hospital for infants born at the threshold of viability. Pediatrics 2000; 106:659-71.
19. Wilson-Costello D, Friedman H, Minich N, et al. Improved neurodevelopmental outcomes for extremely low birth weight infants in 2000-2002. Pediatrics 2007; 119:37-45.
20. Hack M, Taylor HG, Drotar D, et al. Chronic conditions, functional limitations, and special health care needs of school-aged children born with extremely low-birth-weight in the 1990s. JAMA 2005; 294:318-25.
21. Piecuch RE, Leonard CH, Cooper BA, Sehring SA. Outcome of extremely low birth weight infants (500 to 999 grams) over a 12-year period. Pediatrics 1997; 100:633-9.
22. Wood NS, Marlow N, Costeloe K, et al. Neurologic and developmental disability after extremely preterm birth. EPICure Study Group. N Engl J Med 2000; 343:378-84.
23. Keogh J, Sinn J, Hollebone K, et al. Delivery in the 'grey zone': Collaborative approach to extremely preterm birth. Aust N Z J Obstet Gynaecol 2007; 47:273-8.
24. Marlow N, Wolke D, Bracewell MA, et al. Neurologic and developmental disability at six years of age after extremely preterm birth. N Engl J Med 2005; 352:9-19.
25. Goldenberg RL, Rouse DJ. Prevention of premature birth. N Engl J Med 1998; 339:313-20.
26. American College of Obstetricians and Gynecologists. Management of preterm labor. ACOG Practice Bulletin No. 43. Washington DC, ACOG, May 2003. (Obstet Gynecol 2003; 101:1039-47.)
27. Pschirrer ER, Monga M. Risk factors for preterm labor. Clin Obstet Gynecol 2000; 43:727-34.
28. Iams JD, Romero R. Preterm birth. In Gabbe SG, Niebyl JR, Simpson JL, editors. Obstetrics: Normal and Problem Pregnancies. 5th edition. Philadelphia, Churchill Livingstone Elsevier, 2007: 669-712.
29. Menon R. Spontaneous preterm birth, a clinical dilemma: Etiologic, pathophysiologic and genetic heterogeneities and racial disparity. Acta Obstet Gynecol Scand 2008; 87:590-600.
30. Romero R, Espinoza J, Kusanovic JP, et al. The preterm parturition syndrome. Br J Obstet Gynaecol 2006; 113(Suppl 3):17-42.
31. Krupa FG, Faltin D, Cecatti JG, et al. Predictors of preterm birth. Int J Gynaecol Obstet 2006; 94:5-11.
32. Goldenberg RL, Hauth JC, Andrews WW. Intrauterine infection and preterm delivery. N Engl J Med 2000; 342:1500-7.
33. Gibbs RS, Romero R, Hillier SL, et al. A review of premature birth and subclinical infection. Am J Obstet Gynaecol 1992; 166:1515-28.
34. Norwitz ER, Robinson JN, Challis JR. The control of labor. N Engl J Med 1999; 341:660-6.
35. Potkul RK, Moawad AH, Ponto KL. The association of subclinical infection with preterm labor: The role of C-reactive protein. Am J Obstet Gynecol 1985; 153:642-5.
36. Xiong X, Buekens P, Fraser WD, et al. Periodontal disease and adverse pregnancy outcomes: A systematic review. Br J Obstet Gynecol 2006; 113:135-43.
37. Xiong X, Buekens P, Vastardis S, Yu SM. Periodontal disease and pregnancy outcomes: State-of-the-science. Obstet Gynecol Surv 2007; 62:605-15.
38. Yeo BK, Lim LP, Paquette DW, Williams RC. Periodontal disease—the emergence of a risk for systemic conditions: Pre-term low birth weight. Ann Acad Med Singapore 2005; 34:111-6.
39. Dickey RP. The relative contribution of assisted reproductive technologies and ovulation induction to multiple births in the United States 5 years after the Society for Assisted Reproductive Technology/American Society for Reproductive Medicine recommendation to limit the number of embryos transferred. Fertil Steril 2007; 88:1554-61.
40. American College of Obstetricians and Gynecologists. Multiple gestation: Complicated twin, triplet, and high-order multifetal pregnancy. ACOG Practice Bulletin No. 56. Washington, DC, October 2004. (Obstet Gynecol 2004; 104:869-83.)
41. Jackson RA, Gibson KA, Wu YW, Croughan MS. Perinatal outcomes in singletons following in vitro fertilization: A meta-analysis. Obstet Gynecol 2004; 103:551-63.
42. Rudra CB, Frederick IO, Williams MA. Pre-pregnancy body mass index and weight gain during pregnancy in relation to preterm delivery subtypes. Acta Obstet Gynecol Scand 2008; 87:510-7.
43. Nohr EA, Vaeth M, Bech BH, et al. Maternal obesity and neonatal mortality according to subtypes of preterm birth. Obstet Gynecol 2007; 110:1083-90.
44. American College of Obstetricians and Gynecologists. Assessment of risk factors for preterm birth. ACOG Practice Bulletin No. 31. Washington, DC, October 2001. (Obstet Gynecol 2001; 98:709-16.)
45. Dyson DC, Danbe KH, Bamber JA, et al. Monitoring women at risk for preterm labor. N Engl J Med 1998; 338:15-9.
46. Heine RP, McGregor JA, Goodwin TM, et al. Serial salivary estriol to detect an increased risk of preterm birth. Obstet Gynecol 2000; 96:490-7.
47. McGregor JA, Jackson GM, Lachelin GC, et al. Salivary estriol as risk assessment for preterm labor: A prospective trial. Am J Obstet Gynecol 1995; 173:1337-42.
48. Vogel I, Thorsen P, Curry A, et al. Biomarkers for the prediction of preterm delivery. Acta Obstet Gynecol Scand 2005; 84:516-25.
49. Goldenberg RL, Iams JD, Mercer BM, et al. The Preterm Prediction Study: Toward a multiple-marker test for spontaneous preterm birth. Am J Obstet Gynecol 2001; 185:643-51.
50. Feinberg RF, Kliman HJ, Lockwood CJ. Is oncofetal fibronectin a trophoblast glue for human implantation? Am J Pathol 1991; 138:537-43.
51. Goldenberg RL, Mercer BM, Meis PJ, et al. The preterm prediction study: Fetal fibronectin testing and spontaneous preterm birth. Obstet Gynecol 1996; 87:643-8.
52. Smith V, Devane D, Begley CM, et al. A systematic review and quality assessment of systematic reviews of fetal fibronectin and transvaginal length for predicting preterm birth. Eur J Obstet Gynecol Reprod Biol 2007; 133:134-42.
53. Iams JD, Goldenberg RL, Meis PJ, et al. The length of the cervix and the risk of spontaneous premature delivery. N Engl J Med 1996; 334:567-72.
54. Kagan KO, To M, Tsoi E, Nicolaides KH. Preterm birth: The value of sonographic measurement of cervical length. Br J Obstet Gynaecol 2006; 113(Suppl 3):52-6.
55. American College of Obstetricians and Gynecologists. Cervical insufficiency. ACOG Practice Bulletin No. 48. Washington, DC, November 2003. (Obstet Gynecol 2003; 102:1091-9.)
56. Meis PJ, Goldenberg RL, Mercer B, et al. The preterm prediction study: Significance of vaginal infections. Am J Obstet Gynecol 1995; 173:1231-5.
57. Carey JC, Klebanoff MA, Hauth JC, et al. Metronidazole to prevent preterm delivery in pregnant women with asymptomatic bacterial vaginosis. N Engl J Med 2000; 342:534-40.
58. Kiss H, Petricevic L, Husslein P. Prospective randomised controlled trial of an infection screening programme to reduce the rate of preterm delivery. Br Med J 2004; 329:371.
59. Lamont RF, Duncan SL, Mandal D, Bassett P. Intravaginal clindamycin to reduce preterm birth in women with abnormal genital tract flora. Obstet Gynecol 2003; 101:516-22.
60. Ugwumadu A, Manyonda I, Reid F, Hay P. Effect of early oral clindamycin on late miscarriage and preterm delivery in asymptomatic women with abnormal vaginal flora and bacterial vaginosis: A randomised controlled trial. Lancet 2003; 361:983-8.
61. Lamont RF. Can antibiotics prevent preterm birth—the pro and con debate. Br J Obstet Gynaecol 2005; 112(Suppl 1):67-73.
62. Andrews WW, Goldenberg RL, Hauth JC, et al. Interconceptional antibiotics to prevent spontaneous preterm birth: A randomized clinical trial. Am J Obstet Gynecol 2006; 194:617-23.

63. Klebanoff MA, Carey JC, Hauth JC, et al. Failure of metronidazole to prevent preterm delivery among pregnant women with asymptomatic *Trichomonas vaginalis* infection. N Engl J Med 2001; 345: 487-93.
64. Drakeley AJ, Roberts D, Alfirevic Z. Cervical stitch (cerclage) for preventing pregnancy loss in women. Cochrane Database Syst Rev 2003; (1):CD003253.
65. Simcox R, Sin WT, Seed PT, et al. Prophylactic antibiotics for the prevention of preterm birth in women at risk: A meta-analysis. Aust N Z J Gynaecol 2007; 47:368-77.
66. Whitworth M, Quenby S. Prophylactic oral betamimetics for preventing preterm labour in singleton pregnancies. Cochrane Database Syst Rev 2008; (1):CD006395.
67. Meis PJ, Klebanoff M, Thom E, et al. Prevention of recurrent preterm delivery by 17 alpha-hydroxyprogesterone caproate. N Engl J Med 2003; 348:2379-85.
68. da Fonseca EB, Bittar RE, Carvalho MH, Zugaib M. Prophylactic administration of progesterone by vaginal suppository to reduce the incidence of spontaneous preterm birth in women at increased risk: A randomized placebo-controlled double-blind study. Am J Obstet Gynecol 2003; 188:419-24.
69. Dodd JM, Flenady VJ, Cincotta R, Crowther CA. Progesterone for the prevention of preterm birth: A systematic review. Obstet Gynecol 2008; 112:127-134.
70. Rouse DJ, Caritis SN, Peaceman AM, et al. A trial of 17 alpha-hydroxyprogesterone caproate to prevent prematurity in twins. N Engl J Med 2007; 357:454-61.
71. Fonseca EB, Celik E, Parra M, et al. Progesterone and the risk of preterm birth among women with a short cervix. N Engl J Med 2007; 357:462-9.
72. Creasy RK. Preterm birth prevention: Where are we? Am J Obstet Gynecol 1993; 168:1223-30.
73. Schreyer P, Caspi E, Natan NB, et al. The predictive value of fetal breathing movement and Bishop score in the diagnosis of "true" preterm labor. Am J Obstet Gynecol 1989; 161:886-9.
74. Peaceman AM, Andrews WW, Thorp JM, et al. Fetal fibronectin as a predictor of preterm birth in patients with symptoms: A multicenter trial. Am J Obstet Gynecol 1997; 177:13-8.
75. Stan C, Boulvain M, Hirsbrunner-Amagbaly P, Pfister R. Hydration for treatment of preterm labour. Cochrane Database Syst Rev 2002; (2):CD003096.
76. Garite TJ, Keegan KA, Freeman RK, Nageotte MP. A randomized trial of ritodrine tocolysis versus expectant management in patients with premature rupture of membranes at 25 to 30 weeks of gestation. Am J Obstet Gynecol 1987; 157:388-93.
77. Weiner CP, Renk K, Klugman M. The therapeutic efficacy and cost-effectiveness of aggressive tocolysis for premature labor associated with premature rupture of the membranes. Am J Obstet Gynecol 1988; 159:216-22.
78. American College of Obstetricians and Gynecologists. Premature rupture of membranes. ACOG Practice Bulletin No. 80. Washington, DC, April 2007. (Obstet Gynecol 2007; 109:1007-19.)
79. Wright LL, Verter J, Younes N, et al. Antenatal corticosteroid administration and neonatal outcome in very low birth weight infants: The NICHD Neonatal Research Network. Am J Obstet Gynecol 1995; 173:269-74.
80. Andrews EB, Marcucci G, White A, Long W. Associations between use of antenatal corticosteroids and neonatal outcomes within the Exosurf Neonatal Treatment Investigational New Drug Program. Am J Obstet Gynecol 1995; 173:290-5.
81. Murphy K, Aghajafari F, Hannah M. Antenatal corticosteroids for preterm birth. Semin Perinatol 2001; 25:341-7.
82. National Institutes of Health Consensus Development Panel. Antenatal corticosteroids revisited: Repeat courses—National Institutes of Health Consensus Development Conference Statement, August 17-18, 2000. Obstet Gynecol 2001; 98:144-50.
83. Wapner RJ, Sorokin Y, Thom EA, et al. Single versus weekly courses of antenatal corticosteroids: Evaluation of safety and efficacy. Am J Obstet Gynecol 2006; 195:633-42.
84. Wapner RJ, Sorokin Y, Mele L, et al. Long-term outcomes after repeat doses of antenatal corticosteroids. N Engl J Med 2007; 357:1190-8.
85. Elimian A, Garry D, Figueroa R, et al. Antenatal betamethasone compared with dexamethasone (Betacode Trial): A randomized controlled trial. Obstet Gynecol 2007; 110:26-30.
86. Kenyon SL, Taylor DJ, Tarnow-Mordi W. Broad-spectrum antibiotics for spontaneous preterm labour: The ORACLE II randomised trial. ORACLE Collaborative Group. Lancet 2001; 357:989-94.
87. King J, Flenady V. Prophylactic antibiotics for inhibiting preterm labour with intact membranes. Cochrane Database Syst Rev 2002; (4):CD000246.
88. Mercer BM, Miodovnik M, Thurnau GR, et al. Antibiotic therapy for reduction of infant morbidity after preterm premature rupture of the membranes: A randomized controlled trial. National Institute of Child Health and Human Development Maternal-Fetal Medicine Units Network. JAMA 1997; 278:989-95.
89. Kenyon SL, Taylor DJ, Tarnow-Mordi W. Broad-spectrum antibiotics for preterm, prelabour rupture of fetal membranes: The ORACLE I randomised trial. ORACLE Collaborative Group. Lancet 2001; 357:979-88.
90. Berkman ND, Thorp JM Jr, Lohr KN, et al. Tocolytic treatment for the management of preterm labor: A review of the evidence. Am J Obstet Gynecol 2003; 188:1648-59.
91. Crowther CA, Hiller JE, Doyle LW. Magnesium sulphate for preventing preterm birth in threatened preterm labour. Cochrane Database Syst Rev 2002; (4):CD001060.
92. Wray S. Uterine contraction and physiological mechanisms of modulation. Am J Physiol 1993; 264:C1-18.
93. Lopez Bernal A. Overview: Preterm labour: Mechanisms and management. BMC Pregnancy Childbirth 2007; 7(Suppl 1):S2.
94. Breuiller-Fouche M, Charpigny G, Germain G. Functional genomics of the pregnant uterus: From expectations to reality, a compilation of studies in the myometrium. BMC Pregnancy Childbirth 2007; 7(Suppl 1):S4.
95. King JF, Flenady VJ, Papatsonis DN, et al. Calcium channel blockers for inhibiting preterm labour. Cochrane Database Syst Rev 2003; (1):CD002255.
96. Anotayanonth S, Subhedar NV, Garner P, et al. Betamimetics for inhibiting preterm labour. Cochrane Database Syst Rev 2004; (4): CD004352.
97. Husslein P, Cabero Roura L, Dudenhausen JW, et al. Atosiban versus usual care for the management of preterm labor. J Perinat Med 2007; 35:305-13.
98. King J, Flenady V, Cole S, Thornton S. Cyclo-oxygenase (COX) inhibitors for treating preterm labour. Cochrane Database Syst Rev 2005; (2):CD001992.
99. Romero R, Sibai BM, Sanchez-Ramos L, et al. An oxytocin receptor antagonist (atosiban) in the treatment of preterm labor: A randomized, double-blind, placebo-controlled trial with tocolytic rescue. Am J Obstet Gynecol 2000; 182:1173-83.
100. Kashanian M, Akbarian AR, Soltanzadeh M. Atosiban and nifedipine for the treatment of preterm labor. Int J Gynaecol Obstet 2005; 91:10-4.
101. Al-Omari WR, Al-Shammaa HB, Al-Tikriti EM, Ahmed KW. Atosiban and nifedipine in acute tocolysis: A comparative study. Eur J Obstet Gynecol Reprod Biol 2006; 128:129-34.
102. Duckitt K, Thornton S. Nitric oxide donors for the treatment of preterm labour. Cochrane Database Syst Rev 2002; (3):CD002860.
103. Bowes WA Jr. Delivery of the very low birth weight infant. Clin Perinatol 1980; 8:183-95.
104. Low JA, Wood SL, Killen HL, et al. Intrapartum asphyxia in the preterm fetus less than 2000 gm. Am J Obstet Gynecol 1990; 162:378-82.
105. Malloy MH, Rhoads GG, Schramm W, Land G. Increasing cesarean section rates in very low-birth weight infants: Effect on outcome. JAMA 1989; 262:1475-8.
106. Malloy MH, Onstad L, Wright E. The effect of cesarean delivery on birth outcome in very low birth weight infants. National Institute of Child Health and Human Development Neonatal Research Network. Obstet Gynecol 1991; 77:498-503.

107. Grant A, Penn ZJ, Steer PJ. Elective or selective caesarean delivery of the small baby? A systematic review of the controlled trials. Br J Obstet Gynaecol 1996; 103:1197-1200.
108. Wylie BJ, Davidson LL, Batra M, Reed SD. Method of delivery and neonatal outcome in very low-birthweight vertex-presenting fetuses. Am J Obstet Gynecol 2008; 198:640.e1-7.
109. Sciscione AC, Landon MB, Leveno KJ, et al. Previous preterm cesarean delivery and risk of subsequent uterine rupture. Obstet Gynecol 2008; 111:648-53.
110. American College of Obstetricians and Gynecologists. Perinatal care at the threshold of viability. ACOG Practice Bulletin No. 38. Washington, DC, September 2002. (Obstet Gynecol 2002; 100:617-24.)
111. Gravenhorst JB, Schreuder AM, Veen S, et al. Breech delivery in very preterm and very low birthweight infants in The Netherlands. Br J Obstet Gynaecol 1993; 100:411-5.
112. Chervenak FA, Johnson RE, Youcha S, et al. Intrapartum management of twin gestation. Obstet Gynecol 1985; 65:119-24.
113. Boyle RJ, Kattwinkel J. Ethical issues surrounding resuscitation. Clin Perinatol 1999; 26:779-92.
114. Hack M, Friedman H, Fanaroff AA. Outcomes of extremely low birth weight infants. Pediatrics 1996; 98:931-7.
115. Management of the woman with threatened birth of an infant of extremely low gestational age. Fetus and Newborn Committee, Canadian Paediatric Society, Maternal-Fetal Medicine Committee, Society of Obstetricians and Gynaecologists of Canada. Can Med Assoc J 1994; 151:547-53.
116. 2005 American Heart Association (AHA) guidelines for cardiopulmonary resuscitation (CPR) and emergency cardiovascular care (ECC) of pediatric and neonatal patients: Neonatal resuscitation guidelines. Pediatrics 2006; 117:e1029-38.
117. Westgren M, Holmquist P, Svenningsen NW, Ingemarsson I. Intrapartum fetal monitoring in preterm deliveries: Prospective study. Obstet Gynecol 1982; 60:99-106.
118. Luthy DA, Shy KK, van Belle G, et al. A randomized trial of electronic fetal monitoring in preterm labor. Obstet Gynecol 1987; 69:687-95.
119. Shy KK, Luthy DA, Bennett FC, et al. Effects of electronic fetal-heart-rate monitoring, as compared with periodic auscultation, on the neurologic development of premature infants. N Engl J Med 1990; 322:588-93.
120. Thomas J, Long G, Moore G, Morgan D. Plasma protein binding and placental transfer of bupivacaine. Clin Pharmacol Ther 1976; 19:426-34.
121. Rane A, Sjoqvist F, Orrenius S. Cytochrome P-450 in human fetal liver microsomes. Chem Biol Interact 1971; 3:305.
122. Rane A, Sjoqvist F, Orrenius S. Drugs and fetal metabolism. Clin Pharmacol Ther 1973; 14:666-72.
123. Teramo K, Benowitz N, Heymann MA, Rudolph AM. Gestational differences in lidocaine toxicity in the fetal lamb. Anesthesiology 1976; 44:133-8.
124. Pedersen H, Santos AC, Morishima HO, et al. Does gestational age affect the pharmacokinetics and pharmacodynamics of lidocaine in mother and fetus? Anesthesiology 1988; 68:367-72.
125. Smedstad KG, Morison DH, Harris WH, Pascoe P. Placental transfer of local anesthetic in the premature sheep fetus. Int J Obstet Anesth 1993; 2:34-8.
126. Tucker GT, Mather LE. Clinical pharmacokinetics of local anaesthetics. Clin Pharmacokinet 1979; 4:241-78.
127. Biehl D, Shnider SM, Levinson G, Callender K. Placental transfer of lidocaine: Effects of fetal acidosis. Anesthesiology 1978; 48:409-12.
128. Ritter DA, Kenny JD, Norton HJ, Rudolph AJ. A prospective study of free bilirubin and other risk factors in the development of kernicterus in premature infants. Pediatrics 1982; 69:260-6.
129. Morishima HO, Pedersen H, Santos AC, et al. Adverse effects of maternally administered lidocaine on the asphyxiated preterm fetal lamb. Anesthesiology 1989; 71:110-5.
130. Morishima HO, Santos AC, Pedersen H, et al. Effect of lidocaine on the asphyxial responses in the mature fetal lamb. Anesthesiology 1987; 66:502-7.
131. Santos AC, Yun EM, Bobby PD, et al. The effects of bupivacaine, L-nitro-L-arginine-methyl ester, and phenylephrine on cardiovascular adaptations to asphyxia in the preterm fetal lamb. Anesth Analg 1997; 85:1299-306.
132. Arthur GR, Feldman HS, Covino BG. Comparative pharmacokinetics of bupivacaine and ropivacaine, a new amide local anesthetic. Anesth Analg 1988; 67:1053-8.
133. Datta S, Camann W, Bader A, VanderBurgh L. Clinical effects and maternal and fetal plasma concentrations of epidural ropivacaine versus bupivacaine for cesarean section. Anesthesiology 1995; 82:1346-52.
134. Ala-Kokko TI, Alahuhta S, Jouppila P, et al. Feto-maternal distribution of ropivacaine and bupivacaine after epidural administration for cesarean section. Int J Obstet Anesth 1997; 6:147-52.
135. Kuhnert BR, Kuhnert PM, Reese AL, et al. Maternal and neonatal elimination of CABA after epidural anesthesia with 2-chloroprocaine during parturition. Anesth Analg 1983; 62:1089-94.
136. Philipson EH, Kuhnert BR, Syracuse CD. Fetal acidosis, 2-chloroprocaine, and epidural anesthesia for cesarean section. Am J Obstet Gynecol 1985; 151:322-4.
137. Hollmen AI, Jouppila R, Jouppila P, et al. Effect of extradural analgesia using bupivacaine and 2-chloroprocaine on intervillous blood flow during normal labour. Br J Anaesth 1982; 54:837-42.
138. Ontario Perinatal Mortality Study Committee. Second report of the perinatal mortality study in ten university teaching hospitals. Three reports. Toronto, Department of Health, 1967:108-24.
139. Albright GA, Forster RM. Does combined spinal-epidural analgesia with subarachnoid sufentanil increase the incidence of emergency cesarean delivery? Reg Anesth 1997; 22:400-5.
140. Reynolds F. Neurological infections after neuraxial anesthesia. Anesthesiol Clin 2008; 26:23-52.
141. Rolbin SH, Cohen MM, Levinton CM, et al. The premature infant: Anesthesia for cesarean delivery. Anesth Analg 1994; 78:912-7.
142. Khaw KS, Wang CC, Ngan Kee WD, et al. Effects of high inspired oxygen fraction during elective caesarean section under spinal anaesthesia on maternal and fetal oxygenation and lipid peroxidation. Br J Anaesth 2002; 88:18-23.
143. Khaw KS, Ngan Kee WD, Lee A, et al. Supplementary oxygen for elective Caesarean section under spinal anaesthesia: Useful in prolonged uterine incision-to-delivery interval? Br J Anaesth 2004; 92:518-22.
144. Ngan Kee WD, Khaw KS, Ma KC, et al. Randomized, double-blind comparison of different inspired oxygen fractions during general anaesthesia for Caesarean section. Br J Anaesth 2002; 89:556-61.
145. Perouansky M. General anesthetics and long-term neurotoxicity. In Schuttler J, Schwilden H, editors. Modern Anesthetics. (Handbook of Experimental Pharmacology, vol 182.) New York, Springer, 2008:143-57.
146. Jevtovic-Todorovic V, Olney JW. Pro: Anesthesia-induced developmental neuroapoptosis: Status of the evidence. Anesth Analg 2008; 106:1659-63.
147. McClaine RJ, Uemura K, McClaine DJ, et al. A description of the preterm fetal sheep systemic and central responses to maternal general anesthesia. Anesth Analg 2007; 104:397-406.
148. Hearne AE, Nagey DA. Therapeutic agents in preterm labor: Tocolytic agents. Clin Obstet Gynecol 2000; 43:787-801.
149. Tsatsaris V, Papatsonis D, Goffinet F, et al. Tocolysis with nifedipine or beta-adrenergic agonists: A meta-analysis. Obstet Gynecol 2001; 97:840-7.
150. Forman A, Andersson KE, Ulmsten U. Inhibition of myometrial activity by calcium antagonists. Semin Perinatol 1981; 5:288-94.
151. Struyker-Boudier HA, Smits JF, De Mey JG. The pharmacology of calcium antagonists: A review. J Cardiovasc Pharmacol 1990; 15(Suppl 4):S1-10.
152. Glock JL, Morales WJ. Efficacy and safety of nifedipine versus magnesium sulfate in the management of preterm labor: A randomized study. Am J Obstet Gynecol 1993; 169:960-64.
153. Bal L, Thierry S, Brocas E, et al. Pulmonary edema induced by calcium-channel blockade for tocolysis. Anesth Analg 2004; 99:910-1.

154. Oei SG, Oei SK, Brolmann HA. Myocardial infarction during nifedipine therapy for preterm labor. N Engl J Med 1999; 340:154.
155. Blea CW, Barnard JM, Magness RR, et al. Effect of nifedipine on fetal and maternal hemodynamics and blood gases in the pregnant ewe. Am J Obstet Gynecol 1997; 176:922-30.
156. Ducsay CA, Thompson JS, Wu AT, Novy MJ. Effects of calcium entry blocker (nicardipine) tocolysis in rhesus macaques: Fetal plasma concentrations and cardiorespiratory changes. Am J Obstet Gynecol 1987; 157:1482-6.
157. Mari G, Kirshon B, Moise KJ Jr, et al. Doppler assessment of the fetal and uteroplacental circulation during nifedipine therapy for preterm labor. Am J Obstet Gynecol 1989; 161:1514-8.
158. Pirhonen JP, Erkkola RU, Ekblad UU, Nyman L. Single dose of nifedipine in normotensive pregnancy: Nifedipine concentrations, hemodynamic responses, and uterine and fetal flow velocity waveforms. Obstet Gynecol 1990; 76:807-11.
159. Tosone SR, Reves JG, Kissin I, et al. Hemodynamic responses to nifedipine in dogs anesthetized with halothane. Anesth Analg 1983; 62:903-8.
160. Ben-Ami M, Giladi Y, Shalev E. The combination of magnesium sulphate and nifedipine: A cause of neuromuscular blockade. Br J Obstet Gynaecol 1994; 101:262-3.
161. Csapo AI, Puri CP, Tarro S, Henzl MR. Deactivation of the uterus during normal and premature labor by the calcium antagonist nicardipine. Am J Obstet Gynecol 1982; 142:483-91.
162. Schorr SJ, Ascarelli MH, Rust OA, et al. A comparative study of ketorolac (Toradol) and magnesium sulfate for arrest of preterm labor. South Med J 1998; 91:1028-32.
163. Kramer WB, Saade G, Ou CN, et al. Placental transfer of sulindac and its active sulfide metabolite in humans. Am J Obstet Gynecol 1995; 172:886-90.
164. Kramer WB, Saade GR, Belfort M, et al. A randomized double-blind study comparing the fetal effects of sulindac to terbutaline during the management of preterm labor. Am J Obstet Gynecol 1999; 180:396-401.
165. Weitz CM, Ghodgaonkar RB, Dubin NH, Niebyl JR. Prostaglandin F metabolite concentration as a prognostic factor in preterm labor. Obstet Gynecol 1986; 67:496-9.
166. Niebyl JR, Witter FR. Neonatal outcome after indomethacin treatment for preterm labor. Am J Obstet Gynecol 1986; 155:747-9.
167. Kocsis JJ, Hernandovich J, Silver MJ, et al. Duration of inhibition of platelet prostaglandin formation and aggregation by ingested aspirin or indomethacin. Prostaglandins 1973; 3:141-4.
168. Moise KJ Jr, Huhta JC, Sharif DS, et al. Indomethacin in the treatment of premature labor: Effects on the fetal ductus arteriosus. N Engl J Med 1988; 319:327-31.
169. Dudley DK, Hardie MJ. Fetal and neonatal effects of indomethacin used as a tocolytic agent. Am J Obstet Gynecol 1985; 151:181-4.
170. Vermillion ST, Scardo JA, Lashus AG, Wiles HB. The effect of indomethacin tocolysis on fetal ductus arteriosus constriction with advancing gestational age. Am J Obstet Gynecol 1997; 177:256-9.
171. Moise KJ Jr. Effect of advancing gestational age on the frequency of fetal ductal constriction in association with maternal indomethacin use. Am J Obstet Gynecol 1993; 168:1350-3.
172. Kirshon B, Moise KJ Jr, Wasserstrum N, et al. Influence of short-term indomethacin therapy on fetal urine output. Obstet Gynecol 1988; 72:51-3.
173. Kirshon B, Moise KJ Jr, Mari G, Willis R. Long-term indomethacin therapy decreases fetal urine output and results in oligohydramnios. Am J Perinatol 1991; 8:86-8.
174. Anderson RJ, Berl T, McDonald KM, Schrier RW. Prostaglandins: Effects on blood pressure, renal blood flow, sodium and water excretion. Kidney Int 1976; 10:205-15.
175. Wurtzel D. Prenatal administration of indomethacin as a tocolytic agent: Effect on neonatal renal function. Obstet Gynecol 1990; 76:689-92.
176. Loe SM, Sanchez-Ramos L, Kaunitz AM. Assessing the neonatal safety of indomethacin tocolysis: A systematic review with meta-analysis. Obstet Gynecol 2005; 106:173-9.
177. de Swiet M, Redman CW. Aspirin, extradural anaesthesia and the MRC Collaborative Low-dose Aspirin Study in Pregnancy (CLASP). Br J Anaesth 1992; 69:109-10.
178. Horlocker TT, Wedel DJ, Offord KP. Does preoperative antiplatelet therapy increase the risk of hemorrhagic complications associated with regional anesthesia? Anesth Analg 1990; 70:631-4.
179. Horlocker TT, Wedel DJ, Schroeder DR, et al. Preoperative antiplatelet therapy does not increase the risk of spinal hematoma associated with regional anesthesia. Anesth Analg 1995; 80:303-9.
180. Horlocker TT, Wedel DJ, Benzon H, et al. Regional anesthesia in the anticoagulated patient: Defining the risks (the second ASRA Consensus Conference on Neuraxial Anesthesia and Anticoagulation). Reg Anesth Pain Med 2003; 28:172-97.
181. Loudon JA, Groom KM, Bennett PR. Prostaglandin inhibitors in preterm labour. Best Pract Res Clin Obstet Gynaecol 2003; 17:731-44.
182. Bukowski R, Mackay L, Fittkow C, et al. Inhibition of cervical ripening by local application of cyclooxygenase 2 inhibitor. Am J Obstet Gynecol 2001; 184:1374-8.
183. Sawdy RJ, Lye S, Fisk NM, Bennett PR. A double-blind randomized study of fetal side effects during and after the short-term maternal administration of indomethacin, sulindac, and nimesulide for the treatment of preterm labor. Am J Obstet Gynecol 2003; 188:1046-51.
184. Sawdy RJ, Groom KM, Bennett PR. Experience of the use of nimesulide, a cyclo-oxygenase-2 selective prostaglandin synthesis inhibitor, in the prevention of preterm labour in 44 high-risk cases. J Obstet Gynaecol 2004; 24:226-9.
185. Peruzzi L, Gianoglio B, Porcellini G, et al. [Neonatal chronic kidney failure associated with cyclo-oxygenase-2 inhibitors administered during pregnancy]. Minerva Urol Nefrol 2001; 53:113-6.
186. Ali US, Khubchandani S, Andankar P, et al. Renal tubular dysgenesis associated with in utero exposure to nimesulide. Pediatr Nephrol 2006; 21:274-6.
187. Kleinman G, Nuwayhid B, Rudelstorfer R, et al. Circulatory and renal effects of beta-adrenergic-receptor stimulation in pregnant sheep. Am J Obstet Gynecol 1984; 149:865-74.
188. Benedetti TJ. Life-threatening complications of betamimetic therapy for preterm labor inhibition. Clin Perinatol 1986; 13:843-52.
189. Berg G, Andersson RG, Ryden G. Beta-adrenergic receptors in human myometrium during pregnancy: Changes in the number of receptors after beta-mimetic treatment. Am J Obstet Gynecol 1985; 151:392-6.
190. Nanda K, Cook LA, Gallo MF, Grimes DA. Terbutaline pump maintenance therapy after threatened preterm labor for preventing preterm birth. Cochrane Database Syst Rev 2002; (4):CD003933.
191. Benedetti TJ, Hargrove JC, Rosene KA. Maternal pulmonary edema during premature labor inhibition. Obstet Gynecol 1982; 59:33S-7S.
192. Hatjis CG, Swain M. Systemic tocolysis for premature labor is associated with an increased incidence of pulmonary edema in the presence of maternal infection. Am J Obstet Gynecol 1988; 159:723-8.
193. Perry KG Jr, Morrison JC, Rust OA, et al. Incidence of adverse cardiopulmonary effects with low-dose continuous terbutaline infusion. Am J Obstet Gynecol 1995; 173:1273-7.
194. Michalak D, Klein V, Marquette GP. Myocardial ischemia: A complication of ritodrine tocolysis. Am J Obstet Gynecol 1983; 146:861-2.
195. Katz M, Robertson PA, Creasy RK. Cardiovascular complications associated with terbutaline treatment for preterm labor. Am J Obstet Gynecol 1981; 139:605-8.
196. Jacobs MM, Knight AB, Arias F. Maternal pulmonary edema resulting from betamimetic and glucocorticoid therapy. Obstet Gynecol 1980; 56:56-9.
197. Philipsen T, Eriksen PS, Lynggard F. Pulmonary edema following ritodrine-saline infusion in premature labor. Obstet Gynecol 1981; 58:304-8.
198. Benedetti TJ. Maternal complications of parenteral beta-sympathomimetic therapy for premature labor. Am J Obstet Gynecol 1983; 145:1-6.
199. Finley J, Katz M, Rojas-Perez M, et al. Cardiovascular consequences of beta-agonist tocolysis: An echocardiographic study. Obstet Gynecol 1984; 64:787-91.

200. Wagner JM, Morton MJ, Johnson KA, et al. Terbutaline and maternal cardiac function. JAMA 1981; 246:2697-701.
201. Armson BA, Samuels P, Miller F, et al. Evaluation of maternal fluid dynamics during tocolytic therapy with ritodrine hydrochloride and magnesium sulfate. Am J Obstet Gynecol 1992; 167:758-65.
202. Hankins GD, Hauth JC, Kuehl TJ, et al. Ritodrine hydrochloride infusion in pregnant baboons. II. Sodium and water compartment alterations. Am J Obstet Gynecol 1983; 147:254-9.
203. Pisani RJ, Rosenow EC 3rd. Pulmonary edema associated with tocolytic therapy. Ann Intern Med 1989; 110:714-8.
204. Gabel JC, Hansen TN, Drake RE. Effect of endotoxin on lung fluid balance in unanesthetized sheep. J Appl Physiol 1984; 56:489-94.
205. Conover WB, Benumof JL, Key TC. Ritodrine inhibition of hypoxic pulmonary vasoconstriction. Am J Obstet Gynecol 1983; 146:652-6.
206. Perkins RP, Varela-Gittings F, Dunn TS, et al. The influence of intravenous solution content on ritodrine-induced metabolic changes. Obstet Gynecol 1987; 70:892-5.
207. Young DC, Toofanian A, Leveno KJ. Potassium and glucose concentrations without treatment during ritodrine tocolysis. Am J Obstet Gynecol 1983; 145:105-6.
208. Miodovnik M, Peros N, Holroyde JC, Siddiqi TA. Treatment of premature labor in insulin-dependent diabetic women. Obstet Gynecol 1985; 65:621-7.
209. Sato K, Nishiwaki K, Kuno N, et al. Unexpected hyperkalemia following succinylcholine administration in prolonged immobilized parturients treated with magnesium and ritodrine. Anesthesiology 2000; 93:1539-41.
210. Kotani N, Kushikata T, Hashimoto H, et al. Rebound perioperative hyperkalemia in six patients after cessation of ritodrine for premature labor. Anesth Analg 2001; 93:709-11.
211. Kuczkowski KM, Benumof JL. Rebound hyperkalemia after cessation of intravenous tocolytic therapy with terbutaline in the treatment of preterm labor: Anesthetic implications. J Clin Anesth 2003; 15:357-8.
212. Lotgering FK, Lind J, Huikeshoven FJ, Wallenburg HC. Elevated serum transaminase levels during ritodrine administration. Am J Obstet Gynecol 1986; 155:390-2.
213. Nair GV, Ghosh AK, Lewis BV. Bowel distension during treatment of premature labour with beta-receptor agonists (letter). Lancet 1976; 1(7965):907.
214. Rosene KA, Featherstone HJ, Benedetti TJ. Cerebral ischemia associated with parenteral terbutaline use in pregnant migraine patients. Am J Obstet Gynecol 1982; 143:405-7.
215. Catanzarite VA, McHargue AM, Sandberg EC, Dyson DC. Respiratory arrest during therapy for premature labor in a patient with myasthenia gravis. Obstet Gynecol 1984; 64:819-22.
216. Epstein MF, Nicholls E, Stubblefield PG. Neonatal hypoglycemia after beta-sympathomimetic tocolytic therapy. J Pediatr 1979; 94:449-53.
217. Hadders-Algra M, Touwen BC, Huisjes HJ. Long-term follow-up of children prenatally exposed to ritodrine. Br J Obstet Gynaecol 1986; 93:156-61.
218. Laros RK Jr, Kitterman JA, Heilbron DC, et al. Outcome of very-low-birth-weight infants exposed to beta-sympathomimetics in utero. Am J Obstet Gynecol 1991; 164:1657-64.
219. Nuchpuckdee P, Brodsky N, Porat R, Hurt H. Ventricular septal thickness and cardiac function in neonates after in utero ritodrine exposure. J Pediatr 1986; 109:687-91.
220. Friedman DM, Blackstone J, Young BK, Hoskins IA. Fetal cardiac effects of oral ritodrine tocolysis. Am J Perinatol 1994; 11:109-12.
221. Kast A, Hermer M. Beta-adrenoceptor tocolysis and effects on the heart of fetus and neonate: A review. J Perinat Med 1993; 21:97-106.
222. Schoenfeld A, Joel-Cohen SJ, Duparc H, Levy E. Emergency obstetric anaesthesia and the use of beta2-sympathomimetic drugs. Br J Anaesth 1978; 50:969-71.
223. Crowhurst JA. Salbutamol, obstetrics and anaesthesia: A review and case discussion. Anaesth Intensive Care 1980; 8:39-43.
224. Ravindran R, Viegas OJ, Padilla LM, LaBlonde P. Anesthetic considerations in pregnant patients receiving terbutaline therapy. Anesth Analg 1980; 59:391-2.
225. Shin YK, Kim YD. Ventricular tachyarrhythmias during cesarean section after ritodrine therapy: Interaction with anesthetics. South Med J 1988; 81:528-30.
226. Suppan P. Tocolysis and anaesthesia for caesarean section. Br J Anaesth 1982; 54:1007.
227. Shin YK, Kim YD. Anesthetic considerations in patients receiving ritodrine therapy for preterm labor (abstract). Anesth Analg 1986; 65:S140.
228. Chestnut DH, Pollack KL, Thompson CS, et al. Does ritodrine worsen maternal hypotension during epidural anesthesia in gravid ewes? Anesthesiology 1990; 72:315-21.
229. Ralston DH, Shnider SM, DeLorimier AA. Effects of equipotent ephedrine, metaraminol, mephentermine, and methoxamine on uterine blood flow in the pregnant ewe. Anesthesiology 1974; 40:354-70.
230. Chestnut DH, Weiner CP, Wang JP, et al. The effect of ephedrine upon uterine artery blood flow velocity in the pregnant guinea pig subjected to terbutaline infusion and acute hemorrhage. Anesthesiology 1987; 66:508-12.
231. Chestnut DH, Ostman LG, Weiner CP, et al. The effect of vasopressor agents upon uterine artery blood flow velocity in the gravid guinea pig subjected to ritodrine infusion. Anesthesiology 1988; 68:363-6.
232. McGrath JM, Chestnut DH, Vincent RD, et al. Ephedrine remains the vasopressor of choice for treatment of hypotension during ritodrine infusion and epidural anesthesia. Anesthesiology 1994; 80:1073-81.
233. Lee A, Ngan Kee WD, Gin T. A quantitative, systematic review of randomized controlled trials of ephedrine versus phenylephrine for the management of hypotension during spinal anesthesia for cesarean delivery. Anesth Analg 2002; 94:920-6.
234. Cooper DW, Carpenter M, Mowbray P, et al. Fetal and maternal effects of phenylephrine and ephedrine during spinal anesthesia for cesarean delivery. Anesthesiology 2002; 97:1582-90.
235. Slater RM, From RP, Sum Ping JS, Pank JR. Changes in plasma potassium and neuromuscular blockade following suxamethonium in patients pre-treated with terbutaline. Eur J Anaesthesiol 1991; 8:281-6.
236. Bardou M, Rouget C, Breuiller-Fouche M, et al. Is the beta3-adrenoceptor (ADRB3) a potential target for uterorelaxant drugs? BMC Pregnancy Childbirth 2007; 7(Suppl 1):S14.
237. Phaneuf S, Asboth G, MacKenzie IZ, et al. Effect of oxytocin antagonists on the activation of human myometrium in vitro: Atosiban prevents oxytocin-induced desensitization. Am J Obstet Gynecol 1994; 171:1627-34.
238. Goodwin TM, Millar L, North L, et al. The pharmacokinetics of the oxytocin antagonist atosiban in pregnant women with preterm uterine contractions. Am J Obstet Gynecol 1995; 173:913-7.
239. Goodwin TM, Valenzuela GJ, Silver H, Creasy G. Dose ranging study of the oxytocin antagonist atosiban in the treatment of preterm labor. Atosiban Study Group. Obstet Gynecol 1996; 88:331-6.
240. Moutquin JM, Sherman D, Cohen H, et al. Double-blind, randomized, controlled trial of atosiban and ritodrine in the treatment of preterm labor: A multicenter effectiveness and safety study. Am J Obstet Gynecol 2000; 182:1191-9.
241. Worldwide Atosiban versus Beta-agonists Study Group. Effectiveness and safety of the oxytocin antagonist atosiban versus beta-adrenergic agonists in the treatment of preterm labour. Br J Obstet Gynaecol 2001; 108:133-42.
242. European Atosiban Study Group. The oxytocin antagonist atosiban versus the beta-agonist terbutaline in the treatment of preterm labor: A randomized, double-blind, controlled study. Acta Obstet Gynecol Scand 2001; 80:413-22.
243. Papatsonis D, Flenady V, Cole S, Liley H. Oxytocin receptor antagonists for inhibiting preterm labour. Cochrane Database Syst Rev 2005; (3): CD004452.
244. Grimes DA, Nanda K. Magnesium sulfate tocolysis: Time to quit. Obstet Gynecol 2006; 108:986-9.
245. Beall MH, Edgar BW, Paul RH, Smith-Wallace T. A comparison of ritodrine, terbutaline, and magnesium sulfate for the suppression of preterm labor. Am J Obstet Gynecol 1985; 153:854-9.

246. Hollander DI, Nagey DA, Pupkin MJ. Magnesium sulfate and ritodrine hydrochloride: A randomized comparison. Am J Obstet Gynecol 1987; 156:631-7.
247. Chau AC, Gabert HA, Miller JM Jr. A prospective comparison of terbutaline and magnesium for tocolysis. Obstet Gynecol 1992; 80:847-51.
248. Chestnut DH, Thompson CS, McLaughlin GL, Weiner CP. Does the intravenous infusion of ritodrine or magnesium sulfate alter the hemodynamic response to hemorrhage in gravid ewes? Am J Obstet Gynecol 1988; 159:1467-73.
249. Reynolds JD, Chestnut DH, Dexter F, et al. Magnesium sulfate adversely affects fetal lamb survival and blocks fetal cerebral blood flow response during maternal hemorrhage. Anesth Analg 1996; 83:493-9.
250. Mittendorf R, Covert R, Boman J, et al. Is tocolytic magnesium sulphate associated with increased total paediatric mortality? Lancet 1997; 350:1517-8.
251. Cox SM, Sherman ML, Leveno KJ. Randomized investigation of magnesium sulfate for prevention of preterm birth. Am J Obstet Gynecol 1990; 163:767-72.
252. Grether JK, Hoogstrate J, Selvin S, Nelson KB. Magnesium sulfate tocolysis and risk of neonatal death. Am J Obstet Gynecol 1998; 178:1-6.
253. Nelson KB, Grether JK. Can magnesium sulfate reduce the risk of cerebral palsy in very low birthweight infants? Pediatrics 1995; 95:263-9.
254. Scudiero R, Khoshnood B, Pryde PG, et al. Perinatal death and tocolytic magnesium sulfate. Obstet Gynecol 2000; 96:178-82.
255. Farkouh LJ, Thorp JA, Jones PG, et al. Antenatal magnesium exposure and neonatal demise. Am J Obstet Gynecol 2001; 185: 869-72.
256. Rouse DJ, Hirtz DG, Thom E, et al. A randomized, controlled trial of magnesium sulfate for the prevention of cerebral palsy. N Engl J Med 2008; 359:895-905.
257. Mittendorf R, Pryde PG. A review of the role for magnesium sulphate in preterm labour. Br J Obstet Gynaecol 2005; 112(Suppl 1):84-8.
258. Doyle LW, Crowther CA, Middleton P, Marret S. Magnesium sulphate for women at risk of preterm birth for neuroprotection of the fetus. Cochrane Database Syst Rev 2007; (3):CD004661.
259. Vincent RD Jr, Chestnut DH, Sipes SL, et al. Magnesium sulfate decreases maternal blood pressure but not uterine blood flow during epidural anesthesia in gravid ewes. Anesthesiology 1991; 74:77-82.
260. De Vore JS, Asrani R. Magnesium sulfate prevents succinylcholine-induced fasciculations in toxemic parturients. Anesthesiology 1980; 52:76-7.
261. James MF, Cork RC, Dennett JE. Succinylcholine pretreatment with magnesium sulfate. Anesth Analg 1986; 65:373-6.
262. Thompson SW, Moscicki JC, DiFazio CA. The anesthetic contribution of magnesium sulfate and ritodrine hydrochloride in rats. Anesth Analg 1988; 67:31-4.
263. Riley ET, Flanagan B, Cohen SE, Chitkarat U. Intravenous nitroglycerin: A potent uterine relaxant for emergency obstetric procedures: Review of literature and report of three cases. Int J Obstet Anesth 1996; 5:264-8.
264. Bukowski R, Saade GR. New developments in the management of preterm labor. Semin Perinatol 2001; 25:272-94.
265. Bradley KK, Buxton IL, Barber JE, et al. Nitric oxide relaxes human myometrium by a cGMP-independent mechanism. Am J Physiol 1998; 275:C1668-73.
266. Caponas G. Glyceryl trinitrate and acute uterine relaxation: A literature review. Anaesth Intensive Care 2001; 29:163-77.
267. Heymann M, Bootstaylor B, Roman C. Glyceryl trinitrate stops active labour in sheep. In Moncada S, Freelisch M, Busse R, Higgs EA, editors. The Biology of Nitric Oxide, Part 4. London, Portland Press, 1995:201-3.
268. Bootstaylor BS, Roman C, Parer JT, Heymann MA. Fetal and maternal hemodynamic and metabolic effects of maternal nitroglycerin infusions in sheep. Am J Obstet Gynecol 1997; 176:644-50.
269. Buhimschi CS, Buhimschi IA, Malinow AM, Weiner CP. Effects of sublingual nitroglycerin on human uterine contractility during the active phase of labor. Am J Obstet Gynecol 2002; 187:235-8.
270. Bisits A, Madsen G, Knox M, et al. The Randomized Nitric Oxide Tocolysis Trial (RNOTT) for the treatment of preterm labor. Am J Obstet Gynecol 2004; 191:683-90.
271. Smith GN, Walker MC, Ohlsson A, et al. Randomized double-blind placebo-controlled trial of transdermal nitroglycerin for preterm labor. Am J Obstet Gynecol 2007; 196:37.e1-8.

Chapter 35

Abnormal Presentation and Multiple Gestation

BettyLou Koffel, M.D.

The labor and delivery of a parturient with a multiple gestation and/or fetal breech presentation represents a major challenge for the obstetrician and the anesthesia provider. Anesthetic requirements may change from moment to moment, and an obstetric emergency may necessitate immediate intervention. All members of the perinatal care team must communicate directly and clearly with each other as well as with the parturient and her family in order to ensure the best possible outcome for both the mother and the neonate(s).

The **presentation** denotes that portion of the fetus that overlies the pelvic inlet. In most cases, the fetal presenting part can be palpated through the cervix during a vaginal examination. The presentation may be **cephalic, breech,** or **shoulder**. Breech and shoulder presentations occur with increased frequency in patients with multiple gestation. Cephalic presentations are further subdivided into **vertex, brow,** and **face** presentations according to the degree of flexion of the neck.

The **lie** refers to the alignment of the fetal spine with the maternal spine. The fetal lie can be either longitudinal or transverse. A fetus with a vertex or breech presentation has a longitudinal lie. A persistent oblique or transverse lie typically requires abdominal delivery.

The **position** of the fetus denotes the relationship of a specific fetal bony point to the maternal pelvis. The position of the **occiput** defines the position for vertex presentations. Other markers for position are the **sacrum** for breech presentations, the **mentum** for face presentations, and the **acromion** for shoulder presentations. The **attitude** of the fetus describes the relationship of the fetal parts with one another; the term is typically used to refer to the position of the head with regard to the trunk, as in flexed, military, or hyperextended.

ABNORMAL POSITION

During normal labor, the fetal occiput rotates from a transverse or oblique position to a direct **occiput anterior** position. In a minority of patients with an oblique posterior position, the occiput rotates directly posteriorly and results in a **persistent occiput posterior** position. Most cases of persistent occiput posterior position develop through malrotation from an initially occiput anterior position.[1] The occiput posterior position may lead to a prolonged labor that is associated with increased maternal discomfort. Less often, the vertex remains in the **occiput transverse** position; this condition is known as **deep transverse arrest**.

In the past, obstetricians performed manual or forceps rotation to hasten delivery and lessen perineal trauma in women with an abnormal position of the vertex. Today, many obstetricians are reluctant to perform rotational forceps delivery for fear of causing excessive maternal and/or fetal trauma. In cases of persistent occiput posterior position, the contemporary obstetrician is more likely to allow the head to remain in the occiput posterior position at vaginal delivery. One third of nulliparous women and 55% of parous women with a persistent occiput posterior position achieve spontaneous vaginal delivery.[2] Some cases of persistent occiput posterior position, and many cases of deep transverse arrest, require cesarean delivery because of dystocia.

During administration of epidural analgesia in a patient with an abnormal position, it is helpful to add a lipid-soluble opioid to a dilute solution of local anesthetic. This combination provides analgesia while preserving pelvic muscle tone. Relaxation of the pelvic floor and perineum may deter the spontaneous rotation of the vertex during labor. In contrast, profound pelvic floor relaxation is needed to facilitate instrumental vaginal delivery.

BREECH PRESENTATION

Breech presentation describes a longitudinal lie in which the fetal buttocks and/or lower extremities overlie the pelvic inlet. Figure 35-1 shows the three varieties of breech presentation:

- **Frank breech**—lower extremities flexed at the hips and extended at the knees
- **Complete breech**—lower extremities flexed at both the hips and the knees
- **Incomplete breech**—one or both of the lower extremities extended at the hips

Ultrasonographic or radiographic examination typically allows the obstetrician to confirm the type of breech presentation and to exclude the presence of severe congenital anomalies (e.g., anencephaly). The type of breech presentation may influence the obstetrician's decision regarding the mode of delivery. The fetus with a frank breech presentation tends to remain in that presentation throughout labor. In contrast, a complete breech presentation may change to an incomplete breech presentation at any time before or during labor.

Epidemiology

The breech presentation is the most common of the abnormal presentations. Both the incidence and the type of breech presentation vary with gestational age (Table 35-1). Before 28 weeks' gestation, as many as 40% of fetuses are in a breech presentation. Most of these change to a vertex presentation by 34 weeks' gestation, but 3% to 4% of fetuses remain in a breech presentation at term.

Many factors predispose to breech presentation (Box 35-1).[3,4] Abnormalities of the fetus or the maternal pelvis or uterus may play a role. Among patients with pelvic or uterine abnormalities, a breech presentation may allow more room for fetal growth and movement. Likewise, hydrocephalic fetuses are more likely to assume a breech presentation. Multiparity, multiple gestation, hydramnios, and anencephaly also predispose to breech presentation. These conditions may interfere with the normal process of accommodation between the fetal head and the uterine cavity and maternal pelvis. Other factors may also play a role. In a prospective cohort study, low free thyroid hormone (T_4) levels at 12 weeks' gestation were associated with breech presentation at term.[5]

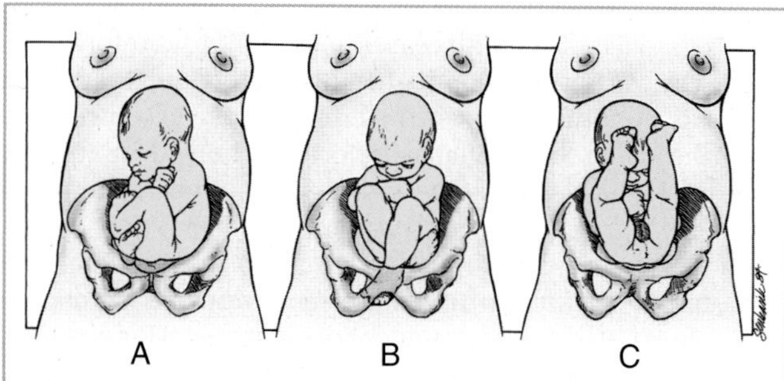

FIGURE 35-1 Three possible breech presentations. **A,** The **complete breech** demonstrates flexion of the hips and flexion of the knees. **B,** The **incomplete breech** demonstrates intermediate deflexion of one or both hips and knees. **C,** The **frank breech** shows flexion of the hips and extension of both knees. (From Lanni SM, Seeds JW. Malpresentations. In Gabbe SG, Niebyl JR, Simpson JL, editors. Obstetrics: Normal and Problem Pregnancies. 5th edition. New York, Churchill Livingstone, 2007:436.)

TABLE 35-1 Types of Breech Presentation

Type of Breech	Percentage of All Breech Presentations	Percentage of Preterm Gestation Breech Presentations
Frank	48-73	38
Complete	5-12	12
Incomplete	12-38	50

Modified from Lanni SM, Seeds JW. Malpresentations. In Gabbe SG, Niebyl JR, Simpson JL, editors. Obstetrics: Normal and Problem Pregnancies. 5th edition. New York, Churchill Livingstone, 2007:436.

Box 35-1 Factors Associated with Breech Presentation

Uterine Distention or Relaxation
- Multiparity
- Multiple gestation
- Hydramnios
- Macrosomia

Abnormalities of the Uterus or Pelvis
- Pelvic tumors
- Uterine anomalies
- Pelvic contracture

Abnormalities of the Fetus
- Hydrocephalus
- Anencephaly

Obstetric Conditions
- Previous breech delivery
- Preterm gestation
- Oligohydramnios
- Cornual-fundal placenta
- Placenta previa

Modified from Cunningham FG, Leveno KJ, Bloom SL, et al. In Williams Obstetrics. 22nd edition. New York, McGraw-Hill, 2005:565-86; and Lanni SM, Seeds JW. Malpresentations. In Gabbe SG, Niebyl JR, Simpson JL, editors. Obstetrics: Normal and Problem Pregnancies. 5th edition. New York, Churchill Livingstone, 2007:428-55.

TABLE 35-2 Incidence of Complications Associated with Breech Presentation

Complication	Incidence
Intrapartum fetal death	Increased 16-fold*
Intrapartum asphyxia	Increased 3.8-fold*
Umbilical cord prolapse	Increased 5- to 20-fold*
Birth trauma	Increased 13-fold*
Arrest of aftercoming head	4.6%-8.8%
Spinal cord injuries with deflexion	21%
Major congenital anomalies	6%-18%
Preterm delivery	16%-33%
Hyperextension of head	5%

*Compared to cephalic presentation.

Modified from Lanni SM, Seeds JW. Malpresentations. In Gabbe SG, Niebyl JR, Simpson JL, editors. Obstetrics: Normal and Problem Pregnancies. 5th edition. New York, Churchill Livingstone, 2007:441.

Obstetric Complications

Obstetric complications are more likely with a breech presentation (Table 35-2). Cesarean delivery decreases the risk for some of these complications. Vaginal breech delivery entails a higher risk of neonatal trauma than delivery of an infant with a vertex presentation, but cesarean delivery does not eliminate the risk of trauma to the infant. Rather, cesarean delivery of a breech presentation can be difficult and traumatic, especially if the skin and uterine incisions are insufficient or maternal muscle relaxation is inadequate.

The risk of umbilical cord prolapse varies with the type of breech presentation (Table 35-3). In the parturient with an incomplete breech presentation, the presenting part does not fill the cervix as well as the vertex or buttocks, allowing the umbilical cord to prolapse into the vagina before delivery. Umbilical cord prolapse typically necessitates prompt cesarean delivery.

MORBIDITY AND MORTALITY

There is a higher risk of **perinatal morbidity** and **mortality** with a breech presentation, even when the risk is adjusted for preterm gestation. The factors that cause breech presentation are often more important than the presentation itself. For example, the severe congenital anomalies that predispose to breech presentation (e.g., hydrocephalus, anencephaly) significantly contribute to neonatal morbidity and mortality. Relative perinatal mortality rates (calculated from data for linked siblings from the Norway Medical Birth Registry) confirm that breech presentation is a marker of perinatal risk, regardless of the mode of delivery.[6] Both nonreassuring fetal heart rate (FHR) tracings and dystocia occur more commonly in patients with a term breech presentation, even those who have undergone successful external cephalic version.[7]

Breech presentation is also associated with an increased risk of **maternal morbidity** and **mortality**. Vaginal breech delivery entails a higher risk of maternal infection, perineal trauma, and hemorrhage.[3] Cesarean delivery is associated with a modest increase in risk of maternal morbidity and mortality,[3,8] especially febrile morbidity.[9] These risks may be even higher for patients who require emergency abdominal delivery. However, in a single-center study of 846 singleton breech deliveries, Schiff et al.[9] did not find a higher risk of maternal morbidity in women who underwent cesarean delivery during labor than in women who underwent planned cesarean delivery.

TABLE 35-3 Risk of Umbilical Cord Prolapse

Type of Breech	Risk of Cord Prolapse (%)
Frank	0.5
Complete	4-6
Incomplete	15-18

Modified from Lanni SM, Seeds JW. Malpresentations. In Gabbe SG, Niebyl JR, Simpson JL, editors. Obstetrics: Normal and Problem Pregnancies. 5th edition. New York, Churchill Livingstone, 2007:436.

Obstetric Management

EXTERNAL CEPHALIC VERSION

The process of external cephalic version converts a breech or shoulder presentation to a vertex presentation. This procedure is successful in 35% to 86% of nonlaboring women at term.[10-12] External cephalic version is most likely to be successful if (1) the presenting part has not entered the pelvis, (2) amniotic fluid volume is normal, (3) the fetal back is not positioned posteriorly, (4) the patient is not obese, (5) the patient is parous, and (6) the presentation is frank breech or transverse.[10-13] Early labor does not preclude successful external cephalic version.[12] External cephalic version is rarely successful when the cervix is fully dilated or when the membranes have ruptured,[10] although anecdotal cases of success in such conditions have been reported.[14]

The optimal timing of external cephalic version is unclear. Compared with external cephalic version at term, external cephalic version at 34 to 35 weeks' gestation may decrease the rate of noncephalic presentation and cesarean delivery.[15] (A large trial is under way to confirm this finding and to assess perinatal outcomes.[15]) However, the fetus may spontaneously return to a breech presentation before the onset of labor. For this reason, many obstetricians prefer to delay external cephalic version until 37 to 39 weeks' gestation. If external cephalic version is successful, the obstetrician may then proceed with amniotomy induction of labor.

Successful external cephalic version helps reduce the risk of perinatal morbidity and mortality associated with breech delivery. The American College of Obstetricians and Gynecologists (ACOG)[16] has suggested that "obstetricians should offer and perform external cephalic version whenever possible." Labor and vaginal delivery occur in 63% to 83% of patients who have undergone successful external cephalic version,[11,17,18] albeit with an increased risk for intrapartum cesarean delivery because of dystocia or a nonreassuring FHR tracing (intrapartum cesarean delivery rate of 27.6% after successful external cephalic version versus 12.5% in women with a spontaneous cephalic presentation).[18]

External cephalic version is associated with a low rate of morbidity in contemporary obstetric practice. Safe external cephalic version requires continuous FHR monitoring. In a systematic review of 44 studies that involved 7377 women,[19] complications included transient (5.7%) and persistent (0.37%) FHR abnormalities, vaginal bleeding (0.47%), and placental abruption (0.12%). Fetomaternal hemorrhage is another potential complication of external cephalic version.[19] In one study, 16 of 89 (18%) patients undergoing external cephalic version had Kleihauer-Betke stains signaling the occurrence of fetomaternal hemorrhage.[20]

Obstetricians often administer a tocolytic agent (e.g., terbutaline) before performing external cephalic version. Two small studies found no difference in success rate of external cephalic version with administration of nitroglycerin and that of terbutaline[21] or placebo.[22]

Several studies have described the use of epidural or spinal anesthesia or analgesia for external cephalic version.[17,23-25] Maternal discomfort may be significant during external cephalic version; greater pain during the procedure is associated with a lower chance of success.[26] Some obstetricians argue that the absence of anesthesia limits the force that the obstetrician can apply during the procedure. They contend that administration of anesthesia may encourage the obstetrician to use excessive force, possibly increasing the risk of perinatal morbidity and mortality.

Schorr et al.[17] randomly assigned 69 women to receive epidural anesthesia (2% lidocaine with epinephrine) or no epidural anesthesia for external cephalic version. The success rate was better in the anesthesia group than in the no-anesthesia group (67% versus 32%, respectively; relative risk 2.1; 95% confidence interval 1.2 to 3.6), and there was no evidence of adverse outcome due to the administration of epidural anesthesia. Similarly, Mancuso et al.[25] randomly assigned 108 women to receive either epidural anesthesia (2% lidocaine and fentanyl) or no anesthesia. The rate of successful version was higher in the anesthesia group (59%) than in the no-anesthesia group (33%) (relative risk 1.8; 95% confidence interval 1.2 to 2.8). Weiniger et al.[23] randomly assigned 70 women to receive either spinal analgesia with bupivacaine 7.5 mg or no anesthesia for external cephalic version. The success rate was 67% in those receiving spinal analgesia, 32% in those without analgesia, and 42% in those who did not consent to enroll in the study. Failure of the procedure was attributed to pain in 15 women in the control group. Eleven of those 15 (73%) women subsequently had successful external cephalic version with spinal analgesia. In contrast, Dugoff et al.[24] found no difference in success rate of external cephalic version between women randomly assigned to receive spinal analgesia (bupivacaine 2.5 mg and sufentanil 10 μg) and the control group without analgesia (44% versus 42%, respectively). Several randomized controlled trials that found no difference in version success rates between women who received neuraxial analgesia/anesthesia and those who received no analgesia/anesthesia have been published as abstracts[27] rather than full reports. This fact suggests the potential for publication bias in the reports of these studies. Additionally, whether or not the *density* of neuraxial analgesia/anesthesia influences the success rate of external cephalic version has not been studied.

Several investigators reported successful outcomes with neuraxial analgesia/anesthesia in women in whom the first attempt at external cephalic version without neuraxial analgesia had been unsuccessful.[28,29] These patients elected to undergo another version attempt with neuraxial analgesia. Neiger et al.[28] reported that 9 of 16 (56%) second procedures were successful, and 7 of those 9 women delivered vaginally. Cherayil et al.[29] reported successful version in 13 of 15 (87%) repeat procedures with neuraxial blockade.

In the Kaiser Permanente Northwest and Providence Health Systems, we do not routinely provide spinal or epidural analgesia during external cephalic version. However, the report by Weiniger et al.,[23] as well as my daughter's description of the discomfort associated with her unsuccessful external cephalic version, have influenced me to advocate for adequate analgesia during this procedure.

MODE OF DELIVERY

A substantial number of obstetricians recommend the routine performance of cesarean delivery in patients with a breech presentation. In contemporary obstetric practice in the United States, most pregnancies with a breech presentation are delivered abdominally.

The Term Breech Trial Collaborative Group enrolled 2088 women from 26 countries with a singleton fetus in a frank or complete breech presentation.[30] These women were randomly assigned to undergo planned cesarean delivery or planned vaginal delivery. Using an intent-to-treat analysis, the investigators noted that perinatal and neonatal mortality rates, and serious neonatal morbidity, were significantly lower in the planned cesarean delivery group. This difference was greatest in those countries with a low perinatal mortality rate (e.g., Canada, United Kingdom, United States).[30] Secondary analysis of perinatal outcomes demonstrated that the lowest risk of adverse outcome occurred when a prelabor cesarean delivery was performed at term gestation. The risk of adverse outcome progressively increased with cesarean delivery performed during early labor and active labor, and was highest with a vaginal birth. Labor augmentation, a longer duration of the second stage, and inexperienced clinicians were associated with perinatal morbidity and mortality.[31] Interestingly, in a 2-year follow-up study in some centers that participated in the Term Breech Trial, there were no differences in death or neurodevelopmental delay between children delivered by planned cesarean and those delivered by planned vaginal delivery.[32] The following two factors may have contributed to the lack of significant differences in outcome at 2 years of age: (1) the sample size may have been inadequate and (2) measures of early neonatal morbidity have a low predictive value for long-term outcomes (i.e., most children with early neonatal morbidity survive and develop normally).[32] Nonetheless, these studies have had worldwide impact on obstetric practice, and the number of planned vaginal breech deliveries has decreased markedly.

Maternal morbidity and mortality in the Term Breech Trial were no different in the two groups for the first 6 postpartum weeks.[30] Women who underwent planned cesarean delivery were less likely to report urinary incontinence at 3 months.[33] Maternal outcomes at 2 years after delivery were similar after planned abdominal delivery and after planned vaginal delivery for singleton breech infants born at term.[34]

Controversy continues within the obstetric community. Some obstetricians believe that vaginal breech delivery still has a place in contemporary obstetric practice.[3,4] For example, obstetricians from the National Maternity Hospital in Dublin reported outcomes from their institution, which has strict prelabor and intrapartum criteria for planned vaginal breech delivery.[35] A review of 641 breech deliveries in that hospital between January 1997 and June 2000 identified 343 (54%) women who underwent elective cesarean delivery and 298 (46%) who underwent a trial of labor. Vaginal delivery occurred in 49% of those who labored. Most (94%) of the intrapartum cesarean deliveries were performed for arrest of labor, and 7 (4.6%) were performed for a nonreassuring FHR tracing. There were no intrapartum or neonatal deaths in normal infants (three infants delivered vaginally had lethal malformations), and no neonates had evidence of neurologic injury or major soft tissue or skeletal trauma. Lanni and Seeds[4] summarized the ongoing controversy surrounding the Term Breech Trial by saying that it "certainly adds to the body of literature on breech vaginal delivery but may not be the final answer to the question of safety of vaginal breech delivery." Glezerman[36] raised important questions about the methodology and design of the Term Breech Trial while recognizing that "the point of no return has been reached as far as planned vaginal breech delivery is concerned." Likewise, results from an Australian survey suggest that "few of the next generation of . . . obstetricians plan to offer vaginal breech delivery to their patients."[37]

In 2006 the American College of Obstetricians and Gynecologists[16] made the following recommendations about mode of singleton breech delivery at term:

The decision regarding mode of delivery should depend on the experience of the health care provider. Cesarean delivery will be the preferred mode for most physicians because of the diminishing expertise in vaginal breech delivery. Planned vaginal delivery of a term singleton breech fetus may be reasonable under hospital-specific protocol guidelines for both eligibility and labor management. Before a vaginal breech delivery is planned, women should be informed that the risk of perinatal or neonatal mortality or short-term serious neonatal morbidity may be higher than if a cesarean delivery is planned, and the patient's informed consent should be documented.[16]

Although a planned trial of labor and vaginal breech delivery occurs uncommonly in most hospitals in North America and the United Kingdom, vaginal breech delivery still occurs because some patients present in advanced labor. Selection criteria such as those listed in Box 35-2 are used by advocates of a trial of labor and vaginal delivery. The availability of personnel experienced in obstetric anesthesia and neonatal resuscitation are prerequisites. Most patients who undergo a trial of labor for breech presentation receive epidural analgesia.[8] Hyperextension of the fetal head remains an absolute contraindication to a trial of labor in the patient with a breech presentation.

BOX 35-2 Criteria for a Trial of Labor and Vaginal Delivery for Patients with Fetal Breech Presentation

- Frank breech presentation
- Adequate pelvis by imaging pelvimetry
- Estimated fetal weight between 2000 and 3500 g by ultrasonography or by two experienced examiners
- Flexion of the fetal head (the neutral position—the so-called military position—is also acceptable)
- Continuous electronic fetal heart rate monitoring
- Spontaneous progression of labor, with timely effacement and dilation of the cervix and timely descent of the breech
- Availability of an individual skilled in vaginal breech delivery and an assistant
- Availability of an individual skilled in the administration of obstetric anesthesia
- Spontaneous delivery to the level of the umbilicus
- Ability to perform an abdominal delivery promptly
- Availability of an individual with skills in neonatal resuscitation

VAGINAL BREECH DELIVERY

Several aspects of the conduct of breech labor differ from those for a vertex presentation. The cervix must be fully dilated before the patient begins to push. Indeed, some obstetricians delay maternal expulsive efforts until 30 minutes after the diagnosis of full cervical dilation. Others delay expulsive efforts until the breech is at the perineum.

There are three varieties of vaginal breech delivery. **Spontaneous breech delivery** is delivery without any traction or manipulation other than support of the infant's body. With **assisted breech delivery** (also known as partial breech extraction), the infant is delivered spontaneously as far as the umbilicus; at that time, the obstetrician assists delivery of the chest and the aftercoming head. With **total breech extraction,** the obstetrician applies traction on the feet and ankles to deliver the entire body of the infant. Except for vaginal delivery of a second twin, obstetricians almost never perform total breech extraction. Total breech extraction increases the likelihood of difficult, traumatic delivery, including entrapment of the fetal head.

During assisted breech delivery or total breech extraction, the obstetrician attempts to maintain flexion of the cervical spine during delivery of the aftercoming head. This may be accomplished manually or by the application of Piper forceps (Figures 35-2 through 35-4). In most cases the obstetrician performs a generous episiotomy to prevent perineal obstruction of the aftercoming head.

CESAREAN DELIVERY

Cesarean delivery does not guarantee an atraumatic delivery, especially if the skin and uterine incisions are inadequate. Before 32 weeks' gestation, the lower uterine segment may be inadequate to allow an atraumatic delivery through a low transverse uterine incision. In such cases, the obstetrician should perform a low vertical incision, which can be extended to facilitate an atraumatic delivery. Unfortunately, such incisions often extend to the body of the uterus, which does not heal as well as the lower uterine segment. It is unclear whether this situation increases the risk of uterine rupture during a trial of labor in a subsequent pregnancy (see Chapter 19).

Anesthetic Management

Benefits of neuraxial analgesia during labor include (1) pain relief, (2) inhibition of early pushing, (3) ability of the parturient to push during the second stage and spontaneously deliver the infant to the level of the umbilicus, (4) a relaxed pelvic floor and perineum at delivery, and (5) the option to

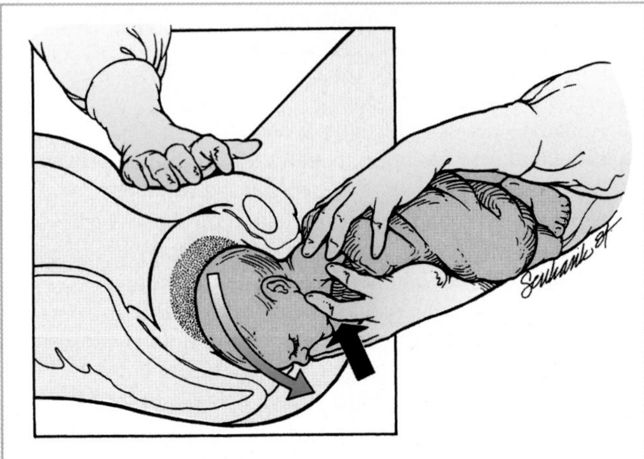

FIGURE 35-2 Vaginal breech delivery. The *black arrow* indicates the direction of pressure from two fingers of the operator's right hand on the fetal maxilla (not the mandible). This maneuver assists in maintaining appropriate flexion of the fetal vertex (*direction of white arrow*), as does moderate suprapubic pressure from an assistant. Delivery of the head may be accomplished with continued maternal expulsive forces and gentle downward traction. (From Lanni SM, Seeds JW. Malpresentations. In Gabbe SG, Niebyl JR, Simpson JL, editors. Obstetrics: Normal and Problem Pregnancies. 5th edition. New York, Churchill Livingstone, 2007:440.)

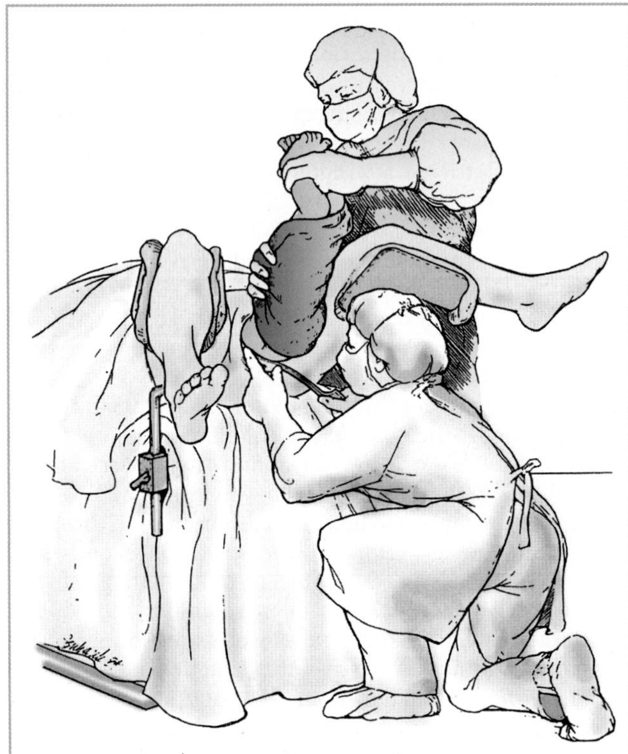

FIGURE 35-3 Vaginal breech delivery. Demonstration of INCORRECT assistance during the application of Piper forceps; the assistant hyperextends the fetal neck. Such positioning increases the risk for neurologic injury. (From Lanni SM, Seeds JW. Malpresentations. In Gabbe SG, Niebyl JR, Simpson JL, editors. Obstetrics: Normal and Problem Pregnancies. 5th edition. New York, Churchill Livingstone, 2007:440.)

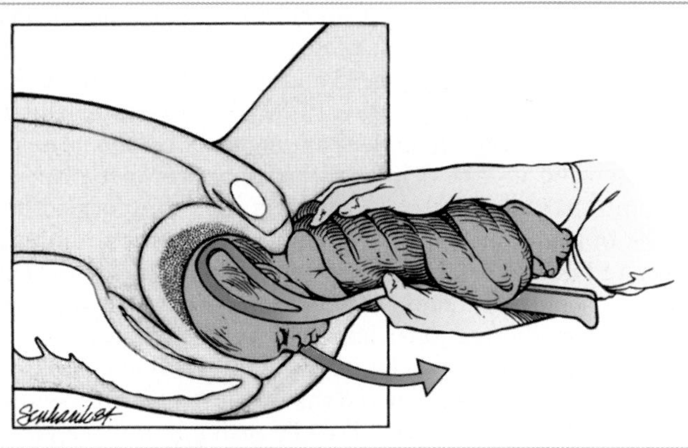

FIGURE 35-4 Vaginal breech delivery. Once the Piper forceps are applied, the fetal trunk is supported by one hand, and gentle traction on the forceps (*arrow*) in the direction of the pelvic axis results in a controlled delivery, as illustrated here. (From Lanni SM, Seeds JW. Malpresentations. In Gabbe SG, Niebyl JR, Simpson JL, editors. Obstetrics: Normal and Problem Pregnancies. 5th edition. New York, Churchill Livingstone, 2007:441.)

extend analgesia to surgical anesthesia for emergency cesarean delivery if needed.

ANALGESIA FOR LABOR

Emergency cesarean delivery may be required at any time during a trial of labor. Epidural analgesia and combined spinal-epidural (CSE) analgesia are excellent choices during a trial of labor in patients with a breech presentation. The anesthesia provider should tailor the analgesic technique to the needs of the individual patient. Patients with a breech presentation often have earlier complaints of rectal pressure than patients with a vertex presentation. It is important to provide sufficient sacral analgesia to inhibit pushing during the first stage of labor. The patient must not push before the cervix is fully dilated; otherwise, the patient might push a lower extremity through her partially dilated cervix, which may result in fetal head entrapment. Early pushing may also increase the risk of a prolapsed umbilical cord. I prefer to add a lipid-soluble opioid (e.g., fentanyl, sufentanil) to a dilute solution of local anesthetic, and I administer that solution by continuous or patient-controlled epidural infusion. Use of a local anesthetic alone to eliminate low back and perineal discomfort results in extensive motor blockade, which may decrease the effectiveness of maternal expulsive efforts during the second stage. The advantages of the epidural administration of both a local anesthetic and a lipid-soluble opioid were confirmed by Benhamou et al.,[38] who observed that a continuous epidural infusion of bupivacaine 0.0625% with sufentanil 0.25 μg/mL produced better maternal analgesia and less motor block than administration of bupivacaine 0.125% in parturients with a breech presentation.

ANESTHESIA FOR VAGINAL BREECH DELIVERY

The patient with a breech presentation should deliver in a room where an emergency abdominal delivery can be performed immediately. I administer a nonparticulate antacid at the time of transfer to the delivery room. The anesthesia provider should be prepared for emergency administration of general anesthesia at any time. Umbilical cord compression is common during the second stage of labor in a patient with a breech presentation. For these reasons, the mother often receives supplemental oxygen during vaginal breech delivery.

Provision of effective analgesia/anesthesia for vaginal breech delivery represents a true challenge for the anesthesia provider. During the second stage of labor, the anesthesia provider is asked to provide analgesia while maintaining adequate maternal expulsive efforts. If the patient is unable to achieve spontaneous delivery of a *vertex* presentation, the obstetrician may perform instrumental vaginal delivery. In contrast, total breech extraction of a singleton fetus is unacceptable in modern obstetric practice. Most obstetricians insist on spontaneous delivery of the infant to the level of the umbilicus.

At any time, the anesthesia provider may be asked to quickly provide dense anesthesia for vaginal or cesarean delivery. Many obstetricians routinely apply Piper forceps to the aftercoming head. This maneuver requires adequate anesthesia and perineal muscle relaxation. Because I typically administer a dilute solution of local anesthetic during the first stage of labor, it often is necessary to administer a more concentrated solution of local anesthetic at the time of delivery. I prefer to maintain analgesia with bupivacaine, but I always have a syringe of 3% 2-chloroprocaine immediately available. To ensure the presence of adequate anesthesia for operative delivery, I begin to inject 3% 2-chloroprocaine at the first evidence of difficulty.

Perhaps the obstetrician's greatest fear is the risk of **fetal head entrapment**. Most cases of this complication involve entrapment of the fetal head behind a partially dilated cervix. The head may also be entrapped by the perineum. Fetal head entrapment is more likely to occur in patients at less than 32 weeks' gestation. Before 32 weeks' gestation, the fetal head is larger than the wedge formed by the fetal buttocks and thighs. The lower extremities, buttocks, and abdomen may deliver before the cervix is fully dilated, and the cervix may then entrap the head. If this complication occurs, the obstetrician may choose one of the following three options: (1) performance of Dührssen incisions in the cervix, (2) request for relaxation of skeletal and cervical smooth muscle, or (3) cesarean delivery.

The performance of **Dührssen incisions** may be technically difficult. The obstetrician makes two or three radial incisions in the cervix at the 2, 6, and 10 o'clock positions.[3] This procedure is associated with a higher risk of maternal morbidity (e.g., genitourinary trauma, hemorrhage). The blood loss may be substantial and concealed. Bleeding within the peritoneal cavity may not be visible externally.

More often, the obstetrician requests that the anesthesia provider establish **relaxation of skeletal and cervical smooth muscle.** Smooth muscle represents only 15% of total cervical tissue,[39] and some physicians argue that it is not possible to provide profound relaxation of the cervix through smooth muscle relaxation. Nonetheless, the provision of both skeletal and smooth muscle relaxation often facilitates vaginal delivery of the aftercoming head. In the past, the technique of choice was rapid-sequence induction of general anesthesia, followed by administration of a high concentration (2 to 3 minimum alveolar concentration [MAC]) of a volatile halogenated agent. It is unnecessary to administer nitrous oxide because such a large dose of the volatile halogenated agent is being given. Moreover, the compromised fetus might benefit from a high inspired concentration of oxygen. This technique results in uterine and cervical relaxation in 2 to 3 minutes. If fetal head entrapment results from perineal obstruction, delivery may soon follow the administration of succinylcholine.

Immediately after delivery, the anesthesia provider should discontinue administration of the volatile halogenated agent and substitute nitrous oxide, with or without an opioid. Administration of a high concentration of a volatile halogenated agent increases the risk of uterine atony after delivery. Prompt discontinuation of the volatile halogenated agent, along with intravenous administration of oxytocin, should provide adequate uterine tone in most patients. Anesthesia should be maintained until the placenta is delivered, the episiotomy and lacerations are repaired, and hemostasis is secured.

In modern practice, intravenous or sublingual administration of nitroglycerin has nearly replaced the use of volatile halogenated agents as agents for uterine relaxation. Administration of nitroglycerin results in the release of nitric oxide, which helps mediate the relaxation of smooth muscle. This common, widespread practice is based on case reports and small series of cases. Well-designed clinical trials on the use of nitroglycerin to provide uterine relaxation in obstetric emergencies are lacking, although the administration of this agent for this purpose appears safe for both the mother and fetus/neonate.[40] Factors such as pregnancy and labor may affect the human myometrial response to nitroglycerin and nitric oxide.

Buhimschi et al.[41] attempted to provide an objective assessment of the effect of nitroglycerin on human uterine tone and contractility in laboring women. In a double-blind fashion, 12 parturients were randomly assigned to receive either placebo or sublingual nitroglycerin (three doses, 800 μg each) 10 minutes apart. Intrauterine pressure was measured with a sensor-tip catheter. Sublingual nitroglycerin did not reduce either uterine activity or tone, despite a significant (20%) reduction in maternal mean arterial pressure. In emergency cases, the lack of maternal hypotension after nitroglycerin administration may reflect intravenous fluid administration, position changes, and maternal anxiety associated with emergency situations.

I prefer to use one or two sublingual sprays of nitroglycerin (400 to 800 μg) rather than intravenous nitroglycerin, because the metered-dose spray is stable and convenient and does not require dilution with crystalloid, with the attendant chance of preparation error. Published reports have described intravenous doses ranging from 50 to 500 μg or more. In my experience, both the sublingual and intravenous routes of administration provide a rapid onset of uterine relaxation, and the effect typically is very brief. I simultaneously prepare for the induction of general anesthesia should nitroglycerin not provide enough relaxation.

The use of epidural analgesia most likely has lowered the incidence of fetal head entrapment during vaginal breech delivery for at least two reasons. First, epidural analgesia inhibits early pushing during the first stage of labor.

Second, although epidural analgesia does not relax the cervix at delivery, it provides effective pain relief and skeletal muscle relaxation. A relaxed pelvic floor and perineum facilitates delivery of the aftercoming head. Moreover, effective analgesia and skeletal muscle relaxation allow an assistant to provide maternal suprapubic pressure, which helps maintain flexion of the fetal cervical spine during delivery.

ANESTHESIA FOR CESAREAN DELIVERY

Spinal, epidural, or general anesthesia can be administered for cesarean delivery. At cesarean delivery, the obstetrician should perform a uterine incision that allows an atraumatic delivery of the infant. Rarely, the obstetrician may request provision of uterine relaxation even when a vertical uterine incision has been performed. Uterine relaxation may be necessary in cases of fetal malformations (e.g., sacral teratoma, hydrocephalus). When general anesthesia is used, the anesthesia provider may increase the concentration of the volatile halogenated agent. When neuraxial anesthesia is used, a small dose of nitroglycerin or a beta-adrenergic tocolytic agent such as terbutaline typically provides adequate relaxation. Rarely, it is necessary to perform intraoperative induction of general anesthesia followed by administration of a high concentration of a volatile halogenated agent.

Regardless of the route of delivery, all members of the obstetric care team should remember that infants with a breech presentation tend to be more depressed than infants with a vertex presentation. An individual skilled in neonatal resuscitation should be immediately available.

OTHER ABNORMAL PRESENTATIONS

Face Presentation

Face presentation occurs in 1 in 500 live births. Approximately 70% to 80% of infants with a face presentation can be delivered vaginally.[4] In general, the infant can be delivered vaginally only if the mentum rotates to an anterior position. Manual efforts to flex the fetal cervical spine or convert an unfavorable mentum posterior position to a more favorable mentum anterior position are rarely successful.[4]

Brow Presentation

In patients with a brow presentation, the cervical spine position is intermediate between the full flexion of a normal vertex presentation and the full extension of a face presentation. Brow presentation occurs in approximately 1 in 1500 deliveries. Persistent brow presentation typically requires cesarean delivery due to dystocia. Spontaneous flexion or extension of the neck may occur during labor, which may allow vaginal delivery.[4]

Compound Presentation

Compound presentation (an extremity is prolapsed alongside the main presenting fetal part) occurs in 1 in 400 to 1 in 1200 deliveries. Most often, an upper extremity presents with the vertex. Umbilical cord prolapse is common (10% to 20%), as is neurologic or musculoskeletal damage to the involved extremity.[4] Labor and delivery may occur safely, but abdominal delivery is needed in patients with cord prolapse or arrest of labor. Manipulation of the prolapsed extremity should be avoided.[4]

Shoulder Presentation

A shoulder presentation (also known as a **transverse lie**) mandates performance of cesarean delivery except in two circumstances. First, successful external cephalic version may allow vaginal delivery. Second, the obstetrician may perform internal podalic version and total breech extraction of a second twin with a shoulder presentation.

Cesarean delivery of a fetus with a **back-down transverse lie** can be especially difficult. This presentation represents one of the few indications in contemporary obstetric practice for a classic uterine incision.

MULTIPLE GESTATION

Epidemiology

Monozygotic twins (which occur when a single fertilized ovum divides into two distinct individuals after a variable number of divisions) exhibit a constant incidence of approximately 4 per 1000 births. The incidence of **dizygotic twins** (which occur when two separate ova are fertilized) varies among races and by maternal age. Dizygotic twins occur most frequently among blacks, least frequently among Asians, and with an intermediate frequency among whites. The incidence increases from 3 per 1000 among women less than 20 years of age to 14 per 1000 among women 35 to 40 years of age. The incidence also increases with parity, independent of maternal age.[42] In the United States the rate of multiple births has risen 70% since 1980.[43] Twin births represented 3% of all births in 2005. Nearly 0.2% of all births were triplets, quadruplets, quintuplets, or other higher-order multiples. The higher rate of multiple births reflects delayed childbearing and greater use of assisted reproductive technologies.

Placentation

Placentas in multiple gestation may be (1) **dichorionic diamniotic,** (2) **monochorionic diamniotic,** or (3) **monochorionic monoamniotic** (Figure 35-5). In all occurrences of dizygotic twins, the placenta is dichorionic diamniotic. A dichorionic diamniotic placenta is also present if monozygotic twinning occurs during the first 2 to 3 days after fertilization. Twinning between 3 and 8 days commonly results in a monochorionic diamniotic placenta. Monochorionic monoamniotic placentas are found when twinning occurs at 8 to 13 days. Embryonic cleavage between 13 and 15 days results in conjoined twins with a monochorionic monoamniotic placenta. Twinning cannot occur beyond 15 days.[44]

The type of placentation determines the likelihood of vascular communications. Vascular communications occur in nearly all monochorionic placentas and are rare in dichorionic placentas.[44] Vascular communications may result in twin-to-twin transfusion syndrome and intrauterine fetal death (IUFD). Monochorionic placentation also increases the risk of intrauterine fetal death from other causes (e.g., cord accident).[44,45]

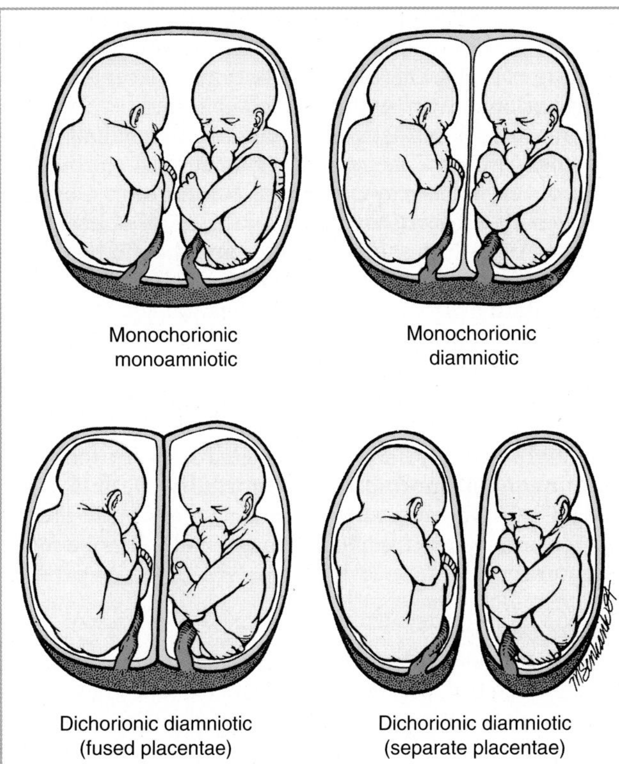

FIGURE 35-5 Placentation in twin pregnancies. (From Cleary-Goldman J, Chitkara U, Berkowitz RL. Multiple gestations. In Gabbe SG, Niebyl JR, Simpson JL, editors. Obstetrics: Normal and Problem Pregnancies. 5th edition. New York, Churchill Livingstone, 2007:736.)

Physiologic Changes

Multiple gestation accelerates and may exaggerate the physiologic and anatomic changes of pregnancy. Of interest to the anesthesia provider, multiple gestation exaggerates the cardiovascular and pulmonary changes of pregnancy. In contrast, the renal, hepatic, and central nervous system changes resemble those that occur in women with a singleton fetus.

Increased uterine size, especially near term, results in reductions in total lung capacity and functional residual capacity (FRC). During periods of hypoventilation or apnea, hypoxemia develops more rapidly because of the decreased FRC and an increased maternal metabolic rate. A cross-sectional study demonstrated no significant difference in respiratory function between 68 women with a twin pregnancy and 140 women with a singleton pregnancy.[46] Maternal weight increases at a greater rate after 30 weeks' gestation in women with multiple gestation,[47] a process that may increase the risk of difficult intubation and ventilation. Greater uterine size displaces the stomach cephalad, decreasing the competence of the lower esophageal sphincter and increasing the risk of pulmonary aspiration of gastric contents.

Maternal blood volume increases by an additional 500 mL with twin gestation.[45] Relative or actual anemia often occurs. Likewise, multiple gestation results in a 20% greater increase in cardiac output than occurs in women with a singleton fetus, owing to a greater stroke volume (15%) and higher heart rate (3.5%).[48] The greater fetal weight and larger volume of amniotic fluid predispose the mother with multiple gestation to aortocaval compression and the supine hypotension syndrome.

BOX 35-3 Fetal Complications Associated with Multiple Gestation

- Preterm delivery
- Congenital anomalies
- Polyhydramnios
- Cord entanglement
- Umbilical cord prolapse
- Intrauterine growth restriction
- Twin-to-twin transfusion
- Malpresentation

Obstetric Complications

FETAL COMPLICATIONS

Fetal complications include those related solely to multiple gestation (e.g., twin-to-twin transfusion syndrome) and those related to abnormal presentation (e.g., prolapsed cord) (Box 35-3).

Twin-to-Twin Transfusion

Nearly all monochorionic twin placentas have vascular anastomoses. Deep arteriovenous anastomoses create a common villous compartment in about half of monochorionic twin placentas.[45] Most of these anastomoses have little fetal consequence. Those with deep arteriovenous vascular communications may result in twin-to-twin transfusion,[49] in which one twin becomes the donor and the other twin becomes the recipient. The donor twin is smaller and is at risk for intrauterine growth restriction (IUGR) and anemia. The recipient twin is plethoric and is at risk for volume overload and cardiac failure. Alternative explanations for the syndrome include unequal blood volumes secondary to compression of a velamentous umbilical cord insertion and higher arterial blood pressure in the donor than in the recipient.[45] Twin-to-twin transfusion increases both the perinatal mortality rate and the risk of adverse neurodevelopmental outcome in survivors.[50]

The therapeutic options most often considered are decompression amniocentesis, interruption of the placental vessel communications, amniotic septostomy, and selective feticide.[51] Selective fetoscopic laser photocoagulation addresses the vascular anastomoses. Decompression amniocentesis or serial amnioreduction may improve circulation to a "stuck" donor twin, allowing restoration of normal amniotic fluid volume and "catch-up" fetal growth. Compared with serial amnioreduction, septostomy has the advantage of requiring only a single procedure.[52] Increasing evidence supports endoscopic laser coagulation to improve perinatal outcome.[51-54]

Intrauterine Growth Restriction

Twin-to-twin transfusion represents only one of the potential etiologies of IUGR in multiple gestation. The polyhydramnios within one fetal sac may limit the growth of the other fetus. In patients with three or more fetuses, limited intrauterine size may restrict fetal growth. Of course, factors that cause IUGR in singleton pregnancies also may cause IUGR in patients with multiple gestation (e.g., uteroplacental insufficiency, chromosomal abnormalities).

Preterm Labor

Patients with multiple gestation are at high risk for preterm labor and delivery. Preterm labor occurs in 52% of women with *in vitro* fertilization (IVF) twins compared with 22% of women with spontaneous twins.[55] Sixty percent of women with twins deliver before 37 weeks' gestation, and only 6% of triplet pregnancies reach term.[43] Routine use of bed rest, prophylactic cerclage, and/or tocolytic therapy has not been shown to improve perinatal outcome in multiple gestation pregnancies.[45] When preterm labor occurs, the patient may receive parenteral tocolytic therapy. Often the anesthesia provider is asked to administer anesthesia after tocolytic therapy has failed. The side effects of the tocolytic agents may affect the response to anesthesia (see Chapter 34) and may increase the risk of postpartum hemorrhage. Multiple gestation most likely increases the risk of pulmonary edema associated with tocolytic therapy.

Abnormal Presentation

Multiple gestation is associated with a higher incidence of abnormal presentation, which results in part from the need to accommodate two or more fetuses within the uterine cavity. Malpresentation increases the risk of umbilical cord prolapse, which may occur either before or after delivery of the first infant.

Morbidity and Mortality

Approximately 10% of all cases of **perinatal mortality** result from multiple gestation. The perinatal mortality rate in twin pregnancies is four times greater than that associated with singleton pregnancies (35 deaths per 1000 births versus 8 per 1000 births, respectively).[45] Preterm delivery accounts for most of this increase, although twins and triplets also have a higher weight-specific mortality, which may be related to twin-to-twin transfusion, congenital malformations, preeclampsia, malpresentation, and/or prolapsed umbilical cord.[56] Some maternal-fetal medicine specialists advocate selective multifetal reduction to reduce the risk of maternal morbidity and the perinatal morbidity and mortality associated with three or more fetuses; this issue is a matter of great controversy, both ethically and medically.[43,45]

Intensive inpatient monitoring may improve perinatal survival of *monoamniotic* twins. In a retrospective analysis of 87 women who had living twins at 24 weeks' gestation, there were no intrauterine deaths among 43 women who were admitted electively for inpatient surveillance (at a median gestational age of 26.5 weeks). In comparison, among women who were monitored as outpatients and admitted only for routine obstetric indications (at a median gestational age of 30.1 weeks), the rate of intrauterine fetal death was 14.8%.[57] Intensive surveillance may also benefit *monochorionic diamniotic* pregnancies.[58] The long-term outcome of the complications of monochorionicity remains an area of limited knowledge.[59]

Johnson and Zhang[60] evaluated outcome for 150,386 sets of twins and 5240 sets of triplets born between 1995 and 1997; fetal death at 20 weeks' gestation or later occurred in 2.6% of twin gestations and 4.3% of triplet gestations. The investigators noted that "survival of the remaining fetuses was inversely related to the time of the first fetal demise."[60] Opposite-gender twins were more likely to survive, possibly reflecting the absence of monochorionic placentation. In monochorionic twin gestations complicated by twin-to-twin transfusion and fetal death, approximately half of the surviving twins experience mortality or serious morbidity.[61] Death of one fetus may occur well before term. Obstetric management decisions are based on the cause of death and the status of both the surviving fetus and the mother. If the cause of death was an abnormality of the fetus rather than maternal or uteroplacental pathology, expectant management of the pregnancy may be warranted.[45,62] Development of maternal intravascular coagulation from dead fetal tissue is a theoretical complication that appears to occur rarely.[62]

Multiple gestation also is associated with an increased risk of **neonatal morbidity and mortality**. Despite a 95% neonatal survival rate, triplets have a significantly greater risk for intraventricular hemorrhage and retinopathy of prematurity.[63]

Order of Delivery

Birth order does not seem to influence perinatal outcome in current obstetric practice.[63,64] Neuraxial anesthesia may improve the outcome for the second twin. In 1987, Crawford[65] observed that among women who received epidural analgesia, the two twins had similar umbilical cord blood pH measurements. In contrast, among women who received general anesthesia, the second twin tended to be more acidotic than the first. Likewise, Jarvis and Whitfield[66] reported no difference in outcome for first and second twins when the mother received epidural analgesia. Administration of general anesthesia is increasingly rare for cesarean delivery in women with multiple gestation.[67]

MATERNAL COMPLICATIONS

Multiple gestation increases the incidence of maternal morbidity and mortality (Box 35-4), even with adjustment of data for confounding factors.[68] The incidence of maternal complications increases in proportion to the number of fetuses. Nearly all triplet gestations are associated with antenatal and/or postnatal maternal complications.[69] Abdominal distention and diaphragmatic elevation can cause respiratory distress and may necessitate early delivery in some patients with three or more fetuses. The increased incidence of cesarean delivery contributes to the higher risk of maternal morbidity and mortality associated with multiple gestation.

BOX 35-4 Maternal Complications Associated with Multiple Gestation

- Preterm premature rupture of membranes
- Preterm labor
- Prolonged labor
- Preeclampsia/eclampsia
- Placental abruption
- Disseminated intravascular coagulation
- Operative delivery (forceps and cesarean)
- Uterine atony
- Obstetric trauma
- Antepartum and/or postpartum hemorrhage

Multiple gestation (and the use of assisted reproductive technologies[70]) increases both the incidence and severity of preeclampsia.[44,45] Preeclampsia prompts delivery by 34 weeks' gestation in as many as 70% of patients with quadruplet pregnancies.[71]

Blood loss with delivery is approximately 500 mL greater in multiple gestation pregnancies.[45] Uterine distention increases the risk of uterine atony and postpartum hemorrhage. Most cases of atony respond to standard pharmacologic therapy (e.g., oxytocin, methylergonovine, 15-methyl prostaglandin $F_{2\alpha}$ [carboprost]). Persistent uterine atony requires the performance of emergency hysterectomy.

Obstetric Management

Twin gestation itself does not contraindicate labor and vaginal delivery. However, multiple gestation is associated with a higher incidence of cesarean delivery. Most obstetricians favor cesarean delivery for all patients with three or more fetuses.[44,45] A meta-analysis of four studies involving 1932 infants found no difference in perinatal or neonatal mortality, neonatal morbidity, or maternal morbidity between twins born through planned cesarean delivery and those born through vaginal delivery unless the first twin (twin A) was in a breech presentation.[72]

Both fetuses have a vertex presentation in 30% to 50% of cases of twin gestation. Approximately 25% to 40% have a vertex/breech combination. The remaining patients have various combinations of vertex, breech, and transverse lie. Most obstetricians allow a trial of labor if both twins have vertex presentation. Similarly, a majority of obstetricians opt for cesarean delivery if the first twin has a breech or shoulder presentation. Controversy remains regarding the ideal management in cases in which twin A has a vertex presentation and twin B has a nonvertex presentation.

TWIN A

Decisions regarding the method of delivery typically revolve around the gestational age and presentation of twin A. An obstetrician who is unwilling to allow a trial of labor in a patient with a singleton breech presentation is unlikely to allow a trial of labor in a patient with a breech presentation for twin A. Moreover, if twin A has a breech presentation and twin B has a vertex presentation, the chins may become interlocked during labor and delivery. This complication occurs infrequently (approximately 1 in 1000 cases of twin delivery), but the consequences can be devastating.[44] Other indications for cesarean delivery of twin A include (1) evidence of discordant growth (especially if twin B is larger than twin A), (2) twin-to-twin transfusion syndrome, (3) selected congenital anomalies, and (4) evidence of uteroplacental insufficiency.[44,45] A trial of labor mandates continuous FHR monitoring of both fetuses. After amniotomy, an electrocardiography lead may be placed on the scalp of twin A, and Doppler ultrasonography may be used to monitor twin B.

The unanticipated case of head entrapment, deflexed head, or locked twins may necessitate emergency abdominal delivery of both twins. The obstetrician proceeds with cesarean delivery while an assistant supports the exteriorized body of twin A. The obstetrician applies gentle traction on the head while the infant's body is guided back into the vagina. This can be accomplished without major injury to the infant or the mother.[73]

TWIN B

If twin A is delivered vaginally, the obstetrician must make a decision about the method of delivery of twin B. If twin B has a vertex presentation and the head is well applied to the cervix, the obstetrician may allow the patient to resume labor and await spontaneous vaginal delivery. Rarely, if twin B has a vertex presentation but the head is not well applied to the cervix, the obstetrician may perform internal podalic version and total breech extraction.

For the twin B with nonvertex presentation, options include (1) external cephalic version followed by a resumption of labor, (2) internal podalic version and total breech extraction, and (3) performance of cesarean delivery. Real-time ultrasonography facilitates the performance of external cephalic version. This procedure is successful in approximately 70% of cases. The likelihood of success is not associated with parity, gestational age, or birth weight.[74] One study noted that mothers who received epidural anesthesia were more relaxed and tolerated the procedure better than those who did not receive epidural anesthesia.[74]

Delivery of twin B is the one situation in contemporary obstetric practice in which internal podalic version and total breech extraction are considered appropriate. Indeed, breech extraction may be preferable to external cephalic version at the time of delivery.[45] After vaginal delivery of twin A, the second twin requires cesarean delivery in approximately 10% of cases.[75] Predictors of emergency cesarean delivery of twin B include malpresentation, nonreassuring FHR tracing, cephalopelvic disproportion, and cord prolapse.[75]

The obstetrician will opt for total breech extraction of twin B only if there is evidence that twin B is not larger than twin A. Antepartum ultrasonographic examination allows the obstetrician to assess the head size and weight of both fetuses. If twin B is not larger than twin A, the pelvis and cervical dilation are probably adequate for vaginal delivery of twin B, provided that the cervix has not begun to contract.

In the past, obstetricians favored the delivery of twin B within 15 to 30 minutes of delivery of twin A. However, most data supporting this practice were obtained before the use of intrapartum FHR monitoring.[44] Using continuous FHR monitoring, Rayburn et al.[76] noted that the interval between deliveries averaged 21 minutes (with a range of 1 to 134 minutes) in 115 patients with live-born twins. A total of 28 infants delivered between 16 and 30 minutes after the delivery of twin A, and 17 delivered more than 30 minutes after the delivery of twin A. All 45 infants who delivered more than 15 minutes after the delivery of twin A did well. In fact, all 17 neonates who delivered after 30 minutes had a 5-minute Apgar score of at least 8. In a review of 118 twin deliveries, Leung et al.[77] demonstrated an association, but not a causal relationship, between the twin-twin delivery interval and the umbilical cord blood gas and pH measurements for twin B. The investigators noted that continuous FHR monitoring is essential; 73% of the second twins not delivered by 30 minutes required operative delivery because of a nonreassuring FHR tracing. A German retrospective analysis of 4110 twin pregnancies suggested that the interval between delivery of twins is an independent risk factor for adverse short-term outcomes for twin B.[78]

Anesthetic Management

LABOR AND VAGINAL DELIVERY

Epidural analgesia provides optimal analgesia and flexibility for subsequent anesthetic needs. The anesthesia provider must be vigilant, because obstetric conditions and anesthetic requirements may change rapidly. Given the greater risk for cesarean delivery in patients with multiple gestation, the anesthesia provider should demand perfect epidural anesthesia. If there is any question regarding the location of the catheter or the efficacy of the block, the catheter should be removed and replaced.

Patients with multiple gestation may be at increased risk for aortocaval compression and hypotension during the administration of neuraxial anesthesia. Use of the full lateral position, both during and after induction of epidural anesthesia, reduces the risk of aortocaval compression. Because these patients are at increased risk for uterine atony and postpartum hemorrhage, establishment of large-bore intravenous access is recommended before delivery.

Patients with multiple gestation should deliver in a room where an emergency abdominal delivery can be performed immediately. As the time for delivery of twin A nears, I augment the intensity of the neuroblockade. I extend the sensory level to approximately T8 to T6 using a solution of local anesthetic that is more concentrated than that used earlier during labor. Effective anesthesia facilitates the performance of internal podalic version and total breech extraction of twin B; it also enables the extension of anesthesia for cesarean delivery if necessary. I prepare a syringe of 3% 2-chloroprocaine to be used if emergency extension of epidural anesthesia is required.

I prefer not to administer single-shot spinal anesthesia for vaginal delivery because of its lack of flexibility in cases of rapidly changing conditions. However, spinal or combined spinal-epidural anesthesia may be appropriate when delivery appears imminent in a patient without preexisting epidural labor analgesia.

VAGINAL DELIVERY OF TWIN A/ABDOMINAL DELIVERY OF TWIN B

The flexibility associated with epidural analgesia is especially advantageous if the obstetrician delivers twin A vaginally and twin B abdominally. I administer a nonparticulate antacid at the first sign of obstetrician distress (not to be confused with fetal distress), and I inject additional local anesthetic to extend the sensory level to approximately T4. In cases of prolonged fetal bradycardia, it may be necessary to administer general anesthesia if adequate neuraxial anesthesia cannot be achieved rapidly. Typically this problem can be avoided if (1) both the level and intensity of anesthesia are augmented at the time of delivery of twin A and (2) the anesthesia provider gives attention to both the FHR tracing and the obstetrician.

If the obstetrician opts for internal podalic version and total breech extraction of twin B, it is better to perform the procedure shortly after the delivery of twin A, before the uterus and the cervix begin to contract. Pain relief and skeletal muscle relaxation (both provided by epidural anesthesia) facilitate internal version and total breech extraction of twin B in most patients. In some cases, pharmacologic uterine relaxation may be required to facilitate internal version and breech extraction of twin B. Sublingual (400 to 800 μg) or intravenous (50 to 250 μg) administration of nitroglycerin may provide adequate relaxation for internal podalic version.[79,80] If this maneuver is unsuccessful, rapid-sequence induction of general anesthesia, followed by administration of a high concentration of a volatile halogenated agent (as discussed earlier), may be needed.

CESAREAN DELIVERY

Epidural, spinal, or general anesthesia can be safely administered for elective abdominal delivery. Spinal anesthesia is increasingly preferred by many anesthesia providers. A historical preference for epidural anesthesia was based on the gradual onset of sympathetic blockade, which was thought to reduce the incidence of severe hypotension. It has been long believed that women with multiple gestation are at higher risk for hemodynamic instability during administration of neuraxial anesthesia than women with a singleton gestation. Ngan Kee et al.[81] compared the incidence of hypotension and vasopressor requirements in women with multiple and singleton gestations undergoing cesarean delivery with spinal anesthesia. There were no differences between groups in maternal and neonatal outcomes.

Comparison of brachial artery and popliteal artery blood pressures allows the detection of occult supine hypotension, which results in reduced uteroplacental perfusion in the presence of a normal brachial artery pressure. If either hypotension or occult supine hypotension is detected, additional left uterine displacement or displacement to the other side may resolve the problem.

Jawan et al.[82] found that women with multiple gestation had a greater cephalad spread of neuroblockade with spinal anesthesia than women with a singleton gestation, whereas Ngan Kee et al.[81] did not. Similarly, Behforouz et al.[83] found no difference in the extent of sensory blockade after administration of epidural anesthesia between women with higher-order multiple gestation pregnancies and women with a singleton gestation. In any case, any difference that may exist is likely to be of little clinical significance. Vallejo and Ramanathan[84] demonstrated that mean umbilical venous (UV) and umbilical arterial (UA) lidocaine concentrations were 35% to 53% higher in twin newborn infants than in singleton infants exposed to epidural anesthesia for cesarean delivery. Mean fetal-to-maternal lidocaine ratios were at least 18% higher in the twin newborns than in the singleton newborns. The investigators speculated that this difference may be a result of the greater maternal cardiac output and plasma volume associated with twin gestation as well as the decreased total plasma protein concentration, which leads to an increase in the free lidocaine concentration.[84]

When general anesthesia is used, the greater oxygen consumption and decreased FRC associated with multiple gestation increase the risk of maternal hypoxemia during periods of apnea. Adequate denitrogenation (preoxygenation) is essential.

The presence of two or more fetuses results in prolonged uterine incision-to-delivery intervals because of the longer time required to deliver multiple infants. A prolonged interval increases the risk of umbilical cord blood acidemia and neonatal depression. Neonatal depression is less likely with neuraxial anesthesia than with general anesthesia.[66] In any case, an individual skilled in neonatal resuscitation should be immediately available.

KEY POINTS

- A higher incidence of breech presentation occurs among patients with preterm labor.
- Both breech presentation and multiple gestation are associated with an increased incidence of perinatal morbidity and mortality, regardless of the method of delivery.
- Epidural analgesia offers several advantages during a trial of labor in the patient with a breech presentation. Specifically, it (1) provides effective pain relief; (2) inhibits early pushing; (3) relaxes the pelvic floor and perineum, facilitating atraumatic delivery of the aftercoming head; and (4) enables provision of anesthesia for emergency cesarean delivery.
- Multiple gestation exaggerates the physiologic and anatomic changes of pregnancy.
- Epidural analgesia is the analgesic technique of choice during labor in the patient with multiple gestation. Provision of pain relief and skeletal muscle relaxation facilitates the vaginal delivery of twin B. Provision of epidural analgesia also facilitates the administration of anesthesia for emergency cesarean delivery if it is needed.
- The obstetrician may request pharmacologic provision of uterine and/or cervical relaxation to facilitate vaginal delivery of twin B or, in cases of breech presentation, to facilitate the delivery of the aftercoming fetal head. Intravenous or sublingual nitroglycerin may provide rapid-onset uterine relaxation of short duration. Rapid-sequence induction of general anesthesia followed by administration of a high concentration of a volatile halogenated agent is another reliable method of providing uterine and cervical relaxation.

REFERENCES

1. Gardberg M, Laakkonen E, Sälevaara M. Intrapartum sonography and persistent occiput posterior position: A study of 408 deliveries. Obstet Gynecol 1998; 91:746-9.
2. Fitzpatrick M, McQuillan K, O'Herlihy C. Influence of persistent occiput posterior position on delivery outcome. Obstet Gynecol 2001; 98:1027-31.
3. Cunningham FG, Leveno KJ, Bloom SL, et al. Williams Obstetrics. 22nd edition. New York, McGraw-Hill, 2005:565-86.
4. Lanni S, Seeds J. Malpresentations. In Gabbe SG, Niebyl JR, Simpson JL, editors. Obstetrics: Normal and Problem Pregnancies. 5th edition. New York, Churchill Livingstone, 2007:428-55.
5. Pop VJ, Brouwers EP, Wijnen H, et al. Low concentrations of maternal thyroxin during early gestation: A risk factor of breech presentation? Br J Obstet Gynaecol 2004; 111:925-30.
6. Albrechtsen S, Rasmussen S, Dalaker K, Irgens LM. Perinatal mortality in breech presentation sibships. Obstet Gynecol 1998; 92:775-80.
7. Lau TK, Lo KW, Rogers M. Pregnancy outcome after successful external cephalic version for breech presentation at term. Am J Obstet Gynecol 1997; 176:218-23.
8. Hofmeyr GJ, Hannah ME. Planned caesarean section for term breech delivery. Cochrane Database Syst Rev 2003; (2):CD000166.
9. Schiff E, Friedman SA, Mashiach S, et al. Maternal and neonatal outcome of 846 term singleton breech deliveries: Seven-year experience at a single center. Am J Obstet Gynecol 1996; 175:18-23.
10. American College of Obstetricians and Gynecologists. External cephalic version. ACOG Practice Bulletin No. 13. Washington, DC, February 2000.
11. Zhang J, Bowes WA Jr, Fortney JA. Efficacy of external cephalic version: A review. Obstet Gynecol 1993; 82:306-12.
12. Fortunato SJ, Mercer LJ, Guzick DS. External cephalic version with tocolysis: Factors associated with success. Obstet Gynecol 1988; 72:59-62.
13. Kok M, Cnossen J, Gravendeel L, et al. Clinical factors to predict the outcome of external cephalic version: A metaanalysis. Am J Obstet Gynecol 2008; 199:630.e1-630.e7.
14. Brost BC, Adams JD, Hester M. External cephalic version after rupture of membranes. Obstet Gynecol 2000; 95:1041.
15. Hutton EK, Hofmeyr GJ. External cephalic version for breech presentation before term. Cochrane Database Syst Rev 2006; (1):CD000084.
16. American College of Obstetricians and Gynecologists Committee on Obstetric Practice. Mode of term singleton breech delivery. ACOG Committee Opinion No. 340. Washington, DC, July 2006. (Obstet Gynecol 2006; 108:235-7.)
17. Schorr SJ, Speights SE, Ross EL, et al. A randomized trial of epidural anesthesia to improve external cephalic version success. Am J Obstet Gynecol 1997; 177:1133-7.
18. Chan LY, Tang JL, Tsoi KF, et al. Intrapartum cesarean delivery after successful external cephalic version: A meta-analysis. Obstet Gynecol 2004; 104:155-60.
19. Collaris RJ, Oei SG. External cephalic version: A safe procedure? A systematic review of version-related risks. Acta Obstet Gynecol Scand 2004; 83:511-8.
20. Fernandez CO, Bloom SL, Smulian JC, et al. A randomized placebo-controlled evaluation of terbutaline for external cephalic version. Obstet Gynecol 1997; 90:775-9.
21. El-Sayed YY, Pullen K, Riley ET, et al. Randomized comparison of intravenous nitroglycerin and subcutaneous terbutaline for external cephalic version under tocolysis. Am J Obstet Gynecol 2004; 191:2051-5.
22. Bujold E, Boucher M, Rinfret D, et al. Sublingual nitroglycerin versus placebo as a tocolytic for external cephalic version: A randomized controlled trial in parous women. Am J Obstet Gynecol 2003; 189:1070-3.
23. Weiniger CF, Ginosar Y, Elchalal U, et al. External cephalic version for breech presentation with or without spinal analgesia in nulliparous women at term: A randomized controlled trial. Obstet Gynecol 2007; 110:1343-50.
24. Dugoff L, Stamm CA, Jones OW, et al. The effect of spinal anesthesia on the success rate of external cephalic version: A randomized trial. Obstet Gynecol 1999; 93:345-9.
25. Mancuso KM, Yancey MK, Murphy JA, Markenson GR. Epidural analgesia for cephalic version: A randomized trial. Obstet Gynecol 2000; 95:648-51.
26. Fok WY, Chan LW, Leung TY, Lau TK. Maternal experience of pain during external cephalic version at term. Acta Obstet Gynecol Scand 2005; 84:748-51.
27. Hofmeyr GJ, Gyte G. Interventions to help external cephalic version for breech presentation at term. Cochrane Database Syst Rev 2004; (1):CD000184.
28. Neiger R, Hennessy MD, Patel M. Reattempting failed external cephalic version under epidural anesthesia. Am J Obstet Gynecol 1998; 179:1136-9.
29. Cherayil G, Feinberg B, Robinson J, Tsen LC. Central neuraxial blockade promotes external cephalic version success after a failed attempt. Anesth Analg 2002; 94:1589-92.
30. Hannah ME, Hannah WJ, Hewson SA, et al. Planned caesarean section versus planned vaginal birth for breech presentation at term: A randomised multicentre trial. Term Breech Trial Collaborative Group. Lancet 2000; 356:1375-83.

31. Su M, McLeod L, Ross S, et al. Factors associated with adverse perinatal outcome in the Term Breech Trial. Am J Obstet Gynecol 2003; 189:740-5.
32. Whyte H, Hannah ME, Saigal S, et al. Outcomes of children at 2 years after planned cesarean birth versus planned vaginal birth for breech presentation at term: The International Randomized Term Breech Trial. Am J Obstet Gynecol 2004; 191:864-71.
33. Hannah ME, Hannah WJ, Hodnett ED, et al. Outcomes at 3 months after planned cesarean vs planned vaginal delivery for breech presentation at term: The international randomized Term Breech Trial. JAMA 2002; 287:1822-31.
34. Hannah ME, Whyte H, Hannah WJ, et al. Maternal outcomes at 2 years after planned cesarean section versus planned vaginal birth for breech presentation at term: The international randomized Term Breech Trial. Am J Obstet Gynecol 2004; 191:917-27.
35. Alarab M, Regan C, O'Connell MP, et al. Singleton vaginal breech delivery at term: Still a safe option. Obstet Gynecol 2004; 103:407-12.
36. Glezerman M. Five years to the Term Breech Trial: The rise and fall of a randomized controlled trial. Am J Obstet Gynecol 2006; 194:20-5.
37. Chinnock M, Robson S. Obstetric trainees' experience in vaginal breech delivery. Obstet Gynecol 2007; 110:900-3.
38. Benhamou D, Mercier FJ, Ben Ayed M, Auroy Y. Continuous epidural analgesia with bupivacaine 0.125% or bupivacaine 0.0625% plus sufentanil 0.25 microg.mL(-1): A study in singleton breech presentation. Int J Obstet Anesth 2002; 11:13-8.
39. Danforth DN. The distribution and functional activity of the cervical musculature. Am J Obstet Gynecol 1954; 68:1261-71.
40. Caponas G. Glyceryl trinitrate and acute uterine relaxation: A literature review. Anaesth Intensive Care 2001; 29:163-77.
41. Buhimschi CS, Buhimschi IA, Malinow AM, Weiner CP. Effects of sublingual nitroglycerin on human uterine contractility during the active phase of labor. Am J Obstet Gynecol 2002; 187:235-8.
42. Hrubec Z, Robinette CD. The study of human twins in medical research. N Engl J Med 1984; 310:435-41.
43. Martin JA, Hamilton BE, Sutton PD, et al. Births: Final data for 2005. Natl Vital Stat Rep 2007; 56:1-103.
44. Cleary-Goldman J, Chitkara U, Berkowitz R. Multiple gestations. In Gabbe SG, Niebyl JR, Simpson JL, editors. Obstetrics: Normal and Problem Pregnancies. 5th edition. New York, Churchill Livingstone, 2007:733-70.
45. Cunningham FG, Leveno KJ, Bloom SL, et al. Williams Obstetrics. 22nd edition. New York, McGraw-Hill, 2005:911-48.
46. McAuliffe F, Kametas N, Costello J, et al. Respiratory function in singleton and twin pregnancy. Br J Obstet Gynaecol 2002; 109:765-9.
47. Pederson AL, Worthington-Roberts B, Hickok DE. Weight gain patterns during twin gestation. J Am Diet Assoc 1989; 89:642-6.
48. Kametas NA, McAuliffe F, Krampl E, et al. Maternal cardiac function in twin pregnancy. Obstet Gynecol 2003; 102:806-15.
49. Bermudez C, Becerra CH, Bornick PW, et al. Placental types and twin-twin transfusion syndrome. Am J Obstet Gynecol 2002; 187:489-94.
50. Lopriore E, Nagel HT, Vandenbussche FP, Walther FJ. Long-term neurodevelopmental outcome in twin-to-twin transfusion syndrome. Am J Obstet Gynecol 2003; 189:1314-9.
51. Roberts D, Neilson JP, Weindling M, Gates S. Interventions for the treatment of twin-twin transfusion syndrome. Cochrane Database Syst Rev 2008; (1):CD002073.
52. Moise KJ, Dorman K, Lamvu G, et al. A randomized trial of amnioreduction versus septostomy in the treatment of twin-twin transfusion syndrome. Am J Obstet Gynecol 2005; 193:701-7.
53. Crombleholme TM, Shera D, Lee H, et al. A prospective, randomized, multicenter trial of amnioreduction vs selective fetoscopic laser photocoagulation for the treatment of severe twin-twin transfusion syndrome. Am J Obstet Gynecol 2007; 197:396.e1-9.
54. Chmait RH, Quintero RA. Operative fetoscopy in complicated monochorionic twins: Current status and future direction. Curr Opin Obstet Gynecol 2008; 20:169-74.
55. Nassar AH, Usta IM, Rechdan JB, et al. Pregnancy outcome in spontaneous twins versus twins who were conceived through in vitro fertilization. Am J Obstet Gynecol 2003; 189:513-8.
56. Buekens P, Wilcox A. Why do small twins have a lower mortality rate than small singletons? Am J Obstet Gynecol 1993; 168:937-41.
57. Heyborne KD, Porreco RP, Garite TJ, et al. Improved perinatal survival of monoamniotic twins with intensive inpatient monitoring. Am J Obstet Gynecol 2005; 192:96-101.
58. Simoes T, Amaral N, Lerman R, et al. Prospective risk of intrauterine death of monochorionic-diamniotic twins. Am J Obstet Gynecol 2006; 195:134-9.
59. Malone FD. Monochorionic pregnancy—where have we been? Where are we going? Am J Obstet Gynecol 2003; 189:1308-9.
60. Johnson CD, Zhang J. Survival of other fetuses after a fetal death in twin or triplet pregnancies. Obstet Gynecol 2002; 99: 698-703.
61. van Heteren CF, Nijhuis JG, Semmekrot BA, et al. Risk for surviving twin after fetal death of co-twin in twin-twin transfusion syndrome. Obstet Gynecol 1998; 92:215-9.
62. American College of Obstetricians and Gynecologists. Multiple gestation: Complicated twin, triplet, and high-order multifetal pregnancy. ACOG Practice Bulletin No. 56. Washington, DC, 2004. (Obstet Gynecol 2004; 104:869-83.)
63. Kaufman GE, Malone FD, Harvey-Wilkes KB, et al. Neonatal morbidity and mortality associated with triplet pregnancy. Obstet Gynecol 1998; 91:342-8.
64. Antoine C, Kirshenbaum N, Young B. Biochemical differences related to birth order in triplets. J Reprod Med 1996; 31:330-2.
65. Crawford JS. A prospective study of 200 consecutive twin deliveries. Anaesthesia 1987; 42:33-43.
66. Jarvis G, Whitfield M. Epidural analgesia and the delivery of twins. J Obstet Gynaecol 1981; 2:90-2.
67. Marino T, Goudas LC, Steinbok V, et al. The anesthetic management of triplet cesarean delivery: A retrospective case series of maternal outcomes. Anesth Analg 2001; 93:991-5.
68. Conde-Agudelo A, Belizan JM, Lindmark G. Maternal morbidity and mortality associated with multiple gestations. Obstet Gynecol 2000; 95:899-904.
69. Malone FD, Kaufman GE, Chelmow D, et al. Maternal morbidity associated with triplet pregnancy. Am J Perinatol 1998; 15:73-7.
70. Lynch A, McDuffie R Jr, Murphy J, et al. Preeclampsia in multiple gestation: The role of assisted reproductive technologies. Obstet Gynecol 2002; 99:445-51.
71. Elliott JP, Radin TG. Quadruplet pregnancy: Contemporary management and outcome. Obstet Gynecol 1992; 80:421-4.
72. Hogle KL, Hutton EK, McBrien KA, et al. Cesarean delivery for twins: A systematic review and meta-analysis. Am J Obstet Gynecol 2003; 188:220-7.
73. Swartjes JM, Bleker OP, Schutte MF. The Zavanelli maneuver applied to locked twins. Am J Obstet Gynecol 1992; 166:532.
74. Tchabo JG, Tomai T. Selected intrapartum external cephalic version of the second twin. Obstet Gynecol 1992; 79:421-3.
75. Wen SW, Fung KF, Oppenheimer L, et al. Occurrence and predictors of cesarean delivery for the second twin after vaginal delivery of the first twin. Obstet Gynecol 2004; 103:413-9.
76. Rayburn WF, Lavin JP Jr, Miodovnik M, Varner MW. Multiple gestation: Time interval between delivery of the first and second twins. Obstet Gynecol 1984; 63:502-6.
77. Leung TY, Tam WH, Leung TN, et al. Effect of twin-to-twin delivery interval on umbilical cord blood gas in the second twins. Br J Obstet Gynaecol 2002; 109:63-7.
78. Stein W, Misselwitz B, Schmidt S. Twin-to-twin delivery time interval: Influencing factors and effect on short-term outcome of the second twin. Acta Obstet Gynecol Scand 2008; 87:346-53.
79. Dufour P, Vinatier D, Vanderstichele S, et al. Intravenous nitroglycerin for internal podalic version of the second twin in transverse lie. Obstet Gynecol 1998; 92:416-9.

80. Vinatier D, Dufour P, Berard J. Utilization of intravenous nitroglycerin for obstetrical emergencies. Int J Gynaecol Obstet 1996; 55:129-34.
81. Ngan Kee WD, Khaw KS, Ng FF, et al. A prospective comparison of vasopressor requirement and hemodynamic changes during spinal anesthesia for cesarean delivery in patients with multiple gestation versus singleton pregnancy. Anesth Analg 2007; 104:407-11.
82. Jawan B, Lee JH, Chong ZK, Chang CS. Spread of spinal anaesthesia for caesarean section in singleton and twin pregnancies. Br J Anaesth 1993; 70:639-41.
83. Behforouz N, Dounas M, Benhamou D. Epidural anaesthesia for caesarean delivery in triple and quadruple pregnancies. Acta Anaesthesiol Scand 1998; 42:1088-91.
84. Vallejo MC, Ramanathan S. Plasma lidocaine concentrations are higher in twin compared to singleton newborns following epidural anesthesia for Cesarean delivery. Can J Anaesth 2002; 49:701-5.

Fever and Infection

Scott Segal, M.D.

Infection and fever are common clinical problems in obstetric patients. The purpose of this chapter is to review the obstetric and anesthetic management of pregnant women with fever and/or infection.

FEVER

Definition and Pathophysiology

In 1868, Carl Wunderlich analyzed more than 1 million axillary temperature measurements from 25,000 patients.[1] He concluded that the average normal temperature of healthy adults was 37.0° C. However, he found a range of temperatures, with a nadir of 36.2° C between 2:00 and 8:00 AM and a zenith of 37.5° C between 4:00 and 9:00 PM. He also observed that women had slightly higher mean temperatures than men. A 1992 study that used modern oral thermometers largely confirmed Wunderlich's original data.[2]

Well-regulated temperature results from hypothalamic integration of afferent thermal information from the skin, spinal cord, and other sites within the central nervous system (CNS). When this integrated temperature deviates from normal, thermoregulatory responses are triggered.[3] In humans, the first (and least metabolically "expensive") response to temperature perturbations is behavioral (e.g., moving to a different environment, putting on appropriate clothing, adjusting room temperature). Such responses obviously are unavailable to an anesthetized patient, although some may be implemented by people caring for the patient. Further responses to temperature perturbations are mediated by the autonomic nervous system. Hypothermia prompts vasoconstriction in peripheral tissues to decrease skin blood flow, reduce heat loss, and retain heat in the core compartment. If vasoconstriction is not adequate to prevent hypothermia, thermoregulatory shivering is triggered to increase heat production. The CNS controls the metabolic activity of skeletal muscle, which converts chemical energy into heat through shivering.

Increased body temperature initially prompts vasodilation. This vasodilation is passive. It results from the release of sympathetic tone, and it is seen in unanesthetized adults exposed to a hot environment before any significant change in central temperature occurs. If vasodilation is not adequate to prevent hyperthermia, thermoregulatory sweating occurs, which increases evaporative heat loss.

An abnormal body temperature can result from drugs or diseases that either change thermoregulatory thresholds or impair thermoregulatory responses. Hypothalamic activity and fever may be triggered by endogenous pyrogens released from immune effector cells in response to invasion by microorganisms (Figure 36-1). Although no single endogenous pyrogen has been identified conclusively as the mediator of the febrile response, tumor necrosis factor seems capable of reproducing many components of the febrile response.[3] Endogenous pyrogen activity appears to depend largely on greater endothelial cell production of prostaglandins. Of interest, many of these products help mediate uterine activity and parturition.[4]

Clinically, temperature measurements exceeding 38° C represent fever. During episodes of fever, the thermoregulatory setpoint is elevated, and the normal thermoregulatory mechanisms are used to maintain the elevated temperature. However, there are circumstances in which an abnormally high temperature is measured in the absence of a change in thermoregulatory setpoint, such as when thermoregulatory responses to hyperthermia are prevented (e.g., block of sympathetically mediated sweating) or

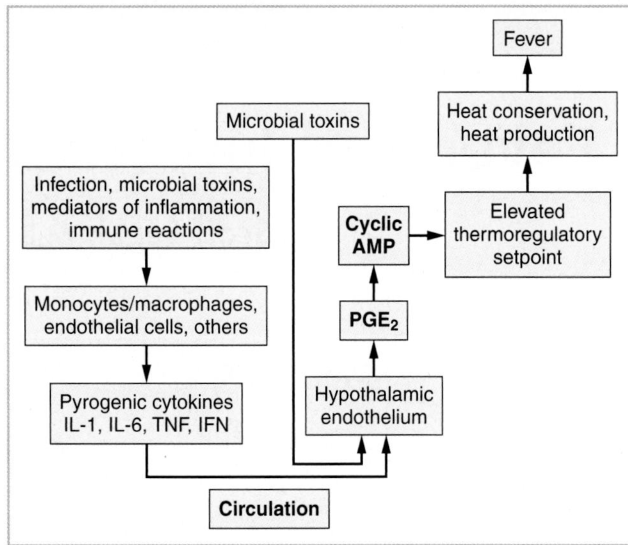

FIGURE 36-1 Chronology of events in the pathophysiology of fever. AMP, adenosine 5′-monophosphate; IFN, interferon; TNF, tumor necrosis factor; IL, interleukin; PGE_2, prostaglandin E_2. (From Faucl AS, Kasper DL, Longo DL, et al. Harrison's Principles of Internal Medicine. 17th edition. The McGraw-Hill Companies. Available at http://www.accessmedicine.com/)

overwhelmed (e.g., immersion in hot water, malignant hyperthermia).

The fetus, by virtue of its intra-abdominal location, has a unique problem with heat elimination. The only anatomic routes for egress of heat are the fetal skin surface (through the amniotic fluid) and the uteroplacental circulation. Current evidence suggests that the fetus relies on heat exchange across the uteroplacental circulation to dissipate most of its metabolic heat. The normal fetus maintains a temperature that is approximately 0.5° C to 0.75° C higher than the maternal temperature.[5]

Interaction with Pregnancy

Maternal-fetal infection is associated with higher perinatal morbidity.[6] The increase in morbidity is the result of many factors, including preterm delivery (perhaps related to a greater release of prostaglandins) and direct effects of the infection. In addition, experimental evidence suggests that extreme levels of fever, independent of the infection itself, may have a deleterious effect on the fetus. Morishima et al.[7] reported increased uterine activity and fetal deterioration during maternal hyperthermia produced by radiant heat in anesthetized baboons. However, the extreme level of hyperthermia (approximately 41.7° C [107° F]) employed in this study produced maternal as well as fetal deaths. Such extreme hyperthermia exceeds the modest fever that often occurs clinically, and the clinical relevance of this study is unclear.

Similarly, Cefalo and Hellegers[8] demonstrated fetal deterioration at levels of hyperthermia that produced maternal cardiovascular collapse in anesthetized gravid ewes. However, these investigators reported greater umbilical blood flow with lesser (more clinically relevant) levels of hyperthermia (approximately 0.5° C to 1.5° C above baseline). They suggested that greater umbilical blood flow (in response to moderate degrees of hyperthermia) might benefit the fetus through an increase in oxygen delivery and heat removal.

Harris et al.[9] demonstrated the preservation of fetal oxygenation and acid-base status during moderate fever (approximately 1° C above baseline) produced by the injection of a bacterial pyrogen in awake pregnant ewes. However, these researchers also observed an increase in fetal heart rate (FHR) and a higher incidence of fetal arrhythmias during fever.

Recently, epidemiologic evidence has suggested that mild maternal fever may not be as benign as has been assumed on the basis of animal studies. Macaulay et al.[10] measured fetal scalp temperature *in utero* using a modified intrauterine pressure catheter. They concluded that fetal core temperature may exceed 40° C (104° F) in some febrile women (Figure 36-2). Lieberman et al.[11] retrospectively reviewed the records of 1218 nulliparous women with singleton, term pregnancies with a vertex presentation and in spontaneous labor, who were afebrile on admission. These investigators found evidence of fever (> 38° C [> 100.4° F]) in 10% of the patients, nearly all of whom had received epidural analgesia. One-minute Apgar scores less than 7 and hypotonia were more common in the babies of febrile mothers. Fever higher than (38.3°C [101° F]) was associated with a more frequent requirement for bag-and-mask ventilation in the delivery room and a greater need for supplemental oxygen in the nursery. There was also a nonsignificant increase in the occurrence of neonatal seizures.[11] The same group performed a case-control follow-up study of unexplained neonatal seizures in term infants

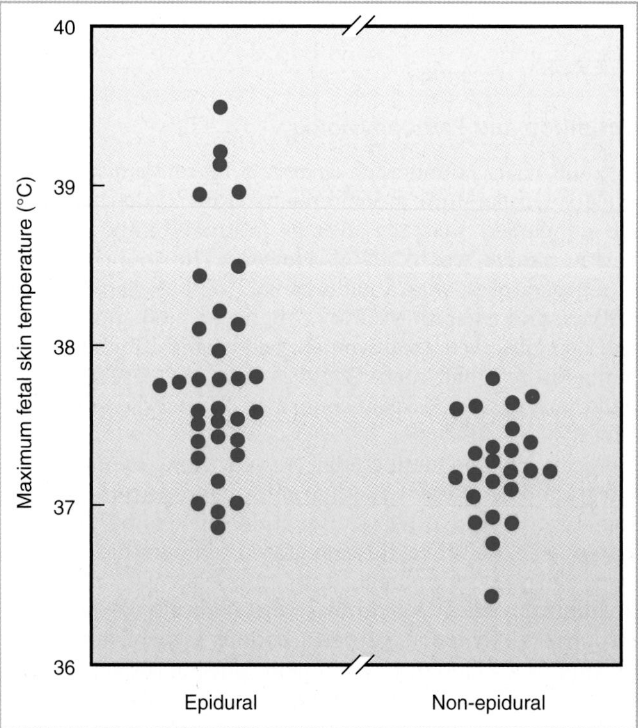

FIGURE 36-2 Fetal scalp temperatures measured *in utero* in women who selected epidural analgesia and those in women selecting other forms of analgesia. (From Macauley JH, Bond K, Steer PJ. Epidural analgesia in labor and fetal hyperthermia. Obstet Gynecol 1992; 80:665-9.)

and found a strong association between intrapartum fever and neonatal seizures (odds ratio = 3.4).[12] A similar finding was reported by Perlman,[13] who found a high incidence of maternal fever among a cohort of infants who had 5-minute Apgar scores of 5 or less or who required chest compressions in the delivery room.

Even more ominous is the suggestion that maternal fever may correlate with neonatal brain injury. In several large epidemiologic studies, otherwise unexplained cerebral palsy was two to nine times more common in babies born to mothers with intrapartum fever (> 38° C) than in those born to afebrile mothers.[14-16] An equally strong association has been observed between maternal fever and neonatal encephalopathy.[17] Dammann et al.[18] reported an increased risk of cognitive deficits (more than 2 SD below the mean on a nonverbal intelligence scale) at age 9 years among children whose mothers had been febrile during labor. The mechanism linking neurologic injuries to maternal fever remains unknown but may involve the liberation of inflammatory cytokines during fever.[19] Animal models of chorioamnionitis suggest that fetal brain lesions can be induced by the infection and blocked by anti-inflammatory cytokines.[20] It remains unclear whether neurologic injury can be produced by temperature elevation itself or whether it requires the additional presence of cytokines or other unknown factors produced by the underlying infection or inflammatory processes.

Fever has significant maternal effects. Elevated temperature is associated with increases in maternal heart rate, cardiac output, oxygen consumption, and catecholamine production. Evidence has also linked post–cesarean delivery fever to the risk of uterine rupture during a subsequent trial of labor.[21] Even low-grade fever may prompt obstetricians to choose instrumental vaginal delivery or cesarean delivery over expectant labor management. In a retrospective analysis of nulliparous women, Lieberman et al.[22] found a twofold higher incidence of both instrumental vaginal delivery and cesarean delivery in women who were afebrile at admission but in whom fever higher than 37.5° C (99.5° F) developed during labor than in women who remained afebrile, even after data were controlled for birth weight, length of labor, and analgesic technique.

Together, these studies suggest that the fetus acutely tolerates modest levels of maternal fever. Transient neonatal depression and, possibly, neonatal seizures and other neurologic disorders may be associated with inflammatory processes that produce maternal fever, although these adverse outcomes are not clearly a result of fever per se. An extremely high fever adversely affects both the mother and fetus.

Infections in Pregnant Women

Fever is most often the result of an infectious process. The most common sites of infection in pregnant women are the fetal membranes, the urinary tract, the respiratory tract, and the postpartum uterine cavity.

CHORIOAMNIONITIS

Chorioamnionitis is one of the most common infections in pregnant women, occurring in approximately 1% of all pregnancies.[6,23-27] The diagnosis of chorioamnionitis is based on clinical signs, which include a temperature higher than 38.0° C (100.4° F) and maternal or fetal tachycardia, uterine tenderness, and/or foul-smelling amniotic fluid. Unfortunately, the laboratory diagnosis of chorioamnionitis is neither sensitive nor specific and may not correlate with the clinical presentation.[6,23-27] Moreover, the classic clinical signs of chorioamnionitis are often absent. Goodman et al.,[28] reviewing the records of 531 women with pathologically proven chorioamnionitis, found that only 10% of the patients had abdominal tenderness, and only 1% had foul-smelling amniotic fluid.

In most cases, bacteria gain access to the amniotic cavity and the fetus by ascending through the cervix after rupture of the membranes. Chorioamnionitis develops in a significant number of parturients with premature rupture of the membranes. Alternatively, infectious agents present in the maternal circulation may undergo transplacental transport and gain access to the amniotic cavity.[6] Like other pelvic infections, chorioamnionitis often is polymicrobial in origin, and bacteria normally present in the genital tract are most likely responsible for most cases of infection. *Bacteroides* species, group B streptococci, and *Escherichia coli* are organisms commonly isolated from the amniotic fluid of parturients with chorioamnionitis.[6] In addition, maternal bacteremia occurs in approximately 10% of women with the clinical diagnosis of chorioamnionitis.[6,23-28] *Candida* species occasionally cause chorioamnionitis, especially in women with preterm labor, and have been associated with severe sequelae, including maternal sepsis and fetal demise.[29] *Ureaplasma urealyticum* has also been implicated in intra-amniotic infection even in patients with intact membranes, and infections with this organism have been associated with preterm labor.[30]

Maternal complications of chorioamnionitis include preterm labor,[31] placental abruption,[32] postpartum infection,[33] uterine atony,[34] postpartum hemorrhage,[35] sepsis, and death. In addition, several studies have noted an increased incidence of cesarean delivery for dystocia in women with chorioamnionitis.[6,23-25,27,35] Some investigators have suggested that infection adversely affects uterine contractility and contributes to a higher risk of cesarean delivery.[24] However, in some cases, chorioamnionitis may represent an ascending infection that develops late in a labor that is already prolonged and dysfunctional.[27] Satin et al.[27] observed no increase in the incidence of cesarean delivery when chorioamnionitis was diagnosed before the administration of oxytocin. However, they also noted a 44% incidence of cesarean delivery when the diagnosis was made after the administration of oxytocin. In this regard, the presence of chorioamnionitis may be seen as influencing the clinical decision-making of the obstetrician rather than as a direct physiologic cause of dystocia.

Neonatal complications of chorioamnionitis include pneumonia, meningitis, sepsis, and death.[23,25] A strong association between chorioamnionitis and **cerebral palsy** has been identified.[14,15,19,36,37] Meta-analyses of more than 20 studies to date have demonstrated relative risks of cerebral palsy of 1.9 to 4.7, respectively, in preterm and term infants born to mothers with clinical chorioamnionitis.[15,37] Neonatal stroke has also been linked to chorioamnionitis.[38] The link between maternal infection and neonatal neurologic injury appears related to intra-amniotic infection or inflammation, particularly when there is evidence of fetal systemic inflammation (funisitis).[19,36] Chorioamnionitis has also been linked epidemiologically to **cystic periventricular leukomalacia,** which often produces devastating neurologic impairment in the child.[37,39] The effect of intra-amniotic inflammation on the fetal lung is complex. Elevated concentrations of amniotic fluid cytokines may reduce the incidence of acute respiratory distress syndrome in preterm neonates by stimulating surfactant production.[40] However, **chronic lung disease** is more common in infants exposed to chorioamnionitis and is apparently also related to inflammatory mediators.[41,42] Studies in African women suggest that chorioamnionitis increases the risk of peripartum vertical transmission of human immunodeficiency virus (HIV) from infected mothers.[43]

Historically, prompt delivery has been the cornerstone of obstetric management of patients with chorioamnionitis. However, Gibbs et al.[23] obtained excellent maternal and neonatal outcomes without the use of arbitrary time limits for delivery. They performed cesarean delivery only for standard obstetric indications and not for the diagnosis of chorioamnionitis alone.[23] No recent studies have reinvestigated this practice as it relates to neonatal neurologic injuries.

For many years pediatricians requested that obstetricians delay antibiotic therapy until after delivery. They cited the theoretical concern that intrapartum therapy might "obscure the results of neonatal blood cultures."[44] However, studies suggest that early, antepartum treatment leads to less maternal and neonatal morbidity than delayed, postpartum treatment.[45,46] Gibbs et al.[45] randomly assigned 45 women with intra-amniotic infection to receive either intrapartum or postpartum antibiotic therapy with ampicillin and gentamicin. Intrapartum antibiotic therapy resulted in a lower incidence of neonatal sepsis and a shorter neonatal hospital stay. Mothers who received intrapartum antibiotics also had a shorter hospitalization, fewer days with fever, and a lower peak postpartum temperature than mothers whose antibiotic therapy was delayed until after delivery. Most obstetricians currently give antibiotics before delivery to women with chorioamnionitis. The early use of antibiotics also may affect the anesthesia provider's decision regarding the administration of neuraxial anesthesia (see later).

UROLOGIC INFECTIONS

Urinary tract infections are common during pregnancy. Increased concentrations of progesterone lead to the relaxation of ureteral smooth muscle. In addition, the gravid uterus causes partial ureteral obstruction. Both factors cause urinary stasis, which increases the risk of urinary tract infection.[6,47,48] Further, these physiologic changes make it more likely that asymptomatic bladder infection will ascend into the kidneys and produce pyelonephritis.

Acute pyelonephritis is a serious threat to maternal and fetal well-being. Symptoms of acute pyelonephritis include fever, chills, flank pain, and other symptoms of lower urinary tract infection. Laboratory tests reveal pyuria and leukocytosis with a left shift. Pregnant women with pyelonephritis may appear severely ill. Approximately 10% of pregnant women with pyelonephritis have transient bacteremia during the course of this infection.[6,46,48] The most common organisms found in such patients are *E. coli*, *Klebsiella*, and *Proteus* species.

Hospitalization is generally required to initiate aggressive parenteral antibiotic treatment of this serious maternal infection, although limited data support outpatient treatment in the first and second trimesters.[49] Pyelonephritis is associated with an increased risk of preterm labor and delivery.[50] Thus obstetricians should observe for evidence of preterm labor.

Obstetricians also should monitor renal and respiratory function. Nearly 20% of affected women have transient renal dysfunction.[48] Cunningham et al.[51] opined that acute pyelonephritis during pregnancy may be associated with pulmonary injury and respiratory failure. They suggested that "this syndrome was probably caused by permeability pulmonary edema, likely mediated by endotoxin-induced alveolar-capillary membrane injury."[51] Towers et al.[52] compared 11 pregnant women who had pyelonephritis and pulmonary injury with 119 women who had pyelonephritis only. They noted that "the presence of a maternal heart rate >110 beats/min and a fever to 103° F (39.4° C) 12 to 24 hours before the occurrence of respiratory symptoms was highly predictive of pulmonary injury."[52] Further, they observed that fluid overload and the use of tocolytic therapy were the most significant predictive factors associated with pulmonary injury. Finally, there was a trend toward a greater risk of pulmonary injury with the use of ampicillin alone for the treatment of pyelonephritis. The investigators concluded:

> *Tocolytic agents should be used only to treat the contractions of those pregnant patients with pyelonephritis who have documented and significant cervical change. The perceived benefit of tocolytic therapy must be weighed against the significant risk of pulmonary injury. Furthermore, strict management of fluids should occur so that patients do not have fluid overload.*[52]

Hemodynamic alterations may be present even in infected women who do not have overt signs of sepsis. Twickler et al.[53] used ultrasonographic techniques to evaluate the central hemodynamic measurements in 37 pregnant women with uncomplicated pyelonephritis. The investigators found lower mean arterial pressure and systemic vascular resistance (SVR), and higher heart rate and cardiac output than in the same patients after they had recovered from their infections.[53]

Reviews now also strongly support the practice of screening and treating pregnant women for asymptomatic bacteriuria, up to 30% of whom will eventually have pyelonephritis. Treatment is associated with a lower incidence of pyelonephritis (odds ratio = 0.23) and low-birth-weight babies (odds ratio = 0.66), although not, as had been previously suggested, with a reduced incidence of preterm delivery.[54] Because pyelonephritis during pregnancy is believed to be preventable, its occurrence may be a marker for poor prenatal care and thus should alert physicians to other potential pregnancy problems.[55]

RESPIRATORY TRACT INFECTION

Most respiratory tract infections during pregnancy are upper respiratory tract viral infections that do not pose a serious threat to the mother or fetus. However, an upper respiratory tract infection precedes approximately 50% of the cases of pneumonia that occur during pregnancy.[56] Pregnancy results in a number of changes that may predispose the pregnant woman to the development of a serious respiratory tract infection. Hyperemia and hypersecretion are characteristic of the respiratory tract mucosa during pregnancy, and these changes may intensify the effect of the initial infection. In the case of a viral infection, the excess secretions may predispose the patient to a bacterial superinfection. Further, the greater oxygen consumption and smaller functional residual capacity characteristic of pregnancy may increase the likelihood that infection will lead to maternal hypoxemia.

Benedetti et al.[57] emphasized the importance of early diagnosis and treatment as well as the assessment of maternal oxygenation in cases of pneumonia during pregnancy. Most community-acquired pneumonias in healthy young women are bacterial in origin. *Streptococcus pneumoniae* is the most common pathogen.[56,57] *Mycoplasma pneumoniae* and influenza are other common pathogens. *Legionella pneumophila*, chlamydia, and varicella are less common pathogens in this population. Varicella pneumonia has been associated with maternal and fetal morbidity. Acyclovir has been used successfully to treat varicella pneumonia during pregnancy.[58] *Pneumocystis carinii* pneumonia represents the most common cause of death related to acquired immunodeficiency syndrome (AIDS) in pregnancy, being associated with mortality as high as 50%.[59] Influenza vaccination is also recommended for most pregnant patients.[60]

POSTPARTUM INFECTION

The most common source of postpartum infection is the genital tract. However, the urinary tract and, less often, the breasts and the lungs may be infected.[6] Postpartum uterine infection typically results in fever, malaise, abdominal pain, and purulent lochia. Bacteremia may occur in as many as 20% of patients with uterine infection after cesarean delivery.[6,26] Although obstetricians typically refer to postpartum uterine infection as *endometritis*, this disease involves the decidua, myometrium, and parametrial tissues. Bacteria that colonize the cervix and vagina gain access to the amniotic fluid during labor and may invade devitalized uterine tissue after delivery.

Patients who undergo cesarean delivery are at higher risk for postpartum endometritis than similar patients who deliver vaginally.[6,26] Prolonged rupture of membranes and/or prolonged duration of labor increases the incidence of postpartum uterine infection. Prophylactic administration of antibiotics decreases the incidence of postpartum uterine infection and wound infection after elective or emergency cesarean delivery in all women.[61] Two reviews found insufficient evidence to recommend administration of prophylactic antibiotics in patients who undergo operative vaginal delivery or manual removal of the placenta after vaginal delivery.[62,63]

Endometritis typically responds to appropriate antibiotic therapy. However, serious complications (e.g., peritonitis, abscess, septic thrombophlebitis) may occur.[6,26] Women who have experienced endometritis are at higher risk for uterine rupture in future pregnancies, and obstetricians and anesthesia providers should demonstrate extra vigilance for this serious complication.[21]

Sepsis and Septic Shock

Sepsis is a rare, life-threatening complication of maternal infection; it complicates approximately 1 in 8000 deliveries.[64] Sepsis is a continuum of syndromes related to severe infection that begins with the **systemic inflammatory response syndrome,** which is characterized by the presence of two or more of the following signs: fever, leukocytosis, increased heart rate, and tachypnea. More severe sepsis involves organ failure of at least one system. Septic shock is characterized by hypotension and multiorgan hypoperfusion and failure.[6,64] Septic shock largely is an effect of the mediators released from immune effector cells, such as endotoxin, nitric oxide, tumor necrosis factor, interleukins, and cyclooxygenase metabolites of arachidonic acid.[65] Antibodies directed against tumor necrosis factor, interleukin-1 antagonists, and nonsteroidal anti-inflammatory agents are being evaluated to determine their efficacy in the treatment of septic shock.[65]

In pregnant women, septic shock is typically associated with gram-negative bacteremia, although it can occur in association with gram-positive aerobic and anaerobic infections. Untreated chorioamnionitis, pyelonephritis, endometritis, wound infection, incomplete abortion, and self-induced abortion may lead to maternal sepsis and septic shock. Rarely, amniocentesis,[66-69] medical abortion,[70] dental procedures, and assisted reproductive technology procedures[71] have been associated with septic shock. The mainstay of therapy is elimination and/or aggressive treatment of the source of infection. Antibiotic therapy should consist of broad-spectrum coverage for bacteria such as *E. coli*, enterococci, and anaerobic organisms. A combination of ampicillin, gentamicin, and clindamycin is an effective regimen, as is a combination of imipenem, cilastatin, and vancomycin.[65]

Laboratory studies have suggested that pregnancy makes laboratory animals more susceptible to infection or products of infection. Beller et al.[72] infused *E. coli* B6 lipopolysaccharide into both nonpregnant and pregnant minipigs. The average length of survival for the nonpregnant animals was 16 hours, whereas the average length of survival for the pregnant animals was only 3.5 hours. The pregnant animals suffered more pronounced cardiovascular abnormalities and metabolic acidosis. The investigators concluded that pregnant minipigs are more susceptible to the harmful effects of lipopolysaccharide than nonpregnant minipigs. They acknowledged that it is unclear whether pregnant women are more susceptible to endotoxin than nonpregnant women. However, clinical studies have noted that once septic shock develops in pregnant patients, the risk of maternal death is high.[73-75]

Only a few reports have described the management of these seriously ill patients. All reports have included single cases or a small number of patients. Lee et al.[74] reviewed 10 cases of septic shock in obstetric patients. Of the 10 women, 8 experienced septic shock during the postpartum period. Risk factors included prolonged rupture of membranes (n = 2), retained products of conception (n = 3), and previous instrumentation of the genitourinary tract (n = 2); 2 of the 10 women died. Other maternal complications included adult respiratory distress syndrome (ARDS) (n = 3), disseminated intravascular coagulation (DIC) (n = 2), pulmonary edema (n = 1), and septic pulmonary embolus (n = 1). The primary hemodynamic abnormalities were decreased systemic vascular resistance and depressed myocardial function; 3 patients, including 1 who died, had markedly depressed myocardial function.

Mabie et al.[75] reported 18 cases of pregnancy-associated septic shock that occurred during 11 years in a single institution, with an incidence of 1 per 8338 deliveries. The most common etiologies were pyelonephritis (n = 6), chorioamnionitis (n = 3), endometritis (n = 2), and toxic shock syndrome (n = 2). Five (28%) patients died. The hemodynamic profiles of the patients in this series were similar to those described by Lee et al.[74]; four of the five patients who died had mildly or severely depressed myocardial function.[75]

In most cases of septic shock, concomitant supportive therapy is required to decrease maternal and fetal morbidity. Physicians must give attention to the maintenance of maternal oxygenation, circulation, and coagulation. These patients are at risk for respiratory, renal, and/or hepatic failure. Both Lee et al.[74] and Mabie et al.[75] as well as the American College of Obstetricians and Gynecologists (ACOG)[65] agree that the mainstay of therapy is eradication of the infectious source. Fluid resuscitation and hemodynamic and respiratory support are also generally required. Controversy surrounds a number of interventions designed to reduce morbidity and mortality from sepsis, and no trials have included pregnant patients and thus considered the unique physiology of pregnancy and its interaction with sepsis. Some evidence supports early institution of "goal-directed therapy" (treatment to achieve targets of cardiopulmonary measurements).[76,77] Evidence from general intensive care unit populations supports aggressive glycemic control in critically ill patients[78]; it is likely but unproven that this would hold true in the diabetogenic pregnant state. Corticosteroid administration has proved very controversial, and empiric corticosteroid therapy may actually worsen outcome. There has been renewed interest, however, in corticosteroid therapy in subsets of septic shock patients who demonstrate impaired adrenal reserve.[79] Excitement has also surrounded the investigational administration of activated protein C, a mediator with anticoagulant and anti-inflammatory properties, in reducing mortality in the most severely ill patients with septic shock.[80]

Although the effects of maternal therapy on the fetus should be considered, treatment of the mother has first priority. Often what is best for the mother is best for the fetus. However, in some cases, maternal sepsis may require preterm delivery before the age of fetal viability. The ACOG recommends early delivery only in cases in which the pregnancy itself is the source of the infection.[65]

EPIDURAL ANALGESIA AND MATERNAL FEVER

Incidence

Epidural anesthesia administered for surgery—including cesarean delivery—typically results in hypothermia. This effect occurs because vasodilation produced by the block causes a redistribution of body heat from the core to the periphery, where it is lost to the environment.[81] Conversely, laboring women who receive neuraxial analgesia may experience a rise in temperature.

In 1989, Fusi et al.[82] first observed that epidural analgesia was associated with progressive intrapartum maternal pyrexia. They reported that the vaginal temperatures of 18 parturients who received epidural analgesia increased approximately 1° C over 7 hours, whereas the temperatures of 15 women who received intramuscular meperidine and metoclopramide remained constant. There was no evidence of infection in any of the women. The investigators suggested that epidural analgesia may cause an "imbalance between the heat-producing and heat-dissipating mechanisms."[82]

Fusi et al.[82] measured maternal vaginal temperature, which may be affected by the sympathectomy and vaginal mucosal vasodilation associated with epidural analgesia. Tympanic membrane temperature, which should not be affected by the local vasodilation associated with epidural analgesia, may provide a more accurate assessment of core temperature. Camann et al.[83] studied the effect of epidural analgesia on maternal oral and tympanic membrane temperature measurements in 53 laboring women. The investigators studied three groups of patients; one group received intravenous nalbuphine, one group received epidural bupivacaine only, and one group received epidural bupivacaine with fentanyl. The patients were not randomly assigned to receive either nalbuphine or epidural analgesia; however, those women who requested epidural analgesia were randomly assigned to receive either epidural bupivacaine only or epidural bupivacaine with fentanyl. The investigators kept the ambient room temperature at 20° C to 22° C. They found that epidural analgesia did not affect maternal temperature during the first 4 hours of the study. At 5 hours and thereafter, the mean tympanic membrane temperatures were significantly higher in both of the epidural groups than in the intravenous nalbuphine group (Figure 36-3). Among women in the bupivacaine-only group, mean tympanic temperature rose from approximately 36.6° C at 1 hour to 37.1° C at 9 hours, a rate of rise of less than 0.07° C per hour. There was no difference between the epidural bupivacaine-only and the epidural bupivacaine-fentanyl groups in maternal tympanic membrane temperature measurements.

Several other investigators have documented similar patterns of temperature elevation and an increased incidence of clinical fever (> 38.0° C) in laboring women receiving

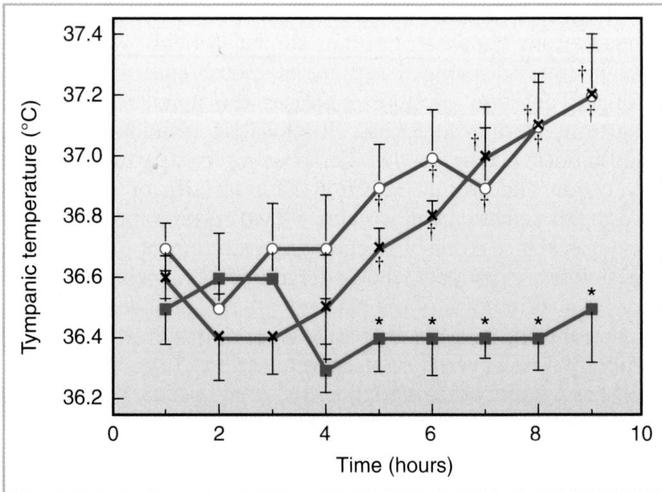

FIGURE 36-3 Mean tympanic temperatures during labor in three groups of patients: Epidural bupivacaine-fentanyl (*open circles*), epidural bupivacaine-only (×), and parenteral opioid (*teal squares*) groups. **P* < .01 compared with the epidural group; †*P* < .01 compared with the pre–epidural analgesia temperature. (From Camann WR, Hortvet LA, Hughes N, et al. Maternal temperature regulation during extradural analgesia for labour. Br J Anaesth 1991; 657:565-8.)

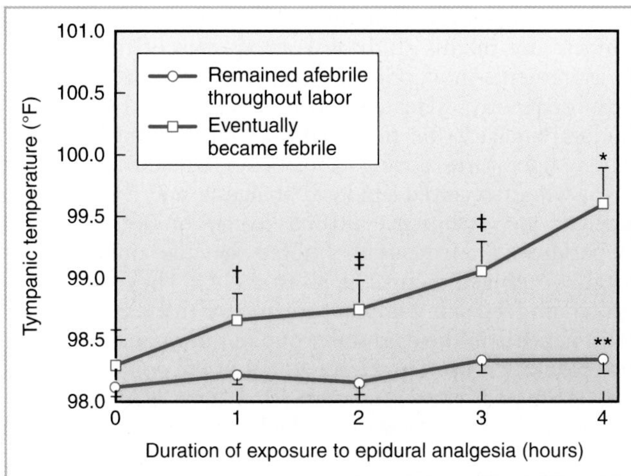

FIGURE 36-4 Mean temperature in labor following epidural analgesia in women in whom clinical fever > 38° C (100.4° F) eventually developed compared with those without fever.*P< .001. †P< .05. ‡P< .01, for difference between afebrile and eventually febrile groups.**P = .26 for change in temperature over time in the afebrile group. (From Goetzl L, Rivers J, Zighelboim I, et al. Intrapartum epidural analgesia and maternal temperature regulation. Obstet Gynecol 2007; 109:687-90.)

epidural analgesia.[84-90] These studies typically have found the rate of temperature increase to be approximately 0.1° C per hour of epidural analgesia, usually after a delay of 4 to 5 hours. However, the incidence of clinical fever has varied strikingly, from 1% to 36%.[85-88,91] Two more recent investigations have suggested that the slow progressive rise observed by Fusi et al.[82] and Camann et al.[83] may actually have been an artifact caused by averaging the temperature curves of women in whom clinical fever developed with those of women who remained afebrile (Figure 36-4).[92,93] This suggestion would imply that an understanding of the nature of the relationship between epidural analgesia and overt fever is the key to understanding hyperthermia during labor in patients with epidural analgesia.

Etiology

The mechanism by which epidural analgesia produces maternal hyperthermia during labor remains unclear. At least three explanations may be relevant—thermoregulatory factors, effect of systemic opioids in patients not receiving epidural analgesia, and inflammation.

THERMOREGULATORY FACTORS

Thermoregulatory factors that may play a role include ambient temperature, impaired heat dissipation, and increased heat production. Fusi et al.[82] attributed the maternal pyrexia to the high ambient temperature (24° C to 26° C) found in most British delivery rooms. However, other investigators have not found an association between ambient temperature and maternal[85] or fetal[10] temperature. Alternatively, epidural analgesia may impair heat-dissipating mechanisms. Decreased sweating and the lack of hyperventilation that follow the provision of effective epidural pain relief may predispose laboring women to pyrexia.[82,83,94] In volunteers, epidural anesthesia raised the sweating threshold by 0.55° C.[95] Moreover, epidural analgesia attenuates but does not eliminate the significant increase in $\dot{V}O_2$ that occurs during uterine contractions and expulsive efforts during the second stage of labor.[96] This decreased ventilation in the setting of greater energy expenditure may manifest as higher temperature in the laboring patient. Finally, the high incidence of shivering among laboring women who receive epidural analgesia may predispose them to the development of fever. Gleeson et al.[97] found that laboring patients who shivered after the administration of epidural analgesia had pyrexia as early as 1 hour after initiation of the block, compared with more than 4 hours after initiation of the block in patients who did not shiver. Moreover, the maximum temperature reached was higher, and the incidence of clinical fever was three times more common, in the women who shivered.[97] Some shivering and sweating in labor have been demonstrated to be nonthermoregulatory (i.e., not accompanied by changes in core temperature or vasomotor tone).[98] However, it is not clear whether shivering is a cause or an effect of increased maternal temperature.

EFFECT OF SYSTEMIC OPIOIDS IN WOMEN NOT RECEIVING EPIDURAL ANALGESIA

Systemic opioids given to women without epidural analgesia might suppress fever that otherwise would have been apparent. In nonpregnant volunteers, injection of interleukin-2 reliably caused fever approximately 4 hours later. Epidural ropivacaine analgesia (with or without epidural fentanyl) did not affect the magnitude of fever, but intravenous fentanyl markedly attenuated the rise in temperature.[99] However, differences in opioid use could not explain the difference in occurrence of fever in one large retrospective study,[100] and Camann et al.[83] did not find a difference in temperature curves between women randomly assigned to receive epidural administration of an opioid-containing and those receiving an opioid-free solution.

INFLAMMATION

Nearly all clinical studies of epidural analgesia–associated fever have been nonrandomized. Women who are more likely to request epidural analgesia during labor also are more likely to have other risk factors for fever during labor, such as nulliparity,[89] prolonged rupture of membranes,[85,89] prolonged labor,[10,83,85,89] higher temperature on admission,[89] early chorioamnionitis,[89] and more frequent cervical examinations.[101] In a case-control study, Vallejo et al.[91] compared women with clinical chorioamnionitis who did not receive epidural analgesia to two groups of women who received epidural analgesia, one with and the other without clinical chorioamnionitis. The diagnosis of chorioamnionitis was confirmed histologically. Not surprisingly, fever was far more common in the infected women. However, the incidence of fever in uninfected women with epidural analgesia was only 1%.[91] Similarly, Dashe et al.[102] examined the placentas and medical records of 149 women who delivered 6 or more hours after membrane rupture. The investigators found a higher incidence of fever (≥ 38° C) in the 54% of their subjects who received epidural analgesia. However, histologic evidence of placental inflammation was also more common among epidural analgesia–exposed women. In the absence of placental inflammation, the incidence of maternal fever was similar in the epidural analgesia–exposed and unexposed patients (11% and 9%, respectively).[102]

Goetzl et al.[103] randomly assigned laboring women who received epidural analgesia to also receive either acetaminophen or placebo during labor. The incidence of fever higher than 38° C (100.4° F) was identical in the two groups. At delivery both maternal and umbilical cord blood levels of interleukin-6 (a marker of inflammation) were higher in febrile women than in afebrile women. Of interest, at the time that epidural analgesia was initiated, maternal levels of interleukin-6 were higher in women who later became febrile, but this difference was not statistically significant. Goetzl et al.[104] subsequently cited this earlier study and stated that "maternal serum levels of interleukin-6 . . . at the initiation of epidural analgesia are predictive of subsequent fever, which suggests an inflammatory basis." In the later study, these investigators demonstrated suppression of epidural analgesia–associated fever with high-dose maternal corticosteroid therapy (methylprednisolone 100 mg every 4 hours).[104] Umbilical cord blood interleukin-6 levels were also lower in the patients treated with high-dose corticosteroids, indicating suppression of inflammation. However, the incidence of asymptomatic neonatal bacteremia was significantly increased by corticosteroid exposure.[104]

The foregoing discussion does not explain a higher incidence of fever in women randomly assigned to receive epidural analgesia in a clinical trial. In the only published trial that specifically assessed maternal fever in women randomly assigned to receive either epidural analgesia or intravenous opioid analgesia during labor, Philip et al.[90] confirmed a higher incidence of fever in women who received epidural analgesia. However, the association was confined to nulliparous patients, and febrile patients also were more likely to have a prolonged labor and to undergo internal fetal monitoring and/or oxytocin augmentation of labor. A systematic review of other randomized trials of epidural versus systemic opioid analgesia, in which the incidence of fever was not a primary outcome measure, has confirmed the association between maternal fever and epidural analgesia.[105]

Consequences

Epidural analgesia–associated maternal hyperthermia has become a subject of significant controversy. In theory, the fetus is at risk for hyperthermia when the mother is febrile, because the fetus dissipates heat by means of its transmission to the amniotic fluid and the maternal blood. In the study by Fusi et al.,[82] although the maximum mean maternal temperature in the epidural group was approximately 37.7° C, the investigators interpreted their results by reference to those of the study by Morishima et al.,[7] in which detrimental maternal and fetal effects were produced by warming pregnant baboons to a temperature of approximately 42° C (107° F). Fusi et al.[82] did not report Apgar scores or umbilical cord blood gas and acid-base measurements. In contrast, Camann et al.[83] argued that the small average temperature rise seen with epidural analgesia is unlikely to affect the fetus. They did not observe any clinically febrile patients in their series, although as noted earlier, it is possible that the small mean rise in maternal temperature in this study was an average of temperature measurements in afebrile and much warmer patients.

Subsequently, Macaulay et al.[10] evaluated the effect of epidural analgesia on maternal oral, intrauterine, and fetal skin temperatures during labor. They studied 57 women, 33 of whom received epidural analgesia and 24 of whom received no analgesia, nitrous oxide, or intramuscular meperidine. The researchers noted that the ambient temperatures ranged from 23.3° C to 29° C. They reported a maximum fetal skin temperature greater than 38.0° C in 10 of 33 patients in the epidural group but in none of 24 in the no-epidural group. Three fetuses (all in the epidural group) had estimated core temperatures higher than 40.0° C. Conversely, only 2 women had an oral temperature higher than 37.5° C during the study. Administration of epidural analgesia did not affect Apgar scores or umbilical cord blood gas and acid-base measurements. The investigators did not report neonatal temperature measurements. Nonetheless, they concluded that "the fetus whose mother has a long labor using epidural analgesia in a hot environment may reach a temperature at which heat-induced neurologic injury can occur."[10] They also cited the study by Morishima et al.,[7] in which detrimental maternal and fetal effects were produced by warming pregnant baboons to near-lethal temperatures. Macaulay et al.[10] did not acknowledge other studies that showed that modest increases in temperature do not cause fetal injury and actually may increase fetal blood flow.[8,9] Nonetheless, the aforementioned epidemiologic association of maternal fever and/or infection with neonatal neurologic injuries[14-18] suggests that efforts to avoid maternal fever, and to reduce it when it occurs, are warranted.

The neonate may also be placed at risk *indirectly* as a result of the interventions triggered by the occurrence of maternal fever.[87,88] Mayer et al.[88] retrospectively analyzed the records of 300 low-risk nulliparous women who received systemic opioids, epidural analgesia, or both (n = 100 per group). They found a 2% incidence of maternal fever in the systemic opioid group, compared with an incidence of 16% to 24% in the two epidural anesthesia groups. The incidence of intrapartum maternal antibiotic administration was 6% in the women who received systemic opioids only, versus 19% to 22% in the women who received epidural analgesia. The investigators noted that among the 10 patients with culture- or pathology-proven chorioamnionitis, none had fever as the *only* presenting sign or symptom. They concluded, "Rather than treating all women with temperature elevations and epidural [analgesia] for presumed chorioamnionitis, it is reasonable to target treatment to those with fetal tachycardia, meconium-stained fluid, or abnormal amniotic fluid studies." Further, they suggested that "by seeking further evidence that the source of the fever is infectious prior to committing both the mother and her neonate to antibiotic therapy, one can limit . . . the use of antibiotics by about 50% without undertreating amnionitis."[88]

In another retrospective study, Lieberman et al.[87] reanalyzed the records of 1657 low-risk nulliparous women originally enrolled in a trial of active management of labor. They also found a higher incidence of maternal temperature higher than 38.0° C in parturients who received epidural analgesia than in those who did not (15% versus

1%, respectively). The investigators reported that neonates in the epidural group had a higher incidence of sepsis evaluation (34% versus 10%, respectively) and antibiotic treatment (15% versus 4%, respectively) than neonates in the no-epidural group. The incidence of actual neonatal sepsis was exceedingly low in both groups (0.3% versus 0.2%, respectively). As in all studies in which women select their analgesia, the women receiving epidural analgesia were already at risk for intrapartum fever; for example, they had larger infants, longer labors, and a twofold higher rate of induction.[87] Moreover, the active labor management protocol mandated frequent cervical examinations and early amniotomy, which may have increased the risk of fever.[106] Unlike in prospective studies of epidural analgesia–associated hyperthermia, Lieberman et al.[87] found fever even in women with labor of less than 6 hours' duration, suggesting the possibility that an increase in maternal temperature may have already begun at the time epidural analgesia was initiated.[101] Of interest, two thirds of the sepsis evaluations occurred in infants of mothers who did *not* have intrapartum fever.[106] Because the investigators did not provide data on the indications for sepsis evaluations, it is not possible to explain the association between these evaluations and the presence of epidural analgesia. In a subsequent study, Goetzl et al.[107] analyzed a cohort in which intrapartum temperature remained below 38° C (100.4° F) throughout labor. Neonatal sepsis evaluations were more common in women with epidural analgesia than in those without (20.4% versus 8.9%, respectively), after data were controlled for gestational age, birth weight, maternal smoking history, active labor management, premature rupture of membranes, and admission cervical dilation. Epidural analgesia was associated with both major (rupture of membranes for longer than 24 hours, fetal heart rate higher than 160 beats/min) and minor criteria (maternal temperature > 37.5° C [99.5° F], rupture of membranes for 12 to 24 hours) for neonatal sepsis evaluation. As with the original study, women were not randomly assigned to receive epidural analgesia, and it is likely that many of the features of labor that led to sepsis evaluations also predisposed women to choose epidural analgesia.

Subsequent work by other investigators has suggested the paramount role of maternal temperature elevation in neonatal sepsis evaluations. In the study by Philip et al.,[90] women randomly assigned to receive epidural analgesia had more fever (> 38° C [100.4° F]) than those assigned to receive intravenous opioid analgesia (15% versus 4%, respectively). Neonatal sepsis evaluations were also far more common in women with fever than in those without (96% versus 13%, respectively). However, within both the febrile and the afebrile cohorts, the incidence of neonatal sepsis evaluation was independent of the type of analgesia. The investigators concluded:

> *Our results indicate that in the absence of maternal fever, epidural analgesia during labor has no bearing on the need for such neonatal management and therefore should not be considered a predictor* per se *for neonatal sepsis evaluations. We attribute this finding to the minimization of ascertainment bias as a result of randomization of analgesia.*[90]

Other investigators have highlighted the importance of neonatal practice style in determining the rate of sepsis evaluations. Yancey et al.[84] studied the rates of maternal fever and neonatal sepsis evaluation during a period in which the rate of epidural analgesia use rapidly rose from 1% to 83% after the introduction of an around-the-clock on-demand epidural analgesia service. The rates of fever higher than 37° C (99.5° F) increased 3-fold, and that of fever higher than 38° C (100.4° F) 18-fold, following the greater use of epidural analgesia, although numerous indices of the patients' admission status and intrapartum obstetric management did not change. The incidence of neonatal laboratory testing (e.g., blood counts, blood cultures) rose modestly (relative risk = 1.5 to 1.7), but there was no change in the incidence of neonatal antibiotic treatment. The investigators contrasted their results with those of Lieberman et al.,[87] attributing the difference to neonatal practice patterns that did not require antibiotic therapy solely on the basis of maternal fever or antibiotic exposure.[84] In an analysis of the records of 1177 nulliparous women and their babies, Kaul et al.[108] also emphasized the practice style of the neonatologists. Women with epidural analgesia had more fever, longer ruptured membrane times, more instrumental and cesarean deliveries, and larger babies. However, the incidence of neonatal sepsis evaluation was no different between women with and without epidural analgesia (7.5% versus 9.4%, respectively). In contrast to Lieberman et al.,[87] these investigators attributed the lower rate of neonatal sepsis evaluation and lack of effect of epidural analgesia to more stringent guidelines for neonatal sepsis evaluation, which do not include maternal fever in the absence of clinical chorioamnionitis.[108]

The link between epidural analgesia and maternal fever is likely a real phenomenon and not purely an artifact of more frequent selection of epidural analgesia by higher-risk patients. Because of the growing evidence that maternal inflammation and infection, which manifest as fever, can be detrimental to the fetal brain, anesthesia providers cannot dismiss this unique physiologic effect as a mere curiosity. Further study to elucidate the relationship between epidural analgesia, labor, and fever is needed to guide development of safe and effective clinical management strategies. In addition, attention must be paid to the indirect effects of maternal fever on the clinical decision-making of obstetricians and neonatologists, in order to minimize unnecessary maternal and fetal interventions. Meanwhile, when maternal pyrexia occurs, good clinical practice dictates that efforts be made to lower maternal temperature and identify and treat a presumed maternal infection.

NEURAXIAL ANESTHESIA IN THE FEBRILE PATIENT

Clinical Studies

Clinicians have long suspected an association between the performance of dural puncture during a period of bacteremia and the subsequent development of meningitis. Some clinicians have feared that diagnostic lumbar puncture may cause meningitis rather than aid in its diagnosis. They reasoned that lumbar puncture might disrupt the rich venous plexus surrounding the spinal cord and allow the direct introduction of infected blood into the CNS by the spinal needle. Alternatively, some have speculated that disruption of the dural barrier may permit hematogenous spread of infection into the CNS without direct vessel trauma. Similar concerns apply to the performance of epidural anesthesia and the development of epidural abscess (see Chapter 32). Administration of continuous epidural analgesia often results in blood vessel trauma and almost always involves the introduction of a foreign body. Theoretically, this technique could produce a nidus for subsequent infection.

At least six retrospective clinical studies have evaluated the risk of diagnostic lumbar puncture.[109-114] (These studies did not evaluate the administration of neuraxial analgesia or anesthesia.) These reports came to conflicting conclusions regarding the risk of meningitis after the performance of dural puncture in bacteremic patients. Two studies suggested an association between dural puncture and meningitis.[109,112] However, both studies had serious methodologic flaws. One study was performed during an epidemic of meningitis.[109] Although the investigators observed a high rate of meningitis after lumbar puncture, they did not evaluate a comparable control group who did not undergo lumbar puncture. In the other study, Teele et al.[112] reported an association between lumbar puncture and meningitis only in bacteremic children younger than 1 year. However, they acknowledged the possibility that clinical judgment might have prompted their pediatricians to perform diagnostic lumbar puncture in children with incipient meningitis before the cerebrospinal fluid (CSF) provided diagnostic evidence of infection.

The remaining four studies clearly did not support an association between dural puncture and meningitis.[110,111,113,114] Shapiro et al.[114] concluded:

The development of bacterial meningitis in children with occult bacteremia is strongly associated with the species of bacteria that causes the infection, but not with a lumbar puncture.... Children with high-density bacteremia may appear to be more severely ill than children who have bacteremia with lower concentrations of bacteria, and therefore may be more likely to undergo a lumbar puncture.

Chestnut[115] stated, "Physicians often perform diagnostic lumbar puncture in patients with fever and/or bacteremia of unknown origin. If dural puncture during bacteremia results in meningitis, one would expect that unequivocal clinical data should exist."

However, no epidemiologic study has clearly established a causal relationship between the performance of dural puncture during bacteremia and the subsequent development of meningitis or epidural abscess. Part of the uncertainty about the risk of dural puncture results from awareness that processes other than meningeal integrity may help protect against the occurrence of CNS infection. For example, as many as 35% of epidural catheters used postoperatively are colonized by bacteria, but epidural abscess is a *very rare* complication.[116] Some anesthesiologists have cited anecdotal reports of meningitis after spinal anesthesia during presumed bacteremia as evidence that dural puncture may cause meningitis.[117-120] In one of these reports, the physicians used reusable equipment, and the source of infection was traced to inadequately sterilized supplies.[117] The use of sterile, disposable equipment and strict attention to aseptic technique have largely eliminated these factors as a source of infection.

However, most evidence points to external contamination, not blood-borne pathogens, as the source of meningitis after spinal anesthesia.[121-126] Kilpatrick and Girgis[119] reported 17 cases of meningitis after spinal anesthesia in nonobstetric patients. In 10 cases CSF culture results were positive, and all cultures grew unusual or nosocomial organisms. Ready and Helfer[127] reported 2 cases of meningitis after the administration of epidural anesthesia in obstetric patients. Both patients were afebrile and without clinical signs of infection at the time of epidural catheter placement, and the epidural catheter was in place for less than 1 hour in one of the patients. Davis et al.[128] reported a case of postpartum meningitis after administration of epidural analgesia during labor. The meningitis apparently was caused by a group B beta-hemolytic streptococcus that was cultured from the patient's blood and vagina. Videira et al.[122] reported 3 cases of meningitis after 38,128 spinal anesthesia procedures (1:12,709). In 2 cases, streptococci presumed to be skin flora were cultured. The investigators concluded that lapses in sterile technique may have been responsible for the meningitis. Poor attention to asepsis was also apparently responsible for 3 cases of meningitis occurring in a 3-year period in a single hospital in another report.[126] In 1 case, the offending organism was cultured from the nose of the anesthesiologist performing the block. Rubin et al.[125] reported 6 cases of meningitis after spinal anesthesia over 5 years, all caused by the same organism; all patients had received care from the same anesthesiologist.

Several reports have described the occurrence of meningitis after the administration of combined spinal-epidural (CSE) analgesia in obstetric patients.[129-131] None of these patients was febrile during administration of CSE analgesia. Further, the investigators concluded that in the cases with positive CSF culture results, contamination by skin flora was the most likely mechanism of infection. Overall, evidence does not support any special risk for meningitis with the CSE technique, but rather, suggests a reporting bias involving complications of a relatively new technique.[132]

Large epidemiologic studies have found a very low incidence of CNS infection after the administration of neuraxial anesthesia. Dripps and Vandam[133] prospectively studied 8460 patients who received 10,098 spinal anesthesia procedures between 1948 and 1951. Similarly, Phillips et al.[134] reported the administration of spinal anesthesia to 10,440 patients between 1964 and 1966. A large number of the patients in both studies underwent obstetric or urologic procedures. Undoubtedly some patients had bacteremia during or after the performance of spinal anesthesia. However, neither study reported a single case of CNS infection.[133,134] Similarly, four reviews of more than 500,000 obstetric patients who received epidural anesthesia reported no cases of meningitis and only two cases of epidural space infection.[135-138] Most likely some of these parturients were bacteremic during the administration of epidural anesthesia, given the frequency with which fever and infection develop during labor. For example, Blanco et al.[26] found a 1% incidence of bacteremia in a random sample of patients on the labor ward. Other studies have noted an 8% to 10% incidence of bacteremia in parturients with chorioamnionitis.[23-25,28] Unfortunately, there are no good predictive factors for identifying the subgroup of febrile patients with chorioamnionitis who are bacteremic at the time of anesthesia. The severity of fever does not reliably predict the likelihood of bacteremia in these patients. For example, Blanco et al.[26] reported that 86 (49%) of 176 patients with documented bacteremia had a temperature below 38.8° C. Furthermore, Bader et al.[139] reported no significant difference between the mean temperatures of bacteremic and nonbacteremic patients with chorioamnionitis. Similarly, in a study of 146 women with chorioamnionitis, Goodman et al.[28] found no differences in temperature, leukocytosis, or maternal symptoms between patients with positive or negative blood culture results.

Bader et al.[139] retrospectively observed no cases of CNS infection after the administration of epidural or spinal anesthesia for labor and/or cesarean delivery in 279 patients with chorioamnionitis. Only 43 of these 279 women received antibiotic therapy before the administration of neuraxial anesthesia. At least three women had positive blood culture results consistent with bacteremia, none of whom received antibiotics before the administration of anesthesia. Similarly, Ramanathan et al.[140] reviewed their experience with administration of epidural anesthesia in 113 parturients with chorioamnionitis. The diagnosis of chorioamnionitis was made before the placement of the epidural catheter in 39 of these 113 women. Antibiotic therapy was begun soon after the diagnosis of chorioamnionitis in most patients; in 16 women, antibiotic therapy was delayed until after delivery. None of these 113 patients had any signs or symptoms of bacterial meningitis or epidural abscess. Goodman et al.[28] found no cases of meningitis or epidural abscess among 531 patients with chorioamnionitis (proven by culture or pathologic examination) who received epidural (n = 517) or spinal (n = 14) anesthesia. Eleven of 45 patients in this study with fever before initiation of the block, and 174 of 229 patients with preexisting leukocytosis, received no antibiotics before instrumentation of the epidural or subarachnoid space.

Together, clinical studies suggest that meningitis and epidural abscess are very rare complications of epidural or spinal anesthesia. Further, bacteremia itself does not appear to increase the risk of CNS infection after the administration of neuraxial anesthesia. However, published studies of neuraxial anesthesia in patients with chorioamnionitis were small and retrospective. Given the infrequent occurrence of CNS infection among noninfected patients receiving neuraxial anesthesia, none of these studies was sufficiently large to exclude the possibility that chorioamnionitis increases the risk of meningitis or epidural abscess. Moreover, the retrospective study design introduces the possibility of selection bias—that is, the anesthesia providers may have avoided neuraxial anesthesia in the sickest patients with chorioamnionitis.

Laboratory Studies

Carp and Bailey[141] performed a study to assess the risk of meningitis after the performance of dural puncture in bacteremic animals. In this study, rats were made bacteremic by producing a flank abscess using *E. coli* bacteria. The bacteremia was similar in magnitude to that occurring during the early phase of sepsis in humans. Cisternal dural puncture was performed after the onset of bacteremia. After 24 hours, the cisterna magna was drained surgically, and the CSF was cultured for evidence of meningitis. Of the 40 animals that underwent dural puncture during *E. coli* bacteremia, 12 had meningitis (Table 36-1). None of the 40 bacteremic animals not subjected to dural puncture had meningitis. Further, dural puncture did not result in infection in the 30 animals without bacteremia. Importantly, *none* of the 30 bacteremic animals given a dose of gentamicin 15 minutes before dural puncture had meningitis.

TABLE 36-1 The Association between Bacteremia and the Recovery of *Escherichia coli* from Cerebrospinal Fluid after Dural Puncture

n	Bacteremia (CFU/mL)*	Gentamicin†	Dural Puncture	CSF *E.coli*‡
40	40 ± 22 (5-100)	No	Yes	12/40§
40	48 ± 25¶ (2-100)	No	No	0/40
30	0(0)	No	Yes	0/30
30	49 ± 35 (5-110)	Yes	Yes	0/30

CFU, colony-forming unit(s); CSF, cerebrospinal fluid; n, number of rats in each group.

*Data expressed as mean ± SD (range in parentheses).

†Gentamicin administered before dural puncture.

‡Data expressed as the number of animals in which *E. coli* cultured from spinal fluid per total number of animals in that group.

§$P < .05$ compared with other groups.

¶Not significantly different from that in the bacteremic groups undergoing cisternal puncture.

Modified from Carp H, Bailey S. The association between meningitis and dural puncture in bacteremic rats. Anesthesiology 1992; 76:739-42.

This study augments earlier laboratory studies that observed the development of meningitis after the performance of dural puncture in bacteremic laboratory animals.[142-144] Although animal models of disease permit careful control of experimental conditions, these studies do not duplicate clinical conditions. Thus there are limitations in the application of this study to clinical practice.[141] First, the level of bacteremia produced in the rats exceeded the transient, low-grade bacteremia that often occurs clinically. Also, these animals most likely had hemodynamic and metabolic changes characteristic of early sepsis. Second, although *E. coli* is a common cause of bacteremia in surgical and obstetric patients, it is an uncommon cause of meningitis. Third, the relative size of the dural tear produced by the 26-gauge needle used in this study is greater in rats compared with that in humans. Fourth, the cisternal site of dural puncture is not used clinically. Fifth, spinal and epidural anesthesia involves the injection of local anesthetics, and these drugs appear to be bacteriostatic.[145] Finally, the investigators knew the identity of the organism (e.g., *E. coli*) and also knew that it was susceptible to gentamicin. In summary, this study suggests that high-grade bacteremia may increase the risk of meningitis after dural puncture. However, antibiotic therapy before dural puncture appears to reduce if not eliminate this risk.

Recommendations

The preponderance of evidence suggests that the anesthesia provider may safely give either spinal or epidural anesthesia to healthy patients at risk for bacteremia. The anesthesia provider need not avoid administration of neuraxial anesthesia in patients at risk for transient, low-grade bacteremia after the administration of anesthesia. Moreover, appropriate antibiotic therapy may lessen the risk of meningitis or epidural abscess in patients with established infection. In my practice, I administer neuraxial anesthesia to patients with evidence of systemic infection, provided that appropriate antibiotic therapy has begun. Thus it is often appropriate for the anesthesia provider to request the institution of antibiotic therapy before administration of anesthesia. Finally, although the choice of anesthesia must be individualized, it seems prudent to avoid neuraxial anesthesia in untreated patients with overt clinical signs of sepsis.

Chestnut,[115] in a review of this subject, concluded as follows:

We do not give regional anesthesia in the absence of other relevant information. Rather, we provide care for febrile patients who require anesthesia for labor, delivery, or emergency surgery. When one considers the risks of infection with regional anesthesia, one should ask: What are the alternatives? What are the consequences of withholding regional anesthesia in a febrile patient? For example, what is the greater risk in a febrile parturient: meningitis or epidural abscess after spinal or epidural anesthesia, or failed intubation and aspiration during general anesthesia?

Finally, both physicians and patients should recognize that most cases of meningitis and epidural abscess occur spontaneously. Eng and Seligman[111] stated, "Even if an appropriate temporal sequence ... is documented ... one cannot differentiate spontaneous meningitis from lumbar puncture-induced meningitis in the individual patient."

GENITAL HERPES INFECTION

Herpes simplex virus type 2 (HSV-2) causes a locally recurring disease that is characterized by asymptomatic periods interrupted by episodes of viral reactivation from sites in the sensory ganglia.[6] Genital herpes infection typically manifests as painful vesicular or papular lesions on the skin or mucous membranes of the genital tract, including the labia, vulva, perineum, cervix, and urethra. Primary maternal HSV-2 infection is associated with transient viremia.[146] Patients with primary infection often have systemic symptoms, including fever, headache, and lymphadenopathy. Hepatitis, aseptic meningitis, encephalitis, and cauda equina syndrome are uncommon complications of primary genital herpes infection. During recurrent (i.e., secondary) infection, maternal antibodies prevent the recurrence of viremia. Thus systemic symptoms are less severe—or do not occur at all—during episodes of recurrent infection. However, recurrent infection may result in severe symptoms localized to the site of the lesions on the external genitalia. Unfortunately, asymptomatic shedding of the virus also may occur in the genital tract.

Interaction with Pregnancy

During the first 20 weeks of pregnancy, primary genital herpes infection may be associated with an increase in the frequency of pregnancy loss and congenital malformations,[147] although more recent cohort studies have disputed the risk of fetal death.[148] However, the major obstetric concern is the potential for transmission of the virus to the infant at the time of birth. The infant may become infected in one of two ways. First, infection can occur as the fetus comes in direct contact with the virus during vaginal delivery. Second, intrauterine infection can occur by ascent of the organism after rupture of membranes. Neonatal HSV infection is a life-threatening infection with the potential for permanent CNS sequelae.[6,146,147] The severity of the neonatal infection may be modified by the early institution of antiviral therapy.[149] Retrospective studies suggest that the risk of neonatal HSV infection associated with a primary maternal infection is much greater than that associated with recurrent maternal infection or asymptomatic shedding of the virus.[147,150-152] Most likely there is a greater risk that the infant will be exposed to the virus during episodes of primary maternal infection.

Obstetric Management

A large epidemiologic study of 58,362 women published in 2003 provided the first direct evidence that cesarean delivery dramatically reduces the overall rate of HSV transmission to the neonate when results of HSV cultures of the cervix and external genitalia from specimens taken at the time of labor are positive. Among women with genital HSV detected at delivery, neonatal herpes occurred in 1.2% of infants delivered by cesarean delivery compared with 7.7% of infants delivered vaginally (odds ratio = 0.14).[153] Other risk factors for neonatal HSV infection were first-episode infection and use of invasive fetal monitoring.[153]

The ACOG[151] has reviewed the obstetric management of parturients with HSV infections and has concluded as follows:

Cesarean delivery is indicated in women with active genital lesions or prodromal symptoms, such as vulvar pain or burning at delivery, because these symptoms may indicate an impending outbreak. The incidence of neonatal disease is low when there is recurrent maternal disease, but cesarean delivery is recommended because of the potentially serious nature of the disease .... In patients with active HSV infection and ruptured membranes at or near term, a cesarean delivery should be performed as soon as the necessary personnel and equipment can be readied. There is no evidence that there is a duration of rupture of membranes beyond which the fetus does not benefit from cesarean delivery. At any time after rupture of membranes, cesarean delivery is recommended.[151]

Of interest, the mothers of most infants infected with HSV have no history of HSV infection and no obvious lesions at the time of delivery.[151,152] Previously, it was thought that antenatal viral cultures could predict asymptomatic viral shedding at the time of delivery and reduce the incidence of neonatal infection. Unfortunately, there is little correlation between antepartum HSV culture results and viral shedding at the time of delivery, even in women with a history of previous HSV infection.[152] However, recent studies support the value of prophylactic acyclovir treatment of the mother with a history of HSV infection in reducing the presence of lesions at the onset of labor.[154-156]

Apparently, asymptomatic shedding is both infrequent and transient, and antenatal cultures may not reflect the situation at the time of delivery. Current clinical recommendations suggest that the route of delivery should be guided by a careful pelvic examination after the onset of labor rather than by antepartum viral cultures. The ACOG has stated that "cesarean delivery is not recommended for women with a history of HSV infection but no active genital disease during labor."[151]

Anesthetic Management

There are at least four published retrospective studies of the use of neuraxial anesthesia in patients with genital herpes infection. These studies reported no serious neurologic sequelae related to the use of neuraxial anesthesia.[140,157-159] However, most of the patients in these studies had recurrent (secondary) infection. Two studies were limited to patients with recurrent infection,[140,158] and a third study did not indicate whether the patients had primary or recurrent infection.[157]

Bader et al.,[159] in reporting outcome for 169 women with genital herpes infection who underwent cesarean delivery, stated, "None of the 164 patients with secondary infections had septic or neurologic complications related to the type of anesthetic administered. Therefore, it is our practice to use either spinal or epidural anesthesia when possible for cesarean delivery in these patients." Only five of the 169 women in this study had primary infections, and three of those women received spinal anesthesia. Of those three women, one had transient, postoperative weakness of the left leg. The investigators also stated, "None of the cases of primary infection had associated systemic symptoms; it is therefore possible that some of these cases were actually misdiagnosed recurrent infections. The safety of regional anesthesia in patients with primary HSV infection remains unclear."[159]

Viremia may accompany primary episodes of genital herpes infection. However, viremia rarely complicates recurrent episodes of genital herpes infection. It is unlikely that a spinal or epidural needle could introduce virus into the CNS in patients with recurrent genital herpes infection. Thus there is consensus that it is safe to give spinal or epidural anesthesia in women with recurrent genital herpes infection and no systemic symptoms. There are insufficient data to allow a definitive recommendation about the safety of neuraxial anesthesia in patients with primary infection who may be viremic. When the anesthesia provider confronts a patient with primary infection, the theoretical risk of CNS infection should be weighed against the risks of alternative methods of analgesia and anesthesia.

Finally, several studies have suggested that spinal or epidural administration of morphine increases the incidence of recurrence of oral HSV infection (e.g., herpes simplex virus type 1 [HSV-1]) in obstetric patients. This phenomenon was confirmed in randomized prospective trials for both epidural[160] and intrathecal[161] morphine. The exact etiology is unknown, but some investigators have speculated that pruritus and scratching play a role. Boyle[162] concluded that facial pruritus is a marker of the migration of morphine to the trigeminal nucleus but not the cause of HSV-1 recrudescence and suggested that immunologic modulation by the opioid within this ganglion is the primary cause of the viral reactivation. To my knowledge, there are no reports suggesting that epidural or intrathecal administration of opioids increases the risk of recurrent *genital* herpes infection.

KEY POINTS

- Fever may be produced by endogenous pyrogens released from immune effector cells in response to infection.
- Fetal temperature typically is slightly higher than maternal temperature.
- Modest maternal fever does not seem to adversely affect the fetus, but maternal infection and other inflammatory states may cause fetal neurologic injury.
- Pyelonephritis and chorioamnionitis are the antepartum infections most likely to result in maternal and perinatal morbidity and mortality. Septic shock is an uncommon but devastating complication of maternal infection that demands aggressive hemodynamic support, broad-spectrum antibiotic therapy, and, in some cases, surgical intervention.
- Epidural analgesia increases the risk of maternal fever during labor. The mechanism is unclear, but evidence now suggests that it is related to inflammation. It is unknown whether epidural analgesia–related fever puts the fetus at risk for neurologic injury. However, no study has directly linked maternal fever associated with epidural analgesia to adverse effects on the fetus. Epidural analgesia-related fever may prompt the neonatologist to evaluate the neonate for possible sepsis.
- The anesthesia provider may safely administer epidural or spinal anesthesia to patients at risk for transient bacteremia.
- The anesthesia provider may safely administer epidural or spinal anesthesia to patients with established infection, provided that there is no evidence of frank sepsis. However, it seems prudent to begin antibiotic therapy before the administration of neuraxial anesthesia.
- Recurrent genital herpes infection does not contraindicate the administration of neuraxial anesthesia.

REFERENCES

1. Wunderlich C. Das Verhalten der Eiaenwarme in Krankenheiten Germany, Ott Wigard, Leipzig, 1868.
2. Mackowiak PA, Wasserman SS, Levine MM. A critical appraisal of 98.6 degrees F, the upper limit of the normal body temperature, and other legacies of Carl Reinhold August Wunderlich. JAMA 1992; 268:1578-80.
3. Beutler B, Beutler AM. The pathogenesis of fever. In Wyngaarden JB, Smith LH, Bennett JC, editors. Textbook of Medicine. 19th edition. Philadelphia, WB Saunders, 1992:1568-71.
4. Novy MJ, Liggins GC. Role of prostaglandins, prostacyclin, and thromboxanes in the physiologic control of the uterus and in parturition. Semin Perinatol 1980; 4:45-66.

5. Walker DW, Wood C. Temperature relationship of the mother and fetus during labor. Am J Obstet Gynecol 1970; 107:83-7.
6. Gibbs RS, Sweet RL. Maternal and fetal infections. In Creasy RK, Resnik R, editors. Maternal-Fetal Medicine: Principles and Practice. 4th edition. Philadelphia, WB Saunders, 1989:656-725.
7. Morishima HO, Glaser B, Niemann WH, James LS. Increased uterine activity and fetal deterioration during maternal hyperthermia. Am J Obstet Gynecol 1975; 121:531-8.
8. Cefalo RC, Hellegers AE. The effects of maternal hyperthermia on maternal and fetal cardiovascular and respiratory function. Am J Obstet Gynecol 1978; 131:687-94.
9. Harris WH, Pittman QJ, Veale WL, et al. Cardiovascular effects of fever in the ewe and fetal lamb. Am J Obstet Gynecol 1977; 128:262-5.
10. Macaulay JH, Bond K, Steer PJ. Epidural analgesia in labor and fetal hyperthermia. Obstet Gynecol 1992; 80:665-9.
11. Lieberman E, Lang J, Richardson DK, et al. Intrapartum maternal fever and neonatal outcome. Pediatrics 2000; 105:8-13.
12. Lieberman E, Eichenwald E, Mathur G, et al. Intrapartum fever and unexplained seizures in term infants. Pediatrics 2000; 106:983-8.
13. Perlman JM. Maternal fever and neonatal depression: Preliminary observations. Clin Pediatr 1999; 38:287-91.
14. Grether JK, Nelson KB. Maternal infection and cerebral palsy in infants of normal birth weight. JAMA 1997; 278:207-11.
15. Wu YW, Colford JM Jr. Chorioamnionitis as a risk factor for cerebral palsy: A meta-analysis. JAMA 2000; 284:1417-24.
16. Wu YW, Escobar GJ, Grether JK, et al. Chorioamnionitis and cerebral palsy in term and near-term infants. JAMA 2003; 290:2677-84.
17. Impey L, Greenwood C, MacQuillan K, et al. Fever in labour and neonatal encephalopathy: A prospective cohort study. Br J Obstet Gynaecol 2001; 108:594-7.
18. Dammann O, Drescher J, Veelken N. Maternal fever at birth and non-verbal intelligence at age 9 years in preterm infants. Dev Med Child Neurol 2003; 45:148-51.
19. Yoon BH, Romero R, Park JS, et al. Fetal exposure to an intra-amniotic inflammation and the development of cerebral palsy at the age of three years. Am J Obstet Gynecol 2000; 182:675-81.
20. Rodts-Palenik S, Wyatt-Ashmead J, Pang Y, et al. Maternal infection-induced white matter injury is reduced by treatment with interleukin-10. Am J Obstet Gynecol 2004; 191:1387-92.
21. Shipp TD, Zelop C, Cohen A, et al. Post-cesarean delivery fever and uterine rupture in a subsequent trial of labor. Obstet Gynecol 2003; 101:136-9.
22. Lieberman E, Cohen A, Lang J, et al. Maternal intrapartum temperature elevation as a risk factor for cesarean delivery and assisted vaginal delivery. Am J Public Health 1999; 89:506-10.
23. Gibbs RS, Castillo MS, Rodgers PJ. Management of acute chorioamnionitis. Am J Obstet Gynecol 1980; 136:709-13.
24. Duff P, Sanders R, Gibbs RS. The course of labor in term patients with chorioamnionitis. Am J Obstet Gynecol 1983; 147:391-5.
25. Yoder PR, Gibbs RS, Blanco JD, et al. A prospective, controlled study of maternal and perinatal outcome after intra-amniotic infection at term. Am J Obstet Gynecol 1983; 145:695-701.
26. Blanco JD, Gibbs RS, Castaneda YS. Bacteremia in obstetrics: Clinical course. Obstet Gynecol 1981; 58:621-5.
27. Satin AJ, Maberry MC, Leveno KJ, et al. Chorioamnionitis: A harbinger of dystocia. Obstet Gynecol 1992; 79:913-15.
28. Goodman EJ, DeHorta E, Taguiam JM. Safety of spinal and epidural anesthesia in parturients with chorioamnionitis. Reg Anesth 1996; 21:436-41.
29. Qureshi F, Jacques SM, Bendon RW, et al. Candida funisitis: A clinicopathologic study of 32 cases. Pediatr Dev Pathol 1998; 1:118-24.
30. Gerber S, Vial Y, Hohlfeld P, Witkin SS. Detection of *Ureaplasma urealyticum* in second-trimester amniotic fluid by polymerase chain reaction correlates with subsequent preterm labor and delivery. J Infect Dis 2003; 187:518-21.
31. Romero R, Espinoza J, Goncalves LF, et al. The role of inflammation and infection in preterm birth. Semin Reprod Med 2007; 25:21-39.
32. Nath CA, Ananth CV, Smulian JC, et al. Histologic evidence of inflammation and risk of placental abruption. Am J Obstet Gynecol 2007; 197:319.e311-6.
33. Tran TS, Jamulitrat S, Chongsuvivatwong V, Geater A. Risk factors for postcesarean surgical site infection. Obstet Gynecol 2000; 95:367-71.
34. Rouse DJ, Leindecker S, Landon M, et al. The MFMU Cesarean Registry: Uterine atony after primary cesarean delivery. Am J Obstet Gynecol 2005; 193:1056-60.
35. Mark SP, Croughan-Minihane MS, Kilpatrick SJ. Chorioamnionitis and uterine function. Obstet Gynecol 2000; 95:909-12.
36. Gaudet LM, Smith GN. Cerebral palsy and chorioamnionitis: The inflammatory cytokine link. Obstet Gynecol Surv 2001; 56:433-6.
37. Wu YW. Systematic review of chorioamnionitis and cerebral palsy. Ment Retard Dev Disabil Res Rev 2002; 8:25-9.
38. Lee J, Croen LA, Backstrand KH, et al. Maternal and infant characteristics associated with perinatal arterial stroke in the infant. JAMA 2005; 293:723-9.
39. Resch B, Vollaard E, Maurer U, et al. Risk factors and determinants of neurodevelopmental outcome in cystic periventricular leucomalacia. Eur J Pediatr 2000; 159:663-70.
40. Shimoya K, Taniguchi T, Matsuzaki N, et al. Chorioamnionitis decreased incidence of respiratory distress syndrome by elevating fetal interleukin-6 serum concentration. Hum Reprod 2000; 15:2234-40.
41. Schmidt B, Cao L, Mackensen-Haen S, et al. Chorioamnionitis and inflammation of the fetal lung. Am J Obstet Gynecol 2001; 185:173-7.
42. Van Marter LJ, Dammann O, Allred EN, et al. Chorioamnionitis, mechanical ventilation, and postnatal sepsis as modulators of chronic lung disease in preterm infants. J Pediatr 2002; 140:171-6.
43. Mwanyumba F, Gaillard P, Inion I, et al. Placental inflammation and perinatal transmission of HIV-1. J Acquir Immune Defic Syndr 2002; 29:262-9.
44. Mead PB. When to treat intra-amniotic infection. Obstet Gynecol 1988; 72:935-6.
45. Gibbs RS, Dinsmoor MJ, Newton ER, Ramamurthy RS. A randomized trial of intrapartum versus immediate postpartum treatment of women with intra-amniotic infection. Obstet Gynecol 1988; 72:823-8.
46. Gilstrap LC 3rd, Leveno KJ, Cox SM, et al. Intrapartum treatment of acute chorioamnionitis: Impact on neonatal sepsis. Am J Obstet Gynecol 1988; 159:579-83.
47. Kass EH. Bacteriuria and pyelonephritis of pregnancy. Arch Intern Med 1960; 205:194-205.
48. Gilstrap LC 3rd, Cunningham FG, Whalley PJ. Acute pyelonephritis in pregnancy: An anterospective study. Obstet Gynecol 1981; 57:409-13.
49. Wing DA. Pyelonephritis in pregnancy: Treatment options for optimal outcomes. Drugs 2001; 61:2087-96.
50. Schaeffer AJ. Experimental gestational pyelonephritis induces preterm births and low birth weights in C3H/HeJ mice. J Urol 2000; 164:260-1.
51. Cunningham FG, Lucas MJ, Hankins GD. Pulmonary injury complicating antepartum pyelonephritis. Am J Obstet Gynecol 1987; 156: 797-807.
52. Towers CV, Kaminskas CM, Garite TJ, et al. Pulmonary injury associated with antepartum pyelonephritis: Can patients at risk be identified? Am J Obstet Gynecol 1991; 164:974-8.
53. Twickler DM, Lucas MJ, Bowe L, et al. Ultrasonographic evaluation of central and end-organ hemodynamics in antepartum pyelonephritis. Am J Obstet Gynecol 1994; 170:814-18.
54. Smaill F, Vazquez JC. Antibiotics for asymptomatic bacteriuria in pregnancy. Cochrane Database Syst Rev 2007; (2):CD000490.
55. Korst LM, Reyes C, Fridman M, et al. Gestational pyelonephritis as an indicator of the quality of ambulatory maternal health care services. Obstet Gynecol 2006; 107:632-40.
56. Leontic EA. Respiratory disease in pregnancy. Med Clin North Am 1977; 61:111-28.
57. Benedetti TJ, Valle R, Ledger WJ. Antepartum pneumonia in pregnancy. Am J Obstet Gynecol 1982; 144:413-17.
58. Landsberger EJ, Hager WD, Grossman JH 3rd. Successful management of varicella pneumonia complicating pregnancy: A report of three cases. J Reprod Med 1986; 31:311-14.
59. Ahmad H, Mehta NJ, Manikal VM, et al. *Pneumocystis carinii* pneumonia in pregnancy. Chest 2001; 120:666-71.

60. Goodnight WH, Soper DE. Pneumonia in pregnancy. Crit Care Med 2005; 33:S390-7.
61. Smaill F, Hofmeyr GJ. Antibiotic prophylaxis for cesarean section. Cochrane Database Syst Rev 2002; (3):CD000933.
62. Chongsomchai C, Lumbiganon P, Laopaiboon M. Prophylactic antibiotics for manual removal of retained placenta in vaginal birth. Cochrane Database Syst Rev 2006; (2):CD004904.
63. Liabsuetrakul T, Choobun T, Peeyananjarassri K, Islam M. Antibiotic prophylaxis for operative vaginal delivery. Cochrane Database Syst Rev 2004; (3):CD004455.
64. Martin SR, Foley MR. Intensive care in obstetrics: An evidence-based review. Am J Obstet Gynecol 2006; 195:673-89.
65. American College of Obstetricians and Gynecologists. Septic shock. ACOG Technical Bulletin No. 204. Washington, DC, April 1995.
66. Ayadi S, Carbillon L, Varlet C, et al. Fatal sepsis due to *Escherichia coli* after second-trimester amniocentesis. Fetal Diagn Ther 1998; 13:98-9.
67. Rode ME, Morgan MA, Ruchelli E, Forouzan I. Candida chorioamnionitis after serial therapeutic amniocenteses: A possible association. J Perinatol 2000; 20:335-7.
68. Winer N, David A, Leconte P, et al. Amniocentesis and amnioinfusion during pregnancy: Report of four complicated cases. Eur J Obstet Gynecol Reprod Biol 2001; 100:108-11.
69. Hamanishi J, Itoh H, Sagawa N, et al. A case of successful management of maternal septic shock with multiple organ failure following amniocentesis at midgestation. J Obstet Gynaecol Res 2002; 28:258-61.
70. Fischer M, Bhatnagar J, Guarner J, et al. Fatal toxic shock syndrome associated with *Clostridium sordellii* after medical abortion. N Engl J Med 2005; 353:2352-60.
71. Slabbert DR, Kruger TF, Siebert TI, Stead P. Endotoxic shock after gamete intrafallopian transfer. Fertil Steril 2005; 83:1041.
72. Beller FK, Schmidt EH, Holzgreve W, Hauss J. Septicemia during pregnancy: A study in different species of experimental animals. Am J Obstet Gynecol 1985; 151:967-75.
73. Ledger WJ, Norman M, Gee C, Lewis W. Bacteremia on an obstetric-gynecologic service. Am J Obstet Gynecol 1975; 121:205-12.
74. Lee W, Clark SL, Cotton DB, et al. Septic shock during pregnancy. Am J Obstet Gynecol 1988; 159:410-16.
75. Mabie WC, Barton JR, Sibai B. Septic shock in pregnancy. Obstet Gynecol 1997; 90:553-61.
76. Rivers E, Nguyen B, Havstad S, et al. Early goal-directed therapy in the treatment of severe sepsis and septic shock. N Engl J Med 2001; 345: 1368-77.
77. Jones AE, Focht A, Horton JM, Kline JA. Prospective external validation of the clinical effectiveness of an emergency department-based early goal-directed therapy protocol for severe sepsis and septic shock. Chest 2007; 132:425-32.
78. van den Berghe G, Wouters P, Weekers F, et al. Intensive insulin therapy in the critically ill patients. N Engl J Med 2001; 345:1359-67.
79. Annane D, Sebille V, Charpentier C, et al. Effect of treatment with low doses of hydrocortisone and fludrocortisone on mortality in patients with septic shock. JAMA 2002; 288:862-71.
80. Bernard GR, Vincent JL, Laterre PF, et al. Efficacy and safety of recombinant human activated protein C for severe sepsis. N Engl J Med 2001; 344:699-709.
81. Matsukawa T, Sessler DI, Christensen R, et al. Heat flow and distribution during epidural anesthesia. Anesthesiology 1995; 83:961-7.
82. Fusi L, Steer PJ, Maresh MJ, Beard RW. Maternal pyrexia associated with the use of epidural analgesia in labour. Lancet 1989; 1(8649): 1250-2.
83. Camann WR, Hortvet LA, Hughes N, et al. Maternal temperature regulation during extradural analgesia for labour. Br J Anaesth 1991; 67:565-8.
84. Yancey MK, Zhang J, Schwarz J, et al. Labor epidural analgesia and intrapartum maternal hyperthermia. Obstet Gynecol 2001; 98:763-70.
85. Vinson DC, Thomas R, Kiser T. Association between epidural analgesia during labor and fever. J Fam Pract 1993; 36:617-22.
86. Ploeckinger B, Ulm MR, Chalubinski K, Gruber W. Epidural anaesthesia in labour: Influence on surgical delivery rates, intrapartum fever and blood loss. Gynecol Obstet Invest 1995; 39:24-7.
87. Lieberman E, Lang JM, Frigoletto F Jr, et al. Epidural analgesia, intrapartum fever, and neonatal sepsis evaluation. Pediatrics 1997; 99:415-19.
88. Mayer DC, Chescheir NC, Spielman FJ. Increased intrapartum antibiotic administration associated with epidural analgesia in labor. Am J Perinatol 1997; 14:83-6.
89. Herbst A, Wolner-Hanssen P, Ingemarsson I. Risk factors for fever in labor. Obstet Gynecol 1995; 86:790-4.
90. Philip J, Alexander JM, Sharma SK, et al. Epidural analgesia during labor and maternal fever. Anesthesiology 1999; 90:1271-5.
91. Vallejo MC, Kaul B, Adler LJ, et al. Chorioamnionitis, not epidural analgesia, is associated with maternal fever during labour. Can J Anaesth 2001; 48:1122-6.
92. Goetzl L, Rivers J, Zighelboim I, et al. Intrapartum epidural analgesia and maternal temperature regulation. Obstet Gynecol 2007; 109:687-90.
93. Gelfand T, Palanisamy A, Tsen LC, Segal S. Warming in parturients with epidurals is an averaging artifact. Anesthesiology 2007; 106:A5.
94. Goodlin RC, Chapin JW. Determinants of maternal temperature during labor. Am J Obstet Gynecol 1982; 143:97-103.
95. Glosten B, Savage M, Rooke GA, Brengelmann GL. Epidural anesthesia and the thermoregulatory responses to hyperthermia—preliminary observations in volunteer subjects. Acta Anaesthesiol Scand 1998; 42:442-6.
96. Hagerdal M, Morgan CW, Sumner AE, Gutsche BB. Minute ventilation and oxygen consumption during labor with epidural analgesia. Anesthesiology 1983; 59:425-7.
97. Gleeson NC, Nolan KM, Ford MR. Temperature, labour, and epidural analgesia. Lancet 1989; 2(8667):861-2.
98. Panzer O, Ghazanfari N, Sessler DI, et al. Shivering and shivering-like tremor during labor with and without epidural analgesia. Anesthesiology 1999; 90:1609-16.
99. Negishi C, Lenhardt R, Ozaki M, et al. Opioids inhibit febrile responses in humans, whereas epidural analgesia does not: An explanation for hyperthermia during epidural analgesia. Anesthesiology 2001; 94:218-22.
100. Gross JB, Cohen AP, Lang JM, et al. Differences in systemic opioid use do not explain increased fever incidence in parturients receiving epidural analgesia. Anesthesiology 2002; 97:157-61.
101. Dolak JA, Brown RE. Epidural analgesia and neonatal fever. Pediatrics 1998; 101:492.
102. Dashe JS, Rogers BB, McIntire DD, Leveno KJ. Epidural analgesia and intrapartum fever: Placental findings. Obstet Gynecol 1999; 93:341-4.
103. Goetzl L, Evans T, Rivers J, et al. Elevated maternal and fetal serum interleukin-6 levels are associated with epidural fever. Am J Obstet Gynecol 2002; 187:834-8.
104. Goetzl L, Zighelboim I, Badell M, et al. Maternal corticosteroids to prevent intrauterine exposure to hyperthermia and inflammation: A randomized, double-blind, placebo-controlled trial. Am J Obstet Gynecol 2006; 195:1031-7.
105. Leighton BL, Halpern SH. The effects of epidural analgesia on labor, maternal, and neonatal outcomes: A systematic review. Am J Obstet Gynecol 2002; 186:S69-77.
106. Tarshis J, Camann WR, Datta S. Epidural analgesia and neonatal fever. Pediatrics 1998; 101:490-1.
107. Goetzl L, Cohen A, Frigoletto F Jr, et al. Maternal epidural use and neonatal sepsis evaluation in afebrile mothers. Pediatrics 2001; 108:1099-102.
108. Kaul B, Vallejo M, Ramanathan S, Mandell G. Epidural labor analgesia and neonatal sepsis evaluation rate: A quality improvement study. Anesth Analg 2001; 93:986-90.
109. Wegefroth P, Lastham JR. Lumbar puncture as a factor in the causation of meningitis. Am J Med Sci 1919; 158:183-5.
110. Pray L. Lumbar puncture as a factor in the pathogenesis of meningitis. Am J Dis Child 1941; 295:62-8.
111. Eng RH, Seligman SJ. Lumbar puncture-induced meningitis. JAMA 1981; 245:1456-9.
112. Teele DW, Dashefsky B, Rakusan T, Klein JO. Meningitis after lumbar puncture in children with bacteremia. N Engl J Med 1981; 305:1079-81.

113. Smith KM, Deddish RB, Ogata ES. Meningitis associated with serial lumbar punctures and post-hemorrhagic hydrocephalus. J Pediatr 1986; 109:1057-60.
114. Shapiro ED, Aaron NH, Wald ER, Chiponis D. Risk factors for development of bacterial meningitis among children with occult bacteremia. J Pediatr 1986; 109:15-19.
115. Chestnut DH. Spinal anesthesia in the febrile patient. Anesthesiology 1992; 76:667-9.
116. Kost-Byerly S, Tobin JR, Greenberg RS, et al. Bacterial colonization and infection rate of continuous epidural catheters in children. Anesth Analg 1998; 86:712-16.
117. Barrie H. Meningitis following spinal anesthesia. Lancet 1941; 1: 242-3.
118. Lee JJ, Parry H. Bacterial meningitis following spinal anaesthesia for caesarean section. Br J Anaesth 1991; 66:383-6.
119. Kilpatrick ME, Girgis NI. Meningitis—a complication of spinal anesthesia. Anesth Analg 1983; 62:513-15.
120. Roberts SP, Petts HV. Meningitis after obstetric spinal anaesthesia. Anaesthesia 1990; 45:376-7.
121. Reynolds F. Infection as a complication of neuraxial blockade. Int J Obstet Anesth 2005; 14:183-8.
122. Videira RL, Ruiz-Neto PP, Brandao Neto M. Post spinal meningitis and asepsis. Acta Anaesthesiol Scand 2002; 46:639-46.
123. Cohen S, Hunter CW, Sakr A, Hijazi RH. Meningitis following intrathecal catheter placement after accidental dural puncture. Int J Obstet Anesth 2006; 15:172.
124. Baer ET. Post-dural puncture bacterial meningitis. Anesthesiology 2006; 105:381-93.
125. Rubin L, Sprecher H, Kabaha A, et al. Meningitis following spinal anesthesia: 6 cases in 5 years. Infect Control Hosp Epidemiol 2007; 28:1187-90.
126. Trautmann M, Lepper PM, Schmitz FJ. Three cases of bacterial meningitis after spinal and epidural anesthesia. Eur J Clin Microbiol Infect Dis 2002; 21:43-5.
127. Ready LB, Helfer D. Bacterial meningitis in parturients after epidural anesthesia. Anesthesiology 1989; 71:988-90.
128. Davis L, Hargreaves C, Robinson PN. Postpartum meningitis. Anaesthesia 1993; 48:788-9.
129. Harding SA, Collis RE, Morgan BM. Meningitis after combined spinal-extradural anaesthesia in obstetrics. Br J Anaesth 1994; 73:545-7.
130. Cascio M, Heath G. Meningitis following a combined spinal-epidural technique in a labouring term parturient. Can J Anaesth 1996; 43: 399-402.
131. Bouhemad B, Dounas M, Mercier FJ, Benhamou D. Bacterial meningitis following combined spinal-epidural analgesia for labour. Anaesthesia 1998; 53:292-5.
132. Rawal N, Holmstrom B, Crowhurst JA, Van Zundert A. The combined spinal-epidural technique. Anesthesiol Clin North America 2000; 18:267-95.
133. Dripps RD, Vandam LD. Long-term follow-up of patients who received 10,098 spinal anesthetics. JAMA 1954; 156:1486-91.
134. Phillips OC, Ebner H, Nelson AT, Black MH. Neurologic complications following spinal anesthesia with lidocaine: A prospective review of 10,440 cases. Anesthesiology 1969; 30:284-9.
135. Hellmann K. Epidural anaesthesia in obstetrics: A second look at 26,127 cases. Can Anaesth Soc J 1965; 12:398-404.
136. Crawford JS. Some maternal complications of epidural analgesia for labour. Anaesthesia 1985; 40:1219-25.
137. Scott DB, Hibbard BM. Serious non-fatal complications associated with extradural block in obstetric practice. Br J Anaesth 1990; 64:537-41.
138. Paech MJ, Godkin R, Webster GS. Complications of obstetric epidural analgesia and anaesthesia: A prospective analysis of 10,995 cases. Int J Obstet Anesth 1998; 7:5-11.
139. Bader AM, Gilbertson L, Kirz L, Datta S. Regional anesthesia in women with chorioamnionitis. Reg Anesth 1992; 17:84-6.
140. Ramanathan S, Sheth R, Turndorf H. Anesthesia for cesarean section in patients with genital herpes infections: A retrospective study. Anesthesiology 1986; 64:807-9.
141. Carp H, Bailey S. The association between meningitis and dural puncture in bacteremic rats. Anesthesiology 1992; 76:739-42.
142. Weed LH, Wegeforth P, Ayer JB, Felton LD. The production of meningitis by release of cerebrospinal fluid during an experimental septicemia: Preliminary note. JAMA 1919; 72:190-3.
143. Idzumi G. Experimental pneumococcus meningitis in rabbits and dogs. J Infect Dis 1920; 26:373-87.
144. Petersdorf RG, Swarner DR, Garcia M. Studies on the pathogenesis of meningitis. II. Development of meningitis during pneumococcal bacteremia. J Clin Invest 1962; 41:320-7.
145. James FM, George RH, Naiem H, White GJ. Bacteriologic aspects of epidural analgesia. Anesth Analg 1976; 55:187-90.
146. Corey L, Adams HG, Brown ZA, Holmes KK. Genital herpes simplex virus infections: Clinical manifestations, course, and complications. Ann Intern Med 1983; 98:958-72.
147. Brown ZA, Vontver LA, Benedetti J, et al. Effects on infants of a first episode of genital herpes during pregnancy. N Engl J Med 1987; 317:1246-51.
148. Eskild A, Jeansson S, Stray-Pedersen B, Jenum PA. Herpes simplex virus type-2 infection in pregnancy: No risk of fetal death: Results from a nested case-control study within 35,940 women. Br J Obstet Gynaecol 2002; 109:1030-5.
149. Whitley RJ, Corey L, Arvin A, et al. Changing presentation of herpes simplex virus infection in neonates. J Infect Dis 1988; 158:109-16.
150. Prober CG, Sullender WM, Yasukawa LL, et al. Low risk of herpes simplex virus infections in neonates exposed to the virus at the time of vaginal delivery to mothers with recurrent genital herpes simplex virus infections. N Engl J Med 1987; 316:240-4.
151. American College of Obstetricians and Gynecologists. Management of herpes in pregnancy. ACOG Practice Bulletin No. 82. Washington, DC, June 2007.
152. Arvin AM, Hensleigh PA, Prober CG, et al. Failure of antepartum maternal cultures to predict the infant's risk of exposure to herpes simplex virus at delivery. N Engl J Med 1986; 315:796-800.
153. Brown ZA, Wald A, Morrow RA, et al. Effect of serologic status and cesarean delivery on transmission rates of herpes simplex virus from mother to infant. JAMA 2003; 289:203-9.
154. Scott LL, Hollier LM, McIntire D, et al. Acyclovir suppression to prevent recurrent genital herpes at delivery. Infect Dis Obstet Gynecol 2002; 10:71-7.
155. Watts DH, Brown ZA, Money D, et al. A double-blind, randomized, placebo-controlled trial of acyclovir in late pregnancy for the reduction of herpes simplex virus shedding and cesarean delivery. Am J Obstet Gynecol 2003; 188:836-43.
156. Sheffield JS, Hill JB, Hollier LM, et al. Valacyclovir prophylaxis to prevent recurrent herpes at delivery: A randomized clinical trial. Obstet Gynecol 2006; 108:141-7.
157. Ravindran RS, Gupta CD, Stoops CA. Epidural analgesia in the presence of herpes simplex virus (type 2) infection. Anesth Analg 1982; 61:714-15.
158. Crosby ET, Halpern SH, Rolbin SH. Epidural anaesthesia for caesarean section in patients with active recurrent genital herpes simplex infections: A retrospective review. Can J Anaesth 1989; 36:701-4.
159. Bader AM, Camann WR, Datta S. Anesthesia for cesarean delivery in patients with herpes simplex virus type-2 infections. Reg Anesth 1990; 15:261-3.
160. Boyle RK. Herpes simplex labialis after epidural or parenteral morphine: A randomized prospective trial in an Australian obstetric population. Anaesth Intensive Care 1995; 23:433-7.
161. Davies PW, Vallejo MC, Shannon KT, et al. Oral herpes simplex reactivation after intrathecal morphine: A prospective randomized trial in an obstetric population. Anesth Analg 2005; 100:1472-6.
162. Boyle RK. A review of anatomical and immunological links between epidural morphine and herpes simplex labialis in obstetric patients. Anaesth Intensive Care 1995; 23:425-32.

Chapter 37

Antepartum and Postpartum Hemorrhage

David C. Mayer, M.D.
Kathleen A. Smith, M.D.

Advances in obstetric care have resulted in progressive decreases in maternal morbidity and mortality. Unfortunately, some parturients sustain profound peripartum blood loss that overwhelms compensatory mechanisms. Severe hemorrhage occurs in 4.5 per 1000 deliveries in the United Kingdom.[1] In *Saving Mothers' Lives: The Seventh Report of the Confidential Enquiries into Maternal Deaths in the United Kingdom 2003-2005*, peripartum hemorrhage was the second leading cause of maternal death.[1] Fourteen women died from obstetric hemorrhage, which represents a rate of 0.66 per 100,000 deliveries and is similar to the rate for the previous triennium. Maternal mortality secondary to hemorrhage has not decreased in the last decade, and hemorrhage remains the most common reason that parturients require admission to an intensive care unit.[1,2] Several contemporary risk factors are noteworthy. Older maternal age at childbirth is associated with a higher incidence of complications from a variety of pregnancy-related disorders. Assisted reproductive technologies have led to a higher incidence of multiple gestation pregnancies. Lastly, cesarean delivery results in uterine scarring and increases the risk of placenta previa and accreta in subsequent pregnancies.[1]

Many adverse outcomes are preventable. The latest triennial report from the United Kingdom noted that 64% of direct maternal deaths were associated with substandard care.[1] Common problems include failure to recognize risk factors, failure to estimate the extent of blood loss accurately, and failure to initiate treatment quickly. Anesthesia providers have the required skills to manage these patients, but an understanding of maternal physiology and an appreciation for the rapidity with which parturients can become unstable are also important. It is essential that anesthesia providers become involved early in the care of bleeding pregnant women. Timely and effective communication among all obstetric caregivers is imperative.

MECHANISMS OF HEMOSTASIS

Following disruption of vascular integrity, mechanisms of hemostasis include (1) platelet aggregation and plug formation, (2) local vasoconstriction, (3) clot polymerization, and (4) fibrous tissue fortification of the clot. Platelet activation and aggregation occur rapidly after endothelial damage. Activated platelets release adenosine diphosphate (ADP), serotonin, catecholamines, and other factors that promote local vasoconstriction and hemostasis. These factors also activate the coagulation cascade. The end result of the cascade is conversion of fibrinogen to fibrin (see Chapter 43).

Contraction of the uterus represents the primary mechanism for controlling blood loss at parturition. Endogenous oxytocic substances effect myometrial contraction after delivery.

Anesthesia providers, obstetricians, and labor nurses frequently underestimate blood loss at delivery.[3] Heavy bleeding may increase the error of the estimate and lead to inadequate replacement of intravascular volume. Various schemes have been developed to help determine the severity of hypovolemia secondary to pathologic blood loss (Table 37-1). The clinical utility of these classification schemes is unclear, and fluid therapy is best guided by continual reassessment of maternal vital signs, urine output, hemoglobin levels, and acid-base balance.

TABLE 37-1 Clinical Staging of Hemorrhagic Shock by Volume of Blood Loss*

Hemorrhage Class	Acute Blood Loss (mL)	% Blood Lost	Physiologic Response
1	900	15	Asymptomatic
2	1200-1500	20-25	Tachycardia and tachypnea Narrowed pulse pressure Orthostatic hypotension Delayed hypothenar refilling
3	1800-2100	30-35	Worsening tachycardia and tachypnea Hypotension Cool extremities
4	>2400	40	Shock Oliguria/anuria

*Total blood volume = 6000 mL.

From Francois KE, Foley MR. Antepartum and postpartum hemorrhage. In Gabbe SG, Niebyl JR, Simpson JL, et al., editors. Obstetrics: Normal and Problem Pregnancies. 5th edition. Philadelphia, Churchill Livingstone, 2007:457.

ANTEPARTUM HEMORRHAGE

Antepartum vaginal bleeding may occur in as many as 20% of pregnant women; fortunately, only a fraction of these patients experience life-threatening hemorrhage. The majority of cases occur during the first trimester.[4] The causes of antepartum hemorrhage range from cervicitis to abnormalities in placentation, including placenta previa and placental abruption. The greatest threat of antepartum hemorrhage is not to the mother but to her fetus. Several decades ago, vaginal bleeding during the second and third trimesters was associated with perinatal mortality rates as high as 80%. More recent data suggest that antepartum bleeding secondary to placenta previa and placental abruption is responsible for perinatal mortality rates of 2.3% and 12%, respectively.[5,6]

Placenta Previa

Placenta previa is present when the placenta implants in advance of the fetal presenting part. Further classification can be made on the basis of the relationship between the cervical os and the placenta. A **total placenta previa** completely covers the cervical os. A **partial placenta previa** covers part but not all of the cervical os. A **marginal placenta previa** lies close to, but does not cover, the cervical os (Figure 37-1).

EPIDEMIOLOGY

The incidence of placenta previa is 3.6 per 1000 pregnancies.[7] The exact etiology is unclear, but prior uterine trauma is a common element in the associated conditions. The placenta may implant in the scarred area, which typically includes the lower uterine segment. Conditions associated with placenta previa include multiparity, advanced maternal age, previous cesarean delivery or other uterine surgery, and previous placenta previa. The presence of placenta previa increases the likelihood that the patient will require a peripartum hysterectomy.[8]

DIAGNOSIS

The classic sign of placenta previa is painless vaginal bleeding during the second or third trimester. The first episode of bleeding typically occurs preterm. (A minority of patients with placenta previa have no vaginal bleeding before term.) With the first episode of bleeding, contractions are usually absent, and the onset of bleeding is not related to any particular event. The lack of abdominal pain and abnormal uterine tone helps distinguish this event from placental abruption. The absence of these factors does not exclude abruption, however, and as many as 10% of patients with placenta previa have coexisting placental abruption.[9] The first episode of bleeding rarely causes shock and characteristically stops spontaneously. Fetal compromise or demise is uncommon with the first episode of hemorrhage.

OBSTETRIC MANAGEMENT

Ultrasonography is the mainstay for confirming the presence of placenta previa. Ultrasonographic examinations are accurate in confirming or excluding the diagnosis of placenta previa and also facilitate the assessment of gestational age.[10] Vaginal examinations are avoided until placenta previa is excluded by ultrasonographic examination. Advances in ultrasonography have made the **double setup examination** (i.e., vaginal examination with all personnel ready for immediate cesarean delivery) nearly obsolete in modern obstetric practice. Magnetic resonance imaging (MRI) is also useful for the diagnosis of placenta previa, but its use is not practical in most cases of antepartum hemorrhage.

Obstetric management is based on the severity of vaginal bleeding and the maturity of the fetus. Active labor, a mature fetus, or persistent bleeding should prompt abdominal delivery.

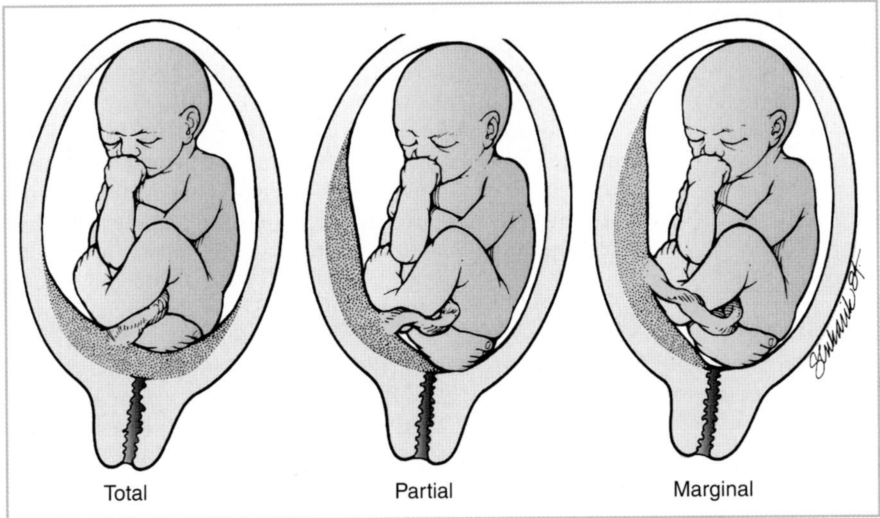

FIGURE 37-1 Three variations of placenta previa. (From Benedetti TJ. Obstetric hemorrhage. In Gabbe SG, Niebyl JR, Simpson JL, editors. Obstetrics: Normal and Problem Pregnancies, 4th edition. New York, Churchill Livingstone, 2001:516.)

The fetus is at risk from two distinct pathophysiologic processes, (1) progressive or sudden placental separation that causes uteroplacental insufficiency and (2) preterm delivery and its sequelae. In the past, delivery was often performed after the second episode of bleeding that required transfusion. Unless the patient has persistent bleeding, most obstetricians now favor expectant management within the hospital. The goal is to delay delivery until the fetus is mature. Maternal vital signs are assessed frequently, and the hemoglobin concentration is checked at regular intervals. Fetal evaluation involves frequent performance of a nonstress test or biophysical profile, ultrasonographic assessment of fetal growth, and fetal lung maturity studies as indicated. Hemorrhage may be prevented by limitations on physical activity and avoidance of vaginal examinations and coitus.

Outpatient management has resulted in good outcome in carefully selected patients.[11] Outpatient management is reserved for stable patients without bleeding in the previous 48 hours who have both telephone access and the ability to be transported quickly to the hospital.[12] Expectant management requires immediate access to a medical center with 24-hour obstetric and anesthesia coverage and a neonatal intensive care unit.

In most cases of placenta previa diagnosed between 24 and 34 weeks' gestation, a corticosteroid (e.g., betamethasone) is administered to accelerate fetal lung maturity. A significant number of patients with placenta previa have preterm labor, which may provoke more bleeding and uterine irritability.[12] Obstetricians must balance the potential cardiovascular consequences of tocolytic therapy in the presence of maternal hemorrhage against the consequences of preterm delivery.[13] In a retrospective study of patients with symptomatic placenta previa, Besinger et al.[14] observed that tocolytic therapy was associated with a clinically significant delay in delivery and an increase in birth weight but did not reduce the frequency or severity of recurrent vaginal bleeding. A small prospective study also demonstrated that use of ritodrine resulted in higher birth weights with no increase in the rate of maternal complications.[15] Tocolytic therapy is not recommended for patients with uncontrolled hemorrhage or those in whom placental abruption is suspected.

The choice of tocolytic drug is controversial. In the past, some maternal-fetal medicine specialists favored magnesium sulfate because of a belief that magnesium sulfate is less likely to cause maternal hypotension during hemorrhage than the beta-adrenergic agents. In addition, the beta-adrenergic agents produce maternal tachycardia, which may make it more difficult to assess maternal intravascular volume. Chestnut et al.[16] evaluated the hemodynamic response to maternal hemorrhage during infusion of either magnesium sulfate or ritodrine in gravid ewes. Magnesium sulfate, but not ritodrine, worsened maternal hypotension during hemorrhage. The fetal pH decreased significantly only in the magnesium sulfate group. The investigators speculated that hypermagnesemia attenuated the maternal compensatory response to hemorrhage. Nifedipine, a calcium entry blocker, is as effective as magnesium sulfate and beta-adrenergic agonists in arresting preterm labor and is associated with fewer maternal side effects.[17,18]

Tocolysis and blood transfusion allow the obstetrician to delay delivery, and assessment of fetal lung maturity helps determine the appropriate timing of delivery. Although expectant management has reduced risks to the neonate, prematurity remains the most common cause of neonatal mortality and morbidity, especially if bleeding begins before 20 weeks' gestation. McShane et al.[19] observed that the onset of bleeding before 20 weeks' gestation was associated with a very poor fetal outcome.

Fetuses of women with placenta previa may be at risk for other problems. Naeye[20] noted an increased incidence of asymmetric intrauterine growth restriction (IUGR) in fetuses of women with placenta previa. Several factors may account for the association between placenta previa and IUGR. First, the lower uterine segment may be less vascular than normal sites of placental implantation. Second, the placenta often is adherent to an area of fibrosis. Third, patients with placenta previa have a higher incidence of first-trimester bleeding, which may promote a partial placental separation, reducing the surface area for placental exchange. Fourth, although the blood loss from placenta previa is almost entirely maternal, trauma to the placenta with vaginal examination or coitus may result in some fetal blood loss, which could retard fetal growth.[21] Some studies have reported a higher incidence of congenital anomalies in the fetuses of women with placenta previa.[22]

ANESTHETIC MANAGEMENT

All patients admitted with antepartum vaginal bleeding should be evaluated by an anesthesia provider on arrival. Special consideration should be given to the airway examination, intravascular volume assessment, and a history of previous cesarean delivery or other procedures that create a uterine scar. At least one large-gauge intravenous catheter should be placed, the patient's hematocrit should be determined, and a blood type and screen should be performed. For women who are actively bleeding, a blood type and cross-match should be performed. Volume resuscitation should be initiated using non–dextrose-containing balanced salt solution (lactated Ringer's or normal saline solution).

Double Setup Examination

The accuracy of ultrasonography for the identification of placenta previa has almost eliminated the need for double setup examination, but a few patients still require it (e.g., morbidly obese patients who cannot be adequately evaluated with ultrasonography). The examination is performed in the operating room. All members of the obstetric care team, including the anesthesia provider, obstetrician, and pediatrician, make full preparation for cesarean delivery. Full preparation consists of application of maternal monitors, insertion of two large-gauge intravenous cannulae, administration of a nonparticulate antacid, and sterile preparation and draping of the abdomen. Two units of packed red blood cells (PRBCs) should be available in the operating room. The obstetrician subsequently performs a careful vaginal examination. A cesarean delivery is performed if significant bleeding occurs or if the obstetrician confirms the presence of placenta previa in a woman with a mature fetus.

Cesarean Delivery

Unless the placenta is more than 2 cm from the internal cervical os, a patient with placenta previa requires abdominal delivery.[12] The choice of anesthetic technique depends on the indication and urgency for delivery, the severity of maternal hypovolemia, and, perhaps, the obstetric history (e.g., prior cesarean delivery).

No consensus exists among anesthesia providers regarding the use of neuraxial anesthesia in patients with a placenta previa *without* active bleeding or intravascular volume deficit. However, surveys of obstetric anesthesiologists show that neuraxial anesthesia is often preferred and performed.[23,24] Patients who have placenta previa—without active preoperative bleeding—remain at risk for increased intraoperative blood loss for at least three reasons. First, the obstetrician may cut into an anteriorly located placenta during uterine incision. Second, after delivery, the lower uterine segment implantation site does not contract as well as the normal fundal implantation site. Third, a patient with placenta previa is at increased risk for placenta accreta, especially if there is a history of previous cesarean delivery.[8] For these reasons, two large-gauge intravenous cannulae should be placed before the start of either elective or emergency cesarean delivery. No consensus exists on the need for blood product availability in these patients, but a blood type and screen should be performed, and some anesthesia providers insist that two units of PRBCs are available in the operating room before the start of surgery. A prospective trial comparing epidural anesthesia with general anesthesia for cesarean delivery in women with placenta previa demonstrated that general anesthesia was associated with a lower postoperative hematocrit. Operative times, estimated blood loss, urine output, and neonatal Apgar scores were similar in the two groups.[25] A reasonable conclusion would be that single-shot spinal anesthesia is also acceptable for this group of patients, provided that there is a low risk of placenta accreta.

Patients with placenta previa and active preoperative bleeding represent a significant challenge for the anesthesia care team. Frequently such patients have just presented to the hospital, and there is minimal time for evaluation. In these cases, patient evaluation, resuscitation, and preparation for operative delivery all proceed simultaneously. Because the placental site is the source of hemorrhage, the bleeding may continue unabated until the placenta is removed and the uterus contracts. Preoperative evaluation requires careful assessment of the parturient's airway and intravascular volume. Two large-gauge intravenous catheters should be placed, and four units of PRBCs should be ordered. Blood administration sets, fluid warmers, and equipment for invasive monitoring should be immediately available. Initially, non–dextrose-containing crystalloid or colloid is infused rapidly. In some cases, the patient requires transfusion prior to completion of the blood cross-match, and type-specific blood or type O, Rh-negative blood must be administered.

Rapid-sequence induction of general anesthesia is the preferred technique for bleeding patients. The choice of intravenous induction agent depends on the degree of cardiovascular instability. In patients with severe hypovolemic shock, endotracheal intubation may require only a muscle relaxant, but this situation is rare. A reduced dose of sodium thiopental should be administered in women with ongoing hemorrhage. In women with *severe* ongoing hemorrhage, it is best to avoid sodium thiopental. Likewise, propofol should not be used in hypovolemic patients.

Ketamine and etomidate are the preferred induction agents for bleeding patients. **Ketamine** (0.5 to 1.0 mg/kg) has an excellent record of safety and efficacy in obstetric anesthesia practice. Postoperative hallucinations and nightmares are uncommon when the dose does not exceed 1 mg/kg. Ketamine may cause myocardial depression in patients with severe hypovolemia. **Etomidate** is an acceptable alternative to ketamine and is safe for use in obstetric patients.[26] When used for induction of anesthesia, etomidate (0.3 mg/kg) causes minimal cardiac depression. A reduced dose is appropriate in patients with severe hemorrhage. Disadvantages of etomidate include venous irritation, myoclonus, and possible adrenal suppression.

For the maintenance of anesthesia, the choice of agents depends on maternal cardiovascular stability. In patients with modest bleeding and no preexisting fetal compromise, 50% nitrous oxide and 50% oxygen can be administered with a low concentration of a volatile halogenated agent to prevent maternal awareness. The concentration of nitrous oxide can be reduced or omitted in cases of fetal compromise. Oxytocin (20 to 30 U/L) should be administered by intravenous infusion immediately after delivery. The lower uterine segment implantation site does not contract as efficiently as the uterine fundus. All uterine relaxants should be eliminated if bleeding continues. Thus, it may be best to eliminate the volatile halogenated agent after delivery and to substitute nitrous oxide (70%) and an intravenous opioid. Small doses of opioid (e.g., fentanyl, remifentanil) and benzodiazepines (e.g., midazolam) can be administered without causing significant cardiovascular depression. Some anesthesia providers contend that bispectral index (BIS) monitoring may be helpful in cases in which the volatile anesthetic agent has been discontinued, although this issue is a matter of some dispute.

If the placenta does not separate easily, a placenta accreta may exist. In such cases, massive blood loss and the need for cesarean hysterectomy should be anticipated (see later). The need for invasive hemodynamic monitoring varies among patients. An indwelling arterial catheter is useful for patients with hemodynamic instability or for those who require frequent determination of hematocrit and blood gas measurements. Occasionally, a central venous catheter can be useful to guide intravascular volume replacement and fluid therapy. Coagulopathy rarely occurs with placenta previa; the most common coagulation deficit is a dilutional thrombocytopenia.

Placental Abruption

Placental abruption is defined as complete or partial separation of the placenta from the decidua basalis before delivery of the fetus. Maternal hemorrhage may be revealed by vaginal bleeding or may be concealed behind the placenta. Fetal compromise occurs because of the loss of placental surface area for maternal-fetal exchange of oxygen and nutrients.[6]

EPIDEMIOLOGY

The etiology is not known, but several conditions are associated with placental abruption. Known risk factors include hypertension, preeclampsia, advanced maternal age and parity, maternal and paternal tobacco use, cocaine use, trauma, premature rupture of membranes, chorioamnionitis, bleeding in early pregnancy, and a history of previous abruption.[27,28] Evidence now suggests that patients hospitalized for both acute and chronic respiratory diseases are at higher risk for placental abruption.[29] Abruption complicates 0.4% to 1.0% of pregnancies, and the incidence is increasing, particularly among black women.[27,28,30-32]

DIAGNOSIS

The classic presentation consists of vaginal bleeding, uterine tenderness, and increased uterine activity. In some cases abruption may manifest as idiopathic preterm labor. Patients may have a variety of nonreassuring fetal heart rate (FHR) patterns, including bradycardia, late or variable decelerations, and/or loss of variability.[6] In cases of concealed abruption, vaginal bleeding may be absent, and a gross underestimation of maternal hypovolemia can occur. The diagnosis of placental abruption is primarily clinical; in a subset of cases, ultrasonography may help confirm it.[33] Ultrasonographic examination often can determine the presence of a retroplacental or subchorionic hematoma, but normal ultrasonographic findings do not exclude the diagnosis. Although ultrasonography is not very sensitive (24%) for abruption, it is highly specific (96%).[33] Ultrasonography is also useful for determining placental location, which can exclude placenta previa as a cause of vaginal bleeding.[6]

PATHOPHYSIOLOGY

The major complications of placental abruption are hemorrhagic shock, acute renal failure (ARF), coagulopathy, and fetal compromise or demise. Abruption is the most common cause of disseminated intravascular coagulation (DIC) in pregnancy.[6] Coagulopathy occurs in 10% of all cases of placental abruption. The incidence of coagulopathy increases with fetal demise.[31]

The rate of IUGR associated with placental abruption suggests that some cases of placental abruption are the result of chronic, long-standing placental abnormalities. Naeye et al.[34] prospectively studied more than 53,000 deliveries and found that decidual necrosis at the placental margin and large placental infarcts were the most common abnormalities. Infants who died had 14% less placental weight, 8% less body weight, and 3% shorter body length than surviving control infants of the same gestational age. In other situations (e.g., trauma), abruption occurs acutely.

The major risks to the fetus are hypoxia and prematurity. Fetal oxygenation depends on adequate maternal oxygen-carrying capacity, uteroplacental blood flow, and transplacental exchange. Separation of all or part of the placenta reduces gas exchange surface area and can lead to fetal death. This situation is made worse by maternal hypotension, which decreases uteroplacental blood flow. Intrauterine bleeding can lead to uterine irritability and preterm labor.[6]

Ananth and Wilcox,[30] reviewing outcomes for 7.5 million pregnancies in the United States, found a 12% perinatal mortality rate associated with placental abruption. The high mortality rate may be due, in part, to the fact that these infants of mothers with placental abruption are five times more likely to be delivered preterm.[30] The extent and location of placental abruption are also important. A placental abruption with a retroplacental hematoma has a less favorable prognosis for fetal survival than a placental abruption with a subchorionic hemorrhage. Large retroplacental bleeding is associated with a perinatal mortality rate of 50% or higher, whereas a similar-sized subchorionic abruption may be associated with a rate of 10%.[35]

OBSTETRIC MANAGEMENT

Once the diagnosis of abruption is suspected, the FHR should be monitored, and if feasible, an internal scalp electrode and intrauterine pressure catheter should be placed. A large-gauge intravenous catheter should be inserted, and blood should be obtained for cross-match and assessment of hematocrit and coagulation. Supplemental oxygen should be administered, and left uterine displacement should be maintained.

The apparent blood loss may not reflect the true extent of intravascular volume deficit, which is often caused by a retroplacental hematoma. Placement of a urethral catheter helps the physician assess the adequacy of renal perfusion.

The definitive treatment is delivery of the infant and placenta, but the degree of maternal and fetal compromise determines the timing and route of delivery. If the patient is preterm, the extent of abruption is minimal, and the fetus shows no signs of compromise, the patient is hospitalized and the pregnancy is allowed to continue to optimize fetal lung maturation. Patients with a term fetus—with no evidence of compromise—may undergo induction of labor. Vaginal delivery is also preferred in patients with intrauterine fetal demise.

More often, a nonreassuring FHR pattern is present. In such cases delivery should proceed without delay, given that longer decision-to-delivery times have been associated with worse perinatal outcomes.[36]

ANESTHETIC MANAGEMENT

The anesthesia provider should consider the severity of the abruption and the urgency of delivery in planning anesthetic management.

Labor and Vaginal Delivery

The patient undergoing induction of labor may receive epidural analgesia if she has normal coagulation studies and no intravascular volume deficit. The appropriateness of epidural analgesia for patients at risk for extension of abruption and further hemorrhage has been questioned. Vincent et al.[37] observed that epidural anesthesia significantly worsened maternal hypotension, uterine blood flow, and fetal PaO_2 and pH during untreated hemorrhage (20 mL/kg) in gravid ewes. Curiously, maternal heart rate decreased during hemorrhage in the epidural anesthesia group but not in the control group (Figure 37-2). However, intravascular volume replacement promptly eliminated the difference between groups in maternal mean arterial pressure (MAP), cardiac output, and fetal PaO_2. The investigators concluded that epidural anesthesia may adversely affect the compensatory response to untreated hemorrhage in pregnant women. Many anesthesia providers offer epidural analgesia to the patient with a partial abruption, provided that her coagulation status is normal and she is not hypovolemic. Close monitoring is required for evidence of further bleeding or changes in intravascular volume status.

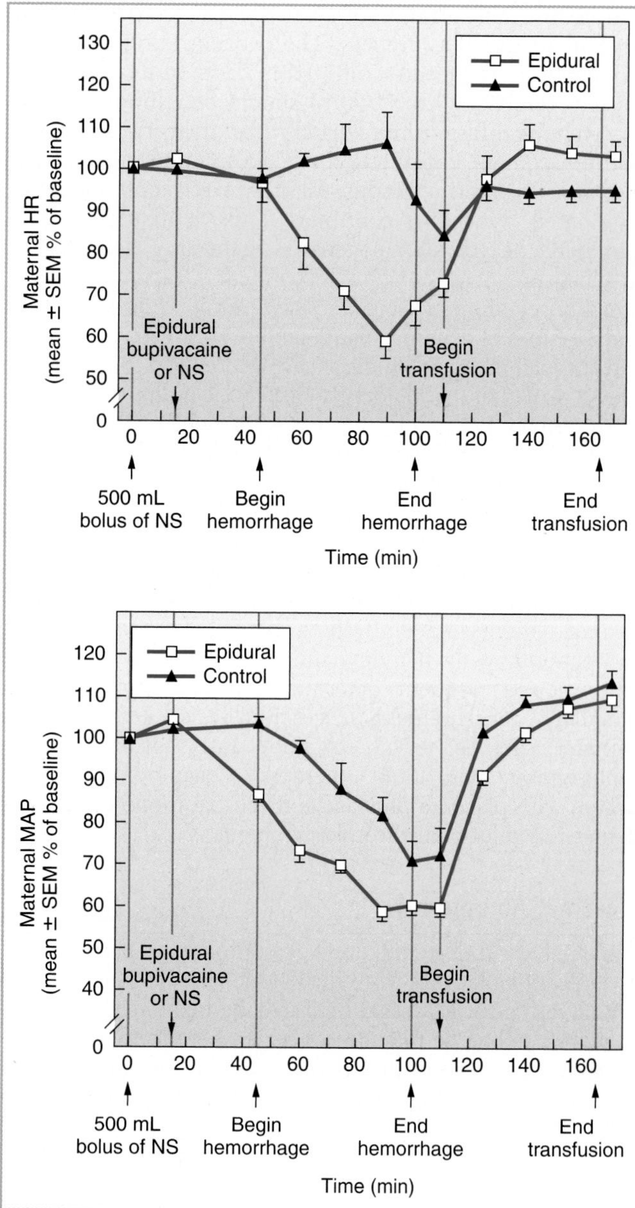

FIGURE 37-2 Maternal heart rate (HR) and mean arterial pressure (MAP) responses over time. Maternal HR was lower during hemorrhage ($P < .05$) in the epidural anesthesia group than in the control group. During transfusion, maternal HR was slightly higher ($P < .05$) in the epidural anesthesia group than in the control group. Maternal MAP was lower during hemorrhage ($P < .05$) in the epidural anesthesia group than in the control group. (Modified from Vincent RD, Chestnut DH, Sipes SL, et al. Epidural anesthesia worsens uterine blood flow and fetal oxygenation during hemorrhage in gravid ewes. Anesthesiology 1992; 76:799-806.)

Cesarean Delivery

General anesthesia is preferred for most cases of urgent cesarean delivery for placental abruption with a nonreassuring FHR pattern. Both propofol and sodium thiopental may precipitate severe hypotension in patients with unrecognized hypovolemia. Ketamine and etomidate are better options for the patient with unknown or decreased intravascular volume. During early gestation, large doses of ketamine may increase uterine tone, which would be deleterious to a compromised fetus.[38] This effect is unlikely, however, with administration of a single dose of ketamine (1 mg/kg) for induction of anesthesia. Severe hypotension after the administration of sodium thiopental or propofol is more likely to be harmful than the possibility of increased uterine tone after administration of a single dose of ketamine.

Aggressive volume resuscitation is critical. Both crystalloid and colloid may be used; the choice is less important than adequate restoration of intravascular volume. In cases of severe hemorrhage, management is aided by the insertion of central venous and arterial catheters. An antecubital vein can be used for central line placement when coagulopathy is suspected or present.

These patients are at risk for persistent hemorrhage resulting from uterine atony or coagulopathy. After delivery, oxytocin (20 to 30 U/L) should be infused promptly to improve uterine tone. Persistent uterine atony requires the administration of other ecbolic drugs (see later). With coagulopathy, coagulation factors should be replaced.

Most parturients recover quickly and completely after delivery. A minority of patients, notably those who have prolonged hypotension or coagulopathy, and who need massive blood volume and blood product replacement, are best monitored and followed in a multidisciplinary intensive care unit.

Uterine Rupture

EPIDEMIOLOGY

Rupture of the gravid uterus can be disastrous to both the mother and the fetus. Fortunately, it does not occur often. Previous uterine trauma increases the risk, although the incidence of true uterine rupture is less than 1% among parturients with a scarred uterus.[39] Uterine rupture is rare in the primigravid woman or the woman with an unscarred uterus.[40] Trauma during attempted forceps delivery may cause uterine rupture in a patient with an unscarred uterus. Box 37-1 lists other conditions associated with uterine rupture.

Because of the variation in nomenclature and severity, accurate determination of the maternal and fetal morbidity secondary to uterine rupture is difficult. The most common variety of disruption is uterine scar separation or dehiscence. Some cases of uterine scar dehiscence are asymptomatic. Uterine scar dehiscence is more common, and is less likely to cause maternal or fetal morbidity, than uterine rupture. **Uterine scar dehiscence** is a uterine wall defect that does not result in FHR abnormalities or excessive hemorrhage and does not require emergency cesarean delivery or postpartum laparotomy. In contrast, **uterine rupture** is a uterine wall defect that results in fetal compromise or maternal hemorrhage sufficient to require cesarean delivery or postpartum laparotomy.

The rupture of a classic uterine scar increases morbidity and mortality because the anterior uterine wall is highly vascular and may include the area of placental implantation. Lateral extension of the rupture can involve the major uterine vessels and is typically associated with massive bleeding. Plauché et al.[41] reviewed 23 cases of catastrophic uterine rupture; they noted no maternal deaths but a fetal mortality rate of 35%. There was one maternal death secondary to uterine rupture in the most recent triennial report from the United Kingdom.[1] Uterine rupture increases the risk of neonatal mortality 60-fold.[39]

BOX 37-1 Conditions Associated with Uterine Rupture

Previous uterine surgery
Trauma
Indirect:
- Blunt (e.g., seat belt injury)
- Excessive manual fundal pressure
- Extension of cervical laceration

Direct:
- Penetrating wound
- Intrauterine manipulation
- Forceps application and rotation
- Postpartum curettage
- Manual placental extraction
- Version and extraction
- External version

Inappropriate use of oxytocin
Grand multiparity
Uterine anomaly
Placenta percreta
Tumors (trophoblastic disease, cervical carcinoma)
Fetal problems (macrosomia, malposition, anomaly)

From Plauché WC. Surgical problems involving the pregnant uterus: Uterine inversion, uterine rupture, and leiomyomas. In Plauché WC, Morrison JC, O'Sullivan MJ, editors. Surgical Obstetrics. Philadelphia, WB Saunders, 1989:224.

DIAGNOSIS

The variable presentation of uterine rupture may cause diagnostic difficulty. True uterine rupture should be suspected when vaginal bleeding, hypotension, cessation of labor, and fetal compromise are present. Historically, obstetricians have considered abdominal pain to be a consistent, sensitive sign of uterine rupture. However, one retrospective study reported the occurrence of pain in less than 10% of patients with either scar dehiscence or true rupture.[42] A nonreassuring FHR pattern is the most reliable sign of uterine scar dehiscence or rupture (see Chapter 19).

In women without previous cesarean delivery, uterine rupture is rare. Risk factors include grand multiparity, fetal malpresentation, bicornuate uterus, prior myomectomy, and induction of labor with oxytocin or prostaglandin.[40] A 2001 study highlighted the high risk of uterine rupture associated with prostaglandin induction and discouraged its use in patients with a previous cesarean delivery.[43] Maternal tachycardia, FHR decelerations, and postpartum hemorrhage may signal uterine rupture. The diagnosis is confirmed by manual exploration of the uterus or during laparotomy.

OBSTETRIC MANAGEMENT

Treatment options include repair, arterial ligation, and hysterectomy. **Uterine repair** is appropriate for most cases of separation of a prior transverse uterine scar and for some cases of rupture of an old classic incision. However, the risk of rupture in a future pregnancy remains. A disadvantage of **arterial ligation** is that it may not control the bleeding and may delay definitive treatment. **Hysterectomy** is the preferred, definitive procedure for most cases of uterine rupture.[41,42] Patients with rupture of an unscarred uterus are more likely to require blood transfusion than patients with rupture of a scarred uterus. The fibrous edges of a scar bleed less readily than the rough edges of a newly ruptured uterus.

ANESTHETIC MANAGEMENT

Patient evaluation and resuscitation are begun while the patient is prepared for emergency laparotomy. If rupture has occurred antepartum, fetal compromise is likely. General anesthesia is often necessary, except in some stable patients with preexisting epidural anesthesia. Aggressive volume replacement and maintenance of urine output are essential. Invasive hemodynamic monitoring is appropriate when there is uncertainty about the intravascular volume status.

Vasa Previa

Vasa previa is defined as the velamentous insertion of the fetal vessels over the cervical os (i.e., the fetal vessels traverse the fetal membranes ahead of the fetal presenting part). Thus, the fetal vessels are not protected by the placenta or the umbilical cord. Rupture of the membranes is often accompanied by tearing of a fetal vessel, which may lead to exsanguination of the fetus.

EPIDEMIOLOGY

Vasa previa occurs rarely (1 in 2500 deliveries).[12] It poses no threat to the mother, but because it involves the loss of fetal blood, vasa previa is associated with one of the highest fetal mortality rates (50% to 75%) of any complication of pregnancy. The fetus at term has approximately 80 to 100 mL/kg of blood. Therefore, the amount of blood that can be lost without fetal death is relatively small. In addition, the vulnerable fetal vessels may be compressed by the presenting part, resulting in fetal hypoxia and death.[12] Vasa previa is associated with multiple gestation, particularly with triplets.

DIAGNOSIS

Vasa previa should be suspected whenever bleeding occurs with rupture of membranes, particularly if the rupture is accompanied by FHR decelerations or fetal bradycardia. Hemorrhage can also occur without rupture of membranes, making the diagnosis more difficult. Early diagnosis and treatment are essential to a good fetal outcome. Rarely, vasa previa can be diagnosed via digital cervical examination or amnioscopy. More commonly, it is detected antenatally with ultrasonography or Doppler imaging. An antenatal diagnosis significantly improves perinatal outcome.[44] Time permitting, the diagnosis of vasa previa can be confirmed through examination of the shed blood for evidence of fetal hemoglobin (e.g., Kleihauer-Betke test).

OBSTETRIC MANAGEMENT

The treatment of vasa previa is directed solely toward ensuring fetal survival. Some obstetricians advocate hospitalization of the patient between 30 and 32 weeks' gestation to ensure prompt delivery if premature rupture of membranes should occur. Otherwise, patients should undergo cesarean delivery at 36 weeks' gestation.[12] Ruptured vasa previa is a true obstetric emergency that requires immediate delivery of the fetus, almost always by the abdominal route. Neonatal resuscitation requires immediate attention to neonatal volume replacement with colloid, balanced salt solutions, and blood.

ANESTHETIC MANAGEMENT

The choice of anesthetic technique depends on the urgency of the cesarean delivery. In many cases, general anesthesia is necessary for prompt delivery.

POSTPARTUM HEMORRHAGE

Postpartum hemorrhage is a major cause of maternal morbidity and mortality worldwide.[45] It occurs in approximately 5% of deliveries, and there is a greater likelihood of recurrence in subsequent pregnancies.[46] Table 37-2 lists predisposing factors for postpartum hemorrhage.

Numerous, and frequently confusing, definitions exist for postpartum hemorrhage. Blood losses of more than 500 mL for vaginal delivery and more than 1000 mL for cesarean delivery are frequently published guidelines. However, these values have low clinical utility because they are only slightly higher than the average blood loss for each type of delivery. Postpartum hemorrhage can also be identified clinically (albeit retrospectively) from a 10% decrease in hematocrit from admission to the postpartum period, or from the need to administer PRBCs.[47]

TABLE 37-2 Factors Predisposing to Postpartum Hemorrhage

Factor	Uterine Atony	Lacerations, Disruptions	Placental Abnormalities	Coagulation Disorders
Precipitous labor	×	×		
Instrumental delivery		×		
General anesthesia	×			
Prolonged labor	×			
Uterine leiomyomas	×	×	×	
Macrosomia	×	×		
Multiple gestation	×	×		
Chorioamnionitis	×			
Multiparity	×		×	
Prior cesarean delivery		×	×	
Prior hysterotomy or curettage		×	×	
Stimulated labor	×	×		
History of postpartum hemorrhage	×		×	×
Fetal demise	×			×
Amniotic fluid embolism	×			×
Tocolytic therapy	×			

Modified from Herbert WNJ, Cefalo R. Management of postpartum hemorrhage. Clin Obstet Gynecol 1984;27:139-47.

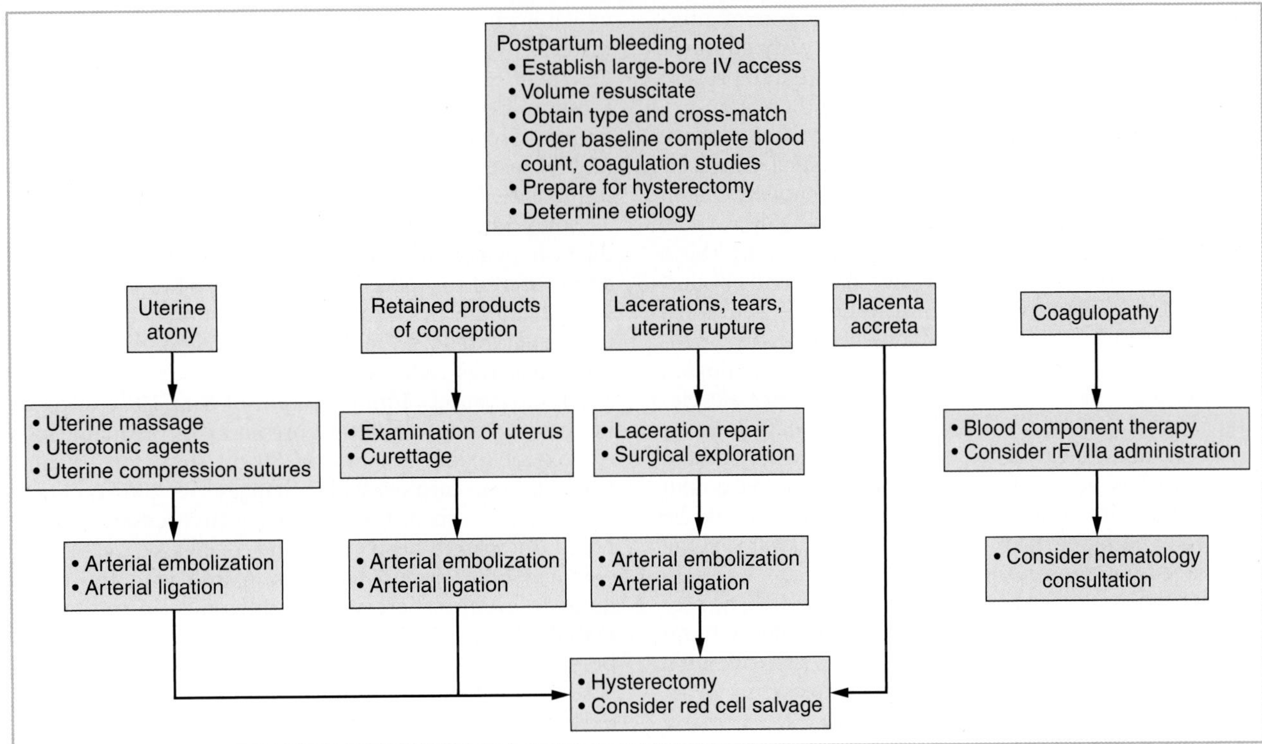

FIGURE 37-3 Management options for postpartum hemorrhage. IV, intravenous.

Results of most studies indicate that physicians and nurses often underestimate the severity of obstetric hemorrhage.[3] In suspected cases of significant postpartum hemorrhage, it is imperative that the clinician use all available modalities to assess the severity of hypovolemia. Urine output monitoring and evaluation of arterial blood gas measurements to ascertain the development of acidosis are advised in these situations. The use of an intra-arterial catheter to measure systolic blood pressure may also be helpful in the assessment of intravascular volume. In some cases postpartum bleeding has resulted in maternal myocardial ischemia. Goals of treatment include early restoration of blood pressure and adequate hemoglobin levels.[48]

Primary postpartum hemorrhage occurs during the first 24 hours, and **secondary** postpartum hemorrhage between 24 hours and 6 weeks after delivery. Primary postpartum hemorrhage is more likely to result in maternal morbidity or mortality. Figure 37-3 provides an overview of the obstetric management of postpartum hemorrhage.

Uterine Atony

EPIDEMIOLOGY

Uterine atony is the most common cause of severe postpartum hemorrhage, and it is the most common indication for peripartum blood transfusion.[49,50] Postpartum hemostasis involves the release of endogenous uterotonic agents in addition to normal hemostatic mechanisms. Contraction of the uterus represents the primary mechanism for controlling blood loss at parturition. Oxytocin and prostaglandins are responsible for uterine contraction and involution during the third stage of labor. Uterine atony represents a failure of this process. Parturients with obstetric hemorrhage may have uterine arteries that are relatively unresponsive to vasoconstrictor substances.[51] Many cases of uterine atony result from overdistention of the uterus. Box 37-2 lists conditions associated with uterine atony.

DIAGNOSIS

A soft postpartum uterus and vaginal bleeding are the most common physical findings in patients with uterine atony. The absence of vaginal bleeding does not exclude this disorder because the atonic, engorged uterus may contain more than 1000 mL of blood. Unrecognized bleeding may manifest as hemodynamic instability secondary to hypovolemia.

OBSTETRIC AND ANESTHETIC MANAGEMENT

Uterine atony accounts for 80% or more of the cases of primary postpartum hemorrhage.[52] Immediate administration of oxytocin after delivery is standard for prevention of uterine atony.[52] A systematic review of published studies identified no advantage to giving an alternative uterotonic

BOX 37-2 Conditions Associated with Uterine Atony

- Multiple gestation
- Macrosomia
- Polyhydramnios
- High parity
- Prolonged labor
- Chorioamnionitis
- Precipitous labor
- Augmented labor
- Tocolytic agents
- High concentration of a volatile halogenated anesthetic agent

agent (rather than oxytocin) for the prevention of uterine atony.[53] Regardless of the agent chosen, early administration of a uterotonic (ecbolic) agent is essential to prevent severe maternal morbidity and mortality.[54,55]

Despite preventive measures, postpartum hemorrhage occurs in 4% to 6% of pregnancies.[52] Bimanual compression, uterine massage, and continued intravenous infusion of oxytocin are successful in most patients. Only a small percentage of these patients with postpartum hemorrhage require transfusion, minimally invasive treatment options, or hysterectomy. Aggressive administration of additional uterotonic agents may help avoid the need for hysterectomy. All patients with uterine atony should be evaluated by an anesthesia provider, who should administer supplemental oxygen, ensure the presence of adequate intravenous access, and make certain that appropriate crystalloid resuscitation has been initiated. A complete blood count, coagulation studies, and a type and cross-match should be performed. The blood bank should be made aware of the possible need for transfusion.

The first-line treatment for postpartum hemorrhage secondary to uterine atony is administration of one or more uterotonic agents.[52] Three classes of drugs are currently available for the treatment of uterine atony: oxytocin, prostaglandins, and ergot alkaloids (Table 37-3).

Oxytocin is the first-line drug for prophylaxis and treatment of uterine atony. The number of uterine high-affinity receptors for oxytocin increases greatly near term. Endogenous oxytocin is a 9–amino acid polypeptide produced in the posterior pituitary. The exogenous form of the drug (Pitocin, Syntocinon) is a synthetic preparation. Older preparations were derived from animal extracts that were contaminated with antidiuretic hormone (ADH). This contamination was problematic during the administration of large doses. Because ADH is also a 9–amino acid polypeptide, even the synthetic form may have a minor ADH effect, which is rarely a problem, especially when the drug is administered with normal saline or lactated Ringer's solution. Oxytocin should not be administered with a hypotonic solution, because doing so might result in dilutional hyponatremia secondary to cross-reactivity with the vasopressin (ADH) receptor in the kidney. The onset of action is almost immediate.[56]

Bolus administration of oxytocin causes peripheral vasodilation, which may result in hypotension. Weis et al.[57] administered oxytocin 0.1 U/kg intravenously to pregnant women in the first trimester. They noted that heart rate increased, MAP decreased by 30%, and total peripheral resistance was reduced by 50%. Secher et al.[58] noted that bolus intravenous administration of 5 or 10 U of oxytocin increased pulmonary artery pressures in pregnant women. An oxytocin infusion rate of 80 mU/min for 10 minutes resulted in no cardiovascular changes.[58] A 2007 randomized trial of 30 women undergoing elective cesarean delivery noted increased heart rate and decreased MAP in the oxytocin bolus group when compared with the oxytocin infusion group. There was no difference in the total estimated blood loss between the two groups.[59] Given the potential for hypotension and the absence of a clear benefit, it seems best to *avoid* bolus intravenous administration of oxytocin as prophylaxis for postpartum hemorrhage.

Various electrocardiographic changes also may occur during the administration of oxytocin, but their significance is unclear. Fortunately, cardiovascular changes are short-lived (less than 10 minutes). The liver, the kidneys, and the enzyme oxytocinase are responsible for the short plasma half-life of oxytocin.

Oxytocin infusion is initiated immediately after umbilical cord clamping at cesarean delivery or after the placenta is delivered at vaginal delivery. Twenty to 30 units of oxytocin are added to a liter of normal saline or lactated Ringer's solution and administered by continuous intravenous

TABLE 37-3 Drug Therapy for Uterine Atony

Agent	Dose and Route	Contraindications	Side Effects	Notes
Oxytocin	20-60 U/L intravenous infusion	None	Decreased systemic vascular resistance and hypotension with bolus intravenous doses Free water retention	Short duration of effect
Methylergonovine (Methergine)	0.2 mg IM	Hypertension Preeclampsia Coronary artery disease	Thromboembolic sequelae? Severe nausea and vomiting Arteriolar constriction	Long duration of action May be repeated once after 1 hr
15-Methylprostaglandin $F_{2\alpha}$ (Hemabate)	250 μg IM or IU	Reactive airway disease Pulmonary hypertension Hypoxemic patients	Bronchoconstriction Shivering Temperature elevation Diarrhea	May be repeated every 15 min up to 2 mg
Misoprostol (Cytotec)	800-1000 μg per rectum	None	Shivering Temperature elevation Diarrhea Nausea/vomiting	Off-label use

IM, intramuscular; IU, intrauterine.

infusion. Increasing the concentration of oxytocin (e.g., 40 U/L) may be indicated in refractory cases of uterine atony. Munn et al.[60] compared two oxytocin regimens (333 mU/min and 2667 mU/min, infused intravenously over 30 minutes) after umbilical cord clamping in laboring women who underwent cesarean delivery. The investigators observed significantly fewer requests for additional uterotonic medications in the high-dose oxytocin group. The incidence of hypotension was similar in the two groups. The clinical advantage associated with administration of oxytocin by the *intramyometrial* route is not well defined.[61]

The **ergot alkaloids** are another class of drugs used for the treatment of uterine atony. The natural ergot alkaloids are produced by a fungus that commonly infests rye and other grains. Ergonovine and methylergonovine (a semisynthetic preparation) are the two ergot alkaloids currently used for treatment of uterine atony. **Ergonovine** (Ergotrate) and **methylergonovine** (Methergine) are identical in their pharmacologic profiles and activity. Both drugs rapidly produce tetanic uterine contraction, and for this reason are restricted to postpartum use. The mechanism of action is poorly understood, but the uterotonic effect is most likely mediated by means of alpha-adrenergic receptor stimulation.[62] Parenteral administration of an ergot alkaloid is associated with a high incidence of nausea and vomiting, an effect that is problematic for the awake patient. Ergonovine and methylergonovine have been reported to be less cardiotoxic than other ergot alkaloids but still may cause serious cardiovascular system derangements, including vasoconstriction, severe hypertension, elevated pulmonary artery pressure, and, possibly, pulmonary edema.[63]

Ergot alkaloids also cause coronary artery vasoconstriction and have been associated with myocardial ischemia or infarction.[62,64] Lin et al.[65] reported one case of maternal death following administration of methylergonovine. Severe hypertension resulting in cerebrovascular accident and seizures has been reported.[66] Patients at greatest risk are those with preexisting hypertension; however, sudden and marked hypertension may also occur in normotensive patients. The combination of an ergot alkaloid followed by a vasopressor has been reported to lead to exaggerated hypertension.[67] Caution is advised when these drugs are administered concurrently. Relative contraindications to the use of ergot alkaloids include hypertension, preeclampsia, peripheral vascular disease, and ischemic heart disease. Treatment of ergot-induced vasoconstriction and hypertension may require administration of a potent vasodilator, such as nitroglycerin or sodium nitroprusside.

Ergot alkaloids are unstable unless refrigerated, and therefore, their use is limited in certain regions of the world. Oxytocin is much more stable than ergot alkaloids.[68]

Ergot alkaloids have a rapid onset when given either intravenously or intramuscularly. Both ergonovine and methylergonovine are dispensed in ampules containing 0.2 mg for intramuscular administration. Bolus intravenous administration is **not** recommended. In cases of life-threatening hemorrhage, 0.2 mg may be diluted in 250 mL of intravenous fluid and then infused with close attention to maternal blood pressure. The uterotonic effect usually lasts for 2 to 3 hours. Regardless of the route of administration, blood pressure and the electrocardiogram should be monitored closely. The latest triennial report from the United Kingdom recommends oxytocin and ergot alkaloids (specifically, ergometrine) as the drugs of first choice in the prevention and treatment of uterine atony.[1]

Prostaglandins of the E and F families have gained wide acceptance as escalation therapy when high-dose oxytocin is inadequate. Concentrations of endogenous prostaglandins increase during labor, but their peak concentrations do not occur until the time of placental separation. In some women, uterine atony may be caused by the failure of prostaglandin concentrations to increase during the third stage of labor.[69,70] Prostaglandins increase myometrial intracellular free calcium concentrations,[71] ultimately leading to an increase in myosin light-chain kinase activity. Patients with chorioamnionitis may show less response to prostaglandin therapy.[72] Common side effects noted after administration of any of the prostaglandins include malaise, fever, chills, explosive diarrhea, nausea, and vomiting.[72]

The preferred prostaglandin for the treatment of refractory uterine atony is **15-methyl prostaglandin $F_{2\alpha}$** (carboprost, Hemabate); its use may succeed in controlling hemorrhage when all other pharmacologic treatments have failed.[72,73] Unfortunately, this valuable ecbolic agent may also result in bronchospasm, abnormal ventilation-perfusion ratios, increased intrapulmonary shunt fraction, and hypoxemia.[74,75] The recommended dose is 250 µg administered intramuscularly or into the uterine muscle. The dose may be repeated every 15 to 30 minutes but should not exceed a total dose of 2 mg (eight doses). One small series reported success with use of this drug as an intravenous infusion, but the safety of this route of administration has not been documented.[76]

Misoprostol (Cytotec) is a prostaglandin E_1 analogue that has been used successfully for cervical priming or the induction of labor at term. Some obstetricians advocate its use in cases of uterine atony unresponsive to conventional uterotonic agents. O'Brien et al.[77] reported 14 cases of successful treatment of postpartum hemorrhage with rectal misoprostol 1000 µg. Abdel-Aleem et al.[78] studied 18 women with unexpected uterine atony and reported a prompt response after rectal misoprostol administration in 16 patients. A randomized controlled trial suggested that misoprostol may be less effective than combined administration of ergometrine and oxytocin for the treatment of postpartum hemorrhage.[79] Although there is no consensus on the optimal dose of misoprostol for this purpose, many clinicians administer 800 to 1000 µg per rectum for cases unresponsive to other uterotonic agents.

Misoprostol is thermostable in tropical conditions and does not require intravenous access for administration. These characteristics make it a desirable alternative to oxytocin and ergot alkaloids in low-resource areas, where the rate of maternal mortality from hemorrhage is high.[50,80] Like other prostaglandins, misoprostol may be associated with significant side effects, such as fever, chills, nausea, vomiting, and diarrhea. High-dose intravaginal misoprostol does not alter maternal cardiac function as measured by transthoracic electrical bioimpedance during midpregnancy.[81] Although studies have shown misoprostol to be an effective uterotonic agent, most clinicians reserve its use for patients in whom other uterotonic agents are ineffective or unavailable.[80] Misoprostol may be used in place of 15-methyl prostaglandin $F_{2\alpha}$ in patients with reactive airway disease or pulmonary hypertension.

Prostaglandin E_2 (dinoprostone) is a third prostaglandin agent used for the treatment of uterine atony. It causes bronchodilation, decreases systemic vascular resistance, and blood pressure, and it increases heart rate and cardiac output in normovolemic patients. Pulmonary vascular resistance does not change.[82,83] One report noted that intravenous administration of a prostaglandin E_2 preparation caused an increase in PaO_2, with no change in $PaCO_2$.[83] In the United States, the only available formulation of prostaglandin E_2 is a 20-mg vaginal suppository, limiting the usefulness of this drug in patients with significant vaginal bleeding. For this reason, some obstetricians prefer rectal administration of the drug. There is limited experience with an intravenous formulation of the drug.[84]

If hemorrhage and atony persist despite aggressive administration of uterotonic drugs, invasive techniques must be considered. Invasive techniques include embolization of the arteries supplying the uterus, surgical ligation of arteries, and cesarean hysterectomy (see later).

Genital Trauma

The most common childbirth injuries are lacerations and hematomas of the perineum, vagina, and cervix. Most injuries have minimal consequence, but some puerperal lacerations and hematomas are associated with significant hemorrhage, either immediate or delayed. Prompt recognition and treatment can minimize morbidity and mortality.[85] Genital tract lacerations should be suspected in all patients who have vaginal bleeding despite a firm, contracted uterus. The cervix and vagina must be inspected carefully in these patients.

Pelvic hematomas may be divided into four types: vaginal, vulvar, vulvovaginal, and retroperitoneal.[85]

Vaginal hematomas result from soft tissue injury during delivery, and they may involve bleeding from the descending branch of the uterine artery. The use of forceps or vacuum extraction increases the risk. A study in Sweden of all cases of vaginal hematoma from 1987 to 2000 found a prevalence of approximately 1 in 1240 deliveries.[86] The investigators concluded that nulliparity, advanced maternal age, and high birth weight are the leading risk factors associated with vaginal hematoma. Other risk factors include a prolonged second stage of labor, multiple gestation, preeclampsia, and vulvovaginal varicosities.[85]

Vulvar hematomas commonly involve branches of the pudendal artery. Injury is usually signified by extreme pain or clinical manifestations of hypovolemia secondary to blood loss.

Small vaginal or vulvar hematomas that are not enlarging may be observed and treated conservatively with ice packs and oral analgesics. Large hematomas should be incised and evacuated. Bleeding vessels should be ligated. Often no specific source can be identified. Broad-spectrum antibiotics and volume resuscitation should be initiated when appropriate.[85]

Retroperitoneal hematomas are the least common and most dangerous hematomas associated with childbirth. A retroperitoneal hemorrhage occurs after laceration of one of the branches of the hypogastric artery. Injury occurs typically during cesarean delivery or rarely after rupture of a low transverse uterine scar during labor. These hematomas may be large and may extend as far as the kidneys.

The symptoms of concealed bleeding depend on the size of the hematoma and the rate at which it forms. In some instances, abrupt hypotension may be the first sign of bleeding. The diagnosis of a retroperitoneal hematoma must be considered whenever a postpartum patient has an unexpected decrease in hematocrit or unexplained tachycardia and hypotension. Other signs and symptoms are restlessness, lower abdominal pain, a tender mass above the inguinal ligament that displaces a firm uterus to the contralateral side, and vaginal bleeding with hypotension out of proportion to the external blood loss. Ileus, unilateral leg edema, urinary retention, and hematuria also may occur.[85] Computed tomography may help determine the location and size of the hematoma. MRI is also useful in detecting the presence, location, and extent of suspected hematoma.[87]

Occasionally a retroperitoneal hematoma may be self-limiting and need no surgical intervention. Life-threatening hematomas require exploratory laparotomy and ligation of the hypogastric vessels. Fliegner[88] reported that 38 of 39 patients with a broad ligament hematoma received a blood transfusion. (The average amount administered was 4000 mL.) Eight (21%) of the patients required an abdominal hysterectomy.

ANESTHETIC MANAGEMENT

Choice of anesthetic technique for the repair of genital lacerations and evacuation of pelvic hematomas depends on the affected area, surgical requirements, physical status of the patient, and urgency of the procedure. Local infiltration and a small dose of intravenous opioid suffice for most vulvar hematomas. Repair of extensive lacerations and drainage of vaginal hematomas require significant levels of analgesia or anesthesia. Previously administered spinal or epidural anesthesia may have regressed. It may be inappropriate to initiate a neuraxial block again because it may cause hypotension in a hypovolemic patient. Pudendal nerve block may not be technically feasible because of anatomic distortion or severe pain from the hematoma. For a brief examination, nitrous oxide (40% to 50%) analgesia can be administered safely and effectively. The analgesia has a rapid onset and is easily reversible. The patient should remain awake and alert, with spontaneous ventilation. The major risk of inhalation analgesia is that the anesthetic depth may change insidiously, especially with previous administration of opioids or sedatives. Loss of laryngeal reflexes may occur, in which case the airway is unprotected. The anesthesia provider must maintain continual verbal contact with the patient. An alternative to nitrous oxide analgesia is ketamine. Low doses of ketamine (10-mg boluses, not exceeding a total dose of 0.5 mg/kg) are sufficient to produce sedation and analgesia and do not alter laryngeal reflexes. A nonparticulate antacid should be administered before administration of either nitrous oxide or ketamine.

Exploratory laparotomy for a retroperitoneal hematoma typically requires the administration of general anesthesia. A rapid-sequence induction is mandatory unless a difficult intubation is expected.

Retained Placenta

Retained placenta is defined as failure to deliver the placenta completely following delivery of the infant, and occurs in as many as 3.3% of deliveries.[89] In some cases, the placenta appears to separate but fragments of the placenta remain within the uterus. Retained placental fragments are a leading cause of both early and late postpartum hemorrhage. The risk of postpartum hemorrhage increases significantly when the interval between delivery of the infant and placental delivery is longer than 30 minutes.[89] The severity of bleeding ranges from minimal to severe, and can be life-threatening. It is difficult to assess the degree of blood loss, because visual estimates are often inaccurate.

OBSTETRIC MANAGEMENT

Treatment of retained placenta during the early postpartum period often involves manual removal and inspection of the placenta. After removal of the placenta, uterine tone should be enhanced with oxytocin, and the patient should be observed for evidence of recurrent hemorrhage. Umbilical venous administration of saline with oxytocin may be helpful in the management of patients with retained placenta.[90]

ANESTHETIC MANAGEMENT

Choice of anesthetic technique depends on the presence or absence of hemorrhage. In patients who are not actively bleeding and are hemodynamically stable, neuraxial anesthesia may be considered. This may be accomplished with either administration of additional local anesthetic through an existing labor epidural catheter or initiation of spinal anesthesia. In some cases, the administration of nitrous oxide (40% to 50%) is effective. An alternative is the administration of small doses of ketamine (10-mg boluses, not exceeding a total dose of 0.5 mg/kg) or fentanyl (50 to 100 μg). Often this is adequate to allow examination and manual placental extraction by a skilled obstetrician. Maintenance of protective airway reflexes is imperative. A nonparticulate antacid should be administered before the procedure.

In some cases, the obstetrician requests uterine relaxation to facilitate manual removal of the placenta. Historically, anesthesia providers have performed rapid-sequence induction of general anesthesia, followed by the administration of a high dose of volatile halogenated agent to relax the uterus. Equipotent doses of halothane, sevoflurane, and desflurane depress uterine contractility equally and in a dose-dependent manner.[91,92] (An equi-anesthetic concentration of isoflurane was a less effective uterine relaxant in a study of isolated human uterine muscle.[92]) Uterine contractility is decreased by 50% with administration of approximately 1.5 minimum alveolar concentration (MAC) of a volatile anesthetic agent. This technique results in a fast onset of uterine relaxation, and discontinuation of the volatile agent results in rapid offset when uterine relaxation is no longer necessary. However, induction of general anesthesia in a parturient entails a risk of failed intubation and/or aspiration.

In an attempt to avoid general anesthesia, many anesthesia providers currently advocate the administration of **nitroglycerin** for uterine relaxation. Nitroglycerin provides reliable smooth muscle relaxation, rapid onset, and a short plasma half-life (1 to 3 minutes).[93,94] Nitroglycerin has been administered for various obstetric emergencies without clinically significant side effects.[94,95] Peng et al.[96] demonstrated successful removal of a retained placenta in 15 parturients following administration of intravenous nitroglycerin 500 μg. DeSimone et al.[97] used a substantially smaller dose of nitroglycerin (50 to 100 μg) with similar results; all patients were managed successfully without the need for induction of general anesthesia and endotracheal intubation. Nitroglycerin may also be administered sublingually via spray or tablet. A prospective, double-blind, randomized, controlled study compared sublingual nitroglycerin with a placebo tablet.[98] All 12 of the parturients who received nitroglycerin successfully delivered their placenta within 5 minutes of administration, compared with only 1 of the 12 who received placebo. Nitroglycerin most likely produces uterine smooth muscle relaxation by releasing nitric oxide, and it may require the presence of placental tissue to be effective.[99]

Placenta Accreta

Placenta accreta is defined as an abnormally adherent placenta. Three types of placenta accreta may occur (Figure 37-4). **Placenta accreta vera** is defined as adherence to the myometrium without invasion of—or passage through—uterine muscle. **Placenta increta** represents invasion of the myometrium. **Placenta percreta** includes invasion of the uterine serosa or other pelvic structures.

EPIDEMIOLOGY

Evidence suggests that the incidence of placenta accreta is rising, primarily because of the increasing cesarean delivery rate.[12,100] The presence of a placenta previa is associated with a greater risk of placenta accreta (even in patients with no antepartum hemorrhage). The combination of one or more previous cesarean deliveries and a current placenta previa (or low-lying placenta) should prompt suspicion of placenta accreta. In a prospective multicenter observational study from academic health centers, Silver et al.[8] noted a 3% incidence of placenta accreta when placenta previa occurred in patients with an unscarred uterus; in patients

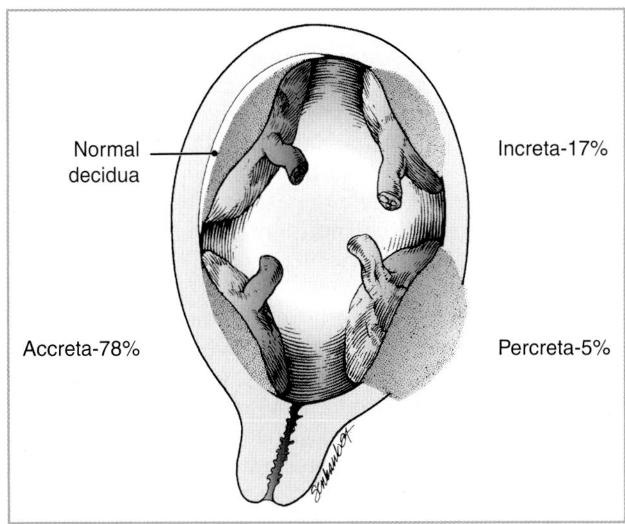

FIGURE 37-4 Uteroplacental relationships found in abnormal placentation. (From Benedetti TJ. Obstetric hemorrhage. In Gabbe SG, Niebyl JR, Simpson JL, editors. Obstetrics: Normal and Problem Pregnancies. 4th edition. New York, Churchill Livingstone, 2001:519.)

TABLE 37-4 Risk of Placenta Accreta in Patients with Current Placenta Previa: Relationship to Number of Prior Cesarean Deliveries

Number of Prior Cesarean Deliveries	% of Patients with Placenta Accreta
0	3
1	11
2	40
3	61
4 or more	67

Modified from Silver RM, Landon MB, Rouse DJ, et al. Maternal morbidity associated with multiple repeat cesarean deliveries. Obstet Gynecol 2006; 107:1226-32.

with one previous cesarean delivery, the incidence of placenta accreta was 11%. The incidence increased to 40% in patients with a history of two previous cesarean deliveries, and two thirds of the patients with placenta previa and four or more previous cesarean deliveries had a placenta accreta (Table 37-4). Patients with placenta previa and previous cesarean delivery are more likely to require cesarean hysterectomy.[8] Another study noted a relationship between the extent of uterine wall invasion and the number of previous cesarean deliveries.[101]

DIAGNOSIS

In some cases the condition is first suspected at vaginal delivery, when the obstetrician notes difficulty in separating the placenta. The definitive diagnosis is then made at laparotomy.

Antenatal diagnosis of placenta accreta facilitates effective planning. Improved imaging techniques allow an antenatal diagnosis of placenta accreta with greater frequency than in the past.[102] Clinicians should have a high index of suspicion for placenta accreta in patients with either a placenta previa or a low-lying placenta and a history of previous cesarean delivery. Ultrasonography is a useful screening tool in patients with placenta previa and previous cesarean delivery,[102] and is the primary imaging modality used for making the diagnosis of placenta accreta.[12] Some evidence suggests that MRI may also help confirm the diagnosis of placenta accreta and assess the extent of uterine wall invasion.[101] However, MRI is no more sensitive than ultrasonography for detecting placenta accreta, and is also more costly and less accessible.

Ultrasonographic and MRI findings may guide preparations for delivery.[101] However, operative management decisions should not be based solely on imaging study results.[85] In cases of suspected placenta accreta, the American College of Obstetricians and Gynecologists (ACOG)[52] has suggested that the following preparatory measures be taken:

- The patient should be counseled about the likelihood of hysterectomy and need for blood transfusion.
- A preoperative anesthesia consultation should be obtained.
- The location and timing of the delivery should be optimized to ensure availability of surgical personnel and equipment.
- Blood products, including clotting factors, should be available.
- Intraoperative blood salvage (cell saver) should be considered, if available (see later).

OBSTETRIC MANAGEMENT

Most patients with placenta accreta require hysterectomy. This condition is currently one of the two most common indications for peripartum hysterectomy; a prompt decision to proceed to hysterectomy without delay enhances the likelihood of an optimal outcome.[55] Attempts to separate and detach the placenta frequently result in massive hemorrhage. Therefore, in cases in which the diagnosis was made before delivery, the obstetrician may proceed directly to hysterectomy without attempting to separate the placenta. Unfortunately, some obstetricians have little or no experience with the performance of peripartum hysterectomy. The presence of two obstetricians for cesarean delivery in women at high risk for placental accreta is recommended. Blood loss in these cases can be substantial. The importance of delivering large amounts of blood products to the operating room quickly cannot be overstated.

Antenatal diagnosis utilizing ultrasonography and MRI may facilitate successful conservative management in some cases.[101] Two forms of conservative therapy have been described. In selected patients with a partial placenta accreta, small focal areas of placental invasion may be managed by curettage and oversewing. Alternatively, in some cases, the obstetrician has left the intact placenta *in situ* and closed the abdomen, and some patients treated in this way have subsequently had successful pregnancies.[103] Currently, this latter procedure is considered a high-risk approach that is seldom used in North America.

Preoperative internal iliac artery balloon placement has been advocated as a means to decrease blood loss and blood component requirements and to allow for a less bloody surgical field.[104] One case-control series described 39% smaller estimated blood loss, 52% smaller red cell transfusion volume, and shorter surgical times in the balloon occlusion group.[104] Other reports have not demonstrated any advantage to this technique, and ischemia of the lower extremities has been reported.[105,106] In one study, 3 of the 19 women who underwent prophylactic placement of an intravascular balloon catheter had a serious complication directly related to placement of the balloon catheter.[106]

Patients with placenta percreta may be at greatest risk for morbidity and mortality. O'Brien et al.[107] reported 109 cases of placenta percreta; 101 cases were managed surgically. Forty-four of the patients received more than 10 units of PRBCs, and eight of the patients died. Prophylactic measures (i.e., balloon occlusion and embolization of the internal iliac arteries) should be considered in patients with placenta percreta, especially when extensive extrauterine involvement is suspected.[108]

ANESTHETIC MANAGEMENT

Preoperative diagnosis of placentation abnormalities, especially those associated with substantial intraoperative blood loss, assists the anesthesia provider as to choice of anesthetic technique. Such knowledge is especially important with regard to patients with placenta percreta (as discussed earlier).

Uterine Inversion

EPIDEMIOLOGY

Uterine inversion, or the turning inside-out of all or part of the uterus, is a rare but potentially disastrous event during the peripartum period. Inversions may be acute or chronic, but only acute peripartum inversions involve the obstetric anesthesia provider. The reported incidence of this disorder varies widely, but acute peripartum inversions most likely occur in 1 in 5000 to 1 in 10,000 pregnancies. Maternal mortality secondary to uterine inversion is very uncommon in the Western world. The latest report of maternal mortality in the United Kingdom cited no maternal deaths secondary to hemorrhage from uterine inversion.[1]

Risk factors for uterine inversion include uterine atony, inappropriate fundal pressure, excessive umbilical cord traction, a short umbilical cord, and uterine anomalies. An abnormally implanted placenta (i.e., placenta accreta) may be first recognized when uterine inversion occurs.

DIAGNOSIS

Many cases of uterine inversion are obvious because of hemorrhage and a mass in the vagina, but others may not be readily apparent. Inversion should be suspected in all cases of postpartum hemorrhage and hypotension. Historically, obstetricians have stated that the shock is out of proportion to the blood loss, but an underestimation of obstetric hemorrhage is more likely. The uterine atony associated with uterine inversion contributes to ongoing blood loss. An incomplete inversion not protruding through the introitus is more likely to result in missed or delayed diagnosis.[85]

OBSTETRIC MANAGEMENT

Immediate replacement of the uterus, even prior to removal of the placenta, is the best treatment.[85] Once the uterus has been replaced, a firm, well-contracted uterus is desired. Oxytocin (20 to 30 U/L) should be infused initially, but additional drugs (e.g., 15-methyl prostaglandin $F_{2\alpha}$, methylergonovine) may be needed. Early diagnosis and prompt correction have greatly reduced the morbidity and mortality associated with uterine inversion.[85]

ANESTHETIC MANAGEMENT

In some cases, uterine tone precludes immediate replacement of the uterus, and uterine relaxation is needed before successful replacement can be performed. The ideal technique should produce rapid uterine relaxation with no side effects and should have a short duration to facilitate restoration of uterine tone after replacement. Administration of general anesthesia with a volatile halogenated agent is the most proven method for producing uterine relaxation. *Endotracheal intubation is mandatory.* Alternatively, some reports have described the use of terbutaline, magnesium sulfate, and organic nitrates to facilitate relaxation and reduction of the inverted uterus. The successful use of intravenous and sublingual nitroglycerin to facilitate relaxation and replacement of the uterus has been reported.[109,110] These anecdotal reports suggest that administration of nitroglycerin may obviate the need for general anesthesia.

Invasive Treatment Options

Regardless of the cause of obstetric hemorrhage, conservative measures may fail to control bleeding. In these cases, invasive procedures must be performed promptly to avoid severe morbidity and mortality. Options include uterine compression sutures, angiographic arterial embolization, uterine artery ligation, internal iliac artery ligation, intrauterine balloon tamponade, and hysterectomy. No randomized controlled trials have assessed the efficacy and safety of these options.[111]

Uterine compression sutures (e.g., B-Lynch) are most useful in cases of refractory uterine atony but have also been used in cases of retained placenta and coagulopathy.[112] Despite high enthusiasm for this procedure, which is performed at cesarean delivery or laparotomy, failure rates of up to 30% have been reported.[111,113] Placement of compression sutures may preserve fertility and may be a useful adjunct to other treatment options. These sutures can be placed quickly and safely by obstetricians of varying experience.

Angiographic arterial embolization is attractive because only local anesthesia is needed, and this procedure has been performed successfully in the presence of a coagulopathy. The uterine arteries, which are branches of the anterior trunk of the internal iliac arteries, provide the primary blood supply to the uterus. The ovarian arteries also make a sizable contribution to uterine blood flow during pregnancy. During angiography the radiologist can identify the vessels responsible for bleeding and embolize these vessels effectively with gelatin sponge pledgets (Gelfoam). The gelatin sponge is a temporary occlusive agent, and flow through these vessels returns over time, preserving both the uterus and fertility.[114] Published success rates in controlling hemorrhage with this approach are as high as 85% to 95%.[111,115] A small percentage of cases may require placement of a metallic coil in addition to gelatin sponges.[116]

In patients with postpartum hemorrhage, successful embolization requires rapid access to an angiography facility and a skilled interventional radiologist. The patient must be observed and monitored carefully while in the angiography suite. Frequently, logistic problems prevent physicians from using this effective technique to full advantage. A 2007 report described three patients with high risk for postpartum bleeding and a strong desire to avoid hysterectomy, whose cesarean deliveries were performed in the interventional radiology suite. After administration of epidural anesthesia, an interventional radiologist placed bilateral uterine artery balloon catheters, which were inflated after delivery in two of the three patients; in one patient, the radiologist also performed embolization of both uterine arteries using a Gelfoam preparation.[117] Given the increasing incidence of placenta accreta, some hospitals may consider the construction of at least one interventional radiology room that meets the size, infection control, and air circulation standards required for a standard operating room.[117]

Ischemic complications of embolization therapy have been reported, but the risk is reduced with use of selective techniques.[111,114] Nonetheless, some physicians have expressed concern about the risks associated with prophylactic placement of intravascular balloon catheters.[105,106] Greenberg et al.[105] stated that if prophylactic internal iliac artery balloon occlusion is used, "intense vascular surveillance is mandatory, and catheters ... should be removed at first opportunity." Further, they suggested that "a patient receiving epidural anesthesia with a balloon catheter should be admitted to a monitored unit for frequent pulse examinations."

Embolization therapy may not be successful if performed after arterial ligation. If embolization fails, options such as arterial ligation and hysterectomy remain.

Bilateral surgical ligation of the uterine, ovarian, and internal iliac arteries may be useful when other measures have failed; surgical ligation permits preservation of fertility when successful. The decrease in pulse pressure distal to the ligature may allow normal hemostatic mechanisms to function. Reported success rates are highly variable, and it appears that internal iliac arterial ligation is being used less often than in the past.[52] Engorgement of pelvic viscera, variability in vascular anatomy, and the increased blood flow during pregnancy increase the risks when this approach is used. Lower extremity ischemia and neuropathy have been reported. Bilateral uterine artery ligation (O'Leary sutures) may be less time consuming and require less surgical expertise than internal iliac arterial ligation.[111] A systematic review noted that the aggregate success rate of ligation therapy was 85% in more than 500 cases.[111] Failure to arrest hemorrhage with this technique may occur in the presence of a rich collateral circulation.[118] Administration of anesthesia for arterial ligation should include preparations for possible hysterectomy (see later).

Intrauterine balloon tamponade is another conservative method for controlling postpartum hemorrhage, especially when uterine atony is suspected.[52,113] Published reports have described a success rate (i.e., avoidance of hysterectomy) as high as 80%.[111,113,119] A variety of devices have been used successfully, and a balloon specifically designed for this purpose is now available.[119] An intrauterine balloon can be deployed quickly, requires minimal analgesia for both insertion and removal, and preserves fertility; failed attempts can be identified quickly.[111] Although intrauterine balloon tamponade has not been proven superior to other methods of controlling postpartum uterine bleeding, its simplicity and lack of significant complications make it an attractive early option in some practice settings.[111]

Cesarean or **postpartum hysterectomy** is often the definitive treatment for postpartum hemorrhage. The two most common indications for this procedure are uterine atony and placenta accreta.[55,120] Peripartum hysterectomy is a technically challenging operation; the uterus is enlarged, the vessels are engorged, exposure may be difficult, and tissues are edematous. Emergency obstetric hysterectomy is associated with increased blood loss. A multicenter review showed that the average blood loss for emergency obstetric hysterectomy was 2526 mL, with an average transfusion requirement of 6.6 units of PRBCs; in elective procedures, the mean blood loss was 1319 mL, and the average replacement was 1.6 units of PRBCs (Table 37-5).[121] A more recent single-center review of 18 emergency peripartum hysterectomies reported a 61% incidence of complications, which included cardiac arrest, pulmonary edema, sepsis, bladder injury, and DIC.[120] The mean transfusion requirement was 10.7 units of PRBCs. In a 13-year review of emergency peripartum hysterectomies, the mean transfusion requirement was 10.1 units of PRBCs for *total* hysterectomy, compared with 6.3 units of PRBCs for *subtotal* hysterectomy.[122] (Total hysterectomy refers to removal of the entire uterus—*not* the ovaries. With a subtotal hysterectomy, the cervix is left *in situ*.) Both surgical techniques have been used successfully in patients with severe postpartum bleeding.

ANESTHETIC MANAGEMENT

Anesthesia for peripartum hysterectomy is frequently challenging. An experienced, skilled team is invaluable during this difficult operation. In emergency cases, massive blood loss can be expected, and large amounts of crystalloid and blood products will likely be needed. General anesthesia should be strongly considered for all patients that require hysterectomy after *vaginal* delivery, even in patients who still have a labor epidural catheter in place. In these cases, all the considerations noted for patients with antepartum hemorrhage should be applied (as discussed earlier). The degree of intravascular volume deficit may be underestimated, and care should be taken in the selection and dosing of induction agents. A second anesthesia provider can be a valuable asset to help operate infusion devices, cross-check blood products, and establish additional vascular access.

If hemorrhage complicates cesarean delivery in a patient with spinal or epidural anesthesia, the anesthesia provider may need to administer general anesthesia to protect the patient's airway. However, an early decision by the obstetrician to proceed with a relatively controlled hysterectomy may obviate the need for general anesthesia, provided that severe hypotension does not occur and the patient remains alert and comfortable. Single-shot spinal anesthesia given for labor is unlikely to provide anesthesia of sufficient duration for the added procedure (hysterectomy), so general anesthesia may be required.

Controversy exists regarding the type of anesthesia that should be administered to the patient who is scheduled for elective cesarean hysterectomy or who is at high risk for emergency hysterectomy during elective cesarean delivery (e.g., the patient with placenta previa, no preoperative bleeding, and a history of two or more previous cesarean deliveries). In a multi-institutional study of peripartum hysterectomy, none of the 12 patients who received continuous epidural anesthesia for elective or emergency hysterectomy required intraoperative induction of general anesthesia.[121] Options for neuraxial anesthesia include continuous spinal anesthesia, combined spinal-epidural anesthesia, and continuous epidural anesthesia. Intraperitoneal manipulation, dissection, and traction may exceed those maneuvers required with cesarean delivery alone, leading to pain, nausea, and vomiting. Maintenance of a T4 sensory level of anesthesia and judicious sedation may reduce the need for intraoperative conversion to general anesthesia.

Most anesthesia providers do not withhold neuraxial anesthesia from normovolemic women undergoing elective, repeat cesarean delivery for placenta previa, despite the risk for placenta accreta and emergency hysterectomy in these

TABLE 37-5 Operative Management and Complications of Elective versus Emergency Obstetric Hysterectomies

	Elective (n = 21)	Emergency (n = 21)	*P*
Anesthesia			
Epidural	8	4	
Spinal	0	1	
General	13	16	
Operative time (min)*	137 ± 55	148 ± 62	NS
Hysterectomy			
Total	21	19	NS
Subtotal	0	2	
Estimated blood loss (mL)*	1319 ± 396	2526 ± 1240	<.001
Intraoperative hypotension	6 (29%)	13 (62%)	<.05
Intraoperative crystalloid (mL)*	4062 ± 1512	5374 ± 2340	<.05
Intraoperative transfusion	7 (33%)	17 (81%)	<.01
Intraoperative or postoperative transfusion	10 (48%)	18 (86%)	<.01
Total units transfused*	1.6 ± 1.9	6.6 ± 5.4	<.001
Discharge hematocrit (%)*	30 ± 4	30 ± 4	NS
Intraoperative injury			
Ureteral	1 (5%)	0	NS
Cystotomy	1 (5%)	0	NS
Reoperation required	0	1 (5%)	NS
Days in hospital*	5.5 ± 1.3	7.3 ± 4.3	<.05
Mortality	0	0	NS

NS, not significant.

*Mean ± SD.

Modified from Chestnut DH, Dewan DM, Redick LF, et al. Anesthetic management for obstetric hysterectomy: A multi-institutional study. Anesthesiology 1989; 70:607-10.

women.[52] However, patients should be informed that severe hemorrhage typically mandates intraoperative administration of general anesthesia so that the airway may be secured.

The presence of a known placenta percreta may greatly increase the risk for significant bleeding, even in comparison with placenta accreta. For these cases, general anesthesia may be preferred. However, if prophylactic bilateral internal iliac (uterine) artery balloon catheters have been placed preoperatively, it may be reasonable to administer neuraxial anesthesia in carefully selected patients.

Regardless of the anesthetic technique used, two large-gauge intravenous catheters should be inserted, and at least four units of PRBCs should be immediately available, with additional blood products readily available without delay. The ACOG recommends consideration of intraoperative blood salvage (cell saver) in cases of placenta accreta (see later).[123] Vasoactive drugs (e.g., phenylephrine, dopamine, epinephrine) should be available. Invasive blood pressure monitoring is suggested, as is the presence of a skilled assistant. A fluid warmer, a forced-air body warmer, and equipment for rapid infusion of fluids and blood products must be readily available when one is anticipating and managing significant blood loss. Teamwork and precise communication are important.

TRANSFUSION THERAPY

Despite advances in the prevention, diagnosis, and treatment of the hemorrhagic complications of pregnancy, the potential for massive blood loss remains a threat. All physicians who provide care for pregnant women should understand the indications, requirements, risks, and benefits of transfusion.

Concerns about blood-borne infectious disease have led to a reevaluation of the indications for and appropriateness of red blood cell (RBC) transfusion, particularly during the peripartum period. Silverman et al.,[124] in a review of 33,795 obstetric-related admissions from 1994 to 2002, found that 0.65% of admitted women received a transfusion. Postpartum hemorrhage was the most common reason for transfusion. Using institutional transfusion guidelines, the investigators concluded that 31.8% of all PRBC transfusions were not appropriate. Despite a definite trend toward more conservative transfusion practices, some parturients will require blood products. Rouse et al.[125] performed a multicenter prospective observational study of approximately 57,000 women undergoing cesarean delivery between 1999 and 2002; 3.2% and 2.2% of patients undergoing primary and repeat cesarean delivery, respectively, required perioperative blood transfusion.

The 2006 American Society of Anesthesiologists (ASA) Practice Guidelines for Perioperative Blood Transfusion state that RBC transfusion is usually unnecessary in patients with a hemoglobin concentration of 10 g/dL or greater, and that RBCs should usually be administered when the hemoglobin concentration is less than 6 g/dL.[126] However, these guidelines must be tailored to the individual patient. In many cases, oxygen delivery is maintained with a low hemoglobin concentration as long as the patient is normovolemic. As the RBC mass decreases, both blood viscosity and resistance to blood flow also markedly drop. These changes lead to an increase in cardiac output and tissue blood flow without a concomitant increase in cardiovascular work. Tissue oxygen delivery is maintained despite the reduced RBC mass. Although anecdotal evidence and case reports suggest that maternal well-being and perinatal outcome are not altered by mild anemia, the higher metabolic rate during pregnancy suggests that the pregnant patient may have less tolerance for the additional cardiovascular stress of severe anemia. The minimum hemoglobin concentration required to sustain a normal pregnancy has not been clearly defined. However, transfusion should be considered in all obstetric patients with clinical evidence of inadequate oxygen-carrying capacity and in most obstetric patients with a hemoglobin concentration less than 7 g/dL. Likewise, ongoing blood loss should prompt the anesthesia provider to begin transfusion in some patients with a hemoglobin concentration greater than 7 g/dL.

The need to obtain an admission blood type and screen for all parturients is controversial. Some clinicians suggest that this test is not necessary in patients with no identifiable risk factors for peripartum hemorrhage. Ransom et al.[127] found that only 0.8 per 1000 low-risk patients undergoing cesarean delivery required a blood transfusion. They concluded that a routine type and screen in low-risk patients is not cost-effective. However, many anesthesia providers believe that the potential need for transfusion and the occasional patient who develops an antibody from fetal antigen exposure during pregnancy warrant the performance of a type and screen. The ASA Practice Guidelines for Obstetric Anesthesia support this recommendation.[128]

It is not necessary for all parturients to undergo a type and cross-match. However, it is prudent to obtain a cross-match for those patients with risk factors for bleeding.[128] Risk factors associated with the need for transfusion in patients undergoing cesarean delivery are preoperative anemia, previous cesarean delivery, placenta previa, abnormal presentation, multiple gestation, chorioamnionitis, placental abruption, preeclampsia, and the HELLP (hemolysis, elevated liver enzymes, low platelet count) syndrome.[125] In addition, patients with a positive antibody screen result should undergo cross-matching, because there could be a delay in obtaining blood for them. If blood is required quickly and the results of antibody screening are not available, the safest option is administration of ABO- and Rh-specific blood. If the blood type is unknown and blood is required immediately, type O Rh-negative blood can be administered.

Autologous Transfusion

The potential advantages of autologous blood transfusion include avoiding the risks of alloimmunization, hemolytic reactions, and viral transmission; reduction of demands on the blood supply; and the psychological benefits to patients of participation in their treatment. The three methods of autologous transfusion are (1) preoperative (antepartum) donation, (2) normovolemic hemodilution, and (3) intraoperative blood salvage. Antepartum donation and normovolemic hemodilution are blood conservation techniques that have been used when blood loss was anticipated before surgery.

ANTEPARTUM DONATION

Although the concept of preoperative autologous donation is not new, the risks of blood-borne infection from donor blood made antepartum donation a popular procedure in the late 1980s and 1990s. In 1992, well over 1 million autologous units of blood were donated prior to elective surgery.[129] Using this technique, a patient may donate up to 4 units of blood preoperatively, which will have a shelf-life of about 35 days. If a perioperative blood transfusion is needed, the patient may then receive one or all of these precollected units. This technique does not have a role in emergency hemorrhage and is useful only in situations in which massive blood loss is anticipated. Therefore, it may be useful in women with a known placenta previa or accreta who will undergo elective cesarean delivery or in patients with a rare blood type for whom there may be great difficulty in locating blood for transfusion. The standards of the American Association of Blood Banks state that the patient's hemoglobin and hematocrit levels should be at least 11 g/dL and 33%, respectively, before donation; these thresholds would exclude some pregnant patients with physiologic or iron deficiency anemia. Some physicians have suggested that a predonation hemoglobin and hematocrit of 10 g/dL and 30%, respectively, are acceptable for pregnant women. However, most published studies of pregnant patients have required a predonation hematocrit of at least 34%.[130-132]

Andres et al.[130] cautioned that antepartum donation by obstetric patients may not be justified. They stated that the commonly accepted risk factors for postpartum hemorrhage and transfusion do not permit physicians to identify correctly the patients who will require blood transfusion and that many patients who donate blood will not require a transfusion. The investigators identified 251 patients with traditionally accepted risk factors for postpartum bleeding, including (1) repeat cesarean delivery, (2) multiple gestation, and (3) placenta previa. Only 4 (1.6%) of these patients required blood transfusion. The investigators suggested that preoperative donation is not beneficial or cost-effective because of the low frequency of blood transfusion in high-risk patients and the difficulty in correctly identifying the patients likely to require transfusion. In addition, their data showed that the transfusion of a single unit of blood is uncommon. Among patients who required transfusion, 12 of 13 (92%) needed more than one unit of RBCs. Many obstetric patients are unable to donate more than one unit of blood. Thus it is likely that homologous blood would be required in addition to autologous transfusion. Preoperative autologous donation therapy is not recommended for nonpregnant patients undergoing uncomplicated hysterectomy,[133] and it has limited use in obstetric practice.

NORMOVOLEMIC HEMODILUTION

The potential advantages of normovolemic hemodilution include (1) no wastage of collected blood, (2) the ability to transfuse fresh blood with active coagulation factors and platelets, and (3) little risk of storage or clerical errors. Limited experience with this technique exists in obstetric practice.[134,135] Grange et al.[135] employed normovolemic hemodilution before cesarean delivery in 38 women at increased risk for significant blood loss (e.g., placenta previa). The investigators collected 500 to 1000 mL of blood from each patient, and the collected blood was re-infused at the end of surgery or earlier, if required. They observed no maternal or fetal complications during or after phlebotomy. One patient also received homologous blood, and 14 patients received previously donated autologous blood. However, as with preoperative autologous donation, evidence does not support the use of normovolemic hemodilution as an effective strategy for avoiding allogeneic transfusion.[136]

INTRAOPERATIVE BLOOD SALVAGE

Intraoperative blood salvage or autotransfusion is a technique of scavenging blood lost during surgery, processing it by centrifugation and washing, and transfusing the scavenged, autologous RBCs.[137] RBCs that are salvaged, processed, and transfused have an excellent survival rate. This procedure, which can rapidly provide large quantities of autologous blood, is widely used in cardiovascular and general surgery and is acceptable to many Jehovah's Witness patients. Many authorities advocate this technique as a potential solution to the worsening shortage of banked blood, increased cost of allogeneic blood transfusion, and concern about transfusion-related infections and clerical errors.[138] Fong et al.[139] have suggested that the use of intraoperative blood salvage might reduce exposure to allogeneic blood in almost half of obstetric patients who require transfusion and might eliminate exposure to allogeneic blood altogether in 14% to 25% of patients.

Malignancy, infection, the presence of old hemolyzed blood, and the use of collagen or hemostatic material are relative contraindications to the use of intraoperative blood salvage. In the past, the use of intraoperative blood salvage in obstetric patients has been limited, in part, by concern that blood processing and washing may not adequately remove amniotic fluid and fetal debris and that transfusion might precipitate amniotic fluid embolism. Studies of *in vitro* washing of scavenged maternal blood mixed with amniotic fluid showed elimination (or greatly reduced concentrations) of alpha-fetoprotein, phospholipids, tissue factor, fetal squamous cells, and other cellular debris.[140,141] The best-washed product for transfusion results from the addition of a leukocyte depletion filter to the system. Even with this added filter, the washed blood is likely to contain fetal RBCs.[140,141] Therefore, isoimmunization of the mother is possible, and anti-D immune globulin should be administered when appropriate. Suction of blood into the cell-washing system should be initiated only after delivery of the infant and the placenta.

In most published obstetric cases, the total volume of transfused salvaged blood was small. In a randomized study of women undergoing cesarean delivery, Rainaldi et al.[142] observed that 34 patients who underwent intraoperative salvage and re-infusion of autologous blood (mean ± SD volume = 363 ± 153 mL) required fewer transfusions of homologous blood and had a shorter hospital stay than a control group. Rebarber et al.[143] performed a retrospective, multicenter study of 139 patients in whom autologous blood transfusion was performed during cesarean delivery between 1988 and 1997. The range of autotransfused volumes was 200 to 11,250 mL. The investigators identified no cases of acute respiratory distress syndrome or amniotic fluid embolism, and they identified no higher incidence of other complications (e.g., DIC) in these patients than in 87 control patients who underwent similar surgical procedures without autotransfusion at the same hospitals.

Advocates of intraoperative blood salvage in obstetric patients argue that amniotic fluid embolism is not an embolic disease but rather is an *anaphylactoid syndrome*. This argument implies that this rare but devastating complication would occur with or without the use of cell salvage, given the fact that amniotic fluid is routinely entrained at the time of delivery.[144] On the other hand, Santrach[145] has offered the following counterarguments: (1) in obstetrics, significant hemorrhage that would benefit from blood salvage is uncommon and often unexpected; (2) because of the low utilization of blood salvage procedures in obstetric practice, ongoing operator (user) competency may be problematic and the risk for error is increased; and (3) the number of patients studied to date is not sufficient to detect adverse events.

Allam et al.[146] reviewed the use of cell salvage in obstetrics and noted that documented use of cell salvage in obstetric patients is limited; at the time of their review (published in 2008), approximately 400 published cases had been reported. They concluded that "no single serious complication leading to poor maternal outcome has been directly attributed to its use." However, they acknowledged that "well-designed large prospective studies to evaluate . . . the balance of clinical effectiveness and safety of cell salvage are clearly needed before wider application in obstetrics."[146]

Intraoperative blood salvage during cesarean delivery is widely regarded as safe in the United Kingdom[138] and is gaining acceptance in the United States, although its practical utility remains a matter of some dispute. The ACOG has stated that in cases of suspected placenta accreta, "cell saver technology should be considered if available."[52] The revised ASA Practice Guidelines for Obstetric Anesthesia recommend that "in cases of intractable hemorrhage when banked blood is not available or the patient refuses banked blood, intraoperative cell salvage should be considered if available."[147] Waters et al.,[148] who performed an economic assessment of the use of cell salvage in obstetrics, noted that its cost-effectiveness may depend, in part, on an institution's case volume.

Because no clear etiology of amniotic fluid embolism has been defined, it seems prudent to limit the use of intraoperative blood salvage to situations in which lifesaving blood transfusion is necessary and banked blood is insufficient or unavailable. Cell salvage may also be indicated for consenting Jehovah's Witness patients who have a major risk factor for hemorrhage (i.e., placenta accreta) and who would otherwise refuse blood product administration. Use of a leukocyte depletion filter may enhance the margin of safety.[140,141]

Treatment of Massive Blood Loss

Postpartum hemorrhage is responsible for 127,000 maternal deaths every year worldwide.[1,49] Early recognition and treatment may prevent this tragic outcome. Successful resuscitation requires adequate intravenous access, aggressive volume replacement with crystalloid or colloid solution, and, on occasion, the administration of large volumes of blood and coagulation factors. In previously healthy parturients, blood pressure may remain near normal until blood loss exceeds 1500 mL. Blood is shifted from venous capacitance vessels to the central circulation by peripheral and splanchnic vasoconstriction. In the initial resuscitation of hemorrhage, warmed non–dextrose-containing crystalloid (e.g., lactated Ringer's solution, normal saline) and colloid solution (e.g., hydroxyethyl starch) are acceptable choices for volume replacement. The crystalloid volume administered should be three times that of the estimated blood loss. When blood replacement therapy is indicated, whole blood would be an ideal choice for maintaining intravascular volume, but few donor units are kept as whole blood in the modern blood bank. The high demand for blood components such as platelets, fresh frozen plasma (FFP), and cryoprecipitate is a major reason that more than 90% of donor blood is fractionated into blood components. **Blood component therapy** provides the patient with only those products that are required and helps extend the shelf-life of each component. Components and derivatives from one unit of blood can be used to treat several patients. A summary of commonly administered blood products is shown in Table 37-6.

RBC units are prepared by removing plasma from whole blood and replacing it with additives to improve red cell survival. This process results in 300 mL of volume with a hematocrit of 70%. Transfusion of one unit of PRBCs increases the hematocrit by approximately 3 percentage points.[149] PRBCs are packaged with preservatives and anticoagulant (citrate, phosphate, dextrose, and adenine) and have a 42-day shelf-life.

A unit of **fresh frozen plasma** has a volume of approximately 250 mL and contains all necessary coagulation factors. Transfusion of FFP is indicated when replacement of coagulation factors is necessary to achieve hemostasis after massive transfusion or in the presence of DIC. Administration of FFP should also be considered when urgent reversal of warfarin is desired and for correction of microvascular bleeding in the presence of a prothrombin time (PT) more than 1.5 times normal or an international normalized ratio (INR) greater than 2.0, and/or an activated partial thromboplastin time (aPTT) more than 2 times normal.[126,149] FFP should not be used to treat hypovolemia or as a protein supplement. One unit of FFP per 20 kg of body weight (or 10 to 15 mL/kg) is an appropriate initial dose.[126,149] The prophylactic use of FFP has not proved to be effective in decreasing blood loss in patients at risk for massive blood loss.[150]

Cryoprecipitate is prepared from thawed FFP and contains factor VIII, fibrinogen, fibronectin, von Willebrand factor, and factor XIII. It is most often used for congenital or acquired deficiencies in fibrinogen and factor XIII, and to treat von Willebrand disease. Administration of 10 bags of cryoprecipitate (10 to 15 mL per bag) will increase the fibrinogen level 65 to 70 mg/dL.[149]

A number of reports have described the administration of **recombinant activated factor VII** (**rFVIIa** [NovoSeven]) for hemorrhage unresponsive to conventional blood product resuscitation. A synthetic vitamin K–dependent glycoprotein, rFVIIa aids in hemostasis via activation of the extrinsic pathway of the coagulation cascade. It was introduced in 1988 for use in patients with hemophilia A and B that was unresponsive to traditional factor replacement owing to a high level of circulating antibodies. Currently the only licensed indications for its use are for treatment of hemophilia A or B, factor VII deficiency, and Glanzmann's thrombasthenia.[151]

Several reports have described off-label use of rFVIIa in the treatment of postpartum hemorrhage.[152-154] Franchini et al.[155] reviewed 65 case reports of rFVIIa administration for postpartum hemorrhage from 1998 to 2006. The most common etiology of postpartum hemorrhage was

TABLE 37-6 Characteristics of Blood Components

Component	Dose	Volume per Dose	Shelf Life	Storage Conditions	Expected Response
Packed red blood cells	1 unit	250-325 mL	21-42 days	1° C to 6° C	1 g/dL increase in hemoglobin concentration
Fresh frozen plasma	Factor replacement: 10-15 mL/kg	200 mL	Frozen: 1 yr Thawed: 24 hr	Frozen: ≤ −18° C Thawed: 1° C to 10° C	Correction of prothrombin time/activated partial thromboplastin time/international normalized ratio by replacement of coagulation factors
Platelets	4-6 units of pooled whole blood–derived platelets or one unit of pheresis platelets	200-250 mL	5 days	20° C to 24° C with continuous and gentle agitation	Increase in platelet count of 30,000-60,000/mm^3
Cryoprecipitate	10 pooled units	100 mL	Frozen: 1 yr Thawed/pooled: 4 hr	Frozen: ≤ −18° C Thawed: 1° C to 10° C	Increases in levels of fibrinogen, von Willebrand factor, factor VIII, factor XIII

Modified from Sanford K, Roseff S. A surgeon's guide to blood banking and transfusion medicine. In Spiess BD, Spence RK, Shander A, editors. Perioperative Transfusion Medicine, 2nd edition. Philadelphia, Lippincott Williams & Wilkins, 2006:179-98.

uterine atony. Among women without congenital factor VII deficiency, the mean dose was 72.9 μg/kg; 73% of women required only a single dose to achieve effective hemostasis. In the largest case series to date, Ahonen and Jokela[152] reported that 11 of 12 parturients with major postpartum hemorrhage responded to rFVIIa administration in doses of 42 to 116 μg/kg; in 5 of these women, hysterectomy was performed before rFVIIa administration. The investigators also observed a significant decrease in units of blood product administered.[152] The dose and frequency of rFVIIa administration for this off-label use are undefined. Review of the literature reveals a wide variation in the dose of rFVIIa administered.[155] In some case reports, the dose was repeated to achieve hemostasis.

Use of rFVIIa should not replace the aggressive use of uterotonic agents, conventional blood product administration, or lifesaving procedures such as arterial ligation, embolization, and hysterectomy. Replacement of blood, platelets, and coagulation factors is paramount to successful treatment. In addition, maintenance of normothermia and correction of acidosis are necessary for optimal rFVIIa activity. There is concern that rFVIIa may increase the likelihood of thromboembolic events.[156] Given the unanswered questions about adverse effects and the high cost of preparation, rFVIIa is not recommended for routine use in obstetric practice. The exact role of rFVIIa as a rescue agent remains undefined. However, ASA guidelines recommend consideration of rFVIIa when "traditional well tested options for treating microvascular bleeding (i.e., coagulopathy) have been exhausted."[126]

Platelets are difficult to store, and inventories in most blood banks are low. One unit of donor platelets increases the platelet count from 5000 to 10,000/mm^3 in the average adult woman. The blood bank typically provides platelets from an ABO- and Rh-compatible donor, although ABO compatibility is not essential.[149] Platelet transfusion may be necessary after massive blood transfusion secondary to a dilutional thrombocytopenia. Patients with dilutional thrombocytopenia often do not have clinical bleeding, even with a low platelet count. A patient undergoing a surgical procedure, including vaginal delivery, is unlikely to benefit from a platelet transfusion unless her platelet count is less than 50,000/mm^3. In nonbleeding patients, a transfusion trigger of 20,000/mm^3 has traditionally been suggested, although many clinicians prefer to give the transfusion before the platelet count drops that low.[157]

A coagulopathy can develop rapidly in the obstetric patient. It may be either a dilutional coagulopathy or true DIC. **Dilutional coagulopathy** results from the replacement of blood loss with crystalloid and PRBCs, which dilutes concentrations of coagulation factors and platelets. Treatment consists of FFP and platelet replacement. Sustained hemorrhagic shock may also lead to DIC, resulting in worsening hemorrhage.[158] Additional pregnancy-related causes of DIC include amniotic fluid embolism, placental abruption, uterine infection, and intrauterine fetal demise.[158]

Confirmatory laboratory tests (e.g., platelet count, PT, aPTT, measurement of fibrinogen concentration and fibrin split products) are required to diagnose coagulopathy. With coagulation factor replacement, the coagulation factor activity need be only 25% of normal to achieve hemostasis. One unit of FFP increases coagulation factor levels by 8%.[149] Cryoprecipitate is indicated in bleeding patients with a fibrinogen level less than 80 to 100 mg/dL, and platelets are indicated when the platelet count is less than 50,000/mm^3. Blood component therapy should be guided by frequent measurements of coagulation parameters. Care must be taken to prevent hypothermia, which often occurs as a result of massive hemorrhage and fluid resuscitation. Hypothermia worsens coagulopathy and increases the risk for cardiac dysrhythmias.

Complications of Transfusion of Blood Products

Transfusion-related complications can be broadly classified as infectious, immunologic, storage-related, and clerical error. The risk of viral transmission due to allogeneic blood transfusion continues to decrease with good donor screening and use of nucleic acid amplification testing (nucleic acid technology [NAT]).[159]

The residual risk of viral transmission after both NAT and serologic testing of donor blood is 1 in 2 million for both human immunodeficiency virus (HIV) and hepatitis C virus (HCV).[160] This is a 10-fold lower risk for HCV transmission than with serologic testing alone. NAT is not routinely used to test for hepatitis B virus (HBV). Donor screening for HB surface antigen (HBsAg) and anti-HBc antibody have greatly reduced the risk of transmission of HBV.[159] The first case of West Nile virus transmitted via a blood transfusion was identified in 2002; since 2003, routine blood screening has been implemented, virtually eliminating this risk.[159] In addition, there have been case reports of transfusion-transmitted Creutzfeldt-Jakob disease. Owing to the long incubation period of this virus, symptoms may not be evident for several years after transfusion.[161]

Cytomegalovirus (CMV) infection may occur as a result of blood transfusion.[162] The virus is carried in the monocytes of asymptomatic donors. Most of these infections are asymptomatic or mild, but infection in the immunocompromised patient and transmission to the fetus can have serious sequelae. The transmission rate may be as high as 30% without preventive techniques. This risk is reduced to 1.3% if seronegative blood is used.[163] Use of leukodepleted red blood cells (latent CMV lives in white blood cells) reduces the risk to approximately 2.5%.[164] In 2000, a Canadian Consensus Conference concluded that these two methods of preventing post-transfusion CMV infection can be used interchangeably.[162] However, because congenitally acquired infection can produce severe infection in some infants, pregnant women should receive blood that is both leukodepleted and seronegative. The presence of yet unknown viruses will continue to present challenges for the field of transfusion medicine.

More common adverse events related to transfusion are bacterial contamination, transfusion-related acute lung injury, and hemolytic transfusion reactions.[126] **Bacterial contamination** of blood products is the leading cause of transfusion-related death. Because platelets may undergo conformational changes at temperatures below 18° C, they are stored at 20° C to 24° C. A warmer storage temperature increases the risk of bacterial proliferation.[126] In 2004, the American Association of Blood Banks mandated testing of all platelets for bacterial contamination. Use of culture-negative platelets has resulted in a reduction in the risk of septic transfusion to 1 in 75,000.[165]

Transfusion-related acute lung injury (TRALI) is noncardiogenic pulmonary edema that results from immune reactivity of leukocyte antibodies a few hours after transfusion. Treatment involves discontinuation of the transfusion and institution of critical care supportive measures.[126]

Transfusion reactions are most commonly caused by accidental administration of ABO incompatible blood.[149] **Acute intravascular hemolysis** typically results in fever, chills, nausea, flushing, and chest and flank pain. These symptoms are masked by general anesthesia. Signs that may manifest during general anesthesia include hypotension, tachycardia, DIC, and hemoglobinuria.[126] Immediate supportive care should consist of discontinuation of the transfusion, treatment of hypotension and hyperkalemia, administration of a diuretic, and alkalinization of the urine. Assays for urine and plasma hemoglobin concentration and antibody screening confirm the diagnosis. A second cross-match must be performed.

The biochemical and additional changes that occur during blood storage can lead to problems in the recipient, particularly when blood is infused rapidly. Plasma potassium concentration increases in stored blood. Transfused potassium usually moves intracellularly or is excreted in the urine.[149] However, rapid infusion of multiple units can lead to **hyperkalemia,** particularly in the hypothermic, acidotic patient. Blood maintained at 4° C also can contribute to **hypothermia,** especially if the patient is anesthetized in a cold operating room. If the temperature of the patient's blood is less than 30° C, ventricular irritability and cardiac arrest may occur.

The decreased pH of stored blood is caused by the addition of citrate-phosphate-dextrose and the accumulation of lactic and pyruvic acids as a result of RBC metabolism and glycolysis. Despite the lower pH, transfusion of large amounts of stored blood rarely causes acidosis as long as tissue perfusion remains normal.[149]

The anticoagulant used for blood collection and storage contains **citrate,** which binds ionized calcium. Citrate is rapidly metabolized in the liver and typically does not lead to significant hypocalcemia. In patients who are cold, who have liver disease, or who require rapid infusion of multiple units of blood, however, citrate may accumulate and cause a decrease in ionized calcium. The **hypocalcemia** results in reduced cardiac contractility, hypotension, and elevated central venous pressure.

KEY POINTS

- The visual estimate of vaginal bleeding often does not reflect the extent of intravascular volume deficit in patients with peripartum bleeding.
- Antepartum hemorrhage represents a greater threat to the fetus than to the mother.
- Uterine atony is the most common cause of postpartum hemorrhage.
- Aggressive drug therapy, including oxytocin, ergot alkaloids, and prostaglandins (carboprost, misoprostol), should be given in cases of severe uterine atony.
- The incidence of placenta accreta is increasing as a result of the higher cesarean delivery rate.
- A history of previous cesarean delivery and current placenta previa increase the risk for placenta accreta.
- Patients with placenta accreta are at high risk for severe postpartum hemorrhage.
- Uterine atony and placenta accreta are the two most common indications for peripartum hysterectomy.
- Prophylactic placement of internal iliac artery balloon catheters by an interventional radiologist may decrease blood loss and morbidity when patients with known placenta accreta are to undergo cesarean delivery.
- Assessment of urine output and laboratory studies (hemoglobin measurement, arterial blood gas analysis) should be used to assess intravascular volume deficits and guide fluid and blood replacement therapy.
- Arterial ligation, uterine compression sutures, and embolization therapy may reduce the need for peripartum hysterectomy.
- Recombinant activated factor VII therapy is expensive, and its safety and efficacy have not been fully evaluated in the treatment of obstetric hemorrhage.

REFERENCES

1. Liston W. Haemorrhage. In Lewis G, editor. The Confidential Enquiry into Maternal and Child Health (CEMACH): Saving Mothers' Lives: Reviewing Maternal Deaths to Make Motherhood Safer—2003-2005. The Seventh Report of the Confidential Enquiries into Maternal Deaths in the United Kingdom. London, CEMACH, 2007:78-85.
2. Heinonen S, Tyrväinen E, Saarikoski S, Ruokonen E. Need for maternal critical care in obstetrics: A population-based analysis. Int J Obstet Anesth 2002; 11:260-4.
3. Bose P, Regan F, Paterson-Brown S. Improving the accuracy of estimated blood loss at obstetric haemorrhage using clinical reconstructions. Br J Obstet Gynaecol 2006; 113:919-24.
4. Axelsen SM, Henriksen TB, Hedegaard M, Secher NJ. Characteristics of vaginal bleeding during pregnancy. Eur J Obstet Gynecol Reprod Biol 1995; 63:131-4.
5. Crane JM, van den Hof MC, Dodds L, et al. Neonatal outcomes with placenta previa. Obstet Gynecol 1999; 93:541-4.
6. Oyelese Y, Ananth CV. Placental abruption. Obstet Gynecol 2006; 108:1005-16.
7. Ananth CV, Savitz DA, Luther ER. Maternal cigarette smoking as a risk factor for placental abruption, placenta previa, and uterine bleeding in pregnancy. Am J Epidemiol 1996; 144:881-9.
8. Silver RM, Landon MB, Rouse DJ, et al. Maternal morbidity associated with multiple repeat cesarean deliveries. Obstet Gynecol 2006; 107:1226-32.
9. Ramin SM. Placental abnormalities: Previa, abruption, and accreta. In Plauché WC, Morrison JC, O'Sullivan MJ, editors. Surgical Obstetrics. Philadelphia, WB Saunders, 1992:203-15.
10. Hertzberg BS, Livingston E, DeLong DM, et al. Ultrasonographic evaluation of the cervix: Transperineal versus endovaginal imaging. J Ultrasound Med 2001; 20:1071-8.
11. Wing DA, Paul RH, Millar LK. Management of the symptomatic placenta previa: A randomized, controlled trial of inpatient versus outpatient expectant management. Am J Obstet Gynecol 1996; 175:806-11.

12. Oyelese Y, Smulian JC. Placenta previa, placenta accreta, and vasa previa. Obstet Gynecol 2006; 107:927-41.
13. Silver R, Depp R, Sabbagha RE, et al. Placenta previa: Aggressive expectant management. Am J Obstet Gynecol 1984; 150:15-22.
14. Besinger RE, Moniak CW, Paskiewicz LS, et al. The effect of tocolytic use in the management of symptomatic placenta previa. Am J Obstet Gynecol 1995; 172:1770-8.
15. Sharma A, Suri V, Gupta I. Tocolytic therapy in conservative management of symptomatic placenta previa. Int J Gynaecol Obstet 2004; 84:109-13.
16. Chestnut DH, Thompson CS, McLaughlin GL, Weiner CP. Does the intravenous infusion of ritodrine or magnesium sulfate alter the hemodynamic response to hemorrhage in gravid ewes? Am J Obstet Gynecol 1988; 159:1467-73.
17. Norwitz ER, Robinson JN, Challis JRG. The control of labor. N Engl J Med 1999; 341:660-6.
18. Glock JL, Morales WJ. Efficacy and safety of nifedipine versus magnesium sulfate in the management of preterm labor: A randomized study. Am J Obstet Gynecol 1993; 169:960-4.
19. McShane PM, Heyl PS, Epstein MF. Maternal and perinatal morbidity resulting from placenta previa. Obstet Gynecol 1985; 65:176-82.
20. Naeye RL. Placenta previa: Predisposing factors and effects on the fetus and surviving infants. Obstet Gynecol 1978; 52:521-5.
21. Dommisse J. Placenta praevia and intra-uterine growth retardation. S Afr Med J 1985; 67:291-2.
22. Crane JMG, van den Hof MC, Dodds L, et al. Neonatal outcomes with placenta previa. Obstet Gynecol 1999; 93:541-4.
23. Oppenheimer L. Society of Obstetricians and Gynaecologists of Canada. Diagnosis and management of placenta previa. J Obstet Gynaecol Can 2007; 29:261-73.
24. Bonner SM, Haynes SR, Ryall D. The anaesthetic management of Caesarean section for placenta praevia: A questionnaire survey. Anaesthesia 1995; 50:992-4.
25. Hong JY, Jee YS, Yoon HJ, Kim SM. Comparison of general and epidural anesthesia in elective cesarean section for placenta previa totalis: Maternal hemodynamics, blood loss and neonatal outcome. Int J Obstet Anesth 2003; 12:12-16.
26. Downing JW, Buley RJ, Brock-Utne JG, Houlton PC. Etomidate for induction of anaesthesia at caesarean section: Comparison with thiopentone. Br J Anaesth 1979; 51:135-40.
27. Tikkanen M, Nuutila M, Hiilesmaa V, et al. Clinical presentation and risk factors of placental abruption. Acta Obstet Gynecol Scand 2006; 85:700-5.
28. Ananth CV, Oyelese Y, Srinivas N, et al. Preterm premature rupture of membranes, intrauterine infection, and oligohydramnios: Risk factors for placental abruption. Obstet Gynecol 2004; 104:71-7.
29. Getahun D, Ananth CV, Peltier MR, et al. Acute and chronic respiratory diseases in pregnancy: Associations with placental abruption. Am J Obstet Gynecol 2006; 195:1180-4.
30. Ananth CV, Wilcox AJ. Placental abruption and perinatal mortality in the United States. Am J Epidemiol 2001; 153:332-7.
31. Saftlas AF, Olson DR, Atrash HK, et al. National trends in the incidence of abruptio placentae, 1979-1987. Obstet Gynecol 1991; 78:1081-6.
32. Ananth CV, Oyelese Y, Yeo L, et al. Placental abruption in the United States, 1979 through 2001: Temporal trends and potential determinants. Am J Obstet Gynecol 2005; 192:191-8.
33. Glantz C, Purnell L. Clinical utility of sonography in the diagnosis and treatment of placental abruption. J Ultrasound Med 2002; 21:837-40.
34. Naeye RL, Harkness WL, Utts J. Abruptio placentae and perinatal death: A prospective study. Am J Obstet Gynecol 1977; 128:740-6.
35. Nyberg DA, Mack LA, Benedetti TJ, et al. Placental abruption and placental hemorrhage: Correlation of sonographic findings with fetal outcome. Radiology 1987; 164:357-61.
36. Kayani SI, Walkinshaw SA, Preston C. Pregnancy outcome in severe placental abruption. Br J Obstet Gynaecol 2003; 110:679-83.
37. Vincent RD Jr, Chestnut DH, Sipes SL, et al. Epidural anesthesia worsens uterine blood flow and fetal oxygenation during hemorrhage in gravid ewes. Anesthesiology 1992; 76:799-806.
38. Oats JN, Vasey DP, Waldron BA. Effects of ketamine on the pregnant uterus. Br J Anaesth 1979; 51:1163-6.
39. Kaczmarczyk M, Sparén P, Terry P, Cnattingius S. Risk factors for uterine rupture and neonatal consequences of uterine rupture: A population-based study of successive pregnancies in Sweden. Br J Obstet Gynaecol 2007; 114:1208-14.
40. Walsh CA, Baxi LV. Rupture of the primigravid uterus: A review of the literature. Obstet Gynecol Surv 2007; 62:327-34.
41. Plauché WC, Von Almen W, Muller R. Catastrophic uterine rupture. Obstet Gynecol 1984; 64:792-7.
42. Farmer RM, Kirschbaum T, Potter D, et al. Uterine rupture during trial of labor after previous cesarean section. Am J Obstet Gynecol 1991; 165:996-1001.
43. Lydon-Rochelle M, Holt VL, Easterling TR, Martin DP. Risk of uterine rupture during labor among women with a prior cesarean delivery. N Engl J Med 2001; 345:3-8.
44. Catanzarite V, Maida C, Thomas W, et al. Prenatal sonographic diagnosis of vasa previa: Ultrasound findings and obstetric outcome in ten cases. Ultrasound Obstet Gynecol 2001; 18:109-15.
45. World Health Organization. WHO Recommendations for the Prevention of Postpartum Haemorrhage. Geneva, WHO, 2007.
46. Ford JB, Roberts CL, Bell JC, et al. Postpartum haemorrhage occurrence and recurrence: A population-based study. Med J Aust 2007; 187:391-3.
47. Combs CA, Murphy EL, Laros RK Jr. Factors associated with hemorrhage in cesarean deliveries. Obstet Gynecol 1991; 77:77-82.
48. Karpati PC, Rossignol M, Pirot M, et al. High incidence of myocardial ischemia during postpartum hemorrhage. Anesthesiology 2004; 100:30-6.
49. World Health Organization. Reducing the global burden: Postpartum haemorrhage: Making pregnancy safer. World Health Organization Hot Topics Issue April 2007; 4:1-8.
50. Bouwmeester FW, Bolte AC, van Geijn HP. Pharmacological and surgical therapy for primary postpartum hemorrhage. Curr Pharm Des 2005; 11:759-73.
51. Nelson SH, Suresh MS. Lack of reactivity of uterine arteries from patients with obstetric hemorrhage. Am J Obstet Gynecol 1992; 166:1436-43.
52. American College of Obstetricians and Gynecologists. Postpartum hemorrhage. Practice Bulletin No. 76. Washington, DC, October 2006. (Obstet Gynecol 2006; 108:1039-47.)
53. Gülmezoglu AM, Forna F, Villar J, Hofmeyr GJ. Prostaglandins for preventing postpartum haemorrhage. Cochrane Database Syst Rev 2007; (3):CD000494.
54. Saito K, Haruki A, Ishikawa H, et al. Prospective study of intramuscular ergometrine compared with intramuscular oxytocin for prevention of postpartum hemorrhage. J Obstet Gynaecol Res 2007; 33:254-8.
55. Knight M, UKOSS. Peripartum hysterectomy in the UK: Management and outcomes of the associated haemorrhage. Br J Obstet Gynaecol 2007; 114:1380-7.
56. Smith JG, Merrill DC. Oxytocin for induction of labor. Clin Obstet Gynecol 2006; 49:594-608.
57. Weis FR Jr, Markello R, Mo B, Bochiechio P. Cardiovascular effects of oxytocin. Obstet Gynecol 1975; 46:211-14.
58. Secher NJ, Arnsbo P, Wallin L. Haemodynamic effects of oxytocin (Syntocinon) and methyl ergometrine (Methergin) on the systemic and pulmonary circulations of pregnant anaesthetized women. Acta Obstet Gynecol Scand 1978; 57:97-103.
59. Thomas JS, Koh SH, Cooper GM. Haemodynamic effects of oxytocin given as i.v. bolus or infusion on women undergoing Caesarean section. Br J Anaesth 2007; 98:116-19.
60. Munn MB, Owen J, Vincent R, et al. Comparison of two oxytocin regimens to prevent uterine atony at cesarean delivery: A randomized controlled trial. Obstet Gynecol 2001; 98:386-90.
61. Rosaeg OP, Cicutti NJ, Labow RS. The effect of oxytocin on the contractile force of human atrial trabeculae. Anesth Analg 1998; 86:40-4.
62. de Groot AN, van Dongen PW, Vree TB, et al. Ergot alkaloids: Current status and review of clinical pharmacology and therapeutic use compared with other oxytocics in obstetrics and gynaecology. Drugs 1998; 56:523-35.

63. Sanders-Bush E. 5-Hydroxytryptamine (serotonin): Receptor agonists and antagonists. In Hardman JG, Limbird LE, Gilman AG, editors. Goodman & Gilman's The Pharmacological Basis of Therapeutics. 10th edition. New York, McGraw-Hill, 2001:269-90.
64. Hayashi Y, Ibe T, Kawato H, et al. Postpartum acute myocardial infarction induced by ergonovine administration. Intern Med 2003; 42:983-6.
65. Lin YH, Seow KM, Hwang JL, Chen HH. Myocardial infarction and mortality caused by methylergonovine. Acta Obstet Gynecol Scand 2005; 84:1022.
66. Abouleish E. Postpartum hypertension and convulsion after oxytocic drugs. Anesth Analg 1976; 55:813-5.
67. Casady GN, Moore DC, Bridenbaugh LD. Postpartum hypertension after use of vasoconstrictor and oxytocic drugs: Etiology, incidence, complications, and treatment. JAMA 1960; 172:1011-5.
68. Hogerzeil HV, Walker GJ. Instability of (methyl)ergometrine in tropical climates: An overview. Eur J Obstet Gynecol Reprod Biol 1996; 69:25-9.
69. Fuchs AR, Husslein P, Sumulong L, Fuchs F. The origin of circulating 13,14-dihydro-15-keto-prostaglandin F2 alpha during delivery. Prostaglandins 1982; 24:715-22.
70. Noort WA, van Bulck B, Vereecken A, et al. Changes in plasma levels of PGF2 alpha and PGI2 metabolites at and after delivery at term. Prostaglandins 1989; 37:3-12.
71. Izumi H, Garfield RE, Morshita F, Shirakawa K. Some mechanical properties of skinned fibres of pregnant human myometrium. Eur J Obstet Gynecol Reprod Biol 1994; 56:55-62.
72. Hayashi RH, Castillo MS, Noah ML. Management of severe postpartum hemorrhage with a prostaglandin F2 alpha analogue. Obstet Gynecol 1984; 63:806-8.
73. Bigrigg A, Chissell S, Read MD. Use of intramyometrial 15-methyl prostaglandin F2 alpha to control atonic postpartum haemorrhage following vaginal delivery and failure of conventional therapy. Br J Obstet Gynaecol 1991; 98:734-6.
74. Andersen LH, Secher NJ. Pattern of total and regional lung function in subjects with bronchoconstriction induced by 15-me PGF2 alpha. Thorax 1976; 31:685-92.
75. O'Leary AM. Severe bronchospasm and hypotension after 15-methyl prostaglandin F(2alpha) in atonic post partum haemorrhage. Int J Obstet Anesth 1994; 3:42-4.
76. Granström L, Ekman G, Ulmsten U. Intravenous infusion of 15 methyl-prostaglandin F2 alpha (Prostinfenem) in women with heavy post-partum hemorrhage. Acta Obstet Gynecol Scand 1989; 68:365-7.
77. O'Brien P, El-Refaey H, Gordon A, et al. Rectally administered misoprostol for the treatment of postpartum hemorrhage unresponsive to oxytocin and ergometrine: A descriptive study. Obstet Gynecol 1998; 92:212-4.
78. Abdel-Aleem H, El-Nashar I, Abdel-Aleem A. Management of severe postpartum hemorrhage with misoprostol. Int J Gynaecol Obstet 2001; 72:75-6.
79. Lokugamage AU, Sullivan KR, Niculescu I, et al. A randomized study comparing rectally administered misoprostol versus Syntometrine combined with an oxytocin infusion for the cessation of primary post partum hemorrhage. Acta Obstet Gynecol Scand 2001; 80:835-9.
80. Blum J, Alfirevic Z, Walraven G, et al. Treatment of postpartum hemorrhage with misoprostol. Int J Gynaecol Obstet 2007; 99:S202-5.
81. Ramsey PS, Hogg BB, Savage KG, et al. Cardiovascular effects of intravaginal misoprostol in the mid trimester of pregnancy. Am J Obstet Gynecol 2000; 183:1100-2.
82. Hughes WA, Hughes SC. Hemodynamic effects of prostaglandin E2. Anesthesiology 1989; 70:713-6.
83. Secher NJ, Thayssen P, Arnsbo P, Olsen J. Effect of prostaglandin E2 and F2alpha on the systemic and pulmonary circulation in pregnant anesthetized women. Acta Obstet Gynecol Scand 1982; 61:213-8.
84. Sarkar PK, Mamo J. Successful control of atonic primary postpartum haemorrhage and prevention of hysterectomy, using i.v. prostaglandin E2. Br J Clin Pract 1990; 44:756-7.
85. You WB, Zahn CM. Postpartum hemorrhage: Abnormally adherent placenta, uterine inversion, and puerperal hematomas. Clin Obstet Gynecol 2006; 49:184-97.
86. Saleem Z, Rydhström H. Vaginal hematoma during parturition: A population-based study. Acta Obstet Gynecol Scand 2004; 83:560-2.
87. Jain KA, Olcott EW. Magnetic resonance imaging of postpartum pelvic hematomas: Early experience in diagnosis and treatment planning. Magn Reson Imaging 1999; 17:973-7.
88. Fliegner JR. Postpartum broad ligament haematomas. J Obstet Gynaecol Br Commonw 1971; 78:184-9.
89. Combs CA, Laros RK Jr. Prolonged third stage of labor: Morbidity and risk factors. Obstet Gynecol 1991; 77:863-7.
90. Carroli G, Bergel E. Umbilical vein injection for management of retained placenta. Cochrane Database Syst Rev 2001; (4):CD001337.
91. Turner RJ, Lambros M, Kenway L, Gatt SP. The in-vitro effects of sevoflurane and desflurane on the contractility of pregnant human uterine muscle. Int J Obstet Anesth 2002; 11:246-51.
92. Yoo K, Lee JC, Yoon MH, et al. The effects of volatile anesthetics on spontaneous contractility of isolated human pregnant uterine muscle: A comparison among sevoflurane, desflurane, isoflurane, and halothane. Anesth Analg 2006; 103:443-7.
93. Caponas G. Glyceryl trinitrate and acute uterine relaxation: A literature review. Anaesth Intensive Care 2001; 29:163-77.
94. Vinatier D, Dufour P, Bérard J. Utilization of intravenous nitroglycerin for obstetrical emergencies. Int J Gynaecol Obstet 1996; 55:129-34.
95. Mayer DC, Weeks SK. Antepartum uterine relaxation with nitroglycerin at caesarean delivery. Can J Anaesth 1992; 39:166-9.
96. Peng AT, Gorman RS, Shulman SM, et al. Intravenous nitroglycerin for uterine relaxation in the postpartum patient with retained placenta. Anesthesiology 1989; 71:172-3.
97. DeSimone CA, Norris MC, Leighton BL. Intravenous nitroglycerin aids manual extraction of a retained placenta. Anesthesiology 1990; 73:787.
98. Bullarbo M, Tjugum J, Ekerhovd E. Sublingual nitroglycerin for management of retained placenta. Int J Gynaecol Obstet 2005; 91:228-32.
99. Segal S, Csavoy AN, Datta S. Placental tissue enhances uterine relaxation by nitroglycerin. Anesth Analg 1998; 86:304-9.
100. Wu S, Kocherginsky M, Hibbard JU. Abnormal placentation: Twenty-year analysis. Am J Obstet Gynecol 2005; 192:1458-61.
101. Palacios Jaraquemada JM, Bruno CH. Magnetic resonance imaging in 300 cases of placenta accreta: Surgical correlation of new findings. Acta Obstet Gynecol Scand 2005; 84:716-24.
102. Warshak CR, Eskander R, Hull AD, et al. Accuracy of ultrasonography and magnetic resonance imaging in the diagnosis of placenta accreta. Obstet Gynecol 2006; 108:573-81.
103. Kayem G, Davy C, Goffinet F, et al. Conservative versus extirpative management in cases of placenta accreta. Obstet Gynecol 2004; 104:531-6.
104. Tan CH, Tay KH, Sheah K, et al. Perioperative endovascular internal iliac artery occlusion balloon placement in management of placenta accreta. Am J Roentgenol 2007; 189:1158-63.
105. Greenberg JI, Suliman A, Iranpour P, Angle N. Prophylactic balloon occlusion of the internal iliac arteries to treat abnormal placentation: A cautionary case. Am J Obstet Gynecol 2007; 470.e1-4.
106. Shrivastava V, Nageotte M, Major C, et al. Case-control comparison of cesarean hysterectomy with and without prophylactic placement of intravascular balloon catheters for placenta accreta. Am J Obstet Gynecol 2007; 197:402.e1-5.
107. O'Brien JM, Barton JR, Donaldson ES. The management of placenta percreta: Conservative and operative strategies. Am J Obstet Gynecol 1996; 175:1632-8.
108. Dubois J, Garel L, Grignon A, et al. Placenta percreta: Balloon occlusion and embolization of the internal iliac arteries to reduce intraoperative blood losses. Am J Obstet Gynecol 1997; 176:723-6.
109. Hong RW, Greenfield MLVH, Polley LS. Nitroglycerin for uterine inversion in the absence of placental fragments. Anesth Analg 2006; 103:511-12.

110. Dufour P, Vinatier D, Puech F. The use of intravenous nitroglycerin for cervico-uterine relaxation: A review of the literature. Arch Gynecol Obstet 1997; 261:1-7.
111. Doumouchtsis SK, Papageorghiou AT, Arulkumaran S. Systematic review of conservative management of postpartum hemorrhage: What to do when medical treatment fails. Obstet Gynecol Surv 2007; 62:540-7.
112. Allam MS, B-Lynch C. The B-Lynch and other uterine compression suture techniques. Int J Gynaecol Obstet 2005; 89:236-41.
113. Brace V, Kernaghan D, Penney G. Learning from adverse clinical outcomes: Major obstetric haemorrhage in Scotland, 2003-05. Br J Obstet Gynaecol 2007; 114:1388-96.
114. Porcu G, Roger V, Jacquier A, et al. Uterus and bladder necrosis after uterine artery embolisation for postpartum haemorrhage. Br J Obstet Gynaecol 2005; 112:122-3.
115. Hansch E, Chitkara U, McAlpine J, et al. Pelvic arterial embolization for control of obstetric hemorrhage: A five-year experience. Am J Obstet Gynecol 1999; 180:1454-60.
116. Eriksson LG, Mulic-Lutvica A, Jangland L, Nyman R. Massive postpartum hemorrhage treated with transcatheter arterial embolization: Technical aspects and long-term effects on fertility and menstrual cycle. Acta Radiol 2007; 48:635-42.
117. O'Rourke N, McElrath T, Baum R, et al. Cesarean delivery in the interventional radiology suite: A novel approach to obstetric hemostasis. Anesth Analg 2007; 104:1193-4.
118. O'Leary JA. Uterine artery ligation in the control of postcesarean hemorrhage. J Reprod Med 1995; 40:189-93.
119. Bakri YN, Amri A, Abdul Jabbar F. Tamponade-balloon for obstetrical bleeding. Int J Gynaecol Obstet 2001; 74:139-42.
120. Smith J, Mousa HA. Peripartum hysterectomy for primary postpartum haemorrhage: Incidence and maternal morbidity. J Obstet Gynaecol 2007; 27:44-7.
121. Chestnut DH, Dewan DM, Redick LF, et al. Anesthetic management for obstetric hysterectomy: A multi-institutional study. Anesthesiology 1989; 70:607-10.
122. Ozden S, Yildirim G, Basaran T, et al. Analysis of 59 cases of emergent peripartum hysterectomies during a 13-year period. Arch Gynecol Obstet 2005; 271:363-7.
123. American College of Obstetricians and Gynecologists Committee on Obstetric Practice. Placenta accreta. ACOG Committee Opinion No. 266. Washington, DC, January 2002. (Obstet Gynecol 2002; 99: 169-70.)
124. Silverman JA, Barrett J, Callum JL. The appropriateness of red blood cell transfusions in the peripartum patient. Obstet Gynecol 2004; 104:1000-4.
125. Rouse DJ, MacPherson C, Landom M, et al. Blood transfusion and cesarean delivery. Obstet Gynecol 2006; 108:891-7.
126. American Society of Anesthesiologists Task Force on Perioperative Blood Transfusion and Adjuvant Therapies. Practice guidelines for perioperative blood transfusion and adjuvant therapies: An updated report. Anesthesiology 2006; 105:198-208.
127. Ransom SB, Fundaro G, Dombrowski MP. Cost-effectiveness of routine blood type and screen testing for cesarean section. J Reprod Med 1999; 44:592-4.
128. American Society of Anesthesiologists Task Force on Obstetric Anesthesia. Practice guidelines for obstetric anesthesia. Anesthesiology 2007; 106:843-63.
129. McCullough J. Transfusion Medicine. New York, McGraw-Hill, 1998:99-118.
130. Andres RL, Piacquadio KM, Resnik R. A reappraisal of the need for autologous blood donation in the obstetric patient. Am J Obstet Gynecol 1990; 163:1551-3.
131. Droste S, Sorensen T, Price T, et al. Maternal and fetal hemodynamic effects of autologous blood donation during pregnancy. Am J Obstet Gynecol 1992; 167:89-93.
132. Kruskall MS, Leonard S, Klapholz H. Autologous blood donation during pregnancy: Analysis of safety and blood use. Obstet Gynecol 1987; 70:938-41.
133. Kanter MH, van Maanen D, Anders KH, et al. Preoperative autologous blood donations before elective hysterectomy. JAMA 1996; 276:798-801.
134. Estella NM, Berry DL, Baker BW, et al. Normovolemic hemodilution before cesarean hysterectomy for placenta percreta. Obstet Gynecol 1997; 90:669-70.
135. Grange CS, Douglas MJ, Adams TJ, Wadsworth LD. The use of acute hemodilution in parturients undergoing cesarean section. Am J Obstet Gynecol 1998; 178:156-60.
136. Bryson GL, Laupacis A, Wells GA. Does acute normovolemic hemodilution reduce perioperative allogeneic transfusion? A meta-analysis. Anesth Analg 1998; 86:9-15.
137. Williamson KR, Taswell HF. Intraoperative blood salvage: A review. Transfusion 1991; 31:662-75.
138. Catling S. Blood conservation techniques in obstetrics: A UK perspective. Int J Obstet Anesth 2007; 16:241-9.
139. Fong J, Gurewitsch ED, Kang HJ, et al. An analysis of transfusion practice and the role of intraoperative red blood cell salvage during cesarean delivery. Anesth Analg 2007; 104:666-72.
140. Catling SJ, Williams S, Fielding AM. Cell salvage in obstetrics: An evaluation of the ability of cell salvage combined with leucocyte depletion filtration to remove amniotic fluid from operative blood loss at caesarean section. Int J Obstet Anesth 1999; 8:79-84.
141. Waters JH, Biscottie C, Potter PS, Phillipson E. Amniotic fluid removal during cell salvage in the cesarean section patient. Anesthesiology 2000; 92:1531-6.
142. Rainaldi MP, Tazzari PL, Scagliarini G, et al. Blood salvage during caesarean section. Br J Anaesth 1998; 80:195-8.
143. Rebarber A, Lonser R, Jackson S, et al. The safety of intraoperative autologous blood collection and autotransfusion during cesarean section. Am J Obstet Gynecol 1998; 179:715-20.
144. Waters JH. Is cell salvage a safe technique for the obstetric patient? Pro. Society for Obstetric Anesthesia and Perinatology Newsletter 2005; Fall:7-8.
145. Santrach PJ. Is cell salvage a safe technique for the obstetric patient? Con. Society for Obstetric Anesthesia and Perinatology Newsletter 2005; Fall:9.
146. Allam J, Cox M, Yentis SM. Cell salvage in obstetrics. Int J Obstet Anesth 2008; 17:37-45.
147. American Society of Anesthesiologists Task Force on Obstetric Anesthesia. Practice guidelines for obstetric anesthesia. Anesthesiology 2007; 106:843-63.
148. Waters JR, Meier HH, Waters JH. An economic analysis of costs associated with development of a cell salvage program. Anesth Analg 2007; 104:869-75.
149. Santoso JT, Saunders BA, Grosshart K. Massive blood loss and transfusion in obstetrics and gynecology. Obstet Gynecol Surv 2005; 60:827-37.
150. O'Shaughnessy DF, Atterbury C, Bolton Maggs P, et al. Guidelines for the use of fresh-frozen plasma, cryoprecipitate and cryosupernatant. Br J Haematol 2004; 126:11-28.
151. Welsby IJ, Monroe DM, Lawson JH, Hoffmann M. Recombinant activated factor VII and the anaesthetist. Anaesthesia 2005; 60:1203-12.
152. Ahonen J, Jokela R. Recombinant factor VIIa for life-threatening post-partum haemorrhage. Br J Anaesth 2005; 94:592-5.
153. Palomino MA, Chaparro MJ, de Elvira MJ, Curiel EB. Recombinant activated factor VII in the management of massive obstetric bleeding. Blood Coagul Fibrinolysis 2006; 17:226-7.
154. Segal S, Shemesh IY, Blumental R, et al. The use of recombinant factor VIIa in severe postpartum hemorrhage. Acta Obstet Gynecol Scand 2004; 83:771-2.
155. Franchini M, Lippi G, Franchi M. The use of recombinant activated factor VII in obstetric and gynaecological haemorrhage. Br J Obstet Gynaecol 2007; 114:8-15.
156. Thomas GOR, Dutton RP, Hemlock B, et al. Thromboembolic complications associated with factor VIIa administration. J Trauma 2007; 62:564-9.

157. Beutler E. Platelet transfusions: The 20,000/microL trigger. Blood 1993; 81:1411-3.
158. Letsky EA. Disseminated intravascular coagulation. Best Pract Res Clin Obstet Gynaecol 2001; 15:623-44.
159. Coste J, Reesink HW, Engelfriet CP, et al. Implementation of donor screening for infectious agents transmitted by blood by nucleic acid technology: Update to 2003. Vox Sang 2005; 88:289-303.
160. Dodd RY, Notari EP, Stramer SL. Current prevalence and incidence of infectious disease markers and estimated window-period risk in the American Red Cross blood donor population. Transfusion 2002; 42:975-9.
161. Llewelyn CA, Hewitt PE, Knight RS, et al. Possible transmission of variant Creutzfeldt-Jakob disease by blood transfusion. Lancet 2004; 363:417-21.
162. Laupacis A, Brown J, Costello B, et al. Prevention of posttransfusion CMV in the era of universal WBC reduction: A consensus statement. Transfusion 2001; 41:560-9.
163. Blajchman MA, Goldman M, Freedman JJ, Sher GD. Proceedings of a consensus conference: Prevention of post-transfusion CMV in the era of universal leukoreduction. Transfus Med Rev 2001; 15:1-20.
164. Boeckh M, Nichols WG. The impact of cytomegalovirus serostatus of donor and recipient before hematopoietic stem cell transplantation in the era of antiviral prophylaxis and preemptive therapy. Blood 2004; 103:2003-8.
165. Eder AF, Kennedy JM, Dy BA, et al. Bacterial screening of apheresis platelets and the residual risk of septic transfusion reactions: The American Red Cross experience (2004-2006). Transfusion 2007; 47:1134-42.

Chapter 38

Embolic Disorders

Kathleen M. Davis, M.D.
Andrew M. Malinow, M.D.

Embolic disease during pregnancy includes pulmonary thromboembolism, amniotic fluid embolism, and venous air embolism. The presentation of each of these entities varies in incidence and clinical course. For example, venous air embolism frequently occurs during cesarean delivery.[1-6] Symptoms, if present, are transient, and the diagnosis often is missed (or dismissed if detected) by the anesthesia provider.[1] In contrast, amniotic fluid embolism is rare, but its clinical presentation is cataclysmic.[7]

In obstetric patients, many embolic events occur intrapartum or postpartum. Together, these disorders represent the most common cause of direct maternal mortality in the Western world.[8] Further, women with inherited or acquired thrombophilia are at risk not only for thromboembolic events, but also for a variety of other adverse pregnancy outcomes, including placental abnormalities and intrauterine growth restriction (IUGR).[9]

Anesthesia providers are often involved in the resuscitation of patients with embolic disorders. Early recognition, diagnosis, and treatment are necessary to reduce associated morbidity and mortality.

THROMBOEMBOLISM

Incidence

Pulmonary thromboembolism (PTE) occurs in approximately 0.01% to 0.05% of all pregnancies.[10,11] The most common etiology is deep vein thrombosis (DVT), but PTE can also occur after superficial vein, puerperal septic pelvic vein, and puerperal ovarian vein thrombosis.

Superficial vein thrombosis occurs during the antepartum period in as many as 0.15% of pregnancies.[10] However, the incidence increases as much as eightfold during the postpartum period. **Deep vein thrombosis** occurs in 0.02% to 0.36% of pregnancies.[10-12] The reported incidence of DVT in pregnant women has risen over the last several decades; this change may represent a true increase as a result of increasing comorbidity or may be a result of improved assessment and diagnosis.[12-17] In the past, the incidence of DVT was fivefold to eightfold higher during the postpartum period.[10,12] Published evidence suggests that the incidence of postpartum DVT has decreased in recent years, most likely because of more aggressive efforts toward early ambulation and the use of other means of thromboembolic prophylaxis after delivery.[11,15,16] As many as half of pregnancy-related episodes of DVT occur by 15 weeks' gestation, and more than two thirds occur by 20 weeks' gestation.[11] **Puerperal ovarian vein thrombosis** and **septic pelvic vein thrombosis** manifest during the early postpartum period with incidences of 0.025% and 0.1%, respectively.[10,18]

Approximately 33% of patients with untreated septic pelvic vein thrombosis experience a pulmonary embolus. However, most cases of PTE during pregnancy result from DVT.[10] Although DVT occurs most commonly during the antepartum period, almost two thirds of all pregnancy-associated cases of PTE occur postpartum. Approximately 15% to 24% of pregnant women with untreated DVT experience a pulmonary embolus, with an associated mortality rate of 12% to 15%.[10,19,20] Appropriate treatment of DVT reduces the incidence of PTE to 0.7% to 4.5%,[12,21] and it reduces the mortality rate to 0.7%.[20,21] Although the incidence of maternal death due to PTE has declined by more than 50% during the last two decades, PTE still accounts for as much as 15% of direct maternal mortality (see Chapter 39).

Etiology

Half of the cases of thromboembolism in women of childbearing age occur during pregnancy or the puerperium.[22] Pregnancy results in a twofold to fivefold increase in the relative risk of thromboembolism.[17,23] The higher frequency of thromboembolic disease during pregnancy is a result of at least three factors: (1) an increase in venous stasis, (2) the hypercoagulable state of pregnancy, and (3) the vascular injury associated with vaginal or cesarean delivery.

VENOUS STASIS

Pregnancy results in an enormous increase in uterine size and blood flow. Maternal blood volume and cardiac output increase approximately 50% during pregnancy. At term, uterine blood flow increases to 700 to 900 mL/min, which represents approximately 10% to 12% of maternal cardiac output.[24] The uterus—normally a pelvic organ—becomes an abdominal organ by term. The gravid uterus compresses the inferior vena cava as well as other anatomic structures (e.g., the ureter). Vena caval compression results in venous stasis distal to the compression in the pelvis and lower extremities.

CHANGES IN COAGULATION

Pregnancy is associated with enhanced platelet turnover, coagulation, and fibrinolysis. It also is associated with an increase in the concentration of clotting factors, including factors I (fibrinogen), V, VII, VIII, IX, X, and XII. Thrombin generation also increases. Platelet count typically remains unchanged (or is decreased by hemodilution) during pregnancy. In summary, pregnancy represents a state of accelerated but compensated intravascular coagulation.

Parturition accelerates platelet activation, coagulation, and fibrinolysis.[25,26] Unlike coagulation activity, fibrinolytic activity decreases during the 48 hours after delivery.[26] Therefore coagulation activity is increased in relation to fibrinolytic activity.

VASCULAR DAMAGE

Both vaginal delivery and separation of the placenta result in vascular trauma, which may initiate a series of physiologic events leading to an acceleration of coagulation activity. This greater coagulation activity is most likely responsible for the higher incidence of PTE during the puerperium. Surgery (e.g., cesarean delivery) results in a further increase in the risk of thromboembolism. The risks of both DVT and PTE are as much as eight times higher after cesarean delivery than after vaginal delivery.[12,27,28] Even tubal ligation after vaginal delivery seems to result in a higher risk of thromboembolism than vaginal delivery alone.[22]

OBSTETRIC CONDITIONS

A population-based study of more than a million deliveries noted a higher risk of PTE in women whose pregnancies were complicated by preeclampsia and multiple gestation (i.e., increased relative risks of sevenfold to eightfold, and twofold to threefold, respectively).[15,27,28] These obstetric conditions—or their management—are associated with risk factors for thromboembolic disease (e.g., bed rest, increased venous stasis, increased risk of operative delivery, vascular injury).

COINCIDENTAL DISEASE

A history of previous thromboembolism increases the risk of PTE during pregnancy. Early in pregnancy, there are higher levels of D-dimer and thrombin/antithrombin complexes in patients with prior thromboembolic events than in normal controls.[29] In addition, coincidental diseases further increase the risk of thromboembolism in obstetric patients. These diseases include heart disease (odds ratio [OR], 7.1), smoking (OR, 1.7), obesity (OR, 4.4), antiphospholipid antibody syndrome (OR, 15.0), and thrombophilias including protein S and C deficiencies, antithrombin III deficiency, hyperhomocysteinemia, and prothrombin gene or factor V Leiden mutation (OR, 25.0 to 50.0).[15,20,22,28]

Pathophysiology

The manifestations and prognosis of PTE depend on the following factors: (1) the size and number of emboli, (2) concurrent cardiopulmonary function, (3) the rate of clot fragmentation and lysis, (4) the presence or absence of a source for recurrent emboli, and (5) the location of the embolism (proximal or main pulmonary artery embolism is more symptomatic than segmental embolization).[30,31] After a pulmonary embolus occurs, respiratory failure results from either extensive occlusion of the pulmonary vasculature (which results in cardiorespiratory decompensation) or pulmonary edema.[32] Pulmonary hypertension may result from direct vascular obstruction by a large embolus (e.g., a saddle embolus). However, a small embolus may also be associated with severe pulmonary hypertension, especially if there is underlying cardiac or pulmonary disease or recurrent pulmonary embolization.[31,32] In any case, right ventricular overload can occur. In addition, disruption of normal capillary integrity may occur.[32] Simultaneous cardiorespiratory compromise may prompt aggressive intravenous volume replacement; the increase in hydrostatic forces and the disruption of normal capillary integrity can lead to pulmonary edema.[32]

Diagnosis

CLINICAL

The diagnosis of a pulmonary embolus requires a high index of suspicion and prompt evaluation (Table 38-1). The patient may complain of dyspnea, palpitations, anxiety, and chest pain, which may be pleuritic. The patient may appear cyanotic and diaphoretic and may have a cough, with or without hemoptysis (i.e., pinkish sputum or frank blood). Physical examination of the patient commonly demonstrates tachypnea, crackles, and decreased breath sounds (more common than rhonchi or wheezing), and tachycardia. Signs of right ventricular failure, including an accentuated or split second heart sound, jugular venous distention, a parasternal heave, and hepatic enlargement, may be seen. The electrocardiogram (ECG) may show signs of right ventricular strain, including a right-axis shift, P pulmonale, ST-T segment abnormalities, T-wave inversion, as well as supraventricular arrhythmias. One or more of the signs of DVT (calf or thigh edema, erythema, tenderness, a palpable cord) generally accompany the pulmonary or cardiovascular findings.[20,30,32]

Embolism leads to a redistribution in pulmonary blood flow. This redistribution of perfusion can lead to

TABLE 38-1 Physical Findings in Pulmonary Embolism

Finding	Patients Affected (%)
Tachypnea	85
Tachycardia	40
Fever	45
Accentuated second heart sound	50
Localized rales	60
Thrombophlebitis	40
Supraventricular dysrhythmia	15

Adapted from Spence TH. Pulmonary embolization syndrome. In Civetta JM, Taylor RW, Kirby RR, editors. Critical Care. Philadelphia, JB Lippincott, 1988:1091-102.

"hyperperfusion" of otherwise low ventilation-perfusion zones in unaffected areas of the lung; in cases of right ventricular failure, a decrease in cardiac output leads to reduced mixed-venous oxygen content, which enhances the effects of ventilation-perfusion mismatch.[33] Arterial hypoxemia often results. However, because as many as 30% of all patients with a pulmonary embolus have a Pa_{O_2} greater than 80 mm Hg, the diagnosis cannot be excluded on the basis of an apparently normal Pa_{O_2}.[30]

Invasive hemodynamic monitoring typically demonstrates (1) normal to low (less than 15 mm Hg) pulmonary artery occlusion pressure, (2) increased mean pulmonary artery pressure (but typically less than 35 mm Hg), and (3) increased (more than 8 mm Hg) central venous pressure.[31,32] Calculated pulmonary vascular resistance typically is more than 2.5 times normal; right ventricular failure occurs when the mean pulmonary artery pressure exceeds 35 to 45 mm Hg.[32] In severe cases, left ventricular failure occurs secondary to poor left ventricular filling and arterial hypoxemia.

DIAGNOSTIC EVALUATION

Clinical assessment should precede imaging studies. Patients are stratified as having low, medium, or high probability of PTE on the basis of the clinical assessment, which helps guide the choice of diagnostic testing. Goals for the diagnosis of PTE during pregnancy include both timely diagnosis and minimization of radiation exposure for fetus and mother.

Enzyme-linked immunosorbent assay (ELISA) for D-dimer has a sensitivity of 95%. A negative D-dimer assay result can be a reassuring diagnostic test in cases with low clinical suspicion. With a negative result, the probability of PTE is less than 2% in a nonpregnant population; no further testing is required, although ultrasonography is optional.[34,35] On the other hand, a positive D-dimer assay result is not specific for PTE in pregnant women; D-dimer levels are detectable during the second trimester and continue to rise in normal pregnancies, returning to baseline by 6 weeks postpartum.[36,37] For a pregnant woman with a positive D-dimer assay result, some physicians recommend proceeding to lower extremity venous ultrasonography before performing tests involving radiation exposure.[35,38] Treatment is instituted immediately if ultrasonography findings are positive for DVT. Unfortunately, the false-negative rate for this modality may be as high as 10%.[39]

Chest radiographs may show atelectasis, pleural effusion, an elevated hemidiaphragm, and a peripheral segmental or subsegmental infiltrate.[10,32] However, chest radiographic findings are neither specific nor sensitive in the diagnosis of PTE; 25% to 40% of patients with pulmonary embolus have normal chest radiographs.[10,31] Nonetheless, chest radiography facilitates the interpretation of a subsequent ventilation-perfusion ($\dot{V}/\dot{Q}$) lung scan because not all perfusion defects that appear in a lung scan are a result of PTE. In addition, chest radiography aids in the diagnosis of other conditions (e.g., pleurisy, pneumothorax, fractured rib) that may mimic PTE.

Ventilation-perfusion scans are a common, efficient, and safe diagnostic tool for use in pregnant women.[40,41] If the perfusion scan is normal (as observed in approximately 75% of pregnant patients in whom there is suspicion of PTE), the diagnosis of PTE can be excluded.[41] Multiple perfusion defects and significant ventilation-perfusion mismatch in the lung scan suggest a high probability of PTE.[32] A high clinical suspicion of PTE and a high-probability lung scan (e.g., segmental perfusion defect with normal ventilation) obviate the need for further diagnostic imaging.[31,32] In such cases, the diagnosis of PTE is most likely correct, and anticoagulation therapy is indicated.

If the ventilation-perfusion lung scan shows subsegmental defects with normal ventilation or matched perfusion and ventilation defects, the probability of PTE is between 10% and 40%.[31] Indeterminate or inconclusive ventilation-perfusion scans occur less often in pregnant women than in nonpregnant patients (24% versus approximately 50%, respectively).[41] Spiral (helical) computed tomography (CT) or pulmonary angiography (preferably performed via the brachial route) should be considered if clinical suspicion is high in a patient with indeterminate lung scan results.[42]

Increasingly, clinicians are using spiral CT with angiography for the initial radiographic evaluation. In nonpregnant patients, spiral CT is very sensitive and specific for a central pulmonary artery embolus. Sensitivity and specificity of spiral CT approach 90% to 100% in evaluations of main, lobar, and segmental pulmonary arteries.[42] The sensitivity of spiral CT for isolated subsegmental PTE is approximately 30%, and such emboli account for approximately 20% of cases of symptomatic PTE.[34] Less than 10% of studies are considered nondiagnostic.[43] Overall, spiral CT may be the most cost-effective study on the basis of its high sensitivity and specificity and the decreased requirement for subsequent testing.[44] Of note, spiral CT involves less radiation exposure of the fetus than ventilation-perfusion scanning during all trimesters, although a higher maternal breast tissue exposure may result.[45] Either study may be modified, however, to reduce radiation exposure (e.g., half-dose radionucleotide protocols for ventilation-perfusion scans, special shielding for CT).[43]

Although the physician should limit unnecessary fetal radiation exposure, small amounts of radiation exposure most likely increase fetal risk to a very limited extent.[32,43,46,47] The absolute risk for childhood cancer in the general population is approximately 0.1%. The greater relative risk for childhood cancer after radiation exposure (e.g., radiographic pelvimetry) *in utero* is 1.2 to 2.4.[46] Most studies suggest that fetal radiation exposure less than 5 rads does not result in a higher incidence of teratogenesis or other adverse outcomes, including pregnancy loss, developmental abnormalities, and malignancies.[32,43,46,47]

Fetal radiation exposure during maternal diagnostic radiologic testing has been estimated (Table 38-2).[32,43,46] It is possible to use a chest radiograph, a ventilation-perfusion scan, and pulmonary angiography to make the diagnosis of PTE, with a total fetal radiation exposure of less than 60 mrads. Even when pulmonary angiography must be performed via the femoral route, total fetal radiation exposure is less than 400 mrads.[47]

There are published case reports of echocardiographic diagnosis of both an intracardiac embolus and a pulmonary artery embolus after cesarean delivery.[48] Although not as sensitive as pulmonary angiography in the detection of a pulmonary artery embolus, echocardiographic confirmation of a clot or the consequent right ventricular dysfunction may obviate the need for a more invasive procedure and may hasten the start of anticoagulation. Prospective Investigation of Pulmonary Embolism Diagnosis II (PIOPED II) investigators have described the efficacy of this bedside method, in addition to lower extremity ultrasonography or portable perfusion scanning, for the patient *in extremis;* both the sensitivity and the negative predictive value for massive PTE are high (97% to 98%) when the procedures are combined.[35,49]

Left-sided proximal iliac or femoral vein occlusion occurs in approximately 70% of all cases of DVT during pregnancy.[8,11,15] It has been suggested that a higher incidence of stasis occurs on the left side than on the right side because the left iliac vein crosses beneath a low bifurcation of the aorta or the right iliac artery.[50] Compression ultrasonography (i.e., comparison of flow before and after compression of a venous segment) is especially effective in diagnosing proximal DVT (iliac or femoral).[50] Compression ultrasonography and color-flow Doppler imaging may substitute for contrast venography in the diagnostic evaluation of symptomatic DVT during pregnancy.[50] ^{125}I-labeled fibrinogen leg scanning is not used during pregnancy, because free ^{125}I crosses the placenta and accumulates in the fetal thyroid gland.

TABLE 38-2 Estimated Doses of Absorbed Fetal Radiation from Procedures Used to Diagnose Maternal Venous Thromboembolism

Procedure	Estimated Fetal Radiation Exposure (mrad)*
Chest radiograph (with shielding)	< 1
Ventilation lung scan (using technetium Tc 99m-sulfur colloid submicronic aerosol)	1-5
Perfusion lung scan (using 1-2 mci technetium Tc 99m-albumin microaggregated)	6-12
Pulmonary angiography:	
Via brachial route	< 50
Via femoral route	< 375
Limited contrast venography (with shielding)	< 50

*1 mrad = 0.01 mGy.

Adapted from Ginsberg JS, Hirsh J, Rainbow AJ, Cuates G. Risks to the fetus of radiologic procedures used in the diagnosis of maternal venous thromboembolic disease. Thromb Haemost 1989; 61:189-96.

Puerperal ovarian vein and septic pelvic vein thromboses appear to represent different manifestations of the same clinical process. These disorders may occur after vaginal or cesarean delivery. Physicians should suspect these entities when a postpartum patient has a prolonged (i.e., greater than 72 hours) fever that is unresponsive to antibiotic therapy. The patient may not complain of pelvic pain or have a pelvic mass, and some women also may have coexistent DVT.[18,20] Therefore, complaints of leg pain, tenderness, and edema may accompany puerperal ovarian vein or septic pelvic vein thrombosis. In the past, the diagnosis of ovarian vein or septic pelvic vein thrombosis was often made after an empirical trial of heparin resulted in the amelioration of signs and symptoms. Rarely, the diagnosis was made at the time of surgery.[18,20] CT (with contrast) and magnetic resonance imaging now often help confirm the diagnosis of these disorders. The physician can also perform sequential imaging studies to follow the clinical resolution of ovarian vein and septic pelvic vein thromboses.[18,51]

Therapy

DEEP VEIN THROMBOSIS

The anesthesia provider must understand whether and how the obstetrician will initiate and maintain anticoagulation therapy. Controversy exists regarding the dose and even the use of anticoagulant therapy in patients with a history of DVT and PTE in a previous pregnancy or in those gravidae who have other risk factors for thromboembolism. The American College of Obstetricians and Gynecologists (ACOG) has published an educational bulletin that presents the scientific rationale for the use of pharmacologic thromboprophylaxis in various scenarios (Table 38-3).[52]

It is clear that prevention of PTE represents the primary focus of therapy for DVT. **Unfractionated heparin** therapy should be initiated immediately following the diagnosis of DVT. During pregnancy, dose requirements may be increased because of higher levels of coagulation factors. The adequacy of heparin therapy is monitored with serial activated partial thromboplastin time (aPTT) measurements. The usual loading dose of heparin is 5000 U (i.e., 80 U/kg) intravenously, followed by an initial intravenous infusion rate of 15 to 20 U/kg/hr (i.e., at least 30,000 U/day); the aPTT should be kept at 1.5 to 2.5 times normal (corresponding to a circulating blood heparin level of approximately 0.3 U/mL or an anti–factor Xa trough blood level of approximately 0.7 U/mL) for 7 to 10 days.[20,52] Intravenous anticoagulation is typically continued for at least 5 to 7 days. Subsequently, subcutaneous heparin administration can be substituted for intravenous administration. Specifically, the daily heparin dose is given subcutaneously in divided doses every 8 hours to keep the aPTT at least 1.5 to 2.5 times control. The subcutaneous route of administration appears to decrease the incidence of bleeding complications.[10]

TABLE 38-3 An Acceptable Regimen for Pharmacologic Thromboprophylaxis in Obstetric Patients

Clinical Situation	Anticoagulation Regimen*
Varicosities	None
Superficial thrombophlebitis	None
Hypercoagulable states	Therapeutic
Previous deep vein thrombosis/pulmonary embolism:	
• Post-trauma	None
• Oral contraceptives	Prophylactic
• Antiphospholipid antibody syndrome	Prophylactic or therapeutic
• Unexplained	Prophylactic
• Recurrent	Prophylactic or therapeutic
Deep vein thrombosis/ pulmonary embolism (current pregnancy)	Therapeutic until 6 to 12 weeks postpartum or therapeutic for 4 to 6 months and then prophylactic until 6 to 12 weeks postpartum
Deep vein thrombosis in a prior pregnancy	Prophylactic beginning in early pregnancy
Pulmonary embolism in a prior pregnancy	Prophylactic or therapeutic

***Prophylactic regimen:** subcutaneous administration of 5000 to 10,000 U of unfractionated heparin bid without prolongation of activated partial thromboplastin time (aPTT). **Therapeutic regimen:** parenteral administration of unfractionated heparin to achieve prolongation of aPTT to 1.5 to 2.5 times control or a circulating blood heparin level of 0.3 U/mL, or low-molecular-weight heparin (to achieve a trough anti–factor Xa level of approximately 0.4 to 0.7 U/mL).

Modified from American College of Obstetricians and Gynecologists. Thromboembolism in Pregnancy. ACOG Practice Bulletin No. 19. Washington, DC, August 2000.

The aPTT is evaluated 6 hours after a subcutaneous dose. The dose of heparin may need to be increased, even by as much as 50%, in the second and third trimesters of pregnancy.[52]

A continuous infusion pump has been used in an effort to improve patient compliance with subcutaneous heparin therapy. Although early reports are conflicting, it appears that infusion pump delivery of subcutaneous heparin (by means of a soft indwelling catheter) helps maintain therapeutic levels of anticoagulation in the ambulatory (and perhaps noncompliant) patient.[53]

Heparin therapy is discontinued when the patient begins active labor, and ideally at least 24 hours before cesarean delivery.[20,54] Operative vaginal or abdominal delivery increases the risk of traumatic hemorrhage. The timing of the last dose of heparin is important, and it may be reassuring to assess anticoagulant activity by determining the aPTT or by directly measuring the blood concentration of heparin. Routine use of protamine is not suggested; it may contribute to bleeding complications owing to possible antithrombin activity. However, if necessary, incremental doses of protamine can be given up to a calculated dose of 1 mg protamine/100 U of heparin. The dose should be titrated to surgical hemostasis[11]; full neutralization may be confirmed by measurement of the activated clotting time (ACT).

Once the postpartum patient is stable and hemostasis has been obtained, heparin therapy can be re-instituted. Warfarin can be administered concurrently. Once warfarin-induced anticoagulation (as monitored by an International Normalized Ratio [INR] of 2.0 to 3.0) is achieved, heparin can be discontinued.[52] Anticoagulation is usually continued for at least 6 weeks postpartum.[10,54] Most evidence suggests that maternal administration of warfarin is compatible with breast-feeding (see Chapter 14).[55]

Over the past decade, the use of **low-molecular-weight heparin (LMWH),** for both *prophylactic* and *therapeutic* anticoagulation during pregnancy has become commonplace.[52] Because LMWH has greater antithrombotic activity (anti–factor Xa) than anticoagulant activity (anti–factor IIa), it does not affect the aPTT. However, it is not clear that the anti–factor Xa level predicts the risk of bleeding, and monitoring of anti–factor Xa activity is not available in all hospitals.

In the United States **enoxaparin** (Lovenox, Rhone-Poulenc Rohrer), injected once or twice daily at a dose of 40 mg (1 mg = 100 U), is often used for thromboprophylaxis during pregnancy.[52] (This is a larger dose than that typically given to nonpregnant patients who have undergone orthopedic surgery.[56]) Peak anti–factor Xa activity occurs within 3 to 5 hours of administration, and 50% of the total anti–factor Xa activity disappears within 6 hours.[56] Enoxaparin is also used for therapeutic anticoagulation in doses of 30 to 80 mg twice daily[52] (or a weight-adjusted dose of 1 mg/kg twice daily[54]). **Dalteparin** (Fragmin, Pfizer Health AB) is another LMWH used in pregnancy. In a dose greater than that given to nonpregnant patients, dalteparin is injected twice daily (i.e., 2500 to 5000 U once or twice daily for thrombo*prophylaxis* and 100 U/kg twice daily for *therapeutic* anticoagulation).[20,52] **Tinzaparin** (Innohep, LEO Pharma) is administered subcutaneously with a *prophylactic* dose of 4500 U daily and a *therapeutic* dose of 175 U/kg daily.[54]

Both the efficacy and the maternal and fetal safety of LMWH have been established. Advantages of LMWH therapy (in comparison with unfractionated heparin) include a decreased risk of heparin-induced thrombocytopenia, allergic skin reactions, osteoporosis, and bleeding. In nonpregnant patients, heparin-induced immune reaction is more common with unfractionated heparin than with LMWH[57,58]; this complication is rare in pregnancy. In cases of heparin-induced immune reaction, substitution of danaparoid (a glycosaminoglycan anticoagulant) or fondaparinux (a pentasaccharide anticoagulant) may be warranted.[54] Osteoporosis is a known complication of long-term heparin administration. Several studies involving pregnant women show significantly less bone demineralization with LMWH than with unfractionated heparin.[59,60] Because of the potential osteoporosis related to long-term heparin use, supplementation with calcium and vitamin D should occur for the duration of heparin therapy.[61] Finally, a systematic review did not find a higher risk of peripartum bleeding in women receiving LMWH than in untreated women.[62,63]

There are several disadvantages of LMWH. The cost can be as much as ten times higher than that of standard unfractionated heparin. As with unfractionated heparin, the pharmacokinetics of LMWH are altered during pregnancy.[64] Therefore, if the drug is being used for therapeutic anticoagulation, anti–factor Xa activity should be monitored, with a desired peak level of 0.7 to 1.2 U/mL measured 3 to 4 hours after dosing and a desired trough level of 0.4 to 0.6 U/mL 12 hours after dosing.[54,65] Thromboelastography (TEG) may provide an alternative, efficient assessment of LMWH activity in the parturient. Carroll et al.[66] demonstrated that this relatively inexpensive and rapid (30 to 60 minutes) test allows for reliable determination of the level of anticoagulation in obstetric patients. Because the parameter of this test, the delta reaction time (ΔR), correlates with anti–factor Xa levels, LMWH doses can be adjusted accordingly to ensure anticoagulation, or conversely, the absence of anticoagulation can be confirmed. LMWH is cleared by the kidney, so its use may be altered or prohibited in patients with renal failure. Finally, it must be remembered that the half-life of LMWH is long; coagulation abnormalities increase the risks of neuraxial analgesia and surgery. It is prudent to establish a plan of care early to minimize risk at the time of delivery; such a plan may include changing from LMWH to unfractionated heparin therapy at 34 to 36 weeks' gestation and/or scheduling an induction of labor before the anticipated date of delivery. If LMWH is continued until term, fresh frozen plasma should be available in the event of hemorrhage.

Protamine does not fully or reliably reverse the effects of LMWH.[67] Protamine reversal of LMWH is not recommended, although it can be argued that serial TEG might guide the use of protamine for attempted reversal of anticoagulation, if time permits.

PULMONARY EMBOLISM

Approximately 10% of all patients with a pulmonary embolus die within the first hour.[68] For pregnant survivors of the acute phase, long-term survival depends on rapid diagnosis and institution of therapy. Therapy focuses on providing (1) adequate maternal and fetal oxygenation; (2) support of maternal circulation, including uteroplacental perfusion; and (3) immediate anticoagulation or venous interruption to prevent recurrence of a (perhaps lethal) pulmonary embolus.[31] Acute decompensation from a pulmonary embolus warrants fibrinolytic therapy or, in severe cases, surgical embolectomy.[10,31,32]

Standard unfractionated heparin is the preferred anticoagulant; therapy should be started immediately. A bolus intravenous dose of 80 to 150 U/kg is followed by a continuous infusion of 15 to 25 U/kg/hr to keep the aPTT at twice-normal values.[10,31,32,52]

Inferior vena caval interruption should be considered in any patient who cannot be anticoagulated or who suffers from recurrent emboli while undergoing anticoagulant therapy.[69] Caval ligation has an operative mortality rate of 10% to 15%. However, in nonpregnant patients, insertion of an inferior vena caval filter has a mortality rate of less than 1% and a rate of recurrence of lethal emboli of less than 1%. Transvenous placement of an inferior vena cava filter has a long-term patency rate of 97%.[69]

Thrombolytic therapy should be considered in the patient with a massive pulmonary embolus.[31,32,70-72] Both urokinase and streptokinase have been used during pregnancy.[22,32,70-72] Urokinase is less antigenic and, in theory, should have fewer side effects.[70,72] A suggested course of urokinase therapy consists of an initial dose of 4400 IU/kg followed by 4400 IU/kg/hr; although increases in aPTT measurements and fibrin degradation product levels can be used to monitor thrombolytic therapy, the most sensitive measure is the thrombin time. The thrombin time should be no greater than five times normal.[72] Nonetheless, the risk of bleeding is always present.[72] Antepartum and intrapartum complications include maternal hemorrhage and placental abruption.[20,70,71]

Recombinant tissue plasminogen activator (rt-PA) has a theoretical advantage over streptokinase and urokinase in that it does not induce systemic fibrinolysis. Instead, rt-PA is active when bound to thrombin and is therefore clot specific.[73] This agent has been used successfully in pregnant women who have experienced massive PTE.[74-77] Bleeding is a risk of rt-PA therapy.[78]

Surgical embolectomy is an extreme measure that is reserved for the rapidly deteriorating patient. In nonpregnant patients, mortality rates as high as 57% have been reported for this procedure.[79]

Anesthetic Management

Cardiopulmonary sequelae of PTE often dictate the anesthetic management for labor and vaginal or cesarean delivery. More often, **asymptomatic women** with a history of DVT present for labor and vaginal or cesarean delivery. If these women are receiving anticoagulation therapy, the anesthesia provider must consider the risks and benefits of neuraxial anesthesia.

The medical literature contains reports of patients who suffered epidural hematoma after epidural anesthesia,[80] after epidural anesthesia and anticoagulation,[81,82] and after anticoagulation alone.[72,83] Vandermeulen et al.[81] reviewed 61 cases of spinal, epidural, or subdural hematoma following spinal or epidural anesthesia that were published between 1906 and 1994. (Approximately 53 of these cases were published during the past 40 years.) Likewise, Wulf[82] reviewed 51 cases of spinal hematoma associated with epidural anesthesia that were published between 1966 and 1995. In contrast, there have been at least 326 published cases of spontaneous epidural or subdural hematoma—not associated with epidural or spinal anesthesia—during the past 40 years.[81] A Swedish report demonstrated lower complication rates for spinal hematoma in obstetric patients (1:200,000) than in the nonpregnant population (1:3600 female orthopedic patients).[84] A review by Ruppen et al.[85] confirms the rarity of spinal hematoma in healthy parturients (1:168,000).

Insertion of an epidural needle causes some bleeding into the epidural space in 10% of healthy patients.[86] However, studies have reported the safe use of epidural or spinal anesthesia in more than 30,000 patients receiving thromboprophylaxis with *unfractionated* heparin during the last 20 years.

In December 1997, the U.S. Food and Drug Administration (FDA) issued a warning calling attention to the risk of epidural or spinal hematoma with concurrent use of LMWH and epidural or spinal anesthesia.[87] At that time, there were at least 30 spontaneous safety reports of patients in the United States in whom epidural or subdural hematoma developed after neuraxial anesthesia or spinal puncture while they were receiving thromboprophylaxis with enoxaparin. Most of these patients were elderly women undergoing orthopedic surgery.[67,87] The risk of hematoma seems to be increased by "traumatic or repeated spinal or epidural punctures."[87] Between 1997 and 2003, 13 additional cases of spinal hematoma following neuraxial techniques were reported, 10 of which occurred in patients undergoing LMWH therapy.[88] The apparent increase in the risk of an neuraxial hematoma following concurrent administration of neuraxial anesthesia and prophylactic LMWH may be related to the relatively greater bioavailability and longer biologic half-life of LMWH than of unfractionated heparin after subcutaneous injection.[81]

The risk of epidural hematoma associated with each specific therapy is unknown. Obviously, both the anesthesia provider and the patient would like reassurance that the risk is the same as or no higher than that for the patient who is not receiving anticoagulation therapy. The Second American Society of Regional Anesthesia and Pain Medicine (ASRA) Consensus Conference on Neuraxial Anesthesia and Anticoagulation published a risk assessment and clinical guidelines in 2003 (Box 38-1).[88] The ASRA document does not specifically address the management of pregnant women; therefore, institution-specific protocols have been developed. The following clinical protocol is used by anesthesia providers at the University of Maryland:

1. Patients who require full anticoagulation receive anticoagulant doses of subcutaneous heparin (approximately 8000 to 10,000 U every 8 to 12 hours) in an effort to keep the aPTT at twice-normal values.
2. Heparin is discontinued with the onset of active labor. In these patients, neuraxial anesthesia is withheld until the aPTT is near normal or the blood heparin concentration is near zero. If these conditions are not met, the patient is offered intravenous opioid analgesia for labor until the aPTT is near normal or the blood heparin concentration is near zero.
3. Many pregnant patients currently receive thromboprophylaxis with LMWH, and some receive *therapeutic* doses of LMWH. Patients and their obstetricians are counseled during early pregnancy that the use of LMWH thromboprophylaxis precludes the use of neuraxial anesthesia until at least 12 hours have elapsed since the time of the last *prophylactic* dose. *Therapeutic* anticoagulation with high-dose LMWH precludes the use of neuraxial anesthesia for 24 hours from the time of the last dose. Standard unfractionated heparin may be substituted for LMWH near term to allow for aPTT monitoring of anticoagulant activity.
4. Protamine reversal of heparin therapy to allow administration of neuraxial anesthesia is not recommended. Further, protamine is unpredictable in reversing the anti–factor Xa activity caused by LMWH.[67] Therefore, protamine reversal of LMWH is not recommended.
5. If cesarean delivery is required in a patient with abnormal coagulation, general anesthesia is administered.
6. The re-institution of anticoagulation therapy after delivery should be discussed with the obstetrician. For postpartum thrombo*prophylaxis* with once-daily doses of LMWH, at least 6 to 8 hours should elapse after spinal or epidural needle placement before the first dose of LMWH is administered; the second postoperative dose should be given no sooner than 24 hours after the first dose.[88] For patients receiving higher (i.e., twice-daily) doses of LMWH, at least 24 hours should elapse after spinal or epidural needle placement before the first postpartum dose of LMWH is given. Similarly, when blood is detected during needle and catheter placement, initiation of LMWH therapy should be delayed for at least 24 hours.

BOX 38-1 Neuraxial Anesthesia in the Anticoagulated Patient: Guidelines for Low-Molecular-Weight Heparin in Nonpregnant Patients

1. Needle placement for single-injection spinal or epidural anesthesia should be delayed at least 10 to 12 hours after the last preoperative *prophylactic* dose of LMWH.
2. For single-dose and continuous-catheter neuraxial techniques, in the presence of adequate hemostasis, the timing of the first postoperative LMWH dose differs between twice-daily and once-daily LMWH regimens. The first postoperative dose of a twice-daily LMWH regimen should not occur earlier than 24 hours after surgery. For once-daily LMWH regimens, the first postoperative dose should be administered 6 to 8 hours after surgery, and the second postoperative dose should not occur sooner than 24 hours after the first dose.
3. Twice-daily LMWH dosing: The epidural catheter may be left indwelling overnight and removed the following day, and the first dose of LMWH may be administered 2 hours after catheter removal.
4. Single daily LMWH dosing: The epidural catheter should be removed a minimum of 10 to 12 hours after the last dose of LMWH. Subsequent LMWH dosing should occur a minimum of 2 hours after catheter removal.
5. In instances where blood is detected during needle and/or catheter placement, initiation of LMWH therapy should be delayed for at least 24 hours postoperatively.
6. NSAIDs alone do not significantly increase the risk of spinal hematoma. Combination therapy with unfractionated heparin, LMWH, oral anticoagulants, and thrombolytics has been demonstrated to increase the frequency of spontaneous hemorrhagic complications, bleeding at puncture sites, and spinal hematoma.
7. The anti-Xa level is not predictive of the risk of bleeding and is, therefore, not helpful in the management of patients undergoing neuraxial blocks and is not recommended.

LMWH, low-molecular-weight heparin; NSAID, nonsteroidal anti-inflammatory drugs; Xa, coagulation factor Xa.

From Horlocker TT, Wedel DJ, Benzon H, et al. Regional anesthesia in the anticoagulated patient: Defining the risks (The Second ASRA Consensus Conference on Neuraxial Anesthesia and Anticoagulation). Reg Anesth Pain Med 2003; 28:172-97.

7. Removal of the epidural catheter may also cause venous disruption and bleeding into the epidural space. The ASRA guidelines state that neuraxial catheters may be "safely maintained" in patients receiving once-daily dosing of LMWH postoperatively.[88] The catheter should be removed at least 10 to 12 hours after the last dose of LMWH, and subsequent doses of LMWH should be given a minimum of 2 hours after catheter removal. For patients receiving twice-daily doses of LMWH, indwelling catheters should be removed before initiation of LMWH thromboprophylaxis. In these women, the first dose of LMWH should not be administered until at least 2 hours have elapsed since catheter removal.

Concomitant fibrinolytic therapy puts the patient at high risk for hemorrhage and contraindicates the administration of epidural anesthesia if delivery has not occurred. There is one published case of a nonpregnant patient in whom an epidural hematoma developed after administration of epidural anesthesia for a vascular surgical procedure that included administration of urokinase.[89] There are case reports describing spontaneous spinal or epidural hematoma following either thrombolytic therapy or combination fibrinolytic and thrombolytic use.[88] Fibrinolytic agents are associated with a significant risk of placental abruption and maternal hemorrhage. Therefore, labor and delivery represent relative contraindications to the use of fibrinolytic therapy, and the question regarding epidural anesthesia is moot.

The peripartum use (before, during, or after the administration of neuraxial anesthesia) of anticoagulation or fibrinolytic therapy requires that the anesthesia provider, obstetrician, and nursing staff remain vigilant for all of the signs and symptoms that herald epidural hematoma. These include (1) severe, unremitting backache; (2) neurologic deficit, including bowel or bladder dysfunction or radiculopathy; (3) tenderness over the spinous or paraspinous area; and (4) unexplained fever.[67,89] Suspicion of epidural hematoma should lead to immediate diagnostic imaging of the spinal cord and neurosurgical consultation for possible spinal cord decompression. To avoid irreversible damage, surgery should occur within 6 to 12 hours.[90,91] According to the American Society of Anesthesiologists (ASA) Closed-Claims database, spinal cord injuries were a leading cause of claims in the last decade, and diagnosis of spinal cord ischemia was frequently delayed because neurologic dysfunction was erroneously attributed to local anesthetic effects.[92]

Risks of general anesthesia in the anticoagulated patient include the risk for airway bleeding. Laryngoscopy and tracheal intubation should be as atraumatic as possible. The anesthesia provider should be aware that placement of nasopharyngeal and oropharyngeal airways, gastric tubes, and other devices (e.g., temperature probes, stethoscopes) carries the tangible risk of traumatic hemorrhage. Emergency surgery may necessitate the administration of protamine or the transfusion of blood products (e.g., plasma, platelets) to reverse anticoagulation and reduce the risk of hemorrhage during and after surgery.

AMNIOTIC FLUID EMBOLISM

Amniotic fluid embolism (AFE) is a devastating condition unique to pregnancy. Although AFE was first reported in 1926,[93] it was not until 1941 that Steiner and Lushbaugh[94] reviewed a series of autopsies and described the syndrome of sudden peripartum shock characterized by pulmonary edema.

Incidence

Reports of incidence vary greatly, in part because AFE is a diagnosis of exclusion that is often assigned only after autopsy. In the United States, the incidence of AFE is 4 to 6 per 100,000 live births.[95] The rate may be higher in multiple gestation births (14.5 per 100,000) than singleton deliveries (6 per 100,000).[96] However, AFE accounts for as many as 12% of maternal deaths.[97] The overall mortality rate for affected parturients is reported to be between 25% and 80%.[7,95,96] Two thirds of these deaths occur within the first 5 hours.[7,98] Among survivors, the incidence of severe and permanent neurologic dysfunction is disappointingly high for this group of young, previously healthy patients. In a U.K. registry, only 7% of survivors had neurologic impairment.[99] However, in a review of 46 cases of AFE reported to an American national registry, only 3 (25%) of 12 patients who had survived a cardiac arrest were judged neurologically intact.[7]

Pathophysiology

The etiology of the AFE syndrome is unclear. In primate models, the injection of autologous amniotic fluid does not produce AFE.[98] The amount of particulate matter found in the lungs does not correlate with the severity of the clinical presentation, and there are many reports of women with clinical features suggestive of AFE whose pulmonary vasculature has not shown classic pathologic evidence (fetal cells).[98] Experimental injection of filtered amniotic fluid has produced the picture of AFE in some animals. Some investigators have suggested that arachidonic acid metabolites, especially leukotrienes, are responsible for the clinical and pathophysiologic features of AFE.[100,101] Others have hypothesized an immune-mediated mechanism with massive complement activation.[102,103] One study suggested the presence of a heat-stable pressor agent in meconium, which enhances the cardiopulmonary response to the infusion of autologous amniotic fluid in goats.[104] In the review of cases reported to the U.S. national registry for AFE, the presence of meconium in the amniotic fluid was associated with a uniformly dismal prognosis, with no neurologically intact survivors.[7]

Experience with hemodynamic monitoring during the resuscitation of parturients with AFE has challenged traditional beliefs garnered from earlier work in nonprimate (and in some cases, nonpregnant) models. Clark[98] has described a **biphasic** response to AFE. The **early phase** consists of transient (but perhaps intense) pulmonary vasospasm, which most likely results from the release of vasoactive substances. This vasospasm may account for the often fatal right heart dysfunction. Low cardiac output leads to increased ventilation-perfusion mismatch, hypoxemia, and hypotension. This phase most likely has a duration of less than 30 minutes. Right heart function and pulmonary artery pressures are typically reported close to "normal" by the time invasive hemodynamic monitoring is begun in humans resuscitated from AFE.[98,105] A report of transesophageal echocardiography initiated within 15 minutes of the onset of symptoms of a fatal AFE confirmed the occurrence of acute, massive right heart failure and severe pulmonary artery hypertension.[106] A **second phase** consisting of left ventricular failure and pulmonary edema occurs in women who survive the initial insult.[98,105,107] Reports of cases in which invasive hemodynamic monitoring was performed have consistently noted the occurrence of left ventricular dysfunction in women with AFE. The etiology of the left ventricular dysfunction remains unclear.[98]

Disruption of the normal clotting cascade occurs in as many as 66% of women with AFE.[95,98] The etiology of the coagulopathy is unclear. Although amniotic fluid contains procoagulant, it is doubtful that this amount of factor X activator is sufficient to cause the clotting abnormalities seen with AFE. Some authorities have suggested that circulating trophoblast may be responsible for the disruption of the normal clotting cascade.[98] In addition, uterine atony occurs in some women (perhaps as a result of a circulating myometrial depressant factor[98] or uterine hypoperfusion). Massive hemorrhage may also contribute to a consumptive coagulopathy.

Clinical Presentation

Amniotic fluid embolism has occurred during first-trimester abortion,[108] in the second trimester,[109] after abdominal trauma,[110] and even in the postpartum period.[95,111,112] In an analysis of the 46 cases reported to the national registry, Clark et al.[7] found that three cases occurred during second-trimester termination of pregnancy. Of the remaining 43 cases, 30 (70%) occurred during labor, and 13 (30%) occurred after cesarean (n = 8) or vaginal (n = 5) delivery. A similar rate was found in a recent review of AFE from Japan in which 21% of cases occurred after cesarean delivery.[113] Of the postpartum patients in the Clark study who experienced AFE, the mean ± SD time from delivery to initial clinical presentation was 8 ± 8 minutes. Nine of the 13 patients who demonstrated AFE after delivery did so within 5 minutes of delivery. Overall, labor was not tumultuous, and analysis of the data suggested "no causative link between hypertonic contractions and the occurrence of AFE."[7] Among the 30 women who had AFE during labor, only 15 (50%) had received oxytocin, and only 1 demonstrated uterine hyperstimulation at the time of the acute event. The investigators concluded that uterine hyperstimulation was a result rather than a cause of AFE (Figure 38-1). Kramer et al.[96] identified an increase in AFE rates in women undergoing medical induction of labor (adjusted odds ratio = 1.8); the association with uterine hyperstimulation was not addressed. Thirty-eight (88%) of 43 patients experienced AFE after spontaneous (n = 12) or artificial (n = 26) rupture of membranes. In 6 of these patients, signs and symptoms of AFE occurred within 3 minutes of artificial rupture of membranes or placement of an intrauterine pressure catheter. Meconium-stained amniotic fluid was noted in a minority of cases.[7]

The diagnosis of AFE is one of exclusion. The clinical presentation often is compatible with other malignant events (Table 38-4). The differential diagnosis should include (1) other obstetric complications (e.g., placental abruption, eclampsia); (2) nonobstetric complications (e.g., PTE, venous air embolism, septic shock, myocardial infarction, anaphylaxis); and (3) anesthetic complications (e.g., total spinal anesthesia, systemic local anesthetic toxicity).[7]

In the past, physicians thought that the detection of fetal squamous cells in the pulmonary circulation was pathognomonic of AFE.[114,115] However, in the cases reported to the national registry, cells of fetal origin were found at autopsy in the pulmonary circulation of only 73% of the patients who died.[7] Further, cells of fetal origin were found in only 50% of patients diagnosed with AFE who underwent aspiration of pulmonary arterial blood. Conversely, obstetricians have detected fetal squamous cells in the pulmonary circulation of both antepartum and postpartum patients with no clinical evidence of AFE.[116,117]

Kobayashi et al.[118] described the use of a monoclonal antibody for detection of an amniotic fluid–specific antigen (fetal mucin) in the maternal circulation of patients with signs and symptoms of AFE. Measurement of the maternal plasma concentration of zinc coproporphyrin, a component of meconium, has also been proposed as a sensitive test for the diagnosis of AFE.[119]

In summary, Clark et al.[7] have concluded that the syndrome of AFE is "not consistent with an embolic event, as it

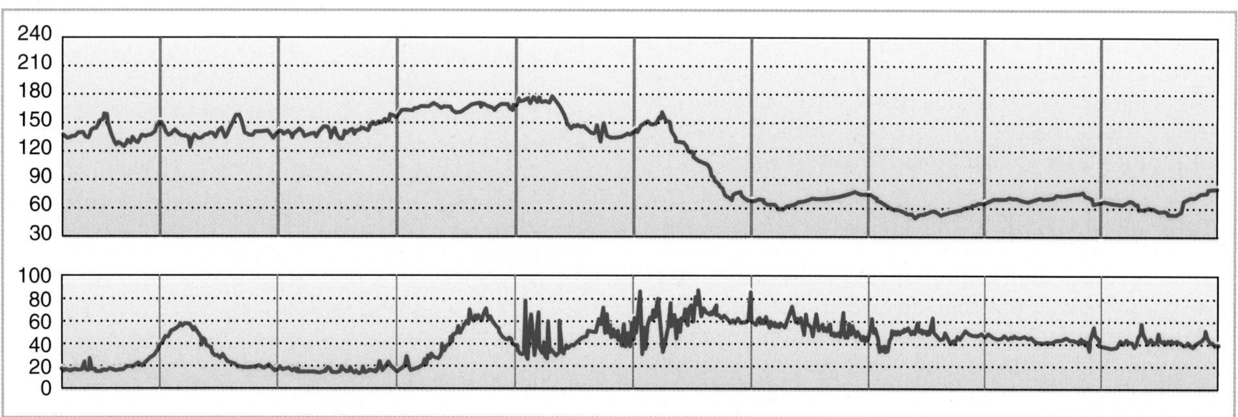

FIGURE 38-1 Fetal heart rate tracing in a patient with amniotic fluid embolism. Maternal symptoms began just *before* the onset of spontaneous uterine hypertonus and fetal bradycardia. (Modified from Clark SL, Hankins GDV, Dudley DA, et al. Amniotic fluid embolism: Analysis of the national registry. Am J Obstet Gynecol 1995; 172:1158-69.)

TABLE 38-4 Signs and Symptoms Noted in 46 Patients with Amniotic Fluid Embolism

Sign or Symptom	Patients Affected No.	Patients Affected Percentage
Hypotension	46	100
Fetal compromise*	30	100
Pulmonary edema or adult respiratory distress syndrome†	28	93
Cardiopulmonary arrest	40	87
Cyanosis	38	83
Coagulopathy‡	38	83
Dyspnea§	22	49
Seizure	22	48
Atony	11	23
Bronchospasm¶	7	15
Transient hypertension	5	11
Cough	3	7
Headache	3	7
Chest pain	1	2

*n = 30; includes all live fetuses *in utero* at time of event.

†n = 30; 16 patients did not survive long enough for these diagnoses to be confirmed.

‡n = 38; 8 patients did not survive long enough for this diagnosis to be confirmed.

§n = 45; 1 patient was intubated at the time of the event and could not be assessed.

¶Difficult ventilation was noted during cardiac arrest in 6 patients, and wheezes were auscultated in 1 patient.

Adapted from Clark SL, Hankins GDV, Dudley DA, et al. Amniotic fluid embolism: Analysis of the national registry. Am J Obstet Gynecol 1995; 172:1158-69.

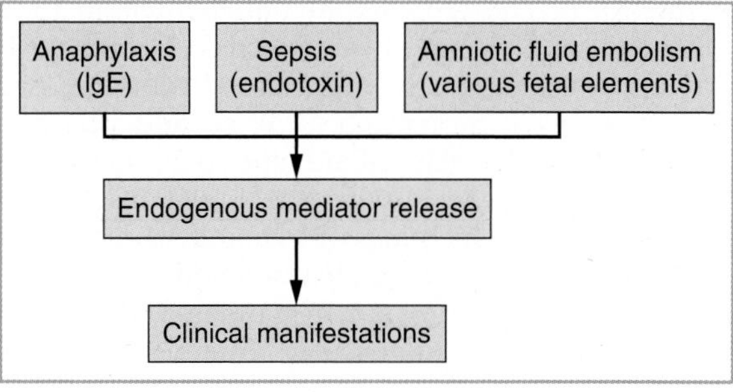

FIGURE 38-2 Proposed pathophysiologic relation between amniotic fluid embolism, septic shock, and anaphylactic shock. Each syndrome may also have specific direct physiologic effects (e.g., fever in endotoxin-mediated sepsis). IgE, immunoglobulin E. (Modified from Clark SL, Hankins GDV, Dudley DA, et al. Amniotic fluid embolism: Analysis of the national registry. Am J Obstet Gynecol 1995; 172:1158-69.)

is commonly understood." Thus, they suggested that the term *amniotic fluid embolism* is a misnomer that should be discarded. They acknowledged that this syndrome seems to occur after maternal intravascular exposure to fetal tissue during normal labor, or during vaginal or cesarean delivery. They suggested that "the syndrome of acute peripartum hypoxia, hemodynamic collapse, and coagulopathy should be [designated] in a more descriptive manner as *anaphylactoid syndrome of pregnancy*."[7] They concluded that "striking similarities between clinical and hemodynamic findings in amniotic fluid embolism and both anaphylaxis and septic shock suggest a common pathophysiologic mechanism for all these conditions" (Figure 38-2).[7]

Anesthetic and Obstetric Management

Prompt recognition and institution of resuscitative measures may influence maternal and fetal outcome (Box 38-2). Most patients require tracheal intubation, mechanical ventilation, and administration of supplemental oxygen. Prompt support of oxygenation and circulation may decrease the severity of neurologic sequelae. Early recognition and communication with the blood bank are necessary to facilitate the provision of the large quantities of blood and blood products required during resuscitation.

Patients are young and typically healthy before the onset of AFE. Resuscitative measures should be aggressive. Devices capable of large-volume, rapid intravenous infusion may be invaluable during resuscitation. Esposito et al.[120] reported the successful use of cardiopulmonary bypass and pulmonary artery thromboembolectomy for the treatment of postpartum shock caused by AFE. Staten et al.[121] used transesophageal echocardiography (TEE) for prompt diagnosis of catastrophic pulmonary vasoconstriction (significant right heart failure) followed by cardiopulmonary bypass to circumvent the lesion. Another case report suggests the benefit of nitric oxide to treat right heart failure and severe pulmonary hypertension.[122,123]

During resuscitation, the obstetrician should make an early decision regarding delivery of the fetus. Among the cases reported to the national registry, at least 28 patients had AFE while the fetus was alive *in utero*.[7] Twenty-two

BOX 38-2 Resuscitation of the Obstetric Patient with Amniotic Fluid Embolism

- Initiate cardiopulmonary resuscitation if necessary.
- Support maternal circulation.
- Perform intravenous volume resuscitation:
  - Establish intravenous access with several large-gauge catheters.
  - Insert an intra-arterial catheter and a pulmonary artery catheter.
  - Begin inotropic support if needed.
- Perform fetal monitoring:
  - Make a decision regarding delivery—either before impending maternal demise or to improve chances of maternal resuscitation.
- Treat the coagulopathy:
  - Decide between component therapy versus fresh whole blood.
  - Obtain early consultation from a hematologist and a blood bank pathologist.
- Manage sequelae of shock (e.g., cardiac failure, pulmonary edema, adult respiratory distress syndrome, renal failure, hepatic failure, neurologic sequelae).
- Anticipate a prolonged intensive care unit stay.

(79%) infants survived, but of those, only 11 were neurologically intact. Among those patients who experienced cardiac arrest while the fetus was *in utero*, a cardiac arrest–to-delivery interval longer than 15 minutes was associated with a lesser likelihood of intact survival. However, the investigators noted some cases of fetal neurologic injury even when delivery occurred within 5 minutes of maternal cardiac arrest. The investigators concluded:

> *Intact maternal survival after cardiac arrest is rare, and delivery may, on theoretical grounds, actually be of benefit to the mother undergoing cardiopulmonary resuscitation. For these reasons we recommend that perimortem cesarean section be initiated as soon as possible after maternal cardiac arrest in patients with clinical amniotic fluid embolism.*[7]

If the patient received neuraxial anesthesia before the onset of AFE, the subsequent coagulopathy should alert physicians and nurses to the potential for bleeding within the epidural space. Neurologic function should be assessed frequently, as allowed by the physical condition of the patient. It has been suggested that an indwelling epidural catheter should be removed as soon as possible, preferably after the transfusion of blood and replacement of coagulation factors has temporarily created a state of normal coagulation.[124-126] An argument can also be made for leaving the catheter *in situ* until coagulation values return to near-normal.

Lastly, Clark[123] reported two cases of successful pregnancy outcomes in women who survived AFE during earlier pregnancies. He stated:

> *This report supports the role of a qualitatively abnormal amniotic fluid, which may be different in a subsequent pregnancy, as opposed to any unusual maternal sensitivity to amniotic fluid per se in the genesis of this condition. Although any conclusions based on two cases must be regarded as tenuous, it appears that on a theoretic basis . . . repeat amniotic fluid embolism syndrome is probably unlikely.*[123]

VENOUS AIR EMBOLISM

Venous air embolism (VAE) is a recognized complication of many surgical procedures. Numerous case reports in obstetric patients have appeared in the medical literature since the early nineteenth century.[127] In 1987, Malinow et al.[1] published the first study of VAE during cesarean delivery. Subsequently, others have confirmed the observation that VAE is a common occurrence during both cesarean delivery[2-5] and vaginal delivery.[128] Venous air embolism may account for transient symptoms (e.g., dyspnea, chest pain) and signs (e.g., sudden decrease in Sa_{O_2}, hypotension, arrhythmias) commonly encountered during cesarean delivery.[1-4]

Incidence

One study determined that subclinical VAE (as determined by analysis of end-tidal nitrogen concentration) occurred in 97% of patients receiving *general* anesthesia for cesarean delivery.[6] Other studies have noted that VAE occurs in as many as 67% of patients receiving *neuraxial* anesthesia for cesarean delivery.[1-5] Precordial Doppler monitoring is able to detect a volume of intracardiac air as small as 0.1 mL. In one study, concurrent transthoracic echocardiography confirmed all episodes of Doppler-detected VAE during cesarean delivery.[2] Together, these studies suggest that either one third of the episodes of VAE during cesarean delivery with *neuraxial* anesthesia are missed when care providers are listening to the Doppler signal, or that general anesthesia during cesarean delivery is associated with a higher risk of VAE.[2,6] In either case, VAE is a common occurrence at any time during delivery.[1-6,129]

Pathophysiology

A pressure gradient as small as −5 cm H_2O between the surgical field and the heart allows a significant amount of air to be entrained into the venous circulation. Routine left uterine displacement and use of the Trendelenburg position (which may be requested during cesarean delivery) increase this gradient. In theory, any cause of reduced central venous pressure (e.g., hemorrhage) also may increase the risk of VAE.

Three studies have provided conflicting data regarding the influence of maternal position on the occurrence of VAE during cesarean delivery.[3,6,130] The steep Trendelenburg position is probably best avoided. Placement of the patient in the reverse Trendelenburg position most likely does not significantly decrease the incidence of VAE. However, at least two studies have observed that uterine exteriorization is associated with a higher incidence of Doppler-detected changes suggestive of VAE during cesarean delivery.[5,131]

Morbidity and mortality from VAE are related to the volume and rate of the infusion of air into the central circulation as well as the site of embolization. Large volumes (more than 3 mL/kg) of air are fatal, most likely because of right ventricular outflow tract obstruction (i.e., "air lock"). Smaller amounts of air can result in ventilation-perfusion mismatch, hypoxemia, right heart failure, arrhythmias, and hypotension. A paradoxical air embolus into the arterial circulation (by means of a patent foramen ovale) can lead to cardiovascular and neurologic sequelae and morbidity.

Clinical Presentation

Massive VAE can manifest as a sudden, dramatic, and devastating event with hypotension, hypoxemia, and even cardiac arrest.[132] However, VAE causes significant hemodynamic compromise (i.e., a more than 20% decrease in blood pressure) in only 0.7% to 2% of parturients at delivery.[2,4] Typically, the clinical picture is much less dramatic. VAE has been associated with chest pain (less than 50% of cases),[1,3-5,129] decreased Sa_{O_2} (25% of cases),[4,5] and dyspnea (20% to 50% of cases).[1,4]

ECG changes, including ST segment depression, are seen in 25% to 50% of all patients undergoing cesarean delivery.[129,133,134] It is unclear whether VAE is responsible for these ECG changes, the clinical significance of which also is unclear. One study used precordial Doppler monitoring, transthoracic echocardiography, and ST segment analysis to supplement ECG monitoring during elective cesarean

BOX 38-3 Resuscitation of the Obstetric Patient with Massive Venous Air Embolism

- Prevent further air entrainment (e.g., flood surgical field, change position).
- Discontinue nitrous oxide and give 100% oxygen.
- Support ventilation as needed.
- Support circulation.
- If hemodynamic instability persists, consider placement of a multi-orifice central venous catheter to attempt aspiration of air.
- Expedite delivery.
- If there is delayed emergence from general anesthesia, consider neurodiagnostic imaging to rule out intracerebral air. Patients with evidence of parodoxic cerebral arterial gas embolism may benefit from hyperbaric oxygen therapy.

delivery. Although decreased ejection fraction as measured by echocardiography was sometimes associated with episodes of ST segment depression, regional wall motion abnormalities were not detected.[129] Doppler evidence of VAE was not associated with ST segment depression in this study, but both modalities were used concurrently in only one fourth of the subjects.[129]

Recommendations

Kaunitz et al.[97] reported that VAE is responsible for 1% of maternal deaths in the United States. However, it is likely that some of these deaths resulted from episodes of VAE during orogenital sex.[135,136] Although there is evidence that VAE is a common occurrence during cesarean delivery, maternal morbidity and mortality are rare. Precordial Doppler monitoring during cesarean delivery is not recommended. However, high-risk patients (those who are hypovolemic or have known intracardiac shunt) may benefit from the use of precordial Doppler monitoring. A high index of suspicion should accompany any complaints of chest pain or dyspnea, decreased Sa_{O_2}, hypotension, or arrhythmia. Early recognition of the signs and symptoms of VAE should prompt the appropriate response (Box 38-3).

KEY POINTS

- Embolic disorders are a major cause of maternal mortality.
- Early recognition, diagnosis, and therapy reduce the incidence of morbidity and mortality associated with embolic disorders.
- Therapy for deep vein thrombosis focuses on the prevention of pulmonary embolism.
- Therapy for a pulmonary embolus focuses on the prevention of a recurrent pulmonary thromboembolic event.
- Amniotic fluid embolism may occur at any time during labor and delivery, although it has been reported both antenatally and in the postpartum period.
- The syndrome of amniotic fluid embolism typically manifests as dyspnea, cyanosis, and sudden cardiovascular collapse. These signs and symptoms are compatible with other embolic phenomena. In some cases, the onset of amniotic fluid embolism may be more insidious and may mimic other obstetric complications (e.g., eclampsia, hemorrhage).
- Venous air embolism is a common occurrence during cesarean delivery. Most of the emboli are small, transient, and benign. Massive venous air embolism is rare during vaginal or cesarean delivery, but it can be fatal.

REFERENCES

1. Malinow AM, Naulty JS, Hunt CO, et al. Precordial ultrasonic Doppler monitoring during cesarean delivery. Anesthesiology 1987; 66:816-9.
2. Fong J, Gadalla F, Piorri MK, Druzin M. Are Doppler detected venous emboli during cesarean section air emboli? Anesth Analg 1990; 71:254-7.
3. Karapurthy VK, Downing JW, Husain FJ, et al. Incidence of venous air embolism during cesarean section is unchanged by 5 to 10 degree head up tilt. Anesth Analg 1989; 69:620-3.
4. Vartikar JV, Johnson MD, Datta S. Precordial Doppler monitoring and pulse oximetry during cesarean delivery and detection of venous air embolism. Reg Anesth 1989; 14:145-8.
5. Handler JS, Bromage PR. Venous air embolism during cesarean delivery. Reg Anesth 1990; 15:170-3.
6. Lew TWK, Tay DHB, Tomas E. Venous air embolism during cesarean section: More common than previously thought. Anesth Analg 1993; 77:448-52.
7. Clark SL, Hankins GDV, Dudley DA, et al. Amniotic fluid embolism: Analysis of the national registry. Am J Obstet Gynecol 1995; 172:1158-69.
8. Bergqvist A, Bergqvist D, Lindhagen A, et al. Late symptoms after pregnancy-related deep vein thrombosis. BJOG 1990; 97:338-41.
9. Alfirevic A, Roberts D, Martlew V. How strong is the association between maternal thrombophilia and adverse pregnancy outcome? A systematic review. Eur J Obstet Gynecol Reprod Biol 2002; 101:6-14.
10. Weiner CP. Diagnosis and management of thromboembolic disease during pregnancy. Clin Obstet Gynecol 1985; 28:107-18.
11. Gherman RB, Goodwin TM, Leung B, et al. Incidence, clinical characteristics, and timing of objectively diagnosed venous thromboembolism during pregnancy. Obstet Gynecol 1999; 94:730-4.
12. Rothbard MJ, Gluck D, Stone ML. Anticoagulation therapy in antepartum pulmonary embolism. N Y State J Med 1976; 76:582-4.
13. James AH, Jamison MG, Brancazio LR, et al. Venous thromboembolism during pregnancy and the postpartum period: Incidence, risk factors, and mortality. Am J Obstet Gynecol 2006; 194:1311-5.
14. Andersen BS, Steffensen FH, Sorensen HT, et al. The cumulative incidence of venous thromboembolism during pregnancy and puerperium: An 11 year Danish population-based study of 63,300 pregnancies. Acta Obstet Gynecol Scand 1998; 77:170-3.
15. James AH, Tapson VF, Goldhaber SZ. Thrombosis during pregnancy and the postpartum period. Am J Obstet Gynecol 2005; 193:216-9.
16. Ray JG, Chan WS. Deep vein thrombosis during pregnancy and the puerperium: A meta-analysis of the period of risk and the leg presentation. Obstet Gynecol Surv 1999; 54:265-71.
17. Stein PD, Hull RD, Kayali F, et al. Venous thromboembolism in pregnancy: 21-year trends. Am J Med 2004; 117:121-5.
18. Brown CEL, Lowe TW, Cunningham FG, et al. Puerperal pelvic thrombophlebitis: Impact on diagnosis and treatment using x-ray

computed tomography and magnetic resonance imaging. Obstet Gynecol 1986; 68:789-94.
19. Rutherford SE, Phelan JP. Deep venous thrombosis and pulmonary embolism in pregnancy. Obstet Gynecol Clin North Am 1991; 18:345-69.
20. Sipes SL, Weiner CP. Venous thromboembolic disease in pregnancy. Semin Perinatol 1990; 14:103-18.
21. Villasanta U. Thromboembolic disease in pregnancy. Am J Obstet Gynecol 1965; 93:142-60.
22. Bonnar J. Venous thromboembolism and pregnancy. Clin Obstet Gynecol 1981; 8:455-73.
23. Heit J, Kobberveg C, Petterson T, et al. Trends in the incidence of deep vein thrombosis and pulmonary embolism during pregnancy or the puerperium: A 30-year population based study. Ann Intern Med 2005; 143:697-706.
24. Palmer SK, Zamudio S, Coffin C, et al. Quantitative estimation of human uterine artery blood flow and pelvic blood flow redistribution in pregnancy. Obstet Gynecol 1992; 80:1000-6.
25. Gerbasi FR, Bottoms S, Farag A, et al. Increased intravascular coagulation associated with pregnancy. Obstet Gynecol 1990; 75:385-9.
26. Gerbasi FR, Bottoms S, Farag A, et al. Changes in hemostatic activity during delivery and the immediate postpartum period. Am J Obstet Gynecol 1990; 162:1158-63.
27. Ros HR, Lichtenstein P, Bellocco R, et al. Pulmonary embolism and stroke in relation to pregnancy: How can high-risk women be identified? Am J Obstet Gynecol 2002; 186:198-203.
28. Lindqvist P, Dahlback B, Marsal K. Thrombotic risk during pregnancy: A population study. Am Coll Obstet Gynecol 1999; 94:595-9.
29. Bremme K, Lind H, Blomback M. The effect of prophylactic heparin treatment in enhanced thrombin generation in pregnancy. Obstet Gynecol 1993; 78:78-83.
30. Stein PD, Beemath A, Matta F, et al. Clinical characteristics of patients with acute pulmonary embolism: Data from PIOPED II. Am J Med 2007; 120:871-9.
31. Spence TH. Pulmonary embolization syndrome. In Civetta JM, Taylor RM, Kirby RR, editors. Critical Care. Philadelphia, JB Lippincott, 1988:1091-2.
32. Hollingsworth HM, Pratter MR, Irwin RS. Acute respiratory failure in pregnancy. J Intensive Care Med 1989; 4:11-34.
33. Gal TJ. Causes and consequences of impaired gas exchange. In Benumof J, Saidman L, editors. Anesthesia and Perioperative Complications. St Louis, Mosby, 1992:203-27.
34. Kearon C. Diagnosis of pulmonary embolism. Can Med Assoc J 2003; 168:183-94.
35. Stein PD, Woodard PK, Weg JG, et al. Diagnostic pathways in acute pulmonary embolism: Recommendations of the PIOPED II investigators. Am J Med 2006; 119:1048-55.
36. Epiney M, Boehlen F, Boulvain M, et al. D-dimer levels during delivery and the postpartum. J Thromb Haemost 2005; 3:268-71.
37. Morse M. Establishing a normal range for D-dimer levels throughout pregnancy to aid in the diagnosis of pulmonary embolism and deep vein thrombosis. J Thromb Haemost 2004; 2:1202-4.
38. Matthews S. Short communication: Imaging pulmonary embolism in pregnancy: What is the most appropriate imaging protocol? Br J Radiol 2006; 79:441-4.
39. Meyerovitz MF, Mannting F, Polak JF, et al. Frequency of pulmonary embolism in patients with low-probability lung scan and negative lower extremity venous ultrasound. Chest 1999; 115:980-2.
40. Boiselle PM, Reddy SS, Villas PA, et al. Pulmonary embolus in pregnant patients: Survey of ventilation-perfusion imaging policies and practice. Radiology 1998; 207:201-6.
41. Chan WS, Ray JG, Murray S, et al. Suspected pulmonary embolism in pregnancy: Clinical presentation, results of lung scanning, and subsequent maternal and pediatric outcomes. Arch Intern Med 2002; 162:1170-5.
42. Ryu JH, Swensen SJ, Olson EJ, et al. Diagnosis of pulmonary embolism with use of computed tomographic angiography. Mayo Clin Proc 2001; 76:59-65.
43. Barron WM. The pregnant surgical patient: Medical evaluation and management. Ann Intern Med 1984; 101:683-91.
44. Doyle NM, Ramirez NM, Mastrobattista JM, et al. Diagnosis of pulmonary embolism: A cost effective analysis. Am J Obstet Gynecol 2004; 191:1019-23.
45. Winer-Muram HT, Boone JM, Brown HL, et al. Pulmonary embolism in pregnant patients: Fetal radiation dose with helical CT. Radiology 2002; 224:487-92.
46. Ginsberg JS, Hirsh J, Rainbow AJ, et al. Risks to the fetus of radiologic procedures used in the diagnosis of maternal venous thromboembolic disease. Thromb Haemost 1989; 61:189-96.
47. Mossman KL, Hill LT. Radiation risks in pregnancy. Obstet Gynecol 1982; 60:237-42.
48. Rosenberg JM, Lefor AT, Kenien G, et al. Echocardiographic diagnosis and surgical treatment of postpartum pulmonary embolism. Ann Thoracic Surg 1990; 49:667-9.
49. Grifoni S, Olivotto I, Cecchini P, et al. Utility of an integrated clinical, echocardiographic, and venous ultrasonographic approach for triage of patients with suspected pulmonary embolism. Am J Cardiol 1998; 82:1230-5.
50. Polak JF, Wilkinson DL. Ultrasonographic diagnosis of symptomatic deep venous thrombosis in pregnancy. Am J Obstet Gynecol 1991; 165:625-9.
51. Mintz MC, Levy DW, Axel L, et al. Puerperal ovarian vein thrombosis: MR diagnosis. Am J Radiol 1987; 149:1273-4.
52. American College of Obstetricians and Gynecologists Committee on Practice. Thromboembolism in Pregnancy. ACOG Practice Bulletin No. 19. Washington, DC, August 2000.
53. Floyd RC, Gookin KS, Hess LW, et al. Administration of heparin by subcutaneous infusion with a programmable pump. Am J Obstet Gynecol 1991; 165:931-3.
54. Bates SM, Greer IA, Pabinger I, et al. Venous thrombembolism, thrombophilia, antithrombolic therapy, and pregnancy: American College of Chest Physicians evidence-based clinical practice guidelines (8th edition). Chest 2008; 133(6 Suppl):844S-886S.
55. American Academy of Pediatrics, Committee on Drugs. The transfer of drugs and other chemicals into human milk. Pediatrics 1994; 93:137-50.
56. Eisenach JC. Safety issues concerning the use of spinal/epidural anesthesia in patients receiving low-molecular-weight heparin prophylaxis. American Society of Regional Anesthesia. ASRA News 1995; Nov:5-6.
57. Lindhoff-Last E, Navok R, Misselwitz F. Incidence and clinical relevance of heparin-induced antibodies in patients with deep vein thrombosis treated with unfractionated or low-molecular-weight heparin. Br J Haematol 2002; 118:1137-42.
58. Warketin TE, Levine MN, Hirsh J, et al. Heparin-induced thrombocytopenia in patients treated with low-molecular-weight heparin or unfractionated heparin. N Engl J Med 1995; 332:1330-5.
59. Nelson-Piercy C, Letsky EA, De Swiet M. Low-molecular-weight heparin for obstetric thromboprophylaxis: Experience of sixty-nine pregnancies in sixty-one women at high risk. Am J Obstet Gynecol 1997; 176:1062-8.
60. Pattila V, Leinonen P, Markkola A, et al. Postpartum bone mineral density in women treated for thromboprophylaxis with unfractionated heparin or LMW heparin. Thromb Haemost 2002; 87:182-6.
61. Duhl AJ, Paidas MJ, Ural SH, et al. Antithrombotic therapy and pregnancy: Consensus report and recommendations for prevention and treatment of venous thromboembolism and adverse pregnancy outcomes. Am J Obstet Gynecol 2007; 197:457.e1-21.
62. Greer I, Nelson-Percy C. Low-molecular-weight heparins for thromboprophylaxis and treatment of venous thromboembolism in pregnancy: A systemic review of safety and efficacy. Blood 2005; 106:104-7.
63. Kominiarek MA, Angelopoulos SM, Shapiro NL, et al. Low-molecular-weight heparin in pregnancy: Peripartum bleeding complications. J Perinatol 2007; 27:329-34.
64. Sephton V, Farquharson RG, Topping J, et al. A longitudinal study of maternal dose response to low-molecular-weight heparin in pregnancy. Obstet Gynecol 2003; 101:1307-11.
65. Katz V. Thrombophilias in Ob/Gyn. Part II: Treatment strategies. Contemp Ob/Gyn 2002; 11:59-70.

66. Carroll RC, Craft RM, Whitaker GL. Thromboelastography monitoring of resistance to enoxaparin anticoagulation in thrombophilic pregnancy patients. Thromb Res 2007; 120:367-70.
67. Horlocker TT, Wedel DJ. Spinal and epidural blockade and perioperative low molecular weight heparin: Smooth sailing on the Titanic (editorial). Anesth Analg 1998; 86:1153-6.
68. Dalen JE, Alpert JS. Natural history of pulmonary embolism. Prog Cardiovasc Dis 1975; 17:259-70.
69. Jones TK, Barnes RW, Greenfield LJ. Greenfield vena caval filter: Rationale and current indications. Ann Thorac Surg 1986; 42:S48-S55.
70. Declos GL, Davies F. Thrombolytic therapy for pulmonary embolism in pregnancy: A case report. Am J Obstet Gynecol 1986; 155: 375-6.
71. Fagher B, Ahlgren M, Astedt B. Acute massive pulmonary embolism treated with streptokinase during labor and the early puerperium. Acta Obstet Gynecol Scand 1990; 69:659-62.
72. Kramer WB, Belfort M, Saade GR, et al. Successful urokinase therapy of massive pulmonary embolism in pregnancy. Obstet Gynecol 1995; 86:660-2.
73. Skerman JH, Huckaby T, Otterson WN. Emboli in pregnancy. In Datta S, editor. Anesthetic and Obstetric Management of High-Risk Pregnancy. St Louis, Mosby, 1991:495-521.
74. Baudo F, Caimi TM, Redaelli R, et al. Emergency treatment with recombinant tissue plasminogen activator of pulmonary embolism in a pregnant woman with antithrombin III deficiency. Am J Obstet Gynecol 1990; 163:1274-5.
75. Blegvad S, Lund O, Nielsen TT, et al. Emergency embolectomy in a patient with massive pulmonary embolism during second trimester pregnancy. Acta Obstet Gynecol Scand 1989; 68:267-70.
76. Ilsaas C, Husby P, Koller ME, et al. Cardiac arrest due to massive pulmonary embolism following caesarean section: Successful resuscitation and pulmonary embolectomy. Acta Anaesthesiol Scand 1998; 42:264-6.
77. Splinter WM, Dwane PD, Wigle RD, et al. Anaesthetic management of emergency cesarean section followed by pulmonary embolectomy. Can J Anaesth 1989; 36:689-92.
78. Nishimura K, Kawaguchi M, Shimokawa M, et al. Treatment of pulmonary embolism during cesarean section with recombinant tissue plasminogen activator. Anesthesiology 1998; 89:1027-8.
79. Digonnet A, Moya-Plana A, Aubert S, et al. Acute pulmonary embolism: A current surgical approach. Interact CardioVasc Thorac Surg 2007; 6:27-9.
80. Stephanov S, dePreux J. Lumbar epidural hematoma following epidural anesthesia. Surg Neurol 1982; 18:351-3.
81. Vandermeulen EP, Van Aken H, Vermylen J. Anticoagulants and spinal-epidural anesthesia. Anesth Analg 1994; 79:1165-77.
82. Wulf H. Epidural anaesthesia and spinal haematoma. Can J Anaesth 1996; 43:1260-71.
83. Harik J, Raichle ME, Reis DJ. Spontaneously remitting spinal epidural hematoma in a patient on anticoagulants. N Engl J Med 1971; 284:1355-7.
84. Moen V, Dahlgren N, Iresstedt L. Severe neurological complications after central neuraxial blockades in Sweden, 1990-1999. Anesthesiology 2004; 101:950-9.
85. Ruppen W, Derry S, McQuay H, et al. Incidence of epidural hematoma, infection, and neurologic injury in obstetric patients with epidural analgesia/anesthesia. Anesthesiology 2006; 105:394-9.
86. Crawford JS. Principles and Practice of Obstetric Anaesthesia. 5th edition. Oxford, Blackwell Scientific, 1984:181-283.
87. Lumpkin M. FDA Public Health Advisory: Reports of epidural or spinal hematomas with the concurrent use of low-molecular-weight heparin and spinal/epidural anesthesia or spinal puncture. Rockville, MD, U.S. Department of Health and Human Services, Public Health Service, Food and Drug Administration, December 15, 1997.
88. Horlocker TT, Wedel DJ, Benzon H, et al. Regional anesthesia in the anticoagulated patient: Defining the risks (The Second ASRA Consensus Conference on Neuraxial Anesthesia and Anticoagulation). Reg Anesth Pain Med 2003; 28:172-97.
89. Dickman CA, Shedd SA, Spetzler RF, et al. Spinal epidural hematoma associated with epidural anesthesia: Complications of systemic heparinization in patients receiving peripheral vascular thrombolytic therapy. Anesthesiology 1990; 72:947-50.
90. Lawton MT, Porter RW, Heiserman JE, et al. Surgical management of spinal epidural hematoma: Relationship between surgical timing and neurological outcome. J Neurosurg 1995; 83:1-7.
91. Kebaish KM, Awad JN. Spinal epidural hematoma causing acute cauda equina syndrome. Neurosurg Focus 2004; 16:e1.
92. Cheney FW, Domino KB, Caplan RA, et al. Nerve injury associated with anesthesia: A closed claims analysis. Anesthesiology 1999; 90:1062-9.
93. Meyer JR. Embolia pulmonar amnio-caseo. Brasil Med 1926; 2:301-3.
94. Steiner PE, Lushbaugh CC. Maternal pulmonary embolism by amniotic fluid. JAMA 1941; 117:1245-54.
95. Gilbert WM, Danielson B. Amniotic fluid embolism: Decreased mortality in a population-based study. Obstet Gynecol 1999; 93:973-7.
96. Kramer MS, Rouleau J, Baskett TF, et al. Amniotic-fluid embolism and medical induction of labour: A retrospective, population-based cohort study. Lancet 2006; 368:1444-8.
97. Kaunitz AM, Hughes JW, Grimes DA, et al. Causes of maternal death in the United States. Obstet Gynecol 1985; 65:605-12.
98. Clark SL. New concepts of amniotic fluid embolism: A review. Obstet Gynecol Surv 1990; 45:360-8.
99. Tufnell DJ. Amniotic fluid embolism. Curr Opin Obstet Gynecol 2003; 15:119-22.
100. Clark SL. Arachidonic acid metabolites and the pathophysiology of amniotic fluid embolism. Semin Reprod Endocrinol 1985; 3:253-7.
101. Azegami M, Mori N. Amniotic fluid embolism and leukotrienes. Am J Obstet Gynecol 1986; 155:1119-24.
102. Benson MD. A hypothesis regarding complement activation and amniotic fluid embolism. Med Hypoth 2007; 68:1019-25.
103. Benson MD, Kobayashi H, Silver RK, et al. Immunologic studies in presumed amniotic fluid embolism. Obstet Gynecol 2001; 97:510-14.
104. Hankins GDV, Snyder RR, Clark SL, et al. Acute hemodynamic and respiratory effects of amniotic fluid embolism in the pregnant goat model. Am J Obstet Gynecol 1993; 168:1113-30.
105. Clark SC, Cotton DB, Gonik B, et al. Central hemodynamic alterations in amniotic fluid embolism. Am J Obstet Gynecol 1988; 158:1124-6.
106. Schechtman M, Ziser A, Markovits R, et al. Amniotic fluid embolism: Early findings of transesophageal echocardiography. Anesth Analg 1999; 89:1456-8.
107. Clark SL, Montz FJ, Phelan JP. Hemodynamic alterations associated with amniotic fluid embolism: A reappraisal. Am J Obstet Gynecol 1985; 151:617-21.
108. Cromley MG, Taslov PJ, Cummings DC. Probable amniotic fluid embolism after first trimester abortion. J Reprod Med 1983; 18:209-11.
109. Kelly MC, Bailie K, McCourt KC. A case of amniotic fluid embolism in a twin pregnancy in the second trimester. Int J Obstet Anesth 1995; 4:175-7.
110. Olcott CO, Robinson AJ, Maxwell TM, et al. Amniotic fluid embolism and disseminated intravascular coagulation after maternal trauma. J Trauma 1973; 13:737-40.
111. Quinn A, Barrett T. Delayed onset of coagulopathy following amniotic fluid embolism: Two case reports. Int J Obstet Anesth 1993; 2:177-80.
112. Margarson MP. Delayed amniotic fluid embolism following cesarean section under spinal anaesthesia. Anaesthesia 1995; 50:804-6.
113. Sakuma M, Sugimura K, Nakamura M. Unusual pulmonary embolism: Septic pulmonary embolism and amniotic fluid embolism. Circ J 2007; 71:772-5.
114. Schaerf RHM, DeCampo T, Civetta JM. Hemodynamic alterations and rapid diagnosis in a case of amniotic-fluid embolus. Anesthesiology 1977; 46:155-7.
115. Dolyniuk M, Orfei E, Vania H, et al. Rapid diagnosis of amniotic fluid embolism. Obstet Gynecol 1983; 61:28-30S.

116. Lee W, Ginsburg KA, Cotton DB, et al. Squamous and trophoblastic cells in the maternal pulmonary circulation identified by hemodynamic monitoring during the peripartum period. Am J Obstet Gynecol 1986; 155:999-1001.
117. Clark S, Pavlova Z, Greenspoon J, et al. Squamous cells in the maternal circulation. Am J Obstet Gynecol 1986; 154:104-6.
118. Kobayashi H, Ohi H, Terao T. A simple, noninvasive, sensitive method for diagnosis of amniotic fluid embolism by monoclonal antibody TKH-2 that recognizes NeuAcalpha2-6GalNAc. Am J Obstet Gynecol 1993; 168:848-53.
119. Kanayama N, Yamazaki T, Naruse H, et al. Determining zinc coproporphyrin in maternal plasma: A new method for diagnosing amniotic fluid embolism. Clin Chem 1992; 38:526-9.
120. Esposito RA, Grossi EA, Coppia G, et al. Successful treatment of postpartum shock caused by amniotic fluid embolism with cardiopulmonary bypass and pulmonary artery thromboembolectomy. Am J Obstet Gynecol 1990; 163:571-4.
121. Staten RD, Iverson LI, Daugherty TM. Amniotic fluid embolism causing catastrophic pulmonary vasoconstriction: Diagnosis by transesophageal echocardiogram and treatment by cardiopulmonary bypass. Am Coll Obstet Gynecol 2003; 102:496-8.
122. McDonnell NJ, Chan BO, Frengley RW. Rapid reversal of critical hemodynamic compromise with nitric oxide in a parturient with amniotic fluid embolism. Int J Obstet Anesth 2007; 16:269-73.
123. Clark SL. Successful pregnancy outcomes after amniotic fluid embolism. Am J Obstet 1992; 167:511-12.
124. Sprung J, Cheng SY, Patel S. When to remove an epidural catheter in a parturient with disseminated intravascular coagulation. Reg Anesth 1992; 17:351-4.
125. Sprung J, Cheng EY, Patel S, et al. Understanding and management of amniotic fluid embolism. J Clin Anesth 1992; 4:235-40.
126. Sprung J, Rakic M, Patel S. Amniotic fluid embolism during epidural anesthesia for cesarean section. Acta Anaesth Belg 1991; 42:225-31.
127. Amussat JZ. Recherches sur l'introduction accidentelle de l'air dans les veins. Paris, Germer Bailliere, 1839:255.
128. Flanagan J, Slimack J, Black D, et al. The incidence of venous air embolism in the parturient (abstract). Reg Anesth 1990; 15:A10.
129. Mathew JP, Fleisher LA, Rinehouse JA, et al. ST segment depression during labor and delivery. Anesthesiology 1992; 77:635-41.
130. Fong J, Gadalla F, Druzin M. Venous emboli occurring during caesarean section: The effect of patient position. Can J Anaesth 1991; 38:191-5.
131. Bromage PR, Hohman WA. Uterine posture and incidence of venous air embolism (VAE) during cesarean section (CS) (abstract). Reg Anesth 1991; 15:S29.
132. Epps SN, Robbins AJ, Marx GF. Complete recovery after near-fatal venous air embolism during cesarean section. Int J Obstet Anesth 1998; 7:131-3.
133. Palmer CM, Norris MC, Giudici MC, et al. Incidence of electrocardiographic changes during cesarean delivery under regional anesthesia. Anesth Analg 1990; 70:36-43.
134. McLintic AJ, Pringle SD, Lilley S, et al. Electrocardiographic changes during cesarean section under regional anesthesia. Anesth Analg 1992; 74:51-6.
135. Aronson ME, Nelson PK. Fatal air embolism in pregnancy resulting from an unusual sexual act. Obstet Gynecol 1967; 30:127-30.
136. Fyke FE, Kazmier FJ, Harms RW. Venous air embolism: Life-threatening complication of orogenital sex during pregnancy. Am J Med 1985; 78:333-6.

Chapter 39

Maternal Mortality

Jill M. Mhyre, M.D.

GLOBAL MATERNAL MORTALITY

Globally, 536,000 women died in 2005 while pregnant or within 42 days of the end of pregnancy.[1] This number corresponds to a ratio of 400 maternal deaths per 100,000 live births and to a 1 in 92 lifetime risk of maternal death for each girl entering her childbearing years (Table 39-1).[1] According to the World Health Organization (WHO), "No issue is more central to global well-being than maternal and perinatal health. Every individual, every family and every community is at some point intimately involved in pregnancy and the success of childbirth. Yet every day, 1500 women and over 10,000 newborns die due to complications that could have been prevented."[2]

Definitions for maternal death are listed in Table 39-2, and measures of maternal mortality are listed in Table 39-3. More than 99% of maternal deaths occur in developing countries, with 86% in either sub-Saharan Africa or South Asia (see Table 39-1). As part of the Millennium Development Goals, the international community has made a commitment to reduce the **maternal mortality ratio (MMR)** by 75% between 1990 and 2015,[1] from 430 to less than 110 per 100,000 live births. Between 1990 and 2005, the global MMR fell 5.4%.[1] Significant reductions were accomplished in many parts of the world,[3] but maternal risk remained stagnant in sub-Saharan Africa, where the lifetime risk of maternal death remains 1 in 22.[1]

According to the WHO 2005 report, the countries with the highest MMRs are Sierra Leone (2100), Niger (1800), Afghanistan (1800), and Chad (1500). The lifetime risk of maternal death is more than 10% in Niger (1 in 7), Afghanistan (1 in 8), and Sierra Leone (1 in 8).[1] There is considerable local variation. The highest MMR ever documented was in Ragh, Badakhshan, a remote region in the Hindu Kush mountains of Afghanistan, where the 2002 MMR was 6500 and the lifetime risk of maternal death was estimated at 1 in 3.[4] In this region, more than half of maternal deaths were attributed to obstructed labor or hemorrhage.[4]

Leading Causes

Hemorrhage, hypertensive disorders of pregnancy, and **sepsis** account for more than half of global maternal deaths, and for slightly more than a third of deaths in the developed world.[5] Hemorrhage is the leading cause of maternal death in both Africa and Asia (more than 30% of deaths). Hypertensive disorders represent the leading cause in Latin America and the Caribbean.[5] Infection and sepsis may be substantially underestimated in regions where laboratory diagnostic tests are unavailable.[6] In one Malawi hospital with full laboratory capabilities, infection played a primary role in almost three quarters of all maternal deaths.[7]

Anemia and **obstructed labor** each cause approximately one tenth of maternal deaths in Asia.[5] Anemia is associated with (1) iron and other micronutrient deficiencies, (2) pregnancy intervals of less than one year, (3) adolescent pregnancy, (4) hemoglobinopathy, (5) urinary tract infection, (6) human immunodeficiency virus (HIV) infection, (7) parasitic infections including malaria, and (8) recurrent antepartum hemorrhage.[8-10] Anemia can cause lethal congestive heart failure in pregnancy.[9] Anemia also increases the risk of maternal death from other complications, particularly hemorrhage and infection.[8]

Obstructed labor is an important cause of maternal death in communities in which early adolescent pregnancy is common, childhood malnutrition leads to small maternal pelves, and operative delivery is unavailable.[11] Maternal mortality from obstructed labor is largely the result of uterine rupture or ascending genital tract infection.[11,12] Prolonged pressure on the pelvic outlet can lead to tissue necrosis and obstetric fistula, which is thought to affect between 2 and 7 million women and girls worldwide.[13,14]

HIV/acquired immune deficiency syndrome (AIDS) is estimated to cause 6% of maternal deaths in sub-Saharan Africa.[5] Because the majority of African women have not been tested for HIV, the true contribution is unknown, and rates are far higher in some regions. In countries most severely affected by HIV, including Malawi, Namibia, South Africa, Uganda, and Zimbabwe, MMRs

TABLE 39-1 Estimates of Maternal Mortality Ratio, Number of Maternal Deaths, Lifetime Risk, and Range of Uncertainty by United Nations MDG Regions, 2005

MDG Region	MMR (Maternal Deaths per 100,000 Live Births)*	Number of Maternal Deaths*	Lifetime Risk of Maternal Death* (1 in:)	Range of Uncertainty for MMR Estimates	
				Lower Estimate	Upper Estimate
World Total	400	536,000	92	220	650
Developed Regions†	9	960	7300	8	17
USA‡	15	620	2700	14	16
Countries of the Commonwealth of Independent States (CIS)§	51	1800	1200	28	140
Developing Regions	450	533,000	75	240	730
Africa	820	276,000	26	410	1400
Northern Africa¶	160	5700	210	85	290
Sub-Saharan Africa	900	270,000	22	450	1500
Asia	330	241,000	120	190	520
Eastern Asia	50	9200	1200	31	80
South Asia	490	188,000	61	290	750
Southeastern Asia	300	35,000	130	160	550
Western Asia	160	8300	170	62	340
Latin America and the Caribbean	130	15,000	290	81	230
Oceania	430	890	62	120	1200

MDG, Millennium Development Goals; MMR, maternal mortality ratio.

*The MMR and the lifetime risk have been rounded according to the following scheme: < 100, no rounding; 100-999, rounded to nearest 10; and > 1000, rounded to nearest 100. The numbers of maternal deaths have been rounded as follows: < 1000, rounded to nearest 10; 1000-9999, rounded to nearest 100; and > 10,000, rounded to nearest 1000.

†Includes Albania, Australia, Austria, Belgium, Bosnia and Herzegovina, Bulgaria, Canada, Croatia, Czech Republic, Denmark, Estonia, Finland, France, Germany, Greece, Hungary, Iceland, Ireland, Italy, Japan, Latvia, Lithuania, Luxembourg, Malta, Netherlands, New Zealand, Norway, Poland, Portugal, Romania, Serbia and Montenegro (Serbia and Montenegro became separate independent entities in 2006), Slovakia, Slovenia, Spain, Sweden, Switzerland, the former Yugoslav Republic of Macedonia, the United Kingdom, and the United States of America.

‡Based on data reported by the U.S. National Center for Health Statistics, 2005. Lifetime risk of maternal death in the United States = $1 - (1 - \text{MMR})^{1.2(\text{TFR})}$, where MMR and TFR (total fertility rate) are expressed as a decimal. The TFR is multiplied by 1.2 to adjust for pregnancies not ending in live births.

§The CIS countries are Armenia, Azerbaijan, Belarus, Georgia, Kazakhstan, Kyrgyzstan, Tajikistan, Turkmenistan, Uzbekistan, the Republic of Moldova, the Russian Federation, and Ukraine.

¶Excludes Sudan, which is included in sub-Saharan Africa.

Adapted from World Health Organization. Maternal Mortality in 2005: Estimates Developed by WHO, UNICEF, and UNFPA. Geneva, Department of Reproductive Health and Research, 2007.

have increased since the mid-1990s owing to AIDS-related complications.[15-19]

Maternal deaths attributed to **unsafe abortion** account for an estimated 66,500 deaths per year globally (i.e., 13% of total maternal deaths).[20,21] The WHO[21] defines *unsafe abortion* as "a procedure for terminating an unintended pregnancy either by individuals without the necessary skills or in an environment that does not conform to minimum medical standards, or both." The incidence of unsafe abortion is highest in South America (38 unsafe abortions per 100 live births).[22] The case-fatality rate (750 maternal deaths per 100,000 unsafe abortions) and the absolute number of maternal deaths per year (35,600) are highest in sub-Saharan Africa.[20,21]

Early marriage (before age 18 years) has been identified as a major health risk for girls, increasing their exposure to domestic violence, sexually transmitted diseases such as HIV/AIDS, and maternal death.[23,24] Girls younger than

TABLE 39-2 Glossary of Terms Used in Discussions of Maternal Mortality

Source	Term	Definition‡
WHO ICD-10*	Maternal death	Death of women while pregnant or within 42 days of termination of pregnancy, irrespective of the duration and site of the pregnancy, from any cause related to or aggravated by the pregnancy or its management, but not from accidental or incidental causes. A34, O00-O95, O98-O99[1,52]
	Direct maternal death	Death resulting from obstetric complications of the pregnant state (pregnancy, labor, and the puerperium), from interventions, omissions, incorrect treatment, or from a chain of events resulting from any of the above. A34, O00-O95[1,52]
	Indirect maternal death	Deaths resulting from previous existing disease or disease that developed during pregnancy and which was not due to direct obstetric causes, but was aggravated by physiologic effects of pregnancy. O98-O99[1,52]
	Late maternal death	The death of a woman from direct or indirect obstetric causes more than 42 days but less than 1 year after termination of pregnancy. O96-O97[1,52]
	Pregnancy-related death	Deaths occurring in women while pregnant or within 42 days of termination of pregnancy, irrespective of the cause of death.
U.S. CDC PMSS†	Pregnancy-associated death	The death of a woman while pregnant or within 1 year of termination of pregnancy, irrespective of cause.
	Pregnancy-related death	The death of a woman while pregnant or within 1 year of termination of pregnancy, irrespective of the duration and site of the pregnancy, from any cause related to or aggravated by her pregnancy or its management, but not from accidental or incidental causes.
	Non-pregnancy-related death	The death of a woman while pregnant or within 1 year of termination of pregnancy, due to a cause unrelated to pregnancy.

*WHO, World Health Organization; ICD-10, International Statistical Classification of Diseases and Related Health Problems, Tenth Revision. (From ICD-10: International Statistical Classification of Disease and Related Health Problems. Geneva, WHO, 1992.)

†U.S. CDC, The United States Center for Disease Control and Prevention PMSS, Pregnancy Mortality Surveillance System. (From Strategies to Reduce Pregnancy-Related Deaths: From Identification and Review to Action. Atlanta, Centers for Disease Control and Prevention, 2001.)

‡Numbers after some definitions indicate cause of death codes, and reference citations at the end of the chapter.

15 years are five times more likely to die in childbirth than women in their 20s, and pregnancy is the leading cause of death worldwide for girls ages 15 to 19.[25]

Anesthesia providers working in the developing world must contend with profound limitations in staffing, equipment, and other resources.[26-31] In addition, patients who labor at home may face a variety of social and environmental obstacles to reach a health facility,[32] and many arrive at these facilities in septic or hemorrhagic shock.[33,34] Emergency cesarean delivery is the most common major surgical procedure in Africa,[35] and perioperative maternal mortality is estimated to be between 1% and 2%.[36,37] As many as one third of deaths that occur within 24 hours of surgery have been attributed to anesthesia, mainly because of airway problems and general anesthesia.[29,38] Peripartum deaths have also been attributed to limited availability or affordability of blood products.[37-39]

Strategies to reduce global maternal mortality include (1) promotion of education, nutrition, and social capital for girls and young women; (2) improvement in family planning services and a reduction in the performance of unsafe abortion; (3) ensuring the presence of a skilled attendant at every birth; and (4) development of the infrastructure needed to provide timely emergency obstetric care, including the performance of indicated cesarean delivery (and safe administration of anesthesia) by trained obstetric care providers, who can also provide resuscitation of women in whom shock develops secondary to hemorrhage or infection.[6,40,41] Randomized controlled trials demonstrating the effectiveness of these strategies are lacking, but their desirability seems self-evident. However, limited human, political, and economic capital mandate more rigorous evaluation of the effectiveness of future programmatic efforts.[42,43]

MATERNAL MORTALITY IN THE DEVELOPED WORLD

In developed regions of the world, the MMR improved from 11 to 9 between 1990 and 2005. More than 40 countries across Europe, East Asia, the Middle East, North America, and the South Pacific now have an MMR lower than 15.[1]

The most comprehensive maternal surveillance system in the world is the **Confidential Enquiry into Maternal and Child Health (CEMACH)** in the United Kingdom. Triennial reports of Confidential Enquiries in England and Wales extend back to 1952 and have covered the

TABLE 39-3 Measures of Maternal Mortality

Maternal Mortality Measure	Definition	Reports Using The Measure
Maternal mortality ratio (MMR)	Direct and indirect maternal deaths, but not late maternal deaths, per 100,000 live births	WHO[1]
Maternal mortality rate	Direct and indirect maternal deaths, but not late maternal deaths, per 100,000 maternities (pregnancies resulting in a live birth or stillbirth ≥ 20 weeks' gestational age)	UK CEMACH[45]
Pregnancy-related mortality ratio (PRMR)	Pregnancy-related deaths per 100,000 live births	US CDC PMSS[59]
Lifetime risk of maternal death	The lifetime risk of maternal death takes into account both the probability of becoming pregnant and the probability of dying as a result of that pregnancy cumulated across a woman's reproductive years.	WHO[1]

PMSS, Pregnancy Mortality Surveillance System; UK CEMACH, The United Kingdom Confidential Enquiries into Maternal and Child Health; US CDC, The United States Center for Disease Control and Prevention; WHO, World Health Organization.

entire United Kingdom since the 1985-1987 report. By government mandate, all maternal deaths are subject to this Confidential Enquiry, and health professionals have a duty to provide all requested information.[44,45] To ensure complete ascertainment, epidemiologists review death certificates for codes that suggest a maternal death and match all death certificates for women of reproductive age with live birth certificates from the previous year.[44,45] Once a case is identified, practitioners are asked to provide (1) a full account of the circumstances leading up to the woman's death, (2) all supporting records, (3) any clinical or other lessons that have been learned, and (4) details of any actions that may have been taken as a result.[44,45] The data are then "de-identified" before regional assessors review the files, all data are digitized, and central assessors compile the cases and produce the triennial reports. The reports focus on both medical and nonmedical recommendations for action to improve safety for future pregnant women.

The CEMACH reports include both the internationally defined MMR and the United Kingdom–defined maternal mortality rate (see Table 39-3). The numerator for the United Kingdom–defined maternal mortality rate includes all deaths that in the opinion of the CEMACH assessors are related to pregnancy, including some causes that are not internationally coded as maternity-related (e.g., suicide attributed to postpartum depression). The denominator includes all pregnancies that resulted in a live birth or stillbirth after 20 weeks' gestation. The international MMR is calculated strictly from data coded on death certificates; the U.K. maternal mortality rate includes all deaths identified through active surveillance. As a result, the 2003-2005 internationally defined MMR for the United Kingdom (6.98 per 100,000 live births) is significantly lower than the 2003-2005 U.K. maternal mortality rate (13.95 per 100,000 maternities).[45]

National confidential enquiry reports are now published by many other countries, including Australia,[46] Canada,[47] France,[48-50] and South Africa.[16]

In the United States, the **National Center for Health Statistics (NCHS)** has provided maternal death counts since 1900 and MMRs since 1915.[51] Accuracy is limited because (1) the system relies on death certificates rather than active surveillance, (2) the certification of death is the legal responsibility of individual states, and (3) the process of maternal death ascertainment varies by state.

The U.S. MMR reported by the NCHS declined from more than 600 deaths per 100,000 live births in 1915 to less than 10 deaths per 100,000 live births by 1980 (Figure 39-1).[51] Throughout the 1980s and 1990s, the MMR ranged between 6.6 and 8.4. Then in 1999, the MMR began to increase, reaching 15.1 by 2005 (Figure 39-2).[52] Improvements in ascertainment explain some of the increase. In 1999, the *International Statistical Classification of Diseases and Related Health Problems, Tenth Revision* (ICD-10) replaced ICD-9 as the coding system for U.S. death certificates and liberalized the criteria by which pregnancy could be linked with death. Growing numbers of states perform electronic matches among women's death certificates, live birth certificates, and fetal death files. In addition, state death certificates increasingly include a specific question about pregnancy status at the time of death.[53] As of 2005, 31 states and the District of Columbia include a pregnancy "check box" on the death certificate; the phrasing of these questions varies by state.[51]

In 1987, the Centers for Disease Control and Prevention (CDC) partnered with state health departments and the American College of Obstetricians and Gynecologists (ACOG) to form the **Pregnancy Mortality Surveillance System (PMSS)**.[54] To more completely capture maternal deaths, the PMSS recommended that states develop an active surveillance system and collect death certificates and matching live birth or fetal death certificates for all pregnancy-associated deaths (see Table 39-2). These are forwarded to the CDC, where clinically experienced epidemiologists manually review the certificates to identify all pregnancy-related deaths (see Table 39-2). Similar surveillance enhancement procedures have been estimated to improve case ascertainment by between 22% and 93%.[55] For the years 1991 to 1999, the PMSS reported a U.S. pregnancy-related mortality ratio (PRMR) of 11.8 per 100,000 live births, which rose from 10.3 in 1991 to 13.2 in 1999 ($P < .001$).[56] Between 1995 and 1997, approximately 6% of

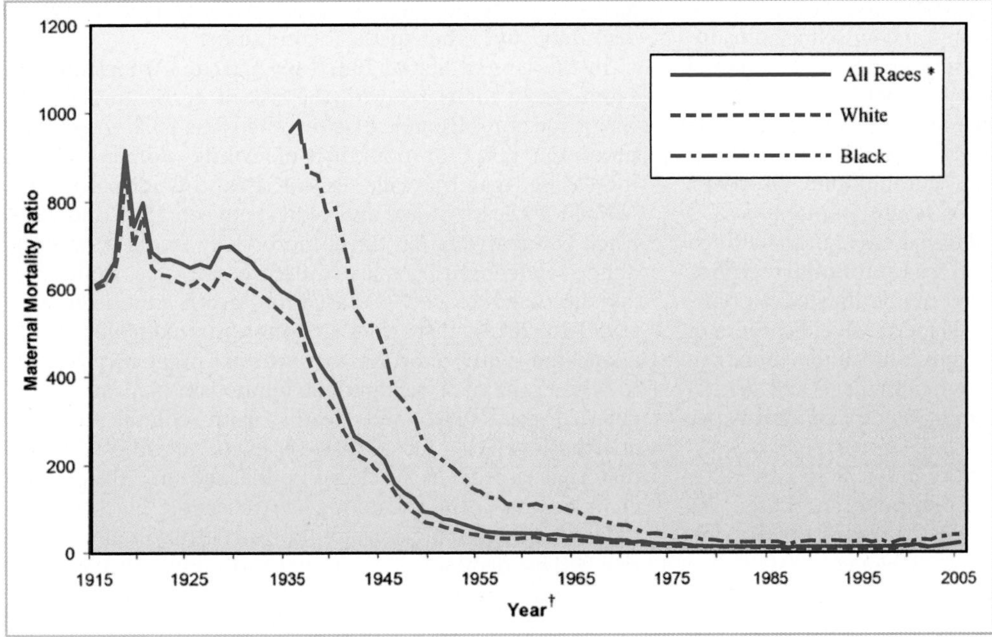

FIGURE 39-1 United States maternal mortality ratios by race, 1915-2005. *Includes races other than white and black. †For 1915-1934, data on black race are not available. (Data from references 51, 52, and 68.)

deaths reported by the NCHS were not identified by the PMSS.[57]

Leading Causes

According to a systematic review of data from France, the United Kingdom, Greece, Romania, and the United States, **hypertensive disorders of pregnancy, embolic disorders,** and **hemorrhage** together account for slightly less than half of maternal deaths in the developed world.[5] **Indirect deaths** account for another 14% and are most commonly attributed to **cardiovascular disease.**[5]

In the United Kingdom, indirect deaths have exceeded direct deaths since the 1997-1999 report, with cardiac disease being the most common single cause in the 2003-2005 report.[45] The mortality ratio attributed to cardiac disease increased from 1 death per 100,000 maternities in 1985-1987 to 2.3 in 2003-2005.[45,58] The leading cardiac cause of maternal death was myocardial infarction or ischemic heart disease.[45] Risk factors included advanced maternal age and maternal obesity. Also, **suicide** emerged as an important cause of death in the 2000-2002 report, when electronic case ascertainment revealed a larger number of suicides than previously recognized through voluntary reporting.[44]

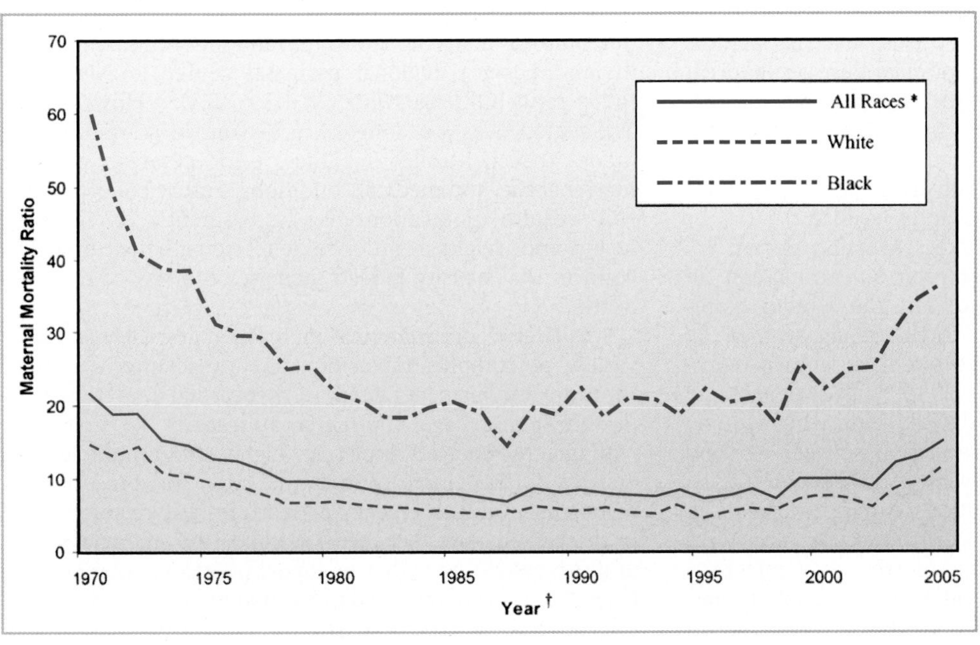

FIGURE 39-2 United States maternal mortality ratios by race, 1970-2005. *Includes races other than white and black. †Beginning in 1989, race for live births was tabulated according to race of mother, not child. (Data from references 51, 52, and 68.)

In response to the high proportion of indirect deaths, CEMACH recommends preconception counseling and support for women with preexisting serious medical or mental health conditions that may be aggravated by pregnancy. These conditions include congenital or acquired cardiac disease, obesity with a body mass index (BMI) of 30 kg/m^2 or higher, epilepsy, diabetes, autoimmune disorders, and a personal or family history of severe mental illness.[45]

The leading direct cause of maternal death in the United Kingdom between 2003 and 2005 was **pulmonary embolism**, with 1.56 deaths per 100,000 maternities (95% confidence interval [CI], 1.11 to 2.19). Hypertensive disorders of pregnancy, genital tract sepsis, amniotic fluid embolism, and the combination of obstetric hemorrhage and genital tract trauma each caused between 0.80 and 0.85 deaths per 100,000 maternities.[45]

According to the PMSS, in the United States between 1991 and 1997, other medical conditions accounted for 18.2% of all pregnancy-related deaths, corresponding to a cause-specific mortality ratio of 2.09 per 100,000 live births. The leading direct cause of death was **hypertensive disorders of pregnancy**, which caused 15.9% of all pregnancy-related deaths (1.83 deaths per 100,000 live births); other causes were infection (1.52), hemorrhage other than ectopic pregnancy (1.44), thrombotic embolism (1.17), amniotic fluid embolism (0.99), cardiomyopathy (0.88), ruptured ectopic pregnancy (0.65), cerebrovascular accidents (0.54), and complications of anesthesia (0.18).[59] Injury-related deaths are considered pregnancy-*associated*, but not pregnancy-related; they are discussed in Chapter 54.

According to the U.S. NCHS, the proportion of deaths attributed to indirect causes rose from 6.1% in 1995 to 25.5% in 2005.[52,60-68] For the years 1999 to 2005, cardiovascular deaths accounted for 13.6% of all maternal deaths, with a cause-specific mortality ratio of 1.7 deaths per 100,000 live births.[69] The leading direct cause, hypertensive disorders of pregnancy, accounted for 12.8% of all deaths, with a cause-specific mortality ratio of 1.6.

Risk Factors

Detailed descriptions of obstetric sepsis, maternal hemorrhage, embolic disorders, cardiovascular disease in pregnancy, and hypertensive disorders of pregnancy are provided in Chapters 36, 37, 38, 41, and 45, respectively. Common clinical and sociodemographic factors that increase the risk of maternal death from all of these complications are discussed in this chapter (see later).

Advanced maternal age increases maternal risk,[70,71] with a linear trend evident for each 5-year increase in maternal age beyond 24 years.[45] In the United States between 1991 and 1997, the PRMR among women 40 years of age and older was 162.6 for black women (compared with 28.9 for black women 25 to 29 years of age) and 29.2 for white women (compared with 6.0 for white women 25 to 29 years of age).[71] The association between age and mortality persisted after data were controlled for parity, prenatal care, race, and education. Among older black women (40 or more years of age), the excess risks were greatest for hypertensive disorders of pregnancy, infection, cerebrovascular accident, and other medical conditions. Among older white women, the greatest excess risks of death were due to hemorrhage, cardiomyopathy, embolic disorders, and other medical conditions.[71]

In the United States, **black or African-American race** significantly correlates with the risk of death. In 2005, the MMR for non-Hispanic black women was 39.2, roughly 3.4 times the ratio for non-Hispanic white women (11.7).[52] Increasing maternal age exacerbates this disparity. For women 40 years of age and older between 1991 and 1997, black women were 5.6 times more likely to die from pregnancy-related causes than white women of a similar age (as discussed earlier).[59] Based on death certificate data (1999 to 2004), disparities are most dramatic for deaths associated with abortion or ectopic pregnancy (black-to-white ratio of 5.7), pulmonary embolism (4.8), cardiovascular disease (4.3), and deaths from complications of anesthesia (4.1).[69] In a case series of anesthesia-related maternal deaths in Michigan published in 2007, six of eight deaths occurred among non-Hispanic black women in Detroit, suggesting a profound concentration of maternal risk.[72] The disparity in maternal mortality between black and white women persists after data are controlled for maternal age, income, and receipt of prenatal care,[73] and appears to be related to a higher case-fatality rate.[74]

Other racial and ethnic groups also face increased risk. In England, black African, black Caribbean, and Middle Eastern women have higher relative risks of death than white women.[45] In the United States, in comparison with non-Hispanic white women, the risk of death is 40% to 70% higher for women who self-identify as Hispanic, Asian, Pacific Islander, American Indian, or Alaska Native.[75,76] The risk is higher for non–U.S.-born Hispanic and Asian/Pacific Islander women than for women of these racial/ethnic groups born in the United States.[59,75,76]

Maternal obesity almost certainly increases the risk of maternal death from a variety of causes, including pulmonary embolism, infection, preeclampsia, and anesthesia-related complications. Remarkably, there are limited epidemiologic data to establish this connection. Obesity is a common feature in case series of maternal deaths. In the 2003-2005 CEMACH report, more than half of women who died were overweight or obese.[45] Obesity (prepregnancy BMI > 29 kg/m^2) has been associated with a composite outcome of maternal mortality and near-miss morbidity in an inner-city regional perinatal center in New York (odds ratio [OR], 3.0; 95% CI, 1.7 to 5.3).[77] However, the association was no longer significant in a multivariate model that controlled for race, prior cesarean delivery, maternal age, and medical conditions. Future cohort studies will require population-level assessments of maternal height and weight in order to generate sufficient power to confirm that obesity indeed increases the risk of maternal death.

Multifetal pregnancies increase maternal risk for a variety of complications, including preeclampsia, venous thromboembolism, heart failure, myocardial infarction, peripartum hemorrhage, and maternal death.[45,78-82] Compared with twin pregnancies, triplet and higher-order multiple pregnancies further increase maternal risk for preeclampsia, hemorrhage, and emergency peripartum hysterectomy.[79,80,82] In the United States between 1991 and 1997, the relative risk of death associated with a multifetal pregnancy was 3.6 (95% CI, 3.1 to 4.1) with threefold to fourfold increases in the cause-specific relative risk of death for embolism, hemorrhage, hypertensive disorders of pregnancy, infection, cardiomyopathy, and other medical conditions.[81]

Cesarean delivery has also been associated with an increased risk of maternal death; however, the association does not always reflect a causal relationship. Death can be a consequence of the indication for the operation rather than the mode of delivery itself. In an attempt to estimate the relative risk of death due to cesarean delivery, a population-based case-control study from France focused on 65 maternal deaths after singleton births among low-risk women in whom complications developed only after delivery.[83] Cases were identified by the French Confidential Enquiry on Maternal Deaths from 1996 through 2000.[48-50] These cases were compared with 10,244 singleton births to low-risk women identified through the French National Perinatal Survey conducted in 1998. After data were controlled for maternal age, nationality, parity, and preterm delivery, the adjusted odds ratio (AOR) for increased risk of death with cesarean delivery was 3.64 (95% CI, 2.15 to 6.19). The increased risk was most dramatic for intrapartum cesarean deliveries (AOR, 4.58; 95% CI, 2.30 to 9.09) but persisted when cesarean delivery preceded labor (AOR, 2.42; 95% CI, 1.14 to 5.13).[83] Among women who underwent cesarean delivery, there was an increased risk of cause-specific maternal mortality from venous thromboembolism, puerperal infection, and complications of anesthesia. There was no difference in risk of death from postpartum hemorrhage or amniotic fluid embolism.

A cohort study of all deliveries in Canada between 1991 and 2005 compared 46,766 planned cesarean deliveries for breech presentation with 2,292,420 planned vaginal deliveries in which labor was either spontaneous or induced. Planned cesarean delivery increased the risk of postpartum cardiac arrest (AOR, 5.1; 95% CI, 4.1 to 6.3), major puerperal infection (AOR, 3.0; 95% CI, 2.7 to 3.4), anesthetic complications (AOR, 2.3; 95% CI, 2.0 to 2.6), and puerperal venous thromboembolism (AOR, 2.2; 95% CI, 1.5 to 3.4), but did not increase the risk of in-hospital maternal death (P = .87).[84]

A medical record review of all in-hospital maternal deaths that occurred in a sample of U.S. hospitals between 2000 and 2006 sought to identify evidence for a causal connection between mode of delivery and the mechanism of maternal death. Among 1,461,270 live births, there were 95 maternal deaths (6.5 per 100,000). Although 61% of the deaths were associated with cesarean delivery, one third of these were perimortem cesarean deliveries in which the surgical procedure followed maternal cardiac arrest. Four deaths were thought to have been directly caused by cesarean delivery (attributed to hemorrhage or infection), with an additional 7 deaths attributed to pulmonary thromboembolism after cesarean delivery. Two deaths were thought to have been causally related to vaginal delivery (one case of uterine inversion and one case of rupture of an unrecognized cerebral berry aneurysm during labor), and 2 deaths were attributed to pulmonary thromboembolism after vaginal delivery. Another 16 deaths were thought to have been potentially preventable had a cesarean delivery or an earlier cesarean delivery been performed (12 due to preeclampsia, 3 due to hemorrhage, and 1 due to sepsis).[85] The investigators concluded that a policy of universal thromboprophylaxis for all patients undergoing cesarean delivery would eliminate the increased risk of maternal death caused by cesarean delivery as opposed to vaginal delivery.[85]

Some **health system characteristics** have been associated with a higher risk of maternal death; they include (1) low maternal-fetal medicine specialist density[86] and (2) a single physician functioning as both the obstetrician and the anesthesia provider.[87]

Severe and Near-Miss Morbidity

Death is considered the extreme outcome of the following continuum of adverse pregnancy events: normal pregnancy → morbidity → severe morbidity → near-miss → death.[88] Approximately half of women experience some **morbidity** during pregnancy, most commonly anemia, urinary tract infection, mental health conditions, hypertensive disorders, and pelvic or perineal trauma.[89] Research has focused on severe morbidity, near-miss events, and maternal deaths in order to elucidate the patient, provider, and health system factors that lead to these adverse outcomes. It is difficult to compare individual studies because no consensus exists as to how to define and distinguish morbidity, severe morbidity, and a near-miss event.[90,91]

Estimates of the incidence of **severe maternal morbidity** in the developed world range from 4 to 15 cases per 1000 deliveries, depending on the health system evaluated, the method of ascertainment, and the definition of severe morbidity used.[92-96] On the basis of a population-level review of ICD-9 codes that reflected severe complications during the delivery hospitalization, Wen et al.[95] estimated the overall rate of severe maternal morbidity at 4.38 per 1000 deliveries in Canada between 1991 and 2001 (95% CI, 4.30 to 4.46). Callaghan et al.,[96] applying a similar list of ICD-9 codes and requiring that the length of hospital stay be at least 3 days, estimated the rate of severe morbidity at 5.1 per 1000 deliveries in the United States between 1991 and 2003 (95% CI, 4.7 to 5.5). Waterstone et al.[92] evaluated pregnancies in France between 1997 and 1998 for the presence of severe preeclampsia, severe hemorrhage, or sepsis; they identified a combined incidence for these three conditions of 12.0 per 1000 deliveries (95% CI, 11.2 to 13.2). Zhang et al.[94] applied the same criteria across Western Europe and identified a combined European incidence for these three conditions as 9.5 per 1000 deliveries (95% CI, 9.1 to 9.9), with the highest incidences identified in Belgium and Finland.

A **near-miss event** occurs when a pregnant or recently pregnant woman survives a life-threatening event, either by chance or because of high-quality (rescue) treatment and care. The concept of a near-miss event evolved from early studies of pregnant patients who required intensive care.[48-50,97-100] The specific criteria used to identify cases vary widely across studies. Mantel et al.[101] proposed a definition that requires evidence of severe organ dysfunction, intensive care unit admission, emergency hysterectomy, or an anesthetic accident such as failed intubation. On the basis of these criteria, there were 3.8 near-miss events per 1000 deliveries in a network of maternity units in Scotland between 2001 and 2002.[93] Geller et al.[102] validated a five-factor scoring system consisting of organ system failure (5 points), intensive care unit admission (4 points), transfusion of more than 3 units of blood products (3 points), extended intubation (2 points), and surgical intervention

(1 point); a total score higher than 7 points defines a near-miss event. According to this scoring system, the incidence of a near-miss event was approximately 0.2 per 1000 deliveries in a perinatal tertiary care center in Chicago between 1995 and 2001.[102]

Evidence suggests that half of U.S. maternal deaths may be preventable through changes in patient, provider, or system factors.[27,45,48-50,103-108] In a case-control study of maternal death, near-miss events, and severe morbidity, Geller et al.[107] determined that 41% of deaths (n = 15/37), 46% of near-miss events (n = 15/33), and 17% of severe morbidities (n = 17/101) were preventable. Preventable severe morbidity or death was most strongly associated with provider factors (e.g., incomplete or inappropriate management) rather than system or patient factors. Cases of near-miss morbidity were more than four times as likely as cases of severe morbidity to have been preventable through changes in provider factors, and cases of maternal mortality were almost twice as likely as cases of near-miss morbidity to have been preventable through changes in provider factors.[107]

TABLE 39-4 Anesthesia-Related Maternal Mortality Ratios in the United States and the United Kingdom, 1979-2005*

Triennium	United States (95% CI)	United Kingdom (95% CI)
1979-81	4.3 (3.1-5.7)	8.7 (5.5-13.2)†
1982-84	3.3 (2.3-4.5)	7.2 (4.3-11.4)†
1985-87	2.3 (1.5-3.4)	2.6 (1.2-5.8)
1988-90	1.7 (1.1-2.7)	1.7 (0.7-4.4)
1991-93	1.4 (0.8-2.2)	3.5 (1.8-6.8)
1994-96	1.1 (0.6-1.9)	0.5 (0.1-2.6)
1997-99	1.2 (0.7-2.0)	1.4 (0.5-4.2)
2000-02	1.0 (0.5-1.7)	3.0 (1.4-6.6)
2003-05	Not available	2.8 (1.3-6.2)

CI, confidence interval.

*Rates reported refer to the risk of anesthesia-related maternal death during pregnancy or up to 1 year after delivery per million live births in the United States or per million maternities in the United Kingdom.

†Rates for England and Wales only.

Data from references 110-136, 147-149.

Anesthesia-Related Maternal Mortality

Anesthesia-related maternal mortality has been defined as "death attributable to anesthesia, either as the result of medications used, method chosen, or the technical maneuvers performed, whether iatrogenic in origin or resulting from an abnormal patient response."[109] A death may be considered anesthesia-related if it can be uniquely attributed to an anesthetic complication.[72] Actual case reports often include layers of comorbidities, anesthetic complications, and problems with nonanesthetic care; these cases may be considered anesthesia-related if ideal anesthetic care would likely have averted the death.[72] If perfect anesthetic care in combination with improvements in obstetric or medical management would likely have saved the woman's life, then the death may be considered anesthesia-contributing.[72] In some cases, the anesthetic complication is tragic but incidental (e.g., failed intubation during advanced cardiac life support for massive pulmonary embolism).

Anesthesia-related maternal death is extremely rare in the developed world (Table 39-4). However, surveillance efforts that rely on death certificate codes may underestimate the rate of anesthesia-related maternal death. CEMACH estimated the anesthesia-related maternal death ratio to be approximately 3.0 per million maternities in the United Kingdom between 2000 and 2005.[110,111]

A number of clinical and sociodemographic factors commonly appear among cases of anesthesia-related maternal death and may play a causal role in the mechanism of death. These include (1) maternal obesity; (2) patient refusal of neuraxial anesthesia; (3) remote anesthetic location; (4) delay in anesthesia provider consultation; (5) insufficient multidisciplinary planning, communication, and coordination; and (6) inadequate supervision of care.[72,109-135] In the United States, the relative risk of anesthesia-related maternal death appears to be increased for African-American women.[69,72,109,136]

Neuraxial anesthesia is considered safer than general anesthesia for cesarean delivery. Case-fatality rates according to mode of anesthesia are presented in Table 39-5. For generation of these estimates, cases were identified from death certificate data collected by the PMSS. Controls were estimated on the basis of the national incidence of cesarean delivery[137] as well as survey estimates of the proportions of cesarean deliveries completed with neuraxial and general anesthesia.[138-140]

Trends in the relative risks of general and neuraxial anesthesia for cesarean delivery reflect three major safety initiatives in anesthesia practice in the United States (see Table 39-5).[141] The first initiative **improved the safety of neuraxial anesthesia.** In the early 1980s, the risk of systemic toxicity of local anesthesia received considerable attention.[142,143] In response, in 1984 the U.S. Food and Drug Administration recommended that bupivacaine 0.75% not be used for epidural anesthesia in obstetric patients. Also, anesthesiologists developed the following series of safety procedures to avoid the unintentional intravascular injection of a local anesthetic (through an epidural catheter) and to identify an intravascular injection before systemic toxicity develops: (1) aspiration of the epidural catheter, (2) administration of an epinephrine-containing test dose, (3) incremental administration of the therapeutic dose of local anesthetic, (4) administration of a dilute solution of local anesthetic for labor analgesia, and (5) in some cases, the addition of epinephrine to the therapeutic solution of local anesthetic in patients undergoing cesarean delivery. More recently, lipid emulsion has become available as a potential rescue therapy[144-146] for the rare patient suffering from severe systemic toxicity as a result of intravascular administration of bupivacaine[111,147] or another local anesthetic agent. Meanwhile, greater recognition of the importance of prompt, aggressive treatment of maternal hypotension has likely improved the safety of both epidural anesthesia and spinal anesthesia for cesarean delivery.

The second initiative involved a shift toward **greater use of neuraxial anesthesia for cesarean delivery.**[139,140]

TABLE 39-5 Case-Fatality Rates per Million Anesthetics for Cesarean Delivery in the United States

Year of Death	General Anesthesia (95% CI)	Neuraxial Anesthesia (95% CI)	Risk Ratio (95% CI)
1979-1984	20.0 (17.7-22.7)	8.6 (7.8-9.4)	2.3 (1.9-2.9)
1985-1990	32.3 (25.9-49.3)	1.9 (1.8-2.0)	16.7 (12.9-21.8)
1991-1996	16.8 (8.9-28.7)	2.5 (1.2-4.5)	6.7 (3.0-14.9)
1997-2002*	6.5 (2.1-15.3)	3.8 (2.3-6.1)	1.7 (0.6-4.6)

CI, confidence interval.

*The data for 1997-2002 were presented in an oral presentation in May 2008, and may yet undergo revision before publication of the final manuscript.

Data from references 136, 147-149.

Between 1985 and 1990, the relative risk of general anesthesia in comparison with neuraxial anesthesia for cesarean delivery was 16.7 (see Table 39-5),[148] and much of the increase in risk was attributed to failed intubation and/or aspiration of gastric contents during induction of general anesthesia.[148,149] In response, anesthesia providers now reserve general anesthesia for specific indications, including (1) emergency cesarean delivery with insufficient time to establish neuraxial anesthesia; (2) medical conditions that make neuraxial anesthesia unsafe, such as maternal coagulopathy, hemorrhagic shock, and septic shock; and (3) failed neuraxial anesthesia with intraoperative pain.

The third initiative introduced a series of **protocols and devices to improve the safety of general anesthesia.**[141] Pulse oximetry and capnography have been widely credited with the decline in the incidence of unrecognized esophageal intubation.[150] (Additional strategies to limit the risk of airway misadventure are discussed in Chapters 29 and 30.) As a result, the relative risk of general anesthesia in comparison with neuraxial anesthesia has fallen since 1990, and was estimated to be 1.7 (95% CI, 0.6 to 4.6) between 1997 and 2002.[147]* Although these data suggest that the higher relative risk of general anesthesia is no longer statistically significant, it must also be acknowledged that a higher proportion of high-risk cesarean deliveries are now performed with neuraxial anesthesia. Later case series continue to report deaths from difficult intubation, unrecognized esophageal intubation, and pulmonary aspiration of gastric contents.[110,147] General anesthesia for cesarean delivery likely remains more hazardous for the mother, but both general anesthesia and neuraxial anesthesia impose remote but real risks of maternal death.

*These data were presented in an oral abstract presentation at the 2008 Annual Meeting of the Society for Obstetric Anesthesia and Perinatology. These data differ from those published in the meeting abstract book because the CDC classification process is ongoing. For example, between January 2008 and May 2008, the CDC reclassified 7 of 49 maternal deaths from anesthesia-related to non–anesthesia-related (e.g., postpartum hemorrhage or indirect cause of maternal death). These data may yet undergo further revision before publication of the final manuscript. Nonetheless, it appears that the relative risk of general anesthesia (versus neuraxial anesthesia) for cesarean delivery has declined during the last two decades.

Why do women die from neuraxial anesthesia? According to the American Society of Anesthesiologists (ASA) Closed-Claims Project, the most common patient injury associated with a claim for death or permanent brain injury among obstetric patients receiving neuraxial anesthesia between 1980 and 1999 was **neuraxial block–associated cardiac arrest** (n = 18/57; 32%), defined as the sudden onset of severe bradycardia or cardiac arrest during neuraxial block with relatively stable hemodynamic measurements preceding the event.[151] Other case series suggest that high spinal anesthesia, hypotensive arrest, and perioperative respiratory arrest may be important mechanisms by which neuraxial anesthesia can lead to cardiac arrest or maternal death.[72,111,115-135]

Anesthesia-related maternal deaths are distributed throughout the perioperative period and follow both neuraxial anesthesia and general anesthesia (see Table 39-5).[72,110,111,115-135,152] These deaths are almost always preventable.[72,110,111,115-135,152] Further efforts to reduce the incidence of anesthesia-related maternal death must include a comprehensive approach to **high-quality perioperative patient care**. Timely preanesthesia evaluation and ongoing communication with obstetric providers are essential to limit the number of patients who require emergency administration of anesthesia without sufficient evaluation and preparation. Problems with postoperative care have long been recognized[112,113,153] but account for a growing proportion of all anesthesia-related maternal deaths.[110,111,115-134] In two case series published in 2007, at least half of anesthesia-related maternal deaths were associated with postoperative airway complications and/or respiratory failure, with death attributed to (1) inadequate postoperative monitoring or (2) failed oxygenation during attempted ventilation or re-intubation.[72,111] Poor postoperative care also contributes to maternal deaths from concealed hemorrhage and maternal sepsis.[45,72] Severe morbidity and mortality are rare in obstetric patients; however, obstetric and anesthesia providers must remain aware that the physiology of pregnancy and the compensatory physiologic responses that occur in young pregnant women may obscure early signs of septic or hemorrhagic shock. Early warning scoring systems are being developed to guide observations and to facilitate diagnosis for women who have, or are beginning to develop, a critical illness.[45,135,154] Chapter 11 details additional strategies to enhance patient safety.

KEY POINTS

- Ninety-nine percent of maternal deaths worldwide occur in developing countries. More than half of global maternal deaths are attributed to direct obstetric causes, including maternal hemorrhage, hypertensive disorders of pregnancy, and infection.
- In the developed world, 9 women die for every 100,000 live births. In the United States, the maternal mortality ratio is increasing; in 2005, 15 U.S. women died per 100,000 live births.
- Advanced maternal age, maternal obesity, multiple gestation, cesarean delivery, and nonwhite race increase the risk of maternal death.
- Hypertensive disorders of pregnancy, embolic disorders, and hemorrhage together account for just under half of maternal deaths in the developed world. Indirect deaths, particularly those attributed to cardiac disease, are increasingly recognized as an important cause of maternal death in the developed world.
- Death is considered the extreme outcome of the following continuum of adverse pregnancy events: normal pregnancy → morbidity → severe morbidity → near-miss → death.
- In the developed world, the anesthesia-related maternal mortality ratio is estimated to range between 1 and 3 per million live births.
- General anesthesia likely remains more hazardous than neuraxial anesthesia for cesarean delivery.
- Anesthesia safety for obstetric patients depends on the provision of high-quality perioperative patient care.

REFERENCES

1. World Health Organization. Maternal Mortality in 2005: Estimates Developed by WHO, UNICEF, and UNFPA. Geneva, Department of Reproductive Health and Research, 2007.
2. World Health Organization. Ensuring Skilled Care for Every Birth. Geneva, Department of Making Pregnancy Safer, 2006.
3. Hill K, Thomas K, AbouZahr C, et al. Estimates of maternal mortality worldwide between 1990 and 2005: An assessment of available data. Lancet 2007; 370:1311-9.
4. Bartlett LA, Mawji S, Whitehead S, et al. Where giving birth is a forecast of death: Maternal mortality in four districts of Afghanistan, 1999-2002. Lancet 2005; 365:864-70.
5. Khan KS, Wojdyla D, Say L, et al. WHO analysis of causes of maternal death: A systematic review. Lancet 2006; 367:1066-74.
6. Costello A, Azad K, Barnett S. An alternative strategy to reduce maternal mortality. Lancet 2006; 368:1477-9.
7. Lema VM, Changole J, Kanyighe C, Malunga EV. Maternal mortality at the Queen Elizabeth Central Teaching Hospital, Blantyre, Malawi. East Afr Med J 2005; 82:3-9.
8. van den Broek N. Anaemia and micronutrient deficiencies. Br Med Bull 2003; 67:149-60.
9. Kavatkar AN, Sahasrabudhe NS, Jadhav MV, Deshmukh SD. Autopsy study of maternal deaths. Int J Gynaecol Obstet 2003; 81:1-8.
10. Kagu MB, Kawuwa MB, Gadzama GB. Anaemia in pregnancy: A cross-sectional study of pregnant women in a Sahelian tertiary hospital in Northeastern Nigeria. J Obstet Gynaecol 2007; 27:676-9.
11. Neilson JP, Lavender T, Quenby S, Wray S. Obstructed labour. Br Med Bull 2003; 67:191-204.
12. Hofmeyr GJ, Say L, Gulmezoglu AM. WHO systematic review of maternal mortality and morbidity: The prevalence of uterine rupture. Br J Obstet Gynaecol 2005; 112:1221-8.
13. United National Population Fund and the University of Aberdeen. Obstetric Fistula Needs Assessment Report: Findings from Nine African Countries. New York, UNFPA, 2003.
14. Wall LL. Obstetric vesicovaginal fistula as an international public-health problem. Lancet 2006; 368:1201-9.
15. Bicego G, Boerma JT, Ronsmans C. The effect of AIDS on maternal mortality in Malawi and Zimbabwe. AIDS 2002; 16:1078-81.
16. Department of Health. Saving Mothers: Third Report on Confidential Enquiries into Maternal Deaths in South Africa, 2002-2004. Pretoria, South Africa, Department of Health, 2006.
17. Fawcus SR, van Coeverden de Groot HA, Isaacs S. A 50-year audit of maternal mortality in the Peninsula Maternal and Neonatal Service, Cape Town, South Africa (1953-2002). Br J Obstet Gynaecol 2005; 112:1257-63.
18. van Dillen J, Meguid T, van Roosmalen J. Maternal mortality audit in a hospital in Northern Namibia: The impact of HIV/AIDS. Acta Obstet Gynecol Scand 2006; 85:499-500.
19. Sewankambo NK, Gray RH, Ahmad S, et al. Mortality associated with HIV infection in rural Rakai District, Uganda. AIDS 2000; 14:2391-400.
20. Grimes DA, Benson J, Singh S, et al. Unsafe abortion: The preventable pandemic. Lancet 2006; 368:1908-19.
21. World Health Organization. Unsafe Abortion: Global and Regional Estimates of the Incidence of Unsafe Abortion and Associated Mortality in 2003. Geneva, Department of Reproductive Health and Research, 2007.
22. Sedgh G, Henshaw S, Singh S, et al. Induced abortion: Estimated rates and trends worldwide. Lancet 2007; 370:1338-45.
23. Clark S. Early marriage and HIV risks in sub-Saharan Africa. Stud Fam Plann 2004; 35:149-60.
24. Jain S, Kurz K. New Insights on Preventing Child Marriage: A Global Analysis of Factors and Programs. Washington, DC, International Center for Research on Women, 2007.
25. United National Population Fund and the University of Aberdeen. Maternal Mortality Update 2004: Delivering into Good Hands. New York, UNFPA, 2004.
26. McKenzie AG. Operative obstetric mortality at Harare Central Hospital, 1992-1994: An anaesthetic view. Int J Obstet Anesth 1998; 7:237-41.
27. Kilpatrick SJ, Crabtree KE, Kemp A, Geller S. Preventability of maternal deaths: Comparison between Zambian and American referral hospitals. Obstet Gynecol 2002; 100:321-6.
28. Rout C. Maternal mortality and anaesthesia in Africa: A South African perspective. Int J Obstet Anesth 2002; 11:77-80.
29. Enohumah KO, Imarengiaye CO. Factors associated with anaesthesia-related maternal mortality in a tertiary hospital in Nigeria. Acta Anaesthesiol Scand 2006; 50:206-10.
30. Hodges SC, Mijumbi C, Okello M, et al. Anaesthesia services in developing countries: Defining the problems. Anaesthesia 2007; 62:4-11.
31. Thoms GM, McHugh GA, O'Sullivan E. The Global Oximetry initiative. Anaesthesia 2007; 62(Suppl 1):75-7.
32. Thaddeus S, Maine D. Too far to walk: Maternal mortality in context. Soc Sci Med 1994; 38:1091-110.
33. Tumwebaze J. Lamula's story. Anaesthesia 2007; 62(Suppl 1):4.
34. Okusanya BO, Okogbo FO, Momoh MM, et al. Maternal mortality and delay: Socio-demographic characteristics of maternal deaths with delay in Irrua, Nigeria. Niger J Med 2007; 16:38-41.
35. Clyburn P, Morris S, Hall J. Anaesthesia and safe motherhood. Anaesthesia 2007; 62(Suppl 1):21-5.
36. Heywood AJ, Wilson IH, Sinclair JR. Perioperative mortality in Zambia. Ann R Coll Surg Engl 1989; 71:354-8.
37. Ouro-Bang'na Maman AF, Tomta K, Ahouangbevi S, Chobli M. Deaths associated with anaesthesia in Togo, West Africa. Trop Doct 2005; 35:220-2.
38. Hansen D, Gausi SC, Merikebu M. Anaesthesia in Malawi: Complications and deaths. Trop Doct 2000; 30:146-9.

39. Cruz JR. Reduction of maternal mortality: The need for voluntary blood donors. Int J Gynaecol Obstet 2007; 98:291-3.
40. Campbell OM, Graham WJ. Strategies for reducing maternal mortality: Getting on with what works. Lancet 2006; 368:1284-99.
41. Paxton A, Bailey P, Lobis S, Fry D. Global patterns in availability of emergency obstetric care. Int J Gynaecol Obstet 2006; 93:300-7.
42. Bullough C, Meda N, Makowiecka K, et al. Current strategies for the reduction of maternal mortality. Br J Obstet Gynaecol 2005; 112:1180-8.
43. Tita AT, Stringer JS, Goldenberg RL, Rouse DJ. Two decades of the safe motherhood initiative: Time for another wooden spoon award? Obstet Gynecol 2007; 110:972-6.
44. Lewis G, editor. The Confidential Enquiry into Maternal and Child Health (CEMACH): Why Mothers Die 2000-2002: The Sixth Report of Confidential Enquiries into Maternal Deaths in the United Kingdom. London, CEMACH, 2004.
45. Lewis G, editor. The Confidential Enquiry into Maternal and Child Health (CEMACH): Saving Mother's Lives: Reviewing maternal deaths to make motherhood safer, 2003-2005. The Seventh Report of the Confidential Enquiries into Maternal Deaths in the United Kingdom. London, CEMACH, 2007.
46. Sullivan EA, Ford JB, Chambers G, Slaytor EK. Maternal mortality in Australia, 1973-1996. Aust N Z J Obstet Gynaecol 2004; 44:452-7.
47. Health Canada. Special Report on Maternal Mortality and Severe Morbidity in Canada—Enhanced Surveillance: The Path to Prevention. Ottawa, Canada, Minister of Public Works and Government Services Canada, 2004.
48. Bouvier-Colle MH, Salanave B, Ancel PY, et al. Obstetric patients treated in intensive care units and maternal mortality. Eur J Obstet Gynecol Reprod Biol 1996; 65:121-5.
49. Bouvier-Colle MH, Varnoux N, Breart G. Maternal deaths and substandard care: The results of a confidential survey in France. Medical Experts Committee. Eur J Obstet Gynecol Reprod Biol 1995; 58:3-7.
50. Bouvier-Colle MH, Ould EL, Joud D, et al. Evaluation of the quality of care for severe obstetrical haemorrhage in three French regions. Br J Obstet Gynaecol 2001; 108:898-903.
51. Hoyert DL. Maternal mortality and related concepts. Vital Health Stat 3 2007; (33):1-13.
52. Kung H-C, Hoyert DL, Xu J, Murphy SL. Deaths: Final data for 2005. Natl Vital Stat Rep 2008; 56:1-120.
53. MacKay AP, Rochat R, Smith JC, Berg CJ. The check box: Determining pregnancy status to improve maternal mortality surveillance. Am J Prev Med 2000; 19:35-9.
54. Berg C, Daniel I, Atrash H, et al., editors. Strategies to Reduce Pregnancy-Related Deaths: From Identification and Review to Action. Atlanta, Centers for Disease Control and Prevention, 2001.
55. Deneux-Tharaux C, Berg C, Bouvier-Colle MH, et al. Underreporting of pregnancy-related mortality in the United States and Europe. Obstet Gynecol 2005; 106:684-92.
56. Chang J, Elam-Evans LD, Berg CJ, et al. Pregnancy-related mortality surveillance—United States, 1991-1999. MMWR Surveill Summ 2003; 52:1-8.
57. MacKay AP, Berg CJ, Duran C, et al. An assessment of pregnancy-related mortality in the United States. Paediatr Perinat Epidemiol 2005; 19:206-14.
58. Malhotra S, Yentis SM. Reports on confidential enquiries into maternal deaths: Management strategies based on trends in maternal cardiac deaths over 30 years. Int J Obstet Anesth 2006; 15:223-6.
59. Berg CJ, Chang J, Callaghan WM, Whitehead SJ. Pregnancy-related mortality in the United States, 1991-1997. Obstet Gynecol 2003; 101:289-96.
60. Peters KD, Kochanek KD, Murphy SL. Deaths: Final data for 1996. Natl Vital Stat Rep 1998; 47:1-100.
61. Hoyert DL, Kochanek KD, Murphy SL. Deaths: Final data for 1997. Natl Vital Stat Rep 1999; 47:1-104.
62. Murphy SL. Deaths: Final data for 1998. Natl Vital Stat Rep 2000; 48:1-105.
63. Hoyert DL, Arias E, Smith BL, et al. Deaths: Final data for 1999. Natl Vital Stat Rep 2001; 49:1-113.
64. Miniño AM, Arias E, Kochanek KD, et al. Deaths: Final data for 2000. Natl Vital Stat Rep 2002; 50:1-119.
65. Arias E, Anderson RN, Kung H-C, et al. Deaths: Final data for 2001. Natl Vital Stat Rep 2003; 52:1-115.
66. Kochanek KD, Murphy SL, Anderson RN, Scott C. Deaths: Final data for 2002. Natl Vital Stat Rep 2004; 53:1-115.
67. Hoyert DL, Heron MP, Murphy SL, Kung H-C. Deaths: Final data for 2003. Natl Vital Stat Rep 2006; 54:1-120.
68. Miniño AM, Heron MP, Murphy SL, Kochanek KD. Deaths: Final data for 2004. Natl Vital Stat Rep 2007; 55:1-119.
69. Centers for Disease Control and Prevention. CDC Wonder. Available at http://wonder.cdc.gov.
70. Panchal S, Arria AM, Labhsetwar SA. Maternal mortality during hospital admission for delivery: A retrospective analysis using a state-maintained database. Anesth Analg 2001; 93:134-41.
71. Callaghan WM, Berg CJ. Pregnancy-related mortality among women aged 35 years and older, United States, 1991-1997. Obstet Gynecol 2003; 102:1015-21.
72. Mhyre JM, Riesner MN, Polley LS, Naughton NN. A series of anesthesia-related maternal deaths in Michigan, 1985-2003. Anesthesiology 2007; 106:1096-104.
73. Harper MA, Espeland MA, Dugan E, et al. Racial disparity in pregnancy-related mortality following a live birth outcome. Ann Epidemiol 2004; 14:274-9.
74. Tucker MJ, Berg CJ, Callaghan WM, Hsia J. The Black-White disparity in pregnancy-related mortality from 5 conditions: Differences in prevalence and case-fatality rates. Am J Public Health 2007; 97:247-51.
75. Hopkins FW, MacKay AP, Koonin LM, et al. Pregnancy-related mortality in Hispanic women in the United States. Obstet Gynecol 1999; 94:747-52.
76. Centers for Disease Control and Prevention. Pregnancy-related deaths among Hispanic, Asian/Pacific Islander, and American Indian/Alaska Native women—United States, 1991-1997. MMWR Morb Mortal Wkly Rep 2001; 50:361-4.
77. Goffman D, Madden RC, Harrison EA, et al. Predictors of maternal mortality and near-miss maternal morbidity. J Perinatol 2007; 27:597-601.
78. Walker MC, Murphy KE, Pan S, et al. Adverse maternal outcomes in multifetal pregnancies. Br J Obstet Gynaecol 2004; 111:1294-6.
79. Day MC, Barton JR, O'Brien JM, et al. The effect of fetal number on the development of hypertensive conditions of pregnancy. Obstet Gynecol 2005; 106:927-31.
80. Francois K, Ortiz J, Harris C, et al. Is peripartum hysterectomy more common in multiple gestations? Obstet Gynecol 2005; 105:1369-72.
81. MacKay AP, Berg CJ, King JC, et al. Pregnancy-related mortality among women with multifetal pregnancies. Obstet Gynecol 2006; 107:563-8.
82. Luke B, Brown MB. Maternal morbidity and infant death in twin vs triplet and quadruplet pregnancies. Am J Obstet Gynecol 2008; 198:401.e1-10.
83. Deneux-Tharaux C, Carmona E, Bouvier-Colle MH, Breart G. Postpartum maternal mortality and Cesarean delivery. Obstet Gynecol 2006; 108:541-8.
84. Liu S, Liston RM, Joseph KS, et al. Maternal mortality and severe morbidity associated with low-risk planned Cesarean delivery versus planned vaginal delivery at term. Can Med Assoc J 2007; 176:455-60.
85. Clark SL, Belfort MA, Dildy GA, et al. Maternal death in the 21st century: Causes, prevention, and relationship to cesarean delivery. Am J Obstet Gynecol 2008; 199:36.e1-5.
86. Sullivan SA, Hill EG, Newman RB, Menard MK. Maternal-fetal medicine specialist density is inversely associated with maternal mortality ratios. Am J Obstet Gynecol 2005; 193:1083-8.
87. Nagaya K, Fetters MD, Ishikawa M, et al. Causes of maternal mortality in Japan. JAMA 2000; 283:2661-7.
88. Geller SE, Rosenberg D, Cox SM, Kilpatrick S. Defining a conceptual framework for near-miss maternal morbidity. J Am Med Womens Assoc 2002; 57:135-9.
89. Bruce FC, Berg CJ, Hornbrook MC, et al. Maternal morbidity rates in a managed care population. Obstet Gynecol 2008; 111:1089-95.

90. Pattinson RC, Hall M. Near misses: A useful adjunct to maternal death enquiries. Br Med Bull 2003; 67:231-43.
91. Minkauskiene M, Nadišauskiene R, Padaiga Ž, Makari S. Systematic review on the incidence and prevalence of severe maternal morbidity. Medicina 2004; 40:299-309.
92. Waterstone M, Bewley S, Wolfe C. Incidence and predictors of severe obstetric morbidity: Case-control study. Br Med J 2001; 322:1089-93.
93. Brace V, Penney G, Hall M. Quantifying severe maternal morbidity: A Scottish population study. Br J Obstet Gynaecol 2004; 111:481-4.
94. Zhang WH, Alexander S, Bouvier-Colle MH, Macfarlane A. Incidence of severe pre-eclampsia, postpartum haemorrhage and sepsis as a surrogate marker for severe maternal morbidity in a European population-based study: The MOMS-B survey. Br J Obstet Gynaecol 2005; 112:89-96.
95. Wen SW, Huang L, Liston R, et al. Severe maternal morbidity in Canada, 1991-2001. Can Med Assoc J 2005; 173:759-64.
96. Callaghan WM, Mackay AP, Berg CJ. Identification of severe maternal morbidity during delivery hospitalizations, United States, 1991-2003. Am J Obstet Gynecol 2008; 199:133.e1-8.
97. Kilpatrick SJ, Matthay MA. Obstetric patients requiring critical care: A five-year review. Chest 1992; 101:1407-12.
98. Wheatley E, Farkas A, Watson D. Obstetric admissions to an intensive therapy unit. Int J Obstet Anesth 1996; 5:221-4.
99. Baskett TF, Sternadel J. Maternal intensive care and near-miss mortality in obstetrics. Br J Obstet Gynaecol 1998; 105:981-4.
100. Mahutte NG, Murphy-Kaulbeck L, Le Q, et al. Obstetric admissions to the intensive care unit. Obstet Gynecol 1999; 94:263-6.
101. Mantel GD, Buchmann E, Rees H, Pattinson RC. Severe acute maternal morbidity: A pilot study of a definition for a near-miss. Br J Obstet Gynaecol 1998; 105:985-90.
102. Geller SE, Rosenberg D, Cox S, et al. A scoring system identified near-miss maternal morbidity during pregnancy. J Clin Epidemiol 2004; 57:716-20.
103. Sachs BP, Brown DA, Driscoll SG, et al. Maternal mortality in Massachusetts: Trends and prevention. N Engl J Med 1987; 316:667-72.
104. Schuitemaker NW, Gravenhorst JB, Van Geijn HP, et al. Maternal mortality and its prevention. Eur J Obstet Gynecol Reprod Biol 1991; 42(Suppl):S31-5.
105. Hoyert DL, Danel I, Tully P. Maternal mortality, United States and Canada, 1982-1997. Birth 2000; 27:4-11.
106. Panting-Kemp A, Geller SE, Nguyen T, et al. Maternal deaths in an urban perinatal network, 1992-1998. Am J Obstet Gynecol 2000; 183:1207-12.
107. Geller SE, Rosenberg D, Cox SM, et al. The continuum of maternal morbidity and mortality: Factors associated with severity. Am J Obstet Gynecol 2004; 191:939-44.
108. Berg CJ, Harper MA, Atkinson SM, et al. Preventability of pregnancy-related deaths: Results of a state-wide review. Obstet Gynecol 2005; 106:1228-34.
109. Endler GC, Mariona FG, Sokol RJ, Stevenson LB. Anesthesia-related maternal mortality in Michigan, 1972 to 1984. Am J Obstet Gynecol 1988; 159:187-93.
110. Cooper GM, McClure JH. Anaesthesia. In Lewis G, editor. Why Mothers Die 2000-2002: The Sixth Report of Confidential Enquiries into Maternal Deaths in the United Kingdom. London, RCOG Press, 2004:122-33.
111. Cooper G, McClure J. Anaesthesia. In Lewis G, editor. Saving Mothers Lives: Reviewing Maternal Deaths to Make Motherhood Safer, 2003-2005: The Seventh Report of the Confidential Enquiries into Maternal Deaths in the United Kingdom. London, CEMACH, 2007:107-16.
112. Maternal deaths associated with anaesthesia. In Turnbull AC, Tindall VR, Robson SG, et al., editors. Report on Confidential Enquiries into Maternal Deaths in England and Wales, 1979-1981. London, HMSO, 1986:83-94.
113. Maternal deaths associated with anaesthesia. In Turnbull AC, editor. Report on Confidential Enquiries into Maternal Deaths in England and Wales, 1982-1984. London, HMSO, 1989:96-106.
114. Deaths associated with anaesthesia. In Tindall V, Beard R, Sykes M, et al., editors. Report on Confidential Enquiries into Maternal Deaths in the United Kingdom, 1985-1987. London, HMSO, 1991:73-87.
115. Deaths associated with anaesthesia. In Hibbard BM, Anderson MM, Drife JO, et al., editors. Report on Confidential Enquiries into Maternal Deaths in the United Kingdom, 1988-1990. London, HMSO, 1994:80-96.
116. Deaths associated with anaesthesia. In Hibbard BM, Anderson MM, Drife JO, et al., editors. Report on Confidential Enquiries into Maternal Deaths in the United Kingdom, 1991-1993. London, HMSO, 1996:87-103.
117. Harmer M. Maternal mortality—is it still relevant? Anaesthesia 1997; 52:99-100.
118. Willatts SM. Confidential enquiries into maternal deaths in the United Kingdom 1991-1993. Int J Obstet Anesth 1997; 6:73-5.
119. Deaths associated with anaesthesia. In Drife J, Lewis G, Neilson J, et al., editors. Why Mothers Die: Report on Confidential Enquiries into Maternal Deaths in the United Kingdom, 1994-1996. London, HMSO, 1998:91-102.
120. Crowhurst JA, Plaat F. Why mothers die—report on confidential enquiries into maternal deaths in the United Kingdom, 1994-96. Anaesthesia 1999; 54:207-9.
121. May AE. The confidential enquiry into maternal deaths, 1994-1996. Int J Obstet Anesth 1999; 8:77-8.
122. Thomas TA, Cooper GM. Anaesthesia. In Drife J, Lewis G, editors. Why Mothers Die: 1997-1999: The Fifth Report on the Confidential Enquiries into Maternal Deaths in the United Kingdom. London, RCOG Press, 2001:134-49.
123. Bolton TJ, Randall K, Yentis SM. Effect of the confidential enquiries into maternal deaths on the use of syntocinon at caesarean section in the UK. Anaesthesia 2003; 58:277-9.
124. Cooper GM, Lewis G, Neilson J. Confidential enquiries into maternal deaths, 1997-1999. Br J Anaesth 2002; 89:369-72.
125. Thomas TA, Cooper GM. Maternal deaths from anaesthesia: An extract from why mothers die 1997-1999, the confidential enquiries into maternal deaths in the United Kingdom. Br J Anaesth 2002; 89:499-508.
126. May A. The confidential enquiries into maternal deaths 1997-1999: What can we learn? Int J Obstet Anesth 2002; 11:153-5.
127. Clyburn PA. Early thoughts on 'why mothers die 2000-2002'. Anaesthesia 2004; 59:1157-9.
128. Edsell MEG, Erasmus PD. Use of the common gas outlet for supplementary oxygen during Caesarean section. Anaesthesia 2005; 60:1152-3.
129. Ngan Kee WD. Confidential enquiries into maternal deaths: 50 years of closing the loop. Br J Anaesth 2005; 94:413-6.
130. Cooper GM, McClure JH. Maternal deaths from anaesthesia: An extract from why mothers die 2000-2002, the confidential enquiries into maternal deaths in the United Kingdom. Chapter 9: Anaesthesia. Br J Anaesth 2005; 94:417-23.
131. Clutton-Brock T. Maternal deaths from anaesthesia: An extract from why mothers die 2000-2002, the confidential enquiries into maternal deaths in the United Kingdom. Chapter 17: Trends in intensive care. Br J Anaesth 2005; 94:424-9.
132. McClure J, Cooper G. Fifty years of confidential enquiries into maternal deaths in the United Kingdom: Should anaesthesia celebrate or not? Int J Obstet Anesth 2005; 14:87-9.
133. Cooper GM, McClure JH. Anaesthesia chapter from saving mothers' lives: Reviewing maternal deaths to make pregnancy safer. Br J Anaesth 2008; 100:17-22.
134. Lyons G. Saving Mothers' lives: Confidential enquiry into maternal and child health, 2003-5. Int J Obstet Anesth 2008; 17:103-5.
135. Dob D, Cooper G, Holdcroft A, editors. Crises in Childbirth—Why Mothers Survive: Lessons from the Confidential Enquiries into Maternal Deaths. Oxford, Radcliffe Publishing, 2007.
136. Hawkins JL, Chang J, Callaghan W, et al. Anesthesia-related maternal mortality in the United States, 1991-1996: An update. Anesthesiology 2002; 96:A1046.
137. Martin JA, Hamilton BE, Sutton PD, et al. Births: Final Data for 2005 National Vital Statistics Reports. Natl Vital Stat Rep 2007; 56:1-104.

138. Gibbs CP, Krischer J, Peckham BM, et al. Obstetric anesthesia: A national survey. Anesthesiology 1986; 65:298-306.
139. Hawkins JL, Gibbs CP, Orleans M, et al. Obstetric anesthesia work force survey, 1981 versus 1992. Anesthesiology 1997; 87:135-43.
140. Bucklin BA, Hawkins JL, Anderson JR, Ullrich FA. Obstetric anesthesia workforce survey: Twenty-year update. Anesthesiology 2005; 103:645-53.
141. D'Angelo R. Anesthesia-related maternal mortality: A pat on the back or a call to arms? Anesthesiology 2007; 106:1082-4.
142. Albright G. Cardiac arrest following regional anesthesia with etidocaine and bupivacaine. Anesthesiology 1979; 51:285-7.
143. Marx GF. Cardiotoxicity of local anesthetics—the plot thickens. Anesthesiology 1984; 60:3-5.
144. Rosenblatt MA, Abel M, Fischer GW, et al. Successful use of a 20% lipid emulsion to resuscitate a patient after a presumed bupivacaine-related cardiac arrest. Anesthesiology 2006; 105:217-8.
145. Litz RJ, Popp M, Stehr SN, Koch T. Successful resuscitation of a patient with ropivacaine-induced asystole after axillary plexus block using lipid infusion. Anaesthesia 2006; 61:800-1.
146. Weinberg GL. Lipid infusion therapy: Translation to clinical practice. Anesth Analg 2008; 106:1340-2.
147. Hawkins JL, Chang J, Palmer SK, et al. Anesthesia-related maternal mortality in the United States, 1997-2002 (abstract). Oral presentation at the Annual Meeting of the Society for Obstetric Anesthesia and Perinatology, Chicago, April 30-May 4, 2008.
148. Hawkins JL, Koonin LM, Palmer SK, Gibbs CP. Anesthesia-related deaths during obstetric delivery in the United States, 1979-1990. Anesthesiology 1997; 86:277-84.
149. Hawkins JL. Anesthesia-related maternal mortality. Clin Obstet Gynecol 2003; 46:679-87.
150. Cheney FW, Posner KL, Lee LA, et al. Trends in anesthesia-related death and brain damage: A closed claims analysis. Anesthesiology 2006; 105:1081-6.
151. Lee LA, Posner KL, Domino KB, et al. Injuries associated with regional anesthesia in the 1980s and 1990s: A closed claims analysis. Anesthesiology 2004; 101:143-52.
152. Kinsella SM, Dob D, Holdcroft A. Anesthesia-related maternal deaths: Where is "regional anesthesia"? Anesthesiology 2008; 108:170.
153. Li XF, Fortney JA, Kotelchuck M, Glover LH. The postpartum period: The key to maternal mortality. Int J Gynaecol Obstet 1996; 54:1-10.
154. Chitre D, Karthikeyan G, Sashidaran R. Severe obstetric morbidity in an inner-city teaching hospital. Anesthesiology 2007; 106:A80.

Part X

The Parturient with Systemic Disease

John Snow, the London physician who twice anesthetized Queen Victoria for childbirth, made the first notes of an anesthetic administered to a parturient with systemic disease. On February 12, 1852, he was called to anesthetize a 23-year-old pregnant woman with osteosarcoma of the left shoulder. Her labor had begun 6 hours earlier. As Snow describes it, "the chloroform was not given to the extent of causing unconsciousness but it removed the suffering and caused fits of laughter in the patient after each time of inhaling it for the first half hour." The child was stillborn, "ill-nourished and small." From the child's condition, Snow believed that it had been dead for some time. He noted that the woman died a few weeks later.[1]

Snow wrote extensively about anesthesia. He was acutely aware that systemic disease affected the patient's response to anesthesia. In his last book, published posthumously, he described in detail various physical conditions that influenced a patient's response. Snow stated, "The comparative strength of debility of the patient has considerable influence on the way in which chloroform acts. Usually the more feeble the patient is, whether from illness, or from any other cause, the more quietly does he become insensible."[2] Snow's approach to patients with systemic disease was the same as that used today. The management of the parturient with severe diseases did not become a significant clinical problem until the twentieth century, when medical care had improved to the point that such a patient could survive into adulthood, and become pregnant with a reasonable chance of carrying a child into the third trimester. Snow's experience with this seriously ill patient was probably unique for his day.[3]

Donald Caton, M.D.

REFERENCES

1. Ellis RH, editor. The Case Books of Dr. John Snow. Med Hist Suppl 1994; 14:218.
2. Snow J. On chloroform and other anaesthetics: Their action and administration. John Churchill 1858:53.
3. Caton D. John Snow's practice of obstetric anesthesia. Anesthesiology 2000; 92:247-52.

Autoimmune Disorders

Robert W. Reid, M.D.

In the late nineteenth century, Ehrlich proposed the dictum of *horror autotoxicus*, the belief that immunity is directed against foreign material and never against one's own body.[1] We now know that autoimmune disorders represent a violation of this dictum—a failure of self-tolerance. The induction of autoimmunity is multifactorial, involving both genetic and environmental factors. More than 40 diseases result from autoimmunity, and many lead to chronic illness and severe disability. Genes within the major histocompatibility complex govern these disorders. Women of childbearing age have the highest incidence of several autoimmune disorders. Occasionally the initial diagnosis is made during pregnancy.

During normal pregnancy, altered immune function allows maternal tolerance of the fetal allograft. Both the mother and fetus produce immunologic factors that inhibit maternal cell-mediated immunity.[2,3] This inhibition helps prevent rejection of the fetus and limit the expression of autoimmunity. However, the high estrogen environment of pregnancy may enhance immune function.[4] Teleologically, this enhancement may be required to protect the mother and fetus from the risks of peripartum infection.

Systemic lupus erythematosus, lupus anticoagulant, scleroderma, and polymyositis/dermatomyositis are discussed in this chapter. Other autoimmune disorders are discussed elsewhere in this text, including insulin-dependent diabetes mellitus (see Chapter 42), autoimmune thrombocytopenic purpura and autoimmune hemolytic anemia (see Chapter 43), rheumatoid arthritis and ankylosing spondylitis (see Chapter 48), and myasthenia gravis (see Chapter 49).

SYSTEMIC LUPUS ERYTHEMATOSUS

Definition and Epidemiology

Systemic lupus erythematosus (SLE) is a multisystem inflammatory disease of unknown etiology that is characterized by the production of autoantibodies against nuclear, cytoplasmic, and cell membrane antigens. Although SLE may occur at any age, it is recognized most commonly in women during their childbearing years, with a female-to-male ratio of 9:1. African-Americans, Asians, and Native

Americans are affected more often than whites.[5] An estimated 1 in 1200 deliveries occur in women with SLE.[6]

Pathophysiology

The etiology of SLE remains unclear, but impaired clearance of apoptotic cells may be involved.[7] Intracellular autoantigens are released by necrotic and apoptotic cells, leading to aberrant sensitization against these antigens. Affected individuals have both hyperactivity of the antibody-producing B cells and defects of the helper and suppressor T cells. Genetic defects in immune regulation and environmental triggers (e.g., toxins, drugs, ultraviolet light, viruses) lead to a proliferation of B cells capable of producing autoantibodies. More than 30 classes of antigens have been identified as targets of these antibodies. Diverse antigen-antibody immune complexes are formed, followed by secondary inflammatory responses. Deposition of immune complexes and continued inflammation within the glomerulus may lead to irreversible renal injury. Deposits also occur within the skin, choroid plexus, and other endothelial surfaces, with or without an inflammatory response. The view of SLE as an immune complex disorder is an oversimplification. For example, some of the autoantibodies actively bind to erythrocytes, granulocytes, lymphocytes, and macrophages, leading to the removal of these cells from the circulation.[5]

Diagnosis

Because of the widespread antigenic targets of SLE, clinical manifestations of this disorder are diverse. Box 40-1 outlines objective criteria for the diagnosis of SLE.[8,9] Although epidemiologic studies require the presence of four or more of these criteria, the clinical diagnosis may be suspected if fewer features are present without another explanation.

BOX 40-1 Diagnostic Criteria for Systemic Lupus Erythematosus

- Malar rash (butterfly rash over malar region)
- Discoid rash (erythematous, raised patches with scaling)
- Photosensitivity
- Oral ulceration
- Arthritis
- Serositis (pleuritis or pericarditis)
- Renal disorder (persistent proteinuria or cellular casts)
- Neurologic disorder (seizures or psychosis)
- Hematologic disorder (hemolytic anemia, leukopenia, lymphopenia, or thrombocytopenia)
- Immunologic disorder (anti-DNA, anti-Sm nuclear antigen, anticardiolipin antibodies, lupus anticoagulant, or false-positive syphilis test)
- Antinuclear antibody

From Tan EM, Cohen AS, Fries JF, et al. The 1982 revised criteria for the classification of systemic lupus erythematosus. Arthritis Rheum 1982; 25:1271-7; and Hochberg MC. Updating the American College of Rheumatology revised criteria for the classification of systemic lupus erythematosus. Arthritis Rheum 1997; 40:1725.

Typically the diagnosis of SLE is made before conception; however, the initial diagnosis is made during pregnancy in 20% of cases.[10]

Effect of Pregnancy

Pregnancy does not worsen the long-term course of SLE.[11,12] The question of whether or not disease activity increases during pregnancy has been debated. Recent studies suggest a twofold to threefold increase in SLE activity during pregnancy.[13,14] Ruiz-Irastorza et al.[15] prospectively assessed disease activity with the Lupus Activity Index during 78 pregnancies in 68 women with previously diagnosed SLE. Sixty-five percent of these patients exhibited worsened disease activity, most often during the second and third trimesters and the puerperium. These flares of SLE activity were not more severe than flares in nonpregnant patients, and most responded to conservative management. Clowse et al.[16] assessed outcome for 265 pregnancies in women with SLE in the Hopkins Lupus Pregnancy Cohort. In this group, the risk of significant disease activity during pregnancy was sevenfold greater if the patient had active disease within 6 months prior to conception.

Effect on the Mother

Most women with SLE do not have renal impairment at conception, probably because renal insufficiency impairs fertility. However, pregnancy may worsen preexisting renal dysfunction. Gestational flaring of lupus nephritis is generally mild and reversible, but approximately 12% of pregnant women with SLE will suffer an irreversible progression of renal dysfunction.[17,18] It is not clear whether preeclampsia occurs more often in patients with SLE. Often it is difficult to distinguish between lupus nephritis and preeclampsia; both may manifest as hypertension, edema, and proteinuria. The difference is a critical one, however, because the corresponding treatments are quite different (i.e., immunosuppressive therapy for lupus nephritis versus delivery for preeclampsia). An increased serum uric acid concentration, proteinuria without active urinary sediment, and liver enzyme abnormalities suggest preeclampsia rather than SLE.

SLE may cause thrombocytopenia. When thrombocytopenia occurs in a pregnant woman, preeclampsia, HELLP syndrome (i.e., hemolysis, elevated liver enzymes, and low platelets), and disseminated intravascular coagulation also must be considered. Although anemia is a common manifestation of SLE, it must be differentiated from nutritional anemia and the physiologic anemia of late pregnancy.

The relaxation of ligaments that often occurs during late pregnancy worsens the pain of lupus arthritis. Patients with SLE occasionally require joint replacement because of osteonecrosis, most commonly of the femoral head. These prostheses may become painful, dislocated, or infected during pregnancy.[19] Finally, neurologic complications of SLE are rare during pregnancy but include seizures, chorea gravidarum, and stroke.

Effect on the Fetus

Maternal SLE impairs fetal survival and increases the risk of preterm delivery. However, Clark et al.[20] demonstrated that improved perinatal management and control of disease activity reduced the rate of fetal loss from 43% (during the years 1960 to 1965) to 17% (in the years 2000 to 2003). In another study, fetal death occurred in 6 of 8 (75%) pregnancies in mothers with SLE and high disease activity, compared with 7 of 51 (14%) pregnancies in mothers with SLE but without active disease.[21] Yasmeen et al.[22] reported data from the California Health Information for Policy Project in which preterm deliveries accounted for 21% of 555 deliveries in women with SLE, a rate six times higher than that found among the general population. In the Hopkins Lupus Pregnancy Cohort, preterm birth occurred in 38 of 57 (67%) pregnancies in women with moderate to severely active SLE, compared with 68 of 210 (32%) pregnancies in women with inactive or mildly active SLE.[16]

Neonatal lupus erythematosus (NLE) is a syndrome that may result when maternal autoantibodies against Ro (SS-A) or La (SS-B) cross the placenta and bind to fetal tissue. These autoantibodies are found in as many as 87% of patients with SLE.[23] However, NLE occurs after only a fraction of these pregnancies. Reversible NLE manifestations—cutaneous lupus, transaminase elevation, and thrombocytopenia—resolve when maternal antibodies disappear from the newborn circulation within 8 months after birth. During fetal cardiac conduction system development, anti-Ro/anti-La antibodies may bind to conduction cells and cause cell death and irreversible fetal heart block. The incidence of congenital heart block is 2% when anti-Ro antibody is detected in the mother.[24] Fetal echocardiography reveals atrioventricular dissociation, cardiac dilation, and pericardial effusion. Treatment includes prompt delivery, newborn cardiac pacing, antepartum administration of dexamethasone, and consideration of apheresis to remove maternal antibodies.[25]

Medical Management

Optimally, women with SLE should delay pregnancy until their disease has been quiet for at least 6 months, and they should be taking "acceptably safe" medications at the time of conception.[18,26-28] Often such planning is not possible, and the physician's focus is to minimize disease activity during gestation by means of medications with acceptable safety.

Hydroxychloroquinine is frequently used to reduce SLE activity. Discontinuation of hydroxychloroquinine just before conception or in early pregnancy leads to a significant increase in disease activity.[29] Thus, hydroxychloroquinine should be continued in all women who were taking it before conception, and it may be used to treat flares during gestation.[29,30]

Similarly, **azathioprine** should be continued if used prior to conception. In contrast, **mycophenolate mofetil** should be discontinued before conception because of the risk of teratogenicity[26,28]; azathioprine is an acceptable substitute. The fetal liver does not express the enzyme necessary to convert azathioprine to its active form.[30] Nevertheless, maternal use of azathioprine has been associated with reversible neonatal lymphopenia, depressed serum immunoglobulin levels, and decreased thymic size in the newborn.[31]

Antenatal exposure to low-dose **prednisone** (less than 20 mg daily) appears to be safe, and most children develop normally. However, there is concern that prolonged fetal exposure to other corticosteroids such as **dexamethasone** or **betamethasone** may lead to decreased intrauterine growth and abnormal neuronal development.[32] Corticosteroid therapy may precipitate gestational diabetes, and patients should be monitored for evidence of glucose intolerance. Striae, gastrointestinal ulceration, and bone demineralization may complicate long-term corticosteroid therapy. Affected patients should receive postprandial and bedtime antacids.[33] The pediatrician should be alerted to the possibility of neonatal adrenal suppression.

Aspirin and other **nonsteroidal anti-inflammatory drugs (NSAIDs)** have been used to manage lupus arthritis and have shown no evidence of teratogenicity.[34] However, NSAIDs can cause premature closure of the ductus arteriosus in the fetus,[35] and they can impair maternal and neonatal hemostasis.[36]

Obstetric Management

Patients with SLE are at increased risk for **intrauterine fetal death** and **preterm delivery**. Estimation of the gestational age is obtained with ultrasonography at the first prenatal visit and again at 20 weeks' gestation. Continued surveillance consists of nonstress testing, biophysical profile measurement, and/or umbilical artery Doppler velocimetry beginning at 26 to 28 weeks' gestation and performed weekly until delivery.[18]

Because the coexistence of antiphospholipid antibodies predicts a much higher fetal risk, maternal serum is obtained to check for these serologic markers. **Thromboprophylaxis** is important in patients with antiphospholipid syndrome (see later). The platelet count, creatinine clearance, 24-hour urine protein level, and presence or absence of anti-Ro/anti-La antibodies should be determined. Platelet count determination is repeated monthly.[37] If anti-Ro/anti-La antibodies are detected or the fetal heart rate is 60 beats per minute without variability in the second trimester, fetal echocardiography and fetal heart rate testing are performed to evaluate for signs of congenital heart block or failure.[38] In normal pregnancy, serial complement levels gradually increase. However, declining levels of C3 and C4 suggest active disease and lupus nephritis.[28] The obstetrician monitors for the onset of preeclampsia with regular assessment of blood pressure, weight gain, and proteinuria.

The timing and route of delivery are individualized. Although vaginal delivery is preferred, the cesarean delivery rate in parturients with SLE is 40%.[6]

Anesthetic Management

The obstetrician, rheumatologist, and anesthesia provider should discuss the condition of both the mother and fetus and should formulate the plan for delivery. Maternal organ system involvement and the current severity of the disease should be evaluated systematically.

Pericarditis is common in patients with SLE; although it typically is asymptomatic, **cardiac tamponade** has been reported.[39] Prolongation of the PR interval or nonspecific T-wave changes may be noted on the electrocardiogram (ECG). A history of dyspnea on exertion or unexplained tachycardia may suggest significant pericarditis or myocarditis. Rarely, coronary artery vasculitis or accelerated atherosclerosis leads to myocardial ischemia and infarction, even in young women.[40] Ozaki et al.[41] reported an episode of myocardial ischemia during emergency anesthesia in an elderly patient with SLE and undiagnosed antiphospholipid syndrome.

Roldan et al.[42] performed echocardiographic studies in 69 patients with SLE and discovered a high incidence of **valvular abnormalities**. Findings included valvular thickening in 51%, vegetations in 43%, regurgitation in 25%, and stenosis in 4% of study subjects. Valvular abnormalities were associated with substantial morbidity and mortality during the follow-up period. In the past, women with SLE and valvular abnormalities received antibiotic prophylaxis for infective endocarditis. Revised American Heart Association guidelines recommend antibiotic prophylaxis only for patients at highest risk for infective endocarditis.[43] Specifically, prophylaxis should be limited to women with previous infective endocarditis, unrepaired cyanotic congenital heart disease, implanted prosthetic material or devices, or a history of cardiac transplantation with cardiac valvulopathy. Prophylactic antibiotics are *not* recommended for women with common valvular lesions undergoing genitourinary procedures, including vaginal delivery.[43]

Winslow et al.[44] studied the prevalence and progression of **pulmonary hypertension** in 28 patients with SLE. The prevalence of pulmonary hypertension was 14% at initial evaluation and 43% 5 years later. Epidural anesthesia for cesarean delivery in parturients with pulmonary hypertension has been reported (see Chapter 41). However, an abrupt onset of sympathetic blockade and subsequent decreased venous return to the right atrium may cause precipitous systemic hypotension and hypoxemia in these patients. One report described the administration of general anesthesia in a parturient with SLE and pulmonary hypertension, with coexisting SLE-related restrictive lung disease, pulmonary edema, and orthopnea.[45] McMillan et al.[46] reported their experience with three parturients with pulmonary hypertension secondary to SLE and antiphospholipid syndrome. Two of these women died from right-sided heart failure within 48 hours of delivery.

Subclinical pleuritis is common, but significant pleural effusions rarely occur. Patients may suffer from infectious pneumonia or lupus pneumonitis. The latter condition is characterized by fleeting hemorrhagic infiltrates that may become consolidated. Pulmonary embolism and diaphragmatic dysfunction have been reported.[40]

Central and peripheral sensorimotor and autonomic neuropathies are observed in as many as 25% of patients with SLE.[47] Vocal cord palsy has been reported in a patient with SLE.[48] These deficits should be documented before the administration of either neuraxial or general anesthesia. **Migraine headache** and **cerebral vasculitis** resulting from SLE must be considered in the differential diagnosis of a postpartum headache. **Psychological disorders** and **frank psychosis** can occur during disease exacerbation.[5,49] **Seizures** can occur, especially if chronic anticonvulsant medications are discontinued inadvertently.

The anesthesia provider should evaluate the parturient for hematologic abnormalities, including **anemia, thrombocytopenia,** and **coagulopathy**. An abnormality of the activated partial thromboplastin time (aPTT), which is not corrected with a 1:1 control plasma mix, suggests the presence of either lupus anticoagulant (a coexistent but separate disease entity) or, more rarely, true autoantibodies against specific coagulation factors (e.g., VIII, IX, XII). Lupus anticoagulant is a laboratory artifact that does *not* cause clinical coagulopathy. True coagulation factor autoantibodies (or inhibitors) may result in a significant bleeding diathesis, which contraindicates the administration of neuraxial anesthesia.

Long-term use of NSAIDs leads to qualitative platelet abnormalities and has rarely been associated with epidural or subdural hematoma.[49-51] However, NSAIDs are widely used, and their potential role in causing spinal epidural hematoma remains conjectural. Horlocker et al.[52] prospectively studied 924 patients undergoing orthopedic procedures with spinal or epidural anesthesia. Preoperative antiplatelet medications were taken by 39% of these patients; however, no cases of spinal epidural hematoma were observed. The same investigators similarly studied 1035 patients undergoing epidural steroid injection.[53] NSAID use was reported by 32% of these patients undergoing chronic pain management. Again, there were no cases of spinal hematoma. In a large, multicenter randomized trial, 9364 pregnant women received either low-dose aspirin (60 mg daily) or placebo for prevention and treatment of preeclampsia.[54] Of 5000 enrollees, at least 1069 patients received epidural analgesia, and no cases of epidural hematoma were observed.[55] In the past, some anesthesia providers have determined the bleeding time in patients taking aspirin or another NSAID. However, the predictive value of the bleeding time measurement is unclear in these patients, and the bleeding time test is no longer recommended to assess risk for spinal epidural hematoma secondary to neuraxial analgesia or anesthesia.

Occasionally, atypical blood antibodies complicate efforts to type and cross-match blood for a patient with SLE. Additional time should be allowed for this possibility.

Prosthetic orthopedic joints should be positioned carefully during vaginal or cesarean delivery. Lupus arthritis rarely involves the cervical spine. Women who have undergone long-term corticosteroid therapy should receive a peripartum stress dose of a corticosteroid.

ANTIPHOSPHOLIPID SYNDROME

Definition and Epidemiology

The antiphospholipid syndrome (also known as Hughes' syndrome[56]) is a *prothrombotic* disorder that results in both arterial and venous thrombosis and is characterized by the presence of two autoantibodies, **lupus anticoagulant** and **anticardiolipin antibody**. The disorder was first recognized in the early 1980s.[57,58] Vilardell, former Dean of Medicine at the University of Barcelona, proclaimed, "There are two 'new' diseases of the late 20th century: AIDS and the antiphospholipid syndrome."[56]

The prevalences of lupus anticoagulant and anticardiolipin antibody among patients with SLE are 34% and 44%, respectively.[59] However, the antiphospholipid syndrome is a distinct and separate entity from SLE. A long-term cohort study found that among patients with antiphospholipid syndrome, only 11 of 128 (8%) had SLE.[60]

The overall prevalence of antiphospholipid syndrome is unclear. In 1990, commenting on the volume of publications on antiphospholipid syndrome, Harris[61] remarked that the syndrome "probably occurs less frequently than the number of papers published on the subject." But in 2007, with greater clinical recognition, Hughes[56] predicted that the prevalence of antiphospholipid syndrome will exceed that of SLE.

Pathophysiology

The antiphospholipid syndrome is characterized by two important misnomers. First, the antibodies do not bind directly to phospholipids. Instead, antiphospholipid antibodies bind to phospholipid-binding plasma proteins such as β_2-glycoprotein I, prothrombin, and annexin V. Second, the lupus anticoagulant has no true anticoagulant activity *in vivo*. Instead, the anticoagulant activity of lupus anticoagulant is a laboratory artifact that affects the phospholipid-dependent coagulation assays: the aPTT, the kaolin clotting time (KCT), the tissue thromboplastin inhibition (TTI) test, and the dilute Russell viper venom time (dRVVT). These times remain prolonged even when the tests are repeated with a 1:1 mixture of the patient's plasma and control plasma. The prothrombin time (PT) typically is normal. Lupus anticoagulant appears to block *in vitro* assembly of prothrombinase (a phospholipid complex), thus preventing the conversion of prothrombin to thrombin. True bleeding caused by lupus anticoagulant is extremely rare and, in most cases, is explained by an underlying factor deficiency or inhibitor.[62,63]

Lupus anticoagulant and anticardiolipin antibody are associated with thrombotic events, both arterial and venous. The current model by which this thrombotic tendency occurs involves antiphospholipid antibodies binding to β_2-glycoprotein I, which then bind to glycoprotein Ibα on platelets, monocytes, and endothelial cells. These complexes cause platelet adhesion, expression of prothrombotic molecules, and local complement activation.[62,64]

Diagnosis

The diagnosis of antiphospholipid syndrome depends on an unexplained clinical history of recurrent venous thrombosis, arterial thrombosis, and/or pregnancy loss as well as on laboratory evidence of anticardiolipin antibody or lupus anticoagulant. The latter is demonstrated by (1) evidence of abnormal phospholipid-dependent coagulation (elevated aPTT); (2) evidence that this abnormality is caused by an inhibitor rather than a factor deficiency (elevated aPTT with 1:1 mix); and (3) proof that the inhibitor is directed against phospholipid rather than specific coagulation factors. Because tests for syphilis are designed to detect the antiphospholipid antibodies present in syphilis, the Venereal Disease Research Laboratory (VDRL) and Wasserman test results often are falsely positive.[63]

Effect on the Mother

The parturient with antiphospholipid antibodies may suffer from **venous and arterial thrombosis,** including **deep vein thrombosis, pulmonary embolism, myocardial infarction,** and **cerebral infarction**. Silver et al.[65] published a historic cohort study of 130 women with antiphospholipid syndrome. During the observation interval (median = 3.2 years), 48% of these women experienced at least one of the following disorders: transient ischemic attack, peripheral thrombosis, stroke, amaurosis fugax, autoimmune thrombocytopenia, and SLE. Twenty-four percent of the thrombotic events occurred during pregnancy and the puerperium. However, women diagnosed with antiphospholipid syndrome on the basis of a history of recurrent pregnancy loss and evidence of antiphospholipid antibody, but without prior thrombotic events, seem rarely to suffer thrombosis during pregnancy.[66] Cuadrado et al.[67] reported a 23% prevalence of thrombocytopenia among 171 patients with antiphospholipid syndrome. Asherson[68] has described a rare syndrome that consists of precipitous multisystem organ thrombosis and failure, known as **catastrophic antiphospholipid syndrome,** which is triggered by pregnancy in 4% of cases.

Effect on the Fetus

Antiphospholipid antibodies may put the fetus at high risk for death *in utero*. In one study of women with lupus anticoagulant, only 13 of 173 (7.5%) pregnancies resulted in the delivery of a live newborn.[69] In a 5-year review of 260 women with a history of recurrent pregnancy loss, 87 (34%) were found to test positive for antiphospholipid antibodies.[66] Most fetal deaths occur during mid- and late pregnancy. Placental infarction is the apparent mechanism of mortality. However, improved understanding and management of the syndrome result in better outcomes. A study of 69 pregnancies in 58 parturients with antiphospholipid syndrome reported 71 live births.[70]

After delivery, most infants of women with antiphospholipid syndrome do not have an increased rate of neonatal or childhood complications.[71] However, from 1987 to 2002, 13 cases of antiphospholipid-related fetal and neonatal thrombosis (mainly cerebral thrombosis) were reported.[72]

Medical and Obstetric Management

Some studies have suggested that fetal survival and maternal thrombotic risk are improved when affected pregnant women are treated with **low-dose aspirin** and **heparin**. A 2005 meta-analysis found that combined treatment with unfractionated heparin and aspirin can reduce pregnancy loss by 54%.[73] The American College of Obstetricians and Gynecologists[63] has made the following recommendations: (1) women with recurrent unexplained pregnancy loss or vascular thrombosis should be tested for antiphospholipid antibodies; (2) women with antiphospholipid syndrome and no thrombotic history should receive prophylactic doses of heparin and low-dose aspirin during pregnancy and for 6 to 8 weeks postpartum; and (3) women with antiphospholipid syndrome and a previous history of thrombosis should receive full anticoagulation throughout pregnancy and the postpartum period. The efficacy of providing prednisone with or without intravenous immunoglobulin is unclear and is not recommended as primary therapy.[63]

The rare occurrence of catastrophic antiphospholipid (Asherson's) syndrome necessitates rapid recognition and aggressive management because of its mortality rate. Full anticoagulation, steroids, repeated plasma exchange, and intravenous immunoglobulin should not be withheld. Severe thrombocytopenia may respond to rituximab.[68]

Anesthetic Management

Management of the patient with antiphospholipid antibodies is similar to that of the patient with SLE. Coexisting autoimmune disorders, secondary organ involvement, and thrombotic phenomena should be evaluated. The anesthesia provider must remain aware that the term *lupus anticoagulant* is a misnomer (as discussed earlier) and does *not* warrant withholding of neuraxial anesthesia. Infrequently, antiphospholipid antibodies can cause coagulation factor deficiencies. In such patients, neuraxial anesthesia is relatively contraindicated. However, in the absence of an underlying coagulation deficit or anticoagulant therapy, the prolonged aPTT does *not* suggest a bleeding tendency, and neuraxial anesthesia may be administered safely.

Ralph[74] reviewed the anesthetic management of 27 pregnancies complicated by antiphospholipid syndrome. All subjects received aspirin (100 to 150 mg daily) throughout pregnancy. Uninterrupted aspirin therapy alone was not considered a contraindication to neuraxial anesthesia. In parturients who had also received thromboprophylaxis with standard unfractionated heparin, the author waited at least 4 hours after the last dose of heparin before administering spinal or epidural anesthesia. He affirmed that the administration of low-molecular-weight heparin (LMWH) for thromboprophylaxis precludes the administration of neuraxial anesthesia until at least 12 hours have elapsed since the time of the last dose. Further, therapeutic anticoagulation with high-dose LMWH precludes the administration of neuraxial anesthesia until at least 24 hours have elapsed since the time of the last dose (see Chapters 38 and 43).[74] A recent report described the use of thromboelastography to document clearance of heparin before administration of neuraxial anesthesia in parturients with lupus anticoagulant.[75]

If there is evidence of fetal compromise secondary to multi-infarct placental insufficiency, hypotension from sympathetic blockade should be prevented. The gradual onset of epidural anesthesia seems preferable to the abrupt onset of single-dose spinal anesthesia. Parturients with antiphospholipid syndrome who undergo general anesthesia are at risk for venous thrombosis. To minimize this risk, compression stockings and warmed fluids should be used.[74,76]

SYSTEMIC SCLEROSIS (SCLERODERMA)

Definition and Epidemiology

Systemic sclerosis or scleroderma is a chronic progressive autoimmune disease of unknown etiology characterized by deposition of fibrous connective tissue in the skin and other tissues. It is a heterogeneous disorder that is separated into **limited cutaneous scleroderma** and **diffuse cutaneous scleroderma**. A subset of patients exhibit systemic sclerosis without cutaneous involvement.[77]

The annual incidence of scleroderma in the United States is 19 per million. The prevalence is 240 per million, which is four to nine times greater than the reported global prevalence.[78,79] Scleroderma is almost five times more common among women than among men, and it occurs primarily between 30 and 50 years of age.[78,79]

Pathophysiology

In systemic sclerosis, fibroblasts produce excess collagen and other matrix constituents through an unknown process or regulatory defect. This excess collagen leads to microvascular obliteration and fibrosis within the skin and other target organs. Endothelial cells undergo vasomotor and permeability changes, which manifest as cyclic vasoconstriction-vasodilation and edema. Patients with scleroderma produce autoantibodies against nuclear and centromere structures, but the significance of these antibodies is unknown.

Scleroderma exhibits a strong female predilection, a steep rise in incidence after the childbearing years, and some clinical similarities to the chronic graft-versus-host disease that may occur after bone marrow transplantation. Because of these observations, some investigators have hypothesized that microchimerism may be involved in the pathogenesis of scleroderma. Fetal cells and DNA have been detected in maternal blood for decades after normal pregnancy and delivery. Nelson et al.[80] sought to determine whether human leukocyte antigen (HLA) compatibility of a child was associated with later development of scleroderma in the mother. They found that HLA class II compatibility between the child and the mother (a condition favorable for microchimerism) was more common among women who experienced scleroderma. This compatibility can allow the fetal cells, which gain access to the maternal circulation during gestation, to remain unrecognized for years or decades. An unknown stimulus may then prompt these fetal cells to differentiate and initiate a graft-versus-host disease–like reaction.[81]

Diagnosis

The triad of Raynaud's phenomenon, nonpitting edema, and hidebound skin establishes the diagnosis of scleroderma. Raynaud's phenomenon is characterized by cyclic pallor and cyanosis of the digits in response to cold or emotion. This phenomenon is a common prodrome to scleroderma, but only 1 in 100 patients with Raynaud's phenomenon progresses to scleroderma. Limited cutaneous scleroderma, also termed **CREST syndrome,** involves calcinosis, Raynaud's phenomenon, esophageal dysfunction, sclerodactyly, and telangiectasia. Skin involvement is limited to the hands, face, and feet in this form of the disease. Clinical manifestations of diffuse cutaneous scleroderma are summarized in Box 40-2.

Effect of Pregnancy

Most patients with scleroderma have slow but progressive skin and organ involvement. More than 70% of patients with diffuse cutaneous scleroderma and more than 90% of those with limited cutaneous scleroderma are still alive 15 years after diagnosis.[82] When death occurs, it most often results from renal failure and malignant hypertension. Steen et al.[83] reviewed the clinical course of 231 women with a history of scleroderma, including 69 with concomitant pregnancy and 162 without. They observed no difference in survival between groups. They reported only one pregnancy-related death. Steen[84] also reported a prospective study of 91 pregnancies among 59 women with systemic sclerosis. In this study, pregnant women indicated

BOX 40-2 Manifestations of Diffuse Cutaneous Systemic Sclerosis

Skin
- Raynaud's phenomenon
- Nonpitting edema
- Hidebound skin (involves all but back and buttocks)

Gastrointestinal
- Hypomotility
- Dysphagia
- Reflux esophagitis
- Postprandial fullness
- Constipation
- Abdominal pain
- Intermittent diarrhea
- Malnutrition
- Ileus

Pulmonary
- Interstitial fibrosis
- Pleuritis
- Pulmonary hypertension

Renal
- Proteinuria
- Renal insufficiency and failure
- Malignant hypertension

Cardiac
- Chronic pericardial effusion
- Myocardial ischemia and infarction
- Conduction disturbances
- Heart failure

Musculoskeletal
- Arthritis (symmetric, small joints)
- Myopathy
- Muscle wasting

Other
- Peripheral or cranial neuropathy
- Facial pain
- Trigeminal neuralgia
- Keratoconjunctivitis sicca
- Xerostomia
- Absence of anticentromere antibodies

From LeRoy EC. Systemic sclerosis (scleroderma). In Wyngaarden JB, Smith LH, Bennett JC, editors. Cecil Textbook of Medicine. 19th edition. Philadelphia, WB Saunders, 1992:1530-5.

that their scleroderma symptoms were unchanged in 57 (62%) of the pregnancies. Eighteen (20%) pregnancies were accompanied with some improvement, usually in the symptoms of Raynaud's phenomenon. In 16 (18%) of the pregnancies, esophageal reflux, cardiac arrhythmias, arthritis, skin thickening, and renal crisis occurred or worsened.

Effect on Pregnancy and the Fetus

The prospective study by Steen[84] revealed no increase in frequency of miscarriage, except in women with long-standing diffuse scleroderma. Preterm birth occurred in 25% of pregnancies (compared with 5% in control pregnancies), and most preterm deliveries occurred in women with unstable diffuse scleroderma of less than 4 years' duration.

Medical Management

No proven treatment exists for the arrest of scleroderma. At best, therapy is directed toward improving existing symptoms and slowing end-organ damage. D-Penicillamine is no longer recommended because of toxicity and minimal evidence of efficacy.[85] Glucocorticoids only ameliorate inflammatory myositis and have no effect on disease progression. The immunosuppressive agents chlorambucil and azathioprine have no beneficial effect.[86,87] Angiotensin-converting enzyme (ACE) inhibitors are the agents of choice for treating scleroderma-associated renal crisis and malignant hypertension. However, the use of ACE inhibitors during pregnancy is associated with teratogenicity (including renal atresia and pulmonary hypoplasia), anhydramnios, and fetopathy. As a general principle, unproven and potentially teratogenic drugs should be discontinued during pregnancy; thus, ACE inhibitors ideally should be avoided during pregnancy in the absence of hypertension or overt renal crisis. Despite these risks, Steen[88] has recommended that an ACE inhibitor should be started immediately with the first evidence of increased maternal blood pressure, because ACE inhibitors provide the only effective control of hypertension during scleroderma-associated renal crisis. Nitric oxide donors and possibly heparin may provide some protection against placental dysfunction in pregnant women with scleroderma.[89]

Obstetric Management

Pregnant women with scleroderma should be evaluated for evidence of renal, pulmonary, and cardiac dysfunction. Some physicians recommend the termination of pregnancy if advanced disease is present.[90] However, intensive antenatal observation for onset of renal disease, systemic hypertension, pulmonary hypertension, cardiac dysfunction, and fetal compromise allows most mothers to deliver healthy infants. Obstructive uropathy may result from an enlarging uterus trapped within a noncompliant abdomen.[91] Uterine and cervical wall thickening may lead to ineffective uterine contractions or cervical dystocia at delivery.[83] Even the tightest abdominal skin usually heals if cesarean delivery is necessary.[88]

Anesthetic Management

The pregnant woman with scleroderma presents several challenges to the anesthesia provider. As with SLE, management is based on a multidisciplinary approach. When possible, an anesthesiologist should evaluate the pregnant woman before labor and delivery.

History and physical examination should be directed toward detection of underlying systemic dysfunction. Laboratory testing consists of a complete blood count, coagulation screen, determination of electrolyte levels and creatinine clearance, arterial blood gas analysis, urinalysis, and urine protein determination. An ECG and pulmonary function testing should be performed in all of these patients. Echocardiography is a useful adjuvant to evaluate ventricular dysfunction, pericardial and pleural effusions, and pulmonary hypertension. In addition, arterial pulses, noninvasive blood pressure measurement, peripheral venous access, extent of Raynaud's phenomenon involvement, and the need for special positioning requirements should be assessed.

A thorough evaluation of the patient's upper airway is necessary. Severe limitation of the oral opening may result from perioral hidebound skin, making direct laryngoscopy impossible. The anesthesia provider should determine the maximal mouth opening, ability to sublux the mandible, visualization of oropharyngeal structures, degree of atlanto-occipital joint extension, and presence of oral or nasal telangiectasias. From this evaluation, the anesthesia provider can determine whether direct laryngoscopy will be difficult if general anesthesia is required.[92] The patient should be prepared for the possibility of an awake intubation. Equipment for fiberoptic intubation and emergency cricothyrotomy must be immediately available in the labor and delivery suite.

Epidural anesthesia has been used successfully in parturients with scleroderma.[93-95] If otherwise appropriate, the anesthesia provider should encourage the early administration of epidural anesthesia in laboring women at risk for difficult intubation. Even when severe, diffuse cutaneous involvement is present, the skin of the lumbar back is spared. Spinal anesthesia for cesarean delivery in a parturient with scleroderma has been reported, although this case was complicated by precipitous hypotension.[96] Full sensation returned 3.5 hours after administration of spinal anesthesia in this woman.

Prolonged duration of regional anesthesia has been observed in some patients with scleroderma. Eisele and Reitan[97] reported a case of an axillary block (performed with 1% lidocaine with epinephrine) that persisted for 24 hours. Lewis[98] reported a case of a digital nerve block (performed with 1% lidocaine without epinephrine) that persisted for 10 hours. Neill[99] reported a case of a sciatic nerve block that lasted 16 hours. Thompson and Conklin[93] used 2% 2-chloroprocaine to establish epidural anesthesia from T6 to S5, which persisted for nearly 6 hours in a laboring woman. Prolonged anesthesia may result from microvasculature changes and diminished uptake of the local anesthetic agent. This does not represent a contraindication to neuraxial anesthesia; rather, it should prompt the anesthesia provider to give small incremental boluses of the local anesthetic agent and to prepare the patient for the possibility of a prolonged block. Incremental bolus injection also seems preferable to the continuous infusion of local anesthetic agent; continuous infusion may result in the administration of an excessive dose with a prolonged block. Epidural anesthesia seems preferable to spinal anesthesia because of the ability to titrate the dose response to the desired level of anesthesia.

If cesarean delivery is required, the decision to use epidural or general anesthesia depends on the urgency of delivery, anticipated airway difficulty, and the anesthesia provider's skills. Gastric hypomotility increases the risk of esophageal reflux and aspiration. Central venous catheterization may be required for venous access in patients with diffuse cutaneous involvement. Extensive skin involvement may lead to inaccurate noninvasive blood pressure cuff measurement, necessitating invasive arterial monitoring. Radial artery catheterization is contraindicated in patients with Raynaud's phenomenon because of the risk of hand ischemia. Brachial artery catheterization may be necessary. Pulmonary artery catheterization may be indicated in the presence of cardiac dysfunction or pulmonary hypertension.[100] The patient—and especially the extremities affected by Raynaud's phenomenon—should be kept warm. Scleroderma reduces tear production, so the eyes should be protected against corneal abrasions.

POLYMYOSITIS AND DERMATOMYOSITIS

Definition and Epidemiology

Polymyositis and dermatomyositis represent two members of a larger disease group, the idiopathic inflammatory myopathic diseases. **Polymyositis** is characterized by nonsuppurative inflammation of muscle, primarily skeletal muscles of the proximal limbs, neck, and pharynx. This inflammation leads to symmetric weakness, atrophy, and fibrosis of affected muscle groups. **Dermatomyositis** represents the same disorder, with the addition of a characteristic heliotrope eruption (blue-purple discoloration of the upper eyelid) and Gottron's papules (raised, scaly, violet eruptions over the knuckles). These disorders are quite rare, with a prevalence of 10 per million and an annual incidence of 5.5 per million. Women are affected twice as often as men. The age of onset is bimodal, with peaks before puberty and during the fifth decade.[101,102]

Pathophysiology

Both polymyositis and dermatomyositis are associated with other autoimmune disorders, notably scleroderma. The etiology of inflammatory muscle disease is unknown and likely multifactorial. An initial insult mediated by viral infection or another infectious agent, or exposure to environmental substances, may lead to initial muscle damage in genetically susceptible individuals. This initial process may then trigger an autoimmune response involving chronic muscle inflammation. A viral etiology is suggested by seasonal and geographic clustering of new cases. However, viral genomic material has not been identified in affected muscle tissue. Many drugs, including lipid-lowering drugs in the statin group and antiretroviral drugs, are associated with the development of myopathy. The presence of cellular infiltrates within affected muscle tissue and complement-mediated capillary damage are features of inflammatory muscle diseases. More than 12 autoantibodies have been identified within affected individuals. Underlying malignancy has been associated with polymyositis and dermatomyositis, although the cause-and-effect relationship is unclear.[101-103]

Diagnosis

Bohan and Peter[104] proposed the diagnostic criteria for polymyositis/dermatomyositis (Box 40-3). The level of serum creatine kinase correlates with disease activity. Electromyography and muscle biopsy provide confirmation of the diagnosis. As with other autoimmune disorders, variable systemic involvement is present. Pharyngeal muscle

BOX 40-3 Diagnostic Criteria for Polymyositis and Dermatomyositis

Polymyositis

- Symmetric weakness of proximal muscles
- Histologic evidence of muscle inflammation and necrosis
- Elevation of serum skeletal muscle enzymes
- Electromyographic evidence of myopathy

Dermatomyositis

- Three or four of the above, plus heliotrope eruption or Gottron's papules

From Bohan A, Peter JB. Polymyositis and dermatomyositis (second of two parts). N Engl J Med 1975; 292:403-7.

involvement leads to **dysphagia** and **reflux**. Most patients exhibit impairment of gastric and esophageal motility.[105] **Chronic aspiration pneumonitis** is the most common pulmonary manifestation of polymyositis/dermatomyositis.[106] **Myositis of the respiratory muscles** may cause respiratory insufficiency. **Interstitial lung disease** has been reported in 5% to 65% of patients.[107] **Cardiac involvement** includes nonspecific repolarization abnormalities, conduction disturbances, arrhythmias, coronary artery vasculitis, and, rarely, heart failure.[108] **Arthritis** generally involves the small hand and finger joints. Renal or hematologic involvement is rare.

Effect of Pregnancy

Reports of polymyositis or dermatomyositis during pregnancy are rare. Ishii et al.[109] reviewed 12 reports of 29 pregnancies during a 30-year period. In 11 (40%) of the patients, the initial diagnosis was made during gestation or during the immediate postpartum period. Pregnancy may be a trigger for induction of dermatomyositis in some women. Among the 18 patients with previously diagnosed disease, the disease remained inactive in 11 (61%) of the patients, and 2 (11%) had an exacerbation of disease activity.

Effect on the Fetus

Fetal survival is affected by concurrent polymyositis/dermatomyositis. Ishii et al.[109] noted that 10 of 29 (32%) pregnancies ended with fetal death or spontaneous abortion; eight infants (26%) were delivered preterm. Fetal outcome was strongly influenced by disease activity. Of the women who had minimal disease activity, nearly 60% delivered healthy babies at term. Silva et al.[110] observed a similar correlation between outcome and disease activity in four pregnancies in four women with polymyositis/dermatomyositis, two with active disease and fetal death, and two with disease remission and uneventful outcome.

Medical and Obstetric Management

Pregnancy should be planned during periods of disease inactivity. Serum creatine kinase, glutamic oxaloacetic transaminase, and aldolase determinations can guide this decision. Glucocorticoid treatment is the mainstay of medical management of the active disease. Although no controlled studies have demonstrated the efficacy of steroids, most clinicians note improvement in muscle strength and decreased creatine kinase levels after 1 to 2 months of steroid therapy. Intravenous immunoglobulin may be beneficial.[111,112] Although methotrexate and azathioprine have been used in nonpregnant patients, their value is unproved. Obstetric management involves frequent monitoring of disease activity and fetal well-being.

Anesthetic Management

Anesthetic management of the pregnant woman with polymyositis/dermatomyositis begins with the evaluation of disease activity and underlying **cardiopulmonary involvement**. If muscle weakness is present, spirometry should be performed to determine whether respiratory muscles are affected. Maximum breathing capacity and peak expiratory flow rate are the most helpful measurements. Pharyngeal weakness may cause chronic aspiration, which may lead to pulmonary diffusion defects. Arterial blood gas analysis and a chest radiograph should be obtained in patients with a history of aspiration. An ECG should be obtained to exclude conduction abnormalities and arrhythmias.

The anesthesia provider must exercise caution when administering neuraxial anesthesia to the patient with muscle weakness. Excessive cephalad spread may further impair intercostal muscle function and lead to ventilatory insufficiency. Abdominal muscle paralysis may slow progress of the second stage of labor. Careful epidural administration of a dilute solution of local anesthetic should provide effective pain relief without adverse effect on the progress of labor. Intrathecal opioid administration is an attractive, alternative method of pain relief during labor in these patients.

Patients with polymyositis/dermatomyositis may exhibit an **atypical response to succinylcholine**. Johns et al.[113] reported a short-lived thumb contracture response after succinylcholine administration in a child with dermatomyositis. Direct laryngoscopy was not impaired, the contracture resolved in 3 minutes, and normal neuromuscular recovery occurred. In this patient, a 20% increase in potassium concentration was observed—a response similar to that seen in normal subjects after succinylcholine administration. Eielsen and Stovner[114] reported a prolonged duration (50 minutes) of paralysis after succinylcholine administration in a patient with dermatomyositis who had homozygous atypical pseudocholinesterase. They obtained dibucaine determinations for four other patients with dermatomyositis and discovered one with heterozygous atypical pseudocholinesterase. Neither the occurrence of benign contractures nor the possibility of atypical pseudocholinesterase precludes the use of succinylcholine if it is required for cesarean delivery. Neuromuscular recovery should be documented before extubation. Some investigators have advocated the avoidance of agents known to trigger malignant hyperthermia in patients with polymyositis/dermatomyositis and elevated creatine kinase levels.[115,116] This approach is speculative and is not supported by published clinical experience.

An **atypical response to nondepolarizing muscle relaxants** has been reported. Flusche et al.[117] published a case of prolonged paralysis (9.5 hours) after the administration of vecuronium in a patient with polymyositis. Underlying malignancy with associated myasthenic syndrome can prolong neuromuscular blockade. Other reports of nondepolarizing neuromuscular blockade in patients with polymyositis/dermatomyositis have indicated a normal response and recovery.[115,118,119] Parturients who have undergone long-term corticosteroid therapy should receive a peripartum stress dose of a corticosteroid.

KEY POINTS

- Pregnancy does not worsen the long-term course of autoimmune disorders.
- Autoimmune disorders can lead to renal, cardiac, and pulmonary dysfunction.
- Systemic lupus erythematosus can result in maternal thrombocytopenia.
- Systemic lupus erythematosus is associated with a higher incidence of spontaneous abortion, intrauterine fetal demise, and preterm delivery.
- Antiphospholipid syndrome is characterized by the presence of the autoantibodies lupus anticoagulant and anticardiolipin antibody.
- The term *lupus anticoagulant* is a misnomer because it has no true anticoagulant activity *in vivo*.
- Patients with lupus anticoagulant do *not* have a bleeding tendency in the absence of an underlying coagulation disorder and can safely receive neuraxial anesthesia.
- Patients with scleroderma are at increased risk for difficult airway management.
- Scleroderma can prolong the duration of neuraxial anesthesia.
- The severity of polymyositis/dermatomyositis affects fetal survival.
- Patients with polymyositis/dermatomyositis may have an atypical response to succinylcholine.
- Neuraxial anesthesia must be administered cautiously to parturients with polymyositis/dermatomyositis and intercostal muscle weakness.

REFERENCES

1. Himmelweit F, Marguardt M, Dale H. The collected papers of Paul Ehrlich. London, Pergamon, 1900:205-12.
2. Rocklin RE, Kitzmiller JL, Carpenter CB, et al. Maternal-fetal relation: Absence of an immunologic blocking factor from the serum of women with chronic abortions. N Engl J Med 1976; 295:1209-13.
3. Olding LB, Murgita RA, Wigzell H. Mitogen-stimulated lymphoid cells from human newborns suppress the proliferation of maternal lymphocytes across a cell-impermeable membrane. J Immunol 1977; 119:1109-14.
4. Dombroski RA. Autoimmune disease in pregnancy. Med Clin North Am 1989; 73:605-21.
5. D'Cruz DP, Khamashta MA, Hughes GR. Systemic lupus erythematosus. Lancet 2007; 369:587-96.
6. Chakravarty EF, Nelson L, Krishnan E. Obstetric hospitalizations in the United States for women with systemic lupus erythematosus and rheumatoid arthritis. Arthritis Rheum 2006; 54:899-907.
7. Munoz LE, Gaipl US, Franz S, et al. SLE—a disease of clearance deficiency? Rheumatology 2005; 44:1101-7.
8. Tan EM, Cohen AS, Fries JF, et al. The 1982 revised criteria for the classification of systemic lupus erythematosus. Arthritis Rheum 1982; 25:1271-7.
9. Hochberg MC. Updating the American College of Rheumatology revised criteria for the classification of systemic lupus erythematosus. Arthritis Rheum 1997; 40:1725.
10. Gimovsky ML, Montoro M, Paul RH. Pregnancy outcome in women with systemic lupus erythematosus. Obstet Gynecol 1984; 63:686-92.
11. Meehan RT, Dorsey JK. Pregnancy among patients with systemic lupus erythematosus receiving immunosuppressive therapy. J Rheumatol 1987; 14:252-8.
12. Tincani A, Balestrieri G, Faden D, DiMario C. Systemic lupus erythematosus in pregnancy. Lancet 1991; 338:756-7.
13. Cortes-Hernandez J, Ordi-Ros J, Paredes F, et al. Clinical predictors of fetal and maternal outcome in systemic lupus erythematosus: A prospective study of 103 pregnancies. Rheumatology 2002; 41:643-50.
14. Petri M. Hopkins Lupus Pregnancy Center: 1987 to 1996. Rheum Dis Clin North Am 1997; 23:1-13.
15. Ruiz-Irastorza G, Lima F, Alves J, et al. Increased rate of lupus flare during pregnancy and the puerperium: A prospective study of 78 pregnancies. Br J Rheumatol 1996; 35:133-8.
16. Clowse ME, Magder LS, Witter F, Petri M. The impact of increased lupus activity on obstetric outcomes. Arthritis Rheum 2005; 52:514-21.
17. Petri M. Systemic lupus erythematosus and pregnancy. Rheum Dis Clin North Am 1994; 20:87-118.
18. Witter FR. Management of the high-risk lupus pregnant patient. Rheum Dis Clin North Am 2007; 33:253-65.
19. Lockshin MD. Pregnancy associated with systemic lupus erythematosus. Semin Perinatol 1990; 14:130-8.
20. Clark CA, Spitzer KA, Laskin CA. Decrease in pregnancy loss rates in patients with systemic lupus erythematosus over a 40-year period. J Rheumatol 2005; 32:1709-12.
21. Georgiou PE, Politi EN, Katsimbri P, et al. Outcome of lupus pregnancy: A controlled study. Rheumatology 2000; 39:1014-9.
22. Yasmeen S, Wilkins EE, Field NT, et al. Pregnancy outcomes in women with systemic lupus erythematosus. J Matern Fetal Med 2001; 10:91-6.
23. Petri M, Watson R, Hochberg MC. Anti-Ro antibodies and neonatal lupus. Rheum Dis Clin North Am 1989; 15:335-60.
24. Brucato A, Doria A, Frassi M, et al. Pregnancy outcome in 100 women with autoimmune diseases and anti-Ro/SSA antibodies: A prospective controlled study. Lupus 2002; 11:716-21.
25. Buyon JP, Clancy RM. Neonatal lupus: Basic research and clinical perspectives. Rheum Dis Clin North Am 2005; 31:299-313.
26. Clowse ME. Lupus activity in pregnancy. Rheum Dis Clin North Am 2007; 33:237-52.
27. Dhar JP, Sokol RJ. Lupus and pregnancy: Complex yet manageable. Clin Med Res 2006; 4:310-21.
28. Petri M. The Hopkins Lupus Pregnancy Center: Ten key issues in management. Rheum Dis Clin North Am 2007; 33:227-35.
29. Clowse ME, Magder L, Witter F, Petri M. Hydroxychloroquinine in lupus pregnancy. Arthritis Rheum 2006; 54:3640-7.
30. Ostensen M, Khamashta M, Lockshin M, et al. Anti-inflammatory and immunosuppressive drugs and reproduction. Arthritis Res Ther 2006; 8:209.
31. Cote CJ, Meuwissen HJ, Pickering RJ. Effects on the neonate of prednisone and azathioprine administered to the mother during pregnancy. J Pediatr 1974; 85:324-8.
32. Scott JR. Risks to the children born to mothers with autoimmune diseases. Lupus 2002; 11:655-60.
33. Samuels P, Pfeifer SM. Autoimmune diseases in pregnancy: The obstetrician's view. Rheum Dis Clin North Am 1989; 15:307-22.
34. Ostensen M, Ostensen H. Safety of nonsteroidal antiinflammatory drugs in pregnant patients with rheumatic disease. J Rheumatol 1996; 23:1045-9.

35. Moise KJ, Huhta JC, Sharif DS, et al. Indomethacin in the treatment of premature labor: Effects on the fetal ductus arteriosus. N Engl J Med 1988; 319:327-31.
36. Stuart MJ, Gross SJ, Elrad H, Graeber JE. Effects of acetylsalicylic-acid ingestion on maternal and neonatal hemostasis. N Engl J Med 1982; 307:909-12.
37. Lockshin MD, Sammaritano LR. Lupus pregnancy. Autoimmunity 2003; 36:33-40.
38. Lockshin MD. Lupus pregnancies and neonatal lupus. Springer Semin Immunopathol 1994; 16:247-59.
39. Averbuch M, Bojko A, Levo Y. Cardiac tamponade in the early postpartum period as the presenting and predominant manifestation of systemic lupus erythematosus. J Rheumatol 1986; 13:444-5.
40. Carette S. Cardiopulmonary manifestations of systemic lupus erythematous. Rheum Dis Clin North Am 1988; 14:135-47.
41. Ozaki M, Minami K, Shigematsu A. Myocardial ischemia during emergency anesthesia in a patient with systemic lupus erythematosus resulting from undiagnosed antiphospholipid syndrome. Anesth Analg 2002; 95:255.
42. Roldan CA, Shively BK, Crawford MH. An echocardiographic study of valvular heart disease associated with systemic lupus erythematosus. N Engl J Med 1996; 335:1424-30.
43. Wilson W, Taubert KA, Gewitz M, et al. Prevention of infective endocarditis: Guidelines from the American Heart Association. Circulation 2007; 116:1736-54.
44. Winslow TM, Ossipov MA, Fazio GP, et al. Five-year follow-up study of the prevalence and progression of pulmonary hypertension in systemic lupus erythematosus. Am Heart J 1995; 129:510-5.
45. Cuenco J, Tzeng G, Wittels B. Anesthetic management of the parturient with systemic lupus erythematosus, pulmonary hypertension, and pulmonary edema. Anesthesiology 1999; 91:568-70.
46. McMillan E, Martin WL, Waugh J, et al. Management of pregnancy in women with pulmonary hypertension secondary to SLE and antiphospholipid syndrome. Lupus 2002; 11:392-8.
47. Huynh C, Ho SL, Fong KY, et al. Peripheral neuropathy in systemic lupus erythematosus. J Clin Neurophysiol 1999; 16:164-8.
48. Lee JH, Sung IY, Park JH, Roh JL. Recurrent laryngeal neuropathy in a systemic lupus erythematosus (SLE) patient. Am J Phys Med Rehabil 2008; 87:68-70.
49. Brey RL, Holliday SL, Saklad AR, et al. Neuropsychiatric syndromes in lupus: Prevalence using standardized definitions. Neurology 2002; 58:1214-20.
50. Locke GE, Giorgio AJ, Biggers SL, et al. Acute spinal epidural hematoma secondary to aspirin-induced prolonged bleeding. Surg Neurol 1976; 5:293-6.
51. Greensite FS, Katz J. Spinal subdural hematoma associated with attempted epidural anesthesia and subsequent continuous spinal anesthesia. Anesth Analg 1980; 59:72-3.
52. Horlocker TT, Wedel DJ, Schroeder DR, et al. Preoperative antiplatelet therapy does not increase the risk of spinal hematoma associated with regional anesthesia. Anesth Analg 1995; 80:303-9.
53. Horlocker TT, Bajwa ZH, Ashraf Z, et al. Risk assessment of hemorrhagic complications associated with nonsteroidal antiinflammatory medications in ambulatory pain clinic patients undergoing epidural steroid injection. Anesth Analg 2002; 95:1691-7.
54. CLASP: A randomised trial of low-dose aspirin for the prevention and treatment of pre-eclampsia among 9364 pregnant women. Collaborative Low-dose Aspirin Study in Pregnancy (CLASP) Collaborative Group. Lancet 1994; 343:619-29.
55. de Swiet M, Redman CW. Aspirin, extradural anaesthesia and the MRC Collaborative Low-dose Aspirin Study in Pregnancy (CLASP). Br J Anaesth 1992; 69:109-10.
56. Hughes G. Hughes syndrome: The antiphospholipid syndrome—a clinical overview. Clin Rev Allergy Immunol 2007; 32:3-12.
57. Carreras LO, Defreyn G, Machin SJ, et al. Arterial thrombosis, intrauterine death and "lupus" anticoagulant: Detection of immunoglobulin interfering with prostacyclin formation. Lancet 1981; 1:244-6.
58. Hughes GR. Thrombosis, abortion, cerebral disease, and the lupus anticoagulant. Br Med J 1983; 287:1088-9.
59. Love PE, Santoro SA. Antiphospholipid antibodies: Anticardiolipin and the lupus anticoagulant in systemic lupus erythematosus (SLE) and in non-SLE disorders: Prevalence and clinical significance. Ann Intern Med 1990; 112:682-98.
60. Gomez-Puerta JA, Martin H, Amigo MC, et al. Long-term follow-up in 128 patients with primary antiphospholipid syndrome: Do they develop lupus? Medicine 2005; 84:225-30.
61. Harris EN. A reassessment of the antiphospholipid syndrome. J Rheumatol 1990; 17:733-5.
62. Vermylen J, Carreras LO, Arnout J. Attempts to make sense of the antiphospholipid syndrome. J Thromb Haemost 2007; 5:1-4.
63. American College of Obstetrics and Gynecologists. Antiphospholipid syndrome. ACOG Practice Bulletin No. 68. Washington, DC, ACOG, November 2005. (Obstet Gynecol 2005; 106:1113-21.)
64. Ware Branch D, Eller AG. Antiphospholipid syndrome and thrombosis. Clin Obstet Gynecol 2006; 49:861-74.
65. Silver RM, Draper ML, Scott JR, et al. Clinical consequences of antiphospholipid antibodies: An historic cohort study. Obstet Gynecol 1994; 83:372-7.
66. Clark CA, Spitzer KA, Crowther MA, et al. Incidence of postpartum thrombosis and preterm delivery in women with antiphospholipid antibodies and recurrent pregnancy loss. J Rheumatol 2007; 34:992-6.
67. Cuadrado MJ, Mujic F, Munoz E, et al. Thrombocytopenia in the antiphospholipid syndrome. Ann Rheum Dis 1997; 56:194-6.
68. Asherson RA. The catastrophic antiphospholipid (Asherson's) syndrome. Autoimmun Rev 2006; 6:64-7.
69. Lubbe WF, Liggins GC. Lupus anticoagulant and pregnancy. Am J Obstet Gynecol 1985; 153:322-7.
70. Tincani A, Lojacono A, Taglietti M, et al. Pregnancy and neonatal outcome in primary antiphospholipid syndrome. Lupus 2002; 11:649.
71. Pollard JK, Scott JR, Branch DW. Outcome of children born to women treated during pregnancy for the antiphospholipid syndrome. Obstet Gynecol 1992; 80:365-8.
72. Boffa MC, Aurousseau MH, Lachassinne E, et al. European register of babies born to mothers with antiphospholipid syndrome. Lupus 2004; 13:713-7.
73. Empson M, Lassere M, Craig J, Scott J. Prevention of recurrent miscarriage for women with antiphospholipid antibody or lupus anticoagulant. Cochrane Database Syst Rev 2005; (2):CD002859.
74. Ralph CJ. Anaesthetic management of parturients with the antiphospholipid syndrome: A review of 27 cases. Int J Obstet Anesth 1999; 8:249-52.
75. Harnett M, Kodali BS. Thromboelastography assessment of coagulation status in parturients with lupus anticoagulant receiving heparin therapy. Int J Obstet Anesth 2006; 15:177-8.
76. Madan R, Khoursheed M, Kukla R, et al. The anaesthetist and the antiphospholipid syndrome. Anaesthesia 1997; 52:72-6.
77. Walker JG, Pope J, Baron M, et al. The development of systemic sclerosis classification criteria. Clin Rheumatol 2007; 26:1401-9.
78. Mayes MD, Lacey JV Jr, Beebe-Dimmer J, et al. Prevalence, incidence, survival, and disease characteristics of systemic sclerosis in a large US population. Arthritis Rheum 2003; 48:2246-55.
79. Moxley G. Scleroderma and related diseases. In Dale DC, Federman DD, Antman K, et al., editors. Scientific American Medicine, Volume 2. New York, WebMD Professional Publishing, 2001:15-V.
80. Nelson JL, Furst DE, Maloney S, et al. Microchimerism and HLA-compatible relationships of pregnancy in scleroderma. Lancet 1998; 351:559-62.
81. Jimenez SA, Artlett CM. Microchimerism and systemic sclerosis. Curr Opin Rheumatol 2005; 17:86-90.
82. Scussel-Lonzetti L, Joyal F, Raynauld JP, et al. Predicting mortality in systemic sclerosis: Analysis of a cohort of 309 French Canadian patients with emphasis on features at diagnosis as predictive factors for survival. Medicine 2002; 81:154-67.
83. Steen VD, Conte C, Day N, et al. Pregnancy in women with systemic sclerosis. Arthritis Rheum 1989; 32:151-7.

84. Steen VD. Pregnancy in women with systemic sclerosis. Obstet Gynecol 1999; 94:15-20.
85. Furst DE, Clements PJ. D-Penicillamine is not an effective treatment in systemic sclerosis. Scand J Rheumatol 2001; 30:189-91.
86. Seibold JR. Scleroderma. In Kelley WN, Harris ED, Ruddy S, Sledge CB, editors. Textbook of Rheumatology. Philadelphia, WB Saunders, 1989:1215-44.
87. Tuffanelli DL. Systemic scleroderma. Med Clin North Am 1989; 73:1167-80.
88. Steen VD. Pregnancy in scleroderma. Rheum Dis Clin North Am 2007; 33:345-58.
89. Carbonne B, Mace G, Cynober E, et al. Successful pregnancy with the use of nitric oxide donors and heparin after recurrent severe pre-eclampsia in a woman with scleroderma. Am J Obstet Gynecol 2007; 197:e6-7.
90. Black CM. Systemic sclerosis and pregnancy. Baillieres Clin Rheumatol 1990; 4:105-24.
91. Moore M, Saffran JE, Baraf HS, Jacobs RP. Systemic sclerosis and pregnancy complicated by obstructive uropathy. Am J Obstet Gynecol 1985; 153:893-4.
92. Benumof JL. Management of the difficult adult airway: With special emphasis on awake tracheal intubation. Anesthesiology 1991; 75:1087-110.
93. Thompson J, Conklin KA. Anesthetic management of a pregnant patient with scleroderma. Anesthesiology 1983; 59:69-71.
94. Erk G, Taspinar V, Donmez F, Ornek D. Neuroaxial anesthesia in a patient with progressive systemic sclerosis: Case presentation and review of the literature on systemic sclerosis. BMC Anesthesiol 2006; 6:11.
95. Picozzi P, Lappa A, Menichetti A. Mitral valve replacement under thoracic epidural anesthesia in an awake patient suffering from systemic sclerosis. Acta Anaesthesiol Scand 2007; 51:644.
96. Bailey AR, Wolmarans M, Rhodes S. Spinal anaesthesia for caesarean section in a patient with systemic sclerosis. Anaesthesia 1999; 54:355-8.
97. Eisele JH, Reitan JA. Scleroderma, Raynaud's phenomenon, and local anesthetics. Anesthesiology 1971; 34:386-7.
98. Lewis GB. Prolonged regional analgesia in scleroderma. Can Anaesth Soc J 1974; 21:495-7.
99. Neill RS. Progressive systemic sclerosis: Prolonged sensory blockade following regional anaesthesia in association with a reduced response to systemic analgesics. Br J Anaesth 1980; 52:623-5.
100. Case records of the Massachusetts General Hospital: Weekly clinicopathological exercises: Case 4-1999: A 38-year-old woman with increasing pulmonary hypertension after delivery. N Engl J Med 1999; 340:455-64.
101. Plotz PH, Dalakas M, Leff RL, et al. Current concepts in the idiopathic inflammatory myopathies: Polymyositis, dermatomyositis, and related disorders. Ann Intern Med 1989; 111:143-57.
102. Olsen NJ. Idiopathic inflammatory myopathies. In Dale DC, Federman DD, Antman K, et al., editors. Scientific American Medicine, Volume 2. New York, WebMD Professional Publishing, 2000:15-VI.
103. Bronner IM, van der Meulen MF, de Visser M, et al. Long-term outcome in polymyositis and dermatomyositis. Ann Rheum Dis 2006; 65:1456-61.
104. Bohan A, Peter JB. Polymyositis and dermatomyositis (second of two parts). N Engl J Med 1975; 292:403-7.
105. Horowitz M, McNeil JD, Maddern GJ, et al. Abnormalities of gastric and esophageal emptying in polymyositis and dermatomyositis. Gastroenterology 1986; 90:434-9.
106. Dickey BF, Myers AR. Pulmonary disease in polymyositis/dermatomyositis. Semin Arthritis Rheum 1984; 14:60-76.
107. Fathi M, Lundberg IE, Tornling G. Pulmonary complications of polymyositis and dermatomyositis. Semin Respir Crit Care Med 2007; 28:451-8.
108. Senechal M, Crete M, Couture C, Poirier P. Myocardial dysfunction in polymyositis. Can J Cardiol 2006; 22:869-71.
109. Ishii N, Ono H, Kawaguchi T, Nakajima H. Dermatomyositis and pregnancy: Case report and review of the literature. Dermatologica 1991; 183:146-9.
110. Silva CA, Sultan SM, Isenberg DA. Pregnancy outcome in adult-onset idiopathic inflammatory myopathy. Rheumatology 2003; 42:1168-72.
111. Mosca M, Strigini F, Carmignani A, et al. Pregnant patient with dermatomyositis successfully treated with intravenous immunoglobulin therapy. Arthritis Rheum 2005; 53:119-21.
112. Williams L, Chang PY, Park E, et al. Successful treatment of dermatomyositis during pregnancy with intravenous immunoglobulin monotherapy. Obstet Gynecol 2007; 109:561-3.
113. Johns RA, Finholt DA, Stirt JA. Anaesthetic management of a child with dermatomyositis. Can Anaesth Soc J 1986; 33:71-4.
114. Eielsen O, Stovner J. Dermatomyositis, suxamethonium action and atypical plasmacholinesterase. Can Anaesth Soc J 1978; 25:63-4.
115. Saarnivaara LH. Anesthesia for a patient with polymyositis undergoing myectomy of the cricopharyngeal muscle. Anesth Analg 1988; 67:701-2.
116. Farag HM, Naguib M, Gyasi H, Ibrahim AW. Anesthesia for a patient with eosinophilic myositis. Anesth Analg 1986; 65:903-4.
117. Flusche G, Unger-Sargon J, Lambert DH. Prolonged neuromuscular paralysis with vecuronium in a patient with polymyositis. Anesth Analg 1987; 66:188-90.
118. Ganta R, Campbell IT, Mostafa SM. Anaesthesia and acute dermatomyositis/polymyositis. Br J Anaesth 1988; 60:854-8.
119. Brown S, Shupak RC, Patel C, Calkins JM. Neuromuscular blockade in a patient with active dermatomyositis. Anesthesiology 1992; 77:1031-3.

Chapter 41

Cardiovascular Disease

Miriam Harnett, M.B., FFARCSI
Lawrence C. Tsen, M.D.

The estimated prevalence of clinically significant cardiac disease in pregnancy has gradually fallen in the past three decades to its current level of less than 1%.[1] This number reflects the successes of early interventions directed toward the correction or treatment of cardiac disorders and infections, particularly rheumatic heart disease. In the developed world, women with congenital heart disease now constitute the majority of pregnant women with heart disease seen at referral centers.[2]

For most women with heart disease, pregnancy is associated with favorable maternal and neonatal outcomes; however, even with modern advances in treatment and monitoring, a high incidence of morbidity and mortality is witnessed in pregnant women with pulmonary hypertension, Eisenmenger's syndrome, and severe cases of Marfan's syndrome.[3-5] These lesions pose a significant risk and may contraindicate pregnancy, regardless of the patient's functional class.

In general, maternal outcomes correlate with the functional classification of the patient as outlined by the New York Heart Association (NYHA) (Box 41-1). NYHA class III or IV, cyanosis, myocardial dysfunction, prior arrhythmia, and prior heart failure or stroke have been identified as risk factors for maternal cardiac events.[1-6] Patients with NYHA class I or II disease have a maternal mortality rate less than 1%, whereas those with class III or IV disease have a mortality rate between 5% and 15%. Overall, cardiac disease accounts for approximately 15% of pregnancy-related maternal mortality in the United States.[7]

The optimal management of women with cardiovascular disease begins before conception, for several reasons. First, if the woman is not examined until she becomes pregnant, the physician may underestimate the severity of the lesion. For example, the murmurs of aortic regurgitation and mitral regurgitation often decrease in intensity during pregnancy, presumably because of a decrease in systemic vascular resistance (SVR). Second, some patients (e.g., women with a prosthetic valve) may require a change in medication before conception. Third, in some cases it may be best for the patient to avoid pregnancy altogether.

BOX 41-1 New York Heart Association Classification of Cardiovascular Disease

- Class I—Patients who are not limited by cardiac disease in their physical activity. Ordinary physical activity does not precipitate the occurrence of symptoms such as fatigue, palpitations, dyspnea, and angina.
- Class II—Patients in whom the cardiac disease causes a slight limitation in physical activity. These patients are comfortable at rest, but ordinary physical activity will precipitate symptoms.
- Class III—Patients in whom the cardiac disease results in a marked limitation of physical activity. These patients are comfortable at rest, but less than ordinary physical activity will precipitate symptoms.
- Class IV—Patients in whom the cardiac disease results in the inability to carry on physical activity without discomfort. Symptoms may be present even at rest, and discomfort is increased by any physical activity.

CONGENITAL HEART DISEASE

Congenital heart disease is now the major cause of cardiac disease in pregnant women in the United States, accounting for 60% to 80% of all cases.[2] Improvements in the early diagnosis and treatment of complex congenital cardiac anomalies have led to an increase in the number of women with congenital heart disease who survive to child-bearing age. In some cases, successful surgery during infancy and childhood results in complete repair and normal cardiovascular function. These women may be asymptomatic and may have relatively normal intracardiac pressures and blood flow patterns. Such patients often require no special treatment. However, the presence of a neonatologist at delivery is desirable because there is a higher incidence of congenital cardiac lesions in the offspring of women with cardiac disease (Table 41-1). Some of the more common lesions that may be repaired successfully in childhood are atrial and ventricular septal defects, patent ductus arteriosus, tetralogy of Fallot, transposition of the great arteries, and tricuspid atresia.

Pregnant women with symptomatic cardiac disease or complex congenital heart repairs may be at risk for significant adverse events during labor and delivery. In a cohort study of 90 pregnancies in 53 women with congenital heart disease, Khairy et al.[8] observed that patients with impaired subpulmonary ventricular ejection fraction and/or severe pulmonary regurgitation were at higher risk for adverse cardiac outcomes, including maternal pulmonary edema (17%), nonsustained arrhythmias (8%), sustained arrhythmias (3%), and need for urgent invasive intervention (6%). Connolly et al.[9] and Therrien et al.[10] reviewed the outcomes of 60 pregnancies in 22 women[9] and 45 pregnancies in 19 women,[10] respectively, with corrected congenital transposition of the great arteries. Overall, 7 patients in these two studies had cardiovascular complications, consisting mainly of congestive heart failure.[9,10]

Pregnancy among women who have undergone a Fontan procedure (diversion of venous blood from the right atrium to the pulmonary arteries) is becoming more common. Canobbio et al.[11] reviewed a series of pregnancies resulting in 15 live births in 14 women who had undergone a Fontan procedure; cardiac problems in these women included atrial flutter in one patient and ventricular dysfunction, aortic regurgitation, and atrioventricular valve regurgitation in another.

In contrast, some women may present during pregnancy with uncorrected or partially corrected cardiac lesions. Obstetric and anesthetic management of these patients is challenging and complex, and a coordinated multidisciplinary approach is preferred.

TABLE 41-1 Familial Recurrence of Congenital Heart Disease

Congenital Heart Defect	Mode of Inheritance	Recurrence Risk (%)
Atrioventricular canal defect	Multifactorial	3-4
	Autosomal dominant	50
Tetralogy of Fallot	Multifactorial	2.5-3
	Autosomal dominant	50
	Autosomal recessive	25
	Three-gene model	2.5-3
Transposition of the great arteries	Multifactorial	1-1.8
	Autosomal dominant	50
Congenitally corrected transposition of the great arteries	Multifactorial	5.8
Left-sided obstructions (hypoplastic left heart syndrome, aortic coarctation, aortic stenosis, and bicuspid aortic valve)	Multifactorial	3
	Autosomal dominant	50
	Autosomal recessive	25
Atrial septal defect	Multifactorial	3
	Autosomal dominant	50

Adapted from Calcagni G, Digilio MC, Sarkozy A, et al. Familial recurrence of congenital heart disease: An overview and review of the literature. Eur J Pediatr 2007; 166:111-6.

Left-to-Right Shunts

Lesions such as a small atrial septal defect, ventricular septal defect, or patent ductus arteriosus may produce a modest degree of left-to-right intracardiac shunting, which is often well tolerated during pregnancy. Left-to-right shunts can eventually lead to pulmonary hypertension and reversal of the shunt flow, with resulting cyanosis. As a consequence, serial examinations of such shunts with echocardiography are recommended during pregnancy. Severe obstetric hemorrhage that leads to acute systemic hypotension can also lead to transient reversal of the shunt flow.[12,13]

Atrial septal defects are sometimes asymptomatic until the reproductive years. Some 20% to 30% of patients have coexisting mitral valve prolapse. Complications can include arrhythmias, pulmonary hypertension, and right ventricular failure; however, these usually develop after the age of 40.[12,13]

Ventricular septal defects are infrequently diagnosed in pregnancy, as they either close spontaneously or are surgically repaired in childhood. Membranous ventricular septal defects are the most common type and can be associated with aortic regurgitation.[14] If closure of a large ventricular septal defect is delayed, irreversible pulmonary hypertension can occur.

Patent ductus arteriosus is uncommonly diagnosed in pregnancy because it either closes spontaneously or is corrected surgically in childhood.

Anesthetic management of patients with these defects should include avoidance of intravenous infusion of air bubbles and use of loss-of-resistance to saline (rather than air) to identify the epidural space. Early administration of epidural labor analgesia should minimize pain-associated increases in maternal plasma catecholamine concentrations and SVR. (These changes can worsen the severity of left-to-right shunting and result in pulmonary hypertension and right ventricular failure.) Incremental injection of neuraxial anesthetic drugs should result in a more gradual onset of sympathetic blockade, which helps avoid the rapid decrease in SVR that can cause an asymptomatic left-to-right shunt to become a right-to-left shunt with maternal hypoxemia. Finally, the patient should receive supplemental oxygen, and it seems prudent to monitor hemoglobin oxygen saturation (Spo_2). Even mild hypoxemia can result in greater pulmonary vascular resistance and reversal of shunt flow. It is also important to avoid hypercarbia and acidosis, which may increase pulmonary vascular resistance.

Coarctation of the Aorta

Coarctation of the aorta is a congenital lesion consisting of a discrete narrowing of the descending aorta, most commonly distal to the left subclavian artery, with proximal hypertension and distal hypoperfusion.[15,16] Eighty percent of cases are detected in childhood, although occasionally the initial diagnosis is made during pregnancy.[17] A maternal arm-to-leg blood pressure gradient less than 20 mm Hg is associated with good pregnancy outcomes,[18] and patients who have normal arm and leg blood pressures after successful corrective surgery do not require special precautions or monitoring. Pregnant women with uncorrected coarctation or residual decrease in aortic diameter are at high risk for left ventricular failure, aortic rupture or dissection, and endocarditis. In such pregnancies, the fetal mortality rate may approach 20% because of reduced uteroplacental perfusion distal to the aortic lesion.[19] Compared with the general population, the patient with aortic coarctation is more likely to have a bicuspid aortic valve (hence the increased risk of endocarditis) or an aneurysm in the circle of Willis. Wide fluctuations in blood pressure during labor may increase the risk for intracranial aneurysm rupture or aortic dissection, which has led some obstetricians to recommend performance of an elective cesarean delivery, particularly if there is gross widening of the ascending aorta on radiologic examinations. In patients who have undergone corrective surgery or who have an arm-to-leg blood pressure gradient less than 20 mm Hg, vaginal delivery is preferred; epidural labor analgesia is recommended to minimize hypertension resulting from pain. A well-functioning catheter-based analgesia/anesthesia technique can also facilitate performance of an instrumental vaginal delivery and consequently minimize the hemodynamic consequences of maternal expulsive efforts and pain.

Beauchesne et al.[16] reviewed the outcome of 118 pregnancies in 50 women with aortic coarctation. Nineteen women (38%) were known to have hemodynamically significant coarctation during pregnancy. The investigators reported one maternal death, one early neonatal death, and a 4% incidence of congenital heart disease in the offspring. Thirty percent of the women (primarily among those with hemodynamically significant coarctation) had hypertension during pregnancy. Vriend et al.,[20] reviewing pregnancy outcomes of 126 pregnancies in 54 women with repaired coarctation, found that 26 pregnancies were complicated by a hypertensive disorder of pregnancy. Overall, the investigators concluded that women with repaired aortic coarctation tolerate pregnancy well.

Tetralogy of Fallot

Tetralogy of Fallot accounts for 5% of cases of congenital heart disease in pregnant women. This lesion has the following four components: (1) a ventricular septal defect, (2) right ventricular hypertrophy, (3) pulmonic stenosis with right ventricular outflow tract obstruction, and (4) an overriding aorta (i.e., the aortic outflow tract receives blood from both the right and left ventricles). Tetralogy of Fallot is the most common congenital heart lesion associated with a right-to-left shunt. Patients typically present with cyanosis.

INTERACTION WITH PREGNANCY

Most pregnant women with tetralogy of Fallot have had corrective surgery. The surgical treatment, typically performed in childhood, involves closure of the ventricular septal defect and widening of the pulmonary outflow tract. This operation is generally successful and leaves the patient without symptoms. In some cases, a small ventricular septal defect may recur, or progressive hypertrophy of the pulmonary outflow tract may occur slowly over the first several decades of life. The cardiovascular changes of pregnancy (e.g., increases in blood volume and cardiac output, reduced SVR) may unmask these previously asymptomatic residua of corrected tetralogy of Fallot. The severity of symptoms depends on the size of the ventricular septal defect, the magnitude of the pulmonic stenosis, and the contractile performance of the right ventricle. Patients with corrected tetralogy of Fallot, even if they have been asymptomatic for many years, should undergo echocardiography before and during early pregnancy.

In the largest and most extensively documented series, Meijer et al.[21] reviewed 63 pregnancies in 29 women with surgically corrected tetralogy of Fallot. Although 13 pregnancies ended in abortion (one elective), 50 successful pregnancies were observed. Fourteen pregnancies (28%) were complicated by severe pulmonic regurgitation, and 6 pregnancies (12%) resulted in arrhythmias that progressed to right-sided heart failure in two patients. No maternal deaths occurred in this case series. The investigators concluded that corrected tetralogy of Fallot is generally well tolerated during pregnancy; however, patients with severe pulmonic regurgitation should consider a pulmonic valve replacement before pregnancy.

Tetralogy of Fallot is also the most common uncorrected cyanotic congenital heart lesion seen in pregnant women. In this situation, pregnancy is discouraged because the decreased SVR of pregnancy increases the volume of the right-to-left shunt and increases cyanosis.[22]

ANESTHETIC MANAGEMENT

Anesthetic management for patients with successful correction of tetralogy of Fallot often does not differ from that for women without this lesion. However, patients with corrected tetralogy of Fallot may demonstrate various atrial and ventricular arrhythmias, owing to surgical injury to the cardiac conduction pathways. Thus it seems prudent to obtain a 12-lead electrocardiogram (ECG), and to monitor the ECG continuously during labor.

Greater attention should be given to the parturient with uncorrected tetralogy of Fallot or corrected tetralogy of Fallot with residua. The anesthesiologist should avoid causing a decrease in SVR, which worsens the severity of the right-to-left shunt. It is also important to maintain adequate intravascular volume and venous return. In the presence of right ventricular compromise, high filling pressures are needed to enhance right ventricular performance and ensure adequate pulmonary blood flow. Administration of neuraxial analgesia during early labor is advisable to limit increases in pulmonary vascular resistance and consequent right-to-left shunting. For cesarean delivery, neuraxial anesthesia should be administered slowly; single-shot spinal anesthesia is a poor choice because the abrupt reduction in SVR with this technique may cause reversal of shunt flow and hypoxemia.

Eisenmenger's Syndrome

A chronic, uncorrected left-to-right shunt may produce right ventricular hypertrophy, elevated pulmonary artery pressures, right ventricular dysfunction, and, ultimately, the syndrome first described by Eisenmenger in 1897.[23] The most common cause of Eisenmenger's syndrome is a large ventricular septal defect, followed by a large patent ductus arteriosus, and less commonly an atrial septal defect. The pulmonary arterial and right ventricular musculature undergoes remodeling in response to chronic pulmonary volume overload. High pulmonary vascular resistance gradually limits flow through the pulmonary vessels, and when pulmonary arterial pressure exceeds that present in the systemic circulation, a reversal of shunt flow occurs. The primary left-to-right shunt becomes a right-to-left shunt. Initially the shunt may be bidirectional, with the primary direction of intracardiac blood flow determined by acute changes in pulmonary vascular resistance or SVR. Eventually, the pulmonary vascular occlusive disease leads to irreversible pulmonary hypertension and permanent right-to-left shunting; at this stage, correction of the primary intracardiac lesion is not helpful.

The clinical manifestations of Eisenmenger's syndrome are the sequelae of arterial hypoxemia and right ventricular failure (e.g., dyspnea, clubbing of the nails, polycythemia, engorged neck veins, peripheral edema).

INTERACTION WITH PREGNANCY

Women with Eisenmenger's syndrome often show inability to respond to the increased demands for oxygen during pregnancy. Maintenance of satisfactory oxygenation requires adequate pulmonary blood flow. The normal pregnancy-related decrease in pulmonary vascular resistance does not occur because the pulmonary vascular resistance is fixed. In addition, the drop in SVR associated with pregnancy tends to exacerbate the severity of the right-to-left shunt. Finally, pregnancy results in a decrease in functional residual capacity. Together, these alterations predispose the pregnant woman with Eisenmenger's syndrome to hypoxemia. Maternal hypoxemia subsequently results in decreased oxygen delivery to the fetus, leading to a high incidence of intrauterine growth restriction (IUGR) and fetal demise.[4] Maternal mortality is as high as 30% to 50% among these patients.[24] Thromboembolic phenomena are responsible for as many as 43% of all maternal deaths in patients with Eisenmenger's syndrome, with many of these deaths occuring as late as 4 to 6 weeks postpartum.

OBSTETRIC MANAGEMENT

A multidisciplinary approach with close communication among the obstetrician, cardiologist, and anesthesiologist is essential. Management during pregnancy consists of bed rest, supplemental oxygen, anticoagulation, and a low threshold for hospitalization if complications arise. Most patients with Eisenmenger's syndrome have an unreactive pulmonary vasculature that does not respond normally to vasodilators such as prostacyclin.[24,25] However, there are limited reports of improved oxygenation with the use of prostacyclin, nifedipine, and inhaled nitric oxide.[26-28] The obstetrician most likely will want to perform an early instrumental vaginal delivery to minimize maternal expulsive efforts.

ANESTHETIC MANAGEMENT

The primary goals of anesthetic management are (1) maintenance of adequate SVR; (2) maintenance of intravascular volume and venous return; (3) avoidance of aortocaval compression; (4) prevention of pain, hypoxemia, hypercarbia, and acidosis, which may increase pulmonary vascular resistance; and (5) avoidance of myocardial depression during general anesthesia.

Inhaled nitric oxide selectively dilates the pulmonary vascular bed with minimal systemic hemodynamic effects. Therefore inhaled nitric oxide may improve right ventricular function; left ventricular function may subsequently improve due to better oxygenation. Experience with inhaled nitric oxide in pregnant women with Eisenmenger's syndrome is limited; however, reductions in pulmonary artery pressure and increased Spo_2 have been noted with its use.[27,28] Unfortunately, in both of the published cases, the patient died within 3 weeks of delivery.

Labor

Supplemental oxygen should be provided at all times. Pulse oximetry is the most useful monitor for detecting acute changes in shunt flow. An intra-arterial catheter facilitates the rapid detection of sudden changes in blood pressure, and a central venous pressure (CVP) catheter can help reveal clinically significant changes in cardiac filling pressures. However, the insertion of a CVP catheter occasionally produces complications (e.g., air emboli, infection, hematoma, pneumothorax) that can be disastrous in patients with Eisenmenger's syndrome.

Although some physicians suggest that a pulmonary artery catheter is "essential" for the intrapartum management of pregnant women with Eisenmenger's syndrome, we disagree for several reasons. First, it is difficult, if not impossible, to properly position the balloon-tipped, flow-directed catheter within the pulmonary artery. Second, if the catheter does go into the pulmonary artery, the risks of pulmonary artery rupture and hemorrhage are great. Third, these patients may not tolerate catheter-induced arrhythmias. Fourth, measurements of cardiac output by thermodilution are uninterpretable in the presence of a large intracardiac shunt. Fifth, pulmonary artery pressure monitoring rarely yields clinically useful information in the presence of severe, fixed pulmonary hypertension. Sixth, the pulmonary artery catheter may predispose to pulmonary thromboembolism. Finally, the risks of placing and using a pulmonary artery catheter include the entire spectrum of complications associated with placement of a CVP catheter.

Effective analgesia is necessary to prevent labor-induced increases in plasma catecholamine levels, which may further increase pulmonary vascular resistance. During the first stage of labor, intrathecal administration of an opioid is ideal, because it produces profound analgesia with minimal sympathetic blockade. For the second stage of labor, epidural or intrathecal injection of both a local anesthetic and an opioid will provide satisfactory analgesia. In some instances, maternal anticoagulation may complicate or contraindicate the use of neuraxial analgesic techniques. In such cases, an intravenous infusion of an opioid, such as fentanyl or remifentanil, with or without patient-controlled analgesia, may be the next best option. However, the quality and reliability of intravenous opioid analgesia are not as good as those provided by a neuraxial analgesic technique.

Cesarean Delivery

Historically, anesthesiologists have avoided neuraxial anesthesia in parturients with Eisenmenger's syndrome because the sympathetic blockade and resulting vasodilation can worsen a right-to-left shunt. However, favorable outcomes have been achieved with epidural anesthesia, which has become the technique of choice for these patients.[29] The key to the safe use of neuraxial anesthesia is the incremental injection of local anesthetic along with careful correction of any adverse hemodynamic sequelae.[30] It is critical to avoid aortocaval compression and to maintain adequate venous return. Intravenous crystalloid and small doses of phenylephrine are administered as needed to maintain maternal preload, SVR, and oxygen saturation.

Several disadvantages are associated with the use of general anesthesia. Positive-pressure ventilation leads to decreased venous return, which compromises cardiac output. The volatile halogenated agents can cause myocardial depression and decreased SVR. Rapid-sequence induction with agents such as thiopental and propofol characteristically reduces both contractility and SVR, which may exacerbate a right-to-left shunt. On the other hand, a slow induction of general anesthesia predisposes to maternal aspiration. This risk notwithstanding, a rapid-sequence induction of general anesthesia is usually avoided in patients with Eisenmenger's syndrome. Although moderate to large doses of opioids are not routinely used for general anesthesia in healthy women undergoing cesarean delivery, an opioid-based induction technique may be appropriate to help maintain hemodynamic stability during induction of general anesthesia in the patient with Eisenmenger's syndrome.

Regardless of the anesthetic technique, these women are at high risk for hemodynamic compromise immediately after delivery. Large blood losses should be replaced promptly with crystalloid, colloid, and/or appropriate blood products. Cautious fluid therapy is important when the blood loss is minimal, because postpartum autotransfusion may cause intravascular volume overload in women with myocardial dysfunction.

PRIMARY PULMONARY HYPERTENSION

The syndrome of primary pulmonary hypertension is characterized by markedly elevated pulmonary artery pressures in the absence of an intracardiac or aortopulmonary shunt.[31] Unlike those with Eisenmenger's syndrome, patients with primary pulmonary hypertension often have a reactive pulmonary vasculature that can respond to vasodilator therapy. Pregnancy and delivery are poorly tolerated by women with severe pulmonary hypertension; in 2005 the maternal mortality rate was reported to be as high as 36%.[32] These patients also have a high incidence of IUGR, fetal loss, and preterm delivery.[33]

The hemodynamic goals of obstetric and anesthetic management are similar to those for patients with Eisenmenger's syndrome; they include (1) prevention of increases in pulmonary vascular resistance by avoiding hypoxemia, acidosis, and hypercarbia; (2) maintenance of intravascular volume and venous return; (3) avoidance of aortocaval compression; (4) maintenance of adequate SVR; and (5) avoidance of myocardial depression during general anesthesia, especially in women with fixed pulmonary hypertension.

Supplemental oxygen acts as a pulmonary vasodilator and should be administered routinely in these patients. Monitoring typically involves placement of both an arterial and a CVP catheter. The use of a pulmonary artery catheter can guide treatment when the pulmonary vascular resistance is responsive to vasodilator therapy; however, any potential benefit must be weighed against the higher risk of pulmonary artery rupture and thrombosis in patients with pulmonary hypertension (as discussed earlier).[32] Transesophageal echocardiography has been used intraoperatively during cesarean delivery.[34]

Agents that have been used to treat primary pulmonary hypertension include nitroglycerin, calcium entry–blocking agents, prostaglandins, endothelial antagonists, inhaled nitric oxide, and inhaled and intravenous prostacyclin.[26,35-40]

The optimal mode of delivery in patients with primary pulmonary hypertension remains controversial. If vaginal delivery is chosen, some means of providing continuous (i.e., catheter-based) neuraxial blockade is important.[32] Epidural analgesia allows for pain-free first and second stages of labor and can facilitate an instrumental vaginal delivery. Elective cesarean deliveries have been successfully performed with use of epidural anesthesia. Slow induction of epidural anesthesia is critical. If hypotension occurs, it should be treated initially with intravenous fluids. Vasopressors should be used with caution because these agents can further increase pulmonary artery pressures. Continuous spinal anesthesia and general anesthesia have also been successfully used in patients with primary pulmonary hypertension.[32] Single-shot spinal anesthesia, which may cause severe hemodynamic instability, should be avoided.

Weeks and Smith,[41] reviewing published cases of intrapartum anesthetic management for women with primary pulmonary hypertension, concluded as follows:

> *Epidural anesthesia has been used with success, but in the presence of preexisting right ventricular failure, any large decrease in systemic vascular resistance may lead to a further decrease in cardiac output. Refractory hypotension may also cause right ventricular ischemia, leading to a further deterioration in right ventricular function. The potential hazards of general anesthesia include increased pulmonary artery pressure during laryngoscopy and intubation, the adverse effects of positive-pressure ventilation on venous return and the negative inotropic effects of certain anesthetic agents. However, these adverse effects can be minimized by the use of a narcotic-based induction and maintenance technique. Any resulting narcotic-induced neonatal depression should be easily treated. Intensive postoperative management is of critical importance and should probably continue for one week because of the high incidence of sudden death during this period.*[41]

Cardiac output and systemic vascular resistance increase immediately after delivery, which is a critical period for patients with pulmonary hypertension.[37] All patients should remain in an intensive care setting for a number of days postpartum, so that changes in systemic and pulmonary vascular resistance can be treated with inhaled nitric oxide and prostacyclin as necessary.

HYPERTROPHIC OBSTRUCTIVE CARDIOMYOPATHY

Hypertrophic obstructive cardiomyopathy (HOCM) is an uncommon form of cardiomyopathy that affects the interventricular septum in the area of the left ventricular outflow tract. This disorder is characterized by left ventricular hypertrophy, decreased left ventricular chamber size, and left ventricular dysfunction. Patients with HOCM require a **slow heart rate** and a **modest expansion of intravascular volume** to ensure adequate ventricular filling. It is important to avoid increases in myocardial contractility and decreases in SVR, which tend to exacerbate the degree of outflow tract obstruction. Patients with HOCM are at increased risk for sudden death from ventricular arrhythmias.

INTERACTION WITH PREGNANCY

Most women with HOCM tolerate pregnancy well.[42] However, the potential for cardiac deterioration and overt cardiac failure remains a concern during the antenatal, intrapartum, and postpartum periods.[42] The greater blood volume of pregnancy helps maintain adequate ventricular filling, which reduces the severity of outflow tract obstruction. However, pregnancy also increases heart rate and myocardial contractility and decreases SVR; independently or together, these physiologic changes may worsen the outflow tract obstruction. Furthermore, aortocaval compression decreases venous return, thereby reducing left ventricular chamber size and worsening the outflow tract obstruction. Thus pregnancy may exacerbate HOCM in some women.

The risk of maternal mortality is higher in women with HOCM than in the general population. However, the absolute risk of maternal mortality is low, and death appears to occur principally among women at high risk.[42] In patients with HOCM, the ability to tolerate pregnancy correlates closely with preconception functional status (see Box 41-1). In a retrospective study, worsening of clinical condition during pregnancy occurred in 4% of patients who were asymptomatic before pregnancy and in 42% of patients who were symptomatic before pregnancy.[42]

MEDICAL MANAGEMENT

Good outcome depends on careful attention to control of heart rate, maintenance of adequate intravascular volume, and prevention of arrhythmias. Medical management includes treatment with a beta-adrenergic receptor antagonist, which should be continued during pregnancy. Women of childbearing age who are symptomatic or have a history of syncope or presyncope should be considered candidates for the insertion of a pacemaker or an automatic implantable cardiac defibrillator (AICD) before conception.

OBSTETRIC MANAGEMENT

Most obstetricians reserve cesarean delivery for obstetric indications in patients with HOCM. These patients typically tolerate the second stage of labor well, given the fact that increased SVR helps maintain ventricular function. If oxytocin is needed after delivery, it should be given slowly; bolus intravenous injection may cause systemic vasodilation and may increase outflow tract obstruction. Methylergonovine may be acceptable as an alternative uterotonic agent.

ANESTHETIC MANAGEMENT

The goals of anesthetic management are (1) maintenance of intravascular volume and venous return, (2) avoidance of aortocaval compression, (3) maintenance of adequate SVR, (4) maintenance of a slow heart rate in sinus rhythm, (5) aggressive treatment of acute atrial fibrillation and other tachyarrhythmias, and (6) prevention of increases in myocardial contractility.

Beta-adrenergic receptor blockade should be maintained during labor and delivery. Neuraxial analgesia techniques, including combined spinal-epidural analgesia using an intrathecal opioid, may be administered during labor. Phenylephrine is the preferred vasopressor for treatment of hypotension in these patients.

An elective cesarean delivery may be performed safely with epidural anesthesia.[43] HOCM represents a relative contraindication to the use of single-shot spinal anesthesia for cesarean delivery because of the rapid onset of a sympathectomy. Patients with HOCM tolerate general anesthesia well.[44] The volatile halogenated agents cause decreased myocardial contractility, which is advantageous in patients with HOCM. The most common adverse occurrence after general anesthesia in patients with HOCM is reversible congestive heart failure.[44] Remifentanil has been used successfully during cesarean delivery in a woman with severe heart dysfunction secondary to HOCM.[45]

ISCHEMIC HEART DISEASE

Acute myocardial infarction is a rare event in women of reproductive age; however, pregnancy increases the risk threefold to fourfold.[46] Ladner et al.[47] reported an overall incidence of acute myocardial infarction of 1 in 35,700 pregnancies during the period from 1991 to 2000; however, the incidence represented an increase from 1 in 73,400 initially to 1 in 24,600 in the final year of the analysis. A total of 151 women had an acute myocardial infarction, with the event occurring antepartum (38%), intrapartum (21%), or 6 weeks postpartum (41%); maternal mortality from the myocardial infarction was 7.3%.[47] In a review of the 2000-2002 data from the Nationwide Inpatient Sample, the largest all-payer inpatient care database in the United States, James et al.[46] found a high incidence (6.2 per 100,000 deliveries) but a relatively low case-fatality rate (5.1%) for pregnancy-related acute myocardial infarction. These data may reflect both an improved ability to identify (with the widespread use of troponin as a marker) and treat pregnant women who have experienced an acute myocardial infarction.

The incidence of myocardial infarction during pregnancy may be increasing for several reasons. First, there is a greater prevalence of delayed and extended childbearing. Assisted reproductive technologies, specifically embryo donation, have resulted in pregnancies in postmenopausal women in their fifth, sixth, and seventh decades of life (see Chapter 15). Second, many young women continue to abuse tobacco. Third, there is a substantial incidence of cocaine abuse among women of childbearing age. Fourth, the use of oral contraceptives after age 35 years may increase the risk of ischemic heart disease.

Risk factors for acute myocardial infarction include hypertension, diabetes mellitus, thrombophilia, smoking, age greater than 35 years, and black race. Obstetric risk factors for acute myocardial infarction include preeclampsia, postpartum hemorrhage, and the requirement of a blood transfusion.[46]

PATHOPHYSIOLOGY

The etiology of myocardial infarction during pregnancy is multifactorial. Coronary artery morphology has been studied in 125 patients who had a myocardial infarction during pregnancy. Coronary atherosclerosis (with or without intracoronary thrombus) was found in 43% of patients, coronary thrombus without atherosclerotic disease in 21%, coronary dissection in 16%, and normal coronary arteries in 29% of patients.[48] An intrapartum myocardial infarction in women with normal coronary arteries may be caused by disorders such as pheochromocytoma, collagen vascular disease, sickle cell anemia, and protracted coronary artery spasm (secondary to cocaine abuse, pregnancy-induced hypertension, or administration of an ergot alkaloid).

INTERACTION WITH PREGNANCY

Pregnancy increases heart rate, myocardial wall tension and contractility, basal metabolic rate, and oxygen consumption. Labor causes a further, progressive increase in oxygen consumption. Pain leads to an increase in maternal concentrations of catecholamines, which increase myocardial oxygen demand. Each uterine contraction results in an autotransfusion of 300 to 500 mL of blood to the central circulation. Autotransfusion increases preload and may further compromise the balance between myocardial oxygen supply and demand. Oxygen consumption peaks at delivery. Maternal expulsive efforts at delivery may result in a 150% increase in oxygen consumption. Oxygen consumption remains 25% higher than nonpregnant levels in the immediate postpartum period. An elective cesarean delivery does not eliminate the cardiovascular stress associated with delivery; cardiac output increases as much as 50% during and after an elective cesarean delivery.

The cardiovascular changes of pregnancy, labor, and delivery may precipitate myocardial ischemia or infarction in women with coronary artery disease or other cardiac lesions (Table 41-2). Cocaine abuse can cause myocardial ischemia as a result of tachycardia, hypertension, arrhythmias, coronary artery spasm, coronary thrombosis, and the acceleration of atherosclerotic disease.[49] Thus the possibility of cocaine abuse should be considered when a pregnant woman experiences myocardial ischemia or infarction (see Chapter 53).

TABLE 41-2 Balance between Myocardial Oxygen Supply and Demand

Parameter	Effect of Pregnancy
Supply	
Diastolic time	Decreased
Coronary perfusion pressure	May be decreased
Arterial oxygen content	
• Arterial oxygen tension	Increased
• Hemoglobin concentration	Decreased
Coronary vessel diameter	Unchanged
Demand	
Basal oxygen requirements	Increased
Heart rate	Increased
Wall tension	
• Preload (ventricular radius)	May be increased
• Afterload	Decreased
Contractility	Increased

DIAGNOSIS

The diagnosis of myocardial ischemia is made from the history, physical findings, and ECG results. Among nonpregnant patients, the most significant symptoms include chest pain, dyspnea, diaphoresis, poor exercise tolerance, and syncope. However, all of these symptoms may occur in normal pregnant women. Measurement of the plasma troponin-1 level is a useful test in patients with suspected peripartum myocardial infarction because it remains within the normal range unless myocardial injury has occurred. The serum creatine kinase MB fraction may increase twofold 30 minutes after delivery in the absence of myocardial ischemia.

The ECG during normal pregnancy may show sinus tachycardia, a leftward axis shift, ST-segment depression, flattened or inverted T waves, and a Q wave in lead III.[50] Because ECG changes can be induced by pregnancy itself, only serial ECG changes are meaningful. Holter monitoring and echocardiography are noninvasive evaluations that remain useful during pregnancy. During early pregnancy, cardiac catheterization is used with caution because of the teratogenic effects of ionizing radiation. However, the risk-to-benefit analysis may favor intrapartum cardiac catheterization with appropriate lead shielding.[51] The simultaneous use of echocardiography may decrease the need for cineangiography, thereby reducing fetal radiation exposure.

The differential diagnosis of chest pain during pregnancy should include preeclampsia, hemorrhage, sickle cell crisis, acute pulmonary embolus, and aortic dissection.

MEDICAL MANAGEMENT

Treatment of myocardial infarction in pregnancy is generally unchanged from that in the nonpregnant patient. Optimal management requires attention to the needs of both mother and fetus. Physicians should treat disease states that may adversely affect myocardial oxygen supply and demand (e.g., anemia, thyrotoxicosis, hypertension, infection, substance abuse).

The pharmacologic agents (e.g., nitrates, beta-adrenergic receptor antagonists, calcium entry antagonists) used in the treatment of myocardial ischemia in nonpregnant patients are also used during pregnancy. Treatment of myocardial ischemia improves cardiac function, which should increase uteroplacental perfusion. Conversely, overly aggressive therapy may adversely affect the fetus. For example, intravenous nitroglycerin can result in a sudden reduction in preload, which may reduce maternal cardiac output and uteroplacental perfusion. It is useful to monitor the fetal heart rate (FHR) in such cases.

Ischemia that is unresponsive to medical management may require percutaneous transluminal coronary angioplasty,[52,53] stent placement,[54] or cardiopulmonary bypass surgery.[55] Cardiac catheterization and interventional procedures are associated with fetal radiation exposure up to 0.1 gray (Gy) units, depending on the extent of the procedure; in general, as long as organogenesis is complete, this level of exposure should not alter maternal management if a catheterization is indicated.

New therapies for the treatment of acute myocardial infarction are being developed. Schumacher et al.[56] reported a case of myocardial infarction that was treated with tissue plasminogen activator (t-PA) at 21 weeks' gestation. Maternal outcome was good, and cesarean delivery for preterm labor was performed at 33 weeks' gestation. This agent has a short half-life, and because of its large molecular weight (65,000 Da), it does not cross the placenta. Nevertheless, t-PA increases the risk of placental abruption, intrauterine hemorrhage, and resultant fetal demise. In addition, the administration of t-PA close to delivery may increase blood loss during operative procedures.

OBSTETRIC MANAGEMENT

The risk of recurrent myocardial infarction in pregnant women with a history of previous myocardial infarction is unknown. Frenkel et al.[57] reviewed 24 published cases of patients who conceived after a myocardial infarction. These investigators noted that "each woman had an uneventful pregnancy with no cardiac or obstetric complications related to the myocardial infarction."[57] Concluding that previous myocardial infarction does not contraindicate labor, they recommended that cesarean delivery be reserved "for situations that are life-threatening to the mother and cannot be corrected immediately."[57] Avila et al.[58] reported 1000 parturients with heart disease, of whom 14 had significant coronary artery disease; the outcome for these women, including 7 who had a prior history of a myocardial infarction, correlated with the severity of the underlying disease and existing myocardial function.

It has been suggested that acute myocardial infarction complicated by refractory congestive heart failure should prompt an early cesarean delivery. Listo and Bjorkenheim[59] described a patient with an acute anterior wall myocardial infarction during labor in whom cardiogenic shock developed, leading to intrapartum fetal death. A rapid resolution of the associated pulmonary edema was observed after cesarean delivery. Mabie et al.[60] reported the case of a 42-year-old woman with no known cardiac risk factors who had an acute myocardial infarction at 32 weeks' gestation and experienced preterm labor. Symptoms of congestive heart failure improved promptly after cesarean delivery, with eventual resolution of the left ventricular dysfunction. The authors of these reports suggested that an early cesarean delivery may help protect stunned but viable myocardium and thereby prevent further damage.

Nonetheless, vaginal delivery is often preferred, with efforts made to decrease myocardial oxygen demand during labor and delivery. Cohen et al.[61] compared the advantages and disadvantages of cesarean and vaginal delivery in patients with a history of recent myocardial infarction. An elective cesarean delivery allows the obstetrician to control the timing of delivery and may avert the prolonged maternal stress of labor and the hyperdynamic circulatory changes associated with maternal expulsive efforts during the second stage of labor. Disadvantages of cesarean delivery are related to (1) a higher risk of blood loss, (2) an increased risk of infection, (3) greater postpartum pain, (4) delayed ambulation, and (5) a greater risk of pulmonary morbidity after delivery.

Intravenous infusion of synthetic oxytocin is considered safe for the induction of labor and treatment of postpartum uterine atony in women with coronary artery disease. However, a bolus injection of oxytocin may cause hypotension, and a prolonged infusion of large doses of oxytocin may result in hyponatremia and congestive heart failure.

Methylergonovine should be avoided in the third stage because it is more likely to cause coronary artery spasm in such patients.

In summary, no consensus exists regarding the optimal method of delivery in patients with ischemic heart disease. Some obstetricians recommend the liberal use of cesarean delivery; however, others argue that the procedure represents major surgery, which does not eliminate maternal hemodynamic stress and predisposes to hemorrhagic and infectious complications. It seems reasonable to reserve cesarean delivery for obstetric indications unless maternal hemodynamic instability mandates immediate delivery.

ANESTHETIC MANAGEMENT

Optimal management of the parturient with ischemic heart disease requires a multidisciplinary approach. The therapeutic options for parturients with coronary artery disease or active ischemia are similar to those for nonpregnant patients. The ECG and SpO_2 should be monitored continuously during labor and vaginal or cesarean delivery. An intra-arterial catheter and, occasionally, a pulmonary artery catheter may facilitate management of women who have recently experienced myocardial infarction or who have left ventricular and/or valvular dysfunction.

Labor

Supplemental oxygen should be administered during labor and delivery. The use of epidural analgesia throughout labor minimizes hyperdynamic circulatory changes associated with vaginal delivery, provides excellent pain relief, prevents hyperventilation, and reduces maternal concentrations of catecholamines. (Hypocapnia and catecholamines both cause coronary artery vasoconstriction.) Amniotomy should be delayed until satisfactory epidural analgesia is established. A dense epidural block ensures total relief of pain during labor, minimizes maternal expulsive efforts during the second stage of labor, and facilitates the rapid achievement of satisfactory anesthesia if urgent cesarean delivery is required.

Epinephrine should not be added to the local anesthetic solution because an unintentional intravascular injection of epinephrine can produce maternal tachycardia, and the systemic absorption of epidural epinephrine can increase the likelihood of maternal hypotension and reduce uteroplacental blood flow. Treatment with ephedrine increases the maternal heart rate, thereby increasing myocardial oxygen demand and possibly aggravating myocardial ischemia. For this reason, phenylephrine is the preferred vasopressor for treatment of hypotension in patients with ischemic heart disease.

Cesarean Delivery

Single-shot spinal anesthesia results in a rapid onset of sympathectomy and a higher risk of severe hypotension. Continuous epidural anesthesia is the preferred technique for cesarean delivery for women with ischemic heart disease. When general anesthesia is required, a modified rapid-sequence induction (e.g., using etomidate, remifentanil, and succinylcholine) can be performed over 1 to 2 minutes without compromising hemodynamic stability.

These women remain at increased risk for cardiovascular instability (myocardial infarction, pulmonary edema) after vaginal or cesarean delivery. Such patients should be monitored in an obstetric intensive care setting for at least 24 hours after delivery. Cardiology consultation is helpful for postpartum management.

VALVULAR DISORDERS

Published guidelines address diagnostic testing, physical activity, thromboprophylaxis, and treatment during pregnancy in patients with valvular heart lesions.[62,63] Valvular heart lesions can be associated with either low or high risk of maternal and fetal morbidity and mortality (Box 41-2).

Aortic Stenosis

Aortic stenosis is classified as valvular, subvalvular, or supravalvular. Aortic stenosis during pregnancy is usually

BOX 41-2 Maternal and Fetal Risk of Morbidity or Mortality Associated with Valvular Heart Lesions during Pregnancy

Low Maternal or Fetal Risk during Pregnancy

- Asymptomatic aortic stenosis with low mean gradient (< 50 mm Hg) in presence of normal LV systolic function (EF > 50%)
- Aortic regurgitation with normal LV systolic function and NYHA functional class I-II symptoms
- Mitral regurgitation with normal LV systolic function and NYHA functional class I-II symptoms
- Mitral valve prolapse with no mitral regurgitation or with mild to moderate mitral regurgitation and normal LV systolic function
- Mild to moderate mitral stenosis (mean valve area > 1.5 cm^2, gradient < 5 mm Hg) without severe pulmonary hypertension
- Mild to moderate pulmonary stenosis

High Maternal Risk or Fetal Risk during Pregnancy

- Severe aortic stenosis with or without symptoms
- Aortic regurgitation with NYHA functional class III-IV symptoms
- Mitral stenosis with NYHA functional class II-IV symptoms
- Mitral regurgitation with NYHA functional class III-IV symptoms
- Aortic or mitral valve disease that results in severe pulmonary hypertension (pulmonary pressure > 75% of systemic pressure)
- Aortic or mitral valve disease with severe LV dysfunction (EF < 40%)
- Mechanical prosthetic valve that requires anticoagulation
- Aortic regurgitation in Marfan's syndrome

EF, ejection fraction; LV, left ventricular; NYHA, New York Heart Association.

Adapted from Bonow RO, Carabello B, de Leon AC, et al. ACC/AHA guidelines for the management of patient with valvular heart disease: A report of the American College of Cardiology/American Heart Association Task Force on Practice Guidelines (Committee on Management of Patients with Valvular Heart Disease). J Am Coll Cardiol 1998; 32:1486-588.

caused by a congenital bicuspid valve.[64] Rheumatic aortic stenosis is less common and occurs in conjunction with mitral valve disease in approximately 5% of women with rheumatic valvular disease.[65-67] Subvalvular aortic stenosis and supravalvular aortic stenosis have also been described in pregnancy.[68,69]

PATHOPHYSIOLOGY

The severity of aortic stenosis can be described by the average valve area or the peak pressure gradient across the valve. Aortic stenosis lesions become hemodynamically significant when the valve diameter is one third of its normal size. Severe aortic stenosis is typically defined as a valve area smaller than 0.8 to 1.0 cm^2 (normal valve area is 2.6 to 3.5 cm^2) and a peak gradient of greater than 40 to 50 mm Hg.[62] Patients with a gradient that exceeds 100 mm Hg are at high risk for myocardial ischemia.

Women with aortic stenosis who are asymptomatic before conception generally tolerate pregnancy well, whereas those with symptoms of severe stenosis are at risk for acute left ventricular failure[70] and are advised to undergo surgical repair before attempting pregnancy.[62] Patients with moderate to severe disease have a relatively fixed stroke volume and so have difficulty achieving the increased cardiac output that is required in pregnancy. These women may be unable to maintain adequate coronary or cerebral perfusion during exertion. Moreover, because the stroke volume is fixed, the heart rate is a key factor in determining cardiac output; bradycardia causes decreased cardiac output and hypotension, whereas tachycardia shortens the time for ventricular filling and also reduces cardiac output.[71] The onset of angina, dyspnea, or syncope is an ominous sign, signaling a life expectancy of less than 5 years.

DIAGNOSIS

A coarse systolic murmur, which reaches its maximal intensity at midsystole and radiates to the apex and the neck, is characteristic of aortic stenosis. The ECG may show evidence of left ventricular hypertrophy, conduction disturbances, and ischemia. In patients with severe aortic stenosis, chest radiographs may demonstrate left ventricular enlargement, aortic valve calcification, and poststenotic dilation of the ascending aorta. Together with clinical symptoms, echocardiographic estimation of the valve area rather than the pressure gradient has been shown to be a better guide to the severity of the disease in pregnancy, during which the hyperdynamic flow can overestimate the valve gradient.[72]

INTERACTION WITH PREGNANCY

The greater blood volume of pregnancy allows women with mild aortic stenosis to tolerate pregnancy well, and management during pregnancy is usually conservative. In patients with suspected bacteremia, prophylactic antibiotics may be administered to decrease the risk of infective endocarditis (see later). Women with severe aortic stenosis have a limited ability to compensate for greater demands during pregnancy and are advised to have corrective surgery before conception. They may experience dyspnea, angina, or syncope. Symptoms early in gestation may warrant the termination of pregnancy to protect the life of the mother. Nonsurgical or surgical intervention (valve replacement) should be considered if a woman's clinical condition worsens or is refractory to medical treatment.[68,69,73-75]

Silversides et al.[69] reported 49 pregnancies in 39 patients with aortic stenosis, all of whom had NYHA class I or II disease at the time of the first prenatal visit. Three of 29 patients with severe aortic stenosis had early complications (pulmonary edema or atrial arrhythmias), which were defined as events that occurred either during pregnancy or after delivery up to the time of hospital discharge. In contrast, none of the 20 patients with mild or moderate aortic stenosis had early complications. In another study from Brazil, patients with moderate to severe aortic stenosis had a 68% incidence of cardiac morbidity, including cardiac failure, angina, need for valve replacement, and sudden death.[58] The differences in these outcomes, including maternal mortality, may reflect differences in access to advanced tertiary care.

OBSTETRIC MANAGEMENT

The preferred obstetric management in a parturient with aortic stenosis is vaginal delivery with an assisted second stage of labor. In the report by Silversides et al.,[69] vaginal delivery was performed successfully in 67% of the 49 pregnancies; of the remaining cases, only one cesarean delivery was performed for cardiac indications. Regardless of the method of delivery, it is critical to maintain intravascular volume, venous return, and sinus rhythm. Aortocaval compression, peripartum hemorrhage, and sympathectomy may reduce cardiac output.

ANESTHETIC MANAGEMENT

The goals of anesthetic management are (1) maintenance of a normal heart rate, sinus rhythm, and adequate SVR; (2) maintenance of intravascular volume and venous return; (3) avoidance of aortocaval compression; and (4) avoidance of myocardial depression during general anesthesia (Box 41-3).[62]

It is important to maintain a normal heart rate and sinus rhythm. Because patients with aortic stenosis have a fixed stroke volume, a slow heart rate decreases cardiac output. Severe tachycardia increases myocardial oxygen demand and shortens time for diastolic perfusion of the hypertrophic left ventricle. Patients with aortic stenosis do not tolerate arrhythmias well. Atrial systole is critical to the maintenance of adequate ventricular filling and cardiac output. Prompt treatment of arrhythmias is essential.

Patients with aortic stenosis do not tolerate a significant decrease in SVR, which results in hypotension and decreased perfusion of the hypertrophic left ventricle. Normal patients compensate for reduced SVR by increasing stroke volume and heart rate. Patients with aortic stenosis have a fixed stroke volume and rely on an increase in heart rate to increase cardiac output; however, severe tachycardia is undesirable and hazardous.

Patients with aortic stenosis also do not tolerate decreases in either venous return or left ventricular filling pressures. Adequate end-diastolic volume is necessary to maintain left ventricular stroke volume. Left uterine displacement must be maintained during the induction and maintenance of anesthesia. Maintenance of venous return and left ventricular end-diastolic volume (LVEDV) is critical.

Hemodynamic monitoring with an intra-arterial line is strongly recommended during labor and delivery in patients

BOX 41-3 Hemodynamic Goals of Anesthetic Management in Patients with Valvular Heart Disease

Goals of Anesthetic Management in Patients with Aortic Stenosis

- Maintain normal heart rate.
- Maintain sinus rhythm.
- Maintain adequate SVR.
- Maintain intravascular volume and venous return.
- Avoid aortocaval compression.
- Avoid myocardial depression during general anesthesia.

Goals of Anesthetic Management in Patients with Aortic Regurgitation

- Maintain normal to slightly elevated heart rate.
- Prevent an increase in SVR.
- Avoid aortocaval compression.
- Avoid myocardial depression during general anesthesia.

Goals of Anesthetic Management in Patients with Mitral Stenosis

- Maintain a slow heart rate.
- Maintain sinus rhythm.
- Aggressively treat acute atrial fibrillation.
- Avoid aortocaval compression.
- Maintain venous return.
- Maintain adequate SVR.
- Prevent pain, hypoxemia, hypercarbia, and acidosis, which may increase pulmonary vascular resistance.

Goals of Anesthetic Management in Patients with Mitral Regurgitation

- Prevent an increase in SVR.
- Maintain a normal to slightly elevated heart rate.
- Maintain sinus rhythm.
- Aggressively treat acute atrial fibrillation.
- Avoid aortocaval compression.
- Maintain venous return.
- Prevent an increase in central vascular volume.
- Avoid myocardial depression during general anesthesia.
- Prevent pain, hypoxemia, hypercarbia, and acidosis, which may increase pulmonary vascular resistance.

SVR, systemic vascular resistance.

with moderate to severe aortic stenosis. During labor, hypovolemia is a greater threat than pulmonary edema. Thus, CVP or pulmonary capillary wedge pressure, when available, should be maintained at high-normal levels (e.g., pulmonary capillary wedge pressure of 18 mm Hg) to protect cardiac output if unexpected peripartum hemorrhage occurs.

Historically, anesthesiologists have avoided spinal and epidural anesthesia in pregnant women with aortic stenosis. Moderate to severe aortic stenosis remains a relative contraindication for single-shot spinal anesthesia. However, numerous reports have described the safe use of continuous epidural or continuous spinal anesthesia for vaginal or cesarean delivery in women with aortic stenosis.[76,77] Slow epidural administration of small bolus doses of local anesthetic with fentanyl allows titration of appropriate volumes of crystalloid and enables the patient to achieve compensatory vasoconstriction above the level of the block. Typically, local anesthetic solutions that contain epinephrine should be avoided in patients with moderate to severe aortic stenosis, because unintentional intravascular injection of epinephrine can precipitate tachycardia, whereas systemic absorption of epinephrine from the epidural space can diminish SVR and lower venous return.

When general anesthesia is needed, a combination of etomidate and a modest dose of opioid is a good choice for the induction of anesthesia and is generally preferable to agents such as sodium thiopental and propofol (which cause myocardial depression and/or vasodilation) and ketamine (which causes tachycardia). Orme et al.[78] reported the successful use of etomidate, remifentanil, and suxamethonium for induction of anesthesia, and isoflurane and remifentanil for maintenance of anesthesia, in four patients with critical aortic stenosis. All patients were extubated at the end of surgery, and all neonates had Apgar scores of 10 at 5 minutes. A combination of low-dose thiopental and ketamine may be a suitable induction regimen if etomidate is unavailable.

Aortic Regurgitation

Aortic regurgitation or insufficiency occurs more frequently than aortic stenosis in women of childbearing age.[79] Aortic regurgitation in young women may be due to a congenital bicuspid valve,[69,80] rheumatic heart disease,[66] endocarditis,[81] or a dilated aortic annulus.[82] Rheumatic heart disease is the etiology in approximately 75% of affected patients. Women with rheumatic aortic regurgitation typically have coexisting mitral valve disease; if an isolated lesion is observed, it is more likely to be of nonrheumatic origin. Traumatic rupture of the aortic valve is an uncommon cause of acute aortic regurgitation. Occasionally, retrograde dissection of the aorta involves the aortic annulus and produces aortic regurgitation. Acute aortic regurgitation is a life-threatening condition. However, in one case, acute dissection in a pregnant woman was managed medically with nifedipine and labetalol, and successful cesarean delivery with epidural anesthesia was accomplished several weeks later.[79]

PATHOPHYSIOLOGY

Regurgitation of blood from the aorta to the left ventricle occurs when the aortic valve fails to close normally. Aortic regurgitation results in left ventricular volume overload, which over time leads to left ventricular dilation and hypertrophy. Initially, the enlarging left ventricle tolerates the increased work. Eventually, however, left ventricular contractility decreases, the ejection fraction and forward stroke volume progressively decline, and LVEDV continues to rise. Deterioration of left ventricular function often precedes the development of symptoms. A competent mitral valve can protect the pulmonary circulation from the initial increases in LVEDV and left ventricular end-diastolic pressure (LVEDP). However, as the ventricle begins to fail, further increases in LVEDV and LVEDP occur, leading to pulmonary edema.

Equilibration between aortic and left ventricular pressures may occur toward the end of diastole, particularly when the heart rate is slow. The LVEDP may reach extremely high levels (greater than 40 mm Hg). Rarely the left ventricular pressure exceeds the left atrial pressure toward the end of diastole. This pressure difference may cause premature closure of the mitral valve or diastolic mitral regurgitation.

Myocardial ischemia occurs in patients with aortic regurgitation because left ventricular dilation and increased left ventricular systolic pressure result in greater myocardial oxygen demand. In addition, diminished coronary blood flow during diastole results in lower myocardial perfusion.

CLINICAL PRESENTATION

Acute aortic regurgitation (secondary to trauma or infective endocarditis) can be heralded by dyspnea, tachycardia, and lightheadedness and is associated with abrupt increases in LVEDV that result in markedly elevated LVEDP. Left atrial and pulmonary artery pressures rise rapidly, and hemodynamic deterioration ensues; emergency surgery is often necessary as a life-saving measure.[79]

With **chronic aortic regurgitation,** the first complaint is often a pounding sensation in the chest, especially when the patient is lying down. Exertional dyspnea is typically the first symptom of diminished cardiac reserve. It is followed by orthopnea, paroxysmal nocturnal dyspnea, and diaphoresis. Symptoms of left ventricular failure are more common than symptoms of myocardial ischemia. However, chest pain may result from coronary insufficiency or excessive pounding of the heart on the chest wall. Late in the course of the disease, peripheral edema, congestive hepatomegaly, and ascites may develop.

DIAGNOSIS

The arterial pulse pressure with aortic regurgitation is typically widened. The severity of aortic regurgitation does not correlate directly with pulse pressure, and some patients with severe aortic regurgitation have normal blood pressures. Patients characteristically have a rapidly rising "water hammer" pulse, which collapses suddenly as arterial pressure plummets during late systole and diastole. Often, a diastolic thrill is palpable along the left sternal border, and a third heart sound is common. The murmur of aortic regurgitation is typically a high-pitched, blowing decrescendo diastolic murmur that is heard best along the left sternal border in the third intercostal space. ECG findings may be normal in patients with mild aortic regurgitation but may show left ventricular hypertrophy and myocardial ischemia in women with severe disease. The presence of atrial fibrillation suggests coexisting mitral valvular disease.

MEDICAL MANAGEMENT

The left ventricular failure of chronic aortic regurgitation initially responds to treatment with digoxin, salt restriction, and diuretics. A direct vasodilator can be used as a substitute for angiotensin-converting enzyme (ACE) inhibitors, which are contraindicated in pregnancy. Cardiac arrhythmias and infections are poorly tolerated and require prompt therapy. Asymptomatic patients with severe aortic regurgitation but normal left ventricular function typically do well and seldom need to have prophylactic valve surgery prior to pregnancy.[83]

OBSTETRIC MANAGEMENT

Aortic regurgitation without left ventricular dysfunction is tolerated well during pregnancy for at least three reasons. First, pregnancy typically results in a modest increase in maternal heart rate, which shortens the time for regurgitant blood flow during diastole. Second, pregnancy decreases SVR, favoring the forward flow of blood and reducing the amount of regurgitant blood flow. Third, the greater blood volume of pregnancy helps maintain adequate filling pressures.

ANESTHETIC MANAGEMENT

The goals of anesthetic management are (1) maintenance of a normal to slightly elevated heart rate, (2) prevention of an increase in SVR, (3) avoidance of aortocaval compression, and (4) avoidance of myocardial depression during general anesthesia (see Box 41-3).[62]

Patients who are symptomatic or have left ventricular dysfunction benefit from hemodynamic monitoring during labor and delivery. Epidural analgesia and anesthesia may decrease afterload and is preferred for either vaginal or cesarean delivery. During labor, early administration of epidural analgesia prevents the pain-associated increase in SVR that can precipitate acute left ventricular volume overload in women with aortic regurgitation. These patients do not tolerate bradycardia, which should be treated promptly. Wadsworth et al.[45] described the use of remifentanil during administration of general anesthesia for cesarean delivery in a woman with aortic regurgitation.

Mitral Stenosis

Mitral stenosis is the most commonly encountered valvular lesion in pregnancy and is almost always associated with rheumatic heart disease.[66,69,84,85] The incidence of rheumatic heart disease has declined in most developed countries but remains an issue in many developing countries. Although mitral stenosis is often accompanied by some mitral regurgitation, pregnancy-related cardiac morbidity is usually related to the valve stenosis.[64]

PATHOPHYSIOLOGY

The normal mitral valve orifice has a surface area of 4 to 5 cm^2, and the severity of mitral stenosis is classified according to the residual valve area; an area greater than 1.5 cm^2 is classified as mild stenosis, an area between 1.0 and 1.5 cm^2 as moderate, and an area of 1 cm^2 or less as severe. Symptoms typically develop when the size of the orifice is 2 cm^2 or less.

Mitral stenosis prevents filling of the left ventricle, which decreases both stroke volume and cardiac output. By definition, mitral stenosis prevents emptying of the left atrium, resulting in left atrial dilation and higher left atrial and pulmonary arterial pressures. Atrial fibrillation may occur, and mural thrombi may develop. Higher pulmonary arterial pressure results in dyspnea, hemoptysis, and pulmonary edema.

Progressive pulmonary hypertension results in compensatory right ventricular hypertrophy. Greater pulmonary vascular resistance worsens with exercise and may lead to right heart failure. Severe, fixed pulmonary hypertension limits the compensatory changes in pulmonary vascular resistance that normally accompany changes in cardiac output and SVR.

DIAGNOSIS

After an acute episode of rheumatic fever, mitral stenosis progresses slowly for 20 to 30 years. Approximately 25% of women with mitral stenosis first experience symptoms during pregnancy. Symptoms and signs associated with mitral stenosis include dyspnea, hemoptysis, chest pain, right heart failure, and thromboembolism. Auscultation may reveal a diastolic murmur, an accentuated first heart sound, an audible fourth heart sound, and an opening snap. The ECG may show left atrial enlargement, atrial fibrillation, and right ventricular hypertrophy. Echocardiography helps confirm the diagnosis, although careful measurements are critical because mitral valve area calculation based on Doppler ultrasonography may be inaccurate during pregnancy.

INTERACTION WITH PREGNANCY

Women with severe mitral stenosis often do not tolerate the cardiovascular demands of pregnancy because (1) the expanded blood volume of pregnancy increases the risk of pulmonary congestion and edema and (2) the physiologic tachycardia of pregnancy shortens the left ventricular filling time, thereby increasing left atrial and pulmonary arterial pressures. Atrial fibrillation is associated with a higher risk of maternal morbidity in women with mitral stenosis. Both the loss of atrial systole and the higher ventricular rate result in diminished cardiac output and an increased risk of pulmonary edema. Approximately 80% of cases of systemic emboli occur in patients with atrial fibrillation.[86]

Hameed et al.[66] described outcome for 46 pregnancies in 44 women with mitral stenosis, 28 and 18 of whom had NYHA class I and II disease, respectively, at the first antenatal visit; 74% of the patients demonstrated clinical deterioration during pregnancy. Women with mild mitral stenosis did well; however, those with moderate or severe mitral stenosis had a higher incidence of maternal morbidity (e.g., development of heart failure, occurrence of arrhythmias, requirement for cardiac medications, need for hospitalization) than healthy controls. Silversides et al.[87] described the outcome of 80 pregnancies in 74 women with mitral stenosis. Maternal cardiac complications, including pulmonary edema and arrhythmias, occurred in 35% of the pregnancies. The incidence of maternal cardiac complications was related to the severity of the mitral stenosis (67% for severe, 38% for moderate, and 26% for mild disease).

Despite the high incidence of morbidity, maternal death associated with mitral stenosis is surprisingly uncommon. In tertiary care hospitals in North America and India, a total of 195 cases of mitral stenosis resulted in no maternal deaths.[66,69,84] Isolated reports have described maternal death in women with critical mitral stenosis and NYHA class III or IV disease.[88]

The sudden increase in preload immediately after delivery may flood the central circulation and result in the development of severe pulmonary edema. For this reason hemodynamic monitoring should be continued for up to 24 hours after delivery in any woman with mitral stenosis.

MEDICAL MANAGEMENT

Beta-adrenergic receptor blockade is useful to prevent tachycardia during pregnancy. al Kasab et al.[89] found that maternal administration of propranolol or atenolol decreased the incidence of maternal pulmonary edema without adverse effects on the fetus or neonate.

Acute atrial fibrillation requires aggressive treatment. If pharmacologic therapy fails to control the ventricular response, cardioversion should be performed. After cardioversion, pulmonary edema typically responds well to bed rest in the left lateral decubitus position and administration of a diuretic.

Patients who have atrial fibrillation should undergo anticoagulation to prevent systemic embolization.[62,90] In the pregnant woman with severe mitral stenosis and an enlarged left atrium, some physicians have advocated the use of prophylactic anticoagulation, even in the absence of atrial fibrillation.[91]

SURGICAL MANAGEMENT

If significant mitral stenosis is recognized before pregnancy, surgery is recommended. A mitral commissurotomy is preferred, unless a valve replacement is required, in which case a bioprosthetic valve is most frequently used.

During pregnancy, some women require percutaneous mitral balloon valvotomy or valvuloplasty to temporarily delay the progression of mitral stenosis and possibly allow the successful completion of pregnancy. The second trimester most likely represents the best time for this palliative procedure. If severe maternal symptoms warrant a more aggressive response, a mitral valve commissurotomy may be performed.

In a historical cohort study, de Souza et al.[92] compared the outcomes of pregnant women with severe mitral stenosis who underwent percutaneous mitral balloon valvuloplasty (n = 21) and those who underwent open mitral valve commissurotomy (n = 24). Percutaneous mitral balloon valvuloplasty decreased the mitral valve gradient, left atrial pressure, and mean pulmonary artery pressure in more than 90% of patients. In addition, the fetal loss rate was significantly lower in the percutaneous mitral balloon valvuloplasty group than in the open surgery group (4% versus 33%, respectively). Percutaneous mitral balloon valvuloplasty presents a relatively safe and highly effective intervention for women with pliable valves and no signs of regurgitation. This procedure circumvents the risks to the mother and fetus associated with an open surgical valve repair or replacement and should be considered in patients with severe mitral stenosis who cannot be further optimized with medical therapy.

OBSTETRIC MANAGEMENT

Parturients with symptomatic mitral stenosis require invasive hemodynamic monitoring during labor and vaginal or cesarean delivery. Mitral stenosis does not affect management of the first stage of labor, except that adequate analgesia is essential. During the second stage, the Valsalva maneuver may result in a sudden, undesirable increase in venous return. Thus, the obstetrician should allow the force of uterine contractions rather than maternal expulsive efforts to facilitate descent of the fetal vertex to a level where low forceps or vacuum extraction delivery can be accomplished.

Silversides et al.[87] reported successful vaginal delivery in 74% of their cohort of pregnancies in patients with mitral stenosis. Among the remaining cases, only one cesarean delivery was prompted by cardiac indications. Similarly, Bhatla et al.[84] reserved cesarean delivery for obstetric indications in their series of patients with mitral stenosis.

ANESTHETIC MANAGEMENT

The goals for the anesthetic management of patients with mitral stenosis are (1) maintenance of a slow heart rate in a sinus rhythm; (2) aggressive treatment of acute atrial fibrillation, if present; (3) avoidance of aortocaval compression; (4) maintenance of adequate venous return; (5) maintenance of adequate SVR; and (6) prevention of pain, hypoxemia, hypercarbia, and acidosis, which may increase pulmonary vascular resistance (see Box 41-3).[62]

A slow heart rate allows longer diastolic filling time through the fixed, obstructed mitral valve. It is important to prevent a significant rise in SVR, given the patient's limited ability to increase cardiac output to maintain perfusion pressure.

Supplemental oxygen administration with pulse oximetry monitoring should be provided to minimize increases in pulmonary vascular resistance. Hemodynamic monitoring during labor and delivery with a pulmonary catheter has been recommended in patients with severe mitral stenosis.[93]

Epidural analgesia is recommended for pain relief during labor and delivery. The risk of hypotension is minimized by careful infusion of crystalloid and the use of a vasoconstrictor without a direct chronotropic effect (i.e., phenylephrine). Intrathecal administration of an opioid provides excellent analgesia during the first stage of labor without causing a sympathetic blockade. An intrathecal opioid with modest doses of a local anesthetic agent may provide satisfactory anesthesia during the second stage of labor. Neuraxial techniques are the most reliable method for providing perineal anesthesia during the second stage of labor.

Epidural anesthesia is preferred for cesarean delivery. Invasive hemodynamic monitoring, judicious intravenous administration of crystalloid, slow induction of anesthesia, and administration of small bolus doses of phenylephrine help ensure maternal hemodynamic stability.

If general anesthesia is required, caution is indicated in the use of drugs that can produce tachycardia (e.g., atropine, ketamine, pancuronium, meperidine). A beta-adrenergic receptor antagonist and a modest dose of opioid should be administered before or during the induction of general anesthesia. Esmolol, with its rapid onset and brief duration of action, is a good choice in patients with mitral stenosis, although it must be used with the acknowledgement that it may cause fetal bradycardia.[94-96] Therefore, the FHR should be monitored until delivery, when possible.

After delivery, care should be taken with the administration of oxytocin, methylergonovine, or 15-methylprostaglandin $F_{2\alpha}$, which may increase pulmonary vascular resistance. Regardless of the method of delivery or anesthetic technique, the patient is at risk for hemodynamic compromise and pulmonary edema during the postpartum period. Cesarean delivery does not eliminate the hemodynamic stress of the puerperium, except that the greater loss of blood during the cesarean delivery may be beneficial for women with mitral stenosis. These patients require intensive care immediately after delivery.

Mitral Regurgitation

The most common causes of noncongenital mitral regurgitation are myxomatous degeneration, ischemic papillary muscle disease, rheumatic fever, and endocarditis. During pregnancy, the usual causes of mitral regurgitation are rheumatic valvular disease and mitral valve prolapse.[66,84,88]

PATHOPHYSIOLOGY

The variable features that influence atrial and ventricular enlargement include the severity of the systolic regurgitant flow and whether the mitral regurgitation is acute or chronic. **Acute mitral regurgitation** may follow rheumatic fever, bacterial endocarditis, blunt chest trauma, myocardial ischemia, or prosthetic valve dysfunction. Acute mitral regurgitation may also occur in patients with Marfan's syndrome and left atrial myxoma. Acute mitral regurgitation imposes a large volume overload on the left atrium. Blood is pumped across the incompetent valve into a noncompliant left atrium. Forward cardiac output decreases, and compensatory peripheral vasoconstriction aggravates the lesion. Pulmonary congestion ensues, resulting in pulmonary edema. If the patient survives the acute episode, pulmonary arterial pressures continue to rise, and right heart failure may develop. In some cases emergency surgery may be necessary.

Chronic mitral regurgitation causes less hemodynamic stress on the left ventricle. The left atrium accommodates the regurgitant blood flow by gradual dilation and increased compliance. Left atrial dilation predisposes to atrial fibrillation. The onset of atrial fibrillation may produce palpitations. However, patients with mitral regurgitation withstand atrial fibrillation better than patients with mitral stenosis because the former have no obstruction to diastolic blood flow. Pulmonary hypertension also is less common in patients with chronic mitral regurgitation than in those with mitral stenosis. Typically, there is only a modest increase in left atrial pressure. Severe, long-standing mitral regurgitation leads to increased left atrial pressure and pulmonary congestion.

DIAGNOSIS

Patients with acute mitral regurgitation complain of dyspnea. Physical examination demonstrates a pansystolic murmur, an accentuated pulmonary component of the second heart sound, and, in severe cases, a third heart sound. ECG findings include left ventricular hypertrophy and atrial arrhythmias. With severe, acute mitral regurgitation, the pulmonary artery catheter tracing includes a V wave with a wide pulse pressure.

Symptoms of chronic mitral regurgitation include chronic weakness and fatigue secondary to a low cardiac output. The ECG may demonstrate atrial fibrillation. Left ventricular dilation and hypertrophy are more common in patients with chronic mitral regurgitation than in those with acute mitral regurgitation. Prominent atrial waves reflect atrial hypertrophy. Chest radiographs may show a moderately enlarged heart and marked left atrial enlargement.

INTERACTION WITH PREGNANCY

The hemodynamic changes of pregnancy are beneficial to patients with mitral regurgitation, even if severe, because the greater blood volume and lower SVR promote forward flow across the regurgitant valve. The uncommon patient with pulmonary congestion can be treated with a diuretic and a vasodilator if there is associated systemic hypertension. There is a higher risk of atrial fibrillation during pregnancy in women with mitral regurgitation.

The hypercoagulability of pregnancy increases the risk for systemic embolization. Anticoagulation may be indicated if cardioversion is planned, if there is a history of embolic phenomena, or if a new onset of atrial fibrillation occurs. Because of the high incidence of fetal loss with cardiac surgery, mitral valve repair should be avoided, if possible, during pregnancy and considered only in patients with severe symptoms not controlled by medical therapy.

ANESTHETIC MANAGEMENT

The goals of anesthetic management for patients with mitral regurgitation include (1) prevention of increases in SVR, (2) maintenance of a normal to slightly increased heart rate in sinus rhythm, (3) aggressive treatment of acute atrial fibrillation, (4) avoidance of aortocaval compression, (5) maintenance of venous return, (6) prevention of increases in central vascular volume, (7) avoidance of myocardial depression during general anesthesia, and (8) prevention of pain, hypoxemia, hypercarbia, and acidosis, which may increase pulmonary vascular resistance (see Box 41-3).[62]

Maternal monitoring during labor should include continuous ECG monitoring. Invasive monitoring is rarely warranted except in cases of severe mitral regurgitation. If pulmonary edema or refractory hypotension develops, the information obtained from a pulmonary artery catheter will help guide treatment.

Continuous epidural analgesia or anesthesia is preferred for labor and vaginal or cesarean delivery. Epidural anesthesia minimizes the increase in SVR associated with pain and may even lead to a modest decrease in SVR, which promotes the forward flow of blood and minimizes pulmonary congestion. However, epidural anesthesia may also decrease venous return. Careful administration of intravenous crystalloid and left uterine displacement are necessary to maintain venous return and left ventricular filling. In contrast to patients with mitral stenosis, patients with mitral regurgitation may benefit from the chronotropic effect of ephedrine if a vasopressor is required.

If general anesthesia is required, the anesthesiologist should give attention to the maintenance of adequate heart rate and decreased afterload. The higher heart rate associated with ketamine and pancuronium may be desirable in patients with mitral regurgitation. Myocardial depression should be avoided. Hypoxemia, hypercarbia, acidosis, and hypothermia produce an undesirable increase in pulmonary vascular resistance, so these perturbations should be avoided.

Acute atrial fibrillation must be treated promptly and aggressively. Hemodynamic instability warrants the immediate performance of cardioversion.

Mitral Valve Prolapse

Mitral valve prolapse (MVP) is the most common cardiac condition encountered during pregnancy; it occurs in approximately 2% to 6% of the general population and 12% to 17% of women of childbearing age.[97] Women with MVP generally tolerate pregnancy very well.[98]

PATHOPHYSIOLOGY

Primary or idiopathic MVP is characterized by a redundant valve that prolapses into the ventricle during systole. MVP can be secondary and associated with an atrial septal defect, endocarditis, or mitral stenosis.[99] MVP is also associated with many medical conditions, including von Willebrand's disease, Ehlers-Danlos syndrome, kyphoscoliosis, pectus excavatum, osteogenesis imperfecta, myotonic dystrophy, and, most notably, Marfan's syndrome. Involvement of the chordae tendineae can lead to chordal rupture and subsequent mitral regurgitation.

DIAGNOSIS

Most patients with MVP are asymptomatic. However, some women experience palpitations, chest pain, anxiety, fatigue, and lightheadedness.

The auscultatory hallmarks are a midsystolic click and a late systolic murmur. The intensity of these auscultatory findings may decrease during pregnancy because of the expansion of the maternal intravascular volume and lower SVR. These conditions increase ventricular volume, enhance forward blood flow, and lessen the prolapse of the mitral valve.

The diagnosis is often made on echocardiography. The most common echocardiographic finding is abrupt posterior movement of both valve leaflets (or only the posterior leaflet) in midsystole. Patients frequently have exaggerated motion of the anterior leaflet; however, actual prolapse into the left atrium appears to be more common with the posterior leaflet.

ECG findings are typically within normal limits in asymptomatic patients. However, nonspecific changes in the inferior and anterolateral leads and a variety of arrhythmias may occur. Paroxysmal supraventricular tachycardia is the most common tachyarrhythmia. Ventricular arrhythmias have been implicated in rare cases of sudden death. There is also a high incidence of MVP among patients with Wolff-Parkinson-White syndrome.

Neurologic complications include acute hemiplegia, transient ischemic attack, cerebellar infarct, amaurosis fugax, and retinal arteriolar occlusion. These complications likely have an embolic etiology. Cardiac arrhythmias may contribute to the likelihood of embolic events.

MEDICAL MANAGEMENT

The prognosis in the patient with MVP depends on the presence or absence of coexisting cardiovascular disease such as HOCM, Marfan's syndrome, atrial septal defect, and coronary artery disease. A beta-adrenergic receptor antagonist may be necessary to treat arrhythmias, chest pain, and palpitations. Because progressive mitral regurgitation occurs in approximately 15% of patients with MVP, treatment of left ventricular failure with digoxin and a diuretic may become necessary.

OBSTETRIC MANAGEMENT

Most patients with MVP tolerate pregnancy very well. A review of 28 pregnant patients with MVP (10 of whom also had mitral regurgitation) found no cardiovascular complications.[100] There appears to be no higher risk for obstetric complications or fetal compromise in patients with MVP. Antibiotic prophylaxis for vaginal delivery is not recommended (see later).[101]

ANESTHETIC MANAGEMENT

The severity of coexisting disease often dictates whether invasive hemodynamic monitoring is required in the patient with MVP. Neuraxial analgesia or anesthesia is an excellent choice for labor and vaginal or cesarean delivery. The sympathectomy and decreased concentrations of catecholamines achieved with this technique are beneficial for these patients. The differential diagnosis of hypotension or neurologic events that occur following neuraxial anesthesia should include cardiac arrhythmias, which occur with greater frequency in patients with MVP.

When general anesthesia is required, sympathomimetic agents (e.g., ketamine, pancuronium) should be avoided because of the high incidence of arrhythmias with their use. It also seems prudent to avoid agents that sensitize the myocardium to catecholamines. Ephedrine may precipitate or exacerbate tachyarrhythmias. Hypotension can be treated with small doses of phenylephrine. Management of the rare patient with MVP and evidence of decreased cardiac reserve is similar to that for the patient with mitral regurgitation.

Prior Prosthetic Valve Surgery

The pregnant woman with a prosthetic valve is at high risk for maternal and fetal complications. Maternal complications include thromboembolic phenomena, valve failure, and infective endocarditis. Although endocarditis is a serious threat to any parturient with a prosthetic heart valve, antibiotic prophylaxis for vaginal delivery is not recommended unless bacteremia is suspected (see later).[62,101]

MATERNAL ANTICOAGULATION

Complications of maternal anticoagulation therapy include fetal teratogenicity and maternal and fetal hemorrhage.[102] Selecting a prosthetic valve for a woman of childbearing age is not an easy matter. The advantage of a bioprosthetic valve is that anticoagulation therapy is avoided unless the woman requires therapy for another condition (e.g., atrial fibrillation, thromboembolism). A major disadvantage of porcine tissue valves is their greater likelihood of failure during the course of a lifetime compared with mechanical valves. Newer-generation mechanical valves have an excellent hemodynamic profile and seldom require replacement,[103] but their use still requires anticoagulation therapy.

Pregnant women are hypercoagulable and at greater risk for the development of thromboembolic complications, particularly if they have mechanical heart valves. Thus it is essential to maintain anticoagulation therapy during pregnancy (Box 41-4).

Warfarin crosses the placenta and is associated with a higher incidence of spontaneous abortion, preterm delivery, intrauterine fetal death, and fetal bleeding. The incidence of fetal embryopathy is estimated to be between 4% and 10%.[104,105] Warfarin is probably safe during the first 6 weeks of pregnancy, but there is a risk of embryopathy if this agent is used between 6 and 12 weeks' gestation. It is considered relatively safe during the second and third trimesters but should be discontinued in favor of heparin at 36 weeks' gestation, which allows easier reversal of anticoagulation before delivery.

Unfractionated heparin (UFH) is a large, water-soluble molecule that does not cross the placenta; thus administration of UFH avoids the risk of warfarin embryopathy.

BOX 41-4 Anticoagulation Regimen for Pregnant Women with a Mechanical Prosthetic Valve

- All pregnant patients with mechanical prosthetic valves must receive continuous therapeutic anticoagulation with frequent monitoring.
- For women requiring long-term warfarin therapy who are attempting pregnancy, pregnancy test results should be monitored with discussions about subsequent anticoagulation therapy, so that anticoagulation can be continued uninterrupted when pregnancy is achieved. The decision about anticoagulant management during pregnancy should include an assessment of additional risk factors for thromboembolism, including valve type, valve position, and history of thromboembolism, and the decision should also be influenced strongly by patient preferences.
- For pregnant women with mechanical heart valves, one of the following anticoagulant regimens should be used:
  - Adjusted-dose, twice-daily LMWH throughout pregnancy. Doses should be adjusted to achieve the manufacturer's recommended peak anti–factor Xa level (approximately 1.0 U/mL) 4 hr after subcutaneous injection.
  - Adjusted-dose UFH throughout pregnancy, administered subcutaneously q12h in doses adjusted to keep the mid-interval aPTT value at least twice the control or to attain an anti–factor Xa heparin level of 0.35 to 0.7 U/mL.
  - Adjusted-dose UFH or LMWH (as above) until the 13th week of gestation, with warfarin substitution until close to delivery, when either UFH or LMWH is resumed.
- In women judged to be at very high risk of thromboembolism in whom concerns exist about the efficacy and safety of UFH or LMWH administered as above (e.g., older-generation prosthesis in the mitral position or history of thromboembolism), vitamin K antagonists should be administered throughout pregnancy, with replacement by UFH or LMWH (as above) close to delivery, after a thorough discussion of the potential risks and benefits of this approach.
- If warfarin is used, the dose should be adjusted to a target INR of 3.0 (range 2.5 to 3.5); a lower therapeutic range, 2.0 to 3.0, can be used in patients with bileaflet aortic valves, provided they do not have atrial fibrillation or left ventricular dysfunction.
- If subcutaneous UFH is used, it should be initiated in high doses (17,500 to 20,000 U q12h) and adjusted to prolong a 6-hr post-injection aPTT into the therapeutic range.
- For pregnant women with prosthetic valves at high risk of thromboembolism, low-dose aspirin (75 to 100 mg/day) should also be administered.

aPTT, activated partial thromboplastin time; INR, International Normalized Ratio; LMWH, low-molecular-weight heparin; UFH, unfractionated heparin.

Information from Bates SM, Greer IA, Pabinger I, et al. Venous thromboembolism, thrombophilia, antithrombotic therapy, and pregnancy: American College of Chest Physicians Evidence-Based Clinical Practice Guidelines (8th edition). Chest 2008; 133:844S-886S.

However, there is a high incidence of thromboembolic events (12% to 24%) in high-risk patients who receive subcutaneous UFH during pregnancy.[104,106,107]

Low-molecular-weight heparin (LMWH) does not cross the placenta and is probably safe for the fetus. In nonpregnant patients, LMWH has a longer half-life and a more predictable dose-response pattern than UFH, which obviates monitoring. However, pregnancy is associated with a greater volume of distribution and accelerated clearance of LMWH; therefore use of LMWH thromboprophylaxis during pregnancy requires adjustments in dose. As pregnancy progresses and the maternal volume of distribution changes, it is necessary to measure plasma anti–factor Xa levels 4 to 6 hours after LMWH administration and adjust the dose to achieve an anti–factor Xa level of 0.7 to 1.2 U/mL. The use of standard doses of LMWH during pregnancy in women with mechanical prosthetic heart valves may not provide adequate anticoagulation; the U.S. Food and Drug Administration has required labeling on these products to specifically indicate that the use of these agents in pregnant women with mechanical prosthetic heart valves has not been adequately studied.

A systematic review of anticoagulation in pregnant women with mechanical heart valves evaluated outcomes with the following anticoagulation regimens: (1) oral anticoagulants (most commonly warfarin) given throughout pregnancy, (2) heparin administered during the first trimester and then warfarin for the duration of pregnancy, and (3) heparin administered throughout pregnancy.[108] The data demonstrated a progressive increase in rates of maternal death with regimens 1, 2, and 3 (i.e., 1.8%, 4.2%, and 15.0%, respectively). The use of warfarin throughout pregnancy was associated with warfarin embryopathy in 6.4% of live-born infants. The substitution of heparin at or before 6 weeks' gestation eliminated that risk.[108]

For pregnant women with prosthetic heart valves, the American College of Chest Physicians (ACCP) has recommended use of one of the following three thromboprophylactic regimens: (1) administration of adjusted-dose, twice-daily LMWH throughout pregnancy; (2) aggressive adjusted-dose UFH throughout pregnancy; or (3) administration of either UFH or LMWH in the first trimester, and then warfarin until close to delivery, when either UFH or LMWH is resumed (see Box 41-4).[63] In high-risk women with prosthetic heart valves, the ACCP suggests the addition of low-dose aspirin to the anticoagulation regimen.[63]

OBSTETRIC MANAGEMENT

Cesarean delivery is reserved for obstetric indications.[102] Some obstetricians may perform an elective instrumental vaginal delivery to shorten the duration of the second stage of labor. The cardiologist may recommend maintenance of anticoagulation during labor and delivery, which may predispose to increased hemorrhage during and after delivery.

ANESTHETIC MANAGEMENT

The maintenance of anticoagulation therapy may contraindicate the administration of neuraxial anesthesia. Long-term use of heparin may also result in thrombocytopenia. Normal or near-normal coagulation parameters and an adequate platelet count should be present both before administration of neuraxial anesthesia in these patients and before the withdrawal of an epidural or spinal catheter. Systemic opioid administration is an alternative form of analgesia for anticoagulated patients; however, the quality of analgesia is not as good as that provided by neuraxial techniques (see Chapter 22).

If cesarean delivery is required, the anticoagulated patient will require general anesthesia. Residual valvular and myocardial dysfunction will affect decisions about the use of invasive hemodynamic monitoring and the choice of anesthetic agents.

The Second American Society of Regional Anesthesia and Pain Medicine (ASRA) Consensus Conference on Neuraxial Anesthesia and Anticoagulation published a risk assessment with clinical guidelines in 2003.[109] Because the ASRA document does not specifically address management of pregnant women, institution-specific protocols have been developed. The following guidelines reflect our current practice:

1. UFH is discontinued with the onset of active labor. Neuraxial analgesia/anesthesia is withheld until the activated partial thromboplastin time (aPTT) value is near normal or the blood heparin concentration is near zero. Until these conditions are met, the patient is offered intravenous opioid analgesia for labor.
2. Patients and their obstetricians are counseled during early pregnancy that the use of LMWH thromboprophylaxis precludes the use of neuraxial analgesic/anesthetic techniques until at least 10 to 12 hours have elapsed since the time of the last *prophylactic* dose. *Therapeutic* anticoagulation with high-dose LMWH precludes the use of neuraxial techniques for 24 hours from the time of the last dose.[109] Standard UFH may be substituted for LMWH by 38 weeks' gestation to allow (1) faster resolution of anticoagulant activity and (2) the ability to monitor anticoagulation activity through measurement of the aPTT.[110]
3. Protamine reversal of heparin therapy to allow administration of neuraxial analgesia/anesthesia is not recommended. Protamine neutralizes approximately 60% of the anti–factor Xa activity caused by LMWH, which may be helpful in patients with life-threatening hemorrhage; however, this effect is unpredictable.[110]
4. For patients who have recently received long-term warfarin therapy, the presence of a normal (or near-normal) prothrombin time (PT) and International Normalized Ratio (INR) should be confirmed before administration of a neuraxial anesthetic technique.[109]
5. If cesarean delivery is required in a patient with abnormal coagulation, general anesthesia is administered.
6. The re-institution of anticoagulation therapy after delivery should be discussed with the obstetrician and cardiologist. The risk of bleeding (including epidural hematoma) should be weighed against the risk of thromboembolic complications. For postpartum *thromboprophylaxis* with once-daily doses of LMWH, we prefer to wait 6 to 8 hours after operative delivery before giving the first dose of LMWH; the second postoperative dose is given no sooner than 24 hours after the first

dose. For patients receiving *therapeutic* (i.e., twice-daily) doses of LMWH, we prefer to wait at least 24 hours after operative delivery before giving the first postpartum dose of LMWH.* Similarly, when blood is detected during needle and catheter placement, initiation of LMWH therapy should be delayed for 24 hours.[109]

7. Removal of the epidural catheter may also cause venous disruption and bleeding into the epidural space. The ASRA guidelines state that neuraxial catheters may be safely maintained in patients receiving single daily doses of LMWH postoperatively.[109] The catheter should be removed at least 10 to 12 hours after the last dose of LMWH, and subsequent doses of LMWH should be administered a minimum of 2 hours after catheter removal. For patients receiving twice-daily doses of LMWH, indwelling catheters should be removed *before* initiation of LMWH thromboprophylaxis. In these women, the first dose of LMWH should not be administered until at least 2 hours have elapsed since catheter removal.[109]
8. For patients in whom warfarin is started after delivery, the neuraxial catheter should be removed while the INR remains less than 1.5.[109]

Cardiac Surgery during Pregnancy

The first reported case of cardiopulmonary bypass during pregnancy occurred in 1958 and consisted of an aortic valvuloplasty at 4 months' gestation.[111] Mortality rates in pregnant women who undergo cardiopulmonary bypass, which are less than 5%, are similar to those in nonpregnant women; however, fetal mortality rates range from 4% to 33%.[112] Possible contributing factors to fetal loss include the severity of the maternal cardiac condition and the effects of cardiopulmonary bypass itself (altered coagulation, complement activation, risk of air embolism, hypotension, nonpulsatile flow, hypothermia).[112]

High pump flow rates (> 2.5 L/min/m^2) and high mean arterial pressures (> 70 mm Hg) are recommended to optimize uteroplacental perfusion. Fetal bradycardia often occurs during the initiation of cardiopulmonary bypass and then normalizes. Several investigators have noted that both the baseline FHR and FHR variability decrease during cardiopulmonary bypass.[113,114] These changes occur in addition to the reduced FHR variability that occurs with the administration of general anesthesia. An increase in pump flow results in a higher FHR in some but not all cases.[114]

Systemic hypothermia is used during cardiopulmonary bypass to help preserve the myocardium and to decrease total-body oxygen demands. It is not clear whether the hypothermia itself is the cause of adverse fetal outcomes. If possible, it seems prudent to maintain normothermia or use only moderate hypothermia (i.e., not less than 32° C).

The second trimester is probably the optimal time for cardiac surgery during pregnancy. Management should focus on the optimization of maternal conditions before, during, and after surgery. Fortunately, women who have undergone successful repair of cardiac lesions can expect good reproductive outcome in subsequent pregnancies.[115]

PERIPARTUM CARDIOMYOPATHY

Peripartum cardiomyopathy is a rare but devastating form of heart failure, which by definition manifests during the last month of pregnancy or during the first 5 postpartum months in patients with no preexisting heart disease and no other obvious reason for heart failure.[116] The incidence is 1 in 3000 to 1 in 15,000 live births in the United States, with an overall higher incidence in Africa (1 in 3000).[117] The presentation is often insidious. Initially, the clinical presentation may be limited to symptoms of a mild upper respiratory infection, chest congestion, and fatigue. These symptoms can rapidly progress to florid cardiac failure with biventricular hypokinesis, low cardiac output, elevated filling pressures, and ventricular ectopy.[118]

Peripartum cardiomyopathy should be distinguished from other causes of cardiomyopathies that tend to present earlier in pregnancy, but are potentially amenable to therapy. These other causes of cardiomyopathy may represent known or previously undiagnosed heart disorders that are revealed by the hemodynamic alterations of pregnancy.

Ejection fraction improves similarly in patients with peripartum cardiomyopathy and patients with other causes of cardiomyopathy, with about half of patients returning to a normal ejection fraction greater than 50%.[119] This improvement in ejection fraction is greater among patients in whom ejection fraction was greater than 30% at the time of diagnosis. Maternal mortality rates are also similar in the two groups.[119]

The etiology of peripartum cardiomyopathy is unknown. Viral myocarditis, immune-mediated injury, and the hemodynamic stress of pregnancy have been suggested as causes.[120-123] Other possible etiologies include nutritional deficiencies, small-vessel coronary artery disease, excessive salt intake, and peripartum fluid shifts.[120,124,125] Peripartum cardiomyopathy appears to occur more commonly in women with multiple gestation,[126] obesity, or advanced maternal age, and also in women who breast-feed.

**Editors' Note:* The timing of the first postpartum dose of LMWH is controversial, given the limited data on bleeding complications following the use of LMWH thromboprophylaxis after delivery. Some anesthesia providers and institutional guidelines advocate a delay in postpartum LMWH administration on the basis of the time elapsed since epidural or spinal needle placement (see Chapter 38). The ASRA guidelines suggest that the delay in LMWH administration should be based on the time elapsed after the completion of surgery, but those guidelines do not specifically address the management of pregnant women.[109] The more conservative approach (namely, that the first dose of LMWH should be determined by the time elapsed since the completion of operative delivery) allows practitioners to evaluate any hemostatic changes that may have occurred during or immediately after delivery. Admittedly, this approach creates some ambiguity in the management of patients who have had an uncomplicated vaginal delivery. Practitioners should weigh the risk of bleeding (including epidural hematoma) against the risk of thromboembolic complications when deciding the timing of the first postpartum dose of LMWH.

The incidence of gestational hypertension in patients with peripartum cardiomyopathy is approximately 43%, which represents a markedly higher presentation than the overall incidence of 8% to 10% in pregnancy.

DIAGNOSIS

The diagnosis is frequently difficult during the late stages of pregnancy because of the overlap with symptoms of pregnancy. Diagnosis should focus on ruling out the other common causes of cardiomyopathy. The role of routine biopsy in the diagnosis is still controversial.[127]

MANAGEMENT

The management of peripartum cardiomyopathy is largely supportive. Patients who are symptomatic should receive the usual treatment for heart failure and should be managed by a multidisciplinary team.

Early studies suggested that the maternal mortality was as high as 30% to 60%; later studies have reported a maternal mortality rate of 9% with a 14% cardiac transplantation rate.[119] More than 50% of patients show normalization of ejection fraction within 6 months; however, in those in whom a substantial improvement is not observed during this period, the mortality rate is 85% at 5 years.[119] Echocardiographic measurements at the time of diagnosis that demonstrate left ventricular fractional shortening of less than 20% and end-diastolic dimensions of 6 cm or greater have been associated with a threefold higher risk for persistent left ventricular dysfunction.[128]

Obstetric management involves expedient delivery of the infant by cesarean or instrumental vaginal delivery. The mode of delivery for patients with peripartum cardiomyopathy is generally based on obstetric indications. In most cases, vaginal delivery can be attempted after stabilization of the mother.[129] Advantages of a vaginal delivery include less blood loss, greater hemodynamic stability, and less chance of postoperative infection and pulmonary complications. Anticoagulation is indicated, given that peripartum cardiomyopathy increases the risk of thromboembolic events.[130,131]

Anesthetic management for vaginal or cesarean delivery in women with peripartum cardiomyopathy should reflect principles similar to those for any patient with severe cardiomyopathy. General anesthesia (e.g., intravenous technique using a combination of remifentanil and propofol),[132] combined spinal-epidural anesthesia,[133] continuous spinal anesthesia,[134] and epidural anesthesia have been described, and in some cases anesthetic management was guided by pulmonary artery pressure measurements.[129] The use of neuraxial analgesia or anesthesia for either vaginal or cesarean delivery is often determined by the anticoagulation regimen (as discussed earlier).

THE PREGNANT PATIENT WITH A TRANSPLANTED HEART

The two most common indications for cardiac transplantation in the adult population are viral cardiomyopathy and ischemic cardiomyopathy. Viral cardiomyopathy is by far the most common indication in women of childbearing age.[135] Other conditions such as congenital heart disease and peripartum cardiomyopathy are less common indications for transplantation.

Current survival rates after cardiac transplantation average approximately 90% at 1 year and 80% at 5 years.[135] A growing number of women have undergone cardiac transplantation for the treatment of end-stage cardiomyopathy and subsequently have had successful pregnancies with uncomplicated vaginal or cesarean delivery.[136]

In patients who have undergone cardiac transplantation, pregnancy presents unique cardiovascular stresses and risks for rejection and infection. The hemodynamic changes of pregnancy are usually well tolerated.[137,138] Despite the fact that pregnancy is considered an immunologically suppressed state, the incidence of rejection is not lower during pregnancy or higher in the postpartum period than in the nonpregnant state.[138] However, the immunosuppression of pregnancy may lead to a higher incidence of infection; therefore, rigorous adherence to asepsis protocols is recommended.

PATHOPHYSIOLOGY

The transplanted heart has no afferent or efferent autonomic or somatic innervation,[139,140] a condition with the following consequences. First, the lack of vagal innervation causes the baseline heart rate to be fast (100 to 120 bpm), and reflex slowing of the heart rate (e.g., oculocardiac reflex, carotid massage) does not occur. In addition, the normal heart rate variation with respiration (sinus arrhythmia) is absent. Drugs that act by means of the vagus nerve (e.g., atropine, neostigmine) have no cardiac effects, although they stimulate peripheral cholinergic receptors. Second, only direct-acting sympathomimetic agents (e.g., isoproterenol) reliably produce chronotropic or inotropic effects. Third, chronic denervation results in the "up-regulation" of cardiac beta-adrenergic receptors,[141] leading to greater sensitivity to beta-adrenergic receptor stimulation.[142] Camann et al.[141] observed profound tachycardia after epidural administration of 12 mL of 2% lidocaine with 1:200,000 epinephrine in a pregnant patient with a transplanted heart. Fourth, the chronotropic response to stress is delayed. Adequate cardiac output depends on maintenance of adequate preload (the Starling mechanism).

INTERACTION WITH PREGNANCY

Women who have undergone heart transplantation tolerate pregnancy well, provided that the function of the transplant was stable before pregnancy.[143] Complications in such pregnancies are related to the immunosuppressive therapy; they include hypertension, preeclampsia, infection, and episodes of acute rejection, preterm delivery, and delivery of a low-birth-weight infant.[144,145] Maternal immunosuppressive therapy does not appear to have an adverse effect on fetal or neonatal outcome.[146] Patients undergoing cyclosporine and prednisone therapy often experience hypertension, which typically requires antihypertensive therapy.[144] The physiologic changes of normal pregnancy (e.g., increases in blood volume and renal blood flow, alteration in drug clearance) may require a change in the dose of cyclosporine.

ANESTHETIC MANAGEMENT

Preanesthetic assessment of the pregnant woman with a heart transplant should include special attention to exercise tolerance after transplantation and during pregnancy. Recent reports of cardiac catheterization and echocardiography should be sought. Most cardiac transplant recipients undergo routine yearly cardiac catheterization for at least the following three reasons: (1) coronary atherosclerosis is accelerated in transplanted hearts, (2) complete afferent denervation prevents the occurrence of angina during myocardial ischemia, and (3) endomyocardial biopsies may provide early evidence of allograft rejection.

The patient with a heart transplant requires an intrapartum "stress" dose of corticosteroids if corticosteroids are part of her immunosuppressive regimen. Regardless of the method of delivery or anesthetic technique, strict aseptic techniques must be employed during performance of invasive procedures in the immunosuppressed patient.

It is essential to avoid aortocaval compression and to maintain adequate intravascular volume and venous return. Some physicians favor the measurement of CVP. However, women with good ventricular function and no evidence of rejection should be able to tolerate the volume changes of labor and delivery.[135] Infection is a major cause of morbidity because of the immunosuppression, and in most cases, the risk of catheter-induced sepsis likely outweighs the benefit of CVP monitoring during labor and vaginal delivery.

Women who have undergone heart transplantation have delivered vaginally with[144] and without[139] epidural anesthesia. Slow induction of epidural analgesia with a dilute solution of local anesthetic with an opioid may decrease the extent of sympathectomy and the incidence and severity of hypotension. If hypotension should occur, small doses of phenylephrine may be administered safely. Ephedrine has both a direct and indirect mechanism of action, and it may be less effective than expected. If a chronotropic agent is required, isoproterenol (not atropine) should be administered.

Epidural anesthesia is the preferred anesthetic technique for cesarean delivery. With slow induction of epidural anesthesia, compensatory mechanisms (e.g., vasoconstriction above the level of sympathetic blockade) reduce the likelihood of severe hypotension. Additional crystalloid can be given to maintain adequate intravascular volume and venous return. Spinal anesthesia has been administered successfully for cesarean delivery in women who have undergone heart-lung transplantation.[147] Both spinal anesthesia and general anesthesia have been used successfully for a wide variety of surgical procedures in nonpregnant patients with a transplanted heart.[135] If general anesthesia is required, it seems reasonable to use ketamine rather than thiopental to preserve sympathetic tone during the induction of anesthesia.

CARDIOPULMONARY RESUSCITATION DURING PREGNANCY

Cardiac arrest during late pregnancy occurs in approximately 1 in 30,000 pregnancies.[148] Major causes are listed in Box 41-5. The outcome depends on the underlying cause of the arrest and the duration of the interval between cardiac arrest and the start of resuscitation. The stage of gestation may affect some management decisions (see later).[149,150]

Advanced cardiac life support (ACLS) protocols are applicable to the pregnant patient, with a few important additional considerations.[150-152] The pregnant woman should be intubated promptly after the initiation of cardiopulmonary resuscitation (CPR), not only to facilitate oxygenation and ventilation but also to protect the airway from the aspiration of gastric contents. Also, chest compressions should be performed "slightly above the center of the sternum to adjust for the elevation of the diaphragm."[151]

BOX 41-5 Major Causes of Cardiac Arrest during Pregnancy

- Amniotic fluid embolism
- Hemorrhage
  - Disseminated intravascular coagulation
  - Placental abruption
  - Placental previa
  - Uterine atony
- Iatrogenic
  - Anesthetic complications
  - Hypermagnesemia
  - Medication errors or allergy
- Preexisting heart disease
  - Congenital
  - Acquired
- Pregnancy-induced hypertension
- Sepsis
- Trauma
- Venous thromboembolism

Adapted from Mallampalli A, Powner DJ, Gardner MO. Cardiopulmonary resuscitation and somatic support of the pregnant patient. Crit Care Clin 2004; 20:747-61.

It is essential to maintain left uterine displacement during CPR. A folded pillow or wedge should be placed beneath the mother's right hip and flank. Alternatively, the uterus can be displaced leftward manually, but this is a less reliable means of relieving aortocaval compression. Cardiac compressions are most efficiently accomplished with the patient on a hard surface. Rees and Willis[149] described the use of a Cardiff wedge, which provides both relief of aortocaval compression and a firm surface for chest compressions. In the absence of a Cardiff wedge, a hard surface and a "human wedge" may be used.[153] A person designated as a human wedge kneels on the floor, sitting on the heels. This person, who need not be medically trained, subsequently uses one arm to stabilize the patient's shoulders and the other arm to stabilize the pelvis (Figure 41-1).

Optimal care of the mother is the best therapy for the fetus. The drug protocols used for ACLS in nonpregnant patients should also be used in pregnant patients.[148,150,152] The American Heart Association (AHA)[150] has stated:

> *The treatments listed in the standard ACLS Pulseless Arrest Algorithm, including recommendations and doses for defibrillation [and] medications ... apply to cardiac arrest in the pregnant woman. ... Vasopressor agents such as epinephrine, vasopressin, and dopamine will decrease blood flow to the uterus. There are no alternatives, however, to using all indicated medications in recommended doses. The mother must be resuscitated or the chances of fetal resuscitation vanish.*[150]

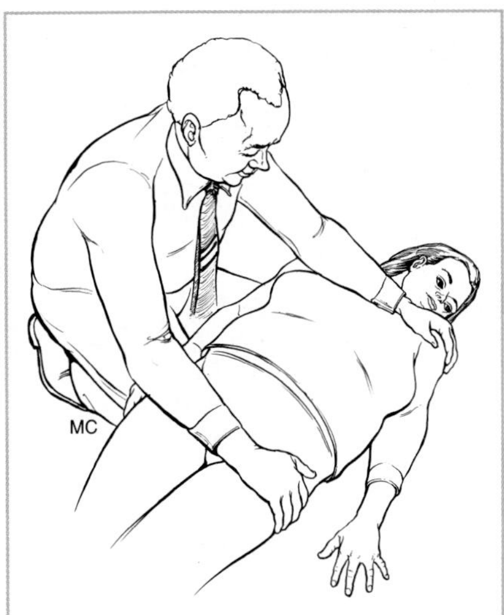

FIGURE 41-1 The human wedge position for cardiopulmonary resuscitation of a pregnant woman.

If initial efforts to restore oxygenation, ventilation, and circulation are unsuccessful in a pregnant woman who has suffered cardiac arrest after 20 weeks' gestation, the physician should consider immediate hysterotomy and delivery.[150,154] Extrauterine survival of the infant is unlikely before 24 weeks' gestation; however, the AHA[150] has endorsed performance of an emergency hysterotomy as early as 20 weeks' gestation to enable successful resuscitation of the mother. Evacuation of the uterus allows relief of aortocaval compression and restoration of venous return to the heart. In a review of 188 perimortem cesarean deliveries performed between 1900 and 1985, Katz et al.[155] identified data on 61 surviving infants. The investigators found that 70% of surviving infants were delivered within 5 minutes of maternal death. This is the basis of the "4-minute rule," which advocates the initiation of cesarean delivery within 4 minutes of cardiac arrest, with neonatal delivery within 5 minutes.[148] Subsequent to the reporting of this 4-minute rule, Katz et al.[156] reviewed 38 cases of perimortem cesarean delivery in which 34 infants survived. Data from the interval between cardiac arrest and delivery was available for 24 infants: 11 were delivered within 5 minutes, 4 between 6 and 10 minutes, 2 between 11 and 15 minutes, and 7 after 15 minutes. Thirteen of 20 mothers with causes of cardiac arrest potentially amenable to resuscitation were discharged from the hospital. Twelve of 18 reports demonstrated an improvement in maternal hemodynamic status after cesarean delivery as a result of relief of aortocaval compression and restoration of venous return, decreased metabolic demands, and provision of more effective chest compressions.

The AHA has concluded:

The resuscitation team leader should consider the need for an emergency hysterotomy (cesarean delivery) protocol as soon as a pregnant woman develops cardiac arrest. The best survival rate for infants >24 to 25 weeks' gestation occurs when the delivery of the infant occurs no more than 5 minutes after the mother's heart stops beating. This typically requires that the provider begin the hysterotomy about 4 minutes after cardiac arrest. Emergency hysterotomy . . . may seem counterintuitive given that the key to salvage of a potentially viable infant is resuscitation of the mother. But the mother cannot be resuscitated unless venous return and aortic output are restored.[150]

If delivery does not facilitate successful maternal resuscitation, physicians should consider other measures, including thoracotomy, open-chest cardiac massage, and cardiopulmonary bypass. Cardiopulmonary bypass has been used as part of maternal resuscitation as a method of rewarming patients who have become hypothermic as a result of rapid, massive volume infusion,[157] in the management of bupivacaine-induced cardiac toxicity,[158] and during the performance of pulmonary embolectomy in patients with a massive pulmonary embolus.[159] Intravenous administration of lipid emulsion has also been described for the treatment of maternal cardiac arrest resulting from systemic local anesthetic toxicity (see Chapters 13 and 23).

Maternal complications that can occur when CPR is performed during pregnancy include laceration of the liver, uterine rupture, hemothorax, and hemopericardium. The newborn infant is likely to be hypoxic and acidotic. Fetal/neonatal hypoxia results from decreased maternal cardiac output, uteroplacental vasoconstriction, and maternal hypoxemia and acidosis.[160]

There are no specific AHA guidelines for CPR in the immediate postpartum period. Right hip displacement should be maintained because the postpartum uterus may still cause significant aortocaval compression. The patient should lie on a firm surface to facilitate chest compressions. Open-chest cardiac massage is used when standard closed-chest resuscitation algorithms fail.

ARRHYTHMIAS

Arrhythmias occur with increased frequency during pregnancy. Robins and Lyons[161] suggested an incidence of symptomatic supraventricular tachycardia during pregnancy of 1 in 8000 pregnancies. Carson et al.[162] found that 39% of healthy asymptomatic pregnant women had sinus tachycardia in the third trimester, the incidence of which was 58% in obese parturients. The most common arrhythmias witnessed in pregnancy are associated with premature atrial and ventricular contractions.

The incidence of arrhythmias is known to increase with labor. An ECG study in normal laboring women found that nearly all the tracings had some abnormality, including premature atrial and ventricular contractions, nodal complexes, sinus tachycardia, and paroxysmal ventricular tachycardia.[163] The higher frequency of arrhythmias during pregnancy may be a result of the associated hemodynamic, hormonal, and autonomic changes. It has been postulated that estrogens may heighten cardiac excitability and may sensitize the myocardium to catecholamines by increasing the number of alpha-adrenergic receptors.[164-166] Silversides et al.[167] determined the recurrence rates of arrhythmias in pregnancy in women with a history of rhythm disorders and examined the impact on fetal and neonatal outcomes. Of women who were in sinus rhythm at baseline, 44% experienced a recurrence of arrhythmias during pregnancy. Adverse fetal and neonatal outcomes

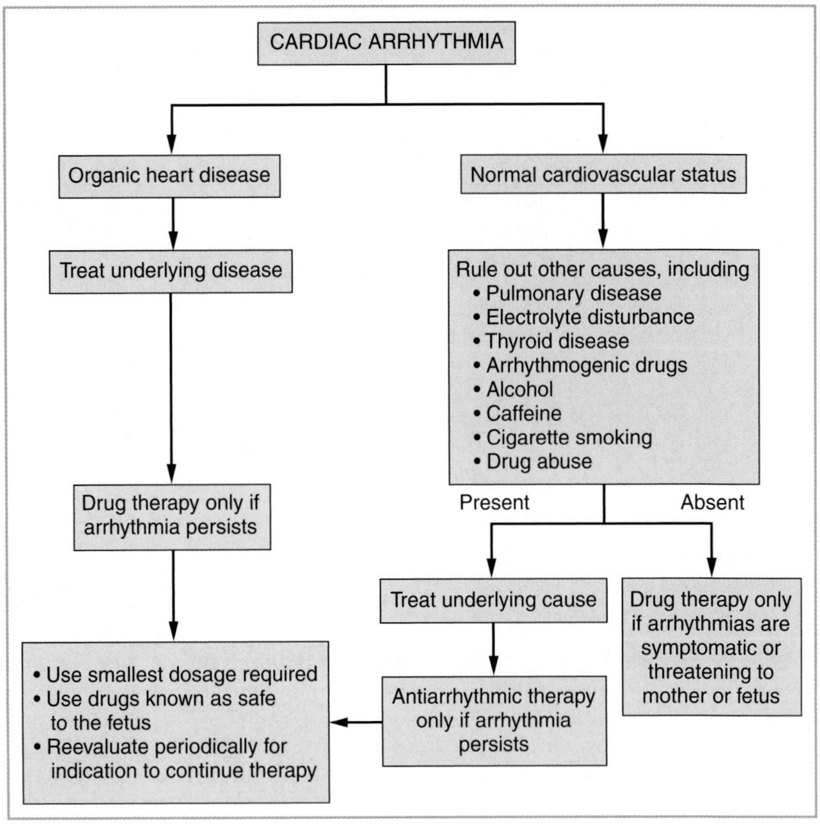

FIGURE 41-2 Management of cardiac arrhythmias during pregnancy. (From Rotmensch HH, Rotmensch S, Elkayam U, et al. Management of cardiac arrhythmias during pregnancy: Current concepts. Drugs 1987; 33:623-33.)

occurred in 17 of 87 births and included preterm delivery, small size for gestational age, fetal demise, respiratory distress syndrome, and intraventricular hemorrhage. Management should be guided by the underlying heart disease, observed rhythm, and available therapies (Figure 41-2).

Antiarrhythmic Medications

DIGITALIS

Digoxin is widely used for the treatment of a variety of maternal atrial tachyarrhythmias and has been used extensively in pregnancy for decades. Enhanced renal function during pregnancy facilitates the excretion of digoxin, although dose requirements are believed to be similar during pregnant and nonpregnant states.[168] Digoxin crosses the placenta and produces drug levels in the fetus that are similar to those found in the mother.[169,170] The maternal digoxin concentration should be monitored at regular intervals, but there is no evidence that therapeutic maternal levels affect the neonatal ECG.[169] In the past, some women received digoxin for treatment of fetal tachyarrhythmias; however, maternal-fetal medicine specialists now give digoxin directly to the fetus. Digoxin is secreted in breast milk but is unlikely to cause any harm to the neonate.[171]

QUINIDINE

Quinidine is used to treat a variety of atrial tachyarrhythmias and has been used safely during pregnancy for decades, without any evidence of teratogenicity. This drug has mild oxytocic properties and may be associated with preterm labor.[172] Quinidine has a high affinity for plasma protein, and it may be necessary to adjust the dose during pregnancy.

BETA-ADRENERGIC RECEPTOR ANTAGONISTS

Propranolol, atenolol, and metoprolol have been widely used during pregnancy for a variety of indications, including hypertension, mitral stenosis, HOCM, and control of heart rate with both atrial and ventricular tachyarrhythmias. The drugs are generally well tolerated.[173] Labetalol has become a popular choice for the treatment of hypertension in women with preeclampsia.

These medications readily cross the placenta. There have been reports of IUGR, fetal bradycardia, and neonatal hypoglycemia during maternal use of a beta-adrenergic receptor antagonist.[174] The incidence of these effects is low. However, the obstetrician and anesthesiologist should be aware of the potential for acute fetal bradycardia during or after intravenous administration of a beta-adrenergic receptor antagonist.[94-96] Esmolol rapidly crosses the placenta but is eliminated rapidly from the plasma of both maternal and fetal sheep. Eisenach and Castro[95] observed that prolonged maternal administration of esmolol resulted in fetal hypoxemia in gravid ewes. It is unclear whether short-term maternal administration of esmolol adversely affects the human fetus. The FHR should be monitored during and after intravenous administration of a beta-adrenergic receptor antagonist.

CALCIUM ENTRY–BLOCKING AGENTS

Verapamil may be administered intravenously to suppress an acute maternal tachyarrhythmia.[175] However, peripheral vasodilation and negative inotropy may occur after intravenous administration, so maternal blood pressure should be monitored closely. Verapamil crosses the placenta to a limited degree. Murad et al.[176] noted that fetal blood concentrations of verapamil were 35% to 45% of maternal blood concentrations; these levels are sufficient to produce a marked slowing of atrioventricular conduction in the fetus.[177] The concentration of verapamil and diltiazem are approximately the same in breast milk as in maternal blood.[178,179] Another calcium entry–blocking agent (nicardipine) has been used for the treatment of hypertension in women with severe preeclampsia.[180]

LIDOCAINE

Lidocaine has been used for the treatment of ectopic ventricular arrhythmias during pregnancy.[172] The patient receiving lidocaine should be monitored for evidence of local anesthetic toxicity (e.g., somnolence, tinnitus, convulsions). Fetal acidosis, if present, may result in the phenomenon of ion trapping, with unexpectedly high fetal blood concentrations of lidocaine (see Chapter 13).

AMIODARONE

Amiodarone is a potentially problematic drug for use during pregnancy; published reports have described adverse fetal effects such as IUGR, preterm delivery, and fetal hypothyroidism.[181,182] Neonatal bradycardia and prolongation of the QT interval in the infant have also been described.[183,184] This medication has been used to treat refractory maternal atrial and ventricular arrhythmias[185,186] as well as fetal tachyarrhythmias.[187] Amiodarone contains iodine, and its long-term use presents a large load of iodine to both maternal and fetal tissues. The exposure to iodine is the proposed mechanism for the high incidence of hypothyroidism in adults using this medication, which presumably has the same effect on the fetus.[181]

Amiodarone is used in pregnant women primarily to treat refractory arrhythmias that are unresponsive to other agents.[188] Amiodarone is now the preferred agent for treatment of life-threatening ventricular arrhythmias in the ACLS algorithm. This agent also now seems to be the drug of choice for treatment of bupivacaine-induced ventricular arrhythmias, although its clinical efficacy in this setting is unproven. (Intravenous administration of lipid emulsion has also been described as an effective treatment of severe systemic local anesthetic toxicity; see Chapters 13 and 23.)

ADENOSINE

Adenosine has become the agent of choice for the acute management of tachyarrhythmias. The primary indication for adenosine is paroxysmal supraventricular tachycardia, the most common arrhythmia in pregnant women.[172] Adenosine is unlikely to affect the fetus adversely because it has such a short plasma half-life. The onset of action is rapid, and the duration of action is brief. Side effects (e.g., hypotension, dizziness, flushing, dyspnea) are common, but they are transient and minor. Numerous case reports and a retrospective study suggest that adenosine is safe and effective.[189,190] Afridi et al.[191] described the use of adenosine to treat hemodynamically significant supraventricular tachycardia associated with Wolff-Parkinson-White syndrome in a patient at 7 months' gestation. In that case, concomitant fetal bradycardia resolved when adenosine converted the maternal tachyarrhythmia to a normal sinus rhythm.

Caution should be exercised in the use of adenosine. Narrow-complex supraventricular rhythms respond well to adenosine, but if atrial fibrillation or flutter is present, conduction through an accessory tract may be enhanced and the rhythm disturbance may actually worsen.

Treatment of Congenital Heart Block and Bradyarrhythmias

Congenital complete heart block is a rare syndrome. There are published cases of asymptomatic women with this syndrome who underwent uncomplicated pregnancy and delivery.[192] Nonetheless, if congenital heart block is recognized in a pregnant woman, a cardiology evaluation is warranted to determine whether placement of a pacemaker (either temporary or permanent) is indicated. Published guidelines for asymptomatic heart block do not support the requirement for a permanent pacemaker.[193] However, for symptomatic patients in the first and second trimesters, permanent pacemaker implantation is the therapy of choice. If the patient is at or near term, temporary pacing immediately before the induction of labor can prevent the complications of prolonged temporary pacing. Because altered hemodynamics can contribute to the patient's symptoms during pregnancy, the patient should be reassessed in the postpartum period before implantation of a permanent pacemaker.[194] Women with permanent pacemakers for symptomatic bradyarrhythmias have had successful pregnancies and deliveries. Pacemakers can be inserted with electrocardiographic or echocardiographic guidance to avoid fetal exposure to ionizing radiation. During labor, the use of epidural analgesia is recommended to minimize maternal expulsive efforts (which might cause a reflex slowing of heart rate) and to facilitate a painless instrumental vaginal delivery.

Prolonged QT Syndrome and Ventricular Tachycardia

Long QT syndrome represents a group of arrhythmogenic cardiovascular disorders originating from cardiac ion channel mutations.[195] Long QT syndrome can be inherited in an autosomal dominant or recessive fashion, or acquired through the presence of drugs, electrolyte imbalances, or metabolic conditions.[196,197] Congenital long QT syndrome is an important cause of sudden death in young people.[196] The annual mortality in untreated patients is 1% to 2%.[198] Prolonged QT syndromes increase the risk for *torsades de pointes* and cardiac arrest during pregnancy.

Therapy with beta-adrenergic receptor antagonists is the mainstay of treatment.[199] Cardiac pacing may be required in patients unresponsive to beta-adrenergic receptor blockade.[200] Critical episodes may be treated with cardioversion or defibrillation. Patients who survive cardiac arrest and are symptomatic despite therapy or have a QT interval longer than 550 msec should be considered for implantation of an AICD.[196,197] AICDs are being utilized more frequently in the obstetric population with good outcomes.[201,202]

Epidural analgesia offers distinct advantages for labor, including (1) preservation of maternal hemodynamic stability, (2) minimization of increases in catecholamine concentrations during labor and delivery, and (3) direct suppression of arrhythmias by pharmacologically active plasma levels of local anesthetic agents.[201] Epidural analgesia may be readily converted to epidural anesthesia for cesarean delivery, if necessary.

Cardioversion

Direct-current cardioversion may be necessary for tachyarrhythmias that are resistant to pharmacologic therapy and/or those that are producing hemodynamic instability. Direct-current cardioversion has been used in parturients at all stages of pregnancy without significant complications.[203] The amount of current reaching the fetus is considered to be negligible.

The risk of pulmonary aspiration of gastric contents should be weighed against the risk of general anesthesia associated with endotracheal intubation. The judicious use of sedation rather than full general anesthesia and endotracheal intubation is usually preferred in this setting. A benzodiazepine, a barbiturate, or propofol can provide satisfactory sedation and amnesia. Women with severe hemodynamic instability may not tolerate the administration of any dose of a sedative drug. Regardless of whether sedation or general anesthesia is selected, a nonparticulate oral antacid should be provided; administration of a histamine (H_2)-receptor antagonist to increase the gastric pH should be considered. The use of metoclopramide in these patients is controversial owing to its possible association with tachyarrhythmias.

The FHR should be monitored because transient FHR abnormalities (and, rarely, sustained fetal bradycardia) may occur during or after cardioversion.[204]

DISEASES OF THE AORTA

Marfan's Syndrome

Marfan's syndrome results from a defect in fibrillin synthesis due to a mutation of its gene on chromosome 15.[205] Patients with the disease who are contemplating pregnancy should be aware of the dominant pattern of inheritance. Patients with Marfan's syndrome have long, slender extremities, joint laxity, and many other musculoskeletal abnormalities. In addition, they have MVP and demonstrate a dilation of the ascending aorta, which may progress to a dissecting aneurysm, aortic incompetence, and rupture of the aorta. Replacement of the ascending aorta in asymptomatic patients is recommended when the root diameter exceeds 5.5 cm.[206] Maternal mortality has been reported to be as high as 50% in pregnant patients with aortic root diameter greater than 4.5 cm, aortic regurgitation, left ventricular dilation, hypertension, or coarctation.[207] However, Meijboom et al.[208] reported pregnancy to be relatively safe in patients with aortic root diameters up to 4.5 cm, although such pregnancies are associated with a high rate of preterm rupture of the membranes and preterm delivery and with increased neonatal mortality.

In general, women with Marfan's syndrome and minimal cardiovascular disease may tolerate pregnancy quite well. Nonetheless, these patients should be carefully observed for symptoms of aortic dissection.[209] Although serial echocardiographic evaluations have been reported to be misleading in the diagnosis of aortic dissection,[210] some physicians have suggested that pregnant patients with Marfan's syndrome should have monthly transthoracic echocardiography to check aortic dimensions. If aortic root involvement is noted, management should be directed toward strict blood pressure control and minimization of shear stress within the aorta.

Some evidence suggests that Marfan's syndrome is associated with cervical incompetence, abnormal placentation, and postpartum hemorrhage.[211]

Aortic Dissection

Acute aortic dissection may occur in association with severe hypertension due to preeclampsia, coarctation of the aorta, or connective tissue disease such as Marfan's and Ehlers-Danlos syndromes. Other risk factors include systemic hypertension (chronic hypertension is present in 70% to 90% of patients with aortic dissection[212]) and a congenitally bicuspid aortic valve.[213] One half of all cases of aortic rupture in women younger than 40 years are associated with pregnancy.[213] Some physicians have suggested that the cardiovascular changes of pregnancy (i.e., increases in blood volume, cardiac output, stroke volume, and heart rate) impose significant stress on the wall of the aorta. Konishi et al.[214] reviewed 51 cases of dissecting aneurysm of the aorta and its branches during pregnancy and the puerperium. Approximately 6% of cases occurred during the first trimester, 10% during the second trimester, and 51% during the third trimester. About 14% of the dissections occurred during labor, and the remaining 20% during the puerperium. In a pregnancy with aortic dissection, maternal mortality is as high as 25%.[206,215]

PATHOPHYSIOLOGY

With aortic dissection, blood moves through a tear in the aortic intima and separates the intima from the adventitia. Most dissections extend distally, but proximal propagation can occur. A false lumen results, which can reconnect with the true lumen anywhere along the course of the dissection. Rupture of the aorta is typically fatal. It occurs most frequently in the pericardial space and left pleural cavity and produces both pericardial tamponade and hemothorax.[216]

The most common point of origin is within the ascending aorta within a few centimeters of the aortic valve. The second most common location is within the descending thoracic aorta just distal to the origin of the left subclavian artery. DeBakey et al.[217] identified three types of aortic dissection (Figure 41-3). A type I dissection extends beyond the ascending aorta into the descending aorta; a type II dissection is confined to the ascending aorta. Type III dissections originate in the descending thoracic aorta; a type IIIA dissection remains above the diaphragm, and a type IIIB dissection extends below the diaphragm. Type I and type II dissections may be complicated by aortic insufficiency, pericardial tamponade, dissection (or obstruction) of major branches of the aortic arch, compression of a mainstem bronchus, and laryngeal nerve compression.

DIAGNOSIS

Prompt medical and surgical management improves the chances of survival in pregnant women with aortic dissection. Aortic dissection should be included in the differential diagnosis whenever a woman complains of severe chest or back pain during pregnancy or the puerperium.

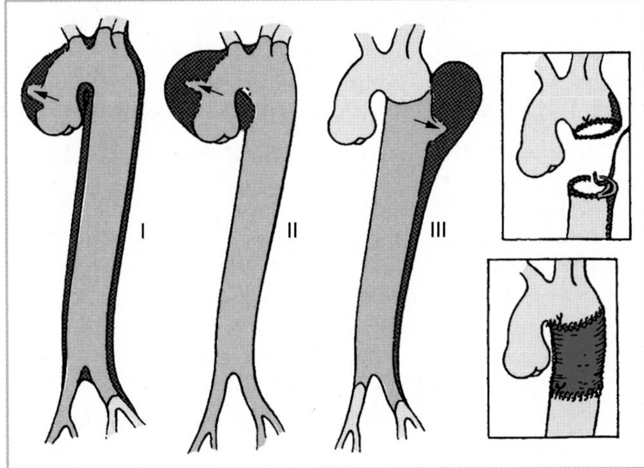

FIGURE 41-3 Classification of aortic dissections. *Arrow* indicates the site of origin for the dissection. Window *insets* illustrate the method of repair. (Courtesy of Dr. Lawrence H. Cohn, Boston.)

Other clinical symptoms and signs are shortness of breath, syncope, tachycardia, and an ischemic extremity. Differential blood pressure in the arms or differential pulses in the lower extremities may be noted.

Chest radiographic examination may show a widening mediastinum or hemothorax. Aortography establishes the definitive diagnosis. Magnetic resonance imaging is a useful technique for the evaluation of aortic disease because it avoids radiation exposure while providing excellent imaging of the aorta.

MANAGEMENT

Pregnancy may affect the choice between medical and surgical therapy. The ultimate goal is to save both the mother and fetus, and the decision to repair is often determined by the maternal clinical condition and the stage of gestation. In almost all cases in which aortic dissection is suspected, aggressive control of blood pressure with a vasodilator agent is essential. The use of a beta-adrenergic receptor antagonist decreases the force of ventricular ejection, which reduces shear stress against the aortic wall. Management should involve placement of an intra-arterial catheter and measurement of CVP. Intravenous opioids are important for minimizing pain, which helps diminish forces that can extend the dissection.

It is generally recommended that for an aortic dissection occurring in a pregnant woman before 28 weeks' gestation, the dissection should be surgically repaired and the pregnancy continued. For a dissection occurring beyond 32 weeks' gestation, a cesarean delivery followed immediately by aortic repair should be considered. For a dissection occurring between 28 and 32 weeks' gestation, an aortic repair is performed, and concurrent cesarean delivery is reserved for patients with evidence of fetal compromise.[215]

INFECTIVE ENDOCARDITIS

Infective endocarditis is an ominous condition that imposes a formidable burden on the cardiovascular demands of pregnancy. Fortunately, it is a rare event during pregnancy. One report suggested that infective endocarditis occurs in approximately 1 in 8000 deliveries.[218] Another study, which included an extensive review of the published literature in English and selected European journals, found only 124 cases during a 40-year period before 1986.[219] Among those cases, the maternal and fetal mortality rates were 29% and 23%, respectively. The most recent systematic evaluation, which identified all reported cases of infective endocarditis in pregnancy, found a total of 68 cases from 1965 to 2002.[220] The overall maternal and fetal mortality rates were 22.1% and 14.7%, respectively.

The incidence of infective endocarditis in the obstetric population appears to be declining; this decrease may be attributable to (1) a diminishing prevalence of rheumatic heart disease, (2) a growing adherence to aseptic practices during obstetric procedures, (3) an increasing practice of early treatment of obstetric infections, and (4) a diminishing incidence of illegal abortion. Intravenous drug abuse has emerged as a major cause of infective endocarditis in women of childbearing age.[221]

PATHOPHYSIOLOGY

Infective endocarditis is defined as the invasion and colonization of cardiac valves, endocardium, and congenital or prosthetic cardiac tissue by an infectious pathogen. Colonization results in the development of friable vegetations, which may produce emboli, hemodynamic compromise, and a fulminant clinical course. Although infective endocarditis typically occurs in association with a preexisting cardiac lesion (which provides a roughened surface for bacterial growth), structurally normal hearts may also be affected.[222] Risk factors for the infection of preexisting cardiac lesions include dental and urologic procedures, prolonged intravenous therapy, and intravenous drug abuse. Risk factors for the infection of normal cardiac tissue include prolonged intravenous therapy or intravenous drug abuse, infection of an arteriovenous shunt, and renal dialysis.[222]

Blood-borne bacteria that adhere to damaged or normal endocardial surfaces may form vegetations. Virtually any pathogen can cause endocarditis.

Seaworth and Durack[219] found that streptococci caused the majority (74%) of infective endocarditis cases that followed obstetric and gynecologic procedures. *Streptococcus viridans* was the predominant pathogen, with enterococci and group B streptococci being uncommon pathogens except after an abortion.[219] Parturients with suppressed or deficient immune systems (e.g., patients with acquired immunodeficiency syndrome) are susceptible to uncommon and less virulent pathogens.

DIAGNOSIS

The clinical outcome of infective endocarditis can be improved by prompt diagnosis and aggressive therapy. The infection is commonly divided into subacute and acute types. **Subacute endocarditis** is characterized by a slow, insidious onset of fever, weakness, malaise, and unexplained embolic phenomena. Blood culture results are positive in 90% of cases. Murmurs typically result from the underlying cardiac lesion. Systemic embolism may develop at any time, giving rise to splinter hemorrhages and mucosal petechiae. Septic abscesses can lead to atrioventricular nodal dysfunction, conduction block, and arrhythmias.

Other manifestations are splenomegaly and nephritis secondary to the deposition of antigen-antibody complexes on the glomerular basement membrane. The latter complication may result in renal failure. The major causes of death include congestive heart failure, embolic cerebral infarction, arrhythmias, and renal failure.

Acute infective endocarditis is heralded by an abrupt onset of symptoms, including high fevers, shaking chills, and early onset of embolic phenomena. Skin and mucosal petechiae may occur. Cardiac decompensation appears early and may worsen suddenly with the erosion of a valve or rupture of the chordae tendineae. Murmurs occur in two thirds of patients with vegetations on the left side of the heart. Aortic ring abscesses may produce conduction disturbances or ventricular septal defects. ECG findings may be normal or may indicate arrhythmias or conduction disturbances. Echocardiography can assist in localizing the valvular vegetations or revealing valvular incompetence or left ventricular failure. The major causes of death in patients with acute infective endocarditis include congestive heart failure, arrhythmias, uncontrolled sepsis, septic emboli, and mycotic aneurysm formation with rupture.

MEDICAL AND SURGICAL MANAGEMENT

The medical management of pregnant women with infective endocarditis is essentially identical to that for nonpregnant patients.[220] The choice of therapy is dictated by the identification of the pathogen and the determination of antibiotic sensitivities. Patients should receive a minimum of 4 to 6 weeks of parenteral antibiotic therapy. Complications such as congestive heart failure and arrhythmias are managed as outlined previously.

Indications for surgical intervention include fungal endocarditis, acquired conduction defects, progressive heart failure, acute hemodynamic deterioration, systemic embolization, and persistent sepsis. Surgical interventions commonly herald the presence of a more severe infective process, which subsequently results in higher morbidity and mortality. Bataskov et al.,[223] reviewing 44 obstetric cases of infective endocarditis that required surgery, found a 30% operative mortality rate.

OBSTETRIC AND ANESTHETIC MANAGEMENT

Obstetric management may include the performance of early instrumental vaginal delivery to minimize maternal expulsive efforts during the second stage of labor. Anesthetic management is dictated by the clinical presentation. Patients with evidence of cardiac decompensation require invasive hemodynamic monitoring. Controversy exists regarding the use of neuraxial anesthesia in patients with systemic infection because of the concern that the procedure may cause meningitis or an epidural abscess (see Chapter 36). Although high-grade bacteremia may increase the risk of meningitis after dural puncture, appropriate antibiotic therapy before dural puncture appears to diminish, if not eliminate, this risk.[224] It may be prudent to avoid neuraxial anesthesia in patients with overwhelming sepsis or acute infective endocarditis; the administration of neuraxial anesthesia can be considered in the hemodynamically stable parturient with infective endocarditis in whom the pathogen has been identified and appropriate therapy initiated. Chestnut[225] suggested that the risks of neuraxial techniques in febrile parturients should be individualized and evaluated in terms of the consequences of withholding these techniques; for example, meningitis or an epidural abscess may represent a lesser risk than failure of intubation and aspiration during general anesthesia.

BOX 41-6 High-Risk Cardiac Conditions Associated with the Highest Risk of Adverse Outcome from Endocarditis, for which Antibiotic Prophylaxis for Deliveries Associated with Infection, or Certain Dental Procedures, Is Reasonable

- Prosthetic cardiac valve or prosthetic material used for cardiac valve repair
- Previous infective endocarditis
- Complex congenital heart disease*
  - Unrepaired cyanotic congenital heart disease, including palliative shunts and conduits
  - Completely repaired congenital heart defect with prosthetic material or device (during the first 6 months after the procedure)†
  - Repaired congenital heart disease with residual defects at the site or adjacent to the site of a prosthetic patch or device (which inhibits endothelialization)
- Cardiac transplantation recipients who develop cardiac valvulopathy

*Except for the conditions listed above, antibiotic prophylaxis is no longer recommended for any other form of congenital heart disease.

†Prophylaxis is reasonable because endothelialization of prosthetic material occurs within 6 months after the procedure.

Editors' Note: The 2007 American Heart Association (AHA) guidelines[226] suggest that antibiotic prophylaxis for uncomplicated vaginal delivery is not necessary, even among patients in the high-risk category. The revised AHA guidelines[226] include the following statement: "The writing group reaffirms that those medical procedures listed as not requiring infective endocarditis prophylaxis in the 1997 statement remain unchanged and extends this view to vaginal delivery, hysterectomy, and tattooing." The American College of Obstetricians and Gynecologists Committee on Obstetric Practice[101] subsequently stated: "Infective endocarditis prophylaxis is no longer recommended for vaginal or cesarean delivery in the absence of infection, regardless of the type of maternal cardiac lesion. Mitral valve prolapse is no longer considered a lesion that ever needs infective endocarditis prophylaxis. Only cardiac conditions associated with the highest risk of adverse outcome from endocarditis are approprite for any infective endocarditis prophylaxis."

Modified from (1) American Heart Association Rheumatic Fever, Endocarditis, and Kawasaki Disease Committee, Council on Cardiovascular Disease in the Young, and the Council on Clinical Cardiology, Council on Cardiovascular Surgery and Anesthesia, and the Quality of Care and Outcomes Research Interdisciplinary Working Group. Prevention of infective endocarditis: Guidelines from the American Heart Association. Circulation 2007; 116:1736-54; and (2) American College of Obstetricians and Gynecologists Committee on Obstetric Practice. Antibiotic prophylaxis for infective endocarditis. ACOG Committee Opinion No. 421. Washington DC, November 2008. (Obstet Gynecol 2008;112:1193-4.)

TABLE 41-3 Antibiotic Prophylaxis Appropriate for Infective Endocarditis

Treatment	Antibiotic	Regimen (preferably 30-60 min before procedure)
Intravenous therapy	Ampicillin or cefazolin or ceftriaxone†	2 g intravenously 1 g intravenously
Allergic to penicillin or ampicillin*	Cefazolin or ceftriaxone† or clindamycin†	1 g intravenously† 600 mg intravenously†
Oral	Amoxicillin	2 g

*Cephalosporins should not be used in patients with a significant sensitivity to pencillins.
†This regimen does not cover enterococcus. Vanomycin can be used if enterococcus is of concern.
From American College of Obstetricians and Gynecologists Committee on Obstetric Practice. Antibiotic prophylaxis for infective endocarditis. ACOG Committee Opinion No. 421. Washington DC, November 2008. (Obstet Gynecol 2008; 112:1193-4.)

ANTIBIOTIC PROPHYLAXIS

Controversy remains regarding the indications for antibiotic prophylaxis against infective endocarditis. From a public health perspective, the indiscriminate use of antibiotics may promote the emergence of bacterial strains that are virulent and resistant to currently available antibiotics. Further, antibiotics may cause maternal allergic reactions and fetal toxicity (see Chapter 14). In an effort to encourage the appropriate use of antibiotics, the AHA[226] has released guidelines for the prevention of infective endocarditis; these guidelines were revised in 1997 and again in 2007 to emphasize the following points: (1) infective endocarditis is much more likely to result from frequent exposure to random bacteremias associated with daily activities than from bacteremia caused by a dental, gastrointestinal tract, or genitourinary tract procedure; (2) prophylaxis may prevent an exceedingly small number of cases of infective endocarditis, if any, in individuals who undergo a dental, gastrointestinal tract, or genitourinary tract procedure; and (3) the risk of antibiotic-associated adverse events exceeds the benefit, if any, from prophylactic antibiotic therapy.[226] Infective endocarditis prophylaxis is not recommended for most patients undergoing vaginal or cesarean delivery.[62,101,226,227] The American College of Obstetricians and Gynecologists (ACOG)[101] recently revised its guidelines, as follows:

Infective endocarditis prophylaxis is no longer recommended for vaginal or cesarean delivery in the absence of infection, regardless of the type of maternal cardiac lesion. Mitral valve prolapse is no longer considered a lesion that ever needs infective endocarditis prophylaxis. Only cardiac conditions associated with the highest risk of adverse outcome from endocarditis are appropriate for any infective endocarditis prophylaxis [Box 41-6]. In patients with one of these conditions and who have an established infection that could cause bacteremia, such as chorioamnionitis or pyelonephritis, the underlying infection should be treated in the usual fashion and the treatment should include a regimen effective for infective endocarditis prophylaxis [Table 41-3]. Prophylaxis should be given intravenously.

Whether clinicians will adopt the revised AHA guidelines for the prevention of infective endocarditis remains to be witnessed. In a review of practices during the intrapartum period at a tertiary referral care hospital over 1 year, Pocock et al.[227] found that only 12% of patients who received infective endocarditis antibiotic prophylaxis met the 1997 AHA/2003 ACOG criteria for infective endocarditis antibiotic prophylaxis.

KEY POINTS

- Heart disease is the primary medical cause of nonobstetric maternal mortality.
- Congenital heart disease represents the etiology of 60% to 80% of cases of cardiac disorders in pregnant women.
- Pulmonary artery catheterization is rarely necessary in pregnant women. The management of most forms of congenital heart disease, including Eisenmenger's syndrome, rarely requires pulmonary artery catheterization.
- Intrathecal administration of a lipophilic opioid represents an excellent choice of intrapartum analgesia for women who may not tolerate decreased systemic vascular resistance and decreased venous return.
- Cardiac lesions do not represent an absolute contraindication to the use of neuraxial anesthesia, assuming that the induction proceeds slowly and the potentially adverse hemodynamic changes are corrected promptly. Single-shot spinal anesthesia can produce circulatory collapse in parturients with severe aortic stenosis, primary pulmonary hypertension, and Eisenmenger's syndrome.
- The treatment of most arrhythmias during pregnancy is similar to that for nonpregnant women.
- When cardiopulmonary resuscitation is required during pregnancy, the standard advanced cardiac life support protocols should be used. Left uterine displacement should be employed to prevent the gravid uterus from compressing the inferior vena cava and the aorta and obstructing venous return and arterial blood flow. Choice of drugs (and doses), as well as indications for defibrillation, are the same as those for nonpregnant adult women. After 20 weeks' gestation, early hysterotomy and uterine evacuation may be necessary to facilitate resuscitation of the mother. Rescuers should be prepared to proceed with cesarean delivery if the resuscitation is not successful within 4 minutes.
- Infective endocarditis prophylaxis is not recommended for vaginal or cesarean delivery in the absence of infection. However, in patients with an underlying cardiac condition associated with the highest risk of adverse outcomes, it may be reasonable to use a prophylactic antibiotic regimen, especially in women at risk for bacteremia.

REFERENCES

1. Hameed AB, Sklansky MS. Pregnancy: Maternal and fetal heart disease. Curr Probl Cardiol 2007; 32:419-94.
2. Siu SC, Colman JM. Heart disease and pregnancy. Heart 2001; 85:710-15.
3. Whittemore R, Hobbins JC, Engle MA. Pregnancy and its outcome in women with and without surgical treatment of congenital heart disease. Am J Cardiol 1982; 50:641-51.
4. Shime J, Mocarski E, Hastings D. Congenital heart disease in pregnancy: Short and long term implications. Am J Obstet Gynecol 1989; 156:312-22.
5. McFaul PB, Dornan JC, Lamki H, Boyle D. Pregnancy complicated by maternal heart disease: A review of 519 women. Br J Obstet Gynaecol 1988; 95:861-7.
6. Siu S, Sermer M, Harrison D, et al. Risk and predictors for pregnancy-related complications in women with heart disease. Circulation 1997; 96:2789-94.
7. Chang J, Elam-Evans L, Berg C, et al. Pregnancy-related mortality surveillance—United States, 1991-1999. MMWR 2003; 52:1-8.
8. Khairy P, Ouyang DW, Fernandes SM, et al. Pregnancy outcomes in women with congenital heart disease. Circulation 2006; 113:517-24.
9. Connolly HM, Grogan M, Warnes C. Pregnancy among women with congenitally corrected transposition of great arteries. J Am Coll Cardiol 1999; 33:1692-5.
10. Therrien J, Barnes I, Somerville J. Outcome of pregnancy in patients with congenitally corrected transposition of the great arteries. Am J Cardiol 1999; 84:820-4.
11. Canobbio MM, Mair DD, van der Velde M, Koos BJ. Pregnancy outcomes after the Fontan repair. J Am Coll Cardiol 1996; 28:763-7.
12. Mendelson MA. Congenital cardiac disease and pregnancy. Clin Perinatol 1997; 24:467-82.
13. Perloff JK. Congenital heart disease and pregnancy. Clin Cardiol 1994; 17:579-87.
14. Stayer SA, Andropoulos DB, Russell IA. Anesthetic management of the adult patient with congenital heart disease. Anesthesiol Clin North Am 2003; 21:653-73.
15. Poppos A. Congenital and acquired heart disease. In Lee R, Rosene-Montella K, Barbour L, editors. Medical Care of the Pregnant Patient. Philadelphia, American College of Physicians, 2000:359-60.
16. Beauchesne LM, Connolly HM, Ammash NM, Warnes CA. Coarctation of the aorta: Outcome of pregnancy. J Am Coll Cardiol 2001; 38:1728-33.
17. Strafford MA, Griffiths SP, Gersony WM. Coarctation of the aorta: A study in delayed detection. Pediatrics 1982; 69:159-63.
18. Saidi AS, Bezold LI, Altman CA, et al. Outcome of pregnancy following intervention for coarctation of the aorta. Am J Cardiol 1998; 82:786-8.
19. Deal K, Wooley CF. Coarctation of the aorta and pregnancy. Ann Intern Med 1973; 78:708-13.
20. Vriend JW, Drenthen W, Pieper PG, et al. Outcome of pregnancy in patients after repair of aortic coarctation. Eur Heart J 2005; 26:2173-8.
21. Meijer JM, Pieper PG, Drenthen W, et al. Pregnancy, fertility, and recurrence risk in corrected tetralogy of Fallot. Heart 2005; 91:801-5.
22. Blanchard DG, Shabetai R. Congenital heart disease and pregnancy. In Creasy RK, Resnik R, Iams JD, editors. Maternal Fetal Medicine. 5th edition. Philadelphia, Saunders, 2004:823-4.
23. Eisenmenger V. Die Angeborenen Defecte der Kammerscheidewand des Herzens. Z Klin Med 1897; 32:1-29.
24. Avila WS, Grinberg M, Snitcowsky R, et al. Maternal and fetal outcome in pregnant women with Eisenmenger's syndrome. Eur Heart J 1995; 16:460-4.
25. Cross J. Obstetric anesthesia in patients with cardiac disease. In Lake C, editor. Advances in Anesthesia. Philadelphia, Mosby, 1999:251-73.
26. Easterling TR, Ralph DD, Schmucker BC. Pulmonary hypertension in pregnancy: Treatment with pulmonary vasodilators. Obstet Gynecol 1999; 93:494-8.
27. Goodwin TM, Gherman RB, Hameed A, Elkayam U. Favorable response of Eisenmenger syndrome to inhaled nitric oxide during pregnancy. Am J Obstet Gynecol 1999; 180:64-7.
28. Lust KM, Boots RK, Dooris M, Wilson J. Management of labor in Eisenmenger syndrome with inhaled nitric oxide. Am J Obstet Gynecol 1999; 181:419-23.
29. Ghai B, Mohan V, Khetarpal M, Malhotra N. Epidural anesthesia for cesarean section in a patient with Eisenmenger's syndrome. Int J Obstet Anesth 2002; 11:44-7.
30. Cole PJ, Cross MH, Dresner M. Incremental spinal anaesthesia for elective caesarean section in a patient with Eisenmenger's syndrome. Br J Anaesth 2001; 86:723-6.
31. Fuster V, Steele PM, Edwards WD, et al. Primary pulmonary hypertension: Natural history and the importance of thrombosis. Circulation 1984; 70:580-7.
32. Bonnin M, Mercier FJ, Sitbon O, et al. Severe pulmonary hypertension during pregnancy: Mode of delivery and anesthetic management of 15 consecutive cases. Anesthesiology 2005; 102:1133-7.
33. Weiss BM, Zemp L, Seifert B, Hess OM. Outcome of pulmonary vascular disease in pregnancy: A systematic overview from 1978 through 1996. J Am Coll Cardiol 1998; 31:1650-7.
34. Palmer CM, DiNardo JA, Hays RL, Van Maren GA. Use of transesophageal echocardiography for delivery of a parturient with severe pulmonary hypertension. Int J Obstet Anesth 2002; 11:48-51.
35. Bildirici I, Shumway JB. Intravenous and inhaled epoprostenol for primary pulmonary hypertension during pregnancy and delivery. Obstet Gynecol 2004; 103:1102-5.
36. Lam GK, Stafford RE, Thorp J, et al. Inhaled nitric oxide for primary pulmonary hypertension in pregnancy. Obstet Gynecol 2001; 98:895-8.
37. Monnery L, Nanson J, Charlton G. Primary pulmonary hypertension in pregnancy: A role for novel vasodilators. Br J Anaesth 2001; 87:295-8.
38. Decoene C, Bourzoufi K, Moreau D, et al. Use of inhaled nitric oxide for emergency cesarean section in a woman with unexpected primary pulmonary hypertension. Can J Anaesth 2001; 48:584-7.
39. Channick RN, Simonneau G, Sitbon O, et al. Effects of the dual endothelin-receptor antagonist bosentan in patients with pulmonary hypertension: A randomised placebo-controlled study. Lancet 2001; 358:1119-23.
40. Rubin LJ, Badesch DB, Barst RJ, et al. Bosentan therapy for pulmonary arterial hypertension. N Engl J Med 2002; 346:896-903.
41. Weeks SK, Smith JB. Obstetric anaesthesia in patients with primary pulmonary hypertension. Can J Anaesth 1991; 38:814-6.
42. Autore C, Conte M, Piccininno MR, et al. Risk associated with pregnancy in hypertrophic cardiomyopathy. J Am Coll Cardiol 2002; 40:1864-9.
43. Paix B, Cyna A, Belperio P, Simmons S. Epidural analgesia for labour and delivery in a parturient with congenital hypertrophic obstructive cardiomyopathy. Anaesth Intensive Care 1999; 27:59-62.
44. Haering JM, Comunale ME, Parker RA, et al. Cardiac risk of noncardiac surgery in patients with asymmetric septal hypertrophy. Anesthesiology 1996; 85:254-9.
45. Wadsworth R, Greer R, MacDonald JM, Vohra A. The use of remifentanil during general anaesthesia for cesarean delivery in two patients with severe heart dysfunction. Int J Obstet Anesth 2002; 11:38-43.
46. James AJ, Jamison MG, Biswas MS, et al. Acute myocardial infarction in pregnancy. Circulation 2006; 113:1564-71.
47. Ladner HE, Danielsen B, Gilbert WM. Acute myocardial infarction in pregnancy and the puerperium: A population-based study. Obstet Gynecol 2005; 105:480-4.
48. Roth A, Elkayan U. Acute myocardial infarction associated with pregnancy. Ann Intern Med 1996; 125:751-62.
49. American College of Obstetricians and Gynecology, Committee on Obstetrics: Maternal and Fetal Medicine: Cocaine in pregnancy. ACOG Committee Opinion No. 114. Washington, DC, ACOG, September 1992.
50. Carruth JE, Mivis SB, Brogan DR, Wenger NK. The electrocardiogram in normal pregnancy. Am Heart J 1981; 102:1075-8.

51. Meltzer RS, Serrvys PW, McGhie J. Cardiac catheterization under echocardiographic control in a pregnant woman. Am J Med 1981; 71:481-4.
52. Ascarelli MH, Grider AR, Hsu HW. Acute myocardial infarction during pregnancy managed with immediate percutaneous transluminal coronary angioplasty. Obstet Gynecol 1996; 88:655-7.
53. Webber MD, Halligan RE, Schumacher JA. Acute infarction, intracoronary thrombolysis, and primary PTCA in pregnancy. Cathet Cardiovasc Diagn 1997; 42:38-43.
54. Cuthill JA, Young S, Greer IA, Oldroyd K. Anaesthetic considerations in a parturient with critical coronary artery disease and a drug-eluting stent presenting for caesarean section. Int J Obstet Anesth 2005; 14:167-71.
55. Garry D, Leikin E, Fleisher AG, Tejani N. Acute myocardial infarction in pregnancy with subsequent medical and surgical management. Obstet Gynecol 1996; 87:802-4.
56. Schumacher B, Belfort MA, Card RJ. Successful treatment of acute myocardial infarction during pregnancy with tissue plasminogen activator. Am J Obstet Gynecol 1997; 176:716-9.
57. Frenkel Y, Barkai G, Reisin L, et al. Pregnancy after myocardial infarction: Are we playing safe? Obstet Gynecol 1991; 77:822-5.
58. Avila W, Rossi E, Ramires J, et al. Pregnancy in patients with heart disease: Experience with 1,000 cases. Clin Cardiol 2003; 26:135-42.
59. Listo M, Bjorkenheim G. Myocardial infarction during delivery. Acta Obstet Gynecol Scand 1966; 45:268-78.
60. Mabie WC, Anderson GD, Addington MB, et al. The benefit of cesarean section in acute myocardial infarction complicated by premature labor. Obstet Gynecol 1988; 71:503-6.
61. Cohen WR, Steinman T, Pastner B. Acute myocardial infarction in a pregnant woman at term. JAMA 1983; 250:2179-81.
62. American College of Cardiology/American Heart Association Task Force on Practice Guidelines. 2006 Guidelines for the management of patients with valvular heart disease. Circulation 2006; 114:e84-231.
63. Bates SM, Greer IA, Pabinger I, et al. Venous thromboembolism, thrombophilia, antithrombotic therapy, and pregnancy: American College of Chest Physicians evidence-based clinical practice guidelines (8th edition). Chest 2008; 133:844S-6S.
64. Elkayam U, Bitar F. Valvular heart disease and pregnancy. J Am Coll Cardiol 2005; 46:223-30.
65. Essop MR, Sareli P. Rheumatic valvular disease and pregnancy. In Elkayam U, Gleicher N, editors. Cardiac Problems in Pregnancy. New York, Wiley-Liss, 1998:55-60.
66. Hameed A, Karaalp IS, Tummala PP, et al. The effect of valvular heart disease on maternal and fetal outcome of pregnancy. J Am Coll Cardiol 2001; 37:893-9.
67. Bhatla N, Lal S, Behera G, et al. Cardiac disease in pregnancy. Int J Gynaecol Obstet 2003; 82:153-9.
68. Hameed AB, Tummala PP, Goodwin TM, et al. Unstable angina during pregnancy in two patients with premature coronary atherosclerosis and aortic stenosis in association with familial hypercholesterolemia. Am J Obstet Gynecol 2000; 182:1152-5.
69. Silversides CK, Colman JM, Sermer M, et al. Early and intermediate-term outcomes of pregnancy with congenital aortic stenosis. Am J Cardiol 2003; 91:1386-9.
70. Naidoo DP, Moodley J. Management of the critically ill cardiac patient. Best Pract Res Clin Obstet Gynaecol 2001; 15:523-44.
71. Cross J. Obstetric Anesthesia in Patients with Cardiac Disease. Philadelphia, Mosby, 1999.
72. Hustead ST, Quick A, Gibbs HR, et al. 'Pseudo-critical' aortic stenosis during pregnancy: Role for Doppler assessment of aortic valve area. Am Heart J 1989; 117:1383-5.
73. Ben-Ami M, Battino S, Rosenfeld T, et al. Aortic valve replacement during pregnancy: A case report and review of the literature. Acta Obstet Gynecol Scand 1990; 69:651-3.
74. Bhargava B, Agarwal R, Yadav R, et al. Percutaneous balloon aortic valvuloplasty during pregnancy: Use of the Inoue balloon and the physiologic antegrade approach. Cathet Cardiovasc Diagn 1998; 45:422-5.
75. Tumelero RT, Duda NT, Tognon AP, et al. Percutaneous balloon aortic valvuloplasty in a pregnant adolescent. Arq Bras Cardiol 2004; 82:98-101.
76. Brian JE, Seifen AB, Clark RB, et al. Aortic stenosis, cesarean delivery, and epidural anesthesia. J Clin Anesth 1993; 5:154-7.
77. Van de Velde M, Budts W, Vandermeersch E, Spitz B. Continuous spinal analgesia for labor pain in a parturient with aortic stenosis. Int J Obstet Anesth 2003; 12:51-4.
78. Orme RM, Grange CS, Ainsworth QP, Grebenik CR. General anaesthesia using remifentanil for caesarean section in parturients with critical aortic stenosis: A series of four cases. Int J Obstet Anesth 2004; 13:183-7.
79. Paulus DA, Layon AJ, Mayfield WR, et al. Intrauterine pregnancy and aortic valve replacement. J Clin Anesth 1995; 7:338-46.
80. Warnes CA, Elkayam U. Congenital heart disease in pregnancy. In Elkayam U, Gleicher N, editors. Cardiac Problems in Pregnancy. New York, Wiley-Liss, 1998:39-55.
81. Takano Y, Matsuyama H, Fujita A, et al. A case of urgent aortic valve replacement for infective endocarditis in pregnancy. Jpn J Anesthesiol 2003; 52:1086-8.
82. Lind J, Eallenburg HC. The Marfan syndrome and pregnancy: A retrospective study in a Dutch population. Eur J Obstet Gynecol Reprod Biol 2001; 98:28-35.
83. Bonow RO, Braunwald E. Valvular heart disease. In Zipes DP, Libby P, Bonow RO, Mann DL, editors. Heart Disease. 7th edition. Philadelphia, Elsevier Saunders, 2005:1553-621.
84. Bhatla N, Lal S, Behera G, Kriplani A, et al. Cardiac disease in pregnancy. Int J Gynaecol Obstet 2000; 82:153-9.
85. Sawhney H, Aggarwal N, Suri V, et al. Maternal and perinatal outcome in rheumatic heart disease. Int J Gynaecol Obstet 2003; 80:9-14.
86. Braunwald E. Valvular heart disease. In Braunwald E, editor. Heart Disease. 4th edition. Philadelphia, WB Saunders, 1992:1011.
87. Silversides CK, Colman JM, Sermer M, Siu SC. Cardiac risk in pregnant women with rheumatic mitral stenosis. Am J Cardiol 2003; 91:1382-5.
88. Lesniak-Sobelga A, Tracz W, Kostkiewicz M, et al. Clinical and echocardiographic assessment of pregnant women with valvular heart diseases—maternal and fetal outcome. Int J Cardiol 2004; 94:15-23.
89. al Kasab SM, Sabag T, al Zaibag M, et al. Beta-adrenergic blockade in the management of pregnant women with mitral stenosis. Am J Obstet Gynecol 1990; 165:37-40.
90. Reimold SC, Rutherford JD. Valvular heart disease in pregnancy. N Engl J Med 2003; 349:52-9.
91. Hameed A, Akhter MW, Bitar F, et al. Left atrial thrombosis in pregnant women with mitral stenosis and sinus rhythm. Am J Obstet Gynecol 2005; 193:501-4.
92. de Souza JA, Martinez EE, Ambrose JA, et al. Percutaneous balloon mitral valvuloplasty in comparison with open mitral valve commissurotomy for mitral stenosis during pregnancy. J Am Coll Cardiol 2001; 37:900-3.
93. Hermmings GT, Whalley DG, O'Connor PH. Invasive monitoring and anesthesia management of patients with mitral stenosis. Can J Anaesth 1987; 34:182-5.
94. Ducey JP, Knape KG. Maternal esmolol administration resulting in fetal distress and cesarean section in a term pregnancy. Anesthesiology 1992; 77:829-32.
95. Eisenach JC, Castro MI. Maternally administered esmolol produces fetal beta-adrenergic blockade and hypoxemia in sheep. Anesthesiology 1989; 71:718-22.
96. Losasso TJ, Muzzi DA, Cucchiara RF. Response of fetal heart rate to maternal administration of esmolol. Anesthesiology 1991; 74:782-4.
97. Savage DD, Garrison RJ, Devereux RB, et al. Mitral valve prolapse in the general population. 1. Epidemiologic features: The Framingham Study. Am Heart J 1983; 106:571-6.
98. Shapiro EP, Trimble EL, Robinson JC, et al. Safety of labor and delivery in women with mitral valve prolapse. Am J Cardiol 1985; 56:806-7.
99. Klein LL, Galan HL. Cardiac disease in pregnancy. Obstet Gynecol Clin North Am 2004; 31:429-59.

100. Chia YT, Yeoh SC, Lim MC, et al. Pregnancy outcome and mitral valve prolapse. Asia Oceania J Obstet Gynaecol 1994; 20:383-8.
101. American College of Obstetricians and Gynecologists Committee on Obstetric Practice. Antibiotic prophylaxis for infective endocarditis. ACOG Committee Opinion No. 421. Washington DC, November 2008. (Obstet Gynecol 2008; 112:1193-4.)
102. Lee CN, Wu CC, Lin PY, et al. Pregnancy following cardiac valve replacement. Obstet Gynecol 1994; 83:353-6.
103. Elkayam U. Pregnancy through a prosthetic heart valve. J Am Coll Cardiol 1999; 33:1642-5.
104. Hirsh J, Fuster V. Guide to anticoagulant therapy. Part 2: Oral anticoagulants. Circulation 1994; 89:1469-80.
105. Salazar E, Izaguirre R, Verdejo J, Mutchinick O. Failure of adjusted doses of subcutaneous heparin to prevent thromboembolic phenomena in pregnant patients with mechanical cardiac valve prostheses. J Am Coll Cardiol 1996; 27:1698-703.
106. Oakley CM. Pregnancy and prosthetic heart valves. Lancet 1994; 344:1643-4.
107. Ginsberg JS, Chan WS, Bates SM, Kaatz S. Anticoagulation of pregnant women with mechanical heart valves. Arch Intern Med 2003; 163:694-8.
108. Chan WS, Anand S, Ginsberg JS. Anticoagulation of pregnant women with mechanical heart valves: A systematic review of the literature. Arch Intern Med 2000; 160:191-6.
109. Horlocker TT, Wedel DJ, Benzon H, et al. Regional anesthesia in the anticoagulated patient: Defining the risks. (The Second ASRA Consensus Conference on Neuraxial Anesthesia and Anticoagulation.) Reg Anesth Pain Med 2003; 28:172-97.
110. Harnett MJ, Walsh ME, McElrath TF, Tsen LC. The use of central neuraxial techniques in parturients with factor V Leiden mutation. Anesth Analg 2005; 101:1821-3.
111. Leyse R, Ofstun M, Dillard DH, Merendino KA. Congenital aortic stenosis in pregnancy, corrected by extracorporeal circulation. JAMA 1961; 176:1109-12.
112. Mahli A, Izdes S, Coskum D. Cardiac operations during pregnancy: Review of factors influencing fetal outcome. Ann Thorac Surg 2000; 69:1622-6.
113. Khandelwal M, Rasanen J, Ludormirski A, et al. Evaluation of fetal and uterine hemodynamics during maternal cardiopulmonary bypass. Obstet Gynecol 1996; 88:667-71.
114. Yun EM, Royak A, Liu X. The effects of cardiopulmonary bypass on uterine blood flow. Anesthesiology 1997; 87:A876.
115. Nunley WC Jr, Kolp LA, Dabinett LN, et al. Subsequent fertility in women who undergo cardiac surgery. Am J Obstet Gynecol 1989; 161:573-6.
116. Pearson GD, Veille JC, Rahimtoola S, et al. Peripartum cardiomyopathy: National Heart, Lung, and Blood Institute and Office of Rare Diseases (National Institutes of Health) Workshop Recommendations and Review. JAMA 2000; 283:1183-8.
117. Murali S, Baldisseri MR. Peripartum cardiomyopathy. Crit Care Med 2005; 33:S340-6.
118. Lampert MB, Lang RM. Peripartum cardiomyopathy. Am Heart J 1995; 130:860-70.
119. Elkayam U, Akhter MW, Singh H, et al. Pregnancy-associated cardiomyopathy: A clinical comparison between early and late presentation. Circulation 2005; 111:2050-5.
120. Ansari AA, Fett JD, Carraway RE, et al. Autoimmune mechanisms as the basis for human peripartum cardiomyopathy. Clin Rev Allergy Immunol 2002; 23:310-24.
121. Ansari A, Neckelmann N, Wang Y, et al. Immunologic dialogue between cardiac myocytes, endothelial cells, and mononuclear cells. Clin Immunol Immunopathol 1993; 68:208-14.
122. Fett JD, Ansari AA, Sundstrom JB, Combs GF. Peripartum cardiomyopathy: A selenium disconnection and an autoimmune connection. Int J Cardiol 2002; 86:311-6.
123. O'Connell JB, Costanzo-Nordin MR, Subramanian R, et al. Peripartum cardiomyopathy: Clinical hemodynamic, histologic and prognostic characteristics. J Am Coll Cardiol 1986; 8:52-6.
124. Adesanya CO, Anjorin FI, Sada IA, et al. Atrial natriuretic peptide, aldosterone, and plasma renin activity in peripartum heart failure. Br Heart J 1991; 65:152-4.
125. Sanderson JE, Adesanya CO, Anjorin FI, Parry EH. Postpartum cardiac failure—heart failure due to volume overload? Am Heart J 1979; 97:613-21.
126. Hogle KL, Hutton EK, McBrien KA, et al. Cesarean delivery for twins: A systematic review and meta-analysis. Am J Obstet Gynecol 2003; 188:220-7.
127. Baughman KL. Peripartum cardiomyopathy. Curr Treat Options Cardiovasc Med 2001; 3:469-80.
128. Chapa JB, Heiberger HB, Weinert L, et al. Prognostic value of echocardiography in peripartum cardiomyopathy. Obstet Gynecol 2005; 105:1303-8.
129. George LM, Gatt SP, Lowe S. Peripartum cardiomyopathy: Four case histories and a commentary on anaesthetic management. Anaesth Intensive Care 1997; 25:292-6.
130. Carlson KM, Browning JE, Eggleston MK, Gherman RB. Peripartum cardiomyopathy presenting as lower extremity arterial thromboembolism. J Reprod Med 2000; 45:351-3.
131. Futterman LG, Lemberg L. Peripartum cardiomyopathy: An ominous complication of pregnancy. Am J Crit Care 2000; 9:362-6.
132. McCarroll CP, Paxton LD, Elliott P, Wilson D. Use of remifentanil in a patient with peripartum cardiomyopathy requiring caesarean section. Br J Anaesth 2001; 86:135-8.
133. Pryn A, Bryden F, Reeve W, et al. Cardiomyopathy in pregnancy and caesarean section: Four case reports. Int J Obstet Anesth 2007; 16:68-73.
134. Velickovic IA, Leicht CH. Continuous spinal anesthesia for cesarean section in a parturient with severe recurrent peripartum cardiomyopathy. Int J Obstet Anesth 2004; 13:40-3.
135. Hosenpud JD, Bennett LE, Keck BM, et al. The Registry of the International Society for Heart and Lung Transplantation: Fourteenth official report—1997. J Heart Lung Transplant 1997; 16:691-712.
136. Miniero R, Tardivo I, Centofanti P, et al. Pregnancy in heart transplant recipients. J Heart Lung Transplant 2004; 23:898-901.
137. Metcalfe J, McAnulty JH, Ueland K. Cardiovascular physiology. Clin Obstet Gynecol 1981; 24:693-5.
138. Hunt SA. Pregnancy in heart transplant recipients: A good idea? J Heart Lung Transplant 1991; 10:499-503.
139. Eskandar M, Gader S, Ong BY. Two successful vaginal deliveries in a heart transplant recipient. Obstet Gynecol 1996; 87:880.
140. Kim KM, Sukhani R, Slogoff S, Tomich PG. Central hemodynamic changes associated with pregnancy in a long-term cardiac transplant recipient. Am J Obstet Gynecol 1996; 174:1651-3.
141. Camann WR, Goldman GA, Johnson MD, et al. Cesarean delivery in a patient with a transplanted heart. Anesthesiology 1989; 71:618-20.
142. Yusuf S, Theodoropoulos S, Mathias C, et al. Increased sensitivity of the denervated transplanted human heart to isoprenaline both before and after beta-adrenergic blockade. Circulation 1987; 75:696-704.
143. Armenti VT, Radomski JS, Moritz MJ, et al. Report from the National Transplantation Pregnancy Registry (NTPR): Outcomes of pregnancy after transplantation. Clin Transpl 2000; 123-34.
144. Morini A, Spina V, Aleandri V, et al. Pregnancy after heart transplant: Update and case report. Hum Reprod 1998; 13:749-57.
145. Scott JR, Wagoner LE, Olsen SL, et al. Pregnancy in heart transplant recipients: Management and outcome. Obstet Gynecol 1993; 82:324-7.
146. Kossoy LR, Herbert CM, Wentz AC. Management of heart transplant recipients: Guidelines for the obstetrician-gynecologist. Am J Obstet Gynecol 1988; 159:490-9.
147. Rigg CD, Bythell VE, Bryson MR, et al. Caesarean section in patients with heart-lung transplants: A report of three cases and review. Int J Obstet Anesth 2000; 9:125-32.
148. Murphy N, Reed S. Maternal resuscitation and trauma. In Damos ES Jr, editor. Advanced Life Support in Obstetrics (ALSO) Provider Course Syllabus. Leawood, KS, American Academy of Family Physicians, 2000:1-25.

149. Rees GA, Willis BA. Resuscitation in late pregnancy. Anaesthesia 1988; 43:347-9.
150. American Heart Association. Cardiac arrest associated with pregnancy. Circulation 2005; 112:IV-150-3.
151. Cohen SE, Dailey PA, and the American Society of Critical Care Anesthesiologists and the American Society of Anesthesiologists Commitee on Critical Care Medicine. Resuscitation of the pregnant woman in cardiac arrest. In Anesthesia Advanced Circulatory Life Support. February 2008. Available at http://www.asahq.org/clinical/AnesthesiologyCentricACLS.pdf.
152. Whitty JE. Maternal cardiac arrest in pregnancy. Clin Obstet Gynecol 2002; 45:377-92.
153. Goodwin AP, Pearce AJ. The human wedge: A maneuver to relieve aortocaval compression during resuscitation in pregnancy. Anaesthesia 1992; 47:433-4.
154. Parker J, Balis N, Chester S, Adey D. Cardiopulmonary arrest in pregnancy: Successful resuscitation of mother and infant following immediate caesarean section in labour ward. Aust N Z J Obstet Gynaecol 1996; 36:207-10.
155. Katz VL, Dotters DJ, Droegemueller W. Perimortem cesarean delivery. Obstet Gynecol 1986; 68:571-6.
156. Katz V, Balderston K, DeFreest M. Perimortem cesarean delivery: Were our assumptions correct? Am J Obstet Gynecol 2005; 192:1916-21.
157. Litwin MS, Loughlin KR, Benson CB, et al. Placenta percreta involving the urinary bladder. Br J Urol 1989; 64:283-6.
158. Long WB, Rosenblum S, Grady P. Successful resuscitation of bupivacaine-induced cardiac arrest using cardiopulmonary bypass. Anesth Analg 1989; 69:403-6.
159. Splinter WM, Dwane PD, Wigle RD, McGrath MJ. Anaesthetic management of emergency caesarean section followed by pulmonary embolectomy. Can J Anaesth 1989; 36:689-92.
160. Lopez-Zeno J, Carlo W, O'Grady J, Fanaroff A. Infant survival following delayed postmortem cesarean delivery. Obstet Gynecol 1990; 76:991-2.
161. Robins K, Lyons G. Supraventricular tachycardia in pregnancy. Br J Anaesth 2004; 92:140-3.
162. Carson MP, Powrie RO, Rosene-Montella K. The effect of obesity and position on heart rate in pregnancy. J Matern Fetal Neonatal Med 2002; 11:40-5.
163. Gowda RM, Khan IA, Mehta NJ, et al. Cardiac arrhythmias in pregnancy: Clinical and therapeutic considerations. Int J Cardiol 2003; 88:129-33.
164. Gleicher N, Meller J, Sandler RZ, Sullum S. Wolff-Parkinson-White syndrome in pregnancy. Obstet Gynaecol 1981; 58:748-52.
165. Roberts JM, Insel PA, Goldfien A. Regulation of myometrial adrenoreceptors and adrenergic response by sex steroids. Mol Pharmacol 1981; 20:52-8.
166. Widerhorn J, Widerhorn AL, Rahimtoola SH, Elkayam U. WPW syndrome in pregnancy: Increased incidence of supraventricular arrhythmias. Am Heart J 1992; 123:796-8.
167. Silversides C, Harris L, Haberer K, et al. Recurrence rates of arrhythmias during pregnancy in women with previous tachyarrhythmia and impact on fetal and neonatal outcomes. Am J Cardiol 2006; 97:1206-12.
168. Conradsson TB, Werko L. Management of heart disease in pregnancy. Prog Cardiovasc Dis 1974; 16:407-19.
169. Rogers MC, Willerson JT, Goldblatt A, Smith TW. Serum digoxin concentrations in the human fetus, neonate and infant. N Engl J Med 1972; 287:1010-13.
170. Saarikoski S. Placental transfer and fetal uptake of 3H-digoxin in humans. Br J Obstet Gynaecol 1976; 83:879-84.
171. Levy M, Granit L, Laufer N. Excretion of drugs in human milk. N Engl J Med 1977; 297:789.
172. Rotmensch HH, Rotmensch S, Elkayam U. Management of cardiac arrhythmias during pregnancy. Drugs 1987; 33:623-33.
173. Frishman WH, Chesner M. Beta-adrenergic blockers in pregnancy. Am Heart J 1988; 115:147-52.
174. Pruyn SC, Phelan JP, Buchanan GC. Long-term propranolol therapy in pregnancy: Maternal and fetal outcome. Am J Obstet Gynecol 1979; 135:485-9.
175. Byerly WG, Hartmann A, Foster DE, Tannenbaum AK. Verapamil in the treatment of maternal paroxysmal supraventricular tachycardia. Ann Emerg Med 1991; 20:552-4.
176. Murad SH, Tabsh KM, Conklin KA, et al. Placental transfer and effects on maternal and fetal hemodynamics and atrioventricular conduction in the pregnant ewe. Anesthesiology 1985; 62:49-53.
177. Wolff F, Brueker KG, Schlensker KH, Bolte A. Prenatal diagnosis and therapy of fetal heart rate anomalies: With a contribution on the placental transfer of verapamil. J Perinatol Med 1980; 8:203-8.
178. Inoue M, Unno N. Excretion of verapamil in breast milk. Br Med J 1983; 287:1596.
179. Okada M, Inoue H, Nakamura Y, et al. Excretion of diltiazem in human milk. N Engl J Med 1985; 312:922-3.
180. Seki H, Takeda S, Kinoshita K. Long-term treatment with nicardipine for severe pre-eclampsia. Int J Obstet Anesth 2002; 76:135-41.
181. Laurent M, Betremieux P, Biron Y, LeHelloco A. Neonatal hypothyroidism after treatment with amiodarone during pregnancy. Am J Cardiol 1987; 60:942.
182. Widerhorn J, Bhandari AK, Bughi S, et al. Fetal and neonatal adverse effects profile of amiodarone treatment during pregnancy. Am Heart J 1991; 122:1162-6.
183. McKenna WJ, Harris L, Rowland E, et al. Amiodarone therapy during pregnancy. Am J Cardiol 1983; 51:1231-3.
184. Penn IM, Barrett PA, Pannikote V, et al. Amiodarone in pregnancy. Am J Cardiol 1985; 56:196-7.
185. Foster CJ, Love HG. Amiodarone in pregnancy: Case report and review of the literature. Int J Cardiol 1988; 20:307-16.
186. Rey E, Bachrach LK, Buttow GN. Effects of amiodarone during pregnancy. Can Med Assoc J 1987; 136:959-60.
187. Arnoux P, Seyral P, Llurens M, et al. Effects of amiodarone during pregnancy. Am J Cardiol 1987; 59:166-7.
188. Schleich JM, Bernard Du Haut Cilly F, Laurent MC, Almange C. Early prenatal management of a fetal ventricular tachycardia treated in utero by amiodarone with long term follow-up. Prenat Diagn 2000; 20:449-52.
189. Elkayam U, Goodwin TM. Adenosine therapy for supraventricular tachycardia during pregnancy. Am J Cardiol 1995; 75:521-3.
190. Harrison JK, Greenfield RA, Wharton JM. Acute termination of supraventricular tachycardia by adenosine during pregnancy. Am Heart J 1992; 5:1386-8.
191. Afridi I, Moise KJ, Rokey R. Termination of supraventricular tachycardia with intravenous adenosine in a pregnant woman with Wolff-Parkinson-White syndrome. Obstet Gynecol 1992; 80:481-3.
192. Dalvi BV, Chaudhuri A, Kulkarni HL, Kale PA. Therapeutic guidelines for congenital complete heart block presenting in pregnancy. Obstet Gynecol 1992; 79:802-4.
193. American College of Cardiology/American Heart Association Task Force on Practice Guidelines (Committee on Pacemaker Implantation). ACC/AHA guidelines for implantation of cardiac pacemakers and antiarrhythmia devices. J Am Coll Cardiol 1998; 31:1175-209.
194. Avasthi K, Gupta S, Avasthi G. An unusual case of complete heart block with triplet pregnancy. Indian Heart J 2003; 55:641-2.
195. Booker PD, Whyte SD, Ladusans EJ. Long QT Syndrome and anaesthesia. Br J Anaesth 2003; 90:349-66.
196. Munger RG, Prineas RJ, Crow R, et al. Prolonged QT interval and risk of sudden death in Southeast Asian men. Lancet 1991; 338:280-81.
197. Wisely NA, Shipton EA. Long QT syndrome and anaesthesia. Eur J Anaesthesiol 2002; 19:853-9.
198. Khan IA. Long QT syndrome: Diagnosis and management. Am Heart J 2002; 143:7-14.
199. Viskin S. Long QT syndrome and torsades de pointes. Lancet 1999; 354:1625-33.
200. Schwartz PJ, Locati EH, Moss AJ, et al. Left cardiac sympathetic denervation in the therapy of congenital long QT syndrome: A worldwide report. Circulation 1991; 84:503-11.
201. Frost DA, Dolak JA. Obstetrical and pediatric anesthesia: Cesarean section in a patient with familial cardiomyopathy and a cardioverter-defibrillator. Can J Anaesth 2006; 53:478-81.

202. Doyle NM, Monga M, Montgomery B, Dougherty AH. Arrhythmogenic right ventricular cardiomyopathy with implantable cardioverter defibrillator placement in pregnancy. J Matern Fetal Neonatal Med 2005; 18:141-4.
203. Klepper I. Cardioversion in late pregnancy. Anaesthesia 1981; 36:611-16.
204. Barnes EJ, Eben F, Patterson D. Direct current cardioversion during pregnancy should be performed with facilities available for fetal monitoring and emergency caesarean section. Br J Obstet Gynaecol 2002; 109:1406-7.
205. Tsipouras P, Del Mastro R, Sarfarazi M, et al. Genetic linkage of the Marfan syndrome, ectopia lentis and congenital contractural arachnodactyly to the fibrillin genes on chromosomes 15 and 5. N Engl J Med 1992; 326:905-9.
206. Lipscomb KJ, Smith JC, Clarke B, et al. Outcome of pregnancy in women with Marfan's syndrome. Br J Obstet Gynaecol 1997; 104:201-6.
207. Pyeritz RE. Maternal and fetal complications of pregnancy in the Marfan syndrome. Am J Med 1981; 71:784-90.
208. Meijboom L, Vos F, Timmermans J, et al. Pregnancy and aortic root growth in the Marfan syndrome: A prospective study. Eur Heart J 2005; 26:914-20.
209. Tritapepe L, Voci P, Pinto G, et al. Anesthesia for cesarean section in the Marfan syndrome. Can J Anaesth 1996; 43:1153-5.
210. Rosenblum NG, Grossman AR, Gabbe SG, et al. Failure of serial echocardiographic studies to predict aortic dissection in a pregnant patient with Marfan syndrome. Am J Obstet Gynecol 1983; 146: 470-1.
211. Paternoster DM, Santarossa C, Vettore N, et al. Obstetric complications in Marfan's syndrome pregnancy. Minerva Ginecol 1998; 50: 441-3.
212. Ergin MA, Lansman SL, Griepp RB. Dissections of the aorta. In Bave AE, Geha AS, Hammond GL, et al., editors. Glenn's Thoracic and Cardiovascular Surgery. 5th edition. Norwalk, CT, Appleton & Lange, 1991: 1955-66.
213. Tobis JM. Aortic dissection in pregnancy. In Elkayam U, Gleicher N, editors. Cardiac Problems in Pregnancy: Diagnosis and Management of Maternal and Fetal Disease. New York, Alan R Liss, 1982:161.
214. Konishi Y, Tatsuta N, Kumada K, et al. Dissecting aneurysm during pregnancy and the puerperium. Jpn Circ J 1980; 44:726-33.
215. Zeebregts CJ, Schepens MA, Hameeteman TM, et al. Acute aortic dissection complicating pregnancy. Thorac Surg 1997; 64:1345-8.
216. Pedowitz P, Perrell A. Aneurysms complicated by pregnancy. Am J Obstet Gynecol 1957; 73:720-35.
217. DeBakey ME, Henly WS, Cooley DA, et al. Surgical management of dissecting aneurysms of the aorta. J Thorac Cardiovasc Surg 1965; 49:130-49.
218. Henry DM, Cotton DB. Bacterial endocarditis in pregnancy associated with septic renal embolization. South Med J 1985; 78:355-6.
219. Seaworth BJ, Durack DT. Infective endocarditis in obstetric and gynecologic practice. Am J Obstet Gynecol 1986; 154:180-8.
220. Campuzano K, Roque H, Bolnick, et al. Bacterial endocarditis complicating pregnancy: Case report and systematic review of the literature. Arch Gynecol 2003; 268:251-5.
221. Cox SM, Leveno KJ. Pregnancy complicated by bacterial endocarditis. Clin Obstet Gynecol 1989; 32:48-53.
222. Karchmer AW. Infective endocarditis. In Braunwald E, Zipes DP, Libby P, editors. Heart Disease. 6th edition. Philadelphia, WB Saunders, 2001:1723-47.
223. Bataskov KL, Hariharan S, Horowitz MD, et al. Gonococcal endocarditis complicating pregnancy: A case report and literature review. Obstet Gynecol 1991; 78:494-5.
224. Carp H, Bailey S. The association between meningitis and dural puncture in bacteremic rats. Anesthesiology 1992; 76:739-42.
225. Chestnut DH. Spinal anesthesia in the febrile patient. Anesthesiology 1992; 76:667-9.
226. American Heart Association Rheumatic Fever, Endocarditis, and Kawasaki Disease Committee, Council on Cardiovascular Disease in the Young, and the Council on Clinical Cardiology, Council on Cardiovascular Surgery and Anesthesia, and the Quality of Care and Outcomes Research Interdisciplinary Working Group. Prevention of infective endocarditis: Guidelines from the American Heart Association. Circulation 2007; 116:1736-54.
227. Pocock SB, Chen KT. Inappropriate use of antibiotic prophylaxis to prevent infective endocarditis in obstetric patients. Obstet Gynecol 2006; 108:280-5.

Chapter 42

Endocrine Disorders

Richard N. Wissler, M.D., Ph.D.

DIABETES MELLITUS

Definition and Epidemiology

Diabetes mellitus (DM) is a common metabolic disorder with a prevalence of 6.8% to 8.2% in the general adult population in the United States.[1,2] DM results from either an absolute deficiency in insulin secretion (type 1) or a combination of resistance to insulin in target tissues and inadequate insulin secretion (type 2).[3] Although a combination of genetic and environmental factors contribute to both types, type 1 DM is primarily an autoimmune disorder. Type 2 DM occurs primarily in obese individuals and accounts for 90% to 95% of cases of DM in the United States.[3] Gestational DM refers to DM or glucose intolerance that is first diagnosed during pregnancy. Gestational DM occurs in approximately 7% of pregnancies in the United States, and its prevalence has been increasing.[4,5]

Pathophysiology

Insulin is a peptide hormone secreted by the beta cells of the islets of Langerhans in the pancreas. Insulin binds to specific cell-surface receptors in insulin-responsive target tissues (e.g., liver, skeletal muscle, fat). The intracellular effects of insulin are mediated by tyrosine kinase in the beta-subunit of the receptor through a cascade of distal protein kinase–mediated phosphorylations.[6,7] Normal hepatic glucose metabolism represents a balance between the effects of insulin and several "counterregulatory" hormones (e.g., glucagon, cortisol, epinephrine, growth hormone).[8] This control system for glucose homeostasis permits rapid adjustments in glucose metabolism in the fed and fasted states. Insulin is also an important anabolic regulator of lipid and amino acid metabolism (Figure 42-1). Insulin deficiency (absolute or relative) associated with DM results in abnormal metabolism of carbohydrates, lipids, and amino acids.

Acute and chronic complications occur in patients with DM (Box 42-1). The three major acute complications are diabetic ketoacidosis, hyperglycemic nonketotic state, and hypoglycemia. **Diabetic ketoacidosis (DKA)** occurs predominantly in patients with type 1 DM. DKA may develop with a new source of insulin resistance (e.g., infection, trauma, stress), and/or as a result of failure to administer usual insulin doses. DKA results from decreased uptake of glucose by insulin-responsive tissues and greater use of free fatty acids as a hepatic energy source. The lack of insulin favors lipolysis, beta-oxidation of free fatty acids in the liver, and hepatic formation of acetoacetate and beta-hydroxybutyrate from the excess acetyl-coenzyme A generated by fatty acid oxidation.[9] These biochemical events result in metabolic acidosis, hyperglycemia, and dehydration secondary to osmotic diuresis. Signs and symptoms of DKA include nausea, vomiting, weakness, tachypnea, hypotension, tachycardia, stupor, and acetone on the breath. The diagnosis of DKA depends on the laboratory findings of hyperglycemia, ketosis, and acidosis.[10]

Hyperglycemic nonketotic state (HNS) occurs predominantly in patients with type 2 DM. Laboratory findings in HNS are hyperglycemia (blood glucose level often greater than 600 mg/dL), hyperosmolarity (greater than 320 mOsm/kg), and moderate azotemia (serum blood urea nitrogen [BUN] often greater than 60 mg/dL), without

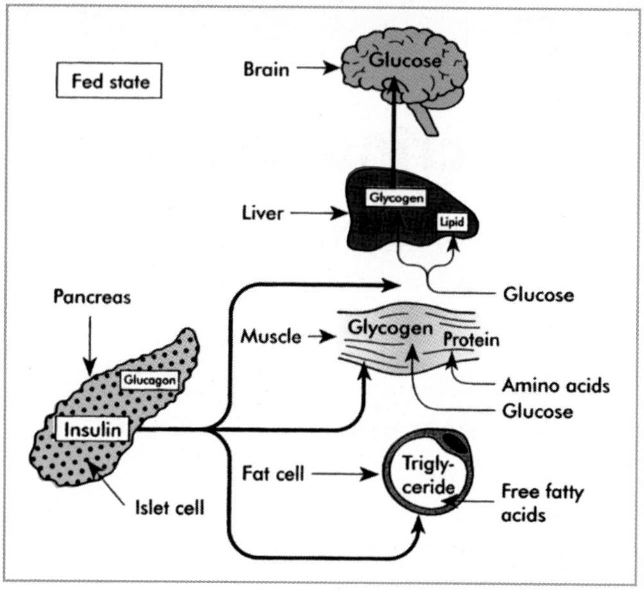

FIGURE 42-1 Substrate use in the fed state, showing the role of insulin in the promotion of fuel storage. (From Kitabchi AE, Murphy MB. Diabetic ketoacidosis and hyperosmolar hyperglycemic nonketotic coma. Med Clin North Am 1988; 72:1545-63.)

ketonemia or significant acidosis.[10] The absence of significant ketosis in HNS may indicate an inhibition of lipolysis by hyperosmolarity or low levels of insulin. DKA and HNS are probably related conditions; inadequate insulin therapy and infection are the most common precipitating events for both.[10]

Hypoglycemia is a continuing health threat in diabetic patients, especially in patients receiving insulin therapy. Hypoglycemia results from an imbalance between insulin or oral hypoglycemic agents and available metabolic fuels. In hospitalized patients with DM, major risk factors for hypoglycemia include renal insufficiency and decreased caloric intake.[11] Symptomatic awareness of hypoglycemia and counterregulatory responses may be inadequate in some diabetic patients with autonomic neuropathy.[12] Problems with hypoglycemia awareness in patients receiving beta-adrenergic receptor antagonists can be minimized by using $beta_1$-adrenergic receptor selective antagonists.[13] In one study, several diabetic pregnant women receiving insulin therapy became hypoglycemic while fasting before cesarean delivery. Factitious hypoglycemia results from a deliberate, inappropriate self-administration of insulin or an oral hypoglycemic agent.[14]

In general, the prevalence of chronic complications increases with the duration of DM.[4,15] The Diabetes Control and Complications Trial, a randomized multicenter study of patients with type 1 DM, demonstrated a positive relationship between tight glucose control and a lowered incidence or rate of progression of **retinopathy, nephropathy,** and **neuropathy.**[16] In a similar study of patients with type 2 DM—the U.K. Prospective Diabetes Study (UKPDS)—intensive glucose control lowered the incidence of microvascular complications but not of macrovascular complications or patient mortality.[17] In contrast, antihypertensive therapy reduced the incidence of macrovascular complications and mortality in patients with both type 2 DM and chronic hypertension.[17] DM may affect **cardiovascular function** as a result of coronary atherosclerosis, autonomic neuropathy, or development of a cardiomyopathy.[18]

Clinical Presentation and Diagnosis

Box 42-2 lists the current diagnostic criteria for DM in *nonpregnant* patients.[4]

Gestational DM is associated with (1) advanced maternal age, (2) obesity, (3) family history of type 2 DM, (4) prior history of gestational DM, (5) history of polycystic ovarian syndrome, (6) glycosuria, and/or (7) history of prior stillbirth, neonatal death, fetal malformation, or macrosomia. The clinical sensitivity of the medical history in detecting gestational DM is only 50%.[19] Box 42-3 lists the current recommendations of the American Diabetes Association

BOX 42-1 Major Complications of Diabetes Mellitus

Acute
- Diabetic ketoacidosis
- Hyperglycemic nonketotic state
- Hypoglycemia

Chronic

Macrovascular (Atherosclerosis)
- Coronary
- Cerebrovascular
- Peripheral vascular

Microvascular
- Retinopathy
- Nephropathy

Neuropathy
- Autonomic
- Somatic

BOX 42-2 Criteria for the Diagnosis of Diabetes Mellitus

Fasting (no caloric intake for at least 8 hours before measurement) plasma glucose ≥ 126 mg/dL (7.0 mmol/L)*

OR

Symptoms of hyperglycemia and casual (measured at any time of day, regardless of time since last meal) plasma glucose ≥ 200 mg/dL (11.1 mmol/L)

OR

2-hour plasma glucose ≥ 200 mg/dL (11.1 mmol/L) during an oral glucose tolerance test*†

*In the absence of unequivocal hyperglycemia, these criteria should be confirmed by further testing on a different day.

†Test should be performed with use of a glucose load containing the equivalent of 75 g anhydrous glucose dissolved in water.

Adapted from American Diabetes Association. Standards of medical care in diabetes—2008. Diabetes Care 2008; 31(Suppl 1):S12-54.

BOX 42-3 Screening and Diagnostic Strategies for Gestational Diabetes Mellitus

- Assess risk at the first prenatal visit.

Low Risk

- Low-risk status does not require screening.
- Criteria for low-risk status (all must be present):
  - Age < 25 years
  - Weight normal before pregnancy
  - Member of an ethnic group with a low prevalence of diabetes
  - No known diabetes in first-degree relatives
  - No history of abnormal glucose tolerance
  - No history of poor obstetric outcome

Very High Risk

- Screen *very-high-risk* women by means of standard diagnostic testing (see Box 42-2) as soon as possible after pregnancy is confirmed.
- Criteria for *very-high-risk* status:
  - Severe obesity
  - Prior history of gestational DM or delivery of large-for-gestational-age infant
  - Presence of glycosuria
  - Diagnosis of polycystic ovarian syndrome
  - Strong family history of type 2 diabetes

Higher than Low Risk

- Screen *higher-than-low-risk* women with one of the following approaches, at 24-28 weeks' gestation:

Two-step approach:

- Perform initial screening by measuring plasma or serum glucose 1 hour after a 50-g oral glucose load (a glucose threshold of ≥ 140 mg/dL identifies ≈80% of women with gestational DM; a threshold of ≥ 130 mg/dL identifies ≈90%).
- If patient exceeds the chosen threshold on 50-g screening, perform a diagnostic 100-g OGTT on a separate day.

One-step approach (may be preferred in clinics with high prevalence of gestational DM):

- Perform a diagnostic 100-g OGTT in all women to be tested at 24-28 weeks' gestation.

Diagnosis of Gestational Diabetes Mellitus

- The 100-g OGTT should be performed in the morning after an overnight fast or a fast of at least 8 hours. A diagnosis of gestational DM requires at least two of the following plasma glucose measurements:
  - Fasting: ≥ 95 mg/dL (> 5.3 mmol/L)
  - 1-hour: ≥ 180 mg/dL (> 10.0 mmol/L)
  - 2-hour: ≥ 155 mg/dL (> 8.6 mmol/L)
  - 3-hour: ≥ 140 mg/dL (> 7.8 mmol/L)

OGTT, oral glucose tolerance test.

Adapted from American Diabetes Association. Standards of medical care in diabetes—2008. Diabetes Care 2008; 31(Suppl 1): S12-54.

for screening and diagnosis of gestational DM.[4] This approach divides pregnant women into three gestational DM risk categories on the basis of history: *low risk*, *very high risk*, and *higher than low risk*. *Low-risk* patients do not require testing; *very-high-risk* patients undergo standard nonpregnant testing. Box 42-3 outlines two different approaches for screening tests at 24 to 28 weeks' gestation for patients in the *higher-than-low-risk* category.

There are some unanswered questions about diagnostic testing for gestational DM. First, is patient history a reliable method for risk stratification prior to testing?[20] Second, is routine testing without risk stratification a cost-effective clinical strategy?[21,22] Any change to the diagnostic threshold for gestational DM changes the number of patients identified and treated for gestational DM. Recent data suggest that women with high plasma glucose measurements that are below the current threshold for diagnosis of gestational DM have larger infants and increased cord-blood serum C-peptide levels, and therefore may benefit from treatment during pregnancy.[23]

Glycosylated hemoglobin (GHb) measurements are used as time-integrated estimates of glycemic control, but not as a diagnostic test for DM. The normal range for hemoglobin A_{1c} in nondiabetic pregnant women is 4.1% to 5.9%.[24]

Interaction with Pregnancy

HOW DOES PREGNANCY AFFECT DIABETES MELLITUS?

Pregnancy is characterized by progressive peripheral resistance to insulin at the receptor and postreceptor levels in the second and third trimesters (Figure 42-2).[25-27] The presumed mechanism involves an increase in counterregulatory hormones (e.g., placental lactogen, placental growth hormone, cortisol, progesterone) during pregnancy. The change in placental lactogen is a plausible mechanism, given that (1) a graph of serum lactogen levels during pregnancy is similar in shape to that of insulin requirements in pregnant women with type 1 DM and (2) placental lactogen has growth hormone–like activity. Also, maternal adipokines probably are important factors in insulin resistance of pregnancy,[26] and they facilitate the provision of maternal fuels for the fetus.[27]

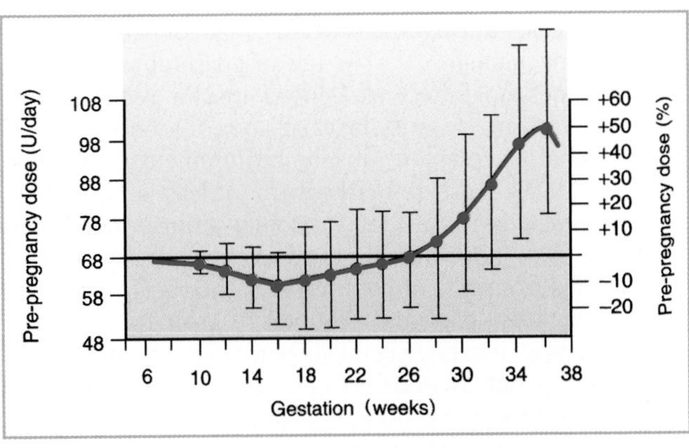

FIGURE 42-2 Insulin requirements in euglycemic women with type 1 diabetes mellitus during pregnancy. (From Crombach G, Siebolds M, Mies R. Insulin use in pregnancy: Clinical pharmacokinetic considerations. Clin Pharmcaokinet 1993; 24:89-100.)

Gestational DM develops when a patient cannot mount a sufficient compensatory insulin response during pregnancy. In some patients, gestational DM can be viewed as a preclinical state of glucose intolerance that is not detectable before pregnancy. After delivery most patients return to normal glucose tolerance but remain at increased risk for DM (predominantly type 2) in later life.[28] The recurrence rate for gestational DM in a subsequent pregnancy is 35% to 70%.[29]

In patients with **pregestational DM,** insulin requirements progressively increase during pregnancy because of peripheral insulin resistance.[30] At term, the daily insulin requirement is approximately 1.0 insulin unit/kg, compared with 0.7 unit/kg before pregnancy.[30] During late pregnancy in normal patients, basal and glucose-stimulated plasma insulin levels are twice the postpartum measurements.[27] These changes reflect pregnancy-related increases in pancreatic islet cell mass and glucose sensitivity, probably secondary to the net effect of competing progesterone and lactogenic hormone stimuli in the endocrine pancreas.[31,32] Near term, maternal overnight insulin requirements may decrease, presumably as a result of a "siphoning of maternal fuels" by the growing fetus during the overnight maternal fast.[33]

Endogenous plasma insulin concentrations during labor and delivery in nondiabetic parturients differ from exogenous insulin requirements in laboring diabetic women. In nondiabetic parturients, the plasma glucose concentration is only one of many factors that affect endogenous insulin secretion; glucose production and utilization are markedly higher during painful labor than postpartum.[34] Plasma insulin concentrations remain unchanged except for a brief increase during the third stage of labor and immediately postpartum.[34,35] This finding suggests that glucose use during labor is largely independent of insulin. The patterns of plasma insulin concentrations are similar in nondiabetic patients with and without analgesia (e.g., nitrous oxide, meperidine).[35]

In patients with type 1 DM, insulin requirements decrease with the onset of the first stage of labor.[36] These patients may require no additional insulin during the first stage of labor, although insulin requirements are modified by (1) the level of metabolic control before labor, (2) the residual effect of prior doses of subcutaneous insulin, and (3) the glucose infusion rate.[36,37] Insulin requirements increase during the second stage of labor via an unknown mechanism.[36,37] The use of epidural analgesia or oxytocin does not affect exogenous insulin requirements during the first and second stages of labor.[36] After delivery—either vaginal or cesarean—insulin requirements in women with type 1 DM decrease markedly for at least several days, although there is significant variability among individuals (Figure 42-3).[25,38] Presumably, the decreased insulin requirement results from loss of counterregulatory hormones produced by the placenta. Pituitary growth hormone responsiveness to hypoglycemia is blunted in late pregnancy and may contribute to impaired counterregulatory responses during the postpartum period.[39] Insulin requirements gradually return to prepregnancy levels within several weeks of delivery in women with type 1 DM.[33]

Before the discovery of insulin in 1921, pregnancies were rare in diabetic patients. Insulin therapy improved the rate of survival in women with severe DM, allowing these

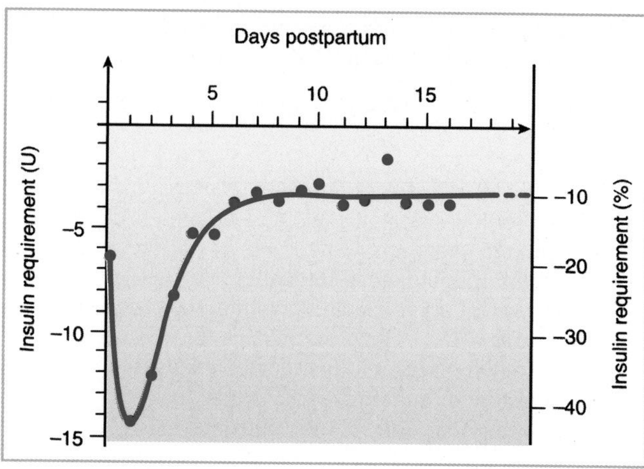

FIGURE 42-3 Insulin requirements in the postpartum period. (From Crombach G, Siebolds M, Mies R. Insulin use in pregnancy: Clinical pharmacokinetic considerations. Clin Pharmcaokinet 1993; 24:89-100.)

women to reach childbearing age and become pregnant. Maternal outcomes improved, but fetal and neonatal morbidity and mortality remained high.[40]

In 1949, White[41] proposed a classification system for DM during pregnancy based on 439 consecutive cases. Physicians caring for pregnant diabetic patients should be familiar with the White system, which has endured with some modifications (Table 42-1). The system emphasizes the relationship among the duration of type 1 DM, vascular complications of type 1 DM, and poor fetal outcome.[42] In the 1950s, fetal survival rates were as follows: class A, 100%; class B, 67%; class C, 48%; class D, 32%, and class F, 3%.[42]

The incidence of **DKA** has decreased from 9% to between 1% and 2% of diabetic pregnancies,[43,44] probably as a result of improvements in medical care and patient education. Similarly, the incidence of perinatal and maternal mortality from DKA during pregnancy has decreased in the past several decades.[44,45] As is true for nonpregnant patients, DKA during pregnancy occurs predominantly in patients with type 1 DM. The higher risk of DKA during pregnancy reflects the metabolic adaptations of pregnancy, including peripheral insulin resistance.[25]

During pregnancy, DKA occurs most commonly during the second and third trimesters.[46] It is associated with (1) emesis, (2) infection, (3) poor compliance or noncompliance, (4) insulin pump failure, (5) use of beta-adrenergic receptor agonists, (6) use of corticosteroids, and (7) poor medical management.[44] The infection rate in pregnant women with pregestational type 1 DM is 3.2 times higher than that in nondiabetic pregnant women.[47] DKA may be the first clinical sign of type 1 DM during pregnancy.[48,49] Beta-adrenergic receptor agonists, which are used to treat preterm labor, and corticosteroids, which are used to accelerate fetal lung maturity, both have counterregulatory pharmacologic effects that oppose insulin action. Beta-adrenergic agonist tocolytic therapy, with or without concurrent corticosteroid therapy, and by any route of administration, can precipitate DKA during pregnancy.[50,51] Beta-adrenergic receptor stimulation worsens glucose intolerance by stimulating glucagon secretion[52]; beta-adrenergic

TABLE 42-1 Modified White Classification of Diabetes Mellitus during Pregnancy

Class	Age of Onset of Diabetes (yrs)		Duration of Diabetes (yrs)	Vascular Disease	Insulin Required
Gestational Diabetes					
A_1	Any		Any	–	–
A_2	Any		Any	–	+
Pregestational Diabetes					
B	> 20		< 10	–	+
C	10-19	or	10-19	–	+
D*	< 10	or	> 20	+	+
F (nephropathy)	Any		Any	+	+
R (proliferative retinopathy)	Any		Any	+	+
T (status post–renal transplantation)	Any		Any	+	+
H (ischemic heart disease)	Any		Any	+	+

–, no; +, yes.

*Vascular disease in D is hypertension or benign retinopathy.

Modified from Landon MB, Gabbe SG. Diabetes mellitus and pregnancy. Obstet Gynecol Clin North Am 1992; 19:633-54.

receptor agonists may be well tolerated in pregnant women with DM if higher insulin requirements are anticipated and doses are adjusted in response to frequent blood glucose determinations.[49,51]

Several case reports have described nonreassuring fetal heart rate patterns during episodes of maternal DKA.[53,54] After appropriate medical management of maternal DKA, preterm uterine contractions stopped and fetal heart rate responses normalized. The mechanism of fetal compromise during DKA is unclear, but it may be related to changes in uterine blood flow. Blechner et al.[55] demonstrated that uterine artery blood flow is reduced by acute maternal metabolic acidosis. A single case report demonstrated reversible redistribution of fetal blood flow during an episode of maternal DKA on the basis of Doppler pulsatility indices of the umbilical and middle cerebral arteries.[56]

There are three case reports of **HNS** during pregnancy.[57-59] No conclusion can be drawn about HNS and pregnancy, except that HNS rarely occurs during pregnancy.

Hypoglycemia is a significant health risk for pregnant women with pregestational type 1 DM, occurring in 33% to 71% of these patients.[60-63] This rate is 3 to 15 times higher than that in similar groups of nonpregnant patients with type 1 DM,[60,61] and 80% to 84% of severe hypoglycemia episodes occur before 20 weeks' gestation.[62,63] In one study, patients with pregestational type 2 DM or gestational DM requiring insulin therapy experienced no episodes of severe hypoglycemia.[61] The risk of hypoglycemia during pregnancy in patients with type 1 DM increases with tight glucose control.[60,62,64] This pattern mirrors the clinical experience in nonpregnant women with type 1 DM, in which a threefold rise in the occurrence of severe hypoglycemia results from tight insulin control.[65] In both pregnant and nonpregnant patients with type 1 DM, counterregulatory hormone responses to hypoglycemia are impaired after intensive insulin therapy.[66,67] Two small series suggest that acute mild to moderate maternal hypoglycemia is not associated with acute alterations in fetal well-being in pregnant women with type 1 DM.[66,68]

The relationship between pregnancy and the development of macrovascular complications of DM is largely unknown. Patients with pregestational type 1 DM have higher systolic and diastolic blood pressures during pregnancy, and they are three times more likely than nondiabetic controls to have **gestational hypertension**.[69,70] In women with pregestational type 1 DM, the risk of preeclampsia is increased with increased severity of diabetes (White classification), and proteinuria early in pregnancy is associated with an increased risk of adverse outcome.[71] **Myocardial infarction** is a rare complication.[72] The effect of gestational hypertension on the progression of **atherosclerotic disease** in diabetic patients is unclear.

Pregnancy may accelerate the development of **proliferative retinopathy,** a microvascular complication of DM; the hyperglycemia and hypertension are also associated with the progression of retinopathy.[73,74] The onset of strict glycemic control may transiently exacerbate diabetic retinopathy in both pregnant and nonpregnant patients with type 1 DM. The Diabetes Control and Complications Trial demonstrated that strict glycemic control is justified in nonpregnant patients.[16]

In contrast to diabetic retinopathy, pregnancy does not accelerate the progression of diabetic **nephropathy**.[75] It is unclear whether pregnancy accelerates the progression of **somatic** or **autonomic neuropathy** in diabetic women.

HOW DOES DIABETES MELLITUS AFFECT THE MOTHER AND FETUS?

Both pregestational and gestational DM are associated with higher rates of gestational hypertension, polyhydramnios, and cesarean delivery.[43,76-78] The incidence of cesarean delivery is higher in women with pregestational DM than in women with gestational DM.[43,76,78] Attempted vaginal birth after cesarean delivery in patients with gestational DM is associated with rates of operative vaginal delivery

BOX 42-4 Fetal Complications of Maternal Diabetes Mellitus

During Pregnancy and the Puerperium

Chronic

- Macrosomia
  - Shoulder dystocia
  - Birth injury or trauma
- Structural malformations
  - Central nervous system: anencephaly, encephalocele, meningomyelocele, spina bifida, holoprosencephaly
  - Cardiac: transposition of great vessels, ventricular septal defect, situs inversus, single ventricle, hypoplastic left ventricle
  - Skeletal: caudal regression
  - Renal: agenesis, multicystic dysplasia
  - Gastrointestinal: anal or rectal atresia, small left colon
  - Pulmonary: hypoplasia

Acute

- Intrauterine or neonatal death
- Neonatal respiratory distress syndrome
- Neonatal hypoglycemia
- Neonatal hyperbilirubinemia

After Pregnancy

- Glucose intolerance
- Possible impairment of cognitive development

and repeat cesarean delivery that are higher than those found in nondiabetic controls.[79] Pregestational DM—but not gestational DM—is associated with a twofold to threefold increase in the incidence of **preterm labor and delivery**.[76,80]

Box 42-4 lists the fetal complications of maternal DM during pregnancy. **Fetal macrosomia** is a well-recognized complication of maternal DM. Most studies suggest that both pregestational DM and gestational DM result in an increased incidence of fetal macrosomia.[81-83] Depending on the definition of macrosomia (4000 g versus 4500 g), pregestational DM results in fetal macrosomia in 9% to 25% of women—a fourfold to sixfold higher rate than in nondiabetic controls.

Macrosomia results in an increased risk of **shoulder dystocia** and **birth trauma** with vaginal delivery.[77,84,85] Moreover, when comparisons are made within birth weight categories above 4000 g, pregnancies in diabetic women have a higher risk of shoulder dystocia than in nondiabetic women.[86] The use of intensive insulin therapy may reduce the risk of birth trauma in women with pregestational DM.[87] Several mechanisms have been suggested for the development of fetal macrosomia in diabetic pregnancy. Maternal hyperglycemia can result in fetal hyperglycemia, with reactive fetal hyperinsulinemia and an anabolic response in the fetus.[88] Shoulder dystocia may reflect the excessive growth of the fetal trunk (relative to the fetal head) in response to fetal hyperinsulinemia.[89]

Women with pregestational DM are at increased risk for **fetal anomalies** (see Box 42-4). The incidence of major anomalies, estimated to be 6% to 10%, is five times higher than in nondiabetic controls.[43,90-92] Overall, cardiovascular anomalies are most common, followed by anomalies of the central nervous system (CNS). The caudal regression syndrome is uncommon, but it is 200 times more likely in diabetic than in nondiabetic pregnancies.[90] The incidence of major congenital anomalies in infants of women with gestational DM is 3% to 8%, which is lower than in infants of women with pregestational DM.[76]

Metabolic factors that may be involved in the development of fetal structural malformations in diabetic pregnancies include hyperglycemia, hypoglycemia, hyperketonemia, somatomedin inhibitors, and zinc deficiency.[92] Most fetal structural malformations that occur during diabetic pregnancies are likely to have a multifactorial etiology. However, hyperglycemia during the period of critical organogenesis before the seventh week after conception is probably the single strongest etiologic factor in diabetic women and may be associated with embryonic oxidative stress.[92,93]

Studies have suggested that patient education and strict glycemic control during the preconception period may reduce the rate of major congenital anomalies from 10% to 1% in patients with pregestational DM.[94] The latter figure is similar to the baseline risk for major structural malformations in the general population. Strict glycemic control initiated during the preconception period also increases the incidence of maternal hypoglycemic episodes. These studies suggest that hypoglycemia is not a significant factor in the etiology of human malformations, because the rate of anomalies decreased tenfold despite hypoglycemic episodes.[94] Similarly, strict glycemic control before conception also has been associated with a threefold decrease in the incidence of spontaneous abortion in women with pregestational DM.[95] Dicker et al.[96] observed normal induced ovulation, *in vitro* fertilization, and early embryonic development in a small series of infertile patients with pregestational DM who attended a preconception diabetes clinic. However, only 36% of women with known pregestational DM receive appropriate medical care before conception.

During the 1950s to 1970s, the **perinatal mortality rate** in women with pregestational DM was 15% to 18%.[43] Subsequent studies noted a decrease to 2%, a rate similar to that in nondiabetic controls.[76] In contrast, one study noted a rate of 8%, three times greater than in nondiabetic controls.[83] When the entire population is considered, the perinatal mortality rate likely remains higher in patients with pregestational DM than in nondiabetic controls. The rate in patients with gestational DM is intermediate between the rate in women with pregestational diabetes and the rate in nondiabetic controls.[76,83]

Historically, **intrauterine fetal death** was responsible for approximately 40% of the perinatal deaths in women with DM; 68% of the stillbirths occurred between 36 and 40 weeks' gestation.[41,83] In contemporary reports, the ratio of intrauterine deaths to neonatal deaths in diabetic pregnancies has varied from 0 to 1.0. Fetal macrosomia is a risk factor for intrauterine fetal demise in both diabetic and nondiabetic pregnancies. Recurrent episodes of intrauterine hypoxia can occur in diabetic pregnancies that end in stillbirth; episodes of hypoxia may reflect reduced uteroplacental blood flow and changes in fetal carbohydrate metabolism. **Congenital anomalies** have now emerged as the leading cause of perinatal mortality in diabetic pregnancies.[92] This change likely reflects better obstetric care during pregnancy, despite the lack of adequate glycemic control before conception.

Two series that involved women who delivered between 1950 and 1979 demonstrated an incidence of **neonatal respiratory distress syndrome (RDS)** in diabetic pregnancies that was 6 to 23 times that in nondiabetic controls.[43,97] Respiratory distress is more common among newborns who are delivered preterm or are surgically delivered without labor. Later studies of patients with both pregestational and gestational DM have not demonstrated a significant difference in the incidence of neonatal respiratory distress syndrome between diabetic and nondiabetic pregnancies.[76,98,99]

The level of glycemic control during pregnancy affects the amniotic fluid phospholipid profile. Poorly controlled diabetic pregnancies may have a higher incidence of immature amniotic fluid fetal lung profiles at 34 to 38 weeks' gestation without an increase in the rate of clinical respiratory distress syndrome.[99,100] In reliably dated diabetic pregnancies, fetal lung maturity testing has little clinical benefit.[101]

Neonatal hypoglycemia occurs in 5% to 12% of cases of pregestational and gestational DM.[76] This represents a 6-fold to 16-fold higher risk of neonatal hypoglycemia than in nondiabetic controls. Neonatal hypoglycemia likely results from sustained fetal hyperinsulinemia in response to chronic intrauterine hyperglycemia. Clinical studies have demonstrated higher fetal insulin levels and exaggerated fetal insulin responses to acute maternal hyperglycemia in diabetic pregnancies.[102,103] An acute increase in maternal glucose concentration, as might occur if a dextrose-containing solution was used for intravenous hydration during administration of neuraxial anesthesia, can lead to reactive neonatal hypoglycemia, even in nondiabetic women.[104]

There is a twofold to fivefold higher incidence of **neonatal hyperbilirubinemia** in women with pregestational and gestational DM than in nondiabetic controls.[76] Other associated factors include the severity of gestational DM and excess maternal weight gain during pregnancy.[105,106] Both the etiology and the clinical significance of neonatal hyperbilirubinemia are unknown, although one study noted the absence of long-term morbidity.[76]

Offspring of diabetic mothers are at increased risk for development of **DM,** likely from a combination of genetic and intrauterine environmental factors. Despite the well-known association of type 1 DM with HLA markers, studies of monozygotic human twins have suggested that genetic factors have a greater role in type 2 DM than in type 1 DM (100% versus 20% to 50% concordance, respectively).[105] In addition, fathers with type 1 DM are five times more likely than mothers with the same disease to have a child with type 1 DM. The intrauterine environment also affects the development of glucose intolerance in offspring.[28]

Some investigators have suggested that **cognitive development** may be impaired in the children of diabetic mothers,[107,108] but this issue remains controversial.

Obstetric Management

Early, strict glycemic control is the best way to prevent fetal structural malformations in women with pregestational DM.[92,94] Determination of hemoglobin A_{1c} concentrations may help the physician determine the adequacy of preconceptional glycemic control.

During pregnancy, the patient should frequently determine capillary blood glucose concentration using a reflectance meter.[109] Continuous glucose monitoring systems (e.g., transdermal, subcutaneous) are more recent approaches.[110,111] Glucose determinations guide adjustments in diet and insulin therapy. In general, insulin requirements increase progressively during the second and third trimesters. Both maternal and perinatal outcomes seem to improve when maternal glycemic control approaches that observed in normal pregnancies. Opinions vary about the optimum target glucose concentration in patients with pregestational DM, but a fasting blood glucose concentration of 60 to 95 mg/dL seems appropriate. Of course, strict glycemic control increases the risk for maternal hypoglycemia.

Therapeutic insulin is available in several forms. Initially, insulin was isolated as a natural product from domestic animals (e.g., cattle, pigs). In the past 20 years, synthetic human insulin has become commercially available and has largely replaced beef and pork insulin in human medicine, with an expected decrease in immune reactions among human recipients.[112,113]

The goal of insulin therapy is to provide plasma insulin concentrations that lead to tight glucose control without hypoglycemia. This goal is facilitated by the availability of several insulin preparations with different subcutaneous absorption rates (Table 42-2).[111] Regular insulin can be administered by the intravenous or subcutaneous route. Regular insulin administered intravenously has a half-life of approximately 4 minutes.[114] Other native insulins listed in Table 42-2 (i.e., neutral protamine Hagedorn [NPH], the zinc suspensions lente and ultralente) represent chemical complexes of regular insulin with protamine or zinc; subcutaneous administration of these insulins is associated with slower absorption and onset of action. Lente and

TABLE 42-2 Pharmacokinetics of Subcutaneous Insulin Administration in Nonpregnant Humans

Insulin Preparations	Onset (hr)	Peak (hr)	Duration (hr)
Short-Acting Class			
Regular	0.5	2-4	5-7
Lispro*	0.25	0.5-1.5	6-8
Aspart*	0.25	1-3	3-5
Glulisine*	0.25	1	4
Intermediate Class			
NPH (neutral protamine Hagedorn)	1-2	6-12	18-24
Lente	1-3	6-12	18-24
Long-Acting Class			
Ultralente	4-6	8-20	>36
Glargine*	1.1	5	24

*Insulin analogue.

Adapted from Gabbe SG, Carpenter LB, Garrison EA. New strategies for glucose control in patients with type 1 and type 2 diabetes mellitus in pregnancy. Clin Obstet Gynecol 2007; 50:1014-24.

ultralente insulins have been replaced clinically by insulin analogues and are of only historical interest. An alternative therapeutic strategy is to administer a rapid-acting insulin by the subcutaneous route using a continuous programmable pump.[110] It is unclear whether continuous subcutaneous pump–administered insulin is clinically superior to intermittent subcutaneous injections of currently available insulins.[115,116]

Human insulin therapy has been fundamentally changed over the past decade by the development of insulin analogues.[117-121] These molecules have specific chemical substitutions in portions of the human insulin protein not involved in receptor binding. Both short-acting and long-acting insulin analogues are in clinical use. **Lispro** and **aspart** are rapid-acting, with a more physiologic onset and offset than regular insulin. **Glargine** is relatively insoluble at neutral pH in the subcutaneous compartment. In contrast to ultralente insulin, subcutaneous glargine has a sustained release without an initial peak of activity. Lispro, aspart, and glargine have all been used safely during human pregnancy. Currently there are no published reports of the use of detemir in human pregnancy, and it is not approved by the U.S. Food and Drug Administration for such use.

Because insulin requirements decrease abruptly at delivery, it is important to verify the times, doses, insulin preparations, and routes of administration in the 24 hours before delivery to avoid maternal postpartum hypoglycemia.

Management of DKA is similar in pregnant and nonpregnant women. It involves (1) intravenous hydration, (2) intravenous insulin, (3) treatment of the underlying cause of DKA, (4) careful monitoring of blood glucose and electrolyte levels, and (5) restriction of bicarbonate therapy to cases of extreme acidosis.[9,10,44] In addition, left uterine displacement should be maintained and supplemental oxygen should be administered. Initial management of the critically ill pregnant woman should focus on the effective management of DKA. Fetal compromise should resolve with appropriate medical management.[53-55]

Diet and exercise are the initial therapeutic approaches for glycemic control in women with gestational DM. Insulin therapy is initiated if the fasting glucose measurement exceeds a threshold of 80 to 105 mg/dL.[22,30,122] In the past, oral hypoglycemic agents were not used extensively in pregnancy, primarily because of concerns about potential teratogenicity and fetal hyperinsulinemia. In current practice, many women with gestational DM are treated with glyburide, glipizide, or metformin.[123,124] A 2008 prospective randomized study that compared metformin (with supplemental insulin as needed) with insulin alone in women with gestational DM found no differences in perinatal complications between the treatment groups.[125]

Timing of delivery is important in the management of diabetic pregnancies. White[42] noted, "Our problem must [be] . . . to prevent premature delivery of the infant of the diabetic mother prior to the period of its viability . . . and, secondly, the termination of the pregnancy at the point of viability and before the dreaded late intrauterine accident can occur." Typically a nonstress test is performed twice weekly in patients with pregestational DM, beginning at 32 weeks' gestation.[30,126,127] A nonreactive nonstress test should prompt the performance of a contraction stress test or a fetal biophysical profile (see Chapter 6). Risk factors for abnormal fetal testing in diabetic pregnancies include maternal nephropathy, hypertension, and poor glycemic control.[128] No consensus exists regarding antepartum testing in women with well-controlled gestational DM.[22] Patients with poorly controlled gestational DM should probably undergo antepartum fetal surveillance similar to that in patients with pregestational DM.[22,122]

In the presence of reassuring fetal testing, delivery can be delayed until after 38 weeks' gestation.[30,126] If fetal testing is abnormal and amniotic fluid analysis indicates fetal pulmonary maturity, the fetus should be delivered as soon as possible. If fetal testing is abnormal but amniotic fluid analysis suggests that the fetal lungs are immature, decisions about the timing of delivery are more difficult.

The decision regarding the method of delivery requires consideration of estimated fetal weight, fetal condition, cervical dilation and effacement, and previous obstetric history. The obstetrician often chooses elective cesarean delivery in the diabetic parturient with evidence of fetal macrosomia to avoid the risk of shoulder dystocia.

Anesthetic Management

Few studies exist of the anesthetic management of pregnant women with DM. In general, clinical decisions about these patients must be guided by logical extensions of studies of nonpregnant diabetic patients and nondiabetic pregnant patients.

Preanesthetic evaluation of the woman with DM should include a history and physical examination that focuses on the identification of the acute and chronic complications of DM (see Box 42-1). There are no published data on the relationship between the complications of DM and responses to anesthetic agents or on anesthetic outcomes in pregnant patients. In a study of nonpregnant diabetic patients, preoperative evidence of **autonomic cardiovascular dysfunction** was predictive of the need for a vasopressor during general anesthesia.[129] Because of the potential for hypotension during neuraxial anesthesia, noninvasive testing of autonomic function may be useful in obstetric patients with pregestational DM. For example, in nonpregnant diabetic patients the corrected QT interval on an electrocardiogram correlates with the severity of autonomic neuropathy.[130] Patients with evidence of autonomic dysfunction may benefit from more frequent blood pressure determinations and more vigorous intravenous hydration before and during the administration of neuraxial anesthesia. **Gastroparesis** is a manifestation of autonomic neuropathy in diabetic patients.[131] In nonpregnant diabetic patients, autonomic neuropathy is associated with a decreased cough reflex threshold and a higher incidence of obstructive sleep apnea.[132,133]

Several studies have examined the maternal, fetal, and neonatal effects of **neuraxial anesthesia** for cesarean delivery for women with pregestational DM.[134-137] Datta and Brown[134] observed that spinal anesthesia was associated with a slightly but significantly lower umbilical cord blood pH measurement at delivery in patients with pregestational DM than in similar patients who received general anesthesia for cesarean delivery. Subsequently, these investigators noted an association between fetal acidosis and peripartum maternal hypotension in patients with pregestational DM who received epidural anesthesia for cesarean delivery.[135]

In both studies, acute maternal hyperglycemia—secondary to intravenous hydration with 5% dextrose before administration of neuraxial anesthesia—was a potentially confounding factor.[134]

Neonatal acidosis is *not* likely to occur during **spinal** or **epidural anesthesia** for cesarean delivery in diabetic parturients, provided that (1) maternal glycemic control is satisfactory, (2) the patient receives aggressive preanesthetic volume expansion with a non–dextrose-containing balanced salt solution, and (3) hypotension is treated promptly and aggressively.[136,137] Some diabetic parturients have chronic uteroplacental insufficiency, so epidural anesthesia may be preferable to spinal anesthesia because the former results in a slower onset of sympathetic blockade. However, no clinical studies have directly addressed this issue in pregnant diabetic women.

Thalme and Engstrom[138] demonstrated normal umbilical arterial blood pH measurements after the administration of **general anesthesia** in a small series of patients with pregestational DM.

After administration of epidural anesthesia for cesarean delivery, Ramanathan et al.[137] observed an increased incidence of neonatal hypoglycemia in patients with pregestational DM compared with nondiabetic controls (35% versus 7%, respectively). In this study, maternal glycemic control was fair (mean fasting plasma glucose level was 127 mg/dL), a non–dextrose-containing solution was used for intravenous hydration, and intravenous insulin therapy was adjusted on the basis of frequent blood glucose determinations. This study illustrates the neonate's vulnerability to hypoglycemia after a diabetic pregnancy despite meticulous anesthesia care at the time of delivery.

Maternal insulin requirements increase progressively during the second and third trimesters of pregnancy.[25] They decrease with the onset of labor, increase again during the second stage of labor, and decrease markedly during the early postpartum period.[36,37] Intravenous insulin therapy is the most flexible method of treatment during this period of rapid change. Absorption of subcutaneous insulin may be unpredictable and may increase the risk of maternal hypoglycemia, especially during the postpartum period.[37] Moreover, strict glycemic control in pregnant women with type 1 DM increases the risk of maternal hypoglycemia as a result of impaired counterregulatory hormone responses (as discussed earlier). Intravenous glucose and insulin infusions during the peripartum period should be titrated to maintain a maternal blood glucose concentration of 70 to 90 mg/dL. During active labor, the glucose requirement is 2.5 mg/kg/min or more.[30,34] Many perioperative strategies have been proposed for metabolic control in nonpregnant patients with DM.[139-141] No convincing evidence suggests that one clinical strategy for perioperative diabetic control is superior in terms of patient outcome. Frequent blood glucose measurements (e.g., at 30- to 60-minute intervals), followed by appropriate adjustment of glucose and insulin infusions, represent the cornerstone of optimal perioperative care in patients with DM.

There are no published data on the effects of DM on the pharmacokinetics and pharmacodynamics of anesthetic agents in pregnant women. In nonpregnant women, DM is associated with (1) a delayed onset of muscle relaxation with tubocurarine and (2) prolonged blockade with vecuronium.[142,143]

The **diabetic stiff-joint syndrome** has been associated with difficult direct laryngoscopy and intubation in patients with DM.[144,145] This syndrome occurs in patients with long-standing type 1 DM and is associated with nonfamilial short stature, joint contractures, and tight skin.[146] Limited movement of the atlanto-occipital joint may result in difficult direct laryngoscopy and intubation. During the preanesthesia evaluation of patients with DM, the anesthesia provider can screen for the stiff-joint syndrome by looking for the "prayer sign" (Figure 42-4). Management is controversial. Some authorities recommend preanesthesia flexion-extension radiographic studies of the cervical spine, followed by awake intubation.[145] Others have expressed doubt about the clinical significance of this syndrome and the reported frequency of airway management problems.[147,148] The term **diabetic scleredema** is synonymous with stiff-joint syndrome. There is one case report of a pregnant patient with pregestational DM and diabetic scleredema who experienced anterior spinal artery syndrome after the administration of epidural anesthesia for cesarean delivery.[149] The author suggested that spinal cord vascular compression resulted from a combination of (1) preexisting microvascular disease, (2) an epidural space that was stiff because of connective tissue disease, and (3) administration of a large volume (i.e., 35 mL) of the local anesthetic agent. In patients with a history and physical examination that suggest diabetic stiff-joint syndrome, the anesthesia provider should consider two potential problems, (1) difficult

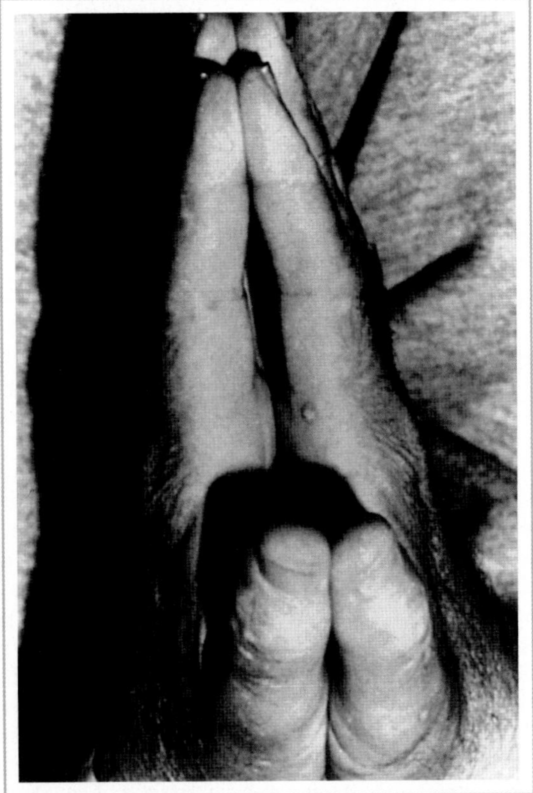

FIGURE 42-4 Inability to approximate the palmar surfaces of the phalangeal joints despite maximal effort, secondary to diabetic stiff-joint syndrome. (From Hogan K, Rusy D, Springman SR. Difficult laryngoscopy and diabetes mellitus. Anesth Analg 1988; 67:1162-5.)

direct laryngoscopy and intubation and (2) a noncompliant epidural space.

Infection is an important cause of morbidity in pregnant women with pregestational DM.[45] There are no published data regarding the incidence of CNS infection after the administration of neuraxial anesthesia in pregnant diabetic patients except for one case of fungal meningitis due to contaminated spinal anesthesia equipment.[150] Strict aseptic technique should be used during the administration of neuraxial anesthesia.

THYROID DISORDERS

Thyroid Hormone Physiology

The follicular cells of the thyroid gland sequester iodine and synthesize thyroglobulin, an iodinated precursor protein. Thyroglobulin is secreted into the lumen of the microscopic thyroid follicles before it undergoes re-uptake, proteolysis, and transfer to lysosomes, where it undergoes degradation.[151] This process results in the systemic release of the thyroid hormones: thyroxine (T_4) and 3,5,3′-triiodothyronine (T_3). Reverse T_3 (3,3′,5′-triiodothyronine) is a structural variant with much less physiologic potency in most target organs.[152]

Thyroid hormone synthesis and release are controlled primarily by thyroid-stimulating hormone (TSH)—a trophic hormone from the pituitary—and the supply of iodine. The thyroid hormones normally participate in a negative feedback loop that regulates TSH secretion (Figure 42-5) and thyrotropin-releasing hormone production in the hypothalamus.[153]

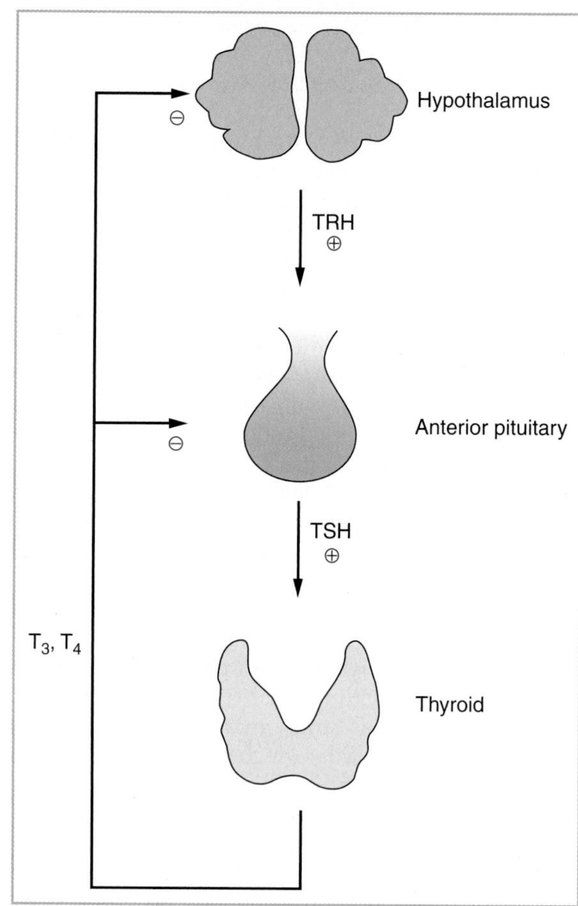

FIGURE 42-5 Normal feedback control of thyroid hormone secretion. TRH, thyrotropin-releasing hormone; TSH, thyroid-stimulating hormone; T_3, triiodothyronine; T_4, thyroxine. (From Davies PH, Franklyn JA. The effects of drugs on tests of thyroid function. Eur J Clin Pharmacol 1991; 40:439-51.)

Thyroid hormones are highly bound to protein in the blood. In euthyroid nonpregnant humans, the normal total serum concentrations of T_4 and T_3 are 50 to 150 nmol/L and 1.4 to 3.2 nmol/L, respectively.[154-156] The unbound or free fractions of T_4 and T_3 are 0.03% and 0.3% of total circulating T_4 and T_3, respectively.[157] Similar proportions of T_4 and T_3 are distributed among the three major plasma proteins that bind thyroid hormones, which are (1) thyroxine-binding globulin (70% to 80%), (2) thyroxine-binding prealbumin or transthyretin (10% to 20%), and (3) albumin (10% to 15%).[158,159] The serum concentration of unbound or free T_4 is typically the major determinant of thyroid hormone activity in target tissues.[160] Thyroid hormones are temporarily inert while bound to plasma proteins. Changes in the concentrations of thyroxine-binding proteins can occur during various physiologic states (e.g., pregnancy) and disease processes. Thyroid hormone action does not change with fluctuations in the total concentration of T_4 as long as the concentration of free T_4 remains constant.

Thyroid hormone is an endocrine regulator in many target organs (e.g., liver, kidneys, skeletal and cardiac muscles, brain, pituitary, placenta).[161] The defined physiologic effects of thyroid hormones are mediated by regulation of specific gene products. These effects include (1) somatic and nervous system development, (2) calorigenesis, (3) augmented skeletal and cardiac muscle performance, (4) intermediary metabolism, and (5) feedback control.[162]

In target tissues, the molecular actions of T_4 begin with the enzymatic deiodination of T_4 to T_3. Iodothyronine deiodinase is widely distributed in the body and occurs in three molecular forms.[163] Only 20% of the daily T_3 production is secreted by the thyroid gland; the rest is formed by peripheral deiodination.[164] In the classic model of thyroid hormone action, T_3 enters the nuclei of target cells, binds to specific thyroid hormone receptors, and alters genomic transcription of specific proteins.[165] Research has now characterized other mechanisms of thyroid hormone action, including mitochondrial transcription and cytoplasmic or cell-surface nontranscriptional effects.[166,167] The thyroid hormone receptor belongs to a family of structurally related, intracellular ligand-binding proteins.[166] Variations in the number and types of thyroid hormone receptors, as well as receptor linkage to development- or tissue-specific genomic expressions, provide additional levels of physiologic control and vulnerability to disease processes.[163]

Figure 42-6 demonstrates the specific sites in thyroid hormone synthesis that are affected by medications. Drugs also may affect (1) the concentrations of binding proteins, (2) deiodinase activity, and (3) peripheral uptake of thyroid hormones.[158,160,168]

Laboratory evaluation of thyroid function consists of two measurements. First, the serum concentration of free T_4 can be directly measured or indirectly calculated. Second, the serum concentration of TSH is measured to assess the negative feedback loop that controls the thyroid gland.

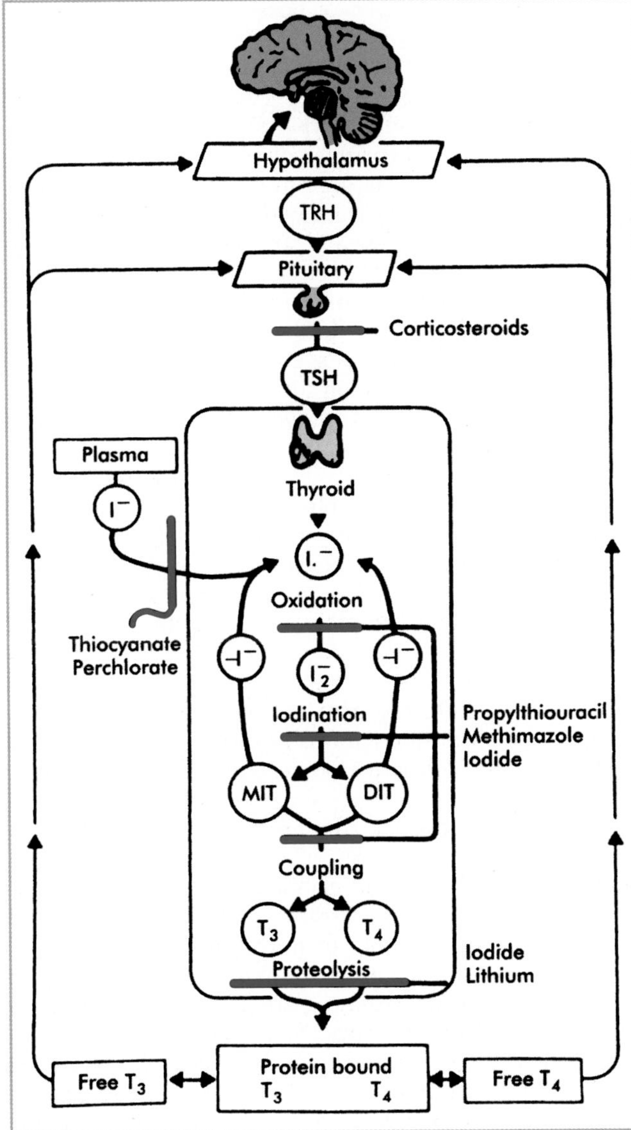

FIGURE 42-6 Effects of antithyroid medications on thyroid hormone synthesis and activity. DIT, diiodotyrosine; I, iodine; MIT, monoiodotyrosine; T_3, triiodothyronine; T_4, thyroxine; TRH, thyrotropin-releasing hormone; TSH, thyroid-stimulating hormone. (From Stehling LC. Anesthetic management of the patient with hyperthyroidism. Anesthesiology 1974; 41:585-95.)

The TSH concentration is judged as appropriate or inappropriate in the context of the serum concentration of free T_4.

During normal human pregnancy, the serum concentration of thyroxine-binding globulin (TBG) steadily increases until it reaches a plateau at 20 weeks' gestation, when it is 50% greater than the nonpregnant level.[154] The greater concentration of TBG results from a prolonged half-life—not higher synthesis—during pregnancy.[159] The normal pregnant woman is euthyroid because the serum concentrations of free T_4 and T_3 are in the normal or low-normal range for nonpregnant humans.[154] However, the increased concentration of TBG means that total serum concentrations of T_4 and T_3 during pregnancy are at or above the upper limit of normal for nonpregnant women.[154,169]

Human chorionic gonadotropin (hCG) is a placental protein that shares some structural features with TSH. The serum concentrations of TSH and hCG have an inverse relationship during normal human pregnancy,[154] reflecting the mild TSH-like activity that results from increased plasma concentrations of hCG during early pregnancy.[170]

Maternal iodine availability is decreased during pregnancy because of greater fetal uptake and increased maternal renal clearance.[171,172] In geographic areas with marginal iodine supplies, the lower availability may predispose the mother to goiter unless she receives dietary iodine supplementation.[154,173,174]

Hyperthyroidism

DEFINITION AND EPIDEMIOLOGY

Hyperthyroidism is defined as an abnormal increase in the serum concentration of unbound or free thyroid hormones. The prevalence of hyperthyroidism in the general population is 0.2% to 1.9%, with a female-to-male ratio of 10:1.[175,176] Etiologies of hyperthyroidism are listed in Box 42-5. Graves' disease is responsible for 70% to 90% of cases; thyroiditis and the combined category of toxic adenoma and toxic multinodular goiter each account for approximately 5% of cases. There are multiple levels of interaction between the thyroid and reproductive endocrine systems in women, with specific implications for patients with hyperthyroidism and hypothyroidism.[177]

PATHOPHYSIOLOGY

Graves' disease is an autoimmune thyroid disease.[175,178] Its etiology is likely multifactorial and includes both **environmental** (e.g., stress, hormones) and **genetic** influences. Several autoantibodies against thyroid tissue have been described in patients with this disease. Autoantibodies directed against the TSH receptor in the thyroid gland may either augment or inhibit TSH action, depending on their binding specificities. These antibodies are called **thyroid receptor antibodies (TRAbs)**. The binding specificities of TRAbs in the blood of each patient with Graves' disease affect the net thyroid-stimulating activity. Autoantibodies against thyroid peroxidase, the

BOX 42-5 Etiologies of Hyperthyroidism

Abnormal Thyroid Stimulator
- Graves' disease
- Gestational trophoblastic neoplasia
- Thyroid-stimulating hormone–secreting pituitary tumor

Intrinsic Thyroid Autonomy
- Toxic adenoma
- Toxic multinodular goiter

Inflammatory Disease
- Subacute thyroiditis

Extrinsic Hormone Source
- Ectopic thyroid tissue
- Thyroid hormone ingestion

Modified from Houston MS, Hay ID. Practical management of hyperthyroidism. Am Fam Physician 1990; 41:909-16.

sodium-iodine cotransporter, and thyroglobulin also have been described in patients with Graves' disease.

Among untreated patients with Graves' disease, approximately 20% undergo spontaneous remission.[178] However, the prognosis for individual patients cannot be predicted from results of clinical or laboratory examinations.

CLINICAL PRESENTATION AND DIAGNOSIS

Hyperthyroidism presents as a physiologic state dominated by an increased metabolic rate. A hyperthyroid symptom scale has been developed on the basis of the following 10 clinical factors: nervousness, sweating, heat intolerance, hyperactivity, tremor, weakness, hyperdynamic precordium, diarrhea, appetite, and level of incapacitation.[168] This symptom scale has been useful to follow the clinical course of patients with Graves' disease. Exophthalmos or infiltrative ophthalmopathy is clinically apparent in most patients.[178-180] Other physical signs may occur at low frequency, including pretibial myxedema or dermopathy (1% to 2%) and nail changes or acropachy (less than 1%). The infiltrative ophthalmopathy in Graves' disease is caused by enlargement of both the extraocular muscle bodies and intraorbital adipose tissue. The pathogenetic mechanism involves abnormal accumulation of hyaluronic acid and edema within these tissues; the orbital fibroblast appears to be the primary target cell of this autoimmune process.[180]

Hyperthyroidism stimulates the cardiovascular system in excess of the underlying increased metabolic rate, resulting in a hyperkinetic circulatory state.[181,182] Myocardial contractility, heart rate, stroke volume, and ventricular size all increase, and peripheral vascular resistance decreases in skin and muscle. Thyroid hormones can affect the ratio of alpha- and beta-adrenergic receptors in the heart.[182] Cardiomyopathy can be demonstrated during exercise in hyperthyroid patients, independent of beta-adrenergic receptors; it is reversible with normalization of thyroid function.[183]

The diagnosis of hyperthyroidism depends on increased serum concentrations of unbound or free T_4. The more common forms of hyperthyroidism (e.g., Graves' disease, toxic adenoma, toxic multinodular goiter) may be differentiated from the less common forms by a radioiodine uptake study.[176] The identification of TSH receptor autoantibodies may have some role in distinguishing Graves' disease from toxic adenoma or multinodular goiter.[178]

INTERACTION WITH PREGNANCY

Normal human pregnancy is a euthyroid state, with normal serum concentrations of unbound or free T_4 despite increased serum concentrations of TBG and total T_4. During pregnancy, hyperthyroidism results from the same etiologies as in nonpregnant patients (see Box 42-5). Graves' disease is the leading cause of hyperthyroidism during pregnancy, with a prevalence of 0.2%, which is lower than in the general population.[184-187] The lower prevalence may reflect a beneficial effect of the immunotolerance of pregnancy on autoimmune disorders such as Graves' disease.[178,187] Human pregnancy is also associated with a change in the specificity of TSH receptor antibody activity from stimulatory to blocking activity.[188]

Gestational trophoblastic neoplasms are frequently associated with elevated serum hCG concentrations. High concentrations of hCG may possess significant thyroid-stimulating bioactivity because of the structural homology between hCG and TSH.[170,189] Transient hyperthyroidism during pregnancy has been reported in association with hyperemesis gravidarum[190]; hyperthyroidism and hyperemesis gravidarum may be parallel disease processes, with elevated hCG as a shared mechanism.[190] Hyperthyroidism can, on rare occasions, result from two coincident disease processes (e.g., Graves' disease and struma ovarii) in both pregnant and nonpregnant women.[191]

Thyroid nodules occur in 4% to 7% of adults. Pregnancy is associated with increases in the number and size of thyroid nodules.[192] Pregnancy probably does not affect the development or progression of thyroid carcinoma, but this conclusion remains controversial.[193,194] Evaluation of a thyroid nodule that presents during pregnancy should include (1) measurement of serum TSH and free T_4 concentrations, (2) ultrasonographic examination to determine whether the lesion is cystic or solid, and (3) fine-needle aspiration or percutaneous needle biopsy. Malignant lesions can be treated surgically during pregnancy. Radioactive iodine therapy may be delayed until the postpartum period.[193]

MEDICAL AND SURGICAL MANAGEMENT

Current therapies for Graves' disease in *nonpregnant* patients include radioactive iodine, antithyroid medications, and surgery.[175,176]

Radioactive iodine is administered orally as ^{131}I, in a dose range of 30 to 75 mCi.[195] All forms of iodine are sequestered by the thyroid gland, and ^{131}I exerts a therapeutic effect in Graves' disease primarily through local emission of beta radiation. In most patients with Graves' disease, hypothyroidism develops after a therapeutic dose of radioactive iodine, necessitating careful follow-up and long-term thyroid hormone replacement therapy. In nonpregnant patients, the long-term health risks of radioactive iodine therapy are minimal.[195] Radioactive iodine therapy is *contraindicated* in pregnancy, because all forms of iodine readily cross the placenta to the fetus. Currently recommended treatment is to delay pregnancy for 4 to 6 months after radioactive iodine therapy, although ^{131}I has a half-life of only 8 days.[195]

Propylthiouracil and **methimazole** are the antithyroid medications used to treat Graves' disease.[196] These drugs interfere with the incorporation of iodine into thyroglobulin and with subsequent coupling reactions in the thyroid gland (see Figure 42-6), and propylthiouracil inhibits iodothyronine deiodinase in peripheral tissues. Propylthiouracil and methimazole may be prescribed alone or, in what is referred to as "block and replace" therapy, at higher doses in combination with thyroxine.[187] Typical oral doses are 5 to 15 mg two times daily for methimazole and 100 to 150 mg three times daily for propylthiouracil. The long-term clinical strategy is to adjust the dose downward as tolerated. Some patients with Graves' disease experience remission after the administration of an antithyroid medication. The major complication of antithyroid medications is asymptomatic agranulocytosis, which has an incidence of 0.03% to 0.5% and typically occurs within 3 months of initiating therapy. If treatment with antithyroid medications is unsatisfactory, *nonpregnant* patients may receive radioactive iodine.

Surgical therapy for Graves' disease is typically reserved for patients unable or unwilling to undergo treatment with radioactive iodine or antithyroid medications.[176,197] Controversy exists about the choice between subtotal and total thyroidectomy; the surgeon must weigh the risk of recurrent hyperthyroidism against that of permanent hypothyroidism requiring supplementation.[197] Perioperative complications of thyroid surgery include (1) unilateral or bilateral vocal cord paralysis secondary to laryngeal nerve injury, (2) wound hematoma, (3) pneumothorax, (4) hypoparathyroidism, and (5) thyroid storm.[197] Hypocalcemia secondary to acute hypoparathyroidism may manifest as laryngospasm during the postoperative period.[198]

Adjunctive therapies for hyperthyroidism include iodine, radiocontrast agents, lithium, and glucocorticoids (see Figure 42-6).[175] Beta-adrenergic receptor antagonists also have been used to decrease cardiovascular responses to higher concentrations of thyroid hormones.

Thyroid Storm

Thyroid storm is a life-threatening exacerbation or decompensation of a preexisting hyperthyroid state.[199-202] It is a clinical diagnosis based on the following signs and symptoms: (1) fever, (2) mental and emotional disturbances, (3) tachycardia, (4) tachypnea, (5) diaphoresis, and (6) diarrhea. Without treatment, thyroid storm may progress to coma, multiorgan system failure, and death. The mortality rate approached 100% in earlier series, but improved therapy has reduced the mortality rate to less than 20%.[202]

In most cases, thyroid storm is associated with a precipitating event in a patient with untreated or incompletely treated hyperthyroidism (Box 42-6). Historically, the precipitating events reflect the common serious medical illnesses of a given era[199-201]; cases of thyroid storm were categorized as "surgical" or "medical" depending on whether or not the exacerbation occurred during the perioperative period. With improved perioperative management, the incidence of *surgical* thyroid storm has decreased markedly, and this terminology is rarely used in contemporary medical practice.

BOX 42-6 Events Associated with Precipitation of Thyroid Storm

- Surgery
- Childbirth
- Trauma
- Iodinated contrast agents
- Treatment with iodide ^{131}I
- Emotional stress
- Pulmonary embolism
- Stroke
- Infection
- Diabetic ketoacidosis
- Hypoglycemia
- Congestive heart failure
- Bowel infarction

From Roth RN, McAuliffe MJ. Hyperthyroidism and thyroid storm. Emerg Med Clin North Am 1989; 7:873-83.

In the past, 2% to 7% of patients hospitalized for hyperthyroidism experienced thyroid storm.[199-201] The current incidence of thyroid storm in hyperthyroid patients is difficult to determine.

The mechanism of thyroid storm development is unknown. On the basis of the clinical presentation and known precipitating events, one hypothesis is that it is caused by increases in thyroid hormone and catecholamine secretion. Limited data suggest that total serum concentrations of T_4 and T_3 do not increase during thyroid storm in hyperthyroid patients,[203] although one case report suggests otherwise.[204] Alternatively, the precipitating event in thyroid storm may augment thyroid hormone action by increasing the circulating free fraction of thyroid hormones. This hypothesis is supported by data that demonstrate higher serum concentrations of free T_4 during thyroid storm as well as by observations of changes in thyroid hormone binding during fever or systemic illness.[205]

Catecholamine secretion may also play a role in the development of thyroid storm. In hyperthyroid patients without thyroid storm, the endogenous secretion of epinephrine and norepinephrine is normal, as are the cardiovascular responses to exogenous epinephrine and isoproterenol.[206,207] These parameters have not been measured during episodes of thyroid storm, but symptoms respond well to medications that block the synthesis or receptor binding of beta-adrenergic receptor agonists.[201] The role of the sympathetic nervous system in thyroid storm is supported by historical observations that spinal anesthesia to the fourth thoracic dermatome level is therapeutic.[208] It is unclear whether thyroid storm can develop with basline catecholamine secretions; a surge of catecholamines may be necessary to trigger this condition.

Box 42-7 outlines the treatment of thyroid storm. Several points merit discussion. Glucocorticoid supplementation is listed as a general supportive measure because endogenous glucocorticoid production is impaired in patients with hyperthyroidism.[209] Glucocorticoids also inhibit both thyroid hormone production and the peripheral conversion of T_4 to T_3.[181] Propylthiouracil and methimazole reduce thyroid hormone production, but only propylthiouracil inhibits the peripheral conversion of T_4 to T_3 (as discussed earlier). In addition to the relief of many symptoms of hyperthyroidism, propranolol inhibits the peripheral conversion of T_4 to T_3. This latter property of propranolol is not related to its beta-adrenergic receptor blocking activity and is not shared by most other beta-blockers.[210,211] Because of its dual action, propranolol is the beta-adrenergic receptor antagonist of choice in cases of thyroid storm. Esmolol also has been used successfully during the treatment of thyroid storm (see later).[212,213]

Thyroid storm is an acute hypermetabolic state that may be difficult to distinguish clinically from malignant hyperthermia; rhabdomyolysis is one of the few features of the latter disorder that has not also been reported in thyroid storm.[214] Three cases of thyroid storm treated with dantrolene have been reported.[215-217] Two patients survived, but the third succumbed to multiorgan system failure that antedated the dantrolene therapy. In another case, a patient with known Graves' disease undergoing subtotal thyroidectomy had an intraoperative hypermetabolic crisis that was initially diagnosed and treated as thyroid storm. The correct diagnosis of malignant hyperthermia

BOX 42-7 Treatment of Thyroid Storm

General supportive measures
- Cooling blanket and ice
- Chlorpromazine (25-50 mg IV) or meperidine (25-50 mg IV) to diminish shivering
- Intravenous hydration
- Glucose and electrolyte replacement
- Oxygen
- Glucocorticoids: dexamethasone (2-4 mg IV q 8 hr) or hydrocortisone (100 mg IV q 8 hr)
- B-complex multivitamins

Reduction of synthesis and secretion of thyroid hormones
- Antithyroid medications: propylthiouracil 200-400 mg orally q 6-8 hr) or methimazole (20-25 mg orally q 6 hr)
- Iodine: sodium iodide (1 g IV or Lugol's solution 4-8 drops orally q 6-8 hr) or supersaturated potassium iodide solution (5 drops orally q 6 hr)
- Glucocorticoids

Reduction of peripheral conversion of thyroxine (T_4) to 3,5,3′-triiodothyronine (T_3)
- Propylthiouracil
- Glucocorticoids
- Radiographic contrast agents
  - Iopanoic acid (Telepaque) (1 g orally q 8 hr for 24 hr, then 500 mg orally q 12 hr)
  - Sodium ipodate (Oragrafin) (1-3 g orally per day)
- Propranolol

Decrease in the metabolic effects of thyroid hormones
- Beta-adrenergic receptor blocking agents
- Propranolol
- Esmolol
- Reserpine
- Guanethidine

Other therapeutic maneuvers
- Plasma exchange
- Dantrolene

Diagnosis and treatment of the underlying illness that precipitated the thyroid storm

IV, intravenous.

Data from Waldstein SS, Slodki SJ, Kaganiec GI, Bronsky D. A clinical study of thyroid storm. Ann Intern Med 1960; 52:626-42; and Mazzaferri EL, Skillman TG. Thyroid storm: A review of 22 episodes with special emphasis on the use of guanethidine. Arch Intern Med 1969; 124:684-90.

was made on the basis of subsequent blood gas analysis, and the patient was successfully treated with dantrolene.[218] Plasma exchange is another unusual but effective therapeutic option in cases of thyroid storm.[219]

In summary, treatment of thyroid storm consists of general supportive measures and the administration of glucocorticoids, propylthiouracil, sodium iodide, and propranolol. It is reasonable to delay iodine treatment until 1 hour after the administration of propylthiouracil to avoid increased iodine use by the thyroid gland.

Preoperative Preparation

The risk of thyroid storm during the perioperative period can be minimized by appropriate preparation of the hyperthyroid patient. Most cases of perioperative thyroid storm involve thyroid surgery. The preoperative therapeutic goals are to inhibit thyroid hormone synthesis and secretion in patients with preexisting hyperthyroidism and to decrease the vascularity of the thyroid gland. The four main therapies used in preoperative preparation are administration of (1) an antithyroid medication (primarily propylthiouracil), (2) a beta-adrenergic receptor antagonist, (3) a glucocorticoid, and (4) iodine.[181,197,220] Iodine inhibits thyroid hormone secretion more effectively in hyperthyroid patients than in euthyroid patients because the latter are capable of mounting a compensatory TSH response as serum T_4 levels decrease.[221]

In some patients, beta-adrenergic receptor blockade may be sufficient to prevent perioperative thyroid storm,[222] although thyroid storm has been reported after preoperative preparation with propranolol alone.[223] In some of these cases, patients probably did not receive effective beta-adrenergic receptor blockade. A 25% reduction in exercise-induced heart rate is a better indication of adequate beta-adrenergic receptor blockade than a change in the resting heart rate.[220] One advantage of beta-adrenergic receptor antagonists over antithyroid medications is the shorter time typically required for preoperative preparation: (i.e., 2 weeks versus 6 to 8 weeks, respectively).[222] Several investigators have recommended preoperative preparation with a beta-adrenergic receptor antagonist, with the addition of iodine beginning 10 days before surgery.[220,224,225] The use of beta-adrenergic receptor antagonists entails a risk of hypoglycemia in hyperthyroid patients, because they have reduced hepatic glucose reserves and nonspecific beta-adrenergic receptor blockade results in a pharmacologic blunting of sympathetic responses.[220]

No prospective randomized studies have compared the efficacy of various methods for preoperative preparation of hyperthyroid patients. A reasonable clinical approach would include the use of multiple therapeutic agents (e.g., a beta-adrenergic receptor antagonist, iodine, and a glucocorticoid), with the doses titrated to the clinical response of each patient. The clinical parameters may include exercise-induced heart rate, fine tremor, weight gain, and recovery of muscle strength.[181]

Elective surgery should not proceed without adequate preoperative preparation of hyperthyroid patients. In cases of emergency surgery, physicians should use the therapies discussed for the treatment of thyroid storm (as discussed earlier) (see Box 42-7).

Medical and Surgical Management during Pregnancy

All of the therapeutic options used in nonpregnant hyperthyroid patients should be efficacious in pregnant women. However, the potential effects on the fetus dictate modifications in the options for treatment of hyperthyroidism during pregnancy.

Radioactive iodine is *contraindicated* during pregnancy because iodine readily crosses the placenta to the fetus. Fetal effects of inadvertent maternal administration of ^{131}I vary with gestational age.[220] Before 10 weeks' gestation, the risk to the fetus is less well-defined and likely approximates that of a low-level dose of radiation during early development[172]; after 10 weeks' gestation, however, the fetal thyroid gland can sequester iodine, and ^{131}I may destroy or significantly damage the gland.

The mainstays of therapy for hyperthyroidism during pregnancy are the antithyroid medications **propylthiouracil** and **methimazole,**[175,184,185,196] which cross the placenta much more easily than the maternal thyroid hormones—potentially inducing fetal hypothyroidism and goiter. Although these agents are similar in efficacy for treatment of hyperthyroidism during pregnancy,[185,196] propylthiouracil has been used more frequently than methimazole. This pattern of therapy is based primarily on the rare but continued observation of fetal congenital scalp defects after maternal methimazole treatment.[196,226] Maintenance therapy for pregnant woman consists of a total daily dose of 100 to 300 mg of propylthiouracil. In a group of patients with Graves' disease who had been treated with methimazole for 1 to 3 years before pregnancy, administration of T_4 (100 μg per day) without methimazole, beginning 5 to 6 months after the onset of pregnancy, resulted in a sixfold reduction in the postpartum rate of recurrent hyperthyroidism.[227] This effect was accompanied by reduced TRAb levels, but the mechanism for the effect was not elucidated.

Surgical therapy (e.g., subtotal thyroidectomy) is generally reserved for pregnant women in whom medical therapy has failed.[187,197] The pregnant woman should receive preoperative preparation with a beta-adrenergic receptor antagonist, a glucocorticoid, and iodine to minimize the risk of thyroid storm. Clinical data suggest that treating maternal Graves' disease with iodine does not result in fetal hypothyroidism[228]; this implies that short-term preoperative maternal treatment with iodine should be safe for the fetus.

There are no published data on the safety of thyroid surgery at various times during pregnancy. It seems prudent to delay surgery during pregnancy until the end of the first trimester, when organogenesis is complete.[197,229] Relative risks and benefits for the mother and fetus should be compared, with an emphasis on the severity of maternal hyperthyroidism and its resistance to medical therapy.

Thyroid storm occurs in 2% to 4% of pregnant patients with hyperthyroidism.[230] Most contemporary cases of thyroid storm during pregnancy occur in patients with undiagnosed or undertreated preexisting hyperthyroidism.[230-234] Precipitating events for thyroid storm during pregnancy include infection, thyroid cancer, normal labor, hemorrhage, cesarean delivery, and eclampsia.[230-235]

Treatment of thyroid storm is identical for both pregnant and nonpregnant patients (as discussed earlier) (see Box 42-7). Despite an association with intrauterine growth restriction (IUGR) or preterm labor,[236] beta-adrenergic receptor antagonists are commonly prescribed during pregnancy. **Propranolol** is the most widely used beta-adrenergic receptor antagonist for treatment of thyroid storm.

Several case reports have described the use of the beta-adrenergic receptor antagonist **esmolol** for treatment of hyperthyroidism in both pregnant and nonpregnant patients,[212,213] although laboratory and clinical observations suggest that maternal administration of esmolol may result in fetal bradycardia and acidosis.[237-240] Esmolol may be considered when propranolol is contraindicated or the patient's hemodynamic status requires the use of a short-acting beta-adrenergic receptor antagonist. Esmolol is preferred for patients with a sensitivity to nonspecific beta-adrenergic receptor blockade (e.g., asthma). Patients with significant cardiomyopathy from hyperthyroidism, who may be very sensitive to beta-adrenergic receptor blockade,[183,241,242] may benefit from esmolol because the dose can easily be titrated to the desired effect.[243] Hyperthyroid cardiomyopathy during pregnancy or the puerperium may require invasive monitoring and the use of multiple medications that require titration.[230,244-246] Esmolol's short half-life allows a rapid reversal of effect if needed. A 2004 case series of hyperthyroid cardiomyopathy in pregnancy described an association with undiagnosed or undertreated hyperthyroidism as well as obstetric complications such as hemorrhage, sepsis, and hypertensive disease.[247]

In general, maternal and fetal interests are best served by optimal maternal therapy. When the physician opts for maternal therapy that could, in theory, adversely affect fetal well-being, the rationale should be documented in the medical record.

OBSTETRIC MANAGEMENT

Poorly controlled hyperthyroidism during pregnancy increases the risks of severe preeclampsia in the mother and of low birth weight in the neonate.[248] The presence of hyperthyroidism does not affect the obstetric management of these problems. In a retrospective study, Davis et al.[230] suggested that early diagnosis and treatment of hyperthyroidism during pregnancy are associated with better maternal and fetal outcomes.

The use of a nonselective beta-adrenergic receptor antagonist may precipitate or aggravate preterm labor. In women with Graves' disease, the placental transfer of antithyroid medications or thyroid-stimulating antibodies may result in the development of fetal goiter,[249] which can interfere with vaginal delivery or lead to airway obstruction in the neonate. Fetal goiter can be diagnosed with ultrasonography; fetal hypothyroidism can be diagnosed with percutaneous umbilical cord blood sampling and can be treated with intra-amniotic injections of thyroxine.[250] In pregnant women with Graves' disease, maternal serum concentrations of TRAbs during the third trimester may predict neonatal thyroid function.[251]

Normal somatic and intellectual development has been reported in the children of hyperthyroid mothers treated with antithyroid medications[252]; such treatment does not contraindicate breast-feeding (see Chapter 14).[196]

ANESTHETIC MANAGEMENT

No prospective randomized studies have evaluated the efficacy or safety of various anesthetic techniques in patients with hyperthyroidism. The following features of hyperthyroidism may affect anesthetic management: (1) the hyperdynamic cardiovascular system and the possibility of cardiomyopathy, (2) partial airway obstruction secondary to an enlarged thyroid gland, (3) respiratory muscle weakness, and (4) electrolyte abnormalities.[181,253]

Describing two patients with uncontrolled hyperthyroidism who required anesthesia for cesarean delivery, Halpern[254] suggested that either neuraxial or general anesthesia can be safely administered in hyperthyroid parturients. On the basis of theoretical concerns, he suggested the omission of epinephrine from the epidural solution of local anesthetic agent and the use of an alpha-adrenergic receptor agonist (e.g., phenylephrine) for the treatment of hypotension. Earlier clinical studies in nonpregnant subjects with spontaneous hyperthyroidism, however, have shown normal hemodynamic responses to exogenous epinephrine, norepinephrine, phenylephrine, and clonidine.[255,256] It therefore appears safe to use epinephrine to minimize local anesthetic uptake and toxicity during the administration of epidural anesthesia in both euthyroid and hyperthyroid patients.

Hyperthyroid women should receive glucocorticoid supplementation because they have a relative deficiency of glucocorticoid reserves.[209] It seems prudent to avoid medications associated with tachycardia (e.g., ketamine, atropine).[181,254] Patients with Graves' disease may have exophthalmos and therefore may require additional care to prevent corneal abrasions during general anesthesia.[254] Clinical data suggest that postoperative hepatic dysfunction after halothane or enflurane anesthesia is unlikely in hyperthyroid patients.[257] Some investigators have emphasized the efficacy of deep preoperative sedation in nonpregnant hyperthyroid patients.[181,208] The routine use of this technique in pregnant patients is not recommended because of the risks of maternal aspiration and neonatal depression.

Adequate preoperative preparation minimizes the risk of perioperative thyroid storm; when time permits, the goal is to make the patient euthyroid. In an emergency, the hyperthyroid patient can be prepared for surgery with oral propylthiouracil, an intravenous glucocorticoid, sodium iodide, and propranolol. The anesthesia provider should be prepared to treat perioperative thyroid storm (see Box 42-7).

BOX 42-8 Causes of Hypothyroidism

Primary

Autoimmune
- Hashimoto's thyroiditis
- Atrophic hypothyroidism

Iatrogenic
- Radioiodine therapy for hyperthyroidism
- Subtotal thyroidectomy

Pharmacologic
- Iodine deficiency or excess
- Lithium
- Amiodarone
- Antithyroid drugs

Congenital
- Dyshormonogenesis
- Thyroid gland dysgenesis or agenesis

Secondary

Pituitary dysfunction
- Irradiation
- Surgery
- Neoplasm
- Sheehan's syndrome
- Idiopathic

Hypothalamic dysfunction
- Irradiation
- Granulomatous disease
- Neoplasm

From Gain LA. The diagnostic dilemmas of hyperthyroxinemia and hypothyroxinemia. Adv Intern Med 1988; 33:185-203.

Hypothyroidism

DEFINITION AND EPIDEMIOLOGY

Hypothyroidism is defined as an abnormal decrease in the serum concentration of unbound or free thyroid hormones. The prevalence of hypothyroidism in the general population is 0.1% to 2%, which is similar to that of hyperthyroidism.[258] Hypothyroidism is more common in women and the elderly. The American College of Physicians has published guidelines suggesting that women older than 50 years undergo laboratory screening for unsuspected but symptomatic thyroid disease.[259] The preferred screening test is a sensitive assay for serum TSH.

PATHOPHYSIOLOGY

Etiologies of hypothyroidism can be divided into primary and secondary categories (Box 42-8); primary hypothyroidism is more common than secondary hypothyroidism. The clinical manifestations of hypothyroidism result from withdrawal of thyroid hormone from its many target organs and tissues.

CLINICAL PRESENTATION AND DIAGNOSIS

The clinical presentation of hypothyroidism is dominated by constitutional signs and symptoms such as dry skin, decreased sweating, hoarseness, paresthesia, periorbital edema, and delayed reflexes.[260] A diagnosis of hypothyroidism may be suggested by detection of the following factors during the preanesthetic history and physical examination: (1) a history of neck irradiation or radioiodine therapy; (2) the use of lithium, iodine, amiodarone, antithyroid medications, or thyroid replacement medications; and (3) a history of thyroid surgery, or the presence of a surgical scar overlying the site of the thyroid gland.

By definition, hypothyroidism is diagnosed by measuring a decreased serum concentration of unbound or free T_4. In the presence of an intact feedback loop, the serum concentration of TSH should be increased in patients with primary hypothyroidism. The serum TSH concentration is a more sensitive indicator of primary hypothyroidism than the serum T_4 concentration and is therefore the best initial laboratory test in a patient with suspected hypothyroidism.[261]

INTERACTION WITH PREGNANCY

The prevalence of hypothyroidism during pregnancy is approximately 0.3% to 0.5%.[262] This estimate is based on laboratory screening of all obstetric patients in a given geographic area. Pregnant women likely exhibit overt or symptomatic hypothyroidism at a much lower rate than nonpregnant women. Hypothyroid women have a lower fertility rate than euthyroid women; this difference reflects neuroendocrine and ovarian dysfunction.[177,263] The immunosuppressive effects of pregnancy may lead to a temporary improvement of Hashimoto's thyroiditis during pregnancy.

MEDICAL MANAGEMENT

Hypothyroidism is treated by replacement therapy with oral thyroid hormones. The medication most commonly used in replacement therapy is **levothyroxine,**[264] which has a half-life of 7 days. Older studies have shown that the required dose of thyroid hormone replacement often increases during pregnancy in hypothyroid women.[184,186,258,262] Newer data suggest that this phenomenon results in part from an inhibition of gastrointestinal absorption of thyroid hormone by prenatal vitamins and supplements.[265] The effect can be minimized by administration of thyroid hormone at least 4 hours apart from vitamins or supplements. Serial measurements of the serum TSH concentration allow titration of the appropriate dose of thyroid hormone.

OBSTETRIC MANAGEMENT

Hypothyroidism is associated with an increased incidence of the following obstetric complications: anemia, preeclampsia, IUGR, placental abruption, and postpartum hemorrhage.[184,262] However, several reports have emphasized successful pregnancy outcomes in some hypothyroid patients.[266-268] Early diagnosis and treatment of hypothyroidism appear to be associated with improved maternal and fetal well-being.

In most instances of maternal hypothyroidism, neonatal thyroid function is normal because fetal thyroid development is typically independent of maternal thyroid function. The fetus, however, depends on maternal thyroxine until the fetal thyroid system is fully functional at approximately 20 weeks' gestation. Therefore, maternal hypothyroidism in the first half of pregnancy may affect fetal brain development. In addition, fetal hypothyroidism during the second half of pregnancy may also affect normal maturation of the CNS.[269] With universal screening of newborns for hypothyroidism, these neonates should be readily identified. Published data suggest that cognitive development is relatively normal in hypothyroid infants who receive appropriate thyroid hormone replacement with an initial dose of 10 to 15 μg/kg per day.[270] Controversy surrounds the routine screening of pregnant women for subclinical hypothyroidism (normal serum free T_4, but elevated serum TSH).[262,271] Because there are no convincing data showing better maternal or fetal outcomes, such screening is not recommended.[272]

A syndrome of proteinuria and hypothyroidism has been described in patients with pregestational type 1 DM.[273] Although the overall clinical implications are unclear, untreated hypothyroidism is associated with reduced insulin requirements in these patients.

ANESTHETIC MANAGEMENT

The clinical manifestations of hypothyroidism that may affect anesthetic management include (1) reversible myocardial dysfunction, (2) coronary artery disease, (3) reversible defects in hypoxic and hypercapnic ventilatory drives, (4) obstructive sleep apnea, (5) paresthesias, (6) prolonged somatosensory-evoked potential central conduction time, (7) increased cerebrospinal fluid protein concentrations, (8) increased peripheral nociceptive thresholds, (9) hyponatremia, (10) decreased glucocorticoid reserves, (11) anemia, and (12) abnormal coagulation factors and platelets.[261,274-286] Hypothyroid patients may have an abnormal response to peripheral nerve stimulation that decreases the clinical utility of a nerve stimulator during neuromuscular blockade.[287] Clinical studies of vasopressors in nonpregnant hypothyroid patients show normal responses to exogenous epinephrine and diminished responses to phenylephrine.[288,289]

Whether elective surgery should or should not be delayed in order to treat hypothyroidism adequately is controversial.[290] Patient safety issues may justify such a delay. For emergency procedures, anesthesia care should include glucocorticoid supplementation. **Myxedema (hypothyroid)** coma is likely the only circumstance in which acute intravenous thyroid hormone replacement is indicated. In most hypothyroid patients, acute intravenous replacement therapy entails a significant risk of myocardial ischemia.[276]

No prospective randomized studies have compared the safety or efficacy of various anesthetic techniques in pregnant or nonpregnant hypothyroid patients. Hypothyroidism is associated with qualitative platelet dysfunction and is a rare cause of acquired von Willebrand's disease.[286,291,292] The anesthesia provider should use findings from the history and physical examination as well as laboratory testing to verify the presence of normal coagulation before administering neuraxial anesthesia to the patient with severe untreated hypothyroidism. Although epidural hematoma represents a theoretical risk in such patients, there are no published reports of this complication in this patient population.

PHEOCHROMOCYTOMA

Definition and Epidemiology

Pheochromocytoma is a tumor of chromaffin cells of neurectodermal origin; 90% of these tumors are located in the medulla of one or both adrenal glands. Most of the remaining 10% arise from para-aortic chromaffin cells within the abdominal cavity (e.g., the organ of Zuckerkandl). Pheochromocytomas have been found, on rare occasions, in extra-abdominal sites.[293] Pheochromocytomas occur bilaterally (e.g., in the medulla of both adrenal glands) in 5% to 10% of cases.[294,295] Approximately 10% of pheochromocytomas are malignant.[293-296]

Approximately 0.1% to 0.2% of hypertensive adults have a pheochromocytoma.[294] Men and women are affected relatively equally, and the peak incidence varies between the third and seventh decades of life.

Pheochromocytoma is one of the tumors found in two of the **multiple endocrine neoplasia** (MEN) syndromes, **MEN 2A** (e.g., medullary thyroid carcinoma, hyperparathyroidism, pheochromocytoma) and **MEN 2B** (e.g., medullary thyroid carcinoma, mucocutaneous neuromas, pheochromocytoma).[297] Other disease processes associated with pheochromocytoma include von Recklinghausen's disease, von Hippel–Lindau disease, Sturge-Weber syndrome, and tuberous sclerosis.[296] Approximately 10% of pheochromocytomas are a familial form of the disease; these tumors are more likely to be bilateral.[294]

Pathophysiology

The pathophysiology of pheochromocytoma is related almost entirely to the systemic effects of its endocrine secretory products, typically norepinephrine and epinephrine. Some pheochromocytomas may, however, secrete other catecholamines (e.g., dopamine, dihydroxyphenylalanine [DOPA]) or peptide hormones (e.g., vasoactive intestinal peptide, endorphins, calcitonin, parathyroid hormone, erythropoietin, adrenocorticotropic hormone, interleukin-6).[297,298] In an individual patient, the clinical manifestations of pheochromocytoma represent the net systemic effects of the tumor's secretory products.

Clinical Presentation and Diagnosis

Pheochromocytoma can present with a variety of common or uncommon symptoms.[293-298] Patients typically have **paroxysmal symptoms** because of the episodic nature of hormone secretion by the tumor (Table 42-3). The attacks may remain the same or the symptoms may evolve over time.[296] Pallor is common, and flushing is uncommon, in patients with pheochromocytoma. Paroxysmal symptoms may be triggered by a wide variety of physical activities that patients learn to avoid.[296] Typically, these activities directly or indirectly increase the pressure around the tumor. One study suggested that the diagnosis of pheochromocytoma can be excluded with 99.9% certainty if a patient does not have attacks of sweating, tachycardia, or headaches.[299] As the tumor grows, the attacks may last longer and occur more frequently.[296]

The ability of pheochromocytomas to mimic other diseases has frustrated and confused several generations of physicians. In one series of patients with pheochromocytoma, 76% of the tumors were not diagnosed before autopsy.[295] Recent publications include numerous examples of pheochromocytomas that were initially confused with other medical or psychiatric disorders.[300-302] In addition to their systemic endocrine effects, pheochromocytomas can occasionally cause local abdominal symptoms.[303]

TABLE 42-3 Symptoms of Pheochromocytoma during Paroxysmal Attacks

Symptom	Patients Affected in Previous Series (%) Mean	Range	Patients Affected in Ross & Griffith Series (%)
Headache	59.9	43-80	57
Sweating	52.2	37-71	61
Palpitations	49.2	44-71	63
Pallor	42.9	42-44	43
Nausea	34.5	10-42	33
Tremor	33.5	30-38	13
Anxiety	28.9	15-72	30
Abdominal pain	25.8	15-62	14
Chest pain	25.0	19-50	0
Weakness	19.4	8-58	25
Dyspnea	17.0	15-39	23
Weight loss	16.5	14-23	7
Flushing	14.8	10-19	4
Visual disturbances	12.4	11-22	19

From Ross EJ, Griffith DN. The clinical presentation of phaeochromocytoma. Q J Med 1989; 71:485-96.

Hypertension is a common but not universal finding, occurring in 77% to 98% of patients with pheochromocytoma.[296,298] Although most patients have paroxysmal episodes of hypertension, half may also experience *sustained* hypertension.[294,298] **Orthostatic hypotension** occurs in 70% of patients.[296-298] The presumed mechanisms for orthostatic hypotension are chronic vasoconstriction with intravascular volume depletion and impaired reflex responses secondary to receptor downregulation or synaptic effects of circulating catecholamines.[296-298]

The current approach to the diagnosis of pheochromocytoma involves the following three steps: (1) biochemical testing for increased catecholamine secretion, (2) anatomic imaging, and (3) functional imaging.[296,298] Catecholamine secretion is evaluated by measuring norepinephrine and epinephrine, or concentrations of their metabolites (normetanephrine, metanephrine, or vanillylmandelic acid), in plasma or urine samples. Although the relative merits of these laboratory tests have been debated, a consensus in favor of measuring the plasma concentration of metanephrines as the initial laboratory test is beginning to emerge.[304-306]

Conversion of norepinephrine and epinephrine to the respective metanephrines by catecholamine-*O*-methyl transferase occurs to a large extent within the pheochromocytoma prior to secretion.[304] Several medical conditions may confound the diagnosis of pheochromocytoma by altering the plasma and urinary concentrations of catecholamine metabolites. These conditions include congestive heart failure, acute myocardial infarction, stroke, cocaine abuse, sleep apnea, and ethanol or clonidine withdrawal.[298,307] Medications that alter normal catecholamine secretion and metabolism include tricyclic antidepressants, acetaminophen, hydralazine, and beta-adrenergic receptor antagonists.[298,308] Chromogranin-A is a protein found with catecholamines inside secretory vesicles within pheochromocytoma and normal adrenal medullary cells. Originally, chromogranin-A was thought to be a packaging protein in secretory vesicles, but it is now recognized as a prohormone for several peptide hormones, including vasostatin.[309] The measurement of plasma concentrations of chromogranin-A is a confirmatory laboratory test for pheochromocytoma.[298,310,311]

For patients in whom initial laboratory findings are equivocal, several pharmacologic tests can be performed. Clonidine fails to suppress catecholamine secretion in pheochromocytoma patients, and glucagon stimulates catecholamine secretion.[298] The baseline plasma catecholamine concentrations dictate which of these pharmacologic tests should be used.[298,308] A stimulatory test carries some risk of provoking a symptomatic attack and hemodynamic instability.[298]

After the laboratory diagnosis is confirmed, the pheochromocytoma is localized with anatomic and functional imaging.[294,298] Functional imaging relies on labeled compounds with a high affinity for pheochromocytoma cells. Meta-iodobenzylguanidine (MIBG) is an analogue of norepinephrine, and ^{123}I-MIBG is commonly used for scintigraphic localization.[294,298,312] Positron emission tomography (PET) with fluorine-18-L-dihydroxyphenylalanine (^{18}F-DOPA) can be used to localize a pheochromocytoma,[294,298,313] although such scans may be less widely available than traditional nuclear medicine imaging.

Interaction with Pregnancy

Pheochromocytoma is rare during pregnancy, with an overall incidence estimated to be less than 0.2 per 10,000 pregnancies.[314] Although pregnancy may accelerate the growth of some tumors, no data suggest that it does so for pheochromocytoma.[315] Both sporadic and familial types of pheochromocytoma, as well as benign and malignant forms, may occur during pregnancy.[316,317]

Clinical signs and symptoms of pheochromocytoma are similar in pregnant and nonpregnant patients.[314,317,318] Noninvasive hemodynamic measurements demonstrated intense vasoconstriction and decreased cardiac output during episodes of hypertension in two pregnant patients with pheochromocytoma.[319,320] The clinical recognition of pheochromocytoma during pregnancy is especially difficult because of its rarity and its similarity to preeclampsia, a common obstetric disease.[319,321,322] The diagnosis of pheochromocytoma before labor and delivery may reduce maternal mortality from 35% to near zero.[314] Easterling et al.[320] demonstrated that either an inverse relationship between blood pressure and heart rate or an increasing hematocrit during treatment with a beta-adrenergic receptor antagonist in a patient with suspected preeclampsia suggests the presence of pheochromocytoma. Pheochromocytoma may also manifest in the early postpartum period after an unremarkable vaginal delivery.[323,324]

Plasma concentrations of epinephrine, norepinephrine, and dopamine in normal pregnant women do not differ significantly from those in nonpregnant controls.[325] These data suggest that the same cutoff levels can be used to interpret most laboratory test results (except urinary norepinephrine and normetanephrine) for the diagnosis of pheochromocytoma in pregnant and nonpregnant patients. During pregnancy, ultrasonography or magnetic resonance imaging is most commonly used for detection of intra-abdominal pheochromocytomas.[317,326]

Medical and Surgical Management

Definitive therapy of pheochromocytoma is surgical resection of the tumor.[295,298,326] The greatest challenge in perioperative management is to prevent or effectively treat wide swings in hemodynamic measurements. The patient is at risk for severe hypertension during induction of anesthesia and surgical manipulation of the tumor; severe hypotension frequently occurs after excision of the tumor because of an abrupt decline in circulating concentrations of catecholamines.

PREOPERATIVE PREPARATION

The preoperative preparation of a patient with pheochromocytoma relies on pharmacologic therapy to return the patient to a near-normal physiologic state. Patients with a norepinephrine-dominant pheochromocytoma have intense peripheral vasoconstriction and severe intravascular volume depletion. In these patients, preoperative preparation includes alpha-adrenergic receptor blockade and intravascular volume repletion.[294,327,328] The most commonly used alpha-adrenergic receptor antagonist is **phenoxybenzamine**. The initial dose is 10 mg orally twice a day, titrated upward to 40 to 50 mg twice a day. **Doxazosin, prazosin,** and **phentolamine** are other alpha-adrenergic receptor antagonists that have been used successfully.[327-329] Beta-adrenergic receptor antagonists may be added to treat arrhythmias, but their use must be preceded by effective alpha-adrenergic receptor blockade to prevent a paradoxical hypertensive response.[293,297,299] Beta-adrenergic receptor blockade must be individualized because patients with pheochromocytoma are at risk for catecholamine-induced cardiomyopathy.[330,331]

The administration of **nicardipine,** a calcium entry–blocking agent, is an alternative approach in the preoperative preparation of these patients.[328,332] **Metyrosine** is another therapeutic option that interferes with catecholamine synthesis; it has been used as an adjunct to preoperative alpha-adrenergic receptor blockade at doses of 250 to 1000 mg orally twice a day.[327,333] Patients whose symptoms or early responses to alpha-adrenergic receptor blockade suggest an epinephrine-dominant pheochromocytoma may need beta-adrenergic receptor blockade as primary preoperative therapy.[334]

Alpha-adrenergic receptor blockade with phenoxybenzamine is the most commonly used technique for preoperative preparation of the patient with pheochromocytoma.[298,317,327] Administration of a long-acting alpha-adrenergic receptor antagonist (e.g., phenoxybenzamine) may be desirable before tumor excision but can contribute to hypotension after tumor removal.[335] Prospective randomized clinical studies comparing different methods of patient preparation have not been performed. A retrospective review of patients with pheochromocytoma who were treated preoperatively with phenoxybenzamine, prazosin, or doxazosin suggests that these agents are effective and safe.[336] Regardless of the method chosen, the patient must be prepared adequately for surgery. Adequate preparation could be the major reason for the recent decline in operative mortality in patients with pheochromocytoma. Hull[334] stated, "Emergency surgery to remove a phaeochromocytoma from an unprepared patient should never be contemplated." Roizen[337] has established four widely accepted criteria for adequate preoperative alpha-adrenergic receptor blockade in patients with pheochromocytoma (Box 42-9). Most patients require 10 to 14 days of treatment to meet these criteria.[337]

INTRAOPERATIVE MANAGEMENT

Intraoperative management includes the treatment of episodic **hypertension** and **tachycardia** *before* excision and treatment of profound **hypotension** *after* excision. Many medications have been used successfully to manage intraoperative hypertension and tachycardia, including calcium entry–blocking agents, nitroprusside, nitroglycerin, esmolol, magnesium sulfate, and adenosine.[328,332,338-341] Because of the episodic nature of catecholamine secretion and the change in cardiovascular status that occurs after tumor excision, the use of agents with a short duration of action may be advantageous. The successful use of various regimens implies that the intraoperative treatment of hypertension and tachycardia depends more on the vigilance and skill of the anesthesia provider than on the specific medication used.

Intraoperative monitoring of a patient with pheochromocytoma should include the use of standard monitors, an intra-arterial catheter, and a Foley catheter. Ongoing assessments of cardiac contractility and cardiac filling

BOX 42-9 Criteria for Adequate Preoperative Alpha-Adrenergic Blockade in Patients with Pheochromocytoma

1. No in-hospital BP reading higher than 165/90 mm Hg should be evident for 48 hours prior to surgery. Arterial BP can be measured every minute for 1 hour in a busy or stressful environment (e.g., postanesthesia care unit). If no BP reading is greater than 165/90 mm Hg, this criterion is considered satisfied.
2. Orthostatic hypotension should be present, but BP on standing should not be lower than 80/45 mm Hg.
3. The electrocardiogram should be free of ST-T changes that are not permanent.
4. No more than one premature ventricular contraction should occur every 5 minutes.

BP, blood pressure.
Modified from Roizen MF. Anesthetic implications of concurrent diseases. In Miller RD, editor. Anesthesia. 5th edition. New York, Churchill Livingstone, 2000:903-1015.

pressures and volumes facilitate the successful treatment of catecholamine-induced cardiomyopathy or postexcision hypotension. This information may be acquired via a pulmonary artery catheter or transesophageal echocardiography.[342] Surgery for resection of pheochromocytoma may be performed by an open or laparoscopic approach; laparoscopic resection is associated with a shorter hospitalization and higher patient satisfaction.[343] In a small prospective randomized study, patients undergoing laparoscopic resection of a pheochromocytoma were subjected to one of two different intra-abdominal pressures during the carboperitoneum (either 8-10 or 15 mm Hg).[344] Patients with lower intra-abdominal pressure had less perioperative catecholamine release and fewer hemodynamic fluctuations than patients with higher intra-abdominal pressure. A retrospective review of 143 patients who underwent resection of pheochromocytoma or paraganglioma at the Mayo Clinic from 1983 to 1996 showed a 25% incidence of sustained intraoperative hypertension but very few serious perioperative complications.[345]

Hypoglycemia may also be a serious problem after the resection of a pheochromocytoma.[346,347] Insulin secretion is inhibited by alpha-adrenergic receptor stimulation, and removal of the tumor may result in a rebound of insulin release. Blood glucose concentration should be measured frequently after pheochromocytoma excision.

Medical therapy of pheochromocytoma is used only as a temporizing measure during pregnancy or in patients with inoperable or metastatic disease. Pheochromocytoma recurs in 6.5% of patients who have undergone complete surgical resection.[348]

MANAGEMENT DURING PREGNANCY

When pheochromocytoma presents during pregnancy, surgical resection of the tumor is the preferred therapy.[314,319,349] A variety of clinical strategies have been associated with successful obstetric and surgical outcomes. They include (1) open or laparoscopic tumor resection at 16 to 21 weeks' gestation followed by vaginal delivery at term,[350-352] (2) cesarean delivery with concurrent open tumor resection,[316,350,353] (3) cesarean delivery with open or laparoscopic tumor resection 2 to 8 weeks later,[318,354,355] and (4) vaginal delivery with laparoscopic tumor resection 6 weeks later.[351] Before 24 weeks' gestation, surgery should proceed as soon as the patient is adequately prepared with adrenergic blockade.[326,356] Anecdotal reports suggest that laparoscopy can be safely used for pheochromocytoma resection during pregnancy.[352] After 24 weeks' gestation, the gravid uterus represents a mechanical obstruction to surgery for most abdominal pheochromocytomas. Women with pregnancy at this gestational age should receive adrenergic blockade for the remainder of the pregnancy, or until the tumor is removed.[326]

Phenoxybenzamine, the most widely used medication for preoperative preparation of the pregnant woman with pheochromocytoma, easily crosses the placenta[356]; a case series suggested that neonates should be monitored closely in an intensive care nursery after intrauterine exposure to phenoxybenzamine.[357] Other alpha-adrenergic receptor antagonists have been used successfully in pregnant patients with pheochromocytoma, including phentolamine, prazosin, and doxazosin.[316,317] Beta-adrenergic receptor blockade may be added if needed to control tachycardia or arrhythmias or to treat an epinephrine-dominant pheochromocytoma. Beta-adrenergic receptor antagonists that have been used successfully in pregnant patients with a pheochromocytoma include propranolol, atenolol, and metoprolol.[354,358,359] Clinical experience with metyrosine during pregnancy is very limited.[314] The current package insert lists metyrosine in "pregnancy category C." Pending further assessment of safety during pregnancy, the use of metyrosine in pregnant women with pheochromocytoma should be restricted to those whose tumors are resistant to adrenergic blockade.

Medications that have been used successfully to control intraoperative hypertension and tachycardia in pregnant patients with pheochromocytoma include phentolamine, nitroprusside, nitroglycerin, magnesium sulfate, propranolol, remifentanil, esmolol, and hydralazine.[318,360,361] Esmolol, however, may not be an ideal medication during pregnancy (as discussed earlier).[237,240] The safety of maternal administration of nitroprusside has also been questioned because of possible fetal cyanide toxicity.[362] Adverse effects were noted in fetal lambs when high doses of nitroprusside were administered in pregnant ewes in which tachyphylaxis had developed.[362] Clinical case reports suggest that a low-dose maternal infusion of nitroprusside (approximately 1 μg/kg/min) should be safe during the peripartum period.[363,364] If maternal tachyphylaxis develops, nitroprusside should be discontinued and a different vasodilator used. Nitroprusside reduces uteroplacental vascular resistance in hypertensive sheep, and it antagonizes norepinephrine-induced uterine artery vasoconstriction in humans and guinea pigs.[365-367] These data suggest theoretical advantages for the perioperative use of nitroprusside in pregnant women with pheochromocytoma.

In summary, early diagnosis of pheochromocytoma during pregnancy and adequate adrenergic receptor blockade are essential to optimize maternal and fetal safety.[314] Phenoxybenzamine is used for preoperative preparation of the pregnant patient. If beta-adrenergic receptor blockade is necessary, metoprolol can be used unless specifically contraindicated.[317] During surgery, short-acting cardiovascular medications are preferred. Monitoring and therapy should be directed toward optimization of preload, afterload, and cardiac contractility for a patient with rapid changes in circulating concentrations of catecholamines. Attention to detail is likely more important than the choice of specific medications.

Obstetric Management

Pheochromocytoma during pregnancy is associated with an increased incidence of fetal death and IUGR.[314] The presumed mechanism is decreased uterine blood flow secondary to catecholamine secretion by the tumor; the metabolic activity of the placenta is an effective barrier to the transplacental passage of maternal catecholamines.[368] When pheochromocytoma is diagnosed and effective maternal alpha-adrenergic receptor blockade is instituted before delivery, the fetal death rate declines from 50% to near zero.[326]

Placental abruption has been reported in patients with pheochromocytoma[369]; from a hemodynamic standpoint, this process may be analogous to the occurrence of placental abruption in patients with acute cocaine intoxication.[370] Pheochromocytoma and preeclampsia may have overlapping clinical presentations; proteinuria, for example, occasionally occurs in patients with pheochromocytoma.[371]

To avoid the increased abdominal pressure on the tumor that can occur during active labor, cesarean delivery is preferred in patients with an unresected pheochromocytoma.[314,369]

Anesthetic Management

Preoperative preparation and intraoperative monitoring and management have already been discussed. A variety of general anesthetic agents as well as spinal and epidural anesthesia have been successfully used in nonpregnant patients with pheochromocytoma.[328,334] A small prospective randomized study of three general anesthetic techniques and one neuraxial anesthetic technique for pheochromocytoma resection in nonpregnant patients did not demonstrate any intraoperative or postoperative differences among groups.[372] Box 42-10 lists perioperative medications that should be avoided to minimize hormone secretion by a pheochromocytoma. A 2008 case series of nonpregnant patients suggested that exogenous glucocorticoids can unpredictably trigger a pheochromocytoma crisis,[373] but this observation requires further confirmation. There are two published cases of nonpregnant patients with pheochromocytoma who were incorrectly diagnosed intraoperatively with malignant hyperthermia.[374,375] Manipulation of a pheochromocytoma during resection may result in a small increase in end-tidal carbon dioxide[376]; it is unlikely, however, that the modest magnitude of this effect would be confused with malignant hyperthermia.

In pregnant women with pheochromocytoma, analgesia during labor is not usually a concern because cesarean delivery is preferred. Cesarean delivery, with or without concurrent tumor resection, has been accomplished safely with **general anesthesia,**[318,353,358,361] **epidural anesthesia,**[354,360,377] and **combined epidural-general anesthesia.**[355] There are no prospective randomized studies of the anesthetic management of pregnant women with pheochromocytoma. It seems reasonable to avoid abrupt hemodynamic changes that can occur during spinal anesthesia and to avoid the medications listed in Box 42-10. Either epidural or general anesthesia for cesarean delivery should be selected on the basis of factors other than the presence or absence of a pheochromocytoma. The care with which anesthesia is administered is probably more important than the specific technique selected.

BOX 42-10 Perioperative Medications to Avoid in Patients with Pheochromocytoma

- Atracurium
- Droperidol
- Glucocorticoids
- Halothane
- Metoclopramide
- Metocurine
- Morphine
- Pancuronium
- Pentazocine
- Succinylcholine
- Tubocurarine
- Vancomycin

These medications may, either directly or indirectly, increase the release of catecholamines by the tumor. Halothane potentiates cardiac arrhythmias in the presence of higher plasma concentrations of catecholamines.

Information from references 293, 334, 373, 374.

KEY POINTS

- Pregnancy is characterized by a progressive increase in peripheral insulin resistance.
- Insulin requirements decrease during the first stage of labor, increase during the second stage, and decrease again after delivery.
- Maternal diabetes mellitus is associated with a higher incidence of polyhydramnios, preterm labor, preeclampsia, fetal macrosomia, neonatal hypoglycemia, and cesarean delivery.
- Fetal structural malformations are the leading cause of perinatal mortality in diabetic parturients; strict glycemic control before conception reduces the risk.
- Normal pregnancy is a euthyroid state because serum concentrations of unbound or free thyroid hormones are within the normal nonpregnant range.
- Thyroid storm is a rare but life-threatening disorder during pregnancy. It is best prevented by effective treatment of preexisting hyperthyroidism and adequate preparation of the patient for surgery.
- The required dose of thyroid hormone replacement medication increases during pregnancy; neonatal thyroid function is normal in most cases of maternal hypothyroidism.

- Maternal and fetal safety is enhanced by early diagnosis of pheochromocytoma and effective adrenergic receptor blockade prior to resection.
- At the time of pheochromocytoma resection, the anesthesiologist should anticipate the potential for (1) episodic hypertension and tachycardia during manipulation of the tumor and (2) severe hypotension after tumor resection.
- For women with an unresected pheochromocytoma, cesarean delivery is preferred.

REFERENCES

1. Ioannou GN, Bryson CL, Boyko EJ. Prevalence and trends of insulin resistance, impaired fasting glucose, and diabetes. J Diabetes Complic 2007; 21:363-70.
2. Bays HE, Bazata DD, Clark NG, et al. Prevalence of self-reported diagnosis of diabetes mellitus and associated risk factors in a national survey in the US population: SHIELD (Study to help improve early evaluation and management of risk factors leading to diabetes). BMC Public Health 2007; 7:277.
3. American Diabetes Association. Diagnosis and classification of diabetes mellitus. Diabetes Care 2008; 31(Suppl 1):S55-60.
4. American Diabetes Association. Standards of medical care in diabetes—2008. Diabetes Care 2008; 31(Suppl 1):S12-54.
5. Hunt KJ, Schuller KL. The increasing prevalence of diabetes in pregnancy. Obstet Gynecol Clin North Am 2007; 34:173-99.
6. Blackshear PJ. Early protein kinase and biosynthetic responses to insulin. Biochem Soc Trans 1992; 20:682-5.
7. Denton RM, Tavare JM, Borthwick A, et al. Insulin-activated protein kinases in fat and other cells. Biochem Soc Trans 1992; 20:659-64.
8. Cohen P. Signal integration at the level of protein kinases, protein phosphatases and their substrates. Trends Biochem Sci 1992; 17:408-13.
9. Wallace TM, Matthews DR. Recent advances in the monitoring and management of diabetic ketoacidosis. Q J Med 2004; 97:773-80.
10. Kitabchi AE, Nyenwe EA. Hyperglycemic crises in diabetes mellitus: Diabetic ketoacidosis and hyperglycemic hyperosmolar state. Endocrinol Metab Clin North Am 2006; 35:725-51, viii.
11. Fisher K, Lees JA, Newman JH. Hypoglycemia in hospitalized patients: Causes and outcomes. N Engl J Med 1986; 315:1245-50.
12. Hoeldtke RD, Boden G, Shuman CR, et al. Reduced epinephrine secretion and hypoglycemia unawareness in diabetic autonomic neuropathy. Ann Intern Med 1982; 96:459-62.
13. Sawicki PT, Siebenhofer A. Beta-blocker treatment in diabetes mellitus. J Intern Med 2001; 250:11-7.
14. Sheehy TW. Case report: Factitious hypoglycemia in diabetic patients. Am J Med Sci 1992; 304:298-302.
15. Santiago JV. Overview of the complications of diabetes. Clin Chem 1986; 32:B48-53.
16. The effect of intensive treatment of diabetes on the development and progression of long-term complications in insulin-dependent diabetes mellitus. The Diabetes Control and Complications Trial Research Group. N Engl J Med 1993; 329:977-86.
17. King P, Peacock I, Donnelly R. The UK Prospective Diabetes Study (UKPDS): Clinical and therapeutic implications for type 2 diabetes. Br J Clin Pharmacol 1999; 48:643-8.
18. Amour J, Kersten JR. Diabetic cardiomyopathy and anesthesia: Bench to bedside. Anesthesiology 2008; 108:524-30.
19. Coustan DR. Screening and diagnosis of gestational diabetes. Semin Perinatol 1994; 18:407-13.
20. Russell MA, Carpenter MW, Coustan DR. Screening and diagnosis of gestational diabetes mellitus. Clin Obstet Gynecol 2007; 50:949-58.
21. Screening for gestational diabetes mellitus. U.S. Preventive Services Task Force recommendation statement. Ann Intern Med 2008; 148:759-65.
22. American College of Obstetricians and Gynecologists. Clinical management guidelines for obstetrician-gynecologists: Gestational diabetes. ACOG Practice Bulletin No. 30. Washington, DC, September 2001. (Obstet Gynecol 2001; 98:525-38.)
23. HAPO Study Cooperative Research Group, Metzger BE, Lowe LP, Dyer AR, et al. Hyperglycemia and adverse pregnancy outcomes. N Engl J Med 2008; 358:1991-2002.
24. O'Kane MJ, Lynch PL, Moles KW, Magee SE. Determination of a diabetes control and complications trial: Aligned HbA1C reference range in pregnancy. Clin Chim Acta 2001; 311:157-9.
25. Crombach G, Siebolds M, Mies R. Insulin use in pregnancy: Clinical pharmacokinetic considerations. Clin Pharmacokinet 1993; 24:89-100.
26. Barbour LA, McCurdy CE, Hernandez TL, et al. Cellular mechanisms for insulin resistance in normal pregnancy and gestational diabetes. Diabetes Care 2007; 30(Suppl 2):S112-9.
27. Lain KY, Catalano PM. Metabolic changes in pregnancy. Clin Obstet Gynecol 2007; 50:938-48.
28. Metzger BE. Long-term outcomes in mothers diagnosed with gestational diabetes mellitus and their offspring. Clin Obstet Gynecol 2007; 50:972-9.
29. Bottalico JN. Recurrent gestational diabetes: Risk factors, diagnosis, management, and implications. Semin Perinatol 2007; 31:176-84.
30. Jovanovic-Peterson L, Peterson CM. Pregnancy in the diabetic woman: Guidelines for a successful outcome. Endocrinol Metab Clin North Am 1992; 21:433-56.
31. Sorenson RL, Brelje TC. Adaptation of islets of Langerhans to pregnancy: Beta-cell growth, enhanced insulin secretion and the role of lactogenic hormones. Horm Metab Res 1997; 29:301-7.
32. Picard F, Wanatabe M, Schoonjans K, et al. Progesterone receptor knockout mice have an improved glucose homeostasis secondary to beta-cell proliferation. Proc Natl Acad Sci U S A 2002; 99:15644-8.
33. Hare JW. Insulin management of type I and type II diabetes in pregnancy. Clin Obstet Gynecol 1991; 34:494-504.
34. Maheux PC, Bonin B, Dizazo A, et al. Glucose homeostasis during spontaneous labor in normal human pregnancy. J Clin Endocrinol Metab 1996; 81:209-15.
35. Holst N, Jenssen TG, Burhol PG, et al. Plasma vasoactive intestinal peptide, insulin, gastric inhibitory polypeptide, and blood glucose in late pregnancy and during and after delivery. Am J Obstet Gynecol 1986; 155:126-31.
36. Jovanovic L, Peterson CM. Insulin and glucose requirements during the first stage of labor in insulin-dependent diabetic women. Am J Med 1983; 75:607-12.
37. Caplan RH, Pagliara AS, Beguin EA, et al. Constant intravenous insulin infusion during labor and delivery in diabetes mellitus. Diabetes Care 1982; 5:6-10.
38. Davies HA, Clark JD, Dalton KJ, Edwards OM. Insulin requirements of diabetic women who breast feed. Br Med J 1989; 298:1357-8.
39. Yen SSC, Vela P, Tsai CC. Impairment of growth hormone secretion in response to hypoglycemia during early and late pregnancy. J Clin Endocrinol Metab 1970; 31:29-32.
40. Feudtner C, Gabbe SG. Diabetes and pregnancy: Four motifs of modern medical history. Clin Obstet Gynecol 2000; 43:4-16.
41. White P. Pregnancy complicating diabetes. Am J Med 1949; 7:609-16.
42. White P. Classification of obstetric diabetes. Am J Obstet Gynecol 1978; 130:228-30.
43. Cousins L. Pregnancy complications among diabetic women: Review 1965-1985. Obstet Gynecol Surv 1987; 42:140-9.
44. Parker JA, Conway DL. Diabetic ketoacidosis in pregnancy. Obstet Gynecol Clin North Am 2007; 34:533-43.
45. Gabbe SG, Mestman JH, Hibbard LT. Maternal mortality in diabetes mellitus: An 18-year survey. Obstet Gynecol 1976; 48:549-51.
46. Miodovnik M, Lavin JP, Harrington DJ, et al. Effect of maternal ketoacidemia on the pregnant ewe and the fetus. Am J Obstet Gynecol 1982; 144:585-93.

47. Stamler EF, Cruz ML, Mimouni F, et al. High infectious morbidity in pregnant women with insulin-dependent diabetes: An understated complication. Am J Obstet Gynecol 1990; 163:1217-21.
48. Montoro MN, Myers VP, Mestman JH, et al. Outcome of pregnancy in diabetic ketoacidosis. Am J Perinatol 1993; 10:17-20.
49. Robertson G, Wheatley T, Robinson RE. Ketoacidosis in pregnancy: An unusual presentation of diabetes mellitus: Case reports. Br J Obstet Gynaecol 1986; 93:1088-90.
50. Bernstein IM, Catalano PM. Ketoacidosis in pregnancy associated with the parenteral administration of terbutaline and betamethasone: A case report. J Reprod Med 1990; 35:818-20.
51. Tibaldi JM, Lorber DL, Nerenberg A. Diabetic ketoacidosis and insulin resistance with subcutaneous terbutaline infusion: A case report. Am J Obstet Gynecol 1990; 163:509-10.
52. Foley MR, Lanon MB, Gabbe SG, et al. Effect of prolonged oral terbutaline therapy on glucose tolerance in pregnancy. Am J Obstet Gynecol 1993; 168:100-5.
53. Rhodes RW, Ogburn PL Jr. Treatment of severe diabetic ketoacidosis in the early third trimester in a patient with fetal distress: A case report. J Reprod Med 1984; 29:621-4.
54. Hughes AB. Fetal heart rate changes during diabetic ketosis. Acta Obstet Gynecol Scand 1987; 66:71-3.
55. Blechner JN, Stenger VG, Prystowsky H. Blood flow to the human uterus during maternal metabolic acidosis. Am J Obstet Gynecol 1975; 121:789-94.
56. Takahashi Y, Kawabata I, Shinohara A, Tamaya T. Transient fetal blood flow redistribution induced by maternal diabetic ketoacidosis diagnosed by Doppler ultrasonography. Prenat Diagn 2000; 20:524-5.
57. Raziel A, Schreyer P, Zabow P, et al. Hyperglycemic hyperosmolar syndrome complicating severe pregnancy-induced hypertension: Case report. Br J Obstet Gynaecol 1989; 96:1355-6.
58. Nayak S, Lippes HA, Lee RV. Hyperglycemic hyperosmolar syndrome (HHS) during pregnancy. J Obstet Gynecol 2005; 25:599-601.
59. Gonzalez JM, Edlow AG, Silber A, Elovitz MA. Hyperosmolar hyperglycemic state of pregnancy with intrauterine fetal demise and preeclampsia. Am J Perinatol 2007; 24:541-3.
60. ter Braak EWM, Evers IM, Erkelens DW, et al. Maternal hypoglycemia during pregnancy in type I diabetes: Maternal and fetal consequences. Diabetes Metab Res Rev 2002; 18:96-105.
61. Lankford HV, Bartholomew SP. Severe hypoglycemia in diabetic pregnancy. Va Med Q 1992; 119:172-4.
62. Kimmerle R, Heinemann L, Delecki A, Berger M. Severe hypoglycemia incidence and predisposing factors in 85 pregnancies of type I diabetic women. Diabetes Care 1992; 15:1034-7.
63. Nielsen LR, Pedersen-Bjergaard U, Thorsteinsson B, et al. Hypoglycemia in pregnant women with type 1 diabetes: Predictors and role of metabolic control. Diabetes Care 2008; 31:9-14.
64. Rosenn BM, Miodovnik M, Holcberg G, et al. Hypoglycemia: The price of intensive insulin therapy for pregnant women with insulin-dependent diabetes mellitus. Obstet Gynecol 1995; 85:417-22.
65. Epidemiology of severe hypoglycemia in the diabetes control and complications trial. The DCCT Research Group. Am J Med 1991; 90:450-9.
66. Diamond MP, Reece EA, Caprio S, et al. Impairment of counterregulatory hormone responses to hypoglycemia in pregnant women with insulin-dependent diabetes mellitus. Am J Obstet Gynecol 1992; 166:70-7.
67. Amiel SA, Sherwin RS, Simonson DC, Tamborlane WV. Effect of intensive insulin therapy on glycemic thresholds for counter regulatory hormone release. Diabetes 1988; 37:901-7.
68. Reece EA, Hagay Z, Roberts AB, et al. Fetal Doppler and behavioral responses during hypoglycemia induced with the insulin clamp technique in pregnant diabetic women. Am J Obstet Gynecol 1995; 172:151-5.
69. Peterson CM, Jovanovic-Peterson L, Mills JL, et al. The diabetes in early pregnancy study: Changes in cholesterol, triglycerides, body weight, and blood pressure. Am J Obstet Gynecol 1992; 166:513-8.
70. Siddiqi T, Rosenn B, Mimouni F, et al. Hypertension during pregnancy in insulin-dependent diabetic women. Obstet Gynecol 1991; 77:514-9.
71. Sibai BM, Caritis S, Hauth J, et al. Risks of preeclampsia and adverse neonatal outcomes among women with pregestational diabetes mellitus. Am J Obstet Gynecol 2000; 182:364-9.
72. Reece EA, Eagan JFX, Coustan DR, et al. Coronary artery disease in diabetic pregnancies. Am J Obstet Gynecol 1986; 154:150-1.
73. Rosenn B, Miodovnik M, Kranias G, et al. Progression of diabetic retinopathy in pregnancy: Association with hypertension in pregnancy. Am J Obstet Gynecol 1992; 166:1214-8.
74. Klein BE, Moss SE, Klein R. Effect of pregnancy on progression of diabetic retinopathy. Diabetes Care 1990; 13:34-40.
75. Landon MB. Diabetic nephropathy and pregnancy. Clin Obstet Gynecol 2007; 50:998-1006.
76. Jacobson JD, Cousins L. A population-based study of maternal and perinatal outcome in patients with gestational diabetes. Am J Obstet Gynecol 1989; 161:981-6.
77. Keller JD, Lopez-Zeno JA, Dooley SL, Socol ML. Shoulder dystocia and birth trauma in gestational diabetes: A five-year experience. Am J Obstet Gynecol 1991; 165:928-30.
78. Kjaer K, Hagen C, Sando SH, Eshoj O. Infertility and pregnancy outcome in an unselected group of women with insulin-dependent diabetes mellitus. Am J Obstet Gynecol 1992; 166:1412-8.
79. Coleman TL, Randall H, Graves W, et al. Vaginal birth after cesarean among women with gestational diabetes. Am J Obstet Gynecol 2001; 184:1104-7.
80. Greene MF, Hare JW, Krache M, et al. Prematurity among insulin-requiring diabetic gravid women. Am J Obstet Gynecol 1989; 161:106-11.
81. Sacks DA. Etiology, detection and management of fetal macrosomia in pregnancies complicated by diabetes mellitus. Clin Obstet Gynecol 2007; 50:980-9.
82. Schaefer-Graf UM, Heuer R, Kilavuz O, et al. Maternal obesity not maternal glucose values correlates best with high rates of fetal macrosomia in pregnancies complicated by gestational diabetes. J Perinat Med 2002; 30:313-21.
83. Johnstone FD, Nasrat AA, Prescott RJ. The effect of established and gestational diabetes on pregnancy outcome. Br J Obstet Gynaecol 1990; 97:1009-15.
84. Iffy L, Brimacombe M, Apuzzio JJ, et al. The risk of shoulder dystocia related permanent fetal injury in relation to birth weight. Eur J Obstet Gynecol Reprod Biol 2008; 136:53-60.
85. Zhang X, Decker A, Platt RW, Kramer MS. How big is too big? The perinatal consequences of fetal macrosomia. Am J Obstet Gynecol 2008; 198:517. e1-6.
86. Langer O, Berkus MD, Huff RW, Samueloff A. Shoulder dystocia: Should the fetus weighing greater than or equal to 4000 grams be delivered by cesarean section? Am J Obstet Gynecol 1991; 165:831-7.
87. Mimouni F, Miodovnik M, Rosenn B, et al. Birth trauma in insulin-dependent diabetic pregnancies. Am J Perinatol 1992; 9:205-8.
88. Beardsall K, Diderholm BMS, Dunger DB. Insulin and carbohydrate metabolism. Best Pract Res Clin Endocrinol Metab 2008; 22:41-55.
89. Modanlou HD, Komatsu G, Dorchester W, et al. Large-for-gestational-age neonates: Anthropometric reasons for shoulder dystocia. Obstet Gynecol 1982; 60:417-23.
90. Tamura RK, Dooley SL. The role of ultrasonography in the management of diabetic pregnancy. Clin Obstet Gynecol 1991; 34:526-34.
91. Sheffield JS, Butler-Koster EL, Casey BM, et al. Maternal diabetes mellitus and infant malformations. Obstet Gynecol 2002; 100:925-30.
92. Reece EA, Homko CJ. Prepregnancy care and the prevention of fetal malformations in the pregnancy complicated by diabetes. Clin Obstet Gynecol 2007; 50:990-7.
93. Ornoy A. Embryonic oxidative stress as a mechanism of teratogenesis with special emphasis on diabetic embryopathy. Reprod Toxicol 2007; 24:31-41.
94. Kitzmiller JL, Gavin LA, Gin GD, et al. Preconception care of diabetes: Glycemic control prevents congenital anomalies. JAMA 1991; 265:731-6.
95. Rosenn B, Miodovnik M, Combs CA, et al. Pre-conception management of insulin-dependent diabetes: Improvement of pregnancy outcome. Obstet Gynecol 1991; 77:846-9.

96. Dicker D, Ben-Rafael Z, Ashkenazi J, Feldberg D. In vitro fertilization and embryo transfer in well-controlled, insulin-dependent diabetics. Fertil Steril 1992; 58:430-2.
97. Robert MF, Neff RK, Hubbell JP, et al. Association between maternal diabetes and the respiratory-distress syndrome in the newborn. N Engl J Med 1976; 294:357-60.
98. Mimouni F, Miodovnik M, Whitsett JA, et al. Respiratory distress syndrome in infants of diabetic mothers in the 1980s: No direct adverse effect of maternal diabetes with modern management. Obstet Gynecol 1987; 69:191-5.
99. Piper JM, Langer O. Does maternal diabetes delay fetal pulmonary maturity? Am J Obstet Gynecol 1993; 168:783-6.
100. Moore TR. A comparison of amniotic fluid fetal pulmonary phospholipids in normal and diabetic pregnancy. Am J Obstet Gynecol 2002; 186:641-50.
101. Kjos SL, Berkowitz KM, Kung B. Prospective delivery of reliably dated term infants of diabetic mothers without determination of fetal lung maturity: Comparison to historical control. J Mat Fetal Neonat Med 2002; 12:433-7.
102. Obenshain SS, Adam PA, King KC, et al. Human fetal insulin response to sustained maternal hyperglycemia. N Engl J Med 1970; 283:566-70.
103. Oakley NW, Beard RW, Turner RC. Effect of sustained maternal hyperglycaemia on the fetus in normal and diabetic pregnancies. Br Med J 1972; 1(5798):466-9.
104. Kenepp NB, Shelley WC, Kumar S, et al. Effects on newborn of hydration with glucose in patients undergoing caesarean section with regional anaesthesia. Lancet 1980; 1(8169):645.
105. Bo S, Menato G, Gallo ML, et al. Mild gestational hyperglycemia, the metabolic syndrome and adverse neonatal outcomes. Acta Obstet Gynecol Scand 2004; 83:335-40.
106. Hedderson MM, Weiss NS, Sacks DA, et al. Pregnancy weight gain and risk of neonatal complications: Macrosomia, hypoglycemia, and hyperbilirubinemia. Obstet Gynecol 2006; 108:1153-61.
107. Hod M, Diamant YZ. The offspring of a diabetic mother: Short and long-range implications. Isr J Med Sci 1992; 28:81-6.
108. Rizzo TA, Ogata ES, Dooley SL, et al. Perinatal complications and cognitive development in 2- and 5-year-old children of diabetic mothers. Am J Obstet Gynecol 1994; 171:706-13.
109. Mazze RS. Measuring and managing hyperglycemia in pregnancy: From glycosuria to continuous blood glucose monitoring. Semin Perinatol 2002; 26:171-80.
110. Kestilä KK, Ekblad UU, Röennemaa T. Continuous glucose monitoring of blood glucose in the treatment of gestational diabetes mellitus. Diabetes Res Clin Practice 2007; 77:174-9.
111. Yogev Y, Hod M. Use of new technologies for monitoring and treating diabetes in pregnancy. Obstet Gynecol Clin North Am 2007; 34:241-53.
112. Zinman B. The physiologic replacement of insulin: An elusive goal. N Engl J Med 1989; 321:363-70.
113. Owens DR, Zinman B, Bolli GB. Insulins today and beyond. Lancet 2001; 358:739-46.
114. Hoffman A, Ziv E. Pharmacokinetic considerations of new insulin formulations and routes of administration. Clin Pharmacokinet 1997; 33:285-301.
115. Mukhopadhyay A, Farrell T, Fraser RB, et al. Continuous subcutaneous insulin infusion vs intensive conventional insulin therapy in pregnant diabetic women: A systematic review and metaanalysis of randomized, controlled trials. Am J Obstet Gynecol 2007; 197:447-56.
116. Pickup JC, Renard E. Long-acting insulin analogs versus insulin pump therapy for the treatment of type 1 and type 2 diabetes. Diabetes Care 2008; 31(Suppl):S140-5.
117. Vajo Z, Fawcett J, Duckworth WC. Recombinant DNA technology in the treatment of diabetes: Insulin analogs. Endocr Rev 2001; 22:706-17.
118. Levien TL, Baker DE, White JR, et al. Insulin glargine: A new basal insulin. Ann Pharmacother 2002; 36:1019-27.
119. Gabbe SG, Carpenter LB, Garrison EA. New strategies for glucose control in patients with type 1 and type 2 diabetes mellitus in pregnancy. Clin Obstet Gynecol 2007; 50:1014-24.
120. Singh C, Jovanovic L. Insulin analogues in the treatment of diabetes in pregnancy. Obstet Gynecol Clin North Am 2007; 34:275-91.
121. Kurtzhals P. Pharmacology of insulin detemir. Endocrinol Metab Clin North Am 2007; 36(Suppl 1):14-20.
122. Gabbe SG, Graves CR. Management of diabetes mellitus complicating pregnancy. Obstet Gynecol 2003; 102:857-68.
123. Langer O. From educated guess to accepted practice: The use of oral antidiabetic agents in pregnancy. Clin Obstet Gynecol 2007; 50:959-71.
124. Feig DS, Briggs GS, Koren G. Oral antidiabetic agents in pregnancy and lactation: A paradigm shift? Ann Pharmacother 2007; 41:1174-80.
125. Rowan JA, Hague WM, Wanzhen G, et al. Metformin versus insulin for the treatment of gestational diabetes. N Engl J Med 2008; 358:2003-15.
126. Landon MB, Gabbe SG, Sachs L. Management of diabetes mellitus and pregnancy: A survey of obstetricians and maternal-fetal specialists. Obstet Gynecol 1990; 75:635-40.
127. American College of Obstetricians and Gynecologists. Pregestational diabetes mellitus. ACOG Practice Bulletin No. 60. Washington DC, March 2005. (Obstet Gynecol 2005; 105:675-84.)
128. Landon MB, Langer O, Gabbe SG, et al. Fetal surveillance in pregnancies complicated by insulin-dependent diabetes mellitus. Am J Obstet Gynecol 1992; 167:617-21.
129. Burgos LG, Ebert TJ, Asiddao C, et al. Increased intraoperative cardiovascular morbidity in diabetics with autonomic neuropathy. Anesthesiology 1989; 70:591-7.
130. Tentolouris N, Katsilambros N, Papazachos G, et al. Corrected QT interval in relation to the severity of diabetic autonomic neuropathy. Eur J Clin Invest 1997; 27:1049-54.
131. Ishihara H, Singh H, Giesecke AH. Relationship between diabetic autonomic neuropathy and gastric contents. Anesth Analg 1994; 78:943-7.
132. Behera D, Das S, Dash RJ, et al. Cough reflex threshold in diabetes mellitus with and without autonomic neuropathy. Respiration 1995; 62:263-8.
133. Ficker JH, Dertinger SH, Siegfried W, et al. Obstructive sleep apnoea and diabetes mellitus: The role of cardiovascular autonomic neuropathy. Eur Respir J 1998; 11:14-9.
134. Datta S, Brown WU. Acid-base status in diabetic mothers and their infants following general or spinal anesthesia for Cesarean section. Anesthesiology 1977; 47:272-6.
135. Datta S, Brown WU, Ostheimer GW, et al. Epidural anesthesia for Cesarean section in diabetic parturients: Maternal and neonatal acid-base status and bupivacaine concentration. Anesth Analg 1981; 60:574-8.
136. Datta S, Kitzmiller JL, Naulty S, et al. Acid-base status of diabetic mothers and their infants following spinal anesthesia for Cesarean section. Anesth Analg 1982; 61:662-5.
137. Ramanathan S, Khoo P, Arismendy J. Perioperative maternal and neonatal acid-base status and glucose metabolism in patients with insulin-dependent diabetes mellitus. Anesth Analg 1991; 73:105-11.
138. Thalme B, Engström L. Acid-base and electrolyte balance in newborn infants of diabetic mothers. Acta Paediatr Scand 1969; 58:133-40.
139. Hirsch IB, McGill JB, Cryer PE, White PF. Perioperative management of surgical patients with diabetes mellitus. Anesthesiology 1991; 74:346-59.
140. Gavin LA. Perioperative management of the diabetic patient. Endocrinol Metab Clin North Am 1992; 21:457-75.
141. McAnulty GR, Robertshaw HJ, Hall GM. Anaesthetic management of patients with diabetes mellitus. Br J Anaesth 2000; 85:80-90.
142. Attallah MM, Daif AA, Saied MMA, Sonbul ZM. Neuromuscular blocking activity of tubocurarine in patients with diabetes mellitus. Br J Anaesth 1992; 68:567-9.

143. Saitoh Y, Kaneda K, Hattori H, et al. Monitoring of neuromuscular block after administration of vecuronium in patients with diabetes mellitus. Br J Anaesth 2003; 90:480-6.
144. Salzarulo HH, Taylor LA. Diabetic "stiff-joint syndrome" as a cause of difficult endotracheal intubation. Anesthesiology 1986; 64:366-8.
145. Hogan K, Rusy D, Springman SR. Difficult laryngoscopy and diabetes mellitus. Anesth Analg 1988; 67:1162-5.
146. Rosenbloom AL. Skeletal and joint manifestations of childhood diabetes. Pediatr Clin North Am 1984; 31:569-89.
147. Meyer RM. Difficult intubation in severe diabetics (letter). Anesth Analg 1989; 69:419.
148. Warner ME, Contreras MG, Warner MA, et al. Diabetes mellitus and difficult laryngoscopy in renal and pancreatic transplant patients. Anesth Analg 1998; 86:516-9.
149. Eastwood DW. Anterior spinal artery syndrome after epidural anesthesia in a pregnant diabetic patient with scleredema. Anesth Analg 1991; 73:90-1.
150. Rodrigo N, Perera KNT, Ranwala R, et al. Aspergillus meningitis following spinal anaesthesia for Caesarean section in Colombo, Sri Lanka. Int J Obstet Anesth 2007; 16:256-60.
151. Lemansky P, Herzog V. Endocytosis of thyroglobulin is not mediated by mannose-6-phosphate receptors in thyrocytes: Evidence for low-affinity-binding sites operating in the uptake of thyroglobulin. Eur J Biochem 1992; 209:111-9.
152. Chopra IJ. Triiodothyronines in health and disease. Monogr Endocrinol 1981; 18:1-14, 58-145.
153. Fliers E, Unmehopa UA, Alkemade A. Functional neuroanatomy of thyroid hormone feedback in the human hypothalamus and pituitary gland. Mol Cell Endocrinol 2006; 251:1-8.
154. Glinoer D, de Nayer P, Bourboux P, et al. Regulation of maternal thyroid during pregnancy. J Clin Endocrinol Metab 1990; 71:276-87.
155. Hohtari H, Pakarinen A, Kauppila A. Serum concentrations of thyrotropin, thyroxine, triiodothyronine and thyroxine binding globulin in female endurance runners and joggers. Acta Endocrinol (Copenh) 1987; 114:41-6.
156. Juan-Pereira L, Navarro MA, Roca M, Fuentes-Arderiu X. Within-subject variation of thyroxin and triiodothyronine concentrations in serum. Clin Chem 1991; 37:772-3.
157. Bartalena L, Robbins J. Variations in thyroid hormone transport proteins and their clinical implications. Thyroid 1992; 2:237-45.
158. Davies PH, Franklyn JA. The effects of drugs on tests of thyroid function. Eur J Clin Pharmacol 1991; 40:439-51.
159. Bartalena L. Recent achievements in studies on thyroid hormone-binding proteins. Endocr Rev 1990; 11:47-64.
160. Mendel CM, Cavalieri RR. Transport of thyroid hormone in health and disease: Recent controversy surrounding the free hormone hypothesis. Thyroid Today 1988; 11:1-9.
161. Sakurai A, Nakai A, DeGroot LJ. Expression of three forms of thyroid hormone receptor in human tissues. Mol Endocrinol 1989; 3:392-9.
162. Glass CK, Holloway JM. Regulation of gene expression by the thyroid hormone receptor. Biochim Biophys Acta 1990; 1032:157-76.
163. Gereben B, Zeoeld A, Dentice M, et al. Activation and inactivation of thyroid hormone by deiodinases: Local action with general consequences. Cell Mol Life Sci 2008; 65:570-90.
164. Schimmel M, Utiger RD. Thyroid and peripheral production of thyroid hormones: Review of recent findings and their clinical implications. Ann Intern Med 1977; 87:760-8.
165. Oetting A, Yen PM. New insights into thyroid hormone action. Best Pract Res Clin Endocrinol Metab 2007; 21:193-208.
166. Psarra AM, Solakidi S, Sekeris CE. The mitochondrion as a primary site of action of steroid and thyroid hormones: Presence and action of steroid and thyroid hormone receptors in mitochondria of animal cells. Mol Cell Endocrinol 2006; 246:21-33.
167. Davis PJ, Leonard JL, Davis FB. Mechanisms of nongenomic actions of thyroid hormone. Front Neuroendocrinol 2008; 29:211-8.
168. Capen CC. Pathophysiology of chemical injury of the thyroid gland. Toxicol Lett 1992; 64-65:381-8.
169. Silva de Sá MF, Maranhão TMO, Iasigi N, et al. Measurement of T_4, T_3 and reverse T_3 levels, resin T_3 uptake, and free thyroxin index in blood from the intervillous space of the placenta, in maternal peripheral blood, and in the umbilical artery and vein of normal parturients and their conceptuses. Gynecol Obstet Invest 1988; 25:223-9.
170. Yoshimura M, Nishikawa M, Yoshikawa N, et al. Mechanism of thyroid stimulation by human chorionic gonadotropin in sera of normal pregnant women. Acta Endocrinol 1991; 124:173-8.
171. Beckmann MW, Wuerfel W, Austin RJ, et al. Suppression of human chorionic gonadotropin in the human placenta at term by human thyroid-stimulating hormone in vitro. Gynecol Obstet Invest 1992; 34:164-70.
172. Burrow GN. Thyroid status in normal pregnancy (editorial). J Clin Endocrinol Metab 1990; 71:274-5.
173. Glinoer D. Regulation of thyroid function in pregnancy: Maternal and neonatal repercussions. Adv Exp Med Biol 1991; 299:197-201.
174. Romano R, Jannini EA, Pepe M, et al. The effects of iodoprophylaxis on thyroid size during pregnancy. Am J Obstet Gynecol 1991; 164:482-5.
175. Nayak B, Hodak SP. Hyperthyroidism. Endocrinol Metab Clin North Am 2007; 36:617-56.
176. Pearce EN. Diagnosis and management of thyrotoxicosis. Br Med J 2006; 332:1369-73.
177. Adlersberg MA, Burrow GN. Focus on primary care: Thyroid function and dysfunction in women. Obstet Gynecol Surv 2002; 57(Suppl):S1-7.
178. Weetman AP. Graves' disease. N Engl J Med 2000; 343:1236-48.
179. Klein I, Trzepacz PT, Roberts M, Levey GS. Symptom rating scale for assessing hyperthyroidism. Arch Intern Med 1988; 148:387-90.
180. Garrity JA, Bahn RS. Pathogenesis of Graves ophthalmopathy: Implications for prediction, prevention, and treatment. Am J Ophthalmol 2006; 142:147-53.
181. Stehling LC. Anesthetic management of the patient with hyperthyroidism. Anesthesiology 1974; 41:585-95.
182. Spaulding SW, Lippes H. Hyperthyroidism: Causes, clinical features, and diagnosis. Med Clin North Am 1985; 69:937-51.
183. Forfar JC, Muir AL, Sawers SA, Toft AD. Abnormal left ventricular function in hyperthyroidism: Evidence for a possible reversible cardiomyopathy. N Engl J Med 1982; 307:1165-70.
184. Casey BM, Leveno KJ. Thyroid disease in pregnancy. Obstet Gynecol 2006; 108:1283-92.
185. Marx H, Amin P, Lazarus JH. Hyperthyroidism and pregnancy. Br Med J 2008; 336:663-7.
186. American College of Obstetricians and Gynecologists. Thyroid disease in pregnancy. ACOG Practice Bulletin No. 37. Washington DC, August 2002. (Obstet Gynecol 2002; 100:387-96.)
187. Lazarus JH, Kokandi A. Thyroid disease in relation to pregnancy: A decade of change. Clin Endocrinol 2000; 53:265-78.
188. Kung AWC, Lau KS, Kohn LD. Epitope mapping of TSH receptor-blocking antibodies in Graves' disease that appear during pregnancy. J Clin Endocrinol Metab 2001; 86:3647-53.
189. Yoshikawa N, Nishikawa M, Horimoto M, et al. Thyroid-stimulating activity in sera of normal pregnant women. J Clin Endocrinol Metab 1989; 69:891-5.
190. Kuscu NK, Koyuncu F. Hyperemesis gravidarum: Current concepts and management. Postgrad Med J 2002; 78:76-9.
191. Kung AWC, Ma JTC, Wang C, Young RTT. Hyperthyroidism during pregnancy due to coexistence of struma ovarii and Graves' disease. Postgrad Med J 1990; 66:132-3.
192. Kung AWC, Chau MT, Lao TT, et al. The effect of pregnancy on thyroid nodule formation. J Clin Endocrine Metab 2002; 87:1010-4.
193. Vini L, Hyer S, Pratt B, et al. Management of differentiated thyroid cancer diagnosed during pregnancy. Eur J Endocrinol 1999; 140:404-6.
194. Driggers RW, Kopelman JN, Satin AJ. Delaying surgery for thyroid cancer in pregnancy: A case report. J Reprod Med 1998; 43:909-12.
195. Kaplan MM, Meier DA, Dworkin HJ. Treatment of hyperthyroidism with radioactive iodine. Endocrinol Metab Clin North Am 1998; 27:205-23.

196. Cooper DS. Antithyroid drugs. N Engl J Med 2005; 352:905-17.
197. Schuessler-Fiorenza CM, Bruns CM, Chen H. The surgical management of Graves' disease. J Surg Res 2006; 133:207-14.
198. Netterville JL, Aly A, Ossoff RH. Evaluation and treatment of complications of thyroid and parathyroid surgery. Otolaryngol Clin North Am 1990; 23:529-52.
199. McArthur JW, Rawson RW, Means JH, Cope O. Thyrotoxic crisis: An analysis of the thirty-six cases seen at the Massachusetts General Hospital during the past twenty-five years. JAMA 1947; 134:868-74.
200. Waldstein SS, Slodki SJ, Kaganiec GI, Bronsky D. A clinical study of thyroid storm. Ann Intern Med 1960; 52:626-42.
201. Mazzaferri EL, Skillman TG. Thyroid storm: A review of 22 episodes with special emphasis on the use of guanethidine. Arch Intern Med 1969; 124:684-90.
202. Nayak B, Burman K. Thyrotoxicosis and thyroid storm. Endocrinol Metab Clin North Am 2006; 35:663-86.
203. Brooks MH, Waldstein SS, Bronsky D, Sterling K. Serum triiodothyronine concentration in thyroid storm. J Clin Endocrinol Metab 1975; 40:339-41.
204. Jacobs HS, Eastman CJ, Ekins RP, et al. Total and free triiodothyronine and thyroxine levels in thyroid storm and recurrent hyperthyroidism. Lancet 1973; 2(7823):236-8.
205. Brooks MH, Waldstein SS. Free thyroxine concentrations in thyroid storm. Ann Intern Med 1980; 93:694-7.
206. Coulombe P, Dussault JH, Letarte J, Simard SJ. Catecholamine metabolism in thyroid diseases. I. Epinephrine secretion rate in hyperthyroidism and hypothyroidism. J Clin Endocrinol Metab 1976; 42:125-31.
207. Coulombe P, Dussault JH, Walker P. Catecholamine metabolism in thyroid disease. II. Norepinephrine secretion rate in hyperthyroidism and hypothyroidism. J Clin Endocrinol Metab 1977; 44:1185-9.
208. Knight RT. The use of spinal anesthesia to control sympathetic overactivity in hyperthyroidism. Anesthesiology 1945; 6:225-30.
209. Mikulaj L, Nemeth S. Contribution to the study of adrenocortical secretory function in thyrotoxicosis. J Clin Endocrinol Metab 1958; 18:539-42.
210. Saunders J, Hall SEH, Crowther A, Soenksen PH. The effect of propranolol on thyroid hormones and oxygen consumption in thyrotoxicosis. Clin Endocrinol 1978; 9:67-72.
211. Aanderud S, Aarbakke J, Sundsfjord J. Effect of different beta-blocking drugs and adrenaline on the conversion of thyroxine to triiodothyronine in isolated rat hepatocytes. Horm Metab Res 1986; 18:110-3.
212. Thorne AC, Bedford RF. Esmolol for perioperative management of thyrotoxic goiter. Anesthesiology 1989; 71:291-4.
213. Vijayakumar HR, Thomas WO, Ferrara JJ. Perioperative management of severe thyrotoxicosis with esmolol. Anaesthesia 1989; 44:406-8.
214. Gronert GA. Malignant hyperthermia. Anesthesiology 1980; 53:395-423.
215. Stevens JJ. A case of thyrotoxic crisis that mimicked malignant hyperthermia. Anesthesiology 1983; 59:263.
216. Christensen PA, Nissen LR. Treatment of thyroid storm in a child with dantrolene. Br J Anaesth 1987; 59:523.
217. Bennett MH, Wainwright AP. Acute thyroid crisis on induction of anaesthesia. Anaesthesia 1989; 44:28-30.
218. Nishiyama K, Kitahara A, Natsume H, et al. Malignant hyperthermia in a patient with Graves' disease during subtotal thyroidectomy. Endocrine J 2001; 48:227-32.
219. Tajiri J, Katsuya H, Kiyokawa T, et al. Successful treatment of thyrotoxic crisis with plasma exchange. Crit Care Med 1984; 12:536-7.
220. Hamilton WFD, Forrest AL, Gunn A, et al. Beta-adrenoceptor blockade and anaesthesia for thyroidectomy. Anaesthesia 1984; 39:335-42.
221. Tan TT, Morat P, Ng ML, Khalid BAK. Effects of Lugol's solution on thyroid function in normals and patients with untreated thyrotoxicosis. Clin Endocrinol 1989; 30:645-9.
222. Caswell HT, Marks AD, Channick BJ. Propranolol for the preoperative preparation of patients with thyrotoxicosis. Surg Gynecol Obstet 1978; 146:908-10.
223. Strube PJ. Thyroid storm during beta blockade. Anaesthesia 1984; 39:343-6.
224. Peden NR, Gunn A, Browning MCK, et al. Nadolol and potassium iodide in combination in the surgical treatment of thyrotoxicosis. Br J Surg 1982; 69:638-40.
225. Feek CM, Sawers JSA, Irvine WJ, et al. Combination of potassium iodide and propranolol in preparation of patients with Graves' disease for thyroid surgery. N Engl J Med 1980; 302:883-5.
226. Chattaway JM, Klepser TB. Propylthiouracil versus methimazole in treatment of Graves' disease during pregnancy. Ann Pharmacother 2007; 41:1018-22.
227. Hashizume K, Ichikawa K, Nishii Y, et al. Effect of administration of thyroxine on the risk of postpartum recurrence of hyperthyroid Graves' disease. J Clin Endocrinol Metab 1992; 75:6-10.
228. Momotani N, Hisaoka T, Noh J, et al. Effects of iodine on thyroid status of fetus versus mother in treatment of Graves' disease complicated by pregnancy. J Clin Endocrinol Metab 1992; 75:738-44.
229. Steinberg ES, Santos AC. Surgical anesthesia during pregnancy. Int Anesth Clin 1990; 28:58-66.
230. Davis LE, Lucas MJ, Hankins GDV, et al. Thyrotoxicosis complicating pregnancy. Am J Obstet Gynecol 1989; 160:63-70.
231. Kamm ML, Weaver JC, Page EP, Chappell CC. Acute thyroid storm precipitated by labor: Report of a case. Obstet Gynecol 1963; 21:460-3.
232. Guenter KE, Friedland GA. Thyroid storm and placenta previa in a primigravida. Obstet Gynecol 1965; 26:403-7.
233. Menon V, McDougall WW, Leatherdale BA. Thyrotoxic crisis following eclampsia and induction of labour. Postgrad Med J 1982; 58:286-7.
234. Pugh S, Lalwani K, Awal A. Thyroid storm as a cause of loss of consciousness following anaesthesia for emergency caesarean section. Anaesthesia 1994; 49:35-7.
235. Tewari K, Balderston KD, Carpenter SE, et al. Papillary thyroid carcinoma manifesting as thyroid storm of pregnancy: Case report. Am J Obstet Gynecol 1998; 179:818-9.
236. Frishman WH, Chesner M. Beta-adrenergic blockers in pregnancy. Am Heart J 1988; 115:147-52.
237. Eisenach JC, Castro MI. Maternally administered esmolol produces fetal beta-adrenergic blockade and hypoxemia in sheep. Anesthesiology 1989; 71:718-22.
238. Losasso TJ, Muzzi DA, Cucchiara RF. Response of fetal heart rate to maternal administration of esmolol. Anesthesiology 1991; 74:782-4.
239. Gilson GJ, Knieriem KJ, Smith JF, et al. Short-acting beta-adrenergic blockade and the fetus: A case report. J Reprod Med 1992; 37:277-9.
240. Ducey JP, Knape KG. Maternal esmolol administration resulting in fetal distress and cesarean section in a term pregnancy. Anesthesiology 1992; 77:829-32.
241. Ikram H. The nature and prognosis of thyrotoxic heart disease. Q J Med 1985; 54:19-28.
242. Ashikaga H, Abreu R, Schneider RF. Propranolol administration in a patient with thyroid storm. Ann Intern Med 2000; 132:681-2.
243. Redahan C, Karski JM. Thyrotoxicosis factitia in a post-aortocoronary bypass patient. Can J Anaesth 1994; 41:969-72.
244. Hankins GDV, Lowe TW, Cunningham FG. Dilated cardiomyopathy and thyrotoxicosis complicated by septic abortion. Am J Obstet Gynecol 1984; 149:85-6.
245. Clark SL, Phelan JP, Montoro M, Mestman J. Transient ventricular dysfunction associated with cesarean section in a patient with hyperthyroidism. Am J Obstet Gynecol 1985; 151:384-6.
246. Valko PC, McCarty DL. Peripartum cardiac failure in a woman with Graves' disease. Am J Emerg Med 1992; 10:46-9.
247. Sheffield JS, Cunningham FG. Thyrotoxicosis and heart failure that complicate pregnancy. Am J Obstet Gynecol 2004; 190:211-7.
248. Millar LK, Wing DA, Leung AS, et al. Low birth weight and preeclampsia in pregnancies complicated by hyperthyroidism. Obstet Gynecol 1994; 84:946-9.
249. Thyroid dysfunction in utero (editorial). Lancet 1992; 339:155.
250. Davidson KM, Richards DS, Schatz DA, Fisher DA. Successful in utero treatment of fetal goiter and hypothyroidism. N Engl J Med 1991; 324:543-6.

251. Mortimer RH, Tyack SA, Galligan JP, et al. Graves' disease in pregnancy: TSH receptor binding inhibiting immunoglobulins and maternal and neonatal thyroid function. Clin Endocrinol (Oxf) 1990; 32:141-52.
252. Messer PM, Hauffa BP, Olbricht T, et al. Antithyroid drug treatment of Graves' disease in pregnancy: Long-term effects on somatic growth, intellectual development and thyroid function of the offspring. Acta Endocrinol (Copenh) 1990; 123:311-6.
253. Nandwani N, Tidmarsh M, May AE. Retrosternal goiter: A cause of dyspnoea in pregnancy. Int J Obstet Anesth 1998; 7:46-9.
254. Halpern SH. Anaesthesia for Caesarean section in patients with uncontrolled hyperthyroidism. Can J Anaesth 1989; 36:454-9.
255. Aoki VS, Wilson WR, Theilen EO. Studies of the reputed augmentation of the cardiovascular effects of catecholamines in patients with spontaneous hyperthyroidism. J Pharmacol Exp Ther 1972; 181:362-8.
256. Del Rio G, Zizzo G, Marrama P, et al. Alpha-2 adrenergic activity is normal in patients with thyroid disease. Clin Endocrinol (Oxf) 1994; 40:235-9.
257. Seino H, Dohi S, Aiyoshi Y, et al. Postoperative hepatic dysfunction after halothane or enflurane anesthesia in patients with hyperthyroidism. Anesthesiology 1986; 64:122-5.
258. Devdhar M, Ousman YH, Burman KD. Hypothyroidism. Endocrinol Metab Clin North Am 2007; 36:595-615.
259. Clinical guideline. Part 1: Screening for thyroid disease. American College of Physicians. Ann Intern Med 1998; 129:141-3.
260. Zulewski H, Muller B, Exer P, et al. Estimation of tissue hypothyroidism by a new clinical score: Evaluation of patients with various grades of hypothyroidism and controls. J Clin Endocrinol Metab 1997; 82:771-6.
261. Nordyke RA, Gilbert FI. Management of primary hypothyroidism. Comp Ther 1990; 16:28-32.
262. Glinoer D, Abalovich M. Unresolved questions in managing hypothyroidism during pregnancy. Br Med J 2007; 335:300-2.
263. Maruo T, Katayama K, Barnea ER, Mochizuki M. A role for thyroid hormone in the induction of ovulation and corpus luteum function. Horm Res 1992; 37(Suppl 1):12-8.
264. Utiger RD. The thyroid: Physiology, thyrotoxicosis, hypothyroidism, and the painful thyroid. In Felig P, Frohman LA, editors. Endocrinology and Metabolism. 4th edition. New York, McGraw-Hill, 2001:261-347.
265. Chopra IJ, Baber K. Treatment of primary hypothyroidism during pregnancy: Is there an increase in thyroxine dose requirement in pregnancy? Metabolism 2003; 52:122-8.
266. Montoro M, Collea JV, Frasier SD, Mestman JH. Successful outcome of pregnancy in women with hypothyroidism. Ann Intern Med 1981; 94:31-4.
267. Balen AH, Kurtz AB. Successful outcome of pregnancy with severe hypothyroidism: Case report and literature review. Br J Obstet Gynaecol 1990; 97:536-9.
268. Tan TO, Cheng YW, Caughey AB. Are women who are treated for hypothyroidism at risk for pregnancy complications? Am J Obstet Gynecol 2006; 194:e1-3.
269. Thilly CH, Delange F, Lagasse R, et al. Fetal hypothyroidism and maternal thyroid status in severe endemic goiter. J Clin Endocrinol Metab 1978; 47:354-60.
270. Fisher DA, Foley BL. Early treatment of congenital hypothyroidism. Pediatrics 1989; 83:785-9.
271. Casey BM, Dashe JS, Wells CE, et al. Subclinical hypothyroidism and pregnancy outcomes. Obstet Gynecol 2005; 105:239-45.
272. American College of Obstetricians and Gynecologists. Subclinical hypothyroidism in pregnancy. ACOG Committee Opinion No. 381. Washington, DC, October 2007. (Obstet Gynecol 2007; 110:959-60.)
273. Jovanovic-Peterson L, Peterson CM. De novo clinical hypothyroidism in pregnancies complicated by type I diabetes, subclinical hypothyroidism, and proteinuria: A new syndrome. Am J Obstet Gynecol 1988; 159:442-6.
274. Bough EW, Crowley WF, Ridgway C, et al. Myocardial function in hypothyroidism: Relation to disease severity and response to treatment. Arch Intern Med 1978; 138:1476-80.
275. Becker C. Hypothyroidism and atherosclerotic heart disease: Pathogenesis, medical management, and the role of coronary artery bypass surgery. Endocr Rev 1985; 6:432-40.
276. Ellyin FM, Kumar Y, Somberg JC. Hypothyroidism complicated by angina pectoris: Therapeutic approaches. J Clin Pharmacol 1992; 32:843-7.
277. Zwillich CW, Pierson DJ, Hofeldt FD, et al. Ventilatory control in myxedema and hypothyroidism. N Engl J Med 1975; 292:662-5.
278. Duranti R, Gheri RG, Gorini M, et al. Control of breathing in patients with severe hypothyroidism. Am J Med 1993; 95:29-37.
279. Rajagopal KR, Abbrecht PH, Derderian SS, et al. Obstructive sleep apnea in hypothyroidism. Ann Intern Med 1984; 101:491-4.
280. Ozkardes A, Ozata M, Beyhan Z, et al. Acute hypothyroidism leads to reversible alterations in central nervous system as revealed by somatosensory evoked potentials. Electroencephalogr Clin Neurophysiol 1996; 100:500-4.
281. Nyström E, Hamberger A, Lindstedt G, et al. Cerebrospinal fluid proteins in subclinical and overt hypothyroidism. Acta Neurol Scand 1997; 95:311-4.
282. Guieu R, Harley JR, Blin O, et al. Nociceptive threshold in hypothyroid patients. Acta Neurol (Napoli) 1993; 15:183-8.
283. Skowsky WR, Kikuchi TA. The role of vasopressin in the impaired water excretion of myxedema. Am J Med 1978; 64:613-21.
284. Ridgway EC, McCammon JA, Benotti J, Maloof F. Acute metabolic responses in myxedema to large doses of intravenous L-thyroxine. Ann Intern Med 1972; 77:549-55.
285. Tudhope GR, Wilson GM. Anaemia in hypothyroidism: Incidence, pathogenesis, and response to treatment. Q J Med 1960; 29:513-37.
286. Hofbauer LC, Heufelder AE. Coagulation disorders in thyroid diseases. Eur J Endocrinol 1997; 136:1-7.
287. Miller LR, Benumof JL, Alexander L, et al. Completely absent response to peripheral nerve stimulation in an acutely hypothyroid patient. Anesthesiology 1989; 71:779-81.
288. Johnson AB, Webber J, Mansell P, et al. Cardiovascular and metabolic responses to adrenaline infusion in patients with short-term hypothyroidism. Clin Endocrinol (Oxf) 1995; 43:747-51.
289. Polikar R, Kennedy B, Ziegler M, et al. Decreased sensitivity to alpha-adrenergic stimulation in hypothyroid patients. J Clin Endocrinol Metab 1990; 70:1761-4.
290. Bennett-Guerrero E, Kramer DC, Schwinn DA. Effect of chronic and acute thyroid hormone reduction on perioperative outcome. Anesth Analg 1997; 85:30-6.
291. Myrup B, Bregengard C, Faber J. Primary haemostasis in thyroid disease. J Intern Med 1995; 238:59-63.
292. Aylesworth CA, Smallridge RC, Rick ME, Alving M. Acquired von Willebrand's disease: A rare manifestation of postpartum thyroiditis. Am J Hematol 1995; 50:217-9.
293. Samaan NA, Hickey RC, Shutts PE. Diagnosis, localization, and management of pheochromocytoma: Pitfalls and follow-up in 41 patients. Cancer 1988; 62:2451-60.
294. Mittendorf EA, Evans DB, Lee JE, Perrier ND. Pheochromocytoma: Advances in genetics, diagnosis, localization, and treatment. Hematol Oncol Clin North Am 2007; 21:509-25.
295. Sutton MG, Sheps SG, Lie JT. Prevalence of clinically unsuspected pheochromocytoma: Review of a 50-year autopsy series. Mayo Clin Proc 1981; 56:354-60.
296. Ross EJ, Griffith DN. The clinical presentation of phaeochromocytoma. Q J Med 1989; 71:485-96.
297. Carney JA. Familial multiple endocrine neoplasia: The first 100 years. Am J Surg Pathol 2005; 29:254-74.
298. Karagiannis A, Mikhailidis DP, Athyros VG, Harsoulis F. Pheochromocytoma: An update on genetics and management. Endocr Relat Cancer 2007; 14:935-56.
299. Bravo EL, Gifford RW Jr. Current concepts: Pheochromocytoma: Diagnosis, localization and management. N Engl J Med 1984; 311:1298-303.
300. Benabarre A, Bosch X, Plana MT, et al. Relapsing paranoid psychosis as the first manifestation of pheochromocytoma (letter). J Clin Psychiatry 2005; 66:949-50.

301. Brouwers FM, Eisenhofer G, Lenders JWM, Pacak K. Emergencies caused by pheochromocytoma, neuroblastoma, or ganglioneuroma. Endocrinol Metab Clin North Am 2006; 35:699-724.
302. Kutluhan S, Kilbas S, Demirci S, et al. Pheochromocytoma presenting with bithalamic infarction, dementia, and increased intraocular pressure. Ophthalmic Surg Lasers Imaging 2007; 38:245-7.
303. Counselman FL, Brenner CJ, Brenner DW. Adrenal pheochromocytoma presenting with persistent abdominal and flank pain. J Emerg Med 1991; 9:241-6.
304. Singh RJ. Advances in metanephrine testing for the diagnosis of pheochromocytoma. Clin Lab Med 2004; 24:85-103.
305. Václavik J, Stejskal D, Lacnák B, et al. Free plasma metanephrines as a screening test for pheochromocytoma in low-risk patients. J Hypertens 2007; 25:1427-31.
306. Unger N, Pitt C, Schmidt IL, et al. Diagnostic value of various biochemical parameters for the diagnosis of pheochromocytoma in patients with adrenal mass. Eur J Endocrinol 2006; 154:409-17.
307. Makino S, Iwata M, Fujiwara M, et al. A case of sleep apnea syndrome manifesting severe hypertension with high plasma norepinephrine levels. Endocr J 2006; 53:363-9.
308. Eisenhofer G, Goldstein DS, Walther MM, et al. Biochemical diagnosis of pheochromocytoma: How to distinguish true- from false-positive test results. J Clin Endocrinol Metab 2003; 88:2656-66.
309. Tota B, Quintieri AM, DiFelice V, Cerra MC. New biological aspects of chromogranin A-derived peptides: Focus on vasostatins. Comp Biochem Physiol A Mol Integr Physiol 2007; 147:11-8.
310. d'Herbomez M, Forzy G, Bauters C, et al. An analysis of the biochemical diagnosis of 66 pheochromocytomas. Eur J Endocrinol 2007; 156:569-75.
311. Algeciras-Schimnich A, Preissner CM, Young WF, et al. Plasma chromogranin A or urine fractionated metanephrines follow-up testing improves the diagnostic accuracy of plasma fractionated metanephrines for pheochromocytoma. J Clin Endocrinol Metab 2008; 93:91-5.
312. Ilias I, Sahdev A, Reznek RH, et al. The optimal imaging of adrenal tumours: A comparison of different methods. Endocr Relat Cancer 2007; 14:587-99.
313. Jager PL, Chirakal R, Marriott CJ, et al. 6-L-18F-fluorodihydroxyphenylalanine PET in neuroendocrine tumors: Basic aspects and emerging clinical applications. J Nucl Med 2008; 49:573-86.
314. Harper MA, Murnaghan GA, Kennedy L, et al. Phaeochromocytoma in pregnancy: Five cases and a review of the literature. Br J Obstet Gynaecol 1989; 96:594-606.
315. Doll DC. Cancer and pregnancy: Introduction. Semin Oncol 1989; 16:335-6.
316. Schreinemakers JMJ, Zonnenberg BA, Höppener JWM, et al. A patient with bilateral pheochromocytoma as part of a Von Hippel-Landau (VHL) syndrome type 2C. World J Surg Oncol 2007; 5:112.
317. Manger WM. The vagaries of pheochromocytomas. Am J Hypertens 2005; 18:1266-70.
318. Dugas G, Fuller J, Watson J. Pheochromocytoma and pregnancy: A case report and review of the literature. Can J Anesth 2004; 51:134-8.
319. Combs CA, Easterling TR, Schmucker BC, Benedetti TJ. Hemodynamic observations during paroxysmal hypertension in a pregnancy with pheochromocytoma. Obstet Gynecol 1989; 74:439-41.
320. Easterling TR, Carlson K, Benedetti TJ, Mancuso JJ. Hemodynamics associated with the diagnosis and treatment of pheochromocytoma in pregnancy. Am J Perinatol 1992; 9:464-6.
321. Oh HC, Koh JM, Kim MS, et al. A case of ACTH-producing pheochromocytoma associated with pregnancy. Endocr J 2003; 50:739-44.
322. Hudsmith JG, Thomas CE, Browne DA. Undiagnosed phaeochromocytoma mimicking severe preeclampsia in a pregnant woman at term. Int J Obstet Anesth 2006; 15:240-5.
323. Cermakova A, Knibb AA, Hoskins C, et al. Post partum phaeochromocytoma. Int J Obstet Anesth 2003; 12:300-4.
324. Kisters K, Franitza P, Hausberg M. A case of pheochromocytoma symptomatic after delivery. J Hypertens 2007; 25:1977.
325. Ratge D, Knoll E, Wisser H. Plasma free and conjugated catecholamines in clinical disorders. Life Sci 1986; 39:557-64.
326. Sam S, Molitch ME. Timing and special concerns regarding endocrine surgery during pregnancy. Endocrinol Metab Clin North Am 2003; 32:337-54.
327. Pacak K. Preoperative management of the pheochromocytoma patient. J Clin Endocrinol Metab 2007; 92:4069-79.
328. Kinney MAO, Narr BJ, Warner MA. Perioperative management of pheochromocytoma. J Cardiothorac Vasc Anesth 2002; 16:359-69.
329. Prys-Roberts C, Farndon JR. Efficacy and safety of doxazosin for perioperative management of patients with pheochromocytoma. World J Surg 2002; 26:1037-42.
330. Sadowski D, Cujec B, McMeekin JD, Wilson TW. Reversibility of catecholamine-induced cardiomyopathy in a woman with pheochromocytoma. Can Med Assoc J 1989; 141:923-4.
331. Hicks RJ, Wood B, Kalff V, et al. Normalization of left ventricular ejection fraction following resection of pheochromocytoma in a patient with dilated cardiomyopathy. Clin Nucl Med 1991; 16:413-6.
332. Proye C, Thevenin D, Cecat P, et al. Exclusive use of calcium channel blockers in preoperative and intraoperative control of pheochromocytomas: Hemodynamics and free catecholamine assays in ten consecutive patients. Surgery 1989; 106:1149-54.
333. Perry RR, Keiser HR, Norton JA, et al. Surgical management of pheochromocytoma with the use of metyrosine. Ann Surg 1990; 212:621-8.
334. Hull CJ. Phaeochromocytoma: Diagnosis, preoperative preparation and anesthetic management. Br J Anaesth 1986; 58:1453-68.
335. Stenstrom G, Haljamae H, Tisell LE. Influence of pre-operative treatment with phenoxybenzamine on the incidence of adverse cardiovascular reactions during anaesthesia and surgery for phaeochromocytoma. Acta Anaesthesiol Scand 1985; 29:797-803.
336. Kocak S, Aydintug S, Canakci N. Alpha blockade in preoperative preparation of patients with pheochromocytomas. Int Surg 2002; 87:191-4.
337. Roizen MF. Anesthetic implications of concurrent diseases. In Miller RD, editor. Anesthesia. 5th edition. New York, Churchill Livingstone, 2000:903-1015.
338. Arai T, Hatano Y, Ishida H, Mori K. Use of nicardipine in the anesthetic management of pheochromocytoma. Anesth Analg 1986; 65:706-8.
339. Zakowski M, Kaufman B, Berguson P, et al. Esmolol use during resection of pheochromocytoma: Report of three cases. Anesthesiology 1989; 70:875-7.
340. James MF. Use of magnesium sulphate in the anaesthetic management of phaeochromocytoma: A review of 17 anaesthetics. Br J Anaesth 1989; 62:616-23.
341. Grondal S, Bindslev L, Sollevi A, Hamberger B. Adenosine: A new antihypertensive agent during pheochromocytoma removal. World J Surg 1988; 12:581-5.
342. Ryan T, Timoney A, Cunningham AJ. Use of transoesophageal echocardiography to manage beta-adrenoceptor block and assess left ventricular function in a patient with phaeochromocytoma. Br J Anaesth 1993; 70:101-3.
343. Gumbs AA, Gagner M. Laparoscopic adrenalectomy. Best Pract Res Clin Endocrinol Metab 2006; 20:483-99.
344. Sood J, Jayaraman L, Kumra VP, Chowbey PK. Laparoscopic approach to pheochromocytoma: Is a lower intraabdominal pressure helpful? Anesth Analg 2006; 102:637-41.
345. Kinney MA, Warner MF, van Heerden JA, et al. Perianesthetic risks and outcomes of pheochromocytoma and paraganglioma resection. Anesth Analg 2000; 91:1118-23.
346. Akiba M, Kodama T, Ito Y, et al. Hypoglycemia induced by excessive rebound secretion of insulin after removal of pheochromocytoma. World J Surg 1990; 14:317-24.
347. Levin H, Heifetz M. Phaeochromocytoma and severe protracted postoperative hypoglycaemia. Can J Anaesth 1990; 37:477-8.
348. van Heerden JA, Roland CF, Carney JA, et al. Long-term evaluation following resection of apparently benign pheochromocytoma(s)/paraganglioma(s). World J Surg 1990; 14:325-9.

349. Fudge TL, McKinnon WM, Geary WL. Current surgical management of pheochromocytoma during pregnancy. Arch Surg 1980; 115:1224-5.
350. Kamari Y, Sharabi Y, Leiba A, et al. Peripartum hypertension from pheochromocytoma: A rare and challenging entity. Am J Hypertens 2005; 18:1306-12.
351. Junglee N, Harries SE, Davies N. Pheochromocytoma in pregnancy: When is operative intervention indicated? J Women's Health 2007; 16:1362-5.
352. Kim PT, Kreisman SH, Vaughn R, et al. Laparoscopic adrenalectomy for pheochromocytoma in pregnancy. Can J Surg 2006; 49:62-3.
353. Kariya N, Nishi S, Hosono Y, et al. Cesarean section at 28 weeks' gestation with resection of pheochromocytoma: Perioperative antihypertensive management. J Clin Anesth 2005; 17:296-9.
354. Bembo SA, Elimian A, Waltzer W, Carlson HE. Pheochromocytoma in a pregnant woman with a history of intracerebral aneurysms. Am J Med Sci 2005; 329:317-9.
355. Browne I, Brady I, Hannon V, et al. Anaesthesia for phaeochromocytoma and sickle cell disease in pregnancy. Int J Obstet Anesth 2005; 14:66-9.
356. Mitchell SZ, Freilich JD, Brant D, Flynn M. Anesthetic management of pheochromocytoma resection during pregnancy. Anesth Analg 1987; 66:478-80.
357. Santiero ML, Stromquist C, Wyble L. Phenoxybenzamine placental transfer during the third trimester. Ann Pharmacother 1996; 30:1249-51.
358. James MF, Huddle KR, Owen AD, van der Veen BW. Use of magnesium sulphate in the anaesthetic management of phaeochromocytoma in pregnancy. Can J Anaesth 1988; 35:178-82.
359. Aplin SC, Yee KF, Cole MJ. Neonatal effects of long-term maternal phenoxybenzamine therapy. Anesthesiology 2004; 100:1608-10.
360. Lyons CW, Colmorgen GH. Medical management of pheochromocytoma in pregnancy. Obstet Gynecol 1988; 72:450-1.
361. Hamilton A, Sirrs S, Schmidt N, et al. Anaesthesia for phaeochromocytoma in pregnancy. Can J Anaesth 1997; 44:654-7.
362. Naulty J, Cefalo RC, Lewis PE. Fetal toxicity of nitroprusside in the pregnant ewe. Am J Obstet Gynecol 1981; 139:708-11.
363. Shoemaker CT, Meyers M. Sodium nitroprusside for control of severe hypertensive disease of pregnancy: A case report and discussion of potential toxicity. Am J Obstet Gynecol 1984; 149:171-3.
364. Stempel JE, O'Grady JP, Morton MJ, Johnson KA. Use of sodium nitroprusside in complications of gestational hypertension. Obstet Gynecol 1982; 60:533-8.
365. Lieb SM, Zugaib M, Nuwayhid B, et al. Nitroprusside-induced hemodynamic alterations in normotensive and hypertensive pregnant sheep. Am J Obstet Gynecol 1981; 139:925-31.
366. Nelson SH, Suresh MS. Comparison of nitroprusside and hydralazine in isolated uterine arteries from pregnant and nonpregnant patients. Anesthesiology 1988; 68:541-7.
367. Weiner C, Liu KZ, Thompson L, et al. Effect of pregnancy on endothelium and smooth muscle: Their role in reduced adrenergic sensitivity. Am J Physiol 1991; 261:H1275-83.
368. Dahia PL, Hayashida CY, Strunz C, et al. Low cord blood levels of catecholamine from a newborn of a pheochromocytoma patient. Eur J Endocrinol 1994; 130:217-9.
369. Davies AE, Navaratnarajah M. Vaginal delivery in a patient with phaeochromocytoma: A case report. Br J Anaesth 1984; 56:913-6.
370. Flowers D, Clark JF, Westney LS. Cocaine intoxication associated with abruptio placentae. J Natl Med Assoc 1991; 83:230-2.
371. Hendee AE, Martin RD, Waters WC. Hypertension in pregnancy: Toxemia or pheochromocytoma. Am J Obstet Gynecol 1969; 105:64-72.
372. Roizen MF, Horrigan RW, Koike M, et al. A prospective randomized trial of four anesthetic techniques for resection of pheochromocytoma (abstract). Anesthesiology 1982; 57:A43.
373. Rosas AL, Kasperlik-Zaluska AA, Papierska L, et al. Pheochromocytoma crisis induced by glucocorticoids: A report of four cases and review of the literature. Eur J Endocrinol 2008; 158:423-9.
374. Allen GC, Rosenberg H. Phaeochromocytoma presenting as acute malignant hyperthermia: A diagnostic challenge. Can J Anaesth 1990; 37:593-5.
375. Crowley KJ, Cunningham AJ, Conroy B, et al. Phaeochromocytoma: A presentation mimicking malignant hyperthermia. Anaesthesia 1988; 43:1031-2.
376. Asai T, Shingu K. Increased carbon dioxide during anaesthesia in patients with phaeochromocytoma. Anaesthesia 2004; 59:830-1.
377. Stonham J, Wakefield C. Phaeochromocytoma in pregnancy: Caesarean section under epidural analgesia. Anaesthesia 1983; 38:654-8.

Chapter 43

Hematologic and Coagulation Disorders

Shiv K. Sharma, M.D., FRCA

ANEMIA

Normal Hemoglobin Morphology

Normal adult hemoglobin consists of four polypeptides (two alpha chains and two beta chains) and the iron-containing prosthetic group (heme or ferroprotoporphyrin IX). In the early embryo, theta (θ) and zeta (ζ) chains are present instead of the alpha (α) chains, and epsilon (ε) chains are present instead of the beta (β) chains. After early embryogenesis, pairs of alpha chains are linked with pairs of either beta, gamma (γ), or delta (δ) chains to form adult hemoglobin (Hgb A = $\alpha_2\beta_2$), fetal hemoglobin (Hgb F = $\alpha_2\gamma_2$), or hemoglobin A_2 (Hgb A_2 = $\alpha_2\delta_2$). By term gestation, the ratio of hemoglobin F to hemoglobin A is approximately 1:1. By 1 year of age, hemoglobin F typically constitutes less than 1% of total hemoglobin. Although hemoglobin A_2 is present, it accounts for less than 2.5% of total adult hemoglobin.

The sequence of amino acids (141 amino acids for alpha chains and 146 for beta chains) defines the **primary structure**. The three-dimensional shape of each chain defines the **secondary structure,** and the relationship between the four chains and the heme prosthetic group defines the **tertiary structure**. The binding of the ligands 2,3-diphosphoglycerate (2,3-DPG) and oxygen defines the **quaternary structure**.

The affinity of hemoglobin for oxygen is expressed as the P_{50} (i.e., the oxygen tension at which half of hemoglobin's oxygen-carrying capacity is used). Increased temperature and increases in hydrogen ion [H^+] and 2,3-DPG concentrations reduce the affinity of hemoglobin for oxygen, leading to an increase in the P_{50} and facilitating the unloading of oxygen at peripheral tissues. In comparison with purified hemoglobin A, purified hemoglobin F has a lower oxygen affinity and a greater response to changes in pH but only a minimal response to changes in 2,3-DPG concentration. The decreased interaction between hemoglobin F and intraerythrocyte 2,3-DPG accounts for the increased affinity of fetal blood for oxygen *in vivo*.

Dilutional Anemia of Pregnancy

During normal pregnancy, plasma volume increases by approximately 50%, but red blood cell (RBC) mass increases by only 30%. This situation results in a dilutional anemia. RBC mass increases linearly after the first trimester until delivery, and plasma volume plateaus or falls slightly near term. Therefore hemoglobin concentrations are lowest between 28 and 34 weeks' gestation. If the hemoglobin concentration falls below 10.5 g/dL, the physician should consider causes other than the dilutional anemia of pregnancy.

Thalassemia

The thalassemias are a diverse group of microcytic, hemolytic anemias that result from the reduced synthesis of one or more of the polypeptide globin chains. This reduced synthesis leads to (1) an imbalance in globin chain synthesis, (2) defective hemoglobin synthesis, and (3) erythrocyte damage resulting from excess globin subunits. In α-thalassemia, alpha-chain production is reduced, and in β-thalassemia, beta-chain production is reduced.

α-THALASSEMIA

There are two alpha-chain loci on each chromosome 16; therefore there are four genes that can produce alpha chains. Because mutations can affect any or all of these genes, four types of α-thalassemia exist, as follows: (1) **silent carrier** (three functioning genes); (2) **α-thalassemia trait** (two functioning genes); (3) **hemoglobin H disease** (one functioning gene); and (4) **α⁰-thalassemia** or **Bart's hydrops** (no functioning genes). As the number of functioning genes decreases from four to zero, the ratio of alpha to beta chains decreases from 0.8:1 to 0.6:1 to 0.3:1 to 0:1. The messenger RNA production from the second alpha gene exceeds that of the first alpha gene by a factor of 1.5 to 3.[1,2] Therefore, deletions of the second alpha gene may produce a greater clinical effect. As beta (or beta-like) chains accumulate, they can form tetramers *in utero* (e.g., hemoglobin Bart's = γ_4) or after delivery (e.g., hemoglobin H = β_4).

In the United States, 30% of black women are **silent carriers** and have only slightly decreased (78 to 80 fL) mean corpuscular volume (MCV); other indices for these women are normal.[3] A chromosome lacking one alpha gene is common in the Mediterranean basin, the Middle East, India, Southeast Asia, Indonesia, and the South Pacific Islands. Women in and from these regions are not at increased risk during pregnancy or surgery.

The **α-thalassemia trait** affects 3% of black women in the United States. These women have an MCV of 70 to 75 fL and mild anemia. They typically are asymptomatic. The diagnosis of α-thalassemia trait should be considered if a black patient with microcytic anemia does not respond to oral iron therapy. The diagnosis is confirmed by alpha-gene analysis. These patients are not at increased risk during pregnancy or surgery.

Patients with **hemoglobin H disease** have moderately severe anemia, splenomegaly, fatigue, and generalized discomfort. Hemoglobin H (β_4) constitutes 2% to 15% of total hemoglobin in these patients. Affected patients do not have a decreased life span, and hospitalization for the treatment of their anemia rarely is required.

α^0-Thalassemia is generally incompatible with life. This disease is relatively common in Southeast Asia, China, and the Philippines. Affected individuals die either *in utero* or shortly after birth of hydrops fetalis, or if transfusions are administered *in utero*, they die in early childhood.

Molecular genetic testing can identify couples at increased risk for offspring with a hemoglobinopathy and provides guidance as to whether to perform prenatal testing. The patient at higher risk for thalassemia who has a low MCV and whose hemoglobin electrophoresis results are inconsistent with β-thalassemia trait should undergo DNA-based testing to detect α-globin gene deletion characteristic of α-thalassemia. Counseling for prenatal genetic testing should be offered if both parents have α-thalassemia trait or if one parent has hemoglobin H disease and the other either is a silent carrier or has α-thalassemia trait.[4]

β-THALASSEMIA

In β-thalassemia, the production of beta chains is reduced. There are more than 50 genetic causes for ineffective beta-chain production, including gene deletion, transcription mutations, and RNA-processing mutations.[5] Unlike the alpha chains, which have four genes (two on each chromosome 16), beta chains have only one gene on each chromosome 11. Production of messenger RNA from the second beta-like gene (i.e., delta) is almost completely suppressed. Therefore, there are only two primary forms of β-thalassemia, **β^0-thalassemia,** in which there is no beta-chain formation, and **β^+-thalassemia,** in which some beta-chain production exists. β^0-thalassemia also is called *β-thalassemia major* or *Cooley's anemia*. Patients who receive β-thalassemia genes from both parents but with mutations of different types often develop a milder form of the disease and require fewer or no transfusions. This condition is known as **thalassemia intermedia**. Finally, **β-thalassemia minor** refers to the heterozygous carrier of β-thalassemia.

β-Thalassemia is found most often in persons from the Mediterranean basin, the Middle East, India, and Southeast Asia. It occurs less frequently among persons from southern Russia, China, and Africa.

Individuals with β-thalassemia have inadequate beta-chain production; thus they have a relative excess of alpha chains. Excess alpha chains precipitate and form inclusion bodies in RBC precursors, resulting in anemia secondary to ineffective erythropoiesis and splenic hemolysis. In the fetus, the gamma chain is unaffected; therefore anemia develops only as gamma-chain production ceases during the first year of life. In some patients, gamma-chain production continues to a variable extent. Thus the ongoing production of hemoglobin F (even in adults) may minimize the effects of decreased beta-chain production.

β-THALASSEMIA MAJOR

In patients with β-thalassemia major, severe anemia develops in the first few months of extrauterine life. The anemia results in tissue hypoxia, increased intestinal absorption of iron, and increased erythropoietin production. The resulting expansion of marrow cavities causes skeletal abnormalities and pathologic fractures. Splenomegaly leads to thrombocytopenia and leukopenia. Transfusions are required to maintain life, and the resulting iron load leads to iron accumulation, first in Kupffer's cells (noncirculating macrophages found in the liver), then in liver parenchymal cells, and finally in endocrine and myocardial cells. Deposition of iron in endocrine tissues may result in diabetes mellitus, adrenal insufficiency, and infertility.[6,7] Myocardial accumulation of iron can lead to conduction abnormalities and intractable heart failure, which is exacerbated by anemia-induced tachycardia.

Heart failure and infection are the most common causes of death.

Patients with β-thalassemia major who present at less than 2 years of age often have hepatomegaly and a hemoglobin concentration as low as 2 g/dL. Patients who present later in life (2 to 12 years of age) typically have a hemoglobin concentration between 4 and 10 g/dL, with marked anisopoikilocytosis and numerous target cells, nucleated RBCs, and inclusion bodies. Levels of hemoglobin F range from 10% to 90% of the total hemoglobin, and hemoglobin A_2 constitutes the remainder of the hemoglobin that is present. Prenatal diagnosis can be accomplished with the use of fetal cells obtained by means of chorionic villus sampling or amniocentesis and subjected to DNA analysis.[4,8]

Treatment includes (1) transfusion of leukocyte-poor RBCs every 2 to 3 weeks to maintain a hemoglobin concentration greater than 10 g/dL, thus preventing endogenous erythropoiesis; (2) splenectomy; and (3) iron chelation therapy to prevent hemosiderosis.[9] Deferoxamine is the most effective chelation agent currently available. It is given by continuous subcutaneous administration or by intermittent intramuscular injection. Oral chelation drugs and bone marrow transplantation are possible future treatment options.

It is unusual for patients with β-thalassemia major to become pregnant. If patients do conceive, the metabolic demands of pregnancy lead to higher transfusion requirements, which may worsen hemosiderosis and cardiac failure. These patients have a higher incidence of spontaneous abortion, intrauterine fetal death, and intrauterine growth restriction.[10]

During pregnancy, the transfusion of 600 mL to 8400 mL of blood is typically required to keep the hemoglobin concentration above 10 g/dL. It is unclear whether chelation therapy should be continued, because the fetal effects of deferoxamine are unknown. A trial of labor is appropriate, and operative delivery should be reserved for obstetric indications. Intraoperative blood salvage has been safely performed during cesarean delivery in a parturient with thalassemia.[11]

Extramedullary hematopoiesis can result in vertebral cortical weakening, pathologic fractures, and, rarely, paraplegia. Although data on this issue are lacking, these skeletal abnormalities do not appear to contraindicate the administration of neuraxial anesthesia. Patients with splenomegaly may have thrombocytopenia. A neuraxial anesthetic can be safely administered for cesarean delivery[12]; however, the anesthesia provider should exclude a history of spontaneous hemorrhage and determine the platelet count prior to the procedure.

β-THALASSEMIA MINOR

In patients with β-thalassemia minor, the clinical course is usually benign. The anemia typically is mild (e.g., hemoglobin concentration of 9 to 11 g/dL) and is characterized by microcytosis and hypochromatosis. Levels of hemoglobin F range from 1% to 3%, and levels of hemoglobin A_2 from 3.5% to 7%.

Moderate anemia develops only during periods of stress, such as pregnancy and severe infection. Nonetheless, most patients with β-thalassemia minor tolerate pregnancy well. Ultrasonographic assessment of fetal weight in the early third trimester facilitates detection of fetal growth restriction.[13] Folate supplementation is recommended. Supplemental iron is administered only to patients with laboratory evidence of iron deficiency. Transfusions are reserved for patients with hemorrhage or a hemoglobin concentration below 8 g/dL. Infection, which can cause bone marrow suppression, must be treated promptly. β-Thalassemia minor typically does not affect anesthetic management during labor or cesarean delivery.

Sickle Cell Disease

More than 380 abnormal alpha, beta, gamma, and delta chains have been identified. Structural hemoglobinopathies result when these abnormal chains are used to form hemoglobin molecules. The most common abnormal hemoglobins are hemoglobin S, hemoglobin C, hemoglobin D, and hemoglobin E. Patients can be homozygous for an abnormal hemoglobin (e.g., **hemoglobin SS** or **sickle cell anemia**), heterozygous for an abnormal hemoglobin (e.g., **hemoglobin SA** or **sickle cell trait**), or doubly heterozygous for an abnormal hemoglobin (e.g., **hemoglobin SC** or **sickle cell hemoglobin C disease**). Both the heterozygous state for the thalassemias and the structural hemoglobinopathies appear to afford some protection against malaria, which may explain their geographic distribution and continued presence in the gene pool.

A **sickle cell disorder** refers to a state in which erythrocytes undergo sickling when they are deoxygenated.[14] Normal erythrocytes have a biconcave shape. Sickle cells are elongated and crescent-shaped, with two pointed ends. **Sickle cell disease** refers to disorders in which sickling results in clinical signs and symptoms; it includes hemoglobin SS disease, hemoglobin SC disease, hemoglobin SD disease, and sickle cell β-thalassemia.

SICKLE CELL ANEMIA

Epidemiology

Table 43-1 lists the prevalence of sickle cell anemia and the other most common hemoglobinopathies in the United States adult black population.[15] In Africa, the prevalence of the sickle cell trait is as high as 20% to 40%.

Pathophysiology

In hemoglobin S molecules, valine is substituted for glutamic acid as the sixth amino acid in the beta chains. This substitution results in a propensity for hemoglobin molecules to aggregate when the hemoglobin is in the deoxygenated state. The hemoglobin molecules stack on top of one another and form microtubules. The primary cause of sickling is the abnormal hemoglobin; however, erythrocyte metabolic and membrane abnormalities may contribute to sickling, a possibility that may explain the variable clinical presentation of patients with hemoglobin SS.

Oxygen tension is the most important determinant in sickling. Hemoglobin S begins to aggregate at a Po_2 of less than 50 mm Hg, and all of the hemoglobin S is aggregated at a Po_2 of approximately 23 mm Hg. The formation of hemoglobin S aggregates is time dependent. Therefore, even though 85% of hemoglobin S would eventually sickle after prolonged exposure to the oxygen tension in venous blood, less than 5% does so because the hemoglobin typically reaches the lungs and becomes oxygenated before aggregates form. If an erythrocyte sickles, it can return to

TABLE 43-1 Prevalence of Hemoglobinopathies in the United States in Persons of African Descent

Type	Estimated Prevalence
Traits	
Hemoglobin AS	1:12.5
Hemoglobin AC	1:33
β-Thalassemia minor	1:67
Persistent hemoglobin F	1:1000
Sickling Disorders	
Hemoglobin SS	1:625
Hemoglobin SC	1:833
Hemoglobin S–β-Thalassemia	1:1667
Hemoglobin S–persistent hemoglobin F	1:25,000
Hemoglobin CC	1:4444
β-Thalassemia major	1:17,778
Hemoglobin C–β-Thalassemia	1:4444

Adapted from Motulsky AG. Frequency of sickling disorders in U.S. Blacks. N Engl J Med 1973; 288:31-3.

its normal shape once the hemoglobin S becomes oxygenated. However, the cellular membrane remains altered, and after it has undergone repeated sickling cycles, it remains sickled regardless of oxygen tension. As a result, the erythrocyte life span is reduced to approximately 12 days.[16]

Other factors that affect sickling are listed in Box 43-1. The sickled cells can form aggregates and cause vaso-occlusive disease. Sickled cells also are cleared more rapidly from the circulation by the reticuloendothelial system, resulting in a reduced erythrocyte life span.

The incidence of pneumonia and pyelonephritis is higher in pregnant patients with sickle cell disease than in other pregnant patients. The clinical picture of sickle cell disease is that of a chronic inflammatory vascular disorder.[14] Marked ventricular hypertrophy can occur in pregnant women with sickle cell disease secondary to increased cardiac output. This may lead to a decrease in ventricular compliance and a deterioration in ventricular diastolic function.[17] The reduced erythrocyte life span results in anemia, jaundice, cholecystitis, and a hyperdynamic cardiac state. Anemia leads to erythroblastic hyperplasia, expansion of medullary spaces, and a loss of cortex in long bones, vertebral bodies, and the skull. Vaso-occlusive events can

BOX 43-1 Factors that Increase Sickling in Women with Sickle Cell Anemia

- Hemoglobin S concentration more than 50% of the total hemoglobin concentration
- Dehydration leading to increased blood viscosity
- Hypotension causing vascular stasis
- Hypothermia
- Acidosis

give rise to **infarctive crises** (which most often occur in the chest, abdomen, back, and long bones), **cerebrovascular accidents,** and, rarely, **peripheral neuropathy**.[18] Aggregate formation in the spleen can result in microinfarcts. **Aplastic crises** can occur from depression of erythropoiesis secondary to infection (especially parvovirus) or from marrow failure secondary to folate deficiency during pregnancy. During an aplastic crisis, the hemoglobin concentration can drop 2 g/dL per day, leading to high-output cardiac failure and death. **Sequestration crises** can result from the massive pooling of erythrocytes, especially in the spleen. This process occurs more frequently in patients with hemoglobin SC disease or sickle cell β-thalassemia than in patients with other forms of sickle cell disease. In general, a major sequestration crisis is one in which the hemoglobin concentration is less than 6 g/dL and has fallen more than 3 g/dL from the baseline measurement.

Diagnosis

In the adult, sickle cell anemia is characterized by (1) a hemoglobin concentration of approximately 6 to 8 g/dL, (2) macrocytosis, (3) elevated reticulocyte count, and (4) the presence of sickle cells on a peripheral blood smear. The diagnosis is confirmed by electrophoresis. Because most hemoglobinopathies are inherited as autosomal recessive conditions, prenatal screening for abnormal hemoglobin by electrophoresis is recommended for couples at high risk for sickle cell disease.[4] *In utero*, the diagnosis can be made through the use of restriction endonucleases specific for the sickle mutation and cells obtained during amniocentesis or chorionic villus sampling.

Interaction with Pregnancy

Pregnancy typically exacerbates the complications of sickle cell anemia. Maternal mortality is as high as 1%.[19] Pulmonary embolism and infection are the leading causes of death. Fetal mortality may approach 20%.[19] Patients with sickle cell anemia have an increased incidence of preterm labor, placental abruption, placenta previa, and hypertensive disorders of pregnancy.[20]

Medical Management

Sickle cell anemia is a chronic anemia, and blood transfusions are given only when they are specifically indicated (e.g., aplastic crisis, pneumonia with hypoxemia, before or during surgery). The goals of transfusion are to achieve a hemoglobin concentration greater than 8 g/dL and to ensure that hemoglobin A represents more than 40% of the total hemoglobin present. Maintaining the hemoglobin concentration above 10 g/dL during pregnancy reduces the incidence of painful crises but does not appear to alter fetal or maternal mortality.[20] If the patient's baseline hemoglobin concentration is less than 6 g/dL, simple transfusions with buffy coat–poor, hemoglobin S–free, washed RBCs should be adequate to meet treatment goals. Otherwise, partial exchange transfusions may be necessary.

Hemoglobin F does not form aggregates with hemoglobin S. Administration of hydroxyurea[21] (or another chemotherapeutic drug) may enhance the production of hemoglobin F, which may in turn decrease the morbidity and mortality of sickle cell anemia. Bone marrow transplantation is another experimental treatment that shows promise.[22]

Obstetric Management

During prenatal visits, the obstetrician should monitor maternal weight gain, blood pressure, and intrauterine fetal growth. Cervical examinations are performed regularly to detect impending preterm labor. Antepartum fetal surveillance is begun at the time of extrauterine viability (i.e., approximately 25 to 26 weeks' gestation). If obstetric complications develop, immediate and aggressive treatment is required. Blood transfusions are reserved for specific indications (e.g., severe anemia, hypoxemia, preeclampsia, septicemia, renal failure, acute chest pain syndrome, anticipated surgery). A hemoglobin concentration of 8 g/dL is adequate for vaginal delivery. It is common practice to increase the hemoglobin concentration to 10 g/dL in patients scheduled for cesarean delivery, but no study has shown that this higher hemoglobin concentration decreases morbidity or mortality.

Anesthetic Management

The anesthetic management of the patient with severe sickle cell anemia resembles that for the patient with high-output heart failure. Pain control during labor is essential, and continuous lumbar epidural analgesia is recommended. For operative delivery, either neuraxial or general anesthesia is acceptable. The choice of anesthetic technique depends on the patient's preference and physical status and the anesthesia provider's preference. Principles of anesthetic management include (1) use of crystalloid to maintain intravascular volume, (2) transfusion of RBCs to maintain oxygen-carrying capacity, (3) administration of supplemental oxygen and the use of a pulse oximeter to monitor oxygen saturation, (4) maintenance of normothermia, and (5) prevention of peripheral venous stasis.[14]

SICKLE CELL DISEASE VARIANTS

If a patient carries one sickle cell gene and another gene for a hemoglobin that has a propensity to sickle, that patient is considered to have sickle cell disease. The resulting diseases form a spectrum between the asymptomatic sickle cell trait (hemoglobin SA) and sickle cell anemia (SS disease). Patients with hemoglobin SD disease tend to have the mildest form, and patients with SC disease or sickle cell β-thalassemia tend to have more severe disease.

As with the hemoglobin S gene, hemoglobin C is most prevalent among persons of West African descent, hemoglobin D is most prevalent among persons of Northwest Indian descent, and hemoglobin E is most prevalent among persons of Southeast Asian descent. Patients with hemoglobin SC and hemoglobin SD disease tend to be asymptomatic during childhood, with only mild anemia. A hemoglobin concentration of 11 to 13 g/dL, with the presence of target cells, is consistent with sickle cell disease in nonpregnant patients. The diagnosis is confirmed with electrophoresis. Typically these individuals do not experience symptoms until the second half of pregnancy. During late pregnancy, they may have severe anemia (secondary to splenic sequestration) and splenomegaly. Patients with hemoglobin SC disease also have a tendency to develop marrow necrosis, which predisposes to fat emboli. The other clinical manifestations are similar to those of sickle cell anemia.

Blood transfusion is recommended only when the hemoglobin concentration is lower than 8 g/dL. Obstetric management and anesthetic management are similar to those for patients with sickle cell anemia.

Patients who are homozygous for hemoglobin C, D, or E typically have mild anemia. Target cells often are seen, and splenomegaly is common. Patients who are heterozygous (i.e., one gene for hemoglobin C, D, or E and one gene for normal hemoglobin) are asymptomatic. The diagnosis is confirmed with electrophoresis. Pregnancy typically is well tolerated, and no specific change in obstetric or anesthetic management is required.

SICKLE CELL TRAIT

Sickle cell trait is the most benign form of the sickle cell disorders. It occurs in approximately 8% of black women in the United States. The RBCs of patients with sickle cell trait do not sickle until the PO_2 falls below 15 mm Hg; therefore erythrocyte life span is normal. A study of 65,000 patients with sickle cell trait found only a slightly higher incidence of renal (hematuria) and pulmonary (embolic) complications than in patients without sickle cell trait.[23] Pregnant women with sickle cell trait are at increased risk for **asymptomatic bacteriuria, pyelonephritis,** and **preeclampsia**.[24] Otherwise, patients with sickle cell trait are not at higher risk during surgery.

Autoimmune Hemolytic Anemia

Patients with autoimmune hemolytic anemia produce antibodies to their own RBCs, resulting in hemolysis and varying levels of anemia. Table 43-2 lists the characteristics of the four main types of autoimmune hemolytic anemia.[25] Warm antibodies react with RBCs at a temperature of 35° C to 40° C, whereas cold antibodies react optimally at a temperature lower than 30° C. The annual incidence of new cases of autoimmune hemolytic anemia is approximately 1 per 80,000 persons. Table 43-3 lists the various etiologies of autoimmune hemolytic anemia.[26]

Patients with warm-reacting antibodies typically respond to treatment with corticosteroids; splenectomy is reserved for patients whose disease is refractory to corticosteroid therapy. After splenectomy, corticosteroid requirements typically decrease, but relapses (that require corticosteroid therapy) are common. Cytotoxic drugs (e.g., cyclophosphamide, 6-mercaptopurine) have not proved to be beneficial in these patients.

In patients with cold-reacting antibodies, the anemia typically is mild, and maintenance of normal body and ambient temperatures usually is all that is required.

COAGULATION

Thrombotic and Thrombolytic Pathways

Hemostasis depends on the normal function of vascular tissue, platelets, and coagulation factors. During the initial response to a loss of vessel integrity, **primary hemostasis** results as platelets adhere to exposed collagen. (This response is facilitated by the von Willebrand factor.) Platelet activation results in the release of substances that constrict the injured vessels and cause other platelets to adhere and form a hemostatic plug. These platelet-released mediators include (1) arachidonic acid, which is converted to thromboxane A_2; (2) 12-hydroxyeicosatetraenoic acid;

TABLE 43-2 Characteristics of Autoimmune Hemolytic Anemias

Disease	Immunoglobulin (Ig)	Complement Involved	Site of Red Blood Cell Destruction	Treatment	Transfusion Requirements
Incomplete warm autoantibodies	Typically IgG Rarely IgA Rarely IgM	No No C4b and C3b	Spleen Spleen Liver	Corticosteroids, splenectomy, gamma-globulin	Rarely needed; if given, combined with corticosteroids
Complete warm autoantibodies:					
Type 1	IgM	C4b and C3b	Liver	Corticosteroids, splenectomy	Rarely needed
Type 2	IgM	C1-9	Intracellular	Plasma exchange, corticosteroids	Frequently needed
Cold autoagglutinins and hemolysins	IgM	No	Intracellular	Corticosteroids, keeping patient warm	Very rarely needed
Biphasic hemolysins:					
Acute	IgG	Yes	Intracellular agglutination	Treatment of underlying infection	Occasionally needed
Chronic	IgG	Yes	Intracellular hemolysis	Plasmapheresis, chlorambucil	Frequently needed

IgA, immunoglobulin A; IgG, immunoglobulin G; IgM, immunoglobulin M.

From Gibson J. Autoimmune hemolytic anemia: Current concepts. Aust NZ J Med 1988: 18:625-37; and Engelfriet CD, Overbeeke MAM, Kr von dem Borne AEG. Autoimmune hemolytic anemia. Semin Hematol 1992; 29:3-12.

(3) serotonin (5-hydroxytryptamine); and (4) adenosine diphosphate.

The platelet plug is not stable, and initiation of the coagulation cascade, followed by deposition and stabilization of fibrin, is required for **secondary hemostasis**. Most coagulation factors circulate in the blood as zymogens, which are converted to active enzymes that in turn convert other zymogens to active enzymes. For example, factor X (a zymogen) is converted to factor Xa (an enzyme), which converts prothrombin to thrombin. A simplified diagram of the coagulation cascade appears in Figure 43-1. In the **intrinsic system,** factor XII binds to negatively charged substrate (e.g., collagen) and may undergo autolysis to form factor XIIa, or it may be converted to XIIa by trace amounts of XIIa. In addition to activating its own zymogen, factor XIIa converts prekallikrein to kallikrein and factor XI to XIa. High-molecular-weight kininogen can bind factor XI and facilitate its conversion to XIa by XIIa. Kallikrein and high-molecular-weight kininogen also can convert factor XII to XIIa. Factor XIa converts factor IX to IXa, which, with factor VIIIa, converts factor X to Xa.

TABLE 43-3 Etiologies of Autoimmune Hemolytic Anemias

Etiology	Approximate Percentage
Primary or idiopathic	43
Secondary:	
• Neoplasms	22
• Drug-related	15
• Infections	8
• Connective tissue diseases	5
• Other diseases	5
• Pregnancy	2

In the **extrinsic system,** tissue damage causes the release of thromboplastin (also known as *factor III* or *tissue factor*). This substance binds with either factor VII or factor VIIa and converts factor X to Xa. The thromboplastin factor VII complex has only 3% of the activity of the thromboplastin factor VIIa complex, but the former may be important in the initiation of coagulation in response to tissue damage. Once factor Xa is formed, it converts factor VII to VIIa, thus increasing the proportion of factor VIIa present, which increases the conversion of factor X to Xa. The thromboplastin factor VII complex also can convert factor IX to IXa, which indicates an interrelation between the intrinsic and extrinsic systems; however, the physiologic significance of this reaction is unclear because it proceeds at a much slower rate than the conversion of factor X to Xa.

Factor Xa promotes platelet aggregation, and it converts factors V and VIII to factors Va and VIIIa, respectively. Factor Xa, combined with factor Va, converts factor II (prothrombin) to factor IIa (thrombin). According to cell-based coagulation theory,[27] activated platelets provide the primary surface for conversion of factor X to Xa and for conversion of prothrombin to thrombin. Thrombin converts factors I (fibrinogen), V, VIII, and XIII to factors Ia (fibrin), Va, VIIIa, and XIIIa, respectively. Thrombin also causes platelet activation. Factor XIIIa is required to cross-link fibrin strands, helping to form a stable clot.

Clot formation is limited by antithrombin III and proteins C and S. Antithrombin III, whose activity is enhanced

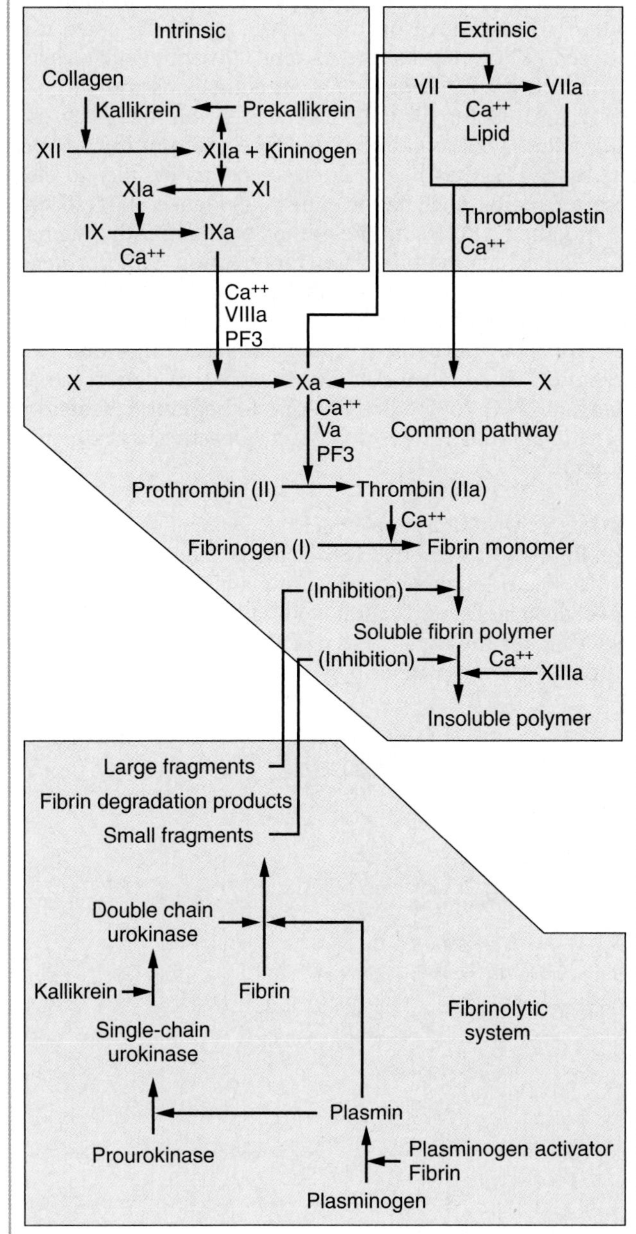

FIGURE 43-1 Components of the extrinsic, intrinsic, and common pathways and the fibrinolytic system. The term *cascade* is a misnomer that stems from the presence of positive and negative feedback loops in both the coagulation and fibrinolytic systems. PF3, Platelet factor 3.

by heparin, inhibits factors IXa and Xa and thrombin. Protein C is activated by a thrombin-thrombomodulin complex. With protein S as a cofactor, protein C breaks down factors Va and VIIIa.

The final component of the hemostatic system is the fibrinolytic system, in which plasmin breaks down fibrin. Tissue-type plasminogen activator (t-PA) circulates as an active protease; however, its activity increases dramatically when it binds to fibrin, at which time it converts plasminogen to plasmin. Urokinase-like plasminogen activator (u-PA) is secreted as the relatively inactive pro-urokinase; it is converted to the active form (single-chain urokinase) by plasmin. Single-chain urokinase is converted to its most active form (double-chain urokinase) by kallikrein, which is released during activation of the coagulation cascade. Plasmin activity is localized to the clot by the local availability of fibrin and by plasminogen activator inhibitors, which are secreted by many cells. The drug epsilon-aminocaproic acid (EACA) inhibits fibrinolysis by binding to plasminogen and plasmin and preventing their binding to fibrin.

Box 2-2 outlines the changes in the concentrations of coagulation factors during pregnancy. The levels of most procoagulants increase during pregnancy, as do the levels of plasminogen and plasminogen activator inhibitors.[28] Deficiencies in these procoagulant factors or an increase in fibrinolytic factors cause **hemorrhagic disorders**. Deficiencies in antithrombin III, protein C or S, or the fibrinolytic system cause **thromboembolic disorders**.

Assessment of Coagulation

ROUTINE HEMATOLOGY

The increase in the concentration of most coagulation factors is associated with shortening of both the prothrombin time (PT) and the activated partial thromboplastin time (aPTT) during *normal* pregnancy (see Chapter 2). In contrast, in severely preeclamptic women with a platelet count of less than 100,000/mm^3, the concentration of coagulation factors may decrease because of their excessive consumption. Therefore, assessment of coagulation in these patients should include the determination of PT, aPTT, and the fibrinogen level.[29]

BLEEDING TIME

The cutaneous bleeding time measurement is used by some physicians to (1) diagnose platelet-related bleeding disorders, (2) predict abnormal bleeding, and (3) monitor therapy for bleeding disorders. However, it is unclear whether the bleeding time correctly predicts the risk of bleeding in an individual patient.

Rodgers and Levin[30] identified and reviewed 862 printed documents that discussed the bleeding time measurement. They constructed receiver operating characteristic (ROC) curves (which characterize the sensitivity and specificity of a test) in every study in which published data were adequate. They made the following conclusions:

1. The utility of the bleeding time measurement has not been enhanced by advances in the standardization of the method.
2. The bleeding time is not a specific indicator of platelet function *in vivo*.
3. No evidence confirms that bleeding from a standardized cut in the skin predicts the risk of hemorrhage elsewhere in the body.
4. No evidence suggests that abnormalities in the test occur sufficiently in advance of other indicators of bleeding to allow actions to be taken that could favorably alter outcome.
5. No evidence confirms that the bleeding time is a useful indicator of the efficacy of therapy.[30]

Others disagree with these conclusions. Burns and Lawrence[31] stated that "patients with known disorders of primary hemostasis, as a result of either hereditary functional platelet disorders or von Willebrand's disease, should be assessed preoperatively with a bleeding time and treated on the basis of the test results."

No evidence suggests that the bleeding time correctly predicts the risk of epidural hematoma after administration of neuraxial anesthesia in a woman with preeclampsia or in a patient who has been taking a nonsteroidal anti-inflammatory drug (NSAID) (e.g., indomethacin, low-dose aspirin). As a result, many anesthesia providers have abandoned the use of the bleeding time measurement before administration of neuraxial anesthesia in such patients.

THROMBOELASTOGRAPHY

Thromboelastography (TEG) is a simple test that measures whole blood coagulation and can rapidly provide information about the adequacy of platelet function and other coagulation factors.[32] Thromboelastographic parameters are interrelated and reflect activities of coagulation proteins, platelets, and their interaction. A simplified diagram of TEG parameters related to intrinsic and extrinsic coagulation appears in Figure 43-2. TEG has been used to determine the coagulation status in healthy and high-risk pregnant women,[33] to manage peripartum coagulopathy,[34] and to assess hemostasis before the administration of epidural anesthesia in pregnant patients with thrombocytopenia.[35] Some investigators have found a correlation between TEG measurements and low-molecular-weight heparin (LMWH) anticoagulation activity, as measured by serum anti–factor Xa (anti-Xa) concentrations. They concluded that TEG might be a useful test to monitor LMWH activity.[36] TEG has been criticized for its inability to diagnose a specific coagulation defect. Evidence suggests that the modified TEG using the monoclonal antibody fragment c7E3 Fab, which inhibits platelet interaction with fibrinogen by binding to glycoprotein IIb/IIIa platelet surface receptors, may provide information about the independent contribution of fibrinogen and platelets to blood clot strength.[37] Further studies are required to determine the ability of TEG to predict the risk for epidural hematoma after the administration of neuraxial anesthesia in pregnant patients.[38]

PLATELET FUNCTION ANALYZER

The PFA-100 (Siemens Healthcare Diagnostics, Deerfield, IL) has been designed to measure platelet function *in vitro*, especially platelet activation and aggregation. This simple test evaluates the capacity of a sodium-citrated whole blood sample to form a platelet plug at the aperture situated on a

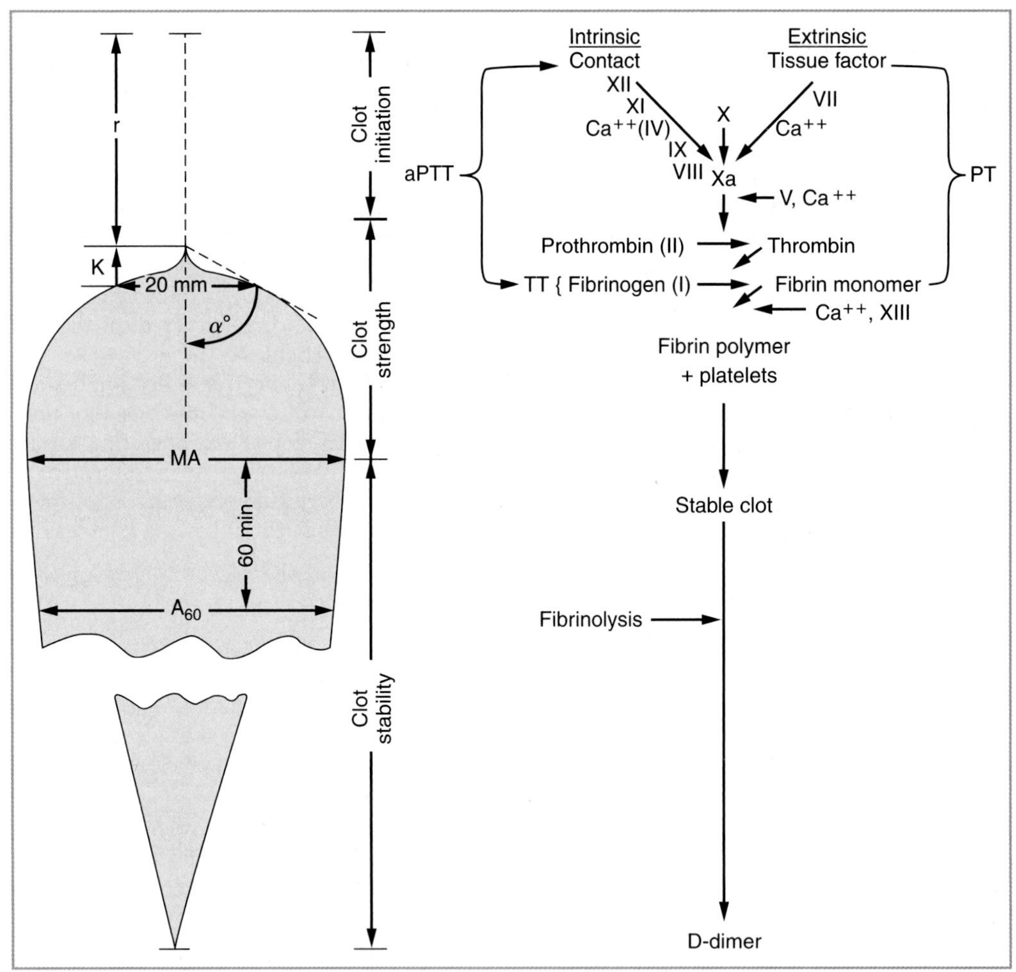

FIGURE 43-2 Simplified side-by-side presentation of thromboelastographic parameters and the routine coagulation profile. α angle, clot formation rate; A60, amplitude 60 minutes after MA; aPTT, activated partial thromboplastin time; K, clot formation time; MA, maximum amplitude; PT, prothrombin time; r, reaction time; TT, thrombin time. (Modified from Sharma SK, Vera RL, Stegall WC, Whitten CW. Management of a postpartum coagulopathy using thromboelastography. J Clin Anesth 1997; 9:243-7.)

collagen/adenosine phosphate or collagen/epinephrine surface under high-shear conditions. The time required for full occlusion of the aperture by the platelet plug is designated as the *closure time*. Some investigators have found this test equally sensitive to platelet aggregometry and more sensitive than the bleeding time for detection of both congenital and acetylsalicylic acid–induced platelet defects.[39] However, evidence suggests that the PFA-100 measurements do not correlate with the platelet count in healthy parturients or in women with preeclampsia.[40-42]

THROMBOCYTOPENIC COAGULOPATHIES

Autoimmune Thrombocytopenic Purpura

Several terms have been used to describe autoimmune thrombocytopenic purpura. *Idiopathic thrombocytopenic purpura* was used first, but the name was changed to *immune thrombocytopenic purpura* when it was discovered that immunoglobulin G (IgG) antibodies were responsible for the greater platelet destruction.[43] Currently the preferred term is **autoimmune thrombocytopenic purpura (ATP)**. This disease should not be confused with neonatal alloimmune thrombocytopenia, in which maternal antibodies to a fetal platelet antigen cause fetal and neonatal thrombocytopenia.

The incidence of mild thrombocytopenia during pregnancy is 4% to 8%,[44,45] but the incidence of ATP is most likely much closer to 0.01%.[46] Antibodies directed against platelet antigens are produced primarily in the spleen, where phagocytosis by macrophages occurs. Antibody production and phagocytosis also can occur in the liver and bone marrow. The binding of complement to platelets can facilitate their clearance, and antibody binding to megakaryocytes can result in the ineffective production of platelets.[47]

DIAGNOSIS

The diagnosis of ATP must be considered if the platelet count is less than 100,000/mm^3 and normal or higher numbers of megakaryocytes are present in the bone marrow. Moreover, the blood smear often reveals the presence of higher platelet volume and greater platelet diameter.[48] Other **nonimmunologic conditions** that must be considered include (1) **gestational** or **essential thrombocytopenia,** (2) **preeclampsia,** (3) **disseminated intravascular coagulation (DIC),** and (4) **thrombotic thrombocytopenic purpura**. Other **immunologic conditions** that must be considered include (1) **drug-induced thrombocytopenia,**[49] (2) **post-transfusion purpura** (in this case, a blood transfusion in the previous 2 weeks is likely),[50] and (3) **pseudothrombocytopenia**. Pseudothrombocytopenia is a laboratory artifact. In cases of pseudothrombocytopenia, chelation of Ca^{++} by ethylenediaminetetraacetic acid (EDTA) exposes antigenic sites that react with antibodies, causing clumping and artificially lowering the platelet count.[51] In these cases, the automated platelet count is normal if citrate anticoagulant is used.

INTERACTION WITH PREGNANCY

If ATP is diagnosed during pregnancy, conservative management is typically sufficient. Corticosteroids are administered if the platelet count is less than 20,000/mm^3 before the onset of labor or less than 50,000/mm^3 at the time of delivery.[52] High-dose intravenous immunoglobulin produces a rapid but transient increase in the platelet count and is administered if there is no response to corticosteroid therapy. In some women with preexisting ATP who become pregnant, thrombocytopenia becomes sufficiently severe that administration of high-dose corticosteroids and immunoglobulin is inadequate, and splenectomy eventually may be necessary.[53]

Some obstetricians have observed significant hemorrhage during the immediate postpartum period in as many as 33% of women with a platelet count less than 100,000/mm^3.[54] In contrast, others have noted no increase in peripartum blood loss in women with a platelet count between 60,000/mm^3 and 100,000/mm^3.[55] Because episiotomies and perineal lacerations pose the greatest potential for intrapartum bleeding, it is preferable to avoid performing an episiotomy in thrombocytopenic women, if possible. Bleeding occurs less often from the placental implantation site.[56] (Contraction of the uterus represents the primary mechanism for postpartum hemostasis.) After delivery, the platelet count often returns to normal in these patients.[57]

OBSTETRIC MANAGEMENT

Maternal IgG can cross the placenta and cause fetal thrombocytopenia, which increases the risk of neonatal hemorrhage. Although there is a correlation between maternal platelet–associated IgG and fetal thrombocytopenia,[56] it is not possible to predict the level of fetal thrombocytopenia on the basis of maternal platelet count[58] or serology results.[59] No study has demonstrated a correlation between the fetal platelet count and intrapartum fetal risk. There are no definitive reports of fetal intracranial hemorrhage secondary to ATP. Neonatal intracranial hemorrhage is rare and is not related to the method of delivery.[60] Thus some obstetricians have concluded that cesarean delivery should be reserved for obstetric indications.[60] Others contend that a fetal platelet count lower than 50,000/mm^3 mandates cesarean delivery.[61] Fetal scalp blood sampling during labor represents a conservative management approach. Percutaneous umbilical cord blood sampling at 38 weeks' gestation has been suggested. However, it is likely that the risk of the procedure is greater than the risk of intrapartum fetal hemorrhage.

Thrombotic Thrombocytopenic Purpura

The classic pentad that defines the syndrome of thrombotic thrombocytopenic purpura (TTP) includes (1) fever; (2) thrombocytopenia (platelet count as low as 20,000/mm^3); (3) microangiopathic hemolytic anemia; (4) neurologic signs such as photophobia, headache, and seizures; and (5) renal failure.[62] These five characteristics need not be present simultaneously. The neurologic and renal changes result from the deposition of platelet emboli and may be of variable intensity in the acute presentation and during recurrences. Diseases that share some of the clinical findings of TTP include DIC, preeclampsia, and hemolytic uremic syndrome.

Disseminated platelet aggregation is a hallmark of TTP.[62,63] Decreased levels of the large multimeric forms of von Willebrand factor are seen in the acute phase of TTP,[64] and these levels return to normal during remission—in contrast to hemolytic uremic syndrome, in which the large multimeric forms of von Willebrand factor are present in normal amounts. The affinity of von Willebrand factor for platelet membrane glycoprotein IIb/IIIa is also increased in TTP.[63] The presence of von Willebrand factor (but not fibrinogen) in platelet aggregates helps differentiate TTP from DIC.[65] (In patients with DIC, fibrinogen but not von Willebrand factor is found in the platelet aggregates.)

Approximately 70% of patients who achieve remission have at least one recurrence.[66] Whether pregnancy affects the incidence of primary or recurrent episodes of TTP is controversial.[67,68] Fetal death typically occurs if TTP develops during the first trimester.[67] Effective treatments include (1) infusion of 30 to 50 mL/kg of plasma, combined with plasmapheresis (approximately 75% plasma exchange); (2) intravenous IgG (400 mg/kg/day); (3) prednisone (1 to 2 mg/kg/day); and (4) infusion of prostacyclin (4 to 9 ng/kg/min).[69-71] Platelet transfusions should be avoided. Termination of pregnancy may be beneficial if the treatment is ineffective[72]; however, evacuation of uterine contents does not always lead to clinical improvement.[67,68] Because of the coagulopathy present in patients with TTP, neuraxial anesthesia is not recommended.

Drug-Induced Platelet Disorders

Drugs can **accelerate platelet destruction** through an immunologic mechanism[73]; however, the drugs that are most likely to result in this complication are not used often in obstetric patients (e.g., quinidine, quinine, gold salts, heparin).

In contrast, drugs that **decrease platelet function** often are used in obstetric patients (Table 43-4). Aspirin irreversibly inactivates cyclooxygenase and prolongs the bleeding time by a factor of 1.5 to 2.[74] The bleeding time is prolonged for 1 to 4 days after the ingestion of aspirin,[75] and *in vitro* platelet function test results can remain abnormal for as long as 1 week.[74] It has been suggested that the maternal ingestion of aspirin may increase the risk of both maternal and neonatal hemorrhage.[76] However, one controlled study demonstrated that doses of aspirin that prolonged the bleeding time did not cause prolonged bleeding after gastric punch biopsy.[77] Therefore, in the absence of a preexisting hemostatic defect (e.g., von Willebrand's disease, hemophilia A, uremia) in which aspirin's effect is more pronounced,[78,79] recent ingestion of aspirin does not contraindicate the administration of neuraxial anesthesia.[80]

Other nonsteroidal anti-inflammatory drugs (e.g., ibuprofen, indomethacin, naproxen) reversibly inhibit cyclooxygenase. These drugs have only a transient effect on the bleeding time[75,81] and have been given to patients with hemostatic diseases (e.g., hemophilia A) without deleterious effect.[82] Maternal ingestion of these drugs should not affect anesthetic management for delivery.

Drugs that increase platelet cyclic adenosine monophosphate (cAMP) levels decrease platelet responsiveness. This increase in cAMP levels can occur after the administration of prostaglandin E_1 or prostacyclin (which stimulates adenyl cyclase)[83] or after the administration of drugs that decrease the destruction of cAMP (e.g., caffeine, theophylline).

Most penicillins and some cephalosporins decrease platelet activity.[84] In addition to its effect on the coagulation system, heparin decreases platelet function by reducing the production of thrombin, a potent platelet activator. Dextran, which is adsorbed onto platelet membranes, can reduce platelet aggregation. Because platelet membranes are a substrate for steps in the coagulation system, clot formation also may be impaired by dextran. Hydroxyethyl starch also appears to decrease platelet function.[85]

TABLE 43-4 Drugs that Affect Platelet Function

Category	Drug(s)
Inhibitors of cyclooxygenase	Aspirin, nonsteroidal anti-inflammatory drugs
Stimulators of adenyl cyclase	Prostaglandin E_1, prostacyclin
Inhibitors of phosphodiesterase	Caffeine, theophylline
Antibiotics	Penicillins, cephalosporins
Anticoagulant	Heparin
Volume expanders	Dextran, hydroxyethyl starch

CONGENITAL COAGULOPATHIES

von Willebrand's Disease

A hemostatic disorder, von Willebrand's disease was named for Erich von Willebrand, who first described it in 1926.[86] The von Willebrand factor is synthesized by endothelial cells and megakaryocytes. The von Willebrand factor subunit is approximately 260 to 275 kDa in size. A dimer is formed by a combination of two subunits, and variable numbers of the dimers are combined to form multimers that range in size from 500 to 200,000 kDa. The von Willebrand factor plays the following two primary roles in coagulation: (1) it forms a complex with factor VIII, which decreases the excretion of factor VIII; and (2) it mediates platelet adhesion by binding to platelets (a reaction enhanced by ristocetin) and collagen. Typically, von Willebrand's disease is inherited as an autosomal dominant trait, and its incidence ranges from 1:100 to 1:2500 for the mild form[87,88] and from 1:200,000 to 1:2,000,000 for the severe homozygous form.[89,90]

Multiple factors control the synthesis of von Willebrand factor. Patients with von Willebrand's disease have variable levels of both von Willebrand factor and factor VIII. Thus some patients with von Willebrand's disease are asymptomatic. Because von Willebrand factor aids in platelet binding to sites of vascular damage, symptoms of von Willebrand's disease (e.g., bleeding from skin and mucosae) can mimic those of platelet disorders. Because von Willebrand factor slows clearance of factor VIII, a deficiency can result in decreased factor VIII levels, and patients with severe disease can present with hemorrhages into muscles and joints similar to those seen in patients with classic hemophilia.

Patients with von Willebrand's disease differ from those with hemophilia in several respects. In von Willebrand's disease, platelet function is affected, and the bleeding time is characteristically prolonged. In contrast, the bleeding time is typically normal in patients with hemophilia. Patients with von Willebrand's disease usually have decreased platelet aggregation in response to ristocetin. In patients with hemophilia, the infusion of small amounts of normal serum or serum from patients with hemophilia has minimal effect on factor VIII levels. Patients with von Willebrand's disease have a prolonged increase in factor VIII levels after the infusion of small amounts of serum from normal patients or patients with hemophilia.

von Willebrand's disease can be divided into several subtypes based on quantitative and qualitative defects in von Willebrand factor.[91] If patients lack the larger multimers, they can have normal factor VIII activity, but they have decreased platelet adhesion and a prolonged bleeding time.

During pregnancy, prophylactic treatment is reserved for patients with a factor VIII level below 25%. For patients with von Willebrand's disease type I or IIa, 0.3 μg/kg of 1-deamino-8-*D*-arginine vasopressin (DDAVP) is administered as labor begins, and the dose is repeated every 12 hours. For patients with no response to DDAVP, fresh frozen plasma or cryoprecipitate (500 to 1500 units of factor VIII activity) should be administered. Most commercial preparations of factor VIII lose von Willebrand factor in the manufacturing process; however, this factor is retained in the processing of Humate-P (CSL Behring, King of Prussia, PA), a pasteurized factor VIII concentrate, which may control hemorrhage in patients with von Willebrand's disease who show no response to cryoprecipitate.[92]

During labor, factor VIII levels should be kept at 50% of normal. If cesarean delivery is required, treatment should be instituted to increase the factor VIII level to 80% of normal. The factor VIII level should be checked daily during the postpartum period, and treatment should be initiated if it falls below 25% or if significant bleeding occurs.[93]

Other Coagulation Factor Deficiencies

In males, the two most common coagulation factor deficiencies are factor VIII (hemophilia A) and factor IX (hemophilia B). Both occur as X-linked traits. A female can have hemophilia if her father is a hemophiliac and her mother is a carrier for hemophilia and passes the abnormal X chromosome to her daughter. A female also can have hemophilia if she is a carrier (i.e., she received one abnormal gene from a carrier mother or an affected father) and she has either a new mutation of the other gene for factor VIII or IX or another X-chromosome abnormality.[94]

In early embryogenesis, half of the X chromosomes are inactivated. Of the gene population, half of the abnormal genes and half of the normal genes are inactivated in females who are heterozygous for hemophilia A or B. On average, these women have half of the normal concentration of factor VIII or IX, which typically is adequate for coagulation. Because the chromosome inactivation is random, more abnormal genes are inactivated in a certain percentage of carriers, and these women have a normal concentration of factor VIII or IX. However, if most of the normal genes are inactivated, the individual can have severely depressed levels of factor VIII or IX. If such a patient becomes pregnant, factor supplementation or plasma exchange (with fresh frozen plasma) may be necessary before or during delivery.

TABLE 43-5 Minimum Coagulation Factor Levels

Coagulation Factor	Plasma Concentration Required for Hemostasis (U or IU/dL)
I	10-25
II	40
V	10-15
VII	5-10
VIII	10-40
IX	10-40
X	10-15
XI	20-30
XIII	1-5

Half of the male children of heterozygous carriers for hemophilia A or B have hemophilia. These infants have an increased incidence of excessive bleeding after circumcision, but the incidence of cephalohematoma does not appear to be increased.[95] It is not clear whether the mode of delivery affects the incidence of cephalohematoma. Heterozygous carriers may undergo a trial of labor and vaginal delivery, but the following procedures should be avoided: (1) placement of a fetal scalp electrode, (2) fetal scalp blood pH determination, (3) vacuum extraction, and (4) difficult forceps delivery.[96] At least one report has described the administration of epidural analgesia during labor in a patient with severe hemophilia A.[97] Maternal considerations should affect the decision to administer (or not administer) neuraxial anesthesia.

Other congenital factor deficiencies occur as autosomal recessive traits and cause symptoms only in the homozygous state. Detailed descriptions of these rare disorders can be found elsewhere.[98,99]

Table 43-5 lists the plasma concentrations of coagulation factors that are required for hemostasis. The patient whose liver disease or vitamin K deficiency is responsible for the coagulopathy may benefit from intramuscular administration of vitamin K. A deficiency can be corrected more rapidly by the administration of 10 to 20 mL/kg of fresh frozen plasma.

ACQUIRED COAGULOPATHIES

Disseminated Intravascular Coagulation

DIC results from an abnormal activation of the coagulation system, which leads to (1) formation of large amounts of thrombin, (2) depletion of coagulation factors, (3) activation of the fibrinolytic system, and (4) hemorrhage. In the obstetric population, the most common causes of DIC are preeclampsia, placental abruption, sepsis, retained dead fetus syndrome, and amniotic fluid embolism.[100]

Laboratory findings consistent with DIC include (1) decreased platelet count; (2) decreased fibrinogen and antithrombin III concentrations; (3) variable increases in prothrombin, partial thromboplastin, thrombin, and reptilase times; and (4) higher concentrations of D dimer, fibrin monomer, and fibrin degradation products.

Therapeutic goals for these patients are to (1) treat or remove the precipitating cause, (2) stop ongoing proteolytic activity (i.e., both the coagulation and fibrinolytic pathways), (3) replace depleted coagulation factors, and (4) provide multisystem support as required. In obstetric patients, evacuation of uterine contents often results in removal of the precipitating cause. A vaginal delivery can be attempted if the mother is stable and delivery can be achieved in a timely manner. If delivery cannot be achieved quickly, cesarean delivery may be required. Rarely, cesarean delivery may be necessary to deliver a dead fetus.

Considerable controversy exists regarding the medical management of patients with DIC. Management may vary according to the etiology of the disorder. If the patient has placental abruption, the physician should give cryoprecipitate or fresh frozen plasma to keep the fibrinogen concentration above 150 mg/dL and to keep the platelet count above 100,000/mm^3.

The use of heparin is controversial. Some physicians have advocated the use of heparin in patients with retained dead fetus syndrome and hypofibrinogenemia,[101] in patients with amniotic fluid embolism who do not have severe hemorrhage,[100] in patients who are septic,[102] and in patients with evidence of peripheral deposition of fibrin.[103] Standard unfractionated heparin can be administered either intravenously or subcutaneously at a dose of 300 to 700 U/hr.[100] LMWH can be given subcutaneously at a rate of 75 U/kg/day.[104] Heparin can cause thrombocytopenia via a nonimmunologic or an immunologic mechanism,[105] but the risk of this problem may be reduced by administration of LMWH.[104,106] Both standard unfractionated heparin and LMWH are effective only in the presence of an adequate concentration of antithrombin III. Patients with DIC may have a depleted concentration of antithrombin III, and administration of fresh frozen plasma may be necessary. In addition to fresh frozen plasma, infusion of cryoprecipitate and platelets may be needed to restore coagulation factors to adequate levels. The use of epsilon-aminocaproic acid, aprotinin, and antithrombin III concentrates as treatment for DIC is controversial. Evidence suggests that administration of antithrombin III is beneficial in the treatment of DIC and sometimes improves organ function.[107]

Patients with DIC often have multi-organ system failure and require mechanical ventilatory support. DIC almost always mandates administration of general anesthesia in patients who require cesarean delivery.

Therapeutic Anticoagulation

Most pregnant women who require long-term anticoagulation receive heparin throughout pregnancy. If warfarin is administered during pregnancy, it is typically discontinued in favor of heparin before the onset of labor. If a patient begins labor while she is still taking warfarin, the effects can be reversed by intramuscular administration of vitamin K. Because reversal of anticoagulation requires time for the synthesis of new procoagulants, acute reversal can be accomplished by the administration of 10 to 20 mL/kg of fresh frozen plasma.

If the patient is receiving standard unfractionated heparin, the drug can be stopped, and the normalization of coagulation can be monitored by following the aPTT or activated coagulation time (ACT). If conditions require immediate reversal, 50 mg of protamine can be administered intravenously, with additional doses given as determined by the aPTT or ACT. Protamine reversal of heparin therapy to allow administration of neuraxial anesthesia is not recommended. Further, protamine is unpredictable in reversing the anti–factor Xa activity caused by LMWH. Therefore, protamine reversal of LMWH is not recommended.

If coagulation is deemed adequate for cesarean delivery, a neuraxial anesthetic technique can be considered. The anesthesia provider should weigh the risks and benefits of neuraxial anesthesia and general anesthesia for the individual patient. It is preferable not to administer neuraxial anesthesia to a patient with a persistent laboratory coagulation abnormality. However, in selected circumstances, neuraxial anesthesia may be offered to a patient with an isolated laboratory abnormality and no clinical evidence of coagulopathy. In such patients, frequent neurologic examinations are performed to facilitate the early detection of an epidural hematoma during the postpartum period.

Other Acquired Coagulopathies

Coagulopathies associated with hypertensive disorders of pregnancy and volume resuscitation after hemorrhage are discussed in Chapters 45 and 37, respectively.

NEURAXIAL ANESTHESIA IN THE PATIENT WITH ONGOING COAGULOPATHY

Concern exists that an epidural hematoma may develop after the administration of neuraxial anesthesia in patients with coagulopathy. There are only a few published cases of epidural or spinal subdural hematoma after the administration of neuraxial anesthesia in pregnant patients.[108,109] This fact suggests that epidural hematoma after neuraxial anesthesia either is very rare (and the risk has been overstated) or is underreported. However, in view of the serious consequences of an epidural hematoma, the risks and benefits of performing neuraxial anesthesia should be carefully assessed in a patient with either clinical or laboratory evidence of coagulopathy.

Frank coagulopathy represents an absolute contraindication to the administration of neuraxial anesthesia. The anesthesia provider can use PT/INR (International Normalized Ratio), aPTT, and ACT measurements or TEG to assess the extent of anticoagulation and the effectiveness of reversal in patients receiving standard unfractionated heparin or oral anticoagulation therapy. If use of a neuraxial anesthetic technique is considered in a patient with a congenital coagulopathy, results of the factor assays (e.g., factor VIII activity and factor VIII ristocetin cofactor activity in patients with von Willebrand's disease; factor VIII and factor IX levels in patients with hemophilia A and B, respectively) should be within the normal range before needle placement.[91]

Through the years, a large number of patients have received neuraxial anesthesia while receiving subcutaneous thromboprophylaxis with **standard unfractionated heparin,** without neurologic complications. Safe practice typically includes the following precautions: (1) proper dosing of heparin, (2) atraumatic placement of the needle or catheter, and (3) measurement of a platelet count in patients undergoing prolonged heparin therapy. Some anesthesia providers prefer to avoid needle/catheter placement or removal within 4 hours of the last dose of standard unfractionated heparin.

In 2002, the American Society of Regional Anesthesia and Pain Medicine (ASRA) convened its second Consensus Conference on Neuraxial Anesthesia and Anticoagulation to provide guidelines for improving the safety of neuraxial anesthesia and analgesia in anticoagulated patients.[110] The ASRA Consensus Conference concluded that subcutaneous (minidose) thromboprophylaxis with standard unfractionated heparin does *not* contraindicate the use of neuraxial anesthetic techniques. However, the platelet count should be assessed before the administration of neuraxial anesthesia or catheter removal in patients who have received standard unfractionated heparin for more than 4 days. In patients receiving long-term *oral* anticoagulation therapy, the anticoagulation therapy should be stopped at least 4 to 5 days before the planned procedure, and the PT/INR should be measured before needle placement.

LMWH (e.g., enoxaparin) is considered to be more efficacious for thromboprophylaxis than standard unfractionated heparin and has been used safely in pregnant women.[106] At least 53 cases of epidural/spinal hematoma after spinal or epidural anesthesia in nonobstetric patients receiving LMWH have been reported.[110,111] In 1997 the U.S. Food and Drug Administration issued a warning that called attention to the risk of epidural or spinal hematoma with the concurrent use of LMWH and epidural or spinal anesthesia. The apparent increase in the risk for an epidural hematoma after concurrent administration of neuraxial anesthesia and prophylactic LMWH may be related to the use of higher doses of LMWH and the relatively greater bioavailability and longer biologic half-life of LMWH after subcutaneous injection in comparison with standard unfractionated heparin.

The ASRA Consensus Conference concluded that in patients receiving preoperative LMWH for thromboprophylaxis, needle placement should occur at least 10 to 12 hours after the last LMWH dose.[110] In patients receiving higher doses of LMWH (e.g., enoxaparin 1 mg/kg every 12 hours, enoxaparin 1.5 mg/kg daily, dalteparin 120 U/kg every 12 hours, dalteparin 200 U/kg daily, or tinzaparin 175 U/kg daily), needle placement should not occur until at least 24 hours after the last dose of LMWH.[110]

In patients receiving a single daily dose of LMWH thromboprophylaxis, the first postoperative LMWH dose should be administered 6 to 8 hours after surgery. An indwelling epidural catheter may be safely maintained in these patients; however, it should be removed at least 10 to 12 hours after the last dose of LMWH, and the next dose of LMWH should be administered at least 2 hours *after* catheter removal. In patients receiving higher (e.g., twice-daily) doses of LMWH, the first dose of LMWH should be delayed for 24 hours postoperatively, and an indwelling catheter should be removed at least 2 hours *before* initiation of LMWH therapy.[110]

The anti-Xa level is not predictive of the risk of bleeding during or after administration of neuraxial anesthesia. Concomitant administration of medications affecting hemostasis (e.g., administration of both LMWH and an antiplatelet drug) further increases the risk of hemorrhagic complications.[110]

The assessment of risk is more problematic in the patient with isolated laboratory evidence of coagulopathy. **Thrombocytopenia** (with variable levels of decreased platelet function) is common in women with severe preeclampsia (see Chapter 45). Asymptomatic thrombocytopenia also may occur in healthy obstetric patients. Some anesthesia providers have reported the safe administration of epidural anesthesia—without any neurologic complications—in healthy pregnant women with thrombocytopenia (i.e., platelet count less than 100,000/mm^3), preeclamptic women, and women with ATP[112]; they contend that in the absence of clinical evidence of bleeding, neuraxial anesthesia should not necessarily be withheld in pregnant women with a platelet count of less than 100,000/mm^3. Published studies of neuraxial anesthesia in thrombocytopenic patients are small and retrospective and do not exclude the possibility that modest thrombocytopenia increases the risk for epidural hematoma. However, no published evidence suggests that a specific platelet count predicts the risk of epidural hematoma in obstetric patients.

When determining whether neuraxial anesthesia is safe in a thrombocytopenic patient, the anesthesia provider should consider the following factors: (1) clinical evidence of bleeding, (2) recent platelet count, (3) a recent change in the platelet count, (4) quality of platelets, (5) adequacy of coagulation factors, and (6) perhaps most important, the risks versus the benefits of performing neuraxial anesthesia. The bleeding time measurement is *not* helpful in determining the risk of epidural hematoma. Although TEG shows some promise, its usefulness in predicting the risk for epidural hematoma is unproven.

Clinical judgment represents the most important means of assessing the risk for epidural hematoma in an individual patient. Clearly, the anesthesia provider would not want to perform neuraxial anesthesia in a patient with clinical evidence of coagulopathy (e.g., bleeding from nasal or oral mucosae or venipuncture sites, presence of petechiae or ecchymoses). In contrast, a patient with severe preeclampsia, severe upper airway edema, a stable platelet count of 100,000/mm^3, and no clinical evidence of coagulopathy may be an appropriate candidate for neuraxial anesthesia. The risk of failed intubation may be greater than the risk of an epidural hematoma in such a patient. Neuraxial analgesia may be offered to such a patient after a thorough discussion of the risks and benefits. In contrast, other anesthesia providers advocate a more conservative approach and recommend alternative methods of analgesia during labor, followed by awake laryngoscopy and intubation if cesarean delivery should become necessary.

Most anesthesia providers no longer obtain a bleeding time measurement in patients who have received **low-dose aspirin** during pregnancy for the prevention of preeclampsia and who have no other risk factors for bleeding. Low-dose aspirin (i.e., 60 to 75 mg) does not significantly prolong the bleeding time in pregnant women.[113] Moreover, a large number of women receiving low-dose aspirin therapy for the prevention or treatment of preeclampsia have undergone epidural analgesia for labor and delivery with no complications.[114]

Several modifications of technique may decrease the risk of venous injury during the administration of epidural analgesia. They are (1) administration of epidural analgesia during early labor before the platelet count or platelet function declines, (2) use of a midline technique, (3) use of a small needle and catheter, and (4) administration of saline through the needle to distend the epidural space before insertion of the catheter. In addition, the epidural catheter may be placed several hours before the patient requires analgesia. This interval allows the anesthesia provider to observe for symptoms and signs of epidural hematoma formation (e.g., back pain, radicular pain, leg weakness) before the administration of an analgesic or anesthetic solution. This last recommendation is impractical in most circumstances. Further, it is unclear that any of these recommendations reduces the likelihood of epidural hematoma in patients with platelet dysfunction or coagulopathy.

During the administration of epidural analgesia, the anesthesia provider can minimize motor blockade by administering a dilute solution of local anesthetic with an opioid (e.g., 0.0625% bupivacaine with 2 μg/mL of fentanyl). The anesthesia provider should subsequently perform a neurologic examination at 1- to 2-hour intervals to look for evidence of neurologic compromise secondary to an epidural hematoma. If unexplained neurologic deficits occur, immediate steps should be taken to exclude an epidural hematoma (see Chapter 32).

Similar precautions should be taken during the administration of postoperative analgesia. Bromage[115] made the following observations:

> *Severe back pain and, later, root pain emanating from the site of compression are the earliest signs calling for urgent neurologic assessment. This implies that postoperative pain management interventions must not distort normal neurologic function. Therefore, intraspinal local anesthetic and opioids should be short acting so that any analgesic intraspinal infusion can be shut off periodically . . . , so that a valid neurologic examination can be carried out and documented at those times. If signs of hematoma arise, the patient is then committed to the serious and costly course of early and appropriate imaging—magnetic resonance imaging or myelography—followed by urgent laminectomy if cord compression is confirmed. This is a formidable contingency plan, costly and risky at best, but with the prospect of catastrophic paralysis if spinal-cord compression is delayed beyond the short period of 6 to 12 hours when full recovery may be expected.*

In some cases, severe thrombocytopenia and coagulopathy may develop *after* the placement of an epidural catheter. In such cases, many anesthesia providers contend that the catheter should *not* be removed until the patient has normal coagulation.[116,117] They argue that movement or removal of the catheter may dislodge a clot, resulting in fresh bleeding and an epidural hematoma. ASRA recommendations (as described earlier) support this view.[110]

HYPERCOAGULABLE STATES

Effective hemostasis is maintained by an appropriate balance of procoagulant and anticoagulant activities. A congenital deficiency in anticoagulant activity occurs in approximately 0.02% of the population and in 2% to 5% of persons with a history of venous thrombosis.[118] Protein C, protein S, and antithrombin III deficiencies and factor V Leiden mutation are the most common causes of hypercoagulability, with plasminogen deficiency and dysfibrinogenemia being less common.[119,120] The incidence of venous thromboses, which are more common than arterial thromboses, increases with surgery, pregnancy, oral contraceptive use, and immobilization.[118] Patients with any of these conditions have an increased incidence of intrauterine growth restriction and preeclampsia, placental abruption, and intrauterine fetal death, perhaps as a result of placental thrombosis and insufficiency.

Protein C Deficiency

Protein C is produced in the liver and requires vitamin K for its synthesis. It acts by inhibiting *activated* factors V and VIII. The incidence of protein C deficiency is approximately 1:15,000.

Protein C levels normally increase by 35% during pregnancy, but this increase is attenuated in patients with protein C deficiency.[121] Thrombosis occurs in 25% of pregnancies in patients with protein C deficiency unless anticoagulation therapy is administered.[122] Two thirds of these episodes occur during the postpartum period. Heparin should be administered during the first and third trimesters, and either heparin or warfarin during the second trimester and postpartum period.

Protein C is a vitamin K–dependent protein with a short half-life (8 hours). If warfarin is administered without prior heparin anticoagulation, the level of protein C falls before the levels of factors II, VII, IX, and X fall. Thrombosis with skin necrosis can result.[118]

Factor V Leiden Mutation

Factor V Leiden mutation is a genetic disorder that occurs from a mutation in a single amino acid in the factor V gene. The mutant factor V Leiden protein persists longer in the circulation as a result of its slower degradation by activated protein C, leading to a hypercoagulable state.[120] The incidence of heterozygous factor V Leiden mutation is about 5% to 8%, which increases the risk of thrombosis fourfold to eightfold. A homozygous mutation is found in 1 in 1600 individuals, and these patients have as much as an 80-fold higher risk for thrombosis. During pregnancy in a patient with factor V Leiden mutation, LMWH thromboprophylaxis should be initiated in the first trimester and maintained until approximately 2 weeks prior to delivery, when a transition from LMWH to standard unfractionated heparin should occur. LMWH thromboprophylaxis should be re-instituted after delivery and continued for up to 6 weeks.[123]

Protein S Deficiency

In contrast to levels of protein C, the plasma levels of protein S normally *decrease* during pregnancy.[121] Protein S also is produced in the liver and depends on vitamin K for its synthesis. Protein S acts as a cofactor for protein C. Circulating protein S binds to C4b-binding protein (a protein of the complement system), but it is the free fraction of protein S that acts as a cofactor for protein C. Immunologic assays measure total protein S concentrations; therefore a diagnosis of protein S deficiency is made either by using a functional assay or by calculating the percentage of protein S bound to C4b-binding protein. The treatment for protein S deficiency is identical to that for protein C deficiency.

Antithrombin III Deficiency

Antithrombin III is synthesized in the liver and endothelial cells. It inactivates thrombin and factors IXa, Xa, XIa, and XIIa. Its activity is potentiated by heparin. Deficiency of antithrombin III occurs in 1 in 5000 persons.[124] Quantitative (type I) and qualitative (type II) deficiencies can exist; thus both immunologic and functional assays are required to detect abnormalities.

The risk of thrombosis during pregnancy increases from 0.1% in normal persons[125] to 55% to 68% in untreated patients with antithrombin III deficiency.[122,126] Anticoagulation or antithrombin III replacement is indicated during pregnancy.[127] Heparin is administered during the first and third trimesters, and heparin or warfarin during the second trimester and postpartum period. Heparin acts by potentiating the activity of antithrombin III. Therefore if antithrombin III levels are reduced, so is heparin's activity. This condition may necessitate the administration of more heparin to patients with antithrombin III deficiency[127] or administration of antithrombin III concentrate (20 to 40 mg/kg) concurrently with the heparin.[118] Alternatively, some experts recommend the administration of antithrombin III only during labor and the postpartum period.[128]

Lupus Anticoagulant

The term *lupus anticoagulant* is a misnomer. Patients with lupus anticoagulant do *not* have a coagulopathy; rather, they are at risk for thromboembolic events. The hypercoagulable state associated with lupus anticoagulant is discussed in Chapter 40.

KEY POINTS

- Neuraxial anesthetic techniques can be used safely during labor and delivery in patients with hemoglobinopathies.
- The first goal in the treatment of disseminated intravascular coagulation is to treat or remove the precipitating cause. In pregnant patients, evacuation of the uterine contents often results in removal of the precipitating cause.
- No evidence suggests that the bleeding time correctly predicts the risk of bleeding within the epidural space in an individual patient.
- Uncorrected, frank coagulopathy represents an absolute contraindication to the administration of neuraxial anesthesia.
- In a patient with an isolated laboratory abnormality and no clinical evidence of coagulopathy, the anesthesia provider should assess the risks and benefits of performing neuraxial anesthesia.

REFERENCES

1. Liebhaber SA, Kan YW. Differentiation of the mRNA transcripts originating from the α_1- and α_2-globin loci in normals and α-thalassemics. J Clin Invest 1981; 68:439-46.
2. Orkin SH, Goff SC. The duplicated human α-globin genes: Their relative expression as measured by RNA analysis. Cell 1981; 24:345-51.
3. Dozy AM, Kan YW, Embury SH, et al. α-Globin gene organisation in blacks precludes the severe form of α-thalassaemia. Nature 1979; 280:605-7.
4. American College of Obstetricians and Gynecologists. Hemoglobinopathies in pregnancy. ACOG Practice Bulletin No. 78. Washington, DC, ACOG, 2007.
5. Weatherall DJ. The Thalassemias. In Williams WJ, Beutler E, Erslev AJ, Lichtman MA, editors. Hematology. New York, McGraw-Hill, 1990:510-39.
6. Lassman MN, O'Brien RT, Pearson HA, et al. Endocrine evaluation in thalassemia major. Ann N Y Acad Sci 1974; 232:226-37.
7. Canale VC, Steinherz P, New M, Erlandson M. Endocrine function in thalassemia major. Ann N Y Acad Sci 1974; 232:333-45.
8. Kazazian HH Jr, Boehm CD. Molecular basis and prenatal diagnosis of β-thalassemia. Blood 1988; 72:1107-16.
9. Piomelli S, Loew T. Management of thalassemia major (Cooley's anemia). Hematol Oncol Clin North Am 1991; 5:557-69.
10. Mordel N, Birkenfeld A, Goldfarb AN, Rachmilewitz EA. Successful full-term pregnancy in homozygous β-thalassemia major: Case report and review of the literature. Obstet Gynecol 1989; 73:837-40.
11. Waters JH, Lukauskiene E, Anderson ME. Intraoperative blood salvage during cesarean delivery in a patient with β thalassemia intermedia. Anesth Analg 2003; 97:1808-9.
12. Butwick A, Findley I, Wonke B. Management of pregnancy in a patient with β thalassaemia major. Int J Obstet Anesth 2005; 14:351-4.
13. Sheiner E, Levy A, Yerushalmi R, Katz M. Beta-thalassemia minor during pregnancy. Obstet Gynecol 2004; 103:1273-7.
14. Firth PG, Head CA. Sickle cell disease and anesthesia. Anesthesiology 2004; 101:766-85.
15. Motulsky AG. Frequency of sickling disorders in U.S. blacks. N Engl J Med 1973; 288:31-3.
16. Solanki DL, McCurdy PR, Cuttitta FF, Schechter GP. Hemolysis in sickle cell disease as measured by endogenous carbon monoxide production: A preliminary report. Am J Clin Pathol 1988; 89:221-5.
17. Veille JC, Hanson R. Left ventricular systolic and diastolic function in pregnant patients with sickle cell disease. Am J Obstet Gynecol 1994; 170:107-10.
18. Tsen LC, Cherayil G. Sickle cell-induced peripheral neuropathy following spinal anesthesia for cesarean delivery. Anesthesiology 2001; 95:1298-9.
19. Poddar D, Maude GH, Plant MJ, et al. Pregnancy in Jamaican women with homozygous sickle cell disease: Fetal and maternal outcome. Br J Obstet Gynaecol 1986; 93:727-32.
20. Koshy M, Burd L, Wallace D, et al. Prophylactic red-cell transfusions in pregnant patients with sickle cell disease: A randomized cooperative study. N Engl J Med 1988; 319:1447-52.
21. Platt OS, Orkin SH, Dover G, et al. Hydroxyurea enhances fetal hemoglobin production in sickle cell anemia. J Clin Invest 1984; 74:652-6.
22. Vermylen C, Fernandez Robles E, Ninane J, Cornu G. Bone marrow transplantation in five children with sickle cell anaemia. Lancet 1988; 1(8600):1427-8.
23. Heller P, Best WR, Nelson RB, Becktel J. Clinical implications of sickle-cell trait and glucose-6-phosphate dehydrogenase deficiency in hospitalized black male patients. N Engl J Med 1979; 300:1001-5.
24. Larrabee KD, Monga M. Women with sickle cell trait are at increased risk for preeclampsia. Am J Obstet Gynecol 1997; 177:425-8.
25. Engelfriet CP, Overbeeke MA, von dem Borne AE. Autoimmune hemolytic anemia. Semin Hematol 1992; 29:3-12.
26. Sokol RJ, Hewitt S. Autoimmune hemolysis: A critical review. Crit Rev Oncol Hematol 1985; 4:125-54.
27. Roberts HR, Monroe DM III, Hoffman M. Molecular biology and biochemistry of the coagulation factors and pathways of hemostasis.

In Beutler E, Lichtman MA, Coller BS, et al, editors. Williams Hematology. 6th edition. New York, McGraw-Hill, 2001:1409-34.
28. Bonnar J, Daly L, Sheppard BL. Changes in the fibrinolytic system during pregnancy. Semin Thromb Hemost 1990; 16:221-9.
29. Leduc L, Wheeler JM, Kirshon B, et al. Coagulation profile in severe preeclampsia. Obstet Gynecol 1992; 79:14-8.
30. Rodgers RP, Levin J. A critical reappraisal of the bleeding time. Semin Thromb Hemost 1990; 16:1-20.
31. Burns ER, Lawrence C. Bleeding time: A guide to its diagnostic and clinical utility. Arch Pathol Lab Med 1989; 113:1219-24.
32. Mallett SV, Cox DJ. Thrombelastography. Br J Anaesth 1992; 69:307-13.
33. Sharma SK, Philip J, Whitten CW, et al. Assessment of changes in coagulation in parturients with preeclampsia using thromboelastography. Anesthesiology 1999; 90:385-90.
34. Sharma SK, Vera RL, Stegall WC, Whitten CW. Management of a postpartum coagulopathy using thromboelastography. J Clin Anesth 1997; 9:243-7.
35. Campos CJ, Pivalizza EG, Abouleish EI. Thromboelastography in a parturient with immune thrombocytopenic purpura (letter). Anesth Analg 1998; 86:675.
36. Klein SM, Slaughter TF, Vail PT, et al. Thromboelastography as a perioperative measure of anticoagulation resulting from low molecular weight heparin: A comparison with anti-Xa concentrations. Anesth Analg 2000; 91:1091-5.
37. Gottumukkala VN, Sharma SK, Philip J. Assessing platelet and fibrinogen contribution to clot strength using modified thromboelastography in pregnant women. Anesth Analg 1999; 89:1453-5.
38. Hunt BJ, Lyons G. Thromboelastography should be available in every labour ward. Int J Obstet Anesth 2005; 14:324-7.
39. Mammen EF, Comp PC, Gosselin R, et al. PFA-100™ system: A new method for assessment of platelet dysfunction. Semin Thromb Hemost 1998; 24:195-202.
40. Vincelot A, Nathan N, Collet D, et al. Platelet function during pregnancy: An evaluation using the PFA-100 analyser. Br J Anaesth 2001; 87:890-3.
41. Beilin Y, Arnold I, Hossain S. Evaluation of the platelet function analyzer (PFA-100®) vs. the thromboelastogram (TEG) in the parturient. Int J Obstet Anesth 2006; 15:7-12.
42. Sharma SK, Warren J, Dadarkar P, et al. The platelet function analyzer (PFA-100) does not predict blood loss during delivery in women with severe preeclampsia. Anesthesiology 2004; 101:A1216.
43. Shulman NR, Marder VJ, Weinrach RS. Similarities between known antiplatelet antibodies and the factor responsible for thrombocytopenia in idiopathic purpura: Physiologic, serologic and isotopic studies. Ann N Y Acad Sci 1965; 124:499-542.
44. Burrows RF, Kelton JG. Incidentally detected thrombocytopenia in healthy mothers and their infants. N Engl J Med 1988; 319:142-5.
45. Kam PC, Thompson SA, Liew ACS. Thrombocytopenia in the parturient. Anaesthesia 2004; 59:255-64.
46. Kessler I, Lancet M, Borenstein R, et al. The obstetrical management of patients with immunologic thrombocytopenic purpura. Int J Gynaecol Obstet 1982; 20:23-8.
47. Gernsheimer T, Stratton J, Ballem PJ, Slichter SJ. Mechanisms of response to treatment in autoimmune thrombocytopenic purpura. N Engl J Med 1989; 320:974-80.
48. Greinacher A, Mueller-Eckhardt C. Hereditary types of thrombocytopenia with giant platelets and inclusion bodies in the leukocytes. Blut 1990; 60:53-60.
49. Mueller-Eckhardt C, Salama A. Drug-induced immune cytopenias: A unifying pathogenetic concept with special emphasis on the role of drug metabolites. Transfus Med Rev 1990; 4:69-77.
50. Waters AH. Post-transfusion purpura. Blood Rev 1989; 3:83-7.
51. Pegels JG, Bruynes EC, Engelfriet CP, von dem Borne AE. Pseudothrombocytopenia: An immunologic study on platelet antibodies dependent on ethylene diamine tetra-acetate. Blood 1982; 59:157-61.
52. Pillai M. Platelets and pregnancy. Br J Obstet Gynaecol 1993; 100:201-4.
53. Laros RK, Sweet RL. Management of idiopathic thrombocytopenic purpura during pregnancy. Am J Obstet Gynecol 1975; 122:182-91.
54. O'Reilly RA, Taber BZ. Immunologic thrombocytopenic purpura and pregnancy: Six new cases. Obstet Gynecol 1978; 51:590-7.
55. Druzin ML, Stier E. Maternal platelet count at delivery in patients with idiopathic thrombocytopenic purpura, not related to perioperative complications. J Am Coll Surg 1994; 179:264-6.
56. Heys RF. Child bearing and idiopathic thrombocytopenic purpura. J Obstet Gynaecol Br Commonw 1966; 73:205-14.
57. Kelton JG, Inwood MJ, Barr RM, et al. The prenatal prediction of thrombocytopenia in infants of mothers with clinically diagnosed immune thrombocytopenia. Am J Obstet Gynecol 1982; 144:449-54.
58. Cines DB, Dusak B, Tomaski A, et al. Immune thrombocytopenic purpura and pregnancy. N Engl J Med 1982; 306:826-31.
59. Aster RH. "Gestational" thrombocytopenia: A plea for conservative management. N Engl J Med 1990; 323:264-6.
60. Payne SD, Resnik R, Moore TR, et al. Maternal characteristics and risk of severe neonatal thrombocytopenia and intracranial hemorrhage in pregnancies complicated by autoimmune thrombocytopenia. Am J Obstet Gynecol 1997; 177:149-55.
61. Scott JR, Cruikshank DP, Kochenour NK, et al. Fetal platelet counts in the obstetric management of immunologic thrombocytopenic purpura. Am J Obstet Gynecol 1980; 136:495-9.
62. Murphy WG, Moore JC, Warkentin TE, et al. Thrombotic thrombocytopenic purpura. Blood Coagul Fibrinolysis 1992; 3:655-9.
63. Moore JC, Murphy WG, Kelton JG. Calpain proteolysis of von Willebrand factor enhances its binding to platelet membrane glycoprotein IIb/IIIa: An explanation for platelet aggregation in thrombotic thrombocytopenic purpura. Br J Haematol 1990; 74:457-64.
64. Murphy WG, Moore JC, Baar RD, et al. Relationship between platelet aggregating factor and von Willebrand factor in thrombotic thrombocytopenic purpura. Br J Haematol 1987; 66:509-13.
65. Asada Y, Sumiyoshi A, Hayashi T, et al. Immunohistochemistry of vascular lesions in thrombotic thrombocytopenic purpura with special reference to factor VIII related antigen. Thromb Res 1985; 38:469-79.
66. Bell WR, Braine HG, Ness PM, Kickler TS. Improved survival in thrombotic thrombocytopenic purpura-hemolytic uremic syndrome. N Engl J Med 1991; 325:398-403.
67. Pinette MG, Vintzileos AM, Ingardia CJ. Thrombotic thrombocytopenic purpura as a cause of thrombocytopenia in pregnancy: Literature review. Am J Perinatol 1989; 6:55-7.
68. Miller JM, Pastorek JG. Thrombotic thrombocytopenic purpura and hemolytic uremic syndrome in pregnancy. Clin Obstet Gynecol 1991; 34:64-71.
69. Rock GA, Shumak KH, Buskard NA, et al. Comparison of plasma exchange with plasma infusion in the treatment of thrombotic thrombocytopenic purpura: Canadian Apheresis Study Group. N Engl J Med 1991; 325:393-7.
70. Finn NG, Wang JC, Hong KJ. High-dose intravenous gamma-immunoglobulin infusion in the treatment of thrombotic thrombocytopenic purpura. Arch Intern Med 1987; 147:2165-7.
71. Tardy B, Page Y, Comtet C, et al. Intravenous prostacyclin in thrombotic thrombocytopenia purpura: Case report and review of the literature. J Intern Med 1991; 230:279-82.
72. Natelson EA, White D. Recurrent thrombotic thrombocytopenic purpura in early pregnancy: Effect of uterine evacuation. Obstet Gynecol 1985; 66(Suppl):54S-6S.
73. Aster RH, George JN. Thrombocytopenia due to enhanced platelet destruction by immunologic mechanisms. In Williams WJ, Beutler E, Erslev AJ, Lichtman MA, editors. Hematology. New York, McGraw-Hill, 1990:1370-98.
74. Weiss HJ, Aledort LM, Kochwa S. The effect of salicylates on the hemostatic properties of platelets in man. J Clin Invest 1968; 47:2169-80.
75. Nadell J, Bruno J, Varady J, Segre EJ. Effect of naproxen and of aspirin on bleeding time and platelet aggregation. J Clin Pharmacol 1974; 14:176-82.

76. Stuart MJ, Gross SJ, Elrad H, Graeber JE. Effects of acetylsalicylic-acid ingestion on maternal neonatal hemostasis. N Engl J Med 1982; 307:909-12.
77. O'Laughlin JC, Hoftiezer JW, Mahoney JP, Ivey KJ. Does aspirin prolong bleeding from gastric biopsies in man? Gastrointest Endosc 1981; 27:1-5.
78. Gaspari F, Viganò G, Orisio S, et al. Aspirin prolongs bleeding time in uremia by a mechanism distinct from platelet cyclooxygenase inhibition. J Clin Invest 1987; 79:1788-97.
79. Kaneshiro MM, Mielke CH, Kasper CK, Rapaport SI. Bleeding time after aspirin in disorders of intrinsic clotting. N Engl J Med 1969; 281:1039-42.
80. Orlikowski CE, Payne AJ, Moodley J, Rocke DA. Thromboelastography after aspirin ingestion in pregnant and non-pregnant subjects. Br J Anaesth 1992; 69:159-61.
81. Buchanan GR, Martin V, Levine PH, et al. The effects of "anti-platelet" drugs on bleeding time and platelet aggregation in normal human subjects. Am J Clin Pathol 1977; 68:355-9.
82. Thomas P, Hepburn B, Kim HC, Saidi P. Nonsteroidal anti-inflammatory drugs in the treatment of hemophilic arthropathy. Am J Hematol 1982; 12:131-7.
83. Fisher CA, Kappa JR, Sinha AK, et al. Comparison of equimolar concentrations of iloprost, prostacyclin, and prostaglandin E_1 on human platelet function. J Lab Clin Med 1987; 109:184-90.
84. Fass RJ, Copelan EA, Brandt JT, et al. Platelet-mediated bleeding caused by broad-spectrum penicillins. J Infect Dis 1987; 155:1242-8.
85. Boldt J, Knothe C, Zickmann B, et al. Influence of different intravascular volume therapies on platelet function in patients undergoing cardiopulmonary bypass. Anesth Analg 1993; 76:1185-90.
86. von Willebrand EA. Hereditors pseudohamofile. Finska Laeksaellsk 1926; 68:87-122.
87. Bloom AL. The von Willebrand syndrome. Semin Hematol 1980; 17:215-27.
88. Rodeghiero F, Castaman G, Dini E. Epidemiological investigation of the prevalence of von Willebrand's disease. Blood 1987; 69:454-9.
89. Mannucci PM, Bloom AL, Larrieu MJ, et al. Atherosclerosis and von Willebrand factor. I. Prevalence of severe von Willebrand's disease in western Europe and Israel. Br J Haematol 1984; 57:163-9.
90. Berliner SA, Seligsohn U, Zivelin A, et al. A relatively high frequency of severe (type III) von Willebrand's disease in Israel. Br J Haematol 1986; 62:535-43.
91. Roqué H, Funai E, Lockwood CJ. von Willebrand disease and pregnancy. J Matern Fetal Med 2000; 9:257-66.
92. Rose E, Forster A, Aledort LM. Correction of prolonged bleeding time in von Willebrand's disease with Humate-P (letter). Transfusion 1990; 30:381.
93. Lipton RA, Ayromlooi J, Coller BS. Severe von Willebrand's disease during labor and delivery. JAMA 1982; 248:1355-7.
94. Mori PG, Pasino M, Rosanda Vadalá C, et al. Haemophilia 'A' in a 46,X,i(Xq) female. Br J Haematol 1979; 43:143-7.
95. Baehner RL, Strauss HS. Hemophilia in the first year of life. N Engl J Med 1966; 275:524-8.
96. Nagey DA, editor. Management of pregnancy in hemophiliac patient. Collected Letters of the International Correspondence Society of Obstetricians and Gynecologists 1982; 23:38-40.
97. Dhar P, Abramovitz S, DiMichele D, et al. Management of pregnancy in a patient with severe haemophilia A. Br J Anaesth 2003; 91:432-5.
98. Roberts HR, Jones MR. Hemophilia and related conditions: Congenital deficiencies of prothrombin (factor II), factor V, and factors VII to XII. In Williams WJ, Beutler E, Erslev AJ, Lichtman MA, editors. Hematology. New York, McGraw-Hill, 1990:1453-73.
99. Gralnick HR. Congenital abnormalities of fibrinogen. In Williams WJ, Beutler E, Erslev AJ, Lichtman MA, editors. Hematology. New York, McGraw-Hill, 1990:1474-90.
100. Brandjes DPM, Schenk BE, Büller HR, ten Cate JW. Management of disseminated intravascular coagulation in obstetrics. Eur J Obstet Gynecol Reprod Biol 1991; 42 (Suppl):S87-9.
101. Thiagarajah S, Wheby MS, Jain R, et al. Disseminated intravascular coagulation in pregnancy: The role of heparin therapy. J Reprod Med 1981; 26:17-20.
102. Risberg B, Andreasson S, Eriksson E. Disseminated intravascular coagulation. Acta Anaesthesiol Scand Suppl 1991; 95:60-71.
103. Feinstein DI. Diagnosis and management of disseminated intravascular coagulation: The role of heparin therapy. Blood 1982; 60:284-7.
104. Oguma Y, Sakuragawa N, Maki M, et al. Treatment of disseminated intravascular coagulation with low molecular weight heparin. Semin Thromb Hemost 1990; 16(Suppl):34-40.
105. Cines DB, Kaywin P, Bina M, et al. Heparin-associated thrombocytopenia. N Engl J Med 1980; 303:788-95.
106. American College of Obstetricians and Gynecologist Committee on Obstretric Practice. Anticoagulation with low-molecular-weight heparin during pregnancy. ACOG Committee Opinion No. 211. Washington, DC, ACOG, November 1998. (Int J Gynaecol Obstet 1999; 65:89-90.)
107. Eisele B, Lamy M, Thijs LG, et al. Antithrombin III in patients with severe sepsis: A randomized placebo-controlled, double-blind multicenter trial plus meta-analysis on all randomized, placebo-controlled, double-blind trials with antithrombin III in severe sepsis. Intensive Care Med 1998; 24:663-72.
108. Vandermeulen EP, Van Aken H, Vermylen J. Anticoagulants and spinal-epidural anesthesia. Anesth Analg 1994; 79:1165-77.
109. Loo CC, Dahlgren G, Irestedt L. Neurological complications in obstetric regional anaesthesia. Int J Obstet Anesth 2000; 9:99-124.
110. Horlocker TT, Wedel DJ, Benzon H, et al. Regional anesthesia in the anticoagulated patient: Defining the risks. (The second ASRA Consensus Conference on Neuraxial Anesthesia and Anticoagulation.) Reg Anesth Pain Med 2003; 28:172-97.
111. Horlocker TT, Wedel DJ. Neuraxial block and low-molecular-weight heparin: Balancing perioperative analgesia and thromboprophylaxis. Reg Anesth Pain Med 1998; 23(Suppl 2):164-77.
112. Beilin Y, Zahn J, Comerford M. Safe epidural analgesia in thirty parturients with platelet counts between 69,000 and 98,000 mm^3. Anesth Analg 1997; 85:385-8.
113. Williams HD, Howard R, O'Donnell N, Findley I. The effect of low dose aspirin on bleeding times. Anaesthesia 1993; 48:331-3.
114. CLASP. A randomized trial of low-dose aspirin for the prevention and treatment of pre-eclampsia among 9364 pregnant women. CLASP (Collaborative Low-dose Aspirin Study in Pregnancy) Collaborative Group. Lancet 1994; 343:619-29.
115. Bromage PR. Epidural anesthesia in the anticoagulated patient. Anesthesiol Rev 1992; 19:22-4.
116. Ruskin KJ, Kaufman BS. Epidural anesthesia in the anticoagulated patient. Anesthesiol Rev 1992; 19:25-6.
117. Rosinia FA. Epidural anesthesia and anticoagulation (letter). Anesthesiology 1993; 79:203.
118. Conard J, Horellou MH, Samama M. Incidence of thromboembolism in association with congenital disorders in coagulation and fibrinolysis. Acta Chir Scand Suppl 1988; 543:15-25.
119. Comp PC. Overview of the hypercoagulable states. Semin Thromb Hemost 1990; 16:158-61.
120. Kujovich JL. Thrombophilia and pregnancy complications. Am J Obstet Gynecol 2004; 191:412-24.
121. Malm J, Laurell M, Dahlbäck B. Changes in the plasma levels of vitamin K-dependent proteins C and S and of C4b-binding protein during pregnancy and oral contraception. Br J Haematol 1988; 68:437-43.
122. Conard J, Horellou MH, Van Dreden P, Samama M. Pregnancy and congenital deficiency in antithrombin III or protein C (abstract). Thromb Haemost 1987; 58:39.
123. Harnett MJ, Walsh ME, McElrath TF, Tsen LC. The use of central neuraxial techniques in parturients with factor V Leiden mutation. Anesth Analg 2005; 101:1821-3.
124. Odegård OR, Abildgaard U. Antithrombin III: Critical review of assay methods: Significance of variations in health and disease. Haemostasis 1978; 7:127-34.

125. Letsky EA, de Swiet M. Thromboembolism in pregnancy and its management. Br J Haematol 1984; 57:543-52.
126. Hellgren M, Tengborn L, Abildgaard U. Pregnancy in women with congenital antithrombin III deficiency: Experience of treatment with heparin and antithrombin. Gynecol Obstet Invest 1982; 14:127-41.
127. Owen J. Antithrombin III replacement therapy in pregnancy. Semin Hematol 1991; 28:46-52.
128. Menache D, O'Malley JP, Schorr JB, et al. Evaluation of the safety, recovery, half-life, and clinical efficacy of antithrombin III (human) in patients with hereditary antithrombin III deficiency. Blood 1990; 75:33-9.

Human Immunodeficiency Virus

David J. Wlody, M.D.

In 1981, a cluster of cases of an unusual disorder, *Pneumocystis carinii* pneumonia (PCP), in five otherwise healthy men, initiated a search that culminated in the characterization of a new disease, acquired immunodeficiency syndrome (AIDS), and the identification of its causative agent, the human immunodeficiency virus (HIV). Subsequently there has been an explosion of this disease in the United States. Geographically, a disease that once was limited to two or three urban areas is now found throughout the country. Further, the number of cases of HIV infection has reached epidemic levels. As of December 2005, more than 984,000 cases of AIDS had been reported to the U.S. Centers for Disease Control and Prevention (CDC). Approximately 475,000 people were reported living with AIDS at that time, and some 550,000 people were reported to have died from AIDS and its complications.[1] The number of asymptomatic individuals who are infected with HIV is undoubtedly more than 1 million. HIV infection has exploded demographically from its initial isolation among homosexual men to its current endemic status among intravenous drug users, their sexual partners, and children born to women infected with HIV.

The impact of HIV infection in the developing world has been nothing less than catastrophic. As of December 2006, the Joint United Nations Programme on HIV/AIDS (UNAIDS) estimated that approximately 40 million people worldwide were infected with HIV, with fully two thirds of these cases seen in sub-Saharan Africa. One third of all worldwide AIDS deaths in 2006 occurred in southern Africa. Also, 75% of women infected worldwide live in sub-Saharan Africa, and most of the new infections occurring in children are seen in this region of the world (Figures 44-1 and 44-2).[2]

In the United States, women represent the fastest growing population of persons with AIDS.[3] One quarter of all new diagnoses of HIV and AIDS are seen in women, and in 2002, HIV was the leading cause of death for black women aged 25 to 34 years.[4] Clearly, anyone providing anesthesia to pregnant women in the United States in the early years of the twenty-first century will care for patients who are infected with HIV. Neither medicolegal concerns nor fear of infection with HIV should prevent anesthesia providers from providing effective intrapartum analgesia and anesthesia to HIV-infected women.

PATHOPHYSIOLOGY

HIV, previously known as lymphadenopathy-associated virus (LAV) and human T-cell lymphotropic virus type III (HTLV-III), is a member of the lentivirus subfamily of human retroviruses. The lentiviruses typically cause indolent infections in their hosts. These infections are notable for central nervous system (CNS) involvement, long periods of clinical latency, and persistent viremia caused by an impaired humoral immune response.[5] HIV is a retrovirus (i.e., it carries the enzyme reverse transcriptase). This enzyme converts the single-stranded viral RNA into double-stranded DNA, which subsequently can be integrated into the DNA of the infected cell. This process is error prone, leading to rapid mutation of the virus, which significantly complicates drug therapy. HIV displays similarity to human immunodeficiency virus type 2 (HIV-2), a

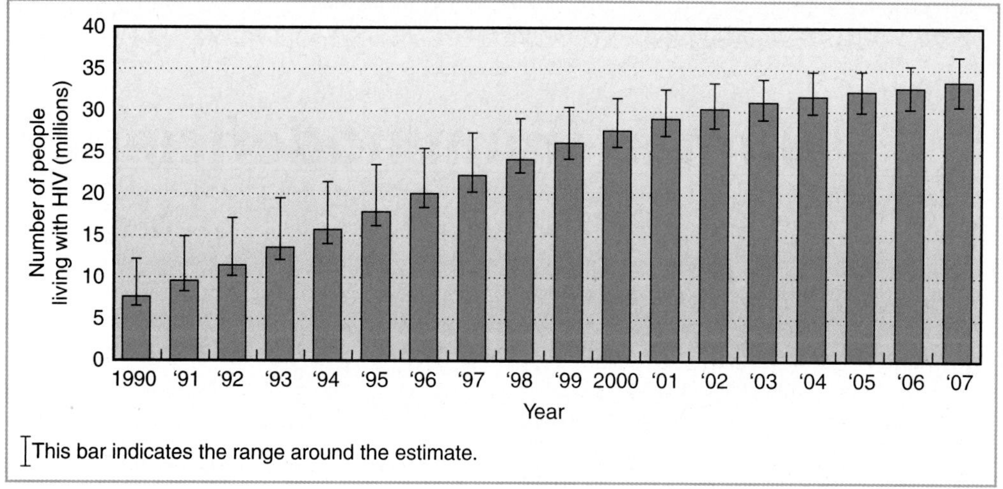

FIGURE 44-1 Estimated number of people living with HIV globally, 1990-2007. (Redrawn from UNAIDS. AIDS Epidemic Update: 2007. Geneva, Joint United Nations Programme on HIV/AIDS [UNAIDS] and World Health Organization, 2007. Available at http://data.unaids.org/pub/EPISlides/2007/2007_epiupdate_en.pdf/)

virus that is endemic in western Africa and that produces a similar syndrome. HIV-2 is even more closely related to the simian immunodeficiency virus (SIV). It has been suggested that HIV arose in human populations through transmission of SIV via infected "bush meat," the meat of chimpanzees and other primates consumed as food.[6]

For infection of the host cell to occur, HIV must bind to a cell-surface receptor, the CD4 antigen complex.[7] This protein molecule was first detected on helper T cells, and it subsequently was identified on B cells, macrophages, and monocytes.[8] It also is found on placental cells[9] and may provide a route of vertical transmission to the fetus during early pregnancy. The interaction between HIV and host cells requires an interaction with an additional cell-surface protein; binding with either the CCR5 or CXCR4 co-receptor is required for infection to occur. A number of potential therapeutic agents target this interaction.[10]

Infection of helper T cells is the key to immune suppression in HIV disease. These cells play a major role in the initial recognition of foreign antigen as well as in the activation of other immune system components.[11] CD4-positive monocytes and macrophages are also targeted by HIV. In addition to these T cell–mediated effects, both neutropenia and disturbances of neutrophil function are common in the later stages of HIV infection.[12] Abnormalities of these elements of the immune system render the HIV patient vulnerable to bacterial, viral, fungal, parasitic, and mycobacterial infection. In addition, for reasons that are not entirely clear, patients infected with HIV are susceptible to several malignancies (e.g., Kaposi's sarcoma, B-cell lymphoma, invasive cervical carcinoma). AIDS-associated Kaposi's sarcoma is almost exclusively limited to homosexual men with HIV or to women whose male sexual partners are bisexual; this fact suggests that the malignancy is related to another sexually transmitted disease. In fact, DNA sequences from human herpesvirus 8 have been identified in AIDS-associated Kaposi's sarcoma.[13,14]

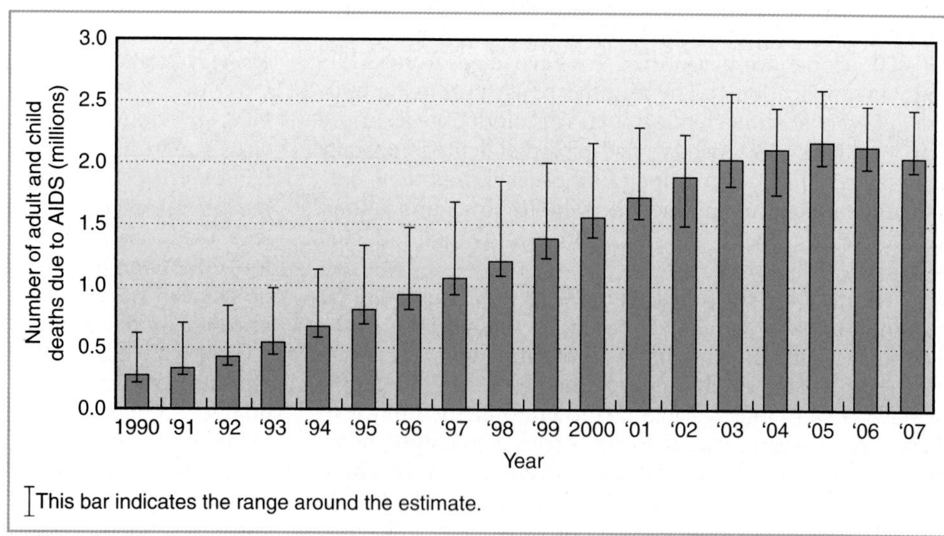

FIGURE 44-2 Estimated number of adult and child deaths due to AIDS globally, 1990-2007. (Redrawn from UNAIDS. AIDS Epidemic Update: 2007. Geneva, Joint United Nations Programme on HIV/AIDS [UNAIDS] and World Health Organization, 2007. Available at http://data.unaids.org/pub/EPISlides/2007/2007_epiupdate_en.pdf/)

DIAGNOSIS

The techniques for diagnosing HIV infection include viral culture, p24 antigen detection tests, nucleic acid amplification tests such as viral polymerase chain reaction (PCR), and immune function tests. Most often, the diagnosis is made on the basis of results of one of two antibody detection tests, enzyme immunoassay (EIA) and the Western blot technique. EIA measures the binding of anti-HIV antibody from the patient's serum to a mixture of antigens that typically have been obtained through recombinant DNA techniques (third-generation test). The use of third-generation tests has improved the reliability of EIA, but false-positive results (caused by autoimmune disorders, influenza or hepatitis B immunization, and/or high parity) and false-negative results (caused by immunosuppressive therapy and various malignancies) can occur.[11] For these reasons, a Western blot test usually is performed after a positive EIA result is obtained. False-positive Western blot tests can also occur, but they are less common than false-positive EIA tests. The Western blot technique allows the identification of antibodies to nine specific HIV antigens. Different organizations have different criteria for a positive Western blot test, but a positive Western blot test generally requires the presence of antibody to at least three different antigens. If there is no detectable antibody to any of these antigens, the result is negative.[11] The finding of any combination of antibodies that does not meet the criteria for a positive result is considered an indeterminant result and an indication for retesting in 4 to 8 weeks.

Nucleic acid amplification tests can detect extremely low levels of infection. This technique can detect viremia as early as 1 to 2 weeks after exposure, during the period of primary symptomatic infection.[11] Although this technique can be used to diagnose acute HIV infection, it is typically used to monitor the response to ongoing antiretroviral therapy.

Both the EIA and the Western blot tests rely on the detection of antibody to HIV antigens. Unfortunately, there may be an interval of several weeks to months after the initial infection before detectable levels of antibody are present. A patient infected with HIV who is tested during this "window period" has a negative test result but is fully capable of infecting others. This is a strong argument for instituting universal precautions. If barrier precautions are instituted only for patients with positive test results, health care workers will be exposed unnecessarily to seronegative but infectious patients.

Patients may be chronically infected with HIV for many years yet appear clinically well or have only minor evidence of immune suppression, such as oral candidiasis or recurrent herpes zoster. The diagnosis of AIDS is made when any one of a number of AIDS-indicator conditions develops (Box 44-1).

BOX 44-1 Acquired Immunodeficiency Syndrome—Indicator Conditions

- Candidiasis of bronchi, trachea, or lungs
- Candidiasis, esophageal
- Cervical cancer, invasive
- Coccidioidomycosis, disseminated or extrapulmonary
- Cryptococcosis, extrapulmonary
- Cryptosporidiosis, chronic intestinal (greater than 1 month's duration)
- Cytomegalovirus disease (other than liver, spleen, or nodes)
- Cytomegalovirus retinitis (with loss of vision)
- Encephalopathy, human immunodeficiency virus–related
- Herpes simplex: chronic ulcer(s) (longer than 1 month's duration); or bronchitis, pneumonitis, or esophagitis
- Histoplasmosis, disseminated or extrapulmonary
- Isosporiasis, chronic intestinal (greater than 1 month's duration)
- Kaposi's sarcoma
- Lymphoma, Burkitt's (or equivalent term)
- Lymphoma, immunoblastic (or equivalent term)
- Lymphoma, primary, of brain
- *Mycobacterium avium* complex or *Mycobacterium kansasii*, disseminated or extrapulmonary
- *Mycobacterium tuberculosis,* any site (pulmonary or extrapulmonary)
- *Mycobacterium,* other species or unidentified species, disseminated or extrapulmonary
- *Pneumocystis carinii* pneumonia
- Pneumonia, recurrent
- Progressive multifocal leukoencephalopathy
- *Salmonella* septicemia, recurrent
- Toxoplasmosis of brain
- Wasting syndrome due to human immunodeficiency virus
- CD4 T lymphocyte count < 200 cells/μL

From 1993 revised classification system for HIV infection and expanded surveillance case definition for AIDS among adolescents and adults. MMWR Recomm Rep 1992; 41(RR-17):1-19.

CLINICAL MANIFESTATIONS

In the early stages of the AIDS epidemic, the predominant symptoms were those of immune suppression (e.g., opportunistic infections, unusual malignancies). Disturbances of gastrointestinal function were also prominent. As improvements in prophylaxis and treatment of opportunistic infections have increased longevity, it has become apparent that HIV eventually affects multiple organ systems. The aggressive use of highly active antiretroviral therapy (HAART) can significantly prolong the symptom-free interval, and it is highly unusual for a pregnant patient to present with significant organ system involvement due to HIV.

Neurologic Abnormalities

Neurologic involvement can occur at any time during HIV infection (Box 44-2). Viral particles can be isolated from the cerebrospinal fluid (CSF) at the time of primary infection.[15] The manifestations of nervous system involvement vary with the stage of the disease.

During **initial systemic HIV infection,** a variety of CNS disorders may occur. Headache, photophobia, and retroorbital pain are common. Cranial and peripheral neuropathies, demyelinating polyneuropathy, and septic meningoencephalitis have been reported.[16] Cognitive and affective changes (e.g., depression, irritability) may

BOX 44-2 Neurologic Manifestations of Human Immunodeficiency Virus Infection

Early (Initial Infection)

- Headache
- Photophobia
- Meningoencephalitis
- Cognitive and affective changes
- Cranial neuropathy
- Peripheral neuropathy

Latent Phase

- Demyelinating neuropathy
- Cerebrospinal fluid abnormalities, even in asymptomatic patients

Late (Clinical Acquired Immunodeficiency Syndrome)

- Meningitis
- Diffuse encephalopathy
- Focal brain lesions
- Myelopathy (segmental or diffuse)
- Peripheral neuropathy
- Myopathy

be noted. Most of these disorders are self-limited, but persistent neurologic dysfunction may occur.[16]

A subset of patients remains neurologically asymptomatic during the **latent phase of HIV infection**. Nevertheless, these patients typically have CSF abnormalities, including the local synthesis of HIV antibody and the presence of HIV particles or viral nucleic acid.[17] This is an important consideration when one is determining the risk of introducing virus into the CNS during the performance of neuraxial anesthesia in an asymptomatic patient. It is almost certain that CNS infection has already occurred.

Finally, the **late stages of HIV infection** are marked by significant neurologic deterioration in almost all patients. **Meningitis** is common, etiologies of which include tuberculosis, *Cryptococcus*, metastatic lymphoma, and direct infection of the meninges by HIV. Diffuse encephalopathy can occur; cytomegalovirus (CMV), herpes simplex virus (HSV), and toxoplasmosis typically produce a simultaneous impairment of both cognition and alertness. **Diffuse encephalopathy** may also be seen as a consequence of systemic disease, such as sepsis or hypoxemia secondary to respiratory disease. Patients with the AIDS dementia complex also present with a diffuse encephalitic picture; however, unlike other forms of encephalitis in which cognitive function is diminished, the level of alertness remains unimpaired. In addition, the complex is associated with impairment of motor function and behavioral changes (apathy, agitation). **Focal brain disorders** can occur, secondary to toxoplasmosis, primary CNS lymphoma, and progressive multifocal leukoencephalopathy (PML), an opportunistic viral infection that causes selective destruction of white matter tracts. **Myelopathy** is common; it can present in an acute, segmental form, as in the transverse myelitis produced by varicella infection, or as a more progressive and diffuse disorder—vacuolar myelopathy—which is marked by a progressive, painless gait disturbance and spasticity. A distal, predominantly sensory **peripheral neuropathy** is quite common in late HIV infection. The etiology is unknown; it has been suggested to occur as a result of cytokine-mediated neurotoxicity.[18] Sensory and motor dysfunction typically are minimal, but pain can be severe enough to prevent walking. CMV infection can also lead to a polyradiculopathy that usually responds to anti-CMV therapy. **Autonomic neuropathy** can present as mild postural hypotension or severe cardiovascular instability during invasive procedures. Autonomic dysfunction also can contribute to the chronic diarrhea that occurs in some patients with AIDS. An inflammatory myopathy resembling dermatomyositis has been reported, although this disorder is less common than the neuropathies.[18] Finally, neurologic side effects of antiretroviral and other therapies also may occur (see later).

Pulmonary Abnormalities

The pulmonary manifestations of HIV disease are caused not by a direct effect of the virus but, rather, by the opportunistic infections associated with the disease. The most prominent of these is *P. carinii*, a fungal organism that is seen in a wide variety of mammals and appears to be carried asymptomatically by many humans.[19] Despite this evidence of widespread exposure to the organism, symptomatic ***Pneumocystis carinii*** **pneumonia** (PCP) is typically seen only in patients with severe immune suppression. The clinical picture is similar to the adult respiratory distress syndrome (ARDS), consisting of severe hypoxemia and a pattern of diffuse interstitial infiltrates on chest radiography. The mortality rate of patients with PCP who require intubation may be as high as 75%.[20] Early initiation of corticosteroid therapy decreases the likelihood of progression to respiratory failure.[21] Patients who survive the disease are at risk for the development of pneumatoceles; subsequent rupture leading to pneumothorax is common. Survivors of PCP also are at risk for developing chronic airway disease, including chronic bronchitis and bronchiectasis.[22]

Reactivation of latent **tuberculosis** is common in patients with HIV infection because of the impairment of cellular immunity that ordinarily keeps the disease in a quiescent state; HIV-infected individuals also may be more susceptible to acquiring tuberculosis when they are exposed to an infectious individual.[23] The impairment of humoral immunity is responsible for a higher incidence of bacterial pneumonia caused by encapsulated organisms (e.g., *Streptococcus pneumoniae, Haemophilus influenzae*).[24] Finally, although less common than PCP, pneumonia secondary to other fungal organisms (e.g., *Aspergillus, Cryptococcus, Coccidioides*) is much more common in patients infected with HIV than in the general population.[24]

Gastrointestinal Abnormalities

Gastrointestinal disturbances occur at some time in almost all patients with HIV infection (Box 44-3). Painful or difficult swallowing is common and is typically caused by herpetic, CMV, or candidal **esophagitis**; the contribution of these disorders to gastroesophageal reflux is unclear.[25,26] **Severe diarrhea** resulting from infection with CMV, HSV, *Shigella, Salmonella, Candida, Cryptosporidia, Giardia, Mycobacterium avium* complex (MAC), or HIV itself can lead to significant cachexia and electrolyte

BOX 44-3 Gastrointestinal Manifestations of Human Immunodeficiency Virus (HIV) Infection

- Esophagitis and dysphagia
- Hepatitis (opportunistic organisms, coexisting hepatitis B)
- Biliary disease (acalculous cholecystitis, sclerosing cholangitis)
- Wasting ("slim disease")
- Chronic diarrhea (HIV infection of bowel, superinfection with bacterial or parasitic pathogens)

abnormalities. Finally, **hepatobiliary disease** is common. Causes of parenchymal liver disease include hepatitis B and C, CMV, mycobacterial infection (both *Mycobacterium tuberculosis* and MAC), and *Cryptococcus*. Kaposi's sarcoma and non-Hodgkin's lymphoma may involve the liver. Biliary tract disease can develop in advanced HIV infection; although several pathogens have been associated with this disorder, treatment of those pathogens is seldom effective. Thus, the etiology of "AIDS cholangiopathy" remains unclear.[27]

Hematologic Abnormalities

HIV infection is associated with hematologic abnormalities that affect each of the peripheral cell lines.[12] **Leukopenia is** a hallmark of the disease, especially the depletion of CD4 lymphocytes; qualitative alterations in the functions of neutrophils and macrophages also occur. **Anemia** is quite common. Causes include direct HIV infection of erythroid precursors, suppression of erythropoiesis due to inappropriate release of tumor necrosis factor, infiltration of bone marrow with MAC or malignancy, and occult gastrointestinal blood loss.

Coagulation disturbances are common in patients with HIV. **Immune thrombocytopenia (ITP)** is common and typically is only mildly symptomatic. Platelet production may be impaired because of direct infection of megakaryocytes with HIV. Thrombocytopenia frequently responds to the initiation of antiretroviral therapy. The response to corticosteroid therapy is variable. Intravenous immune globulin produces a rapid but transient effect, and it may be indicated in patients with life-threatening hemorrhage. The activated partial thromboplastin time (aPTT) may be prolonged because of the presence of the lupus anticoagulant; this finding is linked to a higher incidence of major thromboembolic events in HIV-infected patients. Finally, many of the antiretroviral agents and other drugs used in these patients have hematologic toxicity.

Cardiovascular Abnormalities

When echocardiography and autopsy evidence of lymphocytic infiltration of the myocardium are used as evidence of cardiovascular involvement in patients with HIV, the prevalence of such involvement is as high as 50%.[28] Nevertheless, clinically significant cardiovascular disease is rare in patients with HIV. **Pericarditis** has been reported to be the most prevalent cardiovascular disorder seen in HIV-infected patients. The most common etiology appears to be mycobacterial infection; CMV, HSV, Kaposi's sarcoma, malignant lymphoma, and HIV itself have also been implicated.[29] **Pulmonary hypertension** can develop secondary to repeated episodes of PCP and can also be a consequence of cytokine-mediated endothelial injury.[28] Direct **myocardial involvement**—typically, focal myocarditis—is identified in 15% to 50% of autopsy studies, but clinical myocarditis or cardiomyopathy is rare.[28] **Infective endocarditis** among patients with HIV occurs almost exclusively in intravenous drug users. Finally, the elevations in serum cholesterol and triglyceride concentrations produced by antiretroviral agents appear to increase the risk for coronary artery disease in patients receiving these drugs.[30]

Endocrine Abnormalities

Endocrine dysfunction can result from HIV infection, opportunistic infections, or drug therapy.[31] There is a relatively high incidence of pathologic findings in the adrenal gland at autopsy, yet clinical evidence of glucocorticoid insufficiency is rare. Patients with AIDS frequently have abnormal thyroid function test results, similar to the findings in patients with other chronic illnesses, yet clinical hypothyroidism is unusual. Insulin resistance and diabetes are increasingly recognized as consequences of HIV infection and antiretroviral treatment.[32]

Renal Abnormalities

Patients with HIV are at risk for acute renal failure secondary to sepsis, dehydration, and drug toxicity.[33] A common cause of chronic renal insufficiency is proliferative glomerulonephritis secondary to deposition of immune complexes containing HIV antigen within the glomeruli. Renal failure may also occur because of a specific disorder, **HIV-associated nephropathy** (HIVAN).[34] This entity, seen almost exclusively in black patients, is characterized by a focal segmental glomerulosclerosis. Hypertension is uncommon, deterioration of renal function is extremely rapid, and the long-term prognosis is worse than that seen in renal failure from other causes. The underlying cause appears to be direct infection of renal cells by HIV. Antiretroviral therapy appears to modify the course of the disease.[34]

INTERACTION WITH PREGNANCY

The rapidly rising incidence of HIV infection among heterosexual women limits the credibility of any estimate of the seroprevalence of HIV among pregnant women. In 1991, the CDC reported a nationwide seroprevalence rate of 1.5 per 1000 pregnant women. There was considerable geographic variation in these figures; the highest rates of seroprevalence were found in New York (5.8 per 1000), the District of Columbia (5.5 per 1000), and New Jersey (4.9 per 1000). Seropositive women were identified in all but 2 of the 39 reporting areas.[35] More recently, the nationwide seroprevalence of HIV during pregnancy has been reported to be 1.7 per 1000.[36] In New York City, the prevalence of HIV infection among pregnant women was 6.2 per 1000 in 1999-2000.[37]

The diagnosis of HIV infection in the offspring of HIV-infected mothers has been hampered by the persistence

BOX 44-4 Risk Factors for Vertical Transmission of Human Immunodeficiency Virus

- Severity of maternal disease
- Maternal viral burden
- Viral genotype
- Sexually transmitted disease
- Substance abuse
- Lack of maternal antiviral therapy
- Chorioamnionitis
- Prolonged ruptured membranes
- Invasive fetal monitoring
- Vaginal delivery
- Forceps delivery
- Breast-feeding
- Prematurity

of passively acquired maternal antibody in the newborn for as long as 18 months. Until 18 months of age, an infant's HIV status must be confirmed by viral culture or DNA PCR. Measurement of circulating p24 antigen has been used for rapid diagnosis of neonatal HIV infection,[38] but this test is no longer recommended because it is less sensitive than PCR and is associated with false-positive results.[39]

There is intense interest in the identification of factors that promote perinatal transmission of HIV from mother to infant (i.e., vertical transmission) (Box 44-4).[40] Clinical severity of maternal disease is associated with an increased risk of transmission, as reflected by a higher rate of infection in infants born to women with symptomatic AIDS.[41] Maternal viral burden correlates with transmission. In one study, 13 of 13 women with more than 80,000 viral RNA copies per mL of plasma transmitted the disease, but none of the 63 women with less than 20,000 copies per mL transmitted HIV.[42] Other factors that have been implicated in vertical transmission are the presence of ruptured membranes for more than 4 hours,[43] coexisting sexually transmitted diseases,[44] chorioamnionitis,[45] and invasive procedures such as amniocentesis and cerclage.[44] At least one study has demonstrated that fetal scalp blood sampling and the use of fetal scalp electrodes do not increase vertical transmission[46]; however, the documented presence of HIV in maternal cervical secretions has made some clinicians reluctant to use this monitoring technique.[47] Finally, there is considerable evidence that breast-feeding may double the rate of perinatal transmission in women with established HIV infection.[48] Thus breast-feeding should be discouraged unless bottle-feeding is not a safe alternative, as is true in many developing countries.

In addition to identifying risk factors for vertical transmission, there is a significant effort to determine which active interventions might decrease the transmission of HIV. The first such intervention that was identified is the administration of zidovudine (ZDV, formerly AZT). In a study known as the AIDS Clinical Trial Group (ACTG) Protocol 076, administration of ZDV orally during pregnancy, intravenously during labor, and orally to the infant for the first 6 weeks of life decreased the transmission rate from 25.5% to 8.3%. No significant adverse effects were noted in these infants.[49] Because of the success of HAART in reducing perinatal transmission to 1% to 2%—compared with 10% for ZDV monotherapy[50]—it has been suggested that all HIV-infected pregnant women should receive an aggressive treatment regimen, regardless of viral load.[40]

Because newborn infection rates are low when the time interval between rupture of membranes and delivery is shortened, it has been suggested that cesarean delivery might decrease vertical transmission. At least four studies have suggested that elective cesarean delivery may decrease the rate of transmission by as much as 80%.[51] The American College of Obstetricians and Gynecologists (ACOG) has recommended that HIV-infected women be offered the option of elective cesarean delivery to decrease the rate of transmission below the rate that would be expected with ZDV therapy alone.[52] Although the ACOG acknowledged that the data were insufficient to demonstrate a benefit for women with viral loads less than 1000 viral copies per mL of plasma, there is some evidence that abdominal delivery may be beneficial even in the setting of viral loads below that threshold[53]; thus it has been suggested that elective cesarean delivery be offered to patients in this group as well.[51]

A number of studies have assessed the effect of HIV infection on pregnancy outcome. Alger et al.[54] followed 97 seronegative and 101 seropositive but asymptomatic women throughout pregnancy. There was no difference between groups in the incidence of low-birth-weight (LBW) (less than 2500 g), small-for-gestational-age (SGA) infants, or low 5-minute Apgar scores.[54] However, in a study of 315 seropositive and 311 seronegative women in Kenya, HIV seropositivity was associated with an increased risk of preterm delivery and LBW infants but not with an increased incidence of SGA infants.[55] These different results may reflect the higher incidence of symptomatic HIV disease in the Kenyan patients. Another study noted that the incidence of serious infectious complications (e.g., PCP, CNS toxoplasmosis) is greater than 30% in pregnant women with advanced HIV infection (CD4 lymphocyte counts of less than 300 cells/mm^3).[56] The fetal implications of such infections are obvious. Drug therapy per se does not seem to affect pregnancy outcome; specifically, evidence suggests that there is no higher incidence of preterm delivery, LBW infants, low Apgar scores, or stillbirth in women receiving therapy than in controls.[57]

There also is concern that pregnancy itself may have an adverse effect on the progression of HIV infection. However, no evidence suggests that pregnancy accelerates clinical deterioration in the HIV-infected patient or that viral RNA load changes significantly during pregnancy.[54,58,59]

DRUG THERAPY

There is an ever-increasing number of medications used to treat HIV infection, administered in innumerable multidrug regimens; in addition to HIV medications, patients may receive a number of other drugs to treat or prevent opportunistic infections. The side effects of the most commonly used antiretroviral agents and medications used for prophylaxis and treatment of opportunistic infections are listed in Tables 44-1 and 44-2, respectively.

Fetal Side Effects

There are few published data regarding the use of HIV medications in pregnant women. Fortunately, clinical experience suggests that fetal risk is minimal. This is best demonstrated by ACTG Protocol 076, which showed a significant reduction of vertical transmission of HIV with maternal ZDV therapy.[49] There was no difference between the ZDV and placebo groups in the number and type of birth defects. The only apparent difference in neonatal outcome was a mild transient anemia (which required no treatment) in the ZDV group. Ongoing observation of these infants is planned, but no difference in growth or neurodevelopmental status has been identified in the ZDV group. As of January 2005, the Antiretroviral Pregnancy Registry had collected records of more than 4700 women who had received these agents during pregnancy in the United States; the data suggest that ZDV, lamivudine, nevirapine, abacavir, and nelfinavir are *not* teratogenic.[40]

Historically, physicians have been concerned that the use of trimethoprim-sulfamethoxazole (TMP-SMX) during the third trimester might increase the risk of neonatal kernicterus. This complication has not been reported, and trimethoprim-sulfamethoxazole should be continued until delivery in women who tolerate the drug.[60]

None of the antiretroviral agents or drugs used to treat opportunistic infections during pregnancy are listed in U.S. Food and Drug Administration (FDA) pregnancy category A, which signifies a lack of fetal effect in controlled human trials.[40] Despite the reassuring findings of the Antiretroviral Pregnancy Registry, the use of these drugs requires a full discussion of the risks and benefits with the mother.[61] Minkoff and DeHovitz[60] concluded, "The guiding principle in the use of medications by HIV-infected women who become pregnant is to adhere strictly to standards promulgated for nonpregnant women, unless there are documented and compelling fetal concerns that would justify a modification of those standards."

TABLE 44-1 Side Effects of Antiretroviral Agents

Drug	Side Effects
Zidovudine (AZT, ZDV)	Headache, N&V, bone marrow suppression
Didanosine (ddI, Videx)	N&V, peripheral neuropathy, pancreatitis, lactic acidosis
Zalcitabine (ddC, HIVID)	Peripheral neuropathy, pancreatitis
Stavudine (d4T, Sterit)	Peripheral neuropathy, pancreatitis, lactic acidosis
Lamivudine (3TC, Epivir)	N&V, headache, pancreatitis (children)
Emtricitabine (FTC, Emtriva)	Headache, N&V
Abacavir (ABC, Ziagen)	Systemic hypersensitivity reaction, headache, N&V
Delavirdine (Rescriptor)	Rash, elevated liver function test results
Nevirapine (NVP, Viramune)	Rash, hepatotoxicity
Efavirenz (EFV, Sustiva)	Dizziness, lightheadedness, vivid dreams, rash
Saquinavir (SQV, Invirase)	N&V, diarrhea, abdominal pain, hyperglycemia, increased triglycerides, fat redistribution
Ritonavir (RTV, Norvir)	N&V, diarrhea, abdominal pain, hyperglycemia, increased triglycerides, fat redistribution
Indinavir (IDV, Crixivan)	Nephrolithiasis, gastrointestinal intolerance, hyperglycemia, increased triglycerides, fat redistribution
Nelfinavir (NFV, Viracept)	N&V, diarrhea, hyperglycemia, increased triglycerides, fat redistribution
Amprenavir (APV, Agenerase)	Headache, N&V, hyperglycemia, increased triglycerides, fat redistribution
Lopinavir/ritonavir (LPV/RTV, Kaletra)	N&V, diarrhea, hyperglycemia, increased triglycerides, fat redistribution
Atazanavir (ATV, Reyataz)	N&V, headache, smaller increase in triglycerides than with other protease inhibitors
Tenofovir (TDF, Viread)	N&V, headache
Enfuvirtide (T20, Fuzeon)	Injection site reaction

N&V, Nausea and vomiting.

From Pau Ak, Robertson S. AIDS-related medications. In Dolin R, Masur H, Saag MS, editors. AIDS Therapy. 3rd edition. St. Louis, Churchill Livingstone Elsevier, 2008:1407-40.

ANESTHETIC MANAGEMENT

Coexisting Diseases

Many pregnant women infected with HIV have health problems that are related to the behaviors that led to their infection with HIV. The most significant of these is substance abuse. A significant proportion of women with HIV contract the disease through intravenous drug use. It can be expected that many of these patients also abuse alcohol and crack cocaine.

The HIV-positive parturient is at high risk for harboring other sexually transmitted diseases. From the anesthesia provider's perspective, the most significant of these diseases is syphilis, because of its neurologic effects in later stages. If neuraxial anesthesia is performed, a careful neurologic examination should be completed and documented. Hepatitis B also is a sexually transmitted disease, and it should be investigated in HIV-positive parturients. Severe hepatic impairment affects anesthetic management. Of equal importance are the infectivity of hepatitis B and the high likelihood of its transmission after needlestick injury. For this reason, it is unacceptable for health care workers to remain unvaccinated against hepatitis B.

Neuraxial Anesthesia

Whether HIV-infected patients are more prone to the infectious complications of neuraxial anesthesia is an important concern. This question was addressed in a

TABLE 44-2 Side Effects of Agents Used for Prophylaxis/Treatment of Opportunistic Infections

Opportunistic Infection	Drug	Side Effects
Pneumocystis carinii	Trimethoprim-sulfamethoxazole	Nausea, vomiting, anorexia, rash
	Dapsone	Fever, rash, hepatitis
	Pentamidine	**Intravenous:** nephrotoxicity, leukopenia, hypoglycemia, hyperglycemia **Inhaled:** cough, dyspnea, dizziness
Cytomegalovirus	Ganciclovir	Neutropenia, thrombocytopenia, central nervous system disturbances
	Foscarnet	Nephrotoxicity, electrolyte disturbances
Mycobacterium avium complex	Clarithromycin	Nausea, vomiting, diarrhea
Fungal infections: cryptococcosis, histoplasmosis, coccidiomycosis	Amphotericin	Nephrotoxicity, fever, hypotension
	Fluconazole	Nausea, headache, rash
Herpes simplex virus	Acyclovir	Nephrotoxicity, neurotoxicity

From Pau AK, Robertson S. AIDS-related medications. In Dolin R, Masur H, Saag MS, editors. AIDS Therapy. 3rd edition. St. Louis, Churchill Livingstone Elsevier, 2008:1407-40.

study of 30 HIV-positive pregnant women, of whom 18 received neuraxial anesthesia and 12 did not. There was no evidence of accelerated disease progression or increases in the rate of infectious or neurologic complications in the neuraxial anesthesia group.[62] A later study demonstrated no postoperative changes in viral load or CD4/CD8 lymphocyte ratio, and no increased hemodynamic instability or blood loss in HIV-infected patients undergoing elective cesarean delivery with spinal anesthesia.[63] The lack of infectious complications of neuraxial anesthesia depends, of course, on the maintenance of strict aseptic technique. The American Society of Anesthesiologists (ASA) Subcommittee on Infection Control Policy has recommended that a gown be worn by anyone performing or assisting with invasive procedures in an HIV-infected patient.[64]

Some physicians may question whether it is prudent to administer neuraxial anesthesia to a patient who almost certainly will develop neurologic deficits at some time in the future. Some worry that these deficits might be ascribed to the neuraxial anesthetic technique. Because such deficits are unlikely to be temporally related to the anesthesia, this does not seem to be a significant concern. Further, it seems cruel to deny the most effective intrapartum analgesic techniques to HIV-positive women simply because of fear of future litigation.

Another question is whether an anesthesia provider can ethically or legally refuse to provide care to an HIV-positive patient. Specifically, can an anesthesia provider refuse to provide epidural analgesia during labor? The American Medical Association has taken the position that physicians have an ethical duty to treat HIV-positive patients. Refusing to treat a patient with HIV also places the physician at legal risk, because numerous federal, state, and local statutes prohibit discrimination against patients with HIV disease. Any physician who refuses to provide care for patients with HIV must participate in a referral system ensuring that such patients receive prompt medical care.[65]

Despite the use of small-gauge, pencil-point spinal needles, and despite careful technique during administration of epidural anesthesia, post–dural puncture headache (PDPH) remains a problem in pregnant patients. Clearly, the onset of headache and photophobia in an immunosuppressed patient who has recently undergone a major neuraxial anesthetic can be worrisome, but the typical postural nature of a PDPH should allay fears of bacterial meningitis. Once the diagnosis of PDPH is made, an initial course of conservative therapy is indicated. It typically consists of bed rest, analgesics, and oral hydration. Although dehydration can worsen PDPH, there is no evidence that forced oral or intravenous overhydration has any beneficial effect.

Should conservative therapy for PDPH fail, a number of additional pharmacologic interventions have been proposed, including intravenous or oral caffeine, adrenocorticotropic hormone (ACTH), and the 5-HT receptor agonist sumatriptan; they have varying degrees of success. However, the "gold standard" for treatment of PDPH is the performance of an autologous epidural blood patch. Such treatment can be expected to produce permanent and complete pain relief in the great majority of patients; a second epidural blood patch typically produces relief in most patients for whom the initial procedure fails.

Some physicians have expressed concern that the introduction of HIV-infected blood into the neuraxis might lead to the introduction of HIV into a previously uninfected CNS.[66] The magnetic resonance imaging (MRI) demonstration of subarachnoid extension of an epidural blood patch heightens these concerns.[67] However, it is likely that CNS infection occurs quite early in the course of HIV disease, even in asymptomatic patients. Nevertheless, it seems prudent to acknowledge the possibility that an epidural blood patch could accelerate the CNS manifestations of the disease. This question was addressed in a study of six seropositive patients who experienced PDPH after diagnostic lumbar puncture and who subsequently received an epidural blood patch.[68] These patients subsequently underwent serial neuropsychological testing for as long as 2 years. The investigators stated that "none of these six subjects had a decline in neurocognitive performance or other adverse neurologic or infectious sequelae" during the period of the study. Although these numbers are small, this study provides the best evidence to date of the safety of epidural blood patch in the HIV-infected patient.

An alternative to autologous epidural blood patch is the epidural infusion of normal saline or colloidal solutions such as hetastarch. Unfortunately, the relief obtained from this technique is often transient, lasting only as long as the infusion continues. It may provide palliation until the dural puncture site heals spontaneously. Another proposed alternative is epidural blood patch with fresh homologous blood; however, there are no published data on this technique.

General Anesthesia

As with neuraxial anesthesia, it is appropriate to ask whether patients with HIV might be more susceptible to the infectious (e.g., pulmonary) complications of general anesthesia. No published study has addressed this question. However, it seems appropriate to handle the endotracheal tube in as sterile a manner as possible and to minimize the duration of postoperative ventilation.

Another question involves the effect of general anesthesia on immune function. Several published studies suggest that general anesthesia can transiently depress immune function, but this depression appears to be clinically insignificant in healthy patients.[69] It is appropriate to ask whether this effect might be exaggerated to the point of clinical significance in patients with HIV disease. Studies on this issue are lacking. At present, it would be inappropriate to recommend one anesthetic technique over another on the basis of their effects on immune function.[70]

Evron et al.[71] reviewed anesthetic considerations for patients with HIV.

STRATEGIES TO MINIMIZE TRANSMISSION OF HUMAN IMMUNODEFICIENCY VIRUS

To the Uninfected Patient

Any survey of HIV and anesthesia must include a discussion of those measures that can decrease the risk of HIV transmission to the uninfected patient. The most common iatrogenic cause of such transmission is the transfusion of infected blood. The use of nucleic acid amplification techniques should reduce the risk of transfusing HIV-infected blood. Nonetheless, the most significant impact that anesthesia providers can have on disease transmission is to minimize the transfusion of homologous blood.

In healthy patients, oxygen delivery is satisfactorily maintained at hemoglobin levels much lower than the historical transfusion threshold of 10 g/dL. The Consensus Development Conference on Perioperative Red Blood Cell Transfusion concluded that healthy patients tolerate a hemoglobin concentration as low as 7 g/dL.[72] Patients with chronic anemia have a higher concentration of 2,3-diphosphoglycerate, which allows effective oxygen delivery at low hemoglobin concentrations. New ASA guidelines state the following:

> *The information needed to precisely define when a blood transfusion should be given is not available. . . . Red blood cells should usually be administered when the hemoglobin concentration is low (e.g., less than 6 g/dL in a young, healthy patient), especially when the anemia is acute. Red blood cells are usually unnecessary when the hemoglobin concentration is more than 10 g/dL. . . . The determination of whether intermediate hemoglobin concentrations (i.e., 6 to 10 g/dL) justify or require RBC transfusion should be based on any ongoing indication of organ ischemia, potential or actual ongoing bleeding (rate and magnitude), the patient's intravascular volume status, and the patient's risk factors for complications of inadequate oxygenation. These risk factors include a low cardiopulmonary reserve and high oxygen consumption.*[73]

It is not clear how these guidelines should be applied to pregnant women. An association between preterm delivery and hemoglobin concentrations of less than 10 g/dL has been reported,[74] as has a similar association between LBW infants and hemoglobin concentrations lower than 9 g/dL.[75] However, whether this is a causal relationship or whether anemia serves as a marker of poor nutrition or lower socioeconomic status that may independently lead to perinatal morbidity is unknown. Although it is impossible to designate a minimum acceptable hemoglobin level during pregnancy, anemia is clearly undesirable. Once a cause is determined, appropriate therapy should be initiated, including transfusion if the anemia is life-threatening for the mother or fetus.

Patients often want to use blood specifically donated by friends or relatives for their use (**directed donation**). There are disadvantages of directed donation. First, a directed unit is unavailable to another patient who may need it more urgently. Second, directed donation may discourage the routine voluntary donation of blood. Third, the directed donor sacrifices anonymity and legal protection. More pertinent to the issue of HIV transmission, there is no evidence that blood from designated donors is safer than anonymously donated bank blood[76]; this finding may be related to the slightly higher rate of HIV seropositivity among first-time donors.[77] Further, fatal graft-versus-host disease has been reported in patients receiving blood from first-degree relatives.[78]

Another approach is the use of **autologous blood donation** during pregnancy in patients at high risk of peripartum hemorrhage, such as those with placenta previa or suspected placenta accreta. Several studies have demonstrated the safety of autologous donation in pregnant women with a hematocrit of at least 34%.[79,80] However, it may be impossible to identify the patients who are more likely to require transfusion. In one study, only 4 (1.6%) of 251 high-risk patients eventually required transfusion. Further, only 2 of 13 patients who did receive blood during the peripartum period had identifiable risk factors. These results cast doubt on the benefits and cost-effectiveness of autologous blood donation during pregnancy.[81]

In patients at risk for hemorrhage during cesarean delivery, the use of **acute normovolemic hemodilution** may reduce the need for transfusion. This approach involves the collection of blood immediately before surgery with the simultaneous infusion of an appropriate volume of crystalloid or colloid to maintain normovolemia. In one study of 38 patients at risk for hemorrhage, 750 to 1000 mL of blood was removed with the simultaneous infusion of an equal volume of pentastarch. The hemoglobin concentration dropped from 10.9 to 8.3 g/dL; fetal monitoring revealed no change in the fetal heart rate pattern. The blood was reinfused during surgery. Neonatal outcome was normal, and only 1 patient required homologous blood.[82] In contrast, a meta-analysis in nonpregnant patients did not support the use of normovolemic hemodilution as an effective strategy for avoiding allogeneic transfusion.[83]

A final option for minimizing heterologous transfusion is **intraoperative blood salvage** through the use of a cell saver. In the past, the use of intraoperative blood salvage in obstetric patients has been limited, in part, by concern that transfusion of salvaged blood might precipitate amniotic fluid embolism. But Waters[84] and others have argued that this rare but devastating complication is not an embolic disease but rather an anaphylactoid reaction that would occur with or without transfusion of cell-salvaged blood, given that amniotic fluid is routinely entrained into the maternal circulation at the time of delivery. Santrach[85] has offered the following counter-arguments: (1) in obstetrics, significant hemorrhage that would benefit from blood salvage is uncommon and often unexpected; (2) because of the low utilization of blood salvage procedures in obstetrics, ongoing operator (user) competency may be problematic and the risk for error is increased; and (3) the number of patients studied to date is not sufficient to detect adverse events. Also, the blood salvage procedure does not eliminate fetal red blood cells, so the Rh-negative mother would be at risk for isoimmunization from cell salvage.

Allam et al.,[86] reviewing the use of blood salvage in obstetrics, noted that documented use of cell salvage in obstetric patients is limited; at the time of their review, approximately 400 published cases had been reported. (In most published cases, the total volume of transfused salvaged blood was small.) These investigators concluded that "no single serious complication leading to poor maternal outcome has been directly attributed to its use." However, they acknowledged that "well-designed, large prospective studies to evaluate ... the balance of clinical effectiveness and safety of cell salvage are clearly needed before wider application in obstetrics."[86] The revised ASA Practice Guidelines for Obstetric Anesthesia[87] recommend that "in cases of intractable hemorrhage when banked blood is not available or the patient refuses banked blood, intraoperative cell salvage should be considered if available." And the ACOG[88] has recommended that in patients with an antepartum diagnosis of placenta accreta, "cell saver technology should be considered if available."

Uncertainty remains about the etiology of the syndrome of amniotic fluid embolism (including uncertainty as to which agent[s] trigger[s] the syndrome and which patients are at risk). Thus intraoperative blood salvage should be reserved for those situations in which sufficient banked blood is unavailable or in which homologous blood is unacceptable to the patient, and only after the surgical field has been irrigated and gross contamination with amniotic fluid has been eliminated. Use of a leukocyte depletion filter may enhance the margin of safety. At best, however, intraoperative blood salvage will reduce or eliminate exposure to allogeneic blood in only a fraction of parturients who require transfusion.[89]

STANDARDS FOR EQUIPMENT DISINFECTION

The ASA Subcommittee on Infection Control Policy[64] has made specific recommendations about the disinfection of reusable anesthesia equipment that comes in contact with mucous membranes. In practice, this equipment consists of laryngoscope blades, endoscopes, and face masks. The ASA Subcommittee recommends that such items be washed as soon as possible to remove gross contamination, followed by either high-level disinfection or sterilization. Functionally, each of these procedures kills fungi, viruses, and vegetative bacteria (including mycobacteria). In addition, sterilization kills larger numbers of endospores.[64]

In many institutions, disposable carbon dioxide absorbers and unidirectional valves are used for the anesthetizing of HIV-infected patients. However, no evidence suggests that HIV is transmitted in respiratory aerosols.[90] This practice is unnecessary and is not recommended by the ASA Subcommittee. An exception involves the HIV patient with active pulmonary tuberculosis; if a disposable absorber is not used for such a patient, the entire assembly distal to the fresh gas source must be disassembled and sterilized.

The rate of nosocomial transmission of HIV is negligible, and the only documented cases of such transmission apparently occurred in a setting in which disinfection procedures were notably lax.[90] Commonsense measures should effectively reduce the rate of transmission to zero.

To the Health Care Worker

The primary means of preventing the transmission of HIV to health care workers is the mandatory use of universal blood and body fluid barrier precautions. This policy has three crucial components. First, it must be universal. Establishing a higher level of concern for dealing with known HIV-positive patients implies a lower level of concern in the care of patients not known to be HIV positive. Unfortunately, a patient who is infected with HIV may be living within the window between the acquisition of infection and seroconversion. Further, all care providers should be equally concerned with the transmission of other bloodborne infections of higher infectivity and sometimes equal deadliness, such as hepatitis B and C.

Second, this policy must be followed whenever contact with infectious material is anticipated. Blood obviously is the primary source of exposure, but other potentially infectious body fluids include amniotic fluid, CSF, synovial fluid, pleural fluid, and pericardial fluid. Saliva is not thought to be infectious, but manipulations of the oral mucosa (e.g., laryngoscopy, endotracheal intubation) probably lead to the contamination of saliva with blood.

Third, barrier precautions must be effective. Barriers include gloves, mask, and eye shields. The use of gloves prevents 98% of an anesthesia provider's contact with patient blood.[91] When gross contamination is likely (e.g., during neonatal resuscitation), full-length gowns are indicated.

An additional component of universal precautions is the avoidance of needlestick injuries. The recapping of needles is the most common cause of needlestick injuries. Contaminated needles, including needles that have been injected into intravenous tubing, should not be recapped by hand. If recapping is necessary, a mechanical protective device should be used. The use of needleless systems can be expected to significantly decrease the risk of injury, and the use of such systems should be encouraged.[92]

A challenge that is unique to obstetric anesthesia practice is the appropriate means of removing meconium from the neonate's trachea. The traditional practice of applying direct suction by mouth to an endotracheal tube, even with the interposition of a face mask, is clearly unacceptable. The use of an inline trap can reduce the risk of contamination when oral suction is applied, but unless the trap is kept in the vertical position, it is possible for meconium to be aspirated by the operator. The ideal way of removing meconium consists of the use of a mechanical device that allows direct application of wall suction to the endotracheal tube. The use of extreme negative pressure may cause tracheal invagination.[93] The preferred range of negative pressure is −80 to −120 mm Hg.

POSTEXPOSURE PROPHYLAXIS FOR HEALTH CARE WORKERS

Occupational exposure to HIV is perhaps the most frightening work-related injury that an anesthesia provider can sustain. The risk of seroconversion after percutaneous exposure to HIV-infected blood is approximately 0.3%,[94] but this statistic provides little reassurance to the exposed health care worker in view of the presumed 100% fatality rate of HIV infection. As of June 2000, the CDC had received voluntary reports of 56 United States health care providers with documented HIV seroconversion temporally related to occupational exposure, and an additional 138 reports of seroconversion that were considered possibly a result of occupational exposure.[95]

Certain measures should be taken after any parenteral exposure to potentially infectious body fluids, even those of the HIV-negative patient (Box 44-5). Although it is of uncertain efficacy in preventing HIV seroconversion, local wound care with an antiseptic solution is indicated.[96] In view of the exceedingly high transmission rate of hepatitis B infection, it is mandatory to determine the health care worker's antibody status after parenteral exposure to body fluids from a patient known to have or to be at high risk for hepatitis B. A previously vaccinated health care worker with absence or insufficiency of antibodies to hepatitis B should receive a booster dose of vaccine and hepatitis B immune globulin (HBIG) to provide protection until an adequate antibody response develops. A health care worker with no history of vaccination and absence of antibodies should undergo primary immunization and should receive HBIG.[94]

Several primate studies have demonstrated that the administration of antiretroviral drugs shortly after inoculation with SIV or HIV-2 can prevent seroconversion.[97,98] Further, although prospective data are lacking, a retrospective case-control study demonstrated an 81% reduction in transmission of HIV to exposed health care workers who received ZDV prophylaxis.[99] Finally, the reduction of vertical transmission by ZDV therapy demonstrated by ACTG Protocol 076 was only partly a result of the reduction of maternal viral load; inhibition of viral replication clearly played some role.[94] Altogether, these results suggest that postexposure prophylaxis may play a significant role in preventing seroconversion.

The U.S. Public Health Service has issued postexposure prophylaxis guidelines for health care workers exposed to HIV via both percutaneous injury and mucosal exposure.[94] These recommendations attempt to determine the relative risk of transmission on the basis of (1) the nature of the material to which the worker was exposed, (2) the size of the inoculum, (3) the route of exposure, and (4) the presumed viral titer in the inoculum. Although encouraging results have been obtained, the primary strategy for the prevention of occupational transmission should focus on the prevention of exposure, especially the prevention of needlestick injuries.

BOX 44-5 Treatment of Occupational Exposure to Human Immunodeficiency Virus

- Local wound care
- Administration of tetanus toxoid
- Determination of worker's hepatitis B antibody titers
- Risk stratification
- Chemoprophylaxis as indicated

KEY POINTS

- Women represent the fastest growing population of people with AIDS in the United States.
- The prevalence of HIV seropositivity among pregnant women in the United States has been estimated to be as high as 1.7 per 1000.
- HIV infection eventually can be expected to involve every organ system. Central nervous system involvement occurs as early as the period of initial infection and seroconversion.
- Highly active antiretroviral therapy during pregnancy can reduce the rate of vertical transmission of HIV infection to the fetus to 1% to 2%.
- Elective cesarean delivery can provide further protection in women with more than 1000 copies of viral RNA per mL of plasma and may benefit women with lower viral loads.
- HIV-infected patients often are treated with multiple medications, each of which has side effects that are relevant to anesthetic management.
- Neuraxial anesthesia is safe in the HIV-infected parturient.
- Autologous epidural blood patch is safe in the HIV-infected patient.
- Our greatest contribution to minimizing the spread of HIV to uninfected patients is the minimization of homologous blood transfusion.
- The most effective method of minimizing HIV transmission to health care workers is strict adherence to universal blood and body fluid barrier precautions.
- Postexposure prophylaxis is indicated for all health care workers who experience high-risk exposures to potentially infectious materials.

REFERENCES

1. Centers for Disease Control and Prevention. Cases of HIV infection and AIDS in the United States and Dependent Areas, 2005. HIV/AIDS Surveillance Report, Volume 17, rev ed. Atlanta, GA, United States Department of Health and Human Services, 2007.
2. UNAIDS. AIDS Epidemic Update: 2007. Geneva, Joint United Nations Programme on HIV/AIDS (UNAIDS) and World Health Organization, 2007. Available at http://data.unaids.org/pub/EPISlides/2007/2007_epiupdate_en.pdf/
3. Ahdieh L. Pregnancy and infection with human immunodeficiency virus. Clin Obstet Gynecol 2001; 44:154-66.
4. Centers for Disease Control and Prevention. Twenty-five years of HIV/AIDS—United States, 1981-2006. MMWR Morb Mortal Wkly Rep 2006; 55:585-9.
5. Geleziunas R, Greene WC. Molecular insights into HIV-1 infection and pathogenesis. In Sande MA, Volberding PA, editors. The Medical Management of AIDS. 6th edition. Philadelphia, WB Saunders, 1999:23-39.
6. Hahn BH, Shaw GM, De Cock KM, Sharp PM. AIDS as a zoonosis: Scientific and public health implications. Science 2000; 287:607-14.
7. Kilby JM. Enfuvirtide. In Dolin R, Masur H, Saag MS, editors. AIDS Therapy. 3rd edition. St. Louis, Churchill Livingstone Elsevier, 2008:401-13.
8. Staprans SI, Feinberg MB. Natural history and immunopathogenesis of HIV-1 disease. In Sande MA, Volberding PA, editors. The Medical Management of AIDS. 5th edition. Philadelphia, WB Saunders, 1997:29-56.
9. Maury W, Potts BJ, Rabson AB. HIV-1 infection of first-trimester and term human placental tissue: A possible mode of maternal-fetal transmission. J Infect Dis 1989; 160:583-8.
10. Kuhmann SE, Gulick RM, Moore JP. Inhibiting the entry of R5 and X4 HIV-1 phenotypic variants. In Dolin R, Masur H, Saag MS, editors. AIDS Therapy. 3rd edition. St. Louis, Churchill Livingstone Elsevier, 2008:415-47.
11. Branson BM, McDougal JS. Establishing the Diagnosis of HIV Infection. In Dolin R, Masur H, Saag MS, editors. AIDS Therapy. 3rd edition. St. Louis, Churchill Livingstone Elsevier, 2008:1-22.
12. Moore RD. Hematologic Disease. In Dolin R, Masur H, Saag MS, editors. AIDS Therapy. 3rd edition. St. Louis, Churchill Livingstone Elsevier, 2008:1187-205.
13. Chang Y, Cesarman E, Pessin MS, et al. Identification of herpesvirus-like DNA sequences in AIDS-associated Kaposi's sarcoma. Science 1994; 266:1865-9.
14. Moore PS, Chang Y. Detection of herpesvirus-like DNA sequences in Kaposi's sarcoma in patients with and those without HIV infection. N Engl J Med 1995; 332:1181-5.
15. Denning DW, Anderson J, Rudge P, Smith H. Acute myelopathy associated with primary infection with human immunodeficiency virus. Br Med J (Clin Res Ed) 1987; 294:143-4.
16. Mehandru S, Markowitz M. Acute HIV Infection. In Dolin R, Masur H, Saag MS, editors. AIDS Therapy. 3rd edition. St. Louis, Churchill Livingstone Elsevier, 2008:559-77.
17. Garcia F, Niebla G, Romeu J, et al. Cerebrospinal fluid HIV-1 RNA levels in asymptomatic patients with early stage chronic HIV-1 infection: Support for the hypothesis of local viral replication. AIDS 1999; 13:1491-6.
18. Spudich SS, Price RW. Neurological Disease. In Dolin R, Masur H, Saag MS, editors. AIDS Therapy. 3rd edition. St. Louis, Churchill Livingstone Elsevier, 2008:1075-101.
19. Huang L, Masur H. Pneumocystis pneumonia. In Dolin R, Masur H, Saag MS, editors. AIDS Therapy. 3rd edition. St. Louis, Churchill Livingstone Elsevier, 2008:637-58.
20. Wachter RM, Luce JM, Safrin S, et al. Cost and outcome of intensive care for patients with AIDS, *Pneumocystis carinii* pneumonia, and severe respiratory failure. JAMA 1995; 273:230-5.
21. Bozette SA, Sattler FR, Chiu J, et al. A controlled trial of early adjunctive treatment with corticosteroids for *Pneumocystis carinii* pneumonia in the acquired immunodeficiency syndrome. N Engl J Med 1990; 323:1451-7.
22. Huang L, Stansell JD. *Pneumocystis carinii* pneumonia. In Sande MA, Volberding PA, editors. The Medical Management of AIDS. 6th edition. Philadelphia, WB Saunders, 1999:305-30.
23. Dobbs TE, Kimerling ME. Mycobacterium tuberculosis. In Dolin R, Masur H, Saag MS, editors. AIDS Therapy. 3rd edition. St. Louis, Churchill Livingstone Elsevier, 2008:711-36.
24. Huang L. Respiratory Disease. In Dolin R, Masur H, Saag MS, editors. AIDS Therapy. 3rd edition. St. Louis, Churchill Livingstone Elsevier, 2008:1225-52.
25. Wilcox CM. Diseases of the esophagus, stomach, and small bowel. In Dolin R, Masur H, Saag MS, editors. AIDS Therapy. 3rd edition. Churchill Livingstone, 2008:1337-54.
26. Connolly GM, Hawkins D, Harcourt-Webster JN, et al. Oesophageal symptoms, their causes, treatment, and prognosis in patients with the acquired immunodeficiency syndrome. Gut 1989; 30:1033-9.
27. Martin NM, Chung RT, Sherman KE. Hepatic and Hepatobiliary Diseases. In Dolin R, Masur H, Saag MS, editors. AIDS Therapy. 3rd edition. St. Louis, Churchill Livingstone Elsevier, 2008:1355-81.
28. Cheitlin MD. Cardiovascular complications of HIV infection. In Sande MA, Volberding PA, editors. The Medical Management of AIDS. 6th edition. Philadelphia, WB Saunders, 1999:275-84.
29. Barbaro G. Cardiovascular manifestations of HIV infection. Circulation 2002; 106:1420-5.
30. Lundgren JD, Sjol A. Cardiovascular disease in HIV. In Dolin R, Masur H, Saag MS, editors. AIDS Therapy. 3rd edition. St. Louis, Churchill Livingstone Elsevier, 2008:1207-24.
31. Lo JC, Schambelan M. Adrenal, gonadal, and thyroid disorders. In Dolin R, Masur H, Saag MS, editors. AIDS Therapy. 3rd edition. St. Louis, Churchill Livingstone Elsevier, 2008:1325-36.
32. Hadigan C, Grinspoon S. Diabetes and Insulin Resistance. In Dolin R, Masur H, Saag MS, editors. AIDS Therapy. 3rd edition. St. Louis, Churchill Livingstone Elsevier, 2008:1265-72.
33. Winston JA, Klotman PE. HIV-related renal disease. In Dolin R, Masur H, Saag MS, editors. AIDS Therapy. 3rd edition. St. Louis, Churchill Livingstone Elsevier, 2008:1253-64.
34. Herman ES, Klotman PE. HIV-associated nephropathy: Epidemiology, pathogenesis, and treatment. Semin Nephrol 2003; 23:200-8.
35. Gwinn M, Pappaioanou M, George JR, et al. Prevalence of HIV infection in childbearing women in the United States: Surveillance using newborn blood samples. JAMA 1991; 265:1704-8.
36. U.S. Public Health Service recommendations for human immunodeficiency virus counseling and voluntary testing for pregnant women. MMWR Recomm Rep 1995; 44(RR-7):1-15.
37. Pulver WP, Glebatis D, Wade N, et al. Trends from an HIV seroprevalence study among childbearing women in New York State from 1988 through 2000: A valuable epidemiologic tool. Arch Pediatr Adolesc Med 2004; 158:443-8.
38. Miles SA, Balden E, Magpantay L, et al. Rapid serologic testing with immune-complex-dissociated HIV p24 antigen for early detection of HIV infection in neonates. N Engl J Med 1993; 328:297-302.
39. Pavia AT, Christenson JC. Pediatric AIDS. In Sande MA, Volberding PA, editors. The Medical Management of AIDS. 6th edition. Philadelphia, WB Saunders, 1999:525-35.
40. McIntyre J. Managing Pregnant Patients. In Dolin R, Masur H, Saag M, editors. AIDS Therapy. 3rd edition. St. Louis, Churchill Livingstone Elsevier, 2008:595-635.
41. Ryder RW, Nsa W, Hassig SE, et al. Perinatal transmission of the human immunodeficiency virus type 1 to infants of seropositive women in Zaire. N Engl J Med 1989; 320:1637-42.
42. Dickover RE, Garratty EM, Herman SA, et al. Identification of levels of maternal HIV-1 RNA associated with risk of perinatal transmission: Effect of maternal zidovudine treatment on viral load. JAMA 1996; 275:599-605.
43. Landesman SH, Kalish LA, Burns DN, et al. Obstetrical factors and the transmission of human immunodeficiency virus type 1 from mother to child. N Engl J Med 1996; 334:1617-23.
44. Mandelbrot L, Mayaux MJ, Bongain A, et al. Obstetric factors and mother-to-child transmission of human immunodeficiency

virus type 1: The French perinatal cohorts. SEROGEST French Pediatric HIV Infection Study Group. Am J Obstet Gynecol 1996; 175:661-7.
45. St. Louis ME, Kamenga M, Brown C, et al. Risk for perinatal HIV-1 transmission according to maternal immunologic, virologic, and placental factors. JAMA 1993; 269:2853-9.
46. Viscarello RR, Copperman AB, DeGennaro NJ. Is the risk of perinatal transmission of human immunodeficiency virus increased by the intrapartum use of spiral electrodes or fetal pH sampling? Am J Obstet Gynecol 1994; 170:740-3.
47. Beckerman KP. Conception, pregnancy, and parenthood: Maternal health care and the HIV epidemic. In Sande MA, Volberding PA, editors. The Medical Management of AIDS. 6th edition. Philadelphia, WB Saunders, 1999:555-73.
48. Dunn DT, Newell ML, Ades AE, Peckham CS. Risk of human immunodeficiency virus type 1 transmission through breastfeeding. Lancet 1992; 340:585-8.
49. Connor EM, Sperling RS, Gelber R, et al. Reduction of maternal-infant transmission of human immunodeficiency virus type 1 with zidovudine treatment. Pediatric AIDS Clinical Trials Group Protocol 076 Study Group. N Engl J Med 1994; 331:1173-80.
50. Cooper ER, Charurat M, Mofensen L, et al. Combination antiretroviral strategies for the treatment of pregnant HIV-1-infected women and prevention of perinatal HIV-1 transmission. J Acquir Immune Defic Syndr 2002; 29:484-94.
51. Minkoff H. Human immunodeficiency virus infection in pregnancy. Obstet Gynecol 2003; 101:797-810.
52. American College of Obstetricians and Gynecologists Committee on Obstetric Practice. Scheduled cesarean delivery and the prevention of vertical transmission of HIV infection. ACOG Committee Opinion No. 219. Washington, DC, August 1999. (Int J Gynaecol Obstet 1999; 66:305-6.)
53. Ioannidis JP, Abrams EJ, Ammann A, et al. Perinatal transmission of human immunodeficiency virus type 1 by pregnant women with RNA viral loads <1000 copies/ml. J Infect Dis 2001; 183:539-45.
54. Alger LS, Farley JJ, Robinson BA, et al. Interactions of human immunodeficiency virus infection and pregnancy. Obstet Gynecol 1993; 82:787-96.
55. Temmerman M, Chomba EN, Ndinya-Achola J, et al. Maternal human immunodeficiency virus-1 infection and pregnancy outcome. Obstet Gynecol 1994; 83:495-501.
56. Minkoff H, Willoughby A, Mendez H, et al. Serious infections during pregnancy among women with advanced human immunodeficiency virus infection. Am J Obstet Gynecol 1990; 162:30-4.
57. Tuomala RE, Shapiro DE, Mofenson LM, et al. Antiretroviral therapy during pregnancy and the risk of an adverse outcome. N Engl J Med 2002; 346:1863-70.
58. Burns DN, Landesman S, Minkoff H, et al. The influence of pregnancy on human immunodeficiency virus type 1 infection: Antepartum and postpartum changes in human immunodeficiency virus type 1 viral load. Am J Obstet Gynecol 1998; 178:355-9.
59. Bessinger R, Clark R, Kissinger P, et al. Pregnancy is not associated with the progression of HIV disease in women attending an HIV outpatient program. Am J Epidemiol 1998; 147:434-40.
60. Minkoff HL, DeHovitz JA. Care of women infected with the human immunodeficiency virus. JAMA 1991; 266:2253-8.
61. Minkoff HL, Moreno JD. Drug prophylaxis for human immunodeficiency virus-infected pregnant women: Ethical considerations. Am J Obstet Gynecol 1990; 163:1111-4.
62. Hughes SC, Dailey PA, Landers D, et al. Parturients infected with human immunodeficiency virus and regional anesthesia: Clinical and immunologic response. Anesthesiology 1995; 82:32-7.
63. Avidan MS, Groves P, Blott M, et al. Low complication rate associated with cesarean section under spinal anesthesia for HIV-1-infected women on antiretroviral therapy. Anesthesiology 2002; 97:320-4.
64. American Society of Anesthesiologists Subcommittee on Infection Control Policy. Recommendations for Infection Control for the Practice of Anesthesiology. Park Ridge, IL, ASA, 1994.
65. Kern JMD, Croy BB. AIDS litigation for the primary care physician. In Sande MA, Volberding PA, editors. The Medical Management of AIDS. 3rd edition. Philadelphia, WB Saunders, 1992:477-83.
66. Gibbons JJ. Post-dural puncture headache in the HIV-positive patient (letter). Anesthesiology 1991; 74:953.
67. Griffiths AG, Beards SC, Jackson A, Horsman EL. Visualization of extradural blood patch for post lumbar puncture headache by magnetic resonance imaging. Br J Anaesth 1993; 70:223-5.
68. Tom DJ, Gulevich SJ, Shapiro HM, et al. Epidural blood patch in the HIV-positive patient: Review of clinical experience. San Diego HIV Neurobehavioral Research Center. Anesthesiology 1992; 76:943-7.
69. Schneemilch CE, Schilling T, Bank U. Effects of general anesthesia on inflammation. Best Pract Res Clin Anaesthesiol 2004; 18:493-507.
70. Gershon RY, Manning-Williams D. Anesthesia and the HIV-infected parturient: A retrospective study. Int J Obstet Anesth 1997; 6:76-81.
71. Evron S, Glezerman M, Harow E, et al. Human immunodeficiency virus: Anesthetic and obstetric considerations. Anesth Analg 2004; 98:503-11.
72. Consensus conference. Perioperative red blood cell transfusion. JAMA 1988; 260:2700-3.
73. American Society of Anesthesiologists Task Force on Perioperative Blood Transfusion and Adjuvant Therapies. Practice guidelines for perioperative blood transfusion and adjuvant therapies. Anesthesiology 2006; 105:198-208. Available at http://www2.asahq.org/publications/c-4-practice-parameters.aspx/
74. Klein L. Premature birth and maternal prenatal anemia. Am J Obstet Gynecol 1962; 83:588-90.
75. Kaltreider DF, Johnson JW. Patients at high risk for low-birth-weight delivery. Am J Obstet Gynecol 1976; 124:251-6.
76. Cordell RR, Yalon VA, Cigahn-Haskell C, et al. Experience with 11,916 designated donors. Transfusion 1986; 26:484-6.
77. Cumming PD, Wallace EL, Schorr JB, Dodd RY. Exposure of patients to human immunodeficiency virus through the transfusion of blood components that test antibody-negative. N Engl J Med 1989; 321:941-6.
78. Thaler M, Shamiss A, Orgad S, et al. The role of blood from HLA-homozygous donors in fatal transfusion-associated graft-versus-host disease after open-heart surgery. N Engl J Med 1989; 321:25-8.
79. Herbert WN, Owen HG, Collins ML. Autologous blood storage in obstetrics. Obstet Gynecol 1988; 72:166-70.
80. McVay PA, Hoag RW, Hoag MS, Toy PT. Safety and use of autologous blood donation during the third trimester of pregnancy. Am J Obstet Gynecol 1989; 160:1479-88.
81. Andres RL, Piacquadio KM, Resnik R. A reappraisal of the need for autologous blood donation in the obstetric patient. Am J Obstet Gynecol 1990; 163:1551-3.
82. Grange CS, Douglas MJ, Adams TJ, Wadsworth LD. The use of acute hemodilution in parturients undergoing cesarean section. Am J Obstet Gynecol 1998; 178:156-60.
83. Bryson GL, Laupacis A, Wells GA. Does acute normovolemic hemodilution reduce perioperative allogeneic transfusion? A meta-analysis. Anesth Analg 1998; 86:9-15.
84. Waters JH. Is cell salvage a safe technique for the obstetric patient? Pro. Society for Obstetric Anesthesia and Perinatology Newsletter 2005; Fall:7-8.
85. Santrach PJ. Is cell salvage a safe technique for the obstetric patient? Con. Society for Obstetric Anesthesia and Perinatology Newsletter 2005; Fall:9.
86. Allam J, Cox M, Yentis SM. Cell salvage in obstetrics. Int J Obstet Anesth 2008; 17:37-45.
87. American Society of Anesthesiologists Task Force on Obstetric Anesthesia. Practice guidelines for obstetric anesthesia. Anesthesiology 2007; 106:843-63.
88. American College of Obstetricians and Gynecologists Committee on Obstetric Practice. Placental accreta. ACOG Committee Opinion No. 266. Washington, DC, January 2002.

89. Fong J, Gurewitsch ED, Kang HJ, et al. An analysis of transfusion practice and the role of intraoperative red blood cell salvage during cesarean delivery. Anesth Analg 2007; 104:666-72.
90. Gerberding JL. Limiting the risks to health care workers. In Sande MA, Volberding PA, editors. The Medical Management of AIDS. 5th edition. Philadelphia, WB Saunders, 1997:75-85.
91. Kristensen MS, Sloth E, Jensen TK. Relationship between anesthetic procedure and contact of anesthesia personnel with patient body fluids. Anesthesiology 1990; 73:619-24.
92. Greene ES, Berry AJ, Arnold WP, Jagger J. Percutaneous injuries in anesthesia personnel. Anesth Analg 1996; 83:273-8.
93. Bent RC, Wiswell TE, Chang A. Removing meconium from infant tracheae: What works best? Am J Dis Child 1992; 146:1085-9.
94. Panlilio AL, Cardo DM, Grohskopf LA, et al. U.S. Public Health Service. Updated U.S. Public Health Service guidelines for the management of occupational exposures to HIV and recommendations for postexposure prophylaxis. MMWR Recomm Rep 2005; 54(RR-9):1-17.
95. U.S. Public Health Service; Updated Public Health Service guidelines for the management of occupational exposures to HBV, HCV, and HIV and recommendations for postexposure prophylaxis. MMWR Recomm Rep 2001; 50(RR-11):1-52.
96. Henderson DK, Fahey BJ, Willy M, et al. Risk for occupational transmission of human immunodeficiency virus type 1 (HIV-1) associated with clinical exposures: A prospective evaluation. Ann Intern Med 1990; 113:740-6.
97. Böttiger D, Johansson NG, Samuelsson B, et al. Prevention of simian immunodeficiency virus, SIVsm, or HIV-2 infection in cynomolgus monkeys by pre- and postexposure administration of BEA-005. AIDS 1997; 11:157-62.
98. Otten RA, Smith DK, Adams DR, et al. Efficacy of postexposure prophylaxis after intravaginal exposure of pig-tailed macaques to a human-derived retrovirus (human immunodeficiency virus type 2). J Virol 2000; 74:9771-5.
99. Cardo DM, Culver DH, Ciesielski CA, et al. A case-control study of HIV seroconversion in health care workers after percutaneous exposure. Center for Disease Control and Prevention Needlestick Surveillance Group. N Engl J Med 1997; 337:1485-90.

Hypertensive Disorders

Linda S. Polley, M.D.

Hypertension is the most common medical disorder of pregnancy in the United States, affecting 6% to 8% of pregnant women. It is also a leading cause of maternal and fetal morbidity and mortality worldwide[1]; approximately 63,000 women die every year because of the maternal hypertensive syndromes preeclampsia and eclampsia.[2] Hypertensive disorders also result in fetal complications such as preterm birth, intrauterine growth restriction, and fetal/neonatal death.

CLASSIFICATION OF HYPERTENSIVE DISORDERS

The term **hypertension in pregnancy** encompasses a range of disorders—including preeclampsia and eclampsia, as well as gestational and chronic hypertension—that can be difficult to diagnose, because they often appear similar in clinical presentation despite complex differences in their underlying causes and prognoses. Adding to the challenges for clinicians and researchers alike, a long-standing absence of consensus guidelines for categorizing hypertensive disorders resulted in the use of conflicting definitions that have confounded attempts to compare and interpret data from all but the latest clinical studies. This problem was eventually resolved in 2000, when the National High Blood Pressure Education Program (NHBPEP) Working Group on High Blood Pressure in Pregnancy published a classification scheme establishing definitions that subsequently gained wide international acceptance (Box 45-1). Unfortunately, the utility of much of the currently available data is compromised by the disparities in previous definitions of hypertensive disorders in pregnancy.

Gestational hypertension, the most common cause of hypertension during pregnancy,[3] has outcomes that are generally similar to those of normotensive pregnancies.[4,5] In a woman with no preexisting hypertension or other signs or symptoms of preeclampsia, it manifests as elevated blood pressure after 20 weeks' gestation that resolves by 12 weeks postpartum.[3,6] Most cases of gestational hypertension develop after 37 weeks' gestation. A diagnosis of gestational hypertension is a retrospective diagnosis, because it can be established with certainty only *after* delivery.

Preeclampsia is defined as the new onset of hypertension and proteinuria after 20 weeks' gestation (Table 45-1). The NHBPEP has recommended that clinicians consider the diagnosis of preeclampsia in the absence of proteinuria when any of the following findings are present: (1) persistent epigastric or right upper quadrant pain, (2) persistent cerebral symptoms, (3) fetal growth restriction, (4) thrombocytopenia, and (5) elevated serum liver enzyme concentrations.[7] The term **eclampsia** is used when central nervous system (CNS) involvement results in the new onset of seizures in a woman with preeclampsia. The term **HELLP syndrome** refers to the development of hemolysis, elevated liver enzymes, and low platelets in a woman with preeclampsia. This condition is considered a variant of severe preeclampsia.

Chronic hypertension involves either (1) prepregnancy blood pressure levels ≥ 140 mm Hg systolic or ≥ 90 mm Hg diastolic or (2) elevated blood pressure that fails to resolve after delivery. The pathophysiology of chronic hypertension is better understood than that of preeclampsia (see later), and much of what is known about chronic hypertension in nonpregnant women is also relevant to pregnant women.

BOX 45-1 Classification of Hypertensive Disorders in Pregnancy

- Gestational hypertension
- Preeclampsia:
  - Mild
  - Severe
- Chronic hypertension
- Chronic hypertension with superimposed preeclampsia

From the Report of the National High Blood Pressure Education Program Working Group on High Blood Pressure in Pregnancy. Am J Obstet Gynecol 2000; 183:S1-22.

Table 45-2 compares the clinical findings in chronic hypertension, gestational hypertension, and preeclampsia.

The term **chronic hypertension with superimposed preeclampsia** is used when preeclampsia develops in women who had chronic hypertension before pregnancy. The diagnosis is made in the presence of a new onset of proteinuria or a sudden increase in proteinuria and/or hypertension, or when other manifestations of severe preeclampsia appear. Morbidity with this condition is greater for both mother and fetus than with preeclampsia alone.[8]

PREECLAMPSIA

Preeclampsia is a multisystem disease unique to human pregnancy. Although advances have been made in the understanding of the pathophysiology of the disease, the specific proximal etiology remains unknown. Management is supportive; delivery of the infant and placenta remains the only definitive cure.

The clinical syndrome of preeclampsia is defined as the new onset of hypertension and proteinuria after 20 weeks' gestation. Previous definitions included edema, but edema is no longer part of the diagnostic criteria because it lacks specificity and occurs in many healthy pregnant women.[9] The severity of preeclampsia is categorized as either mild or severe according to clinical criteria (see Table 45-1).

TABLE 45-1 Diagnostic Criteria for Mild and Severe Preeclampsia

Mild Preeclampsia	Severe Preeclampsia
BP $\geq$ 140/90 mm Hg after 20 weeks' gestation	BP $\geq$ 160/110 mm Hg
Proteinuria (300 mg/24 hr or 1+ result on dipstick specimen)	Proteinuria > 5 g/24 hr
	Elevated serum creatinine
	Pulmonary edema
	Oliguria
	Intrauterine growth restriction
	Headache
	Visual disturbances
	Epigastric or right upper quadrant pain
	Signs of HELLP syndrome

BP, blood pressure, shown as systolic/diastolic; HELLP, hemolysis, elevated liver enzymes, and low platelets.

Adapted from the American College of Obstetricians and Gynecologists. Diagnosis and management of preeclampsia and eclampsia. ACOG Practice Bulletin No. 33. Washington DC, ACOG, January 2002. (Obstet Gynecol 2002; 99:159-67.)

Epidemiology

Preeclampsia occurs in approximately 4% of pregnancies in the United States.[10,11] Delivery of the infant and placenta is the only effective treatment; thus preeclampsia is a leading cause of preterm delivery in developed countries.[12] The birth of low-birth-weight and term neonates to preeclamptic mothers results in major medical, social, and economic burdens for families and societies.[13] Preterm delivery is the most common indication for admission to the neonatal intensive care unit.[14] Preeclampsia is also the leading indication for maternal peripartum admission to an intensive care unit.[15]

The clinical findings of preeclampsia manifest as a **maternal syndrome** (e.g., hypertension and proteinuria with or without other systemic abnormalities) with or without a **fetal syndrome** (e.g., fetal growth restriction, oligohydramnios, abnormal oxygenation).[7,16] In approximately 75% of cases, preeclampsia is mild with an onset near term or during the intrapartum period.[3,16] In contrast, disease onset prior to 34 weeks' gestation correlates with greater disease severity and worsened outcomes for both mother and fetus.[1,16] The broad spectrum of disease severity and clinical presentations lends support to the emerging hypothesis that preeclampsia encompasses multiple diseases that may differ in their pathogenic mechanisms.

Significant increases in the incidence of both preeclampsia and gestational hypertension between 1987 and 2004 (Figure 45-1),[17] including an alarming 47% increase in preeclampsia between 1990 and 2005,[18,19] appear to have resulted from major shifts in the demographics of pregnant women in the United States and other developed countries. Average maternal age is rising; older mothers are more likely to have chronic hypertension, a recognized risk factor for preeclampsia. Both the current epidemic of obesity and the greater prevalence of diabetes in the developed world increase the risk of preeclampsia. The growing utilization of assisted reproductive technologies and the use of donated gametes increase risk of the disease by altering the maternal-fetal immune reaction[20] and by increasing the incidence of multiple gestation, another risk factor for preeclampsia. Lastly, improvements in record-keeping and the use of consistent disease definitions since 2000 have likely increased the number of reported cases.[7]

Multiple preconception and pregnancy-related risk factors associated with the development of preeclampsia have been identified (Box 45-2). Preconception risk factors can be divided into **partner-related risk factors,** which depend on a woman's interaction with her sexual partner, and **non–partner-related risk factors,** which depend only on the woman's personal health status.

TABLE 45-2 Hypertensive Disorders of Pregnancy

Clinical Feature	Chronic Hypertension	Gestational Hypertension	Preeclampsia
Time of onset of hypertension	< 20 weeks' gestation	Typically in third trimester	≥ 20 weeks' gestation
Severity of hypertension	Mild or severe	Mild	Mild or severe
Proteinuria*	Absent	Absent	Typically present
Serum urate > 5.5 mg/dL (0.33 mmol/L)	Rare	Absent	Present in almost all cases
Hemoconcentration	Absent	Absent	Present in severe disease
Thrombocytopenia	Absent	Absent	Present in severe disease
Hepatic dysfunction	Absent	Absent	Present in severe disease

*Defined as ≥ 1+ result on dipstick testing on two occasions or ≥ 300 mg in a 24-hour urine collection.

From Sibai BM. Treatment of hypertension in pregnant women. N Engl J Med 1996; 335:257-65.

PARTNER-RELATED RISK FACTORS

The unifying theme among partner-related risk factors is *limited maternal exposure to paternal sperm antigens prior to conception*, suggesting an immunologic role in the pathophysiology of preeclampsia. The leading risk factor for preeclampsia is nulliparity. Long considered a disease of primigravid women, preeclampsia is also more common in (1) teenagers, (2) parous women who have conceived with a new partner, (3) women who have used barrier methods of contraception prior to conception, and (4) women who have conceived with donated sperm.[21,22] Long-term sperm exposure with the same partner appears to be protective; this protective effect is lost in a pregnancy conceived with a new sexual partner.

In a study of 1.7 million births in the Medical Birth Registry of Norway, men who fathered one preeclamptic pregnancy were found to be nearly twice as likely to father a preeclamptic pregnancy in a different woman, irrespective of her previous obstetric history.[23] Therefore, paternal genes (in the fetus) contribute significantly to a pregnant woman's risk of preeclampsia. It is of note that the accuracy of epidemiologic studies is compromised by use of birth certification data, which do not always reflect true paternity.

NON–PARTNER-RELATED RISK FACTORS

Women with a history of preeclampsia in a previous pregnancy are at increased risk for preeclampsia in a subsequent pregnancy.[24] Women of advanced maternal age (older than 35 years) are also at higher risk.[1] A maternal or paternal family history of preeclampsia increases a woman's risk.[23] In addition, women with a history of previous placental abruption, intrauterine growth restriction, or fetal death are at greater risk for preeclampsia in a subsequent pregnancy.[25]

Non-Hispanic blacks constitute a high-risk group, with higher rates of chronic hypertension,[26-28] obesity,[29-33] and preeclampsia.[1,34-38] Black women with severe preeclampsia demonstrate more extreme hypertension, require more antihypertensive therapy,[39] and are more likely to die from the condition than women of other racial backgrounds.[40]

MATERNAL COMORBIDITIES AND LIFESTYLE FACTORS

Obesity is a primary risk factor for preeclampsia, and risk escalates with increasing body mass index (BMI).[41,42]

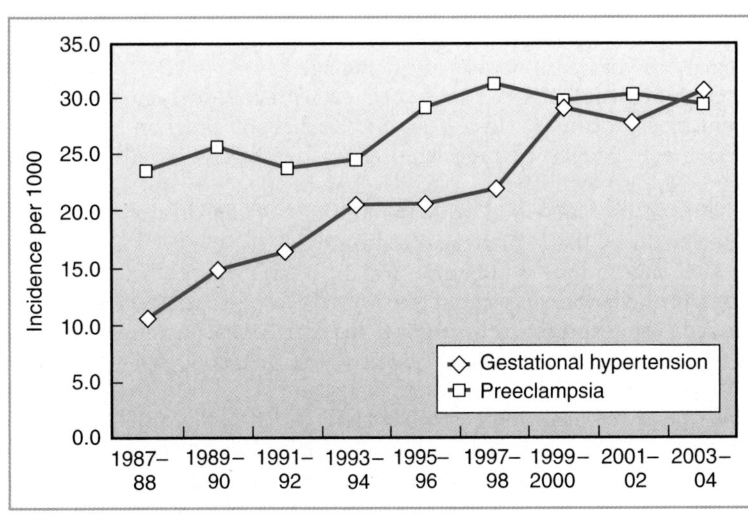

FIGURE 45-1 Age-adjusted incidence per 1000 deliveries for women with gestational hypertension or preeclampsia for 2-year periods, 1987-2004. (Adapted from Wallis AB, Saftlas AF, Hsia J, Atrash HK. Secular trends in the rates of preeclampsia, eclampsia, and gestational hypertension, United States, 1987-2004. Am J Hypertens 2008; 21:521-6.)

BOX 45-2 Risk Factors for Preeclampsia

Preconception

- Partner-related
  - Nulliparity
  - Limited preconceptional exposure to paternal sperm (teenage mother, primipaternity, assisted reproductive technology)
  - Partner who fathered a preeclamptic pregnancy in another woman
- Non–partner-related
  - History of preeclampsia in previous pregnancy
  - Advanced maternal age (> 35 years)
  - Family history of preeclampsia
  - History of placental abruption, intrauterine growth restriction, or fetal death
  - Non-Hispanic black racial background
- Maternal disease–related
  - Obesity
  - Chronic hypertension
  - Diabetes mellitus
  - Thrombotic vascular disease
- Behavioral
  - Cigarette smoking (risk reduction)

Pregnancy-Associated

- Multiple gestation
- Hydatidiform mole

From Eskenazi B, Fenster L, Sidney S. A multivariate analysis of risk factors for preeclampsia. JAMA 1991;266:237-41.

A systematic review found that an increase in body mass index of 5 to 7 kg/m^2 was associated with a twofold higher risk of preeclampsia.[41] Obesity is strongly associated with insulin resistance, another risk factor for preeclampsia. As the prevalence of obesity continues to increase worldwide, the incidence of preeclamptic pregnancies is anticipated to increase as well.

Women with **chronic hypertension** are also at increased risk of preeclampsia. A large case-control study found that preexisting hypertension increased the odds of development of preeclampsia threefold.[43] As women in developed countries delay childbirth, the impact of chronic hypertension will be greater because of the increased prevalence of hypertension with advancing age.[44]

Diabetes mellitus is also associated with the development of preeclampsia. In a study of 334 diabetic pregnancies, the incidence of preeclampsia was 9.9%, compared with 4.3% in nondiabetic controls. The incidence of preeclampsia also increased with the severity of diabetes as determined by the White classification.[45]

The **metabolic syndrome,** which occurs in 7% of women of childbearing age in the United States, is characterized by the presence of obesity, hyperglycemia, insulin resistance, and hypertension.[46] Because the metabolic syndrome increases the risk for both preeclampsia[43] and cardiovascular disease, women with a history of preeclampsia encounter greater risk of premature cardiovascular disease later in life.[47-52] Insulin resistance has been implicated as a common factor in both preeclampsia and cardiovascular disease; microvascular dysfunction may be a predisposing factor for both coronary artery disease and preeclampsia.[53]

Paradoxically, **cigarette smoking** during pregnancy has been associated with a *decreased* risk of preeclampsia,[54-56] an effect consistently observed in studies in various countries. Women who smoke during pregnancy have a 30% to 40% lower risk for development of preeclampsia than women who do not smoke. In a large systematic review, the relative risk was 0.68 (95% confidence interval, 0.67 to 0.69). The protective effect is also dose-related[54,55,57]; heavier smokers have a *lower* incidence of preeclampsia than those who smoke fewer cigarettes.

The duration of this protective effect after smoking cessation has been studied, with conflicting results; the biologic mechanism remains unknown but is thought to involve nicotine inhibition of thromboxane A_2 synthesis, stimulation of nitric oxide release, or a combination of these processes.[55] Further research on the mechanism of this effect may help elucidate the pathogenesis of preeclampsia.

Pathogenesis

The exact pathogenic mechanisms responsible for the initiation and progression of preeclampsia are not known. The placenta is the pathogenetic focus of the disease.

ABNORMAL PLACENTATION AND THE MATERNAL SYNDROME

Preeclampsia is known to be a two-stage disorder.[58] The **asymptomatic first stage** occurs early in pregnancy with a failure of trophoblastic invasion. In normal pregnancy, trophoblasts invade the decidual and myometrial segments of the spiral arteries, causing loss of vascular smooth muscle and the inner elastic lamina (Figure 45-2). The luminal diameter of the spiral arteries increases fourfold, resulting in the creation of flaccid tubes that provide a low-resistance vascular pathway to the intervillous space. Further, the remodeled arteries are unresponsive to vasoactive stimuli.[59,60] These alterations in maternal vasculature ensure adequate blood flow to nourish the growing fetus and placenta.

In contrast, in the preeclamptic woman only the decidual segments undergo change, and the myometrial portions remain small, constricted, and hyperresponsive to vasomotor stimuli. This failure of normal angiogenesis results in superficial placentation. The abnormal maternal response to placentation leads to decreased placental perfusion and placental infarcts, predisposing the fetus to intrauterine growth restriction (Figure 45-3). Placental ischemia worsens throughout pregnancy as narrowed vessels are increasingly unable to meet the needs of the growing fetoplacental unit.

In some women, the reduced perfusion of the intervillous space in the first stage leads to the **symptomatic second stage,** which is characterized by widespread maternal endothelial dysfunction and an accentuated systemic inflammatory response, and may or may not be accompanied by the occurrence of intrauterine fetal growth restriction. In the absence of preeclampsia, healthy endothelium prevents platelet activation, activates circulating anticoagulants, buffers the response to pressors, and keeps fluid in the intravascular compartment. These normal functions are disrupted in preeclampsia. In the symptomatic second

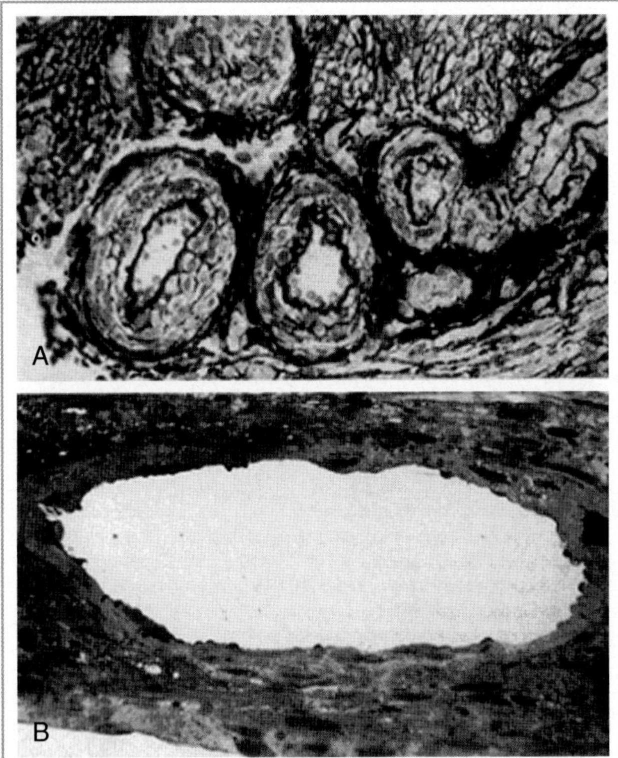

FIGURE 45-2 Sections through spiral arteries (A) at the myometrial-endometrial junction of the nonpregnant uterus and (B) at the myometrial-decidual junction in late normal pregnancy. (×150) (From Sheppard BL, Bonnar J. Uteroplacental arteries and hypertensive pregnancy. In Bonnar J, MacGillivray I, Symonds G, editors. Pregnancy Hypertension. Baltimore, University Park Press, 1980:205.)

stage, the pregnant woman develops hypertension and proteinuria, and is at risk for other manifestations of severe disease (e.g., HELLP syndrome, eclampsia, end-organ damage). Clinical manifestations usually appear after 20 weeks' gestation.

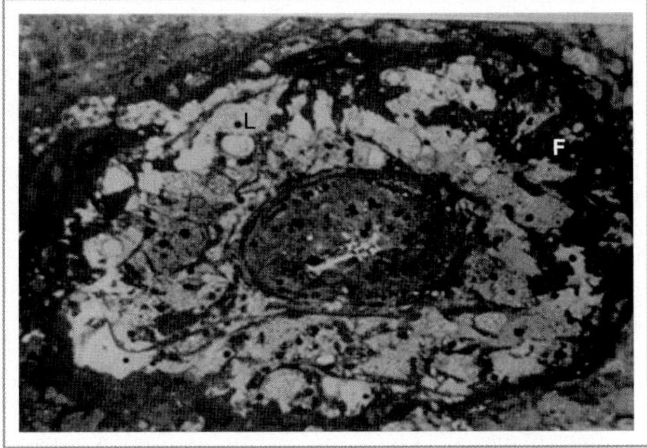

FIGURE 45-3 This figure shows lipid-laden cells (L) and fibrin deposition (F) in this occluded decidual vessel characteristic of both severe preeclampsia and severe intrauterine growth restriction. (×150) (From Sheppard BL, Bonnar J. Uteroplacental arteries and hypertensive pregnancy. In Bonnar J, MacGillivray I, Symonds G, editors. Pregnancy Hypertension. Baltimore, University Park Press, 1980:205.)

Not all women with impaired placental perfusion develop preeclampsia. The same failure of uterine vascular remodeling occurs in women with isolated intrauterine growth restriction[61] and in approximately one third of cases of spontaneous preterm birth without maternal clinical manifestations of preeclampsia.[62]

Numerous theories about the pathogenesis of preeclampsia have been examined and rejected over the years. Currently the most widely accepted explanation is that the placenta fails to embed adequately and, in response to hypoxia caused by poor placental perfusion, releases factors into the circulation that damage the maternal endothelium and give rise to the multisystem manifestations of the maternal syndrome.[11] The placenta but not the fetus is required for the development of preeclampsia; women with molar pregnancy, in which the placenta grows without a fetus, can have severe preeclampsia. The disease syndrome likely occurs in women with specific genetic and immunologic susceptibility.

GENETIC FACTORS

The genetic inheritance of preeclampsia is complex, but a genetic component is likely because the incidence of preeclampsia is higher among family members; a number of susceptibility loci have been reported.[63] Genetic studies of preeclampsia are challenging because the syndrome occurs only in women (i.e., half of the total population) and manifests only during the reproductive years in women who become pregnant. In a summary of inheritance studies, Arngrimsson et al.[64] concluded that, considering these limitations, data support a major dominant gene with variable penetrance or multifactorial inheritance.

Preeclampsia has been classified into the **early form (type I),** with symptom onset before 34 weeks' gestation, and the **late form (type II),** with symptom onset after 34 weeks' gestation (Table 45-3). Early-onset preeclampsia begins with abnormal placentation, has a high rate of recurrence, and has a clear genetic component.[65-67] In contrast, late-onset preeclampsia likely results from the interaction between a normal placenta and a woman genetically or metabolically predisposed to the disease. These women, who often have long-standing hypertension, obesity, diabetes, or other forms of microvascular disease, are challenged to meet the demands of the growing fetoplacental unit and decompensate near term. Decompensation manifests as late-onset or, less frequently, postpartum preeclampsia.[68]

According to **genetic conflict theory,**[69] fetal genes are selected to maximize nutrient transfer to the fetus, and maternal genes are selected to restrict this transfer beyond a specific optimal level. The genetic conflict theory predicts that placental factors (fetal genes) act to increase maternal blood pressure, whereas maternal factors act to reduce blood pressure. In this model, endothelial cell dysfunction may have evolved as a fetal rescue strategy to increase nonplacental vascular resistance when the uteroplacental blood supply is inadequate.[70]

IMMUNOLOGIC FACTORS

The immune system appears to play a major role in the development of preeclampsia. Epidemiologic evidence suggests that long-term exposure to paternal antigens in sperm is protective (as discussed earlier).[71]

TABLE 45-3 Differences between Early- and Late-Onset Preeclampsia

	Early-Onset	Late-Onset
Onset of clinical symptoms	< 34 weeks' gestation	> 34 weeks' gestation
Relative frequency (% of cases)	20	80
Risk for adverse outcome	High	Negligible
Association with intrauterine fetal growth restriction	Yes	No
Clear familial component*	Yes	No
Placental morphology	Abnormal†	Normal†
Etiology	Placental‡	Maternal§
Risk factors (relative risk)	Family history (2.9)	Diabetes (3.56) Multiple pregnancy (2.93) Increased blood pressure at registration (1.38) Increased body mass index (2.47) Maternal age ≥ 40 yr (1.96) Cardiovascular disorders (3.84)

*Defined as recurrence across generations and occurrence within families.

†From Egbor M, Ansari T, Morris N, et al. Morphometric placental villous and vascular abnormalities in early- and late-onset preeclampsia with and without fetal growth restriction. Br J Obstet Gynaecol 2006; 113:580-9.

‡Reduced extravillous trophoblast invasion.

§Predisposed maternal constitution reflecting microvascular disease or predisposed genetic constitution with cis- or trans-acting genomic variations subject to interaction.

From Oudejans CB, van Dijk M, Oosterkamp M, et al. Genetics of preeclampsia: Paradigm shifts. Hum Genet 2007; 120:607-12.

The immune cells that predominate in the decidua—the endometrium in the nonpregnant state becomes the decidua in pregnancy—are a specific group of uterine natural killer cells that interact with fetal trophoblast cell markers via killer immunoglobulin receptors to influence trophoblastic invasion. Specific genotypic combinations of maternal killer immunoglobulin receptors and trophoblastic human leukocyte antigen C (HLA-C) increase the risk of preeclampsia. Normal placentation requires a balance of inhibition and activation of uterine natural killer cells that is mediated by maternal and fetal factors.[72]

Activated autoantibodies to the angiotensin receptor-1 (AT_1) are present in many preeclamptic women in association with defective remodeling of the uteroplacental vasculature.[73,74] These autoantibodies activate AT_1 receptors on cardiac myocytes, trophoblast cells, endothelial cells, and vascular smooth muscle cells.[75-77] Introduction of these autoantibodies into pregnant mice results in hypertension, proteinuria, and greater production of soluble fms-like tyrosine kinase-1 characteristic of the syndrome of preeclampsia in humans (see later). Zhou et al.[78] demonstrated that agonistic autoantibodies (AAs) against the angiotensin receptor-1 (AT_1-AAs), which are recovered from the circulation of women with preeclampsia, can induce preeclampsia-like signs and symptoms in pregnant mice. Although this issue was not addressed specifically, it is possible that AT_1-AAs contribute to the greater sensitivity to angiotensin II that Gant et al.[79] observed several decades ago. AT_1 receptor-activating autoantibodies may induce the production of reactive oxygen species and block trophoblastic invasion[76,77] and thus may play a significant role in the pathophysiology of preeclampsia (see Figure 45-5).

ANTIANGIOGENIC PROTEINS

Two endogenous antiangiogenic proteins of placental origin have now been identified that, on the basis of rodent models, likely play an important role in the pathogenesis of preeclampsia.[80,81] **Soluble fms-like tyrosine kinase-1 (sFlt-1)** is upregulated in the placentas of women with preeclampsia; it antagonizes the angiogenic growth factors, vascular endothelial growth factor (VEGF) and placental growth factor (PlGF).

Maynard et al.[80] demonstrated that sFlt-1 levels rise during gestation and fall after delivery, and that higher circulating sFlt-1 levels reduce circulating levels of free VEGF and PlGF, causing endothelial dysfunction that can be rescued by exogenous VEGF and PlGF. Furthermore, these investigators found that the administration of sFlt-1 to pregnant rats induced hypertension, proteinuria, and glomerular endotheliosis, the last being the classic renal lesion of preeclampsia. VEGF and PlGF cause rat renal arteriolar relaxation *in vitro*, which is blocked by sFlt-1. In response to higher circulating levels of sFlt-1, VEGF and PlGF levels are reduced, resulting in endothelial dysfunction in maternal vessels (Figure 45-4).[58] Levine et al.[82,83] demonstrated that increased sFlt-1 levels and reduced levels of PlGF predicted the subsequent development of preeclampsia prior to the development of any maternal symptoms. Another antiangiogenic protein, **soluble endoglin (sEng)**, is elevated in cases of HELLP syndrome.[81] Of interest, one study has reported that cigarette smoking, known to be protective against preeclampsia, is associated with lower maternal sFlt-1 concentrations during pregnancy than are seen in nonsmokers.[84] The study of antiangiogenic proteins is a

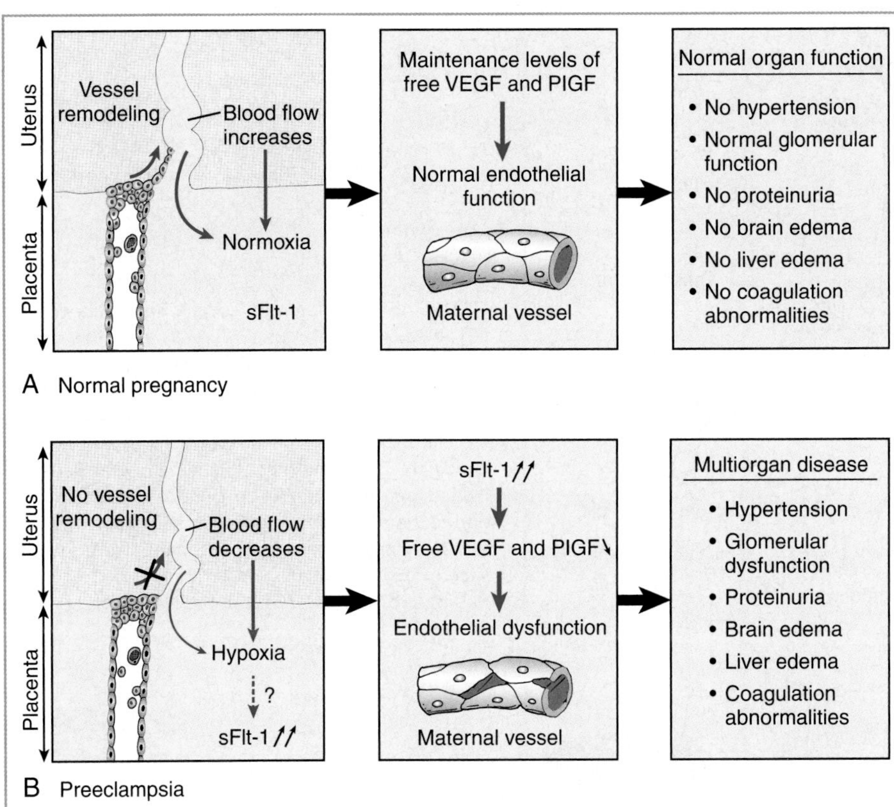

FIGURE 45-4 Hypothesis on the role of soluble fms-like tyrosine kinase-1 (sFlt-1) in preeclampsia. **A,** During normal pregnancy, the uterine spiral arteries are infiltrated and remodeled by endovascular invasive trophoblasts, thereby increasing blood flow significantly in order to meet the oxygen and nutrient demands of the fetus. **B,** In the placenta of preeclamptic women, trophoblast invasion does not occur and blood flow is reduced, resulting in placental hypoxia. In addition, increased amounts of sFlt-1 are produced by the placenta and scavenge vascular endothelial growth factor (VEGF) and placental growth factor (PlGF), thereby lowering circulating levels of unbound VEGF and PlGF. This altered balance causes generalized endothelial dysfunction, resulting in multiorgan disease. It remains unknown whether hypoxia is the trigger for stimulating sFlt-1 secretion in the placenta of preeclamptic mothers and whether the higher sFlt-1 levels interfere with trophoblast invasion and spiral artery remodeling. (From Luttun A, Carmeliet P. Soluble VEGF receptor Flt1: The elusive preeclampsia factor discovered? J Clin Invest 2003; 111:600-2.)

very active area of current research, and rapid progress is being made in understanding the role of these proteins in the pathogenesis of preeclampsia. However, the importance of recent findings is tempered by the knowledge that preeclampsia does not develop in all women with high sFlt-1 and low PlGF levels, and does occur in some women with low sFlt-1 and high PlGF levels.[83,85]

Kanasaki et al.[86] hypothesized that a molecular defect upstream from the soluble factors (released in response to placental hypoxia) contributes to preeclampsia. The investigators have demonstrated that pregnant mice deficient in **catechol-*O*-methyltransferase (COMT)** demonstrate a preeclampsia-like phenotype in response to the absence of **2-methoxyestradiol (2-ME),** a natural metabolite of estradiol that is elevated during the third trimester of normal pregnancy. Administration of 2-ME to COMT-deficient mice suppresses placental hypoxia and sFlt-1 elevation. In addition, women with severe preeclampsia have significantly lower levels of COMT and 2-ME than women with normal pregnancies. The results of this study suggest that 2-ME may have utility both as a diagnostic marker for preeclampsia and as a treatment for the disease.

Current understanding of the pathogenesis of preeclampsia is illustrated in Figure 45-5.[87] In summary, despite exciting new advances, the pathogenesis of preeclampsia is complex and not completely understood. The findings and proposed etiologies might be distinctly different or might be related to one another in ways not yet known. It is likely that preeclampsia is more than one disease.[88]

Prophylaxis

Administration of **low-dose aspirin** has been proposed for the prevention of preeclampsia, on the basis of the observation that **thromboxane** levels are increased relative to **prostacyclin** levels in preeclamptic pregnancies. Aspirin inhibits the synthesis of prostaglandins by the irreversible acetylation and inactivation of cyclooxygenase. Thromboxane and prostacyclin are arachidonic acid metabolites and physiologic antagonists important in vasoregulation. Thromboxane is a potent vasoconstrictor, and prostacyclin is a strong vasodilator. Aspirin inhibits the biosynthesis of platelet thromboxane A_2, and it has been hypothesized that preeclampsia could be prevented by avoiding the imbalance in the thromboxane-to-prostacyclin ratio. Although several small early trials suggested a benefit to aspirin,[89,90] data from subsequent large, randomized, placebo-controlled trials did not confirm these results.[91,92] Despite these findings, some investigators believe that low-dose aspirin may be of benefit in selected women at higher risk for severe early-onset preeclampsia.[93,94] Nearly all existing studies on aspirin prophylaxis have been limited by inconsistent definitions of preeclampsia and a narrow focus on disease *prevention.*[95] Future research may target pharmacologic intervention as a component of *treatment.*

Calcium supplementation has been studied for preeclampsia prophylaxis on the basis of observations that dietary calcium intake and the incidence of preeclampsia have an inverse relationship.[96] A meta-analysis of early trials suggested that prenatal administration of calcium supplementation reduced the incidence of preeclampsia.[97] However, these results were not confirmed in the most definitive trial to date.[98] In a multicenter, randomized,

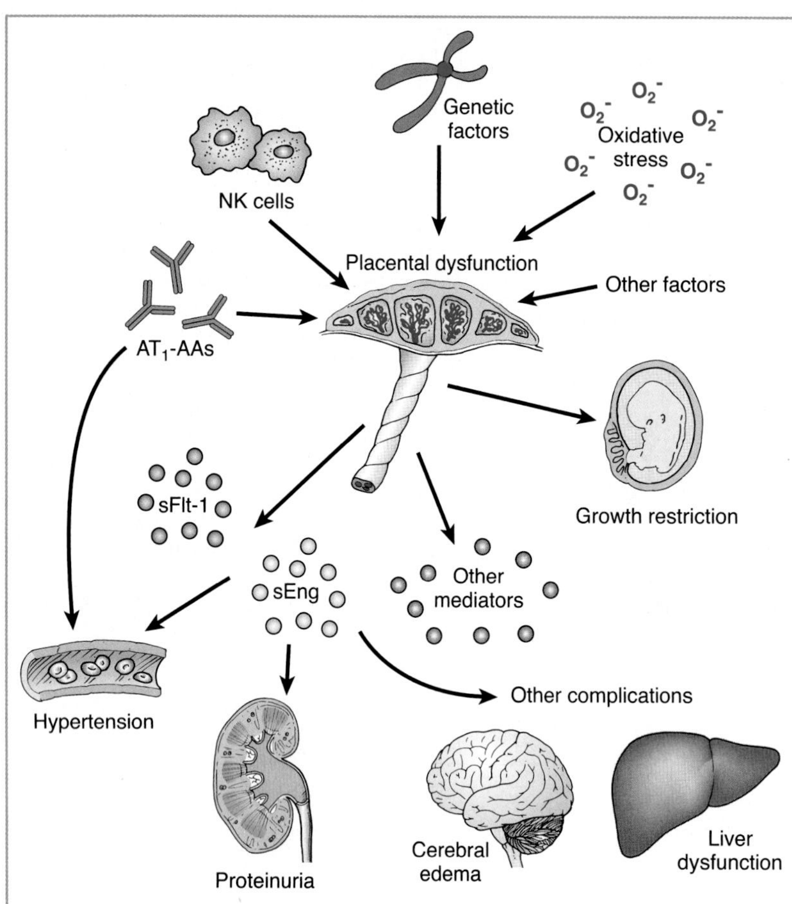

FIGURE 45-5 Angiotensin receptor autoantibodies (AT_1-AAs) in preeclampsia. AT_1-AAs and other factors (such as oxidative stress and genetic factors) may cause placental dysfunction, which in turn leads to the release of antiangiogenic factors (such as soluble fms-like tyrosine kinase-1 [sFlt-1] and soluble endoglin [sEng]) and other inflammatory mediators to induce preeclampsia. AT_1-AAs may also act directly on the maternal vasculature to enhance angiotensin II sensitivity and hypertension. NK, natural killer; O_2^-, superoxide. (From Parikh SM, Karumanchi SA. Putting pressure on preeclampsia. Nat Med 2008; 14:810-2.)

placebo-controlled trial involving 2589 healthy nulliparous women, ingestion of 2 g of elemental calcium daily did not reduce the occurrence of preeclampsia or gestational hypertension either overall or in a subset of women with low baseline calcium intake.[98]

Antioxidant supplementation has also been investigated as prophylaxis because of the oxidative stress observed in preeclampsia. Numerous studies have been conducted to investigate a possible prophylactic or therapeutic role for antioxidant supplementation in the hypertensive disorders of pregnancy. However, in randomized trials, supplementation with 1000 mg of vitamin C and 400 IU of vitamin E did not reduce the incidence of preeclampsia in healthy nulliparous women[99] or in women at increased risk for preeclampsia.[100,101] In a multicenter, randomized, placebo-controlled trial of 2410 women with risk factors for preeclampsia, there was a greater incidence of low birth weight, unexplained fetal death after 24 weeks' gestation, and umbilical cord blood acidosis in patients randomly assigned to the antioxidant group.[101] Conversely, a different multicenter randomized trial did *not* find a higher risk of death or other adverse outcomes in the neonates born to antioxidant-supplemented mothers, although the results concurred about the lack of benefit from vitamin C and E supplementation in healthy nulliparous women.[99] Systematic reviews published in 2005 caution that although vitamin C and E supplementation is not contraindicated in pregnancy, only limited data are available regarding the safety of high doses of these vitamins in pregnant women.[102,103]

Clinical Manifestations

Preeclampsia occurs more frequently in nulliparous women and most commonly manifests during the third trimester, often near term. Women with early-onset disease (prior to 34 weeks' gestation) have worse outcomes than women with late-onset disease. The disease typically regresses rapidly after delivery, with resolution of symptoms within 48 hours. However, preeclampsia can also manifest postpartum with hypertension, proteinuria, or the occurrence of seizures. Postpartum preeclampsia usually manifests within 7 days of delivery.[104]

Disease manifestations of severe preeclampsia occur in all body systems as the result of widespread endothelial dysfunction.

CENTRAL NERVOUS SYSTEM

Although the term *preeclampsia* suggests that eclampsia is the end-stage of preeclampsia, it is more accurate to regard eclampsia as the outward manifestation of disease progression in the brain, similar to other organ involvement. The etiology of eclamptic seizures remains unclear (see later). CNS manifestations include severe headache, visual disturbances, hyperexcitability, hyperreflexia, and coma.[7,105-107]

Noninvasive measurements of cerebral blood flow and resistance suggest that the loss of cerebral vascular autoregulation and vascular barotrauma are the main determinants of the cerebral vascular changes seen in preeclampsia and eclampsia.[108]

AIRWAY

In pregnant women, the internal diameter of the trachea is reduced because of mucosal capillary engorgement. In women with preeclampsia, these changes can be exaggerated along with upper airway narrowing as a result of **pharyngolaryngeal edema,** which may compromise visualization of airway landmarks during direct laryngoscopy. **Subglottic edema** can cause airway obstruction. Signs of airway obstruction include hoarseness, snoring, stridor, and hypoxemia.[109]

PULMONARY

Pulmonary edema is a severe complication that occurs in approximately 3% of women with preeclampsia.[110] It is relatively uncommon in healthy younger women; the risk rises in older multigravid women and in women with preeclampsia superimposed on chronic hypertension or renal disease.

Plasma colloid osmotic pressure is diminished in normal pregnancy because of decreased plasma albumin concentration, and it is reduced even further in preeclamptic women.[111] Women with normal pregnancies have mean osmotic pressures of approximately 22 mm Hg in the third trimester and approximately 17 mm Hg during the early postpartum period. In contrast, a study of women with preeclampsia demonstrated mean colloid osmotic pressures of approximately 18 mm Hg before delivery and 14 mm Hg after delivery.[112] Decreased colloid osmotic pressure, in combination with greater vascular permeability and the loss of intravascular fluid and protein into the interstitium, increases the risk of pulmonary edema and can result in the acute respiratory distress syndrome.[113]

CARDIOVASCULAR

Women with preeclampsia have increased vascular tone and greater sensitivity to vasoconstrictor influences, leading to the clinical manifestations of hypertension, vasospasm, and end-organ ischemia.[114] Preeclampsia is characterized by severe vasospasm as well as exaggerated hemodynamic responses to circulating catecholamines.[79,115-117] Characteristically, blood pressure and systemic vascular resistance are elevated. In mild disease, plasma volume may be normal; however, it may be reduced as much as 40% in women with severe disease.[118]

Severe preeclampsia is usually a **hyperdynamic state**. Many studies have attempted to characterize the hemodynamic characteristics of preeclampsia with the use of invasive monitoring techniques.[119-124] Interpretation and comparison of the results of these studies have been difficult because of variation in patient populations, definitions of preeclampsia, disease severity, prior treatment, and the presence or absence of concomitant comorbid disease. Hemodynamic characteristics in preeclamptic women are more complex than originally thought, in part because hemodynamic measurements change with treatment and disease progression. Overall, studies have found that the majority (approximately 80%) of affected women exhibit hyperdynamic left ventricular function,[122] mild to moderately increased systemic vascular resistance,[122] and normal left and right cardiac filling pressures.[122,123] A smaller group of women constituting a high-risk group present with decreased left ventricular function, markedly reduced systemic vascular resistance, and severely decreased intravascular volume.[122,125]

HEMATOLOGIC

Thrombocytopenia is the most common hematologic abnormality in women with preeclampsia, occurring in 15% to 20% of affected women. Platelet counts less than 100,000/mm^3 occur most commonly in women with severe disease or HELLP syndrome and correlate with both the severity of the disease process and the incidence of placental abruption.[95]

Studies using thromboelastrography have found that women with mild preeclampsia are relatively *hyper*coagulable in comparison with women without preeclampsia, and those with severe disease are relatively *hypo*coagulable.[126]

The syndrome of **disseminated intravascular coagulation** (DIC) occurs in some women with preeclampsia. Activation of the coagulation system is marked by the intravascular disappearance of procoagulants, the intravascular appearance of fibrin degradation products, and end-organ damage secondary to microthrombi formation.[127] In advanced DIC, procoagulants (e.g., fibrinogen, platelets) decrease to a level that permits spontaneous hemorrhage.

HEPATIC

Hepatic manifestations of preeclampsia include periportal hemorrhage and fibrin deposition in hepatic sinusoids. Damage ranges from mild hepatocellular necrosis to the more ominous HELLP syndrome and can be associated with potential subcapsular bleeding and risk of hepatic rupture. Spontaneous hepatic rupture is rare but is associated with a 32% maternal mortality rate.[128]

RENAL

Renal manifestations of preeclampsia include persistent proteinuria, changes in the glomerular filtration rate, and hyperuricemia. The presence of **proteinuria** is a defining element of preeclampsia. The characteristic renal histologic lesion of preeclampsia is glomerular capillary endotheliosis, which manifests as glomerular enlargement and endothelial and mesangial cell swelling. Increasing urinary excretion of protein likely results from changes in the pore size or charge selectivity of the glomerular filter and impaired proximal tubular reabsorption.[129]

During normal pregnancy, the **glomerular filtration rate** (GFR) *increases* by 40% to 60% during the first trimester,[130,131] with a resulting decrease in levels of the serum markers of renal clearance, including blood urea nitrogen (BUN), creatinine, and uric acid. In preeclampsia, the GFR is 34% lower than in normal pregnancy.[129] Notably, women with preeclampsia may have BUN and creatinine measurements in the normal range for nonpregnant women despite significantly decreased GFR relative to normal pregnant women.

The association between preeclampsia and **hyperuricemia** was recognized as early as 1917.[132] Most evidence suggests that decreased renal clearance is the primary mechanism of elevated uric acid concentrations.[133] Because levels of serum uric acid begin to increase as early as 25 weeks' gestation,[134] this process has been investigated as a possible early predictor of preeclampsia. However, a systematic review found that hyperuricemia is a poor predictor of maternal and fetal complications.[135]

Oliguria, a possible late manifestation of severe preeclampsia, parallels the severity of disease. Persistent oliguria (less than 400 mL urine output in 24 hours) requires immediate assessment of intravascular volume status. Progression to renal failure is rare and is typically preceded by hypovolemia, placental abruption, and/or DIC.

UTEROPLACENTAL BLOOD FLOW

Uteroplacental blood flow can be impaired in pregnancies complicated by preeclampsia. In contrast to normal pregnancy, downstream resistance in the uteroplacental bed increases, diastolic flow velocity decreases, and the systolic-to-diastolic flow velocity ratio increases in the woman with preeclampsia.[136] The systolic-to-diastolic blood pressure ratio, calculated from Doppler ultrasonographic determination of blood flow velocities, reflects intrinsic arterial resistance. Pathophysiologic changes can lead to intrauterine fetal growth restriction (the fetal syndrome) in some pregnancies complicated by severe preeclampsia.

Obstetric Management

Optimal management of the woman with preeclampsia requires a team approach. There is considerable overlap in areas of concern to the obstetrician and the anesthesia provider.

Obstetric management of preeclampsia centers on the following: (1) fetal and maternal surveillance, (2) treatment of hypertension, (3) seizure prophylaxis, (4) decisions regarding the timing and route of delivery, and (5) administration of corticosteroids to women with severe preeclampsia or HELLP syndrome. Delivery remains the only cure. Obstetric care of the woman with mild preeclampsia differs little from routine management of healthy pregnant women, with the exception of careful monitoring so as to detect the progression of disease to severe preeclampsia. Pregnancy outcomes for women with mild disease at or beyond 37 weeks' gestation are similar to those for women with uncomplicated pregnancies.[3]

MATERNAL AND FETAL SURVEILLANCE

Maternal surveillance is indicated for all preeclamptic women. In women with mild disease, the goal is early detection of severe disease. In women with severe disease, the goal is detection of the development of organ dysfunction. All women should be evaluated for (1) severe headache, (2) visual disturbances, (3) altered mentation, (4) dyspnea, (5) right upper quadrant or epigastric pain, (6) nausea and vomiting, (7) decreased urine output, and (8) CNS hyperexcitability.[7]

Initial laboratory investigations for the pregnant woman in whom hypertension develops after 20 weeks' gestation are listed in Table 45-4. The admission platelet count is an excellent predictor of subsequent thrombocytopenia.[137] For mildly preeclamptic women with a platelet count exceeding 100,000/mm^3,[137] further coagulation testing is not required because coagulopathy is rarely present in severely preeclamptic women who have a normal platelet count.[137] With a platelet count less than 100,000/mm^3, other hemostatic abnormalities (e.g., prolongation of prothrombin time [PT] and partial thromboplastin time [PTT], and reduced fibrinogen concentration) may be present.[137] Further coagulation studies may be useful, particularly if risk factors for DIC are present (e.g., placental abruption, HELLP syndrome). Liver function tests are obtained in all women with preeclampsia because abnormal levels may prompt delivery. Approximately 20% of preeclamptic women have elevated serum transaminase measurements.[138]

TABLE 45-4 Initial Laboratory Investigations for Pregnant Women in Whom Hypertension Develops after 20 Weeks' Gestation

Test	Rationale
Hemoglobin and hematocrit	Hemoconcentration supports diagnosis of preeclampsia and is an indicator of severity. Measurements are decreased if hemolysis is present.
Platelet count	Thrombocytopenia suggests severe preeclampsia.
Quantification of protein excretion	Pregnancy-associated hypertension with proteinuria should be considered preeclampsia (pure or superimposed) until proven otherwise.
Serum creatinine	Abnormal or rising creatinine level suggests severe preeclampsia, especially in presence of oliguria.
Serum transaminase	Rising serum transaminase measurements suggest severe preeclampsia with hepatic involvement.
Serum uric acid	Increased serum uric acid levels suggest the diagnosis of preeclampsia.

Adapted from the Report of the National High Blood Pressure Education Program Working Group on High Blood Pressure in Pregnancy. Am J Obstet Gynecol 2000; 183:S1-22.

Although there is widespread consensus that fetal surveillance is indicated as part of the expectant management of women with severe preeclampsia, there is no universally accepted regimen of tests. Most obstetricians recommend daily fetal movement counts with either nonstress testing or biophysical profile testing at the time of diagnosis and at regular intervals thereafter.[16] Ultrasonography is used to estimate fetal weight and amniotic fluid volume. Doppler ultrasonography is sometimes used to measure fetal blood flow velocimetry if intrauterine growth restriction is suspected.[139,140]

TREATMENT OF ACUTE HYPERTENSION

Antihypertensive medications are used to treat severe hypertension with the goal of preventing adverse maternal sequelae such as hypertensive encephalopathy, cerebrovascular hemorrhage, myocardial ischemia, and congestive heart failure.[16] There is no evidence to suggest that antihypertensive therapy delays progression of the disease or improves perinatal outcome.[141] The obstetrician usually initiates antihypertensive therapy, although the anesthesia provider may also be involved in acute events.

Although the acute control of maternal blood pressure is critical, rapid changes in maternal perfusion pressure may

TABLE 45-5 Treatment of Acute Severe Hypertension* In Preeclampsia/Eclampsia

Medication	Onset of Action†	Dose
Hydralazine	10-20 min	5 mg IV every 20 min up to maximum dose of 20 mg IV
Labetalol	5-10 min	20 mg IV, then additional doses every 10 min, as needed, up to maximum dose of 220 mg IV
Sodium nitroprusside‡	0.5-1 min	0.25-5 µg/kg/min IV infusion

IV, intravenously.

*Blood pressure ≥ 160 mm Hg systolic, ≥ 105 mm Hg diastolic, or both, if sustained.

†From Stoelting R, Hillier S. Pharmacology & Physiology in Anesthetic Practice. Philadelphia, Lippincott Williams & Wilkins, 2006.

‡Risk of fetal cyanide poisoning with treatment > 4 hours.

Adapted from the Report of the National High Blood Pressure Education Program Working Group on High Blood Pressure in Pregnancy. Am J Obstet Gynecol 2000; 183:S1-22.

adversely affect uteroplacental perfusion and oxygen delivery to the fetus. Antihypertensive medications should be carefully titrated to avoid abrupt changes in maternal blood pressure. The aim of therapy is to lower the mean arterial blood pressure by no more than 15% to 25%, with a target diastolic blood pressure of 100 to 105 mm Hg.[142] Commonly used drugs are hydralazine, labetalol, esmolol, and sodium nitroprusside (Table 45-5); in usual clinical doses, all are considered safe for the fetus.

Hydralazine

Hydralazine has been used safely in pregnant women for decades and has been considered the drug of choice for treating severe hypertension in preeclampsia. Hydralazine exerts a potent and direct vasodilating effect. Plasma volume expansion prior to its administration decreases the risk of maternal hypotension. Other side effects include tachycardia, palpitations, headache, and neonatal thrombocytopenia.[143,144]

Labetalol

Labetalol, formerly considered second-line therapy for severe hypertension, is now also advocated as first-line therapy.[145] It is a combined alpha- and beta-adrenergic receptor antagonist with a 1:7 ratio of alpha- to beta-adrenergic receptor antagonism when administered intravenously. Labetalol should be avoided in women with severe asthma or congestive heart failure.[146]

A systematic review[147] and a meta-analysis[148] of existing small, randomized controlled trials concluded that the efficacy of intravenous labetalol is similar to that of intravenous hydralazine but with fewer maternal side effects. In the largest randomized trial to date, hydralazine was associated with more maternal tachycardia and palpitations but less neonatal bradycardia and hypotension than labetalol.[149] Both antihypertensive drugs are considered safe and effective for the treatment of severe hypertension in pregnant women.

Esmolol

Concerns about the use of esmolol during pregnancy arose in 1989, following reports of dose-dependent prolonged fetal bradycardia in a study of gravid ewes receiving esmolol by stepped infusion.[150] Subsequent human case reports have reported variable responses,[151-153] but in most cases fetal bradycardia was transient and the fetal heart rate (FHR) returned to baseline after discontinuation of the drug. Placental transfer is rapid, and the anesthesia provider should expect to observe the clinical effects of beta-adrenergic receptor blockade in the fetus. Eisenach and Castro[150] demonstrated that maternal administration of esmolol produced similar levels of beta-adrenergic receptor blockade in both gravid ewes and fetal lambs, in contrast to the *lesser* extent of beta-adrenergic blockade observed in fetal lambs after maternal labetalol administration.[154]

Sodium Nitroprusside

Sodium nitroprusside is a powerful smooth muscle vasodilator that interacts with sulfhydryl groups on endothelial cells and results in the release of nitric oxide.[155,156] Occasionally administered to preeclamptic women who show no response to hydralazine or labetalol therapy, sodium nitroprusside relaxes arterial vessels and reduces both afterload and venous return, with an almost instantaneous onset of action.

Sodium nitroprusside is a potent drug that requires careful titration; continuous intra-arterial blood pressure monitoring is mandatory. Because sodium nitroprusside metabolism produces cyanide, which undergoes placental transfer, there is a potential risk of fetal cyanide toxicity. However, fetal harm is unlikely to result from short-term use of sodium nitroprusside in clinical doses of 2 µg/kg/min or less. The drug is typically used for a limited period of time as a bridge to delivery.

Nifedipine

Nifedipine, a calcium entry–blocking drug, lowers blood pressure by relaxing arterial and arteriolar smooth muscle. Although it has been used in pregnant women for the treatment of acute severe hypertension, its sublingual administration has been associated with *cerebral ischemia* and *infarction, myocardial infarction, complete heart block,* and *death.*[157] Sublingual nifedipine has *not* been endorsed by the American College of Obstetricians and Gynecologists (ACOG) for treatment of acute severe hypertension in pregnancy, and the U.S. Food and Drug Administration (FDA) has *not* approved sublingual nifedipine for the treatment of a hypertensive emergency in any patient group.[158]

Nifedipine interactions with magnesium sulfate may have adverse effects in both mother and fetus. Severe hypotension[159,160] and neuromuscular blockade[161,162] have been reported with concurrent use of the two drugs. Nonreassuring FHR patterns have also been reported with concurrent administration of nifedipine and magnesium sulfate.[159,160]

SEIZURE PROPHYLAXIS

The routine use of magnesium sulfate for seizure prophylaxis in women with severe preeclampsia is an established obstetric practice in the United States and has gained popularity throughout the world. There is clear evidence that magnesium sulfate is the best available agent for prevention of recurrent seizures in women with eclampsia[163,164]; thus its use has been extended to seizure prophylaxis in women with preeclampsia.

What is the evidence for the efficacy of magnesium sulfate in the prevention of seizures for women with preeclampsia? Randomized trials have compared the administration of magnesium sulfate to prevent seizures in women with severe preeclampsia with that of placebo[165,166] and with use of the cerebral vasodilator nimodipine.[167] Sibai[168] reviewed available randomized trials and concluded that administration of magnesium sulfate is associated with significantly lower rates of eclampsia. Although this agent is effective at preventing seizures, there is no evidence that administration of magnesium sulfate improves overall outcomes. Specifically, there is no evidence that use of magnesium sulfate lowers the incidence of maternal mortality or placental abruption. In addition, magnesium sulfate was associated with a significant increase in the rate of respiratory depression in all trials.[168]

Similarly, there is no evidence for improved perinatal outcomes with prophylactic magnesium sulfate administration. Prophylactic magnesium sulfate did not reduce the rate of perinatal death in randomized trials,[165,167,169] nor did it increase perinatal morbidity (i.e., respiratory distress, Apgar scores less than 7 at 5 minutes, need for intubation, or days in the neonatal intensive care unit).[166,167] In the past, higher rates of fetal, neonatal, and pediatric deaths have been described with maternally administered magnesium sulfate at higher doses for tocolysis.[170] In contemporary obstetric practice, magnesium is no longer recommended for this indication, and doses used for seizure prophylaxis do not exceed 2 g/hr.

Only two well-controlled trials have evaluated the use of magnesium sulfate for seizure prevention in *mild* preeclampsia. In both studies, there was no difference in the number of women who progressed to *severe* preeclampsia.[171,172] The risk-to-benefit ratio of magnesium sulfate prophylaxis in *mild* preeclampsia is unclear and does not justify its routine use for prevention of seizures.[168]

The mechanism of the anticonvulsant effect of magnesium is not well understood. Eclamptic seizures were previously thought to result from cerebral vasospasm, and it was also believed that the cerebrovasodilating properties of magnesium reduced the rate of eclamptic seizures by relieving vasospasm.[173] However, more recent evidence suggests that abrupt, sustained blood pressure elevation overwhelms myogenic vasoconstriction and causes forced dilation of the cerebral vessels, hyperperfusion, and cerebral edema.[108,173-175] This raises the question of how magnesium sulfate—a vasodilator—could be effective in seizure prophylaxis; magnesium would be expected to worsen cerebral hyperperfusion and edema. Using a rat model, Euser and Cipolla[173] demonstrated that the mesenteric vessels are more sensitive to magnesium-induced vasodilation than cerebral vessels. Their observations suggest that the effectiveness of magnesium sulfate seizure prophylaxis is more closely related to lowering of the systemic blood pressure than to direct effects on cerebral blood flow.

No consensus exists regarding the following issues: (1) the ideal time to initiate treatment with magnesium sulfate, (2) the best loading and maintenance doses, and (3) the optimal duration of therapy. Many obstetricians administer a loading dose of 4 to 6 g over 20 to 30 minutes, followed by a maintenance infusion of 1 to 2 g/hr. The infusion is commonly initiated with the onset of labor and continued for 24 hours postpartum. Sibai[168] has recommended that severely preeclamptic women undergoing cesarean delivery should receive magnesium sulfate at least 2 hours before the procedure, during surgery, and for 12 hours postpartum.

Magnesium sulfate is eliminated almost entirely by renal excretion, and serum levels of this agent may become dangerously high in the presence of renal insufficiency. Side effects include chest pain and tightness, palpitations, nausea, blurred vision, sedation, transient hypotension, and rarely pulmonary edema.[166,176-178] In untreated patients, the normal range for serum magnesium concentrations is 1.7 to 2.4 mg/dL. The therapeutic range lies between 5 and 9 mg/dL.[172] Reflex testing is used as a clinical screen for hypermagnesemia; when deep tendon reflexes are preserved, the more serious side effects are usually avoided. Patellar reflexes are lost at serum magnesium levels of approximately 12 mg/dL. Respiratory arrest occurs at 15 to 20 mg/dL, and asystole occurs when the level exceeds 25 mg/dL.[179] Preeclamptic women with renal impairment should be monitored closely because magnesium toxicity can occur with usual dosing regimens. Serial measurement of serum magnesium levels may be helpful in the management of women with renal dysfunction.

Treatment of suspected magnesium toxicity involves immediate discontinuation of the infusion and the intravenous administration of **calcium gluconate** (1 g) over 10 minutes.[180] In the rare event of respiratory compromise, the patient may require endotracheal intubation and mechanical ventilation until spontaneous ventilation returns.

In the developing world, a lack of infrastructure, equipment, and expertise precludes the timely administration of intravenous magnesium sulfate in most women with severe preeclampsia. A lack of resources for the treatment of systemic magnesium toxicity is also an obstacle to the use of magnesium sulfate. Labetalol has been proposed as a practical, inexpensive, orally administered alternative for women in developing countries.[181]

In summary, published evidence supports the administration of magnesium sulfate for the prevention of eclamptic seizures, but there is no evidence of better maternal or neonatal outcomes as a result of its use.

ROUTE AND TIMING OF DELIVERY

Vaginal delivery should be attempted in all women with mild disease, assuming no other indications for cesarean delivery exist. Vaginal delivery should also be attempted in most women with severe disease, especially those beyond 34 weeks' gestation.[7,182] The Report of the NHBPEP Working Group on High Blood Pressure in Pregnancy[7] states, "Vaginal delivery is preferable to cesarean delivery for women with preeclampsia, because it avoids addition of the stress of surgery to the multiple

TABLE 45-6 Indications for Delivery in Severe Preeclampsia

Maternal	Gestational age ≥ 38 weeks* Platelet count < 100,000/mm^3 Progressive deterioration in hepatic function Progressive deterioration in renal function Suspected placental abruption Persistent severe headaches or visual changes Persistent severe epigastric pain, nausea, or vomiting
Fetal	Severe intrauterine growth restriction Nonreassuring fetal status Oligohydramnios

*Delivery should be based on maternal and fetal conditions as well as on gestational age.

Adapted from Report of the National High Blood Pressure Education Program Working Group on High Blood Pressure in Pregnancy. Am J Obstet Gynecol 2000; 183:S1-22.

physiologic aberrations [of the disease]. Acute palliation for several hours does not increase maternal risk if performed appropriately. Labor induction should be carried out aggressively once the decision for delivery has been made. In gestation remote from term in which delivery is indicated, and with fetal and maternal conditions stable enough to permit pregnancy to be prolonged 48 hours, glucocorticoids can be safely administered to accelerate fetal pulmonary maturity." Cesarean delivery is appropriate when the maternal or fetal condition mandates immediate delivery or when other indications for cesarean delivery exist (Table 45-6).

The timing of delivery can be difficult and requires the obstetrician to weigh the risks and benefits for both the mother and fetus. The primary objective of obstetric management of preeclampsia is the safety of the mother. Delivery is always an appropriate therapeutic option for the mother but may not be in the best interests of the very preterm fetus. Immediate delivery increases neonatal morbidity and mortality and can lead to prolonged neonatal intensive care unit stays for the treatment of the complications of prematurity. Conversely, attempts to prolong pregnancy increase the risk of maternal morbidity and mortality and can also lead to intrauterine fetal asphyxia or death. The obstetric management plan should consider maternal and fetal status at the time of initial assessment, fetal gestational age, the presence or absence of labor, and status of the fetal membranes (i.e., intact versus ruptured).[182]

The clinical course of severe preeclampsia is marked by progressive deterioration of both the maternal and fetal conditions.[183] Because these pregnancies are associated with high rates of maternal morbidity and mortality, there is widespread agreement that delivery is indicated if severe disease develops after 34 weeks' gestation. Women with refractory severe hypertension despite maximum doses of antihypertensive agents *or* women who have persistent cerebral symptoms while receiving magnesium sulfate are delivered within 24 to 48 hours, regardless of gestational age. Other clear indications for delivery include severe intrauterine growth restriction, multiple-organ failure, suspected placental abruption, and nonreassuring fetal testing before 34 weeks' gestation.[183,184] In contrast, the management of severe preeclampsia remote from term—with evidence of both maternal and fetal stability—remains controversial.

Expectant management, an alternative to immediate intervention, refers to the prolongation of pregnancy with close monitoring until (1) the development of maternal or fetal indications for delivery, (2) the attainment of fetal lung maturity, or (3) 34 weeks' gestation. The goal is the safe prolongation of gestation in order to optimize perinatal outcome. Two randomized trials[185,186] have compared the risks and benefits of aggressive and conservative (expectant) management of severe preeclampsia. Aggressive management was defined as corticosteroid therapy followed by delivery within 48 hours, and expectant management consisted of corticosteroid therapy followed by delivery only for specific maternal or fetal indications. Both trials demonstrated that conservative management was associated with better perinatal outcome, with reasonable maternal safety. In the largest trial of expectant management, Sibai et al.[186] studied 95 women with severe preeclampsia at 28 to 32 weeks' gestation, managed either expectantly or aggressively, and found a significant prolongation of pregnancy, shorter stays in the neonatal intensive care unit, and a lower incidence of neonatal respiratory distress syndrome in the expectant management group, without any increase in the incidence of maternal complications.

CORTICOSTEROID ADMINISTRATION FOR SEVERE PREECLAMPSIA OR HELLP SYNDROME

To accelerate fetal lung maturity, all women in whom severe preeclampsia or HELLP syndrome develops between 24 and 34 weeks' gestation should receive a course of corticosteroid therapy. A randomized double-blind trial of 218 women with severe preeclampsia at 26 to 34 weeks' gestation found that those receiving betamethasone, compared with those receiving placebo, had a significantly lower rate of neonatal respiratory distress syndrome as well as reduced rates of neonatal intraventricular hemorrhage, infection, and death.[187]

Complications of Preeclampsia

Severe preeclampsia is associated with an increased risk of maternal morbidity and mortality, including HELLP syndrome, cerebrovascular accident, pulmonary edema, renal failure, placental abruption, and eclampsia. In general, these complications are more common in women with early-onset preeclampsia and in women with prepregnancy medical conditions such as diabetes mellitus, chronic renal disease, and thrombophilia.[1]

CEREBROVASCULAR ACCIDENT

Although the absolute risk of cerebrovascular accident is low, stroke remains the leading cause of death in women with preeclampsia. In the 2003-2005 Confidential Enquiry into Maternal and Child Health (CEMACH) report, 18 deaths were attributed to eclampsia and preeclampsia; 67% resulted from a cerebrovascular accident (10 intracranial hemorrhages and 2 cerebral infarctions).[188] The endothelial dysfunction of preeclampsia can promote edema, vascular tone instability, platelet activation, and local thrombosis. Reversible cerebral edema is the most common CNS feature of preeclampsia or eclampsia. The leading hypothesis regarding the loss of endothelial integrity is that cerebral lesions are caused by a loss of cerebral autoregulation, which results in hyperperfusion that leads to interstitial or vasogenic edema.[189,190] The presence of HELLP syndrome or DIC increases the risk for a hemorrhagic event.

There is growing recognition that mean arterial blood pressure and diastolic blood pressure may not reflect the true risk for stroke. A review of 28 case histories of severely preeclamptic women who suffered a stroke revealed that (1) systolic blood pressure in excess of 160 mm Hg was a far superior predictor of stroke than diastolic hypertension or mean arterial pressure, (2) the majority of strokes were hemorrhagic (93%) as opposed to thrombotic (7%), and (3) the majority of strokes (57%) occurred in the postpartum period.[191] Close attention to blood pressure control throughout the peripartum period is the mainstay of stroke prevention.

PULMONARY EDEMA

Pulmonary edema is a severe complication of preeclampsia that occurs in approximately 3% of affected women.[110] It is relatively infrequent in younger (previously healthy) women; the risk is higher in older multigravid women and in women with preeclampsia superimposed on chronic hypertension or renal disease. The clinical presentation is characterized by worsening dyspnea and orthopnea with concomitant signs of respiratory compromise, such as tachypnea, rales, and hypoxemia. Causes of pulmonary edema include low colloid osmotic pressure, increased intravascular hydrostatic pressure, and greater pulmonary capillary permeability.[192] All of these factors may coexist in a single patient. A large proportion of cases of pulmonary edema occur postpartum, usually within 2 to 3 days of delivery, and management is directed toward the underlying cause (e.g., fluid overload, sepsis, cardiac failure).[193] Echocardiography can be helpful in the diagnosis of cardiogenic causes of pulmonary edema.[194,195] Initial treatment includes administration of supplemental oxygen, fluid restriction, and diuretic therapy (e.g., furosemide). A retrospective study of more than 16,000 deliveries found that although peripartum pulmonary edema was associated with extensive radiographic infiltrates and severe hypoxemia, resolution was typically rapid, with a limited need for intensive care unit admission.[196] Placement of a pulmonary artery catheter can facilitate management of patients with severe refractory pulmonary edema; these women should be managed in an intensive care unit. Notably, in the 2003-2005 CEMACH report, there were no deaths attributed solely to pulmonary causes.[188] Presumably, this trend reflects improvements in the fluid management of women with severe preeclampsia.

RENAL FAILURE

Acute renal failure is a rare but serious complication of severe preeclampsia and HELLP syndrome.[197] The true incidence remains unknown. Acute renal failure is divided into three categories: (1) **prerenal,** which refers to renal hypoperfusion; (2) **intrarenal,** which suggests intrinsic renal parenchymal damage; and (3) **postrenal,** which implies obstructive uropathy.[198] The majority of cases (83% to 90%) of acute renal failure in preeclampsia result from prerenal and intrarenal disease (most commonly acute tubular necrosis) and resolve completely after delivery.[199-201] In contrast, bilateral renal cortical necrosis is a rare and serious condition associated with considerable maternal and perinatal morbidity and mortality. It occurs most commonly in association with known renal parenchymal disease, chronic hypertension with superimposed preeclampsia, placental abruption, or DIC.[202]

PLACENTAL ABRUPTION

Placental abruption occurs in approximately 2% of women with preeclampsia and increases perinatal morbidity and mortality. A retrospective case-control study of 161 women with placental abruption and 2000 women without abruption found a threefold higher risk of placental abruption in women with preeclampsia.[203] The incidence is also increased in women with underlying chronic hypertension.[193] Management depends on the extent of abruption and associated hypotension, coagulopathy, or fetal compromise (see Chapter 37). Placental abruption is also associated with the development of DIC.

HELLP Syndrome

HELLP syndrome is a variant of severe preeclampsia characterized by rapid clinical deterioration. It is associated with a higher risk of maternal death (1%) and increased rates of maternal morbidities, including DIC, placental abruption, pulmonary edema, acute renal failure, liver hemorrhage or failure, acute respiratory distress syndrome, sepsis, and stroke (Table 45-7).[204] Additionally, the syndrome is associated with a 70% rate of preterm delivery[204]; prematurity-related neonatal complications increase the risk of perinatal morbidity and mortality. The onset of HELLP syndrome occurs antepartum in 70% of cases, and postpartum in 30%.[204]

TABLE 45-7 Serious Maternal Complications in a Series of 442 Patients with Hemolysis, Elevated Liver Enzymes, and Low Platelets (HELLP) Syndrome

	Patients Affected	
Complication*	**No.**	**Percentage**
Disseminated intravascular coagulation	92	21
Placental abruption	69	16
Acute renal failure	33	8
Severe ascites	32	8
Pulmonary edema	26	6
Pleural effusions	26	6
Cerebral edema	4	1
Retinal detachment	4	1
Laryngeal edema	4	1
Subcapsular liver hematoma	4	1
Acute respiratory distress syndrome	3	1
Maternal death	4	1

*Some women had multiple complications.

Adapted from Sibai BM, Ramadan MK, Usta I, et al. Maternal morbidity and mortality in 442 pregnancies with hemolysis, elevated liver enzymes, and low platelets (HELLP syndrome). Am J Obstet Gynecol 1993; 169:1000-6.

TABLE 45-8 Diagnostic Criteria for Hemolysis, Elevated Liver Enzymes, and Low Platelets (HELLP) Syndrome

Criteria	Laboratory Findings
Hemolysis	Abnormal peripheral blood smear Bilirubin > 1.2 mg/dL Lactic dehydrogenase > 600 IU/L
Elevated liver enzyme concentrations	Serum glutamic oxaloacetic transaminase (SGOT) ≥ 70 IU/L Lactic dehydrogenase > 600 IU/L
Thrombocytopenia	Platelet count < 100,000/mm^3

From Sibai BM. The HELLP syndrome (hemolysis, elevated liver enzymes, and low platelets): Much ado about nothing? Am J Obstet Gynecol 1990; 162:311-6.

BOX 45-3 Differential Diagnosis of Hemolysis, Elevated Liver Enzymes, and Low Platelets (HELLP) Syndrome

- Acute fatty liver of pregnancy
- Appendicitis
- Cholestasis of pregnancy
- Diabetes insipidus
- Gallbladder disease
- Gastroenteritis
- Glomerulonephritis
- Hemolytic-uremic syndrome
- Hepatic encephalopathy
- Hyperemesis gravidarum
- Idiopathic thrombocytopenia
- Kidney stones
- Peptic ulcer
- Systemic lupus erythematosus
- Thrombotic thrombocytopenic purpura
- Viral hepatitis

From O'Brien JM, Barton JR. Controversies with the diagnosis and management of HELLP syndrome. Clin Obstet Gynecol 2005; 48:460-77.

Because of a lack of universally accepted diagnostic criteria for HELLP syndrome, its incidence cannot be determined accurately. The existence of a subset of cases of preeclampsia complicated by abnormal peripheral blood smear findings, abnormal liver function parameters, and thrombocytopenia has been recognized for decades; in 1982, Weinstein[205] described a series of 29 cases and coined the acronym HELLP. Women who do not demonstrate one or more of these clinical features are said to have "partial" HELLP syndrome.

The definition and diagnosis of HELLP syndrome remain controversial. **Hemolysis,** defined as the presence of microangiopathic hemolytic anemia, is the hallmark of HELLP syndrome; peripheral blood smear demonstrates schistocytes, burr cells, and echinocytes.[206] Common histopathologic findings are periportal hepatic necrosis and hemorrhage.[207] Sibai[206] has proposed standardized laboratory diagnostic criteria, as outlined in Table 45-8. Maternal signs and symptoms include right upper quadrant or epigastric pain, nausea and vomiting, headache, hypertension, and proteinuria. Notably, clinical presentation varies; 12% to 18% of women may be normotensive, and proteinuria is absent in approximately 13%. Diagnosis can be especially challenging because numerous medical and surgical disorders can mimic HELLP syndrome (Box 45-3). Pregnant women who are likely to have preeclampsia, but who demonstrate atypical symptoms, should be screened with a complete blood count, platelet count, and liver enzyme assessment.

The management of HELLP syndrome is also highly controversial. Owing to associated maternal morbidity and mortality, obstetricians have considered HELLP syndrome to be an indication for immediate delivery. There is consensus regarding the need for immediate delivery when HELLP syndrome manifests beyond 34 weeks' gestation or in the presence of complications such as DIC, liver infarction or hemorrhage, renal failure, placental abruption, and nonreassuring fetal status. On the other hand, substantial disagreement exists regarding the management of women with stable maternal and fetal conditions at or before 34 weeks' gestation. Some authorities have recommended the administration of corticosteroids to accelerate fetal lung maturity, followed by delivery 24 hours later,[206,208] and others have recommended prolongation of pregnancy until the development of complications, until fetal lung maturity is achieved, or until 34 weeks' gestation.[209-211] Some reports have suggested that in a select group of women, pregnancy can be prolonged for days—and possibly a few weeks—with associated improvement in laboratory measurements.[209-212]

Women in whom HELLP syndrome is suspected should be immediately hospitalized for observation in a labor and delivery unit; women who have not reached 35 weeks' gestation should be managed in a tertiary care facility with a neonatal intensive care unit capable of caring for a compromised preterm neonate. Clinical management is similar to that for severe preeclampsia and includes intravenous magnesium sulfate for seizure prophylaxis and antihypertensive medications to maintain a systolic blood pressure below 160 mm Hg and a diastolic blood pressure below 105 mm Hg.[206] The first priority is to assess and stabilize the maternal condition, with particular attention given to hypertension and coagulation abnormalities. Next, the fetal condition should be assessed with FHR monitoring, Doppler ultrasonography of fetal vessels, and/or a biophysical profile. Lastly, decisions regarding delivery must be made. If time permits, the mother should receive a course of corticosteroids to accelerate fetal lung maturity.

The platelet count can fall precipitously in the presence of HELLP syndrome, and it should be evaluated prior to the administration of neuraxial anesthesia. Women with a platelet count less than 50,000/mm^3 are at significantly higher risk of bleeding,[213] and general anesthesia is the method of choice for cesarean delivery. O'Brien et al.[208] assessed the impact of corticosteroid administration on the subsequent use of epidural anesthesia in 37 women with HELLP syndrome and a pre-corticosteroid platelet count less than 90,000/mm^3; corticosteroid administration was followed by greater use of epidural anesthesia, particularly in women in whom the interval between corticosteroid administration and delivery was at least 24 hours.

Platelet transfusions are indicated in the presence of significant bleeding and in all parturients with a platelet count lower than 20,000/mm^3. Correction of thrombocytopenia prior to surgery is crucial; for women who have a platelet count less than 40,000/mm^3 and who are scheduled for cesarean delivery, the preincision administration of 6 to 10 units of platelets has been recommended.[214]

Rupture of a subcapsular hematoma of the liver is a life-threatening complication of HELLP syndrome that can manifest as abdominal pain, nausea and vomiting, and headaches; the pain worsens over time and becomes localized to the epigastric area or right upper quadrant. Hypotension and shock typically develop, and the liver is enlarged and tender.[215] Diagnosis is confirmed with ultrasonography, computed tomography, or magnetic resonance imaging of the liver (Figure 45-6). Subcapsular hematoma rupture *with shock* is a surgical emergency that requires immediate multidisciplinary treatment consisting of intravascular volume resuscitation, blood and plasma transfusions, and emergency laparotomy.[215] Prompt surgical intervention and refinements in surgical technique have reduced the maternal mortality rate associated with spontaneous hepatic rupture from 60% in 1976 to 30% in 1997.[128,216] Selective arterial embolization by an interventional radiologist might allow a further reduction in the risk of maternal death.[217-219] The most common causes of death are coagulopathy and exsanguination.[204,220]

Conservative management is recommended for hepatic hemorrhage without hepatic rupture in *stable* women.[214] Careful monitoring is required. An important component of conservative management is to avoid all potential trauma to the liver, including seizures, vomiting, and manual palpation of the abdomen. Patient transport and transfers should be conducted with care to avoid maneuvers that might result in hematoma rupture.

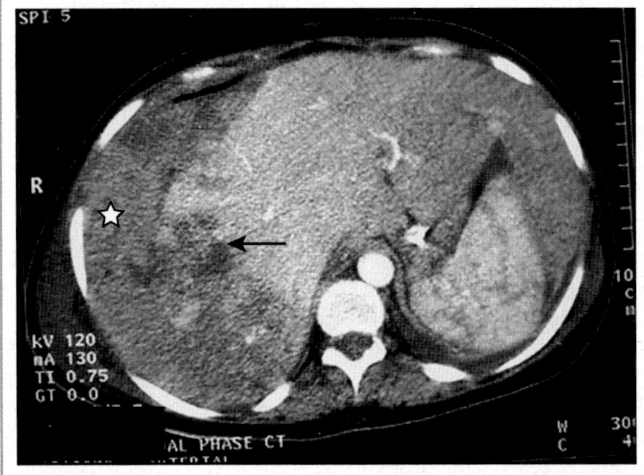

FIGURE 45-6 Contrast-enhanced computed tomography scan showing a large area of parenchymal hemorrhage with hepatic rupture (*arrow*) and subcapsular hematoma (*star*) in the right lobe of the liver. (From Das CJ, Srivastava DN, Debnath J, et al. Endovascular management of hepatic hemorrhage and subcapsular hematoma in HELLP syndrome. Indian J Gastroenterol 2007; 26:244-5.)

Anesthetic Management

The anesthetic management of the woman with mild preeclampsia differs little from the management of a healthy pregnant woman. However, the potential for rapid progression to the severe form of the disease mandates careful observation of the patient. The anesthesia provider must recognize the unpredictability of the development and progression of severe preeclampsia and should be prepared at all times for immediate cesarean delivery.

PREANESTHESIA EVALUATION

The preanesthesia assessment of women with confirmed or suspected preeclampsia should focus on the airway examination, maternal hemodynamic and coagulation status, and fluid balance.

Airway

Generalized edema can involve the airway and obscure visualization of anatomic landmarks at laryngoscopy. The anesthesia provider should anticipate the possibility of a difficult airway (see Chapter 30).

Hemodynamic Monitoring

Systemic arterial blood pressure can change rapidly in women with severe preeclampsia, both as a result of disease progression and in response to the administration of intravenous fluids and antihypertensive drugs. In addition, preeclampsia is associated with variable degrees of intravascular volume depletion, and the clinical assessment of intravascular volume status can be difficult. Therefore, the use of invasive vascular monitoring may be useful in the management of some women with severe preeclampsia.

Indications for continuous arterial blood pressure monitoring are straightforward and well-accepted. The most common indications for radial artery catheter insertion include (1) poorly controlled maternal blood pressure; (2) need for frequent arterial blood gas measurements, especially in the context of pulmonary edema; (3) planned use of a rapid-acting vasodilator (e.g., nitroprusside, nitroglycerin); (4) desire to estimate intravascular volume status with use of calculated systolic pressure variation (SPV);[221] and (5) need for continuous blood pressure monitoring during the induction of general anesthesia in hypertensive women with severe preeclampsia.

Invasive central monitoring has been advocated in the assessment of oliguria and to monitor patient responses to fluid administration. Anesthesiologists have debated the relative merits and risks of placement of a central venous pressure (CVP) catheter compared with a pulmonary artery catheter. The poor correlation between the central venous and pulmonary capillary wedge pressures (in patients with a CVP greater than 6 mm Hg) has been cited as the rationale for the preferential use of the pulmonary artery catheter for accurate assessment of the left ventricular preload.[222,223] However, this lack of correlation is an expected finding in the presence of decreased intravascular volume and varying levels of increased left ventricular afterload.[109]

The use of a pulmonary artery catheter has not been demonstrated to improve patient outcome. Studies in a variety of populations have not found a benefit to therapy directed by pulmonary artery catheter measurements rather than standard care.[224] The American Society of Anesthesiologists (ASA) Task Force on Pulmonary Artery Catheterization has stated:

> *Evidence regarding the effectiveness of pulmonary artery catheterization in obstetrics and gynecology is lacking. Pulmonary catheterization has been recommended for severe preeclampsia, case reports have supported its value, and its use in critical illness seems common, but controlled clinical outcome studies have not been reported.*[225]

Further, the placement of an invasive CVP or pulmonary artery catheter is not a benign procedure. Well-recognized risks include arterial trauma, pneumothorax, venous air embolism, neuropathy, and cardiac arrhythmias. Additional risks of an indwelling pulmonary artery catheter include potentially fatal pulmonary artery hemorrhage, thromboembolism, sepsis, and endocardial damage.[225] The 1991-1993 Report on Confidential Enquiries into Maternal Deaths in the United Kingdom[226] described the postpartum death of a woman after several unsuccessful attempts at internal jugular line placement and a likely carotid artery puncture. Despite digital pressure and application of a pressure dressing after vessel puncture, neck tightness and dyspnea developed 4 hours later. Attempts at re-intubation and resuscitation were unsuccessful, and she expired. In the 2003-2005 CEMACH report, an anesthesia-related maternal death occurred in a woman with fulminant preeclampsia and HELLP syndrome.[188] Shortly after a subclavian line insertion, she had a cardiac arrest and could not be resuscitated. Autopsy showed a large right hemothorax. Because both immediate and delayed[227] maternal deaths have been attributed to the use of invasive central catheters, they should be inserted only after careful consideration of the risks and benefits.

The frequency of pulmonary artery catheter use in obstetric anesthesia practice is low.[228] When invasive central monitoring is desired, a CVP catheter is adequate in the majority of cases. A CVP catheter provides a reliable method of central venous drug administration, and assessment of changes in CVP over time may guide fluid administration.

Timing of the use of invasive central monitoring is important and requires clinical judgment. Many patients are better served by immediate transfer to the operating room for delivery rather than delay of delivery for central line placement. In one study of a critical care unit in an academic hospital, the time from the decision to proceed with placement of a pulmonary artery catheter until the first pressure measurement was obtained was always more than 45 minutes.[229] Insertion time would probably exceed 45 minutes in most labor and delivery settings, where the procedure is rarely performed and qualified assistance may not be available. In the majority of cases, the preoperative placement of an invasive central line will not change the intraoperative anesthetic management. Similarly, many obstetricians prefer to deliver women with persistent oliguria (defined as less than 400 mL of urine output in 24 hours) and to optimize fluid status postoperatively.[230]

In summary, the presence of severe preeclampsia per se is not an indication for CVP or pulmonary artery pressure monitoring. There is no indication for central hemodynamic monitoring that is unique to preeclampsia. Preeclampsia is a disorder of the peripheral circulation, not the central circulation. Indications for invasive central monitoring are similar to those in other multisystem disorders, such as severe sepsis, multisystem organ dysfunction, pulmonary edema, and cardiomyopathy. Some women require transfer to an intensive care unit for specialized nursing care and management directed by a critical care medicine specialist.

NEURAXIAL ANALGESIA FOR LABOR AND DELIVERY

During labor, early administration of epidural analgesia is recommended (1) to avoid general anesthesia and the possibility of airway catastrophe in the event of emergency cesarean delivery, (2) to optimize the timing of epidural catheter placement in the setting of a declining platelet count, and (3) to obtain the beneficial effects of epidural analgesia on uteroplacental perfusion.

Continuous lumbar epidural analgesia and combined spinal-epidural (CSE) analgesia are the preferred methods of pain management during labor in women with preeclampsia. Advantages include (1) provision of high-quality analgesia, which attenuates the hypertensive response to pain[231-233]; (2) a reduction in levels of circulating catecholamines and stress-related hormones[234]; (3) possible improvement in intervillous blood flow[235]; and (4) provision of a means of administering local anesthetic for emergency cesarean delivery, thus obviating the need for general anesthesia with its attendant risks.

One disadvantage of the CSE technique is that epidural catheter function cannot be fully evaluated until after resolution of the intrathecal analgesia. For this reason, many anesthesia providers avoid the CSE technique in favor of a standard epidural technique in women with severe preeclampsia who have a higher risk for emergency cesarean delivery. Use of a standard epidural technique allows for immediate verification of catheter function.

Continuous epidural analgesia has been used in the antepartum period to optimize uteroplacental blood flow in the hope of prolonging pregnancy and avoiding preterm delivery in preeclamptic women remote from term. Kanayama et al.[236] studied 20 severely preeclamptic women at 28 to 32 weeks' gestation, who were assigned by physician choice to receive either long-term epidural bupivacaine combined with routine supportive management or routine supportive management alone. Gestational age at delivery and birth weight were greater in the treatment group, and maternal blood pressure and platelet count were also improved, when compared with the routine management group. Although this study was not well controlled, its results suggest that antepartum epidural analgesia may have the potential to prolong pregnancy and perhaps avoid preterm delivery in women with preeclampsia; further studies are warranted.

For the most part, the clinical administration of epidural analgesia to women with preeclampsia does not differ from that in healthy pregnant women without preeclampsia (see Chapter 23). The choice of local anesthetic, method of epidural space identification, and maintenance of analgesia are not affected by the presence of preeclampsia. However, the following four special considerations apply to preeclamptic women: (1) assessment of coagulation status, (2) intravenous hydration prior to the epidural administration of a local anesthetic, (3) treatment of hypotension, and (4) use of an epinephrine-containing local anesthetic solution.

Coagulation Status

Platelets contribute to coagulation and hemostasis in two important ways. First, their adhesive and cohesive functions lead to the formation of the hemostatic plug. Second, they activate the coagulation process by exposing a phospholipid surface and acting as a catalytic site for subsequent coagulation and consolidation of the initial platelet plug. Activated platelets release adenosine diphosphate, serotonin, thromboxane A_2, and other adhesive proteins, coagulation factors, and growth factors.[237] Women with *mild* preeclampsia are usually hypercoagulable relative to women with an uncomplicated pregnancy and should not be denied neuraxial labor analgesia.

Women with *severe* preeclampsia (particularly those with HELLP syndrome) may have thrombocytopenia, which increases the risk of bleeding into the epidural or spinal space with a neuraxial procedure (see Chapter 32). Neuraxial hematoma formation can have permanent neurologic sequelae. Therefore, documentation of the platelet count is necessary prior to provision of epidural analgesia in women with severe preeclampsia. The incidence of neuraxial hematoma is small but cannot be precisely determined because not all cases are reported and because there is no accurate method to determine the denominator of all preeclamptic women who have received neuraxial anesthesia.

In the past, a platelet count of at least 100,000/mm^3 was considered necessary for the safe administration of neuraxial anesthesia. This threshold probably originated from the results of a 1972 study that correlated platelet counts with bleeding times.[238] Critical appraisal of 1083 human studies concluded that the bleeding time is no longer considered a reliable method of assessing the risk of bleeding for a single individual.[239] In addition, platelet counts of 70,000/mm^3 to 100,000/mm^3 occur during normal pregnancies. A systematic review by Douglas[213] proposed a platelet count threshold of 80,000/mm^3 as adequate for the administration of neuraxial anesthesia in pregnant women without other risk factors. Further coagulation testing is not required for mildly preeclamptic women with a platelet count exceeding 100,000/mm^3, because coagulopathy is rare in preeclamptic women with a normal platelet count.[137] For a woman with a platelet count less than 100,000/mm^3, other hemostatic abnormalities, including prolonged prothrombin time (PT), prolonged partial thromboplastin time (PTT), and reduced fibrinogen concentration can be present.[137] Further coagulation studies may be useful, particularly if risk factors for DIC are present (e.g., placental abruption, HELLP syndrome).[137] In patients at risk for coagulopathy, a normal or nearly normal international normalized ratio (INR) is required for the safe performance of neuraxial anesthesia.[240,241]

Many obstetric anesthesia providers consider a platelet count of 75,000/mm^3 to 80,000/mm^3 to be adequate for administration of neuraxial anesthesia. In this setting, many anesthesia providers believe that spinal needle placement is less traumatic (and less risky) than epidural needle placement because of the smaller size of the spinal needle, although supporting data are lacking.

The trend in the platelet count is also important; a rapidly falling platelet count is a cause for concern because the nadir in the platelet count cannot be identified prospectively. How often should the anesthesia provider obtain a platelet count? Platelet count measurement every 6 hours is adequate when platelet numbers are relatively stable; a measurement obtained as recently as within the last 1 to 3 hours before the neuraxial procedure may be required when the platelet count shows evidence of a significant decline.

The risk of **epidural hematoma** formation exists not only during placement of an epidural catheter but also during its removal. In patients with thrombocytopenia, the catheter should not be withdrawn from the epidural space until there is evidence of an acceptable (and rising) platelet count. A platelet count of 75,000/mm^3 to 80,000/mm^3 seems reasonable for epidural catheter removal. In the absence of corticosteroid administration, the platelet count in women with HELLP syndrome usually reaches a nadir on the second or third postpartum day and then gradually returns to the patient's normal baseline.

Although thromboelastography (TEG) has shown some promise in the assessment of overall coagulation status in pregnant patients with thrombocytopenia,[242] the technique has been criticized for its inability to diagnose a specific coagulation defect. Further, the hypothetical potential of thromboelastography to predict the risk for epidural hematoma after the administration of neuraxial anesthesia in pregnant patients is unproven and requires further study.[243]

There is a consensus among anesthesia providers that a platelet count lower than 50,000/mm^3 precludes the administration of neuraxial anesthesia. For women with a platelet count between 50,000/mm^3 and 80,000/mm^3, the risks and benefits of neuraxial anesthesia must be weighed against the risks of general anesthesia for the individual patient if emergency cesarean delivery is required. If the decision is made to proceed with a neuraxial technique, the following suggestions may help reduce the risk of epidural hematoma and its sequelae:

1. The **most skilled anesthesia provider** available should perform the neuraxial procedure.
2. **A spinal technique may be preferable to an epidural technique** (when appropriate) because of the smaller needle size.
3. **Use of a flexible wire–embedded epidural catheter** may reduce epidural vein trauma.
4. The patient should be carefully monitored after delivery for **neurologic signs that may signal bleeding into the epidural space**.
5. **The platelet count should be checked for evidence of a return toward normal measurements (at least 75,000/mm^3 to 80,000/mm^3) before removal of the epidural catheter.** Epidural vein trauma at the time of catheter discontinuation can result in epidural bleeding and perhaps epidural hematoma.
6. **Imaging studies and neurologic or neurosurgical consultation should be obtained immediately if there is any question of an epidural hematoma.** Prompt surgical intervention may be required to avoid permanent neurologic injury.

Intravenous Hydration

In the past, when higher concentrations of local anesthetic solution (e.g., 0.25% to 0.5% bupivacaine) were administered during labor, intravenous crystalloid hydration preceded epidural local anesthetic administration to prevent or ameliorate post–epidural anesthesia hypotension. In contemporary practice, lower concentrations of local anesthetic are used (e.g., 0.0625% to 0.125% bupivacaine in combination with an opioid), hypotension is less common, and fluid preloading is of less clinical importance. Although the risk of pulmonary edema secondary to fluid preloading has decreased with current techniques for labor analgesia, careful attention to intravenous fluid infusion rates is necessary in women with severe preeclampsia because of the increased risk of pulmonary edema in these patients (as discussed earlier).

Treatment of Hypotension

The incidence of hypotension after the initiation of epidural labor analgesia has declined in modern practice. Women with mild preeclampsia may be treated with routine doses of either ephedrine or phenylephrine. There is an often-expressed concern that severely preeclamptic women may have an exaggerated response to vasopressors that might result in a sharp rise in blood pressure.[244,245] However, supportive data are lacking. The anesthesia provider should initiate treatment with small doses of ephedrine (e.g., 2.5 mg) or phenylephrine (e.g., 25 to 50 μg) to assess maternal blood pressure response before administration of a larger dose. With careful dosing, greater sensitivity to vasopressors is rarely a clinical problem.

Epinephrine

It has been suggested that local anesthetic solutions containing epinephrine (including the standard epinephrine-containing test dose) should be avoided during the administration of epidural analgesia in preeclamptic women. This concern arises from observations that preeclamptic women exhibit a greater sensitivity to vasopressors, including angiotensin II,[79,246] norepinephrine and epinephrine,[117,247] and a thromboxane A_2–mimetic agent.[248] Also, clinical studies have demonstrated that smaller doses of ephedrine and phenylephrine are required to restore maternal blood pressure during spinal anesthesia in preeclamptic women than in pregnant women without preeclampsia.[244,245,249,250] One case has been reported of a hypertensive crisis in a preeclamptic woman after the incremental administration of 30 mL of 2% lidocaine with freshly added epinephrine 5 μg/mL (1:200,000) for planned cesarean delivery.[251] However, the timing of the onset and duration of hypertension was atypical, and a drug error could not be excluded.[251] In contrast, several other case series have used the same solution without adverse effects in women with preeclampsia.[252,253]

No randomized controlled trials have assessed the effects of epidural epinephrine in women with severe preeclampsia. However, epinephrine is unlikely to pose a significant risk of hypertensive crisis, given the absence of confirmed reports after decades of its use in obstetric anesthesia practice. In the absence of malignant hypertension, it seems reasonable to administer the routine epinephrine-containing test dose to exclude intravascular placement of the epidural catheter. Notably, patients who have received beta-adrenergic receptor antagonists (e.g., labetalol) do not demonstrate the typical tachycardic response to intravascular administration of epinephrine.[254]

There is no compelling reason to include epinephrine in epidural labor analgesic solutions because its administration (in combination with epidural bupivacaine) in women *without* preeclampsia has only a modest local anesthetic–sparing effect.[255] In contemporary practice, most anesthesia providers administer an epidural solution of local anesthetic in combination with an opioid when providing epidural labor analgesia.

ANESTHESIA FOR CESAREAN DELIVERY

The administration of neuraxial anesthesia for cesarean delivery in women with preeclampsia does not differ greatly from that in healthy pregnant women (see Chapter 26). Hepatic dysfunction can result in reduced drug clearance but has little clinical impact on choice of anesthetic or analgesic agents.

The choice of local anesthetic, method of epidural space identification, and maintenance of anesthesia are not affected by the presence of preeclampsia. However, there are three special considerations in preeclamptic women undergoing cesarean delivery: (1) choice of anesthetic technique, (2) technique for induction of general anesthesia, and (3) the interaction between magnesium sulfate and nondepolarizing muscle relaxants.

Neuraxial Anesthesia

In the 2003-2005 CEMACH report, the leading cause of death in women with preeclampsia was **intracranial hemorrhage**.[188] Disadvantages of general anesthesia in the presence of preeclampsia include the risk of intracranial hemorrhage from the hypertensive response to intubation and the possibility of difficult intubation secondary to airway edema. Therefore, neuraxial anesthesia is preferred whenever clinical circumstances permit its use.

Epidural anesthesia has long been considered the optimal anesthetic technique for cesarean delivery in women with severe preeclampsia. Its advantages include relatively stable maternal blood pressure (Figure 45-7),[256] optimization of uteroplacental perfusion,[235] and the ability to titrate the administration of local anesthetic and intravenous fluids slowly to achieve the desired level of anesthesia without a precipitous decrease in maternal blood pressure. This method of local anesthetic administration also permits the anesthesia provider to minimize fluid administration to reduce the possibility of fluid overload and pulmonary edema.

The traditional view has been that spinal anesthesia is relatively contraindicated in severe preeclampsia because of the possibility of marked hypotension due to the rapid onset of spinal anesthesia–induced sympathetic blockade. However, there is growing support for the use of spinal anesthesia in women with severe preeclampsia undergoing cesarean delivery, on the basis of results of more recent studies and clinical experience. Wallace et al.[257] randomly assigned 80 women with severe preeclampsia who required cesarean delivery to receive general, epidural, or CSE anesthesia. Notably, the initial spinal dose in the CSE group (hyperbaric bupivacaine 11.25 mg) is a dose comparable to that often used for a single-shot spinal technique. There was no significant difference between the CSE and epidural anesthesia groups in maternal mean arterial pressure over time (Figure 45-8). Another small prospective study randomly assigned women with severe preeclampsia to receive either spinal or epidural anesthesia, with similar results.[258] Hood and Curry, [259] in a retrospective review of cesarean delivery records for 138 women with severe preeclampsia who received either spinal or epidural

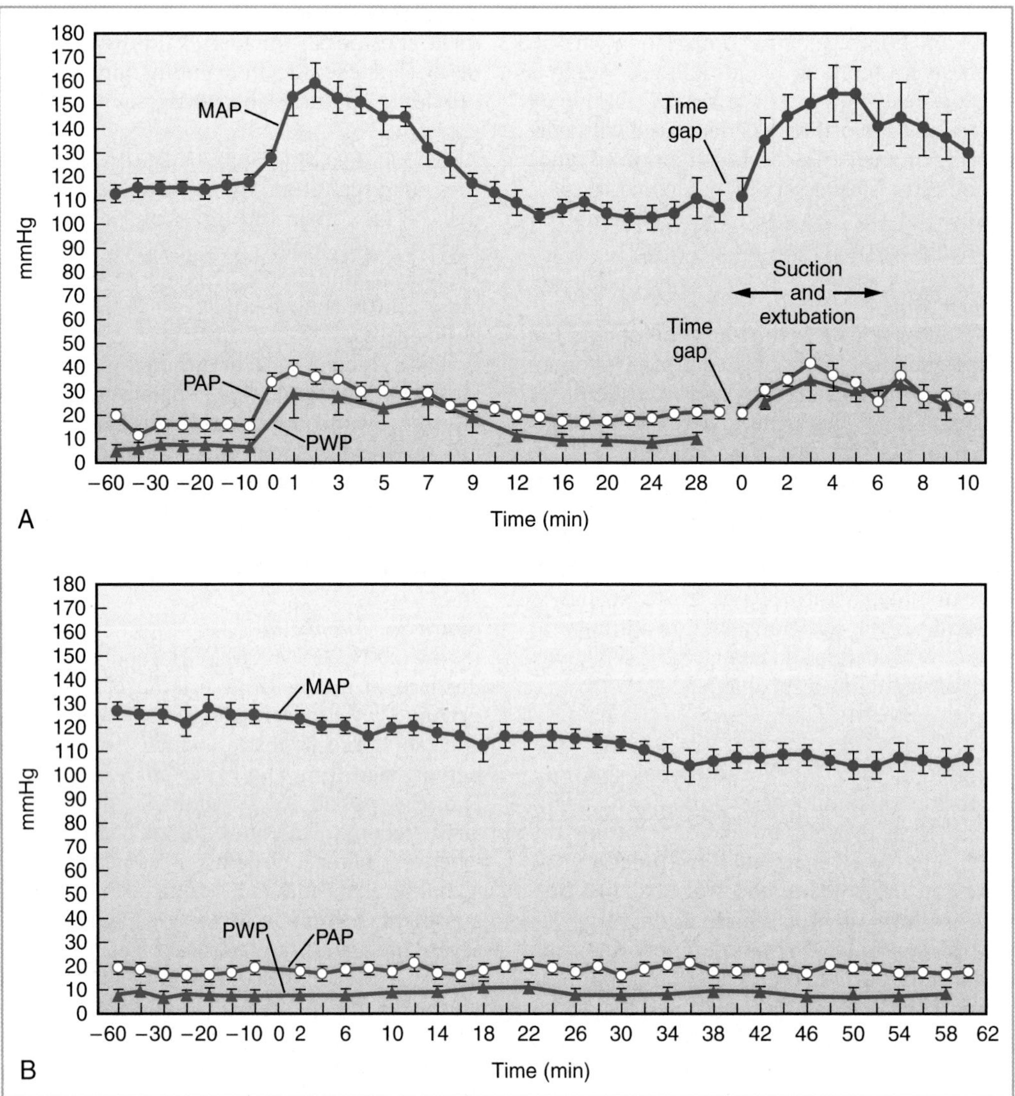

FIGURE 45-7 A, Mean ± SEM of mean arterial pressure (MAP), pulmonary artery pressure (PAP), and pulmonary wedge pressure (PWP) in 10 preeclamptic patients who underwent cesarean delivery under thiopental, nitrous oxide (40%), and halothane (0.5%) anesthesia. Measurements before the induction of anesthesia are indicated at −60 to −10 minutes. The start of induction is indicated by the first 0. The second 0 refers to the start of suction and extubation. *Time gap* refers to the time elapsed between the completion of the first 30 minutes of anesthesia and the start of suction and extubation. **B,** Mean ± SEM of MAP, PAP, and PWP in 10 preeclamptic patients who underwent cesarean delivery under epidural bupivacaine anesthesia. Measurements before epidural injection of bupivacaine (at 0 minutes) are indicated at −60 to −10 minutes, and measurements during epidural anesthesia are indicated at 2 to 60 minutes. (From Hodgkinson R, Husain FJ, Hayashi RH. Systemic and pulmonary blood pressure during caesarean section in parturients with gestational hypertension. Can Anaesth Soc J 1980; 27:389-94.)

anesthesia, found that the lowest mean blood pressure measurements did not differ between the groups. Because of the retrospective study design, the possibility that the groups were dissimilar cannot be excluded (i.e., the anesthesia providers may have chosen to administer epidural anesthesia to the more severely ill women). Nonetheless, the marked hypotension expected after spinal anesthesia did not occur. These studies lend support to the safety of spinal anesthesia in women with severe preeclampsia.

In two prospective cohort studies of women undergoing cesarean delivery, Aya et al.[244,249] compared women with severe preeclampsia to healthy pregnant women (both preterm[244] and at term[249]) and found that the risk of significant spinal anesthesia–induced hypotension (defined as requiring the administration of ephedrine) was significantly lower in the preeclampsia groups than in the control groups. The researchers speculated that the known greater vascular sensitivity to vasoconstrictors may explain the infrequent incidence of post–spinal anesthesia hypotension and the ease with which mean arterial blood pressure can be restored to baseline with small doses of vasopressor.

Lastly, a randomized multicenter study comparing the hemodynamic effects of spinal anesthesia with epidural anesthesia for cesarean delivery in women with severe preeclampsia found that significantly *more* women in the spinal anesthesia group experienced hypotension.[260] However, the duration of hypotension was less than 1 minute in both groups and, although there was more ephedrine use in the spinal group than the epidural

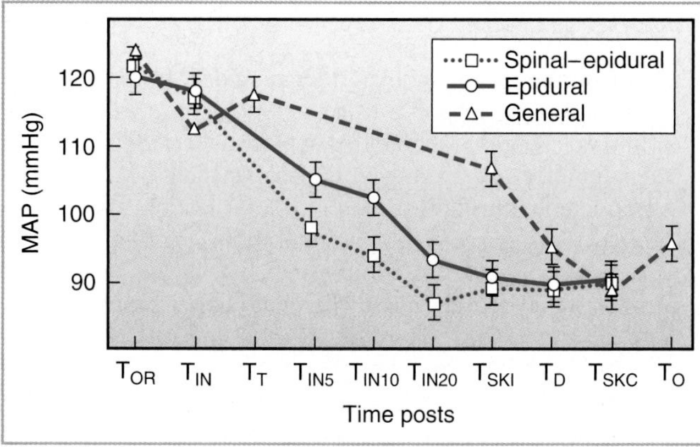

FIGURE 45-8 The profiles of average mean arterial pressure (MAP) were significantly different over the five common time posts ($P < .001$). However, only at skin incision does the general group differ from the two regional groups ($P = .003$). T_{OR}, time into operating room; T_{IN}, time of induction; T_{SKI}, time of skin incision; T_D, time of delivery; T_{SKC}, time of skin closure; T_T, time of intubation; T_O, time of extubation. Regional groups: T_{IN5}, time of induction + 5 minutes; T_{IN10}, time of induction + 10 minutes; T_{IN20}, time of induction + 20 minutes. (From Wallace DH, Leveno KJ, Cunningham FG, et al. Randomized comparison of general and regional anesthesia for cesarean delivery in pregnancies complicated by severe preeclampsia. Obstet Gynecol 1995; 86:193-9.)

group, hypotension was easily treated in both groups. In addition, there was no significant difference in neonatal outcome between infants whose mothers received spinal anesthesia and those whose mothers received epidural anesthesia.[261]

Although the evidence to date is not conclusive, it does suggest that a reappraisal of the use of spinal anesthesia for cesarean delivery in women with severe preeclampsia is appropriate. In the absence of large prospective randomized trials with tight control of inclusion criteria (i.e., antihypertensive medications, magnesium sulfate), it seems reasonable to use spinal anesthesia in women with severe preeclampsia to avoid the risks associated with emergency administration of general anesthesia.[262,263]

General Anesthesia

General anesthesia is less desirable than neuraxial anesthesia because of (1) the possibility of difficult intubation secondary to airway edema and (2) the transient but severe hypertension that accompanies endotracheal intubation (see Figure 45-7). Nonetheless, there are times when general anesthesia is the best anesthetic option. Clinical indications include severe ongoing maternal hemorrhage, sustained fetal bradycardia with a reassuring maternal airway examination, and severe thrombocytopenia or other coagulopathy. The platelet count can fall dramatically with rapidly progressing severe preeclampsia or HELLP syndrome and may mandate administration of general anesthesia. Major placental abruption, intrauterine fetal demise, and preeclampsia all increase the risk of DIC. The safe administration of general anesthesia in women with preeclampsia requires both careful preparation when time permits and an advanced state of readiness when time is limited.

Once the decision has been made to proceed with general anesthesia, the anesthesia provider faces three specific challenges: (1) the potential difficulty of securing the airway, (2) the hypertensive response to direct laryngoscopy and endotracheal intubation, and (3) the effects of magnesium sulfate on neuromuscular transmission and uterine tone. A suggested technique for the administration of general anesthesia is described in Box 45-4.

Airway Considerations Before the induction of general anesthesia, careful airway examination is mandatory. Airway edema may be present even with relatively reassuring airway findings; thus many anesthesia providers try to avoid emergency administration of general anesthesia if there is any suspicion of a difficult airway. Endotracheal tubes in various sizes and difficult airway equipment should be immediately available (see Chapter 30). In unusually difficult situations, it may be prudent to have an otolaryngology surgeon immediately available to establish a surgical airway. One of the dangers of repeated intubation attempts is the risk of traumatic bleeding in the airway, which may make ventilation difficult or impossible. It is wise to avoid repeated attempts and to proceed with insertion of a laryngeal mask airway (LMA)—while maintaining gentle cricoid pressure—before the airway is irretrievably lost. Because the LMA does not protect the patient from pulmonary aspiration of gastric contents, the obstetrician should be encouraged to complete the procedure as quickly as possible.

Hypertensive Response to Laryngoscopy The hemodynamic instability associated with rapid-sequence induction and endotracheal intubation presents a serious problem in the patient with preeclampsia. The transient but severe hypertension that may accompany intubation can result in cerebral hemorrhage or pulmonary edema, both of which are potentially fatal complications. Continuous arterial blood pressure monitoring is required for severely hypertensive women to monitor the effects of antihypertensive drugs administered before and after intubation and to allow rapid detection of adverse hemodynamic responses to laryngoscopy.

Antihypertensive medications that have been used to blunt the hemodynamic response to laryngoscopy include labetalol, esmolol, nitroglycerin, sodium nitroprusside, and remifentanil.[264-268] The goal of treatment is to reduce the arterial blood pressure to approximately 140 mm Hg systolic/90 mm Hg diastolic prior to the induction of general anesthesia. When possible, the FHR should be monitored during intravenous antihypertensive therapy.

Most anesthesia providers regard **labetalol** as the drug of choice for attenuating the hypertensive response to laryngoscopy in women with severe preeclampsia. Ramanathan et al.[266] compared intravenous labetalol with no treatment in a randomized study of preeclamptic women who received general anesthesia for cesarean delivery. Maternal mean arterial pressure rose following intubation in both study groups, but the hypertensive response was significantly less pronounced in the labetalol group. Women in the control group also developed tachycardia (in response to laryngoscopy and intubation), which did not occur in the labetalol group. Labetalol has been administered both via a bolus technique and as a continuous intravenous infusion.

BOX 45-4 Administration of General Anesthesia in Women with Severe Preeclampsia

1. Place a radial arterial cannula for continuous blood pressure monitoring in the woman with severe hypertension.
2. Place an additional intravenous catheter.
3. Make certain that smaller-sized endotracheal tubes and laryngeal mask airways are immediately available. Equipment needed for management of a difficult airway should also be immediately available.
4. Administer an H_2-receptor antagonist and metoclopramide IV between 30 and 60 minutes before induction of anesthesia.
5. Administer 30 mL of 0.3 M sodium citrate by mouth less than 30 minutes before induction of anesthesia.
6. Denitrogenate (3 minutes of tidal-volume breathing or 8 vital capacity breaths with an FIO_2 of 1.0 and a tight-fitting face mask).
7. Give labetalol (10-mg bolus doses) IV; titrate to desired effect before induction of anesthesia.
8. Continue to monitor the fetal heart rate during labetalol administration.
9. Consider alternative antihypertensive agents for patients who showed no response to labetalol (or those with a contraindication to labetalol). Alternatives include remifentanil (1 μg/kg as a single bolus), sodium nitroprusside infusion (starting at 0.5 μg/kg/min and titrated to effect), or nitroglycerin infusion (starting at 0.1 μg/kg/min and titrated to effect).
10. Perform rapid-sequence induction with either propofol 2 to 2.5 mg/kg or sodium thiopental 4 to 5 mg/kg and succinylcholine 1.0 to 1.5 mg/kg.
11. Maintain anesthesia with 50% nitrous oxide and a volatile halogenated agent. After delivery, consider giving an opioid with or without a benzodiazepine. If additional muscle relaxation is required, administer a *reduced dose* of a short-acting nondepolarizing muscle relaxant.
12. At the end of surgery, reverse neuromuscular blockade and give labetalol 5 to 10 mg IV to prevent hypertension during emergence and extubation.

IV, intravenously.

Adapted from Ramanathan J, Bennett K. Preeclampsia: Fluids, drugs, and anesthetic management. Anesthesiol Clin North Am 2003;21:145-63.

There is also evidence of safe short-term administration of **esmolol** in this setting. A randomized double-blind study of 80 hypertensive women presenting for cesarean delivery demonstrated that intravenous esmolol—in doses as high as 2 mg/kg—can be safely used to dampen the hemodynamic response to laryngoscopy and intubation.[269]

Nitroglycerin has many desirable properties for blunting the hypertensive response to intubation. It is a direct vasodilator with a rapid onset, is rapidly metabolized, and has no apparent maternal or fetal toxicity. In a randomized controlled trial, Hood et al.[265] administered intravenous nitroglycerin (200 μg/mL), which was titrated to lower mean arterial blood pressure by 20% prior to induction of general anesthesia. The maximal blood pressure with endotracheal intubation was significantly lower in the nitroglycerin group than in women who did not receive nitroglycerin. Both Apgar scores and umbilical cord blood gas and acid-base measurements were similar in the two groups.

Sodium nitroprusside infusions have also been used to attenuate hemodynamic responses to intubation in women with severe preeclampsia. An intravenous infusion can be initiated at 0.5 μg/kg/min and then titrated to blood pressure response. Short-term infusions are considered safe for the fetus (as discussed earlier).

The short-acting opioid **remifentanil,** which is rapidly metabolized in both mother and neonate by nonspecific blood and tissue esterases, has been administered to preeclamptic women. A clear advantage of remifentanil over other opioids is the rapid onset and short duration of the drug; the limited duration of action should not interfere with the resumption of spontaneous ventilation if intubation is unsuccessful. Ngan Kee et al.[268] randomly assigned 40 pregnant women without preeclampsia who required general anesthesia for cesarean delivery to receive either a one-time intravenous dose of remifentanil 1 μg/kg or saline immediately prior to induction. The primary outcome was the maximum increase in systolic blood pressure (in comparison with a baseline measurement). Administration of remifentanil significantly reduced the maximum increase in maternal systolic pressure. However, remifentanil crosses the placenta, and two neonates in the remifentanil group required naloxone administration for poor respiratory effort.

Effects of Magnesium Sulfate Most severely preeclamptic women present to the operating room after varying durations of exposure to magnesium sulfate for seizure prophylaxis. The primary anesthetic considerations for women receiving magnesium sulfate are (1) interaction with nondepolarizing muscle relaxants, (2) effects on uterine tone, and (3) interaction with calcium entry–blocking agents, specifically nimodipine.

Magnesium inhibits the release of acetylcholine at the neuromuscular junction, decreases the sensitivity of the neuromuscular junction to acetylcholine, and depresses the excitability of the muscle fiber membrane. Magnesium sulfate has been demonstrated to increase the potency and duration of vecuronium, rocuronium, and mivacurium.[270-272] Several case reports have described a requirement for overnight mechanical ventilation after administration of routine doses of vecuronium in women receiving magnesium sulfate.[270,273] Because of this interaction, if nondepolarizing muscle relaxants are used, they should be administered in very small doses and the response should be monitored carefully with a peripheral nerve stimulator.

Even though succinylcholine mimics acetylcholine at the nerve terminal, the onset and duration of a single intubating dose of succinylcholine is not prolonged when administered concurrently with a magnesium sulfate infusion[274]; a routine intubating dose of 1 to 1.5 mg/kg should be used during rapid-sequence induction.

Used for many years as a tocolytic agent, magnesium depresses smooth muscle contractions and inhibits CNS catecholamine release.[275-277] After a prolonged magnesium sulfate infusion, it seems intuitive that the risk of uterine atony and excessive blood loss might be increased.[172] However, studies have not found an increased risk of blood loss in women receiving magnesium sulfate.[166,172] A blood sample for type and screen should be sent to the blood bank prior to cesarean delivery, and uterotonic agents should be immediately available.

The calcium entry–blocking agent nifedipine may interact with magnesium sulfate to have adverse effects. A possibly greater hypotensive effect of nifedipine and neuromuscular blockade has been reported when the drugs were administered concomitantly.[159-162] Severe hypotension and fetal compromise have also been reported with use of the two drugs.[159,160]

Postoperative Analgesia

Options for postoperative analgesia are the same as for uncomplicated pregnancies. They include patient-controlled intravenous opioids, neuraxial opioids (single injection), and continuous epidural infusion of analgesic agents. Many anesthesia providers prefer neuraxial opioid administration for postcesarean analgesia (see Chapter 28). In the rare case of a woman with continuing severe refractory hypertension, continuous epidural analgesia is attractive for its blood pressure–modulating properties.

Regardless of the postoperative analgesic technique, all preeclamptic women should be carefully monitored with pulse oximetry for signs of respiratory depression or airway obstruction.

Postpartum Management

The risks of severe preeclampsia do not end with delivery. Postpartum women are at significant risk for pulmonary edema, sustained hypertension, stroke, venous thromboembolism, airway obstruction, and seizures, and should receive close monitoring of blood pressure, fluid intake, and urine output. In addition, severe preeclampsia, HELLP syndrome, and eclampsia can present for the first time in the postpartum period. A study of almost 4000 women diagnosed with preeclampsia found that the incidence of postpartum disease onset was 5.7%.[104]

The risk of **pulmonary edema** is also highest in the postpartum period. Resolution of preeclampsia usually occurs within 5 days of delivery and is heralded by a marked diuresis that follows mobilization of extracellular fluid and an increase in the intravascular volume. As a consequence, women with severe preeclampsia, particularly those with early-onset disease, renal insufficiency, or pulmonary capillary leak, are at higher risk for the development of pulmonary edema.[16]

In contrast to women with gestational hypertension, who typically become normotensive within a week of delivery, women with severe preeclampsia may have a longer duration of hypertension; the risk of **cerebral vascular accident** is highest during this time.[191,278] Antihypertensive therapy should be started or resumed for these women, and blood pressure should be carefully monitored during therapy.

Venous thromboembolism (VTE) has an estimated incidence of 0.5 per 1000 cesarean deliveries[279] and is a leading cause of maternal death in pregnancy.[280] The risk factors for antepartum and postpartum events differ, suggesting a different pathophysiology for each.[281] Both cesarean delivery[281-284] and preeclampsia[281,282] are independent risk factors for postpartum VTE. An emergency cesarean delivery doubles the risk of VTE compared with a nonemergency cesarean delivery.[285] The 2008 American College of Chest Physicians Evidence-Based Clinical Practice Guidelines recommend that women at increased risk for post–cesarean delivery VTE (because of the presence of an additional risk factor such as preeclampsia) receive either pharmacologic thromboprophylaxis or mechanical prophylaxis (e.g., intermittent pneumatic compression devices) while in the hospital after cesarean delivery.[286]

A review of eight anesthesia-related maternal deaths in Michigan found that all anesthesia-related deaths from **airway obstruction** or **hypoventilation** occurred in the postoperative period and that system errors, lapses in postoperative monitoring, and inadequate supervision by the anesthesia providers played a role in these deaths.[287] One of the women who died had severe preeclampsia and sleep-disordered breathing and was found pulseless and apneic in her hospital room. In another study, investigators found greater upper airway resistance in women with preeclampsia during sleep than in women without preeclampsia.[288] Both studies highlight the need for close monitoring and consistent vigilance in the postoperative care of women with severe preeclampsia—particularly those with generalized edema, known airway swelling, snoring, and obesity.

Long-Term Outcomes

There is mounting evidence that women with a history of preeclampsia are at increased risk of chronic hypertension and cardiovascular disease in later life,[47-49,53,289,290] and for an earlier onset of cardiovascular disease during their lives.[47-49,51,53,289,290] Ischemic heart disease and stroke are the most common manifestations of cardiovascular morbidity. Also, mortality in women with a history of preeclampsia is double that in women whose pregnancies were not complicated by a maternal placental syndrome; Funai et al.[51] concluded that excess risk of death was primarily the result of cardiovascular disease. In the first 10 to 15 years after the occurrence of preeclampsia, the risk of cardiovascular disease and death appears to be low, but it increases markedly thereafter.[52]

In addition, there is evidence of a dose-response relationship between preeclampsia and cardiovascular disease. Women who have severe preeclampsia or early-onset preeclampsia and whose pregnancies are complicated by both preeclampsia (the maternal syndrome) and intrauterine growth restriction (the fetal syndrome) are at higher risk than women with mild preeclampsia or gestational hypertension.[50] Women with preeclampsia in both their first and second pregnancies are at even greater risk for future ischemic heart disease.[49]

The mechanism of the greater risk of cardiovascular disease in preeclampsia is unclear. It is possible that preeclampsia causes permanent damage to the endothelium and hastens the onset of cardiovascular disease. Women with a history of preeclampsia have persistent impairment of brachial artery endothelium-dependent vascular relaxation at 1 to 3 years after delivery, a finding not seen in controls.[291,292] A more likely explanation is that preeclampsia and cardiovascular disease have a common pathogenesis owing to shared risk factors. Common risk factors for preeclampsia and atherosclerosis include hypertension, obesity, insulin resistance, advanced age, hypercholesterolemia, and dyslipidemia.[53,293,294] Cigarette smoking is the notable exception, in that it is an established risk factor for cardiovascular disease but is protective against preeclampsia.[55,56] Preeclampsia may be a cardiovascular risk marker in women with an underlying predisposition to vascular disease; the metabolic stress of pregnancy causes the predisposition to manifest as preeclampsia. After pregnancy women return to a normal state until the threshold for disease development is exceeded in later life. This hypothesis is illustrated in Figure 45-9.

Regardless of the mechanism of increased risk, these observations represent an opportunity for primary disease prevention and risk factor modification. In a 2004 multinational study, 90% of the risk of a first myocardial infarction was attributed to potentially modifiable risk factors.[295] Possible interventions include earlier cardiovascular disease screening and individual counseling about the importance of smoking cessation, regular exercise, and a diet low in saturated fat and high in antioxidants.

In contrast, a history of preeclampsia has been associated with a *decreased* risk of cancer. Several studies have suggested that women who have been diagnosed with preeclampsia have a slightly lower risk for breast cancer in later life than other parous women.[296-300] In contrast, a systematic review and meta-analysis of almost 200,000 women with a history of preeclampsia found no association between preeclampsia and future cancer risk.[52]

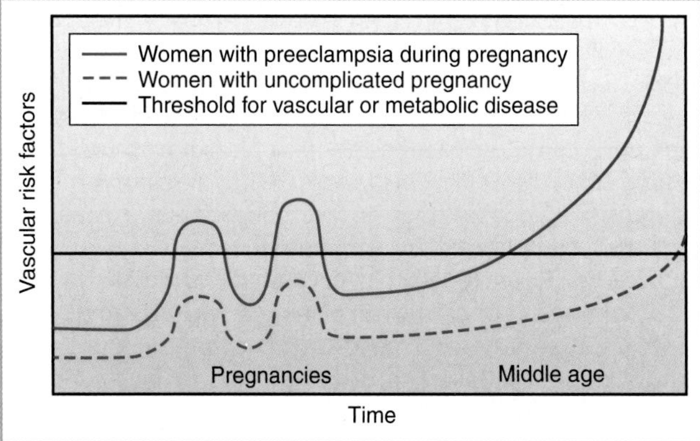

FIGURE 45-9 Vascular risk factors versus time. (From Sattar N, Greer IA. Pregnancy complications and maternal cardiovascular risk: Opportunities for intervention and screening? Br Med J 2002; 325:157-60.)

Preliminary evidence indicates that preeclampsia may also have psychological sequelae. Post-traumatic stress disorder (PTSD) is an anxiety disorder that can develop after exposure to one or more terrifying events that threatened or caused grave physical harm.[301] A woman with a history of severe preeclampsia (particularly with early-onset disease and preterm delivery) has experienced a serious complication that threatened her life and the life of her child. Case reports have described the onset of PTSD after pregnancies complicated by severe preeclampsia or HELLP syndrome.[302] In an exploratory study, approximately one fourth of women experienced PTSD after early-onset preeclampsia.[303] Further research is required to define women at risk for PTSD and to investigate strategies for its prevention and intervention.

ECLAMPSIA

Eclampsia is defined as the new onset of seizures or unexplained coma during pregnancy or the postpartum period in a woman with signs and symptoms of preeclampsia and without a preexisting neurologic disorder.[304-306]

Epidemiology

Findings of population-based studies in the past 10 years suggest that the incidence of eclampsia varies from 0.1 to 5.5 per 10,000 pregnancies in western countries.[1,17,307-310] On average, studies have shown a decrease in the incidence of eclampsia over time (i.e., from 1.04 to 0.8 per 10,000 pregnancies in the United States, and from 4.9 to 2.7 per 10,000 pregnancies in the United Kingdom).[17,309] The variation in rates of eclampsia among studies likely reflects reporting differences among countries or differences in treatment for severe preeclampsia.[309,311]

Eclampsia can occur suddenly at any point in the puerperium; however, most seizures occur intrapartum or within the first 48 hours after delivery. Late eclampsia is defined as seizure onset from 48 hours after delivery to less than 4 weeks postpartum.[305,312] The majority of eclamptic women have evidence of severe preeclampsia, but in 10% to 15% of cases, hypertension is absent or modest and/or proteinuria is not detected.[312] Recent data indicate that an important risk factor for eclampsia is maternal age less than 20 years.[17] Other reported risks include nulliparity, multiple gestation, molar pregnancy, triploidy, preexisting hypertension or renal disease, previous severe preeclampsia or eclampsia, nonimmune hydrops fetalis, and systemic lupus erythematosus.[313] Major maternal complications of eclampsia include pulmonary aspiration, pulmonary edema, cerebral vascular accident, cardiopulmonary arrest, acute renal failure, and death.[9,308,309] Eclampsia is associated with a high perinatal death rate and can be associated with placental abruption, severe intrauterine growth restriction, and extreme prematurity.[304,308,309]

Clinical Presentation and Diagnosis

Any of the pathophysiologic changes of preeclampsia can be present in eclampsia. Premonitory signs and symptoms include persistent occipital or frontal headaches, blurred vision, photophobia, epigastric or right upper quadrant pain, hyperreflexia, and altered mental status[304,312]; these symptoms can occur before or after the onset of seizures.[304]

Seizures have an abrupt onset, typically beginning as facial twitching that is followed by a tonic phase persisting for 15 to 20 seconds. This progresses to a generalized clonic phase characterized by apnea, which lasts approximately 1 minute. Breathing generally resumes with a long stertorous inspiration, and the patient enters a postictal state with a variable period of coma. Cardiorespiratory arrest and pulmonary aspiration of gastric contents can complicate a seizure. Although the definitive diagnosis for eclampsia is a sudden seizure in a pregnant woman who has signs and symptoms of preeclampsia, a woman who lapses into coma without witnessed convulsions can also be classified as eclamptic.[304]

The mechanism of eclamptic seizures remains poorly understood.[95,306] One hypothesis involves a loss of the normal cerebral autoregulatory mechanism that results in hyperperfusion and leads to interstitial or vasogenic cerebral edema and decreased cerebral blood flow.[7,189,190,306] Neuroradiologic studies suggest that eclampsia might be a form of reversible posterior leukoencephalopathy syndrome (PLES)[314] or posterior reversible encephalopathy syndrome (PRES).[315] The difference between PLES and PRES is that significant blood pressure elevations are not necessarily present in PRES.[316]

Until proven otherwise, the occurrence of seizures during pregnancy should be considered eclampsia. Conditions that simulate eclampsia include seizure disorder, stroke, hypertensive encephalopathy, ischemia or hypoxia, cerebral space-occupying lesion, systemic disease (e.g., systemic lupus erythematosus, sickle cell anemia), infection (e.g., meningitis, encephalitis), electrolyte and endocrine disturbances, PRES or PLES, vasculitis or angiopathy, amniotic fluid embolism, medications (withdrawal, illicit drug use), and organ failure.[95,305]

Obstetric Management

Immediate goals are to stop convulsions, establish a patent airway, and prevent major complications (e.g., hypoxemia, aspiration). Further obstetric management consists of antihypertensive therapy, induction or augmentation of labor, and expeditious (preferably vaginal) delivery. Fetal bradycardia typically occurs during and/or immediately after a seizure but does not mandate immediate delivery unless it is persistent.

Resuscitation and Seizure Control

During the seizure, oxygenation may prove impossible, but supplemental oxygen should be delivered by means of an Ambu bag and face mask (Box 45-5). Attempts to insert an oral airway should be withheld until the seizure abates, but insertion of a soft nasopharyngeal airway may facilitate oxygenation. As soon as breathing resumes, ventilation may be gently augmented with a bag-mask device. Pulse oximetry should be used to assess maternal oxygenation. Blood pressure and electrocardiography should be monitored to identify hypertension, arrhythmia, or cardiac arrest. While initial resuscitation is under way, an assistant should establish intravenous access, which can be difficult in a combative postictal woman. Judicious sedation might be required to allow further treatment in some patients.

BOX 45-5 Eclampsia: The ABCs of Seizure Control

Airway
- Turn patient to left side; apply jaw thrust.
- Attempt bag and mask ventilation (F_{IO_2} = 1.0).
- Insert soft nasopharyngeal airway if necessary.

Breathing
- Continue bag and mask ventilation (F_{IO_2} = 1.0).
- Apply pulse oximeter and monitor Sa_{O_2}.

Circulation
- Secure intravenous access.
- Check blood pressure at frequent intervals.
- Monitor electrocardiogram.

Drugs
- Magnesium sulfate:
  - 4 to 6 g IV over 20 minutes
  - 1 to 2 g/hr IV for maintenance therapy
  - 2 g IV, over 10 minutes, for recurrent seizures
- Antihypertensive agents:
  - Labetalol 10 to 20 mg IV or hydralazine 5 to 10 mg IV as needed to treat hypertension

IV, intravenously.

Magnesium sulfate is the preferred drug worldwide for the prevention of further seizures in eclampsia (as discussed earlier).[163,166,317] The administration of magnesium sulfate in eclamptic women is also associated with significantly lower maternal death rates. An initial intravenous bolus of 4 to 6 g is administered, followed by an infusion at 1 to 2 g/hr, assuming the patient has adequate urine output.[318] Recurrent convulsions should prompt administration of an additional bolus of 2 to 4 g, infused over 5 to 10 minutes.[318] The patient should be carefully monitored for signs of magnesium toxicity.

Anesthetic Management

The preanesthetic management of an eclamptic woman parallels that of a patient with severe preeclampsia (as discussed earlier). Management considerations specific to the woman with eclampsia are as follows[180,304,319]:

1. **Assessment of seizure control and neurologic function**. The possibility of increased intracranial pressure is not a cause for concern if the patient remains conscious, alert, and seizure-free. Persistent coma and localizing signs may indicate major intracranial pathology, which could affect anesthetic management (see later).
2. **Maintenance of fluid balance**. Intake should be restricted to 75 to 100 mL/hr to minimize the risk of exacerbating cerebral edema.
3. **Blood pressure control**. Antihypertensive therapy should be instituted if the systolic pressure exceeds 160 mm Hg, or if the diastolic pressure exceeds 110 mm Hg.
4. **Continuous pulse oximetry monitoring** of maternal oxygenation.

5. **Continuous FHR monitoring.**
6. **Laboratory investigations** are the same as in preeclampsia, with the addition of **coagulation studies,** which should be obtained regardless of the platelet count.

The anesthesia plan is tailored to the individual case. In conscious eclamptic women with no evidence of increased intracranial pressure and whose seizures are well-controlled, epidural analgesia/anesthesia can be considered. In a retrospective review of 66 stable South African women with eclampsia, Moodley et al.[320] found no difference in maternal and neonatal outcomes between epidural anesthesia and general anesthesia for cesarean delivery.

Eclamptic seizures are likely associated with an increase in intracranial pressure. In the rare instance of requirement for immediate delivery in a woman with ongoing seizures, a neuroanesthetic technique should be considered. Intravenous induction agents such as propofol[321] and pentothal[322] reduce both cerebral metabolic rate and cerebral blood flow, with consequent decreases in cerebral blood volume and intracranial pressure. These agents are also effective in terminating seizures.[323,324] Because hyperventilation reduces cerebral blood flow without a reduction in cerebral metabolic rate, it should be employed with caution. On the other hand, hypoventilation is associated with hypercarbia, which can lower the seizure threshold. In order to prevent further neurologic injury, it is important not to be overly aggressive in the reduction of systemic pressure, because cerebral perfusion pressure equals mean arterial pressure minus intracranial pressure.[325] Avoidance of hypoxia, hyperthermia, and hyperglycemia are also important in avoiding an exacerbation of neurologic injury.[326] Patients who have not recovered neurologically should remain intubated and should be monitored in an intensive care unit. If unconsciousness persists, further neurologic evaluation, including electroencephalography and computed tomography, should be performed.

Long-Term Outcomes

Neurologic abnormalities occurring in patients with eclampsia (e.g., cortical blindness, focal motor deficits, coma) do not usually result in permanent neurologic deficits.[95] However, a study by Aukes et al.[327] found that formerly eclamptic women had significantly more cognitive failures several (7.6 ± 5.0) years after the index pregnancy; the investigators hypothesized that cognitive failures might be related to some degree of white matter change.

KEY POINTS

- Preeclampsia is a multisystem disorder of pregnancy characterized by a maternal syndrome with or without a fetal syndrome.
- Preeclampsia is a leading cause of maternal and perinatal morbidity and mortality worldwide, particularly in developing countries.
- The etiology of preeclampsia remains unknown.
- The pathophysiology of preeclampsia involves superficial placentation related to abnormal angiogenesis, placental hypoxia, and release of soluble substances toxic to vascular endothelium.
- Management of preeclampsia is supportive, and delivery of the fetus and placenta is the only definitive cure.
- Preeclampsia likely consists of more than one disease; early-onset disease (less than 34 weeks' gestation) carries a worse prognosis than late-onset disease.
- Systemic disease manifestations result from widespread maternal vascular endothelial dysfunction.
- Complications of severe preeclampsia include severe refractory hypertension, cerebrovascular accident, pulmonary edema, placental abruption, renal failure, and HELLP syndrome.
- Important hematologic changes that may occur in preeclamptic women include thrombocytopenia, hypercoagulability (with mild disease), hypocoagulability (with severe disease), and disseminated intravascular coagulation.
- There are no indications for invasive central monitoring that are unique to preeclampsia; indications are similar to those in other multisystem disorders, such as severe sepsis and multisystem organ dysfunction.
- Preeclamptic women are at risk for airway edema. The anesthesia provider should anticipate the possibility of a difficult airway.
- The hypertensive response to direct laryngoscopy and intubation can cause intracranial hemorrhage in women with severe preeclampsia.
- Spinal anesthesia is acceptable for women with severe preeclampsia, especially as an alternative to general anesthesia for emergency cesarean delivery.
- The risks of pulmonary edema, cerebrovascular accident, and venous thromboembolism are higher in the postpartum period.

REFERENCES

1. Zhang J, Meikle S, Trumble A. Severe maternal morbidity associated with hypertensive disorders in pregnancy in the United States. Hypertens Pregnancy 2003; 22:203-12.
2. Duley L. Maternal mortality associated with hypertensive disorders of pregnancy in Africa, Asia, Latin America and the Caribbean. Br J Obstet Gynaecol 1992; 99:547-53.
3. Hauth JC, Ewell MG, Levine RJ, et al. Pregnancy outcomes in healthy nulliparas who developed hypertension. Calcium for Preeclampsia Prevention Study Group. Obstet Gynecol 2000; 95:24-8.
4. Sibai BM, Caritis SN, Thom E, et al. Prevention of preeclampsia with low-dose aspirin in healthy, nulliparous pregnant women. The National Institute of Child Health and Human Development Network of Maternal-Fetal Medicine Units. N Engl J Med 1993; 329:1213-8.
5. Knuist M, Bonsel GJ, Zondervan HA, Treffers PE. Intensification of fetal and maternal surveillance in pregnant women with hypertensive disorders. Int J Gynaecol Obstet 1998; 61:127-33.
6. Barton JR, O'Brien JM, Bergauer NK, et al. Mild gestational hypertension remote from term: Progression and outcome. Am J Obstet Gynecol 2001; 184:979-83.

7. Report of the National High Blood Pressure Education Program Working Group on High Blood Pressure in Pregnancy. Am J Obstet Gynecol 2000; 183:S1-22.
8. Giannubilo SR, Dell'Uomo B, Tranquilli AL. Perinatal outcomes, blood pressure patterns and risk assessment of superimposed preeclampsia in mild chronic hypertensive pregnancy. Eur J Obstet Gynecol Reprod Biol 2006; 126:63-7.
9. Mattar F, Sibai BM. Eclampsia. VIII. Risk factors for maternal morbidity. Am J Obstet Gynecol 2000; 182:307-12.
10. Buhimschi CS, Magloire L, Funai E, et al. Fractional excretion of angiogenic factors in women with severe preeclampsia. Obstet Gynecol 2006; 107:1103-13.
11. Martin J, Hamilton B, Sutton P, et al. Births: Final data for 2004. Natl Vital Stat Rep 2006; 55:1-101.
12. Basso O, Rasmussen S, Weinberg CR, et al. Trends in fetal and infant survival following preeclampsia. JAMA 2006; 296:1357-62.
13. Gilbert WM, Nesbitt TS, Danielsen B. The cost of prematurity: Quantification by gestational age and birth weight. Obstet Gynecol 2003; 102:488-92.
14. Lee SK, McMillan DD, Ohlsson A, et al. Variations in practice and outcomes in the Canadian NICU network: 1996-1997. Pediatrics 2000; 106:1070-9.
15. Umo-Etuk J, Lumley J, Holdcroft A. Critically ill parturient women and admission to intensive care: A 5-year review. Int J Obstet Anesth 1996; 5:79-84.
16. Sibai BM. Diagnosis and management of gestational hypertension and preeclampsia. Obstet Gynecol 2003; 102:181-92.
17. Wallis AB, Saftlas AF, Hsia J, Atrash HK. Secular trends in the rates of preeclampsia, eclampsia, and gestational hypertension, United States, 1987-2004. Am J Hypertens 2008; 21:521-6.
18. Ventura S, Taffel S, Mathews T. Advance report of maternal and infant health data from the birth certificate, 1990. Monthly Vital Stat Rep 1993; 42:1-62.
19. Martin J, Hamilton B, Sutton P, et al. Centers for Disease Control and Prevention, National Center for Health Statistics, National Vital Statistics System. Births: Final data for 2005. Natl Vital Stat Rep 2007; 56:1-103.
20. Keegan DA, Krey LC, Chang HC, Noyes N. Increased risk of pregnancy-induced hypertension in young recipients of donated oocytes. Fertil Steril 2007; 87:776-81.
21. Einarsson JI, Sangi-Haghpeykar H, Gardner MO. Sperm exposure and development of preeclampsia. Am J Obstet Gynecol 2003; 188:1241-3.
22. Smith GN, Walker M, Tessier JL, Millar KG. Increased incidence of preeclampsia in women conceiving by intrauterine insemination with donor versus partner sperm for treatment of primary infertility. Am J Obstet Gynecol 1997; 177:455-8.
23. Lie RT, Rasmussen S, Brunborg H, et al. Fetal and maternal contributions to risk of pre-eclampsia: Population based study. Br Med J 1998; 316:1343-7.
24. Hnat MD, Sibai BM, Caritis S, et al. Perinatal outcome in women with recurrent preeclampsia compared with women who develop preeclampsia as nulliparas. Am J Obstet Gynecol 2002; 186:422-6.
25. Barton JR, Sibai BM. Prediction and prevention of recurrent preeclampsia. Obstet Gynecol 2008; 112:359-72.
26. Gillum RF. Epidemiology of hypertension in African American women. Am Heart J 1996; 131:385-95.
27. Cooper RS, Liao Y, Rotimi C. Is hypertension more severe among U.S. blacks, or is severe hypertension more common? Ann Epidemiol 1996; 6:173-80.
28. Hertz RP, Unger AN, Cornell JA, Saunders E. Racial disparities in hypertension prevalence, awareness, and management. Arch Intern Med 2005; 165:2098-104.
29. Kieffer EC, Carman WJ, Gillespie BW, et al. Obesity and gestational diabetes among African-American women and Latinas in Detroit: Implications for disparities in women's health. J Am Med Womens Assoc 2001; 56:181-7, 96.
30. Ehrenberg HM, Dierker L, Milluzzi C, Mercer BM. Prevalence of maternal obesity in an urban center. Am J Obstet Gynecol 2002; 187:1189-93.
31. Rosenberg TJ, Garbers S, Chavkin W, Chiasson MA. Prepregnancy weight and adverse perinatal outcomes in an ethnically diverse population. Obstet Gynecol 2003; 102:1022-7.
32. Hedley AA, Ogden CL, Johnson CL, et al. Prevalence of overweight and obesity among US children, adolescents, and adults, 1999-2002. JAMA 2004; 291:2847-50.
33. LaCoursiere DY, Bloebaum L, Duncan JD, Varner MW. Population-based trends and correlates of maternal overweight and obesity, Utah, 1991-2001. Am J Obstet Gynecol 2005; 192:832-9.
34. Samadi AR, Mayberry RM, Zaidi AA, et al. Maternal hypertension and associated pregnancy complications among African-American and other women in the United States. Obstet Gynecol 1996; 87:557-63.
35. Sibai BM, Ewell M, Levine RJ, et al. Risk factors associated with preeclampsia in healthy nulliparous women. The Calcium for Preeclampsia Prevention (CPEP) Study Group. Am J Obstet Gynecol 1997; 177:1003-10.
36. Samadi AR, Mayberry RM, Reed JW. Preeclampsia associated with chronic hypertension among African-American and white women. Ethn Dis 2001; 11:192-200.
37. Caughey AB, Stotland NE, Washington AE, Escobar GJ. Maternal ethnicity, paternal ethnicity, and parental ethnic discordance: Predictors of preeclampsia. Obstet Gynecol 2005; 106:156-61.
38. Shen JJ, Tymkow C, MacMullen N. Disparities in maternal outcomes among four ethnic populations. Ethn Dis 2005; 15:492-7.
39. Goodwin AA, Mercer BM. Does maternal race or ethnicity affect the expression of severe preeclampsia? Am J Obstet Gynecol 2005; 193:973-8.
40. Tucker MJ, Berg CJ, Callaghan WM, Hsia J. The black-white disparity in pregnancy-related mortality from 5 conditions: Differences in prevalence and case-fatality rates. Am J Public Health 2007; 97:247-51.
41. O'Brien TE, Ray JG, Chan WS. Maternal body mass index and the risk of preeclampsia: A systematic overview. Epidemiology 2003; 14:368-74.
42. Samuels-Kalow ME, Funai EF, Buhimschi C, et al. Prepregnancy body mass index, hypertensive disorders of pregnancy, and long-term maternal mortality. Am J Obstet Gynecol 2007; 197:490.e1-6.
43. Mazar RM, Srinivas SK, Sammel MD, et al. Metabolic score as a novel approach to assessing preeclampsia risk. Am J Obstet Gynecol 2007; 197:411.e1-5.
44. Roberts JM, Pearson G, Cutler J, Lindheimer M. National Heart, Lung and Blood Institute. Summary of the NHLBI Working Group on Research on Hypertension during Pregnancy. Hypertens Pregnancy 2003; 22:109-27.
45. Garner PR, D'Alton ME, Dudley DK, et al. Preeclampsia in diabetic pregnancies. Am J Obstet Gynecol 1990; 163:505-8.
46. Ford ES, Giles WH, Dietz WH. Prevalence of the metabolic syndrome among US adults: Findings from the third National Health and Nutrition Examination Survey. JAMA 2002; 287:356-9.
47. Smith GC, Pell JP, Walsh D. Pregnancy complications and maternal risk of ischaemic heart disease: A retrospective cohort study of 129,290 births. Lancet 2001; 357:2002-6.
48. Irgens HU, Reisaeter L, Irgens LM, Lie RT. Long term mortality of mothers and fathers after pre-eclampsia: Population based cohort study. Br Med J 2001; 323:1213-7.
49. Wilson BJ, Watson MS, Prescott GJ, et al. Hypertensive diseases of pregnancy and risk of hypertension and stroke in later life: Results from cohort study. Br Med J 2003; 326:845.
50. Ray JG, Vermeulen MJ, Schull MJ, Redelmeier DA. Cardiovascular health after maternal placental syndromes (CHAMPS): Population-based retrospective cohort study. Lancet 2005; 366:1797-803.
51. Funai EF, Friedlander Y, Paltiel O, et al. Long-term mortality after preeclampsia. Epidemiology 2005; 16:206-15.
52. Bellamy L, Casas JP, Hingorani AD, Williams DJ. Pre-eclampsia and risk of cardiovascular disease and cancer in later life: Systematic review and meta-analysis. Br Med J 2007; 335:974.
53. Ramsay JE, Stewart F, Greer IA, Sattar N. Microvascular dysfunction: A link between pre-eclampsia and maternal coronary heart disease. Br J Obstet Gynaecol 2003; 110:1029-31.

54. Zhang J, Klebanoff MA, Levine RJ, et al. The puzzling association between smoking and hypertension during pregnancy. Am J Obstet Gynecol 1999; 181:1407-13.
55. Conde-Agudelo A, Althabe F, Belizan JM, Kafury-Goeta AC. Cigarette smoking during pregnancy and risk of preeclampsia: A systematic review. Am J Obstet Gynecol 1999; 181:1026-35.
56. England LJ, Levine RJ, Qian C, et al. Smoking before pregnancy and risk of gestational hypertension and preeclampsia. Am J Obstet Gynecol 2002; 186:1035-40.
57. Marcoux S, Brisson J, Fabia J. The effect of cigarette smoking on the risk of preeclampsia and gestational hypertension. Am J Epidemiol 1989; 130:950-7.
58. Luttun A, Carmeliet P. Soluble VEGF receptor Flt1: The elusive preeclampsia factor discovered? J Clin Invest 2003; 111:600-2.
59. Brosens I, Robertson WB, Dixon HG. The physiological response of the vessels of the placental bed to normal pregnancy. J Pathol Bacteriol 1967; 93:569-79.
60. Keogh RJ, Harris LK, Freeman A, et al. Fetal-derived trophoblast use the apoptotic cytokine tumor necrosis factor-alpha-related apoptosis-inducing ligand to induce smooth muscle cell death. Circ Res 2007; 100:834-41.
61. Khong TY, De Wolf F, Robertson WB, Brosens I. Inadequate maternal vascular response to placentation in pregnancies complicated by pre-eclampsia and by small-for-gestational age infants. BJOG 1986; 93:1049-59.
62. Arias F, Rodriquez L, Rayne SC, Kraus FT. Maternal placental vasculopathy and infection: Two distinct subgroups among patients with preterm labor and preterm ruptured membranes. Am J Obstet Gynecol 1993; 168:585-91.
63. Zintzaras E, Kitsios G, Harrison GA, et al. Heterogeneity-based genome search meta-analysis for preeclampsia. Hum Genet 2006; 120:360-70.
64. Arngrimsson R, Bjornsson S, Geirsson RT, et al. Genetic and familial predisposition to eclampsia and pre-eclampsia in a defined population. Br J Obstet Gynaecol 1990; 97:762-9.
65. Redman CW, Sargent IL. Latest advances in understanding pre-eclampsia. Science 2005; 308:1592-4.
66. Skjaerven R, Vatten LJ, Wilcox AJ, et al. Recurrence of pre-eclampsia across generations: Exploring fetal and maternal genetic components in a population based cohort. Br Med J 2005; 331:877.
67. Pijnenborg R, Vercruysse L, Hanssens M. The uterine spiral arteries in human pregnancy: Facts and controversies. Placenta 2006; 27:939-58.
68. Oudejans CB, van Dijk M, Oosterkamp M, et al. Genetics of pre-eclampsia: Paradigm shifts. Hum Genet 2007; 120:607-12.
69. Haig D. Genetic conflicts in human pregnancy. Q Rev Biol 1993; 68:495-532.
70. Dekker G, Sibai B. Primary, secondary, and tertiary prevention of pre-eclampsia. Lancet 2001; 357:209-15.
71. Li DK, Wi S. Changing paternity and the risk of preeclampsia/eclampsia in the subsequent pregnancy. Am J Epidemiol 2000; 151:57-62.
72. Roberts JM, Gammill HS. Preeclampsia: Recent insights. Hypertension 2005; 46:1243-9.
73. Wallukat G, Homuth V, Fischer T, et al. Patients with preeclampsia develop agonistic autoantibodies against the angiotensin AT1 receptor. J Clin Invest 1999; 103:945-52.
74. Walther T, Wallukat G, Jank A, et al. Angiotensin II type 1 receptor agonistic antibodies reflect fundamental alterations in the uteroplacental vasculature. Hypertension 2005; 46:1275-9.
75. Dechend R, Homuth V, Wallukat G, et al. AT(1) receptor agonistic antibodies from preeclamptic patients cause vascular cells to express tissue factor. Circulation 2000; 101:2382-7.
76. Xia Y, Wen H, Bobst S, et al. Maternal autoantibodies from preeclamptic patients activate angiotensin receptors on human trophoblast cells. J Soc Gynecol Investig 2003; 10:82-93.
77. Dechend R, Viedt C, Muller DN, et al. AT1 receptor agonistic antibodies from preeclamptic patients stimulate NADPH oxidase. Circulation 2003; 107:1632-9.
78. Zhou CC, Zhang Y, Irani RA, et al. Angiotensin receptor agonistic autoantibodies induce pre-eclampsia in pregnant mice. Nat Med 2008; 14:855-62.
79. Gant NF, Daley GL, Chand S, et al. A study of angiotensin II pressor response throughout primigravid pregnancy. J Clin Invest 1973; 52:2682-9.
80. Maynard SE, Min J-Y, Merchan J, et al. Excess placental soluble fms-like tyrosine kinase 1 (sFlt1) may contribute to endothelial dysfunction, hypertension, and proteinuria in preeclampsia. J Clin Invest 2003; 111:649-58.
81. Venkatesha S, Toporsian M, Lam C, et al. Soluble endoglin contributes to the pathogenesis of preeclampsia. Nat Med 2006; 12:642.
82. Levine RJ, Karumanchi SA. Circulating angiogenic factors in pre-eclampsia. Clin Obstet Gynecol 2005; 48:372-86.
83. Levine RJ, Maynard SE, Qian C, et al. Circulating angiogenic factors and the risk of preeclampsia. N Engl J Med 2004; 350:672-83.
84. Jeyabalan A, Powers RW, Durica AR, et al. Cigarette smoke exposure and angiogenic factors in pregnancy and preeclampsia. Am J Hypertens 2008; 21:943-7.
85. Solomon CG, Seely EW. Preeclampsia—searching for the cause. N Engl J Med 2004; 350:641-2.
86. Kanasaki K, Palmsten K, Sugimoto H, et al. Deficiency in catechol-O-methyltransferase and 2-methoxyoestradiol is associated with pre-eclampsia. Nature 2008; 453:1117-23.
87. Baumwell S, Karumanchi SA. Pre-eclampsia: Clinical manifestations and molecular mechanisms. Nephron Clin Pract 2007; 106:c72-81.
88. Roberts JM. Preeclampsia: Is there value in assessing before clinically evident disease? Obstet Gynecol 2001; 98:596-9.
89. Dekker GA, Sibai BM. Low-dose aspirin in the prevention of pre-eclampsia and fetal growth retardation: Rationale, mechanisms, and clinical trials. Am J Obstet Gynecol 1993; 168:214-27.
90. Hauth JC, Goldenberg RL, Parker CR Jr, et al. Low-dose aspirin therapy to prevent preeclampsia. Am J Obstet Gynecol 1993; 168:1083-91.
91. CLASP: A randomised trial of low-dose aspirin for the prevention and treatment of pre-eclampsia among 9364 pregnant women. CLASP (Collaborative Low-dose Aspirin Study in Pregnancy) Collaborative Group. Lancet 1994; 343:619-29.
92. Caritis S, Sibai B, Hauth J, et al. Low-dose aspirin to prevent pre-eclampsia in women at high risk. N Engl J Med 1998; 338:701-5.
93. Coomarasamy A, Papaioannou S, Gee H, Khan KS. Aspirin for the prevention of preeclampsia in women with abnormal uterine artery Doppler: A meta-analysis. Obstet Gynecol 2001; 98:861-6.
94. Coomarasamy A, Honest H, Papaioannou S, et al. Aspirin for prevention of preeclampsia in women with historical risk factors: A systematic review. Obstet Gynecol 2003; 101:1319-32.
95. Sibai B. Hypertension. In Gabbe S, Niebyl J, Simpson J, editors. Obstetrics: Normal and Problem Pregnancies. 5th edition. Philadelphia, Churchill Livingstone, 2007:864-912.
96. Belizan JM, Villar J, Repke J. The relationship between calcium intake and pregnancy-induced hypertension: Up-to-date evidence. Am J Obstet Gynecol 1988; 158:898-902.
97. Bucher HC, Cook RJ, Guyatt GH, et al. Effects of dietary calcium supplementation on blood pressure: A meta-analysis of randomized controlled trials. JAMA 1996; 275:1016-22.
98. Levine RJ, Hauth JC, Curet LB, et al. Trial of calcium to prevent preeclampsia. N Engl J Med 1997; 337:69-76.
99. Rumbold AR, Crowther CA, Haslam RR, et al. Vitamins C and E and the risks of preeclampsia and perinatal complications. N Engl J Med 2006; 354:1796-806.
100. Beazley D, Ahokas R, Livingston J, et al. Vitamin C and E supplementation in women at high risk for preeclampsia: A double-blind, placebo-controlled trial. Am J Obstet Gynecol 2005; 192:520-1.
101. Poston L, Briley AL, Seed PT, et al. Vitamin C and vitamin E in pregnant women at risk for pre-eclampsia (VIP trial): Randomised placebo-controlled trial. Lancet 2006; 367:1145-54.
102. Rumbold A, Crowther CA. Vitamin C supplementation in pregnancy. Cochrane Database Syst Rev 2005; (2):CD004072.
103. Rumbold A, Crowther CA. Vitamin E supplementation in pregnancy. Cochrane Database Syst Rev 2005; (2):CD004069.
104. Matthys LA, Coppage KH, Lambers DS, et al. Delayed postpartum preeclampsia: An experience of 151 cases. Am J Obstet Gynecol 2004; 190:1464-6.

105. Sibai BM, Spinnato JA, Watson DL, et al. Eclampsia. IV: Neurological findings and future outcome. Am J Obstet Gynecol 1985; 152: 184-92.
106. Thomas SV. Neurological aspects of eclampsia. J Neurol Sci 1998; 155:37-43.
107. Okanloma KA, Moodley J. Neurological complications associated with the pre-eclampsia/eclampsia syndrome. Int J Gynaecol Obstet 2000; 71:223-5.
108. Belfort MA, Varner MW, Dizon-Townson DS, et al. Cerebral perfusion pressure, and not cerebral blood flow, may be the critical determinant of intracranial injury in preeclampsia: A new hypothesis. Am J Obstet Gynecol 2002; 187:626-34.
109. Rout CC. Anaesthesia and analgesia for the critically ill parturient. Best Pract Res Clin Obstet Gynaecol 2001; 15:507-22.
110. Sibai BM, Mabie BC, Harvey CJ, Gonzalez AR. Pulmonary edema in severe preeclampsia-eclampsia: Analysis of thirty-seven consecutive cases. Am J Obstet Gynecol 1987; 156:1174-9.
111. Zinaman M, Rubin J, Lindheimer M. Serial plasma oncotic pressure levels and echoencephalography during and after delivery in severe pre-eclampsia. Lancet 1985; 325:1245-7.
112. Benedetti TJ, Carlson RW. Studies of colloid osmotic pressure in pregnancy-induced hypertension. Am J Obstet Gynecol 1979; 135:308-11.
113. Benedetti TJ, Kates R, Williams V. Hemodynamic observations in severe preeclampsia complicated by pulmonary edema. Am J Obstet Gynecol 1985; 152:330-4.
114. Roberts JM, Cooper DW. Pathogenesis and genetics of pre-eclampsia. Lancet 2001; 357:53-6.
115. Baker PN, Broughton Pipkin F, Symonds EM. Comparative study of platelet angiotensin II binding and the angiotensin II sensitivity test as predictors of pregnancy-induced hypertension. Clin Sci (Lond) 1992; 83:89-95.
116. Kobayashi T, Tokunaga N, Isoda H, et al. Vasospasms are characteristic in cases with eclampsia/preeclampsia and HELLP syndrome: Proposal of an angiospastic syndrome of pregnancy. Semin Thromb Hemost 2001; 27:131-5.
117. VanWijk MJ, Boer K, van der Meulen ET, et al. Resistance artery smooth muscle function in pregnancy and preeclampsia. Am J Obstet Gynecol 2002; 186:148-54.
118. Mushambi MC, Halligan AW, Williamson K. Recent developments in the pathophysiology and management of pre-eclampsia. Br J Anaesth 1996; 76:133-48.
119. Rafferty TD, Berkowitz RL. Hemodynamics in patients with severe toxemia during labor and delivery. Am J Obstet Gynecol 1980; 138:263-70.
120. Benedetti TJ, Cotton DB, Read JC, Miller FC. Hemodynamic observations in severe pre-eclampsia with a flow-directed pulmonary artery catheter. Am J Obstet Gynecol 1980; 136:465-70.
121. Phelan JP, Yurth DA. Severe preeclampsia. I: Peripartum hemodynamic observations. Am J Obstet Gynecol 1982; 144:17-22.
122. Cotton DB, Lee W, Huhta JC, Dorman KF. Hemodynamic profile of severe pregnancy-induced hypertension. Am J Obstet Gynecol 1988; 158:523-9.
123. Mabie WC, Ratts TE, Sibai BM. The central hemodynamics of severe preeclampsia. Am J Obstet Gynecol 1989; 161:1443-8.
124. Visser W, Wallenburg HC. Central hemodynamic observations in untreated preeclamptic patients. Hypertension 1991; 17:1072-7.
125. Clark SL, Cotton DB. Clinical indications for pulmonary artery catheterization in the patient with severe preeclampsia. Am J Obstet Gynecol 1988; 158:453-8.
126. Sharma SK, Philip J, Whitten CW, et al. Assessment of changes in coagulation in parturients with preeclampsia using thromboelastography. Anesthesiology 1999; 90:385-90.
127. Bell WR. Disseminated intravascular coagulation. Johns Hopkins Med J 1980; 146:289-99.
128. Rinehart BK, Terrone DA, Magann EF, et al. Preeclampsia-associated hepatic hemorrhage and rupture: Mode of management related to maternal and perinatal outcome. Obstet Gynecol Surv 1999; 54:196-202.
129. Moran P, Baylis PH, Lindheimer MD, Davison JM. Glomerular ultrafiltration in normal and preeclamptic pregnancy. J Am Soc Nephrol 2003; 14:648-52.
130. Sims EA, Krantz KE. Serial studies of renal function during pregnancy and the puerperium in normal women. J Clin Invest 1958; 37:1764-74.
131. Davison JM, Dunlop W. Renal hemodynamics and tubular function in normal human pregnancy. Kidney Int 1980; 18:152-61.
132. Siemens J, Bogert L. The uric acid content of maternal and fetal blood. J Biol Chem 1917; 32:63-7.
133. Schaffer NK, Dill LV, Cadden JF. Uric acid clearance in normal pregnancy and pre-eclampsia. J Clin Invest 1943; 22:201-6.
134. Powers RW, Bodnar LM, Ness RB, et al. Uric acid concentrations in early pregnancy among preeclamptic women with gestational hyperuricemia at delivery. Am J Obstet Gynecol 2006; 194:160.
135. Thangaratinam S, Ismail KM, Sharp S, et al. Accuracy of serum uric acid in predicting complications of pre-eclampsia: A systematic review. Br J Obstet Gynaecol 2006; 113:369-78.
136. Trudinger BJ, Giles WB, Cook CM, et al. Fetal umbilical artery flow velocity waveforms and placental resistance: Clinical significance. Br J Obstet Gynaecol 1985; 92:23-30.
137. Leduc L, Wheeler JM, Kirshon B, et al. Coagulation profile in severe preeclampsia. Obstet Gynecol 1992; 79:14-8.
138. Romero R, Vizoso J, Emamian M, et al. Clinical significance of liver dysfunction in pregnancy-induced hypertension. Am J Perinatol 1988; 5:146-51.
139. Yoon BH, Lee CM, Kim SW. An abnormal umbilical artery waveform: A strong and independent predictor of adverse perinatal outcome in patients with preeclampsia. Am J Obstet Gynecol 1994; 171:713-21.
140. Pattinson RC, Norman K, Odendaal HJ. The role of Doppler velocimetry in the management of high risk pregnancies. Br J Obstet Gynaecol 1994; 101:114-20.
141. Abalos E, Duley L, Steyn DW, Henderson-Smart DJ. Antihypertensive drug therapy for mild to moderate hypertension during pregnancy. Cochrane Database Syst Rev 2007; (1):CD002252.
142. Barton JR, Sibai BM. Acute life-threatening emergencies in preeclampsia—eclampsia. Clin Obstet Gynecol 1992; 35:402-13.
143. Coppage KH, Sibai BM. Treatment of hypertensive complications in pregnancy. Curr Pharm Des 2005; 11:749-57.
144. Sibai BM. Treatment of hypertension in pregnant women. N Engl J Med 1996; 335:257-65.
145. von Dadelszen P, Menzies J, Gilgoff S, et al. Evidence-based management for preeclampsia. Front Biosci 2007; 12:2876-89.
146. MacCarthy EP, Bloomfield SS. Labetalol: A review of its pharmacology, pharmacokinetics, clinical uses and adverse effects. Pharmacotherapy 1983; 3:193-219.
147. Duley L, Henderson-Smart DJ, Meher S. Drugs for treatment of very high blood pressure during pregnancy. Cochrane Database Syst Rev 2006; (3):CD001449.
148. Magee LA, Cham C, Waterman EJ, et al. Hydralazine for treatment of severe hypertension in pregnancy: Meta-analysis. Br Med J 2003; 327:955-60.
149. Vigil-De Gracia P, Lasso M, Ruiz E, et al. Severe hypertension in pregnancy: Hydralazine or labetalol: A randomized clinical trial. Eur J Obstet Gynecol Reprod Biol 2006; 128:157-62.
150. Eisenach JC, Castro MI. Maternally administered esmolol produces fetal beta-adrenergic blockade and hypoxemia in sheep. Anesthesiology 1989; 71:718-22.
151. Larson CP Jr, Shuer LM, Cohen SE. Maternally administered esmolol decreases fetal as well as maternal heart rate. J Clin Anesth 1990; 2:427-9.
152. Losasso TJ, Muzzi DA, Cucchiara RF. Response of fetal heart rate to maternal administration of esmolol. Anesthesiology 1991; 74:782-4.
153. Ducey JP, Knape KG. Maternal esmolol administration resulting in fetal distress and cesarean section in a term pregnancy. Anesthesiology 1992; 77:829-32.
154. Eisenach JC, Mandell G, Dewan DM. Maternal and fetal effects of labetalol in pregnant ewes. Anesthesiology 1991; 74:292-7.
155. Ignarro LJ, Ross G, Tillisch J. Pharmacology of endothelium-derived nitric oxide and nitrovasodilators. West J Med 1991; 154:51-62.

156. Grossi L, D'Angelo S. Sodium nitroprusside: Mechanism of NO release mediated by sulfhydryl-containing molecules. J Med Chem 2005; 48:2622-6.
157. Grossman E, Messerli FH, Grodzicki T, Kowey P. Should a moratorium be placed on sublingual nifedipine capsules given for hypertensive emergencies and pseudoemergencies? JAMA 1996; 276:1328-31.
158. American College of Obstetricians and Gynecologists. Diagnosis and management of preeclampsia and eclampsia. ACOG Practice Bulletin No. 33. Washington, DC, January 2002. (Obstet Gynecol 2002; 99:159-67.)
159. Waisman GD, Mayorga LM, Camera MI, et al. Magnesium plus nifedipine: Potentiation of hypotensive effect in preeclampsia? Am J Obstet Gynecol 1988; 159:308-9.
160. Impey L. Severe hypotension and fetal distress following sublingual administration of nifedipine to a patient with severe pregnancy induced hypertension at 33 weeks. Br J Obstet Gynaecol 1993; 100:959-61.
161. Snyder SW, Cardwell MS. Neuromuscular blockade with magnesium sulfate and nifedipine. Am J Obstet Gynecol 1989; 161:35-6.
162. Ben-Ami M, Giladi Y, Shalev E. The combination of magnesium sulphate and nifedipine: A cause of neuromuscular blockade. Br J Obstet Gynaecol 1994; 101:262-3.
163. The Eclampsia Trial Collaborative Group. Which anticonvulsant for women with eclampsia? Evidence from the Collaborative Eclampsia Trial. Lancet 1995; 345:1455-63.
164. Witlin A, Sibai B. Randomized trials for prevention and treatment of eclamptic convulsions. In Sibai B, editor. Hypertensive Disorders in Women. Philadelphia, WB Saunders, 2001:221-7.
165. Coetzee EJ, Dommisse J, Anthony J. A randomised controlled trial of intravenous magnesium sulphate versus placebo in the management of women with severe pre-eclampsia. Br J Obstet Gynaecol 1998; 105:300-3.
166. Altman D, Carroli G, Duley L, et al. Do women with pre-eclampsia, and their babies, benefit from magnesium sulphate? The Magpie Trial: A randomised placebo-controlled trial. Lancet 2002; 359:1877-90.
167. Belfort MA, Anthony J, Saade GR, Allen JC Jr. A comparison of magnesium sulfate and nimodipine for the prevention of eclampsia. N Engl J Med 2003; 348:304-11.
168. Sibai BM. Magnesium sulfate prophylaxis in preeclampsia: Lessons learned from recent trials. Am J Obstet Gynecol 2004; 190:1520-6.
169. Moodley J, Moodley VV. Prophylactic anticonvulsant therapy in hypertensive crises of pregnancy—the need for a large, randomized trial. Hypertens Pregnancy 1994; 13:245-52.
170. Crowther C, Hiller J, Doyle L. Magnesium sulphate for preventing preterm birth in threatened preterm labour. Cochrane Database Syst Rev 2002; (4):CD001060.
171. Witlin AG, Friedman SA, Sibai BM. The effect of magnesium sulfate therapy on the duration of labor in women with mild preeclampsia at term: A randomized, double-blind, placebo-controlled trial. Am J Obstet Gynecol 1997; 176:623-7.
172. Livingston JC, Livingston LW, Ramsey R, et al. Magnesium sulfate in women with mild preeclampsia: A randomized controlled trial. Obstet Gynecol 2003; 101:217-20.
173. Euser AG, Cipolla MJ. Resistance artery vasodilation to magnesium sulfate during pregnancy and the postpartum state. Am J Physiol Heart Circ Physiol 2005; 288:H1521-5.
174. Manfredi M, Beltramello A, Bongiovanni LG, et al. Eclamptic encephalopathy: Imaging and pathogenetic considerations. Acta Neurol Scand 1997; 96:277-82.
175. Engelter ST, Provenzale JM, Petrella JR. Assessment of vasogenic edema in eclampsia using diffusion imaging. Neuroradiology 2000; 42:818-20.
176. Cruikshank DP, Pitkin RM, Donnelly E, Reynolds WA. Urinary magnesium, calcium, and phosphate excretion during magnesium sulfate infusion. Obstet Gynecol 1981; 58:430-4.
177. Wilkins IA, Lynch L, Mehalek KE, et al. Efficacy and side effects of magnesium sulfate and ritodrine as tocolytic agents. Am J Obstet Gynecol 1988; 159:685-9.
178. Elliott JP, O'Keeffe DF, Greenberg P, Freeman RK. Pulmonary edema associated with magnesium sulfate and betamethasone administration. Am J Obstet Gynecol 1979; 134:717-9.
179. James MF. Magnesium in obstetric anesthesia. Int J Obstet Anesth 1998; 7:115-23.
180. Royal College of Obstetricians and Gynaecologists. The Management of Severe Pre-Eclampsia/Eclampsia. Guideline 10(A). London, RCOG, March 2006:1-11.
181. Belfort MA, Clark SL, Sibai B. Cerebral hemodynamics in preeclampsia: Cerebral perfusion and the rationale for an alternative to magnesium sulfate. Obstet Gynecol Surv 2006; 61:655-65.
182. Sibai B, Dekker G, Kupferminc M. Pre-eclampsia. The Lancet 2005; 365:785-99.
183. Friedman SA, Schiff E, Lubarsky SL, Sibai BM. Expectant management of severe preeclampsia remote from term. Clin Obstet Gynecol 1999; 42:470-8.
184. Churchill D, Duley L. Interventionist versus expectant care for severe pre-eclampsia before term. Cochrane Database Syst Rev 2002; (3):CD003106.
185. Odendaal HJ, Pattinson RC, Bam R, et al. Aggressive or expectant management for patients with severe preeclampsia between 28-34 weeks' gestation: A randomized controlled trial. Obstet Gynecol 1990; 76:1070-5.
186. Sibai BM, Mercer BM, Schiff E, Friedman SA. Aggressive versus expectant management of severe preeclampsia at 28 to 32 weeks' gestation: A randomized controlled trial. Am J Obstet Gynecol 1994; 171:818-22.
187. Amorim MM, Santos LC, Faundes A. Corticosteroid therapy for prevention of respiratory distress syndrome in severe preeclampsia. Am J Obstet Gynecol 1999; 180:1283-8.
188. Lewis G. The Confidential Enquiry into Maternal and Child Health (CEMACH). Saving Mother's Lives: Reviewing Maternal Deaths to Make Motherhood Safer—2003-2005. London, CEMACH, 2007.
189. Zeeman GG, Fleckenstein JL, Twickler DM, Cunningham FG. Cerebral infarction in eclampsia. Am J Obstet Gynecol 2004; 190:714-20.
190. Schaefer PW, Buonanno FS, Gonzalez RG, Schwamm LH. Diffusion-weighted imaging discriminates between cytotoxic and vasogenic edema in a patient with eclampsia. Stroke 1997; 28:1082-5.
191. Martin JN, Thigpen BD, Moore RC, et al. Stroke and severe preeclampsia and eclampsia: A paradigm shift focusing on systolic blood pressure. Obstet Gynecol 2005; 105:246-54.
192. Perry KG, Martin JN Jr. Abnormal hemostasis and coagulopathy in preeclampsia and eclampsia. Clin Obstet Gynecol 1992; 35:338-50.
193. Dildy GA, Cotton DB. Management of severe preeclampsia and eclampsia. Crit Care Clin 1991; 7:829-50.
194. Mabie WC, Hackman BB, Sibai BM. Pulmonary edema associated with pregnancy: Echocardiographic insights and implications for treatment. Obstet Gynecol 1993; 81:227-34.
195. Desai DK, Moodley J, Naidoo DP, Bhorat I. Cardiac abnormalities in pulmonary oedema associated with hypertensive crises in pregnancy. Br J Obstet Gynaecol 1996; 103:523-8.
196. DiFederico EM, Burlingame JM, Kilpatrick SJ, et al. Pulmonary edema in obstetric patients is rapidly resolved except in the presence of infection or of nitroglycerin tocolysis after open fetal surgery. Am J Obstet Gynecol 1998; 179:925-33.
197. Abraham KA, Kennelly M, Dorman AM, Walshe JJ. Pathogenesis of acute renal failure associated with the HELLP syndrome: A case report and review of the literature. Eur J Obstet Gynecol Reprod Biol 2003; 108:99-102.
198. Singri N, Ahya SN, Levin ML. Acute renal failure. JAMA 2003; 289:747-51.
199. Sibai BM, Villar MA, Mabie BC. Acute renal failure in hypertensive disorders of pregnancy: Pregnancy outcome and remote prognosis in thirty-one consecutive cases. Am J Obstet Gynecol 1990; 162:777-83.
200. Rodriguez Gonzalez D, Godina Gallardo M, et al. Severe pre-eclampsia, HELLP syndrome and renal failure [Spanish]. Ginecol Obstet Mex 1998; 66:48-51.
201. Drakeley AJ, Le Roux PA, Anthony J, Penny J. Acute renal failure complicating severe preeclampsia requiring admission to an obstetric intensive care unit. Am J Obstet Gynecol 2002; 186:253-6.

202. Stratta P, Canavese C, Colla L, et al. Acute renal failure in preeclampsia-eclampsia. Gynecol Obstet Invest 1987; 24:225-31.
203. Lindqvist PG, Happach C. Risk and risk estimation of placental abruption. Eur J Obstet Gynecol Reprod Biol 2006; 126:160-4.
204. Sibai BM, Ramadan MK, Usta I, et al. Maternal morbidity and mortality in 442 pregnancies with hemolysis, elevated liver enzymes, and low platelets (HELLP syndrome). Am J Obstet Gynecol 1993; 169:1000-6.
205. Weinstein L. Syndrome of hemolysis, elevated liver enzymes, and low platelet count: A severe consequence of hypertension in pregnancy. Am J Obstet Gynecol 1982; 142:159-67.
206. Sibai BM. Diagnosis, controversies, and management of the syndrome of hemolysis, elevated liver enzymes, and low platelet count. Obstet Gynecol 2004; 103:981-91.
207. Barton JR, Riely CA, Adamec TA, et al. Hepatic histopathologic condition does not correlate with laboratory abnormalities in HELLP syndrome (hemolysis, elevated liver enzymes, and low platelet count). Am J Obstet Gynecol 1992; 167:1538-43.
208. O'Brien JM, Shumate SA, Satchwell SL, et al. Maternal benefit of corticosteroid therapy in patients with HELLP (hemolysis, elevated liver enzymes, and low platelet count) syndrome: Impact on the rate of regional anesthesia. Am J Obstet Gynecol 2002; 186:475-9.
209. MacKenna J, Dover NL, Brame RG. Preeclampsia associated with hemolysis, elevated liver enzymes, and low platelets—an obstetric emergency? Obstet Gynecol 1983; 62:751-4.
210. Heyborne KD, Burke MS, Porreco RP. Prolongation of premature gestation in women with hemolysis, elevated liver enzymes and low platelets: A report of five cases. J Reprod Med 1990; 35:53-7.
211. Visser W, Wallenburg HC. Temporising management of severe pre-eclampsia with and without the HELLP syndrome. Br J Obstet Gynaecol 1995; 102:111-7.
212. Heller CS, Elliott JP. High-order multiple pregnancies complicated by HELLP syndrome: A report of four cases with corticosteroid therapy to prolong gestation. J Reprod Med 1997; 42:743-6.
213. Douglas M. The use of neuraxial anesthesia in parturients with thrombocytopenia: What is an adequate platelet count? In Halpern S, Douglas M, editors. Evidence-Based Obstetric Anaesthesia. Oxford, Blackwell Publishing, 2005:165-77.
214. Barton J, Sibai B. Diagnosis and management of hemolysis, elevated liver enzymes, and low platelets syndrome. Clin Perinatol 2004; 31:807-33.
215. Sheikh RA, Yasmeen S, Pauly MP, Riegler JL. Spontaneous intrahepatic hemorrhage and hepatic rupture in the HELLP syndrome: Four cases and a review. J Clin Gastroenterol 1999; 28:323-8.
216. Bis KA, Waxman B. Rupture of the liver associated with pregnancy: A review of the literature and report of 2 cases. Obstet Gynecol Surv 1976; 31:763-73.
217. Vujic I, Stanley JH, Gobien RP, et al. Embolic management of rare hemorrhagic gynecologic and obstetrical conditions. Cardiovasc Intervent Radiol 1986; 9:69-74.
218. Boulleret C, Chahid T, Gallot D, et al. Hypogastric arterial selective and superselective embolization for severe postpartum hemorrhage: A retrospective review of 36 cases. Cardiovasc Intervent Radiol 2004; 27:344-8.
219. Chauleur C, Fanget C, Tourne G, et al. Serious primary post-partum hemorrhage, arterial embolization and future fertility: A retrospective study of 46 cases. Hum Reprod 2008; 23:1553-9.
220. Onrust S, Santema JG, Aarnoudse JG. Pre-eclampsia and the HELLP syndrome still cause maternal mortality in the Netherlands and other developed countries: Can we reduce it? Eur J Obstet Gynecol Reprod Biol 1999; 82:41-6.
221. Preisman S, Pfeiffer U, Lieberman N, Perel A. New monitors of intravascular volume: A comparison of arterial pressure waveform analysis and the intrathoracic blood volume. Intensive Care Med 1997; 23:651-7.
222. Newsome LR, Bramwell RS, Curling PE. Severe preeclampsia: Hemodynamic effects of lumbar epidural anesthesia. Anesth Analg 1986; 65:31-6.
223. Cotton DB, Gonik B, Dorman K, Harrist R. Cardiovascular alterations in severe pregnancy-induced hypertension: Relationship of central venous pressure to pulmonary capillary wedge pressure. Am J Obstet Gynecol 1985; 151:762-4.
224. Sandham JD, Hull RD, Brant RF, et al. A randomized, controlled trial of the use of pulmonary-artery catheters in high-risk surgical patients. N Engl J Med 2003; 348:5-14.
225. Practice guidelines for pulmonary artery catheterization: An updated report by the American Society of Anesthesiologists Task Force on Pulmonary Artery Catheterization. Anesthesiology 2003; 99:988-1014.
226. Report on Confidential Enquiries into Maternal Deaths in the United Kingdom, 1991-1993. London, HMSO, 1996.
227. Chestnut DH, Lumb PD, Jelovsek F, Killam AP. Nonbacterial thrombotic endocarditis associated with severe preeclampsia and pulmonary artery catheterization: A case report. J Reprod Med 1985; 30:497-500.
228. Ross V. Invasive hemodynamic monitoring in the management of PIH: A survey of practicing anesthesiologists. Anesthesiology 2000; 92:A89.
229. Lefrant JY, Muller L, Bruelle P, et al. Insertion time of the pulmonary artery catheter in critically ill patients. Crit Care Med 2000; 28:355-9.
230. Haddad B, Sibai BM. Expectant management of severe preeclampsia: Proper candidates and pregnancy outcome. Clin Obstet Gynecol 2005; 48:430-40.
231. Paech MJ. The King Edward Memorial Hospital 1,000 mother survey of methods of pain relief in labour. Anaesth Intensive Care 1991; 19:393-9.
232. Howell CJ, Chalmers I. A review of prospectively controlled comparisons of epidural with non-epidural forms of pain relief during labour. Int J Obstet Anesth 1992; 1:93-110.
233. Simmons SW, Cyna AM, Dennis AT, Hughes D. Combined spinal-epidural versus epidural analgesia in labour. Cochrane Database Syst Rev 2007; (3):CD003401.
234. Ramanathan J, Coleman P, Sibai B. Anesthetic modification of hemodynamic and neuroendocrine stress responses to cesarean delivery in women with severe preeclampsia. Anesth Analg 1991; 73:772-9.
235. Jouppila P, Jouppila R, Hollmen A, Koivula A. Lumbar epidural analgesia to improve intervillous blood flow during labor in severe preeclampsia. Obstet Gynecol 1982; 59:158-61.
236. Kanayama N, Belayet HM, Khatun S, et al. A new treatment of severe pre-eclampsia by long-term epidural anaesthesia. J Hum Hypertens 1999; 13:167-71.
237. Ryan D. Examination of the blood. In Lichtman M, Beutler E, Kipps T, et al, editors. Williams Hematology. 7th edition. New York, McGraw-Hill, 2005.
238. Harker LA, Slichter SJ. The bleeding time as a screening test for evaluation of platelet function. N Engl J Med 1972; 287:155-9.
239. Rodgers RP, Levin J. A critical reappraisal of the bleeding time. Semin Thromb Hemost 1990; 16:1-20.
240. Llau JV, de Andres J, Gomar C, et al. Drugs that alter hemostasis and regional anesthetic techniques: Safety guidelines. Consensus conference [Spanish]. Rev Esp Anestesiol Reanim 2001; 48:270-8.
241. Horlocker TT, Wedel DJ, Benzon H, et al. Regional anesthesia in the anticoagulated patient: Defining the risks. (The second ASRA Consensus Conference on Neuraxial Anesthesia and Anticoagulation.) Reg Anesth Pain Med 2003; 28:172-97.
242. Campos CJ, Pivalizza EG, Abouleish EI. Thromboelastography in a parturient with immune thrombocytopenic purpura. Anesth Analg 1998; 86:675.
243. Watson HG. Thromboelastography should be available in every labour ward. Int J Obstet Anesth 2005; 14:325-7.
244. Aya AG, Vialles N, Tanoubi I, et al. Spinal anesthesia-induced hypotension: A risk comparison between patients with severe preeclampsia and healthy women undergoing preterm cesarean delivery. Anesth Analg 2005; 101:869-75.
245. Dyer RA, Piercy JL, Reed AR, et al. Hemodynamic changes associated with spinal anesthesia for cesarean delivery in severe preeclampsia. Anesthesiology 2008; 108:802-11.
246. Baker PN, Kilby MD, Broughton Pipkin F. The effect of angiotensin II on platelet intracellular free calcium concentration in human pregnancy. J Hypertens 1992; 10:55-60.

247. Nisell H, Hjemdahl P, Linde B. Cardiovascular responses to circulating catecholamines in normal pregnancy and in pregnancy-induced hypertension. Clin Physiol 1985; 5:479-93.
248. Vedernikov YP, Belfort MA, Saade GR, Garfield RE. Inhibition of cyclooxygenase but not nitric oxide synthase influences effects on the human omental artery of the thromboxane A_2 mimetic U46619 and 17beta-estradiol. Am J Obstet Gynecol 2001; 185:182-9.
249. Aya AG, Mangin R, Vialles N, et al. Patients with severe preeclampsia experience less hypotension during spinal anesthesia for elective cesarean delivery than healthy parturients: A prospective cohort comparison. Anesth Analg 2003; 97:867-72.
250. Clark VA, Sharwood-Smith GH, Stewart AV. Ephedrine requirements are reduced during spinal anaesthesia for caesarean section in preeclampsia. Int J Obstet Anesth 2005; 14:9-13.
251. Hadzic A, Vloka J, Patel N, Birnbach D. Hypertensive crisis after a successful placement of an epidural anesthetic in a hypertensive parturient: Case report. Reg Anesth 1995; 20:156-8.
252. Heller PJ, Goodman C. Use of local anesthetics with epinephrine for epidural anesthesia in preeclampsia. Anesthesiology 1986; 65:224-6.
253. Dror A, Henriksen E. Accidental epidural magnesium sulfate injection. Anesth Analg 1987; 66:1020-1.
254. Guinard JP, Mulroy MF, Carpenter RL, Knopes KD. Test doses: Optimal epinephrine content with and without acute beta-adrenergic blockade. Anesthesiology 1990; 73:386-92.
255. Polley LS, Columb MO, Naughton NN, et al. Effect of epidural epinephrine on the minimum local analgesic concentration of epidural bupivacaine in labor. Anesthesiology 2002; 96:1123-8.
256. Hodgkinson R, Husain FJ, Hayashi RH. Systemic and pulmonary blood pressure during caesarean section in parturients with gestational hypertension. Can Anaesth Soc J 1980; 27:389-94.
257. Wallace DH, Leveno KJ, Cunningham FG, et al. Randomized comparison of general and regional anesthesia for cesarean delivery in pregnancies complicated by severe preeclampsia. Obstet Gynecol 1995; 86:193-9.
258. Sharwood-Smith G, Clark V, Watson E. Regional anaesthesia for caesarean section in severe preeclampsia: Spinal anaesthesia is the preferred choice. Int J Obstet Anesth 1999; 8:85-9.
259. Hood DD, Curry R. Spinal versus epidural anesthesia for cesarean section in severely preeclamptic patients: A retrospective survey. Anesthesiology 1999; 90:1276-82.
260. Visalyaputra S, Rodanant O, Somboonviboon W, et al. Spinal versus epidural anesthesia for cesarean delivery in severe preeclampsia: A prospective randomized, multicenter study. Anesth Analg 2005; 101:862-8.
261. Santos AC, Birnbach DJ. Spinal anesthesia for cesarean delivery in severely preeclamptic women: Don't throw out the baby with the bathwater! Anesth Analg 2005; 101:859-61.
262. Santos AC. Spinal anesthesia in severely preeclamptic women: When is it safe? Anesthesiology 1999; 90:1252-4.
263. Santos AC, Birnbach DJ. Spinal anesthesia in the parturient with severe preeclampsia: Time for reconsideration. Anesth Analg 2003; 97:621-2.
264. Stempel JE, O'Grady JP, Morton MJ, Johnson KA. Use of sodium nitroprusside in complications of gestational hypertension. Obstet Gynecol 1982; 60:533-8.
265. Hood DD, Dewan DM, James FM 3rd, et al. The use of nitroglycerin in preventing the hypertensive response to tracheal intubation in severe preeclampsia. Anesthesiology 1985; 63:329-32.
266. Ramanathan J, Sibai BM, Mabie WC, et al. The use of labetalol for attenuation of the hypertensive response to endotracheal intubation in preeclampsia. Am J Obstet Gynecol 1988; 159:650-4.
267. Baker AB. Management of severe pregnancy-induced hypertension, or gestosis, with sodium nitroprusside. Anaesth Intensive Care 1990; 18:361-5.
268. Ngan Kee WD, Khaw KS, Ma KC, et al. Maternal and neonatal effects of remifentanil at induction of general anesthesia for cesarean delivery: A randomized, double-blind, controlled trial. Anesthesiology 2006; 104:14-20.
269. Bansal S, Pawar M. Haemodynamic responses to laryngoscopy and intubation in patients with pregnancy-induced hypertension: Effect of intravenous esmolol with or without lidocaine. Int J Obstet Anesth 2002; 11:4-8.
270. Sinatra RS, Philip BK, Naulty JS, Ostheimer GW. Prolonged neuromuscular blockade with vecuronium in a patient treated with magnesium sulfate. Anesth Analg 1985; 64:1220-2.
271. Kussman B, Shorten G, Uppington J, Comunale ME. Administration of magnesium sulphate before rocuronium: Effects on speed of onset and duration of neuromuscular block. Br J Anaesth 1997; 79:122-4.
272. Hodgson RE, Rout CC, Rocke DA, Louw NJ. Mivacurium for caesarean section in hypertensive parturients receiving magnesium sulphate therapy. Int J Obstet Anesth 1998; 7:12-7.
273. Yoshida A, Itoh Y, Nagaya K, et al. Prolonged relaxant effects of vecuronium in patients with deliberate hypermagnesemia: Time for caution in cesarean section. J Anesth 2006; 20:33-5.
274. Baraka A, Yazigi A. Neuromuscular interaction of magnesium with succinylcholine-vecuronium sequence in the eclamptic parturient. Anesthesiology 1987; 67:806-8.
275. Lipman J, James MF, Erskine J, et al. Autonomic dysfunction in severe tetanus: Magnesium sulfate as an adjunct to deep sedation. Crit Care Med 1987; 15:987-8.
276. James MF, Beer RE, Esser JD. Intravenous magnesium sulfate inhibits catecholamine release associated with tracheal intubation. Anesth Analg 1989; 68:772-6.
277. Sipes SL, Weiner CP, Gellhaus TM, Goodspeed JD. The plasma renin-angiotensin system in preeclampsia: Effects of magnesium sulfate. Obstet Gynecol 1989; 73:934-7.
278. Walters BN, Walters T. Hypertension in the puerperium. Lancet 1987; 2(8554):330.
279. Gherman RB, Goodwin TM, Leung B, et al. Incidence, clinical characteristics, and timing of objectively diagnosed venous thromboembolism during pregnancy. Obstet Gynecol 1999; 94:730-4.
280. Berg CJ, Atrash HK, Koonin LM, Tucker M. Pregnancy-related mortality in the United States, 1987-1990. Obstet Gynecol 1996; 88:161-7.
281. Jacobsen AF, Skjeldestad FE, Sandset PM. Incidence and risk patterns of venous thromboembolism in pregnancy and puerperium—a register-based case-control study. Am J Obstet Gynecol 2008; 198:233.e1-7.
282. Lindqvist P, Dahlback B, Marsal K. Thrombotic risk during pregnancy: A population study. Obstet Gynecol 1999; 94:595-9.
283. Simpson EL, Lawrenson RA, Nightingale AL, Farmer RD. Venous thromboembolism in pregnancy and the puerperium: Incidence and additional risk factors from a London perinatal database. Br J Obstet Gynaecol 2001; 108:56-60.
284. Ros HS, Lichtenstein P, Bellocco R, et al. Pulmonary embolism and stroke in relation to pregnancy: How can high-risk women be identified? Am J Obstet Gynecol 2002; 186:198-203.
285. Macklon NS, Greer IA. Venous thromboembolic disease in obstetrics and gynaecology: The Scottish experience. Scott Med J 1996; 41:83-6.
286. Bates SM, Greer IA, Pabinger I, et al. Venous thromboembolism, thrombophilia, antithrombotic therapy, and pregnancy: American College of Chest Physicians Evidence-Based Clinical Practice Guidelines (8th Edition). Chest 2008; 133:844S-86S.
287. Mhyre JM, Riesner MN, Polley LS, Naughton NN. A series of anesthesia-related maternal deaths in Michigan, 1985-2003. Anesthesiology 2007; 106:1096-104.
288. Bachour A, Teramo K, Hiilesmaa V, Maasilta P. Increased plasma levels of inflammatory markers and upper airway resistance during sleep in pre-eclampsia. Sleep Med 2008; 9:667-74.
289. Hannaford P, Ferry S, Hirsch S. Cardiovascular sequelae of toxaemia of pregnancy. Heart 1997; 77:154-8.
290. Sattar N, Greer IA. Pregnancy complications and maternal cardiovascular risk: Opportunities for intervention and screening? Br Med J 2002; 325:157-60.
291. Chambers JC, Fusi L, Malik IS, et al. Association of maternal endothelial dysfunction with preeclampsia. JAMA 2001; 285:1607-12.

292. Hamad RR, Eriksson MJ, Silveira A, et al. Decreased flow-mediated dilation is present 1 year after a pre-eclamptic pregnancy. J Hypertens 2007; 25:2301-7.
293. Newstead J, von Dadelszen P, Magee LA. Preeclampsia and future cardiovascular risk. Expert Rev Cardiovasc Ther 2007; 5:283-94.
294. Magee LA, von Dadelszen P. Pre-eclampsia and increased cardiovascular risk. Br Med J 2007; 335:945-6.
295. Yusuf S, Hawken S, Ounpuu S, et al. Effect of potentially modifiable risk factors associated with myocardial infarction in 52 countries (the INTERHEART study): Case-control study. Lancet 2004; 364:937-52.
296. Polednak AP, Janerich DT. Characteristics of first pregnancy in relation to early breast cancer: A case-control study. J Reprod Med 1983; 28:314-8.
297. Thompson WD, Jacobson HI, Negrini B, Janerich DT. Hypertension, pregnancy, and risk of breast cancer. J Natl Cancer Inst 1989; 81:1571-4.
298. Troisi R, Weiss HA, Hoover RN, et al. Pregnancy characteristics and maternal risk of breast cancer. Epidemiology 1998; 9:641-7.
299. Cohn BA, Cirillo PM, Christianson RE, et al. Placental characteristics and reduced risk of maternal breast cancer. J Natl Cancer Inst 2001; 93:1133-40.
300. Vatten LJ, Forman MR, Nilsen TI, et al. The negative association between pre-eclampsia and breast cancer risk may depend on the offspring's gender. Br J Cancer 2007; 96:1436-8.
301. National Institute of Mental Health. Post-Traumatic Stress Disorder (PTSD). Available at http://nimh.nih.gov/health/topics/post-traumatic-stress-disorder-ptsd/index.shtml/
302. van Pampus MG, Wolf H, Weijmar Schultz WC, et al. Posttraumatic stress disorder following preeclampsia and HELLP syndrome. J Psychosom Obstet Gynaecol 2004; 25:183-7.
303. Engelhard IM, van Rij M, Boullart I, et al. Posttraumatic stress disorder after pre-eclampsia: An exploratory study. Gen Hosp Psychiatry 2002; 24:260-4.
304. Sibai BM. Diagnosis, prevention, and management of eclampsia. Obstet Gynecol 2005; 105:402-10.
305. Hirshfeld-Cytron J, Lam C, Karumanchi SA, Lindheimer M. Late postpartum eclampsia: Examples and review. Obstet Gynecol Surv 2006; 61:471-80.
306. Shah AK, Rajamani K, Whitty JE. Eclampsia: A neurological perspective. J Neurol Sci 2008; 271:158-67.
307. Wen SW, Huang L, Liston R, et al. Severe maternal morbidity in Canada, 1991-2001. Can Med Assoc J 2005; 173:759-64.
308. Andersgaard AB, Herbst A, Johansen M, et al. Eclampsia in Scandinavia: Incidence, substandard care, and potentially preventable cases. Acta Obstet Gynecol Scand 2006; 85:929-36.
309. Knight M. Eclampsia in the United Kingdom, 2005. Br J Obstet Gynaecol 2007; 114:1072-8.
310. Zwart J, Richters J, Öry F, et al. Severe maternal morbidity during pregnancy, delivery and puerperium in the Netherlands: A nationwide population-based study of 371,000 pregnancies. Br J Obstet Gynaecol 2008; 115:842-50.
311. Ekholm E, Salmi MM, Erkkola R. Eclampsia in Finland in 1990-1994. Acta Obstet Gynecol Scand 1999; 78:877-82.
312. Karumanchi SA, Lindheimer MD. Advances in the understanding of eclampsia. Curr Hypertens Rep 2008; 10:305-12.
313. Sibai BM. Eclampsia. VI: Maternal-perinatal outcome in 254 consecutive cases. Am J Obstet Gynecol 1990; 163:1049-54.
314. Pizon AF, Wolfson AB. Postpartum focal neurologic deficits: Posterior leukoencephalopathy syndrome. J Emerg Med 2005; 29:163-6.
315. Servillo G, Striano P, Striano S, et al. Posterior reversible encephalopathy syndrome (PRES) in critically ill obstetric patients. Intensive Care Med 2003; 29:2323-6.
316. Cipolla MJ. Cerebrovascular function in pregnancy and eclampsia. Hypertension 2007; 50:14-24.
317. Duley L. Evidence and practice: The magnesium sulphate story. Best Pract Res Clin Obstet Gynaecol 2005; 19:57-74.
318. Aagaard-Tillery KM, Belfort MA. Eclampsia: Morbidity, mortality, and management. Clin Obstet Gynecol 2005; 48:12-23.
319. Brodie H, Malinow AM. Anesthetic management of preeclampsia/eclampsia. Int J Obstet Anesth 1999; 8:110.
320. Moodley J, Jjuuko G, Rout C. Epidural compared with general anaesthesia for caesarean delivery in conscious women with eclampsia. Br J Obstet Gynaecol 2001; 108:378-82.
321. Oshima T, Karasawa F, Satoh T. Effects of propofol on cerebral blood flow and the metabolic rate of oxygen in humans. Acta Anaesthesiol Scand 2002; 46:831-5.
322. Kassell NF, Hitchon PW, Gerk MK, et al. Alterations in cerebral blood flow, oxygen metabolism, and electrical activity produced by high dose sodium thiopental. Neurosurgery 1980; 7:598-603.
323. Wood PR, Browne GP, Pugh S. Propofol infusion for the treatment of status epilepticus. Lancet 1988; 1(8583):480-1.
324. Ramsay RE. Treatment of status epilepticus. Epilepsia 1993; 34(Suppl 1):S71-81.
325. Czosnyka M, Pickard JD. Monitoring and interpretation of intracranial pressure. J Neurol Neurosurg Psychiatry 2004; 75:813-21.
326. Bissonnette B. Cerebral protection. Pediatric Anesthesia 2004; 14:403-6.
327. Aukes AM, Wessel I, Dubois AM, et al. Self-reported cognitive functioning in formerly eclamptic women. Am J Obstet Gynecol 2007; 197:365.e1-6.

Chapter 46

Liver Disease

Michael Froelich, M.D., M.S.
Robert W. Reid, M.D.

Liver disease can affect pregnant women in the form of common disorders as well as many disorders that are unique to pregnancy. One common liver disorder, viral hepatitis, is potentially serious during pregnancy and merits special attention from obstetric anesthesia providers. Five liver diseases unique to pregnancy are (1) hyperemesis gravidarum; (2) intrahepatic cholestasis of pregnancy; (3) preeclampsia/eclampsia; (4) hemolysis, elevated liver enzymes, low platelets (HELLP) syndrome; and (5) acute fatty liver of pregnancy (Table 46-1). Preeclampsia/eclampsia and HELLP syndrome are discussed in Chapter 45.

VIRAL HEPATITIS

Definition

Viral hepatitis is an infection that can cause mild nonclinical illness or, when severe, serious conditions such as fulminant hepatic necrosis. It is the most common cause of jaundice. Six types, named hepatitis A, B, C, D, E, and G, have been identified and associated with specific viruses. Types A, B, and C are the most common.[1] Infrequently, hepatitis can also be caused by the herpes simplex, yellow fever, rubella, and Epstein-Barr viruses as well as by cytomegalovirus.

Pathophysiology and Epidemiology

Table 46-2 summarizes the clinical and epidemiologic properties of the six major causative agents.[1-3] **Hepatitis A virus (HAV)** is responsible for nearly half of known cases of viral hepatitis. This virus replicates in the liver, is secreted in the bile, and is then shed through feces. Person-to-person transmission through fecal-oral contamination is the primary means of HAV infection in the United States, occurring most often in the household and extended family setting.[4] Although it is very contagious, the duration of

TABLE 46-1 Liver Diseases Unique to Pregnancy

	Hyperemesis Gravidarum	Intrahepatic Cholestasis of Pregnancy	Preeclampsia/Eclampsia	HELLP Syndrome	AFLP
Incidence	<2%	<10%	2%-8%	0.1%-0.6%	1:10,000-1:15,000
Presentation	1st trimester	2nd or 3rd trimester	2nd or 3rd trimester, or after delivery	2nd or 3rd trimester, or after delivery	3rd trimester
Symptoms, signs, and complications	Nausea/vomiting Ketosis	Pruritus Jaundice	High blood pressure Proteinuria Edema Seizures Renal failure Pulmonary edema Hepatic hematoma/rupture	Abdominal pain Renal dysfunction Hypertension Hepatic hematoma/rupture Liver infarction	Nausea/vomiting Abdominal pain Jaundice Hepatic failure
Laboratory investigation	Elevated aminotransferases	Increased serum bile acid levels Hyperbilirubinemia Mild abnormalities of liver function tests	Low platelet count Proteinuria Increased uric acid level Mildly elevated aminotransferases	Low platelet count Hemolysis Markedly elevated aminotransferases	Low platelet count Hypoglycemia Mildly/moderately elevated aminotransferases
Treatment	Supportive management	Delivery at fetal maturity Ursodeoxycholic acid	Blood pressure control Delivery	Prompt delivery	Prompt delivery
Outcome	Benign for mother and fetus	No increase in maternal death rate Increased risk of preterm delivery and fetal loss May recur with subsequent pregnancies Increased risk of subsequent liver and biliary tract disease	Increased risk of maternal morbidity and mortality Increased risk of perinatal morbidity	Maternal death rate 1%-4% Fetal death rate 1%-30%	Maternal death rate <5% Fetal death rate 1%-23%

AFLP, acute fatty liver of pregnancy; HELLP, hemolysis, elevated liver enzymes, and low platelets.

Adapted from Schutt VA, Minuk GY. Liver diseases unique to pregnancy. Best Pract Res Clin Gastroenterol 2007; 21:771-92; and Ropponen A, Sund R, Riikonen S, et al. Intrahepatic cholestasis of pregnancy as an indicator of liver and biliary diseases: A population-based study. Hepatology 2006; 43:723-8.

TABLE 46-2 Some Agents that Cause Acute Viral Hepatitis

	Hepatitis A	Hepatitis B	Hepatitis C	Hepatitis D	Hepatitis E	Hepatitis G
Virus family	Picornaviridae	Hepadnaviridae	Flaviviridae	Satellite virus or subviral particle	Caliciviridae	Flaviviridae variant
Genomic name	27 nm RNA	42 nm DNA	9.4 kb RNA	36 nm hybrid	7.5 kb RNA	9.4 kb RNA
Typical transmission	Fecal-oral	Parenteral/sexual	Parenteral/sexual	Parenteral/sexual	Fecal-oral	Parenteral/sexual
Proportion of cases	25%	32%	20%	—	—	9%
Incidence in pregnancy	1:1000	1:500	Unknown	Unknown	Unknown	Unknown
Incubation period	15-50 days	60-110 days	37-70 days	Comparable to that of HBV	10-56 days	Unknown
Rate of progression to chronic liver disease	None	1%-5% in adults 80%-90% in children	85%	Chronic liver disease common if HDV superinfection is present in HBV-infected individuals	None	Unknown
Rate of vertical transmission	Rare	10%-20%	2%-10%	Comparable to that of HBV	Common	40%-60%
Immunoglobulin available	Yes	Yes	No	No	No	No
Vaccine	Yes	Yes	No	HBV vaccine	No	No

HBV, hepatitis B virus; HDV, hepatitis D virus; kb, kilobase; nm, nanometer.

TABLE 46-3 Interpretation of Hepatitis B (HB) Marker Test Results

Marker	Acute Infection	Chronic Infection	Past Infection
HB surface antigen (HBsAg)	+	+	–
HB e antigen (HBeAg)	+ early, then –	±	–
Anti–HB surface antigen antibody (anti-HBs)	–	–	+
Anti–HB core immunoglobulin M antibody (anti-HBcIgM)	+	–	–
Anti–HB core immunoglobulin G antibody (anti-HBcIgG)	+	+	+
Anti–HB e-antigen antibody (anti-HBe)	– early, then +	±	+
Hepatitis B virus DNA	+ early, then –	±	–
Alanine aminotransferase	Increased (markedly)	Increased (mildly/ moderately)	Normal

–, absent; +, present.

Adapted from Gitlin N. Hepatitis B: Diagnosis, prevention, and treatment. Clin Chem 1997; 43:1500-6.

viremia is short. Clinical illness is typically mild, is limited to 2 or 3 weeks in duration, and is never associated with a chronic carrier state. Fulminant hepatic necrosis is a rare but devastating complication of HAV infection.

Hepatitis B virus (**HBV**) is caused by a small DNA virus. The intact virus, known as the Dane particle, contains three principal antigens: (1) the hepatitis B surface antigen (HBsAg); (2) the hepatitis B core antigen (HBcAg); and (3) a protein subunit (e-antigen) of the core antigen (HBeAg). The presence of the HBeAg indicates an extremely high viral inoculum and active virus replication (Table 46-3). The virus is transmitted through parenteral or sexual exposure. Women at risk include (1) those with a history of intravenous drug use, multiple sexual partners, sexually transmitted diseases, or exposure to cryoprecipitate; (2) those who work or receive treatment in a hemodialysis unit; (3) those who work in a health or public safety field; (4) those with a recent tattoo; and (5) those who have resided in a prison or in an institution for the developmentally disabled. However, these risk factors identify only half of all HBV-positive pregnant women.[5] In the United States, 0.2% of persons are seropositive for HBV.[6] In contrast to HAV infection, 5% to 10% of those infected with HBV progress to a chronic carrier state, and 30% continue to experience active hepatocellular destruction and are at risk for cirrhosis, hepatocellular carcinoma, and death.

Hepatitis B virus is transmitted by parenteral and sexual contact. Although HBsAg has been detected in a variety of body fluids, only serum, semen, and saliva are infectious.[7] The virus is relatively stable in the environment and can be viable for up to 7 days on surfaces at room temperature; contact with those surfaces can result in infection, even if no blood is visible.[7] Health care–related transmission has long been recognized as an important source of new HBV infections worldwide. A health care worker's risk of infection correlates with his or her exposure to infected blood and contaminated needles. Following needlestick exposure, the risk of HBV infection varies according to the volume and viral concentration of the infectious fluid. The risk of inoculation after a needlestick is at least 30% with HBeAg-positive blood but less than 6% with HBeAg-negative blood.[8]

Most infections with **hepatitis C virus** (**HCV**) are asymptomatic, and many affected people are unaware of their infection. Nevertheless, in up to 90% of infected individuals, cirrhosis, hepatocellular carcinoma, and hepatic failure slowly develop over a period of two decades or longer, leading to death. Women of reproductive age are at particular risk for unrecognized, asymptomatic HCV infection; the risk of perinatal transmission is approximately 1% to 5%.[1]

Hepatitis D virus (**HDV** or **delta agent**) is an incomplete RNA virus that is dependent on co-infection with HBV for transmission. Chronic HDV infection carries an increased risk of fulminant hepatic failure. Although vertical transmission of HDV from mother to infant does occur, measures that protect against HBV infection also protect the neonate against HDV infection.

The **hepatitis E virus** (**HEV**) was identified and cloned in 1990.[9,10] This RNA virus is transmitted by the fecal-oral route and is responsible for major epidemics of viral hepatitis in developing countries. In 1997, Kwo et al.[11] reported the first case of an HEV isolate acquired in the United States. Among nonpregnant patients, HEV infection is typically self-limited and does not lead to a chronic carrier state. However, HEV infection during pregnancy is associated with a high risk of maternal and fetal morbidity and mortality.[12]

A virus tentatively called the **hepatitis F virus** (**HFV**),[13] or **Toga virus,** was isolated in fecal extracts from several patients in France with viral hepatitis not caused by HAV, HBV, HCV, or HEV. Its existence has not been confirmed and is now considered doubtful.[1,14]

Hepatitis G virus (**HGV**; also called **hepatitis GB virus C** or **HGBV-C**) was characterized in 1996.[15] This RNA virus is closely related to the HCV virus. Alter et al.[16] reported that HGV is common among volunteer blood donors, and it can be transmitted by means of blood transfusion. Vertical transmission of HGV from mother to infant has been reported.[17] However, the clinical significance of HGV infection is unknown, and no causal relationship between HGV and hepatitis has been established. In fact, the liver-to-serum concentration ratio of HGV RNA is less than 1, suggesting that HGV may not even be hepatotropic.[18]

Diagnosis

Clinical symptoms of acute viral hepatitis range from vague constitutional symptoms (e.g., malaise, nausea, anorexia) to overt jaundice. Physical examination often reveals tender hepatomegaly. Bilirubinuria and acholic stool are noted. Levels of hepatic transaminase enzymes rise to the 1000-IU range during acute infection.[19] Serologic testing confirms the diagnosis. Acute HAV infection is marked by the presence of immunoglobulin M (IgM) class anti-HAV antibody. Hepatitis B surface antigen (HBsAg) or anti-HBc antibody indicates either an acute HBV infection or the presence of a chronic active infection. The presence of HBeAg suggests a high degree of infectivity and neonatal risk.[20]

The current generation of enzyme immunoassay tests detects anti-HCV antibody with 95% sensitivity. Positive or indeterminant results should be confirmed with recombinant immunoblot assay. Anti-HCV antibodies are not detectable until 15 weeks after acute infection. Hepatitis C viral infection can be detected by qualitative testing for HCV RNA via polymerase chain reaction (PCR).[21]

Hepatitis D viral infection is indicated by serologic evidence for IgM anti-HDV or HDV RNA. Laboratory techniques for the diagnosis of HEV infection include PCR and serologic antibody detection. At this time, there is no reliable serologic assay to diagnose HGV infection; it can be identified only through reverse transcriptase PCR (RT-PCR).[22]

Vertical Transmission

HEPATITIS B

Vertical transmission of HBV from mother to infant remains a significant public health concern. The risk of perinatal infection is 5% to 20% in infants born to HBsAg-positive mothers and 70% to 90% in mothers who are also HBeAg-positive.[7] Because infants do not show evidence of HBV infection until the second or third month after birth, most investigators believe that transmission occurs during the immediate peripartum period, when the infant is exposed to vaginal blood and secretions, rather than by transplacental exposure. In patients with acute hepatitis B, the frequency of vertical transmission also depends on the time during gestation at which maternal infection occurs. For women in whom it occurs in the first trimester, up to 10% of neonates are seropositive for HBsAg. For women acutely infected in the third trimester, 80% to 90% of offspring are infected.[23] The U.S. Centers for Disease Control and Prevention (CDC) recommends universal immunization of all infants born in the United States (see later).[23]

OTHER FORMS OF HEPATITIS

Vertical transmission of HCV is almost always confined to women in whom HCV RNA is detectable.[24] The risk of transmission is increased by the level of maternal HCV viremia and maternal human immunodeficiency virus (HIV) co-infection.[25] Unlike the situation with HBV, currently there are no preventive measures that reduce the risk of vertical HCV infection of neonates. Routine prenatal HCV screening is not recommended. Vertical transmission of HDV has been documented; however, transmission of this virus is uncommon because the measures used to prevent perinatal HBV infection are almost uniformly effective in also preventing HDV infection. Vertical transmission of HEV has been reported, but information is limited.[26]

Medical and Obstetric Management

Management of pregnant women with acute viral hepatitis involves supportive care and prevention of transmission to the newborn. Although most women may be managed at home, hospitalization is indicated for those with severe nausea and vomiting, encephalopathy, coagulopathy, or debilitation. All patients with acute viral hepatitis should avoid strenuous activity and trauma to the upper abdomen. Family contacts should receive immunoprophylaxis.[18,27]

The CDC recommends routine vaccination of children as an effective way to reduce the incidence of hepatitis A in the United States.[28] Only hepatitis A and B can be prevented effectively through vaccination. Nonimmunized patients who have had close personal or sexual contact with an HAV-infected individual should receive postexposure prophylaxis. Immune globulin, which poses no risk to either a pregnant woman or her fetus, should be administered during pregnancy if indicated.

The CDC also recommends HBV vaccination for all newborns, regardless of maternal serologic status. If the mother is HBsAg-*negative*, the newborn is vaccinated with inactivated recombinant hepatitis B vaccine (Recombivax HB, Merck & Co., Inc., Whitehouse Station, NJ, or Engerix-B, GlaxoSmithKline Biologicals, S.A, Rixensart, Belgium) at the following intervals: (1) before hospital discharge, (2) at 1 to 2 months of age, and (3) at 6 to 18 months. If the mother is HBsAg-*positive* or her serologic status is *unknown*, both hepatitis B vaccine and hepatitis B immune globulin (HBIG) should be administered within 12 hours of delivery; the second and third injections of hepatitis B vaccine should be administered at 1 to 2 months and 6 months of age, respectively.[23,29]

No specific therapy is available for treatment of acute HBV infection. Therapeutic agents have been approved by the U. S. Food and Drug Administration (FDA) for treatment of chronic HBV infection. These agents can achieve sustained suppression of HBV replication and remission of liver disease in some patients.[29] In combination with other medications, one of these agents, the antiviral agent lamivudine, is effective for both the treatment of HIV infection and the interruption of vertical HIV transmission. Research has demonstrated the potential benefit of lamivudine treatment in reducing the risk of perinatal transmission of HBV infection from women who were HBV carriers during the last months of pregnancy.[30,31]

Although routine prenatal testing for HCV infection is not yet recommended, women who present with known risk factors should be tested for HCV.[32] Alpha-interferon-2B effectively reduces HCV RNA titers and improves the clinical outcome of patients with chronic HCV infection.[33] Currently the use of interferon is not considered safe during gestation, although at least two reports have described normal pregnancy outcome despite inadvertent interferon therapy.[34,35] No published data support the administration of immune globulin as HCV immunoprophylaxis during labor.[36]

The mode of delivery does not appear to have a significant effect on the efficacy of postpartum hepatitis B vaccine and hepatitis B immune globulin therapy.[37] Maternal-child transmission of HCV is uncommon and occurs only in infants born to mothers with hepatitis C viremia. Transmission of HCV to infants is not influenced by maternal age, mode of delivery, genotype, or type of feeding.[38,39]

INTRAHEPATIC CHOLESTASIS OF PREGNANCY

Definition and Epidemiology

Intrahepatic cholestasis of pregnancy is the second most common cause of jaundice during pregnancy. It is a cholestatic disorder characterized by (1) pruritus with onset in the second or third trimester of pregnancy, (2) markedly elevated serum bile acid levels, and (3) spontaneous relief of signs and symptoms within 2 to 3 weeks after delivery.

Intrahepatic cholestasis of pregnancy has been observed in almost all ethnic groups, but there is geographical variation in its incidence.[40] In most areas, the incidence is less than 0.2% of pregnancies; however, in Scandinavian and South American countries, the disorder occurs in as many as 10% of all pregnancies. Nulliparous women with multiple gestation are at highest risk. In a report from Chile, the prevalence of intrahepatic cholestasis of pregnancy was 21% among women with twin pregnancies and 4.7% among women with singleton pregnancies.[41] Although the disorder resolves promptly after delivery, it commonly recurs in subsequent pregnancies or with the administration of estrogenic oral contraceptives.

The specific etiology of intrahepatic cholestasis of pregnancy is unknown, but it seems to represent an enhanced sensitivity to the cholestatic effects of estrogenic steroids. Sulfation is an important step in reducing the cholestatic potential of estrogens and bile acids. Davies et al.[42] demonstrated decreased sulfotransferase activity during pregnancy.

Diagnosis

The diagnosis of intrahepatic cholestasis of pregnancy is considered in the pregnant woman in whom pruritus develops and is followed by jaundice 2 to 4 weeks later. Pruritus is the most distressing symptom and may lead to irritability, insomnia, and depression. Although physical examination demonstrates mild hepatomegaly, the presence of abdominal pain or hepatic tenderness should exclude the diagnosis of intrahepatic cholestasis of pregnancy. Biochemical abnormalities include markedly elevated serum bile acid concentrations and moderate conjugated hyperbilirubinemia. Serum transaminase enzyme levels may be normal or elevated. Although liver biopsy is rarely indicated, histopathology reveals acinar cholestasis and canalicular bile plugs. Inflammation and necrosis are not observed.[43] Impairment of bile salt excretion causes steatorrhea, fat malabsorption, and mild malnutrition.[44]

Effect on the Mother and Fetus

Intrahepatic cholestasis of pregnancy has minimal impact on maternal health during gestation. However, failure to correct vitamin K malabsorption may lead to clinical coagulopathy. Fisk et al.[45] reported an 11% incidence of postpartum hemorrhage among women with intrahepatic cholestasis of pregnancy.

Although pruritus is distressing, the mother should be assured that the disorder will resolve within 2 weeks after delivery. A 2006 study suggests, however, that some patients with intrahepatic cholestasis of pregnancy are at higher risk for certain liver and biliary diseases such as cirrhosis, hepatitis C, cholelithiasis, and cholecystitis.[46]

Although maternal outcome with intrahepatic cholestasis of pregnancy is generally good, the fetus is at increased risk.[47-49] Intrahepatic cholestasis of pregnancy increases the risk of preterm delivery (as much as 19% to 60%), meconium staining of amniotic fluid (as much as 27%), fetal bradycardia (as much as 14%), nonreassuring fetal heart rate patterns (as much as 22% to 41%), and fetal loss (as much as 0.4% to 4.1%),[48] particularly when associated with fasting serum bile acid levels greater than 40 μmol/L.[49] Early onset of pruritus and high levels of serum bile acids predict a higher risk of preterm delivery in patients with intrahepatic cholestasis of pregnancy and define a subgroup of patients at risk for poor neonatal outcome.[50] Israel et al.[51] demonstrated that myometrial strips from patients with intrahepatic cholestasis of pregnancy exhibit an enhanced contractile response to oxytocin, which correlates with the clinical observation of uterine hypertonus. Neonatal hypoprothrombinemia places the infant at increased risk for intracranial hemorrhage.

Medical and Obstetric Management

Medical management is directed toward improving bile secretion and reducing intestinal reabsorption of bile salts to provide symptomatic relief. Cholestyramine resin relieves the pruritus in many women, but its use has been associated with severe fetal intracranial hemorrhage, and it may aggravate fat malabsorption.[52] Ursodeoxycholic acid modifies the pool of biliary acids and provides marked regression of clinical and biologic markers of intrahepatic cholestasis of pregnancy.[53] Clinical trials have demonstrated better maternal and fetal outcomes after the administration of ursodeoxycholic acid.[54-56] Vitamin K should be administered subcutaneously if prolongation of the prothrombin time (PT) is noted during gestation. Mullally and Hansen[47] have recommended induction of labor and delivery near term (after confirmation of fetal lung maturity), or earlier if fetal compromise is identified.

ACUTE FATTY LIVER OF PREGNANCY (REVERSIBLE PERIPARTUM LIVER FAILURE)

Definition and Epidemiology

Idiopathic acute fatty liver of pregnancy (AFLP), or reversible peripartum liver failure, is an uncommon disorder of late pregnancy that is characterized by impaired hepatic metabolic activity, which may progress to liver failure, disseminated intravascular coagulation (DIC), a profoundly depressed antithrombin III level, hypoglycemia, and renal insufficiency. The liver failure resolves shortly after delivery in all but rare cases. Histologic examination of the liver demonstrates microvesicular fatty infiltration of the liver. Less than 100 cases of AFLP were reported before 1980, and the incidence was estimated at 1 per 1 million pregnancies.[57] With heightened awareness and early recognition, a later study suggested that the disorder may occur in 1 per 6700 gestations.[58]

Pathophysiology

Molecular advances suggest that AFLP may result from mitochondrial dysfunction in the fetal liver.[59] To date, AFLP has been documented in 30% to 80% of pregnancies in which the fetus was found to have a long-chain 3-hydroxyacyl-coenzyme A dehydrogenase (LCHAD) deficiency. It remains unclear why some mothers who give birth to a child with fatty acid oxidation defects develop AFLP, whereas others do not.[3] AFLP is more common in twin than in singleton pregnancies. Davidson et al.[60] reported three cases of AFLP in parturients with triplet gestation. Multiple gestation may further stress the fatty acid oxidation capacity in susceptible pregnant women.

Similarities between AFLP and preeclampsia or eclampsia are intriguing. Both disorders primarily occur near term and are associated with nulliparity and multiple gestation. Hepatic involvement occurs with preeclampsia in the form of the HELLP syndrome.

Diagnosis

The diagnosis of AFLP must be considered in any woman who presents with hepatic dysfunction during late pregnancy. Castro et al.[58] described 28 consecutive cases of AFLP over a 15-year period. Affected parturients recounted a prodromal period of 1 to 21 days (an average of 9 days) with symptoms including nausea and vomiting (71%), malaise (64%), abdominal pain (50%), fever (32%), jaundice or dark urine (29%), headache (21%), pruritus (11%), and sore throat (11%). Pruritus is uncommon and typically suggests the more common disorder intrahepatic cholestasis of pregnancy. Hepatic encephalopathy is a late and ominous finding. In this study, the diagnosis of AFLP was established before delivery in only 36% of cases.[58] Physical examination demonstrates an afebrile patient with mild hypertension and modest peripheral edema and jaundice.

The hallmark laboratory findings are prolonged prothrombin time, profoundly depressed antithrombin III levels, and elevated liver enzyme levels. In the series reported by Castro et al.,[58] all patients exhibited evidence of persistent DIC. Leukocytosis and elevated total bilirubin, creatinine, and alkaline phosphatase concentrations were observed in nearly all cases. Profound hypoglycemia (secondary to impaired hepatic glycogenolysis) was common. Excessive clinical bleeding occurred only in patients with delivery complications such as uterine atony, cesarean delivery, and genital tract injury.[58] Similarly, oliguria is observed only in parturients with hypovolemia caused by hemorrhage. Liver biopsy is rarely required for the diagnosis because clinical findings exclude all other possibilities except preeclampsia. Biopsy findings for preeclampsia are identical to those for AFLP and do not alter treatment (i.e., delivery of the infant). Further, biopsy may be precluded by coagulopathy. Diagnostic imaging rarely contributes to the diagnosis. Fatty infiltration of the liver can be documented by ultrasonography and computed tomography in approximately half of all cases.[58]

Effect on the Mother and Fetus

With improved clinical recognition, prompt delivery of the infant, and aggressive medical management of the parturient, maternal and fetal mortality rates for AFLP have decreased considerably over the last half-century.[58] Maternal complications include DIC, profound hypoglycemia, hepatic encephalopathy, pancreatitis, acute renal failure, and hepatic rupture. Fetal compromise and death may occur secondary to uteroplacental insufficiency. Moise and Shah[61] have cautioned that replacement of maternal coagulation factors may lead to the deposition of fibrin at the choriodecidual interface and subsequent uteroplacental insufficiency.

Among the 30 fetuses (including two sets of twins) reported by Castro et al.,[58] there was one stillbirth and one neonatal death resulting from perinatal asphyxia. Despite aggressive maternal support, fetal compromise occurred frequently. Meconium-stained amniotic fluid was noted in 60% of cases.[58]

Before 1990, it was thought that AFLP did not recur during subsequent pregnancies. Watson and Seeds[62] reviewed the records of 21 women with a history of AFLP during a previous pregnancy. There was no recurrence among the 25 later gestations. However, four cases of recurrent AFLP have subsequently been reported.[63-65]

Medical, Obstetric, and Anesthetic Management

AFLP is a medical emergency that demands rapid evaluation and treatment. Hepatic failure and fetal death may occur within a few days.[57] There are no reported cases of maternal recovery before delivery. As soon as the diagnosis is established and the mother is stabilized, plans must be made for delivery of the infant. Cesarean delivery offers no clear advantage over expeditious vaginal delivery. Immediate maternal supportive care consists of optimization of fluid and electrolytes, treatment of hypoglycemia, and attention to coagulopathy and anemia. The maternal glucose level should be checked every hour[66]; hypoglycemia should be treated by continuous intravenous infusion of 10% dextrose solution.[67] Hepatic encephalopathy may improve with enteral lactulose and a low-protein, high-carbohydrate diet.[57]

The anesthesiologist should anticipate postpartum hemorrhage, establish adequate intravenous access, and ensure that cross-matched blood is immediately available for any parturient with AFLP. In most cases, the maternal condition improves within 24 to 48 hours after delivery, with continued recovery during the subsequent week. Survivors experience no hepatic residua, and subsequent liver biopsies show no evidence of fibrosis.[58] Holzman et al.[68] described the anesthetic management of a patient with AFLP who presented with hepatic dysfunction, coagulopathy, and worsening hepatic encephalopathy. Because of her deteriorating condition, cesarean delivery with general anesthesia was planned. The authors recommended careful documentation of neurologic status both before and after general anesthesia as well as meticulous attention to the coagulopathic state, including adequate venous access and availability of blood products.

Orthotopic liver transplantation is an option for the rare parturient who shows no evidence of recovery within 3 days postpartum.[69-71] This measure must be considered with great caution, because AFLP is a reversible form of acute hepatic failure in nearly all patients. Doepel et al.[72] described a young, previously healthy parturient who was diagnosed with AFLP at delivery. Fulminant hepatic failure with severe encephalopathy and hepatorenal syndrome rapidly ensued. Hepatic imaging showed 90% parenchymal damage, and liver biopsy revealed necrosis. Her name was added to the Scandinavian liver transplant waiting list with high urgent status, but no suitable liver was found. After 8 days, her clinical condition improved, and her name was removed from the transplant waiting list. Four weeks after delivery, the patient was discharged in good condition. Six months later, she was feeling well and clinical parameters were normal.

SPONTANEOUS HEPATIC RUPTURE OF PREGNANCY

Spontaneous hepatic rupture is a rare complication of late pregnancy or the early puerperium. In 2003, Marsh et al.[73] reported that 150 cases of hepatic rupture in pregnancy had been published. Hepatic hematomas are associated with preeclampsia and HELLP syndrome but are also associated with biliary disease, infection, aneurysms, and hepatic neoplasms.[74] The typical presentation is a triad of preeclampsia, right upper quadrant pain, and acute hypotension. Few cases have been diagnosed correctly before laparotomy or autopsy. When cases have been diagnosed at surgery, the preoperative diagnosis usually was placental abruption, uterine rupture, or perforated gastrointestinal ulcer.[75]

By definition, spontaneous hepatic rupture of pregnancy occurs in the absence of antecedent trauma. Instead, rupture is preceded by an intraparenchymal hepatic hematoma. The strong association with preeclampsia suggests that periportal hemorrhagic necrosis, hypertension, and coagulopathy may lead to hematoma formation. With expansion of the hematoma, the hepatic capsule is progressively distended and dissected from the parenchyma, leading to rupture.[75,76]

The mortality rate from hepatic rupture in pregnancy is greater than 60%, but it could be reduced by greater awareness and improved diagnostic modalities.[77] Ultrasonography, computed tomography, magnetic resonance imaging, angiography, technetium scintigraphy, and exploratory laparotomy may demonstrate the expanding hematoma before rupture.[78,79]

Initial management of hepatic rupture typically involves intravenous hydration and transfusion of blood products. Treatment options include open laparotomy, hepatic artery ligation or embolization, and compression of bleeding points with hepatic packing.[77] Shrivastava et al.[77] used an argon beam coagulator to obtain hemostasis in a patient with HELLP syndrome and hepatic rupture; they suggested that this approach represents a "new, potentially superior modality in the management of hepatic rupture in pregnancy." Hepatic transplantation is necessary when the aforementioned maneuvers fail to stop hemorrhage during laparotomy, or when severe hepatic necrosis occurs.[80]

PORTAL HYPERTENSION

Portal hypertension is a disorder that commonly follows cirrhosis of the liver. It may also occur secondary to noncirrhotic portal fibrosis or extrahepatic portal venous obstruction.[81] It is uncommon during pregnancy because it rarely affects women of reproductive age. Chronic liver disease also impairs fertility.[82] Clinical manifestations of portal hypertension include the development of portal-systemic collateral vessels, splenomegaly, and ascites. The portal-systemic collateral vessels of greatest significance are those within the gastric and esophageal mucosae. Hemorrhage from varices is the most significant complication of portal hypertension; it is associated with a 30% to 50% mortality rate per bleeding episode.[83]

Risk of Variceal Hemorrhage during Pregnancy

During normal pregnancy, uterine compression of the inferior vena cava causes diversion of venous return through the azygos and vertebral venous systems.[84] This feature has led some physicians to believe that pregnancy may increase the rate of variceal hemorrhage. In addition, some physicians have advocated cesarean delivery to avoid the straining and variceal rupture that may occur during vaginal delivery.

Schreyer et al.[85] reviewed 99 pregnancies in women with cirrhosis. Pregnancy occurred in 30 women with a portosystemic shunt and 69 without a shunt. The incidence of severe variceal hemorrhage was eight times greater in the patients without shunts (24%) than in patients with shunts (3%). The maternal mortality rate was 13% in the nonshunt group. The investigators recommended consideration of prophylactic portosystemic shunting for cirrhotic women who might become pregnant.

Britton[86] reviewed 83 pregnancies in 53 women with cirrhotic portal hypertension and 77 pregnancies in 38 women with noncirrhotic portal hypertension. When women with prior shunting were excluded, the incidence of variceal hemorrhage was 50%. An 18% mortality rate followed these hemorrhagic events. The majority of bleeding episodes occurred during the second trimester. Only 1 of the 61 patients who underwent vaginal delivery suffered intrapartum variceal bleeding, suggesting that the mode of delivery had little influence on the risk of bleeding.

Kochhar et al.[87] reviewed 116 pregnancies in 44 women with noncirrhotic portal hypertension. The incidence of fetal loss was 8%, which did not differ from the 10% incidence found in an age-matched control group. The incidence of variceal bleeding was 14%. All events were successfully managed with sclerotherapy.

Medical and Obstetric Management

Endoscopic sclerotherapy is the preferred method of managing variceal hemorrhage during pregnancy.[88] It is currently recommended that all women with portal hypertension who wish to conceive should undergo endoscopy and prophylactic sclerotherapy before conception.[89] Endoscopic evaluation should be repeated at least once each trimester. If uncontrolled hemorrhage occurs despite sclerotherapy, portosystemic shunting may be considered.[88,89] Zeeman and Moise[90] reported the use of prophylactic banding in a parturient with severe esophageal varices deemed unmanageable with endoscopic sclerotherapy alone.

The transjugular intrahepatic portosystemic stent-shunt (TIPS) procedure, introduced for the management of portal hypertension in nonpregnant patients,[91] has not achieved better outcomes than traditional endoscopic sclerotherapy.[92] Nevertheless, the procedure is gaining more acceptance, and a 2008 report described its use for the management of acute variceal bleeding in a pregnant woman.[93]

Frequent antenatal assessment of hepatic function, hematologic status, and fetal well-being is recommended. Sodium restriction or diuresis should be approached cautiously during pregnancy. Prophylactic therapy with a histamine H_2-receptor antagonist may prevent reflux esophagitis. Cesarean delivery should be reserved for obstetric indications. Facilities and personnel to manage massive gastrointestinal hemorrhage must be immediately available.

LIVER TRANSPLANTATION DURING PREGNANCY

In 1978, Walcott et al.[94] documented the first pregnancy in a liver transplant recipient. Subsequently, hundreds of such pregnancies have been reported worldwide. Only a few have involved liver transplantation *during* pregnancy. Cases with successful maternal[95,96] and fetal[96] outcomes have been reported.

The need for liver transplantation during pregnancy arises in cases of fulminant hepatic failure, a dramatic clinical event that may result from several diseases.[97-99] Some of these diseases, such as the HELLP syndrome, AFLP, and preeclampsia, are unique to pregnancy. In cases of fulminant hepatic failure, the only alternatives to liver transplantation are living-related right lobe liver transplantation[95,100] and the use of an extracorporeal liver support device such as a molecular adsorbent recirculating system (MARS).[101,102]

Anesthetic considerations for surgery during pregnancy are described in Chapter 17. The primary concerns are preterm delivery and low birth weight,[103] both of which seem to be persistent problems in all solid-organ transplant recipients with immunosuppression.[104]

PREGNANCY AFTER LIVER TRANSPLANTATION

Three large databases track pregnancy in transplant recipients, yielding important information about the effect of pregnancy on the allograft and the obstetric course in pregnant patients with liver transplants. These are the United Kingdom Pregnancy Registry, the European Dialysis and Transplantation Association, and, in the United States, the National Transplantation Pregnancy Registry (NTPR). The NTPR was established in 1991 to study the outcomes of pregnancy in solid organ recipients, including both female recipients and women with pregnancies fathered by male recipients. The NTPR is an active registry that tracks immediate maternal and fetal outcomes as well as long-term follow-up of the recipient and offspring. As of January 2005, the NTPR had reported outcomes in 111 female liver transplant recipients with 187 pregnancies and 189 live-born infants (Table 46-4).[103] The mean gestational age was 37 weeks, and the mean birth weight was 2705 g; 36% of newborns were born preterm, and 34% exhibited low birth weight (defined as birth weight less than 2500 g). The incidence of birth defects in the newborn was not higher than that found in the general population.

Overall, the outcomes of pregnancies in liver transplant recipients appear to be favorable.[105] The live birth rate, between 69% and 73%, appears to be fairly consistent among most studies.[103,105,106] Although the rates of maternal complications—in particular, hypertensive disorders—appear to be higher in pregnancy, no increase in rates of graft loss has been reported. Rejection episodes can be managed with the usual interventions; pregnancy does not appear to increase maternal mortality in this population. Outcomes among newborns appear to be favorable, without significant adverse effects from exposure to

TABLE 46-4 Maternal Outcomes in Liver Transplant Recipients

Maternal Outcomes in Liver Transplant Recipients	
Hypertension during pregnancy	35%
Preeclampsia	23%
Infection during pregnancy	27%
Diabetes during pregnancy	5%
Rejection episode during pregnancy	8%
Graft loss within 2 years of delivery	7%
Outcomes of Live Births of Liver Transplant Recipients	
Mean gestational age	37 weeks
Preterm birth (< 37 weeks)	36%
Mean birth weight	2705 g
Low birth weight (< 2500 g)	34%
Cesarean delivery	35%
Newborn complications	29%
Neonatal deaths (within 30 days of birth)	0%

Adapted from Armenti VT, Radomski JS, Moritz MJ, et al. Report from the National Transplantation Pregnancy Registry (NTPR): Outcomes of pregnancy after transplantation. In Cecka JM, Terasaki PI, editors. Clinical Transplants, 2004. Los Angeles, UCLA Tissue Typing Laboratory, 2004:103-14.

immunosuppressant drugs. Management goals for liver transplant recipients who become pregnant include (1) optimization of maternal health (e.g., graft function, comorbidities); (2) identification and treatment of complications (e.g., preeclampsia); and (3) minimization of the complications of preterm birth.[106] Data from one study suggest that use of the immunosuppressant drug tacrolimus in pregnant women is associated with a lower incidence of new-onset hypertension and preeclampsia than the use of cyclosporine.[104]

ANESTHETIC MANAGEMENT OF THE PARTURIENT WITH LIVER DISEASE

Anesthetic management is determined by the extent of hepatic impairment. Women with inactive viral hepatitis, mild intrahepatic cholestasis of pregnancy, or uncomplicated liver transplantation may be managed in the same manner as healthy parturients, provided that hepatic synthetic and metabolic function are intact; coagulopathy should be excluded or corrected before neuraxial anesthesia is administered. In contrast, the parturient with acute viral hepatitis, advanced cirrhosis, portal hypertension, or AFLP presents the anesthesiologist with many challenges (Box 46-1).

Systemic Abnormalities Associated with Hepatic Disease

Acute and chronic parenchymal liver disease results in impaired synthesis of coagulation factors I, II, V, VII, and X. Cholestasis leads to malabsorption of vitamin K, an important cofactor required for the synthesis of factors II, VII, IX, and X. The plasma half-life of factor VII is 5 hours, so coagulopathy may develop rapidly. Coagulopathy is rapidly corrected by administration of vitamin K if malabsorption is the primary defect, but women with impaired hepatic synthesis do not respond to vitamin K. Fresh frozen plasma or cryoprecipitate may be needed if excessive bleeding occurs.

Cardiovascular manifestations of hepatic insufficiency include increased cardiac output and low systemic vascular resistance (SVR). The latter is caused by extensive arteriovenous shunting. Hepatic insufficiency results in an increase in blood volume greater than that in normal pregnancy. Cardiomyopathy may develop. Although cardiac filling pressures are typically normal, tense ascites may impair venous return. Monitoring of central venous or pulmonary artery pressure should be considered for patients with ascites or cardiomyopathy who require cesarean delivery.

Impaired hypoxic pulmonary vasoconstriction and portopulmonary venous communication lead to significant hypoxemia. Ascites and the gravid uterus cause diaphragmatic elevation, decrease functional residual capacity, and lead to further intrapulmonary shunting. Patients with liver disease exhibit increased 2,3-diphosphoglycerate levels within red blood cells and a rightward shift of the oxyhemoglobin dissociation curve.[107]

Hepatic encephalopathy is a reversible neuropsychiatric disorder that occurs in patients with advanced hepatic failure. Proposed mechanisms include altered gamma-aminobutyric acid levels, increased brain influx of false neurotransmitters, and inadequate hepatic clearance of ammonia and mercaptan toxins.[108] Impairments may range from mild confusion to coma. Patients are at risk for pulmonary aspiration of gastric contents. The integrity of the blood-brain barrier is altered, and anesthetic agents should be titrated carefully.[107]

Metabolic abnormalities associated with hepatic disease include hypoglycemia, hyponatremia, hypokalemia, and acid-base disturbances. Hypoglycemia, which results from impairment of hepatic gluconeogenesis and glycogenolysis, is especially common in patients with AFLP. Glucose concentrations in these patients should be determined frequently.

Albumin is synthesized exclusively by the liver. Its half-life is approximately 15 days; therefore, a change in the serum albumin concentration is not a sensitive marker of hepatic function. Hepatic failure is associated with increased plasma triglyceride and abnormal lipoprotein concentrations.[109] These metabolic changes may be sensitive markers of hepatic function.

Abnormal renal sodium retention often accompanies hepatic disease, contributing to ascites formation. Its pathogenesis, although unclear, seems to involve increases in plasma aldosterone concentration and sympathetic activity, reduction in renal blood flow, and alteration in renal prostaglandins and kinins; it may also involve renal vasoconstriction and central hypovolemia. Overt oliguric renal failure may occur, heralding the onset of the **hepatorenal syndrome.** The prognosis for affected patients is poor.

BOX 46-1 Anesthetic Guidelines for the Parturient with Liver Disease

- Evaluate the extent of hepatic impairment.
- Recognize and evaluate underlying systemic abnormalities.
- Assist the obstetric team with stabilization of maternal condition before delivery.
- Exclude or correct coagulopathy before administration of neuraxial anesthesia.
- Prevent further hepatic injury by optimizing hepatic blood flow and oxygenation.
- Recognize altered pharmacokinetics and pharmacodynamics.
- Prevent transmission of viral hepatitis to the health care team.
- Monitor the patient for evidence of postoperative hepatic dysfunction.

Effect of Anesthesia on Hepatic Blood Flow and Oxygenation

In a parturient with compromised hepatic function, failure to maintain hepatic blood flow or oxygenation may lead to further hepatic necrosis and hepatic failure. Frink et al.[110] examined the effects of four volatile halogenated agents on hepatic blood flow and oxygenation in dogs. Hepatic oxygen delivery was reduced to the following levels of control at 1.0 minimum alveolar concentration (MAC): 86% by sevoflurane, 81% by isoflurane, 57% by enflurane, and 57% by halothane. Kanaya et al.[111] confirmed that isoflurane has a more favorable effect than halothane on liver perfusion.

Adequate hepatic oxygenation is especially important in the presence of halothane because hypoxia forces halothane metabolism into a reductive rather than oxidative pathway. Subsequent reductive metabolites are more reactive and hepatotoxic,[112,113] but no type of general anesthesia has been indisputably proven to cause postoperative hepatic dysfunction.

Neuraxial anesthesia also may reduce hepatic blood flow.[114,115] The reduction largely reflects the effects of systemic arterial hypotension secondary to sympathetic blockade. However, Tanaka et al.[116] demonstrated a reduction in hepatic blood flow during epidural anesthesia despite the maintenance of normotension by continuous infusion of colloid. The decrease in hepatic blood flow was reversed by the addition of a dopamine infusion, suggesting that reduced cardiac output, secondary to sympathetic blockade, was responsible for the observed decrease in hepatic blood flow. Nevertheless, most anesthesiologists believe that judicious hydration, slow induction of epidural anesthesia, and avoidance of systemic hypotension will minimize the chances of a clinically significant reduction in hepatic blood flow.

Neuraxial Anesthesia

In the absence of coagulopathy, neuraxial anesthesia may be administered to the parturient with hepatic disease.[117] Amide-type local anesthetic agents undergo hepatic biotransformation. In patients with cirrhosis, the half-life of lidocaine increases almost threefold (from 108 to 296 minutes), and the volume of distribution increases from 1.3 to 2.3 L/kg.[118] An expanded volume of distribution offers some protection against toxicity despite impaired clearance. 2-Chloroprocaine undergoes hydrolysis with pseudocholinesterase. Although hepatic pseudocholinesterase production may be decreased in patients with liver disease, the effect (if any) on the overall clearance of 2-chloroprocaine is unclear.

In patients with end-stage liver dysfunction being evaluated for liver transplantation, the clearance of ropivacaine was found to be approximately 60% lower than in healthy volunteers, although plasma concentrations were similar.[119] Thus, when repeated doses or continuous infusions of local anesthetic are administered, the accumulation of bupivacaine and ropivacaine (and their metabolites) should be considered, and doses should be reduced accordingly. Even in patients with end-stage liver dysfunction, alpha-1-acid glycoprotein is synthesized, providing some protection against local anesthetic toxicity.[119] Because of the high volume of local anesthetic agent required, some anesthesiologists have discouraged the administration of epidural anesthesia in patients with liver disease, although no studies of drug disposition after such administration have been published.[113] Ascites and portal hypertension lead to engorged epidural veins; the use of a test dose to exclude intravascular injection is essential. Heriot et al.[120] reported the successful administration of epidural anesthesia to a parturient with portal hypertension and esophageal varices. Although one might infer that spinal anesthesia is safer than epidural anesthesia because it requires administration of a smaller dose of local anesthetic, spinal anesthesia also leads to the rapid onset of sympathetic blockade.

General Anesthesia

Coagulopathy, obstetric hemorrhage, severe fetal compromise, and/or altered mental status may necessitate the use of general anesthesia for cesarean delivery. Intravascular volume should be evaluated before the induction of anesthesia. Monitoring of arterial and central venous pressures may be useful in the patient with ascites or cardiovascular compromise. Large-gauge intravenous access should be established. Patients with bleeding esophageal varices should be intubated while awake. Nasogastric suction is contraindicated. Rapid-sequence induction may be facilitated, depending on the patient's hemodynamic status, with thiopental, propofol, ketamine, or etomidate. Liver disease and reduced pseudocholinesterase concentrations may delay the metabolism of succinylcholine, but the delay is of negligible clinical importance.[121] Succinylcholine thus remains the muscle relaxant of choice during rapid-sequence induction of general anesthesia, and it should be administered in the same bolus dose used for healthy parturients. Airway trauma must be avoided in the patient with coagulopathy; profound neuromuscular blockade facilitates atraumatic tracheal intubation. After documentation of neuromuscular recovery, paralysis may be maintained with atracurium or cisatracurium because these agents are metabolized by Hoffman degradation independent of hepatic function. Inhalation anesthesia may be maintained with isoflurane and nitrous oxide. Reversal of neuromuscular blockade must be documented before extubation.

Although clearance is delayed in patients with severe liver disease, opioids may be administered cautiously to provide postoperative analgesia. Advanced liver disease can lead to hepatic encephalopathy.[122] Neurologic deterioration in the postoperative period may result from the residual effects of anesthetic agents, progressive encephalopathy, or elevated intracranial pressure; therefore, regular neurologic observation is essential to the proper management of pregnant women with advanced liver disease.

KEY POINTS

- All pregnant women should be screened for hepatitis B virus, and all newborns should be vaccinated against it.
- Acute fatty liver of pregnancy is a rare but life-threatening complication of pregnancy that demands rapid evaluation and prompt delivery.
- Women with portal hypertension should undergo endoscopy and prophylactic sclerotherapy before conception.
- Pregnancy does not affect the long-term survival of hepatic allografts.
- Post-transplantation immunosuppression is well tolerated during pregnancy.
- Coagulopathy must be excluded or corrected before neuraxial anesthesia is administered to parturients with liver disease.

REFERENCES

1. Keeffe EB. Acute viral hepatitis. In Dale DC, Federman DD, editors. WebMD Scientific American Medicine, 2003 edition. New York City, WebMD Professional Publishing, 2003.
2. American College of Obstetricians and Gynecologists Committee on Gynecologic Practice. Hepatitis B and hepatitis C virus infections in obstetrician-gynecologists. ACOG Committee Opinion No. 332. Washington, DC, ACOG, May 2006.
3. Schutt VA, Minuk GY. Liver diseases unique to pregnancy. Best Pract Res Clin Gastroenterol 2007; 21:771-92.
4. Brundage SC, Fitzpatrick AN. Hepatitis A. Am Fam Physician 2006; 73:2162-8.
5. Jonas MM, Schiff ER, O'Sullivan MJ, et al. Failure of Centers for Disease Control criteria to identify hepatitis B infection in a large municipal obstetrical population. Ann Intern Med 1987; 107:335-7.
6. Arevalo JA, Washington AE. Cost-effectiveness of prenatal screening and immunization for hepatitis B virus. JAMA 1988; 259:365-9.
7. Shepard CW, Simard EP, Finelli L, et al. Hepatitis B virus infection: Epidemiology and vaccination. Epidemiol Rev 2006; 28:112-25.
8. Beltrami EM, Williams IT, Shapiro CN, Chamberland ME. Risk and management of blood-borne infections in health care workers. Clin Microbiol Rev 2000; 13:385-407.
9. Reyes GR, Purdy MA, Kim JP, et al. Isolation of a cDNA from the virus responsible for enterically transmitted non-A, non-B hepatitis. Science 1990; 247:1335-9.
10. Velázquez O, Stetler HC, Avila C, et al. Epidemic transmission of enterically transmitted non-A, non-B hepatitis in Mexico, 1986-1987. JAMA 1990; 263:3281-5.
11. Kwo PY, Schlauder GG, Carpenter HA, et al. Acute hepatitis E by a new isolate acquired in the United States. Mayo Clin Proc 1997; 72:1133-6.
12. Tsega E, Hansson BG, Krawczynski K, Nordenfelt E. Acute sporadic viral hepatitis in Ethiopia: Causes, risk factors, and effects on pregnancy. Clin Infect Dis 1992; 14:961-5.
13. Deka N, Sharma MD, Mukerjee R. Isolation of the novel agent from human stool samples that is associated with sporadic non-A, non-B hepatitis. J Virol 1994; 68:7810-5.
14. Kelly D, Skidmore S. Hepatitis C-Z: Recent advances. Arch Dis Child 2002; 86:339-43.
15. Linnen J, Wages J Jr, Zhang-Keck ZY, et al. Molecular cloning and disease association of hepatitis G virus: A transfusion-transmissible agent. Science 1996; 271:505-8.
16. Alter HJ, Nakatsuji Y, Melpolder J, et al. The incidence of transfusion-associated hepatitis G virus infection and its relation to liver disease. N Engl J Med 1997; 336:747-54.
17. Zanetti AR, Tanzi E, Romanó L, et al. Multicenter trial on mother-to-infant transmission of GBV-C virus. The Lombardy Study Group on Vertical/Perinatal Hepatitis Viruses Transmission. J Med Virol 1998; 54:107-12.
18. Pessoa MG, Terrault NA, Detmer J, et al. Quantitation of hepatitis G and C viruses in the liver: Evidence that hepatitis G virus is not hepatotropic. Hepatology 1998; 27:877-80.
19. Astegiano M, Sapone N, Demarchi B, et al. Laboratory evaluation of the patient with liver disease. Eur Rev Med Pharmacol Sci 2004; 8:3-9.
20. Baumert TF, Thimme R, von Weizsäcker F. Pathogenesis of hepatitis B virus infection. World J Gastroenterol 2007; 13:82-90.
21. Chevaliez S, Pawlotsky JM. Hepatitis C virus serologic and virologic tests and clinical diagnosis of HCV-related liver disease. Int J Med Sci 2006; 3:35-40.
22. Ramezani A, Gachkar L, Eslamifar A, et al. Detection of hepatitis G virus envelope protein E2 antibody in blood donors. Int J Infect Dis 2008; 12:57-61.
23. Mast EE, Margolis HS, Fiore AE, et al. Advisory Committee on Immunization Practices (ACIP). A comprehensive immunization strategy to eliminate transmission of hepatitis B virus infection in the United States: Recommendations of the Advisory Committee on Immunization Practices (ACIP), Part 1: Immunization of infants, children, and adolescents. MMWR Recomm Rep 2005; 54:1-31.
24. Saez A, Losa M, Lo Iacono O, et al. Diagnostic and prognostic value of virologic tests in vertical transmission of hepatitis C virus infection: Results of a large prospective study in pregnant women. Hepatogastroenterology 2004; 51:1104-8.
25. Mariné-Barjoan E, Berrébi A, Giordanengo V, et al. HCV/HIV co-infection, HCV viral load and mode of delivery: Risk factors for mother-to-child transmission of hepatitis C virus? AIDS 2007; 21:1811-5.
26. Sookoian S. Liver disease during pregnancy: Acute viral hepatitis. Ann Hepatol 2006; 5:231-6.
27. Hepatitis in pregnancy. ACOG Technical Bulletin No. 17. Washington, DC, November 1992. (Int J Gynaecol Obstet 1993; 42:189-98.)
28. Advisory Committee on Immunization Practice (ACIP), Fiore AE, Wasley A, Bell BP. Prevention of hepatitis A through active or passive immunization: Recommendations of the Advisory Committee on Immunization Practices (ACIP). MMWR Recomm Rep 2006; 55:1-23.
29. Centers for Disease Control and Prevention, Workowski KA, Berman SM. Sexually transmitted diseases treatment guidelines, 2006. MMWR Recomm Rep 2006; 55:1-94.
30. Xu XW, Chen YG. Current therapy with nucleoside/nucleotide analogs for patients with chronic hepatitis B. Hepatobiliary Pancreat Dis Int 2006; 5:350-9.
31. van Zonneveld M, van Nunen AB, Niesters HG, et al. Lamivudine treatment during pregnancy to prevent perinatal transmission of hepatitis B virus infection. J Viral Hepat 2003; 10:294-7.
32. Burns DN, Minkoff H. Hepatitis C: Screening in pregnancy. Obstet Gynecol 1999; 94:1044-8.
33. Keeffe EB, Hollinger FB. Therapy of hepatitis C: Consensus interferon trials. Consensus Interferon Study Group. Hepatology 1997; 26:101S-7S.
34. Ruggiero G, Andreana A, Zampino R. Normal pregnancy under inadvertent alpha-interferon therapy for chronic hepatitis C. J Hepatol 1996; 24:646.
35. Ozaslan E, Yilmaz R, Simsek H, Tatar G. Interferon therapy for acute hepatitis C during pregnancy. Ann Pharmacother 2002; 36:1715-8.
36. Hunt CM, Carson KL, Sharara AI. Hepatitis C in pregnancy. Obstet Gynecol 1997; 89:883-90.
37. Wang J, Zhu Q, Zhang X. Effect of delivery mode on maternal-infant transmission of hepatitis B virus by immunoprophylaxis. Chin Med J (Engl) 2002; 115:1510-2.
38. Airoldi J, Berghella V. Hepatitis C and pregnancy. Obstet Gynecol Surv 2006; 61:666-72.
39. Syriopoulou V, Nikolopoulou G, Daikos GL, et al. Mother to child transmission of hepatitis C virus: Rate of infection and risk factors. Scand J Infect Dis 2005; 37:350-3.
40. Lammert F, Marschall HU, Glantz A, Matern S. Intrahepatic cholestasis of pregnancy: Molecular pathogenesis, diagnosis and management. J Hepatol 2000; 33:1012-21.
41. Gonzalez MC, Reyes H, Arrese M, et al. Intrahepatic cholestasis of pregnancy in twin pregnancies. J Hepatol 1989; 9:84-90.
42. Davies MH, Ngong JM, Yucesoy M, et al. The adverse influence of pregnancy upon sulphation: A clue to the pathogenesis of intrahepatic cholestasis of pregnancy? J Hepatol 1994; 21:1127-34.
43. Rolfes DB, Ishak KG. Liver disease in pregnancy. Histopathology 1986; 10:555-70.
44. Reyes H, Radrigan ME, Gonzalez MC, et al. Steatorrhea in patients with intrahepatic cholestasis of pregnancy. Gastroenterology 1987; 93:584-90.
45. Fisk NM, Bye WB, Storey GN. Maternal features of obstetric cholestasis: 20 years experience at King George V Hospital. Aust N Z J Obstet Gynaecol 1988; 28:172-6.
46. Ropponen A, Sund R, Riikonen S, et al. Intrahepatic cholestasis of pregnancy as an indicator of liver and biliary diseases: A population-based study. Hepatology 2006; 43:723-8.
47. Mullally BA, Hansen WF. Intrahepatic cholestasis of pregnancy: Review of the literature. Obstet Gynecol Surv 2002; 57:47-52.
48. Fisk NM, Storey GN. Fetal outcome in obstetric cholestasis. Br J Obstet Gynaecol 1988; 95:1137-43.

49. Glantz A, Marschall HU, Mattsson LA. Intrahepatic cholestasis of pregnancy: Relationships between bile acid levels and fetal complication rates. Hepatology 2004; 40:467-74.
50. Kondrackiene J, Beuers U, Zalinkevicius R, et al. Predictors of premature delivery in patients with intrahepatic cholestasis of pregnancy. World J Gastroenterol 2007; 13:6226-30.
51. Israel EJ, Guzman ML, Campos GA. Maximal response to oxytocin of the isolated myometrium from pregnant patients with intrahepatic cholestasis. Acta Obstet Gynecol Scand 1986; 65:581-2.
52. Sadler LC, Lane M, North R. Severe fetal intracranial haemorrhage during treatment with cholestyramine for intrahepatic cholestasis of pregnancy. Br J Obstet Gynaecol 1995; 102:169-70.
53. Glantz A, Reilly SJ, Benthin L, et al. Intrahepatic cholestasis of pregnancy: Amelioration of pruritus by UDCA is associated with decreased progesterone disulphates in urine. Hepatology 2008; 47:544-51.
54. Floreani A, Paternoster D, Melis A, Grella PV. S-adenosylmethionine versus ursodeoxycholic acid in the treatment of intrahepatic cholestasis of pregnancy: Preliminary results of a controlled trial. Eur J Obstet Gynecol Reprod Biol 1996; 67:109-13.
55. Diaferia A, Nicastri PL, Tartagni M, et al. Ursodeoxycholic acid therapy in pregnant women with cholestasis. Int J Gynaecol Obstet 1996; 52:133-40.
56. Berkane N, Cocheton JJ, Brehier D, et al. Ursodeoxycholic acid in intrahepatic cholestasis of pregnancy: A retrospective study of 19 cases. Acta Obstet Gynecol Scand 2000; 79:941-6.
57. Kaplan MM. Acute fatty liver of pregnancy. N Engl J Med 1985; 313:367-70.
58. Castro MA, Fassett MJ, Reynolds TB, et al. Reversible peripartum liver failure: A new perspective on the diagnosis, treatment, and cause of acute fatty liver of pregnancy, based on 28 consecutive cases. Am J Obstet Gynecol 1999; 181:389-95.
59. Ibdah J. Acute fatty liver of pregnancy: An update on pathogenesis and clinical implications. World J Gastroenterol 2006; 12:7397-404.
60. Davidson KM, Simpson LL, Knox TA, D'Alton ME. Acute fatty liver of pregnancy in triplet gestation. Obstet Gynecol 1998; 91:806-8.
61. Moise KJ Jr, Shah DM. Acute fatty liver of pregnancy: Etiology of fetal distress and fetal wastage. Obstet Gynecol 1987; 69:482-5.
62. Watson WJ, Seeds JW. Acute fatty liver of pregnancy. Obstet Gynecol Surv 1990; 45:585-91.
63. Visconti M, Manes G, Giannattasio F, Uomo G. Recurrence of acute fatty liver of pregnancy. J Clin Gastroenterol 1995; 21:243-5.
64. MacLean MA, Cameron AD, Cumming GP, et al. Recurrence of acute fatty liver of pregnancy. Br J Obstet Gynaecol 1994; 101:453-4.
65. Barton JR, Sibai BM, Mabie WC, Shanklin DR. Recurrent acute fatty liver of pregnancy. Am J Obstet Gynecol 1990; 163:534-8.
66. Korula J, Malatjalian DA, Badley BW. Acute fatty liver of pregnancy. Can Med Assoc J 1982; 127:575-8.
67. Mjahed K, Charra B, Hamoudi D, et al. Acute fatty liver of pregnancy. Arch Gynecol Obstet 2006; 274:349-53.
68. Holzman RS, Riley LE, Aron E, Fetherston J. Perioperative care of a patient with acute fatty liver of pregnancy. Anesth Analg 2001; 92:1268-70.
69. Ockner SA, Brunt EM, Cohn SM, et al. Fulminant hepatic failure caused by acute fatty liver of pregnancy treated by orthotopic liver transplantation. Hepatology 1990; 11:59-64.
70. Amon E, Allen SR, Petrie RH, Belew JE. Acute fatty liver of pregnancy associated with preeclampsia: Management of hepatic failure with postpartum liver transplantation. Am J Perinatol 1991; 8:278-9.
71. Franco J, Newcomer J, Adams M, Saeian K. Auxiliary liver transplant in acute fatty liver of pregnancy. Obstet Gynecol 2000; 95:1042.
72. Doepel M, Backas HN, Taskinen EI, et al. Spontaneous recovery of post partum liver necrosis in a patient listed for transplantation. Hepatogastroenterology 1996; 43:1084-7.
73. Marsh FA, Kaufmann SJ, Bhabra K. Surviving hepatic rupture in pregnancy—a literature review with an illustrative case report. J Obstet Gynaecol 2003; 23:109-13.
74. Carlson KL, Bader CL. Ruptured subcapsular liver hematoma in pregnancy: A case report of nonsurgical management. Am J Obstet Gynecol 2004; 190:558-60.
75. Bis KA, Waxman B. Rupture of the liver associated with pregnancy: A review of the literature and report of 2 cases. Obstet Gynecol Surv 1976; 31:763-73.
76. Minuk GY, Lui RC, Kelly JK. Rupture of the liver associated with acute fatty liver of pregnancy. Am J Gastroenterol 1987; 82:457-60.
77. Shrivastava VK, Imagawa D, Wing DA. Argon beam coagulator for treatment of hepatic rupture with hemolysis, elevated liver enzymes, low platelets (HELLP) syndrome. Obstet Gynecol 2006; 107:525-6.
78. Poo JL, Góngora J. Hepatic hematoma and hepatic rupture in pregnancy. Ann Hepatol 2006; 5:224-6.
79. Wilson MW, Fidelman N, Lull RJ, et al. Evaluation of active bleeding into hematomas by technetium-99m red blood cell scintigraphy before angiography. Clin Nucl Med 2002; 27:763-6.
80. Reck T, Bussenius-Kammerer M, Ott R, et al. Surgical treatment of HELLP syndrome-associated liver rupture—an update. Eur J Obstet Gynecol Reprod Biol 2001; 99:57-65.
81. Goyal N, Singhal D, Gupta S, et al. Transabdominal gastroesophageal devascularization without transection for bleeding varices: Results and indicators of prognosis. J Gastroenterol Hepatol 2007; 22:47-50.
82. Cundy TF, O'Grady JG, Williams R. Recovery of menstruation and pregnancy after liver transplantation. Gut 1990; 31:337-8.
83. Friedman SL, Schiano TD. Cirrhosis and its sequelae. In Goldman L, Ausiello D, editors. Cecil Textbook of Medicine. 22nd edition. Philadelphia, Saunders, 2004:936-44.
84. Kerr MG, Scott DB, Samuel E. Studies of the inferior vena cava in late pregnancy. Br Med J 1964; 1(5382):532-3.
85. Schreyer P, Caspi E, El-Hindi JM, Eshchar J. Cirrhosis—pregnancy and delivery: A review. Obstet Gynecol Surv 1982; 37:304-12.
86. Britton RC. Pregnancy and esophageal varices. Am J Surg 1982; 143:421-5.
87. Kochhar R, Kumar S, Goel RC, et al. Pregnancy and its outcome in patients with noncirrhotic portal hypertension. Dig Dis Sci 1999; 44:1356-61.
88. Kochhar R, Goenka MK, Mehta SK. Endoscopic sclerotherapy during pregnancy. Am J Gastroenterol 1990; 85:1132-5.
89. Pauzner D, Wolman I, Niv D, et al. Endoscopic sclerotherapy in extrahepatic portal hypertension in pregnancy. Am J Obstet Gynecol 1991; 164:152-3.
90. Zeeman GG, Moise KJ Jr. Prophylactic banding of severe esophageal varices associated with liver cirrhosis in pregnancy. Obstet Gynecol 1999; 94:842.
91. Rössle M, Haag K, Ochs A, et al. The transjugular intrahepatic portosystemic stent-shunt procedure for variceal bleeding. N Engl J Med 1994; 330:165-71.
92. Conn HO. Transjugular intrahepatic portosystemic shunts versus sclerotherapy: A discussion of discordant results. Ann Intern Med 1997; 126:907-10.
93. Lodato F, Cappelli A, Montagnani M, et al. Transjugular intrahepatic portosystemic shunt: A case report of rescue management of unrestrainable variceal bleeding in a pregnant woman. Dig Liver Dis 2008; 40:387-90.
94. Walcott WO, Derick DE, Jolley JJ, Snyder DL. Successful pregnancy in a liver transplant patient. Am J Obstet Gynecol 1978; 132:340-1.
95. Eguchi S, Yanaga K, Fujita F, et al. Living-related right lobe liver transplantation for a patient with fulminant hepatic failure during the second trimester of pregnancy: Report of a case. Transplantation 2002; 73:1970-1.
96. Jarufe N, Soza A, Pérez-Ayuso RM, et al. Successful liver transplantation and delivery in a woman with fulminant hepatic failure occurring during the second trimester of pregnancy. Liver Int 2006; 26:494-7.
97. Paternoster DM, Gerace PF, Manganelli F, et al. Acute hepatic failure in pregnancy. Eur J Obstet Gynecol Reprod Biol 2004; 112:230-2.
98. Pereira SP, O'Donohue J, Wendon J, Williams R. Maternal and perinatal outcome in severe pregnancy-related liver disease. Hepatology 1997; 26:1258-62.
99. Steingrub JS. Pregnancy-associated severe liver dysfunction. Crit Care Clin 2004; 20:763-76, xi.
100. Tanaka K, Kiuchi T, Kaihara S. Living related liver donor transplantation: Techniques and caution. Surg Clin North Am 2004; 84:481-93.

101. Wu BF, Wang MM. Molecular adsorbent recirculating system in dealing with maternal *Amanita* poisoning during the second trimester of pregnancy: A case report. Hepatobiliary Pancreat Dis Int 2004; 3:152-4.
102. Sen S, Mookerjee RP, Davies NA, et al. Review article: The molecular adsorbents recirculating system (MARS) in liver failure. Aliment Pharmacol Ther 2002; 16:32-8.
103. Armenti VT, Radomski JS, Moritz MJ, et al. Report from the National Transplantation Pregnancy Registry (NTPR): Outcomes of pregnancy after transplantation. In Cecka JM, Terasaki PI, editors. Clinical Transplants, 2004. Los Angeles, UCLA Tissue Typing Laboratory, 2004:103-14.
104. Jain AB, Reyes J, Marcos A, et al. Pregnancy after liver transplantation with tacrolimus immunosuppression: A single center's experience update at 13 years. Transplantation 2003; 76:827-32.
105. Sibanda N, Briggs JD, Davison JM, et al. Pregnancy after organ transplantation: A report from the UK Transplant pregnancy registry. Transplantation 2007; 83:1301-7.
106. Bonanno C, Dove L. Pregnancy after liver transplantation. Semin Perinatol 2007; 31:348-53.
107. Gelman S. Anesthesia and the liver. In Barash P, Cullen B, Stoelting R, editors. Clinical Anesthesia. 2nd edition. Philadelphia, JB Lippincott, 1992:1185-214.
108. Scharschmidt B. Acute and chronic liver failure. In Wyngaarden J, Smith L, Bennet J, editors. Cecil Textbook of Medicine. 19th edition. Philadelphia, WB Saunders, 1992:796-9.
109. Druml W, Fischer M, Pidlich J, Lenz K. Fat elimination in chronic hepatic failure: Long-chain vs medium-chain triglycerides. Am J Clin Nutr 1995; 61:812-7.
110. Frink EJ Jr, Morgan SE, Coetzee A, et al. The effects of sevoflurane, halothane, enflurane, and isoflurane on hepatic blood flow and oxygenation in chronically instrumented greyhound dogs. Anesthesiology 1992; 76:85-90.
111. Kanaya N, Iwasaki H, Namiki A. Noninvasive ICG clearance test for estimating hepatic blood flow during halothane and isoflurane anaesthesia. Can J Anaesth 1995; 42:209-12.
112. McLain GE, Sipes IG, Brown BR Jr. An animal model of halothane hepatotoxicity: Roles of enzyme induction and hypoxia. Anesthesiology 1979; 51:321-6.
113. Ross WT Jr, Daggy BP, Cardell RR Jr. Hepatic necrosis caused by halothane and hypoxia in phenobarbital-treated rats. Anesthesiology 1979; 51:327-33.
114. Greene NM. Anesthesia risk factors in patients with liver disease. Contemp Anesth Pract 1981; 4:87-109.
115. Kennedy WF Jr, Everett GB, Cobb LA, Allen GD. Simultaneous systemic and hepatic hemodynamic measurements during high peridural anesthesia in normal man. Anesth Analg 1971; 50:1069-77.
116. Tanaka N, Nagata N, Hamakawa T, Takasaki M. The effect of dopamine on hepatic blood flow in patients undergoing epidural anesthesia. Anesth Analg 1997; 85:286-90.
117. Feng ZY, Zhang J, Zhu SM, Zheng SS. Is there any difference in anesthetic management of different post-OLT stage patients undergoing nontransplant organ surgery? Hepatobiliary Pancreat Dis Int 2006; 5:368-73.
118. Thomson PD, Melmon KL, Richardson JA, et al. Lidocaine pharmacokinetics in advanced heart failure, liver disease, and renal failure in humans. Ann Intern Med 1973; 78:499-508.
119. Jokinen MJ. The pharmacokinetics of ropivacaine in hepatic and renal insufficiency. Best Pract Res Clin Anaesthesiol 2005; 19:269-74.
120. Heriot JA, Steven CM, Sattin RS. Elective forceps delivery and extradural anaesthesia in a primigravida with portal hypertension and oesophageal varices. Br J Anaesth 1996; 76:325-7.
121. O'Connor CJ, Rothenberg DM, Tuman KJ. Anesthesia and the Hepatobiliary System. In Miller RM, editor. Miller's Anesthesia. 6th edition. Philadelphia, Elsevier, 2005:2209-29.
122. Gregory TL, Hughes S, Coleman MA, De Silva A. Acute fatty liver of pregnancy: Three cases and discussion of analgesia and anaesthesia. Int J Obstet Anesth 2007; 16:175-9.

Chapter 47

Malignant Hyperthermia

M. Joanne Douglas, M.D., FRCPC

Malignant hyperthermia (MH) is an inherited disorder of skeletal muscle. Upon exposure to triggering agents (e.g., succinylcholine, volatile halogenated anesthetic agents), affected individuals demonstrate a hypermetabolic syndrome characterized by hypercapnia, acidosis, muscle rigidity, arrhythmias, and hyperthermia. MH was first described in 1960 by Denborough and Lovell[1] but may have been responsible for some of the earlier deaths attributed to ether and chloroform anesthesia.[2]

EPIDEMIOLOGY

Ording,[3] reviewing the incidence of MH in Denmark, noted that the incidence of the fulminant syndrome (e.g., muscle rigidity, acidosis, hyperkalemia, arrhythmias, hyperthermia, increased creatine kinase [CK] levels, myoglobinuria) was 1 in 220,000 patients who received general anesthesia, and 1 in 62,000 patients in whom succinylcholine was combined with a volatile halogenated agent. MH (either mild or fulminant) was suspected in 1 in 16,000 patients who received anesthesia of any type. The male-to-female ratio was 1.4:1.[3] There is some geographic variation in the incidence of MH.

There are few reports of development of MH during pregnancy and parturition.[4-11] The infrequent occurrence during pregnancy probably reflects both the low frequency of this disorder in the general population and the widespread use of local and regional anesthetic techniques in obstetric patients.

PATHOPHYSIOLOGY

MH is the result of a disorder in the regulation of calcium in skeletal muscle. The precise mechanism by which volatile anesthetics and depolarizing muscle relaxants cause an MH crisis is still unknown.[12] In muscle the sarcoplasmic reticulum is responsible for controlling calcium release and reuptake during muscle contraction.[13] During skeletal muscle excitation-contraction coupling, calcium is released from the terminal sarcoplasmic reticulum via the ryanodine receptor. Dihydropyridine receptors in the T-tubule membrane are alternative calcium release channels. In humans, mutations in both the dihydropyridine receptor and the ryanodine receptor can result in clinical MH. Dantrolene inhibits excitation-contraction coupling, and succinylcholine, caffeine, and volatile halogenated agents increase it.

Wappler et al.[14] have suggested that the 5-hydroxytryptamine (5-HT) system might be involved in the development of MH. *In vivo* and *in vitro* experiments using 5-HT agonists and antagonists demonstrated that 5-HT agonists may initiate MH in MH-susceptible pigs and humans. The precise mechanism is unknown.[14]

GENETICS

MH is a heterogeneous disorder, meaning that more than one gene defect is responsible for expression of the clinical syndrome.[15,16] It is inherited in an autosomal dominant fashion with variable penetrance, although this pattern has been questioned in some families.[17] Porcine MH is transmitted as a recessive gene. The defective gene in MH-susceptible pigs has been localized to a single point mutation in the ryanodine receptor gene responsible for the calcium release channel.[18]

Investigators have found the corresponding point mutation on the human ryanodine receptor in some families with MH (chromosome 19q12.1-13.2; MHS-1), and other mutations in the ryanodine receptor have been linked to MH susceptibility.[19] Other point mutations in the ryanodine receptor are found in patients with central core disease, a myopathy associated with MH.[20] Mutations responsible for MH in some families are located on chromosomes 5p, 17, 7q, 3q, and 1q.[19] Other myopathies may be characterized by a hyperthermic state with muscle damage and metabolic derangements similar to those seen in MH, but their chromosomal abnormality has not been mapped to the same area.[21-25]

TRIGGERS

Known triggers of MH include the depolarizing muscle relaxants (e.g., succinylcholine) and all the volatile halogenated anesthetic agents (i.e., halothane, enflurane, isoflurane, desflurane, sevoflurane) (Box 47-1). The dose and duration of exposure to the triggering agent may influence the onset and severity of a reaction. Previous uneventful administration of general anesthesia with triggering anesthetic agents does not rule out the diagnosis of MH.[26,27]

In contrast to the porcine model, reports of stress-induced MH in humans are rare.[28-30] The sympathetic nervous system is active during an episode of acute MH, but there is insufficient evidence to implicate increased sympathetic activity as a cause in humans. Muscle biopsy testing helps distinguish MH from exercise-induced myolysis, exertional heat stroke, and other myopathies.[31-33] However, evidence is accumulating that some cases of heat stroke and exercise-induced rhabdomyolysis are linked to MH susceptibility.[34-36]

Investigators have explored other possible triggers of MH both in the porcine model and in humans. No evidence suggests that exogenous calcium, digoxin, hypercarbia, potassium,[37] or norepinephrine[38] triggers MH. Exercise[39] and environmental temperature[40-42] may intensify an existing reaction or modify a developing reaction. Sodium thiopental and pancuronium[43] delay the onset in pigs and may modify the reaction in humans. Duke et al.[44] postulated that hypomagnesemia may increase the probability and severity of an MH event in MH-susceptible humans.

There are case reports of the occurrence of MH during regional anesthesia and during general anesthesia with nontriggering agents.[31,45-48] The cases that occurred during regional anesthesia appeared mild and responded readily to treatment. In some cases, however, the diagnosis was not confirmed with muscle biopsy or appropriate laboratory investigation at the time of the event.

CLINICAL PRESENTATION

Individuals who are MH-susceptible may demonstrate the fulminant syndrome when anesthetized with a triggering agent. During an acute episode, the diagnosis is based on the finding of an elevated end-tidal CO_2 concentration, muscle rigidity (generalized and/or masseter), respiratory and metabolic acidosis, and rhabdomyolysis, which causes an elevated CK concentration, hyperkalemia, and myoglobinuria. Hypoxemia, unstable blood pressure, and evidence of sympathetic hyperactivity (e.g., tachycardia, hypertension, arrhythmias) are other signs. Hyperthermia may occur early, but often it is a late sign (Box 47-2). Perioperative rhabdomyolysis, without any of the previously mentioned clinical signs, also may indicate MH susceptibility.[49,50]

With the advent of routine end-tidal CO_2 monitoring, MH may be detected early, often before the development of rhabdomyolysis and hyperthermia.[51] This situation may lead to uncertainty about the clinical diagnosis of MH, given that many of the confirmatory signs and laboratory abnormalities may be absent during the early phase of MH.

BOX 47-1 Triggers for Malignant Hyperthermia (MH)

Factors Known to Trigger MH

- Volatile anesthetic agents
  - Halothane
  - Enflurane
  - Isoflurane
  - Desflurane
  - Sevoflurane
- Succinylcholine

Factors that Do Not Trigger MH

- Exogenous calcium
- Digoxin
- Hypercarbia
- Potassium
- Norepinephrine

BOX 47-2 Signs and Symptoms of Malignant Hyperthermia

- Tachycardia
- Tachypnea
- Masseter spasm
- Generalized rigidity
- Elevated end-tidal CO_2 concentration
- Cyanosis
- Arrhythmias
- Acidosis
- Hyperkalemia
- Hyperpyrexia
- Myoglobinuria
- Increased creatine kinase level

Thus, early treatment of possible MH could present a dilemma as to whether the patient should undergo diagnostic muscle biopsy or should be assumed to be MH susceptible.

Masseter Muscle Rigidity

Masseter muscle rigidity is one of the early signs of MH.[52] The masseter muscles are sensitive to the action of succinylcholine and respond with greater tension in normal individuals.[53,54] Often this greater tension is imperceptible, but in some patients it is impossible to open the mouth for laryngoscopy and intubation. The duration of rigidity parallels the duration of action of succinylcholine. Typically there is no difficulty with mask ventilation. Masseter muscle rigidity rarely occurs after the use of nondepolarizing muscle relaxants such as vecuronium, atracurium, and mivacurium.[55] Patients with myopathies and other neuromuscular disorders also may present with masseter muscle rigidity after the administration of succinylcholine.[23,56]

If masseter muscle rigidity is accompanied by generalized rigidity, anesthesia should be discontinued, dantrolene should be administered, and the patient should be monitored closely.[57] However, there is controversy regarding the management of isolated masseter muscle rigidity.[58] Options include (1) discontinuation of the anesthetic agents and administration of dantrolene; (2) continuation of anesthesia with nontriggering, "safe" agents and close attention to the end-tidal CO_2 concentration; and (3) continuation of anesthesia with triggering agents and careful monitoring. In my judgment, the anesthesia provider should either discontinue anesthesia altogether or continue anesthesia with nontriggering agents. If the anesthesia is continued, the minute ventilation, end-tidal CO_2 concentration, electrocardiogram (ECG), temperature, and arterial blood gases should be monitored. The anesthesia provider also should look for evidence of rhabdomyolysis by monitoring CK levels and looking for myoglobinuria and should recommend that the patient undergo muscle biopsy.[59]

DIAGNOSIS

Several investigators have correlated clinical presentation (i.e., evidence of metabolic and muscle derangements) with muscle biopsy results.[60-62] The greater the number of clinical signs or abnormal laboratory findings, the greater the risk of MH (Table 47-1).[60] An early assessment of the risk of MH allows the anesthesia provider to initiate appropriate treatment. The mortality rate for MH is as high as 80% without dantrolene therapy.[62] Early administration of dantrolene lowers the mortality rate to 4%.[63]

An international group of experts has developed a clinical grading scale to predict MH susceptibility.[64] This scale consists of six processes (rigidity, muscle breakdown, respiratory acidosis, temperature increase, cardiac involvement, family history) and their clinical indicators. Points are assigned for each indicator present in a patient, and the total represents a raw score. A rank is subsequently assigned to this score, which indicates the likelihood of development of MH in the patient.

TESTING

Susceptibility to MH is determined by a positive caffeine-halothane contracture test result. During this test, fresh muscle is exposed to halothane and caffeine, and the extent of contraction is measured. The caffeine-halothane contracture test has been standardized in MH testing centers throughout North America (the North American protocol)[65] and Europe (the European protocol).[66] This test is

TABLE 47-1 Risk of Malignant Hyperthermia (MH) with Associated Signs and Symptoms

Type	Symptoms/Signs	Risk
Fulminant/classic	Metabolic acidosis Muscle rigidity Hyperthermia (> 38.5° C) Arrhythmias Hyperkalemia Myoglobinuria Increased creatine kinase level	0.96
Moderate	Inconclusive signs of MH involving metabolic and muscle abnormalities, with MH the probable diagnosis	0.88
Mild	Signs of metabolic derangement (pH > 7.3, body core temperature < 38.5° C)	0.14
Masseter spasm with rhabdomyolysis	Creatine kinase level > 1500 U/L, myoglobinuria	0.76
Masseter spasm with signs of metabolic disturbance	Arrhythmias, rising core temperature	0.57
Masseter spasm only		0.28
Unexplained perioperative death or cardiac arrest		0.66
Other	Postoperative pyrexia or rhabdomyolysis	0.07

Data from Ellis FR, Halsall PJ, Christian AS, Clinical presentation of suspected malignant hyperthermia during anaesthesia in 402 probands. Anaesthesia 1990; 45:838-41.

the "gold standard" for the diagnosis of MH. The sensitivity and specificity of the North American protocol are 97% and 78%, respectively.[67] Some false-positive results may occur.[68] Patients with a negative caffeine-halothane contracture test result subsequently have received anesthesia with triggering agents without incident.[69-72] Some centers now add ryanodine or 4-chloro-*m*-cresol to the contracture test agents.[73]

Testing for the known genetic mutations associated with MH is now available. However, because all the genetic mutations responsible for MH have yet to be identified, genetic testing is still not sensitive enough to use for routine screening.[74] In the future MH may be detected in most MH-susceptible patients without the more invasive muscle biopsy.[74] Some centers are investigating the use of nuclear magnetic resonance spectroscopy as a noninvasive screening test for MH. Early acidosis and decreased phosphocreatine content occur during graded exercise in MH-susceptible patients.[75] Some of these changes occur with myopathies other than MH, and the investigators have emphasized that further studies are needed to determine whether this technology is suitable for screening for MH susceptibility.

In the absence of muscle biopsy results, a parturient with a positive family history should be treated as if she were MH susceptible.

PREGNANCY AND MALIGNANT HYPERTHERMIA

In 1972, Crawford[76] wondered "whether or not there was a record of a pregnant or newly born patient or animal having developed hyperpyrexia and . . . whether hyperpyrexia has been encountered in a patient undergoing an operation under regional block anesthesia." Subsequently there have been few reports of MH during parturition and fewer reports of maternal mortality attributable to MH. Wadhwa[4] reported the death of a woman with a known family history of MH in whom muscle rigidity developed during twilight sleep for parturition. Douglas et al.[5] subsequently reported one fatal case of MH in a parturient undergoing general anesthesia for cesarean delivery.

There are three published reports of nonfatal MH during cesarean delivery, and one report of MH following cesarean hysterectomy performed because of postpartum hemorrhage.[11] The triggering agents were succinylcholine and halothane,[6] succinylcholine and isoflurane,[11] cyclopropane,[7] and succinylcholine alone (without a volatile halogenated agent).[8] There are several reports of the successful administration of epidural and spinal anesthesia during labor and cesarean delivery in MH-susceptible parturients.[4,11,77-84]

The rarity of these events suggests that pregnancy protects against the occurrence of MH. However, it also may reflect the widespread use of neuraxial anesthesia for labor, vaginal delivery, and cesarean delivery.

Maternal Physiology

Basal metabolic rate, oxygen consumption, and minute ventilation increase during pregnancy.[85] Serum bicarbonate, buffer base, and base excess decrease to maintain normal pH. Thus the pregnant patient typically has a compensated respiratory alkalosis. The reduced buffering capacity could adversely affect the pregnant woman during an episode of MH.

Oxygen consumption and minute ventilation increase further during labor.[86] Maternal lactate and pyruvate concentrations increase steadily during labor, indicating an increase in both aerobic and anaerobic metabolism.[87] Hyperventilation during contractions may result in periods of hypoventilation between contractions, which may adversely affect the Pa_{O_2} of both the mother and the fetus. These metabolic and physiologic responses to pain are similar to those that occur during MH. Effective epidural analgesia decreases oxygen consumption and minute ventilation.[86] If tachycardia and hyperventilation occur despite effective analgesia, they are more likely to signal an episode of MH.

Aortocaval compression from the pregnant uterus results in decreased cardiac output, hypotension, and reduced uteroplacental perfusion. Thus aortocaval compression may accelerate the occurrence of acidosis during an episode of MH. Aortocaval compression hinders resuscitative efforts during cardiac arrest,[88,89] and evacuation of the uterus (i.e., delivery of the fetus) facilitates maternal resuscitation. The same may be true during an episode of MH. The obstetrician may need to deliver the fetus to facilitate maternal resuscitation during a fulminant case of MH.

CK concentrations are not diagnostic of MH. During pregnancy, there is a slight decrease in CK levels during the first trimester. CK levels remain stable until term, when they increase by approximately 50%. At delivery, there is an abrupt rise in the CK concentration, followed by a return to normal by 6 weeks postpartum (Figure 47-1 and Table 47-2).[90] The increased CK concentration results from increases in both the CK-M fraction (skeletal muscle) and the CK-B fraction (myometrium, placenta, and fetal blood). Postpartum CK levels are higher in nulliparous patients regardless of differences in duration of labor.[91] Mean plasma CK activity is approximately 50% higher in African-Americans than in Caucasians or Asians.[90]

Acute cocaine toxicity may mimic MH. Although cocaine does not induce contractures in MH-susceptible

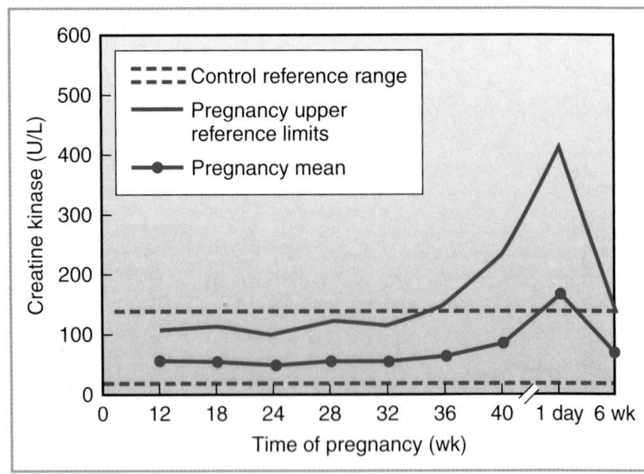

FIGURE 47-1 Changes in creatine kinase activity during and after pregnancy. (Modified from Lockitch G, editor. Handbook of Diagnostic Biochemistry and Hematology in Normal Pregnancy. Boca Raton, FL, CRC Press, 1993:59.)

TABLE 47-2 Gestational Changes in Creatine Kinase Activity

Time of Gestation	Creatine Kinase (U/L)		
	Range	Mean (SD)	% of Control Value
Nonpregnant control	20-137	63 (31)	—
12 weeks	0-111	55 (28)	87
18 weeks	0-113	55 (29)	87
24 weeks	0-100	50 (25)	79
28 weeks	0-122	54 (34)	86
32 weeks	0-114	54 (30)	86
36 weeks	0-145	57 (44)	90
Term	0-227	85 (71)	135
1 day postpartum	0-410	162 (124)	257
6 weeks postpartum	0-139	63 (37)	100

From Lockitch G, editor. Handbook of Diagnostic Biochemistry and Hematology in Normal Pregnancy. Boca Raton, FL, CRC Press, 1993:59.

muscle,[92] elevated CK concentrations and myoglobinemia can occur secondary to rhabdomyolysis and renal failure from cocaine intoxication.[93] Umbilical cord blood CK and myoglobin levels are elevated when cocaine metabolites are present in maternal urine.[94]

Effects on the Fetus and Newborn

MH often is inherited as an autosomal dominant gene. In these cases, there is a 50% chance that the infant of an MH-susceptible parent will also be MH susceptible. All anesthetic agents cross the placenta. Small quantities of succinylcholine also cross the placenta. This knowledge should prompt the anesthesia provider to question the choice of anesthetic agents for an MH-negative mother whose fetus has an MH-susceptible father. In this situation, the anesthesia provider should avoid the use of triggering agents until after delivery.

There is only one published report of suspected MH in a newborn.[95] The condition is rare in infancy, and some reports of infant MH may represent undiagnosed myopathy.[56,96,97]

MANAGEMENT OF THE MALIGNANT HYPERTHERMIA–SUSCEPTIBLE PARTURIENT

Ideally, an anesthesiologist will evaluate every MH-susceptible pregnant patient before she is hospitalized for labor and delivery. Clearly, the obstetrician should consult an anesthesia provider immediately after the admission of each MH-susceptible patient. All hospitals and birthing facilities should be prepared to provide care for MH-susceptible patients. Adequate supplies of dantrolene (at least 36 vials), sterile water, and sodium bicarbonate should be immediately available.

Analgesia for Labor

Soon after admission, a large-gauge intravenous catheter should be placed in each MH-susceptible patient. Maternal temperature, heart rate, and blood pressure should be monitored throughout labor. During early labor, it may be acceptable to monitor temperature and heart rate intermittently to facilitate maternal ambulation, if desired. Once active labor is established, frequent monitoring of the maternal heart rate and temperature should be initiated. Continuous ECG and axillary temperature monitoring are ideal once the parturient is confined to bed. (Measurement of axillary temperature allows placement of a temperature probe in close proximity to large muscle groups.) Of course, aortocaval compression should be avoided throughout labor and delivery.

Most agents used for intrapartum analgesia are considered safe in the MH-susceptible parturient (Table 47-3). Both the obstetrician and the anesthesia provider should encourage the early administration of epidural analgesia. Relief of pain reduces maternal stress (as reflected by decreased catecholamine,[98] cortisol,[99] and adrenocorticotropic hormone [ACTH] concentrations) and decreases maternal metabolism and oxygen consumption.[100] Although experts continue to debate the role of stress in human MH,[101] it is best to diminish stress when possible. Further, the anesthesia provider may extend epidural analgesia for vaginal or cesarean delivery if necessary, thus avoiding administration of general anesthesia.

All local anesthetic agents appear safe for MH-susceptible patients. Epinephrine can be safely added to the local anesthetic agent to improve the quality and duration of analgesia, if clinically appropriate.

Anesthesia for Cesarean Delivery

General anesthesia should be avoided for operative delivery. Spinal or epidural anesthesia using either amide or ester local anesthetic agents can be safely given. Spinal anesthesia entails a greater risk of hypotension, which requires treatment with adrenergic agents such as ephedrine. Ephedrine should be used as required, but it should be avoided during an acute episode of MH. In doses greater than those used clinically, ephedrine exacerbates halothane-induced muscle contractures *in vitro*.[102] Epidural anesthesia may be preferred because slow induction of anesthesia and administration of an adequate volume of intravenous fluid decrease the risk of hypotension.

Rarely, the mother may refuse neuraxial anesthesia. In other cases, neuraxial anesthesia may be contraindicated

TABLE 47-3 Common Anesthetic Drugs and Their Safety in Malignant Hyperthermia (MH)–Susceptible Women

Drug	Route	Use	Safe in MH
Local Anesthetic Agents			
Bupivacaine	Regional	Analgesia/anesthesia	Yes
Lidocaine	Regional	Analgesia/anesthesia	Yes
	Intravenous	Intubation/arrhythmia	Yes
Ropivacaine	Regional	Analgesia/anesthesia	Yes
2-Chloroprocaine	Regional	Analgesia/anesthesia	Yes
Opioids			
Fentanyl	Regional, intravenous	Analgesia	Yes
Meperidine	Regional, intravenous	Analgesia	Yes
Morphine	Regional, intravenous	Analgesia	Yes
Induction Agents			
Sodium thiopental	Intravenous	Induction	Yes
Propofol	Intravenous	Induction	Yes
Etomidate	Intravenous	Induction	Yes
Ketamine	Intravenous	Analgesia/induction	Yes
Benzodiazepines	Intravenous	Amnesia/anxiolysis	Yes
Neuromuscular Blocking Agents			
Succinylcholine	Intravenous	Muscle relaxation	No
Rocuronium	Intravenous	Muscle relaxation	Yes
Atracurium	Intravenous	Muscle relaxation	Yes
Vecuronium	Intravenous	Muscle relaxation	Yes
Pancuronium	Intravenous	Muscle relaxation	Yes
General Anesthetic Agents			
Halothane, enflurane, isoflurane, sevoflurane, desflurane	Inhalation	Anesthesia, uterine relaxation	No
Nitrous oxide	Inhalation	Analgesia/anesthesia	Yes

(e.g., maternal hemorrhage, coagulopathy, prolonged fetal bradycardia). When the anesthesia provider encounters an MH-susceptible parturient, the anesthesia machine and delivery circuit should be flushed of volatile agents. Preparation consists of replacing the carbon dioxide absorbent and the delivery tubing, disabling the vaporizers, and purging the machine of residual anesthetic agent with a 10 L/min flow of oxygen through the circuit (including the ventilator) for 20 minutes.[103] Some of the newer machines with nonmetal internal components require longer purging times.[104]

In cases of general anesthesia, the anesthesia provider should administer a nonparticulate antacid and perform adequate denitrogenation. Unless a difficult intubation is expected, the anesthesia provider should plan a rapid-sequence induction, with application of cricoid pressure, and should administer nontriggering agents (Box 47-3; see Table 47-3). All commonly used induction agents (e.g., thiopental, ketamine, etomidate, propofol) are safe in MH-susceptible patients. Succinylcholine and the volatile halogenated agents (halothane, enflurane, isoflurane, sevoflurane, desflurane) are contraindicated. For intubation, rapid onset (approximately 60 to 90 seconds) of muscle relaxation can be achieved with rocuronium (0.6 to 0.9 mg/kg, which is 2 to 3 times the effective dose in 95% of patients [ED_{95}]).[105] Other options are vecuronium[106] (0.25 mg/kg) and pancuronium (0.15 mg/kg). Nitrous oxide (delivered via a prepared anesthesia machine), opioids, and propofol are safe agents for the maintenance of anesthesia. Midazolam administered after delivery provides amnesia. It is safe to reverse neuromuscular blockade with glycopyrrolate and neostigmine or edrophonium. Atropine may cause an increase in temperature, which could cause a diagnostic dilemma.

At delivery, determination of maternal and umbilical cord blood gas and pH measurements may provide information about an impending reaction in either the mother or the neonate. As well, if the MH-susceptible mother has a known genetic mutation, umbilical cord blood may be used to assess MH susceptibility in the neonate.[107] If uterine relaxation (tocolysis) is required to assist with delivery of the baby or to facilitate the removal of a retained placenta, I prefer to give 100-μg bolus doses of nitroglycerin intravenously[108]; the action of this agent is brief and easily reversed with oxytocin. Clearly, a volatile halogenated agent should *never* be given to effect uterine relaxation in an MH-susceptible patient.

Concern has been raised about administering triggering agents to a non–MH-susceptible mother who is carrying a fetus whose father is MH-susceptible.[109] In this situation many anesthesiologists prefer to treat the mother as MH-susceptible in order to avoid a possible MH reaction in the neonate.

BOX 47-3 General Anesthesia for Cesarean Delivery in the Malignant Hyperthermia–Susceptible Patient

Monitoring
- End-tidal CO_2
- Pulse oximeter
- Electrocardiogram
- Automatic blood pressure monitoring
- Peripheral nerve stimulator
- Temperature (central)

Induction of Anesthesia
- Denitrogenation
- Rapid-sequence induction (thiopental 4 mg/kg, ketamine 1 mg/kg, propofol 2.0 to 2.5 mg/kg)

Muscle Relaxant
- Intubation: rocuronium 0.6 to 0.9 mg/kg
- Maintenance: rocuronium

Maintenance of Anesthesia
- Nitrous oxide/oxygen, propofol, opioid

Amnestic Agent
- Midazolam

Reversal of Neuromuscular Blockade
- Glycopyrrolate and neostigmine

Obstetric Drugs in Malignant Hyperthermia–Susceptible Patients

Information on use of obstetric drugs in MH-susceptible patients is scant (Table 47-4). The beta-sympathomimetic tocolytic agents (e.g., ritodrine, terbutaline) produce anxiety and tachycardia in normal parturients. Such side effects may be confused with MH, but these agents most likely are safe in the MH-susceptible parturient.

Magnesium sulfate attenuates but does not prevent MH in MH-susceptible swine.[110] There is one report of a fatal adverse interaction between dantrolene and the calcium entry–blocking agent diltiazem,[111] and hyperkalemia has been described after the co-administration of dantrolene and verapamil.[112] Administration of calcium entry–blocking agents should be avoided during an episode of MH. These agents also do not prevent the development of MH.[113]

Oxytocin is safe. Some of the commercial preparations of oxytocin contain a preservative (chlorbutol) that has been shown to reverse the development of MH in susceptible pigs *in vitro*.[114] The ergot alkaloids cause vasoconstriction, which may lead to decreased muscle perfusion and a greater tendency toward lactic acidosis. The prostaglandins may be associated with changes in blood pressure and maternal oxygen desaturation.[115] Prostaglandin E_2 and misoprostol also may cause pyrexia, which may lead to confusion about the diagnosis of an MH episode.[116,117] The routine postpartum administration of ergot alkaloids,

TABLE 47-4 Drugs Commonly Used for Labor and Delivery and Their Safety in Malignant Hyperthermia (MH)–Susceptible Women

Drug	Route	Use	Safe in MH
Tocolytics			
Ritodrine	Intravenous	Tocolysis	Yes
Magnesium sulfate	Intravenous	Tocolysis, seizure prophylaxis	Yes
Nitroglycerin	Intravenous	Tocolysis, antihypertensive	Yes
Calcium entry blockers	Intravenous	Tocolysis, antihypertensive	Yes*
Oxytocics			
Oxytocin	Intravenous	Uterine atony	Yes
Prostaglandin $F_{2\alpha}$	Intramuscular, intramyometrial	Uterine atony	Inadequate information available
Misoprostol	Vaginal, rectal	Uterine atony	Inadequate information available
Ergot alkaloids	Intramuscular	Uterine atony	Inadequate information available
Cardiovascular Drugs			
Ephedrine	Intravenous	Vasopressor	Yes
Phenylephrine	Intravenous	Vasopressor	Yes
Epinephrine	Intravenous, regional	Vasopressor, epidural test dose, prolongation of regional block	Yes
Beta-blockers	Oral, intravenous	Antihypertensive	Yes
Antiemetics			
Droperidol	Intravenous	Prophylaxis, therapeutic	Yes
Metoclopramide	Intravenous	Prophylaxis, therapeutic	Yes
Ondansetron	Intravenous	Prophylaxis, therapeutic	Yes

*Do not use during a crisis (see text).

BOX 47-4 Differential Diagnosis of Fever during Parturition

- Infection: chorioamnionitis, urinary tract infection, other infections (e.g., influenza, viral illness)
- Environmental temperature
- Labor epidural analgesia
- Dehydration/labor
- Malignant hyperthermia
- Drug reactions: cocaine, atropine, tricyclic antidepressants, monoamine oxidase (MAO) inhibitors, neuroleptic malignant syndrome, prostaglandins

prostaglandins, or misoprostol probably should not be performed in MH-susceptible patients. However, persistent uterine atony and postpartum hemorrhage may warrant the administration of these agents.

ASSESSMENT OF HYPERTHERMIA AND TACHYCARDIA

The hallmark signs of MH may be present during normal labor (Boxes 47-4 and 47-5). Other causes of fever and tachycardia in the MH-susceptible parturient should be excluded. Tachycardia and tachypnea are normal responses to pain, anxiety, and fever. Fever may be a sign of dehydration and infection. Pain and infection (e.g., chorioamnionitis, urinary tract infection) are much more common during parturition than MH. Normal parturients may have a gradual increase in temperature during epidural analgesia.[118] This may be accompanied by corresponding increases in maternal and fetal heart rates.

The butyrophenones, phenothiazines, thioxanthenes, and other miscellaneous antipsychotic agents may produce tachycardia, fever, and rigidity (i.e., neuroleptic malignant syndrome).[119] There is one published report of neuroleptic malignant syndrome in a pregnant woman.[120] Drugs capable of increasing serotonin in the central nervous system (serotonin reuptake inhibitors [SSRIs]) also can produce a hypermetabolic reaction. Cocaine intoxication causes severe vasoconstriction, fever, and rhabdomyolysis.[121]

TREATMENT

Box 47-6 summarizes the treatment of MH; a more detailed protocol for the management of an MH episode is available online at http://www.mhaus.org. The anesthesia provider should call for help. All triggering agents must be stopped immediately, and the patient should be hyperventilated with 100% oxygen at 10 L/min. The level of volatile agent decreases rapidly with flushing of the machine with 100% oxygen.[103,104] Therefore substitution with a vapor-free machine is not an immediate priority.

BOX 47-5 Differential Diagnosis of Tachycardia during Parturition

- Pain
- Fever
- Anxiety
- Blood loss
- Hypotension
- Drug reactions: cocaine, atropine, beta-adrenergic tocolytic agents
- Malignant hyperthermia

BOX 47-6 Management of Malignant Hyperthermia Crisis

1. Call for help.
2. Discontinue all triggering agents.
3. Hyperventilate with 100% oxygen at high gas flows (>10 L/min).
4. Administer dantrolene 2.5 mg/kg intravenously. Repeat until signs and symptoms resolve.
5. Perform serial blood gas measurements. Treat acidosis with sodium bicarbonate 1 to 2 mEq/kg.
6. Treat hyperkalemia with sodium bicarbonate, glucose, insulin, and calcium.
7. Treat arrhythmias with amiodarone or lidocaine.
8. Cool patient (external cooling blanket, ice packs, cold intravenous solutions, lavage of body cavities with cold solutions).
9. Maintain urine output with fluids, mannitol, and/or furosemide.
10. Call the Malignant Hyperthermia Hotline for assistance (1-800-MH-HYPER).
11. Postoperatively, monitor patient in intensive care unit for 24 to 48 hours. Administer maintenance dantrolene.
12. Counsel patient and family, and refer for caffeine-halothane contracture test.

Modified from Malignant Hyperthermia Association of the United States. Emergency Therapy of Malignant Hyperthermia. May 2008. Available at http://medical.mhaus.org/PubData/PDFs/treatmentposter.pdf/

The anesthesia provider should give dantrolene intravenously in a dose of 2.5 mg/kg, until the signs and symptoms (e.g., tachycardia, hypercarbia, rigidity, fever) have subsided.[122] Although the maximum dantrolene dose is often listed as 10 mg/kg, there are case reports in which higher doses of dantrolene were required to control an MH reaction. Oxygen saturation, end-tidal CO_2, ECG, blood pressure, arterial and venous blood gas measurements, core temperature, potassium levels, lactate concentration, CK levels, coagulation profile, urine output, and urine myoglobin should be monitored.

The anesthesia provider must initiate treatment of acidosis, hyperkalemia, arrhythmias, and hyperthermia. Metabolic acidosis is treated by giving sodium bicarbonate in 1- to 2-mEq/kg increments as guided by blood gas and pH measurements. The anesthesia provider should treat hyperkalemia by administration of bicarbonate, glucose, and insulin. Calcium administration may also be indicated.

Early administration of dantrolene often prevents or successfully treats arrhythmias. If arrhythmias persist, one should follow standard advanced cardiac life support (ACLS) protocols. Amiodarone, lidocaine, procainamide, and adenosine may be used safely. Calcium entry–blocking agents should be avoided because simultaneous administration of dantrolene and a calcium entry blocker may precipitate cardiovascular collapse.

The operating room care team should actively cool the patient. Options for doing so include (1) intravenous administration of iced saline; (2) lavage of stomach, bladder, rectal, peritoneal, and thoracic cavities with iced saline; and (3) surface cooling with ice and/or a hypothermia blanket.

Myoglobin is excreted in the urine. Thus diuresis should be maintained by giving adequate volumes of crystalloid and furosemide 1 mg/kg and/or mannitol 0.25 g/kg. Mannitol is present in dantrolene, and separate administration of a diuretic agent may not be necessary. Sedation should be administered as necessary.

After an acute episode of MH, postoperative administration of dantrolene (1 mg/kg or more intravenously every 4 to 6 hours for 24 to 48 hours) is recommended.[123] In addition, the patient should be monitored closely in an intensive care unit for at least 24 to 48 hours. In a retrospective analysis of data from the North American Malignant Hyperthermia Registry, 20% of patients had recrudescence of MH after the initial MH episode.[124] Recrudesence was associated with increased muscle mass and a longer interval between anesthesia induction and intraoperative reaction. Counseling and diagnostic muscle biopsy should be performed after recovery from the acute episode. The Malignant Hyperthermia Association of the United States (MHAUS) provides a registry and an informative newsletter for MH-susceptible patients. An MH hotline (800-MH-HYPER [800-644-9737] or, outside the United States, 315-464-7079) is available 24 hours a day to assist physicians with questions on treatment, diagnosis, and follow-up.

DANTROLENE IN PREGNANCY

Dantrolene is the drug of choice for the treatment of an MH crisis. It crosses the placenta and can be detected in the fetus after maternal administration.[125] Clinical doses do not adversely affect maternal or fetal cardiovascular and acid-base measurements in gravid ewes. Morison[82] reported a fetal-to-maternal serum dantrolene concentration ratio of approximately 0.4 after prophylactic oral administration of dantrolene. Theoretically, dantrolene may cause neonatal hypotonia if it is administered before delivery.

There is one published report of postpartum uterine atony after the administration of dantrolene.[9] Laboratory testing of the effects of dantrolene sodium on pregnant uterine muscle suggests that the relaxant effect is secondary to the mannitol.[126]

There is no benefit to dantrolene prophylaxis in the MH-susceptible patient when all triggering agents are avoided.[127] However, the anesthesia provider should give dantrolene promptly when an MH crisis is suspected. Using warmed water to mix dantrolene increases the speed of mixing.[128]

Fricker et al.[129] reported serial measurements of dantrolene concentrations in breast milk after administration of dantrolene in a patient with suspected MH during cesarean delivery (Figure 47-2). They estimated that the half-life of dantrolene in breast milk is approximately 9 hours. They concluded that "breast-feeding can be expected to be safe for the newborn 2 days after discontinuation of intravenous dantrolene administration in the mother."[129]

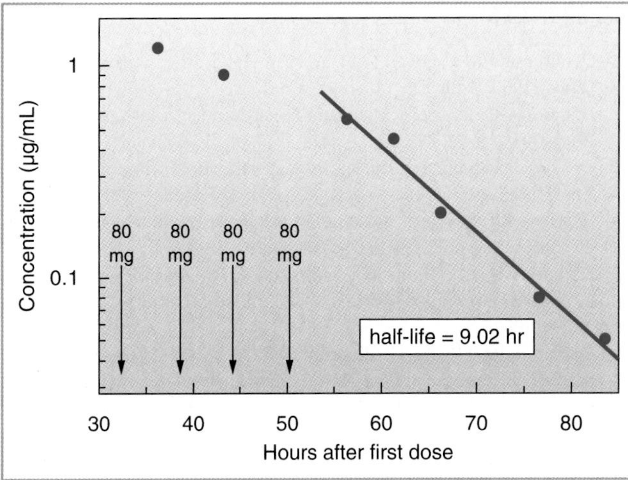

FIGURE 47-2 Estimation of the half-life of dantrolene in breast milk by log-linear fitting of the terminal elimination phase (dantrolene measured in breast milk by high-pressure liquid chromatography [HPLC], reverse-phase high-pressure liquid chromatographic column, by in-line ultraviolet absorption spectrometer; detection limit, 0.02 µg/mL). (From Fricker RM, Hoerauf KH, Drewe J, Kress HG. Secretion of dantrolene into breast milk after acute therapy of a suspected malignant hyperthermia crisis during cesarean section. Anesthesiology 1998; 89:1023-5.)

KEY POINTS

- Malignant hyperthermia is a heterogeneous disorder of skeletal muscle with variable clinical penetrance.
- Affected individuals develop a hypermetabolic syndrome on exposure to triggering agents (succinylcholine, volatile halogenated agents).
- The current diagnostic test is the caffeine-halothane contracture test.
- Current genetic testing has low sensitivity.
- It is unclear whether pregnancy alters susceptibility to MH.
- Both the obstetrician and the anesthesia provider should encourage early administration of epidural analgesia during labor in MH-susceptible patients.
- The anesthesia provider may extend epidural analgesia and thus avoid administration of general anesthesia for emergency cesarean delivery.
- All local anesthetic agents are safe in MH-susceptible patients.
- Intravenous administration of dantrolene is the treatment of choice for an MH crisis.
- Dantrolene crosses the placenta and may result in neonatal hypotonia.
- Dantrolene may cause uterine atony.
- The anesthesia provider need not administer dantrolene prophylactically to MH-susceptible parturients.

REFERENCES

1. Denborough MA, Lovell RRH. Anaesthetic deaths in a family (letter). Lancet 1960; 2:45.
2. Harrison GG, Isaacs H. Malignant hyperthermia: A historical vignette. Anaesthesia 1992; 47:54-6.
3. Ording H. Incidence of malignant hyperthermia in Denmark. Anesth Analg 1985; 64:700-4.
4. Wadhwa RK. Obstetric anesthesia for a patient with malignant hyperthermia susceptibility. Anesthesiology 1977; 46:63-4.
5. Douglas MJ, O'Connor GA, Allanson JE. Malignant hyperthermia in British Columbia. British Columbia Medical Journal 1983; 25:299-300.
6. Liebenschütz F, Mai C, Pickerodt VWA. Increased carbon dioxide production in two patients with malignant hyperpyrexia and its control by dantrolene. Br J Anaesth 1979; 51:899-903.
7. Lips FJ, Newland M, Dutton G. Malignant hyperthermia triggered by cyclopropane during cesarean section. Anesthesiology 1982; 56:144-6.
8. Cupryn JP, Kennedy A, Byrick RJ. Malignant hyperthermia in pregnancy. Am J Obstet Gynecol 1984; 150:327-8.
9. Weingarten AE, Korsh JI, Neuman GG, Stern SB. Postpartum uterine atony after intravenous dantrolene. Anesth Analg 1987; 66:269-70.
10. Tettambel M. Malignant hyperthermia in an obstetric patient. J Am Osteopath Assoc 1980; 79:773-5.
11. Wu Y-C, Ho C-M, Tsou M-Y, et al. Successful management of malignant hyperthermia susceptibility during cesarean hysterectomy for postpartum hemorrhage. Acta Obstet Gynecol Scand 1999; 78:738-9.
12. Wappler F. Malignant hyperthermia. Eur J Anaesthesiol 2001; 18:632-52.
13. Rossi AE, Dirksen RT. Sarcoplasmic reticulum: The dynamic calcium governor of muscle. Muscle Nerve 2006; 33:715-31.
14. Wappler F, Fiege M, Schulte am Esch J. Pathophysiological role of the serotonin system in malignant hyperthermia. Br J Anaesth 2001; 87:794-8.
15. Levitt RC. Prospects for the diagnosis of malignant hyperthermia susceptibility using molecular genetic approaches. Anesthesiology 1992; 76:1039-48.
16. Levitt RC, Nouri N, Jedlicka AE, et al. Evidence for genetic heterogeneity in malignant hyperthermia susceptibility. Genomics 1991; 11:543-7.
17. Fagerlund TH, Islander G, Twetman ER, Berg K. Malignant hyperthermia susceptibility, an autosomal dominant disorder? Clin Genet 1997; 51:365-9.
18. Fujii J, Ostu K, Zorzato F, et al. Identification of a mutation in porcine ryanodine receptor associated with malignant hyperthermia. Science 1991; 253:448-51.
19. Hopkins PM. Malignant hyperthermia: Advances in clinical management and diagnosis. Br J Anaesth 2000; 85:118-28.
20. Wu S, Ibarra MC, Malicdan MC, et al. Central core disease is due to RYR1 mutations in more than 90% of patients. Brain 2006; 129:1470-80.
21. Wang JM, Stanley TH. Duchenne muscular dystrophy and malignant hyperthermia: Two case reports. Can Anaesth Soc J 1986; 33:492-7.
22. Heytens L, Martin JJ, Van de Kelft E, Bossaert LL. In vitro contracture tests in patients with various neuromuscular diseases. Br J Anaesth 1992; 68:72-5.
23. Lehmann-Horn F, Iaizzo PA. Are myotonias and periodic paralyses associated with susceptibility to malignant hyperthermia? Br J Anaesth 1990; 65:692-7.
24. Moslehi R, Langlois S, Yam I, Friedman JM. Linkage of malignant hyperthermia and hyperkalemic periodic paralysis to the adult skeletal muscle sodium channel (SCN4A) gene in a large pedigree. Am J Med Genet 1998; 76:21-7.
25. Lambert C, Blanloeil Y, Krivosic Horber R, et al. Malignant hyperthermia in a patient with hypokalemic periodic paralysis. Anesth Analg 1994; 79:1012-4.
26. Prather Strazis K, Fox AW. Malignant hyperthermia: A review of published cases. Anesth Analg 1993; 77:297-304.
27. Bendixen D, Skovgaard LT, Ørding H. Analysis of anaesthesia in patients suspected to be susceptible to malignant hyperthermia before diagnostic in vitro contracture test. Acta Anaesthesiol Scand 1997; 41:480-4.
28. Britt BA. Combined anesthetic- and stress-induced malignant hyperthermia in two offspring of malignant hyperthermic-susceptible parents. Anesth Analg 1988; 67:393-9.
29. Feuerman T, Gade GF, Reynolds R. Stress-induced malignant hyperthermia in a head-injured patient. J Neurosurg 1988; 68:297-9.
30. Hackl W, Winkler M, Mauritz W, et al. Muscle biopsy for diagnosis of malignant hyperthermia susceptibility in two patients with severe exercise-induced myolysis. Br J Anaesth 1991; 66:138-40.
31. Gronert GA, Thompson RL, Onofrio BM. Human malignant hyperthermia: Awake episodes and correction by dantrolene. Anesth Analg 1980; 59:377-8.
32. Hopkins PM, Ellis FR, Halsall PJ. Evidence for related myopathies in exertional heat stroke and malignant hyperthermia. Lancet 1991; 338:1491-2.
33. Iaizzo PA, Lehmann-Horn F. Anesthetic complications in muscle disorders (editorial). Anesthesiology 1995; 82:1093-6.
34. Wappler F, Fiege M, Steinfath M, et al. Evidence for susceptibility to malignant hyperthermia in patients with exercise-induced rhabdomyolysis. Anesthesiology 2001; 94:95-100.
35. Davis M, Brown R, Dickson A, et al. Malignant hyperthermia associated with exercise-induced rhabdomyolysis or congenital abnormalities and a novel RYR1 mutation in New Zealand and Australian pedigrees. Br J Anaesth 2002; 88:508-15.
36. Tobin JR, Jason DR, Challa VR, et al. Malignant hyperthermia and apparent heat stroke (letter). JAMA 2001; 286:168-9.
37. Gronert GA, Ahern CP, Milde JH, White RD. Effect of CO_2, calcium, digoxin and potassium on cardiac and skeletal muscle metabolism in malignant hyperthermia-susceptible swine. Anesthesiology 1986; 64:24-8.
38. Maccani RM, Wedel DJ, Hofer RE. Norepinephrine does not potentiate porcine malignant hyperthermia. Anesth Analg 1996; 82:790-5.
39. Allsop P, Jorfeldt L, Rutberg H, et al. Delayed recovery of muscle pH after short duration, high intensity exercise in malignant hyperthermia-susceptible subjects. Br J Anaesth 1991; 66:541-5.
40. Nelson TE. Porcine malignant hyperthermia: Critical temperatures for in vivo and in vitro responses. Anesthesiology 1990; 73:449-54.
41. Denborough M, Hopkinson KC, O'Brien RO, Foster PS. Overheating alone can trigger malignant hyperthermia in piglets. Anaesth Intensive Care 1996; 24:348-54.
42. Iaizzo PA, Kehler CH, Carr RJ, et al. Prior hypothermia attenuates malignant hyperthermia in susceptible swine. Anesth Analg 1996; 82:803-9.
43. Gronert GA, Milde JH. Variations in onset of malignant hyperthermia. Anesth Analg 1981; 60:499-503.
44. Duke AM, Hopkins PM, Halsall PJ, Steele DS. Mg^{2+} dependence of Ca^{2+} release from the sarcoplasmic reticulum induced by sevoflurane or halothane in skeletal muscle from humans susceptible to malignant hyperthermia. Br J Anaesth 2006; 97:320-8.
45. Katz JD, Krich LB. Acute febrile reaction complicating spinal anaesthesia in a survivor of malignant hyperthermia. Can Anaesth Soc J 1976; 23:285-9.
46. Kemp DR, Choong LS. Malignant hyperthermia and the conscious patient. Aust N Z J Surg 1988; 58:423-7.
47. Motegi Y, Shirai M, Arai M, et al. Malignant hyperthermia during epidural anesthesia. J Clin Anesth 1996; 8:157-60.
48. Pollock N, Hodges M, Sendall J. Prolonged malignant hyperthermia in the absence of triggering agents. Anaesth Intensive Care 1992; 20:520-3.
49. Fierobe L, Nivoche Y, Mantz J, et al. Perioperative severe rhabdomyolysis revealing susceptibility to malignant hyperthermia. Anesthesiology 1998; 88:263-5.
50. Harwood TN, Nelson TE. Massive postoperative rhabdomyolysis after uneventful surgery: A case report of subclinical malignant hyperthermia. Anesthesiology 1998; 88:265-8.

51. Karan SM, Crowl F, Muldoon SM. Malignant hyperthermia masked by capnographic monitoring. Anesth Analg 1994; 78:590-2.
52. Flewellen EH, Nelson TE. Halothane-succinylcholine induced masseter spasm: Indication of malignant hyperthermia susceptibility? Anesth Analg 1984; 63:693-7.
53. Van Der Spek AFL, Fang WB, Ashton-Miller JA, et al. Increased masticatory muscle stiffness during limb muscle flaccidity with succinylcholine administration. Anesthesiology 1988; 69:11-6.
54. Smith CE, Donati F, Bevan DR. Effects of succinylcholine at the masseter and adductor pollicis muscles in adults. Anesth Analg 1989; 69:158-62.
55. Albrecht A, Wedel DJ, Gronert GA. Masseter muscle rigidity and nondepolarizing neuromuscular blocking agents. Mayo Clin Proc 1997; 72:329-32.
56. Hinkle AJ, Dorsch JA. Maternal masseter muscle rigidity and neonatal fasciculations after induction for emergency cesarean section. Anesthesiology 1993; 79:175-7.
57. O'Flynn RP, Shutack JG, Rosenberg H, Fletcher JE. Masseter muscle rigidity and malignant hyperthermia susceptibility in pediatric patients: An update on management and diagnosis. Anesthesiology 1994; 80:1228-33.
58. Kaplan RF. Clinical controversies in malignant hyperthermia susceptibility. Anesthesiol Clin North Am 1994; 12:537-51.
59. Allen GC, Rosenberg H. Malignant hyperthermia susceptibility in adult patients with masseter muscle rigidity. Can J Anaesth 1990; 37:31-5.
60. Ellis FR, Halsall PJ, Christian AS. Clinical presentation of suspected malignant hyperthermia during anaesthesia in 402 probands. Anaesthesia 1990; 45:838-41.
61. Hackl W, Mauritz W, Schemper M, et al. Prediction of malignant hyperthermia susceptibility: Statistical evaluation of clinical signs. Br J Anaesth 1990; 64:425-9.
62. Larach MG, Rosenberg H, Larach DR, Broennle AM. Prediction of malignant hyperthermia susceptibility by clinical signs. Anesthesiology 1987; 66:547-50.
63. Allen GC. Malignant hyperthermia susceptibility. Anesth Clin North Am 1994; 12:513-35.
64. Larach MG, Localio AR, Allen GC, et al. A clinical grading scale to predict malignant hyperthermia susceptibility. Anesthesiology 1994; 80:771-9.
65. Larach MG. Standardization of the caffeine-halothane muscle contracture test. Anesth Analg 1989; 69:511-5.
66. The European Malignant Hyperpyrexia Group. A protocol for the investigation of malignant hyperpyrexia (MH) susceptibility. Br J Anaesth 1984; 56:1267-9.
67. Allen GC, Larach MG, Kunselman AR. The sensitivity and specificity of the caffeine-halothane contracture test. A report from the North American Malignant Hyperthermia Registry. The North American Malignant Hyperthermia Registry of MHAUS. Anesthesiology 1998; 88:579-88.
68. Serfas KD, Bose D, Patel L, et al. Comparison of the segregation of the RYR1 C1840T mutation with segregation of the caffeine/halothane contracture test results for malignant hyperthermia susceptibility in a large Manitoba Mennonite family. Anesthesiology 1996; 84:322-9.
69. Allen GC, Rosenberg H, Fletcher JE. Safety of general anesthesia in patients previously tested negative for malignant hyperthermia susceptibility. Anesthesiology 1990; 72:619-22.
70. Ørding H, Hedengran AM, Skovgaard LT. Evaluation of 119 anaesthetics received after investigation for susceptibility to malignant hyperthermia. Acta Anaesthesiol Scand 1991; 35:711-6.
71. Islander G, Ranklev-Twetman E. Evaluation of anaesthesias in malignant hyperthermia negative patients. Acta Anaesthesiol Scand 1995; 39:819-21.
72. Scala D, Di Martino A, Cozzolino S, et al. Follow-up of patients tested for malignant hyperthermia susceptibility. Eur J Anaesthesiol 2006; 23:801-5.
73. Rosenberg H, Antognini JF, Muldoon S. Testing for malignant hyperthermia. Anesthesiology 2002; 96:232-7.
74. Litman RS, Rosenberg H. Malignant hyperthermia: Update on susceptibility testing. JAMA 2005; 293:2918-24.
75. Bendahan D, Kozak-Ribbens G, Rodet L, et al. ^{31}Phosphorus magnetic resonance spectroscopy characterization of muscular metabolic anomalies in patients with malignant hyperthermia: Application to diagnosis. Anesthesiology 1998; 88:96-107.
76. Crawford JS. Hyperpyrexia during pregnancy (letter). Lancet 1972; 1:1244.
77. Willatts SM. Malignant hyperthermia susceptibility: Management during pregnancy and labour. Anaesthesia 1979; 34:41-6.
78. Isherwood DM, Ridley J, Wilson J. Creatine phosphokinase (CPK) levels in pregnancy: A case report and a discussion of the value of CPK levels in the prediction of possible malignant hyperpyrexia. Br J Obstet Gynaecol 1975; 82:346-9.
79. Douglas MJ, McMorland GH. The anaesthetic management of the malignant hyperthermia susceptible parturient. Can Anaesth Soc J 1986; 33:371-8.
80. Khalil SN, Williams JP, Bourke DL. Management of a malignant hyperthermia-susceptible patient in labor with 2-chloroprocaine epidural anesthesia. Anesth Analg 1983; 62:119-21.
81. Sorosky JJ, Ingardia CJ, Botti JJ. Diagnosis and management of susceptibility to malignant hyperthermia in pregnancy. Am J Perinatol 1989; 6:46-8.
82. Morison DH. Placental transfer of dantrolene (letter). Anesthesiology 1983; 59:265.
83. Lucy SJ. Anaesthesia for caesarean delivery of a malignant hyperthermia-susceptible parturient. Can J Anaesth 1994; 41:1220-6.
84. Pollock NA, Langton EE. Management of malignant hyperthermia-susceptible parturients. Anaesth Intensive Care 1997; 25:398-407.
85. Cohen SE. Physiological alterations of pregnancy. In Clinics in Anaesthesiology. London, WB Saunders, 1986; 4:33-46.
86. Bonica JJ. Pain of parturition. In Clinics in Anaesthesiology. London, WB Saunders, 1986; 4:1-31.
87. Marx GF, Greene NM. Maternal lactate, pyruvate and excess lactate production during labor and delivery. Am J Obstet Gynecol 1964; 90:786-93.
88. Kasten GW, Martin ST. Resuscitation from bupivacaine-induced cardiovascular toxicity during partial inferior vena cava occlusion. Anesth Analg 1986; 65:341-4.
89. Marx GF. Cardiopulmonary resuscitation of late-pregnant women (letter). Anesthesiology 1982; 56:156.
90. Lockitch G, editor. Handbook of Diagnostic Biochemistry and Hematology in Normal Pregnancy. Boca Raton, FL, CRC Press, 1993:48-59.
91. Abramov Y, Abramov D, Abrahamov A, et al. Elevation of serum creatine phosphokinase and its MB isoenzyme during normal labor and early puerperium. Acta Obstet Gynecol Scand 1996; 75:255-60.
92. Sato N, Brum JM, Mitsumoto H, DeBoer GE. Effect of cocaine on the contracture response to 1% halothane in patients undergoing diagnostic muscle biopsy for malignant hyperthermia. Can J Anaesth 1995; 42:158-62.
93. Lampley EC, Williams S, Myers SA. Cocaine-associated rhabdomyolysis causing renal failure in pregnancy. Obstet Gynecol 1996; 87:804-6.
94. Roby PV, Glenn CM, Watkins SL, et al. Association of elevated umbilical cord blood creatine kinase and myoglobin levels with the presence of cocaine metabolites in maternal urine. Am J Perinatol 1996; 13:453-5.
95. Sewall K, Flowerdew RMM, Bromberger P. Severe muscular rigidity at birth: Malignant hyperthermia syndrome? Can Anaesth Soc J 1980; 27:279-82.
96. Wilhoit RD, Brown RE, Bauman LA. Possible malignant hyperthermia in a 7-week-old infant. Anesth Analg 1989; 68:688-91.
97. Allen G, Rosenberg H. Diagnosis of malignant hyperthermia in infants (letter). Anesth Analg 1990; 70:115.
98. Lederman RP, McCann DS, Work B Jr, Huber MJ. Endogenous plasma epinephrine and norepinephrine in last-trimester pregnancy and labor. Am J Obstet Gynecol 1977; 129:5-8.

99. Thornton CA, Carrie LES, Sayers L, et al. A comparison of the effect of extradural and parenteral analgesia on maternal plasma cortisol concentrations during labour and the puerperium. Br J Obstet Gynaecol 1976; 83:631-5.
100. Pearson JF, Davies P. The effect of continuous lumbar epidural analgesia on the acid-base status of maternal arterial blood during the first stage of labour. J Obstet Gynaecol Br Commonw 1973; 80:218-24.
101. Sessler DI. Malignant hyperthermia. Acta Anaesthesiol Scand Suppl 1996; 109:25-30.
102. Urwyler A, Censier K, Seeberger MD, et al. In vitro effect of ephedrine, adrenaline, noradrenaline and isoprenaline on halothane-induced contractures in skeletal muscle from patients potentially susceptible to malignant hyperthermia. Br J Anaesth 1993; 70:76-9.
103. Rosenbert H, Brandom BW, Sambuughin N, Fletcher JE. Malignant hyperthermia and other pharmacogenetic disorders. In Barash PG, Cullen BF, Stoelting RK, editors. Clinical Anesthesia. 5th edition. Philadelphia, Lippincott Williams & Wilkins, 2006:529-56.
104. Prinzhausen H, Crawford MW, O'Rourke J, Petroz GC. Preparation of the Dräger Primus anesthetic machine for malignant hyperthermia-susceptible patients. Can J Anesth 2006; 53:885-90.
105. Abouleish E, Abboud T, Lechevalier T, et al. Rocuronium (Org 9426) for caesarean section. Br J Anaesth 1994; 73:336-41.
106. Lennon RL, Olson RA, Gronert GA. Atracurium or vecuronium for rapid-sequence endotracheal intubation. Anesthesiology 1986; 64:510-3.
107. Girard T, Jöhr M, Schaefer C, Urwyler A. Perinatal diagnosis of malignant hyperthermia susceptibility. Anesthesiology 2006; 104:1353-4.
108. Mayer DC, Weeks SK. Antepartum uterine relaxation with nitroglycerin at caesarean delivery. Can J Anaesth 1992; 39:166-9.
109. Nanson JK, Sheikh A. Anaesthesia for emergency caesarean section in a parturient with bleeding placenta praevia and a potentially malignant hyperthermia-susceptible fetus. Int J Obstet Anesth 2000; 9:278-88.
110. Lopez JR, Sanchez V, Lopez I, et al. The effects of extracellular magnesium on myoplasmic Ca^{2+} in malignant hyperthermia-susceptible swine. Anesthesiology 1990; 73:109-17.
111. Yoganathan T, Casthely PA, Lamprou M. Dantrolene-induced hyperkalemia in a patient with diltiazem and metoprolol. J Cardiothorac Anesth 1988; 2:363-4.
112. Rubin AS, Zablocki AD. Hyperkalemia, verapamil, and dantrolene. Anesthesiology 1987; 66:246-9.
113. Harrison GG, Wright IG, Morrell DF. The effects of calcium channel blocking drugs on halothane initiation of malignant hyperthermia in MHS swine and on the established syndrome. Anaesth Intensive Care 1988; 16:197-201.
114. Sim ATR, White MD, Denborough MA. The effect of oxytocin on porcine malignant hyperpyrexia-susceptible skeletal muscle. Clin Exp Pharmacol Physiol 1987; 14:605-10.
115. Hankins GDV, Berryman GK, Scott RT, Hood D. Maternal arterial desaturation with 15-methyl prostaglandin F_2 alpha for uterine atony. Obstet Gynecol 1988; 72:367-9.
116. Hughes WA, Hughes SC. Hemodynamic effects of prostaglandin E_2. Anesthesiology 1989; 70:713-6.
117. Hofmeyr GJ, Walraven G, Gülmezoglu AM, et al. Misoprostol to treat postpartum haemorrhage: A systematic review. BJOG 2005; 112:547-42.
118. Mercier FJ, Benhamou D. Hyperthermia related to epidural analgesia during labor. Int J Obstet Anesth 1997; 6:19-24.
119. Heiman-Patterson TD. Neuroleptic malignant syndrome and malignant hyperthermia: Important issues for the medical consultant. Med Clin North Am 1993; 77:477-92.
120. Russell CS, Lang C, McCambridge M, Calhoun B. Neuroleptic malignant syndrome in pregnancy. Obstet Gynecol 2001; 98:906-8.
121. Chan TC, Evans SD, Clark RF. Drug-induced hyperthermia. Crit Care Clin 1997; 13:785-807.
122. Flewellen EH, Nelson TE, Jones WP, et al. Dantrolene dose response in awake man: Implications for management of malignant hyperthermia. Anesthesiology 1983; 59:275-80.
123. Wedel DJ. Malignant hyperthermia: Prevention and treatment. American Society of Anesthesiologists Newsletter 1997; 61:13-5.
124. Burkman JM, Posner KL, Domino KB. Analysis of the clinical variables associated with recrudescence after malignant hyperthermia reactions. Anesthesiology 2007; 106:901-6.
125. Craft JB, Goldberg NH, Lim M, et al. Cardiovascular effects and placental passage of dantrolene in the maternal-fetal sheep model. Anesthesiology 1988; 68:68-72.
126. Shin YK, Kim YD, Collea JV, Belcher MD. Effect of dantrolene sodium on contractility of isolated human uterine muscle. Int J Obstet Anesth 1995; 4:197-200.
127. Krause T, Gerbershagen MU, Fiege M, et al. Dantrolene—a review of its pharmacology, therapeutic use and new developments. Anaesthesia 2004; 59:364-73.
128. Mitchell LW, Leighton BL. Warmed diluent speeds dantrolene reconstitution. Can J Anesth 2003; 50:127-30.
129. Fricker RM, Hoerauf KH, Drewe J, Kress HG. Secretion of dantrolene into breast milk after acute therapy of a suspected malignant hyperthermia crisis during cesarean section. Anesthesiology 1998; 89:1023-5.

Chapter 48

Musculoskeletal Disorders

Roanne Preston, M.D., FRCPC
Edward T. Crosby, M.D., FRCPC

Pregnancy commonly results in musculoskeletal complaints. Although they typically are benign and self-limited, symptoms may be disabling in some women. In addition, preexisting musculoskeletal disorders interact with pregnancy to a variable extent. These interactions range from an ameliorating effect of pregnancy on the course of the disease (e.g., rheumatoid arthritis) to the potential for a significant and possibly life-threatening deterioration in maternal condition (e.g., uncorrected severe thoracic scoliosis). The purpose of this chapter is to discuss the most common musculoskeletal disorders encountered in pregnant women and their implications for obstetric and anesthesia providers.

GESTATIONAL BACK PAIN

Lumbopelvic pain is the most common musculoskeletal complaint during pregnancy; it comprises two distinct areas of discomfort, the lumbar spine area and the posterior pelvic girdle area (from the sacroiliac joints radiating down into the posterior thighs).[1-4] It occurs at some time during gestation in more than 50% of pregnant women and impairs at least one normal activity of daily life.[3] Studies from Scandinavian countries reveal a prevalence as high as 70%, and gestational back or pelvic pain is the most common reason for sick leave during pregnancy.[2] Women with mainly pelvic girdle pain report more disability during pregnancy than those with lumbar pain alone.[4,5] Risk factors include a history of low back pain, young age, hypermobile joints, low socioeconomic class, multiparity, spondylolisthesis, and excessive weight gain during pregnancy.[1-7] Unfortunately, women who suffer from gestational back pain in one pregnancy have a very high risk of experiencing it during subsequent pregnancies.

The etiology includes hormonal and mechanical factors. The corpus luteum synthesizes and releases relaxin, and maternal blood concentrations of this peptide hormone increase 10-fold during gestation. Relaxin induces ligamentous softening and peripheral and pelvic joint laxity, which cause instability of the symphysis pubis and sacroiliac joints; the extent of instability and disability may be related

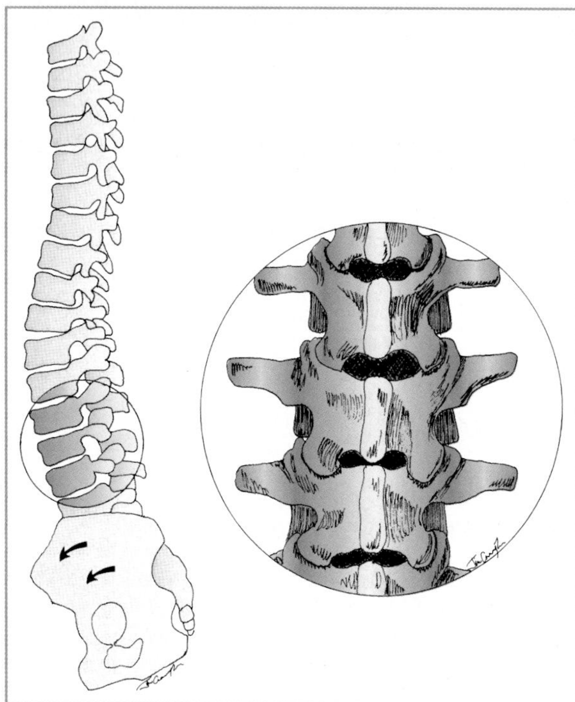

FIGURE 48-1 Musculoskeletal changes of pregnancy. Forward rotation of the pelvis and greater lumbar lordosis increase the load borne by the posterior vertebral elements and tend to close the lumbar interlaminar spaces. *Inset*, Lumbar vertebrae L2 to L4.

to the maternal concentration of relaxin. There is a correlation between mean serum levels of relaxin and the occurrence of back pain during pregnancy, and women with incapacitating symptoms have the highest serum concentrations of relaxin.[8,9]

Mechanical changes have a later onset than hormonal changes. Uterine enlargement results in a forward rotation of the sacrum and an increase in the lumbar lordotic curve, which tends to close the lumbar interlaminar space (Figure 48-1). This change exaggerates the mechanical load borne by both the facet joints and the posterior aspect of the intervertebral discs. These mechanical changes also may compromise nerve root foramina. Sciatica occurs in 1% of pregnant women, and most cases occur late in pregnancy.[10] Sciatica is distinguished from posterior pelvic girdle pain by its extension to the ankle or involvement of the foot, and it may be associated with neurologic changes.[10] Disc herniation is rare in pregnancy but does occur.[11] Incapacitating pain that radiates below the knee, typically accompanied by progressive neurologic deficits or bowel and bladder dysfunction, distinguishes disc herniation from the more common and benign gestational back pain.[5,11]

In summary, hormonal changes cause sacroiliac joint dysfunction, which is responsible for the back pain that occurs early in pregnancy. Mechanical changes are primarily responsible for the back pain that manifests during late gestation, although symphysis pubis and sacroiliac joint instability may also continue to cause pain. Disc herniation is uncommon and is characterized by the presence of neurologic findings.

Obstetric Management

Treatment is conservative in the absence of neurologic compromise.[10] Both structured exercise programs and acupuncture have been shown to be beneficial for women suffering from lumbopelvic pain during pregnancy.[12] Bed rest is reserved for patients with neurologic symptoms or disability secondary to pelvic instability. Patients with severe neurologic signs or symptoms of disc herniation should be assessed by a consultant neurosurgeon who can provide recommendations for intrapartum and postpartum care. Surgical intervention may be required in women with incapacitating pain or progressive neurologic deficits.[11] In a woman with severe symptoms, the obstetrician may choose to perform elective instrumental vaginal delivery to decrease maternal work and back stress during the second stage of labor.

Anesthetic Management

No evidence suggests that epidural or spinal anesthesia is contraindicated in patients with gestational back pain. The anesthesia provider may provide neuraxial anesthesia, even to patients with sciatica. However, neurologic signs and symptoms should be first identified, delineated, and recorded. It seems prudent to administer a dilute solution of local anesthetic, with or without an opioid, to minimize motor block associated with epidural analgesia during labor in order to reduce any further stress on relaxed sacroiliac joints.

All members of the obstetric care team must pay careful attention to the positioning of the patient with back complaints. The patient must not be placed in a position that she could not tolerate before the administration of neuraxial anesthesia. The lithotomy position puts significant stress on the lower back and should be avoided whenever possible. If it is used, care must be taken to raise and lower both legs simultaneously to prevent injury to the lumbar spine and to avoid extremes when positioning the legs. Finally, caregivers should avoid rotational movements of the spine during transfer of the patient between the bed and the operating table.

CHRONIC LOW BACK PAIN

Most instances of acute low back pain do not involve neural structures and represent minor, self-limited injuries. Prolapse of an intervertebral disc occurs in approximately 1% of acute low back injuries, and the resultant compression of neural elements results in sciatica. This injury occurs most commonly in the L4 to L5 or L5 to S1 motion segments in patients 20 to 50 years of age.[13] Approximately 50% of pregnant women with a previous history of back pain or those with chronic low back pain experience a recurrence or exacerbation of their symptoms during pregnancy.[5,7]

Neuraxial anesthesia is more likely to fail in patients with chronic low back pain and in those who have had back surgery.[14-17] Benzon et al.[14] reported a delayed onset of epidural anesthesia in patients with back pain or sciatica; the affected roots were blocked 10 to 70 minutes later than the contralateral roots at the same level. The delay in block onset most likely results from the inability of the local anesthetic agent to diffuse into the area of the injured root. Luyendijk and van Voorthuisen[18] evaluated 600 epidurograms and confirmed that contrast material failed to reach the nerve root in 33% of patients with uncomplicated disc prolapse and did not move beyond the affected disc space in 5% of cases. Schachner and Abram[16] suggested that this finding is caused by epidural scarring and adhesions that may develop during healing after disc injury. During epidurography, they noted that contrast material did not diffuse past the level of an injured disc and exited through the foramina below the abnormal disc. Prolapse of an intervertebral disc may result in relative or total obstruction to the flow of local anesthetic agent within the epidural space. The unblocked area includes the affected segment but also may include all segments (either ipsilateral or bilateral) distal to the affected level.

Sharrock et al.[15] reported a high rate (91%) of successful epidural anesthesia in patients with a history of limited spinal surgery. However, the success rate was lower than that achieved by the same group of anesthesiologists in a population with no history of back surgery (98.7%). They attributed the higher rate of failure to the distortion of surface anatomy and the tethering of the dura to the ligamentum flavum by scar formation, which rendered the epidural space discontinuous or obliterated it entirely. Support for this hypothesis is provided by LaRocca and MacNab's[19] description of the postlaminectomy membrane. They noted the postlaminectomy formation of organized fibrous tissue surrounding the dura and, at times, binding of the nerves to the posterior aspect of the disc and adjacent vertebral body. The fibrous response was proportional to the extent of surgical trauma and was more marked with greater operative exposures. Consequently, a local anesthetic agent injected into the epidural space may not diffuse beyond the area of scarring, and an inadequate block may result.[17] Postlaminectomy spinal stenosis also may lead to attenuation or obliteration of the epidural space, and the most common site of obstructive stenosis is immediately above the fusion mass.[20]

Obstetric Management

It is not uncommon for obstetricians to offer pregnant women who have had persistent chronic low back pain the option of cesarean delivery to decrease the potential for further back injury during labor. There are no data to either encourage or discourage this option.

Anesthetic Management

The anesthesia provider may offer epidural or spinal anesthesia to patients with previous lumbar spine pathology or surgery. A decreased incidence of successful epidural anesthesia may be expected, especially in patients who have had extensive surgery. Nonetheless, the experienced anesthesia provider will administer epidural anesthesia successfully in the majority of patients. Sharrock et al.[15] recommended administration of epidural anesthesia one or two interspaces above the operated segment to improve the likelihood of a successful block. Rarely, a high block may result if there is a total obstruction to flow of the local anesthetic agent at lower spinal levels.[17] Subarachnoid anesthesia is likely to be more reliable than epidural anesthesia in this patient population.

POSTPARTUM BACKACHE

Postpartum backache is a common complaint worldwide, occurring in approximately 25% of women, with 5% to 7% of women seeking medical help.[5] MacArthur et al.,[21,22] citing data obtained from a postal survey of 11,701 women who had delivered 1 to 9 years previously, reported that postpartum backache, starting within 3 months of delivery and persisting for 6 weeks or longer, occurred in 23% of women. Approximately 25% of these women had experienced backache before delivery, but 14% reported new-onset backache. In many women, the pain was persistent; 70% had experienced it for more than 2 years, and 65% had pain at the time of questioning 1 to 9 years later. Back pain was more common in women who delivered vaginally with epidural analgesia than in those who did not have epidural analgesia (18.9% versus 10.5%, respectively). Women who had epidural analgesia also were more likely to have had induced labor, an abnormal fetal position, a multiple pregnancy, a prolonged first or second stage of labor, forceps delivery, episiotomy, cesarean delivery, postpartum hemorrhage, or a large baby. MacLeod et al.[23] also performed a postal survey of 2065 patients 1 year postpartum and reported a 26.2% incidence of postpartum backache in women who had received epidural analgesia, compared with a 1.7% incidence in those who had not; the latter incidence of postpartum backache (1.7%) is the lowest, by far, of any reported by any investigator in a postpartum population in the first year after delivery. Orlikowski et al.,[24] who examined data from 992 women as a secondary analysis of a prospective randomized study on epidural analgesia versus continuous midwifery support, found no relationship between back pain at 6 months postpartum and the use of epidural analgesia.

A number of investigators have carried out prospective evaluations to eliminate the potential for reporting bias that may confound retrospective surveys. Breen et al.[25] performed an assessment of 1042 women at 6 months postpartum. Although 44% of women experienced postpartum backache, there was no difference between those who had received epidural analgesia and those who had not. The most significant predictor of postpartum backache was antenatal back pain. Weight gain was greater in patients with postpartum and new-onset back pain. Groves et al.[26] assessed the incidence of late (12 to 18 months) postpartum backache in this same cohort of patients. The incidence of late postpartum backache was 49%, and as with the Breen study, there was no difference in the incidence between patients who had received epidural analgesia (49%) and those who did not (50%). However, the incidence was higher among women who had reported early postpartum backache (66%) than among those who did not (33%). The incidence of late, new-onset backache after delivery, not present in the first 2 months postpartum, was 21%.

Macarthur et al.[27] also prospectively studied the association between epidural analgesia and early, new-onset postpartum backache in 329 women. In patients who labored without epidural analgesia, the incidence of postpartum backache was 43% at 1 day, 23% at 7 days, and 7% at

6 weeks. The incidence of symptoms in patients who had received epidural analgesia was higher on the first postpartum day (53%), but this increase was not persistent. At 1 year postpartum, 12% of the patients had back pain (9.9% in the epidural group and 13.8% in the control group). Howell et al.[28] performed a randomized controlled trial comparing epidural with nonepidural analgesia during labor in 369 nulliparous women. There was no difference in the incidence or characteristics of postpartum backache at 3 and 12 months postpartum. In a follow-up study, there was no difference between the two groups in the incidence of back pain, disability, or movement restriction more than 2 years after delivery.[29]

The type of epidural analgesia provided has also been reviewed to determine whether alteration of the technique affects the outcome related to postpartum backache. Patel et al.[30] studied 340 nulliparous women and compared women who had received a combined spinal-epidural (CSE) technique for labor analgesia with those who had not received neuraxial analgesia. The incidence of backache at 6 to 8 months postpartum was 33% overall and did not differ between the groups. Russell et al.[31] studied 616 women who requested epidural analgesia for labor and randomly assigned them to one of two study groups; one group received a local anesthetic (0.125% bupivacaine) infusion, and the other received a more dilute solution of local anesthetic with an opioid (0.0625% bupivacaine with either fentanyl 2.5 µg/mL or sufentanil 0.25 µg/mL). A third group who did not wish to have epidural analgesia served as the control group. Thirty-three women reported new-onset postpartum backache after delivery; there was no difference among the three groups. The only factor associated with backache or development of new postpartum backache within the first 3 months postpartum was antenatal backache. Finally, MacArthur and Lewis[32] observed no association between the management of epidural analgesia (e.g., local anesthetic used, infusion type, duration of analgesia, extent of motor and sensory blockade) and the occurrence of postpartum backache.

Both transient and more persistent postpartum backaches are common, but there is little evidence that they are related to the provision of epidural analgesia during labor. Similarly, no evidence suggests that denying a parturient epidural analgesia results in a lower incidence of back problems during the postpartum period. Factors associated with more persistent postpartum backache include the presence of back pain before pregnancy, the presence of gestational backache, and performance of physically demanding work.[5]

SCOLIOSIS

Scoliosis is a lateral deviation in the vertical axis of the spine. The severity of scoliosis is determined by measurement of the angle of the spinal curve, the Cobb angle, which is expressed in degrees (Figure 48-2). The incidence of minor curves is 4 per 1000 in the North American population; larger curves occur less frequently, predominantly in females. Severe scoliosis is relatively rare in pregnant women; it is present in 0.03% of pregnancies.[33] Although women with moderate to severe scoliosis constitute a small population of obstetric patients, pregnancy within this

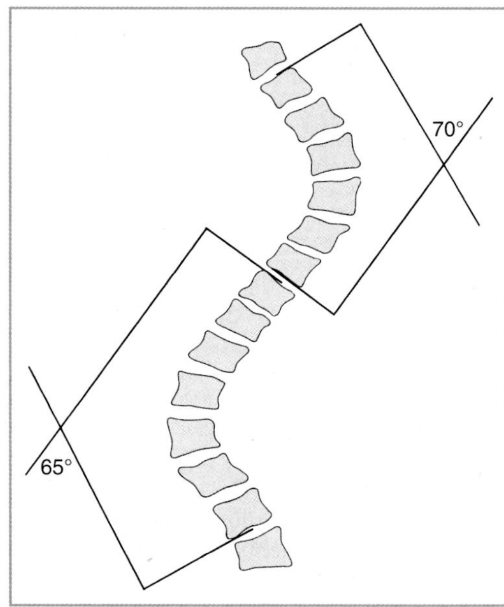

FIGURE 48-2 Schematic representation of the Cobb angle. A line is drawn parallel to the superior cortical plate of the proximal end vertebrae and another line parallel to the inferior cortical plate of the distal end vertebrae. A perpendicular line is drawn to each of these lines. The angle of intersection is the Cobb angle of the curve.

population is common.[34] Most cases of scoliosis are idiopathic, although some are associated with other conditions, most commonly neuromuscular disorders (Box 48-1).

Scoliotic curves can be divided into structural and nonstructural varieties. **Nonstructural curves** are those seen with postural scoliosis, sciatica, and leg-length discrepancies. They do not affect the mobility of the spine and are nonprogressive. **Structural curves** are seen in patients with

BOX 48-1 Conditions Associated with Scoliosis

Congenital (Vertebral) Anomalies
- Hemivertebra
- Spina bifida

Neurologic Disorders
- Cerebral palsy
- Polio
- Neurofibromatosis

Myopathic Disorders
- Myotonic dystrophy
- Muscular dystrophy

Connective Tissue Disorders
- Marfan syndrome
- Rheumatoid disease

Osteochondrodystrophies
- Achondroplasia/hypochondroplasia
- Osteogenesis imperfecta

Infection
- Tuberculosis

Previous Trauma

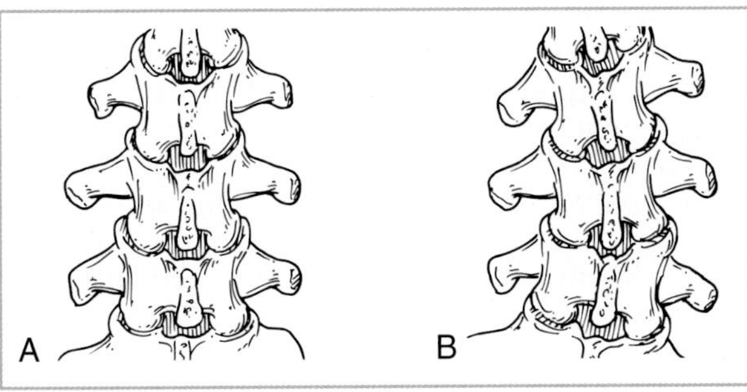

FIGURE 48-3 Spinal rotation with scoliosis. **A,** Posterior anatomy of the midlumbar spine (L2 to L4) in a patient with a normal back. **B,** Anatomy at the same level in a patient with a 30-degree lumbar scoliosis. There is a reduction in the dimensions of the interlaminar space on the concave side of the curve, and an expansion on the convex side. These changes are enhanced with greater severity of the curve. As the curve increases, the spinous processes rotate into the concavity of the curve, further altering the local anatomy.

idiopathic scoliosis and with scoliosis resulting from the conditions listed in Box 48-1. Structural curves lead to reduced spinal mobility, and affected patients typically have a fixed prominence (rib hump) on the convex side of the curve. There is also a rotatory component associated with the structural scoliotic curve. The axial rotation of the vertebral body is such that the spinous processes rotate away from the convexity of the curve and back toward the midline of the patient (Figures 48-3 and 48-4).[35] Deformation of the vertebral bodies results in shorter, thinner pedicles and laminae and a more narrow vertebral canal on the concave side. Vertebral deformation is unusual in patients with a Cobb angle less than 40 degrees.

Scoliosis interferes with the formation, growth, and development of the lungs; the occurrence of scoliosis before lung maturity may reduce the number of alveoli that ultimately form. The pulmonary vasculature develops in parallel with the alveoli; early-onset scoliosis and severe scoliosis may result in greater pulmonary vascular resistance and eventually lead to pulmonary hypertension. Musculoskeletal deformities also affect the mechanical function of the lungs; anatomic findings in scoliosis that are most commonly associated with respiratory compromise include the presence of a thoracic curve, thoracic lordosis, and a rib cage deformity. The most common pulmonary function abnormality is a restrictive pattern with decreases in vital capacity, total lung capacity, and lung compliance. This pattern occurs in all patients with a thoracic curve greater than 65 degrees. The functional residual capacity (FRC) is reduced, and airways may close during normal tidal breathing. If the FRC is reduced to the extent that it falls below the closing capacity, atelectasis may occur in basal alveoli. The most common blood gas abnormality is an increased alveolar-to-arterial oxygen gradient, with reduced $Pa{O_2}$ and a normal $Pa{CO_2}$. It results from both venoarterial shunting and altered regional perfusion. Venous admixture may lead to arterial hypoxemia. The natural history of severe, progressive scoliosis includes early death from cardiopulmonary failure.[36]

Permanent changes of the pulmonary vasculature are common in patients with a curve greater than 65 degrees. Pulmonary hypertension (a resting mean pulmonary artery pressure exceeding 20 mm Hg) occurs in many pàtients with severe deformity long before the onset of right heart failure and is largely attributable to increases in vascular resistance resulting from chronic alveolar hypoxia, hypoxic pulmonary vasoconstriction, and anatomic changes in the vascular bed. Fixed pulmonary hypertension carries a grave prognosis in pregnancy and may prompt a recommendation to avoid or terminate pregnancy.[37,38]

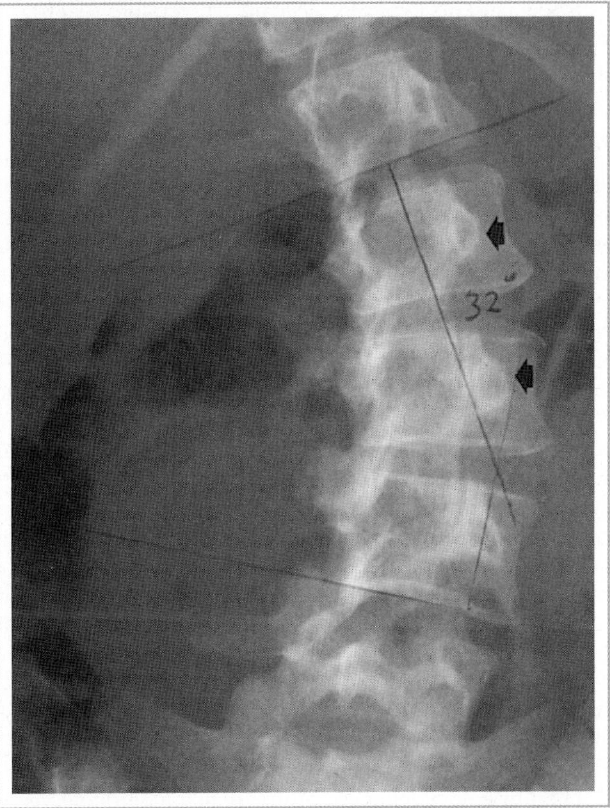

FIGURE 48-4 Radiographic study of the lumbar spine in a 26-year-old woman with idiopathic scoliosis. The spinous processes and pedicles (*arrows*) are rotated away from the convexity and into the concavity of the curve. (The epidural space was entered easily with direction of the needle approximately 15 degrees off the perpendicular at the skin level toward the convexity of the curve.)

Scoliosis Associated with Neuromuscular Disease

When scoliosis develops secondary to a neurologic or myopathic disorder, abnormal respiratory function results not only from the skeletal deformity but also from abnormalities in the central control of respiration and the supraspinal innervation of the respiratory muscles, as well as from the loss of muscle function caused by the underlying disorder. Respiratory function may be further compromised by (1) impairment of the defense mechanisms of the airways due to loss of control of the pharynx and the larynx, (2) an ineffective cough mechanism, and (3) infrequent or reduced large breaths. Recurrent aspiration pneumonitis may result from compromised protective airway reflexes. In general, the prognosis of scoliosis due to neuromuscular disease is worse than that of idiopathic scoliosis and is determined predominantly by progression of the primary disorder.

Affected patients typically develop irreversible respiratory failure at a younger age, and pulmonary hypertension is common; pregnancy is uncommon in this population.

Interaction with Pregnancy

Pregnancy may exacerbate both the severity of spinal curvature and cardiopulmonary abnormalities in women with uncorrected scoliosis. Progression of a curve, defined as an increase in the Cobb angle of 5 degrees or more over subsequent assessments, most likely occurs during periods of rapid growth and in patients with larger curves at the time of diagnosis. Curves that are less than 25 degrees or curves that have been stable before pregnancy typically do not progress during pregnancy.[39,40] In contrast, more severe curves and those that have not stabilized may worsen. Some investigators have described a correlation between the severity of the curve and maternal morbidity and mortality. However, it is likely that the severity of functional cardiopulmonary impairment before pregnancy is a better predictor of maternal outcome than the severity of the curve.[41] Patients with a severe curve (i.e., Cobb angle greater than 60 degrees) but good cardiopulmonary function tolerate pregnancy well, whereas in those with significant cardiopulmonary compromise, and especially in those with pulmonary hypertension, maternal mortality is high.[37,38]

The physiologic changes of pregnancy include decreases in both functional residual and closing capacities and increases in minute ventilation and oxygen demand. The thoracic cage normally increases in circumference during pregnancy as a result of increases in both anteroposterior and transverse diameters. If the chest cage is relatively fixed by scoliosis, the diaphragm is responsible for all increments in minute ventilation. As the enlarging uterus causes elevation of the diaphragm, diaphragmatic activity is restricted and further decreases in residual and closing capacities may occur, which may result in both greater ventilation-perfusion mismatch and decreased arterial oxygen content. The antepartum onset of new symptoms of respiratory compromise or the exacerbation of preexisting symptomatology is associated with higher maternal morbidity and a greater likelihood that assisted ventilation will be required after cesarean delivery.[41]

Minute ventilation typically increases by 45% during pregnancy. In normal pregnancy, the increase is primarily a result of increased tidal volume. In the scoliotic patient with restrictive lung disease, larger tidal volumes may not be possible, and the increased minute ventilation is achieved by means of higher respiratory rates and increased work of breathing. Peak increases in pulmonary activity are reached by the middle of the third trimester, but the uterus continues to grow until term, and it may further encroach on the noncompliant thorax, causing late gestational deterioration despite stabilization of respiratory demand.

Dyspnea on exertion is uncommon in patients with scoliosis who have curves less than 70 degrees, but it becomes more common as the deformity exceeds 100 degrees. In younger patients with a curve less than 70 degrees, exercise capacity is more likely to be impaired because of the lack of regular aerobic exercise and subsequent deconditioning rather than intrinsic ventilatory impairment.[42] Dyspnea is common in many pregnant women, typically begins in the first or second trimester, and is most prevalent at term. Two features help distinguish physiologic from pathologic dyspnea.[43] **Physiologic dyspnea** tends to occur earlier in pregnancy and often plateaus or even improves as term approaches. The **pathologic dyspnea** of cardiopulmonary decompensation more often begins in the second half of pregnancy and is progressive, often becoming most severe as gestation advances and the physiologic loading is maximal. Second, physiologic dyspnea is rarely extreme, and patients can maintain most daily activities. Dyspnea that is extreme or has a limiting effect on normal activity may signal maternal cardiorespiratory decompensation. Dyspnea at rest is also rare in the absence of cardiopulmonary dysfunction, as is dyspnea that is acute in onset or progressive and intractable.

Minute ventilation of the unmedicated parturient increases by a further 75% to 150% in the first stage of labor and by 150% to 300% in the second stage. Oxygen consumption increases above prelabor values by 40% in the first stage and 75% in the second stage. These levels may be unattainable by the scoliotic parturient with restrictive lung disease, and respiratory failure and hypoxemia may result during labor.

Pregnant women with pulmonary hypertension have a limited ability to increase cardiac output. During normal pregnancy, cardiac output increases 40% to 50% above nonpregnant measurements; during labor and delivery, even greater increases are observed. These increases are achieved with both larger stroke volume and a higher heart rate. These demands may put an excessive burden on the cardiovascular system in parturients who had marginal cardiac reserve before pregnancy. If the right ventricle fails in the presence of pulmonary hypertension, left ventricular filling will decrease, and low-output failure and sudden death may occur.[37,38]

Surgical Management

During spinal fusion and instrumentation, the spinal musculature is reflected off the vertebrae over the course of the curve, and the spinous processes and interspinous ligaments are removed. The spine is subsequently extended, correcting the curve. The vertebrae are decorticated throughout the extent of the planned fusion, instrumentation is placed, and bone graft material from the ileum is placed over the decorticated vertebrae. A number of techniques for fusion have been described, but all involve both spinal instrumentation and extensive bone grafting in the axial spine (Figure 48-5).

Obstetric Management

Pregnant women with corrected scoliosis tolerate pregnancy, labor, and delivery well. In the absence of major lumbosacral deformity, there is little alteration of the pelvic cavity, and malpresentation is not more common than in women without scoliosis. Uterine function is normal, and labor is not prolonged. Spontaneous vaginal delivery is anticipated, and cesarean delivery should be reserved for obstetric indications.

One uncontrolled study suggested no difference in the requirement for cesarean delivery in patients with previous Harrington rod instrumentation for correction of idiopathic

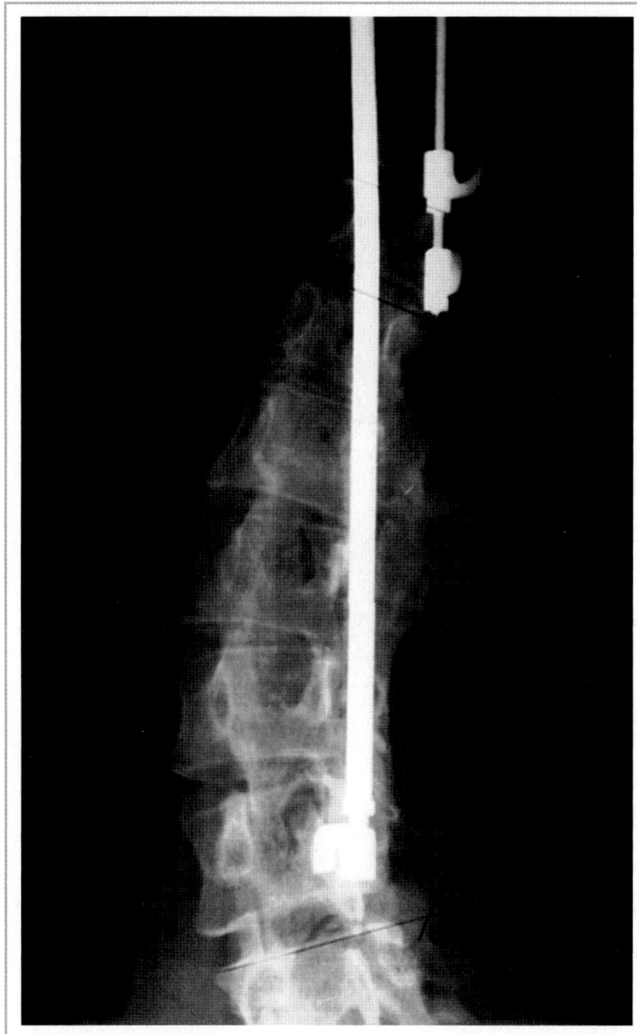

FIGURE 48-5 Harrington rod instrumentation. Radiographic study of the lumbar spine in a 31-year-old woman with thoracolumbar scoliosis corrected with spinal instrumentation. There is rotation of the vertebrae into the curve (toward the rod), and extensive bone grafting is evident adjacent to the rod. Two lumbar interspaces (L4 to L5 and L5 to S1) are not involved in the fusion.

scoliosis; a second and similar study reported a higher incidence of operative delivery.[34,44] The difference in outcomes may be influenced by the severity and etiology of the scoliosis in the populations reviewed and/or differences in the local practice patterns for managing atypical patients. Pelvic abnormalities are more common when scoliosis is associated with neuromuscular disorders and in patients with a severe, uncorrected curve.[45] In addition, abdominal and pelvic muscle weakness predisposes parturients to problems with expulsion of the infant during the second stage of labor and may necessitate instrumental vaginal delivery. The need for instrumental or cesarean delivery seems to be related to the severity of skeletal deformity, the resulting maternal compromise, and cephalopelvic disproportion.

In the second stage of labor, the diaphragm has a nonrespiratory function. With expulsive efforts, maximal isometric contractions may be sustained for 20 seconds or more, and diaphragmatic fatigue has been demonstrated even in normal, laboring women. In parturients whose diaphragmatic function is compromised by neuromuscular disease or severe scoliosis, the potential for fatigue and failure is greater; expulsive forces are decreased, the second stage may be prolonged, and a trial of labor may fail, necessitating instrumental or cesarean delivery. In addition, women with severe cardiopulmonary disease (especially those with gestational decompensation) may require urgent or emergency cesarean delivery because of maternal compromise or nonreassuring fetal status.

Anesthetic Management

Pregnant women who have thoracolumbar scoliosis with a Cobb angle greater than 30 degrees or who have undergone spinal instrumentation and fusion for scoliosis should be referred to an anesthesiologist for antepartum consultation. The anesthesiologist should (1) determine the etiology of the scoliosis, as well as the severity and stability of the curve; (2) obtain a history of maternal musculoskeletal and cardiopulmonary symptoms; and (3) review prior obstetric and anesthetic experiences. For patients with scoliosis secondary to neuromuscular disorders, the anesthesiologist should also become familiar with anesthetic considerations specific to those underlying disorders.

Women with suspected or evident pulmonary compromise should undergo evaluation by a pulmonologist, and pulmonary function studies and arterial blood gas measurements should be obtained. These patients must be reevaluated periodically to ensure that they are tolerating the increasing physiologic demands of pregnancy. Echocardiography is useful to assess right heart function in patients with one or more of the following: (1) a curve of 60 degrees or more, (2) hypoxemia on arterial blood gas measurement, (3) moderate or greater reductions in predicted lung volumes or flows, and/or (4) pulmonary hypertension. Radiographic studies performed before pregnancy and operative notes describing spinal surgical procedures should be reviewed before neuraxial anesthesia is given to any patient with significant scoliosis or previous spinal surgery. The anesthesiologist should also examine the spine and note the surface landmarks and interspaces that are least affected by the deformity. Modes of analgesia and anesthesia for labor and delivery can be discussed during antepartum consultation.

Invasive hemodynamic monitoring is rarely indicated during labor and delivery. Pulmonary function studies that suggest significant respiratory compromise or clinical evidence of impending respiratory failure warrant placement of an arterial catheter and serial assessment of blood gas measurements. Echocardiographic demonstration of significant right heart dysfunction may warrant central venous pressure monitoring. The use of echocardiography may allow for detailed anatomic and physiologic assessment in severely ill mothers with advanced and decompensated cardiopulmonary disease.

The anesthesiologist may offer epidural anesthesia for labor and delivery to patients with severe thoracolumbar scoliosis. Identification of the epidural space is more difficult in such patients, and the anesthesiologist should anticipate a higher incidence of complications. It is useful to remember the presence of the vertebral rotation during the performance of neuraxial anesthesia in a patient with a significant lumbar curve. The midline of the epidural space is deviated toward the convexity of the curve relative to the spinous process palpable at the skin level (see Figures 48-3 and 48-4). The extent of lateral deviation is determined largely by the severity of the deformity. The needle should enter the selected interspace and should be directed toward the concavity of the curve.[46] The experienced anesthesiologist can track the resistance of both the interspinous ligament and the ligamentum flavum to maintain the correct course into the epidural space. The extent of the local anatomic distortion is the limiting factor, and the selection of spaces that are least involved with the curve is advised (Figure 48-6). In patients with scoliosis resulting from myopathic or neurologic disease, distortion of spinal anatomy may be significant enough to prohibit the administration of neuraxial anesthesia. Ultrasonography may be useful in the identification of surgically perturbed anatomy and may assist in the localization of difficult-to-palpate interspaces; there is limited published literature to date on this specific use of ultrasonography, although its application is clearly growing in the practice of regional anesthesia overall.

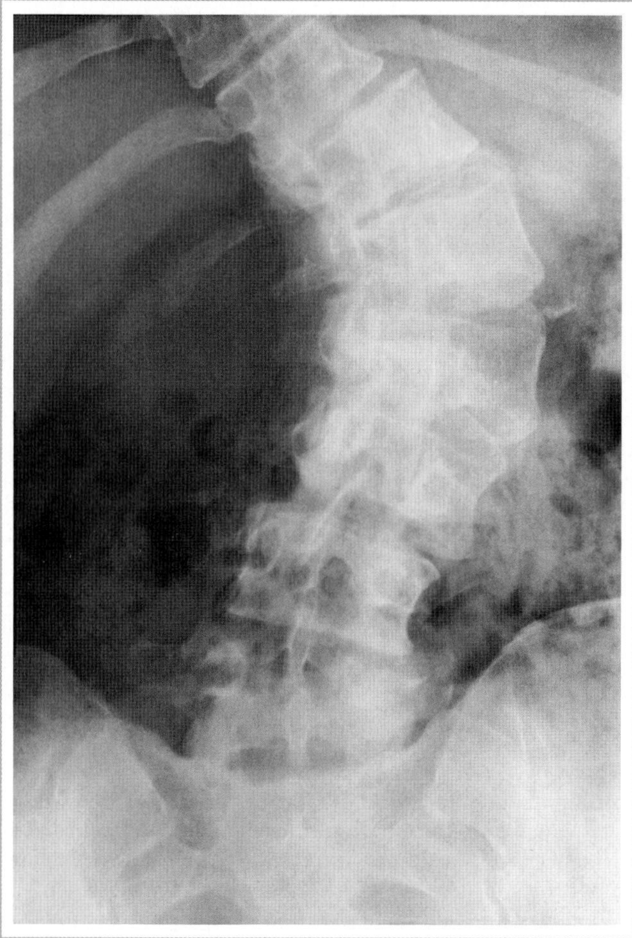

FIGURE 48-6 Radiograph of the lower thoracolumbar spine in a young woman with scoliosis predominantly affecting the lumbar spine and markedly distorting her local anatomy. She received lumbar epidural analgesia for labor during her first pregnancy, after a catheter was placed with some difficulty. She received patient-controlled intravenous nalbuphine for labor analgesia during her second pregnancy after persistent, unsuccessful attempts to insert an epidural catheter. For her third pregnancy, this radiograph directed the practitioner toward the lower lumbar spaces, where anatomic distortion is less pronounced.

Local anesthetic dose requirements for epidural and spinal anesthesia in the patient with scoliosis are variable. Moreover, during administration of spinal anesthesia in a patient with a severe scoliotic curve, hyperbaric local anesthetic solution may pool in dependent portions of the spine, resulting in an inadequate block.[47] Thus, it is preferable to use a continuous technique so that the dose of local anesthetic agent can be titrated to the desired segmental level of anesthesia.

When offering neuraxial anesthesia to patients with a history of corrective surgery, the anesthesiologist must consider the following potential problems:

- Persistent back pain occurs in many patients with corrected scoliosis and correlates with both the extent of fusion and the time since surgery.[48,49]
- Degenerative changes occur in the spine below the area of fusion, and there is a higher incidence of both retrolisthesis and spondylolisthesis.[49]
- Twenty percent of patients undergo fusion to the lowest lumbar levels, limiting the potential for neuraxial anesthesia.[44,50]
- Insertion of an epidural needle in the fused area may not be possible because of the presence of instrumentation, scar tissue, and bone graft material.
- Intraoperative trauma to the ligamentum flavum may result in adhesions in or obliteration of the epidural space, and these changes may interfere with the spread of injected local anesthetic.[19]
- Obliteration of the epidural space may increase the incidence of unintentional dural puncture.
- These patients often manifest a high level of anxiety about their backs and may be reluctant to have neuraxial anesthesia.

Several reports have described the use of epidural anesthesia in obstetric patients with spinal instrumentation and fusion.[44,51] These reports have detailed a higher-than-usual incidence of difficulties encountered during the administration of epidural anesthesia. Complications included (1) unsuccessful identification of the epidural space, (2) multiple attempts before successful identification of the space and insertion of the catheter, (3) false loss-of-resistance, (4) unintentional dural puncture, and (5) failed block or inadequate analgesia. Complications seem to occur more frequently in patients with fusion that extends to the lower lumbar and lumbosacral interspaces than in those with fusion that ends in the upper lumbar spine.

Both the anesthesiologist and the patient should anticipate the possibility that blind attempts to identify the epidural space may fail, and consideration should be given to the use of ultrasonography to guide the performance of a neuraxial block.[52] Although there is limited published experience to date with this specific population, Yeo and French[53] reported the use of ultrasonography to facilitate the administration of neuraxial anesthesia in a patient with Harrington rod instrumentation. Successful subarachnoid

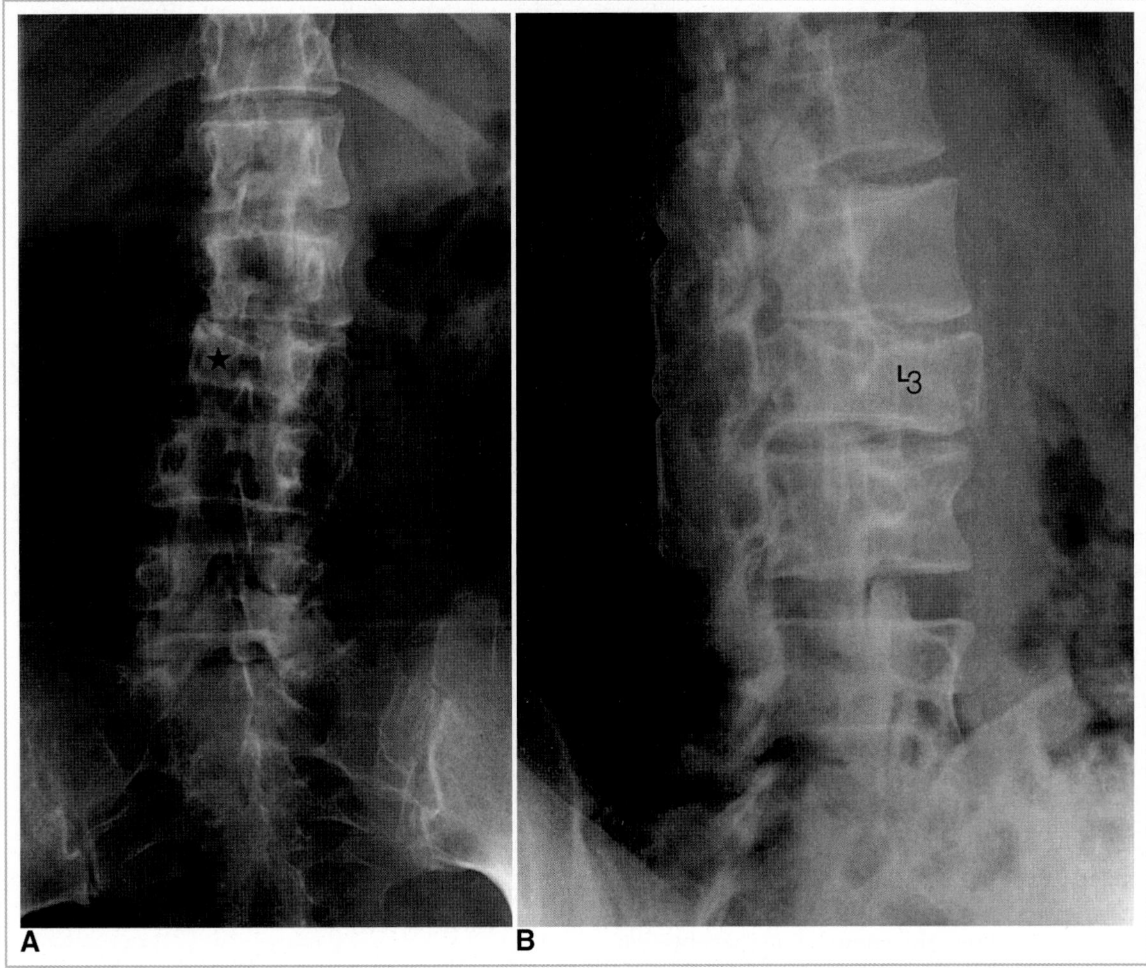

FIGURE 48-7 Radiographs of the lumbar spine in a young woman who had spine fusion after a back injury. **A,** Detailed anteroposterior view, demonstrating vertebral compression at L3 (*star*) and a mild local scoliosis. **B,** Detailed lateral view, demonstrating the considerable bone graft used to create the fusion. After attempts to insert an epidural catheter failed, she was provided labor analgesia with two small-gauge needle (24-gauge Sprotte) dural punctures and injection of bupivacaine 2.5 mg and fentanyl 10 μg.

block occurred, but the epidural catheter functioned poorly and the resulting block was inadequate. Alternative modes of intrapartum analgesia include administration of intraspinal opioids, caudal anesthesia,[54] patient-controlled intravenous opioid analgesia, and inhalation analgesia. Spinal (subarachnoid) analgesia or anesthesia is a reasonable alternative to epidural anesthesia for labor or cesarean delivery in parturients who have undergone major spinal surgery with instrumentation. It is possible to make an intentional dural puncture with a small-gauge needle either through or adjacent to a fusion mass in some patients in whom epidural space identification was previously unsuccessful (Figure 48-7). A catheter may subsequently be passed; alternatively, repeat injections through the same site can be made.

RHEUMATOID ARTHRITIS

Rheumatoid arthritis is a chronic systemic disorder characterized by synovial proliferation that leads to joint destruction and subsequent deformity. The U.S. population prevalence is 0.5% to 1.0%, but the disease occurs more commonly in women.[55]

The lumbosacral spine is affected in only 5% of patients with rheumatoid arthritis. In contrast, the cervical spine is commonly involved, and atlantoaxial subluxation occurs in 25% of patients with rheumatoid arthritis.[56] Although atlantoaxial subluxation may occur early in the course of the disease, it most often occurs in patients with a history of 10 years or more of highly active and erosive disease.[57,58] Atlantoaxial subluxation occurs as a result of an attenuation or disruption of the transverse ligament, which allows anterior movement of C1 on C2 during neck flexion. Radiographically, atlantoaxial subluxation is marked by an increase in the atlas-dens interval, which is best demonstrated on the lateral cervical spine radiograph with the neck flexed (Figure 48-8).

Vertical subluxation of the odontoid process occurs primarily in older patients with severe and long-standing disease. A scoliotic deformity of the trachea and larynx has been reported in patients with vertical subluxation.[59] The deformity is complex, involving both rotation and deviation of the larynx from the midline, and it may make

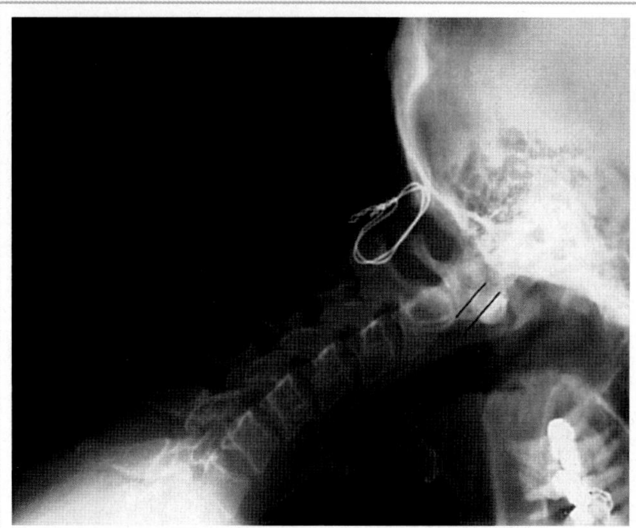

FIGURE 48-8 Lateral radiographic study of the cervical spine (in flexion) in a 32-year-old woman with rheumatoid arthritis. There is isolated atlantoaxial subluxation (6 mm) in the absence of other radiologic changes of rheumatoid arthritis. She presented with neck pain, and a wire was placed between the occiput and the spinous process of C2 to limit the subluxation.

laryngoscopy and endotracheal intubation difficult. However, vertical subluxations occur primarily in older patients with severe, long-standing disease and are unlikely to be seen in women of childbearing age.

Extra-articular features are common in patients with rheumatoid arthritis. Anesthesiologists have a special interest in abnormalities that affect the airway and the cardiovascular and respiratory systems (Box 48-2). These abnormalities occur primarily in patients with long-standing disease and are rarely a problem in young patients.[60]

Interaction with Pregnancy

Rheumatoid arthritis typically does not complicate pregnancy, although a study of U.S. women whose cases were obtained from a database of almost 1 million obstetric hospitalizations showed that women with the disease are more likely to experience intrauterine growth restriction and/or premature rupture of membranes and also are more likely to have a cesarean delivery than women without rheumatoid arthritis.[61] In the absence of vasculitis, fetal outcome is good. Pregnancy has a beneficial, ameliorating effect on the activity of rheumatoid arthritis.[60] Approximately 75% of women note improvement in symptoms during pregnancy, which is typically evident by the end of the first trimester, with a gradual resolution of pain, swelling, and stiffness. The clinical improvement usually continues throughout pregnancy and recurs in future pregnancies. This remission often occurs despite the discontinuation of second-line antirheumatic drugs and a substantial reduction in the dosage of first-line drugs. Relapse occurs postpartum in approximately 90% of women,[60] beginning as early as the second week after delivery. It appears that most patients return to a disease status comparable to their prepregnant state.

BOX 48-2 Extra-articular Features of Rheumatoid Arthritis

Cardiovascular
- Pericarditis
- Pericardial effusions
- Endocardial vegetations
- Myocardial nodules—conduction disturbance
- Arteritis/vasculitis

Airway
- Mandibular hypoplasia
- Cricoarytenoid arthritis
- Temporomandibular joint dysfunction
- Laryngeal deviation and rotation

Pulmonary
- Pleural effusion
- Pulmonary fibrosis
- Pulmonary nodules

Chest Wall
- Costochondritis

Neurologic
- Peripheral nerve compression
- Cervical nerve root compression

Hematologic
- Anemia
- Felty's syndrome

Ophthalmic
- Keratoconjunctivitis

Medical Management

Acetylsalicylic acid (aspirin) is the mainstay of treatment for rheumatoid arthritis.[62] No evidence suggests that it is teratogenic, and it is most likely the safest antirheumatic agent during pregnancy. Potential complications (particularly when high doses are continued until delivery) include anemia, post-term delivery, prolonged labor, antepartum and postpartum hemorrhage, neonatal cephalohematoma, and intracranial hemorrhage in preterm infants.[62] Most of these complications occur at delivery; therefore aspirin should be discontinued near term. Most **nonsteroidal anti-inflammatory drugs (NSAIDs)** do not seem to be a major problem during pregnancy, although dystocia has been attributed to their use. An international consensus conference on the use of NSAIDs in pregnancy concluded that all NSAIDs except low-dose aspirin should be discontinued at 32 weeks' gestation.[62]

Corticosteroids and **antimalarial agents** appear safe and should be continued during pregnancy.[62] Gold and D-penicillamine typically are discontinued, although few problems have been attributed to their use during pregnancy.[62] **Azathioprine** may be used safely during pregnancy at doses less than 2 mg/kg/day, but **other immunosuppressive agents** (e.g., methotrexate, cyclophosphamide, chlorambucil) are highly teratogenic and should be discontinued before conception.[62] Cyclosporin, tacrolimus, and intravenous immunoglobulin may all be used in pregnancy.[62] An attempt is often made to reduce the dose of all antirheumatic agents during pregnancy and, if possible, to discontinue them in the final weeks of gestation.

Obstetric Management

Vaginal delivery is preferred for parturients with rheumatoid arthritis, and cesarean delivery should be reserved for obstetric indications. A major concern is maternal positioning during labor. Rheumatoid joints are unstable because of ligament loosening associated with chronic swelling and because of the destruction of ligaments and cartilage. It is important to determine the permissible range of motion and activity for affected joints. Special emphasis should be given to the hips, knees, and neck. Physicians and nurses should be aware of the potential risks of forcing motion beyond the disease-imposed limits.

Anesthetic Management

The preanesthetic evaluation should include a careful evaluation of the airway. Patients with rheumatoid arthritis may have a small mandible, temporomandibular joint (TMJ) dysfunction, cricoarytenoid arthritis, and laryngeal deviation. In particular, these findings may be present in parturients with juvenile rheumatoid arthritis and may complicate direct laryngoscopy. Cervical spine involvement is not common in young patients but may occur in patients with disease of long duration and in those with severe, deforming disease—typically, patients with juvenile rheumatoid arthritis. Cervical spine radiographs should be evaluated in pregnant women who have severe erosive disease, neck symptoms, or a history of disease of 10 or more years' duration. The cardiac and pulmonary features of rheumatoid arthritis are not common in young patients, but signs and symptoms of pleural and pericardial effusions and pulmonary parenchymal involvement should be sought.

No evidence contraindicates the administration of spinal or epidural anesthesia in patients with rheumatoid arthritis. Care should be taken to avoid excessive manipulation of the neck during administration of general anesthesia. Finally, joints should be padded and protected appropriately during anesthesia.

ANKYLOSING SPONDYLITIS

Ankylosing spondylitis is a chronic inflammatory arthropathy characterized by infiltration of granulation tissue into the bony insertions of ligaments and joint capsules. Subsequent fibrosis, ossification, and ankylosis occur.[63] The sacroiliac, facet, and costovertebral joints are primarily affected. There is progressive flexion and fusion of the spine and fixation of the rib cage. The clinical spectrum is wide, and only a small proportion of patients progress to total spinal ankylosis.[64]

The prevalence of ankylosing spondylitis is 0.1% to 1.4%.[65] Onset is common during the second and third decades, a period of peak childbearing potential.[64] The disease is milder in women than in men, but women are more likely to have peripheral arthritis and involvement of the cervical spine and symphysis pubis.[64] Although clinically significant lesions of the cervical spine may occur early in the course of the disease, they are far more common in patients with long-standing ankylosing spondylitis (Figure 48-9).[66] A slower development of radiologic changes of the dorsolumbar spine occurs in women, and spinal rigidity or deformity and extra-articular manifestations are rare in young patients (Box 48-3).[63,67]

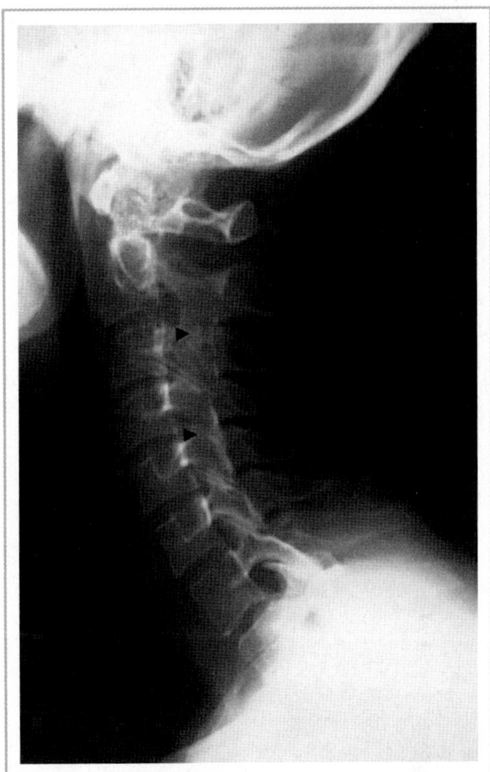

FIGURE 48-9 Lateral radiographic study of the cervical spine in a 31-year-old woman with ankylosing spondylitis. There is evidence of facet joint ankylosis (*arrowheads*), although the lordotic curve remains well preserved. The ligaments of the thoracic spine are undergoing calcification with the spine in flexion, and there is a compensatory increase in the lumbar lordosis to maintain erect posture. (Flexion of the lumbar spine proved difficult, and a paramedian approach was used to enter the epidural space.)

Interaction with Pregnancy

In contrast to rheumatoid arthritis, pregnancy does not seem to reduce the symptoms or slow the progression of disease in patients with ankylosing spondylitis, and a significant number of patients experience an aggravation of morning stiffness and back pain.[64,68] However, one report suggests that there is a mitigation of symptoms in the third trimester despite withdrawal of NSAID therapy.[68] Pregnancy may ameliorate the extra-articular features of this disease (e.g., psoriasis, inflammatory bowel disease, small joint arthritis), but it appears that women with ankylosing spondylitis are more likely than women with rheumatoid arthritis to enter pregnancy with active disease and, hence, to have higher levels of pain at the beginning of pregnancy.[68] Ankylosing spondylitis does not adversely affect pregnancy, labor, or delivery, and in the absence of pelvic joint ankylosis and/or hip joint involvement, an

BOX 48-3 Extra-articular Features of Ankylosing Spondylitis

Systemic
- Fever
- Weight loss
- Fatigue

Cardiovascular
- Aortitis
- Aortic insufficiency
- Conduction disorders—heart block

Pulmonary
- Restrictive lung disease
- Pulmonary fibrosis

Neurologic
- Cauda equina syndrome
- Vertebrobasilar insufficiency
- Peripheral nerve lesions

Hematologic
- Anemia

Urologic
- Prostatitis

Ophthalmic
- Uveitis

uncomplicated vaginal delivery at term should be anticipated in most patients.

Acetaminophen and anti-inflammatory medications (i.e., aspirin and other NSAIDs) represent the mainstays of medical treatment. Most patients require treatment at some point during gestation, especially in the second trimester.[68] At 32 weeks, NSAID therapy should be withdrawn, if possible, because of concerns about premature closure of the fetal ductus arteriosus.[62]

Anesthetic Management

An anesthesiologist should review the patient's history with respect to the duration of the disease, the presence of extra-articular features, and the recent use of analgesics. Temporomandibular joint dysfunction, cervical spine involvement, and cardiopulmonary complications are rare early in the disease course and uncommon in parturients. Severity of back symptoms is often out of proportion to the radiographic appearance of the spine, and calcification of the spinal ligaments is typically not advanced in young patients. The anesthesia provider may administer spinal or epidural anesthesia to patients with ankylosing spondylitis. It is unusual to experience complications during the provision of neuraxial anesthesia to young patients with ankylosing spondylitis. However, calcification of the interspinous ligaments and osteophyte formation may limit the parturient's ability to flex forward, making midline needle placement difficult. A paramedian approach can be considered in this instance.

SPINA BIFIDA

Spina bifida results from the failure of the developing spine to completely enclose the neural elements in a bony canal. There is a wide spectrum with respect to the severity of the deformity and its implications. **Spina bifida occulta** is defined as failed fusion of the neural arch without herniation of the meninges or neural elements. A defect limited to a single vertebra, typically L5 or S1, is so common (occurring in 5% to 36% of the population) that it can be considered a normal variant.[69] Superficial signs of this lesion include a tuft of hair, cutaneous angioma, lipoma, or a skin dimple, but such signs are not common in patients with isolated vertebral arch anomalies and an underlying normal cord. Patients with spina bifida occulta rarely have symptoms related to this anomaly, although they may have a higher incidence of posterior disc herniation.[69]

Spina bifida cystica is defined as failed closure of the neural arch with herniation of the meninges (i.e., meningocele) or the meninges and neural elements (i.e., myelomeningocele) through the vertebral defect. These conditions are relatively uncommon, occurring in 1 to 3 per 1000 births.[70] Neurologic deficits involving the lower extremities and sphincters occur in almost all patients, and these deficits vary primarily in severity. Hydrocephalus is present in many patients, and shunting of the ventricular system is common, with revisions often required during childhood. By puberty as many as 50% of patients who have received shunts have little or no requirement for them.[71] Early and aggressive surgical treatment of spina bifida cystica has improved survival from 45% in the early 1970s to 70% to 90% by the mid-1980s. Obstetric and anesthesia providers can expect to encounter a growing number of pregnant women with spina bifida.[72,73] Unfortunately, many surviving patients have significant residual neurologic impairment and ongoing orthopedic and genitourinary complications. Myelomeningocele is a progressive neurologic disease that eventually produces orthopedic, neurologic, and genitourinary complications. Kyphoscoliosis, which is common in patients with a thoracic lesion, occurs in 20% of patients with a lumbosacral defect.[74] Paralytic scoliosis is the most common type and results from an imbalance of paravertebral muscle tone.

Occult spinal dysraphism is an intermediate group of conditions wherein the bony defect is associated with one or more anomalies of the spinal cord, including intraspinal lipomas, dermal sinus tracts, dermoid cysts, fibrous bands, and diastematomyelia (split cord). These lesions are differentiated from the more benign occulta lesions described previously.[75] Affected patients may have no neurologic symptoms or may have minor sensory, motor, and functional deficits of the lower limbs, bowel, and bladder; they also may have orthopedic issues, such as scoliosis, limb pain, and lower extremity abnormalities.[76,77] Patients with cord abnormalities have cutaneous stigmata in 50% of cases, and 70% have tethered spinal cord.[78]

Tethered Cord and Arnold-Chiari Malformation

Tethered cord syndrome (TCS) is characterized by neurologic deterioration secondary to traction on the conus medullaris, which typically but not invariably is low-lying (L2 to L3).[75,78] Congenital abnormalities of the spinal cord, such as lipoma, tight filum terminale, dermal sinus, meningocele manqué, and diastematomyelia, are found in more than 50% of patients with adult-onset TCS.

A new classification of TCS in adults has been proposed to differentiate tethered cord occurring secondary to spina bifida cystica from the adult-onset neurologic syndrome associated with spinal dysraphism.[79] Magnetic resonance imaging studies suggest that tethering is present in virtually all patients with spina bifida cystica and myelomeningocele and that it is also common in patients with occult spinal dysraphism. Although many of the latter patients do not have obvious neurologic impairment secondary to the tethering, adults with TCS often have a long history of minor neurologic or orthopedic issues.[75,79] Others present with acute symptoms following a precipitating event that stretched the spinal cord, such as heavy lifting or the lithotomy position.[80] Of note, more than 50% of adults with TCS present only with a history of low back and leg pain before a precipitating event that leads to the diagnosis.[75]

Low-lying spinal cords and the possibility of undiagnosed TCS have come to the attention of obstetric anesthesiologists with the publication of several case reports of neurologic injury following spinal or epidural anesthesia for delivery in women subsequently diagnosed with occult spinal dysraphism.[76,77,81] Additionally, in adult TCS, the low-lying cord is located more posteriorly than a normal cord, increasing the likelihood of direct needle trauma during administration of spinal or epidural anesthesia (Figure 48-10).[82] As noted previously, the isolated finding of a defective laminar arch (spinal bifida occulta) is not associated with a low-lying or tethered cord.[75]

More severe forms of spina bifida may also be associated with **Arnold-Chiari malformation,** which is characterized by cerebellar herniation through the foramen magnum and descent of the pons and medulla. Symptoms are more common if the cerebellar herniation exceeds 12 mm or if syringomyelia is present.[83,84]

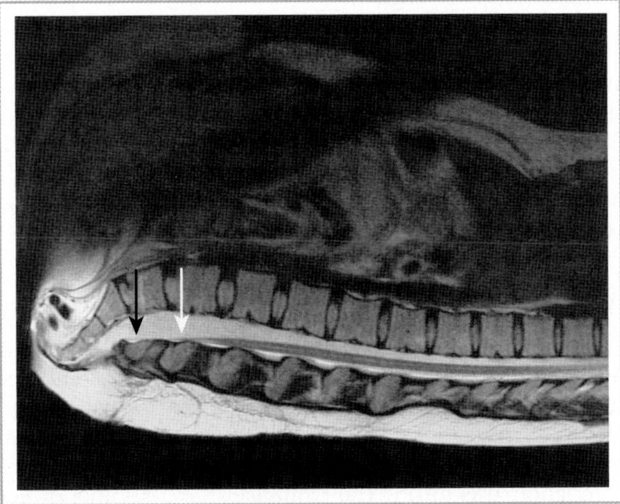

FIGURE 48-10 Magnetic resonance image of the spine in a 27-year-old woman with history of a lumbar myelomeningocele excised as a newborn, with residual bladder dysfunction. A tethered spinal cord is present with a typical posterior low-lying position. The *white arrow* indicates the termination of the conus medullaris at L4 to L5, and the *black arrow* indicates the filum terminale located at L5 to S1. (This patient had a vaginal delivery at term, requiring only nitrous oxide for analgesia.)

Obstetric Management

Pregnancy is not complicated by the presence of a spinal bifida occulta lesion. However, women with known TCS should avoid both the squatting position and prolonged lithotomy position for delivery. Recurrent urinary tract infection is the most common antenatal complication in patients with spina bifida cystica and is associated with preterm labor.[72] Intestinal and urinary tract obstruction, as well as problems related to ileal conduits and stomas, are common during pregnancy, as are pressure sores resulting from greater immobility.[72,73] Uterine enlargement may compromise pulmonary function, especially in patients with kyphoscoliosis. Vaginal delivery is more common in women who are independently mobile and is less common in wheelchair-dependent patients.[73] Pelvic and lower limb anomalies and contractures may obstruct the pelvic outlet and warrant cesarean delivery. The obstetrician should evaluate the adequacy of the pelvis to determine whether a trial of labor is appropriate. Cesarean delivery is reserved for obstetric indications, and its incidence is increased and proportionate to the severity of the underlying defect and its consequences. Cesarean delivery is complicated by the presence of stomas and conduits; postoperative complications and prolonged hospital stays are common.[72,73]

Anesthetic Management

The epidural space may be incomplete or discontinuous across the level of **spina bifida occulta** lesions because of absence of the lamina and variable formation of the ligamentum flavum at this site. An attempt to identify the epidural space at the site of this lesion will likely result in unintentional dural puncture, although successful epidural analgesia has been reported if the catheter is placed within the zone of the lesion. Despite its common occurrence in the population, the isolated finding of a defective laminar arch rarely complicates the administration of neuraxial anesthesia, for two reasons. First, the lesion typically occurs at the L5 to S1 segments, below the level at which most epidural and spinal anesthetics are administered. Second, the most common anomaly is a simple midline split in the lamina, and this defect rarely seems to interfere with either the performance or the development of spinal or epidural anesthesia.

Occult spinal dysraphism is of more concern because of the potential for a low-lying, posteriorly located, and tethered spinal cord. A neurologic history should be taken and a screening neurologic examination should be performed in all women with a known defective laminar arch, preferably antenatally, to determine whether magnetic resonance imaging for spinal dysraphism is necessary.[76,85] The presence of skin dimpling or hair tufts should raise suspicion that an underlying cord abnormality exists. In our judgment, in women with a known low-lying cord, epidural anesthesia performed by an experienced anesthesiologist is safer than spinal anesthesia. If spinal dysraphism is suspected but no imaging studies are available, it would be prudent to avoid neuraxial anesthesia. Women with TCS may prefer to avoid neuraxial anesthesia because of the greater potential for direct neural trauma.

In the patient with a **spina bifida cystica** lesion, the anesthesiologist should determine the level of the lesion and whether the patient has residual spinal cord function below it. Patients with a complete lesion at or above T11 are likely to experience painless labor. However, the risk of autonomic hyperreflexia should be evaluated in patients with thoracic lesions, and prophylaxis should be provided if the patient is deemed to be at risk. This issue is especially important if the lesion is between T5 and T8, but such lesions from any cause are rare in parturients.[86]

If the patient has undergone ventricular shunt placement, the current status of the shunt should be determined. Neurosurgical consultation should be obtained if questions remain about the requirement for—or function of—the shunt. Pulmonary function should be assessed, especially in patients with scoliosis. Baseline renal function also should be determined.

There are published reports of the use of epidural and spinal anesthesia in patients with spina bifida cystica.[70,85,87,88] Unfortunately the experience is limited, and most published series of pregnant women with spina bifida cystica report neither the type of anesthesia provided nor the complications experienced. Tidmarsh and May[87] reported management of intrapartum analgesia in 16 patients with spina bifida, 8 of whom had spina bifida cystica. Five of the latter patients received epidural anesthesia for labor and/or delivery. Three patients had a "normal" block, 1 patient had a somewhat high block (sensory block level of T3 after 10 mL of 0.25% bupivacaine), and 1 patient had poor sacral analgesia.

Limited data exist on the obstetric anesthesia experience in parturients with Arnold-Chiari malformations. The largest series is that of Chantigian et al.,[83] who described their experience with 12 parturients who delivered a total of 30 infants. Nine deliveries were accomplished with neuraxial anesthesia, including six vaginal deliveries with epidural anesthesia, two cesarean deliveries performed with single-shot spinal anesthesia, and one cesarean delivery performed with a spinal catheter in place. No patient experienced postprocedure neurologic sequelae related to the use of neuraxial anesthesia.

In our judgment, administration of epidural or spinal anesthesia may be considered in women with various forms of spina bifida and stable neurologic function. Patients should be informed that there is limited published information on the administration of neuraxial anesthesia (and the risk of neurologic injury) in patients with neural tube defects, and these patients should be actively involved in decision making. In patients with either surgically corrected spina bifida cystica or occult spinal dysraphism, the anesthesiologist should be aware that the terminal portion of the spinal cord typically lies at a vertebral level lower than normal. Imaging studies provide valuable information on neural anatomy and facilitate anesthetic management. In women with spinal dysraphism, a neurologic examination, as well as a full discussion of the risks and benefits of neuraxial anesthesia, should be performed and documented before administration of neuraxial anesthesia. Spinal anesthesia should be performed below the known level of the conus or avoided in favor of epidural anesthesia. In women with spina bifida or occult spinal dysraphism, the epidural space is often abnormal, which increases the likelihood of inadequate epidural anesthesia. In our judgment, spinal anesthesia is not contraindicated in women with negligible function of the lower extremities and sphincters, given that the concern for direct neural trauma to a low-lying spinal cord is not clinically relevant.

ACHONDROPLASIA

Achondroplasia, an inherited disorder of bone metabolism, is the most common cause of disproportionate dwarfism, with a prevalence of 1 in 26,000 live births.[89] Although it is inherited in an autosomal dominant mode, most cases arise from spontaneous mutation.[90] The range of cervical motion may be decreased, lumbar lordosis and thoracic kyphosis are increased, and thoracic kyphoscoliosis occurs.[91-94] The vertebral pedicles are short, and reduced length of the neural arch leads to shortened anteroposterior and transverse diameters of the vertebral canal, resulting in foramen magnum and spinal stenosis.[95,96] Although it may occur earlier, symptomatic spinal stenosis often does not present until the fourth or fifth decade, when kyphosis, scoliosis, osteophytes, and herniated discs typically cause further narrowing of the spinal canal. There is considerable inter-individual variation in the clinical and radiographic characteristics, and skeletal abnormalities often show more variation than consistency.[95,97]

Obstetric Management

The uterus is an abdominal organ in the achondroplastic patient.[98] With advancing pregnancy it may encroach on the small thoracic cage and lead to decreases in the functional residual and closing capacities; severe dyspnea may occur with advancing gestational age. Back discomfort is common during pregnancy, and the reported incidence of sciatica is higher than in normal pregnant women,[99] most likely due to the underlying spinal abnormalities. Typically, an inadequate maternal pelvis combined with a normal-sized (non-achondroplastic) fetus results in cephalopelvic disproportion. Imaging techniques may be used to confirm this situation, and the obstetrician should anticipate the need to deliver most patients with achondroplasia by cesarean delivery.[91,94,95]

Anesthetic Management

The short, obese limbs of the patient with achondroplasia may make it difficult to obtain measurements of blood pressure with a noninvasive cuff, and an intra-arterial catheter may be necessary. Prominent paraspinal muscles and marked lumbar lordosis may complicate attempts to palpate landmarks during the administration of spinal or epidural anesthesia; the use of ultrasonography may help identify landmarks.[94,98] Scoliosis of the spine also may cause technical difficulties with neuraxial anesthesia attempts. The small stature and spinal stenosis reduce the dose of local anesthetic required for major neuraxial anesthesia.[91,94,97,98] It is difficult to estimate the appropriate dose of local anesthetic for single-shot spinal anesthesia. Continuous epidural anesthesia is preferable because it allows the anesthesia provider to titrate the dose of local anesthetic to the desired level of anesthesia. Local anesthetic dose requirements are typically smaller than those in parturients of normal stature; this is not always the case, however, supporting the use of a neuraxial anesthetic technique that may be titrated to the desired effect.[93,99-102]

Difficult intubation has been reported in achondroplastic patients and should be anticipated, although it is not invariable; most reports that comment on the subject note no difficulties in airway management.[89,92,93,103,104]

OSTEOGENESIS IMPERFECTA

Osteogenesis imperfecta is an inherited condition that occurs with an incidence between 1 in 21,000 and 1 in 60,000.[105,106] The genetic defect is within the genome that encodes for type I collagen, the major collagen in tissues that require structural strength. The disease is a generalized connective tissue disorder, and expression ranges from mild osteoporosis to the classical clinical stigmata characterized by multiple bone fractures and skeletal deformities, blue sclera, and middle ear deafness (otosclerosis). Four types may be distinguished clinically, and a system of classification (types I through IV) has been proposed.[107] Type I is the prototype disease. It is inherited as an autosomal dominant trait and is the most common and mildest form of this disease. It typically manifests in childhood as multiple fractures after minor trauma.[107] Types II and III are inherited as autosomal recessive traits and are characterized by extreme bone fragility. Type II is uniformly lethal, and stillbirth or early neonatal death is common; death *in utero* is caused by skeletal collapse, and early neonatal death typically results from chest wall failure and respiratory insufficiency. Infants with type III disease may have fractures at birth and may have progressive skeletal deformities during the first two decades of life. Type IV, also autosomal dominant, is much less common and is variable in expressivity.

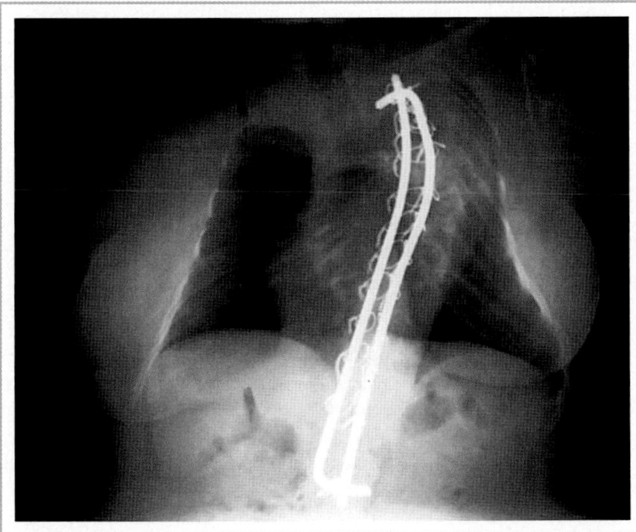

FIGURE 48-11 A chest radiograph of a 30-year-old woman with osteogenesis imperfecta type I. Generalized osteoporosis, corrected thoracic kyphoscoliosis, a restricted thoracic cage, and multiple old fractures are demonstrated. (General anesthesia was provided for cesarean delivery and tubal ligation.)

The majority of pregnant women with osteogenesis imperfecta have type I disease, although pregnancy has been reported in more severe forms of the disease.[108] There is considerable variability among affected patients as to the age of onset and frequency of fractures. Dwarfism is typical, and kyphoscoliosis is common, as are other chest wall abnormalities. These chest and spinal abnormalities result in restrictive lung disorders (Figure 48-11). Other abnormalities include a decrease in the range of motion of the shortened cervical spine, micrognathia, and malformed, brittle teeth.[106,108,109] Poor platelet adhesion may cause platelet dysfunction and a modest bleeding tendency. Hyperthyroidism occurs in 40% of patients with osteogenesis imperfecta; an elevated concentration of thyroxine leads to increases in both oxygen consumption and heat production.[107,108] Hyperthermia may occur, although most patients, when evaluated with the halothane-caffeine contracture test, are not found susceptible to malignant hyperthermia.[110]

Obstetric Management

Platelet dysfunction in osteogenesis imperfecta may result in a higher incidence of intrapartum and postpartum hemorrhage, although this finding is uncommon. Labor and vaginal delivery are associated with an increased risk of uterine rupture and pelvic fracture. These complications are also uncommon and most likely are influenced primarily by the severity of the underlying disease. Cephalopelvic disproportion typically mandates cesarean delivery in severely affected parturients.

Anesthetic Management

The anesthesiologist must be aware of the fragility of the bones, the potential for difficult intubation, and the presence and severity of restrictive lung disease. Transfers, positioning, and any invasive intervention must be accomplished with extreme care. Blood pressure cuffs and tourniquets to facilitate placement of intravenous catheters should be applied gently to prevent fractures. Difficult intubation may occur because of a short neck with limited range of motion and should be anticipated.[108] The anesthesiologist should take care not to hyperextend the neck, and laryngoscopy should be gentle to avoid fractures. Alternatives to direct laryngoscopy may be considered to reduce the applied forces necessary. If succinylcholine is used, a defasciculating dose of a nondepolarizing muscle relaxant should be employed to prevent fasciculations.[109] An alternative to succinylcholine (e.g., rocuronium) may also be administered to prevent fasciculations. Hyperthermia should be anticipated, and there should be provisions to cool the patient if a significant rise in body temperature occurs.

Before administration of neuraxial anesthesia, the anesthesiologist should consider the technical difficulties inherent in performing neuraxial anesthesia in patients with spinal deformities. The anesthesiologist also should be aware of the platelet function defect in these patients. This risk is best evaluated by obtaining a thorough history rather than by laboratory evaluation (e.g., bleeding time) before the administration of neuraxial anesthesia. In the setting of a reassuring history, neuraxial anesthesia need not be withheld. Small stature and spinal abnormalities reduce the local anesthetic dose requirements and increase the risk of both misplaced injection and local anesthetic toxicity. It may be difficult to estimate the appropriate dose for single-shot spinal anesthesia in these patients. Thus continuous epidural or subarachnoid anesthesia is the neuraxial anesthetic technique of choice, barring other contraindications. Yeo and Paech[111] reported the successful use of both epidural and subarachnoid blocks for cesarean delivery on five occasions over 9 years in a single patient with type I osteogenesis imperfecta. The use of ultrasonography may facilitate the administration of neuraxial anesthesia.

SPONDYLOLISTHESIS

Isthmic spondylolisthesis is a condition in which a defect in the pars interarticularis of a vertebra allows anterior slippage of the subjacent portion of the spine. As the body slips forward, it does not carry the neural arch with it; thus there is little tendency toward spinal canal stenosis. Isthmic spondylolisthesis typically occurs at the lumbosacral junction, although it is not uncommon in the lumbar spine. Approximately 38% of cases occur in women.[112] The onset is common in the second and third decades, a period of peak childbearing potential.

Back pain is the presenting feature. Strenuous physical activity often precipitates the onset of pain. Pregnancy increases back symptoms in approximately half of patients with isthmic spondylolisthesis, but obstetric complications are unusual.[112,113] This disorder is not affected by pregnancy.[114]

Degenerative spondylolisthesis occurs when there is a forward slip of one vertebra on the subjacent level with no break in the neural arch.[115] It is four times more common in women than in men and occurs most frequently at the L4 to L5 level. It is not usually diagnosed before the onset of the fourth decade of life and seems to be twice as common in women who have given birth than in women who have not. It is suggested that rotational and sheer stresses on the L4 to L5 joint during gestation may be responsible for the higher incidence of degenerative spondylolisthesis in women who have borne children.

There is no published case of neuraxial anesthesia during labor in a parturient with severe spondylolisthesis (e.g., lumbosacral subluxation). Ideally, an anesthesiologist will see the patient during pregnancy to assess her symptoms and lumbar spinal anatomy. In the absence of evidence of a neurologic deficit, it seems appropriate to administer either epidural or spinal anesthesia.

KEY POINTS

- Low back pain is the most common musculoskeletal complaint during pregnancy. It results from both hormonal and mechanical factors.
- Low back pain does not contraindicate the administration of spinal or epidural anesthesia.
- Corrected idiopathic thoracolumbar scoliosis is the most common major musculoskeletal disorder seen in pregnant women. Prepregnancy pulmonary function is a better predictor of maternal outcome than the severity of the curve.
- Neuraxial anesthesia is more technically challenging in patients with scoliosis, and the anesthesiologist should anticipate a higher incidence of complications and inadequate anesthesia.
- Maternal rheumatoid arthritis and ankylosing spondylitis do not adversely affect the outcome of pregnancy.
- Pregnancy often ameliorates the symptoms of rheumatoid arthritis.
- Spina bifida occulta is a common incidental finding and does not contraindicate the administration of spinal or epidural anesthesia.
- Spina bifida cystica and occult spinal dysraphism are associated with a high incidence of tethered cord, which may complicate the administration of subarachnoid (spinal) anesthesia.
- Cephalopelvic disproportion often mandates cesarean delivery in parturients with achondroplasia or osteogenesis imperfecta.

REFERENCES

1. Orvieto R, Achiron A, Ben-Rafael Z, et al. Low back pain of pregnancy. Acta Obstet Gynecol Scand 1994; 73:209-14.
2. Mogren IM, Pohjanen AI. Low back pain and pelvic pain during pregnancy: Prevalence and risk factors. Spine 2005; 30:983-91.
3. Wang SM, Dezinno P, Maranets I, et al. Low back pain during pregnancy: Prevalence, risk factors, and outcomes. Obstet Gynecol 2004; 104:65-70.
4. Gutke A, Ostgaard HC, Oberg B. Pelvic girdle pain and lumbar pain in pregnancy: A cohort study of the consequences in terms of health and functioning. Spine 2006; 31:E149-55.
5. Wu WH, Meijer OG, Uegaki K, et al. Pregnancy-related pelvic girdle pain (PPP). I. Terminology, clinical presentation, and prevalence. Eur Spine J 2004; 13:575-89.
6. Mogren IM. BMI, pain and hyper-mobility are determinants of long-term outcome for women with low back pain and pelvic pain during pregnancy. Eur Spine J 2006; 15:1093-102.
7. To WWK, Wong MWN. Factors associated with back pain symptoms in pregnancy and the persistence of pain 2 years after pregnancy. Acta Obstet Gynecol Scand 2003; 82:1086-91.
8. Kristiansson P, Svärdsudd K, von Schoultz B. Serum relaxin, symphyseal pain, and back pain during pregnancy. Am J Obstet Gynecol 1996; 175:1342-7.
9. MacLennan AH, Nicolson R, Green RC. Serum relaxin in pregnancy. Lancet 1986; 2(8501):241-3.
10. Ostgaard HC, Zetherström G, Roos-Hansson E, Svanberg B. Reduction of back and posterior pelvic pain in pregnancy. Spine 1994; 19:894-900.
11. Abou-Shameh MA, Dosani D, Gopal D, McLaren AG. Lumbar discectomy in pregnancy. Int J Gynaecol Obstet 2006; 92:167-9.
12. Pennick VE, Young G. Interventions for preventing and treating pelvic and back pain in pregnancy. Cochrane Database Syst Rev 2007; (2):CD001139.
13. Chou R, Qaseem A, Snow V, et al: Diagnosis and treatment of low back pain: A joint clinical practice guideline from the American College of Physicians and the American Pain Society. Ann Intern Med 2007; 147:478-91.
14. Benzon HT, Braunschweig R, Molloy RE. Delayed onset of epidural anesthesia in patients with back pain. Anesth Analg 1981; 60:874-7.

15. Sharrock NE, Urquhart B, Mineo R. Extradural anaesthesia in patients with previous lumbar spine surgery. Br J Anaesth 1990; 65:237-9.
16. Schachner SM, Abram SE. Use of two epidural catheters to provide analgesia of unblocked segments in a patient with lumbar disc disease. Anesthesiology 1982; 56:150-1.
17. Calleja MA. Extradural analgesia and previous spinal surgery: A radiological appraisal. Anaesthesia 1991; 46:946-7.
18. Luyendijk W, van Voorthuisen AE. Contrast examination of the spinal epidural space. Acta Radiol Diagn (Stockh) 1966; 5:1051-66.
19. LaRocca H, MacNab I. The laminectomy membrane: Studies in its evolution, effects and prophylaxis in dogs. J Bone Joint Surg Br 1974; 56:545-50.
20. Brodsky AE. Post-laminectomy and post-fusion stenosis of the lumbar spine. Clin Orthop Relat Res 1976; 115:130-9.
21. MacArthur C, Lewis M, Knox EG, Crawford JS. Epidural anaesthesia and long term backache after childbirth. Br Med J 1990; 301:9-12.
22. MacArthur C, Lewis M, Crawford S. Investigation of longterm problems after obstetric epidural anaesthesia. Br Med J 1992; 304: 1279-82.
23. MacLeod J, MacIntyre C, McClure JH, Whitfield A. Backache and epidural analgesia: A retrospective survey of mothers 1 year after childbirth. Int J Obstet Anesth 1995; 4:21-5.
24. Orlikowski CEP, Dickinson JE, Paech MJ, et al. Intrapartum analgesia and its association with post-partum back pain and headache in nulliparous women. Aust N Z J Obstet Gynaecol 2006; 46:395-401.
25. Breen TW, Ransil BJ, Groves PA, Oriol NE. Factors associated with back pain after childbirth. Anesthesiology 1994; 81:29-34.
26. Groves PA, Breen TW, Ransil BJ, Oriol NE. Natural history of postpartum back pain and its relationship with epidural anesthesia. Anesthesiology 1994; 81:A1167.
27. Macarthur A, Macarthur C, Weeks S. Epidural anaesthesia and low back pain after delivery: A prospective cohort study. Br Med J 1995; 311:1336-9.
28. Howell CJ, Kidd C, Roberts W, et al. A randomised controlled trial of epidural compared with non-epidural analgesia in labour. BJOG 2001; 108:27-33.
29. Howell CJ, Dean T, Lucking L, et al. Randomised study of long term outcome after epidural versus non-epidural analgesia during labour. Br Med J 2002; 325:357.
30. Patel M, Fernando R, Gill P, et al. A prospective study of long-term backache after childbirth in primigravidae—the effect of ambulatory epidural analgesia during labour. Int J Obstet Anesth 1995; 4:187.
31. Russell R, Dundas R, Reynolds F. Long term backache after childbirth: Prospective search for causative factors. Br Med J 1996; 312:1384-8.
32. MacArthur C, Lewis M. Anaesthetic characteristics and long-term backache after obstetric epidural anaesthesia. Int J Obstet Anesth 1996; 5:8-13.
33. To WWK, Wong MWN. Kyphoscoliosis complicating pregnancy. Int J Gynaecol Obstet 1996; 55:123-8.
34. Danielsson AJ, Nachemson AL. Childbearing, curve progression, and sexual function in women 22 years after treatment for adolescent idiopathic scoliosis: A case-control study. Spine 2001; 26:1449-56.
35. White AA, Panjabi MM. Practical biomechanics of scoliosis and kyphosis. In White AA, Panjabi MM, editors. Clinical Biomechanics of the Spine. 2nd edition. Philadelphia, JB Lippincott, 1990:127-68.
36. Pehrsson K, Larsson S, Oden A, Nachemson A. Long-term follow-up of patients with untreated scoliosis: A study of mortality, causes of death, and symptoms. Spine 1992; 17:1091-6.
37. Bonnin M, Mercier FJ, Sitbon O, et al. Severe pulmonary hypertension during pregnancy: Mode of delivery and anesthetic management of 15 consecutive cases. Anesthesiology 2005; 102:1133-7.
38. Warnes CA. Pregnancy and pulmonary hypertension. Int J Cardiol 2004; 97:11-3.
39. Berman AT, Cohen DL, Schwentker EP. The effects of pregnancy on idiopathic scoliosis: A preliminary report on eight cases and a review of the literature. Spine 1982; 7:76-7.
40. Blount WP, Mellencamp DD. The effect of pregnancy on idiopathic scoliosis. J Bone Joint Surg Am 1980; 62:1083-7.
41. Sawicka EH, Spencer GT, Branthwaite MA. Management of respiratory failure complicating pregnancy in severe kyphoscoliosis: A new use for an old technique? Br J Dis Chest 1986; 80:191-6.
42. Kesten S, Garfinkel SK, Wright T, Rebuck AS. Impaired exercise capacity in adults with moderate scoliosis. Chest 1991; 99:663-6.
43. Zeldis SM. Dyspnea during pregnancy: Distinguishing cardiac from pulmonary causes. Clin Chest Med 1992; 13:567-85.
44. Crosby ET, Halpern SH. Obstetric epidural anaesthesia in patients with Harrington instrumentation. Can J Anaesth 1989; 36:693-6.
45. Shneerson JM. Pregnancy in neuromuscular and skeletal disorders. Monaldi Arch Chest Dis 1994; 49:227-30.
46. Liljenqvist UR, Allkemper T, Hackenberg L, et al. Analysis of vertebral morphology in idiopathic scoliosis with use of magnetic resonance imaging and multiplanar reconstruction. J Bone Joint Surg Am 2002; 84:359-68.
47. Moran DH, Johnson MD. Continuous spinal anesthesia with combined hyperbaric and isobaric bupivacaine in a patient with scoliosis. Anesth Analg 1990; 70:445-7.
48. Cochran T, Irstam L, Nachemson A. Long-term anatomic and functional changes in patients with adolescent idiopathic scoliosis treated by Harrington rod fusion. Spine 1983; 8:576-84.
49. Sponseller PD, Cohen MS, Nachemson AL, et al. Results of surgical treatment of adults with idiopathic scoliosis. J Bone Joint Surg Am 1987; 69:667-75.
50. Aaro S, Ohlen G. The effect of Harrington instrumentation on the sagittal configuration and mobility of the spine in scoliosis. Spine 1983; 8:570-5.
51. Daley MD, Rolbin SH, Hew EM, et al. Epidural anesthesia for obstetrics after spinal surgery. Reg Anesth 1990; 15:280-4.
52. Grau T, Leipold RW, Conradi R, et al. Efficacy of ultrasound imaging in obstetric epidural anesthesia. J Clin Anesth 2002; 14:169-75.
53. Yeo ST, French R. Combined spinal-epidural in the obstetric patient with Harrington rods assisted by ultrasonography. Br J Anaesth 1999; 83:670-2.
54. Sudunagunta S, Eckersall SJ, Gowrie-Mohan S. Continuous caudal analgesia in labour for a patient with Harrington rods. Int J Obstet Anesth 1998; 7:128-30.
55. National Institutes of Health, US Department of Health and Human Services. Rheumatoid Arthritis. Bethesda, MD, National Institute of Arthritis and Musculoskeletal and Skin Diseases, 2004.
56. Grantham SA, Lipson SJ. Rheumatoid arthritis and other noninfectious inflammatory diseases: Rheumatoid arthritis of the cervical spine. In the Cervical Spine Research Society Editorial Committee. The Cervical Spine. 2nd edition. Philadelphia, JB Lippincott, 1989:564-98.
57. Wolfe BK, O'Keeffe D, Mitchell DM, Tchang SP. Rheumatoid arthritis of the cervical spine: Early and progressive radiographic features. Radiology 1987; 165:145-8.
58. Santavirta S, Kankaanpaa U, Sandelin J, et al. Evaluation of patients with rheumatoid cervical spine. Scand J Rheumatol 1987; 16:9-16.
59. Keenan MA, Stiles CM, Kaufman RL. Acquired laryngeal deviation associated with cervical spine disease in erosive polyarticular arthritis: Use of the fiberoptic bronchoscope in rheumatoid arthritis. Anesthesiology 1983; 58:441-9.
60. Nelson JL, Ostensen M. Pregnancy and rheumatoid arthritis. Rheum Dis Clin North Am 1997; 23:195-212.
61. Chakavarty EF, Nelson L, Krishnan E. Obstetric hospitalizations in the United States for women with systemic lupus erythematosus and rheumatoid arthritis. Arthritis Rheum 2006; 54:899-907.
62. Ostensen M, Khamashta M, Lockshin M, et al. Anti-inflammatory and immunosuppressive drugs and reproduction. Arthritis Res Ther 2006; 8:209.
63. Sinclair JR, Mason RA. Ankylosing spondylitis: The case for awake intubation. Anaesthesia 1984; 39:3-11.
64. Ostensen M, Ostensen H. Ankylosing spondylitis—the female aspect. J Rheumatol 1998; 25:120-4.
65. Braun J, Sieper J. Ankylosing spondylitis. Lancet 2007; 369:1379-90.
66. Sorin S, Askari A, Moskowitz RW. Atlantoaxial subluxation as complication of early ankylosing spondylitis: Two case reports and a review of the literature. Arthritis Rheum 1979; 22:273-6.

67. Hunter T. The spinal complications of ankylosing spondylitis. Semin Arthritis Rheum 1989; 19:172-82.
68. Ostensen M, Fuhrer L, Mathieu R, et al. A prospective study of pregnant patients with rheumatoid arthritis and ankylosing spondylitis using validated clinical instruments. Ann Rheum Dis 2004; 63:1212-7.
69. Avrahami E, Frishman E, Fridman Z, Azor M. Spina bifida occulta of S1 is not an innocent finding. Spine 1994; 19:12-5.
70. Altamimi Y, Pavy TJG. Epidural analgesia for labour in a patient with a neural tube defect. Anaesth Intensive Care 2006; 34:816-9.
71. Farine D, Jackson U, Portale A, et al. Pregnancy complicated by maternal spina bifida: A report of two cases. J Reprod Med 1988; 33:323-6.
72. Arata M, Grover S, Dunne K, Bryan D. Pregnancy outcome and complications in women with spina bifida. J Reprod Med 2000; 45:743-8.
73. Jackson AB, Sipski MI. Reproductive issues for women with spina bifida. J Spinal Cord Med 2005; 28:81-91.
74. Muller EB, Nordwall A. Prevalence of scoliosis in children with myelomeningocele in western Sweden. Spine 1992; 17:1097-102.
75. Warder DE. Tethered cord syndrome and occult spinal dysraphism. Neurosurg Focus 2001; 10:E1.
76. Ahmad FU, Pandey P, Sharma BS, Garg A. Foot drop after spinal anesthesia in a patient with a low-lying cord. Int J Obstet Anesth 2006; 15:233-6.
77. Wenger M, Hauswirth CB, Brodhage RP. Undiagnosed adult diastematomyelia associated with neurological symptoms following spinal anaesthesia. Anaesthesia 2001; 56:764-7.
78. Warder DE, Oakes WJ. Tethered cord syndrome: The low-lying and normally positioned conus. Neurosurgery 1994; 34:597-600.
79. Yamada S, Won DJ, Pezeshkpour G, et al. Pathophysiology of tethered cord syndrome and similar complex disorders. Neursurg Focus 2007; 23:1-10.
80. Huttmann S, Krauss J, Collmann H, et al. Surgical management of tethered spinal cord in adults: Report of 54 cases. J Neurosurg 2001; 95:173-8.
81. Rees SGO, Collis RE. Spinal cord injury after accidental dural puncture for labour analgesia. Int J Obstet Anesth 2007; 16:193-5.
82. Yamada S, Won DJ, Yamada SM, et al. Adult tethered cord syndrome: Relative to spinal cord length and filum thickness. Neurol Res 2004; 26:732-4.
83. Chantigian RC, Koehn MA, Ramin KD, Warner MA. Chiari I malformation in parturients. J Clin Anesth 2002; 14:201-5.
84. Landau R, Giraud R, Delrue V, Kern C. Spinal anesthesia for cesarean delivery in a woman with a surgically corrected type I Arnold-Chiari malformation. Anesth Analg 2003; 97:253.
85. Wood GG, Jacka MJ. Spinal hematoma following spinal anesthesia in a patient with spina bifida occulta. Anesthesiology 1997; 87:983-4.
86. Crosby E, St-Jean B, Reid D, Elliot RD. Obstetrical anaesthesia and analgesia in chronic spinal cord-injured women. Can J Anaesth 1992; 39:487-94.
87. Tidmarsh MD, May AE. Epidural anaesthesia and neural tube defects. Int J Obstet Anesth 1998; 7:111-4.
88. Kreeger RN, Hilvano A. Anesthetic options for the parturient with a neural tube defect. Int Anesthesiol Clin 2005; 43:65-80.
89. Mayhew JF, Katz J, Miner M, et al. Anaesthesia for the achondroplastic dwarf. Can Anaesth Soc J 1986; 33:216-21.
90. Berkowitz ID, Raja SN, Bender KS, Kopits SE. Dwarfs: Pathophysiology and anesthetic implications. Anesthesiology 1990; 73:739-59.
91. Cohen SE. Anesthesia for cesarean section in achondroplastic dwarfs. Anesthesiology 1980; 52:264-6.
92. Mather JS. Impossible direct laryngoscopy in achondroplasia: A case report. Anaesthesia 1966; 21:244-8.
93. Walts LF, Finerman G, Wyatt GM. Anaesthesia for dwarfs and other patients of pathological small stature. Can Anaesth Soc J 1975; 22:703-9.
94. Carstoniu J, Yee I, Halpern S. Epidural anaesthesia for caesarean section in an achondroplastic dwarf. Can J Anaesth 1992; 39:708-11.
95. Wynne-Davies R, Walsh WK, Gormley J. Achondroplasia and hypochondroplasia: Clinical variation and spinal stenosis. J Bone Joint Surg Br 1981; 63:508-15.
96. Lutter LD, Longstein JE, Winter RB, Langer LO. Anatomy of the achondroplastic lumbar canal. Clin Orthop Relat Res 1977; 126:139-42.
97. Wardall GJ, Frame WT. Extradural anaesthesia for caesarean section in achondroplasia. Br J Anaesth 1990; 64:367-70.
98. Brimacombe JR, Caunt JA. Anaesthesia in a gravid achondroplastic dwarf. Anaesthesia 1990; 45:132-4.
99. Beilin Y, Leibowitz AB. Anesthesia for an achondroplastic dwarf presenting for urgent cesarean section. Int J Obstet Anesth 1993; 2:96-7.
100. Ratner EF, Hamilton CL. Anesthesia for cesarean section in a pituitary dwarf. Anesthesiology 1998; 89:253-4.
101. Morrow MJ, Black IH. Epidural anaesthesia for caesarean section in an achondroplastic dwarf. Br J Anaesth 1998; 81:619-21.
102. DeRenzo JS, Vallejo MC, Ramanathan S. Failed regional anesthesia with reduced spinal bupivacaine dosage in a parturient with achondroplasia presenting for urgent cesarean section. Int J Obstet Anesth 2005; 14:175-8.
103. Bancroft GH, Lauria JI. Ketamine induction for cesarean section in a patient with acute intermittent porphyria and achondroplastic dwarfism. Anesthesiology 1983; 59:143-4.
104. McArthur RDA. Obstetric anaesthesia in an achondroplastic dwarf at a regional hospital. Anaesth Intensive Care 1992; 20:376-8.
105. Cunningham AJ, Donnelly M, Comerford J. Osteogenesis imperfecta: Anesthetic management of a patient for cesarean section: A case report. Anesthesiology 1984; 61:91-3.
106. Carlson JW, Harlass FE. Management of osteogenesis imperfecta in pregnancy: A case report. J Reprod Med 1993; 38:228-32.
107. Sillence D. Osteogenesis imperfecta: An expanding panorama of variants. Clin Orthop Relat Res 1981; 159:11-25.
108. Vogel TM, Ratner EF, Thomas RC Jr, Chitkara U. Pregnancy complicated by severe osteogenesis imperfecta: A report of two cases. Anesth Analg 2002; 94:1315-7.
109. Cho E, Dayan SS, Marx GF. Anaesthesia in a parturient with osteogenesis imperfecta. Br J Anaesth 1992; 68:422-3.
110. Rampton AJ, Kelly DA, Shanahan EC, Ingram GS. Occurrence of malignant hyperpyrexia in a patient with osteogenesis imperfecta. Br J Anaesth 1984; 56:1443-6.
111. Yeo ST, Paech MJ. Regional anaesthesia for multiple caesarean sections in a parturient with osteogenesis imperfecta. Int J Obstet Anesth 1999; 8:284-7.
112. Vebostad A. Spondylolisthesis: A review of 71 patients. Acta Orthop Scand 1974; 45:711-23.
113. Dandy DJ, Shannon MJ. Lumbo-sacral subluxation. (Group 1 spondylolisthesis). J Bone Joint Surg Br 1971; 53:578-95.
114. Saraste H. Spondylolysis and pregnancy—a risk analysis. Acta Obstet Gynecol Scand 1986; 65:727-9.
115. Sanderson PL, Fraser Rd. The influence of pregnancy on the development of degenerative spondylolisthesis. J Bone Joint Surg Br 1996; 78:951-4.

Chapter 49

Neurologic and Neuromuscular Disease

Angela M. Bader, M.D., M.P.H.

The choice of anesthetic technique for pregnant women with neurologic disease requires knowledge of the pathophysiology of the disorder and the controversies involved. If a patient's neurologic condition deteriorates postpartum, the cause may be unclear and the anesthetic technique may be blamed. There are limited published data on specific neurologic and neuromuscular disorders in pregnant women. However, few of these disorders contraindicate the use of neuraxial anesthesia. In most cases, the obstetrician should obtain early antepartum consultation from an anesthesiologist. Early consultation allows accurate antepartum documentation of the extent and pattern of the neurologic deficit as well as discussion and formulation of the anesthetic plan.

MULTIPLE SCLEROSIS

Multiple sclerosis is a major cause of neurologic disability in young adults. The prevalence of the disorder varies with the population, and there appears to be a geographic gradient. The prevalence is less than 1 per 100,000 near the equator but increases to 3 to 8 per 1000 in the northern United States and Canada.[1]

The disease is characterized by variable neurologic disabilities for which the following two general patterns of presentation have been identified: (1) **exacerbating remitting,** in which attacks appear abruptly and resolve over several months, and (2) **chronic progressive**.[2] The relapse rate is approximately 0.3 to 0.4 attacks per year, and the deficits tend to become more progressive and debilitating over time. Environmental factors (e.g., stress, infection, increased body temperature) may provoke a relapse. Most relapses reproduce previous neurologic deficits, which can manifest as pyramidal, cerebellar, or brainstem symptoms.

The etiology remains unclear. There is a clinically significant heritable component, and alleles in the HLA locus have been identified as risk factors for multiple sclerosis.[3] Pathologic findings include inflammation and loss of myelin in the central nervous system (CNS).

The more common symptoms include motor weakness, impaired vision, ataxia, bladder and bowel dysfunction, and emotional lability. Cerebrospinal fluid (CSF) immunoglobulin and lymphocyte concentrations are increased, and magnetic resonance imaging (MRI) studies demonstrate white matter plaques. Lesions may be documented by demonstration of prolonged evoked potentials in the involved areas.

There is no curative treatment. Immunosuppressive therapies may hasten recovery from a relapse, but no evidence suggests that these agents influence the progressive course of the disease. Interferon-beta may significantly reduce the relapse rate and retard disability; however, an increased risk of fetal loss and low birth weight is observed with the use of this therapy during the first trimester of pregnancy.[4] Administration of intravenous immunoglobulin may reduce the risk of relapse, and it has no known adverse effects on pregnancy outcome.[5] Acute relapses during pregnancy can be treated with intravenous corticosteroids, although their use may be associated with maternal glucose intolerance and neonatal adrenal suppression.[6]

Interaction with Pregnancy

Evidence regarding the effect of multiple sclerosis on pregnancy is conflicting. In one cohort study that compared 198 affected women with 1584 normal women, the number of maternal complications was not higher in women with multiple sclerosis.[7] However, infants delivered to women with multiple sclerosis appear to be at greater risk for meconium aspiration, even though the presence of moderate to heavy meconium is not significantly increased.[7] This finding may reflect an intrauterine environment in patients with multiple sclerosis that is more susceptible to acute hypoxic events.[7] A subsequent cohort study of 649 pregnancies in women with multiple sclerosis concluded that infants of these women were more likely to be small for gestational age; this outcome was also attributed to a suboptimal intrauterine environment.[8] Moreover, this study found that mothers with multiple sclerosis were more likely to undergo induction of labor and operative delivery, possibly as a result of neuromuscular weakness and spasticity.

In patients with exacerbating-remitting multiple sclerosis, the relapse rate is slightly decreased during pregnancy; however, the rate then increases during the first 3 to 6 months postpartum.[9] Data from prospective studies have suggested that the mean rate of relapse, in comparison with the year prior to pregnancy, increases during the first 3 months postpartum.[10] Relapse during this period is most probable in women who had higher relapse rates in the year before pregnancy or during pregnancy. Stress, exhaustion, infection, the loss of antenatal immunosuppression, and the postpartum decline in concentrations of reproductive hormones may account for the higher postpartum relapse rate. Treatment with immunologically active agents (e.g., interferon-beta) might result in a decreased postpartum relapse rate, but data are limited.[10]

Pregnancy does not negatively affect the long-term outcome of multiple sclerosis. Rather, at least one study has suggested that parturition may have a slightly favorable effect on long-term disease activity.[11]

Anesthetic Management

The anesthesiologist should assess the patient's level of compromise, document the pattern of deficits, and give special attention to respiratory involvement. Historically, there has been great controversy regarding the administration of anesthesia in patients with multiple sclerosis. Most anesthesia providers have considered general anesthesia to be safe, although published data are limited.[12,13] Many anesthesia providers have been reluctant to administer neuraxial anesthesia because the effect of local anesthetic drugs on the course of the disease is unclear. Some anesthesiologists have expressed concern that neuraxial anesthesia may expose demyelinated areas of the spinal cord to the potential neurotoxic effects of local anesthetic agents. Several animal studies have investigated the histologic effects of local anesthetic agents on the normal spinal cord. In one study, subarachnoid injection of small doses of a local anesthetic agent produced no histologic changes in the cord or meninges. Injection of very large doses caused reversible inflammatory and degenerative changes; all such changes had disappeared by 14 days after injection.[14]

Diagnostic lumbar puncture is not associated with a higher rate of relapse.[15] Two reports have implicated spinal anesthesia in the exacerbation of multiple sclerosis.[13,16] However, these two series included only a small number of relapses. Bamford et al.[13] described only one relapse after nine spinal anesthetics, and Stenuit and Marchand[16] identified only two relapses after the administration of spinal anesthesia in 19 patients. The relationship of these relapses to spinal anesthesia or other postoperative conditions (e.g., stress, infection, hyperpyrexia) known to exacerbate multiple sclerosis is unclear.

There are few published data on the use of epidural anesthesia in patients with multiple sclerosis. Warren et al.[17] reported minor exacerbations after the administration of epidural anesthesia for two separate vaginal deliveries in one patient. Crawford et al.[18] reported only one postoperative relapse in 50 nonobstetric and 7 obstetric patients who received epidural analgesia. Confavreux et al.[9] reported a study of 269 pregnancies in 254 women with multiple sclerosis, of whom 42 received epidural analgesia. They noted that epidural analgesia did not have an adverse effect on the rate of relapse or on the progression of disability in these patients. Bader et al.[19] retrospectively evaluated 32 pregnancies in women with multiple sclerosis; they observed that women who received epidural anesthesia for vaginal delivery did not have a higher incidence of relapse than those who received only local infiltration. Among the 5 patients who underwent cesarean delivery, 1 had a postpartum relapse. The data suggested that the concentration of local anesthetic used for epidural anesthesia may influence the relapse rate because all patients in the relapse group had received higher concentrations of bupivacaine or lidocaine.[19] The concentration of local anesthetic in the CSF progressively increases during prolonged administration of epidural anesthesia, and the higher concentration may overwhelm the protective effect of dilution within the CSF. These observations suggest that anesthesia providers should use dilute solutions of local anesthetic for epidural analgesia during labor. A more recent prospective study in 227 women who had multiple sclerosis for at least 1 year prior to conception, of whom 42 had epidural analgesia during labor, found no adverse effect of epidural analgesia on the rate of relapse or the progression of disability.[10]

The addition of an opioid reduces the total dose of local anesthetic required for epidural analgesia during labor. Berger and Ontell[20] reported the administration of intrathecal morphine, which was added to low-dose tetracaine for surgical anesthesia and postoperative analgesia, and observed no exacerbation of multiple sclerosis at 1 and 6 months after surgery. Leigh et al.[21] described the successful use of intrathecal diamorphine for postoperative analgesia in a patient with multiple sclerosis who underwent a laparotomy.

The administration of neuraxial anesthesia for cesarean delivery is controversial. Because the operation is of limited duration, multiple doses of local anesthetic are typically not needed, so a progressive increase in CSF concentration of local anesthetic over time is less likely. In light of the significant benefits of neuraxial techniques for intraoperative anesthesia and postoperative analgesia, either spinal or epidural anesthesia is the principal anesthetic technique used for cesarean delivery in patients with multiple sclerosis in many institutions, including my own.

In summary, published data do not contraindicate the use of neuraxial anesthetic techniques for labor analgesia or operative anesthesia. The patient should be aware that there is a higher incidence of relapse during the postpartum period, regardless of the type of anesthesia used. However, neither pregnancy nor anesthesia appears to have a negative influence on the long-term course of the disease.

HEADACHE DURING PREGNANCY

Headache is one of the most common neurologic symptoms during pregnancy (Table 49-1). The most common

TABLE 49-1 Headache during Pregnancy

Etiology	Symptoms	Pattern	Treatment
Tension headache	Dull, widespread headache	Increased incidence during peripartum period	Analgesics Tricyclic antidepressants
Migraine headache	Frontotemporal throbbing Prodrome of scotomata	Improvement in 79% of patients during pregnancy	Ergotamine contraindicated during pregnancy Promethazine Beta-blockers for prophylaxis
Preeclampsia	Generalized headache Occasional scotomata and/or blurred vision	Occurrence during pregnancy and occasionally postpartum	Blood pressure control Delivery
Meningeal irritation (subarachnoid hemorrhage, meningitis)	Generalized headache	Increased risk of subarachnoid hemorrhage during pregnancy	Based on etiology
Brain tumor	Variable	No increase in incidence during pregnancy, possible increased growth rate	Based on etiology
Pseudotumor cerebri	Generalized headache Visual symptoms	Increased incidence and worsened symptoms during pregnancy	Typically remits within 1 to 3 months or after childbirth

kinds of headache during pregnancy are tension headache, migraine headache, and headache associated with pregnancy-induced hypertension or preeclampsia.

Tension Headache

Tension or muscle contraction headache is the most common headache during pregnancy.[22] The symptoms typically consist of dull, persistent pain that extends over the entire head. The onset is typically gradual, and the symptoms may persist for long periods. The etiology is unknown, although it is believed to be related to stress rather than hormonal changes. These headaches are more common in women, are frequently associated with anxiety, and may be a symptom of postpartum depression.[23]

TREATMENT

In the nonpregnant patient, treatment may involve acetaminophen, aspirin, opioids, tricyclic antidepressants, and benzodiazepines. In the pregnant patient, acetaminophen should be used as a first-line analgesic. Caffeine, including that contained in combination products (i.e., Fioricet, Fiorinal), should be limited to a total dose less than 300 mg/day to lessen the possibility of intrauterine fetal growth restriction.[24] Limited data suggest that butalbital is not associated with congenital anomalies.[25] Ergot alkaloids (e.g., ergotamine) are contraindicated during pregnancy; these agents may cause marked increases in uterine tone, which may compromise placental perfusion and fetal oxygenation.[26] Use of nonsteroidal anti-inflammatory drugs (NSAIDs) should be limited during the third trimester because of concerns about their association with premature closure of the fetal ductus arteriosus and prolongation of pregnancy. Most obstetricians avoid the administration of benzodiazepines during pregnancy because of conflicting evidence regarding the incidence of orofacial clefts after fetal exposure during the first trimester.[27] Opioids have a long record of safe use during pregnancy. Tricyclic antidepressants also have been used safely during pregnancy; one study suggested that these agents do not have a detrimental effect on the neurodevelopment of children exposed *in utero*.[28]

OBSTETRIC AND ANESTHETIC MANAGEMENT

Pregnancy is not likely to reduce the frequency or severity of tension headache because it is not hormonally mediated. Tension headache may signal a higher risk for postpartum depression.[23] The presence and treatment of tension headache rarely affects obstetric and anesthetic management.

Migraine Headache

Migraine headaches are classically described as unilateral, throbbing headaches sometimes accompanied by nausea and vomiting. The duration varies from hours to days. Visual disturbances (e.g., scotomata) typically precede the onset of these headaches. Focal neurologic symptoms (e.g., aphasia, hemiplegia) may also occur. Most investigators favor neurovascular vasospasm, followed by cerebral vasodilation, as the etiology. It results from either a primary vascular disorder or a disturbance in the noradrenergic nervous system. Patients are also more susceptible to symptoms when serotonin levels are low.[29]

Migraine occurs in 4% to 6% of men and 13% to 17% of women.[30] Symptoms generally occur early in adult life. Headache occurs less frequently with advancing age. Hormonal influences are well known; estrogen withdrawal is associated with an exacerbation of symptoms.[31] Approximately 79% of women with migraine headaches experience improvement during pregnancy, and in 21%, migraine remains unchanged or worsens.[32] After delivery, the drop in hormonal concentrations coincides with an increase in migraine symptoms.[33]

TREATMENT

In nonpregnant patients, therapy often involves ergotamine tartrate, typically in combination with caffeine (Cafergot). However, ergot alkaloids are contraindicated during pregnancy because of associated uterotonic effects and possible (but unproven) teratogenic effects.[26,32,34] In general, acetaminophen is the first-line treatment during pregancy. Combination therapy with agents containing caffeine and/or butalbital can be used with caution; the caffeine component should be limited to a dose less than 300 mg/day to lessen the risk of intrauterine fetal growth restriction. Limited data suggest that butalbital is not associated with congenital anomalies.[25] Use of NSAIDs should be limited during the third trimester because of concerns about their association with premature closure of the ductus arteriosus and prolongation of pregnancy. Beta-adrenergic receptor antagonists (e.g., propranolol) may be used for prophylaxis. However, these agents cross the placenta, and therefore should be used for prophylaxis during pregnancy only when a patient's symptoms are severe. Occasionally, calcium entry–blocking agents are used. The use of sumatriptan or other selective serotonin agonists is controversial. A higher incidence of congenital anomalies has been observed after administration of high doses of sumatriptan in animals[32]; however, in a review of human studies, no evidence that sumatriptan has any specific adverse effect on pregnancy outcome was found.[35]

OBSTETRIC AND ANESTHETIC MANAGEMENT

Data regarding the relationship between the occurrence of migraines and preeclampsia are conflicting. Some evidence suggests that women who have a history of migraines may have a higher risk of preeclampsia; however, other studies have reported no higher incidence of preeclampsia, miscarriage, congenital anomalies, or stillbirth despite the presence and treatment of migraines during pregnancy.[32,36]

Cerebral ischemia has been reported after the administration of terbutaline in pregnant patients with migraine. Rosene et al.[37] recommended that physicians avoid the administration of terbutaline in pregnant women with a history of vascular headache.

There are no published data on the relationship between intrapartum anesthesia and postpartum migraine headaches.

SPINAL CORD INJURY

Spinal cord injuries occur with an incidence of approximately 30 per million population.[38] Improved handling and stabilization of victims at the site of an accident and the availability of extensive rehabilitation services have resulted in a higher number of women who present for obstetric care after spinal cord injury.

Patient disability and residual function depend on the anatomic location of the injury.[39] Cord injuries below S2 involve mainly bladder, bowel, and sexual functions. Affected patients have relaxed perineal muscles, and women with such injuries experience pain during labor. Women with a lesion above T10 do not experience labor pain. Patients with a lesion above T6 have varying levels of respiratory compromise and are at risk for autonomic hyperreflexia (see later).

Spinal shock, defined as transient sensorimotor dysfunction resolving in less than 24 hours, may develop in about half of spinal cord–injured patients.[40] Neurogenic shock consists of hemodynamic abnormalities as well as sensorimotor effects, generally lasts from 1 to 3 weeks, and is characterized by flaccid paralysis with loss of tendon and autonomic reflexes for weeks to months.[40] Patients with neurogenic shock lose vasomotor tone, temperature regulation, sweating, and piloerection in the parts of the body below the lesion. Pulmonary edema, hemodynamic instability, and circulatory collapse can develop in the absence of brainstem regulation of vasomotor tone. The patient is at risk for aspiration, infection, and other pulmonary complications. Paraplegic patients may have a compensatory tachycardia, whereas quadriplegic patients may have bradycardia due to unopposed vagal tone.

After a variable period, the patient progresses to a chronic stage in which reflex activity is regained. In most cases, this return of reflex activity occurs within 1 to 6 weeks after the injury; rarely it may take several months.[41] This stage is characterized by disuse atrophy, flexor spasms, and an exaggeration of reflexes. The **mass motor reflex** results from the absence of central inhibitory mechanisms. A stimulus that normally would cause the contraction of a few muscle units leads to the widespread spasm of entire muscle groups. The mass motor reflex can occur with any level of spinal cord injury. It may occur with autonomic hyperreflexia in a patient with a lesion above T6.[42]

Approximately 85% of patients with chronic spinal cord injuries at or above T6 experience the syndrome of **autonomic hyperreflexia**.[43] This is a life-threatening complication that results from the absence of central inhibition on the sympathetic neurons in the cord below the injury. Noxious stimuli, bladder or bowel distention, and uterine contractions result in afferent transmission by means of the dorsal spinal root (Figure 49-1).[44] These afferent neurons synapse with sympathetic neurons, and the impulse is propagated both cephalad and caudad in the sympathetic chain, without central inhibition. The propagation results in extreme sympathetic hyperactivity and severe systemic hypertension secondary to vasoconstriction below the level of the lesion. In response, the reflex arcs involving the baroreceptors of the aortic and carotid bodies lead to bradycardia and vasodilation above the level of the lesion. In patients with lesions of T6 and above, these compensatory mechanisms are insufficient to compensate for the severe hypertension. Intracranial hemorrhage, arrhythmias, and myocardial infarction occur in some cases. A variety of agents have been used for control of the hypertension of autonomic hyperreflexia (Figure 49-2).[45]

Obstetric Management

Pregnancy may aggravate many of the medical complications of spinal cord injury (Box 49-1).[44] The loss of both functional residual capacity and expiratory reserve volume during pregnancy may increase the likelihood of respiratory compromise associated with spinal cord injury. Pregnancy increases the risks for deep vein thrombosis, thromboembolic phenomena, and urinary tract infection. Loss of sympathetic tone below the level of the lesion renders pregnant patients with spinal cord injury particularly prone to orthostatic hypotension, which may result in a decrease in uteroplacental perfusion. Uterine contractions can stimulate

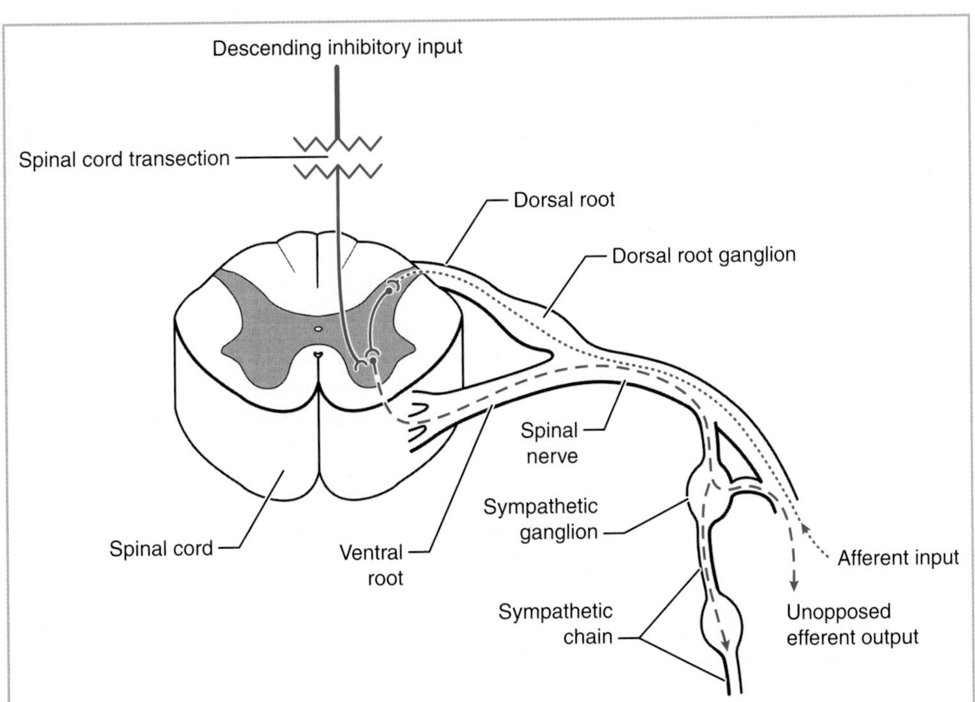

FIGURE 49-1 Noxious stimuli enter the dorsal horn of the spinal cord through the dorsal spinal root (*dotted line*). These afferent neurons synapse either directly or by means of interneurons (*solid line*) with sympathetic neurons in the intermediolateral columns of the lateral horns, which then project through the anterior roots to the paraspinal sympathetic chain (*dashed line*). The impulse is propagated peripherally at that spinal level and also travels both cephalad and caudad in the sympathetic chain, exiting at multiple thoracic and lumbar levels (*dashed line*) and resulting in sympathetic hyperactivity. (Drawing by Naveen Nathan, M.D., Northwestern University Feinberg School of Medicine, Chicago, IL.)

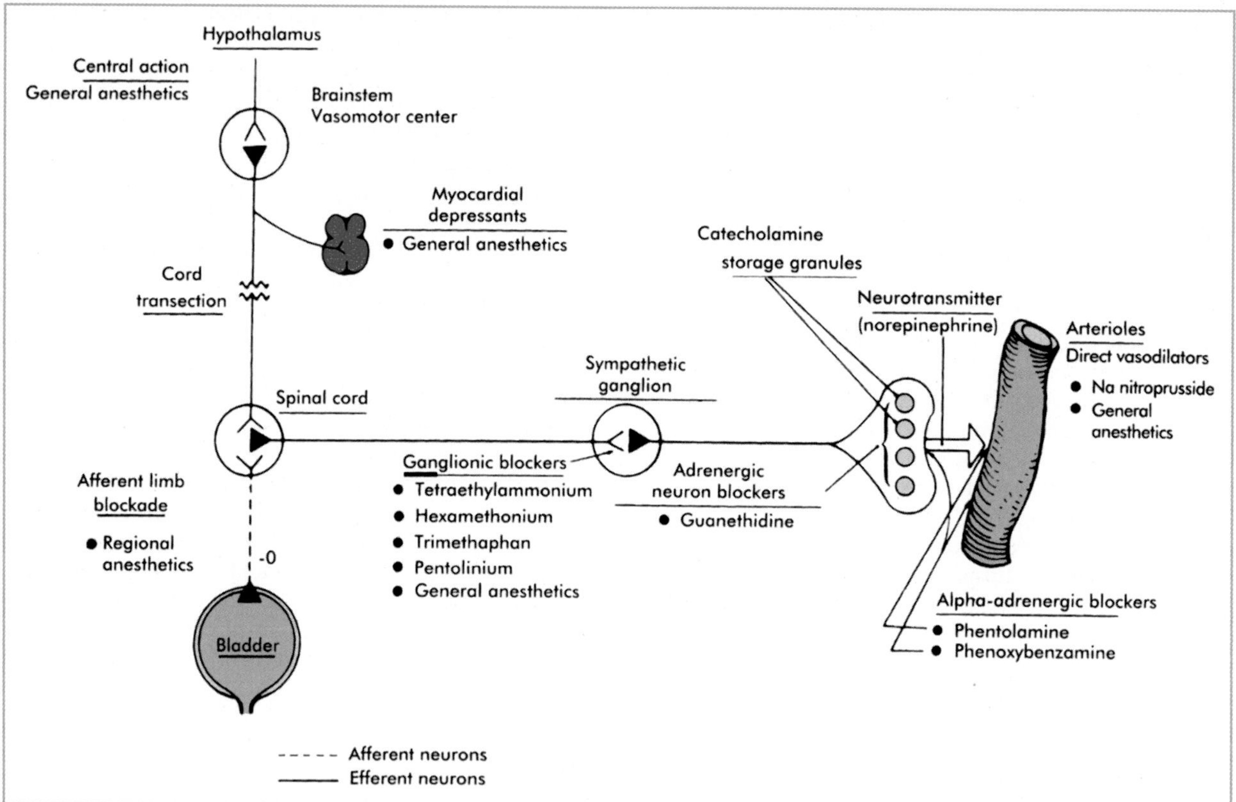

FIGURE 49-2 Sites of action for agents used in the control of hypertension associated with autonomic hyperreflexia. (From Schonwald G, Fish KJ, Perkash I. Cardiovascular complications during anesthesia in chronic spinal cord injured patients. Anesthesiology 1981; 55:550-8.)

autonomic hyperreflexia, and the resultant vasoconstriction can result in fetal hypoxia and bradycardia. In pregnant women, autonomic hyperreflexia occurs most commonly during labor.[40]

Women with a lesion above T11 may have a higher risk of preterm labor.[46] Because these women do not experience labor pain, obstetric management includes weekly cervical examinations during the third trimester. Vaginal delivery is preferred. The use of forceps may be necessary because of the parturient's inability to push.[47] In a study of 52 pregnancies in spinal cord–injured women, 9 of 12 patients with lesions above T5 had symptoms of autonomic hyperreflexia. The cesarean delivery rate was 47% for women with lesions above T5 and 26% for women with lesions at T5 or below.[48] Preterm delivery occurred in 19% of patients.

BOX 49-1 Medical Complications of Spinal Cord Injury Aggravated by Pregnancy

Pulmonary
- Decreased respiratory reserve
- Atelectasis and pneumonia
- Impaired cough

Hematologic
- Anemia
- Deep vein thrombosis
- Thromboembolic phenomena

Urogenital
- Chronic urinary tract infections
- Urinary tract calculi
- Proteinuria
- Renal insufficiency

Dermatologic
- Decubitus ulcers

Cardiovascular
- Hypertension
- Autonomic hyperreflexia

From Crosby E, St. Jean B, Reid D, Elliot RD. Obstetric anaesthesia and analgesia in chronic spinal cord-injured women. Can J Anaesth 1992; 39:487-94.

Anesthetic Management

Women with spinal cord lesions at or above T6 are at risk for autonomic hyperreflexia. This syndrome can be distinguished from other causes of intrapartum hypertension by the occurrence of cyclic hypertension (i.e., blood pressure increases during contractions and decreases between contractions).[49] The American College of Obstetricians and Gynecologists[50] recommends continuous hemodynamic monitoring during labor for all patients at risk for autonomic hyperreflexia.

Administration of neuraxial anesthesia is the most common method for prevention or treatment of autonomic hyperreflexia during labor and delivery. Spinal anesthesia has effectively controlled blood pressure in paraplegic patients undergoing general surgical procedures.[51,52]

Although some anesthesiologists contend that distortion of the vertebral column in paraplegic patients makes it more difficult to predict and control the level of spinal anesthesia, published data do not lend support to this argument.[51,52] If spinal anesthesia is chosen, insertion of an intrathecal catheter and use of a continuous technique may be appropriate; this approach may allow more careful titration of the resulting anesthetic block.

Most obstetric anesthesiologists prefer the use of epidural analgesia for the prevention or treatment of autonomic hyperreflexia during labor and delivery. Case reports have described the successful epidural administration of 0.25% or 0.5% bupivacaine or the administration of combined spinal-epidural (CSE) anesthesia for this purpose.[53-55] Baraka[49] reported the successful epidural administration of meperidine, an opioid with local anesthetic qualities. Abouleish et al.[56] noted that epidural fentanyl alone did not effectively treat the hypertension of autonomic hyperreflexia, but the addition of 0.25% bupivacaine led to a decrease in blood pressure to baseline levels. In one case, the administration of epidural morphine 3 mg (followed by epidural administration of 0.25% bupivacaine during more advanced labor) was effective in the treatment of autonomic hyperreflexia.[57] Maehama et al.[58] described the successful use of magnesium sulfate for management of autonomic hyperreflexia during labor.

The anesthesia provider must remember that the typical epidural test dose will not identify unintentional subarachnoid injection in a patient with spinal cord injury. Therapeutic doses of a local anesthetic agent should be administered cautiously. The cephalad sensory block level can be fully assessed only if it is more cephalad than the level of the spinal cord lesion. Alternatively, a partial assessment can be performed by evaluating segmental reflexes below the level of the lesion. For example, the anesthesia provider can lightly stroke each side of the abdomen above and below the umbilicus, looking for contraction of the abdominal muscles and deviation of the umbilicus toward the stimulus. Reflexes are absent below the level of the block.

Patients with spinal cord injury often have a low baseline blood pressure and some hemodynamic instability. Placement of an intra-arterial catheter allows the continuous assessment of blood pressure. Alternative means of treating autonomic hyperreflexia should be available if neuraxial anesthesia is not successful (see Figure 49-2).

If cesarean delivery is necessary, epidural anesthesia (e.g., 2% lidocaine with 1:200,000 epinephrine) can be administered. Severe respiratory insufficiency or technical difficulties with neuraxial anesthesia may necessitate the use of general anesthesia.[59] If general anesthesia is required, a depolarizing muscle relaxant such as succinylcholine should not be given during the period of denervation injury. By a conservative definition, this period begins 24 hours after the injury and lasts for 1 year. The use of succinylcholine during this period of denervation injury may cause severe hyperkalemia.[60] Rather, a nondepolarizing muscle relaxant should be used to facilitate laryngoscopy and intubation.

MYASTHENIA GRAVIS

Myasthenia gravis is an autoimmune disorder characterized by episodes of muscle weakness that are made worse by activity. Its prevalence is approximately 50 to 125 cases per million. Twice as many women are affected as men, and the onset of the disease peaks earlier, between the second and third decade, versus the sixth and seventh decades in men.[61] Myasthenia gravis has been classified according to severity as follows[61]:

I. Ocular myasthenia
II. Mild generalized myasthenia; may include ocular, oropharyngeal, and respiratory involvement
III. Moderate generalized disease
IV. Severe generalized weakness
V. Defined by requirement for intubation, with or without mechanical ventilation

Myasthenia gravis results from abnormal autoimmune regulation that leads to the production of antibodies against the nicotinic acetylcholine receptor on the neuromuscular end plate of skeletal muscle. The result is receptor destruction as well as antibody-induced blockade of the remaining acetylcholine receptors.[62] Smooth muscle and cardiac muscle are not affected. Thymic hyperplasia is common, and thymic tumors occur in approximately 10% of patients. There is an association between myasthenia gravis and other autoimmune disorders, such as rheumatoid arthritis and polymyositis. In general, an early age of onset and a long duration of purely ocular myasthenia are good prognostic signs.

Medical Management

Treatment involves a thymectomy, administration of anticholinesterase medications and/or immunosuppressive agents, and plasmapheresis. A thymectomy helps approximately 96% of patients; 46% of these have complete remission, and 50% are asymptomatic or experience improvement with therapy.[63] In addition, a thymectomy appears to exert a favorable influence on the outcome of pregnancy. One study noted decreased maternal and perinatal morbidity as well as less frequent clinical exacerbations in patients who had undergone thymectomy.[64]

Anticholinesterase drugs, which inhibit the breakdown of acetylcholine, are the mainstay of therapy. An intravenous dose of edrophonium (10 mg) is administered as a diagnostic test; decreased muscle weakness within minutes after edrophonium administration confirms the diagnosis of myasthenia. Physostigmine crosses the blood-brain barrier and is not used for long-term therapy. Neostigmine and pyridostigmine are quaternary ammonium compounds that do not cross the blood-brain barrier. These drugs may be administered orally or intravenously. In general, pyridostigmine is preferred because it has less severe muscarinic side effects.[65]

Corticosteroids and azathioprine have been used with some success. Plasmapheresis can be especially helpful for patients in crisis. One study noted that preoperative plasmapheresis resulted in less need for mechanical ventilation and less time in the intensive care unit postoperatively.[66]

Myasthenia gravis can manifest in two types of crises. A **cholinergic crisis** results from an excess of the muscarinic effects of anticholinesterase medications combined with a poor response to anticholinesterase therapy. Symptoms are muscle weakness, respiratory difficulty or failure, increased sweating, salivation, bronchial secretions, and miosis. In contrast, a **myasthenic crisis** results from a worsening of the disease; its symptoms include more severe muscle weakness, including greater weakness of respiratory muscles. These two crises can be distinguished by the administration of edrophonium. The symptoms do not improve if a cholinergic crisis is present; an improvement indicates the need for a higher dose of anticholinesterase medication.

Many drugs can cause a worsening of myasthenic symptoms. These patients are extremely sensitive to drugs that can potentiate muscle weakness.[67] These agents include neuromuscular blocking agents, quinidine, propranolol, aminoglycoside antibiotics, and tocolytic agents such as magnesium sulfate,[68,69] terbutaline, and ritodrine.[70] One case report noted worsened symptoms after the maternal administration of betamethasone.[70]

Obstetric Management

The course of myasthenia gravis during pregnancy varies. In general, approximately one third of cases improve, one third worsen, and one third show no change.[71] Approximately 30% of patients experience a relapse postpartum.

Myasthenia gravis causes increases in rates of pregnancy wastage, preterm labor, and maternal mortality and morbidity.[71,72] Plauché[71] noted that maternal mortality is approximately 40 per 1000 live births, and perinatal mortality is approximately 68 per 1000 births. Because the maternal mortality risk is inversely proportional to the duration of myasthenia gravis, with the highest risk occurring in the first year, it is sometimes recommended that myasthenic women delay childbirth for the first few years after diagnosis.[72]

The maternal physiologic changes of pregnancy, including alterations in drug absorption, increases in blood volume, and changes in renal clearance, may require adjustments in the doses of anticholinesterase drugs. Anticholinesterase agents are quaternary ammonium compounds that have minimal placental transfer. Each patient should be monitored carefully for progressive respiratory compromise secondary to diaphragmatic elevation during pregnancy. Aggressive therapy of myasthenic crises is essential. Anticholinesterase drugs have known uterotonic effects[72]; thus uterine activity should be monitored during the administration of these drugs. Vital capacity can be measured to monitor fatigue during labor.[73] Intravenous administration of an anticholinesterase drug may be needed during labor. The treatment of the myasthenic parturient with preeclampsia is problematic. The use of magnesium sulfate for seizure prophylaxis may be associated with a significant increase in muscle weakness and may be contraindicated.[74]

The uterus consists of smooth muscle; therefore myasthenia gravis should not affect the first stage of labor. However, the second stage of labor also requires the use of striated muscle; therefore forceps delivery may be required.

Maternal antibodies to the acetylcholine receptor are transferred across the placenta. Neonatal myasthenia gravis occurs in approximately 16% of infants of mothers with myasthenia gravis.[71] Alpha-fetoprotein blocks the binding of the antibody to the acetylcholine receptor, and therefore varying levels of alpha-fetoprotein may be responsible for variations in the clinical course of myasthenia during pregnancy.[75] The rapid decrease in neonatal alpha-fetoprotein concentrations after birth may be responsible for the onset of transient neonatal myasthenia. The infant demonstrates symptoms of myasthenia (feeding problems, hypotonia, and respiratory difficulty) within the first 4 days of life.[76] Anticholinesterase therapy may be required. The symptoms abate as the antibodies are metabolized, and resolution occurs within 2 to 4 weeks.

Anesthetic Management

Each patient should undergo early antepartum consultation with an anesthesiologist. This evaluation should include an assessment of the extent of bulbar and respiratory involvement. Pulmonary function testing should be performed in patients with evidence of respiratory compromise.

Patients with respiratory compromise may be more susceptible to the respiratory depression associated with opioids. Thus opioids should be used cautiously, if at all, in these patients. Neuraxial analgesic techniques are associated with low pain scores and high rates of maternal satisfaction even without the use of opioids; as a result, these techniques are the preferred method for labor analgesia in patients with myasthenia.[73,77] However, because plasma cholinesterase activity is decreased in patients who are taking anticholinesterase drugs, ester local anesthetic agents may have a prolonged half-life. To avoid the potential risk of local anesthetic toxicity, an amide local anesthetic agent should be given for epidural analgesia. By contrast, with the small doses of local anesthetic agents required for *spinal* analgesia or anesthesia, the anesthesia provider can safely give either an ester or an amide local anesthetic agent intrathecally. D'Angelo and Gerancher[77] reported the administration of CSE analgesia for labor and spontaneous vaginal delivery in a patient with severe myasthenia gravis. The CSE technique offers the advantage of effective analgesia with minimal motor block, but if the intrathecal component contains an opioid, some risk of respiratory depression exists.

For cesarean delivery, neuraxial anesthetic techniques are preferred unless the patient has significant bulbar involvement or respiratory compromise.[78] In these cases, a high level of anesthesia may impair respiratory function. In patients with moderate respiratory compromise, the use of bilevel positive airway pressure (BiPAP) for ventilatory support may improve the safety of neuraxial anesthesia.[79]

In the patient with severe bulbar involvement or respiratory compromise, it may be prudent to secure the airway before surgery. Sodium thiopental, ketamine, and propofol have been used successfully for the induction of general anesthesia in patients with myasthenia gravis.[74,79,80] By contrast, depolarizing muscle relaxants (e.g., succinylcholine) have an unpredictable effect in these patients. In general, muscles affected by the disease are more sensitive to depolarizing agents, whereas unaffected muscles are more resistant.[81] However, because the commonly administered dose of succinylcholine (1 to 1.5 mg/kg) is three to five times the effective dose in 95% of normal patients (ED_{95}), it is likely that this common dose will provide adequate relaxation of resistant normal muscles. Anticholinesterase agents decrease the activity of plasma cholinesterase, as does plasmapheresis, and may cause a delay in succinylcholine hydrolysis.

Myasthenic patients are extremely sensitive to nondepolarizing muscle relaxants. If a nondepolarizing muscle relaxant must be given, the anesthesia provider should administer a small amount of an agent with a short half-life (e.g., rocuronium, atracurium, vecuronium).[63] Volatile halogenated agents potentiate muscle relaxation. Neuromuscular blockade should be monitored continually with a nerve stimulator, with the understanding that myasthenia may prevent a full-strength contraction; therefore, a control train-of-four stimulus test should be performed and its result recorded before paralysis, for later comparison. Small doses of neostigmine may be given cautiously for the reversal of neuromuscular blockade.

After delivery, fluid shifts and a decreased alpha-fetoprotein concentration may necessitate an adjustment of the dose of anticholinesterase drug. Some patients who receive general anesthesia require postoperative ventilation. In earlier studies, the following four factors were associated with a higher risk of postoperative ventilation in nonobstetric myasthenic patients: (1) duration of myasthenia greater than 6 years, (2) history of chronic respiratory disease, (3) pyridostigmine dose higher than 750 mg per day, and (4) vital capacity less than 2.9 L.[82] Later work has not validated these factors, but has identified a different list of factors that predict an increased risk for postoperative ventilation, as follows: (1) female gender, (2) $FEF_{25\%-75\%}$ (forced expiratory flow during the middle half of the forced vital capacity) less than 3.3 L/sec and less than 85% of that predicted, (3) FVC (forced vital capacity) less than 2.6 L/sec and less than 78% of that predicted, and (4) $MEF_{50\%}$ (maximal expiratory flow at 50% of expired vital capacity) less than 3.9 L/sec and less than 80% of that predicted.[83]

EPILEPSY

Epilepsy is a condition in which the patient experiences one of a variety of forms of recurrent seizure activity in the absence of metabolic disorders or acute brain disease. The classification scheme for epileptic seizures is constantly evolving; however, most seizures are grouped into the two major types, partial and generalized.[84,85] In partial seizures, the excess neuronal discharge is thought to originate in one region of the cerebral cortex; in generalized seizures, the discharge occurs bilaterally and involves the entire cortex.

Medical Management

A variety of anticonvulsant drugs are used for seizure therapy, depending on the type of seizure and clinical response.[86] Single-agent therapy is preferred when possible, with the dose adjusted to keep the serum level within the therapeutic range. Classic antiepileptic drugs (e.g., carbamazepine, phenobarbital, phenytoin, valproate) are often used as first-line treatment (Table 49-2). Combination therapy or newer agents (e.g., oxcarbazepine, lamotrigine, gabapentin, pregabalin, topiramate) are used in patients who are unable to remain seizure free with classic drug therapy for a 12-month period.[85] For some of the newer agents, the dose is titrated according to the clinical response, so there is less available information about therapeutic drug levels.

A variety of adverse effects have been reported with antiepileptic drugs, including early-onset events (e.g., somnolence, dizziness, hypersensitivity, rash, gastrointestinal symptoms) and late-onset events (e.g., depression, leukopenia, aplastic anemia, thrombocytopenia, megaloblastic anemia, hyponatremia).[85]

Prognosis for medical control of seizures is good for patients with generalized seizure disorders; 5-year remissions occur in 70% of patients, 50% of whom are able to discontinue their medications.[87] Patients with simple partial seizures also have a good prognosis; as many as 92% of patients are in remission by 8 years.[88] Complex partial seizures (e.g., temporal lobe epilepsy) are more difficult to control.[89]

Interaction with Pregnancy

Approximately 0.5% of all parturients have a chronic seizure disorder.[90] Pregnancy exerts a variable effect on the frequency of seizures. Approximately one third of epileptic women experience an increase in seizure frequency during pregnancy, and about half experience no change.[91]

A variety of etiologies have been proposed for the increase in seizure frequency in some pregnant women (Table 49-3).[86] Higher estrogen concentrations in pregnancy lower the seizure threshold.[92] Greater sodium and water retention, alkalosis secondary to hyperventilation, sleep deprivation, and increased stress and anxiety also have been suggested as mechanisms.[93] In addition, anticonvulsant drug levels can decrease during pregnancy, often despite the administration of a larger dose[90]; this may be partially explained by the decreased plasma protein binding and greater drug clearance observed during pregnancy.[94,95]

Maternal seizures can have devastating consequences. Hypoxia and acidosis that occur during a generalized seizure can result in fetal compromise or intrauterine fetal death.[96] During the past three decades the overall risk of certain obstetric complications in epileptic women has declined. Nonetheless, some studies suggest that epileptic women have a twofold higher incidence of preeclampsia, preterm labor, and placental abnormalities.[97]

Infants of mothers with epilepsy are approximately twice as likely to have adverse pregnancy outcomes, including intrauterine fetal death, cesarean delivery, neonatal and perinatal death, low birth weight, and abnormal development.[97] The risk of congenital malformations is approximately 4% to 6%.[97] Malformations have been associated with all currently used therapeutic modalities; those most often seen are cleft lip and palate, and cardiac, neural tube, and urogenital defects. Certain drugs have been associated with a higher relative risk of congenital defects than others. Data from prospective studies indicate that phenobarbital and valproate are associated with significantly higher rates of major malformations.[86] Animal studies suggest that newer agents (e.g., lamotrigine, gabapentin, felbamate, topiramate, tiagabine, levetiracetam, pregabalin) have less teratogenic effect in animals, but adequate human studies have not been performed.[98] Lamotrigine may be less teratogenic in humans than other antiepileptic agents, although there have been some reports of orofacial clefts in association with its use.[99] The development of collaborative

TABLE 49-2 Classic Antiepileptic Drugs Used during Pregnancy

Drug	Dose	Therapeutic Serum Level	Side Effects	Toxicity	Types of Seizures*		
					Tonic-Clonic	Absence	Complex Partial
Phenytoin (Dilantin)	Average: 400 mg/day Range: 300-1200 mg/day	10-20 μg/mL	Ataxia Drowsiness Gum hyperplasia Hypertrichosis Nystagmus	Rash Serum sickness Pseudolymphoma Stevens-Johnson syndrome Lupus erythematosus Macrocytic anemia Rare hepatic or marrow toxicity Cerebellar degeneration Peripheral neuropathy	+	–	+
Phenobarbital	Average: 120 mg/day Range: 30-210 mg/day	10-35 μg/mL	Drowsiness Ataxia Nystagmus	Rash Possible teratogenicity	+	–	+
Primidone (Mysoline)	Average: 1000 mg/day Range: 500-2000 mg/day	4-12 μg/mL	Drowsiness Nausea Ataxia Nystagmus (Tachyphylaxis typical)	Rash Adenopathy Lupus erythematosus Macrocytic anemia Arthritis Edema	+	–	+
Carbamazepine (Tegretol)	Average: 600 mg/day Range: 200-1200 mg/day	4-8 μg/mL	Drowsiness Dizziness Blurred vision Ataxia Gastrointestinal disturbance	Blood dyscrasia (rare)	+	–	+
Ethosuximide (Zarontin)	Average: 1000 mg/day Range: 500-2000 mg/day	40-100 μg/mL	Nausea Abdominal pain Drowsiness Personality change Headache	Rash Nephropathy Bone marrow depression	–	+	–
Clonazepam	Average: 3 mg/day Range: 1.5-20 mg/day	0.01-0.07 μg/mL	Drowsiness Dizziness Ataxia	Coma	+	+	+

*A plus sign (+) denotes that the drug is useful in the indicated form of seizure; a minus sign (–) indicates that it is not.

Modified from Dalessio DJ. Current concepts: Seizure disorders and pregnancy. N Engl J Med 1985; 312:559-63.

Table 49-3 Possible Causes of Increased Seizure Frequency during Pregnancy

Mechanism	Examples
Hormonal	Changes in levels of estrogen (proconvulsant) and progesterone (anticonvulsant)
Metabolic	Increased water and sodium retention
Psychological	Stress, sleep deprivation
Pharmacokinetics	Increase in liver metabolism, renal clearance, or volume of distribution
Physiologic	Decreased gastrointestinal absorption

international registries is attempting to expand the knowledge base regarding the dose-dependent effects of these agents during pregnancy.

Infants of mothers undergoing long-term antiepileptic therapy are at risk for a deficiency in vitamin K–dependent clotting factors. These infants may have a coagulation defect even when there is no clinical evidence of abnormal maternal coagulation. Antiepileptic agents that are enzyme inducing (e.g., phenytoin, phenobarbital, carbamazepine) are most likely to cause this problem. These drugs cross the placenta and may increase the rate of oxidative degradation of vitamin K in the fetus. Affected infants are at risk for neonatal hemorrhage and respond to vitamin K (1 mg) given intramuscularly at birth. Some physicians believe that women undergoing long-term antiepileptic therapy should receive vitamin K during the final month of pregnancy. However, data now suggest that there is inadequate evidence to support a recommendation of the routine administration of prenatal vitamin K to epileptic women exposed to enzyme-inducing antiepileptic agents.[100]

Anesthetic Management

Serum levels of antiepileptic drugs should be checked if therapeutic levels are known. If the patient experiences a seizure during labor, airway protection and support of ventilation are essential. Small doses of a benzodiazepine or sodium thiopental stop most seizures. Fetal bradycardia may necessitate immediate delivery.

Oral antiepileptic therapies should be continued whenever possible throughout the peripartum period. Unfortunately many of the agents are not available in parenteral forms. If oral agents cannot be taken, conversion to a parenteral agent such as phenytoin may be required. In general these agents have sedating properties, and some are known to induce liver enzymes; this feature could potentially lead to more rapid breakdown of anesthetic agents that are metabolized by the liver.[85]

There is no contraindication to the administration of neuraxial analgesia or anesthesia in epileptic parturients. In a retrospective review of 100 epileptic obstetric patients, 19 received general anesthesia, 48 received spinal anesthesia, 21 received epidural or caudal anesthesia, and 12 received pudendal nerve block.[101] Of the five women who had a postpartum seizure, four had received spinal anesthesia, and one had received general anesthesia with enflurane. No seizures occurred in patients who received epidural or caudal anesthesia. The investigators speculated that alterations in CSF dynamics may have predisposed these patients to postpartum seizures. Merrell and Koch[102] suggested that epidural anesthesia may have an anticonvulsant effect in preeclamptic women.

If general anesthesia is necessary, it seems prudent to avoid drugs such as ketamine, enflurane, and meperidine, which may lower the seizure threshold.[93,103] Sevoflurane has stronger epileptogenic properties than isoflurane, but co-administration of nitrous oxide and hyperventilation both counteract this effect.[104] Low doses of propofol also have been shown to cause activation of the electrocorticogram in epileptic patients, but at higher doses, burst suppression was induced.[105] Induction of general anesthesia can be performed with sodium thiopental and succinylcholine, and anesthesia may be maintained with a mixture of oxygen, nitrous oxide, and isoflurane. One study noted that some patients who receive phenytoin are resistant to vecuronium, but not to atracurium.[106] Some physicians recommend the avoidance of meperidine for postoperative analgesia because of one report of myoclonic seizures in several patients who had received this agent.[93]

MYOTONIA AND MYOTONIC DYSTROPHY

Myotonia is the general term used to describe prolonged contraction of certain muscles after stimulation, followed by a delay in relaxation. **Myotonic dystrophies** are a genetically and phenotypically heterogenous group of neuromuscular disorders caused by expansion defects in nucleotide sequences, principally on chromosome 19.[107-109] As the most common form of myotonic disorders, myotonic dystrophies manifest in two distinct forms with different nucleotide sequences, DM1 and DM2.[107] Both are multisystem disorders characterized by skeletal muscle weakness and myotonia, cardiac conduction abnormalities, cataracts, hypogammaglobulinemia, and insulin resistance. DM1 is generally more severe and exists in congenital, juvenile, and adult forms, whereas only an adult form has been identified for DM2.[108]

Myotonias can involve specific muscles, typically the hand, facial, masseter, and pretibial muscles, which become dystrophic or wasted. The disorder is slowly progressive, and continual deterioration occurs, with gradual involvement of pharyngeal and laryngeal muscles, proximal limb muscles, and the diaphragm. Uterine smooth muscle is affected, and cardiac conduction abnormalities are often present. Patients typically succumb to either pulmonary or cardiac failure.

Congenital myotonic dystrophy is a severe form of myotonic dystrophy (DM1) that manifests early in infancy with hypotonia and feeding difficulties.[110] Myotonia becomes apparent during the first few years of life. In most cases the mother has myotonic dystrophy. **Myotonia congenita** is a milder familial disorder characterized by myotonia of the skeletal muscles; multisystem involvement does not occur.[111] Unlike in myotonic dystrophy, cardiac abnormalities are not present. Smooth muscles are never affected. In some cases, muscle hypertrophy rather than wasting occurs. This disorder can be compatible with long life. It is distinguished from DM1 and DM2 by characteristic clinical features and the absence of significant histopathology in the muscle biopsy specimen. Myotonia congenita is characterized by chloride channel dysfunction.

Central core disease is a rare disorder in which muscle biopsies demonstrate the absence of oxidative enzyme activity in the longitudinal axis of the muscle fiber (i.e., the "central core"). Affected individuals have proximal muscle weakness and often scoliosis. This disease is caused by mutations in the skeletal muscle ryanodine receptor (RYR1) gene at chromosome 19q13.1, which has been implicated in the susceptibility to malignant hyperthermia.[112] Many patients with central core disease test positive for the malignant hyperthermia susceptibility trait on the intravenous contracture test and should therefore be considered at risk for malignant hyperthermia when exposed to triggering agents (i.e., succinylcholine, volatile halogenated agents).[112]

Drugs such as quinine and procainamide are most commonly used to relieve myotonic symptoms.[110,111] Corticosteroids, phenytoin, and tocainide also have been prescribed.

Obstetric Management

In patients with myotonic dystrophy, symptoms of weakness and myotonia usually remain unchanged; in a minority of women, symptoms worsen during pregnancy, but this worsening generally resolves after delivery. Antepartum evaluation should include pulmonary function testing to assess the severity of restrictive lung disease due to muscle wasting. Antepartum evaluation also should include an electrocardiogram, which may demonstrate conduction abnormalities.

There may be a higher risk of spontaneous abortion and preterm labor in patients with myotonic dystrophy.[113] Should preterm labor occur, caution should be used with the administration of pharmacologic tocolysis; Sholl et al.[114] reported that ritodrine tocolysis may provoke symptoms of myotonia. Muscle weakness may result in a prolonged second stage of labor and a higher incidence of instrumental vaginal delivery.[113] Poor uterine contractions may result in prolonged labor, uterine atony, and an increased risk of postpartum hemorrhage.[115,116] The neonate may present with respiratory distress if affected by congenital myotonic dystrophy.

There are reports of patients with myotonia congenita who experience temporary worsening of symptoms during pregnancy.[117] Obstetric problems have not been described, most likely because this disease involves skeletal muscle only; uterine smooth muscle is not affected in patients with myotonia congenita.

Anesthetic Management

Patients with myotonic disorders may be especially sensitive to the respiratory depressant effects of opioid analgesic and general anesthetic agents.[118] All sedatives should be used with caution; in some cases, opioids or sedatives may precipitate apnea. Thus, neuraxial anesthesia is preferred for labor and vaginal or cesarean delivery.

The prolonged contractions witnessed in patients with myotonia are due to an intrinsic muscle disorder that is not relieved by spinal or epidural anesthesia[119]; however, local infiltration with a local anesthetic agent can relieve the contractions. Cold external temperatures and shivering are known triggers of myotonia, so the patient should be kept warm. Although the possibility of respiratory depression may occur with the use of opioids (as discussed earlier), some anesthesiologists recommend the cautious administration of intrathecal or epidural opioids for their reported anti-shivering effect.[120] Patients with myotonic dystrophy have a high incidence of pulmonary complications after general anesthesia.[121]

If general anesthesia is required, depolarizing agents such as succinylcholine should be avoided because fasciculations may trigger myotonia,[122] thereby making ventilation and intubation difficult. By contrast, patients with myotonic dystrophy appear to have a normal response to nondepolarizing muscle relaxants. Regardless, careful neuromuscular monitoring is essential, particularly in those with significant baseline muscle weakness. Patients receiving quinine may require a smaller dose of a nondepolarizing muscle relaxant.[123] Although myotonic dystrophy has not been associated with an increased risk for malignant hyperthermia, some cases of malignant hyperthermia have been reported in patients with myotonia congenita and central core disease.[124] There is some debate regarding the susceptibility of myotonic patients to uncontrolled muscle metabolism and severe rhabdomyolysis in a pattern similar to, but not diagnostic for, malignant hyperthermia. Therefore, some anesthesiologists treat all myopathic patients as malignant hyperthermia-susceptible, whereas others take special precaution only for those myopathies, including central core disease and myotonia congenita, that have a documented association with malignant hyperthermia. Both spinal and epidural anesthesia have been used successfully in patients with myotonic dystrophy.[120,125,126]

MUSCULAR DYSTROPHY

Muscular dystrophy is a group of disorders characterized by a progressive degeneration of skeletal muscle with intact innervation.[127] Research on the subsarcolemmal muscle fiber protein dystrophin has led to a reclassification of these disorders. Analysis of dystrophin quality and quantity can be used diagnostically both before and during pregnancy and, in some cases, can identify carriers.

Duchenne and **Becker muscular dystrophies** are transmitted as X-linked recessive disorders and occur almost exclusively in males. The most common muscular dystrophies affecting females are fascioscapulohumeral dystrophy and limb-girdle dystrophies. **Fascioscapulohumeral dystrophy** is an autosomal dominant, slowly progressive disorder that primarily involves the muscles of the shoulders and face.[127] Over time the pelvic and pretibial muscles may be affected. Tachycardia and arrhythmias have been infrequently reported. **Limb-girdle dystrophies** involve slow degeneration of the shoulder and pelvic muscles.[127] The inheritance pattern and severity of these diseases are variable. Cardiac conduction disorders occur in some affected patients.

Obstetric Management

The classification of the muscular dystrophies is defined by DNA and dystrophin analysis. The presentations of these dystrophinopathies are variable, and the overall management is guided by the presence and severity of symptoms. If significant weakness is present, pulmonary function testing should be obtained to assess the extent of restrictive disease. An antepartum electrocardiogram should also be considered. Pregnant women with muscular dystrophies do not seem to have a higher incidence of adverse pregnancy outcomes, except for an increased incidence of operative delivery; the presence of severe pelvic wasting may necessitate an instrumental vaginal or cesarean delivery.[128,129]

Anesthetic Management

Neuraxial anesthetic techniques are preferred for labor analgesia and cesarean delivery anesthesia. Severe disease may result in both airway abnormalities and spinal deformities, which may complicate the administration of either general or neuraxial anesthesia. Severe kyphoscoliosis during pregnancy can prevent adaptive hyperventilation and might gradually promote respiratory insufficiency.[130] There is one report of the use of CSE anesthesia for cesarean delivery in a parturient who was a manifesting carrier of Duchenne muscular dystrophy. Whereas most females are asymptomatic carriers of the abnormal gene, approximately 2.5% of female carriers have symptoms of the disease—although usually in milder forms than those witnessed in men.[131] These patients are at risk for development of a hypermetabolic syndrome similar to malignant hyperthermia when they are exposed to succinylcholine and/or volatile halogenated anesthetic agents. The mechanism for this response is not well defined but may be related to the ability of these agents to exacerbate the instability and permeability of the dystrophin-deficient muscle membranes.[132] Therefore triggering agents should be avoided in patients with muscular dystrophy who require general anesthesia. In general, these patients have a normal response to nondepolarizing muscle relaxants, but careful neuromuscular monitoring is needed, especially in patients with severe muscle wasting.

THE PHAKOMATOSES (NEUROCUTANEOUS SYNDROMES)

The phakomatoses are congenital disorders that manifest as CNS and cutaneous abnormalities. Structures of ectodermal origin such as skin, nervous system, and eyes are commonly affected.[133] The diseases are classified into three main groups: neurofibromatoses, tuberous sclerosis, and angiomatoses with CNS abnormalities (Box 49-2). The most common phakomatoses are neurofibromatosis types 1 and 2, tuberous sclerosis, Sturge-Weber disease, and von Hippel–Lindau disease. Abnormalities of the brain and the spinal cord can have significant implications for anesthetic management.

BOX 49-2 Neurocutaneous Diseases with Common Ectodermal Derivations

Neurofibromatosis

- Type 1
- Type 2

Tuberous sclerosis

Cutaneous Angiomatosis with Central Nervous System Abnormalities

- Sturge-Weber syndrome: Meningo- or encephalo-facial angiomatosis with cerebral calcification
- Klippel-Trenaunay-Weber syndrome: Dermatomal hemangiomas and spinal vascular malformations, sometimes with limb hypertrophy
- Epidermal nevus syndrome
- Osler-Rendu-Weber disease: Familial telangiectasia
- von Hippel-Lindau disease: Hemangioblastoma of cerebellum and retina
- Louis-Bar disease: Ataxia-telangiectasia
- Fabry disease: Angiokeratosis corporis diffusum

From Adams RD, Victor M, Ropper AH. Principles of Neurology. 7th edition. New York, McGraw-Hill, 2001:1069-79.

Neurofibromatosis

Neurofibromatosis represents the result of excessive proliferation of neural crest elements such as Schwann cells, melanocytes, and fibroblasts. Clinical manifestations include hyperpigmented lesions (café-au-lait spots) accompanied by a variety of cutaneous and subcutaneous tumors. This disorder is now believed to exist in two distinct forms with gene abnormalities on two different chromosomes. The classic form, type 1, has an incidence of approximately 1 per 3000. The severity and progression of the disease is variable, with the neurologic symptoms depending on the location of the tumors. Intracranial tumors and paraspinal neurofibromas are a cause of concern and may require surgical excision. The risk of pheochromocytoma is greater in these patients.[134] Neurofibromatosis type 2, discovered more recently, is a less common form of the disease with fewer cutaneous lesions. Acoustic neuromas as well as other cranial or spinal neurofibromas, meningiomas, and gliomas may be present.

OBSTETRIC MANAGEMENT

Pregnancy may exacerbate the disease and cause an increase in tumor growth.[135] Regression occurs after delivery. Neurofibromatosis has been associated with a poor perinatal outcome[136]; however, a review of 247 pregnancies did not confirm the higher incidence of preeclampsia, preterm delivery, intrauterine growth restriction, and perinatal mortality reported previously.[137] A high cesarean delivery rate (36%) in this population of patients has been observed.[137] The presence of intracranial masses may be problematic during labor and vaginal delivery, particularly with the increased intracranial pressure (ICP) that occurs with the Valsalva maneuver during the second stage of labor.

ANESTHETIC MANAGEMENT

An anesthesiologist should thoroughly assess the patient's current symptoms and known lesions, particularly if they involve neck and laryngeal tumors; such tumors are common, particularly in patients with neurofibromatosis type 1.[138]

Neuraxial anesthetic techniques can be used for labor analgesia and operative anesthesia in most patients with the disorder. However, severe kyphoscoliosis due to the presence of paraspinal tumors may complicate the administration of neuraxial anesthesia in some patients. Patients may have asymptomatic paraspinal or intracranial tumors. For this reason, some authors have opined that neuraxial anesthesia should be administered only after careful clinical and radiographic evaluations have been performed.[139]

If general anesthesia is required, the use of muscle relaxants has been controversial, given the conflicting dose response reports in these patients. Both greater sensitivity and less sensitivity to succinylcholine, as well as an increased sensitivity to nondepolarizing agents, have been reported.[140-142] One study noted minimal alterations in dose response; the investigators recommended no alterations in the use and dose of both depolarizing and nondepolarizing agents in these patients.[140]

Tuberous Sclerosis

Tuberous sclerosis is a phakomatosis characterized by epilepsy, mental retardation, and adenoma sebaceum. The brain shows abnormal growth of glial cells in hamartomas called tubers.[133] Hamartomatous tumors can occur in multiple organs, including the heart, kidneys, liver, and lungs. The inheritance pattern is autosomal dominant with a variable expression, and the disease is slowly progressive.

OBSTETRIC AND ANESTHETIC MANAGEMENT

There are few reports of pregnancy in women with tuberous sclerosis. The obstetrician and anesthesiologist should know the locations of lesions in an individual patient. Hemorrhage into the tumors, renal failure, and hypertension may complicate pregnancy.[143] Renal involvement seems to represent an important prognostic factor during pregnancy, and spontaneous rupture of a renal angiomyolipoma has been reported.[144] Although published reports have included several patients who required cesarean delivery, the authors made no specific mention of anesthetic management or complications.[143,144]

Cutaneous Angiomatosis with Central Nervous System Abnormalities

One group of phakomatoses consists of disorders in which a cutaneous vascular anomaly is accompanied by CNS abnormalities (see Box 49-2).[145] There are few reports of pregnancy in patients with these disorders. Patients may present with neurologic problems related to hemangiomas of the CNS. Cesarean delivery with epidural anesthesia has been reported in a patient with spinal hemangiomas.[146]

LANDRY-GUILLAIN-BARRÉ SYNDROME

Acute idiopathic polyneuritis, also known as *Landry-Guillain-Barré syndrome,* is an inflammatory demyelinating illness with a reported incidence of approximately 1 case per 100,000 persons per year.[147] In 60% of patients a viral illness precedes neurologic symptoms by 1 to 3 weeks. Cases also have occurred after the administration of anti-rabies and influenza vaccines.

Patients present with weakness that involves first the limbs, followed by the trunk, neck, and facial muscles. Loss of reflexes, total motor paralysis, and respiratory failure can occur. Sensory loss typically is not detectable. Symptoms peak at 2 to 3 weeks. The majority of patients recover completely; approximately 10% have severe residual disability. Approximately 3% of patients do not survive.[147]

Nerve conduction studies show a slowing of conduction. Pathologic changes include lymphoid cellular infiltration and areas of demyelination that most likely result from a cell-mediated immunologic reaction against peripheral nerves. Autonomic nervous system involvement and dysfunction may occur.

The treatment is largely supportive and may include mechanical ventilatory support. Plasmapheresis reduces the duration of illness if it is instituted during the evolution phase, and this therapeutic modality has been used safely during pregnancy.[148,149]

Obstetric Management

The incidence of this syndrome appears to be lower in pregnant women than in nonpregnant women. Using data from several nationwide registries, Jiang et al.[150] found that the age-adjusted relative risk of Guillain-Barré syndrome appears to be lower during pregnancy and then increases during the 3 months after delivery. In severe cases, the risk of preterm labor is increased, and neurologic deterioration may occur after delivery.[151] Termination of pregnancy does not appear advantageous for the course of the disease; indications for induction of labor include autonomic dysfunction. Instrumental vaginal delivery may be necessary.[151]

Anesthetic Management

Anesthetic management depends on the status of the patient at the time of delivery. Case reports have documented the use of both epidural and CSE anesthesia in parturients with Guillain-Barré syndrome.[18,152,153] However, some authorities have expressed concern about the use of epidural anesthesia in these patients. Steiner et al.[154] implicated epidural anesthesia as a trigger of Guillain-Barré syndrome in four patients, although a cause-and-effect relationship was not established. Wiertlewski et al.[152] reported the case of a pregnant woman presenting with Guillain-Barré syndrome whose neurologic status worsened immediately after delivery with epidural anesthesia. These authors speculated that the worsening status may have resulted from either immunologic changes associated with pregnancy or anesthetic toxicity.

If general anesthesia is necessary in a patient with Guillain-Barré syndrome, succinylcholine most likely should be avoided because of the risk of hyperkalemia in patients with acute muscle wasting.

The parturient who presents with a history of remote Guillain-Barré syndrome may have persistent diminished respiratory reserve, even in the absence of obvious residual disability.[155] Pulmonary evaluation should be considered before the administration of anesthesia. Approximately 5% of patients experience a relapse, and a small number of these go on to have a chronic disorder.

POLIO

Poliomyelitis is a disease caused by a picornavirus that is transmitted by the fecal-oral route. Most cases are asymptomatic or are accompanied by mild systemic symptoms. More severe symptoms and nervous system involvement occur in approximately 1% of patients.[156] Motor neurons in the cerebral cortex, brainstem, and spinal cord are affected. Asymmetric flaccid paralysis develops over several days. Bulbar paralysis is more common in young adults. The CSF findings are consistent with viral meningitis. Recovery occurs 3 to 4 months after onset, most likely from motor axon terminal sprouting that reinnervates the previously denervated muscle fibers; however, residual deficits often persist.

A slowly progressive syndrome called **postpoliomyelitis muscular atrophy** may develop as many as 40 years after the acute illness. Klingman et al.[157] speculated that the increased functional demands on the surviving neurons or the motor axon terminal sprouts eventually result in their death. Others believe that this syndrome results from a reactivation of the initial viral infection.[158]

Obstetric Management

Currently, polio is a cause for concern only in countries with ineffective vaccination programs. If a woman should require vaccination during pregnancy, oral polio vaccine does not appear to have harmful effects on fetal development.[159]

A history of previous poliomyelitis will affect labor and delivery only if residual deficits have resulted in pelvic asymmetry or an inability to push effectively during the second stage of labor.[160]

Anesthetic Management

In all parturients with a history of polio, a complete preanesthetic evaluation should be performed for the presence of respiratory impairment, sleep apnea, swallowing difficulties, and other neurologic and motor deficits.[161] Some physicians have feared that administration of neuraxial anesthesia might cause reactivation of the virus and postpoliomyelitis muscular atrophy in patients with a history of poliomyelitis. Crawford et al.[18] reported the successful use of epidural analgesia with no adverse complications in patients with a history of polio. There is no evidence that neuraxial analgesia or anesthesia will worsen symptoms in these patients.

For the patient with polio in whom general anesthesia is needed, some anesthesiologists have suggested the use of a decreased dose of a short-acting nondepolarizing muscle relaxant in lieu of succinylcholine, which may provoke the occurrence of severe acute hyperkalemia.[162]

BRAIN NEOPLASMS

Intracranial neoplasms vary in incidence, histology, clinical presentation, and prognosis (Table 49-4).[163] Brain neoplasms in pregnant women appear to occur with the same relative frequency as in nonpregnant women; however, the physiologic alterations that occur during pregnancy can have profound implications for symptomatology and management.

TABLE 49-4 Classification of Brain Tumors in Women

Histologic Type	Percentage of all Diagnosed Tumors
Benign	
Meningioma	35
Schwannoma	7
Pituitary neoplasms	7
Malignant	
Gliomas:	
Low-grade astrocytoma	3
Glioblastoma multiforme (plus high-grade astrocytoma)	23
Other astrocytoma	8
Other	5
Lymphoma	2
Medulloblastoma	2
Other brain neoplasms	8

Gliomas are the most common intracranial neoplasms. They account for approximately 39% of all primary intracranial tumors.[163] These tumors result from anaplasia of astrocytes and vary in invasive potential. This category of tumors includes glioblastoma multiforme, astrocytoma, ependymoma, and oligodendrocytoma. Glioblastoma multiforme is the most lethal, whereas oligodendrocytomas have a better prognosis.

Meningiomas account for 28% of all primary brain tumors.[163] These benign tumors originate from the dura mater or arachnoid. Surgery typically is curative.

Pituitary adenomas account for 7% of diagnosed primary brain neoplasms, but postmortem studies suggest the occurrence of a significantly higher incidence.[163] Only a fraction of these tumors cause symptoms; owing to the location of such tumors, however, the symptoms may include visual field deficits. Tumors may secrete prolactin, growth hormone, or adrenocorticotropic hormone. Growth of pituitary tumors is physically limited by the sella turcica of the sphenoid bone and, in a cephalad orientation, the hypothalamus. Compression of the hypothalamus or pituitary may result in respective decreases in the production or release of vasopressin, leading to diabetes insipidus. Bromocriptine often provides effective medical therapy for prolactin-secreting adenomas. Radiation and surgery also represent effective therapy, and the prognosis is generally good.

Schwannomas, also called **neurinomas,** account for 7% of all brain tumors. These lesions originate in the Schwann cells surrounding the nerve.[163] Clinical presentation depends on the location of the tumor. Acoustic neuromas result when the eighth nerve is involved; these lesions are often seen in patients with neurofibromatosis. The treatment is surgical excision.

Metastatic carcinomas account for a significant number of brain neoplasms.[163] The most common primary cancers are those of the lung, breast, and colon. Prognosis and therapy depend on the tumor of origin.

All brain tumors may share several pathophysiologic features. Neurologic deficits can result from the mass effect, even if the tumor is benign. Tumor enlargement also may result in increased ICP. Brain edema is a prominent feature of cerebral neoplasms; it may result from a combination of vasogenic and cytotoxic mechanisms.

The potential for herniation must be considered in any patient with a mass lesion. The brain is divided into three basic compartments. The falx cerebri separates the cerebrum into right and left halves, and the tentorium isolates the cerebellum. High pressure from a mass can cause shifts from one compartment to another with devastating effects.

Obstetric Management

The incidence of primary brain tumors first manifesting in pregnancy does not appear to be greater than that in aged-matched, nonpregnant women.[164] Approximately 9% of patients with **choriocarcinoma** have brain metastases at the time of diagnosis.[165] In one epidemiologic study, patients with primary brain tumors had a higher incidence of spontaneous abortion, possibly because of hormonal factors.[166]

Although pregnancy does not affect the incidence of brain tumors, some of these lesions appear to grow faster during pregnancy. Visual field defects from pituitary adenomas worsen as a result of tumor enlargement during pregnancy. Symptoms may improve during the postpartum period.[167] Edema and the increased blood volume of vascular tumors may account for some of these observations.[168] Hormonal effects also may play a role because estrogen and progesterone receptors are present in meningiomas and some gliomas.[168]

Diagnosis during pregnancy requires intracranial imaging. In general, MRI is preferred because it avoids the use of ionizing radiation. MRI also uses gadolinium-based contrast agents that do not contain iodine, have a better margin of safety than radiographic contrast agents, and have not been shown to have adverse fetal effects at conventional doses.[164]

Management during pregnancy depends on the nature of the tumor. Surgery for benign tumors (e.g., meningiomas) with mild symptoms can often be delayed until after delivery. Women with more aggressive, malignant tumors or with tumors causing seizures or severe visual impairment may require surgery during pregnancy. Delay in treatment of high-grade CNS tumors can result in acute neurologic deterioration. Delivery may be recommended as soon as reasonable fetal survival can be expected, sometimes by cesarean delivery immediately prior to neurosurgery. For women with pregnancies far from fetal viability, radiation therapy or stereotactic radiosurgery can be considered.[163] Systemic chemotherapy can pose significant hazards to the fetus, especially when administered during the first trimester. Cranial radiotherapy is generally administered first in cases of aggressive neoplasm, but even radiotherapy has some fetal effects, particularly during the first trimester.[164] Some women may opt for surgery after an elective abortion.

In the normal parturient, CSF pressure may increase significantly with painful uterine contractions.[169] In patients with an intracranial mass lesion, this situation could result in an increased risk of herniation. The location and size of the tumor should be assessed in the individual patient so that an appropriate, multispecialty provider plan can be designed. In general, either a pain-free second stage (with instrumental vaginal delivery to avoid pushing) or cesarean delivery may be appropriate.[170]

Anesthetic Management

The optimal anesthetic technique for labor analgesia and cesarean delivery anesthesia in the patient with an intracranial tumor is controversial. Epidural analgesia prevents the increase in ICP that can result with pushing during the second stage of labor.[171] However, there is concern that an unintentional dural puncture might result in herniation in women with increased ICP. Several published reports have described the successful use of epidural analgesia during labor in women with an intracranial neoplasm[171,172]; in addition, the use of spinal anesthesia in a patient with a glioblastoma for an emergency cesarean delivery has been described.[173] However, a fatal brain herniation has been reported in a parturient with an occult brain tumor, which occurred after an unintentional dural puncture associated with an attempted epidural catheter placement.[174] Many anesthesiologists favor general anesthesia for cesarean delivery in the patient with a brain neoplasm[175]; however, potential disadvantages of general anesthesia include (1) the loss of verbal and motor responses that facilitate neurologic assessment and (2) the risks of increased ICP with intubation and extubation.

Wang and Paech[176] have reviewed specific elements of the anesthetic management of the pregnant patient undergoing neurosurgery, many of which are also relevant to the patient with an intracranial tumor undergoing cesarean delivery. For either cesarean delivery or intracranial surgery, the induction of general anesthesia may consist of the administration of sodium thiopental and a rapid-acting nondepolarizing agent. (Some anesthesiologists avoid succinylcholine because it may cause a transient increase in ICP, but others consider this effect to be clinically insignificant.[176]) A combination of isoflurane, nitrous oxide, and low-dose fentanyl is commonly used for maintenance of anesthesia. The fetal heart rate (FHR) should be monitored during nonobstetric (intracranial) surgery when possible.

To preserve cerebral and uteroplacental perfusion, hemodynamic stability should be maintained through appropriate fluid administration, avoidance of aortocaval compression, the prophylactic or early use of vasopressor drugs, and intra-arterial blood pressure monitoring instituted before induction of anesthesia.[176] In general, blood pressure should be kept close to baseline measurements; in the setting of an emergency neurosurgical procedure in a patient with increased ICP, a drop in blood pressure may compromise cerebral perfusion.[176] Fluid management for intracranial surgery should involve administration of isonatremic, isotonic, and glucose-free intravenous solutions to reduce the risk of cerebral edema and hyperglycemia.[177] Mannitol administered to a pregnant woman slowly accumulates in the fetus, leading to fetal hyperosmolality and the subsequent physiologic changes of reduced fetal lung fluid production, decreased fetal urine production, and increased fetal plasma sodium concentrations[178,179]; however, mannitol in doses of 0.25 to 0.5 mg/kg has been used in individual case reports and appears to be associated with good maternal and fetal outcomes.[176] Furosemide is an alternative diuretic that also should be administered cautiously.[176]

There may be some conflict between maternal and fetal interests in the patient with increased ICP. Mechanical hyperventilation often is used to reduce the increased ICP that occurs in nonpregnant patients with a brain tumor or brain injury. However, prophylactic mechanical hyperventilation of head-injured patients to a $PaCO_2$ less than 25 mm Hg has been associated with adverse patient outcomes.[180] Ventilation increases during normal pregnancy, resulting in a maternal $PaCO_2$ of 28 to 32 mm Hg. However, additional hyperventilation and hypocapnia may cause uterine artery vasoconstriction and a leftward shift in the maternal oxyhemoglobin dissociation curve.[181] For pregnant women with an acute increase in ICP, Wang and Paech[176] have suggested a target $PaCO_2$ range of 25 to 30 mm Hg; however, data are insufficient to support evidence-based recommendations specific for pregnant women undergoing intracranial surgery. In pregnant patients with increased ICP, we recommend maintenance of maternal $PaCO_2$ in the middle or at the lower end of the normal range for pregnancy (28 to 32 mm Hg). Management should be individualized according to the clinical setting.

Other ventilatory management measures that assist in the control of ICP include (1) the use of posture (slight head-up position) to potentially reduce peak airway pressures and (2) the use of low tidal volumes during intermittent positive-pressure ventilation.[176]

IDIOPATHIC INTRACRANIAL HYPERTENSION

Idiopathic intracranial hypertension, previously referred to as *pseudotumor cerebri* or *benign intracranial hypertension*, is defined as an increase in ICP with a normal CSF composition, in the absence of hydrocephalus or a mass lesion.[182] The disorder most often occurs in obese women of childbearing age, suggesting that hormonal factors may play a role in the pathophysiology. The majority of patients present with a headache, and in some cases visual symptoms occur. Over time the disorder generally improves, but there is a small risk of recurrence.

Traditional therapies have varied in efficacy; they include serial lumbar punctures and the administration of a carbonic anhydrase inhibitor and/or corticosteroid. Lumboperitoneal shunting may be required in severe cases with visual symptoms. Weight loss appears to improve the condition.

Interaction with Pregnancy

Symptoms of idiopathic intracranial hypertension worsen during pregnancy in 50% of cases and typically improve after delivery.[183] However, in the presence of severe maternal symptoms, the placement of an intracranial shunt can result in clinical improvement and normal perinatal outcomes.[184] Overall, this disorder does not seem to adversely affect maternal and perinatal outcomes.[185]

Anesthetic Management

Deliberate lumbar puncture represents a common form of treatment for idiopathic intracranial hypertension. Cerebellar tonsillar herniation does not occur because of the uniform, global increase in ICP. Paruchuri et al.[186] noted that there are only two published cases of cerebellar tonsillar herniation after diagnostic lumbar puncture in patients with this disorder. Both patients had presented with severe headache, neck pain exacerbated by movement, and focal neurologic deficits. In the absence of these signs and symptoms, the anesthesia provider can safely provide neuraxial analgesia or anesthesia.[187]

Some anesthesiologists recommend the administration of general anesthesia for cesarean delivery in patients with lumboperitoneal shunt. They contend that local anesthetic agents that reach the subarachnoid space may escape into the peritoneum, making it difficult to achieve adequate anesthesia. Moreover, the performance of neuraxial anesthesia may result in trauma to the shunt catheter. However, Bédard et al.[188] reported the successful administration of epidural anesthesia in a preeclamptic patient with a lumboperitoneal shunt that had been placed for the treatment of idiopathic intracranial hypertension. Preoperative radiographic examination may help the anesthesia provider avoid needle placement near the catheter, although such imaging was not used in this published case. Anesthesia via an intrathecal catheter has been used for both vaginal and cesarean delivery in parturients with idiopathic intracranial hypertension and a lumboperitoneal shunt; in one case the intrathecal catheter provided both labor analgesia and temporary control of ICP.[189,190]

MATERNAL HYDROCEPHALUS WITH SHUNT

Hydrocephalus results from a variety of conditions. The most common are intracranial hemorrhage in preterm infants, fetal and neonatal infections, the Arnold-Chiari malformation, aqueductal stenosis, and the Dandy-Walker syndrome.[191] The Arnold-Chiari malformation consists of extension of a portion of cerebellar tissue into the cervical canal, with progressive hydrocephalus. The Dandy-Walker syndrome occurs with failure of development of the midline of the cerebellum, with resultant hydrocephalus of the fourth ventricle.

Ventriculoatrial or ventriculoperitoneal shunt catheters are placed for the treatment of many of these disorders. Because of advances in neonatal and neurosurgical care, hydrocephalic women with CSF shunt catheters are reaching childbearing age in increasing numbers.

Obstetric Management

Obstetric management depends on the presence of other medical and neurologic conditions. In general, although maternal shunt dependency carries a relatively high risk of complications for some patients, proper management can lead to normal pregnancy and delivery.[192] Neurologic complications may occur in as many as 76% of pregnant women with preexisting shunts.[193] They include severe headache, shunt obstruction, and increased ICP. Most symptoms resolve postpartum.

The mother with neurologic stability can undergo labor and vaginal delivery. Elective cesarean delivery is recommended only if the symptoms are severe or lead to neurologic instability.[193]

Anesthetic Management

Anesthetic management of the patient with hydrocephalus may depend on the location of the shunt. There has been concern that some of the local anesthetic agent entering the CSF may escape into the atrium or peritoneum, resulting in inadequate analgesia. However, both epidural and intrathecal anesthesia have been used in patients with lumboperitoneal, ventriculoatrial, and ventriculoperitoneal shunts (as discussed earlier).[188-190] Because of the risk of shunt infection, some physicians recommend preoperative use of a prophylactic antibiotic regimen similar to that used to prevent bacterial endocarditis.

INTRACEREBRAL HEMORRHAGE

Cerebrovascular disease during pregnancy can result from three major mechanisms—hemorrhage, arterial infarction, and venous thrombosis. Intracerebral hemorrhage, which is most commonly associated with an arteriovenous malformation or aneurysm (Figure 49-3), has been calculated to occur with a frequency of 7.1 per 100,000 person-years for pregnant women, compared with 5.0 per 100,000 person-years for nonpregnant women in a large database of inpatient hospitalizations within the age range of 15 to 44 years.[194] Intracerebral hemorrhage accounted for 7.1% of all pregnancy-related deaths in this database.

In a case series of 14 parturients, the major causes of intracerebral hemorrhage were arteriovenous malformation, severe preeclampsia or eclampsia, cocaine use, and primary CNS vasculopathy.[195] Holcomb and Petrie[196] concluded that cerebral aneurysms and arteriovenous malformations manifest in approximately equal proportions during pregnancy. Dias and Sekhar[197] reviewed 154 published cases of intracranial subarachnoid hemorrhage due to identified intracranial lesions during pregnancy. They noted that aneurysms were responsible for intracranial hemorrhage in 77% of the patients, with the remaining cases attributed to arteriovenous malformations.

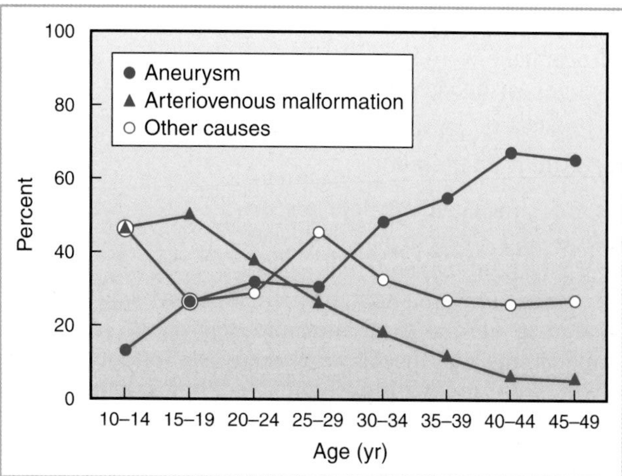

FIGURE 49-3 Relative probability of major causes of subarachnoid hemorrhage for women by age. (From Donaldson JO. Neurology of Pregnancy. 2nd edition. London, WB Saunders, 1989:139.)

Most authors have reported a progressive increase in the incidence of aneurysm bleeding throughout gestation, which appears to correspond with the physiologic increase in blood volume.[197] There is some evidence that aneurysms are most likely to rupture during the late stages of pregnancy and up to 6 weeks postpartum.[197] Because of the risk of rebleeding, a pregnant patient with a history of a bleeding aneurysm that is deemed operable generally is referred for surgical aneurysm clipping. Surgical management of aneurysms during pregnancy has been associated with significantly lower maternal and fetal mortality in affected patients.[197] Once a curative surgical procedure has been performed, it is unnecessary to treat this patient differently from a patient without an aneurysm during labor and delivery. If an aneurysm is found incidentally during pregnancy and has not bled, management should be based on the specific clinical situation, including aneurysm size and location. Two cases of successful endovascular treatment of ruptured intracranial aneurysms in parturients have been reported; this approach avoids a craniotomy.[198]

Bleeding from arteriovenous malformations has been reported to occur with equal or greater frequency with advancing gestational age.[197,199] Whether pregnancy increases the risk of bleeding from an arteriovenous malformation is controversial.[200] Arteriovenous malformations have been reported to have a 25% chance of rebleeding during the same pregnancy.[199] The data regarding surgical management during pregnancy varies, with some reports noting that surgery does not significantly affect maternal or fetal mortality.[197] As with aneurysms, a multidisciplinary decision-making process allows planning based on the location of the lesion, the duration of pregnancy, and the relative risks of interventional and noninterventional methods of management.

Obstetric Management

If the lesion has been treated surgically, the patient requires no special care during labor and delivery. For an untreated aneurysm or arteriovenous malformation, hemodynamic stress during labor and delivery should be minimized. Current data do not demonstrate a definite advantage of cesarean delivery over assisted vaginal delivery.[196,197] For labor and vaginal delivery, epidural analgesia and low outlet forceps or vacuum assistance may be used to shorten the second stage of labor and attenuate fluctuations in blood pressure. The decision about the method of delivery should be based on the individual patient and her pregnancy history.

Anesthetic Management

If the parturient has undergone surgical repair of either an aneurysm or arteriovenous malformation, anesthetic management need not differ from that for other obstetric patients. The parturient with an untreated lesion should be managed to maintain hemodynamic stability and avoid hypertension. Neuraxial analgesic and anesthetic techniques are generally preferred.[201-204] If vaginal delivery is planned, epidural or CSE analgesia should be considered. For cesarean delivery, either epidural or spinal anesthesia can be used. Some anesthesiologists contend that epidural anesthesia provides greater hemodynamic stability and is thus preferred for cesarean delivery.[202]

In some cases, the neurosurgeon may ligate or excise the vascular lesion *during* pregnancy, *before* delivery.[205] There are several published cases of neurovascular intracranial surgery during pregnancy.[206-208] The anesthesiologist should consider the principles of anesthetic management for pregnant women undergoing nonobstetric surgery (see Chapter 17) as well as the special considerations for pregnant women undergoing neurosurgery (as discussed earlier).[176] It is critical to maintain stable blood pressure during induction of anesthesia, laryngoscopy, and intubation. The patient should receive adequate sedation before and after arrival in the operating room. Placement of an intra-arterial catheter is mandatory. The anesthesiologist may attenuate the hypertensive response to laryngoscopy and intubation by intravenous administration of esmolol, labetalol, lidocaine, nitroglycerin, or nitroprusside. An assistant should maintain cricoid pressure during induction of anesthesia.

Succinylcholine can be used for intubation. It seems prudent to give a defasciculating dose of a nondepolarizing muscle relaxant before the administration of succinylcholine. Regardless of the choice of muscle relaxant, it is critical that laryngoscopy and intubation not be performed until the patient is anesthetized adequately. The risks of hypertension and intracranial bleeding as well as the risk of aspiration should be considered during induction of anesthesia.

The anesthesiologist may maintain anesthesia with nitrous oxide and modest doses of isoflurane and an opioid. Aggressive maternal hyperventilation may result in decreased uterine blood flow (as discussed earlier). However, the anesthesiologist may use modest hyperventilation (e.g., Pa_{CO_2} of 28 to 30 mm Hg) as needed to reduce maternal ICP. The anesthesiologist should maintain left uterine displacement in patients beyond 20 weeks' gestation. Intraoperative FHR monitoring allows assessment of the fetal response to maternal general anesthesia and hyperventilation. At many institutions, including my own, intraoperative FHR monitoring is used beginning at 24 weeks' gestation, which corresponds with the onset of extrauterine neonatal viability. Typically an obstetric nurse monitors the FHR tracing during surgery and requests obstetric consultation if needed. An adverse change in the FHR tracing should prompt the anesthesiologist to ensure adequate maternal oxygenation, ventilation, and perfusion.

Use of deliberate hypotension may compromise uteroplacental perfusion. However, several authors have reported the safe use of deliberate hypotension during neurovascular intracranial surgery in pregnant women.[206-208] There is no consensus regarding an acceptable or safe level of hypotension in these patients. There also is no consensus on the ideal method for achieving deliberate hypotension in pregnant women. Prolonged administration of large doses of nitroprusside may result in fetal cyanide toxicity[209]; however, short-term administration of nitroprusside appears safe.[210,211] Intraoperative FHR monitoring allows assessment of the FHR response to deliberate hypotension. Endovascular treatment with general anesthesia avoids the need for craniotomy and deliberate hypotension.[198]

In some cases, the obstetrician and neurosurgeon may perform a combined procedure (e.g., a cesarean delivery followed by ligation or excision of the neurovascular lesion).[212-215] Principles of anesthetic management are similar to those described earlier for intracranial neurovascular surgery during pregnancy.

Rarely, anesthesiologists may provide care for pregnant women who are receiving **extended somatic support** after brain death. Powner and Bernstein[215] reviewed 11 reports of 10 cases of brain death during pregnancy, in which somatic support was provided until successful delivery. Intracranial hemorrhage was the cause of maternal brain death in 6 of the 10 patients. The longest period of support was 107 days, from 15 to 32 weeks' gestation. All 10 infants survived. The authors concluded that preservation of uteroplacental blood flow is the most important priority during extended somatic support, but they acknowledged that this goal is difficult to achieve because of hemodynamic instability, the high prevalence of infection, and other adverse consequences (e.g., diabetes insipidus) associated with brain death.

CEREBRAL VEIN THROMBOSIS

Thrombosis of the cerebral veins and sinuses most often affects young adults and children; approximately 75% of the adult patients are women.[216] Thromboses commonly involve the cavernous sinus, lateral sinus, sagittal sinus, or cortical veins. Thrombosis of the cerebral veins causes venous obstruction with local effects, whereas thrombosis of the major sinuses causes intracranial hypertension. A prothrombotic risk factor or a direct cause can be identified in approximately 85% of patients. An obstetric delivery may be a precipitating factor for sinus thrombosis in a person with a genetically increased risk.[216]

Primary cerebral cortical vein thrombosis is the type of thrombosis most often seen in the parturient. The incidence of cerebral vein thrombosis in the parturient has been estimated to be approximately 12 cases per 100,000 deliveries in developed countries; the incidence appears to be higher in some developing countries. Cerebral vein thrombosis occurs more frequently during the last trimester of pregnancy and in the second and third postpartum weeks.[217,218] The etiology is unclear; however, pregnancy may predispose patients to this condition because of at least two factors.[218] First, traumatic damage to the endothelial lining of vessels may occur during the second stage of labor. Second, pregnancy is a hypercoagulable state. Mechanical causes of sinus thrombosis may include head injury and lumbar puncture.[219,220] It has been postulated that low CSF pressure after a lumbar puncture causes the brain to shift downward, resulting in traction on the cortical veins and sinuses.

Patients with cerebral vein thrombosis may present with headache, nausea and vomiting, and blurred vision. In more severe cases, lateralizing neurologic signs, lethargy, and seizures may occur. In severe cases, transtentorial herniation due to a focal mass effect can occur.

Care should be taken to differentiate cerebral vein thrombosis from post–dural puncture headache (PDPH). In general, the headache associated with cerebral vein thrombosis is more diffuse in location.[219,220] Earlier teaching suggested that the headache does not vary with position, but a 2007 review concluded that the nature of the headache may change over time and that the headache often manifests "as a positional [postural] headache that overlaps the usual timing ... and treatment of PDPH in the parturient."[221]

Diagnosis can be confirmed by MRI with associated venography. Lockhart and Baysinger[221] noted that "anticoagulation seems to be the treatment of choice worldwide, but the indications for its use remain somewhat controversial, given that approximately 50% of cases are associated with hemorrhagic cerebral infarcts." They suggested that the treatment is primarily supportive, although endovascular thrombolysis and surgical thrombectomy may be considered in severe cases. However, some (but not all) studies have suggested that use of anticoagulation is associated with better outcomes, and Wasay et al.[222] have recommended performance of randomized multicenter trials to compare anticoagulation with direct thrombolysis or other interventions.

Some patients with cerebral vein thrombosis may require anticonvulsant therapy. In some cases, residual neurologic deficits and seizures may persist.

Obstetric and Anesthetic Management

Cerebral vein thrombosis rarely occurs before delivery; however, such cases, when associated with maternal neurologic instability and fetal deterioration, may necessitate urgent delivery. Maternal anticoagulation contraindicates the administration of neuraxial anesthesia. The anesthesia provider should avoid systemic hypotension, which may reduce cerebral perfusion pressure and blood flow to injured areas already subjected to marginal perfusion. If the patient has an asymmetric cerebral hematoma, dural puncture may precipitate herniation of the brainstem. Thus it seems preferable to give general anesthesia for cesarean delivery, with special attention to the treatment of increased ICP.

MOTOR NEURON DISORDERS

Motor neuron diseases are a group of disorders characterized by progressive muscular weakness and atrophy. These disorders may affect motor function alone or in conjunction with sensory deficits. There are few data on the course of these disorders in pregnant women. This discussion focuses on three of these disorders, amyotrophic lateral sclerosis and primary spinal muscular atrophy, which are pure motor neuron disorders, and peroneal muscular atrophy, which involves both motor and sensory degeneration. Currently there is no cure for any of these degenerative disorders.

Amyotrophic Lateral Sclerosis

Amyotrophic lateral sclerosis involves progressive degeneration of anterior horn cells with progressive atrophic weakness and hyperreflexia. Patients typically succumb to respiratory failure within 6 years.

This disease is seen more often in patients older than 50 years, but there are several reports of this disorder in pregnant women.[223,224] Physicians should assess and frequently monitor the patient's respiratory compromise during pregnancy and throughout the peripartum period. Epidural analgesia and anesthesia have been used in these patients without evidence of worsened neurologic function postoperatively.[225,226] If general anesthesia is required, patients with amyotrophic lateral sclerosis may be sensitive to the effects of nondepolarizing muscle relaxants.[227]

Spinal Muscular Atrophy

Like amyotrophic lateral sclerosis, primary spinal muscular atrophy involves degeneration of anterior horn cells. However, affected patients tend to be younger, and this disorder progresses more slowly. Some types are hereditary. Spinal muscular atrophy tends to involve mainly the spinal cord, without involvement of the corticospinal tract. Marked kyphoscoliosis combined with truncal and limb weakness, especially involving the proximal musculature, can occur and result in significant ventilatory limitations.

Spinal muscular atrophy may be associated with an increased incidence of preterm labor.[228] One series noted that pregnancy was associated with an exacerbation of muscle weakness in 8 of 12 patients.[228] Epidural and spinal analgesia and anesthesia have been used successfully in patients with this disorder.[229,230]

Peroneal Muscular Atrophy

Peroneal muscular atrophy, also known as *Charcot-Marie-Tooth disease*, includes several inherited peripheral motor and sensory neuropathies and is one of the most common inherited neuromuscular diseases.[231] It involves a progressive sensory and motor degeneration of peripheral nerves and roots. The peroneal nerve is affected early. The disorder progresses to involve all the nerves and muscles of the legs and finally the hands. Paresthesias are typically present. Restrictive pulmonary impairment, phrenic nerve dysfunction, diaphragmatic dysfunction, thoracic cage abnormalities, and sleep apnea have been described in association with peroneal muscular atrophy. Vocal cord dysfunction, possibly due to laryngeal nerve involvement, can also be present. Assessment of peripartum respiratory function is essential.

At least one report has suggested that peroneal muscular atrophy worsens during pregnancy, perhaps because of fluid retention and edema around the nerves.[232] A review of 108 deliveries reported that women with this disorder have higher rates of abnormal fetal presentation, emergency operative delivery, and postpartum bleeding.[233] Both neuraxial anesthesia and general anesthesia have been used for delivery.[234] Careful titration of muscle relaxants is essential if general anesthesia is employed.

ISOLATED MONONEUROPATHIES DURING PREGNANCY

Pregnancy is associated with an increased incidence of several specific mononeuropathies: Bell's palsy, carpal tunnel syndrome, and meralgia paresthetica.

Bell's Palsy

Bell's palsy is a syndrome of acute onset that involves paralysis of the facial nerve. The incidence during pregnancy is approximately 3.3 times higher than that in nonpregnant women, which in turn is 2 to 4 times higher than that in men.[235] Some studies have suggested an association with preeclampsia, which may be based on increased interstitial edema.[236]

One study noted that pregnant patients whose symptoms progressed to complete facial paralysis within 10 days of onset were less likely to experience satisfactory recovery than a comparison group of nonpregnant patients.[237] Patients may benefit from a short course of prednisone.

Dorsey and Camann[238] retrospectively reviewed 36 cases of Bell's palsy associated with pregnancy; 25 women experienced symptoms during the third trimester, and the remaining 11 had symptoms during the first week postpartum. Of the 36 women, 27 received spinal or epidural analgesia or anesthesia. There was no difference in outcome in relation to the type of anesthesia given; therefore neuraxial analgesia or anesthesia does not appear to be contraindicated in patients with Bell's palsy.

Carpal Tunnel Syndrome

Carpal tunnel syndrome is common during pregnancy, occurring in approximately 2% of parturients.[239] This disorder results from compression of the median nerve in the flexor retinaculum at the wrist. Patients typically report paresthesias and weakness in the median nerve distribution. Symptoms are worse on awakening. Patients may be treated with splinting of the wrists. Severe symptoms may require surgery. Most cases resolve spontaneously within the first 2 months postpartum. Reduction in symptoms seems to correlate with loss of the weight gained during pregnancy.[239]

Meralgia Paresthetica

Meralgia paresthetica involves sensory loss and paresthesias in the lateral thigh stemming from compression of the lateral femoral cutaneous nerve. Obesity and the exaggerated lordosis of pregnancy can stretch the nerve.[240] Symptoms of meralgia paresthetica typically resolve within 3 months of delivery.[241] This neurologic deficit, as well as a number of others, are discussed more fully elsewhere (see Chapter 32).

KEY POINTS

- Symptoms of multiple sclerosis may worsen postpartum, regardless of the anesthetic technique used during delivery. However, the long-term prognosis of this disease is most likely unaffected by pregnancy.
- Multiple sclerosis does not contraindicate the use of neuraxial analgesia or anesthesia.
- Continuous epidural anesthesia is the method of choice for the prevention or treatment of autonomic hyperreflexia during labor and delivery in patients with spinal cord injury.
- Patients with myasthenia gravis require close surveillance during labor. Increasing muscle weakness may require an adjustment in the dosage of the anticholinesterase drug. Severe respiratory involvement may preclude the use of neuraxial anesthesia for cesarean delivery.
- The anesthesia provider should avoid succinylcholine in patients with myotonic dystrophy because fasciculations can trigger myotonia.
- Neuraxial analgesia or anesthesia does not appear to precipitate the onset of postpoliomyelitis muscular atrophy.
- Hemodynamic stability should be maintained in the parturient with an untreated intracranial aneurysm or arteriovenous malformation. Epidural anesthesia should be considered during labor and delivery.
- Bell's palsy, carpal tunnel syndrome, and meralgia paresthetica occur at higher rates during pregnancy. Symptoms typically resolve during the first few weeks postpartum.

REFERENCES

1. Kurland LT. The frequency and geographic distribution of multiple sclerosis as indicated by mortality statistics and morbidity surveys in the United States and Canada. Am J Hyg 1952; 55:457-81.
2. Kurtzke JF. Patterns of neurologic involvement in multiple sclerosis. Neurology 1989; 39:1235-8.
3. Hafler DA, Compston A, Sawcer S, et al. Risk alleles for multiple sclerosis identified by a genomewide study. N Engl J Med 2007; 357:851-62.
4. Boskovic R, Wide R, Wolpin J, et al. The reproductive effects of beta interferon therapy in pregnancy: A longitudinal cohort. Neurology 2005; 65:807-11.
5. Achiron A, Kishner I, Dolev M, et al. Effect of intravenous immunoglobulin treatment on pregnancy and postpartum-related relapses in multiple sclerosis. J Neurol 2004; 251:1133-7.
6. Ferrero S, Esposito F, Pretta S, Ragni N. Fetal risks related to the treatment of multiple sclerosis during pregnancy and breastfeeding. Expert Rev Neurother 2006; 6:1823-31.
7. Mueller BA, Zhang J, Critchlow CW. Birth outcomes and need for hospitalization after delivery among women with multiple sclerosis. Am J Obstet Gynecol 2002; 186:446-52.
8. Dahl J, Myhr KM, Daltveit AK, et al. Pregnancy, delivery, and birth outcome in women with multiple sclerosis. Neurology 2005; 65:1961-3.
9. Confavreux C, Hutchinson M, Hours MM, et al. Rate of pregnancy-related relapse in multiple sclerosis. Pregnancy in Multiple Sclerosis Group. N Engl J Med 1998; 339:285-91.
10. Vukusic S, Hutchinson M, Hours M, et al. Pregnancy and multiple sclerosis (the PRIMS study): Clinical predictors of post-partum relapse. Brain 2004; 127:1353-60.
11. Roullet E, Verdier-Taillefer MH, Amarenco P, et al. Pregnancy and multiple sclerosis: A longitudinal study of 125 remittent patients. J Neurol Neurosurg Psychiatry 1993; 56:1062-5.
12. Baskett PJ, Armstrong R. Anaesthetic problems in multiple sclerosis: Are certain agents contraindicated? Anaesthesia 1970; 25:397-401.
13. Bamford C, Sibley W, Laguna J. Anesthesia in multiple sclerosis. Can J Neurol Sci 1978; 5:41-4.
14. Tui C, Preiss A, Barcham I, Nevin M. Local nervous tissue changes following spinal anesthesia in experimental animals. J Pharmacol Exp Ther 1944; 81:209-17.
15. Schapira K. Is lumbar puncture harmful in multiple sclerosis? J Neurol Neurosurg Psychiatry 1959; 22:238.
16. Stenuit J, Marchand P. Sequelae of spinal anesthesia. Acta Neurol Psychiatr Belg 1968; 68:626-35.

17. Warren TM, Datta S, Ostheimer GW. Lumbar epidural anesthesia in a patient with multiple sclerosis. Anesth Analg 1982; 61:1022-3.
18. Crawford J, James F, Nolte H, et al. Regional analgesia for patients with chronic neurological disease and similar conditions. Anaesthesia 1981; 36:821.
19. Bader AM, Hunt CO, Datta S, et al. Anesthesia for the obstetric patient with multiple sclerosis. J Clin Anesth 1988; 1:21-4.
20. Berger J, Ontell R. Intrathecal morphine in conjunction with a combined spinal and general anesthetic in a patient with multiple sclerosis. Anesthesiology 1987; 66:400-2.
21. Leigh J, Fearnley SJ, Lupprian KG. Intrathecal diamorphine during laparotomy in a patient with advanced multiple sclerosis. Anaesthesia 1990; 45:640-2.
22. Marcus DA. Headache in pregnancy. Curr Pain Headache Rep 2003; 7:288-96.
23. Stein G, Morton J, Marsh A, et al. Headaches after childbirth. Acta Neurol Scand 1984; 69:74-9.
24. Berger A. Effects of caffeine consumption on pregnancy outcome: A review. J Reprod Med 1988; 33:945-56.
25. Heinonen O, Slone D, Shapiro S. Birth Defects and Drugs in Pregnancy. Littleton, MA, Publishing Sciences Group, 1977:336-7.
26. Reik LJ. Headaches in pregnancy. Semin Neurol 1988; 8:187-92.
27. Safra MJ, Oakley GP Jr. Association between cleft lip with or without cleft palate and prenatal exposure to diazepam. Lancet 1975; 2(7933):478-80.
28. Nulman I, Rovet J, Stewart DE, et al. Neurodevelopment of children exposed in utero to antidepressant drugs. N Engl J Med 1997; 336:258-62.
29. Marcus DA. Estrogen and chronic daily headache. Curr Pain Headache Rep 2004; 8:66-70.
30. Stewart WF, Shechter A, Rasmussen BK. Migraine prevalence: A review of population-based studies. Neurology 1994; 44:S17-23.
31. Somerville BW. The influence of progesterone and estradiol upon migraine. Headache 1972; 12:93-102.
32. Silberstein SD. Migraine and pregnancy. Neurol Clin 1997; 15:209-31.
33. Chen TC, Leviton A. Headache recurrence in pregnant women with migraine. Headache 1994; 34:107-10.
34. Davis ME, Adair FL, Pearl S. The present status of oxytocics in obstetrics. JAMA 1936; 107:261-7.
35. Fox AW, Chambers CD, Anderson PO, et al. Evidence-based assessment of pregnancy outcome after sumatriptan exposure. Headache 2002; 42:8-15.
36. Marcoux S, Berube S, Brisson J, Fabia J. History of migraine and risk of pregnancy-induced hypertension. Epidemiology 1992; 3:53-6.
37. Rosene KA, Featherstone HJ, Benedetti TJ. Cerebral ischemia associated with parenteral terbutaline use in pregnant migraine patients. Am J Obstet Gynecol 1982; 143:405-7.
38. Kalsbeek WD, McLaurin RL, Harris BS 3rd, Miller JD. The National Head and Spinal Cord Injury Survey: Major findings. J Neurosurg 1980; (Suppl) S19-31.
39. Pereira L. Obstetric management of the patient with spinal cord injury. Obstet Gynecol Surv 2003; 58:678-87.
40. Kang AH. Traumatic spinal cord injury. Clin Obstet Gynecol 2005; 48:67-72.
41. Kuhn RA. Functional capacity of the isolated human spinal cord. Brain 1950; 73:1-51.
42. Marshall J. Observations on reflex changes in the lower limbs in spastic paraplegia in man. Brain 1954; 77:290-304.
43. Kurnick NB. Autonomic hyperreflexia and its control in patients with spinal cord lesions. Ann Intern Med 1956; 44:678-86.
44. Crosby E, St-Jean B, Reid D, Elliott RD. Obstetrical anaesthesia and analgesia in chronic spinal cord-injured women. Can J Anaesth 1992; 39:487-94.
45. Schonwald G, Fish KJ, Perkash I. Cardiovascular complications during anesthesia in chronic spinal cord injured patients. Anesthesiology 1981; 55:550-8.
46. Catanzarite VA, Ferguson JE, Weinstein C, Belton SR. Preterm labor in the quadriplegic parturient. Am J Perinatol 1986; 3:115-8.
47. Greenspoon JS, Paul RH. Paraplegia and quadriplegia: Special considerations during pregnancy and labor and delivery. Am J Obstet Gynecol 1986; 155:738-41.
48. Westgren N, Hultling C, Levi R, Westgren M. Pregnancy and delivery in women with a traumatic spinal cord injury in Sweden, 1980-1991. Obstet Gynecol 1993; 81:926-30.
49. Baraka A. Epidural meperidine for control of autonomic hyperreflexia in a paraplegic parturient. Anesthesiology 1985; 62:688-90.
50. American College of Obstetricians and Gynecologists Committee on Obstetric Practice. Obstetric management of patients with spinal cord injuries. ACOG Committee Opinion No. 275. Washington, DC, September 2002. (Obstet Gynecol 2002; 100:625-7.)
51. Hambly PR, Martin B. Anaesthesia for chronic spinal cord lesions. Anaesthesia 1998; 53:273-89.
52. Thorn-Alquist AM. Prevention of hypertensive crises in patients with high spinal lesions during cystoscopy and lithotripsy. Acta Anaesthesiol Scand Suppl 1975; 57:79-82.
53. Stirt JA, Marco A, Conklin KA. Obstetric anesthesia for a quadriplegic patient with autonomic hyperreflexia. Anesthesiology 1979; 51:560-2.
54. Agostoni M, Giorgi E, Beccaria P, et al. Combined spinal-epidural anaesthesia for Caesarean section in a paraplegic woman: Difficulty in obtaining the expected level of block. Eur J Anaesthesiol 2000; 17:329-31.
55. Kobayashi A, Mizobe T, Tojo H, Hashimoto S. Autonomic hyperreflexia during labour. Can J Anaesth 1995; 42:1134-6.
56. Abouleish EI, Hanley ES, Palmer SM. Can epidural fentanyl control autonomic hyperreflexia in a quadriplegic parturient? Anesth Analg 1989; 68:523-6.
57. Pauzner D, Wolman I, Niv D, David MP. Epidural morphine bupivacaine combination for the control of autonomic hyperreflexia during labor. Gynecol Obstet Invest 1994; 37:215-6.
58. Maehama T, Izena H, Kanazawa K. Management of autonomic hyperreflexia with magnesium sulfate during labor in a woman with spinal cord injury. Am J Obstet Gynecol 2000; 183:492-3.
59. Ahmed AB, Bogod DG. Anaesthetic management of a quadriplegic patient with severe respiratory insufficiency undergoing caesarean section. Anaesthesia 1996; 51:1043-5.
60. Stone WA, Beach TP, Hamelberg W. Succinylcholine—danger in the spinal-cord-injured patient. Anesthesiology 1970; 32:168-9.
61. Stafford IP, Dildy GA. Myasthenia gravis and pregnancy. Clin Obstet Gynecol 2005; 48:48-56.
62. Richman DP, Agius MA. Acquired myasthenia gravis: Immunopathology. Neurol Clin 1994; 12:273-84.
63. Baraka A. Anaesthesia and myasthenia gravis. Can J Anaesth 1992; 39:476-86.
64. Eden RD, Gall SA. Myasthenia gravis and pregnancy: A reappraisal of thymectomy. Obstet Gynecol 1983; 62:328-33.
65. Drachman DB. Myasthenia gravis. N Engl J Med 1994; 330:1797-810.
66. d'Empaire G, Hoaglin DC, Perlo VP, Pontoppidan H. Effect of prethymectomy plasma exchange on postoperative respiratory function in myasthenia gravis. J Thorac Cardiovasc Surg 1985; 89:592-6.
67. Barrons RW. Drug-induced neuromuscular blockade and myasthenia gravis. Pharmacotherapy 1997; 17:1220-32.
68. Cohen BA, London RS, Goldstein PJ. Myasthenia gravis and preeclampsia. Obstet Gynecol 1976; 48:35S-7S.
69. Bashuk RG, Krendel DA. Myasthenia gravis presenting as weakness after magnesium administration. Muscle Nerve 1990; 13:708-12.
70. Catanzarite VA, McHargue AM, Sandberg EC, Dyson DC. Respiratory arrest during therapy for premature labor in a patient with myasthenia gravis. Obstet Gynecol 1984; 64:819-22.
71. Plauché WC. Myasthenia gravis in mothers and their newborns. Clin Obstet Gynecol 1991; 34:82-99.
72. Daskalakis GJ, Papageorgiou IS, Petrogiannis ND, et al. Myasthenia gravis and pregnancy. Eur J Obstet Gynecol Reprod Biol 2000; 89:201-4.
73. Rolbin WH, Levinson G, Shnider SM, Wright RG. Anesthetic considerations for myasthenia gravis and pregnancy. Anesth Analg 1978; 57:441-7.

74. Benshushan A, Rojansky N, Weinstein D. Myasthenia gravis and pre-eclampsia. Isr J Med Sci 1994; 30:229-33.
75. Hatada Y, Munemura M, Matsuo I, et al. Myasthenic crisis in the puerperium: The possible importance of alpha-fetoprotein: Case report. Br J Obstet Gynaecol 1987; 94:480-2.
76. Namba T, Brown SB, Grob D. Neonatal myasthenia gravis: Report of two cases and review of the literature. Pediatrics 1970; 45:488-504.
77. D'Angelo R, Gerancher JC. Combined spinal and epidural analgesia in a parturient with severe myasthenia gravis. Reg Anesth Pain Med 1998; 23:201-3.
78. Mitchell PJ, Bebbington M. Myasthenia gravis in pregnancy. Obstet Gynecol 1992; 80:178-81.
79. Warren J, Sharma SK. Ventilatory support using bilevel positive airway pressure during neuraxial blockade in a patient with severe respiratory compromise. Anesth Analg 2006; 102:910-1.
80. O'Flaherty D, Pennant JH, Rao K, Giesecke AH. Total intravenous anesthesia with propofol for transsternal thymectomy in myasthenia gravis. J Clin Anesth 1992; 4:241-4.
81. Foldes FF, McNall NP. Myasthenia gravis: A guide for anesthesiologists. Anesthesiology 1962; 23:837-72.
82. Leventhal SR, Orkin FK, Hirsh RA. Prediction of the need for post-operative mechanical ventilation in myasthenia gravis. Anesthesiology 1980; 53:26-30.
83. Naguib M, el Dawlatly AA, Ashour M, Bamgboye EA. Multivariate determinants of the need for postoperative ventilation in myasthenia gravis. Can J Anaesth 1996; 43:1006-13.
84. Proposal for revised clinical and electroencephalographic classification of epileptic seizures. From the Commission on Classification and Terminology of the International League Against Epilepsy. Epilepsia 1981; 22:489-501.
85. Elger C, Schmidt D. Modern management of epilepsy: A practical approach. Epilepsy Behav 2008; 12:501-39.
86. Thomas SV. Management of epilepsy and pregnancy. J Postgrad Med 2006; 52:57-64.
87. Annegers JF, Hauser WA, Elveback LR. Remission of seizures and relapse in patients with epilepsy. Epilepsia 1979; 20:729-37.
88. Elwes RD, Johnson AL, Shorvon SD, Reynolds EH. The prognosis for seizure control in newly diagnosed epilepsy. N Engl J Med 1984; 311:944-7.
89. Schmidt D. Prognosis of chronic epilepsy with complex partial seizures. J Neurol Neurosurg Psychiatry 1984; 47:1274-8.
90. Rutherford JM, Rubin PC. Management of epilepsy in pregnancy: Therapeutic aspects. Br J Hosp Med 1996; 55:620-2.
91. Schmidt D, Canger R, Avanzini G, et al. Change of seizure frequency in pregnant epileptic women. J Neurol Neurosurg Psychiatry 1983; 46:751-5.
92. Ramsay RE. Effect of hormones on seizure activity during pregnancy. J Clin Neurophysiol 1987; 4:23-5.
93. Yerby MS. Pregnancy and epilepsy. Epilepsia 1991; 32(Suppl 6):S51-9.
94. Nau H, Kuhnz W, Egger HJ, et al. Anticonvulsants during pregnancy and lactation: Transplacental, maternal and neonatal pharmacokinetics. Clin Pharmacokinet 1982; 7:508-43.
95. Perucca E, Crema A. Plasma protein binding of drugs in pregnancy. Clin Pharmacokinet 1982; 7:336-52.
96. Higgins TA, Comerford JB. Epilepsy in pregnancy. J Ir Med Assoc 1974; 67:317-20.
97. Lowe SA. Drugs in pregnancy: Anticonvulsants and drugs for neurological disease. Best Pract Res Clin Obstet Gynaecol 2001; 15:863-76.
98. Morrell MJ. The new antiepileptic drugs and women: Efficacy, reproductive health, pregnancy, and fetal outcome. Epilepsia 1996; 37(Suppl 6):S34-44.
99. Cunnington M, Tennis P: International Lamotrigine Pregnancy Registry Scientific Advisory Committee. Lamotrigine and the risk of malformations in pregnancy. Neurology 2005; 64:955-60.
100. Yamasmit W, Chaithongwongwatthana S, Tolosa JE. Prenatal vitamin K1 administration in epileptic women to prevent neonatal hemorrhage: Is it effective? J Reprod Med 2006; 51:463-6.
101. Aravapalli R, Abouleish E, Aldrete JA. Anesthetic implications in the parturient epileptic patient. Anesth Analg 1988; 67:S266.
102. Merrell DA, Koch MA. Epidural anaesthesia as an anticonvulsant in the management of hypertensive and eclamptic patients in labour. S Afr Med J 1980; 58:875-7.
103. Modica PA, Tempelhoff R, White PF. Pro- and anticonvulsant effects of anesthetics. Anesth Analg 1990; 70:303-15.
104. Iijima T, Nakamura Z, Iwao Y, Sankawa H. The epileptogenic properties of the volatile anesthetics sevoflurane and isoflurane in patients with epilepsy. Anesth Analg 2000; 91:989-95.
105. Smith M, Smith SJ, Scott CA, Harkness WF. Activation of the electrocorticogram by propofol during surgery for epilepsy. Br J Anaesth 1996; 76:499-502.
106. Ornstein E, Matteo RS, Schwartz AE, et al. The effect of phenytoin on the magnitude and duration of neuromuscular block following atracurium or vecuronium. Anesthesiology 1987; 67:191-6.
107. Cardani R, Mancinelli E, Rotondo G, et al. Muscleblind-like protein 1 nuclear sequestration is a molecular pathology marker of DM1 and DM2. Eur J Histochem 2006; 50:177-82.
108. Arsenault ME, Prevost C, Lescault A, et al. Clinical characteristics of myotonic dystrophy type 1 patients with small CTG expansions. Neurology 2006; 66:1248-50.
109. Shaw DJ, Brook JD, Meredith AL, et al. Gene mapping and chromosome 19. J Med Genet 1986; 23:2-10.
110. Modoni A, Silvestri G, Pomponi MG, et al. Characterization of the pattern of cognitive impairment in myotonic dystrophy type 1. Arch Neurol 2004; 61:1943-7.
111. Heatwole CR, Moxley RT. The nondystrophic myotonias. Neurotherapeutics 2007; 4:238-51.
112. Jungbluth H. Central core disease. Orphanet J Rare Dis 2007; 2:25.
113. Rudnik-Schoneborn S, Schneider-Gold C, Raabe U, et al. Outcome and effect of pregnancy in myotonic dystrophy type 2. Neurology 2006; 66:579-80.
114. Sholl JS, Hughey MJ, Hirschmann RA. Myotonic muscular dystrophy associated with ritodrine tocolysis. Am J Obstet Gynecol 1985; 151:83-6.
115. Arulkumaran S, Rauff M, Ingemarsson I, et al. Uterine activity in myotonia dystrophica: Case report. Br J Obstet Gynaecol 1986; 93:634-6.
116. Blumgart CH, Hughes DG, Redfern N. Obstetric anaesthesia in dystrophia myotonica. Anaesthesia 1990; 45:26-9.
117. Gilchrist JM. Muscle disease in the pregnant woman. In Devinsky O, Feldman E, Hainline B, editors. Advances in Neurology. New York, Raven Press, 1994:193-208.
118. Russell SH, Hirsch NP. Anaesthesia and myotonia. Br J Anaesth 1994; 72:210-6.
119. Donaldson JO. Neurology of Pregnancy. London, WB Saunders, 1989.
120. Camann WR, Johnson MD. Anesthetic management of a parturient with myotonia dystrophica: A case report. Reg Anesth 1990; 15:41-3.
121. Mathieu J, Allard P, Gobeil G, et al. Anesthetic and surgical complications in 219 cases of myotonic dystrophy. Neurology 1997; 49:1646-50.
122. Paterson IS. Generalized myotonia following suxamethonium: A case report. Br J Anaesth 1962; 34:340-2.
123. Hook R, Anderson EF, Noto P. Anesthetic management of a parturient with myotonia atrophica. Anesthesiology 1975; 43:689-92.
124. Rosenbaum HK, Miller JD. Malignant hyperthermia and myotonic disorders. Anesthesiol Clin North Am 2002; 20:623-64.
125. Campbell AM, Thompson N. Anaesthesia for caesarean section in a patient with myotonic dystrophy receiving warfarin therapy. Can J Anaesth 1995; 42:409-14.
126. Cherng YG, Wang YP, Liu CC, et al. Combined spinal and epidural anesthesia for abdominal hysterectomy in a patient with myotonic dystrophy. Reg Anesth 1994; 19:69-72.
127. O'Neill GN. Inherited disorders of the neuromuscular junction. Int Anesthesiol Clin 2006; 44:91-106.

128. Ciafaloni E, Pressman EK, Loi AM, et al. Pregnancy and birth outcomes in women with facioscapulohumeral muscular dystrophy. Neurology 2006; 67:1887-9.
129. Rudnik-Schoneborn S, Glauner B, Rohrig D, Zerres K. Obstetric aspects in women with facioscapulohumeral muscular dystrophy, limb-girdle muscular dystrophy, and congenital myopathies. Arch Neurol 1997; 54:888-94.
130. Gamzu R, Shenhav M, Fainaru O, et al. Impact of pregnancy on respiratory capacity in women with muscular dystrophy and kyphoscoliosis: A case report. J Reprod Med 2002; 47:53-6.
131. Molyneux MK. Anaesthetic management during labour of a manifesting carrier of Duchenne muscular dystrophy. Int J Obstet Anesth 2005; 14:58-61.
132. Denborough M. Malignant hyperthermia. Lancet 1998; 352:1131-6.
133. Lin DD, Barker PB. Neuroimaging of phakomatoses. Semin Pediatr Neurol 2006; 13:48-62.
134. Joffe D, Robbins R, Benjamin A. Caesarean section and phaeochromocytoma resection in a patient with von Hippel-Lindau disease. Can J Anaesth 1993; 40:870-4.
135. Ginsburg DS, Hernandez E, Johnson JW. Sarcoma complicating von Recklinghausen disease in pregnancy. Obstet Gynecol 1981; 58:385-7.
136. Sharma JB, Gulati N, Malik S. Maternal and perinatal complications in neurofibromatosis during pregnancy. Int J Gynaecol Obstet 1991; 34:221-7.
137. Dugoff L, Sujansky E. Neurofibromatosis type 1 and pregnancy. Am J Med Genet 1996; 66:7-10.
138. Hirsch NP, Murphy A, Radcliffe JJ. Neurofibromatosis: Clinical presentations and anaesthetic implications. Br J Anaesth 2001; 86:555-64.
139. Spiegel JE, Hapgood A, Hess PE. Epidural anesthesia in a parturient with neurofibromatosis type 2 undergoing cesarean section. Int J Obstet Anesth 2005; 14:336-9.
140. Richardson MG, Setty GK, Rawoof SA. Responses to nondepolarizing neuromuscular blockers and succinylcholine in von Recklinghausen neurofibromatosis. Anesth Analg 1996; 82:382-5.
141. Mitterschiffthaler G, Maurhard U, Huter O, Brezinka C. Prolonged action of vecuronium in neurofibromatosis. Anaesthesiol Reanim 1989; 14:175-8.
142. Naguib M, Al-Rajeh SM, Abdulatif M, Ababtin WA. The response of a patient with von Recklinghausen's disease to succinylcholine and atracurium. Middle East J Anesthesiol 1988; 9:429-34.
143. Petrikovsky BM, Vintzileos AM, Cassidy SB, Egan JF. Tuberous sclerosis in pregnancy. Am J Perinatol 1990; 7:133-5.
144. Forsnes EV, Eggleston MK, Burtman M. Placental abruption and spontaneous rupture of renal angiomyolipoma in a pregnant woman with tuberous sclerosis. Obstet Gynecol 1996; 88:725.
145. Adams RD, Victor M, Ropper AH. Principles of Neurology. 7th edition. New York, McGraw-Hill, 2001.
146. Ogasawara KK, Ogasawara EM, Hirata G. Pregnancy complicated by von Hippel-Lindau disease. Obstet Gynecol 1995; 85:829-31.
147. Douglas MR, Winer JB. Guillain-Barré syndrome and its treatment. Expert Rev Neurother 2006; 6:1569-74.
148. The Guillain-Barré syndrome Study Group. Plasmapheresis and acute Guillain-Barré syndrome. Neurology 1985; 35:1096-104.
149. Gautier PE, Hantson P, Vekemans MC, et al. Intensive care management of Guillain-Barré syndrome during pregnancy. Intensive Care Med 1990; 16:460-2.
150. Jiang GX, de Pedro-Cuesta J, Strigard K, et al. Pregnancy and Guillain-Barré syndrome: A nationwide register cohort study. Neuroepidemiology 1996; 15:192-200.
151. Rockel A, Wissel J, Rolfs A. Guillain-Barré syndrome in pregnancy—an indication for caesarian section? J Perinat Med 1994; 22:393-8.
152. Wiertlewski S, Magot A, Drapier S, et al. Worsening of neurologic symptoms after epidural anesthesia for labor in a Guillain-Barré patient. Anesth Analg 2004; 98:825-7.
153. Vassiliev DV, Nystrom EU, Leicht CH. Combined spinal and epidural anesthesia for labor and cesarean delivery in a patient with Guillain-Barré syndrome. Reg Anesth Pain Med 2001; 26:174-6.
154. Steiner I, Argov Z, Cahan C, Abramsky O. Guillain-Barré syndrome after epidural anesthesia: Direct nerve root damage may trigger disease. Neurology 1985; 35:1473-5.
155. Sibert KS, Sladen RN. Impaired ventilatory capacity after recovery from Guillain-Barré syndrome. J Clin Anesth 1994; 6:133-8.
156. Lambert DA, Giannouli E, Schmidt BJ. Postpolio syndrome and anesthesia. Anesthesiology 2005; 103:638-44.
157. Klingman J, Chui H, Corgiat M, Perry J. Functional recovery: A major risk factor for the development of postpoliomyelitis muscular atrophy. Arch Neurol 1988; 45:645-7.
158. Sharief MK, Hentges R, Ciardi M. Intrathecal immune response in patients with the post-polio syndrome. N Engl J Med 1991; 325:749-55.
159. Harjulehto-Mervaala T, Aro T, Hiilesmaa VK, et al. Oral polio vaccination during pregnancy: Lack of impact on fetal development and perinatal outcome. Clin Infect Dis 1994; 18:414-20.
160. Daw E, Chandler G. Pregnancy following poliomyelitis. Postgrad Med J 1976; 52:492-6.
161. Lambert D, Giannouli E, Schmidt B. Postpolio syndrome and anesthesia. Anesthesiology 2005; 103:638-44.
162. Connelly N, Abbott T. Successful use of succinylcholine for cesarean delivery in a patient with postpolio syndrome. Anesthesiology 2008; 108:1151-2.
163. Swensen R, Kirsch W. Brain neoplasms in women: A review. Clin Obstet Gynecol 2002; 45:904-27.
164. Stevenson CB, Thompson RC. The clinical management of intracranial neoplasms in pregnancy. Clin Obstet Gynecol 2005; 48:24-37.
165. Soper JT, Spillman M, Sampson JH, et al. High-risk gestational trophoblastic neoplasia with brain metastases: Individualized multidisciplinary therapy in the management of four patients. Gynecol Oncol 2007; 104:691-4.
166. Choi NW, Schuman LM, Gullen WH. Epidemiology of primary central nervous system neoplasms. II. Case-control study. Am J Epidemiol 1970; 91:467-85.
167. Enoksson P, Lundberg N, Sjostedt S, Skanse B. Influence of pregnancy on visual fields in suprasellar tumors. Acta Psychiatr Scand 1961; 36:524-38.
168. Isla A, Alvarez F, Gonzalez A, et al. Brain tumor and pregnancy. Obstet Gynecol 1997; 89:19-23.
169. Marx GF, Zemaitis MT, Orkin LR. Cerebrospinal fluid pressures during labor and obstetrical anesthesia. Anesthesiology 1961; 22:348-54.
170. Finfer SR. Management of labour and delivery in patients with intracranial neoplasms. Br J Anaesth 1991; 67:784-7.
171. Kepes ER, Andrews IC, Radnay PA, et al. Conduct of anesthesia for delivery with grossly raised cerebrospinal fluid pressure. N Y State J Med 1972; 72:1155-6.
172. Goroszeniuk T, Howard RS, Wright JT. The management of labour using continuous lumbar epidural analgesia in a patient with a malignant cerebral tumour. Anaesthesia 1986; 41:1128-9.
173. Atanassoff PG, Alon E, Weiss BM, Lauper U. Spinal anaesthesia for caesarean section in a patient with brain neoplasma. Can J Anaesth 1994; 41:163-4.
174. Su TM, Lan CM, Yang LC, et al. Brain tumor presenting with fatal herniation following delivery under epidural anesthesia. Anesthesiology 2002; 96:508-9.
175. Chang L, Looi-Lyons L, Bartosik L, Tindal S. Anesthesia for cesarean section in two patients with brain tumours. Can J Anaesth 1999; 46:61-5.
176. Wang L, Paech M. Neuroanesthesia for the pregnant woman. Anesth Analg 2008; 107:193-200.
177. Bharti N, Kashyap L, Mohan V. Anesthetic management of a parturient with cerebellopontine-angle meningioma. Int J Obstet Anesth 2002; 11:219-21.
178. Burns PD, Linder RO, Drose VE, Battaglia F. The placental transfer of water from fetus to mother following the intravenous infusion of hypertonic mannitol to the maternal rabbit. Am J Obstet Gynecol 1963; 86:160-7.
179. Lumbers E, Stevens A. Changes in fetal renal function in response to infusions of a hyperosmotic solution of mannitol to the ewe. J Physiol 1983; 343:439-46.

180. Muizelaar J, Marmarou A, Ward J. Adverse effects of prolonged hyperventilation in patients with severe head injury: A randomized clinical trial. J Neurosurg 1991; 75:731-9.
181. Low J, Boston R, Cerveneko F. Effect of low maternal carbon dioxide tension on placental gas exchange. Am J Obstet Gynecol 1970; 106:132-41.
182. Friedman DI, Jacobson DM. Diagnostic criteria for idiopathic intracranial hypertension. Neurology 2002; 59:1492-5.
183. Koontz WL, Herbert WN, Cefalo RC. Pseudotumor cerebri in pregnancy. Obstet Gynecol 1983; 62:324-7.
184. Bagga R, Jain V, Das CP, et al. Choice of therapy and mode of delivery in idiopathic intracranial hypertension during pregnancy. MedGenMed 2005; 7:42.
185. Digre KB, Varner MW, Corbett JJ. Pseudotumor cerebri and pregnancy. Neurology 1984; 34:721-9.
186. Paruchuri SR, Lawlor M, Kleinhomer K, et al. Risk of cerebellar tonsillar herniation after diagnostic lumbar puncture in pseudotumor cerebri. Anesth Analg 1993; 77:403-4.
187. Palop R, Choed-Amphai E, Miller R. Epidural anesthesia for delivery complicated by benign intracranial hypertension. Anesthesiology 1979; 50:159-60.
188. Bédard JM, Richardson MG, Wissler RN. Epidural anesthesia in a parturient with a lumboperitoneal shunt. Anesthesiology 1999; 90:621-3.
189. Kaul B, Vallejo MC, Ramanathan S, et al. Accidental spinal analgesia in the presence of a lumboperitoneal shunt in an obese parturient receiving enoxaparin therapy. Anesth Analg 2002; 95:441-3.
190. Aly EE, Lawther BK. Anaesthetic management of uncontrolled idiopathic intracranial hypertension during labour and delivery using an intrathecal catheter. Anaesthesia 2007; 62:178-81.
191. Paciorkowski AR, Greenstein RM. When is enlargement of the subarachnoid spaces not benign? A genetic perspective. Pediatr Neurol 2007; 37:1-7.
192. Liakos AM, Bradley NK, Magram G, Muszynski C. Hydrocephalus and the reproductive health of women: The medical implications of maternal shunt dependency in 70 women and 138 pregnancies. Neurol Res 2000; 22:69-88.
193. Wisoff JH, Kratzert KJ, Handwerker SM, et al. Pregnancy in patients with cerebrospinal fluid shunts: Report of a series and review of the literature. Neurosurgery 1991; 29:827-31.
194. Bateman BT, Schumacher HC, Bushnell CD, et al. Intracerebral hemorrhage in pregnancy: Frequency, risk factors, and outcome. Neurology 2006; 67:424-9.
195. Kittner SJ, Stern BJ, Feeser BR, et al. Pregnancy and the risk of stroke. N Engl J Med 1996; 335:768-74.
196. Holcomb WL, Petrie RH. Cerebrovascular emergencies in pregnancy. Clin Obstet Gynecol 1990; 33:467-72.
197. Dias MS, Sekhar LN. Intracranial hemorrhage from aneurysms and arteriovenous malformations during pregnancy and the puerperium. Neurosurgery 1990; 27:855-65.
198. Piotin M, de Souza Filho CB, Kothimbakam R, Moret J. Endovascular treatment of acutely ruptured intracranial aneurysms in pregnancy. Am J Obstet Gynecol 2001; 185:1261-2.
199. Sadasivan B, Malik GM, Lee C, Ausman JI. Vascular malformations and pregnancy. Surg Neurol 1990; 33:305-13.
200. Mas JL, Lamy C. Stroke in pregnancy and the puerperium. J Neurol 1998; 245:305-13.
201. Hudspith MJ, Popham PA. The anaesthetic management of intracranial haemorrhage from arteriovenous malformations during pregnancy: Three cases. Int J Obstet Anesth 1996; 5:189-93.
202. Viscomi CM, Wilson J, Bernstein I. Anesthetic management of a parturient with an incompletely resected cerebral arteriovenous malformation. Reg Anesth 1997; 22:192-7.
203. Sharma SK, Herrera ER, Sidawi JE, Leveno KJ. The pregnant patient with an intracranial arteriovenous malformation: Cesarean or vaginal delivery using regional or general anesthesia? Reg Anesth 1995; 20:455-8.
204. Yih PS, Cheong KF. Anaesthesia for caesarean section in a patient with an intracranial arteriovenous malformation. Anaesth Intensive Care 1999; 27:66-8.
205. Stoodley MA, Macdonald RL, Weir BK. Pregnancy and intracranial aneurysms. Neurosurg Clin North Am 1998; 9:549-56.
206. Donchin Y, Amirav B, Sahar A, Yarkoni S. Sodium nitroprusside for aneurysm surgery in pregnancy: Report of a case. Br J Anaesth 1978; 50:849-51.
207. Dhamee MS, Goh M. Deliberate hypotension for clipping of cerebral aneurysm during pregnancy. Anesthesiol Rev 1985; 12:20-2.
208. Newman B, Lam AM. Induced hypotension for clipping of a cerebral aneurysm during pregnancy: A case report and brief review. Anesth Analg 1986; 65:675-8.
209. Naulty J, Cefalo RC, Lewis PE. Fetal toxicity of nitroprusside in the pregnant ewe. Am J Obstet Gynecol 1981; 139:708-11.
210. Ellis SC, Wheeler AS, James FM, et al. Fetal and maternal effects of sodium nitroprusside used to counteract hypertension in gravid ewes. Am J Obstet Gynecol 1982; 143:766-70.
211. Nelson SH, Suresh MS. Comparison of nitroprusside and hydralazine in isolated uterine arteries from pregnant and nonpregnant patients. Anesthesiology 1988; 68:541-7.
212. Conklin KA, Herr G, Fung D. Anaesthesia for caesarean section and cerebral aneurysm clipping. Can Anaesth Soc J 1984; 31:451-4.
213. Jaeger K, Ruschulte H, Muhlhaus K, Tatagiba M. Combined emergency Caesarean section and intracerebral aneurysm clipping. Anaesthesia 2000; 55:1138-40.
214. Whitburn RH, Laishley RS, Jewkes DA. Anaesthesia for simultaneous caesarean section and clipping of intracerebral aneurysm. Br J Anaesth 1990; 64:642-5.
215. Powner DJ, Bernstein IM. Extended somatic support for pregnant women after brain death. Crit Care Med 2003; 31:1241-9.
216. Stam J. Thrombosis of the cerebral veins and sinuses. N Engl J Med 2005; 352:1791-8.
217. Lanska DJ, Kryscio RJ. Peripartum stroke and intracranial venous thrombosis in the National Hospital Discharge Survey. Obstet Gynecol 1997; 89:413-8.
218. Cantu C, Barinagarrementeria F. Cerebral venous thrombosis associated with pregnancy and puerperium: Review of 67 cases. Stroke 1993; 24:1880-4.
219. Wilder-Smith E, Kothbauer-Margreiter I, Lammle B, et al. Dural puncture and activated protein C resistance: Risk factors for cerebral venous sinus thrombosis. J Neurol Neurosurg Psychiatry 1997; 63:351-6.
220. Chisholm ME, Campbell DC. Postpartum postural headache due to superior sagittal sinus thrombosis mistaken for spontaneous intracranial hypotension. Can J Anaesth 2001; 48:302-4.
221. Lockhart EM, Baysinger CL. Intracranial venous thrombosis in the parturient. Anesthesiology 2007; 107:652-8.
222. Wasay M, Bakshi R, Bobustuc G, et al. Cerebral vascular thrombosis: Analysis of a multicenter cohort from the United States. J Stroke Cerebrovasc Dis 2008; 17:49-54.
223. Leveck DE, Davies GA. Rapid progression of amyotrophic lateral sclerosis presenting during pregnancy: A case report. J Obstet Gynaecol Can 2005; 27:360-2.
224. Jacka MJ, Sanderson F. Amyotrophic lateral sclerosis presenting during pregnancy. Anesth Analg 1998; 86:542-3.
225. Hara K, Sakura S, Saito Y, et al. Epidural anesthesia and pulmonary function in a patient with amyotrophic lateral sclerosis. Anesth Analg 1996; 83:878-9.
226. Kochi T, Oka T, Mizuguchi T. Epidural anesthesia for patients with amyotrophic lateral sclerosis. Anesth Analg 1989; 68:410-2.
227. Rosenbaum KJ, Neigh JL, Strobel GE. Sensitivity to nondepolarizing muscle relaxants in amyotrophic lateral sclerosis: Report of two cases. Anesthesiology 1971; 35:638-41.
228. Pugh CP, Healey SK, Crane JM, Young D. Successful pregnancy and spinal muscular atrophy. Obstet Gynecol 2000; 95:1034.
229. Weston LA, DiFazio CA. Labor analgesia and anesthesia in a patient with spinal muscular atrophy and vocal cord paralysis: A rare and unusual case report. Reg Anesth 1996; 21:350-4.
230. Harris SJ, Moaz K. Caesarean section conducted under subarachnoid block in two sisters with spinal muscular atrophy. Int J Obstet Anesth 2002; 11:125-7.

231. Aboussouan LS, Lewis RA, Shy ME. Disorders of pulmonary function, sleep, and the upper airway in Charcot-Marie-Tooth disease. Lung 2007; 185:1-7.
232. Rudnik-Schoneborn S, Rohrig D, Nicholson G, Zerres K. Pregnancy and delivery in Charcot-Marie-Tooth disease type 1. Neurology 1993; 43:2011-6.
233. Hoff JM, Gilhus NE, Daltveit AK. Pregnancies and deliveries in patients with Charcot-Marie-Tooth disease. Neurology 2005; 64:459-62.
234. Greenwood JJ, Scott WE. Charcot-Marie-Tooth disease: Peripartum management of two contrasting clinical cases. Int J Obstet Anesth 2007; 16:149-54.
235. Cohen Y, Lavie O, Granovsky-Grisaru S, et al. Bell palsy complicating pregnancy: A review. Obstet Gynecol Surv 2000; 55:184-8.
236. Shmorgun D, Chan WS, Ray JG. Association between Bell's palsy in pregnancy and pre-eclampsia. QJM 2002; 95:359-62.
237. Gillman GS, Schaitkin BM, May M, Klein SR. Bell's palsy in pregnancy: A study of recovery outcomes. Otolaryngol Head Neck Surg 2002; 126:26-30.
238. Dorsey DL, Camann WR. Obstetric anesthesia in patients with idiopathic facial paralysis (Bell's palsy): A 10-year survey. Anesth Analg 1993; 77:81-3.
239. Finsen V, Zeitlmann H. Carpal tunnel syndrome during pregnancy. Scand J Plast Reconstr Surg Hand Surg 2006; 40:41-5.
240. Van Diver T, Camann W. Meralgia paresthetica in the parturient. Int J Obstet Anesth 1995; 4:109-12.
241. Massey EW. Mononeuropathies in pregnancy. Semin Neurol 1988; 8:193-6.

Obesity

Robert D'Angelo, M.D.
David D. Dewan, M.D.

The prevalence of obesity in the general population is growing at an alarming rate and is reaching epidemic proportions (Table 50-1). Data from the National Center for Health Statistics show that in 2004, 66% of Americans were overweight and 32% were obese.[1] It has been estimated that complications of obesity lead to approximately 300,000 preventable deaths in the United States each year.[2] The World Health Organization (WHO) estimates that by 2020, two thirds of the global burden of disease will be attributable to chronic noncommunicable diseases associated with diet; the WHO has therefore encouraged a concerted multinational effort to address the ramifications of overnutrition.[3] On the other hand, there is some evidence that the prevalence of obesity among women in the United States may have reached a plateau; Ogden et al.[1] noted that the prevalence among women did not increase significantly between 1999 and 2004.

Although no definition of obesity specific to pregnancy exists, a pregnant woman is generally considered *obese* when her body mass index (BMI) is 30 kg/m^2 or greater, and *morbidly obese* when her BMI equals or exceeds 40 kg/m^2 (see Table 50-1).

Obesity is associated with an increased risk of maternal morbidity and mortality.[4] In obese pregnant women, there are higher rates of hypertension, coronary artery disease, cerebrovascular disease, diabetes mellitus, gallbladder disease, and nonalcoholic fatty liver disease.[5-7] Providing anesthesia for these patients presents unique challenges that can best be met through an understanding of the pathophysiologic changes associated with obesity and with use of techniques that maximize benefits while reducing the risks of complications.

PHYSIOLOGIC CHANGES OF OBESITY

Obesity is a complex disorder with neuronal, hormonal, neuroendocrine, genetic, hereditary, and psychosocial components.[8] These components produce physiologic changes in obese pregnant women that lead to greater maternal, neonatal, surgical, and anesthetic risks.

Pulmonary Changes

Obesity increases the demands on the pulmonary system. As energy expenditure increases proportionate to the increase in body mass,[9] oxygen consumption and carbon dioxide (CO_2) production also increase proportionate to the increase in work performed.[10] Minute ventilation then increases owing to the elevated respiratory demand, except in the 5% to 10% of patients with pickwickian syndrome, who display a reduced sensitivity to CO_2.[11] Obesity affects the body's ability to meet these demands by changing pulmonary mechanics, altering lung volumes, and impairing oxygen consumption.

PULMONARY MECHANICS

Obesity increases the weight of the chest wall; thus, greater energy expenditure is required during ventilation to move this greater mass. Several prospective studies have demonstrated that morbidly obese patients, in comparison with controls, expend a disproportionately high percentage of total oxygen consumption on respiratory work—even during quiet breathing.[12,13] The weight gain associated with pregnancy further increases the work of breathing in obese patients. In obese individuals, frequent shallow

TABLE 50-1 Weight of U.S. Women Ages 20-39 According to World Health Organization Classification

Classification	Body Mass Index (kg/m²)	Percentage of Women	
Underweight	<18.5	2.6	
Normal weight	18.5-24.9	32.9	
Overweight	25.0-29.9	27.3	
Obesity I	30.0-34.9	17.3	34.4
Obesity II	35.0-39.9	9.7	
Obesity III	≥40.0	5.4	

Data from World Health Organization. Diet, Nutrition, and the Prevention of Chronic Diseases: Report of a Joint WHO/FAO Expert Consultation. WHO Technical Report Series 916. Geneva, 2002; and Centers for Disease Control and Prevention. National Health and Nutrition Examination Survey, 2005-2006. Hyattsville, MD, CDC, 2006. Available at http://www.cdc.gov/nchs/about/major/nhanes/nhanes2005-2006/nhanes05_06.htm

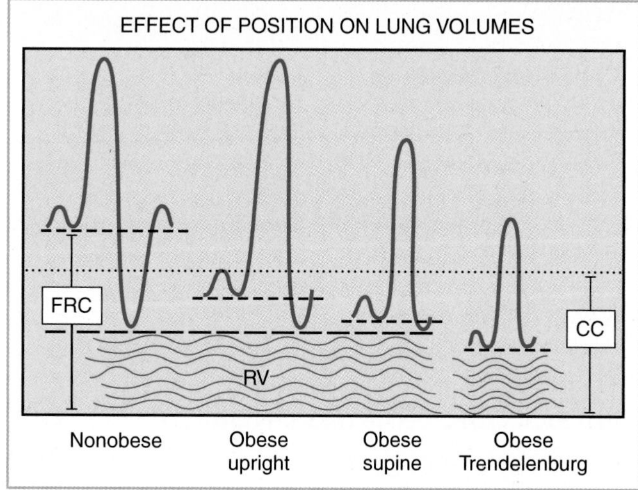

FIGURE 50-1 Effect of position change on various lung volumes in a markedly obese subject compared with a nonobese subject. FRC, functional residual capacity; RV, residual volume; CC, closing capacity. (Adapted from Vaughan RW. Pulmonary and cardiovascular derangements in the obese patient. In Brown BR, editor. Anesthesia and the Obese Patient. Philadelphia, FA Davis, 1982:26.)

respirations may represent a more efficient breathing pattern than a pattern characterized by large tidal volumes. Noble[14] documented increased tidal volumes in obese patients after weight loss, suggesting that obese patients conserve energy by decreasing tidal volume. This pattern of frequent shallow respirations contrasts with the increased tidal volumes that typically accompany pregnancy. Although the Pa_{CO_2} in most morbidly obese pregnant women is not different from that in nonobese pregnant women, pulmonary reserve is reduced in morbidly obese pregnant women.

LUNG VOLUMES

Greater abdominal weight restricts diaphragm movement, especially in the supine or Trendelenburg position, thus encouraging smaller tidal volumes. Functional residual capacity (FRC) decreases at the expense of expiratory reserve volume and may be less than closing capacity. In morbidly obese patients, this difference can result in airway closure during tidal ventilation (Figure 50-1). Similarly, expiratory reserve volume, vital capacity, inspiratory capacity, total lung capacity, and maximum minute ventilation all decrease in morbidly obese patients. Both chest wall and lung compliance decrease, but airway resistance increases.[15,16]

Pregnancy also alters lung volumes. In nonobese pregnant women, expiratory reserve volume and FRC both decline approximately 20% to 25% by term. Eng et al.,[17] examining a series of pregnant women whose estimated prepregnancy weights ranged from 50% to 140% above normal, measured lung volumes during the third trimester and again at 2 months postpartum. With the exception of FRC, the lung volume changes resembled those that occur in nonobese pregnant women. However, FRC decreased less in obese pregnant women than in nonobese pregnant women. Perhaps this lesser decrease may confer some protection from premature airway closure in the obese pregnant woman.

OXYGENATION

Pulmonary diffusion typically remains normal in most women with morbid obesity. Decreased chest wall compliance and greater abdominal weight promote airway closure in the dependent portion of the lung.[18] Ventilation preferentially occurs in the more compliant, nondependent portion of the lung. In contrast, pulmonary blood flow preferentially occurs in the dependent portion of the lung, resulting in ventilation-perfusion mismatch and hypoxemia.[18,19] Barrera et al.[19] suggested that there is relative hyperperfusion of poorly ventilated alveoli in obese patients.

Consistent with the positional deterioration of lung volumes, oxygenation worsens in obese persons in the supine and Trendelenburg positions. Although oxygenation does not necessarily correlate linearly with weight,[20] massive weight loss improves Pa_{O_2} and expiratory reserve volume. Weight loss does not, however, improve forced expiratory volume in 1 second, forced vital capacity, or maximum mid-expiratory flow.[21]

The greater ventilation and cardiac output that occur during pregnancy may confer some protection to the obese patient. A small study measured a mean Pa_{O_2} of 85 mm Hg in obese pregnant women breathing room air.[17] Although this Pa_{O_2} is lower than measurements seen in normal pregnant women, it exceeds measurements in morbidly obese nonpregnant patients presenting for gastric bypass surgery.

Cardiovascular Changes

Obesity increases blood volume and cardiac output. A weight gain from 70 to 170 kg results in a doubling of cardiac output and blood volume in nonpregnant women.[22] The cardiac index remains normal. Increased cardiac output results primarily from increased stroke volume. The systemic arteriovenous oxygen difference remains normal.[23]

Pulmonary blood volume increases in proportion to increases in cardiac output and total blood volume. **Pulmonary hypertension** can occur and may be position dependent. Paul et al.[24] observed an 11% increase in oxygen consumption and a 44% increase in pulmonary capillary wedge pressure when morbidly obese patients were placed in a supine position. Hypoxemia, if present, increases pulmonary vascular resistance. Airway obstruction may also increase pulmonary artery pressure. Teeple and Ghia,[25] in their examination of an obese patient, noted a decline in pulmonary capillary wedge pressure from 38 to 5 mm Hg after endotracheal intubation and relief of airway obstruction.

Hypertension occurs more frequently among obese pregnant women. A BMI of 30 or more is associated with a threefold higher incidence of hypertension during pregnancy than a BMI less than 30.[5] Mabie et al.[26] described a subset of obese, hypertensive pregnant women with increased left ventricular mass, normal systolic function, and abnormal diastolic function. The investigators suggested that these findings reflect volume overload in the presence of inadequate left ventricular relaxation. Primary therapy for these patients includes reducing the expanded blood volume via vigorous diuretic therapy.

A clear relationship exists between obesity and **death from cardiovascular causes.**[4,27] Drenick et al.[27] demonstrated a 12-fold higher mortality among obese patients between the ages of 25 and 34 than in nonobese patients in the same age range; cardiovascular disease was the most common cause of death. Tsueda et al.[28] reported two cases of cardiac arrest in morbidly obese patients who had been placed in the supine position. The authors speculated that the sudden circulatory changes associated with this change in position accounted for the sudden death of these patients. Although the relative risk of mortality associated with obesity has decreased since 1971, Flegal et al.[29] estimated that obesity was associated with more than 111,000 excess deaths in 2000. They speculated that this lower relative risk is a result of improved public health policies and better medical care.

Messerli et al.[30] documented a 30-fold increase in premature ventricular contractions in obese patients with **eccentric left ventricular hypertrophy** in comparison with lean subjects. There is an association between increased left ventricular mass and greater weight, even after data are controlled for age and blood pressure, especially in patients with a BMI greater than 30.[31] Among morbidly obese pregnant women, left atrial size, left ventricular thickness, interventricular septal thickness, and left ventricular mass increase; however, left ventricular function remains similar to that in nonobese pregnant women.[32] Alexander[23] concluded that excess epicardial fat is not a prominent feature in obese patients with cardiac enlargement. Fatty infiltration of the heart can occur, especially in the right ventricle and perhaps in the conduction system, but eccentric left ventricular hypertrophy is the major cause of an enlarged heart.

Gastrointestinal Changes

It is unclear whether a combination of pregnancy and obesity increases gastric volume and decreases gastric pH. Vaughan et al.[33] observed that 88% of obese nonpregnant patients presenting for surgery had a gastric pH less than 2.5, and 86% had a gastric volume exceeding 25 mL. These findings resemble those in a cohort of healthy pregnant patients who presented for elective cesarean delivery.[34]

Hiatal hernia is more common in obese patients than in nonobese patients, but the effect of obesity on pregnancy-associated changes in lower esophageal sphincter tone is unclear.[35-37] It seems likely, however, that morbidly obese patients are at higher risk for pulmonary aspiration of gastric contents.

Endocrine Changes

Gestational diabetes and **diabetes mellitus** occur more frequently in obese patients.[5,38] Farmer et al.[39] identified a relative insulin insufficiency and reduced insulin sensitivity among obese women during pregnancy. It has been estimated that as many as 92% of women with gestational diabetes progress to type 2 diabetes mellitus, depending on ethnicity, the diagnostic criteria used, and the duration of surveillance.[6]

Coagulation Changes

The obese patient may be at higher risk for **deep vein thrombosis** and **pulmonary thromboembolism.**[40,41] It is likely that obesity increases the risks for thromboembolic disease associated with pregnancy, especially in patients who are relatively inactive, although this issue is a matter of some dispute.[42]

INTERACTION WITH PREGNANCY

In 2000, 34.4% of women in the United States between the ages of 20 and 39 years were considered obese (see Table 50-1). The median weight gain during pregnancy in the United States is 30.5 lb,[43] and 20.6% of pregnant women gain more than 40 lb.[44] The incidence of morbid obesity among pregnant women varies according to the definitions used.

Obesity results in greater utilization of health care resources. Chu et al.[45] reported that obese pregnant women require significantly more prenatal tests, ultrasonographic examinations, medications, and prenatal visits with a physician, and are at greater risk of having a high-risk pregnancy, cesarean delivery, and prolonged hospitalization than pregnant women of normal weight.

Obesity is associated with higher risks for chronic hypertension, gestational hypertension, and diabetes mellitus during pregnancy.[5-7,38,46-48] A study of 117 morbidly obese patients found a 14-fold higher incidence of chronic hypertension (24% versus 2%, respectively) among patients whose weight exceeded 300 lb (136.4 kg) at the time of delivery than in a control group of nonobese patients.[49] The greater risk of chronic hypertension may result, in part, because obese pregnant patients typically are older than nonobese pregnant patients.

Morbidly obese women have a two- to eight-fold higher risk of acquiring diabetes mellitus during pregnancy than nonobese women.[6,7,46] Obesity also is associated with an increased risk for development of type 2 diabetes mellitus after pregnancy.[6]

Most importantly, obesity increases the risk of death during pregnancy.[4,50-52] Kaunitz et al.[50] suggested that advanced age and a higher incidence of hypertension, diabetes, thromboembolic disease, and infection are factors that increase the risk of maternal death in obese pregnant women.

The American College of Obstetricians and Gynecologists (ACOG)[53,54] has recommended a multidisciplinary approach to treatment of obesity in pregnancy, and has suggested that obstetricians (1) evaluate all women for obesity by calculating BMI, (2) offer preconception counseling to obese women, and (3) refer obese pregnant patients for antepartum preanesthetic consultation.

The obstetric care team also may encounter patients who have undergone bariatric surgery. Bariatric surgery offers the most effective treatment for morbid obesity; approximately 50,000 women of reproductive age in the United States have the surgery each year.[55] After surgery, anatomic and physiologic changes may affect future pregnancies. Although fertility improves after the surgery, the women have a higher risk of gastrointestinal malabsorption and intestinal obstruction.

Progress of Labor and Method of Delivery

Higher BMI, increased prepregnancy weight, and excessive maternal weight gain increase the risk for cesarean delivery.[46,47,56] Reasons for the higher cesarean delivery rate among obese patients are not clear but may include a higher incidence of abnormal presentation, fetal macrosomia, and/or prolonged labor. These factors may also contribute to the greater risk of a failed trial of labor and uterine rupture in obese parturients with a history of previous cesarean delivery.[57]

Cedergren[38] found a higher incidence of fetal compromise and need for cesarean delivery in morbidly obese patients. Conversely, an earlier study found that the indications for cesarean delivery—with the exception of failed induction of labor—were remarkably similar in normal-weight and morbidly obese patients.[49]

Hypertension and diabetes often prompt elective induction of labor, which increases the risk of cesarean delivery. Garbaciak et al.[47] reviewed the records of 9667 patients who were subdivided into four weight categories: *underweight*, *normal weight*, *overweight*, and *morbidly obese*. The investigators found that as weight increased, so did the frequency of antenatal medical complications, including hypertension, preeclampsia, and diabetes mellitus. The need for cesarean delivery was increased by the presence of such complications in the normal weight and overweight groups, but not in the morbidly obese group; the investigators suggested that other factors must also account for the higher cesarean delivery rate among obese women.

Obese women are also at increased risk of experiencing abnormal labor.[56,58] They have a higher incidence of meconium-stained amniotic fluid and late fetal heart rate (FHR) decelerations.[56] The frequent diagnosis of dystocia in obese women is consistent with the observed decrease in the incidence of preterm delivery and low-birth-weight infants and the increase in the incidence of fetal macrosomia and postterm gestation.[5-7,38,47,48]

Maternal diabetes and obesity may independently increase the likelihood of fetal macrosomia.[5,8] Weight gain during pregnancy also may affect the risk of fetal macrosomia.[5,38] It has been suggested that weight gain *during* pregnancy is more likely than absolute weight *before* pregnancy to increase the need for a cesarean delivery. Bianco et al.[59] suggested that restricting maternal weight gain to less than 25 lb during pregnancy reduces the risk of delivering a large-for-gestational-age infant and improves neonatal outcome. Others have not confirmed that excess maternal weight gain increases the risk of fetal macrosomia.[60]

Abrams and Laros[61] noted that maternal weight gain significantly increased newborn birth weight for underweight, ideal-weight, and moderately overweight women but not for women whose prepregnancy weights were greater than 135% of the ideal. These investigators and others have suggested that recommending a minimum weight gain for morbidly obese women is unnecessary. Klebanoff et al.[62] noted that a *maternal* birth weight in excess of 8 lb was second only to maternal weight gain during pregnancy as a predictor of macrosomia in her baby. Crane et al.[63] speculated that prepregnancy weight loss can decrease the risk of needing a cesarean delivery and suggested counseling as a way to encourage this weight loss. The ACOG[53] has recommended similar counseling. In summary, the morbidly obese patient, with or without diabetes, and with or without excessive weight gain during pregnancy, is at increased risk for having a macrosomic infant.

Johnson et al.[60] observed a higher incidence of cesarean delivery among obese patients even when patients with hypertension, diabetes, and macrosomic infants were excluded from analysis. Further, medicolegal considerations may increase the likelihood of cesarean delivery in obese patients (i.e., obstetricians may perform a cesarean delivery to avoid the risk of shoulder dystocia during a vaginal delivery). Others have suggested that soft tissue dystocia increases the risk of cesarean delivery in obese patients.[64] Prough et al.[65] speculated that perineal fat and intrapelvic fat deposits near the sigmoid colon and lateral pelvic sidewalls may alter the shape of the vaginal canal and mechanically impede the progress of labor in obese women. Garbaciak et al.[47] also suggested that the increase in maternal pelvic soft tissue narrows the birth canal in obese women.

Excessive blood loss during cesarean delivery has been noted in obese patients.[60] Prolonged, difficult surgery may be responsible for this observation, although one series did not observe an increase in blood loss during cesarean delivery among patients who weighed more than 300 lb (136.4 kg).[49]

Perinatal Outcome

Obese women are at lower risk for both preterm delivery and delivery of a low-birth-weight infant.[38,60] However, pregnant women with a prepregnancy BMI greater than 30 have an increased risk of fetal death with advancing gestation. Nohr et al.[66] estimated the relative risk of fetal death to be 4.6 times higher at 40 weeks' gestation for obese women than in women with normal prepregnancy weight; placental dysfunction may be a contributing factor. Infants of obese women also may have a higher risk of neural tube defects and other congenital malformations.[67]

Fetal macrosomia may predispose obese women to trauma at delivery and increase the likelihood of shoulder dystocia during vaginal delivery.[46,56] Johnson et al.[56] observed an association between fetal macrosomia and a higher incidence of shoulder dystocia in obese parturients. Perlow et al.[48] observed a greater frequency of neonatal intensive care unit admissions among infants born to obese women. Although Rahaman et al.[68] reported a tenfold increase in perinatal mortality among obese parturients, other investigators have not confirmed these findings.[56,57] No neonatal deaths among women who weighed more than 300 lb (136.4 kg) at delivery were observed in the Hood and Dewan series,[49] despite the fact that 46% of patients had antenatal complications.

ANESTHETIC MANAGEMENT

Preanesthetic Assessment

The high incidence of comorbid conditions among obese pregnant women necessitates early, careful preanesthetic assessment (as discussed earlier).

Unless the length of the sphygmomanometer cuff exceeds the circumference of the arm by 20%, systolic and diastolic blood pressure measurements may overestimate true maternal blood pressure. Use of an appropriately sized blood pressure cuff and an automated blood pressure measurement device often obviate the need for intra-arterial monitoring in the obese parturient. However, an intra-arterial catheter may be beneficial in patients with chronic hypertension or preeclampsia and in those requiring frequent arterial blood gas measurements during and after cesarean delivery.

Pulse oximetry may be used to assess the adequacy of maternal oxygenation; however, arterial blood gas measurements are invaluable in assessing maternal ventilation when there is cause for concern. The presence of preeclampsia makes platelet count assessment necessary. Unless there is clinical evidence of coagulopathy or rapid patient deterioration, other coagulation tests are not indicated.

When administering neuraxial anesthesia in obese patients, the anesthesia provider should anticipate the need for a longer spinal needle.[69] In the majority of obese parturients, the epidural space can be identified with a standard-length epidural needle. In contrast, for spinal anesthesia in morbidly obese patients, longer-than-normal needles are more frequently required.

Appropriately sized labor beds, transportation gurneys, and operating tables, and sufficient personnel to assist with patient transport, are imperative. Although standard operating tables are generally rated for persons weighing up to 500 lb (227.3 kg), this rating may be insufficient for morbidly obese patients, especially when the table is articulated. Regardless of the weight rating of the table, it is critical that the obese patient be centered over the operating table pedestal at all times.

Labor and Vaginal Delivery

Because it may be difficult in some obese patients, intravenous access should be established early in labor. Ultrasonographic guidance may be useful; however, if intravenous access remains unsuccessful, central venous cannulation may be necessary.

Options for analgesia are the same as those for nonobese patients. Although some obese women may not require analgesia for labor and spontaneous vaginal delivery, obesity does not affect the severity of labor pain,[70] and most obese women desire analgesia during labor.

The potential for neonatal depression complicates the administration of systemic opioids during labor. For delivery, a pudendal nerve block may be more technically difficult in obese patients. Inhalation analgesia is useful in some patients; however, nitrous oxide has limited effectiveness and is no longer available in many birthing rooms. Further, inhalation analgesia could lead to loss of consciousness, which can precipitate disaster in an obese woman with a difficult airway. Given the greater risks for fetal macrosomia and shoulder dystocia in obese patients, satisfactory anesthesia may be necessary to facilitate an atraumatic vaginal delivery.

Lumbar epidural analgesia is an excellent choice for labor and vaginal delivery in obese parturients. Epidural analgesia reduces oxygen consumption and attenuates the increase in cardiac output that occurs during labor and delivery. In addition, the use of epidural analgesia during labor allows the anesthesia provider to extend epidural anesthesia for cesarean delivery when necessary, and avoid the risks of general anesthesia.

Buckley et al.[69] reported a 20% incidence of failed epidural anesthesia in morbidly obese patients. Although the investigators reported 1 patient with an inadequate block and 10 patients in whom they were unable to identify the epidural space, other experience suggests that a high rate of success with epidural analgesia can be achieved in obese pregnant women. In the Hood and Dewan series,[49] 94% of patients who weighed more than 300 lb (136.4 kg) experienced adequate analgesia for delivery, compared with 98% of controls. However, more attempts were required to identify the epidural space in obese women, there was a significantly higher initial failure rate, and placement of a second or third epidural catheter was more often required.

The greater depth of the epidural space in obese patients contributes to a higher failure rate of epidural analgesia; some authorities have speculated that the greater depth exaggerates minor directional errors and increases the likelihood of identifying a lateral portion of the epidural space.[71,72] Although ultrasonographic guidance has been suggested as a means of identifying the epidural space,[73] not all anesthesia providers are proficient in this technique. Placing the patient in the sitting position facilitates identification of the midline of the spinal column, which is helpful in locating the subarachnoid or epidural space. Further, the distance from the skin to the epidural space is minimized when the patient is in the sitting flexed position.[74,75] Conversely, when the patient moves from the sitting flexed position to the lateral decubitus position, the soft tissue of the back is redistributed, the distance from the skin to the epidural space becomes longer, and an unsecured catheter will appear to be drawn inward. As demonstrated by Hamilton et al.,[75] a catheter secured with tape to the back of a patient in the sitting flexed position can be unintentionally dislodged from the epidural space when she assumes the lateral decubitus position. Their observations were most striking in obese patients. These investigators recommended having the patient assume the lateral position *before* the epidural catheter is secured to the skin.

Ideally, epidural labor analgesia provides excellent pain relief with little motor block. Epidural administration of a dilute solution of bupivacaine with fentanyl provides analgesia for labor while minimizing adverse effects such as motor blockade.[76] However, the administration of both a local anesthetic and an opioid to initiate labor analgesia can mask the malposition of an epidural catheter because opioid administration by any route provides some pain relief. If the patient subsequently requires cesarean delivery, a malpositioned catheter may result in inadequate anesthesia. Some anesthesia providers document satisfactory epidural analgesia before adding an opioid to the local anesthetic solution in morbidly obese patients.

Similarly, the intrathecal component of a combined spinal-epidural (CSE) technique can provide high-quality analgesia despite an incorrectly positioned epidural catheter. Because delayed recognition of an incorrectly positioned epidural catheter is a significant shortcoming of CSE analgesia, many anesthesia providers prefer to use a standard epidural technique when providing labor analgesia in morbidly obese parturients.

The epidural block should be bilateral and *near perfect*. Otherwise, the epidural catheter should be removed and replaced. In a study of morbidly obese parturients, the initial administration of local anesthetic through the epidural catheter resulted in failure of analgesia/anesthesia in 42% of the women, a rate sevenfold higher than that in controls.[49] However, careful evaluation of the epidural block and early replacement of malpositioned catheters resulted in a high rate of success, so that only 1 of 55 cesarean deliveries attempted with epidural anesthesia required conversion to general anesthesia because of inadequate anesthesia.[49] In this retrospective study, positioning and position changes were not controlled, a fact that may have contributed to the high initial failure rate (as discussed earlier).

In cases of unintentional dural puncture, continuous spinal analgesia can be used to provide labor analgesia.[77] As with epidural analgesia, continuous spinal analgesia may be extended for emergency cesarean delivery. Unintentional administration of an epidural dose of a local anesthetic through the spinal catheter increases the risk of high spinal block and loss of the airway in the birthing room.

Cesarean Delivery

In the Hood and Dewan series,[49] 48% of patients weighing more than 300 lb (136.4 kg) who underwent a trial of labor subsequently required cesarean delivery. Among nonobese patients, cesarean delivery has been associated with a higher risk of maternal mortality,[78] especially when performed as an *emergency* procedure.[79] Morbid obesity further increases the risks of maternal morbidity, fetal injury,[56,80] and anesthesia-related maternal death during and after cesarean delivery.[4,81]

A careful, thorough airway assessment is essential. Large breasts, the greater anteroposterior diameter of the chest, airway edema, and reduced chin-to-chest distance increase the likelihood of difficult laryngoscopy and failed intubation in obstetric patients.[82] Obesity exaggerates many of the anatomic changes of pregnancy. Increased fat in the neck and shoulders increases the difficulty of positioning the patient for intubation. Further, the fat pads on the back of the shoulders often restrict the range of motion of the neck, exacerbating the difficulty of mask ventilation, laryngoscopy, and intubation. Neck extension may increase upper airway obstruction in these women.

All morbidly obese parturients undergoing cesarean delivery should be placed in a ramped position with left uterine displacement, regardless of the planned anesthetic technique. This position has been demonstrated to improve laryngoscopic view in morbidly obese parturients undergoing elective bariatric surgery.[83] Folded blankets are placed under the chest and head to achieve horizontal alignment between the external auditory meatus and the sternal notch (Figure 50-2).[84] This position aligns the oral, pharyngeal, and tracheal axes to facilitate intubation and has been shown to improve hemodynamic and respiratory parameters during laparoscopic gastric bypass surgery.[85]

It may be difficult to position the obese patient appropriately and safely. The protuberant abdomen may shift markedly with left uterine displacement. The patient must be secured to the operating table before the table is tilted leftward; however, it is important to initiate left uterine displacement as soon as possible. Tsueda et al.[28] described two obese patients who experienced acute cardiovascular collapse after assuming the supine position. A morbidly obese parturient in a ramped position (see Figure 50-2) with a leftward tilt may be unstable on the operating table. The anesthesia provider should (1) confirm that the patient's weight does not exceed the weight limits of the table,[84] (2) consider use of lateral table extenders if required, and (3) use foam or blankets to ensure that the shoulders and arms are on a horizontal plane. Correct arm position will maximize patient comfort, improve stability, and avoid upper extremity neurologic injury.[86]

The anesthesia care team may be asked to participate in cephalad retraction of the large panniculus by tethering retractors to an object such as the ether screen. Both the obstetrician and the anesthesia provider must remain cognizant of the risks of hypotension, difficulty with ventilation, and fetal compromise during cephalad retraction of the panniculus in morbidly obese patients. Hodgkinson and Husain[80] reported an intraoperative fetal death in a morbidly obese patient who had received epidural anesthesia for cesarean delivery. The death was attributed to prolonged hypotension associated with cephalad retraction of a large panniculus.

Use of a supraumbilical midline skin incision has been advocated in obese women undergoing cesarean delivery, both to prevent potential cardiopulmonary compromise and to avoid making a Pfannenstiel skin incision in the anaerobic area beneath the panniculus, which may predispose the patient to postoperative infection.[87,88] Larger studies in parturients, however, have not demonstrated a lower infection rate in association with a supraumbilical incision than with a low transverse skin incision.[89,90]

Difficult mask ventilation is often accompanied by gastric distention with air, which increases the risk of regurgitation and pulmonary aspiration of gastric contents. It may be difficult to identify the cricoid cartilage accurately in obese patients; thus, the assistant may have trouble applying cricoid pressure correctly during rapid-sequence induction of general anesthesia. Finally, in cases of failed intubation, obesity can increase the difficulty of cricothyrotomy and the likelihood of unsuccessful transtracheal jet ventilation.

Obese pregnant patients require aggressive pharmacologic aspiration prophylaxis. A total of 30 mL of a 0.3 M

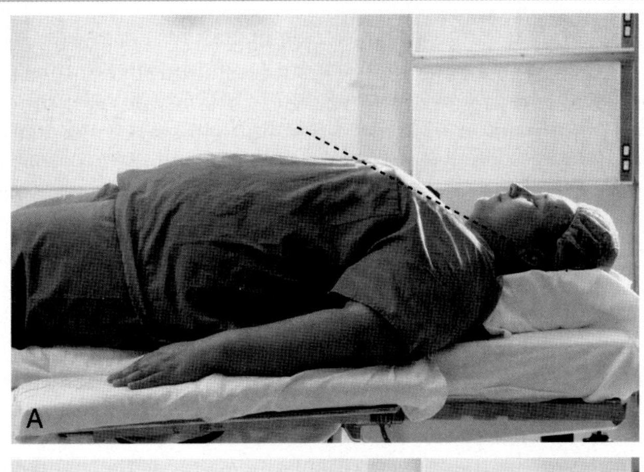

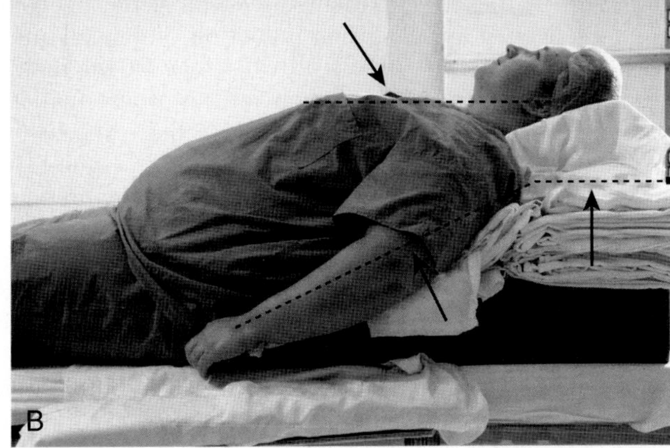

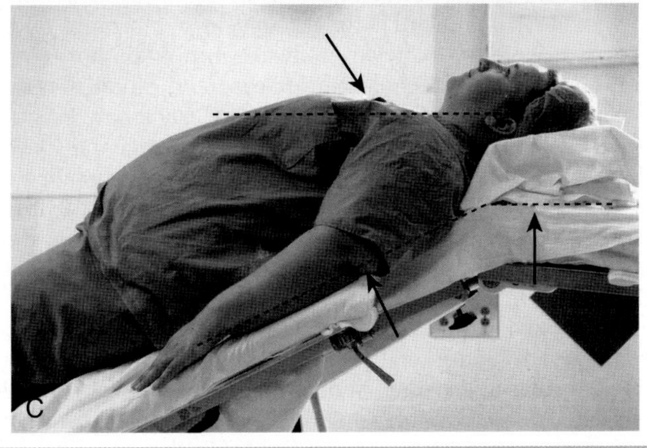

FIGURE 50-2 Positioning the obese patient to facilitate intubation of the trachea. **A,** A patient in the supine position using standard head support. Note that the *dashed line* (see **B**) is not parallel to the floor. **B,** Elevating the patient's head with neck and shoulder supports so that an imaginary line drawn through the external auditory meatus and the sternal notch (*upper dashed line*) is parallel to the floor may facilitate tracheal intubation. **C,** Similar positioning achieved by repositioning the operating table. Note the similarity of the *upper* and *lower dashed lines* with use of the second and third positioning techniques.

solution of sodium citrate effectively increases gastric pH within 5 minutes.[91] Administration of a histamine H_2-receptor antagonist and metoclopramide provides additional protection[92]; however, metoclopramide may be less effective in the presence of preexisting anticholinergic or opioid therapy.[93] The anesthesia provider must be aware that the patient remains at risk for aspiration at the end of surgery; the efficacy of sodium citrate wanes 45 to 60 minutes after administration.[34]

SPINAL ANESTHESIA AND COMBINED SPINAL-EPIDURAL ANESTHESIA

Concerns about the use of spinal anesthesia in obese patients include technical difficulties, potential for an exaggerated cephalad spread of anesthesia, and insufficient duration of anesthesia.

Spinal anesthesia is technically feasible in morbidly obese pregnant women, although a longer spinal needle may be required. The distribution of adipose tissue varies among obese patients. Spinal needle placement can be uneventful in women who do not have excessive adipose tissue over the midline of the back. However, a single-shot spinal anesthetic may not have sufficient duration if surgery is prolonged.

Obesity may result in an unpredictable, exaggerated spread of local anesthetic during administration of spinal or epidural anesthesia. Hormonal and mechanical factors may be responsible for a smaller local anesthetic dose requirement in pregnant women. Magnetic resonance imaging (MRI) has confirmed that obese patients have a reduced cerebrospinal fluid (CSF) volume.[94] Pregnancy-associated engorgement of the epidural veins and inward movement of soft tissue through the intervertebral foramina as a result of increased abdominal pressure may be responsible for the reduced CSF volume in these patients. A separate study using magnetic resonance imaging demonstrated an inverse correlation between block height and lumbar CSF volume[95]; this finding suggests that reduced CSF volume in obese patients increases the risk of a high spinal block. Additionally, Greene[96] has suggested that excess adipose tissue in the buttocks may result in relative Trendelenburg positioning of the vertebral column in the supine position, which can lead to an exaggerated cephalad spread of anesthesia. Other studies have suggested that the maximal spread of anesthesia does not correlate with weight or BMI.[97,98] Norris[98] administered hyperbaric bupivacaine 12 mg intrathecally and found no correlation between height, weight, BMI, and the spread of spinal anesthesia. However, only one woman in this study had a BMI greater than 34, so these results may not be applicable to heavier parturients. In contrast, McCulloch and Littlewood[99] administered 4 mL of 0.5% bupivacaine to a group of obese patients and found a correlation between the spread of anesthesia and the severity of obesity. In summary, it is likely that obese parturients are at increased risk of a high spinal block.

The consequences of extensive neuroblockade dictate caution when selecting spinal anesthesia for an obese patient with an anticipated difficult airway. Loss of thoracic motor function may be hazardous in morbidly obese patients; spinal anesthesia results in a more profound thoracic motor blockade than epidural anesthesia, and so could adversely affect oxygenation and ventilation of the obese parturient. Moreover, von Ungern-Sternberg et al.[100] found that spinal anesthesia impairs respiratory function significantly more in obese patients than in nonobese patients.

The potential for prolonged surgery must be considered in the planning of anesthesia for the obese woman undergoing cesarean delivery. Johnson et al.[60] noted that the duration of cesarean delivery exceeded 2 hours in 55% of women who weighed more than 250 lb (113.6 kg). Mean operative time in another study was 77 ± 31 minutes.[49] Because intraoperative induction of general anesthesia is undesirable and potentially hazardous in morbidly obese pregnant women, a continuous neuraxial technique (i.e., epidural, CSE, or continuous spinal anesthesia) is preferable to single-shot spinal anesthesia.[77,101]

EPIDURAL ANESTHESIA

Epidural anesthesia is preferred if (1) a functioning catheter is already in place, (2) surgery duration may exceed 2 hours, (3) the airway examination is worrisome, or (4) cardiopulmonary function is impaired. Identification of the epidural space with a large-gauge epidural needle is often technically easier than identification of the subarachnoid space with a small-gauge spinal needle. The ability to titrate the dose of local anesthetic and the unlimited duration of anesthesia with repeated injections of local anesthetic are other significant advantages of epidural anesthesia.

In 1980, Hodgkinson and Husain[102] administered 20 mL of 0.75% epidural bupivacaine at the L3 to L4 interspace over a period of 40 seconds (which, of course, is neither safe nor acceptable in contemporary obstetric anesthesia practice). The patients remained supine for 40 minutes after drug injection. None of the patients whose BMI exceeded 28 required additional local anesthetic for the achievement of surgical anesthesia. Although the sensory level reached C5 in some parturients, no patient needed positive-pressure ventilation, and hypotension occurred in only 12% of the patients. The height of the block was proportional to BMI and weight but not to height. In contrast, another study found that neither patient position nor obesity affected the height of the sensory block when 12 mL of 0.25% bupivacaine was administered for epidural analgesia during labor.[103] In fact, an up-down sequential allocation study found that obese women required significantly less epidural bupivacaine for labor than women of normal weight.[104]

The ability to administer incremental doses of drug through an epidural catheter allows the anesthesia provider to titrate the dose to the desired dermatomal level while maintaining hemodynamic stability. The desired sensory level to touch for cesarean delivery is T5.[105,106] An indwelling epidural catheter also facilitates the epidural administration of an opioid and/or local anesthetic for postoperative analgesia. Further, there is evidence that epidural administration of bupivacaine decreases the risk of deep vein thrombosis in patients undergoing total hip replacement,[107] although no studies have documented this advantage in obstetric patients.

GENERAL ANESTHESIA

Endotracheal intubation is essential during administration of general anesthesia for cesarean delivery, but it may be difficult or impossible (via direct laryngoscopy) in morbidly obese patients. The association between obesity and a short neck can make endotracheal intubation difficult in this population.[108] Buckley et al.[69] reported 9 difficult intubations among 68 morbidly obese, nonpregnant patients (13%). In a later series of patients who had received general anesthesia for cesarean delivery, the incidence of difficult intubation was 33% among women who weighed more than 300 lb (136.4 kg).[49] Difficult intubation occurred in 1 patient who had undergone successful intubation during a previous cesarean delivery. Clearly, the history of a previous successful intubation does not guarantee the same result during a subsequent procedure. Lee et al.[109] reported their experience with difficult intubation in 284 morbidly obese patients who underwent gastric bypass surgery. The incidence of difficult intubation was 2.4% among patients between 1.5 and 1.75 times the ideal weight, and the incidence of difficult intubation tripled to 7.3% in patients whose weight was 1.75 to 2 times the ideal. Correct positioning improves the success rate for endotracheal intubation (as discussed earlier).

The potential for failed intubation and difficult mask ventilation in the obese patient underscores the need for an experienced assistant during induction of general anesthesia. The primary anesthesia provider may fatigue rapidly with attempted mask ventilation of an obese patient. Further, the jaw-thrust maneuver may require the use of both hands, and additional personnel will be required to provide positive-pressure ventilation and cricoid pressure. A short-handled laryngoscope, assorted laryngoscope blades, various sizes of endotracheal tubes and laryngeal mask airways, and equipment for percutaneous cricothyrotomy and transtracheal jet ventilation should be readily available.[110]

Awake intubation, via either direct visualization or fiberoptic laryngoscopy, is an alternative method of securing the airway. Successful awake intubation also has been performed with a Bullard laryngoscope in a morbidly obese pregnant woman.[111] However, awake intubation poses several challenges. Catecholamine release and blood pressure elevation during awake procedures may exacerbate existing hypertension and adversely affect uteroplacental blood flow.[112] Further, women requiring urgent performance of cesarean delivery are not ideal candidates for awake intubation. In these women, it is difficult to perform an awake laryngoscopy and intubation successfully unless the anesthesia provider has adequate time to prepare the patient's airway. However, the mother's well-being should not be endangered to deliver a compromised fetus. Specifically, the anesthesia provider should not proceed with rapid-sequence induction of general anesthesia if intubation is expected to be difficult or impossible. In this scenario, the anesthesia provider should consider the administration of neuraxial anesthesia.

When preanesthetic assessment suggests that intubation will *not* be difficult, rapid-sequence induction is indicated. The administration of general anesthesia begins with effective pulmonary denitrogenation (or so-called preoxygenation). During apnea, pregnant women become hypoxemic more rapidly than nonpregnant women.[113] Similarly, during apnea, obese patients become hypoxemic more rapidly than nonobese patients.[114] Therefore, adequate denitrogenation is essential prior to the administration of general anesthesia in obese pregnant women (see Chapter 30).

One study demonstrated that 4 maximal inspirations of 100% oxygen within 30 seconds provide benefit similar to that provided by 3 minutes of tidal-volume breathing of 100% oxygen before rapid-sequence induction of general anesthesia for cesarean delivery.[115] However, another study reported a more-rapid onset of hypoxemia in patients who underwent 4 maximal inspirations of 100% oxygen than in similar patients who underwent 3 minutes of tidal-volume breathing of 100% oxygen.[116] Goldberg et al.[92] evaluated the use of both techniques in morbidly obese nonpregnant patients undergoing gastric bypass surgery. The techniques provided similar increases in Pa_{O_2}, but patients who used the 3-minute technique showed evidence of a slight retention of CO_2. The investigators speculated that a blunted ventilatory response to CO_2 contributed to the increase in Pa_{CO_2}. In contrast, other studies have suggested that obese patients have a normal ventilatory response to CO_2.[11] Later data from a study in 20 pregnant volunteers (at 36 to 38 weeks' gestation) compared 3 minutes of tidal-volume breathing with methods involving 4 deep breaths (4 DB) in 30 seconds or 8 deep breaths (8 DB) in 1 minute of 100% oxygen by measuring end-tidal fractional oxygen concentration (F_{ETO_2}) following preoxygenation. An F_{ETO_2} value of 90% or greater was achieved in 76% of women after either the 3-minute or the 8 DB method, compared with only 18% of women after the 4 DB method of preoxygenation.[117] The investigators concluded that for emergency cesarean delivery using general anesthesia, the 8 DB method was as effective as the 3-minute tidal-volume method of preoxygenation and was more quickly performed.

It is wise to apply a tight-fitting face mask and administer 100% oxygen as soon as the patient is moved onto the operating table; this maneuver helps achieve denitrogenation while other preparations are being made. It then seems reasonable to let circumstances dictate the selected method of denitrogenation. When the 3-minute tidal-volume breathing technique is selected, the anesthesia provider should encourage the patient to take several deep breaths. In urgent situations, such as emergency cesarean delivery for maternal hemorrhage, the patient should be instructed to take 8 deep breaths (the 8 DB method) to extend the safe interval before oxyhemoglobin desaturation occurs. When time allows, the 8 DB method is preferred over the 4 DB method.

Obesity alters the distribution of anesthetic drugs; a larger volume of distribution prolongs the elimination half-life of thiopental in obese patients.[118] The clinical significance of these findings in obstetric patients is unclear.

Kumar et al.[119] observed similar times to eye opening after administration of either methohexital or Althesin in obese patients. The investigators suggested that in the absence of complicating medical disease, the choice of intravenous agent is relatively unimportant. Ketamine is an excellent induction agent in nonobese patients; however, no study has specifically evaluated the use of ketamine in obese pregnant women, and this agent is relatively contraindicated in hypertensive parturients. The choice of drug and dose remains a matter of clinical judgment. If the anesthesia provider chooses to give thiopental, administration of less than 4 mg/kg may increase the risk of maternal awareness, hypertension, and decreased uteroplacental blood flow during light anesthesia. Administration of a larger dose may be associated with delayed arousal in the event of failed intubation. Similar concerns apply to other commonly used induction agents (e.g., propofol, etomidate).

Succinylcholine remains the muscle relaxant of choice for rapid-sequence induction, and doses of 1.0 to 1.5 mg/kg are commonly used for general anesthesia and endotracheal intubation in obese parturients. Adequate relaxation is essential, and the anesthesia provider should not attempt laryngoscopy in the presence of incomplete muscle relaxation. On the other hand, administration of a large dose of succinylcholine likely delays the return of spontaneous ventilation in cases of failed intubation. In morbidly obese nonpregnant patients, Lemmens et al.[120] compared the efficacy of succinylcholine in dosing regimens of 1 mg/kg based on (1) ideal body weight, (2) lean body weight, and (3) total body weight. The third regimen (1 mg per kg total body weight) was demonstrated to be superior for providing complete neuromuscular paralysis and predictable laryngoscopy conditions. The investigators also noted that "none of these dosing regimens will provide . . . a safe (short) duration of apnea."[120] Thus the anesthesia provider must be prepared to use alternative airway management techniques in cases of failed intubation (see Chapter 30).

Neuromuscular blockade should be carefully monitored after intubation. Adequate muscle relaxation is essential because cesarean delivery can be technically difficult in the morbidly obese patient. Morbidly obese women likely have a normal response to nondepolarizing muscle relaxants, although Weinstein et al.[121] observed a prolonged duration of action after administration of vecuronium in nonpregnant obese patients. The investigators speculated that impaired hepatic clearance may have contributed to the prolonged duration of neuromuscular blockade. In contrast, the administration of atracurium, which does not require hepatic metabolism, is associated with a normal duration of action in obese patients. The time required to reverse atracurium-induced neuromuscular blockade is not affected by total body weight or BMI.[122]

No evidence suggests that obesity alters the minimum alveolar concentration (MAC) of volatile halogenated anesthetic agents in pregnant women. However, obesity does affect blood-gas partition coefficients. The blood-gas partition coefficient for enflurane, which is 2.03 with normal body weight, is 1.76 with obesity, whereas for halothane, the blood-gas partition coefficient is higher with obesity.[123] These changes are unlikely to be clinically significant, however.

In theory, increased body fat serves as a reservoir for inhalational and intravenous agents. Likewise, the body fat reservoir could increase the threat of biotransformation of volatile halogenated agents, which would increase the risk of organ toxicity. Bentley et al.[124] have reported higher serum fluoride and bromide concentrations after 2 hours of halothane anesthesia in nonpregnant obese patients than in nonobese patients. Rice and Fish[125] suggested that obese patients might be at risk for fluoride-induced nephrotoxicity after prolonged administration of enflurane; this is a potential concern in obese parturients with severe preeclampsia and abnormal renal function. Isoflurane, which has largely supplanted halothane and enflurane in clinical practice, is an appropriate choice for morbidly obese parturients due to its limited biotransformation.[126,127] The newer agents, desflurane and sevoflurane, are associated with shorter time-to-extubation than isoflurane in obese patients.[128,129] However, metabolic degradation of sevoflurane may result in release of fluoride ions, and at least one study has shown that fluoride levels increase more rapidly in obese patients.[130]

High concentrations of a volatile halogenated agent increase the likelihood of neonatal depression, uterine atony, and maternal blood loss. In contrast, low concentrations of a volatile agent increase the risk of maternal awareness, catecholamine release, hypertension, and decreased uteroplacental blood flow. Most anesthesia providers administer nitrous oxide to nonobese pregnant patients to allow administration of a lower concentration of a volatile halogenated agent. However, morbidly obese patients may require administration of a higher inspired concentration of oxygen and may not tolerate usual concentrations of nitrous oxide. Moreover, general anesthesia reduces FRC. The supine and Trendelenburg positions further decrease FRC, thus increasing the risk of intraoperative hypoxemia.

Techniques that may improve intraoperative oxygenation in the obese patient include administration of a higher inspired oxygen concentration, use of a large tidal volume, administration of positive end-expiratory pressure (PEEP), and elevation of the panniculus to relieve thoracoabdominal compression.[131] Salem et al.[132] questioned the wisdom of using a large tidal volume and PEEP in the obese patient after they observed better oxygenation after the discontinuation of PEEP. Eriksen et al.,[133] comparing a 35% increase in tidal volume with PEEP, found that although both techniques increased maternal Pa_{O_2}, neither technique increased oxygen delivery. Additionally, PEEP may reduce cardiac output.[134] This reduction, in turn, could diminish uteroplacental blood flow and result in fetal compromise when the induction-to-delivery interval is prolonged. Nonetheless, it is imperative to maintain adequate maternal oxygenation in the morbidly obese patient.

Finally, airway obstruction may increase pulmonary capillary wedge pressure and precipitate cardiovascular decompensation.[24,25] All efforts should be directed toward avoiding airway obstruction during induction of and emergence from anesthesia.

POSTOPERATIVE COMPLICATIONS

Obesity increases the risk of postoperative complications such as endometritis, urinary tract infection, wound infection, wound dehiscence, peripheral nerve injury, hemorrhage, deep vein thrombosis, pulmonary thromboembolism, atelectasis, pneumonia, asthma, respiratory depression, hypoxemia, tracheal reintubation, sleep apnea, myocardial infarction, cardiac arrest, and maternal death.[7,135-137] In one study, all major postpartum complications in morbidly obese women were associated with cesarean delivery.[49] Prolonged surgery and greater operative blood loss during cesarean delivery may increase the risk of postoperative morbidity.[138]

The obesity epidemic has resulted in a higher prevalence of sleep-disordered breathing and obstructive sleep apnea in the United States.[139,140] The combination of obesity, obstructive sleep apnea, general anesthesia, and opioid administration increases the risk of anesthesia-related postoperative complications. In a report on maternal mortality in Michigan, Mhyre et al.[81] found that all anesthesia-related maternal deaths from airway obstruction or hypoventilation occurred during emergence and recovery. No maternal deaths were associated with aspiration or difficult intubation during induction of general anesthesia. Obesity was identified as a significant risk factor for anesthesia-related maternal mortality. Although whether any of the women who died had obstructive sleep apnea is unknown, there is cause for concern that anesthesia-related maternal mortality will increase in the future unless measures are taken to reduce risk in morbidly obese patients and in patients with obstructive sleep apnea.[141] The American Society of Anesthesiologists (ASA) has addressed these concerns in its Practice Guidelines for the Perioperative Management of Patients with Obstructive Sleep Apnea, with recommendations for the preoperative, intraoperative, and postoperative management of these patients.[142] Although the published literature is often insufficient to establish definite relationships between interventions and outcomes, the Task Force consultants made the recommendations listed in Box 50-1. These recommendations are not intended specifically for pregnant women, but they do provide some guidance for the care of the obese parturient undergoing cesarean delivery.

Postoperative Analgesia

Effective pain management after cesarean delivery may improve maternal outcome, although the ideal method of administration in obese patients remains unclear. Postoperative analgesia reduces the incidence of atelectasis and pulmonary complications; nevertheless, opioids must be used with caution in obese patients because they decrease the central ventilatory response to CO_2. Intramuscular administration of an opioid can result in variable, unpredictable absorption of the drug—especially in morbidly obese patients—and is therefore not recommended. Intravenous administration of an opioid either by intermittent bolus injection or by patient-controlled analgesia may provide more consistent pain relief,[143] but it also increases the risk of respiratory depression in obese parturients. Intravenously administered sufentanil, and theoretically any lipid-soluble opioid, is eliminated slowly in obese patients, and the anesthesia provider should consider reduction of the maintenance dose.[144] Nonsteroidal anti-inflammatory drugs (NSAIDs) should be used to supplement analgesia and decrease total opioid requirements when appropriate.

Thoracic epidural anesthesia reduces oxygen consumption, arterial-venous oxygen difference, and left ventricular stroke work in morbidly obese patients.[145] Rawal et al.[146] observed that administration of epidural morphine resulted in earlier ambulation, fewer pulmonary complications, and shorter hospitalization than did intramuscular morphine in morbidly obese patients recovering from abdominal surgery. Although epidural morphine has been successfully administered in a nonpregnant patient with obstructive sleep apnea,[147] a respiratory arrest has also been reported after neuraxial morphine administration in a patient with sleep apnea.[148]

It is important to recognize that morbidly obese parturients may have undiagnosed obstructive sleep apnea. The ASA practice guidelines encourage the use of regional techniques for postoperative analgesia to reduce or eliminate the requirement for systemic opioids in patients at increased perioperative risk from obstructive sleep apnea.[142] For obstetric patients undergoing cesarean

BOX 50-1 American Society of Anesthesiologists Practice Guidelines for Perioperative Management of Patients with Obstructive Sleep Apnea

Preoperative

- Preoperative initiation of continuous positive airway pressure (CPAP) should be considered, particularly if obstructive sleep apnea (OSA) is severe.
- Patients with known or suspected OSA may have a difficult airway and therefore should be managed according to the ASA Practice Guidelines for Management of the Difficult Airway.*

Intraoperative

- The potential for postoperative respiratory compromise should be considered.
- Patients at increased perioperative risk from OSA should be extubated while awake.
- Full reversal of neuromuscular blockade should be verified before extubation.
- When possible, extubation and recovery should be carried out in the lateral, semi-upright, or other nonsupine position.

Postoperative

- [For postoperative analgesia], regional analgesic techniques should be considered to reduce or eliminate the requirement for systemic opioids in patients at increased perioperative risk from OSA.
- If neuraxial analgesia is planned, [the anesthesiologist should] weigh the benefits (improved analgesia, decreased need for systemic opioids) and risks (respiratory depression from rostral spread) of using an opioid or opioid–local anesthetic mixture as compared to a local anesthetic alone.
- If patient-controlled systemic opioids are used, continuous background infusions should be used with extreme caution or avoided entirely.
- Nonsteroidal anti-inflammatory agents and other modalities should be considered if appropriate to reduce opioid requirements.
- Supplemental oxygen should be administered continuously to all patients who are at increased perioperative risk from OSA until they are able to maintain their baseline oxygen saturation while breathing room air.
- Hospitalized patients at increased risk of respiratory compromise from OSA should be monitored with continuous pulse oximetry after discharge from the recovery room.

*American Society of Anesthesiologists Task Force on Management of the Difficult Airway. Practice guidelines for management of the difficult airway. Anesthesiology 2003; 98:1269-77.

Selected recommendations from American Society of Anesthesiologists Task Force on Perioperative Management of Patients with Obstructive Sleep Apnea. Practice guidelines for the perioperative management of patients with obstructive sleep apnea. Anesthesiology 2006;104:1081-93; published with permission.

delivery, regional analgesia most often refers to the use of a neuraxial technique. The applicability and efficacy of other regional analgesic techniques (e.g., local anesthetic infiltration, continuous incisional infusion of local anesthetic, ilioinguinal nerve block) for post–cesarean delivery analgesia in morbidly obese patients are unclear. A systematic review of randomized controlled trials (including both obstetric and nonobstetric patients) found that continuous infusion of local anesthetic through catheters placed at the incisional site led to an improvement in analgesia and patient satisfaction as well as to reductions in opioid use, side effects, and duration of hospital stay, in comparison with administration of systemic opioids alone.[149] In light of their efficacy, technical simplicity, and low side-effect profile, instillation catheters placed at the incisional site should probably be used more frequently for post–cesarean delivery analgesia, especially in patients who are not candidates for neuraxial analgesia and/or those who are sensitive to opioids administered by any route (see Chapter 27).

Morbidly obese patients at risk for obstructive sleep apnea who have undergone cesarean delivery should be monitored with continuous pulse oximetry after being discharged from the post–anesthesia care unit.

KEY POINTS

- The presence of coexisting disease(s) complicates obstetric and anesthetic management of the morbidly obese pregnant woman.
- The obese pregnant woman is at increased risk for obstetric, anesthetic, neonatal, surgical, and postoperative complications.
- Airway complications constitute the most common cause of anesthesia-related maternal death, and they occur most commonly in the postoperative period.
- The anesthesia provider should perform a careful, thorough assessment of the airway in every obese pregnant woman, and should consider securing the airway prior to induction of general anesthesia when a difficult airway is anticipated.
- Early administration of epidural analgesia is advised in obese patients undergoing a trial of labor; anesthesia providers should critically evaluate the quality of the epidural block and replace any catheter that does not provide excellent analgesia.
- Continuous spinal anesthesia should be considered in emergency settings involving potentially difficult

intubation, and in cases of unintentional dural puncture in morbidly obese patients.

- Morbidly obese parturients are at high risk for obstructive sleep apnea; therefore, they should be carefully monitored with continuous pulse oximetry for postoperative hypoxemia resulting from airway obstruction and/or respiratory depression after discharge from the postanesthesia care unit.

REFERENCES

1. Ogden CL, Carroll MD, Curtin LR, et al. Prevalence of overweight and obesity in the United States, 1999-2004. JAMA 2006; 295:1549-55.
2. Allison DB, Fontaine KR, Manson JE, et al. Annual deaths attributable to obesity in the United States. JAMA 1999; 282:1530-8.
3. Chopra M, Galbraith S, Darnton-Hill I. A global response to a global problem: The epidemic of overnutrition. Bull World Health Organ 2002; 80:952-8.
4. Samuels-Kalow ME, Funai EF, Buhimschi C, et al. Prepregnancy body mass index, hypertensive disorders of pregnancy, and long-term maternal mortality. Am J Obstet Gynecol 2007; 197:490.e1-6.
5. Weiss JL, Malone FD, Emig D, et al. Obesity, obstetric complications and Cesarean delivery rate—a population-based screening study. Am J Obstet Gynecol 2004; 190:1091-7.
6. Kaaja RJ, Greer IA. Manifestations of chronic disease during pregnancy. JAMA 2005; 294:2751-7.
7. Catalano PM. Management of obesity in pregnancy. Obstet Gynecol 2007; 109:419-33.
8. Broberger C. Brain regulation of food intake and appetite: Molecules and networks. J Intern Med 2005; 258:301-27.
9. Lafortuna CL, Agosti F, Galli R, et al. The energetic and cardiovascular response to treadmill walking and cycle ergometer exercise in obese women. Eur J Appl Physiol 2008; 103:707-17.
10. Dempsey JA, Reddan W, Balke B, Rankin J. Work capacity determinants and physiologic cost of weight-supported work in obesity. J Appl Physiol 1966; 21:1815-20.
11. Lourenco RV. Diaphragm activity in obesity. J Clin Invest 1969; 48:1609-14.
12. Kress JP, Pohlman AS, Alverdy J, Hall JB. The impact of morbid obesity on oxygen cost of breathing (VO(2RESP)) at rest. Am J Respir Crit Care Med 1999; 160:883-6.
13. Babb TG, Ranasinghe KG, Comeau LA, et al. Dyspnea on exertion in obese women: Association with an increased oxygen cost of breathing. Am J Respir Crit Care Med 2008; 178:116-23.
14. Noble AB. The problem of obesity in anaesthesia for abdominal surgery. Can Anaesth Soc J 1962; 9:6-14.
15. Parameswaran K, Todd DC, Soth M. Altered respiratory physiology in obesity. Can Respir J 2006; 13:203-10.
16. Pelosi P, Croci M, Ravagnan I, et al. The effects of body mass on lung volumes, respiratory mechanics, and gas exchange during general anesthesia. Anesth Analg 1998; 87:654-60.
17. Eng M, Butler J, Bonica JJ. Respiratory function in pregnant obese women. Am J Obstet Gynecol 1975; 123:241-5.
18. Holley HS, Milic-Emili J, Becklake MR, Bates DV. Regional distribution of pulmonary ventilation and perfusion in obesity. J Clin Invest 1967; 46:475-81.
19. Barrera F, Reidenberg MM, Winters WL, Hungspreugs S. Ventilation-perfusion relationships in the obese patient. J Appl Physiol 1969; 26:420-6.
20. Lee J, Larsen R, Buckley J, Roberts R. Pulmonary function and its correlation to the degree of obesity of 294 patients. Anesthesiol Rev 1981; 8:28-32.
21. Vaughan RW, Cork RC, Hollander D. The effect of massive weight loss on arterial oxygenation and pulmonary function tests. Anesthesiology 1981; 54:325-8.
22. Alexander JK, Dennis EW, Smith WG, et al. Blood volume, cardiac output, and distribution of systemic blood flow in extreme obesity. Cardiovasc Res Cent Bull 1962; 1:39-44.
23. Alexander JK. The cardiomyopathy of obesity. Prog Cardiovasc Dis 1985; 27:325-34.
24. Paul DR, Hoyt JL, Boutros AR. Cardiovascular and respiratory changes in response to change of posture in the very obese. Anesthesiology 1976; 45:73-8.
25. Teeple E, Ghia JN. An elevated pulmonary wedge pressure resulting from an upper respiratory obstruction in an obese patient. Anesthesiology 1983; 59:66-8.
26. Mabie WC, Ratts TE, Ramanathan KB, Sibai BM. Circulatory congestion in obese hypertensive women: A subset of pulmonary edema in pregnancy. Obstet Gynecol 1988; 72:553-8.
27. Drenick EJ, Bale GS, Seltzer F, Johnson DG. Excessive mortality and causes of death in morbidly obese men. JAMA 1980; 243:443-5.
28. Tsueda K, Debrand M, Zeok SS, et al. Obesity supine death syndrome: Reports of two morbidly obese patients. Anesth Analg 1979; 58:345-7.
29. Flegal KM, Graubard BI, Williamson DF, Gail MH. Excess deaths associated with underweight, overweight, and obesity. JAMA 2005; 293:1861-7.
30. Messerli FH, Nunez BD, Ventura HO, Snyder DW. Overweight and sudden death: Increased ventricular ectopy in cardiopathy of obesity. Arch Intern Med 1987; 147:1725-8.
31. Lauer MS, Anderson KM, Kannel WB, Levy D. The impact of obesity on left ventricular mass and geometry: The Framingham Heart Study. JAMA 1991; 266:231-6.
32. Veille JC, Hanson R. Obesity, pregnancy, and left ventricular functioning during the third trimester. Am J Obstet Gynecol 1994; 171:980-3.
33. Vaughan RW, Bauer S, Wise L. Volume and pH of gastric juice in obese patients. Anesthesiology 1975; 43:686-9.
34. Dewan DM, Floyd HM, Thistlewood JM, et al. Sodium citrate pretreatment in elective Cesarean section patients. Anesth Analg 1985; 64:34-7.
35. Ulmsten U, Sundstrom G. Esophageal manometry in pregnant and nonpregnant women. Am J Obstet Gynecol 1978; 132:260-4.
36. Van Thiel DH, Wald A. Evidence refuting a role for increased abdominal pressure in the pathogenesis of the heartburn associated with pregnancy. Am J Obstet Gynecol 1981; 140:420-2.
37. Nilsson M, Lundegardh G, Carling L, et al. Body mass and reflux oesophagitis: An oestrogen-dependent association? Scand J Gastroenterol 2002; 37:626-30.
38. Cedergren MI. Maternal morbid obesity and the risk of adverse pregnancy outcome. Obstet Gynecol 2004; 103:219-24.
39. Farmer G, Hamilton-Nicol DR, Sutherland HW, et al. The ranges of insulin response and glucose tolerance in lean, normal, and obese women during pregnancy. Am J Obstet Gynecol 1992; 167:772-7.
40. Blaszyk H, Wollan PC, Witkiewicz AK, Bjornsson J. Death from pulmonary thromboembolism in severe obesity: Lack of association with established genetic and clinical risk factors. Virchows Arch 1999; 434:529-32.
41. Tsai AW, Cushman M, Rosamond WD, et al. Cardiovascular risk factors and venous thromboembolism incidence: The longitudinal investigation of thromboembolism etiology. Arch Intern Med 2002; 162:1182-9.
42. Kerstein MD, McSwain NE Jr, O'Connell RC, et al. Obesity: Is it really a risk factor in thrombophlebitis? South Med J 1987; 80:1236-8.
43. Martin J, Hamilton B, Ventura S, et al. Births: Final data for 2001. Natl Vital Stat Rep 2002; 51:1-102.
44. Martin J, Brady E, Sutton P, et al. Births: Final data for 2005. Natl Vital Stat Rep 2007; 56:1-103.
45. Chu SY, Bachman DJ, Callaghan WM, et al. Association between obesity during pregnancy and increased use of health care. N Engl J Med 2008; 358:1444-53.
46. Abrams B, Parker J. Overweight and pregnancy complications. Int J Obes 1988; 12:293-303.
47. Garbaciak JA Jr, Richter M, Miller S, Barton JJ. Maternal weight and pregnancy complications. Am J Obstet Gynecol 1985; 152:238-45.

48. Perlow JH, Morgan MA, Montgomery D, et al. Perinatal outcome in pregnancy complicated by massive obesity. Am J Obstet Gynecol 1992; 167:958-62.
49. Hood DD, Dewan DM. Anesthetic and obstetric outcome in morbidly obese parturients. Anesthesiology 1993; 79:1210-8.
50. Kaunitz AM, Hughes JM, Grimes DA, et al. Causes of maternal mortality in the United States. Obstet Gynecol 1985; 65:605-12.
51. Rochat RW, Koonin LM, Atrash HK, Jewett JF. Maternal mortality in the United States: Report from the Maternal Mortality Collaborative. Obstet Gynecol 1988; 72:91-7.
52. Endler GC, Mariona FG, Sokol RJ, Stevenson LB. Anesthesia-related maternal mortality in Michigan, 1972 to 1984. Am J Obstet Gynecol 1988; 159:187-93.
53. American College of Obstetricians and Gynecologists Committee on Obstetric Practice. The role of obstetrician-gynecologist in the assessment and management of obesity. ACOG Committee Opinion No. 319. Washington, DC, ACOG, October 2005. (Obstet Gynecol 2005;106:895-9.)
54. American College of Obstetricians and Gynecologists Committee on Obstetric Practice. Obesity in pregnancy. ACOG Committee Opinion No. 315. Washington, DC, September 2005. (Obstet Gynecol 2005; 106:671-5.)
55. Wax JR, Pinette MG, Cartin A, Blackstone J. Female reproductive issues following bariatric surgery. Obstet Gynecol Surv 2007; 62:595-604.
56. Johnson JW, Longmate JA, Frentzen B. Excessive maternal weight and pregnancy outcome. Am J Obstet Gynecol 1992; 167:353-70.
57. Hibbard JU, Gilbert S, Landon MB, et al. Trial of labor or repeat Cesarean delivery in women with morbid obesity and previous Cesarean delivery. Obstet Gynecol 2006; 108:125-33.
58. Buhimschi CS, Buhimschi IA, Malinow AM, Weiner CP. Intrauterine pressure during the second stage of labor in obese women. Obstet Gynecol 2004; 103:225-30.
59. Bianco AT, Smilen SW, Davis Y, et al. Pregnancy outcome and weight gain recommendations for the morbidly obese woman. Obstet Gynecol 1998; 91:97-102.
60. Johnson SR, Kolberg BH, Varner MW, Railsback LD. Maternal obesity and pregnancy. Surg Gynecol Obstet 1987; 164:431-7.
61. Abrams BF, Laros RK Jr. Prepregnancy weight, weight gain, and birth weight. Am J Obstet Gynecol 1986; 154:503-9.
62. Klebanoff MA, Mills JL, Berendes HW. Mother's birth weight as a predictor of macrosomia. Am J Obstet Gynecol 1985; 153:253-7.
63. Crane SS, Wojtowycz MA, Dye TD, et al. Association between prepregnancy obesity and the risk of Cesarean delivery. Obstet Gynecol 1997; 89:213-6.
64. Roman H, Goffinet F, Hulsey TF, et al. Maternal body mass index at delivery and risk of Cesarean due to dystocia in low risk pregnancies. Acta Obstet Gynecol Scand 2008; 87:163-70.
65. Prough SG, Aksel S, Wiebe RH, Shepherd J. Continuous estrogen/progestin therapy in menopause. Am J Obstet Gynecol 1987; 157:1449-53.
66. Nohr EA, Bech BH, Davies MJ, et al. Prepregnancy obesity and fetal death: A study within the Danish National Birth Cohort. Obstet Gynecol 2005; 106:250-9.
67. Waller DK, Mills JL, Simpson JL, et al. Are obese women at higher risk for producing malformed offspring? Am J Obstet Gynecol 1994; 170:541-8.
68. Rahaman J, Narayansingh GV, Roopnarinesingh S. Fetal outcome among obese parturients. Int J Gynaecol Obstet 1990; 31:227-30.
69. Buckley FP, Robinson NB, Simonowitz DA, Dellinger EP. Anaesthesia in the morbidly obese: A comparison of anaesthetic and analgesic regimens for upper abdominal surgery. Anaesthesia 1983; 38:840-51.
70. Ranta P, Jouppila P, Spalding M, Jouppila R. The effect of maternal obesity on labour and labour pain. Anaesthesia 1995; 50:322-6.
71. Narang VP, Linter SP. Failure of extradural blockade in obstetrics: A new hypothesis. Br J Anaesth 1988; 60:402-4.
72. Clinkscales CP, Greenfield ML, Vanarase M, Polley LS. An observational study of the relationship between lumbar epidural space depth and body mass index in Michigan parturients. Int J Obstet Anesth 2007; 16:323-7.
73. Whitty RJ, Maxwell CV, Carvalho JC. Complications of neuraxial anesthesia in an extreme morbidly obese patient for Cesarean section. Int J Obstet Anesth 2007; 16:139-44.
74. Hamza J, Smida M, Benhamou D, Cohen SE. Parturient's posture during epidural puncture affects the distance from skin to epidural space. J Clin Anesth 1995; 7:1-4.
75. Hamilton CL, Riley ET, Cohen SE. Changes in the position of epidural catheters associated with patient movement. Anesthesiology 1997; 86:778-84.
76. Douglas MJ, Flanagan ML, McMorland GH. Anaesthetic management of a complex morbidly obese parturient. Can J Anaesth 1991; 38:900-3.
77. Bell E. Decreased incidence of postdural puncture headache in morbidly obese parturients following continuous spinal using 17 gauge Tuohy needle (abstract). Anesthesiology 1997; 87:A886.
78. Hood D, Dewan D. Obstetric anesthesia. In Brown D, editor. Risk and Outcome in Anesthesia. 2nd edition. Philadelphia, JB Lippincott, 1992:356-413.
79. Moldin P, Hokegard KH, Nielsen TF. Cesarean section and maternal mortality in Sweden 1973-1979. Acta Obstet Gynecol Scand 1984; 63:7-11.
80. Hodgkinson R, Husain FJ. Caesarean section associated with gross obesity. Br J Anaesth 1980; 52:919-23.
81. Mhyre JM, Riesner MN, Polley LS, Naughton NN. A series of anesthesia-related maternal deaths in Michigan, 1985-2003. Anesthesiology 2007; 106:1096-104.
82. Honarmand A, Safavi MR. Prediction of difficult laryngoscopy in obstetric patients scheduled for Caesarean delivery. Eur J Anaesthesiol 2008; 25:714-20.
83. Brodsky JB, Lemmens HJ, Brock-Utne JG, et al. Anesthetic considerations for bariatric surgery: Proper positioning is important for laryngoscopy. Anesth Analg 2003; 96:1841-2.
84. Brodsky JB, Lemmens HJ, Brock-Utne JG, et al. Morbid obesity and tracheal intubation. Anesth Analg 2002; 94:732-6.
85. Artuso D, Wayne M, Cassaro S, et al. Hemodynamic changes during laparoscopic gastric bypass procedures. Arch Surg 2005; 140: 289-92.
86. Brunette KE, Hutchinson DO, Ismail H. Bilateral brachial plexopathy following laparoscopic bariatric surgery. Anaesth Intensive Care 2005; 33:812-5.
87. Greer BE, Cain JM, Figge DC, et al. Supraumbilical upper abdominal midline incision for pelvic surgery in the morbidly obese patient. Obstet Gynecol 1990; 76:471-3.
88. Gal D. A supraumbilical incision for gynecologic neoplasms in the morbidly obese patient. J Am Coll Surg 1994; 179:18-20.
89. Wall PD, Deucy EE, Glantz JC, Pressman EK. Vertical skin incisions and wound complications in the obese parturient. Obstet Gynecol 2003; 102:952-6.
90. Houston MC, Raynor BD. Postoperative morbidity in the morbidly obese parturient woman: Supraumbilical and low transverse abdominal approaches. Am J Obstet Gynecol 2000; 182:1033-5.
91. O'Sullivan GM, Bullingham RE. Noninvasive assessment by radiotelemetry of antacid effect during labor. Anesth Analg 1985; 64:95-100.
92. Goldberg ME, Norris MC, Larijani GE, et al. Preoxygenation in the morbidly obese: A comparison of two techniques. Anesth Analg 1989; 68:520-2.
93. Schmidt JF, Jorgensen BC. The effect of metoclopramide on gastric contents after preoperative ingestion of sodium citrate. Anesth Analg 1984; 63:841-3.
94. Hogan QH, Prost R, Kulier A, et al. Magnetic resonance imaging of cerebrospinal fluid volume and the influence of body habitus and abdominal pressure. Anesthesiology 1996; 84:1341-9.
95. Carpenter RL, Hogan QH, Liu SS, et al. Lumbosacral cerebrospinal fluid volume is the primary determinant of sensory block extent and duration during spinal anesthesia. Anesthesiology 1998; 89:24-9.
96. Greene NM. Distribution of local anesthetic solutions within the subarachnoid space. Anesth Analg 1985; 64:715-30.

97. Pitkanen MT. Body mass and spread of spinal anesthesia with bupivacaine. Anesth Analg 1987; 66:127-31.
98. Norris MC. Height, weight, and the spread of subarachnoid hyperbaric bupivacaine in the term parturient. Anesth Analg 1988; 67:555-8.
99. McCulloch WJ, Littlewood DG. Influence of obesity on spinal analgesia with isobaric 0.5% bupivacaine. Br J Anaesth 1986; 58:610-4.
100. von Ungern-Sternberg BS, Regli A, Bucher E, et al. Impact of spinal anaesthesia and obesity on maternal respiratory function during elective Caesarean section. Anaesthesia 2004; 59:743-9.
101. Jacobs LL, Berger HC, Fierro FE. Obesity and continuous spinal anesthesia: A case report. Anesth Analg 1963; 42:547-9.
102. Hodgkinson R, Husain FJ. Obesity and the cephalad spread of analgesia following epidural administration of bupivacaine for Cesarean section. Anesth Analg 1980; 59:89-92.
103. Milligan KR, Cramp P, Schatz L, et al. The effect of patient position and obesity on the spread of epidural analgesia. Int J Obstet Anesth 1993; 2:134-6.
104. Panni MK, Columb MO. Obese parturients have lower epidural local anaesthetic requirements for analgesia in labour. Br J Anaesth 2006; 96:106-10.
105. Russell IF. Levels of anaesthesia and intraoperative pain at caesarean section under regional block. Int J Obstet Anesth 1995; 4:71-7.
106. Yentis SM. Height of confusion: Assessing regional blocks before Caesarean section. Int J Obstet Anesth 2006; 15:2-6.
107. Henny CP, Odoom JA, ten Cate H, et al. Effects of extradural bupivacaine on the haemostatic system. Br J Anaesth 1986; 58:301-5.
108. Rocke DA, Murray WB, Rout CC, Gouws E. Relative risk analysis of factors associated with difficult intubation in obstetric anesthesia. Anesthesiology 1992; 77:67-73.
109. Lee J, Larson R, Buckley J, Roberts R. Airway maintenance in the morbidly obese. Anesthesiol Rev 1980; 7:33-6.
110. American Society of Anesthesiologists Task Force on Obstetric Anesthesia. Practice guidelines for obstetric anesthesia. Anesthesiology 2007; 106:843-63.
111. Cohn AI, Hart RT, McGraw SR, Blass NH. The Bullard laryngoscope for emergency airway management in a morbidly obese parturient. Anesth Analg 1995; 81:872-3.
112. Shnider SM, Wright RG, Levinson G, et al. Uterine blood flow and plasma norepinephrine changes during maternal stress in the pregnant ewe. Anesthesiology 1979; 50:524-7.
113. Byrne F, Oduro-Dominah A, Kipling R. The effect of pregnancy on pulmonary nitrogen washout: A study of pre-oxygenation. Anaesthesia 1987; 42:148-50.
114. Berthoud MC, Peacock JE, Reilly CS. Effectiveness of preoxygenation in morbidly obese patients. Br J Anaesth 1991; 67:464-6.
115. Norris MC, Dewan DM. Preoxygenation for Cesarean section: A comparison of two techniques. Anesthesiology 1985; 62:827-9.
116. Gambee AM, Hertzka RE, Fisher DM. Preoxygenation techniques: Comparison of three minutes and four breaths. Anesth Analg 1987; 66:468-70.
117. Chiron B, Laffon M, Ferrandiere M, et al. Standard preoxygenation technique versus two rapid techniques in pregnant patients. Int J Obstet Anesth 2004; 13:11-4.
118. Jung D, Mayersohn M, Perrier D, et al. Thiopental disposition in lean and obese patients undergoing surgery. Anesthesiology 1982; 56:269-74.
119. Kumar V, Harvey J, Cooper GM. Does obesity affect recovery? A study using intravenous methohexitone and Althesin for short procedures. Anaesthesia 1983; 38:968-71.
120. Lemmens HJ, Brodsky JB. The dose of succinylcholine in morbid obesity. Anesth Analg 2006; 102:438-42.
121. Weinstein JA, Matteo RS, Ornstein E, et al. Pharmacodynamics of vecuronium and atracurium in the obese surgical patient. Anesth Analg 1988; 67:1149-53.
122. Kirkegaard-Nielsen H, Lindholm P, Petersen HS, Severinsen IK. Antagonism of atracurium-induced block in obese patients. Can J Anaesth 1998; 45:39-41.
123. Borel JD, Bentley JB, Vaughan RW, Gandolfi AJ. Enflurane blood-gas solubility: Influence of weight and hemoglobin. Anesth Analg 1982; 61:1006-9.
124. Bentley JB, Vaughan RW, Gandolfi AJ, Cork RC. Halothane biotransformation in obese and nonobese patients. Anesthesiology 1982; 57:94-7.
125. Rice SA, Fish KJ. Anesthetic metabolism and renal function in obese and nonobese Fischer 344 rats following enflurane or isoflurane anesthesia. Anesthesiology 1986; 65:28-34.
126. Carpenter RL, Eger EI, Johnson BH, et al. The extent of metabolism of inhaled anesthetics in humans. Anesthesiology 1986; 65: 201-5.
127. Strube PJ, Hulands GH, Halsey MJ. Serum fluoride levels in morbidly obese patients: Enflurane compared with isoflurane anaesthesia. Anaesthesia 1987; 42:685-9.
128. Torri G, Casati A, Comotti L, et al. Wash-in and wash-out curves of sevoflurane and isoflurane in morbidly obese patients. Minerva Anestesiol 2002; 68:523-7.
129. Juvin P, Vadam C, Malek L, et al. Postoperative recovery after desflurane, propofol, or isoflurane anesthesia among morbidly obese patients: A prospective, randomized study. Anesth Analg 2000; 91:714-9.
130. Higuchi H, Satoh T, Arimura S, et al. Serum inorganic fluoride levels in mildly obese patients during and after sevoflurane anesthesia. Anesth Analg 1993; 77:1018-21.
131. Wyner J, Brodsky JB, Merrell RC. Massive obesity and arterial oxygenation. Anesth Analg 1981; 60:691-3.
132. Salem MR, Dalal FY, Zygmunt MP, et al. Does PEEP improve intraoperative arterial oxygenation in grossly obese patients? Anesthesiology 1978; 48:280-1.
133. Eriksen J, Andersen J, Rasmussen JP, Sorensen B. Effects of ventilation with large tidal volumes or positive end-expiratory pressure on cardiorespiratory function in anesthetized obese patients. Acta Anaesthesiol Scand 1978; 22:241-8.
134. Santesson J. Oxygen transport and venous admixture in the extremely obese: Influence of anaesthesia and artificial ventilation with and without positive end-expiratory pressure. Acta Anaesthesiol Scand 1976; 20:387-94.
135. Bamgbade OA, Rutter TW, Nafiu OO, Dorje P. Postoperative complications in obese and nonobese patients. World J Surg 2007; 31:556-60.
136. Soens MA, Birnbach DJ, Ranasinghe JS, van Zundert A. Obstetric anesthesia for the obese and morbidly obese patient: An ounce of prevention is worth more than a pound of treatment. Acta Anaesthesiol Scand 2008; 52:6-19.
137. Hendler I, Schatz M, Momirova V, et al. Association of obesity with pulmonary and nonpulmonary complications of pregnancy in asthmatic women. Obstet Gynecol 2006; 108:77-82.
138. Wolfe HM, Gross TL, Sokol RJ, et al. Determinants of morbidity in obese women delivered by Cesarean. Obstet Gynecol 1988; 71:691-6.
139. Young T, Palta M, Dempsey J, et al. The occurrence of sleep-disordered breathing among middle-aged adults. N Engl J Med 1993; 328:1230-5.
140. Tishler PV, Larkin EK, Schluchter MD, Redline S. Incidence of sleep-disordered breathing in an urban adult population: The relative importance of risk factors in the development of sleep-disordered breathing. JAMA 2003; 289:2230-7.
141. D'Angelo R. Anesthesia-related maternal mortality: A pat on the back or a call to arms? Anesthesiology 2007; 106:1082-4.
142. American Society of Anesthesiologists Task Force on Perioperative Management of Patients with Obstructive Sleep Apnea. Practice guidelines for the perioperative management of patients with obstructive sleep apnea. Anesthesiology 2006; 104:1081-93.
143. Levin A, Klein SL, Brolin RE, Pitchford DE. Patient-controlled analgesia for morbidly obese patients: An effective modality if used correctly (letter). Anesthesiology 1992; 76:857-8.
144. Schwartz AE, Matteo RS, Ornstein E, et al. Pharmacokinetics of sufentanil in obese patients. Anesth Analg 1991; 73:790-3.

145. Gelman S, Laws HL, Potzick J, et al. Thoracic epidural vs balanced anesthesia in morbid obesity: An intraoperative and postoperative hemodynamic study. Anesth Analg 1980; 59:902-8.
146. Rawal N, Sjostrand U, Christoffersson E, et al. Comparison of intramuscular and epidural morphine for postoperative analgesia in the grossly obese: Influence on postoperative ambulation and pulmonary function. Anesth Analg 1984; 63:583-92.
147. Pellecchia DJ, Bretz KA, Barnette RE. Postoperative pain control by means of epidural narcotics in a patient with obstructive sleep apnea. Anesth Analg 1987; 66:280-2.
148. Lamarche Y, Martin R, Reiher J, Blaise G. The sleep apnoea syndrome and epidural morphine. Can Anaesth Soc J 1986; 33:231-3.
149. Liu SS, Richman JM, Thirlby RC, Wu CL. Efficacy of continuous wound catheters delivering local anesthetic for postoperative analgesia: A quantitative and qualitative systematic review of randomized controlled trials. J Am Coll Surg 2006; 203:914-32.

Renal Disease

Yaakov Beilin, M.D.
Robert W. Reid, M.D.

"Children of women with renal disease used to be born dangerously or not at all—not at all if their doctors had their way."[1] This statement describes early experiences with maternal renal disease and pregnancy outcome. It remains true that renal disease, either preexisting or occurring during gestation, may impair maternal and fetal health. Experience and investigations during the last three decades have significantly improved the outcome for pregnant women with renal disease.[2]

PHYSIOLOGIC CHANGES IN PREGNANCY

A review of the renal physiologic changes that occur during normal pregnancy is helpful to the understanding and evaluation of coexisting renal disorders. Early in gestation, increased vascular volume leads to renal enlargement. Hormonal changes result in dilation of the renal pelvis and ureters; dilation often is accompanied by decreased ureteral peristalsis. Dilated uterine and ovarian veins, and the gravid uterus, may obstruct ureter drainage at the pelvic brim. Together, these changes predispose pregnant women to vesicoureteric reflux and ascending infection. Alterations in glomerular hemodynamics and tubular function also occur. Increased cardiac output and decreased intrarenal vascular resistance cause an 80% increase in renal blood flow and a 50% increase in glomerular filtration rate (GFR) during pregnancy. These changes are somewhat less pronounced near term. Because of the increased GFR, a serum creatinine concentration greater than 0.8 mg/dL and a blood urea nitrogen (BUN) concentration greater than 13 mg/dL (which are normal values for the nonpregnant patient) suggest renal insufficiency in the pregnant woman. Tubular sodium reabsorption and osmoregulation are reset, allowing a "physiologic hypervolemia" during gestation. Modest proteinuria also occurs during pregnancy (e.g., up to 300 mg in 24 hours).[3]

Urinary tract infections (see Chapter 36) and hypertensive disorders of pregnancy (see Chapter 45) are discussed elsewhere in this text.

RENAL PARENCHYMAL DISEASE

Definition and Pathophysiology

Renal parenchymal disease consists of two general groups of disorders, **glomerulopathies** and **tubulointerstitial disease**. Glomerulopathies are further subdivided into disorders that involve inflammatory or necrotizing lesions—the **nephritic syndromes**, and disorders that involve abnormal permeability to protein and other macromolecules—the **nephrotic syndromes**. More than 20 specific glomerulopathies exist. The nomenclature for these glomerulopathies is confusing, and specific diseases are not discussed in detail here.

Tubulointerstitial diseases are disorders characterized by abnormal tubular function. They result in abnormal urine composition and concentration but are not characterized by decreased GFR until late in the disease course. The disorders in this category include interstitial nephritis, renal cystic disease, renal neoplasia, and functional tubular defects.

Patients with renal parenchymal disorders may remain asymptomatic for years, and they may exhibit only proteinuria and microscopic hematuria, with little if any evidence of reduced renal function. Spontaneous recovery or improvement with treatment occurs with many glomerulopathies. However, other patients exhibit progressive nephropathy, hypertension, and renal insufficiency. Approximately 120,000 patients in the United States have chronic renal failure; in two thirds of these patients, the disorder results from glomerulopathy, and in one third, from tubulointerstitial disease.

Diagnosis

Women with preexisting disease may choose to become pregnant without the counsel of their nephrologist. When such patients become pregnant, the obstetrician and nephrologist seek to define the extent of renal involvement. Serial blood pressure measurements are obtained to define the severity of hypertension and the efficacy of current antihypertensive therapy. Creatinine clearance and the level of proteinuria should be determined. Urinalysis yields information about the presence of renal casts and bacteriuria. The determination of serum creatinine and BUN concentrations defines the extent of renal insufficiency. A serum creatinine concentration greater than 0.8 mg/dL, although normal in the nonpregnant woman, may represent significant renal insufficiency during pregnancy. Alternatively, the obstetrician may first detect renal dysfunction through routine prenatal screening tests. If proteinuria, hematuria, or azotemia is detected, a complete biochemical evaluation should be performed.

Both preeclampsia and renal disease may manifest as hypertension, proteinuria, and edema. The distinction between the two disorders is often unclear, especially after 20 weeks' gestation. Fisher et al.[4] evaluated 176 renal biopsy specimens obtained from hypertensive women immediately postpartum, most of whom had a clinical diagnosis of preeclampsia. The clinicopathologic correlation was poor. Histologic evidence of preeclampsia (e.g., glomerular endotheliosis without hypercellularity) was present in only 65% of these hypertensive women. Primary renal disease was present in 20%, and hypertensive nephrosclerosis in 11%. Nulliparous women (84%) were more likely to have a correct diagnosis of preeclampsia than parous women (38%).

Renal tissue biopsy is often used to establish a diagnosis in nonpregnant patients. Chen et al.[5] reported a series of 15 percutaneous renal biopsies performed in 15 pregnant women with onset of renal dysfunction of unknown cause during pregnancy. All patients underwent biopsy before 30 weeks' gestation. No biopsy-related complications occurred, except in 1 patient who experienced gross hematuria. Histologic results provided useful clinical guidance that facilitated successful fetal outcome in 14 of the pregnancies. In contrast, Kuller et al.[6] reviewed 18 renal biopsies performed during pregnancy (n = 15) or in the immediate postpartum period (n = 3). In this series, renal hematoma was identified in 7 (39%) patients, and 2 (11%) patients required blood transfusion following the biopsy. Four intrauterine fetal deaths occurred, although none was a direct result of the biopsy. Because renal biopsy exposes the pregnant woman to potential complications, many maternal-fetal medicine physicians recommend biopsy only when sudden deterioration in renal function or symptomatic nephrotic syndrome occurs before 32 weeks' gestation, at which time definitive diagnosis may guide appropriate treatment. For problems beyond 32 weeks' gestation, maternal-fetal medicine physicians typically prefer to delay biopsy until the postpartum period.

Effect of Pregnancy

The extent to which pregnancy affects preexisting renal disease depends on the level of renal insufficiency before pregnancy. Among women with mild antenatal renal insufficiency, pregnancy does not substantially alter the natural course of renal disease. In contrast, pregnant women with moderate or severe antenatal renal insufficiency often experience deterioration of renal function and exacerbation of hypertension. Katz et al.[7] studied the outcome of 121 pregnancies in 89 women with mild renal insufficiency (i.e., serum creatinine concentration less than 1.4 mg/dL). Hypertension complicated 23% of these pregnancies, and renal function decreased during 16% of these pregnancies, most often in women with diffuse glomerulonephritis. However, the decrease in renal function was modest, and renal function returned to baseline after delivery. Only 5 (6%) women progressed to end-stage renal failure, which occurred as many as 8 years after pregnancy. Jungers et al.[8] evaluated the effect of pregnancy on renal function among 360 women with primary glomerulonephritis. During the study period, 171 (48%) of 360 women became pregnant. All study subjects had normal renal function at the time of entry into this study, and all of the patients who became pregnant had normal renal function at conception. In this case-control study, pregnancy was not identified as a risk factor for progression to end-stage renal failure.

In contrast, Jones and Hayslett[9] analyzed the outcome of 82 pregnancies in 67 women with preexisting moderate or severe renal insufficiency (i.e., serum creatinine greater than 1.4 mg/dL before pregnancy or at the first antepartum visit). The mean ± SD serum creatinine concentration increased from 1.9 ± 0.8 mg/dL in early pregnancy to 2.5 ± 1.3 mg/dL in the third trimester. The prevalence of hypertension rose from 28% at baseline to 48% during late pregnancy. Pregnancy-related loss of maternal renal function occurred in 43% of cases. A woman with a serum creatinine concentration greater than 2.0 mg/dL who became pregnant had a one-in-three chance of developing dialysis-dependent end-stage renal disease during or shortly after pregnancy.[10]

The pathophysiology by which pregnancy exacerbates renal disease is unknown. One hypothesis is that increased glomerular perfusion, which normally accompanies pregnancy, paradoxically causes further injury to the kidneys in patients with preexisting impairment of function. However, this hypothesis is unsupported by published data, which demonstrate no evidence of hyperfiltration (i.e., an initial decline in serum creatinine concentration) during early pregnancy in patients with renal disease. Epstein[10] outlined an alternative hypothesis in which preexisting renal disease may induce a cascade of platelet aggregation, microvascular fibrin thrombus formation, and endothelial dysfunction that leads to microvascular injury in the already tenuous kidneys.

Effect on the Mother and Fetus

Obstetric complications from chronic renal disease include intrauterine growth restriction (IUGR), preterm delivery, hypertension, preeclampsia, an increased cesarean delivery rate, and a higher risk of neonatal mortality.[11] The incidence of obstetric complications is proportionate to the extent of preexisting maternal renal disease. Among pregnant women with mild antenatal renal insufficiency, the rate of preterm delivery is 20%, and that of IUGR is 24%.[7] When the mother has preexisting moderate to severe renal insufficiency, these rates increase to 59% and 37%, respectively.[9] Ramin et al[12] recently reviewed the effect of renal disease on pregnancy outcome. Fetal survival ranged from 64% to 98% depending on the extent of renal insufficiency and the presence or absence of hypertension.

Alexopoulos et al.[13] described the outcome of 24 pregnancies in 17 women with biopsy-proven glomerular disease. All but two patients had normal renal function at the onset of pregnancy. The fetal survival rate was 75%. There were six preterm deliveries, three newborns that were small for gestational age (SGA), one stillbirth, and five elective abortions. Impaired renal function at conception portended worse fetal outcome. Bar et al.[14] evaluated maternal and neonatal outcomes in 38 women (46 pregnancies) with primary renal disease. They, too, observed an increase in complications (Figure 51-1), and they developed a logistic regression model to predict successful pregnancy outcome. Interestingly, they found that the absence of preexisting hypertension and a low preconception serum uric acid level predicted successful pregnancy outcome. Other factors (e.g., degree of preexisting renal impairment) did not.

Medical and Obstetric Management

During pregnancy, the nephrologist and the obstetrician monitor maternal renal function, blood pressure, and fetal development at frequent intervals. Monthly determination of serum creatinine concentration, creatinine clearance, and proteinuria allows the recognition of renal deterioration. Some glomerulopathies respond to corticosteroids, and corticosteroid therapy should be continued during pregnancy. Rapid deterioration of renal function that occurs before 32 weeks' gestation may require renal biopsy to exclude rapidly progressive glomerulopathies that need treatment. Antihypertensive therapy should be instituted (see Chapter 45). Recombinant human erythropoietin improves maternal anemia during pregnancy.[15]

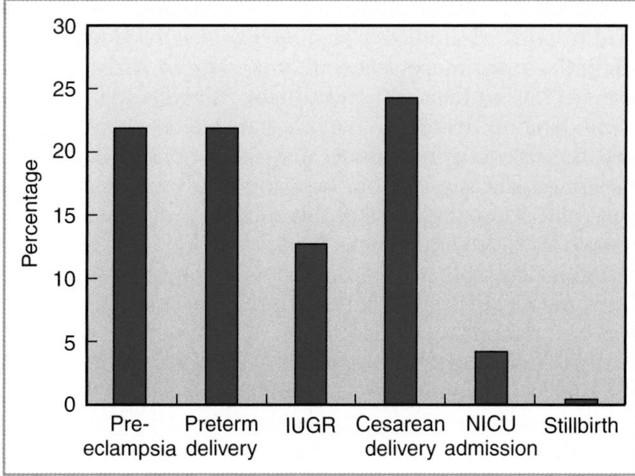

FIGURE 51-1 Short-term pregnancy outcome in women with primary renal disease. IUGR, intrauterine growth restriction; NICU, neonatal intensive care unit. (From Bar J, Orvieto R, Shalev Y, et al. Pregnancy outcome in women with primary renal disease. Isr Med Assoc J 2000; 2:178-81.)

Protein restriction puts the fetus at risk for IUGR and is not utilized. Deterioration of maternal renal function, the onset of preeclampsia, or evidence of fetal compromise may necessitate preterm delivery.

Hemodialysis and Long-Term Ambulatory Peritoneal Dialysis

When renal disease has progressed to end-stage renal failure (i.e., the GFR is less than 5 mL/min), fertility is suppressed and conception and pregnancy are rare. Less than 10% of premenopausal patients undergoing dialysis have regular menses. Luteinizing hormone and follicle-stimulating hormone concentrations assume an anovulatory pattern, which causes 40% of affected women to be amenorrheic. Half of all female patients undergoing dialysis exhibit hyperprolactinemia because of reduced clearance and hypothalamic disturbances.[16] The European Dialysis and Transplant Association reported only 16 pregnancies among 13,000 women of childbearing age who were undergoing dialysis.[17] Toma et al.[18] surveyed 2504 dialysis units in Japan and reported 172 pregnancies among 38,889 women who were undergoing dialysis.

There are two modalities of dialysis, extracorporeal hemodialysis and intracorporeal peritoneal dialysis. **Hemodialysis** is complicated by (1) the need for vascular access, (2) cardiovascular instability, (3) large fluid and electrolyte shifts, (4) the need for anticoagulation of the extracorporeal circuit, and (5) the risk of hepatitis. Hypotension may compromise uteroplacental perfusion and cause fetal compromise. Even when hypotension and major fluid shifts are avoided, Doppler ultrasonographic examination of uterine and umbilical artery flow during hemodialysis suggests the occurrence of a redistribution of arterial flow away from the uteroplacental vascular bed.[19] Fetal heart rate monitoring is recommended during dialysis.[20] Rapid removal of maternal solutes and reduced oncotic pressure with attendant free-water diffusion into the amniotic cavity may lead to polyhydramnios.[20] Hemodynamic consequences are minimized by more frequent but shorter dialysis runs. Long-term ambulatory **peritoneal dialysis** allows less hemodynamic trespass, a more stable fetal environment, and the freedom to undergo dialysis at home.[21] However, peritoneal dialysis may not be associated with greater fetal survival.[22] Complications of this modality include peritonitis and catheter difficulties.

Published reports have noted a wide range of successful outcomes in dialysis-dependent pregnant women, regardless of the modality of dialysis.[18,20,21] Toma et al.[18] reported that 90 (52%) of 172 pregnancies in women undergoing long-term hemodialysis were successful. More recently, the success rate appears to be improving. Chou et al.[22] pooled data from 10 published case series and 12 case reports, and they found that 71% of women undergoing hemodialysis and 64% of women undergoing peritoneal dialysis had a successful delivery. The birth weight, however, was significantly greater if hemodialysis was started before conception (1529 g) than after conception (1245 g). Yoo et al.[23] reported successful triplet pregnancy in a woman on hemodialysis, and Bamberg et al.[24] described successful pregnancies with a mean gestation of 32 weeks in five consecutive women who received an intensified hemofiltration scheme combined with intensive fetal surveillance, including nonstress testing and Doppler ultrasonography.

Maternal complications include malnutrition, anemia, and hypertension. Fetal complications include IUGR, fetal death, and preterm labor. BUN levels are kept below 80 mg/dL before dialysis and below 30 mg/dL after dialysis.[25] At birth, azotemia in the neonate is similar to that in the mother. Although these infants born to mothers on dialysis often have low 1-minute Apgar scores, they typically respond to resuscitative efforts and are vigorous at 5 minutes. The long-term effects of intrauterine azotemia on newborn cognitive development are unknown.[20]

Patients undergoing hemodialysis have a high prevalence of viral hepatitis, a greater frequency of active tuberculosis, and a higher rate of infection with vancomycin-resistant enterococci, human immunodeficiency virus (HIV), and methicillin-resistant *Staphylococcus aureus* (MRSA). A 1995 survey of 2647 long-term hemodialysis centers in the United States revealed that 76% of these centers reuse disposable dialyzers.[26] The prevalence of hepatitis C virus (HCV) antibody was 10% among patients and 2% among staff at these hemodialysis centers. With greater surveillance for HCV and the decline in the reuse of dialysis equipment, these infection risks are likely to decline. In 2002, Harmankaya et al.[27] presented encouraging data from a single hemodialysis unit. This group used dedicated, isolated dialysis machines for HCV-seropositive patients. Only 8 (4.8%) of 168 patients showed HCV seroconversion during an 8-year observation period. Four patients became HCV seropositive after they had undergone hemodialysis in other dialysis centers while on holiday, and 2 patients had undergone blood transfusion within the 6 months preceding seroconversion.

Anesthetic Management

Anesthetic management is influenced by the extent of renal dysfunction and hypertension. The parturient with stable renal disease, mild to moderate renal insufficiency, well-controlled hypertension, and euvolemia requires minimal special consideration. In contrast, the dialysis patient with end-stage renal failure presents many anesthetic challenges (Box 51-1). Poorly controlled hypertension leads to left ventricular hypertrophy and dysfunction. Symptoms of cardiovascular compromise should prompt echocardiography to evaluate ventricular function. Uremic pericarditis, cardiomyopathy, and accelerated atherosclerosis are rarely seen until advanced uremia has been present for several years.

NEURAXIAL ANESTHESIA

Uremic toxins cause functional platelet defects and a prolonged bleeding time. These abnormalities are reversed by dialysis. Thrombocytopenia also may occur as a result of increased peripheral destruction of platelets.

Uremic patients may be hypervolemic or hypovolemic, depending on the time elapsed since their last

BOX 51-1 Chronic Renal Failure: Abnormalities that May Affect Anesthetic Management

Cardiovascular
- Hypertension
- Fluid overload
- Ventricular hypertrophy
- Accelerated atherosclerosis
- Uremic pericarditis
- Uremic cardiomyopathy

Pulmonary
- Increased risk of difficult airway
- Recurrent pulmonary infections

Metabolic and Endocrine
- Hyperkalemia
- Metabolic acidosis
- Hyponatremia
- Hypocalcemia
- Hypermagnesemia
- Decreased protein binding of drugs
- Hypoglycemia

Hematologic
- Anemia
- Platelet dysfunction
- Decreased coagulation factors
- Leukocyte dysfunction

Neurologic
- Autonomic neuropathy
- Mental status changes
- Peripheral neuropathy
- Restless legs syndrome
- Seizure disorder

Gastrointestinal
- Delayed gastric emptying
- Increased gastric acidity
- Hepatic venous congestion
- Hepatitis (viral or drug-induced)
- Malnutrition

dialysis session. Hypovolemia and autonomic neuropathy may lead to profound hypotension during the initiation of sympathetic blockade. This risk may be minimized through proper prehydration and slow induction of epidural anesthesia.[28] Preexisting peripheral neuropathy should be documented before the administration of neuraxial anesthesia.

There are reports of systemic local anesthetic toxicity after bupivacaine brachial plexus blockade in patients with chronic renal failure.[29,30] However, Rice et al.[31] found no significant difference in the pharmacokinetic profile of bupivacaine after brachial plexus blockade in a group of uremic patients and in patients with normal renal function. There are no published data on the pharmacokinetics of epidurally administered local anesthetic agents in patients with chronic renal failure. Orko et al.[32] administered spinal anesthesia with 0.75% bupivacaine to 20 nonpregnant patients with chronic renal failure and 20 control patients. Maximal segmental anesthesia occurred more rapidly in the patients with renal disease (21 versus 35 minutes). Further, the extent of sensory blockade was two segments higher in the patients with renal disease.

GENERAL ANESTHESIA

Patients with chronic uremia exhibit delayed gastric emptying and hyperacidity, which increase the risk of aspiration pneumonitis. In addition to sodium citrate, the anesthesia provider also should give a histamine H_2-receptor antagonist and metoclopramide when time allows. Recommended single doses for patients with renal failure are ranitidine 50 mg and metoclopramide 10 mg intravenously. Weir and Chung[33] suggested that patients with chronic renal failure present greater difficulties with tracheal intubation than otherwise healthy patients; however, an objective analysis of airway difficulty has not been performed in this population.

Patients with chronic renal failure frequently have normochromic, normocytic anemia secondary to impaired erythropoietin production, chronic gastrointestinal bleeding, and vitamin deficiency. Typically the anemia is well tolerated and does not require transfusion, unless excessive surgical bleeding occurs. Intravascular volume must be assessed before induction of anesthesia. Central venous pressure monitoring should be considered when the hemodynamic condition is unclear. An intra-arterial catheter also may aid the management of the parturient with poorly controlled hypertension. Hemodialysis fistulas should be padded carefully to prevent thrombosis in both the operating and recovery rooms. Blood pressure cuffs should not be placed on these extremities.

Propofol and thiopental exhibit normal volume of distribution and elimination in patients with renal failure. Protein binding of propofol is unaffected by renal failure.[34] However, decreased albumin binding of thiopental allows a higher concentration of free drug.[35] Uremia increases blood-brain barrier permeability to many drugs.[36] These changes may warrant a small reduction in the dose of propofol or thiopental for induction. The serum potassium concentration should be determined before induction of anesthesia. If the potassium concentration is greater than 5.5 mEq/L, dialysis should be performed before an elective procedure. Succinylcholine will cause a 0.5 to 0.7 mEq/L increase in potassium concentration, which is similar to the increment that occurs in patients without renal disease.[37] If the patient is already hyperkalemic, this mild elevation may be sufficient to precipitate cardiac dysrhythmias. Plasma cholinesterase concentrations are normal, even after dialysis.[38]

After delivery, neuromuscular blockade can be maintained with atracurium, which undergoes Hofmann (nonenzymatic) degradation and nonspecific esterase metabolism. Cisatracurium represents a good alternative neuromuscular blocker for patients with renal disease. Cisatracurium undergoes Hofmann degradation, but it undergoes little (if any) nonspecific esterase hydrolysis. Unlike atracurium, cisatracurium does not cause histamine release. The duration of action of atracurium or cisatracurium is not prolonged in patients with renal failure. Magnesium-containing antacids may lead to hypermagnesemia, which potentiates neuromuscular blockade.[39] Although anticholinesterase agents undergo renal elimination and have a prolonged duration in patients with renal insufficiency, the volume of distribution remains the same and standard doses are used for the reversal of neuromuscular blockade.

ACUTE RENAL FAILURE

Definition and Epidemiology

Acute renal failure (ARF) is an uncommon but serious complication of pregnancy. Rapid deterioration of renal function leads to an accumulation of fluid and nitrogenous waste products with impaired electrolyte regulation. In the mid-twentieth century, nearly a quarter of all cases of ARF were obstetric. Fortunately, during the last five decades, the incidence of ARF in developed countries has fallen significantly.[40,41] Stratta et al.[40] reported a steady decline in the incidence of ARF from 1 in 3000 to 1 in 18,000 pregnancies from 1958 to 1994. With respect to all ARF cases, the proportion related to pregnancy fell from 43% to 0.5%. This progress has resulted from improved obstetric care and fewer septic abortions.

Pathophysiology and Diagnosis

ARF is suggested by a sharp increase in the plasma creatinine (greater than 0.8 mg/dL) and BUN (greater than 13 mg/dL) concentrations. In complete renal failure, the serum creatinine concentration rises at the rate of 0.5 to 1.0 mg/dL/day. Urine output typically falls to less than 400 mL/day (oliguria), but some patients may be nonoliguric. Frank anuria is rare.[42] ARF is subdivided according to underlying etiology (i.e., prerenal, postrenal, intrarenal causes) (Box 51-2). The inciting disorders vary among countries.[40,41,43-49] In countries where access to elective abortion is restricted, septic abortion is the leading cause of pregnancy-related ARF. In other countries severe preeclampsia-eclampsia, acute pyelonephritis of pregnancy, and bilateral renal cortical necrosis are the most common underlying disorders.

PRERENAL CAUSES

The most common prerenal causes of ARF—hyperemesis gravidarum[50] and obstetric hemorrhage—lead to hypovolemia and inadequate renal perfusion. Urinary indices show urinary osmolality greater than 500 mOsm/kg water, urine

BOX 51-2 Causes of Acute Renal Failure during Pregnancy

Prerenal

- Hyperemesis gravidarum
- Uterine hemorrhage
- Heart failure

Postrenal

- Urolithiasis
- Ureteral obstruction by the gravid uterus

Intrarenal

- Acute tubular necrosis
- Septic abortion
- Amniotic fluid embolism
- Drug-induced acute interstitial nephritis
- Acute glomerulonephritis
- Bilateral renal cortical necrosis
- Acute pyelonephritis
- Preeclampsia/eclampsia
- Hemolysis, elevated liver enzymes, and low platelets (HELLP) syndrome
- Acute fatty liver of pregnancy
- Idiopathic postpartum renal failure

sodium less than 20 mEq/L, fractional sodium excretion less than 1%, and a urinary-to-plasma creatinine ratio greater than 40.[42] Concealed uterine hemorrhage from placental abruption may remain unrecognized until hypotension and renal failure ensue.[51] Women with preeclampsia may be more likely to develop ARF after hemorrhage because of preexisting intravascular contraction and widespread maternal endothelial dysfunction.[47]

POSTRENAL CAUSES

The postrenal causes of ARF include nephrolithiasis and ureteral obstruction by the gravid uterus.[52] The latter complication is more likely in pregnant women with polyhydramnios or multiple gestation.[53] Preexisting ureteral dilation and impaired peristalsis increase the risk of obstructive uropathy during pregnancy. Flank pain and decreased urine output during late gestation should alert the clinician to this possibility. Courban et al.[54] reported an unusual case of obstructive uropathy leading to ARF in a pregnant woman with multiple uterine leiomyomas.

INTRARENAL CAUSES

Once prerenal and postrenal causes of ARF have been excluded, intrarenal processes remain. In general, oliguric intrarenal ARF is not easily reversed and must run its course. Causes include acute tubular necrosis, interstitial nephritis, and acute glomerulonephritis as well as a few causes unique to pregnancy. These last causes include renal cortical necrosis, acute pyelonephritis, severe preeclampsia-eclampsia, acute fatty liver of pregnancy, and idiopathic postpartum renal failure. A thorough history, review of medications, and urinalysis typically help determine the specific initiating factor.

Acute tubular necrosis results from nephrotoxic drugs, amniotic fluid embolism, rhabdomyolysis, intrauterine fetal death, and prolonged renal ischemia secondary to hemorrhage or septic shock. Urinalysis demonstrates dirty brown epithelial cell casts and coarse granular casts. Urinary indices show urine osmolality less than 350 mOsm/kg water, urine sodium greater than 40 mEq/L, fractional sodium excretion greater than 1%, and a urinary-to-plasma creatinine ratio less than 20.[42]

Acute interstitial nephritis is caused by nonsteroidal anti-inflammatory drugs (NSAIDs) and various antibiotics. Patients typically have fever, rash, eosinophilia, and urine eosinophils.

Acute glomerulonephritis is rare during pregnancy. It is suggested by hematuria, red cell casts, and proteinuria. Urinary indices of acute glomerulonephritis are similar to those of prerenal ARF.

Bilateral renal cortical necrosis, which is rarely observed in the nonobstetric patient, is responsible for 10% to 38% of cases of obstetric ARF.[48,51,55-57] It may occur during both early and late pregnancy. Placental abruption is the most common precipitating event. The pathogenesis of this disorder is unclear but may involve renal hypoperfusion or endothelial damage by endotoxins imposed on the normal hypercoagulable state of pregnancy. A single dose of endotoxin may precipitate bilateral renal cortical necrosis in pregnant animals and has led some investigators to view this disorder as a clinical analogue of the experimental Sanarelli-Shwartzman reaction.[47] Extensive microthrombi are found within the glomeruli and renal arterioles. Diagnosis is made by selective renal arteriography, which reveals absence or patchiness of the cortex. Renal biopsy also may be performed in the absence of active coagulopathy.[51]

Acute pyelonephritis is one of the most common infectious complications of pregnancy (see Chapter 36). Although acute pyelonephritis rarely leads to ARF in the nongravid patient, it accounts for 5% of cases of ARF among pregnant women.[58] The reason for this greater susceptibility is unclear. Whalley et al.[59] noted that acute pyelonephritis causes a marked reduction of GFR in pregnant women. In contrast, pyelonephritis causes little reduction in GFR in nonpregnant patients. The kidney may be more sensitive to bacterial endotoxins during pregnancy.

Severe preeclampsia-eclampsia has been blamed for 20% of cases of obstetric ARF.[58] However, many cases of renal dysfunction and failure may only mimic preeclampsia and may actually result from other factors.[4] Other causes of ARF should be considered before preeclampsia is considered to be the basis of renal failure.

Sibai and Ramadan[60] reported 32 cases of ARF associated with **HELLP syndrome** (hemolysis, elevated liver enzymes, and low platelets). The majority of patients had a derangement of multiple organ systems and other obstetric complications (e.g., placental abruption, intrauterine fetal death, disseminated intravascular coagulation, postpartum hemorrhage, sepsis). Renal histology demonstrates thrombotic microangiopathy and acute tubular necrosis, suggesting pathogenesis of acute renal failure associated with HELLP syndrome.[61] In the Sibai and Ramadan[60] report, a total of 4 (13%) parturients died, and 10 (31%) required dialysis. The perinatal mortality rate was 34%, with 72% of deliveries occurring preterm. Celik et al.[62] reviewed 13 patients with HELLP syndrome and found that 36% had ARF. Of interest, Flynn et al.[63] reported the successful use of cadaveric kidneys procured from a parturient who died following HELLP syndrome and ARF. Both recipients had acceptable graft function 2 years after transplantation.

Acute fatty liver of pregnancy (reversible peripartum liver failure)—a rare but life-threatening disorder of pregnancy—is associated with a 60% to 100% incidence of ARF. Specific clinical features of acute fatty liver of pregnancy are discussed in Chapter 46.

The syndrome of **idiopathic postpartum renal failure** was initially described by Robson et al.[64] in 1968. Subsequently, approximately 200 cases have been reported. This syndrome is characterized by ARF, microangiopathic hemolytic anemia, and thrombocytopenia occurring 2 days to 10 weeks after an uncomplicated delivery. It appears closely related to the hemolytic uremic syndrome. Idiopathic postpartum renal failure is typically preceded by an upper respiratory or gastrointestinal viral syndrome that rapidly progresses to ARF. The use of ethinyl estradiol as a contraceptive may also be causally related to this syndrome.[65] Spontaneous bleeding, congestive heart failure, hypertension, and seizures have been reported.[66,67] Some investigators believe that this syndrome represents a clinical analogue to the generalized Shwartzman reaction, a condition induced in laboratory animals by two successive injections of endotoxin, which results in factor XII activation, thrombin generation, and fibrin deposition. Others consider the platelet deposition to be the primary event that leads to microvascular thrombi.[66]

Management involves plasma infusion and antiplatelet therapy. The role of heparin therapy in idiopathic postpartum renal failure is controversial. The mortality rate among affected patients is high. In a review of 67 patients, 31 (46%) died, 8 (12%) required chronic dialysis or renal transplantation, 10 (15%) had residual renal impairment, and only 13 (19%) had complete recovery.[68] In another review of 25 patients, 8 (32%) patients survived, 1 (4%) recovered normal renal function, 4 (16%) recovered with moderate chronic renal impairment, and 3 (12%) required long-term hemodialysis.[67] Marcovici and Marzano[69] described the clinical course of a woman in whom postpartum renal failure and acute pancreatitis developed. The authors recommended that diuretics should be cautiously administered because they may increase the risk of pancreatitis.

Effect on the Mother and Fetus

Maternal mortality from ARF ranges from none to 34%.[40] This prognosis is better than that for ARF in the nonobstetric population because most obstetric patients are otherwise young and healthy. Stratta et al.[40] reported 84 cases of pregnancy-related ARF, of which 6% required hemodialysis. Although maternal prognosis has improved significantly in developed countries, mortality remains high (16%) among inner city populations.[70] The prognosis for the fetus is worse than that for the mother, and more than 40% of pregnancies in women with ARF end in fetal death.[45,57,71,72]

Medical and Obstetric Management

Management is directed toward rapid recognition of the underlying abnormality. Reversible disorders such as hypovolemia, concealed uterine hemorrhage, urinary tract infection, ureteral obstruction, and drug-induced ARF must be excluded. The urine-to-plasma osmolality ratio is a useful laboratory test to identify reversible prerenal causes. Intravascular volume should be optimized. Electrolyte and acid-base status should be monitored carefully. Hypertension must be managed aggressively. Many obstetric causes of ARF also may cause disseminated intravascular coagulation; therefore, coagulation abnormalities should be excluded.[40]

Because urea and other metabolic products cross the placenta, hemodialysis or peritoneal dialysis should be directed toward maintaining the postdialysis BUN concentration at or below 30 mg/dL. Fluid shifts during hemodialysis should be minimized by short but frequent periods of dialysis. If the fetus is mature, delivery should be accomplished when the maternal condition is stabilized. The pediatrician must be alerted to the presence of high fetal BUN levels, which may lead to an osmotic diuresis and neonatal dehydration. Ertürk et al.[73] reported the first known delivery of a healthy infant during a hemodialysis session.

Anesthetic Management

A multidisciplinary approach involving anesthesiologists, obstetricians, and nephrologists should be employed to optimize the maternal condition before the induction of labor or performance of cesarean delivery in a woman with ARF. Evaluation of maternal intravascular volume may require central venous or pulmonary artery pressure monitoring.[74] The level of azotemia, electrolyte balance, and hematologic status should be assessed. If the BUN level is higher than 80 mg/dL or the serum potassium concentration higher than 5.5 mEq/L, dialysis should be performed before elective vaginal or cesarean delivery. Neuraxial anesthesia may be administered in the absence of coagulopathy, thrombocytopenia, and hypovolemia. Occult uterine hemorrhage should be excluded. Epidural anesthesia may be preferred over spinal anesthesia when the intravascular volume status is in question; under these circumstances the level of sympathetic blockade may be established more slowly while an appropriate volume of intravenous fluid is administered, although this recommendation has not been validated in a controlled study. Normal saline (without potassium) should be administered. As the sympathetic blockade dissipates, the mother should be monitored for evidence of volume overload and pulmonary edema. General anesthesia may be required for urgent cesarean delivery or in patients with coagulopathy or hemorrhage.

RENAL TRANSPLANTATION

Fewer than 1 in 800 women of childbearing age who are undergoing long-term dialysis for renal failure become pregnant.[17] However, successful renal transplantation improves the fertility rate to more than 1 in 50. Since 1963, when Murray et al.[75] reported the first pregnancy after renal transplantation, many women with renal transplants have completed successful pregnancies.

Renal Hyperfiltration

When a kidney is removed from a donor and is transplanted into an anephric recipient, it undergoes a process of hyperfiltration. This is a maladaptive response that, in the short term, attempts to bring the GFR toward the rate of a binephric system. In the long term, this hyperfiltration may lead to glomerular sclerosis and loss of renal function if it is associated with increased glomerular or capillary pressure.[76] In normal pregnancy, the GFR increases by 30% to 50% during the first and second trimesters and subsequently decreases somewhat during the third trimester. Theoretically, this additional hyperfiltration of pregnancy predisposes the patient to a loss of renal function.

Baylis et al.[77,78] allayed many of these concerns by demonstrating that gestational hyperfiltration is not associated with increased glomerular pressure because of matching afferent and efferent arteriolar vasodilation. They produced hyperfiltration in rodent kidneys by performing uninephrectomy, maintaining the animals on a high-protein diet, and subjecting them to five consecutive pregnancies. The investigators observed no functional impairment or renal histologic changes in this animal model. In addition, they demonstrated that glomerular pressure is lower in female rats than in male rats 10 months after uninephrectomy. Hakim et al.[79] have shown a similar gender advantage in humans after uninephrectomy.

TABLE 51-1 Effect of Pregnancy on Long-Term Function of Renal Allografts*

Parameter	Pregnant Group (n = 18)	Nonpregnant Control Group (n = 18)
Plasma creatinine (mg/dL)	1.26 ± 0.83 (19% increase)	1.44 ± 0.59 (8% increase)
Glomerular filtration rate (mL/min)	58 ± 29 (18% decrease)	56 ± 32 (7% decrease)
Mean arterial pressure (mm Hg)	96 ± 12 (1% decrease)	101 ± 9 (5% increase)
Graft loss or chronic rejection	2 (11%)	2 (11%)

*Percentage increase or decrease represents change from initial assessment to end of follow-up. No statistically significant differences were noted.

From Sturgiss SN, Davison JM. Effect of pregnancy on long-term function of renal allografts. Am J Kidney Dis 1992; 19:167-72.

Effect of Pregnancy on the Renal Allograft

Attempts to evaluate the impact of pregnancy on renal allograft function and survival are limited by the inability to randomly assign transplant recipients to pregnancy or no pregnancy. Davison[80] surveyed 2309 pregnancies in 1594 women. Forty percent of the pregnancies did not progress beyond the first trimester (the spontaneous abortion rate was 13%, and the elective abortion rate was 27%). Pregnancies that progressed beyond the first trimester were complicated by IUGR (25%), preterm delivery (50%), and hypertensive disorders of pregnancy (30%). In most women, allograft function was enhanced during early pregnancy and deteriorated briefly during late pregnancy. Only 15% of the women studied experienced persistent renal impairment.[80]

Sturgiss and Davison[81] performed a case-control study of 36 renal transplant recipients, 18 of whom became pregnant and 18 did not. Groups were matched according to age, early rejection episodes, primary renal function, time since transplantation, and extent of histocompatibility. The investigators noted no significant difference between the two groups in plasma creatinine concentration, GFR, mean arterial blood pressure, or the number who suffered graft loss or chronic rejection over a mean follow-up period of 12 years (Table 51-1).

Rahamimov et al.[82] compared long-term graft survival, kidney function, and patient survival between women who became pregnant after renal transplantation (n = 39) with those who did not (n = 117). Each pregnant woman was matched with three controls for 12 factors that may affect graft survival. These investigators did not find a significant difference between groups in any of the outcome measures during the 15-year follow-up period. Kashanizadeh et al.[83] also compared graft survival, allograft function, and patient survival between transplant recipients who conceived (n = 85) and those who did not (n = 125). They, too, did not find a difference in 5-year graft or patient survival between groups. Interestingly, Kashanizadeh et al.[83] noted a smaller increase in creatinine levels in women who had conceived, suggesting that pregnancy might exert a protective effect; this finding has not been confirmed by others.[84] Mahanty et al.[85] proposed an intriguing hypothesis that mothers receiving renal allografts from offspring might have a better graft survival than either fathers receiving allografts from offspring or mothers receiving allografts from non-offspring. Fetal cells and DNA have been detected in maternal blood for decades after normal pregnancy and delivery. The investigators suggested that this microchimerism of fetal cells might induce tolerance and improve renal allograft survival in offspring donor–maternal recipient combinations. However, an initial study failed to support this hypothesis.

Effect on the Fetus

Although intercurrent pregnancy seems to have minimal effect on maternal health or allograft survival in renal transplant recipients, fetal outcome is less favorable. The Toronto Renal Transplant Program reviewed 44 consecutive pregnancies in 26 women who had undergone renal transplantation.[86] Of these, 12 (27%) pregnancies ended with abortion or intrauterine death, and 32 (73%) pregnancies resulted in live-born infants. The mean infant weight in this group was 2540 g, versus 3590 g in a control group. In Singapore, Tan et al.[87] reported abortion or stillbirth among 13 (31%) of 42 pregnancies after renal transplantation. The remaining successful pregnancies were complicated by preterm delivery (45%) and IUGR (86%). Toma et al.[18] surveyed 194 pregnancies in renal transplant recipients. Spontaneous or elective abortion occurred in 28 (14%) of these gestations, and successful delivery of surviving infants occurred in 159 (82%). The National Transplantation Pregnancy Registry reported 53 (11%) fetal deaths in 461 pregnancies following renal transplantation.[88]

Most post-transplantation protocols consist of a primary immunosuppressant (cyclosporine or tacrolimus) and one or two adjunctive agents (azathioprine, mycophenolate mofetil, sirolimus, and/or corticosteroids).[89] Despite transplacental exposure to these immunosuppressant drugs, congenital anomalies and other adverse effects are infrequent.[88,90-92] Kainz et al.[93] reported the outcome of 100 pregnancies in 84 women treated with tacrolimus following solid organ transplantation (27% kidney and 66% liver). In the 68 resulting live births, 4 (6%) neonates presented with malformation of varied nature. Intrauterine exposure to cyclosporine impairs development and function of T, B, and NK cells in neonates. This effect, as well as depressed levels of serum immunoglobulin, persists during the first year of life.[94] These factors place the infant at risk for a suboptimal immunologic response after administration of classic vaccines, and for adverse effects after administration of live, attenuated vaccines. Delay of vaccination (until after 6 months of life) is recommended for infants exposed to immunosuppressant agents *in utero*.

Transplant recipients may become infected with cytomegalovirus (CMV) at the time of transplantation, or they may experience reactivation secondary to immunosuppression. Active CMV infection during pregnancy is associated with congenital anomalies (e.g., cerebral cysts, microcephaly, mental retardation). In addition, active neonatal CMV infection may lead to serious illness or death.

Following renal transplantation, residual impairment of renal function may lead to false-positive results of biochemical screening for trisomy 21. Karidas et al.[95] demonstrated a significant correlation between free beta-human chorionic gonadotropin (β-hCG) and serum urea and creatinine concentrations. Similar alterations in alpha-fetoprotein (AFP) levels were not observed. In this setting, the double-marker biochemical test may be interpreted inaccurately. In patients with altered serum urea and creatinine concentrations, first-trimester nuchal translucency measurement—in combination with second-trimester ultrasonography—may be a more useful screening regimen (see Chapter 6).

Medical and Obstetric Management

Discontinuation of immunosuppressant therapy, even years after transplantation, may lead to acute rejection. Thus, the renal transplant recipient's immunosuppressant regimen must be continued during pregnancy unless toxicity results. Cyclosporine requirements increase during pregnancy, most likely because of enhanced metabolism.[96] The pregnant patient must be intensively monitored for any evidence of acute or chronic allograft rejection, infection, ureteral and renal artery obstruction, impaired renal function, hypertension, fluid volume disturbances, anemia, or any combination of these symptoms. Recombinant human erythropoietin has been used safely and has successfully improved anemia in a few pregnant transplant recipients.[97]

Initial laboratory studies include (1) complete blood count, (2) renal function tests, (3) determination of serum electrolyte and glucose concentrations, and (4) viral serologic testing for CMV, hepatitis B virus, HCV, and HIV. Serial ultrasonographic assessments allow the recognition of fetal anomalies and the evaluation of fetal growth.

Cultures of the lower genital tract should be obtained in women with lesions that suggest herpes simplex virus infection. A patient who presents in labor and with evidence of active genital herpes simplex virus infection should undergo cesarean delivery (see Chapter 36).

Vaginal examinations are minimized and always performed in a strict aseptic manner. The renal allograft is typically implanted in the extraperitoneal iliac fossa and does not impair vaginal delivery. Prophylactic antibiotics and stress-dose corticosteroids are indicated in patients who undergo cesarean delivery.

Anesthetic Management

In the absence of renal dysfunction and hypertension, anesthetic management of the parturient with a renal transplant is similar to that of the otherwise healthy parturient. Strict aseptic technique is maintained during the placement of intravascular catheters and the performance of neuraxial anesthetic techniques. Sowter et al.[98] reported an epidural abscess that occurred 23 days after epidural anesthesia in a nonpregnant patient undergoing corticosteroid therapy for rheumatoid arthritis. Fortunately, this complication is exceedingly rare. In the absence of systemic infection, immunosuppression itself should not be considered a contraindication to administration of epidural or spinal anesthesia.

UROLITHIASIS

Definition and Epidemiology

Urolithiasis is characterized by the abnormal formation of calculi within the renal calyces or pelvis. Calculi may lodge within the ureters or bladder. Most stones are calcium oxalate (70%) or calcium phosphate (10%). The disorder affects 1% to 5% of the general U.S. population, but it is more common in the southeastern "stone belt" and mountainous regions. Symptomatic urolithiasis occurs during 1 in 240 to 1 in 3300 pregnancies[99,100] and is more common among whites than African-Americans. Because pregnancy does not affect the rate of urolithiasis, this incidence approximates that observed among nonpregnant young women during a 9-month period.

Pathophysiology

The presence of urolithiasis presumes an underlying physiologic abnormality that leads to persistent supersaturation of the particular minerals involved. Supersaturation may occur secondary to acidic urine, oliguria, or an increased excretion of the stone constituents. During pregnancy, an elevated plasma 1,25-dihydroxyvitamin D level causes greater intestinal absorption of calcium, net mobilization of calcium from bone, and a state of absorptive hypercalciuria.[101] Ultimately, these changes provide calcium for the fetal skeleton. The fact that pregnant women rarely have urolithiasis implies the occurrence of other physiologic changes during pregnancy that offset this stone-forming tendency. Calcium stone inhibitors such as citrate, magnesium, and glycoprotein are excreted in the urine to a greater extent during pregnancy.[102]

Diagnosis

Urolithiasis most commonly manifests during the second or third trimester. Only 20% of affected pregnant women recount a prior history of renal calculi.[103] More than 80% of cases of gestational urolithiasis are diagnosed in parous women, possibly reflecting the higher incidence of this disease with advanced age.[104] Among 72 cases of urolithiasis reported by Lewis et al.,[99] 60% were right-sided, 36% were left-sided, and 4% were bilateral.

The diagnosis of urolithiasis during pregnancy must be differentiated from that of ectopic pregnancy, preterm labor, appendicitis, pyelonephritis, and benign hematuria of pregnancy. A history of previous urolithiasis, recurrent urinary tract infections, or urologic surgery is suggestive. Symptoms include flank and abdominal pain, urgency, dysuria, nausea, and fever. Examination reveals costovertebral tenderness, abdominal tenderness, pyuria, and hematuria. Urolithiasis must be considered in patients with pyelonephritis who remain febrile or have continued bacteriuria despite 48 hours of parenteral antibiotics.

The initial imaging modality for the evaluation of urolithiasis during pregnancy is transabdominal ultrasonography. This technology has evolved so that most cases of gestational urolithiasis may be diagnosed confidently without exposing the fetus to ionizing radiation. Specifically, color Doppler ultrasonography allows the identification of ureteral jets during pregnancy, and the asymmetry or absence of these jets indicates the presence of urinary calculi.[105-107] Vaginal ultrasonography may augment suboptimal transabdominal ultrasonographic images. However, 40% of calculi are missed when the urinary tract is imaged with ultrasonography alone.[104]

If urinary calculi are not successfully visualized with ultrasonography and clinical suspicion for urolithiasis remains high, limited intravenous pyelography may be utilized.[103,104] Fetal radiation exposure during excretory urography is less than 1.5 rads. Exposure to 5 to 10 rads during the embryogenic period confers a 1% to 3% increase in the risk of congenital anomalies.[108] Of greater concern is the risk for childhood malignancies following radiation exposure *in utero*. Harvey et al.[109] studied 32,000 twins born in Connecticut from 1930 to 1969 (a time when twin gestations were diagnosed with limited abdominal radiography). The average radiation dose to which the fetuses were exposed was 1 rad (range of 0.16 to 4 rads). These children subsequently were found to have a 1.6-fold increase in the relative risk for leukemia and a 3.2-fold increase in the relative risk for childhood malignancies. These risks must be considered in the selection of urologic imaging techniques. Magnetic resonance urography, with strongly T2-weighted sequences, also may show the site and type of obstruction without exposing the fetus to ionizing radiation.[106]

Effect of Pregnancy

In an effort to determine any effect of pregnancy on the natural history of urolithiasis, Coe et al.[110] reviewed the records of 58 pregnancies in women with the preexisting diagnosis of urolithiasis. The stone recurrence rate in this group was 0.49 stone per patient-year, which was not significantly different from the rate of 0.44 stone per patient-year in the general population.[111] The authors concluded that pregnancy does not alter the activity or severity of stone disease.

Effect on the Mother and Fetus

In a retrospective cohort study, Swartz et al.[112] compared women with nephrolithiasis (n = 2339) with randomly selected women without nephrolithiasis (n = 6729). The investigators found that women with nephrolithiasis had an almost twofold higher rate of preterm delivery. However, these women were not at increased risk for other adverse outcomes, including premature rupture of the membranes, low birth weight, and infant death. Honoré[113] suggested that there is a higher incidence of renal stones among women who have a spontaneous abortion. He hypothesized that abnormalities of calcium hemostasis may lead to myometrial hyperirritability or abnormal hormonal secretion by the corpus luteum, the placenta, or both. Rare cases of ureteral rupture[114] and obstructed labor caused by a vesicular[115] or bladder calculus[116] have been reported.

Urologic and Obstetric Management

During pregnancy, 70% of calculi pass spontaneously with conservative management (e.g., hydration, antibiotics if the patient is febrile, bed rest, analgesia).[100] Urologic intervention is indicated in the patient with persistent pyelonephritis, deterioration of renal function, massive hydronephrosis, persistent pain, or sepsis. Ureteral stent placement with ureteroscopy and ultrasonographic guidance is required in 29% of affected pregnant women, and percutaneous nephrostomy in 3%.[100] Open ureterolithotomy or nephrectomy is required infrequently. Holmium:yttrium-aluminum-garnet (YAG) laser lithotripsy, using state-of-the-art ureteroscopes, is an emerging technique for stone management in pregnancy.[117] Extracorporeal lithotripsy is not approved for use during pregnancy.[118]

Women with a history of urolithiasis should increase their intake of fluids. Calcium supplementation through prenatal vitamins should be avoided in women with recurrent urolithiasis. Medical management of stone disease may have untoward fetal effects. Thiazides are associated with fetal hyponatremia, hypoglycemia, and thrombocytopenia.[119] Although D-penicillamine, which is used to treat cystinuric urolithiasis, has been associated with congenital connective tissue defects,[120] some physicians consider this risk to be overstated if a low-methionine diet is avoided when this agent is used.[121] Adverse effects of xanthine oxidase inhibitors are unknown.[122]

The following conditions may raise suspicion of the presence of **primary hyperparathyroidism** in a pregnant woman: (1) urolithiasis with or without pancreatitis, (2) hyperemesis beyond the first trimester, (3) a history of recurrent spontaneous abortion or intrauterine fetal death, (4) neonatal hypocalcemia or tetany, and/or (5) a total serum calcium concentration greater than 10.1 mg/dL during the second trimester or 8.8 mg/dL during the third trimester.[123,124]

Anesthetic Management

The ureters receive sensory innervation through the renal, ovarian, and hypogastric plexuses (T11 to L1 spinal segments). During conservative management of urolithiasis, epidural analgesia provides the patient with significant pain relief and facilitates the passage of the calculus, possibly through decreased ureteral spasm.[125-127] Ready and Johnson[125] reported the use of epidural analgesia in a patient with severe renal colic at 23 weeks' gestation. Analgesia that was maintained for 16 hours allowed the passage of the stone. Neuraxial analgesia allows the anesthesia provider to avoid systemic opioids, which impair normal peristalsis in ureteric smooth muscle. Improved maternal pain control may also decrease endogenous catecholamine release and improve uteroplacental blood flow.

KEY POINTS

- Pregnant women with moderate or severe renal insufficiency are at increased risk for deterioration of renal function, exacerbation of hypertension, and other obstetric complications, including intrauterine fetal growth restriction and preterm delivery.
- Pregnancy does not affect the long-term survival of a renal allograft.
- Immunosuppressive therapy must be continued during pregnancy in the patient with a renal transplant. The anesthesia provider should maintain strict aseptic technique during the placement of intravascular catheters and the performance of neuraxial anesthetic techniques.
- Epidural analgesia may facilitate the spontaneous passage of renal calculi.

REFERENCES

1. Pregnancy and renal disease. Lancet 1975; 2(7939):801-2.
2. Lindheimer MD, Davison JM, Katz AI. The kidney and hypertension in pregnancy: Twenty exciting years. Semin Nephrol 2001; 21:173-89.
3. Davison JM. Kidney function in pregnant women. Am J Kidney Dis 1987; 9:248-52.
4. Fisher KA, Luger A, Spargo BH, Lindheimer MD. Hypertension in pregnancy: Clinical-pathological correlations and remote prognosis. Medicine (Baltimore) 1981; 60:267-76.
5. Chen HH, Lin HC, Yeh JC, Chen CP. Renal biopsy in pregnancies complicated by undetermined renal disease. Acta Obstet Gynecol Scand 2001; 80:888-93.
6. Kuller JA, D'Andrea NM, McMahon MJ. Renal biopsy and pregnancy. Am J Obstet Gynecol 2001; 184:1093-6.
7. Katz AI, Davison JM, Hayslett JP, et al. Pregnancy in women with kidney disease. Kidney Int 1980; 18:192-206.
8. Jungers P, Houillier P, Forget D, et al. Influence of pregnancy on the course of primary chronic glomerulonephritis. Lancet 1995; 346:1122-4.
9. Jones DC, Hayslett JP. Outcome of pregnancy in women with moderate or severe renal insufficiency. N Engl J Med 1996; 335:226-32.
10. Epstein FH. Pregnancy and renal disease. N Engl J Med 1996; 335:277-8.
11. Reddy SS, Holley JL. Management of the pregnant chronic dialysis patient. Adv Chronic Kidney Dis 2007; 14:146-55.
12. Ramin SM, Vidaeff AC, Yeomans ER, Gilstrap LC. Chronic renal disease in pregnancy. Obstet Gynecol 2006; 108:1531-9.
13. Alexopoulos E, Bili H, Tampakoudis P, et al. Outcome of pregnancy in women with glomerular diseases. Ren Fail 1996; 18:121-9.
14. Bar J, Orvieto R, Shalev Y, et al. Pregnancy outcome in women with primary renal disease. Isr Med Assoc J 2000; 2:178-81.
15. McGregor E, Stewart G, Junor BJ, Rodger RS. Successful use of recombinant human erythropoietin in pregnancy. Nephrol Dial Transplant 1991; 6:292-3.
16. Lim VS. Reproductive function in patients with renal insufficiency. Am J Kidney Dis 1987; 9:363-7.
17. Successful pregnancies in women treated by dialysis and kidney transplantation: Report from the Registration Committee of the European Dialysis and Transplant Association. Br J Obstet Gynaecol 1980; 87:839-45.
18. Toma H, Tanabe K, Tokumoto T, et al. Pregnancy in women receiving renal dialysis or transplantation in Japan: A nationwide survey. Nephrol Dial Transplant 1999; 14:1511-6.
19. Krakow D, Castro LC, Schwieger J. Effect of hemodialysis on uterine and umbilical artery Doppler flow velocity waveforms. Am J Obstet Gynecol 1994; 170:1386-8.
20. Hou S. Pregnancy in women requiring dialysis for renal failure. Am J Kidney Dis 1987; 9:368-73.
21. Jakobi P, Ohel G, Szylman P, et al. Continuous ambulatory peritoneal dialysis as the primary approach in the management of severe renal insufficiency in pregnancy. Obstet Gynecol 1992; 79:808-10.
22. Chou CY, Ting IW, Lin TH, Lee CN. Pregnancy in patients on chronic dialysis: A single center experience and combined analysis of reported results. Eur J Obstet Gynecol Reprod Biol 2008; 136:165-70.
23. Yoo J, Unnikrishnan D, Lwin LN, et al. Successful triplet pregnancy in a patient on chronic haemodialysis. Nephrol Dial Transplant 2004; 19:994-7.
24. Bamberg C, Diekmann F, Haase M, et al. Pregnancy on intensified hemodialysis: Fetal surveillance and perinatal outcome. Fetal Diagn Ther 2007; 22:289-93.
25. Asrat T, Nageotte MP. Renal failure in pregnancy. Semin Perinatol 1990; 14:59-67.
26. Tokars JI, Miller ER, Alter MJ, Arduino MJ. National surveillance of dialysis associated diseases in the United States, 1995. ASAIO J 1998; 44:98-107.
27. Harmankaya O, Cetin B, Obek A, Seber E. Low prevalence of hepatitis C virus infection in hemodialysis units: Effect of isolation? Ren Fail 2002; 24:639-44.
28. Tighe KE, Smith ID, Bogod DG. Caesarean section in chronic renal failure. Eur J Anaesthesiol 1995; 12:185-7.
29. Gould DB, Aldrete JA. Bupivacaine cardiotoxicity in a patient with renal failure. Acta Anaesthesiol Scand 1983; 27:18-21.
30. Lucas LF, Tsueda K. Cardiovascular depression after brachial plexus block in two diabetic patients with renal failure. Anesthesiology 1990; 73:1032-5.
31. Rice AS, Pither CE, Tucker GT. Plasma concentrations of bupivacaine after supraclavicular brachial plexus blockade in patients with chronic renal failure. Anaesthesia 1991; 46:354-7.
32. Orko R, Pitkanen M, Rosenberg PH. Subarachnoid anaesthesia with 0.75% bupivacaine in patients with chronic renal failure. Br J Anaesth 1986; 58:605-9.
33. Weir PH, Chung FF. Anaesthesia for patients with chronic renal disease. Can Anaesth Soc J 1984; 31:468-81.
34. Costela JL, Jimenez R, Calvo R, et al. Serum protein binding of propofol in patients with renal failure or hepatic cirrhosis. Acta Anaesthesiol Scand 1996; 40:741-5.
35. Ghoneim MM, Pandya H. Plasma protein binding of thiopental in patients with impaired renal or hepatic function. Anesthesiology 1975; 42:545-9.
36. Freeman RB, Sheff MF, Maher JF, Schreiner GE. The blood-cerebrospinal fluid barrier in uremia. Ann Intern Med 1962; 56:233-40.

37. Miller RD, Way WL, Hamilton WK, Layzer RB. Succinylcholine-induced hyperkalemia in patients with renal failure? Anesthesiology 1972; 36:138-41.
38. Ryan DW. Preoperative serum cholinesterase concentration in chronic renal failure: Clinical experience of suxamethonium in 81 patients undergoing renal transplant. Br J Anaesth 1977; 49:945-9.
39. Ghoneim MM, Long JP. The interaction between magnesium and other neuromuscular blocking agents. Anesthesiology 1970; 32:23-7.
40. Stratta P, Besso L, Canavese C, et al. Is pregnancy-related acute renal failure a disappearing clinical entity? Ren Fail 1996; 18:575-84.
41. Selcuk NY, Tonbul HZ, San A, Odabas AR. Changes in frequency and etiology of acute renal failure in pregnancy (1980-1997). Ren Fail 1998; 20:513-17.
42. Mitch WE. Acute renal failure. In Goldman L, Bennett JC, editors. Cecil Textbook of Medicine. 22nd edition. Philadelphia, WB Saunders, 2000:567-71.
43. Diaz JH, De Gordon G, Hernandez L, Medina R. Acute kidney insufficiency of obstetric origin: Experience at the Santo Tomas Hospital (1966-1981) [Spanish]. Rev Med Panama 1990; 15:35-41.
44. Turney JH, Ellis CM, Parsons FM. Obstetric acute renal failure 1956-1987. Br J Obstet Gynaecol 1989; 96:679-87.
45. Randeree IG, Czarnocki A, Moodley J, et al. Acute renal failure in pregnancy in South Africa. Ren Fail 1995; 17:147-53.
46. Bamgboye EL, Mabayoje MO, Odutola TA, Mabadeje AF. Acute renal failure at the Lagos University Teaching Hospital: A 10-year review. Ren Fail 1993; 15:77-80.
47. Grunfeld JP, Pertuiset N. Acute renal failure in pregnancy: 1987. Am J Kidney Dis 1987; 9:359-62.
48. Prakash J, Tripathi K, Pandey LK, et al. Renal cortical necrosis in pregnancy-related acute renal failure. J Indian Med Assoc 1996; 94:227-9.
49. Utas C, Yalçindag C, Taskapan H, et al. Acute renal failure in Central Anatolia. Nephrol Dial Transplant 2000; 15:152-5.
50. Hill JB, Yost NP, Wendel GD. Acute renal failure in association with severe hyperemesis gravidarum. Obstet Gynecol 2002; 100:1119-21.
51. Krane NK. Acute renal failure in pregnancy. Arch Intern Med 1988; 148:2347-57.
52. Khanna N, Nguyen H. Reversible acute renal failure in association with bilateral ureteral obstruction and hydronephrosis in pregnancy. Am J Obstet Gynecol 2001; 184:239-40.
53. Homans DC, Blake GD, Harrington JT, Cetrulo CL. Acute renal failure caused by ureteral obstruction by a gravid uterus. JAMA 1981; 246:1230-1.
54. Courban D, Blank S, Harris MA, et al. Acute renal failure in the first trimester resulting from uterine leiomyomas. Am J Obstet Gynecol 1997; 177:472-3.
55. Chugh KS, Jha V, Sakhuja V, Joshi K. Acute renal cortical necrosis—a study of 113 patients. Ren Fail 1994; 16:37-47.
56. Seedat YK, Grant W, Chetty S. Bilateral renal cortical necrosis: A report of 2 cases. S Afr Med J 1976; 50:933-6.
57. Ventura JE, Villa M, Mizraji R, Ferreiros R. Acute renal failure in pregnancy. Ren Fail 1997; 19:217-20.
58. Grunfeld JP, Ganeval D, Bournerias F. Acute renal failure in pregnancy. Kidney Int 1980; 18:179-91.
59. Whalley PJ, Cunningham FG, Martin FG. Transient renal dysfunction associated with acute pyelonephritis of pregnancy. Obstet Gynecol 1975; 46:174-7.
60. Sibai BM, Ramadan MK. Acute renal failure in pregnancies complicated by hemolysis, elevated liver enzymes, and low platelets. Am J Obstet Gynecol 1993; 168:1682-7; discussion 1687-90.
61. Abraham KA, Kennelly M, Dorman AM, Walshe JJ. Pathogenesis of acute renal failure associated with the HELLP syndrome: A case report and review of the literature. Eur J Obstet Gynecol Reprod Biol 2003; 108:99-102.
62. Celik C, Gezginc K, Altintepe L, et al. Results of the pregnancies with HELLP syndrome. Ren Fail 2003; 25:613-8.
63. Flynn MF, Power RE, Murphy DM, et al. Successful transplantation of kidneys from a donor with HELLP syndrome-related death. Transpl Int 2001; 14:108-10.
64. Robson JS, Martin AM, Ruckley V, Macdonald MK. Irreversible postpartum renal failure: A new syndrome. Q J Med 1968; 37:423-35.
65. Hayslett JP. Current concepts: Postpartum renal failure. N Engl J Med 1985; 312:1556-9.
66. Sun NC, Johnson WJ, Sung DT, Woods JE. Idiopathic postpartum renal failure: Review and case report of a successful renal transplantation. Mayo Clin Proc 1975; 50:395-401.
67. Segonds A, Louradour N, Suc JM, Orfila C. Postpartum hemolytic uremic syndrome: A study of three cases with a review of the literature. Clin Nephrol 1979; 12:229-42.
68. Li PK, Lai FM, Tam JS, Lai KN. Acute renal failure due to postpartum haemolytic uraemic syndrome. Aust N Z J Obstet Gynaecol 1988; 28:228-30.
69. Marcovici I, Marzano D. Pregnancy-induced hypertension complicated by postpartum renal failure and pancreatitis: A case report. Am J Perinatol 2002; 19:177-9.
70. Nzerue CM, Hewan-Lowe K, Nwawka C. Acute renal failure in pregnancy: A review of clinical outcomes at an inner-city hospital from 1986-1996. J Natl Med Assoc 1998; 90:486-90.
71. Naqvi R, Akhtar F, Ahmed E, et al. Acute renal failure of obstetrical origin during 1994 at one center. Ren Fail 1996; 18:681-3.
72. Lindheimer MD, Katz AI, Ganeval D, Grünfeld JP. Acute renal failure in pregnancy. In Brenner BM, Lazarus JM, editors. Acute Renal Failure. New York, Churchill Livingstone, 1988:597-620.
73. Ertürk S, Akar H, Uckuyu A, et al. Delivery of healthy infant during hemodialysis session. J Nephrol 2000; 13:75-7.
74. Gilbert WM, Towner DR, Field NT, Anthony J. The safety and utility of pulmonary artery catheterization in severe preeclampsia and eclampsia. Am J Obstet Gynecol 2000; 182:1397-403.
75. Murray JE, Reid DE, Harrison JH, Merrill JP. Successful pregnancies after human renal transplantation. N Engl J Med 1963; 269:341-3.
76. Terasaki PI, Koyama H, Cecka JM, Gjertson DW. The hyperfiltration hypothesis in human renal transplantation. Transplantation 1994; 57:1450-4.
77. Baylis C, Wilson CB. Sex and the single kidney. Am J Kidney Dis 1989; 13:290-8.
78. Baylis C, Reckelhoff JF. Renal hemodynamics in normal and hypertensive pregnancy: Lessons from micropuncture. Am J Kidney Dis 1991; 17:98-104.
79. Hakim RM, Goldszer RC, Brenner BM. Hypertension and proteinuria: Long-term sequelae of uninephrectomy in humans. Kidney Int 1984; 25:930-6.
80. Davison JM. Dialysis, transplantation, and pregnancy. Am J Kidney Dis 1991; 17:127-32.
81. Sturgiss SN, Davison JM. Effect of pregnancy on long-term function of renal allografts. Am J Kidney Dis 1992; 19:167-72.
82. Rahamimov R, Ben-Haroush A, Wittenberg C, et al. Pregnancy in renal transplant recipients: Long-term effect on patient and graft survival: A single-center experience. Transplantation 2006; 81:660-4.
83. Kashanizadeh N, Nemati E, Sharifi-Bonab M, et al. Impact of pregnancy on the outcome of kidney transplantation. Transplant Proc 2007; 39:1136-8.
84. Armenti VT, Radomski JS, Moritz MJ, et al. Report from the National Transplantation Pregnancy Registry (NTPR): Outcomes of pregnancy after transplantation. Clin Transpl 2004; 103.
85. Mahanty HD, Cherikh WS, Chang GJ, et al. Influence of pretransplant pregnancy on survival of renal allografts from living donors. Transplantation 2001; 72:228-32.
86. Sgro MD, Barozzino T, Mirghani HM, et al. Pregnancy outcome post renal transplantation. Teratology 2002; 65:5-9.
87. Tan PK, Tan AS, Tan HK, et al. Pregnancy after renal transplantation: Experience in Singapore General Hospital. Ann Acad Med Singapore 2002; 31:285-9.
88. Armenti VT, Coscia LA, McGrory CH, Moritz MJ. National Transplantation Pregnancy Registry: Update on pregnancy and renal transplantation. Nephrol News Issues 1998; 12:19-23.
89. Gaston RS. Maintenance immunosuppression in the renal transplant recipient: An overview. Am J Kidney Dis 2001; 38:S25-35.

90. Bar J, Stahl B, Hod M, et al. Is immunosuppression therapy in renal allograft recipients teratogenic? A single-center experience. Am J Med Genet A 2003; 116:31-6.
91. Scott JR, Branch DW, Holman J. Autoimmune and pregnancy complications in the daughter of a kidney transplant patient. Transplantation 2002; 73:815-6.
92. Willis FR, Findlay CA, Gorrie MJ, et al. Children of renal transplant recipient mothers. J Paediatr Child Health 2000; 36:230-5.
93. Kainz A, Harabacz I, Cowlrick IS, et al. Review of the course and outcome of 100 pregnancies in 84 women treated with tacrolimus. Transplantation 2000; 70:1718-21.
94. Schen FP, Stallone G, Schena A, et al. Pregnancy in renal transplantation: Immunologic evaluation of neonates from mothers with transplanted kidney. Transpl Immunol 2002; 9:161-4.
95. Karidas CN, Michailidis GD, Spencer K, Economides DL. Biochemical screening for Down syndrome in pregnancies following renal transplantation. Prenat Diagn 2002; 22:226-30.
96. Biesenbach G, Zazgornik J, Kaiser W, et al. Cyclosporin requirement during pregnancy in renal transplant recipients. Nephrol Dial Transplant 1989; 4:667-9.
97. Al Shohaib S. Erythropoietin therapy in a pregnant post-renal transplant patient. Nephron 1999; 81:81-3.
98. Sowter MC, Burgess NA, Woodsford PV, Lewis MH. Delayed presentation of an extradural abscess complicating thoracic extradural analgesia. Br J Anaesth 1992; 68:103-5.
99. Lewis DF, Robichaux AG, Jaekle RK, et al. Urolithiasis in pregnancy: Diagnosis, management and pregnancy outcome. J Reprod Med 2003; 48:28-32.
100. Cormier CM, Canzoneri BJ, Lewis DF, et al. Urolithiasis in pregnancy: Current diagnosis, treatment, and pregnancy complications. Obstet Gynecol Surv 2006; 61:733-41.
101. Gertner JM, Coustan DR, Kliger AS, et al. Pregnancy as state of physiologic absorptive hypercalciuria. Am J Med 1986; 81:451-6.
102. Loughlin KR, Ker LA. The current management of urolithiasis during pregnancy. Urol Clin North Am 2002; 29:701-4.
103. Butler EL, Cox SM, Eberts EG, Cunningham FG. Symptomatic nephrolithiasis complicating pregnancy. Obstet Gynecol 2000; 96:753-6.
104. Horowitz E, Schmidt JD. Renal calculi in pregnancy. Clin Obstet Gynecol 1985; 28:324-38.
105. Burke BJ, Washowich TL. Ureteral jets in normal second- and third-trimester pregnancy. J Clin Ultrasound 1998; 26:423-6.
106. Grenier N, Pariente JL, Trillaud H, et al. Dilatation of the collecting system during pregnancy: Physiologic vs obstructive dilatation. Eur Radiol 2000; 10:271-9.
107. Asrat T, Roossin MC, Miller EI. Ultrasonographic detection of ureteral jets in normal pregnancy. Am J Obstet Gynecol 1998; 178:1194-8.
108. Swartz HM, Reichling BA. Hazards of radiation exposure for pregnant women. JAMA 1978; 239:1907-8.
109. Harvey EB, Boice JD, Honeyman M, Flannery JT. Prenatal x-ray exposure and childhood cancer in twins. N Engl J Med 1985; 312:541-5.
110. Coe FL, Parks JH, Lindheimer MD. Nephrolithiasis during pregnancy. N Engl J Med 1978; 298:324-6.
111. Coe FL, Keck J, Norton ER. The natural history of calcium urolithiasis. JAMA 1977; 238:1519-23.
112. Swartz MA, Lydon-Rochelle MT, Simon D, et al. Admission for nephrolithiasis in pregnancy and risk of adverse birth outcomes. Obstet Gynecol 2007; 109:1099-104.
113. Honoré LH. The increased incidence of renal stones in women with spontaneous abortion: A retrospective study. Am J Obstet Gynecol 1980; 137:145-6.
114. Eaton A, Martin PC. Ruptured ureter in pregnancy: A unique case? Br J Urol 1981; 53:78-9.
115. Drago JR, Rohner TJ, Chez RA. Management of urinary calculi in pregnancy. Urology 1982; 20:578-81.
116. Ait Benkaddour Y, Aboulfalah A, Abbassi H. Bladder stone: Uncommon cause of mechanical dystocia. Arch Gynecol Obstet 2006; 274:323-4.
117. Watterson JD, Girvan AR, Beiko DT, et al. Ureteroscopy and holmium:YAG laser lithotripsy: An emerging definitive management strategy for symptomatic ureteral calculi in pregnancy. Urology 2002; 60:383-7.
118. Streem SB. Contemporary clinical practice of shock wave lithotripsy: A reevaluation of contraindications. J Urol 1997; 157:1197-203.
119. Gray MJ. Use and abuse of thiazides in pregnancy. Clin Obstet Gynecol 1968; 11:568-78.
120. Mjolnerod OK, Dommerud SA, Rasmussen K, Gjeruldsen ST. Congenital connective-tissue defect probably due to D-penicillamine treatment in pregnancy. Lancet 1971; 1(7701):673-5.
121. Gregory MC, Mansell MA. Pregnancy and cystinuria. Lancet 1983; 2(8360):1158-60.
122. Maikranz P, Coe FL, Parks J, Lindheimer MD. Nephrolithiasis in pregnancy. Am J Kidney Dis 1987; 9:354-8.
123. Carella MJ, Gossain VV. Hyperparathyroidism and pregnancy: Case report and review. J Gen Intern Med 1992; 7:448-53.
124. Schnatz PF, Curry SL. Primary hyperparathyroidism in pregnancy: Evidence-based management. Obstet Gynecol Surv 2002; 57:365-76.
125. Ready LB, Johnson ES. Epidural block for treatment of renal colic during pregnancy. Can Anaesth Soc J 1981; 28:77-9.
126. Romagnoli A. Continuous epidural block in the treatment of impacted ureteric stones (letter). Can Med Assoc J 1973; 109:968.
127. Lloyd JW, Carrie LES. A method of treating renal colic. Proc R Soc Med 1965; 58:634.

Chapter 52

Respiratory Disease in Pregnancy

Karen S. Lindeman, M.D.

ASTHMA

Definition

Asthma is defined by the presence of the following three characteristic findings: (1) reversible airway obstruction, (2) airway inflammation, and (3) airway hyperresponsiveness. **Airway obstruction** produces the clinical manifestations of wheezing, cough, and dyspnea. **Airway inflammation** modulates the course of asthma by independently producing airway obstruction and enhancing airway hyperresponsiveness. **Airway hyperresponsiveness** is marked by exaggerated responses to a wide variety of bronchoconstrictor stimuli, including histamine, methacholine, prostaglandin $F_{2\alpha}$, hypo-osmotic solutions, and cold air.

Epidemiology

Asthma is an increasingly common problem among young, otherwise healthy women of childbearing age. Morbidity and mortality rates from this disease increased during the 1980s and 1990s. The prevalence of asthma, rates of hospitalization due to asthma, and death rates from asthma increased from 1980 until 1996 but have stabilized since 1997.[1]

The prevalence of asthma in women of childbearing age continues to rise. From 1988 to 1994, asthma affected approximately 3.2% of pregnant women in the United States, but the estimate increased to between 3.7% and 8.4% from 1997 to 2001.[2] The greatest effect appeared in younger women, 18 to 24 years; the prevalence increased threefold between the periods 1976 to 1980 and 1988 to 1994.[2]

Pathophysiology

Asthma is thought to occur under a variety of environmental influences in the presence of genetic susceptibility.[3] The underlying defect that produces the clinical syndrome of asthma is unknown. The most important potential mechanisms are (1) an enhancement of contractility or an impairment of relaxation of airway smooth muscle, (2) a neural imbalance, (3) airway inflammation, and (4) changes in the function of the airway epithelium.

AIRWAY SMOOTH MUSCLE

Contraction of airway smooth muscle is thought to be the most important factor in producing acute airway obstruction. For many years, an enhancement of airway smooth muscle responsiveness to contractile agonists was assumed to be a major mechanism of asthma. To test this hypothesis, investigators attempted to correlate airway responsiveness *in vivo* and *in vitro* in human subjects[4-8] and in the Basenji-greyhound dog model of asthma.[9] These studies did not demonstrate a significant correlation between the airway response to histamine or cholinergic agonists *in vivo* and airway smooth muscle contraction *in vitro*. Some studies actually demonstrated a negative correlation between the *in vivo* and *in vitro* responses,[8,9] suggesting that diminished responsiveness may represent a chronic adaptive response of airway smooth muscle.

Instead of an enhancement in responsiveness to contractile stimuli, a reduction in responsiveness to relaxant stimuli may contribute to airway obstruction. One study demonstrated impaired relaxant responses to isoproterenol in airway smooth muscle from human asthmatic subjects in comparison with the responsiveness of airway smooth muscle from controls.[10] Other evidence substantiates the presence of impaired airway relaxation in asthmatic subjects *in vivo*.[11] Although the mechanism for this effect is poorly understood, a reduction in airway sensitivity to beta-adrenergic agonists could contribute to airway hyperresponsiveness by altering the balance between constricting and dilating influences.

NEURAL COMPONENTS

A balance between constricting and dilating influences also exists with respect to the autonomic nervous system. A shift in this balance, with an increase in constricting influences, may be a mechanism of asthma.

The parasympathetic nervous system provides the dominant constrictor input to the airways (Figure 52-1). Efferent cholinergic fibers travel in the vagus nerve to synapse in ganglia within the airway wall.[12] Postganglionic fibers release acetylcholine to activate muscarinic receptors and stimulate airway smooth muscle contraction. A negative feedback system limits release of acetylcholine from nerve terminals. Muscarinic autoreceptors, or receptors on the nerve ending,[13] also are activated by acetylcholine and inhibit further release of acetylcholine from the nerve terminal.

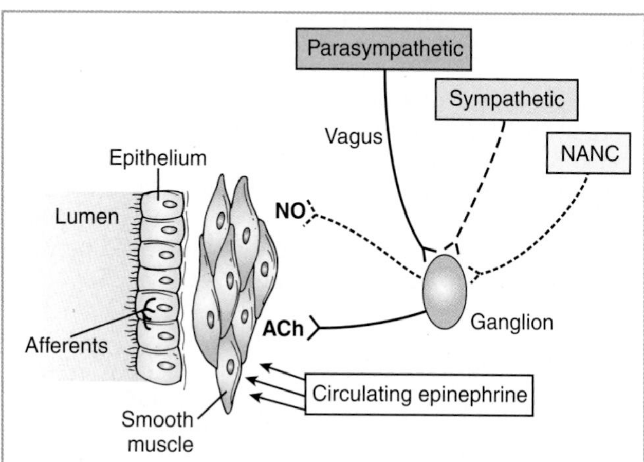

FIGURE 52-1 Neural control of the airway. Parasympathetic, sympathetic, and nonadrenergic, noncholinergic (NANC) efferents innervate ganglia within the airway wall. Postganglionic cholinergic efferents release acetylcholine (ACh) to constrict airway smooth muscle. Postganglionic NANC efferents release nitric oxide (NO) to relax airway smooth muscle. Circulating epinephrine relaxes the airway. Afferents from the airway originate in the epithelium, and are activated by airway irritation, as occurs with endotracheal intubation.

The importance of exaggerated cholinergic efferent activity in the pathogenesis of airway hyperreactivity has been debated extensively. The relatively limited efficacy of anticholinergic agents in relieving clinical bronchospasm, as well as growing evidence supporting other mechanisms, suggests that this pathway has a limited role in the pathophysiology of asthma. However, this mechanism appears to be very important in the perioperative management of asthmatic subjects. Reflex stimulation of airway smooth muscle by placement of an endotracheal tube represents one of the most important causes of bronchospasm in the perioperative period.

An alternative mechanism by which the parasympathetic nervous system may contribute to airway hyperresponsiveness is through dysfunction of the muscarinic autoreceptors. Dysfunction of these receptors allows increased postganglionic release of acetylcholine after reflex stimulation.[14] This mechanism is well established in a guinea pig model of viral infection[15] and may explain the airway hyperresponsiveness that occurs for several weeks after an upper respiratory tract infection, although additional autoreceptor-independent mechanisms may also be present.[16] The role of this mechanism in the pathophysiology of clinical asthma is unclear.

The sympathetic nervous system primarily acts to decrease airway tone. In contrast to the parasympathetic nervous system, sympathetic innervation of airway smooth muscle in human subjects is either sparse or absent.[17] Circulating catecholamines activate beta-adrenergic receptors in airway smooth muscle and provide the primary sympathetic efferent input to human airways. Because airways of normal human subjects do not become hyperresponsive after beta-adrenergic blockade,[18] it is unlikely that impaired catecholamine secretion contributes significantly to the pathogenesis of asthma.

The alpha-adrenergic system is thought to play a relatively minor role in determining the state of airway responsiveness. Although alpha-adrenergic receptors are present in human airways,[19] the protective effects of alpha-adrenergic antagonists have been disappointing and can be attributed to other properties, such as antihistamine activity.

In addition to cholinergic and adrenergic input, a third neural system, the nonadrenergic, noncholinergic (NANC) system, provides efferent nerves to the airways. Both constricting and dilating pathways have been identified.[20] Nitric oxide serves as the inhibitory NANC neurotransmitter in human airways.[21] Potentially, a relative increase in constricting influences or a decrease in dilating influences in the NANC system could contribute to asthma. However, asthmatic subjects demonstrated no deficit in NANC inhibitory pathways,[22] and inhibition of NANC excitatory neurotransmission did not improve airway hyperresponsiveness.[23] Thus, current evidence does not support imbalance of the NANC system as a major mechanism of asthma.

AIRWAY INFLAMMATION

Airway inflammation appears to serve primarily as a modulating influence in asthma. Inflammation is certainly present in some but not all asthmatic subjects.[24] The process of inflammation involves the occurrence of airway wall edema and infiltration of the mucosa by a variety of inflammatory cells, including neutrophils, mast cells, helper T lymphocytes, macrophages, and eosinophils.[25] These cells produce and release mediators of inflammation, such as histamine, leukotrienes, platelet-activating factor, prostaglandins, thromboxanes, cytokines, serotonin, and nitric oxide.[25] Mediators can modulate airway responsiveness by stimulating airway smooth muscle contraction,[26] directing migration of inflammatory cells,[27] modifying neural control of the airways,[28] increasing mucosal permeability,[29] or disrupting airway epithelium.[30] In addition, airway inflammation can reduce airway diameter. Airway hyperresponsiveness is correlated with increased baseline airway tone.[31] The overall importance of inflammation in asthma has been debated. Although inflammation appears to modulate the course of asthma, other factors certainly contribute to the pathogenesis.

AIRWAY EPITHELIUM

The epithelium provides a barrier to protect the subepithelial layers against stimuli that could provoke bronchospasm. Airways of asthmatic subjects demonstrate areas of epithelial destruction,[32] and the clinical significance of this finding has been demonstrated.[33]

The epithelium not only serves as a barrier but also plays an active role in the maintenance of airway tone. The epithelium produces constricting and dilating factors.[34,35] An alteration in the balance between these factors could alter airway responsiveness. The relative importance of alterations in epithelial function in the pathogenesis of asthma is unknown.

Diagnosis

MEDICAL HISTORY

The classic symptoms of asthma include wheezing, cough, dyspnea, and chest tightness. A patient's medical history also should include information about the pattern and severity of the symptoms, precipitating and aggravating factors, and the duration and course of these symptoms.

PHYSICAL EXAMINATION

Physical examination is directed to the respiratory tract. Auscultation of the chest may reveal wheezing and a prolonged phase of expiration.

LABORATORY STUDIES

Laboratory studies that aid in the diagnosis of asthma depend on findings from the medical history and physical examination. In general, pulmonary function tests are useful to document the severity and establish the reversibility of obstruction (Box 52-1). In the absence of additional findings, other tests are not as useful in establishing the diagnosis of asthma. Bronchoprovocation tests (with agents such as methacholine or histamine) are used when the history and physical examination strongly suggest the presence of asthma but spirometry does not show airway obstruction.

BOX 52-1 Pulmonary Function Tests in Patients with Asthma

Forced vital capacity (FVC)
- The volume of gas exhaled after maximal inspiration
- May be reduced in asthma

Forced expiratory volume in 1 second (FEV_1)
- The volume exhaled in the first second after maximal inspiration
- May be reduced in asthma

FEV_1/FVC $<$ 0.75 in asthma

Interaction with Pregnancy

EFFECTS OF PREGNANCY ON ASTHMA

The overall course of asthma has been reported to improve, worsen, or remain the same during pregnancy.[36,37] Some of the variability in these reports may reflect differences in baseline asthma severity, because patients with more severe asthma seem more likely to experience deterioration during pregnancy.[37] Another reason for the variation in these studies is the difference in methods of assessing the severity of asthma. Most studies have used either clinical symptoms or requirements for pharmacologic therapy as indicators of the course of the disease. These measures do not correlate with objective measures of airway obstruction.[38] Juniper et al.[39] measured methacholine sensitivity before, during, and after pregnancy. Measurements of sensitivity to methacholine made during the second and third trimesters were lower than preconception or postpartum measurements (Figure 52-2). Although these findings suggest a reduction in airway hyperresponsiveness during pregnancy, the limited study population (16 subjects) makes extrapolation of the data to the general population unclear. Exacerbations of asthma during labor and delivery occur in as many as 20% of subjects,[37] and occur more frequently after cesarean delivery than after vaginal delivery (41% and 4%, respectively).[40]

A number of mechanisms may be responsible for the changes in the clinical course of asthma during pregnancy (Box 52-2). An increase in the progesterone level is thought to be one mechanism that improves asthma during pregnancy. Progesterone relaxes uterine and gastrointestinal smooth muscle and may or may not have similar effects on airway smooth muscle. However, Juniper et al.[39] did not demonstrate a strong association between methacholine responsiveness and progesterone levels during pregnancy, suggesting that progesterone does not play a central role in attenuating airway hyperresponsiveness. In contrast, progesterone may actually worsen asthma by enhancing inflammation.[41] Thus, effects of pregnancy on asthma appear to involve a number of factors other than direct effects of hormones on airway smooth muscle.

EFFECTS OF ASTHMA ON THE PARTURIENT AND FETUS

Many investigators have questioned whether maternal asthma adversely affects perinatal outcome. Differences in study design (e.g., retrospective or prospective) and differences in severity and treatment of asthma may account for different study results. Some studies have reported an

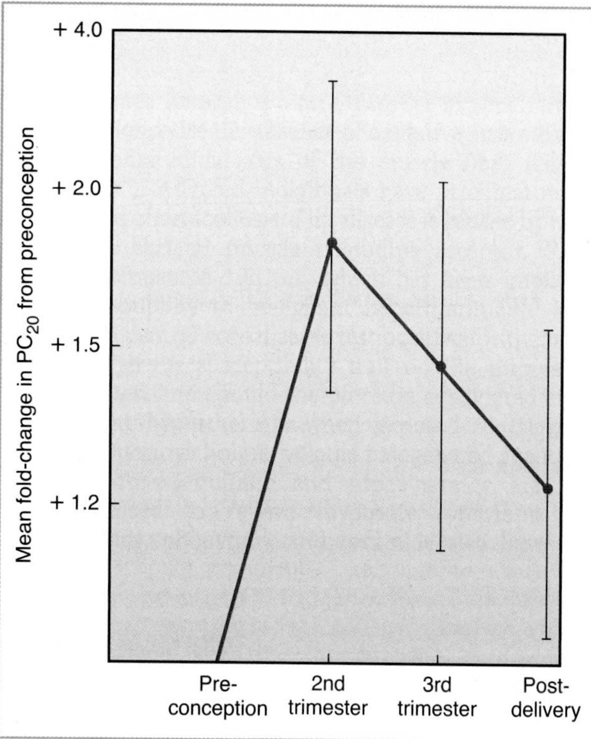

FIGURE 52-2 Airway responsiveness before, during, and after pregnancy expressed as fold change in PC_{20}—dose of methacholine needed to reduce FEV_1 (forced expiratory volume in 1 second) by 20%—compared with values before conception (n = 16; *P* =.033 for the effect of pregnancy on airway responsiveness). (From Juniper EF, Daniel EE, Roberts RS, et al. Improvement in airway responsiveness and asthma severity during pregnancy. Am Rev Respir Dis 1989; 140:924-31.)

increased incidence of preeclampsia,[42,43] cesarean delivery,[44-46] low-birth-weight (LBW) infants,[47] preterm labor,[45,48] antepartum and postpartum hemorrhage,[49] and perinatal mortality.[50] Diabetes mellitus appears to be more common among asthmatic patients treated with corticosteroids.[51] A number of studies have shown an association between severe or poorly controlled asthma and the probability of an adverse outcome.[40,52,53] No controlled studies have documented better perinatal outcome with aggressive asthma treatment. Potential mechanisms of increased perinatal morbidity and mortality in patients with uncontrolled asthma include hypoxemia and hypocapnia, inflammation, and altered placental function from asthma-associated mediator release.[54] Siddiqui et al.[55] have documented an association between preeclampsia and airway hyperresponsiveness and have proposed that the mechanism involves an interaction between mast cells and smooth muscle. A large prospective study is needed to confirm this association.

BOX 52-2 Factors that May Improve or Worsen Asthma during Pregnancy

Factors that May Improve Asthma

- Progesterone-induced relaxation of airway smooth muscle
- Increased production of bronchodilating prostaglandins
- Higher circulating cortisol level

Factors that May Worsen Asthma

- Decreased sensitivity to beta-adrenergic agonists
- Increased production of bronchoconstricting prostaglandins
- Reduced sensitivity to circulating cortisol because of binding of steroid hormones (e.g., progesterone) to cortisol receptors

Medical Management

Pharmacologic therapy of asthma during pregnancy is directed toward avoiding acute exacerbations and episodes of status asthmaticus. Ideally, management should begin before conception. Although general principles typically dictate that unnecessary medication should be avoided during pregnancy, studies investigating the effects of asthma on perinatal outcome suggest that the risks of uncontrolled asthma are significantly higher than medication-associated risks.[56] Medications that are currently used to treat asthma fall into two general categories, bronchodilators and anti-inflammatory agents. These agents generally are safe for the fetus. The prophylactic use of antibiotics is unnecessary.

BRONCHODILATORS

Beta-adrenergic agonists exert beneficial effects in asthmatic patients by activation of $beta_2$-adrenergic receptors, which mediate a number of processes (Box 52-3). Short-acting beta-adrenergic agonists represent the most effective therapy for acute exacerbations of asthma.[57,58] Daily use of long-acting beta-adrenergic agonists is controversial. Long-acting beta-adrenergic agonist therapy is associated with a significant increase in the risk of death,[59] but controlled studies have not confirmed a cause-and-effect relationship.[60] Although regular use of beta-adrenergic agonists in asthma may be beneficial in conjunction with other forms of therapy, these agents do not appear to provide optimal control when used alone. Conversely, no compelling evidence requires that beta-adrenergic agonists be discontinued after conception or that their use be reserved for treatment of an acute exacerbation.

These agents may be administered as aerosols, orally, or parenterally. The aerosol route is generally preferred during pregnancy because high concentrations of the medication can be delivered directly to the site of activity in the airways, with relatively less drug delivered to the uteroplacental circulation.

The limited number of human studies investigating the fetal safety of long-term administration of a beta-adrenergic agonist have not shown significant adverse neonatal

BOX 52-3 Mechanisms of Beneficial Effects of Beta-Adrenergic Agonists in Asthma

- Direct airway smooth muscle relaxation
- Enhanced mucociliary transport
- Decreased airway edema
- Inhibition of cholinergic neurotransmission

outcomes.[61,62] In addition, the long history of use of these agents without reports of teratogenicity suggests that their use should not be restricted because of fetal concerns. Optimal control of maternal symptoms of asthma appears to be more important for the fetus than potential detrimental effects of beta-adrenergic agonists.

On the basis of the potential risks of long-term single-agent therapy with a beta-adrenergic agonist, a novel and paradoxical approach to the treatment of asthma may involve long-term administration of a beta-adrenergic antagonist.[63] This approach is analogous to the paradigm based in the cardiovascular system, in which long-term administration of a beta-adrenergic antagonist is beneficial in patients with congestive heart failure. Studies in asthmatic patients are ongoing.

Methylxanthines (e.g., theophylline, aminophylline) were used for many years in the long-term treatment of asthma. Although their mechanism of action is controversial, relaxation of airway smooth muscle is the most prominent effect. The ability of the agents to inhibit intracellular phosphodiesterase and increase concentrations of cyclic adenosine monophosphate (cAMP) is not the mechanism of bronchodilation, because these effects do not occur at clinically relevant concentrations *in vivo*.[64] Furthermore, in the patient taking anti-inflammatory agents and beta-adrenergic agonists, methylxanthines add little to optimal asthmatic control.[65] Although their use is now limited to patients whose asthma responds poorly to other forms of therapy, methylxanthines do not appear to cause significant adverse fetal outcomes.[62] Serum concentrations of theophylline should be monitored carefully, especially in the third trimester, when theophylline clearance decreases.[66]

Bronchodilation with **anticholinergic agents** occurs through the blockade of muscarinic receptors on airway smooth muscle. Overall, anticholinergic agents alone are not as effective as beta-adrenergic agonists, but some patients show better response to anticholinergic agents.[67] The effects of adding anticholinergic agents to beta-adrenergic agonists for acute[68] and chronic[69] asthma were evaluated in meta-analyses of randomized trials. Anticholinergic agents improved lung function in acute asthma[68] but had little benefit in chronic asthma.[69] The **quaternary anticholinergic agent ipratropium bromide** can be delivered as an aerosol, allowing higher concentrations in the lung with reduced systemic absorption and potential effects on the fetus. Human data on the safety of anticholinergic agents and on potential teratogenicity are lacking, but ipratropium bromide is not associated with teratogenicity in animal studies.[70]

Magnesium sulfate relaxes airway smooth muscle, most likely via its antagonism of calcium entry into airway smooth muscle cells.[71] Its use is limited primarily to acute bronchospasm.[72]

ANTI-INFLAMMATORY AGENTS

Proposed mechanisms of action for corticosteroids are (1) decreases in cellular infiltration and mediator release, (2) reductions in airway permeability, and (3) up-regulation of the beta-adrenergic system.[73] Unlike bronchodilators, corticosteroids not only reduce airway sensitivity to a constrictor stimulus[74] but also decrease the maximal extent of airway narrowing, a feature that may predict severity of an acute asthmatic episode.[75]

The use of **inhaled corticosteroids** has gained popularity. This route of administration is effective and may limit fetal side effects. Effects of systemic and inhaled corticosteroids on the fetus are controversial. Neither systemic nor inhaled corticosteroids have been proven to increase the risk of congenital malformations in humans. Although some older studies observed an increased incidence of preterm and LBW infants in corticosteroid-dependent mothers,[52,76] these studies did not distinguish between severe, poorly controlled disease and the effects of the pharmacologic agent. When these factors were controlled, inhaled corticosteroid use during pregnancy was not associated with increased perinatal risk.[77] Furthermore, a meta-analysis did not show an association between corticosteroid use and any adverse perinatal outcome.[78]

Corticosteroids may increase perinatal morbidity by exacerbating maternal glucose intolerance, especially in women who also receive treatment with a beta-adrenergic agonist.[79] Thus, careful monitoring of maternal glucose concentration is indicated in asthmatic women who require treatment with a corticosteroid during pregnancy. However, because of the efficacy of corticosteroids in controlling severe asthma during pregnancy, these agents should not be withheld from the medical regimen.

Some authorities have recommended that corticosteroid-dependent asthmatic women receive large doses of parenteral corticosteroids during labor to prevent complications related to adrenal suppression.[56,80,81] The scientific basis for this recommendation is questionable. Although physiologic glucocorticoid replacement reduced hemodynamic instability and mortality in adrenalectomized primates that underwent surgery, supraphysiologic doses provided no additional benefit.[82] Furthermore, inhaled corticosteroids in moderate doses do not produce adrenocortical suppression.[83] There is little information about the benefit of corticosteroid replacement therapy during labor. The potential for adrenal insufficiency in infants of asthmatic mothers taking inhaled or oral corticosteroids appears to be very low,[81] most likely due to the widespread use of either prednisone or prednisolone. In the mother, prednisone is converted rapidly to prednisolone, which crosses the placental barrier to a very limited extent.

Cromolyn sodium and **nedocromil sodium** belong to a class of drugs that are thought to reduce inflammation and mediator release primarily by stabilizing mast cells and perhaps other inflammatory cells. Nedocromil also inhibits cellular chloride ion flux, a feature that may explain its ability to affect a range of airway cells, including nerve cells.[84]

Cromolyn and nedocromil are administered as aerosols. Limited studies suggest that cromolyn is safe during pregnancy,[85] and clinical experience is greater with cromolyn than with nedocromil. Thus, use of cromolyn is preferred.

On the basis of the observation that leukotrienes are released into the airways by immune cells and contribute to the inflammatory process, other forms of anti-inflammatory therapy are **leukotriene receptor antagonists** and **leukotriene synthesis inhibitors**. Safety data for the use of these agents in pregnancy are scarce. Bracken et al.[47] did not observe adverse neonatal outcomes in nine women exposed to these agents. A later prospective study of 96 women showed that use of leukotriene receptor antagonists was not associated with a specific pattern of congenital abnormalities, but the investigators cautioned that extrapolation of the data to a large population would require additional studies because of the limited sample size of the study.[85]

Obstetric Management

The following aspects of obstetric management of the asthmatic parturient may differ from that of the nonasthmatic patient: (1) induction of labor, (2) management of postpartum hemorrhage, and (3) treatment of hypertension.

For induction of labor, prostaglandins should be administered cautiously in women with asthma. Prostaglandin $F_{2\alpha}$ constricts airways *in vivo*[86] and *in vitro*.[87] Airways of asthmatic subjects demonstrate greater sensitivity to prostaglandin $F_{2\alpha}$, and its use to induce labor is associated with bronchospasm.[88] Prostaglandin E_2 can have either dilating or constricting effects on the airways, perhaps because of its ability to activate a variety of different types of prostaglandin receptors.[89] Because of the known risk of bronchospasm after exposure to prostaglandin $F_{2\alpha}$ and the possible risk after exposure to prostaglandin E_2, alternative methods of induction of labor are preferred in asthmatic women.

Likewise, asthma represents a relative contraindication to the administration of 15-methyl prostaglandin $F_{2\alpha}$ (carboprost, Hemabate) for the treatment of postpartum hemorrhage. The use of ergot alkaloids to treat postpartum hemorrhage in asthmatic women has also been questioned. Although controlled studies have not been performed, ergot alkaloids have been associated with episodes of acute bronchospasm,[90,91] on the basis of either their tryptaminergic actions or their ability to activate alpha$_1$-adrenergic receptors on airway smooth muscle cells. Oxytocin, which does not significantly affect airway tone, is the preferred ecbolic agent in asthmatic patients.

Beta-adrenergic receptor antagonists are used to treat hypertension in some pregnant women. In asthmatic women, these agents may provoke bronchospasm when used acutely.[92] Other antihypertensive agents, such as hydralazine and sodium nitroprusside, do not seem to enhance airway responsiveness.

Anesthetic Management

PREOPERATIVE ASSESSMENT

During the preoperative evaluation, the anesthesia provider should assess the severity of the disease and whether an acute asthmatic episode is present. The medical history should include information about symptoms of wheezing, dyspnea, and cough. Further information should be sought about the frequency and severity of symptoms, the course of these symptoms during pregnancy, and the date of the most recent exacerbation. Patients who have frequent, severe attacks are at increased risk for morbidity in the peripartum period.

Physical examination should focus on the pulmonary system. Chest auscultation may demonstrate wheezing with or without a prolonged expiratory phase. However, wheezing may not be audible if air movement is markedly reduced. Additional signs of an acute exacerbation of asthma include tachypnea, an exaggerated (greater than 20 mm Hg) pulsus paradoxus, and the use of accessory respiratory muscles.

In a pregnant woman with stable asthma, laboratory tests add little to anesthetic management. However, if an acute exacerbation is suspected, chest radiographic examination, arterial blood gas measurements, and pulmonary function tests may assist with diagnosis and therapy. **Chest radiographic examination** helps diagnose precipitating or complicating conditions such as pneumonia, pneumothorax, and heart failure. During an episode of acute asthma, **arterial blood gas measurements** often show hypoxemia and respiratory alkalosis. After a prolonged, severe episode, arterial carbon dioxide tension increases as a result of fatigue. **Spirometry** measures the volume of gas exhaled over time (see Box 52-1). The most convenient indirect measurement for assessing airway obstruction during labor is the **peak expiratory flow rate,** which can be measured at the bedside with a Wright peak-flow meter.[93]

MANAGEMENT DURING LABOR AND VAGINAL DELIVERY

The goals of analgesia for labor and delivery in asthmatic women include (1) provision of pain relief, (2) reduction in the stimulus to hyperpnea, and (3) prevention or relief of maternal stress. The goal of adequate pain relief does not differ for asthmatic women. It is important to prevent hyperpnea and stress in women who describe asthmatic episodes triggered by exercise or stress. These goals should be accomplished with minimal sedation, minimal paralysis of the muscles of respiration, and minimal depression of the fetus. Possible analgesic regimens include systemic opioids, paracervical block, pudendal nerve block, lumbar sympathetic block, and epidural or spinal analgesia using local anesthetic agents, opioids, or both.

Systemic opioids may provide reasonable pain relief and reduce the stimulus to hyperpnea, especially during the early part of the first stage of labor. In theory, opioids reduce the risk of bronchospasm in asthmatic subjects. Opiate receptors are thought to be present in the respiratory tract[94] and to inhibit release of excitatory neuropeptides. The clinical relevance of these findings is unknown, because moderate doses of inhaled morphine do not significantly alter airway tone.[95] Conversely, high doses of opioids may increase the risk of bronchospasm by releasing histamine. The risk of using moderate doses of morphine does not seem excessive, because airway tone does not change in subjects with moderate to severe asthma after inhalation of morphine.[95] High doses of opioids are not desirable in subjects with active wheezing because of the risks of maternal and neonatal respiratory depression (see Chapter 22).

Paracervical block and **pudendal nerve block** performed by an obstetrician are acceptable choices for analgesia during the first and second stages of labor, respectively. These techniques provide analgesia without sedation or paralysis of the respiratory muscles. The problems with these techniques in asthmatic women are similar to those in nonasthmatic parturients (see Chapter 24).

Lumbar sympathetic block also provides pain relief without sedation or motor block during the first stage of labor. This technique has the same limitations as for women without asthma (see Chapter 24).

Intrathecal and **epidural opioid** techniques are useful during the first stage of labor and do not produce motor block (see Chapter 23). The advantage of the absence of motor block should be weighed against the risk of respiratory depression in asthmatic subjects.

Advantages of the use of local anesthetic agents for **lumbar epidural analgesia** in asthmatic patients include continuous pain relief and a reduction in the stimulus to hyperventilation. These goals typically are achieved without maternal sedation or neonatal depression. Unlike other analgesic techniques, continuous lumbar epidural analgesia adds a margin of safety by providing the opportunity to extend the sensory block for cesarean delivery. The possibility of extension allows the anesthesia provider to avoid some of the risks of general endotracheal anesthesia. The most significant disadvantage of epidural local anesthetics in an asthmatic subject is the risk of a high thoracic motor block and respiratory insufficiency. Use of an appropriate epidural catheter test dose and maintenance of a sensory level at the tenth thoracic dermatome minimize this risk. In addition, the use of a dilute concentration of local anesthetic combined with a modest dose of an opioid produces satisfactory analgesia with less motor block than local anesthetic alone.[96]

MANAGEMENT DURING CESAREAN DELIVERY

The choice between neuraxial anesthesia and general anesthesia for cesarean delivery depends on obstetric considerations and the respiratory status of the parturient. In general, avoidance of airway instrumentation is desirable, because endotracheal intubation markedly increases airway tone in asthmatic subjects.[97]

The most significant advantage of neuraxial anesthesia in the asthmatic patient is that this technique obviates the necessity of endotracheal intubation. Neuraxial anesthesia is associated with a lower incidence of bronchospasm than general anesthesia in asthmatic subjects.[98] Stable asthmatic patients can undergo either spinal anesthesia or epidural anesthesia. In unstable asthmatic patients who require the use of accessory muscles of respiration, neuraxial anesthesia may be hazardous because of impaired ventilatory capacity in the presence of a high thoracic motor block.

The adrenal medulla receives innervation from preganglionic sympathetic fibers arising from the sixth thoracic to the second lumbar spinal segment.[99] Some authors have postulated that neuraxial anesthesia and the ensuing sympathectomy could precipitate or potentiate bronchospasm during cesarean delivery in asthmatic subjects by reducing adrenal output of epinephrine.[100] This possibility seems remote. First, although epinephrine infusion can reduce airway reactivity in asthmatic subjects,[101] epinephrine concentrations do not decrease during nonobstetric surgery performed with neuraxial anesthesia that achieves high thoracic sensory levels.[102,103] Second, the idea that neuraxial anesthesia may prevent increases in circulating epinephrine that are required to compensate for stress-induced bronchospasm does not appear to be valid. Bronchoconstriction does not stimulate epinephrine secretion in human asthmatic subjects.[104] Thus neuraxial anesthesia is appropriate for cesarean delivery in stable asthmatic subjects.

General anesthesia for asthmatic women undergoing cesarean delivery requires a balance between the competing considerations of aspiration and intraoperative bronchospasm. Although airway instrumentation provides a great stimulus for bronchospasm, the high risk of aspiration mandates endotracheal intubation during administration of general anesthesia in parturients.

Most commonly, options for endotracheal intubation include awake intubation and rapid-sequence induction, although mask induction of general anesthesia with sevoflurane has been described in a parturient with status asthmaticus.[105] Indications for awake intubation in asthmatic subjects are similar to those for nonasthmatic patients, and pretreatment with a local anesthetic and a beta-adrenergic agonist can attenuate reflex-induced bronchoconstriction following awake intubation.[97] The benefits of topical local anesthetics and airway nerve blocks for awake intubation should be weighed against a possible increase in the risk of aspiration from the loss of protective airway reflexes. Rapid-sequence induction for cesarean delivery in asthmatic patients is most often accomplished using either **propofol** or **ketamine**. A sympathomimetic agent, ketamine has long been considered the intravenous induction agent of choice for asthmatic subjects. Ketamine relaxes airway smooth muscle and inhibits neural reflexes.[106] Propofol provides better protection than thiopental against bronchospasm associated with endotracheal intubation in asthmatic patients,[107] but propofol has not been compared directly with ketamine in human subjects. Beneficial airway effects of propofol, like those of ketamine, also appear to occur via inhibition of airway reflexes.[106] Intravenous **lidocaine,** which also inhibits airway reflexes, attenuates irritant-induced bronchoconstriction,[108] including endotracheal intubation, and produces an additional protective effect above that of beta-adrenergic agonist pretreatment alone.[109]

In patients *without* asthma, maintenance of general anesthesia typically includes administration of a low concentration of a volatile halogenated anesthetic agent, with or without nitrous oxide, before delivery of the infant. After delivery, maintenance of anesthesia typically consists of nitrous oxide and an intravenous opioid, with or without a low concentration of a volatile halogenated agent. In *asthmatic* parturients, the **volatile halogenated anesthetic agents** are considered the agents of choice for the maintenance of anesthesia. These agents attenuate airway responsiveness through direct effects on airway smooth muscle,[110-112] inhibition of airway reflexes,[113] and effects on the epithelium.[114]

A high concentration of a volatile halogenated anesthetic agent has salutary effects on the airways but also increases the risk of hemorrhage during cesarean delivery by causing dose-dependent uterine relaxation.[115] Alternatively, nitrous oxide, an intravenous opioid, and a low concentration of a volatile halogenated agent may be given. Although halothane and isoflurane are approximately equipotent bronchodilators at high concentrations, halothane produces greater bronchodilation at lower concentrations[116] and therefore may be preferable for anesthesia for cesarean delivery. Sevoflurane acts as a bronchodilator in large and small airways[117] and reverses airway constriction associated with endotracheal intubation.[118] Effects of desflurane are controversial. Desflurane protects against a direct stimulus to the airways[119] but may be less effective against reflex stimuli, such as endotracheal intubation.[120]

A bronchodilator can be added if bronchospasm occurs. The potential disadvantage of this technique is that the most effective bronchodilators (i.e., the beta-adrenergic agonists) also relax uterine smooth muscle. The administration of a beta-adrenergic agonist by aerosol delivers a relatively greater dose of drug to the airways and minimizes uterine relaxation.

Emergence from general anesthesia, as with induction, requires a balance between reducing the risk of aspiration and lowering the risk of bronchospasm. Extubation of the trachea when the patient is awake minimizes the risk of aspiration, but the endotracheal tube may stimulate reflexes and precipitate bronchospasm as the depth of anesthesia is reduced. If bronchospasm occurs during emergence, bronchodilators can be administered. For refractory bronchospasm, continued mechanical ventilation in an intensive care unit may be required.

CIGARETTE SMOKING

Epidemiology

Cigarette smoking is a significant, preventable cause of maternal morbidity and prenatal mortality.[121] Although the prevalence of smoking among pregnant women has declined since 1965, approximately 16.5% of pregnant women in the United States smoke cigarettes.[122] Approximately 40% of women who smoke quit smoking during pregnancy.[123]

Pathophysiology

Cigarette smoke contains a large number of separate components that have a variety of biologic effects. Nonrespiratory effects of cigarette smoking are described in Chapter 53.

The primary respiratory effects of cigarette smoking include alterations in small airway function, increased mucus secretion, and impairment of ciliary transport.[124] The precise mechanisms for these effects are unknown. Smoking also is associated with an increase in nonspecific airway reactivity,[125] possibly through epithelial damage or altered airway geometry due to increased mucus secretion. These changes lead to a marked increase in the incidence of postoperative pulmonary complications.[124]

Interaction with Pregnancy

Few studies have documented the respiratory effects of cigarette smoking during pregnancy. In one study, reductions in forced expiratory flow rates suggested that pregnant women who smoke cigarettes have greater small airway resistance than those who do not smoke.[126] These and other abnormalities were similar to the changes in airway function observed in nonpregnant smokers. Although further studies are warranted, other respiratory effects of cigarette smoking in pregnant women are likely to be similar to those effects in nonpregnant women.

Cigarette smoking adversely affects pregnancy in a number of ways. Studies have shown associations between smoking and fetal growth restriction, preterm birth, and perinatal mortality.[127] Most of these studies were observational and did not include a control group. Further details regarding adverse maternal and fetal effects are described in Chapter 53.

Medical Management

Cessation of smoking is the preferred form of medical management. Smoking cessation programs are effective in pregnant women.[128] Nonpharmacologic methods are preferred to pharmacologic methods (e.g., nicotine patches) because of insufficient safety information for the latter.[123] Das et al.[129] demonstrated that smoking cessation before or early in pregnancy results in prompt improvement in maternal airway function. Smoking cessation reduces perioperative complications in the setting of nonobstetric surgery,[130] but no controlled studies have evaluated effects of smoking cessation on peripartum outcome.

Anesthetic Management

Endotracheal intubation is associated with bronchospasm in smokers.[131] For vaginal delivery, any of the analgesic techniques described earlier for asthmatic parturients are acceptable. For cesarean delivery, neuraxial anesthesia achieves the goal of avoiding airway instrumentation and is therefore preferable to general anesthesia, although no controlled studies have documented differences in peripartum morbidity. If general anesthesia is required, the methods for reducing the risk of intraoperative bronchospasm described previously may be considered. During induction of general anesthesia in smokers, the formulation of propofol containing sulfite results in greater respiratory resistance after endotracheal intubation than the formulation containing ethylenediaminetetraacetic acid (EDTA).[132] The clinical significance of this finding is unknown. One study noted that respiratory resistance did not decrease after endotracheal intubation in smokers anesthetized with desflurane,[120] suggesting that other volatile halogenated anesthetic agents might be preferable.

CYSTIC FIBROSIS

Epidemiology

Cystic fibrosis, a lethal genetic disorder that is transmitted as an autosomal recessive trait, affects approximately 1 in 3200 white newborns in the United States.[133] Because of improvements in diagnosis and therapy, a growing number of women with cystic fibrosis survive to reproductive age. The number of pregnancies reported to a national cystic fibrosis registry increased from fewer than 100 in the 1980s[134] to approximately 140 at present.[135]

Pathophysiology

Clinical features of cystic fibrosis result from abnormalities of epithelial tissues, especially in the respiratory, digestive, and reproductive tracts. The underlying mechanism is a defect in cAMP-mediated activation of the chloride (Cl^-) conductance in the epithelium.[136,137] Normal epithelial cells secrete Cl^- in response to an increase in intracellular cAMP. In cystic fibrosis, a genetic mutation makes epithelial cells unable to alter Cl^- permeability in response to changes in cAMP. The gene responsible for cystic fibrosis is located on chromosome 7 and encodes a protein known as the *cystic fibrosis transmembrane regulator* (CFTR).[138,139] The CFTR acts as a Cl^- channel but also has a number of other actions.[140] Cystic fibrosis is characterized by obstruction of exocrine glands with mucus, but the precise molecular mechanism is not well understood. In sweat glands, however, patients with cystic fibrosis show abnormalities that can be readily explained by impairment of the CFTR, which limits reabsorption of Cl^- and therefore of salt. In the airways, two opposing hypotheses, one in which the airway epithelium behaves similarly to the sweat duct epithelium and one in which the airway epithelium "behaves in a fashion essentially opposite to that of the sweat duct," have been proposed to explain alterations in fluid and electrolyte composition of airway secretions in patients with cystic fibrosis.[140]

In the lungs, abnormalities of electrolyte transport alter the composition of airway secretions. Inflammation, with infiltration of polymorphonuclear leukocytes, also contributes to changes in airway secretions.[141] Large numbers of disintegrating neutrophils release DNA in quantities sufficient to overwhelm the ability of deoxyribonuclease I (DNAse I), an endogenously released enzyme, to digest extracellular DNA. Undigested DNA increases the viscosity of airway secretions, which causes obstruction of small airways and reduced lung volumes. The ensuing ventilation-perfusion inequalities produce arterial hypoxemia. Some patients have hyperreactive airways. Spontaneous pneumothorax often occurs. Chronic airway obstruction and impaired mucus clearance increase the frequency of pulmonary infection. Most patients become colonized or infected with *Pseudomonas aeruginosa*. Eventually, tissue damage leads to bronchiectasis and pulmonary insufficiency. Chronic hypoxemia and lung destruction may produce pulmonary hypertension and cor pulmonale. Nonrespiratory manifestations of cystic fibrosis include pancreatic exocrine insufficiency, intestinal obstruction, and infertility.

Diagnosis

Clinical criteria for the diagnosis of cystic fibrosis include (1) the presence of chronic obstructive lung disease and colonization with *P. aeruginosa* before age 20 years, (2) exocrine pancreatic insufficiency, and (3) a family history of cystic fibrosis. Laboratory findings include (1) sweat Cl^- concentrations greater than 60 mEq/L, (2) CFTR genotype with two known cystic fibrosis mutations, and (3) detection of CFTR dysfunction by nasal potential difference test.[142] Chest radiographic examination often demonstrates hyperinflation, and arterial blood gas measurements may show hypoxemia. Pulmonary function tests, which can reveal obstructive or restrictive lung patterns, are useful to assess the severity of the disease. With serial measurements, clinicians should look for evidence of an increased residual volume and a reduced FEV_1 (forced expiratory volume in 1 second).[143]

Interaction with Pregnancy

EFFECT OF PREGNANCY ON CYSTIC FIBROSIS

The following factors may contribute to the deterioration of pulmonary function during pregnancy: (1) increased airway responsiveness and obstruction (as can occur in patients with asthma), (2) increased work of breathing, and (3) cardiovascular changes such as congestive heart failure and pulmonary hypertension associated with the increased blood volume of pregnancy.

In spite of potential negative effects of pregnancy on the course of cystic fibrosis, long-term survival does not appear to be affected.[144] However, enthusiasm for these results should be tempered by the knowledge that pregnant women with cystic fibrosis require more intensive medical care than healthy pregnant women.[145,146]

EFFECT OF CYSTIC FIBROSIS ON PREGNANCY

Cystic fibrosis is associated with a higher risk for LBW infants and preterm delivery.[146,147] The mechanisms are thought to include chronic hypoxemia and poor maternal nutrition.

Medical Management

Respiratory management of cystic fibrosis is primarily symptomatic. Patients with large volumes of mucus production undergo mechanical airway clearance. Some patients inhale recombinant human deoxyribonuclease I to reduce viscosity of lung secretions caused by accumulating DNA.[133] Recent studies have reported that 7% hypertonic saline inhalation aids clearance of airway mucus.[133] Bronchodilators may help those patients who manifest a reversible component of airway obstruction. Continuous oxygen therapy may benefit patients with hypoxemia and cor pulmonale.

Long-term antibiotic therapy with inhaled tobramycin reduces both the incidence of recurrent pulmonary infection and the frequency of exacerbations in patients with cystic fibrosis.[148] Long-term administration of oral azithromycin also decreases exacerbations from cystic fibrosis[149] through either its antibiotic or its anti-inflammatory properties. Effects of long-term antibiotic therapy on the fetus are unknown.

Other forms of therapy include gene therapy and lung transplantation. Gene therapy uses recombinant adeno-associated viral vectors to transfer the normal CFTR to airway epithelium of patients with cystic fibrosis.[150] Significant pulmonary deterioration sometimes leads to double lung transplantation,[151] although it is unclear whether transplantation alters survival.[152]

Obstetric Management

Because of the influence of pregravid maternal health on pregnancy outcome, the primary obstetric issue centers on the advisability of pregnancy in patients with cystic fibrosis. Criteria for the termination of pregnancy are not clearly defined. Genetic counseling regarding the risks of cystic fibrosis in the offspring is another important component of obstetric management.

Anesthetic Management

Considerations for anesthetic management focus primarily on the pulmonary system. Because of the high incidence of hypoxemia in patients with cystic fibrosis, continuous monitoring of oxygen saturation and appropriate oxygen therapy are advisable.

The goals of pain relief during labor are to provide adequate analgesia and to prevent maternal hyperventilation while avoiding high thoracic motor block and respiratory depression. High thoracic motor block may impair the parturient's ability to cough and eliminate thick secretions. Hyperventilation increases the work of breathing and may cause decompensation in patients with severe pulmonary dysfunction. For pain relief during labor, parenteral opioid analgesia may worsen pulmonary function by depressing respiratory drive and inhibiting cough. Intrathecal opioids have been used successfully,[153] but patients should be monitored carefully for respiratory depression. An ideal way to deliver a short-acting intrathecal opioid might be through a microcatheter, which would provide a margin of safety by allowing repeated administration of small doses of the opioid.[154] Alternatively, continuous lumbar epidural analgesia, with a sensory nerve block maintained at the level of the tenth thoracic dermatome, can provide excellent pain relief and reduce the stimulus for hyperventilation, with minimal motor block of the thorax. A dilute solution of bupivacaine, with or without an opioid, provides sensory analgesia with minimal motor block and is therefore nearly ideal in this setting.[155,156] In healthy parturients, this technique actually improves respiratory function slightly.[157]

Cesarean delivery necessitates the choice between general anesthesia and neuraxial anesthesia. Among patients with cystic fibrosis, no studies have documented differences in outcome between general anesthesia and neuraxial anesthesia. Neuraxial anesthesia offers the advantage of avoiding endotracheal intubation, which may be associated with bronchospasm or obstruction of the endotracheal tube with secretions. Neuraxial anesthesia also avoids positive-pressure ventilation, which may enlarge a preexisting pneumothorax. The primary consideration for neuraxial anesthesia during cesarean delivery is to avoid a high thoracic motor block, which may impair ventilation and the ability to cough. Effective spinal anesthesia for cesarean delivery slightly decreases vital capacity.[158] Methods for reducing the risk of excessively high motor block include the use of a continuous catheter technique, which allows titration of the local anesthetic agent to achieve the desired sensory level, and the use of the lowest concentration of local anesthetic (with or without an opioid) that provides surgical anesthesia. The use of both epidural anesthesia[159] and combined spinal-epidural anesthesia[160,161] has been reported in parturients with cystic fibrosis.

For general anesthesia, techniques to reduce the risk of bronchospasm, as described for patients with asthma (see earlier), may be warranted. Additional considerations include (1) humidification of gases to prevent inspissation of mucus, (2) frequent suctioning to remove excess secretions, and (3) use of ventilator settings that allow an appropriately long expiratory phase to prevent air trapping and pneumothorax. It may also be prudent to avoid nitrous oxide in the parturient with cystic fibrosis, because of the risk of pneumothorax. Patients with cystic fibrosis should be allowed to awaken fully before extubation of the trachea. Chest physiotherapy may be required in the immediate postoperative period.

RESPIRATORY FAILURE

Epidemiology

The prevalence of respiratory failure during pregnancy is unknown. A significant subset of patients with respiratory failure suffers from **acute respiratory distress syndrome** (ARDS). The prevalence of ARDS in pregnancy has been estimated at approximately 1 in 6000 to 7000 deliveries.[162,163] Mortality from respiratory failure during pregnancy is high.[164]

Pathophysiology

The pathophysiology of respiratory failure depends on the underlying disorder. ARDS results from a group of predisposing conditions, but a common final pathway leads to similar manifestations.[165] Damage to the alveolar and capillary membranes initiates a cascade of events leading to fluid transudation that often is accompanied by pulmonary venoconstriction. Direct injury to the alveolar and capillary membranes can result from pulmonary aspiration of gastric contents and perhaps oxygen toxicity. Indirect toxicity can result from humoral and cellular mechanisms caused by triggers such as sepsis and amniotic fluid embolism. Transudation of fluid leads to atelectasis, airway obstruction, reduced lung compliance, and altered ventilation-perfusion relationships. Both physiologic dead space and shunt fractions are increased.

Diagnosis

A variety of disorders can cause acute respiratory failure during pregnancy (Box 52-4). Specific diagnostic criteria depend on the disorder.

The diagnosis of ARDS requires the exclusion of other disorders. Prominent characteristics of ARDS include arterial hypoxemia, radiographic evidence of pulmonary

BOX 52-4 Etiology of Respiratory Failure during Pregnancy

Adult Respiratory Distress Syndrome (ARDS)

- Infection
  - Bacterial or viral pneumonia
  - Endometritis
  - Pyelonephritis
  - Sepsis
  - Preeclampsia
- Hemorrhage
  - Multiple transfusions
  - Disseminated intravascular coagulation
- Aspiration of gastric contents
- Embolism
- Drugs
  - Salicylates
  - Opioids

Pulmonary Embolism

- Thromboembolism
- Amniotic fluid embolism
- Venous air embolism

Cystic Fibrosis

Pulmonary Edema

- Beta-adrenergic receptor agonists (e.g., ritodrine, terbutaline)
- Cardiogenic

infiltrates, and reduced lung compliance in the setting of a recognized predisposing condition.[166]

Interaction with Pregnancy

Pregnancy is not known to alter the overall course of respiratory failure. However, differences in outcome between pregnant and nonpregnant patients have been observed in subsets of patients with respiratory failure. In a series of patients with **severe acute respiratory syndrome** (SARS), pregnant patients had greater morbidity.[167] Mortality rates are similar in pregnant and nonpregnant subjects.[164]

The most significant effect of respiratory failure on pregnancy is a reduction in oxygen delivery to the fetus. This reduction results most commonly from maternal arterial hypoxemia or maternal hypotension, which often accompanies respiratory failure. Hypotension may result from associated underlying conditions or from elevated mean airway pressures during mechanical ventilation. High rates of prenatal complications with or without preterm delivery have been reported.[162,163]

Medical Management

Therapeutic strategies for managing respiratory failure during pregnancy do not differ qualitatively from those in nonpregnant patients. The primary goals of medical management are to (1) eliminate predisposing conditions, (2) limit fluid transudation, and (3) maintain maternal oxygen delivery. Fluid restriction and diuretics help limit fluid transudation, although this therapy must be used cautiously when the underlying cause of respiratory failure is associated with intravascular fluid depletion. The goals for maintenance of oxygen delivery may differ quantitatively during pregnancy. Oxygen delivery to the fetus worsens significantly when Pa_{O_2} decreases below 70 mm Hg or oxygen saturation (Sa_{O_2}) falls below 95%.[162,167] Standard methods of maintaining oxygen delivery include (1) administration of a higher inspired concentration of oxygen, (2) administration of bronchodilators in the presence of reversible airway obstruction, (3) administration of pharmacologic agents to support the circulation as needed, and (4) mechanical ventilation. A higher inspired oxygen concentration, delivered by face mask, is relatively safe during pregnancy and may obviate the necessity of endotracheal intubation and its risks of aspiration and difficult airway management. Bronchodilator therapy can also be used for respiratory failure as described earlier for asthma. Pharmacologic agents for circulatory support include agents with both alpha- and beta-adrenergic activity.

Indications for endotracheal intubation and mechanical ventilation are similar for pregnant and nonpregnant patients with respiratory failure.[168,169] Maternal and fetal effects of current approaches to mechanical ventilation, including use of low tidal volumes and passive hypercapnia, have not been studied in pregnant patients. Positive end-expiratory pressure may be used if cardiac output is maintained to allow sufficient blood flow to the uterus.

Some pregnant patients with respiratory failure do not show adequate response to conventional methods of treatment. For these patients, treatment options include extracorporeal membrane oxygenation (ECMO),[170] high-frequency oscillatory ventilation,[171] and inhaled **nitric oxide**.[172,173] Nitric oxide relaxes vascular smooth muscle. Rapid inactivation of nitric oxide by binding to hemoglobin in the circulation allows inhaled nitric oxide to produce pulmonary vasodilation without systemic vascular effect. Selective pulmonary vasodilation in well-ventilated areas of the lung presumably would improve oxygen delivery. The safety of these alternative forms of treatment in pregnancy is unknown because reports of their use are anecdotal.

Obstetric Management

Because the beneficial effects of delivery on the course of respiratory failure have not been proved, indications for induction of labor or cesarean delivery in this setting are not well defined. Small observational studies have not clearly shown an association between delivery and improved respiratory status in pregnant women with respiratory failure.[163,174,175] Furthermore, data to support decisions as to mode of delivery are limited. Vaginal delivery is possible during mechanical ventilation[176,177] and may avoid complications of major intra-abdominal surgery in a critically ill woman.

Anesthetic Management

The anesthetic management of patients with respiratory failure requires appropriate medical management. During labor, analgesia for mechanically ventilated patients can be achieved with intravenous opioids, which are often used for sedation during mechanical ventilation. Lumbar epidural analgesia provides pain relief without the neonatal respiratory depression associated with high doses of opioids. Labor epidural analgesia also reduces oxygen consumption,[178] which may be beneficial in hypoxemic patients. The use of labor epidural analgesia in patients with respiratory failure depends on underlying conditions and ongoing therapy. Close attention should be paid to intravascular volume, adequacy of coagulation, and presence or absence of infection.

In mechanically ventilated patients, general endotracheal anesthesia is often the most convenient choice for cesarean delivery. Aside from the issues of medical management (as discussed earlier), the techniques and pharmacologic agents do not differ substantially from those used in patients without respiratory failure.

KEY POINTS

- Patients with asthma, infection, respiratory failure, or cystic fibrosis and patients who smoke cigarettes may have reversible airway obstruction.
- In patients with airway hyperresponsiveness, endotracheal intubation provides one of the most significant stimuli for bronchospasm during the perioperative period.
- Inhaled $beta_2$-adrenergic agonists are the most effective therapy for perioperative bronchospasm.
- Most bronchodilators also produce uterine relaxation. However, their administration by aerosol should minimize their effects on uterine tone.
- Neuraxial anesthesia is often the anesthetic technique of choice in patients with respiratory

disease because it does not require endotracheal intubation.

- Techniques of neuraxial anesthesia should be modified to reduce the likelihood of a high thoracic motor block in patients with significant respiratory disease.

REFERENCES

1. Moorman JE, Rudd RA, Johnson CA, et al. National surveillance for asthma—United States, 1980-2004. MMWR Surveill Summ 2007; 56:1-54.
2. Kwon HL, Belanger K, Bracken MB. Asthma prevalence among pregnant and childbearing-aged women in the United States: Estimates from national health surveys. Ann Epidemiol 2003; 13:317-24.
3. Wenzel SE. Asthma: Defining of the persistent adult phenotypes. Lancet 2006; 368:804-13.
4. Vincenc KS, Black JL, Yan K, et al. Comparison of in vivo and in vitro responses to histamine in human airways. Am Rev Respir Dis 1983; 128:875-9.
5. Armour CL, Lazar NM, Schellenberg RR, et al. A comparison of in vivo and in vitro human airway reactivity to histamine. Am Rev Respir Dis 1984; 129:907-10.
6. Roberts JA, Raeburn D, Rodger IW, Thomson NC. Comparison of in vivo airway responsiveness and in vitro smooth muscle sensitivity to methacholine in man. Thorax 1984; 39:837-43.
7. Roberts JA, Rodger IW, Thomson NC. Airway responsiveness to histamine in man: Effect of atropine on in vivo and in vitro comparison. Thorax 1985; 40:261-7.
8. Goldie RG, Spina D, Henry PJ, et al. In vitro responsiveness of human asthmatic bronchus to carbachol, histamine, β-adrenoceptor agonists and theophylline. Br J Clin Pharmacol 1986; 22:669-76.
9. Downes H, Austin DR, Parks CM, Hirshman CA. Comparison of drug responses in vivo and in vitro in airways of dogs with and without airway hyperresponsiveness. J Pharmacol Exp Ther 1986; 237:214-9.
10. Cerrina J, Le Roy Ladurie MR, Labat C, et al. Comparison of human bronchial muscle responses to histamine in vivo with histamine and isoproterenol agonists in vitro. Am Rev Respir Dis 1986; 134:57-61.
11. Skloot G, Permutt S, Togias A. Airway hyperresponsiveness in asthma: A problem of limited smooth muscle relaxation with inspiration. J Clin Invest 1995; 96:2393-403.
12. Richardson JB. State of the art: Nerve supply to the lungs. Am Rev Respir Dis 1979; 119:785-802.
13. Starke K, Göthert M, Kilbinger H. Modulation of neurotransmitter release by presynaptic autoreceptors. Physiol Rev 1989; 69:864-989.
14. Barnes PJ. Muscarinic autoreceptors in the airways: Their possible role in airway disease. Chest 1989; 96:1220-1.
15. Fryer AD, Jacoby DB. Parainfluenza virus infection damages inhibitory M2 muscarinic receptors on pulmonary parasympathetic nerves in the guinea pig. Br J Pharmacol 1991; 102:267-71.
16. Sorkness R, Clough JJ, Castleman WL, Lemanske RF Jr. Virus-induced airway obstruction and parasympathetic hyperresponsiveness in adult rats. Am J Respir Crit Care Med 1994; 150:28-34.
17. Nadel JA, Barnes PJ. Autonomic regulation of the airways. Annu Rev Med 1984; 35:451-67.
18. Tattersfield AE, Leaver DG, Pride NB. Effects of β-adrenergic blockade and stimulation on normal human airways. J Appl Physiol 1973; 35:613-9.
19. Spina D, Rigby PJ, Paterson JW, Goldie RG. α_1-Adrenoceptor function and autoradiographic distribution in human asthmatic lung. Br J Pharmacol 1989; 97:701-8.
20. Krishnakumar S, Holmes EP, Moore RM, et al. Non-adrenergic non-cholinergic excitatory innervation in the airways: Role of neurokinin-2 receptors. Auton Autacoid Pharmacol 2002; 22:215-24.
21. Belvisi MG, Stretto CD, Yacoub M, Barnes PJ. Nitric oxide is the endogenous neurotransmitter of bronchodilator nerves in humans. Eur J Pharmacol 1992; 210:221-2.
22. Lammers JW, Minette P, McCusker MT, et al. Capsaicin-induced bronchodilation in mild asthmatic subjects: Possible role of nonadrenergic inhibitory system. J Appl Physiol 1989; 67:856-61.
23. Kraan J, Vink-Klooster H, Postma DS. The NK-2 receptor antagonist SR 48968C does not improve adenosine hyperresponsiveness and airway obstruction in allergic asthma. Clin Exp Allergy 2001; 31:274-8.
24. Hogg JC, James AL, Paré PD. Evidence for inflammation in asthma. Am Rev Respir Dis 1991; 143:S39-42.
25. Tattersfield AE, Knox AJ, Britton JR, Hall IP. Asthma. Lancet 2002; 360:1313-22.
26. Veerappan A, Reid AC, Estephan R, et al. Mast cell renin and a local renin-angiotensin system in the airway: Role in bronchoconstriction. Proc Natl Acad Sci U S A 2008; 105:1315-20.
27. Luster AD, Tager AM. T-cell trafficking in asthma: Lipid mediators grease the way. Nat Rev Immunol 2004; 4:711-24.
28. Black JL. Control of human airway smooth muscle. Am Rev Respir Dis 1991; 143:S11-12.
29. Schwartz LB. Cellular inflammation in asthma: Neutral proteases of mast cells. Am Rev Respir Dis 1992; 145:S18-21.
30. Nadel JA. Biologic effects of mast cell enzymes. Am Rev Respir Dis 1992; 145:S37-41.
31. Bergner A, Kellner J, Kemp da Silva A, et al. Bronchial hyperreactivity is correlated with increased baseline airway tone. Eur J Med Res 2006; 11:77-84.
32. Hogg JC. Pathology of asthma. J Allergy Clin Immunol 1993; 92:1-5.
33. Knight DA, Holgate ST. The airway epithelium: Structural and functional properties in health and disease. Respirology 2003; 8:432-46.
34. Zietkowski Z, Skiepko R, Tomasiak MM, Bodzenta-Lukaszyk A. Endothelin-1 in exhaled breath condensate of allergic asthma patients with exercise-induced bronchoconstriction. Respir Res 2007; 8:76.
35. Qin XQ, Xiang Y, Liu C, et al. The role of bronchial epithelial cells in airway hyperreponsiveness. Sheng Li Xue Bao 2007; 59:454-64.
36. Kircher S, Schatz M, Long L. Variables affecting asthma course during pregnancy. Ann Allergy Asthma Immunol 2002; 89:463-6.
37. Schatz M, Dombrowski MP, Wise R, et al. Asthma morbidity during pregnancy can be predicted by severity classification. J Allergy Clin Immunol 2003; 112:283-8.
38. Teeter JG, Bleecker ER. Relationship between airway obstruction and respiratory symptoms in adult asthmatics. Chest 1998; 113:272-7.
39. Juniper EF, Daniel EE, Roberts RS, et al. Improvement in airway responsiveness and asthma severity during pregnancy: A prospective study. Am Rev Respir Dis 1989; 140:924-31.
40. Mabie WC, Barton JR, Wasserstrum N, Sibai BM. Clinical observations on asthma in pregnancy. J Matern Fetal Med 1992; 1:45-50.
41. Hellings PW, Vandekerckhove P, Claeys R, et al. Progesterone increases airway eosinophilia and hyper-responsiveness in a murine model of allergic asthma. Clin Exp Allergy 2003; 33:1457-63.
42. Martel MJ, Rey E, Beauchesne MF, et al. Use of inhaled corticosteroids during pregnancy and the risk of pregnancy induced hypertension: Nested case-control study. Br Med J 2005; 330:230.
43. Enriquez R, Griffin MR, Carroll KN, et al. Effect of maternal asthma and asthma control on pregnancy and perinatal outcomes. J Allergy Clin Immunol 2007; 120:625-30.
44. Dombrowski MP, Schatz M, Wise R, et al. Asthma during pregnancy. Obstet Gynecol 2004; 103:5-12.
45. Sorensen TK, Dempsey JC, Xiao R, et al. Maternal asthma and risk of preterm delivery. Ann Epidemiol 2003; 13:267-72.
46. Sheiner E, Mazor M, Levy A, et al. Pregnancy outcome of asthmatic patients: A population-based study. J Matern Fetal Neonatal Med 2005; 18:237-40.
47. Bracken MB, Triche EW, Belanger K, et al. Asthma symptoms, severity, and drug therapy: A prospective study of effects on 2205 pregnancies. Obstet Gynecol 2003; 102:739-52.
48. Getahun D, Ananth CV, Oyelese Y, et al. Acute and chronic respiratory diseases in pregnancy: Associations with spontaneous premature rupture of membranes. J Matern Fetal Neonatal Med 2007; 20:669-75.

49. Tata LJ, Lewis SA, McKeever TM, et al. A comprehensive analysis of adverse obstetric and pediatric complications in women with asthma. Am J Respir Crit Care Med 2007; 175:991-7.
50. Sobande AA, Archibong EI, Akinola SE. Pregnancy outcome in asthmatic patients from high altitudes. Int J Gynaecol Obstet 2002; 77:117-21.
51. Källén B, Otterblad Olausson P. Use of anti-asthmatic drugs during pregnancy. 1. Maternal characteristics, pregnancy and delivery complications. Eur J Clin Pharmacol 2007; 63:363-73.
52. Perlow JH, Montgomery D, Morgan MA, et al. Severity of asthma and perinatal outcome. Am J Obstet Gynecol 1992; 167:963-7.
53. Jana N, Vasishta K, Saha SC, Khunnu B. Effect of bronchial asthma on the course of pregnancy, labour and perinatal outcome. J Obstet Gynaecol 1995; 21:227-32.
54. Murphy VE, Gibson PG, Smith R, Clifton VL. Asthma during pregnancy: Mechanisms and treatment implications. Eur Respir J 2005; 25:731-50.
55. Siddiqui S, Goodman N, McKenna S, et al. Pre-eclampsia is associated with airway hyperresponsiveness. Br J Obstet Gynaecol 2008; 115:520-2.
56. Rey E, Boulet LP. Asthma in pregnancy. Br Med J 2007; 334:582-5.
57. Pauwels RA, Löfdahl CG, Postma DS, et al. Effect of inhaled formoterol and budesonide on exacerbations of asthma. N Engl J Med 1997; 337:1405-11.
58. Najafizadeh K, Sohrab Pour H, Ghadyanee M, et al. A randomised, double-blind, placebo-controlled study to evaluate the role of formoterol in the management of acute asthma. Emerg Med J 2007; 24:317-21.
59. Nelson HS, Weiss ST, Bleecker ER, et al. The Salmeterol Multicenter Asthma Research Trial: A comparison of usual pharmacotherapy for asthma or usual pharmacotherapy plus salmeterol. Chest 2006; 129:15-26.
60. Oppenheimer J, Nelson HS. Safety of long-acting β-agonists in asthma: A review. Curr Opin Pulm Med 2008; 14:64-9.
61. Osur SL. The management of asthma and rhinitis during pregnancy. J Womens Health (Larchmt) 2005; 14:263-76.
62. Gluck JC, Gluck PA. Asthma controller therapy during pregnancy. Am J Obstet Gynecol 2005; 192:369-80.
63. Bond RA, Spina D, Parra S, Page CP. Getting to the heart of asthma: Can "beta blockers" be useful to treat asthma? Pharmacol Ther 2007; 115:360-74.
64. Bukowskyj M, Nakatsu K, Munt PW. Theophylline reassessed. Ann Intern Med 1984; 101:63-73.
65. Lam A, Newhouse MT. Management of asthma and chronic airflow limitation: Are methylxanthines obsolete? Chest 1990; 98:44-52.
66. Carter BL, Driscoll CE, Smith GD. Theophylline clearance during pregnancy. Obstet Gynecol 1986; 68:555-9.
67. Chhabra SK, Pandey KK. Comparison of acute bronchodilator effects of inhaled ipratropium bromide and salbutamol in bronchial asthma. J Asthma 2002; 39:375-81.
68. Lanes SF, Garrett JE, Wentworth CE III, et al. The effect of adding ipratropium bromide to salbutamol in the treatment of acute asthma: A pooled analysis of three trials. Chest 1998; 114:365-72.
69. Westby M, Benson M, Gibson P. Anticholinergic agents for chronic asthma in adults. Cochrane Database Syst Rev 2004; (3):CD003269.
70. Barsky HC. Asthma and pregnancy: A challenge for everyone concerned. Postgrad Med 1991; 89:125-30, 132.
71. Gourgoulianis KI, Chatziparasidis G, Chatziefthimiou A, Molyvdas PA. Magnesium as a relaxing factor of airway smooth muscles. J Aerosol Med 2001; 14:301-7.
72. Rowe BH, Camargo CA Jr. The role of magnesium sulfate in the acute and chronic management of asthma. Curr Opin Pulm Med 2008; 14:70-6.
73. Barnes PJ. Molecular mechanisms and cellular effects of glucocorticosteroids. Immunol Allergy Clin North Am 2005; 25:451-68.
74. Berry M, Morgan A, Shaw DE, et al. Pathological features and inhaled corticosteroid response of eosinophilic and non-eosinophilic asthma. Thorax 2007; 62:1043-9.
75. Bel EH, Timmers MC, Zwinderman AH, et al. The effect of inhaled corticosteroids on the maximal degree of airway narrowing to methacholine in asthmatic subjects. Am Rev Respir Dis 1991; 143:109-13.
76. Fitzsimons R, Greenberger PA, Patterson R. Outcome of pregnancy in women requiring corticosteroids for severe asthma. J Allergy Clin Immunol 1986; 78:349-53.
77. Schatz M, Dombrowski MP, Wise R, et al. The relationship of asthma medication use to perinatal outcomes. J Allergy Clin Immunol 2004; 113:1040-5.
78. Rahimi R, Nikfar S, Abdollahi M. Meta-analysis finds use of inhaled corticosteroids during pregnancy safe: A systematic meta-analysis review. Hum Exp Toxicol 2006; 25:447-52.
79. Bernstein IM, Catalano PM. Ketoacidosis in pregnancy associated with parenteral administration of terbutaline and betamethasone: A case report. J Reprod Med 1990; 35:818-20.
80. Greenberger PA. Asthma during pregnancy. J Asthma 1990; 27:341-7.
81. Chung KF, Barnes PJ. Treatment of asthma. Br Med J Clin Res Ed 1987; 294:103-5.
82. Udelsman R, Ramp J, Gallucci WT, et al. Adaptation during surgical stress: A reevaluation of the role of glucocorticoids. J Clin Invest 1986; 77:1377-81.
83. Barnes NC. The properties of inhaled corticosteroids: Similarities and differences. Prim Care Respir J 2007; 16:149-54.
84. Alton EW, Norris AA. Chloride transport and the actions of nedocromil sodium and cromolyn sodium in asthma. J Allergy Clin Immunol 1996; 98:S102-5.
85. Bakhireva LN, Jones KL, Schatz M, et al. Safety of leukotriene receptor antagonists in pregnancy. J Allergy Clin Immunol 2007; 119:618-25.
86. Mathé AA, Hedqvist P. Effect of prostaglandins F2 alpha and E2 on airway conductance in healthy subjects and asthmatic patients. Am Rev Respir Dis 1975; 111:313-20.
87. Ishimura M, Kataoka S, Suda M, et al. Effects of KP-496, a novel dual antagonist for leukotriene D4 and thromboxane A2 receptors, on contractions induced by various agonists in the guinea pig trachea. Allergol Int 2006; 55:403-10.
88. Kreisman H, Van de Weil W, Mitchell CA. Respiratory function during prostaglandin-induced labor. Am Rev Respir Dis 1975; 111:564-6.
89. Tilley SL, Hartney JM, Erikson CJ, et al. Receptors and pathways mediating the effects of prostaglandin E2 on airway tone. Am J Physiol Lung Cell Mol Physiol 2003; 284:L599-606.
90. Sellers WF, Long DR. Bronchospasm following ergometrine. Anaesthesia 1979; 34:909.
91. Crawford JS. Bronchospasm following ergometrine. Anaesthesia 1980; 35:397-8.
92. Leff AR. Endogenous regulation of bronchomotor tone. Am Rev Respir Dis 1988; 137:1198-216.
93. Wright BM, McKerrow CB. Maximum forced expiratory flow rate as a measure of ventilatory capacity: With a description of a new portable instrument for measuring it. Br Med J 1959; 2:1041-7.
94. Belvisi MG, Rogers DF, Barnes PJ. Neurogenic plasma extravasation: Inhibition by morphine in guinea pig airways in vivo. J Appl Physiol 1989; 66:268-72.
95. Otulana B, Okikawa J, Linn L, et al. Safety and pharmacokinetics of inhaled morphine delivered using the AERx system in patients with moderate-to-severe asthma. Int J Pharmacol Ther 2004; 42:456-62.
96. Chestnut DH, Owen CL, Bates JN, et al. Continuous infusion epidural analgesia during labor: A randomized, double-blind comparison of 0.0625% bupivacaine/0.0002% fentanyl versus 0.125% bupivacaine. Anesthesiology 1988; 68:754-9.
97. Groeben H, Schlicht M, Stieglitz S, et al. Both local anesthetics and salbutamol pretreatment affect reflex bronchoconstriction in volunteers with asthma undergoing awake fiberoptic intubation. Anesthesiology 2002; 97:1445-50.
98. Shnider SM, Papper EM. Anesthesia for the asthmatic patient. Anesthesiology 1961; 22:886-92.
99. Bonica JJ. Autonomic innervation of the viscera in relation to nerve block. Anesthesiology 1968; 29:793-813.
100. Mallampati SR. Bronchospasm during spinal anesthesia. Anesth Analg 1981; 60:839-40.

101. Knox AJ, Campos-Gongora H, Wisniewski A, et al. Modification of bronchial reactivity by physiological concentration of plasma epinephrine. J Appl Physiol 1992; 73:1004-7.
102. Pflug AE, Halter JB. Effect of spinal anesthesia on adrenergic tone and the neuroendocrine responses to surgical stress in humans. Anesthesiology 1981; 55:120-6.
103. Shimosato S, Etsten BE. The role of the venous system in cardiocirculatory dynamics during spinal and epidural anesthesia in man. Anesthesiology 1969; 30:619-28.
104. Emerman CL, Cydulka RK. Changes in serum catecholamine levels during acute bronchospasm. Ann Emerg Med 1993; 22:1836-41.
105. Que JC, Lusaya VO. Sevoflurane induction for emergency cesarean section in a parturient in status asthmaticus. Anesthesiology 1999; 90:1475-6.
106. Brown RH, Wagner EM. Mechanisms of bronchoprotection by anesthetic induction agents: Propofol versus ketamine. Anesthesiology 1999; 90:822-8.
107. Pizov R, Brown RH, Weiss YS, et al. Wheezing during induction of general anesthesia in patients with and without asthma: A randomized, blinded trial. Anesthesiology 1995; 82:1111-6.
108. Groeben H, Schwalen A, Irsfeld S, et al. Intravenous lidocaine and bupivacaine dose-dependently attenuate bronchial hyperreactivity in awake volunteers. Anesthesiology 1996; 84:533-9.
109. Groeben H, Silvanus MT, Beste M, Peters J. Combined intravenous lidocaine and inhaled salbutamol protect against bronchial hyperreactivity more effectively than lidocaine or salbutamol alone. Anesthesiology 1998; 89:862-8.
110. Mercier FJ, Naline E, Bardou M, et al. Relaxation of proximal and distal isolated human bronchi by halothane, isoflurane and desflurane. Eur Respir J 2002; 20:286-92.
111. Jones KA, Housmans PR, Warner DO, et al. Halothane alters cytosolic calcium transient in tracheal smooth muscle. Am J Physiol 1993; 265:L80-6.
112. Duracher C, Blanc FX, Gueugniaud PY, et al. The effects of isoflurane on airway smooth muscle crossbridge kinetics in Fisher and Lewis rats. Anesth Analg 2005; 101:136-42.
113. Warner DO, Vettermann J, Brichant JF, Rehder K. Direct and neurally mediated effects of halothane on pulmonary resistance in vivo. Anesthesiology 1990; 72:1057-63.
114. Park KW, Dai HB, Lowenstein E, Sellke FW. Epithelial dependence of the bronchodilatory effect of sevoflurane and desflurane in rat distal bronchi. Anesth Analg 1998; 86:646-51.
115. Gultekin H, Yildiz K, Sezer Z, Dogru K. Comparing the relaxing effects of desflurane and sevoflurane on oxytocin-induced contractions of isolated myometrium in both pregnant and nonpregnant rats. Adv Ther 2006; 23:39-46.
116. Brown RH, Zerhouni EA, Hirshman CA. Comparison of low concentrations of halothane and isoflurane as bronchodilators. Anesthesiology 1993; 78:1097-101.
117. Burburan SM, Xisto DG, Ferreira HC, et al. Lung mechanics and histology during sevoflurane anesthesia in a model of chronic allergic asthma. Anesth Analg 2007; 104:631-7.
118. Rooke GA, Choi JH, Bishop MJ. The effect of isoflurane, halothane, sevoflurane, and thiopental/nitrous oxide on respiratory system resistance after tracheal intubation. Anesthesiology 1997; 86:1294-9.
119. Lele E, Petak F, Fontao F, et al. Protective effects of volatile agents against acetylcholine-induced bronchoconstriction in isolated perfused rat lungs. Acta Anaesthesiol Scand 2006; 50:1145-51.
120. Goff MJ, Arain SR, Ficke DJ, et al. Absence of bronchodilation during desflurane anesthesia: A comparison to sevoflurane and thiopental. Anesthesiology 2000; 93:404-8.
121. Cnattingius S. The epidemiology of smoking during pregnancy: Smoking prevalence, maternal characteristics, and pregnancy outcomes. Nicotine Tob Res 2004; 6:S125-40.
122. 2006 National Survey on Drug Use and Health. Rockville, MD, Substance Abuse and Mental Health Services Administration, Office of Applied Studies, 2006. Available at http://nsduhweb.rti.org/ and http://oas.samhsa.gov/nsduh/2k6nsduh/2k6Results.pdf/
123. American College of Obetetricians and Gynecologists Committees on Healthcare for Underserved Women and Obstetric Practice. Smoking cessation during pregnancy. ACOG Committee Opinion No. 316. Washington, DC, October 2005. (Obstet Gynecol 2005; 106:883-8.)
124. Pearce AC, Jones RM. Smoking and anesthesia: Preoperative abstinence and perioperative morbidity. Anesthesiology 1984; 61:576-84.
125. Gerrard JW, Cockcroft DW, Mink JT, et al. Increased nonspecific bronchial reactivity in cigarette smokers with normal lung function. Am Rev Respir Dis 1980; 122:577-81.
126. Das TK, Moutquin JM, Parent JG. Effect of cigarette smoking on maternal airway function during pregnancy. Am J Obstet Gynecol 1991; 165:675-9.
127. Shea AK, Steiner M. Cigarette smoking during pregnancy. Nicotine Tob Res 2008; 10:267-78.
128. Pollak KI, Oncken CA, Lipkus IM, et al. Nicotine replacement and behavioral therapy for smoking cessation in pregnancy. Am J Prev Med 2007; 33:297-305.
129. Das TK, Moutquin JM, Lindsay C, et al. Effects of smoking cessation on maternal airway function and birth weight. Obstet Gynecol 1998; 92:201-5.
130. Warner DO. Perioperative abstinence from cigarettes: Physiologic and clinical consequences. Anesthesiology 2006; 104:356-67.
131. Kim SE, Bishop MJ. Endotracheal intubation but not laryngeal mask airway insertion, produces reversible bronchoconstriction. Anesthesiology 1999; 90:391-4.
132. Rieschke P, LaFleur BJ, Janicki PK. Effects of EDTA- and sulfite-containing formulations of propofol on respiratory system resistance after tracheal intubation in smokers. Anesthesiology 2003; 98:323-8.
133. Saeed Z, Wojewodka G, Marion D, et al. Novel pharmaceutical approaches for treating patients with cystic fibrosis. Curr Pharm Des 2007; 13:3252-63.
134. Kotloff RM, FitzSimmons SC, Fiel SB. Fertility and pregnancy in patients with cystic fibrosis. Clin Chest Med 1992; 13:623-35.
135. Tonelli MR, Aitken ML. Pregnancy in cystic fibrosis. Curr Opin Pulm Med 2007; 13:537-40.
136. Hwang TC, Lu L, Zeitlin PL, et al. Cl^- channels in CF: Lack of activation by protein kinase C and cAMP-dependent protein kinase. Science 1989; 244:1351-3.
137. Li M, McCann JD, Liedke CM, et al. Cyclic AMP-dependent protein kinase opens chloride channels in normal but not cystic fibrosis airway epithelium. Nature 1988; 331:358-60.
138. Riordan JR, Rommens JM, Kerem B, et al. Identification of the cystic fibrosis gene: Cloning and characterization of complementary DNA. Science 1989; 245:1066-73.
139. Rommens JM, Iannuzzi MC, Kerem B, et al. Identification of the cystic fibrosis gene: Chromosome walking and jumping. Science 1989; 245:1059-65.
140. Rowe SM, Miller S, Sorscher EJ. Cystic fibrosis. N Engl J Med 2005; 352:1992-2001.
141. Konstan MW, Hilliard KA, Norvell TM, Berger M. Bronchoalveolar lavage findings in cystic fibrosis patients with stable, clinically mild lung disease suggest ongoing infection and inflammation. Am J Respir Crit Care Med 1994; 150:448-54.
142. Boyle MP. Adult cystic fibrosis. JAMA 2007; 298:1787-93.
143. Kerem E, Reisman J, Corey M, et al. Prediction of mortality in patients with cystic fibrosis. N Engl J Med 1992; 326:1187-91.
144. Goss CH, Rubenfeld GD, Otto K, Aitken ML. The effect of pregnancy on survival in women with cystic fibrosis. Chest 2003; 124:1460-8.
145. Cheng EY, Goss CH, McKone EF, et al. Aggressive prenatal care results in successful fetal outcomes in CF women. J Cyst Fibros 2006; 5:85-91.
146. McMullen AH, Pasta DJ, Frederick PD, et al. Impact of pregnancy on women with cystic fibrosis. Chest 2006; 129:706-11.
147. Ødegaard I, Stray-Pedersen B, Hallberg K, et al. Maternal and fetal morbidity in pregnancies of Norwegian and Swedish women with cystic fibrosis. Acta Obstet Gynecol Scand 2002; 81:698-705.

148. Ramsey BW, Pepe MS, Quan JM, et al. Intermittent administration of inhaled tobramycin in patients with cystic fibrosis. N Engl J Med 1999; 340:23-30.
149. McArdle JR, Talwalkar JS. Macrolides in cystic fibrosis. Clin Chest Med 2007; 28:347-60.
150. Flotte TR. Adeno-associated virus-based gene therapy for inherited disorders. Pediatr Res 2005; 58:1143-7.
151. Liou TG, Adler FR, Huang D. Use of lung transplantation survival models to refine patient selection in cystic fibrosis. Am J Respir Crit Care Med 2005; 171:1053-9.
152. Liou TG, Adler FR, Cox DR, Cahill BC. Lung transplantation and survival in children with cystic fibrosis. N Engl J Med 2007; 357:2143-52.
153. Hyde NH, Harrison DM. Intrathecal morphine in a parturient with cystic fibrosis. Anesth Analg 1986; 65:1357-8.
154. Arkoosh VA, Palmer CM, Yun EM, et al. A randomized, double-masked, multicenter comparison of the safety of continuous intrathecal labor analgesia using a 28-gauge catheter versus continuous epidural labor analgesia. Anesthesiology 2008; 108:286-98.
155. Howell PR, Kent N, Douglas MJ. Anaesthesia for the parturient with cystic fibrosis. Int J Obstet Anesth 1993; 2:152-8.
156. Deshpande S. Epidural analgesia for vaginal delivery in a patient with cystic fibrosis following double lung transplantation. Int J Obstet Anesth 1998; 7:42-5.
157. von Ungern-Sternberg BS, Regli A, Bucher E, et al. The effect of epidural analgesia in labour on maternal respiratory function. Anaesthesia 2004; 59:350-3.
158. von Ungern-Sternberg, Regli A, Bucher E, et al. Impact of spinal anaesthesia and obesity on maternal respiratory function during elective Caesarean section. Anaesthesia 2004; 59:743-9.
159. Bose D, Yentis SM, Fauvel NJ. Caesarean section in a parturient with respiratory failure caused by cystic fibrosis. Anaesthesia 1997; 52:578-82.
160. Cameron AJD, Skinner TAJ. Management of a parturient with respiratory failure secondary to cystic fibrosis. Anaesthesia 2005; 60:77-80.
161. Muammar M, Marshall P, Wyatt H, Skelton V. Caesarean section in a patient with cystic fibrosis. Int J Obstet Anesth 2005; 14:70-3.
162. Catanzarite V, Willms D, Wong D, et al. Acute respiratory distress syndrome in pregnancy and the puerperium: Causes, courses, and outcomes. Obstet Gynecol 2001; 97:760-4.
163. Mabie WC, Barton JR, Sibai BM. Adult respiratory distress syndrome in pregnancy. Am J Obstet Gynecol 1992; 167:950-7.
164. Vasquez DN, Estenssoro E, Canales HS, et al. Clinical characteristics and outcomes of obstetric patients requiring ICU admission. Chest 2007; 131:718-24.
165. Ware LB, Matthay MA. The acute respiratory distress syndrome. N Engl J Med 2000; 342:1334-49.
166. Nunn JF. Applied Respiratory Physiology. London, Butterworth-Heinemann, 1987:450-9.
167. Lam CM, Wong SF, Leung TN, et al. A case-controlled study comparing clinical course and outcomes of pregnant and non-pregnant women with severe acute respiratory syndrome. Br J Obstet Gynaecol 2004; 111:771-4.
168. Cole DE, Taylor TL, McCullough DM, et al. Acute respiratory distress syndrome in pregnancy. Crit Care Med 2005; 33:S269-78.
169. Deblieux PM, Summer WR. Acute respiratory failure in pregnancy. Clin Obstet Gynecol 1996; 39:143-52.
170. Cunningham JA, Devine PC, Jelic S. Extracorporeal membrane oxygenation in pregnancy. Obstet Gynecol 2006; 108:792-5.
171. Raphael JH, Bexton MD. Combined high frequency ventilation in the management of respiratory failure in late pregnancy. Anaesthesia 1993; 48:596-8.
172. Huang S, DeSantis ER. Treatment of pulmonary arterial hypertension in pregnancy. Am J Health Syst Pharm 2007; 64:1922-6.
173. Bugge JF, Tanbo T. Nitric oxide in the treatment of fulminant pulmonary failure in a young pregnant woman with varicella pneumonia. Eur J Anaesthesiol 2000; 17:269-72.
174. Collop NA, Sahn SA. Critical illness in pregnancy: An analysis of 20 patients admitted to a medical intensive care unit. Chest 1993; 103:1548-52.
175. Tomlinson MW, Caruthers TJ, Whitty JE, Gonik B. Does delivery improve maternal condition in the respiratory-compromised gravida? Obstet Gynecol 1998; 91:108-11.
176. Jenkins TM, Troiano NH, Graves CR, et al. Mechanical ventilation in an obstetric population: Characteristics and delivery rates. Am J Obstet Gynecol 2003; 188:549-52.
177. Pacheco LD, Gei AF, VanHook JW, et al. Burns in pregnancy. Obstet Gynecol 2005; 106:1210-2.
178. Ackerman WE III, Molnar JM, Juneja MM. Beneficial effect of epidural anesthesia on oxygen consumption in a parturient with adult respiratory distress syndrome. South Med J 1993; 86:361-4.

Substance Abuse

Lisa R. Leffert, M.D.

Abuse of licit and illicit substances by pregnant women poses a significant risk to maternal and fetal health. Estimates of the prevalence of substance abuse in pregnant women range from 4% to 17%, depending on the substance and data source (Table 53-1); however, there is a consensus that the actual prevalence is significantly higher, and the adverse effects are of great consequence.[1-8] Pregnant women who ingest these substances experience a myriad of acute and chronic adverse effects, including the development of (1) cardiovascular, pulmonary, and neurologic complications and (2) obstetric complications (e.g., decreased intrauterine fetal growth, preterm labor, placental abruption, fetal death).[6,9-17] Anesthesia providers often care for these patients during the provision of analgesia and anesthesia for labor and vaginal or cesarean delivery as well as during other obstetric procedures before and after delivery. Patients with substance abuse may have abnormal pain sensitivity, and anesthesia providers are often consulted for treatment of acute postoperative pain.

DRUG DETECTION

Optimal care requires the identification of the substances that have been taken. The anesthesia provider should ask questions in a respectful and nonjudgmental manner. It may be necessary to speak to the patient without family or friends present in order to encourage more accurate self-reporting. Maternal self-reporting typically underrepresents the true incidence of substance abuse[18-20]; therefore health care providers should be familiar with the characteristic signs and symptoms that should raise the index of suspicion. A myriad of methods are available to test pregnant patients and their babies for the presence of these drugs, including the analysis of urine, blood, hair, meconium, and umbilical cord tissue. The analysis of amniotic fluid or neonatal gastric aspirate has also been reported to be useful (Tables 53-2 and 53-3).[18-23] Immunoassays are the most commonly used drug testing methods, but these assays can have false-positive or false-negative results in the presence of structurally related drugs or additives. Gas chromatography with mass spectrometry is often used to provide confirmation of positive results.[19]

LICIT DRUGS

Alcohol

EPIDEMIOLOGY

Alcohol (ethanol) abuse represents a significant problem for pregnant women and their offspring. Since 1981, official advisories have warned against the use of alcohol by pregnant women or women considering pregnancy[2]; however, alcohol use is still common in this population. The 2006 National Survey on Drug Use and Health[24] noted that 11.8% of pregnant women 15 to 44 years old reported current alcohol use, 2.9% reported binge drinking, and 0.7% reported heavy drinking. These rates are significantly lower than those of nonpregnant women in the same age brackets (53.0%, 23.6%, and 5.4%, respectively). Survey data indicate that among heavy drinkers, more than 30% also use illicit drugs.[24]

PHARMACOLOGY

Alcohol, usually ingested orally, is absorbed through the gastrointestinal tract, primarily within the small intestine. Ingested alcohol is metabolized by alcohol and acetaldehyde dehydrogenases. This process leads to the production of acetaldehyde and the reduction of nicotinamide adenine dinucleotide (NAD) to its reduced form, NADH; the excess reduced form relative to NAD results in metabolic derangements. A small residual amount (2% to 8%) of alcohol is excreted via the lungs, urine, and sweat.[25-27]

TABLE 53-1 Data Sources for Prevalence of Substance Abuse

Study*	Study Design	Participants	Dates of Data Collection	Focus	Instrument(s) of Analysis
Maternal Lifestyle Study[160]	Survey (observational study)	Four clinical centers National scope 11,811 mother/infant dyads	1993-1995	Prenatal effect of cocaine and/or opioid exposure	Maternal self-report Meconium gas chromatography/mass spectroscopy
National Survey on Drug Use and Health[161]	Survey (random sampling)	National scope ≈70,000 subjects/year	Yearly	Broad-based licit and illicit drug use	Computerized questionnaire administered by professional field interviewer
National Pregnancy and Health Survey[162]	Survey (two-stage)	Samples from U.S. hospitals with > 200 births/year 2613 subjects	1992-1993	Methamphetamine use; included prenatal alcohol, tobacco, and marijuana exposure	Personal interviews Self-enumerated answer sheets Medical records Hair assays Urine tests
Infant Development, Environmental, and Lifestyle (IDEAL) Study[70]	Survey (observational study)	Four clinical centers Geographic areas with high prevalence of substance abuse 1618 subjects	Yearly, with longitudinal cohort first enrolled in 2002-2003	Prevalence and correlates of alcohol, tobacco, and other substance use during pregnancy	Maternal self-report Gas chromatography/mass spectroscopy confirmation of amphetamine metabolites in meconium
DC Metropolitan Area Drug Study[163]	Survey (16 separate studies)	Urban population (predominantly black women in Washington, D.C.)	1991-1992	Prevalence of tobacco, alcohol, and drug use	Household survey

*Superscript numbers indicate reference citations listed at the end of the chapter.

SYSTEMIC EFFECTS

According to legal statutes, the definition of "intoxication" requires a blood alcohol level of at least 80 to 100 mg/dL, although behavioral, cognitive, and psychomotor changes can occur at levels of 20 to 30 mg/dL (e.g., after 1 to 2 drinks) (Table 53-4).[25-27]

Alcohol has complex effects on the central nervous system (CNS); it acts as both a depressant and a stimulant through a variety of neurotransmitter pathways.[27] When alcohol is consumed in conjunction with barbiturates or benzodiazepines, these effects can be compounded. Endogenous opioids interact with alcohol to "reinforce" further alcohol use; this effect is blunted by opioid antagonists.[27]

Alcohol and its metabolites (e.g., acetaldehyde) can be directly toxic to brain tissue.[25,26] Chronic alcoholism is associated with brain atrophy that results in impairments of memory, abstract problem-solving, verbal learning, and visual-spatial processing.[25] Additional adverse neurologic effects result from vitamin (thiamine, B_{12}) deficiencies.[25]

Heavy alcohol consumption also damages other organs, either singly or together. Over time, hepatic cirrhosis can develop, which in turn can lead to encephalopathy, coagulopathy, and esophageal varices (Table 53-5). Gastrointestinal mucosa injury, pancreatitis, and cardiomyopathy may also occur.[13,14,26,28]

Women who abuse alcohol are at increased risk for depression, suicide, and accidents.[11,29] Symptoms of acute alcohol withdrawal (e.g., nausea, vomiting, tachycardia, hypertension, arrhythmias, tremor, hallucinations, agitation, seizures) usually occur within 6 to 48 hours after cessation of alcohol consumption (Table 53-6).[13,14,30] Pharmacologic therapy to minimize the signs and symptoms of alcohol withdrawal includes the use of benzodiazepines and $alpha_2$-adrenergic agonists (e.g., clonidine).[13] The most severe form of withdrawal symptoms, **delirium tremens,** manifests as agitation, disorientation, hallucinations, and fever combined with autonomic instability. Delirium tremens occurs rarely in pregnant women, but it can lead to maternal and fetal death if untreated.[10,31]

EFFECTS ON PREGNANCY AND THE FETUS

Intrauterine alcohol exposure is the leading cause of preventable birth defects in the United States.[32,33] No safe level of alcohol consumption by pregnant women has been identified.[2,31,33] **Fetal alcohol syndrome** is defined as the

TABLE 53-2 Drug Detection: Overview

Specimen	Advantages	Limitations
Urine	Detection of diverse group of illicit substances (except volatile alcohols) Specimen and test readily available Short turnaround time (30 minutes at point of care; 2 hours for laboratory specimens) More sensitive test (compared with meconium and hair) for cannabis	Underrepresents most illicit drug use Significant false-positive rate for phencyclidine (PCP) Narrow detection window compared with that for meconium and hair
Blood	Most commonly used for volatile alcohols (can detect other illicit substances) Specimen and test readily available	Narrow detection window compared with that for urine, meconium, and hair
Meconium	Highly sensitive (compared with urine testing) for cocaine and opioids Wide detection window No false-positive results for cocaine	Specimen may not be readily available Low sensitivity for detecting cannabinoids
Hair	Highly sensitive test for detecting cocaine (three times that of urine) and opioids Wide detection window (reflects chronic cumulative use) Samples can be stored at room temperature Samples can be analyzed remote from collection	Multiple hairs required; harvested close to scalp Environmental contamination may cause false-positive result Low sensitivity for detecting tetrahydrocannabinol
Umbilical cord blood	Comparable to meconium with more rapid results	Specimen not available before delivery

Data from references 18-20, 22, 80.

presence of particular neonatal facial features (small palpebral fissures, flat midface with a short upturned nose, thin upper lip) and significant impairment in neurodevelopment and physical growth.[13,14,33-35] **Fetal alcohol spectrum disorders** refer to the wide range of possible adverse effects of fetal exposure to alcohol.[33] The extent to which an individual fetus is affected is related to the characteristics of the exposure, genetic variables, and the intrauterine environment.[36]

Alcohol exposure is also associated with pregnancy loss. Harlap et al.[37] reported an increased risk of second-trimester fetal loss in pregnant women who consumed

TABLE 53-3 Drug Detection Window in Urine*

Drug	Analyte	Detection Window
Tobacco	Cotinine Nicotine	19 hr (urine $T_{1/2}$) 2 hr (urine $T_{1/2}$)
Cocaine	Cocaine Benzoylecgonine	3-6 hr 1-2 days, if used IV; 2-3 days, if used intranasally
Amphetamines	Amphetamine Methamphetamine	1-3 days 60 hr, if smoked
Methylenedioxymethamphetamine (MDMA, ecstasy)	MDMA	1-3 days
Marijuana (cannabis)	Tetrahydrocannabinol (THC) THCCOOH	10 hr, if smoked Up to 25 days
Lysergic acid diethylamide (LSD)	LSD 2-Oxo-3OH-LSD	24 hr 96 hr
Heroin	6-Acetyl morphine Morphine	2-4.5 hr, if used IV 19-35 hr

IV, intravenously; $T_{1/2}$, half-life.

*Average values based on recent use; precise values may vary according to method of ingestion, assay employed, and duration of use.

Data from references 9, 23, 81, 164.

TABLE 53-4 Acute Intoxication and Organ Dysfunction

Substance	Neurologic	Cardiovascular	Pulmonary	Gastrointestinal	Hematologic	Other
Alcohol	↓ Cognition	—	↑ risk of aspiration	—	—	↑ Cortisol ↓ Glucose
Tobacco	—	↑HR, BP, myocardial work	↓ Tissue oxygenation secondary to ↑ carboxyhemoglobin ↓ Mucociliary clearance ↑ Airway irritability	—	—	Impaired wound healing
Caffeine	—	Mild ↑ BP in low doses		—	—	Diuresis
Marijuana (cannabis)	↓ Cognitive and motor performance	Biphasic autonomic effect ST segment and T wave changes on electrocardiogram	↑ HR **If smoked:** effects similar to those of tobacco	Appetite stimulation	—	Conjunctival vasodilation and reddening
Cocaine	Subarachnoid or intracranial hemorrhage Cerebral infarct Seizures	Hemodynamic instability, arrhythmias Acute myocardial infarction Aortic dissection	**If free-based:** pulmonary edema & pulmonary hemorrhage **If smoked:** see "Tobacco" **If snorted:** nasal septal injury & epistaxis	↑ AST & ALT	↓ Platelets (?)	Infection ↑ Temperature ↑ Cortisol ↑ Glucose
Amphetamines	Seizures Stroke Paranoia Hallucinations	Similar to effects associated with cocaine	—	—	—	Proteinuria ↑ Temperature
Hallucinogens	Hallucinations Paranoia Intracerebral hemorrhage (rare) Seizures (rare)	Supraventricular tachycardia (rare) Acute myocardial infarction (rare)	—	—	—	—
Opioids	—	↓HR ↓BP	Respiratory depression	—	—	—
Solvents	Encephalopathy Seizures	Arrhythmias Acute myocardial infarction	Hypoxemia Bronchospasm Acute respiratory distress syndrome	Mucosal injury		Ethylene glycol ingestion: Metabolic acidosis Renal failure

ALT, alanine aminotransferase; AST, aspartate aminotransferase; BP, blood pressure; HR, heart rate; ↑, increase in; ↓, decrease in.

TABLE 53-5 Effects of Chronic Substance Abuse

	Neurologic	Cardiac	Pulmonary	Gastrointestinal	Hematologic	Other
Alcohol	Peripheral neuropathy Brain atrophy Encephalopathy	Cardiomyopathy	—	Hepatitis Cirrhosis Gastric mucosal injury Pancreatitis	Anemia (± leukopenia, thrombocytopenia) Coagulopathy	↑ Cortisol
Tobacco	—	Atherosclerosis	Diffusion capacity abnormalities ↓ Pulmonary immune function ↑ Incidence of bronchitis, COPD ↑ Airway irritability ↑ Risk of lung cancer	—	—	—
Caffeine	Cessation may produce withdrawal headache	Does *not* negatively affect cardiac health at moderate dose	—	—	—	↑ Risk of bladder dysfunction with high intake
Marijuana (cannabis)	↓ Attention, memory ↓ Ability to process complex information	—	**If smoked:** effects similar to those associated with tobacco	↑ Rare forms of oropharyngeal cancer	—	—
Cocaine	Brain atrophy	Cardiomyopathy Myocarditis Blood vessel occlusion	**If smoked:** effects similar to those associated with tobacco **If snorted:** mucosal & nasal septal injury	Gastrointestinal ischemia/ulceration ↑ AST & ALT	↓ Platelets (?)	Renal failure
Amphetamines	Paranoid psychosis Impaired memory	—	—	—	—	↑ Tooth decay ("meth mouth")
Hallucinogens (episodic use)	Delayed hallucinations	—	—	—	—	—
Opioids	Abnormal pain sensitivity	Infective endocarditis	—	—	—	Hepatitis or human immunodeficiency virus infection with exposure to contaminated needles
Solvents	Visual loss Cranial neuropathy Peripheral neuropathy Autonomic dysfunction Ataxia Brain atrophy Encephalopathy	Cardiomyopathy Acute myocardial infarction	—	Nonviral hepatitis Hepatocellular carcinoma	Aplastic anemia	"Glue-sniffer's" rash Renal failure

ALT, alanine aminotransferase; AST, aspartate aminotransferase; ↑, increase in; ↓, decrease in.

TABLE 53-6 Symptoms of and Treatment for Substance Abuse Withdrawal

Substance	Symptoms	Therapy
Alcohol (ethanol)	Nausea Vomiting Tachycardia Hypertension Tremor Hallucinations Agitation	Benzodiazepines and $alpha_2$-drenergic agonist (e.g., clonidine)
	Delirium tremens: • Autonomic instability/arrhythmias • Seizures • Severe tremors • Disorientation • Fever	Benzodiazepines and $alpha_2$-adrenergic agonist (e.g., clonidine) Antiarrhythmics Anticonvulsants (e.g., phenytoin)
Tobacco	Cravings Irritability Headache Cough Insomnia	Nicotine replacement therapies, including patch, gum, and inhalers
Caffeine	Headache Anxiety Depressed mood Fatigue	Supportive care Caffeine ingestion
Cannabis	Mild abstinence syndrome Headache Restlessness Tremor Anxiety Autonomic effects	Supportive care
Cocaine	Prolonged sleep phase Hunger Anxiety Weakness Headaches Tremors and seizures	Supportive care Re-introduction of drug, if necessary, with slow taper
Amphetamines	Fatigue Depression Hunger Intense cravings	Tricyclic antidepressants, dopaminergic agents (e.g., bromocriptine), and amino acid therapy (no therapy has proved to be successful)
Hallucinogens (e.g., phencyclidine, [PCP], lysergic acid diethylamide [LSD])	No clearly associated withdrawal symptoms, although psychological dependence can occur	Not applicable
Opioids (e.g., heroin)	Flulike symptoms, such as fatigue, weakness, restlessness, rhinorrhea, perspiration, fever, diarrhea	Supportive therapy $Alpha_2$-adrenergic agonist (e.g., clonidine) Doxepin Re-introduction of drug, if necessary, with slow taper
Solvents (e.g., ethylene glycol, toluene, glue)	Not applicable	Not applicable

alcohol early in pregnancy (relative risk 1.98 for those consuming 1 to 2 drinks/day, and 3.53 for those consuming more than 3 drinks/day, in comparison with nondrinkers). Identification of mothers at risk can facilitate treatment and perhaps improve pregnancy outcomes.[33]

ANESTHETIC MANAGEMENT

Alcohol-intoxicated parturients are at increased risk for behavioral problems, electrolyte abnormalities, greater gastric acid secretion, and co-intoxication with other substances.[13,14,31,38] Determining whether the patient can protect her airway is of paramount importance, because acute intoxication increases the risk of pulmonary aspiration of gastric contents. In addition, these patients may have intravascular volume depletion secondary to vomiting, inadequate oral intake, diuresis, and hypoalbuminemia. Significant alcohol ingestion in the setting of poor oral intake may also manifest as severe hypoglycemia.[26,38,39]

Neuraxial analgesia or anesthesia can be safely administered for labor or cesarean delivery provided that (1) the patient is cooperative, (2) there is no evidence of coagulopathy (as a result of liver disease), (3) the patient is volume replete, and (4) baseline neurologic deficits (e.g., peripheral neuropathy, cognitive deficits) are assessed and documented.[13]

If emergency delivery is required and the patient is either uncooperative or too sedated to protect her airway, general anesthesia will be necessary. The patient should receive pharmacologic aspiration prophylaxis (i.e., nonparticulate antacid, histamine H_2-receptor antagonist, metoclopramide) and should undergo a rapid-sequence induction of general anesthesia.[40]

Evidence from published reports is inconclusive about predictable differences in anesthetic requirements in patients with acute and chronic alcohol use.[38] Acute alcohol intoxication is believed to decrease a patient's anesthetic requirements, in part because of the additive effect of alcohol and other CNS depressants. The notion that chronic alcoholics require more anesthesia than their non–alcohol-using counterparts is based primarily on data from an abstract published by Han,[41] who demonstrated that the mean minimum alveolar concentration (MAC) for halothane in 6 chronic alcoholic patients who had been heavy drinkers for more than 10 years was significantly higher than that for 6 healthy adult subjects. Subsequently, Swerdlow et al.[42] assessed the response to thiopental in 11 nonpregnant, chronic alcohol users. After eliminating potential confounders such as acute intoxication, withdrawal, polysubstance abuse, and end-organ dysfunction, these investigators found that chronic alcohol intake did not alter thiopental dose requirements, pharmacokinetics, or pharmacodynamics. No large population studies have assessed dose requirements for volatile anesthetic agents or hypnotic agents in patients who chronically abuse alcohol.

Short-term consumption of alcohol inhibits the metabolism of drugs by the liver (through competition for cytochrome P-450), which results in higher plasma concentrations of drugs metabolized by the liver. *Long-term* consumption of alcohol increases the levels of cytochrome P-450, resulting in decreased levels of medications such as diazepam and labetalol, and increased levels of toxic metabolites that occur from hepatic degradation of illicit drugs such as cocaine.[26] Both pregnancy and liver disease can lead to decreased plasma concentrations of pseudocholinesterase; however, this decrease does not seem to have a clinically significant effect on the degradation of succinylcholine and ester local anesthetics.[38]

These patients are at risk for intravascular volume depletion, hypoalbuminemia, and cardiomyopathy. Further, high concentrations of volatile anesthetic agents depress uterine tone and may increase blood loss at cesarean delivery. Therefore anesthesia providers should avoid making an arbitrary conclusion that pregnant women who abuse alcohol require higher doses of anesthetic drugs. On the other hand, the anesthesia provider must give attention to the risk of awareness during administration of general anesthesia for emergency cesarean delivery.

Tobacco

EPIDEMIOLOGY

Cigarette smoking is the most common form of substance abuse during pregnancy. Greater public awareness exists regarding the hazards of smoking during pregnancy,[43] and the prevalence of cigarette smoking during pregnancy has declined over the past 40 years. An estimated 18.0% of pregnant women reported being smokers in 2003,[4] compared with 16.5% in 2006[24]; the prevalence of smoking in nonpregnant women was 29.5% in 2006.[24] Unfortunately, among the approximately 40% of patients who stop smoking when they discover that they are pregnant, 60% to 80% return to smoking by 6 months postpartum.[44]

PHARMACOLOGY

More than 4000 chemicals are found in tobacco, including nicotine, carbon monoxide, and cyanides.[27,45] Tobacco is most often smoked, but it can also be chewed or sniffed. Nicotine, the principal drug of abuse in tobacco, acts at peripheral and central nicotinic (acetylcholine) receptors throughout the body to effect the release of catecholamines.[27] Nicotine's effects begin immediately upon exposure; it is then rapidly metabolized in the liver and the lungs, and excreted by the kidneys. The half-life is typically a few hours. The duration of the acute effects of nicotine is shorter in heavy smokers than in light smokers.[27]

Carbon monoxide, another constituent of cigarette smoke, interferes with oxygen delivery to the cells by competitively binding to hemoglobin, thereby decreasing the oxygen-binding capacity and shifting the oxyhemoglobin dissociation curve to the left.[46] Depending on the extent of smoke inhalation, carbon monoxide may occupy 3% to 15% (or more) of the oxygen-carrying capacity of the blood.[47]

SYSTEMIC EFFECTS

Smoking alters maternal physiology through both the acute pharmacologic actions of tobacco's chemical constituents and their contribution to comorbid disease. Peripherally, nicotine increases sympathetic tone, thereby increasing maternal heart rate, blood pressure, and cardiac work (see Table 53-4).[48] Nicotine affects neurotransmitter release in different areas of the brain, producing feelings of alertness, euphoria, and, ultimately, dependence.[27,48]

Increased production of carboxyhemoglobin is thought to be a major factor in the impaired wound healing observed in smokers.[46] Smoking also promotes atherosclerosis. The effects of tobacco smoking on the lungs include changes in the volume and composition of mucus, impaired mucociliary clearance, and an increased incidence of bronchitis and chronic obstructive pulmonary disease (see Table 53-5).[48]

Tobacco is addictive, and cessation of its use produces withdrawal symptoms, including cravings, irritability, headache, cough, and insomnia (see Table 53-6). Smoking cessation interventions may consist of counseling and therapy, hypnosis, acupuncture, and pharmacologic therapy.[4]

The use of nicotine replacement therapy (e.g., nicotine gum, patch, inhaler) has not undergone sufficient evaluation of safety during pregnancy; thus the American College of Obstetricians and Gynecologists (ACOG)[4] has recommended that nicotine replacement therapy be used only when nonpharmacologic interventions have failed. The physiologic benefits to the parturient of smoking cessation are progressive; even brief smoke-free intervals can result in a reduction in the carboxyhemoglobin concentration, improved ciliary function, and decreased small airway obstruction.[49]

EFFECTS ON PREGNANCY AND THE FETUS

Nicotine has a low molecular weight and readily crosses the placenta.[6] Smoking may result in decreased fetal oxygenation as a result of increased concentrations of carboxyhemoglobin and reduced uteroplacental perfusion. It also leads to decreased uptake of nourishing amino acids by the placenta.[45] Smoking is associated with a higher incidence of ectopic pregnancy, spontaneous fetal loss, placental abruption, and sudden infant death syndrome (SIDS).[4,37,50] Smoking seems to protect against the occurrence of preeclampsia (see Chapter 45).[51]

Smoking adversely affects fetal growth.[45,52-56] Low birth weight (LBW) is associated with increased neonatal and infant mortality.[45,52,53] Mello et al.[54] studied the effects of tobacco smoke on pregnant female rats and found that offspring exposed to cigarette smoke weighed less and were shorter at birth than their nonexposed counterparts. In a retrospective cohort study of more than three million births, Salihu et al.[53] documented that infant mortality was 40% higher in the offspring of pregnant women who smoked than in the offspring of nonsmoking pregnant women; this risk increased in a dose-dependent fashion for the infants who were small for gestational age (SGA). In a prospective study of 7470 pregnant women, Shiono et al.[55] showed that cigarette smoking was associated with LBW. Smoking cessation before the third trimester ameliorates the smoking-associated reduction in birth weight.[4]

Intrauterine exposure to smoking (tobacco and/or marijuana) may also have long-term effects. Fried et al.[57] examined the cognitive performance in 145 adolescents (13 to 16 years of age) from a low-risk, middle-class population; after controlling data for socioeconomic status and polysubstance abuse, they found that measures of overall intelligence and auditory memory were negatively related to prenatal maternal smoking in a dose-related fashion.

ANESTHETIC MANAGEMENT

Smoking is a risk factor for several perioperative complications, including respiratory sequelae and impaired wound healing.[46,48] Smoking results in increased airway secretions, decreased ciliary motility, and impaired gas exchange.[13,48] Smoking is also associated with an increase in nonspecific airway reactivity, and endotracheal intubation may provoke bronchospasm. Wilkes et al.[58] observed that coughing upon exposure to desflurane was more pronounced in smokers. By contrast, Kim and Bishop[59] observed that although most patients coughed as they awakened from general anesthesia maintained with isoflurane, smokers were not more likely to cough than nonsmokers.

Six months of abstinence may be required before the function of alveolar macrophages and pulmonary cytokines during and after general anesthesia in former smokers is similar to that of nonsmokers.[49] Administration of neuraxial anesthesia avoids airway manipulation and is typically preferred in parturients who smoke.[13]

Caffeine

EPIDEMIOLOGY

Approximately 80% to 98% of women drink caffeine-containing beverages on a daily basis.[13,60] The prevalence of consumption of caffeine-containing beverages during pregnancy is unknown.

PHARMACOLOGY

Caffeine (1,3,7-trimethylxanthine) is a naturally occurring alkaloid found in coffee, tea, cocoa, and some soft drinks and medicines.[13,60,61] The primary sources of caffeine in the adult diet are coffee (56 to 100 mg/100 mL if brewed) and tea (20 to 73 mg/100 mL). Caffeine is readily absorbed through the gastrointestinal tract, and maximum blood concentrations of caffeine are attained 1 to 1.5 hours after ingestion.[60] Caffeine undergoes hepatic metabolism and is then excreted in the urine.[60,61] The elimination half-life of caffeine is 3 to 7 hours. In pregnancy, the half-life increases from 4 hours in the first trimester to 18 hours by the third trimester.[60,62] Caffeine crosses the placenta and can also be found in breast milk. Habitual use of caffeine at levels greater than 500 to 600 mg/day is defined as abuse.[60]

The half-life of caffeine in the neonate is prolonged in comparison with that in children and nonpregnant women.[60]

SYSTEMIC EFFECTS

Caffeine acts as an antagonist at the adenosine receptor. In the absence of the inhibitory effects of adenosine, the neurotransmitters norepinephrine, dopamine, and serotonin are released in increased concentrations.[60,62] Systemic effects of caffeine include CNS stimulation, changes in blood pressure and metabolic rate, and diuresis (see Table 53-4).[61] The side effects commonly attributed to caffeine vary among individuals, in part related to the doses ingested and the degree of chronic use. Studies of the effects of caffeine on alertness, vigilance, mood, and memory have produced inconsistent results.[60]

Moderate caffeine intake ($\leq$ 400 mg/day or $\leq$ 4 cups of coffee/day) does not seem to negatively affect cardiovascular health in most people. Although some people who ingest caffeine report tachycardia and palpitations, doses lower than 450 mg/day do not appear to increase significant cardiac arrhythmias in either healthy patients or in those with ischemia or ventricular ectopy.[60] Caffeine doses as low as 250 mg have been reported to have a hypertensive effect after acute ingestion (an increase in systolic blood pressure of 5 to 15 mm Hg, and an increase in diastolic blood pressure of 5 to 10 mm Hg), particularly in caffeine-naïve individuals; however, epidemiologic studies have produced inconsistent results.[60] In general, people who ingest caffeine on a long-term and frequent basis are less likely than occasional users to have difficulty sleeping.[60]

Caffeine appears to affect bladder function in women. Moderate caffeine intake may exacerbate preexisting bladder symptoms, and excessive intake (> 400 mg/day) increases the risk of bladder dysfunction.[60]

Evidence suggests that caffeine is not a human carcinogen.[60,61] The lethal dose of caffeine in human beings has been estimated to be 10 g; however, only a few such cases have been reported.[60]

Caffeine withdrawal is associated with headache, anxiety, depressed mood, and fatigue (see Table 53-6).[13,60] Typically, symptoms begin 12 to 24 hours after cessation of use, peak at 20 to 48 hours, and last up to 7 days. The severity and likelihood of symptoms are not predictable.

EFFECTS ON PREGNANCY AND THE FETUS

Caffeine readily crosses the placenta. Whereas animal studies have shown that very high doses can have a teratogenic effect, moderate doses do not appear to result in teratogenesis in humans.[60,63,64] Nawrot et al.[60] recommended that "caffeine intake for women who plan to become pregnant and for women during gestation should not exceed 300 mg/day."

Caffeine consumption of 300 mg/day or more may reduce fertility[60]; whether this effect persists when confounding factors such as maternal age, smoking, and parity are considered is unknown.[61,65] Most studies have not shown an association between caffeine intake less than 300 mg/day and a higher risk of spontaneous abortion or preterm delivery, particularly when confounding factors are eliminated.[60,61,65]

Although the results are conflicting, there is some evidence that caffeine doses of 300 mg/day or higher may result in intrauterine growth restriction (IUGR) and decreased birth weight, particularly in women who also smoke or drink significant amounts of alcohol.[60] In a randomized, controlled, double-blind study, Bech et al.[62] found that a moderate reduction in caffeine intake during the second half of pregnancy had no effect on birth weight or length of gestation. Moderate intake of caffeine in pregnant and lactating women does not adversely affect postnatal development.[60,61]

Two studies have suggested that moderate caffeine intake during pregnancy may actually have beneficial effects on the mother and the fetus. Adeney et al.[66] found that women who consumed caffeinated coffee before conception had a significantly lower risk for development of gestational diabetes mellitus than women who did not consume coffee. No reduction in risk was associated with ingestion of tea or soda. Back et al.[67] showed that newborn mice exposed to caffeine and subsequently subjected to hypoxia seemed to have less neurologic injury (i.e., less ventriculomegaly, less disruption in myelination) than non–caffeine-exposed mice.

ANESTHETIC MANAGEMENT

Caffeine may enhance the side effects of beta-adrenergic receptor agonists, such as epinephrine and albuterol. Caffeine may also increase the risk of a hypertensive crisis in patients taking monoamine oxidase (MAO) inhibitors. Caffeine slows the elimination of theophylline and acetaminophen, thus resulting in higher drug concentrations in the blood. In contrast, serum concentrations of lithium may be decreased secondary to caffeine-enhanced elimination.[61]

Perhaps of greatest significance to the anesthesia provider is the potential for **caffeine withdrawal headache.** In preparation for labor or elective cesarean delivery, parturients often abruptly decrease their usual caffeine intake; they may subsequently experience a headache that may be confused with a post–dural puncture headache. Caffeine withdrawal should be considered in a postpartum patient who presents with a nonspecific, nonpositional headache without associated lateralizing neurologic findings (see Chapter 31).

Evidence for the efficacy of caffeine in the treatment of post–dural puncture headache is scant (see Chapter 31).[68] On the other hand, resumption of caffeine ingestion may be considered for treatment of caffeine withdrawal headache.

ILLICIT DRUGS

Marijuana (Cannabis)

Use of marijuana for medical and recreational indications can be traced back thousands of years.[69] In 2006 approximately 2.1 million people in the United States used marijuana for the first time.[24] Although precise estimates of marijuana use in the pregnant population vary (6% to 7%),[20,70] it is thought to be the illicit drug most commonly used for recreational purposes by pregnant women.[69]

PHARMACOLOGY

Marijuana contains more than 400 compounds, including 60 cannabinoids. Most of the psychotropic effects are caused by 9-tetrahydrocannabinol (THC).[69,71] Non-cannabinoid constituents of marijuana are similar to those in tobacco, with the exception of nicotine.[71] Inhaled THC is absorbed through the lungs and reaches the brain within minutes. Oral ingestion of marijuana results in blood THC concentrations that are 25% to 30% of those obtained by smoking, with a delayed onset of action (up to 2 hours). Cannabinoids are highly lipid-soluble compounds that are sequestered in fatty tissues and are gradually released into other tissues. Thus, a single ingestion can have an elimination half-life of up to 7 days; complete elimination of the inactive metabolite THCCOOH requires as long as 25 to 30 days. Metabolism occurs in the liver, with excretion in the urine. Measured concentrations of THC and other cannabinoid metabolites in the blood and urine correlate poorly with the degree of intoxication.[71]

SYSTEMIC EFFECTS

Cannabis interacts with specific cannabinoid receptors in the brain and peripheral nerves. Psychoactive effects include anxiolysis, analgesia, appetite stimulation, euphoria, and, in some instances, dysphoria (see Table 53-4).[71] Marijuana intoxication impairs cognitive and psychomotor function. Impairment of memory, attention, and the ability to process complex information occurs with long-time heavy use (see Table 53-5); it is unclear whether these effects are reversible.[72]

Acute intoxication with marijuana appears to have a biphasic effect on the autonomic nervous system; low doses cause tachycardia and higher cardiac output owing to increased sympathetic tone and decreased parasympathetic tone. In contrast, high doses produce sympathetic inhibition and parasympathetic stimulation, resulting in bradycardia and hypotension.[9,69] Although ventricular ectopy can occur, life-threatening arrhythmias in patients without preexisting cardiac disease are rare, and autonomic disturbances are generally well tolerated.[9] Reversible ST segment and T wave abnormalities may occur, perhaps as a result of the higher heart rate associated with marijuana use.[9]

As with tobacco, the respiratory consequences of smoking marijuana include mucociliary dysfunction, increased susceptibility to bronchitis, and chronic obstructive pulmonary disease (see Table 53-5). Acute intoxication may cause conjunctival vasodilation and associated visible reddening of the eyes.[71] Although high doses of marijuana can cause hallucinations and psychosis, fatal overdose has not been documented.[10,71]

Withdrawal from long-time marijuana use may produce a mild abstinence syndrome that includes headache, restlessness, tremor, anxiety, and autonomic effects similar to those of withdrawal from use of benzodiazepines and hypnotic drugs (see Table 53-6).[9,69,72]

EFFECTS ON PREGNANCY AND THE FETUS

It is difficult to ascertain specific effects of marijuana on pregnancy, as women who use marijuana often engage in polysubstance abuse.[69] In a prospective study of more than 3800 pregnancies, Hatch et al.[72] showed that regular marijuana use by white women was associated with an increased risk of delivering an LBW and/or SGA infant, but occasional use was not. The risk for these adverse outcomes in non-white marijuana-using women was not elevated above their baseline level of increased risk. In a prospective multicenter study of more than 7000 multiethnic pregnant women, marijuana use was not associated with increased risk of LBW, preterm delivery, or placental abruption.[55]

Intrauterine exposure to marijuana causes subtle postnatal neurologic derangements such as infant inattention, hyperactivity, and disturbed sleep.[69] Fried et al.[57] did not find an association between maternal marijuana use and overall IQ and verbal memory in exposed offspring; however, certain aspects of cognition, such as memory at 4 years of age, attention at 6 years, attention and visually related cognition at 9 to 12 years, and stability of attention at 13 to 16 years, were negatively associated with prenatal marijuana exposure.

ANESTHETIC MANAGEMENT

Neuraxial analgesia is typically preferred during labor and delivery. Drug-related changes in heart rate and blood pressure are usually well tolerated in otherwise healthy patients who are acutely intoxicated.[69] However, the administration of atropine, pancuronium, and ketamine can exacerbate existing tachycardia,[69] and it is tempting to speculate that such exacerbation could occur after epidural administration of an epinephrine-containing local anesthetic.

Long-time marijuana users are at risk for many of the same respiratory complications during and after general anesthesia as are tobacco cigarette smokers; these patients may have increased airway secretions, impaired mucociliary clearance, and perhaps increased airway reactivity.[48,71] White[73] reported a case of persistent, postextubation laryngospasm in a patient with a history of heavy marijuana smoking.

Acute intoxication with marijuana can have additive effects with those of sedative agents and volatile anesthetic agents[28]; careful titration to clinical effect is recommended.

The effect of marijuana on pain perception has been explored. Wallace et al.[74] presented a model of human experimental pain in which smoked marijuana had a biphasic effect on pain scores; a low dose had no effect, a medium dose reduced pain, and a high dose significantly increased pain. The clinical implications of these findings are unclear.

Cocaine

The use of cocaine, extracted from the leaf of the South American *Erythroxylon coca* bush,[75] can be dated as far back as 600 AD.[76] Cocaine was introduced into clinical practice as a local anesthetic in the 1880s. During this period, Sigmund Freud also experimented with cocaine's ability to combat hunger and fatigue and with its use in the treatment of opiate addiction.[76,77] Because of its unique vasoconstrictive and local anesthetic properties, cocaine is still employed in some clinical settings. The local anesthetic activity of cocaine occurs as a result of its ability to block sodium channels during depolarization.

EPIDEMIOLOGY

The prevalence of cocaine use during pregnancy is difficult to estimate; studies using a variety of detection techniques have reported rates that range from 1.8% to 18%, depending on the method and the population studied.[76] Survey data show that cocaine abuse in pregnancy is distributed broadly across ethnic and socioeconomic groups. In addition, an estimated 60% to 90% of pregnant cocaine users engage in polysubstance abuse, including the use of tobacco.[78,79] As with other illicit substances, the self-reporting of cocaine use results in identification of fewer drug users than urine testing and use of other biologic markers.[80] There is an association between cocaine use and an increased risk of sexually transmitted diseases, preterm labor, and failure to obtain prenatal care.[80]

PHARMACOLOGY

Cocaine (benzoylmethylecgonine) is an ester of benzoic acid and the base ecgonine, which is the parent compound of atropine and scopolamine.[77,81] Cocaine is consumed in a variety of forms. When dissolved in hydrochloric acid to form a water-soluble powder (cocaine hydrochloride), it can be chewed, administered intravenously ("mainlined"), or taken intranasally ("snorted").[75] Intrarectal and intravaginal use has also been reported.[82] When cocaine is processed with either sodium bicarbonate ("crack") or ammonia and ether ("freebase"), the resulting cocaine alkaloid can be smoked.[75-77,83] The amount (dose) and duration of exposure are more important determinants of the effects of cocaine than the particular chemical formulation.[84] Smoked cocaine (crack or freebase) is rapidly absorbed through the lungs and reaches the brain in 6 to 8 seconds, intravenous cocaine reaches the brain in 12 to 16 seconds, and snorted cocaine reaches the brain in 3 to 5 minutes.[83] The typical half-life of cocaine is 30 to 90 minutes, and its effects can last as long as 6 hours.[77]

Cocaine is metabolized to ecgonine esters and benzoylecgonine (biologically inactive) by plasma and hepatic cholinesterases, and to norcocaine (biologically active) by nonenzymatic hydrolysis. Cocaine is almost completely metabolized, with only small amounts excreted unchanged in the urine.[75,76,83] In the presence of alcohol, cocaine is transesterified to cocaethylene, which has a longer half-life and greater physiologic effects than cocaine.[75,76]

SYSTEMIC EFFECTS

Cocaine has complex actions on the central and peripheral nervous systems and on nerve conduction. The powerful sympathomimetic effects of cocaine occur secondary to the drug's inhibition of the reuptake of norepinephrine, dopamine, and serotonin, thus allowing these neurotransmitters to accumulate at the synaptic clefts and produce sustained stimulation.[75,76,83,85] This process may result in as much as a fivefold increase in circulating concentrations of catecholamines,[9] which may then lead to euphoria, increased energy, and decreased feelings of fear.[76,83] Repetitive use of cocaine eventually leads to depletion of neurotransmitter stores, up-regulation of receptors, and a higher dose requirement to achieve the desired euphoric effects.[77]

The peripheral nervous system effects of cocaine and its derivatives also result from binding to tissue receptors involved in monoamine reuptake, thus resulting in hypertension and/or labile blood pressure and tachycardia. Cocaine produces widespread small and large vessel occlusion through vasospasm, thrombosis, and endothelial injury, which may result in significant end-organ damage.[77]

Cocaine has profound effects on the **cardiovascular** system, and pregnancy appears to enhance these effects. Acute administration of cocaine increases peripheral vascular resistance, cardiac contractility, and myocardial oxygen demand (see Table 53-4).[77,86] Coronary vasoconstriction also occurs; a greater effect occurs in diseased vessel segments than in nondiseased segments.[75] Studies *in vitro* have indicated that cocaine can have a procoagulant effect in small and large vessels,[9] which may lead to thrombus formation and coronary plaque rupture in the setting of cocaine-induced hypertension.[77,87]

Cocaine-induced chest pain is a common complaint among young people presenting to the emergency room.[88] Mittleman et al.[87] found that cocaine use was associated with a significant, abrupt, and transient increase in the risk of acute myocardial infarction in patients who were otherwise at low risk. Although cocaine abusers who suffer a myocardial infarction have fewer postinfarction sequelae than the general population, the incidence of major cardiovascular complications is not trivial; 5% to 7% have congestive heart failure, 4% to 17% have ventricular arrhythmias, and up to 2% die.[75]

The occurrence of cocaine-induced electrocardiographic changes is not unusual and is not necessarily associated with true ischemia.[75,89] Measurement of troponin I levels is suggested if acute myocardial infarction is suspected, because creatinine kinase levels are elevated in pregnant patients and in half of cocaine-abusing patients for other reasons.[90] In addition, treatment with supplemental oxygen, aspirin, vasodilators, and reperfusion therapy may be indicated.[9,88]

Prompt recognition of acute cocaine-induced cardiovascular toxicity facilitates management.[79] However, not all cocaine-induced hypertension in pregnant women requires intervention. Beta-adrenergic receptor blockade may result in unopposed alpha receptor–mediated vasoconstriction, which can lead to coronary artery vasoconstriction and myocardial failure. If a beta-adrenergic receptor antagonist is used, then labetalol, which is both an alpha- and a beta-adrenergic receptor antagonist, is preferred. Of note, labetalol does not ameliorate the cocaine-induced coronary artery vasoconstriction.[75] Direct vasodilators (e.g., nitrates, hydralazine) can be used, but may cause further tachycardia.[9,75] Vertommen et al.[91] noted that hydralazine treated the hypertension in cocaine-intoxicated pregnant ewes but did not restore uterine blood flow. Calcium entry–blocking agents can potentiate the toxic effects of cocaine.[92] In addition, verapamil may cause fetal bradycardia, heart block, and depression of myocardial contractility.[93] The adjunct use of sedatives (e.g., benzodiazepines) and magnesium sulfate may ameliorate the cardiovascular effects.[9,75]

Other acute cardiovascular effects of cocaine include QT prolongation, bradycardia, and arrhythmias, including supraventricular or ventricular tachycardia and ventricular fibrillation.[77] Severe bradycardia can be treated with atropine or electrical pacing. If supraventricular tachycardia occurs and is well tolerated, close observation, vagal maneuvers, and/or the use of adenosine are warranted.[93,94] In the unstable patient with supraventricular tachycardia, direct current (DC) cardioversion may be required.[94]

The use of lidocaine as an antiarrhythmic agent appears to be acceptable in patients who have used cocaine. In a retrospective multicenter study, Shih et al.[95] found that the use of lidocaine in nonpregnant patients with cocaine-induced myocardial infarction was not associated with significant cardiovascular or CNS toxicity. Although the use of amiodarone therapy for maternal and fetal arrhythmias has been described as having only minor adverse effects in some patients, there are reports of associated fetal hypothyroidism and IUGR.[94,96,97] Thus the use of amiodarone in pregnant women is reserved for malignant arrhythmias that are refractory to other therapies.

Long-time cocaine abuse can cause left ventricular hypertrophy and dilated cardiomyopathy with accompanying systolic dysfunction (see Table 53-5).[75,77] Aortic dissection has also been reported.[75] Intravenous use of cocaine and other injectable drugs increases the risk for development of infective endocarditis. Noncardiogenic pulmonary edema, pulmonary hypertension, and right heart failure can also occur in the setting of cocaine abuse.[9,77]

The **neurologic** complications of cocaine may be transient or permanent. Morbidity and mortality may result from subarachnoid hemorrhage, intracerebral hemorrhage, cerebral vasculitis, and/or transient ischemic attacks.[12,98,99] Many cocaine-abusing patients in whom cerebral infarct(s) and hemorrhage developed had additional risk factors for stroke, including hypertension, alcohol abuse, and smoking. Cocaine-induced seizures, when they are self-limited, are typically treated with supportive care and benzodiazepines, if needed.[98]

Respiratory complications occur in 25% of cocaine users. As with tobacco, smoking cocaine can have profound respiratory effects, which include bronchospasm, chronic cough, and diffusion capacity abnormalities.[83,100] Cocaine-abusing parturients are at increased risk for peripartum wheezing.[12] Inhaled cocaine vapor can produce thermal burns throughout the patient's airway. "Snorting" cocaine can lead to epistaxis, oral ulcers, and nasal septal injury.[77] The intense pulmonary and bronchial arterial vasoconstriction produced by cocaine can cause interstitial and alveolar hemorrhage. Pneumothorax, pneumomediastinum, and pneumopericardium have also been reported.[77]

Cocaine ingestion can result in serious **gastrointestinal** complications, such as ischemia, ulceration, and perforation.[83] In addition, cocaine's anticholinergic effects include delayed gastric emptying and an increased risk of aspiration.[77] Although some cocaine users have abnormal liver enzyme levels, cocaine is not clearly hepatotoxic.[83]

Hematologic consequences of cocaine exposure during pregnancy may include thrombocytopenia.[101,102] Cocaine-induced thrombocytopenia has a clinical course similar to that of idiopathic thrombocytopenic purpura, with platelet counts normalizing after termination of drug exposure, therapy with corticosteroids, and, in one published case, splenectomy.[102] Kain et al.[101] examined the prevalence of cocaine-associated thrombocytopenia in an inner-city obstetric hospital; the rate of thrombocytopenia was higher in the cocaine group than in the drug-free group (6.7% versus 1.5%, respectively), even when human immunodeficiency virus (HIV)–positive patients were excluded. However, Gershon et al.[103] compared the platelet count measurements in a group of more than 7000 pregnant patients, 671 of whom tested positive for cocaine; only 2.5% of the cocaine-positive women had a platelet count lower than 140,000/mm^3, compared with 4.7% in the cocaine-negative group.

Renal failure can result from cocaine abuse on the basis of rhabdomyolysis, renal infarction, and impaired immunologic function.[77] Cocaine-abusing patients have a higher prevalence of syphilis, HIV infection, and other **infectious diseases** compared with non–cocaine-using patients, even after controlling for intravenous drug abuse.[83,104] Studies of the **endocrine system** in gravid ewes have shown that cocaine exposure results in increases in maternal adrenocorticotropic hormone and cortisol as well as maternal and fetal plasma glucose and lactate.[105,106]

Cocaine also impairs cutaneous vasodilation and sweating. The lethal effects of cocaine are related, in part, to the drug's tendency to produce **hyperthermia,** particularly in hot weather.[107]

In summary, cocaine use has been associated with **sudden death** from a variety of factors, including cardiac arrhythmias, respiratory arrest, status epilepticus, and impaired thermoregulation.

Cocaine withdrawal can be difficult to recognize because its signs and symptoms are nonspecific; they consist of a prolonged sleep phase followed by hunger, anxiety, weakness, headaches, tremors, and seizures (see Table 53-6).[28] Recommended therapy involves supportive care, and re-introduction of the drug, if necessary, followed by a slow taper of the dose over days to weeks.[28]

EFFECTS ON PREGNANCY AND THE FETUS

Pregnant women metabolize cocaine to norcocaine to a greater extent than their nonpregnant counterparts, exposing both mother and fetus to this more potent metabolite.[76,81] Cocaine has a low molecular weight and high lipophilicity, and it is mostly un-ionized at physiologic pH; thus, it readily crosses the placenta.[12,76]

Woods et al.[108] demonstrated that cocaine increases both heart rate and myocardial oxygen consumption and decreases cardiac output to a greater extent in gravid ewes than in nonpregnant ewes. Cocaine also increases maternal blood pressure and decreases uterine blood flow in gravid ewes.[109]

Obstetric complications associated with maternal cocaine use include a higher incidence of placental abruption and preterm labor; the latter occurs in 17% to 29% of women who use cocaine.[110] IUGR and LBW occur in 25% to 48% of all infants exposed to cocaine *in utero*.[76] Kuhn et al.[111] found that heavier, but not lighter, use of cocaine, together with exposure late in pregnancy, was associated with IUGR.

One study noted that the most common indications for cesarean delivery in cocaine-abusing patients were fetal compromise (48%) and placental abruption (21%); in contrast, the most common indications for cesarean delivery in a drug-free control group were failed progress of labor and a request for repeat cesarean delivery.[12] Acute cocaine toxicity can mimic preeclampsia or eclampsia when pregnant women present with hypertension, headache, blurred vision, and/or seizures.[112] In one case series, cocaine-induced changes were distinguished through a positive test result for cocaine, the presence of normal laboratory measurements, and rapid resolution of symptoms in the absence of delivery.

The impact of maternal use of cocaine (particularly "crack") on the fetus has been the subject of intense legal, political, and scientific debate since the 1980s.[113] Animal data and retrospective human studies have suggested an increased risk of major congenital anomalies such as genitourinary and abdominal wall defects in fetuses exposed to cocaine. However, these reports are confounded by concurrent use of other drugs and low statistical power.[114] Two studies found no significant difference in type or number of congenital anomalies between infants who had and those who had not been exposed to cocaine, after accounting for confounding variables.[78,115]

Frank et al.[116] reviewed studies published between 1984 and 2000 to assess the possible relationships between maternal cocaine use during pregnancy and childhood outcome. After controlling the data for possible confounding factors, these investigators found no consistent negative association between intrauterine cocaine exposure and physical growth, developmental test scores within the first 6 years of life, or the presence of expressive or receptive language skills. They observed less optimal motor performance up to 7 months of age, but after this age, these effects did not appear to persist. They also indicated that there were insufficient data to comment on cocaine's effects on developmental scores in infants born preterm.[116]

Subsequently, Mayes et al.[117] examined the trajectories of motor and mental development between the ages of 3 and 36 months in an impoverished high-risk population. These authors found (1) a general decline (compared with age-adjusted equivalents) in motor performance for these high-risk children and a trend toward a greater decrease in performance in cocaine-exposed children; (2) a decline in performance on mental tasks until 24 months, with a similar trajectory of decline for the cocaine-exposed and non–cocaine-exposed cohorts; and (3) evidence of lower mental performance in cocaine-exposed children compared with non–cocaine-exposed children at all assessment ages.[117] Messinger et al.[118] studied high-risk infants and found that prenatal exposure to cocaine (and opiates) was not associated with motor, mental, or behavioral deficits after data were controlled for covariables. Lumeng et al.[119] examined physical growth patterns, excluding children with fetal alcohol syndrome identified at birth;

intrauterine cocaine exposure affected infant weight, height, and head circumference at birth, but "catch-up" growth in cocaine-exposed infants occurred by 6 months for all of these parameters.

Bauer et al.[78] found that infectious complications, such as hepatitis, syphilis, and, to a lesser extent, HIV infection, were significantly more common in infants of cocaine-abusing mothers. Finally, Bae and Zhang[120] used a rat model to show that prenatal cocaine exposure induced abnormal apoptosis and myocyte hypertrophy in the post-natal heart, which might result in greater susceptibility to myocardial ischemia and reperfusion injury.

ANESTHETIC MANAGEMENT

Cocaine-abusing patients are at risk for acute and chronic multiorgan system dysfunction[104] and the need for urgent cesarean delivery. During labor, neuraxial anesthesia may be administered provided that the patient is cooperative, is able to protect her airway, and has a platelet count above the threshold of concern for the anesthesia provider.[79] The use of neuraxial anesthesia can reduce levels of circulating catecholamines and thereby may mitigate the systemic effects of cocaine.[12] Early administration of epidural analgesia is encouraged; existing epidural analgesia facilitates the extension to anesthesia for emergency cesarean delivery.

In one study, cocaine users had a greater incidence of hypotension during administration of epidural anesthesia for cesarean delivery; however, there was no difference between cocaine users and nonusers in the incidence of hypotension during spinal anesthesia.[12] Treatment of hypotension should include volume resuscitation, and, if needed, careful titration of vasopressors. Depending on the level of circulating catecholamines, cocaine-intoxicated patients can be either more or less responsive to ephedrine; thus, phenylephrine may be a better choice for treatment of hypotension.[16,79]

Jatlow et al.[121] found that subjects who were presumed to be homozygous for atypical cholinesterase on the basis of a low dibucaine number and a history of prolonged apnea after succinylcholine administration had impaired ability to metabolize cocaine *in vitro*. When an ester local anesthetic or succinylcholine is administered to a patient who has ingested cocaine, the medication might compete with cocaine for available plasma cholinesterase.[12,81] Kain et al.[12] described a prolonged response to succinylcholine in a parturient who had abused cocaine chronically and had a normal dibucaine number but a low level of pseudocholinesterase.

Changes in μ- and κ-opioid receptors and altered baseline endorphin levels may result in an increased perception of pain in cocaine-abusing patients, despite the presence of an apparently satisfactory level of neuraxial anesthesia.[13] Ross et al.[122] observed a reduction in duration of intrathecal sufentanil analgesia during labor in cocaine-abusing women, although the quality of analgesia was not diminished.

If general anesthesia is required, premedication with a benzodiazepine may help attenuate the acute physiologic effects of cocaine.[9] The anticholinergic effects of cocaine can delay gastric emptying and subsequently increase the risk of aspiration; pharmacologic prophylaxis and a rapid-sequence induction of general anesthesia are indicated. Ketamine should be avoided; anesthetic agents that sensitize the myocardium to catecholamines (e.g., halothane) should also be avoided.[79,81] Cocaine-abusing patients who receive general anesthesia are at greater risk for hypertension and tachycardia during and after laryngoscopy and endotracheal intubation.[12,13] Some authorities advocate pretreatment with a benzodiazepine, an opioid, and/or nitroglycerin.[9,79]

Despite the risk of altered metabolism of succinylcholine (see earlier), a standard intubating dose of succinylcholine should be administered.[79] Early studies in dogs demonstrated that acute cocaine intoxication was associated with a dose-dependent increase in halothane dose requirements.[123]

Cocaine can cause hyperthermia in both laboratory animals and humans[77,107]; core temperature should be monitored in cocaine-abusing patients. However, given the propensity for nasal septal defects in such patients, temperature probes (and other tubes and monitors) should *not* be inserted intranasally. Measures that provide active warming should be used only if needed.

Amphetamines

Owing to their high potential for abuse, amphetamines have been categorized by the U.S. Drug Enforcement Agency as schedule II stimulants since 1971.[70] Methamphetamine is thought to be the most widely abused amphetamine.[70]

EPIDEMIOLOGY

A 2005 survey estimated that 4.3% of the U.S. population 12 years or older have used methamphetamine at some point in their lives.[124] In 2006, there were a reported 259,000 new users.[24] Arria et al.[70] observed that 5.2% of high-risk pregnant women had used methamphetamine at some time during pregnancy. Polydrug use in women who use methamphetamine and 3,4-methylenedioxymethamphetamine (MDMA; ecstasy) appears to be common.[70,125] Amphetamines have been prescribed as components of nasal decongestants, bronchodilators, weight loss drugs, and therapies for narcolepsy and attention deficit-hyperactivity disorder (ADHD).[124]

PHARMACOLOGY

Amphetamines (and related compounds) are amines that exist as either salts of various acids or free bases. Used illicitly, they can be ingested orally, inhaled, or, less commonly, injected, resulting in significant CNS penetration.[27] The plasma half-life ranges from 5 to 30 hours. Metabolism is variable; up to 30% of the parent compound can be found in the urine. Detection of these compounds and their metabolites in the urine may be feasible up to several days after ingestion.[9]

Methamphetamine ("speed" or "crystal meth") is a congener of amphetamine that contains a methyl radical.[70] This white, odorless, bitter-tasting powder can be smoked, snorted, ingested orally, or administered rectally.[125] Methamphetamine is more potent than amphetamine and has a longer half-life; 50% of the drug is cleared in 12 hours. When it is smoked or injected intravenously, the "flash" from this drug is intense and of short duration. Snorting produces euphoria within 5 minutes, and oral ingestion does so within 20 minutes.[124]

The amphetamine analogue, MDMA, has been steadily growing in popularity, particularly in young women.[126] The methylenedioxy group that is attached to the aromatic ring of the amphetamine molecule confers some of the pharmacologic hallucinogenic effects.[127] The effects of MDMA typically begin approximately 20 minutes after ingestion and last approximately 6 hours; large doses have effects for up to 2 days. MDMA is metabolized by the liver and is then excreted by the kidneys.[9]

SYSTEMIC EFFECTS

Acute amphetamine ingestion leads to indirect sympathetic activation through the release of norepinephrine, dopamine, and serotonin from adrenergic nerve terminals (see Table 53-4).[9,128] The physiologic effects of amphetamines are similar to those of cocaine, with the following two important differences: (1) amphetamines and their derivatives lack local anesthetic properties, and (2) amphetamine can inhibit monoamine oxidase activity, leading to decreased degradation of catecholamines.[9]

Long-term use of high doses of amphetamines has a number of adverse maternal effects, including damage to the cardiovascular and neurologic systems, and behavioral changes such as hostility, violence, hallucinations, and paranoid psychosis (see Table 53-5).[125]

The **cardiovascular** effects of amphetamines and their derivatives are similar to those of cocaine.[9] Methamphetamine has a much longer duration of action than cocaine, because a smaller fraction of the former drug is metabolized.[124] Drug-induced effects include vasoconstriction, tachycardia, and labile blood pressure[28]; patients typically become hypertensive, although catecholamine depletion over time can result in hypotension.[9] Arrhythmias, myocardial ischemia, endothelial damage, and acceleration of atherosclerosis can also occur. Recommendations for the management of cardiovascular complications are similar to those previously described for cocaine toxicity.[9]

The pleasurable effects of methamphetamine and the deleterious **neurologic** sequelae are thought to be the result of high levels of dopamine in the brain. In addition to the positive feelings of well-being,[124] patients who have taken methamphetamine may experience anxiety, mood disturbances, paranoia, and hallucinations.[10] Severe intracranial hypertension has been reported in the setting of acute abuse.[10] Long-time use has been associated with impairment of motor function and verbal learning as well as significant changes in the areas of the brain associated with memory and emotion (see Table 53-5).[124] Volkow et al.[129] observed that prolonged abstinence (12 to 17 months) resulted in significant recovery of brain dopamine transporters, although performance on neuropsychological tests did not improve to the same extent. In addition, psychotic features of long-time amphetamine use may be precipitated by stress in former users (after months or even years of abstinence).[124]

Psychostimulant withdrawal causes fatigue, depression, hunger, and intense cravings (see Table 53-6).[130] Among the medications that have been tried for treatment of stimulant withdrawal (e.g., tricyclic antidepressants, dopaminergic agents [e.g., bromocriptine], amino acid replacement therapy), none has been completely successful.[130] In the setting of methamphetamine overdose, the ensuing seizures, severe hypertension, and hyperthermia can be fatal. Treatment goals include provision of a calm environment (with or without a benzodiazepine) and airway protection. Active cooling, antihypertensives, and anticonvulsants should be used as needed.[124]

EFFECTS ON PREGNANCY AND THE FETUS

Ingestion of amphetamines results in high levels of circulating catecholamines, which may lead to vasoconstriction and decreased uteroplacental blood flow.[125,131] Animal studies have suggested that intrauterine exposure to methamphetamine is associated with an increased incidence of retinal defects, cleft palate, and rib malformations and a decreased overall rate of growth and motor development.[125] Human studies are limited by small sample sizes, and the results may be confounded by polysubstance abuse.[125,132] Oro and Dixon[131] examined neonates born with positive maternal or fetal toxicology results; neonates with intrauterine exposure to methamphetamine, cocaine, or both were smaller than those in a comparable, high-risk drug-free cohort. In addition, the cocaine/amphetamine group had higher rates of preterm delivery, retroplacental hemorrhage, and fetal compromise. Exposure to cocaine/amphetamine was associated with significant newborn neurologic derangements, including abnormal sleep patterns, tremors, poor feeding, sneezing, and high-pitched cry.

Cernerud et al.[133] conducted long-term follow-up of 65 Swedish children with intrauterine exposure to amphetamines; a higher percentage of these children were in a grade lower than their chronological age, and their performance on mathematics, language, and sports was significantly below that of their peers.

ANESTHETIC MANAGEMENT

Amphetamines cause (indirect) sympathetic activation; intoxicated patients are at risk for dangerous cardiovascular events, including hemodynamic instability and cardiac arrest during administration of anesthesia. Recommendations for management are similar to those for patients with cocaine toxicity (as discussed earlier).[9]

A cooperative patient may be a candidate for neuraxial analgesia/anesthesia. Refractory hypotension has been reported in a long-time amphetamine user undergoing neuraxial anesthesia with intravenous propofol sedation; it was thought to be a result of down-regulation of beta-adrenergic receptors and catecholamine depletion.[134] Phenylephrine may be a better choice than ephedrine for the treatment of hypotension in amphetamine-intoxicated patients.

Parturients who are amphetamine abusers may be at increased risk for urgent cesarean delivery requiring general anesthesia. Evidence suggests that acute ingestion of amphetamines increases the MAC for volatile halogenated anesthetic agents, whereas chronic ingestion of amphetamines decreases the MAC of volatile agents.[135,136] Johnston et al.[135] found that the acute intravenous administration of dextroamphetamine in dogs receiving halothane anesthesia was associated with a significant increase in MAC; these dogs also showed an increase in blood pressure and body temperature. In addition, dogs pretreated with amphetamine had a decreased duration of action of thiopental. In contrast, dogs chronically exposed to amphetamine had a decreased MAC of halothane.[135]

There is a well-recognized association between methamphetamine abuse and severe tooth decay (i.e., "meth mouth"), which may present a hazard during laryngoscopy. The preanesthesia airway assessment should include attention to the presence of fragile or loose teeth that might be dislodged during laryngoscopy.

Hallucinogens

LSD (lysergic acid diethylamide), PCP (phencyclidine), psilocybin, and mescaline are drugs of abuse that are considered to be hallucinogens.[130] 3,4-Methylenedioxymethamphetamine (MDMA) also has hallucinogenic effects.

EPIDEMIOLOGY

Hallucinogen use is usually episodic.[13,137] In 2006, 1.1 million Americans 12 years or older used hallucinogens for the first time; more than 75% of these encounters involved the hallucinogen MDMA.[124] The prevalence of hallucinogen use during pregnancy is unknown.

PHARMACOLOGY

These diverse drugs are notable for their complex mechanism of actions, which include agonist, partial agonist, and antagonist effects at serotonergic, dopaminergic, and adrenergic receptors.[9] Overall, the adrenergic effects of these drugs are mild compared with those of cocaine and amphetamine.

Both **psilocybin,** the hallucinogen in some wild mushrooms, and **LSD,** which is manufactured synthetically,[130] are indole derivatives that chemically resemble serotonin.[9] When ingested, they evoke auditory, visual, and tactile hallucinations. Clinical effects usually develop over 15 to 60 minutes and last for 6 to 12 hours.[13,130] LSD is 100 times more potent than psilocybin and can be detected in urine or plasma for up to 3 days. LSD is metabolized by the liver and has a plasma half-life of 100 minutes.[9] The potency of individual samples of psilocybin varies, although the physiologic effects typically occur at doses of 20 to 60 mg.[130] Animal studies indicate that 65% of psilocybin is excreted in urine and 15% to 20% is excreted in bile or feces. Most of the drug is excreted in the first 8 hours, although small amounts are excreted for up to a week.[130]

Phencyclidine, initially developed as a general anesthetic agent, was removed from the legal market in 1978. **Ketamine,** a related compound, is a clinically used anesthetic agent that is also a drug of abuse.[130] In powder form, these drugs can be ingested orally, intranasally, intravenously, or rectally, and can be smoked. The psychological effects of PCP typically last 12 to 48 hours. Ketamine has a shorter duration of action.[130]

The phenethylamines include MDMA (as discussed earlier) and mescaline. **Mescaline,** the active ingredient in peyote cactus buttons, is typically eaten or drunk as a tea.[130] The effects of mescaline include visual hallucinations, nausea, and vomiting and typically last approximately 12 hours.[130]

SYSTEMIC EFFECTS

Ingestion of hallucinogens causes **activation of the sympathetic nervous system,** which results in hypertension, tachycardia, dilated pupils, and increased core body temperature (see Table 53-4).[13] The cardiovascular effects of these drugs are rarely serious, although some instances of supraventricular tachycardia and acute myocardial infarction have been reported. Myocardial infarction may result from vasospasm and increased platelet aggregation.[9]

Carotid artery occlusion has been reported following the use of LSD. Use of PCP has been associated with seizures, delayed hypertensive crisis, and intracerebral hemorrhage.[10] Overdose with PCP can be associated with confusion and combativeness, which may progress to seizures and catatonia.

Some users of LSD experience a "bad trip," which is likely to be a manifestation of an acute anxiety reaction. Other users report "flashbacks" of systemic effects of these drugs that occur months or even years after ingestion; some of these episodes are believed to be related to delayed release of small amounts of drug from fatty tissues. The use of LSD may unmask an underlying psychiatric disorder in some vulnerable patients.[130]

The psychological effects of psilocybin ("magic mushrooms") include giddiness, visual hallucinations, and gastrointestinal dysfunction. Morbidity is associated primarily with inadvertent ingestion of toxic species of mushrooms.[130] Although psychological dependence on these drugs has been observed, no clearly associated withdrawal symptoms occur with abstinence (see Table 53-6).[13]

A direct causal relationship between abuse of these drugs and death has not been documented; however, hallucinogens can cause feelings of paranoia and panic that can lead to accidents or fatalities.[10,13]

EFFECTS ON PREGNANCY AND THE FETUS

There is conflicting evidence as to whether intrauterine PCP exposure has deleterious fetal effects. Mvula et al.[138] found that PCP-positive women had smaller and more preterm infants compared with non–PCP-positive women. The PCP-positive women were also more likely to have syphilis and diabetes and to use tobacco, alcohol, and marijuana. Early reports of chromosomal damage secondary to LSD were not confirmed by later studies.[10]

ANESTHETIC MANAGEMENT

Management of a hallucinogen-intoxicated patient is primarily supportive and noninterventional.[9] Stressful situations can provoke panic attacks, which in turn can intensify the physiologic effects of these drugs. Specific recommendations include provision of a quiet, supportive environment and administration of a benzodiazepine if needed.[9,13] Neuroleptic medications are relatively contraindicated in such a patient, because they can intensify toxic reactions.[9]

Hemodynamic perturbations are usually relatively mild and well tolerated. Occasionally patients experience supraventricular tachycardia, hypertension, or myocardial ischemia.[9] If hypotension requiring vasopressor therapy occurs, the acutely intoxicated patient may have an exaggerated response to ephedrine[13]; phenylephrine may be preferable and should be titrated to effect. LSD may have some intrinsic anticholinesterase activity, but the clinical significance is unclear.

Either neuraxial or general anesthesia can be administered for vaginal or cesarean delivery as the clinical situation warrants.

Opioids

Opioids refer to the class of naturally occurring and synthetic drugs that are structurally and functionally related to morphine. The term *opiate* specifically describes any of the narcotic alkaloids found in the juice of poppy plants, including morphine and codeine.[27]

EPIDEMIOLOGY

The estimated prevalence of opioid use during pregnancy varies from 1.6% to 7.2%, depending on the methodology used and the population studied.[7] The National Survey on Drug Use and Health[24] estimated that more than 300,000 Americans 12 or older used heroin in 2006, including approximately 90,000 who used it for the first time that year. Between 2002 and 2004, an estimated 6.0% of pregnant women reported the nonmedical use of prescription drugs; more than two thirds of these women were using pain relievers such as oxycodone.[139]

PHARMACOLOGY

The naturally occurring opioids are metabolized first to morphine,[27] which has a plasma half-life of 2 to 3 hours. Morphine then undergoes rapid metabolism in the liver and is excreted in the urine, where both active and inactive metabolites can be detected for up to 2 days in occasional users, and longer in chronic users.[9,27]

Heroin (diacetylmorphine or diamorphine), a commonly abused semisynthetic analogue of morphine, is highly addictive and can be smoked, snorted, or injected intravenously or intramuscularly.[9,27,140] Most fatal overdoses occur in users of intravenous heroin.[140] The speed of onset varies from less than 1 minute to 15 minutes, depending on the delivery method; the elimination half-life is typically 1 to 2 hours. Heroin is metabolized by the liver and excreted in the urine.[9,27,28,140] The formulation of street heroin has become increasingly pure. In 1990, a typical 100-mg bag of powder had up to 8 mg of heroin mixed with inert, often toxic additives; subsequently the drug has become available with a purity as high as 45% to 90%. Heroin is more lipid soluble than other opioids; thus it rapidly crosses the blood-brain barrier and has significant and toxic CNS effects.[140]

Rapidly acting semisynthetic opioids such as **oxycodone** and **hydrocodone** have become available for both legitimate prescribed use and illicit distribution. The oral bioavailability of oxycodone is higher than that of morphine, and its potency, with oral ingestion, is greater.[27]

Methadone is a synthetic compound that is structurally unrelated to the other opioids but has similar effects.[27,141] It is formulated as a racemic mixture of two enantiomers: R-methadone, which is a potent μ- and δ-opioid receptor agonist, and S-methadone, which is a noncompetitive *N*-methyl-D-aspartate (NMDA) antagonist that prevents the reuptake of 5-hydroxytryptamine and norepinephrine.[142] Typically available in powder form, methadone can be reconstituted for oral, rectal, or intravenous use.[143] Bioavailability of methadone (ingested orally) is typically three times that of morphine.[142,143] There is significant interindividual variability in its clinical effect and duration of action; when methadone is taken orally, its peak effect occurs at roughly 3 hours, and its half-life varies from 15 to 40 hours.[27,28,139,142-144] Because of its long elimination half-life, life-threatening complications may result from the cumulative effects of successive doses.[142]

Unlike morphine, methadone undergoes biotransformation (rather than conjugation) in the liver and is excreted primarily by the fecal route.[142] Methadone has been used since the 1960s for stabilization and maintenance therapy for patients suffering from opioid-addictive disorders, and since the 1970s for the same reason in pregnant patients.[144] It is also used for analgesic therapy in patients with chronic pain.[142] Pregnancy is associated with greater methadone metabolism and reduced methadone bioavailability because of greater maternal blood volume and changes in hepatic enzymatic activity and glomerular filtration rate.[27,144,145]

SYSTEMIC EFFECTS

Opioids mimic the activity of endogenous peptides and exert their effects through binding to μ-, δ-, and κ-opioid receptors. Morphine and heroin exert their euphoric, analgesic, and reinforcing effects primarily through stimulation of the μ receptors. Long-time opioid use causes neuroadaptations in the brain that may explain the manifestations of withdrawal.[27,140]

Opioids act in the CNS to reduce sympathetic activity and increase parasympathetic activity; these compounds also promote histamine release from mast cells. The resulting cardiovascular effects include bradycardia, hypotension, and, in some cases, potentially lethal tachyarrhythmias and bradyarrhythmias (see Table 53-4).[9] Noncardiogenic pulmonary edema has been observed in some cases of overdose and is believed to be caused by hypoxia, intense pulmonary vasoconstriction, and, perhaps, the use of reversal agents.[9]

Opioid-induced respiratory depression occurs through a direct effect on the brainstem that reduces the ventilatory response to hypercarbia.[140] Opioid overdose can progress from miosis and respiratory depression to obtundation and death.[10,14] Treatment of overdose includes maintenance of a patent and protected airway, provision of hemodynamic support, and, if necessary, administration of an opioid antagonist (e.g., naloxone).[9]

Women who abuse opioids or other drugs intravenously are at risk for infective endocarditis (usually right-sided valves), HIV infection, viral hepatitis, septic emboli, and pulmonary abscess formation.[9,28] In addition, hilar adenopathy may develop as a result of ingestion of additives such as quinine and starch.

Animal studies have found an association between opioid administration and abnormal pain sensitivity, including hyperalgesia and allodynia (see Table 53-5).[146] Patients receiving methadone maintenance therapy often have diminished pain tolerance.[147] Opioid tolerance develops with chronic use and is related to duration and amount of drug exposure; tolerance results from changes in drug distribution and metabolism (pharmacokinetics) and in receptor density and activity (pharmacodynamics).[141]

Acute opioid withdrawal results from sympathetic hyperactivity, resulting in flu-like signs and symptoms such as fatigue, weakness, restlessness, rhinorrhea, perspiration, fever, and diarrhea (see Table 53-6).[10,28] These systemic effects can persist for several days if not treated. The onset and duration of withdrawal symptoms vary according to the opioid ingested; morphine or heroin withdrawal is associated with symptoms that begin within 6 to 18 hours after the last dose, reach their peak intensity by 3 days, and last for 7 to 10 days. Methadone withdrawal symptoms are delayed— with an onset within 24 to 48 hours, a peak intensity within 3 to 21 days, and duration of up to 6 to 7 weeks.[141] Clonidine, an alpha$_2$-adrenergic agonist, can modulate symptoms of withdrawal, although postural hypotension may result.[28] Doxepin, a tricyclic antidepressant that inhibits the reuptake of serotonin and noradrenaline, has also been administered in this setting. Acute withdrawal can also be treated by administration of an opioid and institution of a gradual dose taper.[13]

Substitution pharmacology (e.g., **methadone maintenance therapy**) has been recommended for the treatment of opioid dependency if abstinence is not attainable and withdrawal is not feasible.[6,116,144] Typically, long-acting μ agonists (e.g., methadone) or partial agonists (e.g., buprenorphine) are substituted for the opioid of abuse in combination with behavioral modification therapy. Drug maintenance therapy decreases withdrawal symptoms and attenuates both craving and the positive rewards associated with subsequent opioid use.[6,116]

The U.S. Food and Drug Administration (FDA) guidelines for methadone administration in pregnancy were developed in 1970.[6,144] Subsequently, a number of studies have shown that methadone maintenance therapy in heroin-addicted pregnant women is beneficial for both the mother and the infant.[148] Specific benefits include better medical and prenatal care,[148] a lower incidence of unplanned pregnancies,[149] decreased neonatal abstinence symptoms and days of hospitalization,[143,145] and less maternal illicit drug use at delivery.[145]

McCarthy et al.[145] compared the effect of higher doses of methadone ($\geq$ 100 mg/day) with lower doses of methadone ($<$ 100 mg/day) in pregnant women; there was no difference in the rate of medical therapy for neonatal abstinence symptoms or days of infant hospitalization, and the high-dose mothers had less illicit drug use at delivery.

Hulse et al.[150] evaluated obstetric and neonatal outcomes in 17 pregnant women managed with naltrexone implant treatment and in 90 women who were managed with methadone maintenance. Mean gestational age and birth weight did not differ between groups, although the methadone group had higher proportions of deliveries before 37 weeks' gestation and LBW infants, in comparison with Australian national data.

Hensel et al.[151] described an ultrarapid opioid detoxification protocol involving the administration of naltrexone (via a nasogastric tube) to opiate-addicted, nonpregnant patients receiving general endotracheal anesthesia (propofol infusion) in an intensive care unit. They observed minor instances of bradycardia and hypotension, but no major anesthetic complications occurred. The application of this technique to pregnant patients has not been described.

EFFECTS ON PREGNANCY AND THE FETUS

Heroin use during pregnancy is associated with first-trimester spontaneous abortion, preterm delivery, and IUGR, in part as a result of poor maternal nutrition.[6,143,148,152] Maternal and neonatal infection and neonatal abstinence syndrome have also been described.[6,152] **Neonatal abstinence syndrome,** which occurs in neonates repeatedly exposed to opioids *in utero*, is characterized by irritability, poor feeding, abnormal sleep patterns, diarrhea, fever, and seizures. Affected neonates may also have autonomic symptoms such as yawning and mottling. If prolonged and untreated, neonatal abstinence syndrome can result in death.[6] Children born to women using heroin or methadone have been found to have normal development at the time of entry into school.[6]

ANESTHETIC MANAGEMENT

Opioid-dependent patients may have end-organ damage and infectious diseases, and may exhibit opioid tolerance, physical dependence, and withdrawal.[141] Evidence suggests that opioid-addicted patients are more likely to report inadequate analgesia during labor, vaginal or cesarean delivery, and postpartum.[153]

Preanesthesia Assessment and Communication

Establishing trust and effective communication is critical in the care of methadone-maintained or opioid-addicted patients, and may improve the ability to elicit a more complete drug history. Ideally, before the patient presents for delivery, a thorough anesthesia consultation, which incorporates a mutually agreeable strategy for pain management and appropriate goals for pain intensity scores, should be conducted. Patient monitoring (e.g., drug screens, pill counts) may be necessary.[141]

Opioid Maintenance Requirements

Opioids used on a regular basis for chronic pain or methadone maintenance should be continued, with additional therapies added for acute pain as needed. As the analgesic conversion of methadone to equipotent forms of opioids may not be predictable, it is prudent to continue the current methadone dose regimen during and after hospitalization.[116,141-143] The precise dose of methadone prescribed should be confirmed with the dispenser, because improper dosing can result in inadequate analgesia, withdrawal phenomena, or life-threatening overdose.[142]

When these patients present in labor, they may have recently ingested opioids illicitly, sometimes in addition to methadone maintenance therapy. Although the precise calculation of these patients' long-term requirements is usually not feasible, knowledge of the potential implications of their drug use, adequate treatment of withdrawal, and use of additional resources such as social and addiction services may improve care.

Alterations of Drug Levels

Sedative medications can increase the depressant effects of chronically ingested opioids. Methadone has a long half-life and is metabolized by cytochrome P-450; thus women receiving methadone are particularly vulnerable to changes in metabolism that result from administration of other medications. Anticonvulsants (e.g., phenobarbital, phenytoin) increase methadone clearance, and selective serotonin reuptake inhibitors decrease it. Methadone dose requirements are typically established by titrating to effect; thus the discontinuation of these other medications can have unintended consequences.[141]

Opioid Antagonists and Mixed Agonists/Antagonists

The use of opioid antagonists (e.g., naloxone, naltrexone) and mixed agonists/antagonists (e.g., nalbuphine) in opioid-using patients is considered to be appropriate in only two circumstances: (1) in the acutely intoxicated patient who is unresponsive and (2) in the addicted patient who is undergoing detoxification under direct supervision of a physician. (With the exception of an ultrarapid detoxification regimen, detoxification often involves slow titration of an opioid antagonist to minimize withdrawal signs and symptoms.) Otherwise the use of opioid antagonists is relatively contraindicated, because they may precipitate severe withdrawal symptoms.[141]

Mixed agonists/antagonists (e.g., nalbuphine) are commonly employed for labor analgesia or treatment of neuraxial opioid-induced pruritus in patients *without* a history of opioid abuse. These agents should be *avoided* in patients with a history of opioid abuse. Thus it is important to identify patients at risk for opioid withdrawal.

Potential Relapse

Providers, family, and patients often express concern that exposing a previously addicted patient to opioids or other sedatives will prompt cravings or a frank relapse. However, anxiety and pain have also been identified as precipitants of relapse[116]; therefore withholding appropriate analgesic and anxiolytic medications from such a patient cannot be justified.

Anesthetic Technique and Dose Requirements

In a review of publications on opioid-dependent parturients, Cassidy and Cyna[153] catalogued the needs of this patient population across a broad range of anesthetic techniques and modes of delivery. They found no significant difference in the proportion of opioid-dependent women who required general anesthesia for cesarean delivery or the number who requested labor epidural analgesia in comparison with non–opioid-dependent women. However, a significant incidence of pain management problems was observed, particularly after cesarean delivery; 26% of the patients required consultation for inpatient pain management in addition to usual labor analgesia, and 74% of the patients had difficulties with post–cesarean delivery analgesia. These patients also presented significant vascular access problems and generated more emergency calls for fainting and collapse.

Neuraxial analgesia or anesthesia is the technique of choice for a methadone-maintained or other opioid-addicted patient undergoing vaginal or cesarean delivery, assuming that the patient is cooperative and has no evidence of coagulopathy. Meyer et al.[149] specifically investigated whether pregnant women who received methadone maintenance therapy differed from matched controls in intrapartum or postpartum analgesic requirements. The two groups had similar pain scores and analgesia requirements during labor, but the methadone-maintained patients required 70% more opioid analgesia after cesarean delivery.

Providers should not assume that the etiology of inadequate pain relief is solely a result of the patient's addiction. Opioid-addicted patients can have objectively inadequate (failed) neuraxial analgesia and anesthesia just like their nonaddicted counterparts.

If neuraxial techniques are contraindicated for labor, intravenous patient-controlled analgesia (PCA) can be employed. Patients who use either physician-prescribed or illicit opioids over the long term demonstrate a relative insensitivity to opioids. Their opioid dose requirements for intraoperative and postoperative analgesia may be 30% to 100% higher than those of opioid-naive patients.[141] It is important to administer the parturient's baseline opioid requirements to avoid opioid withdrawal, and to provide additional analgesia for treatment of acute pain.

During administration of general anesthesia for cesarean delivery, the anesthesia provider should consider the potential for decreased MAC in a patient with acute opioid intoxication as well as the potential for cross-tolerance with CNS depressants in a patient with a history of long-time opioid use.[13]

Postpartum Analgesia

In one study, methadone-maintained women had higher pain scores but did not receive higher doses of opioids after vaginal delivery. However, methadone-maintained women had higher pain scores and did receive higher doses of opioids after cesarean delivery.[149] Multimodal therapy, including nonsteroidal anti-inflammatory drugs (NSAIDs), is recommended for post–cesarean delivery analgesia.[141]

Solvents

Solvents are a chemically diverse group of readily available substances (e.g., toluene, ethylene glycol) that can be sniffed, aerosolized, or ingested to produce feelings of euphoria, excitement, and invulnerability.[9,154,155]

EPIDEMIOLOGY

In 2006 an estimated 783,000 individuals in the United States used an inhalant for the first time.[24] The prevalence of solvent abuse in pregnant patients has not been reported.

PHARMACOLOGY

Inhalants are quickly absorbed through the lungs and typically are rapidly metabolized in the liver. The precise mechanism of action of inhalants is variable and is not completely understood.

Detection, though difficult, can be facilitated by the presence of the "glue sniffer's" facial rash[28] or the odor of the abused inhalant.[155] Laboratory assays can detect many solvents in the blood within 10 hours of exposure; urine assays are available only for certain volatile substances (e.g., toluene, chlorinated solvents) but may provide a longer window of detection.[9]

Ethylene glycol, a bittersweet-tasting component of antifreeze, brake fluids, and industrial solvents, is sometimes ingested by substance-abusing adults as an inexpensive substitute for alcohol. Readily absorbed via the gastrointestinal tract with ingestion, this solvent reaches maximal blood concentrations within 1 to 4 hours. It is metabolized by the hepatic enzyme alcohol dehydrogenase to four toxic organic acids.[156] The primary screening test findings for ethylene glycol intoxication include serum anion-gap metabolic acidosis, high urine osmolality with an osmol gap, and the presence of calcium oxylate crystals in the urine.[156,157]

SYSTEMIC EFFECTS

Typically the user of inhalants feels an initial sense of euphoria followed by a brief period of disinhibition and impulsivity.[155] Intoxication can be prolonged through repeated inhalation of the solvent. As the dose increases, dizziness, diplopia, and disorientation manifest, followed by headache, drowsiness, and sleep.[155]

Mucous membrane irritation often occurs and can result in rhinorrhea, epistaxis, excessive salivation, and conjunctival redness. Gastrointestinal symptoms, such as nausea, vomiting, and diarrhea, can also be seen.[155] Ingestion of volatile substances can lead to potentially lethal tachyarrhythmias, likely secondary to sympathetic stimulation, or bradyarrhythmias, which are believed to occur from decreased sinoatrial node automaticity or direct vagal stimulation and myocardial depression (see Table 53-4).[9] Hypoxemia may occur as a result of formation of carboxyhemoglobinemia, methemoglobinemia, or suffocation.[9,155,158]

Chronic inhalant abuse can result in multiorgan system disease, with **cardiac** (cardiomyopathy, arrhythmias, myocardial infarction), **pulmonary** (wheezing, acute respiratory distress syndrome, pulmonary hypertension), **central and peripheral nervous system** (cognitive impairment, ataxia, muscle weakness, peripheral neuropathy), and **autonomic dysfunction** (see Table 53-5).[9,10] Renal toxicity, aplastic anemia, and hepatocellular carcinoma have also been reported.[130,155] Imaging studies have demonstrated loss of brain mass, white matter degeneration, and subcortical abnormalities in long-term users.[155,158] Significant methemoglobinemia with attendant cyanosis can also occur from exposure to some compounds.[9,155,158]

Cessation of chronic use can lead to reversal of many of the pathophysiologic changes, although the CNS effects may persist. Death from inhalant use typically occurs from suffocation, aspiration, or accidental injury. **Sudden sniffing death syndrome,** thought to be secondary to a fatal arrhythmia in the setting of a sensitized myocardium, electrolyte abnormalities, and hypoxemia, has been reported in both new and long-term users.[155]

Ingestion of ethylene glycol has inebriating effects similar to those of alcohol (see earlier), with more devastating consequences. Accumulation of the toxic metabolite glycolic acid occurs, resulting in CNS depression and seizure activity. Cardiopulmonary manifestations are often delayed (12 to 24 hours after ingestion) and may be fatal. If the patient survives, she will likely experience **renal failure** 24 to 72 hours after ingestion.[156] The estimated lethal dose of undiluted ethylene glycol is 1.4 mL/kg.[156] The treatment of ethylene glycol ingestion can require the induction of emesis with ipecac in the alert and awake patient, or the use of gastric lavage.[156] The conversion of ethylene glycol to its toxic metabolites can be prevented with the use of the antidote **fomepizole** or **ethanol**. (Alcohol dehydrogenase has 100 times greater affinity for ethanol than for ethylene glycol.) Hemodialysis may be warranted.

EFFECTS ON PREGNANCY AND THE FETUS

Solvent abuse has been associated with IUGR, preterm delivery, and perinatal mortality.[13] Babies born of inhalant-abusing women exhibit abstinence syndrome symptoms, including excessive and high-pitched crying, sleep disorders, CNS irritability, and poor feeding.[159] Phenobarbital can be somewhat effective in ameliorating these manifestations.[159]

Kralova et al.[157] reported a case in which ethylene glycol intoxication was misdiagnosed as eclampsia when the patient presented at 26 weeks' gestation with hypertension and seizures followed by coma. After an emergency cesarean delivery, her postoperative course was complicated by hemodynamic instability, severe metabolic acidosis, and acute renal failure, which prompted suspicion of substance intoxication. Toxicology investigation confirmed ethylene glycol poisoning. Subsequently, the patient was successfully treated with hemodialysis and intravenous ethanol; her newborn was treated with diuresis and replacement transfusion. Prior to discharge, the mother admitted that she had ingested 400 mL of ethylene glycol.

ANESTHETIC MANAGEMENT

Identification of solvent abuse in the parturient is critical to safe anesthetic care.[30,158] If inhalation abuse is suspected, then the parturient's skin and clothing should be decontaminated.[155] A careful physical examination, including documentation of preexisting sensory or motor deficits, should be undertaken.[13] Electrolyte abnormalities should be identified early and corrected as necessary.

If the patient is cooperative and able to protect her airway, neuraxial labor analgesia can be administered. It may be prudent to avoid administration of an epinephrine-containing local anesthetic solution, given the risk for arrhythmias in these patients. The treatment of hypotension should include the use of intravenous fluids and small doses of phenylephrine (which may cause bradycardia) or ephedrine (which may cause tachycardia). Atropine should be readily available but used with caution.[9] In stable patients with sustained tachyarrhythmias, beta-adrenergic receptor antagonists should be the first line of therapy.[9]

In intoxicated or otherwise uncooperative patients, rapid-sequence induction of general anesthesia for cesarean delivery may be indicated.[13]

KEY POINTS

- Substance abuse by pregnant women results in significant risks of maternal and fetal morbidity and mortality.
- Anesthesia providers often care for substance-abusing patients during labor or emergency cesarean delivery.
- Patients with substance abuse may have abnormal pain sensitivity. Anesthesia providers are often consulted for treatment of acute postoperative pain.
- Anesthesia providers should ask patients questions about substance abuse in a respectful and nonjudgmental manner.
- Maternal self-reporting underestimates the true incidence of substance abuse. Drug testing (urine, blood, hair, meconium) should be employed if substance abuse is suspected.
- Intrauterine alcohol exposure is the leading cause of preventable birth defects in the United States.

- Smoking during pregnancy negatively affects fetal growth. Pregnant women who smoke are more likely to suffer respiratory complications and impaired wound healing.
- Moderate maternal caffeine intake (< 300 mg/day) does not appear to have adverse maternal or fetal effects.
- Smoking marijuana increases maternal respiratory comorbidities. The long-term effects on exposed offspring are unclear.
- Cocaine use has been associated with sudden death from a variety of factors, including cardiac arrhythmias, respiratory arrest, status epilepticus, and impaired thermoregulation. Maternal cocaine use increases the likelihood of placental abruption and urgent cesarean delivery.
- Acute cocaine intoxication can mimic preeclampsia, eclampsia, or malignant hyperthermia.
- Ingestion of amphetamines results in high levels of circulating catecholamines, leading to hemodynamic instability and, in some cases, cardiac arrest.
- There is conflicting evidence as to whether intrauterine hallucinogen exposure has deleterious effects on the fetus.
- Care of the opioid-dependent patient should involve maintenance of long-term opioid requirements, multimodal management of acute pain, and avoidance of opioid antagonists and mixed-agonists/antagonists (unless the patient shows signs of overdose or is undergoing medically supervised detoxification).
- Inhalant abuse can lead to severe maternal hypoxemia and potentially lethal arrhythmias.
- For most patients with a history of substance abuse, neuraxial analgesia may be administered for a trial of labor and vaginal delivery, provided that the patient is cooperative, is able to protect her airway, and does not have a coagulopathy or a platelet count below the threshold of concern for the anesthesia provider.

REFERENCES

1. The National Survey on Drug Use and Health. NSDUH Report: Substance Use During Pregnancy: 2002 and 2003 Update. DHHS Publication No. SMA-04-3964, NSDUH Series H-25 and SMA-03-3836, NSDUH Series H-22. Rockville, MD, Office of Applied Studies, Substance Abuse and Mental Health Services Administration, 2005:3.
2. Alcohol consumption among pregnant and childbearing-aged women—United States, 1991 and 1995. MMWR Morb Mortal Wkly Rep 1997; 46:346-50.
3. Alcohol consumption among women who are pregnant or who might become pregnant—United States, 2002. MMWR Morb Mortal Wkly Rep 2004; 53:1178-81.
4. American College of Obstetricians and Gynecologists Committees on Healthcare for Underserved Women and Obstetric Practice. Smoking cessation during pregnancy. ACOG Committee Opinion No. 316. Washington, DC, ACOG, October 2005. (Obstet Gynecol 2005; 106:883-8.)
5. Kaskutas LA. Understanding drinking during pregnancy among urban American Indian and African Americans: Health messages, risk beliefs, and how we measure consumption. Alcohol Clin Exp Res 2000; 24:121-50.
6. Huestis MA, Choo RE. Drug abuse's smallest victims: In utero drug exposure. Forensic Sci Int 2002; 128:20-30.
7. Crome IB, Kumar MT. Epidemiology of drug and alcohol use in young women. Semin Fetal Neonatal Med 2007; 12:98-105.
8. Ebrahim SH, Gfroerer J. Pregnancy-related substance use in the United States during 1996-1998. Obstet Gynecol 2003; 101:374-9.
9. Ghuran A, Nolan J. Recreational drug misuse: Issues for the cardiologist. Heart 2000; 83:627-33.
10. Brust JC. Neurologic complications of substance abuse. J Acquir Immune Defic Syndr 2002; 31(Suppl 2):S29-34.
11. Curet LB, Hsi AC. Drug abuse during pregnancy. Clin Obstet Gynecol 2002; 45:73-88.
12. Kain ZN, Mayes LC, Ferris CA, et al. Cocaine-abusing parturients undergoing cesarean section: A cohort study. Anesthesiology 1996; 85:1028-35.
13. Kuczkowski KM. Anesthetic implications of drug abuse in pregnancy. J Clin Anesth 2003; 15:382-94.
14. Khan HN. Substance abuse. In Pian-Smith MCM, Leffert L, editors. Obstetric Anesthesia. New York, Cambridge University Press, 2007:694-704.
15. Bishai R, Koren G. Maternal and obstetric effects of prenatal drug exposure. Clin Perinatol 1999; 26:75-86, vii.
16. Bloomstone JA. The drug-abusing parturient. Int Anesthesiol Clin 2002; 40:137-50.
17. Birnbach DJ. Anesthetic management of the drug-abusing parturient: Are you ready? J Clin Anesth 2003; 15:325-7.
18. Ostrea EM Jr, Knapp DK, Tannenbaum L, et al. Estimates of illicit drug use during pregnancy by maternal interview, hair analysis, and meconium analysis. J Pediatr 2001; 138:344-8.
19. Montgomery D, Plate C, Alder SC, et al. Testing for fetal exposure to illicit drugs using umbilical cord tissue versus meconium. J Perinatol 2006; 26:11-4.
20. Lester BM, El Sohly M, Wright LL, et al. The Maternal Lifestyle Study: Drug use by meconium toxicology and maternal self-report. Pediatrics 2001; 107:309-17.
21. Lester BM, Andreozzi L, Appiah L. Substance use during pregnancy: Time for policy to catch up with research. Harm Reduct J 2004; 1:5.
22. Musshoff F, Madea B. Review of biologic matrices (urine, blood, hair) as indicators of recent or ongoing cannabis use. Ther Drug Monit 2006; 28:155-63.
23. Verstraete AG. Detection times of drugs of abuse in blood, urine, and oral fluid. Ther Drug Monit 2004; 26:200-5.
24. 2006 National Survey on Drug Use and Health. Rockville, MD, Substance Abuse and Mental Health Services Administration, Office of Applied Studies, 2006. Available at http://nsduhweb.rti.org/ and http://oas.samhsa.gov/nsduh/2k6nsduh/2k6Results.pdf/
25. Spampinato MV, Castillo M, Rojas R, et al. Magnetic resonance imaging findings in substance abuse: Alcohol and alcoholism and syndromes associated with alcohol abuse. Top Magn Reson Imaging 2005; 16:223-30.
26. Lieber CS. Medical disorders of alcoholism. N Engl J Med 1995; 333:1058-65.
27. Reynolds EW, Bada HS. Pharmacology of drugs of abuse. Obstet Gynecol Clin North Am 2003; 30:501-22.
28. Wood PR, Soni N. Anaesthesia and substance abuse. Anaesthesia 1989; 44:672-80.
29. Gomberg ES. Suicide risk among women with alcohol problems. Am J Public Health 1989; 79:1363-5.
30. Kuczkowski KM. Labor analgesia for the drug abusing parturient: Is there cause for concern? Obstet Gynecol Surv 2003; 58:599-608.
31. Kuczkowski KM. Labor analgesia for the tobacco and ethanol abusing pregnant patient: A routine management? Arch Gynecol Obstet 2005; 271:6-10.
32. Wright A, Walker J. Management of women who use drugs during pregnancy. Semin Fetal Neonatal Med 2007; 12:114-8.
33. Floyd RL, O'Connor MJ, Sokol RJ, et al. Recognition and prevention of fetal alcohol syndrome. Obstet Gynecol 2005; 106:1059-64.
34. Baumbach J. Some implications of prenatal alcohol exposure for the treatment of adolescents with sexual offending behaviors. Sex Abuse 2002; 14:313-27.

35. Kuczkowski KM. Drug misuse in pregnancy. Br J Psychiatry 2004; 184:182.
36. Mayes LC. Genetics of childhood disorders: IV. Prenatal drug exposure. J Am Acad Child Adolesc Psychiatry 2003; 42:1258-61.
37. Harlap S, Shiono PH. Alcohol, smoking, and incidence of spontaneous abortions in the first and second trimester. Lancet 1980; 2(8187):173-6.
38. Bruce DL. Alcoholism and anesthesia. Anesth Analg 1983; 62:84-96.
39. Ackland GL, Smith M, McGlennan AP. Acute, severe hypoglycemia occurring during general anesthesia in a nondiabetic adult. Anesth Analg 2007; 105:553-4.
40. American Society of Anesthesiologists Task Force on Obstetric Anesthesia. Practice guidelines for obstetric anesthesia. Anesthesiology 2007; 106:843-63.
41. Han YH. Why do chronic alcoholics require more anesthesia? Anesthesiology 1969; 30:2.
42. Swerdlow BN, Holley FO, Maitre PO, et al. Chronic alcohol intake does not change thiopental anesthetic requirement, pharmacokinetics, or pharmacodynamics. Anesthesiology 1990; 72:455-61.
43. Kuczkowski KM. Smoking in pregnancy: A need for improving information available to pregnant women on deleterious effects of smoking on pregnancy outcome. J Gynecol Obstet Biol Reprod (Paris) 2004; 33:259.
44. Lerman C, Patterson F, Berrettini W. Treating tobacco dependence: State of the science and new directions. J Clin Oncol 2005; 23:311-23.
45. Sastry BV. Placental toxicology: Tobacco smoke, abused drugs, multiple chemical interactions, and placental function. Reprod Fertil Dev 1991; 3:355-72.
46. Hlastala MP, McKenna HP, Franada RL, et al. Influence of carbon monoxide on hemoglobin-oxygen binding. J Appl Physiol 1976; 41:893-9.
47. Klausen K, Andersen C, Nandrup S. Acute effects of cigarette smoking and inhalation of carbon monoxide during maximal exercise. Eur J Appl Physiol Occup Physiol 1983; 51:371-9.
48. Warner DO. Perioperative abstinence from cigarettes: Physiologic and clinical consequences. Anesthesiology 2006; 104:356-67.
49. Kotani N, Kushikata T, Hashimoto H, et al. Recovery of intraoperative microbicidal and inflammatory functions of alveolar immune cells after a tobacco smoke-free period. Anesthesiology 2001; 94:999-1006.
50. Kistin N, Handler A, Davis F, et al. Cocaine and cigarettes: A comparison of risks. Paediatr Perinat Epidemiol 1996; 10:269-78.
51. Klonoff-Cohen H, Edelstein S, Savitz D. Cigarette smoking and preeclampsia. Obstet Gynecol 1993; 81:541-4.
52. Visscher WA, Feder M, Burns AM, et al. The impact of smoking and other substance use by urban women on the birthweight of their infants. Subst Use Misuse 2003; 38:1063-93.
53. Salihu HM, Aliyu MH, Pierre-Louis BJ, et al. Levels of excess infant deaths attributable to maternal smoking during pregnancy in the United States. Matern Child Health J 2003; 7:219-27.
54. Mello PR, Pinto GR, Botelho C. [The influence of smoking on fertility, pregnancy and lactation]. J Pediatr (Rio J) 2001; 77:257-64.
55. Shiono PH, Klebanoff MA, Nugent RP, et al. The impact of cocaine and marijuana use on low birth weight and preterm birth: A multicenter study. Am J Obstet Gynecol 1995; 172:19-27.
56. Bada HS, Das A, Bauer CR, et al. Low birth weight and preterm births: Etiologic fraction attributable to prenatal drug exposure. J Perinatol 2005; 25:631-7.
57. Fried PA, Watkinson B, Gray R. Differential effects on cognitive functioning in 13- to 16-year-olds prenatally exposed to cigarettes and marihuana. Neurotoxicol Teratol 2003; 25:427-36.
58. Wilkes AR, Hall JE, Wright E, et al. The effect of humidification and smoking habit on the incidence of adverse airway events during deepening of anaesthesia with desflurane. Anaesthesia 2000; 55:685-9.
59. Kim ES, Bishop MJ. Cough during emergence from isoflurane anesthesia. Anesth Analg 1998; 87:1170-4.
60. Nawrot P, Jordan S, Eastwood J, et al. Effects of caffeine on human health. Food Addit Contam 2003; 20:1-30.
61. Higdon JV, Frei B. Coffee and health: A review of recent human research. Crit Rev Food Sci Nutr 2006; 46:101-23.
62. Bech BH, Obel C, Henriksen TB, et al. Effect of reducing caffeine intake on birth weight and length of gestation: Randomised controlled trial. Br Med J 2007; 334:409.
63. Browne ML. Maternal exposure to caffeine and risk of congenital anomalies: A systematic review. Epidemiology 2006; 17:324-31.
64. Browne ML, Bell EM, Druschel CM, et al. Maternal caffeine consumption and risk of cardiovascular malformations. Birth Defects Res Part A Clin Mol Teratol 2007; 79:533-43.
65. Hey E. Coffee and pregnancy. Br Med J 2007; 334:377.
66. Adeney KL, Williams MA, Schiff MA, et al. Coffee consumption and the risk of gestational diabetes mellitus. Acta Obstet Gynecol Scand 2007; 86:161-6.
67. Back SA, Craig A, Luo NL, et al. Protective effects of caffeine on chronic hypoxia-induced perinatal white matter injury. Ann Neurol 2006; 60:696-705.
68. Halker RB, Demaerschalk BM, Wellik KE, et al. Caffeine for the prevention and treatment of postdural puncture headache: Debunking the myth. Neurologist 2007; 13:323-7.
69. Kuczkowski KM. Marijuana in pregnancy. Ann Acad Med Singapore 2004; 33:336-9.
70. Arria AM, Derauf C, Lagasse LL, et al. Methamphetamine and other substance use during pregnancy: Preliminary estimates from the Infant Development, Environment, and Lifestyle (IDEAL) study. Matern Child Health J 2006; 10:293-302.
71. Ashton CH. Pharmacology and effects of cannabis: A brief review. Br J Psychiatry 2001; 178:101-6.
72. Hatch EE, Bracken MB. Effect of marijuana use in pregnancy on fetal growth. Am J Epidemiol 1986; 124:986-93.
73. White SM. Cannabis abuse and laryngospasm. Anaesthesia 2002; 57:622-3.
74. Wallace M, Schulteis G, Atkinson JH, et al. Dose-dependent effects of smoked cannabis on capsaicin-induced pain and hyperalgesia in healthy volunteers. Anesthesiology 2007; 107:785-96.
75. Lange RA, Hillis LD. Cardiovascular complications of cocaine use. N Engl J Med 2001; 345:351-8.
76. Fajemirokun-Odudeyi O, Lindow SW. Obstetric implications of cocaine use in pregnancy: A literature review. Eur J Obstet Gynecol Reprod Biol 2004; 112:2-8.
77. Shanti CM, Lucas CE. Cocaine and the critical care challenge. Crit Care Med 2003; 31:1851-9.
78. Bauer CR, Langer JC, Shankaran S, et al. Acute neonatal effects of cocaine exposure during pregnancy. Arch Pediatr Adolesc Med 2005; 159:824-34.
79. Kuczkowski KM. Peripartum care of the cocaine-abusing parturient: Are we ready? Acta Obstet Gynecol Scand 2005; 84:108-16.
80. Kline J, Ng SK, Schittini M, et al. Cocaine use during pregnancy: Sensitive detection by hair assay. Am J Public Health 1997; 87:352-8.
81. Fleming JA, Byck R, Barash PG. Pharmacology and therapeutic applications of cocaine. Anesthesiology 1990; 73:518-31.
82. Ettinger TB, Stine RJ. Sudden death temporally related to vaginal cocaine abuse. Am J Emerg Med 1989; 7:129-31.
83. Warner EA. Cocaine abuse. Ann Intern Med 1993; 119:226-35.
84. Hatsukami DK, Fischman MW. Crack cocaine and cocaine hydrochloride: Are the differences myth or reality? JAMA 1996; 276:1580-8.
85. Kuczkowski KM. Cardiovascular complications of recreational cocaine use in pregnancy: Myth or reality? Acta Obstet Gynecol Scand 2005; 84:100-1.
86. Feng Q. Postnatal consequences of prenatal cocaine exposure and myocardial apoptosis: Does cocaine in utero imperil the adult heart? Br J Pharmacol 2005; 144:887-8.
87. Mittleman MA, Mintzer D, Maclure M, et al. Triggering of myocardial infarction by cocaine. Circulation 1999; 99:2737-41.
88. Hollander JE, Henry TD. Evaluation and management of the patient who has cocaine-associated chest pain. Cardiol Clin 2006; 24:103-14.
89. Kuczkowski KM. More on the idiosyncratic effects of cocaine on the human heart. Emerg Med J 2007; 24:147.

90. Livingston JC, Mabie BC, Ramanathan J. Crack cocaine, myocardial infarction, and troponin I levels at the time of cesarean delivery. Anesth Analg 2000; 91:913-5.
91. Vertommen JD, Hughes SC, Rosen MA, et al. Hydralazine does not restore uterine blood flow during cocaine-induced hypertension in the pregnant ewe. Anesthesiology 1992; 76:580-7.
92. Derlet RW, Albertson TE. Potentiation of cocaine toxicity with calcium channel blockers. Am J Emerg Med 1989; 7:464-8.
93. Mason BA, Ricci-Goodman J, Koos BJ. Adenosine in the treatment of maternal paroxysmal supraventricular tachycardia. Obstet Gynecol 1992; 80:478-80.
94. Gowda RM, Khan IA, Mehta NJ, et al. Cardiac arrhythmias in pregnancy: Clinical and therapeutic considerations. Int J Cardiol 2003; 88:129-33.
95. Shih RD, Hollander JE, Burstein JL, et al. Clinical safety of lidocaine in patients with cocaine-associated myocardial infarction. Ann Emerg Med 1995; 26:702-6.
96. Widerhorn J, Bhandari AK, Bughi S, et al. Fetal and neonatal adverse effects profile of amiodarone treatment during pregnancy. Am Heart J 1991; 122:1162-6.
97. Schleich JM, Bernard Du Haut Cilly F, Laurent MC, et al. Early prenatal management of a fetal ventricular tachycardia treated in utero by amiodarone with long term follow-up. Prenat Diagn 2000; 20:449-52.
98. Spivey WH, Euerle B. Neurologic complications of cocaine abuse. Ann Emerg Med 1990; 19:1422-8.
99. Jacobs IG, Roszler MH, Kelly JK, et al. Cocaine abuse: Neurovascular complications. Radiology 1989; 170:223-7.
100. Ettinger NA, Albin RJ. A review of the respiratory effects of smoking cocaine. Am J Med 1989; 87:664-8.
101. Kain ZN, Mayes LC, Pakes J, et al. Thrombocytopenia in pregnant women who use cocaine. Am J Obstet Gynecol 1995; 173:885-90.
102. Orser B. Thrombocytopenia and cocaine abuse. Anesthesiology 1991; 74:195-6.
103. Gershon RY, Fisher AJ, Graves WL. The cocaine-abusing parturient is not at an increased risk for thrombocytopenia. Anesth Analg 1996; 82:865-6.
104. Kain ZN, Rimar S, Barash PG. Cocaine abuse in the parturient and effects on the fetus and neonate. Anesth Analg 1993; 77:835-45.
105. Owiny JR, Jones MT, Sadowsky D, et al. Cocaine in pregnancy: The effect of maternal administration of cocaine on the maternal and fetal pituitary-adrenal axes. Am J Obstet Gynecol 1991; 164:658-63.
106. Owiny JR, Sadowsky D, Jones MT, et al. Effect of maternal cocaine administration on maternal and fetal glucose, lactate, and insulin in sheep. Obstet Gynecol 1991; 77:901-4.
107. Crandall CG, Vongpatanasin W, Victor RG. Mechanism of cocaine-induced hyperthermia in humans. Ann Intern Med 2002; 136:785-91.
108. Woods JR, Scott KJ, Plessinger MA. Pregnancy enhances cocaine's actions on the heart and within the peripheral circulation. Am J Obstet Gynecol 1994; 170:1027-33.
109. Woods JR, Plessinger MA, Clark KE. Effect of cocaine on uterine blood flow and fetal oxygenation. JAMA 1987; 257:957-61.
110. Little BB, Snell LM, Trimmer KJ, et al. Peripartum cocaine use and adverse pregnancy outcome. Am J Hum Biol 1999; 11:598-602.
111. Kuhn L, Kline J, Ng S, et al. Cocaine use during pregnancy and intrauterine growth retardation: New insights based on maternal hair tests. Am J Epidemiol 2000; 152:112-9.
112. Towers CV, Pircon RA, Nageotte MP, et al. Cocaine intoxication presenting as preeclampsia and eclampsia. Obstet Gynecol 1993; 81:545-7.
113. Shankaran S, Lester BM, Das A, et al. Impact of maternal substance use during pregnancy on childhood outcome. Semin Fetal Neonatal Med 2007; 12:143-50.
114. Richardson GA, Hamel SC, Goldschmidt L, et al. Growth of infants prenatally exposed to cocaine/crack: Comparison of a prenatal care and a no prenatal care sample. Pediatrics 1999; 104:e18.
115. Behnke M, Eyler FD, Garvan CW, et al. The search for congenital malformations in newborns with fetal cocaine exposure. Pediatrics 2001; 107:E74.
116. Frank DA, Augustyn M, Knight WG, et al. Growth, development, and behavior in early childhood following prenatal cocaine exposure: A systematic review. JAMA 2001; 285:1613-25.
117. Mayes LC, Cicchetti D, Acharyya S, Zhang H. Developmental trajectories of cocaine-and-other-drug-exposed and non-cocaine-exposed children. J Dev Behav Pediatr 2003; 24:323-35.
118. Messinger DS, Bauer CR, Das A, et al. The maternal lifestyle study: Cognitive, motor, and behavioral outcomes of cocaine-exposed and opiate-exposed infants through three years of age. Pediatrics 2004; 113:1677-85.
119. Lumeng JC, Cabral HJ, Gannon K, et al. Prenatal exposures to cocaine and alcohol and physical growth patterns to age 8 years. Neurotoxicol Teratol 2007; 29:446-57.
120. Bae S, Zhang L. Prenatal cocaine exposure increases apoptosis of neonatal rat heart and heart susceptibility to ischemia-reperfusion injury in 1-month-old rat. Br J Pharmacol 2005; 144:900-7.
121. Jatlow P, Barash PG, Van Dyke C, et al. Cocaine and succinylcholine sensitivity: A new caution. Anesth Analg 1979; 58:235-8.
122. Ross VH, Moore CH, Pan PH, et al. Reduced duration of intrathecal sufentanil analgesia in laboring cocaine users. Anesth Analg 2003; 97:1504-8.
123. Stoelting RK, Creasser CW, Martz RC. Effect of cocaine administration on halothane MAC in dogs. Anesth Analg 1975; 54:422-4.
124. Methamphetamine Abuse and Addiction. National Institute on Drug Abuse Research Report Series. NIH Publication Number 06-4210. Washington, DC, U.S. Health and Human Services, National Institutes of Health, National Institute on Drug Abuse, 1998, revised 2006.
125. Wouldes T, LaGasse L, Sheridan J, et al. Maternal methamphetamine use during pregnancy and child outcome: What do we know? N Z Med J 2004; 117:U1180.
126. Ho E, Karimi-Tabesh L, Koren G. Characteristics of pregnant women who use ecstasy (3, 4-methylenedioxymethamphetamine). Neurotoxicol Teratol 2001; 23:561-7.
127. Kalant H. The pharmacology and toxicology of "ecstasy" (MDMA) and related drugs. Can Med Assoc J 2001; 165:917-28.
128. Samuels SI, Maze A, Albright G. Cardiac arrest during cesarean section in a chronic amphetamine abuser. Anesth Analg 1979; 58:528-30.
129. Volkow ND, Chang L, Wang GJ, et al. Loss of dopamine transporters in methamphetamine abusers recovers with protracted abstinence. J Neurosci 2001; 21:9414-8.
130. Sajo E. Pharmacology of substance abuse. Prim Care Pract 2000; 4:319-35.
131. Oro AS, Dixon SD. Perinatal cocaine and methamphetamine exposure: Maternal and neonatal correlates. J Pediatr 1987; 111:571-8.
132. Smith LM, LaGasse LL, Derauf C, et al. The infant development, environment, and lifestyle study: Effects of prenatal methamphetamine exposure, polydrug exposure, and poverty on intrauterine growth. Pediatrics 2006; 118:1149-56.
133. Cernerud L, Eriksson M, Jonsson B, et al. Amphetamine addiction during pregnancy: 14-year follow-up of growth and school performance. Acta Paediatr 1996; 85:204-8.
134. Hanzawa S, Nemoto M, Etoh S, et al. [A case of amphetamine-induced down-regulation of beta-adrenoceptor]. Masui 2001; 50:1242-5.
135. Johnston RR, Way WL, Miller RD. Alteration of anesthetic requirement by amphetamine. Anesthesiology 1972; 36:357-63.
136. Michel R, Adams AP. Acute amphetamine abuse: Problems during general anaesthesia for neurosurgery. Anaesthesia 1979; 34:1016-9.
137. The National Survey on Drug Use and Health. NSDUH Report: Patterns of Hallucinogen Use and Initiation: 2004 and 2005. DHHS Publication No. SMA 07-4293, NSDUH Series H-32. Rockville, MD, Substance Abuse and Mental Health Services Administration, Office of Applied Studies, 2007.
138. Mvula MM, Miller JM Jr, Ragan FA. Relationship of phencyclidine and pregnancy outcome. J Reprod Med 1999; 44:1021-4.
139. The National Survey on Drug Use and Health. Substance Abuse and Mental Health Services Administration. Results from the 2005 National Survey on Drug Use and Health: National Findings.

NSDUH Series H-30, DHHS Publication No. SMA 06-4194. Rockville, MD, Substance Abuse and Mental Health Services Administration, Office of Applied Studies, 2006. Available at http://www.oas.samhsa.gov/prescription/Ch2.htm/

140. Sporer KA. Acute heroin overdose. Ann Intern Med 1999; 130:584-90.
141. Mitra S, Sinatra RS. Perioperative management of acute pain in the opioid-dependent patient. Anesthesiology 2004; 101:212-27.
142. Peng PW, Tumber PS, Gourlay D. Review article: Perioperative pain management of patients on methadone therapy. Can J Anaesth 2005; 52:513-23.
143. Fajemirokun-Odudeyi O, Sinha C, Tutty S, et al. Pregnancy outcome in women who use opiates. Eur J Obstet Gynecol Reprod Biol 2006; 126:170-5.
144. Kandall SR, Doberczak TM, Jantunen M, et al. The methadone-maintained pregnancy. Clin Perinatol 1999; 26:173-83.
145. McCarthy JJ, Leamon MH, Parr MS, et al. High-dose methadone maintenance in pregnancy: Maternal and neonatal outcomes. Am J Obstet Gynecol 2005; 193:606-10.
146. Mao J. Opioid-induced abnormal pain sensitivity: Implications in clinical opioid therapy. Pain 2002; 100:213-7.
147. Compton P, Charuvastra VC, Ling W. Pain intolerance in opioid-maintained former opiate addicts: Effect of long-acting maintenance agent. Drug Alcohol Depend 2001; 63:139-46.
148. Fischer G. Treatment of opioid dependence in pregnant women. Addiction 2000; 95:1141-4.
149. Meyer M, Wagner K, Benvenuto A, et al. Intrapartum and postpartum analgesia for women maintained on methadone during pregnancy. Obstet Gynecol 2007; 110:261-6.
150. Hulse GK, O'Neil G, Arnold-Reed DE. Methadone maintenance versus implantable naltrexone treatment in the pregnant heroin user. Int J Gynaecol Obstet 2004; 85:170-1.
151. Hensel M, Kox WJ. Safety, efficacy, and long-term results of a modified version of rapid opiate detoxification under general anaesthesia: A prospective study in methadone, heroin, codeine and morphine addicts. Acta Anaesthesiol Scand 2000; 44:326-33.
152. Sinha C, Ohadike P, Carrick P, et al. Neonatal outcome following maternal opiate use in late pregnancy. Int J Gynaecol Obstet 2001; 74:241-6.
153. Cassidy B, Cyna AM. Challenges that opioid-dependent women present to the obstetric anaesthetist. Anaesth Intensive Care 2004; 32:494-501.
154. Kuczkowski KM. Ethylene glycol and other solvent use in pregnancy: A new phenomenon and a new diagnostic dilemma. Acta Anaesthesiol Scand 2006; 50:1037.
155. Williams JF, Storck M. Inhalant abuse. Pediatrics 2007; 119:1009-17.
156. Leth PM, Gregersen M. Ethylene glycol poisoning. Forensic Sci Int 2005; 155:179-84.
157. Kralova I, Stepanek Z, Dusek J. Ethylene glycol intoxication misdiagnosed as eclampsia. Acta Anaesthesiol Scand 2006; 50:385-7.
158. Kuczkowski KM. Solvents in pregnancy: An emerging problem in obstetrics and obstetric anaesthesia. Anaesthesia 2003; 58:1036-7.
159. Tenenbein M, Casiro OG, Seshia MM, et al. Neonatal withdrawal from maternal volatile substance abuse. Arch Dis Child Fetal Neonatal Ed 1996; 74:F204-7.
160. Lester B. The Maternal Lifestyle Study (MLS). 1993. Available at http://clinicaltrials.gov/show/NCT00059540/
161. National Survey on Drug Use and Health (NSDUH). 2006. Available at www.oas.samhsa.gov/nhsda.htm/
162. National Pregnancy and Health Survey: Drug Use Among Women Delivering Live Births, 1992. Available at http://www.icpsr.umich.edu/cocoon/SAMHDA/STUDY/02835.xml/
163. Substance Abuse and Mental Health Services Administration. (Washington) DC Metropolitan Area Drug Study (DC*MADS) Series. Rockville, MD, Substance Abuse and Mental Health Services Administration, Office of Applied Studies, 1991. Available at http://www.icpsr.umich.edu/cocoon/SAMHDA/SERIES/00108.xml/
164. Haufroid V, Lison D. Urinary cotinine as a tobacco-smoke exposure index: A minireview. Int Arch Occup Environ Health 1998; 71:162-8.

Trauma

Paul Howell, M.B.Ch.B., FRCA

Trauma is the leading cause of death for people under 45 years of age in the United States. Data on pregnancy-associated deaths (collected by the U.S. Centers for Disease Control and Prevention) are incomplete, but trauma is widely recognized to be the leading cause of nonobstetric maternal mortality.[1] Almost one third of maternal deaths reported to the U.S. Pregnancy Mortality Surveillance System between 1991 and 1999 were injury-related, and the leading single cause of pregnancy-associated maternal death was motor vehicle accident.[2]

EPIDEMIOLOGY

Trauma occurs in as many as 8% of all pregnancies,[3] and as many as 20% of affected women require emergency surgery.[4] The rate of trauma admissions rises with each trimester of pregnancy; 8% occur in the first trimester, 40% in the second trimester, and 52% in the third trimester.[5,6] Trauma admissions are most common in urban areas and peak in the summer months.[7]

Pregnant women appear to encounter a lower threshold for hospital admission than nonpregnant women; pregnant women are admitted more frequently than nonpregnant women when presenting with trauma injuries of similar or lesser severity.[8,9] Although most pregnant trauma victims are eventually able to continue their pregnancies at home, as many as 38% remain hospitalized until delivery.[4,10-12]

The most common type of injury to pregnant women is blunt trauma.[9] Data from the American College of Surgeons National Trauma Data Bank (NTDB) suggest that motor vehicle accidents (MVAs) cause 70% of such injuries; the other major causes are domestic violence (12%) and falls (9%).[13] Falls cause 17% to 39% of trauma-associated emergency department visits during pregnancy,[14] and the majority of these falls are probably preventable.[13] Falls can result from an unstable gait during pregnancy; pregnant women also experience an increased risk of falling during physical activity. Penetrating injuries, although uncommon in pregnancy, often cause more serious harm, accounting for a disproportionate number of maternal deaths.[15] The rates of injury are higher in pregnant women than in nonpregnant women of reproductive age; they include higher risk ratios for assault (2.56; 95% confidence interval [CI], 2.33 to 2.82), MVAs (1.88; 95% CI, 1.78 to 1.98), firearm injury (1.54; 95% CI, 1.23 to 1.94), and falls (1.50; 95% CI, 1.41 to 1.59).[16]

Trauma has both direct and indirect effects. For example, **direct tissue injury** from penetrating trauma, blunt trauma, or burns can also result in **indirect tissue injury** from shock, disseminated intravascular coagulation, and acute respiratory distress syndrome (ARDS). Limited data suggest that the incidence, severity, and outcome of maternal **burn injuries** do not differ from those in the nonpregnant population, and that fetal survival of burn injuries typically accompanies maternal survival.[17,18]

Domestic Violence

The impact of domestic violence as a major cause of maternal death is increasingly recognized in both the United States[19] and the United Kingdom.[20] The latest Report of the Confidential Enquiry into Maternal and Child Health (CEMACH) in the United Kingdom suggests that domestic violence is significantly underreported.[20] Physical abuse during pregnancy is a strong predictor of subsequent abuse.[21] Gazmararian et al.[22] concluded that the prevalence of violence in pregnancy is as high as 20%. Domestic violence is also a problem in the developing world; a 2006 report from Uganda showed that domestic violence was associated with a fourfold increase in the incidence of low birth weight and a 37% higher rate of maternal obstetric complications.[23] CEMACH and others have urged the development and implementation of programs to screen women for risk of violence during pregnancy.[20,22]

Motor Vehicle Accidents

Morbidity and mortality for the mother and fetus involved in MVAs are both greatly increased when automobile safety restraints (safety belts) are not used—or are used incorrectly—by vehicle occupants. Published guidelines recommend using safety belts "above and below the bump,"[20,24] and proper safety belt use, with or without airbag deployment, is associated with better fetal outcome in lower-severity crashes that account for the majority of MVAs.[24] Metz and Abbott[25] observed abnormal abdominal findings in 90% of women involved in MVAs who were not wearing safety belts, and fetal death is approximately three times more likely if the mother does not wear a safety belt.[26] Improper positioning of a safety belt has also been implicated in a death from amniotic fluid embolism following blunt abdominal trauma in an MVA.[27]

Despite frequent public health messages emphasizing the advantages of correctly using safety belts, approximately one third of pregnant women in the United States either do not use them at all or use them improperly.[3,9,25] In Japan, the proportion of women who always wear safety belts declines from more than 70% before pregnancy to less than 40% in the third trimester.[28] These data suggest that the importance of properly using automobile safety restraints should be reinforced in childbirth preparation classes.

Suicide

Inadequate attention has been given to the altered pattern of suicide in pregnant and postpartum women and the considerable contribution of depressive illness to maternal deaths. CEMACH data indicate that suicides are more likely to be violent when committed by women who are pregnant or postpartum; more than half of these deaths involve hanging or jumping from a lethal height.[20]

Substance Abuse

An NTDB study of trauma patients compared cohorts of 1195 pregnant and 76,126 nonpregnant women. The pregnant cohort was significantly more likely to show evidence of alcohol or drug use than the nonpregnant cohort ($P < .0001$); 13% of the pregnant patients had consumed alcohol prior to their injuries, and 20% tested positive for illegal drugs.[9] Another study in Tennessee tested 82 of 160 pregnant MVA patients for intoxicants; 46% tested positive for intoxicant drugs (e.g., alcohol, opiates, cannabis, cocaine, ethanol), and 73% who tested positive had been driving under the influence of intoxicants prior to their injuries.[3]

COMPLICATIONS AND OUTCOMES

Maternal Outcome

Head injury and hemorrhagic shock account for most maternal deaths from trauma during pregnancy.[29] Pelvic and acetabular fractures are also associated with a high risk of maternal death.[30,31] The maternal mortality rate from trauma appears to be higher in pregnant than in nonpregnant women even for less severe injuries.[3]

The vast majority of injuries that occur during pregnancy are minor, and many women do not seek medical care following injury. In a review from Virginia, blunt trauma accounted for 88% of hospitalizations in pregnant trauma victims; 52% of women were discharged home from the emergency department, but 18% required emergency surgery.[4] The most common injuries were fractures, dislocations, sprains, and strains, which usually do not put the pregnancy at risk.[9]

Several studies have demonstrated that trauma in pregnancy is associated with a significant increase in the risk of obstetric complications, both **immediate** (e.g., uterine rupture, placental abruption, maternal mortality) and **delayed** (e.g., preterm labor).[12,32] Studies have also shown that even women who suffer minor injuries are at higher risk for obstetric complications.[11,12] Even in situations in which pregnant women appear to have been *uninjured* after an MVA, there is an eightfold increase in risk of preterm labor and a sixfold increase in risk of placental abruption later in the pregnancy.[11]

Severe abdominal trauma can cause **uterine rupture,** which occurs in 0.6% of all injuries during pregnancy.[33] Although rare, uterine rupture can be life-threatening. Maternal mortality rates are as high as 10%, and fetal mortality rates approach 100%.

Placental abruption complicates 1% to 5% of minor injuries in pregnancy and 20% to 50% of major injuries. It can cause overt or occult maternal hemorrhage and coagulopathy. Risk increases with the severity of injury. However, pregnant women experience a higher risk of placental abruption even when their injuries are relatively minor.[34,35]

Preterm labor can be triggered by trauma, possibly due to the release of arachidonic acid and prostaglandins from myometrial injury. Preterm labor occurs in approximately 25% of cases of trauma in pregnant women.[11,12,36] Premature rupture of membranes also increases the risks of infection and preterm labor.

The etiology of **amniotic fluid embolism** (AFE) is unclear; some physicians have suggested that uterine injury or rupture of membranes may be associated with an increased risk of AFE, although this is unproved. There have been a few reports of AFE occurring in association with blunt abdominal trauma.[37-39] One report included immunohistochemical evidence of an anaphylactoid reaction, which supported the diagnosis of AFE.[27]

Fetomaternal hemorrhage can occur after trauma when injury to the uteroplacental circulation permits fetal red blood cells to enter the maternal circulation.[40,41] In cases of abdominal trauma, uterine tenderness should increase the index of suspicion for fetomaternal hemorrhage.[40] Fetomaternal hemorrhage can cause **Rhesus isosensitization** in the Rh-negative mother and can also induce preterm labor.

Fetal and Neonatal Outcome

In early pregnancy the uterus is thick-walled, and the pelvis protects the fetus from external injury relatively well. The two primary risks in this period are spontaneous abortion and maternal isoimmunization from fetomaternal hemorrhage. In the second trimester, the uterus emerges from the pelvis into the abdomen, and the fetus is protected by the large volume of amniotic fluid. Toward term, the abdominal viscera are displaced and the uterus becomes thin-walled, providing less protection from direct injury to the fetus. Case reports have described direct fetal injuries as well as isolated injuries to the umbilical cord and placenta.[42-44] Fetal skull fracture and intracranial hemorrhage can occur as a result of blunt trauma during late pregnancy (after the fetal head has entered the pelvis) in association with pelvic fractures.[44,45] The most common causes of fetal death are placental abruption and maternal death.

Motor vehicle accidents account for 82% of fetal deaths related to maternal trauma.[13] There is a strong correlation between crash severity and maternal injury, and the more severe the maternal injury, the greater the risk of fetal morbidity or mortality. Not infrequently, however, fetal outcome is poor in mothers who have sustained minor injuries.[6,46] Fetal/neonatal death rates often exceed maternal death rates, especially after penetrating abdominal trauma. Relatively few fetal deaths are caused by maternal injuries due to firearms (6%) and falls (3%).[13]

Analysis of outcomes for 1195 pregnant trauma victims in the NTDB identified the most important risk factors for fetal death as (1) an Injury Severity Scale (ISS) score of more than 15 (on a scale of 0 to 75, with 0 indicating no injury and 75 indicating an unsurvivable injury); (2) major injury to the maternal thorax, abdomen, or lower extremities; and (3) severe maternal head injury with a score of 8 or lower on the Glasgow Coma Scale.[9] These results provide an organizational framework for the findings of others who have identified the following risk factors for fetal death: (1) maternal ejection from a vehicle, (2) motorcycle collisions, (3) failure to wear safety belts, (4) abnormal fetal heart rate (FHR) tracing at hospital admission, (5) maternal tachycardia, and (6) death of the mother.[47] Other investigators have also found that poor fetal outcomes are associated with maternal hypotension, fetal bradycardia, advanced maternal age, trauma during early gestation, and a maternal serum lactate level greater than 2 mEq/L.[4,6] Pelvic and acetabular fractures are associated with the particularly high fetal fatality rate of 35% (Box 54-1).[30] Severe hemorrhage can result in fetal hypoxia or exsanguination, and surviving neonates can be anemic.

The fetus remains at increased risk of delayed complications following hospital discharge of the mother. Delayed complications include a twofold increase in risk of preterm delivery and low birth weight,[41] and a ninefold increase in risk of fetal death.[11] Risks increase with more serious maternal injuries,[36] but even when the mother experiences only minor trauma in pregnancy, the fetus is at risk for late (delayed) complications.[11] El Kady et al.[48] observed a 46% increase in the risk of low birth weight when mothers sustained simple fractures during pregnancy.

There are growing concerns about late effects of minor trauma in pregnancy on childhood development as well as reports of a higher incidence of cerebral palsy in children born to mothers who experienced even minor trauma during pregnancy.[49]

BOX 54-1 Factors Associated with Poor Fetal Outcome in the Pregnant Trauma Victim

- Maternal death
- High Injury Severity Scale score (>15)
- Pelvic fractures
- Motor vehicle accident with ejection from vehicle
- Failure to use safety belts
- Motorcycle collision
- Maternal hypotension
- Maternal tachycardia
- First-trimester trauma
- Advanced maternal age
- Maternal serum lactate level > 2 mEq/L

Information from references 4,6,9,30, and 47.

INJURY SCALES

Determination of the severity of injuries is necessary for prehospital triage, clinical management, and statistical evaluation of outcome. There is at present no completely reliable assessment tool for the prediction of maternal and fetal outcome after trauma. Currently used scoring systems include (1) **anatomic injury scales** that rely on findings of physical examination and diagnostic procedures (e.g., ISS), (2) **physiologic injury scales** (e.g., Champion Trauma Score, Glasgow Coma Scale) that rely on assessment of physiologic responses and function, and (3) **combination injury scales**.

The Glasgow Coma Scale is the most widely used physiologic scoring system, but it correlates poorly with fetal outcome.[3] The ISS largely correlates with the risks of preterm delivery and low birth weight,[36] but it is an unreliable predictor of placental abruption, fetal death, or other adverse outcomes.[6,9,34] In the critical care setting, neither APACHE II nor APACHE III (Acute Physiology, Age, and Chronic Health Evaluation) scores correlate well with maternal mortality; these scores overestimate the risk of dying.[20,50]

CEMACH has recommended the use of Modified Early Obstetric Warning Scores (MEOWS) as a means of identifying the critically ill or deteriorating obstetric patient.[20] CEMACH has emphasized the significance of maternal tachycardia and tachypnea as markers of severe illness in pregnancy. However, the organization stresses that MEOWS "can only be part of the solution, as it is the response to the abnormal score that will determine any real change in outcome."[20]

RESUSCITATION AND OBSTETRIC MANAGEMENT

Management of obstetric trauma requires multidisciplinary teamwork as well as an awareness of the particular needs of the pregnant woman and the fetus that is based on an understanding of the normal changes in anatomy and physiology during pregnancy (Table 54-1) and the pathophysiologic effects produced by injuries. Potential disruptions in uteroplacental perfusion and the possibility of direct fetal injury can result in fetal compromise.

New Strategies in Resuscitation

New approaches in the prehospital and early in-hospital phases of trauma resuscitation have gained acceptance. The **"scoop and run"** approach provides only minimal lifesaving treatment at the accident site and transfers the patient as quickly as possible to a trauma unit appropriately staffed and equipped to treat the injuries. In the United States, helicopter retrieval is well established, providing rapid transfer to Level 1 trauma units.

Relative fluid restriction (hypovolemic resuscitation) is another new approach to trauma resuscitation. This technique employs permissive hypotension and aims for a systolic blood pressure of 80 to 90 mm Hg until hemorrhage is controlled.[51] Small boluses of intravenous fluids are titrated to maintain a radial pulse (equivalent to a systolic blood pressure of 80 mm Hg) in a conscious patient. This concept stems from evidence that, in the absence of head injury (in which maintenance of cerebral blood flow is critical), early aggressive resuscitation in the presence of uncontrolled hemorrhage is associated with higher mortality. It is presumed that increasing blood pressure hinders clot formation and contributes to the ongoing hemorrhage, and that rapid administration of fluid dilutes endogenous clotting factors and aggravates hypothermia.[51] No data are available regarding the applicability of this approach to resuscitation of pregnant trauma victims. Because fluid restriction is likely to impair uteroplacental perfusion, it is not recommended in pregnant patients.[52]

Similarly, there is a trend toward allowing **relative anemia** (hemoglobin concentration of 7 to 9 g/dL) in the early stages of resuscitation before hemostasis has been achieved in nonpregnant trauma victims.[53] These levels are not far outside the range experienced by healthy pregnant women because of the physiologic anemia of pregnancy. However, there is no evidence to suggest that this technique is safe in pregnant women.

Damage control surgery is a major change in surgical practice in the last 20 years. Surgeons have been slow to accept the principles of damage control surgery, because its principles contravene historic surgical teaching practices (i.e., the best operation for a patient is a single definitive procedure). Damage control surgery was developed after clinical observations that the main cause of death in bleeding trauma patients is metabolic failure and consequent coagulopathy, hypothermia, and metabolic acidosis. Once this metabolic failure is established, it is very difficult to control hemorrhage and correct the metabolic derangements. The patients do not survive long complex surgery, and damage control surgery aims to perform an initial quick and effective surgical procedure to stop the hemorrhage, followed by a period of further resuscitation and stabilization, which involves correction of the acidosis, coagulopathy, hypoxemia, and hypothermia in a critical care unit. Once the patient is stable, definitive surgery is performed as a semi-elective staged procedure. As with other trauma techniques, little data have been published with respect to damage control surgery in pregnant patients; because the goal is rapid hemodynamic stabilization and metabolic normalization, it might be appropriate for obstetric patients.

Some authorities advocate conservative, **nonoperative management of solid visceral injury** (e.g., spleen or liver injury) in selected patients; evidence now suggests that this approach may reduce morbidity and mortality in nonobstetric patients. Criteria for this conservative approach include good response to initial resuscitation, relative hemodynamic stability, and limited transfusion requirements.[52]

Depending on the nature and extent of the injuries, as well as the capabilities and expertise of the receiving hospital and physicians, transfer of the injured patient to a specialized unit may be necessary. The American College of Surgeons guidelines list pregnancy among the comorbid factors that may prompt early transfer from a rural hospital to a facility with a higher level of trauma care.[54] Similarly, the Advanced Life Support Group (ALSG) in the United Kingdom has issued guidelines outlining a structured approach to safe patient transfer.[55]

ABCs of Resuscitation

The primary goal in the initial management of the injured pregnant woman is the stabilization of the mother. As the American College of Obstetricians and Gynecologists (ACOG) has stated, "If attention is drawn to the fetus before the woman is stabilized, serious or life-threatening maternal injuries might be overlooked."[56] Obvious injuries demand attention, but a thorough physical examination of the patient should focus on looking for other, less obvious injuries.

Maternal resuscitation is the most effective method of fetal resuscitation. Evaluation and resuscitation should occur simultaneously. Standard resuscitation and trauma guidelines[57,58] apply in the pregnant patient, with two caveats: First, beginning at 18 to 20 weeks' gestation, the effect of aortocaval compression must be considered, and the patient must not be allowed to lie supine without left uterine displacement. Second, uterine evacuation may (or may not) increase the likelihood of fetal survival, depending on gestational age, but physicians should understand that uterine evacuation may also be necessary to facilitate resuscitation of the mother.[52]

AIRWAY

Airway evaluation and management is always the first priority during resuscitation, and it is the anesthesia provider's primary responsibility. Some patients require the simplest airway maintenance maneuvers (e.g., relief of obstruction, chin lift, jaw thrust), whereas others need endotracheal intubation and full ventilatory support. All patients should

TABLE 54-1 Physiologic Changes of Pregnancy*

Parameter	Effect of Pregnancy	Implications
Cardiovascular		
Cardiac output	↑ by 35%-50%	Aortocaval compression may markedly decrease cardiac output
Blood pressure	↓ by 5%-15% in second trimester; subsequently approaches baseline at term	
Systemic vascular resistance	↓ by 35% at midpregnancy; then increases slightly but remains ↓ by 20% at term	
Heart rate	↑ by 15%-25%	Early diagnosis of hypovolemia is more difficult
Central venous pressure	Unchanged	
Hematologic		
Blood volume	↑ by 30%-50%	Significant blood loss may occur before signs of hypovolemia and shock are apparent
Hemoglobin	↓ to 10-12 g/dL	Physiologic anemia of pregnancy
White blood cell count	↑ by 10%-50%, marked ↑ in labor	Increase may be mistaken for infection
Coagulation factors	↑ I, VII, VIII, IX, X, XII	Hypercoagulable state
Respiratory		
Functional residual capacity	↓ by 20%	Hypoxemia occurs more rapidly during periods of apnea
Tidal volume	↑ by 35%-45%	Normal hyperventilation
Respiratory rate	No change or slightly ↑	
Chest radiograph	Elevated diaphragm, leftward rotation of heart, no lung field changes	Chest tubes should be inserted at a higher level
Metabolic		
Oxygen consumption	↑ by as much as 60%	Reflects both maternal and fetal oxygen demands
pH	↑ to 7.42-7.46	Incomplete compensatory respiratory alkalosis
$Pa{O_2}$	↑ to 100-107 mm Hg (may decrease near term)	
$Pa{CO_2}$	↓ to 28-32 mm Hg	Reflects normal hyperventilation
HCO_3	↓ to 19-22 mEq/L	Reduced buffering capacity
Base deficit	↑ by 2-3 mEq/L	
Gastrointestinal		
Gastric emptying	Normal, but ↓ with labor and opioids	↑ risk of pulmonary aspiration of gastric contents
Lower esophageal sphincter	↓ competence	↑ risk of gastric reflux and pulmonary aspiration
Renal		
Renal blood flow	↑ by 60%-75%	
Glomerular filtration rate	↑ by 50%	
Blood urea nitrogen	↓ to 8-9 mg/dL	High (for pregnancy) measurements often overlooked
Serum creatinine	↓ 0.5-0.6 mg/dL	High (for pregnancy) measurements often overlooked
Musculoskeletal		
Symphysis pubis	Widened	May mislead interpretation of pelvic radiographs/computed tomography scans
Sacroiliac joints	Widened	May mislead interpretation of pelvic radiographs/computed tomography scans

*See Chapter 2 for greater detail.

↑, increase; ↓, decrease.

receive supplemental oxygen through a high-performance mask or bag-valve-mask system.

The anatomic and physiologic changes of pregnancy (e.g., mucosal edema, decreased functional residual capacity, increased oxygen consumption) increase the difficulty and decrease the safety margin of airway management. Trauma itself can produce a wide range of airway management problems, including facial fractures, airway burns, and cervical spine injuries. A decreased level of consciousness (e.g., from hypoxia, hypotension, eclampsia, poisoning, alcohol intoxication, or intracranial pathology) increases the risks of airway obstruction and aspiration. Similarly, the patient who tolerates an oral (Guedel) airway is unlikely to have an adequate level of consciousness to protect her own airway. Endotracheal intubation is required if injuries result in any one of the following: (1) airway obstruction, (2) compromised protective laryngeal reflexes and decreased ability to clear blood and secretions from the airway, (3) decreased adequacy of ventilatory efforts, and (4) hypoxemia despite the administration of supplemental oxygen. Some women require cricothyrotomy or tracheostomy. Early consultation with an otolaryngologist should be obtained if airway examination suggests that endotracheal intubation might be difficult or impossible. In emergency circumstances, cricothyrotomy or tracheostomy can also be difficult.

All pregnant patients involved in trauma should be considered at increased risk for pulmonary aspiration of gastric contents, and if intubation is considered necessary (or if the level of consciousness deteriorates), appropriate precautions should be taken. The technique chosen will depend on the anesthesia provider's individual skills, but in most situations rapid-sequence induction of anesthesia is performed. Awake fiberoptic intubation is an alternative option, although it may be difficult if the patient is combative or if there is blood in the airway. The nasotracheal route should be avoided if there is suspicion of a basilar skull fracture (e.g., presence of cerebrospinal fluid rhinorrhea).

Airway management of patients with cervical spine injuries requires special skill and attention, given that flexion, extension, or rotation of the head and neck can worsen injuries. Victims of blunt trauma are at risk for cervical spine injury, so the cervical spine should be immobilized until cleared by clinical appraisal and cervical spine and odontoid view radiographs or computed tomography (CT) scan. Immobilization does not preclude provision of left uterine displacement, but care must be taken to maintain inline support and immobilization.

Immobilization of the neck in a neutral position (by manual inline stabilization or cervical collar) can make intubation difficult. Additional airway equipment to assist intubation should be available; it may include a gum elastic bougie, an intubating stylet, a McCoy levered laryngoscope, a light wand, an intubating laryngeal mask airway, and/or a video laryngoscope. If intubation is not possible, the laryngeal mask airway may enable ventilation, albeit with limited protection from aspiration.

BREATHING

Once airway patency is confirmed, adequacy of ventilation should be assessed. Ventilatory drive can be reduced in patients with head injury, poisoning, or alcohol intoxication. Ventilatory ability can be diminished by pneumothorax, hemothorax, lung contusion, or chest wall injury. Respiratory failure is the most common cause of death in patients in whom neck injuries involve the cervical spinal cord.[59]

Management may involve chest drainage, endotracheal intubation, and positive-pressure ventilation, as appropriate. Because the diaphragm is displaced in a cephalad direction by the gravid uterus, chest tubes (e.g., for hemothorax or pneumothorax) should be inserted at a higher dermatomal level than in the nonpregnant patient to avoid damage to abdominal organs.

European guidelines suggest that hyperventilation in severely hypovolemic intubated patients is associated with a higher mortality than normal ventilation,[53] but the normal physiologic hyperventilation of pregnancy should be respected. It seems reasonable to maintain Pa_{CO_2} within the normal range for pregnancy, with use of the lowest possible airway pressures to minimize the risks of hypotension and barotrauma. Unless required for oxygenation, positive end-expiratory pressure (PEEP) should not be used because it has been shown to reduce cardiac output in nonpregnant trauma patients.[53]

CIRCULATION

Pregnancy-associated increases in circulating blood volume and cardiac output along with decreased systemic vascular resistance provide some maternal protection from hemorrhage. The pregnant woman compensates well, and can lose as much as 1.5 to 2 L of blood (35% of her circulating blood volume) before exhibiting the classic signs of hypovolemia. Therefore, when compensation fails, she will have lost significantly more blood from hemorrhage than a nonpregnant woman with similar findings. Because of the concomitant physiologic anemia of pregnancy, the pregnant woman with signs of hypovolemia is likely to have a serious deficit in oxygen-carrying capacity. Maternal compensation often occurs at the expense of the fetoplacental unit, and a nonreassuring FHR tracing may be the first sign of maternal hypovolemia. Aortocaval compression is never more hazardous than in the hypovolemic, hypotensive pregnant woman, highlighting the importance of continuous left uterine displacement.

Depending on the type of trauma, hemorrhage can be **compressible** (e.g., leg trauma) or **noncompressible** (e.g., splenic rupture, placental abruption). If possible, compressible hemorrhage should be stopped. Concealed losses from fractures are often underestimated; for example, a fractured pelvis can result in a blood loss of 3 L, and a closed femoral fracture can conceal a blood loss of 1.5 L.

Cardiac tamponade can occur with blunt or penetrating trauma to the chest and can be difficult to detect clinically. Ultrasonography can confirm the diagnosis quickly and should be part of an initial assessment process involving the focused assessment with sonography for trauma (FAST) examination.[60] Recommended treatment consists of needle paracentesis with ultrasonographic guidance and continuous electrocardiographic monitoring.

Venous Access

The upper extremities are the preferred sites for initial venous access; two large-bore peripheral venous catheters should be inserted as quickly as possible. In cases of hypovolemic shock, access to the central venous circulation can be critical but difficult to obtain in the hypovolemic, cold, vasoconstricted patient. Use of the Seldinger technique is recommended, and ultrasonographic visualization can be valuable. The internal jugular vein is the preferred site because the subclavian approach can result in hemothorax. Catheterization of the femoral vessels may be difficult in pregnant patients, increases the risk of thromboembolism and sepsis, and should be used only as a last resort. Formal cutdown of peripheral veins is another option for emergency intravenous access.

Fluids

Pregnant women in hypovolemic shock should be treated aggressively with rapid restoration of circulating volume and oxygen-carrying hemoglobin.[52] Crystalloids are recommended for initial resuscitation, although the intravenous "crystalloid versus colloid" debate continues.[48,52] The Saline versus Albumin Fluid Evaluation (SAFE) study demonstrated no difference in overall mortality between nonpregnant patients who received albumin and those who received normal saline, but mortality in patients with traumatic brain injury was *higher* if they received albumin.[61]

Crystalloids In general, crystalloid solutions induce an inflammatory response, produce hypercoagulability, and involve a higher risk of abdominal compartment syndrome than colloid solutions. Normal saline (in volumes exceeding 2 L) can produce a hyperchloremic acidosis.[62] The Advanced Trauma Life Support (ATLS) "gold standard" solution—lactated Ringer's solution—is superior but acidic (pH 6.0), and the usual racemic solution contains D-lactate, which has proinflammatory effects.[63] Newer buffered solutions such as Ringer's ethyl pyruvate and Ringer's hydroxybutyrate might have an effect on the inflammatory response and may be clinically useful, but outcome data are lacking.

Colloids Colloids, which have not been shown to be superior to crystalloids for improving maternal survival, are a heterogeneous group of very different solutions. Dextran solutions can cause anaphylaxis and have adverse effects on coagulation. Gelatin solutions have a higher rate of anaphylaxis than the hydroxyethyl starches (HES) and are probably of limited value in patients with ongoing hemorrhage. The effects and side effects of the starches depend on their mean molecular weight, concentration, and level of substitution. In general, they are associated with very low risks of anaphylaxis. Voluven (HES 130/0.4; Fresenius Kabi Norge A.S., Halden, Norway), which has gained U.S. Food and Drug Administration (FDA) approval for resuscitation after massive blood loss, might prove to be the best currently available choice of colloid.

Hypertonic Solutions The role of hypertonic saline in trauma resuscitation is controversial, and there is no convincing evidence that use of hypertonic saline improves patient survival. Initial studies suggested that a combination of hypertonic saline and colloid might be beneficial; two clinical trials are under way.[64] However, hypertonic solutions cannot be recommended for use in pregnant women until further results are published and their applicability to the pregnant trauma victim is made clear.

Blood Products

All facilities that provide care for obstetric trauma patients must have rapid access to a supply of group O, Rh-negative blood for emergency use before type-specific or cross-matched blood is available. Military experience now suggests that in cases of massive hemorrhage, aggressive use of blood components is associated with lower mortality, and a 1:1 rule, by which one unit of fresh frozen plasma is transfused for each unit of red blood cells, has been recommended for nonpregnant trauma victims.[65]

In the setting of uncontrollable hemorrhage in nonobstetric patients, the use of tranexamic acid and recombinant factor VIIa (rFVIIa) has been advocated.[53] Recombinant factor VIIa is a relatively new agent that has gained popularity in management of both trauma and obstetric hemorrhage, despite the paucity of data supporting its use. Numerous case reports have suggested that rFVIIa may reduce blood requirements in patients with massive hemorrhage. Hypothermia and acidosis may diminish its effect, and some clotting factors, particularly fibrinogen, must be present for it to be effective. However, guidelines developed by a multidisciplinary Israeli group (based on the use of rFVIIa in 36 severely injured trauma victims with uncontrollable hemorrhage) suggest that it is effective in controlling hemorrhage, and that hypothermia does not necessarily affect its usefulness.[66] European consensus guidelines also advocate the use of rFVIIa in patients with major bleeding (following blunt trauma) that persists despite best-practice use of blood components.[53] However, concerns regarding increased risks of thromboembolism highlight the need for more data before definitive recommendations can be made about the appropriate clinical use of rFVIIa in pregnant patients. It should be considered in a pregnant woman only if all standard therapies have failed.

Cell salvage has proved useful during surgery in nonobstetric patients, particularly for elective surgical cases in which there are predictably large blood losses. There is a growing consensus that cell salvage is safe in obstetric patients,[67] although debate continues regarding the utility of cell salvage in the obstetric setting.

Warming

Hypothermia aggravates coagulopathy and is a major contributor to poor outcome. Fluid warmers should be available and used for trauma victims. Rapid-volume fluid warmers can be useful in patients with major hemorrhage.

TRAUMATIC BRAIN INJURY

Neurologic assessment is important because a reduced level of consciousness can reflect intracranial pathology, intoxication, metabolic disorders (e.g., diabetes), the postictal state of eclampsia, or hypovolemia. Of particular concern is a changing level of consciousness. Thus frequent re-evaluation is required.

Head trauma, the most common severe injury among MVA victims, is a leading cause of maternal deaths secondary to trauma.[68] Increased intracranial pressure (ICP) frequently accompanies serious head injuries. CT is the investigation of choice in patients with known head injury and should be performed within an hour of hospital admission.

The SAFE study suggested that resuscitation with crystalloids is preferable to that with colloids in patients with traumatic brain injury (as discussed earlier).[61] Specific maneuvers can help promote venous drainage to decrease ICP. These include elevating the head 30 to 45 degrees and minimizing flexion and rotation of the head.[69,70]

Hypoventilation should be avoided because it increases ICP. Mechanical hyperventilation to a $Pa{CO_2}$ between 25 and 30 mm Hg only provides a short-lived reduction in ICP in nonpregnant patients. Similarly, the beneficial effects of mannitol and furosemide are transient, and generally all these maneuvers are reserved for acute reduction of ICP prior to more definitive management. Hypertonic saline-dextran solutions are currently being tested for this purpose.[71] Corticosteroids are no longer recommended in patients with traumatic brain injury and their use significantly increases mortality. On the other hand, barbiturates (e.g., thiopental, pentobarbital) effectively decrease cerebral blood flow and metabolism.

Hyperventilation is disadvantageous for the fetus because it can decrease uterine blood flow by decreasing maternal cardiac output and blood pressure, and perhaps by causing uteroplacental vasoconstriction. Both mannitol and furosemide cross the placenta and, theoretically, could increase fetal plasma osmolality and decrease intravascular volume.[72,73] In general, however, concern regarding fetal effects should be overridden by the immediate needs of the mother. It seems reasonable to maintain maternal $Pa{CO_2}$ within the normal range for pregnancy, with use of the lowest possible airway pressures to minimize the risks of hypotension and barotrauma.

In patients with traumatic brain injury, hypotension and hypoxia can cause rapid deterioration, and aggressive management, including rapid replacement of circulatory volume and cardiovascular pressor support, is required to maintain perfusion of the brain and other vital organs.

Maternal Monitoring

Standard noninvasive monitoring consists of pulse oximetry, electrocardiography, blood pressure, and temperature as well as FHR and uterine activity monitoring. A urethral catheter should be inserted, and hourly urine output should be monitored. An invasive arterial cannula is indicated for labile or low blood pressure or persistent hypoxemia; it permits direct measurement of blood pressure and easy access for arterial blood gas analysis.

If endotracheal intubation becomes necessary, the usual ventilatory parameters should be monitored; these include (1) tidal volume, (2) airway pressure, and (3) end-tidal carbon dioxide monitoring to confirm endotracheal intubation and monitor the level of ventilation. If a volatile halogenated agent is used to maintain anesthesia, the end-tidal concentration of the volatile agent should be monitored.

The use of pulmonary artery catheters in the critically ill has declined and, in some centers, has been replaced by transesophageal echocardiography (TEE). Alternative minimally invasive techniques for cardiac output monitoring (e.g., pulse contour analysis, use of a LiDCO monitor [lithium dilution technique; LiDCO Ltd., London]), may also be useful, depending on local availability and experience.

Fetal Monitoring

A nonreassuring FHR tracing may be the first sign of significant maternal hypovolemia; the FHR should be monitored continuously, and both baseline FHR and FHR variability should be assessed. The FHR variability is reduced when the pregnant woman receives opioid analgesia. The physician should look for evidence of uterine contractions, ruptured membranes, and placental abruption (abdominal pain, uterine tenderness, and vaginal bleeding). Fetal heart ST analysis (STAN) is a new method of fetal assessment that is currently undergoing evaluation.[74,75]

Diagnostic Tests

Indicated laboratory investigations are listed in Box 54-2. Laboratory results should be evaluated with knowledge of normal laboratory measurements in pregnancy (see Table 54-1).

BLOOD TESTING

Although blood tests may provide useful information in isolation, they are generally most valuable in serial assays to monitor the effectiveness (or failure) of treatment. Near-patient (bedside) testing can provide rapid and accurate assessment of many clinical parameters, and results are available more quickly than those of formal laboratory testing.

Complete blood counts include hemoglobin and hematocrit measurements, which help estimate the need for blood, but should not be the sole basis for decision-making, because they are influenced by the volume of previously administered resuscitation fluids. An elevated white blood cell (WBC) count can be an indicator of sepsis; in a small retrospective review, a high WBC count was shown to be predictive of placental abruption.[76] However, the WBC count is normally elevated by 10% to 40% during pregnancy, making interpretation difficult in the pregnant woman.

Similarly, a decreased platelet count can be a marker of hemorrhage or a sign of HELLP (hemolysis, elevated liver enzymes, low platelets) syndrome. Blood group typing is

BOX 54-2 Initial Laboratory Analyses for the Pregnant Trauma Victim

- Blood type, cross-match, and Rh status
- Complete blood count (hemoglobin measurement, white blood cell count, platelet count)
- Prothrombin and partial thromboplastin times
- Fibrinogen (or fibrin degradation products) concentration
- Serum electrolyte and urate levels
- Liver function tests
- Serum amylase level
- Blood glucose level
- Blood lactate level
- Toxicology screen
- Arterial blood gas measurements (pH, $Pa{O_2}$, $Pa{CO_2}$, bicarbonate, base deficit)
- Kleihauer-Betke assay
- Urinary protein, blood, bilirubin, and glucose levels
- Urine osmolality or specific gravity

important for detection of women who are Rh-negative and at risk of isoimmunization. Antibody screening is important for assessment of cross-match compatibility.

Arterial blood gas analysis provides information about oxygen tension, ventilation, and acid-base status. Bicarbonate levels in pregnant women are reduced because of compensation for the normal respiratory alkalosis of pregnancy. Determination of base deficit helps estimate and monitor the extent of bleeding and shock in nonpregnant patients[53] and can be followed in pregnant women (with recognition that normal pregnancy is associated with an increase in base deficit of 2 to 3 mEq/L). Plasma lactate measurement is also a sensitive test to estimate the severity of hemorrhage and shock and is an indirect measure of oxygen debt and tissue hypoperfusion.[77]

Assessment of serum electrolytes allows detection of hypernatremia or hyperkalemia. Blood urea nitrogen (BUN) and serum creatinine levels provide an index of renal function (normal values in pregnancy must be considered in interpretation of results). Serum urate measurement can be useful in patients with suspected preeclampsia, but it is an unreliable test after administration of large volumes of intravenous fluid during resuscitation. Blood glucose assay will detect or exclude hypoglycemia and hyperglycemia. Measurements of liver enzymes and amylase are also indicated in trauma patients, and a toxicology screen will identify any involvement of drugs or alcohol.

Coagulopathy can develop from blood loss, hemodilution, or disseminated intravascular coagulation triggered by uterine trauma or placental abruption. Coagulation test results (prothrombin time, partial thromboplastin time, assessments of fibrinogen and fibrin degradation products, platelet count) guide the administration of coagulation factors (fresh frozen plasma, cryoprecipitate, platelets). In addition, coagulation test results may be predictive of maternal outcome.[3]

The Kleihauer-Betke acid elution assay is used to detect and quantify the extent of fetomaternal hemorrhage (i.e., fetal blood entering the maternal circulation). It is traditionally used in Rh-negative women to detect transplacental hemorrhage that can lead to Rhesus isosensitization if Rh(D) immune globulin is not administered. Sequential Kleihauer-Betke testing helps detect ongoing fetomaternal hemorrhage and the need for multiple doses of Rh(D) immune globulin. Additionally, in a retrospective study of 71 pregnant trauma patients, the Kleihauer-Betke test was a useful and sensitive test for predicting the development of preterm labor[78]; therefore it may be useful in the management of all pregnant trauma victims, regardless of Rh status.

URINE TESTING

Urine should be routinely tested for protein, blood, bilirubin, and glucose. Assessment of urinary osmolality (or specific gravity) provides information about renal function, and hourly urine output monitoring helps determine the effectiveness of resuscitation.

RADIOGRAPHIC IMAGING

The pregnant trauma patient often requires a radiographic skeletal survey and may also need special radiographic procedures to diagnose specific injuries. Despite fears about potential harm to the developing fetus from exposure to ionizing radiation, the risks of radiation-induced teratogenesis, malignancy, or gene mutation are small.[79] The fetus is at greatest risk for teratogenesis during the first trimester. When possible, lead shielding should be used over the pelvis to protect the fetus during radiographic investigations. The small fetal risk is almost always outweighed by the potential benefit to the mother (and, by extension, the fetus) of appropriate imaging.

Fetal risk of malformations is considered to be low with total radiation exposures of less than 50 to 100 mGy (5 to 10 rads).[80] Individual radiographic examinations produce very low levels of exposure. Intravenous pyelography subjects the fetus to as much as 1.4 rads of exposure but can provide critically important functional information about the kidneys, ureters, and bladder. CT produces higher levels of radiation exposure than plain radiographs, but even abdominal and pelvic CT scanning usually produces estimated fetal exposures below those typically associated with adverse fetal/neonatal outcomes (see Table 17-2). Despite the logistic difficulties of transferring the injured patient into the CT scanner, the speed and usefulness of the information obtained usually justifies its use in the patient who is reasonably stable. The CT scan is the definitive radiographic study in most patients with trauma. CT of the abdomen, pelvis, chest, and head is the most sensitive and accurate noninvasive diagnostic tool for identification of soft tissue injury and fractures.

Modern multidetector (multislice) CT (MDCT) scanners result in higher fetal radiation exposure but have significant advantages in terms of speed and quality. Modern 64-slice CT scanners can perform whole-body scanning within 30 seconds, although some repositioning of different body parts might be required for optimal images. In most instances, the whole process can be completed in minutes. MDCT scanning is clearly superior to plain radiography in trauma imaging; overall, MDCT has been shown to have a sensitivity of 94%, a specificity of 100%, and an accuracy of 97%.[81] As a result, MDCT is now the gold standard imaging tool for trauma patients, if available.

The risks of transferring a potentially unstable patient to and from a remote CT scanning unit must be weighed against the potential benefits, but risks are minimized if the scanner is close to (or within) the emergency department. Deaths have occurred in the CT scanner; therefore careful assessment of the patient's stability must be made prior to transfer into the scanner, and the patient should be accompanied by a physician. The avoidance of aortocaval compression in pregnant trauma patients is essential, and radiology staff unfamiliar with the need for left uterine displacement in pregnant patients might need encouragement to use a wedge or lateral position.

Magnetic resonance imaging (MRI) avoids the risk of fetal radiation exposure, but it is too slow and impractical for the seriously injured, unstable patient who needs ongoing resuscitation and monitoring.

ULTRASONOGRAPHY

Ultrasonography is a useful diagnostic tool in patients with blunt abdominal trauma and has largely replaced diagnostic peritoneal lavage for the detection of intra-abdominal hemorrhage.[82] It detects free fluid in the hepatorenal and splenorenal spaces, the pouch of Douglas in the pelvis, and the pericardium, and it can also detect hemopneumothorax. Free fluid in the abdomen or pelvis is associated with intra-abdominal injury.[83] Sensitivity and specificity of ultrasonography in pregnant patients are similar to that seen in nonpregnant patients,[84] although the technique is less sensitive in detecting retroperitoneal and hollow viscus injuries. Patients without intraperitoneal fluid are considered to be at low risk for an intra-abdominal injury requiring surgical intervention.[84] As a screening test for intra-abdominal hemorrhage, ultrasonography is most sensitive in the first trimester,[85] but it has also proved useful in a limited number of third-trimester patients, despite the greater uterine size and displaced intra-abdominal viscera.[84] An additional advantage is the ability to image the fetal heart or detect a previously undiagnosed intrauterine pregnancy.

DIAGNOSTIC PERITONEAL LAVAGE

Diagnostic peritoneal lavage has become a largely obsolete investigation with the better availability of reliable and noninvasive ultrasonography and rapid CT scanning. If this evaluation is necessary in a pregnant patient, the needle should be inserted above the umbilicus.[57]

Other Management Issues

ANALGESIA

Pregnant women with traumatic injuries should not be denied effective analgesia simply because they are pregnant. In most serious injuries, intravenous opioids are the mainstay of analgesia, just as in the nonpregnant population. Opioids typically cause a reduction in FHR variability, which does not necessarily signal fetal compromise; therefore the obstetrician should be notified of opioid administration. Nonsteroidal anti-inflammatory drugs (NSAIDs) should generally be avoided in patients with major trauma because of their deleterious effects on platelet function and renal perfusion. Intravenous acetaminophen (known as paracetamol, and approved for use, in the United Kingdom) has an opioid-sparing effect. Other analgesic techniques are peripheral nerve blocks, with or without an indwelling catheter, and intercostal blocks for rib fractures.

RISK OF THROMBOSIS

Pregnancy is a hypercoagulable state, and once acute coagulopathy due to trauma has resolved, the patient is at increased risk of thromboembolic events, especially if the injuries cause immobility. Pregnant women with fractures have a ninefold higher risk of thrombotic events.[48] Therefore, thromboprophylaxis must be considered after hemostasis is secured and the patient is hemodynamically stable.

PREECLAMPSIA AND ECLAMPSIA

Blood pressure generally falls slightly in pregnancy, but it can be elevated in patients with chronic hypertension or preeclampsia. Although hypertension is one of the cardinal features of preeclampsia, it is not always apparent early in the disease process, and it can also be masked by hypovolemia. Unexpectedly high (or normal) blood pressure measurements in the presence of significant blood loss, proteinuria, elevated serum urate or liver enzyme levels, unexplained thrombocytopenia, or the new onset of seizures should raise the suspicion of underlying preeclampsia or eclampsia.

Seizures after traumatic head injury in a pregnant woman present a difficult diagnostic problem because eclamptic seizures are a clinical diagnosis of exclusion. Supportive evidence for eclampsia includes proteinuria (although this could result from trauma), increased serum urate and liver enzyme levels, thrombocytopenia not explained by hemorrhage, and a previous diagnosis of preeclampsia. Whenever eclampsia is strongly suspected, intravenous magnesium sulfate should be administered.

EVACUATION OF THE UTERUS

There are two distinct reasons to empty the uterus in pregnant trauma victims. First, fetal compromise can result from inadequate uteroplacental perfusion due to hypovolemia, placental abruption, or uterine rupture. The presence of a nonreassuring FHR pattern that does not resolve with initial resuscitation of the mother (including adequate left uterine displacement) may prompt immediate delivery for fetal indications. Second, uterine evacuation may improve hemodynamic stability in an unstable mother (e.g., one who is unresponsive to resuscitation, continues to bleed, or requires laparotomy). In these situations, delivery is performed as part of maternal resuscitation, and also offers a better chance of survival for the viable fetus.

CARDIAC ARREST AND PERIMORTEM CESAREAN DELIVERY

When cardiac arrest occurs in a pregnant woman, standard Advanced Cardiac Life Support (ACLS) resuscitation guidelines apply, with two important modifications. First, attempts must be made to minimize aortocaval compression by maintaining left uterine displacement. However, this position change might interfere with effective chest compression. Various solutions to this problem have been advocated, including use of (1) a sandbag under the right hip, (2) a human wedge (i.e., tilting the patient on the bent knees of a kneeling rescuer), and (3) the Cardiff wedge, a large wedge-shaped board on which resuscitation takes place. In the presence of potential neck injury, particular care should be taken to stabilize the head and neck if the patient is turned to her side.

Second, as part of the process of maternal resuscitation in the second half of pregnancy, the infant should be delivered, usually by cesarean delivery. Katz et al.[86] first advocated the "4-minute rule," which calls for perimortem cesarean delivery to begin within 4 minutes of maternal cardiac arrest, so that the infant is delivered within 5 minutes of cardiac arrest. This approach increases the likelihood of both maternal and neonatal survival.[86] In general, when cesarean delivery is performed outside this 5-minute window, outcome for mother and baby is very poor. However, isolated case reports of infant survival after more than 20 minutes of maternal cardiac arrest support the performance of a perimortem cesarean delivery in any case of maternal cardiac arrest, with continued evidence of fetal cardiac activity, beyond 24 weeks' gestation.

In cases of cardiac arrest during the second half of pregnancy, cesarean delivery aids resuscitation of the mother by (1) minimizing the aortocaval compression from the pregnant uterus, thereby increasing venous return; (2) reducing maternal oxygen consumption; (3) aiding ventilation; and (4) allowing cardiopulmonary resuscitation (CPR) to be performed with the patient in the supine position.[20,52] If CPR has not been effective within 4 minutes in the tilted position, cesarean delivery should be performed immediately. CPR should continue during and after surgery, and unless the operating room is very close to the area of maternal collapse, it is likely that the delivery will have to be performed where the cardiac arrest occurred (e.g., labor and delivery room, emergency department). The benefits of rapid intervention outweigh the practical limitations of working outside the operating room. Because of the rarity of maternal cardiac arrest, drills are needed to maintain staff skills and preparedness for the event.

If cesarean delivery is required, endotracheal intubation is not likely to require anesthetic drugs. However, if cardiac output improves after further resuscitation, awareness can occur, and anesthesia should be provided as needed and tolerated. The presence of hypotension does not uniformly prevent awareness in young patients, and administration of anesthetic and/or amnestic agents should be considered after a positive hemodynamic response has been observed.

COMA, PERSISTENT VEGETATIVE STATE, AND BRAINSTEM DEATH

Several case reports have noted that it is possible, in a pregnant woman with irreversible brain damage or brainstem death, for the pregnancy to be prolonged to achieve delivery of a viable infant, usually by cesarean delivery.[87,88] Three women with MVA-associated traumatic brain injury during the first or second trimester received between 107 and 189 days of life support prior to delivery at 31 to 35 weeks' gestation.[89-91] Hyperthermia or thermovariability was a problem in all of these cases. Guidelines for the management of hypotension and mechanical ventilation in pregnancies complicated by fatal maternal brain injury have been published.[92]

Education and Training

Since its inception in 1978, the Advanced Trauma Life Support (ATLS) course has provided a structured, reproducible, systemized approach to trauma care that has been adopted by more than 50 countries.[57] A section of the course titled "Trauma in Women" explores the anatomic and physiologic alterations of pregnancy and establishes assessment and treatment priorities for both mother and baby.

ATLS focuses on the interventions of a physician working with limited resources in a community hospital setting. As trauma care has evolved, and with specialized providers (including anesthesia providers for airway management) present at more centers, there is a growing call for the development of a course to better reflect modern multidisciplinary practice using a team approach.[93,94]

In the United Kingdom, the Managing Obstetric Emergencies and Trauma (MOET) course is offered in collaboration with the Royal College of Obstetricians and Gynaecologists.[52] Designed for senior anesthesia providers and obstetricians, it provides training, similar to that of the ATLS course, in the management of trauma in pregnant women. The course is now offered in 14 centers in the United Kingdom as well as in several other countries in the developed and developing world.[52,95] CEMACH has endorsed and recommended the MOET course for all health care providers involved in obstetric emergencies.[20]

TABLE 54-2 Web Resources

Advanced Trauma Life Support Course	http://www.facs.org/trauma/atls/index.html
ALS Group (for Managing Obstetric Emergencies and Trauma Course)	http://www.alsg.org
Primary Trauma Care Foundation	http://www.primarytraumacare.org
European Resuscitation Council (for European Trauma Course)	http://www.erc.edu
National Confidential Enquiry into Patient Outcome and Death	http://www.ncepod.org.uk
Confidential Enquiry into Maternal and Child Health	http://www.cemach.org.uk
Trauma.org	http://www.trauma.org

The European Trauma Course (ETC) is a new simulator-based course being developed by the European Resuscitation Council to cover both prehospital and in-hospital care.[58] The ETC approaches initial management not as a fixed, rigid sequence of interventions but rather as a variable set of processes that occur simultaneously and adapt to the severity of the patient's condition. The ETC specifically addresses trauma in early and late pregnancy, and it considers physiologic changes of pregnancy and their consequences for the ABCs of resuscitation as well as fetomaternal hemorrhage, domestic abuse, nonreassuring FHR tracings, and the difficulties in distinguishing between head injury and preeclampsia (Table 54-2).

ANESTHETIC MANAGEMENT

The anesthetic management of pregnant trauma patients incorporates the principles of anesthesia for nonpregnant trauma victims with those for pregnant patients undergoing nonobstetric surgery. The primary goals are to maintain maternal hemodynamic stability and optimize uteroplacental perfusion (Box 54-3). Most drugs commonly used in anesthetic practice are considered safe for use during pregnancy. As previously stated, neonatal outcomes depend on resuscitation and stabilization of the mother. Therefore, optimization of maternal condition is the best strategy for optimizing fetal condition.

The anesthetic technique depends on the nature of the maternal injuries and the preference of the anesthesia provider, and does not diverge greatly from that in the nonpregnant trauma patient. To minimize the adverse effects of aortocaval compression, left uterine displacement (or leftward tilt of the operating table) should be maintained, beginning at 18 to 20 weeks' gestation. Surgeons unfamiliar with obstetric patients might need reassurance that the tilted position is necessary to optimize maternal cardiac output.

BOX 54-3 General Principles for Management of the Pregnant Trauma Victim

- Optimization of gas exchange
- Early restoration of tissue perfusion and oxygenation
- Restoration of blood volume
- Maintenance of uteroplacental circulation and fetal oxygenation
- Detection of unrecognized injuries
- Protection of the brain and spinal cord
- Minimization of the biochemical effects of trauma
- Maintenance of normothermia
- Correction of coagulopathy
- Maintenance of renal function
- Maintenance of gastrointestinal function
- Avoidance of transfusion complications
- Prevention of maternal awareness during surgery
- Avoidance of teratogenic drugs during the first trimester
- Prevention of preterm labor

Patients are often hypothermic on arrival in the operating room. Because surgery and anesthesia result in further heat loss, aggressive warming measures (e.g., warming mattress, warm air blanket, fluid warmer, raised ambient temperature) are recommended.

Standard noninvasive hemodynamic monitoring can be supplemented with central venous and invasive arterial pressure monitoring, and patients in critical condition might benefit from TEE to guide fluid therapy. Temperature measurement is important to monitor the effectiveness of active warming. Some anesthesia providers contend that bispectral index monitoring may reduce the risk of maternal awareness, although its utility in this setting is unproved.

Induction and Intubation

Pregnant women are at increased risk for pulmonary aspiration and should receive antacid prophylaxis if possible and if time permits. Following intubation, a gastric tube should be passed to empty or decompress the stomach. The oral route for gastric intubation is preferred if basilar skull fracture is suspected.

Following denitrogenation (so-called preoxygenation) with 100% oxygen, rapid-sequence induction of anesthesia with cricoid pressure is preferred, although awake fiberoptic intubation is an option in some instances. Alternative airway tools (e.g., gum elastic bougie, McCoy laryngoscope, laryngeal mask airway in various sizes) should be available for management of the difficult airway.

Succinylcholine remains the muscle relaxant of choice for rapid-sequence induction in most trauma victims. In some cases **rocuronium** is administered for this purpose and might become an even more useful alternative if the U.S. FDA joins European regulators in approving the clinical use of suggamadex (a rocuronium reversal agent; Schering-Plough Corporation, Kenilworth, NJ). Once endotracheal intubation is achieved, muscle relaxation is maintained with a nondepolarizing muscle relaxant and guided by peripheral nerve stimulator monitoring.

Although hypovolemia precludes the administration of usual doses of anesthetic agents, young patients might experience intraoperative awareness during paralysis and light anesthesia, even in the presence of severe hypotension. Standard doses of **etomidate** (0.3 mg/kg) or **ketamine** (1 to 1.5 mg/kg) provide better blood pressure support than thiopental. Propofol is relatively contraindicated in bleeding trauma victims because of its vasodilatory and hypotensive effects. Administration of a bolus of fluid prior to induction of anesthesia might ameliorate the hypotensive effects of induction agents.

Ketamine is unique among anesthetic agents because its sympathomimetic qualities result in cardiovascular stimulation. It is often used in trauma patients, but it can cause myocardial depression in patients with severe hypovolemia and might increase ICP in patients with head injury. Large doses (greater than 2 mg/kg) may increase uterine tone and decrease uteroplacental perfusion,[96] but smaller doses are less likely to have adverse effects on the uteroplacental circulation.

Opioids (e.g., fentanyl) can be used to supplement a reduced dose of hypnotic agent. Although contrary to the historic practice of rapid-sequence induction, this modified approach can provide a smoother induction with less risk of maternal awareness. Light anesthesia is also bad for the fetus because higher levels of circulating maternal catecholamines can reduce uteroplacental blood flow. If delivery is planned as part of the surgical procedure, opioid-induced respiratory depression in the neonate can be reversed with naloxone.

Ventilation can be difficult in patients with chest trauma, and techniques to minimize barotrauma should be employed (e.g., small tidal volumes, minimal peak inspiratory pressures, avoidance of PEEP). A pressure-controlled ventilator may be necessary in cases of severe lung injury or when ARDS develops.

Maintenance of Anesthesia

Many anesthesia providers favor a balanced anesthetic technique, using a volatile halogenated anesthetic agent, opioids, and neuromuscular blockade, for the maintenance of hemodynamic stability during trauma surgery. In unstable hypotensive patients, small doses of amnestic agents (e.g., midazolam) and opioids (e.g., fentanyl) should be administered until the patient's hemodynamic status permits the use of a volatile halogenated agent.

In pregnant patients, volatile halogenated agents provide distinct advantages, because they are easily titrated, reduce the risk of intraoperative awareness, and decrease uterine activity by relaxing uterine smooth muscle. Little evidence guides the specific choice of agent (isoflurane, sevoflurane, or desflurane). In patients undergoing cesarean delivery, uterine contractility typically can be maintained with a small concentration of a volatile agent (and concurrent infusion of oxytocin), but in the presence of obstetric hemorrhage due to uterine atony, it seems prudent to minimize the concentration of the volatile halogenated agent or convert to an intravenous anesthetic technique.

The use of nitrous oxide may be limited or avoided because of the need for a high inspired oxygen fraction or by the presence (or risk) of air-filled cavities such as pneumothorax.

Worsening hypotension, hypoxemia, and difficulty with ventilation may indicate a tension pneumothorax.

Unless necessary for oxygenation, PEEP is not advisable because it increases the risks of pneumothorax and reduces cardiac output in patients with hypovolemia.[53]

Fetal Monitoring

Electronic FHR monitoring should be performed before and after surgery to assess fetal well-being. Intraoperative monitoring is recommended when possible, particularly when gestational age exceeds 24 weeks and cesarean delivery is likely to result in a viable fetus. During general anesthesia, decreased FHR variability reflects the transplacental transfer of anesthetic agents and is not necessarily a cause for concern. However, sustained fetal tachycardia or bradycardia or recurrent FHR decelerations suggest fetal compromise.

The ACOG[97] has acknowledged that there are no data to allow specific recommendations for FHR monitoring in obstetric patients undergoing nonobstetric surgery. The ACOG has stated, "The decision to use fetal monitoring should be individualized, and, if used, may be based on gestational age, type of surgery, and facilities available."[97]

Fetal heart rate abnormalities can signal the need to (1) optimize maternal oxygenation, ventilation, and acid-base status; (2) expand maternal blood volume; (3) increase maternal perfusion pressure by administration of a vasopressor; (4) increase maternal oxygen-carrying capacity through transfusion of red blood cells; (5) relieve aortocaval compression by increasing left uterine displacement or repositioning surgical retractors; and/or (6) perform cesarean delivery.

Uterine activity should be monitored in the perioperative period to facilitate the early diagnosis of preterm labor, which may be treated with a tocolytic agent.

An experienced obstetric care provider should be present to monitor and interpret the FHR tracing and uterine activity when the fetus is continuously monitored. An obstetrician should be immediately available to perform cesarean delivery of a viable fetus when severe fetal compromise occurs during surgery or if the maternal condition demands it.

Cesarean Delivery

If cesarean delivery is performed, an oxytocic agent is required to restore uterine tone after delivery of the infant, but care must be taken with the use of intravenous oxytocin. A widely publicized maternal death in the United Kingdom highlighted the dangers of administering oxytocin as a single 10-unit bolus dose in the presence of circulatory compromise,[98] and even a 5-unit dose might be excessive and cause cardiovascular collapse.[20] In a hypovolemic patient, oxytocin is best administered as a slow intravenous infusion.[20] To minimize relaxant effects on the uterus, high concentrations of volatile halogenated agents should be avoided.

Fluids

Fluid management is based on estimated preoperative fluid status, observed intraoperative blood loss, maternal hemodynamic status, and information obtained from central venous pressure monitoring, TEE, and/or urine output monitoring. Coagulopathy requires aggressive management, and the blood bank should be notified of the presence of a patient with massive hemorrhage and anticipated transfusion requirements. In cases of massive blood loss, the use of a cell salvage system, if available, should be considered. If cell salvage is used at cesarean delivery, attempts must be made to limit the collection of amniotic fluid, and a leukocyte depletion filter should be used.[67]

Pulmonary Edema

Pulmonary edema, due to either iatrogenic fluid overload or ARDS, can complicate the postresuscitation, postoperative course in obstetric patients. Women with severe injuries after trauma, particularly with major fluid shifts or continuing blood loss, unresolved coagulopathy, or multiorgan injury, should remain intubated, ventilated, and anesthetized at the end of the procedure and should be transferred to a critical care unit for subsequent management.

KEY POINTS

- Trauma occurs in 5% to 10% of all pregnancies and ranks first among nonobstetric causes of maternal mortality.
- Head injury and hemorrhagic shock account for most maternal deaths secondary to trauma.
- Placental abruption and maternal death are the most common causes of fetal death secondary to trauma.
- Even minor trauma increases the risk of placental abruption, preterm labor, and low birth weight.
- Domestic violence and depressive illness should be considered in the evaluation of maternal trauma.
- Maternal resuscitation is the most effective method of fetal resuscitation.
- Beginning at 18 to 20 weeks' gestation, left uterine displacement is required in all injured pregnant women to avoid or minimize aortocaval compression.
- In severely injured pregnant women, a low threshold for uterine evacuation maximizes the chances of survival for both the mother and the fetus.
- Standard resuscitation guidelines apply in cases of maternal cardiac arrest.
- Perimortem cesarean delivery should begin within 4 minutes of maternal cardiac arrest, and the fetus should be delivered within 5 minutes of maternal cardiac arrest.
- Electronic fetal heart rate monitoring helps guide anesthetic and obstetric management during maternal resuscitation, surgery, and postoperative management.

REFERENCES

1. Harper M, Parsons L. Maternal deaths due to homicide and other injuries in North Carolina: 1992-1994. Obstet Gynecol 1997; 90:920-3.
2. Chang J, Berg CJ, Saltzman LE, Herndon J. Homicide: A leading cause of injury deaths among pregnant and postpartum women in the United States, 1991-1999. Am J Public Health 2005; 95:471-7.

3. Patteson SK, Snider CC, Meyer DS, et al. The consequences of high-risk behaviors: Trauma during pregnancy. J Trauma 2007; 62: 1015-20.
4. Aboutanos SZ, Aboutanos MB, Dompkowski D, et al. Predictors of fetal outcome in pregnant trauma patients: A five-year institutional review. Am Surg 2007; 73:824-7.
5. Buchsbaum H. Penetrating injury of the abdomen. In Buchsbaum H, editor. Trauma in Pregnancy. Philadelphia, WB Saunders, 1979:82-100.
6. Baerga-Varela Y, Zietlow SP, Bannon MP, et al. Trauma in pregnancy. Mayo Clin Proc 2000; 75:1243-8.
7. Redelmeier DA, Drucker A, Venkatesh V. Major trauma in pregnant women during the summer. J Trauma 2005; 59:112-6.
8. Weiss HB, Lawrence BA, Miller TR. Pregnancy-associated assault hospitalizations. Obstet Gynecol 2002; 100:773-80.
9. Ikossi DG, Lazar AA, Morabito D, et al. Profile of mothers at risk: An analysis of injury and pregnancy loss in 1,195 trauma patients. J Am Coll Surg 2005; 200:49-56.
10. Kuo C, Jamieson DJ, McPheeters ML, et al. Injury hospitalizations of pregnant women in the United States, 2002. Am J Obstet Gynecol 2007; 196:161e, 1-6.
11. Schiff MA, Holt VL. Pregnancy outcomes following hospitalization for motor vehicle crashes in Washington State from 1989 to 2001. Am J Epidemiol 2005; 161:503-10.
12. El Kady D, Gilbert WM, Anderson J, et al. Trauma during pregnancy: An analysis of maternal and fetal outcomes in a large population. Am J Obstet Gynecol 2004; 190:1661-8.
13. Weiss HB, Songer TJ, Fabio A. Fetal deaths related to maternal injury. JAMA 2001; 286:1863-8.
14. Dunning K, LeMasters G, Levin L, et al. Falls in workers during pregnancy: Risk factors, job hazards, and high risk occupations. Am J Ind Med 2003; 44:664-72.
15. Desjardins G. Management of the injured pregnant patient. Trauma.org. Available at http://www.trauma.org/archive/resus/pregnancytrauma.html/
16. Weiss HB. Pregnancy associated assault hospitalizations, selected U.S. states, 1997: Exploring the incidence and risk for hospitalized assaults against women during pregnancy. Rockville, MD, National Institute of Justice, 2003.
17. Mabrouk AR, el-Feky AE. Burns during pregnancy: A gloomy outcome. Burns 1997; 23:596-600.
18. Guo SS, Greenspoon JS, Kahn AM. Management of burn injuries during pregnancy. Burns 2001; 27:394-7.
19. Shadigian E, Bauer ST. Pregnancy-associated death: A qualitative systematic review of homicide and suicide. Obstet Gynecol Surv 2005; 60:183-90.
20. Lewis G, editor. The Confidential Enquiry into Maternal and Child Health (CEMACH): Saving Mothers' Lives: Reviewing Maternal Deaths to Make Motherhood Safer—2003-2005. The Seventh Report of the Confidential Enquiries into Maternal Deaths in the United Kingdom. London, CEMACH, 2007.
21. Martin SL, Mackie L, Kupper LL, et al. Physical abuse of women before, during, and after pregnancy. JAMA 2001; 285:1581-4.
22. Gazmararian JA, Lazorick S, Spitz AM, et al. Prevalence of violence against pregnant women. JAMA 1996; 275:1915-20.
23. Kaye DK, Mirembe FM, Bantebya G, et al. Domestic violence during pregnancy and risk of low birthweight and maternal complications: A prospective cohort study at Mulago Hospital, Uganda. Trop Med Int Health 2006; 11:1576-84.
24. National Highway Transportation Administration. Should pregnant women wear seatbelts? Available at http://www.nhtsa.dot.gov/staticfiles/DOT/NHTSA/Communication%20&%20Consumer%20Information/Articles/Associated%20Files/BUA_PregnancyNHTSAchange.pdf/
25. Metz TD, Abbott JT. Uterine trauma in pregnancy after motor vehicle crashes with airbag deployment: A 30-case series. J Trauma 2006; 61:658-61.
26. Hyde LK, Cook LJ, Olson LM, et al. Effect of motor vehicle crashes on adverse fetal outcomes. Obstet Gynecol 2003; 102:279-86.
27. Rainio J, Penttila A. Amniotic fluid embolism as cause of death in a car accident—a case report. Forensic Sci Int 2003; 137:231-4.
28. Ichikawa M, Nakahara S, Okubo T, Wakai S. Car seatbelt use during pregnancy in Japan: Determinants and policy implications. Inj Prev 2003; 9:169-72.
29. Rothenberger D, Quattlebaum FW, Perry JF Jr, et al. Blunt maternal trauma: A review of 103 cases. J Trauma 1978; 18:173-9.
30. Leggon RE, Wood GC, Indeck MC. Pelvic fractures in pregnancy: Factors influencing maternal and fetal outcomes. J Trauma 2002; 53:796-804.
31. Pape HC, Pohlemann T, Gansslen A, et al. Pelvic fractures in pregnant multiple trauma patients. J Orthop Trauma 2000; 14:238-44.
32. El Kady D, Gilbert WM, Xing G, Smith LH. Maternal and neonatal outcomes of assaults during pregnancy. Obstet Gynecol 2005; 105:357-63.
33. Fries MH, Hankins GD. Motor vehicle accident associated with minimal maternal trauma but subsequent fetal demise. Ann Emerg Med 1989; 18:301-4.
34. Schiff MA, Holt VL. The injury severity score in pregnant trauma patients: Predicting placental abruption and fetal death. J Trauma 2002; 53:946-9.
35. Schiff MA, Holt VL, Daling JR. Maternal and infant outcomes after injury during pregnancy in Washington state from 1989 to 1997. J Trauma 2002; 53:939-45.
36. Sperry JL, Casey BM, McIntire DD, et al. Long-term fetal outcomes in pregnant trauma patients. Am J Surg 2006; 192:715-21.
37. Olcott C IV, Robinson AJ, Maxwell TM, Griffin HA. Amniotic fluid embolism and disseminated intravascular coagulation after blunt abdominal trauma. J Trauma 1973; 13:737-40.
38. Ellingsen CL, Eggebo TM, Lexow K. Amniotic fluid embolism after blunt abdominal trauma. Resuscitation 2007; 75:180-3.
39. Judich A, Kuriansky J, Engelberg I, et al. Amniotic fluid embolism following blunt abdominal trauma in pregnancy. Injury 1998; 29:475-7.
40. Pak LL, Reece EA, Chan L. Is adverse pregnancy outcome predictable after blunt abdominal trauma? Am J Obstet Gynecol 1998; 179:1140-4.
41. Rose PG, Strohm PL, Zuspan FP. Fetomaternal hemorrhage following trauma. Am J Obstet Gynecol 1985; 153:844-7.
42. Crosby WM, Costiloe JP. Safety of lap-belt restraint for pregnant victims of automobile collisions. N Engl J Med 1971; 284:632-6.
43. Pepperell RJ, Rubinstein E, MacIsaac IA. Motor-car accidents during pregnancy. Med J Aust 1977; 1:203-5.
44. Lane PL. Traumatic fetal deaths. J Emerg Med 1989; 7:433-5.
45. Klinich KD, Flannagan CA, Rupp JD, et al. Fetal outcome in motor-vehicle crashes: Effects of crash characteristics and maternal restraint. Am J Obstet Gynecol 2008; 198:450, e1-9.
46. Klinich KD, Schneider LW, Moore JL, Pearlman MD. Investigations of crashes involving pregnant occupants. Annu Proc Assoc Adv Automot Med 2000; 44:37-55.
47. Curet MJ, Schermer CR, Demarest GB, et al. Predictors of outcome in trauma during pregnancy: Identification of patients who can be monitored for less than 6 hours. J Trauma 2000; 49:18-25.
48. El Kady D, Gilbert WM, Xing G, Smith LH. Association of maternal fractures with adverse perinatal outcomes. Am J Obstet Gynecol 2006; 195:711-6.
49. Hayes B, Ryan S, Stephenson JB, King MD. Cerebral palsy after maternal trauma in pregnancy. Dev Med Child Neurol 2007; 49:700-6.
50. Stevens TA, Carroll MA, Promecene PA, et al. Utility of acute physiology, age, and chronic health evaluation (APACHE III) score in maternal admissions to the intensive care unit. Am J Obstet Gynecol 2006; 194:e.13-5.
51. Fowler R, Pepe PE. Fluid resuscitation of the patient with major trauma. Curr Opin Anaesthesiol 2002; 15:173-8.
52. Grady K, Howell C, Cox C, editors. Managing Obstetric Emergencies and Trauma. London, Royal College of Obstetricians and Gynaecologists Press, 2007.
53. Spahn DR, Cerny V, Coats TJ, et al. Management of bleeding following major trauma: A European guideline. Crit Care 2007; 11:R17.
54. American College of Surgeons Committee on Trauma. Interfacility Transfer of Injured Patients: Guidelines for Rural Communities. Chicago, ACS, 2002.

55. Advanced Life Support Group. Safe Transfer and Retrieval (STaR) Course. Manchester, UK, ALSG Centre for Training & Development, 2008.
56. American College of Obstetricians and Gynecologists. Obstetric aspects of trauma management. ACOG Educational Bulletin No. 251. Washington, DC, September 1998. (Int J Gynaecol Obstet 1999; 64:87-94.)
57. American College of Surgeons Committee on Trauma. Trauma in Women. In Advanced Trauma Life Support for Doctors: Student Course Manual. Chicago, American College of Surgeons, 2004.
58. European Trauma Course. Antwerp, European Resuscitation Council, 2008.
59. Hastings RH, Marks JD. Airway management for trauma patients with potential cervical spine injuries. Anesth Analg 1991; 73:471-82.
60. Helling TS, Wilson J, Augustosky K. The utility of focused abdominal ultrasound in blunt abdominal trauma: A reappraisal. Am J Surg 2007; 194:728-32.
61. The SAFE Study Investigators. Saline or albumin for fluid resuscitation in patients with traumatic brain injury. N Engl J Med 2007; 357:874-84.
62. Vincent JL. Fluid resuscitation: Colloids vs crystalloids. Acta Clin Belg Suppl 2007; (2):408-11.
63. Jaskille A, Koustova E, Rhee P, et al. Hepatic apoptosis after hemorrhagic shock in rats can be reduced through modifications of conventional Ringer's solution. J Am Coll Surg 2006; 202:25-35.
64. Brasel KJ, Bulger E, Cook AJ, et al. Hypertonic resuscitation: Design and implementation of a prehospital intervention trial. J Am Coll Surg 2008; 206:220-32.
65. Borgman MA, Spinella PC, Perkins JG, et al. The ratio of blood products transfused affects mortality in patients receiving massive transfusions at a combat support hospital. J Trauma 2007; 63:805-13.
66. Martinowitz U, Michaelson M. Guidelines for the use of recombinant activated factor VIII (rFVIIa) in uncontrolled bleeding: A report by the Israeli Multidisciplinary rFVIIa Task Force. J Thromb Haemost 2005; 3:640-8.
67. Allam J, Cox M, Yentis SM. Cell salvage in obstetrics. Int J Obstet Anesth 2008; 17:37-45.
68. Luce JM. Medical management of head injury. Chest 1986; 89:864-72.
69. Mayer SA, Chong JY. Critical care management of increased intracranial pressure. J Intensive Care Med 2002; 17:55-67.
70. Stocchetti N, Longhi L, Valeriani V. Bilateral cannulation of internal jugular veins may worsen intracranial hypertension. Anesthesiology 2003; 99:1017-8.
71. Battison C, Andrews PJ, Graham C, Petty T. Randomized, controlled trial on the effect of a 20% mannitol solution and a 7.5% saline/6% dextran solution on increased intracranial pressure after brain injury. Crit Care Med 2005; 33:196-202.
72. Burns PD, Linder RO, Drose VE, Battaglia F. The placental transfer of water from fetus to mother following the intravenous infusion of hypertonic mannitol to the maternal rabbit. Am J Obstet Gynecol 1963; 86:160-7.
73. Witter FR, King TM, Blake DA. Adverse effects of cardiovascular drug therapy on the fetus and neonate. Obstet Gynecol 1981; 58:100S-5S.
74. Rosen K, Blad S, Larsson D, et al. Assessment of the fetal bioprofile during labor by fetal ECG analysis. Expert Rev Obstet Gynecol 2007; 2:609-20.
75. Neilson J. Fetal electrocardiogram (ECG) for fetal monitoring during labour. Cochrane Database Syst Rev 2006; (3):CD000116.
76. Shah S, Miller PR, Meredith JW, Chang MC. Elevated admission white blood cell count in pregnant trauma patients: An indicator of ongoing placental abruption. Am Surg 2002; 68:644-7.
77. Dunham CM, Siegel JH, Weireter L, et al. Oxygen debt and metabolic acidemia as quantitative predictors of mortality and the severity of the ischemic insult in hemorrhagic shock. Crit Care Med 1991; 19:231-43.
78. Muench MV, Baschat AA, Reddy UM, et al. Kleihauer-Betke testing is important in all cases of maternal trauma. J Trauma 2004; 57:1094-8.
79. Toppenberg KS, Hill DA, Miller DP. Safety of radiographic imaging during pregnancy. Am Fam Physician 1999; 59:1813-20.
80. McCollough CH, Schueler BA, Atwell TD, et al. Radiation exposure and pregnancy: When should we be concerned? Radiographics 2007; 27:909-18.
81. Ahvenjarvi L, Mattila L, Ojala R, Tervonen O. Value of multidetector computed tomography in assessing blunt multitrauma patients. Acta Radiol 2005; 46:177-83.
82. Brown MA, Sirlin CB, Farahmand N, et al. Screening sonography in pregnant patients with blunt abdominal trauma. J Ultrasound Med 2005; 24:175-81.
83. Ormsby EL, Geng J, McGahan JP, Richards JR. Pelvic free fluid: Clinical importance for reproductive age women with blunt abdominal trauma. Ultrasound Obstet Gynecol 2005; 26:271-8.
84. Goodwin H, Holmes JF, Wisner DH. Abdominal ultrasound examination in pregnant blunt trauma patients. J Trauma 2001; 50:689-93, discussion 94.
85. Richards JR, Ormsby EL, Romo MV, et al. Blunt abdominal injury in the pregnant patient: Detection with US. Radiology 2004; 233:463-70.
86. Katz VL, Dotters DJ, Droegemueller W. Perimortem cesarean delivery. Obstet Gynecol 1986; 68:571-6.
87. Chiossi G, Novic K, Celebrezze JU, Thomas RL. Successful neonatal outcome in 2 cases of maternal persistent vegetative state treated in a labor and delivery suite. Am J Obstet Gynecol 2006; 195:316-22.
88. Feldman DM, Borgida AF, Rodis JF, Campbell WA. Irreversible maternal brain injury during pregnancy: A case report and review of the literature. Obstet Gynecol Surv 2000; 55:708-14.
89. Sampson MB, Petersen LP. Post-traumatic coma during pregnancy. Obstet Gynecol 1979; 53:2S-3S.
90. Ben Aderet N, Cohen I, Abramowicz JS, et al. Traumatic coma during pregnancy with persistent vegetative state: Case report. Br J Obstet Gynaecol 1984; 91:939-41.
91. Bernstein IM, Watson M, Simmons GM, et al. Maternal brain death and prolonged fetal survival. Obstet Gynecol 1989; 74:434-7.
92. Field DR, Gates EA, Creasy RK, et al. Maternal brain death during pregnancy: Medical and ethical issues. JAMA 1988; 260:816-22.
93. Driscoll P, Wardrope J. ATLS: Past, present, and future. Emerg Med J 2005; 22:2-3.
94. Nolan JP. Advanced trauma life support in the United Kingdom: Time to move on. Emerg Med J 2005; 22:3-4.
95. Johanson RB, Menon V, Burns E, et al. Managing Obstetric Emergencies and Trauma (MOET): Structured skills training in Armenia, utilising models and reality based scenarios. BMC Med Educ 2002; 2:5.
96. Craft JB Jr, Coaldrake LA, Yonekura ML, et al. Ketamine, catecholamines, and uterine tone in pregnant ewes. Am J Obstet Gynecol 1983; 146:429-34.
97. American College of Obstetricians and Gynecologists Committee on Obstetric Practice. Nonobstetric surgery in pregnancy. ACOG Committee Opinion No. 284. Washington, DC, ACOG August 2003. (Obstet Gynecol 2003; 102:431.)
98. Thomas TA, Cooper GM. Anaesthesia. In Drife J, Lewis G, editors. Why Mothers Die: 1997-1999: The Fifth Report on the Confidential Enquiries into Maternal Deaths in the United Kingdom. London, RCOG Press, 2001:134-49.

American Society of Anesthesiologists Guidelines for Regional Anesthesia in Obstetrics*

These guidelines apply to the use of regional anesthesia or analgesia in which local anesthetics are administered to the parturient during labor and delivery. They are intended to encourage quality patient care but cannot guarantee any specific patient outcome. Because the availability of anesthesia resources may vary, members are responsible for interpreting and establishing the guidelines for their own institutions and practices. These guidelines are subject to revision from time to time as warranted by the evolution of technology and practice.

GUIDELINE I
REGIONAL ANESTHESIA SHOULD BE INITIATED AND MAINTAINED ONLY IN LOCATIONS IN WHICH APPROPRIATE RESUSCITATION EQUIPMENT AND DRUGS ARE IMMEDIATELY AVAILABLE TO MANAGE PROCEDURALLY RELATED PROBLEMS.

Resuscitation equipment should include, but is not limited to: sources of oxygen and suction, equipment to maintain an airway and perform endotracheal intubation, a means to provide positive pressure ventilation, and drugs and equipment for cardiopulmonary resuscitation.

GUIDELINE II
REGIONAL ANESTHESIA SHOULD BE INITIATED BY A PHYSICIAN WITH APPROPRIATE PRIVILEGES AND MAINTAINED BY OR UNDER THE MEDICAL DIRECTION[1] OF SUCH AN INDIVIDUAL.

Physicians should be approved through the institutional credentialing process to initiate and direct the maintenance of obstetric anesthesia and to manage procedurally related complications.

GUIDELINE III
REGIONAL ANESTHESIA SHOULD NOT BE ADMINISTERED UNTIL: 1) THE PATIENT HAS BEEN EXAMINED BY A QUALIFIED INDIVIDUAL[2]; AND 2) A PHYSICIAN WITH OBSTETRICAL PRIVILEGES TO PERFORM OPERATIVE VAGINAL OR CESAREAN DELIVERY, WHO HAS KNOWLEDGE OF THE MATERNAL AND FETAL STATUS AND THE PROGRESS OF LABOR AND WHO APPROVES THE INITIATION OF LABOR ANESTHESIA, IS READILY AVAILABLE TO SUPERVISE THE LABOR AND MANAGE ANY OBSTETRIC COMPLICATIONS THAT MAY ARISE.

Under circumstances defined by department protocol, qualified personnel may perform the initial pelvic examination. The physician responsible for the patient's obstetrical care should be informed of her status so that a decision can be made regarding present risk and further management.[2]

GUIDELINE IV
AN INTRAVENOUS INFUSION SHOULD BE ESTABLISHED BEFORE THE INITIATION OF REGIONAL ANESTHESIA AND MAINTAINED THROUGHOUT THE DURATION OF THE REGIONAL ANESTHETIC.

GUIDELINE V
REGIONAL ANESTHESIA FOR LABOR AND/OR VAGINAL DELIVERY REQUIRES THAT THE PARTURIENT'S VITAL SIGNS AND THE FETAL HEART RATE BE MONITORED AND DOCUMENTED BY A QUALIFIED INDIVIDUAL. ADDITIONAL MONITORING APPROPRIATE TO THE CLINICAL CONDITION OF THE PARTURIENT AND THE FETUS SHOULD BE EMPLOYED WHEN INDICATED. WHEN EXTENSIVE REGIONAL BLOCKADE IS ADMINISTERED FOR COMPLICATED VAGINAL DELIVERY, THE STANDARDS FOR BASIC ANESTHETIC MONITORING[3] SHOULD BE APPLIED.

GUIDELINE VI
REGIONAL ANESTHESIA FOR CESAREAN DELIVERY REQUIRES THAT THE STANDARDS FOR BASIC ANESTHETIC MONITORING[3] BE APPLIED AND THAT A PHYSICIAN WITH PRIVILEGES IN OBSTETRICS BE IMMEDIATELY AVAILABLE.

---

*Approved by the ASA House of Delegates on October 12, 1988, and last amended on October 17, 2007.

[1]The Anesthesia Care Team (Approved by ASA House of Delegates 10/26/82 and last amended 10/18/2006).

[2]American Academy of Pediatrics and American College of Obstetricians and Gynecologists. Guidelines for Perinatal Care, 5th Edition. Elk Grove Village, IL: AAP; Washington, DC: ACOG, 2002.

[3]Standards for Basic Anesthetic Monitoring (Approved by ASA House of Delegates 10/21/86 and last amended 10/25/2005).

GUIDELINE VII

QUALIFIED PERSONNEL, OTHER THAN THE ANESTHESIOLOGIST ATTENDING THE MOTHER, SHOULD BE IMMEDIATELY AVAILABLE TO ASSUME RESPONSIBILITY FOR RESUSCITATION OF THE NEWBORN.[3]

The primary responsibility of the anesthesiologist is to provide care to the mother. If the anesthesiologist is also requested to provide brief assistance in the care of the newborn, the benefit to the child must be compared to the risk to the mother.

GUIDELINE VIII

A PHYSICIAN WITH APPROPRIATE PRIVILEGES SHOULD REMAIN READILY AVAILABLE DURING THE REGIONAL ANESTHETIC TO MANAGE ANESTHETIC COMPLICATIONS UNTIL THE PATIENT'S POSTANESTHESIA CONDITION IS SATISFACTORY AND STABLE.

GUIDELINE IX

ALL PATIENTS RECOVERING FROM REGIONAL ANESTHESIA SHOULD RECEIVE APPROPRIATE POSTANESTHESIA CARE. FOLLOWING CESAREAN DELIVERY AND/OR EXTENSIVE REGIONAL BLOCKADE, THE STANDARDS FOR POSTANESTHESIA CARE[4] SHOULD BE APPLIED.

1. A postanesthesia care unit (PACU) should be available to receive patients. The design, equipment and staffing should meet requirements of the facility's accrediting and licensing bodies.
2. When a site other than the PACU is used, equivalent postanesthesia care should be provided.

GUIDELINE X

THERE SHOULD BE A POLICY TO ASSURE THE AVAILABILITY IN THE FACILITY OF A PHYSICIAN TO MANAGE COMPLICATIONS AND TO PROVIDE CARDIOPULMONARY RESUSCITATION FOR PATIENTS RECEIVING POSTANESTHESIA CARE.

[4]Standards for Postanesthesia Care (Approved by ASA House of Delegates 10/12/88 and last amended 10/27/04).

Practice Guidelines for Obstetric Anesthesia

*An Updated Report by the American Society of Anesthesiologists Task Force on Obstetric Anesthesia**

PRACTICE guidelines are systematically developed recommendations that assist the practitioner and patient in making decisions about health care. These recommendations may be adopted, modified, or rejected according to clinical needs and constraints and are not intended to replace local institutional policies. In addition, practice guidelines are not intended as standards or absolute requirements, and their use cannot guarantee any specific outcome. Practice guidelines are subject to revision as warranted by the evolution of medical knowledge, technology, and practice. They provide basic recommendations that are supported by a synthesis and analysis of the current literature, expert opinion, open forum commentary, and clinical feasibility data.

This update includes data published since the ''Practice Guidelines for Obstetrical Anesthesia'' were adopted by the American Society of Anesthesiologists in 1998; it also includes data and recommendations for a wider range of techniques than was previously addressed.

Methodology

A. Definition of Perioperative Obstetric Anesthesia

For the purposes of these Guidelines, *obstetric anesthesia* refers to peripartum anesthetic and analgesic activities performed during labor and vaginal delivery, cesarean delivery, removal of retained placenta, and postpartum tubal ligation.

B. Purposes of the Guidelines

The purposes of these Guidelines are to enhance the quality of anesthetic care for obstetric patients, improve patient safety by reducing the incidence and severity of anesthesia-related complications, and increase patient satisfaction.

C. Focus

These Guidelines focus on the anesthetic management of pregnant patients during labor, nonoperative delivery, operative delivery, and selected aspects of postpartum care and analgesia (*i.e.*, neuraxial opioids for postpartum analgesia after neuraxial anesthesia for cesarean delivery). The intended patient population includes, but is not limited to, intrapartum and postpartum patients with uncomplicated pregnancies or with common obstetric problems. The Guidelines do not apply to patients undergoing surgery during pregnancy, gynecologic patients, or parturients with chronic medical disease (*e.g.*, severe cardiac, renal, or neurologic disease). In addition, these Guidelines do not address (1) postpartum analgesia for vaginal delivery, (2) analgesia after tubal ligation, or (3) postoperative analgesia after general anesthesia (GA) for cesarean delivery.

D. Application

These Guidelines are intended for use by anesthesiologists. They also may serve as a resource for other anesthesia providers and healthcare professionals who advise or care for patients who will receive anesthetic care during labor, delivery, and the immediate postpartum period.

E. Task Force Members and Consultants

The American Society of Anesthesiologists (ASA) appointed a Task Force of 11 members to (1) review the published evidence, (2) obtain the opinion of a panel of consultants including anesthesiologists and nonanesthesiologist physicians concerned with obstetric anesthesia and analgesia, and (3) obtain opinions from practitioners likely to be affected by the Guidelines. The Task Force included anesthesiologists in both private and academic practices from various geographic areas of the United States and two consulting methodologists from the ASA Committee on Standards and Practice Parameters.

The Task Force developed the Guidelines by means of a seven-step process. First, they reached consensus on the criteria for evidence. Second, original published research studies from peer-reviewed journals relevant to obstetric anesthesia were reviewed. Third, the panel of expert consultants was asked to (1) participate in opinion surveys on the effectiveness of various peripartum management strategies

*Excerpted from Practice Guidelines for Obstetric Anesthesia: An Updated Report by the American Society of Anesthesiologists Task Force on Obstetric Anesthesia. Anesthesiology 2007; 106:843-63. ©2007, Americian Society of Anesthesiologists, Inc. Lippincott Williams & Wilkins, Inc. A copy of the full text can be obtained from American Society of Anesthesiologists, 520 N. Northwest Highway, Park Ridge, IL 60068-2573.

Developed by the American Society of Anesthesiologists Task Force on Obstetric Anesthesia: Joy L. Hawkins, MD (Chair), Denver, Colorado; James F. Arens, MD, Houston, Texas; Brenda A. Bucklin, MD, Denver, Colorado; Richard T. Connis, PhD, Woodinville, Washington; Patricia A. Dailey, MD, Hillsborough, California; David R. Gambling, MBBS, San Diego, California; David G. Nickinovich, PhD, Bellevue, Washington; Linda S. Polley, MD, Ann Arbor, Michigan; Lawrence C. Tsen, MD, Boston, Massachusetts; David J. Wlody, MD, Brooklyn, New York; and Kathryn J. Zuspan, MD, Stillwater, Minnesota.

Submitted for publication October 31, 2006. Accepted for publication October 31, 2006. Supported by the American Society of Anesthesiologists under the direction of James F. Arens, MD, Chair, Committee on Standards and Practice Parameters. Approved by the House of Delegates on October 18, 2006. A list of the references used to develop these Guidelines is available by writing to the American Society of Anesthesiologists.

and (2) review and comment on a draft of the Guidelines developed by the Task Force. Fourth, opinions about the Guideline recommendations were solicited from active members of the ASA who provide obstetric anesthesia. Fifth, the Task Force held open forums at two major national meetings[†] to solicit input on its draft recommendations. Sixth, the consultants were surveyed to assess their opinions on the feasibility of implementing the Guidelines. Seventh, all available information was used to build consensus within the Task Force to finalize the Guidelines (Appendix 1).

F. Availability and Strength of Evidence

Preparation of these Guidelines followed a rigorous methodologic process. To convey the findings in a concise and easy-to-understand fashion, these Guidelines use several descriptive terms. When sufficient numbers of studies are available for evaluation, the following terms describe the strength of the findings.

Support: Meta-analysis of a sufficient number of randomized controlled trials[‡] indicates a statistically significant relationship ($P < 0.01$) between a clinical intervention and a clinical outcome.

Suggest: Information from case reports and observational studies permits inference of a relationship between an intervention and an outcome. A meta-analytic assessment of this type of qualitative or descriptive information is not conducted.

Equivocal: Either a meta-analysis has not found significant differences among groups or conditions, or there is insufficient quantitative information to conduct a meta-analysis and information collected from case reports and observational studies does not permit inference of a relationship between an intervention and an outcome.

The *lack* of scientific evidence in the literature is described by the following terms.

Silent: No identified studies address the specified relationship between an intervention and outcome.

Insufficient: There are too few published studies to investigate a relationship between an intervention and outcome.

Inadequate: The available studies cannot be used to assess the relationship between an intervention and an outcome. These studies either do not meet the criteria for content as defined in the Focus section of these Guidelines, or do not permit a clear causal interpretation of findings due to methodologic concerns.

Formal survey information is collected from consultants and members of the ASA. The following terms describe survey responses for any specified issue. Responses are solicited on a five-point scale ranging from 1 (strongly disagree) to 5 (strongly agree), with a score of 3 being equivocal. Survey responses are summarized based on median values as follows:

Strongly Agree: Median score of 5 (at least 50% of the responses are 5).

Agree: Median score of 4 (at least 50% of the responses are 4 or 4 and 5).

Equivocal: Median score of 3 (at least 50% of the responses are 3, or no other response category or combination of similar categories contain at least 50% of the responses).

Disagree: Median score of 2 (at least 50% of the responses are 2 or 1 and 2).

Strongly Disagree: Median score of 1 (at least 50% of the responses are 1).

Guidelines

I. Perianesthetic Evaluation

History and Physical Examination. Although comparative studies are insufficient to evaluate the peripartum impact of conducting a focused history (*e.g.*, reviewing medical records) or a physical examination, the literature reports certain patient or clinical characteristics that may be associated with obstetric complications. These characteristics include, but are not limited to, preeclampsia, pregnancy-related hypertensive disorders, HELLP syndrome, obesity, and diabetes.

The consultants and ASA members both strongly agree that a directed history and physical examination, as well as communication between anesthetic and obstetric providers, reduces maternal, fetal, and neonatal complications.

Recommendations. The anesthesiologist should conduct a focused history and physical examination before providing anesthesia care. This should include, but is not limited to, a maternal health and anesthetic history, a relevant obstetric history, a baseline blood pressure measurement, and an airway, heart, and lung examination, consistent with the ASA "Practice Advisory for Preanesthesia Evaluation."[§] When a neuraxial anesthetic is planned or placed, the patient's back should be examined.

Recognition of significant anesthetic or obstetric risk factors should encourage consultation between the obstetrician and the anesthesiologist. A communication system should be in place to encourage early and ongoing contact between obstetric providers, anesthesiologists, and other members of the multidisciplinary team.

Intrapartum Platelet Count. The literature is insufficient to assess whether a routine platelet count can predict anesthesia-related complications in uncomplicated parturients. The literature suggests that a platelet count is clinically useful for parturients with suspected pregnancy-related hypertensive disorders, such as preeclampsia or HELLP syndrome, and for other disorders associated with coagulopathy.

The ASA members are equivocal, but the consultants agree that obtaining a routine intrapartum platelet count does *not* reduce maternal anesthetic complications. Both the consultants and ASA members agree that, for patients with suspected

[†]International Anesthesia Research Society, 80th Clinical and Scientific Congress, San Francisco, California, March 25, 2006; and Society of Obstetric Anesthesia and Perinatology 38th Annual Meeting, Hollywood, Florida, April 29, 2006.

[‡]A prospective nonrandomized controlled trial may be included in a meta-analysis under certain circumstances if specific statistical criteria are met.

[§]American Society of Anesthesiologists Task Force on Preanesthesia Evaluation: Practice advisory for preanesthesia evaluation. Anesthesiology 2002; 96:485–96.

preeclampsia, a platelet count reduces maternal anesthetic complications. The consultants strongly agree and the ASA members agree that a platelet count reduces maternal anesthetic complications for patients with suspected coagulopathy.

Recommendations. A specific platelet count predictive of neuraxial anesthetic complications has not been determined. The anesthesiologist's decision to order or require a platelet count should be individualized and based on a patient's history, physical examination, and clinical signs. A routine platelet count is not necessary in the healthy parturient.

Blood Type and Screen. The literature is insufficient to determine whether obtaining a blood type and screen is associated with fewer maternal anesthetic complications. In addition, the literature is insufficient to determine whether a blood cross-match is necessary for healthy and uncomplicated parturients. The consultants and ASA members agree that an intrapartum blood sample should be sent to the blood bank for all parturients.

Recommendations. A routine blood cross-match is not necessary for healthy and uncomplicated parturients for vaginal or operative delivery. The decision whether to order or require a blood type and screen, or cross-match, should be based on maternal history, anticipated hemorrhagic complications (*e.g.*, placenta accreta in a patient with placenta previa and previous uterine surgery), and local institutional policies.

Perianesthetic Recording of the Fetal Heart Rate. The literature suggests that anesthetic and analgesic agents may influence the fetal heart rate pattern. There is insufficient literature to demonstrate that perianesthetic recording of the fetal heart rate prevents fetal or neonatal complications. Both the consultants and ASA members agree, however, that perianesthetic recording of the fetal heart rate reduces fetal and neonatal complications.

Recommendations. The fetal heart rate should be monitored by a qualified individual before and after administration of neuraxial analgesia for labor. The Task Force recognizes that *continuous* electronic recording of the fetal heart rate may not be necessary in every clinical setting and may not be possible during initiation of neuraxial anesthesia.

II. Aspiration Prevention

Clear Liquids. There is insufficient published evidence to draw conclusions about the relationship between fasting times for clear liquids and the risk of emesis/reflux or pulmonary aspiration during labor. The consultants and ASA members both agree that oral intake of clear liquids during labor improves maternal comfort and satisfaction. Although the ASA members are equivocal, the consultants agree that oral intake of clear liquids during labor *does not* increase maternal complications.

Recommendations. The oral intake of modest amounts of clear liquids may be allowed for uncomplicated laboring patients. The uncomplicated patient undergoing elective cesarean delivery may have modest amounts of clear liquids up to 2 h before induction of anesthesia. Examples of clear liquids include, but are not limited to, water, fruit juices without pulp, carbonated beverages, clear tea, black coffee, and sports drinks. The volume of liquid ingested is less important than the presence of particulate matter in the liquid ingested. However, patients with additional risk factors for aspiration (*e.g.*, morbid obesity, diabetes, difficult airway) or patients at increased risk for operative delivery (*e.g.*, nonreassuring fetal heart rate pattern) may have further restrictions of oral intake, determined on a case-by-case basis.

Solids. A specific fasting time for solids that is predictive of maternal anesthetic complications has not been determined. There is insufficient published evidence to address the safety of *any* particular fasting period for solids in obstetric patients. The consultants and ASA members both agree that the oral intake of solids during labor increases maternal complications. They both strongly agree that patients undergoing either elective cesarean delivery or postpartum tubal ligation should undergo a fasting period of 6–8 h depending on the type of food ingested (*e.g.*, fat content).[‖] The Task Force recognizes that in laboring patients the timing of delivery is uncertain; therefore, compliance with a predetermined fasting period before nonelective surgical procedures is not always possible.

Recommendations. Solid foods should be avoided in laboring patients. The patient undergoing elective surgery (*e.g.*, scheduled cesarean delivery or postpartum tubal ligation) should undergo a fasting period for solids of 6–8 h depending on the type of food ingested (*e.g.*, fat content)[‖].

Antacids, H_2 Receptor Antagonists, and Metoclopramide. The literature does not sufficiently examine the relationship between reduced gastric acidity and the frequency of emesis, pulmonary aspiration, morbidity, or mortality in obstetric patients who have aspirated gastric contents. Published evidence supports the efficacy of preoperative nonparticulate antacids (*e.g.*, sodium citrate, sodium bicarbonate) in decreasing gastric acidity during the peripartum period. However, the literature is insufficient to examine the impact of nonparticulate antacids on gastric volume. The literature suggests that H_2 receptor antagonists are effective in decreasing gastric acidity in obstetric patients and supports the efficacy of metoclopramide in reducing peripartum nausea and vomiting. The consultants and ASA members agree that the administration of a nonparticulate antacid before operative procedures reduces maternal complications.

Recommendations. Before surgical procedures (*i.e.*, cesarean delivery, postpartum tubal ligation), practitioners should consider the timely administration of nonparticulate antacids, H_2 receptor antagonists, and/or metoclopramide for aspiration prophylaxis.

III. Anesthetic Care for Labor and Vaginal Delivery

Overview. Not all women require anesthetic care during labor or delivery. For women who request pain relief for labor and/or delivery, there are many effective analgesic techniques available. Maternal request represents sufficient justification for pain relief. In addition, maternal medical and obstetric conditions may warrant the provision of neuraxial techniques to improve maternal and neonatal outcome.

The choice of analgesic technique depends on the medical status of the patient, progress of labor, and resources at the facility. When sufficient resources (*e.g.*, anesthesia and nursing staff) are available, neuraxial catheter techniques should be one of the analgesic options offered. The choice of a specific neuraxial block should be individualized and based on anesthetic risk factors, obstetric risk factors, patient preferences, progress of labor, and resources at the facility.

[‖]American Society of Anesthesiologists Task Force on Preoperative Fasting: Practice guidelines for preoperative fasting and the use of pharmacologic agents to reduce the risk of pulmonary aspiration. Anesthesiology 1999; 90:896–905.

When neuraxial catheter techniques are used for analgesia during labor or vaginal delivery, the primary goal is to provide adequate maternal analgesia with minimal motor block (*e.g.*, achieved with the administration of local anesthetics at low concentrations with or without opioids).

When a neuraxial technique is chosen, appropriate resources for the treatment of complications (*e.g.*, hypotension, systemic toxicity, high spinal anesthesia) should be available. If an opioid is added, treatments for related complications (*e.g.*, pruritus, nausea, respiratory depression) should be available. An intravenous infusion should be established before the initiation of neuraxial analgesia or anesthesia and maintained throughout the duration of the neuraxial analgesic or anesthetic. However, administration of a fixed volume of intravenous fluid is not required before neuraxial analgesia is initiated.

Timing of Neuraxial Analgesia and Outcome of Labor. Meta-analysis of the literature determined that the timing of neuraxial analgesia does not affect the frequency of cesarean delivery. The literature also suggests that other delivery outcomes (*i.e.*, spontaneous or instrumented) are also unaffected. The consultants strongly agree and the ASA members agree that early initiation of epidural analgesia (*i.e.*, at cervical dilations of less than 5 cm vs. equal to or greater than 5 cm) improves analgesia. They both *disagree* that motor block or maternal, fetal, or neonatal side effects are increased by early administration.

Recommendations. Patients in early labor (*i.e.*, < 5 cm dilation) should be given the option of neuraxial analgesia when this service is available. Neuraxial analgesia should not be withheld on the basis of achieving an arbitrary cervical dilation, and should be offered on an individualized basis. Patients may be reassured that the use of neuraxial analgesia does not increase the incidence of cesarean delivery.

Neuraxial Analgesia and Trial of Labor after Previous Cesarean Delivery. Nonrandomized comparative studies suggest that epidural analgesia may be used in a trial of labor for previous cesarean delivery patients without adversely affecting the incidence of vaginal delivery. Randomized comparisons of epidural *versus* other anesthetic techniques were not found. The consultants and ASA members agree that neuraxial techniques improve the likelihood of vaginal delivery for patients attempting vaginal birth after cesarean delivery.

Recommendations. Neuraxial techniques should be offered to patients attempting vaginal birth after previous cesarean delivery. For these patients, it is also appropriate to consider early placement of a neuraxial catheter that can be used later for labor analgesia, or for anesthesia in the event of operative delivery.

Early Insertion of a Spinal or Epidural Catheter for Complicated Parturients. The literature is insufficient to assess whether, when caring for the complicated parturient, the early insertion of a spinal or epidural catheter, with later administration of analgesia, improves maternal or neonatal outcomes. The consultants and ASA members agree that early insertion of a spinal or epidural catheter for complicated parturients reduces maternal complications.

Recommendations. Early insertion of a spinal or epidural catheter for obstetric (*e.g.*, twin gestation or preeclampsia) or anesthetic indications (*e.g.*, anticipated difficult airway or obesity) should be considered to reduce the need for GA if an emergent procedure becomes necessary. In these cases, the insertion of a spinal or epidural catheter may precede the onset of labor or a patient's request for labor analgesia.

Continuous Infusion Epidural Analgesia.

CIE Compared with Parenteral Opioids. The literature suggests that the use of continuous infusion epidural (CIE) local anesthetics with or without opioids provides greater quality of analgesia compared with parenteral (*i.e.*, intravenous or intramuscular) opioids. The consultants and ASA members strongly agree that CIE local anesthetics with or without opioids provide improved analgesia compared with parenteral opioids.

Meta-analysis of the literature indicates that there is a longer duration of labor, with an average duration of 24 min for the second stage, and a lower frequency of spontaneous vaginal delivery when continuous epidural local anesthetics are administered compared with *intravenous* opioids. Meta-analysis of the literature determined that there are no differences in the frequency of cesarean delivery. Neither the consultants nor ASA members agree that CIE local anesthetics compared with parenteral opioids significantly (1) increase the duration of labor, (2) decrease the chance of spontaneous delivery, (3) increase maternal side effects, or (4) increase fetal and neonatal side effects.

CIE Compared with Single-injection Spinal. There is insufficient literature to assess the analgesic efficacy of CIE local anesthetics with or without opioids compared to *single-injection spinal opioids* with or without local anesthetics. The consultants are equivocal, but the ASA members agree that CIE local anesthetics improve analgesia compared with single-injection spinal opioids; both the consultants and ASA members are equivocal regarding the frequency of motor block. The consultants are equivocal, but the ASA members disagree that the use of CIE compared with single-injection spinal opioids increases the duration of labor. They both *disagree* that CIE local anesthetics with or without opioids compared to single-injection spinal opioids with or without local anesthetics decreases the likelihood of spontaneous delivery or increases maternal, fetal, or neonatal side effects.

CIE with and without Opioids. The literature supports the *induction* of analgesia using epidural local anesthetics combined *with opioids* compared with equal concentrations of epidural local anesthetics *without opioids* for improved quality and longer duration of analgesia. The consultants strongly agree and the ASA members agree that the addition of opioids to epidural local anesthetics improves analgesia; they both disagree that fetal or neonatal side effects are increased. The consultants disagree, but the ASA members are equivocal regarding whether the addition of opioids increases maternal side effects.

The literature is insufficient to determine whether induction of analgesia using local anesthetics with opioids compared with *higher concentrations* of epidural local anesthetics without opioids provides improved quality or duration of analgesia. The consultants and ASA members are equivocal regarding improved analgesia, and they both disagree that maternal, fetal, or neonatal side effects are increased using lower concentrations of epidural local anesthetics with opioids.

For *maintenance of analgesia*, the literature suggests that there are no differences in the analgesic efficacy of *low concentrations* of epidural local anesthetics with opioids compared with *higher concentrations* of epidural local anesthetics without opioids. The Task Force notes that the addition of an opioid to a local anesthetic infusion allows an even lower concentration of local anesthetic for providing equally effective analgesia. However, the literature is insufficient to examine whether a bupivacaine infusion concentration of *less than or equal to 0.125%* with an opioid provides comparable or improved analgesia compared with a bupivacaine concentration *greater than 0.125%* without an opioid.[#] Meta-analysis of the literature determined that low concentrations of epidural local anesthetics with opioids compared with higher concentrations of epidural local anesthetics without opioids are associated with reduced motor block. No differences in the duration of labor, mode of delivery, or neonatal outcomes are found when epidural local anesthetics with opioids are compared with epidural local anesthetics without opioids. The literature is insufficient to determine the effects of epidural local anesthetics with opioids on other maternal outcomes (*e.g.*, hypotension, nausea, pruritus, respiratory depression, urinary retention).

The consultants and ASA members both agree that maintenance of epidural analgesia using *low* concentrations of local anesthetics with opioids provides improved analgesia compared with *higher* concentrations of local anesthetics without opioids. The consultants agree, but the ASA members are equivocal regarding the improved likelihood of spontaneous delivery when lower concentrations of local anesthetics with opioids are used. The consultants strongly agree and the ASA members agree that motor block is reduced. They agree that maternal side effects are reduced with this drug combination. They are both equivocal regarding a reduction in fetal and neonatal side effects.

Recommendations. The selected analgesic/anesthetic technique should reflect patient needs and preferences, practitioner preferences or skills, and available resources. The continuous epidural infusion technique may be used for effective analgesia for labor and delivery. When a continuous epidural infusion of local anesthetic is selected, an opioid may be added to reduce the concentration of local anesthetic, improve the quality of analgesia, and minimize motor block.

Adequate analgesia for uncomplicated labor and delivery should be administered with the secondary goal of producing as little motor block as possible by using dilute concentrations of local anesthetics with opioids. The lowest concentration of local anesthetic infusion that provides adequate maternal analgesia and satisfaction should be administered. For example, an infusion concentration greater than 0.125% bupivacaine is unnecessary for labor analgesia in most patients.

Single-injection Spinal Opioids with or without Local Anesthetics. The literature suggests that spinal opioids with or without local anesthetics provide effective analgesia during labor without altering the incidence of neonatal complications. There is insufficient literature to compare spinal opioids with parenteral opioids. There is also insufficient literature to compare single-injection spinal opioids *with* local anesthetics *versus* single-injection spinal opioids *without* local anesthetics.

[#]References to bupivacaine are included for illustrative purposes only, and because bupivacaine is the most extensively studied local anesthetic for continuous infusion epidural analgesia. The Task Force recognizes that other local anesthetics are appropriate for continuous infusion epidural analgesia.

The consultants strongly agree and the ASA members agree that spinal opioids provide improved analgesia compared with parenteral opioids. They both disagree that, compared with parenteral opioids, spinal opioids increase the duration of labor, decrease the chance of spontaneous delivery, or increase fetal and neonatal side effects. The consultants are equivocal, but the ASA members disagree that maternal side effects are increased with spinal opioids.

Compared with spinal opioids *without* local anesthetics, the consultants and ASA members both agree that spinal opioids *with* local anesthetics provide improved analgesia. They both disagree that the chance of spontaneous delivery is decreased and that fetal and neonatal side effects are increased. They are both equivocal regarding an increase in maternal side effects. However, they both agree that motor block is increased when local anesthetics are added to spinal opioids. Finally, the consultants disagree, but the ASA members are equivocal regarding an increase in the duration of labor.

Recommendations. Single-injection spinal opioids with or without local anesthetics may be used to provide effective, although time-limited, analgesia for labor when spontaneous vaginal delivery is anticipated. If labor is expected to last longer than the analgesic effects of the spinal drugs chosen or if there is a good possibility of operative delivery, a catheter technique instead of a single injection technique should be considered. A local anesthetic may be added to a spinal opioid to increase duration and improve quality of analgesia. The Task Force notes that the rapid onset of analgesia provided by single-injection spinal techniques may be advantageous for selected patients (*e.g.*, those in advanced labor).

Pencil-point Spinal Needles. The literature supports the use of pencil-point spinal needles compared with cutting-bevel spinal needles to reduce the frequency of post-dural puncture headache. The consultants and ASA members both strongly agree that the use of pencil-point spinal needles reduces maternal complications.

Recommendations. Pencil-point spinal needles should be used instead of cutting-bevel spinal needles to minimize the risk of post-dural puncture headache.

Combined Spinal–Epidural Analgesia. The literature supports a faster onset time and equivalent analgesia with combined spinal–epidural (CSE) local anesthetics with opioids *versus* epidural local anesthetics with opioids. The literature is equivocal regarding the impact of CSE versus epidural local anesthetics with opioids on maternal satisfaction with analgesia, mode of delivery, hypotension, motor block, nausea, fetal heart rate changes, and Apgar scores. Meta-analysis of the literature indicates that the frequency of pruritus is increased with CSE.

The consultants and ASA members both agree that CSE local anesthetics with opioids provide improved early analgesia compared with epidural local anesthetics with opioids. They are equivocal regarding the impact of CSE with opioids on overall analgesic efficacy, duration of labor, and motor block. The consultants and ASA members both disagree that CSE increases the risk of fetal or neonatal side effects. The consultants disagree, but the ASA members are equivocal regarding whether CSE increases the incidence of maternal side effects.

Recommendations. Combined spinal–epidural techniques may be used to provide effective and rapid onset of analgesia for labor.

Patient-controlled Epidural Analgesia. The literature supports the efficacy of patient-controlled epidural analgesia (PCEA) *versus* CIE in providing equivalent analgesia with reduced drug consumption. Meta-analysis of the literature indicates that the duration of labor is longer with PCEA compared with CIE for the first stage (*e.g.*, an average of 36 min) but not the second stage of labor. Meta-analysis of the literature also determined that mode of delivery, frequency of motor block, and Apgar scores are equivalent when PCEA administration is compared with CIE. The literature supports greater analgesic efficacy for PCEA with a background infusion compared with PCEA without a background infusion; meta-analysis of the literature also indicates no differences in the mode of delivery or frequency of motor block. The consultants and ASA members agree that PCEA compared with CIE improves analgesia and reduces the need for anesthetic interventions; they also agree that PCEA improves maternal satisfaction. The consultants and ASA members are equivocal regarding a reduction in motor block, an increased likelihood of spontaneous delivery, or a decrease in maternal side effects with PCEA compared with CIE. They both agree that PCEA with a background infusion improves analgesia, improves maternal satisfaction, and reduces the need for anesthetic intervention. The ASA members are equivocal, but the consultants disagree that a background infusion decreases the chance of spontaneous delivery or increases maternal side effects. The consultants and ASA members are equivocal regarding the effect of a background infusion on the incidence of motor block.

Recommendations. Patient-controlled epidural analgesia may be used to provide an effective and flexible approach for the maintenance of labor analgesia. The Task Force notes that the use of PCEA may be preferable to fixed-rate CIE for providing fewer anesthetic interventions and reduced dosages of local anesthetics. PCEA may be used with or without a background infusion.

IV. Removal of Retained Placenta

Anesthetic Techniques. The literature is insufficient to assess whether a particular type of anesthetic is more effective than another for removal of retained placenta. The consultants strongly agree and the ASA members agree that, if a functioning epidural catheter is in place and the patient is hemodynamically stable, epidural anesthesia is the preferred technique for the removal of retained placenta. The consultants and ASA members both agree that, in cases involving major maternal hemorrhage, GA is preferred over neuraxial anesthesia.

Recommendations. The Task Force notes that, in general, there is no preferred anesthetic technique for removal of retained placenta. However, if an epidural catheter is in place and the patient is hemodynamically stable, epidural anesthesia is preferable. Hemodynamic status should be assessed before administering neuraxial anesthesia. Aspiration prophylaxis should be considered. Sedation/analgesia should be titrated carefully due to the potential risks of respiratory depression and pulmonary aspiration during the immediate postpartum period. In cases involving major maternal hemorrhage, GA with an endotracheal tube may be preferable to neuraxial anesthesia.

Uterine Relaxation. The literature suggests that nitroglycerin is effective for uterine relaxation during the removal of retained placenta. The consultants and ASA members both agree that the administration of nitroglycerin for uterine relaxation improves success in removing a retained placenta.

Recommendations. Nitroglycerin may be used as an alternative to terbutaline sulfate or general endotracheal anesthesia with halogenated agents for uterine relaxation during removal of retained placental tissue. Initiating treatment with incremental doses of intravenous or sublingual (*i.e.*, metered dose spray) nitroglycerin may relax the uterus sufficiently while minimizing potential complications (*e.g.*, hypotension).

V. Anesthetic Choices for Cesarean Delivery

Equipment, Facilities, and Support Personnel. The literature is insufficient to evaluate the benefit of providing equipment, facilities and support personnel in the labor and delivery operating suite comparable to that available in the main operating suite. The consultants and ASA members strongly agree that the available equipment, facilities, and support personnel should be comparable.

Recommendations. Equipment, facilities, and support personnel available in the labor and delivery operating suite should be comparable to those available in the main operating suite. Resources for the treatment of potential complications (*e.g.*, failed intubation, inadequate analgesia, hypotension, respiratory depression, pruritus, vomiting) should also be available in the labor and delivery operating suite. Appropriate equipment and personnel should be available to care for obstetric patients recovering from major neuraxial anesthesia or GA.

General, Epidural, Spinal, or Combined Spinal–Epidural Anesthesia. The literature suggests that induction-to-delivery times for GA are lower compared with epidural or spinal anesthesia and that a higher frequency of maternal hypotension may be associated with epidural or spinal techniques. Meta-analysis of the literature found that Apgar scores at 1 and 5 min are lower for GA compared with epidural anesthesia and suggests that Apgar scores are lower for GA *versus* spinal anesthesia. The literature is equivocal regarding differences in umbilical artery pH values when GA is compared with epidural or spinal anesthesia.

The consultants and ASA members agree that GA reduces the time to skin incision when compared with either epidural or spinal anesthesia; they also agree that GA increases maternal complications. The consultants are equivocal and the ASA members agree that GA increases fetal and neonatal complications. The consultants and ASA members both agree that epidural anesthesia increases the time to skin incision and decreases the quality of anesthesia compared with spinal anesthesia. They both disagree that epidural anesthesia increases maternal complications.

When spinal anesthesia is compared with epidural anesthesia, meta-analysis of the literature found that induction-to-delivery times are shorter for spinal anesthesia. The literature is equivocal regarding hypotension, umbilical pH values, and Apgar scores. The consultants and ASA members agree that epidural anesthesia increases time to skin incision and reduces the quality of anesthesia when compared with spinal anesthesia. They both disagree that epidural anesthesia increases maternal complications.

When CSE is compared with epidural anesthesia, meta-analysis of the literature found no differences in the frequency of hypotension or in 1-min Apgar scores; the literature is insufficient to evaluate outcomes associated with the use of CSE compared with spinal anesthesia. The consultants and ASA members agree that CSE anesthesia improves anesthesia and reduces time to skin incision when compared with *epidural* anesthesia. The ASA members are equivocal, but the consultants disagree that maternal side effects are reduced. The consultants and ASA members both disagree that CSE improves anesthesia compared with *spinal* anesthesia. The ASA members are equivocal, but the consultants disagree that maternal side effects are reduced. The consultants strongly agree and the ASA members agree that CSE compared with spinal anesthesia increases flexibility of prolonged procedures, and they both agree that the time to skin incision is increased.

Recommendations. The decision to use a particular anesthetic technique for cesarean delivery should be individualized, based on several factors. These include anesthetic, obstetric, or fetal risk factors (*e.g.*, elective vs. emergency), the preferences of the patient, and the judgment of the anesthesiologist. Neuraxial techniques are preferred to GA for most cesarean deliveries. An indwelling epidural catheter may provide equivalent onset of anesthesia compared with initiation of spinal anesthesia for urgent cesarean delivery. If spinal anesthesia is chosen, pencil-point spinal needles should be used instead of cutting-bevel spinal needles. However, GA may be the most appropriate choice in some circumstances (*e.g.*, profound fetal bradycardia, ruptured uterus, severe hemorrhage, severe placental abruption). Uterine displacement (usually left displacement) should be maintained until delivery regardless of the anesthetic technique used.

Intravenous Fluid Preloading. The literature supports and the consultants and ASA members agree that intravenous fluid preloading for spinal anesthesia reduces the frequency of maternal hypotension when compared with no fluid preloading.

Recommendations. Intravenous fluid preloading may be used to reduce the frequency of maternal hypotension after spinal anesthesia for cesarean delivery. Although fluid preloading reduces the frequency of maternal hypotension, initiation of spinal anesthesia should not be delayed to administer a fixed volume of intravenous fluid.

Ephedrine or Phenylephrine. The literature supports the administration of ephedrine and suggests that phenylephrine is effective in reducing maternal hypotension during neuraxial anesthesia for cesarean delivery. The literature is equivocal regarding the relative frequency of patients with breakthrough hypotension when infusions of ephedrine are compared with phenylephrine; however, lower umbilical cord pH values are reported after ephedrine administration. The consultants agree and the ASA members strongly agree that ephedrine is acceptable for treating hypotension during neuraxial anesthesia. The consultants strongly agree and the ASA members agree that phenylephrine is an acceptable agent for the treatment of hypotension.

Recommendations. Intravenous ephedrine and phenylephrine are both acceptable drugs for treating hypotension during neuraxial anesthesia. In the absence of maternal bradycardia, phenylephrine may be preferable because of improved fetal acid–base status in uncomplicated pregnancies.

Neuraxial Opioids for Postoperative Analgesia. For improved postoperative analgesia after cesarean delivery during epidural anesthesia, the literature supports the use of epidural opioids compared with intermittent injections of intravenous or intramuscular opioids. However, a higher frequency of pruritus was found with epidural opioids. The literature is insufficient to evaluate the impact of epidural opioids compared with intravenous PCA. In addition, the literature is insufficient to evaluate spinal opioids compared with parenteral opioids. The consultants strongly agree and the ASA members agree that neuraxial opioids for postoperative analgesia improve analgesia and maternal satisfaction.

Recommendations. For postoperative analgesia after neuraxial anesthesia for cesarean delivery, neuraxial opioids are preferred over intermittent injections of parenteral opioids.

VI. Postpartum Tubal Ligation

There is insufficient literature to evaluate the benefits of neuraxial anesthesia compared with GA for postpartum tubal ligation. In addition, the literature is insufficient to evaluate the impact of the timing of a postpartum tubal ligation on maternal outcome. The consultants and ASA members both agree that neuraxial anesthesia for postpartum tubal ligation reduces complications compared with GA. The ASA members are equivocal but the consultants agree that a postpartum tubal ligation within 8 h of delivery *does not* increase maternal complications.

Recommendations. For postpartum tubal ligation, the patient should have no oral intake of solid foods within 6–8 h of the surgery, depending on the type of food ingested (*e.g.*, fat content).[‖] Aspiration prophylaxis should be considered. Both the timing of the procedure and the decision to use a particular anesthetic technique (*i.e.*, neuraxial vs. general) should be individualized, based on anesthetic risk factors, obstetric risk factors (*e.g.*, blood loss), and patient preferences. However, neuraxial techniques are preferred to GA for most postpartum tubal ligations. The anesthesiologist should be aware that gastric emptying will be delayed in patients who have received opioids during labor, and that an epidural catheter placed for labor may be more likely to fail with longer postdelivery time intervals. If a postpartum tubal ligation is to be performed before the patient is discharged from the hospital, the procedure should not be attempted at a time when it might compromise other aspects of patient care on the labor and delivery unit.

VII. Management of Obstetric and Anesthetic Emergencies

Resources for Management of Hemorrhagic Emergencies. Observational studies and case reports suggest that the availability of resources for hemorrhagic emergencies may be associated with reduced maternal complications. The consultants and ASA members both strongly agree that the availability of resources for managing hemorrhagic emergencies reduces maternal complications.

Recommendations. Institutions providing obstetric care should have resources available to manage hemorrhagic

‖American Society of Anesthesiologists Task Force on Preoperative Fasting: Practice guidelines for preoperative fasting and the use of pharmacologic agents to reduce the risk of pulmonary aspiration. Anesthesiology 1999; 90:896–905.

TABLE 1 Suggested Resources for Obstetric Hemorrhagic Emergencies

- Large-bore intravenous catheters
- Fluid warmer
- Forced-air body warmer
- Availability of blood bank resources
- Equipment for infusing intravenous fluids and blood products rapidly. Examples include, but are not limited to, hand-squeezed fluid chambers, hand-inflated pressure bags, and automatic infusion devices

The items listed represent suggestions. The items should be customized to meet the specific needs, preferences, and skills of the practitioner and health-care facility.

emergencies (table 1). In an emergency, the use of type-specific or O negative blood is acceptable. In cases of intractable hemorrhage when banked blood is not available or the patient refuses banked blood, intraoperative cell-salvage should be considered if available.

Central Invasive Hemodynamic Monitoring. There is insufficient literature to examine whether pulmonary artery catheterization is associated with improved maternal, fetal, or neonatal outcomes in patients with pregnancy-related hypertensive disorders. The literature is silent regarding the management of obstetric patients with central venous catheterization alone. The consultants and ASA members agree that the routine use of central venous or pulmonary artery catheterization does not reduce maternal complications in severely preeclamptic patients.

Recommendations. The decision to perform invasive hemodynamic monitoring should be individualized and based on clinical indications that include the patient's medical history and cardiovascular risk factors. The Task Force recognizes that not all practitioners have access to resources for use of central venous or pulmonary artery catheters in obstetric units.

Equipment for Management of Airway Emergencies. Case reports suggest that the availability of equipment for the management of airway emergencies may be associated with reduced maternal, fetal, and neonatal complications. The consultants and ASA members both strongly agree that the immediate availability of equipment for the management of airway emergencies reduces maternal, fetal, and neonatal complications.

Recommendations. Labor and delivery units should have personnel and equipment readily available to manage airway emergencies, to include a pulse oximeter and qualitative carbon dioxide detector, consistent with the ASA Practice Guidelines for Management of the Difficult Airway.** Basic airway management equipment should be immediately available during the provision of neuraxial analgesia (table 2). In addition, portable equipment for difficult airway management should be readily available in the operative area of labor and delivery units (table 3). The anesthesiologist should have a preformulated strategy for intubation of the difficult airway. When tracheal intubation has failed, ventilation with mask and cricoid pressure, or with a laryngeal mask airway or supraglottic airway device (*e.g.*, Combitube®, Intubating LMA [*Fastrach*™]) should be considered for maintaining an airway and ventilating the lungs. If it is not possible to ventilate or awaken the patient, an airway should be created surgically.

TABLE 2 Suggested Resources for Airway Management during Initial Provision of Neuraxial Anesthesia

- Laryngoscope and assorted blades
- Endotracheal tubes, with stylets
- Oxygen source
- Suction source with tubing and catheters
- Self-inflating bag and mask for positive-pressure ventilation
- Medications for blood pressure support, muscle relaxation, and hypnosis
- Qualitative carbon dioxide detector
- Pulse oximeter

The items listed represent suggestions. The items should be customized to meet the specific needs, preferences, and skills of the practitioner and health-care facility.

Cardiopulmonary Resuscitation. The literature is insufficient to evaluate the efficacy of cardiopulmonary resuscitation in the obstetric patient during labor and delivery. In cases of cardiac arrest, the American Heart Association has stated that 4–5 min is the maximum time rescuers will have to determine whether the arrest can be reversed by Basic Life Support and Advanced Cardiac Life

TABLE 3 Suggested Contents of a Portable Storage Unit for Difficult Airway Management for Cesarean Delivery Rooms

- Rigid laryngoscope blades of alternate design and size from those routinely used
- Laryngeal mask airway
- Endotracheal tubes of assorted size
- Endotracheal tube guides. Examples include, but are not limited to, semirigid stylets with or without a hollow core for jet ventilation, light wands, and forceps designed to manipulate the distal portion of the endotracheal tube.
- Retrograde intubation equipment
- At least one device suitable for emergency nonsurgical airway ventilation. Examples include, but are not limited to, a hollow jet ventilation stylet with a transtracheal jet ventilator, and a supraglottic airway device (*e.g.*, Combitube®, Intubating LMA [*Fastrach*™])
- Fiberoptic intubation equipment
- Equipment suitable for emergency surgical airway access (*e.g.*, cricothyrotomy)
- An exhaled carbon dioxide detector
- Topical anesthetics and vasoconstrictors

The items listed represent suggestions. The items should be customized to meet the specific needs, preferences, and skills of the practitioner and health-care facility.

Adapted from Practice guidelines for management of the difficult airway: An updated report by the American Society of Anesthesiologists Task Force on Management of the Difficult Airway. Anesthesiology 2003; 98:1269–77.

**American Society of Anesthesiologists Task Force on Management of the Difficult Airway: Practice guidelines for management of the difficult airway: An updated report. Anesthesiology 2003; 98:1269–77.

Support interventions.[††] Delivery of the fetus may improve cardiopulmonary resuscitation of the mother by relieving aortocaval compression. The American Heart Association further notes that "the best survival rate for infants >24 to 25 weeks in gestation occurs when the delivery of the infant occurs no more than 5 min after the mother's heart stops beating. This typically requires that the provider begin the hysterotomy about 4 min after cardiac arrest."[††] The consultants and ASA members both strongly agree that the immediate availability of basic and advanced life-support equipment in the labor and delivery suite reduces maternal, fetal, and neonatal complications.

Recommendations. Basic and advanced life-support equipment should be immediately available in the operative area of labor and delivery units. If cardiac arrest occurs during labor and delivery, standard resuscitative measures should be initiated. In addition, uterine displacement (usually left displacement) should be maintained. If maternal circulation is not restored within 4 min, cesarean delivery should be performed by the obstetrics team.

Appendix 1: Summary of Recommendations

I. Perianesthetic Evaluation

- Conduct a focused history and physical examination before providing anesthesia care
  - -Maternal health and anesthetic history
  - -Relevant obstetric history
  - -Airway and heart and lung examination
  - -Baseline blood pressure measurement
  - -Back examination when neuraxial anesthesia is planned or placed
- A communication system should be in place to encourage early and ongoing contact between obstetric providers, anesthesiologists, and other members of the multidisciplinary team
- Order or require a platelet count based on a patient's history, physical examination, and clinical signs; a routine intrapartum platelet count is not necessary in the healthy parturient
- Order or require an intrapartum blood type and screen or cross-match based on maternal history, anticipated hemorrhagic complications (*e.g.*, placenta accreta in a patient with placenta previa and previous uterine surgery), and local institutional policies; a routine blood cross-match is not necessary for *healthy and uncomplicated* parturients
- The fetal heart rate should be monitored by a qualified individual before and after administration of neuraxial analgesia for labor; *continuous* electronic recording of the fetal heart rate may not be necessary in every clinical setting and may not be possible during initiation of neuraxial anesthesia

II. Aspiration Prophylaxis

- Oral intake of modest amounts of clear liquids may be allowed for uncomplicated laboring patients
- The uncomplicated patient undergoing elective cesarean delivery may have modest amounts of clear liquids up to 2 h before induction of anesthesia
- The volume of liquid ingested is less important than the presence of particulate matter in the liquid ingested
- Patients with additional risk factors for aspiration (*e.g.*, morbid obesity, diabetes, difficult airway) or patients at increased risk for operative delivery (*e.g.*, nonreassuring fetal heart rate pattern) may have further restrictions of oral intake, determined on a case-by-case basis
- Solid foods should be avoided in laboring patients
- Patients undergoing elective surgery (*e.g.*, scheduled cesarean delivery or postpartum tubal ligation) should undergo a fasting period for solids of 6–8 h depending on the type of food ingested (*e.g.*, fat content)
- Before surgical procedures (*i.e.*, cesarean delivery, postpartum tubal ligation), practitioners should consider timely administration of non-particulate antacids, H_2 receptor antagonists, and/or metoclopramide for aspiration prophylaxis

III. Anesthetic Care for Labor and Delivery

Neuraxial Techniques: Availability of Resources.

- When neuraxial techniques that include local anesthetics are chosen, appropriate resources for the treatment of complications (*e.g.*, hypotension, systemic toxicity, high spinal anesthesia) should be available
- If an opioid is added, treatments for related complications (*e.g.*, pruritus, nausea, respiratory depression) should be available
- An intravenous infusion should be established before the initiation of neuraxial analgesia or anesthesia and maintained throughout the duration of the neuraxial analgesic or anesthetic
- Administration of a fixed volume of intravenous fluid is not required before neuraxial analgesia is initiated

Timing of Neuraxial Analgesia and Outcome of Labor.

- Neuraxial analgesia should not be withheld on the basis of achieving an arbitrary cervical dilation, and should be offered on an individualized basis when this service is available
- Patients may be reassured that the use of neuraxial analgesia does not increase the incidence of cesarean delivery

Neuraxial Analgesia and Trial of Labor after Previous Cesarean Delivery.

- Neuraxial techniques should be offered to patients attempting vaginal birth after previous cesarean delivery
- For these patients, it is also appropriate to consider early placement of a neuraxial catheter that can be used later for labor analgesia or for anesthesia in the event of operative delivery

Early Insertion of Spinal or Epidural Catheter for Complicated Parturients.

- Early insertion of a spinal or epidural catheter for obstetric (*e.g.*, twin gestation or preeclampsia) or anesthetic indications (*e.g.*, anticipated difficult airway or obesity) should be considered to reduce the need for general anesthesia if an emergent procedure becomes necessary
  - -In these cases, the insertion of a spinal or epidural catheter may precede the onset of labor or a patient's request for labor analgesia

---

[††] 2005 American Heart Association guidelines for cardiopulmonary resuscitation and emergency cardiovascular care. Circulation 2005; 112(suppl):IV1–203.

Continuous Infusion Epidural (CIE) Analgesia.

- The selected analgesic/anesthetic technique should reflect patient needs and preferences, practitioner preferences or skills, and available resources
- CIE may be used for effective analgesia for labor and delivery
- When a continuous epidural infusion of local anesthetic is selected, an opioid may be added to reduce the concentration of local anesthetic, improve the quality of analgesia, and minimize motor block
- Adequate analgesia for uncomplicated labor and delivery should be administered with the secondary goal of producing as little motor block as possible by using dilute concentrations of local anesthetics with opioids
- The lowest concentration of local anesthetic infusion that provides adequate maternal analgesia and satisfaction should be administered

Single-injection Spinal Opioids with or without Local Anesthetics.

- Single-injection spinal opioids with or without local anesthetics may be used to provide effective, although time-limited, analgesia for labor when spontaneous vaginal delivery is anticipated
- If labor is expected to last longer than the analgesic effects of the spinal drugs chosen or if there is a good possibility of operative delivery, a catheter technique instead of a single injection technique should be considered
- A local anesthetic may be added to a spinal opioid to increase duration and improve quality of analgesia

Pencil-point Spinal Needles.

- Pencil-point spinal needles should be used instead of cutting-bevel spinal needles to minimize the risk of post–dural puncture headache

Combined Spinal–Epidural (CSE) Anesthetics.

- CSE techniques may be used to provide effective and rapid analgesia for labor

Patient-controlled Epidural Analgesia (PCEA).

- PCEA may be used to provide an effective and flexible approach for the maintenance of labor analgesia
- PCEA may be preferable to CIE for providing fewer anesthetic interventions, reduced dosages of local anesthetics, and less motor blockade than fixed-rate continuous epidural infusions
- PCEA may be used with or without a background infusion

IV. Removal of Retained Placenta

- In general, there is no preferred anesthetic technique for removal of retained placenta

  -If an epidural catheter is in place and the patient is hemodynamically stable, epidural anesthesia is preferable

- Hemodynamic status should be assessed before administering neuraxial anesthesia
- Aspiration prophylaxis should be considered
- Sedation/analgesia should be titrated carefully due to the potential risks of respiratory depression and pulmonary aspiration during the immediate postpartum period
- In cases involving major maternal hemorrhage, general anesthesia with an endotracheal tube may be preferable to neuraxial anesthesia
- Nitroglycerin may be used as an alternative to terbutaline sulfate or general endotracheal anesthesia with halogenated agents for uterine relaxation during removal of retained placental tissue

  -Initiating treatment with incremental doses of intravenous or sublingual (*i.e.*, metered dose spray) nitroglycerin may relax the uterus sufficiently while minimizing potential complications (*e.g.*, hypotension)

V. Anesthetic Choices for Cesarean Delivery

- Equipment, facilities, and support personnel available in the labor and delivery operating suite should be comparable to those available in the main operating suite

  -Resources for the treatment of potential complications (*e.g.*, failed intubation, inadequate analgesia, hypotension, respiratory depression, pruritus, vomiting) should be available in the labor and delivery operating suite
  -Appropriate equipment and personnel should be available to care for obstetric patients recovering from major neuraxial or general anesthesia

- The decision to use a particular anesthetic technique should be individualized based on anesthetic, obstetric, or fetal risk factors (*e.g.*, elective vs. emergency), the preferences of the patient, and the judgment of the anesthesiologist

  -Neuraxial techniques are preferred to general anesthesia for most cesarean deliveries

- An indwelling epidural catheter may provide equivalent onset of anesthesia compared with initiation of spinal anesthesia for urgent cesarean delivery
- If spinal anesthesia is chosen, pencil-point spinal needles should be used instead of cutting-bevel spinal needles
- General anesthesia may be the most appropriate choice in some circumstances (*e.g.*, profound fetal bradycardia, ruptured uterus, severe hemorrhage, severe placental abruption)
- Uterine displacement (usually left displacement) should be maintained until delivery regardless of the anesthetic technique used
- Intravenous fluid preloading may be used to reduce the frequency of maternal hypotension after spinal anesthesia for cesarean delivery
- Initiation of spinal anesthesia should not be delayed to administer a fixed volume of intravenous fluid
- Intravenous ephedrine and phenylephrine are both acceptable drugs for treating hypotension during neuraxial anesthesia

  -In the absence of maternal bradycardia, phenylephrine may be preferable because of improved fetal acid–base status in uncomplicated pregnancies

- For postoperative analgesia after neuraxial anesthesia for cesarean delivery, neuraxial opioids are preferred over intermittent injections of parenteral opioids

VI. Postpartum Tubal Ligation

- For postpartum tubal ligation, the patient should have no oral intake of solid foods within 6–8 h of the surgery, depending on the type of food ingested (*e.g.*, fat content)

- Aspiration prophylaxis should be considered
- Both the timing of the procedure and the decision to use a particular anesthetic technique (*i.e.*, neuraxial *vs.* general) should be individualized, based on anesthetic risk factors, obstetric risk factors (*e.g.*, blood loss), and patient preferences
- Neuraxial techniques are preferred to general anesthesia for most postpartum tubal ligations

    -Be aware that gastric emptying will be delayed in patients who have received opioids during labor and that an epidural catheter placed for labor may be more likely to fail with longer postdelivery time intervals

- If a postpartum tubal ligation is to be performed before the patient is discharged from the hospital, the procedure should not be attempted at a time when it might compromise other aspects of patient care on the labor and delivery unit

VII. Management of Obstetric and Anesthetic Emergencies

- Institutions providing obstetric care should have resources available to manage hemorrhagic emergencies

    -In an emergency, the use of type-specific or O negative blood is acceptable
    -In cases of intractable hemorrhage when banked blood is not available or the patient refuses banked blood, intraoperative cell-salvage should be considered if available
    -The decision to perform invasive hemodynamic monitoring should be individualized and based on clinical indications that include the patient's medical history and cardiovascular risk factors

- Labor and delivery units should have personnel and equipment readily available to manage airway emergencies, to include a pulse oximeter and qualitative carbon dioxide detector, consistent with the ASA Practice Guidelines for Management of the Difficult Airway

    -Basic airway management equipment should be immediately available during the provision of neuraxial analgesia
    -Portable equipment for difficult airway management should be readily available in the operative area of labor and delivery units
    -The anesthesiologist should have a preformulated strategy for intubation of the difficult airway
    -When tracheal intubation has failed, ventilation with mask and cricoid pressure, or with a laryngeal mask airway or supraglottic airway device (*e.g.*, Combitube®, Intubating LMA [*Fastrach*™]) should be considered for maintaining an airway and ventilating the lungs
    -If it is not possible to ventilate or awaken the patient, an airway should be created surgically

- Basic and advanced life-support equipment should be immediately available in the operative area of labor and delivery units
- If cardiac arrest occurs during labor and delivery, standard resuscitative measures should be initiated

    -Uterine displacement (usually left displacement) should be maintained
    -If maternal circulation is not restored within 4 min, cesarean delivery should be performed by the obstetrics team

Optimal Goals for Anesthesia Care in Obstetrics*

This joint statement from the American Society of Anesthesiologists (ASA) and the American College of Obstetricians and Gynecologists (ACOG) has been designed to address issues of concern to both specialties. Good obstetric care requires the availability of qualified personnel and equipment to administer general or regional anesthesia both electively and emergently. The extent and degree to which anesthesia services are available varies widely among hospitals. However, for any hospital providing obstetric care, certain optimal anesthesia goals should be sought. These include:

1. Availability of a licensed practitioner who is credentialed to administer an appropriate anesthetic whenever necessary. For many women, regional anesthesia (epidural, spinal, or combined spinal epidural) will be the most appropriate anesthetic.
2. Availability of a licensed practitioner who is credentialed to maintain support of vital functions in any obstetric emergency.
3. Availability of anesthesia and surgical personnel to permit the start of a cesarean delivery within 30 minutes of the decision to perform the procedure.
4. Immediate availability of appropriate facilities and personnel, including obstetric anesthesia, nursing personnel, and a physician capable of monitoring labor and performing cesarean delivery, including an emergency cesarean delivery in cases of vaginal birth after cesarean delivery (VBAC).[1] The definition of immediately available personnel and facilities remains a local decision based on each institution's available resources and geographic location.
5. Appointment of a qualified anesthesiologist to be responsible for all anesthetics administered. There are many obstetric units where obstetricians or obstetrician-supervised nurse anesthetists administer labor anesthetics. The administration of general or regional anesthesia requires both medical judgment and technical skills. Thus, a physician with privileges in anesthesiology should be readily available.

Persons administering or supervising obstetric anesthesia should be qualified to manage the infrequent but occasionally life-threatening complications of major regional anesthesia such as respiratory and cardiovascular failure, toxic local anesthetic convulsions, or vomiting and aspiration. Mastering and retaining the skills and knowledge necessary to manage these complications require adequate training and frequent application.

To ensure the safest and most effective anesthesia for obstetric patients, the Director of Anesthesia Services, with the approval of the medical staff, should develop and enforce written policies regarding provision of obstetric anesthesia. These include:

1. A qualified physician with obstetric privileges to perform operative vaginal or cesarean delivery should be readily available during administration of anesthesia. Readily available should be defined by each institution within the context of its resources and geographic location. Regional and/or general anesthesia should not be administered until the patient has been examined and the fetal status and progress of labor evaluated by a qualified individual. A physician with obstetric privileges who concurs with the patient's management and has knowledge of the maternal and fetal status and the progress of labor should be readily available to deal with any obstetric complications that may arise. A physician with obstetric privileges should be responsible for midwifery back up in hospital settings that utilize certified nurse midwives/certified midwives as obstetric providers.
2. Availability of equipment, facilities, and support personnel equal to that provided in the surgical suite. This should include the availability of a properly equipped and staffed recovery room capable of receiving and caring for all patients recovering from major regional or general anesthesia. Birthing facilities, when used for analgesia or anesthesia, must be appropriately equipped to provide safe anesthetic care during labor and delivery or postanesthesia recovery care.
3. Personnel, other than the surgical team, should be immediately available to assume responsibility for resuscitation of the depressed newborn. The surgeon and anesthesiologist are responsible for the mother and may not be able to leave her to care for the newborn, even when a regional anesthetic is functioning adequately. Individuals qualified to perform neonatal resuscitation should demonstrate:
    - 3.1. Proficiency in rapid and accurate evaluation of the newborn condition, including Apgar scoring.
    - 3.2. Knowledge of the pathogenesis of a depressed newborn (acidosis, drugs, hypovolemia, trauma,

*Approved by the House of Delegates on October 22, 2008 as a joint statement of the American Society of Anesthesiologists and the American College of Ostetricians and Gynecologists.

anomalies, and infection), as well as specific indications for resuscitation.

3.3. Proficiency in newborn airway management, laryngoscopy, endotracheal intubations, suctioning of airways, artificial ventilation, cardiac massage, and maintenance of thermal stability.

In larger maternity units and those functioning as high-risk centers, 24-hour in-house anesthesia, obstetric and neonatal specialists are usually necessary. Preferably, the obstetric anesthesia services should be directed by an anesthesiologist with special training or experience in obstetric anesthesia. These units will also frequently require the availability of more sophisticated monitoring equipment and specially trained nursing personnel.

A survey jointly sponsored by ASA and ACOG found that many hospitals in the United States have not yet achieved the goals mentioned previously. Deficiencies were most evident in smaller delivery units. Some small delivery units are necessary because of geographic considerations. Currently, approximately 34% of hospitals providing obstetric care have fewer than 500 deliveries per year.[2] Providing comprehensive care for obstetric patients in these small units is extremely inefficient, not cost-effective and frequently impossible. Thus, the following recommendations are made:

1. Whenever possible, small units should consolidate.
2. When geographic factors require the existence of smaller units, these units should be part of a well-established regional perinatal system.

The availability of the appropriate personnel to assist in the management of a variety of obstetric problems is a necessary feature of good obstetric care. The presence of a pediatrician or other trained physician at a high-risk cesarean delivery to care for the newborn or the availability of an anesthesiologist during active labor and delivery when VBAC is attempted and at a breech or multifetal delivery are examples. Frequently, these physicians spend a considerable amount of time standing by for the possibility that their services may be needed emergently, but may ultimately not be required to perform the tasks for which they are present. Reasonable compensation for these standby services is justifiable and necessary.

A variety of other mechanisms have been suggested to increase the availability and quality of anesthesia services in obstetrics. Improved hospital design, to place labor and delivery suites closer to the operating rooms, would allow for safer and more efficient anesthesia care, including supervision of nurse anesthetists. Anesthesia equipment in the labor and delivery area must be comparable to that in the operating room.

Finally, good interpersonal relations between obstetricians and anesthesiologists are important. Joint meetings between the two departments should be encouraged. Anesthesiologists should recognize the special needs and concerns of the obstetrician and obstetricians should recognize the anesthesiologist as a consultant in the management of pain and life-support measures. Both should recognize the need to provide high quality care for all patients.

References:

1. Vaginal birth after previous cesarean delivery. ACOG Practice Bulletin No. 54. American College of Obstetricians and Gynecologists. Obstet Gynecol 2004;104:203-12.
2. Bucklin BA, Hawkins JL, Anderson JR, et al. Obstetric anesthesia workforce survey: Twenty-year update. Anesthesiology 2005; 103:645-53.

Online Resources for Obstetric Anesthesia Providers

William Camann, M.D.

A variety of Internet-based resources exist for obstetric anesthesia providers. These websites offer information regarding clinical practice, ongoing research, and recent publications. This appendix includes a brief guide to some of these resources.

These sites were active at the time that this guide was prepared (September 2008). The author of this appendix, and the editors and publisher of this textbook, bear no responsibility for the accuracy (or lack thereof) of any information found in these sites. Publication of this list does not imply endorsement of these sites.

OBSTETRIC ANESTHESIOLOGY SOCIETIES

The Obstetric Anaesthetists Association (OAA)

http://www.oaa-anaes.ac.uk

The OAA provides both education and training for anaesthetists and other practitioners in the United Kingdom and other countries, and serves as a resource for women seeking information about analgesia for labour and anaesthesia for caesarean delivery. Significant amounts of educational material are freely available for all users.

The Society for Obstetric Anesthesia and Perinatology (SOAP)

http://www.soap.org

The SOAP is a United States-based subspecialty anesthesiology society that promotes excellence in research and the clinical practice of obstetric anesthesiology and perinatology. Significant amounts of educational material are freely available for all users.

OTHER PROFESSIONAL SOCIETIES OF INTEREST

The American Academy of Pediatrics (AAP)

http://www.aap.org

The AAP promotes the attainment of optimal physical, mental, and social health and well-being for all infants, children, adolescents, and young adults. Significant amounts of educational material are freely available for all users.

The American College of Obstetricians and Gynecologists (ACOG)

http://www.acog.org

The ACOG promotes health care for women through policy and guideline development, education, and advocacy. A password is required for access to much of the online information, including committee opinions and practice bulletins and guidelines.

The American Society of Anesthesiologists (ASA)

http://www.asahq.org

The ASA encourages education, research, and scientific progress in anesthesiology. The ASA strives to be an advocate for all patients who require anesthesia or relief from pain. The majority of documents, policies, and guidelines are freely available; some sections require a password for access.

The ASA practice guidelines for obstetric anesthesia can be found at the following site: http://www2.asahq.org/publications/pc-119-4-practice-guidelines-for-obstetric-anesthesia.aspx

The American Society of Regional Anesthesia and Pain Medicine (ASRA)

http://www.asra.com

The ASRA provides clinical and professional education for physicians and scientists with an interest in regional anesthesia and pain medicine. The ASRA also promotes excellence in patient care and encourages research to advance the scientific basis of regional anesthesia and pain medicine.

The ASRA consensus statement on regional (neuraxial) anesthesia in the anticoagulated patient can be found at the following site: http://www.asra.com/consensus-statements/2.html

The ASRA consensus statements regarding infectious complications of neuraxial blockade can be found at the following site: http://asra.com/consensus-statements/3.html

The Anesthesia Patient Safety Foundation (APSF)

http://www.apsf.org/

The APSF seeks to improve patient safety during anesthesia care by encouraging and conducting research and education, programs and campaigns, and national and international exchange of information and ideas. Significant amounts of educational material are freely available for all users.

The *APSF Newsletter* can be found at the following site: http://www.apsf.org/resource_center/newsletters.mspx

The Association of Women's Health, Obstetric and Neonatal Nurses (AWHONN)

http://www.awhonn.org/awhonn/

The AWHONN seeks to improve the health of women and newborns and to strengthen the nursing profession through advocacy, research, education, and provision of other professional and clinical resources for nurses and other healthcare professionals. Some content is freely available for all users.

The AWHONN position statement on the role of the registered nurse in the care of the pregnant woman receiving analgesia/anesthesia by neuraxial catheter techniques is available at the following site: http://www.awhonn.org/awhonn/content.do?name=05_HealthPolicyLegislation/5H_PositionStatements.htm

The Canadian Anesthesiologists' Society (CAS)

http://www.cas.ca/

The CAS promotes science, vigilance, and compassion in the practice of anesthesiology. Significant amounts of information (including practice guidelines) are freely available for all users.

The CAS guidelines for regional (neuraxial) analgesia in obstetric patients can be found at the following site: http://www.cas.ca/members/sign_in/guidelines/practice_of_anesthesia/default.asp?load=obstetrical_regional_analgesia

The International Anesthesia Research Society (IARS)

http://www.iars.org

The IARS encourages the development and dissemination of current, state-of-the-art basic and clinical research data, as well as the newest advances in all areas of clinical anesthesia care.

The International Fetal Medicine and Surgery Society (IFMSS)

http://www.ifmss.org

The IFMSS promotes education and research related to the field of fetal diagnosis and therapy.

The North American Society of Obstetric Medicine (NASOM)

http://www.nasom.org

The NASOM promotes and supports research collaboration, communication, and teaching concerning the medical care of pregnant women. General internists from the United States and Canada form the core membership of the society.

The Society for Maternal-Fetal Medicine (SMFM)

http://www.smfm.org

The SMFM seeks to promote and expand education and research in maternal-fetal medicine, and encourages the exchange of new ideas and research concerning the most recent approaches and treatments for obstetric problems.

The Society of Obstetric Medicine of Australia and New Zealand (SOMANZ)

http://www.somanz.org

The SOMANZ seeks to advance clinical and scientific knowledge of hypertensive diseases and medical disorders in pregnancy, and to foster collaboration with other regional and international societies interested in hypertension in pregnancy and obstetric medicine.

GOVERNMENTAL REGULATORY AND INFORMATIONAL WEBSITES

The Centers for Disease Control and Prevention (CDC)

http://www.cdc.gov/

The CDC provides extensive information on most health-related subjects. For example, information is available on assisted reproductive technologies, birth rates, birth defects, breast-feeding, medication use during pregnancy, nutrition in pregnancy, preterm labor, maternal mortality, and various disease processes in pregnancy.

Confidential Enquiries into Maternal and Child Health (CEMACH)

http://www.cemach.org.uk

The CEMACH provides extensive information on maternal and perinatal mortality statistics, including anesthesia-related deaths, in the United Kingdom.

JOURNALS AND SCIENTIFIC LITERATURE

American Journal of Obstetrics and Gynecology (the official journal of the SMFM)

http://www.ajog.org

A subscription is required for most text.

Anesthesiology (the official journal of the ASA)

http://www.anesthesiology.org

Content more than 6 months old is freely available without a subscription or password.

Anesthesia & Analgesia (the official journal of the IARS and the SOAP)

http://www.anesthesia-analgesia.org

Content more than 12 months old is freely available without a subscription or password.

Canadian Journal of Anesthesia (the official journal of the CAS)

http://www.cja-jca.org/

Content more than 12 months old is freely available without a subscription or password.

The Cochrane Collaboration

http://www.cochrane.org

The Cochrane Collaboration provides frequently updated reviews of current literature in a variety of medical specialties, including anesthesiology and obstetrics. Most information in abstract form is freely available; however, a subscription is required for access to full-text documents.

International Journal of Obstetric Anesthesia (the official journal of the OAA)

http://www.elsevier.com/wps/find/journaldescription.cws_home/623045/description#description

This is the only peer-reviewed journal devoted solely to obstetric anesthesia. A subscription is required for most text.

Obstetric Anesthesia Digest

http://www.obstetricanesthesia.com

Recent publications of interest to obstetric anesthesia providers are cited, reviewed, and discussed by a panel of experts. A subscription is required for access to full text.

Obstetrics & Gynecology (the official journal of the ACOG)

http://www.greenjournal.org

New or updated ACOG practice bulletins and committee opinions are frequently published in *Obstetrics & Gynecology*. A subscription is required for most text.

Pediatrics (the official journal of the AAP)

http://pediatrics.aappublications.org/

Content more than 12 months old is freely available without a subscription or password (for a rolling 8-year period).

PubMed (a medical literature search resource supported by the National Institutes of Health)

http://www.pubmed.gov or http://www.ncbi.nlm.nih.gov/sites/entrez

This site provides citations and abstracts; the user must go to the original source to obtain the full text of most articles.

Index

Note: Page numbers followed by **b** refer to boxes; page numbers followed by **f** refer to figures; and page numbers followed by **t** refer to tables.

B

C

G

H

I

N

O

T

U

V

W

Z